KUMAR & CLARK'S

Clinical Medicine

Kumar & Clark's
Clinical Medicine

Tenth Edition

Edited by

Adam Feather MBBS, FRCP, FAcadMEd
Consultant Physician and Clinical Director
St Mary's Hospital
The Isle of Wight, UK

David Randall MA, MRCP
Clinical Research Fellow
Barts and The London School of Medicine and
 Dentistry, QMUL;
Specialty Registrar in Renal Medicine
Barts Health NHS Trust
London, UK

Mona Waterhouse MA (Oxon), MRCP
Consultant Physician and Endocrinologist
St Bartholomew's Hospital, Barts Health NHS Trust
London, UK

Foreword by

**Professor Dame Parveen J Kumar CBE,
BSc, MD, DM(HC), FRCP (L&E), FRCPath**
Professor of Medicine and Education
Barts and The London School of Medicine and
 Dentistry, QMUL;
Honorary Consultant Physician and
 Gastroenterologist
Barts Health NHS Trust and Homerton University
 Hospital NHS Foundation Trust
London, UK

Michael L Clark MD, FRCP
Honorary Senior Lecturer
Barts and The London School of Medicine and
 Dentistry, QMUL, and Princess Grace Hospital
London, UK

Use the PIN code on the inside front cover to access additional online content.

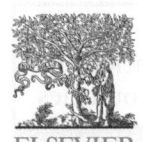

ELSEVIER London New York Oxford Philadelphia St Louis Sydney 2021

First edition 1987
Second edition 1990
Third edition 1994
Fourth Edition 1998
Fifth Edition 2002
Sixth Edition 2005
Seventh Edition 2009
Eighth Edition 2012
Ninth Edition 2017
Tenth Edition 2021

Notices

Practitioners and researchers must always rely on their own experience and knowledge in evaluating and using any information, methods, compounds or experiments described herein. Because of rapid advances in the medical sciences, in particular, independent verification of diagnoses and drug dosages should be made. To the fullest extent of the law, no responsibility is assumed by Elsevier, authors, editors or contributors for any injury and/or damage to persons or property as a matter of products liability, negligence or otherwise, or from any use or operation of any methods, products, instructions, or ideas contained in the material herein.

ISBN: 978-0-7020-7868-2
International ISBN: 978-0-7020-7869-9

For Elsevier:
Content Strategists: Pauline Graham, Alex Mortimer
Senior Content Development Specialists: Kim Benson, Louise Cook, Helen Leng, Joanne Scott
Project Managers: Anne Collett, Julie Taylor
Design: Amy Buxton
Illustration Manager: Paula Catalano
Illustrators: Ethan Danielson, Bruce Hogarth, Richard Morris, MPS North America LLC
Marketing Manager: Deborah Watkins

Printed in Scotland

Last digit is the print number: 9   8   7   6   5   4   3   2

Working together
to grow libraries in
developing countries

www.elsevier.com • www.bookaid.org

Contents

vi Contents

See your e-book for new Clinical Overviews, plus MCQs, videos, audio, Clinical Cases and Special Topics from the International Advisory Board.

Foreword to the Tenth Edition

After 35 years and nine editions of Kumar and Clark's *Clinical Medicine*, we felt it was time for the younger generation to continue with this 10th edition. The book has been described as the 'gold standard, thorough guide to clinical medicine', and is used by the majority of medical schools around the world. This would not have been possible without the dedication of our expert authors and specialists, who have written many chapters over the years. This 10th edition certainly maintains the high standard of its predecessors.

When we started those many years ago, our aim was to produce a comprehensive book of medicine which had a sound grounding in the basic sciences for understanding the mechanisms of diseases. This has proven to be a valuable concept for young students, doctors and practising health professionals. It contains sufficient knowledge and detail to be of great value in the day-to-day care of patients in hospitals and clinics, and in the field. It is used not only by the medical profession but also by all professions related to medicine. Pharmacists and consultant nurses are now taking a bigger role in patient care, and *Clinical Medicine* is the book used by many of these professionals as a source of evidence-based medical information.

Over the years, to keep up to date and advance with the times, we have travelled widely across the world, visiting many countries and developing lifelong friendships. This has enabled us to see different styles of education, along with different ways in which medicine is practised. The result has been the production of a textbook designed for a 'doctor of the world'. This is essential, as with the swiftness of travel, diseases spread with ease and rapidity, as seen with the recent epidemics. Our International Advisory Board members have provided much useful advice and written articles for the online version to help us with this task.

We have taken much advice, as well as criticisms (!) and suggestions, from our readers so that *Clinical Medicine* remains a comprehensive reference book, as well as being practical and user-friendly.

We are delighted to welcome the new editors for this edition, who are all in current clinical posts with research activities. They have produced a book with a slightly different approach but still maintaining the high standards of previous editions.

We would like to give our warm thanks to all our readers and friends across the world. They should take credit for the way that this book has developed over the years, and no doubt will continue to help over future editions.

Lastly, on a personal note, we have both enormously enjoyed our time as authors and editors of *Clinical Medicine*. It is hard to believe that, 35 years ago, a few of us sat down to think and design a new textbook of medicine. We endeavoured to produce a new book with colour, tables and algorithms, changing the old, staid texts into a lively, easy-to-learn and user-friendly book. It has been very hard work but also a huge responsibility to assemble the correct medical facts to inspire the next generation of young doctors. We would like to thank all those with whom we have had the pleasure to work over the years, particularly the many dedicated staff at Elsevier, who have worked tirelessly with us to come up with the final products.

Parveen Kumar and Michael Clark
2020

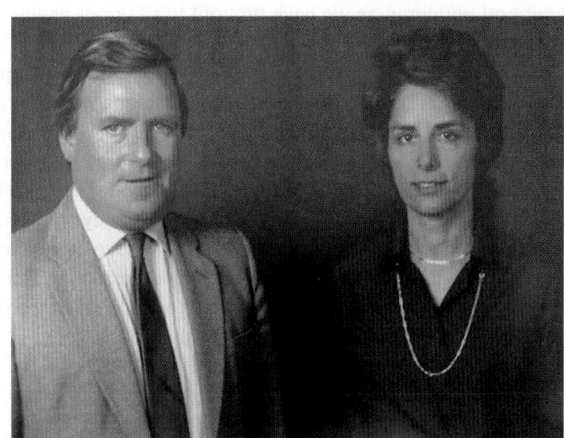

Dr Michael L Clark and Professor Dame Parveen J Kumar on the occasion of the publication of the first edition of *Clinical Medicine* in 1987.

Preface to the Tenth Edition

'There must be a good reason to write a new textbook of medicine when there are already a good number on the market.' So began the preface to the First Edition of *Clinical Medicine*, published 33 years ago this year. Edited by Professor Dame Parveen Kumar and Dr Michael Clark, 'Kumar and Clark' has become synonymous not just with a medical textbook, but with the combination of excellence and accessibility they sought to provide. Their desire to empower clinical students and doctors has been the driving ambition behind the book ever since – 'to strike a balance between exciting new developments in medical research and the vast quantity of established fact that needs to be absorbed… so that the management of disease can be based on sound physiological concepts'.

The book they produced has become an international medical best-seller, and has played a crucial part in the education of a generation of doctors – among them a new team of editors, humbled to be standing on the shoulders of these medical giants. Taking over is an honour and a great responsibility, and we are grateful for the legacy they have left, as well as for their continued support and input as we have brought this current edition to production.

Clinical Medicine has always attempted to bridge the gap between basic introductory texts and larger reference works: to be as comprehensible as it is comprehensive. The pace at which medical science continues to develop is astounding. The present generation of junior doctors and undergraduates must provide high-quality, patient-centred care in the context of a burgeoning body of medical research, patients presenting with multimorbidity and resulting polypharmacy, continuing inequalities in society and across the world, and a medical culture that expects doctors to work within teams, bridging traditional specialty and professional divides.

For this reason, we have introduced into this edition a number of new chapters to equip readers to address these new challenges: Evidence-based practice (Ch. 4), Surgery (Ch. 11), Public health (Ch. 14), Geriatric medicine, frailty and multimorbidity (Ch. 15), Haematological oncology (Ch. 17) and Men's health (Ch. 40). In some cases, we have divided up larger chapters to highlight conditions that straddle traditional subspecialty boundaries but require a joined-up approach: Sepsis and the treatment of bacterial infection, (Ch. 8), Venous thromboembolic disease (Ch. 29), Hypertension (Ch. 31) and Obstetric medicine (Ch. 38).

We have included new clinical skills content at the beginning of most of the chapters to try to fulfil the historic aims of this book: bringing the clinical sciences to bear on the problems experienced by patients in day-to-day medical practice. We hope readers will learn not just to take generic histories and perform routine physical examinations, but to tailor their approach according to the presentation of the individual patient in front of them. We offer our own take on the clinical method and the importance of building a therapeutic relationship with patients in a new first chapter, describing what we believe remains key to the art of medicine: diagnosis (Ch. 1).

Online, readers will find a range of additional resources, including self-assessment questions, bite-sized overview topic pages covering major conditions, clinical skills videos and expanded coverage of subjects with particular international or regional relevance.

We hope you will find this edition helpful in your efforts to learn and practise medicine. Any suggestions you may wish to make are warmly welcomed and will help us to ensure that this book continues to meet the needs of its readers.

Adam Feather, David Randall and Mona Waterhouse
2020

HOW TO USE THIS BOOK

There is a broad movement through the book from early chapters which focus on general principles of clinical practice, to later chapters that deal with individual organ systems and clinical subspecialties.

These later chapters, based around individual subspecialties, begin by offering a tailored approach to basic clinical skills such as history-taking and examination. We have tried to encourage generic skills to be applied thoughtfully to the specialty in question: to encourage learners to adopt the approach taken by experts in the field, so that relevant questions are asked and key physical signs are carefully sought.

Most chapters then cover basic sciences, including the anatomy and physiology of the relevant organs in question, before dealing with individual conditions in order. Within the text:

- **Pink subheadings** introduce individual conditions,
- Green subheadings introduce the scientific background to the condition (e.g. 'Aetiology' or 'Clinical features'), and
- Orange subheadings introduce clinical material, such as 'Investigations' or 'Management'.

Boxes have been classified by the type of information they provide and have the following symbols:

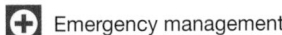 Emergency management

i Clinical information

? Differential diagnosis

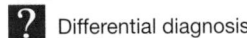 Practical procedures

'Emergency' boxes are in red.

E-Book extras

Clinical Overviews, Special Topics, Clinical Cases and more in the Learning Resources, Videos and Assessments chapters online, accessible via the PIN page in the front of this book.

Prescribing

We have used the Recommended International Non-proprietary Names (rINNs) for all drugs. In some diseases where a particular formulation of a drug is required, the proprietary name is used. Drugs spellings follow international usage, e.g. bendroflumethiazide and not bendrofluazide, and amfetamine and not amphetamine. For adrenaline and noradrenaline, we have added epinephrine and norepinephrine in brackets, as these names are often used in emergency guidelines across the world.

Dosages have been given where appropriate but we recommend that all readers check with their national formularies for the exact dosages.

Units of measurement

We have used the International System of Units (SI units) throughout the book. On occasion, if there is a possibility for confusion, we have also used non-SI units and given a conversion factor.

Also in the Kumar & Clark family of books:
- *Essentials of Kumar & Clark's Clinical Medicine, 6e*
- *Kumar & Clark's Cases in Clinical Medicine, 3e*
- *Clinical Surgery, 3e*
- *Essentials of Paediatrics, 2E*

Online Clinical Overviews

Acid–base disorders

Anaemia: investigations

Arrhythmias: supraventricular tachycardia (SVT) and atrial fibrillation (AF)

Arrhythmias: bradycardia and heart block

Asthma

Blood transfusion

Breast cancer

Central nervous system infections

Chronic obstructive pulmonary disease (COPD)

Cirrhosis

Colorectal carcinoma

Dementia

Diabetes: complications

Diabetes: emergencies

Diabetes: management

Eczema/dermatitis

Epilepsy

Extracellular fluid volume: disorders

Falls, instability, osteoporosis and fractures

Frailty and ageing

Gastrointestinal bleeding

Heart disease: acute coronary syndrome (ACS)

Heart failure

Hepatitis: B and C

HIV: clinical approach to the patient

Hypertension

Inflammatory bowel disease (IBD)

Leukaemias: acute

Leukaemias: chronic

Lung cancer

Lymphoma

Malaria

Malnutrition

Movement disorders

Multiple sclerosis (MS)

Myeloma and other plasma cell disorders

Myeloproliferative neoplasms

Nephrotic syndrome, nephritic syndrome and glomerulonephritis

Obesity

Osteoarthritis

Pituitary disease

Pneumonia

Potassium concentration: disorders

Prostate cancer

Renal disease: acute kidney injury (AKI)

Renal disease: chronic kidney disease (CKD)

Renal replacement therapy

Rheumatoid arthritis

Sepsis

Sickle syndromes

Skin: malignant disease

Sodium concentration: disorders

Stroke

Systemic lupus erythematosus (SLE)

Thyroid disorders: hypo- and hyperthyroidism

Venous thromboembolic disease

Online Special Topics
From the International Advisory Board

Editors: *Professor H Janaka de Silva* and *Professor Senaka Rajapakse*

Online Clinical Cases

List of Contributors

The editors would like to acknowledge and offer grateful thanks for the input of all previous editions' contributors, without whom this new edition would not have been possible.

Ajit Abraham MBBS, MS, MA(Med Ethics & Law), FRCS, FRCS (General Surgery)
Consultant HPB, Trauma & General Surgeon, Honorary Clinical Senior Lecturer, QMUL, The Royal London Hospital, Barts Health NHS Trust, London, UK
Surgery

Jane Anderson BSc, PhD, MBBS, FRCP
Consultant Physician and Director, Centre for the Study of Sexual Health and HIV, Homerton University Hospital NHS Foundation Trust; Professor, Institute of Cell and Molecular Science, Barts and The London School of Medicine and Dentistry, QMUL, UK
Sexually transmitted infections and human immunodeficiency virus

Neil Ashman PhD, FRCP
Consultant Nephrologist, Department of Renal Medicine and Transplantation, Barts Health NHS Trust, London, UK
Kidney and urinary tract disease

Simona Baracaia BSc (Hons), BM BCh, MSc, MFPH
Specialty Registrar in Public Health Medicine, Public Health Team, Barts Health NHS Trust, London, UK
Public Health

Gavin Barlow MBChB, DTM&H, MD, FRCP
Consultant Physician in Infectious Diseases/General Medicine, Hull and East Yorkshire Hospitals NHS Trust; Clinical Associate, Centre for Immunology and Infection, University of York, UK
Infectious disease

Helen Barratt MBBS, PhD, MSc, MA, BSc
Senior Clinical Research Associate, Honorary Consultant in Public Health, Department of Applied Health Research, University College London, London, UK
Evidence-based practice

Ian Basnett MBBS, MSc, FFPHM
Public Health Director, Public Health Team, Barts NHS Trust, London, UK
Public Health

Sara Booth MD, FRCP
Macmillan Consultant in Palliative Medicine, Clinical Director of Palliative Care, Palliative Care Service, Addenbrooke's Hospital, Cambridge University Hospitals NHS Foundation Trust, UK
Palliative care and symptom control

Julius Bourke MBBS, MRCPsych
Consultant Liaison Psychiatrist and Neuropsychiatrist; Honorary Clinical Senior Lecturer, Centre for Psychiatry, Wolfson Institute of Preventive Medicine, Barts and The London School of Medicine and Dentistry, QMUL, UK
Liaison psychiatry

Deborah Bowman BA, MA (Oxon), PhD (London), FRSA
Professor of Bioethics, Clinical Ethics and Medical Law and Deputy Principal, St George's, University of London, UK
Ethical practice and clinical communication

Sally M Bradberry BSc, MD, FRCP, FAACT, FEAPCCT
Deputy Director, National Poisons Information Service (Birmingham Unit); Director, West Midlands Poisons Unit, City Hospital, Birmingham, UK
Prescribing, therapeutics and toxicology

Matthew Buckland MSc, PhD, FRCP, FRCPath, FHEA
Consultant in Clinical Immunology, Royal London Hospital, Barts Health NHS Trust, UK
Immunity

Nicholas H Bunce BSc, MBBS, MD
Consultant Cardiologist, St George's Healthcare NHS Trust, London, UK
Cardiology

Chloe Chin BSc (Hons), MSc, MBBS, MPhil (Cantab)
Consultant in Palliative Medicine, Department of Palliative Medicine, Cambridge University Hospitals NHS Foundation Trust, Cambridge, UK
Palliative care and symptom control

Francis Chinegwundoh MBE MBBS, MS, MML FRCS(Eng), FRCS(Ed), FRCS(Urol), FEBU
Consultant Urological Surgeon, Barts Health NHS Trust, London, UK; Visiting Professor, School of Health Sciences, City University of London, UK; Honorary Clinical Senior Lecturer, Wolfson Centre of Preventative Medicine, Queen Mary College, University of London, London, UK
Men's health

Michael L Clark
Honorary Senior Lecturer, Barts and The London School of Medicine and Dentistry, QMUL, and Princess Grace Hospital, London, UK
Environmental medicine

Richard Conway MD BCh, BAO, PhD, MRCPI
Consultant Rheumatologist, St James's Hospital, Dublin, Ireland
Bone disease

Silvie Cooper PhD, FHEA
Teaching Fellow, NIHR ARC North Thames Academy, Department of Applied Health Research, University College London, London, UK
Online content for Evidence-based practice

Colette Coyle MBBS, BSc Hons Physiotherapy, FFICM, MRCP
Consultant in Intensive Care Medicine, Adult Critical Care Unit, The Royal London Hospital, London, UK
Critical care medicine

xiii

Annie Cushing PhD (London), FDSRCS(Eng), BDS(Hons)
Professor of Clinical Communication, Head of Unit of Clinical and Communication Skills, Institute of Health Sciences Education, Barts and The London School of Medicine and Dentistry, QMUL, UK
Ethical practice and clinical communication

Marinos Elia BSc(Hons), MD, FRCP
Professor of Clinical Nutrition and Metabolism, Institute of Human Nutrition, University of Southampton, UK
Nutrition

Vanessa Foggo MA, MBBS, MRCP, FRCPath
Consultant Haematologist, Department of Haemato-Oncology, St Bartholomew's Hospital, London, UK
Haematological oncology

Graham Foster BA, FRCP, PhD
Professor of Hepatology, Barts and The London School of Medicine and Dentistry, QMUL; Consultant, Barts Health NHS Trust, UK
Liver disease

Ian Giles BSc, MBBS, PhD, FRCP, SFHEA
Professor in Rheumatology, Centre for Rheumatology, Department of Medicine, University College London, UK
Rheumatology

Helena Gleeson MBBS, MRCP(UK), MD
Consultant in Endocrinology, Department of Endocrinology, Queen Elizabeth Hospital, Birmingham, UK
Endocrinology

Robin D Hamilton MBBS, DM, FRCOphth
Consultant Ophthalmologist, Moorfields Eye Hospital, London, UK
Ear, nose and throat and eye disease

Damiete Harry MBBS, MRCS
Higher Specialist Trainee in Urology, Barts Health NHS Trust, London, UK
Men's health

Adam Harper MBBS, MSc, FRCP
Consultant Geriatrician and Honorary Clinical Senior Lecturer, Department of Geriatric Medicine, Brighton and Sussex University Hospitals NHS Trust, Brighton, UK
Geriatric medicine, frailty and multimorbidity

Richard Ian Gregory Holt MA, MBBChir, PhD, FRCP
Professor in Diabetes and Endocrinology, Faculty of Medicine, University of Southampton, UK; Honorary Consultant Physician, Diabetes and Endocrinology, University Hospital Southampton NHS Foundation Trust, UK
Diabetes mellitus

William L Irving MA, PhD, MBBChir, MRCP, FRCPath
Professor of Virology, University of Nottingham, UK
Infectious disease

Paul Jarman MA, MBBS(Hons), PhD
Consultant Neurologist, National Hospital for Neurology and Neurosurgery, London, UK
Neurology

Noor Jawad MBBS, BSc, PhD, MRCP(UK), MRCP (Gastro)
Consultant Gastroenterologist, Department of Gastroenterology, Bart's Health NHS Trust, London, UK
Gastroenterology

Vikas Kapil MA (Cantab), MBBS, PhD, FRCP
Clinical Senior Lecturer in Clinical Pharmacology and Therapeutics, William Harvey Research Institute, Barts and the London School of Medicine and Dentistry, QMUL, London, UK; Consultant Physician in Cardiovascular Medicine, Barts BP Centre of Excellence, Barts Heart Centre, Barts Health NHS Trust, London, UK
Prescribing, therapeutics and toxicology
Hypertension

David P Kelsell PhD
Professor of Human Molecular Genetics, Centre for Cell Biology and Cutaneous Research, Blizard Institute, Barts and The London School of Medicine and Dentistry, QMUL, UK
Human genetics

Klaartje Bel Kok
Gastroenterologist, Gastrointestinal and Liver Services, Barts Health NHS Trust, London, UK
Nutrition

Parveen June Kumar DBE, BSc, MD, DSc, DEd, DMhc, FRCP, FRCPE, FRCPI, FRCPG, FRCPath
Professor Dame, Department of Gastroenterology, Wingate Institute, Barts and the London School of Medicine and Dentistry, QMUL, London, UK
Global health
Environmental medicine

Susan A Lanham-New BA, MSc, PhD, RNutr, FAfN, FSB
Professor of Nutrition, Head of Department of Nutritional Sciences, School of Biosciences and Medicine, University of Surrey, Guildford, UK
Nutrition

Andrew William Leitch MA (Cantab), MBBS, FRCA, FFICM
Consultant in Intensive Care Medicine and Anaesthesia, Adult Critical Care Unit, The Royal London Hospital, London, UK
Sepsis and the treatment of bacterial infection
Critical care medicine

Miles J Levy MD, FRCP
Consultant Physician and Endocrinologist, Leicester Royal Infirmary, University Hospitals of Leicester NHS Trust, UK
Endocrinology

Rachel Lewis MBBS, BSc, MRCP, FRCR
Consultant Clinical Oncologist, Radiotherapy Department, Barts Health NHS Trust, London, UK
Malignant disease

Peter MacCallum MD, FRCP, FRCPath
Doctor, Wolfson Institute of Preventive Medicine, QMUL, London, UK
Venous thromboembolic disease

Kieran McCafferty MA, MBBChir, MRCP MD(res)
Consultant Nephrologist, Department of Nephrology, Barts Health NHS Trust; Senior Lecturer, Department of Nephrology, Barts and The London School of Medicine and Dentistry, QMUL, UK
Water balance, fluids and electrolytes

Nishchay Mehta PhD, FRCS (ORL-HNS)
Consultant Ear, Nose and Throat Surgeon, Royal National ENT Hospital, University College London Hospitals, UK
Ear, nose and throat and eye disease

Mark Melzer MA (Cantab), FRCP, FRCPath, MSc (Microbiology), DTM&H
Consultant in Microbiology and Infectious Diseases, Whipps Cross Hospital and Royal London Hospitals, Barts Health NHS Trust, London, UK; Senior Lecturer in Infection, QMUL, London, UK
Sepsis and the treatment of bacterial infection

Catherine Moffat BSc (Hons)
Clinical Specialist Physiotherapist, Palliative Care, Cambridge University Hospitals NHS Foundation Trust, Cambridge, UK
Palliative care and symptom control

Peter J Moss MBChB, MD, FRCP, DTMH
Consultant in Infectious Diseases, Department of Infection and Tropical Medicine, Director of Infection Prevention and Control, and Deputy Medical Director, Hull and East Yorkshire Hospitals NHS Trust, UK
Infectious disease

Edward WS Mullins PhD, MRCOG
NIHR Academic Clinical Lecturer, Imperial College and Queen Charlotte's and Chelsea Hospital, London, UK
Women's health

Michael F Murphy MD, FRCP, FRCPath
Professor of Blood Transfusion Medicine, University of Oxford; Consultant Haematologist, NHS Blood and Transplant and Department of Haematology, Oxford University Hospitals NHS Trust, UK
Haematology

Catherine Nelson-Piercy MA, FRCP, FRCOG
Professor of Obstetric Medicine, Women's Health Academic Centre, St Thomas' Hospital; Consultant Obstetric Physician, Guy's and St Thomas' NHS Foundation Trust, London, UK
Obstetric medicine

Alastair O'Brien MBBS, BSc, MRCP, PhD
Professor of Experimental Hepatology, University College London, UK
Liver disease

K John Pasi MBChB, PhD, FRCP, FRCPath, FRCPCH
Professor of Haemostasis and Thrombosis, Barts and The London School of Medicine and Dentistry, QMUL; Consultant Haematologist, Barts Health NHS Trust, London, UK
Haematology
Venous thromboembolic disease

Hitesh Patel BSc, MBBS, PhD, MRCP, CCDS
Interventional Heart Failure Cardiologist, Alfred Hospital, Melbourne, Australia
Cardiology

Mark Peakman MBBS, BSc, MSc, PhD, FRCPath
Professor of Clinical Immunology, King's College London School of Medicine, UK
Immunity

Munir Pirmohamed
MBChB(Hons), PhD, FRCP, FMedSci
David Weatherall Chair of Medicine and NHS Chair of Pharmacogenetics, Department of Molecular and Clinical Pharmacology, The Wolfson Centre for Personalised Medicine, University of Liverpool, UK
Prescribing, therapeutics and toxicology

Piers N Plowman MA, MD, FRCP, FRCR
Consultant Clinical Oncologist, St Bartholomew's Hospital, London, UK
Malignant disease

Joanna Preston MBBS, MRCP(UK) (Geriatric Medicine), MSc
Consultant Geriatrician, Senior Health Department, St George's NHS University Hospitals Foundation Trust, London, UK
Geriatric medicine, frailty and multimorbidity

Anisur Rahman MA, PhD, BMBCh, FRCP
Professor of Rheumatology, Centre for Rheumatology, Department of Medicine, University College London, UK
Rheumatology

Rosalind Raine BSc, MBBS, MSc, PhD
Professor, Department of Applied Health Research, University College London, UK
Evidence-based practice

Neil Rajan MBBS, PhD
Senior Lecturer and Honorary Consultant Dermatologist, Translational and Clinical Research Institute, Newcastle University, Newcastle upon Tyne, UK
Human genetics

Radha Ramachandran MBBS, MRCP, MSc, FRCPath, PhD
Consultant, Adult Inherited Metabolic Diseases, Guys and St Thomas' Hospitals NHS Foundation Trust; Consultant, Chemical Pathology and Metabolic Medicine, Guys and St Thomas' Hospitals NHS Foundation Trust, London, UK
Lipid and metabolic disorders

Robin Ray MBBS MA(Oxon), MRCP, PhD
Consultant in Heart failure and Cardiac Imaging, St George's University Hospitals NHS Foundation Trust, London, UK
Cardiology

Narendra Reddy MD, FRCP, CCT (Oxf)
Consultant Endocrinologist, Diabetes and Endocrinology, University Hospitals of Leicester, Leicester, UK; Honorary Senior Lecturer, University of Leicester, UK
Endocrinology

Lesley Regan MD, DSC, FRCOG, FACOG
Professor of Obstetrics and Gynaecology, Imperial College at St Mary's Hospital, London, UK
Women's health

Noémi Roy MBChB, DPhil
Honorary Senior Clinical Lecturer, Weatherall Institute of Molecular Medicine, University of Oxford, UK; Consultant Haematologist, Department of Haematology, Oxford University Hospitals NHS Foundation Trust, UK
Haematology

Prina Ruparelia MBChB, MSc, FRCP, MD
Respiratory medicine, St Bartholomew's Hospital, London, UK
Respiratory disease

Babulal Sethia BSc, MB BS, FRCS, FRCP
Past President, Royal Society of Medicine, London, UK
Global health

Jonathan Shamash MBChB, MD, FRCP
Consultant Medical Oncologist, Barts Health NHS Trust, London, UK
Malignant disease

Stephen Shepherd MBBS, MRCP, FRCA, FFICM
Consultant in Anaesthesia and Intensive Care, Department of Perioperative Medicine, St Bartholomew's Hospital, London, UK
Critical care medicine

Jonathan Sive BSc (Hons), MBChB, PhD, MRCP, FRCPath
Consultant Haematologist, Department of Haematology, University College London Hospital, London, UK
Haematological oncology

Charlotte Skinner BM BCh, MA (Cantab), MRCP (Gastro)
Doctor, Gastroenterology, Barts Health NHS Trust, London, UK
Gastroenterology

Francis Vaz MBBS, BSc(Hons), FRCS(ORL-HNS)
Consultant Ear, Nose and Throat/Head and Neck Surgeon, Department of ENT/Head and Neck Surgery, University College London Hospital, UK
Ear, nose and throat and eye disease

Umesh Vivekananda MA, MRCP, PhD
Neurology Academic Clinical Lecturer, National Hospital for Neurology and Neurosurgery, London, UK and University College London, UK
Neurology

Christopher Wadsworth MBBS, PhD, MRCP
Consultant Gastroenterologist and Hepato-Pancreato-Biliary Physician, Hammersmith Hospital, Imperial College Healthcare NHS Trust, London, UK
Biliary tract and pancreatic disease

Sarah H Wakelin BSc, MBBS, FRCP
Consultant Dermatologist, Imperial College Healthcare NHS Trust, London, UK
Dermatology

David W Wareham MBBS, MSc, PhD, MRCP, FRCPath
Consultant Microbiologist, Department of School of Medicine and Dentistry, QMUL, London, UK
Sepsis and the treatment of bacterial infection

Veronica White BSc, MBBS, MSc, MD, FRCP
Consultant Physician, Department of Respiratory Medicine, Barts Health NHS Trust, London, UK
Respiratory disease

Anthony S Wierzbicki DM, DPhil, FRCPath
Consultant in Metabolic Medicine/Chemical Pathology, Department of Metabolic Medicine, Guy's & St Thomas' Hospitals, London, UK
Lipid and metabolic disorders

Iain Wilkinson MBBS, MA, FRCP, FHEA
Consultant Orthogeriatrician, Medicine for the Elderly, Surrey and Sussex Healthcare NHS Trust, Surrey, UK; Honorary Senior Lecturer, Brighton and Sussex Medical School, Brighton, UK
Geriatric medicine, frailty and multimorbidity

Janet D Wilson MBChB, FRCP
Consultant in Genitourinary Medicine and HIV, Leeds Sexual Health, Leeds Teaching Hospitals NHS Trust, UK
Sexually transmitted infections and human immunodeficiency virus

Sarah Elizabeth Winchester MB BChir, MSc, MA (Cantab), MFPH
Specialty Registrar in Public Health Medicine, Public Health Team, Barts Health NHS Trust, London, UK
Public Health

M Magdi Yaqoob MD, FRCP
Professor of Nephrology, William Harvey Research Institute, Barts and The London School of Medicine and Dentistry, QMUL; Consultant, Department of Renal Medicine and Transplantation, Barts Health NHS Trust, London, UK
Kidney and urinary tract disease
Water balance, fluids and electrolytes

Parjam Zolfaghari MBBS, PhD, FRCA, FFICM, FHEA
Consultant in Intensive Care Medicine and Anaesthesia, Barts Health NHS Trust; Honorary Senior Lecturer, QMUL; Adult Critical Care Unit, The Royal London Hospital, London, UK
Critical care medicine

International Advisory Board

Acknowledgements for the Tenth Edition

As always, this book is made what it is by the diligence and expertise of the individual chapter authors, who have worked hard to ensure that the content they provided is up to date, well presented and reflective of modern practice. We are grateful to them for their efforts.

The process of editing has been made much easier by the high standards and clear priorities set out by Parveen Kumar and Mike Clark through their careful editorial work on an astonishing previous nine editions of this book. We are now in a better position than many to appreciate the sheer amount of hard work this involved, and on behalf of the medical profession – our thanks.

We would like to acknowledge and offer grateful thanks for the input of all previous editions' contributors, without whom this new edition would not have been possible. As well as welcoming a number of new contributors to this edition, we would like to thank various others who have stepped down this time around – especially those who have had a long association with the book. Much of their work is reflected in the text of this edition, and so we thank them for their input:

- John V Anderson (Diabetes mellitus and metabolic disorders)
- Rachel Buxton-Thomas (Respiratory medicine)
- Sarah R Doffman (Respiratory medicine)
- Gail E Eva (Palliative medicine)
- Anthony J Frew (Respiratory medicine)
- Edwin AM Gale (Diabetes mellitus and metabolic disorders)
- Christopher J Gallagher (Malignant disease)
- Charles J Hinds (Critical care medicine)
- Katharine Hurt (Respiratory medicine)
- Miriam J Johnson (Palliative medicine)
- Louise Langmead (Gastroenterology)
- James Lindsay (Gastroenterology)
- Kenneth J Linton (Molecular cell biology)
- Adam Mead (Haematology)
- Michael J O'Dwyer (Critical care medicine)
- Donncha O'Gradaigh (Bone disease)
- David G Paige (Skin disease)
- Rupert M Pearse (Critical care medicine)
- Sean L Preston (Gastroenterology)
- Michael Rawlins (Clinical pharmacology)
- Matthew Smith (Malignant disease)
- J Allister Vale (Poisoning)
- David Westaby (Biliary tract and pancreatic disease)
- Peter D White (Psychological medicine)

We were saddened to hear of the untimely death of Anthony J Frew (Respiratory medicine), who made a major contribution to this book but also to the wider practice of medicine.

We are grateful to the International Advisory Board, who have supplied a significant amount of online material that helps to ensure this book maintains the global relevance it has always striven to enjoy.

We would like to thank Dr Robert Stephenson and Dr Joseph Davies for their radiological input and figures.

The team at Elsevier have worked extremely hard in bringing this project to fruition. We are particularly grateful to Pauline Graham and Helen Leng, the commissioning and development editors, who did so much to drive this project forward before they left Elsevier. We owe them much gratitude and wish them every success in their future ventures. Pauline in particular has worked on a number of previous editions of this book and the recent success of *Clinical Medicine* owes much to her oversight.

Thanks to Alex Mortimer, who took over as commissioning editor relatively late in the project, and from a standing start provided helpful guidance and direction in the final stages of production. Thanks to Louise Cook, who completed various aspects of development with a close eye for detail. Thanks to our copy-editors, Wendy Lee and Lynn Watt, who checked thoroughly, detected error and redundancy, and acted pre-emptively to offer helpful suggestions. Julie Taylor and Anne Collett acted as production managers and we are grateful to them for their experience and efficiency in bringing a large and spreading project together into a finished piece of work. Thanks to Kim Benson for her work in putting together the online content in a way that will maximize its usefulness to readers around the world.

Finally, thanks to our long-suffering families, who have endured much absence and distraction as we have worked at antisocial hours on manuscripts at various stages of development. This would not have been possible without your patience and support, and we are most grateful.

Diagnosis: the art of being a doctor

David Randall, Adam Feather and Mona Waterhouse

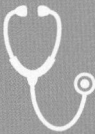

CORE SKILLS AND KNOWLEDGE

Being a doctor is a privilege; our patients allow us to share in their troubles and triumphs, and place their faith in our judgement and skill.

In the 21st century, professional roles and responsibilities are rapidly changing, and so defining what it means to be a doctor is difficult. Healthcare is provided by teams, not individuals, and other healthcare professionals now perform tasks in assessing and managing patients that were previously carried out exclusively by doctors. The use of artificial intelligence, which applies vast, unsorted clinical and academic datasets to produce algorithms that can inform diagnostic and management questions, provides a fundamental challenge to the historically crucial role of doctors in these areas.

While the process of diagnosis will be increasingly augmented by artificial intelligence, it is unlikely ever to be replaced by it because at the centre of any diagnostic conundrum is a human being. Working out what is wrong with a patient involves not just technical skills, such as the assimilation of information, interpretation of data and use of clinical reasoning to reach a diagnosis. It also requires compassion, empathy, trust, respect and humour: the stuff that makes up a relationship between human beings. And it brings into play an ethical code developed to ensure that the great power of medical knowledge is used for the good of individual patients and of society as a whole.

Once a diagnosis is made, the human tasks continue. Doctors tailor their explanations to the needs and understanding of their patients. They negotiate a management strategy and share clinical decision-making with the person under their care. However medicine evolves in the future, at the centre of everything we do must remain the huge privilege and pleasure of caring for, supporting, empowering and helping people so that their health and social needs are optimally met.

DIAGNOSIS IN THE CLINICAL CONSULTATION

In many patient interactions, the forming of a diagnosis stands as a turning point in the therapeutic journey: the focus shifts from the gathering of information and the performance of tests to planning of treatment and discussion of outcomes. Forming a diagnosis is a complex process, which always starts with taking a history. The initial patient story is first developed into a set of problems, which in turn becomes a list of differential diagnoses. Data-gathering, further information, initial treatment and the passage of time help to form and confirm a definitive diagnosis.

Fig. 1.1 shows how diagnosis is often an iterative process, in which information is gathered, interpreted and integrated to form a working diagnosis, and then communicated and acted on through treatment; all the time the working diagnosis is refined or revised using newly gathered information, including the patient's response to treatment.

THE MEDICAL CONSULTATION

The initial interaction – forming a rapport

First impressions matter. A clinical interaction that begins badly often runs into problems later on. Patients need to be able to share their most intimate and worrying problems and this will be impossible if they cannot develop confidence and trust in their clinicians. The clinician should always ask, 'How would I wish my own doctor to behave?' The physical environment can also be improved to help the interaction go well: always ensure patients' privacy, dignity and comfort, treating them and their carers with respect.

A warm greeting is always worthwhile. Introduce yourself (and any other health professionals present), explaining your role and the purpose of the encounter. A healthcare system is generally busy and confusing, so help patients understand where they are in their journey through it. The 'Hello, my name is ...' campaign, supported by the Department of Health in the UK, highlights the importance of basic introductions on the part of staff members (**Box 1.1**). Further

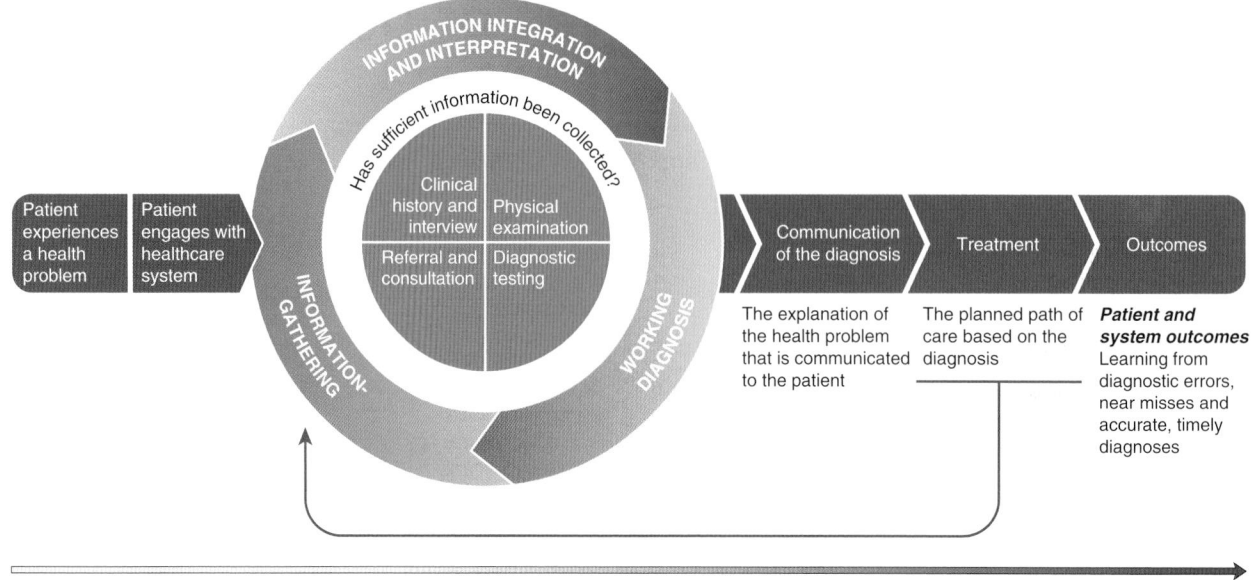

Fig. 1.1 A conceptualization of the diagnostic process. *(From National Academies of Sciences, Engineering, and Medicine. Improving Diagnosis in Health Care. Washington, DC: The National Academies Press; 2015. https://doi.org.10.17226/21794.)*

> ### Box 1.1 The 'Hello, my name is ...' campaign
>
> In 2011, geriatrician Dr Kate Granger was diagnosed with metastatic sarcoma, from which she eventually died in 2016. Noticing that many of the healthcare staff treating her during her illness failed to introduce themselves, she created the 'Hello, my name is ...' campaign. Describing why an initial introduction is so important, she said, 'I firmly believe it is not just about common courtesy, but it runs much deeper. Introductions are about making a human connection between one human being who is suffering and vulnerable, and another human being who wishes to help. They begin therapeutic relationships and can instantly build trust in difficult circumstances.'
>
>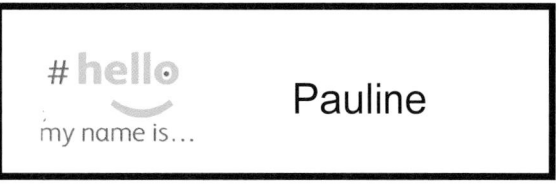
>
> The campaign encourages healthcare staff to greet and introduce themselves to patients and encourages the wearing of easy-to-read name badges like this one.

comments expressing empathy, support or care for the patient at this point can be very helpful in ensuring that a good rapport is established, before proceeding to talk about the problem that has led the patient to seek medical help (**Box 1.2**).

Information-gathering

Once a rapport has been established, the consultation is generally divided into three parts: *history*, *examination* and *investigations/management*. Depending on the context and the acuity of the situation, these may occur in isolation, follow on from one another or, in severely ill patients, happen synchronously.

The history

In the construction of an accurate diagnosis, nothing is more important than taking a full history from the patient. It is estimated

that up to 80% of the diagnosis can be made on the basis of a careful history alone. In addition to information-gathering, eliciting the history is key to the therapeutic relationship. If it goes well, the patient knows they have been listened to, has had an opportunity to convey all of their concerns, and knows that the clinician cares for them and will act as their advocate. This builds mutual trust and respect, and helps the patient to undergo invasive or intimate procedures and adhere to therapeutic interventions in the future.

A meeting of two experts

It has been said that a medical consultation is a meeting of two experts. A good consultation is based on mutual respect, rejecting a traditional paternalistic view of medicine ('doctor knows best'), and assisting joint exploration of the biomedical and the patient perspectives on the problem. This will lead to shared understanding, where clinician and patient jointly grasp what is wrong, what impact it is having on the patient's life, what the patient expects from medical intervention, and which options would be best for investigating and treating the problem (see **Fig. 5.1**).

The golden minute

At the start of the consultation the clinician should avoid interrupting the patient for as long as possible. Patients often mentally rehearse a script relating to the symptoms or problems they wish to describe. An early interruption may throw them off course and cause them to forget key points, leaving them feeling dissatisfied with the interaction. The term '*the golden minute*' has been coined to encourage clinicians to allow patients to tell their story uninterrupted for at least 1 minute. This gives them time to describe their symptoms as they have experienced them, including information that might be missed if the clinician jumps in too soon with closed, focused questions.

Allowing the patient freedom to tell their own story aids clinicians in achieving their primary objective of making a diagnosis, but ultimately forms and reinforces the therapeutic relationship and increases both patient and clinician satisfaction. **Box 1.3** summarizes some techniques that can be used to help patients share information in a way that is accurate and comprehensive. Some will

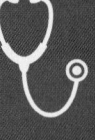

Box 1.2 Good practice for using the medical history to build a therapeutic relationship

- Allow the patient to tell their story, without jumping in prematurely with questions.
- Ask the patient specifically about their ideas, concerns and expectations (ICE):
  - **Ideas:** What do they think might be going on? Have they done any reading about their symptoms or asked anyone they know?
  - **Concerns:** Are they feeling anxious or worried about their symptoms? What is causing them concern? Are there any particular areas where their symptoms might be making life difficult?
- **Expectations:** What are they hoping for from this consultation?
- Try to develop an understanding of who the patient is as a person. Where, and with whom, do they live? What is their occupation? What things do they enjoy? Moments of human connection, such as a shared interest in a place or activity, can be powerful in building a relationship between clinician and patient.
- Try to convey empathy and concern, reinforcing to the patient that you are their advocate and will do your best to help them.

Box 1.3 Strategies in history-taking

- **Begin with open questions** ('Could you tell me more about the pain?'): do this before moving to closed questions to help rule certain key problems in or out ('Did the pain get worse after eating?').
- **Emphasize your active listening:** maintain eye contact, nod, acknowledge key points, and respond to comments the patient might make that are humorous or sad.
- **Respond to the patient's body language:** note whether the patient becomes distressed or embarrassed. If so, acknowledge this and look for ways to address it.

- **Empathize:** try to show the patient that you care about what they are going through. Put yourself in their shoes: how might they be feeling? Communicate this: 'Thanks for sharing this – it must be difficult not knowing what is going on.'
- **Summarize:** run through what the patient has told you, to make sure nothing has been missed out.
- **Signpost:** explain what you have just covered and what you are now going on to explore, and why.
- **Use plain English:** avoid medical jargon or complicated vocabulary, unless it is clear that the patient is able to understand this.

Box 1.4 A structured approach to information-gathering in the medical history

- Presenting complaint: why has the patient sought medical advice?
- History of the presenting complaint: further information about the patient's main problem
- Past medical and surgical history
- Drug history and allergies
- Family history
- Social history: information on the patient's present living arrangements and relevant risk factors

Box 1.5 Using the time course of symptoms to suggest an underlying cause

Onset of symptoms	Possible causes
Immediate (seconds to minutes)	Vascular – thrombotic or embolic Anatomical – e.g. perforation of a viscus Electrical – e.g. dysrhythmias, seizures
Hours to days	Bacterial or viral infections Inflammatory and autoimmune diseases
Weeks to months	Malignant disease Inflammatory and autoimmune diseases Chronic infections, e.g. mycobacterial
Months to years	Degenerative conditions Fibrotic diseases

have given a lot of thought to their symptoms and come with a well-thought-through story; others may not have reflected much on what has been going on, and key information may need to be drawn out by sensitive questioning.

Structuring the medical history

Over the last 150 years a formal structure for the recording of the patient's history has evolved. This has several subsections (**Box 1.4**). While facts may be recorded in this very stylized manner, the patient will rarely, if ever, present them in this structure. It is up to the interviewing clinician to assimilate and interpret the information fully and to form a considered diagnostic narrative, so that when it is presented to others, either verbally or in written form, sense can be made of the diagnostic reasoning and conclusions.

History of the presenting complaint

The aim is to provide a thorough account of the symptoms that led the patient to seek medical attention. It is vital to listen closely to how the symptoms are described and not to miss any clues that can be followed up with direct questioning. For each symptom the patient presents with, additional questioning should be used to identify:

- **Time course**: When did the problem begin? Does it come and go? Is there anything that triggers it? Is there any variation in the symptoms during the day or night? Has the patient ever had anything like this in the past? Establishing the pattern in which symptoms have developed is often one of the most helpful parts of the history in helping to form a diagnosis (**Box 1.5**).

- **Associated symptoms**: What else has the patient noticed? Begin with an open question, and then proceed to asking about the presence or absence of relevant symptoms that may help to determine the cause of the problem.
- **Severity, site, radiation and character** of any pain: How would the patient rate it on a scale from 1 to 10? Do they describe it as tight, dull, electric or burning? Is it getting worse, staying the same or starting to improve?
- **Responses**: What has the patient done about the symptoms? Have they sought medical advice or used medication that they have at home?

The 'Clinical skills' sections at the beginning of many of the chapters in this book present additional questioning techniques relevant to particular medical specialties. At this point in the history, asking questions to form a review of systems can be valuable in eliciting further symptoms that the patient may not have mentioned or not thought relevant (**Box 1.6**).

Past medical and surgical history

This should include all significant medical conditions, including hospital admissions, long-term conditions, life-threatening or life-changing conditions, and important investigations, procedures and therapeutic interventions (operations, endoscopies, biopsies and significant courses of treatment such as chemo- or radiotherapy).

---

i **Box 1.6 Review of systems**

Conducting a brief but comprehensive 'review of systems' may be a particularly useful schema when the patient has non-specific symptoms, e.g. weight loss, tiredness and weakness, or when someone reports 'I just don't feel right, doctor'.

Respiratory

Cough, sputum (volume, frequency, consistency, colour, offensive taste or smell), haemoptysis (volume, frequency, consistency, colour, freshness, altered nature, clots), shortness of breath, exercise tolerance, orthopnoea, wheeze, chest pain

Cardiovascular

Chest pain, shortness of breath, cough, sputum, orthopnoea, swelling of ankles (peripheral oedema) or abdomen (ascites), paroxysmal nocturnal dyspnoea, palpitations

Gastrointestinal

General – normal and present weight, appetite, oral intake

Upper – dysphagia (level: high – base of neck, mid and lower chest), consistency of food tolerated/not tolerated), dyspepsia, odynophagia, upper abdominal pain, early satiety, nausea/vomiting (volume, frequency, consistency – unaltered food (regurgitation), altered food, blood), haematemesis (volume, frequency, consistency, colour, freshness, altered nature, clots)

Lower – lower abdominal pain, altered bowel habit, constipation, diarrhoea (volume, frequency, consistency, colour), blood per rectum, mucus per rectum, anal pain

Hepatobiliary and pancreatic

Jaundice, associated pain, pruritus, symptoms of encephalopathy, abdominal swelling (ascites)

Renal

Urine (frequency, volume, colour, offensive odour), dysuria, haematuria (volume, frequency, colour, freshness, clots), symptoms of bladder outflow tract obstruction (hesitancy, frequency, small volume, terminal dribbling)

Musculoskeletal

Bone pains, back pain and stiffness, joint stiffness, swelling, pain, erythema, patterns of joints involved, muscular pain, weakness, acute pain suggesting pathological or fragility fractures

Dermatological

Rashes, blisters, ulcers

Endocrine

Diabetic symptoms and complications, sexual function, menstruation, symptoms of thyroid dysfunction

Neurological

Seizures, muscle weakness, involuntary movements, loss of sensation, altered gait, speech and swallowing dysfunction

Ophthalmic

Eye pain, redness, dryness or grittiness, changes in vision, flashing lights

Ear, nose and throat

Changes in smell, taste or hearing, pain in ears, nose, throat or sinuses, nasal discharge or crusting

Haematological

Easy bleeding or bruising, tiredness, lymph node swelling, abdominal fullness (splenomegaly)

Mental health

Mood (suicidality when relevant), anxiety, altered perceptions (hallucinations), abnormal beliefs (delusions)

Genitourinary

Urethral or vaginal discharge, pain or itching, pain during sexual intercourse, sexual function, in women – menstrual cycle, use of contraception, history of pregnancies and childbirth

---

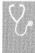 **Box 1.7 Five questions for the patient with a long-term condition**

1. *Diagnosis* – HOW, WHY, WHERE and WHEN was your condition first diagnosed?
2. *Progression* – How has it progressed since?
3. *Control* – How do you monitor your condition? Which healthcare professionals are involved with your care? When did you last have a check-up? What medications do you take? What are your biggest challenges in controlling your condition?
4. *The good and the bad* – What is the BEST and WORST your condition has ever been? How does it have an impact on your life?
5. *Today/recently* – How have you been? If unwell, have you ever been this unwell before? What happened when you were last this unwell?

If the patient has had any surgical interventions a comprehensive anaesthetic history should be sought and recorded. Five good questions to ask about chronic conditions are listed in **Box 1.7**.

Drug history

Document all medications the patient has been taking, including prescribed, over-the-counter and herbal or traditional treatments. Record when each was started, along with the dosing regimen; ask about side-effects and adherence to treatment. When you are unsure or ignorant of a drug, it is essential to research and record the class, common side-effects and interactions. Medication error is a common cause of morbidity and mortality, and ignorance is no defence. Ask about and record **drug allergies**, including the timing and nature of any reactions.

Family history

This is particularly relevant when assessing younger patients or when the differential diagnosis includes possible genetic conditions. It is essential to record the structure of the patient's family in detail, including the patient's and parents' siblings, any 'half-siblings' (genetically related to only one of the patient's parents), and where relevant, a history of consanguinity. Once this is completed, confirm which of these relatives have been affected by a given condition or by premature death (see p. 13).

Social history

The social history has two key purposes:

- **Establishing whether there are any environmental factors** that may be causative or exacerbating the patient's symptoms. Always ask about housing, occupation, tobacco smoking, alcohol intake, and use of recreational and illicit drugs. Where relevant, draw up a travel history, including animal and insect bites, a sexual history (if a sexually transmitted disease, including HIV infection, is suspected), and hobbies, leisure activities and pets.
- **Understanding more about the lifestyle** of the patient. Where do they live? How active are they? Are they limited in any daily activities by physical or mental health problems? Do they have informal or formal carers? If so, how often do the carers attend and what do they do for the patient?

Physical examination

The physical examination, including any objective observations, should be used to confirm or refute the initial diagnosis/diagnoses made from the history. It is a key part of all medical interactions but its duration and extent will be guided by the patient's history and the acuity of the presentation.

Even in the era of complex technological investigations a careful physical examination performs a number of key functions, including:

- Providing objective evidence (physical signs) to complement subjective evidence (symptoms) from the history. Sometimes a

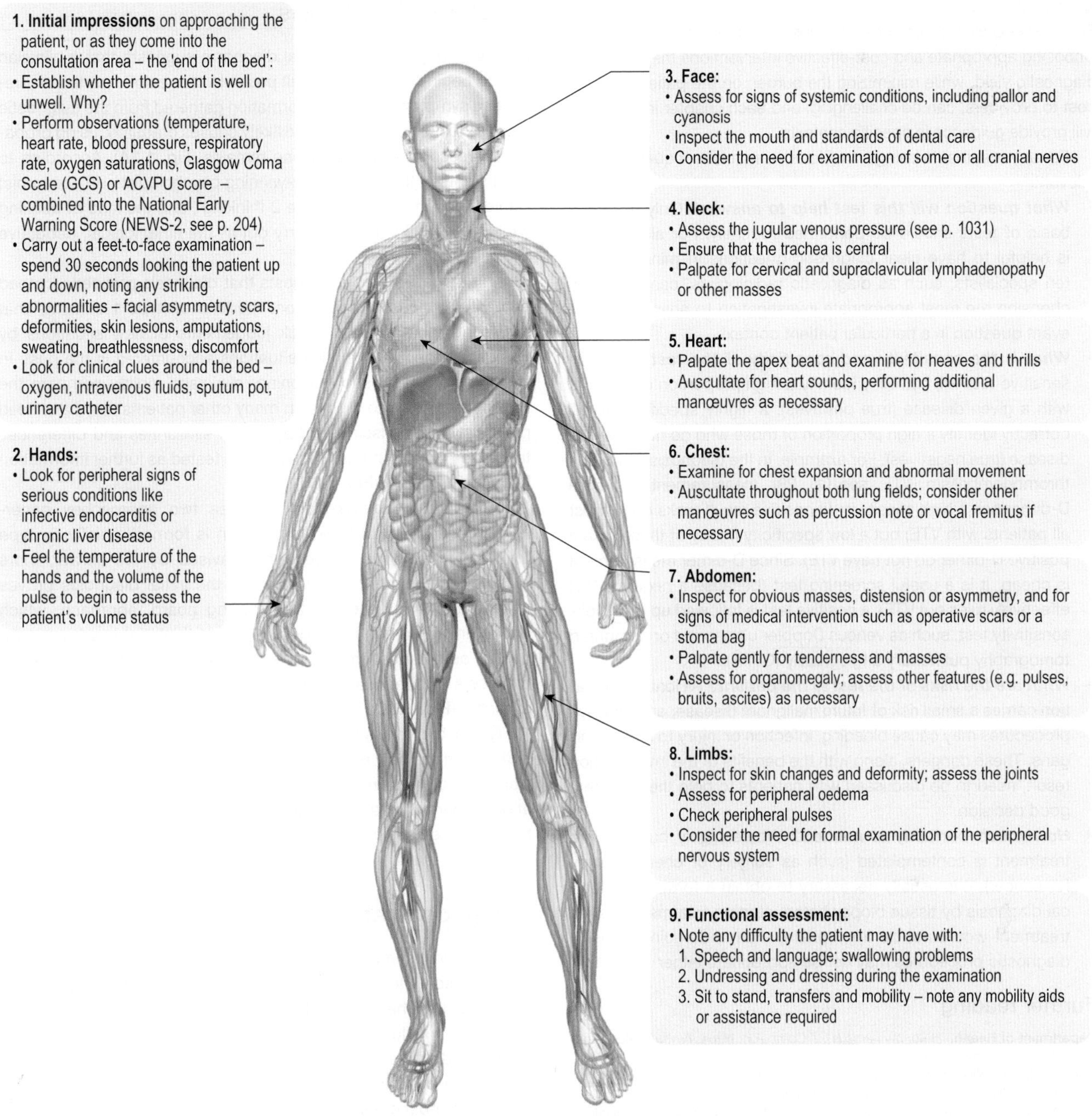

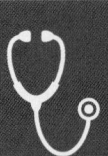

1. Initial impressions on approaching the patient, or as they come into the consultation area – the 'end of the bed':
- Establish whether the patient is well or unwell. Why?
- Perform observations (temperature, heart rate, blood pressure, respiratory rate, oxygen saturations, Glasgow Coma Scale (GCS) or ACVPU score – combined into the National Early Warning Score (NEWS-2, see p. 204)
- Carry out a feet-to-face examination – spend 30 seconds looking the patient up and down, noting any striking abnormalities – facial asymmetry, scars, deformities, skin lesions, amputations, sweating, breathlessness, discomfort
- Look for clinical clues around the bed – oxygen, intravenous fluids, sputum pot, urinary catheter

2. Hands:
- Look for peripheral signs of serious conditions like infective endocarditis or chronic liver disease
- Feel the temperature of the hands and the volume of the pulse to begin to assess the patient's volume status

3. Face:
- Assess for signs of systemic conditions, including pallor and cyanosis
- Inspect the mouth and standards of dental care
- Consider the need for examination of some or all cranial nerves

4. Neck:
- Assess the jugular venous pressure (see p. 1031)
- Ensure that the trachea is central
- Palpate for cervical and supraclavicular lymphadenopathy or other masses

5. Heart:
- Palpate the apex beat and examine for heaves and thrills
- Auscultate for heart sounds, performing additional manœuvres as necessary

6. Chest:
- Examine for chest expansion and abnormal movement
- Auscultate throughout both lung fields; consider other manœuvres such as percussion note or vocal fremitus if necessary

7. Abdomen:
- Inspect for obvious masses, distension or asymmetry, and for signs of medical intervention such as operative scars or a stoma bag
- Palpate gently for tenderness and masses
- Assess for organomegaly; assess other features (e.g. pulses, bruits, ascites) as necessary

8. Limbs:
- Inspect for skin changes and deformity; assess the joints
- Assess for peripheral oedema
- Check peripheral pulses
- Consider the need for formal examination of the peripheral nervous system

9. Functional assessment:
- Note any difficulty the patient may have with:
  1. Speech and language; swallowing problems
  2. Undressing and dressing during the examination
  3. Sit to stand, transfers and mobility – note any mobility aids or assistance required

Fig. 1.2 A basic approach to clinical examination.

firm diagnosis can be made almost solely on the basis of examination findings, such as in a number of skin disorders.
- Assessing the severity or extent of problems.
- Identifying unexpected findings that patients themselves have not noticed.
- Building rapport with patients. The value of performing a physical examination can be significant in reinforcing to patients that they have been dealt with thoroughly and compassionately.

Typically a general assessment will be made as the history is being elicited (Is the patient well or unwell? Are there any obvious clinical signs?). This will be aided by a set of formal observations (blood pressure, heart rate, oxygen saturation, respiratory rate, level of consciousness, capillary blood glucose and temperature). A more detailed assessment is then carried out, including a 'general examination' (hands, upper limbs, face and neck), examination of the likely affected system(s) as suggested by the history, and finally a wider examination of other organ systems.

Fig. 1.2 outlines a typical general and systematic examination routine suitable for use in patients presenting with a wide range of medical conditions. The 'Clinical skills' sections at the beginning of many of the chapters in this book offer tailored versions of this basic routine relevant to patients with specific types of complaint.

Discussion and negotiation around investigations

In the modern era, there are a huge number of investigations available to the clinician, ranging from simple bedside tests such as spirometry or urine dipstick analysis, through to complex radiological imaging and invasive procedures such as endoscopy or angiography. Some tests may combine both diagnostic and therapeutic potential. Choosing appropriate and cost-effective interventions that maximize diagnostic yield, while minimizing the burden on the patient and the cost to providers, can be challenging, and each chapter in this book will provide guidance in specific contexts.

For any test that is being considered, a number of questions are relevant:

- *What question will this test help to answer?* Only the most basic of tests should be performed routinely. For all others, it is helpful to have clear diagnostic questions in mind, and often specialists, such as diagnostic radiologists, can help with choosing the most appropriate investigation to answer the relevant question in a particular patient context.
- *What is the sensitivity and specificity of the test?* A highly sensitive test will correctly identify a high proportion of patients with a given disease (true positives); a highly specific test will correctly identify a high proportion of those who do not have the disease (true negatives). For example, in the diagnosis of venous thromboembolism (VTE, see Ch. 29), measurement of serum D-dimer has a high sensitivity (a positive result picks out almost all patients with VTE) but a low specificity (many of those with a positive D-dimer do not have VTE). Since D-dimer measurement is cheap, it is a useful screening test (because a negative test effectively rules out VTE); a positive test is followed up by a high-sensitivity test, such as venous Doppler ultrasound or computed tomography pulmonary angiography (CTPA).
- *What are the risks of the test to the patient?* All ionizing radiation carries a small risk of future malignant disease, and invasive procedures may cause bleeding, infection or injury to internal organs. These dangers, along with the benefits of the investigation result, need to be discussed with patients to help them make a good decision.
- *How much certainty is needed?* Where highly burdensome treatment is contemplated (such as surgery or chemotherapy for cancer), it is usually necessary to obtain a formal histological diagnosis by tissue biopsy before starting treatment. If such treatment would not be appropriate, then undergoing invasive diagnostic procedures may not be appropriate either.

Further reading

Department of Health. *'Hello, my name is …' Campaign*. https://www.health-ni.gov.uk/articles/hello-my-name.
Glynn M, Drake WM (eds). Hutchinson's Clinical Methods: An Integrated Approach to Clinical Practice. Edinburgh: Elsevier; 2018.
Kurtz S, Silverman J, Benson J et al. Marrying content and process in clinical method teaching: enhancing the Calgary-Cambridge guides. *Acad Med* 2003; 78:802–809.
McKelvey I. The consultation hill: a new model to aid teaching consultation skills. *Br J Gen Pract* 2010; 60:538–540.
National Academies of Sciences, Engineering, and Medicine. *Improving Diagnosis in Health Care*. Washington, DC: The National Academies Press; 2015.

CLINICAL DIAGNOSTIC REASONING

Forming a diagnosis involves a complex process of reasoning. Large amounts of information gathered from the history, examination and available investigation results need to be assimilated and synthesized into a working diagnosis. Each piece of evidence should be weighed according to the degree of confidence you have in its accuracy, and no significant findings should remain unexplained. If you, as the treating clinician, are unable to make sense of the information presented to you, you should be humble and insightful enough to seek help from others.

Models of diagnosis

A traditional model of medical diagnosis suggests that a clinician should begin by considering all possible causes of a particular presenting symptom, and use information gathered from the diagnostic process to include and exclude likely causes gradually, using probabilistic reasoning, until only one remains (**Fig. 1.3A**). According to the insights of the Nobel Prize-winning psychologist and economist Daniel Kahneman, this is 'type 2 thinking', and the kind of thinking we like to imagine that we carry out all the time: logical, deductive and rational.

An alternative model suggests that diagnosis proceeds instead primarily by pattern recognition, the kind of 'type 1 thinking' that allows humans to make quick judgements of new situations by comparing them with similar situations encountered in the past. In this form of diagnostic reasoning, clinicians rapidly compare the patient presenting to them with many other patients they have seen previously, subconsciously drawing on similarities and differences to form an initial impression that is then tested as further information becomes available (**Fig. 1.3B**).

In reality, a combination of these two approaches generally occurs: an initial rapid impression is formed, chiefly by type 1 thinking, which is subsequently revised by the slower, more reason-based type 2 thinking where the initial diagnosis proves inadequate. This 'back to the drawing board' approach, which draws on the strengths of both types of thinking, has been suggested as the best model for safe diagnosis – where a working diagnosis is continually re-evaluated as new evidence becomes available (**Fig. 1.3C**).

Type 1 thinking is prone to bias (see later), where it is assumed that everything new must be similar to things seen before. It is crucial for doctors to re-evaluate an initial diagnosis actively in situations where things 'don't quite fit' rather than persisting with a hastily formed assumption that may prove incorrect.

Diagnostic error and patient safety

It has been estimated that 10–15% of medical diagnoses are wrong. Misdiagnosis or delayed diagnosis can be the cause of significant patient harm, including adverse effects from unnecessary treatment or failure to receive an appropriate timely intervention. While misdiagnosis may occur as a result of inadequate clinical knowledge or (particularly in resource-poor settings) through a lack of diagnostic resources, it also arises as a direct result of one or more cognitive biases. **Box 1.8** lists a number of common cognitive biases, applied to the field of diagnostic reasoning, which together form a key avoidable source of medical harm, termed 'human error'.

Strategies for avoiding bias

Various strategies can be employed in order to reduce the chances of making an incorrect diagnosis:

- *Adopting an iterative approach*, in which all previous diagnoses are subjected to appropriate re-evaluation, especially if evidence appears that brings them into question.
- *Team discussions*, where all team members are empowered to challenge the reasoning of more senior clinicians. Multidisciplinary team meetings bring clinicians from different specialties together with allied healthcare professionals to ensure that all relevant

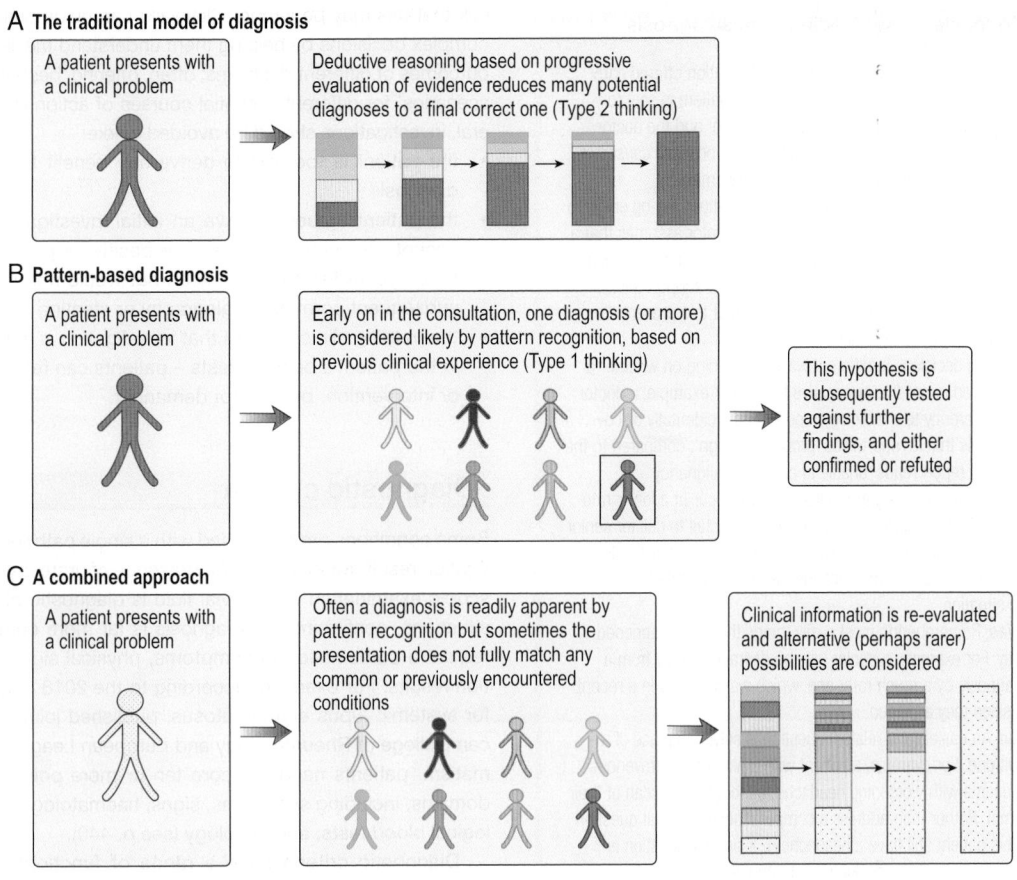

Fig. 1.3 Approaches to diagnosis. (A) The traditional model of diagnosis. **(B)** Pattern-based diagnosis. **(C)** A combined approach.

knowledge and expertise is shared in a collaborative environment. Leaders of healthcare teams have a particular responsibility to 'flatten the authority gradient' and empower more junior members to contribute knowledge and ideas to team discussions.

- ***Diagnostic criteria and guidelines***, where robust standards are outlined to ensure that potential diagnoses are correctly assigned and similar conditions are differentiated from each other.
- ***Considering patient problems in language devoid of assumption***, as far as possible, seeking to describe a patient's problems succinctly and objectively without recourse to previous diagnostic reasoning.
- ***Using lists of disease classes to avoid jumping to conclusions***: simple *aides-mémoire* encourage clinicians to consider, for example, malignant, infectious, vascular, metabolic, inflammatory and degenerative causes of a particular problem.

Levels of diagnostic depth

A clinical impression is formed by taking a comprehensive history and undertaking a relevant physical examination. Drawing on the information gathered, clinicians may typically assign a widely understood umbrella term to categorize a collection of signs and symptoms into a clinical entity: for example, 'acute coronary syndrome', 'delirium', 'upper respiratory tract infection' or 'sepsis'. Some patient presentations do not fall neatly into boxes, and so sticking with a narrative description of the patient's problems is appropriate in some cases. However, naming a clinical impression in a few simple words is often vital in moving towards a final diagnosis.

An impression formed at the end of a clinical consultation can often be refined by simple, quick and relatively non-invasive tests; but it might require complex, expensive or potentially hazardous investigations to produce a definitive diagnosis. Likewise, additional tests might be needed in order to demonstrate the extent, severity or treatment-responsiveness of the condition (**Fig. 1.4**).

Often, it is appropriate to stop at the level of a syndrome or clinical impression rather than continuing with investigations to demonstrate a precise histopathological cause. This might be the case if:

- the patient is satisfied with this level of explanation and declines further diagnostic work-up
- the problem is mild or self-limiting
- further investigation is unlikely to yield a specific cause, e.g. where a patient with acute but resolving diarrhoea or vomiting is diagnosed with likely viral gastroenteritis without a specified pathogen
- further investigation is unlikely to influence management, e.g. if none of the specific pathological processes that cause the condition is amenable to active management
- treatment is possible, but the patient is very frail and the proposed investigations or treatments are felt, after discussion with the patient, to be inappropriate.

The role of watchful waiting

All diseases have a natural history. Some progress inexorably, some are self-limiting and some relapse and remit. Where there is diagnostic uncertainty, there can be a role for waiting to see how events develop before reaching for a diagnostic label. Indeed, this is sometimes necessary, as the diagnostic criteria for some diseases stipulate that symptoms must have been present for a certain length of time before a diagnostic label can be assigned. For instance, in multiple sclerosis, where an initial presentation with symptoms suggestive of a demyelinating illness is usually termed a 'clinically isolated syndrome', some patients will suffer no further episodes while others will progress to multiple sclerosis. In other cases, it is wise to defer risky or burdensome investigations until the clinical course of the disease makes it clear that such investigations are justified. Watching and waiting can be a valid approach only if, firstly, the patient's clinical condition allows it; and secondly, it does not involve withholding treatment that would otherwise be of benefit (**Box 1.9**). Discussion with the patient is crucial.

When not to investigate

Decisions about whether and how to pursue a formal diagnosis are often complex and should be made in conjunction with the patient. Everyone is different and individuals differ in their willingness to tolerate uncertainty, with some wanting to seek a firm diagnosis at all costs, and others happy to accept a presumed diagnosis and run the

risk that this may be wrong. Clinicians can guide patients in making complex decisions by helping them understand the likely or possible outcomes of different decisions; often, offering 'best- and worst-case scenarios' for different potential courses of action is helpful. In general, investigations should be avoided where:
- the patient is too frail to derive any benefit from confirming a diagnosis
- the patient agrees to have an initial investigation, but will not accept intervention if the result is positive, e.g. the patient agrees to a myocardial perfusion scan but would not want to undergo subsequent coronary angiography or stenting
- the treating clinician feels that investigation is not deemed to be in the patient's best interests – patients can refuse investigation or intervention, but cannot demand it.

Diagnostic criteria

Some conditions are diagnosed with a single pathognomonic investigation result: for example, the presence of urate crystals on microscopic examination of synovial fluid is diagnostic of gout. In other situations, confirming the diagnosis is far more complex and may require a combination of symptoms, physical signs and investigation results. For example, according to the 2018 diagnostic criteria for systemic lupus erythematosus, published jointly by the American College of Rheumatology and European League Against Rheumatism, patients need to score ten or more points from different domains, including symptoms, signs, haematological and immunological blood tests, and histology (see p. 440).

Diagnostic criteria have a range of functions beyond treating individual patients, including a role in public health (in the compilation of statistics for monitoring trends in the incidence and distribution of diseases), research (to allow study of diseases and treatments in well-defined disease populations), and remuneration or reimbursement (in many health systems, payment to healthcare providers is on the basis of diagnostic codes assigned to patients receiving care). The *International Statistical Classification of Diseases* (ICD), now in its 11th edition, is produced by the World Health Organization in order to provide a standardized set of coding and diagnostic criteria across the world. Although useful at a population level, and for the research and administrative purposes described, these criteria are rarely used in routine clinical practice.

Overdiagnosis

Overdiagnosis refers to a diagnosis that is correctly assigned on the basis of a screening programme, but is inappropriate because it is unlikely ever to cause harm to the patient in question. It is the inevitable result of population health screening and poses risks to patients because of the potential for unnecessary further diagnostic procedures, therapy, or insurance charges.

For example, a frail 93-year-old man with dementia is visited at home by his GP at the request of his daughter. A routine check reveals a heart rate of 66 bpm and a blood pressure of 168/96 mmHg. A diagnosis of hypertension is made and the elderly man is started on an antihypertensive. This diagnosis may be considered inappropriate on a number of grounds:
- While blood pressure rises with age, 'normal' blood pressure in a 93-year-old is not clearly defined; neither is an acceptable target blood pressure to guide intervention.

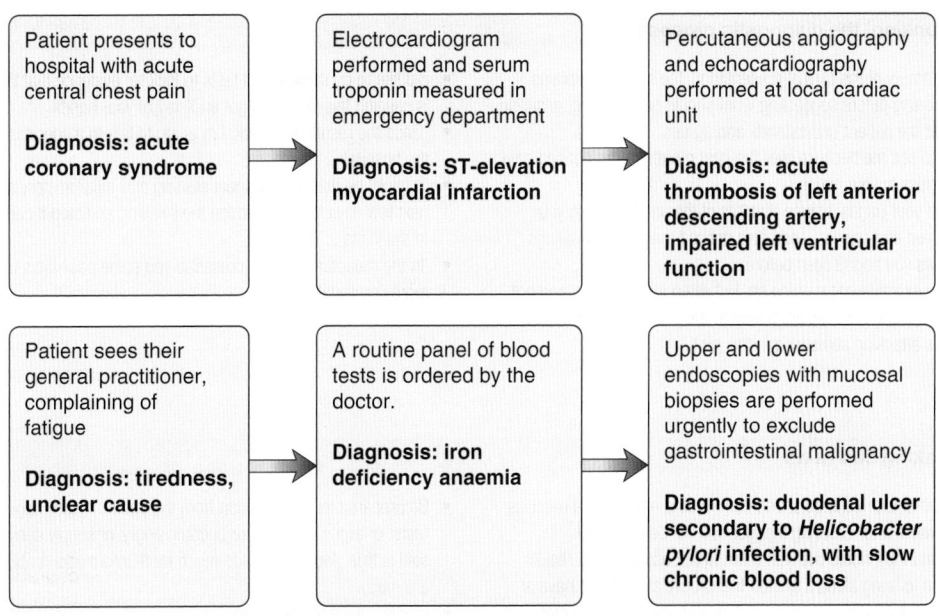

Fig. 1.4 Examples of different levels of diagnosis.

Box 1.9 The role of watchful waiting in diagnosis

- **A 77-year-old woman is undergoing CT scanning of the coronary arteries after an episode of chest pain.** A small (<10 mm) pulmonary nodule is incidentally noted. She is at high risk for lung cancer because of a long smoking history. In accordance with the British Thoracic Society's 'Guidelines for the Investigation and Management of Pulmonary Nodules', she is offered computed tomography screening at 3 months and 1 year. These reveal stable appearances with no increase in size, so she is reassured and discharged from further follow-up of this nodule.
- **A 34-year-old man is found to have abnormal liver function tests and is referred to a hepatology clinic.** A set of blood tests screening for common causes of liver disease, including viral hepatitis antibodies, are all normal. A liver biopsy is discussed with the patient, but because his liver function tests are not rapidly deteriorating, a decision is made in favour of watchful waiting. Two months later, his liver function tests return to normal ranges and remain normal after another 6 months. He is discharged from clinic without a diagnosis for his transient liver injury.
- **An 18-year-old woman with a history of presumed minimal change disease** as a child presents to the renal outpatient department with recurrent nephrotic syndrome. She is commenced on a loop diuretic and high-dose corticosteroids, but after 2 months remission has not been achieved. Because it is atypical for minimal change disease to fail to remit by this point, and because the diagnosis had never before been histologically proven, a renal biopsy is carried out. This revealed a different but related renal disorder: focal segmental glomerulosclerosis.

- A one-off high blood pressure measurement may have several confounding factors, including stress on being examined by the doctor. It would require further follow-up to corroborate this finding.
- Hypertension is known to increase the risk of cardiovascular disease and stroke significantly when left untreated for a period of years in younger patients, but it is far from certain that this pattern is seen in newly diagnosed hypertension in the elderly.
- All medications have side-effects: those of commonly used antihypertensive drugs include postural dizziness that may lead to falls, and increased susceptibility to acute kidney injury. These may significantly outweigh any benefits of treatment.

Some have argued that there is no such thing as overdiagnosis, only 'overtreatment'. Certainly, in this clinical scenario, little

evidence exists to support the diagnosis or treatment. As any good geriatrician will confirm, there is art as well as science involved in intervening wisely in a complex situation such as this.

Further reading

Bulliard JL, Chiolero A. Screening and overdiagnosis: public health implications. *Public Health Rev* 2015; 36:8.
Kahneman D. *Thinking, Fast and Slow.* New York: Strauss and Giroux; 2012.
Norman G, Barraclough K, Dolovich L et al. Iterative diagnosis. *BMJ* 2009; 339:b3490.
O'Sullivan ED, Schofield SJ. Cognitive bias in clinical medicine. *J R Coll Physicians Edinb* 2018; 48:225–232.
Saposnik G, Redelmeier D, Ruff CC et al. Cognitive biases associated with medical decisions: a systematic review. *BMC Med Inform Decis Mak* 2016; 16:138.

COMMUNICATING A DIAGNOSIS

Towards the end of a clinical consultation, the clinician will need to explain their diagnostic reasoning to the patient, along with their plans for further investigation and intervention. Explaining and teaching is a key part of working in medicine, and this part of the consultation is crucial in laying the foundation on which decisions for the future can be made.

Explaining diagnoses to patients

Some patients will have little difficulty in understanding complex medical explanations; this should never be assumed, however. While it is wise to avoid patronizing patients with a good understanding, it is generally worth assuming that patients understand less rather than more about their condition, and explaining all parts of the reasoning process, at least in brief. Using a phrase like 'I know you understand lots about this already, but I'm just going to go over things right from the beginning so we both understand each other' can be a good way of giving simple explanations without causing embarrassment.

Explaining a patient's diagnosis is best done in chunks, waiting between each chunk to ensure they have understood (**Box 1.10**). It is wise to work chronologically through the symptoms, employing

Box 1.10 'Chunking' the diagnostic process

Beginning with a summary of the clinical presentation, the clinician explains their diagnostic reasoning before suggesting what should happen next, ensuring after each chunk that the patient understands and agrees.
- 'So you came in to see me because over the past month you've noticed pain, swelling and stiffness in your hands ...'
- 'When I examined your hands, I found that lots of the small joints in your fingers were hot, red and swollen, and I also noticed these new swellings behind your elbows you hadn't seen before ...'
- 'Now I don't know exactly what is going on, but when joints get red and hot like this, it often means there is inflammation in the joints – often the body's immune system is attacking something in the joint ...'

- 'I'd like to do some blood tests to look for evidence that the immune system is causing this, and also get an X-ray of your hands ...'
- 'Once the results are back, I'm going to talk to a specialist rheumatologist at the hospital ...'
- 'It might be that they suggest starting anti-inflammatory medication over the next few days to try to reduce the swelling and stop it causing any damage to the joints ...'
- 'In the meantime, let me prescribe you some painkillers to try to make things more comfortable.'

Box 1.11 Breaking bad news

- Choose a setting that is private, quiet and comfortable – perhaps a relatives' room off a main ward, after ensuring that you will not be disturbed.
- Ask the patient who they would like with them to discuss their test results – encourage them to bring along a trusted friend or relative. Try to have at least two members of clinical staff present, e.g. a senior treating doctor and a nurse caring for the patient.
- Set aside time – ideally, at least 20 minutes – to ensure that the discussion is not rushed and that questions can be dealt with.
- Introduce yourself and others present and explain the purpose of the meeting, e.g. to go through recent test results.
- Ask how the patient has been since the last time you spoke with them.
- Briefly (in not more than two or three sentences) recap their history – what symptoms they presented with and why certain tests were done.
- Fire a warning shot: explain that things are looking more serious than first thought.
- Pause.
- Clearly, briefly and in plain English, describe the findings, e.g. 'I'm afraid that the CT scan revealed there is a lump in your left lung, and the doctor reporting the scan thinks that this could be lung cancer.'
- Pause.

- Be prepared for any reaction from the patient – they might break down in tears, or argue with you, or become angry, or simply deny that what you have said is true. Avoid giving too much more information until they indicate they are ready.
- Briefly outline the likely diagnosis, any areas of uncertainty and the next steps (e.g. further investigations or referral to a specialist).
- Pause.
- Invite questions.
- Be ready to answer the question 'How long have I got?' It is often impossible to say at this stage, and it is generally misleading and inappropriate to give specific figures. It can sometimes be helpful to outline whether a condition is survivable, or to give best- and worst-case scenarios.
- Give hope: explain what can be done, even it is simply a matter of care, support and symptom control. Try to help patients to maintain some control over their life, but never make false promises.
- Empathize: e.g. some patients like to be touched, with a reassuring hand placed on theirs, while others do not. Always try to convey concern and support explicitly.
- Outline a brief plan: what happens now? What should they do if they think of questions over the next few hours?

causal explanations and tying symptoms to the underlying pathological processes. This helps patients to understand the clinician's diagnostic reasoning and future priorities in management.

Breaking bad news

Sometimes, clinicians have to tell patients that they have a severe, chronic or life-limiting disease. This might be expected news for the patient or it might come as a complete surprise. This is one of the most difficult things a clinician has to do. It is never a pleasant task but having a good structure enables a clinician to be sensitive and kind, and leaves the patient knowing that they are not on their own (**Box 1.11**).

Traditionally, it was commonplace to withhold bad news from patients, telling it only to their families. Such an approach will often cause far greater distress to the patient (as a result of being deceived) and is now considered unacceptable. Where patients do not wish to be told about their diagnosis, this should be respected, and information can be given to family members instead if the patient consents; often, in such cases, the patient may understand that the news is not good and may wish to be spared the full details. If major treatment decisions need to be made and the patient has mental capacity to make them, clinicians should do their best to persuade patients of the importance of understanding what is wrong with them.

Box 1.12 Example of a 'problem list' in an elderly patient admitted to hospital

1. Right lower lobe pneumonia (presumed aspiration pneumonia, no positive microbiology)
2. Impaired swallow, awaiting speech and language therapy assessment
3. Previous stroke, right-sided hemiparesis, bedbound
4. Acute kidney injury probably secondary to sepsis and hypotension – resolving
5. Previously struggling to cope at home despite four-times-daily care package; may require residential nursing care

Team communication

Communication of a diagnosis between members of the healthcare team should be succinct and accurate. Technical terms are appropriate, alongside abbreviations, as long as they are widely understood. Often, patients with complex medical histories may present with multiple problems, and so clinicians treating them may compile a '***problem list***' outlining currently unresolved issues (**Box 1.12**). This can help to highlight issues that need to be resolved, guide investigations and management, and be used in communicating a patient's needs between members of the healthcare team.

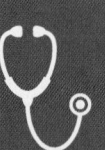

 Box 1.13 Benefits of shared decision-making

Benefits for the patient
- Better understanding of the different treatment options available and their benefits and risks
- A feeling of empowerment as different options are explored
- A treatment plan tailored to the patient's individual needs

Benefits for the healthcare provider
- A better understanding of what things are most important to this individual patient
- Better patient engagement with the illness and its management
- Better adherence to prescribed medication

The SBAR tool

Reviews of serious incidents occurring in hospital often highlight poor communication between team members as playing a key role in subsequent patient harm. For example, a member of the nursing staff may notice a deteriorating patient and summon the on-call doctor, who may fail to appreciate the severity of the situation and therefore not respond in a timely manner.

To address this problem, the SBAR tool has been developed to help formalize such communication. Staff members are encouraged to use this to structure their communication, in order to emphasize the need for full attention and an adequate response from the professional receiving the call.

- *S*ituation: who is making the call, which patient does it relate to and where are they in the hospital?
- *B*ackground: why was the patient admitted and what have been the recent events?
- *A*ssessment: why are you calling, what are the patient's current problems and what assessment have you made of them?
- *R*esponse: what do you need the person receiving the call to do?

Shared decision-making

Generally a diagnosis will be reached that incorporates information from the history, physical examination and relevant investigations. This will be communicated to the patient by the clinician treating them, who should check their understanding and discuss the implications. As with history-taking, the patient must be regarded and treated as an equal partner. The concept of shared decision-making has been developed to emphasize just how important joint involvement is, with benefits for both the healthcare provider and the patient (**Box 1.13**).

For patients to participate as equal partners, it is crucial for them to be provided with all the necessary information about their condition and the various treatment options available, presented in language that is easily understood. Information leaflets and online materials, often produced by patient support groups and charities, are available to help achieve this.

Managing uncertainty

Sometimes, it is not possible to make a definitive, corroborated diagnosis. This may be because:
- the investigations available are unable to provide definitive proof, for example if medicine is being delivered in a resource-poor setting

- definitive investigation is avoided because of the dangers or burdens involved
- the patient declines investigation
- investigations have commenced but will not reach a conclusion for some time.

This can be very difficult for both patients and clinicians. Without a confirmed diagnosis, it is impossible to produce a confident prognosis, and this can be profoundly challenging for patients. It can also be unnerving to clinicians to be taken to the point at which science can offer nothing more and they are forced to acknowledge their limitations. At this point, the clinician should help the patient deal with this lack of closure and uncertainty. It might be relevant to establish what gives the patient's life meaning, to enquire about their religious or spiritual beliefs, or to ask what most concerns them about facing their current illness.

In the meantime, plans can be built on the available evidence relating to the patient's underlying illness, guided by key concerns expressed by the patient:
- Symptomatic treatment (such as pain relief or anti-sickness drugs) is always appropriate when required, and may be a way of restoring a sense of control in an uncertain situation (see Ch. 7).
- Empirical treatment can be instituted on the basis of a suspected underlying pathology, even if a firm diagnosis is not possible. However, this needs clear discussion with the patient about the likelihood that the proposed treatment may cause side-effects, and may be ineffective or even harmful if the suspected diagnosis is incorrect.
- If a rapidly life-limiting condition, such as advanced malignancy, is suspected, then discussions should begin early about end-of-life care. What is important to the patient? Where would they like to be cared for in their final months or weeks?
- Help from psychologists or chaplains can be of great benefit and is often readily available.

Further reading

Baile WF, Buckman R, Lenzi R et al. SPIKES – a six-step protocol for delivering bad news: application to the patient with cancer. *Oncologist* 2000; 5:302–311.
Hatch S. Uncertainty in medicine. *BMJ* 2017; 357:j2180.
NHS Improvement. *SBAR Communication Tool*. https://improvement.nhs.uk/documents/2162/sbar-communication-tool.pdf.
NICE. *Shared Decision Making Guidelines*. https://www.nice.org.uk/about/what-we-do/our-programmes/nice-guidance/nice-guidelines/shared-decision-making.

DIAGNOSIS, ARTIFICIAL INTELLIGENCE AND THE FUTURE OF MEDICINE

Artificial intelligence (AI) describes the ability of machines to perform tasks traditionally believed to require higher cognitive skills. Examples include natural language processing, learning, executive planning and pattern recognition. Although multiple predictions are made about the future powers of self-conscious computers and 'super-intelligences', all the AI technology available currently, and in the near future, may be described as 'narrow AI' or 'weak AI': that is, systems designed to augment specified tasks within limited and well-defined fields of activity. The basis of all AI systems lies in the ability of high-capacity computer systems to analyse and utilize trends in large datasets that correlate with predefined outputs, 'seeing' patterns in data that possess predictive significance but are invisible to human observers. AI systems are 'fed' data and use this to develop and refine rules that predict the outputs they are designed to detect.

AI systems in healthcare

A number of such narrow AI systems have been trialled with encouraging results in different areas of medical practice:

- **'Computer vision'.** These AI systems review large numbers of medical images with appropriate diagnostic labels supplied by experts, and build diagnostic algorithms based on features of the image that correlate with the assigned diagnosis. Such systems have been shown to perform as well as, or better than, human experts in a number of clinical settings, including the interpretation of electrocardiograms, the diagnosis of skin cancers, the recognition of abnormalities on retinal screening photographs, and the reporting of chest X-rays and other radiological images.
- **Risk prediction.** These AI systems consider large sets of patient data (age, sex, ethnicity, environmental risk factors, physiological observations, results of blood tests and other investigations, administered medications) and correlate these with patient outcomes to form powerful predictive tools. Patterns are detected that may have previously been overlooked by human researchers, such as beat-to-beat heart rate variation, which correlates strongly with mortality and development of sepsis in patients in critical care settings. Similar algorithms have been shown to be effective in predicting in-hospital complications and mortality, out-of-hospital events (such as 10-year cardiovascular mortality) and even less obvious outcomes (such as suicide risk).
- **Individualized treatment.** No two patients suffer exactly the same disease and yet patients with the same diagnosis are generally, at present, offered the same treatment options. AI systems have been developed that analyse a large volume of patient data (relating, for example, to patients' whole-genome sequences or samples from tumours), allowing genetic variants to be identified that predict the likely responses to different types of treatment. These allow treatment regimens to be tailored to individual patients, maximizing efficacy and minimizing toxicity.

Future uses of AI

All of the currently and imminently available AI systems simply present clinicians with suggestions: probabilities that might suggest a diagnosis, or quantify a set of risks, or identify treatments most likely to be of benefit. As such, these AI systems provide doctors with a helpful '**second opinion**', from a unique, non-human perspective. The key ethical issue of deciding what to do next falls to the patient and doctor, working collaboratively.

However, other AI technologies are being developed that pose far greater ethical questions about the role that machines should play in healthcare. Although these are presently far off, some developers envisage robotic systems that would almost completely replace human doctors: patients would tell a computer system their symptoms, undergo whatever investigations were required, and receive an automated, algorithm-driven diagnosis and management plan. These systems would use natural language processing to review all relevant medical literature, and make use of this data to identify exactly which treatment would be most appropriate for the patient in question.

In the social care sector, robotic systems are already being designed that provide 'care' and 'companionship' for elderly, disabled or cognitively impaired people. Other systems administer talking-based therapy to patients with mood disorders such as depression. Does this represent a good use of technology, reducing the cost and improving the quality of care? Or is there something fundamental about caring for people that requires a human to do it?

The role and goals of medicine

Predictions about the future implications of technology are notoriously difficult to make and prone to embarrassingly high degrees of error. It is right for doctors to welcome rigorously tested narrow AI as it is currently available, and to appraise future developments critically to ensure that they maintain the safety and dignity of the patients they are designed to help.

However, technology can never replace the human-to-human interaction at the heart of every medical consultation. While we strive to use all available technology to refine diagnosis and improve management, this must never be at the expense of the relationship that has always formed the cornerstone of effective medical care. We are increasingly able to provide our patients with the most incredible therapeutic interventions that deliver invaluable improvements in quality and quantity of life. But we are also always able to give them our attention, comfort, compassion and care. There can be no greater privilege than having a patient trust you with their life and health, and we shoulder a heavy responsibility when seeking to act as their doctors.

Further reading

Academy of Medicine Royal Colleges. *Artificial Intelligence in Healthcare*, 2018; https://www.aomrc.org.uk/wp-content/uploads/2019/01/Artificial_intelligence_in_healthcare_0119.pdf.
Nuffield Council on Bioethics. *Artificial Intelligence (AI) in Healthcare and Research*, 2018; http://nuffieldbioethics.org/wp-content/uploads/Artificial-Intelligence-AI-in-healthcare-and-research.pdf.

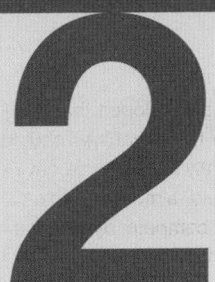

2

Human genetics

Neil Rajan and David P. Kelsell

CORE SKILLS AND KNOWLEDGE

The clinical practice of diagnosing and managing genetic disease is an expanding and evolving field. Increasingly, this is carried out by experts in organ-based subspecialties (e.g. neurologists and dermatologists), in partnership with clinical genetics teams. Hence, a working knowledge of skills such as documenting a family history and understanding basic genetic investigations is relevant across a range of disciplines. Typically, clinical geneticists are qualified adult or paediatric physicians who undertake postgraduate training in the specialty, often including a period of laboratory-based research. Genetics services are usually delivered in specialist centres in the outpatient setting.

Key skills in clinical genetics include:

- Obtaining a comprehensive history. A careful family history is essential.
- Drawing and interpreting a family tree.
- Estimating the risk of a future pregnancy being affected or carrying a disorder, based on common patterns of inheritance.
- Understanding the principles of genetic testing, and the ethical challenges this may entail.

Exposure to genetics multidisciplinary team meetings and genetics clinics represent opportunities for medical students and training clinicians to gain insights into how to ask relevant questions when taking a history from a patient with genetic disease. This has to be coupled with thorough clinical examination, which may lead to the selection of appropriate radiological imaging tests and invasive tests such as tissue biopsies.

CLINICAL SKILLS FOR GENETIC MEDICINE

Taking a genetic family history

A genetic family history consists of information describing how family members are related to each other (their biological relationships) and any medical conditions they may have.

Establishing such a family history can:

- reveal patterns of inheritance
- help make or refine a diagnosis
- help assess the likelihood of genetic disease in relatives
- affect testing, treatment and management strategies
- highlight the need for referral to specialist services
- help in building rapport with patients.

Information is usually gathered by asking a series of questions about each member of the family in a systematic order (**Box 2.1**) and recording the information pictorially as a family tree (a pedigree; see opposite). Family history can be an important risk factor for cancer and a wide range of conditions with monogenic or complex polygenic aetiology. Some national clinical guidelines therefore highlight the importance of taking and recording a genetic family history.

Drawing a pedigree

A set of agreed symbols is used when drawing a pedigree (**Fig. 2.1**). In order to show how individuals are related to each other, lines are drawn between symbols. The correct placement of these lines is a key skill to ensure that the pedigree gives an accurate picture of family relationships.

A dominantly inherited example is presented in **Fig. 2.2**. Affected males and females are filled in with black, and unaffected are left white. Males and females are equally affected, and both can transmit the disease to their offspring, who carry a 50% chance of inheriting the 'faulty' gene. More examples of patterns of inheritance are shown on page 28.

 Box 2.1 How to take a genetic family history

Immediate family

In adult patients, information is typically obtained first on which members of the immediate family are affected by a disorder. Begin drawing a pedigree with the patient towards the bottom of the page (allowing space below for any children).

- Ask about their spouse or partner.
- Ask about any children the patient may have.
- Enquire sensitively about stillbirths and miscarriages.

Where any individual is affected, try to determine the age at which they were diagnosed and the severity of their disease.

Patient's siblings and parents

Siblings are drawn alongside the patient and the parents are placed above, with lines indicating family relationships (which can be complex):

- Ask whether the patient's parents are alive, and about any illnesses they have at present or have been diagnosed with in the past. If the parents are deceased, record the stated cause of death and the age at which this happened.
- Ask how many siblings and half-siblings the patient has, and their ages. Enquire about their health.

Sometimes, patients may not know the family members' cause of death, which may, in some cases, reflect medical uncertainty (e.g. in conditions that cause sudden death); this uncertainty should be recorded.

Father's side of the family

Typically, these family members will be drawn above and to the left of the patient, and include the father's siblings and parents. Information on a minimum of three generations should be obtained.

Mother's side of the family

Typically, these family members will be drawn above and to the right of the patient, and include the mother's siblings and parents. Information on a minimum of three generations should be obtained.

Family history questionnaire

Sometimes, patients may find it difficult to recall information in a clinical consultation. A family history questionnaire can aid information-gathering, as the patient can fill this in at home, with the help of family. These questionnaires can be verified against cancer registry data, which is important as patients sometimes may not know which specific cancers affected their relatives. Increasingly, online forms are being piloted, which can be filled in electronically.

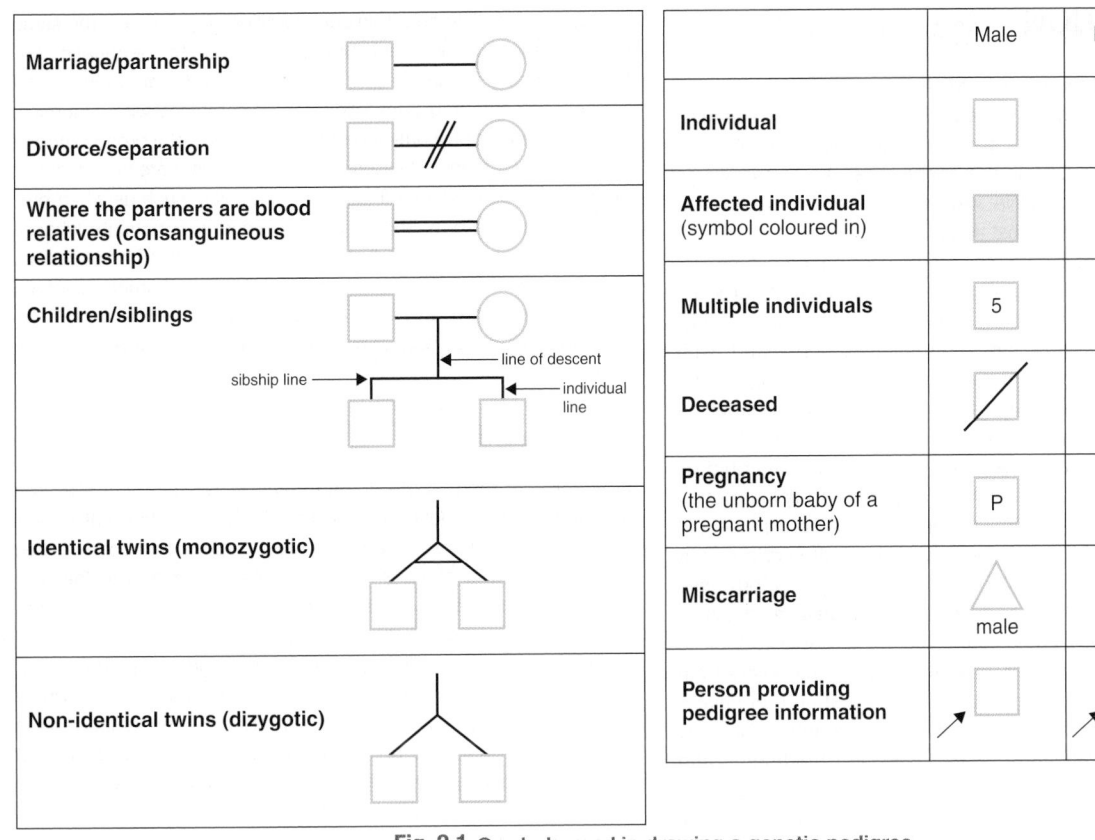

Fig. 2.1 Symbols used in drawing a genetic pedigree.

Autosomal dominant

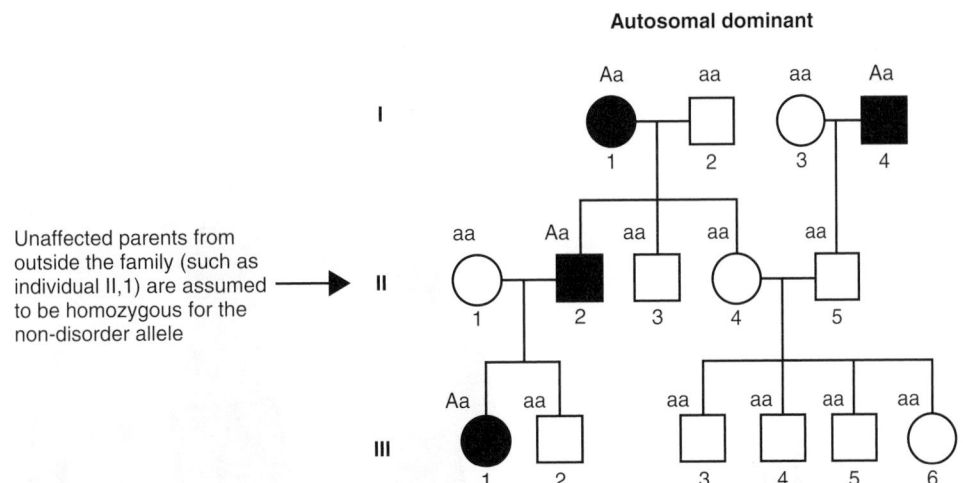

Fig. 2.2 An autosomal dominant pattern of inheritance. Affected males and females are shown in black. Capital 'A' indicates the allele associated with the disorder in question and lower case 'a' the non-disorder allele.

INTRODUCTION

The genetic code that forms the instruction manual for humans can now be sequenced in less than a day. From a clinical perspective, this brings an enormous range of new possibilities and challenges to the practice of medicine. In this chapter, we aim to provide an overview of key concepts in DNA, when we can use it to predict with confidence, and the caveats that apply.

DNA is an efficient means of storing information. Three billion base-pairs (bp) sit in the nucleus of each cell and carry the instructions to make all the parts of any cell in the human body. When a cell divides, all of this information is duplicated, with systems designed to prevent mistakes from occurring during this process. Nonetheless, errors do arise, which can either be harmless or cause disease, depending on the nature and the timing of the change. The discovery that the genetic code could be 'read' or sequenced allowed changes in parts of this instruction manual to be sought as an explanation for inherited diseases. In addition, the study of how the genetic code is altered in malignant cells has provided new insights into cancer biology (see Ch. 6). Progressive advances in deoxyribonucleic acid (DNA) sequencing technology have meant that we are able to look at the human genome of an individual at multiple time points from conception to the grave (**Fig. 2.3**). This information can have a range of implications, from pre-implantation genetic diagnosis to predicting and stratifying disease, selecting treatments and assessing drug response and the risk of adverse side-effects. An understanding of how this new information fits into clinical medicine is immensely relevant for patient care. As the cost of DNA sequencing drops, adoption of this technology is likely to become more widespread. In the UK, the 100,000 Genomes Project aims to study patients with rare diseases and cancer. Commercially available testing is accessible simply by supplying a saliva sample in the post.

However, while we are able to sequence DNA rapidly, much bigger challenges lie ahead. For example, it can be difficult to interpret changes in DNA found in apparently healthy individuals. Until recently, genetic changes in rare diseases were studied in the context of affected individuals and their families. A genetic change that can cause disease within such families may not have the same effect in other people. This is thought to be due to the genetic context in which the change presents. It is hoped that when careful phenotyping and long-term follow-up are combined with genomics, we can advise appropriately on the implications of a broad range of such genetic changes. Currently, in some areas there is consensus on 'actionable' incidental findings in genomics: such as when preventative mastectomy should be discussed with patients when a genetic change is found that may predict early-onset breast cancer. But work remains to be done to capture how the human genotype predicts phenotype, and large consortia efforts such as the Human Phenotype Ontology project aim to achieve this across all diseases.

Gene editing

In addition to reading the human genome, we can now also edit and change the genetic code, using very precise molecular tools such as CRISPR (see **Fig. 2.18**). By 2018, reports had been verified of gene editing in humans, which can be transmitted to the next generation. There is much discussion about how gene-editing technologies should and should not be used.

Here we aim to highlight selected genetic advances that exemplify concepts of genetic disease and to describe cases where genetic information has been clinically relevant to patients, either in routine care or in the context of clinical trials. The ability to interpret and contextualize genetic information in clinical care is becoming increasingly relevant as genomics is mainstreamed across clinical specialties.

CLINICAL GENETICS

Genetic disorders pose considerable health and economic problems and early diagnosis is crucial. While individual diseases are rare, it is estimated that almost 6000 genetic disorders are recognized, and as a collective, 1 in 25 children may be affected with a genetic disorder. In any pregnancy, the risk of a serious developmental abnormality is approximately 1 in 50 pregnancies, and around 15% of

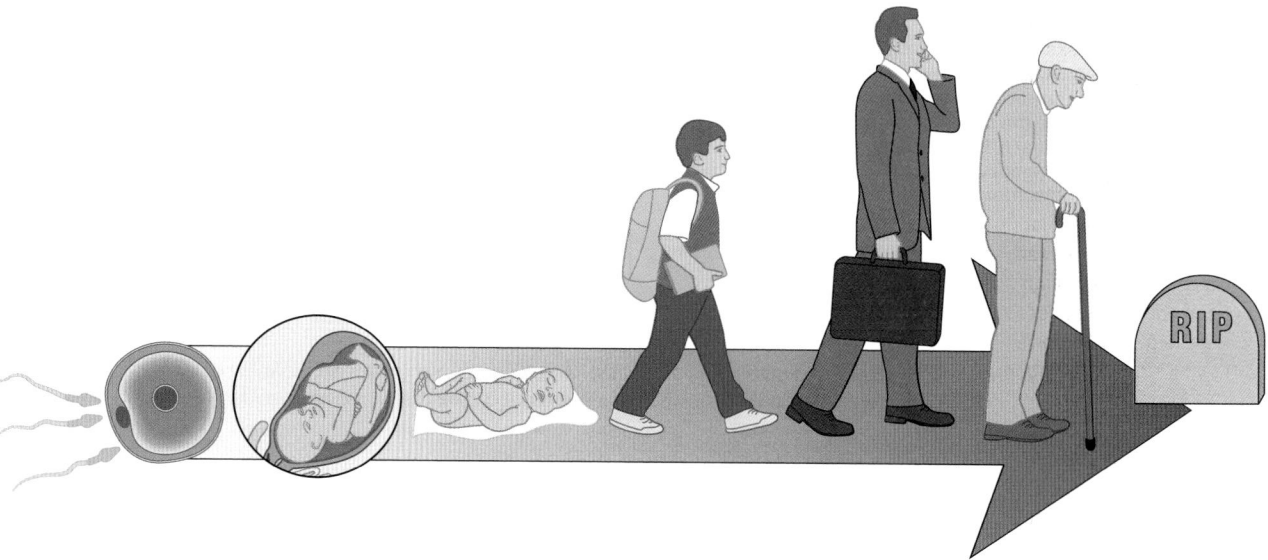

Fig. 2.3 Genotype and phenotype. Sequencing the human genome throughout our lifetime can give insights into disease susceptibility and healthcare management.

paediatric inpatients have a multifactorial disorder with a predominantly genetic element. In addition, 50% of clinical genetics referrals are adults with late-onset disease, including neurological, endocrine and gastrointestinal conditions, along with cancer.

Approach to the patient with a suspected genetic disease

Genetic services routinely coordinate clinical diagnosis, genetic testing, information-giving, family planning and targeted screening for a range of genetic disorders. Clinicians assessing a patient with a genetic disorder should keep in mind the following aims:

- *Obtaining a full history.* The pregnancy history, drug and alcohol ingestion during pregnancy, and maternal illnesses (e.g. diabetes) should be detailed.
- *Establishing an accurate diagnosis.* Examination may help in diagnosing a genetically abnormal child with characteristic features (e.g. trisomy 21) or ascertaining whether a genetically normal fetus was damaged *in utero*.
- *Drawing a family tree.* This is essential. Questions should be asked about abortions, stillbirths, deaths, marriages, consanguinity, and medical history of family members. Diagnoses may need verification from other hospital reports.
- *Estimating the risk of a future pregnancy being affected or carrying a disorder.* Estimation of risk should be based on the pattern of inheritance. Disorders caused by mutations in single genes carry a high risk; chromosomal abnormalities other than translocations typically carry a low risk. Empirical risks may be obtained from population or family studies.
- *Information-giving.* Information on prognosis and management should be supplied, with adequate time allowed for it to be discussed openly and freely, and repeated as necessary.
- *Continued support and follow-up.* An explanation should be provided of the implications for other siblings and family members.
- *Genetic screening.* This includes prenatal diagnosis or pre-implantation genetic diagnosis (*in vitro* fertilization followed by testing of embryos before implantation) and, if requested, carrier detection. A large number of molecular genetic tests are available.

Genetic counselling should be non-directive, with the couple making their own decisions on the basis of an accurate presentation of the facts and risks in a way they can understand.

Further details on taking a genetic history and drawing a family tree can be found on pages 2–3.

Ethical considerations

Ethical considerations must be taken into account in any discussion of clinical genetics. For example, prenatal diagnosis with the option of termination may be unacceptable on moral or religious grounds. In the case of diseases for which there is no cure and currently no treatment (e.g. Huntington's chorea), genetic tests can accurately predict which family members will be affected; many people, however, would rather not have this information. One very serious outcome of new genetic information is that disease susceptibility may be predictable – for example, in Alzheimer's disease – and so medical insurance companies can decline to issue policies for individuals at high risk. In some countries, a moratorium is in place to prevent insurers from using such data against patients in this way. It remains to be decided who should have access to an individual's genetic information and to what extent privacy should be preserved.

Testing for genetic disease

Genetic testing is extremely powerful, as it can reveal changes in DNA that explain why a patient has a clinical disease. Once such information is acquired, it can, for example, guide the selection of screening tests, aid prognostication and influence treatment. In some instances, it can elegantly replace the multiple radiological tests that were previously required to make a diagnosis of a genetic disease. In some situations, where the diagnosis is unknown and a strong clinical suspicion of genetic disease exists, genetic tests can provide the necessary clues to exclude certain differentials and aid the process of making and refining a diagnosis.

There will increasingly be a temptation simply to order whole-genome sequencing (see p. 33) for any genetic disease but this may have negative outcomes. For example, it may reveal unexpected findings that patients may not necessarily have wanted to know, such as a predisposition to early-onset dementia or cancer. Changes in disease genes may also be detected and cause anxiety, yet the genetic changes may not give rise to the expected disease in that patient. In some situations, incomplete knowledge may make any form of prognostication or reassurance impossible. The individual responses of each patient to such uncertainty can be difficult to predict, and more dialogue is needed to understand how to make better decisions for comprehensive testing in partnership with patients.

The importance of taking a comprehensive personal and family history and performing a clinical examination should be highlighted. This information may identify a single gene that needs to be tested if a particular disorder is suspected. In some conditions, where a selection of genes may account for a phenotype, a panel of 10–20 relevant genes can be tested. Some genomic centres favour this approach, in which only clinically relevant genes are studied in a tiered manner, with further comprehensive testing carried out only in cases that are negative.

From a technical perspective, this increasingly involves a single test (such as whole-exome or genome sequencing) with reporting on relevant genes only. Genetic testing is a rapidly changing field and exposure to clinical genetics clinics and multidisciplinary meetings will be crucial in training clinicians to select and implement the 'right' test.

Further reading

Middleton A, Wright CF, Morley KI et al. Potential research participants support the return of raw sequence data. *J Med Genet* 2015; 52:571–574.
Wright CF, FitzPatrick DR, Firth HV. Paediatric genomics: diagnosing rare disease in children. *Nat Genet* 2018; 19:253–268.
Wright CF, Hurles ME, Firth HV. Principle of proportionality in genomic data sharing. *Nat Genet* 2015; 17:1–2.

THE CELLULAR BASIS OF GENETICS

DNA and the genetic code

Hereditary information is contained in the sequence of the building blocks of double-stranded DNA (**Fig. 2.4**). Each strand of DNA is made up of a deoxyribose–phosphate backbone and a series of purine (adenine (A) and guanine (G)) and pyrimidine (thymine (T) and cytosine (C)) bases. Because of the way in which the sugar–phosphate backbone is chemically coupled, each strand has a polarity, with a phosphate at one end (the 5′ end) and a hydroxyl at the other (the 3′ end). The two strands of DNA are held together by hydrogen bonds between the bases. T can pair only with A, and G can pair only with C; therefore, each strand is the antiparallel complement of the other (see **Fig. 2.4**). This is key to DNA replication because each strand can be used as a template to synthesize the other.

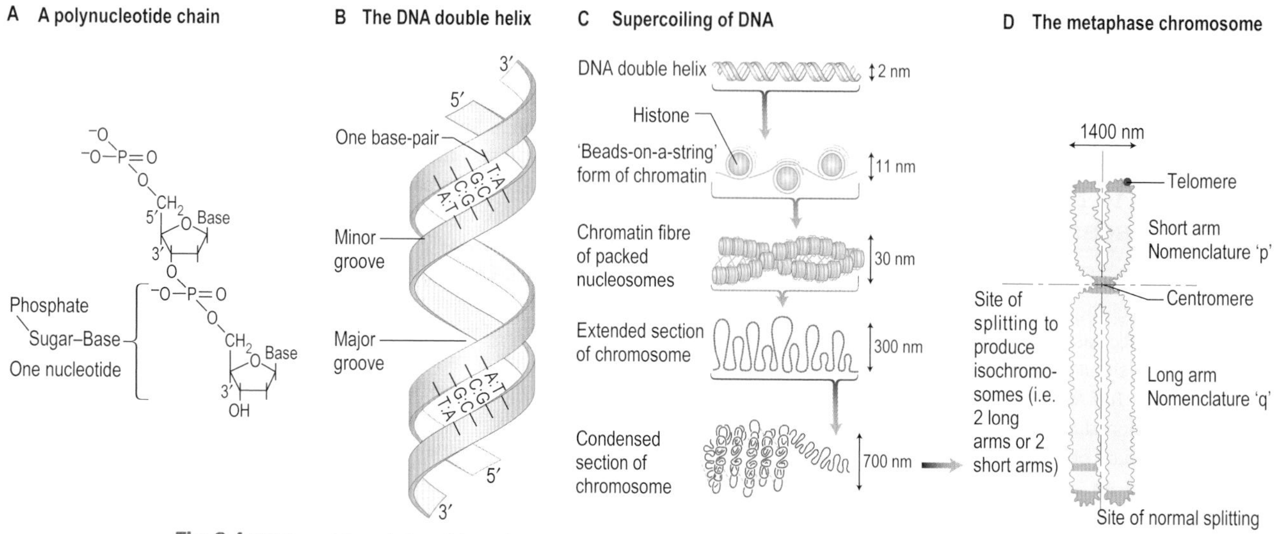

A   A polynucleotide chain

B   The DNA double helix

C   Supercoiling of DNA

D   The metaphase chromosome

Fig. 2.4 DNA and its relationship to human chromosomes. (A) Individual nucleotides form a *polymer* linked via the deoxyribose sugars to form a single-strand DNA (ssDNA). The 5′ carbon of the sugar is covalently joined to phosphate. The 3′ carbon links the phosphate on the 5′ carbon of the ribose of the next nucleotide, forming the sugar–phosphate backbone of the nucleic acid. The 5′ to 3′ linkage gives orientation to a sequence of DNA. (B) *Double-stranded DNA*. The two strands of DNA are held together by hydrogen bonds between the bases. T pairs with A, and G with C. The orientation of the complementary ssDNA is thus complementary and antiparallel. The helical three-dimensional structure has major and minor grooves, and a complete turn of the helix contains 12 base-pairs. The grooves are structurally important: DNA-binding proteins predominantly interact with the major grooves. (C) *Supercoiling of DNA*. The large helical DNA is coiled into nucleosomes by winding around nuclear proteins (histones), and further condensed by coiling and supercoiling into the chromosomes that are visible at metaphase. (D) *At the end of the metaphase, DNA replication* results in a twin chromosome joined at the centromere. Chromosomes are assigned a number (or the letter X or Y for the sex chromosomes), plus short arm (p) or long arm (q). The region or subregion is defined by the transverse light and dark bands observed when staining with Giemsa (see Fig. 2.17) (hence G-banding) or quinacrine, and numbered from the centromere outwards. *Chromosome constitution = chromosome number + sex chromosomes + abnormality*; e.g. 46XX = normal female; 47XX + 21 = Down's syndrome (trisomy 21); 46XYt (2;19) (p21; p12) = male with a normal number of chromosomes but a translocation between chromosome 2 and 19 with breakages at short-arm bands 21 and 12 of the respective chromosomes.

The two strands twist to form a double helix with a major and a minor groove, and the large stretches of helical DNA are coiled around histone proteins to form nucleosomes (see **Fig. 2.4**). They can be condensed further into the chromosomes that can be visualized by light microscopy at metaphase (see **Figs 2.4** and **2.11**).

Human chromosomes

Chromosomes are complex structures containing one linear molecule of DNA that is wound around histone proteins into small units called nucleosomes, and these are further wound to make up the structure of the chromosome itself.

Diploid human cells have 46 chromosomes, 23 inherited from each parent; thus there are 23 'homologous' pairs of chromosomes (22 pairs of '*autosomes*' and two '*sex chromosomes*'). The sex chromosomes, called X and Y, are not homologous but are different in size and shape. Males have an X and a Y chromosome; females have two X chromosomes. (Primary male sexual characteristics are determined by the *SRY* gene – sex-determining region on the Y chromosome.)

The chromosomes are classified according to their size and shape, the largest being chromosome 1. The constriction in the chromosome is the *centromere*, which can be in the middle of the chromosome (metacentric) or at one extreme end (acrocentric). The centromere divides the chromosome into a short arm and a long arm, referred to as the *p arm* and the *q arm*, respectively (see **Fig. 2.4**).

Chromosomes can be stained when they are in the metaphase stage of the cell cycle and are very condensed. The stain gives a different pattern of light and dark *bands* that is diagnostic for each chromosome. Each band is given a number, and gene-mapping techniques allow genes to be positioned within a band within an arm of a chromosome. For example, the *CFTR* gene (a defect in which gives rise to cystic fibrosis) maps to 7q21: that is, on chromosome 7 in the long arm in band 21.

During cell division (mitosis), each chromosome divides into two so that each daughter nucleus has the same number of chromosomes as its parent cell. During gametogenesis, however, the number of chromosomes is halved by meiosis, so that, after conception, the number of chromosomes remains the same and is not doubled. In the female each ovum contains one or other X chromosome, but in the male the sperm bears either an X or a Y chromosome.

Chromosomes can be seen easily only in actively dividing cells. Typically, lymphocytes from the peripheral blood are stimulated to divide and are processed to allow the chromosomes to be examined. Cells from other tissues can also be used for chromosomal analysis: for example, amniotic fluid, placental cells from chorionic villus sampling, or bone marrow and skin cells (**Box 2.2**).

The mitochondrial chromosome

In addition to the 23 pairs of chromosomes in the nucleus of every diploid cell, the mitochondria in the cytoplasm of the cell also have

Antenatal
- Positive maternal serum screening test for aneuploid pregnancy
- Ultrasound features consistent with an aneuploid fetus or genetic syndrome (e.g. skeletal dysplasia)
- Severe fetal growth retardation
- Sexing of fetus in X-linked disorders

In the neonate
- Congenital malformations
- Suspicion of trisomy or monosomy
- Suspicion of microdeletion syndrome
- Ambiguous genitalia

In children and adolescents
- Primary amenorrhoea or failure of pubertal development
- Growth retardation
- Malignant disorders (e.g. haematological malignancies, Wilms' tumour, neuroblastoma)

In the adult
- Screening of parents of a child with a chromosomal abnormality for further genetic counselling
- Learning difficulties
- Certain malignant disorders (e.g. haematological malignancies)

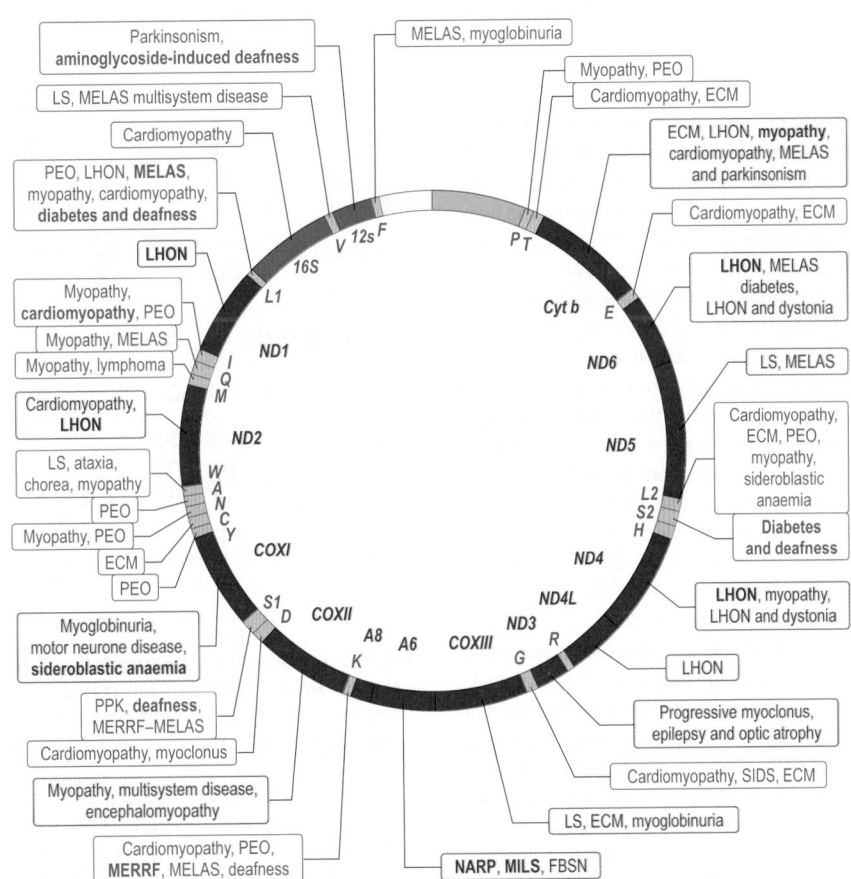

Fig. 2.5 Mitochondrial chromosome abnormalities. Disorders that are frequently or prominently associated with mutations in a particular gene are shown in bold. Diseases due to mutations that impair mitochondrial protein synthesis are shown in blue. Diseases due to mutations in protein-coding genes are shown in red. ECM, encephalomyopathy; FBSN, familial bilateral striatal necrosis; LHON, Leber's hereditary optic neuropathy; LS, Leigh's syndrome; MELAS, mitochondrial encephalomyopathy, lactic acidosis and stroke-like episodes; MERRF, myoclonic epilepsy with ragged-red fibres; MILS, maternally inherited Leigh's syndrome; NARP, neuropathy, ataxia and retinitis pigmentosa; PEO, progressive external ophthalmoplegia; PPK, palmoplantar keratoderma; SIDS, sudden infant death syndrome.

their own genome. The mitochondrial chromosome is a circular DNA (mtDNA) molecule of approximately 16 500 bp, and every base-pair makes up part of the coding sequence. These genes principally encode proteins or RNA molecules involved in mitochondrial function. These proteins are components of the mitochondrial respiratory chain involved in oxidative phosphorylation, producing adenosine triphosphate (ATP). They also have a critical role in apoptotic cell death. Every cell contains several hundred mitochondria, and therefore several hundred mitochondrial chromosomes.

Virtually all mitochondria are inherited from the mother, as the sperm head contains no (or very few) mitochondria. Disorders mapped to the mitochondrial chromosome are shown in **Fig. 2.5**.

DNA transcription

To express the information in the genome, cells transcribe the code into the single-stranded ribonucleic acid (RNA). RNA is similar to

DNA in that it comprises four bases – A, G and C but with uracil (U) instead of T – and a sugar–phosphate backbone with ribose instead of deoxyribose. Several types of RNA are made by the cell. Messenger RNA (mRNA) codes for proteins that are translated on ribosomes. Ribosomal RNA (rRNA) is a key catalytic component of the ribosome, and amino acids are delivered to the nascent peptide chain on transfer RNA (tRNA) molecules.

A gene is usually 20–40 kilobases of DNA that contains the code for a polypeptide sequence (but lengths vary – the muscle protein dystrophin is 2.4 megabases long). Three adjacent nucleotides (a codon) specify a particular amino acid, such as AGA for arginine. There are only 20 common amino acids, but 64 possible codon combinations make up the genetic code (see **Fig. 2.7**). This redundancy means that most amino acids are encoded by more than one triplet, and additional codons are used to signal initiation or termination of polypeptide-chain synthesis.

RNA is transcribed from the DNA template by an enzyme complex of more than 100 proteins, including RNA polymerase, transcription factors and enhancer proteins. Promoter regions upstream of the gene dictate the start point and direction of transcription. The complex binds to the promoter region, the nucleosomes are remodelled to allow access, and a DNA helicase unwinds the double helix. RNA, like DNA, is synthesized in the 5′ to 3′ direction as ribonucleotides are added to the growing 3′ end of a nascent transcript. RNA polymerase does this by base-pairing the ribonucleotides to the DNA template strand it is reading in the 3′ to 5′ direction. Messenger RNA is modified as it is synthesized (**Fig. 2.6**). It is capped at the 5′ end with a modified guanine that is required for efficient processing of the mRNA and translation. The 3′ end of the mRNA is modified with up to 200 A nucleotides by the enzyme poly-A polymerase. This 3′ poly-A tail is essential for nuclear export (through the nuclear pores), stability and efficient translation into protein by the ribosome. Human protein coding sequences (exons) are interrupted by intervening sequences that are non-coding (introns) at multiple positions (see **Fig. 2.6**). These are spliced from the nascent message in the nucleus by an RNA/protein complex called a spliceosome. Differential splicing can cause exons to be spliced alongside their intervening introns. This contributes significantly to the complexity of the human transcriptome, as proteins translated from these messages lack particular domains and therefore have different activity.

There are also a variety of RNAs that regulate gene expression or RNA processing. The non-coding RNAs (ncRNAs) include a group that regulate gene expression. These include microRNA (miRNA) and small interfering RNA (siRNA), which typically bind to a subset of mRNAs and inhibit their translation and/or initiate their degradation (siRNA only initiates degradation). Micro RNAs and siRNAs are short ncRNAs (19–29 bp) that together regulate expression of approximately 30% of genes by degradation of transcripts or repression of protein synthesis. A growing range of additional regulatory ncRNA classes are being identified, many of which control gene expression by epigenetic mechanisms (see later).

Control of gene expression

The genome of all cells in the body encodes the same genetic information, yet different cell types express very different subsets of proteins. Gene expression is controlled at many steps from transcription to protein degradation. However, for many genes, transcription is the key point of regulation. This is controlled primarily by proteins, which bind to short sequences within the promoter regions that either repress or activate transcription, or to more distant

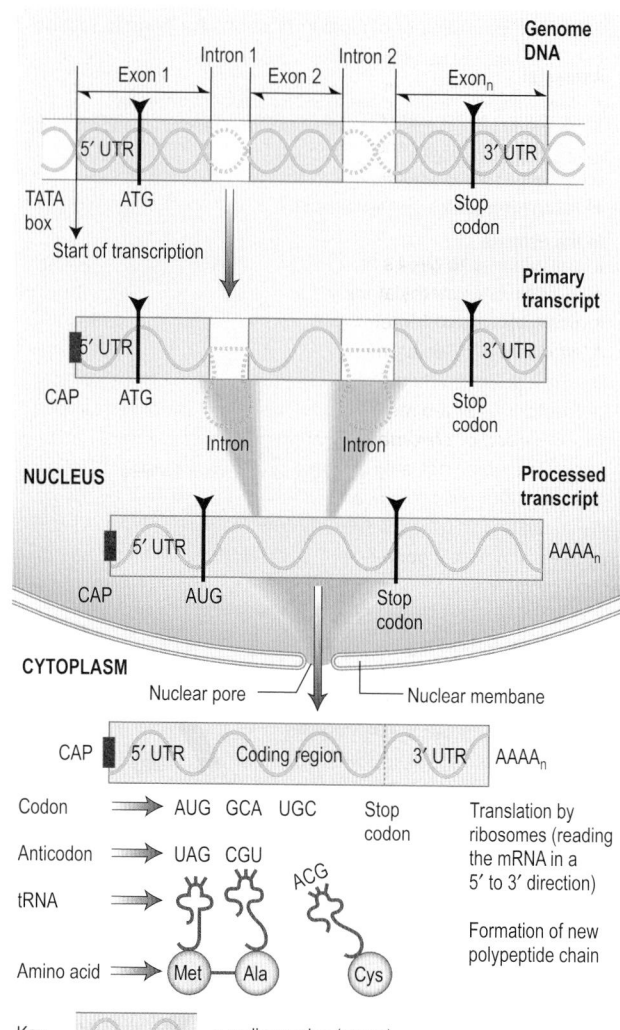

Fig. 2.6 Transcription and translation (DNA to RNA to protein). *RNA polymerase* transcribes an RNA copy of the DNA gene sequence. The *transcript* is capped at the 5′ end by the addition of an inverted guanine residue, which is then methylated to form 7-methylguanosine. At the 3′ end, the sequence AAUAAA is recognized by endonuclease, and the transcript is then cleaved 20 base-pairs further downstream. *Poly-A polymerase* then adds adenosine residues to the 3′ end, forming a poly-A tail (polyadenylation). The *introns* are then spliced to produce the mature messenger RNA (mRNA), which is trafficked to the cytosol via nuclear pores. *Ribosomal subunits* assemble on the 5′ end of the mRNA to translate the message into protein, for which transfer RNAs (tRNAs) deliver the amino acid building blocks (see also **Fig. 2.7**). UTR, untranslated region.

sequences where proteins bind to enhance expression. These transcription factors and enhancers are often the end-points of signalling pathways that transduce extracellular signals to change gene expression. This level of regulation often involves the translocation of an activated factor from the cytoplasm to the nucleus. In the nucleus, these DNA-binding proteins recognize the shape and position of hydrogen bond acceptor and donor groups within the major and minor grooves of the double helix (i.e. the double helix does not need to unwind). There are several classes of DNA-binding protein that differ in the protein structural motif that allows them to interact with the double helix. More permanent control of gene expression patterns can be achieved epigenetically.

Epigenetics

Although the importance of the genetic code has been emphasized, normal function and disease can occur, despite a particular DNA sequence being exactly the same. The term '**epigenetics**' is used to explain changes that arise due to differing gene expression but do not involve changes in the underlying DNA sequence. Despite not altering the genetic sequence, the effects of epigenetic changes are stable over rounds of cell division. A number of systems initiate and sustain these changes:

- **Modifications to DNA's surface structure** but not its base-pair sequence: DNA methylation. Enzymes called methyltransferases modify cytosine to 5-methylcytosine. This 'tag' occurs mainly in sites where a cytosine molecule is next to a guanidine nucleotide, a CpG site. When CpG islands (groups of CpG sites) in the promoter region are methylated, gene expression is repressed.
- **Modification of chromatin proteins** (in particular, acetylation of histones), which not only support DNA but also bind it so tightly as to regulate gene expression. At the extreme, such binding can permanently prevent the DNA sequences being exposed to, let alone acted on by, gene transcription (DNA-binding) proteins.

  Some epigenetic modifications are also 'transmissible', meaning that a dividing liver cell, for example, can give rise to two daughter cells with the same epigenetic signals, such that they express the appropriate transcriptome for a liver cell. Epigenetic change forms the basis of genomic imprinting (see p. 29).

  Epigenetic changes in gene expression also occur in cancer. An example is DNA methylation repressing tumour suppressor genes. Targeted therapy is already playing a big role in the control of malignant disease.

The X chromosome and inactivation

Although females have two X chromosomes (XX), they do not have two doses of X-linked genes (compared with just one dose for a male XY) because of the phenomenon of X inactivation or **lyonization** (after its discoverer, Dr Mary Lyon). In this process, one of the two X chromosomes in the cells of females is epigenetically (see earlier) silenced through the action of a regulatory ncRNA, so the cell has only one dose of the X-linked genes. Inactivation is random and can affect either X chromosome.

Protein synthesis and secretion

While the instructions are essentially the same in every cell, in different tissues the regions that are transcribed are cell-specific, and so are the ensuing proteins. For example, in skeletal muscle, the RNA transcripts involve the generation of proteins that are needed for muscle, such as myosin. Conversely, in the cells of the cornea, specific keratins that are transparent are expressed. The actual working parts of the cell are protein, and the translation of the nucleic acid sequence to protein involves the ribosome.

Protein translation

Mature mRNA is transported through the nuclear pore into the cytoplasm for translation into protein by ribosomes (**Fig. 2.7A**).

- The two subunits of ribosomes (40S and 60S) are formed in the nucleolus from multiple proteins and several rRNAs, before transport to the cytoplasm.
- In the cytoplasm, the two ribosomal subunits interact on an mRNA molecule, usually via ribosome-binding sites encoded in the untranslated 5′ region of the message. The mRNA is then pulled through the ribosome until a translation initiation codon is encountered (usually an AUG).

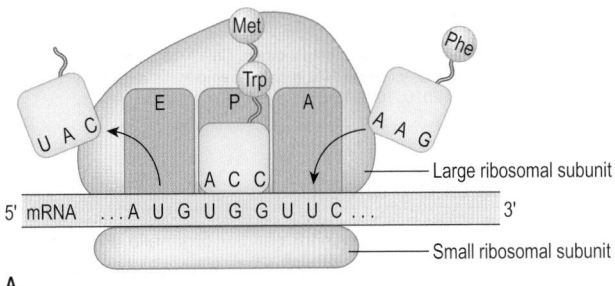
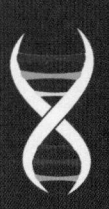

A

	Second letter			
First letter	U	C	A	G	Third letter

B

Fig. 2.7 **Protein translation.** (A) Ribosomal assembly of amino acid chains. (B) The genetic code and amino acids.

- As the mRNA is pulled through the ribosome in the 5′ to 3′ direction, codons distal to the AUG are recognized by complementary sequences, or anticodons, in tRNA molecules that dock on the ribosome. Each tRNA molecule carries an amino acid specific to the anticodon (**Fig. 2.7B**). The amino acids are transferred from tRNA molecules and sequentially linked to the carboxy-terminus of the growing polypeptide by the peptidyl transferase activity of the ribosome. The poly-A tail of the mRNA is not translated (3′ untranslated region (UTR)) and is preceded by a translational stop codon: UAA, UAG or UGA.

Protein structure

The amino acid sequence of a polypeptide chain (its **primary structure**) ultimately determines its shape. The weak bonds (hydrogen bonds, electrostatic and van der Waals interactions) formed between the side-chains of the different amino acids and/or the peptide backbone provide the **secondary structure** (α-helices, β-strands, loops). These, in turn, are folded into a three-dimensional, **tertiary structure** to provide functional protein domains of 40–350 amino acids. The modular nature of domains allows their functionality to be combined in protein complexes of different proteins. This final level of organization is the **quaternary structure**.

The folding of polypeptides into fully functional proteins is facilitated by an assortment of molecular chaperones, which bind to partially folded polypeptides and prevent the formation of inappropriate bonds.

Further reading

Rivera CM, Ren B. Mapping human epigenomes. *Cell* 2013; 155:39–55.
Zhou H, Hu H, Lai M. Non-coding RNAs and their epigenetic regulatory mechanisms. *Biol Cell* 2010; 102:645–655.

Genetics and the cell

The nucleus is the most prominent cellular organelle (**Fig. 2.8**) and has a double membrane enclosing the human genome (the outer membrane is continuous with the endoplasmic reticulum). The double membrane contains nuclear pores, through which gene regulatory proteins, transcription factors and mRNA that has been transcribed from DNA are transported. The nuclear matrix is highly organized. Microscopically dense regions of heterochromatin represent highly compacted chromosomal DNA, which tends to be transcriptionally repressed. Lighter regions of euchromatin contain extended chromosomes, which tend to be transcriptionally active. Outside the nucleus, mRNA is translated into amino acid chains in the endoplasmic reticulum (see p. 20 for how the trinucleotide code is converted to the corresponding amino acids that are the building blocks of proteins).

Embryonic development and stem cells

It is critical to recognize that all of the estimated 37 trillion cells that form a person are derived from a single cell. Genetic changes that involve this first cell, whether due to natural variation or artificial manipulation via gene-editing techniques like CRISPR (clusters of regularly interspaced short palindromic repeats), are carried forward to every subsequent cell. These changes are also passed on to future generations. The gravity of intervening at this moment is captured in the ethical debates around interventions such as pre-implantation genetic diagnosis and mitochondrial replacement therapy (see p. 36).

Following fertilization, the newly formed zygote and the cells it forms following the first few divisions are totipotent, meaning that they can differentiate into any cell type in the adult body (**Fig. 2.9A**). At the blastula stage of embryonic development, these cells undergo a primary differentiation event to become either the trophectoderm or the inner cell mass (ICM) (see **Fig. 2.9A**). The trophectoderm gives rise to the fetal cells of the placenta, while the ICM cells are pluripotent and give rise to all other cell types of the body (except

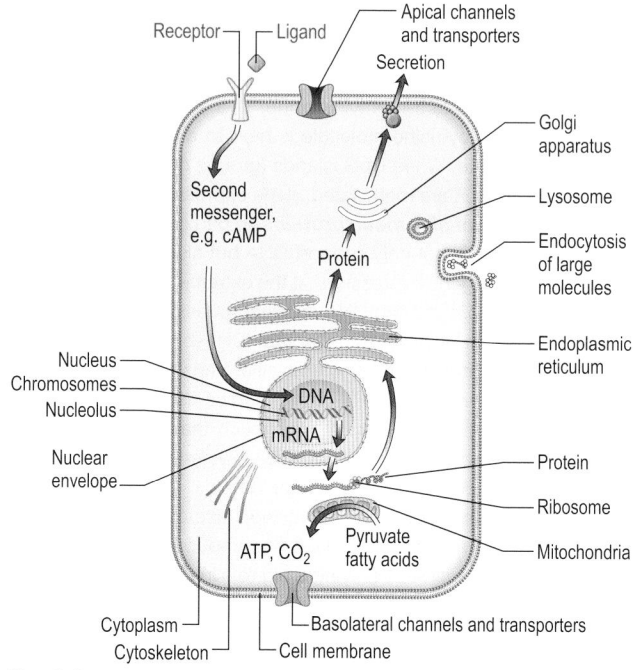

Fig. 2.8 The cell. The major organelles and receptor activation, intracellular messengers, protein formation and secretion, endocytosis of large molecules and production of adenosine triphosphate (ATP) are shown. cAMP, cyclic adenosine monophosphate; DNA, deoxyribonucleic acid; mRNA, messenger RNA.

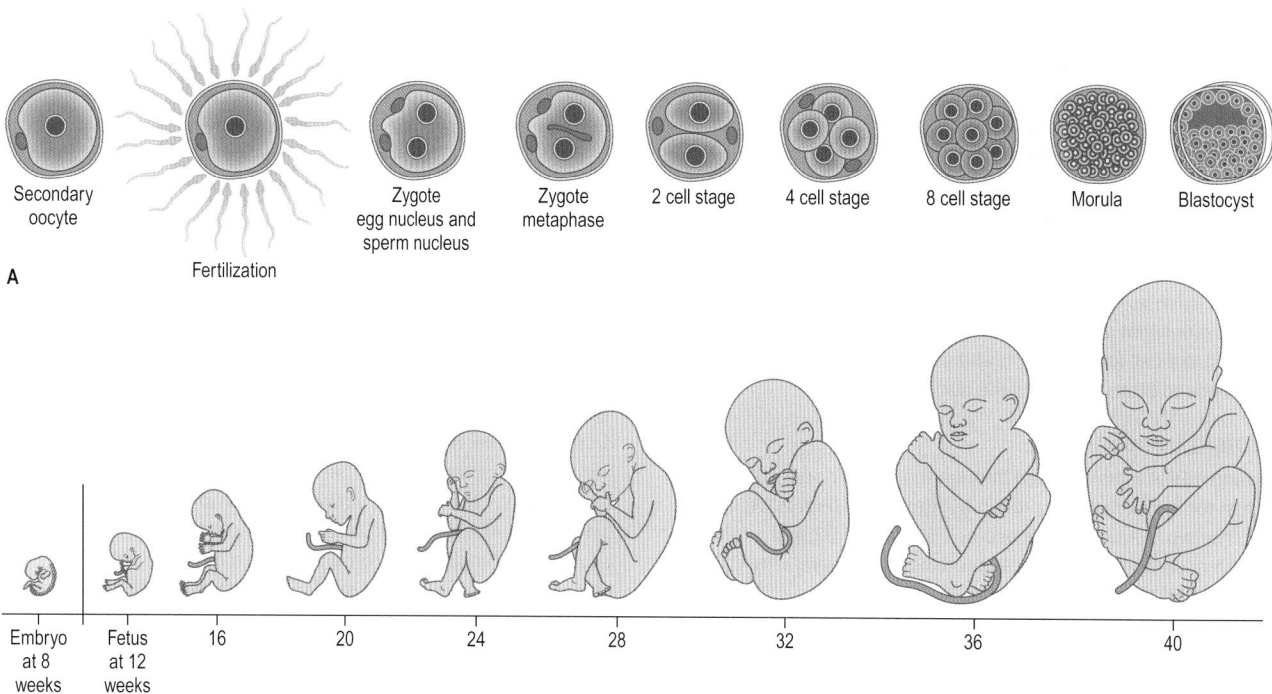

Fig. 2.9 Cell division, embryogenesis and fetal development. (A) Early stages of cell division leading to the formation of the blastocyst. **(B)** Stages of fetal development.

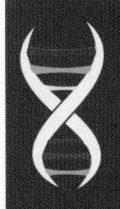

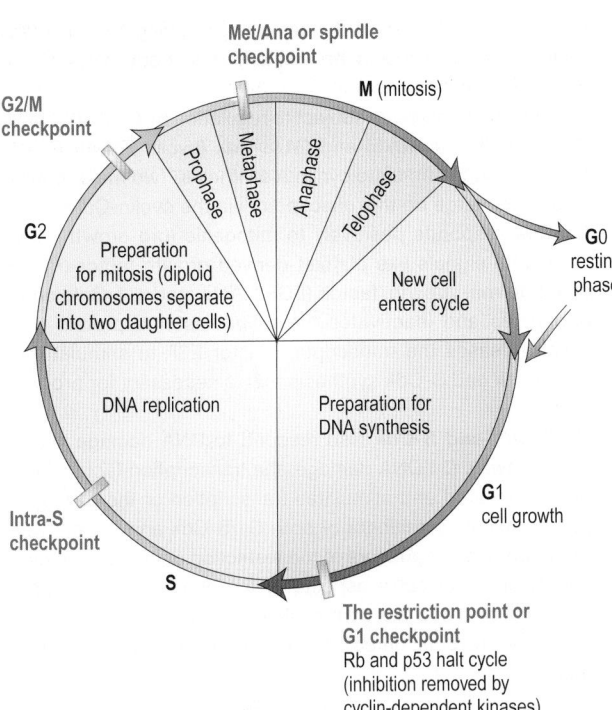

Fig. 2.10 The cell cycle. Cells are stimulated by growth factors to leave non-cycle **G0** to enter G1 phase. **During G1**, transcription of the DNA synthesis molecules occurs. Rb is a 'checkpoint' (inhibition molecule) between G1 and S phases and must be removed for the cycle to continue. This is achieved by the action of the cyclin-dependent kinase produced during G1. During the **S phase**, any DNA defects will be detected and p53 will halt the cycle (see p. 24). Following DNA synthesis (S phase), cells enter **G2**, a preparation phase for cell division. Mitosis takes place in the **M phase**. The new daughter cells can now either enter **G0** and differentiate into specialized cells, or re-enter the cell cycle.

those of the placenta); they are more commonly called embryonic stem (ES) cells. Stem cells have two properties:

- **self-renewal**: the ability to divide indefinitely without differentiating
- **pluripotency** or **totipotency**: the capability to differentiate, given the appropriate signals, into any cell type (except fetal placental cells).

During embryogenesis, a carefully orchestrated programme ensues, with this ball of cells ultimately forming the early embryo, recognizable as human with the formation of organs such as the heart and the development of limbs (**Fig. 2.9B**).

As they begin to differentiate, adult progenitor cells (sometimes referred to erroneously as stem cells) retain their ability to self-renew but their potency is reduced; with this limited ability to self-renew they can differentiate into multiple related lineages (multipotent, like haemopoietic 'progenitor cells') or single lineages (unipotent, like muscle satellite cells). The body uses these partially differentiated progenitor cells to replace or repair damaged cells and tissues, even into adulthood.

Stem cells have great therapeutic potential and can be obtained from blood from the umbilical cord, which contains embryo-like stem cells (which are not as primitive as ES cells but can differentiate into many more cell types than adult progenitor cells). Alternatively, adult cells, such as skin fibroblast cells, can be reprogrammed to regain stem-like properties (induced pluripotent stem cells, IPSC).

Further reading

Ben-David U, Benvenisty N. The tumorigenicity of human embryonic and induced pluripotent stem cells. *Nat Rev Cancer* 2011; 11:268–277.
Doudna JA, Charpentier E. The new frontier of genome engineering with CRISPR-Cas9. *Science* 2014; 346:1258096.
Forraz N, McGuckin CP. The umbilical cord: a rich and ethical stem cell source to advance regenerative medicine. *Cell Prolif* 2011; 44(Suppl 1):60–69.
Rice CM, Kemp K, Wilkins A et al. Cell therapy for multiple sclerosis: an evolving concept with implications for other neurodegenerative diseases. *Lancet* 2013; 382:1204–1213.
Wu SM, Hochedlinger K. Harnessing the potential of induced pluripotent stem cells for regenerative medicine. *Nat Cell Biol* 2011; 13:497–505.

Control of cell division

The division of cells is central to the development, growth and maintenance of humans. At each division, a duplication of the entire genetic code occurs and is passed to the next generation of daughter cells. When this process goes awry, cancer can follow. The cell duplication cycle has four phases called **G1**, **S**, **G2** and **mitosis** (**Fig. 2.10**), and takes about 20–24 hours to complete for a rapidly dividing adult cell. G1, S and G2 are collectively known as interphase, during which the cell doubles in mass (the two gap phases are for growth) and duplicates its 46 chromosomes (S phase). Mitosis describes, in four subphases (prophase, metaphase, anaphase and telophase; see **Fig. 2.10**), the process of chromosome separation and nuclear division before cytokinesis (division of the cytoplasm into two daughter cells).

G1 – S – G2 – synthesis phase: DNA replication

To undergo duplication of the genetic code, a robust mechanism for DNA duplication is initiated. DNA synthesis by a multi-enzyme complex is initiated simultaneously at multiple foci across the genome known as replication forks. The key components of the replication machinery are DNA helicase, DNA primase, DNA polymerase and single-stranded DNA binding proteins.

DNA helicase unwinds the double helix and exposes each strand as a template for replication. The two strands are antiparallel, and DNA is extended by addition of nucleotide triphosphates to the end of the growing chain. DNA primase synthesizes a short (approximately ten-nucleotide) RNA molecule annealed to the DNA template, which acts as a primer for DNA polymerase. DNA polymerase extends the primer by adding nucleotides to the 3′ end.

The phases of mitosis (M)

Once a copy of the entire genetic code has been made, there is careful separation of these two copies, such that one copy goes into each daughter cell. With a light microscope, it is possible to see that two copies have been made by counting chromosomal bodies, which rise from 46 to 92. The next steps are described at the level of a single chromosome pair (or sister chromatids) for simplicity (**Fig. 2.11**).

Prophase

The two sister chromatids condense in the nucleus. The two centrosomes, at the centre of each chromatid, are the sites between which the microtubules of the mitotic spindle will form; they then move apart in the cytoplasm. At the end of prophase, the nuclear membrane breaks down. A protein complex called the kinetochore then orchestrates the movement of these chromosomes.

Metaphase

The chromosomes are aligned on a central plane, with the two centrosomes at opposite poles. The sister chromatids are attached to microtubules from different centrosomes via the kinetochore.

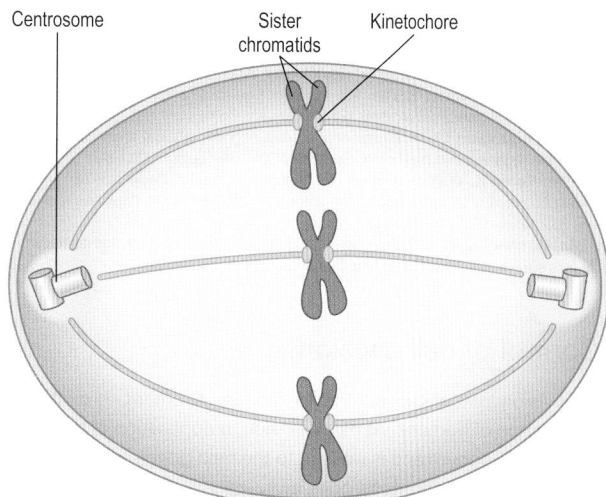

Fig. 2.11 The mitotic spindle at metaphase.

Anaphase

The sister chromatids are pulled in opposite directions as the microtubules shorten towards their respective spindle poles.

Telophase

Each set of daughter chromosomes is held at a spindle pole and the nuclear envelope reforms around the genome of each new daughter cell.

Cytokinesis

Splitting of the cytoplasm begins in telophase, before the completion of mitosis, with the appearance of a ring of actin and myosin filaments around the equator of the cell. Cytokinesis is completed as the ring contracts to create a cleavage furrow and separate the two daughter cells.

When to divide? Control of the cell cycle and checkpoints

Cells can exit the cell cycle and become quiescent. Indeed, most terminally differentiated adult cells are in a phase termed G0, in which the cycling machinery is switched off. In some cell types, the switch is irreversible (e.g. in neurones), but others, like hepatocytes, retain the ability to re-enter the cell cycle and proliferate. This gives the liver a significant ability to regenerate following damage.

Cyclin-dependent kinases

Progression through the cell cycle is tightly controlled and punctuated by three key checkpoints, where the cell interprets environmental and cellular signals to determine whether it is appropriate or safe to proceed (see **Fig. 2.11**). The switches that allow progression beyond these checkpoints are a family of small protein complexes called cyclin-dependent kinases (Cdks), which phosphorylate serines or threonines in key target proteins at each stage.

Checkpoints, retinoblastoma protein and p53
Restriction point (G1 checkpoint)

The restriction point works to ensure that the cell cycle does not progress into S phase unless growth conditions are favourable and the genomic DNA is undamaged. The cyclin-Cdk complexes active early in S phase are denoted S-Cdk (cyclin A with Cdk1 or Cdk2).

S-Cdks have two roles:
- to phosphorylate their target proteins to initiate helix unwinding of the DNA at origins of replication, allowing the replication complex to begin DNA synthesis

- to prevent re-initiation at the same origin during the same cell cycle (because it would be deleterious to copy parts of the genome more than once).

S-Cdks are themselves subject to regulation by G1-Cdk (cyclin D1–3 with Cdk4 or Cdk5) and G1/S-Cdk (cyclin E with Cdk2), both of which can stimulate cyclin A synthesis. Two major cancer pathways converge on this checkpoint via the cyclin-Cdks:

- **G1-Cdk** responds positively to mitogenic (pro-growth) environmental signals like platelet-derived growth factor (PDGF) or epidermal growth factor (EGF). Activated G1-Cdk phosphorylates and inactivates the retinoblastoma protein (Rb), which releases the transcription factor E2F to stimulate the G1/S-Cdk and S-Cdk synthesis that is necessary for progression.

- **G1/S-Cdk and S-Cdk** also respond to DNA damage via the p53 pathway. On DNA damage, the transcription factor p53 is phosphorylated and stimulates transcription of the *p21* gene. p21 protein is an inhibitor of both G1/S-Cdk and S-Cdk. Both Rb and p53 are regulators of the restriction point. Loss of function of either disables aspects of the negative control pathways. *RB* and *p53* are commonly mutated in cancer and both are therefore considered 'tumour suppressor genes' (see p. 38).

G2/M checkpoint

The G2/M checkpoint prevents entry into mitosis in the presence of DNA damage or non-replicated DNA. M-Cdk (cyclin B with Cdk1) accumulates towards the end of G2 and is activated following dephosphorylation by the phosphatase Cdc25. Activated M-Cdk has three roles at the G2/M checkpoint:
- to initiate chromosome condensation
- to promote breakdown of the nuclear membrane
- to initiate assembly of the mitotic spindle.

DNA damage and the presence of non-replicated DNA negatively regulate M-Cdk and prevent entry into mitosis. The kinases that phosphorylate p53 in response to DNA damage and block progression through the restriction point can also phosphorylate and inhibit Cdc25, inactivating M-Cdk. Thus DNA damage also blocks cell cycle progression at this checkpoint.

Met/Ana checkpoint

The metaphase to anaphase checkpoint is regulated by protein degradation. The anaphase-promoting complex APC/C is a ubiquitin ligase that transfers a small protein, ubiquitin, to other proteins, marking them for degradation. The primary targets are securin, and the S- and M-cyclins of the cyclin-Cdks present at the start of mitosis. The degradation of securin results in the digestion of cohesin, which holds the two sister chromatids together, allowing them to be pulled apart by the mitotic spindle.

Review of cellular genetics

According to the fundamental paradigm in genetics, information to create a human is stored in the genetic code in a cell. This code is identically replicated in every cell from conception onwards. In different cells, different parts of the code are needed, specific to that cell type, to make proteins required for the functioning of that cell; this control of gene expression is achieved through a number of mechanisms affecting gene transcription, processing of RNA and translation of mRNA into protein.

In the next section, we describe examples of what happens when there are specific changes in the genetic code that have been associated with the presentation of specific genetic disorders.

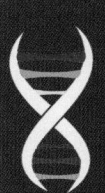

Genetic disease

- 0.5% of all newborns have a chromosomal abnormality
- 7% of all stillborns have a chromosomal abnormality
- 20–30% of all infant deaths are due to genetic disorders
- 11% of paediatric hospital admissions are for children with genetic disorders
- 12% of adult hospital admissions are due to genetic causes
- 15% of all cancers have an inherited susceptibility
- 10% of chronic diseases of the adult population (heart, diabetes, arthritis) have a significant genetic component

Congenital malformation

- 3–5% of all births result in congenital malformations
- 30–50% of post-neonatal deaths are due to congenital malformations
- 18% of paediatric hospital admissions are for children with congenital malformations

European incidences per 1000 births

Single-gene disorders: 10
- Dominant: 7.0
- Recessive: 1.66
- X-linked: 1.33

Chromosomal disorders: 3.5
- Autosomes: 1.69
- Sex chromosomes: 1.80

Congenital malformations: 31
- Genetically determined: 0.6
- Multifactorial: 30
- Non-genetic: ~0.4

[a]Although individual genetic diseases are rare, regional variation is enormous; the incidence of Down's syndrome varies from 1/1000 to 1/100 worldwide. Single-gene diseases collectively comprise over 15 500 recognized genetic disorders. The global prevalence of all single-gene diseases at birth is approximately 10/1000.

Condition	Mechanism responsible
Down's syndrome	Trisomy 21
Cystic fibrosis	Recessive
Haemophilia	Dominant or recessive
BRCA	Dominant
Xeroderma pigmentosum	Recessive
Huntington's disease	Anticipation
Angelman's syndrome	Imprinting
Myoclonic epilepsy with ragged-red fibres (MERRF)	Mitochondrial

GENETIC DISORDERS

Inherited genetic disorders occur due to mutations in genetic code; their prevalence is indicated in **Box 2.3**. They can arise because of new mutations in sperm or ova, or as a result of an inherited mutation passed down a family line. These disorders can stem from a single base-pair change, alteration of a region of a chromosome, or even duplication or omission of an entire chromosome (**Box 2.4**). The pattern of inheritance in a family tree depends on which chromosome the mutation occurs in, and whether both copies need to be affected to cause the disease. Somatic mutations typically occurring after birth can be responsible for benign and malignant tumours, and are discussed on page 37.

To start, we will consider conditions for which chromosomal changes are responsible. These were among the first to be studied, as the technique known as karyotyping allowed for visualization of differences in chromosomes using a light microscope.

Chromosomal disorders

Chromosomal abnormalities are much more common than is generally appreciated (see **Box 2.3**). Over half of spontaneous abortions have chromosomal abnormalities, compared with only 4–6 abnormalities per 1000 live births. Specific chromosomal abnormalities can lead to well-recognized and severe clinical syndromes; autosomal aneuploidy (a differing from the normal diploid number) is usually more severe than the sex chromosome aneuploidies (**Box 2.5**). Abnormalities may occur in either the number or the structure of the chromosomes.

Abnormal chromosome numbers

If a chromosome or chromatids fail to separate ('non-disjunction') in either meiosis or mitosis, one daughter cell will receive two copies of that chromosome and one daughter cell will receive no copies of the chromosome. If this non-disjunction occurs during meiosis, it can lead to an ovum or sperm having:

- ***an extra chromosome***, resulting in a fetus that is 'trisomic' and has three instead of two copies of the chromosome
- ***no chromosome***, resulting in a fetus that is 'monosomic' and has one instead of two copies of the chromosome.

Non-disjunction can occur with autosomes or sex chromosomes. However, only individuals with trisomy 13, 18 and 21 survive to birth, and most children with trisomy 13 and trisomy 18 die in early childhood. **Trisomy 21 (Down's syndrome)** is observed with a frequency of 1 in 650 live births, regardless of geography or ethnic background. This rate is reduced with widespread screening and selective termination of pregnancy (see p. 27). Full **autosomal monosomies** are extremely rare and generally incompatible with survival to full gestation. **Sex chromosome trisomies** (e.g. Klinefelter's syndrome, XXY) are relatively common. The **sex chromosome monosomy** in which the individual has one X chromosome only and no second X or Y chromosome (i.e. X0) is known as **Turner's syndrome** and is estimated to occur in 1 in 2500 live-born girls.

Occasionally, non-disjunction can occur during mitosis shortly after two gametes have fused. It will then result in the formation of two cell lines, each with a different chromosome complement; the person is termed a 'mosaic' as only some of his or her cells carry an incorrect number of chromosomes (see p. 29).

Very rarely, the entire chromosome set will be present in more than two copies, so the individual may be triploid rather than diploid and have a chromosome number of 69. Triploidy and tetraploidy (four sets) is not usually compatible with life and results in spontaneous abortion.

Abnormal chromosome structures

As well as abnormal numbers of chromosomes, chromosomes can have abnormal structures, and the disruption to the DNA and gene sequences may give rise to a genetic disease.

- ***Deletions*** of a portion of a chromosome may give rise to a disease syndrome if two copies of the genes in the deleted region are necessary, and with just the one normal copy remaining on the non-deleted homologous chromosome the individual will not be normal. Many deletion syndromes have been well described. For example, ***Prader–Willi syndrome*** is

Box 2.5 Chromosomal abnormalities: examples of a few syndromes

Syndrome	Chromosome karyotype	Incidence and risks	Clinical features	Mortality
Autosomal abnormalities				
Trisomy 21 (Down's syndrome)	47,+21 (95%) Mosaicism translocation 5%	1:650 (overall) (risk with a 20- to 29-year-old mother 1:1000; >45-year-old mother 1:30)	Flat face, slanting eyes, epicanthic folds, small ears, simian crease, short and stubby fingers, hypotonia, variable learning difficulties, congenital heart disease (up to 50%)	High in first year but many survive to adulthood
Trisomy 13 (Patau's syndrome)	47,+13	1:5000	Low-set ears, cleft lip and palate, polydactyly, micro-ophthalmia, learning difficulties	Rarely survive for more than a few weeks
Trisomy 18 (Edwards' syndrome)	47,+18	1:3000	Low-set ears, micrognathia, rocker-bottom feet, learning difficulties	Rarely survive for more than a few weeks
Sex chromosome abnormalities				
Fragile X syndrome	46,XX, fra (X) 46,XY, fra (X)	1:2000	Most common inherited cause of learning difficulties, predominantly in males Macro-orchidism	Typically survive to adulthood
Female				
Turner's syndrome	45,XO	1:2500	Infantilism, primary amenorrhoea, short stature, webbed neck, cubitus valgus, normal IQ	Typically survive to adulthood
Triple X syndrome	47,XXX	1:1000	No distinctive somatic features, learning difficulties	Typically survive to adulthood
Male				
Klinefelter's syndrome	47,XXY (or XXYY)	1:1000 (more in sons of older mothers)	Decreased crown–pubis:pubis–heel ratio, eunuchoid, testicular atrophy, infertility, gynaecomastia, learning difficulties (20%; related to number of X chromosomes)	Typically survive to adulthood
Double Y syndrome	47,XYY	1:800 High incidence in tall criminals	Tall, fertile, minor mental and psychiatric illness	Typically survive to adulthood

the result of deletion of part of the long arm of chromosome 15; **Wilms' tumour** is characterized by deletion of part of the short arm of chromosome 11; and microdeletions in the long arm of chromosome 22 give rise to **DiGeorge's syndrome** (see p. 60).

- **Duplications** occur when a portion of the chromosome is present on the chromosome in two copies, so the genes in that chromosome portion are present in an extra dose. A form of neuropathy, **Charcot–Marie–Tooth disease** (see p. 891), is due to a small duplication of a region of chromosome 17.
- **Inversions** involve an end-to-end reversal of a segment within a chromosome, e.g. 'abcdefgh' becomes 'abcfedgh', as in **haemophilia** (see p. 375).
- **Translocations** occur if two chromosome regions join together, when they would not do so normally. Chromosome translocations in somatic cells may be associated with tumorigenesis (see p. 38 and **Fig. 2.23**).

Translocations can be very complex, involving more than two chromosomes, but most are simple and fall into one of two categories:

- **Reciprocal translocations** occur when any two non-homologous chromosomes break simultaneously and rejoin, swapping ends. In this case, the cell still has 46 chromosomes but two of them are rearranged. Someone with a balanced translocation is likely to be normal (unless a translocation breakpoint interrupts a gene); however, at meiosis, when the chromosomes separate into different daughter cells, the translocated chromosomes will enter the gametes, and any resulting fetus may inherit one abnormal chromosome and have an unbalanced translocation with physical manifestations.
- **Robertsonian translocations** occur when two acrocentric chromosomes join and the short arm is lost, leaving only 45 chromosomes. This translocation is balanced, as no genetic material is lost and the individual is healthy. However, any offspring have a risk of inheriting an unbalanced arrangement. This risk depends on which acrocentric chromosome is involved. The 14/21 Robertsonian translocation is clinically relevant. A woman with this karyotype has a 1 in 8 risk of having a baby with Down's syndrome (a male carrier has a 1 in 50 risk). However, they have a 50% risk of producing a carrier like themselves; hence the necessity for genetic family studies. Relatives should be alerted to the increased risk of Down's syndrome in their offspring, and should have their chromosomes checked.

Mitochondrial chromosome disorders

The mitochondrial chromosome (see **Fig. 2.5**) carries its genetic information in a very compact form; for example, there are no introns in the genes. Therefore, any mutation has a high chance of having an effect. However, as every cell contains hundreds of mitochondria, a single altered mitochondrial genome will not be noticed. As mitochondria divide, there is a statistical likelihood that there will be more mutated mitochondria and, at some point, this will give rise to a mitochondrial disease.

Most mitochondrial diseases are myopathies and neuropathies with a maternal pattern of inheritance. Other abnormalities include retinal degeneration, diabetes mellitus and hearing loss. **Myopathies** include chronic progressive external ophthalmoplegia (CPEO); encephalomyopathies include myoclonic epilepsy with ragged-red fibres (MERRF) and mitochondrial encephalomyopathy, lactic acidosis and stroke-like episodes (MELAS) (see p. 897).

- **Kearns–Sayre syndrome** includes ophthalmoplegia, heart block, cerebellar ataxia, deafness and learning difficulties due to long deletions and rearrangements.
- **Leber's hereditary optic neuropathy** (LHON) is the most common cause of blindness in young men, with bilateral loss of central vision and cardiac arrhythmias, and is an example of a mitochondrial disease caused by a point mutation in one gene.
- **Multisystem disorders** include **Pearson's syndrome** (sideroblastic anaemia, pancytopenia, exocrine pancreatic failure, subtotal villous atrophy, diabetes mellitus and renal tubular dysfunction). In some families, hearing loss is the only symptom, and one of the mitochondrial genes implicated may predispose patients to aminoglycoside cytotoxicity.

Analysis of chromosomal disorders

Historically, karyotyping involved growing cells from patient samples and studying the chromosomes. The cell cycle can be arrested at mitosis with the use of colchicine and, following staining, the chromosomes with their characteristic banding can be seen and any abnormalities identified. This is an automated process with computer scanning software searching for metaphase spreads and then automatic binning of each chromosome to allow easy scoring of chromosome number and banding patterns.

Current approaches utilize genome-wide array-based platforms (called single nucleotide polymorphism (SNP) arrays) to identify changes in chromosome copy number and can identify very small interstitial deletions and insertions. The presence of translocations cannot be detected using SNP arrays, but instead is studied in a targeted way using fluorescence *in situ* hybridization (FISH). Large, region-specific probes are labelled with fluorescently tagged nucleotides and used to allow rapid identification of metaphase chromosomes. As whole-genome sequencing is becoming more accessible and coverage increases, it will increasingly be used to identify deletions, insertions and translocation breakpoints.

Point mutations, insertions and deletions

The advent of Sanger sequencing rapidly accelerated the discovery of base-pair level changes. These mutations can have various effects on the expression of the gene and many cause a dysfunction of the protein product. In contrast to the previous section, where changes were described that affect millions of base-pairs in a cell, point mutations can involve just one critical base-pair. These are small but important changes.

Mutations

Although DNA replication is a very accurate process, mistakes occasionally occur and produce changes or mutations. These changes can also arise because of other factors, such as radiation, ultraviolet light or chemicals. Mutations in gene sequences or in the sequences that regulate gene expression (transcription and translation) may alter the amino acid sequence in the protein encoded by that gene. In some cases, protein function will be maintained; in other cases, it will change or cease, perhaps producing a clinical disorder. Many different types of mutation occur.

Point mutation

This is the simplest type of change and involves the substitution of one nucleotide for another, so changing the codon in a coding sequence and leading to an amino acid substitution (assuming the new sequence is non-synonymous with the former). For example, in *sickle cell disease*, a mutation within the globin gene changes one codon from GAG to GTG so that, instead of glutamic acid, valine is incorporated into the polypeptide chain, which radically alters its properties. However, substitutions may have no effect on the function or stability of the proteins produced, as several codons code for the same amino acid (synonymous – see **Fig. 2.7**).

Insertion or deletion

Insertion or deletion of one or more bases is a more serious change, particularly if the inserted or deleted DNA is not a multiple of three bases, as this will cause the following sequence to be out of the reading frame and can result in a premature stop codon.

Splicing mutations

If the DNA sequences that direct the splicing of introns from mRNA are mutated, then abnormal splicing may occur. In this case, the processed mRNA that is translated into protein by the ribosomes may carry intron sequences or miss exons, so altering amino acid sequence and affecting protein function.

Nonsense mutations

A nonsense mutation is a point mutation in a sequence of DNA that results in a premature stop codon.

Prenatal diagnosis of congenital anomalies

Prenatal screening should be offered to *all* pregnant women. In England, screening for the three most common trisomies (Down's, Edwards' and Patau's) is offered to all pregnant women. The risk increases disproportionately for children born to mothers older than 35 years. Infants born to mothers with a history or family history of other conditions due to chromosomal abnormalities may also be at increased risk.

Personal choice

There should be a detailed discussion with all mothers about the possible consequences of each screening test before they are offered it. In particular, they should have an understanding of the failure rates, detection rates, and false-positive and false-negative rates of each test so that they can exercise choice properly.

Investigations

The choice of investigation depends on gestational age:

7–11 weeks (vaginal ultrasound)

Ultrasound is used to confirm viability, fetal number and gestation by crown–rump measurement. This scan is not a screening test for aneuploidy.

10–13 weeks and 6 days (combined test)

The combined test comprises:
- ultrasound for nuchal translucency measurement; nuchal translucency is also increased in Turner's syndrome)
- testing of maternal serum for pregnancy-associated plasma protein-A (PAPP-A from the syncytial trophoblast) and β-human chorionic gonadotrophin for trisomy 21.

All serum marker measurements are corrected for gestational ages, a multiple of the mean (MOM) value for the appropriate week of gestation. If abnormalities are detected, it is necessary to continue to discuss whether further investigation is desired or not. The next option is chorionic villus sampling (CVS) at 11–13 weeks under ultrasound guidance to sample the placental site, or amniocentesis at 15 weeks to sample amniotic fluid and obtain the fetal cells necessary for cytogenetic testing.

The combined test is more accurate than the triple test alone at 16 weeks.

14–20 weeks (serum triple or quadruple test)

A serum triple or quadruple test is done if the pregnancy is too advanced for the earlier tests or if the combined test was not offered.

The triple test for chromosomal abnormalities consists of testing maternal serum for levels of:

- α-fetoprotein (low)
- unconjugated oestradiol (low)
- human chorionic gonadotrophin (high) for Down's syndrome and for neural tube defects.

The α-fetoprotein is high for neural tube defects.

The quadruple test also measures inhibin A (high in Down's syndrome).

18–20 weeks

Ultrasound detects structural abnormalities (e.g. neural tube defects and congenital heart defects).

Reported detection rates for congenital anomalies varies: for example, from 14–61% for hypoplastic ventricle to 97–100% for anencephaly.

Non-invasive prenatal testing

It is possible to sequence fetal DNA in the maternal bloodstream to measure the copies of chromosomes that inform the risk of the child having a chromosomal disorder. Known as non-invasive prenatal testing (NIPT), it is more accurate than standard combined or quadruple testing. NIPT has been evaluated in the UK's National Health Service and there is a plan to introduce it as a follow-on screening test in some women.

Further reading

Archer SL. Mitochondrial dynamics – mitochondrial fission and fusion in human diseases. *N Engl J Med* 2013; 369:2236–2251.

Bodurtha J, Strauss JF. Genomics and perinatal care. *N Engl J Med* 2012; 366:64–73.

NHS. *Screening Tests in Pregnancy: Your Pregnancy and Baby Guide*. https://www.nhs.uk/conditions/pregnancy-and-baby/screening-tests-abnormality-pregnant/.

Park CB, Larsson N.G. Mitochondrial DNA mutations in disease and aging. *J Cell Biol* 2011; 193:809–818.

RCOG. https://www.rcog.org.uk/globalassets/documents/guidelines/scientific-impact-papers/sip_15_04032014.pdf/. *Royal College of Obstetrics and Gynaecology guidelines on non-invasive prenatal testing (NIPT) for Down's syndrome.*

Patterns of inheritance of single-gene diseases

Monogenetic disorders involving single genes can be inherited in a dominant, recessive or sex-linked manner.

Autosomal dominant disorders

Each diploid cell contains two copies of all the autosomes. An autosomal dominant disorder (**Fig. 2.12A**) occurs when one of the two copies has a mutation and the protein produced by the normal form of the gene cannot compensate. In this case, a heterozygous individual who has two different forms (or alleles) of the same gene will manifest the disease. The offspring of heterozygotes have a 50% chance of inheriting the chromosome carrying the disease allele, and therefore also of having the disease. However, estimation of risk to offspring for counselling families can be difficult because of three factors:

- Some disorders have a great variability in their manifestation. 'Incomplete penetrance' may occur if patients have a dominant

A Autosomal dominant

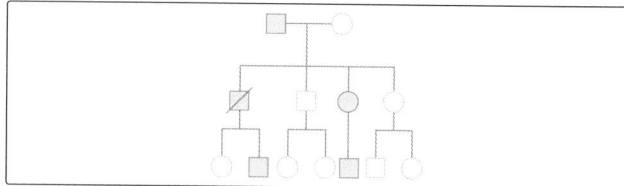

B Autosomal recessive

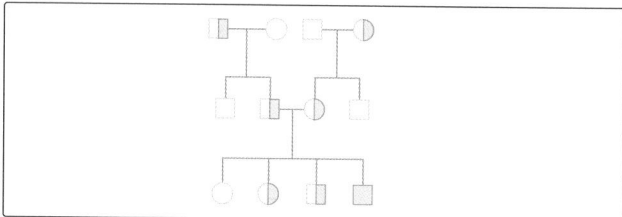

C X-linked dominant

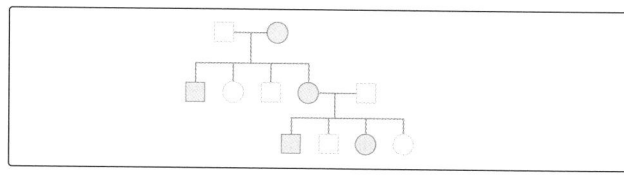

D X-linked recessive

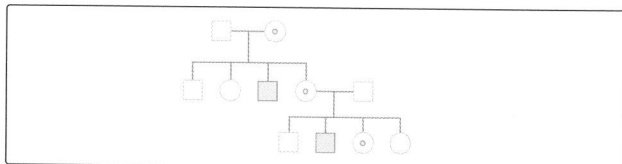

E Mitochondrial

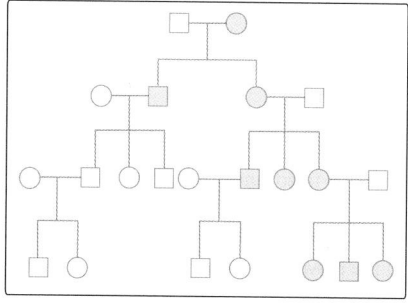

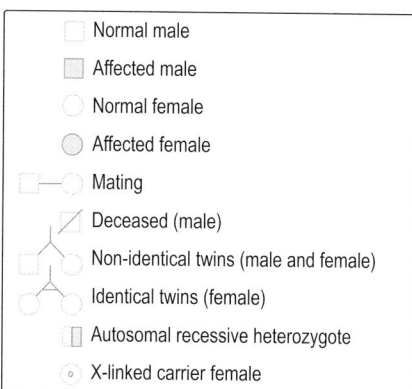

- ☐ Normal male
- ◼ Affected male
- ○ Normal female
- ● Affected female
- ☐—○ Mating
- ⧄ Deceased (male)
- Non-identical twins (male and female)
- Identical twins (female)
- Autosomal recessive heterozygote
- ⊙ X-linked carrier female

Fig. 2.12 Modes of inheritance of simple gene disorders and mitochondrial inheritance.

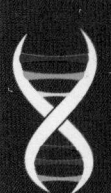

disorder but it does not manifest itself clinically in them. This gives the appearance of the gene having 'skipped' a generation.

- Dominant traits are extremely variable in severity (variable expression) and a mildly affected parent may have a severely affected child.
- New cases in a previously unaffected family may be the result of a new mutation. In this case the risk of a further affected child is negligible. Most cases of achondroplasia, for example, are due to new mutations.

Autosomal recessive disorders

These disorders (**Fig. 2.12B**) manifest themselves only when an individual is homozygous or a compound heterozygote for the disease allele: that is, both chromosomes carry the same gene mutation (homozygous) or two different mutations in the same gene (compound heterozygote). The parents are unaffected carriers (heterozygous for the disease allele). If carriers marry, the offspring have a 1 in 4 chance of carrying both mutant copies of the gene and being affected, a 1 in 2 chance of being a carrier, and a 1 in 4 chance of being genetically normal. Parental relatedness increases the risk.

Sex-linked disorders

Genes carried on the X chromosome are said to be 'X-linked' and can be dominant or recessive in the same way as autosomal genes (**Fig. 2.12C,D**).

X-linked recessive disorders

These disorders present in males and only in homozygous females (usually rare). X-linked recessive diseases are transmitted by healthy female carriers or affected males if they survive to reproduce. An example of an X-linked recessive disorder is **haemophilia A** (see p. 375), which is caused by a mutation in the X-linked gene for factor VIII. It has been shown that in 50% of cases there is an intrachromosomal rearrangement (inversion) of the tip of the long arm of the X chromosome (one breakpoint being within intron 22 of the factor VIII gene).

Of the offspring from a carrier female and a normal male:

- 50% of the girls will be carriers, as they inherit a mutant allele from their mother and the normal allele from their father; the other 50% of the girls inherit two normal alleles and are themselves normal
- 50% of the boys will have haemophilia, as they inherit the mutant allele from their mother (and the Y chromosome from their father); the other 50% of the boys will be normal, as they inherit the normal allele from their mother (and the Y chromosome from their father).

The male offspring of a male with haemophilia and a normal female will not have the disease, as they do not inherit his X chromosome. However, all the female offspring will be carriers, as they all inherit his X chromosome.

X-linked dominant disorders

These are rare. Females who are heterozygous for the mutant gene and males who have one copy of the mutant gene on their single X chromosome will manifest the disease. Half the male or female offspring of an affected mother and all the female offspring of an affected male will have the disease. Affected males tend to have the disease more severely than the heterozygous female.

Mitochondrial inheritance

The pattern of inheritance associated with alterations in the mtDNA involves both males and females, but always with the condition passed on through the female line (maternal inheritance). Since many mitochondria are passed into the egg from the cells in the ovary, all the offspring of an affected woman would be expected to inherit the condition. An affected male does not pass his mitochondria on to his children, so his children will be unaffected (see **Fig. 2.12E**). Note that not all mitochondrial diseases will show this pattern of inheritance. As these conditions arise due to incorrectly functioning mitochondria, they may also be caused by an alteration in the nuclear DNA that has an impact on mitochondrial function, and not just be caused directly by a mitochondrial mutation. Hence, some mitochondrial diseases may demonstrate dominant patterns of inheritance.

Special presentations of genetic disease

These are disorders that may be due to mutations in single genes but which do not manifest as simple monogenic disorders. They can arise from a variety of mechanisms.

Mosaicism

Genetic mosaicism arises when a mutation occurs in a cell during embryonic development. This cell and its progeny are then genetically distinct from the rest of the fetus. This can give rise to a less severe form of recognized genetic disease, sometimes referred to historically as a 'forme fruste'. Equally, some mutations are not compatible with life if every cell in the fetus is affected, but may be rescued if the fetus is mosaic. Schimmelpenning's syndrome is an example, where patients carry a mosaic *HRAS* gene mutation.

Triplet repeat mutations and genetic anticipation

In the gene responsible for myotonic dystrophy (see p. 896), the mutated allele was found to have an expanded 3′ UTR region in which three nucleotides, CTG, were repeated up to about 200 times. In families with myotonic dystrophy, people with the late-onset form of the disease had 20–40 copies of the repeat, but their children and grandchildren who presented with the disease from birth had vast increases in the number of repeats – up to 2000 copies. It is thought that some mechanism during meiosis causes this 'triplet repeat expansion' so that the offspring inherit an increased number of triplets. The number of triplets affects mRNA and protein function, and patients with more repeats present earlier (**Box 2.6**). The phenomenon has also been recognized with Huntington's chorea, where patients with more repeats present earlier and with progressively worse symptoms. This 'anticipation' is due to unstable mutations occurring within the disease gene. Trinucleotide repeats, such as CTG (dystrophia myotonica) and CAG (Huntington's disease), expand within the disease gene with each generation, and somatic expansion with cellular replication is also observed. This type of genetic mutation can occur within the translated region or untranslated (and presumably regulatory) regions of the target genes. This genetic distinction has been used to subclassify a number of genetic diseases that have now been shown to be caused by trinucleotide repeat expansion and display phenotypic 'anticipation' (see **Box 2.6**).

Imprinting

It is known that normal humans need a diploid number of chromosomes: that is, 46. However, the maternal and paternal contributions can be different. The mechanism that regulates the differential expression of two alleles of the same gene is termed *genetic imprinting*.

Imprinting is relevant to human genetic disease because different phenotypes may result, depending on whether the mutant chromosome is maternally or paternally inherited. A deletion of part of the long

Box 2.6 Examples of trinucleotide repeat genetic disorders

Syndrome inheritance pattern	Disease prevalence	Gene, product, location and disorder	Genetic test detection rate (%)
Friedreich's ataxia – AR	2–4/100 000	*FRDA* (frataxin) 9q13 – GAA trinucleotide repeat expansion disorder in intron 1 of *FRDA*	96
Fragile X syndrome – X-linked	16–25/100 000	*FMR1* (fragile X mental retardation 1 protein) Xq27.3 – CGG trinucleotide repeat expansion and methylation changes in the 5′ untranslated region of *FMR1* exon 1	99
Huntington's disease – AD	3–15/100 000	*HD* (Huntingtin protein) 4p16.3 – CAG trinucleotide repeat expansion within the translated protein, giving rise to long tracts of repeat glutamine residues in *HD*	98
Myotonic dystrophy – AD	1/20 000	*DMPK* (myotonin–protein kinase) 19q13.2–13.3 – CTG trinucleotide repeat expansion in the 3′ untranslated region of the *DMPK* gene (dystrophia myotonica 1, DM1). Less common form – expanded. CCTG repeat in zinc finger protein 9 (*ZNF9*) gene (DM2)	100

AD, autosomal dominant; AR, autosomal recessive.

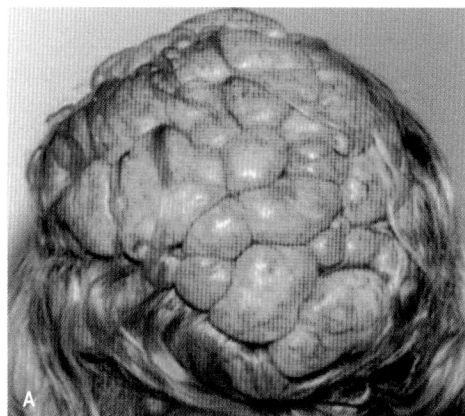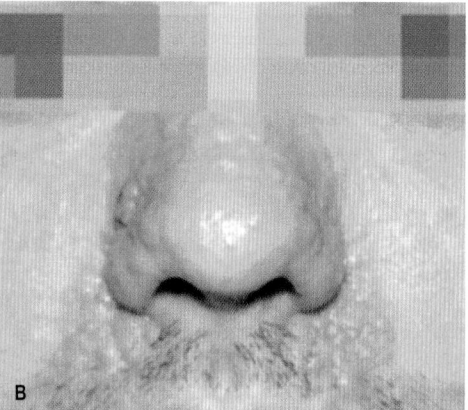

Fig. 2.13 *CYLD* **cutaneous syndrome.** Distinct phenotypes seen with identical genetic mutations reflect the impact of the genetic background on disease presentation. **(A)** Scalp cylindromas. **(B)** Trichoepitheliomas around the nasal fold.

arm of chromosome 15 (15q11–q13) will give rise to **Prader–Willi syndrome**, if it is paternally inherited. A deletion of a similar region of the chromosome gives rise to **Angelman's syndrome** if it is maternally inherited. The affected gene has been identified as ubiquitin (*UBE3A*).

Different genes that cause the same disease

Although classically divided into autosomal dominant, recessive or X-linked disorders, many syndromes show multiple forms of inheritance pattern. For example, in **Ehlers–Danlos syndrome**, there is autosomal dominant, recessive and X-linked inheritance. This has now been explained by the finding that mutations in different genes that contribute to a common function can have the same clinical presentation. In addition, in some recessive disorders, even having just one defective allele gives a mild form of the disease (semidominant), while having both alleles with the mutation results in a more severe form of the syndrome.

Different diseases caused by the same gene

The following are two examples of how different mutations in a gene can cause different diseases, referred to as genotype–phenotype correlation.

CYLD

In patients with germline mutations in *CYLD*, two strikingly different phenotypes are seen. Patients can develop tumours on the head or on the face, previously categorized as two separate diseases. It

is now known that these different presentations can occur within a family where the same pathogenic variant has been documented, so genetic changes may manifest differently based on the genetic background in which they arise (**Fig. 2.13**).

STAT3

The transcription factor signal transducer and activator of transcription 3 (*STAT3*) is a critical regulator of multiple and diverse cellular processes. Heterozygous, germline, loss-of-function mutations in *STAT3* lead to the primary immune deficiency hyper-IgE syndrome. Recently, germline, heterozygous mutations in *STAT3* that confer a gain of function have been discovered and result in early-onset, multiorgan autoimmunity.

Complex traits: multifactorial and polygenic inheritance

Characteristics resulting from a combination of genetic and environmental factors are said to be multifactorial; those involving multiple genes are said to be polygenic. There has been an explosion in genetic discoveries about these complex traits with the development of high-throughput genome-wide SNP arrays, which has allowed cost-effective and unbiased screening of large case–control cohorts (in excess of 1000 cases). These studies are known as genome-wide association studies (GWAS) and are discussed later. They have permitted unequivocal identification of SNPs associated with a variety of traits and diseases. For

Box 2.7 Examples of disorders that may have a polygenic inheritance

Disorder	Frequency (%)	Heritability (%)[a]
Hypertension	5	62
Asthma	4	80
Schizophrenia	1	85
Congenital heart disease	0.5	35
Neural tube defects	0.5	60
Congenital pyloric stenosis	0.3	75
Ankylosing spondylitis	0.2	70
Cleft palate	0.1	76

[a]Percentage of the total variation of a trait that can be attributed to genetic factors.

example, over 30 SNPs in immune-related gene loci have been associated with coeliac disease, with over half also associated with other immune-mediated or inflammatory diseases. This indicates that there are many low-risk genetic risk factors associated with complex traits, and common pathways are implicated in different diseases.

Most human diseases, such as heart disease, diabetes and common mental disorders, are multifactorial traits (**Box 2.7**).

Further reading

De Matteis MA, Luine A. Mendelian disorders of membrane trafficking. *N Engl J Med* 2011; 365:927–938.
Manolio TA. Genomewide association studies and assessment of the risk of disease. *N Engl J Med* 2010; 363:166–176.
Vogel TP, Milner JD, Cooper MA. The ying and yang of STAT3 in human disease. *J Clin Immunol* 2015; 35:615–623.
https://ukgtn.nhs.uk/ *Genetic testing.*
https://www.ebi.ac.uk/gwas/ *A catalogue of published genome-wide association studies.*
http://www.ncbi.nlm.nih.gov/omim *Autosomal single-gene disorders.*

TECHNIQUES FOR STUDYING THE GENETIC CODE

Polymerase chain reaction

Polymerase chain reaction (PCR) is a core technique in genetics, which has revolutionized genetic research because small regions of interest in a sample of DNA – for example, the *BRCA1* gene – can be amplified over a million times within a few hours. The DNA is amplified between two short (generally 17–25 bases) single-stranded DNA fragments ('oligonucleotide primers') that are complementary to the sequences on different strands at each end of the DNA of interest (**Fig. 2.14**). These short lengths of amplified DNA can then be sequenced to obtain identification of the exact nucleotide sequence using Sanger sequencing (named after its inventor).

Sanger sequencing

This involves a chemical process known as dideoxy-sequencing. Once the sequence of interest is amplified, this is used as a template for the Sanger sequencing reaction. An oligonucleotide primer is designed to anneal adjacent to the region of interest. This primer acts as the starting point for a DNA polymerase to build a new DNA chain that is complementary to the sequence under investigation. Chain extension is prematurely interrupted when a fluorescently labelled dideoxynucleotide becomes incorporated

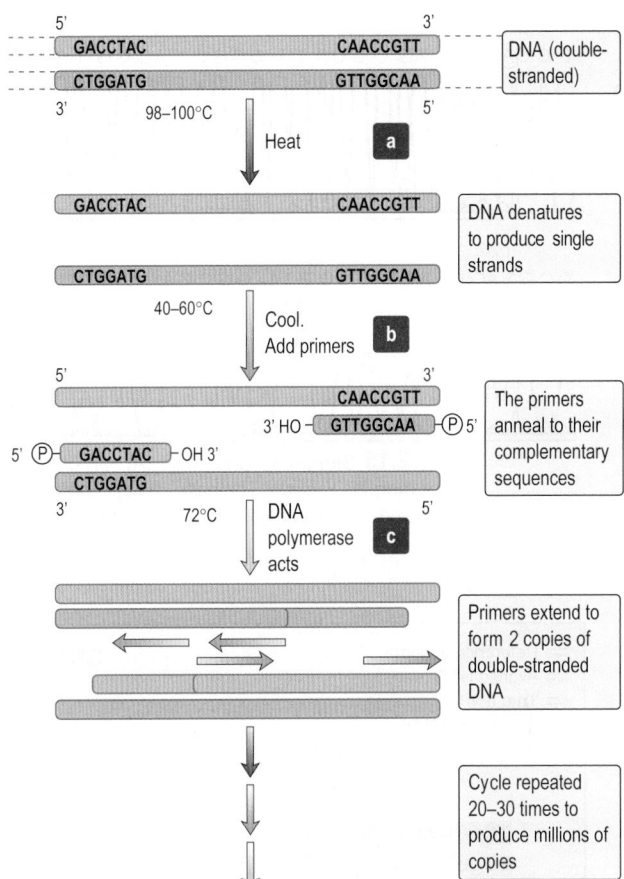

Fig. 2.14 Polymerase chain reaction. The technique is based on thermal cycling and has three basic steps. (a) The double-stranded genomic DNA is heat-denatured into single-stranded DNA. (b) The sample is cooled to favour annealing of the primers to their target DNA. (c) A thermostable DNA polymerase extends the primers over the target DNA. After one cycle, there are two copies of double-stranded DNA, after two cycles there are four copies, and so on.

(this happens because it lacks the necessary 3′-hydroxyl group needed for extension). Each base dideoxynucleotide (G, C, T, A) has a different fluorochrome attached, and thus each termination base can be identified by its fluorescent colour. As each strand can be separated efficiently by capillary electrophoresis according to its size or length, simply monitoring the fluorescence as the reaction products elute from the capillary tube will give the gene sequence (**Fig. 2.15**). This is a widely used but relatively low-throughput method, which is increasingly being replaced with high-throughput methods.

Next-generation sequencing

Sequencing technology has developed such that it is now possible to sequence DNA molecules in a high-throughput manner ('next-generation sequencing', NGS) and new, faster and cheaper methods are being developed. For under £200 (2019 price), it is possible to sequence all the coding genes in an individual's human genome (termed the 'exome') to catalogue all possible disease-associated and non-disease-associated variants in every human gene. If necessary, whole genomes (including non-coding regions) can also be sequenced in this way, although this involves a greater cost. The

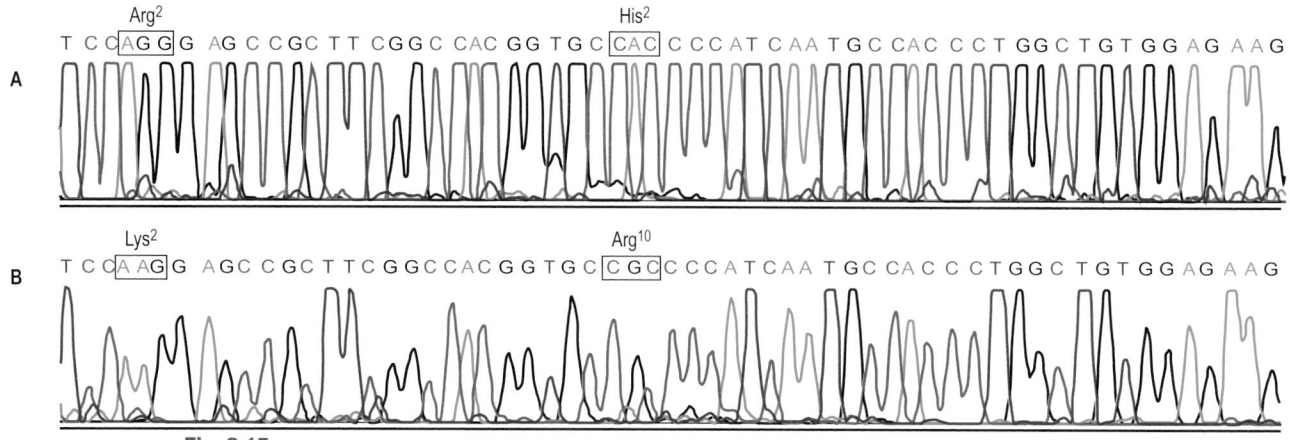

Fig. 2.15 Sanger sequencing. (A) Part of the normal luteinizing hormone beta chain gene. **(B)** Two polymorphic variants. The base changes and consequential alterations from arginine to lysine, and histidine to arginine amino acid residues are indicated.

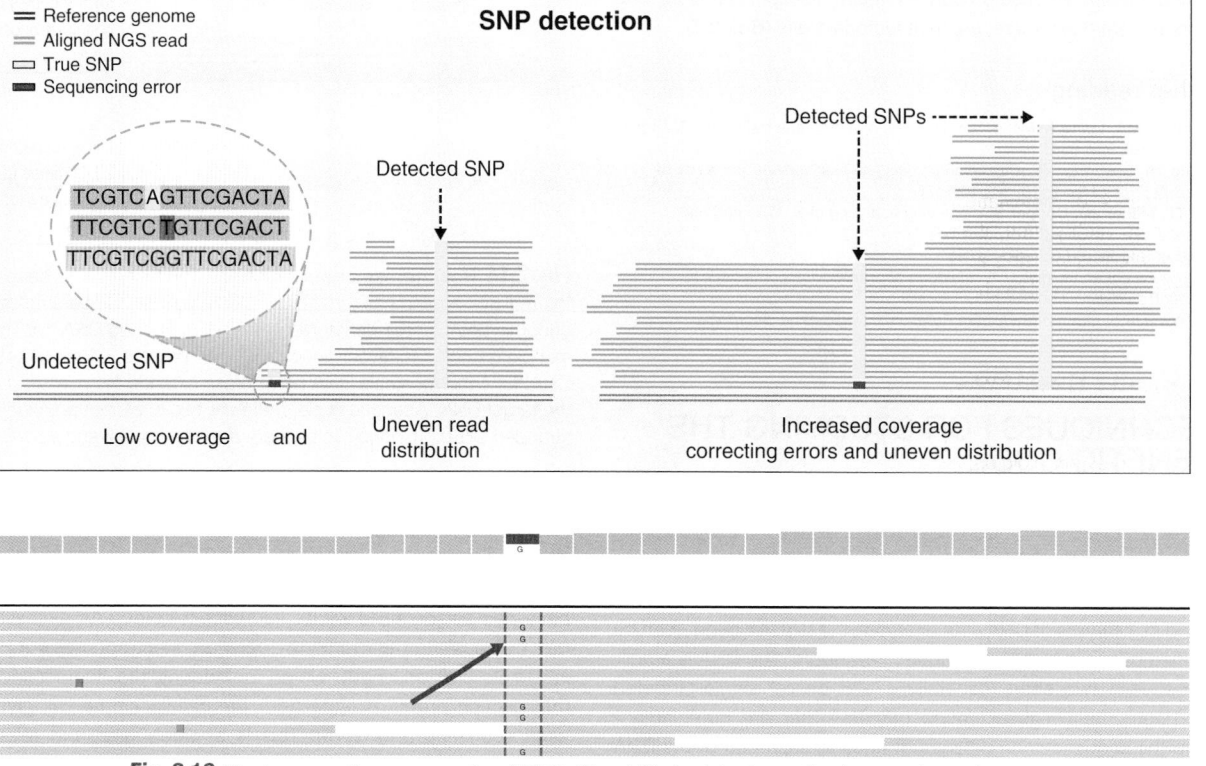

Fig. 2.16 Next-generation sequencing (NGS). The ability to detect genetic changes depends on good coverage of the region of interest, and the depth allows for true calls of variants over sequencing artefacts. SNP, single-nucleotide polymorphism.

sequences are typically generated as short runs of sequences between 75 and 200 bp long, known as reads, which are aligned to the reference human genome (**Fig. 2.16**).

Differences from the reference genome are called 'variants' and are catalogued for each sample. The computational requirements for processing data from NGS experiments are significant and are usually performed on dedicated computer clusters. Whole-genome sequencing has the advantage over whole-exome sequencing of being able to detect intronic changes, structural variants and changes in DNA copy number.

Hybridization arrays

This technique employs a fundamental property of DNA: when two strands are separated – for example, by heating – they will always reassociate and stick together again because of their complementary base sequences. The presence or position of a particular gene can therefore be identified using a gene 'probe' consisting of DNA or RNA, with a base sequence that is complementary to that of the sequence of interest. A DNA probe is thus a piece of single-stranded DNA that can locate and bind to its complementary sequence. Almost 1 million

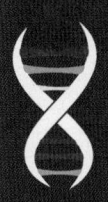

such probes can be placed on a chip in an array, and can be used to interrogate samples to obtain clinically relevant information such as SNP data for GWAS studies (see below) at a low cost per sample.

Transcriptomics

As well as sequencing genomic DNA, NGS technology can be used to sequence RNA (termed 'RNAseq') to assess gene expression levels accurately, in addition to determining all splice variations and allelic copy number. Analysis of all the RNA transcripts in a sample, or 'transcriptomics', allows for the comprehensive study of disease states. A limitation of this approach is that there may be a difference between levels of RNA transcripts and corresponding proteins that are encoded, warranting validation using additional techniques. Note that, in addition to carrying out such work on whole-tissue samples, such as liver or skin, it is now possible to sequence single cells. This represents an opportunity to investigate disease states at unprecedented resolution; the Human Cell Atlas is one such project that aims to capture representative transcriptomes of human cells from all tissues.

Epigenetic techniques

NGS can also be used to study epigenetic changes. Changes in methylation can be studied using a technique that converts the unmethylated cytosines across the whole genome using a chemical process called bisulphite conversion, allowing for the absence and presence of methylation to be comprehensively detected. In addition to methylation, it is possible to determine the accessibility of chromatin using additional techniques such as assay for transposase-accessible chromatin sequencing (ATAC-seq).

Genome databases

Information arising from human genome sequencing is publicly available, providing biological information on every gene in the human genome. Information on any gene describing its protein product, function, tissue-specific expression, disease association and sequence variation/mutation can be easily obtained by searching and manipulating computer databases. In addition to genotype, it is necessary to consider databases that couple genotype with phenotype, such as DECIPHER. Phenotyping is difficult to do, although frameworks to aid this have been developed, such as the Human Phenotype Ontology (HPO).

Further reading

Biesecker LG, Green RC. Diagnostic clinical genome and exome sequencing. *N Engl J Med* 2014; 370:2418–2425.
Feinberg AP. The key role of epigenetics in human disease prevention and mitigation. *N Engl J Med* 2018; 378:1323–1334.
Firth HV, Richards HM, Bevan AP et al. DECIPHER: Database of Chromosomal Imbalance and Phenotype in Humans using Ensembl Resources. *Am J Hum Genet* 2009; 84:524–533.

Research techniques

Discovery of disease-causing genes
Sequencing trios using whole-exome and whole-genome sequencing (WES/WGS)

The ability to study whole genomes is being used in work such as the 100,000 Genomes Project to discover new disease-causing genes. The aims of gene discovery include diagnosis, genetic counselling and targeted screening. Typically, affected and unaffected individuals are studied, and variants that segregate with the disease are filtered. The DNA from both parents and the affected individual, known as a 'trio', is the minimum, and usually the suspected gene in the affected individual will be found in other families with the same disease, strengthening the association. These advances have made it possible to find novel disease-causing genes in smaller pedigrees.

Genetic polymorphisms and linkage studies

Linkage analysis has provided many breakthroughs in mapping the positions of genes that cause genetic diseases, such as the gene for cystic fibrosis, which was found to be tightly linked to a marker on chromosome 7.

These studies relied on finding markers that segregate with the disease in large families and are typically used in rare monogenic disease. Techniques that identify and quantitate genetic polymorphisms, such as SNPs (see p. 30), microsatellites and copy number variants (CNVs), are essential, as these serve as markers. Polymorphisms that are closer together are more likely to have alleles that move together in a block during meiosis than those further apart. This phenomenon is called 'linkage disequilibrium' and enables, for example, one SNP variant (tag SNP) in this block to act as a marker for the presence of other SNP variants.

Genome-wide association studies (GWAS)

Breakthroughs in complex polygenic disease are increasingly being achieved by studying large numbers (typically several thousands) of affected and unaffected patients. Many of these studies use SNP arrays, which provide informative data on hundreds of thousands of SNPs across the entire genome of an individual. Using these markers, statistical testing of association is applied and changes that are linked with disease are typically plotted on a Manhattan plot (so called because the graph can look like the skyline of Manhattan: **Fig. 2.17**). This plot has genomic coordinates on the x-axis, and a measure of the statistical likelihood that the association detected has occurred by chance on the y-axis. SNPs that are likely to be associated with the disease have a low p-value, and as the y-axis values are plotted as negative logarithmic transformations of these p-values, a peak is displayed for such changes. These SNPs may not necessarily sit within in the causative gene but may, for example, lie nearby, such as in the promoter of the gene affecting expression. GWAS can highlight regions of interest for polygenic diseases, which can then be studied in more detail, with the aim of gaining genetic insights into disease pathogenesis.

Identification of gene function

Following the finding of genes of interest in either rare or common disease, the challenge is to understand the function of these protein-coding genes. To gain insights into gene function, the genetic changes found in disease can be modelled in cells or in animals. Most studies rely on the comparison of a cell's or an animal's phenotype in the presence or absence of the genetic change in question. Each approach has its respective merits and faults.

Cell culture models
DNA transfection

Human cells can be grown in cell culture flasks in the laboratory and their behaviour (growth rate, morphology, motility, gene expression profile and biochemistry) characterized. A specific gene can then be

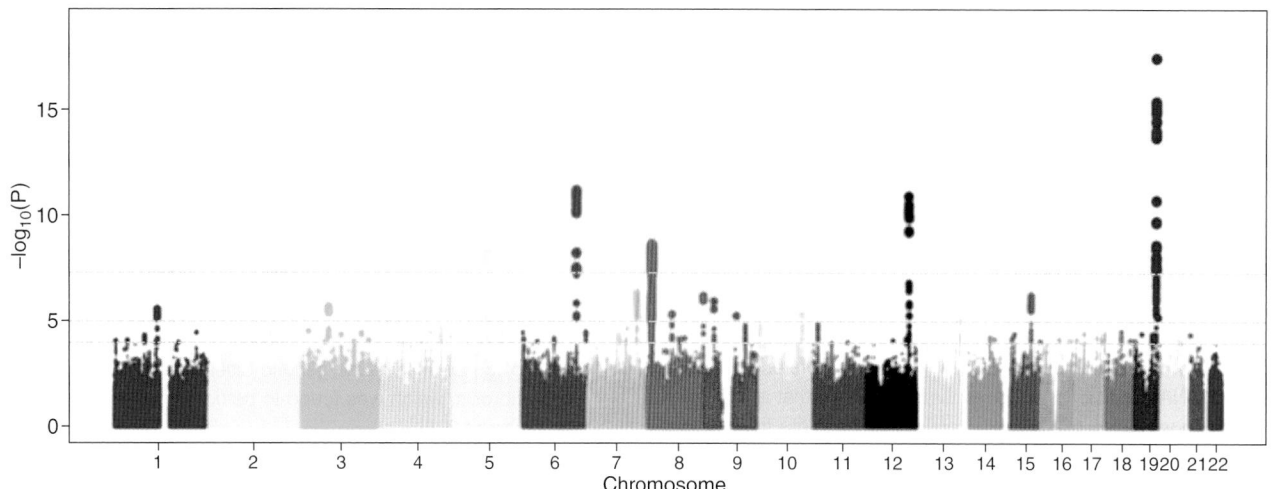

Fig. 2.17 **A Manhattan plot of a genome-wide association study.** Single-nucleotide polymorphisms (SNPs) at genetic loci that associate with the disease being studied are indicated: in this case, regions of interest lie in chromosomes 5, 6, 8, 12 and, most strongly, 19. Such regions can then be studied further.

introduced in a small plasmid (a circle of DNA from which the gene of interest can be expressed) or incorporated into a virus, and the change in cell behaviour assessed to provide an indication of gene function.

A recent advance is the use of CRISPR (clusters of regularly interspaced short palindromic repeats) gene editing to introduce the genetic change found in humans into cell lines (**Fig. 2.18**). This has the advantage of achieving physiological levels of gene expression over plasmids, where genes may be expressed at higher levels due to the presence of viral promoters in plasmid DNA. CRISPR can be used to introduce patient mutations into cells or to knock out genes completely to study their function.

RNA interference

Alternatively, if the cell line in question already expresses the gene of interest, its expression can be knocked down by RNA interference (RNAi). RNAi takes advantage of the cellular machinery that allows microRNAs encoded by the genome to regulate the expression of many genes at the level of mRNA stability and translation (see p. 20). This phenomenon has been exploited in the laboratory to study the function of a gene of interest or, on a much larger scale, the function of each gene in the genome. In such an RNAi screen, an siRNA specific for each gene in the genome is introduced into cells grown *in vitro*, in effect knocking down expression of each gene in approximately 20 000 separate experiments. The phenotype of the cells in each experiment is then monitored to test the effect of loss of gene expression.

Animal models

The effect of a gene at organism level can also be tested by misexpression/over-expression or knockout of a particular gene in a model animal. Nematode worms (*Caenorhabditis*), fruit flies (*Drosophila*), zebrafish and rodents have all been genetically engineered to identify the function of a gene of interest. Knockout models of the higher organisms can be particularly helpful for medical research in providing a model of disease for exploration of therapeutic intervention. Large-scale mutagenesis programmes are knocking out every gene or regulatory element in the mouse genome. However, note that the physiology of rodents and humans can differ.

GENOMIC MEDICINE

Gene therapy

A clinical aim of genetics has been to correct the disease-causing mutation and to treat the disease.

There are many technical problems to overcome in gene therapy, particularly in finding delivery systems to introduce DNA into a mammalian cell. Very careful control and supervision of gene manipulation is necessary because of its potential hazards and the attendant ethical issues.

Two major factors are involved in gene therapy:
- the introduction of the functional gene sequence into target cells
- the expression and permanent integration of the transfected gene into the host cell genome.

Haemophilia

These approaches have been gaining ground with conditions such as haemophilia, where recent trials of gene therapy have meant that some patients no longer need transfusions to maintain normal clotting function. This approach has involved using a virus to deliver a DNA construct with a normal sequence of factor VIII (haemophilia A) or factor IX (haemophilia B) to cells in the patient, administered as an infusion. Due to the design of this DNA construct, liver cells selectively express and produce functional clotting factors, with clinical improvement measured as reduction of bleeding episodes in the absence of regular transfusions of coagulation factors (**Fig. 2.19**).

Cystic fibrosis

Restoring function in diseases affecting solid organs rather than blood poses different challenges. In cystic fibrosis (CF), rather than trying to restore the altered sequence of the gene in every affected cell, a different approach is used. *CFTR*, the cystic fibrosis transmembrane regulator (see also p. 984), is an unusual ABC transporter in that it does not function as a primary active transporter but as a ligand-gated chloride channel (**Fig. 2.20**). The common CF mutation is a 3 bp deletion in exon 10 that results in the removal of a codon specifying phenylalanine (F508del). In this mutation, the CFTR protein is misfolded,

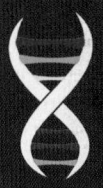

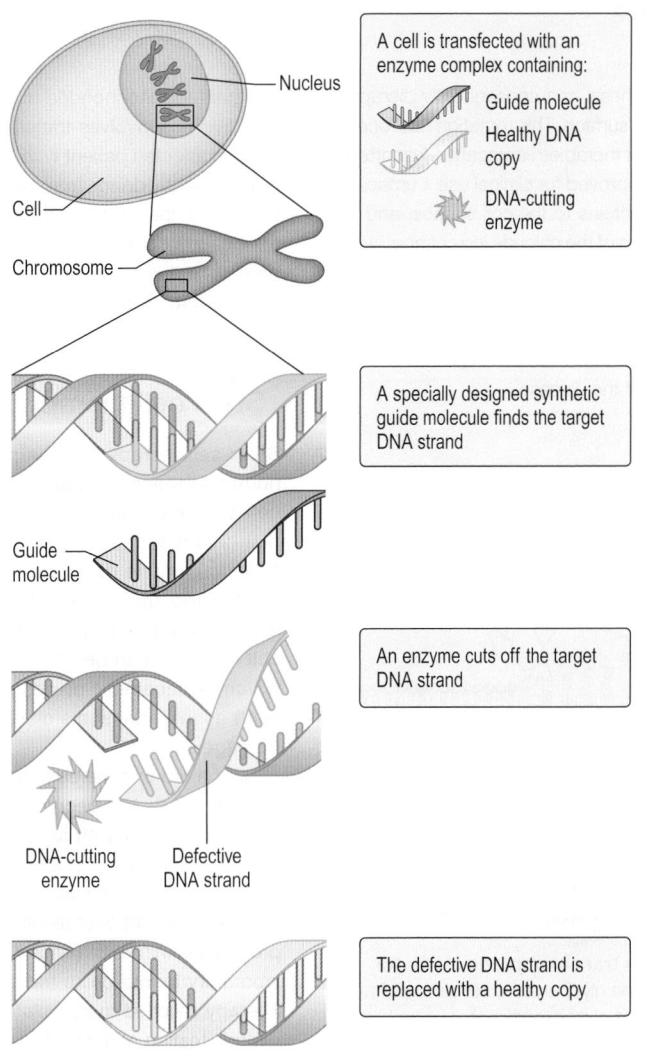

Fig. 2.18 Gene editing using technologies such as CRISPR (clusters of regularly interspaced short palindromic repeats).

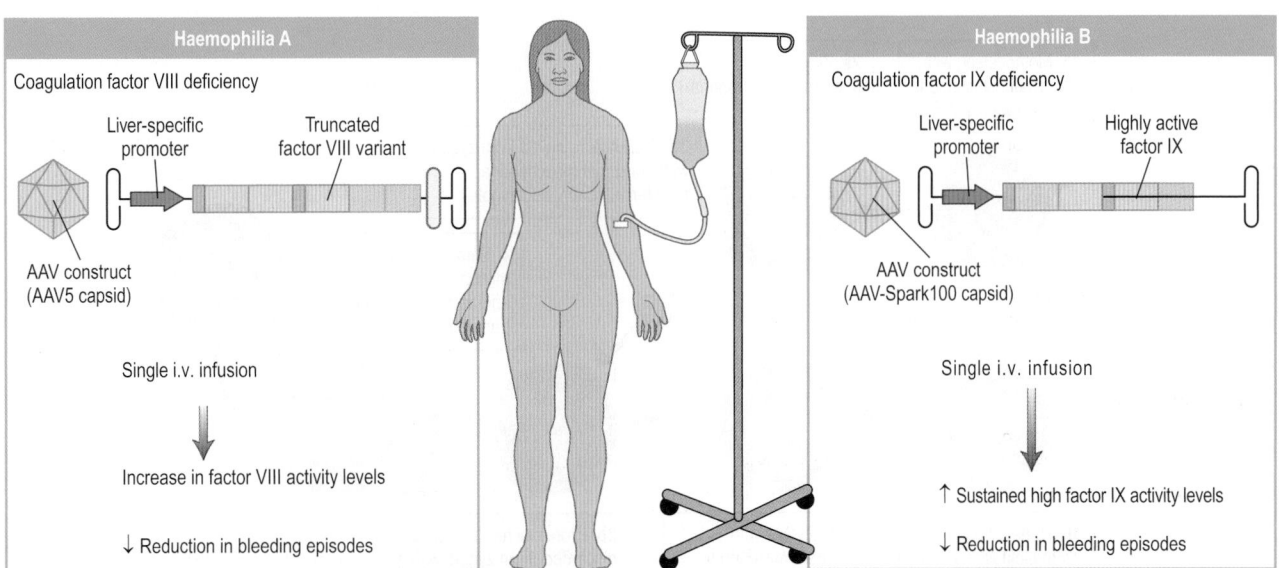

Fig. 2.19 Haemophilia targeted with gene therapy. Virally delivered DNA constructs with liver-specific promoters restore hepatic production of functioning coagulation factors in patients with haemophilia. Trial results shown are from Rangarajan S, Walsh L, Lester W et al. AA5-Factor VIII gene transfer in severe haemophilia A. *N Engl J Med* 2017; 317(26):2519–2530, and George LA, Sullivan SK, Giermasz A et al. Hemophilia B gene therapy with a high-specific-activity Factor IX variant. *N Engl J Med* 2017; 377(23):2215–2227. AAV, adeno-associated virus.

thereby causing ineffective biosynthesis and consequently disrupting the delivery of the protein to the cell surface. This mutation has recently been targeted with a combination of therapies (lumacaftor–ivacaftor) in phase 3 clinical trials, and is now approved for clinical use. Lumacaftor brings more mutant CF channel proteins to the cell surface, and ivacaftor aids by prolonging the opening of the chloride ion channel, which restores partial function to the mutated protein. Early clinical results are encouraging, with patients demonstrating increased pulmonary function as measured by improved forced expiratory volume. More recent trials are being carried out to determine whether early intervention in childhood may modify the course of the disease.

Mitochondrial replacement therapy

In mitochondrial diseases arising due to mutations in the mitochondrial DNA, it is possible to avoid transmission of these maternally

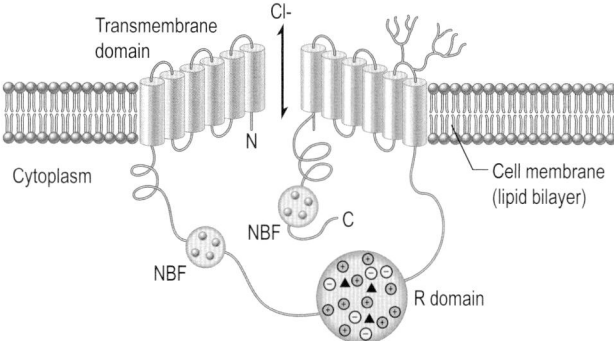

Fig. 2.20 Model of cystic fibrosis transmembrane regulator (CFTR). This is an integral membrane glycoprotein, consisting of two repeated elements. The cylindrical structures represent six membrane-spanning helices in each half of the molecule. The *nucleotide-binding folds (NBFs)* are in the cytoplasm. The *regulatory (R)* domain links the two halves and contains charged individual amino acids and protein kinase phosphorylation sites (black triangles). *N* and *C* are the amino and carboxy termini of the protein, respectively. The branched structure top right represents potential glycosylation sites.

transmitted mitochondria using a technique known as pro-nuclear transfer. This involves transferring the nucleus from a fertilized cell from an affected patient with mitochondrial disease to a fertilized cell from a healthy donor, from which the nucleus has been removed. By doing this, the developing embryo will have mitochondria only from the healthy donor, while retaining nuclear DNA from the biological parents. In the UK, this process is under way in a small number of families (**Fig. 2.21**).

Stem cell therapy

Stem cell therapy has the potential to change the treatment of human disease radically (see p. 23). A number of adult stem cell therapies already exist, particularly bone marrow transplants in immune deficiencies. In this context, a patient with a genetic immune deficiency receives a transplant from a healthy donor, and these normally functioning cells confer immunity. It is currently anticipated that technologies derived from stem cell research can be used to treat a wider variety of diseases in which replacement of destroyed specialist tissues is required, such as in Parkinson's disease, spinal cord injuries and muscle damage.

In the era of gene editing, the possibility of restoring genetically corrected cells has become a reality in some genetic blistering skin disorders. A boy with junctional epidermolysis bullosa developed blisters, with epidermal loss affecting 80% of his total body surface area. Skin cells were taken from this patient and transduced with a DNA construct that resulted in the production of the necessary protein, laminin 332. These corrected stem cells were grown in the laboratory before being transplanted back on to the patient's skin. Therapy resulted in complete coverage of the patient's skin, with genetic testing of the skin confirming the presence of the corrected cells.

These examples are indicative of the potential for using genetic information for clinical benefit, and also of the length of time it takes to achieve meaningful outcomes.

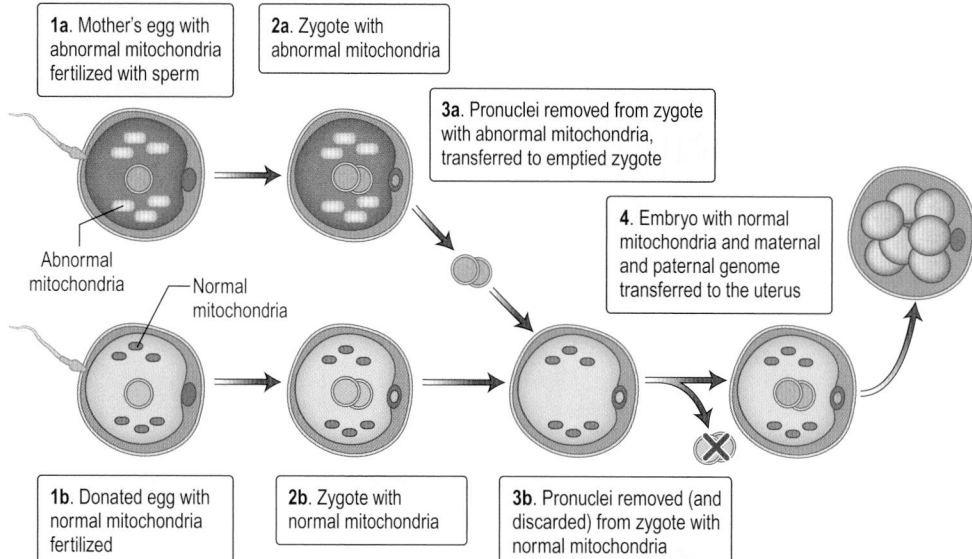

Fig. 2.21 Mitochondrial replacement therapy. Parents with transmissible mitochondrial disease provide fertilized eggs that carry abnormal mitochondria (1a, 2a). A healthy donor produces a fertilized egg, with normal mitochondria (1b, 2b). The nucleus from the affected parents' egg is transferred to the donor egg (3) and this is then transferred to the uterus to develop (4).

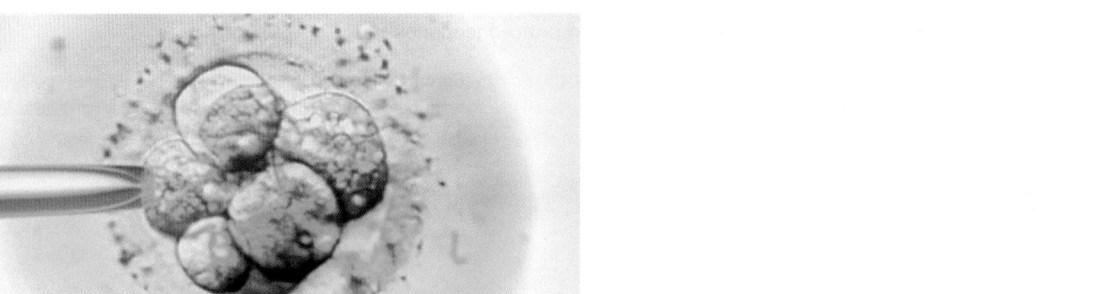

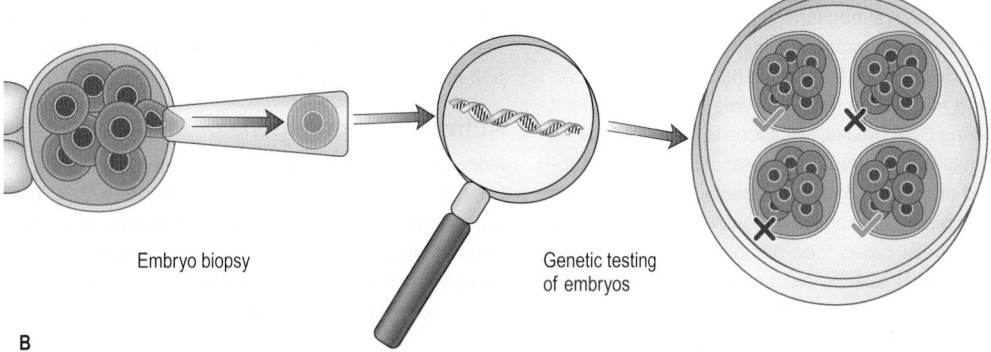

Embryo biopsy   Genetic testing
                                 of embryos

B

Fig. 2.22 Pre-implantation genetic diagnosis. (A) An early-stage blastocyst being sampled for genetic testing. **(B)** Each cell is tested, and only embryos without the screened mutation are selected for implantation.

Pre-implantation genetic diagnosis

Genetic diagnosis in a family can also be used to prevent transmission of a disease. This process requires knowledge of the genetic mutation that runs in the family. Early stage 8 cell embryos can have a cell removed and continue to form into a normal baby (**Fig. 2.22A**). It is possible to take such a cell and use it to genotype an embryo. Only embryos that do not carry the mutation are taken forward for implantation (**Fig. 2.22B**). This approach has been used to prevent transmission of cancer genes such as *BRCA*.

Further reading

Charo RA. Rogues and regulation of germline editing. *N Engl J Med* 2019; 380:976–980.

Dietz HC. New therapeutic approaches to Mendelian disorders. *N Engl J Med* 2010; 363:852–863.

Hirsch T, Rothoeft T, Teig N et al. Regeneration of the entire human epidermis using transgenic stem cells. *Nature* 2017; 551:327–332.

Hyslop LA, Blakeley P, Craven L et al. Towards clinical application of pronuclear transfer to prevent mitochondrial DNA disease. *Nature* 2016; 534:383–386.

Keating D, Marigowda G, Burr L et al. VX-445–tezacaftor–ivacaftor in patients with cystic fibrosis and one or two Phe508del alleles. *N Engl J Med* 2018; 379:1612–1620.

McDermott U, Downing JR, Stratton MR. Genomics and the continuum of cancer care. *N Engl J Med* 2011; 364:340–350.

Pickar AK, Gersbach CA. Gene therapies for hemophilia hit the mark in clinical trials. *Nature* 2018; 24:121–122.

Porteus MH. A new class of medicines through DNA editing. *N Engl J Med* 2019; 380:947–959.

Wang L, McLeod HL, Weinshilboum RM. Genomics and drug response. *N Engl J Med* 2011; 364:1144–1153.

THE GENETIC BASIS OF CANCER

The preceding sections have given an outline of how the genetic code gives rise to human health and disease. Cancers are genetic diseases and involve changes to the genetic code that result in abnormal function of cellular genes. The Cancer Genome Project set out to map the variety of mutations seen across human cancers, and these changes are detailed in online repositories (the Catalogue of Somatic Mutations in Cancer, COSMIC). Multiple gene mutations interact during oncogenesis and a progression of genetic defects gives a cancer cell a survival advantage over surrounding normal cells, famously termed the 'hallmarks of cancer' (see **Fig. 6.2**). These hallmarks include processes like increased proliferation, avoidance of control mechanisms such as apoptosis (programmed cell death) and the ability to evade immune detection. In the vast majority of cancer cases (especially those arising later in life), the multiple genetic changes that occur are somatic: that is, they occur *de novo* and are not inherited. In the next section, the impact of inheriting mutations in cancer predisposition genes, such as early-onset and multiple cancers, is exemplified.

Inherited cancer syndromes

In some cancers (normally those that occur at an earlier age), an inherited single-gene defect can give rise to an almost Mendelian trend with lifetime risks of nearly 90%.

Autosomal dominant inheritance of cancer syndromes

The development of cancers at an earlier age and the occurrence of multiple tumours in these individuals highlight how genetic mutations facilitate the development of cancer. The following are examples of cancer syndromes (see **Box 6.1**) that exhibit dominant inheritance:

• *Retinoblastoma.* This eye tumour is found in young children. It occurs in both hereditary (40%) and non-hereditary (60%) forms. In the hereditary form, there is a germline mutation in the retino-

> ### Box 2.8 Examples of acquired/somatic mutations and proto-oncogenes
>
> **Point mutation**
> - *K-RAS*: colorectal and pancreatic cancer
> - *B-RAF*: melanoma, thyroid cancer
> - *ALK*: lung cancer
>
> **DNA amplification**
> - *MYC*: neuroblastoma
> - *HER2*-neu: breast cancer
>
> **Chromosome translocation**
> - *BCR/ABL*: chronic myeloid leukaemia, acute lymphoblastic leukaemia
> - *PML/RARA*: acute promyelocytic leukaemia
> - *BCL2/IGH*: follicular lymphoma
> - *IGH/CCND1*: mantle cell lymphoma
> - *MYC/IgH*: Burkitt's lymphoma

blastoma gene (*RB1*) and people are also at risk of developing other tumours, particularly osteosarcoma. Knudson studied these patients and this led to the 'two-hit hypothesis' (see p. 39).

- **Breast and ovarian cancer.** Two major genes have been identified: *BRCA1* and *BRCA2*. A strong family history along with germ-line mutation of these genes accounts for most cases of familial breast cancer and over half of familial ovarian cancers. BRCA1 and 2 proteins bind to the DNA repair enzyme Rad51 to make it functional in repairing DNA breaks. Mutations in the *BRCA* genes will lead to accumulation of unrepaired mutations in tumour suppressor genes and crucial oncogenes. Recently, treatments that block the remaining repair mechanism of double-stranded breaks in these cells, a process called 'non-homologous end joining', have been used to treat *BRCA*-deficient cancers. This paradoxically increases the mutational load in these cells, resulting in cell death. The process is described as synthetic lethality and, in the case of *BRCA*-deficient tumours, is achieved by inhibitors of an enzyme called poly-ADP ribose polymerase (PARP).
- **Neurofibromatosis.** Inactivation of the *NF1* gene will lead to constitutive activation of Ras proteins and the development of multiple tumours in the nervous system (see p. 886).
- **Lynch's syndrome** (see p. 1215). Patients with defects in a group of genes that encode proteins involved in DNA mismatch repair are at increased risk of colorectal cancer. This syndrome has recently been highlighted as one instance where chemoprevention with aspirin can reduce the development of colorectal cancer by as much as 63%.

Autosomal recessive inheritance of cancer syndromes

Some relatively rare autosomal recessive diseases associated with abnormalities of DNA repair predispose to the development of cancer:

- **Xeroderma pigmentosum.** There is an inability to repair DNA damage caused by ultraviolet light and by some chemicals, leading to a high incidence of skin cancer.
- **Ataxia telangiectasia.** Mutation results in an increased sensitivity to ionizing radiation and a higher incidence of lymphoid tumours.
- **Bloom's syndrome and Fanconi's anaemia.** An increased susceptibility to lymphoid malignancy is seen.

The majority of individuals who develop cancer do not have a genetic predisposition. In these people, somatic changes in DNA drive cancer. Studies of cancer where such changes are amplified have led to the discovery of selected genes that repeatedly cause cancer when mutated. These include oncogenes and tumour suppressor genes.

Oncogenes

The genes coding for growth factors, growth factor receptors, secondary messengers or even DNA-binding proteins would act as promoters of abnormal cell growth if mutated. This concept was verified when viruses were found to carry genes that promoted oncogenesis when integrated into the host cell. These were originally termed viral or 'v-oncogenes'; later, their normal cellular counterparts, c-oncogenes, were found. Thus, oncogenes encode proteins that are known to participate in the regulation of normal cellular proliferation: for example, *erb-A* on chromosome 17q11–q12 encodes for the thyroid hormone receptor.

Activation of oncogenes

Non-activated oncogenes, which are functioning normally, have been referred to as 'proto-oncogenes' (**Box 2.8**). Their transformation to oncogenes can occur by mutation. A range of patterns of genetic mutations have been shown to cause cancer, and additional mechanisms such as 'chromothripsis', or chromosomal shattering, have been recently described.

Mutation

Carcinogens, such as those found in cigarette smoke, ionizing radiation and ultraviolet light, can cause point mutations in genomic DNA encoding tumour suppressor genes or oncogenes.

Chromosomal translocation

If an error occurs during cell division and two chromosomes translocate, so that a portion swaps over, the translocation breakpoint may occur in the middle of two genes, resulting in a mutation. If this happens, then the end of one gene is translocated on to the beginning of another gene, giving rise to a 'fusion gene'. Therefore, sequences of one part of the fusion gene are inappropriately expressed because they are under the control of the other part of the gene. An example of such a fusion gene (the Philadelphia chromosome) occurs in **chronic myeloid leukaemia** (**Fig. 2.23**).

Viral activation

There are different ways in which viruses can cause cancer. When viral RNA is transcribed by reverse transcriptase into viral cDNA and, in turn, is spliced into the cellular DNA, the viral DNA may integrate within an oncogene and activate it. Alternatively, the virus may pick up cellular oncogene DNA and incorporate it into its own viral genome. Subsequent infection of another host cell might result in expression of this viral oncogene. For example, the Rous sarcoma virus of chickens was found to induce cancer because it carried the *Ras* oncogene.

Tumour suppressor genes

These genes restrict undue cell proliferation (in contrast to oncogenes), and induce the repair or self-destruction (apoptosis) of cells containing damaged DNA. Therefore, mutations in these genes, which disable their function, lead to uncontrolled cell growth in cells with active oncogenes.

The **RB gene** was the first tumour suppressor gene to be described. In inherited retinoblastoma, the first mutation in the *RB* gene is inherited; by chance, a second somatic mutation in the remaining normal

soft tissue sarcomas, brain tumours and leukaemia. Mutations in *p53* have been also found in almost all sporadic human cancers, suggesting that somatic mutations in *p53* are driver mutations. The protein encoded by *p53* plays a role in DNA repair and synthesis, in the control of the cell cycle, cell differentiation and apoptosis. Four p53 protein molecules assemble into a tetramer that is functionally active.

p53 is a DNA-binding protein that activates many gene expression pathways but it is normally only short-lived. In some cancers, there is loss of *p53* from both chromosomes, accounting for loss of normal function of *p53* and ensuing tumour formation. In many tumours, mutations that disable *p53* function also prevent its cellular catabolism. Thus, even a mutation in a single copy of the gene can promote tumour formation because a heterotetramer of mutated and normal *p53* subunits would still be dysfunctional.

Many other genes have been identified that function as tumour suppressor genes, including those found in Lynch's syndrome, which are responsible for repairing DNA mismatches (see p. 1216).

Genetic diagnostics for cancer

The ability to detect cancer-specific DNA sequences has led to the development of monitoring tests that can detect levels of circulating cell-free DNA in the blood. In addition, cancer cells can circulate in the bloodstream, and tests are being developed to detect these.

Targeted treatments for cancer

The ability to sequence cancers rapidly has supported the development of targeted treatments. These aim to be selective, and ideally have few side-effects compared to conventional chemotherapy. Tyrosine kinase inhibitors, such as imatinib, are examples of targeted treatments in selected haematological malignancies that carry the Philadelphia chromosome, and even some solid cancers such as gastrointestinal stromal tumours. A shift heralded by cancer sequencing is the concept of orphan molecular entities. Rather than treating cancer of a tissue such as breast or lung, sequencing allows the detection of drivers in a cancer, for which a selected cocktail of treatments may apply. This may lead to the increased personalization of cancer therapy. Resistance to such treatments is well recognized, however, as cancers mutate further to become resistant to these drugs. An example is seen in metastatic melanoma, where drugs that target mutant *BRAF* in melanoma cells offered temporary but non-sustained remission for patients.

Further reading

Burn J, Gerdes AM, Macrae F et al. Long-term effect of aspirin on cancer risk in carriers of hereditary colorectal cancer: an analysis from the CAPP2 randomised controlled trial. *Lancet* 2011; 378:2081–2087.
Hanahan D, Weinberg RA. Hallmarks of cancer: the next generation. *Cell* 2011; 144:646–674.
Knudson AG. Mutation and cancer: statistical study of retinoblastoma. *Proc Natl Acad Sci USA* 1971; 68:820–823.

Bibliography

Alberts B, Johnson A, Lewis J et al. *Molecular Biology of the Cell*, 5th edn. New York: Garland Science; 2007.
Lodish H, Berk A, Kaiser CA et al. *Molecular Cell Biology*, 6th edn. New York: WH Freeman; 2007.

Significant websites

http://genome.ucsc.edu *University of California at Santa Cruz Genome Bioinformatics*.
http://www.ensembl.org/index.html *Ensembl*.
http://www.ncbi.nlm.nih.gov *National Center for Biotechnology Information*.
http://www.ncbi.nlm.nih.gov/omim *McKusick's Online Mendelian Inheritance in Man (OMIM), for information on gene products and their disease association*.
https://cancer.sanger.ac.uk/cosmic *Catalogue of somatic mutations in cancer*.
https://decipher.sanger.ac.uk/ *DECIPHER*.

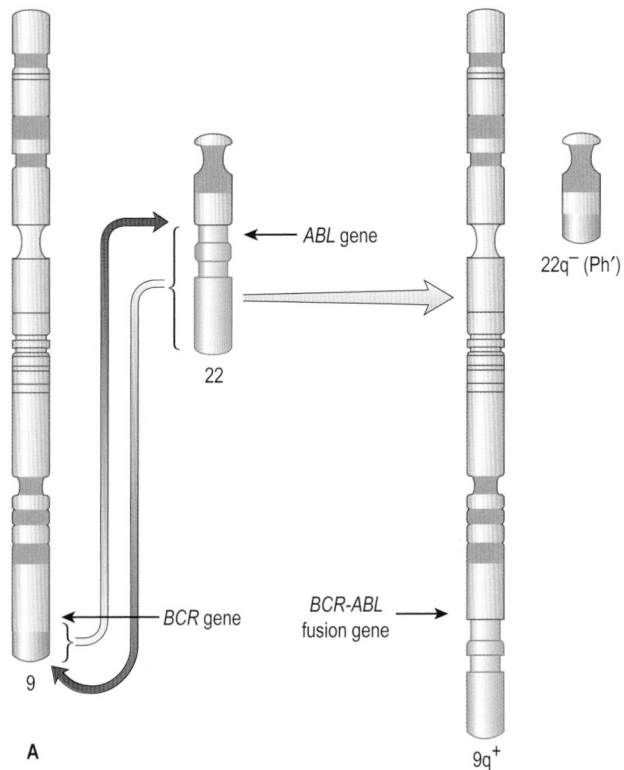

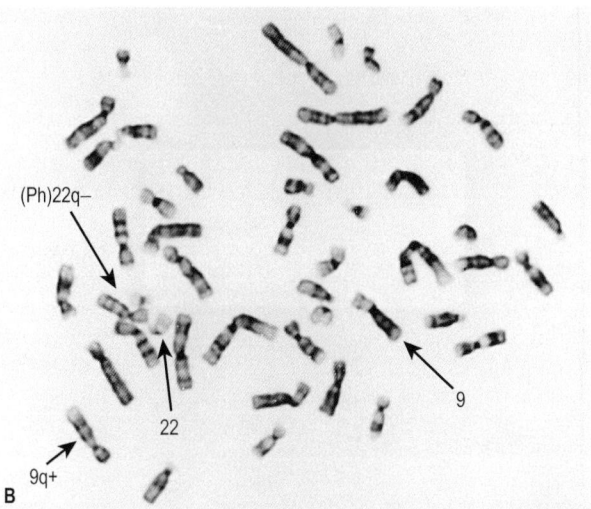

Fig. 2.23 The Philadelphia chromosome (Ph). (A) The long arm (q) of chromosome 22 has been shortened by a reciprocal translocation with chromosome 9. **(B)** The Philadelphia chromosome is formed by a reciprocal translocation of part of the long arm (q) of chromosome 22 to chromosome 9. It is seen in 90–95% of patients with chronic myeloid leukaemia. The karyotype is expressed as 46XX, (9; 22)(q34; q11).

copy of the *RB* gene then occurs, with the formation of a tumour. In the sporadic variety, mutations occur in both of the *RB* genes in a single cell. Knudson described this phenomenon as the 'two-hit' hypothesis, which accounts for the earlier and bilateral presentation of tumours in patients with germline *RB* mutations. *RB* is involved in normal regulation of the cell cycle, and loss of control of the cell cycle in *RB*-deficient retinal cells contributes to tumour formation.

Since the finding of *RB*, other tumour suppressor genes have been described, including the gene ***p53***, known as the 'guardian of the genome'. Rarely, patients are born with an inherited change in *p53*, giving rise to Li–Fraumeni syndrome. These patients have an increased predisposition to a range of types of cancer, including breast cancer,

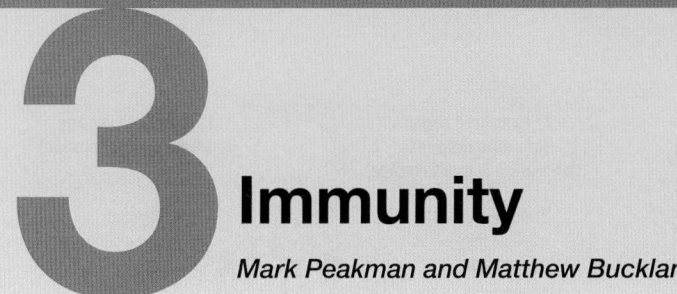

3 Immunity

Mark Peakman and Matthew Buckland

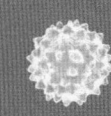

CORE SKILLS AND KNOWLEDGE

Aspects of immunity have an impact on all areas of medicine, from diagnosis and treatment through to diseases that arise when the immune system goes wrong. There are more than 80 different autoimmune diseases, which affect 1 in 20 individuals at some point in their life; allergic disease is even more common, affecting 1 in 10.

The role of a clinical immunologist is to manage immune-mediated diseases and provide specialist advice and guidance to primary care physicians and hospital practitioners on diagnostic testing, interpretation and treatment. Clinical immunologists run clinics for severe or complex allergy, and patients with inborn errors of immunity (IEI) that can lead to severe immunodeficiency.

Key skills in clinical immunology include:

- recognizing the possibility of an immunodeficiency syndrome in patients presenting with recurrent or severe infections such as meningitis or pneumonia, and understanding appropriate ways to investigate and manage this
- assessing patients with complex allergy, including food and drug allergy, and undertaking provocation testing and desensitization when appropriate.

Opportunities to learn clinical immunology in general medical contexts include seeking to apply basic immunological principles to understand patients with autoimmune conditions or those receiving immunosuppressant medications. Attending specialist immunology clinics gives insight into how patients live with chronic disease, how parenteral therapies such as immunoglobulins are administered, and how immunologically mediated conditions, including urticaria, angioedema, allergic rhinitis and anaphylaxis, can be managed.

INTRODUCING THE TISSUES, CELLS AND MOLECULES OF THE IMMUNE SYSTEM

Immunity can be defined as protection from infection, whether this is bacterial, viral, fungal or due to multicellular parasites. The immune system is composed of cells and molecules organized into specialized tissues and acts in concert to orchestrate an immune response (**Fig. 3.1**).

The **primary lymphoid organs** (thymus and bone marrow) are where the cells originate. Cells and molecules of the immune system circulate in the blood; immune responses do not take place there but are initiated at the site of infection (typically the mucosa or skin). Immunity is then propagated and refined in the **secondary lymphoid organs** (e.g. lymph nodes). Following resolution of the infection, immunological memory specific for the pathogen is generated and resides in cells (lymphocytes) in the spleen and lymph nodes, as well as being widely secreted in a molecular form (antibodies). Secondary lymphoid organs also include adenoids, tonsils, spleen, Peyer's patches in the small intestine, peripheral lymph nodes (cervical, axillary, inguinal) and the thoracic duct, which drains the lymph (containing immune cells) into the right subclavian vein.

Immune response: location and dynamics

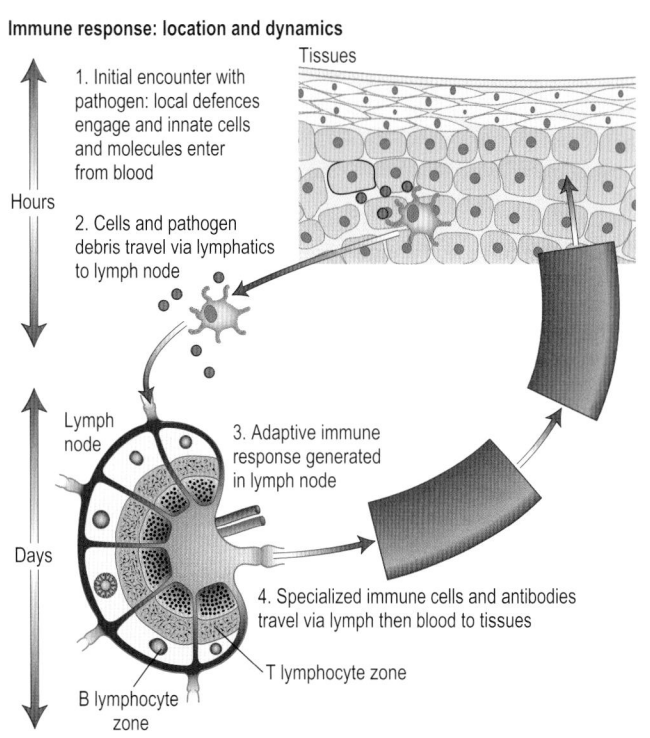

1. Initial encounter with pathogen: local defences engage and innate cells and molecules enter from blood

Hours

2. Cells and pathogen debris travel via lymphatics to lymph node

Tissues

Lymph node

3. Adaptive immune response generated in lymph node

Days

4. Specialized immune cells and antibodies travel via lymph then blood to tissues

T lymphocyte zone

B lymphocyte zone

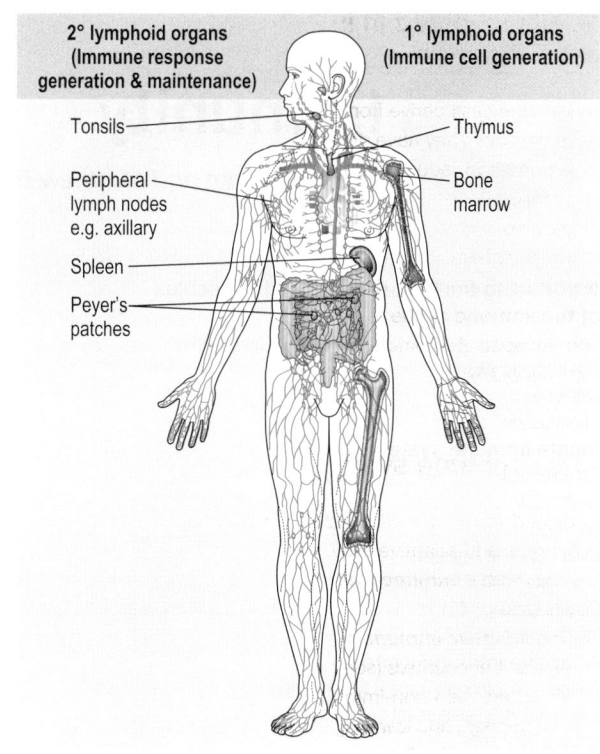

| 2° lymphoid organs (Immune response generation & maintenance) | 1° lymphoid organs (Immune cell generation) |

Tonsils
Peripheral lymph nodes e.g. axillary
Spleen
Peyer's patches
Thymus
Bone marrow

Cells involved in the immune response

Category	Cells	Main functions	Origin	Special features
Myeloid	Neutrophils	Immunity to bacteria and fungi	Bone marrow	Major first-line defence against pathogens
	Eosinophils, mast cells and basophils	Immunity to parasites	Bone marrow	Role in allergy
	Monocytes and macrophages	Immunity to bacteria, fungi, parasites	Bone marrow	Specialized phagocytes; cytokine secretion
Lymphoid	Dendritic cells	Antigen presentation to T lymphocytes	Bone marrow	Key role in activating T lymphocytes
	B lymphocytes	Antibody production	Bone marrow	Have specific receptor for antigen (called 'antibody'). Mature into plasma cells that are 'antibody factories'
	T lymphocytes	Orchestration of immune response against bacteria, fungi, parasites and viruses	Precursors come from bone marrow and undergo selection process in the thymus to avoid self-reactivity	Have specific receptor for antigen (called T-cell receptor). Two major subsets: CD4 ('helper' and 'regulatory') and CD8 ('cytotoxic')

Non-immune host defence mechanisms

Normal barriers	Events that compromise barrier function
Physical barriers	
Cough reflex	Suppression, e.g. by opiates, neurological disease
Skin and mucous membranes	Trauma, burns, i.v. cannulae
Mucosal function	Ciliary paralysis (e.g. smoking)
	Increased mucus production (e.g. asthma)
	Abnormally viscid secretions (e.g. cystic fibrosis)
	Decreased secretions (e.g. sicca syndrome)
Urine flow	Stasis (e.g. prostatic hypertrophy)
Chemical barriers	High gastric pH (gastric acid secretion inhibitors)
Resistance to pathogens provided by commensal skin and gut organisms	Changes in flora (e.g. broad-spectrum antibiotics)

Fig. 3.1 Overview of the cells, molecules and tissues of the immune system. Lymphocytes are generated as precursors in the bone marrow and differentiate into T (thymus) or B (bone marrow) lymphocytes in the primary lymphoid tissue. Once differentiated, 98% of lymphocytes reside in the secondary lymphoid tissue, where the adaptive immune response takes place. Other types of immune cells originate in the bone marrow (left-hand box). Non-immune host defence mechanisms (right-hand box) are occasionally insufficient and an immune response is initiated by infection in the tissues (1). There are rapid local responses that include ingress of cells (e.g. neutrophils) from the blood. Immune cells and pathogen debris migrate via lymphatics to the local lymph node (2), where an adaptive immune response is generated (3). Effector cells travel by lymph and then blood to the infected tissue (4).

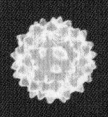

Cells involved in immune responses: origin and function

All immune cells derive from pluripotent stem cells generated in the bone marrow. They have diverse functions (see **Fig. 3.1**). **T lymphocytes** undergo 'education' in the thymus to avoid self-recognition, and populate the peripheral lymphoid tissue, where B lymphocytes also reside. Both sets of lymphocytes undergo activation in the peripheral tissue, to become mature effector cells. **B lymphocytes** may further differentiate into antibody-secreting plasma cells. Lymphoid tissue is frequently found at mucosal surfaces in non-encapsulated patches, termed **mucosa-associated lymphoid tissue (MALT)**.

The immune system

Cells and molecules involved in immune responses are classified into innate and adaptive systems:

- The **innate immune system** is inborn and operates throughout life (see p. 43).
- The **adaptive immune system** changes in response to the pathogens it encounters (see p. 48).

There are also non-immunological barriers that are involved in host protection, and lowering of these may allow a pathogen to gain a foothold (see **Fig. 3.1**).

The immune system is immensely powerful, in terms of its ability to inflame, damage and kill, and it has a capacity to recognize a myriad of molecular patterns in the microbial world. However, immune responses are not always beneficial. They can give rise to a range of autoimmune and inflammatory diseases, known as **immunopathologies**. Conversely, the immune system may fail, giving rise to immune deficiency states. These conditions are grouped under the umbrella of clinical immunology.

A major feature of the immune system is the complexity of its surface-bound, intracellular and soluble mediators. In particular, it is necessary to be aware of the clusters of differentiation (CD) classification (**Box 3.1**) and the functions of cytokines and chemokines. The CD classification is like a barcode for defining a cell.

Cytokines

Cytokines are small polypeptides released by a cell in order to change the function of the same or another cell. These chemical messengers are found in many organ systems but especially the immune system. Cytokines have become markers in the

---

---

investigation of disease pathogenesis; they are also therapeutic agents in their own right, as well as the targets of therapeutic agents (see p. 67). The key features of a cytokine are:

- **pleiotropy**: has different effects on different cells
- **autocrine function**: modulates the cell secreting it
- **paracrine function**: modulates adjacent cells
- **endocrine effects**: modulates cells and organs at remote sites
- **synergistic activity**: acts in concert with other cytokines to achieve effects greater than the summation of their individual actions.

The main immune cytokines are the **interferons** (IFNs) and the **interleukins** (ILs). The IFNs are limited to a few major types (α, β and γ), whereas there are 40 interleukins.

Chemokines

The defining feature of chemokines is their function as chemotactic molecules: that is, they attract cells along a gradient of low to high chemical concentration, particularly from the blood into the tissues, and from the tissues into lymphatics. They also have the ability to activate immune cells. All chemokines have a similar structure relating to the configuration of cysteine residues, which gives rise to four families (**Box 3.2**).

Cell-surface receptors for chemokines are denoted by 'R'. CCR5 is a co-receptor for the human immunodeficiency virus (HIV; see p. 1441), and drugs to block this and other chemokine receptors are under active development to combat inflammation.

INNATE IMMUNE SYSTEM

Innate immunity provides immediate, first-line host defence. The key features of this system (as well as the adaptive system, p. 48) are shown in **Box 3.3**. It is present at birth and remains operative at comparable intensity into old age. Innate immunity

---

> *i* **Box 3.2 Features of chemokine mediators and receptors**

Chemokine family	Structure	Receptor family	Pathological or therapeutic target
CXC	Two cysteines (C) separated by any other amino acid residue (X)	CXCR	CXCR4 – co-receptor for late HIV infection
CC	Two cysteines next to each other	CCR	CCR5 – co-receptor for early HIV infection and blocked by 'entry inhibitors'
C	One cysteine	CR	XCR1 – target of Kaposi's sarcoma human virus protein
CX3C	Two cysteines separated by any three amino acids	CX3CR	Possible survival factor in myeloma

R, receptor.

Innate	Adaptive
No memory: quality and intensity of response invariant	Memory: response adapts with each exposure
Recognition of limited number of non-varying, generic molecular patterns on, or made by, pathogens	Recognition of vast array of specific antigens[a] on, or made by, pathogens
Pattern recognition mediated by a limited array of receptors	Antigen recognition mediated by a vast array of antigen-specific receptors
Response immediate on first encounter	Response on first encounter takes 1–2 weeks; on second encounter, 3–7 days

[a]Antigen is a molecular structure (protein, peptide, lipid, carbohydrate) that generates an immune response.

Molecules	Name (examples)	Function	Provide immunity against
Complement	Cascade of >50 proteins	Lyse bacteria; opsonize[a] bacteria; promote inflammation; recruit and activate immune cells	Bacteria, viruses
Collectins	Mannose-binding lectin	Bind bacteria; activate complement	Bacteria
Pentraxins	C-reactive protein[b]	Opsonize bacteria	Bacteria
Enzymes	Lysozyme	Present in secretions; cleave bacterial cell wall	Bacteria

[a]Opsonize means coat bacteria to enhance phagocytosis by granulocytes and monocytes/macrophages. [b]C-reactive protein (CRP) is an acute phase protein. Blood level rises 10–100-fold within hours of the start of an infective or inflammatory process, making it extremely useful in monitoring infective or inflammatory diseases and their response to treatment.

is mediated by a variety of cells and molecules (**Box 3.4**). Activation of innate immune responses is mediated through interaction between:

- the ***pathogen side***, comprising a relatively limited array of molecules (pathogen-associated molecular patterns, PAMPs)
- the ***host side***, comprising a limited portfolio of receptors (pattern recognition receptors, PRRs).

Activation of certain cells in the innate immune system leads in turn to activation of the ***adaptive immune response*** (see p. 48).

The ***dendritic cell*** is especially involved in this process, and forms a bridge between innate and adaptive systems.

Complement

Complement proteins are produced in the liver and circulate in an inactive form. When triggered, complement molecules become enzymatically active and trigger several molecules of the next stage in a series. This ***complement cascade*** is initiated via three distinct

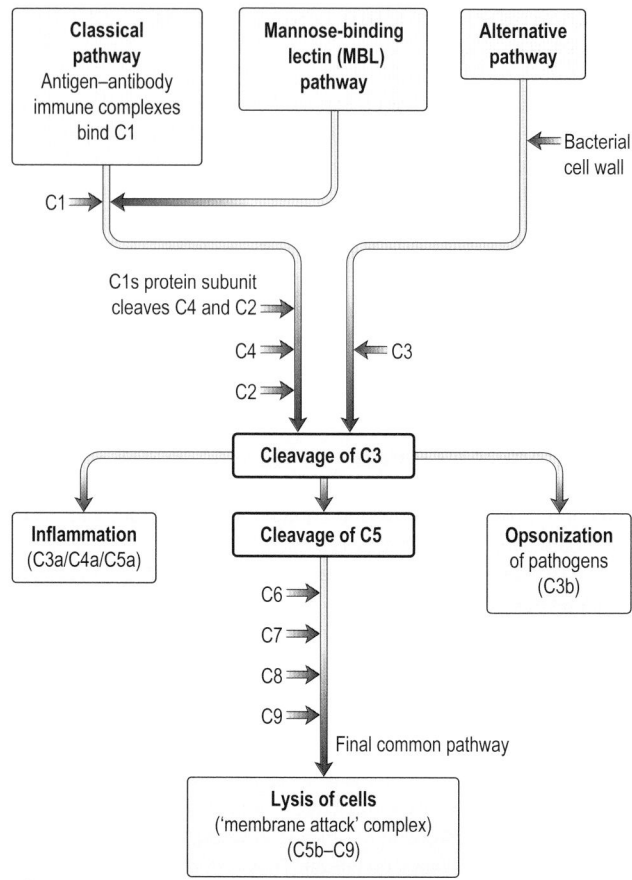

Fig. 3.2 The complement pathways and their effector functions.

pathways: alternative, classical and lectin (**Fig. 3.2**). Each pathway culminates in the cleavage of C3 and C5. Cleavage of C3 has a number of biological consequences; breakdown of C5 achieves the same and, in addition, provides the triggering stimulus to the final common ('membrane attack') pathway, which provides most of the biological activity (see **Fig. 3.2**).

The main functions of complement activation are to:

- promote inflammation (e.g. through the actions of the anaphylatoxins C3a, C4a and C5a)
- recruit cells (e.g. through chemoattractants)
- kill targeted cells, such as bacteria
- solubilize antigen–antibody ('immune') complexes and remove them from the circulation.

During an immune response, removal of immune complexes protects unaffected tissues from the deposition of these large, insoluble composites, which could result in unwanted inflammation. Failure of this protective mechanism can result in immunopathology: for example, in the joints, kidney and eye.

Neutrophils

Neutrophils (see also p. 363) phagocytose and kill microorganisms by releasing antimicrobial compounds (e.g. defensins). They are derived from the bone marrow, which can produce between 10^{11} (healthy state) and 10^{12} (during infection) new cells per day. In health, neutrophils are rarely seen in the tissues.

Neutrophil phagocytosis is activated by interaction with bacteria, either directly or after bacteria have been coated (opsonized)

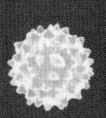

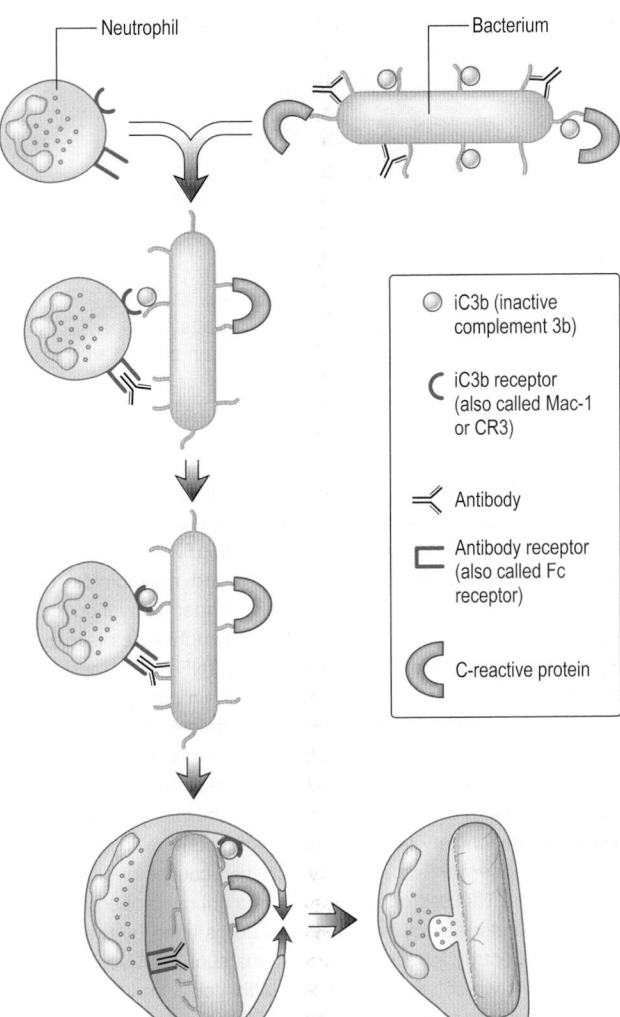

Neutrophil   Bacterium

iC3b (inactive complement 3b)

iC3b receptor (also called Mac-1 or CR3)

Antibody

Antibody receptor (also called Fc receptor)

C-reactive protein

Fig. 3.3 Opsonization. Bacteria are coated with a variety of soluble factors from the innate immune system (opsonins), which enhance phagocytosis. This leads to engulfment of the bacteria into phagosomes and fusion with granules to release antibacterial agents.

> **_i_** **Box 3.5** Contents and function of key neutrophil granules
>
> | Function | Primary or azurophilic granules | Secondary or specific granules |
> |---|---|---|
> | **Antibacterial** | Lysozyme
Defensins
Myeloperoxidase (MPO)
Proteinase-3
Elastase
Cathepsins
Bactericidal/ permeability increasing protein (BPI) | Respiratory burst components (e.g. cytochrome b_{558}) producing reactive oxygen metabolites, such as hydrogen peroxide, hydroxyl radicals and singlet oxygen
Lysozyme
Lactoferrin |
> | **Cell movement** | | Collagenase
CD11b/CD18 (adhesion molecule)
N-formyl-methionyl-leucylphenylalanine receptor (FMLP-R) |

Eosinophils

Eosinophils release pro-inflammatory mediators to provide immunity against parasites. In contrast to neutrophils, several hundred times more eosinophils are present in the tissues than in the blood, particularly at epithelial surfaces, where they survive for several weeks. The main role of eosinophils is protection against multicellular parasites such as worms (helminths). This is achieved by the release of pro-inflammatory mediators, which are toxic, cationic proteins. In populations and societies in which such parasites are rare, eosinophils contribute mainly to allergic disease, particularly asthma (see p. 949). Eosinophils have two types of granule:

- **_Specific granules_** (95%) contain the cationic proteins, of which there are four main types: **_major basic protein (MBP), eosinophil cationic protein (ECP)_** and **_eosinophil neurotoxin_**, which are all potently toxic to helminths; and **_eosinophil peroxidase_**, similar to neutrophil myeloperoxidase.
- **_Primary granules_** (5%) synthesize and release **_leukotrienes C_4 and D_4_** and **_platelet-activating factor (PAF)_**, which alter airway smooth muscle and vasculature).

Eosinophils are activated and recruited by a variety of mediators via specific surface receptors, including complement factors and LTB_4. In addition, the chemokines eotaxin-1 (CCL11) and eotaxin-2 (CCL24) are highly selective in eosinophil recruitment. There are surface receptors for the cytokines IL-3 and IL-5, which promote the development and differentiation of eosinophils.

Mast cells and basophils

Mast cells release pro-inflammatory and vasoactive mediators, and have a role in allergy. Mast cells and basophils share features in common, especially in that they contain:

- histamine-containing granules
- high-affinity receptors for immunoglobulin E (IgE, an antibody type that is involved in allergic disease, see Box 3.10).

Mast cells are found in tissues (especially skin and mucosae) and basophils in the blood. Both mast cells and basophils release pro-inflammatory mediators, which are either pre-formed or synthesized _de novo_ (**Box 3.6**).

Histamine is a low-molecular-weight amine (111 Da) with a blood half-life of less than 5 minutes; it constitutes 10% of the mast cell's

to make them more ingestible (**Fig. 3.3**). The contents of neutrophil granules are released both intracellularly (predominantly azurophilic granules) and extracellularly (specific granules) following fusion with the plasma membrane. Approximately 100 different molecules in neutrophil granules (**Box 3.5**) kill and digest microorganisms, for example:

- **_Myeloperoxidase and cytochrome b_{558}_** are key components of major oxygen-dependent bactericidal systems.
- **_Cathepsins, proteinase-3 and elastase_** are deadly to Gram-positive and Gram-negative organisms, as well as some _Candida_ species.
- **_Defensins_** are naturally occurring cysteine-rich antibacterial and antifungal polypeptides (29–35 amino acids).
- **_Collagenase and elastase_** break down fibrous structures in the extracellular matrix, facilitating progress of the neutrophil through the tissues.

Granule release is initiated by the products of bacterial cell walls, certain complement proteins, leukotrienes (LTB_4) and chemokines (e.g. CXCL8), and cytokines such as tumour necrosis factor-alpha (TNF-α). A further defence mechanism is the formation of **_neutrophil extracellular traps (NETs)_** from DNA, which bind pathogens to facilitate killing.

Mediators	Effects
Pre-formed	
Histamine	Vasodilation Vascular permeability ↑ Smooth muscle contraction in airways
Proteases	Digestion of basement membrane causes ↑ vascular permeability and aids migration
Proteoglycans (e.g. heparan)	Anticoagulant activity
Synthesized *de novo*	
Platelet-activating factor (PAF)	Vasodilation
Leukotriene B_4 (LTB$_4$), LTC$_4$, LTD$_4$	Neutrophil and eosinophil activation and chemoattraction Vascular permeability ↑ Bronchoconstriction
Prostaglandins (mainly PGD$_2$)	Vascular permeability ↑ Bronchoconstriction Vasodilation

weight. When injected into the skin, histamine induces the typical 'weal and flare' or 'triple' response: reddening (erythema) due to increased blood flow, swelling (weal) due to increased vascular permeability, and distal vascular changes (flare) due to effects on local axons.

The ***complement-derived anaphylatoxins*** C3a, C4a and C5a activate basophils and mast cells, as does IgE. The mast cell also has a role in the early response to bacteria through release of TNF-α, in cell recruitment to inflammatory sites such as arthritic joints, in promotion of tumour growth by enhancing neovascularization and in allograft tolerance.

Monocytes and macrophages

Monocytes (in blood) and macrophages (in tissue) ingest and kill bacteria, release pro-inflammatory molecules, present antigen to T lymphocytes, and are necessary in immunity to intracellular pathogens such as mycobacteria.

Cells of the monocyte/macrophage lineage are highly sophisticated phagocytes. ***Monocytes*** are the blood form of a cell that spends a few days in the circulation before entering into the tissues to differentiate into ***macrophages***, and some types of dendritic cell. Blood monocytes can be divided into subsets according to expression of CD14 (a receptor for lipopolysaccharide, a bacterial cell wall component) and CD16 (a receptor for IgG antibodies).

A key role of tissue macrophages is the maintenance of tissue homeostasis through clearance of cellular debris, especially following infection or inflammation. They are responsive to a range of pro-inflammatory stimuli, using their PRRs to recognize PAMPs. Once activated, they engulf and kill microorganisms, especially bacteria and fungi, and release a range of pro-inflammatory cytokines. Evidence suggests that evolutionarily conserved molecular patterns in mitochondria (organelles that were originally derived from bacteria) can also activate monocytes. These damage-associated molecular patterns (DAMPs) could play a major role in the systemic inflammatory response that follows extensive tissue damage (e.g. following ischaemic injury).

It has been observed that some PAMPs induce the cytoplasmic assembly of large oligomeric structures of PRRs termed ***inflammasomes***. There are numerous examples: members of the Nod-like receptor (NLR) family can be activated by stimuli such as viruses,

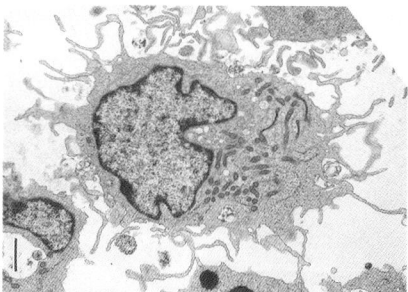

Fig. 3.4 Mature dendritic cell. The cell ingests pathogens, migrates to lymph nodes and presents pathogen-derived antigen to T lymphocytes to enable adaptive immunity.

bacterial toxins and, interestingly, crystallized endogenous molecules, including urate. Inflammasomes have potent effects in activating caspases, leading to processing and secretion of pro-inflammatory cytokines such as IL-1β and IL-18.

Macrophages have pro-inflammatory and microbicidal capabilities similar to those of neutrophils. Under activation conditions, macrophages present antigen to T-lymphocytes (see p. 56) and secrete a range of cytokines, notably TNF-α, IL-1 and IFN-γ. These are necessary for the removal of certain pathogens that live within mononuclear phagocytes (e.g. mycobacteria). Macrophages and related cells may also undergo a process termed ***autophagy***. Autophagy is a lysosomal degradative process that removes abnormal organelles, protein aggregates and intracellular pathogens. The autophagy machinery targets an autophagosome with the relevant material to fuse with lysosomes, which then causes degradation of the contents. This self-cannibalization is a critical property of many cell types under starvation conditions, but is used by the immune system to destroy intracellular pathogens such as *Mycobacterium tuberculosis*, which otherwise persist within cells and block normal antibacterial processes. Autophagy is also a means of enhancing antigen presentation pathways. Dysregulation of the autophagic pathway has been associated with a number of diseases, including cancer, inflammatory disease and infections.

Tissue macrophages involved in chronic inflammatory foci may undergo terminal differentiation into multinucleated giant cells, typically found at the site of the granulomata characteristic of tuberculosis and sarcoidosis (see pp. 968 and 985).

Dendritic cells

The function of dendritic cells is activation of naive T lymphocytes to initiate adaptive immune responses (see p. 48); they are the only cells capable of this. The definition of a dendritic cell is one that has:
- dendritic morphology (**Fig. 3.4**)
- machinery for sensing pathogens
- the ability to process and present antigens to CD4 and CD8 T lymphocytes, coupled with the ability to activate these T lymphocytes from a naive state
- the ability to dictate the T lymphocyte's future function and differentiation.

This is a powerful cell type that functions as a critical bridge between the innate and adaptive immune systems.

Types of dendritic cell

The major types are the ***conventional DC (cDC)***, the ***plasmacytoid DC (pDC)*** and a variety of specialized DCs found in tissues

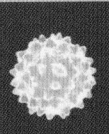

Box 3.7 Molecules on dendritic cells

	Conventional dendritic cell		Plasmacytoid dendritic cell	
	Immature	Mature	Immature	Mature
CD1c	+	++	−	−
CD123 (interleukin 3 receptor)	−	−	+	++
Molecules involved in co-stimulation of T lymphocytes (CD80, CD86)	+	+++	+	+++
Human leucocyte antigen (HLA) class I and II molecules for antigen presentation to T lymphocytes	+	+++	+	+++

Box 3.8 Toll-like receptors (TLRs)

Pattern recognition receptor (PRR)	Pathogen-associated molecular pattern (PAMP)	Pathogen	PRR expressed by
TLR2	Peptidoglycan	Gram-positive bacteria	cDC
TLR3	Double-stranded RNA	Viruses	cDC
TLR4	Lipopolysaccharide	Gram-negative bacteria	cDC
TLR7	Single-stranded RNA	Viruses	pDC
TLR9	Double-stranded DNA	Viruses	pDC

cDC, conventional dendritic cell; pDC, plasmacytoid dendritic cell.

Box 3.9 Conventional dendritic cell (cDC) maturation

Immature cDC	Mature cDC
Is highly pinocytotic	Ceases pinocytosis
Has low-level expression of molecules required for T lymphocyte activation	Upregulates CD80, CD86 and HLA molecules
Has low-level expression of machinery required to process and present microbial antigens	Begins to process microbial antigens (break down into small peptides) in readiness to present them to T lymphocytes (using HLA molecules)
Is generally localized and sedentary	Begins active migration to local lymph node
Minimally secretes cytokines	Actively secretes cytokines in readiness to stimulate T lymphocytes, in particular IL-12

CD, cluster of differentiation; HLA, human leucocyte antigen; IL-12, interleukin 12.

that resemble cDCs (e.g. the Langerhans cell in the skin; see **Ch. 22**). DCs have several distinctive cell surface molecules, some of which have pathogen-sensing activity (e.g. the antigen uptake receptor DEC205 on cDCs), while others are involved in interaction with T lymphocytes (**Box 3.7**). Immature cDCs and pDCs are present in the blood but at very low levels (<0.5% of lymphocyte/ monocyte cells).

Pathogen-sensing is a key component of the function of immature DCs, as well as monocytes/macrophages, and is achieved through expression of a limited array of specialized PRR molecules capable of binding to structures common to pathogens, aided by long cell dendrites and pinocytosis (constant ingestion of soluble material).

PRRs include **mannose-binding lectin**, which initiates complement activity, inducing opsonization (see Fig. 3.3), and **signalling receptors**, such as the PRR known as Toll-like receptor 4 (TLR4), which binds lipopolysaccharide, a molecular pattern found in the cell walls of many Gram-negative bacteria (**Box 3.8**). Other TLRs bind double-stranded and single-stranded RNA from viruses and other non-self antigens. Innate immunity critically depends on TLR signalling. The key principle at play is that the immune system has devised a means of identifying most types of invading microorganisms by using a limited number of PRRs recognizing common molecular patterns, or PAMPs. This recognition event has been termed a '**danger signal**'; it alerts the immune system to the presence of a pathogen. Sensing danger is a key role of the DC and a key first step towards activation of the adaptive immune system.

Dendritic cells and T-cell activation

In a sequence of events that spans 1–2 days, immature DCs are activated by PAMPs or DAMPs in the tissues binding to PRRs. The immature pDC is a small, rounded cell that develops dendrites on activation and secretes enormous quantities of IFN-α, a potent antiviral and pro-inflammatory cytokine; this seems to be the major role of pDCs. In contrast, the activated cDC migrates to the local lymph node with the engulfed pathogen. During migration, the cDC matures, changing its shape, gene and molecular profile and function within a matter of hours to take on a mature form, with altered capabilities (**Box 3.9** and **Fig. 3.5**), the most important of which is upregulating the machinery required to activate T

lymphocytes. Once in the lymph node, the mature cDC interacts with naive T lymphocytes (antigen presentation), resulting in two key outcomes:

- activation of T cells with the ability to recognize peptide fragments (termed epitopes) of the pathogen
- polarization of the T cell towards a functional phenotype (see below) that is tailored to the particular pathogen.

The mature cDC provides three major signals to naive T cells (see **Fig. 3.5**):

- **signal 1**: presentation of peptide fragments from the pathogen bound to surface human leucocyte antigen (HLA) molecules
- **signal 2**: co-stimulation through CD80 and CD86 interacting with CD28 on T cells
- **signal 3**: secretion of cytokines, notably IL-12.

Natural killer cells

Natural killer (NK) cells are described on page 53.

Innate lymphoid cells

Innate lymphoid cells (ILCs) were identified relatively recently as a lymphoid cell type that resembles T lymphocytes in terms of function

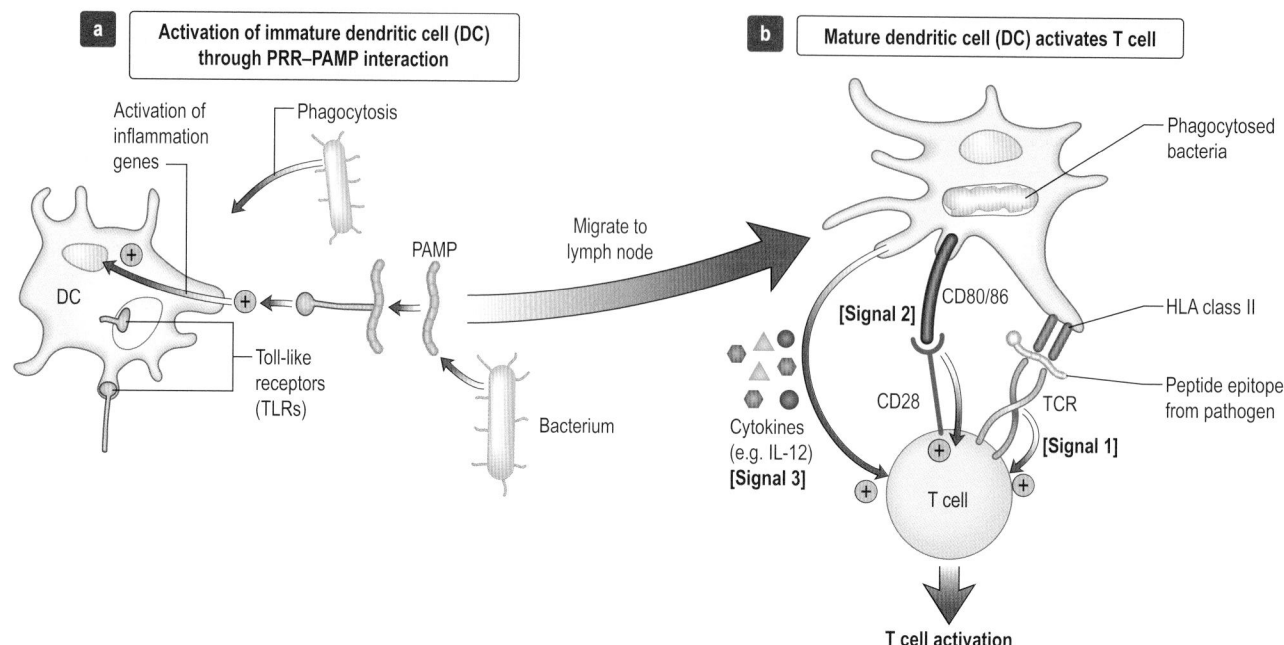

Fig. 3.5 Dendritic cell activation of T lymphocytes. (a) Immature dendritic cells (DCs) in the tissues are activated by pathogens through pathogen-associated molecular pattern–pattern recognition receptor (PAMP–PRR) interaction. **(b)** Multiple rapid changes in gene expression lead to migration to the lymph node as the DC takes on the mature phenotype. During migration, there is synthesis of the machinery required for activation of T lymphocytes, shown here in response to **signals 1–3**. CD, cluster of differentiation; HLA, human leucocyte antigen; IL-12, interleukin 12; TCR, T-cell receptor.

but differs in that it lacks any form of specific receptor to recognize targets such as pathogens. The role of these cells in immunity and pathology is the subject of intense interest.

Further reading

Guilliams M, Mildner A, Yona S. Developmental and functional heterogeneity of monocytes. *Immunity* 2018; 49:595–613.

Ley K, Hoffman HM, Kubes P et al. Neutrophils: new insights and open questions. *Sci Immunol* 2018; 3:pii: eaat4579.

Ravin KA, Loy M. The eosinophil in infection. *Clin Rev Allergy Immunol* 2016; 50:214–227.

Waisman A, Lukas D, Clausen BE et al. Dendritic cells as gatekeepers of tolerance. *Semin Immunopathol* 2017; 39:153–163.

ADAPTIVE IMMUNE SYSTEM

The information gained by cDCs that interact with a pathogen is passed on, in the form of signals 1–3 (see **Fig. 3.5b**). These activate T lymphocytes in the adaptive immune system, which recognize the same pathogen. T lymphocytes may be involved in pathogen removal directly (e.g. by killing) or indirectly (e.g. by recruiting B lymphocytes to make specific antibody). Lymphocytes orchestrate immune responses via cell-to-cell interactions and cytokine release.

Antigen receptors on T and B lymphocytes

One of the key features of the adaptive immune system is specificity for antigen. For example, if a person is immunized against the measles virus, that person does not have immunity to hepatitis B, and vice versa. This specificity is conferred by two types of receptor: the T-cell receptor (TCR) on T lymphocytes and an equivalent on B lymphocytes, the B-cell receptor (BCR). BCRs are also termed surface immunoglobulin (sIg); they differ from TCRs in also being secreted in large quantities by end-stage B lymphocytes (plasma cells) as soluble immunoglobulins, also known as antibodies.

To maintain protection against the multiplicity of pathogens in our environment, each of us generates great diversity among TCRs and antibodies. This is achieved through a mechanism shared by both TCR and antibody, in which distinct families of genes are encoded in the germline, each family (called constant, variable, diversity and joining) contributing a sequence to part of the receptor. Recombination between randomly selected members of each family ensures diversity in the end product. Recombination frequently involves base deletions and additions, adding to the diversity. In the case of antibodies, the result is a potential capacity of more than 10^{14} different antibody molecules; for TCRs, it may be as high as 10^{18}.

Immunoglobulins

In structural terms, antibodies have four chains: two identical heavy and two identical light chains (**Fig. 3.6**). Each chain contains both highly variable and essentially constant regions. The variable parts of the heavy and light chains pair to form the potentially diverse part of the antibody molecule that binds antigen. The constant region of the heavy chain dictates the function of the antibody and belongs to one of the classes M, G1–4, A1–2, D and E, giving rise to antibodies called IgM, IgG1–4, IgA1–2, IgD and IgE. The characteristics of these different isotypes are shown in **Box 3.10**. As it matures, and under the instruction of T lymphocytes, a B lymphocyte may change the class (class switching), but never the specificity, of the antibody it makes; minor changes in antibody gene sequence can take place (somatic mutation), potentially allowing antibodies with higher affinity to arise and be selected for the effector response (affinity maturation).

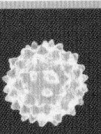

Antibody function

In host defence, antibodies target, neutralize and remove infectious organisms and toxins from the circulation and tissues, often through recruitment of innate host effector mechanisms such as complement, phagocytes and mast cells (by binding to specific surface receptors on these cells).

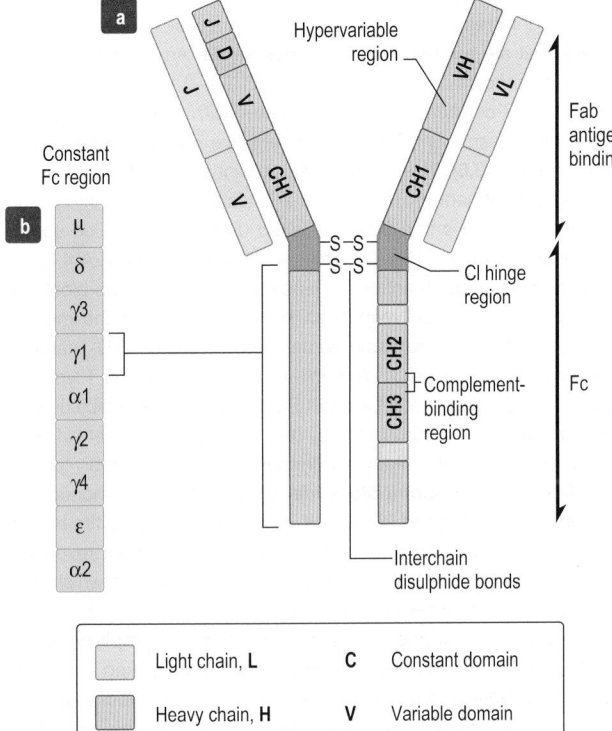

Fig. 3.6 **Immunoglobulin structure.** Basic subunit consisting of two heavy and two light chains (**a**). Genes on the Fab and Fc regions of an immunoglobulin (**b**). The chain is made up of a V (variable) gene, which is translocated to the J (joining) chain. The VJ segment is then spliced to the C (constant) gene. Heavy chains have an additional D (diversity) segment, which forms the VDJ segment that bears the antigen-binding site determinants.

In clinical medicine, specific anti-pathogen antibody levels are used in diagnosing/monitoring infectious disease, and may also be administered as serum pools to provide host protection passively.

Antibodies can be raised in animals to generate monoclonal antibodies, which are commonly used in diagnostic immunology tests and increasingly employed as therapeutics (***immunotherapy***; e.g. to target cancer cells, or to target immune cells and molecules to suppress or activate immune responses), often after 'humanization' (see later).

T-cell receptor genes and receptor diversity

The genomic organization of T-cell receptor (TCR) genes and principles of generation of receptor diversity are similar to those of immunoglobulin genes. The TCR exists as a heterodimer, with a similar overall structure to that of the antibody molecule. There are two TCR types:

- *α and β chains* ($\alpha\beta$ TCR). These are expressed on all CD4 T lymphocytes and approximately 90% of CD8 T lymphocytes; they play a role in adaptive immune responses.
- *γ and δ chains* ($\gamma\delta$ TCR). These are fewer in number and are expressed mainly on intraepithelial lymphocytes; they are involved in epithelial defence.

The chains of each type of TCR are divided into variable and constant domains, each domain being encoded by separate gene pools. Like the B lymphocyte producing a single clone of immunoglobulin molecules, the T lymphocyte expresses only one form of TCR once the genes have been rearranged. Unlike antibodies, TCRs do not undergo somatic hypermutation and are not secreted.

T lymphocyte development and activation

T lymphocytes are generated from precursors in the bone marrow, which migrate to the thymus (**Fig. 3.7**). Only 1% of the cells that enter the thymus will leave it as naive T lymphocytes to populate the lymph nodes. This process (termed thymic selection) leads to a cohort of cells (**Box 3.11**) with:

- functionally rearranged genes allowing surface expression of a receptor for antigen (the TCR) alongside the CD3 accessory molecule involved in transducing the antigen-specific signal

Box 3.10 Characteristics of the immunoglobulins (Igs)

	IgG	IgM	IgA	IgE	IgD
Description	Dominant class of antibody	Produced first in immune response	Found in mucous membrane secretions	Responsible for symptoms of allergy: used in defence against nematode parasites	Found almost solely on B lymphocyte surface membranes
Heavy chain	γ	μ	α	ε	δ
Mean adult serum levels (g/L)	IgG (total) = 8–16 G1 = 6.5 G2 = 2.5 G3 = 0.7 G4 = 0.3	0.5–2	IgA (total) = 1.4–4 A1 = 1.5 A2 = 0.2	17–450 ng/mL	0–0.4
Half-life (days)	21	10	6	2	3
Complement fixation					
Classical	++	+++	–	–	–
Alternative	–	–	+/–	–	–
Binding to mast cells	–	–	–	+	–
Crosses placenta	+	–	–	–	–

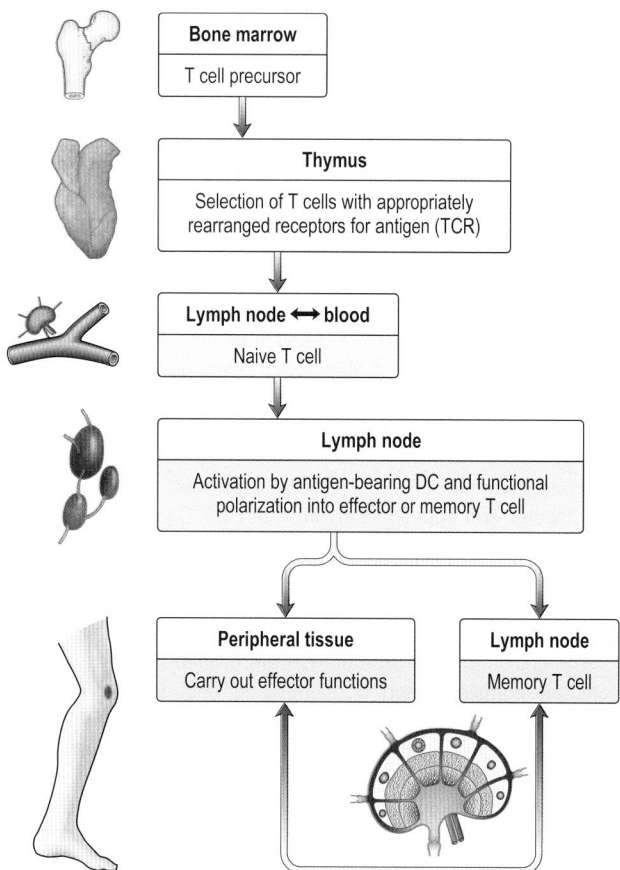

Fig. 3.7 Development of T lymphocytes in the thymus and life cycle in the secondary lymphoid tissue. DC, dendritic cell; TCR, T-cell receptor.

> **i** **Box 3.11** Identification of T lymphocytes

T-cell population	Marker	Typical percentages in blood	Additional information
T lymphocytes	T-cell receptor CD3	100% of T cells (70% of lymphocytes)	All T cells are thymus-derived
Helper T lymphocytes (Th)	CD4	66% of T cells	Th interact with antigen presented by MHC class II molecules
Cytotoxic T lymphocytes (CTL)	CD8	33% of T cells	CTL interact with antigen presented by MHC class I molecules

CD, cluster of differentiation; MHC, major histocompatibility complex.

- selection of a co-receptor, either CD4 or CD8, to stabilize the interaction between TCR and peptide-HLA:
  - CD4 T-cell responses require presentation of peptide antigens by *self* HLA class II molecules
  - CD8 T-cell responses require presentation of peptide antigens by *self* HLA class I molecules
- a reduced or absent tendency of the selected TCR to recognize self antigens (thus avoiding autoimmunity).

Thus, during thymic education, most TCRs are rejected for further use (negative selection), either because they are unable to bind

self HLA molecules, or because they bind with too strong an affinity, which would run the risk of self-reactivity and autoimmune disease. The chosen TCRs (positive selection) have low/intermediate affinity for self HLA molecules. During post-thymic activation of T lymphocytes in the lymph node, TCR interaction with HLA has to be bolstered by additional signals (called co-stimulation) provided by cDCs. This ensures that T lymphocytes are activated by a mature cDC; this happens only in the presence of pathogens.

Co-stimulation of T cells is such a critical event in immune responses that it is tightly regulated. One level of control relies on molecular interactions that are termed ***immune checkpoints***. An example is cytotoxic T-lymphocyte-associated antigen 4 (CTLA-4), which is expressed shortly after T-cell activation and competes with CD80 and CD86 for CD28, at the same time providing a negative signal, reducing T-cell activation (**Fig. 3.8**). This immune checkpoint is exploited in a highly successful treatment for rheumatoid arthritis, in which the interaction between CD80/86 and CD28 is blocked using a drug called abatacept (also known as CTLA-4Ig, being a soluble form of CTLA-4 fused to the Fc portion of an antibody), leading to co-stimulation blockade and suppression of T-cell responses. A further example is the immune checkpoint involving programmed cell death protein-1 (PD-1) and its ligands (PD-L1/L2). Like CTLA-4, PD-1 is upregulated after T lymphocyte activation, and interaction with PD-L1/L2 leads to inhibition of T lymphocyte function. PD-L1/L2 may be expressed on a variety of cells, including cDCs but also many non-immune cells, most notably tumour cells. ***Immune checkpoint blockade*** (see **Fig. 3.8**) using monoclonal antibodies focused on to PD-1/PD-L interactions releases the brakes on the immune system and is at the heart of the recent revolution in cancer immunotherapy (see p. 112), the discovery of which was awarded the 2018 Nobel Prize for Medicine.

Most naive T lymphocytes are resident in the lymph nodes or spleen, while 2% are present in the blood, representing a recirculating pool. Naive T lymphocytes are activated for the first time in the lymph node by antigens presented to their TCRs as short peptides bound to major histocompatibility complex (MHC) molecules on the surface of DCs (see **Fig. 3.5**). Provision of signals 1–3 (see p. 47) sets off an intracellular cascade of signalling molecule activation, leading to induction of gene transcription in T lymphocytes.

The outcome is T lymphocyte activation, cell division and functional polarization, which is the acquired ability to promote a selected type of adaptive immune response. These processes take several days to achieve. The best-described polarities of T-cell responses (**Box 3.12**) are:
- CD4⁺ pro-inflammatory T lymphocytes; T helper 1 (Th1), Th2 and Th17
- CD8⁺ cytotoxic T lymphocytes (CTLs) (**Box 3.13**)
- CD4⁺ regulatory responses (Treg).

Through cell division, a proportion of the T lymphocytes that are activated in response to a pathogen undertake these effector or regulatory functions, while a proportion is assigned to a memory pool. Once established, effector and memory T lymphocytes have lesser requirements for subsequent activation, which can be mediated by monocytes, macrophages and B lymphocytes.

CD4 T lymphocyte functions

As the pivotal cell in immune responses, the CD4 T lymphocyte influences most aspects of immunity, either through the release of cytokines or via direct cell–cell interaction, a process often termed 'licensing'. Licensing critically involves the pairing of CD40 on a specialized subset of cDC (cDC1) with CD40 ligand (CD40L, CD154) on the CD4 T lymphocyte; defects in this process result in antibody deficiency (see later).

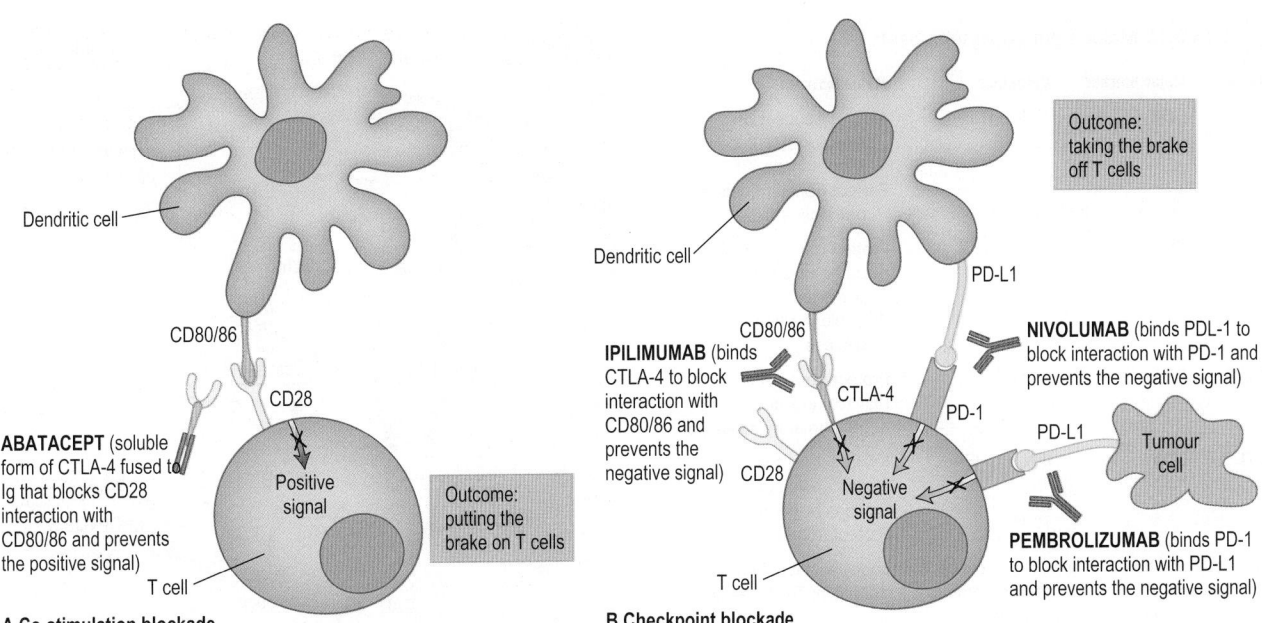

Fig. 3.8 **Understanding immune checkpoints for immunotherapy.** **(A)** T cells require co-stimulation, as well as recognition of antigen, to undergo full activation (see also **Fig. 3.5b**). CD80/86 on the dendritic cell binds CD28 on the T-cell receptor, providing a positive co-stimulatory signal. The drug abatacept is a soluble fusion of the cytotoxic T-lymphocyte-associated antigen 4 (CTLA-4) molecule with an immunoglobulin stalk. Since CTLA-4 has a higher affinity for CD80/86 than CD28, abatacept blockades co-stimulation and suppresses T-cell responses. **(B)** Soon after activation, T cells express CTLA-4 and programmed cell death protein-1 (PD-1), which deliver negative signals. Monoclonal antibodies aimed at blocking the interactions of these receptor/ligand pairs are thus able to take the brakes off the T-cell response. This can be critical for promoting anti-tumour responses.

---

i | **Box 3.12** Identification of CD4 T lymphocyte subsets by function

T-cell type	Main cytokines causing polarization	Main cytokines produced	Functions	Major role in physiological immune response
T helper 1 (Th1) cells	IL-12	IFN-γ, IL-2, TNF-α	Pro-inflammatory	Organize killing of bacteria, fungi and viruses; activate macrophages to kill intracellular bacteria; instruct cytotoxic T-cell responses
T helper 2 (Th2) cells	IL-4	IL-4, IL-5, IL-13	Pro-inflammatory	Organize killing of parasites by recruiting eosinophils; promote antibody responses, especially switching to IgE
T helper 17 (Th17) cells	IL-6, IL-23, TGF-β	IL-17	Pro-inflammatory	Not yet fully defined; capable of recruiting cells and damaging targets; may be more resistant to Treg than Th1/Th2 cells
Regulatory T cells (Treg)	IL-10, TGF-β	IL-10, TGF-β	Regulatory	Regulation of inflammation

IFN-γ, interferon-gamma; IgE, immunoglobulin E; IL, interleukin; TGF-β, transforming growth factor beta; TNF-α, tumour necrosis factor alpha.

Major functions of CD4 T lymphocytes are:

- **licensing of cDCs** during antigen presentation to activate CD8 T lymphocytes and generate cytotoxic cells
- **licensing of B lymphocytes** to initiate and mature antibody responses, leading to class switching, affinity maturation of antibodies, and generation of plasma cells or memory cells
- **secretion of cytokines** responsible for growth and differentiation of a range of cell types, especially other T lymphocytes, macrophages and eosinophils
- **regulation of immune reactions**.

T helper 1 cells

T helper 1 cells (Th1) are the main effector subtype of CD4 T lymphocytes. In physiology, they drive activation of monocytes/macrophages and CTLs. In pathology, they have a key role in protection against intracellular pathogens such as viruses and mycobacteria. Th1 cells are recognized by secretion of the pro-inflammatory cytokines IFN-γ and TNF-α (**Box 3.13**).

T helper 2 cells

In physiology, Th2 cells drive antibody responses, especially IgE, and also promote eosinophil granulocyte functions. In pathology, they have a key role in protection from extracellular parasites (helminths) and also in the immune responses that underlie allergic disease. Th2 cells are recognized by secretion of IL-4, IL-5 and IL-13.

T helper 17 cells

In physiology, Th17 cells drive inflammatory responses, especially via recruitment of neutrophil granulocytes. In pathology, they are

Name	Major marker	Cytokines	Major features
Th1	CD4	IFN-γ, TNF-α	Are main subset of effector CD4 T lymphocytes Protect from intracellular pathogens
Th2	CD4	IL-4, IL-5, IL-13	Protect from extracellular pathogens such as parasites Play role in allergic disease
Th17	CD4	IL-17	Protect from fungi Play role in autoimmune inflammatory diseases
CTL	CD8	IFN-γ, TNF-α	Kill target cells via recognition of HLA class I+ peptide Protect from viruses

CD, cluster of differentiation; CTL, cytotoxic T lymphocytes; HLA, human leucocyte antigen; IFN-γ, interferon-gamma; IL, interleukin; Th, T helper; TNF-α, tumour necrosis factor alpha.

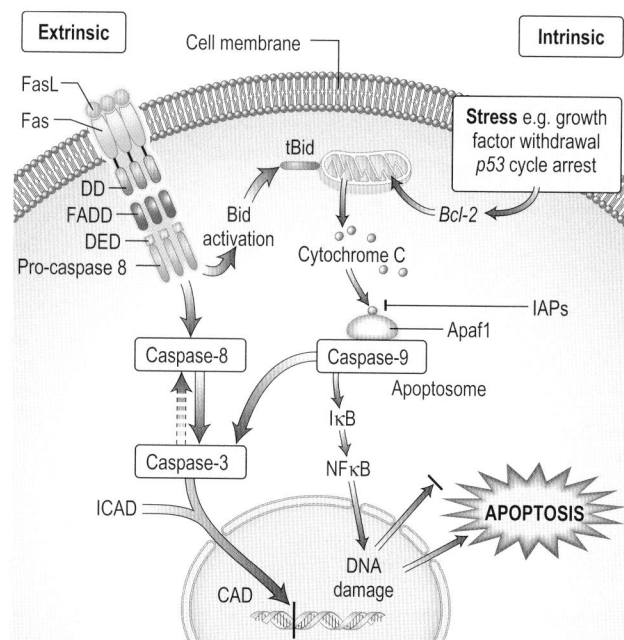

Fig. 3.9 Extrinsic and intrinsic apoptotic signalling network. The Fas protein and Fas ligand (FasL) are two proteins that interact to activate an apoptotic pathway: that is, a process of programmed cell death that removes cells that are infected or contain damaged DNA. Fas and FasL are both members of the tumour necrosis factor (TNF) family; Fas is part of the transmembrane receptor family and FasL is part of the membrane-associated cytokine family. When the homotrimer of FasL binds to Fas, it causes Fas to trimerize and brings together the death domains (DD) on the cytoplasmic tails of the protein. The adaptor protein FADD (Fas-associating protein with death domain) binds to these activated death domains and they bind to pro-caspase 8 through a set of death effector domains (DED). When pro-caspase 8s are brought together, they transactivate and cleave themselves to release caspase 8, a protease that cleaves protein chains after aspartic acid residues. Caspase 8 then cleaves and activates other caspases, which eventually leads to activation of caspase 3. Caspase 3 cleaves ICAD, the inhibitor of caspase activated DNase (CAD), which frees CAD to enter the nucleus and cleave DNA. Although caspase 3 is the pivotal execution caspase for apoptosis, the processes can be initiated by intrinsic signalling, which always involves mitochondrial release of cytochrome C and activation of caspase 9. Apaf1, apoptotic protease activating factor 1; Bid, family member of Bcl-2 protein; IAPs, inhibitor of apoptosis proteins; IκB, inhibitor of kappa B; NFκB, nuclear factor kappa B.

necessary for protection from fungal infections, and are increasingly recognized as having a role in chronic inflammatory diseases such as multiple sclerosis, rheumatoid arthritis and inflammatory bowel disease. They are recognized by secretion of IL-17.

T follicular helper cells

T follicular helper cells (Tfh) express CXCR5, the inducible T-cell co-stimulator molecule (ICOS), and secrete IL-21. They are responsible for licensing B lymphocytes for antibody production (see earlier).

Regulatory T lymphocytes

The generation of B and T lymphocytes provides a potentially vast array of rearranged antigen receptors. Although there are selection processes to remove lymphocytes with 'dangerous' avidity for 'self', these are not foolproof and the potential for autoreactivity remains. The fact that there is no self-destruction in the vast majority of people implies that the norm is a state of immunological self-tolerance: the controlled inability to respond to self. Several mechanisms operate to maintain this state, including CD4 T lymphocytes that respond to antigenic stimulation by suppressing ongoing immune responses. These regulatory T lymphocytes (Treg) express high levels of CD25, the receptor for IL-2; regulate other T lymphocytes by cell–cell contact; and also secrete the immune-suppressive cytokines IL-10 and TGF-β. They can be generated in the thymus or post-thymically in the periphery. Their key feature is high expression of the transcription factor Foxp3.

Evidence that Tregs are clinically relevant is provided by rare cases of genetic defects in the *Foxp3* gene, leading to IPEX (**i**mmune **d**ysregulation, **p**olyendocrinopathy, **e**nteropathy, **X**-linked) syndrome. Patients with this rare syndrome have defective Tregs and develop a range of conditions soon after birth, including organ-specific autoimmune disease such as type 1 diabetes. Much research effort is directed at harnessing this natural regulatory potential in new immunotherapies: for example, to control organ graft rejection and autoimmune disease.

CD8 T lymphocyte functions

Cytotoxic CD8 T lymphocytes (CTLs) are involved in defence against viruses. CTLs kill virus-infected cells following recognition

of viral peptide-HLA class I complexes. CTLs must be activated first in the lymph node by a specialized cDC subset (called cDC1) that cross-presents the *same* viral peptide that is seen on infected cells, and is licensed by a CD4 T lymphocyte recognizing viral peptide-HLA class II complexes. The same defence mechanism may also apply in tumour surveillance. This is a checkpoint that ensures that CTL responses, which have great destructive power, are activated only against a target for which there is also a CD4 T-cell response. CTLs kill via three mechanisms:

- cytotoxic granule proteins (cytolysins such as perforin, granzyme B)
- toxic cytokines (e.g. IFN-γ, TNF-α)
- death-inducing surface molecules (e.g. Fas ligand binds Fas on target cells mediating apoptosis via caspase activation, **Fig. 3.9**).

Natural killer cells

Natural killer (NK) cells are bone marrow-derived, present in the blood and lymph nodes, and represent 5–10% of lymphoid cells. The name reflects two features. Unlike B and T lymphocytes, NK cells are able to:

- mediate their effector function *spontaneously* (i.e. *killing* of target cells through release of perforin, a pore-forming protein) in the absence of previous known sensitization to that target
- achieve this with a very limited repertoire of germline-encoded receptors that do not undergo somatic recombination.

For identification purposes, the main surface molecules associated with NK cells are CD16 (see later) and CD56 (note that NK cells are CD3- and TCR-negative). The role of NK cells is to kill 'abnormal' host cells, typically cells that are virus-infected, or tumour cells. Killing is achieved in similar ways to CTLs. NK cells also secrete copious amounts of IFN-γ and TNF-α, through which they can mediate cytotoxic effects and activate other components of the innate and adaptive immune systems. To become activated, NK cells integrate the signal from a potential target cell through a series of receptor–ligand pairings (**Box 3.14**). These pairings provide activating and inhibitory signals, and it is the overall balance of these that determines the outcome for the NK cell. The balance can be abnormal on a virus-infected or tumour cell, which might have altered expression of HLA molecules, for example, that mark them out for NK cytotoxicity.

In addition, through CD16, which is the low-affinity receptor for IgG (FcgRIIIA), NK cells can kill IgG-coated target cells in a process termed antibody-dependent cellular cytotoxicity (ADCC).

Further reading
Cepika AM, Sato Y, Liu JM et al. Tregopathies: monogenic diseases resulting in regulatory T-cell deficiency. *J Allergy Clin Immunol* 2018; 142:1679–1695.
Diefenbach A, Colonna M, Romagnani C. The ILC world revisited. *Immunity* 2017; 46:327–332.
Freud AG, Mundy-Bosse BL, Yu J et al. The broad spectrum of human natural killer cell diversity. *Immunity* 2017; 47:820–833.
Halle S, Halle O, Förster R. Mechanisms and dynamics of T cell-mediated cytotoxicity in vivo. *Trends Immunol* 2017; 38:432–443.
Schmitt N, Ueno H. Regulation of human helper T cell subset differentiation by cytokines. *Curr Opin Immunol* 2015; 34:130–136.

CELL MIGRATION

Immune cells are mobile. They can migrate into the lymph node to participate in an evolving immune response (e.g. a pathogen-loaded DC from the skin or a recirculating naive T lymphocyte) or

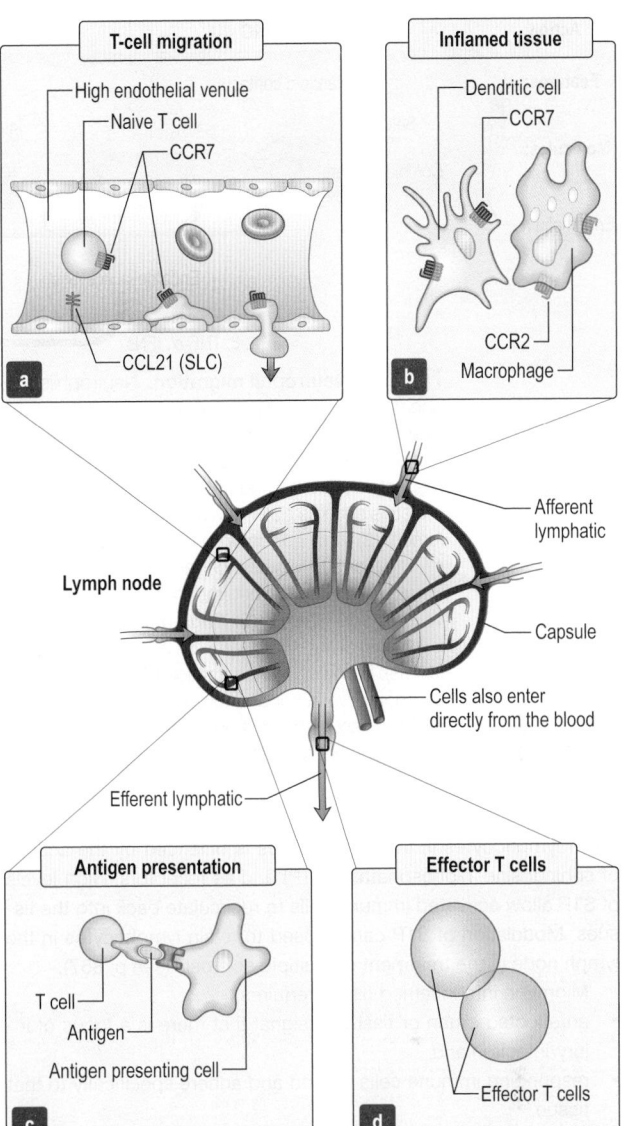

Fig. 3.10 Migration of an immune cell through a lymph node. **(a)** *T lymphocytes* migrate through endothelial venules, which express the chemokine CCL21 (secondary lymphoid tissue chemokine, or SLC). **(b)** *Dendritic cells* (expressing CCR7) and macrophages (expressing CCR2) enter lymph nodes via afferent lymphatics and localize in the paracortex. **(c)** *Antigen presentation* (see also **Figs 3.14** and **3.15**) results in activation of T lymphocytes. **(d)** *Effector T lymphocytes* leave the lymph node via efferent lymphatics.

can migrate from the lymph node, via the blood, to the site of a specific infection in the tissues. Such migration takes place along blood and lymphatic vessels and is a highly regulated process.

To take the example of a DC migrating into the lymph node from the tissues via the lymphatics (**Fig. 3.10**), this is highly dependent on expression of the chemokine receptor CCR7 by the migrating cell, and of its ligand (CCL21) by the target tissue. Likewise, circulating naive lymphocytes are CCR7+ and migrate with ease into the lymph nodes from the blood or via tissue recirculation. In addition, naive lymphocytes express L-selectin, which binds a glycoprotein cell adhesion molecule (GlyCAM-1), found on the high endothelial venules of lymph nodes. This system can be upregulated in an inflamed lymph node, leading to an influx of naive lymphocytes and the typical symptom of a swollen node. The ability of CCR7 to

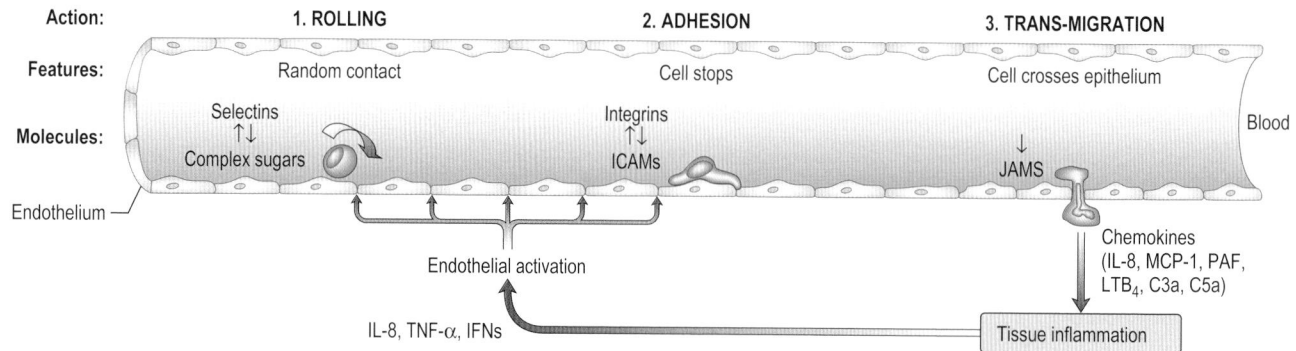

Fig. 3.11 Neutrophil migration. Neutrophils arrive at the site of the inflammation, attracted by various chemoattractants. **(1)** They *roll* along the blood vessel wall through interaction between L-selectin, on their surface, binding to a carbohydrate structure (e.g. sialyl-Lewis^X) on the endothelium. E-selectin on the endothelium mediates a similar effect. P-, E- and L-selectin (**p**latelet, **e**ndothelium and **l**eucocyte, respectively) are named after the predominant cell type that expresses them and bind to carbohydrate moieties such as sialyl-Lewis^X (CD15s) on immune cells, inducing them to slow and roll along the vessel lumen. **(2)** *Firm adhesion* is then mediated via interaction between integrins on the neutrophil and intercellular and vascular cell adhesion molecules (ICAM-1 and VCAM-1) on the endothelium. The best-known integrin is the heterodimer of CD11a/CD18 (leucocyte function associated antigen-1 – LFA-1), which binds ICAM-1. **(3)** *Trans-migration* (diapedesis) then occurs: this is a complex process that involves platelet-endothelial cell adhesion molecule-1 (PECAM-1) and junctional adhesion molecules (JAMs). Following transmigration (diapedesis), mediators such as interleukin-8 (IL-8), macrophage-chemotactic factor and tumour necrosis factor alpha (TNF-α) attract and activate the neutrophil to the infected tissue, where it phagocytoses and destroys the C3b-coated bacteria. IFNs, interferons; LTB$_4$, leukotriene B$_4$; MCP-1, monocyte chemoattractant protein-1 (CCL2); PAF, platelet-activating factor.

retain lymphocytes in the lymph nodes is balanced by the activity of sphingosine-1-phosphatase (S1P) and its receptors. High levels of S1P allow activated immune cells to recirculate back into the tissues. Modulation of S1P can be used to retain lymphocytes in the lymph node in the treatment of multiple sclerosis (see p. 867).

Migration into inflamed tissue requires:

- an affected organ or tissue to signal that there is a focus of injury/infection *and*
- responding immune cells to bind and adhere specifically to that tissue.

This process is highly organized and has a similar basis for all immune cells, involving three basic steps: rolling, adhesion and transmigration. Each of these is dependent on specialized adhesion molecules (**Fig. 3.11**).

The expression of these molecules (e.g. leucocyte function associated antigen-1, LFA-1) is upregulated on T lymphocytes after activation in the lymph node. Intercellular cell adhesion molecule 1 (ICAM-1) expression on tissue endothelium is sensitive to numerous pro-inflammatory molecules and allows immune cells to be guided from the blood into the tissues. Once there, cells move along a gradient of increasing concentration of mediators such as chemokines in the process of chemotaxis.

HLA MOLECULES AND ANTIGEN PRESENTATION

On the short arm of chromosome 6 is a collection of genes termed the major histocompatibility complex (MHC; known as the human leucocyte antigens, or HLA, in humans), which plays a critical role in immune function. MHC genes code for proteins expressed on the surface of a variety of cell types that are involved in antigen recognition by T lymphocytes. The T lymphocyte receptor for antigen recognizes its ligand as a short antigenic peptide

embedded within a physical groove at the extremity of the HLA molecule (**Fig. 3.12**).

The HLA genes are particularly interesting for clinicians and biologists. First, differences in HLA molecules between individuals are responsible for tissue and organ graft rejection (hence the name 'histo'(*tissue*)-compatibility). Second, possession of certain HLA genes is linked to susceptibility to particular diseases (**Box 3.15**).

The human major histocompatibility complex

The human MHC comprises three major classes (I, II and III) of genes involved in the immune response (**Fig. 3.13**).

HLA classes

Classical HLA class I genes

Classical HLA class I genes (also termed Ia) are designated *HLA-A*, *HLA-B* and *HLA-C*. Each encodes a class I α chain, which combines with a β chain to form the class I HLA molecule (see **Fig. 3.12**). While there are several types of α chain, there is only one type of β chain: β$_2$ microglobulin. The HLA class I molecule has the role of presenting short (8–10 amino acid) antigenic peptides to the T-cell receptor on the subset of T lymphocytes that bear the co-receptor CD8. As an example of HLA polymorphism, there are nearly 200 allelic forms at the *A* gene locus. Class I HLA molecules are expressed on all nucleated cells.

Non-classical HLA class I genes

Non-classical HLA class I genes are less polymorphic, have a more restricted expression on specialized cell types, and present a restricted type of peptide or none at all. These are the *HLA-E, F* and *G* (Ib genes) and MHC class I-related (MIC, or class Ic) genes, *A* and *B*. The products of these genes are predominantly found

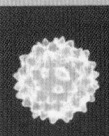

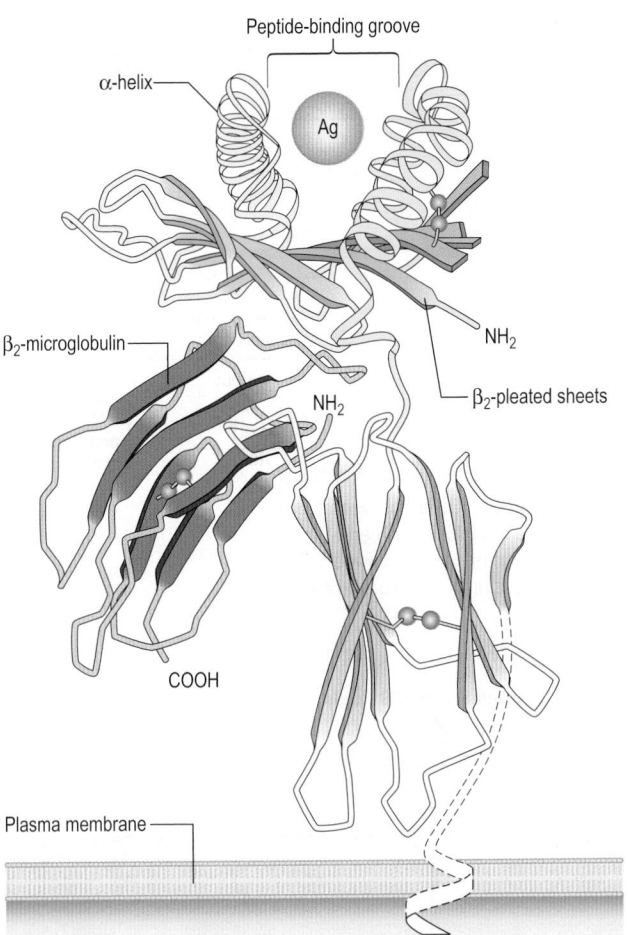

Fig. 3.12 Structure of human leucocyte antigen (HLA) class I molecule. The peptide-binding groove is used to present antigen (Ag) to T lymphocytes.

on epithelial cells, signal cellular stress and interact with lymphoid cells, especially natural killer cells (see p. 53).

HLA class II genes

The class II genes have three major subregions: *DP*, *DQ* and *DR*. In these subregions are genes encoding *A* and *B* genes that combine to form dimeric αβ molecules that present short (12–15 amino acid) peptides to T lymphocytes that bear the CD4 co-receptor. Class II HLA genes (apart from *DRA*) are highly polymorphic. Other genes in this region encode proteins with key roles in antigen presentation (e.g. TAP, HLA-DM, HLA-DO, proteasome subunits; see later). Class II HLA genes are expressed on a restricted cohort of cells that go by the general term of antigen presenting cells (APCs; DCs, monocyte/macrophages, B lymphocytes).

HLA class III genes

HLA class III genes encode proteins that can regulate or modify immune responses; they include tumour necrosis factor (TNF), heat shock protein (HSP) and complement protein (C2, C4).

HLA genotypes and the range of their protein products

HLA genotype is denoted first by the letters that designate the locus (e.g. *HLA-A*, *HLA-DR*, *HLA-DQ*). For class I alleles, this is followed by an asterisk and then a two- to four-digit number defining the

---

	Box 3.15 HLA associations with immune-mediated and infectious diseases	
Disease process	**Disease**	**HLA type**
Autoimmunity	Type 1 diabetes	Class II: *DQA1*03:01/DQB1*03:02* (susceptibility) *DQA1*05:01/DQB1*02:01* (susceptibility) *DQA1*01:02/DQB1*06:02* (protection) Class I: *HLA-A*24, HLA-B*18, HLA-B*39*
	Multiple sclerosis	*HLA-DRB1*15:01* (susceptibility)
	Myasthenia gravis	*HLA-A*01, HLA-B*08* and *HLA-DRB1*03* extended haplotype (susceptibility) predominates in younger females *HLA-B*07-DRB1*15* (susceptibility) predominates in older males *HLA-DRB1*16, HLA-DRB1*14, HLA-DQB1*05* (susceptibility) for MUSK variant myasthenia
	Behçet's syndrome	*HLA-B*51:01* (susceptibility)
	Rheumatoid arthritis	*HLA-DRB1*0404* (susceptibility)
	Autoimmune hepatitis	*HLA-DRB1*03, HLA-DRB1*04* (susceptibility)
	Goodpasture's syndrome (anti-glomerular basement membrane disease)	*HLA-DRB1*15:01* (susceptibility)
	Pemphigus vulgaris	*HLA-DRB1*04:02, HLA-DQB1*05:03* (susceptibility)
Inflammatory	Coeliac disease	*HLA-DQA1*05:01/DQB1*02:01* (susceptibility)
	Ankylosing spondylitis	*HLA-B*27* (susceptibility)
	Psoriasis	*HLA-Cw*06:02* (susceptibility)
	Idiopathic membranous nephropathy	*HLA-DQA1* (susceptibility)
Infectious	Human immunodeficiency virus infection	*HLA-B*27, HLA-B*51, HLA-B*57* (associated with slow progression of disease) *HLA-B*35* (associated with rapid progression)
Other	Narcolepsy	*HLA-DQA1*01:02, HLA-DQB1*06:02* (susceptibility) *HLA-DQB1*03:01* (worsens) *HLA-DQB1*05:01, HLA-DQB1*06:01* (protect)

allelic variant at that locus, often called the HLA type (e.g. *HLA-A*02* is the 02 variant of the *HLA-A* gene). The class II nomenclature is the same, except that both *A* and *B* genes are named (although HLA-DR molecules require only the name of the *B* gene because the *A* gene is the same in all of us).

Some general principles apply to the HLA genes and their protein products:

- The presence of multiple genes on each chromosome, and the fact that both maternal and paternal genes are co-dominantly expressed, allow considerable breadth in the number of HLA molecules that an individual expresses.

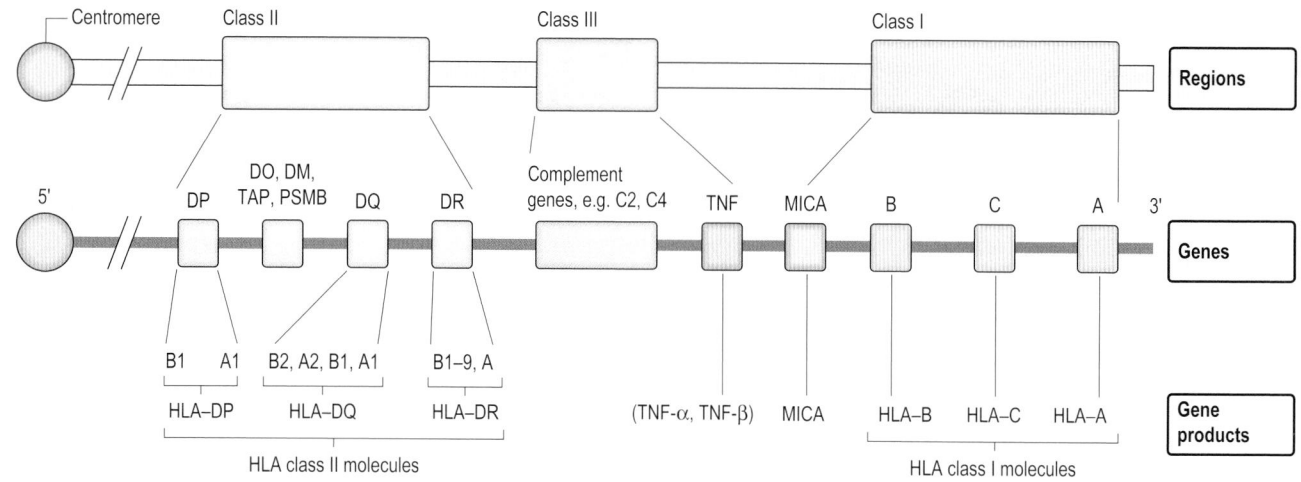

Fig. 3.13 The human leucocyte antigen (HLA) system in humans. On chromosome 6 are three major HLA regions (classes I–III), including genes that encode the HLA class I and II molecules, complement genes, the cytokine tumour necrosis factor (TNF) and other genes involved in antigen presentation (HLA-DO, HLA-DM; transporter associated with processing, TAP; proteasome subunit beta, PSMB; and the non-classical HLA class Ic molecule, MICA).

• The existence of polymorphisms at each locus provides great breadth in the number of HLA molecules expressed at a population level. The polymorphic forms of HLA molecules differ predominantly in the peptide-binding groove (see **Fig. 3.12**).

Overall, then, each human can bind a range of peptide epitopes from pathogens to enhance individual protection; similarly, the population has an even greater range of protection, to ensure population survival.

Antigen presentation

HLA molecules bind short peptide fragments that are processed ('chopped up') from larger proteins (antigens) derived from pathogens. The peptide–HLA complex is presented on APCs for recognition by TCRs on T lymphocytes. There are three major routes to antigen processing and presentation:

• **The endogenous route** (**Fig. 3.14**) is a property of all nucleated cells; the internal milieu is sampled to generate peptide–HLA class I complexes for display ('presentation') on the cell surface. In a healthy cell, the peptides are derived from self proteins in the cytoplasm (see **Fig. 3.14**) and are ignored by the immune system. In a virus-infected cell, viral proteins are processed and presented. The resulting viral peptide–HLA class I complex is presented to CD8 T lymphocytes that have cytotoxic (killer) function. In an immune response against a virus infection, CD8 T lymphocytes recognizing viral peptide–HLA complexes on the surface of an infected cell will kill it as a means to limit and eradicate infection.

• **The exogenous route** (**Fig. 3.15**) is a property of APCs; the external milieu is sampled. Antigens are internalized, either in the process of phagocytosis of a pathogen, through pinocytosis, or through specialized surface receptors (e.g. for antigen/antibody/complement complexes). The antigen is broken down by a combination of low pH and proteolytic enzymes for 'loading' into HLA class II molecules. At the APC surface, the pathogen peptide–HLA class II complex is presented to, and able to interact with, CD4 T lymphocytes. Presentation by DCs can initiate an adaptive immune

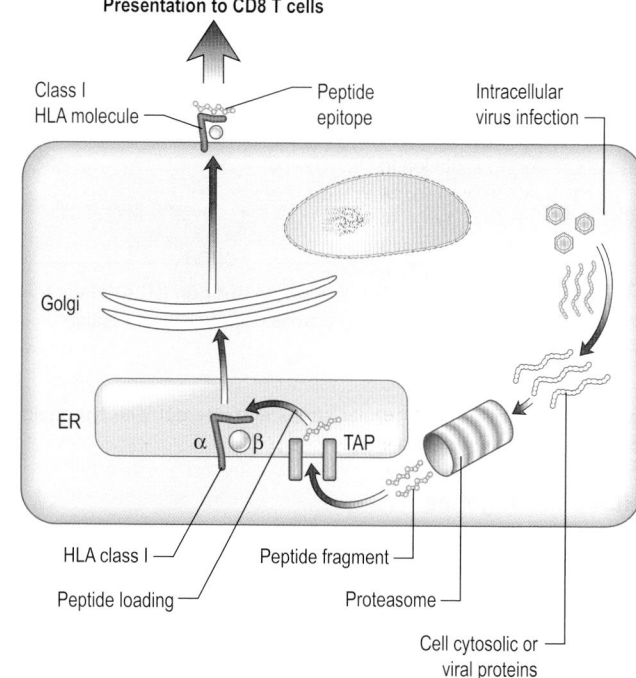

Presentation to CD8 T cells

Fig. 3.14 The endogenous route of antigen presentation. Antigen is presented to CD8 T lymphocytes. Cytosolic proteins derived from self (resting cells) or viruses (virus-infected cells) are broken down by the proteasome (a sort of 'protein recycler') into fragments 2–25 amino acids long. Some of these are taken into the endoplasmic reticulum (ER) by a transporter (TAP), trimmed, and loaded into empty human leucocyte antigen (HLA) class I molecules. These are exported to the surface membrane for presentation to CD8 T lymphocytes.

response by activating a naive, pathogen-specific CD4 T lymphocyte. Presentation by monocyte/macrophages and B lymphocytes can maintain and enhance this response by activating effector and memory pathogen-specific CD4 T lymphocytes.

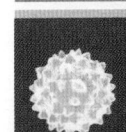

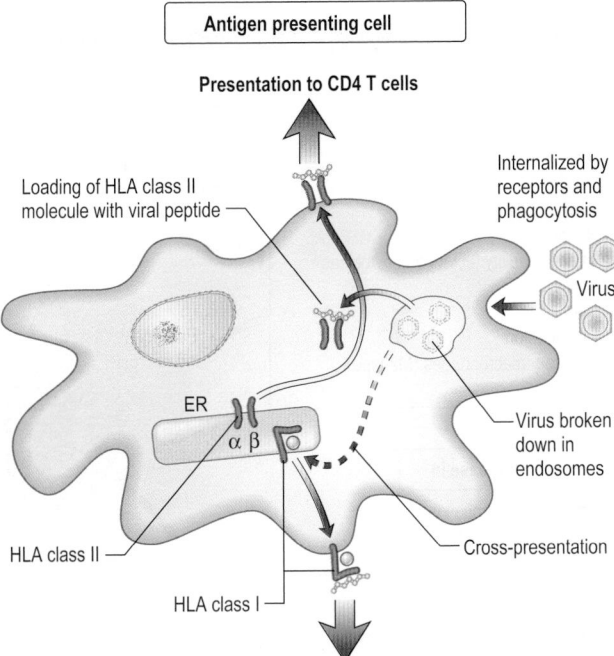

Antigen presenting cell

Presentation to CD4 T cells

Loading of HLA class II
molecule with viral peptide

Internalized by
receptors and
phagocytosis

Virus

ER

α β

Virus broken
down in
endosomes

HLA class II

Cross-presentation

HLA class I

Presentation to CD8 T cells

Fig. 3.15 The exogenous route of antigen presentation and cross-presentation. External material (e.g. virus particles) is taken into an antigen presenting cell and broken down into specialized compartments by a combination of low pH and proteolysis. Peptides are then loaded into human leucocyte antigen (HLA) class II molecules for presentation to CD4 T lymphocytes. Material may also be transferred across the cell so that it is loaded on to HLA class I molecules for presentation to CD8 T lymphocytes. This process of cross-presentation is restricted to specialized antigen presenting cells such as dendritic cells. ER, endoplasmic reticulum.

- **Cross-presentation** refers to the ability of some APCs (mainly cDC1s) to internalize exogenous antigens and process them through the endogenous route (see **Fig. 3.14**). This is an essential component in the activation of CD8 cytotoxic T-cell responses against a virus.

Further reading

Jurewicz MM, Stern LJ. Class II MHC antigen processing in immune tolerance and inflammation. *Immunogenetics* 2019; 71:171–187.
Lézaro S, Gamarra D, Del Val M. Proteolytic enzymes involved in MHC class I antigen processing: a guerrilla army that partners with the proteasome. *Mol Immunol* 2015; 68:72–76.
Sadegh-Nasseri S, Kim A. Exogenous antigens bind MHC class II first, and are processed by cathepsins later. *Mol Immunol* 2015; 68:81–84.
Worbs T, Hammerschmidt SI, Förster R. Dendritic cell migration in health and disease. *Nat Rev Immunol* 2017 17:30–48.
http://hla.alleles.org/ *Information on the human MHC.*

THE IMMUNE SYSTEM IN CONCERT

Acute inflammation: events and symptoms

This is the early and rapid host response to tissue injury. To take a bacterial infection as the classic example:

- Local expansion of pathogen numbers leads to direct activation of complement in the tissues, with ensuing degranulation of mast cells.

- Inflammatory mediators (from mast cells and complement) change the blood flow and attract and activate granulocytes (neutrophils).
- Concomitantly, there are the local symptoms of heat, pain, swelling and redness, and perhaps more systemic symptoms such as fever due to the effect of circulating cytokines (IL-1, IL-6, TNF-α) on the hypothalamus. Indeed, gene mutations that lead to excessive actions of IL-1 (e.g. mutation of the *IL1RN* gene, which encodes a natural IL-1 antagonist) give rise to rare disease with just these symptoms, as well as bone erosion and skin rashes, which are treatable with IL-1 blockade using soluble IL-1 receptor antagonist (anakinra) or monoclonal anti-IL-1β antibody.
- Systemically active mediators (especially IL-6) also initiate the production of C-reactive protein (CRP) in the liver.
- Bacterial lysis follows through the actions of complement and neutrophils, leading to formation of fluid in the tissue space containing dead and dying bacteria and host granulocytes ('pus').
- At the site of pathogen entry, there is often relative tissue hypoxia. The low oxygen tension has the effect of amplifying the responses of innate immune cells and suppressing the response of adaptive immune cells. This is probably an effective means of preventing excessive immune activation, which can result in collateral damage (**Fig. 3.16**).
- The inflammation may become organized and walled off through local fibrin deposition to protect the host.
- Antigens from the pathogen travel via the lymphatics (which may become visible as red tracks in the superficial tissues – lymphangitis) in soluble form or are carried by DCs to establish an adaptive immune response, which, at the first host–pathogen encounter, takes approximately 7–14 days. DCs are activated via the PRR–PAMP system (see **Fig. 3.5**).
- The adaptive immune response leads to activation of pathogen-specific T lymphocytes and of B lymphocytes, and production of pathogen-specific antibody, initially of the IgM class and of low to moderate affinity, and subsequently of the IgG class (or IgA if the infection is mucosal) and of high affinity.
- Resolution of the infection is aided by the scavenging activity of tissue macrophages.

Chronic inflammation: events and symptoms

Inflammation arising in response to immunological insults that cannot be resolved in days or weeks gives rise to chronic inflammation. Examples include infectious agents (viruses that cause chronic infections such as hepatitis B and C, or intracellular bacteria such as mycobacteria) and environmental toxins (such as asbestos and silicon). At the intracellular level, key processes of inflammasome generation (see p. 46) and autophagy (see p. 46) serve to enhance the chronic inflammatory process. Chronic inflammation is also a hallmark of some forms of allergic disease, autoimmune disease and organ graft rejection.

The common feature of these pathological processes is the difficulty of removing the inciting stimulus. For example, some viruses and mycobacteria remain hidden intracellularly. In many ways, the pathology that results is inadvertent: the immune system is caught between the repercussions of not dealing with the infection or insult and the tissue damage that is caused by chronic activation of lymphoid and mononuclear cells.

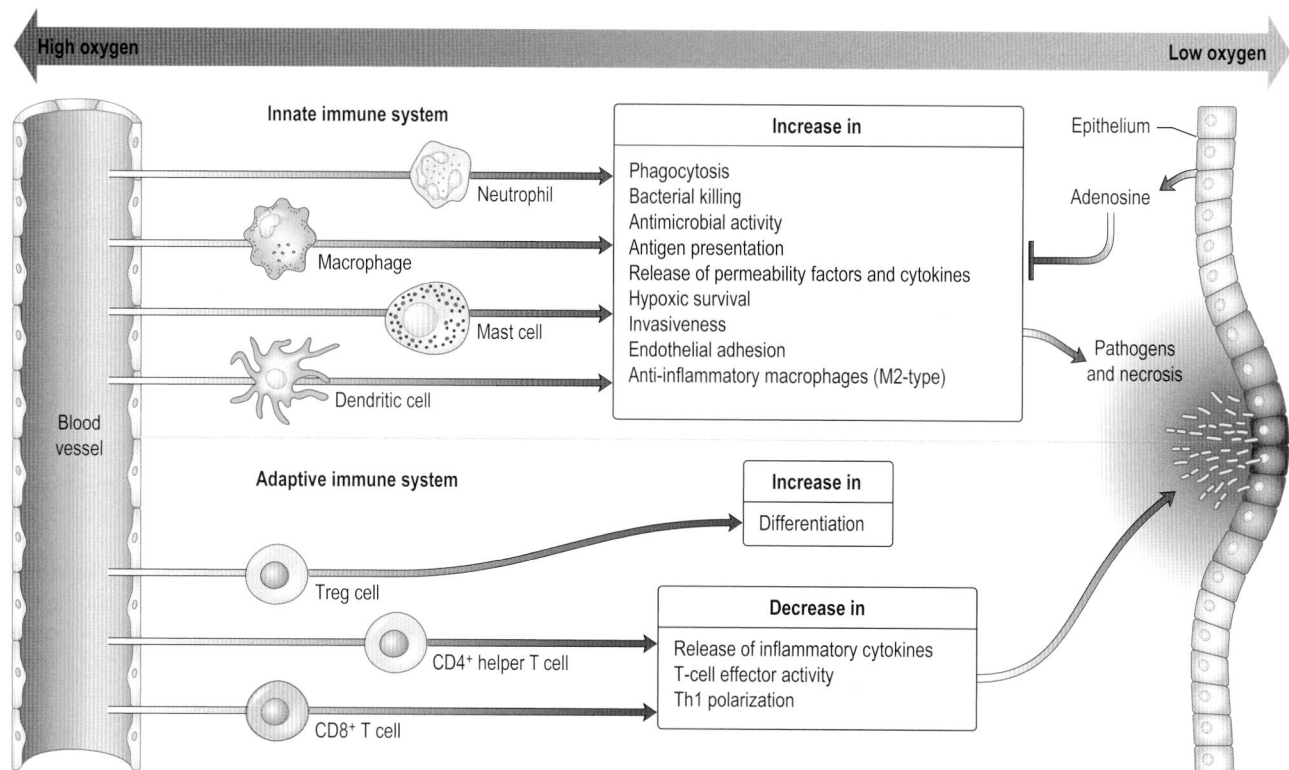

Fig. 3.16 Hypoxia and inflammation. At the site of pathogen invasion and necrosis, the oxygen tension is low. Hypoxia acts on the inflammatory process by amplifying innate immune cell responses and dampening down the adaptive response. Overall, this benefits the host by avoiding an excessive, uncontrolled immune response.

Mycobacterium leprae

In *Mycobacterium leprae* infection (leprosy, p. 550) this feature is well demonstrated. With the same infecting organism, two very different forms of disease are seen: lepromatous or tuberculous. In the tuberculous form, there is a good immune response to chronic infection but the immune response causes nerve damage and numb patches of skin. In the lepromatous form, Th1 responses are less pronounced and infection is widespread but there is less nerve damage.

In both of these forms of mycobacterial disease, the chronic inflammation may lead to permanent organ damage or impaired vascular function, and can be fatal. If the inciting stimulus is removed, inflammation resolves. With leprosy, this is achieved with antibiotics. However, inflammation can return rapidly (24–48 hours) on re-exposure. This rapid recall response is the basis for patch testing to identify the cause of contact dermatitis, another form of chronic inflammation, and also for the Mantoux (skin) or the interferon gamma release (IGRA) blood test of tuberculosis immunity.

The main immunological event is the presence of a pro-inflammatory focus comprising T and B lymphocytes and APCs, especially macrophages. If antigen persists, inflammation becomes chronic and the macrophages in the lesion fuse to form giant cells and epithelioid cells. Both Th1 and Th2 reactivity is recognized but specific syndromes may be polarized towards one or the other (e.g. chronic mycobacterial or viral infection initiates Th1 responses, chronic allergic inflammation Th2).

When the inflammation is sufficiently chronic, it may take on the appearance of organized lymphoid tissue resembling a lymph node germinal centre (e.g. in the joints in rheumatoid arthritis, p. 456).

There is massive cytokine production by T lymphocytes and APCs, which contributes to local tissue damage. Granulomata, which 'wall off' the inciting stimulus, may also arise and result in fibrosis and calcification. Symptoms typically relate to the site of the inflammation and the type of pathology, but there may also be systemic effects such as fever and weight loss.

Crohn's disease

Chronic inflammation is a hallmark of several immune-mediated and autoimmune diseases but it is often unclear what kick-starts or maintains the inflammatory process. Large-scale studies that identify the genetic basis for these disorders (genome-wide association studies (GWAS), p. 33) are beginning to provide some clues. A good example is Crohn's disease (see p. 1198). Several of the polymorphisms associated with Crohn's disease reside in genes known to be involved in inflammasome induction, such as *NOD2*. Cytokine regulation has also emerged as a critical disease pathway in GWAS studies on Crohn's disease: most notably, *IL-23R* (the IL-23 receptor gene), which influences Th17 cell differentiation. Clues like these point to patients with Crohn's disease having impaired ability to control or terminate inflammasome activity, as well as a predisposition to make polarized pro-inflammatory cytokine responses. This information can now be exploited to devise novel therapeutic approaches, such as monoclonal antibodies that target the key cytokines.

Further reading

Eltzschig HK, Carmeliet P. Hypoxia and inflammation. *N Engl J Med* 2011; 364:656–665.

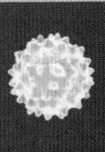

Box 3.16 Examining the immune system in the clinical immunology laboratory

	Measurement	Interpretation
Proteins	C-reactive protein	Raised levels indicate infection or inflammation
	Total immunoglobulins	Low levels indicate antibody deficiency, usually a result of underlying disease or primary immunodeficiency. High levels, e.g. ↑ IgM, are seen in acute viral infection (e.g. hepatitis A)
	IgG subclasses	Specific reductions in IgG subclasses (1–4) may indicate immune deficiency. High levels of IgG4 are observed in IgG4 disease
	Complement level and function	Low levels indicate consumption of complement in immune complex disease or primary complement deficiency, which can be confirmed with testing of the alternative or classical pathway function
	IgE	Raised levels are seen in allergy; allergen-specific IgE is useful to pinpoint the inciting stimulus (e.g. pollen, grass), component allergens may be useful in assessing anaphylaxis risk or cross-reactivity between allergens
Cells	Neutrophils	High levels are seen in bacterial infection; low levels in secondary immune deficiency
	Eosinophils	High levels are seen in allergic or parasitic disease
	CD4 T lymphocytes	Low levels are seen in HIV infection
Function	Neutrophil respiratory burst	Absent in immune deficiency chronic granulomatous disease
	T lymphocyte proliferation	Abnormally low in primary T-cell immune deficiency disease
Autoantibodies (see also **Box 3.23** and **Box 18.6**)	Rheumatoid factor, anti-citrullinated peptide antibodies (ACPA)	Rheumatoid arthritis
	Double-stranded DNA autoantibodies	Systemic lupus erythematosus
	Acetylcholine receptor antibodies	Myasthenia gravis
	Anti-neutrophil cytoplasmic antibodies (ANCA)	Vasculitis
	Mitochondrial	Primary biliary cholangitis

LABORATORY INVESTIGATIONS OF THE IMMUNE SYSTEM

In the clinical immunology laboratory, proteins and cells can be measured to ascertain the status of the immune system. The results

Box 3.17 Classification of immunodeficiencies and the main diseases in each category[a]

Immune component	Examples of diseases
T lymphocyte deficiency	DiGeorge's syndrome
	Acquired immunodeficiency syndrome (AIDS)/ human immunodeficiency virus (HIV) infection
	T-cell activation defects (e.g. CD3γ chain mutation)
	X-linked hyper-IgM syndrome (XHIM; CD40L deficiency)
B lymphocyte deficiency	X-linked agammaglobulinaemia (XLA)
	Common variable immunodeficiency (CVID)
	Selective IgA deficiency (IgAD)
Combined T- and B-cell defects	Severe combined immunodeficiency (SCID) (e.g. due to defects in common γ chain receptor for IL-2, 4, 7, 9, 15)
T-cell–antigen presenting cell interactions	IFN-γ receptor deficiency
	IL-12 deficiency and IL-12 receptor deficiency
Neutrophil defects	Chronic granulomatous disease (CGD)
	Leucocyte adhesion deficiency (LAD)
Deficiency of complement components	Classical pathway
	Alternative pathway
	Common pathway
	Regulatory proteins
	Mannose-binding lectin

[a]Apart from AIDS, all the diseases shown here are primary immunodeficiencies.

may indicate an undiagnosed inflammatory or infectious disease (e.g. high CRP level); a state of immune deficiency (e.g. low concentration of IgG); or a state of immune pathology (e.g. the presence of autoantibodies or allergen-specific IgE).

Examples of the more common tests and their interpretation are shown in **Box 3.16**.

CLINICAL IMMUNODEFICIENCY

Secondary (acquired) versus primary immunodeficiency

Most forms of immunodeficiency are secondary to infection (mainly HIV) or therapy (e.g. corticosteroids, monoclonal antibody therapy, cytotoxic anticancer drugs, bone marrow ablation pre-transplant). Examples of other secondary immunodeficiencies are:

- *Acquired neutropenias*, which are common (e.g. due to myelosuppression by disease or drugs, or the increased rate of destruction in hypersplenism or autoimmune neutropenia) and carry a high risk of infection once the neutrophil count falls below 0.5×10^9/L.
- *Acquired reductions in levels of immunoglobulins* (hypogammaglobulinaemia), which are seen in patients with myeloma and chronic lymphocytic leukaemia or lymphoma.
- *Impairment of defence against capsulated bacteria*, especially pneumococcus, following splenectomy; such patients should receive pneumococcal, meningococcal and Hib vaccinations as a matter of course (see **Box 16.18**).

Primary immunodeficiency is rare and arises at birth as the congenital effect of a developmental defect or as a result of genetic abnormalities (**Box 3.17**). Gene defects may not become

---

> ℹ️ **Box 3.18** Immune defects and associated infections

Neutropenia and defective neutrophil function
- *Staphylococcus aureus*
- *Staphylococcus epidermidis*
- *Escherichia coli*
- *Klebsiella pneumoniae*
- *Proteus mirabilis*
- *Pseudomonas aeruginosa*
- *Serratia marcescens*
- *Bacteroides* spp.
- *Aspergillus fumigatus*
- *Candida* spp. (systemic)

Opsonin defects (antibody/complement deficiency)
- Pneumococcus
- *Haemophilus influenzae*
- Meningococcus
- *Streptococcus* spp. (capsulated)

Antibody deficiency only
- *Campylobacter* spp.
- *Mycoplasma* spp.
- *Ureaplasma* spp.
- Echovirus
- *Pseudomonas* spp.

Complement lytic pathway defects (C5–9)
- Meningococcus
- Gonococcus (disseminated)

Defect in T-cell or T-cell–antigen presenting cell responses
- *Listeria monocytogenes*
- *Legionella pneumophilae*
- *Salmonella* spp. (non-*typhi*)
- *Nocardia asteroides*
- *Mycobacterium tuberculosis*
- Atypical mycobacteria, especially *M. avium-intracellulare*
- *Candida* spp. (mucocutaneous)
- *Cryptococcus neoformans*
- *Histoplasma capsulatum*
- *Pneumocystis jiroveci*
- *Toxoplasma gondii*
- Herpes simplex
- Herpes zoster
- Cytomegalovirus
- Epstein–Barr virus

---

manifest until later in infancy or childhood, and some forms of immunodeficiency typically present in adolescence or adulthood.

Clinical features of immunodeficiency

The infections associated with immunodeficiency have several typical features:
- They are often chronic, severe or recurrent.
- They resolve only partially with antibiotic therapy or return soon after cessation of therapy.
- The organisms involved are often unusual ('opportunistic' or 'atypical').

The pattern of infection, in terms of the type of organism involved, is indicative (**Box 3.18**):
- **'Opportunistic' organisms** are of low virulence but become invasive in immunodeficient states, e.g. atypical mycobacteria, *Pneumocystis jiroveci*, *Staphylococcus epidermidis*.
- **Phagocyte defects** cause deep skin infections, abscesses and osteomyelitis, for example.
- **Defective antibody** producers experience infections with pyogenic ('pus-forming') bacteria.
- **T lymphocyte deficiency** causes infection with fungi, protozoa and intracellular microorganisms.
- **Congenital deficiencies** of antibody production are not revealed for several months after birth, due to the 28-day half-life of maternal IgG.

The family history may reveal unexplained sibling death, the fact that only males of the family are affected (X-linked), or consanguinity; each of these makes a primary genetic syndrome more likely. Graft-versus-host disease (GVHD) may arise as a complication of primary or secondary T lymphocyte immunodeficiency. For GVHD to occur, there must be impaired T lymphocyte function in the recipient and the transfer of immunocompetent T lymphocytes from an HLA non-identical donor (see later). GVHD is usually caused by therapeutic interventions such as transfusions or transplantation, but may be due to transfer of maternal cells across the placenta, in which case it is called **materno-fetal engraftment**.

Primary immunodeficiency

T lymphocyte deficiency

Complete DiGeorge's syndrome

DiGeorge's syndrome arises in 1–5 per 100 000 of the population due to deletions on the long arm of chromosome 22. It has a highly variable presentation, including **c**ardiac abnormalities, **a**bnormal facies, **t**hymic dysfunction, **c**left deformities and **h**ypocalcaemia/hypoparathyroidism, remembered by the acronym 'CATCH-22'. In those DiGeorge individuals born without a thymus, the lack of a location for T lymphocyte development means that they have reduced or absent T lymphocyte number and proliferation responses. Apart from calcium supplementation, correction of cardiac abnormalities and prophylactic antibiotics, cure has been reported with thymic transplantation using fetal tissue or stem cell transplant (SCT) from HLA identical siblings. Other athymic conditions include Foxn1 deficiency and CHARGE syndrome (**c**oloboma, **h**eart defects, choanal **a**tresia, **r**etardation of **g**rowth and development, **e**ar abnormalities) caused by CHD7 mutations.

Other T lymphocyte deficiencies

Other T lymphocyte deficiencies caused by single-gene defects have been characterized and typically present from the age of 3 months with candidal infections of the mouth and skin, protracted diarrhoea, fever and failure to thrive. These disorders are similar in presentation and management to the combined (T and B lymphocyte) immunodeficiencies.

T and B lymphocyte deficiency

Severe combined immunodeficiencies

Severe combined immunodeficiencies (SCID) are a heterogeneous group of rare (1–2 live births per 100 000), genetically determined disorders resulting from impaired T, NK and B lymphocyte immunity. The most common form of SCID is an X-linked defect in the IL-2 receptor γ chain, interfering with the function not just of IL-2 but also of IL-4, IL-7, IL-9 and IL-15, which share

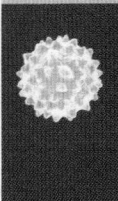

this component in their receptors. Clinical features are similar to those of pure T lymphocyte deficiency and, in the blood, T and NK cells are lacking while B lymphocyte numbers may be normal. The most successful treatment for all forms of SCID is SCT, preferably from HLA-identical donors such as siblings. For a few disorders such as ADA (adenosine deaminase) and γ chain-deficient SCID, gene therapy is possible if no appropriate HLA-matched donor can be found.

Hyper-IgM syndrome

This mixed or combined immunodeficiency may not be diagnosed until later in life. It usually results from an X-linked defect in the gene encoding CD40 ligand (CD40L, also called CD154). Signalling between CD40 on B cells and CD40L on T cells is necessary for the generation of class-switched B cells bearing high-affinity immunoglobulin, and for mature T-cell responses. In CD40L deficiency, B lymphocytes are unable to class-switch, producing only IgM. Levels of other types of immunoglobulin, IgG and IgA, are absent or low and there are mild defects in T-cell function. Autosomal forms are also seen with defects in CD40, activation-induced cytidine deaminase (AID) and uracil-DNA glycosylase (UNG).

Opportunistic infections occur: for example, with *Pneumocystis*, *Cryptosporidium*, *Candida*, *Cryptococcus* and herpes viral infections. Treatment is with replacement immunoglobulin, antifungals, antibiotics and avoidance of *Cryptosporidium* by boiling water. SCT is used in some patients.

Wiskott–Aldrich syndrome

This is an X-linked defect (at Xp11–23) in a gene involved in signal transduction and cytoskeletal function. It is associated with eczema and thrombocytopenia; a mainly cell-mediated defect with falling immunoglobulins is seen, and autoimmune manifestations and lymphoreticular malignancy may develop. Activating mutations in the same gene have been described that cause severe congenital neutropenia, highlighting the key role of Wiskott–Aldrich serine protease (WASP) in immune regulation.

Ataxia telangiectasia

Patients with this disease have defective DNA repair mechanisms and have cell-mediated defects with low IgA and IgG$_2$. Lymphoid malignancy is common and a shortened life expectancy often results from the neurological disease.

Epstein–Barr virus-associated immunodeficiencies

Apparently normal but genetically predisposed individuals develop overwhelming Epstein–Barr virus (EBV) infection, polyclonal EBV-driven lymphoproliferation, combined immunodeficiency, aplastic anaemia and lymphoid malignancy. EBV appears to act as a trigger for the expression of a hitherto silent immunodeficiency. Many genetic susceptibilities to EBV have now been described, including X-linked lymphoproliferative disease 1 and 2 (XLP1 and XLP2), which demonstrate defects in the *SH2D1A* and *XIAP* genes, respectively, and may also present with Crohn's-like gut inflammation (see p. 1198). Other genetic causes include mutations in *CD70*, *CD27*, *ITK* and *CARD11*.

Antibody deficiencies

Antibody deficiency syndromes may be caused by intrinsic defects in B lymphocyte development, resulting in absence of B lymphocytes or specific subsets. Antibody deficiency due to inborn errors of immunity (IEI) also occur when normal antibody production is not well sustained. Intrinsic developmental defects tend to present 6 months after birth when transplacentally transferred maternal IgG has declined, while other syndromes may present variably throughout childhood and adult life. The clinical features of antibody deficiency are severe, recurrent sinopulmonary infection leading to bronchiectasis and persistence of gut pathogens (e.g. *Giardia*) with resultant chronic diarrhoea and malabsorption. Morbidity and mortality are high if the conditions are untreated, mainly due to chronic lung disease and central nervous system infections with enteroviruses.

X-linked agammaglobulinaemia

X-linked agammaglobulinaemia (XLA) is an intrinsic defect in B lymphocyte maturation. The cause is a loss-of-function mutation of Bruton's tyrosine kinase, which is involved in cell activation and maturation. B lymphocyte development is arrested at the pre-B stage, and B lymphocytes are absent in the blood. Clinical presentation follows the fall in protective maternal IgG.

Common variable immunodeficiencies

Common variable immunodeficiencies (CVID) are a heterogeneous group of disorders arising during late childhood and early adulthood, with very low IgG levels. Although rare (1/50 000) it is the most common severe primary immune deficiency and carries a significant risk of morbidity and mortality. Autoimmunity and granulomatous disease are found in up to 15% of cases. Genetic defects underlying the condition have revealed mutations in multiple genes: in Europe the most common is haploinsufficiency of *NFKB1*. In most patients, the underlying defect remains unknown.

Selective IgA deficiency

Selective IgA deficiency (IgAD; serum IgA <0.05 g/L), with normal levels of IgG and IgM, is found in approximately 1/600 Northern Europeans. Most individuals are asymptomatic but numerically this is the most common primary immunodeficiency. The underlying defect is unknown. Patients may present at any age with recurrent infections caused by pyogenic organisms, particularly affecting mucosal sites.

Treatment of antibody deficiencies

Treatment of IgAD is not usually required; when it is, antibiotics are used. Some IgAD patients produce anti-IgA antibodies of the IgG and IgE classes, and so infusion of exogenous IgA (e.g. during a blood transfusion) could result in anaphylaxis. IgAD patients should therefore be screened for anti-IgA antibodies if there is a history of transfusion reaction, and transfused with appropriate precautions if positive.

For patients with XLA, CVID or another major antibody deficiency, treatment is with replacement immunoglobulins (intravenous or subcutaneous, IVIg or SCIg) to a level that controls infections. Trough IgG concentrations should remain well within normal limits (i.e. >6 g/L), and infections should be treated promptly and aggressively with antibiotics. Prognosis has improved in recent years as more patients survive into adulthood, but chronic lung disease and lymphomas remain life-threatening complications.

Defects in antigen presenting cell function

A series of rare genetic defects have been uncovered in which APCs demonstrate an inability to mount protective responses to intracellular bacteria, particularly low-virulence mycobacteria and salmonella. The axis affected is the interplay between CD4 T lymphocytes and APCs that drives Th1 responses, and therefore in turn activates mononuclear cells such as macrophages to kill and eradicate intracellular pathogens. Defective genes so far identified include those encoding a component chain of IL-12; a component chain of the IL-12 receptor; and IFN-γ receptor chains 1 or 2 or the intracellular signalling pathway (STAT 1).

Neutrophil defects

Chronic granulomatous disease

Chronic granulomatous disease (CGD) is a rare (1/250 000) immunodeficiency that is caused by a defect in neutrophil killing; it is characterized by deep-seated infections. The functional defect is an inability to generate antibacterial metabolites through the respiratory burst (see **Box 3.5**). X-linked and autosomal forms are described. Typical onset is at toddler age. Neutrophil numbers are normal or increased. A simple respiratory burst test of neutrophil function is diagnostic. The dysfunctional neutrophils' inability to clear infection adequately and frustrated apoptosis lead to granulomatous inflammation, and CGD may also present with a Crohn's-like gut disease (see p. 1198).

Treatment of infections and prophylactic antibiotic and antifungal therapy are required. In many cases, SCT is necessary. For the X-linked form, gene therapy is a treatment option when a suitably matched donor cannot be found.

Leucocyte adhesion deficiency

Leucocyte adhesion deficiency (LAD) results from defects in integrins (see **Fig. 3.11**). Numerous underlying defects in the genes encoding one of the component chains, *CD18*, have been described in LAD-1. LAD-1 has an autosomal recessive inheritance, presenting almost immediately after birth with delayed umbilical cord separation. In later life, there is a characteristic failure to lose primary dentition and severe gingivitis. Recurrent infections appear during the first decade of life. Blood neutrophil levels are high but cells are absent from the sites of infection, which require aggressive antimicrobial and antifungal treatment, and SCT for cure.

Hyper-IgE syndrome (Job's syndrome)

This is an autosomal dominant (occasionally sporadic) immune disorder with high serum IgE levels, dermatitis, boils, pneumonias with cyst formation, and bone and dental abnormalities. Mutations in *STAT3*, *DOCK8* and *ZNF341* have been found.

Schwachman–Diamond syndrome

This can resemble cystic fibrosis clinically, with exocrine pancreatic insufficiency and pyogenic infections. A mild neutropenia is associated with a defect of neutrophil migration.

Chédiak–Higashi syndrome

This rare recessive disorder is caused by a mutation in the lysosomal trafficking regulator gene (*LYST*) on chromosome 1q42–45. There are defects in neutrophil function with defective phagolysosome fusion, and large lysosome vesicles are seen in phagocytes. Patients have recurrent infections, neutropenia, anaemia and hepatomegaly. As with Schwachman–Diamond syndrome, tissue infiltration with histiocytes is usually seen, including in bone marrow, and Chédiak–Higashi syndrome is one of several genetic causes of primary haemophagocytic lymphohistiocytosis (HLH). Similar genetic abnormalities in melanocytes cause partial oculocutaneous albinism.

Complement deficiency

The consequences of deficiency of complement proteins can be predicted from their functions (see **Fig. 3.2**):

- Failures in innate response components (e.g. the alternative pathway) lead to impaired non-specific immunity with an increase in bacterial infections.

- Failure of the classical pathway results in a tendency towards infection and also towards diseases in which immune complex deposition causes inflammation, such as systemic lupus erythematosus (e.g. C1 and C4 deficiency), vasculitis and glomerulonephritis.

Neisserial infections (e.g. meningitis due to *N. meningitidis*) are often encountered in patients with complement defects of the membrane attack complex (C6–9). Lectin pathway deficiency in isolation rarely causes major ill health.

Complement regulatory proteins

Deficiency of C1 inhibitor (***C1 esterase deficiency***; see also p. 668) is relatively rare. Since this enzyme is involved in regulation of several plasma enzyme systems (e.g. the kinin system) and is continuously consumed, a single parental chromosome defect resulting in 50% of normal production barely copes with the demand and fails under stress (hence has an autosomal dominant effect). As a result, uncontrolled activation of low-molecular-weight kinins may occur, leading to oedema of the deep tissues affecting the face, trunk, viscera and airway, and explaining the alternative name of hereditary angio-oedema (HAE). Treatment is with C1 inhibitor concentrate or a selective bradykinin-2 receptor antagonist (icatibant). Steroids and antihistamines are not useful in this form of angio-oedema. Prophylaxis may be with attenuated androgens or specific kallikrein inhibitors. A rarer acquired form (acquired angio-oedema, AAE) may be seen in lymphoproliferative disease or complicating autoimmunity. The treatment is largely as for HAE.

Further reading

Boufiha A, Jeddane L, Picard C et al. The 2017 IUIS phenotypic classification for primary immunodeficiencies. *J Clin Immunol* 2018; 38:129–143.
Maurer M, Magerl M, Ansotegui I et al. The international WAO/EAACI guideline for the management of hereditary angioedema – the 2017 revision and update. *World Allergy Organ J* 2018; 11:5.

ALLERGIC DISEASE (IMMEDIATE HYPERSENSITIVITY)

Normally, host defence can cope with potentially harmful cells and molecules. Under some circumstances a harmless molecule can initiate an immune response that can lead to tissue damage and death. Such exaggerated, inappropriate responses are termed hypersensitivity reactions or allergic disease.

In ***allergic hypersensitivity***, the binding of an antigen to specific IgE bound to its high-affinity receptor on a mast cell surface results in massive and rapid cell degranulation and the inflammatory response outlined on page 45. The antigens involved are typically inert molecules present in the environment (these are termed allergens, p. 949).

The immediate effects of allergen exposure are often very florid (***early phase response***). Allergic disorders also have a second phase, occurring a few hours after exposure and lasting up to several days. These '***late phase responses***' (LPRs) are mediated by Th2 cells recognizing peptide epitopes of the allergen. Recruitment of eosinophils is often a prominent feature.

From a pathological and therapeutic viewpoint, the LPR gives rise to chronic inflammation, which is difficult to control. In ***asthma***, the LPR causes prolonged wheezing, which can be fatal. Immediate hypersensitivity is usually responsive to antihistamines but the LPR is not, requiring powerful immune modulators such as corticosteroids.

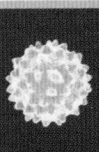

In immunopathological terms, in the LPR:

- Neutrophils and eosinophils are prominent in the first 6–18 hours and may persist for 2–3 days.
- Th2 cells accumulate around small blood vessels and persist for 1–2 days.
- Mediators responsible for the cellular infiltrate include platelet-activating factor and leukotrienes (**Box 3.19**).
- Th2 cytokines IL-4 and IL-5 and chemokines such as eotaxin act as growth and activation stimuli for eosinophils, which are capable of extensive tissue damage. Th2 cytokines are also responsible for the class switch of Ig production towards IgE, maintaining the cycle of immediate and late responses.

What makes an allergen so powerful?

Several allergens are proteolytic enzymes, allowing them to cross skin and mucosal barriers. They are often contained within small, aerodynamic particles (e.g. pollen grains) that gain access to nasal and bronchial mucosa.

Why do some people react and others do not?

The tendency to develop allergic responses (known as atopy) shows strong heritability. Between 20% and 30% of the UK population is atopic, and two, one or no atopic parents pass on the atopic trait to their children with a risk of 75%, 50% and 15%, respectively. In developing nations, the tendency to allergy is estimated at one-tenth of the rate in industrialized countries. Among the predisposing genes are those encoding the β chain of the high-affinity receptor for IgE and IL-4, both strongly associated with Th2 pathways. The presence of Th2 cells recognizing allergens is the pathological hallmark of allergy.

What environmental factors are involved?

Early exposure to allergens (even *in utero*) may be a factor in developing atopy. Over-zealous attention to cleanliness (the hygiene hypothesis) in developed societies (use of antibiotics, reduced exposure to pathogens that might favour a Th1-like environment) may favour a reduction in Treg activity. This environmental factor is demonstrated by the rapid increase of allergy in the eastern part of Germany following reunification in 1990.

In clinical terms, approximately two-thirds of atopic individuals (who can be identified as those with circulating allergen-specific IgE) have **clinical allergic disease** (equating to 15–20% of the UK population). Allergy accounts for up to one-third of school absences because of chronic illness. Allergic disorders include allergic rhinitis (hay fever), allergic eczema, bee and wasp venom allergy, some forms of food allergy, urticaria and angio-oedema.

Diagnosis

Diagnosis of allergic disease is usually made on the history and backed up by skin-prick testing (insertion of a tiny quantity of allergen under the skin and measurement of the size of the weal) and/or measurement of serum allergen-specific IgE. Mast cell tryptase serum levels peak 1–2 hours after an event, remaining high for 24 hours.

Treatment

Avoidance is the first line of therapy. Other measures are as follows:

- **Antihistamines** are effective for many immediate hypersensitivity reactions (but have no role in the treatment of asthma).
- **Corticosteroids** have several well-identified modifying actions in the allergic process: production of prostaglandin and leukotriene mediators is suppressed, inflammatory cell recruitment and migration are inhibited, and vasoconstriction leads to reduced cell and fluid leakage from the vasculature.
- **Cysteinyl leukotriene receptor antagonists** (**LTRAs**) inhibit leukotrienes (LTs) by blocking the type I receptor (e.g. montelukast, used in asthma, particularly the aspirin-induced type).
- **Omalizumab** is a monoclonal antibody that binds IgE. It is used in severe asthma (see p. 953) that cannot be controlled with a corticosteroid plus a long-acting β_2 agonist. Treatment must be initiated in a specialist centre where staff have experience of treating severe, persistent asthma.
- **Dupilumab** is a monoclonal antibody that inhibits the biological activity of both IL-4 and IL-13. It has been shown to be beneficial in severe atopic eczema and asthma.
- **Desensitization** (**allergen immunotherapy**) works on the principle that allergy can be prevented by inoculation if the allergen is given in a controlled way. Desensitization is indicated for disorders in which the hypersensitivity is IgE-mediated, e.g. life-threatening allergy to insect stings, drug allergy and allergic rhinitis. An induction course of subcutaneous injections of increasing doses of the allergen extract, given once every 1–2 weeks, is followed by maintenance injections monthly for 2–3 years. A systematic review of 51 published randomized, placebo-controlled clinical trials, enrolling a total of nearly 3000 participants, showed a low risk of adverse events with consistent clinical benefit. From an immunological viewpoint, desensitization seems capable of modifying the allergic response at several levels (**Box 3.20**). Sublingual allergen

---

_i_ | **Box 3.19 Mediators involved in the allergic response**

Pre-formed mediators
- Histamine and serotonin:
  - Bronchoconstriction
  - Increased vascular permeability
- Neutrophil chemotactic factor (NCF) and eosinophil chemotactic factor (ECF):
  - Induction of inflammatory cell infiltration

Newly formed mediators (membrane-derived)
- Leukotriene (LT) B_4:
  - Chemoattractant
- LTC_4, LTD_4, LTE_4 (slow-reacting substance of anaphylaxis, SRS-A):
  - Sustained bronchoconstriction and oedema
- Prostaglandins and thromboxanes:
  - Platelet-activating factor (PAF)
  - Prolonged airway hyperactivity

_i_ | **Box 3.20 Mechanism of action of desensitization for allergy**

Probable mechanism	Effect
IgG blocking antibodies	During repeated exposure to desensitizing allergen, IgG class antibodies develop (especially IgG4 subclass); these compete with the pathogenic IgE for allergen binding and/or prevent IgE–allergen complexes from binding to mast cell high-affinity IgE receptors
Regulation	Exposure to repeated desensitizing allergen induces Treg cells, which recognize allergen but invoke regulatory immune responses, dampening down migration, infiltration and inflammation
Immune deviation	A shift away from Th2- to Th1-producing CD4 cells results in the generation of cytokines (e.g. interferon-gamma) that are inhibitory to IgE production

> **Box 3.21 Sources of allergens known to provoke anaphylaxis**
>
> **Foods**
> - Nuts: peanuts (protein – *Arachis hypogaea* Ara h 2), Brazil, cashew
> - Shellfish: shrimp (allergen Met e 1), lobster
> - Dairy products
> - Egg
> - More rarely: citrus fruits, mango, strawberry, tomato
>
> **Venoms**
> - Wasps, bees, yellow-jackets, hornets
>
> **Medications**
> - Antisera (tetanus, diphtheria), dextran, latex, some antibiotics

> **Box 3.22 Treatment of acute anaphylaxis**
>
> **Clinical features**
> - Bronchospasm
> - Facial and laryngeal oedema
> - Hypotension
> - Nausea, vomiting and diarrhoea
>
> **Management**
> - ABCDE (airway, breathing, circulation, disability, exposure)
> - Position the patient lying flat with the feet raised
> - Ensure the airway is free
> - Give oxygen
> - Monitor blood pressure
> - Establish venous access
> - Administer 0.5 mg *intramuscular* adrenaline (epinephrine) 0.5 mL of 1 : 1000 adrenaline, i.e. 1 mg/mL, and repeat after 5 min if shock persists (dose reduced for children or adults on beta-blockers)
> - Administer intravenous antihistamine (e.g. 10–20 mg chlorphenamine) slowly
> - Administer 100 mg intravenous hydrocortisone.
>   - If hypotension persists, give 1–2 L of intravenous fluid
>   - If hypoxia is severe, assisted ventilation may be required
>   - Take blood for tryptase levels (aids diagnosis)

immunotherapy (using grass pollen extract tablets of Phl p 5 from timothy grass) is used in hay fever that has not responded to anti-allergic drugs (the first dose is given under medical supervision) (see p. 947).

Anaphylaxis

Anaphylaxis is a serious allergic reaction that is rapid in onset and may cause death. It arises as an acute, generalized IgE-mediated immune reaction involving specific antigen, mast cells and basophils. The reaction requires priming by the allergen, followed by re-exposure. To provoke anaphylaxis, the allergen must be systemically absorbed, after either ingestion or parenteral injection. A range of allergens that provoke anaphylaxis has been identified (**Box 3.21**).

Anaphylaxis is rare, but the symptom/sign constellation ranges from widespread urticaria to cardiovascular collapse, laryngeal oedema, airway obstruction and respiratory arrest leading to death:

- Fatal reactions to penicillin occur once every 7.5 million injections.
- Between 1 in 250 and 1 in 125 individuals have severe reactions to bee and wasp stings, and a death takes place every 6.5 million stings, with 60–80 deaths per year in North America and 5–10 in the UK.

Central to the pathogenesis of anaphylaxis is the activation of mast cells and basophils, with systemic release of some mediators and generation of others. The initial symptoms may appear innocuous: tingling, warmth and itchiness. The ensuing effects on the vasculature lead to vasodilatation and oedema. The consequence may be no more than a generalized flush, with urticaria and angiooedema. More serious sequelae are hypotension, bronchospasm, laryngeal oedema and cardiac arrhythmia or infarction. Death may occur within minutes.

Serum platelet-activating factor (PAF) levels correlate directly with the severity of anaphylaxis, whereas PAF acetylhydrolase (the enzyme that inactivates PAF) correlates inversely and is significantly lower in peanut-sensitive patients with fatal anaphylactic reactions.

Management

Early recognition and treatment are essential (**Box 3.22**).

The best treatment is prevention. Avoidance of triggering foods, particularly nuts and shellfish, may require almost obsessive self-discipline. Patient education is necessary and many are instructed in the self-administration of adrenaline (epinephrine) and carry preloaded syringes. Desensitization has a well-established place in the management of this disorder, particularly if exposure is unavoidable or unpredictable, as in insect stings. In peanut allergy (see p. 1257), it has been shown that early introduction of peanuts in children modulates the response in later life, and this benefit extends to high-risk

children with atopic eczema or allergy to another food. Further studies have shown that it is possible to give graded peanut exposure to those already sensitized and that oral desensitization can reduce the risk of anaphylaxis associated with inadvertent exposure in children with a history of peanut allergy. The addition of modified peanut peptides further enhances the success and tolerability of this approach.

Further reading

Du Toit G, Roberts G, Sayre PH et al. Randomised trial of peanut consumption in infants at risk for peanut allergy. *N Engl J Med* 2015; 372:803–813.
The PALISADE Group of Clinical Investigators. AR101 oral immunotherapy for peanut allergy. *N Engl J Med* 2018; 379:1991–2001.
http://www.allergen.org *Allergen nomenclature.*

AUTOIMMUNE DISEASE

Autoimmunity is when the immune response turns against self, i.e. recognizes 'self' antigens. The vast array of possible TCRs and antibodies that can be generated by the host make it highly probable that at least a small proportion can recognize self (i.e. are autoreactive). Moreover, a degree of autoreactivity is physiological: the TCR is designed to interact both with the peptide epitope in the HLA molecule binding groove *and* with the HLA molecule itself.

The critical event in the development of autoimmune disease is when T and B lymphocytes bearing these receptors for 'self' become activated: this leads to loss of immunological tolerance. The major checkpoints that the immune system has in place to prevent this are:

1. removal of TCRs with very strong affinity for 'self' in the thymus
2. the presence of naturally arising regulatory T lymphocytes (Tregs)
3. the requirement for a danger signal to license dendritic cells to activate CD4 T lymphocytes.

Failure of immune tolerance checkpoint 1: thymic education

During thymic education, TCRs with a dangerously high affinity for self are deleted. It has become apparent that this process relies on

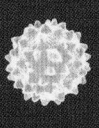

the thymic expression of self antigens. Situations that compromise the expression of a self protein would be expected to favour the development of autoimmunity. Indeed, in a rare group of patients who develop multiple autoimmune disorders affecting the adrenal and parathyroid glands (autoimmune polyglandular syndrome type 1, p. 648), there is a defect in the autoimmune regulator (*AIRE*) gene, which controls thymic expression of a host of self genes. When the gene malfunctions, there is reduced expression of self proteins in the thymus and autoimmune disease is a consequence.

Failure of immune tolerance checkpoint 2: regulatory T lymphocytes

An example of Treg failure is the defect in the gene encoding Foxp3, a critical transcription factor in Tregs, which leads to IPEX (see p. 52). IPEX is very rare but it serves to indicate how Treg defects can lead to autoimmune disease. Laboratory studies in this area are revealing subtle Treg defects in several autoimmune diseases (e.g. type 1 diabetes, multiple sclerosis, rheumatoid arthritis). The role of FoxP3 in regulating peripheral immune responses highlights the control of immune expansion and regulation of immunological 'space'. Another component of this process is the contraction of an immune response once the infection has been dealt with. Autoimmune lymphoproliferative syndrome (ALPS) is a disorder with defects in either Fas, its ligand (FasL or CD95) or the associated intracellular signalling pathway. Individuals develop multiple cytopenias, organ-specific autoimmunity, and lymphoproliferation that may mimic lymphoma. The common problem is the inability to 'switch off' activated T cells. Treatment is with haemopoietic SCT if the disorder is severe. Many patients with multiple cytopenias, including Evans' syndrome (autoimmune thrombocytopenia and haemolytic anaemia), are revealed to have ALPS defects when appropriately tested.

Failure of immune tolerance checkpoint 3: CD4 T lymphocyte activation against an autoantigen (or its mimic)

For an autoimmune disease to develop, there must be presentation of autoantigens to a naive, potentially autoreactive CD4 T lymphocyte by activated cDCs. Several theories exist to explain this:

- Tissue damage due to infection leads to both the release of hidden self antigens and the provision of sufficient danger signals to activate cDCs, which in turn activate autoreactive CD4 T lymphocytes, as well as pathogen-specific ones. This is often termed 'bystander activation'.
- A pathogen mimics a self antigen. In the process of mounting an entirely appropriate immune response against the pathogen, T or B lymphocytes are generated that also have the capacity to recognize self. This is termed molecular mimicry.
- Post-translational modification. Self proteins and peptides are modified in such a way that they appear foreign. A good example is an antibody found in patients with rheumatoid arthritis, which recognizes citrulline-modified forms of self peptides.

It is unlikely that, for the common autoimmune diseases (**Box 3.23**), there is a 'single tolerance checkpoint' explanation. Rather, it is likely that multiple subtle defects, at various checkpoints, are at play.

Mechanisms of tissue damage in autoimmune disease

Figure. 3.17 illustrates potential mechanisms of immune damage in autoimmune disease.

> *i*   **Box 3.23 Some autoimmune diseases and their autoantigens**

Disease	Antigens
Addison's disease	21 α-hydroxylase
Goodpasture's syndrome	Alpha-3 chain of type IV collagen
Granulomatosis with polyangiitis	Neutrophil proteinase 3
Graves' thyroiditis	Thyroid-stimulating hormone receptor
Hashimoto's thyroiditis	Thyroid peroxidase, thyroglobulin
Multiple sclerosis	Myelin basic protein Myelin oligodendrocyte glycoprotein
Myasthenia gravis	Acetylcholine receptor, muscle-specific kinase (MuSK)
Pemphigus vulgaris	Desmoglein-3
Pernicious anaemia	H^+/K^+-ATPase, intrinsic factor
Polymyositis/dermatomyositis	Transfer RNA synthases (e.g. Jo-1, PL7, PL12)
Primary biliary cholangitis	Pyruvate dehydrogenase complex
Rheumatoid arthritis	Citrullinated cyclic peptide, IgM
Scleroderma	Topoisomerase
Sjögren's syndrome	Ro/La ribonuclear proteins
Systemic lupus erythematosus	Sm/RNP, Ro/La (SS-A/SS-B), histone and native double-stranded DNA
Type 1 diabetes	Pro-insulin, glutamic acid decarboxylase, IA-2, ZNT8
Vitiligo	Pigment cell antigens

Tissue damage via chronic inflammation

In a number of autoimmune diseases (e.g. type 1 diabetes, multiple sclerosis), autoreactive T lymphocytes are likely to be the main drivers of disease and tissue damage. Th1 cells, CTLs and Th17 cells induce chronic inflammation and release cytokines that recruit other effector cells (macrophages) or are directly toxic (e.g. insulin-producing β cells are susceptible to the combined effects of IL-1β, IFN-γ and IL-17 in type 1 diabetes).

IgG4 disease

IgG4 disease is a fibro-inflammatory condition with the formation of swellings at multiple sites infiltrated with IgG4-producing plasma cells and a tendency to high circulating levels of IgG4. Unlike many autoimmune disorders, IgG4-related disease is driven by Th2 T cells in association with high numbers of FoxP3+ T cells. The first recognized form of this disorder was autoimmune pancreatitis, but lesions in the biliary tree, salivary glands, periorbital tissues, kidneys, lungs, lymph nodes, meninges, aorta, breast, prostate, thyroid, pericardium and skin are recognized (**Box 3.24**). The current hypothesis is that Th2 cells drive the activation of macrophages and myofibroblasts, leading to fibrosis and IgG4 plasma cell proliferation.

Tissue damage via autoantibodies

Examples of damage through direct binding to a target cell or structure, with recruitment of complement and other destructive processes, include:

- ***myasthenia gravis*** (autoantibodies against the acetylcholine receptor cause damage to the neuromuscular junction)
- ***autoimmune haemolytic anaemia*** (autoantibody targets red blood cell autoantigens, leading to lysis)

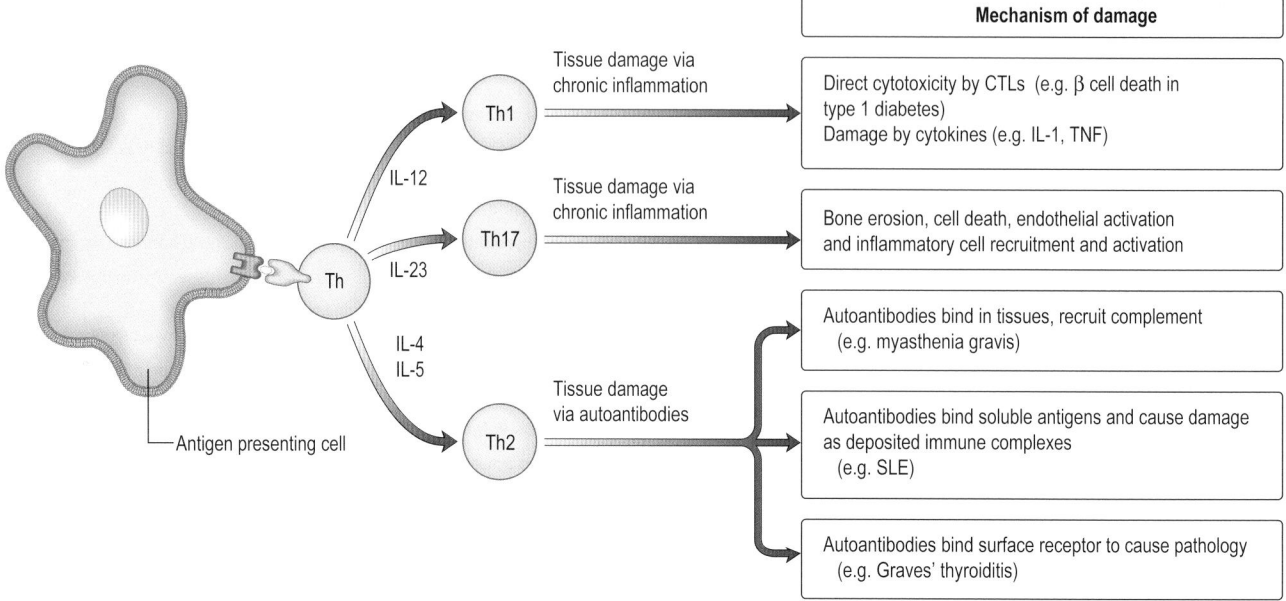

Fig. 3.17 Potential mechanisms of immune damage in autoimmune disease. CTL, cytotoxic T lymphocyte; IL, interleukin; SLE, systemic lupus erythematosus; Th, helper T lymphocyte; TNF, tumour necrosis factor.

Box 3.24 IgG4-related disease

Condition	Affected organ or tissue
Chronic stenotic sialadenitis	Submandibular glands
Eosinophilic angiocentric fibrosis	Orbits, upper respiratory tract
Fibrosing mediastinitis	Mediastinum
Hypertrophic pachymeningitis	Dura mater
Idiopathic hypocomplementaemic tubulointerstitial nephritis with extensive tubulointerstitial deposits	Kidney
Inflammatory aortic aneurysm	Aorta
Inflammatory pseudotumour	Orbits, lungs, kidneys and other organs
Mikulicz's syndrome	Salivary and lacrimal glands
Multifocal fibrosclerosis	Orbits, thyroid gland, retroperitoneum, mediastinum, and other tissues and organs
Periaortitis and periarteritis	Aorta and large blood vessels
Retroperitoneal fibrosis (Ormond disease)	Retroperitoneum
Riedel's thyroiditis	Thyroid
Sclerosing mesenteritis	Mesentery
Sclerosing pancreatitis	Pancreas

(After Mahajan VS, Mattoo H, Deshpande V et al. IgG4-related disease. Ann Rev Pathol 2014; 9:315–347.)

- **Goodpasture's syndrome** (anti-glomerular basement membrane autoantibodies damage glomerular integrity).

Autoantibodies can also bind their antigen in the circulation to form immune complexes. When these are deposited in the tissues, complement- and cell-mediated immune reactions are initiated. Immune complexes preferentially deposit in sites such as the kidney glomerulus, leading to chronic kidney disease. This is a feature of systemic lupus erythematosus, in which the autoantigen within the immune complexes is DNA.

Autoantibody binding may act by binding to surface receptors. In Graves' thyroiditis, for example, the anti-thyroid stimulating hormone receptor antibody stimulates follicular cells to produce thyroid hormones, leading to hyperthyroidism.

Common autoimmune diseases

Over 80 diseases are now classified as autoimmune. The autoimmune origin of some of these diseases is very clear-cut but that is not so for others, and both major and minor factors must be defined.

Major criteria

- There is evidence of autoreactivity (e.g. activated or memory autoreactive T lymphocytes or autoantibodies).
- A clinical response to immune suppression can be demonstrated.
- Passive transfer of the putative immune effector (e.g. autoreactive T lymphocyte or autoantibody) causes the disease (this is the hardest criterion to satisfy in humans but is the most stringent).

Minor criteria

- An animal model exists that resembles the human condition, and in which there is a similar loss of immunological tolerance to self.
- There is evidence that, in the animal model, passive transfer of the putative immune effectors reproduces the disease in a naive animal.
- There is an HLA association (a frequent indicator that a disease is autoimmune).

Further reading

Atkinson MA, Roep BO, Posgai A et al. The challenge of modulating β-cell autoimmunity in type 1 diabetes. *Lancet Diabetes Endocrinol* 2019; 7:52–64.
Cho JH, Gregerson PK. Genomics and the multifactorial nature of human autoimmune disease. *N Engl J Med* 2011; 365:1621–1623.
Goodnow C. Multistep pathogenesis of autoimmune disease. *Cell* 2007; 130:25–35.
Harbige J, Eichmann M, Peakman M. New insights into non-conventional epitopes as T cell targets: the missing link for breaking immune tolerance in autoimmune disease? *J Autoimmun* 2017; 84:12–20.
Kamisawa T, Zen Y, Pillai S et al. IgG4-related disease. *Lancet* 2015; 385:1460–1470.

ORGAN REJECTION IN CLINICAL TRANSPLANTATION

The outcome of an allograft (i.e. a graft between genetically non-identical members of the same species) in the absence of adequate immunosuppressive therapy is *immunological rejection*. Histological analysis of rejected organs shows a range of immunological processes in action (**Box 3.25**). With modern tissue-matching approaches, hyperacute rejection is rare and acute rejection can usually be prevented or treated with immunosuppression. The process of chronic rejection typically takes place over several years and is the main reason for organ graft failure.

The antigens recognized in acute and chronic graft responses are donor HLA molecules (alloantigens):

- In acute rejection, it is thought that the predominant response is against intact HLA molecules (**direct allorecognition**) and is mediated by CD4+ and CD8+ T lymphocytes.
- As the rejection process becomes more chronic, peptides from donor HLA molecules are processed and presented to T lymphocytes by host HLA molecules (**indirect allorecognition**).

IMMUNE-BASED THERAPIES

Manipulation of the immune response in a therapeutic setting has seen many successes, as evidenced by the control of organ rejection in clinical transplantation through targeted immunosuppression (**Box 3.25**). Monoclonal antibodies offer the opportunity to neutralize the unwanted effects of cytokines, or to direct immune responses, drugs, toxins or irradiation against a specific target, whether it be a tumour cell or an immune cell involved in a damaging autoimmune response. Natural antiviral mediators, such as the interferons, are already in the clinic as therapies for chronic viral infection, among other things. Genetic manipulation of T lymphocytes has generated a new class of cellular therapies.

Monoclonal antibody therapy (targeted therapy)

The combined power of monoclonal antibody (MAb) and recombinant DNA technology has led to a series of 'designer' drugs, which have been engineered so that they:

- are exquisitely targeted
- have optimal effector function
- do not carry antigenic segments that may incite a neutralizing response in the host.

In general, this has meant a process of 'humanizing' antibodies of mouse origin and selecting an appropriate effector function. For example, a MAb designed to remove a subpopulation of lymphocytes from the patient should have good complement-fixing ability or bind well to receptors on phagocytes, whereas a MAb designed to 'modulate' a cell without depletion should have these functions removed. Many examples of MAbs in current use are described in individual chapters. Therapeutic MAbs are potent modifiers of essential components of immune responses and therefore carry both predictable and unpredictable risks. For example, anti-TNF therapies increase the risk of invasive viral and mycobacterial infection. The new inhibitors of integrins, such as natalizumab, have been associated with JC virus reactivation in patients, leading to progressive multifocal leukoencephalopathy (PML). Since integrins

i **Box 3.25 Classification of rejection**

Description	Timing of response	Immunological mechanism	Management
Hyperacute	Minutes to hours	Pre-formed antibodies (e.g. anti-blood group, anti-HLA)	Prevention with typing to avoid mismatch, or depleting antibodies for 'high-risk' transplants
Accelerated acute	1–5 days	T lymphocytes	Combinations of immune suppression used prophylactically and as required, e.g. corticosteroids, ciclosporin, tacrolimus, sirolimus, polyclonal antibodies (e.g. against all T lymphocytes) and monoclonal antibodies (e.g. against activated T lymphocytes expressing CD25)
Acute	7–14 days onwards	T lymphocytes	
Chronic	Months to years	Antibodies, complement, endothelial cell changes	Chronic oral immunosuppression

HLA, human leucocyte antigen.

are essential for the migration of T cells into tissues, the blockade prevents egress into inflammatory sites but also reduces immune surveillance of infection.

Chimeric antigen receptor T-cell therapy

Chimeric antigen receptor (CAR) T-cell therapy is an exciting new approach to the treatment of haematological malignancy. In the first licensed product of its kind (tisagenlecleucel) for B lymphocyte leukaemia and lymphoma, blood is taken from the patient and T lymphocytes are separated out. Using a retrovirus, the T lymphocytes are modified to express the CAR (which comprises a receptor for CD19 coupled to a powerful intracellular co-stimulation molecule). The CD19 target is expressed on all B lymphocytes (including lymphomas and B-cell leukaemias). The CAR-modified T lymphocytes are infused back into the patient and will then kill all target B lymphocytes. The main risk of this therapy is massive cytokine release from CAR T lymphocyte activation. Since all B lymphocytes (and not just the tumour cells) are removed, the patients develop antibody deficiency and require life-long immunoglobulin replacement. Specific co-stimulation domains in the CAR T cells have been shown to aid long-term persistence, correlating with prolonged protection against disease relapse. Further targets and approaches are now in clinical trials.

Immunosuppressive drugs

- *Glucocorticosteroids* (cortisone, hydrocortisone, prednisone and prednisolone) are the most commonly used steroids and have a variety of effects on immune function, including:
  - potent effects on monocyte production of the pro-inflammatory cytokines IL-1 and TNF-α

- o blockade of T lymphocyte production of IL-2 and IFN-γ
- o reduced activation and migration of a range of innate and adaptive immune cells.
- *Ciclosporin, tacrolimus and sirolimus (rapamycin)* have similar effects on T lymphocyte function. Ciclosporin and tacrolimus are calcineurin inhibitors and inhibit Ca^{2+}-dependent second messenger signals in T lymphocytes following activation via TCRs. By contrast, sirolimus achieves a similar effect but acts at the level of post-activation events in the nucleus.
- *Purine analogues* such as azathioprine are also frequently used as anti-inflammatory drugs in conjunction with steroids and act by inhibiting DNA synthesis in dividing adaptive immune cells. Similar in mode of action, but more powerful, is mycophenolate mofetil (MMF).
- *Alkylating agents* that interfere with DNA synthesis, such as cyclophosphamide, are also used for immunosuppression.
- *Kinase inhibitors* have profoundly improved the treatment of some malignancies with previously very poor outcomes. Tyrosine kinases (TYK) are ubiquitous regulators of cell activation, promoting cell division and proliferation in response to growth factors and cytokines. Inhibition of the signalling pathways can lead to immune suppression. In immune cells, the relevant kinases include the Janus kinases (JAK) that signal through the STAT pathway. Inherited mutations in JAK-STAT pathway molecules can lead to immunodeficiency or, if the mutation causes constant (constitutive) activation, can give rise to uncontrolled cell division independent of growth factors: that is, cancer. Specific inhibitors of TYK have been developed for a range of cancers and as T- and B-cell immune suppressants.

Cytokines and anticytokines

Cytokines are pleiotropic agents with powerful pro-inflammatory and immunosuppressive effects, and are attractive targets for therapies that inhibit or enhance their function. TNF-α targeting agents (cytokine modulators) have been tested in rheumatoid arthritis, as has the recombinant IL-1 receptor antagonist anakinra, although with much less success. None the less, the good safety profile of anakinra has prompted its use in other diseases, and a beneficial effect has been shown in type 2 diabetes, which may have an innate inflammatory component. IL-2 and its receptor (CD25) are also obvious candidates for immune therapies. Interferons are successfully used to boost pro-inflammatory immunity in chronic virus infection.

Restoring tolerance in autoimmune diseases and allergy

One of the goals of immune-based therapies for autoimmune disease is not simply to achieve immunosuppression, but also to restore immunological tolerance against the relevant autoantigens. In animal models, an effective means of achieving this is to administer the autoantigen itself, or key peptide epitopes from it. This is known as antigen-specific or peptide immunotherapy and is under trial for several autoimmune diseases, where it appears to induce Tregs. The diseases that have the most advanced clinical data are in the field of allergy. For example, administration of cocktails of peptides of the cat allergen Fel d 1 has led to a reduction in detectable skin-prick responses and improved clinical scores.

Intravenous immunoglobulin

Intravenous immunoglobulin (IVIg) is a preparation of polyspecific IgG chemically purified from the plasma of large numbers (>20 000) of healthy donors. IVIg is used as a replacement therapy in patients with primary and secondary antibody deficiencies. When it is used for inflammatory conditions, however, there is also a therapeutic benefit, although randomized, placebo-controlled studies are few. In the USA, IVIg is recommended only for a small number of diseases in addition to antibody deficiency. These include immune-mediated thrombocytopenia, Kawasaki's disease, chronic inflammatory demyelinating polyneuropathy and post-transfusion purpura.

The mechanism of action is not known, but may include:

- blockade of Fc receptors to prevent pathogenic antibodies binding to phagocytes
- inhibition of autoantibody synthesis by B lymphocytes
- modulation of dendritic cell function
- inhibition of complement activation
- inhibition of specific cytokines
- induction of T-cell regulation.

Further reading

Bluestone JA. Interleukin-mediated immunotherapy. *N Engl J Med* 2011; 365:2129–2139.

De Benedetti F, Gattorno M, Anton J et al. Canakinumab for the treatment of autoinflammatory recurrent fever syndromes. *N Engl J Med* 2018; 378:1908–1919.

Gelfand EW. Intravenous immunoglobulin in autoimmune and inflammatory diseases. *N Engl J Med* 2012; 367:2015–2025.

Maude SL, Laetsch TW, Buechner J et al. Tisagenlecleucel in children and young adults with B-cell lymphoblastic leukemia. *N Engl J Med* 2018; 378:439–448.

O'Shea JJ, Holland SM, Staudt LM. JAKs and STATs in immunity, immunodeficiency and cancer. *N Engl J Med* 2013; 368:161–170.

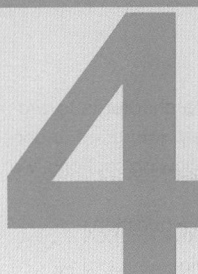

4 Evidence-based practice

Rosalind Raine and Helen Barratt

CORE SKILLS AND KNOWLEDGE

Estimates from various countries suggest that up to 40% of patients do not receive evidence-based healthcare. For example, despite the evidence for the effectiveness of prompt corticosteroids for Bell's palsy, almost half of patients (44%) do not receive this treatment, and provision is even lower for patients over the age of 60. Furthermore, 20% or more of healthcare is unnecessary or potentially harmful. For example, antibiotics for acute respiratory tract infection continue to be widely prescribed, despite being ineffective.

Evidence-based practice offers a framework to assist clinicians in making efficient and appropriate use of the available literature and taking informed decisions about its application. All doctors need to develop key skills in applying this framework to clinical scenarios, including:

- converting real-life clinical and population health problems into answerable questions
- locating the best available evidence
- appraising the evidence critically
- applying the evidence in practice.

Opportunities for developing skills in evidence-based medicine include attending (or setting up) a journal club where research papers are critically appraised, following the PICO approach – described later in this chapter – to apply evidence to particular dilemmas presenting in patients seen in clinical practice, visiting a local public health team to see how evidence is applied at a population level, or helping to write a local clinical guideline where evidence is applied at an institutional level.

INTRODUCTION

The evidence-based medicine movement emerged over 30 years ago and is widely accepted as the gold standard for medical decision-making. It was defined in 1996 as 'the conscientious, explicit, and judicious use of current best evidence in making decisions about the care of individual patients', with evidence in this case referring to peer-reviewed research literature. The focus has since expanded to include an emphasis on the importance of the patient and carer perspective in decision-making, alongside research evidence. We therefore refer in this chapter to evidence-based practice (EBP), which we define as '***an approach to decision-making in which the clinician uses the best scientific evidence available, in consultation with the patient, to decide upon the option that suits the patient best***'. This chapter will also embrace evidence-based public health practice, which applies evidence to wider populations, as well as individual patients.

The need for EBP

A number of factors have driven the rapid expansion of EBP. These include a growing awareness among health professionals of the gap between the large amount of good-quality research evidence available in the published literature and its often limited use in clinical practice. For example, thrombolysis using tissue plasminogen activator (tPA) is an evidence-based treatment that is effective in acute stroke. However, despite the potential benefits offered by thrombolysis, achieving and sustaining high rates of tPA delivery to eligible patients has proved problematic. EBP also has a role in ensuring that treatments offered by healthcare providers are of high value and accrue the most benefits for patients and the public – especially where escalating demands for care result in constrained resources.

Barriers to EBP

A multitude of barriers exist that lead to research evidence not being taken up into clinical practice, or to its being implemented in a delayed or patchy manner.

Knowledge barriers and the use of clinical guidelines

The most obvious barrier is lack of knowledge. It is estimated that general physicians would need to read 20 articles a day, all year round, to keep abreast of emerging knowledge in their specialist field. As research evidence continues to expand, clinical guidelines have become an important mechanism for informing day-to-day practice and helping clinicians keep up to date. Clinical guidelines identify, evaluate and summarize the best available research evidence relating to the management of specific conditions.

Consequently, they are a useful first port of call when seeking information on which to base decision-making. Guidelines are usually produced at national or international level by medical associations or government bodies. In the UK, the National Institute for Health and Care Excellence (NICE) provides recommendations about care for patients with specific conditions. In the USA, the National Guideline Clearing House maintains a catalogue of guidelines published by various health and medical associations, including the Agency for Healthcare Research and Quality.

While clinical guidelines are not legally binding, doctors are expected to take them into account, and yet the extent to which this happens in practice varies. For example, UK clinical guidelines recommend that patients with high blood pressure and raised cholesterol should receive antihypertensives, antiplatelet drugs and lipid-lowering drugs for the secondary prevention of ischaemic stroke. However, one study demonstrated that only 25.6% of men and 20.8% of women receive appropriate treatment, and the likelihood of 80–89-year-olds receiving secondary prevention is nearly half that of 50–59-year-olds.

Other factors limiting the implementation of EBP

These include:

- doubts about the accuracy of the research evidence being promoted
- national and local political values
- priorities and pressures from industry, patients, the public and clinicians
- cost.

These often interconnecting factors can lead to health policies being implemented *despite* the availability of contradictory evidence. For example, a programme of five-yearly preventative health checks for 40–74-year-olds is now mandatory across the National Health Service in England. It had been argued that the scheme would help prevent 1600 heart attacks yearly, saving at least 650 lives; prevent over 4000 people from developing diabetes; and detect at least 20 000 cases of diabetes or kidney disease earlier. However, the evidence suggests that general health checks:

- do not, in fact, reduce morbidity or mortality
- increase the number of diagnoses made, with consequent costs to the health service.

For example, although health checks lead to more diagnoses and more medical treatment for hypertension, this does not improve mortality or morbidity. Consequently, this intervention could be considered inappropriate, as the potential harms outweigh the expected benefits.

A framework for applying evidence to clinical problems

EBP offers a framework to assist clinicians in making efficient and appropriate use of the available literature and in reaching considered decisions about its application. The goal of this chapter is to promote ways in which evidence can be used wisely, with good understanding of its value and its limitations. In the following sections, we describe four essential steps:

- converting information needs into answerable questions
- locating the best available evidence
- appraising the evidence critically
- applying the evidence in practice.

Further reading

Krogsbøll LT, Jørgensen KJ, Grønhøj Larsen C et al. General health checks in adults for reducing morbidity and mortality from disease: Cochrane systematic review and meta-analysis. *BMJ* 2012; 345:e7191.

Muir Gray JA. *Evidence-Based Healthcare: How to Make Health Policy and Management Decisions*, 2nd edn. London: Churchill Livingstone; 2001.

Paul CL, Ryan A, Rose S et al. How can we improve stroke thrombolysis rates? A review of health system factors and approaches associated with thrombolysis administration rates in acute stroke care. *Implement Sci* 2016; 11:51.

Raine R, Wong W, Ambler G et al. Socio-demographic variations in the contribution of secondary drug prevention to stroke survival at middle and older ages: a cohort study. *BMJ* 2009; 338:b1279.

Sackett DL, Rosenberg WM, Gray JA et al. Evidence based medicine: what it is and what it isn't. *BMJ* 1996 13; 312:71–72.

ASKING ANSWERABLE QUESTIONS

Every day, doctors make multiple decisions that involve asking implicit and explicit questions. Evidence-based care protocols, pathways and clinical guidelines are available that cover the management of a wide range of both common and rare conditions, and these should generally be a clinician's first port of call.

Sometimes, however, a literature search is required – perhaps where a patient does not fit well into the categories dealt with by clinical guidelines, or where a condition is rare and not covered by good evidence-based summaries. The first step is to turn the information need into a focused question. This must be directly relevant to the patient at hand and incorporate the key issues that need to be present in research articles to inform the decision-making process. Identification of these key issues will allow formulation of a focused literature search strategy.

The *PICO approach* facilitates this process (**Box 4.1**), where *p*atient, *i*ntervention, *c*omparison and *o*utcome (PICO) are considered the four most key parts of a well-built clinical question.

SEARCHING FOR THE EVIDENCE

The next step is to identify relevant research evidence that will provide an answer to the clinical question. There are two main sources of evidence available.

Primary sources of evidence

These are comprised of the thousands of original articles published every year in research journals. Research papers are catalogued in a variety of databases, which are searchable on the Internet.

ℹ Box 4.1 Components of clinical questions structured using the PICO approach

Patient or problem (P)
- Who is the relevant patient?
- What is the condition or problem of interest?
- What are the most important characteristics of the patient?

Intervention (I)
- What is the management strategy of interest (e.g. diagnostic test, treatment)?

Comparison of interventions (C)
- What is the main alternative management strategy being considered, if any?

Outcome (O)
- What will the management strategy accomplish, measure, improve or affect?
- What are the patient-relevant consequences?

For many medical queries, Medline is the best-known database of health-related literature and makes a good starting place. The size and breadth of databases mean that a systematic searching approach is required to identify the best evidence available.

Secondary sources of evidence

In order to deal with the growing volume of primary research, secondary sources of evidence are increasingly consulted. Secondary sources are summaries and analyses of evidence derived from and based on primary sources. The Cochrane Library (UK) was one of the first online collections of databases relevant to medicine and other healthcare specialties, and includes the Cochrane Database of Systematic Reviews. Other organizations producing systematic reviews and other evidence syntheses to inform practice and policy include the Joanna Briggs Institute and the Campbell Collaboration.

How to conduct a search

Although biomedical databases vary in terms of their structure, the principles of using them are largely the same. Using the PICO approach to generate a clinical question is helpful, as the components can then be employed to select search terms for conducting a search in Medline. Text-word searching involves seeking specific words or

---

> ### *i* Box 4.2 Searching for evidence – worked example
>
> Charlie is a 20-year-old student who has attended his GP practice with a sore throat. You wonder whether antibiotics might help improve his symptoms.
>
> **Answerable clinical question**
> Are antibiotics effective in reducing the duration of symptoms in patients with upper respiratory tract infections?
>
> **PICO**
> *Patient problem or population*: Patients with a sore throat
> *Intervention or exposure*: Antibiotics
> *Comparison or control*: None
> *Outcome measure*: Duration of symptoms
>
> **Search terms in evidence/database (e.g. Medline)**
> "sore throat" AND antibiotics – 1032 articles
> "sore throat" AND antibiotics AND "symptom duration" – 6 articles
>
> **Answer**
> Antibiotics shorten the duration of symptoms by about 16 hours overall (Spinks A, Glasziou PP, Del Mar CB. Antibiotics for sore throat. *Cochrane Database of Systematic Reviews* 2013; 11. Art. No.: CD000023. https://doi.org/10.1002/14651858.CD000023.pub4.)

---

phrases, usually in the title or abstract of an article. The first step is to break the clinical question down into its individual components. **Box 4.2** contains a worked example, using the PICO approach.

Practical tips for searching databases include:

- Searching only for articles that include a full phrase, rather than individual words on their own, by putting double quotation marks around a group of words (e.g. "sore throat").
- Narrowing the search and reducing the number of citations identified by using AND in the database search function.
- Avoiding narrowing too far. Using the example question in **Box 4.2**, entering "*sore throat*" AND *antibiotics* in the search function will identify articles that contain both terms, whereas including "*sore throat*" AND *antibiotics* AND "*symptom duration*", theoretically yielding the highest concentration of relevant articles, may also miss others. Consequently, for routine clinical queries, using two terms in a search strategy is usually sufficient to focus the search.
- Engaging the help of expert health sciences librarians. This may be valuable in developing search strategies for more complex queries.
- Remembering the dangers of publication bias. Studies with negative results may not have made it as far as publication. On the other hand, studies may be in progress that could inform decision-making.

APPRAISING THE EVIDENCE

Once some potentially relevant research articles have been identified, the next step is to decide whether the studies described were undertaken in a way that makes their findings reliable and valid, and to consider the relevance of any articles to the clinical question identified. This process is known as critical appraisal.

The hierarchy of evidence

Ethically, patients should receive the best-evidenced treatment available, and the 'hierarchy of evidence' is a core principle of EBP that helps to ensure this. The hierarchy is formed by ***ranking study types based on the extent to which the reader can be confident that the results and estimates of a treatment effect are correct***. In most hierarchies, meta-analyses and systematic reviews are at the top of the pyramid, followed by experimental and observational studies, with case reports or case series at the bottom (**Fig. 4.1**). The hierarchy encourages a top-down approach to locating the best

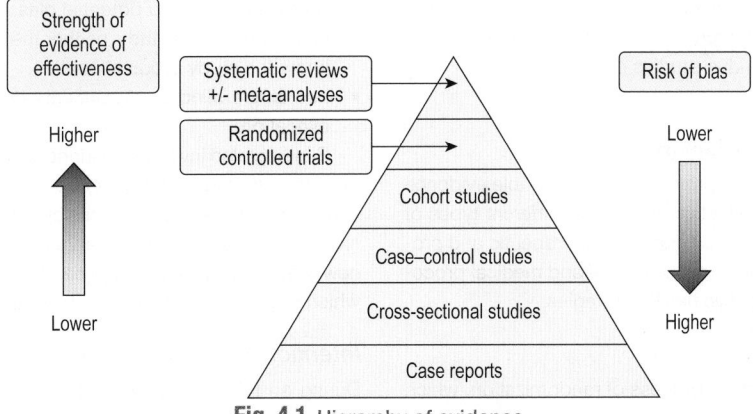

Fig. 4.1 Hierarchy of evidence.

evidence, which involves first searching for evidence at the top (e.g. a recent meta-analysis), and if that is not available, moving down to the next level of evidence.

Whatever the study design, when reading papers it is important to remain vigilant for poorly conducted research, as this diminishes the confidence that can be placed in the results.

Systematic reviews and meta-analyses
Systematic reviews

These synthesize the results of all available studies in a particular area, identified via comprehensive, systematic literature searches. They therefore provide a summary of current evidence about a topic, including an analysis of study results, strengths and weaknesses. Systematic reviews also highlight remaining gaps in knowledge or a lack of robust evidence. Data from all the included studies are combined to build up a broader picture of the evidence.

Systematic reviews aim to locate as much as possible of the research relevant to a particular research question. Explicit methods are then used to identify what can reliably be said about the topic, drawing on the findings of all the included studies. All study types can be included in a systematic review, including randomized controlled trials (RCTs) and observational studies, which are described later. A well-conducted review will assign a quality score to included studies so that the conclusions provide an overview of the status of the research field. For example, where there is a lot of robust evidence available to answer a question, clear recommendations can be made about patient care, or – in contrast – where there is a limited amount of low-quality evidence available, reliable recommendations cannot be made.

As systematic reviews draw together the findings of multiple studies, they lie at the top of the evidence hierarchy, though this position is not an absolute. For example, findings might quickly be superseded by evidence that is more recent. A large, well-conducted RCT may also provide more convincing evidence of effect than a systematic review of smaller RCTs.

Meta-analyses

These represent an extension of a systematic review. Data from each of the included studies are combined statistically to give a single estimate of effect. To conduct a meta-analysis, the included studies must address the same research question and make use of the same outcome measure. It can be carried out only when the relevant numerical data are presented in enough detail in the individual research papers.

An estimate of effect is calculated using weighted averages of all the results. The weighting given to individual studies is based on their sample size, with larger studies contributing more to the final meta-analysis than smaller ones. As meta-analyses pool findings from all the included studies, and therefore draw on data from a larger number of patients, they provide a stronger and more accurate estimate of a treatment effect than individual studies on their own.

Interventional studies
Randomized controlled trials (RCTs)

RCTs are generally considered to provide the most reliable evidence of whether an intervention is effective. A range of different types of intervention can be tested in an RCT, including therapeutic and prophylactic agents (e.g. drugs, vaccines), surgical and medical procedures, or health service and public health strategies.

Randomization

The strength of the RCT lies in the process of randomization, which is characteristic of this type of study design. Study participants are randomly assigned to one of two study groups: the experimental group who will receive the intervention being tested, and a comparison group (known as controls) who may receive:

- a conventional treatment (referred to as usual care)
- no intervention
- a placebo: a substance that resembles the intervention in all respects, except that it contains no active ingredients.

Every participant has an equal chance of being in the treatment group or the control group. The two groups are then followed up prospectively over time, to assess the effectiveness of the intervention compared with the conventional or placebo treatment.

The goal of randomization is to ensure that the two study groups are as similar as possible in all respects, apart from the treatment or intervention. Any other factors that might also have an impact on the outcome, known as confounders, should be distributed equally and randomly between the two groups. Consequently, any observed differences between the study groups are more likely to be due to differences in the treatment alone.

Those responsible for recruiting participants into a study must not influence the process of randomization. A common method of achieving this is randomization by telephone, where the investigator calls a central randomization service to obtain information about which study arm the participant should be allocated to.

Confounding factors

These are factors that could potentially influence both the exposure and the outcome in a study, leading to inaccurate results. For example, when the relationship between alcohol consumption (the exposure) and coronary heart disease (CHD; the outcome) is under examination, smoking may be a confounding factor. Smoking is correlated with alcohol consumption but is also associated with CHD, so may mask the true relationship between alcohol and CHD. Randomization is a way of trying to control for confounders, by ensuring that these factors are randomly (and, one hopes, fairly equally) divided between control and intervention groups.

Blinding

When a participant has been randomized, the investigator may or may not be aware of which group the participant has been allocated to. If they know which treatment the participant is receiving, this might influence (intentionally or unintentionally) the way in which they measure or interpret the outcome data, introducing bias into the study. For example, they may interpret information more favourably if it comes from participants who they know to be receiving the drug under investigation. Similarly, if a participant knows that they have been allocated to the placebo group, this may influence the way in which they participate in the trial. Therefore, blinding can be seen as a way to avoid potential bias.

- In a double-blind study, neither the patients nor the investigators know the study group allocation.
- In a single-blind study, patients do not know their study group allocation.

Blinding also involves ensuring that, as far as possible, the intervention and standard or placebo treatment both appear the same, although this may not be possible for non-drug interventions. For example, if the intervention involves physiotherapy exercises or a new way of delivering a service, it is often not feasible to conceal which group participants have been allocated to.

Intention-to-treat analysis

During an RCT, participants may be lost to follow-up for a range of reasons. Individuals may be unable to continue participating,

or may stop taking their allocated treatment – perhaps because of adverse side-effects or because they felt it was not working. If these individuals are subsequently excluded from the analysis of the results, the effectiveness of the drug may be overestimated. In the real world, patients do not always take their medication as prescribed, so RCT data are often examined using intention-to-treat analysis. The final results are analysed based on the treatment arm to which participants were initially allocated, and not on the treatment they actually received.

Limitations of RCTs

Although RCTs are considered to provide the most reliable evidence of effectiveness, by minimizing the possibility of bias, they are not without their limitations.

Patients to whom the results might subsequently be applied in real clinical practice may often be excluded from RCTs in order to minimize differences between experimental groups. For example, strict inclusion and exclusion criteria may mean that patients with co-morbidities are excluded, as this might affect their response to the intervention. However, many patients in the real world will have more than one condition. Patients recruited to trials are also more likely to be receiving care in teaching hospitals, where care may differ from that provided in district general hospitals. This reduces the external validity or generalizability of the trial, or the extent to which the findings can be applied in other settings.

Additionally, although RCTs are the gold standard for evaluating the effectiveness of interventions, randomization may not always be required. For example, an RCT may be unnecessary when the effect of an intervention is dramatic (e.g. vaccination for smallpox or penicillin for bacterial infections). In these cases, the likelihood of unknown confounding factors affecting the outcome is so small that they can be ignored.

An RCT may be unfeasible when the outcome of greatest interest occurs rarely (e.g. death), and may be too costly if the outcome of greatest interest occurs far in the future (e.g. loosening of artificial hip joints). Observational methods, such as cohort studies, may be the only practical means of obtaining such information in these cases.

Finally, the use of RCTs raises several ethical issues. RCTs are based on the premise that there is sufficient doubt about the particular intervention being tested to justify not giving it to half of the participants. At the same time, there must be sufficient belief in its potential benefit to justify exposing the remaining half of the patients. This is known as **clinical equipoise**, and requires careful consideration to be given to the intervention that is received by the control group. If an effective treatment already exists, participants in the control group should have this rather than a placebo, in order to make a transparent assessment of the novel intervention in comparison to usual care. Informed consent is required in all study designs but particularly so in RCTs. Participants need to understand that they are participating in an experiment and, consequently, may not receive the treatment under investigation.

Observational studies

Cohort studies

Cohort studies follow a group of individuals over a period of time (often years) to examine whether they benefit from a healthcare or public health intervention, or develop a disease or other outcome of interest. A cohort is a group of individuals who have a common characteristic. Cohorts are selected on the basis that individuals share similar, relevant characteristics, such as receiving cancer screening or being exposed to cigarette smoking. For example, the

British Doctors Study, which ran from 1951 to 2001, was a cohort made up of doctors, including both smokers and non-smokers. It provided convincing proof of the association between smoking and lung cancer, and led to a dramatic decline in smoking from the 1970s onwards.

Cohort studies are a type of observational study, meaning that no adjustments are made to participants' treatments or lifestyle. However, detailed information is collected about the interventions they receive, their sociodemographic characteristics, lifestyles and behaviours, and their outcomes, using questionnaires, interviews, physical examinations and investigations such as blood tests, and taking information from existing sources such as medical records. Cohort studies can therefore be prospective, involving the collection of new data, or retrospective, looking back in time and using existing data such as medical records. Retrospective studies are cheaper and faster to conduct because the data have already been collected and stored. However, because it was not collected for research purposes, information in patients' medical records may be incomplete, inaccurate and inconsistently recorded.

Cohort studies can also vary significantly in terms of their size and complexity. At one extreme, a large population may be studied over decades. For example, the Millennium Cohort Study (MCS) follows the lives of around 19 000 young people born across England, Scotland, Wales and Northern Ireland in 2000-1. Families were first assessed when children were 9 months old and have been followed up at regular intervals. Interviews are carried out with the main parent and the child, and a range of information is collected, including employment and income; housing; family structure; ethnicity; parenting activities such as reading to the child; developmental indicators; and both parental and child mental health. At the other extreme, some cohort studies follow up relatively small groups for a few days or weeks.

Cohort studies are particularly valuable in situations where RCTs cannot be performed because randomization is either unethical or impractical. They also allow rare or long-term outcomes to be assessed: for example, in the UK, the National Joint Registry collects information on a nationwide cohort of patients who have undergone joint replacement operations. Implants that fail earlier than expected can be identified and the information acted on. External validity (also referred to as generalizability) will be higher in large cohort studies such as this because a broad range of patients, from different settings, are included, without the restricted inclusion criteria required in an RCT.

A limitation of the cohort method is losses to follow-up. Cohort members may decline to continue participation in the study or fail to maintain contact. Such events may (or may not) be related to the exposure, the outcome or both. For example, a study looking at the effect of high-impact exercise on risk factors for osteoporosis had greater loss to follow-up in the group assigned to exercise. Women who dropped out may have had inherently lower bone strength that made the exercise less tolerable for them. If so, this would have produced selective loss of women more likely to develop osteoporosis from the active treatment group, and this would cause a biased estimate: specifically, an overestimate of the benefit of exercise.

Case–control studies

In a case–control study, patients who have received a healthcare intervention or developed a disease are identified. Their past history is then compared with that of individuals – or controls – who did not receive the intervention or do not have the disease. For example, participants with a disease of interest (e.g. lung cancer) may be tracked back in time, sometimes for many years, to determine whether they were exposed to a risk factor of interest (e.g. second-hand tobacco smoke). In another example, a study used primary healthcare records to look at service use in the previous year, in order to identify factors associated with frequent attendance at hospital emergency departments.

Researchers try to ensure that the cases and controls are as similar as possible with respect to other factors. This can be done either on an individual basis (e.g. by pairing each case with a control of the same age and sex) or in groups (e.g. choosing a control group with an overall age and sex distribution similar to that of the cases). Unknown differences may still exist between the cases and controls, however, which could influence the results.

A particular limitation of case–control studies is the risk of recall bias. Case participants are usually keen to find out what caused their illness, or may ascribe their positive and adverse outcomes to an intervention. As a result, they may be better motivated to remember details of their past than controls with no special interest in the study question. Assessing the exposure of controls may therefore be challenging, especially if this relies only on their personal recall. This risk can be lessened by using data from electronic medical records.

Case–control studies are another form of observational study because no intervention takes place. Since the assessment is retrospective and the risk of recall bias is high, case–control studies lie towards the bottom of the EBP hierarchy. However, they can provide interesting insights. For example, case–control studies start with people who are known to have a disease of interest, rather than looking at a population free of disease and waiting to see who develops it. This approach therefore lends itself to studying groups of patients with rare conditions. For example, in 1955, Richard Doll published a case–control study demonstrating a significant excess of the rare lung cancer mesothelioma among asbestos workers. This study was the first to identify asbestos as one of the world's most dangerous industrial carcinogens.

Cross-sectional surveys

These observational studies provide a snapshot of a particular group of patients or people at a single point in time, and can be used to assess the prevalence of illness or a risk factor, or the range of perceived symptoms in a given population. Examples include the proportion of patients with bladder cancer who smoke, or patient-reported outcomes on discharge from hospital.

As cross-sectional data describe only what is happening at a single moment in time, they cannot be used to answer questions about the causes of disease or the impact of treatment. They also do not provide information about changes over time, unless they are repeated. Consequently, they are ranked low in the EBP hierarchy of evidence.

Nevertheless, cross-sectional surveys can provide key information: for example, in planning services and ensuring that they are equipped to meet the needs of the local population. They may also be used to draw inferences about possible relationships between factors or outcomes, or to gather preliminary data to support further research and experimentation.

Case series or case reports

These describe a group of patients or a single individual with an outcome of interest, or novel and unusual features. Due to their descriptive nature, they provide little evidence about causality. Their small size and lack of representativeness also mean that they cannot be assumed to have relevance for the wider population of patients with the same condition. Therefore, they are regarded as the weakest form of evidence in the EBP hierarchy.

Nevertheless, they can still provide useful information, particularly in the very early stages of research into a disease area. For example, in 1985, the Centers for Disease Control in the USA published a report describing five cases of *Pneumocystis* pneumonia in previously healthy, gay men in Los Angeles. This was the first official reporting of what became known as the AIDS epidemic. However, case reports can also be misused: for example, the now discredited case series published in *The Lancet* in 1998, which posited a link between the measles, mumps and rubella vaccine, colitis and autism.

Problems with the 'hierarchy of evidence'

Although the evidence hierarchy has become widely accepted, concerns have been raised about ranking evidence in this way. As has been outlined, study designs traditionally ranked lower down the hierarchy may be more appropriate if, for example, outcomes of interest are rare or occur far into the future. Observational studies also produce results with higher external validity because inclusion and exclusion criteria are usually less restrictive. Additional concerns, including the extent to which the findings of RCTs can be applied to patients in other settings, are explored in the final section of this chapter.

The hierarchy focuses only on research addressing the question of the effectiveness of interventions. Other questions are equally salient, however, such as:
- prognosis (what is likely to happen?)
- harm (is this substance likely to have adverse effects?)
- experience (what is it like to receive this intervention?)
- implications for services (staff workload, the need for additional monitoring and so on).

Different types of question require different study designs (**Box 4.3**):
- Determining the number of patients living with a condition at a given point in time (a ***prevalence question***) may be best achieved using a cross-sectional survey. However, because it provides only a snapshot of that single time point, it cannot explain the likely duration between diagnosis and death.
- The design needed for a ***prognosis question*** is a cohort study – a study that follows up recently diagnosed patients and records what happens to them.
- To answer ***experience questions*** (what it is like to live with a particular condition, or whether a certain intervention is acceptable to patients), qualitative approaches, such as interviews or focus groups, are often also needed.

Combined approaches

Although there are big differences between the underlying assumptions of quantitative and qualitative research, the most comprehensive, generalizable and useful research is that which brings the two approaches together. For example, qualitative approaches can helpfully be used within an RCT to explore how an intervention was implemented and what was actually delivered, compared with what was intended. This is known as a ***process evaluation***, as it documents the process that took place. Process evaluation can explain discrepancies between expected and observed outcomes, help us to understand how local context influences outcomes, and provide insights to aid implementation in other settings.

Critical appraisal

Critical appraisal aims to:
- identify the methodological strengths and weaknesses of a piece of research

Box 4.3 Key messages about study design

Randomized controlled trials (RCTs)

- *Randomization* aims to ensure that the study groups are as similar as possible, apart from whether or not they receive the treatment being studied. Consequently, observed differences are more likely to be due to differences in the treatment alone.
- *Blinding* ensures that there are no differences in the way participants in each study arm are managed or their progress and outcome is measured. In a double-blind study, neither patients nor investigators know the study arm to which the participant has been allocated.
- In an *intention-to-treat analysis*, RCT findings are analysed based on the treatment arm to which participants were initially allocated, regardless of whether they dropped out of the study.
- Ensuring that RCT participants are as similar as possible enhances the *internal validity* of the results (i.e. their accuracy in the study context) but may reduce their *external validity* (i.e. their generalizability to the diverse range of patients with the condition under study).
- RCTs are a form of *experimental study*. The researcher manipulates exposure to the intervention (e.g. a new drug treatment) by allocating participants to the intervention or control group.

Observational studies

- In an *observational study*, the researcher measures exposures (e.g. new surgical procedures) that the participants are already receiving. Outcomes (e.g. postoperative complications) are then observed as they occur.
- In a *cohort study*, a group of participants (the cohort) is followed over time. Researchers observe which individuals develop outcomes of interest (e.g. breast cancer), and collect information about factors that might be relevant to the development of the outcome (e.g. smoking, alcohol consumption). Cohort studies can provide valuable evidence when conducting an RCT is unfeasible. The findings may have greater generalizability because inclusion and exclusion criteria are usually less restrictive.
- In a *case–control study*, patients who have an outcome of interest are identified (i.e. cases). Their past history is then compared with that of individuals – or controls – who do not. Cases and controls should be as similar as possible with respect to other factors. A particular limitation of case–control studies is the risk of recall bias because cases may be better motivated to remember details of their past than controls.

- assess whether the researchers used the right design for their study
- make informed decisions about the quality of the evidence being appraised
- establish how useful the piece of research is for wider decision-making.

A range of tools and checklists exist to help assess the quality of each design (see 'Further reading'). However, these checklists should merely supplement the level of careful thought and judgement required whenever reading a paper. Regardless of the study type, critical appraisal involves some overarching questions (**Box 4.4**); the three main steps involved are described below.

Question 1: Are the results of the study valid?

Validity refers to the soundness or methodological rigour of a study. A study is considered valid if the way it has been designed and carried out means that the results provide a trustworthy estimate of clinical effectiveness. A study that is **sufficiently free from bias** has internal validity.

Bias is a consistently occurring error in a study that results in an incorrect estimate of the association between an exposure and an outcome. For example, in a case–control study, recall bias may occur because a patient with an outcome of interest (e.g. lung cancer) may report their exposure experience (e.g. smoking) differently to a control without the outcome. This would then lead to an incorrect assessment of the relationship between smoking and lung cancer.

No study is perfect and free from all bias. A systematic check should be carried out to ensure that the researchers have done all they can to minimize it. Different study designs are prone to different types of bias but observational studies (and especially case–control studies) are particularly susceptible. More than 50 types of research bias have been identified but, for simplicity, they can be broadly grouped into two categories:

- *Information bias.* This results from systematic differences in the way in which data are collected from the various study groups, including data relating to either the exposure (i.e. factors that may be associated with an outcome of interest, such as weight) or the outcome (e.g. type 2 diabetes). For example, has participants' weight been recently recorded or does the study rely on information collected at the time they registered in primary care?

Box 4.4 Key questions in critical appraisal

Why was the study done?

- A clearly focused question should address population, intervention and outcomes.

What type of study was done?

- The study design must match the question asked.

What are the study characteristics?

- Use the PICO question format to help answer this question.

Are the results of the study valid?

- Was the assignment of patients to treatments in a controlled trial (RCT) randomized? If another design was used, how were participants allocated?
- Were patients, health workers and study personnel 'blind' to treatment allocation?
- Were all the patients who entered the study properly accounted for at its conclusion? Look for follow-up tables and whether patients in an RCT were analysed in the groups to which they were randomized.
- Were the groups similar at the start of the study?
- Aside from the experimental intervention, were the groups treated equally?

What were the results?

- How large was the treatment effect? How precise was the estimate of the treatment effect?
- Look for confidence limits and p-values.

Will the results help?

- Can these results be applied locally? Are these findings applicable to other patients?
- Were all relevant outcomes considered, including those relevant to patients?
- Are the benefits worth the harms and costs?

In this case, information might be systematically more accurate for patients with diabetes than for patients without weight-related conditions, leading to an incorrect estimate of the association between exposure and outcome.

- *Selection bias.* This occurs when there is a systematic difference between either:
  - those who participate in the study and those who do not *or*
  - those in the treatment arm of a study and those in the control group.

Patients and clinicians who have strong treatment preferences are often excluded from RCTs. While these steps increase the internal validity of an RCT, they often lead to selection bias and an overestimation of the benefits of treatment, especially for patient-centred outcomes. For example, some women with early breast cancer have a strong preference for less invasive lumpectomy, whereas others prefer the reassurance of knowing that all potentially cancerous tissue has been removed by a mastectomy. In one series of RCTs, only women without a strong preference for a particular treatment were recruited. However, as few as 10% subsequently agreed to have their treatment chosen at random, significantly reducing the extent to which the findings could be generalized to the wider population.

Similarly, telehealth interventions are becoming a prominent part of healthcare delivery, with examples including online cognitive behavioural therapy or home monitoring of health parameters such as blood pressure. There is some evidence of their effectiveness from RCTs. However, in several trials a large number of eligible individuals (over 75% in some cases) have declined to take parti. As well as compromising external validity, this may also indicate problems with the acceptability of the intervention, which may have a negative impact on uptake if it is later introduced into routine practice. In the case of telehealth, issues might include physical barriers in terms of accessing technology, as well as psychological barriers such as low confidence in using it.

Question 2: What are the results?

The second step of critical appraisal is to consider the results. A range of statistical methods are available to help determine whether an intervention is effective. Results are presented in many different ways but are typically expressed in terms of likely harms or benefits. In RCTs, cohort studies and case–control studies, two groups are compared and the results are often expressed as ratios. These are calculated by dividing the outcome in the intervention group by the outcome in the control group.

- If the outcome is measured as the ***likelihood*** or odds of an event occurring in a group (those with the event/those without the event), then this comparison is known as the odds ratio (OR).
- If the outcome is the ***frequency*** with which an event occurs in a group (those with the event/the total number in that group), then this is known as the relative risk or risk ratio (RR). A worked example is provided in **Box 4.5.**

When there is no difference between the groups, the OR and the RR are 1. A ratio of more than 1 means that the outcome occurred more frequently in the intervention group, compared with the control group. If this is a desired outcome, such as stopping smoking or using a new medicine, then the intervention worked. If the outcome is not desired – for example, death – then the control group performed better. Similarly, if the ratio is less than 1, then the outcome occurred less frequently in the intervention group.

Results may be more helpful when they are presented as absolute, rather than relative, numbers. For example, a relative risk reduction as large as 50% is likely to influence decision-making. However, decision-makers also need to understand whether this represents an absolute difference in risk of, say 0.1-0.2%, rather than 10-20%. To express a result in terms of absolute numbers, the proportion of events in the control group is subtracted from that in the intervention group. The risk difference can also be presented as the number needed to treat (NNT, **Box 4.6**).

Confidence intervals and p-values

The results of many tests that examine the relationship between an intervention and an outcome are expressed using confidence intervals and p-values (**Box 4.7**). There will always be some uncertainty about the true result because trials provide us with only a sample of possible results. However, the confidence interval (CI) gives the range of where the 'true' value in the population can be found. CIs are usually expressed for a given degree of certainty, usually 95%. This means that we can be 95% confident that the true value lies within those limits.

In contrast, p-values report the probability of seeing a result, such as the one obtained, if, in fact, the intervention had no real effect. In other words, how likely is the result to have occurred by chance? p-values can range from 0 (absolutely impossible) to 1 (absolutely certain). A p-value of less than 0.05 means that a result, such as the one seen, would occur by chance on less than 1 in 20 occasions. In this circumstance, a result is described as statistically significant. However, judgement should be applied to the p-value because a statistically significant result may not be clinically significant, if, for example, the effect size is too small to make a meaningful difference to patients.

CIs are more informative than p-values because they provide a range of values that are likely to include the true effect. Statistical non-significance may occur because the study sample size was too small. This is often indicated by very wide CIs. A bigger sample will result in small CIs and hence a more precise estimate of the effect of the intervention. As we have seen, however, statistical significance does not necessarily equal clinical significance. The best-quality studies first define and then examine evidence of an effect that is meaningful to patients and their clinicians.

Question 3: Will the results help?

The final step of critical appraisal is considering whether the study is applicable to the decision being made for a particular patient. There are three issues to consider here.

First, are there any ***important differences*** between the participants in the study and the patient in question? These must be identified, as they could have an impact on the effectiveness of an intervention. Check the study inclusion and exclusion criteria, which are usually reported in the methods section. Would the patient in your care have been eligible for inclusion in the study? Identify any characteristics that the patient has that were not considered in the study.

Second, many interventions and processes used in everyday clinical practice have both benefits and ***adverse consequences***, and these should be weighed against each other. For example, breast cancer screening programmes in the UK currently invite women aged 50–70 years to undergo mammography every 3 years. Breast screening helps identify breast cancer early. The earlier the condition is found, the better the chances of surviving it, and the less likely patients are to need a mastectomy or adjuvant therapy (chemotherapy and/or radiotherapy). However, for each woman with breast cancer whose death is prevented by screening, three women will be over-diagnosed. Over-diagnosis refers to the detection of cancers through screening that would not have become clinically apparent in the woman's lifetime. Although their cancer would not have caused their death, these women will undergo treatment, such as surgery, which may result in side-effects and complications, as well as psychological, social and financial consequences. Of the 307 000 UK women aged 50–52 years who are invited to begin screening every year, just over 1% will be over-diagnosed with cancer in the next 20 years. This risk of unnecessary treatment, and the potential associated harms, means that the appropriateness of breast cancer screening is hotly debated.

> *i*   **Box 4.5** Interpreting odds ratios, relative risk, confidence intervals and p-values – worked example

A randomized controlled trial was conducted to examine the benefits of prescribing the antiplatelet agent clopidogrel in addition to aspirin in patients with an ST-elevation myocardial infarction (MI). A total of 45 852 patients admitted to hospital within 24 h of suspected acute MI onset were randomly allocated to a group receiving clopidogrel 75 mg daily (n = 22 961) or a group receiving a matching placebo (n = 22 891). Both groups also received aspirin 162 mg daily. Treatment was continued until discharge or up to 4 weeks in hospital (mean 15 days in survivors). One of the pre-specified primary outcome measures was death from any cause during the scheduled treatment period. Some 1726 (7.5%) of the participants in the clopidogrel group died during the treatment period, compared with 1845 (8.1%) in the placebo arm. OR = 0.93 (95% CI 0.87–0.99, p = 0.03 (COMMIT Collaborative Group. Addition of clopidogrel to aspirin in 45,852 patients with acute myocardial infarction: randomised placebo-controlled trial. *Lancet* 2005; 366:1607–1621).

The findings of the trial can be summarized in a 2 × 2 table.

	Event *Death from any cause*	No event *No death/alive*	Total
Intervention arm *Clopidogrel group*	D_I *1726*	A_I *21 235*	N_I *22 961*
Control arm *Placebo group*	D_C *1845*	A_C *21 046*	N_C *22 891*

D_I, D_C, A_I and A_c are the numbers of participants with each outcome ('D' or 'A') in each group ('I' or 'C'). Text in italics refers to the study described earlier.

Odds ratios (OR)

An odds ratio is a relative measure of effect, which allows comparison of the intervention group of a study to the comparison or placebo group.

The trial compared participants who had received clopidogrel (intervention arm) with participants who had received a placebo (control arm). The outcome – or event – of interest was mortality from any cause, and the findings were as follows:

Odds of all-cause mortality in clopidogrel group (intervention arm):
= Number of participants with an event/Number of participants with no event
= Number of participants who died/Number of participants who remained alive
= D_I/A_I
= 1726/21 235 = 0.0812 (4 decimal places)

Odds of all-cause mortality for placebo group (control arm):
= Number of participants with an event/Number of participants with no event
= Number of participants who died/Number of participants who remained alive
= D_C/A_C
= 1845/21 046 = 0.0877 (4 decimal places)

Odds ratio:
= Odds of event in intervention arm/Odds of event in control arm
= $(D_I/A_I)/(D_C/A_C)$
= 0.0813/0.0877 = 0.93

An odds ratio of 0.93 means that the odds of death in the clopidogrel group (intervention arm) are 7% less than in the placebo group (control arm).
Here, the OR is <1, so the intervention is better than the control.
If the OR were >1, the control would be better than the intervention.

If the OR were = 1, there would be no difference between the two study groups, as the outcome is the same in both.

Relative risk (RR)

Risk of event in clopidogrel group (intervention arm):
= Number of participants with an event/Total number of participants
= D_I/N_I
= 1726/ 22 961
= 0.0752 (4 decimal places)

Risk of event in placebo group (control arm):
= Number of participants with an event/Total number of participants
= D_C/N_C
= 1845/22 891
= 0.0806 (4 decimal places)

Risk ratio:
= Risk of event in intervention group/Risk of event in control arm
= $(D_I/N_I)/(D_C/N_C)$
= 0.0752/0.0806 = 0.93

A risk ratio, also known as the relative risk, of 0.93 means that the risk of death in the clopidogrel group (intervention arm) is 7% less than in the placebo group (control arm). The RR is <1, so again the intervention is better than the control.

If an outcome is relatively rare (e.g. death in this study), then the odds ratio will be very similar to the risk ratio.

Confidence intervals (CI)

The confidence interval indicates the level of uncertainty around a measure of effect (i.e. the precision of the effect estimate), which in this study was expressed as an odds ratio. Confidence intervals are used because a study recruits only a small sample of the overall population. By interpreting upper and lower confidence limits, we can infer that the true population effect lies between these two points. Most studies report the 95% confidence interval (95% CI).

If the confidence interval crosses 1 (e.g. 95% CI 0.9–1.1), this implies that there is no difference between the two arms of the study. If it does not (e.g. 95% CI 0.7–0.8), then a difference exists.

In the trial comparing clopidogrel to placebo, OR = 0.93 (95% CI 0.87–0.99). This can be interpreted as follows: the odds of death in the clopidogrel arm are 7% less than in the placebo arm, and we can be 95% confident that the true population effect lies between 13% and 1%.

p-values

The p-value in this study is 0.03. This means that if clopidogrel actually had no effect, compared to the placebo, there is a 3% of chance that the study result (i.e. the observed difference) occurred by chance.

A p-value of <0.05 indicates that there is a statistically significant difference between groups. A p-value of >0.05 indicates that the difference is not statistically significant.

Conclusion

The trial comparing clopidogrel to placebo stated OR = 0.93 (95% CI 0.87–0.99, p = 0.03). This means that the odds of death in the clopidogrel arm are 7% less than in the placebo arm, and we can be 95% confident that the true population effect lies between 13% and 1%. This result was statistically significant (https://ebm.bmj.com/content/ebmed/11/3/82.full.pdf).

Finally, ***cost-effectiveness*** is commonly not reported in the analysis of clinical trials. If a treatment is effective but provides only a small benefit and is very expensive, it may not be a good use of resources. Equally, even if a treatment is shown to be cost-effective, it may not be affordable. In the UK, NICE uses the cost per quality-adjusted life-year (QALY) to judge the cost-effectiveness of new technologies. This is the estimated cost of each additional year of life gained by a treatment or procedure, measured not just in terms of extra months or years of life, but in terms of the quality of that life. This is defined, for example, as

freedom from or reduction in pain, or the ability to carry out the basic activities of daily living. Currently, NICE uses a threshold of £20 000–£30 000 per QALY. Treatments that come in at or below the threshold are usually approved. Those that come in above tend not to be judged cost-effective and so are not recommended for adoption by the NHS. Again, however, affordability to the healthcare system is not taken into account by this approach. For example, a treatment may result in significant quality of life gains, but be very expensive and applicable only to a small subset of patients with a particular condition.

Box 4.6 Relative risk, absolute risk and number needed to treat – worked example

A study compared the incidence of dyskinesia after treatment with either ropinirole (ROP) or levodopa (LD) in patients with early Parkinson's disease.[a] A total of 17 of 179 patients who took ROP (treatment group) and 23 of 89 who took LD (control group) developed dyskinesia. The risk of developing dyskinesia among patients who took ROP was 17/179 = 0.095, whereas the risk of developing dyskinesia among patients who took LD was 23/89 = 0.258.

The *relative risk* of a treatment equals the risk in the treated group divided by the risk in the control group (i.e. the risk ratio).

Absolute risk reduction (ARR) is the difference between the risk of an event in the treated group and the risk of an event in the control group (i.e. risk in treatment group minus risk in control group).

In the Parkinson's trial, the relative risk was 0.095/0.258 = 0.368. This means that the risk of dyskinesia was 63.2% lower in the ROP group. However, the ARR was 0.258 − 0.095 = 0.163. This means that, by using ROP rather than LD, the risk of developing dyskinesia was reduced by 16%. While the RR is useful for summarizing the trial findings, the ARR provides a better indication of the likely clinical benefit of using ROP, rather than LD.

Based on the ARR, the *number needed to treat (NNT)* is the reciprocal of the absolute risk reduction (i.e. 1/ARR). This measure indicates the number of patients that need to be treated to achieve the desired outcome in 1 patient who would not have benefited otherwise.

In the trial, the number needed to treat = 1/ARR = 1/0.163 = 6.13. This means that at least 6 patients would need to be treated with ROP, rather than LD, to achieve the desired outcome in 1 patient who would not have benefited otherwise.

[a]Rascol O, Brooks D, Korczyn AD et al. A five-year study of the incidence of dyskinesia in patients with early Parkinson's disease who were treated with ropinirole or levodopa. *N Engl J Med* 2000; 342:1484–1491.

 Box 4.7 Estimating confidence in research findings

95% confidence interval
We can be 95% confident that the true value lies within the limits given.

p-value
The likelihood that a given result has occurred by chance alone (e.g. if $p < 0.001$, then the result would occur only 1:1000 times by chance).

Further reading

Black N. Why we need observational studies to evaluate the effectiveness of health care. *BMJ* 1996; 312:1215–1218.
Greenhalgh T. *How to Read a Paper: The Basics of Evidence-Based Medicine*. London: Wiley–Blackwell; 2014.
Petrie A, Sabin C. *Medical Statistics at a Glance*. London: Wiley–Blackwell; 2009.
Straus SE, Glasziou P, Richardson WS et al. *Evidence-Based Medicine*. Edinburgh: Elsevier/Churchill Livingstone; 2018.
http://www.casp-uk.net/casp-tools-checklists *Critical Appraisal Skills Programme (CASP) checklists*.

APPLYING THE EVIDENCE

The medical literature is continuously expanding, with new information published every day that could help to improve care for patients and population health. However, there are often major challenges involved in implementing the findings of research in clinical practice, with some estimates suggesting that the process takes an average of 17 years. The gap leads not only to the under-use of effective interventions, but also to the incorrect use of others, as well as the over-use of unhelpful or unproven interventions. All of this means negative outcomes for patients and for population health. It is also a waste of health service resources and of costly and time-consuming research. Consequently, considerable effort has been put into improving the routine use of research findings.

Challenges of implementing evidence

Trial design

RCTs are designed to minimize the possibility of bias in the results, so that any observed variation can be interpreted as a causal relationship. They may achieve this internal validity at the expense of external validity or generalizability. There are three reasons why RCTs in many areas of healthcare may have low external validity:

- *The provider.* The healthcare professionals who participate may be unrepresentative. They may have a particular interest in the topic or be enthusiasts and innovators.
- *The setting.* This also may be atypical: a teaching hospital, for example.
- *The patients.* All trials exclude certain categories of patients: for example, older patients or those with more than one illness. Often the exclusion criteria are so restrictive that the patients who are eligible for inclusion represent only a small proportion of the patients being treated in normal practice.

The outcome of drug treatment is likely to be unaffected by the characteristics of the prescribing doctor or the setting in which it is administered. On the other hand, the outcome of activities such as surgery and physiotherapy may be highly dependent on the characteristics of the provider, setting and patients. As a result, RCTs generally offer an indication of the *efficacy* of an intervention, rather than its actual *effectiveness* in everyday practice. For successful implementation, however, both external validity and effectiveness are required if the findings are to be generalized to different patients and different settings.

Pragmatic RCTs

In a conventional RCT, the principal aim is to establish whether a treatment works. As outlined, because of the emphasis placed on internal validity, these 'explanatory' RCTs generally provide evidence of efficacy, or what can be achieved in ideal circumstances.

However, the ultimate goal is to improve the health of real people in real settings, so it is crucial also to know whether an intervention is going to be effective in the real world. In contrast to explanatory trials, pragmatic RCTs place the emphasis on effectiveness rather than efficacy, and seek to measure the benefit that the treatment produces in routine clinical practice; they therefore provide better evidence for decision-making.

There are some key differences between explanatory and pragmatic trials:

- Explanatory trials recruit as homogeneous a population as possible. In contrast, the design of a pragmatic trial reflects variations between patients that occur in real clinical practice.
- It may not be possible to blind participants and investigators to the treatment that is being given. Such biases are not necessarily viewed as detrimental in a pragmatic trial.
- In pragmatic trials, outcome measures should represent the full range of health gains relevant to patients and clinicians, e.g. both a reduction in mortality after stroke and an improvement in quality of life.
- The two approaches to trial design will sometimes arrive at different conclusions about the benefit of a treatment because a treatment that works in an ideal setting may not work in real life.

The difference could also stem from the fact that improvement in a biomedical end-point does not produce the expected health gain. For example, although fluoride treatment for osteoporosis increases a commonly measured biomedical end-point (non-vertebral bone density), it actually raises fracture rates (an important clinical end-point) because it increases skeletal fragility. Consequently, it is not effective treatment for postmenopausal osteoporosis.

Patient-centred outcome measures

Research only has external validity if it reflects the wider priorities of patients and, for population health research, the public. For this reason, the outcomes of most relevance to patients must be included in trials. In one study, for example, patients with multiple sclerosis and their doctors were independently asked to select the three aspects of the disease that had the greatest effect on quality of life. Doctors focused mainly on the physical effects of the disease, whereas patients were more concerned about mental health, emotional wellbeing, general health and vitality, which are often not measured in RCTs. Similarly, in RCTs of anticonvulsants, individuals with epilepsy are much more interested in the proportion of patients rendered free of seizures than they are in changes in mean seizure frequency (a commonly used measure of benefit in RCTs).

Barriers and facilitators to change

Almost all healthcare interventions are complex and involve several interacting components. For example, a new drug therapy may superficially seem simple to implement and yet the process might actually require additional patient monitoring or allow management to move from an inpatient to a community setting, requiring a change in care pathways. Other new interventions may necessitate amendments to referral processes (e.g. by allowing direct access to hospital care) or involve care provision by different staff (e.g. allied health professionals rather than doctors). These changes may involve modification of working practices, equipment and care setting, and entail additional unforeseen costs. It is often not clear which of the specific components of these complex interventions represent the 'active ingredient' for bringing about the intervention's effect.

If interventions are to be rolled out in other settings, careful consideration should be given to ensuring that interventions are designed in such a way as to be easily and successfully replicated. This involves trying to identify not only the key 'ingredients' that must be included, but also whether or not the intervention might be sensitive to particular features of the local setting.

Intervention context

Barriers to change can arise at different levels in the healthcare system: the patient, their carer and family, the individual care professional, the healthcare team, the healthcare organization (e.g. its resources, capabilities, structure, culture and politics) and wider society (e.g. the economic, social and political environment). Each of these components makes up the context of the intervention (**Fig. 4.2**). When a new intervention is being implemented, consideration should be given to what will happen when these individual contextual factors interact. Because of the complexity and diversity of each of these factors, the effect is likely to differ in different settings.

For example, reduction in hospital-acquired infections is a healthcare priority in many countries. Hand-washing plays a key role. However, concordance on the part of healthcare workers in general, and doctors in particular, is known to be poor. Doctors

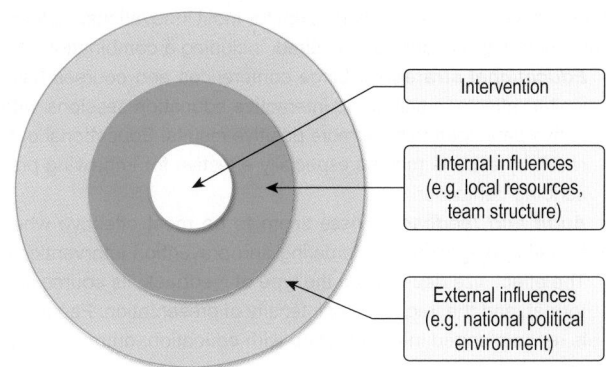

Fig. 4.2 Contextual factors that influence the implementation of evidence.

are generally aware of the evidence but overestimate their own hand-washing practices. Most countries and many hospitals have guidelines on prevention of infections but they are frequently not followed. This means that, despite well-established evidence that has been properly disseminated, performance remains poor.

What is the problem? Research has shown that a range of competing demands reduce the likelihood of doctors washing their hands. These include a high workload; organization of the ward and access to facilities; concerns about skin irritation; lack of knowledge of the evidence; a lack of leadership to encourage change and mutual accountability; and an absence of institutional policies. Even if doctors are aware of the evidence and are willing to change, altering well-established patterns of care is difficult, if the clinical environment is not conducive to change. These factors will be present to differing extents in different settings. The key ones should be identified in each location to ensure that change comes about.

Leadership

Local leadership has been identified as key to ensuring that evidence is used in practice. Leadership includes the actions taken by formal leaders in an organization to influence change. The attributes and qualities of leaders that appear to facilitate the use of research evidence to change practice include:

- valuing research
- being knowledgeable about research
- role-modelling evidence-based practice
- involving other staff in decision-making
- supporting changes in practice
- ensuring that policy and procedures are evidence-based and up-to-date.

Resistant leadership that fails to support change reduces the likelihood that evidence will be applied in practice.

Improving the uptake of evidence

There is a growing body of evidence relating to the effectiveness of different interventions to improve the uptake of evidence and change clinical and public health practice, which includes synthesizing and disseminating evidence in more accessible formats. For example, information graphics (or 'infographics') utilize images and data visualizations (pie charts, bar graphs, line graphs) to present research in an engaging way. Infographics add value by enhancing understanding and the reach of research. Information is more likely to be retained if it has been learned from an infographic than from text alone. However, although this may help ensure the uptake of some simple changes, it is insufficient for most innovations. Instead, multifaceted approaches are required, including a combination of:

- **Educational strategies.** Large conferences and courses have limited effects; small group interactive education sessions with active participation have more positive results. Educational outreach by experts may be especially effective for improving prescribing behaviour.
- **Audit and feedback.** These seem to be most effective when targeting diagnostic test ordering and prevention interventions. The effect size depends on the type of feedback, its source and format, and the frequency or intensity of presentation. Feedback is recommended in combination with education, outreach visits or reminders.
- **Use of reminders and computers.** Computer prompts, for example, may be one of the most effective interventions. They have been shown to be particularly effective for increasing the use of prevention interventions, e.g. vaccination and cancer screening reminders.

All of these interventions have the potential to help facilitate the effective transfer of evidence to practice, although the evidence base for them is still emerging. More than one approach may be needed. Further research is on-going to increase understanding of the processes and elements behind successful change.

Further reading

Bauer M, Damschroder L, Hagedorn H et al. An introduction to implementation science for the non-specialist. *BMC Psychol* 2015; 3:32.

Grol R, Grimshaw J. From best evidence to best practice: effective implementation of change in patients' care. *Lancet* 2003; 362:1225–1230.

Wensing M. Implementation science in healthcare: introduction and perspective. *J Evid Training Qual Health Care* 2015; 109:97–102.

Online material at StudentConsult.com includes a significant amount of additional content, including practical exercises based on published clinical evidence, to help readers put into practice the principles described in this chapter.

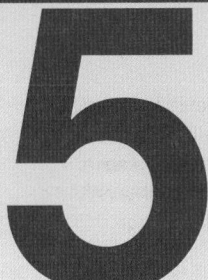

5 Ethical practice and clinical communication

Deborah Bowman and Annie Cushing

CORE SKILLS AND KNOWLEDGE

At its heart, the practice of medicine is a human endeavour concerned with forming therapeutic relationships with patients. It is crucial for everyone practising medicine to understand the moral and legal framework that underlies and regulates their work. Likewise, effective communication is fundamental to achieving optimal patient-centred care, maintaining safety and ensuring optimal health outcomes. Patients expect humanity and empathy from their doctors, as well as competence.

In routine practice, ethical and legal decisions are made on a daily basis by clinical teams working with patients and, where appropriate, involving their families. Sometimes an ethics committee's view or a legal opinion may be sought. If situations are contested and disagreement seems intractable, the courts will occasionally make a decision. Many clinicians have qualifications in ethics and law, and further study can lead to academic, policy, legal, ethical and leadership roles.

All doctors should develop:

- an awareness of key *moral theories* and ethical tools
- an understanding of legal concepts and principles
- the cognitive skills necessary for reasoning, critiquing and communicating ethical decisions
- a range of advanced communications skills for listening and speaking to all types of people in a range of different settings.

Communication ability is not just innate. There is an evidence base for effective skills that can be developed by training and experience. Reflect carefully about your practice and seek feedback. Remain informed about changes in the law, ethical guidance and professional standards. University departments, specialist sections in general medical journals and, in the UK, the General Medical Council, the British Medical Association's ethics team and the Institute of Medical Ethics are good starting points for further exploration.

ETHICS AND THE LAW

Ethics: what it includes and why it matters

The subject of ethics incorporates knowledge, cognitive skills such as reasoning, critique and logical analysis, and skills for integrating abstract ethical learning with other clinical learning and applying it appropriately. Unless students and clinicians are able to draw on learning in ethics to enhance daily practice and better serve their patients, ethics education has ultimately failed.

The practice of medicine is inherently moral:

- Biomedical expertise and clinical science have to be applied by and to people.
- Medical decisions are underpinned by values and principles.
- Potential courses of action will have implications that are often uncertain.
- Technological advancements sometimes have unintended or unforeseen consequences.

The profession has to agree on its collective purpose, aims and standards. People are much more than a collection of symptoms and signs – they have preferences, priorities, fears and hopes. Doctors, too, are much more than interpreters of symptoms and signs – they also have preferences, priorities, fears and hopes. Ethics is part of practice; it is a practical pursuit.

Ethical reasoning may sound grand or even off-putting but it is simply thinking through the available options and weighing the relative merits logically and thoroughly. Becoming, and practising as, a doctor demands an awareness of, and reflection on, our ethical attitudes. All of us have personal *values* and moral intuitions. In the field of ethics, a necessary part of learning is becoming aware of the assumptions on which these personal values are based, reflecting on them critically, and listening and responding to challenging or opposing beliefs.

A frequently heard complaint about ethics is that there is 'no right answer'. While ethics often incorporates diverse analyses, leading sometimes to a number of different conclusions, there are ways of approaching an ethical issue that are dependent on an accurate understanding of the **relevant law, professional guidance** and clear elucidation of the relevant moral questions. In other words, there is information to learn and there are ways of expressing views that provide structure and rigour. Personal views are important, but need to acknowledge other perspectives, be supported by reasoning and be located in an accurate understanding of the current law and relevant professional guidance.

Ethics is commonly characterized as the consideration of big moral questions that preoccupy the media. Questions about cloning, stem cells and euthanasia are what many immediately think of when the words 'medical ethics' are used. However, ethics pervades all of medicine. The daily and routine workload is rife with ethical questions, choices and dilemmas; introductions to patients, dignity on the wards, the use of resources in clinic, the choice of antibiotic; knowing whether and when to challenge a colleague, how to balance one's own wellbeing in a demanding clinical practice, or whether to provide a medical report for a third party – all of these are as central to ethics as the issues that pervade the common representation of this area.

Ethics and law are a core part of most medical curricula and postgraduate training programmes. Formal teaching ranges from didactic lectures to small group discussions, and from sessions led by specialists in ethics to those led by patients. There are plenty of specialist books, journals and online resources to provide additional material to supplement the core curriculum. Much of what is learned in ethics will, like other areas of clinical practice, develop by watching others. **Role models**, both positive and less so, are influential, and most students and doctors will be exposed to a wide range of approaches, ethical engagement and practice. Noting when you admire or are discomfited by someone will teach you much about what you value and what kind of a practitioner you want to be (and remain).

Ethical practice: sources, resources and approaches

Engaging with an ethical issue in clinical practice depends on:
- discerning the relevant moral question(s)
- looking at the relevant **ethical theories** and/or tools
- identifying applicable guidance (e.g. from a professional body)
- integrating the **ethical analysis** with an accurate account of the law (both national and international).

Personal views must be taken into account, but other perspectives should also be acknowledged and supported by reasoning, and reflect an accurate understanding of the current law and relevant professional guidance.

Key ethical theories that you might encounter are summarized in **Box 5.1**.

Many people find that frameworks and tools that focus on the application of ethical theory to clinical problems are useful. Perhaps the best known is the **'Four Principles'** approach:
- **autonomy**: allowing 'self-rule', i.e. letting patients make their own choices and decide what happens to them
- **beneficence**: doing good, i.e. acting in a patient's best interests
- **non-maleficence**: avoiding harm
- **justice**: treating people equitably and fairly.

For others, a consistent process, almost like a checklist, that incorporates the best of each theoretical approach works well. For example, whatever the ethical question, one should:
- summarize the problem and state the moral dilemma(s)
- identify the assumptions being made or that are to be made

> **i   Box 5.1 Key ethical theories**
>
> - **Deontology**: a universally applicable rule or duty-based approach to morality, e.g. a deontologist would argue that one should always tell the truth, irrespective of the consequences.
> - **Consequentialism**: an approach that argues that morality is located in consequences. Such an approach will focus on likely risks and benefits.
> - **Virtue ethics**: an approach in which particular traits or behaviours are identified as desirable.
> - **Rights theory**: an assessment of morality with reference to the justified claims of others. Rights are either 'natural' and arise from being human, or legal and therefore enforceable in court. Positive rights impose a duty on another to act, while negative rights prohibit interference by others.
> - **Narrative ethics**: an approach that argues that morality is embedded in the stories shared between patient and clinician, and allows for multiple perspectives.

- analyse with reference to ethical principles, consequences, professional guidance and the law
- acknowledge other approaches and state the preferred one with explanation.

Do not be afraid to experiment with ways of thinking about and approaching ethics. Whatever approach you favour, the steps set out at the beginning of this section provide a structure. What this means in practice is shown in the scenario in **Box 5.2**.

Professional guidance and codes of practice

As well as ethical theories and frameworks, there are **codes of practice and professional guidelines**. For example, in the UK, the standards set out by the General Medical Council (GMC) inform doctors' regulation; if a doctor falls below the expectations of the GMC, disciplinary procedures may follow, irrespective of the harm caused or whether legal action ensues. In other countries, similar professional bodies license doctors and regulate healthcare. All clinicians should be aware of the regulatory framework and professional standards in the country within which they practise.

Ethical practice and professionalism are significant from the earliest days of medical study and training. In the UK, the GMC defines the standards expected of medical students, and all medical schools are required to have 'fitness to practise' procedures. Students should be aware of their professional obligations from the beginning. All medical schools are effectively vouching for a student's suitability for provisional registration at graduation. Medical students commonly work with patients from the earliest days of their training and are privileged in the access they have to vulnerable people, confidential information and sensitive situations. As such, medical schools have particular responsibilities to ensure that students behave professionally and are fit to study, and eventually to practise, medicine.

The Hippocratic Oath, although well known, is outdated and rarely, if ever, sworn. The symbolic value of taking an oath remains, however, and many medical schools expect students to make a formal commitment to maintain ethical standards.

Further reading

General Medical Council. *Good Medical Practice*. London: GMC; 2013, updated 2019.
General Medical Council. *Medical Students: Professional Values and Fitness to Practise*. London: GMC; 2016.
General Medical Council. *Outcomes for Graduates*. London: GMC; 2018.

Box 5.2 Vignette 1

Malik is a junior doctor who works on a busy ward where junior doctors frequently care for large numbers of patients. He regularly stays on to complete tasks after his shift was due to end and this evening is no exception. As he is leaving, Malik is approached by a patient's son, who is concerned that his father, Mr Homa, who has dementia and was admitted following a fall, is 'in unacceptable distress'. Specifically, he tells Malik that his father is 'too often in pain' and 'the staff seem too busy to respond'.

Commentary
Discerning the moral question(s)
There are several moral problems or questions that arise, even from this short vignette. They include:
- What is Malik's responsibility, given that he is already working beyond his contracted hours on the ward?
- Are there considerations of **confidentiality** in talking to the patient's son?
- What particular characteristics and considerations apply to Mr Homa and what might that mean for a clinician's duty of care?
- Does Mr Homa have **capacity**? If not, on what basis is care being provided, both in general and in relation to the administration of medication?
- What systemic factors might contribute to the situation described by the patient's son? What is Malik's role, as an individual within a complex system, in terms of raising and addressing those factors?
- Is Mr Homa vulnerable in ways that potentially mean he is being, or should be, treated differently?

Looking at the relevant ethical theories and/or tools
- What **duties** does Malik have and to whom?
- What might be the **consequences** of his options and choices, and for whom?
- What would a **virtuous** doctor do in this situation? Which virtues are most relevant and why?
- What would it look like for Malik to demonstrate **values-based practice** in responding to this situation?
- Does Malik need to think about using an ethical decision-making tool or approach to inform and structure his approach?

Identifying applicable professional guidance
- What does national and professional guidance on **consent,** prescribing and confidentiality say that might be relevant?
- Is there other relevant guidance, e.g. from the hospital or an appropriate health organization, on responding to complaints?
- Are there any **safeguarding** considerations and, if so, which guidance is relevant?

Integrating the ethical analysis with an accurate account of the law
- What does the law relating to mental capacity and decision-making say about working with patients who may lack capacity?
- What criteria should Malik use to evaluate Mr Homa's capacity, and have they been used appropriately here?
- What limits are there to sharing confidential information, even with a family member?
- Might the patient's son be Mr Homa's legal proxy? How would Malik know, and what might it mean?
- What legal obligations apply to individual clinicians working for a large NHS organization, and what does this mean for Malik's responsibilities in this case?
- If Malik had concerns about Mr Homa's care, how would he raise those lawfully and effectively?
- How might Malik's response relate to the law concerning medical negligence?

Malik is unlikely to think about all of these things at the same time and, depending on where he is working and who is available to support him, some areas will be more relevant or constitute greater priorities than others. Of course, Malik is also a busy junior doctor who needs to make a decision and get home! With an ethical disposition and an internal capacity to think about a situation from different perspectives and perhaps make time to reflect on it afterwards, Malik is well placed to make a considered choice that is grounded in both principle and the practicalities of a demanding clinical service. He can also, if asked, explain why he responded as he did, which, as a junior doctor, is an essential skill.

The law

As it pertains to medicine, the law establishes boundaries for what is deemed to be acceptable professional practice. The law that applies to medicine is both national and international: for example, the European Convention on Human Rights (**Box 5.3**). In the UK, along with other jurisdictions, both **statutes and common law** apply to the practice of medicine (**Box 5.4**). There are legal differences between England and Wales, Scotland and Northern Ireland.

The majority of cases involving healthcare arise in the civil system. Occasionally, a case is subject to criminal law: for example, when a patient dies in circumstances that could constitute manslaughter.

Respect for autonomy: capacity and consent

Capacity

Capacity is central to ethical decision-making because it is the gateway to self-determination (**Box 5.5**). People can make choices only if they have the capacity to do so. The presumption is that adult patients have capacity to make their own decisions. Assessing capacity is a significant ethical undertaking; a patient's freedom to choose depends on it. In England and Wales, the Mental Capacity Act 2005 sets out the criteria for evaluating whether a person has the capacity to make a decision

(see p. 800). In Scotland, the Adults with Incapacity (Scotland) Act 2000 applies. In Northern Ireland, there is no statute but common law applies.

Evaluating capacity is not a one-off judgement. Capacity can fluctuate and assessments should be regularly reviewed. Capacity should be understood as decision- and time-specific, and task-oriented. People may have capacity to make some choices but not others, and capacity is not precluded by specific diagnoses or impairments such as dementia. How a doctor communicates can enhance or diminish a patient's capacity, as can pain, fatigue and the environment.

Consent

Consent is integral to ethical and lawful practice. To act without, or in opposition to, a patient's valid consent is, in many jurisdictions, to commit an assault or battery. Obtaining consent fosters choice and gives meaning to autonomy. Valid consent is:
- given by a patient with capacity
- voluntary, i.e. free from undue pressure, coercion or persuasion
- sufficiently informed
- continuing, i.e. patients should know that they can change their mind at any time.

The basis of consent

Those seeking consent for a particular intervention must be competent in applying the procedure or treatment and be familiar with its problems. While it is good practice for written information to be

**Box 5.3 European Convention on Human Rights:
         substantive rights that apply to evaluating good
         medical practice**

- Right to life (Article 2)
- Prohibition of torture, inhuman or degrading treatment or punishment (Article 3)
- Prohibition of slavery and forced labour (Article 4)
- Right to liberty and security (Article 5)
- Right to a fair trial (Article 6)
- No punishment without law (Article 7)
- Right to respect for private and family life (Article 8)
- Freedom of thought, conscience and religion (Article 9)
- Freedom of expression (Article 10)
- Right to marry (Article 12)
- Prohibition of discrimination (Article 14)

---

i **Box 5.4 Statutes and common law**

Statutes

- Primary legislation made by the state, e.g. Acts of Parliament in the UK, such as the Mental Capacity Act 2005
- Secondary (or delegated) legislation: supplementary law made by an authority given the power to do so by the primary legislation
- Implementation (or statutory) guidance, e.g. the Mental Health Act Code of Practice

Common law

- Judicial decisions made in cases: these establish precedents, which are then applied to future cases
- Precedent: whether a decision constitutes a precedent depends on which court made the decision – higher-level courts have authority over lower-level courts

---

i **Box 5.5 Principles of self-determination[a]**

- Every adult has the right to make their own decisions and to be assumed to have capacity unless proved otherwise.
- Everyone should be encouraged and enabled to make their own decisions, or to participate as fully as possible in decision-making.
- Individuals have the right to make eccentric or unwise decisions.
- Proxy decisions should consider best interests, prioritizing what the patient would have wanted, and should be the 'least restrictive of basic rights and freedoms'.

[a]Principles underlying the Mental Capacity Act 2005 (England and Wales), which applies to patients over the age of 16 years.

---

provided, offering leaflets and using a consent form do not remove the responsibility to talk to the patient. The information that is given should be that which a reasonable person in the patient's situation would require and doctors must be alert to the particular priorities and concerns of individuals. Information shared should:

- cover potential harms and benefits, considering how these might be perceived by the individual patient, e.g. whether some elements matter more than others
- explain possible consequences of treatment and non-treatment
- explain options
- disclose uncertainty; this should be as much part of the discussion as sharing what is well understood.

Patients should be encouraged to ask questions and express their concerns, values and preferences. Since it is the health and lives of patients that are at stake, the moral focus of such disclosure should be on what is acceptable to patients rather than to the professionals.

Consent in educational settings

Medical education and training often take place in clinical environments. Future doctors have to learn new skills and apply their knowledge to real patients. However, patients must be given a choice as to whether they wish to participate in educational activities. The principles of seeking consent for education are identical to those applied to clinical situations.

Advance decisions

Many countries have laws that allow people to make decisions about their future care. In the UK, these are called advance decisions (sometimes colloquially described as 'living wills' or, more formally, as 'advance decisions to refuse treatment'). An advance decision enables someone to express their wishes about future care. Advance decisions are made in anticipation of someone losing capacity. An advance decision may refuse treatment but cannot request specific treatment. Where the treatment is life-saving, the advance decision must be made in a specific way. Countries have differing approaches to advance decision-making and the relevant law where medicine is being practised must be understood. In the UK, legislation governs advance decisions. For example, the Mental Capacity Act 2005 applies in England and Wales, where a legally valid advance decision must be:

- made by someone with capacity
- made voluntarily
- based on appropriate information
- specific and applicable to the situation in which it is being considered.

In practice, it is often the specificity requirement that is difficult to satisfy because inevitable uncertainty surrounds future illness and potential treatments or interventions. For some people, the difficulty in anticipating the future and how they are likely to feel about that future informs an ethical objection to advance decision-making.

Format

Advance decisions can be made orally or in writing. However, decisions about withdrawing or withholding life-sustaining treatment must be in writing and witnessed. The decision should state explicitly that it is intended to include life-saving situations. The more informal and non-specific an advance decision is, the more likely it is to be challenged or disregarded. If working in a country where advance decisions are recognized, clinicians should make reasonable attempts to establish whether a valid advance decision exists. The presumption is to save life where there is ambiguity about either the existence or the content of an advance decision. Advance decisions should be periodically reviewed; amendments, revocations or additions are possible, provided an individual still has capacity.

Ethical and practical rationale

The ethical rationale for advance decisions is usually said to be respect for **patient autonomy** and extension of the right to make choices about healthcare to the future. Respect for autonomy necessarily involves supporting people to make choices that others might consider misguided. Some suggest that advance decisions foster trust and effective clinical relationships. However, others argue that none of us can have the capacity to make decisions about our future care because the person we become when ill differs from who we are when we are healthy.

Advance statements

Advance statements are broader than advance decisions and allow patients to express preferences and priorities without specifically

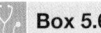

ruling out an intervention or treatment. For example, a patient may wish to be more lucid than not towards the end of life or may like to retain the ability to eat with their family for as long as possible. A birth plan is often comprised of advance statements in which women express their wishes for their labour and delivery. These preferences are not about choosing or ruling out specific treatments but are advance statements of wishes regarding the details of future care.

Lasting power of attorney

Some countries allow for the appointment of a *proxy*: that is, someone else to make decisions for patients lacking capacity. In England and Wales, consent to or refusal of treatment can be expressed by someone who has been granted lasting power of attorney (LPA) by a patient at a point when the patient still has the capacity to decide on this. The attorney gains the power to represent the patient's interests only when the patient loses capacity and this is registered with the Public Guardian. Establish whether there is a valid LPA for an incapacitous patient and adhere to the attorney's wishes. The only exception is where the attorney appears not to be acting in the patient's best interests, in which case the matter should be referred to the Court of Protection. Like advance decisions, the ethical rationale for LPAs is that prospective autonomy is desirable and facilitates informed care, rather than second-guessing patient wishes.

Best interests of patients who lack capacity

Where an adult lacks capacity to give consent and there is no valid advance decision or LPA, clinicians must act in the patient's best interests, which encompasses more than someone's best *medical* interests. In practice, determining best interests is likely to involve several people: for example, members of the healthcare team, professionals with whom the patient had a longer-term relationship, clinical ethicists, relatives and carers.

In England and Wales, an Independent Mental Capacity Advocacy Service advocates for patients without capacity who have no family or friends to represent their interests. In such a situation, people, including Independent Mental Capacity Advocates (IMCAs), are not making decisions; rather, they are giving an informed sense of the patient and their likely preferences.

If someone lacks capacity, it is meaningless to seek consent. **Box 5.6** shows how decisions for someone who may lack capacity are made in practice, as the ethical dimensions of Mr Homa's care and Malik's response unfold further.

Further reading

General Medical Council. *Decision Making and Consent: Supporting Patient Choices about Health and Care*. London: GMC; 2019.

Provision or cessation of life-sustaining treatment

For a patient who lacks capacity and has neither an advance decision nor an LPA, it is considered acceptable not to use medical means to prolong life where:

- the team believes, based on good evidence, that further treatment will not save the patient's life
- the patient is already imminently and irreversibly close to death
- the patient is so permanently or irreversibly brain-damaged that they will always be incapable of any future self-directed activity or intentional social interaction.

Moral beliefs vary and, in general, decisions not to provide or continue life-sustaining treatment should be made with as much consensus as possible among the clinical team and those close to the patient. Where there is unresolvable conflict, a court should be consulted. In the UK, judges are available in the relevant court, even in emergencies.

Where clinicians decide not to prolong the lives of imminently dying and/or extremely brain-damaged patients, the legal conceptualization is that they are acting in the patient's **best interests** by seeking to minimize suffering rather than intending to kill. Ethically, the significance of intention, along with the moral status of **acts and omissions**, is integral to debates about assisted dying and euthanasia.

Assisted dying

The language surrounding assisted dying can be confusing and disputed. Assisted dying is a term that describes what happens when someone helps another person to die. Other terms that are used include **euthanasia**, which can be categorized as 'active' or 'passive', and 'voluntary' or 'involuntary'. Active and passive refer to the distinction sometimes drawn between 'killing' and 'letting die'. The terms 'active' and 'passive' are used infrequently in contemporary medical practice. Voluntary and involuntary euthanasia refer to whether an individual has requested or sought an assisted death. *Assisted dying* is the term that is more commonly used. Physician-assisted dying is where a doctor helps an individual to die; it is a subcategory of 'assisted dying'.

In many countries, such as the UK, assisted dying is illegal. In contrast, some jurisdictions, including the Netherlands, Switzerland, Belgium and certain US states, allow assisted dying. Where

---

Box 5.6 Vignette 2

Malik visits Mr Homa. He finds signs of infection, including a high temperature, and notes that Mr Homa appears to be in distress. Malik talks to Mr Homa about his symptoms and what he believes is happening. He notes that Mr Homa is not able to understand or remember information, and he shows no ability to weigh things up when Malik explains that he wants to begin treatment with antibiotics and do further investigations. Malik recognizes that Mr Homa's confusion might be related to his acute symptoms or his dementia but is clear that he should continue to evaluate his capacity, irrespective of the diagnosis. Malik concludes that Mr Homa lacks capacity and asks to speak to the patient's concerned son. Malik asks him whether his father has a legal proxy or whether Mr Homa made an advance statement or decision before he became unwell. Mr Homa's son says that neither applies. Malik explains that he would like to investigate and treat Mr Homa in his **best interests**. Mr Homa's son is relieved and asks when his father is likely to be more comfortable. Malik obtains a chest X-ray, blood cultures and blood tests, and starts Mr Homa on a broad-spectrum antibiotic pending further information. He also checks with his consultant whether Mr Homa's medication and care plan should be reviewed following his new symptoms. Malik asks Mr Homa's son to let him know if there is anything else that might be comforting or supportive for his father while he is in hospital. Malik arranges for Mr Homa to be reviewed regularly and for that to include consideration of his capacity.

Commentary

Malik follows the steps to manage Mr Homa's care ethically and lawfully. He evaluates his capacity using the criteria set out in the Mental Capacity Act and records his findings in a timely way and relating to the specific decision. Malik does not assume that Mr Homa lacks capacity because he has dementia, and he recognizes that he must assess function and review that assessment. Malik asks whether Mr Homa has a lasting power of attorney or has made an advance decision about future care. On learning that neither is applicable, Malik proceeds on the basis of Mr Homa's best interests. His question about Mr Homa's on-going comfort and wellbeing after he has arranged investigations and begun treatment show that he is alert to best interests beyond the merely medical. Finally, he arranges for the evaluation of capacity to be revisited as part of reviewing the patient.

assisted dying is not lawful, withholding and withdrawing treatment are usually acceptable in strictly defined circumstances, where the intention of the clinician is to minimize suffering, not to cause death. The doctrine of **double effect** remains in law, but its clinical application is limited because of improved practice and understanding in palliative and supportive care. Double effect is the legal doctrine that allows clinicians to prescribe medication that has, as its principal aim, the reduction of suffering but which may have side-effects that potentially shorten someone's life. Such prescribing is legally justifiable because the intention is benign and the side-effects, while foreseen, are not the primary aim. End-of-life care pathways are discussed in Chapter 7.

Although assisted dying is unlawful in the UK, the Director of Public Prosecutions (DPP) provides guidance on how prosecution decisions are made following an action brought by right-to-die campaigner Debbie Purdy. Those guidelines indicate what circumstances are likely to weigh either in favour of, or against, a prosecution and make reference to an individual who has a professional role, such as a doctor or nurse. Nevertheless, the law itself is clear: for a clinician to end a patient's life is a criminal offence.

The legalization of assisted dying remains a matter of debate in the UK, including among doctors and the organizations that represent them, such as the Royal Colleges and medical associations. Those who support a change in the law emphasize patient autonomy and choice, arguing that it is morally right that people can determine the extent to which they can tolerate illness and suffering. Those who oppose assisted dying express concerns about vulnerability, the potential for a slippery slope whereby regulation is unable to prevent abuse, and arguments that such legislative change undermines what they believe to be the inherent sanctity of life. For some doctors, there is a question about whether assisting another to die is contrary to the medical role as they perceive it. When someone does help a patient to die – for example, by supporting their travel to a jurisdiction where assisted dying is lawful – the DPP will use guidance to determine whether there should be a prosecution. There have been a number of cases where relatives have been interviewed by the police as part of a formal investigation but no prosecutions have yet followed.

How the legal and ethical framework apply in practice is shown in **Box 5.7**.

Further reading

General Medical Council. *Treatment and Care Towards the End of Life*. London: GMC; 2010.

Mental health and consent

The majority of people being treated for psychiatric illness have capacity. However, mental illness sometimes compromises an individual's capacity to make his or her own decisions. Many countries have specific legislation that enables people to be treated without consent on the basis that they pose a risk to themselves and/or to others.

People who have, or are suspected of having, a mental disorder may be detained for assessment and treatment in England and Wales under the **Mental Health Act 2007**. The Act was reviewed in 2018, but at the time of writing, no changes to the law have yet been made. The law defines a mental disorder as 'any disorder or disability of the mind'. Addiction to drugs and alcohol is excluded. Appropriate medical treatment should be available to those admitted under the Mental Health Act. In addition, the legislation provides for **Supervised Community Treatment Orders**. The law sets out

Box 5.7 Vignette 3

Ten days have passed and Malik is concerned about Mr Homa. He has sadly not responded to treatment. He deteriorates further, requiring high-flow oxygen and developing multiorgan failure. Mr Homa's son tells Malik and the consultant on the ward round that he 'hates to see his father suffering' and asks, 'What can you do to bring Dad's distress to an end?' Malik's consultant raises Mr Homa's care at the multidisciplinary team meeting. He explains that he is concerned that on-going treatment is no longer in Mr Homa's best interests. The team agree that Mr Homa is increasingly unwell and note his son's concern about his father. They agree that there should be an urgent discussion with Mr Homa's son about next steps. During that conversation, Mr Homa's son says that his Dad 'would have hated to be in this state and always said "just let me go with dignity when the time comes". Can't you give him an injection to help him on his way?' The consultant explains that they cannot do anything to hasten Mr Homa's death deliberately but they can withdraw active treatment, such as antibiotics and breathing assistance. They would also want to ensure that Mr Homa is comfortable by prescribing sedative drugs that might have an effect on his breathing but would help avoid him being distressed. His son agrees that this is the best course of action and asks if he can sit with his Dad. The team agrees and arranges for Mr Homa to be transferred to a side-room on the ward, where Mr Homa's son can stay with his father. They ask if there is anything else they can do to support either of them.

Commentary

The team is right to consider Mr Homa's best interests together and to discuss the next steps with his son. Mr Homa's son is able to give a clear sense of his father's values and wishes. The consultant is clear that any action, such as an injection, to assist dying is unlawful, but explains that it is possible to withdraw active treatment that is no longer in Mr Homa's best interests. He also explains that he may prescribe medication to alleviate suffering but with the potential to depress respiratory effort. The care provided is intended to allow a peaceful dying process that supports both the patient and his son, who wishes to stay until the end.

multiple checks and limitations that are essential, given the ethical implications of detaining and treating someone against their will.

Even in situations in which it is lawful to give a detained patient psychiatric treatment compulsorily, consent should be sought and obtained if possible. For concurrent physical illness, capacity should be evaluated as usual. If the patient has capacity, consent should be obtained for treatment of the physical illness. If a patient lacks capacity because of the severity of a psychiatric illness, treatment for physical illness should be given on the basis of best interests or with reference to a proxy or advance decision. If treatment can be postponed without compromising the patient's interests, consent should be sought when the patient has capacity.

Consent and children

Where a child does not have the capacity to make decisions, treatment will usually depend upon obtaining proxy consent. In the UK, consent is sought on behalf of the child from someone with 'parental responsibility'. In the absence of someone with parental responsibility – for example, in emergencies, where urgent treatment is indicated – clinicians proceed on the basis of the child's best interests.

Sometimes parents and doctors disagree about the care of a child who is too young to make their own decisions. Both national and European case law demonstrate that the courts are prepared to override parental beliefs if they are perceived to compromise the child's best interests. However, the courts have also emphasized that a child's best *medical* interests are not necessarily the same as a child's **best overall interests or welfare**. Whenever the patient is a child, clinicians interact with a family unit. Sharing decisions and attending to the child as a member of a family are the most effective and ethical ways of practising.

As children mature, whether a young person has capacity to make his or her own decisions is evaluated using principles derived from a case called *Gillick v. West Norfolk and Wisbech Area Health Authority*, which determined that a young person can make a choice about their own health where:

- the patient, although under 16, can understand medical information sufficiently
- the doctor cannot persuade the patient to inform, or give permission for the doctor to inform, the parents
- a young person is seeking contraception and is likely to have sexual intercourse with or without adequate contraception
- the patient's mental or physical health (or both) is likely to suffer if treatment is not provided
- it is in the patient's best interests for the doctor to treat without parental consent.

The *Gillick* case recognized that young people differ in their abilities to make decisions and established that function, not age, matters when considering whether a child can give consent. Situations should be approached on a case-by-case basis, taking into account the individual young person's level of understanding of a particular treatment. It is possible (and perhaps likely) that someone may be considered to have capacity to consent to one treatment but not another. Even where a child does not have capacity to make their own decision, clinicians should respect the child's dignity by discussing the proposed treatment with the child, even if the consent of the parents also has to be obtained.

In the UK, once a child reaches the age of 16, the Mental Capacity Act 2005 states that they should be treated as an adult, except for the purposes of advance decision-making and appointing an LPA.

Further reading

General Medical Council. *0–18 Years: Guidance for All Doctors*. London: GMC; 2018.
General Medical Council. *Protecting Children and Young People: The Responsibilities of All Doctors*. London: GMC; 2012, updated 2018.

Confidentiality

Confidentiality is essential to therapeutic relationships. If clinicians violate the privacy of their patients, they risk harm, disrespect autonomy, undermine trust and call the medical profession into disrepute. The diminution of trust is significant ethically, with potentially serious consequences. Within the UK, confidentiality is protected by common and statutory law. Some jurisdictions make legal provision for privacy. Doctors who breach the confidentiality of patients may face professional and legal sanctions.

Respecting confidentiality in practice

Patients should understand that information about them will be shared with other professionals involved in their treatment. Usually, by giving consent for investigations or treatment, patients are deemed to give their implied consent for information to be shared within the clinical team. Rarely, patients might object to information being shared, even within a team. In such situations, the advice is that the patient's wish should be respected, unless it compromises treatment. In almost all clinical circumstances, therefore, the confidentiality of patients must be respected. Confidentiality can be breached inadvertently. For example, clinical conversations take place in lifts, corridors and cafés. Even on wards, confidentiality may be compromised by the proximity of beds and the visibility of whiteboards containing medical information. Everyone should be alert to incidental breaches of confidentiality and seek to minimize their role in unwittingly revealing sensitive information.

> **i** **Box 5.8 Examples of circumstances in which a doctor is required to share confidential information**
>
> - Notifiable diseases, which, by virtue of public health legislation, must be notified to the relevant consultant in communicable disease control
> - Court orders
> - Road traffic accidents that lead to requests from the police
> - Actual or suspected terrorist activity

When confidentiality must or may be breached

The duty of confidence is not absolute. Sometimes, the law requires that clinicians must reveal information about patients to others, even if they wish it were otherwise (**Box 5.8**). There are also circumstances in which a doctor has the discretion to share confidential information within defined terms. Such circumstances highlight the ethical tension between the rights of individuals and the public interest.

Aside from legal obligations, there are three situations in which information may be shared, namely:

- The patient has given consent.
- It is in the patient's best interests to share the information, but it is impracticable or unreasonable to seek consent.
- It is in the public interest.

These three categories are a useful framework within which to think about the duty of confidentiality. They also require ethical judgement, particularly where sharing confidential information might be in the *'public interest'*. In England and Wales, there is legal guidance on what constitutes sufficient 'public interest' to justify sharing confidential information, which is derived from the case of *W v. Egdell*. In that case, the Court of Appeal held that only the 'most compelling circumstances' could justify a doctor acting contrary to the patient's perceived interest in the absence of consent. The court stated that it would be in the public interest to share confidential information where:

- there is a real and serious risk of harm
- the risk is of physical harm
- there is a risk to an identifiable individual or individuals.

Consent should be sought wherever possible, and disclosure on the basis of the 'public interest' should be a last resort. Each case must be weighed on its own merits and a clinician who discloses confidential information on the grounds of 'public interest' must be prepared to justify the decision. Even where disclosure is justified, confidential information must be shared only with those who need to know.

If there is a perceived risk to the public interest, does a doctor have a duty to warn others of potential risk? In some jurisdictions there is a duty to warn, but in England and Wales there is no professional duty to do so. The judgement in *W v. Egdell* provides a justification for breaches of confidence in the public interest but it does not impose an obligation on clinicians to warn third parties about potential risks posed by their patients.

Further reading

British Medical Association. *Confidentiality and Disclosure of Health Information: Toolkit*. London: BMA; 2009.
General Medical Council. *Confidentiality: Good Practice in Handling Patient Information*. London: GMC; 2017.

Resource allocation

Resources encompass all aspects of clinical care: that is, they include time, knowledge, skills and space, as well as treatment. In circumstances of scarcity, waste and inefficiency of any resource are of ethical concern.

Access to healthcare is considered to be a fundamental right and has been captured in international law since it was included in the *Universal Declaration of Human Rights*. However, the question of how to allocate limited resources is a perennial ethical question. Within the UK, the courts have made it clear that they will not force National Health Service (NHS) Trusts to provide treatments that are beyond their means. Nevertheless, the courts also demand that decisions about resources must be made on reasonable grounds.

Fairness

Both ethically and legally, prejudice or favouritism is unacceptable. Methods for allocating resources should be fair and just. In practice, this means that scarce resources should be allocated to patients on the basis of need and the time at which they sought treatment. It is respect on the part of clinicians for these principles of equality – equal need and equal chance – that fosters fairness and justice in the delivery of healthcare. For example, a well-run emergency department will draw on the principles of equality of need and chance to:

- decide who to treat first and how
- offer treatment that has been shown to deliver optimal results for minimal expense
- use triage to determine which patients are most in need and ensure that they are seen first, the queue (or waiting list) being based on need and time of presentation.

People should not be denied potentially beneficial treatments on the basis of their lifestyles. Such decisions are almost always prejudicial. For example, why single out smokers or the obese for blame, as opposed to those who engage in dangerous sports? Patients are not equal in their abilities to lead healthy lives and to make wise healthcare choices. Education, information, economic worth, confidence and support are all variables that contribute to, and socially determine, health and wellbeing. As such, to regard all people as equal competitors and to reward those who, in many ways, are already better off is unjust and unfair.

Global perspectives

Increasingly, resource allocation is being considered from an international or global perspective. Beyond the boundaries of the NHS and the borders of the UK, moral questions about the availability of, and access to, effective healthcare are rightly attracting the attention of ethicists and clinicians. Anyone who is training for, or working in, medicine in the 21st century should consider fundamental moral questions about resource allocation, in particular those being raised by issues such as:

- the role and work of pharmaceutical companies
- the mobility of trained clinicians
- the preoccupation of funded and commercial biomedical research with diseases that are prevalent in developed countries
- notions of rights to health and life
- the status of those seeking asylum
- persistent inequalities in health.

Professional competence and mistakes

Doctors must practise to an acceptable professional standard. There are essentially three sources that inform what it means to be a 'competent' doctor, namely:

- the law
- professional guidance from bodies such as the GMC
- local policy.

In practice, there is often overlap and interaction between the categories: for example, a doctor may be both a defendant in a negligence action and the subject of fitness to practise procedures. Professional bodies are established by, and work within, a legal framework and, in order to implement policy, legislation is required and interpretative case law will often follow.

Standards and the law

In most countries, the law provides the statutory framework within which the medical profession is regulated. For example, in the UK, it is the function of the GMC to maintain the register of medical practitioners, provide ethical guidance, guide and quality-assure medical education and training, and conduct fitness-to-practise procedures. It is the GMC that defines standards of professional practice and has responsibility for investigation when a doctor's standard of practice is questioned.

Clinicians have a responsibility not only to reflect on their own practice, but also to be aware of and, if necessary, respond to the practice of colleagues, even in the absence of formal 'line management' responsibilities.

Conscientious objection

Doctors are human beings who will have their own views about what is and is not acceptable ethically. Any student or doctor should feel able to express concerns, raise questions and challenge constructively. However, the GMC is clear that doctors must not allow their own beliefs or judgements to compromise clinical care or discriminate against patients.

In the UK (apart from Northern Ireland), there is one situation in which the law provides for a right of conscientious objection: namely, in the provision of terminations of pregnancy and some reproductive medicine involving embryos. The right of conscientious objection allows doctors to choose not to be involved in providing terminations, including making referrals to specialist services. However, doctors must not convey their beliefs in a judgemental way to a patient and should arrange for colleague to see the patient without delay. In an emergency, which is likely to be extremely rare in contemporary Western practice, a doctor would have to act if no one else was available.

The law is silent on whether the provision applies to medical students, although most medical schools will offer guidance and accommodate students who have a conscientious objection to terminations.

Clinical negligence

Negligence is a civil claim where damage or loss has arisen as a result of an alleged breach of professional duty, such that the standard of care was not, on the balance of probabilities, that which could be reasonably expected.

Of the components of negligence, duty is the simplest: all doctors have a **duty of care** to their patients. Whether a doctor has discharged their professional duty adequately is determined by expert opinion on the standards that can reasonably be expected and an individual's conduct in relation to those standards. If doctors have acted in a way that is consistent with a reasonable body of their peers and their actions or omissions withstand logical analysis, they are likely to meet the expected standards of care. Lack of experience is not taken into account in legal determinations of negligence.

The most common reason for a clinical negligence action to fail is **causation**. For example, the alleged harm may have occurred against the background of a complex medical condition or course of treatment, making it difficult to establish the actual cause.

Clinical negligence remains relatively rare and undue fear of litigation can lead to defensive and poor practice. All doctors make mistakes and these do not necessarily constitute negligence or indicate incompetence. Inherent in the definition of incompetence is time: that is, on-going review of a doctor's practice to see whether there are patterns of error or repeated failure to learn from error. Regulatory bodies and medical defence organizations require doctors to be honest about their mistakes and to apologize, remembering that to do so is not necessarily an admission of negligence. Such honesty and humility, aside from its inherent moral value, have been shown to reduce the prospect of patient complaints or litigation. Being open is recognized as good practice internationally, and examples of an open approach in the USA, Australia and Singapore have actually reduced the costs of complaints.

Professional bodies

Professional bodies have diverse but often overlapping roles in developing, defining and revising standards for doctors. The principal publications in which the GMC sets out standards and obligations relating to competence and performance are *Duties of a Doctor* and *Good Medical Practice*.

Policy

There have been an exponential number of policy reforms that have shaped the ways in which the medical competence and accountability agendas have evolved. One of the most notable is the increase in the number of organizations concerned broadly with 'quality' and performance. The increased scrutiny of doctors' competence has found further policy translation in the development of appraisal schemes and the revalidation process. There have been other policy initiatives that adopt the rhetoric of 'quality', such as increased use of clinical and administrative targets and the development of specialist facilities.

Professional accountability is a hot topic. The law, professional guidance and policy documentation provide a starting point for clinicians. Complaints and possible litigation are often brought by patients who feel aggrieved for reasons that may be unconnected with the clinical care that they have received. When patients are asked about their decisions to complain or to sue doctors, it is common for poor communication, insensitivity, administrative errors and lack of responsiveness to be cited as motivation. Doctors should offer an apology and explain fully and promptly what has happened, along with the likely short-term and long-term effects of any harm. Reluctance to say 'sorry' comes from a fear that it is an admission of fault, which later implies liability, but guidelines from medical defence organizations emphasize that this is not so. There is less to fear than doctors sometimes believe. The courts and professional bodies are concerned neither with best practice, nor with unfeasibly high standards of care. What is expected is that doctors behave in a way that accords with the practice of a reasonable doctor – and the reasonable doctor is not perfect. As long as clinicians adhere to some basic principles, it is possible to practise *defensible* rather than *defensive* medicine. Good habits begin in medical school. In particular, effective communication is a potent weapon in preventing complaints and, ultimately, encounters with the legal and regulatory systems. Having a clear framework helps resolve complaints, reduces clinicians' stress and develops their professional reputation for handling difficult situations properly (**Box 5.9**).

Further reading

National Patient Safety Agency. Being Open: Communicating Patient Safety Incidents, Their Families and Carers; 2009. https://webarchive.natio nalarchives.gov.uk.
Parliamentary and Health Service Ombudsman. Principles of Good Complaint Handling. London: HMSO; 2009.
World Health Organization. Patient Safety: Curriculum Guide for Medical Schools. Topic 8. Engaging with patients and carers. Geneva: WHO; 2009; pp. 183–199.
https://www.gmc-uk.org/ethical-guidance/ethical-guidance-for-doctors/good-medical-practice/duties-of-a-doctor. *Duties of a doctor*.

COMMUNICATION IN MEDICINE

Worldwide changes in society, together with evidence relating to improved health outcomes, are the forces driving expectations of *patient partnership* in care. While ethics and law underpin the context of healthcare, it is through communication processes that evidence-based and *patient-centred care* is delivered. Doctors conduct around 200 000 consultations during their careers. Specific skills contribute to a consulting style that fosters trust and demonstrates flexibility, openness, partnership, respect for autonomy and collaboration with the patient. Medical schools all over the world now include the learning skills of communication as a core part of the curriculum

What is patient-centred communication?

Patient-centred communication aims to reach a common understanding with the patient about the illness, its treatment, and the roles that the clinician and the patient will assume (**Fig. 5.1**). Both the biomedical facts relating to the patient's illness and the patient's ideas, concerns, expectations and feelings are needed in order to diagnose what is the matter with the patient and to discover what matters to them (see Ch. 1).

This requires a good balance between:

- clinicians asking all the questions needed to include or exclude diagnoses
- patients being asked to express their thoughts, ideas, concerns and expectations
- clinicians explaining and advising in ways that patients can understand so that they can be involved in decisions about their care.

This does not mean that clinicians totally abdicate power but rather that they share it. Patients want their doctors' expert opinions and, in some cases, may still prefer to leave matters to the clinician.

Understanding patient concerns and expectations is always important because clinicians can offer practical help; even when they cannot, they can always listen supportively. *Empathy* has been described as 'imagination for others'. It is different from sympathy

---

Box 5.9 Responding to complaints

- Remember that the complainant is still a patient, to whom there is a duty of care.
- Do not delay.
- Listen and express regret for distress.
- Acknowledge when things have gone wrong – be objective, not resentful or defensive.
- Apologize for actual or perceived shortcomings.
- Provide easily understood information or explanations.
- Explain what has happened and the likely short-term and long-term effects of any harm.
- Offer appropriate redress.
- Explain how things will improve.
- Leave medical records strictly unaltered.

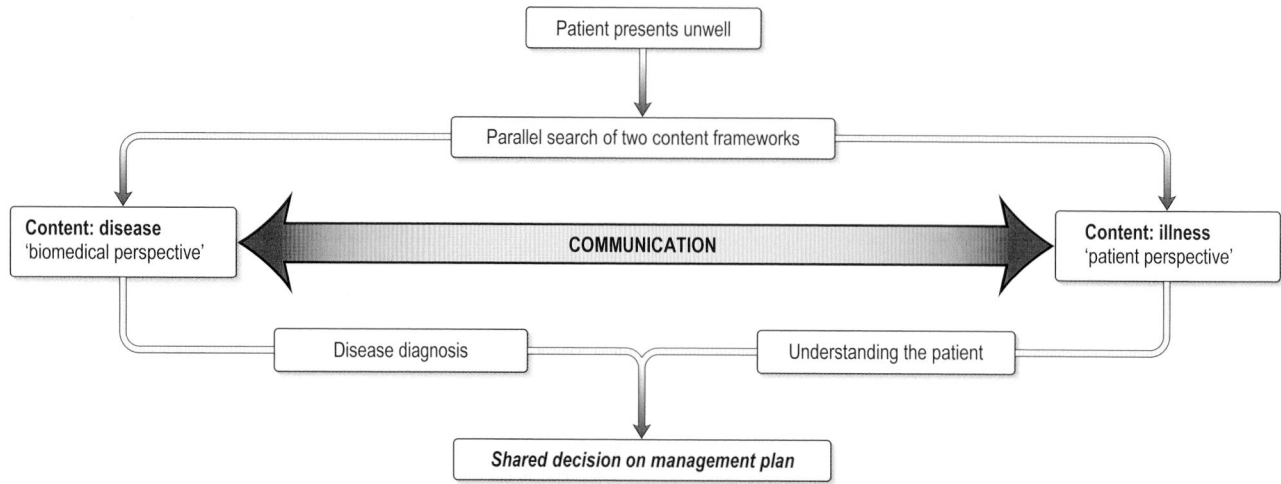

Fig. 5.1 The patient-centred clinical interview: content and skills. *(Adapted from McWhinney IR, Levenstein JH. In: Stewart M, Roter D, eds.* Communicating with Medical Patients. *Thousand Oaks, CA: Sage; 1989.)*

(feeling the same as the patient), which rarely helps and can lead to clinician burnout. Empathy is a key skill in building the patient–clinician relationship and is itself highly therapeutic. The essential starting point is attentive listening and observation of patients to try to understand their particular predicament and respond in a supportive way. Empathy can be developed with practice, but it has to be genuine and cannot be counterfeited by a repertoire of routine mannerisms.

The majority of health problems in industrialized countries are long-term conditions that cannot be cured. In 2018 in the UK, people with long-term conditions accounted for about 50% of all GP appointments, 64% of all outpatient appointments and over 70% of all inpatient bed days. To manage their conditions well on a daily basis, patients have to become experts in self-care and try to reduce their risks from lifestyle habits. All of these factors support the need for ***person-centred communication***.

Patient-centredness has evolved in the West and English-speaking countries, and may not align well with societies where cultural norms prioritize collectivism over individualism. In the latter, people are seen as part of their wider social group (family-oriented), and harmony, obedience and respect for seniors are valued over open expression of difference in opinion and egalitarianism. In recent years, research on professional–patient communication in parts of East Asia and India has revealed complexity and variability of clinical encounters and patient preferences due to such culturally specific influences. Nevertheless, there are increasing signs that patient and professional preferences in these societies are moving towards active patient involvement in discussions about treatment. A more ***participatory style*** of healthcare is likely to grow with worldwide access to the Web and societal expectations.

What are the effects of communication?

Communication can have an effect on ***health outcomes*** in a variety of ways (**Fig. 5.2**). Decades of research evidence show which aspects of communication improve diagnostic accuracy and efficiency, patients' ability to follow treatment advice, patient and clinician satisfaction and, ultimately, health outcomes. Poor communication results in missed problems and concerns, strained relationships, distress for patients, complaints and litigation. In the

USA, surgeons exhibiting an authoritarian style and tone of communication are more likely to be sued.

Some patients may not understand or remember what doctors said, while others actively decide not to follow advice and commonly do not tell their doctors, resulting in poor management. Skilful communicators routinely check patients' understanding as they explain and ask what patients think of the advice they are given (**Box 5.10**). ***Errors*** in use of medications are costly and risk patient safety.

Improved time management and costs

Integrating patient-centred communication into all interviews actually saves time in the long term and reduces non-essential investigations and referrals, which waste resources. Patients given the latest evidence of benefits and risks in treatment options commonly choose more conservative managements, without detriment to health. This has potential for considerable savings for health budgets.

Barriers and difficulties in communication

Communication is not straightforward. Time constraints can prevent both doctors and patients from feeling that they have each other's attention and that they fully understand the problem from each other's perspective. Under-estimation of the influence of psychosocial issues on illness and their costs to healthcare means clinicians may resort to avoidance strategies, such as switching topic, premature reassurance or jollying patients along when they fear the discussion will unleash emotions that are too difficult to handle, upset the patient or take too much time. Patients, for their part, may not disclose concerns if they are anxious and embarrassed, or sense that the clinician is not interested or thinks that their complaints are trivial.

Oral and written information is often so complex that it exceeds many people's functional skills in language and numeracy. ***Health literacy*** is the ability to understand health information well enough to access and use information and services in order to make decisions. Many patients have poor knowledge of how their body works and struggle to understand new information provided by doctors. Some concepts may be too unfamiliar to make sense of, even if

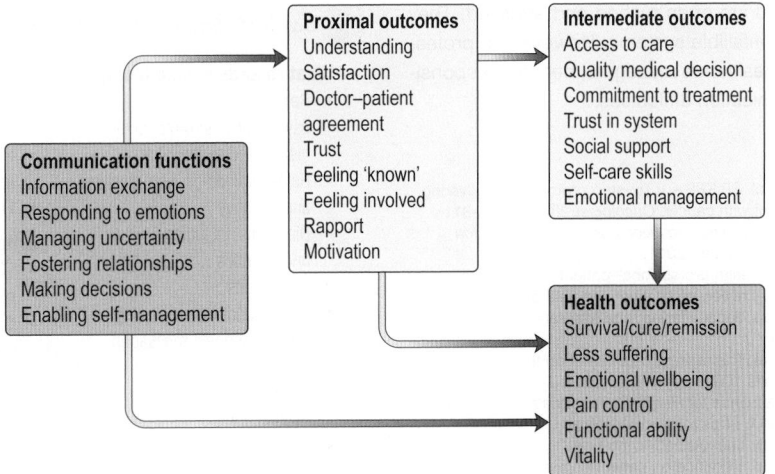

Fig. 5.2 Pathways from communication to health. *(From Street RL Jr, Makoul G, Arora NK et al. How does communication heal? Pathways linking clinician–patient communication to health outcomes. Patient Educ Couns 2009; 74:295–301 with permission.)*

 Box 5.10 Giving information and 'teach back'

Explore

- *Ask.* Establish what the patient already knows or thinks is wrong. This allows you to confirm, correct or add new information.

Explain

- *Chunk and check.* Give information in chunks that are easy to assimilate, one thing at a time. Check after each chunk that the patient understands.
- *Signpost.* 'I'll explain first of all'; 'Can I move on now to explain treatment options …?'
- *Link.* Explain the cause and effect of the condition in the context of the patient's symptoms, e.g. 'The reason you

are experiencing … is because …'

- *Use plain language.* Use clear, concise language; 'translate' any unavoidable medical terms and write them down.
- *Aid recall.* Make use of simple diagrams and leaflets; recommend websites and support organizations.

Explore

- *'Teach back'.* Use the universal precaution of always asking patients to recap to you so you check you have explained it clearly enough.
- *Acknowledge feelings.* Check what patient feels about the information.

 Box 5.11 'ATTEND': a mnemonic for patient–physician communication using the electronic medical record

Acquaint yourself with the medical record

- Look at the patient's record beforehand, allowing for less review 'screen time' while in the patient's presence

Take a minute

- Start the visit technology-free, giving the patient and their concerns your full attention

Triangulate placement of computer, patient, clinician

- Arrange the room so that it allows you to look at both the screen and the patient, and the patient to look at you and the screen

Engage, explain, educate

- Engage the patient in your use of the computer as a tool during the visit
- Explain what you are doing when you are both entering data and looking for information on the computer (signposting)
- Educate the patient by letting them see what you are seeing on the screen, especially graphs and images

No more screen

- When discussing sensitive issues, completely disengage from the screen (look at the patient, turn away from the screen, take your hands off the keys)

Describe the discharge/Don't forget to log out

- Be explicit about what orders you are entering in the computer at the end of the visit and what the patient should expect (e.g. scheduling, tests)

Rosenbaum M, Jansen KL, Shen W et al. University of Iowa Carver College of Medicine, 2014. Personal communication.

---

described simply. For example, when fasting blood sugar levels are explained to newly diagnosed diabetics, many do not realize and are puzzled by the fact that there is sugar in their blood. Patients may be too embarrassed to say they do not understand. Cultural factors and language barriers also impede mutual understanding. The computer can act as a further barrier to communication with patients and guidelines exist for best practice in its use in consultations (**Box 5.11**).

Anxiety and *emotions* are major blocks to communication. Breaking bad news about a serious medical condition presents particular challenges (see p. 10). The way that news is broken has an immediate and long-term effect. When skilfully performed, it helps the patient and family to understand, cope and make the best of even very bad circumstances. These interviews are difficult because biomedical measures are sometimes of limited help, and patients are upset and can react unpredictably. The clinician may also feel upset – more so if there is an element of medical mishap. The two most difficult things that clinicians report are how to be honest with

the patient while not destroying hope, and how to deal with the patient's emotions. Guidelines on communicating bad news provide help to do these well.

Managing uncertainty is part of medical practice (see p. 11). Around 20% of GP consultations in the UK are for persistent bodily complaints where adequate examination does not reveal a structural or pathological explanation. In secondary care, 50% of outpatients fulfil criteria for such medically unexplained symptoms. Guidelines and training are available for doctors on how best to communicate and manage this difficult situation for patients in order to reduce futile and costly investigations or interventions and help patients cope with symptoms.

Clinicians are human and are often rushed and stressed. They work against the clock and infallible systems. However, as professionals, they, together with healthcare managers, bear the responsibility for addressing communication difficulties.

Further reading

Baile WF, Lenzi R, Kudelka AP et al. SPIKES – a six-step protocol for delivering bad news: application to the patient with cancer. *Oncologist* 2000; 5:302–311.

Coulter A, Collins A. *Making Shared Decision-making a Reality. No Decision About Me Without Me*. London: King's Fund; 2011.

Pun JKH, Chan EA, Wang S et al. Health professional–patient communication practices in East Asia: an integrative review of an emerging field of research and practice in Hong Kong, South Korea, Japan, Taiwan and Mainland China. *Pat Educ Couns* 2018; 101:1193–1206.

Roter DL, Frankel RM, Hall JA et al. The expression of emotion through nonverbal behaviour in medical visits. *J Gen Intern Med* 2006; 21:S28–S34.

Royal College of Psychiatrists. *Guidance for Health Professionals on Medically Unexplained Symptoms (MUS)*; 2011. https://www.rcpsych.ac.uk/mental-health/problems-disorders/medically-unexplained-symptoms.

Stewart M, Brown JB, Boon H et al. Evidence on patient communication. *Cancer Prev Control* 1999; 3:25–30.

World Health Organization. *Health Literacy – Stepping up Impact*; 2017. https://www.who.int/global-coordination-mechanism/working-groups/hl_kickbusch.pdf.

Teamwork

Modern healthcare is complex, with patients being looked after by multiple healthcare professionals working in shifts. Problems arise when information is not transmitted, is misunderstood or is not recorded. A shared sense of ethical endeavour and effective communication are essential, especially when people are busy or a patient is critically ill.

Most complaints in teams relate to communication. Communication styles vary. Some people are indirect and more elaborate in their speech, while others come straight to the point, leaving out detail and their own rationale. Each type can feel irritated, offended or puzzled by the other. *Hierarchies* make it harder for people to speak up. The multidisciplinary team meeting is a space to establish norms, model inclusivity and enact ethical practice by listening, valuing and involving all members of the team. A functional team is an ethical team that recognizes that good care begins with the way colleagues treat each other. Poor communication and inattention to ethical norms can be dangerous if, for example, someone feels unable to point out an error, offer information or ask a question. Hinting and hoping is not good communication. Team leaders who 'flatten' the hierarchy by knowing and using people's names, routinely having briefings and debriefings, do not let their own self-image override doing the right thing, and positively encourage colleagues to speak up reduce the number of adverse events. Teamwork requires collaboration, open sharing of ideas and a readiness to discuss weaknesses and errors. Lessons from industries such as aviation have been used to show how to reduce errors caused by poor communication.

Contexts for team communication include ward handovers, requests for help, acceptance of referrals and communication in the operating theatre.

Handover between teams is helped when everyone adopts a clear system. Frameworks such as **SBAR** (**s**ituation – **b**ackground – **a**ssessment – **r**ecommendation) use standardized prompt questions in four sections to ensure team members share concise and focused information at the correct level of detail (see p. 11). This increases patient safety.

Communication on discharge is just as essential, and primary care physicians need sufficient information, including details of medication, to continue care safely. Patients in some countries now receive copies of letters sent to their doctors to ensure that

---

Box 5.12 Essentials of record-keeping

What records should include
- Relevant clinical and psychosocial information – history and examination
- Relevant findings, both positive and negative
- Diagnosis, including uncertainties
- Test results
- Correspondence, including e-mails and text messages
- Decisions made, actions agreed and identification of who is making and agreeing decisions
- Information given to patients
- Consent – details of patient's capacity (or lack of capacity) to consent
- Drugs prescribed or other investigations or treatments
- Follow-up and referrals

Criteria for good records[a,b]
- Clear, accurate, legible and contemporaneous
- Dated and signed with printed name
- Original – never altered (using a signed, dated additional note alongside any mistake)
- Kept secure

[a]General Medical Council. *Good Medical Practice*. London: GMC; 2012.
[b]Medical Protection Society. *An Essential Guide to Medical Records*; 2018. https://www.medicalprotection.org/uk/articles/an-mps-essential-guide-to-medical-records.

---

information is shared. This requires some skill to enable meaning to be clear to all parties.

Clinical records

All medical interviews should be well documented. Good records are vital in providing best care, reducing error and ensuring patient safety. They are the responsibility of everyone in the healthcare team (**Box 5.12**).

In many countries, patients have the right to see their records, which provide essential information when a complaint or claim for negligence is made. They are also valuable as part of audit to improve standards of healthcare.

Electronic patient records are increasingly replacing written ones. They include more information, overcome problems of legibility, and reduce prescription error by 66% compared to handwritten ones. With adequate data protection, they offer immense potential for unifying record systems and allowing access across the healthcare team in primary, secondary and tertiary care sectors. Increasingly, patients will have access and even contribute to their records.

Further reading

British Medical Association. *Safe Handover: Safe Patients. Guidance on Clinical Handover for Clinicians and Managers*. London: BMA; 2009; http://www.bma.org.uk.

Royal College of Physicians. *A Clinician's Guide to Record Standards*. 2009; http://www.rcplondon.ac.uk.

Royal College of Physicians. *Ward Rounds in Medicine*. London: RCP; 2012; https://www.rcplondon.ac.uk.

World Health Organization. *The WHO Surgical Safety Checklist*. 2009; http://www.who.int.

Culture, diversity and communication

Culture is a broad term that extends beyond language and includes values, beliefs, behaviours, practices, institutions and the way people communicate. Clinicians commonly express anxiety and uncertainty about how to respond to cultural diversity, how to work with interpreters and how to avoid causing offence. Doctors strive to treat all patients equally; however, research reveals that those from minority cultures receive poorer healthcare, even when they speak the same language as the clinician. They experience fewer expressions of empathy, shorter consultations and less inclusion in shared decision-making. They also tend to say less in consultations.

Beliefs

We all take our culture for granted but it can profoundly affect ideas about symptoms, causes of illness, and appropriate behaviour and treatment. Beliefs influence when a patient seeks medical assistance, what patients and doctors expect of the consultation, and how they communicate. In some cultures, for example, it is very difficult for a woman to be seen by a male doctor. Talking about death is strongly taboo in others, thus inhibiting discussions about end-of-life care. Some cultures regard it as the family members' duty to speak for the patient, while the doctor, respecting patient autonomy, will expect to talk directly with the patient. Sensitive topics may be more difficult but avoidance could jeopardize care. It helps to apologize if inadvertent offence occurs and explain why such questions are required. Clinicians vary too. Those from traditional cultures may have a more paternalistic style than some patients want.

Language

Patients sometimes bring a family member or friend to interpret. The latter may not understand medical questions and may be censoring sensitive matters or expressing their own views rather than those of the patient. Confidentiality cannot be guaranteed and patients may feel restricted in what they can say. On the other hand, patients may want a trusted family member to translate. Children should not be used to interpret.

For these reasons a trained interpreter who follows best practice guidelines should be used. Ask for the correct pronunciation of a patient's name and about any beliefs and concerns that are relevant in the patient's culture, as well as cultural differences in body language. Patients may be more or less culturally traditional, so check out assumptions.

Arrange seating to see both the patient and the interpreter but always look and speak directly to the patient. Speak in short phrases, avoid jargon and find out the patient's ideas, concerns and expectations. Watch for non-verbal communication and check that the patient understands.

Clinicians sometimes worry that interpreters are editing when long exchanges are followed by only a short summary back to them. It helps to ask interpreters to translate exactly what has been said. The interpreter can stand outside the curtain during examination. If professional interpreters are not available, telephone language lines can be used. Advocates are more than just language interpreters in that they understand cultural beliefs and practices. They also help patients to understand the workings of the healthcare system.

Non-verbal communication

Awareness of cultural taboos is helpful in maintaining dignity and respect. For example, hand-shaking, eye contact, personal space and sensitive subjects vary across cultures.

Paraverbal communication – the way things are said rather than what is said – also differs and influences rapport and relationships. We infer things from tone of voice, stress on words and phrases, silence, pace and the politeness conventions that are used. Some cultures are more open, direct and assertive than others. Some languages do not differentiate gender in common nouns and pronouns, so 'he' and 'she' may be used interchangeably. It is hardly surprising that misunderstandings occur and it can be much harder to create

a rapport. It is worth remembering that smiling is a universal expression of kindness and warmth.

Further reading

Cooper LA, Roter DL, Carson KA et al. The associations of clinicians' implicit attitudes about race with medical visit communication and patient ratings of interpersonal care. *Am J Public Health* 2012; 102:979–987.
Kai J. Enhancing consultations with interpreters: learning more about how. *Br J Gen Pract* 2013; 63:66–67.

Patients with impaired communication faculties

All healthcare professionals need patience, ingenuity and willingness to learn to be able to communicate effectively with patients who have impaired communication faculties.

Impaired hearing

Some 55% of people over 60 are deaf or hard of hearing. Patients may be accompanied by a signer but fewer than 1% of hearing-impaired people sign. Many hard-of-hearing people lip-read and some common-sense tips are listed in **Box 5.13**. Clinicians who mumble, speak fast or have strong accents have a responsibility to make particular efforts to be understood. Conversation aids may be available or patients can be asked how best to communicate with them.

Impaired vision

Patients who have visual impairment can miss non-verbal cues in communication. It may sound obvious but it helps to make more conscious efforts to use patients' names so they know they are being spoken to. Clinicians should avoid sudden touch, explain what they are about to do, and say what they are doing as they go along. Large-print information sheets should be available. Email and SMS text communication is increasingly used by blind and partially sighted people who have a smartphone, tablet or computer equipped with assistive technology.

Patients with limited understanding or speech

Aphasia is a communication disorder following strokes. Even though hearing and thought processes are unaffected, patients find it hard to understand, or they know what they want to say but cannot find the words; they are literally 'lost for words'. This also affects their ability to write, gesture, draw or mime their thoughts.

Patients may have a strength in one area – for example, ability to understand – with a weakness in another other area – for example, expression – or vice versa. It helps to find a quiet place without distractions, to make eye contact and attract the person's attention. Speak slowly and clearly, use simple phrases, try different words, and leave plenty of time between sentences to allow for extra processing time. Make it obvious when changing the subject.

 Box 5.13 Communicating with people who are deaf or hard of hearing

- Ask if they need to lip-read when you are speaking
- Position yourself on the better-hearing side
- Smile and use eye contact
- Face the light
- Do not cover your face or mouth
- Use plain language
- Speak clearly but not too slowly
- Do not shout
- If stuck, write it down
- Check for understanding
- Never say 'Forget it'!

https://www.actiononhearingloss.org.uk/ *Action on Hearing Loss.*

Closed questions requiring 'yes' or 'no' answers are easier. Write down key words or headings, to which both the patient and the clinician can refer. This helps because the auditory memory needed to 'hold on to' the spoken word taxes the patient's language system. Use pictures and have pen and paper to hand if the patient can use them. Gestures, pointing and more facial expression can help. Do not interrupt or pretend to understand. Seek advice from carers and speech and language therapists.

Technology

The Internet

The Internet has revolutionized ready access to information. Research reveals that people feel more able to ask informed questions and have less fear of the unknown. Most doctors support Internet use in enhancing consultations, especially post diagnosis, when it helps patients understand and manage their illness. They also worry that patients access poor-quality information. Directing patients to trustworthy, reputable Internet sites is recommended. Telemedicine and artificial intelligence are growing areas within healthcare. They call for adaptation of communication and the need for research on its impact on health outcomes.

Decision aids

Weighing up treatment benefits and risks where both may be substantial but not guaranteed is very hard for patients. Decision aids that are evidence-based, are written in non-technical language and include visual representations help people digest complex statistical information. They are available in a variety of media (online, print, video). Decision aids from reliable and independent sources help people think through what is important to them, so that they can make choices from the evidence that reflect their own values and preferences.

These aids can improve communication between doctors and patients, and support patient autonomy in decisions over management. If they are to become part of routine clinical practice, they need to be embraced by the clinical community, established as part of the clinical workflow, and included in education, training and development programmes for healthcare professionals.

Training in communication skills

This chapter has covered principles and some practical advice on communication in healthcare. There is clear evidence that communication ability is not just innate. It is a professional skill and responsibility that can be learned. Skills cannot be learned from books, and the opportunity to practise and receive constructive feedback on performance is essential.

Further reading

Drug and Therapeutics Bulletin. An introduction to patient decision aids. *BMJ* 2013; 346:f4147.

Pletneva N, Cruchet S, Simonet MA et al. Results of the 10th HON Survey on Health and Medical Internet Use. *Stud Health Technol Inform* 2011; 169:73–77.

Robertson K, updated by Cushing A. *Communication Skills*. BMJ Learning Online; 2016. https://learning.bmj.com/learning/module-intro/communication-skills-guide.

Silverman J, Kurtz Z, Draper J. The Calgary–Cambridge guide: a guide to the medical interview. In: *Skills for Communicating with Patients*, 3rd edn. Abingdon: Radcliffe Medical Press; 2013. http://www.skillscascade.com.

Significant websites

https://decisionaid.ohri.ca/ *Patient decision aids*.
https://www.actiononhearingloss.org.uk/ *Action on Hearing Loss*.
http://www.bma.org.uk/ethics *British Medical Association ethics*.
http://www.each.eu/ *International Association for Communication in Healthcare*.
https://www.england.nhs.uk/rightcare/useful-links/shared-decision-making/ *NHS Shared Decision Making programme*.
http://www.gmc-uk.org/ *General Medical Council*.
http://www.rnib.org.uk *Royal National Institute of Blind People*.
http://www.stroke.org.uk *Stroke Association*.

Reliable Internet information for patients/patient experiences

http://www.healthtalk.org *Provides advice and information by sharing people's experiences*.
http://www.HON.ch *Health On the Net*.
http://www.nhs.uk *UK National Health Service*.

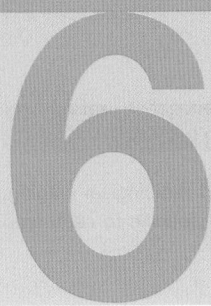

6

Malignant disease

Rachel Lewis, Piers N. Plowman and Jonathan Shamash

CORE SKILLS AND KNOWLEDGE

In developed countries, more than one-third of the population will develop cancer at some time during their life, and it is second only to cardiovascular disease as a cause of death. Many advances have been made in recent years, in terms of both the molecular understanding and the targeted treatment of different cancers.

Patients are diagnosed with cancer in a number of different settings: by screening, via the GP, as an emergency admission, or in a routine hospital outpatient or inpatient encounter. Many professionals are involved in the care of patients with cancer, and management decisions are made at multidisciplinary team meetings (usually tumour site-specific), with input from surgeons, oncologists, radiologists, pathologists, palliative care physicians, clinical nurse specialists and allied health professionals.

Oncologists are trained to deliver radiotherapy and/or systemic therapy. They must combine clinical skill and knowledge with empathy and excellent communication skills, as they often see patients when they are at their most vulnerable.

Key learning outcomes in malignant disease include:

- understanding the biology of cancer, including its presentation and natural history
- understanding the goals of treatment – cure, active management and palliation – and the principles underlying the main classes of cancer intervention: surgery, chemotherapy, radiotherapy, hormonal therapy, targeted therapy and immunotherapy
- being able to assess a patient with a malignant disease, understanding where they are in the course of their disease and treatment, and communicating likely outcomes
- managing emergencies caused by the cancers themselves (such as spinal cord compression) or by anti-cancer treatment (such as neutropenic sepsis).

Opportunities for learning about malignant disease include reviewing patients undergoing urgent investigation for malignant disease (e.g. in urgent referral outpatient clinics), attending cancer multidisciplinary team meetings, visiting chemo- and radiotherapy day units, attending clinics with the treating clinicians, and shadowing clinical nurse specialists.

CLINICAL SKILLS FOR MALIGNANT DISEASE

History

This needs to be tailored to the clinical setting: in a patient being investigated for malignant disease the diagnostic questions will be crucial, as will the patient's performance status. In a patient already undergoing active therapy, questions about treatment-related symptoms and general fitness will be more relevant. At all stages, it is necessary to consider how the patient is coping with the emotional challenges of confirmed or suspected malignancy, and to adopt an empathetic and caring approach.

The questions in **Box 6.1** are grouped into different sections that can be brought together according to the clinical setting. Patients often present with non-specific systemic symptoms such as weight loss, malaise and lethargy, pains all over, 'not feeling great' – for these patients it can be worth using 'review of systems' questions to slowly tease out specific system-based problems.

Investigations

Cancers require both radiological and histological evaluation for a complete diagnosis (**Box 6.2** and see pp. 102 and 107). The findings are used to establish histological grade and radiological staging, according to internationally agreed systems specific to each type of malignancy.

Formulating a management plan

A diagnosis of cancer can have different implications for a patient. After seeing patients with a confirmed or suspected malignancy, it is crucial to establish where they are in the disease process. Are they previously fit and well but recently diagnosed with a potentially curable disease? Or are they into their third cycle of chemotherapy for metastatic malignancy, with few additional treatment options left? Asking the questions in **Box 6.3** will shed light on the patient's perspective, and the answers can then be supplemented by reviewing medical records for investigation results and details of multidisciplinary team discussions.

---

i **Box 6.1 Taking a history in malignant disease**

General symptoms of malignancy
- Weight loss
- Anorexia/loss of appetite
- Malaise, weakness and tiredness
- Paraneoplastic syndromes

Common site-specific symptoms
- Brain: seizures, any focal neurological symptoms, personality change
- Lung: cough, haemoptysis, chest wall pain (if invasive), breathlessness
- Oesophagus and stomach: mechanical dysphagia, early satiety, regurgitation, symptoms of anaemia due to occult blood loss
- Hepatobiliary tract: upper abdominal pain and heaviness, jaundice
- Colon and rectum: altered bowel habit, rectal bleeding, tenesmus, symptoms of anaemia from blood loss
- Breast: breast lump, skin changes, nipple discharge
- Prostate: obstructive lower urinary tract symptoms (see p. 1477)
- Ovary: abdominal discomfort and bloating
- Cervix and endometrium: postmenopausal, intramenstrual or postcoital bleeding
- Thyroid: neck swelling, thyrotoxicosis
- Urinary tract: painless haematuria
- Bone: dull bony pain, pathological fractures, back pain

- Mouth and throat: non-healing ulcer, voice change and hoarseness
- Skin: progressive moles or ulcers
- Metastases: may present with any of the above symptoms and are most common to the long bones, spine, liver, lung and brain

Risk factors
- Smoking
- Obesity
- Air pollution
- Industrial exposure: asbestos, chemicals, dyes, dusts
- Viral infection: hepatitis viruses, human immunodeficiency virus, HPV, Epstein–Barr virus
- Lack of engagement with screening: breast, cervix, bowel

Common chemotherapy related side-effects
- Nausea and vomiting
- Oral mucositis
- Anorexia/loss of appetite
- Diarrhoea
- Peripheral neuropathy
- Fever: if present, always consider neutropenic sepsis, which is a medical emergency

---

i **Box 6.2 Investigation of malignant disease**

Radiology
- Typically, a computed tomography (CT) scan of the chest, abdomen and pelvis is performed to assess the local tumour site for the size of the tumour and for signs of localized invasion.
- ^{18}Fluorodeoxyglucose positron emission tomography (^{18}FDG-PET)–CT scanning may be used if there is evidence of lymphadenopathy, to assess whether lymph nodes are metabolically active, which may suggest malignant spread.
- Other forms of imaging are used if symptoms are suggestive of malignancy, e.g. a contrast-enhanced CT scan of the head to look for brain metastases, or a radiolabelled technetium bone scan to assess for bony metastases.

Histology
- Tissue biopsy is generally required for all forms of malignancy before treatment is considered.
- Basic histology confirms the tumour type (classified by the original cell type, e.g. adenocarcinoma from glandular epithelium), the degree of differentiation (poor differentiation is a bad prognostic sign) and local neurovascular invasion.
- More advanced techniques may look for expression of cell-surface molecules predictive of response to treatment, e.g. the oestrogen receptor in breast cancer.
- Genetic sequencing of tumour material has the potential to allow therapeutic regimens to be designed that target the particular genetic abnormalities in the malignant cells present.

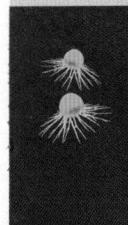

Examination

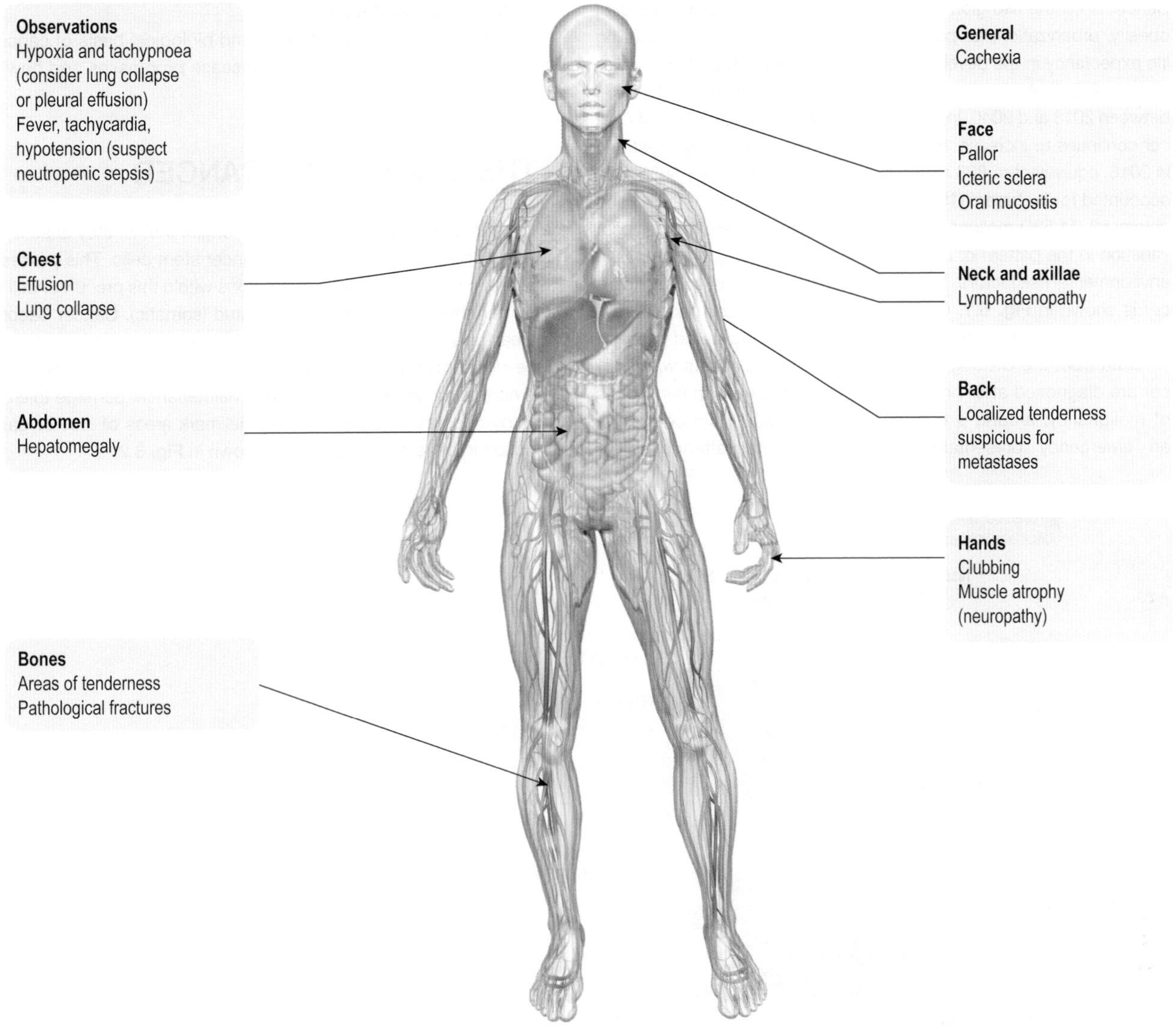

Observations
Hypoxia and tachypnoea
(consider lung collapse
or pleural effusion)
Fever, tachycardia,
hypotension (suspect
neutropenic sepsis)

Chest
Effusion
Lung collapse

Abdomen
Hepatomegaly

Bones
Areas of tenderness
Pathological fractures

General
Cachexia

Face
Pallor
Icteric sclera
Oral mucositis

Neck and axillae
Lymphadenopathy

Back
Localized tenderness
suspicious for
metastases

Hands
Clubbing
Muscle atrophy
(neuropathy)

Box 6.3 Implications of a cancer diagnosis for the patient

- When was the patient diagnosed?
- What do they understand about the condition?
- Have they been offered surgery, chemotherapy, radiotherapy or other forms of treatment?
- What do they understand about the aims of the treatment – cure or palliation?

- What do they understand about the likely outcomes of their disease?
- How do they feel about further courses of treatment?
- Who is supporting them through their disease, and what other sources of support (social networks, religious faith etc.) do they have?
- Do they have late effects from their curative treatment?

INTRODUCTION

Cancer is on the rise globally, driven by a range of factors including obesity, urbanization, air pollution, tobacco smoking and increasing life expectancy in the developing world. The Global Cancer Observatory predicts that the worldwide incidence of cancer will rise by 62% between 2018 and 2040. In England, the number of new cases of cancer continues to increase, with over 300,000 new cancers registered in 2016, equivalent to 828 new cases a day. Of these, over 50% were accounted for by breast (15.3%), prostate (13.4%), lung (12.7%) and colorectal (11.5%) malignancies, although globally there is significant variation in the pattern of malignant disease, reflecting differences in environmental risk factors. The global burden of different types of cancer is shown in **Fig. 6.1**. Cancer is a disease of older people, with those over 65 years accounting for 65.3% of total registered cancers.

Data from the UK suggests that whilst most patients with cancer are diagnosed after presenting to primary care with symptoms of malignancy, around a quarter are diagnosed in the context of an emergency presentation requiring hospital attendance or admission. Patients diagnosed in an emergency situation tend to have a worse outcome, as the cancer is more aggressive or is more advanced at presentation.

An appreciation of the genetic and biological basis of cancer is crucial in understanding how the disease progresses and how different modalities of treatment work.

THE BIOLOGY OF CANCER

Most human neoplasms are clonal in origin: that is, they arise from a single population of precursor or cancer stem cells. This process is typically initiated by genetic aberrations within this precursor cell that may be inherited (germline) or acquired (somatic). Cancer becomes increasingly common with increasing age, and can be related to a time-dependent accumulation of DNA damage that is not repaired by the normal mechanisms of genome maintenance, damage tolerance and by checkpoint pathways. The hallmark areas of loss or gain in function in developing cancer are shown in **Fig. 6.2**.

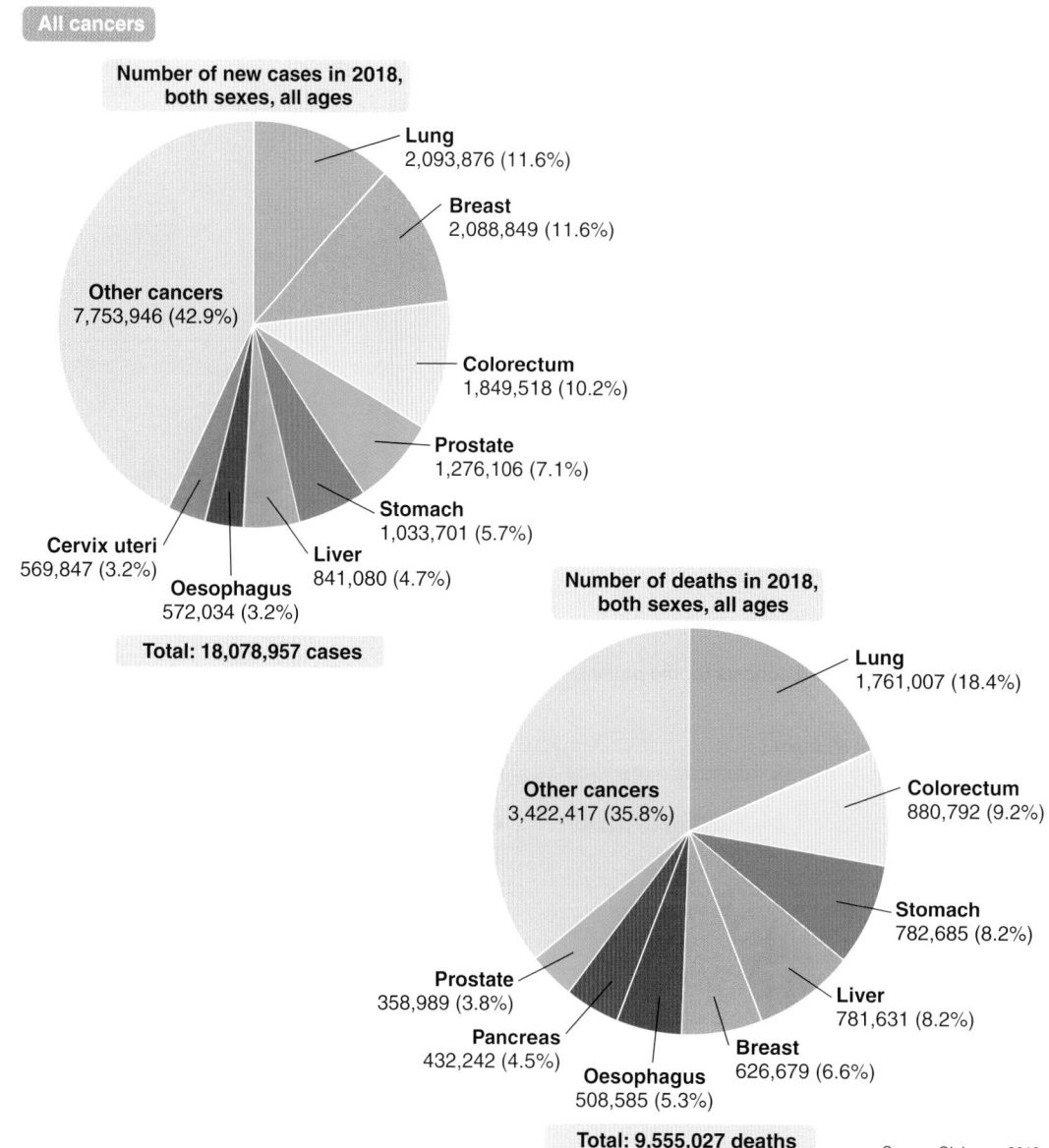

Fig. 6.1 The worldwide burden of cancer: new cases and deaths in 2018. *(GLOBOCAN 2018 Graph production: IARC (http://gco.iarc.fr/today) World Health Organization.)*

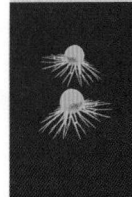

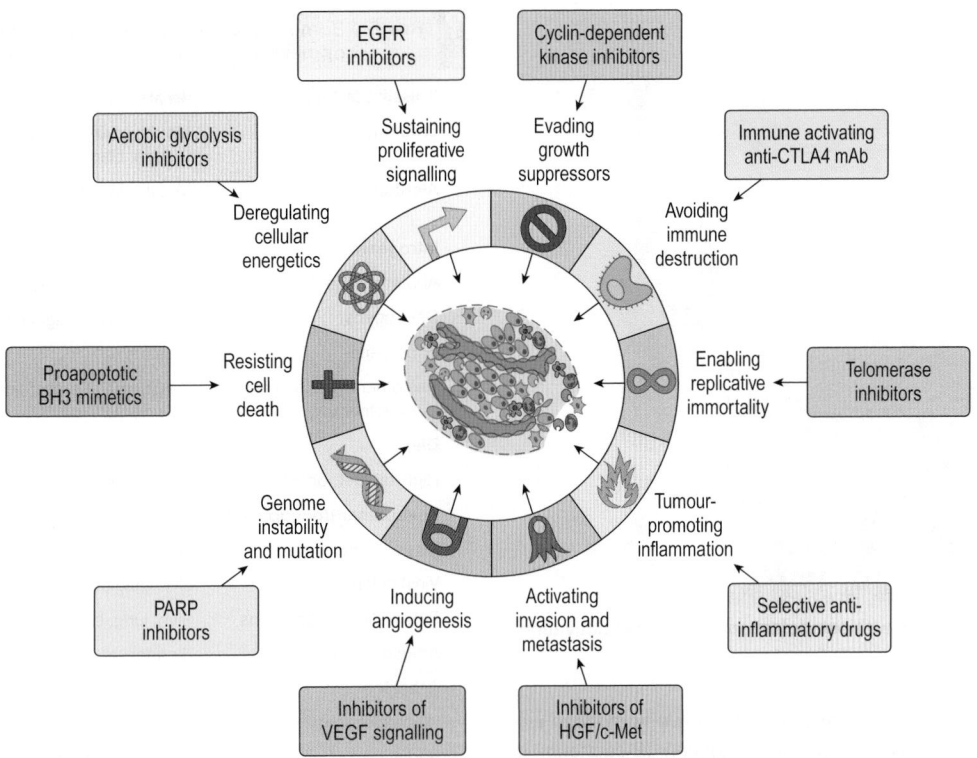

Fig. 6.2 **The hallmarks of cancer.** Ten biologically damaging capabilities are acquired during the multistep development of human tumours. Different colours indicate different actions of malignant cells, as depicted in the circle. Each of these can be targeted by anti-cancer drugs, as shown by the different-coloured rectangular boxes. In multitargeting, toxicity to normal healthy tissue is a major challenge. BH3, member of bcl2 family of proteins/homologue BH3; CTLA4, cytotoxic T lymphocyte-associated antigen; EGFR, epidermal growth factor receptor; HGF/c-Met, hepatocyte growth factor/c-Met receptor complex; PARP, poly-ADP ribose polymerase; VEGF, vascular endothelial growth factor. *(From Hanahan D. The cancer wars 2: rethinking the war on cancer. Lancet 2014; 383:558–563, with permission. Adapted from Hanahan D, Weinberg PA. The hallmarks of cancer: the next generation. Cell 2011; 144:646–474).*

Whole-genome sequencing experiments are now identifying significant clonal genetic heterogeneity within tumours, including 'passenger' (inactive) and 'driver' (active) mutations. This heterogeneity is a potential source of treatment-resistant clones and is temporally variable, so that, at relapse, the predominant founder clone that has not been eradicated is seen to have acquired new mutations on its return; alternatively, a subclone, selected out by treatment pressure, has gained further mutations and led to a recurrence. A fuller description of the genetic basis of cancer is found in Chapter 2.

Evading growth suppression

Tumour cells are usually not recognized and killed by the immune system, for two main reasons:

- There is a failure to express molecules such as human leucocyte antigen (HLA) and co-stimulatory B7 molecules that are required for activation of cytotoxic, or 'killer', T lymphocytes.
- Tumours may also actively secrete immunosuppressive cytokines and cause a generalized immunosuppression.

Successful strategies for tumour vaccines that overcome these obstacles are developing in renal cancer and prostate cancer. The monoclonal antibody (MAb) ipilimumab, which works against the inhibitory cytotoxic T lymphocyte-associated antigen 4 (CTLA4) molecule expressed after T-cell activation, is used in melanoma (see p. 113). There is increasing interest in the programmed death pathway (PD/PD-ligand), a checkpoint inhibitor (see p. 50) that negatively affects the immune response. Blocking of either PD-1 (on T

cells) or its ligand, PDL-1, which is present in some tumours, has recently been associated with an immune response capable of producing tumour shrinkages that may be durable. Common tumours, such as squamous lung cancer and transitional cell carcinomas, have responded, as have those tumours expected to be susceptible to immunological therapies (melanoma and renal cancer).

Inducing angiogenesis

There is a progressive slowing of the rate of growth as many tumours become larger. This occurs for many reasons but outgrowing the blood supply to the tumour is a crucial factor. New vessel formation (angiogenesis) is stimulated by a variety of peptides produced both by tumour cells and by host inflammatory cells, such as basic fibroblast growth factor (bFGF), angiopoietin 2 and vascular endothelial growth factors (VEGFs), which are stimulated by hypoxia. The anti-VEGF-receptor MAb, bevacizumab, has had some success in the treatment of colorectal and ovarian cancer. Alternatively, small molecules that target post-receptor response (tyrosine kinase inhibitors, TKIs) may be used; examples include sunitinib and pazopanib.

Invasion and metastasis

Solid cancers spread by both local invasion and distant metastasis (**Fig. 6.3**), through the vessels of the blood and lymphatic systems. Infiltration into surrounding tissues is associated with loss

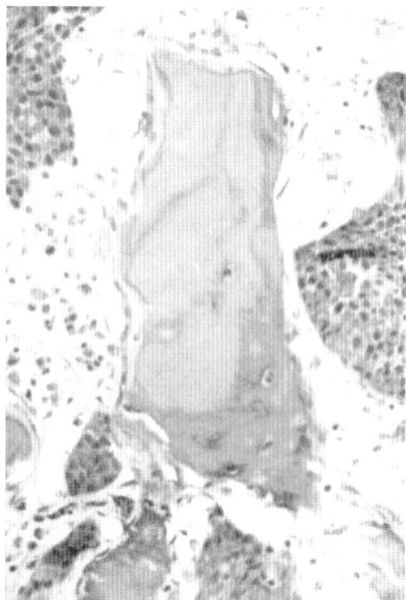

Fig. 6.3 Bone metastasis with osteoclast and osteoblast activation.

of cell–cell cohesion, which is mediated by active homotypic cell adhesion molecules (CAMs). Epithelial cadherin (E-cadherin) is expressed by many carcinomas and mutated in some, such as familial gastric carcinoma (see p. 1178).

Invasion is also determined by the balance of activators and inhibitors of proteolysis. The matrix metalloproteinases (MMPs) and their tissue inhibitors (TIMPs) are involved in tumour growth, invasion, metastasis and angiogenesis, and are being targeted by new therapeutic drugs for cancer treatment.

Dissemination of tumour cells occurs through intravasation into the vascular and lymphatic vessels and dissemination to distant sites, partly by chance, but also because of specific interactions between receptors and cytokines found on stromal and tumour cells, such as tumour necrosis factor (TNF), interleukin 6 (IL-6) and chemokines.

Further reading

Aparicio S, Caldas C. The implications of clonal genome evolution for cancer medicine. *N Engl J Med* 2013; 368:842–851.
Ding L, Ley TJ, Larson DE et al. Clonal evolution in relapsed acute myeloid leukaemia revealed by whole-genome sequencing. *Nature* 2012; 481:506–510.
Hanahan D. Rethinking war on cancer. *Lancet* 2014; 383:558–563.
Hanahan D, Weinberg RA. The hallmarks of cancer. *Cell* 2000; 100:57–70.
Hodi FS, O'Day SJ, McDermott DF et al. Improved survival with ipilimumab in patients with metastatic melanoma. *N Engl J Med* 2010; 363:711–723.
Pritchard CC, Grady WM. Colorectal cancer molecular biology moves into clinical practice. *Gut* 2011; 60:116–129.

AETIOLOGY AND EPIDEMIOLOGY

In most patients the cause of cancer is unknown, probably representing a multifactorial interaction between individual genetic predispositions and environmental factors.

Aetiology

Genetic factors

These are outlined on pages 37–8.

Environmental factors

A wide range of environmental factors has been identified as being associated with the development of malignancy (**Box 6.4**) and may

? Box 6.4 Some causative factors associated with the development of cancer

Causative factors	Neoplasms
Smoking	Mouth, pharynx, oesophagus, larynx, lung, bladder, lip
Alcohol	Mouth, pharynx, larynx, oesophagus, colorectal
Iatrogenic	
Alkylating agents	Bladder, bone marrow
Oestrogens	Endometrium, vagina, breast, cervix
Androgens	Prostate
Radiotherapy (e.g. mantle radiotherapy)	Carcinoma of breast and bronchus
Diet	
High-fat diet, obesity	Colorectal
Environment/occupation	
Air pollution	Lung cancer
Vinyl chloride	Liver (angiosarcoma)
Polycyclic hydrocarbons	Skin, lung, bladder
Aromatic amines	Bladder
Asbestos	Lung, mesothelium
Ultraviolet light	Skin, lip
Radiation	e.g. Leukaemia, thyroid cancer
Aflatoxin	Liver
Biological agents	
Hepatitis B virus	Liver (hepatocellular carcinoma)
Hepatitis C virus	Liver (hepatocellular carcinoma)
Epstein–Barr virus	Nasopharyngeal carcinoma
Human papillomavirus types 16 and 18	Cervix
	Oral cancer (type 16)
Schistosoma japonicum	Bladder
Helicobacter pylori	Stomach

be amenable to preventative action, such as smoking cessation, dietary modification and antiviral immunization (**Box 6.5**). Environmental factors interact with genetic predisposition. For example, subsequent generations of people moving from countries with a low incidence of breast or colon cancer to those with a high incidence acquire the cancer incidence of the country to which they have moved, while Northern Europeans exposed to strong ultraviolet radiation have the highest risk of developing melanoma.

Tobacco

Since the mid-1990s the incidence of lung cancer, in both men and women, has increased dramatically worldwide but is falling in many high-income countries. The association of smoking with lung cancer is indisputable and causative mechanisms have been identified; cigarette tobacco is responsible for one-third of all deaths from cancer in the UK. Smoking not only causes lung cancer, but also is associated with cancer of the mouth, larynx, oesophagus and bladder. Smoking is discussed on page 963.

Alcohol

Alcohol is associated with cancers of the upper respiratory and gastrointestinal tracts, and also interacts with tobacco in the aetiology of these tumours. It may be associated with an increased risk of breast cancer.

- Stop smoking
- Moderate alcohol consumption
- Maintain a healthy weight
- Take moderate exercise
- Eat healthily (fruit and vegetables, high fibre, low fat/salt/sugar)

- Limit sun exposure
- Minimize occupational risk
- Minimize radiation exposure
- Vaccinate against hepatitis B and human papillomavirus

Diet

One-third of cancer deaths have been attributed to dietary factors, although it is often difficult to differentiate these from other epidemiological causes. For example, the incidence of stomach cancer is particularly high in the Far East, while breast and colon cancers are more common in Western, high income countries. Many associations have been observed, without a causative link being identified, between the incidence of cancer and the consumption of dietary fibre, red meat, saturated fats, salted fish, vitamin E, vitamin A and many others. Food and its role in the causation of gastrointestinal cancer are discussed on in Chapter 33. Higher levels of obesity in the developed world have been linked with increases in cancers associated with oestrogenic stimulation of the breast and endometrium in women.

Ultraviolet light

Ultraviolet (UV) light is known to increase the risk of skin cancer (basal cell, squamous cell and melanoma). The incidence of melanoma is therefore particularly high in the white Anglo-Celtic population of Australia, New Zealand and South Africa, where exposure to UV light is combined with a genetically predisposed population.

Arsenic contamination

Arsenic contamination of water supplies has been linked to a high incidence of lung and colon cancers in South-east Asia, particularly where boreholes are the main water source.

Occupational factors

In 1775, Percival Pott described the association between carcinogenic hydrocarbons in soot and the development of scrotal epitheliomas in chimney sweeps. The principal causes nowadays are **asbestos** (lung and mesothelial cancer) and **polycyclic hydrocarbons** from fossil fuel combustion (skin, lung and bladder cancers). **Organic chemicals**, such as benzene, may cause the development of bone marrow conditions, such as myelodysplastic syndrome or acute myeloid leukaemia.

Infectious agents

The geographical distribution of some rare malignancies suggests that they might be caused by, or associated with, an infective agent. Chronic persistent infection provides growth stimulation, while many viruses contain transforming viral oncogenes.

T-cell leukaemia, seen almost exclusively in residents of the southern island of Japan and in the West Indies, is caused by infection with the locally endemic retrovirus human T-cell leukaemia (or lymphotropic) virus type 1 (HTLV-1) and integration of the oncogene, *TAX*, into the cellular genome.

Hepatocellular carcinoma occurs in patients with hepatitis B and C virus infections, and Burkitt's lymphoma and nasopharyngeal carcinoma are associated with the Epstein–Barr virus (EBV). EBV is also linked with Hodgkin lymphoma (see p. 399).

Patients with human immunodeficiency (HIV) infection or immunosuppression from organ transplantation have an increased incidence of EBV-related lymphoma and herpesvirus-8-associated Kaposi's sarcoma.

Human papillomavirus (HPV) infection types 16 and 18, for which an effective vaccine is now available, is an established cause

i **Box 6.6** Radiation exposure from common diagnostic radiological procedures[a]

Procedure	mSv
Chest X-ray	0.02
Computed tomogram (CT) chest	7
CT abdomen	8–10
Whole-body CT	20
Percutaneous coronary intervention	15
Myocardial perfusion imaging	15.6

[a]UK background radiation is 2.6 mSv per year. 1 mSv carries a lifetime cancer risk of 1 in 17 500, and 5 mSv a risk of 1 in 3500.
(Modified from Smith-Bindman R, Lipson J, Marcus R et al. Arch Intern Med *2009; 169: 2078–2086 and Fazel R, Krumholz HM, Wang Y et al.* N Engl J Med *2009; 361:849–857.)*

of the rise in cervical cancer among sexually active women; more recently, it has also been associated with an increase in head and neck cancers. Bacterial infection with *Helicobacter pylori* predisposes to the development of gastric cancer and gastric lymphoma, while *Schistosoma japonicum* infection predisposes to the development of squamous cell carcinomas in the bladder.

Medication

Oestrogens have been implicated in the development of vaginal, endometrial and breast carcinoma. Certain cytotoxic drugs, such as those given for Hodgkin lymphoma (see p. 401), are themselves associated with an increased incidence of secondary acute myeloid leukaemia, and bladder and lung cancer. Androgens have been linked with both benign and malignant liver tumours.

Radiation
Accidental

The nuclear disasters of Hiroshima, Nagasaki and Chernobyl led to an increased incidence of leukaemia after 5–10 years in the exposed population, as well as greater incidences of thyroid and breast cancer. Radiation workers are at a higher risk of malignancy due to occupational exposure, unless precautions are taken to minimize the danger by using personal and environmental shielding, and to record and limit the amount of personal exposure.

Therapeutic

Long-term survivors who have been treated with radiotherapy, such as those with Hodgkin lymphoma, for which patients were historically treated with wide radiation fields, have an increased incidence of cancer, particularly at the radiation field margins. These patients should have regular surveillance follow-up: for example, for the early identification of breast malignancy in the Hodgkin cohort of patients.

Diagnostic

Imaging procedures involving radiation exposure are associated with an increased risk of cancer. This risk is cumulative, dose-dependent and time-dependent, and so children are at higher risk than adults. The cancer risk of various common investigations is shown in **Box 6.6**. All doctors should strive to minimize diagnostic exposure to radiation

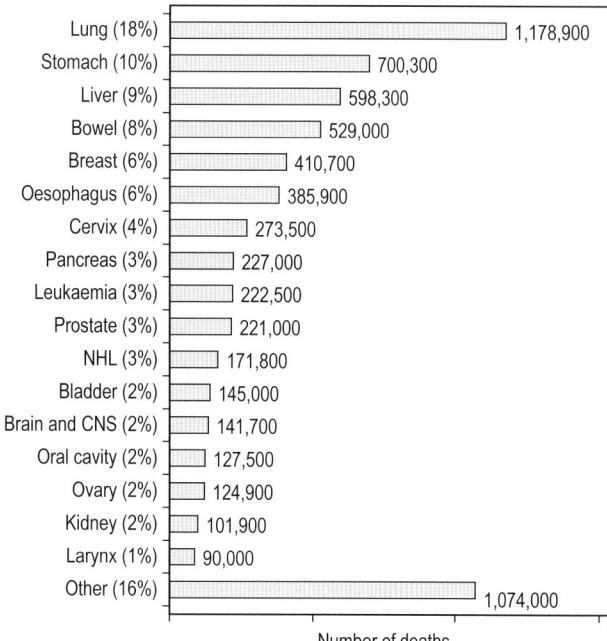

Fig. 6.4 The most common causes of death from cancer world-wide: 2002 estimates. Non-melanoma skin cancers are excluded. CNS, central nervous system; NHL, non-Hodgkin lymphoma. *(From http://info.canceresearchuk.org/cancerstats/world/the-global-picture/.)*

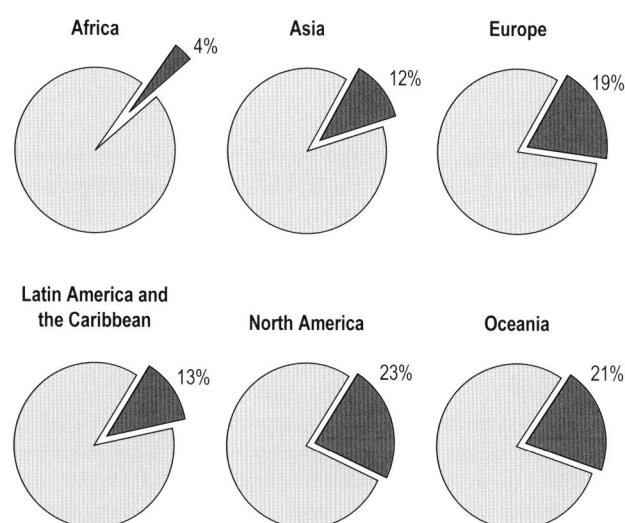

Fig. 6.5 Percentage of all deaths due to cancer in different regions of the world. *(From http://info.canceresearchuk.org/cancerstats/world/the-global-picture/.)*

where possible by using alternative modalities such as ultrasound or magnetic resonance imaging (MRI). Good documentation of radiation doses is required, particularly in children and pregnant women.

Epidemiology

The incidence and mortality from cancer vary by tumour type and geographical region across the world.

Geographical distribution

The incidence of cancer across the world is dependent on local environmental factors, diet and the genetics of the population (see earlier) (**Figs 6.4 and 6.5**). Age is also a factor, as most cancers

occur in those over the age of 65, who comprise 3.3% of the population in Africa, compared with 15.2% in Europe. Reproductive patterns influence the incidence of breast cancer. Migrating individuals often take on the risks associated with local environmental factors.

Other factors

Incidence and mortality are closely linked for those cancers for which treatment has yet to make significant improvements, such as lung, stomach and liver. However, in countries with effective screening programmes, there is an increasing incidence, but decreasing mortality, for breast, cervix, bowel and prostate cancers.

Further reading

Hoeijmakers JH. DNA damage, aging and cancer. *N Engl J Med* 2009; 361:1475–1485.
McDermott U, Downing JR, Stratton MR. Genomics and the continuum of cancer care. *N Engl J Med* 2011; 364:340–350.
Pearce MS, Salotti JA, Little MP et al. Radiation exposure from CT scans in childhood and subsequent risk of leukaemia and brain tumours: a retrospective cohort study. *Lancet* 2012; 380:499–505.

SCREENING AND INVESTIGATIONS

Asymptomatic detection through screening

Most common cancers start as focal microscopic clones of transformed cells, and diagnosis becomes likely only once sufficient tumour bulk has accumulated to cause symptoms or signs. In order to try to make an earlier diagnosis and enhance the curative possibilities, an increasing number of screening programmes are being developed that either target the asymptomatic or pre-invasive stages of the cancer, as in cervix, breast and colon, or use serum tumour markers, as in prostate and ovarian cancers. Genetic screening can be used to target screening to those groups at most risk of developing cancer, such as *BRCA1*-positive individuals who may develop breast cancer (**Box 6.7**).

The aim of screening programmes is to improve individual and/or population survival by detecting cancer in its very early stages, when the patient is asymptomatic. This strategy is dependent on finding tests that are sufficiently sensitive and specific, using detection methods that identify cancer before it has spread, and having curative treatments that are practical and consistent with maintenance of a normal lifestyle and quality of life.

In the UK, population screening is provided for breast, cervical and colon cancer and also to individuals via annual check-ups; alternatively, it may be opportunistic, when patients see their doctor for other reasons.

Unfortunately, earlier diagnosis does not necessarily mean longer survival and randomized trials are necessary to prove benefit. With lead-time bias, the patient is merely treated at an earlier date and hence the survival appears longer; death still occurs at the same time from the point of genesis of the cancer (**Fig. 6.6**). With length-time bias, a greater number of slowly growing tumours are detected when asymptomatic individuals are screened, leading to a false impression of an improvement in survival.

The characteristics of effective screening programmes are shown in **Box 6.8**.

Cervical cancer

The cervical cancer screening test (smear test) is cheap and safe but requires a well-trained cytologist to identify the early changes (dyskaryosis and cervical intraepithelial neoplasia, CIN). However, developments in liquid cytology and co-testing for HPV DNA may overcome this. Effective treatment for high-risk, pre-invasive,

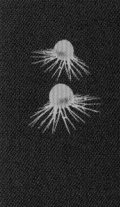

i **Box 6.7 Familial cancer syndromes for which genetic screening may be relevant**

Syndrome	Gene	Neoplasms
Autosomal dominant		
Retinoblastoma	*RB1*	Eye
Wilms' tumour	*WT1*	Kidney
Li–Fraumeni	*p53*	Sarcoma/brain/leukaemia
Neurofibromatosis type 1	*NF1*	Neurofibromas/leukaemia
Familial adenomatous polyposis (FAP)	*APC*	Colon
Lynch's syndrome (previously hereditary non-polyposis colon cancer, HNPCC)	*MLH1* and *MSH2*	Colon, endometrium
Hereditary diffuse gastric cancer syndrome	E-cadherin	Stomach
Breast/ovary families	*BRCA1*	Breast/ovary
	BRCA2	
	p53	
Melanoma	*p16*	Skin
Von Hippel–Lindau	*VHL*	Renal cell carcinoma and haemangioblastoma
Multiple endocrine neoplasia type 1	*MEN1*	Pituitary, pancreas, parathyroid
Multiple endocrine neoplasia type 2	*RET*	Thyroid, adrenal medulla
Autosomal recessive		
Xeroderma pigmentosa	*XP*	Skin

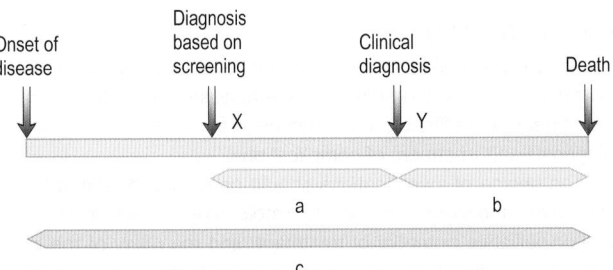

Fig. 6.6 Lead-time bias. Earlier diagnosis, at X, made by screening tests before the clinical diagnosis, at Y, suggests an increased survival time of a + b. The actual survival time (c) remains unchanged.

malignant changes reduces the incidence and mortality from cervical cancer, although there are no randomized trials. Screening will continue to be required, despite the introduction of vaccination against HPV infection for women before they become sexually active, because the lag time between infection and the appearance of disease can be in the order of 40–50 years. In the UK, women are offered screening every 3 years from the age of 25 to 64.

Breast cancer

The UK National Health Service Breast Screening Programme (involving biplanar mammography every 3 years for women aged 50–70 years) has been shown to reduce mortality from breast cancer in randomized controlled studies. The test is acceptable to most

i **Box 6.8 Characteristics of an effective screening programme**

- It must be affordable for the healthcare system
- It must be acceptable to all social groups so that they attend for screening
- It must have a good discriminatory index between benign and malignant lesions
- It must show a reduction in mortality from the cancer

women, with 50–75% of individuals attending for screening when sufficiently educated about the benefits. In North America, there is continuing debate about whether annual mammography from a younger age is more effective.

The cost is estimated to be between £250 000 and £1.3 million per life saved; money which, according to critics, could be used more appropriately for better treatment.

Women from families with *BRCA1*, *BRCA2* and *p53* mutations require intensive screening starting at an earlier age, when mammography is inaccurate due to greater breast density and MRI scanning is preferred.

Colorectal cancer

Faecal occult blood is a cheap test for the detection of colorectal cancer. Large randomized studies have shown a reduction in cancer-related mortality of 15–33%. However, the false-positive rates are high, meaning many unnecessary colonoscopies (see p. 1219). The UK has introduced a national screening programme using faecal occult blood in patients aged 60–64 years, in which positive tests have identified that 10% have cancer and 40% have adenomas. A randomized trial in Norway has found an increased number of early-stage cancers in the screened population but a high incidence of interval cancers, arising between biennial screens. Patients with an increased risk of developing bowel cancer (those with a family history of familial adenomatous polyposis or Lynch's syndrome (hereditary non-polyposis colorectal cancer)) will have a more intensive screening programmed, starting at an earlier age.

Colonoscopy is the 'gold standard' technique for examination of the colon and rectum and is the investigation of choice for high-risk patients. Universal screening strategies have been recommended in the USA, but the shortage of skilled endoscopists, the expense, the need for full bowel preparation and the small risk of perforation make colonoscopy impractical as a population screening tool at present; CT colonography ('virtual colonoscopy') (see **Fig. 32.8B**) may become an alternative, along with genetic testing and stool DNA tests.

Prostate cancer

Screening for prostate cancer using serum prostate specific antigen (PSA) is discussed on page 294 and page 1480.

Epithelial ovarian cancer

Serum CA125 can be used for the early detection of this cancer and is the subject of on-going trials. An improvement in survival of a screened population can be shown but at the cost of many unnecessary laparotomies, so that further enhancements are being investigated by serial testing and in combination with transvaginal ultrasound scans.

The symptomatic patient with cancer

Patients may offer information about predisposing conditions and family history that alerts the clinician to the likelihood of a cancer diagnosis. Many present with a history of tumour site-specific symptoms, such as

Box 6.9 Symptoms and signs of malignant disease

Degree of spread	Anatomical location	Examples of clinical problems
Local	Mass	Thyroid nodule, pigmented naevus, breast lump, abdominal mass, testicular mass
	Local infiltration of skin	Dermal nodules, peau d'orange, ulceration
	Local infiltration of nerve	Neuropathic pain and loss of function
		Horner's syndrome, cord compression, Pancoast tumour, focal CNS deficit, hypopituitarism
	Local infiltration of vessel	Venous thrombosis, tumour emboli, haemorrhage, e.g. gastrointestinal
	Obstruction of viscera or duct	Small or large bowel obstruction, dysphagia, SVC obstruction
		Obstructive uropathy, acute kidney injury, urinary retention, stridor, lobar collapse, pneumonia, cholestatic jaundice
Nodal	Peripheral	Supraclavicular fossa, Virchow's node, lymphoedema
	Central	Mediastinum – SVC obstruction; porta hepatis – obstructive jaundice, para-aortic nodes and back pain
Metastatic	Lung	Pleuritic pain, cough, shortness of breath, lymphangitis and respiratory failure, recurrent pneumonia
	Liver	RUQ pain, anorexia, fever, raised serum liver enzymes, jaundice
	Brain	Headache and vomiting of raised intracranial pressure, focal deficit, coma, seizure
	Bone	Bone pain, cord compression, fracture, hypercalcaemia
	Pleura	Effusion, pain, shortness of breath
	Peritoneum	Ascites, Krukenberg tumours
	Adrenal	Addison's disease (hypoadrenalism)
	Umbilicus	Sister Mary Joseph's nodule

CNS, central nervous system; RUQ, right upper quadrant; SVC, superior vena cava.

pain, and physical signs, such as a mass, which readily identify the primary site of the cancer (**Box 6.9**). Cancer symptoms typically increase with time and do not respond to measures such as antibiotics. However, some patients seek medical attention only when more systemic and non-specific symptoms occur, such as weight loss, night sweats, fever, fatigue, recurrent infections and anorexia. These usually indicate a more advanced stage of disease, except in some paraneoplastic and ectopic endocrine syndromes. Other patients are diagnosed only on discovery of established metastases, such as the abdominal distension of ovarian cancer, the back pain of metastatic prostatic cancer, or the liver enlargement of metastatic gastrointestinal cancer

Paraneoplastic syndromes are indirect effects of cancer (**Box 6.10** and **Fig. 6.7**) that are often associated with specific types of cancer and may be reversible with treatment of the cancer. The effects and mechanisms can be very variable. For example, in the Lambert–Eaton syndrome (see p. 895), there is cross-reactivity between tumour antigens and the normal tissue acetylcholine receptors at neuromuscular junctions.

The *coagulopathy of cancer* may present with thrombophlebitis, deep venous thrombosis and pulmonary emboli, particularly in association with cancers of pancreas, stomach and breast. Some 18% of patients with recurrent pulmonary embolus will be found to have an underlying cancer and many cancer patients are at increased risk of venous thromboembolism (VTE) following diagnosis. Trousseau's syndrome – superficial thrombophlebitis migrans – refers to this process in the superficial venous system. All patients with active cancer admitted to hospital are at high risk of VTE and should be given prophylaxis with, for example, subcutaneous low-molecular-weight heparin in the absence of any contraindications (see p. 1014).

Other symptoms are related to peptide or hormone release, such as in carcinoid or Cushing's syndrome.

Cachexia of advanced cancer is thought to be due to release of chemokines such as TNF, as well as the fact that patients lose their appetite. The unexplained loss of more than 10% of a patient's body weight should always stimulate a search for an explanation.

Cancer-associated immunosuppression can lead to reactivation of latent infections such as herpes zoster (**Fig. 6.8**) and tuberculosis.

Serum tumour markers

Tumour markers are intracellular proteins or cell surface glycoproteins released into the circulation and detected by immunoassays. Examples are given in **Box 6.11**. Values in the normal range do not necessarily equate with the absence of disease and a positive result must be corroborated by histology, as these markers can be seen in many benign conditions. They are most useful in the serial monitoring of response to treatment. MicroRNA may be more tumour-specific and offer the possibility of increased sensitivity compared to classical tumour markers.

Cancer imaging

Radiological investigation by experts is required at various stages: at initial diagnosis and staging of the disease, during the monitoring of treatment efficacy, at the detection of recurrence, and for the diagnosis and treatment of complications.

The choice of investigations should be guided by the patient's symptoms and signs, the site and histology of the cancer, the curative or palliative potential of treatment, and the utility of the information in guiding treatment. Specific investigations are described under each tumour type in the relevant chapter of this book.

Contrast agents are used for increased structural discrimination in cross-sectional imaging and can be further enhanced with functional specificity for metabolically active tissue with ^{18}FDG-PET–CT scan, as used extensively in head and neck cancer, lung cancer and lymphoma. *Radionuclide imaging* of sentinel lymph nodes is used to guide lymphatic surgery in breast cancer and melanoma. Tumour-targeted contrast agents can improve detection rates; examples include the radiolabelled MAb rituximab for lymphoma, or radiolabelled small molecules such as octreotide for neuroendocrine tumours. Research into the use of reporter agents that become visible only on activation within the tumour environment holds the promise of greater sensitivity and specificity in the future.

Biopsy and histological examination

A diagnosis of cancer may be suspected by both patient and doctor, but advice about treatment can usually be given only on the basis of a tissue diagnosis. This may be obtained by endoscopic,

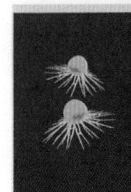

i Box 6.10 Paraneoplastic syndromes

Syndrome	Tumour	Serum antibodies
Neurological		
Lambert–Eaton syndrome	Lung (small-cell) carcinoma	Anti-VGCC
Peripheral sensory neuropathy	Lung (small-cell), breast and ovary lymphoma	Anti-Hu
Cerebellar degeneration	Lung (particularly small-cell) lymphoma	Anti-Yo
Opsoclonus/myoclonus	Breast, lung (small-cell)	Anti-Ri
Stiff person syndrome	Breast, lung (small-cell)	Anti-amphiphysin
Limbic, hypothalamic or brainstem encephalitis	Lung	Anti-Ma protein
	Testicular	Anti-NMDAR
Endocrine/metabolic		
SIADH	Lung (small-cell)	
Ectopic ACTH secretion	Lung (small-cell)	
Hypercalcaemia	Renal, breast, myeloma, lymphoma	
Fever	Lymphoma, renal	
Musculoskeletal		
Hypertrophic pulmonary osteoarthropathy	Lung (non-small-cell)	
Clubbing	Lung	
Skin		
Dermatomyositis/polymyositis	Lung and upper gastrointestinal	
Acanthosis nigricans	Mainly gastric	
Velvet palms	Gastric, lung (non-small-cell)	
Hyperpigmentation	Lung (small-cell)	
Haematological		
Erythrocytosis	Renal cell carcinoma, hepatocellular carcinoma, cerebellar haemangioblastoma	
Thrombocytosis	Ovarian cancer	
Migratory thrombophlebitis	Pancreatic adenocarcinoma	
DVT	Adenocarcinoma	
DIC	Adenocarcinoma	
Renal		
Membranous nephropathy (frequently presenting with nephrotic syndrome)	Lung, stomach and colon cancers	
Amyloidosis (presenting with nephrotic syndrome)	Myeloma	

ACTH, adrenocorticotrophic hormone; DIC, disseminated intravascular coagulation; DVT, deep venous thrombosis; NMDAR, N-methyl-D-aspartate receptors; SIADH, syndrome of inappropriate antidiuretic hormone secretion; VGCC, voltage-gated calcium channels.

radiologically guided or surgical biopsy, or by cytology (e.g. lung cancer may be diagnosed by sputum cytology). Malignant lesions can be distinguished morphologically from benign ones by the pleomorphic nature of the cells, increased numbers of mitoses, nuclear abnormalities of size, chromatin pattern and nucleolar organization, and evidence of invasion into surrounding tissues, lymphatics or vessels. The degree of differentiation of the tumour has prognostic significance: generally speaking, well-differentiated tumours have a better prognosis than poorly differentiated or anaplastic ones. In some tumours, diagnosis and treatment may be combined within a single surgical procedure, with the exact nature of the procedure being carried out varying depending on the presence of malignancy. An intraoperative provisional histological opinion can be rapidly obtained with a tissue sample processed using 'frozen section' techniques, rather than having the sample paraffin embedded, which takes more than a day.

Immunocytochemistry, using MAbs against tumour antigens, is very helpful in differentiating between lymphoid and epithelial tumours, and between some subsets of these (see **Box 6.18**). However, there is much overlap in the expression of many of these

tissue tumour markers, and some adenocarcinomas and squamous carcinomas do not bear any distinctive immunohistochemical markers that are diagnostic of their primary site of origin.

Molecular markers of genetic abnormalities have long been available in the haematological cancers and are increasingly available in solid cancers. For example, *fluorescence in situ hybridization* (FISH; see p. 27) can be used to look for characteristic chromosomal translocations, as in lymphoma and leukaemia, as well as deletions or amplifications, as in breast cancer (see p. 38). The development of the new targeted MAbs and TKIs has been guided by increasing use of mutation analysis of common oncogenes, such as *RAS* and *RAF* in colon cancer and melanoma. *Tissue microarrays* can identify patterns of multiple genomic alterations and single nucleotide polymorphisms (SNPs), as in breast cancer and lymphoma (see p. 27), and *RNA assays* with reverse transcriptase polymerase chain reaction (RT-PCR) can be used to identify tissue of origin with prognostic and predictive relevance.

Genomics and proteomics are being investigated in order to target new (and expensive) therapies, such as imatinib in chronic myeloid leukaemia and gastrointestinal stromal tumours (GIST);

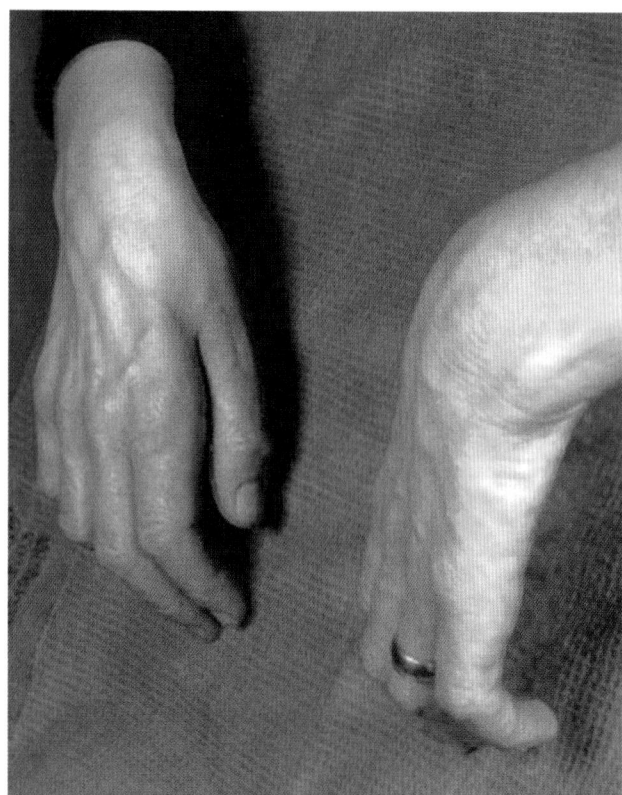

Fig. 6.7 Paraneoplastic peripheral neuropathy. There is wasting of the small muscles of the hands.

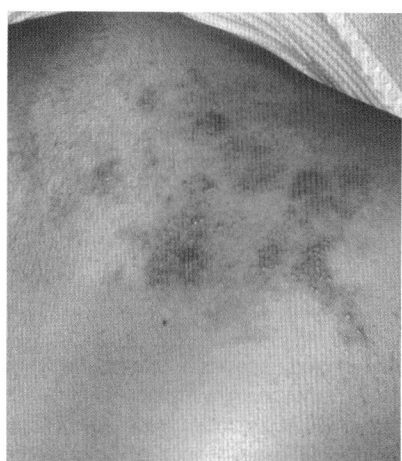

Fig. 6.8 Reactivated herpes zoster (shingles).

trastuzumab and lapatinib in breast cancer; erlotinib and crizotinib in lung cancer; and cetuximab and bevacizumab in colon cancer.

Further reading

Fearon KCH. Cancer cachexia and fat–muscle physiology. *N Engl J Med* 2011; 365:565–567.

Hugosson J, Carlsson S, Aus G et al. Mortality results from the Göteborg randomised population-based prostate-cancer screening trial. *Lancet Oncol* 2010; 11:725–732.

Ilic D, Neuberger MM, Djulbegovic M et al. *Screening for Prostate Cancer* (Cochrane Review). Chichester: Cochrane Library; 2013; issue 1.

Paimela H, Malila N, Palva T et al. Early detection of colorectal cancer with faecal occult blood test screening. *Br J Surg* 2010; 97:1567–1571.

Schröder FH, Hugosson J, Roobol MJ et al. Prostate cancer mortality at 11 years of follow-up. *N Engl J Med* 2012; 366:981–990.

Box 6.11 Serum tumour markers

Serum tumour marker	Neoplasms
α-Fetoprotein (AFP)	Hepatocellular carcinoma and non-seminomatous germ cell tumours of the gonads
β-Human chorionic gonadotrophin (β-hCG)	Choriocarcinomas, germ cell tumours (testicular) and lung cancers
Prostate-specific antigen (PSA)	Carcinoma of the prostate
Carcinoembryonic antigen (CEA)	Gastrointestinal cancers
CA125	Ovarian cancer
CA19–9	Gastrointestinal cancers, particularly pancreatic cancer
CA15–3	Breast cancer
Osteopontin	Many cancers, including mesothelioma
Calcitonin	Medullary carcinoma of the thyroid
Thyroglobulin	Papillary and follicular thyroid cancer

PRINCIPLES OF CANCER TREATMENT

Aims of treatment

Optimal cancer treatment is delivered by a multidisciplinary team that coordinates the delivery of the appropriate anticancer treatment, supportive and symptomatic care, and psychosocial support.

Establishment of agreed patient pathways has enabled more effective and timely delivery of care and post-treatment rehabilitation. Central to this endeavour is the involvement of the patient, through education as to the nature of their disease and the treatment options available.

A curative approach

For most solid tumours, local control is necessary, but not sufficient, for cure, because of the presence of systemic (microscopic) disease; while haematological cancers are usually disseminated from the outset. Improvement in the rate of cure of most cancers is thus dependent on earlier detection to increase the success of local treatment and effective systemic response. The likelihood of cure of the systemic disease rests on the type of cancer and its expression of appropriate treatment targets, its drug sensitivity and tumour bulk (microscopic or clinically detectable). A few rare cancers are so chemosensitive that even bulky metastases can be cured: for example, leukaemia, lymphoma, gonadal germ cell tumours and choriocarcinoma. For most common solid tumours, such as lung, breast and colorectal cancer, there is no current cure of bulky (clinically detectable) metastases, but micrometastatic disease treated by adjuvant systemic therapy (see below) after surgery can be cured in 10–20% of patients.

Adjuvant therapy for solid tumours

Micrometastatic spread by lymphatic or haematological dissemination often occurs early in the development of the primary tumour and can be demonstrated by molecular biological methods capable of detecting the small numbers (1 in 10^6) of circulating cells. Studies correlating prognosis with histological features of the primary cancer, such as differentiation, invasion of blood vessels or regional

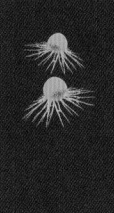

> **Box 6.12** Staging and survival of colorectal cancers: TNM and Dukes' systems

TNM classification	Description	Notation	Modified Dukes' classification	5-year survival (%)
Stage I (N0, M0)	Tumours invade submucosa	T1	A	90
	Tumours invade muscularis propria	T2		
Stage IIA (N0, M0)	Tumours invade into subserosa	T3	B	70
Stage IIB	Tumours invade directly into other organs	T4		65
Stage III (M0)	T1, T2 + 1–3 regional lymph nodes involved	N1	C	60
Stage IIIB	T3, T4 + 1–3 regional lymph nodes involved	N1		35
Stage IIIC	Any T + 4 or more regional lymph nodes	N2	C	25
Stage IV	Any T, any N + distant metastases	M1	D	7

---

lymph nodes, and molecular markers like human epidermal growth factor receptor 2 (HER2) in breast cancer, enable risk stratification and increasing individualization of therapy.

- **_Adjuvant therapy_** is defined as treatment given, in the absence of macroscopic evidence of metastases, to patients at risk of recurrence from micrometastases, following treatment given for the primary lesion.
- **_'Neoadjuvant' therapy_**, alternatively, is given before primary surgery, both to shrink the tumour in order to improve local excision, and to treat any micrometastases as soon as possible.

The success of adjuvant treatment across many tumour types relies on careful selection of patients according to defined risk criteria, and reduction of treatment toxicity to reach a balanced risk/benefit ratio. However, the majority who receive such treatment do not benefit, either because they were already cured or because the cancer is resistant to the treatment. Better tests, such as gene arrays and circulating tumour cells, are being developed to identify those with micrometastases, who really do benefit from treatment.

A palliative approach

When cure is no longer possible, palliation – that is, relief of tumour symptoms, preservation of quality of life and prolongation of life – is possible in many cancers in proportion to their drug and radiation sensitivity. There is, on average, a 2–18-month prolongation in median life expectancy with treatments for solid tumours (see specific tumour types for details); those individuals with the most responsive tumours experiencing the greatest benefit. In addition, through early assessment during treatment, it is possible to stop if no evidence of benefit is demonstrable early on, so as to minimize exposure to toxic and unsuccessful treatment.

Assessment before treatment

Staging

Before a decision about treatment can be made, not only does the type of tumour need to be established, but also its extent and distribution (see **Box 6.2**). Various 'staging investigations' are therefore performed before a treatment decision is made. To be useful clinically, the staging system must subdivide the patients into groups with different prognoses, which can guide treatment selection. The TNM (tumour, node, metastases) classification (**Box 6.12**) can be adapted for application to most common cancers.

Performance status

In addition to anatomical staging, the person's age and general state of health need to be taken into account when planning treatment. The latter has been called 'performance status' and is of great prognostic significance for all tumour types (**Box 6.13**). Performance status

> **Box 6.13** Eastern Cooperative Oncology Group (ECOG) performance status scale

Status	Description
0	Asymptomatic, fully active and able to carry out all pre-disease performance without restrictions
1	Symptomatic, fully ambulatory but restricted in physically strenuous activity and able to carry out performance of a light or sedentary nature, e.g. light housework, office work
2	Symptomatic, ambulatory and capable of all self-care but unable to carry out any work activities. Up and about >50% of waking hours; in bed <50% of day
3	Symptomatic, capable of only limited self-care, confined to bed or chair >50% of waking hours but not bedridden
4	Completely disabled, cannot carry out any self-care, totally bedridden

reflects the effects of the cancer on the patient's functional capacity. An alternative performance rating scale is provided by Karnofsky. With a performance status of 2 or more, response to, and survival following, treatment are greatly reduced for most tumour types.

Assessment of the benefits of treatment

A measurable response to treatment can serve as a useful early surrogate marker when deciding whether to continue a given treatment for an individual patient. Trials to assess response to treatment in advanced disease have identified active agents for use in the more curative setting of adjuvant treatment of early-stage disease.

Response to treatment can be subjective or objective.

A subjective response is one perceived by the patient in terms of, for example, relief of pain and dyspnoea, or improvement in appetite, weight gain or energy. Such a subjective response is a major aim of most palliative treatments. Quantitative measurements of these subjective symptoms (**p**atient-**r**eported **o**utcome **m**easures, PROMs) form a part of the assessment of response to chemotherapy, especially in those situations where cure is not possible and where the aim of treatment is to provide prolongation of good-quality life. In these circumstances, measures of quality of life enable an estimate of the balance of benefit and side-effects to be made.

An objective response to treatment is assessed clinically and radiologically (**Fig. 6.9**). The term 'remission' is often used synonymously with 'response', which, if complete, means an absence of detectable disease without necessarily implying a cure of the cancer. The terms used to evaluate the responses of tumours are

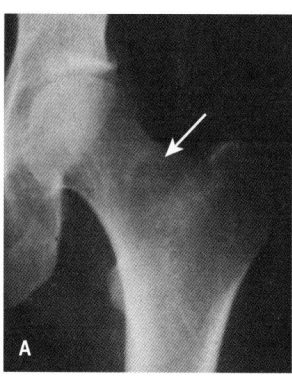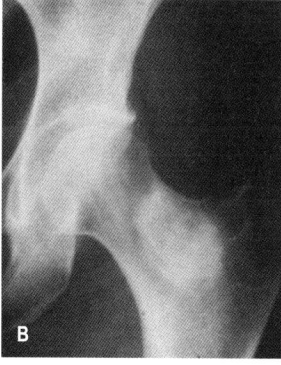

Fig. 6.9 Radiological response to chemotherapy and radiotherapy: X-rays showing response to chemotherapy and radiotherapy. (**A**) Arrow pointing to lytic bone metastasis. (**B**) Bone metastasis showing response to chemotherapy and radiotherapy with sclerotic new bone formation.

> ℹ **Box 6.14 RECIST criteria for assessing response to treatment in solid tumours**
>
> | Criterion | Description |
> |---|---|
> | **Complete response** | Disappearance of all target lesions |
> | **Partial response** | ≥30% decrease in the baseline sum of the longest diameters of all target lesions |
> | **Progression** | ≥20% increase in the sum of the longest diameters of all target lesions compared with the smallest recorded sum since treatment started, or the appearance of any new lesions |
> | **Stable disease** | All values between partial response and progressive disease |
> | **Target lesions** | Measurable lesions up to 5 per organ and 10 in total, selected on size and replicable measurement |
> | **Non-target lesions** | Non-measurable lesions recorded as present or absent at baseline and on follow-up |
> | **Measurable** | Lesions with the longest diameter in one dimension of ≥2.0 cm or ≥1.0 cm if assessed by spiral CT scan |
> | **Non-measurable** | e.g. Bone lesions, meningeal disease, ascites, pleural effusion, inflammatory breast cancer, lymphangitis cutis and pulmonis, cystic lesions |
>
> RECIST, Response Evaluation Criteria in Solid Tumours.

defined in **Box 6.14**. For a complete response, all previous clinical abnormalities should have resolved and this needs to be confirmed by clinical examination or sampling of the primary disease site, or by detection of serum tumour markers. Radiologically, a partial response, defined since 1999 by the **R**esponse **E**valuation **C**riteria **i**n **S**olid **T**umours (RECIST) convention, is a reduction of 30% of more in the sum of all measurable lesion diameters.

The increasing use of PET-CT has meant that metabolic responses (reduction in tracer avidity with or without a reduction in the size of the mass) may predict long-term outcome more accurately; this is particularly the case in lymphoma, where a classification of metabolic response exists, as well as in gastrointestinal stromal tumour (GIST).

The final assessment of treatment outcome is the impact of the therapy on remission duration and survival: that is, the **cure rate**. Such survival figures are increasingly incorporating quality-of-life assessments and a health economic assessment to calculate the number of quality-adjusted life years (QALYs) gained for the cost of the treatment, and judgements are made about health system affordability (see p. 77).

Further reading

Biggi A, Gallamini A, Chauvie S et al. International validation study for interim PET in ABVD-treated, advanced-stage Hodgkin lymphoma: interpretation criteria and concordance rate among reviewers. *J Nucl Med* 2013; 54:683–690.

Principles of chemotherapy

Cytotoxic chemotherapy employs systemically administered drugs that directly damage cellular DNA (and RNA). It kills cells by promoting apoptosis and, sometimes, frank necrosis. Different cytotoxic drugs work at different stages in the cell cycle (**Fig. 6.10**; see also **Fig. 2.10**).

There is a narrow therapeutic window between doses necessary for effective treatment of the cancer and those that cause normal tissue toxicity, because cytotoxic drugs are not cancer-specific (unlike some of the targeted biological agents) and the increased proliferation in cancers is often not much greater than in normal tissues. The dose and schedule of the chemotherapy are limited by normal tissue tolerance, especially in those more proliferative tissues of the bone marrow and gastrointestinal tract mucosa. All tissues can be affected, however, depending on the pharmacokinetics of the drug and its affinity for particular tissues (e.g. heavy metal compounds for kidneys and nerves).

The therapeutic effect on the cancer is achieved by a variety of mechanisms that seek to exploit differences between normal and transformed cells. While most drugs in the past (such as alkylating agents) have been derived by empirical testing of many different compounds, new molecular biology is leading to targeted approaches to particular genetic defects in the cancer (see p. 113).

Toxicity to normal tissue can be limited in some instances by supplying growth factors such as granulocyte colony-stimulating factor (G-CSF) or by infusing stem cell preparations to diminish bone marrow toxicity. The use of more specific targeted biological agents with relatively weak pro-apoptotic effects, in combination with general cytotoxics, has also improved the therapeutic ratio (e.g. trastuzumab and breast cancer; see p. 122). Certain cytotoxic therapies may also be administered into the pleural space, peritoneum or cerebrospinal fluid (CSF), or into the arterial supply of a tumour.

Most tumours rapidly develop resistance to single agents given on their own, through changes in membrane transport and DNA repair pathways. For this reason, the principle of intermittent combination chemotherapy was developed. Several drugs are combined, chosen on the basis of differing mechanisms of action and non-overlapping toxicities. These drugs are given over a period of a few days, followed by a rest of a few weeks, during which time the normal tissues have the opportunity for regrowth. If the normal tissues are more proficient at DNA repair than the cancer cells, it may be possible to deplete the tumour while allowing the restoration of normal tissues between chemotherapy cycles (**Fig. 6.11**).

In many experimental tumours, it has been shown that there is a log–linear relationship between drug dose and number of cancer cells killed, and that the maximum effective dose is very close to the maximum tolerated dose at which dose-limiting toxicity is reached. With a chemosensitive tumour, relatively small increases in dose may have a large effect on tumour cell kill. It is therefore apparent that, where cure is a realistic option, the dose administered is critical and may need to be maintained despite toxicity. In situations where cure is not a realistic possibility and palliation is the aim, a sufficient dose to exceed the

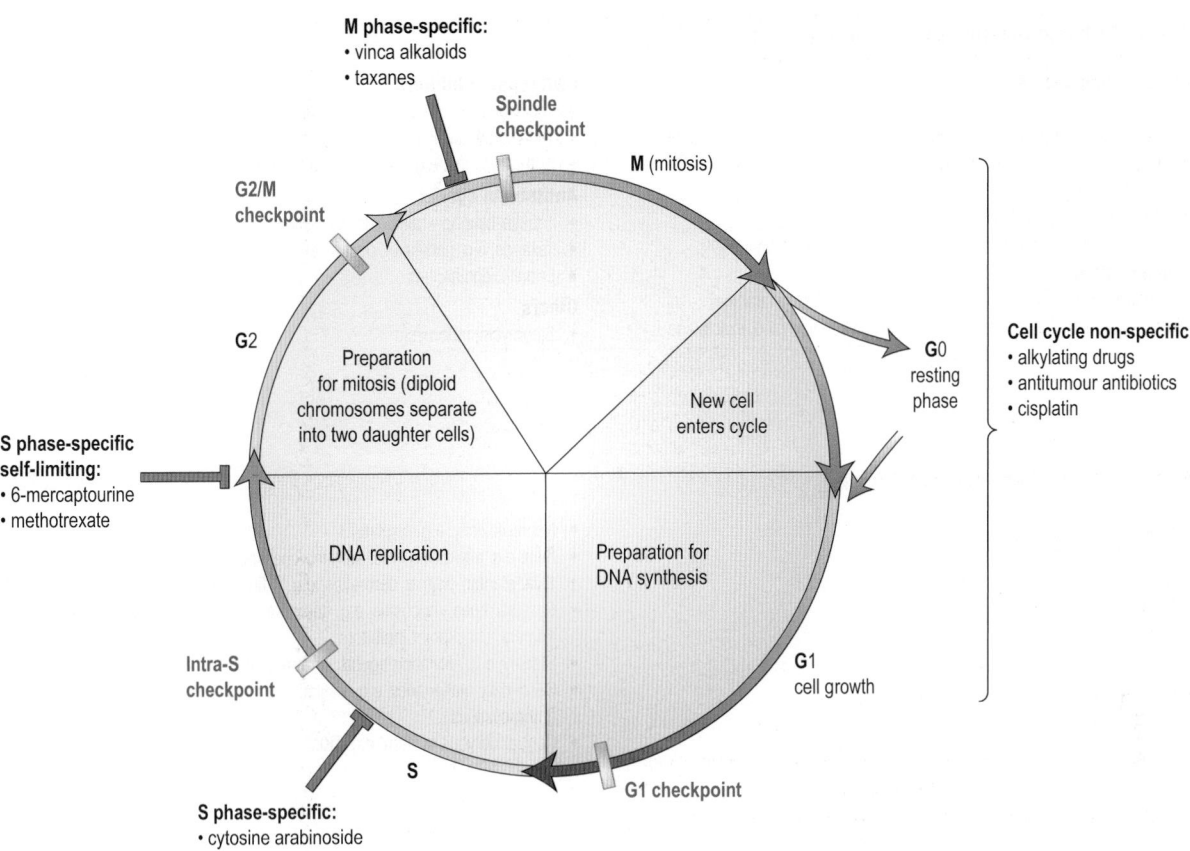

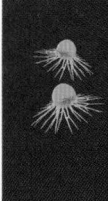

M phase-specific:
• vinca alkaloids
• taxanes

Spindle
checkpoint

M (mitosis)

G2/M
checkpoint

G2

Preparation
for mitosis (diploid
chromosomes separate
into two daughter cells)

Cell cycle non-specific:
• alkylating drugs
• antitumour antibiotics
• cisplatin

G0
resting
phase

New cell
enters cycle

**S phase-specific
self-limiting:**
• 6-mercaptourine
• methotrexate

DNA replication

Preparation for
DNA synthesis

Intra-S
checkpoint

G1
cell growth

S

G1 checkpoint

S phase-specific:
• cytosine arabinoside
• fluorouracil

Fig. 6.10 Cell cycle and chemotherapy drugs. See also **Figure 2.10**.

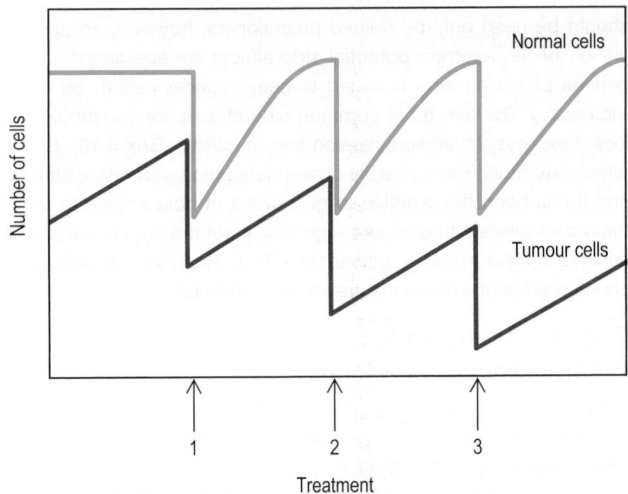

Number of cells

Normal cells

Tumour cells

1   2   3

Treatment

Fig. 6.11 Effects of multiple courses of cytotoxic chemotherapy. The decrease in the number of cells with each course is shown.

therapeutic threshold, but not cause undue toxicity, is required, as the short-term quality of life becomes a major consideration.

Classification of cytotoxic drugs

See **Box 6.15**.

DNA-damaging drugs

Alkylating agents

These act by covalently binding alkyl groups. Their major effect is to cross-link DNA strands, interfering with DNA synthesis and causing strand breaks. Examples include bendamustine and cyclophosphamide.

Platinum compounds

Cisplatin, carboplatin and oxaliplatin cause interstrand cross-links of DNA and are often regarded as non-classical alkylating agents. They have transformed the treatment of testicular cancer (cisplatin) and play a major role against many other tumours.

Antimetabolites

Antimetabolites are usually structural analogues of naturally occurring metabolites that interfere with normal synthesis of nucleic acids by falsely substituting purines and pyrimidines in metabolic pathways.

Folic acid antagonists

This class includes methotrexate, which is structurally very similar to folic acid and binds preferentially to dihydrofolate reductase, the enzyme responsible for the conversion of folic acid to folinic acid. It is used widely in the treatment of solid tumours and haematological malignancies. Folinic acid is often given to 'rescue' normal tissues from the effects of high doses of methotrexate. A related drug, pemetrexed, targets the enzyme thymidylate synthase, as well as glycinamide ribonucleotide formyltransferase (GARFT).

Pyrimidine antagonists

5-Fluorouracil (5-FU) consists of a uracil molecule with a substituted fluorine atom. It acts by blocking thymidylate synthase, which is essential for pyrimidine synthesis. Oral capecitabine is metabolized to 5-FU, as is tegafur with uracil.

---

i **Box 6.15** Chemotherapy: some cytotoxic drugs

DNA-damaging agents
- Free radicals:
  - Alkylators, e.g. cyclophosphamide, melphalan, chlorambucil, ifosfamide
  - Nitrosoureas, e.g. carmustine (BCNU), bendamustine, lomustine (CCNU), busulfan
  - Tetrazines, e.g. dacarbazine, temozolomide
- DNA cross-linking – platinum, e.g. cisplatin, carboplatin, oxaliplatin

Antimetabolites
- Pyrimidine synthesis, e.g. 5-fluorouracil, capecitabine, cytarabine, fludarabine, gemcitabine, cladribine, clofarabine, nelarabine, azacitidine
- Purine synthesis, e.g. mercaptopurine, tioguanine
- Antifolates, e.g. methotrexate, pemetrexed

DNA repair inhibitors
- Topoisomerase-I inhibitors, e.g. irinotecan
- Topoisomerase-II inhibitors, e.g. etoposide
- Anthracyclines, e.g. daunorubicin, doxorubicin, epirubicin

Antitubulin agents
- Tubulin-binding – alkaloids, e.g. vincristine, vinorelbine
- Taxanes, e.g. paclitaxel, docetaxel
- Eribulin, epothilones

Others
- Bleomycin, mitomycin

---

i **Box 6.16** Side-effects of chemotherapy

Common
- Nausea and vomiting
- Hair loss
- Myelosuppression
- Mucositis
- Fatigue

Drug-specific
- Cardiotoxicity, e.g. anthracyclines
- Progressive pulmonary fibrosis, e.g. bleomycin, busulfan
- Neurotoxicity, e.g. cisplatin, vinca alkaloids, taxanes

- Nephrotoxicity, e.g. cisplatin
- Skin, e.g. anti-EGFR TKIs, immune checkpoint inhibitors
- Skin: plantar–palmar dermatitis, e.g. 5-fluorouracil, liposomal doxorubicin
- Gut: diarrhoea, mucositis, e.g. fluorouracil, methotrexate, etoposide, TKIs, immune checkpoint inhibitors
- Sterility, e.g. alkylating agents, anthracyclines
- Secondary malignancy, e.g. alkylating agents, epipodophyllotoxins, anthracyclines
- Central nervous system, e.g. TKIs

EGFR, epidermal growth factor receptor; TKI, tyrosine kinase inhibitor.

Arabinosides

Arabinosides inhibit DNA synthesis by inhibiting DNA polymerase. Cytarabine is used almost exclusively in the treatment of acute myeloid leukaemia, where it remains the backbone of therapy.

Purine antagonists

This class includes 6-mercaptopurine and 6-tioguanine, which are both used almost exclusively in the treatment of acute leukaemia.

DNA repair inhibitors
Epipodophyllotoxins

These are semisynthetic derivatives of podophyllotoxin, which inhibit the topoisomerase enzymes that allow unwinding and uncoiling of supercoiled DNA, and maintain DNA strand breaks.

Cytotoxic antibiotics

The anthracyclines act by intercalating adjoining nucleotide pairs on the same strand of DNA and by inhibiting topoisomerase-II DNA repair. They have a wide spectrum of activity in haematological and solid tumours.

Antitubulin agents
Vinca alkaloids

Drugs such as vincristine, vinblastine and vinorelbine act by binding to tubulin and inhibiting microtubule formation during mitosis (see p. 23). They are associated with neurotoxicity due to their antimicrotubule effect and must never be given intrathecally, as this is lethal.

Taxanes

Paclitaxel and docetaxel bind to tubulin dimers and prevent their assembly into microtubules.

Side-effects of chemotherapy

Chemotherapy carries many potentially serious side-effects and should be used only by trained practitioners; however, an appreciation of its common potential side-effects is necessary for any general physician who is called to see a cancer patient on chemotherapy. The five most common side-effects are vomiting, hair loss, tiredness, myelosuppression and mucositis (**Box 6.16**). Side-effects are much more directly dose-related than anticancer effects and it has been the practice to give drugs at doses close to their maximum tolerated dose, although this is not always necessary to achieve their maximum anticancer effect. Common combination chemotherapeutic regimens are shown in **Box 6.17**.

Common side-effects
Extravasation of intravenous drugs

Cytotoxic drugs should be given only by trained personnel. They cause severe local tissue necrosis if leakage occurs outside the vein. Stop the infusion immediately and institute local measures: for example, aspirate as much of the drug as possible from the cannula, infiltrate the area with 0.9% saline and apply warm compresses. Antihistamines and corticosteroids may give symptomatic relief.

Nausea and vomiting

The severity of these common side-effects varies with the cytotoxicity and are particular problems with platinum analogues. They can be eliminated in 75% of patients by using modern antiemetics. A stepped policy, with antiemetics such as metoclopramide and domperidone, followed by 5-HT$_3$ (5-hydroxytrypamine, serotonin) antagonists (e.g. ondansetron, granisetron) combined with dexamethasone, should be used to match the emetogenic potential of the chemotherapy. **Apreitant**, a neurokinin receptor antagonist, is helpful in preventing acute and delayed nausea and vomiting. It is

Cancer	Abbreviation[a]	Regimen
Breast	AC	Adriamycin (doxorubicin), cyclophosphamide
Lung	PE	Cisplatin, etoposide
Stomach	ECF	Epirubicin, cisplatin, 5-fluorouracil
Colorectal	FOLFOX	Oxaliplatin, 5-fluorouracil, folinic acid

[a]Some abbreviations are related to trade names.

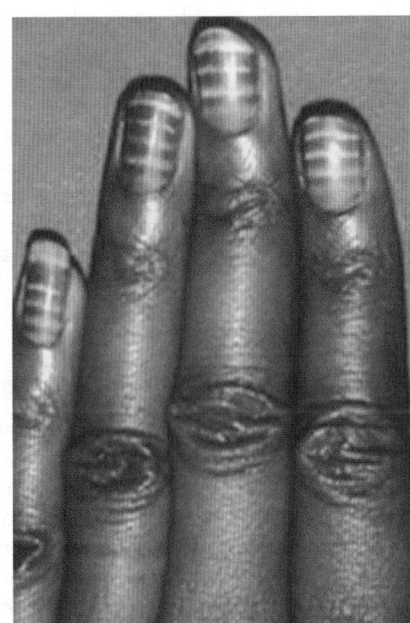

Fig. 6.12 Nail growth cessation with each drug cycle (Beau's lines).

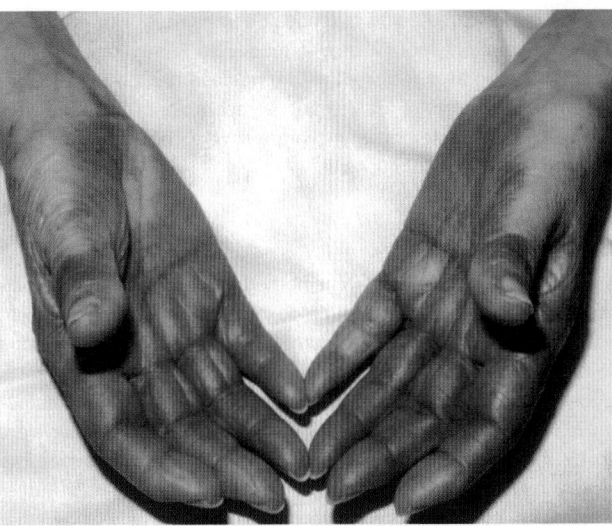

Fig. 6.13 Hands showing palmar–plantar skin toxicity.

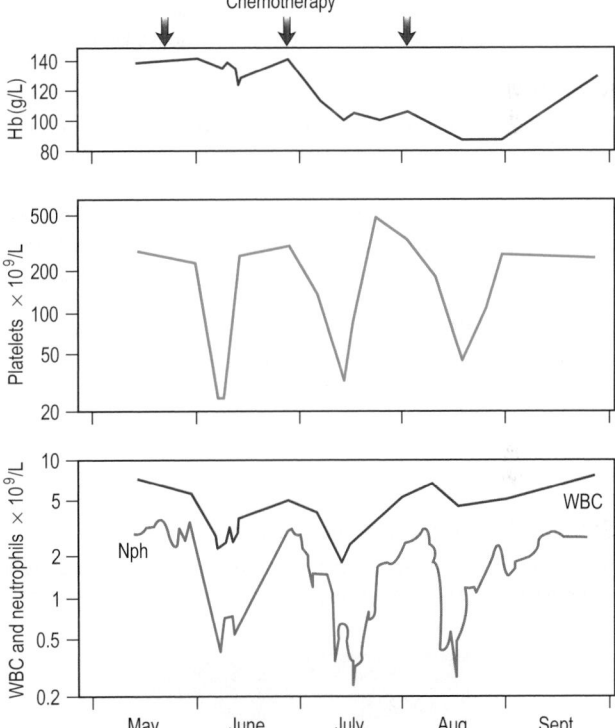

Fig. 6.14 Cyclical myelosuppression from chemotherapy (arrowed). Hb, haemoglobin; Nph, neutrophils; WBC, white blood cells.

used with dexamethasone and a 5-HT$_3$ antagonist. Drugs such as cyclizine, olanzapine and levomepromazine, and benzodiazepines, can be used to control persistent nausea.

Effects on hair, skin and nails

Many, but not all, cytotoxic drugs are capable of causing hair loss. Scalp cooling can sometimes be used to reduce hair loss but, in general, this side-effect can be avoided only by selection of drugs, where this is possible. Hair regrows on completion of chemotherapy. Nails will demonstrate banding, reflecting periods of cessation of growth during each chemotherapy cycle (**Fig. 6.12**), and skin toxicity may be particularly pronounced with 5-FU, capecitabine and docetaxel (**Fig. 6.13**).

Fatigue

This is often significant and may continue beyond completion of therapy. Other problems, such as anaemia or depression, may exacerbate fatigue. Attention should be paid to nutrition, hydration, sleep hygiene, gentle exercise, task prioritization, pacing, realistic target setting and scheduling of rest within the day.

Bone marrow suppression and immunosuppression

Suppression of the production of red blood cells, white blood cells and platelets occurs with most cytotoxic drugs and is a dose-related phenomenon (**Fig. 6.14**). Severely myelosuppressive chemotherapy may be required if treatment is to be given with curative intent, despite the potential for rare but fatal infection or bleeding. Anaemia and thrombocytopenia are managed by red cell or platelet

transfusions. (Neutropenic infection is discussed on p. 116.) The risk of infective problems can be ameliorated by the use of prophylactic antimicrobials, such as ciprofloxacin, or the use of G-CSF as primary prophylaxis in those chemotherapy regimens that carry a significant risk of febrile neutropenia or in those patients on less intensive therapies who are at higher risk due to age or co-morbidity.

Mucositis

This common side-effect of chemotherapy reflects the sensitivity of the mucosa to antimitotic agents. Mucositis causes severe pain in the oropharyngeal region and problems with swallowing and nutrition. It can be generalized throughout the intestinal tract and can cause life-threatening diarrhoea. Treatment is with antiseptic and anti-candidal mouthwash; if mucositis is severe, fluid and antibiotic support is required, as the mucosa is a portal for entry of enteric organisms. Palifermin, a recombinant keratinocyte-derived growth factor, may ameliorate severe chemotherapy- and radiotherapy-induced mucositis.

Other toxicities

Cardiotoxicity

This is a rare side-effect of chemotherapy and is usually associated with anthracyclines such as doxorubicin; effects can present as an acute arrhythmia during administration or cardiac failure due to cardiomyopathy after chronic exposure (**Fig. 6.15**). This effect is dose-related and can largely be prevented by restricting the cumulative total dose of anthracyclines within the safe range (equivalent to $450\,mg/m^2$ body surface area cumulative doxorubicin dose). The risk of anthracycline cardiomyopathy is also dependent on other treatments, such as trastuzumab or radiotherapy, as well as other cardiac risk factors, such as hypertension, smoking and hypercholesterolaemia. Cardiotoxicity can also be reduced by using the analogue epirubicin or by reducing peak drug concentrations through delayed-release preparations, such as liposomal doxorubicin. 5-FU and its prodrug, capecitabine, can cause cardiac ischaemia.

Neurotoxicity

This occurs predominantly with the vinca alkaloids, taxanes and platinum analogues (but not carboplatin). It is dose-related and cumulative. Chemotherapy is usually stopped before the development of a significant polyneuropathy, which, once established, is only partially reversible. *Vinca alkaloids, such as vincristine, must never be given intrathecally*, as the neurological damage is progressive and fatal.

Nephrotoxicity

Cisplatin (but not oxaliplatin or carboplatin), methotrexate and ifosfamide can potentially cause renal damage. This can usually be prevented by maintaining an adequate diuresis during treatment to reduce drug concentration in the renal tubules, and by monitoring of renal function.

Sterility and premature menopause

Some anticancer drugs, particularly alkylating agents but also anthracyclines and docetaxel, may cause gonadal damage, resulting in sterility and, in women, the loss of ovarian oestrogen production, which may be irreversible.

In males, storage of sperm prior to chemotherapy should be offered to the patient when chemotherapy is given with curative intent.

In females, collection of oocytes to be fertilized *in vitro* and cryopreserved as embryos for subsequent implantation is most successful; however, it is also possible to collect and freeze by vitrification of unstimulated oocytes. Cryopreservation of ovarian tissue and retrieval of viable oocytes for subsequent fertilization are still experimental. The recovery of gonadal function is dependent on the status before treatment; in women, this is mostly related to age since menarche, with those under 40 years having significantly more ovarian reserve.

Secondary malignancies

Anticancer drugs have mutagenic potential and the development of secondary malignancies, predominantly acute leukaemia, is an uncommon but particularly unwelcome long-term side-effect in patients otherwise cured of their primary malignancies. The alkylating agents, anthracyclines and epipodophyllotoxins are particularly implicated.

Principles of endocrine therapy

Oestrogens are capable of stimulating the growth of breast and endometrial cancers, and androgens can stimulate the growth of prostate cancer. Removal of these growth factors by manipulation of the hormonal environment may result in apoptosis and regression of the cancer. Endocrine therapy can be curative in a proportion of patients treated for micrometastatic disease in the adjuvant setting for breast and prostate cancer, and provides a minimally toxic, non-curative (palliative) treatment in advanced or metastatic disease. The presence of detectable cellular receptors for the hormone is strongly predictive of response. However, this is also modified by the many molecular interactions between the activation pathways of, for example, epidermal growth factor receptor (EGFR), the androgen receptor (AR (see p. 128)) and oestrogen receptor (ER) (see p. 122).

Principles of biological and targeted therapy

Immunotherapy

Certain antigens that are specific to cancer cells, such as sequences of tumour immunoglobulin from melanoma antigens, have been used as tumour vaccines, together with manipulation of the immune system to overcome tolerance. Engineered chimeric antigen receptors (CARs) that direct T cells to specific antigenic targets are emerging as a powerful potential tool in the treatment of a wide range of cancers.

Interferons

Interferons are naturally occurring cytokines that mediate the cellular immune response. Interferon-alpha (IFN-α) has been used to treat advanced melanoma and renal cell carcinoma.

Treatment with IFN has side-effects (see p. 1281): most commonly, influenza-like symptoms, which tend to diminish with time, and fatigue, which generally does not and can be treatment-limiting. IFN used to be given as a daily subcutaneous injection, but conjugation with polyethylene glycol (PEG interferon) has led to a reduction in frequency of injection and severity of side-effects.

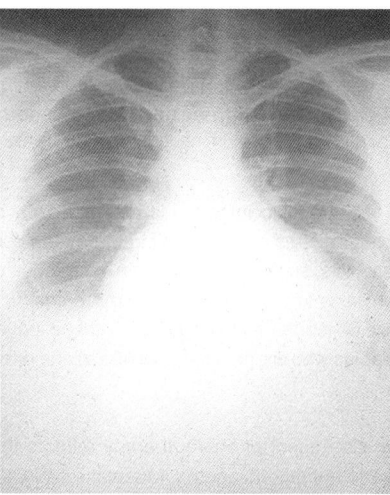

Fig. 6.15 Anthracycline dilated cardiomyopathy with congestive heart failure.

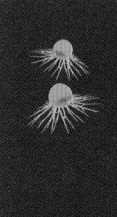

Interleukins

Interleukin 2 (IL-2), a recombinant protein, is used to activate T-cell responses, often in conjunction with IFN-stimulated B-cell activation. Anti-tumour activity has been observed in renal cell carcinoma and melanoma, with responses in 10–20% of patients, occasionally for prolonged periods. Toxicity is common; acutely, this includes the capillary leak syndrome with hypotension and pulmonary oedema, while autoimmune thyroiditis and vitiligo occur later.

Immune checkpoint inhibitors

These new agents directly interfere with the relationship between T cells and antigen-presenting cells or tumour cells to overcome the common problems of immune tolerance and anergy. Ipilimumab is a MAb that blocks the CD152 (CTLA4) receptor responsible for downregulating T-cell responses, and is active in the treatment of melanoma. The inhibitors of the programmed death (PD-1) receptor or its ligands, PD-L1 and L2, on activated T cells, further reactivate tumour-specific cytotoxic T cells, so that ipilimumab plus nivolumab (a PD-1 receptor blocker) doubled the response rate from 20% to 40% in metastatic melanoma. Many clinical trials are now examining these agents in the context of a variety of other cancers.

Immunomodulatory drugs: thalidomide, lenalidomide, pomalidomide

This family of immunomodulatory drugs (IMIDs) is increasingly being used in a range of malignancies, such as myeloma, chronic lymphocytic leukaemia and myelodysplastic syndrome, as well some solid tumours. They have anti-angiogenic functions, as well as effects on cytokine production, tumour/stromal interactions and T-cell co-stimulatory functions. They are all considered teratogenic and should be avoided in women of reproductive potential, unless extra precaution is taken against conception. There is increasing evidence that IMIDs work through binding of the E3 ligase protein, cereblon, which acts to degrade two specific B-cell transcription factors, IKZF1 and IKZF3.

Targeted therapies

The fast-developing field of targeted therapies includes MAbs, receptor kinase inhibitors and small molecule receptor blockers. Expression of the targeted molecule is not sufficient of itself to indicate that use of the corresponding drug will be therapeutic because it is also necessary for the drug to be able to interrupt a growth-critical pathway in that cancer.

Monoclonal antibodies

Monoclonal antibodies (MAbs; **Box 6.18**) directed against tumour cell surface antigens are 'humanized' by being genetically engineered to have a range of functions, including:

- acting as a carrier molecule to target toxins or radioisotopes to the tumour cells, e.g. trastuzumab or trastuzumab emtansine for breast cancer
- acting as anti-growth factor agents added to chemotherapy by inhibiting dimerization of the extracellular receptor molecules.

Side-effects are those of hypersensitivity to the foreign protein and specific cross-reactivities: for example, trastuzumab for the myocardium, bevacizumab for the mucosa and renal tubule, and cetuximab for the skin follicles.

Intracellular signal inhibitors

Many cancer cells are transformed by the activity of the protein products of oncogenes that signal growth by phosphorylation of tyrosine residues on the intracellular portion of growth factor receptors. Small molecule inhibitors (**Box 6.19**) have many

Box 6.18 Monoclonal antibodies (MAbs) in cancer

Antigen	Mutation/ amplification	Tumour type	MAb
EGFR	cERBB2/HER2 amplification	Breast, gastric	**Trastuzumab**
	cERBB2/HER2 amplification	Breast	**Pertuzumab**
	RAS/BRAF wt	Colorectal, oropharyngeal	**Cetuximab**
	RAS/BRAF wt	Colorectal	**Panitumumab**
CTLA-4	+	Melanoma	**Ipilumumab**
VEGFR	+	Colorectal, ovarian	**Bevacizumab**
PD-1	+	Melanoma, Hodgkin lymphoma, NSCLC	**Nivolumab**
RANKL	+	Bone metastases	**Denosumab**

CTLA-4, Cytotoxic T-lymphocyte associated protein 4; EGFR, epidermal growth factor receptor; NSCLC, non-small-cell lung cancer; PD-1, programmed cell death protein 1; RANKL, receptor activator of nuclear factor kappa-B ligand; VEGFR, vascular endothelial growth factor receptor.

Box 6.19 Intracellular signal inhibitor therapies in cancer

Gene	Genetic alteration	Tumour type	Therapeutic agent
Receptor tyrosine kinase			
EGFR	Mutation, amplification	Lung	**Gefitinib, erlotinib, afatinib**
ERBB2	Amplification	Breast	**Lapatinib**
PDGFRA	Mutation	GIST	**Sunitinib, imatinib, nilotinib**
PDGFRB	Translocation	Chronic myelomonocytic leukaemia	**Sunitinib, sorafenib, imatinib**
ALK	Mutation or amplification	Lung, neuroblastoma	**Crizotinib, alectinib**
c-Met	Amplification	Gefitinib-resistant NSCLC, gastric	**Crizotinib**
c-Kit	Mutation	GIST	**Sunitinib, imatinib**
RET	Mutation, translocation	Thyroid medullary carcinoma	**Vandetanib**
Serine–threonine–lipid kinase			
BRAF	Mutation (V600E)	Melanoma	**Vemurafenib**
mTOR	Increased activation	Renal cell carcinoma, breast	**Everolimus**
DNA damage or repair			
BRCA1 and BRCA2	Mutation (synthetic lethal effect)	Breast, ovarian	**Olaparib (PARP inhibitors)**

GIST, gastrointestinal stromal tumour; NSCLC, non-small-cell lung cancer.

pharmacokinetic advantages over the MAb inhibitors. The first example was the TKI imatinib, which specifically inhibits the BCR-ABL fusion oncoprotein and c-Kit. This compound is an extremely effective treatment for chronic myeloid leukaemia and GIST, which are characterized by the presence of the c-Kit target. Lapatinib, which inhibits HER2, has increased survival in breast cancer. The less specific TKIs, sunitinib and pazopanib, which inhibit signalling by EGFR and vascular endothelial growth factor receptor (VEGFR), have proved effective in metastatic renal cancer, while afatinib, erlotinib and gefitinib have shown activity in lung cancer. Vemurafenib is a kinase inhibitor and has a specificity for BRAF-V600, as used in malignant melanoma (see p. 691). Many other similar molecules are in pre-clinical or early clinical development, but heterogeneity within a single tumour occurs and genomic anomalies may not all be represented in a single biopsy specimen. Vandetanib, a combined VEGF and C-RET inhibitor, is useful in the treatment of medullary thyroid cancer.

Proteasome inhibitors

The proteasome degrades redundant or damaged proteins that have been labelled by a process called ubiquitination. Such proteins include cyclins and cyclin-dependent kinases, as well as factors in the nuclear factor kappa-B (NFκB) pathway. Inhibition of the proteasome leads to apoptosis in cancer cells and is synergistic with other treatments such as steroids and chemotherapy. Bortezomib is the first of such inhibitors to reach clinical practice and is used in myeloma, as well as some types of non-Hodgkin lymphoma. There are also recent additions to this class, including carfilzomib and ixazomib.

Gene therapy

Antisense oligonucleotides are short sequences of DNA bases that specifically inhibit complementary sequences of either DNA or RNA. As a result, they can be generated against genetic sequences, which are specific for tumour cells. Their clinical development has been hampered by poor uptake by tumour cells and rapid degradation by natural endonucleases. However, one antisense sequence directed against the *Bcl-2* oncogene has been shown to have an anti-tumour effect in patients with non-Hodgkin lymphoma. Viral vectors for the transfection of tumour cells *in vivo* are being tested as a way of delivering specific replacement gene therapy in head and neck cancers.

Further reading

Longo DL. Tumor heterogeneity and personalized medicine. *N Engl J Med* 2010; 366:956–957.

Lu G, Middleton RE, Sun H et al. The myeloma drug lenalidomide promotes the cereblon-dependent destruction of Ikaros proteins. *Science* 2014; 343:305–309.

Maus MV, Grupp SA, Porter DL et al. Antibody-modified T cells: CARS take the front seat for haematologic malignancies. *Blood* 2014; 123:2625–2635.

Touchefeu Y, Montassier E, Nieman K et al. Systematic review: the role of the gut microbiota in chemotherapy- or radiation-induced gastrointestinal mucositis. *Aliment Pharmacol Ther* 2014; 40:409–421.

Wolchok JD, Kluger H, Callahan MK et al. Nivolumab plus ipilimumab in advanced melanoma. *N Engl J Med* 2013; 369:122–133.

Principles of radiation therapy

Radiation is an important modality for the treatment of cancer and can be used with radical, adjuvant or palliative intent. More than 50% of patients with a cancer diagnosis are treated with radiotherapy. In order to justify radiotherapy treatment, it is important to have histological confirmation of cancer and to perform relevant imaging. All treatment options should be discussed with the patient; they should be aware of treatment intentions and side-effects, and must consent to treatment.

Radical radiotherapy aims to deliver a tumouricidal treatment dose to a well-defined target volume with curative intent, sparing the surrounding normal tissues as much as possible. It is usually given as a fractionated course over a number of weeks, with patients receiving daily treatment. Carcinoma of the cervix, for example, can be cured with 5.5 weeks of daily radiotherapy delivered Monday to Friday with concurrent cisplatin chemotherapy.

Adjuvant radiotherapy is used to reduce the risk of tumour recurrence after primary surgery. The aim of treatment is to eradicate occult micrometastatic disease that cannot be demonstrated on imaging, as occurs in a significant percentage of patients. In breast cancer, for example, a patient may have radiotherapy after wide local excision surgery, and this reduces the risk of recurrence to the same level as if they had had a mastectomy.

Palliative radiotherapy can be used to alleviate symptoms of local disease (such as haematuria) or distant metastases (such as bone pain). Treatment is usually given with a small number of fractions, and effective results can also be achieved with a single fraction of radiotherapy.

Theoretical background

Radiotherapy is the therapeutic use of ionizing radiation. X-rays were first used in the treatment of cancer at the end of the 19th century. Since that time, our understanding of the effects of ionizing radiation on malignant and normal tissues has progressed with increased knowledge of radiobiology. In parallel, our knowledge of radiation physics has advanced and there have been significant technological developments in treatment planning and delivery.

Radiation physics

Radiation, used therapeutically, exerts its effects through the ionization of intracellular molecules; the radiation can be electromagnetic or particulate. The two types of *electromagnetic radiation* used in radiotherapy are X-rays and gamma rays, and both of these can also be described by the term 'photon'. Gamma rays are produced from the nuclear decay of radioactive isotopes, whereas X-rays are produced artificially by electrical means, usually in a linear accelerator, accelerating electrons to a high energy and then stopping them abruptly in a heavy metal target. *Particulate radiation* consists of subatomic particles, including alpha particles, protons and neutrons.

Interactions of X-rays with matter

The process by which photons are absorbed depends principally on their energy and the chemical composition of the absorbing material. The radiation effect depends on the intensity of the radiation source, measured as the linear energy transfer or frequency of ionizing events per unit of path, which is subject to the inverse square law as the energy diminishes with distance from the source. The depth of penetration of biological tissues by the photons depends on the energy of the beam. Low-energy photons from an 85 kV source are suitable for superficial treatments, while high-energy 15 mV sources produce a beam with deeper penetration, lower dose at the initial skin boundary (skin-sparing), sharper edges and less absorption by bone. Superficial radiation may also be delivered by electron beams from a linear accelerator, from which the target electrode that generates the X-rays has been removed. The radiation dose is measured in Gray (Gy), 1 Gray being equal to 1 joule (J) absorbed per kilogram of absorbing tissue. There are differing processes of energy absorption, depending on the energy of the photons delivered, but all share in common the fact that the photon causes excitation of electrons within the targeted tissue.

Biological effect

The resultant biological damage is caused in either an indirect or a direct way. X-rays and gamma rays mainly interact with target biological molecules in an indirect way. The interaction is initially with

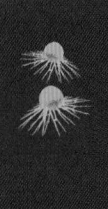

other atoms and molecules within the cells, producing free radicals, which are highly reactive molecules generated from water and oxygen. These free radicals exert a biological effect through the generation of single- and double-strand DNA breaks, inducing apoptosis of cells as they progress through the cell cycle.

The biological effect is dependent on the dose rate, duration, volume irradiated and tissue sensitivity. Sensitivity to photon damage is greatest during the G2–M phase of the cell cycle (see p. 23) and is also dependent on the DNA repair capacity of the cell.

Radiobiology is the study of the actions of ionizing radiation on living things. The effects of radiation on normal and malignant tissues evolve through a series of steps. Classical radiobiology describes the 'five Rs' of the radiation response:

- **Repair.** This is the ability of cells to repair DNA damaged by ionizing radiation using different DNA repair mechanisms. Delivery of small daily doses of radiotherapy enables repair of DNA in the cells of normal tissues.
- *Redistribution.* When radiation is delivered, cells in the G2–M phase of the cell cycle are most radiosensitive. Cells in the more radioresistant phases (e.g. S phase) survive and progress through the cell cycle and are then in the more radiosensitive phase when the next fraction of radiotherapy is delivered.
- *Reoxygenation.* Oxygenated cells are more susceptible to DNA damage by radiation. Due to irregular blood supplies, tumour cells may be hypoxic. After radiation, the more oxygenated cells die, and the surviving hypoxic cells are reoxygenated as oxygen diffuses into these areas, making these cells more susceptible to radiation with the next fraction of treatment.
- *Repopulation.* During a course of fractionated radiotherapy, viable tumour cells continue to divide and repopulate the tumour. In some cancers – for example, those of the head and neck or cervix – it is important not to extend the overall treatment time if there are gaps in treatment, as the tumour will repopulate.
- *Radiosensitivity.* Some tumours are more sensitive to radiation than others. For example, squamous cell carcinomas and lymphomas are radiosensitive, whereas melanomas and brain tumours are radioresistant.

Clinical application of radiation therapy

Radiotherapy planning involves both detailed physics of the applied dose and knowledge of the biology of the cancer; it is also necessary to establish whether the intention is to treat the tumour site alone or to include the likely loco-regional patterns of spread. Normal tissue tolerance will determine the extent of the side-effects and, therefore, the total achievable dose to the tumour. A balanced decision is made according to the curative or palliative intent of the treatment and the likely early or late side-effects. The clinician outlines on the planning scan the areas that they wish to treat using all the clinical information available. They also delineate the critical structures that they do not wish to receive a dose. The physicist then uses planning algorithms to enable the best delivery of dose to the tumour, avoiding critical structures as far as possible. Depending on the site of the tumour, the patient is immobilized to allow reproducibility of position for each fraction of treatment. For example, if the brain is being treated, they will wear a mask that keeps them still on the treatment couch.

The cancers for which radiotherapy is usually employed in a primary curative approach, when the tumour is anatomically localized, are listed in **Box 6.20**, along with those in which radiotherapy has curative potential when added to surgery (adjuvant radiotherapy).

> *i* **Box 6.20** Curative radiotherapy treatment
>
> | **Primary modality** | **Adjuvant to primary surgery** |
> |---|---|
> | • Retina | • Lung |
> | • Central nervous system | • Breast |
> | • Skin | • Uterus |
> | • Pharynx and larynx | • Bladder |
> | • Cervix and vagina | • Rectum |
> | • Prostate | • Testis |
> | • Lymphoma | • Sarcoma |

> *i* **Box 6.21** Palliative benefits of radiotherapy
>
> - Pain relief, e.g. bone metastases
> - Reduction of headache and vomiting in raised intracranial pressure from central nervous system metastases
> - Relief of obstruction of bronchus, oesophagus, ureter and lymphatics
> - Preservation of skeletal integrity from metastases in weight-bearing bones
> - Reversal of neurological impairment from spinal cord or optic nerve compression by metastases

---

Palliative treatments are frequently used to provide relief of symptoms and to improve quality, if not duration, of survival (**Box 6.21**). Palliative treatment is usually given in as few fractions as possible over as short a time as possible.

Radiotherapy planning with CT guidance has been complemented by the introduction of three-dimensional planning and volumetric modulated arc therapy (VMAT), which can deliver curved dose distributions to improve the therapeutic ratio. This allows a greater differential in dose between the tumour and critical normal structures, in turn permitting dose escalation or a reduced risk of toxicity.

Four-dimensional radiotherapy planning is also becoming widely available. It varies radiation dose over time: for example, the respiratory cycle during lung cancer treatment.

Types of radiation therapy

Fractionated external beam radiotherapy uses photons generated in a linear accelerator. The radiation dose is delivered in increments separated by at least 4–6 hours to try to exploit any advantage in DNA repair between normal and malignant cells.

Stereotactic radiosurgery/radiotherapy (γ-knife, CyberKnife or linear accelerator-based treatment) can concentrate X-rays or gamma radiation from multiple sources on to a small volume to generate an ablative dose of radiation with rapid dose fall-off, minimizing the dose to surrounding tissues. Small lung cancers can be treated in this way, and it allows for the more aggressive treatment of cancer that has spread to the brain.

Proton beam therapy is an alternative type of external beam radiotherapy that uses charged proton particles. Due to their larger mass the protons have little side-scatter and so offer a much more focused beam with less dose to surrounding structures. Proton therapy is particularly recommended for the treatment of children, in whom radiotherapy can affect normal growth and development.

Brachytherapy is the use of radiation sources in close contact with the tissue to provide intense exposure over a short distance to a restricted volume. Such techniques have been used to treat localized breast, prostatic and cervical carcinoma.

Systemic radionuclides, such as ^{131}iodine- (in thyroid cancer) or radioisotope-labelled MAbs (e.g. anti-CD20 for lymphoma) and hormones (e.g. somatostatin for carcinoid tumours), can be administered by intravenous or intracavitary routes to provide radiation targeted to particular tissue uptake via surface antigens or receptors.

Radiotherapy in combination with systemic therapy

The local efficacy of radiotherapy can be increased by the simultaneous but not serial addition of chemotherapy with agents such as cisplatin, mitomycin and 5-FU for cancers of the head and neck, lung, oesophagus, stomach, rectum, anus, cervix and bladder. Reduced local recurrence rates have translated into survival benefits and further research is investigating the concurrent use of biological agents (e.g. EGFR inhibitors) and immunotherapy with radiation. The **abscopal effect** occurs when localized radiotherapy induces the regression of non-irradiated metastatic lesions at a distance from the primary site of irradiation by a systemic immune-mediated response, which may be augmented by giving immunotherapy with the radiotherapy. This is an exciting area of oncology that is being explored in a number of tumour sites.

Side-effects of radiotherapy

Early radiotherapy side-effects may occur within days to weeks of treatment; at this point, they are usually self-limiting but associated with general systemic disturbance (**Box 6.22**). The side-effects depend on tissue sensitivity, fraction size and treatment volume, and are managed with supportive measures until normal tissue repair occurs. The toxicity may also be enhanced by exposure to other radiation-sensitizing agents, especially some cytotoxics, such as bleomycin, actinomycin, anthracyclines, cisplatin and 5-FU.

Later side-effects occur months to years later and are unrelated to the severity of the acute effects because they have a different mechanism. Late effects reflect both the loss of slowly proliferating cells and a local endarteritis that produces ischaemia and proliferative fibrosis. The risks of late side-effects are related to the fraction size and total dose delivered to the tissue. Growth may be arrested if bony epiphyses are not yet fused and are irradiated, leading to distorted skeletal growth in later life.

Secondary malignancies following radiotherapy may appear 10–20 years after cure of the primary cancer. Haematological malignancies tend to occur sooner than solid tumours from the irradiated tissues. The latter are very dependent on the status of the tissue at the time of treatment; for example, the pubertal breast is up to 300 times more sensitive to malignant transformation than the breast tissues of a woman in her thirties. Patients who smoke are more liable to develop lung cancer. Treatment of these secondary cancers can be successful, provided there is normal bone marrow to reconstitute the haematopoietic system, or the whole tissue at risk can be resected (e.g. thyroid after mantle radiotherapy for lymphoma).

ACUTE ONCOLOGY

The acute care of all patients admitted to hospital with a cancer diagnosis has become known as acute oncology; it aims to ensure coordinated patient care with access to all facets of the multidisciplinary team, and thus the most efficient use of high-cost inpatient facilities. In addition, there are a number of common oncological emergencies to which urgent treatment is critical for success (**Box 6.23**).

Neutropenic sepsis

This is the most common cause of attendance in the emergency department for any cancer patient and must always be considered in anyone who is unwell within a month of chemotherapy. Neutropenic patients are at high risk of bacterial and fungal infections, most often from enteric bowel flora; hence, some units will advocate a specific neutropenic diet that is low in bacterial and fungal contamination (**Box 6.24**). Patients must be warned of the possibility of neutropenic fever occurring. Non-specific symptoms are also common, such as nausea, diarrhoea, drowsiness and breathlessness. A fever may not always be present. The critical test is the full blood count. Patients with neutrophils $<1.0 \times 10^9$/L are managed by the

---

⊕ Box 6.23 Acute oncology: problems and common causes

Problem	Common causes
Fever	Neutropenic sepsis
Breathlessness	Pulmonary embolus, pleural effusion Neutropenic sepsis Bronchial obstruction and lobar collapse Tense ascites
Hypotension	Neutropenic sepsis Pulmonary embolus, pericardial tamponade
Swollen face	Superior vena caval obstruction
Leg weakness	Spinal cord compression
Mental deterioration	Hypercalcaemia Raised intracranial pressure
Renal failure	Obstructive uropathy, sepsis Drugs: non-steroidal anti-inflammatory drugs, methotrexate, cisplatin Metabolic: calcium, uric acid, myeloma protein, tumour lysis
Haemorrhage	Tumour erosion, thrombocytopenia, disseminated intravascular coagulation
Bone pain	Pathological fracture
Acute abdomen	Intestinal obstruction and perforation
Jaundice	Obstructing mass liver, parenchymal destruction by tumour or drugs

---

ⓘ Box 6.22 Side-effects of radiotherapy

Acute temporary side-effects/dependent on region being treated
- Anorexia, nausea, malaise
- Mucositis, oesophagitis, diarrhoea
- Alopecia
- Myelosuppression

Late side-effects
- Skin: ischaemia, ulceration
- Bone: necrosis, fracture, sarcoma
- Mouth: xerostomia, ulceration

- Bowel: stenosis, fistula, diarrhoea
- Bladder: fibrosis, frequency, incontinence
- Vagina: dyspareunia, stenosis
- Lung: fibrosis, breathlessness
- Heart: pericardial fibrosis, cardiomyopathy, vasculopathy
- Central nervous system: myelopathy
- Gonads: infertility, menopause
- Secondary malignancies: e.g. leukaemia, cancer (e.g. thyroid)
- Other: carotid artery stenosis

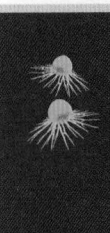

immediate introduction of broad-spectrum antibiotics. Signs of systemic illness, such as tachycardia, hypotension or oliguria, mandate urgent admission and resuscitation with intravenous treatment (**Box 6.25**). Initial empirical therapy should be reviewed following microbiological results.

All such patients need to be discussed with the appropriate specialist oncology team and hospitals should have clear protocols for the rapid institution of antibiotics within an hour of arrival in the emergency department. In units practised in the assessment of febrile neutropenia, it is possible to follow a more risk-stratified antibiotic policy and to avoid or curtail admission with oral co-amoxiclav plus ciprofloxacin when low-risk features are present: that is, absence of tachycardia, hypotension, hypoxia and mucositis, and an expected short duration of myelosuppression.

Pulmonary embolus

This is a common complication of the coagulopathy of cancer and is a side-effect of chemotherapy (**Fig. 6.16**). It often presents with unexplained breathlessness and episodic exacerbations from multiple small emboli, rather than chest pain. A high level of suspicion should be maintained in any cancer patient with breathlessness, hypoxia or chest pain. CT pulmonary angiography is the investigation of choice. Prophylactic anticoagulation is given to all immobilized patients (see p. 1013). Warfarin is ineffective (and direct oral anticoagulants are unlicensed) in reversing the coagulopathy of cancer; low-molecular-weight heparin is preferred.

Superior vena caval obstruction

Superior vena caval obstruction (**Fig. 6.17**) can arise from any upper mediastinal mass but is most commonly associated with lung cancer and lymphoma. The patient presents with difficulty breathing and/or swallowing, stridor, a swollen, oedematous face and arms, venous congestion in the neck, and dilated veins in the upper chest

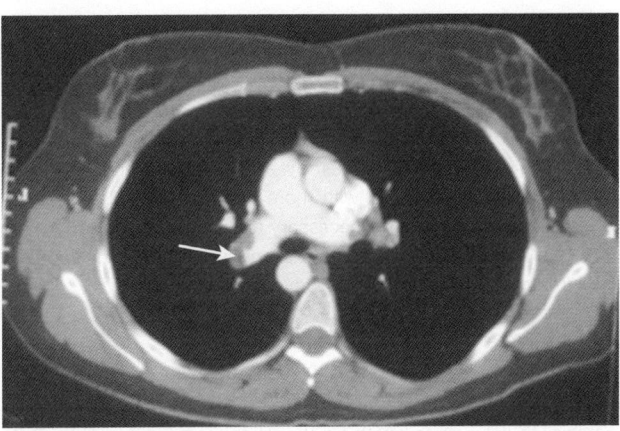

Fig. 6.16 Pulmonary embolism (arrowed) (seen as a filling defect on CT pulmonary angiogram).

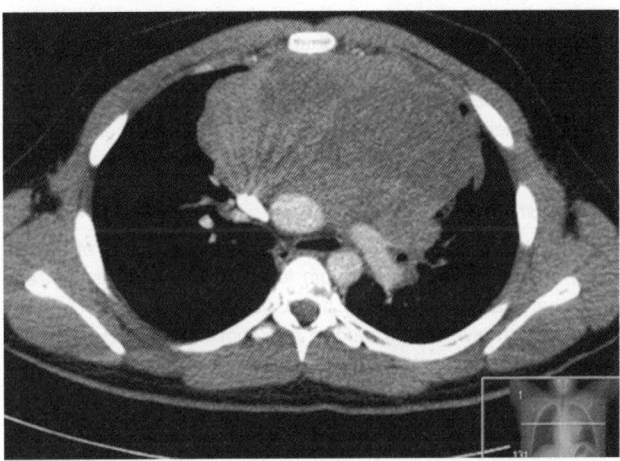

Fig. 6.17 Bulky anterior mediastinal mass in a patient presenting with superior vena caval obstruction in T-lymphoblastic lymphoma.

ⓘ Box 6.24 Neutropenic diet

Foods and drinks that should be avoided
- All uncooked vegetables and most fruits – peel off thick skin from foods like oranges and bananas
- Raw or rare meat
- Fish
- Uncooked or undercooked eggs
- Foods from salad bars and delicatessen counters
- Soft blue/mould cheeses, e.g. brie, camembert, stilton
- 'Well' water – or boil it for 1 min before drinking

Foods and drinks that are safe
- Cooked vegetables
- Canned fruits and juices
- Well-done meat
- Hard-boiled eggs (no runny yolks)
- Vacuum-packed lunch meats (not freshly sliced meats)
- Pasteurized milk, cheese, yogurt and other dairy products only
- Tap water if the source is known – or boil it; bottled water

---

Box 6.25 Management of febrile neutropenia

- Febrile neutropenia is classed as a one-off reading of ≥38.5°C or a reading of ≥38°C sustained for 1 h
- Patients on antipyretics/steroids and elderly patients may not mount a febrile response
- Hypothermia or clinical deterioration may be the first sign

Immediate intervention is essential
- Resuscitate with intravenous fluids to restore circulatory function; monitor urine output, Glasgow Coma Scale score and central venous pressure
- Take cultures of blood, urine, sputum and stool
- Consider the need for admission to critical care and consider inotropic support at an early stage
- Give empirical antibiotics as per local policy and sensitivities:
  - Commonly used antibiotics should include activity against enteric Gram-negative bacteria and *Pseudomonas*, e.g. ceftazidime or piperacillin–tazobactam with gentamicin; or meropenem monotherapy

- Antibiotics against staphylococci may be needed, e.g. vancomycin, especially with indwelling venous access lines
- Change antibiotics according to culture results, or empirically increase Gram-negative cover and consider adding Gram-positive cover, if the patient deteriorates clinically and/or temperature is still elevated after 48 h; discuss with the microbiology department
- Consider imaging, e.g. chest CT, if fever is not responding to broad-spectrum antibiotics, to detect an occult source of fever; consider adding treatment for opportunistic infections:
  - Liposomal amphotericin B or voriconazole – *Candida* and *Aspergillus*
  - High-dose co-trimoxazole – *Pneumocystis*
  - Clarithromycin – *Mycoplasma* and *Legionella*
  - Anti-tuberculous therapy – *Mycobacterium tuberculosis*

and arms. Treatment is with immediate steroids, chemotherapy where the tumour is expected to respond, and possibly mediastinal radiotherapy. Sometimes, vascular stents and anticoagulation are also required. Some tumours, such as lymphomas, small-cell lung cancers and germ cell tumours, are so sensitive to chemotherapy that this is preferred to radiotherapy, as the masses are likely to be both large and associated with more disseminated disease elsewhere. An early decision is necessary and should be based on the patient's likely prognosis, as ventilatory support may be required until treatment has had time to relieve the obstruction.

Spinal cord compression

Spinal cord compression (see p. 823) needs to be rapidly diagnosed, and urgent treatment arranged within 24 hours of onset of paresis, to salvage as much functional capacity as possible. Early neurological clinical features may be incomplete, more subjective than objective, and gradual in onset. Whole spine MRI scanning is the investigation of choice. Treatment should begin with high-dose steroids and both neurosurgical and oncological opinions, with a neurosurgeon advising on spinal stability, the need for spinal precautions for movement, and the role of decompressive surgery and external bracing for limited-extent disease. In the absence of surgery, radiotherapy alone may be used.

Tumour lysis syndrome

This occurs if treatment triggers a massive breakdown of tumour cells, leading to increased serum levels of urate, potassium and phosphate, and a secondary hypocalcaemia. These biochemical changes can give rise to cardiac arrhythmias and seizures. Urate deposition in the renal tubules can cause renal failure (hyperuricaemic nephropathy). Vigorous hydration, often with diuretics, is crucial to maintain high urine outputs in such patients; however, a proportion will require dialysis for uraemia, oliguria or severe electrolyte disturbances. The xanthine oxidase inhibitor allopurinol should be given before treatment is started in low-risk patients. Intravenous rasburicase, a recombinant urate oxidase, is used for prophylaxis in high-risk patients and in the treatment of tumour lysis syndrome.

Acute hypercalcaemia

This presents with vomiting, confusion, constipation and oliguria. Treatment is by resuscitation with intravenous fluids first, to establish a saline diuresis, and then an intravenous bisphosphonate, such as pamidronate or the more potent zoledronic acid (see **Box 21.56**). Treating the cause is crucial. Denosumab and calcitonin can be used in intractable cases.

Raised intracranial pressure

Raised intracranial pressure due to intracerebral metastases presents classically with headache, nausea and vomiting. There are often no localizing neurological signs and almost never papilloedema until very late in the disease. However, for many, there is a slower onset with non-specific symptoms such as drowsiness or mental deterioration. Treatment is by high-dose steroids and investigation by MRI. Surgery is appropriate if the condition is unifocal and/or threatening the fourth ventricle; otherwise, whole-brain or local stereotactic CyberKnife radiotherapy is required.

Malignant bile duct obstruction

This presents with cholestatic jaundice. Lymphomatous obstruction responds very well to prompt initiation of therapy. A small proportion of pancreatic and bile duct tumours are surgically resectable, more commonly those in the distal bile duct as compared to those in the

hilar region. However, in the greater proportion of patients, treatment is palliative. In recent years, endoscopic techniques have allowed the insertion of stents into the biliary tree to re-establish bile flow. Self-expanding metal stents have long periods of patency but are at risk of ascending infection. In the small proportion of patients in whom bile duct drainage is not possible endoscopically, the percutaneous route offers an alternative. Endoscopic photodynamic laser therapy with a photoporphyrin sensitizer can also prolong patency.

Further reading

Howard SC, Jones DP, Pui CH. The tumor lysis syndrome. *N Engl J Med* 2011; 364:1844–1854.

COMMON SOLID TUMOUR TREATMENT

Common cancer mortality is listed in **Box 6.26**; improvements in survival in recent years have stemmed from advances in prevention, diagnosis and treatment. The presentation, diagnosis, natural history and systemic treatment of the common cancers are described in the relevant chapters of this book; haematological malignancy is presented in Chapter 17. The decision to treat and the aim of that treatment, whether palliation or cure, require knowledge of the natural history of the disease, prognostic and predictive factors, the patient's performance status and the potential efficacy of treatment. Management should be carried out by a multidisciplinary team, which will usually be led by an oncologist.

Box 6.26 Index of net survival of all cancers at 5 years after diagnosis

Cancer type	5-year survival (%)	
	Men	Women
Pancreas	3.6	3.1
Lung	8.4	11.6
Oesophagus	15.6	14.7
Stomach	19.5	17.7
Brain	17.8	19.5
Multiple myeloma	50	43.8
Ovary		46.4
Leukaemia	53.3	49.1
Kidney	56.7	55.6
Colon	59.2	57.3
Rectum	56.6	59.8
Non-Hodgkin lymphoma	68.1	69.7
Prostate	84.8	
Bladder	56.5	45.3
Cervix		67.5
Melanoma	87.8	92.4
Breast		86.7
Hodgkin lymphoma	84.1	86.3
Testis	98	
All cancers	49.2	59.2

(From Quaresma M, Coleman MP, Rachet B. 40-year trends in an index of survival for all cancers combined and survival adjusted for age and sex for each cancer in England and Wales, 1971–2011: a population-based study. Lancet 2015; 385:1206–1218, with permission.)

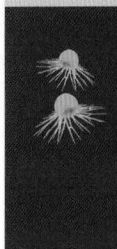

LUNG CANCER

The presentation and diagnosis of lung cancer are covered more fully in Chapter 28. Current treatment reflects the fact that the majority of patients are diagnosed at an advanced stage with a poor prognosis; there are therefore many trials assessing different screening strategies to try to achieve earlier diagnosis that would permit more curative treatment.

Prognosis

Lung cancer histology is divided into two main types (**Box 6.27**):
- *Small-cell lung cancers (SCLC)*, which derive from neuroendocrine tissue and which tend to disseminate early in their development.
- *Non-small-cell lung cancers (NSCLC)*, which are more likely to be diagnosed in a localized form. As treatments have improved, it has become clear that what previously was simply called non-small-cell lung cancer needs to be separated into individual pathological entities, as management varies and some therapies are effective only in particular subtypes.

Tumour stage and patient performance status are used in selecting treatment and predicting response and prognosis. While overall 5-year survival has remained approximately 10%, treatment is beginning to have an impact in selected groups.

Staging

Where the technology is available, staging is normally based on PET–CT. In the absence of distant metastases, further evaluation of local/regional lymph nodes is frequently undertaken if:
- lymph nodes are enlarged but of low glucose avidity, *or*
- lymph nodes do not appear enlarged but do show significant glucose avidity.

In these cases, confirmatory tests are required to yield histological samples: for example, endobronchial ultrasound (EBUS) and biopsy or, in the case of central nodes closer to the oesophagus, endoscopic ultrasound (EUS)-based biopsy.

General approach to management

This is based on the stage of disease, the histological subtype, the presence of particular genetic mutations, the patient's performance status (see **Box 6.13**) and, crucially, the patient's own wishes.
- For *stage 1–2 disease* the treatment of choice is surgical resection by lobectomy or pneumonectomy, with stereotactic ablative radiotherapy (SABR) when surgery is contraindicated.
- Selected patients with *stage 3A disease* can be managed surgically, but the alternative approach is a combination of chemotherapy and radiotherapy, directed by histological subtype and molecular testing.
- For patients with *more advanced disease*, a variety of agents can prolong survival, and specific palliative measures can relieve symptoms and improve quality of life.

Non-small-cell lung cancer

Staging of NSCLC is classified according to the TNM system (see **Box 6.12** and **Box 28.53**); this system divides the disease into local, locally advanced and advanced stages, with 5-year survival varying from 55–67% to 23–40% and 1–3%, respectively.

Management

Surgery

Surgery can be curative in NSCLC (T1,N0,M0) but only 5–10% of all cases are suitable for resection; about 70% of these survive for 5 years. Surgery is rarely appropriate in those over 65 years, as the operative mortality rate in these patients often exceeds the 5-year survival rate. Trial data suggest that neoadjuvant chemotherapy may downstage tumours to render them operable and may also improve 5-year survival in patients whose tumours are operable at presentation.

In operable disease of stages T1,N0 to T3,N2 (stage I–IIIa), adjuvant radiotherapy and chemotherapy following surgery can improve prognosis in patients of good performance status, as shown by the International Adjuvant Lung Cancer Trial and a meta-analysis of 12 randomized controlled trials. Cisplatin-based combination chemotherapy induced a response in 60% and produced a relative risk reduction of 11% with an absolute improvement in 5-year survival for stage II and IIIa disease of 4%, from 40.4% to 44.5%. There appears to be no difference in survival if chemotherapy is given before (neo-adjuvant) or after surgery.

Preoperative assessment includes lung function testing and walking oximetry, which is used to predict postoperative potential. An active life after pneumonectomy is unlikely if the gas transfer is reduced below 50%.

Radiation therapy for cure

In patients who are fit and who have a stage 1 NSCLC, high-dose radiotherapy (65 Gy or 6500 rads) can result in a 27-month median survival and a 22% 5-year survival. It is the treatment of choice if surgery is not appropriate; however, poor lung function can also be a relative contraindication to radiotherapy. *Radiation pneumonitis* (defined as an acute infiltrate precisely confined to the radiation area and occurring within 3 months of radiotherapy) develops in 10–15% of cases. *Radiation fibrosis*, a fibrotic change occurring within a year or so of radiotherapy and not precisely confined to the radiation area, occurs to some degree in all cases but is usually asymptomatic.

Tyrosine kinase inhibitors

Increasingly, tissue obtained at biopsy is investigated using next-generation sequencing (NGS, p. 31) to seek the presence of specific oncogenic (activating) mutations (**Box 6.28**). These are more common in non-smokers, although they account for less than 5% of cases in unselected series. Where mutations are identified, targeting these driver mutations with an appropriate TKI is the first-line treatment (see **Box 6.19**).

For example, for EGFR mutants, either a first- or second-generation drug may be selected: afatinib or erlotinib. High initial response rates are seen but progression within 1–2 years is usual. At this point, genetic sequencing of circulating blood DNA may reveal

---

Box 6.27 Histological subtypes of lung cancer

Histological subtype	Percentage of all lung cancers
Small-cell lung cancer (SCLC)	15%
Non-small-cell lung cancer (NSCLC)	85%:
Adenocarcinoma	40%
Squamous cell carcinoma	35%
Large cell carcinoma	10%
Other (including carcinoid tumours and sarcomatoid carcinomas)	3%

(Adapted from Wistuba I, Brambilla E, Noguchi M. Classic anatomic pathology and lung cancer. In: Pass HI, Ball D, Scagliotti GV, eds. IASLC Thoracic Oncology, 2nd edn. Philadelphia: Elsevier; 2018, pp. 143–146.)

> **Box 6.28 Activating mutations seen in non-small-cell lung cancer**
>
> | | EGFR | ALK | ROS-1 | PDL-1 | BRAF | NTRK |
> |---|---|---|---|---|---|---|
> | Adenocarcinoma/ large-cell neuroendocrine tumours | Y | Y | Y | Y | Y | Y |
> | Squamous cell carcinoma in never smokers | Y | Y | | Y | | Y |
> | Squamous cell carcinoma in smokers | | | | Y | | |

the presence of the T790 mutation, which generates resistance to first-line TKIs. The third-generation drug osimertinib overcomes this mechanism of resistance.

Immunotherapy

Programmed death ligand 1 (PDL-1) and its receptor, programmed death protein 1 (PD-1), are often overexpressed in NSCLC, allowing cancer cells to evade destruction by the body's immune system. In patients who are PDL-1-positive but lack the driver mutations described earlier, pembrolizumab (a MAb that acts as a PD-1 antagonist) is used, sometimes alongside conventional chemotherapy, with significant improvements in survival. The PDL-1 antagonist durvalumab, used every 2 weeks for 1 year alongside cisplatin-based chemotherapy, has been shown to raise the median time to progression or death from 16 to 28 months in NSCLC.

Conventional chemotherapy

This is used in the absence of specific driver mutations. Cisplatin (or carboplatin) plus gemcitabine remains the standard treatment (and is superior in this group to regimes based on cisplatin and pemetrexed). An alternative, particularly in older patients, is carboplatin and paclitaxel. Single-agent docetaxel may be offered as second-line therapy if patients are fit.

Small-cell lung cancer

Prognosis

SCLC is an aggressive neuroendocrine tumour. It is staged in the same way as NSCLC, and stage 1 tumours may benefit from surgery. For non-operable cases, disease is classified as limited- or extensive-stage disease.

Management

Limited-stage disease is confined to one anatomical area and is present in approximately 30% of patients. It is best treated with concurrent chemotherapy and radiotherapy using either cisplatin or carboplatin, with either etoposide or irinotecan, which increases survival at 5 years from 15% to 25%, compared with radiotherapy alone. Recurrence is usual within 6–12 months; for those who remain fit, further chemotherapy is appropriate. A similar degree of improvement can also be achieved with hyperfractionated radiotherapy. Prophylactic whole-brain radiation to prevent cerebral metastases can reduce symptomatic central nervous system disease and improve overall survival by 5%.

For **extensive disease**, concurrent chemoradiotherapy with cisplatin and etoposide chemotherapy over four cycles, followed by prophylactic cranial irradiation, is considered optimal. This can increase median survival from 6 months to 9–13 months, and the 2-year survival to 20%. Second-line chemotherapy can provide further palliation for patients with good performance status.

Symptomatic care for lung cancer patients

The prognosis for the majority of patients remains poor because the disease is diagnosed at an advanced stage and the co-morbidity from other smoking-related diseases compromises treatment. Therefore, much of the treatment, whether symptomatic or anticancer, is delivered with palliative intent. (General palliative care is discussed in Chapter 7.) Specific issues for lung cancer are the relief of bronchial obstruction and breathlessness, and the alleviation of local pain, for which radiotherapy is often employed alongside appropriate opiate analgesia. Laser therapy, endobronchial irradiation and tracheobronchial stents are used (see p. 980).

Metastases in the lung

Metastases are very common and usually present as round shadows (1.5–3.0 cm in diameter). They are usually detected on chest X-ray in patients already diagnosed as having cancers at other sites but may be the initial presentation of disease. Typical sites for the primary tumour include the kidney, prostate, breast, bone, gastrointestinal tract, cervix or ovary.

Metastases usually develop in the parenchyma or pleura and are often relatively asymptomatic, even when the chest X-ray shows extensive disease. Rarely, metastases may develop within the bronchi and present with haemoptysis.

Metastatic carcinomas (particularly of the stomach, pancreas and breast) can involve the mediastinal lymph nodes and spread along the lymphatics of both lungs (**lymphangitis carcinomatosa**), leading to progressive and severe breathlessness. Chest X-ray signs of hilar lymphadenopathy and basal shadowing are unreliable, compared with the characteristic signs on CT scan of irregular thickening of the interlobular septa in a polygonal pattern around a thick-walled central vessel.

Occasionally, a pulmonary metastasis may be detected as a solitary round shadow on chest X-ray in an asymptomatic patient. The most common primary tumour that presents in this way is a renal cell carcinoma.

The differential diagnosis includes:

* primary bronchial carcinoma
* tuberculoma
* benign tumour of the lung
* hydatid cyst.

Single pulmonary metastases can be removed surgically, but as CT scans usually show the presence of small metastases that remain undetected on chest X-ray, detailed imaging, including PET scanning and assessment, is essential before undertaking surgery.

Further reading

Gandhi L, Rodríguez-Abreu D et al., **KEYNOTE-189 Investigators**. Pembrolizumab plus chemotherapy in metastatic non-small-cell lung cancer. *N Engl J Med* 2018; 378:2078–2092.

Rosell R, Bivona T, Karachaliou N. Genetics and biomarkers in personalisation of lung cancer treatment. *Lancet* 2013; 382:720–731.

Soloman BJ, Mok T, Kim DW et al. First-line crizotinib versus chemotherapy in ALK-positive lung cancer. *N Engl J Med* 2014; 371:2167–2177.

Soria JC, Ohe Y, Vansteenkiste J et al., FLAURA Investigators. Osimertinib in untreated EGFR-mutated advanced non-small-cell lung cancer. *N Engl J Med* 2018; 378:113–125.

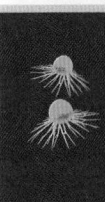

BREAST CANCER

Breast cancer is the most common cancer in women who do not smoke. The screening programme in the UK has improved the detection of early and curable breast cancer and is a model for other screening programmes. Improvements in multimodality treatment have also increased overall cure rates. Breast-conserving surgery for selected early-disease patients has greatly ameliorated the psychosexual impact of the disease.

Aetiology and pathology

The majority of breast cancers arise from the epithelial cells of the milk ducts and lobules. They reproduce their histological features in a variety of patterns (**Box 6.29**), of which the most common is an infiltrating ductal carcinoma.

Hormonal effects

At the time of menarche, oestrogen receptors in breast tissue react to ovarian oestrogen secretion. This stimulation causes milk duct epithelial cells to divide (mainly through activation of the cyclin D1/cyclin-dependent phosphorylating enzyme complex, which phosphorylates the retinoblastoma suppressor of G1- to S-phase progression of the cell cycle) and allows the breast to develop physiologically. This pathway for controlling cell division in the breast remains important throughout life and its dysregulation is a key 'driver' in the progression of oestrogen receptor (ER)-positive breast cancer (i.e. breast cancers that retain the expression of the oestrogen receptor) – a point of great interest in therapy.

Long-term exposure to the mitotic effects of oestrogens is a predisposing factor to breast cancer development because mutations are more likely to occur at times of DNA replication, and long-term hyperplasia due to oestrogen exposure predisposes to this. Thus, women with early menarche and late menopause, and those on hormone replacement therapy for long periods, are at greater risk of developing breast cancer.

Genetic predisposition

Approximately 5% of patients with breast cancer have a genetic predisposition. The best known are the familial *BRCA* mutant carriers, who have a very high risk of breast cancer and also ovarian cancer. Men who are positive for *BRCA* are at risk of male breast cancer and – for *BRCA2* mutants – prostate cancer. The BRCA protein product, a tumour suppressor, plays a role in DNA repair. Other familial breast cancer genes are often involved in DNA repair, and if deficient, may leave the cells more sensitive to DNA-damaging events. This phenomenon can be exploited in therapy, and a class of drugs called poly-ADP-ribose polymerase (PARP) inhibitors causes double-stranded DNA breaks to occur. In normal tissue these DNA strand breaks are repaired, but in cancer cells (e.g. those lacking effective BRCA action) repairs cannot be made and so the cell dies – a phenomenon described as 'synthetic lethality'.

Young breast cancer patients, those with a strong family history of breast cancer in near relatives and those with male breast cancer all require genetic counselling (**Box 6.30**).

Screening

There may be a long period between induction of breast cancer and invasion. The term '*in situ*' cancer refers to the development of cancerous changes in milk duct epithelial cells that have not yet breached the basement membrane of the ducts (and hence have no access to routes of spread by lymphatics). This 'pre-cancer' stage of the disease can be picked up on mammography when it is still highly curable, usually by breast-conserving surgery (unless changes are widespread in the breast, in which case more radical surgery may be required). In the UK, all women aged 50–70 are offered screening by biplanar digital mammography, often in designated clinics or mobile screening units, every 3 years. Patients with abnormal mammograms are recalled for further assessment.

Clinical features

Most women with symptomatic (rather than screen-detected) breast cancer present with a painless, increasing mass that may also be associated with nipple discharge, skin tethering, ulceration and, in inflammatory cancers, oedema and erythema. Where the cancer may be deeply tethered to pectoralis, the clinician asks the patient to tense the muscle by putting their hands on their iliac crests and pressing inwards; in deep tethering the mass loses its mobility.

The clinician should document:
- the position of the lesion(s) in the breast
- its/their size in centimetres

> **Box 6.29 Breast cancer histology**
>
> **Non-invasive**
> - Ductal cancer *in situ*
> - Lobular cancer *in situ*
>
> **Invasive**
> - Infiltrating ductal cancer
> - Infiltrating lobular cancer
> - Metaplastic cancer
> - Mucinous cancer
>
> - Medullary cancer
> - Papillary cancer
> - Tubular cancer
>
> **Other**
> - Adenoid cystic, secretory, apocrine cancers
> - Paget's disease of the nipple
> - Phyllodes tumour (sarcoma)

> **Box 6.30 Familial patterns of breast and ovarian cancer with increased risk of inherited *BRCA* mutations**
>
> - A mother or sister diagnosed with breast cancer before the age of 40
> - Two close relatives from the same side of the family diagnosed with breast cancer; at least one must be a mother, sister or daughter
> - Three close relatives diagnosed with breast cancer at any age
> - A father or brother diagnosed with breast cancer at any age
> - A mother or sister with breast cancer in both breasts, the first cancer diagnosed before the age of 50
>
> - One close relative with ovarian cancer and one with breast cancer, diagnosed at any age; at least one must be a mother, sister or daughter
> - A close relative of Ashkenazi Jewish origin with breast or ovarian cancer
> - A close relative with pancreatic cancer and breast or ovarian cancer

- the presence or absence of tethering (superficial or deep)
- any other relevant signs, such as nipple discharge, skin oedema (a so-called 'peau d'orange' appearance) or inflammatory changes
- the presence or absence of axillary lymphadenopathy.

Where effective screening programmes exist, most breast cancers are detected early; in other settings, including many developing countries, a much higher percentage of patients are likely to present with advanced disease.

Investigations

The **triple assessment** of any symptomatic breast mass is by:
- palpation
- radiology (mammography, ultrasound and MRI scan)
- fine needle aspiration cytology.

This combination is effective in differentiating breast cancer from benign breast masses, which are 15 times more common. Where cancer is considered likely, large-bore core needle biopsy should follow, to provide histological confirmation and to assess for factors predictive of prognosis and response to treatment. These features include:
- **grade of tumour**
- **Ki-67 proliferation index**, by which the proportion of cells staining positive for Ki-67 protein (a marker of cellular proliferation) is measured
- **oestrogen, progesterone and HER2 receptor status**
- **molecular profiling**, using an assay such as the Oncotype DX, which compares a number of molecular markers to assess risk of recurrence and benefit of chemotherapy.

Assessment should be carried out in a dedicated one-stop clinic that is able to provide appropriate support and arrange for referral. Staging considers:
- **Tumour size and evidence of local invasion.**
- **Axillary lymph node status**, through scanning (and potentially sampling) the 'sentinel' nodes that drain the area of the breast in which the cancer lies, identified by dye or radioactive tracer injection. At present, only 20% of patients are diagnosed with no evidence of microscopic nodal metastases.
- **Examination of common sites of metastasis** in advanced disease, PET–CT being the most sensitive modality of investigation.

Management of early disease

Surgery

In early disease, surgical options include wide local excision and segmental mastectomy with breast conservation for masses of less than 3 cm in diameter; simple mastectomy, with or without reconstruction, is used for larger tumours. The choice is dictated by the location and extent of the breast mass, and patient preference. Clear histological margins around the cancer are important for cure.

In the absence of clinical or ultrasound evidence of lymphadenopathy, surgery to the axilla can be minimized if sentinel lymph node-guided sampling excludes local spread; otherwise, dissection to level three is required if there are clinically involved nodes, in order to gain local control and provide prognostic information to guide adjuvant treatment. The greater the amount of axillary surgery, the greater is the risk of postoperative lymphoedema.

Radiotherapy

All patients who undergo breast-conserving surgery for early breast cancer require postoperative radiotherapy to the breast to provide security of local control equivalent to that conferred by mastectomy (**Box 6.31**). Those undergoing mastectomy who have disease close

Box 6.31 Indications for adjuvant radiotherapy in breast cancer

- Breast-conserving surgery
- Large, high-grade primary tumour
- Proximity to surgical margins
- Lymph node metastases

to resection margins also require radiotherapy to the chest wall and regional nodes. The axillary nodes are spared radiotherapy if the axilla has been dissected (to avoid arm lymphoedema) but supraclavicular nodes are included, and internal mammary node irradiation is occasionally given in selected higher-risk cases.

Systemic therapy

For locally advanced breast cancers, systemic therapy ('**neoadjuvant therapy**') is sometimes given to downstage the cancer before locoregional treatment with surgery and radiotherapy. This may allow safe breast-conserving therapy in a patient with disease that, at presentation, would have required full mastectomy.

The term '**adjuvant therapy**' applies to systemic treatment that is given after definitive locoregional therapy in a patient who is perceived to have a significant risk of future relapse. The aim is to destroy microscopic residual disease that may have disseminated elsewhere in the body, and trials have shown benefit from both endocrine treatment and chemotherapy. Typical chemotherapy regimens are discussed later in 'Management of advanced breast cancer'. Those with node-positive breast cancer, large primaries, oestrogen receptor-negative cancers and HER2 cancers are good examples of patients who would usually derive a significant survival advantage from adjuvant systemic therapy.

Targeted therapy

A range of agents can be used, depending on the receptor status of the underlying disease:

HER2-positive disease

The human epidermal growth factor receptor 2 (HER2) is over-expressed in 20% of all breast cancers and acts as an oncogene, 'driving' the cancer to grow. HER2-positive cancers tend to behave aggressively but respond to treatment with HER2 inhibitors such as trastuzumab and pertuzumab; endocrine therapy is used subsequently if tumours are also ER-positive. If indicated, radiotherapy is usually given following systemic therapy, the logic being that the systemic therapy is most likely to cure any microscopic disease when the tumour burden is lowest, and that systemic therapy also treats regional disease and so should be given as soon as possible.

Oestrogen receptor-positive disease

For cancers that present a lesser risk and are ER-positive, adjuvant endocrine therapy is delivered, often for as long as 10 years after surgery. There are two strategies for endocrine therapy:
- **oestrogen receptor blockade** using tamoxifen (a competitive inhibitor of the oestrogen receptor) or fulvestrant (which also causes degradation of the oestrogen receptor)
- **oestrogen deprivation** using aromatase inhibitors such as letrozole (which blocks non-ovarian oestrogen synthesis); aromatase inhibitors are not active in premenopausal women.

In a head-to-head study, a slight advantage was proven for use of aromatase inhibitors as adjuvant therapy in postmenopausal

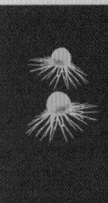

women with ER-positive breast cancer when compared to tamoxifen; consequently, this is now first-line endocrine therapy in this group. In premenopausal women with higher-risk ER-positive disease, there is an advantage for complete ovarian suppression (laparoscopic oophorectomy or luteinizing hormone-releasing hormone (LHRH) agonist therapy) plus aromatase inhibition.

In ER-positive breast cancer the effector pathway that stimulates cellular proliferation is mediated via a cyclin D/cyclin-dependent kinase phosphorylating holoenzyme, which regulates the RB protein (a suppressor of G1- to S-phase progression). The addition of cyclin inhibitors (e.g. palbociclib, abemaciclib) to an aromatase inhibitor or fulvestrant significantly enhances the response rate and duration of this endocrine-based therapy in ER-positive breast cancer.

Follow-up

After the end of therapy (or during the on-going adjuvant endocrine therapy or on-going anti-HER2 therapy), patients are reviewed clinically every 3–6 months by examination and enquiry into weight, energy and general wellbeing. Health economic studies have not supported the usefulness of proactive scanning in patients who have negative follow-ups based on these clinical assessments. However, an annual mammogram – both for the index breast and the contralateral side (where, irrespective of the genetics, there is an increased risk of a new cancer) – is recommended for at least the first decade of follow-up.

Management of advanced disease

The management of patients presenting with metastatic disease depends on the extent and location of disease.

Widespread visceral disease

Patients are advised to have systemic chemotherapy (with or without HER2-directed therapy), followed by endocrine therapy if the cancer is ER-positive. Treatment is unlikely to be curative but may well delay death by long periods, during which quality of life may be good.

The chemotherapy advised for this situation (and, indeed, the adjuvant therapy discussed earlier) is based on combinations of drugs, thereby reducing resistance (the same premise as is applied with multidrug antibiotic therapy for tuberculosis infection). Combinations of drugs are selected for their anti-tumour activity in breast cancer and their non-overlapping toxicities. Anthracyclines, taxanes, alkylating agents, 5-FU and vinca alkyloids all feature in first-line regimens. For triple-negative breast cancer (ER-negative, PR-negative, HER2 non-amplified) the platins also have a role, possibly in combination with a DNA repair inhibitor. Interestingly, the triple-negative group tend to carry a high mutational load and are the only group of breast cancers that may respond well to immunotherapy with checkpoint inhibitors and perhaps other such drugs.

Limited metastatic disease

For patients who present with one or only a few sites of metastatic disease (oligometastatic disease), there may still be a chance of cure. Aggressive treatment with ablative focal therapy to those oligometastatic sites (e.g. radiofrequency ablation, stereotactic radiation or surgical metastatectomy) may be worth pursuing in a fit patient.

Indolent metastatic disease that is not immediately life-threatening

If the cancer is ER-positive, primary endocrine therapy may hold the disease at bay for long periods; chemotherapy may be delayed until the cancer progresses despite this endocrine-based therapy. Breast cancers driven by HER2 or mammalian target of rapamycin (mTOR) may also benefit from cyclin inhibitors or mTOR inhibitors such as everolimus. Such an approach does not prejudice overall survival, and in a situation where therapy is not ultimately curative, there are big advantages to recommend it.

Metastatic disease confined to regional lymph nodes

An aggressive regime of neoadjuvant chemotherapy, surgery to breast and axillary nodes, regional radiotherapy and long-term endocrine or HER2-directed therapy offers a chance of cure.

Relapsed disease after previous systemic therapy

The systemic therapy previously received has to be carefully considered before new therapy is instituted. The timing between the previous therapy and relapse is important, as re-introduction of agents may be sensible only if the cancer has not been exposed to a particular group of drugs for a number of years. New agents (i.e. ones to which the cancer has not been exposed) are preferable, and eribulin is a chemotherapy agent that has value in this situation. In *BRCA*-driven cancer, the PARP inhibitors (DNA repair inhibitors that seem to augment the defect of *BRCA* mutation in a lethal way) may enhance the efficacy of certain drugs, such as the platins, or be active as single agents. It is sometimes worth obtaining a biopsy at the time of relapse for further genomic analysis of the 'new' tumour, as the constant mutational events in a progressing cancer throw up new driver mutations, some of which can be blocked. For example, the phosphoinositide 3-kinase (PI3K) escape pathway may become a driving force in progressing breast cancer and there are now inhibitors of this common escape pathway in multiple relapsing breast cancer. This type of emerging new mutation can sometimes be detected from peripheral blood draw and cancer cell-free DNA (cfDNA) analysis.

Further reading

Baselga J, Cortés J, Kim SB et al. Pertuzumab plus trastuzumab plus docetaxel for metastatic breast cancer. *N Engl J Med* 2012; 366:109–119.
Burstein HJ, Morrow M. Nodal irradiation after breast cancer surgery in the era of effective adjuvant therapy. *N Engl J Med* 2015; 373:379–381.
Coudert B, Asselain B, Campone M et al. Extended benefit from sequential administration of docetaxel after standard fluorouracil, epirubicin, and cyclophosphamide regimen for node positive breast cancer: the 8-year follow-up results of the UNICANCER-PACS01 trial. *Oncologist* 2012; 17:900–909.
Donker M, van Teinhoven G, Straver ME et al. Radiotherapy or surgery of the axilla after a positive sentinel node in breast cancer (EORTC 10981-22023 AMROS): a randomized, multicenter, open-label, phase 3 non-inferiority trial. *Lancet Oncol* 2014; 15:1303–1310.
EBCTG (Early Breast Cancer Trialists Collaborative Group). Effect of radiotherapy after mastectomy and axillary surgery on 10-year recurrence and 20-year breast cancer mortality: meta-analysis of individual patient data for 8135 women in 22 randomised trials. *Lancet* 2014; 383:2127–2135.
Reis-Filho JS, Pusztai L. Gene expression profiling in breast cancer: classification, prognostication and prediction. *Lancet* 2011; 378: 1812–1823.

UPPER GASTROINTESTINAL CANCERS

Oesophageal cancer

Presentation and diagnosis are described on page 1171. Early diagnosis, as pioneered in Japan, where there is a particularly high incidence, has shown that it is possible to improve the prognosis of a disease that otherwise is typically diagnosed only when local metastases have already occurred.

Prognosis and management

Pre-treatment histology, stage, age and performance status are critical prognostic factors for treatment decisions, which should be made by a multidisciplinary team in designated units with the surgical expertise to avoid treatment mortality. The prognosis for the majority of symptomatic patients is poor: 50% have distant metastases at the time of diagnosis, and the majority of the remainder having locoregional spread into adjacent mediastinal structures. Staging with endoscopic ultrasound, CT scan and PET–CT scan has improved the selection of patients of good performance status with truly localized disease, for whom curative treatment may be attempted. The overall 5-year survival figures are poor (see p. 1172), only attaining 4% for stage 4 cancers, because 70% of patients present late with stage 3 or higher disease.

Treatment of early-stage disease

Surgery provides the best chance of cure particularly for distal primaries but should be used as the primary modality only when imaging has shown that the tumour has not infiltrated outside the oesophageal wall (stage 1). Patients with locally advanced disease that is potentially resectable are recommended to have neoadjuvant chemotherapy with cisplatin/5-FU prior to surgery; neoadjuvant chemoradiotherapy prior to surgery has recently been shown to improve overall survival further. Response to neoadjuvant therapy is a strong prognostic factor. Radical chemoradiotherapy alone is an alternative approach for patients with squamous cell carcinoma of the thoracic oesophagus, and avoids the morbidity associated with surgery. Those with adenocarcinoma of the oesophago-gastric junction can be treated with perioperative chemotherapy in a combination of docetaxel, oxaliplatin, fluorouracil and leucovorin (FLOT).

Treatment of advanced or metastatic disease

This can be palliated with 5-FU or capecitabine chemotherapy in approximately 30%, increasing to 45–55% with the addition of oxaliplatin or irinotecan for a median duration of 6–8 months.

Palliative approaches

Distressing symptomatic problems with dysphagia can be partially relieved by endoscopic insertion of expanding metal stents, percutaneous endoscopic gastrostomy tubes to support liquid enteral feeding and endoscopic ablation to help control bleeding. The patient and family need considerable support and explanation to enable them to understand that feeding, including parenteral methods, does not improve survival beyond that dictated by the underlying cancer, and may introduce its own complications with adverse effects on quality of life.

Gastric cancer

The presentation and diagnosis of gastric cancer are described on page 1179.

Prognosis and management

The majority of patients are still diagnosed at an advanced stage, except in Japan, which has an active surveillance policy. Thus, in the West, the overall prognosis has not improved above 10% survival at 5 years. Selected groups may do much better and the histological grade and staging, with respect to the presence of serosal involvement (T3), nodal involvement (N1–2) and performance status, are the main factors in determining prognosis and selecting treatment.

Treatment of early-stage disease

Early non-ulcerated, mucosal lesions can be removed endoscopically. Otherwise, surgery remains the most effective form of treatment if the patient is considered 'operable' in terms of lack of direct invasion and nodal spread: selection based on operability has reduced the numbers undergoing surgery and significantly improved the overall surgical 5-year survival rates. Perioperative chemotherapy with FLOT improves 3-year overall survival in this patient group from 35% to 57%. If a patient has not had neoadjuvant treatment, adjuvant chemotherapy or chemoradiotherapy can be used.

Treatment of advanced disease

This may be palliated with chemotherapy, such as oxaliplatin and capecitabine combined with cisplatin and infusional 5-FU for patients with squamous cell carcinoma, with a response in 40–50% for a median of 8–12 months in those patients with good performance status (see p. 107). The addition of trastuzumab a and pertuzumab for tumours overexpressing HER2 (see p. 122) has improved median survival from 11 to 16 months. For patients with deficient mismatch repair, high levels of microsatellite instability or PDL-1 overexpression, immune checkpoint inhibitors targeting PD-1 (pembrolizumab) have activity in this tumour type and may be considered in the future for patients who have relapsed. Trifluridine/tipiracil, which interferes with tumour DNA synthesis, may also have activity in the relapsed setting.

Palliative approaches

Supportive care for patients with upper gastrointestinal cancers, more than cancers in any other site, must include attention to nutrition with the use of endoscopic stents to relieve obstruction, nasojejunal and percutaneous gastrostomy feeding tubes, and occasionally parenteral nutrition. When the disease progresses and active anti-cancer treatment is no longer appropriate, management of distressing obstructive symptoms can include octreotide to reduce secretions and, if necessary, a venting gastrostomy.

Gastrointestinal stromal tumours

Gastrointestinal stromal tumours (GISTs) are rare, slow-growing neoplasms that may arise in the stomach or small or large intestine. Prognosis depends on size, site, Ki-67 proliferation index (see p. 1180) and association with neurofibromatosis type 1 (see p. 886). Immunohistochemistry for CD117 and DOG-1 is usually positive; if negative, diagnosis can be reached by analysis of the known mutational sites in *c-Kit* or *PDGFRA* oncogenes. These mutations predict response to TKIs such as imatinib (see p. 113). Surgery is potentially curative for localized disease, and imatinib adjuvant therapy for 3 years prolongs survival. In metastatic disease, imatinib treatment should continue until relapse and can induce remissions in 50–80% for a median of 2 years; further responses are possible with alternative TKIs such as sunitinib and nilotinib.

Further reading

Al-Batran SE, Homann N, Schmalemberg H et al. Perioperative chemotherapy with docetaxel, oxaliplatin, and fluorouracil/leucovorin (FLOT) versus epirubicin, cisplatin, and fluorouracil or capecitabine (ECF/ECX) for resectable gastric or gastroesophageal junction (GEJ) adenocarcinoma (FLOT4-AIO): a multicenter, randomized phase 3 trial. *J Clin Oncol* 2017; 35(suppl; abstr 4004).

Rubenstein JH, Shaheen NJ. Epidemiology, diagnosis, and management of esophageal adenocarcinoma. *Gastroenterology* 2015; 149:642–643.

Shapiro J, van Lanschot JJ, Hulshof MC et al. Neoadjuvant chemoradiotherapy plus surgery versus surgery alone for oesophageal or junctional cancer (CROSS): long-term results of a randomised controlled trial. *Lancet Oncol* 2015; 16:1090–1098.

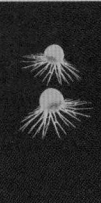

LOWER GASTROINTESTINAL CANCERS

Small intestinal cancer

Predisposing factors for small intestinal cancer, and its presentation and treatment, are described on page 1196. The principles of treatment are determined by extrapolation from management of the more common colorectal cancers.

Colorectal cancer

Presentation and diagnosis of colorectal cancer are described on page 1218.

Prevention

A *low-fat, high-fibre diet* for the prevention of sporadic colorectal cancer, along with endoscopic screening, is recommended for at-risk patients with a strong family history and for inherited syndromes (e.g. familial adenomatous polyposis, Lynch's syndrome).

   Non-steroidal anti-inflammatory drugs (NSAIDs) or aspirin may play a role in prevention. After 5 years' treatment with daily aspirin, there is a 35% reduction in all gastrointestinal cancers, although caution must be exercised because of the risk of gastric erosion.

Screening

See pages 294 and 1219.

Prognosis

The site of the disease (above or below the pelvic peritoneal reflection), TNM stage (see **Box 6.11**), surgical margins and the patient's performance status (see **Box 6.2**) are the main clinical prognostic factors (**Box 6.32**). Gene expression profiling, using Oncotype DX and Coloprint, for example, can identify prognostic subgroups, but is not predictive of treatment benefit. High microsatellite instability (MSI) predicts a better prognosis and can be used to identify low-risk patients for whom adjuvant therapy is unlikely to be of benefit. Mutations in *BRAF* occur in 6–8% and indicate a poor prognosis, as do mutations with predictive effect in *KRAS* in 40% and *NRAS* in 10–15% of cancers.

Management

Management should be undertaken by multidisciplinary teams working in specialist units. About 80% of patients with colorectal cancer undergo surgery, although fewer than half of these survive for more than 5 years. The operative procedure depends on the cancer site. The TNM staging system has now largely replaced the older Dukes' staging system.

Surgery

Rectal cancer

Total mesorectal excision (TME) is used for careful removal of the entire package of mesorectal tissue surrounding the cancer.

A low rectal anastomosis is then performed. Abdomino-perineal excision, which requires a permanent colostomy, is reserved for very low tumours within 5 cm of the anal margin. Local trans-anal surgery is used very occasionally for early superficial rectal cancers.

Colon cancer

A segmental resection and restorative anastomosis, with removal of the draining lymph nodes as far as the root of the mesentery, is employed for cancer elsewhere in the colon. Surgery in patients with obstruction carries greater morbidity and mortality. Where technically possible, preoperative decompression by endoscopic stenting with a mesh-metal stent relieves obstruction; surgery can therefore be elective rather than emergency, and is probably associated with a decrease in morbidity and mortality.

Neoadjuvant chemotherapy and radiotherapy

Neoadjuvant chemoradiation treatment of locally advanced rectal cancers, using 5-FU or capecitabine with 5 weeks of radiotherapy and then a 2-month wait, has increased the proportion of locally advanced tumours that can be resected with clear surgical margins and has improved the local control rate, but has not had a beneficial effect on distant metastatic relapse and overall survival. Preoperative, rather than postoperative, treatment has reduced toxicity to the other pelvic structures due to preservation of the normal anatomical relations. Alternatives include short-course radiotherapy over 1 week with immediate or delayed surgery, and total neoadjuvant treatment with chemotherapy prior to or after chemoradiotherapy in those patients most at risk of metastatic disease, although this has not been proven in large randomized trials. In 20–30% of patients, there is a complete clinical and radiological response to treatment after chemoradiotherapy, and in these individuals it may be possible to avoid surgery with stringent follow-up.

Adjuvant chemotherapy and radiotherapy

Adjuvant chemotherapy with oxaliplatin and 5-FU or capecitabine chemotherapy increases survival in patients with node-positive colorectal cancer, with a 5-year overall survival of 73%. Recent data have demonstrated that in those with lower-risk stage III disease it is possible to give 3 months of adjuvant therapy rather than 6 without reducing survival, sparing patients the neuropathy that is associated with oxaliplatin. Less benefit is seen with adjuvant treatment for stage II, node-negative patients. Those with higher-risk features can be considered for adjuvant single-agent capecitabine. If the tumour is deficient in one of the mismatch repair genes, adjuvant chemotherapy in this patient cohort has been shown not to be effective. Immunotherapy could be considered for these individuals in a trial setting.

Follow-up

In all patients who have surgery a total colonoscopy should be performed before surgery to look for additional lesions. If total colonoscopy cannot be achieved before surgery, a second 'clearance' colonoscopy within 6 months of surgery is essential. Patients with stage II or III disease should be followed up with regular colonoscopy and carcinoembryonic antigen (CEA) measurements; rising levels of CEA suggest recurrence. CT scanning to detect operable liver metastases should be performed for up to 5 years post surgery.

> *i* **Box 6.32 Prognostic and predictive factors for colorectal cancer**
>
> - Site above or below pelvic peritoneal reflection
> - TNM stage and performance status
> - Surgical margins
>
> - Favourable mutational profile:
>   - Low microsatellite instability
>   - *BRAF* wild type
>   - *RAS* wild type

Metastatic colorectal cancer

Patients with colorectal cancer can present with liver metastases. With appropriate selection of patients who have a good performance status and in whom MRI and PET–CT scans do not demonstrate disease elsewhere, local treatment can prolong good-quality survival. A variety of methods are used, including surgical resection, stereotactic body radiotherapy, radiofrequency ablation, cryoablation or hepatic artery embolization. Small lesions can be ablated but larger ones are best managed by partial hepatectomy or a combination approach, so that embolization is followed by hepatic regeneration before final resection. Patient selection is critical; long-term survival without recurrence is reported in up to 20% at 5 years with a single lesion of less than 4 cm amenable to resection presenting more than a year from initial diagnosis. More patients can be rendered suitable with perioperative chemotherapy, such as FOLFOX (oxaliplatin, 5-FU, folinic acid) or FOLFIRI (irinotecan and 5-FU) with cetuximab if *RAS* is wild-type. A similar approach is utilized for patients with lung metastases.

Untreated advanced colorectal cancer has an overall survival of 5–6 months. With sequential chemotherapy regimens (including FOLFOX, CAPOX (oxaliplatin and 5-FU or capecitabine), FOLFIRI and LONSURF (trifluridin–tipiracil)), this can increase to over 2 years. Patients without mutations in the *KRAS* gene can be considered for treatment with EGFR-targeted agents such as cetuximab and panitumumab. Immunotherapy can be of use in patients with loss of function of one or more of the mismatch repair genes.

Anal cancer

Anal squamous cell carcinoma is radically treated with chemoradiotherapy with mitomycin C and 5-FU or capecitabine. This is organ-preserving treatment, enabling the patient to avoid surgery that would result in a colostomy. Salvage abdominoperineal resection is possible if the tumour recurs. Metastatic anal cancer is treated with carboplatin and paclitaxel chemotherapy. Immune checkpoint inhibitors may have activity in these tumours, as they do in squamous cell carcinoma of the head and neck.

Further reading

Boland CR, Goel A. Prognostic subgroups among patients with stage II colon cancer. *N Engl J Med* 2016; 374:277–278.
Fiorica F, Cartei F, Licata A et al. Can chemotherapy concomitantly delivered with radiotherapy improve survival of patients with resectable rectal cancer? A meta-analysis of literature data. *Cancer Treat Rev* 2010; 36:539–549.
O'Connell MJ, Lavery I, Yothers G et al. Relationship between tumor gene expression and recurrence in four independent studies of patients with stage II/III colon cancer treated with surgery alone or surgery plus adjuvant fluorouracil plus leucovorin. *J Clin Oncol* 2010; 28:3937–3944.
Rothwell PM, Fowkes FG, Belch JF et al. Effect of daily aspirin on long-term risk of death due to cancer: analysis of individual patient data from randomised trials. *Lancet* 2011; 377:31–41.

HEPATOBILIARY AND PANCREATIC CANCERS

Liver

Hepatocellular carcinoma

Hepatocellular carcinoma (HCC; see p. 1308) arises in a cirrhotic liver in 95% of cases and can be screened and detected by cross-sectional imaging and a rise in serum α-fetoprotein.

Prognosis and management

Surgical resection of isolated lesions of less than 5 cm in diameter or up to three lesions of less than 3 cm in diameter is associated with a median survival of 5 years, although the remaining liver remains at risk of further recurrence. Liver transplantation offers the only opportunity for cure for patients with a small primary tumour, but is often limited by the underlying cause of the hepatitis and cirrhosis. Other focal treatments include transarterial embolization and chemoembolization, radioembolization, radiofrequency ablation and stereotactic body radiotherapy in patients with small primaries and adequate liver function; these prolong survival, though less successfully than surgery.

In progressive disease, antiangiogenic compounds are being evaluated: sorafenib prolongs survival to 10 months in patients with non-resectable tumours, and lenvatinib is an alternative TKI that is used to treat patients in the first-line advanced setting.

Biliary tract

Cancer of the biliary tract may be intra- or extrahepatic. These malignancies represent approximately 1% of all cancers. A number of associations have been identified, such as choledochal cyst and chronic infection of the biliary tract with, for example, *Clonorchis sinensis*. There are also associations with autoimmune disease processes, such as primary sclerosing cholangitis and inflammatory bowel disease.

Carcinoma of the gall bladder

See page 1322.

Cholangiocarcinoma

Cholangiocarcinoma (see also p. 1322) usually presents with jaundice and is detected by imaging: initially ultrasound, and most importantly, magnetic resonance cholangiopancreatography (MRCP). Spread is usually by local lymphatics or local extension. Cholangiocarcinoma of the common bile duct may be resectable at presentation but local extension precludes such management in the majority of more proximal lesions. Localized disease justifies an aggressive surgical approach, including partial hepatic resection. Hepatic transplantation for selected stage 1 and 2 disease has achieved 80% 5-year survival.

Palliative chemotherapy for patients with good performance status and advanced disease, using gemcitabine and cisplatin, effects a response in 50% with a median survival of 12 months. Chemoradiation has been used to treat localized small hilar cholangiocarcinomas and radiotherapy can provide good analgesia.

Pancreas

Pancreatic adenocarcinoma

The presentation and initial investigation of pancreatic cancer are covered on page 1333.

Prognosis

The 5-year survival rate for carcinoma of the pancreas is approximately 2–5%, with surgical intervention representing the only chance of long-term survival. Approximately 20% of all cases have a localized tumour suitable for resection, but in an elderly population many individuals have co-morbid factors that preclude such major surgery.

Management

Borderline-resectable tumours can be considered for neoadjuvant therapy to downstage the tumour, but this should generally be

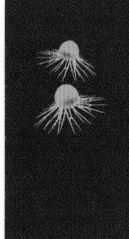

contemplated only as part of a clinical trial. Adjuvant gemcitabine and capecitabine chemotherapy can be used where tumours have been removed. Locally advanced pancreatic cancer can be treated with combination chemotherapy, followed by chemoradiotherapy with concurrent capecitabine. This can achieve a response in 30% and a median survival of 17 months.

In the majority of cases, management is palliative. Obstruction of the biliary tree and jaundice is a debilitating complication, often associated with severe pruritus and also non-specific malaise, lethargy and anorexia. Endoscopic placement of endoprostheses (stents) offers excellent palliation.

Palliative surgery has a role in duodenal obstruction (a complication seen in 10% of cases), but in advanced disease, self-expanding metal stents can be placed across the duodenal obstruction with excellent short-term results.

Palliative chemotherapy for advanced disease can be managed with combination chemotherapy. First-line treatment for patients with a good performance status is FOLFIRINOX (5-FU, leucovorin, irinotecan and oxaliplatin). This combination treatment was found to lead to a median overall survival of 11.1 months. An alternative regimen for patients who are not fit enough for this treatment is gemcitabine and nab-paclitaxel (paclitaxel as albumin-bound nanoparticles). With disease progression, abdominal pain is a frequent complicating factor; it may prove extremely difficult to treat but can sometimes be helped by radiotherapy.

Further reading

Al-Rajabi R, Patel S, Ketchum NS et al. Comparative dosing and efficacy of sorafenib in hepatocellular cancer patients with varying liver dysfunction. *J Gastrointest Oncol* 2015; 6:259–267.

Caplin ME, Pavel M, Ćwikła JB et al. Lanreotide in metastatic enteropancreatic neuroendocrine tumors. *N Engl J Med* 2014; 371:224–233.

El-Serag HB. Hepatocellular carcinoma. *N Engl J Med* 2011; 365:1118–1127.

Grossman EJ, Millis JM. Liver transplantation for non-hepatocellular carcinoma malignancy: indications, limitations, and analysis of the current literature. *Liver Transpl* 2010; 16:930–942.

Raymond E, Dahan L, Raoul JL et al. Sunitinib malate for the treatment of pancreatic neuroendocrine tumors. *N Engl J Med* 2011; 364:501–513.

UROLOGICAL CANCERS

Renal cancer

Clinical features and diagnosis

See page 1407.

Investigations and management

At diagnosis, renal cancers are staged using CT and/or MRI to assess operability and the presence or absence of metastases.

Disease confined to the kidney

A nephrectomy is performed unless bilateral tumours are present, in which case conservative surgery may be indicated. Preservation of as many nephrons as possible is beneficial in the long term, and a partial nephrectomy should be undertaken where possible.

Metastatic disease

For patients with metastatic disease, prognosis is predicted on the basis of the International Metastatic renal cell carcinoma Database Consortium (IMDC or Heng) criteria. A point is scored for each of the following poor prognostic features:

- impaired fitness (<80% on the Karnofsky performance status score)
- haemoglobin below the lower limit of normal
- neutrophils above the upper limit of normal
- platelets above the upper limit of normal
- serum calcium above the upper limit of normal
- <12 months from diagnosis to the requirement for systemic chemotherapy.

Those with no adverse prognostic factors have a 2-year survival of more than 75% and are considered to have a good prognosis; those with one or two factors are regarded as having an intermediate prognosis and have an approximately 50% chance of surviving for 2 years; and those with three factors or more have a poor prognosis and a 2-year survival of 7%. Patients with a good prognosis may benefit from a debulking palliative nephrectomy, which is sometimes followed by regression of metastases. Adjuvant therapy reduces the risk of progression but benefit must be weighed against toxicity.

Systemic therapy

TKIs are the mainstay of therapy for metastatic disease. When the prognosis is good, either sunitinib or pazopanib is given as first-line treatment. For patients with an intermediate or poor prognosis but preserved performance status, the combination of the MAb pembrolizumab (which targets PD-1) and the TKI axitinib increases survival compared to sunitinib (hazard ratio (HR) –0.53). An alternative in these patients is the combination of the MAbs ipilimumab and nivolumab (HR –0.68 compared to sunitinib). Good-risk patients may benefit from high-dose IL-2, which appears to increase survival by 5–10%. Sequential use of other drugs, such as cabozantinib, lenvatinib and everolimus, can produce further responses and improvement in disease control. Isolated metastases may be amenable to surgery or stereotactic irradiation.

Urothelial (bladder and ureteric) cancer

These cancers are usually transitional cell carcinomas (TCCs), associated with smoking and exposure to a range of chemical agents, although squamous cell carcinomas are common in areas where schistosomiasis is endemic. Their clinical presentation is described on page 1407.

Superficial cancers

Superficial TCC of the bladder without invasion through the basement membrane may be treated by transurethral resection or local diathermy. The risk of recurrence varies according to the degree of differentiation, and follow-up check cystoscopies and cytological examination of the urine are required. Recurrent superficial TCCs can be treated with bladder installation of the mycobacterium BCG (bacille Calmette–Guérin), which activates immune destruction of cancer cells; alternatively, a cytotoxic drug may be used: either gemcitabine or mitomycin.

Invasive bladder cancer

For invasive cancers, the strongest evidence is for neoadjuvant chemotherapy followed by either surgery (cystectomy) or chemoradiotherapy:

- ***Neoadjuvant chemotherapy*** is usually cisplatin-based, most commonly with gemcitabine. It improves absolute survival by 10%, the prognosis ranging from a 5-year survival of 80–90% for lesions not involving bladder muscle to 5–10% for those presenting with metastases.
- ***Surgical treatment*** involves cystectomy, generally followed by ileal conduit and stoma formation; in some cases, however, a neobladder can be constructed, allowing more normal micturition. This very much depends on the position of the tumour and the absence of extensive carcinoma *in situ*.

- **Bladder preservation strategies** for those with T1 with grade 3 histology, or T2–T4 tumours can alternatively be offered with chemoradiotherapy using mitomycin and fluorouracil. In many patients, this can achieve complete disease response, bladder preservation with a good quality of life, and comparable long-term survival (30–50% at 5 years) to cystectomy.

Metastatic urothelial cancer

Patients with metastatic disease may be palliated by chemotherapy (cisplatin- or carboplatin-based) or immunotherapy (using a PD-1/PDL-1 checkpoint inhibitor such as pembrolizumab or atezolizumab). Responses are seen in approximately 25% of cases with PDL-1 expression. In the UK, these treatments are currently approved in patients who are ineligible for cisplatin treatment or in whom cisplatin-based therapy has failed.

Upper tract tumours

Early-stage tumours are treated by nephro-ureterectomy. The addition of adjuvant therapy with cisplatin and gemcitabine in the management of non-metastatic T2 tumours has been shown to reduce the risk of recurrence by half (HR 0.49).

Prostate cancer

Clinical features and diagnosis

The pathogenesis, presentation, diagnosis and initial investigation of prostate cancer are discussed on page 1480.

Prognosis

The histological appearances are graded and accorded a Gleason score (see **Fig. 40.5**). Together with the serum PSA level, and accurate staging of the local extent of disease with pelvic MRI (dynamic contrast) and transrectal ultrasound, this score can identify prognostic groups (**see Box 40.6**). Treatment decisions must balance the age and performance status of the patient with the predicted behaviour of the cancer, which is becoming more objectively identifiable with advances in gene profiling. This allows the selection of patients with a good prognosis for no active treatment; they may reasonably choose to be kept under surveillance and die with, but not because of, their prostate cancer, as do 75% of men over the age of 80. In experienced hands, pre-biopsy MRI may allow targeted biopsy of the prostate and prediction of those who will have clinically significant prostate cancer.

Management
Disease localized to the prostate

This can be managed by surgical resection, brachytherapy, radiotherapy or watchful waiting with regular surveillance. The optimum approach depends on both features of the disease and the wider patient context. Management of localized disease is discussed on page 1481.

Locally advanced disease

Locally advanced prostate cancer (T3,N0) without distant metastases is best treated with combined androgen deprivation (see later) and radiotherapy; this improves 10-year survival, compared with endocrine treatment alone, from 61% to 71%.

Metastatic disease

Metastatic prostate cancer is normally treated initially with androgen deprivation to achieve medical castration (see later), and this may effectively palliate 70% of patients for a median duration of 2 years.

Once this fails, the disease is termed 'castration-resistant'; further palliative options are more potent hormonal drugs (such as androgen receptor blockers; see later) or conventional chemotherapy. If chemotherapy fails, a return to hormonal therapy may prolong disease control. The timing of chemotherapy remains unclear; rather as in breast cancer, it may be deferred until all available hormonal therapy has failed or it may be used earlier.

Endocrine therapy

Prostate cancer is the most hormone-sensitive malignancy, with the androgen receptor playing a critical role. However, prostate cancer tissue is able to trap circulating androgens so that tissue levels of androgens are maintained, even despite very low levels of circulating androgens. This means that resistance to endocrine therapy often develops over time, commonly involving receptor super-sensitivity and altered ligand binding, allowing other steroids to act as agonists and eventually bypassing the androgen receptor. A number of strategies are employed to reduce or abolish androgen stimulation of cancer cells:

- **Gonadotrophin releasing hormone (GnRH) agonists**, e.g. goserelin and leuprorelin, are as effective as orchidectomy at lowering circulating androgens and inducing responses in prostate cancer. However, in the first week, GnRH agonists produce a rise in luteinizing hormone (LH) and testosterone, which can result in a tumour flare in metastatic disease; they must therefore be combined with an antiandrogen, e.g. flutamide, in the initial phases. An alternative is to use a gonadorelin antagonist, e.g. degarelix. Physical castration, achieved by bilateral orchidectomy, achieves very effective androgen deprivation but is invasive, often unacceptable to patients and generally unnecessary.
- **Androgen receptor blockers** include drugs such as bicalutamide and the more potent antagonist, enzalutamide. They directly block the action of testosterone on prostate cancer cells.
- **Androgen synthesis inhibitors**, such as abiraterone, act by inhibiting CYP17, a key enzyme in the testosterone production pathway.
- **Corticosteroids and oestrogens** may also be helpful in disease that has become refractory to castration.

Hormonal agents may also be used after chemotherapy for prostate cancer, and both enzalutamide and abiraterone have been shown to prolong life in this situation. Adjuvant androgen deprivation treatment, such as monthly depot goserelin, has not improved survival following surgery, but when given before and during radiotherapy, can extend the overall survival at 3 years for T1–T3 tumours from 62% to 78%.

Non-hormonal therapy

Non-hormonal approaches are frequently used for metastatic disease:

- **Conventional chemotherapy.** The use of docetaxel in the early management of metastatic castration-sensitive disease has led to an improvement in overall survival. The hazard ratio for benefit from docetaxel is constant but when it is used early at a point when survival is greater, this translates into a greater absolute benefit in overall survival than when it is used after failure of hormonal therapy. The timing of chemotherapy versus hormonal treatment is currently not clear in prostate cancer: early use of the androgen synthesis inhibitor abiraterone, as an alternative to docetaxel, in the management of metastatic, castration-sensitive disease seems to confer similar benefits. It is not known whether combining the two approaches will lead to further improvements. If chemotherapy fails, a return to hormonal therapy may prolong disease control. Currently, there is no consensus as to whether chemotherapy should be deferred until all available hormonal therapy has failed, or be used earlier in disease control.

- **PARP inhibitors.** It is clear that a proportion of prostate cancers have deficits in DNA repair, often associated with carriage of the *BRCA2* gene. These patients seem to respond to PARP inhibitors such as olaparib, which prevent repair of DNA strand breaks and cause the death of cancer cells.
- **Bone-targeted therapy.** Drugs such as alpharadin ([223]radium), zoledronic acid and denosumab, alongside palliative radiotherapy, can be used to target painful metastases.

Penile cancer

Penile cancer is described on page 1482).

Testicular and ovarian germ cell tumours

Germ cell tumours are the most common cancers in men aged 15–35 years but comprise only 1–2% of all cancers. They are much less common in women. There are two main histological types: *seminoma* (termed '*dysgerminoma*' in women) and *non-seminoma*. Non-seminomas may be comprised of varying proportions of mature and immature elements; the mature elements are now known as teratoma (previously, this term referred to all non-seminomas). Teratomas in women present as dermoid cysts with low malignant potential (**Box 6.33**). Germ cell tumours may rarely occur in extragonadal sites in the midline, such as the pituitary, mediastinum or retroperitoneum, but should be treated in a similar manner.

Clinical features

Most men present with a testicular mass. In women, the mass presents with vague pelvic symptoms but at a younger age than the more common epithelial ovarian cancers (see later).

Investigations

- **Ultrasound or MRI scanning** of the testicle or ovary is required. Ultrasound is very sensitive and inexpensive, and should be performed in all suspected cases. MRI scanning is more sensitive and specific than ultrasound; however, expense and limited availability reduce its use as an initial diagnostic tool.
- **Assay of serum tumour markers** includes α-fetoprotein (AFP), β-human chorionic gonadotrophin (β-hCG) and lactate dehydrogenase (LDH). A urinary pregnancy test for hCG in the emergency department has saved the lives of young men with metastatic germ cell cancer.
- **CT or MRI scanning** is performed to seek distant metastases.

Management
Surgery
- **In men**, surgery is by the inguinal approach, so-called radical inguinal orchidectomy, to avoid spillage of highly metastatic tumour in the scrotum.
- **In women**, surgery for diagnosis and staging should always be conservative, compared to the approach in epithelial ovarian cancer, with preservation of fertility because of the efficacy of chemotherapy.

> **i** | **Box 6.33** Germ cell histology: WHO classification

- Seminoma
- Non-seminoma
  - Embryonal carcinoma
  - Choriocarcinoma
  - Yolk sac tumour
  - Teratoma

Seminomas

Seminomas are very radiosensitive and chemosensitive. They are associated with a raised serum LDH but only rarely a mildly raised β-hCG and never a raised AFP. Stage I disease limited to the gonad is associated with a 10–30% 5-year risk of recurrence with surgery alone, and so adjuvant therapy, with either chemotherapy or radiotherapy to the para-aortic lymph nodes, is preferred as it leads to a cure rate of more than 95% in early-stage disease. Carboplatin is the first choice because of convenience, reduced acute side-effects, and absence of the long-term risks of secondary malignancy that are associated with radiotherapy. Alternatively, post-surgical surveillance can be undertaken, with treatment reserved for those who relapse; this approach carries an equally high cure rate, since combination chemotherapy (e.g. cisplatin, etoposide and bleomycin, BEP) will cure over 90% of those with visible metastatic disease.

Non-seminomas
Early disease
The risk of relapse after surgery for stage I disease varies from 5% to 50%, depending on the prognostic factors of histological differentiation, presence of embryonal elements, and extent of local and vascular invasion. For those at moderate to high risk, adjuvant chemotherapy with a single cycle of BEP carries a 97% cure rate.

Metastatic disease
This commonly involves para-aortic lymph nodes and lungs but may spread rapidly (especially if trophoblastic, β-hCG-producing elements are present) and cause life-threatening respiratory or other organ failure. A rapid diagnosis can be made in the presence of gynaecomastia and a positive urinary pregnancy test before the institution of potentially life-saving treatment. About 80% of teratomas will express either β-hCG or AFP, and almost all metastatic disease will be associated with an elevation of the less specific serum marker, LDH.

The percentage cure rate depends on the height of the tumour markers (AFP >10 000 and β-hCG >100 000 IU/L) and the sites of metastases; it ranges from 50% to 95%. The most established regimen is BEP and 3–4 cycles are usually given. More intensive regimens appear to yield higher progression-free survival rates and may be preferred in some patients.

Relapsed disease
Patients who relapse following initial chemotherapy may well be cured by subsequent chemotherapy: this is most commonly with further cisplatin-based chemotherapy or high-dose chemotherapy, usually with carboplatin and etoposide, and a stem cell transplant. The timing of high-dose chemotherapy is uncertain: some clinicians prefer to defer it and use it only after standard-dose salvage treatment has failed. Others feel that the best results are seen if it is used on first relapse.

Although approximately 20% of men will be infertile due to azoospermia at the time of diagnosis, the majority of the remainder will retain their fertility after chemotherapy and be able to father children normally. Similarly, most women retain their fertility, although less is known about the association with infertility at presentation owing to the much lower frequency of germ cell tumours in women.

Further reading
Attard G, Parker C, Eeles RA et al. Prostate cancer. *Lancet* 2016; 387:70–82.
Beer TM, Armstrong AJ, Rathkopf DE et al. and PREVAIL Investigators. Enzalutamide in metastatic prostate cancer before chemotherapy. *N Engl J Med* 2014; 371:424–433.
Mateo J, Carreira S, Sandhu S et al. DNA-repair defects and olaparib in metastatic prostate cancer. *N Engl J Med* 2015; 373:1697–1708.

Quinn DI, Lara PN Jr. Renal cell cancer – targeting an immune checkpoint or multiple kinases. *N Engl J Med* 2015; 373:1872–1874.

Ryan CJ, Smith MR, de Bono JS et al. and COU-AA-302 Investigators. Abiraterone in metastatic prostate cancer without previous chemotherapy. *N Engl J Med* 2013; 368:138–148.

Sweeney CJ, Chen YH, Carducci M et al. Chemohormonal therapy in metastatic hormone-sensitive prostate cancer. *N Engl J Med* 2015; 373:737–746.

GYNAECOLOGICAL CANCERS

The main gynaecological cancers are those of the cervix, the body of the uterus (endometrium) and ovary. The presentation and investigation of these cancers are introduced in **Box 39.8**. All are important and enormous progress has been made in therapy.

Cervical cancer

In high-income countries the incidence of invasive cervical cancer has diminished substantially in recent years due to positive effects of screening and the HPV vaccine; worldwide, however, the incidence remains high.

Aetiology and pathophysiology

Infection with high-risk types of HPV is the most important risk factor for developing cervical cancer. HPV 16 and 18 are the main predisposing viruses and account for 70% of cases in the UK. Infection may be related to a high number of sexual partners and social deprivation, but HPV infection is very common in many populations. Other predisposing factors include smoking and immunodeficiency.

Cervical cancer derives from the squamous epithelium of the cervix. It has a long pre-cancerous phase, when it is termed a 'carcinoma intraepithelial neoplasm' (CIN), at which point the cancer has not breached the basement membrane.

Screening

The long pre-invasive phase makes cervical cancer ideal for screening because, at the CIN stage, it is almost universally curable. The cervical screening programme has great importance in cancer prevention worldwide, and even when screening takes place at extended intervals (e.g. in India) it confers great benefit in terms of preventing invasive disease. In the UK the recommendations are that screening should be performed 3-yearly from age 25 to 50, and 5-yearly from age 50 to 64.

Management and prognosis

CIN is classified into three grades, according to the thickness of the cervical epithelium involved: CIN1, CIN2 and CIN3. Removal of abnormal cells is recommended in most CIN2 and all CIN3 disease, and is most commonly achieved by a colposcopic loop electrosurgical excision procedure (LEEP).

Localized disease

Early-stage cancer may be treated using limited surgical techniques that preserve the function of the cervix and are compatible with future fertility. More deeply invasive disease that remains non-metastatic is still highly curable by more major resection of the uterus, ovaries and pelvic nodes (which are the first site of metastatic disease in most cases); this is termed the Wertheim hysterectomy. When disease is more advanced or surgery is contraindicated for reasons of age or co-morbidity, pelvic radiotherapy (usually with concomitant chemotherapy with cisplatin and a transvaginal radiation brachytherapy boost to the cervix) is advised; this confers a similarly high chance of cure.

Metastatic disease

There are no curable options but platin-based chemotherapy, often together with a taxane, is recommended for fitter patients and will delay progression for some time in many. Immunotherapy trials in progress aim to quantify the advantages of this type of therapy for advanced disease.

Endometrial cancer

Cancer of the body of the uterus is less common than cervical cancer, and arises from the endometrial lining of the uterine body. It is almost exclusively a postmenopausal cancer, and patients nearly always present with postmenopausal vaginal bleeding – a 'red flag' symptom.

Aetiology

Predisposing factors include a long menstrual life (early menarche and late menopause), endometrial hyperplasia (the partial oestrogen agonist tamoxifen can be a precipitating cause) and obesity (which, in itself, can lead to higher levels of oestrogen, largely oestrone, in postmenopausal women). There is no link to smoking but a weak familial tendency has been observed.

Diagnosis and management

Urgent gynaecological investigation is required for women with postmenopausal bleeding. Transvaginal ultrasound shows a thickened endometrium, and this is followed by cervical dilation and curettage to allow histological diagnosis. Patients usually present at an early stage, as bleeding occurs early.

Early disease

When the cancer is diagnosed at an early stage and is confined to the uterus, hysterectomy is the recommended treatment. The 5-year survival rate exceeds 80%.

Advanced and metastatic disease

When disease is more advanced, postoperative pelvic radiotherapy lowers the risk of local recurrence when the cancer has penetrated deep into the myometrium. For those with disease outside the uterus, chemotherapy may delay progression for some time. Genomically targeted therapy may be useful (the mTOR pathway may be one such 'driver' cancer path, targetable using the mTOR inhibitor everolimus), and progestogens may have a small retarding role for those with advanced disease or those too frail to benefit from systemic chemotherapy.

Ovarian cancer

Ovarian cancer arising from the surface epithelial cells ('epithelial ovarian carcinoma', EOC) is discussed in this section; other rarer cancers arising from the ovary include stromal cell tumours or germ cell tumours (see earlier and **Box 6.34**).

Aetiology and epidemiology

Ovarian carcinoma is the seventh most common cancer in women and accounts for 30 cases per 100 000 of the UK population. Most occur in older women, with half of new cases arising in patients above the age of 63 years.

In younger patients, a familial cause (inherited mutation) should be suspected. Mutations of the *BRCA1* or *BRCA2* gene are the most common familial cause, present in 10% overall, and a genetics review of those with a family history of ovarian or breast cancer should be

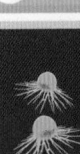

Box 6.34 Ovarian cancer pathology

- Serous cystadenocarcinoma
- Papillary cystadenocarcinoma
- Endometrioid cancer
- Adenocarcinoma
- Mucinous cancer
- Clear cell cancer
- Mixed mesodermal Müllerian tumours
- Granulosa cell tumours

- Germ cell cancers:
  - Dysgerminoma
  - Embryonal cancer
  - Endodermal sinus tumour
  - Choriocarcinoma
  - Teratoma – immature/mature
- Brenner, Sertoli–Leydig tumour, carcinoid tumours
- Other stromal cell tumours

considered. Prophylactic oophorectomy in *BRCA* carriers, after they have had their family, is recommended (along with bilateral mastectomies) because the risk of developing cancer is so high (**Box 6.35**).

There is a consistent relationship between the risk of EOC and the frequency and duration of ovulation. While not fully understood, this provides an explanation for the reduced risk of EOC with early pregnancy and use of the oral contraceptive pill.

Clinical features

Ovarian cancer often presents late, as its early progress is clinically silent. It arises from the surface epithelial cells and these have a tendency to shed when malignant; transcoelomic spread (across the peritoneum) therefore occurs early, and this peritoneal disease evokes ascites. When significant, the ascites leads to abdominal swelling, discomfort, bloating and other abdominal symptoms: indigestion, early satiety, acid reflux and shortness of breath, due to increasing pressure within the abdomen (**Box 6.36**). Symptoms of irritable bowel syndrome can be confused with those of ovarian cancer but rarely present for the first time over the age of 50, and so the presence of new-onset symptoms should stimulate investigation for ovarian cancer.

Diagnosis

The majority of patients present with a pelvic mass and advanced stage III (spread within the peritoneal cavity) or IV (extraperitoneal) disease. Imaging may reveal ascites, an ovarian mass and peritoneal deposits. Usually, transvaginal ultrasound is performed first, with MRI being the definitive imaging technique for the pelvis, and PET–CT scans assisting in staging the patient. The risk of malignancy index (RMI) (**Box 6.37**) can predict the chances of an adnexal mass being malignant, but confirmation with ascitic fluid cytology or with surgically obtained tissue is required for diagnosis.

Screening (see pp. 102–3) with the serum tumour marker CA125 and transvaginal ultrasound scan does detect some early cancers, with improved survival; however, it is being further refined with serial tests to avoid too many negative laparotomies and is thus still considered a research tool.

Prognosis

Histological subtype (clear cell and mucinous are worse), grade/differentiation, stage, extent of residual disease following surgery (macroscopic versus microscopic or none) and performance status are all significant independent prognostic factors for survival (**Box 6.38**).

BRCA mutation status should be assessed in patients with a positive family history (see **Box 6.30**) and in those with high-grade serous adenocarcinoma histology under the age of 50. Five-year survival rates for stage III disease vary with *BRCA* mutational status: 44% with *BRCA1* and 61% with *BRCA2* mutations, compared to 25% in *BRCA*-negative disease. *BRCA* status is also a predictive marker for increased sensitivity to platinum and anthracycline cytotoxics, and to PARP inhibitors like olaparib.

Box 6.35 Risk of cancer associated with *BRCA1* or *BRCA2* germline mutation

Cancer	General population	*BRCA1* mutated	*BRCA2* mutated
Breast	12%	50–80%	40–70%
Breast second primary	3.5% at 5 years	27% at 5 years	12% at 5 years
Ovary	1–2%	24–40%	11–18%
Prostate	15% (North European) 18% (African American)	<30%	<39%
Pancreas	0.5%	1–3%	2–7%

(From http://www.ncbi.nlm.nih.gov/books/NBK1247/)

Box 6.36 Symptoms associated with ovarian cancer that need investigation

- Persistent abdominal distension (women often refer to this as bloating)
- Feeling full when eating or early satiety and loss of appetite
- Pelvic or abdominal pain
- Increased urinary urgency or frequency

Box 6.37 Risk of ovarian malignancy index (RMI)

- RMI combines three presurgical features and is a product of the ultrasound scan score (U), menopausal status (M) and serum CA125 level (CA125):
  $$RMI = U \times M \times CA125$$
- The ultrasound result is scored as 1 point for each of the following characteristics: multilocular cysts, solid areas, metastases, ascites and bilateral lesions: U = 0 (for an ultrasound score of 0), U = 1 (for an ultrasound score of 1), U = 3 (for an ultrasound score of 2–5).
- The menopausal status is scored as 1 = premenopausal and 3 = postmenopausal. The classification of 'postmenopausal' relates to women who have had no period for more than 1 year or women over the age of 50 who have had a hysterectomy.
- Serum CA125 is measured in IU/mL and can vary between 0 and hundreds or even thousands of units.
- If the RMI is >250, a strong suspicion of ovarian cancer should be maintained.

Management

Early disease

Curative treatment inevitably requires radical surgery (laparotomy with bilateral salpingo-oophorectomy, hysterectomy and omentectomy). Because of the high risk of peritoneal dissemination, all but patients with very early, ovary-confined cancers benefit from postoperative adjuvant chemotherapy, which is given despite complete macroscopic resection of all visible disease. Clinical trials have

i **Box 6.38 Survival rates in invasive epithelial ovarian cancer**

Stage	Relative 5-year survival rate
I	89%
IA	94%
IB	91%
IC	80%
II	66%
IIA	76%
IIB	67%
IIC	57%
III	34%
IIIA	45%
IIIB	39%
IIIC	35%
IV	18%

(From Heintz AP, Odicino F, Maisonneuve P et al. Carcinoma of the ovary. FIGO 26th Annual Report on the Results of Treatment in Gynecological Cancer. Int J Gynaecol Obstet 2006; 95(Suppl 1):S161–192, with permission.)

shown that such postoperative chemotherapy reduces the chance of subsequent relapse when the subsequent relapse risk is high.

Advanced disease

In patents presenting with widespread peritoneal disease, or metastatic disease beyond the abdomen and pelvis, neoadjuvant chemotherapy is usually used first to shrink the cancer down to minimal proportions before debulking surgery is attempted. Among the chemotherapy options used for treating ovarian cancer – adjuvantly or for advanced disease – the platinum group are the best single agents and a taxane is usually the partnering cytotoxic. A good majority of advanced cancers respond to these agents. The VEGF inhibitor bevacizumab may be usefully added in advanced disease cases.

Relapsed disease

Response to therapy may be assessed clinically, by scanning and by measurement of the useful ovarian tumour marker CA125: rising CA125 suggests relapse. Drugs used for relapsed disease include other cytotoxics but new agents too are making an impact on therapy. The realization that ovarian cancer is driven by DNA repair faults and that the protein PARP1 is significant in this repair has led to the use of PARP inhibitors to treat advanced ovarian cancer, particularly in cancers that have a known DNA repair deficit such as *BRCA* or *PALB2* mutations. PARP inhibitors used in combination with a DNA 'toxin' that causes strand breaks, such as platin chemotherapy, achieves a 'synthetic lethality' – a new concept in cancer therapy that made its first inroads in ovarian cancer. It is also predicted that immunotherapy will have a role in advanced ovarian cancer but it is too early to review the data.

Palliative approaches

Up to 30% of those with metastatic disease may be alive after 5 years, although this falls to 5–10% if it is not possible to debulk the cancer at operation or if it has spread outside the peritoneal cavity. Bulky disease in the peritoneum commonly causes progressive bowel obstruction, which may require palliative surgery or expert palliative care support to manage the terminal phases of the illness.

Further reading

Jayson GC, Kohn EC, Kitchener HC et al. Ovarian cancer. *Lancet* 2014; 384:1376–1388.

BRAIN TUMOURS

The most common intracranial tumours are secondary brain metastases, which can be solitary or multifocal. Primary brain tumours account for 3% of total cancer cases in the UK. The clinical presentation and initial investigation of brain tumours are on pages 875–876.

Brain metastases

Any cancer can metastasize to the brain but the most common tumours to do so are those arising from:

- lung
- breast
- skin (melanoma)
- kidney.

Management

Cerebral oedema surrounding the tumours responds to steroid therapy. Many systemic therapies for the primary tumour do not cross the blood–brain barrier and therefore do not control brain metastases. There has therefore been a move in recent years to treat brain metastases more aggressively, and it is possible to resect some brain metastases neurosurgically. An alternative option is to employ stereotactic radiotherapy (gamma knife/CyberKnife or linear accelerator-based therapy). In these techniques, focused high-dose radiotherapy is delivered to small areas within the brain, leading to an improvement in overall survival. There is still occasionally a role for whole-brain radiotherapy when there are large numbers of brain metastases or they are too large to treat with stereotactic radiotherapy.

Primary brain tumours

Glioma

Gliomas can be low- or high-grade; this has an impact on prognosis, although low-grade tumours nearly always transform into high-grade tumours eventually. Survival is generally limited, with a median overall duration of 12–18 months (with treatment) in glioblastoma (grade 4 astrocytoma).

Knowledge of molecular pathology can also inform prognosis, predict response to treatment, and may direct therapy in the future:

- ***Mutations in isocitrate dehydrogenase 1 or 2 (IDH1 or IDH2)*** indicate that a tumour may be slower-growing. If they are found in a patient with a high-grade tumour, it may indicate that the tumour has transformed from a low-grade one rather than arising *de novo*.
- ***Loss of heterozygosity of 1p and 19q genes*** is associated with oligodendrogliomas, and a better prognosis and response to treatment.
- ***Promoter methylation of the O6-methylguanine-DNA methyl-transferase (MGMT) gene*** causes inactivation of the gene and predicts a better response to temozolomide chemotherapy, conferring a better prognosis.

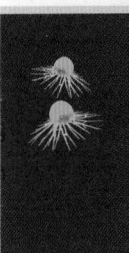

Management

The management of gliomas depends on the grade, the molecular pathology (if known), the site of the tumour and the patient's performance status and wishes. Options include:

- **Surveillance.** Low-grade tumours were traditionally followed up with serial imaging alone, but a more proactive approach with earlier intervention is now also considered an option.
- **Surgery.** Craniotomy and maximum debulking surgery are carried out, if possible. This depends on the site of the glioma, as it is not possible to resect a tumour in an area of the brain that would cause significant disability if removed. As gliomas spread along white matter tracts, full resection of a high-grade glioma is never possible. A stereotactic biopsy via a burr hole to inform diagnosis may be a preferable option to debulking surgery.
- **Adjuvant treatment.** Treatment after surgery can include radiotherapy with or without chemotherapy. The chemotherapy must cross the blood–brain barrier: options include temozolomide (an oral alkylating agent), which is commonly used both during radiotherapy (in the case of high-grade tumours) and after radiotherapy.

At relapse, further surgery, radiotherapy or chemotherapy (temozolomide or procarbazine, lomustine and vincristine (PCV)) may all play a part. The role of immunotherapy in the treatment of patients with gliomas is still under investigation, as are agents targeting *IDH1* and PARP inhibitors, which sensitize cancers to the effect of radiotherapy. Anti-angiogenic agents may also have a role in the relapse setting but have not been shown to improve survival.

Meningioma

The majority of meningiomas are low-grade but may not behave in a 'benign' manner, as they can cause significant disability to the patient: for instance, by causing mass effect, eroding adjacent structures or obstructing the flow of CSF. Surgery is the definitive treatment but may not be feasible due to the location of the tumour. There is a role for fractionated external beam radiotherapy and also stereotactic radiosurgery in the management of inoperable, recurrent and residual meningiomas.

Neurofibroma/schwannoma

Stereotactic radiosurgery is commonly used to treat these tumours and prevent hearing loss; otherwise, surgery may be required.

HEAD AND NECK CANCER

The term 'head and neck cancer' generally describes squamous cell cancers arising from the mucosa lining the aerodigestive tract. (Thyroid cancer is discussed on pages 621–622.)

Aetiology and pathophysiology

Constant stimulation of the squamous mucosa to divide and repair is an important precancerous phenomenon; mitosis is the most vulnerable time in the cell cycle for DNA replication errors to creep in, and some of these escape DNA repair mechanisms. The accumulation of these mutations in the genome of the daughter cells can lead to eventual cancer formation.

Predisposing factors for head and neck cancer include those that stimulate mucosal division and repair, and those that directly cause damage to DNA. They include:

- the irritant effects of spices, spirits and tobacco smoking
- poor oral hygiene, leading to chronic low-grade periodontal inflammation, or irritation of the tongue as it rubs against a sharp tooth
- the mutagenic effects of air pollution or tobacco smoking
- the effects of viruses (HPV for oropharyngeal cancer and EBV for nasopharyngeal cancer)
- some chronic inflammatory conditions (such as lichen planus of the mouth).

Squamous head and neck cancer describes a group of cancers that spread 'logically': first to regional lymph nodes (the horizontal group – occipital, post-auricular, pre-auricular, facial, submandibular and submental, or the vertical deep cervical chain) before spreading elsewhere – often to the lung. Furthermore, a considerable time frequently elapses before disease spreads beyond the primary site and nodes. This provides a greater chance for cure in the form of local and regional therapy, such as surgical resection with local radiotherapy. Most cases of early head and neck cancer are curable.

Clinical features

Presenting symptoms depend on the cancer's site of origin. Hoarseness of the voice is a 'red flag' for general practitioners, as it is an early symptom of laryngeal cancer, while a persistent lump or ulcer in the mouth is a 'red flag' for dentists, in that it may be an early symptom of oral cancer. An enlarged lump in the neck (that persists after an obvious upper respiratory tract infection) similarly needs to be regarded with suspicion. Ear, nose and throat clinic review is warranted, with consideration of biopsy or cytology.

Staging

Biopsy-proven cancer requires staging using the TNM system. PET scanning is often useful for staging distant disease, while MRI is best for obtaining anatomical detail of local spread and depth of invasion. Viral status (HPV or EBV) may have implications for therapy. Genomic analysis and predictive tests for immunotherapy have roles in the relapsed patient.

Management
Early disease

Where early cases are easily operable with margins clear of disease, surgery is usually curative. Elective dissection of the deep cervical chain is sometimes indicated to treat 'one step ahead of the cancer's spread': that is, resecting the next most likely site to harbour microscopic disease. Where surgical resection of the primary may lead to great morbidity (e.g. laryngectomy for early laryngeal cancer), and radiotherapy, to which this type of cancer is sensitive, has an equivalent chance of cure, radiotherapy is preferred. Where the cancer is invading cartilage or bone, it is considered to be more radiotherapy-resistant and surgery may be the better option.

Locally advanced disease

In more locally advanced cases for which radiotherapy is chosen, chemotherapy (usually cisplatin) in conjunction with the radiotherapy enhances the radiation effect. The EGFR inhibitor cetuximab can be used to inhibit signal transduction within cancer cells, again in conjunction with radiotherapy.

Metastatic disease

The lungs and bones are the most common sites for spread after local lymph node groups. Chemotherapy with cisplatin-based regimens, often given alongside 5-FU, is first-line therapy, and again, cetuximab may have a role. Immunotherapy agents, such as the PD-1 inhibitor nivolumab, may have significant efficacy and can induce remarkable remissions in some cases, presumably due to the high mutational load and PDL-1 expression of these squamous cancers.

METASTATIC CANCER OF UNKNOWN PRIMARY

Patients presenting with symptoms of metastases, or with an incidental finding on imaging without a clinically obvious primary cancer after investigation, represent a common clinical problem and comprise 5–10% of patients in a specialist oncological centre. Clinical guidelines are based on several systematic studies, some with postmortem follow-up. Patients predicted to have a poor prognosis (based on performance status, histology, and site and extent of disease) can be spared the discomfort of intensive investigation and be given more appropriate palliative care.

Diagnosis

Diagnosis requires histology first and foremost, as it will lead to the identification of several distinct groups.

- **Squamous cancers** mostly present in the lymph nodes of the cervical region; 80% are associated with an occult head and neck primary, the remainder arising from the lung. Inguinal

> ### i Box 6.39 Adenocarcinoma of unknown primary: where search for the primary is of therapeutic benefit
>
> - Breast, e.g. isolated axillary lymphadenopathy
> - Ovary, e.g. peritoneal carcinomatosis
> - Prostate, e.g. pelvic lymphadenopathy
> - Colon, e.g. liver metastases

nodes usually point to a primary of the genital tract or anal canal. Treatment with radiotherapy and chemotherapy may have curative potential, especially in the head and neck area, and even in the absence of an identifiable primary on pan-endoscopy.

- **Poorly differentiated or anaplastic cancers** include a number of potentially curable cancers, such as high-grade lymphomas and germ cell tumours, and should be suspected in all young patients with midline masses. They are sometimes identifiable by their immunocytochemistry and tumour markers. Gene markers, such as i12p for germ cell tumours in cancer of unknown primary, and BCL-2 for lymphomas, are increasingly available to aid diagnosis. Treatment and prognosis are as outlined for lymphoma (see Ch. 17) and germ cell tumours (p. 129).
- **Adenocarcinomas** form the majority of cases of metastatic cancer of unknown primary. Their investigation should be guided by the desire to identify the most treatable options, and the knowledge that the largest proportion will have arisen from the lung or pancreas, with relatively poor treatment prospects.

Investigations

Investigations should always start with a thorough review of the histology and imaging, such as CT of the chest, abdomen and pelvis. In men, further investigations should include serum PSA and rectal ultrasound to identify prostate cancers; in women, mammography and breast MRI to identify occult breast cancer, and pelvic MRI to identify ovarian cancer should be undertaken (**Box 6.39**).

Tissue tumour markers can be helpful (**Box 6.40**) and, increasingly, gene profiles are able to identify the primary site of origin by

i Box 6.40 Carcinoma of unknown primary

Immunohistochemistry marker	Most probable (but not exclusive) tissue of origin
Epithelial membrane antigen (EMA)	Epithelial
Leucocyte common antigen (LCA)	Lymphoid
Cytokeratin 7+ 20+	Pancreas 65%, cholangiocarcinoma 65%
	Gastric 40%, transitional cell 65%, ovarian mucinous 90%
Cytokeratin 7+ 20–	Ovarian (except mucinous) 100%, breast 90%, lung adenocarcinoma 90%, uterus endometrioid 85%, transitional cell 35%, pancreas adenocarcinoma 30%, cholangiocarcinoma 30%, thyroid 100%, mesothelioma 65%
Cytokeratin 7– 20+	Colorectal adenocarcinoma 80%, gastric adenocarcinoma 35%, Merkel cell 70%
Cytokeratin 7– 20–	Hepatocellular 80%, carcinoid 80%, lung small-cell and squamous 75%, prostate 85%, renal adenocarcinoma 80%, adrenal 100%, germ cell 95%, squamous cancer of head and neck, and oesophagus 70%, mesothelioma 35%
Thyroid transcription factor 1 (TTF-1)	Lung, thyroid
Thyroglobulin	Thyroid
Oestrogen receptor (ER), progesterone receptor (PR) and HER2 receptor	Breast
Prostate-specific antigen (PSA)	Prostate, breast
Carcinoembryonic antigen (CEA)	Gastrointestinal
CDX2	Colorectal, small intestinal
Villin	Gastrointestinal
CA125 peritoneal antigen	Ovarian, fallopian tube and primary peritoneal and breast
WT1	Ovarian serous cancer, mesothelioma, desmoplastic tumours, Wilms' tumours
S100, melanin and HMB45	Melanoma
Myosin, desmin and factor VIII	Soft tissue sarcoma
Chromogranin and neurone-specific enolase (NSE)	Neuroendocrine
α-Fetoprotein (AFP)	Germ cell tumours, hepatocellular carcinoma
β-Human chorionic gonadotrophin (β-hCG)	Germ cell and trophoblastic tumours
CD117	Gastrointestinal stromal tumours

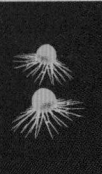

gene expression microarray and RT-PCR. Mutation analysis is more easily available to identify potential targets for treatment, such as *RAS*, *EGFR* and *RET*; however, clinical trials are still needed to establish whether specific pathway inhibitors have a therapeutic effect.

For good-prognosis patients wishing to have palliative chemotherapy, investigations such as endoscopy to identify lung, colon or stomach primaries are indicated to guide the choice of chemotherapy agents, although the diagnostic yield of 4–5% must be set against the discomfort and risks. Serum tumour markers for other solid cancers, although highly sensitive, are too non-specific and unreliable to be useful as diagnostic aids in this situation.

Further investigation may require PET–CT for head and neck, lung and possibly other primaries, and radio-isotope scans for thyroid and carcinoid tumours. PET–CT may also be used to seek other metastatic sites if surgery is being considered for unifocal disease.

Prognosis

Most large series report an overall median survival of 12 weeks but a considerably better rate among subgroups, such as patients presenting with isolated nodal metastases, who have a significantly better prognosis than the majority with visceral and/or bone metastases. These better-prognosis patients may warrant more extensive investigation.

Management

If investigations have not identified a primary site, surgery may be considered for unifocal adenocarcinoma of unknown primary (ACUP) metastases in lymph nodes, lung, liver and brain, especially if due to suspected melanoma and so having the potential for long-term survival.

In women, an isolated axillary lymph node metastasis should be treated as for lymph node-positive breast cancer; this has a similar prospect for long-term cure, though without the need for breast surgery. Malignant ascites in women should be treated with a trial of chemotherapy, as for primary peritoneal, fallopian tube or epithelial ovarian cancer. The prognosis for those responding to the therapeutic trial is similar to that in disease of known primary origin. Primary chemotherapy that achieves an excellent response on imaging and CA125 criteria should be followed by debulking surgery; if successful, this carries a median survival in excess of 4 years.

For men, the occasional occult prostatic cancer found because of a raised serum PSA offers some palliative treatment prospects.

For the patient presenting with hepatic metastases, which are most commonly associated with an occult gastrointestinal primary, there is increasing choice and efficacy of chemotherapy agents for gastrointestinal cancers that have the potential to improve their palliation.

If there is an excellent response, suitable patients may even be considered for hepatic ablation or resection. If, after all efforts, no primary has been identified, palliative chemotherapy can achieve responses in 20–40% in highly selected series, with a median survival of 9–10 months, and 5–10% surviving to 5 years.

Further reading

Greco FA, Spigel DR, Yardley DA et al. Molecular profiling in unknown primary cancer: accuracy of tissue of origin prediction. *Oncologist* 2010; 15:500–506.
Varadhachary GR, Raber MN. Cancer of unknown primary site. *N Engl J Med* 2014; 371:757–763.

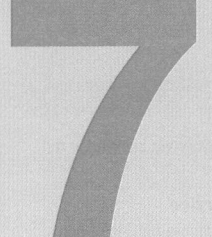

7 Palliative care and symptom control

Chloe Chin, Catherine Moffat and Sara Booth

CORE SKILLS AND KNOWLEDGE

Palliative care is the active total care of patients who have advanced, progressive, life-shortening disease. It is based on needs and not diagnosis, and is required in non-malignant diseases as well as in cancer. Knowledge of the principles of palliative medicine is essential for all healthcare professionals, and can be applied throughout medical practice so that all patients, across all care settings, receive and have access to good palliative care.

Palliative care is delivered by multidisciplinary teams that include doctors, nurses, therapists, chaplains, psychologists and social workers. It may be given in the patient's own home, during acute hospital admissions, and through hospices, which typically provide both inpatient and outpatient services. There is a focus on addressing all aspects of a patient's care needs, promoting independence, and supporting patients and their families through the dying process.

Key skills to acquire in palliative care include:
- learning to talk openly and sensitively with patients about disability, uncertainty, deterioration and death
- learning about the range of interventions used in managing common symptoms such as pain and nausea
- working within a multidisciplinary team to provide holistic care for patients.

Opportunities for learning these skills include visiting a hospice and talking with patients and those close to them, shadowing different members of a palliative care team as they visit patients, and attending palliative care clinics to observe how healthcare professionals communicate with patients and address their needs.

INTRODUCTION AND GENERAL ASPECTS

Palliative care is an approach that has relevance in medicine well beyond the final weeks of death from malignant disease. Patients with chronic non-malignant disease, such as organ failures (heart, lung and kidney) and neurodegenerative diseases, have been shown to have a similar or greater symptom burden than people with cancer, may live many years with these difficulties, and may therefore benefit from an early palliative care approach with access to specialist palliative care (SPC) for complex problems (**Box 7.1**). Additionally, increasing numbers of cancer patients are surviving longer but experiencing long-term sequelae of their cancer and its treatment. There may be a less clear end-stage of disease but the principles of symptom control are the same: holistic assessment, treatment of reversible factors and multiprofessional support.

The *goal* of palliative care is to achieve the best possible quality of life for patients and their carers by:
- managing physical, psychological, social and spiritual problems to provide excellent symptom control
- enabling patients to be cared for and to have the best chance of dying in their preferred place

- enabling the acceptance of death as a normal process when life-prolonging treatments no longer improve or maintain quality of life
- providing the opportunity to say goodbye and reduce complicated grief.

Throughout the course of illness, careful open discussion of the patient's possible future options and their wishes is essential. Early discussion of difficult choices and management of the potential uncertainty surrounding their condition(s) is helpful. These discussions are ideally held when the patient is relatively well and outside an acute episode of care. Discussions delayed until the crisis of acute admission may lead to acceptance of invasive and potentially non-beneficial treatment that is later regretted by the patient and/or their loved ones (**Box 7.2**).

Who provides palliative care?

A hallmark of palliative care is the multiprofessional team, as single professionals cannot provide the breadth of necessary expertise. The emotional demands of working in this area require team support to enable balanced, compassionate and professional care. Members of the team can include, but are not restricted to, clinical nurse specialists, doctors, psychologists, therapists (occupational, physical, music and creative), chaplains and social workers. In some centres the term *supportive care* is used instead of palliative care.

Key points in palliative care
- Patients should always be involved in decisions about their care.
- Quality of life is increased when treatment goals are clearly understood by everyone, including patient and carer.
- The multidisciplinary team provide a high standard of care but there must be realism and honesty about what can be achieved.
- End-of-life care is delivered in all settings: the patient's usual place of residence, hospitals and hospices.
- Care at home should be encouraged for as long as possible, even if the patient's preferred place of death is elsewhere.
- Discussions about end-of-life care planning are best held outside times of crisis, with clinicians with whom the patient has a good relationship. An unplanned admission can be a trigger for advance care planning discussions.

- Discussions must be recorded and made known to everyone involved in the patient's care.

Key components of a modern palliative care service
- Management based on *needs*, not diagnosis: the symptom burden of non-malignant disease often equals that of cancer.
- Care that is independent of the patient's location and that helps patients to remain at home if possible, avoiding unwanted admissions to hospital.
- Rehabilitation for people with advanced disease.
- Support for carers.
- Bereavement care for people with complicated grief.
- Advice for other clinicians; dissemination of palliative care knowledge.
- Education (surrounding palliative and end-of-life care) for clinicians of all disciplines and all levels.

- There is insufficient time to achieve good symptom control by combining non-pharmacological and pharmacological components.
- Specialist palliative care services are deemed less acceptable by patient and family, being associated with 'dying', 'giving up' or 'giving in' to illness.
- Psychological distress and physical symptoms become intractable and contribute to complex grief.
- It becomes too late to adopt a rehabilitative approach or teach/use non-pharmacological interventions that need a degree of training and patient motivation (e.g. cognitive behavioural approaches, mindfulness meditation, attendance at day therapy).

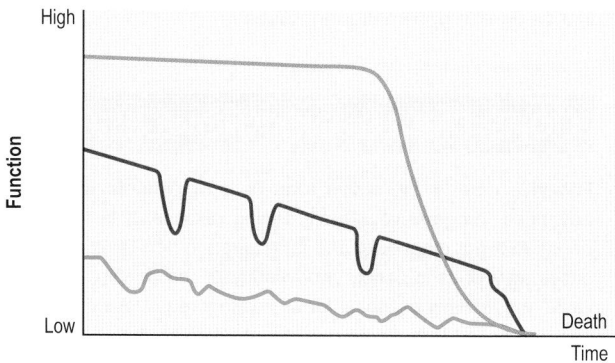

Fig. 7.1 Trajectories of different disease types. Green = cancer, red = chronic non-malignant disease, blue = multimorbidity and increasing frailty. *(From Murray SA, Kendall M, Boyd K et al. Illness trajectories and palliative care.* BMJ *2005; 330:1007.)*

All healthcare providers should have basic palliative care skills and know how to access SPC advice. The latter may come from teams based in hospitals, hospices or in the community, as palliative care crosses all healthcare settings. Clinicians should be aware of the services that their local SPC teams offer and recognize when referral is appropriate. Palliative care can be used from the time of diagnosis of potentially life-threatening or life-limiting illness, even when cure is considered possible ('hoping for the best, preparing for the worst'). A problem-based approach to disease management will ensure that patients and carers obtain access to appropriate support services, including SPC, and avoid an either/or approach ('either curative treatment or palliative care').

Patients may have very close relationships with their usual medical team and an integrated approach is needed to allow optimization of disease-directed intervention as well as palliation. Excellent communication between all members of the healthcare team, and between patient and carer, underpins the successful management of advanced disease and end-of-life care. Effective liaison between the hospital, primary care centre and hospice is also essential.

When should palliative care needs be assessed – problems rather than prognosis?

Early assessment of needs is crucial to achieving the best outcome for maintaining or improving quality of life for both patient and carer. Palliative care is most effective when included as part of routine care as soon as possible after diagnosis, alongside disease-specific therapy. Early referral links palliative care with quality-of-life improvements; positive associations increase the likelihood that patients and families continue to use palliative care services when they need them over the course of the illness. In cancer, there is good evidence that integrating palliative care and anti-tumour

Would you be surprised if this patient died within the next 12 months?

Further resources
Downar J, Goldman R, Adhikari N. The 'surprise question for predicting death' in seriously ill patients: a systematic review and meta-analysis. *CMAJ* 2017; 189:E484–493.
https://www.goldstandardsframework.org.uk/ *The Gold Standards Framework, 2011*

treatment soon after diagnosis reduces long-term distress and even increases survival in selected cases.

If palliative care is seen as relevant only to the end-of-life phase, patients may be denied expert help for complex symptoms. Timely management of physical and psychosocial issues earlier in the course of disease prevents intractable problems later (see **Box 7.2**). It can be difficult to know when to consider palliative care in non-malignant conditions due to their variable disease trajectories (**Fig. 7.1**) but using the 'Surprise Question' (**Box 7.3**) may help clinicians decide; it is the basis of the Gold Standards Framework tool that is commonly used to help tailor care to the right time and place. Anyone with symptoms or complex family issues, whatever their prognosis, may benefit from support from the palliative care team.

What are the patient's needs and what is the patient's understanding?

The causes of a patient's symptoms are often multifactorial, and a holistic assessment (**Box 7.4**) is central to optimum management. Assessment of the patient's grasp of the disease, understanding

i **Box 7.4** Domains of a holistic assessment[a]

Mnemonic	Domain	Things to consider
P	Physical	Symptom assessment: may involve specific symptom assessment tools or assessment by other professionals, e.g. physiotherapists, specialist clinicians
E	Emotional	Psychological assessment, including understanding patient expectations: may involve psychological assessment tools, e.g. distress thermometer, and onward referral for appropriate support
P	Personal	Cultural, ethnic, spiritual and religious needs
S	Social support	Work and finance, family and close relationships, recreational activities: may benefit from social services referral or occupational therapy advice
I	Information and communication	Patient understanding of the plan, multidisciplinary team outcomes communicated, identification of key workers
C	Control and autonomy	Mental capacity to make decisions, patient choice regarding treatment options/plans, preferred place of care and death
O	Out of hours	Advance care planning, awareness of where to access services out of hours
L	Living with your illness	Rehabilitation, management of activities of daily living, future expectations and end-of-life care planning
A	Aftercare	Funeral arrangements, bereavement needs, future support for family

[a]In each domain the tool identifies potential anticipated patient issues and concerns, cue questions to ask patients and carers, and resources for professionals to signpost to. Adapted from the Gold Standards Framework.

their wishes and acknowledging their concerns, will help the team plan and implement effective support. Validated questionnaires, such as the integrated Palliative care Outcome Scale (iPOS), have been developed and are routinely used to aid this. Patients will have differing needs for information and will deal with 'bad news' in different ways. A sensitive approach, respecting individual requirements, is crucial.

How can patients use palliative care services?

Changes in the provision of SPC services have been forced by the increase in the number of patients who survive malignant disease ('living with and beyond cancer'), and the ageing and increasing rates of multimorbidity in the population, as well as recognition of the needs of patients who have non-malignant disease. Palliative care services can be accessed for specialist symptom management and psychological support, not just care in the last few weeks and days of life, and patients should be informed of this. They may use inpatient SPC services for a limited period (days to weeks) for complex problems to be intensively addressed, and then may be discharged with community palliative care follow-up. They have the opportunity for re-referral if help is required later. Many patients are managed at home by community palliative care in close conjunction with primary care services.

Further reading

Etkind S, Bone A, Gomes B et al. How many people will need palliative care in 2040? Past trends, future projections and implications for services. *BMC Medicine* 2017; 15:102–112.
Kelley AS, Morrison RS. Palliative care for the seriously ill. *N Engl J Med* 2015; 373:747–755.
Temel J, Greer J, Muzikansky A et al. Early palliative care for patients with metastatic non-small-cell lung cancer. *N Engl J Med* 2010; 363:733–742.

SYMPTOM CONTROL

Good palliative care integrates non-pharmacological approaches, such as anxiety management and rehabilitation, with pharmacological control of symptoms. Medications should be rationalized to reduce polypharmacy. A key, and usually initial, component of palliative care is actively identifying and managing reversible problems that could be contributing to inadequate symptom control (**Box 7.5**). Symptom management runs in parallel with these active treatments.

Pain

Pain is the most feared symptom at the end of life. At least two-thirds of people with cancer suffer significant pain. Pain has a number of causes, and not all pains respond equally well to opioid analgesics. It may be related to the tumour either directly (e.g. pressure on surrounding structures) or indirectly (e.g. due to weight loss or pressure ulcers), and can result from co-morbidity such as arthritis. Various scales can be used to assess a patient's pain (**Fig. 7.2**). Emotional and spiritual distress may be expressed as, and can exacerbate, physical pain.

The term 'total pain' encompasses a variety of influences that contribute to pain:

- *biological*: the disease itself, disease-modifying therapy (drugs, surgery, radiotherapy)
- *social*: family distress, loss of independence, financial problems
- *psychological*: fear of dying, of pain, or of being in hospital; anger at dying or at the process of diagnosis and perceived delays, with anxiety and/or depression stemming from all of these
- *spiritual*: fear of death, questions about life's meaning, guilt, why me?

i **Box 7.5** Examples of reversible problems that can be treated to improve symptoms

Patient 1
Mr K has metastatic prostate cancer with known spinal metastases at multiple levels. He complains of worsening back pain and leg weakness. This warrants urgent magnetic resonance imaging to rule out metastatic spinal cord compression, which could be treated with steroids and radiotherapy leading to an improvement in his symptoms and functioning.

Patient 2
Mrs S has metastatic breast cancer. She describes a history of general deterioration, nausea, abdominal pain, constipation and low mood. This warrants a set of blood tests that may reveal hypercalcaemia, which can improve with intravenous fluids and bisphosphonates; there may even be resolution of symptoms.

Patient 3
Mrs B has metastatic ovarian cancer. She has a similar history to that of Mrs S. A thorough clinical examination may reveal tense ascites as a cause of abdominal discomfort, nausea and constipation, which could be alleviated by paracentesis.

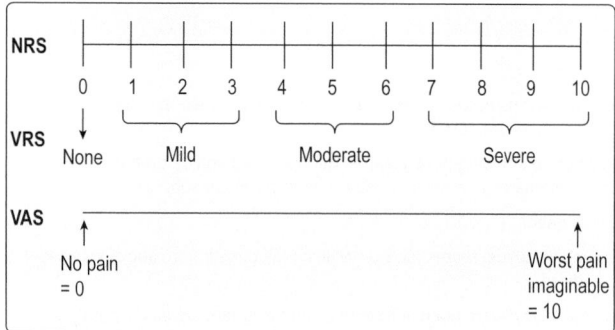

Fig. 7.2 Commonly used one-dimensional scales for pain assessment. An 11-point numerical rating scale (NRS), visual analogue scale (VAS, which can be 0–10 or 0–100) and verbal rating scale (VRS). *(Adapted from Breivik H, Borchgrevink PC, Allen SM et al. Assessment of pain.* Br J Anaesthesia *2008; 101:17–24.)*

The WHO analgesic ladder

Most cancer pain can be managed with oral or commonly used transdermal preparations. The World Health Organization (WHO) cancer pain relief ladder guides the choice of analgesic according to pain *severity* (**Fig. 7.3**).

If *regular* use of optimum dosing (e.g. paracetamol 1 g four times daily) for step 1 does not control pain, then an analgesic from the next step of the ladder is prescribed. As pain has different physical aetiologies, an adjuvant analgesic may be needed: for example, a gabapentinoid for neuropathic pain (see **Box 7.9**).

Strong opioid drugs
Dose titration and route

Morphine is the drug of choice and, in most circumstances, should be given regularly by mouth. The dose should be tailored to the individual's needs by allowing 'as required' doses up to every 1–2 hours. Morphine for cancer pain does not have a 'ceiling' effect but there may be a limit to the usefulness of opioids in chronic non-cancer pain. If a patient has needed further doses in addition to the regular daily dose *and* they have been effective, then the amount in the additional doses can be added to the following day's regular dose. This up-titration can be repeated until the daily requirement becomes stable (**Box 7.6**). When a stable daily dose requirement has been established, the morphine can be changed to a modified-release preparation and the patient given 'as required' doses of immediate-release morphine, which are usually one-sixth of their total daily morphine dose.

The starting dose of morphine is usually 5–10 mg every 4 hours, depending on patient size, renal function and whether a weak opioid is already being given. If an individual is already on step 2 of the WHO ladder, explaining conversions between medications can be helpful to gain patient confidence. For example, maximum-dose codeine (60 mg four times daily) is equivalent to a total of 24 mg morphine per day (**Box 7.7**). If there is renal dysfunction, morphine should be used in low doses, or oxycodone considered in mild to moderate renal dysfunction (hepatic metabolism). Modified-release preparations ought to be avoided. However, if renal dysfunction is significant (estimated glomerular filtration rate <30 mL/min), an alternative opioid, such as alfentanil, should be considered because of the risk of metabolite accumulation. If there is concurrent significant hepatic dysfunction, oxycodone should be avoided. Dosing is not an exact science in palliative care: Advice can be sought from the SPC team.

Strong opioids come in transdermal preparations, such as buprenorphine or fentanyl *patches* (**Box 7.8**). These are useful in

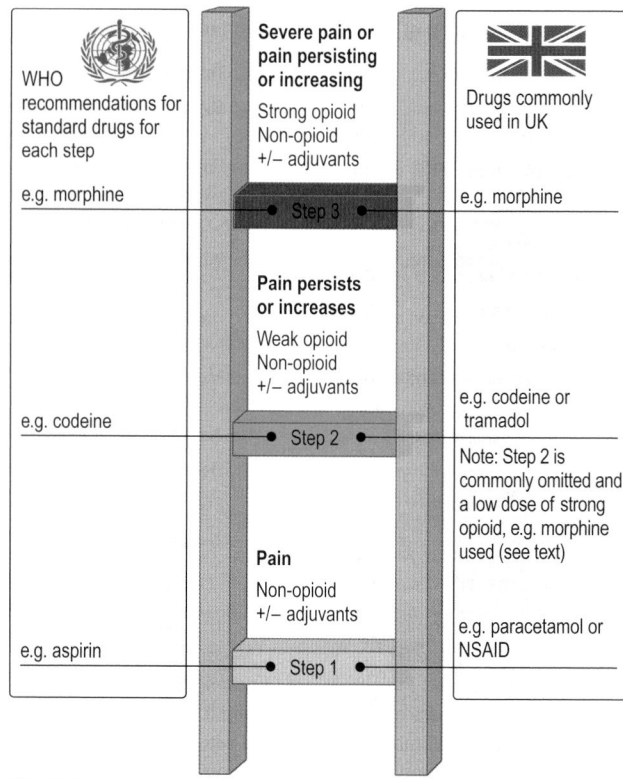

Fig. 7.3 The World Health Organization analgesic ladder for cancer and other chronic pain. Adjuvant drugs are listed in **Box 7.9**. NSAID, non-steroidal anti-inflammatory drug.

Box 7.6 Opioid titration examples

Scenario 1

A patient regularly takes 20 mg morphine sulphate immediate release every 4 hours. What long-acting preparation could they be started on?

    20 mg every 4 hours = 120 mg morphine per day

    = 60 mg twice daily of a 12-h morphine sulphate modified-release (MR) preparation

Scenario 2

The same patient has started morphine sulphate MR 60 mg twice a day with 'as required' immediate-release morphine 20 mg every 1–2 hours. A few months later, their pain escalates due to disease progression and they require an additional 4 doses per day of immediate-release morphine. What should their long-acting morphine be increased to?

    20 mg × 4 = additional 80 mg morphine per day

    Total daily morphine dose including morphine MR = 200 mg

    = 100 mg twice daily of a 12-h morphine sulphate MR

Top tip: Always thoroughly check dose conversions. Dosing is not an exact science - discuss with SPC if unsure.

patients with stable pain. Serum levels do not change quickly with transdermal patches; they can therefore be hazardous if the pain stimulus is removed, and are cumbersome to titrate in patients with escalating or unstable pain. The patient should be reassessed and reasons for the escalation in pain sought; if necessary, advice should be requested. Be aware that transdermal patches may be administered every 72 hours or weekly, depending on the dose and brand – always check this when prescribing.

If a patient is unable to take oral medication due to weakness, swallowing difficulties or nausea and vomiting, the opioid should be given parenterally. This may be via continuous subcutaneous infusion, whereby the opioid dose is administered continuously via a syringe pump over the course of 24 hours.

Box 7.7 Opioid equivalences

Drug/route	Dose	Potency to oral morphine equivalent
Codeine/p.o.	100 mg	1:10
Diamorphine/s.c.	3 mg	3:1
Morphine/p.o.	10 mg	1:1
Morphine/s.c.	5 mg	2:1
Oxycodone/p.o.	6.6 mg	1.5–2:1
Oxycodone/s.c.	3.3 mg	3:1
Tramadol/p.o.	100 mg	1:10
Alfentanil/s.c.	0.3 mg	30:1

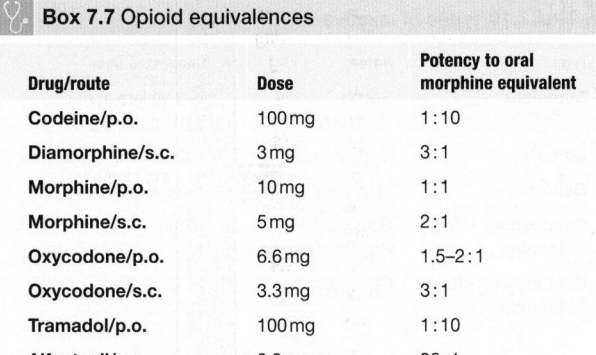

p.o., per os (orally); s.c., subcutaneous. *(Adapted from https://bnf.nice.org.uk/guidance/prescribing-in-palliative-care.html.)*

Box 7.8 Buprenorphine and fentanyl patches

Oral morphine equivalent/day	Patch
12 mg	Buprenorphine 5 µg/h
24 mg	Buprenorphine 10 µg/h
36 mg	Buprenorphine 15 µg/h
30 mg	Fentanyl 12 µg/h
60 mg	Fentanyl 25 µg/h
120 mg	Fentanyl 50 µg/h
180 mg	Fentanyl 75 µg/h

(Adapted from https://bnf.nice.org.uk/guidance/prescribing-in-palliative-care.html.)

Doctors and patients may have worries, such as the fear of addiction, which mean that adequate doses of opioids are not prescribed or taken. Iatrogenic addiction is very rare (<0.01% risk), but the adverse effects and morbidity from uncontrolled pain are much higher. Patients and carers should be reassured about their medications and the rationale for their use, and it is good practice to provide written information regarding opioids. Regular review is necessary to achieve optimal pain control, including regular assessment to distinguish pain severity from distress due to pain.

The opioid epidemic

In 2018 there were 6000 deaths from opioid overdose in the USA. These deaths were mainly in young people who had first become addicted to opioids in the form of legally available drugs, some then switching to other, more potent, opioids from illegal sources. Many of those involved came from stable, middle-class backgrounds. The epidemic of addiction has had profound societal consequences and is beginning to affect the status of opioids for medical use: for example, there is shorter postoperative prescription of drugs, and opioids for non-malignant pain have been withdrawn. It may yet have a further impact, as legal action is being taken against drug companies for providing misleading information in the 'selling' of opioids: for example, their statement that modified-release oxycodone is not addictive. Be aware of the dependency potential of longer-term opioids and ensure that family members know the dangers of using the patient's pain and breathlessness medication.

Side-effects

The most common side-effects of strong opioids are:
- *Nausea and vomiting*. These can be managed with use of antiemetics.
- *Constipation*. This is common and should be anticipated; best practice guidelines advocate that *all* opioids should be co-prescribed with laxatives. Newer laxatives for opioid-induced constipation – e.g. naloxegol or methylnaltrexone, peripherally acting opioid receptor antagonists – can be used if response to other laxatives is poor.

If side-effects are intractable, a change of opioid is often helpful. Some patients find transdermal preparations of opioids less constipating.

Toxicity

Confusion, persistent and undue drowsiness, myoclonus, nightmares and hallucinations indicate opioid toxicity. This may follow rapid dose escalation and responds to dose reduction and slower retitration. It may indicate pain that is poorly responsive to opioids and the need for adjuvant analgesics. Patients should be assessed for reversible factors contributing to reduced tolerance of opioids, such as sepsis. Importantly, respiratory depression (respiratory rate <8 breaths/min) is a late sign and indicates significant toxicity that needs management as an emergency. Consider stopping any long-acting opioid preparation and administering naloxone if respiratory depression is severe. Dependency on opioids used in the longer term does occur and means that sudden reversal (with naloxone) or withdrawal of opioids is not advisable, unless absolutely necessary.

Antipsychotics such as haloperidol may help settle the patient's distress while waiting for toxicity to resolve. Some individuals will tolerate an alternative opioid such as oxycodone better, or an alternative route such as subcutaneous injection.

Adjuvants and alternatives

Box 7.9 outlines the most commonly used adjuvant analgesics. Neuropathic pain often responds well to adjuvants in the antiepileptic or tricyclic antidepressant class. Other treatments, such as radio- or chemotherapy, interventional pain strategies (e.g. nerve blocks, epidurals) and transcutaneous electrical nerve stimulation (TENS), may be useful in selected patients. Multidisciplinary team working is essential to manage patients' pain optimally, and joint working between palliative care and pain teams helps to achieve this.

Additionally, to improve their symptoms and wellbeing, patients facing incurable illness are increasingly turning to less conventional therapies to complement, and serve as alternatives to, prescribed medical treatments. These include acupuncture and herbal and massage therapies. Although there may not be a strong evidence base to support some of these, this does not mean that they do not have a beneficial contribution to make to the holistic care of patients. There has been significant recent interest in certain agents, such as cannabinoids. Evidence is mounting that points to the benefits of medicinal cannabis in a wide variety of conditions, and it has a good risk:benefit profile. This has led certain countries to legalize cannabis and allow its prescription. As ever, more research is needed into these compounds and therapies to demonstrate their effectiveness clearly, and the picture will evolve over time. Institutions and organizations are increasingly developing guidance and policies.

Further reading

Caraceni A, Hanks G, Kaasa S et al. Use of opioid analgesics in the treatment of cancer pain: evidence-based recommendations from the EAPC. *Lancet Oncol* 2012; 13:e58–e68.
National Institute for Health and Care Excellence. *NICE Clinical Guideline CG140: Palliative Care for Adults: Strong Opioids for Pain Relief*. NICE 2016; https://www.nice.org.uk/Guidance/CG140.

Box 7.9 Commonly used adjuvant analgesics

Drugs	Indication
Non-steroidal anti-inflammatory drugs (NSAIDs), e.g. naproxen (250–500 mg twice daily)	Bone pain, inflammatory pain
Antiepileptics, e.g. gabapentin (300–2400 mg daily in divided doses) or pregabalin (50–600 mg daily in divided doses)	Neuropathic pain
Tricyclic antidepressants, e.g. amitriptyline (10–75 mg daily)	Neuropathic pain
Bisphosphonates, e.g. zoledronic acid, denosumab (a RANKL inhibitor)	Metastatic bone disease
Dexamethasone	Neuropathic pain, inflammatory pain (e.g. liver capsule pain), headache from cerebral oedema due to brain metastases

RANKL, receptor activator of nuclear factor kappa-B ligand.

Gastrointestinal symptoms

Nausea and vomiting

These symptoms are common and may have numerous causes: both physical and psychological factors can contribute. Careful choice of antiemetic targeted towards the underlying cause of the nausea and/or vomiting is essential.

Nausea and vomiting are associated with:

- **Chemotherapy.** Certain agents, e.g. cisplatin, confer a high risk of nausea and vomiting. A 5-hydroxytryptamine$_3$ (5-HT$_3$) antagonist, such as ondansetron 8 mg three times daily, may help. Aprepitant, a neurokinin-1 (NK-1) antagonist, is increasingly being used as an adjunct in chemotherapy-induced nausea and vomiting.
- **Chemical causes**, e.g. hypercalcaemia, hepatic failure, uraemia or drugs. Haloperidol 0.5–1.5 mg as required every 4 hours, up to a maximum of 5 mg daily, is the first choice.
- **Gastric stasis and distension.** Metoclopramide 10 mg three times daily is a prokinetic and promotes gastric emptying. The prokinetic effects can also ameliorate constipation.
- **Raised intracranial pressure**, e.g. brain tumour. Cyclizine 50 mg three times daily is most useful.
- **Mechanical causes of vomiting.** It may be necessary to start antiemetic therapy parenterally by continuous subcutaneous infusion to gain control. If the patient has gastrointestinal obstruction or poor oral/gastrointestinal absorption, this route may need to be continued. Levomepromazine is a second-line antiemetic if initial therapy is not successful; 6.25 mg as required, up to a maximum of 25 mg per day, is recommended. Other medications to aid nausea and vomiting include corticosteroids, particularly in the case of bowel obstruction, where reducing tumour oedema may alleviate the obstruction and improve symptoms.

Constipation

This is common, occurring in up to 45% of hospice patients and 90% of patients on opioids. It is best managed with a combination of pharmacological and non-pharmacological strategies. Non-pharmacological measures can include maintaining hydration, mobility, dietary advice, optimal positioning, privacy and comfort to aid relaxation when trying to open bowels.

Box 7.10 Types of laxative

Type	Name	Suggested dose
Stimulant	Senna	2–4 tablets at night
	Bisacodyl	5–10 mg at night
Softener	Docusate sodium	100–200 mg twice daily
Osmotic	Macrogol	1–3 sachets daily
Suppository – soft-loading	Bisacodyl	10 mg
	Phosphate enema	1
Suppository – hard-loading	Glycerol	1

Pharmacological strategies – that is, laxatives (**Box 7.10**) – are targeted to the cause of the constipation and a careful history is required. Often, opioid-induced constipation responds to a combination of stool softener and stimulant, e.g. docusate and senna. Doses will require individual titration. Some patients may need suppositories or enemas. Those with reduced sensation and mobility – for example, due to spinal cord compression – may require a bowel regimen of regular suppositories and maintenance of a relatively firm stool to facilitate best care. Many are likely to need to continue regular laxatives, as they will develop troublesome constipation again on cessation of these medications.

Bowel obstruction

This is common in advanced cancer (3%), and especially so in gynaecological and colorectal cancers. It is caused by mechanical obstruction of the bowel lumen and/or peristaltic failure due to infiltration of the nerves. Presenting symptoms include pain, vomiting, colic and constipation. It can be partial or complete, at single or multiple sites, and carries a poor prognosis. Palliative management of bowel obstruction focuses on medications to improve symptoms, as opposed to the surgical approach, which uses a large-bore nasogastric tube (to decompress) and intravenous fluids, coupled with keeping the patient nil by mouth. Consideration should be paid to nutrition, including parenteral. The patient's prognosis and further treatment options, among other things, should be taken into account.

Metoclopramide's prokinetic effect can be employed in partial obstruction to encourage the bowels to function again. However, it should be avoided in complete obstruction where the bowel is physically blocked, as it will worsen colic. In this situation, an antispasmodic, such as hyoscine butylbromide, is preferred, along with regular analgesia and an antiemetic such as haloperidol. A dose of 60–120 mg/24 h s.c. is usually recommended but much higher doses (300–480 mg) may be needed, as parenteral hyoscine butylbromide can be rapidly inactivated.

Octreotide (a somatostatin analogue) is used as second-line treatment in bowel obstruction to improve symptoms, which it does by reducing gut secretions and the volume of vomitus. However, there is only low-level evidence of benefit in management of symptoms, and a small number of randomized controlled trials have failed to show any benefit. Further studies are needed. **Ranitidine** may have a role in reducing gastric secretions.

Physical measures, such as a defunctioning colostomy or a venting gastrostomy, may be helpful. Occasionally, a lower bowel obstruction is resolved with insertion of a stent or transrectal resection of tumour in selected individuals. Steroids can shorten the length of episodes of obstruction, if resolution is possible.

In **advanced disease**, where the obstruction is irreversible, patients should be encouraged to drink and take small amounts of soft diet for comfort as they wish. With good mouth care (see later),

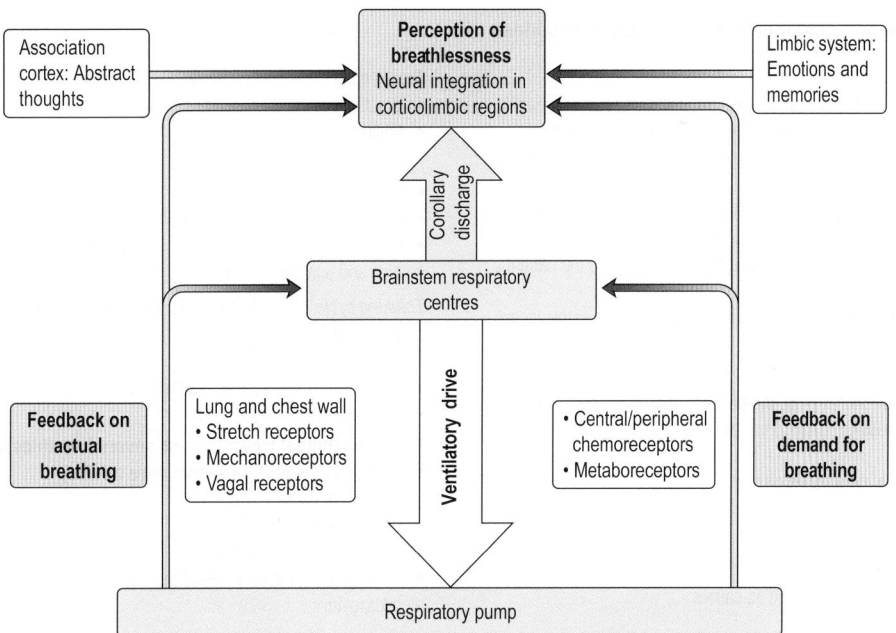

Fig. 7.4 Genesis of breathlessness. *(Adapted from Moosavi S, Booth S. The genesis of breathlessness. In:* Cambridge Breathlessness Intervention Service Treatment Manual. *Cambridge: Cambridge University Hospitals NHS Foundation Trust; 2011.)*

the sensation of thirst can be managed and parenteral fluids may not be needed. If these are indicated, they should be introduced as a trial to improve symptoms and patients counselled about the benefits and risks, including their possible contribution to increased gut secretions and volume of vomitus; in this case the fluids may be ceased.

Anorexia, weight loss and malaise

These result from the cachexia syndrome of advanced disease and are poor prognostic factors. Although attention must be paid to nutrition, the syndrome is mediated through chronic stimulation of the acute phase response and tumour-secreted substances. Thus, calorie–protein support alone gives limited benefit; parenteral feeding has been shown to make no difference to patient survival or quality of life.

Management is generally supportive and advice from dieticians may be helpful. Patients and their carers should be reassured that decreased appetite is to be expected, and advising 'little and often' and 'what you want, when you want' can be useful.

Corticosteroids are occasionally used as appetite stimulants. However, the weight gained is usually fluid retention, and muscle catabolism is accelerated, causing proximal myopathy. Any benefit in appetite stimulation tends to be short-lived, which must be explained clearly to patients and carers. Thus, use of corticosteroids should be limited to the short term and reviewed regularly.

Other interventions – for example, a rehabilitative palliative care programme encompassing nutritional supplementation and exercise in advanced cancer – are being trialled.

Further reading

Obita GP, Boland EG, Currow DC et al. Somatostatin analogues compared with placebo and other pharmacologic agents in the management of symptoms of inoperable malignant bowel obstruction: a systematic review. *J Pain Symp Manage* 2016; 52:901–919.

Roila, F, Molassiotis A, Herrstedt et al on behalf of the participants of the MASCC/ESMO Consensus Conference Copenhagen 2015. 2016 MASCC and ESMO guideline update for the prevention of chemotherapy- and radiotherapy-induced nausea and vomiting and of nausea and vomiting in advanced cancer patients. *Annals Onc* 2016; 27(Suppl 5):v119–v133.

Respiratory symptoms

Breathlessness

Chronic breathlessness (dyspnoea) is a common but frightening symptom of many advanced malignant and non-malignant diseases but often goes unrecognized and untreated. Its features have been described as 'breathlessness that persists despite optimal treatment of the underlying pathophysiology and that results in disability'. It is also terrifying for carers, who often feel helpless. Carer anxiety may exacerbate a patient's breathlessness and it is therefore essential to involve them in treatment strategies and support them in their own right. Recent advances have helped to establish effective treatments to reduce the impact of breathlessness, but palliative care or specialist breathlessness services are often needed to provide optimal care.

The sensation of being breathless is generated in the central nervous system through the integration of peripheral and central signals by a complex network involving structures in the mid brain, higher cortical regions and the limbic system (**Fig. 7.4**). Individual assessment is key, as is reversal of any contributory factors, such as optimizing treatment of underlying medical conditions, although in advanced disease many of these are irreversible.

The first step in assessing breathlessness (**Box 7.11**) is to ask directly about it, as many patients with severe breathlessness will not be troubled at rest. Best practice in managing breathlessness rests on a complex intervention comprised of a number of non-pharmacological and pharmacological approaches (**Boxes 7.11** and **7.12**). Careful assessment of the patient – for example, utilizing the 'Breathing, Thinking, Functioning' clinical model (**Fig. 7.5**) – guides the choice of initial non-pharmacological approach (**Box 7.12**). Pharmacological measures should be reserved for those with severe breathlessness on exertion or at rest, or with advanced progressive disease such as untreatable lung cancer or heart failure. Morphine is the drug with the best evidence base; other treatments, such as mirtazapine, are being

Box 7.11 Assessment and management of breathlessness

Step 1
- Ask directly about breathlessness: 'Are you troubled by breathlessness?'
- Ask about other respiratory symptoms: 'Are you troubled by a cough?'
- Ask about fatigue: 'Are you troubled by fatigue or extreme tiredness that does not go away with rest or sleep?'
- Take a full history of each symptom, particularly if the patient is breathless at rest or on the most minimal exertion, such as brushing the hair or eating
- Ask about the carer's views, thoughts and feelings relating to the patient's breathlessness
- Find out what happens when the patient has an 'attack' of breathlessness

Step 2
- Assess whether breathing dysfunction ('Breathing'), deconditioning and lack of exercise ('Functioning'), or the patients' thoughts and feelings about being breathless ('Thinking') are the most troubling/disabling for the patient
- Choose an initial treatment based on that

Initial treatment
All patients
- Hand-held fan
- Education about breathlessness and its causes

Breathing cycle – dysfunctional, inefficient breathing
- Breathing techniques and breathing retraining from physiotherapist
- Positioning

Functioning cycle
- Pulmonary rehabilitation
- Individual exercise programme from palliative care
- Pacing and prioritizing from occupational therapist
- Aids and adaptations for mobility and activities of daily living

Thinking cycle – beliefs, thoughts and feelings about breathlessness (also carer beliefs)
- Address misconceptions
- Relaxation exercises and mindfulness
- Specialist psychological help

Pharmacological treatment for severe breathlessness or at end of life (seek specialist palliative care advice)
- Use oral or parenteral opioids
- Consider mirtazapine
- Consider benzodiazepines
- Dying patients with breathlessness will need subcutaneous opioids and midazolam

---

i **Box 7.12 Key non-pharmacological interventions for breathlessness**

Intervention	Putative mechanism of action	Most useful
Hand-held fan	Cools area served by second and third branches of trigeminal nerve	For reducing length of episodes of SOB on exertion or at rest
	Reduces temperature of air flowing over nasal receptors, altering signal to brainstem respiratory complex and so changing respiratory pattern	For giving patient and carer confidence by having an intervention they can use Use needs to be explained
Exercise	Stops spiral of disability developing	In patients who are still quite mobile
	Changes muscle structure: less lactic acid produced	In patients who have not developed onset of SOB, lessening/deferring symptoms by reducing deconditioning
Anxiety reduction, e.g. CBT (needs skilled clinician to administer) or simple relaxation therapy	Works on central perception of breathlessness, reducing impact	In people with higher levels of anxiety at baseline (i.e. when first seen)
	Interrupts panic–anxiety cycle	In patients willing to persevere with learning a new skill
Carer support	Reduces carer anxiety and distress, which are part of 'total' anxiety–panic cycle	Where carer is isolated, under extra pressures (e.g. looking after elderly parent, going through divorce)
Breathing retraining	Improves mechanical effectiveness of respiratory system	Where breathlessness is disproportionate to disease severity due to dysfunctional breathing pattern or anxiety
Pacing (finding a balance between activity and rest, prioritizing daily activities)	Avoids over-exertion, which can lead to exhaustion, inactivity and subsequent deconditioning	In patients who are able and willing to modify daily routines
Neuromuscular electrical stimulation	Increases muscle bulk, simulating effect of exercise	In patients who: live alone, are unable to attend a rehabilitation group, have a short prognosis, or who have co-morbidities that prevent exercise

CBT, cognitive behavioural therapy; SOB, shortness of breath (breathlessness).

---

investigated. Benzodiazepines should not be used routinely to manage breathlessness, as there is no evidence of their benefit; they may, however, be prescribed in those at the end of life or when there is a limited prognosis. Oxygen is not helpful in relieving the sensation of breathlessness but may be essential in managing the underlying medical condition and improving exercise capacity. There are specific assessment tools, such as the Dyspnoea-12 and numerical rating scales (NRS), which can help initial management and subsequent monitoring of treatment strategies.

Cough

This is an unpleasant symptom that can affect the lives of both patient and carer. Drug approaches (e.g. opioids or gabapentin) have limited impact but may be needed. Recently, specialist multidisciplinary non-pharmacological approaches have been developed for both non-malignant and malignant disease.

Secretions

Excessive respiratory secretions at the end of life can be treated with **glycopyrronium** 200–400 µg every 2–4 hours, maximum 1.2–2.4 mg per

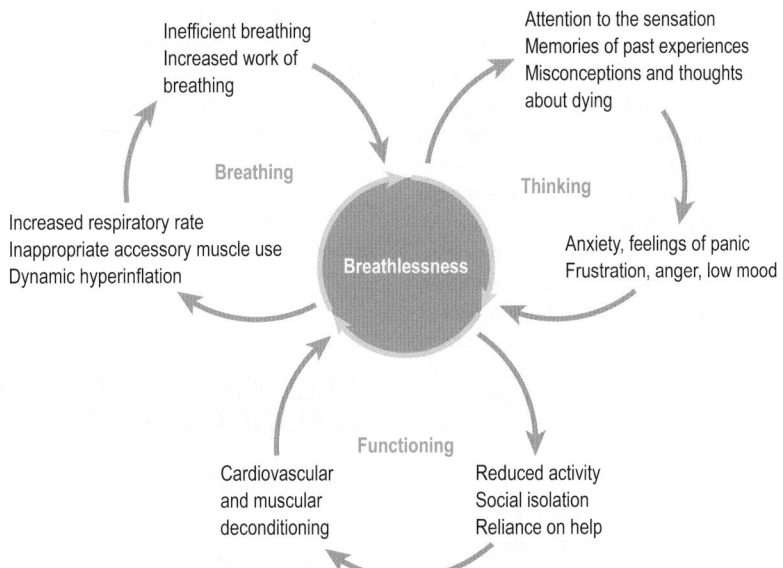

Fig. 7.5 The Breathing, Thinking, Functioning clinical model. *(From Spathis A, Booth S, Moffat C et al. The Breathing, Thinking, Functioning clinical model: a proposal to facilitate evidence-based breathlessness management in chronic respiratory disease. NPJ Prim Care Respir Med 2017; 27:27. Reproduced with kind permission of Dr Anna Spathis, University of Cambridge and Cambridge University Hospitals NHS Foundation Trust.)*

24 hours, or **hyoscine butylbromide** 20 mg every 1–2 hours, maximum 120 mg per 24 hours. These can be given by continuous subcutaneous infusion. Both give a dry mouth and care must be taken not to dry secretions significantly in a patient who is still able to cough well, as they may become too sticky to expectorate, leading to significant discomfort.

Further reading

Johnson MJ, Yorke J, Currow D. A delphi process defining 'chronic breathlessness syndrome': A distinct clinical entity. *Eur Resp J* 2016; 48:PA3754.
Parshall MB, Schwartzstein RM, Adams L et al. An official American Thoracic Society statement: update on the mechanisms, assessment, and management of dyspnea. *Am J Respir Crit Care Med* 2012; 185:435–452.
Spathis A, Booth S, Moffat C et al. The Breathing, Thinking, Functioning clinical model: a proposal to facilitate evidence-based breathlessness management in chronic respiratory disease. *NPJ Prim Care Respir Med* 2017; 27:27.

Other physical symptoms

People with cancer may develop other physical symptoms caused by the tumour directly (e.g. hemiplegia due to brain metastases) or indirectly (e.g. bleeding or venous thromboembolism due to coagulopathy). Symptoms may also result from treatment, such as lymphoedema in breast cancer, or heart failure secondary to chemotherapy. The principles of holistic assessment, treatment of reversible factors, and appropriate involvement of the multiprofessional team should be applied.

Fatigue

Fatigue is a significant and debilitating problem for palliative patients. It has physical, cognitive and affective components; unlike normal tiredness, it is not relieved by usual sleep or rest. An assessment for reversible contributory factors, such as anaemia, hypokalaemia or over-sedation due to poorly optimized medication, should be undertaken. Management strategies are mainly non-pharmacological: relaxation, sleep hygiene, resting 'proactively' rather than collapsing

when exhausted, and planning, pacing and prioritizing daily activities. Trials of pharmacological agents – such as methylphenidate, a central nervous system stimulant – are currently under way but drug-free approaches remain best practice, as previous randomized controlled trials have proved drugs to be ineffective.

Mouth symptoms

Dry mouth is common in advanced disease and may be a result of medications used to treat other symptoms, such as pain or nausea. It can be managed with artificial saliva substitutes and good mouth care to keep mucous membranes moist. Careful inspection of the mouth identifies any reversible causes contributing to oral discomfort: for example, candidiasis, which is common in the immunocompromised but treatable with antifungals. As patients lose weight, dentures may become ill-fitting, causing ulceration to the gums. This can be managed with analgesia, denture cushions, and topical treatments to numb the sore parts of the mouth.

Patients receiving courses of radiotherapy for haematological disorders or head and neck cancers can develop painful mucositis (pain and inflammation of the mucous membrane, which may present as painful mouth ulceration affecting any or all intraoral surfaces). This is a common reason for referral to hospital palliative care teams, even when the treatment aims are curative. Management is with meticulous mouth care, including mouthwashes to maintain oral hygiene, as well as to provide pain relief. Some patients with severe mucositis will require enteral feeding and management of their pain with continuous subcutaneous infusion until it settles.

Loss of function, disability and rehabilitation

Some of the most pressing concerns include increasing physical frailty, loss of independence, and perception of being a burden on others. Evidence suggests that functional problems are not routinely assessed, and not as well managed as other symptoms.

Palliative rehabilitation in long-term incurable illness aims to enable patients to achieve their functional and social priorities in the context of physical decline, as well as to adjust to change in physical ability, role and sense of self. Patients and carers often appreciate a focus on what is still possible, rather than what is lost.

Rehabilitation may include exercise to address reversible physical decline and fatigue, which may be especially evident following an exacerbation or relapse. Understandably, sustaining motivation to maintain physical activity can be difficult. Setting small and achievable goals may help maintain motivation and promote self-efficacy. Involving carers in rehabilitation sessions may reduce over-protectiveness.

Rehabilitation includes supporting adaptation by encouraging patients to do things differently, including the use of mobility aids or equipment. Aids and adaptations may be seen as symbols of 'giving up' by some patients. They need to be presented in a positive light as 'enablers' that assist people to achieve their goals and that may also reduce carer burden. Psychological support to accept change may be required.

Hospices take a 'rehabilitative approach', with most having physical and occupational therapists and exercise equipment. Referral to hospice day therapy, pulmonary rehabilitation, community exercise groups or community physical or occupational therapy may be appropriate. However, patients have to have an active desire to engage in rehabilitation. Some may see therapy as an additional unwanted drain on their time and their wishes should be ascertained, as well as discussing the merits and disadvantages of engaging.

Functional problems and fatigue should not be seen as inevitable, unavoidable and insoluble. All healthcare professionals have a role in promoting the benefits of patients keeping as active as they are able, to help maintain their strength and ability in long-term incurable illness. Barriers to this, including misconceptions about exercise and activity being harmful, should be discussed and addressed, as well as considering psychological barriers such as anxiety and depression. Throughout illness, there is a need to take into account changing performance status, as well as changes in goals and priorities.

Poor sleep

This is common, and patients may have longstanding difficulties with sleep that worsen during their illness. Discomfort in bed, leading to worsening symptoms and psychological concerns surrounding their condition and the future, can compound the problem. Eliciting and listening to patients' concerns, explaining the concept of sleep hygiene and discouraging lengthy day-time naps, can be helpful, as well as therapy team review of the bed and provision of equipment that will optimize symptom management. Pharmacological measures – for example, hypnotics such as zopiclone or melatonin – should be used only temporarily and are not long-term solutions to sleep problems. Complementary therapies are available in hospices and some hospitals, and may offer relaxation to patients to aid sleep.

Psychosocial issues

Depression is a common feature of life-limiting and disabling illness, and is often missed or dismissed as 'understandable'. However, it may respond to antidepressant drugs and/or to non-pharmacological measures such as cognitive behavioural therapy, increased social support and support for family relationships. Antidepressants can take several weeks to take effect and a patient's prognosis must therefore be considered if they are initiated. The 'side-effects' of certain antidepressant medications

are sometimes utilized to benefit patients. For example, mirtazapine can improve sleep, anxiety, appetite and low mood, but may also be helpful to treat pain and nausea; evidence is also emerging for its benefits in gastroparesis. Such interventions can make a big difference to the patient's quality of life and ability to manage their situation.

Further reading

Hudson PL, Remedios C, Thomas K. A systematic review of psychosocial interventions for family carers of palliative care patients. *BMC Palliat Care* 2010; 9:17.

PALLIATIVE CARE IN NON-MALIGNANT DISEASE

Heart failure

There are special considerations with respect to cardiac medication in advanced disease:

- *Drugs*. Many commonly used palliative care medications can prolong the QT interval and are therefore contraindicated in heart failure; they include amitriptyline and many antiemetics. Others may precipitate worsening symptoms: for example, non-steroidal anti-inflammatory drugs (NSAIDs) may exacerbate fluid retention. However, use of certain medications that can be harmful in the long term may become appropriate when the patient is dying, and the risks and benefits are weighed up and discussed with the patient and family.

- *Sudden death*. This is more common than in patients with malignancy. An implanted defibrillator may be in place and, if present, the device should be reprogrammed to pacemaker mode in people with advanced disease. Implanted defibrillators have not been shown to improve survival in severe heart failure and it will be distressing for patient, carer and staff if the defibrillator discharges as the patient is dying.

- *Peripheral oedema*. This can become a major problem and may be more resistant to diuretic therapy; careful balancing of medication regimens is required. Ultimately, symptom relief is prioritized over renal function.

- *Medications*. Drugs prescribed to reduce long-term secondary risk (e.g. statins) can be stopped but those that help with symptom control (including angiotensin-converting enzyme inhibitors, which also benefit survival) can be continued, thus rationalizing medications and reducing polypharmacy. Beta-blockers may have to be stopped if the patient can no longer maintain non-symptomatic hypotension. A randomized trial of withdrawal versus continuation of statins in those thought to be in the last year of life showed no detrimental effect on quality of life with withdrawal.

Chronic respiratory disease

Chronic obstructive pulmonary disease (COPD) is the most common chronic respiratory disease. Patients with COPD may live increasingly restricted lives for years, rather than months or weeks, once they become breathless. This can lead to depression, isolation, frustration and sometimes guilt associated with previous smoking habits. As with many chronic conditions, patients can reach older age before becoming very disabled, and an elderly spouse often has to carry significant physical carer burdens.

Palliative care breathlessness support services can be very helpful for patients unable to manage pulmonary rehabilitation or those with complex psychosocial needs that require individual assessment. Emergency admissions to hospital for non-medical reasons are often due to severe anxiety (in patient and/or carer), and the support offered by community palliative care services and/or breathlessness services working with respiratory teams can help reduce these.

In advanced disease, patients may be using non-invasive ventilation (NIV) regularly at home. This may provide considerable symptom relief but early discussions should take place regarding management of NIV during exacerbations of COPD and at the end of life.

Pulmonary fibrosis, another chronic respiratory illness that often requires palliative care, has a trajectory similar to that of cancer, with rapidly developing breathlessness and cough. The breathlessness of pulmonary fibrosis can be particularly frightening but may respond well to opioids; early access to hospice services is particularly relevant to help with symptom control and anxiety. Long-term oxygen therapy may be necessary to manage severe hypoxaemia and maintain function in these patients.

Opioid titration in non-malignant respiratory disease

In non-malignant respiratory disease, opioid titration may need to follow a different pattern from that used in malignant disease, in which many patients are already on opioids for pain control before they develop breathlessness. Individual assessment is essential. Some clinicians recommend a cautious approach in starting opioids in chronically breathless patients who have non-malignant disease, but the evidence indicates that those with *adequate renal function* and without type 2 respiratory failure may safely be started on 5–10 mg per day modified release morphine, given appropriate monitoring. Significant respiratory depression has not been noted in various trials of opioids in advanced respiratory disease.

Further reading

Johnson MJ, Booth S. Palliative and end-of-life care for patients with chronic heart failure and chronic lung disease. *Clin Med (London)* 2010; 10:286–289.

Renal disease

All care for patients who have end-stage chronic kidney disease (CKD) is directed towards maintenance or improvement of renal function. Prescribing is complicated, particularly in those receiving dialysis. Drugs are variably removed by dialysis and this must be taken into account; the renal drug database (see 'Further reading') is helpful. Care must be taken not to cause inadvertent renal damage with potentially nephrotoxic medication, and close liaison with renal physicians is mandatory.

In patients who have CKD, co-morbidities such as cardiovascular disease, diabetes or osteoporosis may cause greater problems than the renal disease itself. Those with a fluctuant course of symptoms, such as the 25–33% who have coexisting cardiac disease, bear disproportionately greater physical and psychological burdens.

Withdrawal of dialysis

Withdrawal of dialysis is necessary when the effort of attendance becomes burdensome, there is little improvement in quality of life and the impact of other co-morbidities becomes intrusive.

If there is no residual renal function (i.e. the patient is anuric), survival after withdrawal of dialysis is likely to be a few days at most. In contrast, patients who have some residual function may live for months or even a year after withdrawal. Patients and carers need to understand these differences in order to make informed choices.

Patients who are not on dialysis

There may not be any survival benefit conferred by starting dialysis as opposed to conservative management of renal dysfunction in the elderly. Conservative management may allow more time out of hospital and better quality of life for these patients. Maximizing and preserving remaining renal function are critical considerations in deciding which medications can or should be prescribed.

- Medication that accelerates loss of renal function, such as NSAIDs, may markedly reduce survival in patients who can live with very little remaining renal function.
- The renal impact of both dose and drug choice must be taken into account. For example, morphine and diamorphine metabolites accumulate in end-stage renal dysfunction; thus alternative opioids such as alfentanil or fentanyl should be used instead. These may have to be given parenterally.

Further reading

Kane PM, Vinen K, Murtagh FE. Palliative care for advanced renal disease: a summary of the evidence and future direction. *Palliat Med* 2013; 27: 817–821.
https://renaldrugdatabase.com *Prescribing guide for renal practitioners*.

Neurological disease

People with chronic degenerative neurological diseases have a considerable burden of palliative care needs, which may include:

- difficulties in swallowing (e.g. in motor neurone disease and multiple sclerosis)
- excessive difficulty clearing secretions, and weak cough leading to fear of choking
- progressive loss of physical function with associated pain and vulnerable pressure areas
- loss of mental capacity (see p. 83), anxiety and depression.

The multidisciplinary team is vital to the care of these patients, and may provide physiotherapy and occupational therapy to manage loss of function, as well as speech and language therapy to optimize communication. Discussions regarding the patient's care preferences and practical wishes (e.g. writing a will) should take place early so that these can be supported, if the patient is able to participate and when communication is easier.

Motor neurone disease

Motor neurone disease is usually rapidly progressive, often requiring hospice support. Percutaneous endoscopic gastrostomy feeding may be needed. Secretions, such as excess saliva, can be problematic and treatment may entail careful balancing of antisecretory medication: for example, hyoscine hydrobromide, which is available as a transdermal preparation. In addition, if ventilatory failure develops, NIV may be offered. Patients and their carers need to understand:

- why this treatment has been offered (to prevent hypercapnia and associated morning headache and confusion; it can confer a survival benefit)
- when this treatment will be withdrawn (when it is no longer helping to maintain or improve quality of life in the face of advancing disease; guidelines are widely available to help with these specialist discussions).

Patients need to have a clear understanding of what alternative symptom control will be offered at withdrawal.

Multiple sclerosis

Pain is often prominent in multiple sclerosis because of muscle spasm. This is managed with regular physiotherapy, medications and, in severe cases, botulinum toxin, nerve blocks or surgery. Patients may become too disabled to attend outpatient clinics and then receive little surveillance or support. Hospice day therapy services, rehabilitation, and support for the family can have a huge impact on quality of life. A person can live for many years disabled and symptomatic, and regular surveillance and support are essential.

Dementia

Dementia-related palliative care needs arise in the context of neurological conditions that:
- tend to occur in older people (Alzheimer's disease and vascular dementia)
- also affect younger people (e.g. Parkinson's disease, multiple sclerosis, Huntington's disease).

It is often difficult to ascertain whether these patients are in pain. An assessment tool that assesses behavioural response to pain can be useful, such as the Abbey or Doloplus pain scale; these are based on vocalization (e.g. groaning), facial expression (e.g. frowning), and body language (fidgeting, rocking), behaviour (e.g. confusion, refusal to eat) and physical changes.

Mental capacity orders and Deprivation of Liberty Safeguards (DoLS) may need to be considered where a patient is effectively 'deprived' of their liberty in a care home or hospital.

Further reading

Hussain J, Allgar V, Oliver D. Palliative care triggers in progressive neurodegenerative conditions: an evaluation using a multi-centre retrospective case record review and principle component analysis. *Palliat Med* 2018; 32:716–725.

Children and young people

Increasing numbers of children are living with life-threatening and life-limiting illness, such as cystic fibrosis and severe cerebral palsy. Palliative care supports these children and their families to achieve the best possible quality of life and care. The model of palliative care in young people is different to that in adult services, as many children are supported for years by hospices; generally, they are cared for in their own homes and the number of deaths is small compared to that in adults. Many conditions are extremely rare and may be familial. As well as symptom management, hospices can provide short respite breaks for families caring for seriously ill children. An increasing number of these patients will now survive to adulthood, and ensuring a smooth transition to adult services is an evolving area of development.

Further reading

https://www.togetherforshortlives.org.uk *Help to support seriously ill children who are expected to have short lives.*

CARE OF THE DYING

Most people express a wish to die in their own homes, provided their symptoms are controlled and their carers are supported. However, patients die in any setting and all healthcare professionals should therefore be proficient in end-of-life care.

Hospitals and communities have developed individualized or personalized care plans for the last days of life that help to prompt discussions surrounding the dying process, and how physical, psychological, social, spiritual and carer concerns will be addressed (**Box 7.13**). The decision to provide support through a personalized care plan for the last days of life is reached by a multiprofessional team through careful assessment of the patient, exclusion of reversible causes of deterioration, and excellent communication with carers or family.

Hospitals in England take part in yearly national audits to assess end-of-life care. The data are used to allow development of quality improvement initiatives to continuously improve end of life care.

Do not attempt resuscitation orders and treatment escalation plans

The resuscitation status of every patient should be discussed by senior doctors at the time of admission to hospital, or when deterioration is noted that is not thought to be reversible. This decision must be clearly documented in the notes. Treatment escalation plans and 'ceilings of care' determining what treatments are likely to be beneficial or futile should be discussed at the same time in line with patient wishes.

Hospitals and communities have specific 'do not attempt resuscitation' (DNAR) forms. Deciding a person's resuscitation status is a careful balance of risk versus benefit. Co-morbidities, pre-morbid quality of life and the patient's wishes should be taken into account.

DNAR orders and treatment escalation plans are medical treatment decisions. However, the patient and family must be involved in discussions, unless they have specifically requested not to be, and the reasoning behind decisions should be explained. In the UK in 2014 the Court of Appeal ruled in the case of *Tracey* vs *Cambridge University Hospitals NHS Foundation Trust* that a failure to discuss the making of a DNAR order with a patient who had expressed a wish to be involved in decision-making around their care constitutes a breach of their human rights. Concern regarding possible patient distress is no justification for not discussing resuscitation, though it will guide the way the subject is considered with the patient. Only if it is felt that there will be significant psychological or physical harm resulting from the discussion can it be postponed. If the patient requests that cardiopulmonary resuscitation is not performed in the event of cardiopulmonary arrest, this should be respected.

Remember that a decision not to resuscitate a patient is not the same as a decision to withhold other treatment. A patient who is 'not for resuscitation' may still be eligible for, and benefit from, antibiotics, fluids, endoscopy and even surgery. Management should remain positive and proactive, allowing the patient to die free of distress and with dignity.

ℹ️ **Box 7.13 Components of personalized care plans for the last days of life**

- Recognition of the dying phase and communication with patient and carers
- Initial assessment (which includes the patient's and carers' understanding, wishes and psychological state)
- Resuscitation status and treatment escalation plans
- Discussion surrounding how symptoms will be managed
- Discussion about feeding and fluids
- Ongoing assessment and monitoring
- Support for the carers after the patient's death

ReSPECT (Recommended Summary Plan for Emergency Care and Treatment) is starting to be implemented in many hospitals. It is a process that creates and records personalized recommendations for a person's clinical care in a future emergency in which they are unable to make or express choices. It is likely to be useful in those with complex health needs, integrating discussion surrounding DNAR and treatment escalation.

Further reading

Etheridge Z, Gatland E. When and how to discuss 'do not resuscitate' decisions with patients. *BMJ* 2015; 350:h2640.

General Medical Council. *Treatment and Care Towards the End of Life: Good Practice in Decision Making*. London: GMC; 2010.

National Institute for Health and Care Excellence. *NICE Guideline NG31: Care of Dying Adults in the Last Days of Life*. NICE 2015; https://www.nice.org.uk/guidance/ng31.

Bibliography

British National Formulary. *Guidance on Prescribing: Prescribing in Palliative Care. British National Formulary*. London: BMJ Group and RPS Publishing; http://www.bnf.org.

Twycross R, Wilcock A, Howard P. *Palliative Care Formulary*, 6th edn; 2018; www.pharmpress.com.

Watson M, Armstrong P, Back I et al. *Palliative Adult Network Guidelines*, 4th edn; 2016; https://book.pallcare.info.

Significant websites

http://uk.sagepub.com/en-gb/eur/journal/palliative-medicine *Palliative medicine*.

http://www.cancerresearchuk.org *UK charity*.

http://www.cuh.org.uk *Cambridge University Hospitals breathlessness information*.

http://www.macmillan.org.uk *UK patient organization*.

http://www.palliativedrugs.com *Palliative drugs information*.

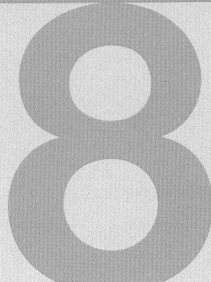

8 Sepsis and the treatment of bacterial infection

Mark Melzer, Andrew Leitch and David Wareham

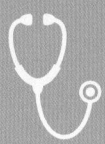

CORE SKILLS AND KNOWLEDGE

Sepsis is a serious complication of infection in which a dys-regulated immune response leads to organ dysfunction and sometimes death. It is the final common pathophysiological pathway in patients who die from infection. It is estimated that, worldwide, 49 million people develop sepsis every year, and 11 million die.

Sepsis is a medical emergency; antibiotics must be empiri-cally prescribed within 1 hour of presentation and then reviewed at 72 hours when culture results become available.

All healthcare staff should be aware of sepsis, which may present via the hospital emergency department or develop on general medical or surgical wards. Specialist care for patients with severe complications of sepsis may be provided in a critical care unit. Infectious Diseases (ID) physicians become involved in managing patients with complex or disseminated infections,

and may run Outpatient Antibiotic Treatment (OPAT) services and specialist ID clinics.

Key skills in this chapter area include:

- identifying sepsis and instituting emergency management us-ing the Sepsis Six care bundle
- appreciating the potential complications of sepsis, and rec-ognizing the need for appropriate escalation of care in acutely unwell or deteriorating patients
- becoming familiar with the appropriate use of antibiotics to treat commonly encountered infections.

Opportunities for students to learn about sepsis and infec-tion are gained by reviewing patients with suspected infection in the emergency department or acute assessment units, ID wards or critical care settings, or those deteriorating on general wards who may be identified by attending critical care outreach rounds. Observing specialist ID and OPAT clinics (including multidisci-plinary team meetings) provides an insight into the longer-term follow-up of patients with infection.

CLINICAL SKILLS FOR INFECTION AND SEPSIS

History

When taking a history, this should be tailored to cover the points in **Box 8.1**, which are highly relevant to a presentation with sus-pected sepsis or infection.

Management of sepsis

Sepsis is a medical emergency, and an approach based on the Sepsis Six care bundle ensures that management and investigation proceed hand in hand, and patients are cared for in the most appro-priate location for their needs. See **Fig. 8.1**.

Box 8.1 Features in the history relevant to sepsis

Symptoms
- Duration
- Symptoms of inflammatory response: fevers, chills, rigors, malaise, confusion, vomiting
- Localizing symptoms indicating site of infection:
  - Chest: cough, sputum, shortness of breath
  - Urinary tract: dysuria, urgency, flank pain
  - Central nervous system: headache, meningism
  - Biliary tract: upper abdominal pain, jaundice, vomiting
  - Skin and soft tissue: signs of cellulitis, pain

Past medical history
- Immunosuppression (diabetes, asplenism, human immunodeficiency virus, etc.)
- Previous sepsis

Drug history
- Immunosuppressant medication
- Recent courses of antibiotics

Risk factors for specific pathogen types
- Recent contact with medical institutions
- Previous infection with antibiotic-resistant organisms
- Travel history

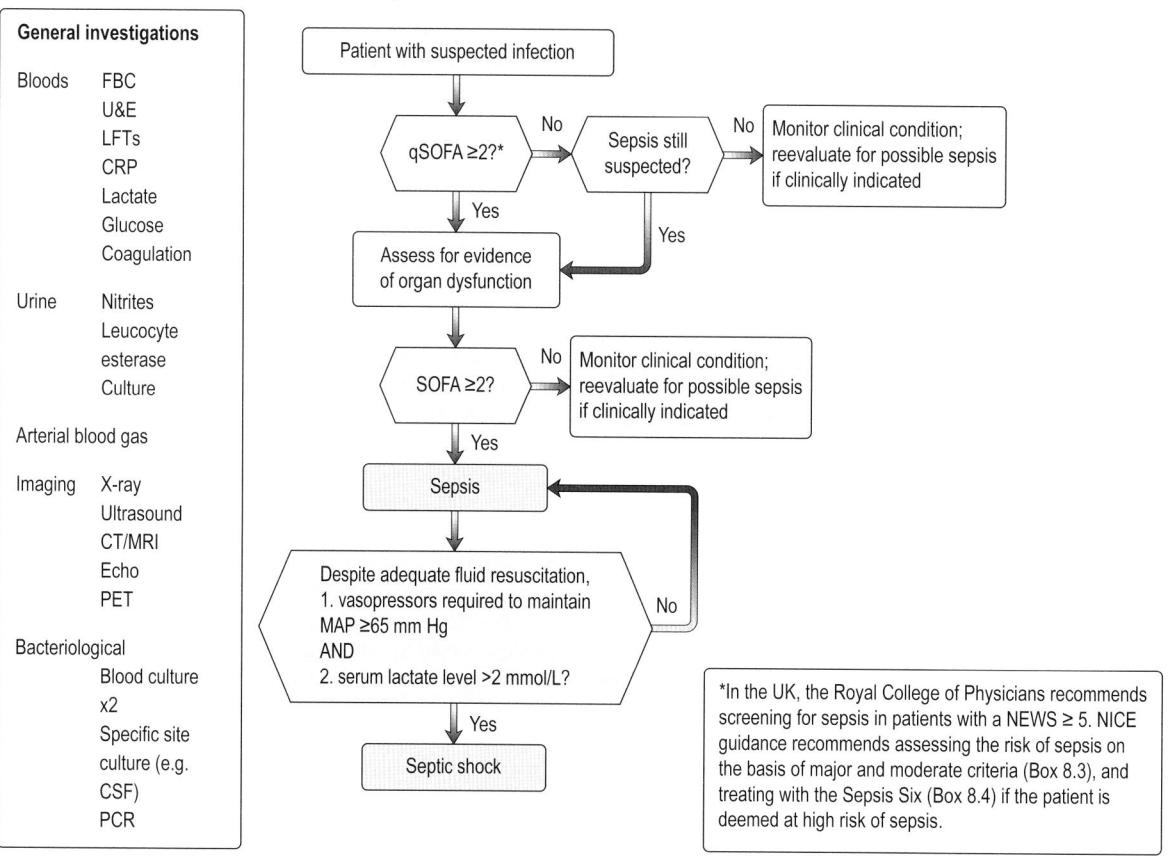

General investigations

Bloods FBC
        U&E
        LFTs
        CRP
        Lactate
        Glucose
        Coagulation

Urine   Nitrites
        Leucocyte esterase
        Culture

Arterial blood gas

Imaging X-ray
         Ultrasound
         CT/MRI
         Echo
         PET

Bacteriological
         Blood culture x2
         Specific site culture (e.g. CSF)
         PCR

*In the UK, the Royal College of Physicians recommends screening for sepsis in patients with a NEWS ≥ 5. NICE guidance recommends assessing the risk of sepsis on the basis of major and moderate criteria (Box 8.3), and treating with the Sepsis Six (Box 8.4) if the patient is deemed at high risk of sepsis.

End-organ failure

- Systolic blood pressure (SBP) <90 mmHg or >40 mmHg fall from baseline or mean arterial pressure (MAP) <65 mmHg
- Bilateral pulmonary infiltrates with no new need for oxygen to maintain saturations >90% or with PaO_2/FiO_2 ratio <300 mmHg or 39.9 kPa
- Serum lactate >2.0 mmol/L

- Serum creatinine >170 μmol/L or urine output <0.5 mL/kg per hour for 2 successive hours
- INR >1.5 or an (activated) partial thromboplastin time (PTT) >60 sec
- Platelet count <100 × 10⁹/L
- Bilirubin >32 μmol

Fig. 8.1 Management of suspected sepsis. CCU, critical care unit; GCS, Glasgow Coma Scale score; CRP, C-reactive protein; CT, computed tomography; ESR, erythrocyte sedimentation rate; FBC, full blood count; FiO_2, fraction of inspired oxygen; Hb, haemoglobin; INR, international normalized ratio; LFTs, liver function tests; MAP, mean arterial pressure; MRI, magnetic resonance imaging; MSU, mid-stream specimen of urine; NAAT, nucleic acid amplification technique; PaO_2, arterial oxygen tension; PCR, polymerase chain reaction; PET, positron emission tomography; SOFA, sequential organ failure assessment; WBC, white cell count. *(Modified from Singer M, Deutschman CS, Seymour CW et al. The Third International Consensus Definitions for Sepsis and Septic Shock (Sepsis-3). JAMA 2016; 315:801–810.)*

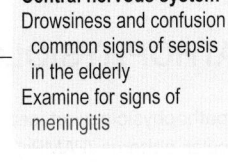

Examination

Highlighted in red are sites of infection that are common causes of sepsis, with associated clinical signs. This list is not exhaustive and, in a patient with the sepsis syndrome but no clear source, careful examination is vital to establish the underlying diagnosis.

SITES AND SIGNS OF INFECTION

Observation chart
Fever
Tachypnoea (a key sign of clinical deterioration)
Tachycardia and hypotension
Hypoxia (may suggest lower respiratory tract infection)

General observation
Appears 'unwell'
Hot to touch
Confused or reduced consciousness

Pulse
Tachycardia common; acute atrial fibrillation possible
May be high-volume ('bounding') due to vasodilation
May be low-volume if 'peripherally shut down' due to relative hypovolaemia

Chest
Tachypnoea
Consolidation may be present in lower respiratory tract infection

Back
Localized tenderness may indicate discitis or spinal abscess
Loin tenderness common in pyelonephritis

Genital examination
Males – signs of epididymo-orchitis
Females – pelvic inflammatory disease; consider retained tampons causing toxic-shock syndrome

Feet
Infected ulcers (especially in patients with diabetes)

Central nervous system
Drowsiness and confusion common signs of sepsis in the elderly
Examine for signs of meningitis

Jugular venous pressure
May be reduced in dehydration/volume depletion

Heart
New or changed murmur may indicate infective endocarditis

Indwelling devices (e.g. Hickman lines)
Examine for signs of intravenous device infection such as discharge or induration
Obtain additional culture from line where possible

Abdomen
Examine for signs of peritonitis
Right upper quadrant tenderness common in biliary sepsis
Right lower quadrant tenderness seen in appendicitis, pelvic inflammatory disease and cystitis
Left-sided tenderness common in diverticulitis

Extremities
Coolness (may indicate hypotension or intravascular volume depletion)
Cellulitis or soft tissue infection (consider devastating infection such as necrotizing fasciitis – see p. 669)
High index of suspicion for septic arthritis if any joints are swollen

INTRODUCTION

Sepsis is a rare but serious complication of infection. The syndrome arises when the adaptive immune response to infection becomes maladaptive, leading to organ dysfunction. Multi-organ failure in septic shock is the final common pathway for most patients who die from infection.

PATHOPHYSIOLOGY

The pathophysiology of sepsis is complex. Pathogen-associated molecular patterns (PAMPs) include components of bacterial, fungal and viral pathogens; these activate the innate immune system, which is chiefly comprised of macrophages, monocytes, granulocytes, natural killer cells and dendritic cells (see p. 43). This activation occurs through Toll-like and C-type lectin receptors on cell surfaces and nucleotide-binding oligomerization domain (NOD)-like and retinoic acid-inducible gene-I (RIG-I) like receptors in the cytosol. The downstream effects of these activation events, mediated through the upregulation of multiple genes, include the production of pro-inflammatory cytokines such as tumour necrosis factor-alpha (TNF-α) and interleukins 1 (IL-1) and 6 (IL-6). Further effects include increased innate immune activity, production of hepatic acute phase proteins (e.g. complement, fibrinogen and C-reactive protein (CRP)), release of microparticles containing inflammatory, pro-oxidant and procoagulant lipids and proteins, and elaboration of neutrophil extracellular traps (NETs), which are scaffolds of DNA and antimicrobial proteins and enzymes. The release of microparticles and NETs, combined with increased intravascular tissue factor expression, leads to the phenomenon of 'immunothrombosis', whereby microbes are trapped in microthrombi, which in turn attract and further activate leucocytes.

This highly preserved innate response is usually very effective at controlling and neutralizing local infection. When the response exceeds a certain threshold, damage to the host becomes clinically evident. This may be mediated through mitochondrial dysfunction, leading to deficient adenosine triphosphate (ATP) production, and through widespread immunothrombosis as complement activation increases vascular permeability and causes disseminated intravascular coagulation (DIC); this leads to further inflammation, impaired microvascular function and subsequent organ dysfunction. Sepsis becomes a self-reinforcing pathophysiological phenomenon, associated with fierce catabolism to fuel it.

Organ dysfunction

At organ level, sepsis represents a systemic loss of homeostasis, the dysfunction of each organ system adversely affecting the function of every other. The physiological demand requires an increased cardiac output, which most patients achieve after fluid resuscitation. However, the syndrome itself, and associated acidosis, can exert a negatively inotropic influence on the heart. Vasoplegia leads to reduced total peripheral resistance, and capillary leak of plasma and protein-rich fluid causes tissue oedema, which in turn impairs oxygen delivery to cells. In the lungs, it can cause acute lung injury and adult respiratory distress syndrome. Epithelial disruption in the gut can lead not only to malabsorption, but also to translocation of bacteria into the bloodstream, further amplifying the septic insult. Acute kidney injury is common and associated with an increased risk of death. Brain dysfunction manifests as septic encephalopathy, ranging from mild drowsiness and confusion to coma.

Consensus definition (Sepsis-3)

The complexity of the sepsis syndrome does not lend itself to a simple diagnostic test. Many biomarkers have been proposed but none is specific enough to be used to define the condition.

In 1991, the first consensus conference to agree a definition of sepsis allied it to the concept of the systemic inflammatory response syndrome (SIRS). This definition was modestly revised in 2001. In the light of intercurrent research and growing knowledge, the latest definition was published in 2016. In anticipation of further updates as our understanding of the syndrome evolves, it was given the name 'Sepsis-3'.

Sepsis is currently defined as '*life-threatening organ dysfunction caused by a dysregulated host response to infection*'. 'SIRS' is no longer used to define sepsis; the term 'sepsis' is reserved for the syndrome described above, as opposed to simple infection. Clinicians must be clear about the diagnosis. Inappropriate use of the term 'urosepsis' to describe a simple urinary tract infection (UTI), for example, is misleading and distorts healthcare statistics.

Examination of a large dataset of electronic patient records enabled the authors of the Sepsis-3 definition to construct clinical criteria that best predicted which patients with infection developed life-threatening organ dysfunction, for which the surrogate measure of in-hospital mortality was used. In intensive care this consisted of changes in the Sequential Organ Failure Assessment (SOFA) score (**Box 8.2**). The best predictor of death or a requirement for 3 days or more of intensive care for ward patients was a new construct, the 'quick SOFA' (qSOFA). Patients are deemed positive for qSOFA if they have two of:

- Glasgow Coma Scale score of <15 (see **Box 26.28**)
- respiratory rate of ≥22 breaths/min
- systolic blood pressure of ≤100 mmHg.

In the UK, the Royal College of Physicians recommends using a National Early Warning Score (NEWS 2) of 5 or more as an indicator that a patient is at high risk of having sepsis (see **Fig. 10.1**). Remember that neither the qSOFA nor the NEWS 2 is diagnostic of sepsis; they merely indicate that a patient is at higher risk of having sepsis and should be assessed for the condition.

Septic shock

The term 'septic shock' is reserved for the subset of patients with sepsis whose circulatory and metabolic dysfunction is such that their risk of death is significantly increased. Clinically, patients are identified as septic who require vasopressor support to maintain a mean arterial pressure of 65 mmHg or more, and who have an elevated serum lactate concentration (>2 mmol/L) despite adequate volume resuscitation.

Further reading

Singer M, Deutschman CS, Seymour CW et al. The third international consensus definitions for sepsis and septic shock (Sepsis-3). *JAMA* 2016; 315:801–810.

RECOGNITION OF SEPSIS

At-risk groups

Whether a simple infection will progress to sepsis or not depends on a range of factors, including the virulence of the pathogen, the microbial load, the site of infection and the host response. The latter

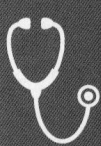

i **Box 8.2 Sequential Organ Failure Assessment (SOFA) score[a]**

	0	1	2	3	4
Respiratory P/F (kPa[b])	≥53.3	<53.3	<40	<26.7 and MV	<13.3 and MV
Coagulation Platelet count (×10⁹/L)	≥150	<150	<100	<50	<20
Liver Bilirubin (µmol/L)	<20	20–32	33–101	102–204	>204
Cardiovascular	MAP ≥70 mmHg	MAP <70 mmHg	Dopamine < 5 µg/kg per min or dobutamine (any dose)	Dopamine 5.1–15 µg/kg per min or adrenaline (epinephrine) or noradrenaline (norepinephrine) ≤0.1 µg/kg per min	Dopamine > 15 µg/kg per min or adrenaline (epinephrine) or noradrenaline (norepinephrine) >0.1 µg/kg per min
Central nervous system Glasgow Coma Scale score	15	13–14	10–12	6–9	<6
Renal Creatinine (µmol/L) Urine output (mL/day)	<110 –	110–170 –	171–299 –	300–440 <500	>440 <200

[a]An increase in SOFA score of ≥2 points identifies patients with organ dysfunction for the purposes of the Sepsis-3 definition. Any such patients should be considered for admission to the critical care unit.
[b]PaO_2/FiO_2 (FiO_2 as a fraction ≤1).
MAP, mean arterial pressure; MV, mechanically ventilated.

is influenced by genetic make-up, co-morbidities, past medical history and chronic treatments. Groups at higher risk of developing sepsis include:

- older people (>65 years of age) and the very young (neonates)
- people who have previously had sepsis
- people with immunosuppressive medical conditions (such as HIV, asplenism, cirrhosis, autoimmune diseases)
- people who are iatrogenically immunosuppressed (those on immunosuppressive drugs, including systemic corticosteroids)
- patients with indwelling devices, especially if they breach normal barriers against infection
- pregnant women
- people who abuse alcohol or intravenous drugs.

In-hospital surveillance

Inpatients have a higher risk of developing sepsis that patients in the community. Hospitals should therefore have systems in place to identify deteriorating patients early, aligned with processes that enable a prompt medical response. In the UK the NEWS 2 score (see earlier) assigns a numerical score to patients' observations, weighted according to the degree of deviation from normal values. It has long been known that cardiac arrest is usually preceded by several hours of increasingly deranged physiology, reflected by an increasing NEWS 2 score.

Most hospitals empower ward staff to call for help at certain NEWS 2 thresholds. In many instances this will be on the basis of a total NEWS 2 of 5 or more, or on clinical concern, which should always trump a numerical score. The request for assistance (conveyed using the SBAR approach, for example; see p. 11) should prompt an urgent medical review, including screening for sepsis.

There is no binary test for sepsis. Screening consists of a risk assessment, carried out by an experienced and informed clinician, of the likelihood that a deteriorating patient is developing sepsis. That likelihood is increased in the presence of extreme physiological derangement, highly suspicious elements of recent medical history, acute kidney injury or raised serum lactate, as incorporated into a recent NICE guideline (**Box 8.3**). The diagnosis should

be made on the basis of bedside observations and limited point-of-care testing, in order to minimize the time to treatment. Given that early antimicrobial therapy may alter the natural history of the syndrome, waiting for laboratory blood tests and other investigations to confirm the presence of organ dysfunction is counterproductive. Where available, point-of-care lactate measurement can be especially useful. Lactate level is prognostic in patients with sepsis; a raised lactate should never be ignored and is usually a sign of organ dysfunction, even in patients who might otherwise seem relatively well.

Origins of sepsis

Sepsis may be either community-acquired, healthcare-associated or hospital-acquired. Community-acquired disease is defined as sepsis occurring within 48 hours of hospital admission, whereas in hospital-acquired disease sepsis occurs after 48 hours. Healthcare-associated sepsis, a subset of community-onset sepsis, is defined as sepsis occurring in:

- patients within 30 days of hospital discharge
- nursing home residents but not those living in residential homes
- patients accessing medical treatment in the community (e.g. patients on haemodialysis).

Community-acquired infection tends to be severe and is likely to be caused by virulent but more antibiotic-sensitive organisms. Examples include *Staphylococcus aureus*, *Streptococcus pneumoniae*, *Escherichia coli*, *Klebsiella pneumoniae* and *Neisseria meningitidis*. The most common sites of infection are the urinary tract, biliary tract and lower respiratory tract (pneumonia); rarely, there may be infective endocarditis or meningitis.

In contrast, organisms causing ***hospital-acquired infection*** are less virulent but often multidrug-resistant; they are therefore harder to treat. Examples include *Stenotrophomonas maltophilia* and *Acinetobacter baumannii*. Infection is often procedure- or medical device-related. The risk of procedure-related sepsis (e.g. following surgical procedures or tissue biopsy) can be minimized by appropriate antibiotic prophylaxis, and where sepsis is associated with a medical device (e.g. a blocked urinary catheter or infected intravascular catheter), this should be removed (termed 'source control').

Box 8.3 Risk stratification tool for adults, children and young people aged 12 years and over with suspected sepsis

Category	High-risk criteria	Moderate to high-risk criteria	Low-risk criteria
History	Objective evidence of new altered mental state	History from patient, friend or relative of new onset of altered behaviour or mental state History of acute deterioration of functional ability Impaired immune system (illness or drugs, including oral steroids) Trauma, surgery or invasive procedures in previous 6 weeks	Normal behaviour
Respiratory	Raised respiratory rate: ≥25 breaths/min New need for oxygen (40% more) to maintain saturation >92% (or >88% in known chronic obstructive pulmonary disease)	Raised respiratory rate: 21–24 breaths/min	No high-risk or moderate to high-risk criteria met
Blood pressure	Systolic blood pressure: ≤90 mmHg, or systolic blood pressure >40 mmHg below normal	Systolic blood pressure: 91–100 mmHg	No high-risk or moderate to high-risk criteria met
Circulation and hydration	Raised heart rate: more than 130 beats/min Not passed urine in previous 18 h Catheterized patients: passed <0.5 mL/kg of urine per hour	Raised heart rate: 91–130 beats/min (for pregnant women 100–130 beats/min) or new-onset arrhythmia Not passed urine in previous 12–18 h Catheterized patients: passed 0.5–1 mL/kg of urine per hour	No high-risk or moderate to high-risk criteria met
Temperature		Tympanic temperature <36°C	
Skin	Mottled or ashen appearance Cyanosis of skin, lips or tongue Non-blanching skin rash	Signs of potential infection, including redness, swelling or discharge at surgical site, or breakdown of wound	No non-blanching rash

Clinical features

Early sepsis can be difficult to diagnose. Signs and symptoms evolve in variable fashion along a continuum from those of localized infection (e.g. cough, dysuria) to more systemic evidence of organ dysfunction (e.g. confusion, oliguria, petechial haemorrhage). Some patients' organ dysfunction evolves gradually, while others may exhibit a precipitous deterioration from minor symptoms to multi-organ failure in a matter of hours. No symptom is pathognomonic but patients typically complain of rigors, breathlessness, muscle pain, vomiting, mottled skin and a feeling of being extremely unwell, in addition to the symptoms relating to their underlying infection. Signs correspond to those of the infective source, together with those of systemic inflammation, such as tachycardia, tachypnoea, hypotension, warm, dilated peripheries, oliguria, confusion or drowsiness. Immunosuppressed patients may display relatively few signs and symptoms of inflammation, although those relating to the physiological response should still be present.

Investigations reveal non-specific evidence of inflammation and organ dysfunction, such as raised white cell count and CRP, rising creatinine and bilirubin, falling platelet count, possible infiltrates on chest X-ray, and dysrhythmias on the electrocardiogram (ECG). Imaging may help identify the site of infection.

Sepsis in special situations

Returning travellers

A detailed history is required, with dates of travel, areas visited and onset of symptoms. Exposures that put travellers at risk of tropical infections (e.g. insect bites or fresh-water swimming) should be elicited, and enquiry should be made as to whether patients took malaria prophylaxis or were immunized prior to travel. Assessments should be carried out for viral haemorrhagic fever (in patients with fever within 21 days of return from an endemic region, see p. 531) and Middle East respiratory syndrome coronavirus (MERS-CoV) (in patients with onset of respiratory symptoms within 14 days of arrival from the Middle East, see p. 521). Minimum investigations include blood cultures and a malaria screen, in addition to routine blood tests. The approach to a returned traveller is covered more fully in **Chapter 20**.

People who inject drugs

Most episodes of sepsis are related to infected thrombophlebitis or local abscesses at or around injection sites. The most common causative bacteria are meticillin-sensitive and meticillin-resistant *S. aureus* (MSSA and MRSA, respectively) and *Streptococcus pyogenes*. Occasionally, staphylococcal infections can disseminate to distant sites, including heart valves, the vertebral column and joints (see **Box 20.23**). If the tricuspid valve becomes infected, embolization to the lungs may occur, resulting in multiple lung abscesses. In addition to source control (e.g. drainage of paraspinal collections, washout of peripheral joints and, rarely, tricuspid valve replacement), patients often require weeks of antibiotic treatment.

People who inject drugs are more prone to aspiration pneumonia or empyema because of diminished cough reflex and fluctuating levels of consciousness. Rarely, when lemon juice is used as a solvent, yeasts in the blood may cause ocular endophthalmitis. Optimal management requires vitreal amphotericin implants and prolonged antifungal treatment.

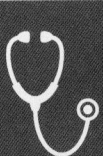

Neutropenic patients

Most commonly, sepsis occurs in haematological oncology patients post chemotherapy (see **Ch. 17**). Due to the risk of overwhelming pseudomonal infection, most empirical treatment includes piperacillin/tazobactam (tazocin) with or without an aminoglycoside.

Paralysed patients

Acutely, these patients are most commonly cared for in a critical care setting. The greatest risk is that posed by medical devices (e.g. central venous catheters, urinary catheters and endotracheal tubes). Implementation of care bundles around the placement and aftercare of such devices minimizes the risk of infection, which may be caused by multidrug-resistant organisms that, consequently, are often harder to treat. Pressure sores can be prevented by use of appropriate mattresses and regular turning the patient. Individuals with spinal cord injuries may present with signs and symptoms of autonomic dysreflexia rather than infection if the site is below the level of injury.

Further reading

National Institute for Health and Care Excellence. *NICE Guideline 51: Sepsis: Recognition, Diagnosis and Early Management.* NICE 2016; https://www.nice.org.uk/guidance/NG51.
Royal College of Physicians. *National Early Warning Score (NEWS 2): Standardising the Assessment of Acute-illness Severity in the NHS. Updated Report of a Working Party.* London: RCP, 2017.

MANAGEMENT OF SEPSIS

Surviving Sepsis Campaign guidelines

The cornerstones of management for sepsis are urgent treatment of the infection and support of failing organs. It is likely the patient will need to be admitted to a critical care unit in order to access specialized organ support. Suspected sepsis is a medical emergency, however, so initial treatment and resuscitation should start without delay. The Sepsis Six is a suggested bundle of care, which includes early broad-spectrum antibiotics (**Box 8.4**).

The Surviving Sepsis Campaign (SSC) produces regularly updated international guidelines on the management of sepsis and septic shock. The various recommendations and suggestions are graded according to the quality of research evidence available. The key recommendations are given in **Box 8.5**.

Supporting a failing circulation: fluid resuscitation

Fluid resuscitation is a first step in supporting organ perfusion. The SSC recommends infusing at least 30 mL/kg of crystalloid solution within 3 hours of diagnosis. Such early high-volume resuscitation is common practice in well-resourced healthcare systems. However, trial evidence is emerging that bolus resuscitation is not beneficial in all populations. Two high-quality trials conducted in low-income countries demonstrated that fluid resuscitation in patients with sepsis increased mortality, despite early improvement in indices of perfusion. Proposed explanations for these unexpected findings include lack of critical care support to counteract harmful side-effects of high-volume fluid resuscitation, and excessive reperfusion injury, which may be worse in a population that presents later in the natural history of the condition.

Aborting the microbial driver: antimicrobials and source control

A retrospective study of patients with sepsis found that, after the onset of hypotension, for every hour's delay in the administration of broad-spectrum antibiotics, the risk of death rose by 7.6%. More recent data from 49 331 emergency department patients in New York State confirm a directly proportional rise in mortality with time to first antibiotic administration. This finding is biologically plausible, given that it is the microbial burden that is driving the immune response, which is, in turn, giving rise to the sepsis syndrome.

Not every infection can be cured with antimicrobials alone. Infected collections with an inadequate or absent blood supply, such as deep abscesses, infected prostheses or intravascular devices, need physical removal. This process, whether it requires open surgery or percutaneous drainage, is termed source control (see later).

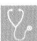 **Box 8.4 The Sepsis Six**

1. Give oxygen to maintain SpO_2 >94%
2. Take blood cultures
3. Give broad-spectrum intravenous antibiotics
4. Give a fluid challenge
5. Measure lactate
6. Measure urine output and chart hourly fluid balance

 Box 8.5 Surviving Sepsis Campaign: main recommendations for early management

Initial resuscitation
- Instigate i.v. fluid resuscitation with 30 mL/kg crystalloid within the first 3 h
- Give further fluid guided by haemodynamic assessment and use of dynamic variables to ascertain fluid responsiveness
- Target mean arterial pressure to 65 mmHg
- Guide resuscitation to normalize lactate in patients with raised lactate

Screening
- Have in place systems to screen acutely ill high-risk patients for sepsis

Diagnosis
- Obtain cultures before starting antibiotic treatment

Antimicrobial therapy
- Give i.v. antibiotics within 1 h of recognition of sepsis
- Start with broad-spectrum empirical therapy, with the aim of de-escalating once the pathogen and its sensitivities are known; assess for de-escalation daily

Source control
- Establish anatomical diagnosis and arrangements for emergency source control as soon as possible
- Remove potentially infected vascular access devices as soon as new access is obtained

Fluid therapy
- Apply a fluid challenge technique when on-going fluid administration is required
- Use crystalloids, the recommended fluid of choice
- Consider human albumin solution in addition, when large volumes of fluid are required
- Avoid hydroxyethyl starches

Useful diagnostic samples and laboratory processing

There is always time to obtain blood cultures before starting empirical antibiotic treatment. This is critical, even in an acutely septic or unstable patient. In adults, a minimum of 5 mL of blood should be inoculated into both aerobic and anaerobic blood culture bottles. The one exception is in suspected meningococcal septicaemia, where antibiotic administration should never be delayed. Administration of antibiotics prior to sample collection may result in sterile blood cultures, but polymerase chain reaction (PCR) testing for bacterial DNA in whole blood may still enable detection of the causative bacterial pathogen (**Box 8.6**).

For other acute infections, the ability to take further samples before antibiotics will depend on the stability of the patient. Examples include mid-stream urine (MSU), cerebrospinal fluid (CSF), stool, intravenous line tips and pus. Where bacteria are cultured in pure growth, these samples can help to define sites of infection. The laboratory can also provide susceptibility data for bacteria, particularly when resistance to commonly used antibiotics is unpredictable. An example is a UTI associated with Gram-negative bacteraemia, typically with *E. coli* or *K. pneumoniae*, in which susceptibility to beta-lactams, quinolones and aminoglycosides, often used as empirical therapy, is highly unpredictable. In stable patients whose site of infection remains undefined, imaging may reveal collections that require drainage or surgical intervention.

Culture-independent molecular methods of identifying pathogens may improve the speed and sensitivity of microbiological diagnosis, although the use of these technologies is not yet widespread (see **Box 8.6**). For example, if samples from a tissue collection are culture-negative post antibiotic exposure, they should be processed additionally for 16S PCR, a molecular test capable of identifying bacterial DNA.

In established chronic infections (e.g. diabetic foot infection, osteomyelitis and chronic respiratory disorders), where patients rarely exhibit signs of sepsis, empirical treatment can be delayed while deep-tissue, pus or sputum samples are obtained. Superficial swabs are rarely useful and may confuse management. Samples should always be transported to the laboratory in a timely fashion. As most results are available within 72 hours, this is the point when they may help with rationalizing antibiotic choices.

Source control

Management of infection requires not only appropriate antibiotic treatment but also an understanding of the site of infection. Occasionally, interventions at these sites are required and this is termed 'source control'. For example:

- Biomedical devices are commonly associated with infection and source control necessitates the removal of infected intravascular and urinary catheters, particularly when these are blocked.
- Obstructed biliary and urinary tract systems are common causes of sepsis and, under these circumstances, placement of a common bile duct stent, urinary catheter or nephrostomy tube may be required.
- Intra-abdominal collections require drainage, as do empyemas and paraspinal collections.
- If a native peripheral joint is infected, an arthroscopic washout is required, and an infected prosthetic joint may require debridement and removal of the prosthesis.
- Valvectomy is increasingly used to optimize management of infective endocarditis, particularly for acute infections caused by *S. aureus*.
- Surgical debridement of infected tissue is required for optimal management of monomicrobial necrotizing fasciitis caused by *S. pyogenes* or Fournier's gangrene.

Further reading

Andrews B, Semler MW, Muchemwa L et al. Effect of an early resuscitation protocol on in-hospital mortality among adults with sepsis and hypotension: a randomized clinical trial. *JAMA* 2017; 318:1233–1240.

Harris PNA, Tambyah PA, Lye DC et al. Effect of piperacillin-tazobactam versus meropenem on 30-day mortality for patients with E. coli or K. pneumoniae bloodstream infection and ceftriaxone resistance: a randomised clinical trial. *JAMA* 2018; 320:984–994.

Kumar A, Roberts D, Wood KE et al. Duration of hypotension before initiation of effective antimicrobial therapy is the critical determinant of survival in human septic shock. *Crit Care Med* 2006; 34:1589–1596.

Maitland K, Kiguli S, Opoka RO et al. Mortality after fluid bolus in African children with severe infection. *N Engl J Med* 2011; 364:2483–2495.

Rhodes A, Evans LE, Alhazzani W et al. Surviving sepsis campaign: international guidelines for management of sepsis and septic shock: 2016. *Crit Care Med* 2017; 45:486–552.

Thwaites GE, Scarborough M, Szubert A et al. Adjunctive rifampicin for *Staphylococcus aureus* bacteraemia (ARREST): a multicentre, randomised, double-blind, placebo-controlled trial. *Lancet* 2018; 391:668–678.

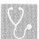 **Box 8.6 Molecular identification of infectious agents causing sepsis**

While traditional culture-based methods remain the gold standard, their disadvantages include:

- delay in obtaining results (it generally takes around 24 h for cultures to become positive, and 48 h for a firm bacterial identification to be made)
- the fact that cultures may be negative if antibiotics were administered before samples were taken.

Two methods have become widely accepted into clinical practice:

16S polymerase chain reaction (PCR) sequencing

- 16S ribosomal RNA is a component of the 30S small subunit of all prokaryotic ribosomes
- Due to the slow evolution of 'conserved' areas within the gene, to which DNA primers can anneal (allowing PCR amplification), sequencing of the hypervariable regions can be used to detect and speciate bacteria from a variety of clinical specimens (e.g. pus and deep tissue samples)

- Unlike culture, this diagnostic test does not provide susceptibility data but is of particular value for clinical samples that are culture-negative due to antibiotic exposure

Matrix-assisted laser desorption/ionization-time of flight (MALDI-TOF) mass spectroscopy

- Bacterial isolates are fixed in a matrix, which is then fragmented and subjected to mass spectroscopy
- Each protein-containing fragment of matrix has a different mass/charge profile, allowing a spectral profile to be generated that is unique to individual bacterial species
- Sometimes, genes conferring antibiotic resistance are detectable by MALDI-TOF, e.g. meticillin-resistant *Staphylococcus aureus* (MRSA) produces a different spectral profile to that of meticillin-sensitive *Staphylococcus aureus* (MSSA)

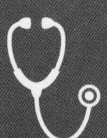

ANTIMICROBIAL STEWARDSHIP

Antimicrobial stewardship, or the prudent use of antibiotics, is a key component in the fight against the emergence of multidrug-resistant organisms. It is both a national and an international public health priority. In lay terms, it can be summarized as administering the right antibiotic for the right condition, given at the right dose, for the right duration.

UK-based targets

In 2017, Commissioning for Quality and Innovation (CQUIN) targets were introduced in the UK for hospital-based National Health Service (NHS) trusts. Key performance indicators (KPIs) were a reduction in total antibiotic prescribing, particularly of carbapenems and tazobactam–piperacillin (tazocin), and a documented antibiotic review at 72 hours. In subsequent years the reduction in total prescribing and carbapenem usage targets has continued but hospital doctors are now required to specify different prescribing options at 72 hours (see later). In general practice, KPIs are based on reductions in ciprofloxacin and amoxicillin/clavulanate usage and, for uncomplicated UTIs, prescribing nitrofurantoin rather than trimethoprim (as it is more effective against common urinary pathogens, including multidrug-resistant *E. coli*).

Considerations before starting empirical antibiotics

Most hospitals will have an empirical antimicrobial policy. Policies differ, depending on the local prevalence of antimicrobial resistance to key surveillance organisms. To prescribe appropriately, the likeliest site of infection must be determined, based on clinical assessment and other investigations. Previous microbiology results, such as previous infection/colonization with extended-spectrum beta-lactamase (ESBL)-producing Enterobacteriaceae, may help to determine appropriate choices of antimicrobial: for example, whether or not to prescribe a carbapenem.

Considerations that should be documented when choosing an initial antibiotic regimen include:
- route of administration
- frequency
- duration of treatment
- monitoring for potential toxicity
- where appropriate, drug levels (e.g. pre-dose gentamicin or amikacin levels)
- dose adjustment in renal/hepatic failure
- need for adjuvant therapy (e.g. rifampicin or fusidic acid for severe *S. aureus* infection)
- alternative antibiotics for severe or non-severe penicillin allergy.

Antimicrobial decision-making at 72 hours

At 72 hours, when most culture results are available, one of the following five decisions should be made:
- ***Stop antibiotic treatment.*** Symptoms of sepsis, such as confusion, may be caused by many different factors. After a period of observation and review of investigations, cessation of antibiotics is the appropriate action when patients are thought not to have had an infection after all.
- ***Step down to an oral alternative.*** For uncomplicated infections, e.g. pneumonia or pyelonephritis, treatment can normally be switched from intravenous to oral after 2–3 days if the patient is clinically stable and is showing signs of clinical improvement.
- ***Switch treatment.*** This may be necessary because of an unanticipated site of infection (e.g. infective endocarditis requiring prolonged intravenous antibiotic treatment) or unanticipated resistance (such as urosepsis and bacteraemia caused by an ESBL-producing *E. coli* requiring treatment with an intravenous carbapenem).
- ***Continue with intravenous treatment.*** The patient has a more complicated or difficult-to-treat infection, such as meningitis or septic arthritis.
- ***Discharge on outpatient parenteral antibiotic treatment.*** This is defined as the provision of intravenous antibiotics to patients out of hospital in either the community or an ambulatory care setting. For conditions such as skin and soft tissue infection, urinary tract infections and bone and joint infection, where the patient is otherwise well, treatment may be continued in the community, provided proper governance arrangements are in place (see later).

Where a switch or step down to an oral alternative is made, a key component of good antimicrobial stewardship is the choice of a narrow-spectrum agent when culture results are available. This reduces the risk of *Clostridium difficile* infection and colonization with multidrug-resistant organisms, and is therefore both safe for patients and cost-effective.

Outpatient parenteral antimicrobial treatment

Outpatient parenteral antimicrobial treatment (OPAT) has been cited as one of five antimicrobial prescribing decision options in UK Department of Health guidance on antibiotic stewardship after 72 hours of treatment. It may be accessed via several routes:
- through the hospital emergency or ambulatory care department, where patients can be clinically assessed, investigated and commenced on intravenous antibiotics for conditions such as lower limb cellulitis without hospital admission; OPAT is increasingly used for admission avoidance
- following a hospital admission for infections requiring inpatient admission (such as severe community-acquired pneumonia requiring supplementary oxygen), after the patient improves clinically but still requires intravenous antibiotics
- following a hospital admission required for source control (e.g. surgical removal of an infected joint prosthesis); OPAT is an option for carefully selected groups of patients, as it allows hospital discharge earlier than expected.

OPAT is associated with high levels of patient satisfaction, as most prefer to be treated out of hospital. Because there is less clinical supervision, governance arrangements around patient care are important, and clinical guidelines, published in both the UK and USA, should be complied with.

Conditions suitable for OPAT services

Skin and soft tissue infections – in particular, lower limb cellulitis – are the most common medical conditions referred to OPAT services. Patients are typically treated for 3–5 days with intravenous antibiotics but those with lymphoedema or underlying skin conditions typically require longer courses. Increasingly, multidrug-resistant

UTIs may be treated in the community with intravenous antibiotics, and patients may be recruited for OPAT by direct laboratory referral after a multi-resistant organism is grown. Those with bone and joint infection, such as vertebral osteomyelitis or native or prosthetic joint infection, invariably require prolonged intravenous antibiotic courses. Other conditions suitable for OPAT include infected diabetic foot ulcers (with or without osteomyelitis), infective endocarditis, empyema and abscesses of the brain and liver, once patients are deemed clinically stable.

The suitability of a patient to receive OPAT needs careful assessment and is dependent on age, co-morbidities and severity of infection. OPAT also requires patients to engage reliably with therapy. Therefore, intravenous drug users and patients with serious mental health problems are generally not suitable.

Delivery of OPAT services

Commonly used antibiotics are given once daily and reduce nursing time, although some teams can administer intravenous antibiotics four times per day. Examples of antibiotics suitable for once-daily dosing include ceftriaxone, ertapenem, amikacin, teicoplanin and daptomycin. Some services insist on the first dose of antibiotic being given in hospital when there is a history of antibiotic allergy, but many now give the first dose of intravenous antibiotics in the community. OPAT teams may need to monitor drug levels (e.g. pre-dose teicoplanin levels for efficacy, or pre-dose amikacin levels for nephrotoxicity). For most intravenous antibiotics, full blood count, urea and electrolytes, CRP and liver function tests should be monitored on a weekly basis at least.

Antibiotics can be administered through a peripheral intravenous cannula, but for longer durations of treatment (>7 days) administration through a Hickman line or a peripherally inserted central catheter (PICC) is preferable. Insertion by a suitably trained healthcare professional or interventional radiologist reduces the risk of line infection. Patients can also be taught to self-administer or attach 'infusion devices', commonly known as elastomeric devices, which save district nurse time.

There are different models for delivering OPAT services. These are **community-based** (nurses deliver treatment within the patient's home) or **hospital-based** (patients attend hospital or an ambulatory care centre on a daily basis for intravenous antibiotic treatment). Ideally, an OPAT multidisciplinary team should consist of doctors, hospital-based nurses, community nurses and a pharmacist.

Monitoring patients in OPAT services

Patients must be appropriately monitored with clinical assessments, blood tests and, where relevant, imaging at appropriate intervals. Some NHS trusts capture patients on virtual wards, which facilitates clinical ownership and follow-up. Good practice includes regular multidisciplinary team meetings (where cases are discussed with an infection specialist), the taking of blood tests and organization of other investigations. While many conditions can be managed exclusively by a clinical microbiologist or ID physician, joint care is required for orthopaedic or neurosurgical cases. The treatment of lower limb cellulitis can be managed by nurses and requires minimal involvement from medical staff.

Because of there being less clinical supervision there are risks associated with OPAT, unless strict governance arrangements are in place. Adverse drug reactions are not uncommonly reported and central venous access can be associated with access site infections and thrombophlebitis. Overuse of broad-spectrum intravenous antibiotics can be associated with *C. difficile* infection and, depending on the condition being treated, relapse and hospital re-admission

can occur. There should therefore be formal re-admission pathways to secondary care. Evidence suggests that OPAT is safe, provided it is administered through a formal service, designed to minimize risk, with doctors and nurses working together across primary and secondary care. OPAT services are likely to expand in the UK, driven by good safety data, high levels of patient satisfaction and healthcare efficiencies.

Assessment of allergy risk

Around 10% of the population report a history of penicillin allergy but data show that the true figure is only around 1%. In some infections, penicillins are the first-choice antibiotic and other agents are associated with a worse outcome.

Anaphylaxis to penicillins or any antibiotic can be fatal, so careful evaluation is required. The timing of the reaction is of paramount importance:

- **Immediate hypersensitivity reactions**, which include anaphylaxis, are immunoglobulin E (IgE)-mediated and classically begin within 1 h of the dose, and often within minutes. Typically, they are characterized by facial swelling, rash and severe shortness of breath.
- **Delayed reactions** appear after multiple doses of treatment, typically after days or weeks. While they may be immune-mediated, they are not associated with anaphylaxis, although in some rare cases they can lead to severe or life-threatening conditions such as Stevens–Johnson syndrome and toxic epidermal necrolysis (see p. 697).

When a patient reports an antibiotic allergy, the following information should be ascertained:

- the name(s) of the antibiotic(s) they report an allergy to
- the timing between starting the antibiotic and the symptoms or signs
- the nature of the symptoms or signs, asking specifically about rash, wheeze, swelling and loss of consciousness
- time to resolution of the symptoms
- whether they tried the same or similar antibiotics since.

Severe allergy is typically a hypersensitivity reaction but occasionally can also be a delayed reaction. In type 1 (IgE-mediated, p. 62) and other severe penicillin allergies, cephalosporins and carbapenems should also be avoided.

Non-severe allergy is typically non IgE-mediated and is commonly described as a mild rash. In these circumstances, cephalosporins, carbapenems and monobactams can be cautiously used. Other antibiotic classes are safe alternatives.

Selected patients reporting a penicillin allergy should be referred to allergy services for formal testing. These include:

- patients with a history of an allergic reaction when on multiple drugs, e.g. during general anaesthesia
- patients allergic to multiple antibiotics
- patients for whom there is no reliable alternative antibiotic
- patients in whom there is a current requirement for a prolonged course of antibiotics and an allergy to 'gold standard' treatment
- patients with an absolute requirement for penicillin, e.g. those with central nervous system syphilis, immunodeficiency or cardiac valve disorders requiring prophylaxis, or post splenectomy
- patients likely to need repeated courses of antibiotics, e.g. those with haematological malignancies, cystic fibrosis or inflammatory bowel disease.

It is possible to desensitize patients with carefully introduced, gradually increasing doses of specific antibiotics. For example, a

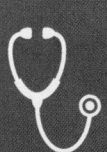

well-recognized protocol for co-trimoxazole sensitization has been used since the late 1990s.

Antibiotic chemoprophylaxis

The value of antibiotic chemoprophylaxis has been questioned, as there are relatively few controlled trials to prove efficacy. The evidence for chemoprophylaxis against infective endocarditis is an example. National Institute for Health and Care Excellence (NICE) guidelines recognize that procedures can cause bacteraemia but without a significant risk of infective endocarditis. Even patients at 'high risk', such as those with previous infectious endocarditis, prosthetic heart valves and surgical shunts, do not always require prophylaxis (**Box 8.7**). However, there are a number of indications for which the prophylactic use of antibiotics is still advised. These include surgical procedures carrying a high risk of infection (ie colon surgery), or with potentially serious consequences of infection (organ transplantation, post-splenectomy sepsis). The choice of agent(s) is determined by the likely infectious risk and the established efficacy and safety of the regimen. Antibiotic prophylaxis for the vast majority of surgical or radiological procedures should not extend for more than 24 hours post procedure and, for most operations, a single dose at induction is all that is required.

Further reading

National Institute for Health and Care Excellence. *NICE Guideline 15: Antimicrobial Stewardship: Systems and Processes for Effective Antimicrobial Medicine Use.* NICE 2015; https://www.nice.org.uk/guidance/ng15.

ANTIBIOTIC THERAPIES

Timely administration of antibiotics that are active against the infecting pathogen is critical in the effective management of sepsis. Delays in administration of antimicrobial therapy are well documented as having an impact on the survival and outcome of patients with septic shock.

The selection of an antibiotic, either empirically or as definitive therapy, requires knowledge of standard pharmacokinetic considerations of absorption, distribution, metabolism and excretion (see p. 253). Parenteral administration is usually indicated in the severely ill patient to ensure rapid, high and consistent blood and tissue concentrations. Whether an antibiotic is able to kill bacteria (bactericidal) or can only inhibit the growth of the organism (bacteriostatic) at the infection site is another factor used for antibiotic selection. Therapy should be given at the optimal dosing regimen based on pharmacokinetic/pharmacodynamic indices, summarized for drugs commonly used to treat sepsis in **Box 8.8**.

Antibiotics commonly used in the treatment of sepsis

Beta-lactams (penicillins, cephalosporins, monobactams) and carbapenems

Beta-lactams are the most widely used antimicrobials in human medicine. They are naturally derived compounds that share a

---

ⓘ Box 8.7 Antibiotic chemoprophylaxis

Clinical problem	Aim	Drug regimen[a]
General		
Splenectomy/spleen malfunction	To prevent serious pneumococcal sepsis	Phenoxymethylpenicillin 500 mg twice daily
Rheumatic fever	To prevent recurrence and further cardiac damage	Phenoxymethylpenicillin 250 mg twice daily or sulfadiazine 1 g if allergic to penicillin
Meningitis:		
Due to meningococci	To prevent infection in close contacts	Adults: rifampicin 600 mg twice daily for 2 days Children: <1 year: 5 mg/kg; >1 year: 10 mg/kg Alternative (single-dose) ciprofloxacin 500 mg (p.o.) or ceftriaxone 250 mg (i.m.)
Due to *Haemophilus influenzae* type b	To reduce nasopharyngeal carriage and prevent infection in close contacts	Adults: rifampicin 600 mg daily for 4 days Children: <3 months 10 mg/kg; >3 months 20 mg/kg
Tuberculosis	To prevent infection in exposed (close contacts) tuberculin-negative individuals, infants of infected mothers, and immunosuppressed patients	Oral isoniazid 300 mg daily for 6 months Children: 5–10 mg/kg daily

Endocarditis[b]

Antibacterial prophylaxis and chlorhexidine mouthwash are *not* recommended for the prevention of endocarditis in patients undergoing dental procedures

Antibacterial prophylaxis is *not* recommended for the prevention of endocarditis in patients undergoing procedures of the:
    upper and lower respiratory tract (including ear, nose and throat procedures and bronchoscopy)
    genitourinary tract (including urological, gynaecological and obstetric procedures)
    upper and lower gastrointestinal tract

Any infection in patients at risk of endocarditis should be investigated promptly and treated appropriately to reduce the risk of endocarditis

If patients at risk of endocarditis are undergoing a gastrointestinal or genitourinary tract procedure at a site where infection is suspected, they should receive appropriate antibacterial therapy that includes cover against organisms that cause endocarditis

Patients at risk of endocarditis should be:
    advised to maintain good oral hygiene
    told how to recognize signs of infective endocarditis and advised when to seek expert advice

[a] Unless stated, doses are those recommended in adults. For surgical procedure, see individual procedures in text.
[b] NICE guidelines for adults and children undergoing interventional procedures, March 2008, updated in 2016.
(*Adapted from Joint Formulary Committee.* British National Formulary, *70th edn. London: BMJ Group and RPS Publishing; 2015.*)

Box 8.8 Dosages for drugs commonly used to treat sepsis

Drug	Standard dose	High dose	Special situations
Penicillins			
Amoxicillin i.v.	1 g × 3–4 i.v. (under review)[a]	2 g × 6 i.v.	Meningitis: 2 g × 6 i.v.
Amoxicillin oral	0.5 g × 3[a]	0.75 g–1 g × 3[a]	*H. influenzae:* High dose only
Amoxicillin–clavulanic acid i.v.	(1 g amoxicillin + 0.2 g clavulanic acid) × 3-4 i.v. (under review)[a]	(2 g amoxicillin + 0.2 g clavulanic acid) × 3 i.v.	
Amoxicillin–clavulanic acid oral	(0.5 g amoxicillin + 0.125 g clavulanic acid) × 3[a]	(0.875 g amoxicillin + 0.125 g clavulanic acid) × 3[a]	*H. influenzae:* High dose only
Piperacillin–tazobactam	(4 g piperacillin + 0.5 g tazobactam) × 3 i.v.	(4 g piperacillin + 0.5 g tazobactam) × 4 i.v.	*Pseudomonas* spp.: High dose only
Flucloxacillin	1 g × 3 oral or 2 g × 4 i.v. (or 1 g × 6 i.v.)[a]	1 g × 4 oral or 2 g × 6 i.v.	
Cephalosporins			
Cefotaxime	1 g × 3 i.v.	2 g × 3 i.v.	Meningitis: 2 g × 4 i.v. *S. aureus:* High dose only
Ceftazidime	1 g × 3 i.v.	2 g × 3 i.v. *or* 1 g × 6 i.v.[a]	*Pseudomonas* spp.: High dose only
Cefuroxime i.v.	0.75 g × 3 i.v.	1.5 g × 3 i.v.	*E. coli, Klebsiella* spp. (except *K. aerogenes*), *Raoultella* spp. and *P. mirabilis:* High dose only
Cefuroxime oral	0.25–0.5 g × 2 oral depending on species and/or infection type	None	
Carbapenems			
Ertapenem	1 g × 1 i.v. over 30 min	None	
Imipenem	0.5 g × 4 i.v. over 30 min	1 g × 4 i.v. over 30 min	*Pseudomonas* spp.: High dose only
Meropenem	1 g × 3 i.v. over 30 min	2 g × 3 i.v. over 3 h[a]	Meningitis: 2 g × 3 i.v. over 30 min (or 3 h)
Fluoroquinolones			
Ciprofloxacin	0.5 g × 2 oral or 0.4 g × 2 i.v.	0.75 g × 2 oral or 0.4 g × 3 i.v.	*Pseudomonas* spp.: High dose only *Staphylococcus* spp.: High dose only + combination
Levofloxacin	0.5 g × 1 oral or 0.5 g × 1 i.v.	0.5 g × 2 oral or 0.5 g × 2 i.v.	*Pseudomonas* spp.: High dose only *Streptococcus* groups A, B, C and G: High dose only *S. pneumoniae:* High dose only
Aminoglycosides			
Amikacin	20 mg/kg × 1 i.v.	30 mg/kg × 1 i.v.	Enterobacterales: High dose only *Pseudomonas* spp.: High dose only *Acinetobacter* spp.: High dose only
Gentamicin	5 mg/kg × 1 i.v.	7 mg/kg × 1 i.v.	Enterobacterales: High dose only *Pseudomonas* spp.: High dose only *Acinetobacter* spp.: High dose only
Glycopeptides and lipoglycopeptides			
Teicoplanin	0.4 g × 1 i.v.	0.8 g × 1 i.v.[a]	
Vancomycin	0.5 g × 4 i.v. or 1 g × 2 i.v. *or* 2 g × 1 by continuous infusion	None	Based on body weight. Therapeutic drug monitoring should guide dosing
Macrolides, lincosamides and streptogramins			
Azithromycin	0.5 g × 1 oral *or* 0.5 g × 1 i.v.	None	Gonorrhoea: 2 g oral as a single dose
Clarithromycin	0.25 g × 2 oral	0.5 g × 2 oral	
Tetracyclines			
Doxycycline	0.1 g × 1 oral	0.2 g × 1 oral	
Oxazolidinones			
Linezolid	0.6 g × 2 oral *or* 0.6 g × 2 i.v.	None	
Miscellaneous agents			
Fosfomycin oral	3 g × 1 oral as a single dose	None	
Metronidazole	0.4 g × 3 oral *or* 0.4 g × 3 i.v.	0.5 g × 3 oral *or* 0.5 g × 3 i.v.	
Nitrofurantoin	50–100 mg × 3-4 oral[a]	None[a]	Dosing is dependent on drug formulation
Trimethoprim	0.16 g × 2 oral	None	
Trimethoprim–sulfamethoxazole	(0.16 g trimethoprim + 0.8 g sulfa) × 2 oral *or* (0.16 g trimethoprim + 0.8 g sulfa) × 2 i.v	(0.24 g trimethoprim + 1.2 g sulfa) × 2 oral *or* (0.24 g trimethoprim + 1.2 g sulfa) × 2 i.v.	*Stenotrophomonas maltophilia:* High dose only

[a]European Committee on Antimicrobial Susceptibility Testing (EUCAST) breakpoints are based on these dosages. Alternative dosing regimens that result in equivalent exposure are acceptable. The table should not be considered exhaustive guidance for dosing in clinical practice, and does not replace specific local, national or regional dosing guidelines.

common ring structure. Modifications to the β-lactam ring and/or the side-chain may expand the antimicrobial spectrum to include many Gram-negative and positive organisms. Following the discovery of penicillin, dozens of β-lactam-based drugs (first to fifth generations) have been developed for clinical use, either from bacterial or fungal sources (e.g. cephalosporins, carbapenems) or by chemical engineering of the β-lactam ring. All β-lactams block bacterial cell-wall synthesis by binding to and inactivating specific penicillin-binding proteins, peptidases, which are involved in the final stages of cell-wall assembly and division. They are generally bactericidal to susceptible bacterial cells in a time-dependent manner.

Many bacteria produce β-lactamase enzymes, which inactivate antibiotics of this class. The emergence of Gram-negative organisms producing extended-spectrum β-lactamases (ESBLs) and carbapenemases (see below) has rendered some bacteria resistant to all β-lactams.

Penicillins

Benzylpenicillin can only be given parenterally and is still the drug of choice for some serious infections. However, due to increasing antimicrobial resistance, it should not be used empirically in serious infections without laboratory confirmation that the organism is penicillin-sensitive. Uses include serious streptococcal infections (including infective endocarditis), group A streptococcus (*Streptococcus pyogenes*) necrotizing fasciitis and gas gangrene (usually combined with other antibiotics).

Flucloxacillin is used in infections caused by penicillinase-producing staphylococci and remains the drug of choice for serious infections caused by MSSA.

Amoxicillin is susceptible to β-lactamase but its antimicrobial activity includes streptococci, pneumococci and enterococci, as well as Gram-negative organisms such as *Salmonella* spp., *Shigella* spp., *E. coli*, *Haemophilus influenzae* and *Proteus* spp. The extended-spectrum penicillin **ticarcillin** is active against *Pseudomonas* infections, as is the acylureidopenicillin **piperacillin** in combination with tazobactam (tazocin).

Pivmecillinam is used for the treatment of UTI and has activity against Gram-negative bacteria, including ESBL-producing *E. coli*, *Klebsiella*, *Enterobacter* and *Salmonella* spp. but not *Pseudomonas aeruginosa*.

Temocillin is active against Gram-negative bacteria only, including many ESBL producers. It appears to be less relatively likely to trigger *C. difficile* infection, and is increasingly used because of resistance but also as a carbapenem-sparing agent. It is not active against *Pseudomonas* or *Acinetobacter* spp.

Generally, the penicillins are safe. Hypersensitivity (skin rash, urticaria and anaphylaxis), encephalopathy and tubulointerstitial nephritis can occur. Amoxicillin and ampicillin produce a hypersensitivity rash in approximately 90% of patients with infectious mononucleosis (glandular fever) who receive this drug. Amoxicillin/clavulanate (co-amoxiclav) (see below) causes cholestatic jaundice six times more frequently than amoxicillin, as does flucloxacillin.

Cephalosporins

The cephalosporins (**Fig. 8.2**) have an advantage over penicillins in that they are not inactivated by staphylococcal penicillinases. Except for the newer fifth-generation cephalosporins **ceftaroline** and **ceftobiprole**, they are not active against MRSA. Activity extends to many Gram-negative and positive organisms, except for

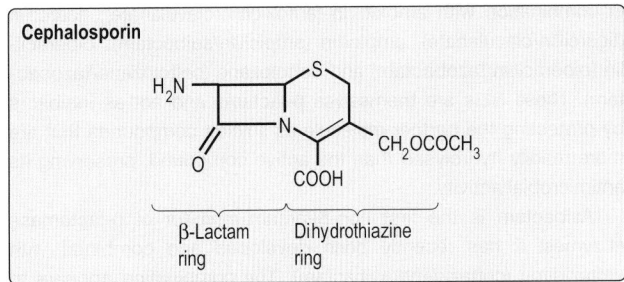

Fig. 8.2 The structure of a cephalosporin.

enterococci and Gram-negative anaerobic bacteria. Only certain cephalosporins (e.g. **ceftazidime** and **cefepime**) are active against *P. aeruginosa*.

Second- and third-generation cephalosporins are reserved for the treatment of specific serious infections, as empirical use against Gram-negative infections can be rendered ineffective due to ESBL production, and has been associated with an increased risk of *C. difficile* infection.

The toxicity is similar to that of the penicillins but is less commonly encountered. Some 10% of patients allergic to one group are also allergic to the other. The early cephalosporins caused proximal tubule damage, although the newer derivatives have fewer nephrotoxic effects.

Monobactams

Aztreonam is the only member of this class available. It is a synthetic β-lactam and, unlike the penicillins and cephalosporins, has no ring other than the β-lactam one: hence its description as a monobactam. Aztreonam's spectrum of activity is limited to aerobic Gram-negative bacilli. It is a useful alternative to aminoglycosides in combination therapy, largely for the treatment of intra-abdominal sepsis, as it has activity against some carbapenem-resistant strains that produce metallo-β-lactamases. It is also used in *P. aeruginosa* infection (including lung infection in cystic fibrosis).

Carbapenems

The carbapenems are semi-synthetic β-lactams and include **imipenem**, **meropenem**, **doripenem** and **ertapenem**. They currently have the broadest spectrum of the antibiotics, being active against the majority of Gram-positive, Gram-negative and anaerobic bacterial pathogens (but not against MRSA). Ertapenem, unlike the others, is not active against *Pseudomonas* or *Acinetobacter* spp. They differ in their dosage and frequency of administration. Imipenem is partially inactivated in the kidney by enzymatic inactivation and is therefore administered in combination with cilastatin.

Carbapenems are the mainstay of treatment for severe ESBL-producing Gram-negative infections (e.g. urinary tract or biliary tract sepsis) and are also used for severe hospital-acquired infections when multidrug-resistant Gram-negative bacilli or mixed aerobic and anaerobic infections are suspected.

Their side-effect profile is similar to that of β-lactam antibiotics. Nausea, vomiting and diarrhoea occur in less than 5% of cases. Imipenem and ertapenem may cause seizures and should not be used to treat meningitis. Meropenem is safe for this indication.

β-lactam/β-lactamase inhibitor combinations

One approach to the problem of β-lactamase-mediated resistance is to combine β-lactams with 'inhibitor' molecules (BLIs). Classical 'inhibitors' include clavulanic acid, sulbactam and tazobactam given in combination with amoxicillin (amoxicillin/clavulanate), ticarcillin (ticarcillin/clavulanate), ampicillin (ampicillin/sulbactam), piperacillin (piperacillin/tazobactam) and ceftolozane (ceftolozane/tazobactam). These BLIs are themselves β-lactams and act as inhibitors by protecting the partner molecule as suicide compounds that are more readily hydrolysed than the active compound, preserving its antimicrobial activity.

Avibactam is the first non-β-lactam inhibitor of β-lactamase enzymes; it has recently been developed and combined with ceftazidime (ceftazidime/avibactam). The combination appears to be stable to most ESBLs and some carbapenemase (KPC, OXA-48) enzymes in Enterobacterales.

Quinolones

The quinolone group of drugs inhibits bacterial DNA synthesis by inhibiting topoisomerase IV and DNA gyrase, the enzymes responsible for maintaining the super-helical twists in DNA.

Extended-spectrum quinolones such as **ciprofloxacin** have activity against Gram-negative bacteria, including *P. aeruginosa*, and some Gram-positive bacteria. They are useful in Gram-negative bloodstream infections, bone and joint infections, urinary and respiratory tract infections, meningococcal carriage, some sexually transmitted diseases such as gonorrhoea and non-specific urethritis due to *Chlamydia trachomatis*, as well as in severe cases of travellers' diarrhoea. The newer oral quinolones (e.g. **levofloxacin**, **moxifloxacin**) provide an alternative to β-lactams in the treatment of community-acquired lower respiratory tract infections and are effective against *S. pneumoniae*, *H. influenzae* and the 'atypical' respiratory pathogens. They can also be used in the treatment of tuberculosis.

In many countries, a high proportion of *E. coli* and *Klebsiella* spp. are now resistant (>80%). Resistance is also an emerging problem among *Salmonella*, *Vibrio cholerae*, *S. pneumoniae* and *S. aureus*.

Gastrointestinal disturbances, photosensitive rashes and occasional neurotoxicity can occur. Use should be avoided in pregnancy and childhood, and in patients taking corticosteroids, unless the benefit outweighs the risk. Tendon damage, including rupture, can occur within 48 hours of use. MRSA and *C. difficile* infections in hospitals have been linked to high prescribing rates of quinolones, particularly when the O27 hypervirulent strain of *C. difficile* was endemic in most UK hospitals. Use is discouraged where an effective alternative is available. There is concern about QTc prolongation, and concomitant prescribing with other QTc prolongation drugs should be avoided whenever possible.

Aminoglycosides

Aminoglycosides (**Fig. 8.3**) interrupt bacterial protein synthesis by inhibiting ribosomal function (messenger RNA reading and transfer RNA binding). **Gentamicin** and **tobramycin** are given parenterally. They are highly effective against many Gram-negative organisms,

including *Pseudomonas* spp. They are synergistic at low doses with penicillins against *Enterococcus* spp. and *Streptococcus viridans*, and are therefore often used in endocarditis. **Amikacin** has a similar spectrum but is more resistant to the aminoglycoside-modifying enzymes (phosphorylating, adenylating or acetylating) produced by some bacteria, in particular ESBL-producing Enterobacterales. Its use should be restricted to gentamicin-resistant organisms.

Dose-related nephrotoxicity and ototoxicity (vestibular and auditory) can occur, particularly in the elderly. Enhanced nephrotoxicity occurs with other nephrotoxic drugs, and enhanced ototoxicity with some diuretics. The m.1555A>G mutation has been associated with gentamicin ototoxicity but appears to occur in less than 1% of the general population. Monitoring is necessary to ensure therapeutic and non-toxic drug concentrations. Once-daily dosing is used for most indications, with a serum drug level taken at 6–14 hours post dose, followed by application of an appropriate nomogram to determine the subsequent frequency of dosing (e.g. every 24 or 48 hours). When aminoglycosides are used for endocarditis, low doses are prescribed every 12 hours with different target pre- and post-dose level ranges than for once-daily dosing. Alternatively, and more simply, a pre-dose level can be checked prior to drug administration and appropriate drug adjustments made with subsequent doses. Neuromuscular blockade can occur with curariform drugs and aminoglycosides should be avoided in patients with myasthenia gravis.

Glycopeptides

The glycopeptides are active against Gram-positive bacteria and act by inhibiting cell-wall synthesis.

Vancomycin is given intravenously for MRSA and other multi-resistant, Gram-positive organisms. It is only slowly bactericidal (in contrast to β-lactams). It is also used for treatment of and prophylaxis against Gram-positive infections in penicillin-allergic patients. It is given in *S. pneumoniae* meningitis, in combination with other effective antibiotics, when disease is caused by penicillin-resistant strains.

Vancomycin can cause ototoxicity and nephrotoxicity, and thus pre-dose (trough) serum levels should be monitored regularly. Serum levels at 1 hour post dose (peak) are also monitored to optimize drug efficacy. Care must be taken to avoid extravasation at the injection site, as this causes necrosis and thrombophlebitis. Too rapid infusion can produce symptomatic release of histamine (red man syndrome).

Teicoplanin is less nephrotoxic than vancomycin. It has more favourable pharmacokinetic properties, allowing once-daily or thrice-weekly dosage. It is given intravenously and pre-dose (trough) serum levels are monitored to optimize efficacy.

Lipopeptides

Daptomycin is a lipopeptide with a similar spectrum to that of vancomycin, and is given by the intravenous route. It is used particularly for complicated skin and soft tissue infections, including those caused by MRSA, and is also a useful alternative agent for endocarditis, bone and joint infections, and Gram-positive bloodstream infections. Lipopeptides with very long elimination times, such as **dalbavancin**, are used as single-dose therapies for skin and soft tissue infections.

Oxazolidinones

Linezolid was the first oxazolidinone antibacterial to be developed. **Tedizolid** has recently been approved for use in skin and skin structure infections. These drugs act by inhibiting protein synthesis,

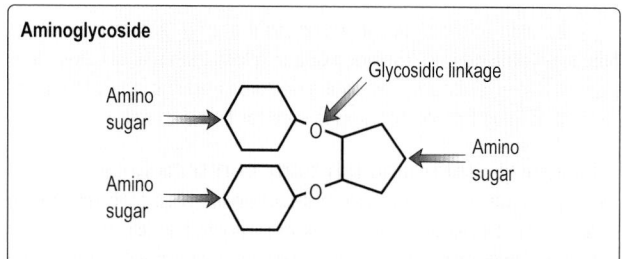

Fig. 8.3 The structure of an aminoglycoside.

binding to the bacterial 23S ribosomal RNA of the 59S subunit, thereby preventing the formation of a functional 70S complex that is essential to bacterial translation.

Oxazolidinones are active against a variety of Gram-positive pathogens, including vancomycin-resistant *Enterococcus faecium* (although resistant organisms have been reported), MRSA and penicillin-resistant *S. pneumoniae*. They are also active against group A and group B streptococci. Clinical experience with linezolid has demonstrated efficacy in a variety of hospitalized patients with severe to life-threatening infections, including bacteraemia, hospital-acquired pneumonia, skin and soft tissue infection, and bone and joint infection. These drugs can be given both intravenously and by mouth, and are almost 100% bioavailable by the oral route in patients with normal gastrointestinal absorption.

Oxazolidinones interact reversibly as non-selective inhibitors of monoamine oxidase and have the potential for interacting with serotoninergic and adrenergic agents. Side-effects include gastrointestinal disturbances, headache, rash, hypertension, reversible but potentially severe cytopenias, and occasional reports of optic and peripheral neuropathy in patients receiving linezolid for longer than 28 days. Tedizolid is less myelotoxic and can also be given once daily (in contrast to twice-daily linezolid). Weekly monitoring of the full blood count for cytopenias, and for other serious adverse effects, is mandatory. Safety has not yet been shown in pregnancy but linezolid has been used successfully for serious infections in children.

Tetracyclines

These are bacteriostatic drugs possessing a four-ring hydronaphthacene nucleus (**Fig. 8.4**). Included among the tetracyclines are **tetracycline**, **oxytetracycline**, **doxycycline** and **minocycline**. **Tigecycline** is an injectable glycylcycline that is structurally related to the tetracyclines.

Tetracyclines inhibit bacterial protein synthesis by interrupting ribosomal function (transfer RNA binding) and are active against Gram-positive and Gram-negative bacteria. Tigecycline is active against many organisms resistant to tetracycline, as it avoids common bacterial efflux pump systems. This includes vancomycin-resistant enterococci, MRSA and Gram-negative bacilli, such as *Acinetobacter baumannii*, but not *Pseudomonas* or *Proteus* spp. Tigecycline is increasingly used in combination with other antibiotics (e.g. polymyxins) to treat infections caused by highly resistant, carbapenemase-producing, Gram-negative bacteria. The licensed indications are complicated skin and soft tissue infections and intra-abdominal sepsis. Tigecycline is also used to treat spirochaetal and rickettsial infections, and also has a role as malaria prophylaxis. However, a 2010 US Food and Drug Administration (FDA) alert raised concerns about the efficacy of tigecycline in some serious infections (notably ventilator-associated pneumonia) and it should be used only on expert advice. The efficacy of tetracyclines is reduced by antacids and oral iron-replacement therapy.

Tetracyclines are generally safe drugs but they may enhance established or incipient renal failure, although doxycycline is safer than others in this group. They cause brown discoloration of growing teeth and thus are not given to children or pregnant women. Photosensitivity occurs in approximately 1 in 20 patients. Nausea and vomiting are the most frequent adverse effects of tigecycline.

Macrolides

Macrolides inhibit protein synthesis by interrupting ribosomal function. **Erythromycin** has a similar (but not identical) antibacterial spectrum to that of penicillin and may be useful in individuals with penicillin allergy, especially in the management of bacterial respiratory infections. It can be given orally or parenterally, but oral intake is associated with significant gastrointestinal side-effects, while the intravenous formulation is very irritant and causes phlebitis. For these reasons, **clarithromycin** (which has similar antimicrobial properties but fewer side-effects) is often preferred. These drugs are useful in the treatment of pneumonias caused by *Legionella* and *Mycoplasma* spp. They are also effective in the treatment of infections due to *Bordetella pertussis* (whooping cough), *Campylobacter* and *Chlamydia* spp. Macrolides are otherwise not usually used for life-threatening or serious infections, such as endocarditis and meningitis.

Other macrolides include **azithromycin** and **telithromycin**. They have a broad spectrum of activity that covers selective Gram-negative organisms (*Salmonella*, *Shigella*). Compared with erythromycin, they have superior pharmacokinetic properties with enhanced tissue and intracellular penetration and a longer half-life that allows once-daily dosage. Concern has been raised about the use of azithromycin in bloodstream infections (bacteraemia) because of low serum bioavailability. Azithromycin is also employed for trachoma, cholera and some sexually transmitted infections.

Erythromycin and other macrolides interact with theophyllines, carbamazepine, digoxin and ciclosporin, occasionally necessitating dose adjustment of these agents. Diarrhoea, vomiting and abdominal pain are the main side-effects of erythromycin (less so with clarithromycin and azithromycin) as a consequence of the intestinal prokinetic properties of the macrolides. QTc prolongation is a recognized cardiac effect of the macrolides and may lead to the potentially life-threatening syndrome of 'torsades de pointes' (see p. 1064). Concomitant use of other drugs that cause QTc prolongation should be avoided unless absolutely essential.

Polymyxins (polymyxin B, colistimethate sodium (polymyxin E))

This is an old antibiotic class that, until recently, was rarely used in clinical practice because of concerns about neuro- and nephrotoxicity. The emergence of multidrug-resistant Gram-negative bacteria, in particular carbapenemase-producing Enterobacterales, has resulted in the increased use of drugs in this class as an agent of last resort, often in combination with other antibiotics. Colistimethate sodium (CMS) is an inactive prodrug, metabolized *in vivo* to the active component **colistin**. This complicates dosing strategies and increases the potential for toxicity. The mechanism of bacterial killing of polymyxins is thought to be disruption of the bacterial cell membrane following binding to the lipopolysaccharide (LPS) component. They are active against most Gram-negative bacilli (except *Proteus* and *Providencia* spp.) and are administered intravenously for serious infections. Plasmid-mediated resistance, due to the

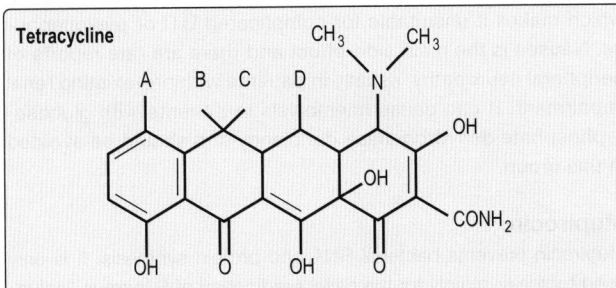

Fig. 8.4 The structure of a tetracycline. Substitution of CH_3, OH or H at positions A–D produces variants of tetracycline.

MCR-1 phosphoethanolamine enzyme that modifies bacterial LPS, has recently been described, although mostly in veterinary strains in South and South-east Asia.

Sodium fusidate

Sodium fusidate has a structure resembling that of bile salts and is a potent inhibitor of bacterial protein synthesis. Its entry into cells is facilitated by the detergent properties inherent in its structure. It is mainly used for penicillinase-producing *S. aureus* infections, such as osteomyelitis (it is well concentrated in bone) or endocarditis, and as an adjunctive agent for other staphylococcal infections accompanied by septicaemia. The drug is well absorbed orally but must be given in combination with another staphylococcal agent to prevent resistance, which may occur rapidly.

Sodium fusidate commonly causes gastrointestinal adverse effects and may occasionally be hepatotoxic; however, it is generally a safe drug and can be given during pregnancy if necessary. Concomitant statin use is avoided. Sodium fusidate is also available in topical preparations for use in minor skin conditions (impetigo) but these should be avoided to limit the risk of emerging resistance.

Sulphonamides and trimethoprim

The sulphonamides are all derivatives of the prototype sulfanilamide, and act by blocking thymidine and purine synthesis by inhibiting microbial folic acid synthesis. Trimethoprim is a 2,4-diaminopyrimidine, which prevents the bacterial reduction of dihydrofolate to tetrahydrofolate.

Sulfamethoxazole is mainly used in combination with trimethoprim (as **co-trimoxazole**). Because of its adverse effect profile, use in developed countries was largely restricted to the treatment and prevention of *Pneumocystis jiroveci* infection and listeriosis; however, it is increasingly being prescribed in hospitals again for other infections, such as acute exacerbations of chronic bronchitis and UTI, as it appears to carry a relatively lower risk for triggering *C. difficile* infection and remains useful for some resistant Gram-negative infections. It may also be given for toxoplasmosis and nocardiosis. **Trimethoprim** alone is often used for empirical treatment of UTIs.

Resistance to sulphonamides is often plasmid-mediated and results from the production of a sulphonamide-resistant dihydropteroate synthase. Sulphonamides potentiate oral anticoagulants and some hypoglycaemic agents.

The adverse effects of co-trimoxazole are most commonly due to the sulphonamide component. Sulphonamides cause a variety of skin eruptions, including toxic epidermal necrolysis, the Stevens–Johnson syndrome, thrombocytopenia, folate deficiency and megaloblastic anaemia with prolonged usage. They can provoke haemolysis in individuals with glucose-6-phosphate dehydrogenase deficiency and therefore should not be used in such people. Trimethoprim is similar in molecular structure to the potassium-sparing diuretic amiloride; monitoring of renal function is required when using trimethoprim or co-trimoxazole, particularly when the patient is prescribed other potassium-sparing drugs (e.g. angiotensin-converting enzyme (ACE) inhibitors) and during prolonged therapy to avoid hyperkalaemia.

Nitroimidazoles

These agents are active against anaerobic bacteria and some pathogenic protozoa. The most widely used drug is **metronidazole** (Fig. 8.5). Others include **tinidazole** and **nimorazole.** After

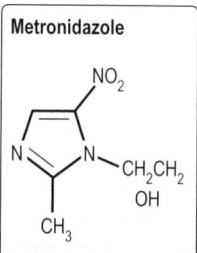

Fig. 8.5 The structure of metronidazole, a nitroimidazole.

reduction of their 'nitro' group to a nitrosohydroxyl amino group by microbial enzymes, nitroimidazoles cause strand breaks in microbial DNA.

Metronidazole plays a major role in the treatment of anaerobic bacterial infections, particularly those due to *Bacteroides* spp. It is also used prophylactically in colonic surgery. It may be given orally, by suppository (well absorbed and cheap) or intravenously (more expensive). It is also the treatment of choice for mild *C. difficile* infection, amoebiasis, giardiasis and infection with *Trichomonas vaginalis*.

Nitroimidazoles can produce a disulfiram-like reaction with ethanol and enhance the anticoagulant effect of warfarin; patients should be warned not to drink alcohol while taking them. They are tumorigenic in animals and mutagenic for bacteria, although carcinogenicity has not been described in humans. They cause a metallic taste and polyneuropathy with prolonged use. High-dose regimens should be avoided in pregnancy and during breast-feeding, unless the benefit is deemed to outweigh the risk.

Other antibiotics
Clindamycin

This is not widely used because of its strong association with *C. difficile* infection. It is active against Gram-positive cocci, including some penicillin-resistant staphylococci, and is a useful agent for severe streptococcal or staphylococcal cellulitis. It has the added effect of inhibiting staphylococcal toxic shock syndrome toxin 1 (TSST-1) and alpha toxin production, and has a role in infections caused by *S. aureus*-secreting Panton Valentine leukocidin (PVL). It is also active against anaerobes, especially *Bacteroides*. It is well concentrated in bone and used for osteomyelitis.

Nitrofurantoin

This is an old agent that is still widely used as an oral treatment for uncomplicated UTI. It is active against almost all the common urinary pathogens, with the exception of *Proteus* spp., and resistance remains rare. It is extensively metabolized, with only about 20% of the active component excreted in the urine, which makes it unsuitable for complicated UTI or pyelonephritis. Nausea is the main side-effect and there are rare reports of peripheral neuropathy, usually in patients with pre-existing renal impairment. It can cause haemolysis in patients with glucose-6-phosphate dehydrogenase deficiency and should be avoided in this group.

Mupirocin

Mupirocin prevents bacterial RNA and protein synthesis. It is only used topically, mainly for the nasal eradication of *S. aureus*, including MRSA, but can also be employed for minor skin infections and

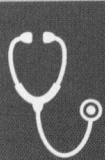

treatment of peritoneal dialysis catheter site infection. High-level resistance to mupirocin in MRSA due to plasmid-encoded MupA may lead to failure of topical therapies.

Fosfomycin

This is a relatively old antibiotic that has been used in some European countries for many years. It inhibits bacterial peptidoglycan biosynthesis. It requires a functional sugar transport system (glucose-6-phosphate) for uptake by Enterobacterales, thus requiring modifications to standard susceptibility testing methods. It is active against many Gram-positive organisms and *E. coli*, but many other Gram-negative bacteria have been slow to produce an enzyme (FosA) that is able to destroy the drug. The clinical significance of FosA-mediated resistance is unclear. Fosfomycin retains activity against many ESBL-producing *E. coli* and is therefore the subject of renewed interest. It is increasingly used in the UK, particularly for resistant UTI, and is available in oral and intravenous formulations.

Rifaximin

This is a rifamycin with poor gastrointestinal absorption. It is used in portosystemic encephalopathy (see p. 1297) and the prevention of travellers' diarrhoea; it may be of short-term benefit in irritable bowel syndrome.

Treatment of infection caused by multidrug-resistant organisms

Meticillin-resistant *Staphylococcus aureus*

Meticillin resistance is mediated through changes in the cell-wall penicillin-binding protein 2a, an enzyme that catalyses cell-wall cross-linking, which meticillin or flucloxacillin is unable to inhibit. In the UK, most MRSA infections are healthcare-associated. Uncomplicated infections are typically associated with intravascular catheters or devices; in these cases, line removal (source control) should form part of management. In approximately 5% of cases, infection may disseminate, with haematogenous spread to bones, joints and heart valves.

For decades, the treatment drug of choice has been intravenous **vancomycin**; pre-levels of 15–20 mg/L are required for maximum therapeutic efficacy. Renal function should be closely monitored, as vancomycin is nephrotoxic. Treatment is for a minimum of 2 weeks and, for complicated infection, the addition of a second agent should be considered (e.g. fusidic acid, rifampicin, gentamicin or ciprofloxacin). There is, however, no good evidence that this improves clinical outcomes: recently, a large UK trial of adjunctive rifampicin demonstrated no clinical benefit in staphylococcal bacteraemic infection.

An alternative to intravenous vancomycin is the oxazolidanone **linezolid**. The major advantage is that it can be taken orally and is not nephrotoxic. However, it can cause reversible myelosuppression, in particular thrombocytopenia, and so weekly full blood count monitoring is required. In the longer term, there is a smaller risk of peripheral neuropathy or optic neuritis.

While MRSA is primarily seen in the UK in association with intravascular devices, in the USA it has been described as frequently causing severe skin and soft tissue infections. Empirical treatment therefore includes antibiotics such as linezolid, clindamycin or co-trimoxazole.

Vancomycin-resistant enterococci

Vancomycin resistance in enterococci is mediated through changes in the peptidoglycan precursor from D-Ala-D-Ala to D-Ala-D-Lac, preventing glycopeptides (vancomycin and teicoplanin) binding to these cell-wall precursors and inhibiting cell-wall synthesis. Most infections caused by vancomycin-resistant enterococci (VRE) are healthcare-associated. This organism is of low virulence but is difficult to treat, and with the exception of infective endocarditis, infection with VRE is generally of low consequence. More common sites of infection include the urinary and biliary tracts. The only oral treatment is **linezolid**; intravenous options include **daptomycin** and **tigecycline**.

Carbapenem-resistant *Pseudomonas*

The most common cause of carbapenem resistance in *Pseudomonas* is increased expression of efflux systems or increased impermeability due to decreased porin expression. Most commonly, carbapenem-resistant *Pseudomonas* causes device-related infections or infection of the lower respiratory tract. If disease is mono-resistant, treatment options include **ciprofloxacin**, **gentamicin**, **ceftazidine** and **piperacillin/tazobactam** (tazocin). Often, however, isolates are multidrug-resistant, with the exception of intravenous **colistin**. This needs to be dosed appropriately and pre-drug levels should be taken, to minimize the risk of both nephrotoxicity and neurotoxicity. More recently, ceftolazone/tazobactam has become available, and is effective against multidrug-resistant *Pseudomonas*, as well as less toxic than colistin.

Extended-spectrum β-lactamase-producing Enterobacteriaceae

ESBLs are inactivating enzymes that confer resistance to most β-lactam antibiotics, including penicillins, cephalosporins and aztreonam. In the UK, ESBL-producing *E. coli* of the CTX-M-15 type suddenly emerged in 2004 and approximately 15% of all *E. coli* bacteraemic isolates are now ESBL producers. Other Enterobacteriaceae, most commonly *K. pneumoniae*, can also be ESBL producers. The most common sites of infection for ESBL-producing Enterobacteriaceae are the urinary tract and, less frequently, the gastrointestinal or hepatobiliary tract. For both organisms, these isolates are often multidrug-resistant, and may express resistance to antibiotics such as ciprofloxacin, co-trimoxazole and gentamicin. The mainstay of treatment is a carbapenem, either intravenous **meropenem** three times daily or, if OPAT is considered, once-daily intravenous **ertapenem**. Potential carbapenem-sparing options include intravenous **amikacin** or intravenous **temocillin** but the suitability of these choices depends on sites of infection. Even when the infecting organism is shown to be susceptible to penicillins by minimum inhibitory concentration (MIC), a carbapenem should be used, as piperacillin/tazobactam has been found to be inferior to carbapenems in a recent trial.

Carbapenem-resistant Enterobacteriaceae

Carbapenem resistance is mediated through the production of enzymes that inactivate carbapenems, together with most β-lactams, and are therefore called carbapenemases. Like ESBL-producing Enterobacteriaceae, carbapenem-resistant Enterobacteriaceae (CRE) most frequently cause UTIs. Worldwide, the five most common types of carbapenemase are *K. pneumoniae* carbapenemases (KPC), New Delhi metallo-β-lactamases (NDM), Verona integron-encoded metallo-β-lactamase (VIM), imipenemase (IMP) metallo-β-lactamase and the oxacillin carbapenemase (OXA). In the UK, the most common CRE types are OXA-48, NDM and

KPC. Carbapenem-resistant isolates with OXA-48 or KPC production may be susceptible to quinolones and aminoglycosides, and so other commonly used therapeutic options are available for treatment. Resistance to ceftazidine/avibactam in KPC and OXA-48 producers has been reported but remains rare. Isolates that produce NDMs tend to be pan-resistant, with the exception of **colistin**, **fosfomycin** and **tigecycline**. Susceptibility testing for each of these drugs against CRE isolates is not well standardized. Genetic analysis suggests that *Klebsiella* is intrinsically resistant to fosfomycin and that heteroresistance to colistin and tigecycline can emerge during therapy. In these circumstances, colistin is the mainstay of treatment, with tigecycline and sometimes fosfomycin used as adjuvant therapy, depending on susceptibility data. Meropenem, given as a bolus or an infusion, is also of benefit as targeted therapy when organisms demonstrate intermediate sensitivity, as evidenced by a MIC of 8–16 mg/L. An understanding of the mechanisms of CRE production is therefore helpful when choosing different treatment options.

Further reading

Tängdén T, Ramos Martín V, Felton TW et al. The role of infection models and PK/PD modelling for optimising care of critically ill patients with severe infections. *Intensive Care Med* 2017; 43:1021–1032.

http://www.eucast.org *European Committee on Antimicrobial Susceptibility Testing.*

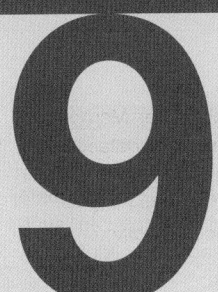

9

Water balance, fluids and electrolytes

M. Magdi Yaqoob and Kieran McCafferty

CORE SKILLS AND KNOWLEDGE

Learning about fluid and electrolyte disorders and acid–base physiology can be a daunting experience for medical students and practising physicians alike. However, these disorders form some of the most common presentations to hospital and may complicate a wide range of other conditions, and so all doctors need to be confident when approaching them.

This chapter reviews the physiology that underpins normal fluid, electrolyte and acid–base balance, and discusses disorders of blood chemistry caused by dietary factors, underlying medical conditions, and medical treatments. These imbalances may be acute or chronic, may occur with varying degrees of severity, and may or may not be partially compensated by the body's regulatory mechanisms.

Key skills to master for undergraduates include:
- comprehensively assessing a patient's fluid status and gaining confidence in prescribing intravenous fluids and diuretics appropriately
- developing an appropriate diagnostic approach to abnormalities of common electrolytes including sodium and potassium
- understanding the implications of an abnormal blood pH and diagnosing the common causes of acidosis and alkalosis.

These skills can be best learned by experience – particularly in assessing patients presenting to the hospital emergency department or who have been admitted to critical care units. Take the opportunity to review patients' fluid balance charts on ward rounds and try (with supervision) to practise prescribing intravenous fluids appropriately. Review the results of blood gas analyses and work through any abnormalities shown.

CLINICAL SKILLS FOR WATER BALANCE, FLUIDS AND ELECTROLYTES

Assessing a patient's fluid status is a key skill for all doctors, requiring key clinical skills in history-taking (**Box 9.1**), examination (figure at bottom of this page), and data interpretation (**Box 9.2**). Many patients are hypovolaemic on admission to hospital as a result of acute illness. The algorithm on page 182 helps guide decision-making regarding intravenous fluid therapy in such patients. Others will exhibit signs of increased extracellular volume and require diuretic therapy (see p. 173).

Assessing a patient's fluid status

Box 9.1 Clues to volume status in the history

	Increased extracellular volume	Decreased extracellular volume
Symptoms	Peripheral oedema Breathlessness on exercise Orthopnoea Paroxysmal nocturnal dyspnoea	Thirst Dizziness
Medical history	Heart failure Cirrhosis Advanced chronic kidney disease Intravenous fluid administration	Recent diarrhoea or vomiting Symptoms suggesting sepsis Use of diuretics

Box 9.2 Clues to volume status on basic investigations

Evidence for increased extracellular volume
- 'Haemodilution': fall in blood haemoglobin concentration and packed cell volume (haematocrit)
- Fluid overload on chest X-ray (see p. 928)
- Evidence of volume overload or cardiac dysfunction on transthoracic echocardiogram

Evidence for decreased extracellular volume
- 'Haemoconcentration': rise in blood haemoglobin and packed cell volume (haematocrit)
- Acute kidney injury (see p. 1387)
- Disproportionate rise in serum urea compared with serum creatinine
- Rise in serum sodium and osmolality
- Concentrated urine: specific gravity (measured on dipstick) >1.025

Clues to volume status on clinical examination

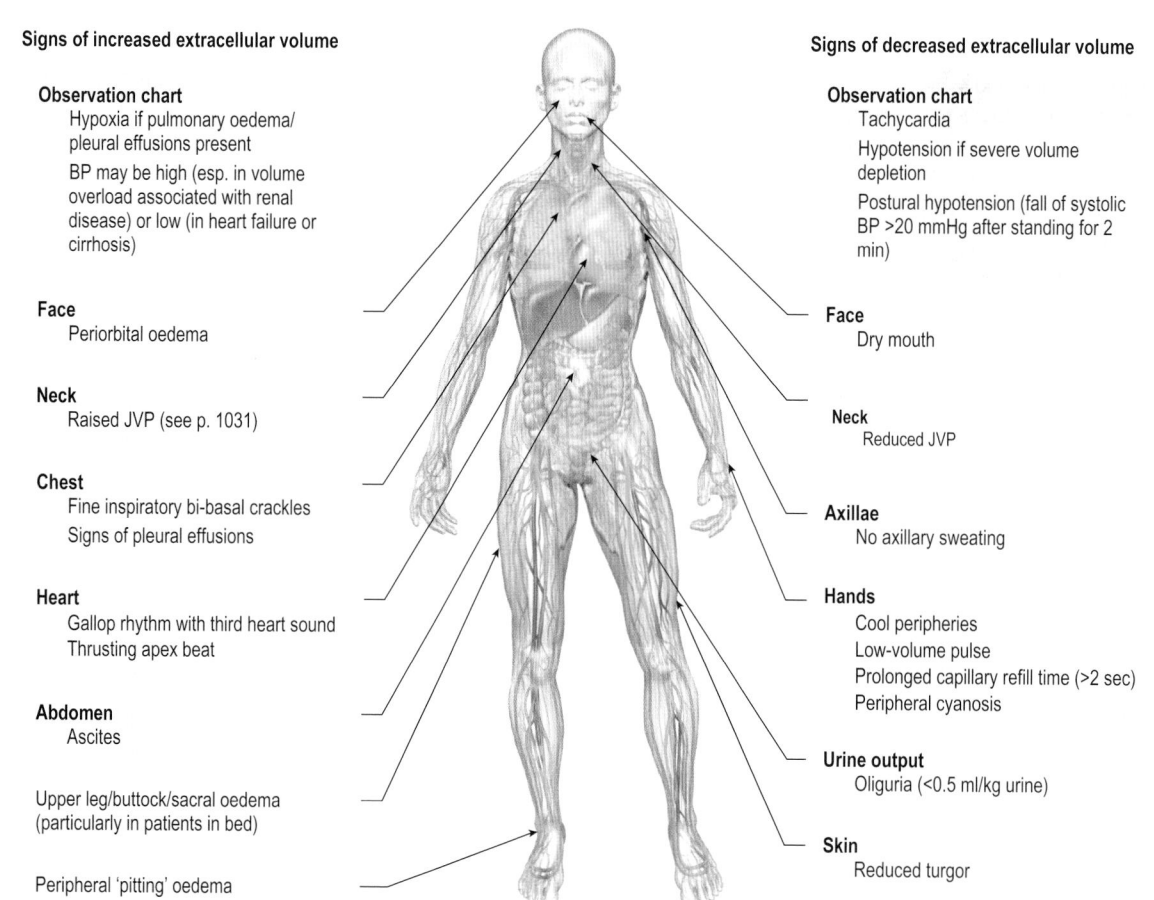

Signs of increased extracellular volume

Observation chart
Hypoxia if pulmonary oedema/pleural effusions present
BP may be high (esp. in volume overload associated with renal disease) or low (in heart failure or cirrhosis)

Face
Periorbital oedema

Neck
Raised JVP (see p. 1031)

Chest
Fine inspiratory bi-basal crackles
Signs of pleural effusions

Heart
Gallop rhythm with third heart sound
Thrusting apex beat

Abdomen
Ascites

Upper leg/buttock/sacral oedema (particularly in patients in bed)

Peripheral 'pitting' oedema

Signs of decreased extracellular volume

Observation chart
Tachycardia
Hypotension if severe volume depletion
Postural hypotension (fall of systolic BP >20 mmHg after standing for 2 min)

Face
Dry mouth

Neck
Reduced JVP

Axillae
No axillary sweating

Hands
Cool peripheries
Low-volume pulse
Prolonged capillary refill time (>2 sec)
Peripheral cyanosis

Urine output
Oliguria (<0.5 ml/kg urine)

Skin
Reduced turgor

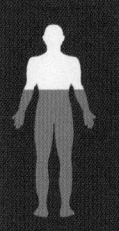

Assessing acid-base disturbance

Arterial or venous blood gas analysis is readily carried out in most hospitals using table-top blood gas analysers (**Fig. 9.1**), which measure:

- blood pH
- partial pressures of carbon dioxide (PCO_2) and oxygen (PO_2)
- calculated base excess (BE) and bicarbonate (HCO_3^-)
- blood electrolytes including sodium and potassium concentrations
- other molecules including glucose and lactate.

This information is vital in assessing respiratory failure, critical illness (failure to maintain blood pH in the normal range is often a poor prognostic marker) as well as chronic disorders affecting acid–base homeostasis.

A stepwise approach to interpreting blood gas analyses is shown in **Fig. 9.2**. It is always worth going through a blood gas analysis report fully, describing all the abnormalities present, before pulling the different abnormalities together into a complete description.

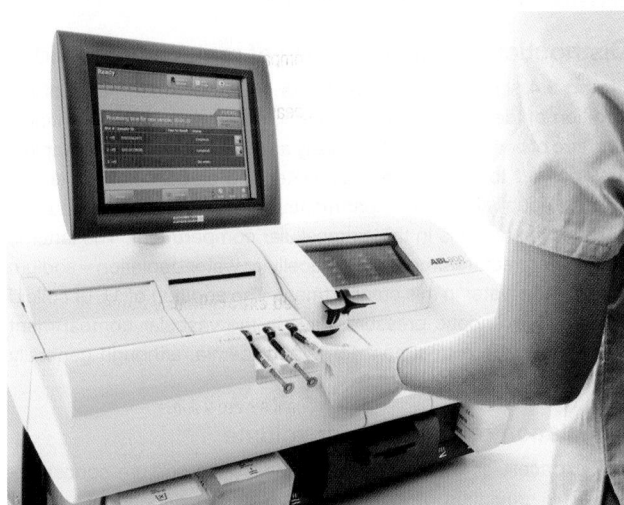

Fig. 9.1 The ABL800FLEX blood gas analyser. (*From Al-Shaikh B, Stacey SG. Essentials of Equipment in Anaesthesia, Critical Care and Peri-Operative Medicine, 5th edn. Edinburgh: Elsevier, 2019, Fig. 13.5, courtesy Radiometer Ltd.*)

1: What is the blood pH?

- <7.35 constitutes acidaemia
- >7.45 constitutes alkalaemia
- 7.35–7.45 may be normal, or may represent full correction of an underlying abnormality by a compensatory mechanism

↓

2: What is the respiratory component?

- PCO_2>6.0 kPa constitutes **respiratory acidosis**
- PCO_2<4.5 kPa constitutes **respiratory alkalosis**

↓

3: What is the metabolic component?

- HCO_3^-<22 mmol/L constitutes **metabolic acidosis**
- HCO_3^->28 mmol/L constitutes **metabolic alkalosis**

If metabolic acidosis is present, use the available electrolytes to calculate the serum **anion gap** (see p. XXX), which may be normal or high

↓

4: Is there evidence of respiratory failure?

- Type 1 respiratory failure: PO_2 <8.0 kPa with PCO_2<6.0 kPa
- Type 2 respiratory failure: PO_2 <8.0 kPa with PCO_2>6.0 kPa

↓

5: What other information is available?

Modern blood gas analysers may offer a range of other useful diagnostic tests:

- Raised serum lactate implies **lactic acidosis**
- Raised glucose in a type 1 diabetic may suggest **diabetic ketoacidosis**
- Raised creatinine may imply metabolic acidosis due to **renal failure**

↓

Bring it all together:

- Determine the primary abnormality present, which will almost always be the one driving an abnormal pH – it is generally impossible to 'overcompensate', although if the pH is normal it can occasionally be more complicated to determine which is the primary and which the compensatory process

- It is possible (and not uncommon) for different primary abnormalities to coexist, e.g. combined respiratory and metabolic acidosis, particularly in severely unwell patients

- Try to determine the cause of any primary abnormality identified, using lists of common causes or diagnostic algorithms based on additional tests, e.g. urinary chloride in metabolic alkalosis

- Always think about the need for emergency management: an abnormal pH always implies a failure of physiology, which may require urgent corrective measures

Fig. 9.2 Stepwise approach to interpreting blood gas analysis.

WATER AND ELECTROLYTES

In normal healthy people, the total body water constitutes 50–60% of lean body weight in men and 45–50% in women. In a healthy 70 kg male, total body water is approximately 42 L. This is contained in three major compartments:

- intracellular fluid (28 L, about 35% of lean body weight)
- extracellular – the interstitial fluid that bathes the cells (9.4 L, about 12%)
- plasma (also extracellular) (4.6 L, about 4–5%).

In addition, small amounts of water are contained in bone, dense connective tissue and epithelial secretions, such as the digestive secretions and cerebrospinal fluid (CSF).

The intracellular and interstitial fluids are separated by the cell membrane; the interstitial fluid and plasma are separated by the capillary wall (**Fig. 9.3**). In the absence of solute, water molecules move randomly and in equal numbers in either direction across a semipermeable membrane. However, if solutes are added to one side of the membrane, the intermolecular cohesive forces reduce the activity of the water molecules. As a result, water tends to stay in the solute-containing compartment because there is less free diffusion across the membrane. This ability to hold water in the compartment can be measured as the osmotic pressure.

Osmotic pressure

Osmotic pressure is the primary determinant of the distribution of water among the three major compartments. The concentrations of the major solutes in the compartments differ, each having one solute that is primarily limited to that compartment and therefore determines its osmotic pressure:

- The **intracellular fluid** contains mainly potassium (K^+) (most intracellular Mg^{2+} is bound and osmotically inactive).
- In the extracellular compartment, Na^+ salts predominate in the **interstitial fluid**, and proteins in the plasma.

Regulation of the plasma volume is somewhat more complicated because of the tendency of the plasma proteins to hold water in the vascular space by an oncotic effect that is partly counterbalanced by the hydrostatic pressure in the capillaries that is generated by

cardiac contraction (see **Fig. 9.3**). The composition of intracellular and extracellular fluids is shown in **Box 9.3**.

Osmotically active solutes cannot freely leave their compartment. The capillary wall, for example, is relatively impermeable to plasma proteins, and the cell membrane is 'impermeable' to Na^+ and K^+ because the Na^+/K^+-adenosine triphosphatase (ATPase) pump largely restricts Na^+ to the extracellular fluid and K^+ to the intracellular fluid. By contrast, Na^+ freely crosses the capillary wall and achieves similar concentrations in the interstitium and plasma; as a result, it does not contribute to fluid distribution between these compartments. Similarly, urea crosses both the capillary wall and the cell membrane, and is osmotically inactive. Thus, the retention of urea in renal failure does not alter the distribution of the total body water.

Body Na^+ stores are the primary determinant of the extracellular fluid volume. Thus, the extracellular volume – and therefore tissue perfusion – are maintained by appropriate alterations in Na^+ excretion. For example, if Na^+ intake is increased, the extra Na^+ will initially be added to the extracellular fluid. The associated increase in extracellular osmolality will cause water to move out of the cells, leading to extracellular volume expansion. Balance is restored by excretion of the excess Na^+ in the urine.

Distribution of different types of replacement fluid

Figure 9.4 shows the relative effects on the compartments of the addition of identical volumes of water, saline and colloid solutions. One litre of water given intravenously as 5% glucose (which is rapidly metabolized to generate energy, water and carbon dioxide) is distributed equally into all compartments, whereas the same amount of 0.9% saline remains in the extracellular compartment. The latter is thus the correct treatment for extracellular water depletion – sodium keeping the water in this compartment. The addition of 1 L of colloid with its high oncotic pressure stays in the vascular compartment and used to be a treatment for hypovolaemia, although generally 0.9% saline is now used.

Regulation of extracellular volume

The extracellular volume is determined by the sodium concentration. The regulation of extracellular volume is dependent upon a tight control of sodium balance, which is exerted by normal kidneys (**Fig. 9.5**). Renal Na^+ excretion varies directly with the effective circulating volume. In a 70-kg man, plasma fluid constitutes one-third of extracellular volume (4.6 L); of this, 85% (3.9 L) lies in the venous circulation and only 15% (0.7 L) resides in the arteries.

The fullness of the arterial vascular compartment (**effective arterial blood volume**, EABV) is the primary determinant of renal

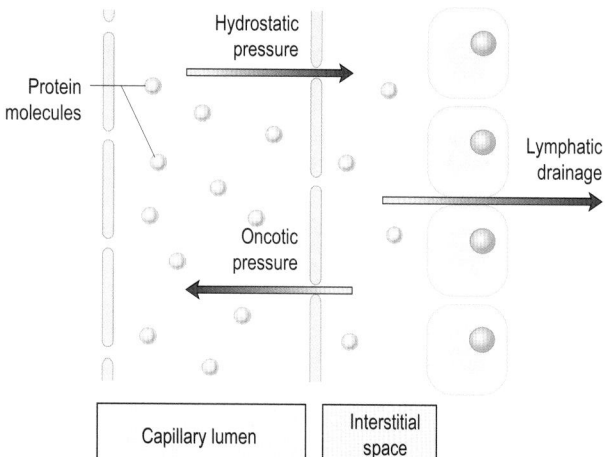

Fig. 9.3 Distribution of water between the vascular and extravascular (interstitial) spaces. This is determined by the equilibrium between hydrostatic pressure, which tends to force fluid out of the capillaries, and oncotic pressure, which acts to retain fluid within the vessel. The net flow of fluid outwards is balanced by 'suction' of fluid into the lymphatics, which returns it to the bloodstream. Similar principles govern the volume of the peritoneal and pleural spaces.

	Plasma	Interstitial fluid	Intracellular fluid
Na⁺	142	144	10
K⁺	4	4	160
Ca²⁺	2.5	2.5	1.5
Mg²⁺	1.0	0.5	13
Cl⁻	102	114	2
HCO₃⁻	26	30	8
PO₄²⁻	1.0	1.0	57
SO₄²⁻	0.5	0.5	10
Organic acid	3	4	3
Protein	16	0	55

Box 9.3 Electrolyte composition of intracellular and extracellular fluids (mmol/L)

sodium and water excretion: that is, the **effective circulatory volume** for the purposes of body fluid homeostasis.

The fullness of the arterial compartment depends upon a relationship between cardiac output and peripheral arterial resistance. Thus, diminished EABV is initiated by a fall in cardiac output or a fall in peripheral arterial resistance (an increase in the holding capacity of the arterial vascular tree). When the EABV is expanded, the urinary Na^+ excretion is increased and can exceed 100 mmol/L. By contrast, the urine can be rendered virtually free of Na^+ in the presence of EABV depletion and normal renal function.

These changes in Na^+ excretion can result from alterations both in the filtered load, determined primarily by the glomerular filtration rate (GFR), and in tubular reabsorption, which is affected by multiple factors. In general, changes in tubular reabsorption constitute the main adaptive response to fluctuations in the effective circulating volume. How this occurs can be appreciated from **Box 9.4** and **Fig. 9.6**, and from **Fig. 36.3**, which depicts the sites and determinants of segmental Na^+ reabsorption. Although the loop of Henle and distal tubules make a major overall contribution to net Na^+ handling, transport in these segments primarily varies with the amount of Na^+ delivered; that is, reabsorption is flow-dependent. In comparison, the neurohumoral regulation of Na^+ reabsorption according to body needs occurs primarily in the proximal tubules and collecting ducts.

A Water

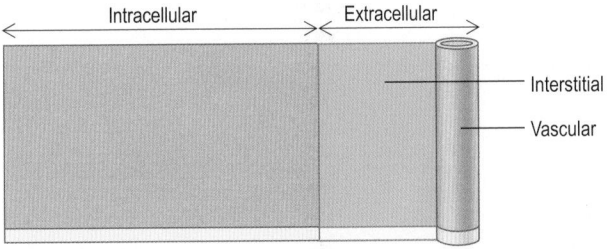

B Saline

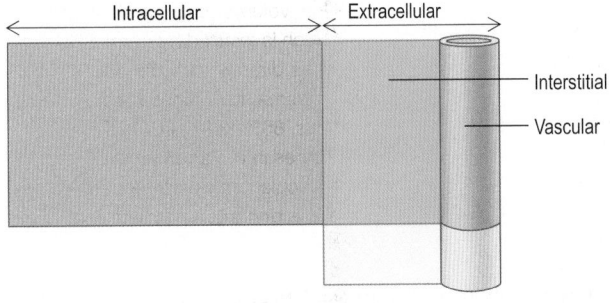

C Colloid

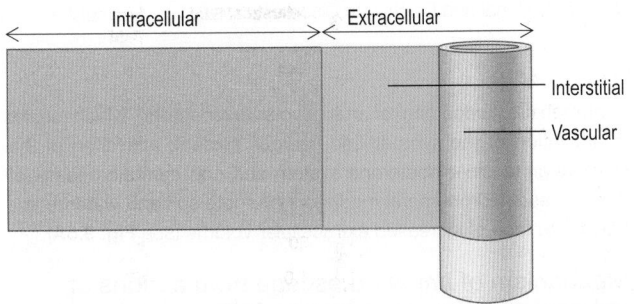

Fig. 9.4 Relative effects of the addition of 1 L of **(A)** water, **(B)** saline 0.9% and **(C)** a colloid solution. See text for a fuller explanation.

The diseases associated with malfunction of each section of the tubule are shown in **Box 9.5**.

Neurohumoral regulation of extracellular volume

This is mediated by volume receptors that sense changes in the EABV rather than alterations in the sodium concentration. These receptors are distributed in both the renal and cardiovascular tissues.

- **Intrarenal receptors.** Receptors in the walls of the afferent glomerular arterioles respond, via the juxtaglomerular apparatus, to changes in renal perfusion, and control the activity of the renin–angiotensin–aldosterone system (see p. 1347). In addition, sodium concentration in the distal tubule and sympathetic nerve activity alter renin release from the juxtaglomerular cells. Prostaglandins I_2 and E_2 are also generated within the kidney in response to angiotensin II, acting to maintain GFR and sodium and water excretion, and modulating the sodium-retaining effect of this hormone.
- **Extrarenal receptors.** These are located in the vascular tree in the left atrium and major thoracic veins, and in the carotid sinus body and aortic arch. These volume receptors respond to a slight reduction in effective circulating volume and this results in increased sympathetic nerve activity and a rise in catecholamines. In addition, volume receptors in the cardiac atria control the release of a powerful natriuretic hormone – atrial natriuretic peptide (ANP) – from granules located in the atrial walls (see p. 1346).

High-pressure arterial receptors (carotid, aortic arch, juxtaglomerular apparatus) predominate over low-pressure volume receptors in volume control in mammals.

Aldosterone and possibly ANP are responsible for day-to-day variations in Na^+ excretion, through their respective ability to augment and diminish Na^+ reabsorption in the collecting ducts.

- A **salt load**, for example, leads to an increase in the effective circulatory and extracellular volume, raising both renal perfusion pressure, and atrial and arterial filling pressure. The increase in the renal perfusion pressure reduces the secretion of renin, and subsequently that of angiotensin II and aldosterone (see **Fig. 36.6**), whereas the rise in atrial and arterial filling pressure increases the release of ANP. These factors combine to reduce Na^+ reabsorption in the collecting duct, thereby promoting excretion of excess Na^+.
- By contrast, in patients with a **low Na^+** intake or in those who become volume-depleted as a result of vomiting or diarrhoea, the ensuing decrease in effective volume enhances the activity of the renin–angiotensin–aldosterone system and reduces the secretion of ANP. The net effect is enhanced Na^+ reabsorption in the collecting ducts, leading to a fall in Na^+ excretion. This increases the extracellular volume towards normal.

With **more marked hypovolaemia**, a decrease in GFR leads to an increase in proximal and thin ascending limb Na^+ reabsorption, which contributes to Na^+ retention. This is brought about by enhanced sympathetic activity acting directly on the kidneys and indirectly by stimulating the secretion of renin/angiotensin II (see **Fig. 9.5B**) and non-osmotic release of antidiuretic hormone (ADH), also called vasopressin. The pressure natriuresis phenomenon may be the final defence against changes in the effective circulating volume. Marked persistent hypovolaemia leads to systemic hypotension and increased salt and water absorption in the proximal tubules and ascending limb of Henle. This process is partly mediated by changes in renal interstitial hydrostatic pressure and local prostaglandin and nitric oxide production. Recurrent episodes of hypovolaemia may, over time, lead to chronic kidney disease (CKD), such as in the recently described syndrome Mesoamerican nephropathy, where recurrent episodes of

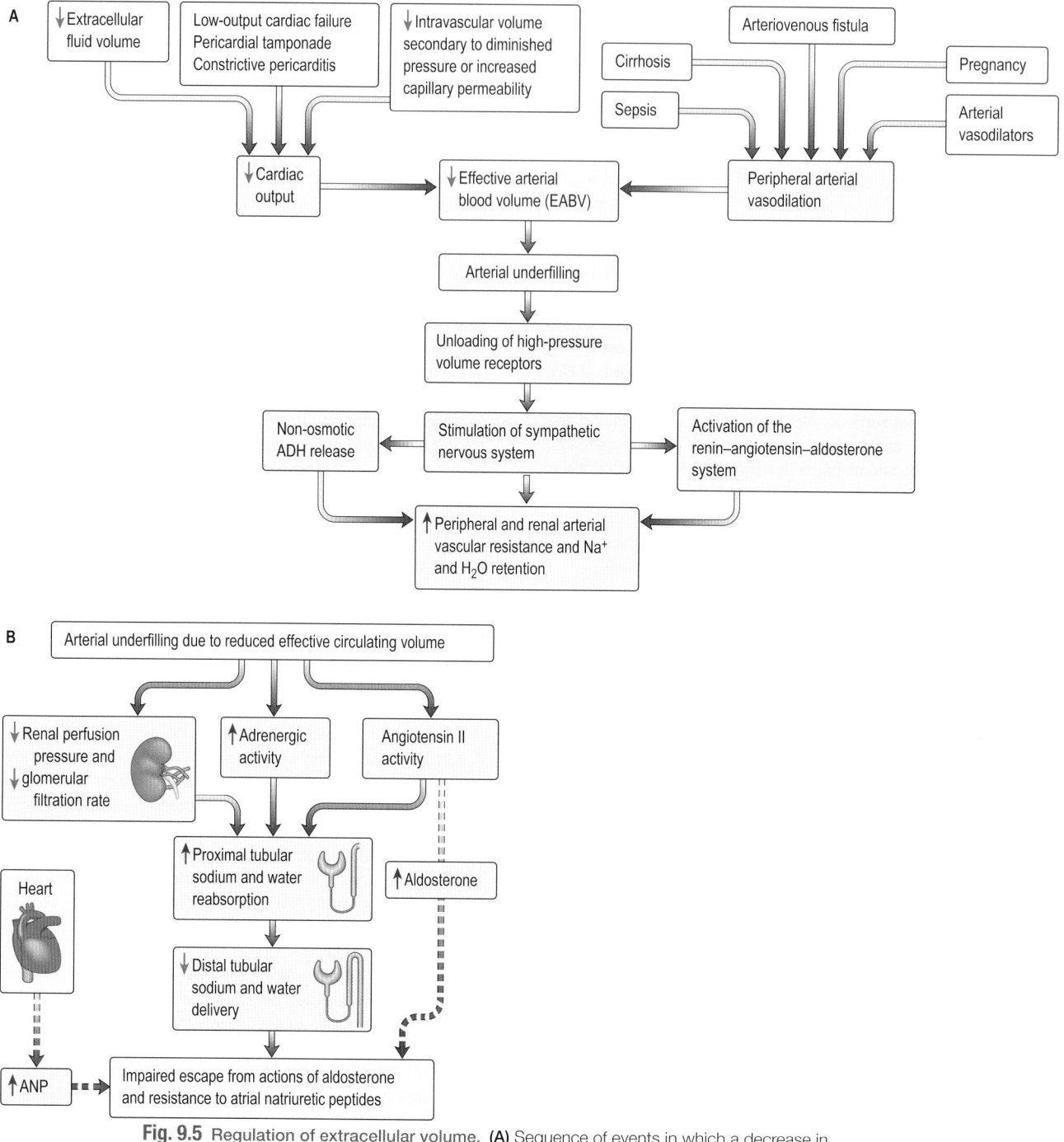

Fig. 9.5 Regulation of extracellular volume. **(A)** Sequence of events in which a decrease in cardiac output or peripheral arterial dilation initiates renal sodium and water retention. **(B)** Mechanism of impaired escape from the actions of aldosterone and resistance to atrial natriuretic peptides (ANP). ADH, antidiuretic hormone. *(Modified with permission from Schrier RW. Renal and Electrolyte Disorders, 7th edn. Philadelphia: Lippincott Williams & Wilkins, 2010.)*

heat-stress in young to middle-aged male agricultural workers along the Pacific coast in Central America is thought to be a cause.

Volume regulation in oedematous conditions

Sodium and water are retained despite increased extracellular volume in oedematous conditions such as cardiac failure, hepatic cirrhosis and hypoalbuminaemia. Here the principal mediator of salt and water retention is the concept of arterial underfilling due to either reduced cardiac output or diminished peripheral arterial resistance. Arterial underfilling in these settings leads to reduction of pressure

or stretch (i.e. 'unloading' of arterial volume receptors), which results in activation of the sympathetic nervous system, activation of the renin–angiotensin–aldosterone system and non-osmotic release of ADH. These neurohumoral mediators promote salt and water retention in the face of increased extracellular volume (see **Fig. 9.5A**).

Mechanism of impaired escape from actions of aldosterone and resistance to ANP

Not only is the activity of the renin–angiotensin–aldosterone system increased in oedematous conditions such as cardiac failure, hepatic

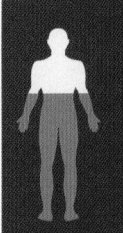
i Box 9.4 Mechanisms of sodium transport in the various nephron segments			
	Filtered Na reabsorbed (%)	**Major mechanisms of luminal Na⁺ entry**	**Major factors regulating transport**
Proximal tubule	60–70	Na^+–H^+ exchange and co-transport of Na^+ with glucose, phosphate and other organic solutes	Angiotensin II Noradrenaline (norepinephrine)
Loop of Henle	20–25	Na^+–K^+–$2Cl^-$ co-transport	Flow Pressure natriuresis mediated by nitric oxide
Distal tubule	5	Na^+–Cl^- co-transport	Flow
Collecting ducts	4	Na^+ channels	Aldosterone Atrial natriuretic peptide

i Box 9.5 Major functions of each section of the tubule and associated diseases		
Site	**Function**	**Diseases associated with this section of nephron**
Proximal convoluted tubule (PCT)	Early PCT: Solute reabsorption: glucose, amino acids, bicarbonate, phosphate, low-molecular-weight proteins Late PCT: Urate secretion/absorption Straight PCT: Secretion of drugs (loop and thiazide diuretics) and drug metabolites	Fanconi's syndrome: failure to reabsorb solutes and low-molecular-weight proteins. Leads to glycosuria, phosphaturia, aminoaciduria and low-molecular-weight proteinuria. May be caused by drugs, myeloma, Wilson's disease and rare genetic diseases Type 2 renal tubular acidosis (see p. 199)
Loop of Henle	Site of counter-current multiplier, which sets up loop, enabling control of final urine concentration	Bartter's syndrome (see p. 187)
Distal convoluted tubule	Involvement in sodium and chloride transport, and calcium and magnesium reabsorption	Gitelman's syndrome (see p. 188) Gordon's syndrome (see p. 189)
Collecting ducts	Na^+ and water reabsorption Secretion of potassium Secretion of bicarbonate or H^+	Liddle's syndrome (see p. 188) Pseudohypoaldosteronism type 1 (see p. 189) Nephrogenic diabetes insipidus: resistance to actions of vasopressin. Leads to large volume of dilute urine with polyuria/polydipsia Syndrome of inappropriate antidiuretic hormone secretion (SIADH; see p. 643) Type 1 renal tubular acidosis (see p. 199)

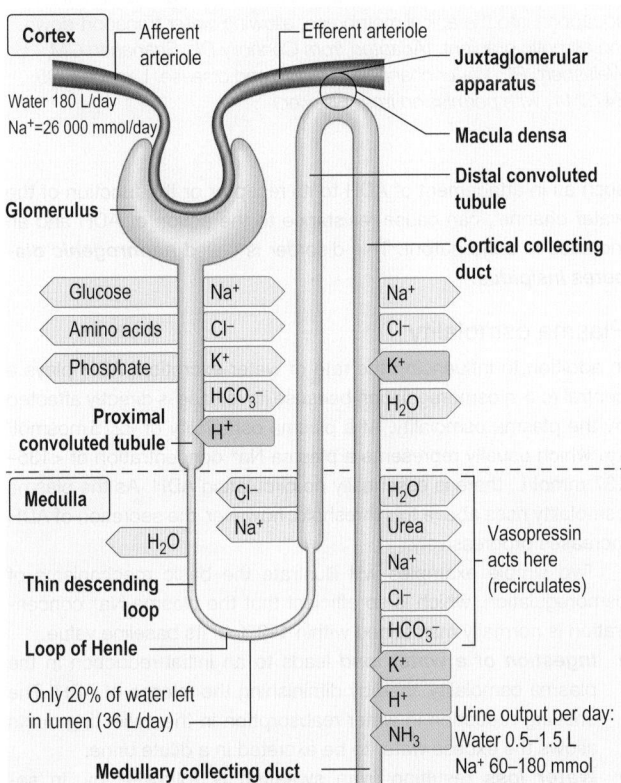

Fig. 9.6 The nephron – electrolyte and water exchange. Some 180 L of water and 26 000 mmol of sodium/day enter the nephrons via the afferent arterioles to the kidneys. Removal or addition of electrolytes results in the excretion of approximately 1 L of water and 60–180 mmol of sodium/day.

This escape from mineralocorticoid-mediated sodium retention explains why oedema is not a characteristic feature of primary hyperaldosteronism. The escape is dependent on an increased delivery of sodium to the site of action of aldosterone in the collecting ducts. The increased distal sodium delivery is achieved by high extracellular volume-mediated arterial overfilling. This suppresses sympathetic activity and angiotensin II generation, and increases cardiac release of ANP with resultant increase in renal perfusion pressure and GFR. The net result of these events is reduced sodium absorption in the proximal tubules and increased distal sodium delivery, which overwhelms the sodium-retaining actions of aldosterone.

In patients with the oedematous conditions described, such as heart failure, escape from the sodium-retaining actions of aldosterone does *not* occur and therefore they continue to retain sodium in response to aldosterone. Accordingly, they have substantial natriuresis when given spironolactone, which blocks mineralocorticoid receptors. Alpha-adrenergic stimulation and elevated angiotensin II increase sodium transport in the proximal tubule, and reduced renal perfusion and GFR further increase sodium absorption from the proximal tubules by presenting less sodium and water in the tubular fluid. Sodium delivery to the distal portion of the nephron, and thus the collecting duct, is reduced. Similarly, increased cardiac ANP

cirrhosis and hypoalbuminaemia, but also the action of aldosterone is more persistent than in normal subjects and patients with primary hyperaldosteronism (Conn's syndrome), who have increased aldosterone secretion (see p. 606).

In normal subjects, high doses of mineralocorticoids initially increase renal sodium retention so that the extracellular volume is increased by 1.5–2 L. However, renal sodium retention then ceases, sodium balance is re-established, and there is no detectable oedema.

release in these conditions requires optimum sodium concentration at the site of its action in the collecting duct for its desired natriuretic effects. Decreased sodium delivery to the collecting duct is therefore the most likely explanation for the persistent aldosterone-mediated sodium retention, absence of escape phenomenon and resistance to natriuretic peptides in these patients (see **Fig. 9.5B**).

Regulation of water excretion

Body water homeostasis is affected by thirst and the urine-concentrating and diluting functions of the kidney. These, in turn, are controlled by intracellular osmoreceptors, principally in the hypothalamus, to some extent by volume receptors in capacitance vessels close to the heart, and via the renin–angiotensin system. Of these, the major and best-understood control is via osmoreceptors. Changes in the plasma Na^+ concentration and osmolality are sensed by osmoreceptors that influence both thirst and the release of ADH (vasopressin) from the supraoptic and paraventricular nuclei of the anterior hypothalamus.

ADH plays a central role in urinary concentration by increasing the water permeability of the normally impermeable cortical and medullary collecting ducts. There are three major G-protein coupled receptors for vasopressin (ADH):

- **V_{1A}** found in vascular smooth muscle cells: activation induces vasoconstriction.
- **V_{1B}** in the anterior pituitary and throughout the brain: this mediates the effect of ADH on the pituitary, leading to adrenocorticotrophic hormone (ACTH) release.
- **V_2** receptors in the principal cells of the kidney distal convoluting tubule and collecting ducts: these mediate the ADH response.

The ability of ADH to increase the urine osmolality is related indirectly to transport in the ascending limb of the loop of Henle, which reabsorbs NaCl without water. This process, which is the primary step in the counter-current mechanism, has two effects: it makes the tubular fluid dilute and the medullary interstitium concentrated. In the absence of ADH, little water is reabsorbed in the collecting ducts, and a dilute urine is excreted. By contrast, the presence of ADH promotes water reabsorption in the collecting ducts down the favourable osmotic gradient between the tubular fluid and the more concentrated interstitium. As a result, there is an increase in urine osmolality and a decrease in urine volume.

The cortical collecting duct has two cell types (see also p. 1343) with very different functions:

- **Principal cells** (about 65%) have sodium and potassium channels in the apical membrane and, as in all sodium-reabsorbing cells, Na^+/K^+-ATPase pumps in the basolateral membrane.
- **Intercalated cells**, in comparison, do not transport NaCl (since they have a lower level of Na^+/K^+-ATPase activity) but play a role in hydrogen and bicarbonate handling and in potassium reabsorption in states of potassium depletion.

The ADH-induced increase in collecting duct water permeability occurs primarily in the principal cells. ADH acts on V_2 (vasopressin) receptors located on the basolateral surface of principal cells, resulting in the activation of adenyl cyclase. This leads to protein kinase activation and to pre-formed cytoplasmic vesicles that contain unique water channels (called aquaporins) moving to, and then being inserted into, the luminal membrane. The water channels span the luminal membrane and permit water movement into the cells down a favourable osmotic gradient (**Fig. 9.7**). This water is then rapidly returned to the systemic circulation across the basolateral membrane. When the ADH effect has worn off, the water channels are removed from the luminal membrane by endocytosis and returned to the cytoplasm. A defect in any step in this pathway,

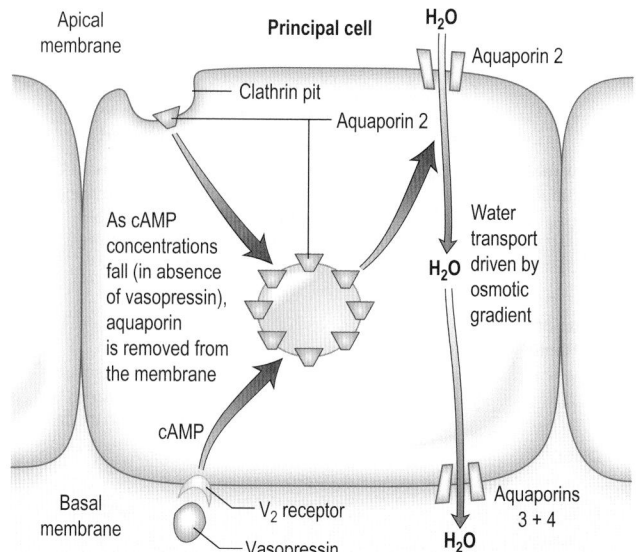

Fig. 9.7 Aquaporin-mediated water transport in the renal collecting duct. Stimulation of the vasopressin 2 receptor causes cyclic adenosine monophosphate (cAMP)-mediated insertion of the aquaporin into the apical membrane, allowing water transport down the osmotic gradient. *(Adapted from Connolly DL, Shanahan CM, Weissberg PL. Water channels in health and disease. Lancet 1996; 347:211, with permission from Elsevier.)*

such as in attachment of ADH to its receptor or the function of the water channel, can cause resistance to the action of ADH and an increase in urine output. This disorder is called **nephrogenic diabetes insipidus**.

Plasma osmolality

In addition to influencing the rate of water excretion, ADH plays a central role in osmoregulation because its release is directly affected by the plasma osmolality. At a plasma osmolality of <275 mosmol/kg, which usually represents a plasma Na^+ concentration of <135–137 mmol/L, there is essentially no circulating ADH. As the plasma osmolality rises above this threshold, however, the secretion of ADH increases progressively.

Two simple examples will illustrate the basic mechanisms of osmoregulation, which is so efficient that the plasma Na^+ concentration is normally maintained within 1–2% of its baseline value.

- **Ingestion of a water load** leads to an initial reduction in the plasma osmolality, thereby diminishing the release of ADH. The ensuing reduction in water reabsorption in the collecting ducts allows the excess water to be excreted in a dilute urine.
- **Water loss** resulting from sweating is followed by, in sequence, a rise in both plasma osmolality and ADH secretion, enhanced water reabsorption, and the appropriate excretion of a small volume of concentrated urine. This renal effect of ADH minimizes further water loss but does not replace the existing water deficit. Thus, optimal osmoregulation requires an increase in water intake, which is mediated by a concurrent stimulation of thirst. The importance of thirst can also be illustrated by studies in patients with central diabetes insipidus, who are deficient in ADH. These patients often complain of marked polyuria, which is caused by the decline in water reabsorption in the collecting ducts. However, they do not typically become hypernatraemic because urinary water loss is offset by the thirst mechanism.

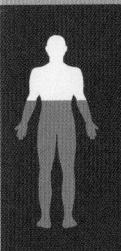

Osmoregulation versus volume regulation

A common misconception is that regulation of the plasma Na⁺ concentration is closely correlated with the regulation of Na⁺ excretion. It is, however, related to volume regulation, which has different sensors and effectors (volume receptors) from those involved in water balance and osmoregulation (osmoreceptors).

The roles of these two pathways should be considered separately when evaluating patients.

- A **water load** is rapidly excreted (in 4–6 h) by inhibition of ADH release so that there is little or no water reabsorption in the collecting ducts. This process is normally so efficient that volume regulation is not affected and there is no change in ANP release or in the activity of the renin–angiotensin–aldosterone system. Thus, a dilute urine is excreted and there is little alteration in the excretion of Na⁺.
- **0.9% saline** administration, by contrast, causes an increase in volume but no change in plasma osmolality. In this setting, ANP secretion is increased, aldosterone secretion is reduced and ADH secretion does not change. The net effect is the appropriate excretion of the excess Na⁺ in a relatively iso-osmotic urine.

In some cases, both volume and osmolality are altered and both pathways are activated. For example, if a person with normal renal function eats salted crisps or peanuts without drinking any water, the excess Na⁺ will increase the plasma osmolality, leading to osmotic water movement out of the cells and increased extracellular volume. The rise in osmolality will stimulate both ADH release and thirst (the main reason why many restaurants and bars supply free salted foods), whereas the hypervolaemia will enhance the secretion of ANP and suppress that of aldosterone. The net effect is increased excretion of Na⁺ without water.

This principle of separate volume and osmoregulatory pathways is also evident in the **syndrome of inappropriate antidiuretic hormone secretion** (**SIADH**). Patients with SIADH (see p. 643) have impaired water excretion and hyponatraemia (dilutional) caused by the persistent presence of ADH. However, the release of ANP and aldosterone is not impaired and, thus, Na⁺ handling remains intact. These findings have implications for the correction of the hyponatraemia in this setting, which initially requires restriction of water intake. ADH is also secreted by non-osmotic stimuli such as stress (e.g. surgery, trauma), markedly reduced effective circulatory volume (e.g. cardiac failure, hepatic cirrhosis), psychiatric disturbance and nausea, irrespective of plasma osmolality. This is mediated by the effects of sympathetic overactivity on supraoptic and paraventricular nuclei. In addition to water retention, ADH release in these conditions promotes vasoconstriction owing to the activation of V₁ₐ (vasopressin) receptors distributed in the vascular smooth muscle cells.

Increased extracellular volume

Increased extracellular volume occurs in numerous disease states. The physical signs depend on the distribution of excess volume and on whether the increase is local or systemic. According to Starling principles, distribution depends on:

- venous tone, which determines the capacitance of the blood compartment and thus hydrostatic pressure
- capillary permeability
- oncotic pressure – mainly dependent on serum albumin
- lymphatic drainage.

Depending on these factors, fluid accumulation may result in expansion of interstitial volume, blood volume or both.

Clinical features

Peripheral oedema is caused by expansion of the extracellular volume by at least 2 L (15%). The ankles are normally the first part of the body to be affected. Oedema may be noted in the face, particularly in the morning, or if the patient is in bed, oedema may accumulate in the sacral area. Expansion of the interstitial volume also causes pulmonary oedema, pleural effusions, pericardial effusion and ascites. Expansion of the blood volume causes a raised jugular venous pressure, cardiomegaly, added heart sounds and basal crackles, as well as a raised arterial blood pressure.

Aetiology

Extracellular volume expansion is due to renal sodium chloride retention. Increased oral salt intake does not normally cause volume expansion because of rapid homeostatic mechanisms that increase salt excretion. However, a rapid intravenous infusion of a large volume of saline will cause volume expansion.

Heart failure

Reduction in cardiac output and the consequent fall in effective circulatory volume and arterial filling lead to activation of the renin–angiotensin–aldosterone system, non-osmotic release of ADH, and increased activity of the renal sympathetic nerves via volume receptors and baroreceptors (see **Fig. 9.5B**). Sympathetic overdrive also indirectly augments ADH and renin–angiotensin–aldosterone response in these conditions. The cumulative effect of these mediators results in increased peripheral and renal arteriolar resistance and water and sodium retention. These factors lead to extracellular volume expansion and increased venous pressure, causing oedema formation.

Hepatic cirrhosis

The mechanism is complex but involves peripheral vasodiltation, due to increased nitric oxide generation, resulting in reduced EABV and arterial filling. This leads to an activation of a chain of events common also to other conditions with marked peripheral vasodilation and heart failure (see **Fig. 9.5**). The cumulative effect results in increased water and sodium retention, and oedema formation.

Nephrotic syndrome

Interstitial oedema is a common clinical finding with hypoalbuminaemia, particularly in the nephrotic syndrome. Expansion of the interstitial compartment is secondary to the accumulation of sodium in the extracellular compartment. This is due to an imbalance between oral (or parenteral) sodium intake and urinary sodium loss, as well as alterations of fluid transfer across capillary walls. The intrarenal site of sodium retention is the cortical collecting duct (CCD), where Na⁺/K⁺-ATPase expression and activity are increased threefold along the basolateral surface (see **Fig. 9.6**). In addition, amiloride-sensitive epithelial sodium channel activity is also increased in the CCD. The renal sodium retention should normally be counterbalanced by increased secretion of sodium in the inner medullary collecting duct, brought about by the release of ANP. This regulatory pathway is altered in patients with nephrotic syndrome by enhanced **kidney-specific** catabolism of cyclic guanosine monophosphate (cGMP, the second messenger for ANP) following phosphodiesterase activation.

Oedema generation was classically attributed to the decrease in plasma oncotic pressure and the subsequent increase in the transcapillary oncotic gradient. However, the oncotic pressure and transcapillary oncotic gradient remain unchanged and the transcapillary hydrostatic pressure gradient is not altered.

The mechanism for oedema seen in nephrotic syndrome is increased capillary hydraulic conductivity (a measure of permeability). In addition, increased circulating ANP can increase capillary hydraulic conductivity by altering the permeability of intercellular junctional complexes. Furthermore, reduction in effective circulatory volume and the consequent fall in cardiac output and arterial filling can lead to a chain of events, as in cardiac failure and cirrhosis (see earlier and **Fig. 9.2**). These factors result in extracellular volume expansion and oedema formation.

Sodium retention

A decreased GFR decreases the renal capacity to excrete sodium. This may be acute, as in the acute nephritic syndrome (see p. 1360), or may occur as part of the presentation of CKD. In end-stage renal failure, extracellular volume is controlled by the balance between salt intake and its removal by dialysis.

Numerous drugs cause renal sodium retention, particularly in patients whose renal function is already impaired:

*   **Oestrogens** cause mild sodium retention, due to a weak aldosterone-like effect. This is the reason for weight gain in the premenstrual phase.
*   **Mineralocorticoids and liquorice** (the latter potentiates the sodium-retaining action of cortisol) have aldosterone-like actions.
*   **Non-steroidal anti-inflammatory drugs (NSAIDs)** cause sodium retention in the presence of activation of the renin–angiotensin–aldosterone system by heart failure, in cirrhosis and in renal artery stenosis.
*   **Thiazolidinediones (TZDs**; see p. 718) are widely used to treat type 2 diabetes. Their mechanism of action is attributed to binding and activation of the peroxisome proliferator-activated receptor gamma (PPAR-γ) system. PPARs are nuclear transcription factors, essential to the control of energy metabolism, which are modulated via binding with tissue-specific fatty acid metabolites. Of the three PPAR isoforms, γ has been extensively studied and is expressed at high levels in adipose and liver tissues, macrophages, pancreatic β cells and principal cells of the collecting duct. These drugs have been associated with salt and water retention and are contraindicated in patients with heart failure. TZD-induced oedema is also due to upregulation of epithelial Na transporter channel (ENaC) but by different pathways. The diuretics of choice for TZD-induced oedema are amiloride and triamterene.

Substantial amounts of sodium and water may accumulate in the body without clinically obvious oedema or evidence of raised venous pressure. In particular, several litres may accumulate in the pleural space or as ascites; these spaces are then referred to as 'third spaces'. Bone may also act as a 'sink' for sodium and water.

Other causes of oedema

*   Initiation of insulin treatment for type 1 diabetes and re-feeding after malnutrition are both associated with the development of transient oedema. The mechanism is complex but involves upregulation of ENaC in the principal cell of the collecting duct. This transporter is amiloride-sensitive, which makes amiloride or triamterene the diuretic of choice in insulin-induced oedema.
*   Oedema may result from increased capillary pressure owing to relaxation of pre-capillary arterioles. The best example is the peripheral oedema caused by dihydropyridine calcium-channel blockers such as amlodipine, which affects up to 10% of patients. Oedema is usually resolved by stopping the offending drug.
*   Oedema is also caused by raised interstitial oncotic pressure as a result of increased capillary permeability to proteins. This can occur as part of a rare complement-deficiency syndrome; with therapeutic use of interleukin 2 in cancer chemotherapy; or in ovarian hyperstimulation syndrome (see p. 632).

Idiopathic oedema

This tends to occur in women without heart failure, hypoalbuminaemia, and renal or endocrine disease. Oedema is intermittent and often worse in the premenstrual phase. The condition remits after the menopause. Patients complain of swelling of the face, hands, breasts and thighs, and a feeling of being bloated. Sodium retention during the day and increased sodium excretion during recumbency are characteristic; an abnormal fall in plasma volume on standing, caused by increased capillary permeability to proteins, may be the cause of this. The oedema may respond to diuretics but returns when they are stopped. A similar syndrome of diuretic-dependent sodium retention can be caused by abuse of diuretics – for instance, as part of an attempt to lose weight – and the syndrome was described before diuretics were introduced for clinical use, so the cause remains unclear.

Local increase in oedema

This does not reflect disturbances of extracellular volume control *per se* but can cause clinical confusion. Examples are ankle oedema due to venous or lymphatic damage following thrombosis or surgery, ankle or leg oedema due to immobility, oedema of the arm due to subclavian thrombosis, and facial oedema due to superior vena caval obstruction.

Management

The underlying cause should be treated where possible. Heart failure, for example, should be treated and offending drugs such as NSAIDs withdrawn.

Sodium restriction has only a limited role but is useful in patients who are resistant to diuretics. Sodium intake can easily be reduced to approximately 100 mmol (2 g) daily; reductions below this are often difficult to achieve without affecting the palatability of food.

Manoeuvres that increase venous return (e.g. strict bed rest or water immersion) stimulate salt and water excretion by effects on cardiac output and ANP release, but they are seldom of practical value.

The mainstay of treatment is the use of **diuretic agents**, which increase sodium, chloride and water excretion in the kidney (**Box 9.6**). These agents act by interfering with membrane ion pumps that are present on numerous cell types; they mostly achieve specificity for the kidney by being secreted into the proximal tubule, resulting in much higher concentrations in the tubular fluid than in other parts of the body.

Clinical use of diuretics

Loop diuretics

These potent diuretics are useful in the treatment of any cause of systemic extracellular volume overload. They stimulate excretion of both sodium chloride and water by blocking the sodium–potassium-2-chloride (NKCC2) channel in the thick ascending limb of Henle (**Fig. 9.8**) and are useful in stimulating water excretion in states of relative water overload. They also act by causing increased venous capacitance, resulting in rapid clinical improvement in patients with left ventricular failure, preceding the diuresis. Unwanted effects include:

*   urate retention, causing gout
*   hypokalaemia
*   hypercalciuria leading to increased risk of calcium-based renal stones
*   hypomagnesaemia
*   decreased glucose tolerance
*   allergic tubulointerstitial nephritis and other allergic reactions
*   myalgia – especially with high-dose bumetanide

Box 9.6 Types and clinical uses of diuretics

Class	Major action	Examples	Clinical uses	Potency
Loop diuretics	↓ Na⁺-Cl⁻-K⁺ co-transport in thick ascending limb of loop of Henle	Furosemide Bumetanide Torasemide	Volume overload (CCF, nephrotic syndrome, CKD) SIADH	+++
Thiazide and related diuretics	↓ Na⁺-Cl co-transport in early distal convoluted tubule	Bendroflumethiazide Chlortalidone Metolazone Indapamide	Hypertension Volume overload (CCF) Hypercalciuria	++
Potassium-sparing diuretics	↓ Na⁺ reabsorption (in exchange for K⁺) in collecting duct (principal cells)	Aldosterone antagonists, e.g. spironolactone, eplerenone Others: amiloride, triamterene	Hyperaldosteronism (primary and secondary) Bartter's syndrome Heart failure Cirrhosis with fluid overload Prevention of K⁺ deficiency in combination with loop or thiazide	+
Carbonic anhydrase inhibitors	↓ Na⁺ HCO₃⁻ reabsorption in proximal collecting duct ↓ Aqueous humour formation	Acetazolamide	Metabolic alkalosis Glaucoma	±
Vasopressin/ADH receptor blockers (aquaretics)	Block V₂ receptor in collecting ducts producing free water diuresis	Lixivaptan Tolvaptan Satavaptan I.v. conivaptan (also blocks V₁A)	Heart failure, cirrhosis, SIADH	+

CCF, congestive cardiac failure; CKD, chronic kidney disease; SIADH, syndrome of inappropriate antidiuretic hormone secretion.

- ototoxicity (due to an action on sodium pump activity in the inner ear) – particularly with furosemide
- interference with excretion of lithium, resulting in toxicity.

There is little to choose between the drugs in this class. Bumetanide has a better oral bioavailability than furosemide, particularly in patients with severe peripheral oedema, and has more beneficial effects than furosemide on venous capacitance in left ventricular failure.

Thiazide diuretics

Thiazide diuretics (see p. 1073) are less potent than loop diuretics. They act by blocking a sodium chloride channel in the ***distal convoluted tubule*** (producing an induced form of Gitelman's syndrome, which is associated with reduced function of this channel; see p. 188) (**Fig. 9.9**). They cause relatively more urate retention, glucose intolerance and hypokalaemia than loop diuretics. They interfere with water excretion and may cause hyponatraemia, particularly if combined with amiloride or triamterene. This effect is clinically useful in diabetes insipidus. Thiazides reduce peripheral vascular resistance by mechanisms that are not completely understood but do not appear to depend on their diuretic action, and are widely used in the treatment of essential hypertension. They are also used extensively in mild to moderate cardiac failure. Thiazides reduce calcium excretion. This effect is useful in patients with idiopathic hypercalciuria but may cause hypercalcaemia. Numerous agents are available, with varying half-lives but little else to choose between them. Metolazone is not dependent for its action on glomerular filtration, and therefore retains its potency in renal impairment.

Potassium-sparing diuretics

Potassium-sparing diuretics (**Fig. 9.10**) are of two types:

- ***Aldosterone antagonists***, which compete with aldosterone in the collecting ducts and reduce sodium absorption, e.g. spironolactone and eplerenone (which has a shorter half-life). Spironolactone is used in patients with heart failure because it significantly reduces the mortality in these individuals by antagonizing the fibrotic effect of aldosterone on the heart. Eplerenone may be preferred because it is devoid of antiandrogenic or antiprogesterone properties.
- ***Amiloride and triamterene***, which inhibit sodium uptake by blocking epithelial sodium channels in the collecting duct and

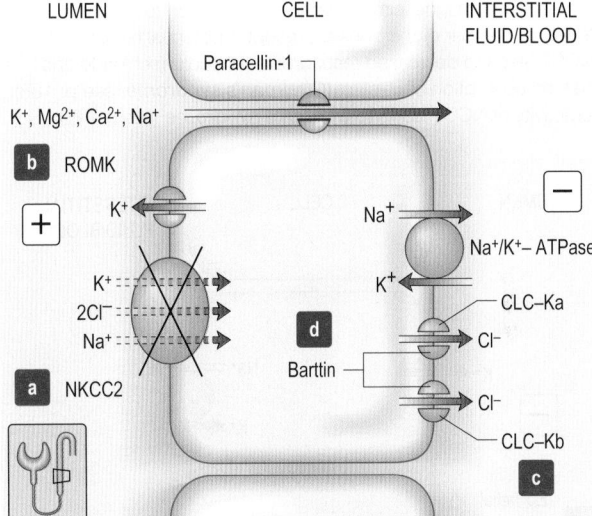

Fig. 9.8 Transport mechanisms in the thick ascending limb of the loop of Henle. Sodium chloride is reabsorbed in the thick ascending limb by the bumetanide-sensitive sodium–potassium-2–chloride co-transporter (NKCC2), which is the target of loop diuretics such as furosemide. The electroneutral transporter is driven by the low intracellular sodium and chloride concentrations generated by the Na⁺/K⁺-ATPase and the kidney-specific basolateral chloride channel (CLC-Kb). The availability of luminal potassium is rate-limiting for NKCC2, and recycling of potassium through the ATP-regulated potassium channel (renal outer medulla K⁺ channel, ROMK) ensures the efficient functioning of the NKCC2 and generates a lumen-positive transepithelial potential. Calcium and magnesium, along with potassium and sodium, are also absorbed paracellularly in the thick ascending loop. ***Bartter's syndrome:*** loss of function mutations for the different types of syndrome. **(a)** NKCC2 (type I). **(b)** ROMK (type II). **(c)** CLC-Kb (type III). **(d)** Barttin (type IV). In addition, type V may be caused by a gain-of-function mutation of the calcium-sensing receptor (not shown).

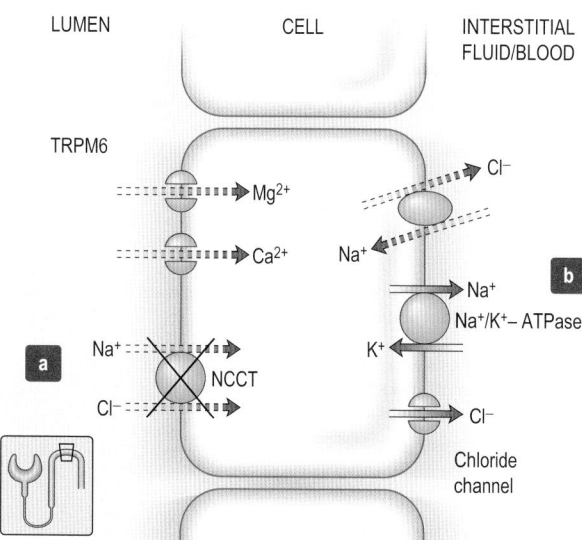

Fig. 9.9 Transport mechanisms in the distal convoluted tubule. **(a)** Sodium chloride is usually reabsorbed by the apical *thiazide-sensitive* sodium–chloride co-transporter *(NCCT)* in the distal convoluted tubule. **(b)** The electroneutral transporter is driven by the low intracellular sodium and chloride concentrations generated by the Na^+/K^+-ATPase, and an undefined basolateral chloride channel. In this nephron segment, there is an apical calcium channel and a basolateral sodium-coupled exchanger. The mechanisms for the transport of magnesium are similar to those for calcium, involving *TRPM6*, a member of the transient receptor potential family. Mutation of NCCT leads to decreased reabsorption of sodium chloride and increased absorption of calcium (*Gitelman's syndrome*, see p. 188). Overactivity of NCCT leads to *Gordon's syndrome* (see p. 189).

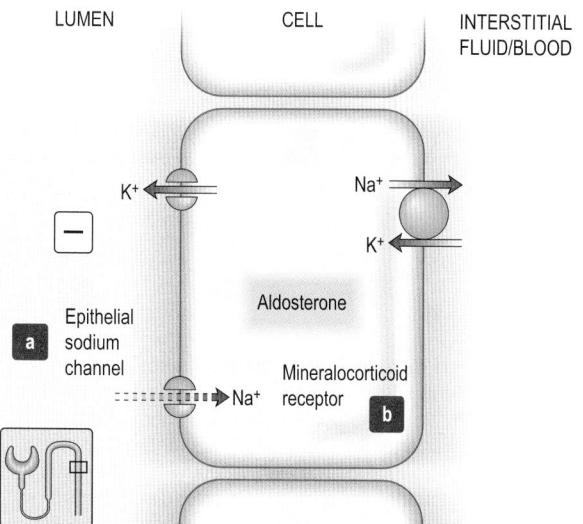

Fig. 9.10 Aldosterone-regulated transport in the cortical collecting ducts. Under normal conditions, the *epithelial sodium channel* is the rate-limiting barrier for the normal entry of sodium from the lumen into the cell. The resulting lumen-negative transepithelial voltage (indicated by the minus sign) drives potassium secretion from the principal cells and proton secretion from the α-intercalated cells (see **Fig. 9.15**). **(a)** Site of action of amiloride and triamterene: mutation of the epithelial sodium channel gene (*Liddle's syndrome*) produces reabsorption of sodium and increased secretion of potassium (not shown). **(b)** Site of action of aldosterone antagonists: mutation of the gene encoding mineralocorticoid receptor leads to salt wasting and decreased secretion of potassium.

reduce renal potassium excretion by reducing lumen-negative transepithelial voltage. They are mainly used as potassium-sparing agents with thiazide or loop diuretics.

Carbonic anhydrase inhibitors

These are relatively weak diuretics and are seldom used, except in the treatment of glaucoma. They cause metabolic acidosis and hypokalaemia.

Aquaretics (vasopressin or ADH antagonists)

Vasopressin V_2 receptor antagonists are very useful agents in the treatment of conditions associated with elevated levels of vasopressin, such as heart failure, cirrhosis and SIADH (see p. 643). Non-peptide vasopressin V_2 receptor antagonists are efficacious in producing free water diuresis in humans. Studies in patients with heart failure and cirrhosis suggest that such agents will allow normalization of serum osmolality with less water restriction (see p. 186).

Sodium–glucose co-transporter 2 (SGLT2) inhibitors

This recently developed class of medications for type 2 diabetes have demonstrated significant cardiac and renal protection in large clinical trials and act by blocking glucose and sodium reabsorption in the proximal tubule leading to an osmotic diuresis and a naturesis. SGLT2 inhibitors therefore lead to glycosuria (with a modest caloric deficit) and an improvement in diabetic control along with a modest diuretic and antihypertensive effect, which may in part be responsible for their favourable cardiovascular protection data.

Resistance to diuretics

Resistance may occur as a result of:
- poor bioavailability
- reduced GFR, which may be due to decreased circulating volume despite oedema (e.g. nephrotic syndrome, cirrhosis with ascites) or intrinsic renal disease
- activation of sodium-retaining mechanisms, particularly aldosterone.

Intravenous administration of diuretics may be required to establish a diuresis, and high doses of loop diuretics are needed to achieve adequate concentrations in the tubule if GFR is depressed. However, the daily dose of furosemide must be limited to a maximum of 2 g for an adult because of ototoxicity. Intravenous albumin solutions restore plasma oncotic pressure temporarily in the nephrotic syndrome and allow mobilization of oedema but do not increase the natriuretic effect of loop diuretics.

Combinations of various classes of diuretics are extremely helpful in patients with resistant oedema. A loop diuretic plus a thiazide inhibit two major sites of sodium reabsorption; this effect may be further potentiated by addition of a potassium-sparing agent. Metolazone in combination with a loop diuretic is particularly useful in refractory congestive cardiac failure because its action is less dependent on glomerular filtration. However, this potent combination can cause severe electrolyte imbalance.

Effects on renal function

All diuretics may increase plasma urea concentrations by increasing urea reabsorption in the medulla. Thiazides may also promote protein breakdown. In certain situations, diuretics also decrease GFR:
- Excessive diuresis causes volume depletion and pre-renal failure.
- Diuretics can cause allergic tubulointerstitial nephritis.
- Thiazides may directly cause a drop in GFR; the mechanism is complex and not fully understood.

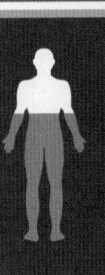

Further reading

Baum M. Inherited disorders of tubular transport. *Curr Opin Pediatr* 2017; 29:165–167.

Ellison DH, Felker GM. Diuretic treatment in heart failure. *N Engl J Med* 2017; 16:1964–1975.

Knepper MA, Kwon T-H, Nielson S. Molecular physiology of water balance. *N Engl J Med* 2015:1349–1358.

Peri A, Grohé C, Berardi R et al. SIADH: differential diagnosis and clinical management. *Endocrine* 2017; 55:311–319.

Decreased extracellular volume

Deficiency of sodium and water causes shrinkage both of the interstitial space and of the blood volume, and may have profound effects on organ function.

Clinical features

Symptoms

Thirst, muscle cramps, nausea and vomiting, and postural dizziness occur. Severe depletion of circulating volume causes hypotension and impairs cerebral perfusion, causing confusion and eventual coma.

Signs

Signs can be divided into those due to loss of interstitial fluid and those due to loss of circulating volume.

- **Loss of interstitial fluid** leads to loss of skin elasticity ('turgor') – the rapidity with which the skin recoils to normal after being pinched. Skin turgor decreases with age, particularly at the peripheries. The turgor over the anterior triangle of the neck or on the forehead is less dependent on age and so may be more useful.
- **Loss of circulating volume** leads to decreased pressure in the venous and (if severe) arterial compartments. Loss of up to 1 L of extracellular fluid in an adult may be compensated for by venoconstriction and may cause no physical signs.

  Loss of more than this amount causes the following:
- **Postural hypotension** Normally, the blood pressure rises if a subject stands up, as a result of increased venous return due to venoconstriction (this maintains cerebral perfusion). Loss of extracellular fluid (underfill) prevents this and causes a fall in blood pressure. This is one of the earliest and most reliable signs of volume depletion, as long as the other causes of postural hypotension are excluded (**Box 9.7**).
- **Low jugular venous pressure** In hypovolaemic patients, the jugular venous pulsation can be seen only with the patient lying completely flat, or even head down, because the right atrial pressure is lower than 5 cmH₂O.
- **Peripheral venoconstriction** This causes cold skin with empty peripheral veins (which are difficult to cannulate just when the patient needs intravenous therapy the most!) This sign is often absent in sepsis, where peripheral vasodilation contributes to effective hypovolaemia.
- **Tachycardia** This is not always a reliable sign. Beta-blockers and other antiarrhythmics may prevent tachycardia, and hypovolaemia may activate vagal mechanisms and actually cause bradycardia.

Aetiology

Salt and water may be lost from the kidneys, the gastrointestinal tract or the skin (**Box 9.8**).

In addition, there are a number of situations where signs of volume depletion occur despite a normal or increased body content of sodium and water:

- Septicaemia causes vasodilation of both arterioles and veins, resulting in greatly increased capacitance of the vascular space. In addition, increased capillary permeability to plasma proteins leads to loss of fluid from the vascular space to the interstitium.
- Diuretic treatment of heart failure or nephrotic syndrome may lead to rapid reduction in plasma volume. Mobilization of oedema may take much longer.
- There may be inappropriate diuretic treatment of oedema (e.g. when the cause is local rather than systemic), causing systemic hypovolaemia.

Investigations

Blood tests are, in general, not helpful in the assessment of extracellular volume. Plasma urea may be raised owing to increased urea reabsorption and, later, to pre-renal failure (when the creatinine rises as well), but this is very non-specific. Urinary sodium is low if the kidneys are functioning normally, but is misleading if the cause of the volume depletion involves the kidneys (e.g. diuretics, intrinsic renal disease). Urine osmolality is high in volume depletion (owing to increased water reabsorption) but may also often mislead.

Assessment of volume status is shown in **Box 9.9**.

Management

The overriding principle is to replace what is missing.

Haemorrhage

The rational treatment of acute haemorrhage is the infusion of a combination of red cells and a plasma substitute or (if unavailable)

? Box 9.7 Postural hypotension: some causes of a fall in blood pressure from lying to standing

Decreased circulating volume (hypovolaemia)	Interference with peripheral vasoconstriction by drugs
Autonomic failure	• Nitrates
• Diabetes mellitus	• Calcium-channel blockers
• Systemic amyloidosis	• α-Adrenoceptor-blocking drugs
• Shy–Drager syndrome	**Prolonged bed rest (cardio-vascular deconditioning)**
• Parkinson's disease	
• Ageing	
Interference with autonomic function by drugs	
• Tricyclic antidepressants	

? Box 9.8 Causes of extracellular volume depletion (hypovolaemia)

Haemorrhage	Renal losses
• External	• Diuretic use
• Concealed, e.g. leaking aortic aneurysm	• Impaired tubular sodium conservation
Burns	• Reflux nephropathy
Gastrointestinal losses	• Papillary necrosis
• Vomiting	- Analgesic nephropathy
• Diarrhoea	- Diabetes mellitus
• Ileostomy losses	- Sickle cell disease
• Ileus	

whole blood. (Chronic anaemia causes salt and water retention rather than volume depletion by a mechanism common to conditions with peripheral vasodilation.)

Loss of plasma

Loss of plasma, as occurs in burns or severe peritonitis, should be treated with human plasma or a plasma substitute (see p. 221).

? Box 9.9 Assessment of volume status

Best achieved by simple clinical observations, which you should carry out yourself (see figure on p. 170). Check:

- Jugular venous pressure
- Central venous pressure: both basal and after intravenous fluid challenge (see p. 210)
- Postural changes in blood pressure
- Chest X-ray
- Serial weights of the patient
- Urine output measurements at regular intervals

Loss of water and electrolytes

Loss of water and electrolytes, as occurs with vomiting, diarrhoea or excessive renal losses, should be treated by replacement of the loss. If possible, this should be with oral water and sodium salts. These are available as slow sodium (600 mg, approximately 10 mmol each of Na^+ and Cl^- per tablet), the usual dose of which is 6–12 tablets/day with 2–3 L of water. They are used in mild or chronic salt and water depletion, such as that associated with renal salt wasting.

Sodium bicarbonate (500 mg, 6 mmol each of Na^+ and HCO_3^- per tablet) is given in doses of 6–12 tablets/day with 2–3 L of water. This is used in milder chronic sodium depletion with acidosis (e.g. CKD, post-obstructive renal failure, renal tubular acidosis). Sodium bicarbonate is less effective than sodium chloride in causing positive sodium balance. Oral rehydration solutions are described in **Box 20.36**.

Intravenous fluids

Intravenous fluids are sometimes required (**Box 9.10, Fig 9.11**). Rapid infusion (e.g. 1000 mL per hour or even faster) of 0.9% NaCl

---

i Box 9.10 Intravenous fluid preparations for treating fluid and electrolyte disturbances

I.v. fluid	Na$^+$ (mmol/L)	K$^+$ (mmol/L)	HCO$_3^-$ (mmol/L)	Cl$^-$ (mmol/L)	Indication[a]
Normal plasma values	142	4.5	26	103	
Sodium chloride 0.9%	150	–	–	150	1
Sodium chloride 0.18% + glucose 4%	30	–	–	30	2
Glucose 5% + potassium chloride 0.3%	–	40	–	40	3
Sodium bicarbonate 1.26%	150	–	150	–	4
Hartmann's[b]	131	5	29 (as lactate)	111	4,5
Plasma-Lyte	140	5	27 (as acetate) 23 (as gluconate)	98	4,5

[a]1. Volume expansion in hypovolaemic patients. Rarely, to maintain fluid balance when there are large losses of sodium. The sodium (150 mmol/L) is higher than in plasma and hypernatraemia can result. It is often necessary to add KCl 20–40 mmol/L.
2. Maintenance of fluid balance in normovolaemic, normonatraemic patients.
3. To replace water. Can be given with or without potassium chloride. May be alternated with 0.9% saline as an alternative to (2).
4. For volume expansion in hypovolaemic, acidotic patients, alternating with (1). Occasionally, for maintenance of fluid balance combined with (2) in salt-wasting, acidotic patients.
5. For volume expansion in hypovolaemic patients. May be better than 0.9% saline for patients with sepsis and relative hypovolaemia.
[b]Hartmann's solution also contains 2 mmol/L of calcium.

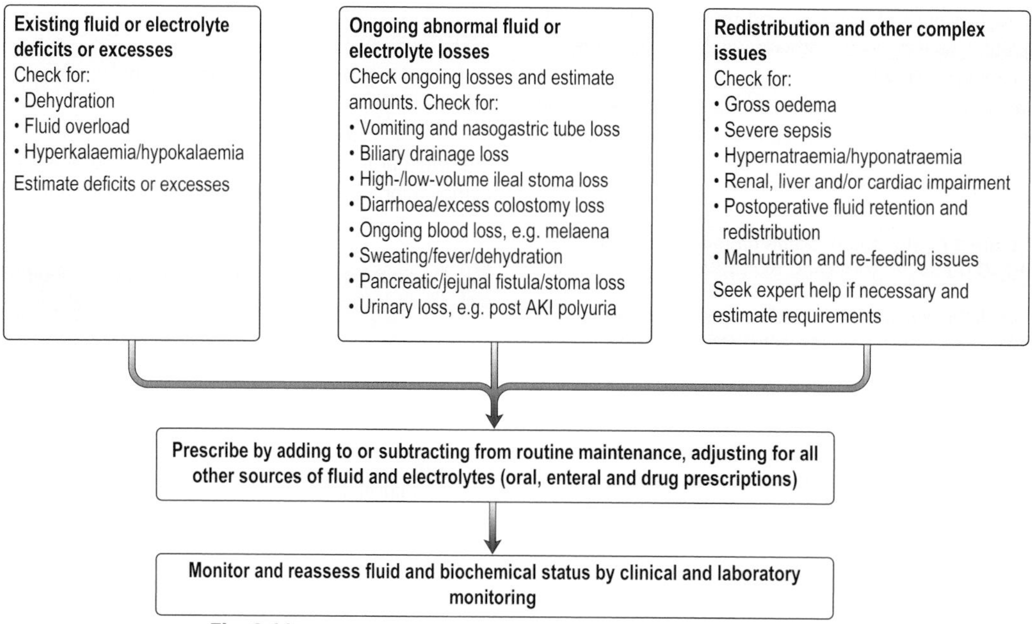

Existing fluid or electrolyte deficits or excesses
Check for:
- Dehydration
- Fluid overload
- Hyperkalaemia/hypokalaemia

Estimate deficits or excesses

Ongoing abnormal fluid or electrolyte losses
Check ongoing losses and estimate amounts. Check for:
- Vomiting and nasogastric tube loss
- Biliary drainage loss
- High-/low-volume ileal stoma loss
- Diarrhoea/excess colostomy loss
- Ongoing blood loss, e.g. melaena
- Sweating/fever/dehydration
- Pancreatic/jejunal fistula/stoma loss
- Urinary loss, e.g. post AKI polyuria

Redistribution and other complex issues
Check for:
- Gross oedema
- Severe sepsis
- Hypernatraemia/hyponatraemia
- Renal, liver and/or cardiac impairment
- Postoperative fluid retention and redistribution
- Malnutrition and re-feeding issues

Seek expert help if necessary and estimate requirements

↓

Prescribe by adding to or subtracting from routine maintenance, adjusting for all other sources of fluid and electrolytes (oral, enteral and drug prescriptions)

↓

Monitor and reassess fluid and biochemical status by clinical and laboratory monitoring

Fig. 9.11 Adult intravenous fluid therapy. AKI, acute kidney injury.

is necessary if there is hypotension and evidence of impaired organ perfusion (e.g. oliguria, confusion). However, in critically ill patients the use of balanced crystalloids (Hartmann's solution or Plasma-Lyte, which have lower chloride concentrations than saline) have been shown to result in a lower rate of the composite outcome of death from any cause, new renal-replacement therapy or persistent renal dysfunction than the use of saline, particularly if large volumes of replacement fluids are given.

Repeated clinical assessments are vital in this situation. Severe hypovolaemia induces venoconstriction, which maintains venous return; over-rapid correction does not give time for this to reverse, resulting in signs of circulatory overload (e.g. pulmonary oedema), even if a total body extracellular fluid deficit remains. In less severe extracellular fluid depletion, the fluid should be replaced at a rate of 1000 mL every 4–6 h, again with repeated clinical assessment. If all that is required is avoidance of fluid depletion during surgery, 1–2 L can be given over 24 h, remembering that surgery is a stimulus to sodium and water retention and that over-replacement may be as dangerous as under-replacement. Regular monitoring by fluid balance charts, body weight and plasma biochemistry is crucial.

Loss of water alone

This causes extracellular volume depletion only in severe cases because the loss is spread evenly among all the compartments of body water. In the rare situations where there is a true deficiency of water alone, as in diabetes insipidus or in a patient who is unable to drink (e.g. after surgery), the correct treatment is to give water.

If intravenous treatment is required, water is given as 5% glucose with K[+] because pure water would lead to osmotic lysis of blood cells.

Further reading

El Gkotmi N, Kosmeri C, Filippatos TD et al. Use of intravenous fluids/solutions: a narrative review. *Curr Med Res Opin* 2017; 33:459–471.
Huang L, Zhou X, Yu H. Balanced crystalloids vs 0.9% saline for adult patients undergoing non-renal surgery: a meta-analysis. *Int J Surg* 2018; 51:1–9.
Semler MW, Self WH, Wanderer JP et al. SMART Investigators and the Pragmatic Critical Care Research Group. Balanced crystalloids versus saline in critically ill adults. *N Engl J Med* 2018; 378:829–839.

DISORDERS OF SODIUM CONCENTRATION

These are generally best thought of as disorders of body water content. As discussed above, sodium content is regulated by volume receptors; water content is adjusted to maintain, in health, a normal osmolality and (in the absence of abnormal osmotically active solutes) a normal sodium concentration. Disturbances of sodium concentration are caused by disturbances of water balance.

However, recently non-invasive quantitative sodium magnetic resonance imaging (Na-MRI) studies in patients have shown that:

- remarkable amounts of Na are stored in muscle, bones and skin without water
- fluids in the skin interstitium are hypertonic compared with plasma
- interstitial osmotic stress induces local immune cell and lymphatic-capillary driven mechanisms for electrolyte clearance and maintenance of the internal environment, suggesting that Na homeostasis requires additional extrarenal regulatory mechanisms.

Hyponatraemia

Hyponatraemia (Na <135 mmol/L) is the most common biochemical abnormality in hospitalized patients, with up to 35% of inpatients developing hyponatraemia during their stay. The causes depend on the associated changes in extracellular volume:

- hyponatraemia with hypovolaemia
- hyponatraemia with euvolaemia
- hyponatraemia with hypervolaemia.

Rarely, hyponatraemia may be a 'pseudo-hyponatraemia'. This occurs in hyperlipidaemia (either high cholesterol or high triglyceride) or hyperproteinaemia where there is a spuriously low measured sodium concentration, the sodium being confined to the aqueous phase but having its concentration expressed in terms of the total volume of plasma. In this situation, plasma osmolality is normal and therefore treatment of 'hyponatraemia' is unnecessary. Note that artefactual 'hyponatraemia', caused by taking blood from the limb into which fluid of low sodium concentration is being infused, should be excluded.

Hyponatraemia with hypovolaemia

This is due to salt loss in excess of water loss; the causes are listed in **Box 9.11**. In this situation, ADH secretion is initially suppressed (via the hypothalamic osmoreceptors) but, as fluid volume is lost, volume receptors override the osmoreceptors and stimulate both thirst and the release of ADH. This is an attempt by the body to defend circulating volume at the expense of osmolality.

With extrarenal losses and normal kidneys, the urinary excretion of sodium falls in response to the volume depletion, as does water excretion, leading to concentrated urine containing <10 mmol/L of sodium. However, in salt-wasting kidney disease, renal compensation cannot occur and the only physiological protection is increased water intake in response to thirst.

Clinical features

With sodium depletion, the clinical picture is usually dominated by features of volume depletion (see p. 181). The diagnosis is usually obvious where there is a history of gut losses, diabetes mellitus with significant hyperglycaemia, or diuretic abuse. Examination of the patient is often more helpful than the biochemical investigations, which include plasma and urine electrolytes and osmolality.

Box 9.12 shows the potential daily losses of water and electrolytes from the gut. Losses due to renal or adrenocortical disease may be less easily identified but a urinary sodium concentration of >20 mmol/L, in the presence of clinically evident volume depletion, suggests a renal loss.

? **Box 9.11 Causes of hyponatraemia with decreased extracellular volume (hypovolaemia)**

Extrarenal (urinary sodium <20 mmol/L)	Kidney (urinary sodium >20 mmol/L)
- Vomiting	- Osmotic diuresis (e.g. hyperglycaemia, severe uraemia)
- Diarrhoea	- Diuretics
- Haemorrhage	- Adrenocortical insufficiency
- Burns	- Tubulointerstitial renal disease
- Pancreatitis	- Recovery phase of acute tubular necrosis

> **Box 9.12** Average concentrations and potential daily losses of water and electrolytes from the gut

	Na⁺ (mmol/L)	K⁺ (mmol/L)	Cl⁻ (mmol/L)	Volume (mL in 24 h)
Stomach	50	10	110	2500
Small intestine				
Recent ileostomy	120	5	110	1500
Adapted ileostomy	50	4	25	500
Bile	140	5	105	500
Pancreatic juice	140	5	60	2000
Diarrhoea	130	10–30	95	1000–2000⁺

> **Box 9.13** Causes of hyponatraemia with normal extra-cellular volume (euvolaemia)
>
> **Abnormal antidiuretic hormone (ADH) release**
> - Vagal neuropathy (failure of inhibition of ADH release)
> - Deficiency of adrenocortico-trophic hormone (ACTH) or glucocorticoids (Addison's disease)
> - Hypothyroidism
> - Severe potassium depletion
>
> **Syndrome of inappropriate antidiuretic hormone secretion (SIADH)**
> - See Box 21.54
>
> **Psychiatric illness**
> - 'Psychogenic polydipsia'
>
> - Antidepressant therapy
>
> **Increased sensitivity to ADH**
> - Chlorpropamide
> - Tolbutamide
>
> **ADH-like substances**
> - Oxytocin
> - Desmopressin
>
> **Unmeasured osmotically active substances stimulating osmotic ADH release**
> - Glucose
> - Chronic alcohol misuse
> - Mannitol
> - Sick-cell syndrome (leakage of intracellular ions)

Management

This is directed at the primary cause whenever possible.

In a healthy patient:
- Give oral electrolyte–glucose mixtures (see p. 543).
- Increase salt intake with slow sodium 60–80 mmol/day.

In a patient with vomiting or severe volume depletion:
- Give intravenous fluid with potassium supplements, that is 1.5–2 L 5% glucose (with 20 mmol K⁺) and 1 L 0.9% saline over 24 h *plus* measurable losses.
- Correction of acid–base abnormalities is usually not required.

Hyponatraemia with euvolaemia

Hyponatraemia with euvolaemia (**Box 9.13**) results from an intake of water in excess of the kidneys' ability to excrete it (dilutional hyponatraemia); there is no change in body sodium content but the plasma osmolality is low.
- With normal kidney function, dilutional hyponatraemia is uncommon even if a patient drinks approximately 1 L per hour.
- The most common iatrogenic cause is over-generous infusion of 5% glucose into postoperative patients; in this situation, it is exacerbated by an increased ADH secretion in response to stress.
- Postoperative hyponatraemia is a common clinical problem (seen in almost 1% of patients) with *symptomatic* hyponatraemia occurring in 20% of these patients.
- Marathon runners who drink excess water can become hyponatraemic. Even so-called 'isotonic sports drinks' can lead to hyponatraemia, as they contain little sodium, their osmolality being made up with carbohydrates, which are metabolized into energy and water.
- Premenopausal females are at most risk for developing hyponatraemic encephalopathy postoperatively, with postoperative ADH values in young females being 40 times higher than in young males.

To prevent hyponatraemia, avoid using hypotonic fluids postoperatively and administer 0.9% saline unless clinically contraindicated. The serum sodium should be measured daily in any patient receiving continuous parenteral fluid.

Some degree of hyponatraemia is usual in acute oliguric kidney injury, while in CKD it is most often due to ill-given advice to 'push' fluids.

Syndrome of inappropriate ADH secretion

This is described on page 643. There is inappropriate secretion of ADH, causing water retention and hyponatraemia.

Clinical features

Symptoms of dilutional hyponatraemia are common when hyponatraemia develops *acutely* (<48 h, often postoperatively). Overt neurological symptoms rarely occur until the serum sodium is less than 125 mmol/L, and are more usually associated with values around 115 mmol/L or lower, particularly when *chronic*. In elderly patients, however, even mild hyponatraemia with a serum sodium of 130–135 mmol/L has been associated with increased falls risk and subtle changes in cognition. They are due to the movement of water into brain cells in response to the fall in extracellular osmolality.

Hyponatraemic encephalopathy

Symptoms and signs include headache, confusion and restlessness leading to drowsiness, myoclonic jerks, generalized convulsions and eventually coma. Magnetic resonance imaging (MRI) of the brain may reveal cerebral oedema but, in the context of electrolyte abnormalities and neurological symptoms, can help to make a confirmatory diagnosis.

Risk factors for developing hyponatraemic encephalopathy

The brain's adaptation to hyponatraemia initially involves extrusion of blood and CSF, as well as sodium, potassium and organic osmolytes, in order to decrease brain osmolality. Various factors can interfere with successful adaptation. These factors, rather than the absolute change in serum sodium, predict whether a patient will suffer hyponatraemic encephalopathy.
- *Children* under 16 years are at increased risk due to their relatively large brain-to-intracranial volume ratio compared with adults.
- *Premenopausal women* are more likely to develop encephalopathy than postmenopausal females and males because of inhibitory effects of sex hormones and the effects of vasopressin on cerebral circulation, resulting in vasoconstriction and hypoperfusion of the brain.
- *Hypoxaemia* is a major risk factor for hyponatraemic encephalopathy. Patients with hyponatraemia who develop hypoxia, from any cause, have a high risk of mortality. Hypoxia is the strongest predictor of mortality in patients with symptomatic hyponatraemia.

Investigations

The cause of hyponatraemia with apparently normal extracellular volume requires investigation:

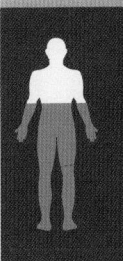

- *Plasma and urine electrolytes and osmolalities.* The plasma concentrations of sodium, chloride and urea are low, giving a low osmolality. The urine sodium concentration is usually high and the urine osmolality is typically higher than the plasma osmolality.
- *Further investigations.* These are needed to exclude Addison's disease, hypothyroidism, syndrome of inappropriate ADH secretion (SIADH) and water retention induced by drugs, e.g. chlorpropamide.

Potassium depletion and magnesium depletion potentiate ADH release and are causes of diuretic-associated hyponatraemia.

SIADH is often over-diagnosed. Some causes are associated with a lower set-point for ADH release, rather than completely autonomous ADH release; an example is chronic alcohol use.

Management

The underlying cause should be corrected where possible (**Box 9.14**).

- *Most patients.* Most cases are simply managed by restriction of water intake (to 1000 or even 500 mL/day) with review of diuretic therapy. Magnesium and potassium deficiency must be corrected. In mild sodium deficiency, 0.9% saline given slowly (1 L over 12 h) is sufficient.
- *Acute onset with symptoms.* The most common cause of acute hyponatraemia in adults is postoperative iatrogenic hyponatraemia. Excessive water intake associated with psychosis, marathon running and use of Ecstasy (a recreational drug) are other causes. All are acute medical emergencies and should be treated aggressively and immediately. In patients who demonstrate severe neurological signs, such as fits, coma or cerebral oedema, **hypertonic saline** (3%, 513 mmol/L) should be used. It must be given very slowly (not more than 70 mmol/h), the aim being to increase the serum sodium by 4–6 mmol/L in the first 4 h, but the absolute change should not exceed 15–20 mmol/L over 48 h. In general, the plasma sodium should not be corrected to >125–130 mmol/L. Assuming that total body water comprises 50% of total body weight, 1 mL/kg of 3% sodium chloride will raise the plasma sodium by 1 mmol/L.
- *Symptomatic hyponatraemia in patients with intracranial pathology.* This should be managed aggressively and immediately with 3% saline, as for acute hyponatraemia.
- *Chronic/asymptomatic hyponatraemia.* If hyponatraemia has developed slowly, as it does in the majority of patients, the brain will have adapted by decreasing intracellular osmolality and the hyponatraemia must be corrected slowly.

However, clinically, it can be difficult to know how long the hyponatraemia has been present for and 3% hypertonic saline may still be required.

Osmotic demyelination syndrome
Avoiding osmotic demyelination syndrome

A rapid rise in extracellular osmolality, particularly if there is an 'overshoot' to high serum sodium and osmolality, will result in the osmotic demyelination syndrome (ODS), formerly known as central pontine demyelination, which is a devastating neurological complication. Plasma sodium concentration in patients with hyponatraemia should not rise by more than 8 mmol/L per day. The rate of rise of plasma sodium should be even lower in patients at higher risk for ODS: for example, those with alcohol excess, cirrhosis, malnutrition or hypokalaemia. Other factors predisposing to demyelination are pre-existing hypoxaemia and central nervous system radiation. ODS is diagnosed by the appearance of characteristic hypointense

> **Box 9.14 Key points in the management of hyponatraemia**
>
> - Always treat the underlying cause
> - What is the volume status of the patient?
>   - If hypovolaemic: rehydrate with 0.9% saline
>   - If euvolaemic (SIADH): restrict fluid to 500–700 mL/day
>   - If hypervolaemic (chronic kidney disease/heart failure): restrict fluid and salt, consider loop diuretic
> - Does the patient have symptomatic hyponatraemia (seizures/coma)?
>   - Yes: involve critical care input early; 3% saline 1 mL/kg over 1 h
> - Is the hyponatraemia acute or chronic?
>   - If acute: more likely to develop symptomatic hyponatraemia
>   - If chronic: increased risk of osmotic demyelination due to rapid correction
>   - If unsure: give 3% saline very slowly
> - Check sodium levels frequently: may need to check Na every 1–2 h
> - Correction must not exceed 8 mmol in first 24 h and 18 mmol in 48 h

lesions on T_1-weighted images and hyperintense lesions on T_2-weighted images on MRI; these can take 2 weeks or more to appear.

The pathophysiology of ODS is not fully understood. The most plausible explanation is that the brain loses organic osmolytes very quickly in order to adapt to hyponatraemia so that osmolarity is similar between the intracellular and extracellular compartments. However, neurons take up organic osmolytes slowly in the phase of rapid correction of hyponatraemia, resulting in a hypo-osmolar intracellular compartment and shrinkage of cerebral vascular endothelial cells. Consequently, the blood–brain barrier is functionally impaired, allowing lymphocytes, complement and cytokines to enter the brain, damage oligodendrocytes, activate microglial cells and cause demyelination.

The most crucial issue in the treatment of hyponatraemia is to *prevent rapid correction* as it can be fatal. A rapid rise in plasma sodium is almost always due to a water diuresis, which happens when vasopressin (ADH) action stops suddenly; for example, with volume repletion in patients with intravascular volume depletion, cortisol replacement in patients with Addison's disease, or resolution of non-osmotic stimuli for vasopressin release such as nausea or pain. Sometimes, however, chronic hyponatraemia can develop in the absence of vasopressin excess. Even in these cases, water diuresis due to *increased distal delivery of filtrate* is the main cause of rapid rise in plasma sodium.

In the absence of vasopressin, it is *generally assumed* that the total urine volume is equal to the volume of filtrate delivered to the distal nephron, which is the GFR minus the volume reabsorbed in the proximal convoluted tubule. Approximately 80% of the GFR is reabsorbed in proximal convoluted tubule under normal circumstance (and this increases even more in the presence of intravascular volume depletion). However, *in real life*, water excretion will be less than the volume of distal delivery of filtrate, even in the absence of vasopressin, because a significant degree of water is reabsorbed in the inner medullary collecting duct through its residual water permeability, prompted by a very high osmotic force in the interstitium (see **Fig. 36.3**).

Even a modest water diuresis in the elderly with reduced muscle mass is large enough to cause a rapid rise in plasma sodium. Moreover, there is a higher risk for ODS if hypokalaemia is present. In such cases, if plasma sodium rises too quickly due to anticipated water diuresis, administration of desmopressin to stop the water diuresis is beneficial. If plasma sodium rises regardless, then lowering plasma sodium to the maximum limit of correction (<8 mmol/L per day) with the administration of 5% glucose solution is the best strategy.

Reversible hyponatraemia culminating in hypernatraemia

In many patients, the cause of water retention is reversible (e.g. hypovolaemia, thiazide diuretics). On correction of the cause, vasopressin levels fall and plasma sodium rises by up to 2 mmol/L per hour as a result of excretion of dilute urine. This excessive water diuresis should be anticipated and prevented by use of desmopressin.

Patients who are chronically hyponatraemic with concomitant hypokalaemia are especially susceptible to overcorrection. Plasma sodium is a function of the ratio of exchangeable body sodium plus potassium to total body water, so potassium administration increases sodium concentration. For example, a mildly symptomatic hyponatraemic patient with a plasma sodium of <120 mmol/L and potassium of <2 mmol/L can potentially develop ODS as a result of overcorrection of hyponatraemia simply as a direct result of replacing the large potassium deficit.

Antidiuretic hormone antagonists (vasopressin antagonists)

Vasopressin V_2 receptor antagonists (see p. 180), which produce a free water diuresis, are being used in clinical trials for the treatment of hyponatraemic encephalopathy. Three oral agents, lixivaptan, tolvaptan and satavaptan, are selective for the V_2 (antidiuretic) receptor, while conivaptan blocks both V_{1A} and V_2 receptors.

These agents produce a selective water diuresis without affecting sodium and potassium excretion; they raise the plasma sodium concentration in patients with hyponatraemia caused by SIADH, heart failure and cirrhosis.

The efficacy of oral tolvaptan in ambulatory patients has been demonstrated in individuals with hyponatraemia (mean plasma sodium 129 mmol/L) caused by SIADH, heart failure or cirrhosis who had a sustained rise in plasma sodium to 136 mmol/L for 4 weeks. Tolvaptan is now approved for use in patients with euvolaemic hyponatraemia and those with SIADH. In addition, intravenous conivaptan is available and is also approved for the treatment of euvolaemic hyponatraemia (i.e. SIADH) in some countries. The approved dosing for conivaptan is a 20 mg bolus followed by continuous infusion of 20 mg over 1–4 days. The continuous infusion increases the risk of phlebitis, which requires the use of large veins and change of infusion site every 24 h.

Hyponatraemia with hypervolaemia

The common causes of hyponatraemia due to water excess are shown in **Box 9.15**. In all these conditions, there is usually an element of reduced GFR with avid reabsorption of sodium and chloride in the proximal tubule. This leads to reduced delivery of chloride to the 'diluting' ascending limb of the loop of Henle and a reduced ability to generate 'free water', with a consequent inability to excrete dilute urine. This is commonly compounded by the administration of diuretics that block chloride reabsorption and interfere with the dilution of filtrate either in the loop of Henle (loop diuretics) or distally (thiazides).

Hypernatraemia

This is much rarer than hyponatraemia and nearly always indicates a water deficit. Causes are listed in **Box 9.16**.

Hypernatraemia is always associated with increased plasma osmolality, which is a potent stimulus to thirst. None of the factors listed in **Box 9.16** causes hypernatraemia unless thirst sensation is abnormal or access to water limited. For instance, a patient with diabetes insipidus will maintain a normal serum sodium concentration by maintaining a high water intake until an intercurrent illness prevents this. Thirst is frequently deficient in elderly people, making them more prone to water depletion. Hypernatraemia may occur in the presence of normal, reduced or expanded extracellular volume, and does not necessarily imply that total body sodium is increased.

Clinical features

Symptoms of hypernatraemia are non-specific. Nausea, vomiting, fever and confusion may occur. A history of longstanding polyuria, polydipsia and thirst suggests diabetes insipidus. Assessment of extracellular volume status guides resuscitation. Mental state should be assessed. Convulsions occur in severe hypernatraemia.

Investigations

Simultaneous urine and plasma osmolality and sodium should be measured. Plasma osmolality is high in hypernatraemia. Passage of urine with an osmolality lower than that of plasma in this situation is clearly abnormal and indicates diabetes insipidus. In pituitary diabetes insipidus, urine osmolality will increase after administration of desmopressin; the drug (a vasopressin analogue) has no effect in nephrogenic diabetes insipidus (see p. 643). If urine osmolality is high, this suggests either an osmotic diuresis due to an unmeasured solute (e.g. in parenteral feeding) or excessive extrarenal loss of water (e.g. heat stroke).

Management

Treatment is that of the underlying cause. For example:
- In ADH deficiency, replace ADH in the form of desmopressin, a stable non-pressor analogue of ADH.
- Remember to withdraw nephrotoxic drugs where possible and replace water either orally or, if necessary, intravenously.

> **? Box 9.16 Causes of hypernatraemia**
>
> **Antidiuretic hormone (ADH) deficiency**
> - Pituitary diabetes insipidus (see p. 641)
>
> **Iatrogenic**
> - Administration of hypertonic sodium solutions
> - Administration of drugs with a high sodium content (e.g. piperacillin)
> - Use of 8.4% sodium bicarbonate after cardiac arrest
>
> **Insensitivity to ADH (nephrogenic diabetes insipidus)**
> - Lithium
> - Tetracyclines
>
> - Amphotericin B
> - Acute tubular necrosis
> - Osmotic diuresis
> - Total parenteral nutrition
> - Hyperosmolar hyperglycaemic state (see p. 725)
>
> **Plus**
> - Deficient water intake: impaired thirst or consciousness
> - Excessive water loss through skin or lungs

> **? Box 9.15 Causes of hyponatraemia with increased extracellular volume (hypervolaemia)**
>
> - Heart failure
> - Liver failure
> - Oliguric kidney injury
> - Hypoalbuminaemia

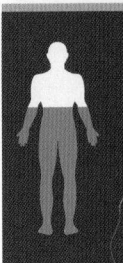

In **severe** (>170 mmol/L) hypernatraemia, 0.9% saline (150 mmol/L) should be used initially. Avoid too rapid a drop in serum sodium concentration; the aim is correction over 48 h, as over-rapid correction may lead to cerebral oedema.

In **less severe** (e.g. >150 mmol/L) hypernatraemia, the treatment is 5% glucose or 0.45% saline; the latter is obviously preferable in hyperosmolar diabetic coma. Very large volumes – 5 L/day or more – may need to be given in diabetes insipidus.

If there is clinical evidence of volume depletion (see p. 181), this implies that there is a sodium deficit as well as a water deficit. Treatment of this is discussed on page 185.

Further reading

Cuesta M, Garrahy A, Thompson CJ. SIAD: practical recommendations for diagnosis and management. *J Endocrinol Invest* 2016; 39:991–1001.
Dineen R, Thompson CJ, Sherlock M. Hyponatraemia – presentations and management. *Clin Med (Lond)* 2017; 17:263–269.
Fogarty J, Loughrey C. Hyponatraemia in hospitalised adults: a guide for the junior doctor. *Ulster Med J* 2017; 86:84–89.
Hofmeister LH, Perisic S, Titze J. Tissue sodium storage: evidence for kidney-like extrarenal countercurrent systems? *Pflugers Arch* 2015; 467: 551–558.
Liamis G, Filippatos TD, Elisaf MS. Evaluation and treatment of hypernatremia: a practical guide for physicians. *Postgrad Med* 2016; 128:299–306.
Sterns RH. Disorders of plasma sodium – causes, consequences and correction. *N Engl J Med* 2015; 372:55–65.

DISORDERS OF POTASSIUM CONCENTRATION

Regulation of serum potassium concentration

The World Health Organization (WHO) recommends a dietary intake of 90 mmol/day to reduce blood pressure; most people have a dietary intake of between 80 and 150 mmol daily, depending upon fruit and vegetable intake. Most of the body's potassium (3500 mmol in an adult) is intracellular. Serum potassium levels are controlled by:

- uptake of K^+ into cells
- renal excretion
- extrarenal losses (e.g. gastrointestinal).

Uptake of potassium into cells is governed by the activity of the Na^+/K^+-ATPase in the cell membrane and by H^+ concentration.

Uptake is **stimulated** by:

- insulin
- β-adrenergic stimulation
- theophyllines.

Uptake is **decreased** by:

- α-adrenergic stimulation
- acidosis – K^+ exchanged for H^+ across cell membranes
- cell damage or cell death – resulting in massive K^+ release.

The **kidney** plays the pivotal role in the maintenance of potassium balance by varying its secretion with changes in dietary intake. Over 90% of the filtered potassium is reabsorbed in the proximal tubule and the loop of Henle and only <10% of the filtered load is delivered to the early distal tubule. Potassium absorption in the proximal tubule is entirely passive and follows that of sodium and water, while its reabsorption in the thick ascending limb of the loop of Henle is mediated by the sodium–potassium-2–chloride co-transporter. However, potassium is secreted by the principal cells in the cortical and outer medullary collecting tubule. Secretion in these segments is very tightly regulated in health and can be varied according to individual needs; it is responsible for most of urinary potassium excretion.

Renal excretion of potassium is increased by aldosterone, which stimulates K^+ and H^+ secretion in exchange for Na^+ in the principal cells of the collecting duct (see **Fig. 9.10**). Because H^+ and K^+ are interchangeable in the exchange mechanism, acidosis decreases and alkalosis increases the secretion of K^+. Aldosterone secretion is stimulated by hyperkalaemia and increased angiotensin II levels, as well as by some drugs, and this acts to protect the body against hyperkalaemia and against extracellular volume depletion. The body adapts to dietary deficiency of potassium by reducing aldosterone secretion. However, because aldosterone is also influenced by volume status, conservation of potassium is relatively inefficient, and significant potassium depletion may therefore result from prolonged dietary deficiency.

A number of drugs affect K^+ homeostasis by affecting aldosterone release (e.g. heparin, NSAIDs) or by directly affecting renal potassium handling (e.g. diuretics).

Other endogenous proteins and metabolites also affect potassium homeostasis. Klotho, an anti-ageing protein expressed in the distal tubule (and other organs), increases potassium excretion. CD63, a tetra-spanning protein, inhibits its excretion. Moreover, protein kinase A- and C-mediated phosphorylation inhibits conductance of K^+ channels in the principal cells of the collecting duct but the cytochrome P450-epoxygenase-mediated metabolite of arachidonic acid (11–12-epoxyeicosatrienoic acid) activates these channels and plays a role in overall potassium homeostasis.

Normally, only about 10% of daily potassium intake is excreted in the gastrointestinal tract. Vomit contains around 5–10 mmol/L of K^+, but prolonged vomiting causes hypokalaemia by inducing sodium depletion, stimulating aldosterone, which increases renal potassium excretion. Potassium is secreted by the colon, and diarrhoeal fluid contains 10–30 mmol/L of K^+; profuse diarrhoea can therefore induce marked hypokalaemia. Colorectal villous adenomas may rarely produce profuse diarrhoea and marked K^+ loss.

Hypokalaemia

Aetiology
Common causes

The most common causes of chronic hypokalaemia are diuretic treatment (particularly thiazides) and hyperaldosteronism. In hospitalized patients acute hypokalaemia is most often caused by diuretic (thiazide or loop) use and intravenous fluids without potassium, and redistribution into cells, particularly in the case of diabetic ketoacidosis (see p. 722), where the use of fluids without potassium combined with insulin treatment can cause a rapid fall in the serum potassium. The common causes are shown in **Box 9.17**.

Rare causes

These rare causes are discussed in detail because they show the mechanisms of how diuretics can affect the kidney.

Bartter's syndrome

Bartter's syndrome (clinically similar to the effects of treatment with loop diuretics) consists of metabolic alkalosis, hypokalaemia, hypercalciuria, occasionally hypomagnesaemia (see p. 191), normal blood pressure, and an elevated plasma renin and aldosterone. The primary defect in this disorder is an impairment in sodium and chloride reabsorption in the thick ascending limb of the loop of Henle (see **Fig. 9.8**). Mutation in the genes encoding either the sodium–potassium-2–chloride co-transporter (*NKCC2*), the ATP-regulated

? Box 9.17 Causes of hypokalaemia

Increased renal excretion
(Urinary K^+ >20 mmol/day)
- Diuretics:
  - Thiazides
  - Loop diuretics

Increased aldosterone secretion
- Liver failure
- Heart failure
- Nephrotic syndrome
- Cushing's syndrome
- Conn's syndrome
- Adrenocorticotrophic hormone (ACTH)-producing tumours

Exogenous mineralocorticoid
- Corticosteroids
- Liquorice (potentiates renal actions of cortisol)

Renal disease
- Renal tubular acidosis types 1 and 2
- Renal tubular damage (diuretic phase)
- Acute leukaemia
- Nephrotoxicity:
  - Amphotericin
  - Aminoglycosides
  - Cytotoxic drugs

- Release of urinary tract obstruction
- Bartter's syndrome
- Liddle's syndrome
- Gitelman's syndrome

Reduced intake of K+
- Intravenous fluids without K^+
- Dietary deficiency

Redistribution into cells
- β-Adrenergic stimulation
- Acute myocardial infarction
- Beta-agonists, e.g., salbutamol, fenoterol
- Insulin treatment, e.g. treatment of diabetic ketoacidosis
- Correction of megaloblastic anaemia, e.g. B_{12} deficiency
- Alkalosis
- Hypokalaemic periodic paralysis

Gastrointestinal losses
(Urinary K^+ <20 mmol/day)
- Vomiting
- Severe diarrhoea
- Purgative abuse
- Villous adenoma
- Ileostomy or ureterosigmoidostomy
- Fistulae
- Ileus/intestinal obstruction

renal outer medullary potassium channel (*ROMK*) or kidney-specific basolateral chloride channels (*CLC-Kb*) – Bartter's syndrome types I, II and III, respectively – causes loss of function of these channels, with consequent impairment of sodium and chloride reabsorption. Loss-of-function mutations of the protein Barttin cause type IV Bartter's syndrome, which is associated with sensorineural deafness and renal failure.

In summary, these defects in sodium chloride transport initiate the following sequence, which is almost identical to that seen with chronic ingestion of a loop diuretic: the initial salt loss leads to mild volume depletion, resulting in activation of the renin–angiotensin–aldosterone system; the combination of hyperaldosteronism and increased distal flow (owing to the reabsorptive defect) enhances potassium and hydrogen secretion at the secretory sites in the collecting tubules, leading to hypokalaemia and metabolic alkalosis.

Diagnostic pointers include high urinary potassium and chloride despite low serum values, as well as increased plasma renin. (N.B. In primary aldosteronism, renin levels are low.) Hyperplasia of the juxtaglomerular apparatus is seen on renal biopsy (exclusion of diuretic abuse is necessary). Hypercalciuria is a common feature but magnesium wasting, though rare, also occurs.

Treatment is with combinations of potassium supplements, amiloride and rarely indometacin to block prostaglandin, which then restores vasoresponsiveness to angiotensin II and potassium.

Gitelman's syndrome

Gitelman's syndrome (similar to the effects of treatment with thiazide diuretics) is a phenotype variant of Bartter's syndrome characterized by hypokalaemia, metabolic alkalosis, hypocalciuria, hypomagnesaemia, normal blood pressure, and elevated plasma renin and

aldosterone. There are striking similarities between Gitelman's syndrome and the biochemical abnormalities induced by chronic thiazide diuretic administration. Thiazides act in the distal convoluted tubule to inhibit the function of the apical sodium–chloride co-transporter (NCCT) (see **Fig. 9.9**). Analysis of the gene encoding the NCCT has identified loss-of-function mutations in Gitelman's syndrome.

As in Bartter's syndrome, defective NCCT function leads to increased solute delivery to the collecting duct, with resultant solute wasting, volume contraction and an aldosterone-mediated increase in potassium and hydrogen secretion. Impaired function of NCCT causes hypocalciuria, as does thiazide administration. Impaired sodium reabsorption across the apical membrane, coupled with continued intracellular chloride efflux across the basolateral membrane, causes the cell to become hyperpolarized. This in turn stimulates calcium reabsorption via apical, voltage-activated calcium channels. Decreased intracellular sodium also facilitates calcium efflux via the basolateral sodium–calcium exchanger. The mechanism for urinary magnesium losses is described on pages 190–192.

Treatment consists of potassium and magnesium supplementation ($MgCl_2$) and a potassium-sparing diuretic. Volume resuscitation is usually not necessary, because patients are not dehydrated.

Liddle's syndrome

This is characterized by potassium wasting, hypokalaemia and alkalosis, but is associated with low renin and aldosterone production, and high blood pressure. There is a mutation in the gene encoding for the amiloride-sensitive epithelial sodium channel in the distal tubule/collecting duct. This constitutive activation of the epithelial sodium channel results in excessive sodium reabsorption with coupled potassium and hydrogen secretion. Unregulated sodium reabsorption across the collecting tubule causes volume expansion, inhibition of renin and aldosterone secretion, and development of low-renin hypertension (see **Fig. 9.10**).

Treatment consists of sodium restriction, along with amiloride or triamterene administration. Both are potassium-sparing diuretics that directly close the sodium channels. The mineralocorticoid antagonist spironolactone is ineffective, since the increase in sodium-channel activity is not mediated by aldosterone.

Clinical features

Hypokalaemia is usually asymptomatic but severe hypokalaemia (<2.5 mmol) causes muscle weakness. Potassium depletion may also cause symptomatic hyponatraemia (see p. 184).

Hypokalaemia is associated with an increased frequency of atrial and ventricular ectopic beats. This association may not always be causal because adrenergic activation (for instance, after myocardial infarction) results in both hypokalaemia and increased cardiac irritability. Hypokalaemia in patients without cardiac disease is unlikely to lead to serious arrhythmias.

Hypokalaemia seriously increases the risk of digoxin toxicity by increasing binding of digoxin to cardiac cells, potentiating its action and decreasing its clearance.

Chronic hypokalaemia is associated with interstitial renal disease but the pathogenesis is not completely understood.

Management

The underlying cause should be identified and treated where possible. **Box 9.18** shows some examples.

Acute hypokalaemia may correct spontaneously. In most cases, withdrawal of oral diuretics or purgatives, accompanied by the oral administration of potassium supplements in the form of slow-release

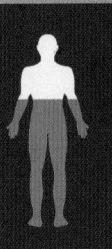

Box 9.18 Treatment of hypokalaemia

Cause	Treatment
Dietary deficiency	Increase intake of fresh fruit/vegetables or oral potassium supplements (20–40 mmol daily) (Potassium supplements can cause gastrointestinal irritation)
Hyperaldosteronism, e.g. cirrhosis, thiazide therapy	Spironolactone/eplerenone Co-prescription of a potassium-sparing diuretic with a similar onset and duration of action
Intravenous fluid replacement	Add 20 mmol of K+/L of fluid with monitoring Ensure potassium is checked at least daily until 48 h after potassium supplementation stopped

Box 9.19 Causes of hyperkalaemia

Decreased excretion
- Acute kidney injury[a]
- Drugs:[a]
  - Amiloride
  - Triamterene
  - Spironolactone/eplerenone
  - ACE inhibitors/ACE blockers
  - NSAIDs
  - Ciclosporin
  - Heparin
- Aldosterone deficiency
- Hyporeninaemic hypoaldosteronism (RTA type 4)
- Addison's disease
- Acidosis[a]
- Gordon's syndrome

Increased release from cells
(Decreased Na+/K+-ATPase activity)
- Acidosis
- Diabetic ketoacidosis
- Rhabdomyolysis/tissue damage

- Tumour lysis
- Succinylcholine (amplified by muscle denervation)
- Digoxin poisoning
- Vigorous exercise (α-adrenergic; transient)

Increased extraneous load
- Potassium chloride
- Salt substitutes
- Transfusion of stored blood[a]

Spurious
- Increased *in vitro* release from abnormal cells
- Leukaemia
- Infectious mononucleosis
- Thrombocytosis
- Familial pseudohyperkalaemia, e.g. haemolysis in syringe
- Increased release from muscles
- Vigorous fist clenching during phlebotomy

ACE, angiotensin-converting enzyme; NSAIDs, non-steroidal anti-inflammatory drugs; RTA, renal tubular acidosis.
[a]Common causes.

potassium or effervescent potassium, is all that is required. Intravenous potassium replacement is needed only in conditions such as cardiac arrhythmias, muscle weakness or severe diabetic ketoacidosis. When intravenous therapy is used in the presence of poor renal function, replacement rates <2 mmol per hour should only be used, with hourly monitoring of serum potassium and electrocardiogram changes. Ampoules of potassium should be thoroughly mixed in 0.9% saline; do not use a glucose solution, as this would make hypokalaemia worse.

The treatment of adrenal disorders is described in Chapter 21.

Failure to correct hypokalaemia may be due to concurrent hypomagnesaemia. Serum magnesium should be measured and any deficiency corrected.

Hyperkalaemia

Aetiology
Common causes

Acute self-limiting hyperkalaemia occurs normally after vigorous exercise and is of no pathological significance. Hyperkalaemia in all other situations is due either to increased release from cells or to failure of excretion (**Box 9.19**). The most common causes are renal impairment and drug interference with potassium excretion. The combination of angiotensin-converting enzyme (ACE) inhibitors with potassium-sparing diuretics or NSAIDs is particularly dangerous.

Rare causes
Hyporeninaemic hypoaldosteronism

This is also known as type 4 renal tubular acidosis (see p. 199). Hyperkalaemia occurs because of acidosis and hypoaldosteronism.

Pseudohypoaldosteronism type 1 (autosomal recessive and dominant types)

This is a disease of infancy, apparently due to resistance to the action of aldosterone. It is characterized by hyperkalaemia and evidence of sodium wasting (hyponatraemia, extracellular volume depletion). Autosomal recessive forms result from loss of function because of mutations in the gene for epithelial sodium-channel activity (the opposite to Liddle's syndrome). Pseudohypoaldosteronism type 1 involves multiple organ systems and is especially marked in the neonatal period. With aggressive salt replacement

and control of hyperkalaemia, these children can survive and the disorder appears to become less severe with age. The autosomal dominant type is due to mutations affecting the mineralocorticoid receptor (see **Fig. 9.10**). These patients present with salt wasting and hyperkalaemia but do not have other organ-system involvement.

Hyperkalaemic periodic paralysis

Hyperkalaemic periodic paralysis (see p. 897) is precipitated by exercise, and is caused by an autosomal dominant mutation of the skeletal muscle sodium-channel gene.

Gordon's syndrome (familial hyperkalaemic hypertension, pseudohypoaldosteronism type 2)

This appears to be a mirror image of Gitelman's syndrome (see p. 188), in which primary renal retention of sodium causes hypertension, volume expansion, low renin/aldosterone, hyperkalaemia and metabolic acidosis. There is also an increased sensitivity of sodium reabsorption to thiazide diuretics, suggesting that the thiazide-sensitive sodium–chloride co-transporter (NCCT) is involved (see **Fig. 9.9**). Genetic analyses, however, have excluded abnormalities in NCCT. The involvement of two loci on chromosomes 1 and 12 and further genetic heterogeneity have also been found. These genes do not correspond to ionic transporters but to unexpected proteins, WNK (*w*ith *n*o lysine *k*inase) 1 and WNK 4, which are two closely related members of a novel serine–threonine kinase family. WNK 4 normally inhibits NCCT by preventing its membrane translocation from the cytoplasm. Loss-of-function mutation in *WNK 4* results in escape of NCCT from normal inhibition and its overactivity, as seen from the patient's phenotype. WNK 1 is an inhibitor of WNK 4 and, in some patients with Gordon's syndrome, gain-of-function mutation in *WNK 1* results in functional deficiency of WNK 4 and overactivity of NCCT. Use of calcineurin inhibitors can cause hypertension due to an acquired Gordon's syndrome-type phenotype, and may respond to thiazide diuretics.

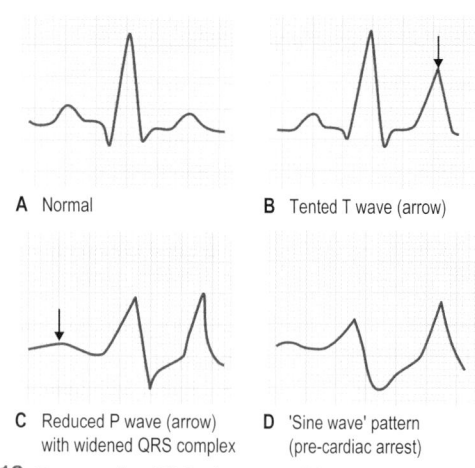

A Normal   B Tented T wave (arrow)

C Reduced P wave (arrow) D 'Sine wave' pattern
   with widened QRS complex (pre-cardiac arrest)

Fig. 9.12 Progressive ECG changes with increasing hyperkalaemia.

Suxamethonium and other depolarizing muscle relaxants

These cause release of potassium from cells. Induction of muscle paralysis during general anaesthesia may result in a rise of plasma potassium of up to 1 mmol/L. This is not usually a problem unless there is pre-existing hyperkalaemia.

Clinical features

Serum potassium of >7.0 mmol/L is a medical emergency and is associated with ECG changes (**Fig. 9.12**). Severe hyperkalaemia may be asymptomatic and may predispose to sudden death from asystolic cardiac arrest. Muscle weakness is often the only symptom, unless (as is commonly the case) the hyperkalaemia is associated with metabolic acidosis, causing Kussmaul respiration. Hyperkalaemia causes depolarization of cell membranes, leading to decreased cardiac excitability, hypotension, bradycardia and eventual asystole.

Management

Hyperkalaemia is a potentially life-threatening emergency all too commonly encountered in routine hospital practice.

Treatment for severe hyperkalaemia requires emergency, acute and subacute measures to prevent cardiac arrest and to keep potassium down, as summarized in **Box 9.20**. The cause of the hyperkalaemia should be found and treated.

High potassium levels are cardiotoxic, as they inactivate sodium channels. Divalent cations, e.g. calcium, restore the voltage dependability of the channels. **Calcium ions** protect the cell membranes from the effects of hyperkalaemia but do not alter the potassium concentration.

Supraphysiological intravenous insulin (10–20 units) drives potassium into the cell and lowers plasma potassium by 1 mmol in 60 min, but must be accompanied by intravenous glucose to avoid hypoglycaemia. Regular measurements of blood glucose for at least 6 h after use of insulin should be performed and extra glucose must be available for immediate use. The use of glucose alone in non-diabetic patients, to stimulate endogenous insulin release, does not produce the high levels of insulin required and therefore is not recommended.

Intravenous or nebulized salbutamol (10–20 mg) has not yet found widespread acceptance and may cause disturbing muscle tremors at the doses required.

Box 9.20 Correction of severe hyperkalaemia

This is a potentially life-threatening emergency. Management is divided into emergency, acute and subacute management

Emergency management
- ECG monitor and i.v. access

Protect the myocardium
- 10 mL of 10% calcium gluconate i.v. over 5 min
- Effect is temporary but dose can be repeated after 15 min

Acute management

Drive K⁺ into cells
- Insulin 10 units + 50 mL of 50% glucose i.v. over 10–15 min, followed by regular checks of blood glucose and plasma K⁺. Note: be aware of risk of hypoglycaemia in the following 1–2 h post insulin/dextrose repeat as necessary:
- Consider correction of severe acidosis (pH <6.9) – infuse $NaHCO_3$ (1.26%)
- Consider salbutamol 0.5 mg in 100 mL of 5% glucose over 15 min (rarely used)
- Stop all potassium supplements, and drugs reducing urinary excretion of potassium

Sub-acute

Deplete body K⁺ (to decrease plasma K⁺ over the next 24 h)
- Novel potassium binders (patiromer or sodium zirconium cyclosilicate)
  - May have faster action of onset/may be better tolerated
- Older potassium binders
  - Polystyrene sulphonate resins (e.g. calcium resonium): 15 g orally up to three times daily with laxatives; 30 g rectally followed 9 h later by an enema
- Haemodialysis or peritoneal dialysis if the above fails

Correction of acidosis with hypertonic (8.4%) sodium bicarbonate causes volume expansion due to the high sodium concentration, and should only be used in emergency situations; 1.26% is used with severe acidosis (pH <6.9). Gastric aspiration will remove potassium and leads to alkalosis.

Patiromer and ***sodium zirconium cyclosilicate*** (ZS9) are new non-absorbed agents that bind potassium in the gastrointestinal (GI) tract to facilitate faecal excretion. Clinical trials of patiromer and ZS9 have demonstrated clear evidence of a dose-dependent potassium-lowering effect. Patiromer and ZS9 have improved upon the age-old standard ion-exchange resins for the treatment of hyperkalemia, and are now used particularly in patients with heart failure and CKD to attenuate ACE inhibitor/ARB-induced hyperkalaemia.

Ion-exchange resins (polystyrene sulphonate resins, SPS, such as calcium resonium) are an older form of gut-acting maintenance therapy to keep potassium down after emergency treatment. They make use of the ion fluxes that occur in the gut to remove potassium. They may cause fluid overload (resonium contains Na⁺) or hypercalcaemia (calcium resonium). Resins do not appear to enhance the excretion of potassium significantly, beyond the effect of diarrhoea induced by osmotic or secretory cathartics, and their use has now been superseded by the newer gut-acting potassium binders described above.

In general, all of these measures are simply ways of buying time either to correct the underlying disorder or to arrange removal of potassium by dialysis, which is the definitive treatment for hyperkalaemia in severe acute or chronic renal failure.

Further reading

Beccari MV, Meaney CJ. Clinical utility of patiromer, sodium zirconium cyclosilicate, and sodium polystyrene sulfonate for the treatment of hyperkalemia: an evidence-based review. *Core Evid* 2017; 23:11–24.
Seyberth HW, Weber S, Kömhoff M. Bartter's and Gitelman's syndrome. *Curr Opin Pediatr* 2017; 29:179–186.
Tutakhel OAZ, Moes AD, Valdez-Flores MA et al. NaCl cotransporter abundance in urinary vesicles is increased by calcineurin inhibitors and predicts thiazide sensitivity. *PLoS One* 2017; 21:e0176220.

DISORDERS OF MAGNESIUM CONCENTRATION

Magnesium (Mg^{2+}) plays a pivotal role in many biological processes such as enzymatic reactions, gene transcription, bone remodelling and neuromuscular stability. Approximately 99% of the Mg^{2+} in the body is in the intracellular compartment, mainly in bone (approximately 85%) and in muscle and soft tissues (approximately 14%). The other 1% is in the extracellular fluid.

Plasma magnesium levels are normally maintained within the range 0.7–1.1 mmol/L (1.4–2.2 mEq/L). The average daily magnesium intake is 15 mmol, which is absorbed mainly in the small intestine and, to a lesser extent, in the colon. In the healthy adult, there is no net gain or loss of magnesium from bone, so that balance is achieved by the urinary excretion of the net magnesium absorbed. The kidney reabsorbs between approximately 95% and 98% of the filtered Mg^{2+} and plays a major role in maintaining plasma Mg^{2+} concentrations within the normal range.

Control and renal handling of magnesium
Cortical thick ascending limb of Henle

Approximately 30% of Mg^{2+} is bound to plasma proteins but the remaining fraction is freely filterable. The major site of magnesium transport is the cortical thick ascending limb of the loop of Henle, where 65–70% of the filtered load is reabsorbed, with only 10–20% being reabsorbed in the proximal tubule (see **Fig. 9.8**). This transport is passive, paracellular and carried out by tight junction proteins (paracellin-1 and claudins). This process is driven by the lumen-positive electrochemical gradient, characteristic of this segment. This voltage gradient is created by the apical disproportionate net transport of two Cl^- to one Na^+ (by the bumetanide-sensitive sodium–potassium-2–chloride transporter) and the secretion of K^+ (via the ROMK) (see **Fig. 9.8**). Loss-of-function mutations in these key reabsorptive processes lead to hypomagnesaemia as part of the distinctive clinical syndromes described later.

Bartter's syndrome

Hypomagnesaemia is rare in Bartter's syndrome (see p. 187). This is because the transepithelial voltage, which is responsible for magnesium reabsorption, is preserved and any additional filtered magnesium will be offset by a compensatory increase in absorption in the distal convoluted tubule.

Familial hypomagnesaemia, hypercalciuria and nephrocalcinosis

Familial hypomagnesaemia, hypercalciuria and nephrocalcinosis (FHHNC) is characterized by excessive renal magnesium and calcium wasting; the main defect lies in cTAL. Ten different mutations have been identified in a novel gene that encodes for paracellin-1 and claudins 16/19 complex, in the tight junction proteins.

Individuals develop bilateral nephrocalcinosis and progressive CKD. Patients also have elevated parathyroid hormone levels, which precedes any reduction in GFR. A substantial proportion of patients show incomplete distal renal tubular acidosis, hypocitraturia and hyperuricaemia. Extrarenal involvement, such as myopia, nystagmus and chorioretinitis, has been reported.

Distal convoluted tubule

The reabsorption rate in the distal convoluted tubule (DCT) – 10% – is much lower than in the cTAL, but it defines the final urinary excretion, as there is no significant reabsorption in the collecting duct; 3–5% of filtered magnesium is finally excreted in the urine. Magnesium reabsorption in the DCT is transcellular and active (see **Fig. 9.9**). The DCT has a slight lumen-negative voltage of approximately −5 mV. The luminal Mg^{2+} concentration in the DCT ranges between 0.2 and 0.7 mmol/L, whereas the intracellular concentration of Mg^{2+} is estimated to be maintained at around 0.2–1.0 mmol/L. Therefore, the voltage difference across the apical membrane plays a key role in Mg^{2+} transport within the DCT.

Magnesiotropic proteins
These include the following:

- **TRPM6**, the *t*ransient *r*eceptor *p*otential channel *m*elastatin member 6, is an Mg^{2+}-permeable channel that is also expressed in the luminal membrane of the intestinal epithelium.
- **The pro-epidermal growth factor (EGF)** resides on the basolateral surface of the DCT cells. It markedly stimulates the activity of TRPM6. Cancer therapies that inhibit EGF also cause hypomagnesaemia by the above mechanism.
- **Thiazide-sensitive Na^+–Cl^+ co-transporter in the DCT** plays a role in sodium and chloride absorption and maintenance of lumen-negative voltage. Loss-of-function mutation in this co-transporter results in **Gitelman's syndrome** (see p. 188 and **Fig. 9.9**). Hypomagnesaemia is likely to be due to a reduced abundance of TRPM6. The observed hypocalciuria is caused by an increased proximal tubular reabsorption, a process that occurs in response to the mild volume depletion.
- **The γ-subunit of the Na^+/K^+-ATPase** on the basolateral aspect of the DCT plays a pivotal role in the sodium and chloride absorption and maintenance of lumen-negative voltage (a key requirement for magnesium absorption) in this segment of the nephron.
- **ATP-sensitive inward rectifier potassium channel 10 (Kir4.1)** is present on the basolateral surface of the DCT. It allows K^+ ions to recycle across the basolateral membrane, thereby maintaining an adequate supply of K^+ to sustain the high Na^+/K^+-ATPase activity observed in this segment.

Hypomagnesaemia

In addition to the familial causes described earlier, hypomagnesaemia most often develops as a result of deficient intake, defective gut absorption (associated with the use of proton pump inhibitors), or excessive gut or urinary loss (**Box 9.21**). It can also occur with acute pancreatitis, possibly owing to the formation of magnesium soaps in the areas of fat necrosis and drug treatment with aminoglycosides and cisplatinum compounds. Due to the severe effects of hypomagnesaemia, routine measurements of serum Mg^{2+} should be conducted in the critically ill, as well as in patients who are exposed to drugs and other conditions associated with Mg^{2+} deficiency.

Clinical features

Symptoms and signs (indicating a deficit of 0.5–1 mmol/kg) include irritability, tremor, ataxia, carpopedal spasm, hyper-reflexia, confusional and hallucinatory states, and epileptiform convulsions. An ECG may show a prolonged QT interval, broad flattened T waves and occasional shortening of the ST segment.

Management

This involves the withdrawal of precipitating agents such as diuretics or purgatives. If symptomatic (or with hypocalcaemia), give a parenteral infusion of 50 mmol of magnesium chloride in 1 L of 5% glucose or other isotonic fluid over 12–24 h. This should be

Box 9.21 Causes of hypomagnesaemia

Decreased magnesium absorption
- Malabsorption (severe)
- Malnutrition
- Alcohol excess
- Proton pump inhibitors

Increased renal excretion
- Drugs:
  - Loop diuretics
  - Thiazide diuretics
  - Digoxin
- Diabetic ketoacidosis
- Hyperaldosteronism
- SIADH
- Alcohol excess
- Hypercalciuria
- 1,25-(OH)-vitamin D_3 deficiency
- Drug toxicity:
  - Amphotericin
  - Aminoglycosides
  - Cisplatin
  - Ciclosporin

Gut losses
- Prolonged nasogastric suction
- Excessive purgation
- Gastrointestinal/biliary fistulae
- Severe diarrhoea

Inherited tubular wasting
- Bartter's syndrome
- Familial hypomagnesaemia, hypercalciuria and nephrocalcinosis
- Isolated dominant hypomagnesaemia
- Gitelman's syndrome (see p. 188)
- Isolated recessive hypomagnesaemia
- Hypomagnesaemia with secondary hypocalcaemia
- EAST syndrome (*E*pilepsy, *A*taxia, *S*ensorineural deafness and *T*ubulopathy)

Miscellaneous
- Acute pancreatitis,

repeated daily and continued for 2 days after normal plasma levels have been achieved.

Relationship between hypomagnesaemia and plasma calcium

Calcium deficiency usually, but not always, develops with hypomagnesaemia. Hypomagnesaemia can be further subdivided into three main groups:

- **Hypercalciuria with hypomagnesaemia.** This occurs from defects in Mg^{2+} absorption in cTAL, such as in several forms of Bartter's syndrome, loop diuretic administration and FHHNC.
- **Normocalciuria.** This includes autosomal dominant hypomagnesaemia due to mutations in the *EGF* gene.
- **Hypocalciuria with hypomagnesaemia.** This is a hallmark feature of thiazide diuretic use and Gitelman's syndrome, and has also been reported in EAST syndrome, due to mutations in *NCC* and *Kir4.1*, respectively. Genetic defects of β-cell function and isolated dominant hypomagnesaemia (IDH) also lead to hypomagnesaemia with accompanying hypocalciuria.

Relationship between hypomagnesaemia and plasma potassium

Magnesium depletion can lead to refractory hypokalaemia. The normal concentration of intracellular magnesium usually blocks secretory K^+ currents through ROMK channels. Magnesium depletion promotes K^+ loss by releasing ROMK from magnesium-mediated inhibition. Close monitoring, with potassium supplements if necessary, is required in patients presenting with primary symptomatic low plasma magnesium levels.

Hypermagnesaemia

This primarily occurs in patients with acute or CKD given magnesium-containing laxatives or antacids. It can also be induced by magnesium-containing enemas. Mild hypermagnesaemia may occur in patients with adrenal insufficiency. Causes are given in **Box 9.22**.

Box 9.22 Causes of hypermagnesaemia

- Impaired renal excretion:
  - Chronic kidney disease
  - Acute kidney injury
- Increased magnesium intake:
  - Purgatives, e.g. magnesium sulphate
  - Antacids, e.g. magnesium trisilicate
- Haemodialysis with high $[Mg^{2+}]$ dialysate

Clinical features

Symptoms and signs relate to neurological and cardiovascular depression, and include weakness with hyporeflexia proceeding to narcosis, respiratory paralysis and cardiac conduction defects. Symptoms usually develop when the plasma magnesium level exceeds 2 mmol/L (4 mEq/L).

Management

Treatment requires withdrawal of any magnesium therapy. An intravenous injection of 10 mL of calcium gluconate 10% (2.25 mmol calcium) is given to antagonize the effects of hypermagnesaemia, along with glucose and insulin (as for hyperkalaemia; see p. 189) to lower the plasma magnesium level. Dialysis may be required in patients with severe kidney disease.

Further reading

Ayuk J, Gittoes NJ. Contemporary view of the clinical relevance of magnesium homeostasis. *Ann Clin Biochem* 2014; 51(Pt 2):179–188.
Wolf MT. Inherited and acquired disorders of magnesium homeostasis. *Curr Opin Pediatr* 2017; 29:187–198.

DISORDERS OF PHOSPHATE CONCENTRATION

Phosphate forms an essential part of most biochemical systems. The regulation of plasma phosphate level is both directly and closely linked to that of calcium.

About 85% of all body phosphorus is within bone, plasma phosphate normally ranging from 0.80 to 1.15 mmol/L (2.5–3.6 mg/dL) and accounting for only 1% of the total body phosphate. However, plasma phosphate levels correlate in most circumstances with total body sodium. Phosphate reabsorption from the glomerular filtrate occurs entirely and actively in the renal proximal tubule and is hormonally regulated. It is decreased by parathyroid hormone (PTH), mediated by a cyclic adenosine monophosphate (cAMP)-dependent mechanism; thus, primary hyperparathyroidism is associated with low plasma levels of serum phosphate. Other factors that are known to control phosphate reabsorption in the proximal tubule are 1,25-dihydroxyvitamin D_3, sodium delivery to the proximal tubule, serum concentrations of calcium, bicarbonate, carbon dioxide tension, glucose, alanine, serotonin, dopamine and sympathetic activity.

Osteoblast-secreted phosphaturic factors (phosphatonins), such as fibroblast growth factor 23 (FGF23), matrix extracellular phosphoglycoprotein (MEPG) and frizzled-related protein 4 (FRP-4), play a role in phosphate homeostasis. FGF23 is the most extensively investigated phosphatonin. It binds to its receptor, FGFR1, in the kidney and causes phosphaturia; it also regulates vitamin D by inactivation of 1α-hydroxylase (CYP27B1) and upregulation of 24 hydroxylase (CYP24A1) enzymes, with the net result of low 1,25-vitamin D synthesis. Serum FGF23 is also the earliest marker of abnormal phosphate handling in CKD patients, occurring before changes in serum phosphate, calcium or PTH (**Fig. 9.13**). Moreover,

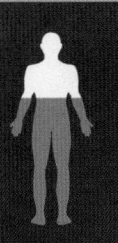

FGF23 requires Klotho (see p. 187) to act as a co-receptor with FGFR1 for its activity. Loss-of-function mutation in either FGF23 or Klotho results in a similar phenotype of shortened lifespan, premature ageing and hyperphosphataemia, and, as expected from the mode of action, increases 1,25 vitamin D levels. Klotho can also inhibit phosphate absorption directly in the absence of FGF23 or PTH.

Phosphate absorption is an active process carried out by a family of sodium–phosphate co-transporters (NPT) in the gut and kidneys. NPT2a and NPT2c are expressed in the brush border of the renal proximal tubule while NPT2b is expressed in lungs and intestine. NPT2a plays a central role in the renal reabsorption of phosphate but requires a companion protein called sodium hydrogen exchanger regulatory factor 1 (NHERF1) for membrane sorting. Intestinal absorption is carried out by NPT2b but its mutation does not cause any alteration in serum phosphate due to compensation by the renal expression of NPT2a and possibly NPT2c. Under normal circumstances, plasma phosphate levels are kept constant; for example, after a phosphate-rich meal, the bone releases FGF23,

which inhibits NPT2a and causes phosphate excretion. Moreover, phosphate in the plasma causes the release of PTH, either directly or indirectly by lowering ionized calcium. PTH also inhibits NPT2a, NPT2C and NHERF1, resulting in phosphaturia (see **Fig. 9.13**). These two principal mechanisms keep plasma phosphate levels within normal limits on a daily basis.

Hypophosphataemia

Significant hypophosphataemia (<0.4 mmol/L or <1.25 mg/dL) occurs in a number of clinical situations, owing to redistribution into cells, renal losses or decreased intake (**Box 9.23**).

Clinical features include:

- muscle weakness, e.g. diaphragmatic weakness, decreased cardiac contractility, skeletal muscle rhabdomyolysis
- a left shift in the oxyhaemoglobin dissociation curve (reduced 2,3-bisphosphoglycerate, 2,3-BPG) and rarely haemolysis
- confusion, hallucinations and convulsions.

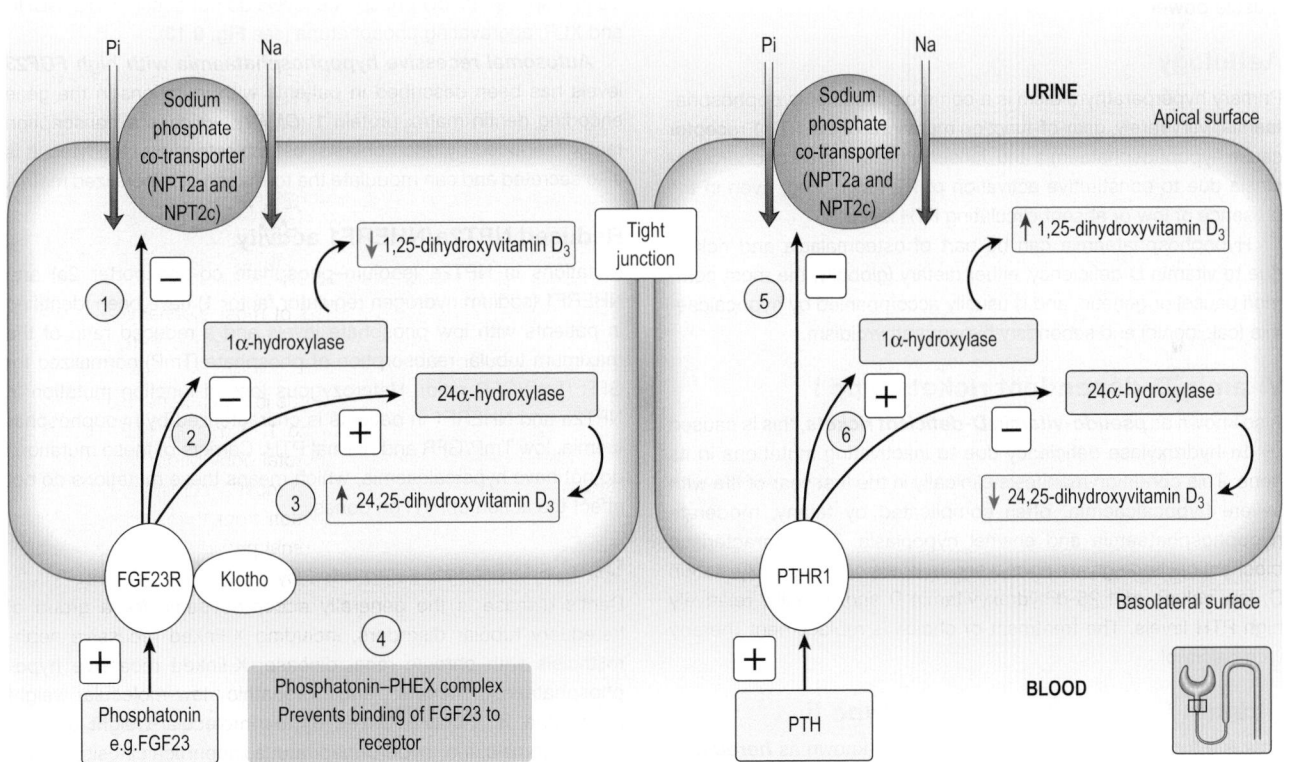

Fig. 9.13 *PHEX* and PTH regulation of phosphate transport and vitamin D metabolism in the proximal tubule.

(1) *Fibroblast growth factor 23 (FGF23)* inhibits the sodium–phosphate co-transporter (NPT2a, c), causing phosphaturia.
(2) *Binding of FGF23 to the FGFR1–Klotho complex* leads to lower levels of the active form of *vitamin D* (1,25-vitamin D) by inhibiting 1α-hydroxylase.
(3) It also increases levels of *inactive vitamin D* (24,25-vitamin D) by stimulating 24α-hydroxylase.
(4) *PHEX (phosphate-regulating gene with homologies to endopeptidase on the X chromosome)* acts as a competitive inhibitor, binding FGF23 and blocking its action.
(5) *Parathyroid hormone (PTH)* also inhibits NPT2a, which leads to phosphaturia.
(6) *PTH has opposite effects on vitamin D metabolism* compared with FGF23 by stimulating 1α-hydroxylase and inhibiting 24α-hydroxylase.

? Box 9.23 Causes of hypophosphataemia

Redistribution
- Respiratory alkalosis
- Treatment of diabetic ketoacidosis (insulin drives phosphate into cells)
- Re-feeding (particularly with carbohydrate) after fasting or starvation
- After parathyroidectomy (hungry bone disease)

Decreased intake/absorption
- Diet
- Malabsorption
- Vomiting
- Gut phosphate binders, e.g. sevelamer

- Vitamin D deficiency
- Alcohol withdrawal

Renal losses
- Hyperparathyroidism
- Renal tubular defects
- Diuretics
- Tenofovir treatment

Hypophosphataemic rickets
- Vitamin D-dependent rickets types I and II
- Tumour-induced osteomalacia (TIO)
- Autosomal dominant and recessive
- X-linked dominant rickets (XLR)
- Dent's disease

Mild hypophosphataemia often resolves without specific treatment. However, diaphragmatic weakness may be severe in acute hypophosphataemia, and may impede the weaning of a patient from a ventilator. Interestingly, chronic hypophosphataemia (in X-linked hypophosphataemia) is associated with normal muscle power.

Aetiology

Primary hyperparathyroidism is a common cause of hypophosphataemia. Very rarely, gain-of-function mutations of the PTH1 receptor cause hypophosphataemia and Jansen's metaphyseal chondrodysplasia due to constitutive activation of PTH signalling, even in the presence of low or absent circulating PTH levels.

Hypophosphataemia can be part of osteomalacia and rickets due to vitamin D deficiency, either dietary (globally, the most common cause) or genetic, and is usually accompanied by hypocalcaemia (calcipenic) and secondary hyperparathyroidism.

Vitamin D-dependent rickets type I

Also known as **pseudo-vitamin D-deficient rickets**, this is caused by 1α-hydroxylase deficiency due to inactivating mutations in its gene. This condition manifests clinically in the first year of life with severe hypocalcaemia, often complicated by tetany, moderate hypophosphataemia and enamel hypoplasia. The characteristic biochemical findings are normal serum levels of 25-hydroxyvitamin D, low values of 1,25-dihydroxyvitamin D and, usually, relatively high PTH levels. The treatment of choice is replacement therapy with calcitriol.

Vitamin D-dependent rickets type II

This is a form of vitamin D resistance and is known as **hereditary vitamin D-resistant rickets**. It is an autosomal recessive disorder and is usually caused by loss-of-function mutations in the gene encoding the vitamin D receptor. The clinical manifestations vary widely, depending upon the type of mutation within the vitamin D receptor and the amount of residual vitamin D receptor activity. Affected children usually develop rickets within the first 2 years of life, with alopecia in two-thirds of cases, which is due to lack of vitamin D receptor action within keratinocytes. The treatment involves a therapeutic trial of calcitriol and calcium supplementation. Long-term infusion of calcium into a central vein is a possible alternative for severely resistant patients. Oral calcium therapy may be sufficient once radiographic healing has been observed.

Decreased renal reabsorption of phosphate
Excessive phosphatonins (FGF23)

This condition also occurs in patients with **tumour-induced osteomalacia** (TIO), **X-linked dominant hypophosphataemic rickets** (XLR) and **autosomal dominant hypophosphataemic rickets** (ADHR). These syndromes have similar biochemical and osseous phenotypes. Patients have osteomalacia or rickets, reduced tubular phosphate reabsorption, hypophosphataemia, normal or low serum calcium, normal PTH and PTH-related protein concentrations, and normal or low 1,25-dihydroxyvitamin D_3. Urinary cAMP levels are generally in the normal range.

In **TIO**, there is excessive production of phosphaturic agents (which are normally produced by osteoblasts and function as hormones by acting on kidneys and regulating phosphate absorption and vitamin D activation): for example, FGF23, MEPG and FRP-4. The result is excess inhibition of the sodium–phosphate cotransporter in the proximal tubule and phosphaturia.

In **ADHR**, FGF23 is mutated so that it is resistant to PHEX (phosphate-regulating gene with homologies to endopeptidases on the X chromosome) proteolysis.

In **XLR**, mutations in PHEX prevent binding to FGF23 and FRP-4, resulting in a net relative excess of phosphatonins.

Normal adaptive increases in 1,25-dihydroxyvitamin D_3 synthesis in response to low phosphate levels do not occur in TIO, ADHR and XLR, aggravating phosphaturia (see **Fig. 9.13**).

Autosomal recessive hypophosphataemia with high FGF23 levels has been described in patients with mutations in the gene encoding dentin matrix protein 1 (**DMP1**), which is a transcription factor produced by odontoblasts, osteoblasts and osteocytes. It is also secreted and can modulate the formation of mineralized matrix.

Reduced NPT2a/NHERF1 activity

Mutations in NPT2a (sodium–phosphate co-transporter 2a) and NHERF1 (sodium hydrogen regulator factor 1) have been identified in patients with low phosphate levels and a reduced ratio of the maximum tubular reabsorption of phosphate (TmP) normalized for GFR (TmP/GFR ratio). Heterozygous loss-of-function mutation in NPT2a and NHERF1 in patients is characterized by hypophosphataemia, low TmP/GFR and normal PTH. Carriers of these mutations do not have hypercalcaemia, which means these mutations do not affect the action of PTH on bones.

Dent's disease

Dent's disease is the generally accepted name for a group of hereditary tubular disorders, including X-linked recessive nephrolithiasis with chronic renal disease, X-linked recessive hypophosphataemic rickets, and idiopathic low-molecular-weight proteinuria. It is characterized by low-molecular-weight proteinuria, hypercalciuria, hyperphosphaturia, nephrocalcinosis, kidney stones and eventual renal failure, with some patients developing rickets or osteomalacia.

Dent's disease is caused, in 60% of cases, by loss-of-function mutation of a proximal tubular endosomal chloride channel, CLC5. Mutations in OCRL1 occur in 15% of cases. This chloride channel, along with the proton pump, is essential for acidification of proximal tubular endosomes. The process is linked with normal endocytosis, degradation and recycling of absorbed proteins, vitamins and hormones. Defective endosomal acidification (owing to the mutated CLC5 gene) results in impaired endosomal degradation and recycling of endocytosed hormones such as PTH, with the clinical phenotype of hyperparathyroidism.

Moreover, the receptors for reabsorption of low-molecular-weight proteins and albumin in the proximal tubules (megalin and cubilin) are decreased in Dent's disease. This explains the low-molecular-weight proteinuria and excessive urinary leaks of cytokines, hormones and chemokines. This urinary profile is associated with progressive renal fibrosis and more rapid decline in renal function.

Re-feeding syndrome

Hypophosphataemia may also occur as part of the 're-feeding syndrome' (see p. 1253), which occurs in significantly malnourished patients (e.g. in people with anorexia nervosa) who rapidly recommence feeding via oral, enteral or parenteral routes.

Following starvation, the body's stores of phosphate are low due to reduced intake. After a carbohydrate load, insulin is released, which causes rapid cellular uptake of phosphate, along with potassium and magnesium, leading to a fall in the serum concentrations of these electrolytes.

Furthermore, insulin stimulates production of adenosine triphosphate (ATP) thus increasing the cellular requirement for phosphate. The inability to phosphorylate ADP to ATP due to inadequate phosphate concentrations leads to cardiac dysfunction and arrhythmias, respiratory failure due to weakness of the diaphragm, rhabdomyolysis and seizures.

Re-feeding syndrome can be prevented by correcting electrolyte disturbances before re-feeding and avoiding rapid increases of caloric intake above the resting energy requirements.

Management is essentially supportive; patients may require hospitalization for electrolyte replacement and monitoring.

Diagnosis

Patients with hypophosphataemia should have their urinary fractional excretion of phosphate measured. A value of <0.7 mmol/L indicates renal phosphate wasting. If PTH levels are high, then the patient is very likely to have hyperparathyroidism, either primary or secondary to vitamin D deficiency (acquired or genetic) or Dent's disease. If PTH levels are low, then the only possibility is gain-of-function mutation in PTH1R. If PTH levels are normal, then assess FGF23 levels. High FGF23 serum levels will indicate possible mutated genes in FGF23/Klotho, PHEX and DMP1. Normal FGF23 and PTH levels point to mutations in NPT2a, NPT2c and NHERF1.

Management

Oral phosphate supplementation and calcitriol (1,25-dihydroxy vitamin D) administration is required if there is vitamin D deficiency. Treatment of *acute hypophosphataemia* is with intravenous phosphate at a maximum rate of 9 mmol every 12 h. Repeated measurements of calcium and phosphate are required, as over-rapid administration of phosphate may lead to severe hypocalcaemia, particularly in the presence of alkalosis. *Chronic hypophosphataemia* can be corrected with oral effervescent sodium phosphate. The anti-FGF23 neutralizing antibody (burosumab) is a novel therapeutic agent that has successfully reversed biochemical and clinical phenotypic manifestations in patients with genetically elevated FGF23, and may become standard care for such patients.

Hyperphosphataemia

Hyperphosphataemia is common in patients with CKD (see p. 1394; **Box 9.24**). Hyperphosphataemia is usually asymptomatic but may

> **? Box 9.24** Causes of hyperphosphataemia
>
> - Acute kidney injury
> - Chronic kidney disease
> - Phosphate-containing enemas
> - Hyperparathyroidism/pseudo-hyperparathyroidism
> - Tumour lysis
> - Rhabdomyolysis
> - Familial tumoural calcinosis

result in precipitation of calcium phosphate, particularly in the presence of a normal or raised calcium level or of alkalosis. Uraemic itching may be caused by a raised calcium phosphate product. Prolonged hyperphosphataemia causes hyperparathyroidism and periarticular and vascular calcification.

Familial tumoural calcinosis is characterized by calcifications of muscles, skin, eyelids and vessels, as well as hyperostosis. In this condition, absence of glycosylation of FGF23 makes it unstable and more sensitive to proteolysis. This results in its deficiency and hyperphosphataemia due to increased renal phosphate reabsorption through increased NPT2a activity.

Usually, no treatment is required for acute hyperphosphataemia, as the causes are self-limiting. Treatment of chronic hyperphosphataemia is with gut phosphate binders and dialysis (see p. 1395).

Further reading

Insogna KL, Briot K, Imel EA et al. A randomized, double-blind, placebo-controlled, phase 3 trial evaluating the efficacy of burosumab, an anti-FGF23 antibody, in adults with X-linked hypophosphatemia: week 24 primary analysis. *J Bone Miner Res* 2018; 33:1383–1393.
Wagner CA, Rubio-Aliaga I, Biber J et al. Genetic diseases of renal phosphate handling. *Nephrol Dial Transplant* 2014; 29(Suppl 4):iv45–54.

ACID–BASE DISORDERS

The concentration of hydrogen ions in both extracellular and intracellular compartments is extremely tightly controlled, and very small changes lead to major cell dysfunction. The blood pH is tightly regulated and is normally maintained at between 7.38 and 7.42. Any deviation from this range indicates a substantial change in the hydrogen ion concentration [H^+] because blood pH is the negative logarithm of [H^+] (**Box 9.25**). The [H^+] at a physiological blood pH of 7.40 is 40 nmol/L. An increase in the [H^+] (a fall in pH) is termed acidaemia. A decrease in [H^+] (a rise in the blood pH) is termed alkalaemia. The disorders that cause these changes in the blood pH are acidosis and alkalosis, respectively.

> **i Box 9.25** Relationship between [H+] and pH
>
> | pH | [H+] (nmol/L) |
> | --- | --- |
> | 6.9 | 126 |
> | 7.0 | 100 |
> | 7.1 | 79 |
> | 7.2 | 63 |
> | 7.3 | 50 |
> | 7.4 | 40 |
> | 7.5 | 32 |
> | 7.6 | 25 |

Normal acid–base physiology

The normal adult diet contains 70–100 mmol of acid (H^+). Throughout the body there are buffers that minimize any changes in blood pH that these ingested hydrogen ions might cause. Such buffers include intracellular proteins (e.g. haemoglobin) and tissue components (e.g. the calcium carbonate and calcium phosphate in bone), as well as the bicarbonate–carbonic acid buffer pair generated by the hydration of carbon dioxide. This buffer pair is clinically most relevant, in part because its contribution can be measured and because alterations in this buffer pair reveal changes in all other buffer systems. Bicarbonate ions [HCO_3^-] and carbonic acid (H_2CO_3) exist in equilibrium; and in the presence of carbonic anhydrase, carbonic acid dissociates to carbon dioxide and water, as expressed in the following equation:

$$H^+HCO_3^- \rightleftarrows H_2CO_3 \xleftarrow{\text{carbonic anhydrase}} CO_2 + H_2O.$$

The addition of hydrogen ions drives the reaction to the right, decreasing the plasma bicarbonate concentration [HCO_3^-] and increasing the arterial carbon dioxide pressure (P_aCO_2). As shown in the following **Henderson–Hasselbalch equation**, a fall in the plasma [HCO_3^-] increases [H^+] and thus lowers blood pH:

$$[H^+] = 181 \times P_aCO_2[HCO_3^-]$$

where [H^+] is expressed in nmol/L, P_aCO_2 in kilopascals, [HCO_3^-] in mmol/L and 181 is the dissociation coefficient of carbonic acid. Alternatively, the equation can be expressed as:

$$pH = pK + \frac{\log[HCO_3^-]}{[H_2CO_3]}$$

where $pK = 6.1$. Thus, the bicarbonate used in the buffering process must be regenerated to maintain normal acid–base balance.

Although the acidaemia stimulates an increase in ventilation, which blunts this change in pH, increased ventilation does not regenerate the bicarbonate used in the buffering process. Consequently, the kidney must excrete hydrogen ions to return the plasma [HCO_3^-] to normal. Maintenance of a normal plasma [HCO_3^-] under physiological conditions depends not only on daily regeneration of bicarbonate but also on reabsorption of all bicarbonate filtered across the glomerular capillaries.

Renal reabsorption of bicarbonate

The plasma [HCO_3^-] is normally maintained at approximately 25 mmol/L. In individuals with a normal GFR (120 mL/min), about 4500 mmol of bicarbonate is filtered each day. If this filtered bicarbonate were not reabsorbed, the plasma [HCO_3^-] would fall, along with blood pH. Thus, maintenance of normal plasma [HCO_3^-] requires that essentially all of the bicarbonate in the glomerular filtrate be reabsorbed (**Fig. 9.14**).

The proximal convoluted tubule reclaims 85–90% of filtered bicarbonate; by contrast, the distal nephron reclaims very little. This difference is caused by the greater quantity of luminal (brush border) carbonic anhydrase in the proximal tubule than in the distal nephron. As a result of these quantitative differences, bicarbonate that escapes reabsorption in the proximal tubule is excreted in the urine.

Proximal tubular bicarbonate reabsorption is catalyzed by the Na^+/K^+-ATPase pump located in the basolateral cell membrane. By exchanging peritubular potassium ions for intracellular sodium ions, the pump keeps the intracellular sodium concentration low, allowing sodium ions to enter the cell by moving down the sodium

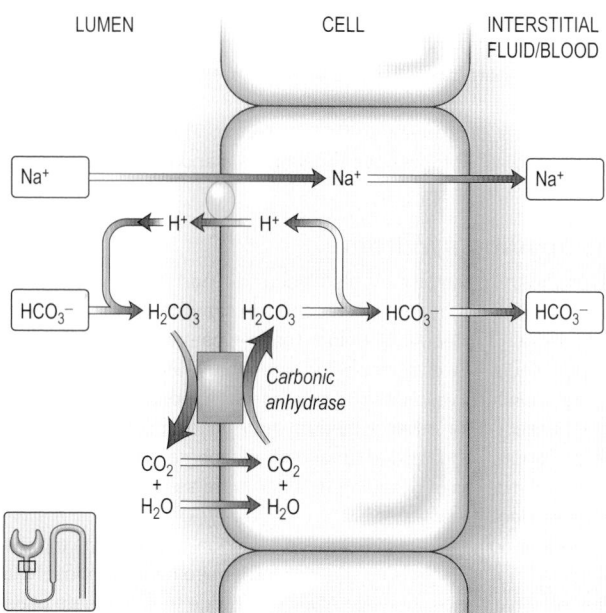

Fig. 9.14 Resorption of sodium bicarbonate in the renal (mainly proximal) tubule. Bicarbonate is reclaimed by the secretion of H^+ in exchange for Na^+ into the tubule. This results in the formation of H_2CO_3, which is then broken down to CO_2. This is reabsorbed and converted back to H_2CO_3, which now dissociates into H^+ and HCO_3^-. The net result is reabsorption of Na^+ and HCO_3^-. This process is dependent on carbonic anhydrase within the cells and on the luminal surface of the tubular cell.

concentration gradient from the tubule lumen to the cell interior. Hydrogen ions are transported in the opposite direction (at the Na^+–H^+ antiporter), thereby maintaining electroneutrality. Before bicarbonate enters the proximal tubule, it combines with secreted hydrogen ions, forming carbonic acid. In the presence of luminal carbonic anhydrase (CA-IV), carbonic acid rapidly dissociates into carbon dioxide and water, which can then rapidly enter the proximal tubular cell. In the cell, carbon dioxide is hydrated by cytosolic carbonic anhydrase (CA-II), ultimately forming bicarbonate, which is then transported down an electrical gradient from the cell interior, across the membrane into the peritubular fluid, and into the blood. In this process, each hydrogen ion secreted into the proximal tubule lumen is reabsorbed and can be resecreted; there is no net loss of hydrogen ions or net gain of bicarbonate ions.

Renal excretion of [H^+]

More acid is secreted into the proximal tubule (up to 4500 nmol of hydrogen ions each day) than in any other nephron segment (**Fig. 9.15**). However, the hydrogen ions secreted into the proximal tubule are almost completely reabsorbed with bicarbonate; consequently, proximal tubular hydrogen ion secretion does not contribute significantly to hydrogen ion elimination from the body. The excretion of the daily acid load requires hydrogen ion secretion in more distal nephron segments.

Most dietary hydrogen ions come from sulphur-containing amino acids that are metabolized to sulphuric acid (H_2SO_4), which then reacts with sodium bicarbonate as follows:

$$H_2SO_4 + 2NaHCO_3 \rightarrow Na_2SO_4 + 2CO_2 + 2H_2O.$$

Excess sulphate is excreted in the urine, whereas excess hydrogen ions are buffered by bicarbonate and lower the plasma [HCO_3^-].

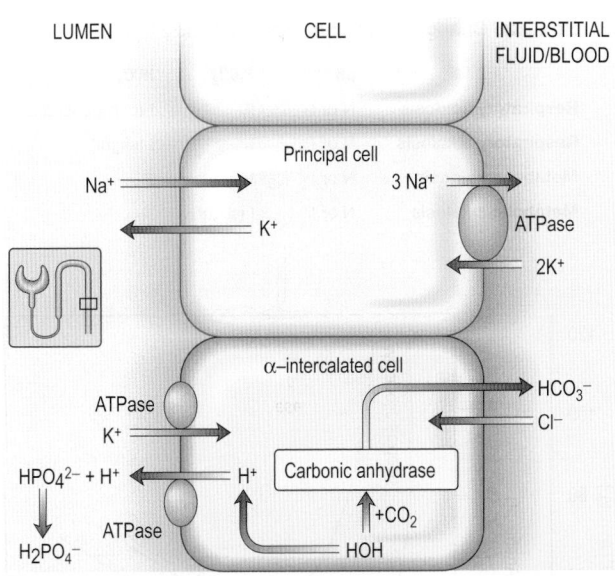

Fig. 9.15 Renal excretion of H^+. H^+ excretion is indirectly controlled by aldosterone in the cortical collecting ducts. Aldosterone enhances sodium absorption and potassium excretion by opening sodium channels and enhancing the activity of the Na^+/K^+-ATPase in the principal cell. These actions set up an electrochemical gradient favouring H^+ excretion. Aldosterone also facilitates H^+ excretion by stimulating H^+-ATPase in the intercalated cell.

This fall in plasma $[HCO_3^-]$ leads to a slight decrease in the blood pH, although a smaller decrease than would have occurred if buffer were unavailable. The subsequent excretion of hydrogen ions takes place primarily in the collecting duct and results in the regeneration of 1 mmol of bicarbonate for every mmol of hydrogen ions excreted in the urine.

The **collecting duct** has three types of cell:

- The **principal cells** with an aldosterone-sensitive Na^+ absorption site. These cells reabsorb Na^+ and H_2O and secrete K^+ under the influence of aldosterone.
- The **α-intercalated cells**, which possess the proton pump for the active secretion of hydrogen ions in exchange for reabsorption of K^+ ions. Aldosterone increases H^+ ion secretion.
- The **β-intercalated cells** are mirror images of α-intercalated cells. Here the H^+-ATPase pump is located in the basolateral rather than the apical membrane, whereby H^+ ions are secreted into the peritubular capillary. The HCO_3^- ions, on the other hand, are secreted into the tubular lumen by an anion exchanger in the apical membrane. The identity of this transporter is uncertain, however, as it does not appear to represent the same Cl^--HCO_3^- exchanger that is present in the basolateral membrane of the H^+-secreting intercalated cells.

Secretion of hydrogen ions from the CCD is indirectly linked to sodium reabsorption.

- Aldosterone has several facilitating effects on hydrogen ion secretion. Aldosterone opens sodium channels in the luminal membrane of the **principal cell** and increases Na^+/K^+-ATPase activity. The subsequent movement of cationic sodium into the principal cell creates a negative charge within the tubule lumen. Potassium ions from the principal cells and hydrogen ions from the α-intercalated cells move out from the cells down the electrochemical gradient and into the lumen.
- Aldosterone also stimulates directly the H^+-ATPase in the α-intercalated cell, further enhancing hydrogen ion secretion. The H^+ to be secreted arises from the reassociation of H_2O and CO_2 in the presence of carbonic anhydrase; thus, a bicarbo-

nate molecule is regenerated each time an H^+ is eliminated in the urine.

When hydrogen ions are secreted into the lumen of the collecting tubule, a tiny, but physiologically critical, fraction of these excess hydrogen ions remains in solution. Here, they increase the urinary $[H^+]$ and lower urinary pH below 4.0. Nevertheless, below this urine pH, inhibition of proton-secreting pumps, such as H^+-ATPase, severely restricts kidney secretion of more hydrogen ions. Consequently, secretion of hydrogen ions depends on the presence of buffers in the urine that maintain the urine pH at a level higher than 4.0.

In the presence of alkali excess, the homeostatic needs are reversed. Although the kidney can excrete excess alkaline load by reducing reabsorption of filtered bicarbonate in the proximal and distal tubule, the collecting ducts also contribute by secreting bicarbonate brought about by switching to β-intercalated cells. This switch enables kidneys to secrete bicarbonate and conserve H^+ ions.

Buffer systems in acid excretion

Two buffer systems are involved in acid excretion: the titratable acids, such as phosphate, and the ammonia system. Each system is responsible for excreting about half of the daily acid load of 50–100 mmol under physiological conditions (see **Fig. 9.15**).

Titratable acid

A titratable acid is a filtered buffer substance having a conjugate anion that can be titrated within the pH range occurring physiologically in the urine. Phosphoric acid (pK_a 6.8) is the usual titratable urinary buffer. Hydrogen ions bind to the conjugate anions of the titratable acids and are excreted in the urine. For each hydrogen ion excreted in this form, a bicarbonate ion is regenerated within the cell and returned to the blood (see **Fig. 9.15**).

Ammonium (NH_4^+)

In the setting of metabolic acidosis, titratable acids cannot increase significantly because the availability of titratable acid is fixed by the plasma concentration of the buffer and by the GFR. The ammonia buffer system, by contrast, can increase several hundred-fold when necessary. Consequently, impaired renal excretion of hydrogen ions is always associated with a defect in ammonium excretion (**Fig. 9.16**).

All ammonia used to buffer urinary hydrogen ions in the collecting tubule is synthesized in the proximal convoluted tubule. Glutamine is the primary source of ammonia. It undergoes deamination catalyzed by glutaminase, resulting in α-ketoglutaric acid (see **Fig. 9.16**) and ammonia. Once formed, ammonia can diffuse into the proximal tubule lumen and become acidified, forming ammonium. Once in the proximal tubule lumen, ammonium flows along the tubule to the thick ascending limb of the loop of Henle. Here, it is transported out of the tubule into the medullary interstitium. Ammonium then dissociates to ammonia, leading to a high interstitial ammonia concentration. The notion that ammonia diffuses down its concentration gradient into the lumen of the collecting tubule has been challenged by the discovery of rhesus (Rh)-associated glycoproteins acting as ammonia transport proteins, also called RhCG/Rhcg, which are expressed in the basolateral and apical surfaces of the DCT, inner medullary collecting duct and type α-intercalated cells. These proteins play a fundamental role in renal ammonia excretion under both basal and acidotic states. Once secreted, NH_3 reacts with the hydrogen ions secreted by the collecting tubular cells to form ammonium. Because ammonium (NH_4) is not lipid-soluble, it is trapped in the lumen and excreted in the urine as ammonium

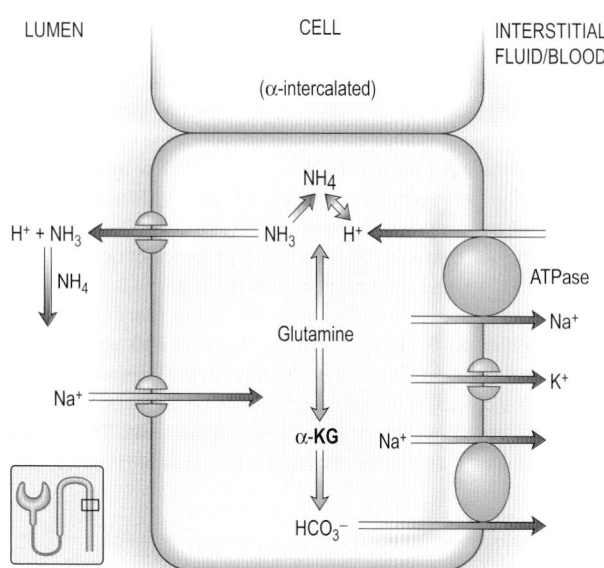

Fig. 9.16 The ammonia buffering system in the kidney. All ammonia used to buffer H^+ in the collecting duct is synthesized in the proximal convoluted tubule, and glutamine is the main source of this ammonia. As glutamine is metabolized, α-ketoglutarate (α-KG) is formed, which ultimately breaks down to bicarbonate that is then secreted into the peritubular fluid at an Na^+-HCO_3^- co-transporter.

chloride. Two conditions predominantly promote ammonia synthesis by the proximal tubular cell: systemic acidosis and hypokalaemia.

Aetiology of acid–base disturbance

Acid–base disturbance may be caused by:

- abnormal CO_2 removal in the lungs ('respiratory' acidosis and alkalosis)
- abnormalities in the regulation of bicarbonate and other buffers in the blood ('metabolic' acidosis and alkalosis).

Both may, and usually do, coexist. For instance, metabolic acidosis causes hyperventilation (via medullary chemoreceptors, see **Fig. 28.5**), leading to increased removal of CO_2 in the lungs and partial compensation for the acidosis. Conversely, respiratory acidosis is accompanied by renal bicarbonate retention, which could be mistaken for primary metabolic alkalosis. The situation is even more complex if a patient has both respiratory disease and a primary metabolic disturbance.

Diagnosis

Clinical history and examination usually point to the correct diagnosis. **Box 9.26** shows the typical blood changes, but in complicated patients the acid–base nomogram (**Fig. 9.17**) is invaluable. The [H^+] and $P_a CO_2$ are measured in arterial blood (for precautions), as well as the bicarbonate. If the values from a patient lie in one of the bands in the diagram, it is likely that only one abnormality is present. If the [H^+] is high (pH low) but the $P_a CO_2$ is normal, the intercept lies between two bands: the patient has respiratory dysfunction, leading to failure of CO_2 elimination, but this is partly compensated for by metabolic acidosis, stimulating respiration and CO_2 removal (this is the most common 'combined' abnormality in practice).

Box 9.26 Changes in arterial blood gases

	pH	$P_a CO_2$	HCO_3^-
Respiratory acidosis	N or ↓	↑↑	↑ (compensated)
Respiratory alkalosis	N or ↑	↓↓	↓ (slight)
Metabolic acidosis	N or ↓	↓	↓↓
Metabolic alkalosis	N or ↑	↑ (slight)	↑↑

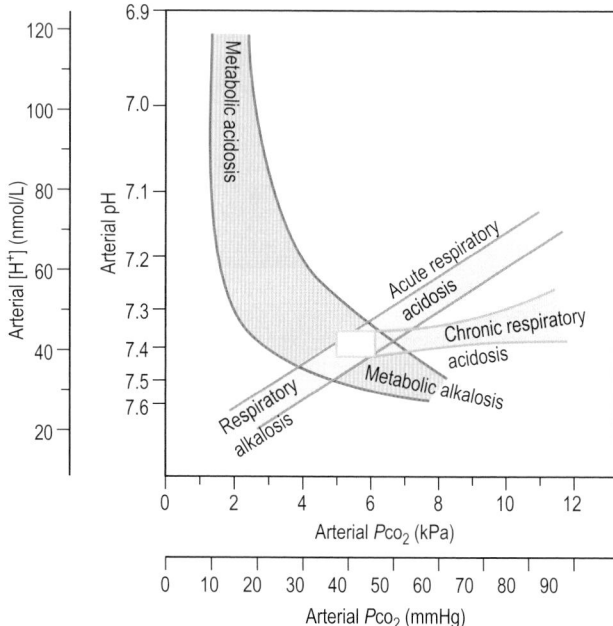

Fig. 9.17 The Flenley acid–base nomogram. This was derived from a large number of observations in patients with 'pure' respiratory or metabolic disturbances. The bands show the 95% confidence limits representing the individual varieties of acid–base disturbance. The central white box shows the approximate limits of arterial pH and PCO_2 in normal individuals.

Respiratory acidosis and alkalosis

Respiratory acidosis

This is caused by retention of CO_2, commonly seen in chronic obstructive pulmonary disease (COPD). The $P_a CO_2$ and [H^+] rise. Renal retention of bicarbonate may partly compensate, returning the [H^+] towards normal (see p. 214).

Respiratory alkalosis

Increased removal of CO_2 is caused by hyperventilation, so there is a fall in $P_a CO_2$ and [H^+] (see p. 214).

Metabolic acidosis and alkalosis

Metabolic acidosis

This is due to the accumulation of any acid other than carbonic acid, and there is a primary decrease in the plasma [HCO_3^-]. Several disorders can lead to metabolic acidosis: acid administration, acid generation (e.g. lactic acidosis during shock or cardiac arrest), impaired acid excretion by the kidneys, or bicarbonate losses from the gastrointestinal tract or kidneys. Calculation of the plasma anion gap is extremely useful in narrowing this differential diagnosis.

Anion gap

The first step is to identify whether the acidosis is due to retention of H^+Cl^- or to another acid. This is achieved by calculation of the anion gap.

- The normal cations present in plasma are Na^+, K^+, Ca^{2+} and Mg^{2+}.
- The normal anions present in plasma are Cl^-, HCO_3^- and negative charges present on albumin, phosphate, sulphate, lactate and other organic acids.
- The sums of the positive and negative charges are equal.
- Measurement of plasma $[Na^+]$, $[K^+]$, $[Cl^-]$ and $[HCO_3^-]$ is usually easily available.

As there are more unmeasured anions than cations, the **normal anion gap** is 12–16 mmol/L, although calculations with more sensitive methods place this at 3–9 mmol/L. Albumin normally makes up the largest portion of these unmeasured anions. As a result, a fall in the plasma albumin concentration from the normal value of about 40 g/L to 20 g/L may reduce the anion gap by as much as 6 mmol/L because each 1 g/L of albumin has a negative charge of 0.2–0.28 mmol/L.

Metabolic acidosis with a normal anion gap

If the anion gap is normal in the presence of acidosis, this suggests that H^+Cl^- is being retained or that $Na^+HCO_3^-$ is being lost. Causes of a normal-anion-gap acidosis are given in **Box 9.27**. In these conditions, plasma bicarbonate decreases and is replaced by chloride to maintain electroneutrality. Consequently, these disorders are sometimes referred to collectively as hyperchloraemic acidosis.

Renal tubular acidosis

The term 'renal tubular acidosis' (RTA) refers to systemic acidosis caused by impairment of the ability of the renal tubules to maintain acid–base balance. This group of disorders is uncommon and only rarely a cause of significant clinical disease.

Type 4 renal tubular acidosis

This results from a deficiency or unresponsiveness to aldosterone and, as such, type 4 RTA is also called 'hyporeninaemic hypoaldosteronism'. This is the most common form of RTA. The cardinal features are hyperkalaemia and acidosis occurring in a patient with mild CKD, usually caused by tubulointerstitial disease (e.g. reflux nephropathy) or diabetes. Hyperkalaemia maintains the acidosis through impairment of ammonia production in the proximal tubule leading to a reduction in net acid excretion. Gordon's syndrome (see p. 189) shares biochemical abnormalities but differs in having normal GFR and hypertension. Plasma renin and aldosterone are found to be low, even after measures that would normally stimulate their secretion. Features of type 4 RTA are shown in **Box 9.28**. An identical syndrome is caused by chronic ingestion of NSAIDs, which impair renin and aldosterone secretion. In the presence of acidosis, urine pH may be low. Treatment is with fludrocortisone, sodium bicarbonate, diuretics or gut-acting potassium binders, or a combination of these. Resolution of hyperkalaemia may correct the metabolic acidosis through increased ammonium excretion. Dietary potassium restriction alone is ineffective.

Type 3 renal tubular acidosis

This condition is vanishingly rare, and represents a combination of type 1 and type 2 RTA. Inherited type 3 RTA is caused by mutations

Increased gastrointestinal bicarbonate loss
- Diarrhoea
- Ileostomy
- Ureterosigmoidostomy

Increased renal bicarbonate loss
- Acetazolamide therapy
- Proximal (type 2) renal tubular acidosis
- Hyperparathyroidism
- Tubular damage, e.g. drugs, heavy metals, paraproteins

Decreased renal hydrogen ion excretion
- Distal (type 1) renal tubular acidosis
- Type 4 renal tubular acidosis (aldosterone deficiency)

Increased HCl production
- Ammonium chloride ingestion
- Increased catabolism of lysine, arginine

resulting in carbonic anhydrase type II deficiency, which is characterized by osteopetrosis, RTA of mixed type, cerebral calcification and mental retardation.

Type 2 ('proximal') renal tubular acidosis

This is very rare in adult practice. It is caused by failure of sodium bicarbonate reabsorption in the proximal tubule. The cardinal features are acidosis, hypokalaemia, an inability to lower the urine pH below 5.5 despite systemic acidosis, and the appearance of bicarbonate in the urine despite a subnormal plasma bicarbonate. This disorder normally occurs as part of a generalized tubular defect, together with other features such as glycosuria and amino-aciduria. Inherited forms of isolated type 2 RTA are described as both autosomal dominant and recessive patterns of inheritance, where putative mutations are in the Na^+–H^+ antiporter in the apical membrane and Na^+–HCO_3^- co-transporter in the basolateral membrane of proximal tubular cells, respectively (see **Fig. 9.10**). Treatment is with sodium bicarbonate; massive doses may be required to overcome the renal 'leak'.

Type 1 ('distal') renal tubular acidosis

This is due to a failure of H^+ excretion in the distal tubule (**Box 9.29**). It consists of:
- acidosis
- hypokalaemia (few exceptions)
- inability to lower the urine pH below 5.3 despite systemic acidosis
- low urinary ammonium production.

These features may be present only in the face of increased acid production, hence the need for an acid load test in diagnosis (**Box 9.30**). Other features include:
- low urinary citrate (owing to increased citrate absorption in the proximal tubule, where it can be converted to bicarbonate)
- hypercalciuria.

These abnormalities result in osteomalacia, renal stone formation and recurrent urinary infections:
- **Osteomalacia** is caused by buffering of H^+ by Ca^{2+} in bone, resulting in depletion of calcium from bone.
- **Renal stone formation** is caused by hypercalciuria, hypocitraturia (citrate inhibits calcium phosphate precipitation) and alkaline urine (which favours precipitation of calcium phosphate).
- **Recurrent urinary infections** are caused by renal stones.

Both autosomal dominant and recessive inheritance patterns have been reported in primary distal RTA. In autosomal recessive

> **Box 9.28** Features of type 4 renal tubular acidosis (hyporeninaemic hypoaldosteronism)
>
> - Hyperkalaemia (in the absence of drugs known to cause hyperkalaemia)
> - Low plasma bicarbonate and hyperchloraemia
> - Normal adrenocorticotrophic hormone (ACTH) stimulation test (see p. 590)
> - Low basal 24 h urinary aldosterone
> - Subnormal response of plasma renin and plasma aldosterone to stimulation: samples taken over 2 h supine and again after 40 mg furosemide (80 mg if creatinine >120 μmol/L) and 4 h upright posture
> - Correction of hyperkalaemia by fludrocortisone 0.1 mg daily

> **Box 9.29** Causes of type 1 distal renal tubular acidosis
>
> **Primary**
> - Idiopathic
> - Genetic
> - Marfan's syndrome
> - Ehlers–Danlos syndrome
> - Sickle cell anaemia
>
> **Nephrocalcinosis**
> - Chronic hypercalcaemia
> - Medullary sponge kidney
>
> **Hypergammaglobulinaemic states**
> - Amyloidosis[a]
> - Cryoglobulinaemia
> - Chronic liver disease
>
> **Drugs and toxins**
> - Amphotericin B
> - Lithium carbonate
> - NSAIDs
>
> [a]May also cause proximal renal tubular acidosis.

> **Box 9.30** Diagnosis of renal tubular acidosis
>
> Plasma HCO_3^- <21 mmol/L, urine pH >5.3 = renal tubular acidosis.
>
> *Distal RTA: defect in dietary acid excretion. Urine pH always >5.5*
>
> *Proximal RTA: defect in bicarbonate reabsorption. Urine pH variable*
>
> **Bicarbonate infusion test**
> Differentiates between proximal and distal RTA:
> - Use a bicarbonate infusion (0.5–1 mmol/kg per hour) to raise serum bicarbonate to 18–20 mmol/L.
> - If urine pH rises to >7.5 and the fractional excretion of bicarbonate (Fe HCO_3^-)[a] rises to >15%, the defect is bicarbonate reabsorption and the diagnosis is proximal RTA.
>
> - If there is little change in urine pH and fractional excretion of bicarbonate remains low, the diagnosis is distal RTA.
>
> **Acid load test**
> Required if plasma HCO_3^- is >21 mmol/L but there is suspicion of partial RTA (e.g. nephrocalcinosis-associated diseases):
> - Give 100 mg/kg ammonium chloride by mouth.
> - Check urine pH hourly and plasma HCO_3^- at 3 h.
> - Plasma HCO_3^- should drop below 21 mmol/L unless the patient vomits (in which case the test should be repeated with an antiemetic).
> - If urine pH remains >5.3 despite a plasma HCO_3^- of 21 mmol/L, the diagnosis is confirmed.

distal RTA, a substantial proportion of patients have sensorineural deafness, and this is associated with a loss-of-function mutation in the H^+-ATPase at the apical surface of intercalated cells.

Treatment is with sodium bicarbonate, potassium supplements and citrate. Thiazide diuretics are useful because they cause volume contraction and increased proximal sodium bicarbonate reabsorption.

Urinary anion gap

Another useful tool in the evaluation of metabolic acidosis with a normal anion gap is the urinary anion gap:

$$URINARY\,ANION\,GAP = \{urinary\ [Na^+] + urinary\ [K^+]\} - urinary\ [Cl^-].$$

This calculation can be used to distinguish the normal-anion-gap acidosis caused by diarrhoea (or other gastrointestinal alkali loss) from that caused by distal RTA. In both disorders, the plasma $[K^+]$ is characteristically low. In patients with RTA, urinary pH is always greater than 5.3.

Although excretion of urinary hydrogen ions in the patient with diarrhoea should acidify the urine, hypokalaemia leads to enhanced ammonia synthesis by the proximal tubular cells. Despite acidaemia, the excess urinary buffer increases the urine pH to a value above 5.3 in some patients with diarrhoea. Whenever urinary acid is excreted as ammonium chloride, the increase in urinary chloride excretion decreases the urinary anion gap. Thus, the urinary anion gap should be negative in the patient with diarrhoea regardless of the urine pH. On the other hand, although hypokalaemia may result in enhanced proximal tubular ammonia synthesis in distal RTA, the inability to secrete hydrogen ions into the collecting duct in this condition limits ammonium chloride formation and excretion; thus, the urinary anion gap is positive in distal RTA.

Metabolic acidosis with a high anion gap

If the anion gap is increased, there is an unmeasured anion present in increased quantities. This is either one of the acids normally present in small but unmeasured quantities, such as lactate, or an exogenous acid. See later and **Box 9.31** for causes of a high-anion-gap acidosis.

Chronic kidney disease

Chronic acidosis is most often caused by CKD, in which there is a failure to excrete fixed acid. Up to 40 mmol of hydrogen ions may accumulate daily. These are buffered by bone, in exchange for calcium. Chronic acidosis is therefore a major risk factor for renal osteodystrophy and hypercalciuria.

Chronic acidosis has also been shown to be a risk factor for muscle wasting in renal failure, and may also contribute to the inexorable progression of some types of renal disease.

Kidney disease causes acidosis in several ways:
- Reduction in the number of functioning nephrons decreases the capacity to excrete ammonia and H^+ in the urine.
- Tubular disease may cause bicarbonate wasting.

Acidosis is a particular feature of those types of CKD in which the tubules are particularly affected, such as reflux nephropathy and chronic obstructive uropathy.

Uraemic acidosis should be corrected because of the effects on growth, muscle turnover and bones. Oral sodium bicarbonate 2–3 mmol/kg daily is usually enough to maintain serum bicarbonate above 20 mmol/L but may contribute to sodium overload. Calcium carbonate improves acidosis and also acts as a phosphate binder and calcium supplement, and is commonly used. Acidosis in end-stage kidney disease is usually fully corrected by adequate dialysis.

Lactic acidosis

Increased lactic acid production occurs when cellular respiration is abnormal, because of either a lack of oxygen in the tissues (*'type A'*) or a metabolic abnormality, such as that induced by drugs such as metformin (*'type B'*). The most common cause in clinical practice is type A lactic acidosis, occurring in septic or cardiogenic shock (see p. 218). Significant acidosis can occur despite a normal blood pressure and P_aCO_2, owing to splanchnic and peripheral vasoconstriction. Acidosis worsens cardiac function and vasoconstriction further, contributing to a downward spiral and fulminant production of lactic acid.

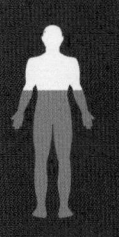

Raised serum D-lactate occurs with fermentation of glucose by abnormal bowel flora in the short gut syndrome.

Ketoacidosis

See also page 722. There is a high-anion-gap acidosis due to the accumulation of acetoacetic and hydroxybutyric acids, owing to increased production and some reduced peripheral utilization in diabetic ketoacidosis. Ketoacidosis without hyperglycaemia occurs in starvation and after alcohol overdose.

Mixed metabolic acidosis

Both types of acidosis may coexist. For instance, cholera would be expected to cause a normal-anion-gap acidosis owing to massive gastrointestinal losses of bicarbonate, but the anion gap is often increased owing to renal failure and lactic acidosis as a result of hypovolaemia.

To help ascertain if there is an additional normal-anion-gap acidosis as well as, for example, a ketoacidosis, the delta anion gap can be calculated. This is the difference between the upper reference value of the anion gap and the calculated anion gap. This value should equal the fall in the bicarbonate concentration from the lower limit of normal. If the bicarbonate is significantly *lower* than predicted (>5 mmol/L), then an additional normal-anion-gap *acidosis* must be present. Similarly, if the bicarbonate is >5 mmol/L *higher* than expected, an additional normal-anion-gap *alkalosis* must be present.

Clinical features of acidosis

Clinically, the most obvious effect is stimulation of respiration, leading to the clinical sign of 'air hunger', or Kussmaul respiration. Interestingly, patients with profound hyperventilation may not complain of breathlessness, although in others it may be a presenting complaint.

Acidosis increases delivery of oxygen to the tissues by shifting the oxyhaemoglobin dissociation curve to the right, but it also leads to inhibition of 2,3-BPG production, which returns the curve towards normal (see **Fig. 10.3**) Cardiovascular dysfunction is common in acidotic patients, although it is often difficult to dissociate the numerous possible causes of this. Acidosis is negatively inotropic. Severe acidosis also causes venoconstriction, resulting in redistribution of blood from the peripheries to the central circulation, and increased systemic venous pressure, which may worsen pulmonary oedema caused by myocardial depression. Arteriolar vasodilatation also occurs, further contributing to hypotension.

Cerebral dysfunction is variable. Severe acidosis is often associated with confusion and fits, but numerous other possible causes are usually present.

As mentioned earlier, acidosis stimulates potassium loss from cells, which may lead to potassium deficiency if renal function is normal, or to hyperkalaemia if renal potassium excretion is impaired.

General treatment of acidosis

Treatment should be aimed at correcting the primary cause. In lactic acidosis caused by poor tissue perfusion ('type A'), treatment should be aimed at maximizing oxygen delivery to the tissues by protecting the airway, and improving breathing and circulation. This usually requires inotropic agents, mechanical ventilation and invasive monitoring. In 'type B' lactic acidosis, treatment is directed at the underlying disorder – for example:

- insulin in diabetic ketoacidosis
- treatment of methanol and ethylene glycol poisoning with ethanol
- removal of salicylate by dialysis.

The question of whether severe acidosis should be treated with bicarbonate is extremely controversial:

- Rapid correction of acidosis may result in tetany and fits owing to a rapid decrease in ionized calcium.
- Administration of sodium bicarbonate (8.4%) provides 1 mmol/mL of sodium, which may lead to extracellular volume expansion, exacerbating pulmonary oedema.
- Bicarbonate therapy increases CO_2 production and will therefore correct acidosis only if ventilation can be increased to remove the added CO_2 load.
- The increased amounts of CO_2 generated may diffuse more readily into cells than bicarbonate, worsening intracellular acidosis.

Administration of sodium bicarbonate (50 mmol, as 50 mL of 8.4% sodium bicarbonate i.v.) is still occasionally given during cardiac arrest and is often necessary before arrhythmias can be corrected. Correction of hyperkalaemia associated with acidosis is also of undoubted benefit. In other situations, there is no clinical evidence to show that correction of acidosis improves outcome, but it is standard practice to administer sodium bicarbonate when [H+] is above 126 nmol/L (pH <6.9), using intravenous 1.26% (150 mmol/L) bicarbonate infused over 2–3 hours with electrolyte and pH monitoring. Intravenous sodium lactate should never be given.

Metabolic alkalosis

Metabolic alkalosis is common, comprising half of all the acid–base disorders in hospitalized patients. This observation should not be surprising since vomiting, the use of diuretics and nasogastric suction are common among hospitalized patients. The mortality associated with metabolic alkalosis is substantial; the mortality rate is 45% in patients with an arterial pH of 7.55 and 80% when the pH is over 7.65. Although this relationship is not necessarily causal, severe alkalosis should be viewed with concern.

Classification and definitions

Metabolic alkalosis has been classified on the basis of underlying pathophysiology (**Box 9.32**):

- *chloride depletion*, the most common cause, which can be corrected without potassium repletion
- *potassium depletion*, usually with mineralocorticoid excess
- *metabolic alkalosis*, due to both potassium and chloride depletion.

Chloride may be lost from the gut, kidney or skin. The loss of gastric fluid rich in acid results in alkalosis because bicarbonate generated during the production of gastric acid returns to the circulation. In Zollinger–Ellison syndrome (see p. 1336) or gastric outflow

Box 9.32 Causes of metabolic alkalosis

Chloride depletion
- Gastric losses: vomiting, mechanical drainage, bulimia
- Chloruretic diuretics, e.g. bumetanide, furosemide, chlorothiazide, metolazone
- Diarrhoeal states: villous adenoma, congenital chloridorrhoea
- Cystic fibrosis (high sweat chloride)

Potassium depletion/ mineralocorticoid excess
- Primary aldosteronism
- Secondary aldosteronism
- Apparent mineralocorticoid excess: primary deoxycorticosterone excess: 11α- and 17α-hydroxylase deficiencies

- Drugs: liquorice (glycyrrhizic acid) as a confection or flavouring, carbenoxolone
- Liddle's syndrome
- Bartter's and Gitelman's syndromes and their variants
- Laxative abuse, clay ingestion

Hypercalcaemic states
- Hypercalcaemia of malignancy
- Acute or chronic milk–alkali syndrome

Others
- Amoxicillin or penicillin therapy
- Bicarbonate ingestion: massive or smaller ingestion with kidney disease
- Recovery from starvation
- Hypoalbuminaemia

obstruction, these losses can be massive. Although sodium and potassium loss in the gastric juice is variable, the obligate urinary loss of these cations is intensified by bicarbonaturia, which occurs during disequilibrium.

Chloruretic agents all directly produce loss of chloride, sodium and fluid in the urine. These losses in turn promote metabolic alkalosis by several mechanisms:

- Diuretic-induced increases in sodium delivery to the distal nephron enhance potassium and hydrogen ion secretion.
- Extracellular volume contraction stimulates renin and aldosterone secretion, which blunts sodium losses but accelerates potassium and hydrogen ion secretion.
- Potassium depletion augments bicarbonate reabsorption in the proximal tubule and stimulates ammonia production, which in turn will increase urinary net acid excretion.

Urinary losses of chloride exceed those for sodium and are associated with alkalosis, even when potassium depletion is prevented. The cessation of events that generate alkalosis is not necessarily accompanied by resolution of the alkalosis. A widely accepted hypothesis for the maintenance of alkalosis is chloride depletion rather than volume depletion. Although normal functioning of the proximal tubule is essential for bicarbonate absorption, the collecting duct appears to be the major segment of the nephron for altered electrolyte and proton transport in both maintenance and recovery from metabolic alkalosis. During maintenance, the α-intercalated cells in the CCD do not secrete bicarbonate because insufficient chloride is available for bicarbonate exchange. When chloride is administered and luminal or cellular chloride concentration increases, bicarbonate is promptly excreted and alkalosis is corrected.

Metabolic alkalosis in **hypokalaemia** is generated primarily by an increased intracellular shift of hydrogen ion, causing intracellular

acidosis. Potassium depletion is also associated with enhanced ammonia production and increased obligate net acid excretion. This is the corollary to the acidosis seen with hyperkalaemia in type 4 RTA. Infusion of potassium alone can correct systemic alkalosis and intracellular acidosis as cells exchange extracellular potassium for intracellular hydrogen, which can then buffer extracellular bicarbonate.

Milk–alkali syndrome, in which both bicarbonate and calcium are ingested, produces alkalosis by vomiting, calcium-induced bicarbonate absorption and reduced GFR.

Clinical features

The symptoms of metabolic alkalosis *per se* are difficult to separate from those of chloride, volume or potassium depletion. Tetany (see **Box 21.58**), apathy, confusion, drowsiness, cardiac arrhythmias and neuromuscular irritability are common when alkalosis is severe. The oxyhaemoglobin dissociation curve is shifted to the left. Respiration may be depressed.

Management
Chloride-responsive metabolic alkalosis

Although replacement of the chloride deficit is essential in chloride depletion states, selection of the accompanying cation – sodium, potassium or proton – is dependent on the assessment of extracellular fluid volume status (see p. 182), the presence or absence of associated potassium depletion, and the degree and reversibility of any depression of GFR. If kidney function is normal, bicarbonate and base equivalents will be excreted with sodium or potassium, and metabolic alkalosis will be rapidly corrected as chloride is made available.

If chloride and extracellular depletion coexist, then isotonic saline solution is appropriate therapy.

In the clinical setting of fluid overload, saline is contraindicated. In such situations, intravenous hydrochloric acid or ammonium chloride can be given. If GFR is adequate, acetazolamide, which causes bicarbonate diuresis by inhibiting carbonic anhydrase, can also be used. When the kidney is incapable of responding to chloride repletion, dialysis is necessary.

Chloride-resistant metabolic alkalosis

Metabolic alkalosis due to potassium depletion is managed by correction of the underlying cause (see 'Hypokalaemia', p. 187). Mild to moderate alkalosis requires oral potassium chloride administration. However, the presence of a cardiac arrhythmia or generalized weakness requires intravenous potassium chloride.

Further reading

Berend K. Diagnostic use of base excess in acid-base disorders. *N Engl J Med* 2018; 378:1419–1428.

Berend K. Review of the diagnostic evaluation of normal anion gap metabolic acidosis. *Kidney Dis (Basel)* 2017; 3:149–159.

Kraut JA, Madias NE. Lactic acidosis. *N Engl J Med* 2015; 372:1078–1079.

Seifter JL, Chang HY. Disorders of acid-base balance: new perspectives. *Kidney Dis (Basel)* 2017; 2:170–186.

Weiner ID, Verlander JW. Ammonia transporters and their role in acid-base balance. *Physiol Rev* 2017; 97:465–494.

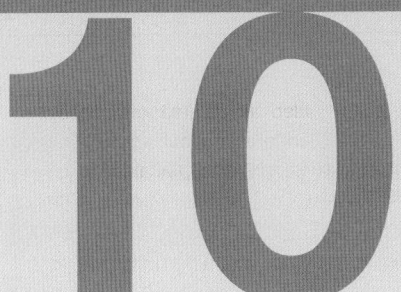

10

Critical care medicine

Stephen Shepherd, Colette Coyle, Andrew Leitch and Parjam Zolfaghari

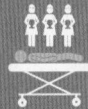

CORE SKILLS AND KNOWLEDGE

Critical care medicine is concerned predominantly with the management of patients with acute life-threatening conditions in specialized units. In addition to emergency cases, intensive care units (ICUs) electively admit high-risk patients after major surgery. The proportion of a hospital's resources dedicated to intensive care varies widely internationally, with the UK providing 6.6 ICU and high-dependency unit (HDU) beds per 100 000 population, and Germany providing 29.2.

ICU staff also provide care throughout the hospital in the form of medical emergency and outreach teams. These teams recognize critically ill patients and provide resuscitation and safe transport to the ICU. They also identify patients who are deteriorating on the ward and intervene early, potentially preventing the need for intensive care admission.

Key skills provided by specialists in critical care medicine include:

- recognizing and managing acutely ill and deteriorating patients, and implementing basic resuscitation with advanced medical care and organ support
- working as part of a multidisciplinary team that includes medical, nursing and allied health professionals
- developing an ability to communicate effectively, taking into consideration the risks and benefits of critical care management and advanced life support, especially when these treatments may be futile and not in the best interest of the patient.

Opportunities for learning critical care medicine include attending ward rounds on ICUs and HDUs, accompanying critical care outreach teams who are reviewing deteriorating patients on the wards, observing key procedures such as endotracheal intubation or central venous catheter insertion, and observing the titration of organ support systems as patients' clinical parameters change.

INTRODUCTION

Critical care medicine describes the care given to some of the sickest patients in the hospital (**Box 10.1**). This might be provided initially by outreach teams in clinical areas such as the emergency department or general medical or surgical wards, but appropriate patients are transferred to either an ICU or an HDU.

ICUs are usually reserved for patients with established or impending organ failure and provide facilities for the diagnosis, prevention and treatment of multiple organ dysfunction. They are fully equipped with monitoring and technical facilities, including an adjacent laboratory and 'near-patient testing' devices for the rapid determination of blood gases and simple biochemical data such as serum potassium, blood glucose and serum lactate levels. Technological advances have introduced more compact and complex devices to manage ventilation and cardiac and renal support. Portable ultrasound and echocardiography equipment is commonly available. Most importantly, patients receive continuous expert nursing care and the constant attention of appropriately trained medical staff.

HDUs offer a level of care between that available on the general ward and that provided in an ICU. They ensure monitoring of and support for patients with acute (or acute-on-chronic) single-organ failure and for those who are at risk of developing organ failure. They can also provide a 'step-down' facility for patients being discharged from intensive care.

CLINICAL APPROACH TO THE CRITICALLY ILL PATIENT

Recognition and diagnosis of critical illness

Early recognition, immediate resuscitation and stabilization are fundamental to the successful management of the critically ill. In order to facilitate identification of 'at-risk' patients on the ward and early referral to the critical care team, a number of early warning systems have been devised (e.g. the Modified Early Warning Score, MEWS). These are based primarily on bedside recognition of deteriorating physiological variables and can be used to supplement clinical

---

> ⓘ **Box 10.1 Some common indications for admission to intensive care**
>
> **Surgical emergencies**
> - Acute intra-abdominal catastrophe:
>   - Perforated viscus, especially with faecal soiling of peritoneum (often complicated by sepsis/septic shock)
>   - Ruptured/leaking abdominal aortic aneurysm
> - Trauma (often complicated by hypovolaemic shock and later sepsis/septic shock):
>   - Multiple injuries
>   - Massive blood loss
>   - Severe head injury
>
> **Medical emergencies**
> - Respiratory failure:
>   - Exacerbation of chronic obstructive pulmonary disease (COPD)
>   - Acute severe asthma
>   - Severe pneumonia (often complicated by sepsis/septic shock)
>
> - Cardiac failure (cardiogenic shock) often following myocardial infarction, arrhythmias and cardiac arrest
> - Meningococcal infection
> - Status epilepticus
> - Severe diabetic ketoacidosis
> - Coma
>
> **Elective surgical admissions**
> - Extensive/prolonged procedure (e.g. oesophagogastrectomy)
> - Cardiothoracic surgery
> - Major head and neck surgery
> - Coexisting cardiovascular or respiratory disease
>
> **Obstetric emergencies**
> - Severe pre-eclampsia/eclampsia
> - Haemorrhage
> - Amniotic fluid embolism

intuition. The MEWS score been superseded by the National Early Warning Score (NEWS2) in the UK, which has been optimized to recognize sepsis and new-onset confusion (**Fig. 10.1**).

These early warning systems are not infallible and have not been universally implemented. It is therefore imperative that clinicians are trained to recognize critically ill patients at the bedside. The initial assessment may elicit obvious signs. The patient may be unduly agitated or, perhaps more worryingly, unresponsive. Of particular concern is the obtunded patient who is unable to protect their own airway from aspiration of gastric or oral contents. Snoring, grunting or other respiratory sounds may indicate an obstructed airway, which can be caused by posterior displacement of the tongue due to lax oropharyngeal musculature in a comatose patient, or perhaps by secretions pooling in the oropharynx in a patient with a depressed cough reflex. Obvious use of the accessory respiratory muscles and a tracheal tug are sensitive signs of impending respiratory decompensation. Patients in severe respiratory distress frequently sit forwards, grip the sides of the bed and cannot complete sentences in a single breath. Review of the nursing observations may reveal a sudden deterioration in recorded variables, such as a sharp rise in temperature, increasing heart rate, a fall in blood pressure or decreased urine output.

On examination, cool peripheries in conjunction with diaphoresis indicate increased sympathetic drive and may be a sign of cardiogenic shock, hypovolaemia or hypoglycaemia. In contrast, flushed, warm peripheries may be a sign of a hyperdynamic circulation consistent with sepsis (see Ch. 8). **Abdominal catastrophes** are a common cause of an acute deterioration; an abdominal examination should always be performed and may reveal a distended, tender abdomen and often absent or altered bowel sounds consistent with a perforated viscus or ischaemic bowel. **Blood gas analysis** should be performed as soon as possible. Acid–base status, haemoglobin concentration, blood glucose and electrolyte levels obtained from an arterial blood gas sample are helpful when assessing the cause and severity of acute illness. Increased lactate levels usually indicate severe illness. An **electrocardiogram** (**ECG**) can allow the rapid diagnosis of treatable conditions, as can a portable **chest X-ray**.

Frequently, the precise underlying diagnosis is initially unclear but, in all cases, the immediate objective is to preserve life and prevent, reverse or minimize damage to vital organs such as the lungs, brain, kidneys and liver. A systematic approach to the recognition and initial treatment of acute illness should be adopted, as well as the performance of investigations to search for the underlying cause. A rapid assessment following the ABC approach (*Airway, Breathing, Circulation*; see **Fig. 10.24**) should be undertaken, with simultaneous institution of treatment. In practice, resuscitation, assessment and diagnosis usually proceed in parallel.

General aspects of managing the critically ill

Critically ill patients require multidisciplinary care that should include the following elements.

Intensive skilled nursing care

In the UK, this usually entails a 1:1 nurse to patient ratio in an ICU (level 3 care) or 1:2 in an HDU (level 2 care). Frequent clinical observations and treatment are required.

Specialized physiotherapy

This should include chest physiotherapy, mobilization and rehabilitation.

Management of pain and distress

There should be judicious administration of analgesics and sedatives (see p. 227).

Constant reassurance and support

Critically ill patients easily become disorientated; delirium (a transient alteration in consciousness, attention, orientation, perception or behaviour) is common. Delirium may be hypoactive, agitated (hyperactive) or a combination of the two. Pain, advanced age, sleep/sensory deprivation, sedative administration (especially benzodiazepines), alcohol/drug withdrawal, neurological injury, severe illness and medical co-morbidities all play a role. Patients with delirium are more difficult to wean from ventilation, require larger doses of sedatives and have an associated increased mortality and length of hospital stay. Treatment focuses on effective pain control, minimizing sensory deprivation, early mobilization, avoidance of benzodiazepines and limiting sedative administration. Newer sedative agents, such as the α_2 agonist dexmedetomidine, may reduce the incidence of delirium and time on the ventilator.

Gastric protection

H_2-receptor antagonists or proton pump inhibitors reduce gastric acidity and prevent stress-induced ulceration. They may, however, encourage bacterial overgrowth in the upper gastrointestinal tract and predispose patients to ventilator-associated pneumonia; they are also associated with *Clostridium difficile* colitis.

Physiological parameter	3	2	1	Score 0	1	2	3
Respiration rate (per minute)	≤8		9–11	12–20		21–24	25
SpO₂ Scale 1 (%)	≤91	92–93	94–95	≥96			
SpO₂ Scale 2 (%)	≤83	84–85	86–87	88–92 ≥93 on air	93–94 on oxygen	95–96 on oxygen	≥97 on oxygen
Air or oxygen?		Oxygen		Air			
Systolic blood pressure (mmHg)	≤90	91–100	101–110	111–219			≥220
Pulse (per minute)	≤40		41–50	51-90	91–110	111–130	≥131
Consciousness				Alert			CVPU
Temperature (°C)	≤35.0		35.1–36.0	36.1–38.0	38.1–39.0	≥39.1	

Fig. 10.1 The National Early Warning Score (NEWS2) system. SpO₂ Scale 1 should be used in all patients except those where there is previously confirmed and documented hypercapnoeic respiratory failure demonstrated on blood gas analysis. Aggregate scores of 0–4 (low clinical risk) require a ward-based response, and those of 5–6 (medium risk) require an urgent response from the clinical team. Aggregate scores of 7 or more (high clinical risk) should receive an urgent emergency response from critical care staff. CVPU, confusion, voice, painful stimulus, unresponsive. *(Reproduced from: Royal College of Physicians. National Early Warning Score (NEWS) 2: Standardising the assessment of acute-illness severity in the NHS. Updated report of a working party. London: RCP, 2017.)*

Deep vein thrombosis prevention

This should be instigated with use of compression stockings, pneumatic compression devices and subcutaneous low-molecular-weight heparin.

Mouth care, tooth-brushing and oropharyngeal suction

These measures help to reduce hospital-acquired infections and ventilator-associated pneumonia by reducing the burden of pathogenic oral flora that may be aspirated into the respiratory tree. Chlorhexidine body washes may reduce the total carriage of resistant microorganisms.

Prevention of constipation and pressure ulcers

Steps should be taken to prevent constipation and pressure ulcers developing.

Organ support

For example, inotropes and vasopressors may be required for cardiovascular support, invasive and non-invasive ventilation for respiratory failure, and dialysis for renal failure. Specialized units may provide extracorporeal membrane oxygenation (ECMO) for severe respiratory failure, mechanical support of the circulation for cardiac failure, and advanced liver support in the form of liver dialysis (e.g. the molecular adsorbent recirculation system, MARS).

Nutritional support

(See p. 1231.) Protein–energy malnutrition is common in critically ill patients and is associated with muscle wasting, weakness, delayed mobilization, difficulty weaning from ventilation, immune compromise and impaired wound healing. ***Enteral nutrition***, usually delivered via a fine-bore nasogastric tube, is preferred because it is less expensive, preserves gut mucosal integrity, is more physiological and is associated with fewer complications. However, the value of enteral nutrition early in the course of an acute illness remains uncertain. If enteral feeding is not possible due to the gut dysmotility and malabsorption associated with critical illness, the alternative is ***intravenous (parenteral) nutrition*** (see p. 1255). This is more invasive and expensive, and can be complicated by deranged liver function tests, hypertriglyceridaemia, hyperglycaemia and an increased susceptibility to hospital-acquired infections. Hypocaloric enteral nutrition is usually continued for up to a week in previously well-nourished patients before parenteral nutrition is considered. Administering parenteral nutrition early in order to maintain caloric input and prevent an energy deficit may be detrimental.

Although all nutrition should contain carbohydrate, protein, lipids and some micronutrients, the precise optimal formulation is unclear. Supplementation with the amino acid glutamine has theoretical advantages in some conditions (burns and trauma) but not in multiorgan failure. The omega-3 fatty acids derived from fish oils also have potentially beneficial antioxidant activity but have not been convincingly shown to improve outcome, as has been the case for micronutrient supplementation with selenium, copper, manganese, zinc, iron and vitamins.

Many critically ill patients are at risk of developing a '***re-feeding syndrome***' (see p. 1235) when nutritional support is first initiated and should be monitored closely.

Insulin treatment

Treatment should be given for critical illness-induced hyperglycaemia. Insulin is often required in high doses, to combat insulin resistance and hyperglycaemia (which is associated with hospital-acquired infections, renal impairment and poor wound healing, see p. 738). Although the use of intensive insulin therapy to achieve 'tight glycaemic control' (blood glucose level between 4.4 and 6.1 mmol/L) was initially shown to improve outcome, subsequent studies found that this approach is associated with an unacceptably high incidence of hypoglycaemia, and possibly increased mortality. Current recommendations suggest that blood glucose levels should be maintained below 10 mmol/L.

Discharge from the ICU/HDU

Discharge of patients from intensive care should normally be planned in advance and ideally take place during normal working hours. Frequently, when the condition of critically ill patients improves, they are initially 'stepped down' to HDU (level 2) care. Premature or unplanned discharge from the ICU or HDU, especially during the night, has been associated with higher hospital mortality and is best avoided. A discharge summary, including 'points to review', should be included in the clinical notes, with a detailed handover to the receiving team (medical and nursing). The intensive care team should continue to review the patient (who might deteriorate following discharge) on the ward and be available for advice on further management (e.g. tracheostomy care, nutritional support). In this way, deterioration and re-admission to intensive care (which is associated with a particularly poor outcome), or even cardiorespiratory arrest, might be avoided.

This chapter concentrates on cardiovascular, respiratory, renal and neurological problems. Many patients also have failure of other organs, such as the liver; treatment of these is dealt with in more detail in the relevant chapters.

Further reading

Adhikari NKJ, Fowler RA, Bhagwanjee S et al. Critical care and the global burden of critical illness. *Lancet* 2010; 376:1339–1341.
Arabi YM, Aldawood AS, Haddad SH et al. Permissive underfeeding or standard enteral feeding in critically ill adults. *N Engl J Med* 2015; 372:2398–2408.
Casaer MP, Van den Berghe G. Nutrition in the acute phase of critical illness. *N Engl J Med* 2014; 370:1227–1236.
Frost PJ, Wise MP. Early management of acutely ill ward patients. *BMJ* 2012; 345:e5677.
Fullerton JN, Perkins GD. Who to admit to intensive care? *Clin Med* 2011; 11:601–604.
NICE–SUGAR Study Investigators. Intensive versus conventional glucose control in critically ill patients. *N Engl J Med* 2009; 360:1293–1297.
Reade MC, Finfer S. Sedation and delirium in the intensive care unit. *N Engl J Med* 2014; 370:444–454.
Royal College of Physicians. National Early Warning Score (NEWS) 2: Standardising the assessment of acute-illness severity in the NHS. Updated report of a working party. London: RCP, 2017.
Singer P, Blaser AR, Berger MM et al. ESPEN guideline on clinical nutrition in the intensive care unit. *Clin Nutr* 2019; 38:48–79.
Vincent JL. Critical care – where have we been and where are we going? *Crit Care* 2013; 17(Suppl 1):S2.

APPLIED CARDIORESPIRATORY PHYSIOLOGY

Oxygen delivery and consumption

Normal cellular, tissue and organ functions depend on adequate delivery of oxygen and fuel to mitochondria, a process requiring the heart, lungs, vascular and haematological systems. Adequate blood flow needs proper functioning of the three components of the circulation: that is, the muscle pump, circulating volume and arterial resistance to flow to perfuse distal tissues; each area has its own regulatory system and may develop pathology.

The term oxygen delivery (DO_2) describes the total amount of oxygen supplied to the body per unit time (**Fig. 10.2**). Its main determinants are the amount of blood pushed through the microcirculation by the cardiac output (Q_t) and the amount of oxygen carried in that blood (i.e. arterial oxygen content, C_aO_2). Oxygen is transported primarily in combination with haemoglobin: the amount combined is determined by its oxygen capacity (usually 1.34 mL of oxygen per gram) and percentage saturation (SO_2). Oxygen is also carried dissolved in plasma; this depends on the partial pressure of oxygen (PO_2) and is usually insignificant.

'Global' oxygen delivery as a concept is of limited clinical value, as differing tissues have differing metabolic requirements and blood flow. Generally, delivery is matched to individual metabolic requirements. Some organs (such as the heart) have high oxygen requirements relative to their blood flow and may receive insufficient oxygen, even if overall delivery appears adequate. Microcirculatory flow is also reduced by increased blood viscosity.

Oxygenation of the blood
Oxyhaemoglobin dissociation curve

The saturation of haemoglobin with oxygen is determined by the partial pressure of oxygen (PO_2), this relationship being described by the oxyhaemoglobin dissociation curve (**Fig. 10.3**). The sigmoid shape of this curve is significant for a number of reasons:

- Modest falls in the partial pressure of oxygen in arterial blood (P_aO_2) have little effect on oxygen content, provided percentage saturations remain above about 92%.
- Increasing the P_aO_2 to above normal has only a minimal effect on oxygen content, unless hyperbaric oxygen is administered (when the amount of oxygen in solution in plasma becomes significant).
- On the slope of the curve (percentage saturation below 90%), a small decrease in P_aO_2 can cause large falls in oxygen content, whereas increasing P_aO_2 only slightly, e.g. by administering 28% oxygen to a patient with chronic obstructive pulmonary disease (COPD), can lead to a useful increase in oxygen saturation and content.

If the PCO_2 increases, the oxyhaemoglobin curve moves to the right, facilitating oxygen unloading to the tissues (Bohr effect).

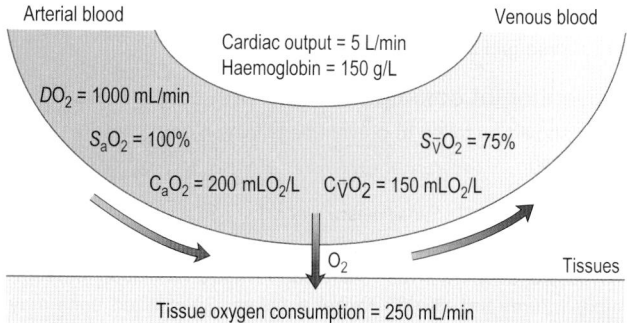

Fig. 10.2 Tissue oxygen delivery and consumption in a normal 70 kg person breathing air. Oxygen delivery (DO_2) = cardiac output × (haemoglobin concentration × oxygen saturation (S_aO_2) × 1.34). In normal adults, oxygen delivery is roughly 1000 mL/min, of which 250 mL is taken up by tissues. Mixed venous blood is thus 75% saturated with oxygen. C_aO_2, arterial oxygen content; $C_{\bar{v}}O_2$, mixed venous oxygen content; $S_{\bar{v}}O_2$, mixed venous oxygen saturation.

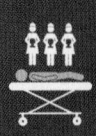

The P_aO_2 is influenced, in turn, by the alveolar oxygen tension (P_AO_2), the efficiency of pulmonary gas exchange, and the partial pressure of oxygen in mixed venous blood ($P_{\bar{v}}O_2$).

Alveolar oxygen tension (P_AO_2)

The partial pressures of inspired gases are shown in **Fig. 10.4**. By the time the inspired gases reach the alveoli, they are fully saturated with water vapour at body temperature (37°C), which has a partial pressure of 6.3 kPa (47 mmHg), and contain CO_2 at a partial pressure of approximately 5.3 kPa (40 mmHg); the P_AO_2 is thereby reduced to approximately 13.4 kPa (100 mmHg).

The clinician can influence P_AO_2 by administering oxygen or by increasing the barometric pressure (hyperbaric therapy).

Pulmonary gas exchange

In *normal* subjects, a small alveolar–arterial oxygen difference ($P_{A-a}O_2$) exists due to:
- a small (0.133 kPa (1 mmHg)) pressure gradient across the alveolar membrane
- a small amount of blood (2% of total cardiac output) bypassing the lungs via the bronchial and thebesian veins
- a small degree of ventilation/perfusion mismatch.

There are three pathological causes of an increased $P_{A-a}O_2$ difference:
- ***Diffusion defect.*** This is *not* a major cause of hypoxaemia, even in conditions such as lung fibrosis, in which the alveolar–capillary membrane is considerably thickened. Carbon dioxide is also not affected, as it is more soluble than oxygen.
- ***Right-to-left shunts.*** In cyanotic congenital heart disease or following collapse of a lung segment, a proportion of venous blood passes to the left side of the heart without taking part in gas exchange, causing arterial hypoxaemia that cannot be corrected by administering oxygen to increase the P_AO_2 because blood leaving normal alveoli is already fully saturated; further increases in PO_2 will not, therefore, significantly affect its oxygen content. On the other hand, because of the shape of the carbon dioxide dissociation curve (**Fig. 10.5**), the high PCO_2 of the shunted blood is compensated for by overventilating patent alveoli; hence many patients with acute right-to-left shunts hyperventilate, producing a low or normal P_aCO_2.
- ***Ventilation/perfusion mismatch*** (see p. 933). This happens when parts of the lung ventilate without much blood flow (e.g. pulmonary embolism), or when there is blood flow but no ventilation, such as in parenchymal lung disease (pneumonia, pulmonary oedema). Both of these states result in hypoxaemia. The increased dead space can be compensated for by increasing overall ventilation. In contrast to the hypoxia resulting from a true right-to-left shunt, that due to areas of low $\dot{V}/\dot{Q}$ can be partially corrected by administering oxygen and thereby increasing the P_AO_2.

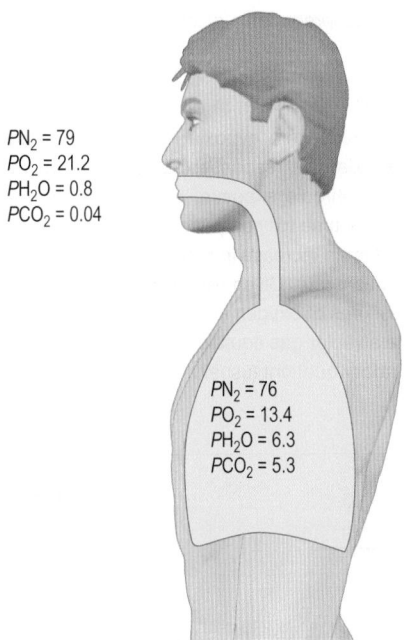

Fig. 10.4 The composition of inspired and alveolar gas. (Partial pressures in kPa.)

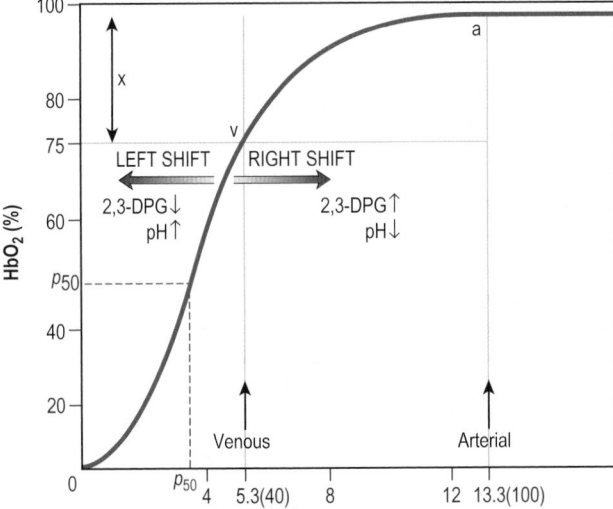

Fig. 10.3 The oxyhaemoglobin dissociation curve. HbO₂ (%) is the percentage saturation of haemoglobin with oxygen. The curve will move to the right in the presence of acidosis (metabolic or respiratory), pyrexia or an increased red cell 2,3-diphosphoglycerate (2,3-DPG) concentration. For a given arteriovenous oxygen content difference, the mixed venous PO_2 will then be higher. Furthermore, if the mixed venous PO_2 is unchanged, the arteriovenous oxygen content difference increases, and more oxygen is off-loaded to the tissues (see p. 326). P_{50} (the PO_2 at which haemoglobin is half-saturated with O₂) is a useful index of these shifts – the higher the P_{50} (i.e. shift to the right), the lower the affinity of haemoglobin for O₂. a, arterial point; v, venous point; x, arteriovenous oxygen content difference.

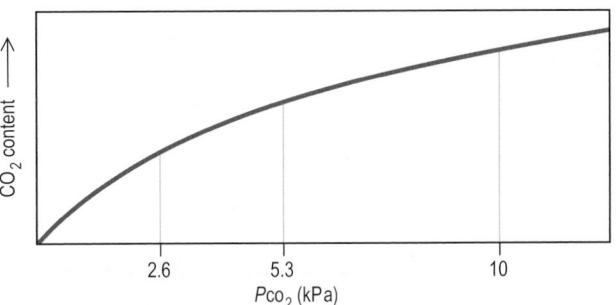

Fig. 10.5 The carbon dioxide dissociation curve. Note that, in the physiological range, the curve is essentially linear.

Oxygen cascade

Oxygen levels fall further as it is unloaded into the tissues and diffuses to the mitochondria. Tissue oxygen content varies, depending on the distance travelled from the local capillary network. Some mitochondria continue to function at a PO_2 as low as 0.07 kPa (0.5 mmHg) (**Fig. 10.6**).

Mixed venous oxygen tension and saturation

Mixed venous oxygen tension ($P_{\bar{v}}O_2$) is the partial pressure of oxygen in pulmonary arterial blood that has been thoroughly mixed in the right heart. Assuming P_aO_2 remains constant, both $P_{\bar{v}}O_2$ and mixed venous oxygen saturation $S_{\bar{v}}O_2$) fall as more oxygen is extracted by tissues. Low $S_{\bar{v}}O_2$ therefore indicates either inadequate oxygen delivery or a rise in tissue requirements beyond compensations in cardiac output. This may exacerbate pulmonary shunting; hence, worsening hypoxaemia does not necessarily indicate declining pulmonary function. Conversely, rises in venous oxygen content may reflect impaired tissue extraction due to microcirculatory abnormalities and/or reduced utilization due to mitochondrial dysfunction, as in severe sepsis or certain poisons (see later). Monitoring central venous oxygen saturation from the superior vena cava ($S_{cv}O_2$) rather than the pulmonary artery is less invasive and approximates $S_{\bar{v}}O_2$ to within around 5% in most situations, although this relationship becomes less predictable at the extremes of physiology (see p. 224).

Adaptation to hypoxia

Acute exposure to severe hypoxia may lead to sudden death if the immediate adaptive responses fail to maintain mitochondrial oxygen delivery. Chronic exposure to low oxygen tension, on the other hand, allows time for compensatory mechanisms to develop. Among the first is an increase in cardiac output, achieved primarily by increasing heart rate. Given the reciprocal relationship between the partial pressures of oxygen and carbon dioxide in the alveoli, as defined by the alveolar gas equation ($P_AO_2 = P_IO_2 - P_ACO_2/R$, where R is the respiratory quotient (usually 0.8)), an increase in respiratory

rate serves to decrease alveolar PCO_2 and thereby increase alveolar PO_2 (see also **Fig. 10.4**). Over time, increased erythropoietin production stimulates haemoglobin synthesis, leading to a marked increase in haematocrit. Over the longer term, capillary bed density in specific tissues adjusts to the physiological demand. In those residing at altitude over generations, the hypoxic ventilatory drive and pulmonary vasoconstrictor response evolve to maximize oxygen uptake. In 2007 a series of arterial blood samples were obtained by a group of critical care doctors on the summit of Mount Everest (see 'Further reading'). The project included a 4-month acclimatization period at altitude and the samples were eventually obtained at an altitude of 8400 m while breathing air. The average P_aO_2 was 3.2 kPa (24.6 mmHg). These figures neatly demonstrate features of both acute (hyperventilation) and chronic (increased haematocrit) acclimatization to hypobaric hypoxia.

Further reading

Grocott MPW, Martin DS, Levett DZH et al. Arterial blood gases and oxygen content in climbers on Mount Everest. *N Engl J Med* 2009; 360:140–149.

Cardiac output

Cardiac output is the product of heart rate and stroke volume (**Fig. 10.7**). When the heart rate increases, the duration of systole is largely unchanged but diastole, and thus time for ventricular filling, progressively shortens and stroke volume eventually falls. In normal hearts this occurs at rates of more than about 160 beats per minute, but in those with cardiac pathology, particularly restricted ventricular filling (e.g. mitral stenosis), it may be seen at much lower rates. Tachycardia increases myocardial oxygen consumption and may precipitate ischaemia in areas with restricted coronary perfusion. Conversely, when heart rate falls, the compensatory increase in stroke volume eventually becomes insufficient and cardiac output falls. Furthermore, rhythm disturbances (e.g. atrial fibrillation, complete heart block) may prevent atrial augmentation of ventricular filling, exacerbating the fall in stroke volume.

Stroke volume

The volume of blood ejected in a single contraction is the difference between the ventricular end-diastolic volume (VEDV) and ventricular end-systolic volume (VESV) (i.e. stroke volume = VEDV – VESV). The ejection fraction describes the stroke volume as a percentage of VEDV (i.e. ejection fraction = (VEDV – VESV)/VEDV × 100%) and is an indicator of myocardial performance.

Three interdependent factors determine the stroke volume (see p. 1025).

Preload

This is defined as the tension of the myocardial fibres at the end of diastole, and is related to the degree of stretch of the fibres. As the end-diastolic volume of the ventricle increases, tension in the

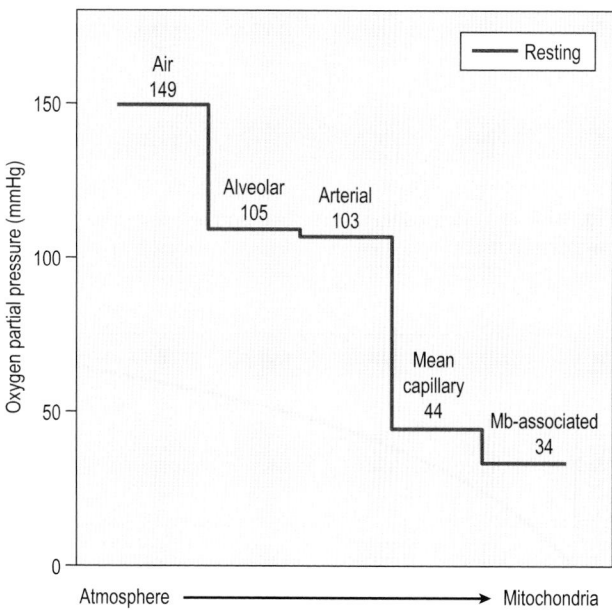

Fig. 10.6 The oxygen cascade. Oxygen levels decrease (shown in graph) as oxygen is unloaded into the tissues and diffuses to the mitochondria. Mb, myoglobin.

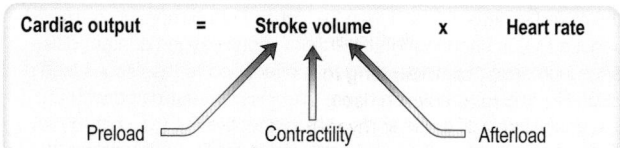

Fig. 10.7 The determinants of cardiac output.

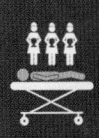

myocardial fibres is increased and stroke volume rises (**Fig. 10.8**). Myocardial oxygen consumption ($\dot{V}_mO_2$) increases only slightly with an increase in preload (produced, for example, by a 'fluid challenge', see later) and this is therefore the most efficient way of improving cardiac output.

Myocardial contractility

This refers to the ability of the heart to perform work, independent of changes in preload and afterload. The state of myocardial contractility determines the response of the ventricles to changes in preload and afterload. Contractility is often reduced in critically ill patients, as a result of either pre-existing myocardial damage (e.g. ischaemic heart disease) or the acute disease process itself (e.g. sepsis). Changes in myocardial contractility alter the slope and position of the Starling curve; worsening ventricular performance is manifested as a depressed, flattened curve (see **Figs 10.8** and **30.5**). Inotropic drugs are used to increase myocardial contractility (see later).

Afterload

This is defined as the myocardial wall tension developed during systolic ejection. In the case of the left ventricle, the resistance imposed by the aortic valve, the peripheral vascular resistance and the elasticity of the major blood vessels are the major determinants of afterload. Ventricular wall tension will also be increased by ventricular dilation, an increase in intraventricular pressure or a reduction in ventricular wall thickness.

Decreasing the afterload (through vasodilation due to exercise, sepsis or vasodilating agents) can increase the stroke volume achieved at a given preload (**Fig. 10.9**), while reducing $\dot{V}_mO_2$. The reduction in wall tension also leads to an increase in coronary blood flow, thereby improving the myocardial oxygen supply/demand ratio. Excessive reductions in afterload will cause hypotension.

Increasing the afterload (vasoconstriction due to increased sympathetic activity, vasoconstrictor agents), on the other hand, can cause a fall in stroke volume and an increase in $\dot{V}_mO_2$.

Right ventricular afterload is normally negligible because the resistance of the pulmonary circulation is very low but is increased in pulmonary hypertension. Unlike the left ventricle, the right is poorly tolerant of acute changes in this parameter and acutely elevated pulmonary vascular resistance may cause shock.

Cardiovascular assessment and monitoring of critically ill patients

Monitoring helps establish or confirm a diagnosis, gauge severity of a condition, follow its evolution, guide interventions and assess response to treatment. Invasive monitoring is usually indicated in critically ill patients and those unresponsive to initial resuscitation. These techniques carry a risk of significant complications, are costly and may lead to patient discomfort. They should be used only when potential benefits outweigh their dangers, and for the minimum time necessary.

Assessment of tissue perfusion

- *Pale, cold skin*, delayed capillary refill and the absence of visible veins in the hands and feet indicate poor perfusion. Although peripheral skin temperature measurements can help clinical evaluation, the earliest compensatory response to hypovolaemia or a low cardiac output, and the last to resolve after resuscitation, is splanchnic vasoconstriction.
- *Metabolic acidosis with raised lactate concentration* suggests that tissue perfusion is sufficiently compromised to cause cellular hypoxia and anaerobic glycolysis. Persistent, severe lactic acidosis is associated with a very poor prognosis. In addition to serving as a screen for cardiovascular insufficiency and poor tissue perfusion, lactate levels are frequently used to guide resuscitation. High lactate levels that do not respond to resuscitation suggest reduced splanchnic blood flow and bowel ischaemia. In sepsis, lactic acidosis can also be caused by metabolic disorders unrelated to tissue hypoxia and exacerbated by reduced clearance owing to hepatic or renal dysfunction, as well as the administration of adrenaline (epinephrine).
- *Urinary flow* is a sensitive indicator of renal perfusion and haemodynamic performance.

Blood pressure

Alterations in blood pressure are often interpreted as reflecting changes in cardiac output. However, if there is vasoconstriction with a high peripheral resistance, the blood pressure may be normal,

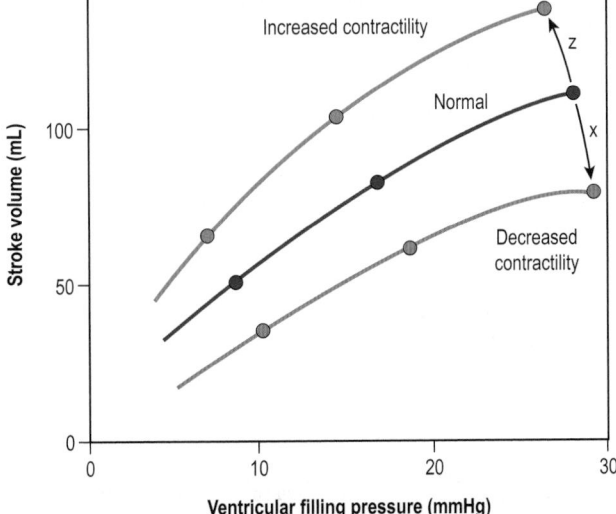

Fig. 10.8 The Frank–Starling relationship: as preload is increased, stroke volume rises. If the ventricle is overstretched, stroke volume will fall (x). In myocardial failure, the curve is depressed and flattened. Increasing contractility, such as that due to sympathetic stimulation, shifts the curve upwards and to the left (z).

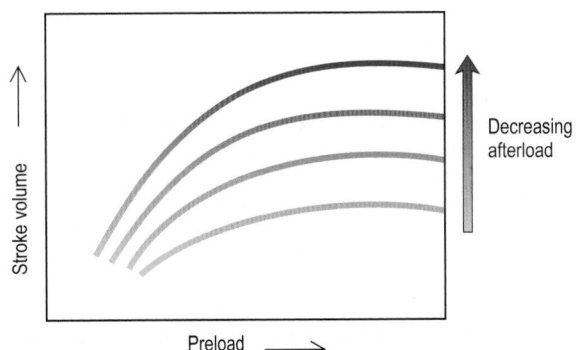

Fig. 10.9 The effect of changes in afterload on the ventricular function curve. At any given preload, decreasing afterload increases the stroke volume.

even when the cardiac output is low. Conversely, the vasodilated patient may be hypotensive, despite a very high cardiac output.

Hypotension jeopardizes perfusion of vital organs. The adequacy of blood pressure in an individual patient must always be assessed in relation to the pre-morbid value. Blood pressure is traditionally measured using a sphygmomanometer, but if rapid alterations are anticipated, continuous monitoring using an intra-arterial cannula is indicated (**Box 10.2** and **Fig. 10.10**).

Central venous pressure

Assessment of central venous pressure (CVP) provides a fairly simple, but approximate, method of gauging the adequacy of a patient's circulating volume and preload. The absolute value of the CVP is not as informative as its response to a fluid challenge (the infusion of 100–200 mL of fluid over a few minutes; **Fig. 10.11**). The hypovolaemic patient will initially respond to transfusion with little or no change in CVP but will exhibit some improvement in cardiovascular function (falling heart rate, rising blood pressure, increased peripheral temperature and urine output). As the normovolaemic state is approached, the CVP may rise slightly and reach a plateau, while other cardiovascular values begin to stabilize. At this stage, volume replacement should be slowed or even stopped. In cardiac failure, the venous pressure is usually high; the patient will not improve in response to volume replacement, which will cause a further, sometimes dramatic, rise in CVP.

However, the use of CVP to assess cardiovascular function is controversial and newer methods, particularly pulse contour analysis and oesophageal Doppler techniques, have largely replaced it (see later).

Central venous catheters are usually inserted via percutaneous puncture of the subclavian or internal jugular vein using a guidewire technique (**Box 10.3**; **Figs 10.12** and **10.13**). The objective is to place the tip of the catheter approximately at the junction of the superior vena cava and the right atrium. Usually, these catheters consist of more than one lumen, some of which may be used for drug or fluid administration. Central venous cannulae may also be inserted via the femoral vein; when this route is used, the tip of the cannula will lie in the inferior vena cava. Guidewire techniques can also be employed for inserting double-lumen cannulae for haemofiltration or pulmonary artery catheter introducers. The routine use of ultrasound to guide central venous cannulation reduces complication rates.

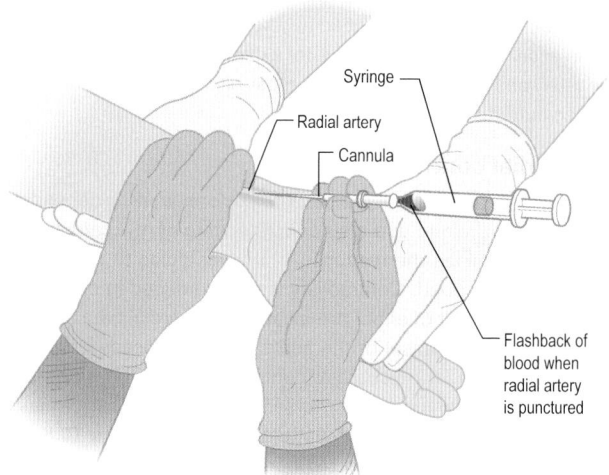

Fig. 10.10 Percutaneous cannulation of the radial artery.

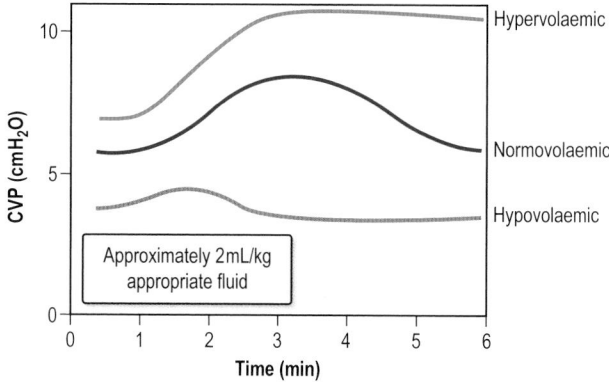

Fig. 10.11 The effects on the central venous pressure (CVP) of rapid administration of a 'fluid challenge' to patients with a CVP within the normal range.

 Box 10.2 Radial artery cannulation

Technique

1. Explain the procedure to the patient and, if possible, obtain consent.
2. Ask an assistant to support the patient's arm, with the wrist extended. (Gloves should be worn.)
3. Clean the skin with chlorhexidine. Take sterile precautions throughout the procedure.
4. Palpate the radial artery where it arches over the head of the radius.
5. In conscious patients, inject local anaesthetic to raise a weal over the artery, taking care not to puncture the vessel or obscure its pulsation.
6. Make a small skin incision over the proposed puncture site.
7. Use a small, parallel-sided cannula (20 gauge for adults, 22 gauge for children) in order to allow blood flow to continue past the cannula.
8. Insert the cannula over the point of maximal pulsation and advance it in line with the direction of the vessel at an angle of approximately 30 degrees.
9. Look for 'flashback' of blood into the cannula, which indicates that the radial artery has been punctured.
10. To ensure that the shoulder of the cannula enters the vessel, lower the needle and cannula and advance them a few millimetres into the vessel.
11. Thread the cannula off the needle into the vessel and withdraw the needle.
12. Connect the cannula to a non-compliant manometer line filled with saline. Then connect this via a transducer and continuous flush device to a monitor, which records the arterial pressure.

Possible complications

- Thrombosis
- Loss of arterial pulsation
- Distal ischaemia, e.g. digital necrosis (rare)
- Infection
- Accidental injection of drugs – can produce vascular occlusion
- Disconnection – rapid blood loss

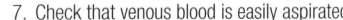

Box 10.3 Internal jugular vein cannulation

Technique

1. Explain the procedure to the patient and, if possible, obtain consent.
2. Place the patient head down to distend the central veins (this facilitates cannulation and minimizes the risk of air embolism, but may exacerbate respiratory distress and is dangerous in those with raised intracranial pressure).
3. Clean the skin with an antiseptic solution such as chlorhexidine. Take sterile precautions throughout the procedure.
4. Inject local anaesthetic (1% plain lidocaine) intradermally to raise a weal at the apex of a triangle formed by the two heads of sternomastoid with the clavicle at its base.
5. Make a small incision through the weal.
6. Insert the cannula or needle through the incision and direct it laterally, downwards and backwards, in the direction of the nipple, until the vein is punctured just beneath the skin and deep to the lateral head of sternomastoid. *Ultrasound-guided puncture is recommended to reduce the incidence of complications.*

7. Check that venous blood is easily aspirated.
8. Thread the cannula off the needle into the vein or pass the guidewire through the needle (see **Fig. 10.13**).
9. Connect the central venous pressure manometer line to a manometer/transducer.
10. Take a chest X-ray to verify that the tip of the catheter is in the superior vena cava and to exclude pneumothorax.

Possible complications

- Haemorrhage
- Accidental arterial puncture (carotid or subclavian)
- Pneumothorax
- Damage to thoracic duct on left
- Air embolism
- Thrombosis
- Catheter-related sepsis

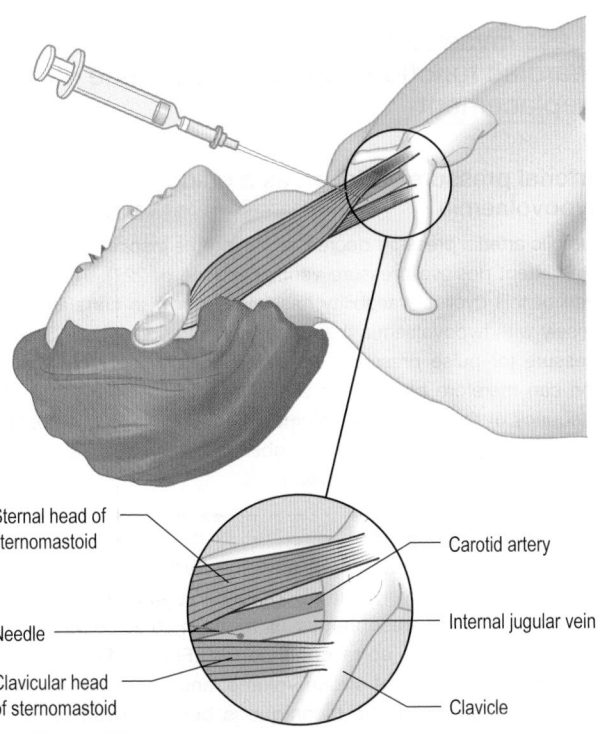

Sternal head of sternomastoid

Needle

Clavicular head of sternomastoid

Carotid artery

Internal jugular vein

Clavicle

Fig. 10.12 Cannulation of the right internal jugular vein.

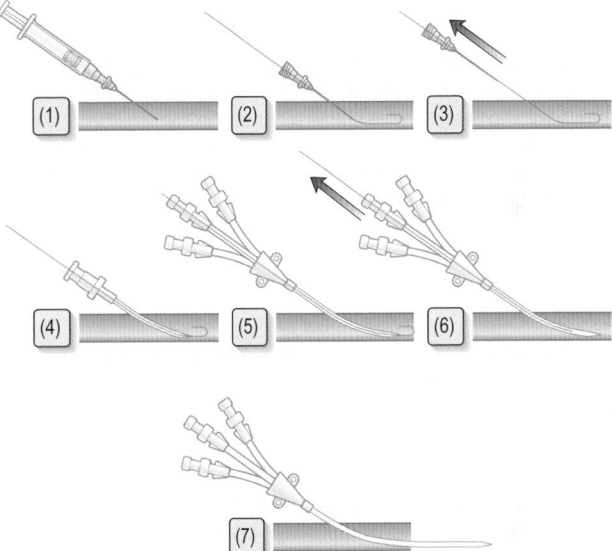

Fig. 10.13 Seldinger technique – insertion of a catheter over guidewire. **(1)** Puncture vessel. **(2)** Advance guidewire. **(3)** Remove needle. **(4)** Dilate vessel. **(5)** Advance catheter over guidewire. **(6)** Remove guidewire. **(7)** Catheter *in situ*.

The CVP is usually displayed continuously using a transducer and bedside monitor but can also be recorded intermittently using a manometer system. It is essential for the recorded pressure always to be related to the level of the right atrium. Various landmarks are advocated (e.g. sternal notch with the patient supine; sternal angle or mid-axilla when the patient is at 45 degrees), but the choice is largely immaterial, provided the landmark is used consistently in an individual patient.

Left atrial pressure

In uncomplicated cases, careful interpretation of the CVP may provide a reasonable guide to the filling pressures of both sides of the heart. In some critically ill patients, however, there is a disparity in function between the two ventricles. Most commonly, left ventricular performance is worse, so that the left ventricular function curve

is displaced downwards and to the right (**Fig. 10.14**). High right ventricular filling pressures, with normal or low left atrial pressures, are less common but occur with right ventricular dysfunction and with raised pulmonary vascular resistance (i.e. right ventricular afterload), such as in acute respiratory failure and pulmonary embolism.

Pulmonary artery pressures

A 'balloon flotation catheter' enables reliable catheterization of the pulmonary artery. These 'Swan–Ganz' catheters are inserted centrally (see **Fig. 10.12**). Passage of the catheter from the major veins, through the chambers of the heart into the pulmonary artery and into the wedged position, is monitored and guided by the pressure waveforms recorded from the distal lumen (**Box 10.4** and **Fig. 10.15**). A chest X-ray should always be obtained to check the final position of the catheter (**Fig. 10.16**).

Once in position, the catheter measures pulmonary artery mean, systolic and end-diastolic pressures (PAEDP). The pulmonary artery

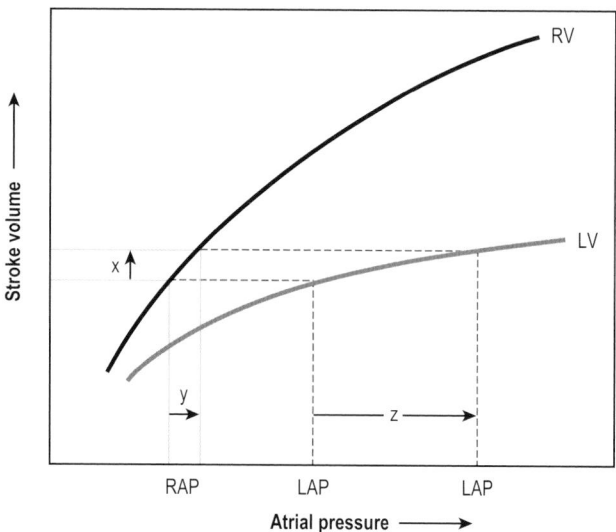

Fig. 10.14 Left ventricular (LV) and right ventricular (RV) function curves in a patient with left ventricular dysfunction. Since the stroke volume of the two ventricles must be the same (except, perhaps, for a few beats during a period of circulatory adjustment), left atrial pressure (LAP) must be higher than right atrial pressure (RAP). Moreover, an increase in stroke volume (x) produced by expanding the circulatory volume may be associated with a small rise in RAP (y) but a marked increase in LAP (z).

Box 10.4 Passage of a pulmonary artery balloon flotation catheter

The catheter is passed through the chambers of the heart into the 'wedged' position.
1. Explain the procedure to the patient and, if possible, obtain consent. Place the patient in a 'head down' position.
2. Insert a balloon flotation catheter through a large vein (see text).
3. Look for respiratory oscillations once the catheter is in the thorax. Advance it further towards the lower superior vena cava/right atrium (see **Fig. 10.15A**), where pressure oscillations become more pronounced. Then inflate the balloon and advance the catheter.
4. When the catheter is in the right ventricle (see **Fig. 10.15B**), there is no dicrotic notch and the diastolic pressure is close to 0. Return the patient to the horizontal or slightly head-up position before advancing the catheter further.
5. When the catheter reaches the pulmonary artery (see **Fig. 10.15C**), a dicrotic notch appears and there is elevation of the diastolic pressure. Advance the catheter further with the balloon inflated.
6. Reappearance of a venous waveform indicates that the catheter is 'wedged'. Deflate the balloon to obtain the pulmonary artery pressure. Inflate the balloon intermittently to obtain the pulmonary artery occlusion pressure (also known as pulmonary artery or capillary 'wedge' pressure, see **Fig. 10.15D**).

occlusion pressure (PAOP, or capillary 'wedge' pressure) is measured by inflating the balloon at the tip of the catheter. This creates a continuous column of fluid between the distal lumen of the catheter and the left atrium, so that the PAOP is usually a reasonable reflection of left atrial pressure.

The technique is generally safe; the majority of complications, such as 'knotting', valve trauma and pulmonary artery rupture (which can be fatal), are related to user inexperience.

Cardiac output

The gold standard cardiac output monitor uses a modified pulmonary artery catheter that transmits low-energy heat from a heating element in the catheter into the surrounding blood. A 'thermodilution curve' is constructed by measuring dissipation of the heat using a thermistor located distal to the heating coil. The dissipation of heat is directly proportional to the cardiac output. These catheters also optically measure and continuously display $S_{\bar{v}}O_2$.

In general, pulmonary artery catheters may help the clinician to optimize cardiac output and oxygen delivery, while minimizing the risk of volume overload. They guide the rational use of inotropes and vasoactive agents, particularly in patients with pulmonary hypertension. The unselective use of this monitoring device in the absence of evidence-based haemodynamic goals does not, however, lead to improved outcomes, and less invasive techniques are preferred, except in the most complex cases (e.g. high-risk cardiac surgery).

Less invasive techniques for assessing cardiac function and guiding volume replacement

Arterial pressure variation as a guide to hypovolaemia

Systolic arterial pressure decreases during the inspiratory phase of intermittent positive pressure ventilation (see p. 227). The magnitude of this cyclical variability has been shown to correlate more closely with hypovolaemia than other monitored variables. Systolic pressure (or pulse pressure) variation during mechanical ventilation can therefore be used as a simple and reliable guide to the adequacy of the circulatory volume. The response to fluid loading can also be predicted simply by observing the changes in pulse pressure during passive leg-raising.

Oesophageal Doppler

Stroke volume, cardiac output and myocardial function can be assessed non-invasively using Doppler ultrasonography. A probe is passed into the oesophagus to monitor velocity waveforms from the descending aorta continuously (**Fig. 10.17**). Although reasonable estimates of stroke volume, and hence cardiac output, can be obtained, the technique is best reserved for trend analysis rather than for making absolute measurements. It is particularly valuable for perioperative optimization of the circulating volume and cardiac performance in the unconscious patient. It is contraindicated in patients with oropharyngeal/oesophageal pathology.

Arterial waveform analysis

Lithium dilution/pulse contour analysis does not require pulmonary artery catheterization or instrumentation of the oesophagus and is suitable for use in conscious patients. A bolus of lithium chloride is administered via a central venous catheter and the change in arterial plasma lithium concentration is detected by a lithium-sensitive electrode. This sensor can be connected to an existing arterial cannula via a three-way tap. The cardiac output determined in this way can be used to calibrate an arterial pressure waveform ('pulse contour') analysis programme that will continuously monitor changes in cardiac output. Devices that employ uncalibrated pulse contour analysis to estimate cardiac output are also available.

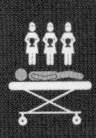

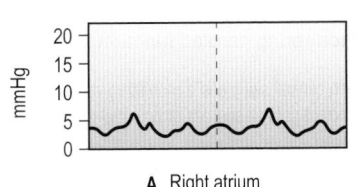

A Right atrium

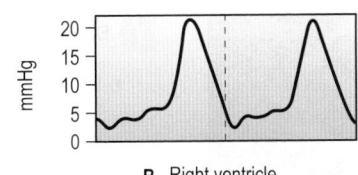

B Right ventricle

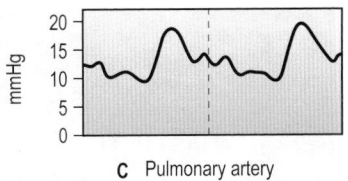

C Pulmonary artery

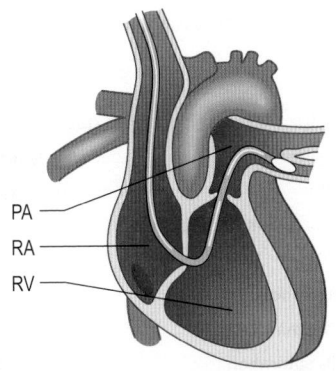

PA
RA
RV

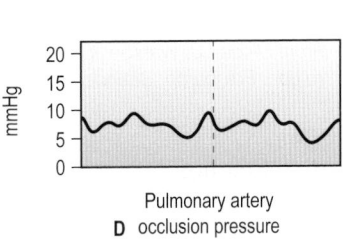

Pulmonary artery
D occlusion pressure

Fig. 10.15 Passage of pulmonary artery balloon flotation catheter through the chambers of the heart. The catheter is passed into the 'wedged' position to measure the pulmonary artery occlusion pressure (see **Box 10.4**). PA, pulmonary artery; RA, right artery; RV, right ventricle.

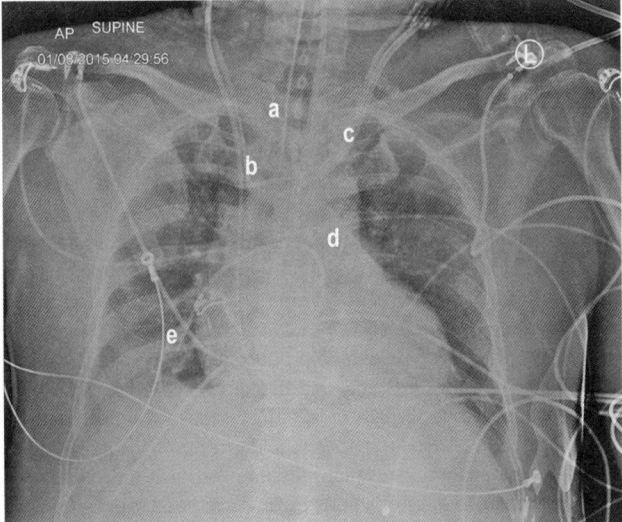

Fig. 10.16 Chest X-ray of a critically ill, mechanically ventilated patient. The X-ray shows **(a)** endotracheal tube; **(b)** end of central venous line seen here medial to the proximal end of the pulmonary artery catheter; **(c)** double-lumen catheter for continuous renal replacement therapy placed via the left internal jugular vein; **(d)** tip of the intra-aortic balloon pump travelling superiorly from a femoral artery; and **(e)** pulmonary artery catheter. Note that the tip of the catheter is too distal; it was therefore subsequently withdrawn by a few centimetres.

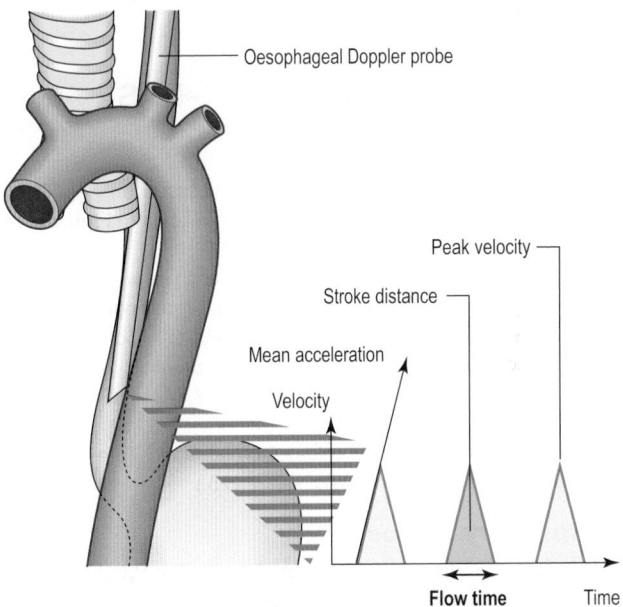

Fig. 10.17 Doppler ultrasonography. Velocity waveform traces are obtained using oesophageal Doppler ultrasonography. *(Reproduced from Singer M, Bennett, ED. Noninvasive optimization of left ventricular filling using esophageal Doppler. Crit Care Med 1991;19:1132-1137, with permission. © 1991 The Williams & Wilkins Co., Baltimore.)*

Other devices utilize a thermodilution technique, where a small volume of cold fluid is injected into a large central vein and a temperature washout curve is detected via a sensor in a modified arterial line. Following this calibration, beat-to-beat cardiac output is generated by computer-based analysis of the arterial pressure waveform.

As with pulse pressure variation, stroke volume variation, determined by oesophageal Doppler or arterial waveform analysis, can be used to guide fluid replacement.

Echocardiography

Focused echocardiography is increasingly used to provide immediate diagnostic information about cardiac structure and function (myocardial contractility, ventricular filling) in the critically ill patient. Although transoesophageal echocardiography (TOE) may be preferred because of its superior image clarity (**Fig. 10.18**), transthoracic echocardiography is non-invasive and more readily available.

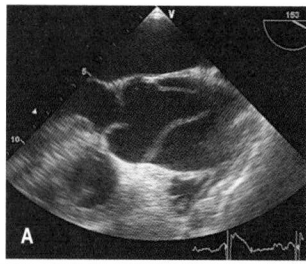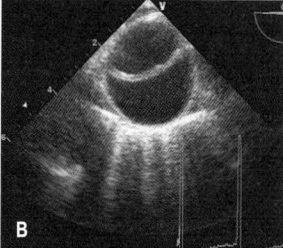

Fig. 10.18 Aortic dissection (transoesophageal echocardiography, TOE). **(A)** Mid-oesophageal, long-axis view showing type A aortic dissection. **(B)** Short-axis view of descending aorta showing intimal flap with false and true lumen. *(From Hinds CJ, Watson JD. Intensive Care: A Concise Textbook, 3rd edn. Edinburgh: Saunders; 2008. Courtesy of Dr C. Rathwell.)*

Key points in monitoring cardiac function

These are shown in **Box 10.5**.

Further reading

Lamperti M, Bodenham AR, Pittiruti M et al. International evidence-based recommendations on ultrasound-guided vascular access. *Intensive Care Med* 2012; 38:1105–1117.
Marik PE, Monnet X, Teboul JL. Hemodynamic parameters to guide fluid therapy. *Ann Intensive Care* 2011; 1:1.
Saugel B, Vincent JL. Cardiac output monitoring: how to choose the optimal method for the individual patient. *Curr Opin Crit Care* 2018; 24:165–172.

DISTURBANCES OF ACID–BASE BALANCE

The physiology of acid–base control is discussed on page 196. Acid–base disturbances can be described in relation to **Figure 9.14** (which shows P_aCO_2 plotted against arterial [H+]).

Both acidosis and alkalosis can occur, each of which is either metabolic (primarily affecting the bicarbonate component of the system) or respiratory (primarily affecting P_aCO_2). Compensatory changes may also be apparent. In clinical practice, arterial [H+] values outside the 18–126 nmol/L (pH 6.9–7.7) range are rarely encountered.

Blood gas and acid–base values (normal ranges) are shown in **Box 10.6**. (For blood gas analysis, see p. 225.)

Respiratory acidosis

This is caused by retention of carbon dioxide. The P_aCO_2 and [H+] rise. A chronically raised P_aCO_2 is compensated by renal retention of bicarbonate and the [H+] returns towards normal. A constant arterial bicarbonate concentration is then usually established within 2–5 days. This represents a primary respiratory acidosis with a compensatory metabolic alkalosis (see p. 198). Common causes of respiratory acidosis include ventilatory failure and COPD (type II respiratory failure, where there is a high P_aCO_2 and a low P_aO_2, see p. 224).

Respiratory alkalosis

In this case, the reverse occurs and there is a fall in P_aCO_2 and [H+], often with a small reduction in bicarbonate concentration. If hypocarbia persists, some degree of renal compensation may occur, producing a metabolic acidosis, although in practice this is unusual. A respiratory alkalosis may be produced, intentionally or unintentionally, when patients are mechanically ventilated; it may also be seen in patients with hypoxaemic (type I) respiratory failure (see

- If there is disagreement between clinical signs and a monitored variable, assume that the monitor is incorrect until all sources of potential error have been checked and eliminated
- Remember that changes and trends in monitored variables are more informative than a single reading
- Use non-invasive monitoring where possible
- Remove invasive devices as soon as possible

i **Box 10.6** Arterial blood gas and acid–base values

Analyte	Normal reference range
H+	35–45 nmol/L (pH 7.35–7.45)
PO_2 (breathing room air)	10.6–13.3 kPa (80–100 mmHg)
PCO_2	4.8–6.1 kPa (36–46 mmHg)
Base deficit	±2.5
Plasma HCO_3^-	22–26 mmol/L
O_2 saturation	95–100%

p. 224), those with spontaneous hyperventilation and those living at high altitudes.

Metabolic acidosis

Metabolic acidosis (see p. 198) may be due to excessive acid production, often lactic acid (lactic acidosis), as a consequence of anaerobic metabolism during an episode of shock or following cardiac arrest. A metabolic acidosis may develop as a consequence of chronic renal failure or in diabetic ketoacidosis. It can also follow the loss of bicarbonate from the gut or from the kidney in renal tubular acidosis. Respiratory compensation for a metabolic acidosis is usually slightly delayed because the blood–brain barrier initially prevents the respiratory centre from sensing the increased blood [H+]. Following this short delay, however, the patient hyperventilates and 'blows off' carbon dioxide to produce a compensatory respiratory alkalosis. There is a limit to this respiratory compensation since, in practice, values for P_aCO_2 of less than about 1.4 kPa (11 mmHg) are rarely achieved. Spontaneous respiratory compensation cannot occur if the patient's ventilation is controlled or if the respiratory centre is depressed: for example, by drugs or head injury.

Metabolic alkalosis

This can be caused by loss of acid – for example, from the stomach with nasogastric suction, or in high intestinal obstruction, or excessive administration of absorbable alkali. Over-zealous treatment with intravenous sodium bicarbonate is sometimes implicated. Respiratory compensation for a metabolic alkalosis is often slight, and it is rare to encounter a P_aCO_2 above 6.5 kPa (50 mmHg), even with severe alkalosis.

SHOCK, SEPSIS AND ACUTE DISTURBANCES OF HAEMODYNAMIC FUNCTION

Shock is the term used to describe acute circulatory failure with inadequate or inappropriately distributed tissue perfusion, resulting in generalized cellular hypoxia and/or an inability of the cells to utilize oxygen.

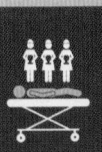

Aetiology of shock

Abnormalities of tissue perfusion can result from:

- failure of the heart to act as an effective pump
- mechanical impediments to forward flow
- loss of circulatory volume
- abnormalities of the peripheral circulation.

The causes of shock are shown in **Box 10.7**; see also page 154 for definitions of sepsis. Often, shock can result from a combination of these factors (e.g. in sepsis, distributive shock is frequently complicated by hypovolaemia and myocardial depression).

Pathophysiology

The sympatho-adrenal response to shock

Hypotension stimulates baroreceptors, and to a lesser extent chemoreceptors, causing increased sympathetic nervous activity with 'spill-over' of noradrenaline (norepinephrine) into the circulation. Later, this is augmented by the release of catecholamines (predominantly adrenaline (epinephrine)) from the adrenal medulla. The resulting vasoconstriction,

together with increased myocardial contractility and heart rate, help to restore blood pressure and cardiac output (**Fig. 10.19**).

Reduced perfusion of the renal cortex stimulates the juxtaglomerular apparatus to release renin. This converts angiotensinogen to angiotensin I, which, in turn, is converted in the lungs and by the vascular endothelium to the potent vasoconstrictor angiotensin II. Angiotensin II also stimulates secretion of aldosterone by the adrenal cortex, causing sodium and water retention (see p. 1346). This helps to restore the circulating volume (see p. 173).

The neuroendocrine response

- ***Release of pituitary hormones*** includes adrenocorticotrophic hormone (ACTH), vasopressin (antidiuretic hormone, ADH) and endogenous opioid peptides. (In septic shock, there may be a relative deficiency of vasopressin.)
- ***Release of cortisol*** causes fluid retention and antagonizes insulin.
- ***Release of glucagon*** raises the blood sugar level.

? **Box 10.7 Causes of shock**

Hypovolaemic
- Exogenous losses (e.g. haemorrhage, burns)

Cardiogenic
- 'Myocardial failure' (e.g. ischaemic myocardial injury)

Obstructive
- Obstruction to cardiac outflow (e.g. pulmonary embolus)
- Restricted cardiac filling (e.g. cardiac tamponade, tension pneumothorax)

Distributive
- Vascular dilation (eg sepsis, anaphylaxis)
- Sequestration
- Arteriovenous shunting
- Maldistribution of flow

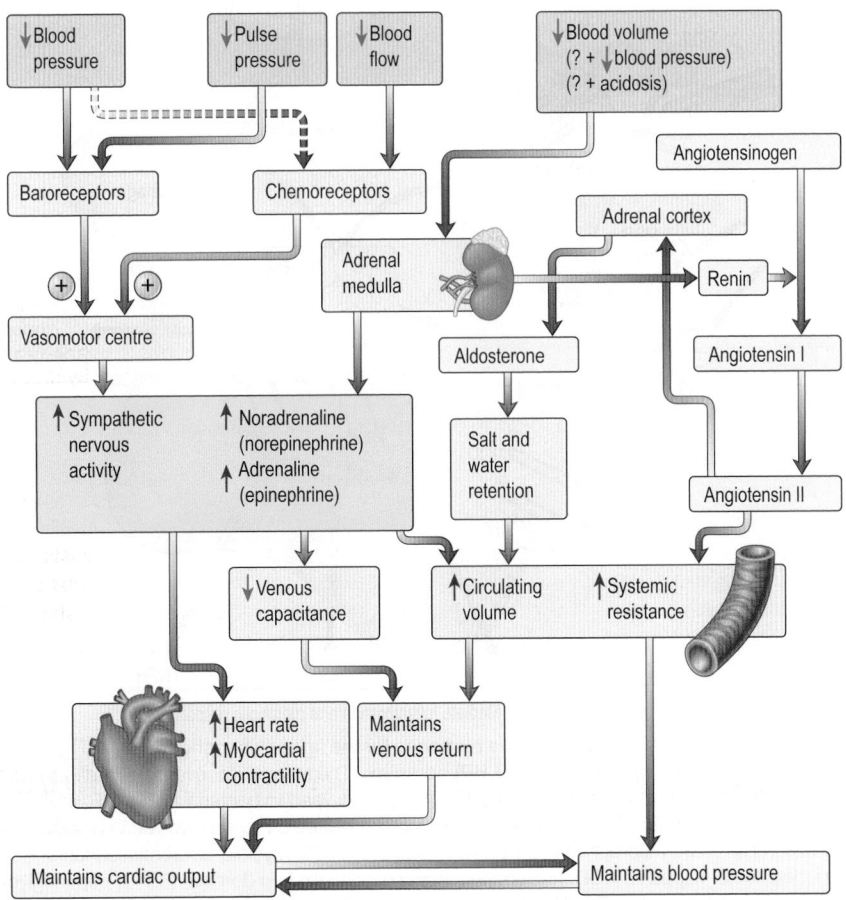

Fig. 10.19 The sympatho-adrenal response to shock. The effect of increased catecholamines is shown on the left, and the release of angiotensin and aldosterone on the right. Both mechanisms help to maintain cardiac output and blood pressure in shock.

Although absolute adrenocortical insufficiency (e.g. due to bilateral adrenal haemorrhage or necrosis in meningococcal infection) is rare, a blunted response to exogenous ACTH (so-called '*relative*' or '*occult*' *adrenocortical insufficiency*) has been observed in septic shock patients with impaired vasoconstrictor response to noradrenaline (norepinephrine). Steroid supplementation improves vasomotor response with a rise in blood pressure but without mortality benefit.

Release of immune mediators

Severe infection (often with bacteraemia or endotoxaemia), the presence of large areas of damaged tissue (e.g. following trauma or extensive surgery), hypoxia or prolonged/repeated episodes of hypoperfusion can all trigger a dysfunctional immune response with alterations in leucocyte activation and release of a variety of potentially damaging 'mediators' (see also p. 57). Although an appropriate immune response is clearly beneficial, the disseminated, dysregulated response observed in some patients can lead to shock and organ failure. This immune response is complex, with upregulation and downregulation of both the innate and the adaptive immune pathways at different stages of the illness. Characteristically, the later phase is typified by a period of immune suppression, during which the patient is at increased risk of developing secondary infections.

Microorganisms and their toxic products

In sepsis/septic shock, the innate immune response (**Fig. 10.20**) and inflammatory cascade are triggered by the recognition of pathogen-associated molecular patterns (PAMPs), including bacterial and fungal DNA, cell-wall components (e.g. endotoxin) and/or exotoxins (antigenic proteins produced by bacteria such as staphylococci, streptococci and *Pseudomonas*) (see also p. 154).

Endotoxin is a lipopolysaccharide (LPS) derived from the cell wall of Gram-negative bacteria and a potent trigger of the immune

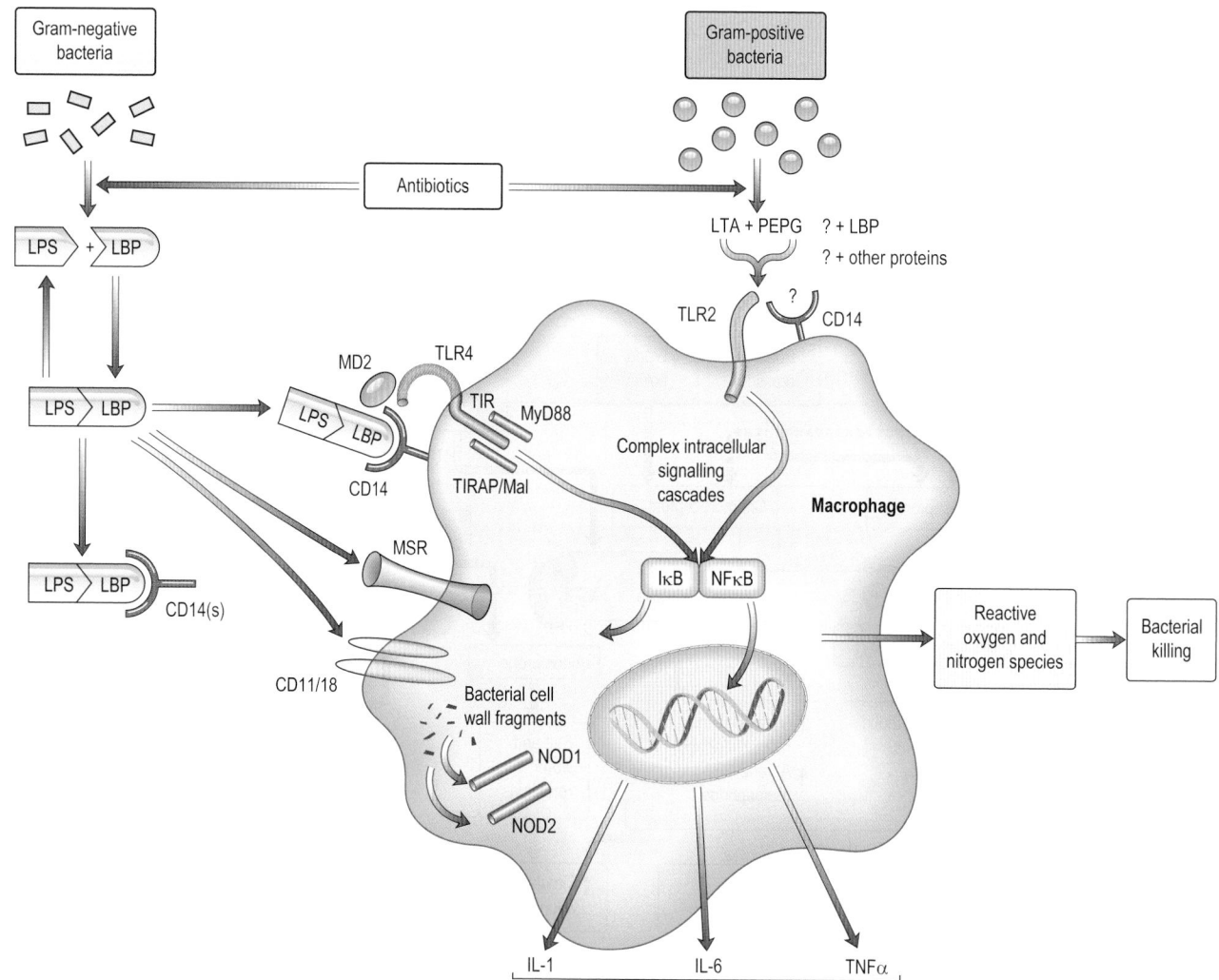

Fig. 10.20 Induction of the innate immune response by the lipopolysaccharide–lipopolysaccharide-binding protein (LPS–LBP) complex. The intracellular events (simplified) initiated by Gram-negative and Gram-positive bacteria, which eventually lead to bacterial killing. IκB, inhibitory factor kappa B; IL, interleukin; LTA, lipoteichoic acid; MD2, a secreted protein involved in binding liposaccharide with TLR4; MSR, macrophage scavenger receptor; MyD88, myeloid differentiation factor 88; NFκB, nuclear factor kappa B; NOD, nucleotide-binding oligomerization domain; PEPG, peptidoglycan-N; TIR, Toll-interleukin receptor; TIRAP, Toll-interleukin 1 receptor adaptor protein; TIRAP/Mal, an adaptor protein for TLR2 and TLR4; TLR, Toll-like receptors; TNF-α, tumour necrosis factor-alpha.

response. The lipid A portion of LPS is bound by a serum protein known as lipopolysaccharide-binding protein (LBP). The LBP–LPS complex attaches to the cell surface marker CD14 and, combined with a secreted protein (MD2), then binds to a member of the Toll-like receptor family (TLR4), which transduces the activation signal into the cell. Activation of these receptors promotes the synthesis of a wide variety of immune mediators. Gram-positive bacteria have cell-wall components that are similar in structure to LPS (e.g. lipoteichoic acid), and can also trigger an inflammatory response through similar pathways (see **Fig. 10.20**).

Toxic products of tissue injury (surgery and trauma)

Following traumatic or surgical tissue injury, inflammatory pathways may be triggered by damage-associated molecular patterns (DAMPS), such as DNA fragments. Of particular importance is circulating mitochondrial DNA (mtDNA), which is similar to bacterial DNA and can be 'mistaken' by the immune system for bacteria. This initiates an immune response identical to that observed following bacterial invasion. This is why distributive shock secondary to infection can be difficult to distinguish clinically from that caused by a 'sterile' insult such as severe trauma or surgery.

Cytokines and other immune mediators

An array of cytokines and chemokines (small proteins that orchestrate immune cell behaviour), prostaglandins, leukotrienes, heat shock proteins, adhesion molecules and endothelial derived vasoactive factors are induced, particularly during distributive shock. These include pro-inflammatory cytokines (tumour necrosis factor-alpha (TNF-α) and interferon-gamma (IFN-γ)), anti-inflammatory cytokines (interleukin 10 (IL-10)), mediators promoting extracellular extravasation (intracellular adhesion molecule 1 (ICAM-1), see **Fig. 3.10**) and vasodilation (inducible nitric oxide synthase (iNOS), **Fig. 10.21**). Although there was initial enthusiasm for treatments

that dampened the immune response in septic shock (e.g. high-dose steroids and anti-TNF-α compounds), these strategies failed to improve survival and some worsened it (**Box 10.8**).

Activation of the complement cascade

Fragments of C3 act as opsonins and co-stimulatory molecules that assist lymphocytes with the adaptive immune response, while small peptides derived from C3, C4 and C5 cause leucocyte chemotaxis, release of cytokines and increased vascular permeability (see p. 44).

Influence of genetic variation

Individuals vary considerably in their susceptibility to infection, as well as their ability to recover from apparently similar infections, illnesses or traumatic insults; this is explained in part by genetic variations.

Haemodynamic and microcirculatory changes

The dominant haemodynamic feature of severe sepsis/septic shock is peripheral vascular failure with:

- vasodilation
- maldistribution of regional blood flow
- abnormalities in the microcirculation (**Fig. 10.22**):
  - 'stop-flow' capillaries (flow is intermittent)
  - 'no-flow' capillaries (capillaries are obstructed)
  - failure of capillary recruitment
  - increased capillary permeability with interstitial oedema.

Although these **vascular and microvascular abnormalities** may partly account for the reduced oxygen extraction seen in septic shock, there is also a **primary defect of cellular oxygen utilization** caused by mitochondrial dysfunction (see earlier). These changes may be associated with impaired oxygen consumption, a reduced arteriovenous oxygen content difference, an increased $S_{\bar{v}}O_2$ and a lactic acidosis (so-called '**tissue dysoxia**'). Similar vasodilation and increased vascular permeability also occur in anaphylactic shock.

The glycocalyx consists of a tight, negatively charged, extremely thin meshwork of proteoglycans on the luminal surface of the vascular endothelium. Oxidative stress, free radicals and endotoxaemia all have specific detrimental effects on the glycocalyx that promote

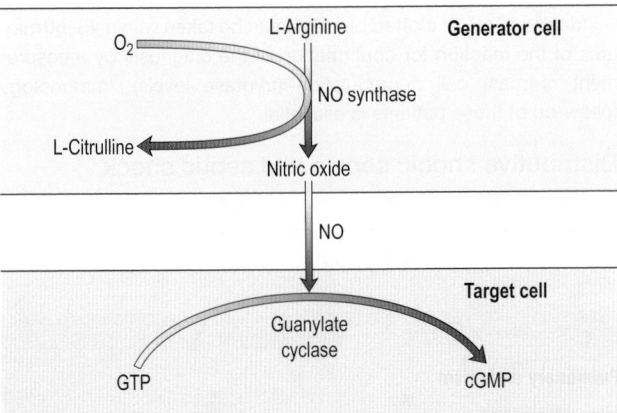

Fig. 10.21 Synthesis and biochemical action of nitric oxide (NO). cGMP, cyclic guanosine monophosphate; GTP, guanosine triphosphate.

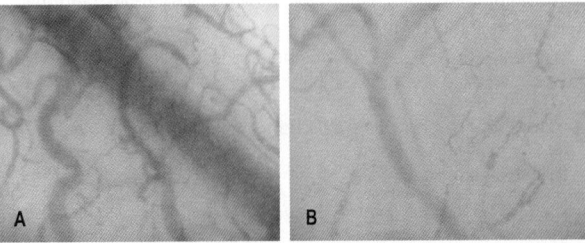

Fig. 10.22 Still side-stream dark field (SDF) images of the microcirculation. **(A)** Normal subject. **(B)** Septic shock.

---

i **Box 10.8 Some therapeutic strategies for sepsis tested in randomized, controlled, phase II/III trials**

- Granulocyte–monocyte colony stimulating factor
- Toll-like receptor/endotoxin antagonists
- Bactericidal permeability-increasing protein
- Tissue necrosis factor (TNF) antibodies
- Soluble TNF receptors
- Interleukin-1 receptor antagonists

- Platelet-activating factor antagonists
- Nitric oxide synthase inhibition
- Antithrombin III
- Activated protein C
- Low-dose steroids

fluid movement into the tissues. Hence, 'pitting' peripheral oedema is often seen in the most seriously ill patients.

Activation of the coagulation system

The immune response to shock, tissue injury and infection is frequently associated with systemic activation of the clotting cascade, leading to platelet aggregation and widespread microvascular thrombosis, resulting in turn in reduced tissue perfusion.

Initially, the production of prostaglandin I$_2$ (PGI$_2$) by the capillary endothelium is impaired. Vascular endothelial injury leads to exposure to tissue factor (see p. 368), which triggers coagulation. In severe cases, these changes are compounded by impairment of fibrinolysis, as well as by deficiencies in physiological inhibitors of coagulation (including antithrombin, proteins C and S, and tissue factor-pathway inhibitor). This procoagulant state can lead to end-artery thrombosis and digital and mesenteric ischaemia. Following clot formation, plasminogen is converted to plasmin, which breaks down thrombus, liberating fibrin/fibrinogen degradation products (FDPs). These processes continue in parallel, leading to a 'consumptive' coagulopathy known as **disseminated intravascular coagulation (DIC)**. Circulating levels of FDPs and D-dimers are therefore increased, the thrombin time, partial thromboplastin time (PTT) and prothrombin time (PT) are prolonged, and platelet and fibrinogen levels fall. Clinically, the patient will bleed from trivial venepuncture sites but, paradoxically, may still be at risk of thrombosis. The development of DIC is often associated with multiple organ failure. In some cases, a microangiopathic haemolytic anaemia develops. DIC is relatively uncommon but is associated particularly with septic shock, especially when due to meningococcal infection (see p. 545). Management targets the **underlying cause**, as well as supportive treatment with fresh frozen plasma, platelets and cryoprecipitate when fibrinogen levels are low and the patient is bleeding.

Clinical features of shock and sepsis

Although many clinical features are common to all types of shock, the causes may be distinguished by the associated haemodynamic changes (**Box 10.9**) and by examination.

Hypovolaemic shock

- **Inadequate tissue perfusion**:
  - Skin: cold, pale, slate-grey, slow capillary refill, 'clammy'.
  - Kidneys: oliguria, anuria.
  - Brain: drowsiness, confusion and irritability.

- **Increased sympathetic tone**:
  - Tachycardia, narrowed pulse pressure, 'weak' or 'thready' pulse.
  - Sweating.
  - Blood pressure: may be maintained initially (despite up to a 25% reduction in circulating volume if the patient is young and fit) but hypotension later supervenes.
- **Lactic acidosis:** compensatory tachypnoea.
  Extreme hypovolaemia may be associated with bradycardia.

Cardiogenic shock

The signs in cardiogenic shock (see Box 30.28) are the same as those in hypovolaemic shock, with the addition of myocardial failure: for example, raised jugular venous pressure (JVP), pulsus alternans, 'gallop' rhythm, basal crackles and pulmonary oedema.

Obstructive shock

Again, the signs are as in hypovolaemic shock with the following additions:
- elevated JVP
- pulsus paradoxus and muffled heart sounds in cardiac tamponade
- signs of pulmonary embolism (see p. 1003).

Distributive shock: anaphylactic shock

(See p. 65.)
- Signs of profound vasodilation:
  - warm peripheries
  - low blood pressure
  - tachycardia.
- Erythema, urticaria, angio-oedema, pallor, cyanosis.
- Bronchospasm, rhinitis.
- Oedema of the face, pharynx and larynx.
- Pulmonary oedema.
- Hypovolaemia due to vascular leak.
- Nausea, vomiting, abdominal cramps, diarrhoea.
  Ideally, 10 mL of clotted blood should be taken within 45–60 minutes of the reaction for confirmation of the diagnosis by measurement of mast cell degranulation (tryptase levels). Immunology follow-up of these patients is essential.

Distributive shock: sepsis and septic shock

Sepsis and **septic shock** are defined on page 154. The **Sequential Organ Failure Assessment score (SOFA)**, used to identify organ dysfunction, is shown in **Box 8.2**.

> ### i Box 10.9 Haemodynamic changes in shock
>
> **Hypovolaemic shock**
>
> *Low central venous pressure (CVP) and pulmonary artery occlusion pressure (PAOP)*
> - Low cardiac output
> - Increased systemic vascular resistance
>
> **Cardiogenic shock**
>
> *Signs of myocardial failure*
> - Increased systemic vascular resistance
> - CVP and PAOP high (except when hypovolaemic)
>
> **Cardiac tamponade**
>
> *Parallel increases in CVP and PAOP*
> - Low cardiac output
> - Increased systemic vascular resistance
>
> **Pulmonary embolism**
>
> *Low cardiac output*
> - High CVP, high pulmonary artery pressure but low PAOP
> - Increased systemic vascular resistance
>
> **Anaphylaxis**
>
> *Low systemic vascular resistance*
> - Low CVP and PAOP
> - High cardiac output
>
> **Septic shock**
>
> *Low systemic vascular resistance*
> - Low CVP and PAOP
> - Cardiac output usually high
> - Myocardial depression – low ejection fraction
> - Stroke volume maintained by ventricular dilation
> - Cardiac output maintained or increased by tachycardia

Symptoms and signs of sepsis include:

- pyrexia and rigors, or hypothermia (unusual, but more common in the elderly and associated with worse prognosis)
- nausea, vomiting
- vasodilation, warm peripheries
- bounding pulse
- rapid capillary refill
- hypotension, low diastolic pressure, widened pulse pressure
- occasionally, signs of cutaneous vasoconstriction
- other signs
  - jaundice
  - coma, stupor
  - bleeding due to coagulopathy (e.g. from vascular puncture sites, gastrointestinal tract and surgical wounds)
  - rash and meningism
  - hyperglycaemia; in more severe cases, hypoglycaemia.

The ***diagnosis of sepsis*** is easily missed, particularly in the elderly. Clues include mild confusion, tachycardia, tachypnoea, unexplained hypotension, a reduction in urine output, a rising plasma creatinine and glucose intolerance.

Sepsis and multiple organ failure (multiple organ dysfunction syndrome)

Sepsis is being diagnosed with increasing frequency and is now the most common cause of death in non-coronary adult ICUs. The estimated incidence of severe sepsis is 77–300 cases per 100 000 of the population. The most common cause is community-acquired pneumonia (**Fig. 10.23**). Mortality rates are high (between 20% and 60%) and are closely related to the severity of illness and the number of organs that fail. Although some early deaths are caused by cardiovascular collapse, advances in ICU care and supportive therapy have reduced early deaths, and most of those who die are overwhelmed by persistent or recurrent sepsis, with fever, intractable hypotension and failure of several organs.

Sequential failure of vital organs occurs progressively over days or weeks, although the pattern of organ dysfunction is variable. In many cases, the lungs are the first to be affected (acute respiratory distress syndrome, ARDS; see later) in association with cardiovascular instability and deteriorating renal function. Secondary pulmonary infection, complicating ARDS, frequently acts as a further stimulus to the immune response.

Liver dysfunction may develop later. Gastrointestinal failure, with an inability to tolerate enteral feeding and paralytic ileus, is common. Ischaemic colitis, acalculous cholecystitis, pancreatitis and gastrointestinal haemorrhage may also occur. Features of central nervous system dysfunction include impaired consciousness and disorientation, progressing to coma. Characteristically, these patients initially have a hyperdynamic circulation with vasodilation and a high cardiac output, associated with an increased metabolic rate. Eventually, however, cardiovascular collapse supervenes. It is often possible to support such patients for weeks or months; most die following a decision to withdraw or not to escalate treatment (see p. 236).

Metabolic response to trauma, major surgery and severe infection

This is initiated and controlled by the neuroendocrine system and various cytokines (e.g. IL-6) acting in concert, and is characterized initially by an increase in energy expenditure ('hypermetabolism'; **Box 10.10** and see also p. 1253). Gluconeogenesis is stimulated by increased glucagon and catecholamine levels, while hepatic mobilization of glucose from glycogen is increased. Catecholamines inhibit insulin release and reduce peripheral glucose uptake. Combined with elevated circulating levels of other insulin antagonists such as cortisol, and downregulation of insulin receptors, these changes mean that the majority of patients are hyperglycaemic ('insulin resistance'). Later, hypoglycaemia may be precipitated by depletion of hepatic glycogen stores and inhibition of gluconeogenesis. Free fatty acid synthesis is also increased, leading to hypertriglyceridaemia.

Protein breakdown is initiated to provide energy from amino acids, and hepatic protein synthesis is preferentially augmented to produce the 'acute phase reactants'. The amino acid glutamine (which is indispensable in this situation) is mobilized from muscle for use as a metabolic fuel in rapidly dividing cells such as leucocytes and enterocytes. Glutamine is also required for hepatic production of the free radical scavenger glutathione. When severe and prolonged, this catabolic response can lead to considerable weight loss. Protein breakdown is associated with wasting and weakness of skeletal and respiratory muscle, prolonging the need for mechanical

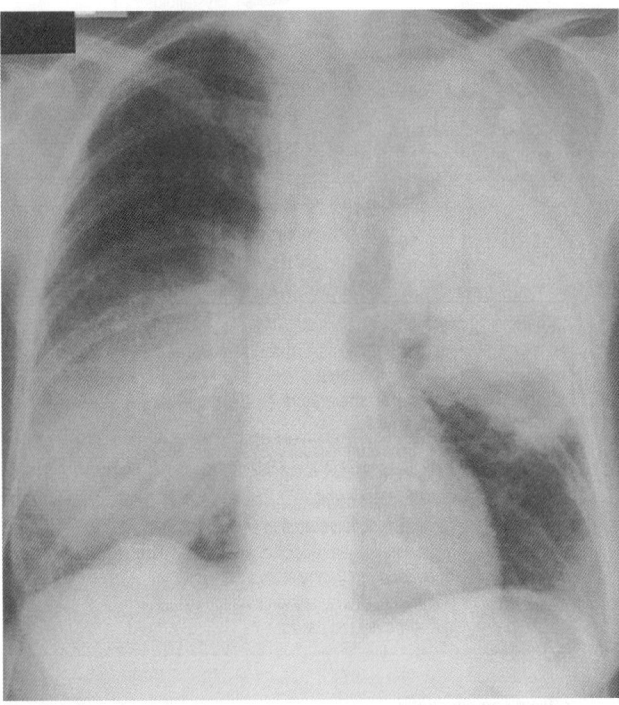

Fig. 10.23 Bilateral pneumococcal pneumonia. Community-acquired pneumonia is the most common cause of sepsis requiring admission to intensive care. *(From Hinds CJ, Watson JD.* Intensive Care: A Concise Textbook, *3rd edn. Edinburgh: Saunders; 2008. Courtesy of Dr SPG Padley.)*

---

i | **Box 10.10** The metabolic response to trauma, major surgery and severe infection

- ↑ Energy expenditure
- ↑ Gluconeogenesis
- ↑ Mobilization of glucose from glycogen
- Insulin resistance and hyperglycaemia

- ↑ Free fatty acid synthesis
- ↑ Protein breakdown
- ↑ Liver synthesis of acute phase reactants

ventilation and delaying mobilization. Tissue repair, wound healing and immune function are also compromised.

Management of shock and sepsis

Delays in recognizing sepsis and initiating resuscitation and treatments (**Fig. 10.24**) (particularly antibiotics when infection is the underlying cause) are associated with substantially increased morbidity and mortality.

A patent airway must be maintained and oxygen given, as is standard for any acutely ill patient. Some may require endotracheal intubation and those with impending respiratory arrest will require immediate mechanical ventilation.

The underlying cause of shock should be sought and corrected where possible; for example, haemorrhage should be controlled or infection eradicated. In patients with septic shock, every effort must be made to identify the source of infection and isolate the causative organism. A thorough history, clinical examination and imaging (X-rays, ultrasonography or computed tomography (CT) scanning) should be undertaken. Appropriate samples (blood, urine, sputum, cerebrospinal fluid (CSF), pus drained from

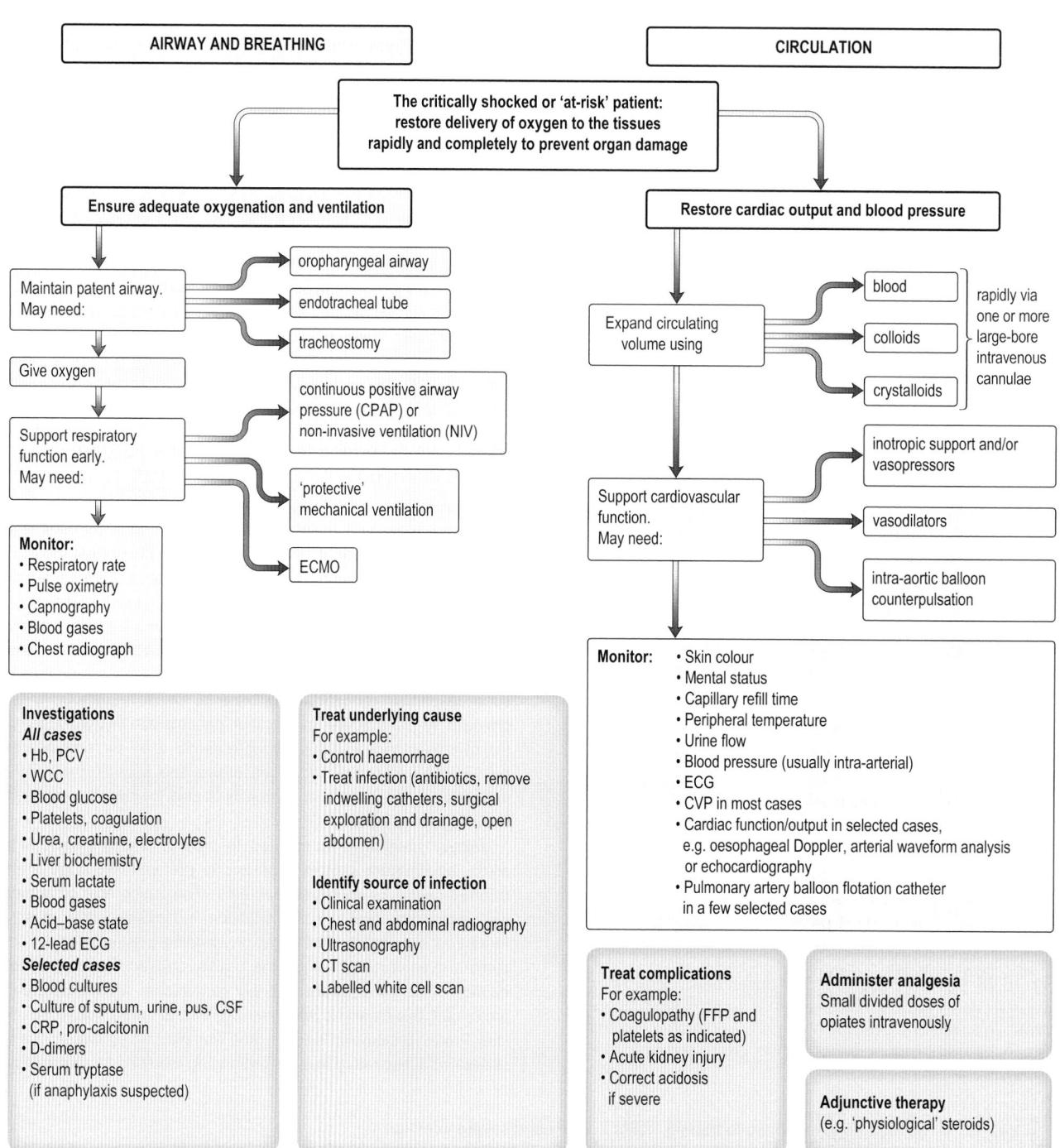

Fig. 10.24 Management of the critically ill, shocked or 'at-risk' patient. CRP, C-reactive protein; CSF, cerebrospinal fluid; CT, computed tomography; CVP, central venous pressure; ECG, electrocardiogram; ECMO, extracorporeal membrane oxygenation; FFP, fresh frozen plasma; Hb, haemoglobin; PCV, packed cell volume; WCC, white cell count.

abscesses) should be taken for microscopy, culture and sensitivities. Empirical, broad-spectrum antibiotic therapy (see p. 161) should be commenced *within the first hour* of recognition of sepsis. If an organism is isolated later, therapy can be adjusted appropriately. The choice of antibiotic depends on the likely source of infection, previous antibiotic therapy and known local resistance patterns, as well as on whether infection was acquired in hospital or in the community. Abscesses must be drained, and infected indwelling catheters removed.

Whatever the aetiology of the haemodynamic abnormality:

- *Tissue blood flow* must be restored promptly by achieving and maintaining an adequate cardiac output.
- *Arterial blood pressure* must be sufficient to maintain perfusion of vital organs.
- *Published guidelines* for adult patients suffering septic shock should be followed. These advocate targeting a MAP of >65 mmHg, a CVP of 8–12 mmHg (>12 mmHg if mechanically ventilated), a urine output of >0.5 mL/kg per hour and an $S_{CV}O_2$ of ≥70% as the initial goals of resuscitation.
- The *aim of current sepsis guidelines* (see 'Further reading') is to combine evidence-based interventions with early effective resuscitation (aimed especially at achieving an adequate circulating volume, combined with the rational use of inotropes and/or vasoactive agents to maintain blood pressure, cardiac output and oxygen transport), in order to create 'bundles of care' delivered within specific time limits.

Preload and volume replacement

Optimizing preload is the most efficient way of increasing cardiac output. Volume replacement is obviously essential in hypovolaemic shock but is also required in anaphylactic and septic shock because of vasodilation, sequestration of blood and loss of circulating volume because of vascular leak.

In obstructive shock, high filling pressures may be required to maintain an adequate stroke volume. Even in cardiogenic shock, careful volume expansion may, on occasion, lead to a useful increase in cardiac output. On the other hand, patients with severe cardiac failure, in whom ventricular filling pressures are markedly elevated, often benefit from measures to reduce preload (and afterload), such as the administration of vasodilators and diuretics (see later). Adequate perioperative volume replacement also reduces morbidity and mortality in high-risk surgical patients.

The circulating volume must be replaced quickly in order to reduce tissue damage and prevent acute kidney injury. Continuous observation of clinical signs, biochemical variables (acid–base and lactate levels) and stroke volume are vital for management and avoidance of volume overload. Pulmonary and peripheral oedema is more likely in seriously ill patients receiving large-volume fluid resuscitation because of a low colloid osmotic pressure (usually due to a low serum albumin), disruption of the alveolar–capillary membrane, microcirculatory changes and destruction of the endothelial glycocalyx.

Choice of fluid for volume replacement
Blood

This is conventionally given for haemorrhagic shock as soon as it is available. In extreme emergencies, group-specific crossmatch can be performed in minutes (see p. 358). When available and not contraindicated, blood salvage may be employed for those with severe ongoing bleeding. Unmatched blood is frequently administered in trauma patients presenting *in extremis* to the emergency department.

Transfusion of whole blood has largely been replaced by that of red cell concentrates (see p. 363). The use of leucodepleted blood is considered to be safer in terms of immune-mediated transfusion reactions, disease transmission and immune suppression. Although red cell transfusion can augment oxygen-carrying capacity, and hence global oxygen delivery, transfusion of old stored red blood cells, which become spherical rather than biconcave, and poorly deformable with increased adhesiveness, can compromise microvascular flow. In the case of traumatic or intraoperative haemorrhagic shock, many now favour 'hypotensive resuscitation' with blood and blood products until surgical control of the bleeding has been achieved. This partial resuscitation has been shown to reduce the rate of bleeding and allows the surgeon a greater chance of achieving definitive haemostasis. Once the patient is stable, higher haemoglobin and blood pressure targets may be pursued.

The absolute haemoglobin target in critically ill patients has changed with increasing awareness of the subtle detrimental immune effects associated with transfusing blood. In patients not actively bleeding and without significant cardiovascular risk factors, it is usual to transfuse in order to achieve a target haemoglobin level of 70 g/L or more ('restrictive transfusion strategy'). In patients with significant coronary artery disease or limited respiratory reserve, a target level of 90 g/L ('liberal transfusion strategy') may be more appropriate but remains controversial. Previously healthy individuals can tolerate haemoglobin levels as low as 40 g/L before displaying signs of cardiac ischaemia.

Massive blood transfusion can be defined as a volume of more than 8–10 units of red cells transfused within a 24-hour period, and *massive haemorrhage* as a loss of 50% or more of blood volume within 3 hours or a rate of blood loss exceeding 150 mL/min.

Complications of blood transfusion are discussed on page 359. Special problems arise as a result of massive transfusion:

- *Temperature changes.* Bank blood is stored at 4°C; transfusion may result in hypothermia, peripheral venoconstriction and arrhythmias. Blood should be warmed during massive transfusion and in those at risk of hypothermia (e.g. prolonged major surgery with open body cavity).
- *Coagulopathy.* Stored blood has virtually no effective platelets or clotting factors. Massive blood transfusions are now accompanied by administration of fresh frozen plasma and platelet concentrates in a balanced ratio of 1:1:1, especially in the treatment of severe traumatic haemorrhage. Cryoprecipitate also plays a key role in securing haemostasis. Recombinant factor VIIa is rarely indicated in those with uncontrollable bleeding, and prothrombin complex concentrates have the advantage that they do not need to be crossmatched or thawed, but are expensive.
- *Hypocalcaemia.* Citrate is used to stop coagulation in stored blood by binding calcium ions. As a result, during large transfusion, total body ionized calcium levels often drop, causing myocardial depression and exacerbating coagulation defects. This is corrected by administering 10 mL of 10% calcium chloride intravenously.
- *Increased oxygen affinity.* In stored blood, the red cell 2,3-diphophoglycerate (2,3-DPG) content is reduced, so that the oxyhaemoglobin dissociation curve is shifted to the left. The oxygen affinity of haemoglobin is therefore increased and oxygen unloading is impaired. Red cell levels of 2,3-diphophoglycerate (2,3-DPG) are substantially restored within 12 hours of transfusion.

- *Hyperkalaemia.* Plasma potassium levels rise progressively as blood is stored. However, hyperkalaemia is rarely a problem, as rewarming of the blood increases red cell metabolism; the sodium pump becomes active and potassium levels fall.
- *Microembolism.* Microaggregates in stored blood may obstruct the pulmonary capillaries. This process is thought by some to contribute to acute lung injury.
- *Immunity.* Blood transfusion has subtle detrimental effects on the host immune system and has been implicated in a greater susceptibility to nosocomial infections and an increase in the risk of cancer recurrence.

Crystalloids and colloids

The choice of intravenous fluid for resuscitation and the relative merits of crystalloids or colloids have long been controversial. Crystalloid solutions are cheap and convenient to use. However, they are not completely free of side-effects, as large volumes of solutions with high chloride content, such as 0.9% saline, can cause a hyperchloraemic acidosis and are associated with a greater risk of renal impairment. Balanced solutions, such as compound sodium lactate or Plasma-Lyte 148, may be preferred (see **Box 9.10**).

In critically ill patients, resuscitation with equivalent volumes of either 0.9% saline or the colloid 4% albumin has been shown to result in similar outcomes.

Polygelatin solutions have an average molecular weight of 35 000, which is iso-osmotic with plasma. They are cheap and do not interfere with crossmatching. Clinically significant coagulation defects are unusual and renal function is not significantly impaired. However, because they readily cross the glomerular basement membrane, their half-life in the circulation is only approximately 4 hours and they can promote an osmotic diuresis. These solutions may be useful during the acute phase of resuscitation, especially when volume losses are continuing. Allergic reactions can, however, occur.

Hydroxyethyl starches (HES) are available as numerous preparations with differing half-lives. Elimination of HES occurs primarily via the kidneys following hydrolysis by amylase. HES are stored in the reticuloendothelial system, apparently without causing functional impairment, but skin deposits have been associated with persistent pruritus. HES, especially the higher-molecular-weight fractions, have anticoagulant properties, can increase the risk of acute kidney injury and have been associated with an increased mortality. *HES should no longer be used in critically ill patients.*

Human albumin solution (HAS) is a natural colloid that has been used for volume replacement in shock and burns, and for the treatment of hypoproteinaemia. HAS is not generally recommended for routine volume replacement because supplies are limited and other cheaper solutions are equally effective. It may have a role in the treatment of hepatorenal syndrome in patients with liver cirrhosis or low albumin.

Myocardial contractility and inotropic agents

Myocardial contractility can be impaired by many factors, such as hypoxaemia and hypocalcaemia, as well as by some drugs (e.g. beta-blockers, antiarrhythmics and sedatives).

Severe metabolic acidosis is conventionally said to depress myocardial contractility and limit the response to vasopressor agents. Attempted correction of acidosis with intravenous sodium bicarbonate, however, generates additional carbon dioxide, which diffuses across cell membranes, producing or exacerbating intracellular acidosis. Other disadvantages of bicarbonate therapy include sodium overload and a left shift of the oxyhaemoglobin dissociation curve. Ionized calcium levels may be reduced and, combined with the fall in intracellular pH, this may impair myocardial performance.

Treatment of lactic acidosis should therefore concentrate on correcting the cause. Bicarbonate should be administered only to correct *extreme persistent metabolic acidosis* (see p. 201).

If the signs of shock persist, despite adequate volume replacement, and perfusion of vital organs is jeopardized, inotropic/vasopressor agents should be administered to improve cardiac output and blood pressure. Vasopressor therapy may also be required to maintain perfusion in those with life-threatening hypotension, even when volume replacement is incomplete. All inotropes increase myocardial oxygen consumption, particularly if a tachycardia develops, and this can lead to an imbalance between myocardial oxygen supply and demand, with the development or extension of ischaemic areas. Inotropes should therefore be used with especial caution, particularly in cardiogenic shock following myocardial infarction and in known ischaemic heart disease.

Many of the most seriously ill patients become increasingly resistant to the effects of pressor agents, an observation attributed to 'downregulation' of adrenergic receptors and nitric oxide-induced 'vasoplegia' (see later).

All inotropic agents should be administered via a large central vein and their effects continually monitored (**Box 10.11**).

Adrenaline (epinephrine)

Adrenaline stimulates both α- and β-adrenergic receptors but β effects predominate at low doses. Heart rate and cardiac index increase, while peripheral resistance is reduced. If there is an associated increase in perfusion pressure, urine output may improve. Adrenaline at higher doses can cause excessive (α-mediated) vasoconstriction with reductions in splanchnic flow, and cardiac output may fall. Prolonged high-dose administration can cause peripheral gangrene and lactic acidosis. The minimum effective dose of adrenaline should therefore be used for as short a time as possible.

Noradrenaline (norepinephrine)

This is predominantly an α-adrenergic agonist. It is particularly useful in patients with hypotension and a low systemic vascular resistance, such as is seen in septic shock. There is a risk of producing excessive vasoconstriction with impaired organ perfusion and increased afterload, particularly if noradrenaline is administered when fluid resuscitation is inadequate, and the circulating volume is reduced.

Dopamine

The haemodynamic effects of dopamine are dose-dependent. At low doses, dopamine is a positive inotrope with vasodilator actions on the renal and splanchnic circulation. Higher doses may be complicated by tachycardia, arrhythmias and vasoconstriction. Dopamine may be used as an alternative to noradrenaline in patients with bradycardia and a low risk of tachyarrhythmia.

Dopexamine

Dopexamine is an analogue of dopamine that activates β_2 receptors, as well as DA_1 and DA_2 receptors. Dopexamine is a weak positive inotrope but a powerful splanchnic vasodilator, reducing afterload and improving blood flow to vital organs, including the kidneys. It has been used as an adjunct to the perioperative management of high-risk surgical patients (see below).

Dobutamine

Dobutamine is closely related to dopamine and has predominantly β_1 activity. Dobutamine has no specific effect on the renal vasculature but urine output often increases as cardiac

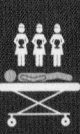

i **Box 10.11 Receptor actions of sympathomimetic and dopaminergic agents**

Agent	Receptor						Dose dependence
	β_1	β_2	α_1	α_2	DA_1	DA_2	
Adrenaline (epinephrine)							++++
Low-dose	++	+	+	±	−	−	
Moderate-dose	++	+	++	+	−	−	
High-dose	++(+)	+(+)	++++	+++	−	−	
Noradrenaline (norepineph-rine)	++	0	+++	+++	−	−	+++
Isoprenaline	+++	+++	0	0	−	−	
Dopamine							+++++
Low-dose	±	0	±	+	++	+	
Moderate-dose	++	+	++	+	++(+)	+	
High-dose	+++	++	+++	+	++(+)	+	
Dopexamine	+	+++	0	0	++	+	++
Dobutamine	++	+	±	?	0	0	++
Action	*Postsynaptic:* positive inotropism and chronotropism; renin release	*Presynaptic:* stimulation of noradrenaline release *Postsynaptic:* positive inotropism and chronotropism; vascular dilation; relaxation of bronchial smooth muscle	*Postsynaptic:* constriction of periph-eral, renal and coronary vascular smooth muscle; positive inotropism; antidiuresis	*Presynaptic:* inhibition of noradrenaline release; vasodilation *Postsynaptic:* constriction of coronary arteries; promotion of salt and water excretion	*Postsynaptic:* dilation of renal, mesenteric and coronary vessels; renal tubular effect (natriuresis, diuresis)	*Presynaptic:* inhibition of adrenaline release	

output and blood pressure improve. It reduces systemic vascular resistance, as well as improving cardiac performance, thereby decreasing afterload and ventricular filling pressures. Dobutamine is therefore useful in patients with cardiogenic shock and cardiac failure.

Phosphodiesterase inhibitors (e.g. milrinone, enoximone)

These agents have both inotropic and vasodilator properties. Because the phosphodiesterase type III inhibitors bypass the β-adrenergic receptor they cause less tachycardia and fewer arrhythmias than β agonists. They are useful in patients with recep-tor 'downregulation', those receiving beta-blockers, those being weaned from cardiopulmonary bypass and those with cardiac failure.

Vasopressin

Low-dose vasopressin can increase blood pressure and systemic vascular resistance in patients with vasodilatory septic shock and a high cardiac output unresponsive to other vasopressors ('vaso-plegia'). Low-dose vasopressin is sometimes added to conventional vasopressors in patients with septic shock.

Levosimendan

Levosimendan is a myofilament calcium sensitizer. Unlike other ino-tropes, levosimendan does not exert its action through increases in intracellular Ca^{2+} and, as a result, does not impair diastolic relax-ation of the heart. Levosimendan has phosphodiesterase inhibitor actions but these are not thought to be clinically significant. The

dose is usually infused over 24 hours but, significantly, a long-acting metabolite of levosimendan has similar calcium-sensitizing actions, maintaining the inotropic effect of levosimendan once an infusion is stopped. Adverse cardiovascular effects of levosimendan include tachycardia and hypotension; as a consequence, the addition of a vasopressor may be required.

Summary for use of inotropic and vasopressor agents

A combination of dobutamine and noradrenaline (norepinephrine) is used for the management of patients who are **shocked with a low systemic vascular resistance** (e.g. septic shock).

- Dobutamine is given to achieve optimal cardiac output.
- Noradrenaline, sometimes supplemented by vasopressin, is used for restoration of an adequate blood pressure by reducing vasodilation.

In **vasodilated septic patients** with an adequate cardiac out-put, noradrenaline can be used alone. There is evidence to suggest that adrenaline (epinephrine) may be equally safe and effective as a dobutamine/noradrenaline combination. Because of its potency, adrenaline is particularly useful in patients with **refractory hypo-tension**. Phosphodiesterase inhibitors can be used in the manage-ment of cardiac failure, especially when associated with pulmonary hypertension, and perioperatively in those undergoing cardiac surgery. Dobutamine is an alternative that is also used in septic patients with fluid overload or myocardial failure. Dopamine is used much less frequently than in the past. The role of levosimendan in the management of shock is less clear due to high cost and lack of mortality benefit, but it may be useful in resistant cardiogenic shock.

> *i* **Box 10.12 Patients at risk of developing perioperative multiorgan failure**
>
> - The elderly
> - Patients with co-morbidity, especially limited cardiorespiratory reserve
> - Patients with trauma to two body cavities requiring multiple blood transfusions
> - Patients undergoing surgery involving extensive tissue dissection, e.g. oesophagectomy, pancreatectomy, aortic aneurysm surgery
> - Patients undergoing emergency surgery for intra-abdominal or intra-thoracic catastrophic states, e.g. faecal peritonitis, oesophageal perforation

Targeting haemodynamics and oxygen transport

Although resuscitation has conventionally aimed at achieving normal haemodynamics, many of the critically ill patients that survive have raised values for cardiac output, DO_2 and VO_2. However, elevation of DO_2 and VO_2 to these 'supranormal' levels following admission to intensive care produces no benefit and may be harmful. Despite its initial promise, early goal-directed therapy to resuscitate patients in the emergency room, aimed at maintaining a central venous oxygen saturation of more than 70%, does not appear to improve outcome in patients with severe sepsis or septic shock.

High-risk surgical patients

These patients benefit from intensive perioperative monitoring and circulatory support in a critical care area (**Box 10.12**): in particular, maintenance of oxygenation, adequate circulating volume and blood pressure. Circulating volume replacement and administration of inotropes or vasopressors should be guided by monitoring of stroke volume/cardiac output. The value of the routine use of inodilators such as dopexamine remains unclear.

Vasodilator therapy

In selected cases, afterload reduction is used to increase stroke volume and decrease myocardial oxygen requirements by reducing the systolic ventricular wall tension. Vasodilation (see p. 1075) also decreases heart size and the diastolic ventricular wall tension, so that coronary blood flow is improved. Vasodilators also improve microcirculatory flow.

Vasodilator therapy can be particularly helpful in patients with cardiac failure in whom the ventricular function curve is flat (see **Figs 10.8** and **10.9**), so that falls in preload have only a limited effect on stroke volume. This form of treatment, combined in selected cases with inotropic support, is therefore useful in the management of patients with cardiogenic shock and in those with cardiogenic pulmonary oedema or mitral regurgitation.

Nitroglycerine (NTG), at low doses, is predominantly a venodilator, but as the dose is increased it also causes arterial dilation, thereby decreasing both preload and afterload. Nitrates are particularly useful in the treatment of cardiac failure with pulmonary oedema and are usually given in combination with intravenous furosemide. NTG reduces pulmonary vascular resistance, an effect that can be exploited in patients with a low cardiac output secondary to pulmonary hypertension.

Sodium nitroprusside (SNP) dilates arterioles and venous capacitance vessels, as well as the pulmonary vasculature, by donating nitric oxide. SNP therefore reduces the afterload and preload of both ventricles and can improve cardiac output and the myocardial oxygen supply/demand ratio. The effects of SNP are rapid in onset and spontaneously reversible within a few minutes of discontinuing the infusion. Cyanide poisoning is a risk with high-dose, prolonged infusions.

Mechanical support of the myocardium

Intra-aortic balloon counterpulsation (IABCP) is the technique used most widely for mechanical support of the failing myocardium. It is discussed on page 1050. In specialized centres, ventricular assist devices and veno-arterial ECMO (see below) may be used in the treatment of cardiac failure.

Further reading

Angus DC, Barnato AE, Bell D et al. A systematic review and meta-analysis of early goal-directed therapy for septic shock: the ARISE, ProCESS and ProMISe Investigators. *Intensive Care Med* 2015; 41:1549–1560.

De Backer D, Biston P, Devriendt J et al. Comparison of dopamine and norepinephrine in the treatment of shock. *N Engl J Med* 2010; 362:779–789.

Haase N, Perner A, Hennings LI et al. Hydroxy ethyl starch 130/0.38-0.45 versus crystalloid or albumin in patients with sepsis: systematic review with meta-analysis and trial sequential analysis. *BMJ* 2013; 346:1839.

Hunt BS. Bleeding and coagulopathies in critical care. *N Engl J Med* 2014: 370:847–859.

Lilly CM. The ProCESS trial – a new era of sepsis management. *N Engl J Med* 2014; 370:18:1750–1751.

Patel A, Laffan MA, Waheed U et al. Randomised trials of human albumin for adults with sepsis: systematic review and meta-analysis with trial sequential analysis of all-cause mortality. *BMJ* 2014; 349:g4561.

Pearse RM, Harrison DA, MacDonald A et al. Effect of a perioperative, cardiac output-guided hemodynamic therapy algorithm on outcomes following major gastrointestinal surgery: a randomized clinical trial and systematic review. *JAMA* 2014; 311:2181–2190.

Rautanen A, Mills TC, Gordon AC et al. Genome-wide association study of survival from sepsis due to pneumonia: an observational cohort study. *Lancet Respir Med* 2015; 3:53–60.

Rhodes A, Evans LE, Alhazzani W et al. Surviving Sepsis Campaign: international guidelines for management of sepsis and septic shock: 2016. *Intensive Care Med* 2017; 43:304–377.

Russell JA. Is there a good MAP for septic shock? *N Engl J Med* 2014; 370:1649–1651.

Singer M, Deutschman CS, Seymour CW et al. The Third International Consensus Definition for Sepsis and Septic Shock (Sepsis-3). *JAMA* 2016; 315:801–810.

Venet F, Lukaszewicz AC, Payen D et al. Monitoring the immune response in sepsis: a rational approach to administration of immunoadjuvant therapies. *Curr Opin Immunol* 2013; 25:477–483.

Venkatesh B, Finfer S, Cohen J et al. Adjunctive glucocorticoid therapy in patients with septic shock (ADRENAL study). *N Engl J Med* 2018; 378:797–808.

Zhang D, Raoof M, Chen Y et al. Circulating mitochondrial DAMPs cause inflammatory responses to injury. *Nature* 2010; 464:104–107.

http://www.survivingsepsis.org *Surviving Sepsis campaign*.

RESPIRATORY FAILURE

(See also Chapter 28.)

Classification and aetiology

The respiratory system consists of a gas-exchanging organ (the lungs) and a ventilatory pump (respiratory muscles/thorax), either or both of which can fail and precipitate respiratory failure. Respiratory failure occurs when pulmonary gas exchange is sufficiently impaired to cause hypoxaemia with or without hypercarbia. In practical terms, respiratory failure is present when the P_aO_2 is below 8 kPa (60 mmHg) or the P_aCO_2 is above 7 kPa (55 mmHg). It can be divided into:

- type I respiratory failure, in which the P_aO_2 is low and the P_aCO_2 is normal or low
- type II respiratory failure, in which the P_aO_2 is low and the P_aCO_2 is high.

Type I or 'acute hypoxaemic' respiratory failure occurs with diseases that damage lung tissue. Hypoxaemia is due to right-to-left shunts or $\dot{V}/\dot{Q}$ mismatch. Common causes include pneumonia, acute lung injury, cardiogenic pulmonary oedema, pulmonary embolism and lung fibrosis.

Type II or 'ventilatory failure' occurs when alveolar ventilation is insufficient to remove the volume of carbon dioxide being produced by tissue metabolism. Inadequate alveolar ventilation may be due to reduced ventilatory effort, inability to overcome an increased resistance to ventilation, failure to compensate for an increase in dead space and/or carbon dioxide production, or a combination of these factors. The most common cause is COPD. Other causes include chest-wall deformities, respiratory muscle weakness (e.g. Guillain–Barré syndrome) and depression of the respiratory centre (e.g. drug overdose).

Deterioration in the mechanical properties of the lungs and/or chest wall increases the work of breathing and the oxygen consumption/carbon dioxide production of the respiratory muscles. Respiratory muscle fatigue is a factor in the pathogenesis of respiratory failure.

Clinical features

A clinical assessment of respiratory distress should be made on the following criteria:
- the use of accessory muscles of respiration
- intercostal recession
- tachypnoea
- tachycardia
- sweating
- pulsus paradoxus (rarely present)
- inability to speak, unwillingness to lie flat
- agitation, restlessness, diminished conscious level
- asynchronous respiration (a discrepancy in the timing of movement of the abdominal and thoracic compartments)
- paradoxical respiration (abdominal and thoracic compartments move in opposite directions)
- respiratory alternans (breath-to-breath alteration in the relative contribution of the intercostal/accessory muscles and the diaphragm).

Investigations

Blood gas analysis should be performed to guide oxygen therapy and to provide an objective assessment of the severity of the respiratory failure. The **most sensitive clinical indicator** of increasing respiratory difficulty is a rising respiratory rate. **Vital capacity** is a better guide to deterioration, particularly in patients with respiratory inadequacy due to neuromuscular problems such as the Guillain–Barré syndrome or myasthenia gravis, in which the vital capacity decreases as weakness worsens. Measurement of **forced expiratory volume in 1 second (FEV$_1$)** is useful in the assessment of patients suffering from acute asthma or COPD.

Monitoring

Pulse oximetry

Pulse oximeters applied to a finger or earlobe measure the changing amount of light transmitted through the pulsating arterial blood and provide a continuous, non-invasive measurement of arterial oxygen saturation (S_pO_2). These devices are reliable and easy to use, and do not require calibration.

Pulse oximetry is not a sensitive guide to *changes* in oxygenation. An S_pO_2 within normal limits in a patient receiving supplemental oxygen does not exclude the possibility of hypoventilation with carbon dioxide retention. Readings can be inaccurate in those with poor peripheral perfusion.

Blood gas analysis

Normal values of blood gas analysis are shown in **Box 10.6**. Disposable pre-heparinized syringes are available for blood gas analysis.
- The sample should be analysed immediately. Alternatively, the syringe should be immersed in iced water to prevent the con-

tinuing metabolism of white cells from causing a reduction in PO_2 and a rise in PCO_2.
- Air almost inevitably enters the sample and air bubbles should be ejected immediately. The gas tensions within these air bubbles will equilibrate with those in the blood, thereby lowering the PCO_2 and usually raising the PO_2 of the sample.

Interpretation of the results of blood gas analysis can be considered in two separate parts:
- disturbances of acid–base balance (see p. 214)
- alterations in oxygenation.

Correct interpretation requires a knowledge of the patient's clinical history and age, the inspired oxygen concentration, patient temperature and any other relevant treatment (e.g. the ventilator settings for those on mechanical ventilation or the administration of sodium bicarbonate). The oxygen content of the arterial blood is determined by the percentage saturation of haemoglobin with oxygen. The relationship between the latter and the P_aO_2 is determined by the oxyhaemoglobin dissociation curve (see **Fig. 10.3**).

P_aO_2/F_iO_2 ratio

This calculated variable is a simple approximation to the $P_{A–a}O_2$ and can be used to assess the severity of respiratory failure, particularly in patients with ARDS (see p. 232). It is calculated by taking the arterial PO_2 in mmHg and dividing by the F_iO_2 expressed as a fraction of 1.

Capnography

Continuous breath-by-breath analysis of the expired carbon dioxide concentration can be used to:
- confirm tracheal intubation
- continuously monitor end-tidal PCO_2, which approximates to P_aCO_2 in normal subjects, and is used to assess effectiveness of ventilation
- detect acute airway problems, e.g. blocked or dislodged tracheal tube/tracheostomy, in all mechanically ventilated patients (essential when transporting the critically ill)
- detect acute alterations in cardiorespiratory function (e.g. a sudden fall in cardiac output).

Management

Standard management of patients with respiratory failure includes:
- administration of supplemental oxygen through a patent airway
- treatment for distal airways obstruction
- measures to limit pulmonary oedema
- control of secretions
- treatment of pulmonary infection.

The load on the respiratory muscles should be reduced by improving lung mechanics. Correction of abnormalities that may lead to respiratory muscle weakness, such as hypophosphataemia and malnutrition, is also necessary.

Oxygen therapy
Methods of oxygen administration

Oxygen is initially given via a face mask. In the majority of patients (except those with COPD with chronically elevated P_aCO_2), the precise concentration of oxygen given is not vital and oxygen can therefore be delivered by a 'variable performance' device such as a simple face mask or nasal cannula (**Fig. 10.25**).

With these devices, the inspired oxygen concentration varies from about 35% to 55%, with oxygen flow rates of 6–10 L/min. Nasal cannulae are often preferred because they are less claustrophobic and do not interfere with feeding or speaking, but can cause ulceration of

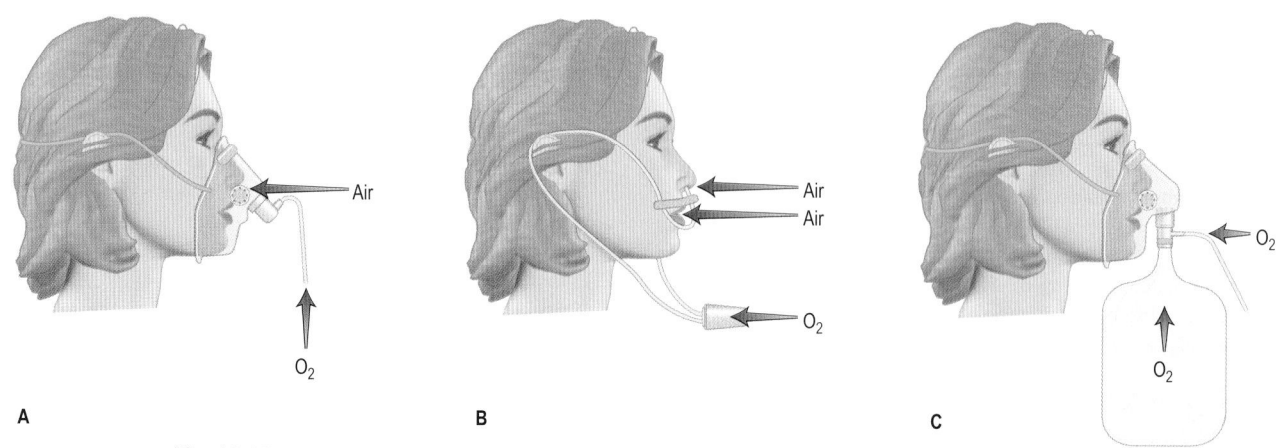

Fig. 10.25 Methods of administering supplemental oxygen to the unintubated patient. **(A)** Simple face mask. **(B)** Nasal cannulae. **(C)** Mask with reservoir bag and non-rebreathing valve.

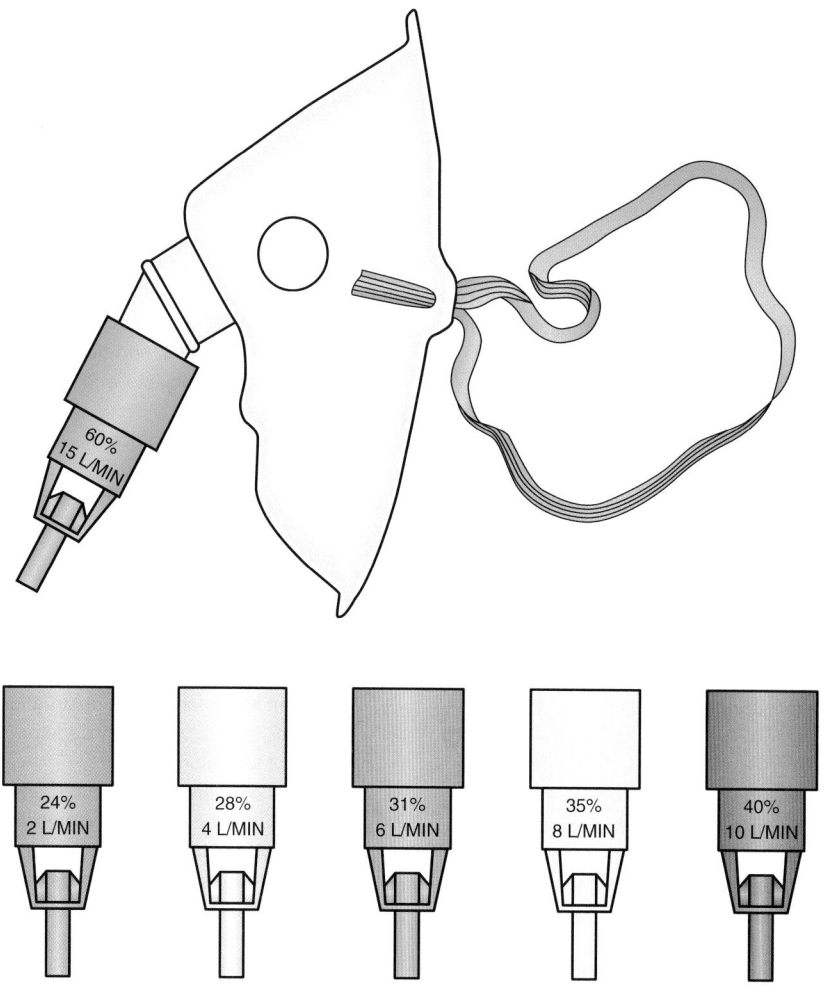

Interchangeable Venturi valves

Fig. 10.26 Fixed performance Venturi valves attached to a face mask to deliver a fixed percentage of oxygen.

the nasal mucosa and the inspired oxygen concentration is diluted by mouth breathing. Higher concentrations of oxygen can be administered by using a mask with a reservoir bag attached (**Fig. 10.25C**). **Fig. 10.25** should be compared with the fixed-performance mask shown in **Fig. 10.26**. The latter allows the oxygen concentration to be controlled and is used in patients with COPD and chronic type II failure who rely on their hypoxic drive to stimulate respiration. The hazards of reducing hypoxic drive can at times be overemphasized and are less dangerous when the patient is in a critical care unit. *Remember*, severe hypoxaemia is more dangerous than hypercapnia.

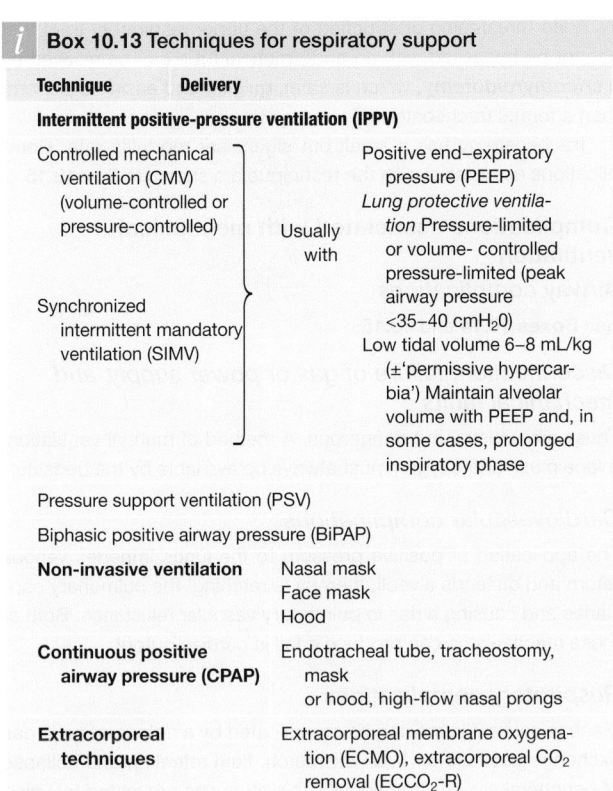

Box 10.13 Techniques for respiratory support

Technique	Delivery
Intermittent positive-pressure ventilation (IPPV)	
Controlled mechanical ventilation (CMV) (volume-controlled or pressure-controlled)	Usually with
Synchronized intermittent mandatory ventilation (SIMV)	Positive end–expiratory pressure (PEEP) *Lung protective ventilation* Pressure-limited or volume- controlled pressure-limited (peak airway pressure <35–40 cmH$_2$0) Low tidal volume 6–8 mL/kg (±'permissive hypercarbia') Maintain alveolar volume with PEEP and, in some cases, prolonged inspiratory phase
Pressure support ventilation (PSV)	
Biphasic positive airway pressure (BiPAP)	
Non-invasive ventilation	Nasal mask Face mask Hood
Continuous positive airway pressure (CPAP)	Endotracheal tube, tracheostomy, mask or hood, high-flow nasal prongs
Extracorporeal techniques	Extracorporeal membrane oxygenation (ECMO), extracorporeal CO$_2$ removal (ECCO$_2$-R)

Oxygen toxicity

Hyperoxia can cause pulmonary damage due to increased oxygen free radicals and oxidative damage to the lung tissue. Although dangerous hypoxia through fear of pulmonary oxygen toxicity should never be tolerated, oxygen saturations between 90% and 92% are probably adequate for most patients and there is some suggestion that targeting higher oxygen saturations using greater concentrations of inspired oxygen may be detrimental (e.g. post myocardial infarction). Recent evidence suggests that even a brief period of hyperoxia may increase mortality compared with normoxia, even hyperoxia following emergency intubations for any cause in the emergency department.

Respiratory support

If, despite the above measures, the patient continues to deteriorate or fails to improve, the institution of some form of respiratory support is necessary (**Box 10.13**). *Non-invasive ventilation* via a mask or hood (see p. 230) can be used, but in many critically ill patients *invasive ventilation* through an endotracheal tube or tracheostomy is required.

Invasive mechanical ventilation (IMV) is achieved by intermittently inflating the lungs with positive pressure delivered by a mechanical ventilator through an endotracheal or tracheostomy tube, commonly carried out in the absence of spontaneous breaths. This is called *intermittent positive pressure ventilation (IPPV)* or controlled mechanical ventilation (CMV). However, technological development has meant that it is now more commonly carried out by augmenting the patient's own spontaneous breaths (see p. 229). This has the advantage of maintaining the patient's own respiratory muscle activity and function, thereby avoiding muscle atrophy.

Indications for mechanical ventilation

Acute respiratory failure, with signs of severe respiratory distress (e.g. respiratory rate >40 breaths/min, inability to speak, patient exhaustion) persisting despite maximal therapy, requires mechanical ventilation. Confusion, restlessness, agitation, a decreased conscious level, a rising P_aCO$_2$ (>8 kPa, >60 mmHg) and extreme hypoxaemia (<8 kPa, <60 mmHg), despite oxygen therapy, are further indications.

In *acute ventilatory failure* due, for example, to myasthenia gravis, Guillain–Barré syndrome or high spinal cord injuries, mechanical ventilation should usually be instituted when the vital capacity has fallen to 10 mL/kg or less. This will avoid complications such as atelectasis and infection, as well as preventing respiratory arrest. The tidal volume and respiratory rate are relatively insensitive indicators of respiratory failure in these conditions and change late in the course of the disease. A high P_aCO$_2$ (particularly if rising) is an indication for urgent mechanical ventilation.

Not all patients with respiratory failure and/or a reduced vital capacity require ventilation; clinical assessment of each individual case is essential. The patient's general condition, degree of exhaustion, level of consciousness and ability to protect the airway are often more useful than blood gas values.

Other indications include:
- postoperative ventilation in high-risk patients
- head injury: to avoid hypoxia and hypercarbia, which increase cerebral blood flow and intracranial pressure (see later)
- trauma: chest injury with lung contusions and high spinal cord injuries
- severe left ventricular failure with pulmonary oedema
- coma with airway compromise or breathing difficulties, e.g. following drug overdose.

Institution of invasive respiratory support

This requires tracheal intubation, which should be performed under anaesthesia only by experienced staff. If the patient is conscious, the procedure should be fully explained and consent obtained. The complications of tracheal intubation are given in **Box 10.14**.

Intubating a critically ill patient is very different to intubating a patient in the operating theatre for elective surgery. The patient is usually hypoxic and hypercarbic, with increased sympathetic activity; the stimulus of laryngoscopy and intubation can precipitate dangerous arrhythmias, bradycardia and even cardiac arrest. In extreme emergencies, it may be necessary to ventilate the patient by hand using a bag-valve mask (supplemented with high-flow oxygen) and an oropharyngeal airway or a laryngeal mask airway, until experienced help arrives.

The ECG and oxygen saturation should be monitored, and the patient pre-oxygenated with 100% oxygen before intubation. Resuscitation drugs should be immediately available. If time allows, the circulating volume should be optimized and, if necessary, inotropes commenced before intubation is attempted. In some cases, it is appropriate to establish intra-arterial and CVP monitoring before instituting mechanical ventilation, although many patients will not tolerate the supine or head-down position. In some deeply comatose patients no sedation may be required, but in the majority a short-acting intravenous anaesthetic agent, usually with an opiate followed by muscle relaxation, will be necessary. Capnography must be used to confirm tracheal intubation.

Sedation, analgesia and muscle relaxation

Most critically ill patients require analgesia and many will receive sedatives. The combination of an opiate with a benzodiazepine or propofol is often used to facilitate mechanical ventilation. Heavy

i **Box 10.14 Complications of tracheal intubation**

Complication	Comments
Immediate	
Trauma to the upper airway	Affects lips, teeth, gums, trachea
Tube in oesophagus	Gives rise to hypoxia and abdominal distension Detected by absence of capnography trace Requires immediate removal, bag-mask ventilation with oxygen and re-insertion of tracheal tube
Tube in one or other (usually the right) main bronchus	Avoid by checking both lungs are being inflated, i.e. both sides of chest move, and air entry is heard bilaterally on auscultation Obtain chest X-ray to check position of tube and to exclude lung collapse
Early	

Migration of tube out of trachea
Leaks around tube
Obstruction of tube because of kinking or secretions
	These are dangerous complications
	Patient becomes distressed and cyanosed, and has poor chest expansion
	The following should be performed immediately:
	    Manual inflation with 100% oxygen
	    Tracheal suction
	    Check position of tube
	    Deflation of cuff
	    Check tube for 'kinks' or blockage with secretions or blood (common)
	If no improvement, remove tube, ventilate with face mask and then insert new endotracheal tube

Late	
Sinusitis Mucosal oedema and ulceration Laryngeal injury Tracheal narrowing and fibrosis Tracheomalacia	

sedation is indicated in those with severe respiratory failure, especially since 'lung-protective' ventilatory strategies (see later) are inherently uncomfortable. A few may require neuromuscular blockade. It is recognized, however, that minimizing sedation levels using 'sedation scores' and 'daily wakening', or even the avoidance of sedatives altogether, often in combination with spontaneous breathing modes of respiratory support (see later), is associated with reductions in the duration of mechanical ventilation and more rapid discharge from the ICU and hospital.

Tracheostomy

Tracheostomy may be required for long-term control of the airway in some patients with persistent reduced conscious state, to manage excessive bronchial secretions, facilitate respiratory weaning, reduce sedation requirements and improve patient comfort.

Tracheostomy is now performed most commonly on the ICU by the intensivist, adopting a percutaneous dilational approach. This approach is quicker, less resource-intensive, safe and associated with a greatly reduced wound infection rate than surgical tracheostomy performed in the operating theatre. Surgical tracheostomy is reserved for when anatomical factors preclude a percutaneous approach or when there are concerns regarding abnormal coagulation that may require surgical haemostasis.

A life-threatening obstruction of the upper respiratory tract that cannot be bypassed with an endotracheal tube can be relieved by a **cricothyroidotomy**, which is safer, quicker and easier to perform than a formal tracheostomy.

Tracheostomy has a small but significant mortality rate. Complications associated with the technique are shown in **Box 10.15**.

Complications associated with mechanical ventilation

Airway complications

See **Boxes 10.14** and **10.15**.

Disconnection, failure of gas or power supply, and mechanical faults

These are unusual but dangerous. A method of manual ventilation, a face mask and oxygen must always be available by the bedside.

Cardiovascular complications

The application of positive pressure to the lungs impedes venous return and distends alveoli, thereby 'stretching' the pulmonary capillaries and causing a rise in pulmonary vascular resistance. Both of these mechanisms can produce a fall in cardiac output.

Respiratory complications

Mechanical ventilation can be complicated by a deterioration in gas exchange because of $\dot{V}/\dot{Q}$ mismatch, fluid retention and collapse of peripheral alveoli. Traditionally, the latter was prevented by using high tidal volumes (10–12 mL/kg) but high inflation pressures, with over-distension of compliant alveoli, perhaps exacerbated by the repeated opening and closure of distal airways, can disrupt the alveolar–capillary membrane. There is an increase in microvascular permeability and release of inflammatory mediators, leading to **'ventilator-associated lung injury'**. This **'barotrauma'** and **'volutrauma'** can result in rupture of the alveoli and may be complicated by pneumomediastinum, subcutaneous emphysema, pneumothorax and intra-abdominal air. The risk of pneumothorax is increased in those with destructive lung disease (e.g. necrotizing pneumonia, emphysema), asthma or fractured ribs.

A **tension pneumothorax** can be rapidly fatal in ventilated patients. Signs include the development or worsening of hypoxia, hypercarbia, respiratory distress and an unexplained increase in airway pressure, as well as hypotension and tachycardia, sometimes accompanied by a rising CVP. Examination may reveal unequal chest expansion, mediastinal shift away from the side of the pneumothorax (deviated trachea, displaced apex beat) and a hyper-resonant hemithorax. Although breath sounds are often diminished over the pneumothorax, this sign can be misleading in ventilated patients. If there is time, the diagnosis can be confirmed by chest X-ray. In a rapidly deteriorating patient with a high index of suspicion for a tension pneumothorax, a needle decompression into the second intercostal space in the mid-clavicular line may be indicated, followed by insertion of a definitive chest drain.

Ventilator-associated pneumonia

Hospital-acquired pneumonia occurs in as many as one-third of patients receiving mechanical ventilation and is associated with a significant increase in length of stay and mortality. The diagnosis can be controversial, as pyrexia and infiltrates on the chest X-ray that may not be infective in origin are common. Organisms commonly isolated are aerobic Gram-negative bacilli (e.g. *Pseudomonas aeruginosa*, *Klebsiella pneumoniae*, *Escherichia coli*, *Acinetobacter* spp.) and *Staphylococcus aureus*, including meticillin-resistant

The complications for tracheal intubation shown in **Box 10.14** *plus*:

Early
- Death
- Pneumothorax
- Haemorrhage
- Hypoxia
- Hypotension
- Cardiac arrhythmias
- Tube misplaced in pretracheal subcutaneous tissues
- Subcutaneous emphysema

Intermediate
- Mucosal ulceration
- Erosion of tracheal cartilages (can cause tracheo-oesophageal fistula)
- Erosion of innominate artery (occasionally leads to fatal haemorrhage)
- Stomal infection
- Pneumonia

Late
- Failure of stoma to heal
- Tracheal granuloma
- Tracheal stenosis at level of stoma, cuff or tube tip
- Collapse of tracheal rings at level of stoma
- Cosmetic factors

Staphylococcus aureus (MRSA). Deciding whether an organism that has been isolated is causing ventilator-associated pneumonia or is simply colonizing the respiratory tract can also be difficult. Leakage of infected oropharyngeal secretions past the tracheal tube cuff is thought to be largely responsible for ventilator-associated pneumonia and many ICUs now utilize endotracheal tubes with modern tube cuffs and subglottic aspiration ports to minimize the risk. Bacterial colonization of the oropharynx may be promoted by regurgitation of colonized gastric fluid and so the risk of ventilator-associated pneumonia can be reduced by nursing patients in the semi-recumbent position and by oropharyngeal decontamination. Treatment is with an appropriate broad-spectrum antibiotic, which can be modified if a causative organism is isolated.

Techniques for respiratory support
(See **Box 10.13**.)

Controlled mechanical ventilation
Controlled mechanical ventilation (CMV) is used when respiratory efforts are absent or have been abolished. It involves one of two types:
- **Volume-controlled ventilation**. The tidal volume and respiratory rate are preset on the ventilator. The airway pressure varies according to both the ventilator setting and the patient's lung mechanics (airways resistance and compliance).
- **Pressure-controlled ventilation**. Both the inspiratory pressure and the respiratory rate are preset but the tidal volume varies according to the patient's lung mechanics.

Positive end-expiratory pressure
A positive airway pressure can be maintained at a chosen level throughout expiration using a threshold resistor valve in the expiratory limb of the circuit. Positive end-expiratory pressure (PEEP) re-expands under-ventilated lung units, and redistributes lung water from the alveoli to the perivascular interstitial space, thereby reducing shunt and increasing P_aO_2. The inevitable rise in mean intrathoracic pressure associated with the application of PEEP may, however, further impede venous return, increase pulmonary vascular resistance and reduce cardiac output. The fall in cardiac output can be ameliorated by expanding the circulating volume, although inotropic or vasopressor support is required in some cases. Thus, although arterial oxygenation is often improved by the application of PEEP, a simultaneous fall in cardiac output can lead to a reduction in total oxygen delivery.

Low levels of PEEP (5–8 cmH$_2$O) are used in the majority of mechanically ventilated patients in order to maintain lung volume, as well as in those with basal atelectasis and in selected cases with airways obstruction.

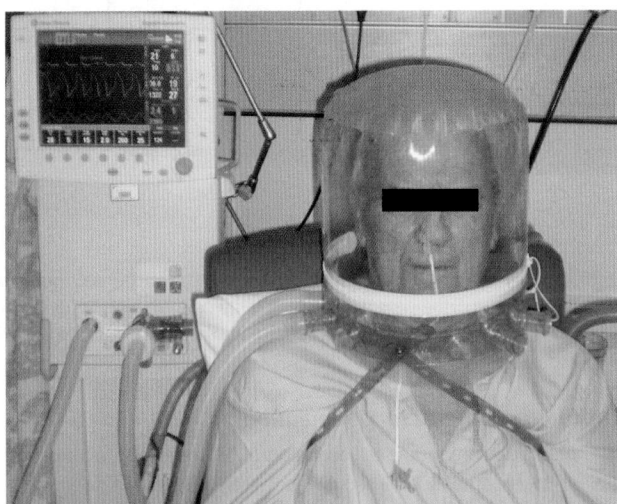

Fig. 10.27 Use of a continuous positive airway pressure (CPAP) hood.

Continuous positive airway pressure
The application of continuous positive airway pressure (CPAP) achieves for the spontaneously breathing patient what PEEP does for the ventilated patient. Oxygen and air are delivered under pressure via an endotracheal tube, a tracheostomy, a tightly fitting face mask or a hood (**Fig. 10.27**). Not only can CPAP improve oxygenation, but also the lungs become more compliant and the work of breathing is reduced.

An alternative is to use a very high flow of oxygen and air delivered via large-diameter nasal prongs to create a modest amount of CPAP. This high-flow nasal oxygen (HFNO) system is often better tolerated, as the patient is able to cough, expectorate, communicate and eat. Commencing therapy with HFNO in patients with type I respiratory failure may be equivalent to, and in some circumstances more effective than, non-invasive ventilation in preventing patient deterioration and avoiding subsequent invasive ventilation.

Pressure support ventilation
In pressure support ventilation (PSV), spontaneous breaths are augmented by a preset level of positive pressure (usually between 5 and 20 cmH$_2$O), triggered by the patient's spontaneous respiratory effort and applied for a given fraction of inspiratory time or until inspiratory flow falls below a certain level. Tidal volume is determined by the set pressure, the patient's effort and pulmonary mechanics. The level of pressure support can be reduced progressively as the patient improves.

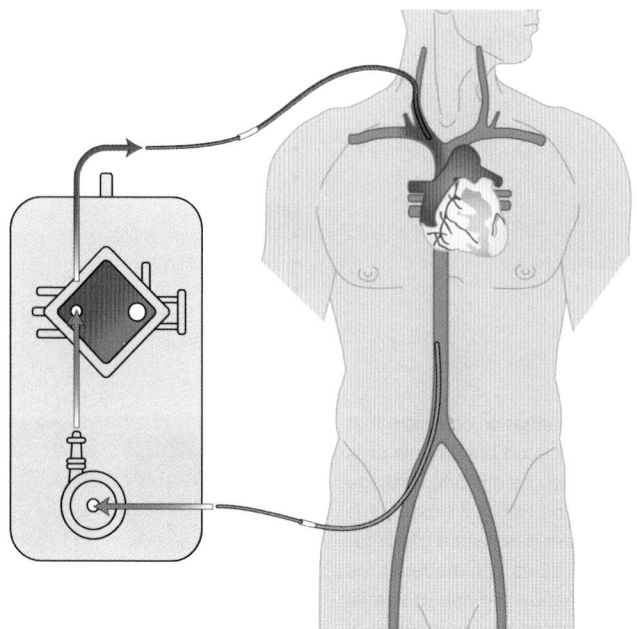

Fig. 10.28 Veno-venous extracorporeal membrane oxygenation (ECMO). A pump pulls blood off the patient through a large cannula with tip in the inferior vena cava. The blood then passes through a membrane oxygenator and is returned to the superior vena cava fully oxygenated and with CO_2 removed.

Intermittent mandatory ventilation

The intermittent mandatory ventilation (IMV) technique allows the patient to breathe spontaneously between the 'mandatory' tidal volumes delivered by the ventilator. These mandatory breaths are timed to coincide with the patient's own inspiratory effort (synchronized intermittent mandatory ventilation, or SIMV). SIMV can be used with or without CPAP, and spontaneous breaths may be assisted with pressure support ventilation.

'Lung-protective' ventilation

This is an ideal method of mechanical ventilation that avoids over-distension of alveoli, as well as repeated energetic opening and closing of distal airway and alveoli. Alveolar volume is maintained with PEEP, and sometimes by prolonging the inspiratory phase, while tidal volumes are limited to 4–8 mL/kg ideal body weight (ideally, 6 mL/kg). Plateau pressures (P_{Plat}) should not exceed 30 cmH$_2$O. Respiratory rate can be increased to improve CO_2 removal and avoid severe acidosis (pH >7.2), but permissive hypercarbia is common and acceptable. Ventilation with low tidal volumes has been shown to improve outcome in patients with ARDS (see later). Lung-protective ventilation should be used in almost all patients undergoing mechanical ventilation.

High-frequency oscillation

High-frequency oscillation (HFO) is administered using a purpose-designed ventilator. With HFO, there is no bulk flow of gas; rather, gas oscillates to and fro at rates of 4–15 Hz in a CPAP circuit set at a high mean airway pressure (often 20–30 cmH$_2$O). The mechanism of gas exchange is not fully understood but lung volume is well maintained and oxygenation may be improved. Recent evidence has shown, however, that HFO does not offer any mortality benefit in adults, and one trial suggested increased mortality.

Extracorporeal gas exchange

In patients with severe refractory respiratory failure, pumped, high-flow, veno-venous blood flow through an artificial lung is used in specialized centres to achieve adequate oxygenation and CO_2 removal (extracorporeal membrane oxygenation, ECMO; **Fig. 10.28**). Extracorporeal carbon dioxide removal (ECCO$_2$-R) is more easily administered, and uses lower blood flow rates to provide effective CO_2 removal but less efficient oxygenation. Both techniques have been used to reduce ventilation requirements, thereby minimizing further ventilation-induced lung damage and encouraging resolution of the lung injury.

Non-invasive ventilation

Non-invasive ventilation (NIV) is suitable for patients who are conscious, cooperative and able to protect their airway; they must also be able to expectorate effectively. Positive pressure is applied to the airways using a tight-fitting full-face/nasal mask or a hood. Modern ventilators are cheap, easy to use and flexible. They deliver bi-level positive airway pressure (BiPAP) with inspiratory (IPAP) and expiratory (EPEP) pressure levels, and times are set independently. Unrestricted spontaneous respiration is possible throughout the respiratory cycle. BiPAP can also be patient-triggered. There is a reduced risk of ventilator-associated pneumonia and improved patient comfort, with preservation of airway defence mechanisms, speech and swallowing (which allows better nutrition). Spontaneous coughing and expectoration are not hampered, permitting effective physiotherapy, and sedation is usually unnecessary. Institution of non-invasive respiratory support can rest the respiratory muscles, reduce respiratory acidosis and breathlessness, improve clearance of secretions and re-expand collapsed lung segments. The intubation rate, length of ICU and hospital stay, and, in some categories of patient, mortality may all be reduced. NIV is particularly useful in acute hypercapnic respiratory failure associated with COPD,

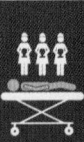

> **_i_ Box 10.16 Indications for/contraindications to use of non-invasive ventilation**
>
> **Some indications**
> - Acute exacerbation of chronic obstructive pulmonary disease (H^+ >44 nmol/L; pH <7.35)
> - Cardiogenic pulmonary oedema
> - Chest wall deformity/neuromuscular disease (hypercapnic respiratory failure)
> - Obstructive sleep apnoea
> - Severe pneumonia (with caution – see **Box 28.29**)
>
> - Asthma (occasionally)
> - Weaning patients from invasive ventilation
>
> **Some contraindications**
> - Facial or upper airway surgery
> - Reduced conscious level
> - Inability to protect the airway

---

provided the patient is not profoundly hypoxic or obtunded. NIV is also valuable in immunocompromised patients with acute respiratory failure, and following extubation of hypercapnic patients with respiratory disorders to reduce the risk of subsequent respiratory failure and mortality. **Box 10.16** lists some indications and contraindications for the use of NIV when standard medical treatment has failed.

Weaning

Weakness and wasting of respiratory muscles are inevitable consequences of the catabolic response to critical illness and the disuse atrophy that will occur as a result of mechanical ventilation. Often, abnormalities of gas exchange and lung mechanics persist. Not surprisingly, therefore, many patients experience difficulty in resuming unsupported spontaneous ventilation.

Neuromuscular weakness complicating critical illness

Polyneuromyopathies have most often been described in association with persistent sepsis and multiple organ failure.

Critical illness polyneuropathy is characterized by a primary axonal neuropathy involving both motor and, to a lesser extent, sensory nerves. Clinically, the initial manifestation is often difficulty in weaning the patient from respiratory support. There is muscle wasting, the limbs are weak and flaccid, and deep tendon reflexes are reduced or absent. Cranial nerves are relatively spared. Nerve conduction studies confirm axonal damage. The CSF protein concentration is normal or minimally elevated. These findings differentiate critical illness neuropathy from Guillain–Barré syndrome, in which nerve conduction studies nearly always provide evidence of demyelination and CSF protein is usually high.

The cause of critical illness polyneuropathy is not known and there is no specific treatment. Weaning from respiratory support and rehabilitation are likely to be prolonged. With resolution of the underlying critical illness, recovery can be expected after 1–6 months but weakness and fatigue frequently persist.

Critical illness myopathies can also occur, often in association with a neuropathy. A severe quadriplegic myopathy has been associated in particular with the administration of steroids and muscle relaxants to mechanically ventilated patients who have acute, severe asthma.

Criteria for weaning patients from mechanical ventilation

Clinical assessment is the best way of deciding whether a patient can be weaned from the ventilator. A key part of the assessment is deciding whether the precipitating need for mechanical ventilation is no longer present or has vastly improved, to allow a trial without ventilation. The patient's conscious level and cardiovascular performance, as well as the effects of drugs, must all be taken into account. A subjective evaluation by an experienced clinician of the patient's response to a short period of spontaneous breathing (spontaneous breathing trial) is the most reliable predictor of weaning success or failure. Objective criteria are based on an assessment of pulmonary gas exchange (blood gas analysis), lung mechanics and muscular strength.

Techniques for weaning

Patients who have received mechanical ventilation for less than 24–48 hours – after elective major surgery, for example – can usually resume spontaneous respiration immediately and no weaning process is required. This procedure can also be adopted for those who have been ventilated for longer periods but who tolerate a spontaneous breathing trial and clearly fulfil objective criteria for weaning.

Techniques of weaning include the following:

- The traditional method is to allow the patient to breathe entirely spontaneously for a short time, following which respiratory support is resumed. These periods of spontaneous breathing are gradually increased and the periods of respiratory support are progressively reduced. Initially, it is usually advisable to ventilate the patient throughout the night. This method can be stressful and tiring for both patients and staff, although it is sometimes successful when other methods have failed.
- SIMV (see earlier) involves a progressive reduction in the frequency of mandatory breaths. Spontaneous breaths are usually pressure-supported.
- Gradual reduction of the level of pressure support is thought to be the preferred technique.
- CPAP (see above) can prevent the alveolar collapse, hypoxaemia and fall in compliance that might otherwise occur when patients start to breathe spontaneously. It is therefore used during weaning with SIMV or pressure support, during spontaneous breathing trials and in spontaneously breathing patients prior to extubation.
- Tracheostomy is often used to facilitate weaning from mechanical ventilation.
- Non-invasive respiratory support (BiPAP, CPAP) can be used following extubation to prevent respiratory failure and re-intubation.

Extubation and tracheostomy decannulation

These should not be performed until patients can cough, swallow and protect their own airway, and are sufficiently alert to be cooperative. Patients who fulfil these criteria can be extubated, provided their respiratory function has improved sufficiently to sustain spontaneous ventilation indefinitely. Similar considerations guide the elective removal of tracheostomy tubes.

The 'rapid shallow breathing index' – the ratio of respiratory rate (in breaths/minute) to tidal volume (in litres) – can be used to predict successful extubation, provided all other preconditions have also been met. A score of less than 100 is a relatively good predictor of extubation success and represents a patient who breathes slowly and comfortably with adequate tidal volumes.

Further reading

Bouadma L, Luyt CE, Tubach F et al. Use of procalcitonin to reduce patients' exposure to antibiotics in intensive care units. *Lancet* 2010; 375:463–474.

Davidson AC, Banham S, Elliott M et al. BTS/ICS guideline for the ventilatory management of acute hypercapnic respiratory failure in adults. *Thorax* 2016; 71 (Suppl. 2):1–35.

Frat JP, Thille AW, Mercat A et al. High-flow oxygen through nasal cannula in acute hypoxemic respiratory failure. *N Engl J Med* 2015; 372:2185–2196.

Malhotra A, Drazen JM. High-frequency oscillatory ventilation on shaky ground. *N Engl J Med* 2013; 368:863–865.

Nava S, Hill N. Non-invasive ventilation in acute respiratory failure. *Lancet* 2009; 374:250–259.

Page D, Ablordeppey E, Wessman B et al. Emergency department hyperoxia is associated with increased mortality in mechanically ventilated patients: a cohort study. *Critical Care* 2018; 22:9

Peek GJ, Mugford M, Tinwoipati R et al. Efficacy and economic assessment of conventional ventilatory support versus extracorporeal membrane oxygenation for severe adult respiratory failure (CESAR): a multicentre randomised controlled trial. *Lancet* 2009; 374:1351–1363.

Strom T, Martinussen T, Toft P. A protocol of no sedation for critically ill patients receiving mechanical ventilation: a randomized trial. *Lancet* 2010; 375:475–480.

ACUTE RESPIRATORY DISTRESS SYNDROME

Definition and aetiology

The acute respiratory distress syndrome (ARDS, **Box 10.17**) can be defined as follows:

- Respiratory distress.
- Stiff lungs: reduced pulmonary compliance resulting in high inflation pressures.
- Chest X-ray: new bilateral, diffuse, patchy or homogeneous pulmonary infiltrates.
- Non-cardiac origin: no apparent cardiogenic cause of pulmonary oedema (pulmonary artery occlusion pressure <18 mmHg, or normal echocardiogram and cardiac indices).
- Gas exchange abnormalities, all with a PEEP ≥5 cmH$_2$O (**Berlin definition**):
  - mild: P_aO_2/F_iO_2 ratio 300–200 mmHg (40-26.6 kPa)
  - moderate: P_aO_2/F_iO_2 200–100 mmHg (26.6-13.3 kPa)
  - severe: P_aO_2/F_iO_2 ratio <100 mmHg (<13.3 kPa).

ARDS can occur as a non-specific reaction of the lungs to a wide variety of direct pulmonary and indirect non-pulmonary insults. Approximately 10% of admissions to critical care fit the Berlin definition for ARDS, and the classifications above predict mortality which ranges from 27% in mild, 32% in moderate and 45% in severe ARDS. By far the most common predisposing factor is sepsis, and 20–40% of patients with severe sepsis will develop ARDS (see **Box 10.17**).

Pathogenesis and pathophysiology

ARDS can be viewed as an early manifestation of a generalized inflammatory response with endothelial dysfunction and therefore is frequently associated with the development of multiple organ dysfunction syndrome (MODS, see p. 219).

Non-cardiogenic pulmonary oedema

This is the cardinal feature of ARDS and is the first and clinically most evident sign of a generalized increase in vascular permeability, caused by the microcirculatory changes and release of immune mediators described earlier, with activated neutrophils playing a key role. The pulmonary epithelium is also damaged in the early stages, reducing surfactant production and predisposing to alveolar collapse.

Box 10.17 Disorders associated with acute respiratory distress syndrome

Direct lung injury	Indirect lung injury
Common causes	
Pneumonia	Sepsis
Aspiration of gastric contents	Severe trauma with shock and multiple transfusions
Less common causes	
Pulmonary contusion	Cardiopulmonary bypass
Blast injury	Drug overdose (heroin, barbiturates)
Fat embolism	Acute pancreatitis
Near-drowning	Transfusion-associated lung injury (TRALI)
Inhalational injury (smoke or corrosive gases)	
Reperfusion lung injury after lung transplantation or pulmonary embolectomy	Eclampsia
	High altitude
	Severe burns
Amniotic fluid embolism	Pulmonary vasculitis

Pulmonary hypertension

Pulmonary hypertension, sometimes complicated by right ventricular failure (see p. 1115), is a common feature of ARDS. Initially, mechanical obstruction of the pulmonary circulation may occur as a result of vascular compression by interstitial oedema, while local activation of the coagulation cascade leads to thrombosis and obstruction in the pulmonary microvasculature. Later, pulmonary vasoconstriction may develop in response to increased autonomic nervous activity and circulating substances such as catecholamines and thromboxane. Those vessels supplying alveoli with low oxygen tensions constrict (the 'pulmonary hypoxic vasoconstrictor response'), diverting pulmonary blood flow to better-oxygenated areas of lung and thus limiting the degree of shunt.

Haemorrhagic intra-alveolar exudate

This exudate is rich in platelets, fibrin, fibrinogen and clotting factors, and may inactivate surfactant and stimulate inflammation, as well as promoting hyaline membrane formation and the migration of fibroblasts into the air spaces.

Resolution, fibrosis and repair

Within days of the onset of lung injury, formation of a new epithelial lining is under way and activated fibroblasts accumulate in the interstitial spaces. In some cases, there is progressive interstitial fibrosis. In those who recover the lungs are substantially remodelled.

Physiological changes

Shunt and dead space increase, compliance falls and there is evidence of airflow limitation. Although the lungs in ARDS are diffusely injured, the pulmonary lesions, when identified as densities on a CT scan, are predominantly located in dependent regions (**Fig. 10.29**). This is partly explained by the effects of gravity on the distribution of extravascular lung water and areas of lung collapse. Pleural effusions are common.

Clinical features

The first sign of the development of ARDS is often an unexplained tachypnoea, followed by increasing hypoxaemia and breathlessness. Fine crackles are heard throughout both lung fields. Later, the chest X-ray shows bilateral diffuse shadowing, interstitial at first, but subsequently with an alveolar pattern and air bronchograms (**Fig. 10.30**). The differential diagnosis includes cardiac failure and lung fibrosis.

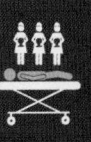

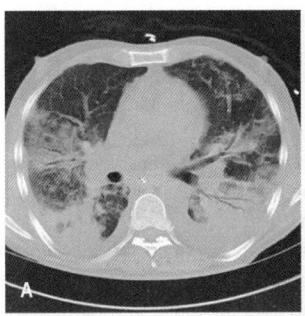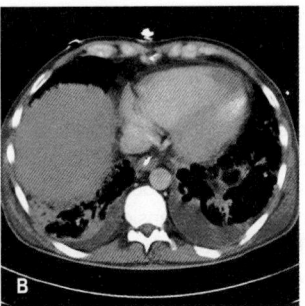

Fig. 10.29 Acute respiratory distress syndrome. (A) Computed tomography scan of the lung showing ground-glass opacification in non-dependent regions, with atelectasis and consolidation in dependent regions. There are small pleural effusions. **(B)** The same patient as shown in (A) using soft tissue window settings to demonstrate small bilateral effusions layering in the dependent region of both hemithoraces. *(From Hinds CJ, Watson JD. Intensive Care: A Concise Textbook, 3rd edn. Edinburgh: Saunders; 2008, with permission. Courtesy of Dr SPG Padley.)*

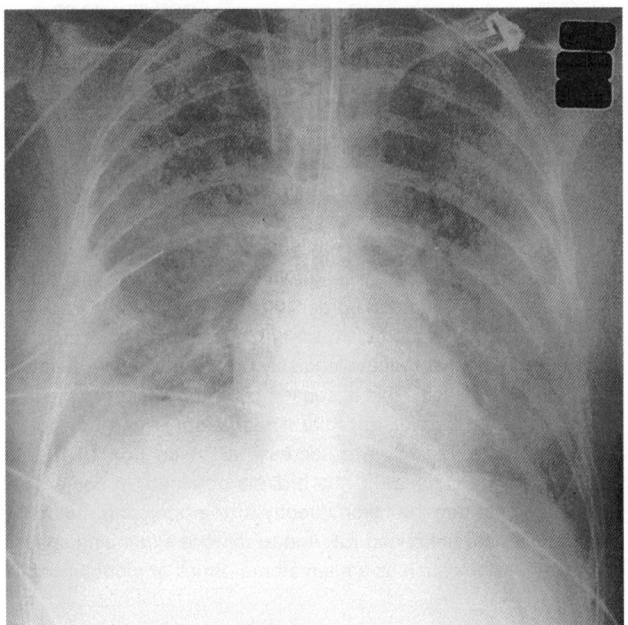

Fig. 10.30 Chest X-ray appearances in acute respiratory distress syndrome. Bilateral diffuse alveolar shadowing with air bronchograms and no cardiac enlargement.

Management

This is based on treatment of the underlying condition (e.g. eradication of sepsis), supportive measures, and avoidance of complications such as ventilator-induced lung injury and ventilator-associated pneumonia.

Mechanical ventilation

This is the cornerstone of management; strategies designed to minimize ventilator-induced lung injury and encourage lung healing should be used (see earlier).

Pulmonary oedema limitation

Pulmonary oedema formation should be limited by fluid restriction, the use of diuretics and, if these measures fail, prevention of fluid overload by haemofiltration. The aim should be to achieve a consistently negative fluid balance.

Prone position

When the patient is changed from the supine to the prone position, lung densities in the dependent region are redistributed and shunt fraction is reduced. More uniform alveolar ventilation, caudal movement of the diaphragm, redistribution of perfusion and recruitment of collapsed alveoli all contribute to the improvement in gas exchange. Recent findings suggest that proning early in the course of the disease process and spending longer periods prone than supine are associated with substantial mortality benefits.

Inhaled nitric oxide

This vasodilator, when inhaled, may improve ventilation-perfusion matching by increasing perfusion of ventilated lung units, as well as reducing pulmonary hypertension. It has been shown to improve oxygenation in so-called 'responders' with ARDS but has not been shown to enhance survival.

Aerosolized prostacyclin

This appears to have similar effects to inhaled nitric oxide and is easier to deliver. As with inhaled nitric oxide, the response to aerosolized prostacyclin is variable: although it improves oxygenation, its effect on outcome is unclear.

Steroids

Administration of steroids to patients with persistent ARDS may improve lung function but does not appear to improve outcome. Their use remains controversial.

Prognosis

Mortality from ARDS has fallen over the last two decades, from around 60% to 20–40%, perhaps as a consequence of improved general care, lung-protective ventilation strategies, the increasing use of management protocols, and attention to infection control and nutrition. Prognosis is, however, still very dependent on aetiology. When ARDS occurs in association with intra-abdominal sepsis, mortality rates remain very high, whereas much lower mortality is to be expected in those with 'primary' ARDS (pneumonia, aspiration, lung contusion). Mortality rises with increasing age and failure of other organs. Most of those dying with ARDS do so as a result of MODS and haemodynamic instability rather than impaired gas exchange.

Further reading

ARDS Definition Task Force. Acute respiratory distress syndrome: the Berlin definition. *JAMA* 2012; 307:2526–2533.

Bellani G, Laffey J, Pham T et al. Epidemiology, patterns of care and mortality for patients with acute respiratory distress syndrome in intensive care units in 50 countries. *JAMA* 2016; 315:788–800.

Guérin C, Reignier J, Richard JC et al. Prone positioning in severe acute respiratory distress syndrome. *N Engl J Med* 2013; 368:2159–2168.

Faculty of Intensive Care Medicine/Intensive Care Society. *Guidelines on the Management of Acute Respiratory Distress Syndrome*, version 1, 2018; https://www.ficm.ac.uk/sites/default/files/ficm_ics_ards_guideline_-_july_2018.pdf.

Hall JP, Kress JP. The burden of functional recovery from ARDS. *N Engl J Med* 2011; 364:1360–1366.

Herridge MS, Tansey CM, Matté A et al. Functional disability 5 years after acute respiratory distress syndrome. *N Engl J Med* 2011; 364:1293–1304.

Kress JP, Hall JB. ICU-acquired weakness and recovery from critical illness. *N Engl J Med* 2014; 370:1626–1635.

Sud S, Sud M, Friedrich JP. High-frequency oscillation in patients with acute lung injury and acute respiratory distress syndrome (ARDS): systematic review and meta-analysis. *BMJ* 2010; 340:C2327.

Young D, Lamb S, Shah S et al. High-frequency oscillation for acute respiratory distress syndrome. *N Engl J Med* 2013; 368:806–813.

ACUTE KIDNEY INJURY

Acute kidney injury (AKI) is a common and serious complication of critical illness, and is strongly associated with increased morbidity and mortality. The presence and severity of AKI are now formally classified by relative increases in serum creatinine and/or a persistent reduction in urine output (see **Box 36.30**).

The importance of preventing renal injury with rapid and effective resuscitation, the avoidance of nephrotoxic drugs (especially non-steroidal anti-inflammatory drugs, NSAIDs), and control of infection cannot be overemphasized. While shock and sepsis are the most common causes of AKI in the critically ill, causes requiring specific treatment should be excluded, especially urinary tract obstruction and acute intrinsic renal disease such as rapidly progressive glomerulonephritis (see p. 1360).

Acutely, oliguria often accompanies shock and renal hypoperfusion, and should prompt attempts to optimize cardiovascular function by expanding the circulating volume and restoring blood pressure; restoration of urine output is a good indicator of successful resuscitation. However, when AKI is established, urine output is often normal or high due to impaired concentrating capacity, so that development of oliguria then implies almost complete loss of renal function; in this case, continued fluid resuscitation will be ineffective and potentially harmful.

There is no evidence to support specific pharmacological interventions to prevent or treat AKI; in particular, low-dose dopamine is ineffective for preventing or reversing renal impairment in sepsis (see p. 1390). Thus, treatment of those developing or at risk of AKI should focus on prompt resuscitation with fluid and/or vasopressor therapy, as well as treatment of the underlying causes of shock and sepsis. If these measures fail to reverse oliguria, loop diuretics such as furosemide (see p. 178) may be used to treat or prevent fluid overload. However, there is no evidence that diuretics alter the clinical course of AKI, and renal replacement therapy (RRT) should not be delayed if indicated.

In AKI, RRT is indicated for refractory fluid overload, major electrolyte disturbances (especially hyperkalaemia), severe acidosis and, less often, uraemia. There is no evidence to support commencement of RRT for less severe AKI in the absence of these indications. Continuous renal replacement therapy (RRT, see p. 1398) is associated with greater haemodynamic stability and better control of fluid balance than intermittent haemodialysis, while use of peritoneal dialysis is unsatisfactory in critically ill patients (although this may be an option in resource-limited environments). Thus, continuous RRT is now the preferred method of renal support in the critically ill.

In critical illness complicated by AKI, if the underlying problems resolve, renal function usually recovers over a period of a few days to several weeks. However, there is good evidence to suggest that, after recovery, subtle defects in renal function persist, so that patients requiring RRT in the ICU have a significantly increased risk of developing chronic kidney disease in the months and years after critical illness.

Further reading

Bellomo R, Kellum JA, Ronco C. Acute kidney injury. *Lancet* 2012; 380:756–766.
RENAL Replacement Therapy Study Investigators. Intensity of continuous renal-replacement therapy in critically ill patients. *N Engl J Med* 2009; 361:1627–1638.

NEUROCRITICAL CARE

Physiology

Neurones are particularly susceptible to acute ischaemic/hypoxic insults, as they have very limited capacity for anaerobic metabolism and are irreversibly lost when blood flow is restricted for as little as 3–8 minutes.

The intracranial contents – brain parenchyma, blood and CSF – are contained in the rigid skull vault. Intracranial pressure (ICP, pressure within the skull) is approximately 7–15 mmHg in a resting, supine adult. Changes in intra-abdominal and intrathoracic pressures, such as occur during coughing or a Valsalva manoeuvre, may result in transient increases in ICP that are of no consequence. The **Monro–Kellie doctrine** states that, because the intracranial volume is fixed, any increase in the volume of one of the intracranial constituents must be compensated by a decrease in volume of the others. As space-occupying lesions expand or brain tissue swells, the rise in ICP is limited by displacement of CSF and venous blood from the intracranial compartment. Once these compensatory mechanisms are exhausted, further increases in intracranial volume cause exponentially greater increases in ICP (**Fig. 10.31**).

In health, **autoregulation** maintains constant cerebral blood flow over a range of blood pressures. However, these mechanisms are lost following significant intracranial injury, and cerebral blood flow then becomes directly dependent on cerebral perfusion pressure (CPP). CPP is calculated as the MAP minus the ICP. Occasionally, a very high CVP, greater than the ICP, will also reduce CPP (**Fig. 10.32**).

Clinical features and investigations

The causes of coma are listed in **Box 26.29**. Conscious level should be documented regularly. The Glasgow Coma Scale (GCS) score (**Box 26.28**) is widely used as a semi-quantitative, yet crude, means of gauging the level of consciousness. Assessment of the airway is of particular importance. Patients with airway obstruction due to lax oropharyngeal musculature should be managed as discussed on page 220. Patients without a cough or gag reflex may need to be intubated in order to protect the airway. Pupillary size and reactivity is a crucial part of the assessment. A unilaterally dilated pupil that reacts sluggishly or not at all is frequently a sign of increasing ICP. This is caused by compression of the IIIrd cranial nerve by herniating brain; if untreated, it can be rapidly fatal. Immediate measures to decrease ICP (see **Box 10.18**) are required while a CT scan of the brain is obtained. In some situations, patients may be taken directly to the operating theatre in order to alleviate the raised ICP and to remove expanding space-occupying lesions such as a haematoma. Small or pinpoint pupils

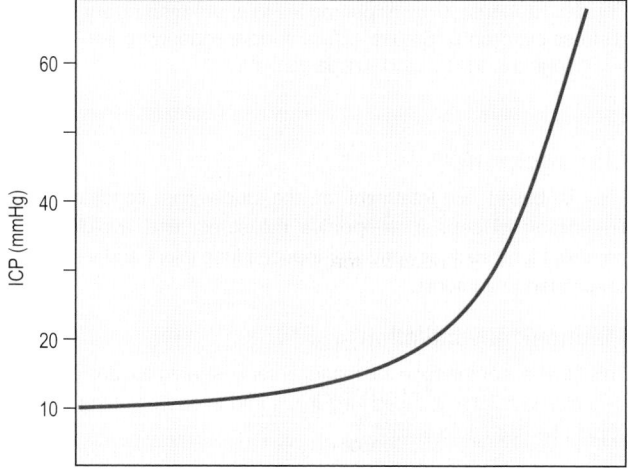

Fig. 10.31 Intracranial compliance curve. ICP, intracranial pressure. *(From Hinds CJ, Watson JD. Intensive Care: A Concise Handbook, 3rd edn. Edinburgh: Saunders; 2008, with permission.)*

may be a sign of mid-brain injury or opioid overdose. New focal neurological signs should be sought, such as cranial nerve palsies, limb weakness or hemiparesis. Seizures should be recognized and treated appropriately (see p. 856).

Monitoring

Regular clinical assessments by the bedside nurse are essential, including GCS score and pupillary size and reaction to light at least every hour. Neurological assessments are inevitably limited

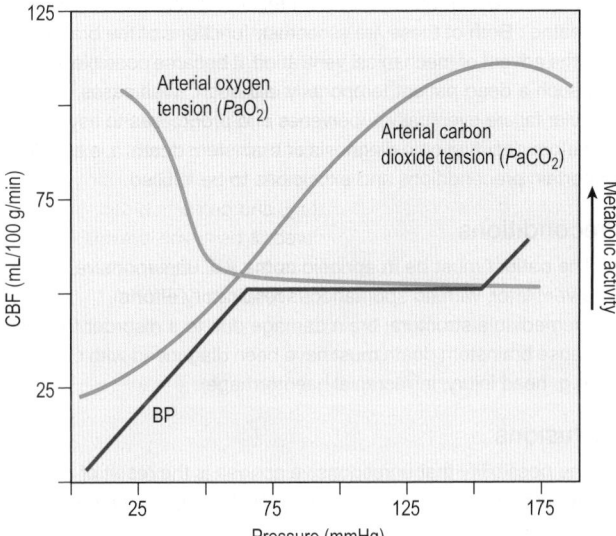

Fig. 10.32 Factors influencing cerebral blood flow (CBF). BP, mean arterial blood pressure.

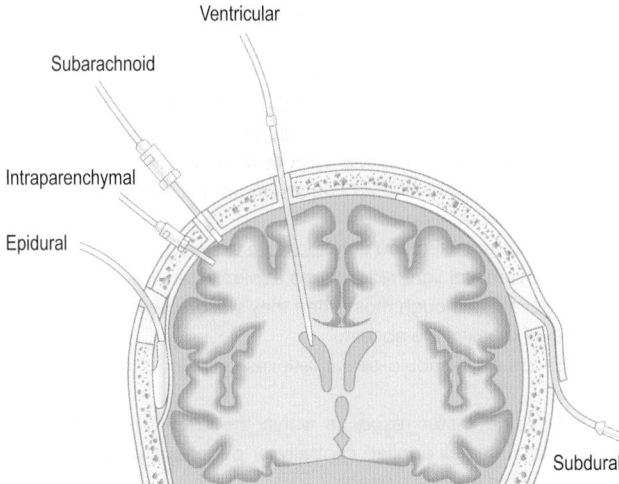

Fig. 10.33 Methods for measuring intracranial pressure.

in patients requiring sedation and mechanical ventilation. In these individuals, invasive monitoring of ICP may be necessary.

Invasive ICP monitoring devices may be extradural, subdural, subarachnoid, intraparenchymal or intraventricular (**Fig. 10.33**). The external ventricular drain (EVD) is the most difficult to insert, particularly when increased ICP causes the ventricles to collapse. EVDs are normally placed through the non-dominant (usually right) hemisphere into the lateral ventricle in the operating theatre. Their main advantage over the other monitoring devices is that they can also be used to treat raised ICP by draining CSF from the ventricular system. They are more prone to infection, however.

Multi-electrode electroencephalography (EEG) monitors give both a waveform and an analogue display that can help in the diagnosis of non-convulsive seizures and are also useful in monitoring the depth of sedation.

Oximeter-tipped catheters can be placed via the internal jugular vein and advanced in a cranial direction to lie in the jugular bulb just external to the skull. These 'jugular bulb oximetry' catheters monitor venous saturation in blood leaving the brain and give an indication of the balance between cerebral oxygen supply and demand. Measurements can be interpreted similarly to the mixed venous oxygen content (see p. 208).

Cerebral oximetry uses near-infrared spectroscopy (NIRS) technology to estimate the oxygenation of a small portion of the cerebral cortex. Adhesive pads that both emit and capture near-infrared light waves are placed over the frontal cortex. Cerebral oximetry can provide an early warning of decreased cerebral oxygen delivery.

Management

Little can be done to reverse the immediate primary brain injury and irreversible loss of neurones that occur as a direct consequence of intracerebral haemorrhage, infarct or traumatic brain injury. ICU care is focused on minimizing secondary brain injury (**Box 10.18**). This commonly occurs as a result of increases in ICP and consequent decreases in CPP. Cerebral oedema, expanding mass lesions (e.g. haemorrhage), prolonged seizure activity and hypercarbia (which causes cerebral vasodilation) are all examples of mechanisms leading to secondary injury. Neurocritical care has therefore focused on monitoring ICP and maintaining CPP. The Brain Trauma Foundation (BTF) guidelines state that an ICP of 22 mmHg or less and a CPP of between 60 and 70 mmHg should be the aim, with vasopressors and fluid given as required in conjunction with supportive care; the latter should include airway protection, maintenance of normocarbia, reduction of the risk of nosocomial infections and prevention of thromboembolic complications.

Further reading

http://www.braintrauma.org *Brain Trauma Foundation.*

---

i **Box 10.18 Measures to control raised intracranial pressure and prevent secondary brain injury**

- Control/restoration of blood pressure
- Control of intracranial pressure:
  - Reduction of intracranial blood volume
  - Mechanical ventilation
  - Sedation
  - Unobstructed venous drainage
  - Control of cerebral oedema

- Osmotic diuretics (e.g. mannitol)
- Loop diuretic (e.g. furosemide)
- Other measures:
  - Removal of cerebrospinal fluid via intraventricular catheter
  - Decompressive craniectomy
  - Excision of brain tissue
- Control of seizure activity

OUTCOMES

Withholding and withdrawing treatment

(See also Ch. 7.)

For many critically ill patients, intensive care is undoubtedly life-saving and resumption of a normal lifestyle is to be expected. It is also widely accepted that the elective admission of high-risk patients into an ICU or HDU, particularly in the immediate post-operative period, can minimize morbidity and mortality and lower costs, as well as reducing the demands on medical and nursing personnel on general wards. In the most seriously ill patients, however, mortality rates are high, and a significant number die soon after discharge from the ICU. Mortality rates are particularly high in those who require readmission to intensive care. Moreover, patients surviving a prolonged ICU admission often do not regain their pre-morbid functional status, and longer-term mortality rates (for at least 10 years post discharge) remain higher than in a general population matched for age and illness severity.

Inappropriate use of intensive care facilities has other implications. The patient may experience unnecessary suffering and loss of dignity, while relatives may also have to endure considerable emotional pressures. In some cases treatment may simply prolong the process of dying, and in others the risks of interventions outweigh the potential benefits. Lastly, intensive care is expensive, particularly for those with the worst prognosis, and resources are limited.

To ensure both a humane approach to the management of critically ill patients and the appropriate use of limited resources, it is necessary to:

- avoid admitting patients who cannot benefit from intensive care
- limit further aggressive therapy when the prognosis is clearly hopeless.

Such decisions are extremely difficult; each case is assessed individually, taking into account previous health and quality of life, the patient's expressed wishes, the primary diagnosis, medium- and long-term prognosis of the underlying condition, and survivability of the acute illness. Age alone should not be the sole consideration. When in doubt, active measures should continue but with regular review in light of response to treatment and any other changes.

Decisions to limit therapy, not to resuscitate or to withdraw treatment should be made jointly by the ICU medical staff, the primary physician or surgeon, nursing staff and, if possible, the patient, normally in consultation with the patient's family. Limitation of active treatment is *not* the cessation of medical or nursing care; rather, a caring approach must be adopted to ensure a dignified death, free of pain and distress, with support for family and friends (see p. 148).

Scoring systems

A variety of scoring systems have been developed to evaluate the severity of critical illness. Some include an assessment of the patient's previous state of health and the severity of the acute disturbance of physiological function (***acute physiology, age, chronic health evaluation***, or ***APACHE***; and the ***simplified acute physiology score***, or ***SAPS***). Other systems have been designed for particular categories of patient (e.g. the Injury Severity Score (ISS) for trauma victims).

The APACHE and SAPS scores are widely applicable and have been extensively validated. They can accurately quantify the severity of illness and predict the overall mortality for large groups of critically ill patients, and are therefore useful for defining the 'case mix' of patients when auditing a unit's clinical activity, for comparing results nationally or internationally, and for characterizing groups of patients in clinical studies. Although the APACHE and SAPS methodologies can also estimate mortality risk, no scoring system has yet been devised that can predict with certainty the outcome in an individual patient. They must not, therefore, be used in isolation as a basis for limiting or discontinuing treatment.

Brain death and organ donation

Traditionally, death is thought of as cessation of breathing and the heartbeat. Brain death means 'the irreversible loss of the capacity for consciousness combined with the irreversible loss of the capacity to breathe'. Both of these are essentially functions of the brainstem. With the advent of mechanical ventilation, it became possible to support such a dead patient temporarily, although, in all cases, cardiovascular failure eventually supervenes and progresses to asystole.

Before deciding on a diagnosis of brainstem death, it is essential for certain preconditions and exclusions to be fulfilled.

Preconditions

- The patient must be in apnoeic coma (i.e. unresponsive and on a ventilator, with no spontaneous respiratory efforts).
- Irremediable structural brain damage due to a disorder that can cause brainstem death must have been diagnosed with certainty (e.g. head injury, intracranial haemorrhage).

Exclusions

- The possibility that unresponsive apnoea is the result of poisoning, sedative drugs or neuromuscular blocking agents must be excluded.
- Hypothermia must be excluded as a cause of coma (core temperature >34°C).
- There must be no significant circulatory, metabolic or endocrine disturbance that could produce or contribute to coma or cause it to persist (including acid–base, electrolyte and glucose abnormalities).

Diagnostic tests for the confirmation of brainstem death

All brainstem reflexes are absent in brainstem death.

The following tests should not be performed in the presence of seizures or abnormal postures.

- The pupils are fixed and unresponsive to bright light. Both direct and consensual light reflexes are absent. The size of the pupils is irrelevant, although most often they will be dilated.
- Corneal reflexes are absent.
- There are no vestibulo-ocular reflexes on caloric testing (see p. 816).
- There is no motor response within the cranial nerve territory to painful stimuli applied centrally or peripherally. Spinal reflex movements may be present.
- There is no gag or cough reflex in response to pharyngeal, laryngeal or tracheal stimulation.
- Spontaneous respiration is absent. The patient should be ventilated with 100% O_2 for 10 minutes and then temporarily disconnected from the ventilator for 5 minutes. Oxygenation is maintained by insufflation with 100% oxygen via the endotracheal tube. The patient is observed for any signs of spontaneous respiratory efforts. A blood gas sample should be obtained during this period to ensure that the P_aCO_2 is sufficiently high to stimulate spontaneous respiration (starting P_aCO_2 ≥6.0 kPa and pH <7.4, with P_aCO_2 rise of >0.5 kPa after 5 minutes).

The examination should be performed and repeated by two senior doctors.

In the UK, it is not considered necessary to perform confirmatory tests, such as EEG or carotid and vertebral angiography. The primary purpose of establishing a diagnosis of brainstem death is to demonstrate beyond doubt that ongoing treatment is futile. In many jurisdictions, brainstem death is legally equivalent to cardiac death.

In suitable cases, and provided the assent of relatives has been obtained (easier if the patient is a registered organ donor), the organs of those in whom brainstem death has been established may be retrieved while the heart is still beating and be used for transplantation.

Organ donation may be possible in situations where ongoing life-sustaining treatment is deemed futile and a decision is reached in conjunction with the family (and, in rare circumstances, the patient) to withdraw treatments such as invasive ventilation and inotropes that are simply delaying an inevitable death. If the patient and family wish to consider organ donation, then withdrawal of life-sustaining therapies usually occurs in a planned fashion and often in the operating department suite. If death occurs relatively quickly, then organ retrieval may proceed immediately following cardiac death.

Both of these situations require rapport and trust to be established with the family. In the UK, there are separate teams of nurse specialists to help the families through these very difficult situations and coordinate organ retrieval. A local and regional transplant coordinator can help with the process, as well as providing information, training and advice about organ donation. The medical teams involved in the ICU care of the patient and those involved in the organ retrieval process must remain completely independent.

Further reading

Academy of Royal Medical Colleges. *A Code of Practice for the Diagnosis and Confirmation of Death*. London: Academy of Royal Medical Colleges; 2008.
Curtis JR, Vincent JL. Ethics and end of life care for adults in the intensive care unit. *Lancet* 2010; 376:1347–1353.
Finfer S, Vincent JL. Dying with dignity in the intensive care unit. *N Engl J Med* 2014; 370:2506–2514.

Bibliography

Bersten AD, Soni N. Oh's Intensive Care Manual, 7th edn. Oxford: Butterworth–Heinemann; 2014.

Significant websites

http://www.esicm.org *European Society of Intensive Care Medicine*.
http://www.ficm.ac.uk *Faculty of Intensive Care Medicine*.
http://www.icnarc.org *Intensive Care National Audit & Research Centre*.
http://www.ics.ac.uk *UK Intensive Care Society*.
http://www.sccm.org/Research *Society of Critical Care Medicine guidelines*.

11 Surgery

Ajit Abraham

CORE SKILLS AND KNOWLEDGE

Around 313 million surgical procedures are carried out worldwide each year, though fewer than 6% of these procedures are performed in low- and low-middle income countries. Although local patterns vary, general surgeons tend to focus on surgical problems of the intra-abdominal organs, and typically subspecialize within fields such as colorectal, hepatobiliary, upper gastrointestinal or trauma surgery. Other major surgical specialties include orthopaedic, cardiothoracic, vascular, plastic and paediatric surgery, neurosurgery and urology.

Elective surgery is discussed and planned with patients in the outpatient setting and often carried out as a day-case procedure, with only major operations requiring an inpatient stay. Most general surgeons will participate in on-call work, in which patients presenting to hospital with surgical problems are admitted and treated on surgical wards, sometimes undergoing emergency surgery.

Keys skills to learn in surgery include:

- appreciating the benefits and risks of operative management compared with medical management in a range of conditions, and the patient factors that make different approaches appropriate in different situations
- understanding the physiological responses to surgery, and knowing how to instigate the appropriate anaesthetic and perioperative management to prevent harm
- recognizing common postoperative complications and understanding how to prevent and treat them.

Opportunities for learning surgery include observing operations and 'scrubbing in' to assist, attending surgical outpatient clinics to observe surgery being discussed with patients, pre-assessing patients on surgical day-stay units who are due to undergo elective surgery, and reviewing the role of surgical versus conservative management in patients on surgical assessment units who have presented with a range of acute surgical problems.

CLINICAL SKILLS FOR SURGERY

History

A good history is the bedrock of diagnosis in the surgical patient, and along with a focused, diagnostic clinical examination, shapes and guides the subsequent investigations and management (**Box 11.1**).

Examination

The general examination and a review of vital signs and systems are just as they are for any medical patient. However, the typical surgical patient often presents with a swelling or lump that benefits from a more surgical approach to examination, based on the time-tested methods of *inspection*, *palpation*, *percussion* and *auscultation* (**Box 11.2**).

Box 11.1 Key elements in surgical history-taking

History of the presenting complaint
- A clear account of each problem experienced by the patient, including its duration
- The sequence of events leading up to the present illness or injury

Past medical and drug history
- Other medical problems
- Previous operations, including any reaction to anaesthesia
- Use of antiplatelet or anticoagulant medication

- Last menstrual period (LMP), always considering ectopic pregnancy in women of childbearing age

Fitness for surgery
- Time of last meal
- Social circumstances of patient, including baseline functional status:
  – How far can the patient walk along the flat on a good day?
  – Can they climb a flight of stairs?

 Box 11.2 The surgical approach to examining a swelling or lump

LOOK (observe)
- Site or location of the lump
- Size, shape and number of lumps
- Surface and colour
- Prominent veins
- Visible expansive or transmitted pulsations
- Previous scars
- Cough impulse
- Pressure or infiltrative effects, including vascular or nerve involvement:
  – Oedema
  – Ischaemia
  – Muscular atrophy
- Lymph node enlargement

FEEL (palpate and percuss)
Always ask if the lump is painful BEFORE gently seeking to elicit tenderness!
- Consistency
- Fluctuation (suggests fluid content)

- Pulsations, thrills and compressibility (suggests vascular lesions)
- Cough impulse and reducibility (in possible hernias)
- Relationship/fixity of the lump to adjacent structures, including skin, muscle and bone
- Percuss for tympanic, resonant or dull notes
- Palpate the relevant draining lymph node groups

LISTEN (auscultate)
Auscultate over the lump or swelling for peristaltic sounds, bruits and murmurs
- High-pitched tinkling of trapped bowel suggests an obstructed hernia
- Sluggish or absent peristaltic sounds suggest paralytic ileus or generalized peritonitis
- Bruits and murmurs are suggestive of arteriovenous fistulae, arterial stenosis or aneurysms

Box 11.3 Preoperative investigation

Establishing the diagnosis
- Sometimes this is possible with simple or more complex imaging techniques, e.g. ultrasound, magnetic resonance imaging (MRI) or positron emission tomography (PET)
- Diagnostic angiography is minimally invasive and allows visualization of vascular pathology
- Often tissue samples are required for histological diagnosis: these may be obtained by a range of more or less invasive tests, including endoscopy, endoscopic retrograde cholangiopancreatography (ERCP), endoscopic ultrasound (EUS), fine needle aspiration (FNA) and Trucut core biopsy

Clarifying anatomy and guiding surgical approach
- Cross-sectional imaging, e.g. contrast-enhanced CT scanning allows excellent visualization of tissue pathology and is used to plan operative approaches, e.g. by assessing whether a tumour is resectable

Determining the fitness of the patient
- A basic surgical preoperative work-up could include a full blood count, serum creatinine and electrolytes, liver function tests, clotting profile, group and save/crossmatch anticipating possible transfusion requirements and urine testing, as well as electrocardiography (ECG) and chest X-ray
- Older people, or those with pre-existing co-morbidities, may also require echocardiography, cardiac stress tests, pulmonary function tests and cardiopulmonary exercise testing (CPET), to allow preoperative optimization of patients

Investigations

A thorough surgical history and examination are routinely supported by a variety of investigations and interventions performed for different purposes (**Box 11.3**).

Surgical pathology and nomenclature

These are described in (**Box 11.4**).

i   **Box 11.4** Surgical nomenclature

Abscess
- A collection of pus

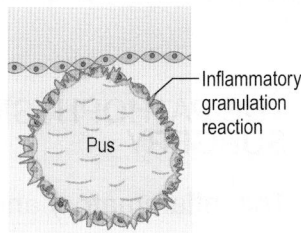

Pus — Inflammatory granulation reaction

Cyst
- A collection of fluid lined by epithelium
- May be complicated by bleeding, infection, rupture, local pressure effects and sometimes malignant change, e.g. thyroid, ovarian and liver cysts
- Pancreatic pseudocysts are collections of inflammatory pancreatic fluid lined by granulation tissue; they can cause all of the complications listed except malignancy, as a lining epithelium is absent

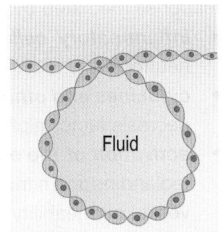

Fluid

Sinus
- A blind-ending tract lined by epithelium
- Pilonidal sinuses, for example, are typically found in the internatal cleft and are prone to infection and abscess formation

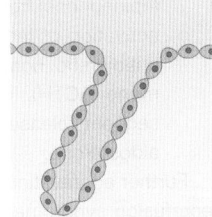

Obstruction
- Blockage or occlusion of a hollow viscus or structure
- Obstruction can occur:
  - From within the lumen of any tubular structure, e.g. gallstones in the common bile duct causing jaundice, or a ureteric stone causing renal colic
  - From the wall or lining epithelium of a structure, e.g. an inflammatory stricture of the terminal ileum in Crohn's disease, or malignant adenocarcinoma of the colon
  - From extrinsic pressure, e.g. a massive ovarian cyst causing pelvic vein congestion and bowel obstruction

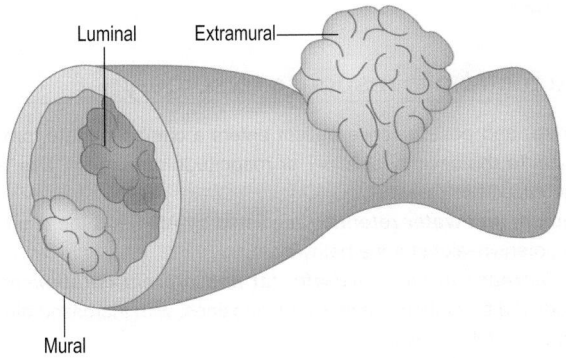

Luminal   Extramural

Mural

Fistula
- An abnormal communication between two epithelial surfaces
- Fistulae may be formed due to embryological, infective, inflammatory, traumatic and malignant processes; they persist because of undrained sepsis, distal obstruction, malignancy, high-volume throughput, epithelialization of the fistula tract, and presence of a foreign body
- They can heal with careful attention to fluid and electrolyte balance, nutrition, protection of surfaces, and optimally timed surgery to drain all pus, excise malignancy when feasible, remove foreign bodies and relieve obstruction
- Examples of intentionally permanent fistulae include arteriovenous fistulae, colostomies and ileostomies

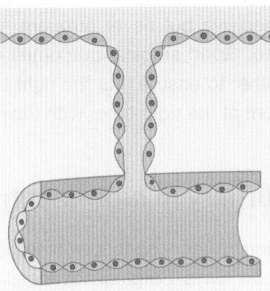

Hernia
- An abnormal protrusion of part or all of a viscus through a defect in the wall of its containing cavity

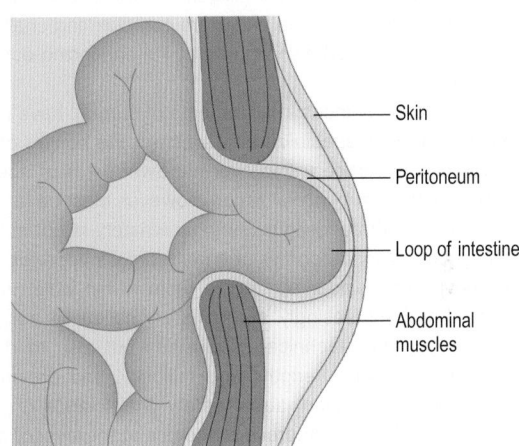

Skin

Peritoneum

Loop of intestine

Abdominal muscles

Tumour
- Typically, a solid lump arising as a consequence of a neoplastic process
- Benign tumours may cause pain, bleeding, infection and obstruction
- Malignant tumours may also invade locally and metastasize

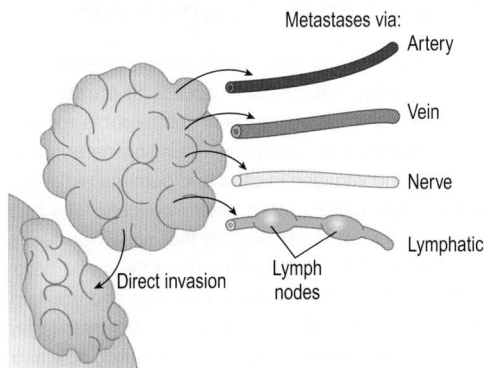

Metastases via:
Artery

Vein

Nerve

Lymphatic

Direct invasion   Lymph nodes

INTRODUCTION

Surgery is the branch of medicine that employs manual techniques to treat injury, deformity and disease. The word 'surgery' derives from the Greek *kheirourgia*, meaning 'labour of the hands'. Diseased tissue or organs are removed, repaired, manipulated or replaced, and more so than anywhere else in medicine, patients commit their lives to surgeons' hands, consenting to bodily incursion and placing their trust in the surgeon's technical skills.

Performing an operation demands a particular mix of knowledge and skills: deep knowledge of anatomy, a profound respect for tissues, extreme task absorption, and the courage and confidence to be decisive but never arrogant – to know when to cut and when not to. Good surgical outcomes depend on many people working together to ensure that the right operation is performed in the right patient at the right time, with the right team and the right tools.

Surgery in high-income countries

Modern surgery continues to improve, innovate and evolve in exciting new ways. Surgical advances over the last 150 years have been facilitated by breakthroughs in medical science and technology: safe anaesthesia, aseptic technique and antibiotic therapy, cross-sectional imaging, minimal-access surgical instruments, endoscopy and robotics, three-dimensional printing, virtual and augmented reality simulation, and artificial intelligence. Where healthcare systems are well resourced, more and more complex and challenging operations can be undertaken with safer, life-enhancing outcomes for patients.

Technological advances in all aspects of surgery have inevitably required surgical specialization to permit the honing of technical skills and expertise within ever narrower fields of specialist focus. This move to subspecialization, however, must be tempered by the realization that individual surgical mastery is not sufficient to achieve exemplary outcomes of care. Success depends on the effectiveness of the wider healthcare team within which surgery is practised and, increasingly, surgeons are called on not just to refine their individual technical capabilities but also to develop insight into their own strengths and fallibility, and dependence on others. They must learn about safety, the science of clinical improvement and how to improve outcomes at the level of healthcare systems. They must provide clinical leadership and work effectively in multidisciplinary teams, supporting and empowering each team member to achieve the best possible outcomes for patients and their families.

Global provision of surgical care

The World Health Organization (WHO) estimates that 5 billion of the global population currently lack access to timely, safe and effective surgical care, which remains unaffordable for up to 90% of people in low-income countries. Changing demographics, ageing populations and variation in need and demand make access to safe surgery a major global public health concern. The health inequity and the global burden of suffering that arise from untreated surgical conditions in less wealthy regions of the world have substantial negative impacts on human health, welfare and economic development. The surgical challenge of the 21st century is to provide surgical healthcare for all that is high-quality, timely, safe and affordable.

Further reading

Alkire BC, Raykar NP, Shrime MG et al. Global access to surgical care: a modelling study. *Lancet Glob Health* 2015; 3:e316–323.
World Alliance for Patient Safety. *The Second Global Patient Safety Challenge: Safe surgery saves lives*. Geneva: World Health Organization; 2008.

THE PATHOPHYSIOLOGY OF SURGERY

The inflammatory and stress response

A major operation constitutes a significant injury to the body. The metabolic response is characterized by an acute inflammatory response mediated by:

- *inflammatory cells*, including macrophages, monocytes and neutrophils
- *cytokines and other inflammatory mediators*, such as tumour necrosis factor-alpha (TNF-α) and various interleukins
- *activation of the endothelium* with production of kinins, prostaglandins and nitric oxide, leading to vasodilation and increased vessel permeability
- *release of stress hormones*, mediated primarily via:
  - the sympathetic nervous system, through noradrenaline (norepinephrine) from sympathetic nerve endings and adrenaline (epinephrine) from the adrenal glands
  - activation of the hypothalamic–pituitary axis with release of antidiuretic hormone (ADH) and adrenocorticotrophic hormone (ACTH), leading to direct effects, as well as the subsequent release of other hormones such as glucagon and aldosterone.

Further aggravation of the injury may occur through ischaemia–reperfusion syndrome or superadded bacterial infection, which in turn may cause sepsis (see **Chapter 8**).

Fluid balance in surgical conditions

Significant fluid losses may result from surgery and trauma, and further complicate the physiological challenge to body homeostasis. These losses include:

- *loss of blood* (haemorrhage)
- *direct loss of body fluids* (through vomiting, diarrhoea, sweating, and exudative losses in drains and catheters)
- *loss of fluid that is sequestered or shifted into 'third spaces'*, often as a result of increased capillary permeability due to the acute inflammatory response.

For example, in patients with bowel obstruction, large volumes of fluid can rapidly be secreted into the gut, causing intravascular hypovolaemia.

The metabolic response to surgery

The intra- and postoperative patient enters a catabolic state, proportional to the severity of injury or magnitude of surgery. This is characterized by:

- *sodium and water retention* mediated by ADH and the renin–angiotensin–aldosterone pathway
- *an increase in carbohydrate, fat and protein catabolism*, mediated by catecholamines and cytokines, with increased glucose and fat turnover

- *the breakdown of adipose tissue and catabolism of skeletal muscle proteins* to provide amino acids for both gluconeogenesis and acute-phase proteins by the liver
- *hypercoagulopathy*, typically in the first 24–48 hours after surgery and mediated via endothelial injury and activation, which increases the risk of thromboembolism.

Wound healing

Stages of healing

In simple terms, the body's response to a breach in the integrity of an internal or external body surface follows three phases (**Fig. 11.1**).

Haemostatic phase

Vasoconstriction restricts rapid blood loss and a primary platelet plug forms. Secondary platelet/fibrin clot formation through activation of the coagulation pathway stops bleeding and plugs the breach in surface integrity within minutes.

Inflammatory phase

An inflammatory response is mediated primarily by scavenger macrophages and neutrophils, which swarm around the wound and release cytokines with 12–48 hours of injury. This causes the classic features of inflammation, including redness (*rubor*), heat (*calor*), swelling (*tumor*) and pain (*dolor*), with consequent restriction of function (*functio laesa*).

Resolution phase

Cytokines, including VEGF, PDGF and EGF, stimulate formation of granulation tissue from underlying mesoderm-derived connective tissue at the base of the wound. A matrix of new capillary networks is formed that nourishes and supports migratory myo-fibroblasts, which enable physiological wound contraction, collagen deposition and scar formation. Concurrent re-epithelialization occurs from the edges of the wound by epithelial cells derived from ectoderm or endoderm. The epithelium grows over the underlying granulation tissue scaffold and this continues until epithelial cover is established and the breach repaired.

Surgical closure

Surgical skin closure may be by primary, delayed primary and secondary intention, depending on the type of wound encountered. Closure by primary intention produces the best aesthetic and functional outcomes for the patient and is appropriate for most clean wounds (such as those made during an operation); closure by secondary intention or delayed primary intention is appropriate where a wound is contaminated or irregular, or where there is insufficient surrounding skin to allow closure by primary intention (**Fig. 11.2**).

Further reading

Doherty M, Buggy DJ. Intraoperative fluids: how much is too much? *Br J Anaesth* 2012; 109:69–79.
Finnerty CC, Mabvuure NT, Ali A et al. The surgically induced stress response. *J Parenter Enteral Nutr* 2013; 37(5 Suppl):21S–29S.

MANAGEMENT OF THE PERIOPERATIVE PATIENT

A systematic and evidence-based approach to the perioperative care of surgical patients has been brought together by international collaborators in Enhanced Recovery After Surgery (ERAS) protocols. These highlight the role of basic interventions before, during and after surgery that have been shown to improve patient outcomes. Implementation of these protocols has been shown to reduce complication rates, length of stay and re-admission rates after surgery, as well as the costs of treatment.

Fluid and electrolyte balance

All patients undergoing surgery require careful attention to their fluid and electrolyte balance (see Ch. 9). Appropriate management requires:

- *relevant maintenance fluids* for patients who are 'nil by mouth' ahead of surgical procedures
- *prediction of likely shifts in body fluids* in response to the particular disease process, e.g. where 'third space' fluid sequestration (see earlier) can be predicted to occur in conditions such as

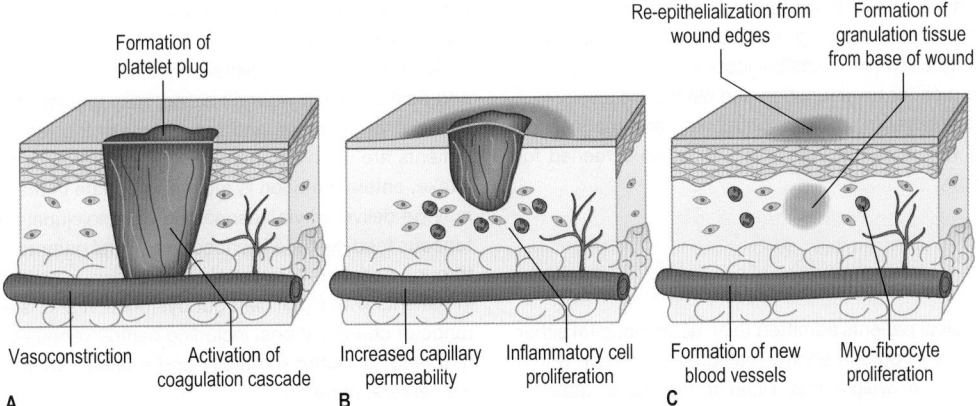

Formation of platelet plug

Re-epithelialization from wound edges

Formation of granulation tissue from base of wound

Vasoconstriction   Activation of coagulation cascade

Increased capillary permeability   Inflammatory cell proliferation

Formation of new blood vessels   Myo-fibrocyte proliferation

A   B   C

Fig. 11.1 The stages of wound healing. (A) Haemostatic phase with formation of a platelet plug followed by secondary platelet/fibrin scab. **(B)** Inflammatory phase with proliferation of macrophages and fibroblasts, leading to the classic features of inflammation. **(C)** Resolution phase with neovascularization, myo-fibrocyte activity, collagen deposition and scar formation from the base on the wound. Re-epithelialization occurs from the wound margins.

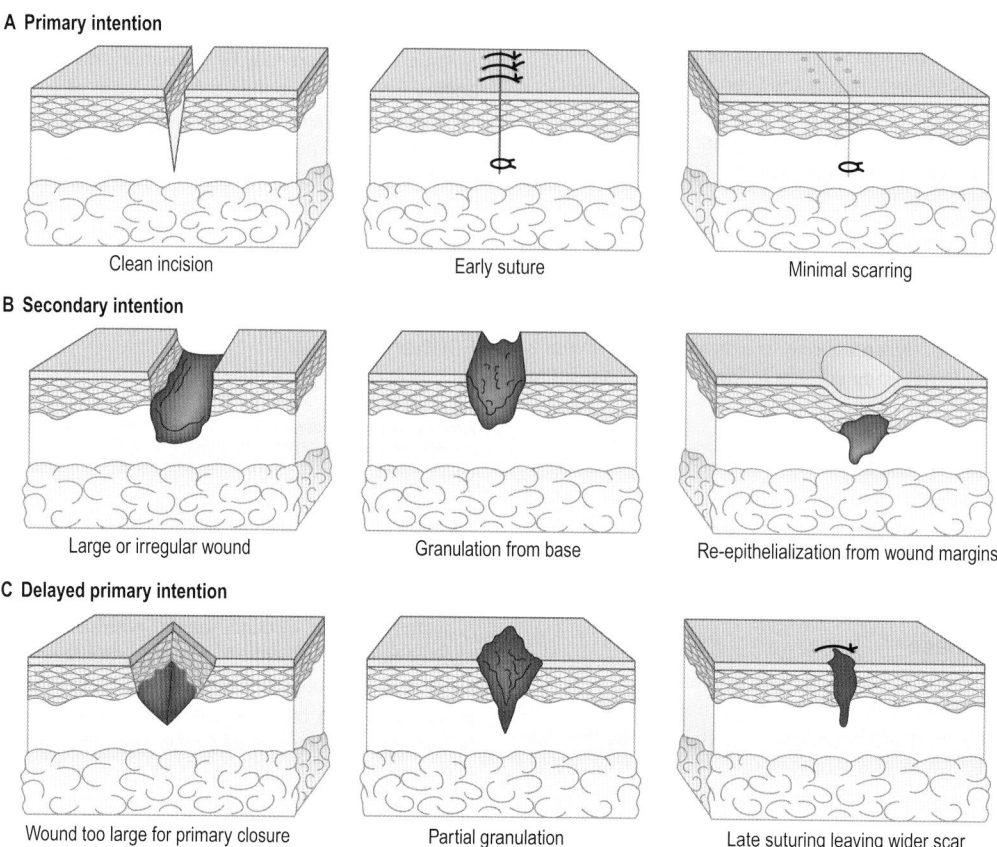

A Primary intention

Clean incision   Early suture   Minimal scarring

B Secondary intention

Large or irregular wound   Granulation from base   Re-epithelialization from wound margins

C Delayed primary intention

Wound too large for primary closure   Partial granulation   Late suturing leaving wider scar

Fig. 11.2 Wound closure techniques in surgery. (**A**) Closure by primary intention. (**B**) Closure by secondary intention. (**C**) Closure by delayed primary intention.

acute pancreatitis, paralytic ileus and bowel obstruction; where significant losses occur through surgical drains and high-output ileostomies; or where widespread skin injury, such as that after burns, can cause gross fluid losses

- **recognition of increased insensible fluid losses** in all febrile and catabolic patients
- **careful assessment of the patient's fluid status** through clinical examination (see p. 170)
- **review of fluid input and output charts**, noting urine output, and fluid losses from surgical drains and nasogastric tubes, and calculating cumulative fluid balance (total input minus total output), which should generally be positive by about 500 mL over a 24-hour period to allow for insensible losses
- **blood tests** to monitor renal function and electrolyte levels.

Imbalances of potassium, sodium, phosphate and magnesium concentration, as well acid–base disorders, must be screened for and treated promptly.

Nutrition

The majority of surgical patients admitted to an acute hospital either present with evidence of protein-energy malnutrition or leave with a degree of malnutrition or weight loss. Patients may have depleted reserves because of prior infection, anorexia, starvation or malignancy. They may then experience further exacerbation through poor nutrition in hospital related to restricted intake or to intestinal malabsorption from obstruction, inflammation or short gut syndrome; typically, they have increased catabolic rates.

Nutrition can be formally assessed using composite measures that include body mass index (BMI), skinfold (subcutaneous fat) thickness, skeletal muscle wasting, and biochemical parameters such as pre-albumin and 24-hour urinary urea excretion. In routine practice, the Malnutrition Universal Screening Tool (MUST) is widely used for screening inpatients at risk of malnutrition (see p. 1233).

Daily energy and protein requirements after surgery vary between 30 and 40 kcal/kg per day and 1 and 2 g/kg per day respectively, depending on whether the surgery is uncomplicated or complicated. Dietician and nutrition team input is invaluable in the care of the surgical patient.

Malnutrition has adverse effects on patients' mood, mobility and postoperative wound healing, may predispose to wound infection and pneumonia, and may increase the length of stay. Where patients are unable to meet their energy requirements through oral intake, enteral nutrition is most appropriate in the first instance and may be delivered via nasogastric or nasojejunal tubes, or a percutaneous feeding-tube jejunosotomy. Total parenteral nutrition (TPN), through peripheral or central venous lines, is typically indicated only in patients with significant gut dysfunction and is associated with a range of complications, including central venous catheter infection, that lead to higher morbidity and mortality than those associated with enteral nutrition.

The use of preoperative nutritional supplementation in the weeks prior to major surgery, and carbohydrate preloading the night before, delivered as part of the ERAS programme, have accounted for some of the significant improvements in surgical outcomes after major surgery in recent decades.

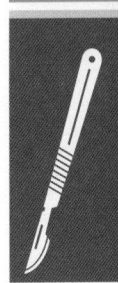

Coagulation, bleeding and transfusion

Massive blood transfusion is defined as the replacement of the equivalent of the circulating blood volume (4.5–6 L) by transfusion within 24 hours. It is not uncommonly required in major surgical emergencies, including major exsanguinating trauma, massive gastrointestinal bleeding and obstetric complications. Blood transfusion and its complications are covered comprehensively on pages 357–362.

Blood is a precious resource, dependent on the good will of voluntary donors, meaning that every effort must be made to avoid unnecessary transfusions. In the elective setting, triggers for transfusion include a haemoglobin level of <70 g/L (or 90 g/L in patients with cardiovascular disease). Transfusion in the context of a haemoglobin level >100 g/L is unjustified. Transfusion requirements may be reduced by:

- **preoperative use of erythropoietin and intravenous iron** to raise haemoglobin concentrations prior to elective surgery
- **preoperative blood donation** by healthy patients in advance of their own surgery, which can then be 'given back' as required during or after surgery
- **acute normovolaemic haemodilution**, where whole blood is removed from patients immediately prior to surgery and replaced with the same volume of other intravenous fluids; surgery then takes place with a normal blood volume containing a reduced red cell mass, and the stored blood is restored to the patient postoperatively
- **meticulous intraoperative haemostasis**, based on good surgical technique, use of diathermy and other energy devices, antifibrinolytics such as tranexamic acid and aprotinin, and fibrin sealants and other topical haemostats
- **intraoperative red cell salvage**, where medical devices operated by the surgeon retrieve, wash and then re-infuse a patient's own blood that has been lost during a procedure.

In the future, synthetic or biologically engineered blood substitutes may become available.

Trauma

The Advanced Trauma and Life Support (ATLS) guidelines provide a systematic approach to patients presenting after major trauma, and pay careful attention to the relative immediacy of threats to life. The 'ABCDE' approach used in critically ill patients elsewhere in medicine is adapted to trauma, recognizing the physiological consequences of different types of traumatic injury:

- The **airway** is assessed while also **protecting the cervical spine**, which may have been injured during the incident that led to the trauma.
- **Breathing** may be compromised by massive haemothorax or tension pneumothorax, requiring urgent chest drain insertion.
- **Circulatory compromise** from haemorrhagic shock or cardiac tamponade may occur, and **haemorrhage control** is undertaken before proceeding to further evaluation.
- **Disability** may occur from traumatic brain or spine injury.
- **Exposure and environmental control** is carried out to exclude other injuries not immediately obvious on initial assessment, and steps are taken to warm the patient and prevent hypothermia.

The metabolic response to injury is aggravated in major trauma by what has been termed an 'unholy triad' of **hypothermia**, **acidosis** and **coagulopathy**. Together, these can have devastating consequences for a rapidly exsanguinating, severely injured patient. While massive blood transfusion is often required, emergency surgery to achieve control of a catastrophic bleed and '**turn off the tap**' is an immediate and life-saving intervention. Studies have revealed that a degree of hypotension can be permitted until surgical control can be achieved, in order to limit the loss of blood. Excessive crystalloid resuscitation must be avoided in the severely injured patient and this may exacerbate coagulopathy; instead, use of antifibrinolytics such as tranexamic acid, and transfusion of packed cells, fresh frozen plasma, platelets and cryoprecipitate in 1:1:1 ratios, form part of major transfusion protocols in trauma.

Care has been revolutionized by a focus on early transfusion in the management of massive haemorrhage in trauma, in combination with damage control surgery. The availability of less invasive but equally effective radiological angio-embolization techniques has facilitated a more conservative approach to blunt trauma in particular. The outcomes for severely injured patients continue to improve.

The key principles of major trauma are based around the principle of **damage control** – operating early to avert life-threatening complications, leaving definitive surgical management until the patient is more stable (**Box 11.5**).

The critically ill surgical patient

Surgical patients may be critically ill at the time of presentation to hospital (e.g. if suffering from a life-threatening surgical emergency such as intestinal perforation, ruptured aortic aneurysm or necrotizing fasciitis), or may become critically ill as a consequence of major surgery or its complications.

Shock is characterized by inadequate tissue perfusion and oxygenation. If uncorrected, shock will lead to cellular dysfunction and organ damage, and eventually irreversible organ failure and death. Causes of shock in the surgical patient include haemorrhage or hypovolaemia, sepsis and anaphylaxis. Prompt recognition and resuscitation (see p. 203), along with early management with blood products or intravenous antibiotics, is critical.

Early transfer to the high-dependency/intensive care unit may improve outcomes. This allows intensive physiological monitoring (including intra-arterial blood pressure and invasive cardiac monitoring), as well as the institution of inotropic support using agents such as noradrenaline (norepinephrine), adrenaline (epinephrine) and vasopressin. Respiratory support, including artificial ventilation and renal replacement therapy (haemofiltration), may be required to help patients survive critical illness, and often high-risk individuals are moved directly to critical care units for intensive monitoring and treatment directly after major surgery.

⊕ Box 11.5 Key principles of treatment for major trauma

- **Haemorrhage control** by surgical or radiological intervention, combined with rapid use of appropriate blood products and antifibrinolytics
- **Elimination of contamination** by thorough washout of wounds and repair of perforated gut
- **Limited surgery** initially, doing only what is necessary to achieve the objectives above, while seeking to limit operative duration
- **Temporary abdominal closure** or **laparostomy**, where the abdominal cavity is left open and protected using a vacuum device, in order to reduce the risk of abdominal compartment syndrome and allow easy access for repeat surgery

Cancer

Cancer is a pathological condition that is characterized by the proliferation of neoplastic cells, which display unregulated growth and resistance to programmed cell death (see also Ch. 6). Cancers can directly invade adjoining organs and tissues, or may metastasize. Metastasis occurs in one of several ways:

- via lymphatics to draining lymph nodes
- haematogenously via veins and arteries to distant sites
- along the nerves (perineurally)
- across body cavities such as the peritoneum (transcoelomic spread).

Cancer results in general systemic symptoms, including anorexia and weight loss, as well as local symptoms. The latter may include specific surgical pathology (**Box 11.6**).

Most cancers can be TNM-staged according to:

- the size of the tumour (T)
- the extent of lymph node involvement (N)
- the presence or absence of distant metastases (M) (see **Box 6.12**).

Surgery remains the only potentially curative therapeutic option for the majority of solid and hollow organ cancers, and complete cure is often possible only in the early stages. The key principle of oncologically curative surgery is to ensure that the cancer has been excised completely: that is to achieve an 'R0' resection. If microscopic tumour remains at the pathology excision margins (R1) or is macroscopically present (R2), then cancer recurrence is either highly likely (R1 resection margins) or inevitable (R2).

All patients being considered for cancer treatment must be discussed in multidisciplinary meetings where radiologists, pathologists, oncologists, palliative physicians, surgeons and allied health professionals with cancer expertise are present to plan optimal therapy. Survival outcomes for patients undergoing cancer surgery have been immensely enhanced over the last few decades, through improvements in surgery and anaesthesia, progress in understanding tumour biology and genetics, and related advances in medical oncology and radiotherapy. Surgery in potentially curable disease is often supplemented by chemotherapy and radiotherapy, provided by clinical oncologists. This may be:

- **neoadjuvant** (preoperative), to reduce tumour mass prior to resection
- **adjuvant** (postoperative), to kill any remaining cancer cells and prevent recurrence.

Surgery, alongside other interventional techniques including interventional radiology and endoscopy, also has a role to play in the palliation of cancer. For example, large-volume tumours causing symptoms as a result of mass effect may be 'debulked', or expansile stents may be inserted into obstructed hollow viscera such as the duodenum or the biliary tract.

Further reading

Lamb CM, MacGoey P, Navarro AP et al. Damage control surgery in the era of damage control resuscitation. *Br J Anaesth* 2014; 113:242–249.
Weimann A, Braga M, Carli F et al. ESPEN guideline: Clinical nutrition in surgery. *Clin Nutr* 2017; 36:623–650.
https://www.facs.org/quality-programs/trauma/atls *American College of Surgeons' Advanced Trauma Life Support programme.*

---

i   Box 11.6 Surgical pathology in cancer patients

Pathology	Examples
Obstruction	Bowel obstruction, biliary tract dilation, hydronephrosis or hydrocephalus
Haemorrhage	Acute or chronic gastrointestinal bleeding, a common presenting complaint of oesophageal, stomach and colorectal cancer
Fistulation	Colorectal cancers, which may erode and create an abnormal opening into adjacent organs such as the bladder (colovesical fistula)
Pain	May result from: Direct invasion of adjoining tissues Metastases to structures such as bone Mass effect causing stretching of organs, e.g. liver capsule pain arising in the presence of primary and secondary liver tumours
Infection	Unexplained bacteraemia with commensal gut bacteria, e.g. *Streptococcus milleri*, which should prompt investigation for an occult colorectal cancer that is allowing translocation of bacteria into the circulation

---

THE PATIENT JOURNEY IN SURGERY

The patient journey through surgical treatment is best understood in terms of three phases: preoperative, intraoperative and postoperative. Surgery may be elective, expedited, urgent or immediate (**Box 11.7**). For example, a patient with colon cancer could present with life-threatening haemorrhage (requires immediate surgical intervention), perforation and peritonitis (requires urgent surgery), impending bowel obstruction (requires expedited surgery), or for a planned colonic resection of the tumour (elective surgery).

An increasing number of minor and intermediate-complexity elective procedures, and even some emergency operations, are being carried out in the day surgery or short overnight-stay setting. Inpatient stays are reserved for more major procedures or for patients with more complex co-morbidity.

---

i   Box 11.7 Confidential Enquiry into Perioperative Death (CEPOD) classification of intervention

Immediate
- Life-, limb- or organ-saving intervention
- Resuscitation is carried out simultaneously with the intervention
- Surgery occurs within minutes of the decision to operate

Urgent
- Intervention for acute-onset, clinically deteriorating and potentially life-threatening conditions, including those that may threaten survival of a limb or organ, or for fixation of many fractures and relief of pain or other distressing symptoms
- Surgery occurs within hours of the decision to operate

Expedited
- Patients requiring early treatment, but the condition is not an immediate threat to life, limb or organ survival
- Surgery is undertaken within days of the decision to operate

Elective
- Intervention is planned or booked in advance of a routine admission to hospital
- The timing is arranged to suit the patient, hospital and staff

Preoperative phase

Fitness for surgery

One of the aims of the preoperative assessment is to evaluate a patient's fitness for surgery, often graded using the American Society of Anesthesiologists (ASA) criteria (**Box 11.8**). Once risk has been estimated, a second focus is to optimize a patient's physical state in terms of nutrition and pre-existing medical conditions, in order to minimize this risk.

The preoperative assessment seeks to:
- establish the status of known pre-existing co-morbidities, e.g. respiratory and cardiovascular disease
- screen for undiagnosed conditions, e.g. diabetes and hypertension
- identify drug allergies
- document current medications and identify the need for these to be modified perioperatively, e.g. withholding anticoagulants and antiplatelet drugs that could increase bleeding risk
- note previous anaesthesia history and any related problems
- identify modifiable risk factors, e.g. smoking, alcohol use and obesity.

If there are factors that are not modifiable in the necessary time-scale, and that place the patient at high risk of operative or anaesthetic complications, assignment of an appropriate postoperative high-dependency/intensive care setting is critical.

Preoperative ERAS principles include optimization of nutritional status: for example, by using dietary supplements, intensive physiotherapy and pre-habilitation ('pre-hab') for deconditioned patients with poor functional reserves undergoing major surgery.

Patients must be appropriately fasted for expedited/elective procedures, taking no food for 4–6 hours and no liquids for 2 hours prior to the procedure. Appropriate premedication, as determined by the anaesthetist, may be administered to alleviate anxiety and pain.

Deciding when to operate

A critical skill in surgery is judging whether or not to operate on a patient. A simple series of questions can facilitate sensible decision-making.

Is the patient willing?

The surgeon must ensure that the patient is willing to have the surgery and has sufficient mental capacity to make an informed decision (see p. 83). The patient must have an understanding of the rationale for the operation; the likely benefits in terms of recovery of function, quality of life, survival and prognosis; and the predicted risks in terms of morbidity and mortality. Operative risk can be quantified using scoring systems such as the Preoperative Risk Calculator (PoRC) and Physiological and Operative Severity Score for the enUmeration of Mortality and morbidity (POSSUM). Patients should be aware of alternative treatment options, the role of non-intervention and the likely outcomes of different approaches. They must be given an idea of what they can expect in the immediate postoperative period, including the likelihood of an intensive care/high-dependency unit stay, and should be warned about postoperative drains, vascular access lines, catheters and the predicted course of recovery. Patients should be offered a second opinion, and indeed encouraged to seek one, particularly for complex major interventions.

Is the patient fit enough?

The preoperative physiological reserve of the patient who is to undergo the proposed surgery must be determined and optimized, both in elective and emergency situations, to minimize surgical risk (see earlier). The expertise of colleagues in other specialties such as anaesthesia, intensive care and cardiovascular, respiratory, renal, metabolic and geriatric medicine, as well as the input of allied health professionals, including physiotherapists and nutritionists, should be sought, in order to mitigate against pre-existing illness and deconditioning.

Is the operation doable?

The operation must be technically feasible. For example, a proposed cancer resection must be capable of accomplishing satisfactory resection margins if it is to achieve its curative intent.

Who is the right person to do the operation?

The operating surgeon has the responsibility to ensure that they have the necessary skills to perform the operation to the highest possible standard. The team and the organization in which they

---

i Box 11.8 American Society of Anesthesiologists (ASA) grading

ASA grade[a]	Assessment	Description
I	A normal healthy patient	Healthy, non-smoking, no or minimal alcohol use
II	A patient with mild systemic disease	Mild diseases only, without substantive functional limitations. Examples include: current cigarette smoking, social alcohol drinking, pregnancy, obesity (BMI 30–40), well-controlled diabetes or hypertension, mild lung disease
III	A patient with severe systemic disease	Substantive functional limitations; one or more moderate to severe diseases. Examples include: poorly controlled diabetes or hypertension, COPD, morbid obesity (BMI ≥40), active hepatitis, alcohol dependence or abuse, moderate reduction of ejection fraction, end-stage renal failure undergoing regular dialysis, recent (but >3 months) myocardial infarction or stroke
IV	A patient with severe systemic disease that is a constant threat to life	Examples include: recent (<3 months) myocardial infarction, stroke or coronary intervention (such as coronary angioplasty), on-going cardiac ischaemia or severe valve dysfunction, severe reduction of ejection fraction, sepsis, advanced renal impairment not on dialysis
V	A moribund patient who is not expected to survive without the operation	Examples include: ruptured abdominal/thoracic aortic aneurysm, massive trauma, intracranial bleed with mass effect, ischaemic bowel, multiple organ/system dysfunction
VI	A declared brain-dead patient whose organs are being removed for donor purposes	

[a]The addition of 'E' denotes emergency surgery (when delay in treatment would lead to a significant increase in the threat to life or body part). BMI, body mass index; COPD, chronic obstructive pulmonary disease.

work must be similarly equipped. Where appropriate, patients with complex problems ought to be referred elsewhere, if greater expertise is available. Surgical outcomes improve based on the number of particular procedures performed by the surgeon each year, and so uncommon procedures may be best performed in tertiary referral centres where experience can be pooled.

Is it sensible to proceed?

Having confirmed all of the above, the surgeon must still make a holistic judgement in partnership with the patient on the overall wisdom of proceeding with surgery.

Intraoperative phase

Anaesthesia

Anaesthesia seeks to achieve three goals for a patient undergoing surgery:
- hypnosis
- analgesia
- muscle relaxation.

The phases of general anaesthesia include induction, maintenance and recovery. Anaesthetists make use of induction agents, muscle relaxants, analgesics and inhalational anaesthetic agents to allow endotracheal intubation, mechanical ventilation and complete muscle relaxation during major surgery. Depending on the type of surgery, regional anaesthesia using a spinal, epidural or regional nerve block can be used, or procedures may be performed under local anaesthesia. Avoiding a general anaesthetic can be important where a patient's co-morbidity or lack of physiological reserve mean that sedation, ventilation and the subsequent haemodynamic fluctuations that they entail could carry significant risk.

Operating theatre safety

The successful outcome of any surgical procedure relies on constant attention to patient safety. The five-step surgical checklist published by the WHO in 2008 (**Box 11.9**) has been shown to reduce 30-day mortality after emergency abdominal surgery by 38% in a study carried out in 58 different countries.

Operative technique

Meticulous intraoperative attention to surgical technique is required to ensure optimal outcomes for the surgical patient. Good pre- and postoperative care cannot compensate for intraoperative surgical failures. Although all operations differ, some basic techniques are common to almost all procedures

Access

Accurate placement of an appropriate surgical incision, based on relevant anatomical considerations, is critical to the success of any open surgical procedure. Similar principles remain valid for laparoscopic and robotic surgery, as laparoscope port placement can determine both the ease and the success of minimally invasive procedures.

Exposure

The use of retractors to expose the surgical field adequately is critical to safe surgery. During laparoscopic procedures, endosufflators safely create a CO_2 pneumoperitoneum to enable adequate exposure.

Visibility

This is critical for safe surgery. High-quality theatre lighting enables the surgeon to see the key organs and structures clearly and to determine relevant anatomy in open surgery. Laparoscopic and robotic surgery is dependent on high-quality light sources and laparoscopic camera systems of increasing sophistication.

Haemostasis

Achieving meticulous surgical control of bleeding throughout a procedure, aided by sophisticated modern electrocautery and other energy devices, can reduce transfusion requirements, enable a smooth postoperative recovery and prevent complications.

Respect for tissues

Gentle handling of all tissue by the surgeon is vital, with the utmost care being required to respect anatomical planes, avoid bruising, prevent crushing, tension and ischaemia, and minimize the need for surgical drains where possible. These steps reduce postoperative infection and ensure better surgical outcomes.

Postoperative phase

Postoperative care is informed by ERAS principles and requires excellent analgesia, careful attention to fluid and electrolyte balance, early mobilization of the patient, early fluids and feeding (as soon as tolerated by the patient), and removal of drains, tubes and

---

ⓘ Box 11.9 The World Health Organization 'five-step' surgical checklist

Team brief
- All team members should be present, and should introduce themselves and explain their roles
- Everyone should understand the planned sequence of events, the skill levels of different team members, likely equipment and staffing requirements, and anticipated problems

Sign in
- Prior to induction of anaesthesia, a check is made with the patient about drug allergies and the site of surgery (and appropriate markings made)
- Consent is confirmed

Time out
- A final check is made before commencing operation to ensure the correct patient identity, operation site, positioning and preparation
- Any other concerns are raised

Sign out
- This is done at the end of the procedure before the patient leaves theatre for recovery, to ensure that:
  - All swabs and instruments are accounted for
  - Specimens have been collated and labelled
  - Operation notes have been written
  - The patient has an assigned bed on an appropriate ward or critical care area

Team debrief
- All members of the multidisciplinary surgical team participate in a discussion of good points of the operating process and any issues that arose, answer any concerns, and identify areas for learning and future improvement

catheters as soon as safely possible, with nutritional support and post-habilitation if required.

Postoperative care has:

- an '***immediate phase***' within the recovery room, where the focus is on ensuring safe and full return of consciousness with careful attention to airway, breathing and circulation
- a '***return to surgical ward care***' phase (unless transfer to the high-dependency or intensive care unit is indicated)
- a possible '***late rehabilitation/convalescence***' phase, depending on the pre-morbid status of the patient, the magnitude of surgery and the development of related complications.

Direct complications of surgery

Some complications arise directly as a result of the surgical procedure and may require further surgical intervention:

Haemorrhage

This can occur during the operation ('primary haemorrhage'); or within 24 hours or so of surgery when it is often due to a dislodged surgical tie or displacement of a diathermy eschar or clot when the waking patient's blood pressure rises ('reactive haemorrhage'); or in the later period of recovery, often 7–10 days after the operation and frequently caused by infection and erosion of a blood vessel ('secondary haemorrhage'). Haemorrhage often requires an immediate return to the operating theatre for control, although radiological intervention may also be employed.

Anastomotic leaks

Leaks from breakdown of surgically created anastomoses, typically related to gastrointestinal surgery, can lead to gastric, biliary, pancreatic, small intestinal and colonic contents leaking into the peritoneum. This can cause sepsis and peritonitis, and the formation of abscesses and fistulae.

Wound infections

These may progress to cause superficial or deep wound dehiscence and subsequent incisional herniation.

Paralytic ileus

This commonly occurs after intraperitoneal surgery as a result of significant displacement and handling of bowel. Patients present with symptoms that are similar to those of bowel obstruction, including constipation, vomiting, abdominal discomfort and bloating. Management is conservative, with nasogastric drainage, antiemetics, intravenous fluids, and a slow and gradual introduction of oral feeding.

Pain

Pain at the operative site is common after surgery. Standard analgesia using paracetamol, non-steroidal anti-inflammatory drugs (NSAIDs), and weak and strong opiates can sometimes be supplemented with local interventions at the site of surgery, such as transversus abdominis plane (TAP) block after abdominal surgery.

Medical complications in the postoperative patient

Other complications arise indirectly as a result of surgery but are common and potentially life-threatening. Typically, surgical teams identify these problems and commence initial management, calling on the expertise of relevant physicians where appropriate.

Venous thromboembolic disease

Venous thromboembolic disease (including deep vein thrombosis and pulmonary embolus) is common in the postoperative period, especially after abdominal or lower limb orthopaedic surgery. Prophylaxis with low-molecular-weight heparin is almost always indicated (see p. 1006).

Pulmonary complications

These include lower lobe atelectasis and pneumonia, which are common following surgery and are often a result of under-breathing caused by pain and sedation. Good analgesia and the use of incentive spirometry to encourage deep breathing and re-expansion of basal lung segments can help to prevent these complications.

Cardiac complications

Cardiac complications, including acute myocardial infarction, can be seen postoperatively, often complicating pre-existing cardiac disease.

Delirium

This is common after surgery, especially in elderly patients or those with pre-existing cognitive impairment. Contributory factors include pain, constipation and use of opiate analgesia. Careful management uses the principles outlined on page 310, and in many hospitals geriatric physicians provide a surgical liaison service to help manage the medical needs of elderly patients undergoing surgical procedures.

Acute kidney injury

This is common in the postoperative period and can be multifactorial, causes including fluid losses, sepsis, use of NSAID analgesia and urinary retention. Monitoring of urine output is crucial in the postoperative period, and oliguria should prompt an assessment of fluid status and current medications. Abrupt anuria often indicates urinary retention, a common complication of spinal and general anaesthesia.

Further reading

Haynes AB, Weiser TG, Berry WR et al. A surgical safety checklist to reduce morbidity and mortality in a global population. *N Engl J Med* 2009; 360:491–499.
Ljungqvist O, Hubner M. Enhanced recovery after surgery–ERAS–principles, practice and feasibility in the elderly. *Aging Clin Exp Res* 2018; 30:249–252.
Mayhew D, Mendonca V, Murthy BVS. A review of ASA physical status – historical perspectives and modern developments. *Anaesthesia* 2019; 74:373–379.

SURGICAL ETHICS, CONSENT AND THE LAW

The four principles of clinical ethics are crucial in ensuring that surgery is performed in a patient's best interests through shared decision-making (see also p. 82).

- ***Autonomy*** is typically reflected in the critical importance of obtaining properly informed patient consent before surgery, and providing information about different courses of action and their likely outcomes to allow patients to make their own choice of treatment.
- ***Non-maleficence*** manifests as a commitment to patient safety, driving clinical improvement to avoid causing unnecessary harm.
- ***Beneficence*** requires on-going surgical commitment to the highest quality of surgical outcomes, improving patient experience and encouraging continuous surgical quality improvement.
- ***Justice*** demands a surgical understanding of equity and fairness in terms of access and allocation of finite resources for healthcare and health.

Consent in surgery

Consent must be understood as a process, not merely the one-off signing of a document. Through the consent process, a surgeon empowers, enables and assists the patient to make a fully informed decision regarding treatment by providing all necessary information in a comprehensible way, including a description of all the available alternatives to surgery, such as medical treatment or non-intervention.

Where patients lack mental capacity to consent to a procedure, emergency surgery (to save 'life or limb') is often carried out on the basis of a surgical decision that it is in a patient's best interests. When elective or non-urgent procedures are contemplated, a careful safeguarding process is followed, where views expressed by the patient are weighed alongside surgical opinions about a patient's best interests, and other opinions: for instance, those of family members or carers. Sometimes, independent advocates or even the courts can be required to make decisions. These principles are explained more fully in Chapter 5.

Surgical audit and quality improvement

Surgical outcomes should be monitored in an attempt to provide continuous quality improvement. Both the performance of individual surgeons, and hospital or departmental surgical outcomes in terms of complications and mortality should be tracked. Local 'mortality and morbidity' meetings allow lessons to be learned where avoidable harm has been done to patients, and local surgical outcomes should be contributed to relevant national specialty audits to benchmark local services against national or international equivalents.

Further reading

Royal College of Surgeons. *Consent*. https://www.rcseng.ac.uk/standards-and-research/gsp/domain-3/3-5-1-consent/.

Royal College of Surgeons. *Morbidity and Mortality Meetings: A Guide to Good Practice*. https://www.rcseng.ac.uk/standards-and-research/standards-and-guidance/good-practice-guides/morbidity-and-mortality-meetings/.

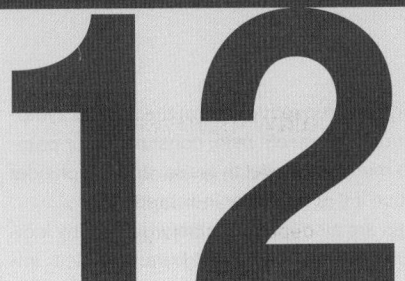

12 Prescribing, therapeutics and toxicology

Vikas Kapil, Sally M. Bradberry and Munir Pirmohamed

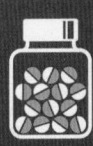

CORE SKILLS AND KNOWLEDGE

All doctors need to learn how to prescribe medications safely and effectively. This requires mastery of the principles in the first half of this chapter, which cover key concepts including pharmacokinetics, pharmacodynamics, drug interactions and adverse drug reactions. Pharmacists play a critical role in helping doctors make safe and effective choices when prescribing.

The second half of the chapter covers poisoning: a significant global health problem most commonly seen in the context of deliberate self-harm, but with a substantial proportion of inadvertent poisoning globally. Patients who have taken a drug overdose, a substance of abuse or who have been accidentally poisoned will usually present to a hospital emergency department. Fortunately most can be managed with supportive care alone, although a few require critical care admission. Poisoning with rare agents may require the expertise of clinical toxicologists in a specialist poisons unit.

Key skills related to prescribing, therapeutics and toxicology include:

- developing a systematic approach to prescribing, using key pharmacological principles to select and administer an appropriate drug, avoiding interactions and anticipating or preventing toxicity
- understanding treatment algorithms for patients poisoned by one of the 'top ten poisons' described in this chapter.

There are many practical ways to learn prescribing skills: reviewing patients' medication charts on ward rounds, rewriting medication charts under supervision, observing annual medication reviews in primary care, reporting adverse drug reactions (e.g. using the 'Yellow Card' scheme in the UK), or working with pharmacists reviewing inpatient or outpatient prescriptions. The initial assessment and management of patients who have been poisoned, either intentionally or accidentally, is best observed in the emergency department. Subsequent management may be observed in the intensive care setting or on medical wards.

PRESCRIBING

INTRODUCTION

Prescribing a medicine is the most common healthcare intervention performed by doctors and hence the correct choice of medication and the act of prescribing are key skills required by all doctors. The 1984 'Nairobi Declaration' emphasized that prescribing should be to the **right patient** with the **right drug** at the **right dose**, and at an **affordable cost**. Thus, the prescription of a medicine needs to take into account the potential benefits and harms of that medicine, and ensure that every step is taken to maximize the benefit:harm ratio. The key principles of prescribing are described in **Box 12.1**.

WHY DO PATIENTS NEED DRUGS?

There are many reasons for prescribing drugs to patients. These are as follows:

- **Disease treatment**. A reliable diagnosis is crucial before starting treatment to ensure that a patient is not exposed unnecessarily to the hazards of a particular intervention (rational). However, a prior diagnosis may not be possible in every circumstance. For example, in sepsis, the initiation of **blind** (empirical) antimicrobial therapy is justified, as delay would expose a patient to serious hazard (see p. 159).

- **Symptom relief**. Drugs are frequently used in the relief of symptoms; e.g. in the treatment of severe pain, constipation or pruritus. It is imperative to monitor for effectiveness, and to consider stopping the medication if it is no longer indicated.
- **Prevention**. Medicines are also given to otherwise healthy individuals. In such circumstances, there must be a very clear imperative to ensure that the benefits to the individual outweigh the harm. Examples include:
  - ○ primary cardiovascular prevention with lipid-lowering therapy (i.e. statins)
  - ○ oral contraceptives for prevention of pregnancy.

THE CHOICE OF DRUG

The choice of the drug often depends on clinical factors (such as age of the patient, concomitant disease and concurrent therapy), pharmaceutical factors (the availability of other medicines and relative cost-effectiveness) and, increasingly, individual (host) factors.

Selecting the right drug (therapeutics) involves three elements:
- the drug's clinical efficacy for the proposed use
- the balance between the drug's efficacy and safety
- patient preference.

The most common approach to assessing a drug's efficacy is the randomized controlled trial **(RCT) (Box 12.2)**, although other approaches can be informative (see Ch. 4). Although common

---

 Box 12.1 Key principles of prescribing

- **Be clear about the reasons for prescribing.** Obtain an accurate diagnosis and have clear aims of what the benefits will be from prescribing the drug
- **Obtain an accurate drug history.** Patients should be asked about their current medications, over-the-counter herbal medicines, and illicit drug usage. A past history of intolerances, including true allergic reactions, is also required.
- **Obtain an accurate history of other factors that might affect the benefit:harm ratio of drugs.** Take note of liver and renal impairment, age, whether patient is pregnant or breast-feeding, and co-morbidities.
- **Establish what the patient expects from the drug, and deal with any concerns.** Provide good information for the patient and answer any questions clearly.
- **Select the most clinically effective, cost-effective and safe medicine for the patient, based on an assessment of the individual.** Optimize the benefit:harm balance by choosing the right dose and frequency, and the right drug, in the best formulation, route of administration and duration of treatment. Prescribe within the licence of the medicine, except when no alternative is available.

- **Adhere to guidelines and local and national formularies.** Based on the needs of the individual patient, use the most reliable information to identify the medicine most suited to the patient.
- **Write prescriptions legibly using the correct documents, or prescribe electronically, depending on availability.** Take care to avoid medication errors.
- **Monitor the patient for both efficacy and safety after starting the drug.** This is essential to optimize dose, identify adverse reactions, and determine when to stop the medicine. Report adverse reactions using spontaneous reporting schemes, if appropriate.
- **Communicate clearly with other healthcare professionals and patients about the reasons for prescribing decisions.** Communication is essential to optimize the benefit:harm ratio of drugs, particularly when there are multiple prescribers for a single patient.
- **Prescribe within your competencies.** Prescribing should be within the limits of your knowledge and experience. Do not be afraid to ask for advice and ensure that complex prescriptions are checked (e.g. when calculating doses).

Adapted from British Pharmacological Society; https://www.bps.ac.uk/education-engagement/teaching-pharmacology/ten-principles-of-good-prescribing.

---

i   Box 12.2 Evaluation of new drugs

Phase I: Healthy human subjects (usually men)
- First use in humans
- Evaluation of safety and toxicity
- Pharmacokinetic assessment
- Sometimes pharmacodynamic assessment
- Approximately 100 subjects

Phase II: First assessment in patients
- Safety and toxicity evaluated
- Dose range identified
- Pharmacokinetic and pharmacodynamic monitoring
- Approximately 500 subjects

Phase III: Use in wider patient population
- Efficacy main objective
- Safety and toxicity also monitored
- Often multicentre trials
- Approximately 2000 patients involved

Phase IV: Post-marketing surveillance
- All patients prescribed drug monitored
- Efficacy, safety and toxicity measured
- Quantification of unusual drug adverse effects
- Yellow Card and spontaneous reports of adverse reactions
- Often very large numbers of patients observed

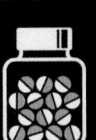

adverse reactions are usually identified in early-phase drug development studies and RCTs, rare (often serious) adverse reactions are often only discovered after drugs are licensed by post-marketing surveillance studies (pharmacovigilance) (see **Box 12.2**). All patients should be offered the opportunity to be involved in making decisions about their medical treatment, including those about medications, so-called **shared decision-making** (see p. 11). Patients' own preferences should be discussed to enable them to be equal partners in decision-making about whether, and how, they wish to be treated. This approach improves 'concordance' with treatment regimens.

Further reading

Aronson JK. Rational prescribing, appropriate prescribing. *Br J Clin Pharmacol* 2004; 57:229–230.

THE DOSE

The dose administered to the patient is crucial in determining both efficacy and safety of medicines. Appropriate drug dosages will usually have been determined from the results of so-called '**dose-ranging**' studies during the drug development programme (see **Box 12.2**).

In some cases, drug doses are **fixed**, with all patients being given the same dose: for example, levonorgestrel for emergency contraception (see p. 1469). However, these situations are unusual. Although most patients take 75 mg aspirin daily, doses of up to 300 mg daily have been used for the secondary prevention of myocardial infarction (see p. 1086).

More commonly, doses are **titrated**. For many drugs, there are wide inter-individual variations in response. As a consequence, while a particular dose may, in one person, lack any therapeutic effect, the same dose in another may cause serious toxicity. This is because the concentration of drug reaching the systemic circulation – that is, exposure – varies between individuals even for the same dose, and it is exposure that determines the response to drugs, in terms of both efficacy and safety. Pharmacokinetic factors (including differences in the rates of drug absorption, metabolism and excretion) are the main determinants of such variability in exposure between individuals.

Variability in response, at an equivalent exposure, can also be due to **pharmacodynamic factors**, where there are differences in the sensitivity of the drug target that generally fall into the categories of receptors, enzymes, ion channels, transporters, DNA or transcription factors.

Because it is not easy to measure exposure, we use the dose as a proxy. Furthermore, it is not always possible to predict pharmacodynamic variability. For these two reasons, prescribers should thus start most drugs at a low dose and titrate to the **lowest effective dose**. This can help overcome the inter-individual variability in the dose (concentration)–response curve, whereby there is an increase in response with an increase in dose, until a plateau effect is reached (**Fig. 12.1**).

Pharmacokinetics

Pharmacokinetics is the study of **what the body does to a drug**. This can be divided into four different processes: absorption, distribution, metabolism and excretion. Age, body weight, renal and hepatic function, concomitant drugs, co-morbidities, diet, smoking and alcohol are all known to affect the pharmacokinetics and so increase inter-individual variation in required drug dose. Genetic factors affecting drug pharmacokinetics also play a role in determining how individuals respond to drugs.

Absorption

Drugs can be administered by various different routes (**Box 12.3**) but oral administration is the most common. The main determinants of a drug's plasma concentration after oral administration are its bioavailability (**Box 12.4**) and its rate of systemic clearance (by hepatic metabolism or renal excretion). A drug's oral bioavailability depends on the extent to which it is:

- **Destroyed in the gastrointestinal tract**, especially by gastric acid.
- **Unable to cross the gastrointestinal epithelium.** Drugs can cross either by passive diffusion or by active uptake by gut epithelial transporters. Transporters can generally be divided into influx transporters, which increase uptake of drug (e.g. the PEPT1 influx transporter is required for the uptake of penicillins), and efflux transporters, which limit the absorption of a drug (e.g. P-glycoprotein is an efflux transporter that limits digoxin absorption).
- **Metabolized by the liver** before reaching the systemic circulation ('first-pass' metabolism). First-pass metabolism can be avoided by non-enteral routes.

Distribution

This is the process by which drugs are distributed from the bloodstream to organs and cells. Most drugs will circulate in the bloodstream bound to plasma proteins, most commonly albumin. Free drug, which is the active drug, is usually in dynamic equilibrium with protein-bound drug, with the latter being released as the free drug concentration decreases.

Metabolism

Metabolism takes place in many different organs, the liver being the most common site. Drug metabolism converts lipid-soluble drugs to water-soluble drugs for excretion by the kidneys. Metabolism usually inactivates a drug, but in some cases, it can convert a pro-drug into an active drug (e.g. enalapril to enalaprilat) or lead to the formation of toxic metabolites (N-acetyl-para-benzoquinoneimine in paracetamol overdose). Drug metabolism occurs in two stages:

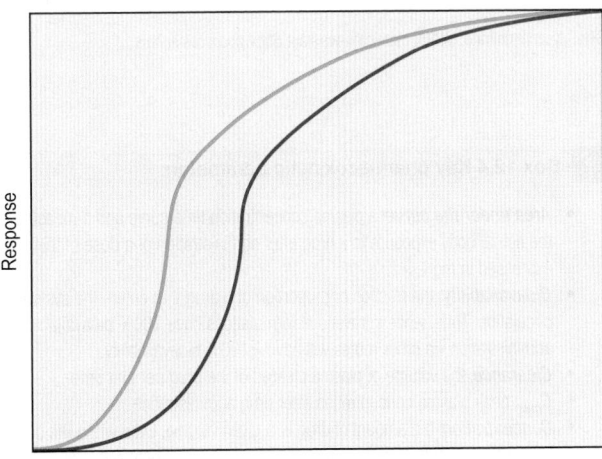

Fig. 12.1 Dose–response curve, showing the variable response of the same dose in different patients. The patient represented by the red line requires a higher dose to achieve the same desired effect than the patient represented by the green line, and may therefore be at risk of experiencing more adverse effects.

Box 12.3 Routes of drug administration

Route	Description	Example
Buccal	Rapid absorption, avoids first-pass metabolism	Midazolam for status epilepticus
Epidural	Administration of drug into epidural space around the spinal cord	Epidural anaesthetic for pain relief during labour
Inhaled	Achieves high concentrations at site of disease with limited systemic absorption	Salbutamol for acute asthma relief
Intra-muscular	Easier than intravenous route but absorption is less predictable	Adrenaline (epinephrine) in anaphylaxis
Intranasal	Often used for local delivery	Intranasal corticosteroids in allergic conditions
Intrathecal	Used to achieve high local levels	Methotrexate in acute lymphoblastic leukaemia
Intravenous	100% of dose enters systemic circulation but invasive and inconvenient	Intravenous teicoplanin for treatment of invasive MRSA infections
Oral	Most common route, convenient, but subject to first-pass metabolism for certain drugs	Ramipril for hypertension
Per rectum	For local administration: for rectal/colonic disorders For systemic absorption: when oral or intravenous routes not possible	Prednisolone enema for rectal inflammatory bowel disease Diazepam for seizures
Subcutaneous	Good absorption, can be self-administered	Insulin for diabetes
Sublingual	Rapid absorption, avoids first-pass metabolism	GTN for acute relief of angina chest pain
Topical	Used for local application of cutaneous or joint diseases	Corticosteroids for eczema
Transdermal	Absorption through the skin via a patch	Nicotine replacement therapy for smoking cessation

GTN, glyceryl trinitrate; MRSA, methicillin-resistant *Staphylococcus aureus*.

- **Phase I**: oxidation, reduction or hydrolysis. This is largely undertaken by a family of isoenzymes known as the cytochrome P450 system. Inhibition or induction of cytochrome P450 isoenzymes is a major cause of drug–drug interactions (see p. 259).
- **Phase II**: conjugation with glucuronate, sulphate or other substances. This renders drugs more water-soluble.

Variability in the genes that encode drug-metabolizing enzymes (**Box 12.5**) is a major determinant of the inter-individual differences in the therapeutic and adverse responses to drug treatment. One-quarter of all licensed medicines are substrates for a single P450 isoenzyme, CYP2D6. The poor metabolizer (reduced function) CYP2D6 phenotype increases the risk of toxicity, for example, with those antidepressants (e.g. selective serotonin reuptake inhibitors, SSRIs) or antipsychotics (e.g. risperidone) that undergo CYP2D6 metabolism.

Reduced conversion of a prodrug to active metabolite may also compromise efficacy in some patients; for example, poor metabolizers of CYP2D6 do not experience analgesic benefit with codeine, which is a prodrug converted to morphine by CYP2D6. In individuals with more than two copies of the normal *CYP2D6* gene (ultra-rapid metabolizers), there is increased drug metabolism and therapeutic failure at conventional doses. Ultra-rapid metabolism can also lead to increased toxicity with prodrugs such as codeine, because there is increased conversion of morphine, thereby increasing the risk of respiratory depression at therapeutic doses, particularly in children with upper airways obstruction, for example with enlarged tonsils/adenoids.

Warfarin is predominantly metabolized by CYP2C9. Up to 10% of most populations have reduced CYP2C9 activity. Such individuals metabolize warfarin more slowly, leading to higher plasma levels, a greater risk of bleeding, and require lower doses if the international normalized ratio (INR) is to be maintained appropriately. When combined with the genetic polymorphisms in the vitamin K epoxide reductase complex (*VKORC1*) genes (a pharmacodynamic variation), and age and body mass index (BMI), over 50% of the variation in individual daily-dose requirement can be predicted. Pre-prescription genotyping for *CYP2C9* and *VKORC1* has been shown to improve anticoagulation control.

Individual differences in the activity of thiopurine methyltransferase (TPMT), a phase II enzyme, are used to determine safe dosing of the immunosuppressants, mercaptopurine and azathioprine. TPMT inactivates these drugs and testing for TMPT activity is therefore undertaken routinely to determine appropriate starting doses to reduce the risk of bone marrow suppression associated with these drugs.

Box 12.4 Key pharmacokinetic parameters

- *Area under the curve*: a plasma concentration time curve and a measure of the actual body exposure to a drug after administration of a dose of the drug; expressed in mg/L × h.
- *Bioavailability*: the fraction or proportion of a drug that enters the systemic circulation. Thus, while intravenous formulations have 100% bioavailability, administration via other routes will have <100% bioavailability.
- *Clearance*: the volume of plasma cleared of the drug per unit time.
- C_{max}: peak plasma concentration after drug administration.
- *Concentration*: the amount of drug in a given volume. Even when the dose is similar, concentrations (and thus exposure) will vary between individuals.
- *Dose*: the amount of drug administered. This may be micrograms, milligrams or grams. Occasionally, drugs are administered per body weight or body surface area.
- *Loading dose*: an initial larger dose to achieve immediate therapeutic plasma or tissue drug concentration. It is usually reserved for medical

emergencies, but can also be used for drugs with long-half-lives, which would otherwise take a long time to reach desired therapeutic steady-state concentration.
- *Elimination half-life*: the time required for the drug concentration to reach half its original value. With repeat dosing, for most drugs, it takes 4–5 half-lives to approach steady state.
- *Steady state:* the situation for most drugs where drug intake is in dynamic equilibrium with drug elimination.
- T_{max}: time to reach C_{max}.
- V_d: volume of distribution – the apparent volume in which a drug is distributed. Drugs with low V_d are predominantly in the circulation, while drugs with a high V_d have diffused into the peripheral tissue compartment, such as body fat. Drugs with a low Vd are amenable to removal by haemodialysis in overdose, while drugs that have a high Vd are not.

> ℹ **Box 12.5 Genetic polymorphisms affecting drug response**
>
> | Organ or system involved | Associated gene/allele | Drug/drug response phenotype | Pharmacokinetic/pharmacodynamic |
> |---|---|---|---|
> | **Blood** | | | |
> | Red blood cells | G6PD | Primaquine and others | Pharmacodynamic |
> | | TPMT*2 | Azathioprine/6MP-induced neutropenia | Pharmacokinetic |
> | Neutrophils | UGT1A1*28 | Irinotecan-induced neutropenia | Pharmacokinetic |
> | Platelets | CYP2C19*2 | Stent thrombosis | Pharmacokinetic |
> | Coagulation | CYP2C9*2, *3, VKORC1 | Warfarin dose requirement | Mixed |
> | **Brain and peripheral nervous system** | | | |
> | CNS depression | CYP2D6*N | Codeine-related sedation and respiratory depression | Pharmacokinetic |
> | Anaesthesia | Butyrylcholinesterase | Prolonged apnoea | Pharmacokinetic |
> | Peripheral nerves | NAT-2 | Isoniazid-induced peripheral neuropathy | Pharmacokinetic |
> | **Drug hypersensitivity and liver injury** | | | |
> | | HLA-B*57:01 | Abacavir hypersensitivity | Pharmacodynamic |
> | | HLA-B*15:02 | Carbamazepine-induced Stevens–Johnson syndrome (in some Asian groups) | Pharmacodynamic |
> | | HLA-A*31:01 | Carbamazepine-induced hypersensitivity in Caucasians and Japanese | Pharmacodynamic |
> | | HLA-B*58:01 | Allopurinol-induced serious cutaneous reactions | Pharmacodynamic |
> | | HLA-B*57:01 | Flucloxacillin hepatotoxicity | Pharmacodynamic |
> | **Malignancy** | | | |
> | Breast cancer | CYP2D6 | Response to tamoxifen | Pharmacokinetic |
> | Chronic myeloid leukaemia | BCR-ABL | Imatinib and other tyrosine kinase inhibitors | Pharmacodynamic |
> | Colon cancer | KRAS | Cetuximab efficacy | Pharmacodynamic |
> | Gastrointestinal stromal tumours | c-kit | Imatinib efficacy | Pharmacodynamic |
> | Lung cancer | EGFR | Gefitinib efficacy | Pharmacodynamic |
> | | EML4-ALK | Crizotinib efficacy | Pharmacodynamic |
> | Malignant melanoma | BRAF V600E | Vemurafenib efficacy | Pharmacodynamic |
> | **Muscle** | | | |
> | General anaesthetics | Ryanodine receptor | Malignant hyperthermia | Pharmacodynamic |
> | Statins | SLCO1B1 | Myopathy/rhabdomyolysis | Pharmacokinetic |
>
> (Adapted from Pirmohamed M. Pharmacogenetics: past, present and future. Drug Discov Today 2011; 16:852–861.)

Excretion

Excretion of drugs and their metabolites occurs most commonly via the kidneys, although faeces, breath and sweat represent other routes of excretion. In the kidney, free drug is filtered through the glomerulus and excreted in the urine as long as it is water-soluble. Lipid-soluble drugs are usually reabsorbed in the renal tubules. Some drugs, such as benzylpenicillin, are actively excreted by cells in the proximal convoluted tubule. Renal impairment reduces the elimination of water-soluble drugs, and thus reduction of the maintenance dose must be undertaken to avoid toxicity.

Pharmacodynamics

Pharmacodynamics is the study of **what the drug does to the body**. Pharmacodynamic sources of variation in drug action can be due to changes in the expression of the drug target, their affinity or their selectivity. This can be caused by genetic factors and also by disease. For example, in hepatic impairment, pharmacodynamic factors can determine the sensitivity to a drug, adding to changes in pharmacokinetics.

Genetic factors affecting drug pharmacodynamics also play a role in determining how individuals respond to drugs. For example, variation in the β_2-adrenoceptor gene can affect response to the most common bronchodilator (salbutamol) in asthma. Glucose-6-phosphate dehydrogenase deficiency, the most common enzyme deficiency, can predispose patients to acute red cell haemolysis with certain drugs such as primaquine, dapsone, sulphonamides and rasburicase. The biggest clinical advances in this area have occurred in two therapeutic areas: targeted cancer therapies and drug safety. Sequencing the cancer genome has identified novel driver mutations, leading to the development of targeted therapies. These have seen remarkable success, for instance, trastuzumab is only of value in women with breast cancer whose malignant cells express the HER2 epidermal growth factor receptor. Some immune-mediated reactions involving the skin and liver can now be predicted by genotyping for certain human leucocyte antigen (HLA) polymorphisms. For example, pre-prescription genotyping for HLA-B*57:01 has largely eliminated hypersensitivity to the anti-human immunodeficiency virus (HIV) drug abacavir. Similarly, HLA-B*15:02 predisposes patients from South-east Asia to Stevens–Johnson syndrome with carbamazepine.

As we learn more about the human genome, and the fact that many drugs undergo metabolism via many pathways and act on a number of targets, most of which show polymorphic expression, it may be possible in the future to utilize this information to personalize drug therapy to improve both efficacy and safety of drugs. The prospect for personalized prescribing will be enhanced when the interplay between pharmacokinetics and pharmacodynamics is better understood, which will then permit drug selection and dosing to become much more precise. With the advent of national programmes to increase the availability of whole genome sequencing in routine clinical practice (such as Genomics England 100,000 Genomes Project), this represents a key component of the drive towards **personalized medicine**.

Further reading

Relling MV, Evans ME. Pharmacogenomics in the clinic. *Nature* 2015; 326:343–350.
Wang L, McLeod JL, Weinshilboum RM. Genomics and drug response. *N Engl J Med* 2011; 364:1144–1153.

PRESCRIBING IN SPECIAL POPULATIONS

Most medications are evaluated in clinical trials, and therefore licensed for use, in adult patients. Therefore, healthcare professionals need to consider the specific issues relating to prescribing in other special populations.

For example, the use of drugs in young people poses special problems. Young people have different drug pharmacokinetics:
- **Absorption**: reduced intestinal motility, gastric emptying and acidity.
- **Distribution**: increased total body water (and relative less body fat) increases the volume of distribution for water-soluble drugs; immature blood–brain barrier.
- **Metabolism**: immature hepatic metabolic pathways (up to 1 year old).
- **Excretion**: immature renal excretory pathways (up to 6 months old).

Thus, extrapolating from adult dosage regimens, merely adjusting for weight, can lead to excessive (and potentially toxic) prescribing.

Other issues pertinent to prescribing in young people include administration:
- **Oral**: unreliable in ill newborn babies due to slow gastric transit, while precise oral dosing on liquids may be difficult due to refusal/spitting out.
- **Intramuscular** (IM): reduced muscle mass may lead to slower absorption from IM injections.
- **Intravenous** (IV): risk of volume overload, need for slow infusion rates.

In addition, many treatments have never been subject to formal trials in either children or adolescents and therefore their benefits and risks have not been appropriately assessed in these age groups. Adverse effect profiles of medicines may be different in children compared with adults for example Reye's syndrome in children given aspirin or suicidal ideas in depressed adolescents treated with SSRIs (see p. 780).

Pregnant women

Four in five pregnant women use an over-the-counter or prescribed medicine while pregnant. There is little published evidence for the safety of most drugs in pregnancy. Clinicians should be extremely cautious about prescribing drugs to pregnant women and only essential treatments should be given. There are significant changes in maternal physiology that have consequences for the prescribing of medications.

Pharmacokinetics
- **Absorption**: decreased intestinal motility and gastric emptying, increased gastric reflux and emesis.
- **Distribution**: increased total plasma volume (up to 40% higher), increased total body fat, decreased albumin.
- **Metabolism**: no major changes.
- **Excretion**: increased glomerular filtration rate (GFR) (up to 50% higher).

There is also significant drug transfer to the fetal circulation. Blood flow to the placenta increases 1000% over the last 6 months of gestation. Total placental surface (and therefore drug transfer) is greatest at term. Drugs that are small (<1 kDa) can cross the placenta and the main determinant of fetal drug concentration is maternal drug concentration.

Up to 1% of fetal malformations may be due to drug effects. In addition to the pharmacokinetic and pharmacodynamic differences in a young person (see p. 256), additional issues are encountered when there is significant fetal *in utero* drug exposure. Organ structure and function is most susceptible to perturbation during gestation, especially during organogenesis between 2 and 14 weeks' gestation, which may include a period where the woman is unaware of being pregnant. Many drugs are known to cause developmental abnormality, known as teratogenesis (**Box 12.6**). Furthermore, there is increased exposure to drugs that are renally excreted in the amniotic fluid as this is reswallowed and recirculated in the fetus *in utero*.

When a known teratogen is needed during pregnancy (e.g. an anticonvulsant drug or lithium), the potential adverse effects should be discussed with the parents, preferably before conception. Teratogens are best known for causing structural malformations; for example, congenital heart disease. However, teratogens can also lead to neurodevelopmental problems without any obvious structural damage. For example, exposure to sodium valproate *in utero* can lead to developmental neurotoxicity, which is manifested as cognitive and behavioural problems. The relevant drug literature should be consulted when prescribing for pregnant women.

Box 12.6 Some human teratogens

Drug or drug class	Effect
ACE inhibitors	Oligohydramnios
Retinoids, e.g. isotretinoin	Multiple abnormalities
Carbimazole	Neonatal hypothyroidism Abnormalities of bone growth
Fluconazole	Fallot's tetralogy
Antiepileptics: carbamazepine, lamotrigine, phenytoin, valproate	Cleft palate, facial abnormalities, neural tube defect, neurodevelopmental delay
NSAIDs	Delayed closure of the ductus arteriosus
Cytotoxic drugs	Most are presumed teratogens
Lithium	Ebstein's anomaly
Misoprostol	Moebius' syndrome (rare neurological condition)
Thalidomide (and possibly lenalidomide)	Phocomelia

Note: All drugs should be avoided in pregnancy unless benefit clearly outweighs the risk.

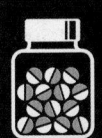

Breast-feeding women

Although most drugs can be detected in breast milk, the quantity is generally small. This is because, for most drugs, the concentration in milk is in equilibrium with plasma water (i.e. the non-protein-bound fraction). A few drugs (e.g. aspirin, carbimazole, methotrexate) may, however, cause harm to the infant if ingested in breast milk. This is especially the case for drugs that cause idiosyncratic reactions where there is little or no concentration–effect relationship (type B adverse events (see p. 258). The relevant drug literature should be consulted when prescribing for nursing mothers.

Prescribing in old age

Prescribing in old age has additional considerations. Old age alters drug pharmacokinetics:

- *Absorption*: diminished due to reductions in intestinal motility and blood flow.
- *Distribution*: reduced total body water affects the volume of distribution for water-soluble drugs; increased total body fat affects volume of distribution of fat-soluble drugs.
- *Metabolism*: decreased hepatic blood flow and enzyme function.
- *Excretion*: renal function declines with age at the rate of approximately 1 mL/min after the age of 40 years.

Old age alters pharmacodynamics:

- *Exaggerated pharmacodynamic effects* of drugs acting on the central nervous, cardiovascular and gastrointestinal systems are common.

Examples of common problems encountered in the use of drugs among older people are shown in **Box 12.7**. *Extrapolation of drug dosages* from those appropriate in younger adults may therefore lead to toxic plasma levels in older patients.

Additional considerations include:

- *Co-morbidity*, often associated with polypharmacy, leads to increased opportunities for disease–drug and drug–drug interactions.
- *Concordance with treatment regimens* diminishes as the number of prescribed drugs increases and is especially poor in the face of cognitive impairment (see p. 315).

---

i **Box 12.7** Common adverse reactions to drugs in the elderly

Drug or drug class	Effect
Nitrates α-Adrenoceptor-blockers Loop diuretics	Postural hypotension
Diuretics (thiazides)	Glucose intolerance, gout
Antimuscarinic drugs Tricyclic antidepressants Neuroleptics Anticonvulsants Hypnotics Opioids	Confusion, cognitive dysfunction
Non-steroidal anti- inflammatory drugs (NSAIDs)	Gastric erosions Small bowel and colonic lesions (less frequently than gastric) Upper gastrointestinal bleeding Perforated peptic ulcer Salt and water retention Renal impairment

Patients with renal disease

Prescribing drugs that require renal excretion as a major form of drug clearance can be problematic in patients with coexisting chronic kidney disease.

In chronic kidney disease there is less glomerular filtration of drugs leading to reduced renal clearance, enhanced drug half-life and potential for drug accumulation. As well as these significant pharmacokinetic considerations, patients with chronic kidney disease appear to be more susceptible and sensitive to adverse drug effects. Furthermore, some medications, such as thiazide and thiazide-like diuretics, work from the luminal side of the collecting duct, and therefore are ineffective in advanced chronic kidney disease.

The level of renal function below which the dose of a drug must be reduced depends on the proportion of the drug eliminated by renal excretion and its toxicity. For many drugs with only minor or no dose-related side-effects very precise modification of the dose regimen is unnecessary and a simple scheme for dose reduction is sufficient. For more toxic drugs with a small safety margin or patients at extremes of weight, dose regimens based on renal function should be used. When both efficacy and toxicity are closely related to plasma drug concentration, dosage must be adjusted according to clinical response and plasma drug concentration.

Renal function can be measured in different ways. Renal function varies with age. Term infants have 30% of adult renal capacity and adult function is reached by 9–12 months. From the fourth decade onwards, GFR decreases by approximately 1 mL/min per year. Serum creatinine is a simple measure of renal function but is dependent on muscle mass and is only elevated once 50% of renal function is lost. Estimates of GFR are better, as they take into account age and sex (and some formulas take into account other factors such as weight and ethnicity). Most drug adjustments are recommended to use estimated GFR (eGFR) or creatinine clearance (usually calculated by the Cockcroft–Gault formula). Although there is a good correlation between these two measures, at the extremes of weight there can be significant differences and so the relevant drug literature should be checked when prescribing for patients with chronic kidney disease to be sure which measure is recommended.

Various patterns of drug-induced nephrotoxicity can occur:

- *Pre-renal*: diuretics (volume), angiotensin-converting enzyme (ACE) inhibitors (renal perfusion), antihypertensive medications (hypotension).
- *Intrinsic*: glomerular (non-steroidal anti-inflammatory drugs, NSAIDs), immune (PPIs), tubular (lithium).
- *Post-renal*: drug crystallization (aciclovir), oxalate crystallization (allopurinol).

It is good practice to advise avoidance where possible of nephrotoxic drugs, especially over-the-counter drugs such as NSAIDs, in patients with chronic kidney disease.

Patients with liver disease

Prescribing drugs that require hepatic metabolism as a major form of drug clearance can be problematic in patients with coexisting chronic liver disease.

In chronic liver disease, there is less first-pass metabolism. In addition, there are often portosystemic shunts. Therefore, after oral dosing these combine to increase the proportion of drug that enters the systemic circulation, increasing drug exposure for a fixed-given dose.

However, some drugs require hepatic metabolism for efficacy (prodrugs, such as clopidogrel). For prodrugs, the presence of chronic liver disease and/or portosystemic shunts reduces the proportion of orally ingested drug that undergoes hepatic activation and therefore there is relatively less circulating active drug per oral dose.

The assessment of severity of chronic liver disease that requires dose-adjustment is more nebulous than when dose adjusting in renal failure. Although there are validated scoring systems for predicting outcome in chronic liver disease, such as Child–Pugh and MELD (see p. 1290), these have not been routinely used to make decisions on drug-dose adjustment. Holistic clinical assessment is preferred and the relevant drug literature should be consulted when prescribing for patients with chronic liver disease.

Drugs can cause liver injury in various patterns, for example:
- **hepatitis**: paracetamol, amiodarone, azathioprine
- **fatty change**: tetracyclines
- **cholestasis**: co-amoxiclav, nifedipine.

Therefore, for patients with chronic liver disease, avoid hepatotoxins if possible or reduce doses. For example, it is common to restrict paracetamol dosing to 2 g/day in chronic liver disease, compared with 4 g/day in patients without liver injury.

MONITORING DRUG THERAPY

The combination of pharmacokinetic and pharmacodynamic causes of variability makes monitoring of the effects of treatment essential. Three approaches are used:
- **Pre-treatment dose selection.** In patients who have known, or suspected, impaired renal or liver function, it is usually possible to predict dose requirements from their eGFR (see p. 1346) or clinical assessment of severity of chronic liver disease (see p. 1268).
- **Measuring plasma drug concentrations (therapeutic drug monitoring).** For a few drugs, dosages can be effectively monitored by reference to their plasma concentrations (**Box 12.8**). This technique, however, is useful only if both of the following criteria are fulfilled:
  - There is a reliable and available drug assay.
  - Plasma concentrations correlate well with both therapeutic efficacy and toxicity.

Therapeutic drug monitoring refers to the individualization of dosage by maintaining plasma or blood drug concentrations

within a target range (therapeutic range, therapeutic window). Using this pharmacokinetic approach, therapeutic drug monitoring is used in two major situations:
- when drugs are used prophylactically to maintain the **absence** of a condition, such as seizures, cardiac arrhythmias, depressive or manic episodes, asthma relapses or organ rejection
- to avoid serious toxicity, as with the aminoglycoside antibiotics which, unlike most antibiotics, have a narrow therapeutic range.

Measuring drug effects

For many drugs, dosage adjustments are made in line with patients' responses (pharmacodynamics approach). Monitoring can involve dose titration against a therapeutic end-point or a toxic effect. Objective measures (such as monitoring antihypertensive therapy by measuring blood pressure, or cytotoxic therapy with serial white blood cell counts) are most helpful, but subjective ones are necessary in many instances (as with antipsychotic therapy in people with schizophrenia). Pharmacodynamic tests can be used in clinical practice to target therapy or to avoid undue sensitivity. Examples are use of the INR or prothrombin time to titrate warfarin dosage to find the targeted level of anticoagulation for different diseases (see p. 1006).

Further reading

Pirmohamed M, Burnside G, Eriksson N et al. A randomized trial of genotype-guided dosing of warfarin. *N Engl J Med* 2013; 369:2294–2303.

ADVERSE DRUG REACTIONS

Adverse drug reactions (ADRs), defined as 'the unwanted effects of drugs occurring under normal conditions of use', are a significant cause of morbidity and mortality. The burden of ADRs is huge in both adults and children: ADRs account for about 6.5% of hospital admissions, affecting 15% of adult inpatients. In addition, about 1 in 4 patients in primary care will have an adverse reaction but fortunately these are mild in most cases. Unwanted effects of drugs are 5–6 times more likely in the elderly than in young adults, and the risk of an ADR rises sharply with the number of drugs administered. ADRs are also more common in women than in men.

Classification

Two types of ADR are recognized: type A (augmented) reactions and type B (idiosyncratic) reactions (**Box 12.9**).

Diagnosis

All ADRs mimic some naturally occurring disease, and drawing a distinction between an iatrogenic aetiology and an event unrelated to the drug is often difficult. The patient should be asked not only about prescription drugs but also about over-the-counter medicines, herbal medicines and illicit drugs. Although some effects are obviously iatrogenic (e.g. acute anaphylaxis occurring a few minutes after intravenous penicillin), many are less so.

Causality assessment of a suspected ADR can be difficult, particularly in patients on multiple drugs. The temporal relationship between drug exposure and suspected adverse events should be

---

i	**Box 12.8 Some drugs for which therapeutic drug monitoring is used**		

Drug	Therapeutic plasma concentration range	Toxic level	Optimum post-dose sampling time (h)
Carbamazepine	20–50 µmol/L	>50 µmol/L	>8
Ciclosporin	50–200 µg/L	>200 µg/L	Pre-dose
Digoxin	1.3–2.6 nmol/L	>2.6 nmol/L	>8
Gentamicin	Trough <2 mg/L	>2 mg/L	Pre-dose
	Peak 5–10 mg/L	>12 mg/L	>1
Lithium	0.6–1.0 mmol/L	>1.5 mmol/L	>10
Phenytoin	40–80 µmol/L	>80 µmol/L	>10
Theophylline	55–110 µmol/L	>110 µmol/L	>4
Vancomycin	15–20 mg/L	>20 mg/L	Pre-dose

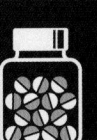

appropriate, and other causes of the suspected adverse events should be excluded. Rechallenge with the suspected drug and dechallenge (i.e. stopping the suspected drug to see if the adverse effect disappears) may be appropriate in certain circumstances. Some ADRs are so typical, such as cough or angio-oedema following initiation of ACE inhibitors, that identification of such as an ADR is likely.

Management

As a general rule, type A reactions can usually be managed by a reduction in dosage, while type B reactions almost invariably require the drug to be withdrawn (and never re-instituted). Most ADRs resolve spontaneously when the drug is withdrawn, but specific therapy is sometimes required for ADRs that cause acute patient harm (see p. 64). For example, bleeding with anticoagulants is actively reversed (vitamin K and prothrombin complex can be used for warfarin) and drug-induced anaphylaxis is a medical emergency, such that patients are given their own supply of adrenaline (epinephrine) to self-inject in such cases). When a patient suffers an ADR, this should be reported to the regulatory agency; for example, through the UK's **Yellow Card reporting** scheme to the Medicines Healthcare Products Regulatory Agency. The criteria for reporting vary across the world but, in general, all ADRs to new drugs or drugs used outside their licence should be reported, while only the serious ADRs to established drugs (i.e. those that have been on the market for usually more than 2 years) should be reported.

Further reading

Coleman JJ, Pontefract SK. Adverse drug reactions. *Clin Med* 2016; 16:481–485.

DRUG INTERACTIONS

Drugs can interact with each other (drug–drug interactions, DDIs), with food (drug–food interactions) and with herbal medicines (drug–herbal interactions) (**Box 12.10**). These interactions, in general, can be either pharmacokinetic (affecting the processes of absorption, distribution, metabolism and excretion), pharmacodynamic (synergistic or antagonistic) or mixed. Approximately 1% of all ADRs that lead to hospital admission are due to DDIs. A major risk factor for DDIs is polypharmacy, which is becoming more common because of the co-morbidities associated with an ageing population (see p. 305). About 57% of patients above the age of 65 years are on more than five drugs, with 12% being on more than ten drugs.

Food–drug interactions are also becoming increasingly recognized. A common example is grapefruit juice that inhibits CYP3A4 in the intestinal wall, increasing the bioavailability of drugs metabolized by CYP3A4 (see **Box 12.10**), resulting in higher exposure and toxicity.

Herbal medicines are taken by almost 20% of the population but are rarely asked about when a patient's clinical history is taken. Many different herbal–drug interactions have been described, the best recognized of which is with St John's Wort (SJW), which is an inducer of P450 enzymes and drug transporters, such as P-glycoprotein. SJW can lead to increased drug metabolism, reduction in drug concentration, and failure of therapeutic effect. An example is interaction with immunosuppressants such as prednisolone and ciclosporin, where the use of SJW has led to allograft rejection.

Reliable sources of information (see next section) must be used when prescribing new drugs to patients who already are taking other medications to ensure that no significant DDI exist.

Further reading

Bailey DG, Dresser G, Arnold JM. Grapefruit–medication interactions: forbidden fruit or avoidable consequences? *CMAJ* 2013; 185:309–316.
Magro L, Moretti U, Leone R. Epidemiology and characteristics of adverse drug reactions caused by drug–drug interactions. *Expert Opin Drug Saf* 2012; 11:83–94.

> **i   Box 12.9 Classification and examples of adverse drug reactions**
>
> **Type A (augmented)**
> - Common but only occasionally serious
> - Qualitatively normal, but quantitatively abnormal, manifestations of known pharmacology
> - Show a clear dose–response relationship
> - May occur after a single dose (hypotension with atenolol), or may develop after months (dependence with opioids), or years (second malignancies with anticancer drugs)
> - Usually reproducible in animal models
>
> | Type of drug (or drug class) | Type A adverse reaction |
> | --- | --- |
> | Anticoagulants, e.g. warfarin | Gastrointestinal bleeding
Intracerebral haemorrhage |
> | Antipsychotics, e.g. haloperidol | Acute dystonia/dyskinesia
Parkinsonian symptoms
Tardive dyskinesia |
> | Cytotoxic agents, e.g. 5-fluorouracil | Bone marrow dyscrasias
Cancer |
> | Diuretics, e.g. furosemide | Dehydration, renal impairment |
> | Insulin | Hypoglycaemia |
>
> **Type B (idiosyncratic)**
> - Usually rare and are often serious
> - Qualitatively abnormal responses to the drug (not predictable from its known pharmacology)
> - Show a dose–response relationship that is complex and not easily discernible
> - Not reproducible in animal models
>
> | Type of drug (or drug class) | Type B adverse reaction |
> | --- | --- |
> | Benzylpenicillin
Radiological contrast media | Anaphylaxis |
> | Broad-spectrum penicillins. e.g. co-amoxiclav | Maculopapular rash |
> | Phenytoin
Sulphonamides | Toxic epidermal necrolysis
Stevens–Johnson syndrome |
> | Diclofenac
Isoniazid | Hepatotoxicity |
> | Isotretinoin | Depression, suicidal ideation |

INFORMATION SOURCES

Pharmacotherapy moves at a very rapid pace and it is impossible for anyone to keep up with contemporary advances. Reliable prescribing advice can be found in:

- The **Summary of Product Characteristics (SmPCs)** produced by manufacturers and vetted by drug regulatory authorities.
- **The relevant national formulary.** Many countries have their own formularies: e.g. the UK has the *British National Formulary* (BNF).
- **Guidance** produced by national health technology agencies such as the UK's *National Institute for Health and Care Excellence (NICE)*.

Further reading

http://bnf.nice.org.uk *British National Formulary.*
http://www.guideline.gov *National Guideline Clearinghouse clinical guidelines in the USA.*
https://www.medicines.org.uk/emc *Electronic Medicines Compendium.*
http://www.nice.org.uk *National Institute for Health and Care Excellence (NICE) clinical guidelines.*

Box 12.10 Some examples of drug interactions

Implicated drug(s)	Affected drug(s)	Mechanism	Clinical effect
Pharmacokinetic: absorption			
Colestyramine	Digoxin	Binding of colestyramine to digoxin	Reduced digoxin plasma concentration and reduced efficacy
Pharmacokinetic: enzyme induction			
Carbamazepine	Oral contraceptive	CYP3A4 induction	Contraceptive failure
Phenytoin	Warfarin	CYP2C9 induction	Thrombosis
Rifampicin	Ciclosporin	CYP3A4 and P-glycoprotein induction	Allograft rejection
Pharmacokinetic: enzyme inhibition			
Amiodarone	Warfarin	CYP2C9 inhibition	Haemorrhage
Ciprofloxacin	Theophylline	CYP1A2 inhibition	Arrhythmias
Grapefruit juice	Simvastatin	CYP3A4 inhibition	Myopathy
Ritonavir	Inhaled fluticasone	CYP3A4 inhibition	Cushing's syndrome
Pharmacokinetic: excretion			
Naproxen	Methotrexate	Inhibition of methotrexate excretion	Methotrexate toxicity
Bendroflumethiazide	Lithium	Inhibition of lithium excretion	Lithium toxicity
Pharmacodynamic: synergistic interaction			
Verapamil	Atenolol	Atrioventricular node block	Bradycardia, heart block
Ramipril	Spironolactone	Reduced excretion of potassium	Hyperkalaemia
Pharmacodynamic: antagonistic interaction			
Salbutamol	Atenolol	Opposing effects at the β-receptor	Lack of bronchodilation
Furosemide	Digoxin	Hypokalaemia	Digoxin toxicity

POISONING

INTRODUCTION

In developed countries, poisoning is responsible for approximately 10% of acute hospital medical presentations and 1% of admissions. Most cases involve self-administration of prescribed or over-the-counter medicines, and/or illicit drugs.

- **Poisoning in children** aged <6 months is usually iatrogenic. Children between 8 months and 5 years of age may ingest poisons accidentally (due to inappropriate storage of prescribed or illicit medicines intended for use by an older family member/carer). Drugs may also be administered deliberately to cause harm (abuse by proxy).
- **Self-poisoning in adults** is commonly a 'cry for help', particularly among females <35 years old who are otherwise in good physical health. The overdose is taken in circumstances where they are likely to be found, often in the presence of others. In the over-55s, there is a preponderance of men who are suffering from mental and/or physical ill health.
- **Occupational poisoning** due to dermal or inhalational exposure to chemicals is more common in the developing world.
- Poisoning may be **iatrogenic**, and common in drugs with a narrow therapeutic window, e.g. lithium, digoxin, theophylline or phenytoin.
- The **type of agent** taken in overdose is influenced by availability and culture. In the UK, paracetamol poisoning remains the most common drug taken, whereas in Sri Lanka, for example, the agents ingested are more often pesticides (e.g. organophosphorus insecticides) or plants (e.g. oleander). In addition, ingestion of heating fuels, antimalarials, anti-tuberculous drugs and traditional medicines are common in the developing world. Poisoning from snake venoms is also a problem in rural areas.

Most patients taking an overdose reach for a drug, or a combination of drugs, that is easily available. To this end, **Box 12.11** lists some significant aspects of poisoning prevention. Acute overdoses often involve more than one agent, particularly alcohol. There is often a poor correlation between the patient's history (which itself may change over time) and subsequent analytical findings.

The majority of patients do not require intensive medical management, but all require a sympathetic and caring approach, with a psychiatric and social assessment. Fatalities in the UK are due predominantly to antidepressants, paracetamol, or analgesic combinations containing paracetamol and an opioid, heroin, methadone or cocaine. In North America there has been a substantial increase in recent years in fatal poisonings from prescription and illicit opioids (including fentanyl).

CLINICAL APPROACH TO THE POISONED PATIENT

History

More than 80% of adults are conscious on arrival at hospital and the diagnosis of self-poisoning can usually be made from the history (**Box 12.12**). Acute poisoning should be considered in the differential diagnosis of any patient presenting with impaired consciousness.

Examination

Box 12.13 provides a quick examination guide. The 'cluster of features' on presentation may be distinctive and diagnostic; for example, sinus tachycardia, fixed dilated pupils, exaggerated tendon reflexes, extensor plantar responses and coma suggest tricyclic antidepressant poisoning (**Box 12.14**).

Box 12.11 Prevention of self-poisoning

Patients usually take what is readily available at home:

- Only small amounts of drugs should be sold
- Foil-wrapped drugs are less likely to be taken in overdose
- Drugs should always be kept in a safe place
- Drugs and liquids should be kept in their original containers

- Child-resistant drug containers should be used
- Care should be taken in prescribing all drugs
- Prescriptions for any susceptible patient (e.g. the depressed) must be monitored
- Household products should be labelled and kept safely away from children

Box 12.12 History-taking in poisoning (record in notes)

- Obtain history (if possible) from patient, relatives, friends, paramedics, witnesses
- Seek evidence of overdose
- Establish whether suicide note was left
- Ascertain what drugs/poisons were taken
- Establish time/route taken

- Ask about additional drugs, e.g. alcohol
- Seek details from GP, e.g. prescribed medicines
- Assess suicide risk
- Assess capacity to make decisions
- Record a general history – past history, allergies, family history, social history

Box 12.13 Quick examination guide for the poisoned patient

- A B C D E (see p. 833)
- Level of consciousness (Glasgow Coma Scale; see p. 832)
- Ventilation – pulse oximetry
- Blood pressure and pulse rate

- Pupil size and reaction to light
- Temperature
- Head injury complicating poisonings
- If patient is unconscious, check cough and gag reflex

Box 12.14 Common feature clusters in acute poisoning

Feature clusters	Poisons
Coma, hypertonia, hyper-reflexia, extensor plantar responses, myoclonus, strabismus, mydriasis, sinus tachycardia	Tricyclic antidepressants; less commonly, antihistamines, particularly diphenhydramine
Coma, hypotonia, hyporeflexia, plantar responses flexor or non-elicitable, hypotension	Benzodiazepines, with or without alcohol
Coma, miosis, reduced respiratory rate	Opioid analgesics
Nausea, vomiting, tinnitus, deafness, sweating, hyperventilation, vasodilation, tachycardia	Salicylates
Hyperthermia, tachycardia, delirium, agitation, mydriasis	Ecstasy (MDMA) or other amfetamines, cathinones, cocaine
Miosis, hypersalivation, rhinorrhoea, bronchorrhoea	Organophosphorus and carbamate insecticides, nerve agents

PRINCIPLES OF MANAGEMENT OF POISONING

Most people with self-poisoning require only general care and support of the vital systems (**Box 12.15**). However, for a few poisons additional therapy is required.

Care of the unconscious patient

(See also page 833.) In all cases, the initial priority is to ensure that basic resuscitative measures are instituted promptly, establishing a clear airway and supporting breathing as necessary. Remember that pulse oximetry alone will not detect hypercapnia. Loss of the cough or gag reflex is the prime indication for intubation. In many severely poisoned patients, the reflexes are depressed sufficiently to allow intubation without the use of sedatives or relaxants.

Immediate catheterization of the bladder is not usually required. Insertion of a venous cannula is usual, but administration of intravenous fluids is unnecessary unless the patient has been unconscious for more than 12 hours, is dehydrated or is hypotensive.

Cardiovascular support

Severe hypotension and shock are unusual in the acutely poisoned patient but may be caused by:

- *a direct cardio-depressant action* of the poison (e.g. beta-blockers, calcium-channel blockers, tricyclic antidepressants)
- *vasodilation and venous pooling* in the lower limbs (e.g. ACE inhibitors, phenothiazines)
- *a decrease in circulating blood volume* because of gastrointestinal losses (e.g. profuse vomiting), increased sweating, increased renal losses and/or increased capillary permeability.

Hypotension may be exacerbated by coexisting hypoxia, acidosis and dysrhythmias. Volume expansion with intravenous crystalloids is usually sufficient to restore blood pressure. Volume replacement and the use of inotropes are discussed on pages 221–222. All patients with cardiogenic shock should have electrocardiographic (ECG) monitoring.

Systemic hypertension may occur in poisoning with drugs such as amfetamines and cocaine. If this is mild and associated with agitation, treatment with a benzodiazepine may suffice. In more severe cases there may be a risk of arterial rupture, particularly intracranial. To prevent this, intravenous nitrates such as glyceryl trinitrate are given, starting at a dose of 1–2 mg/h, gradually increasing the dose to a maximum of 12 mg/h until blood pressure is controlled. Calcium antagonists, such as verapamil 240–480 mg daily in divided doses, are an alternative second-line therapy. Sodium nitroprusside 0.5–1.5 μg/kg/min (to a maximum of 8 μg/kg/min) is an option for patients with increased blood pressure when there is no evidence of cardiac ischaemia, but caution is required as it may cause a rapid fall in blood pressure.

Arrhythmias can occur, such as tachyarrhythmias following ingestion of a tricyclic antidepressant, or bradyarrhythmias with digoxin poisoning. Known arrhythmogenic factors, such as hypoxia, acidosis and hypokalaemia, should be corrected.

Box 12.15 Management strategy in acute poisoning

Immediate decisions
- Supportive treatment
- Is an antidote appropriate? (see **Box 12.16**)
- Is it appropriate to try to reduce poison absorption?
- Is it appropriate to perform toxicological investigations?
- Is it appropriate to try to enhance elimination?

Practical points – contact with poison

Eyes
- Remove contact lenses
- Wash eyes with 0.9% saline or water for about 15 min
- Assess corneal damage (if necessary) with slit lamp and fluorescein stain

Skin
- Remove clothing
- Wash thoroughly with soap and water if, e.g., chemical exposure

Other problems

Hypothermia

A rectal temperature below 35°C is a recognized complication of poisoning, especially in older patients or in those who are comatose. The patient should be covered with a 'space blanket' and, if necessary, given intravenous fluids at normal body temperature. The administration of heated (37°C), humidified oxygen delivered by face mask is also useful.

Hyperthermia

Body temperature can, rarely, increase to being potentially fatal after poisoning with central nervous stimulants such as cocaine, and amfetamines, including 'ecstasy' (MDMA) and the weight-loss/body-building agent dinitrophenol (DNP). Muscle tone is often increased and convulsions and rhabdomyolysis are common. Cooling measures, sedation with diazepam and, in severe cases, intravenous dantrolene (a skeletal muscle relaxant) 1 mg/kg body weight should be given.

Skin blisters

Skin blisters may be found in poisoned patients who are, or have been, unconscious and do not move. Such lesions are not diagnostic of specific poisons but are sufficiently common in poisoned patients (and sufficiently uncommon in patients unconscious from other causes) to be of diagnostic value.

Rhabdomyolysis

Rhabdomyolysis can occur from pressure necrosis in drug-induced coma, or it may complicate poisoning in the absence of coma, such as in ecstasy (MDMA) abuse. People with rhabdomyolysis are at risk of developing acute kidney injury from myoglobinaemia, particularly if they are hypovolaemic and have a metabolic acidosis. Severe rhabdomyolysis may lead to the development of a compartment syndrome (see p. 427), which can cause serious tissue damage if not treated promptly.

Convulsions

These may occur in poisoning from many drugs, including tricyclic antidepressants, mefenamic acid and opioids. Usually seizures are short-lived but, if they are prolonged, intravenous diazepam 10–20 mg or lorazepam 4 mg should be administered. Persistent fits must be controlled rapidly to prevent severe hypoxia, brain damage and laryngeal trauma. If diazepam or lorazepam in repeated dose is ineffective, second-line treatments include intravenous phenytoin (loading dose 20 mg/kg at not more than 50 mg/min) or intravenous phenobarbital sodium (10 mg/kg at not more than 100 mg/min). Phenytoin is contraindicated in cases of poisoning with sodium channel-blocking drugs (such as tricyclic antidepressants) and is relatively contraindicated in all cases of poisoning with cardiotoxic drugs.

Stress ulceration and bleeding

An intravenous PPI should be given to prevent stress ulceration of the stomach in the elderly and patients with a previous history of ulceration.

Body 'packers' and body 'stuffers'

Body 'packers' (sometimes called 'mules' or 'swallowers') are those who swallow a substantial number of packages containing illicit drugs as a means of smuggling. Heroin used to be the drug of choice but this has been superseded by cocaine. Although each package contains a potentially lethal amount of drug, packets are now usually machine-manufactured using a material that does not leak. Body packers may ingest up to 100–200 packages.

Body 'stuffers' swallow a small number of packages containing an illicit drug, usually heroin, cocaine, cannabis or an amfetamine, in an unplanned attempt to conceal evidence when on the verge of being arrested. These drugs are usually either unpackaged or poorly packaged and, as a consequence, leakage may occur over the ensuing 3–6 hours and cause significant symptoms. Some also hide illicit drug packages in their rectum or vagina with the same intent (these are sometimes known as **body 'pushers'**).

The **role of imaging** is usually confined to body packers; imaging has little role in the care of body stuffers or pushers. Ultrasound is of similar accuracy to abdominal X-ray in locating packages but is less accurate than computed tomography (CT). A urine screen for drugs of misuse should be performed. A screen that is positive for one or more drugs of misuse suggests that either the patient has used the drug in the previous few days, or at least one packet is leaking. A negative screen strongly suggests that no packet is leaking. Screens should be repeated daily, or immediately if the patient develops features of intoxication, to confirm the diagnosis.

Management

Packages can be removed most expeditiously in body stuffers by employing whole-bowel irrigation (see p. 263). Indications for urgent surgery in body packers include evidence of acute intestinal obstruction, radiological confirmation of many packets and clinical or analytical evidence to suggest package leakage, particularly if the drug involved is cocaine.

Packets in the vagina can usually be removed manually.

Specific management of the poisoned patient

Antidotes

Specific antidotes are available for a small number of poisons only (**Box 12.16**).

Antidotes may exert a beneficial effect by:

- *forming an inert complex* with the poison (e.g. desferrioxamine, dicobalt edetate, digoxin-specific antibody fragments, dimercaprol, HI-6, hydroxocobalamin, obidoxime, pralidoxime, sodium calcium edetate, succimer (dimercaptosuccinic acid; DMSA), Unithiol (dimercaptopropanesulphonate; DMPS))
- *accelerating detoxification* of the poison (e.g. acetylcysteine, sodium thiosulphate)
- *reducing the rate of conversion* of the poison to a more toxic compound (e.g. ethanol, fomepizole)
- *competing with the poison* for essential receptor sites (e.g. oxygen, naloxone, phytomenadione)
- *blocking essential receptors* through which the toxic effects are mediated (e.g. atropine)
- *bypassing the effect* of the poison (e.g. oxygen, glucagon).

Gut decontamination

Although it seems logical to assume that removal of unabsorbed drug from the gastrointestinal tract will be beneficial (gut decontamination), the efficacy of gastric lavage and syrup of ipecacuanha (to induce vomiting) remains unproven and efforts to remove small amounts of non-toxic drugs are clinically not worthwhile or appropriate.

Gastric lavage should only be performed if a patient has ingested a potentially life-threatening amount of a poison, e.g. iron, and the procedure can be undertaken within 60 minutes of ingestion. Ensure the airway is protected. Lavage is contraindicated if a hydrocarbon with high aspiration potential or a corrosive substance has been ingested.

Syrup of ipecacuanha to induce vomiting should *not* be used, as the amount of drug recovered is highly variable and diminishes with time; there is no evidence that it improves outcome.

Single-dose activated charcoal can adsorb a wide variety of compounds. Exceptions are strong acids and alkalis, ethanol, ethylene glycol, iron, lithium, mercury and methanol. In studies in volunteers given 50 g activated charcoal, the mean reduction in absorption was 40%, 16% and 21%, at 60 min, 120 min and 180 min, respectively, after ingestion. Administration of oral activated charcoal (50 g for an adult, 1 g/kg for a child) should be considered following ingestion of a potentially toxic amount of a poison (except those listed above) if this is possible within 1 hour of ingestion. There are insufficient data to support or exclude its use after 1 hour. There is no evidence that administration of activated charcoal improves clinical outcome.

Cathartics have no role in the management of the poisoned patient.

Whole-bowel irrigation requires the insertion of a nasogastric tube into the stomach and the introduction of polyethylene glycol electrolyte solution 1500–2000 mL/h in an adult, which is continued until the rectal effluent is clear. Whole-bowel irrigation may be used for potentially toxic ingestions of sustained-release or enteric-coated drugs, or to remove illicit drug packets.

Increasing poison elimination

Multiple-dose activated charcoal (MDAC) involves the repeated administration of oral activated charcoal to increase elimination of

Box 12.16 Antidotes of value in poisoning

Poison	Antidotes
Aluminium	Desferrioxamine
Arsenic	Succimer (DMSA), dimercaprol
Benzodiazepines	Flumazenil
β-Adrenoceptor-blocking drugs	Atropine, glucagon
Calcium-channel blockers	Atropine
Carbamate insecticides	Atropine
Carbon monoxide	Oxygen
Cyanide	Oxygen, dicobalt edetate, hydroxocobalamin, sodium nitrite, sodium thiosulphate
Digoxin and digitoxin	Digoxin-specific antibody fragments
Ethylene glycol	Fomepizole, ethanol
Hydrogen sulphide	Oxygen
Iron salts	Desferrioxamine
Lead (inorganic)	Succimer (DMSA), sodium calcium edetate
Methaemoglobinaemia	Methylthioninium chloride (methylene blue)
Methanol	Fomepizole, ethanol
Mercury (inorganic)	Unithiol (DMPS)
Nerve agents	Atropine, HI-6, obidoxime, pralidoxime
Opioids	Naloxone
Organophosphorus insecticides	Atropine, HI-6, obidoxime, pralidoxime
Paracetamol	Acetylcysteine
Warfarin and similar anticoagulants	Phytomenadione (vitamin K)

DMPS, dimercaptopropanesulphonate; DMSA, dimercaptosuccinic acid.

a drug that has already been absorbed. Most absorbed drugs re-enter the gut from the villi capillaries by passive diffusion (a few by an active process) if the concentration in the gut is lower than that in the blood (this is called the entero-enteric circulation). Some drugs are also secreted in the bile (enterohepatic circulation). Activated charcoal will bind any drug that is in the gut lumen, so keeping the concentration in the gut low and favouring further diffusion from blood to gut lumen.

Elimination of drugs with a small volume of distribution (<1 L/kg), low pK_a (which maximizes transport across membranes), low binding affinity and prolonged elimination half-life following overdose is particularly likely to be enhanced by MDAC. MDAC also improves total body clearance of the drug when endogenous processes are compromised by liver and/or renal failure.

Although MDAC has been shown to increase drug elimination significantly, it has not reduced morbidity and mortality in controlled studies. At present, MDAC should be used only in patients who have ingested a life-threatening amount of carbamazepine, dapsone, phenobarbital, quinine or theophylline.

In *adults*, charcoal should be administered in an initial dose of 50–100 g and then at a rate of not less than 12.5 g/h, preferably via a nasogastric tube; usually, 200 g is sufficient. Intravenous ondansetron 4–8 mg is an effective antiemetic and facilitates MDAC administration if vomiting is a problem.

Urine alkalinization enhances elimination of salicylate, phenobarbital and chlorophenoxy herbicides (e.g. 2,4-dichlorophenoxyacetic acid) by mechanisms that are not clearly understood. Urine alkalinization is a metabolically invasive procedure requiring frequent biochemical monitoring and medical and nursing expertise. Advice should be sought from those familiar with the procedure before urine alkalinization is commenced. Plasma volume depletion, electrolytes (notably plasma potassium since sodium bicarbonate exacerbates pre-existing hypokalaemia) and metabolic abnormalities should be corrected first. Sufficient bicarbonate is then administered to ensure that urine pH is over 7.5 and preferably close to 8.5. In one study, sodium bicarbonate 225 mmol was the mean amount required initially. This can be administered intravenously as 225 mL of an 8.4% solution (1 mmol bicarbonate/mL) over 1 hour but great care must be taken to avoid extravasation if given via a peripheral line.

Haemodialysis and haemodiafiltration are of little value in patients poisoned with drugs that have large volumes of distribution (e.g. tricyclic antidepressants) because the plasma contains only a small proportion of the total amount of drug in the body. These methods are indicated in patients with severe clinical features and high plasma concentrations of ethanol, ethylene glycol, isopropanol, lithium, methanol and salicylate: that is, drugs with small volumes of distribution.

Lipid emulsion therapy involves the intravenous administration of 20% Intralipid (fractionated soya oil) 1.5 mL/kg, followed by 0.25–0.5 mL/kg per minute for 30-60 minutes to an initial maximum of 500 mL. Use of lipid emulsion as an antidote for severe poisoning with highly lipid-soluble drugs is based on experience of its efficacy in local anaesthetic poisoning. It is believed to increase the intravascular lipid phase, so creating a 'lipid sink' to reduce the amount of active drug in plasma. Other proposed mechanisms of benefit include increasing myocardial fatty acid energy substrate and improving the function of cell membrane-bound ion channels (particularly Ca^{2+} and Na^+). The role of Intralipid in the management of poisoning with highly lipid-soluble drugs is not well defined but case reports suggest some benefit in life-threatening cardiotoxicity that is resistant to other measures.

Investigations

Box 12.17 (and see also **Box 12.20**) sets out investigations that may be helpful in poisoned patients. On admission, or at an appropriate time post overdose, a timed blood sample should be taken if it is suspected that aspirin, digoxin, ethylene glycol, iron, lithium, methanol, paracetamol, paraquat, quinine or theophylline has been ingested (**Box 12.18**). The determination of the concentrations of these drugs will be valuable in management. Drug screens on blood and urine are occasionally indicated in severely poisoned patients in whom the cause of coma is unknown. A poison information service will advise.

> **ℹ Box 12.17 Investigations that may be helpful in poisoned patients**
>
> - Serum creatinine and electrolytes, estimated glomerular filtration rate
> - Creatine kinase activity
> - Acid–base assessment (arterial gas, unless no concern regarding ventilation)
> - Blood for specific poisons (see later)
> - Electrocardiography (see p. 265)
> - Urine saved (plain tube) for possible drug screen
> - Radiology (see p. 265)

Some routine investigations (**Box 12.19**) are of value in the differential diagnosis of coma or the detection of poison-induced hypokalaemia, hyperkalaemia, hypoglycaemia, hyperglycaemia, hepatic or renal failure or metabolic acidosis (**Box 12.20**). Measurement of carboxyhaemoglobin, methaemoglobin and cholinesterase activities are of assistance in the diagnosis and management of cases of poisoning due to carbon monoxide, methaemoglobin-inducing agents, such as nitrites, and organophosphorus insecticides, respectively.

ECG

Routine ECG is of limited diagnostic value, but continuous ECG monitoring should be undertaken in those ingesting potentially cardiotoxic drugs; for example, sinus tachycardia with prolongation of the PR and QRS intervals in an unconscious patient suggests tricyclic antidepressant overdose. QT interval prolongation is an adverse effect of several drugs (e.g. quetiapine).

> **ℹ Box 12.18 Laboratory analysis for toxins**
>
> - Carbon monoxide (carboxyhaemoglobin) concentrations are available on most blood gas analysers
> - Ethanol (when monitoring treatment in glycol and methanol poisoning)
> - Ethylene glycol
> - Iron
> - Lithium
> - Methanol
> - Paracetamol
> - Salicylate
> - Theophylline

> **ℹ Box 12.19 Relevant non-toxicological investigations with examples**
>
> | Investigation | Situation |
> |---|---|
> | **Serum sodium concentration** | Hyponatraemia in ecstasy (MDMA) poisoning |
> | **Serum potassium concentration** | Hypokalaemia in theophylline poisoning
Hyperkalaemia in digoxin poisoning |
> | **Serum creatinine concentration** | Estimated glomerular filtration rate (eGFR) in acute kidney injury in ethylene and diethylene glycol poisoning |
> | **Acid–base disturbances** | Including metabolic acidosis (see **Box 12.20**) |
> | **Blood glucose concentration** | Hypoglycaemia in insulin poisoning
Hyperglycaemia in salicylate poisoning |
> | **Serum calcium concentration** | Hypocalcaemia in ethylene glycol poisoning |
> | **Liver function (prothrombin time)** | In paracetamol poisoning |
> | **Carboxyhaemoglobin concentration** | In carbon monoxide poisoning |
> | **Methaemoglobin concentration** | In nitrite poisoning |
> | **Cholinesterase activity** | Organophosphorus insecticide and nerve agent poisoning |
> | **ECG** | Wide QRS in tricyclic antidepressant poisoning |
> | **X-ray** | Detection of radio-opaque toxins, e.g. elemental mercury |

> **Box 12.20** Some poisons that induce metabolic acidosis

- Carbon monoxide
- Cyanide
- Ethanol
- Ethylene glycol
- Iron
- Metformin
- Methanol
- Paracetamol
- Salicylates
- Tricyclic antidepressants

> **Box 12.21** Regimen for acetylcysteine

- Acetylcysteine 150 mg/kg in 200 mL 5% glucose over 60 min
- Then 50 mg/kg in 500 mL of 5% glucose over the next 4 h
- Then 100 mg/kg in 1000 mL of 5% glucose over the ensuing 16 h
- Total dose 300 mg/kg over 21 h

Radiology

Routine radiology is of little diagnostic value. It can confirm ingestion of metallic objects (e.g. coins, button batteries) or injection of globules of metallic mercury. Some enteric-coated or sustained-release drugs or ingested packets of illicit substances may be seen on plain abdominal X-rays. Radiology can confirm complications of poisoning, such as aspiration pneumonia, non-cardiogenic pulmonary oedema (salicylates) and acute respiratory distress syndrome (ARDS).

SPECIFIC POISONS

- *All patients must be reviewed by senior medical staff.*
- *All **patients** should have relevant blood tests and monitoring when appropriate.*
- The general principles of management of self-poisoning outlined earlier will always need to be applied.

In this section, only the specific treatment regimens are outlined. The first section covers the 'top ten' drug types encountered in poisoning; paracetamol, NSAIDs, opiates/opioids, antidepressants, benzodiazepines, stimulants (including cocaine), ethanol, neuroleptics, cannabis/synthetic cannabinoids and anticonvulsants. All doctors working in an acute setting should be familiar with the clinical presentation and principles of management of poisoning with these agents.

The top ten

Paracetamol (acetaminophen)

In ***therapeutic doses***, paracetamol is conjugated with glucuronide and sulphate. A small amount of paracetamol is metabolized by mixed-function oxidase enzymes to form a highly reactive toxic compound (*N*-acetyl-*p*-benzoquinoneimine; NAPQI), which is then immediately conjugated with glutathione and subsequently excreted as cysteine and mercapturic conjugates.

In ***overdose***, large amounts of paracetamol are metabolized by oxidation because of saturation of the sulphate conjugation pathway. Liver glutathione stores become depleted so that the liver is unable to deactivate NAPQI. Paracetamol-induced kidney injury probably results from a mechanism similar to that responsible for hepatotoxicity.

Clinical features

Following the ingestion of an overdose of paracetamol, patients usually remain asymptomatic for the first 24 hours or, at the most, develop anorexia, nausea and vomiting. Liver damage is not usually detectable by routine liver function tests until at least 18 hours after ingestion of the drug. Liver damage usually reaches a peak, as assessed by measurement of alanine transferase (ALT) activity and prothrombin time (INR), at 72–96

hours after ingestion. Without treatment, a small percentage of patients will develop fulminant hepatic failure. Acute kidney injury due to acute tubular necrosis occurs in 25% of patients who have severe hepatic damage and in a few without evidence of serious disturbance of liver function.

Management

Acetylcysteine is an effective protective agent, provided that it is administered within 8–10 hours of ingestion of the overdose. It acts by replenishing cellular glutathione stores, though it may also repair oxidation damage caused by NAPQI. The treatment regimen is shown in **Box 12.21**.

There are now two main approaches to treatment worldwide. In the UK, following a decision by the Medicines and Healthcare products Regulatory Agency (MHRA) in 2012 to abandon a detailed risk assessment in the decision to treat, it is deemed that patients with concentrations above a 'treatment line' starting at 100 mg/L 4 hours after ingestion (**Fig. 12.2**) should be given treatment with acetylcysteine. In most other countries, a parallel line starting at 150 mg/L 4 hours after ingestion is used, though some still follow the original treatment line starting at 200 mg/L 4 hours after ingestion. The treatment lines (see **Fig. 12.2**) are uncertain if the patient presents 15 hours or more after ingestion or has taken a modified-release preparation of paracetamol. Although these lines are often extended to 24 hours (dotted lines), the concentrations are not based on clinical trial data.

A summary of single acute paracetamol overdose management at different times post ingestion is given in **Box 12.22**. Note that patients whose paracetamol overdose is staggered over more than 1 hour or who take repeated therapeutic excess are at greater risk of liver damage, and decisions to treat are generally based on the dose ingested/24 hours. In the UK, treatment with acetylcysteine is considered if more than 75 mg/kg has been ingested in 24 hours.

Up to 15% of patients treated with intravenous acetylcysteine develop a rash, angio-oedema, hypotension and/or bronchospasm. These reactions, which are histamine-mediated and related to the initial bolus, are seldom serious and discontinuing the infusion is usually all that is required. In more severe, adult cases, intravenous chlorphenamine 10–20 mg should be given.

If liver or renal failure ensues, this should be treated conventionally, although there is evidence that a continuing infusion of acetylcysteine (continue 16-h infusion until recovery) will improve the morbidity and mortality. Liver transplantation has been performed successfully in patients who have paracetamol-induced acute hepatic failure (see **Box 34.13**).

Non-steroidal anti-inflammatory drugs

Self-poisoning with non-steroidal anti-inflammatory drugs (NSAIDs), other than salicylates, has increased, particularly now that ibuprofen is available without prescription, over the counter, in many countries. Poisoning with salicylates is considered on page 271.

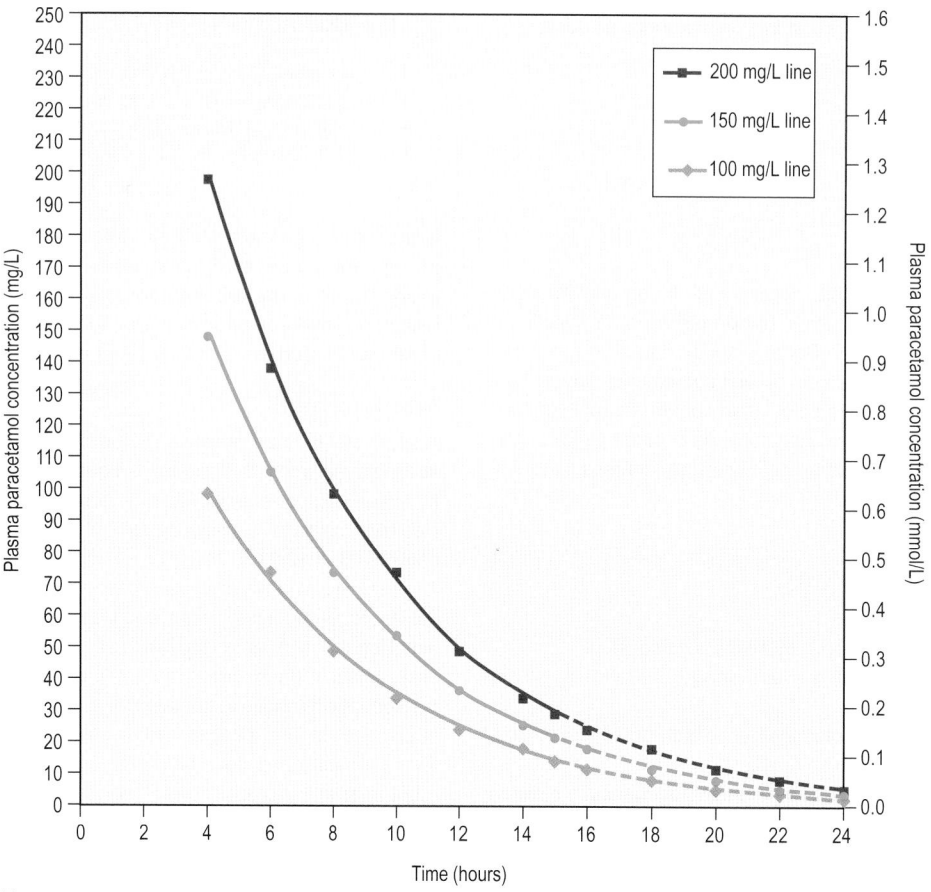

Fig. 12.2 Nomogram for treatment of paracetamol poisoning. Note that the treatment lines are uncertain if the patient presents 15 hours or more after ingestion, or has taken a modified-release preparation of paracetamol. Although these lines are often extended to 24 hours (dotted lines), the concentrations are not based on clinical trial data.

 Box 12.22 Summary of management of single acute paracetamol overdose

All patients

- Clarify date, time, formulation and dose of paracetamol taken
- Weigh the patient
- Calculate the paracetamol dose ingested in mg/kg

Patients presenting 0–8 hours since last paracetamol ingestion

- Wait until 4 h post ingestion then take venous blood for plasma paracetamol concentration, serum creatinine and electrolytes, bicarbonate, liver function and INR
- If the blood results will not be available until after 8 h post ingestion *AND* patient has ingested >150 mg/kg, commence acetylcysteine immediately
- When the plasma paracetamol concentration is available, assess need for antidotal treatment with acetylcysteine using the treatment nomogram (see **Fig. 12.2**)
- Administer acetylcysteine if required. If already commenced but not required, acetylcysteine can be discontinued at this stage
- Seek specialist advice if plasma paracetamol concentration is below the treatment line but LFTs or clotting are abnormal
- At end of acetylcysteine course take venous blood for serum creatine and electrolytes, liver function and INR
- Consider need for further acetylcysteine if post-treatment bloods are abnormal

Patients presenting between 8 h and 24 h after paracetamol ingestion

- Take venous blood for urgent measurement of plasma paracetamol concentration, serum creatinine and electrolytes, bicarbonate, liver function, INR
- Commence acetylcysteine immediately if ingested paracetamol dose is >150 mg/kg
- If ingested dose <150 mg/kg, await blood results and assess need for acetylcysteine using treatment nomogram

- Administer acetylcysteine if required. If already commenced but not required, acetylcysteine can be discontinued at this stage
- BEWARE that for patients presenting >12 h after ingestion, the plasma paracetamol concentration at which treatment is required may be close to the laboratory's limit of detection. If borderline, treat with acetylcysteine
- Seek specialist advice if plasma paracetamol concentration is below the treatment line but LFTs or clotting are abnormal
- At end of acetylcysteine course take venous blood for serum creatinine and electrolytes, bicarbonate, liver function and INR
- Consider need for further acetylcysteine if post-treatment bloods are abnormal

Patients presenting more than 24 h post overdose

- Commence acetylcysteine if the patient is jaundiced or has hepatic tenderness
- Measure the plasma paracetamol concentration (before NAC is administered if possible), serum creatinine and electrolytes, bicarbonate, LFTs, glucose, FBC and INR
- Treat with acetylcysteine if the ALT is above the upper limit of normal, *OR* INR is >1.3 (in the absence of another cause, e.g. warfarin) *OR* paracetamol concentration is detectable
- If the paracetamol concentration is not detectable, the INR and ALT are normal, and the patient is asymptomatic, no treatment with an antidote is indicated. If acetylcysteine has been started it may then be discontinued
- At end of acetylcysteine course take venous blood for serum creatinine and electrolytes, bicarbonate, liver function and INR
- Consider need for further acetylcysteine if post treatment bloods are abnormal

ALT, alanine transferase; FBC, full blood count; LFTs, liver function tests; INR, international normalized ratio; NAC, N-acetyl cysteine.

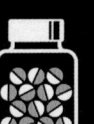

Clinical features and management

In most cases, minor gastrointestinal disturbance is the only feature but, in more severe cases, coma, convulsions and acute kidney injury have occurred. Transient renal impairment is common after ibuprofen overdose. Poisoning with mefenamic acid commonly results in convulsions, though these are usually short-lived.

Treatment is symptomatic and supportive.

Opiates and opioids

Clinical features

Cardinal signs of opiate poisoning are pinpoint pupils, reduced respiratory rate and coma. Hypothermia, hypoglycaemia and convulsions are occasionally observed in severe cases. Non-cardiogenic pulmonary oedema has been reported in severe heroin overdose. See page 141 for more information about the worldwide opioid crisis.

Management

Intravenous naloxone will reverse respiratory depression and coma, at least partially. In severe poisoning, an initial dose of 1.2 mg is likely to be required and repeat doses necessary. Lower doses (0.4–0.8 mg) may suffice in less severe cases and if precipitating opioid withdrawal is a concern. The duration of action of naloxone is often less than the drug taken in overdose; for example, methadone, which has a very long half-life. For this reason, an infusion of naloxone is often required. Non-cardiogenic pulmonary oedema should be treated with mechanical ventilation.

Antidepressants: tricyclics and selective serotonin reuptake inhibitors

Tricyclic antidepressants block the reuptake of monoamines (e.g. norepinephrine (noradrenaline) and serotonin) into peripheral and intracerebral neurones, thereby increasing the concentration of these neurotransmitters in these areas. They also have antimuscarinic actions and class 1 antiarrhythmic (quinidine-like) sodium-channel-blocking activity.

Selective serotonin reuptake inhibitors (SSRIs) (e.g. citalopram, escitalopram, fluoxetine, fluvoxamine, paroxetine and sertraline) lack the antimuscarinic and sodium-channel-blocking actions of tricyclic antidepressants.

Clinical features

Tricyclic antidepressants. Mild poisoning commonly causes drowsiness, sinus tachycardia, dry mouth, dilated pupils, urinary retention (all antimuscarinic effects), and increased reflexes and extensor plantar responses. Severe intoxication leads to coma, convulsions and, occasionally, divergent strabismus. Plantar, oculocephalic and oculovestibular reflexes may be abolished temporarily. An ECG will often show a wide QRS interval and there is a reasonable correlation between the width of the QRS complex and the severity of poisoning. Life-threatening arrhythmias may ensue. Metabolic acidosis and cardiorespiratory depression are observed in severe cases.

SSRIs. Even in large overdoses, SSRIs appear to be relatively safe unless potentiated by ethanol. Most patients will show no signs of toxicity but drowsiness, nausea, diarrhoea and sinus tachycardia have been reported. Rarely, junctional bradycardia, seizures and hypertension have been encountered and influenza-like symptoms may develop.

Serotonin syndrome occasionally occurs (see p. 781).

Venlafaxine is a serotonin norepinephrine reuptake inhibitor (SNRI) with a similar toxicity profile to the SSRIs but with greater risk of cardiac arrhythmias and convulsions. Mirtazapine, an antidepressant that acts via presynaptic alpha blockade to increase central serotonin release, is probably the safest antidepressant in overdose, causing mainly only sedation.

Management

The majority of patients recover with supportive therapy alone (adequate oxygenation, control of convulsions and correction of acidosis), although a small percentage who ingest a tricyclic will require assisted ventilation for 24–48 hours. The onset of supraventricular tachycardia and ventricular tachycardia should be treated with intravenous sodium bicarbonate (8.4%) 50 mmol, even if there is no acidosis present; a second bolus may be required.

Benzodiazepines

Benzodiazepines are commonly taken in overdose but rarely produce severe poisoning, except in the elderly or those with chronic respiratory disease.

Clinical features

Benzodiazepines produce drowsiness, ataxia, dysarthria and nystagmus. Coma and respiratory depression develop in severe intoxication.

Management

If respiratory depression is present in patients who have severe benzodiazepine poisoning, intravenous flumazenil 0.5–1.0 mg is given in an adult and this dose often needs repeating. Flumazenil use often avoids the need for assisted ventilation. It is relatively contraindicated in patients with mixed proconvulsant (e.g. tricyclic antidepressants)/benzodiazepine poisoning and those with a history of epilepsy because it may cause convulsions.

Stimulants

The most commonly abused stimulants are the amfetamines, cocaine and the synthetic cathinones.

Amfetamines are central nervous system (CNS) and cardiovascular stimulants. These effects are mediated by increasing synaptic concentrations of adrenaline (epinephrine) and dopamine. The *N*-methylated derivative, metamfetamine (the crystalline form of this salt is known as 'crystal meth' or 'ice'), and 3,4-methylenedioxymetamfetamine (MDMA), known as ecstasy, are common examples.

Cocaine hydrochloride ('street' cocaine, 'coke') is a water-soluble powder or granule that can be taken orally, intravenously or intranasally ('snorting'). 'Freebase' or 'crack' cocaine comprises crystals ('rocks') of relatively pure cocaine without the hydrochloride moiety. Crack cocaine is more suitable for smoking in a pipe or mixed with tobacco; it can also be heated on foil and the vapour inhaled (approximately 35 mg of drug per 'line' or a 'rail'). The effects of cocaine are experienced almost immediately after intravenous administration or smoking, about 10 minutes following intranasal administration and 45–90 minutes after ingestion. The effects start to resolve in about 20 minutes but may last up to 90 minutes. In severe poisoning, death occurs in minutes, and death rarely occurs more than 3 hours after exposure.

Cocaine blocks the reuptake of biogenic amines:

- Inhibition of dopamine reuptake is responsible for psychomotor effects.
- Blockade of noradrenaline (norepinephrine) reuptake produces tachycardia.
- Inhibition of serotonin reuptake induces hallucinations.
- CNS arousal is enhanced by potentiating the effects of excitatory amino acids.
- Cocaine is a powerful local anaesthetic and vasoconstrictor.

Cathinone (khat) is a naturally occurring stimulant derived from the plant *Catha edulis*. The drug is released during prolonged chewing of plant leaves. An increasing number of synthetic cathinone derivatives are available, the best-known of which is mephedrone (4-methyl methcathinone). While typically sold as 'plant foods' or 'bath salts', these 'legal highs' are purchased for their recreational abuse potential. Synthetic cathinones may be taken by mouth, nasal insufflation or injection.

Clinical features

Stimulants cause dilated pupils, tachycardia and hypertension, sweating, euphoria, extrovert behaviour, and a lack of desire to eat or sleep. More severe intoxication is associated with agitation, paranoid delusions, hallucinations and violent behaviour. Convulsions, rhabdomyolysis, hyperthermia, metabolic acidosis and cardiac arrhythmias may develop. Rarely, dissection of the aorta, myocarditis, myocardial infarction, dilated cardiomyopathy, subarachnoid haemorrhage, or cerebral haemorrhage or infarction may occur and can be fatal. Disseminated intravascular coagulation and acute kidney injury are recognized. If a young person presents with a stroke or myocardial infarction, poisoning with a stimulant should be considered in the differential diagnosis.

Management

Agitation is best controlled by intravenous diazepam 10–20 mg. Hypertension and tachycardia also usually respond to sedation but if hypertension persists, consider intravenous glyceryl trinitrate starting at 1–2 mg/h and gradually increase the dose (maximum 12 mg/h) until the blood pressure is controlled. The peripheral sympathomimetic actions of amfetamines can be antagonized by β-adrenoceptor-blocking drugs but these are rarely required. The use of beta-blockers in cocaine poisoning is controversial. Active external cooling should be employed for hyperthermia and if uncontrolled, intravenous dantrolene 1 mg/kg body weight should be considered (see p. 262). Early use of a benzodiazepine is often effective in relieving stimulant-associated non-cardiac chest pain. Myocardial ischaemia/infarction should be treated conventionally.

Ethanol

Ethanol is commonly ingested in beverages and deliberately with other substances in overdose. It is also present in many cosmetic and antiseptic preparations. Following absorption, ethanol is oxidized to acetaldehyde and then to acetate. Ethanol is a CNS depressant and the features of ethanol intoxication are generally related to blood concentrations (**Box 12.23**).

Box 12.23 Clinical features of ethanol poisoning

Blood (ethanol)		Clinical features
mg/L	mmol/L	
500–1500	11.0–32.5	Emotional lability Mild impairment of coordination
1500–3000	32.5–65.0	Visual impairment Incoordination Slowed reaction time Slurred speech
3000–5000	65.0–108.5	Marked incoordination Blurred or double vision Stupor Occasionally, hypoglycaemia, hypothermia and convulsions
>5000	>108.5	Depressed reflexes Respiratory depression Hypotension Hypothermia Death (from respiratory or circulatory failure, or from aspiration)

Clinical features

In children in particular, severe hypoglycaemia may accompany alcohol intoxication due to inhibition of gluconeogenesis. Hypoglycaemia is also observed in those who are malnourished or who have fasted in the previous 24 hours. In severe cases of intoxication, coma and hypothermia are often present, and lactic acidosis, ketoacidosis and acute kidney injury have been reported.

Management

Supportive care is paramount. Intravenous glucose may be required to treat hypoglycaemia. Haemodialysis should be considered if the blood ethanol concentration exceeds 7500 mg/L and if a severe metabolic acidosis (see p. 198) is present, which has not been corrected by fluids and intravenous bicarbonate.

Neuroleptics and atypical neuroleptics

Neuroleptic (antipsychotic) drugs are thought to act predominantly by blockade of dopamine D_2 receptors. The ***first-generation neuroleptics*** include the phenothiazines (chlorpromazine), the butyrophenones (benperidol, haloperidol) and the substituted benzamides (sulpiride). More ***selective second-generation (or 'atypical') antipsychotics*** include amisulpride, aripiprazole, clozapine, olanzapine, quetiapine and risperidone.

Clinical features

These include impaired consciousness, hypotension, respiratory depression, hypothermia or hyperthermia, antimuscarinic effects such as tachycardia, dry mouth and blurred vision, occasionally seizures, rhabdomyolysis, cardiac arrhythmias (both atrial and ventricular) and ARDS. Extrapyramidal effects, including acute dystonic reactions, occur but are not dose related. Most 'atypical' antipsychotics have less profound sedative actions than the older neuroleptics.

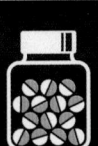

QT interval prolongation and subsequent ventricular arrhythmias (including torsades de pointes) have occurred following overdose with the atypical neuroleptics. Unpredictable fluctuations in conscious level, with variations between agitation and marked somnolence, have been particularly associated with olanzapine overdose.

Management

Intravenous procyclidine 5–10 mg in an adult can occasionally be required for the treatment of dyskinesia and oculogyric crisis. After acidosis has been corrected with sodium bicarbonate, the preferred treatment for arrhythmias caused by antipsychotic drugs (including torsades de pointes) is intravenous magnesium (see p. 1065) or cardiac pacing (p. 1049).

Cannabis (marijuana) and synthetic cannabinoids

Cannabis is usually smoked but may be ingested as a 'cake', made into a tea or injected intravenously. The major psychoactive constituent is δ-11-tetrahydrocannabinol (THC). THC possesses activity at the benzodiazepine, opioid and cannabinoid receptors.

Synthetic cannabinoids emerged onto the drug scene around 2009, initially sold as herbal incense or 'spice'. There are now hundreds of derivatives and most are considerably more potent than THC.

Clinical features

Cannabis intoxication initially causes euphoria followed by distorted and heightened images, colours and sounds, altered tactile sensations and sinus tachycardia. Visual and auditory hallucinations and acute psychosis are particularly likely to occur after substantial ingestion in naive users. Heavy users suffer impairment of memory and attention, and poor academic performance. There is an increased risk of anxiety and depression. Regular users are at risk of dependence. Cannabis use results in an overall increase in the relative risk for later schizophrenia and psychotic episodes (see p. 793). Cannabis smoke is probably carcinogenic.

The clinical features observed following intoxication with synthetic cannabinoids are variable, reflecting the numerous derivatives available. Tachycardia and agitation are the most consistent effects but psychosis, seizures, respiratory failure, coma, acute kidney injury, stroke and myocardial infarction have all been reported and fatalities have occurred.

Management

Reassurance is usually the only treatment required, although sedation with intravenous diazepam (10–20 mg in an adult) or intramuscular or oral haloperidol (2–5 mg in an adult) is sometimes required if agitation is severe. Occasionally, agitation is sufficiently severe for patients to require sedation in a critical care environment.

Anticonvulsants
Clinical features

The clinical features of poisoning with anticonvulsant drugs are summarized in **Box 12.24**.

Management

Elimination of carbamazepine can be significantly increased by multiple-dose activated charcoal.

If hepatotoxicity and encephalopathy develop in severe valproate poisoning, early intravenous supplementation with L-carnitine

Box 12.24 Clinical features of poisoning with anticonvulsant drugs

Anticonvulsant drug	Clinical features of poisoning
Carbamazepine and oxcarbazepine (a prodrug of carbamazepine)	Dry mouth, coma, convulsions, ataxia, incoordination, hallucinations (particularly in the recovery phase) Ocular: nystagmus, dilated pupils (common), divergent strabismus, complete external ophthalmoplegia (rare)
Phenytoin	Nausea, vomiting, headache, tremor, cerebellar ataxia, nystagmus, loss of consciousness (rare)
Sodium valproate	Most frequent: drowsiness, impairment of consciousness, respiratory depression Uncommon complications: liver damage, hyper-ammonaemia, metabolic acidosis Very severe poisoning: myoclonic jerks, seizures, cerebral oedema
Gabapentin and pregabalin	Lethargy, ataxia, slurred speech, gastrointestinal symptoms
Lamotrigine	Lethargy, coma, ataxia, nystagmus, seizures, cardiac conduction abnormalities
Levetiracetam	Lethargy, coma, respiratory depression
Tiagabine	Lethargy, facial grimacing, nystagmus, posturing, agitation, coma, hallucinations, seizures
Topiramate	Lethargy, ataxia, nystagmus, myoclonus, coma, seizures, metabolic acidosis (secondary to carbonic anhydrase inhibition)

will reduce the formation of ammonia and other toxic metabolites of valproic acid. Haemodialysis increases the elimination of valproate and should be instituted if severe hyper-ammonaemia and electrolyte and acid–base disturbances occur.

Other drugs of importance in poisoning

For ease of reference these are arranged in alphabetical order and include antidiabetic drugs, antimalarial drugs, beta-blockers, calcium-channel blockers, digoxin, iron salts, lithium salts and salicylates.

Antidiabetic drugs

Insulin (if injected but not if ingested) and **sulphonylureas** cause hypoglycaemia. This is not seen with **metformin**, since its mode of action is to increase glucose utilization, but lactic acidosis is a potentially serious complication of metformin poisoning.

Clinical features

Features of severe hypoglycaemia include drowsiness, coma, convulsions, depressed limb reflexes, extensor plantar responses and cerebral oedema. Hypokalaemia also occurs. Cranial (neurogenic) diabetes insipidus and persistent vegetative states are possible long-term complications if hypoglycaemia is prolonged.

Management

The blood or plasma glucose concentration should be measured urgently and intravenous glucose given, if necessary. Glucagon produces only a slight rise in blood glucose, although it can reduce the amount of glucose required (see p. 717).

Severe insulin poisoning

A continuous infusion of 10–20% glucose (with K+ 10–20 mmol/L) is required, together with carbohydrate-rich meals, though there may be difficulty in maintaining normoglycaemia.

Sulphonylurea poisoning

The administration of glucose increases already high circulating insulin concentrations. Intravenous octreotide (50 µg), which inhibits insulin release, should be given as well as glucose.

Antimalarials

Chloroquine

Severe poisoning may present with hypotension, cardiac failure, pulmonary oedema and cardiac arrest. Agitation, acute psychosis, convulsions and coma may occur. Hypokalaemia is common and is due to chloroquine-induced potassium-channel blockade. Bradyarrhythmias and tachyarrhythmias are common, and ECG conduction abnormalities are similar to those seen in quinine poisoning.

Quinine

Cinchonism (tinnitus, deafness, vertigo, nausea, headache and diarrhoea) is common. In more severe poisoning, convulsions, hypotension, pulmonary oedema and cardiorespiratory arrest are seen (due to ventricular arrhythmias that are often preceded by ECG conduction abnormalities, particularly QT prolongation). Quinine cardiotoxicity is due to sodium-channel blockade. Patients may also develop ocular features, including blindness, which can be permanent.

Primaquine

The main concern is primaquine's propensity to cause methaemoglobinaemia and haemolytic anaemia.

Management

Multiple-dose oral activated charcoal increases quinine and probably chloroquine clearance. Hypokalaemia should be corrected. Intravenous sodium bicarbonate 50–100 mmol is given if the ECG shows QRS prolongation but it will exacerbate hypokalaemia, which should be corrected first. Mechanical ventilation, the administration of an inotrope (see p. 222) and high doses of diazepam (1 mg/kg as a loading dose and 0.25–0.4 mg/kg per hour maintenance) may reduce the mortality in severe chloroquine poisoning. Overdrive pacing may be required if torsades de pointes (see p. 1065) occurs in quinine poisoning and does not respond to intravenous magnesium sulphate (see p. 1065). If clinically significant methaemoglobinaemia (generally above 30%) develops in primaquine poisoning, methylthioninium (methylene blue) 1–2 mg/kg body weight should be administered.

Beta-adrenoceptor-blocking drugs

In mild poisoning, sinus bradycardia is the only feature, but if a substantial amount has been ingested, coma, convulsions and hypotension develop. Less commonly, delirium, hallucinations and cardiac arrest supervene. Bronchospasm and hypoglycaemia are rare complications.

Management

Glucagon 50–150 µg/kg (typically 5–10 mg in an adult), followed by an infusion of 5–10 mg/h, is the most effective agent. It acts by bypassing the blocked beta-receptor, thus activating adenyl cyclase and promoting formation of cyclic adenosine monophosphate (cAMP) from adenosine triphosphate (ATP); cAMP, in turn, exerts a direct beta-stimulant effect on the heart. Intravenous atropine 0.6–1.2 mg can be used to treat bradycardia but is usually less effective. High-dose insulin (initial intravenous bolus of 1.0 IU/kg, followed by 1-10 IU/kg per hour) with hypertonic glucose to avoid hypoglycaemia, has been shown to improve myocardial contractility and systemic perfusion.

Calcium-channel blockers

Calcium-channel blockers all act by blocking voltage-gated calcium channels. Dihydropyridines (e.g. amlodipine, felodipine, nifedipine) are predominantly peripheral vasodilators, while verapamil (a phenylalkylamine) and diltiazem (a benzothiazepine) also have significant cardiac effects. Poisoning, particularly with verapamil and diltiazem, causes heart block and hypotension; in severe poisoning, there is a substantial fatality rate. When a sustained-release preparation has been ingested, the onset of severe features is delayed, sometimes for more than 12 hours. Overdose with even small amounts can have profound effects.

Clinical features

Hypotension occurs due to peripheral vasodilation, myocardial depression and conduction block. The ECG may progress from sinus bradycardia through first, then higher, degrees of block, to asystole. Cardiac and non-cardiac pulmonary oedema may ensue in severely poisoned patients. Other features include nausea, vomiting, seizures and a lactic acidosis.

Management

Intravenous atropine 0.6–1.2 mg, repeated as required, should be given for bradycardia and heart block. The initial dose can be repeated every 3–5 min, but if there is no response in pulse rate or blood pressure after three doses, it is unlikely that further boluses will be helpful. The response to atropine is sometimes improved following intravenous 10% calcium chloride, 5–10 mL (at 1–2 mL/min). If there is an initial response to calcium, a continuous infusion is warranted as 10% calcium chloride, 1–10 mL/h.

Cardiac pacing has a role if there is evidence of atrioventricular conduction delay but failure to capture occurs.

Hypotension that persists despite volume replacement may respond to IV glucagon, which activates myosin kinase independent of calcium. An initial bolus of 50–150 µg/kg can be repeated as necessary or an infusion of 5–10 mg/h can be commenced.

Insulin–glucose euglycaemia has been shown to improve myocardial contractility and systemic perfusion, and should be considered in cases of resistant hypotension. Insulin is given as a bolus dose of 1 IU/kg, followed by an infusion of 1–10 IU/kg per hour with hypertonic glucose and frequent monitoring of blood glucose and potassium.

Digoxin

Toxicity occurring during chronic administration is common, though acute poisoning is infrequent.

Clinical features

These include nausea, vomiting, dizziness, anorexia and drowsiness. Rarely, confusion, visual disturbances and hallucinations occur. Initial sinus bradycardia may be followed by supraventricular arrhythmias with or without heart block, ventricular premature beats and ventricular tachycardia. Hyperkalaemia occurs due to inhibition of the sodium–potassium activated ATPase pump.

Management

- *Intravenous atropine* 1.2–2.4 mg is given to reduce sinus bradycardia, atrioventricular block and sinoatrial standstill.
- *Digoxin-specific antibody fragments* (digoxin-Fab) should be given intravenously for significant hyperkalaemia, marked arrhythmias (usually severe bradycardia compromising the cardiac output) and asystole. In both acute and chronic poisoning, only half the estimated dose required for full neutralization (calculated from amount of drug taken or serum digoxin concentration) need be given initially; a further dose is given if clinically indicated.

Iron salts

Unless more than 60 mg of elemental iron per kg of body weight is ingested (a ferrous sulfate tablet contains 60 mg of iron), features are unlikely to develop. As a result, poisoning is seldom severe but deaths still occur. Iron salts have a direct corrosive effect on the upper gastrointestinal tract.

Clinical features

Initial features include nausea, vomiting (the vomit may be grey or black in colour), abdominal pain and diarrhoea. Severely poisoned patients develop haematemesis, hypotension, coma and shock at an early stage. Usually, however, most patients suffer only mild gastrointestinal symptoms. A small minority deteriorate 12–48 hours after ingestion and develop shock, metabolic acidosis, acute tubular necrosis and hepatocellular necrosis. Rarely, up to 6 weeks after ingestion, intestinal strictures occur due to corrosive damage. The serum iron concentration should be measured some 4 hours after ingestion; if the concentration exceeds the predicted normal iron-binding capacity (usually >5 mg/L; 90 μmol/L), free iron is circulating and treatment with desferrioxamine should be considered.

Management

The majority of patients ingesting iron do not require desferrioxamine therapy. If a patient develops coma or shock, desferrioxamine should be given without delay in an intravenous dose of 15 mg/kg per hour (the total amount of infusion usually not to exceed 80 mg/kg in 24 h). If the recommended rate of administration is continued for several days, adverse effects, including pulmonary oedema and ARDS (see p. 232), have been reported.

Lithium salts

Lithium poisoning usually results from impaired renal elimination in an individual on lithium therapeutically; that is, chronic toxicity rather than deliberate self-poisoning (acute toxicity). Lithium has a narrow therapeutic index (target plasma range 0.8–1.2 mmol/L).

Clinical features

Features of intoxication include diarrhoea and vomiting, tremor, thirst, polyuria and, in more serious cases, impairment of consciousness, hypertonia and convulsions; irreversible neurological damage may occur. Measurement of the serum lithium concentration confirms the diagnosis. However, in chronic poisoning the plasma lithium concentration may not be markedly above the upper end of the therapeutic range despite the presence of severe neurological features (which are due to accumulation of lithium in the CNS). Conversely, acute massive overdose may produce high plasma concentrations with few toxic features.

Management

The plasma lithium concentration must always be interpreted in association with the clinical features present. Since lithium is

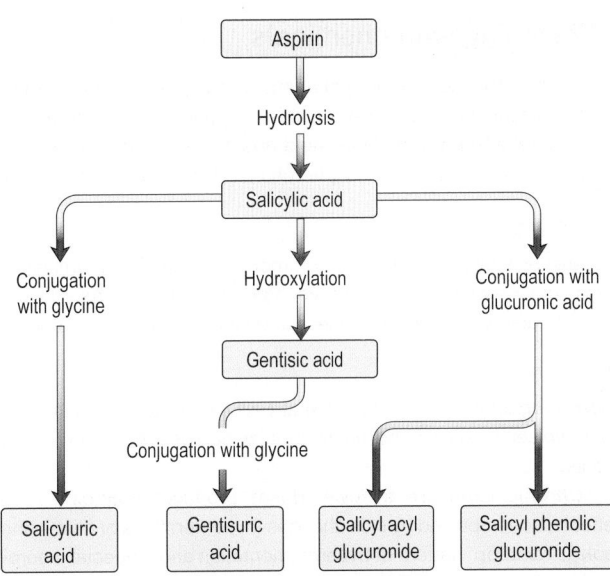

Fig. 12.3 The metabolism of aspirin.

eliminated unchanged via the kidneys, diuresis with sodium chloride 0.9% is effective in increasing clearance. Haemodialysis is far superior and is used if neurological features are present and/or if renal function is impaired. It is employed particularly in cases of chronic toxicity.

Salicylates

Aspirin is metabolized to salicylic acid (salicylate) by esterases present in many tissues, especially the liver, and subsequently to salicyluric acid and salicyl phenolic glucuronide (**Fig. 12.3**); these two pathways become saturated, with the consequence that the renal excretion of salicylic acid increases after overdose; this excretion pathway is extremely sensitive to changes in urinary pH.

Clinical features

Salicylates stimulate the respiratory centre, increase the depth and rate of respiration, and induce a respiratory alkalosis. Compensatory mechanisms, including renal excretion of bicarbonate and potassium, result in a metabolic acidosis. Salicylates also interfere with carbohydrate, fat and protein metabolism, and disrupt oxidative phosphorylation, producing increased concentrations of lactate, pyruvate and ketone bodies, all of which contribute to the acidosis.

Common features of poisoning include tachypnoea, sweating, vomiting, epigastric pain, tinnitus and deafness. Respiratory alkalosis and metabolic acidosis supervene and a mixed acid–base disturbance is typical. Rarely, in severe poisoning, non-cardiogenic pulmonary oedema, coma and convulsions ensue.

The severity of salicylate toxicity is dose-related.

Management

Fluid and electrolyte replacement are required with prompt correction of dehydration and hypokalaemia. Mild cases of salicylate poisoning are managed with parenteral fluid and electrolyte replacement only. Patients whose plasma salicylate concentrations are in excess of 500 mg/L (3.6 mmol/L) should receive urine alkalinization (see p. 264). Haemodialysis is the treatment of choice for severely poisoned patients (plasma salicylate concentration >700 mg/L; >5.1 mmol/L), particularly those with coma and metabolic acidosis.

Poisoning with chemicals

Included in this section, in alphabetical order, are arsenic, carbamate insecticides, carbon monoxide, copper sulfate, corrosives, cyanide, ethylene glycol, household agents, lead, mercury, methanol, nerve agents, organophosphorus insecticides and phosphides.

Arsenic

Arsenic poisoning worldwide is commonly caused by contamination of the ground water by inorganic arsenates, particularly in Asia. Occasionally, arsenic is found in Chinese and Indian traditional remedies.

Clinical features

Acute ingestion causes abdominal pain, vomiting and diarrhoea. Hypovolaemic shock and acute tubular necrosis occur in severe cases.

Chronic exposure to lower doses produces gastrointestinal effects, accompanied by skin changes (hyperkeratosis of palms and soles, 'raindrop' pattern of hyperpigmentation and alopecia), neurological features (headache, sensorimotor neuropathy), abnormal liver biochemistry (non-cirrhotic portal hypertension is recognized), peripheral vascular arteriosclerosis and haematological abnormalities (pancytopenia).

Management

The identification of, and removal from, the source of exposure to arsenic is vital. Chelation therapy with oral DMSA 30 mg/kg per day or intravenous DMPS 30 mg/kg per day may be indicated.

Carbamate insecticides

Carbamate insecticides inhibit acetylcholinesterase but the duration of this inhibition is comparatively short-lived in comparison with organophosphorus insecticides (see p. 275), since the carbamate–enzyme complex tends to dissociate spontaneously.

Clinical features

Although carbamate insecticide poisoning is generally less severe than organophosphorus insecticide poisoning, acute poisoning with a carbamate can be severe and fatal. Cholinergic symptoms usually develop within a few minutes. In the most severe cases, muscle twitching, profound weakness, profuse sweating, incontinence, mental confusion and progressive cardiac and respiratory failure ensue. In less severe cases, cholinergic symptoms are usually evident within 2 hours and typically resolve within 24 hours. Seizures are relatively uncommon, since carbamate penetration into the CNS is limited.

Management

Mild cases require no specific treatment other than the removal of soiled clothing. Intravenous atropine 2 mg should be given every 3–5 minutes, if necessary, to reduce increased secretions, rhinorrhoea and bronchorrhoea. If this measure fails, the patient should be intubated and mechanical ventilation instituted. Since carbamates have a shorter duration of action than organophosphorus insecticides, pralidoxime should be used only rarely in carbamate poisoning. If intoxication is life-threatening, give intravenous pralidoxime chloride 30 mg/kg body weight over 5–10 minutes, followed by an infusion of 8–10 mg/kg per hour.

Carbon monoxide

The most common source of carbon monoxide is an improperly maintained and poorly ventilated heating system. In addition, inhalation of methylene chloride (found in paint strippers) may also lead to carbon monoxide poisoning, as methylene chloride is metabolized *in vivo* to carbon monoxide. Carbon monoxide has a greater affinity for haemoglobin and forms carboxyhaemoglobin (COHb), thereby reducing the oxygen-carrying capacity. The affinity of the remaining haem groups for oxygen is increased. This shifts the oxyhaemoglobin dissociation curve to the left, impairing liberation of oxygen to the cells and leading to tissue hypoxia. In addition, carbon monoxide also inhibits cytochrome oxidase a_3.

Clinical features

Symptoms of mild to moderate exposure to carbon monoxide may be mistaken for a viral illness.
- A peak COHb concentration of <10% is not normally associated with symptoms.
- A peak COHb concentration of 10–30% usually causes headache and mild exertional dyspnoea.
- Higher concentrations of COHb are associated with coma, convulsions and cardiorespiratory arrest. Metabolic acidosis, myocardial ischaemia, hypertonia, extensor plantar responses, retinal haemorrhages and papilloedema also occur.

Neuropsychiatric features may develop after apparent recovery from carbon monoxide exposure.

Management

In addition to removing the patient from carbon monoxide exposure, high-flow oxygen should be administered using a tightly fitting face mask (see p. 230). Endotracheal intubation and mechanical ventilation are required in those who are unconscious. Several controlled studies of hyperbaric oxygen have been published but none has shown long-term clinical benefit.

Copper sulphate

Copper sulphate is used in fungicides, algicides, electroplating, dyes, inks, disinfectants and wood preservatives.

Clinical features

Ingestion causes vomiting, abdominal pain, diarrhoea, headache, dizziness and a metallic taste. Gastrointestinal haemorrhage, intravascular haemolysis, methaemoglobinaemia, rhabdomyolysis, coma, convulsions and hepatorenal failure may ensue and fatalities have occurred. Body secretions may be blue/green.

Management

Treatment is supportive with replenishment of lost fluids/blood. Blood copper concentrations correlate with the severity of poisoning; a copper concentration of >8 mg/L is indicative of severe poisoning. Early endoscopy (or CT scan with contrast if endoscopy is not possible) is recommended if corrosive damage is suspected. Methaemoglobinaemia of >30% should be treated with intravenous methylthioninium chloride 1-2 mg/kg. Renal failure may require extracorporeal support.

Corrosive agents

Strong acids and alkalis cause chemical burns. Inorganic acids such as hydrochloric and sulphuric acid are generally more toxic than organic acids such as acetic acid. Hydrofluoric acid is considered separately (see p. 273). Some household products, such as water-sterilizing tablets, are strong alkalis. Following corrosive ingestion, the vital aspects of management are early (within 24 h) assessment of the severity of injury (ideally with endoscopy, or alternatively with CT imaging) and prompt surgical intervention to remove necrotic tissue, if indicated.

Cyanide

Cyanide and its derivatives are used widely in industry. Hydrogen cyanide is also released during the thermal decomposition of polyurethane foams, such as that in mattresses. Cyanide reversibly inhibits cytochrome oxidase a_3, so that cellular respiration ceases.

Clinical features

Inhalation of hydrogen cyanide produces symptoms within seconds and death within minutes. By contrast, the ingestion of a cyanide salt may not produce features for 1 hour. After exposure, initial symptoms are non-specific and include a feeling of constriction in the chest and dyspnoea. Coma, convulsions and metabolic acidosis may then supervene.

Management

Oxygen should be administered and, if it is available, dicobalt edetate 300 mg should be administered intravenously; the dose is repeated in severe cases. Dicobalt edetate (and the free cobalt contained in the preparation) complexes free cyanide. An alternative but expensive antidote is intravenous hydroxocobalamin (5 g), which enhances endogenous cyanide detoxification; a second dose may be required in severe cases. If these two antidotes are not available, intravenous sodium thiosulphate 12.5 g, which acts by enhancing endogenous detoxification, and intravenous sodium nitrite 300 mg should be administered. Sodium nitrite produces methaemoglobinaemia; methaemoglobin combines with cyanide to form cyanmethaemoglobin.

Ethylene glycol

Ethylene glycol is found in a variety of common household products, including antifreeze, windshield washer fluid, brake fluid and lubricants. The features observed in poisoning are due to metabolites predominantly, not the parent chemical. Ethylene glycol (**Fig. 12.4**) is metabolized to glycolate, the cause of the acidosis. A small proportion of glyoxylate is metabolized to oxalate. Calcium ions chelate oxalate to form insoluble calcium oxalate, which is responsible for renal toxicity.

Clinical features

Initially, the features of ethylene glycol poisoning are similar to those of ethanol intoxication (though there is no ethanol on the breath). Coma and convulsions follow and a variety of neurological abnormalities, including nystagmus and ophthalmoplegias, are seen. Severe metabolic acidosis, hypocalcaemia and acute kidney injury are well-recognized complications.

Management

If the patient presents early after ingestion, the priority is to inhibit metabolism using either intravenous fomepizole or ethanol; the former does not require monitoring of blood concentrations.

- **Fomepizole**: 15 mg/kg body weight should be administered, followed by four 12-hourly doses of 10 mg/kg, then 15 mg/kg every 12 h until glycol concentrations are not detectable. Following a substantial ingestion, haemodialysis or haemodiafiltration should be employed to remove the glycol and metabolites. If dialysis is used, the frequency of fomepizole dosing should be increased to 4-hourly because fomepizole is dialysable.
- **Ethanol**: alternatively, a loading dose of ethanol 50 g can be administered, followed by an intravenous infusion of ethanol 10–12 g/h to produce blood ethanol concentrations of 500–1000 mg/L (11–22 mmol/L). The infusion is continued until the glycol is no longer detectable in the blood. If haemodialysis is employed, the rate of ethanol administration will need to be increased to 17–22 g/h, as ethanol is dialysable.

Supportive measures to combat shock, hypocalcaemia and metabolic acidosis should be instituted.

Household products

The agents most commonly involved are bleach, cosmetics, toiletries, detergents, disinfectants, and petroleum distillates such as paraffin and white spirit. Ingestion of household products is usually accidental and is most common among children less than 5 years of age.

Clinical features

If ingestion is accidental, features very rarely occur, except in the case of petroleum distillates where aspiration is a recognized complication because of their low surface tension. Powder detergents, sterilizing tablets, denture cleaning tablets and industrial bleaches (which contain high concentrations of sodium hypochlorite) are corrosive to the mouth and pharynx if ingested. Nail polish and nail polish remover contain acetone, which may produce a coma if ingested in substantial quantities. Inhalation by small children of substantial quantities of talcum powder has occasionally given rise to severe pulmonary oedema and death.

Hydrofluoric acid and hydrogen fluoride

Hydrofluoric acid, a solution of hydrogen fluoride in water, is a colourless, fuming liquid that is widely used in industry. It is particularly dangerous because of its unique ability among acids to penetrate tissue.

Clinical features

Dermal exposure to hydrofluoric acid results in rapid liquefactive necrosis and erosion of bone. If more than 1% of the body surface area is contaminated with a 50% or higher solution of hydrofluoric acid, there is a high risk of hypocalcaemia from the formation of calcium fluoride. This may lead to cardiac conduction disturbances, notably QT interval prolongation and an increased risk of ventricular arrhythmias, particularly torsades de pointes (see p. 1065).

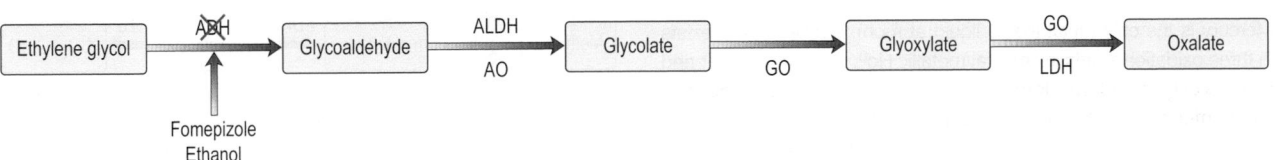

Fig. 12.4 The metabolism of ethylene glycol. Fomepizole and ethanol inhibit ADH. ADH, alcohol dehydrogenase; ALDH, aldehyde dehydrogenase; AO, aldehyde oxidase; GO, glycolate oxidase; LDH, lactate dehydrogenase.

Ingestion of hydrofluoric acid causes severe corrosive injury to the gastrointestinal tract.

Inhalation of hydrogen fluoride causes irritation of the eyes and nose, with sore throat, cough, chest tightness, headache, ataxia and confusion. Dyspnoea and stridor due to laryngeal oedema may follow, depending on the concentration of hydrogen fluoride. Haemorrhagic pulmonary oedema with increasing breathlessness, wheeze, hypoxia and cyanosis may take up to 36 hours to develop.

Management

- **Dermal exposure.** Immediate irrigation of the skin with copious volumes of water is the priority, followed by the prompt application of calcium gluconate gel to reduce pain and limit skin damage.
- **Ingestion.** This is a medical emergency with the need for immediate assessment for surgery after endoscopy or CT.
- **Inhalation.** If the patient has clinical features of bronchospasm after inhalation, then treat conventionally with nebulized bronchodilators and steroids. Treat pulmonary oedema and/or ARDS (see p. 232) with continuous positive airway pressure (CPAP) or, in severe cases, with intermittent positive pressure ventilation (IPPV).

Lead

Exposure to lead occurs occupationally, children may eat lead-painted items in their homes (pica), and the use of lead-containing cosmetics or 'drugs' has also resulted in poisoning.

Clinical features

Mild intoxication may result in no more than lethargy and occasional abdominal discomfort, though abdominal pain, vomiting, constipation and encephalopathy (seizures, delirium, coma) may develop in more severe cases. Encephalopathy is more common in children than in adults but is rare in the developed world. Typically, though very rarely, lead poisoning results in foot drop attributable to peripheral motor neuropathy.

Anaemia (normally normochromic normocytic) occurs due both to inhibition by lead of several enzymes involved in haem synthesis and to haemolysis. The latter results from damage to the red cell membrane by aggregates of RNA that accumulate owing to inhibition by lead of pyrimidine-5-nucleotidase, causing characteristic 'basophilic stippling' of erythrocytes.

Management

The social and occupational dimensions of lead poisoning must be recognized. Simply giving patients chelation therapy and then returning them to a contaminated environment is of no value.

The decision to use chelation therapy is based not only on the blood lead concentration but also on the presence of symptoms. Parenteral sodium calcium edetate 75 mg/kg per day or oral succimer (DMSA) 30 mg/kg per day is of similar efficacy. At least 5 days' treatment is usually required. As chelation of zinc may occur with sodium calcium edetate, serum zinc concentrations should be checked.

Mercury

Mercury is the only metal that is liquid at room temperature. It exists in three oxidation states (elemental/metallic Hg^0, mercurous Hg_2^{2+} and mercuric Hg^{2+}) and can form inorganic (e.g. mercuric chloride) and organic (e.g. methylmercury) compounds. Metallic mercury is very volatile; when spilled, it has a large surface area so that high atmospheric concentrations may be produced in enclosed spaces, particularly when environmental temperatures are high. Thus, great care should be taken in clearing up a spillage. If ingested, metallic mercury will usually

be eliminated per rectum, though small amounts may settle in the appendix and remain there for years. Mercury salts are well absorbed following ingestion, as is mercury vapour following inhalation.

Clinical features

Acute inhalation of mercury vapour causes headache, nausea, cough, chest pain and, occasionally, a chemical pneumonitis. Proteinuria and nephrotic syndrome are observed rarely.

Ingestion of inorganic or organic mercury compounds causes an irritant gastroenteritis. Mercurous (Hg_2^{2+}) compounds are less corrosive and less toxic than mercuric (Hg^{2+}) salts.

Systemic accumulation of mercury from any source and by any route of exposure leads to characteristic neurological features, including a fine tremor, lethargy, memory loss, insomnia, personality changes and ataxia. Peripheral nerve damage has also been observed, as has renal tubular damage.

Management

Unithiol (DMPS) is the antidote of choice and is given in an intravenous dose of 30 mg/kg per day. At least 5 days' treatment is usually required.

Methanol

Methanol is used widely as a solvent and is found in antifreeze solutions. Methanol is metabolized to formaldehyde and formate (**Fig. 12.5**). The concentration of formate increases greatly and is accompanied by accumulation of hydrogen ions, leading to metabolic acidosis.

Clinical features

Methanol causes inebriation and drowsiness. After a latent period, coma supervenes. Blurred vision and diminished visual acuity occur due to formate accumulation. The presence of dilated pupils that are unreactive to light suggests that permanent blindness is likely to ensue. A severe metabolic acidosis may develop and be accompanied by hyperglycaemia and a raised serum amylase activity. A blood methanol concentration of 500 mg/L (15.6 mmol/L) confirms severe poisoning. The mortality correlates well with the severity and duration of metabolic acidosis. Survivors may show permanent neurological sequelae, including parkinsonian-like signs as well as blindness.

Management

Treatment is similar to that of ethylene glycol poisoning (see p. 273) with the addition of intravenous folinic acid 30 mg 6-hourly for 48 hours, which accelerates formate metabolism, thereby reducing ocular toxicity.

Nerve agents

Nerve agents are related chemically to organophosphorus insecticides (see below) and have a similar mechanism of toxicity but a much higher mammalian acute toxicity, particularly via the dermal

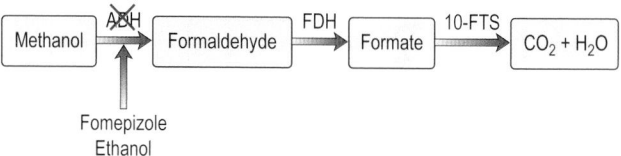

Fig. 12.5 The metabolism of methanol. Fomepizole and ethanol inhibit ADH. ADH, alcohol dehydrogenase; FDH, formaldehyde dehydrogenase; 10-FTS, 10-formyl tetrahydrofolate synthetase.

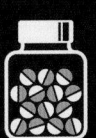

route. In addition to inhibition of acetylcholinesterase, a chemical reaction known as 'ageing' also occurs rapidly and more completely than in the case of insecticides. This makes the enzyme resistant to spontaneous reactivation or treatment with oximes (pralidoxime, obidoxime or HI-6).

Several classes of nerve agent are recognized: G agents (named after *Gerhard Schrader*, who synthesized the first agents) and V agents (V allegedly standing for venomous). G agents include tabun, sarin, soman and cyclosarin. The V agents, for example VX, were introduced later. The G agents are both dermal and respiratory hazards, whereas the V agents, unless aerosolized, are contact poisons. The latest class of nerve agents to receive notoriety are the Novichok agents, which are potent contact poisons.

Clinical features

Systemic features include increased salivation, rhinorrhoea, bronchorrhoea, miosis (which is characteristic) and eye pain, abdominal pain, nausea, vomiting and diarrhoea, involuntary micturition and defecation, muscle weakness and fasciculation, tremor, restlessness, ataxia and convulsions. Bradycardia, tachycardia and hypotension occur, depending on whether muscarinic or nicotinic effects predominate. Death occurs from respiratory failure within minutes but individuals with mild or moderate exposure usually recover completely. Diagnosis is confirmed by measuring the erythrocyte cholinesterase activity.

Management

The administration of intravenous atropine 2 mg repeated every 3–5 min as necessary to patients presenting with rhinorrhoea and bronchorrhoea may be lifesaving. In addition, an oxime should be given to all those requiring atropine as soon as possible after exposure before 'aging' has occurred; for example, intravenous pralidoxime chloride 30 mg/kg, followed by an infusion of pralidoxime chloride 8–10 mg/kg per hour. Alternatively, boluses of pralidoxime chloride 30 mg/kg may be given 4- to 6-hourly. Intravenous diazepam 10–20 mg, repeated as required, is useful in controlling apprehension, agitation, fasciculation and convulsions.

Organophosphorus insecticides

Organophosphorus (OP) insecticides are used widely throughout the world and are a common cause of poisoning, leading to thousands of deaths annually in the developing world. Intoxication may follow ingestion, inhalation or dermal absorption. OP insecticides inhibit acetylcholinesterase, causing accumulation of acetylcholine at central and peripheral cholinergic nerve endings, including neuromuscular junctions. Many OP insecticides require biotransformation before becoming active and so the features of intoxication may be delayed.

Clinical features

Poisoning is characterized by anxiety and restlessness, which is typically followed by nausea, vomiting, abdominal colic, diarrhoea (particularly if exposure is by ingestion), tenesmus, sweating, hypersalivation and chest tightness. Respiratory failure will ensue in severe cases and is exacerbated by the development of bronchorrhoea and pulmonary oedema. Miosis is characteristic. Muscle fasciculation and flaccid paresis of limb muscles, and, occasionally, paralysis of extraocular muscles is observed. Coma and convulsions occur in severe poisoning.

Diagnosis is confirmed by measuring the erythrocyte acetylcholinesterase activity; plasma cholinesterase activity is less specific but may also be depressed.

The *intermediate syndrome* usually becomes established 1–4 days after exposure, when the symptoms and signs of the acute cholinergic syndrome are no longer obvious. The characteristic features of the syndrome are weakness of the muscles of respiration (diaphragm, intercostal muscles and accessory muscles, including neck muscles) and of proximal limb muscles. Accompanying features often include weakness of muscles innervated by some cranial nerves.

Delayed polyneuropathy is a rare complication of acute exposure to some OP insecticides not marketed in most countries. It presents with glove and stocking paraesthesiae some 1–4 weeks after exposure, followed by an ascending motor polyneuropathy in many cases. It is initiated by phosphorylation, and subsequent ageing, of at least 70% of an esterase – neuropathy target esterase (NTE) – in peripheral nerves. Most mild cases improve with time but severe cases can be left with an upper motor neurone syndrome and permanent disability.

Management

Mild cases require no specific treatment other than the removal of soiled clothing. Intravenous atropine 2 mg should be given every 3–5 minutes if necessary, to reduce increased secretions, rhinorrhoea and bronchorrhoea.

Symptomatic patients should also be given an oxime (pralidoxime, obidoxime) to reactivate inhibited acetylcholinesterase; for example, pralidoxime chloride 30 mg/kg by slow intravenous injection, followed by an infusion of pralidoxime chloride 8–10 mg/kg per hour. There is no specific treatment for the intermediate syndrome apart from supportive care, including prolonged ventilation, though a prospective trial suggested that early treatment with oximes could reduce the likelihood of the syndrome developing. Most patients recover in 2–3 weeks.

Phosphides

Aluminium and zinc phosphides are used as rodenticides and insecticides. They react with moisture in the air (and the gastrointestinal tract) to produce phosphine, the active pesticide. Acute poisoning with these compounds may be direct, due to ingestion of the salts, or indirect, from accidental inhalation of phosphine generated during their approved use.

Clinical features

Ingestion causes vomiting, epigastric pain, peripheral circulatory failure, severe metabolic acidosis, acute kidney injury and disseminated intravascular coagulation, in addition to the features induced by phosphine.

Exposure to phosphine causes lacrimation, rhinorrhoea, cough, breathlessness, chest tightness, dizziness, diplopia, headache, nausea, drowsiness, intention tremor and ataxia. Acute pulmonary oedema, hypertension, cardiac arrhythmias, convulsions and jaundice have been described in severe cases.

Management

Treatment is symptomatic and supportive. Gastric lavage should not be used, as it can speed up the rate of disintegration of the product ingested and increase toxicity. Activated charcoal may bind metal phosphides. The mortality is high, despite supportive care.

Poisons in the natural world

Numerous biological organisms produce or contain substances that are toxic to humans, including animals (snakes, insects, spiders and marine creatures), and some species of plants and fungi. Space precludes discussion of all of these poisons and toxins here, where only snake bite is covered because of its relatively high prevalence and potential severity. An online supplement covers these other naturally occurring poisons in detail, alongside much more detailed description of the treatment of different subtypes of snake envenomation.

Venomous snakes

Approximately 15% of the 3000 species of snake found worldwide are considered to be dangerous to humans. Snake bite is common in some tropical countries; rural areas of West Africa, Southeast Asia, the Indian subcontinent, New Guinea and the Amazon region are particularly affected. Bites by venomous snakes cause more than 100 000 deaths and many permanent sequelae each year (some 46 000 people are killed each year in India alone).

There are three main groups of venomous snakes, representing some 200 species, which have in their upper jaws a pair of enlarged teeth (fangs) that inject venom into the tissues of their victim. These are:
- **Viperidae** (with two subgroups: Viperinae – European adders and Russell's vipers; and Crotalinae – American rattlesnakes, moccasins, lance-headed vipers and Asian pit vipers)
- **Elapidae** (African and Asian cobras, Asian kraits, African mambas, American coral snakes, Australian and New Guinean venomous snakes, including the death adder – *Acanthophis antarcticus* – and sea snakes)
- **Hydrophiidae** (sea snakes).

In addition, some members of the family Colubridae are mildly venomous (mongoose snake).

Clinical features

The main effects of envenoming are:
- local swelling, bruising, blistering, regional lymph node enlargement and necrosis
- anti-haemostatic defects: consumption coagulopathy and spontaneous systemic bleeding from gums, nose, skin, gut, genitourinary tract and intracranial haemorrhage
- shock (hypotension) and myocardial damage
- descending paralysis: progressing from ptosis and external ophthalmoplegia to bulbar, respiratory muscle and total flaccid paralysis
- generalized rhabdomyolysis with myoglobinuria
- intravascular haemolysis
- acute kidney injury.

Viperidae (Viperinae and Crotalinae)

Russell's viper causes most of the snake-bite mortality in India, Pakistan and Myanmar. There is local swelling at the site of the bite, which may become massive. Local tissue necrosis may occur. Evidence of systemic involvement (**envenomation**) occurs within 30 minutes, including vomiting, shock and hypotension. Haemorrhage due to incoagulable blood can be fatal. Envenomation by European adders (*Vipera berus*) is rarely fatal.

Elapidae

There is not usually any swelling at the site of the bite, except with Asian cobras and African spitting cobras; in these cases, the bite is painful and is followed by local tissue necrosis. Vomiting occurs first, followed by shock and then neurological symptoms and muscle weakness, with paralysis of the respiratory muscles in severe cases. Cardiac muscle can be involved.

Hydrophiidae

Envenomation produces muscle involvement, myalgia and myoglobinuria, which can lead to acute kidney injury. Cardiac and respiratory paralysis may occur.

Management

Following a snake bite, all efforts should be made to transport the patient quickly to a hospital or dispensary. Traditional methods should be discouraged, as they are often ineffective and may harm the patient. Arterial tourniquets should *not* be used, and incision or excision of the bite area should *not* be performed.

As a first aid measure, a firm pressure bandage should be placed over the bite and the limb immobilized, as this may delay the spread of the venom. Local wounds often require little treatment. If necrosis is present, antibiotics should be given. Skin grafting may be required later. Anti-tetanus prophylaxis must be given. The type of snake should be identified, if possible.

In about 50% of cases, no venom has been injected by the bite but, nevertheless, careful observation for 12–24 hours is necessary in case envenomation develops. General supportive measures should be carried out, as necessary. These include intravenous fluids with volume expanders for hypotension and diazepam for anxiety. Treatment of acute respiratory, cardiac and kidney injury is instituted as necessary.

Antivenoms are not generally indicated unless envenomation is present, as they can cause severe allergic reactions. Antivenoms can rapidly neutralize venom, but only if an amount in excess of the amount of venom is given. Large quantities of antivenom may be required; as antivenoms cannot reverse the effects of the venom, they must be given early to minimize some of the local effects and may prevent necrosis at the site of the bite. Antivenoms should be administered intravenously by slow infusion, the same dose being given to children and adults.

Allergic reactions are frequent, and adrenaline (epinephrine) 1 in 1000 solution should be available. In severe cases, the antivenom infusion should be continued even if an allergic reaction occurs, with subcutaneous injections of adrenaline being given as necessary. Some forms of neurotoxicity, such as those induced by the death adder, respond to anticholinesterase therapy with neostigmine and atropine.

Further reading

Vale JA, Bradberry S. Poisoning (parts 1 and 2). *Medicine* 2016; 44:75–204.
Warrell DA. Snake bite. *Lancet* 2010; 375:77–88.
Warrell DA. Venomous animals. *Medicine* 2016; 44:120–124.

See StudentConsult.com for additional online content on naturally occurring poisons.

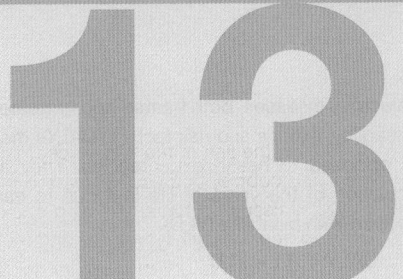

13

Global health

Babulal Sethia and Parveen Kumar

CORE SKILLS AND KNOWLEDGE

Global health can be defined as 'an area of study, research and practice that places a priority on improving health and achieving equity in health for all people worldwide'. It recognizes that health is determined by challenges that transcend national boundaries, and looks at healthcare needs across the world as well as within individual nations. Such needs are complex, may be triggered by natural disasters or armed conflict, and must be addressed using a multiprofessional approach.

Efforts to improve global health are championed by non-governmental organizations such as the World Health Organization (WHO), the United Nations Children's Fund (UNICEF) and the World Food Programme, alongside individual charities and local government health systems, and interventions are often directed by international targets such as the United Nations' Sustainable Development Goals.

Opportunities for developing an understanding of global health include:

- engaging actively in debates about the global economic and political determinants of health
- considering the evidence for community-level interventions in improving health outcomes
- travelling to see medicine being practised in a radically different context (e.g. as part of a medical school elective, see p. 283), and reflecting on the successes and ongoing challenges of local healthcare provision.

INTRODUCTION

Complex individual and community health needs are present in high-, as well as low- and middle-income countries (LMICs), but may be particularly acute in times of crisis, for example during or after armed conflict. Effective delivery of global health (GH) requires multiprofessional collaboration between healthcare workers, politicians, economists and scientists in pursuit of both individual wellbeing and population-based prevention and care.

Examples of successful interventions include campaigns for the provision of vaccines by the Global Alliance for Vaccines and Immunization (GAVI) and initiatives to reduce the economic exploitation of child labour. The African Programme for Onchocerciasis Control (APOC) has transformed the lives of millions of people by the administration of a single, annual dose of the drug *ivermectin*. Similarly, the use of *praziquantel* by the Schistosomiasis Control Programme, funded by many organizations, has in many areas significantly reduced the prevalence of schistosomiasis (bilharzia), one of the most common but neglected tropical diseases.

The scale of the problem worldwide

Although global life expectancy has increased by 5.5 years since 2000 (mean 69.8 years in males and 74.2 years in females; WHO 2017/18), several unacceptable facts remain:

- Around 5.4 million children under the age of 5 die each year.
- Preterm birth (before 37 weeks' gestation) accounts for >1 million deaths per year.
- Each day, 830 women die from preventable causes related to pregnancy and childbirth.
- Cardiovascular diseases are the leading cause of death globally.
- Some 36.9 million people are living with human immunodeficiency virus/acquired immunodeficiency syndrome (HIV/AIDS), and 65% of deaths from HIV/AIDS occur in the WHO African region.
- Mental health disorders, e.g. depression, are among the 20 leading causes of disability worldwide.
- Tobacco use kills more than 7 million people each year and 80% of users live in an LMIC.
- More than 1.9 billion adults, 41 million children below 5 years of age and 340 million children and adolescents (aged 5–19 years) were obese or overweight in 2016.

- Approximately 1.6 million deaths were due to diabetes mellitus in 2016. The number of people living with diabetes increased from 108 million in 1980 to 422 million in 2014.
- Nearly 1.35 million people die from road traffic collisions every year.

Further reading

HM Government. *Health is Global: An Outcomes Framework for Global Health 2011–2015.* London: Department of Health; 2011.

MILLENNIUM AND SUSTAINABLE DEVELOPMENT GOALS

In 2000, world leaders from 189 countries adopted a series of goals, the *Millennium Development Goals (MDGs)*, to be achieved by 2015. Several of these goals aimed to reduce poverty, improve the health of women and children, and combat HIV/AIDS, malaria and other diseases. The MDGs were only partially achieved and were succeeded by a new set of *Sustainable Development Goals (SDGs)* in the 2030 United Nations Agenda for Sustainable Development. The 17 SDGs (**Fig. 13.1**) cover a vast area for improvement and emphasize the fact that achievement of the good health and wellbeing goal (SDG 3) is inextricably linked to other major areas such as politics, economics and agriculture. SDG 3 now also includes non-communicable diseases, mental health, road accident injuries and universal health coverage (**Box 13.1**).

GLOBAL BURDEN OF DISEASE

There is a gross global mismatch in the use of funds, research and development with the majority (90%) going to high-income countries (**Fig. 13.2**), which only have 10% of the disease burden (2006). *The Global Burden of Disease (GBD) Study 2010* provided critical data for guiding prevention and other interventions by retrospectively reviewing and updating data using the same methodology. This gives an accurate understanding of health trends and future health priorities for the global community and for individual countries.

The 2010 GBD study introduced a new metric that gave a single measure to quantify the burden of diseases, injuries and risk factors. This *disability-adjusted life year (DALY)* metric allowed the comparison of burden across diseases, both treated and untreated, mortality, morbidity, disability, injuries and risk factors. DALYs measure health gaps, as opposed to health expectancies. They are derived from the calculation of the years of life lost due to early death (YLL) and years lived with disability (YLD).

$$DALY = YLL + YLD$$

Unfortunately, this GBD equation has some limitations: for example, it does not incorporate rapid demographic changes such as changing age, causes of death and disability. Any change in DALYs can be a useful indicator of health outcomes but must be interpreted with care. Both a decrease and an increase in DALYs may reflect improved outcomes. A decrease in DALYs for maternal and neonatal deaths can be accounted for by better education, nutrition or obstetric facilities. However, an increase in DALYs is seen when an ageing population requires treatment for chronic ill health, despite a reduction in mortality.

Further reading

Murray CJL, Lopez AD. Measuring the global burden of disease. *N Engl J Med* 2013; 369: 448–457.
The Global Burden of Disease Study 2017. *Lancet* 2018; 392:1683–2138, e14–e18.

POVERTY

In 2018, nearly half of the world population lived on less than US$ 5.50 per day (compared with US$ 2.50 in 2003). Extreme poverty (defined as <US$ 1.90) was seen in 385 million children, and in 2015 only 10% of the world population lived in extreme poverty (compared with 33% in 1990). Poverty is on the rise in sub-Saharan Africa and in conflict-affected states. Efforts continue to reduce the incidence of extreme poverty to less than 3% by 2030. SDGs 1, 2, 12, 13 and 15 (see **Box 13.1**) relate to this ambition.

Poverty, hunger, agriculture and climate change

These issues are inextricably interdependent. Food production is compromised when agricultural land is directed towards alternative priorities, such as industrial development. Astonishingly, 25%

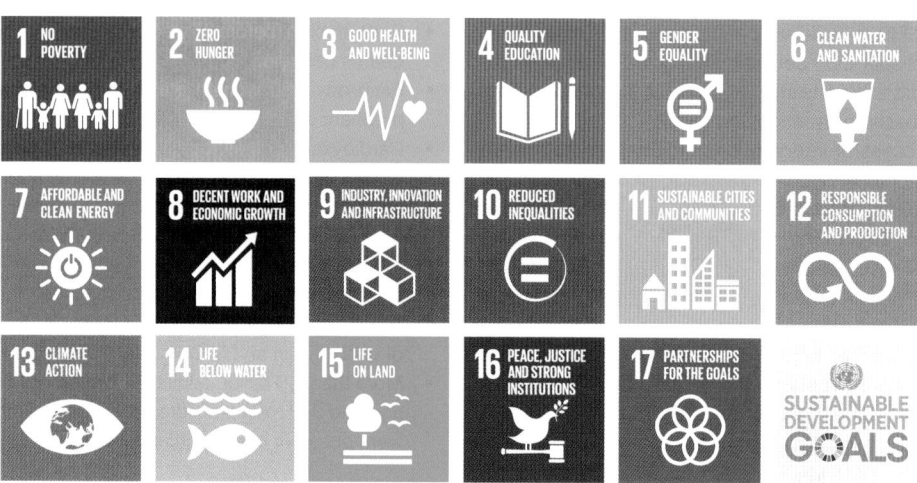

Fig. 13.1 The 17 Sustainable Development Goals.

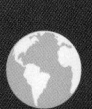

of food is wasted in LMICs by crop deterioration due to deficiencies in transport and storage. Globally, one-third of all food produced, equivalent to 1.3 billion tonnes, is wasted each year.

In 2009, the UCL-Lancet Commission on 'Managing the health effects of climate change' called climate change 'the biggest global threat of the 21st century'. Changes in climate pose major threats to human health either directly (heatwaves, floods, fires, droughts) or indirectly (agricultural losses, mass migration); for example, a 1ºC rise in mean temperature in India would result in the loss of 7 million tons of wheat (**Fig. 13.3**). The 2015 Paris accord, ratified by 195 parties, agreed to target a reduction in global temperature rise to below 2°C by 2100. The 2018 report of the Intergovernmental Panel on Climate Change (IPCC) emphasized the urgent need to further reduce global warming by reporting the beneficial effects in combating climate change of a lower, 1.5°C rise in global temperatures (**Fig. 13.4**).

Chronic illness and disease in LMICs cause much pain and suffering due to the incurred massive expenditure, accentuated by food shortages and dramatic changes in climate. In 2010, 808 million people experienced catastrophic health spending (where health spending exceeded 10% of household consumption).

Further reading

Intergovernmental Panel on Climate Change (IPCC). Global warming of 1.5°C. *Special Report 2018*; http://www.ipcc.ch.
Watts N, Adger WN, Agnolucci P et al. Health and climate change: policy responses to protect public health. *Lancet* 2015; 386:1861–1914.

WATER AND SANITATION

Poor water and sanitation are major causes of early mortality, particularly in children. More than 800 children under the age of 5 years die each day as a result of diarrhoea caused by poor water and sanitation. In 2018, 848 million people still lacked access to safe drinking water, and 1 billion people had access to very basic drinking water services. A total of 892 million people were forced to defecate outside in the open. The MDG target to halve the proportion of people without sustainable access to safe drinking water and sanitation by 2015 was not met and is now in *SDG 6*. Water is usually collected by women, often from distant sources; this can be a hazardous journey, as the women are unprotected and open to abuse. A secondary effect of improved access to water is that the time saved in collecting water can be spent on income generation, food production, education, and activities that lead to social and health benefits.

ORGANIZATIONS AND THE GLOBAL HEALTH AGENDA

International support for GH initiatives may be directed at disease-specific projects (vertical care models) or allied to national health system development. A vast number of organizations (**Box 13.2**) cover the key areas for health development and infrastructural support, including the response to emergency situations (war and natural disasters). The areas encompass service delivery, patient care, education and training, research, equipment, medicines and human

---

> ℹ️ **Box 13.1 The nine main targets of the Sustainable Development Goal for Health (Goal 3)**
>
> 1. By 2030, reduce global maternal mortality ratio to less than 70 per 100 000 live births
> 2. End preventable deaths of newborns and children under 5 years of age
> 3. End the epidemics of AIDS, tuberculosis, malaria and neglected tropical diseases
> 4. Reduce premature mortality from non-communicable diseases by one-third while promoting mental health and wellbeing
> 5. Strengthen the prevention and treatment of substance abuse
> 6. Ensure universal access to sexual and reproductive healthcare
> 7. Substantially reduce the number of deaths and illnesses from hazardous chemicals and air, water soil pollution and contamination
> 8. By 2020, halve the number of deaths and injuries from road traffic accidents
> 9. Achieve universal health coverage including access to essential medicines and vaccines

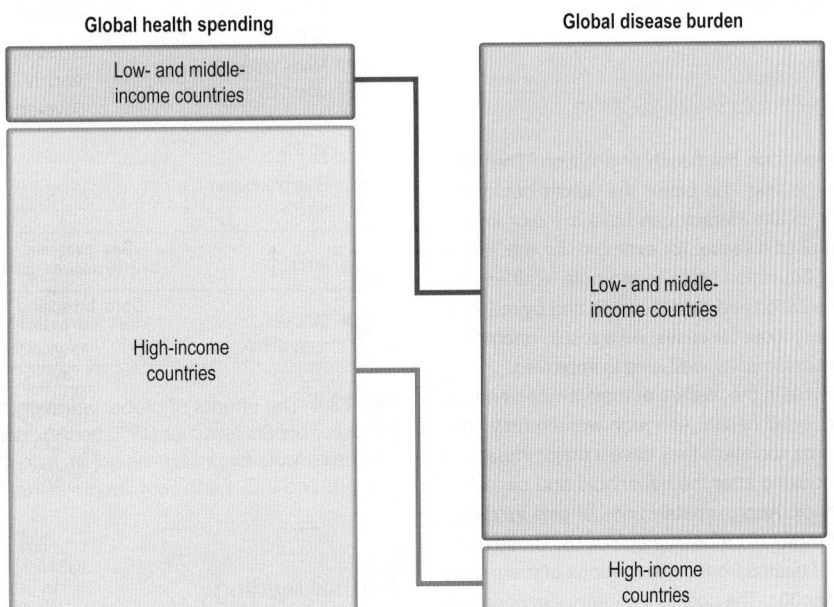

Fig. 13.2 Mismatch between health spending and resources. *(From Gottet P, Schieber G.* Health Financing Revisited: A Practitioner's Guide. *Washington: World Bank; 2006.)*

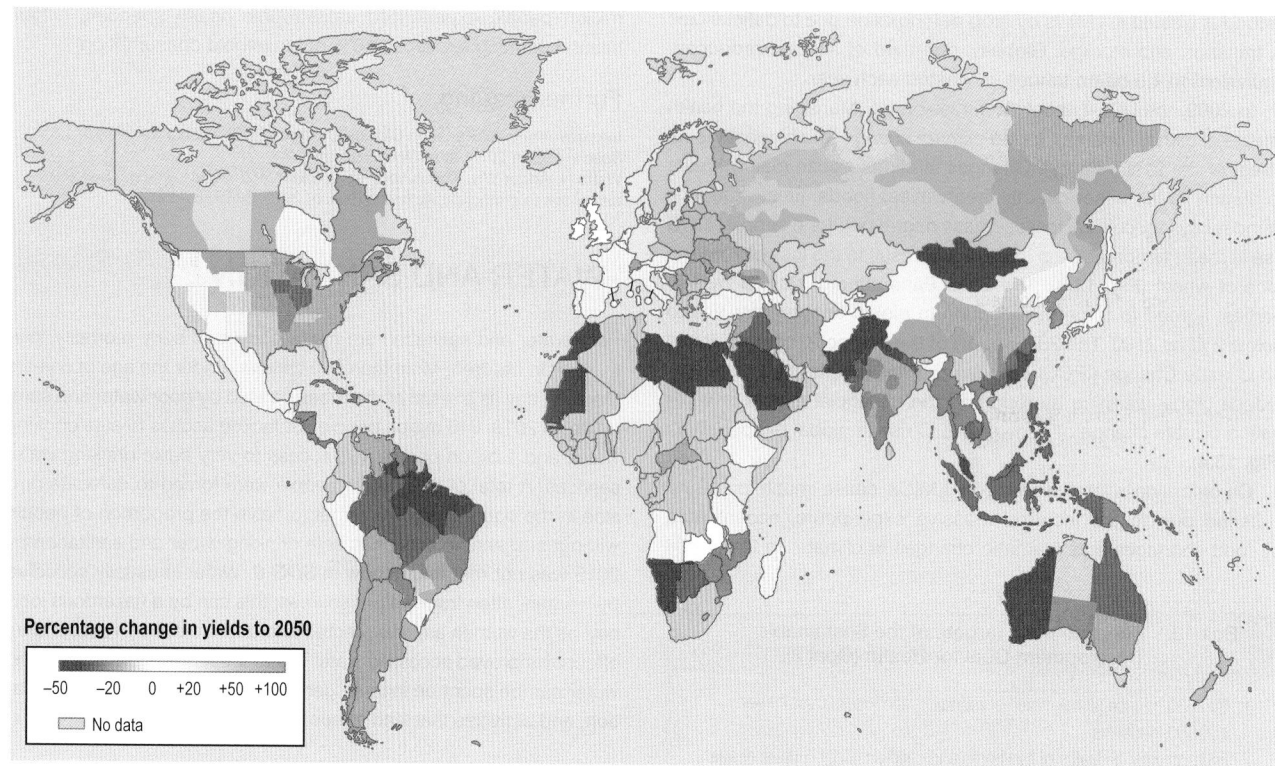

Fig. 13.3 Climate change and modelled cereal grain yields to 2050. A rise in global temperature will make currently 'hot' countries (red) hotter, decreasing their grain yield. Alternatively, current cold countries (green) will get warmer with an increased yield of grain. *(From UN Development Programme 2009.)*

Percentage change in yields to 2050

−50   −20   0   +20   +50   +100

No data

resources. Investment in healthcare systems promotes public health benefits by the provision of vaccination, hygiene and sanitation, as well as major infrastructural projects including technology and communications, such as building roads.

Empowering the local population to help themselves by delivering locally appropriate education and training is of paramount importance.

Further reading

http://www.ghets.org *Global Health through Education, Training and Service.*
http://www.thet.org *Tropical Health and Education Trust.*

EDUCATION

Education has a major impact on the health of a nation. The more years that are spent in schooling, the better the health outcomes. Literacy and, in particular, health literacy can have a major impact on nutrition and the control of disease: for example, by the simple process of hand washing. Education helps to promote healthier lifestyles, both by improving nutrition and development, and by reducing the risks associated with infectious diseases. As a result, unemployment falls while family and community wellbeing is improved.

Women have a crucial role in the welfare of their families and the development of a nation's good health. Although women may have a lower social status in some societies, they have a major impact on the health of a family by looking after the household and caring for the children, elderly and sick. Approximately 25% of girls in 'developing countries' become mothers before the age of 18. These pregnancies have a high rate of deaths from complications of pregnancy and childbirth (see **Chapter 30**). The cost to a country's economy of adolescent pregnancy, as a share of gross domestic product (GDP), can be as high as 30%. The education and welfare of women should be major issues in any developing society.

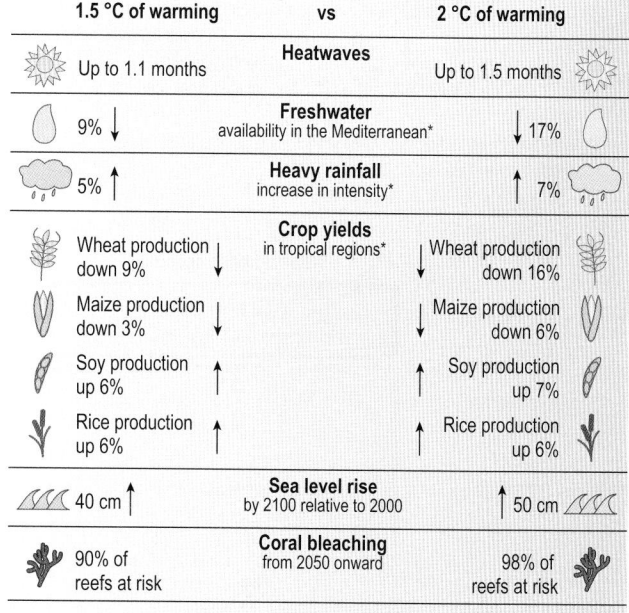

1.5 °C of warming	vs	2 °C of warming
Up to 1.1 months	**Heatwaves**	Up to 1.5 months
9% ↓	**Freshwater** availability in the Mediterranean*	↓ 17%
5% ↑	**Heavy rainfall** increase in intensity*	↑ 7%
	Crop yields in tropical regions*	
Wheat production down 9%	↓	↓ Wheat production down 16%
Maize production down 3%	↓	↓ Maize production down 6%
Soy production up 6%	↑	↑ Soy production up 7%
Rice production up 6%	↓	↓ Rice production up 6%
40 cm ↑	**Sea level rise** by 2100 relative to 2000	↑ 50 cm
90% of reefs at risk	**Coral bleaching** from 2050 onward	98% of reefs at risk

Fig. 13.4 The effects of global warming. *Relative to 1986–2005. *(All data from Schleussner CF, Tabea K, Lissner EM et al. Differential climate impacts for policy-relevant limits to global warming: the case of 1.5°C and 2°C. Earth Syst Dynam 2016; 7:327–351.)*

Further reading

Chaaban J, Cunningham W. Measuring the economic gain of investing in girls: the girls effect dividend. Policy Research working paper 5753: *World Bank* 2011; http://documents.worldbank.org/curated/en/730721468326167343/Measuring-the-economic-gain-of-investing-in-girls-the-girl-effect-dividend.

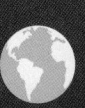

> **i Box 13.2 Some organizations involved in global aid**
>
> **International organizations**
> - World Health Organization (WHO)
> - Global Fund to fight AIDS, tuberculosis and malaria
> - Joint United Nations Programme on HIV/AIDS (UNAIDS)
> - World Bank
> - Department for International Development (DFID; UK)
> - President's Emergency Plan for AIDS Relief (PEPFAR; USA)
> - Global Alliance for Vaccines and Immunization (GAVI)
>
> **Scientific and educational organizations**
> - Mainly disease-specific, e.g. microbiology, diabetes, infectious diseases
> - Consortium of Universities for Global Health (CUGH)
> - Global Health through Education, Training and Service (GHETS)
>
> **Advocacy and policy organizations**
> - Centre for Strategic and International Studies (CSIS)
> - Global Health Policy Centre
> - Global Alliance for Chronic Diseases (GACD)
> - Global Health Council
>
> - Global Health Technologies Coalition (GHTC)
> - The Earth Institute (Columbia University)
> - Kaiser Family Foundation (KFF)
> - US Global Health Policy
> - Tropical Health and Education Trust (THET)
>
> **Foundations**
> - Bill and Melinda Gates Foundation
> - Wellcome Trust
> - UN Foundation (UNF)
> - Accordia Global Health Foundation
>
> **Other non-governmental organizations**
> - Save the Children
> - United Nations International Children's Emergency Fund (UNICEF)
> - Red Cross
> - Oxfam
> - International Rescue Committee (IRC)
> - Médecins Sans Frontières (MSF)

MATERNAL AND CHILD HEALTH

Maternal health

(See also Chapter 39.) Women remain disadvantaged in many parts of the world. Although maternal mortality dropped by about 44% between 1990 and 2015, approximately 830 women die from preventable causes related to pregnancy and childbirth every day, 99% of these in LMICs. Every second, 380 women become pregnant; approximately half of these are unplanned or unwanted pregnancies (e.g. from rape). These stark data support the arguments for women to control their own health and fertility.

Of major concern, 303 000 women die in childbirth every year and 80% of these deaths are avoidable (WHO). Maternal mortality figures are more than 100 times greater in low-income countries (LICs) compared with high-income countries (HICs). The risk of maternal mortality is highest in adolescent girls under 15 years old. The major medical causes of death are haemorrhage, hypertensive disease of pregnancy and infections. Hypertensive disease can be complicated by pre-eclampsia (see p. 1454). Infections can be caused, for example, by bacteria, HIV, malaria and syphilis. Obstructed labour is another potentially fatal complication and can be due to the fibrosis caused by female genital mutilation (FGM), which is still traditionally or illegally practised in some countries. As most maternal and neonatal deaths occur around the time of delivery, the need for basic and emergency care before and during labour and delivery is paramount. The presence of a skilled birth attendant has been shown to reduce both maternal and neonatal mortality in many LMICs.

Child health

Globally, the under 5 years mortality rate has fallen mainly due to the prevention of pneumonia, diarrhoea and malaria by organizations and governments working together. Nevertheless, over 50% of these deaths could have been prevented by access to simple and affordable interventions. Most of these deaths are caused by preterm complications, birth asphyxia, diarrhoea, pneumonia and malaria. Almost 50% of them are linked to malnutrition and children die from common, otherwise non-fatal, childhood ailments. Deaths in children under 5 years of age are mainly concentrated in

South-east Asia and in sub-Saharan Africa, where children are 15 times more likely to die in comparison to children in HICs. In the rest of the world, mortality figures in children dropped from 12.6 million in 1990 to 5.4 million in 2017 and so there remains a need for global and concerted action to improve the survival chances for children.

Vaccination

The World Health Assembly produced a framework to prevent millions of deaths by more equitable access to vaccines and developed a 'Decade of Vaccines Global Vaccine Action Plan 2011–2020'. GAVI plays a critical role in this area by financing and facilitating the delivery of vaccine platforms, and by 2017 85% of infants worldwide had received the diphtheria–tetanus–pertussis vaccine.

Child labour

The global number of children engaged in child labour declined by 38% between 2012 and 2017 (246 million dropping to 152 million). Some 48% of these children (73 million) were engaged in hazardous work, mainly in agriculture.

Child nutrition

Improving child nutrition remains a global imperative as nearly half of the deaths in children under 5 years of age are attributable to malnutrition.

According to data from UNICEF (2017), stunting affects 151 million children under 5 years of age. This problem can be mitigated by appropriate interventions during maternal pregnancy and increased access to food before the child is 2 years old.

Further reading

Bustreo F, Okwo-Bele JM, Kamara L. World Health Organization perspectives on the contribution of the Global Alliance for Vaccines and Immunization on reducing child mortality. *Arch Dis Child* 2015; 100: S34–S37.
International Labour Organization (ILO). *Ending Child Labour by 2025: A Review of Policies and Programmes.* Geneva: ILO 2017.
UNICEF Data. *Malnutrition in Children.* https://data.unicef.org/topic/nutrition/malnutrition/.

MENTAL HEALTH

Mental health (including psychological and neurological problems) or substance abuse disorders affect 15.5% of the global

---

Box 13.3 International guidelines for essential trauma care ('rights of the injured')

- Obstructed airways cleared and maintained
- Impaired breathing supported until the injured person is self-ventilating
- Pneumothorax and haemothorax promptly relieved
- Bleeding stopped promptly
- Shock recognized and treated with intravenous fluid replacement
- Traumatic brain injury treated with timely decompression of space-occupying lesions

- Intestinal and other abdominal injuries promptly addressed
- Disabling extremity injuries corrected
- Unstable spinal cord injuries managed appropriately with early immobilization
- Appropriate rehabilitative services available
- Medications for the above and for pain control readily available

(Adapted from Mock C, Joshipura M, Goosen J et al. Overview of the Essential Trauma Care Project. World J Surg *2006; 30:919–929.)*

---

population. Mental health is thus the second leading cause of long-term disability.

Depression and anxiety disorders remain major clinical challenges with approximately 600 million sufferers worldwide. Additionally, it is estimated that suicide will account for 1.5 million deaths each year by 2020, with a further 15–30 million people attempting suicide.

Globally, the incidence of dementia is rising. In 2017, 50 million people were living with dementia worldwide and this is predicted to increase to 152 million by 2050; 60% of people with dementia live in LMICs. All of these data represent a major worldwide social and financial burden, especially for poorer countries.

Further reading

Collins PY, Patel V, Joestl SS et al. Grand challenges in global mental health. *Nature* 2011;475:27–30.
Ritchie H, Roser M. Mental health. *Our World in Data* 2018; https://ourworldindata.org/mental-health.

ACCIDENTS AND TRAUMA

We are currently in the midst of a global trauma epidemic. It is estimated that 5.8 million people die each year as a result of injury and trauma. At least 2 million of these deaths are potentially avoidable.

Injuries are a significant and increasing cause of mortality and morbidity; more than 90% of injury-related deaths occur in LMICs.

Around 5 billion people do not have access to safe and affordable surgical and anaesthesia care when needed, especially in LMICs. Many of those who do access care risk personal financial ruin. The WHO estimates that, by 2030, trauma from road traffic accidents will be the third most common cause worldwide of both mortality and disability (as measured in DALYs).

The Guidelines for Essential Trauma Care (WHO 2004) established a core list of 11 essential trauma services (**Box 13.3**). Although the implementation of these recommendations has been hampered by deficiencies in planning and infrastructure that need to be addressed by national governments, recent (2018) evaluation of these guidelines suggests that they remain appropriate recommendations for trauma system development.

Further reading

Haagsma JA, Graetz N, Bolliger I et al. Global burden of injury: incidence, mortality, disability-adjusted life years and time trends from the Global Burden of Disease Study 2013. *Inj Prev* 2016; 22:3–18.
Mock C, Joshipura M, Lormand J et al. Strengthening trauma systems globally: the Essential Trauma Care Project. *J Trauma* 2005; 59:1243–1246.

CONFLICT AND CATASTROPHE

Recent years have seen a number of natural disasters; examples include earthquakes in Nepal (2015) and Indonesia (2018), tsunamis in Sri Lanka (2004) and Japan (2011), and hurricanes in the Caribbean (2019). Conflicts also persist in Syria, Yemen and numerous other parts of the world. Effective global action following these unexpected events is frequently compromised by deficiencies in the disaster response. Many of these deficiencies can be rectified through appropriate training whilst addressing long-term structural challenges.

Conflicts and catastrophes severely disrupt healthcare provision, especially for women and children. The use of rape as a weapon of war magnifies this tragedy. Furthermore, disruption to education, along with the physical and psychological sequelae of conflict, leads to increased long-term societal healthcare burdens, especially in the field of mental health.

ECONOMICS AND POLITICS IN GLOBAL HEALTH

Funding for initiatives in the GH development of LMICs (also known as Development Assistance for Health, DAH) has, historically, originated from multiple sources (see **Box 13.3**). While these initiatives may have been beneficial for specific diseases like malaria (see p. 563), tuberculosis (p. 967) and HIV/AIDS (p. 1425), health systems development has frequently lagged behind such high-profile schemes. The consequences of this were seen in the slow response of the WHO and others to the 2014 outbreak of Ebola virus in Africa.

Improvements in healthcare result in economic growth. For example, a 10% reduction of malaria in endemic areas is associated with a 0.3% increase in GDP. Treatment of HIV-positive patients with anti-retroviral drugs results in net economic benefit through increased productivity and a reduction in the costs of medical care. Any failure to invest in health and health systems is a threat to future global prosperity, particularly in poor countries. Transnational collaboration is especially necessary in the face of pandemic threats.

Surgical care is currently a neglected component of the health systems in many countries (see p. 242). The cumulative loss of economic productivity between 2015 and 2030, in the absence of a significant scaling up of global surgical services, is estimated at US$ 12.3 trillion.

Political decisions regarding investment in healthcare and health systems also need to focus on infrastructure, including food and agriculture, the environment and human rights issues, especially the rights of women. In essence, the pursuit of 'pro-poor' policies that place the poor at the centre of development policy is essential for future global prosperity.

Further reading

Figuera J, McKee M. *Health Systems, Health, Wealth and Societal Well-being.* Maidenhead: McGraw Hill/Open University Press; 2012.

Meara JG, Leather AJM, Hagander L et al and the Lancet Commission on Global Surgery. Global Surgery 2030; evidence and solutions for achieving health, welfare, and economic development. *Lancet* 2015; 386:569–624.
Resch S, Korenromp E, Stover J et al. Economic returns to investment in AIDS treatment in low and middle income countries. *PLoS One* 2011; 6:e25310.

SOCIAL DETERMINANTS OF HEALTH

The drivers of health inequities reside in the social, economic and political environments. The WHO (2008) defined the social determinants of health as 'the conditions in which people are born, grow, work, and age. These circumstances are shaped by the distribution of money, power and resources at global, national and local levels.'

The social gradient of health follows the socioeconomic pattern from the top to the bottom: that is, the lower the individual is within their socioeconomic position, the worse their health. This is seen globally in HICs, as well as in LMICs. The socioeconomic status of a person is their social position in society, which is determined by their education, income and occupation.

There is now clear evidence to justify national policies that aim to reduce health inequity and the health divide across all countries. It has also been suggested that reduction in health inequities should become one of the main criteria used to assess the effectiveness of health systems and governments as a whole.

Further reading

Donkin A, Goldblatt P, Allen J et al. Global action on the social determinants of health. *BMJ Global Health* 2018; 3:e000603.
Marmot M, Allen J, Bell R et al and World Health Organization. European review of social determinants of health and health divide. *Lancet* 2012; 38:1011–1029.

HUMAN RIGHTS AND THE VALUE OF ENGAGEMENT IN GLOBAL HEALTH

The Universal Declaration of Human Rights (1948), while not legally binding, serves as a 'common standard for all peoples and all nations'. It has given rise to two new legally binding covenants: the International Covenant on Civil and Political Rights and the International Covenant on Economic, Social and Cultural Rights.

The WHO is a specialized agency of the United Nations with a remit for international public health. Its constitution enshrines 'the highest attainable standard of health' as a fundamental right of every human being. The right to health contains four elements: availability (of programmes of public health), accessibility (of health facilities and services in a non-discriminatory fashion), acceptability (ethical and cultural requirements), and good-quality care.

The healthcare workforce

There is a worldwide shortage of healthcare workers from all disciplines (**Fig. 13.5**). Current estimates suggest that an additional 40 million healthcare workers will be required by 2030 to meet global demand. Engagement in GH challenges helps to promote patterns of behaviour that benefit healthcare workers and their recipients. These behaviours include altruism, team-working and appreciation of cultural diversity.

Medical electives

Many medical students and doctors undertake periods of time visiting and working in unfamiliar environments, whether in their home

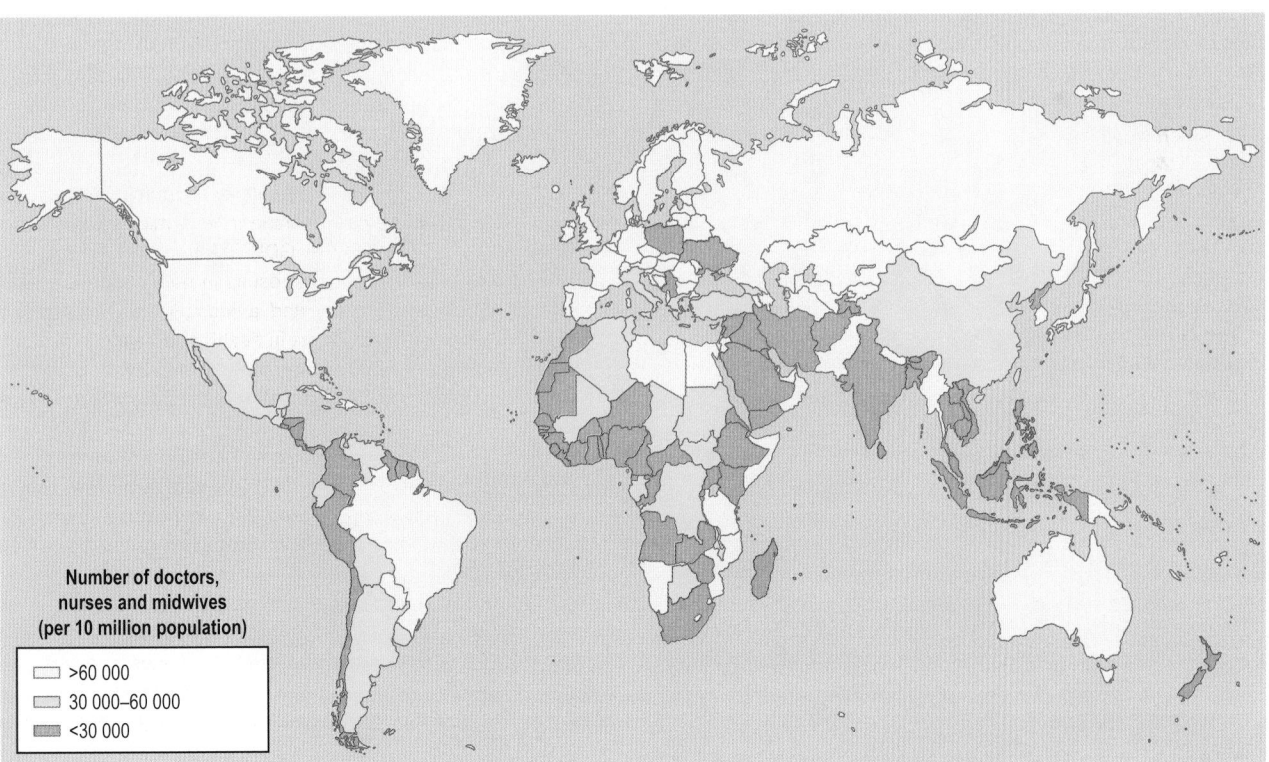

Number of doctors, nurses and midwives (per 10 million population)

- >60 000
- 30 000–60 000
- <30 000

Fig. 13.5 **Worldwide shortage of healthcare workers.** There are 57 countries with a critical shortage of 2.4 million health service providers (doctors, nurses and midwives). Africa has 25% of the world's healthcare burden and 1.3% of the providers. *(From Crisp N, Cheng L. Global supply of health professionals. N Engl J Med 2014; 370:950–957 [Figure 1], with permission.)*

country or abroad. This is mutually beneficial to all participants, provided that a culture of shared learning is embraced. All such visits, commonly termed 'medical electives', should have clear objectives and measurable educational outcomes. They promote altruistic behaviours and should not compromise the working arrangements for host organizations. Pre-departure preparation should include consideration of culture, ethical challenges and security issues. All visitors must work within their approved competencies, be appropriately supervised and comply with national guidance on good medical practice. Maximum benefit from medical electives is achieved when there is a mutual commitment to long-term partnership.

Further reading

http://www.ohchr.org *International Bill of Human Rights.*
http://www.un.org *Universal Declaration of Human Rights.*

Bibliography

Crisp N. *Turning the World Upside Down. The Search for Global Health in the 21st Century*. London: Royal Society of Medicine Press; 2010.
Global Burden of Disease Study 2013 Collaboration. Global, regional, and national incidence, prevalence, and years lived with disability for 301 acute and chronic diseases and injuries in 188 countries, 1990–2013: a systematic analysis for the Global Burden of Disease Study 2013. *Lancet* 2015; 386:743–800.
Marmot M. *The Health Gap: The Challenge of an Unequal World*. London: Bloomsbury Publishing; 2015.
Sethia B, Kumar P. *Essentials of Global Health*. Edinburgh: Elsevier; 2018.

Public health

Sarah Winchester, Simona Baracaia and Ian Basnett

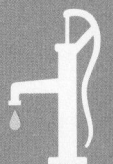

CORE SKILLS AND KNOWLEDGE

Factors that influence health stretch from climate change through to health behaviours. A multiprofessional approach, incorporating the epidemiological study of disease alongside practical health interventions, is required to address these complex and high-level challenges. When John Snow analysed cases of cholera in 1854, he not only mapped the distribution of cases and the possible link to a water pump, but also dealt with the source of the outbreak by removing the pump.

The core workforce includes doctors within the medical specialty of public health, working alongside epidemiologists, analysts, commissioners, nurses, health visitors and environmental health officers. Clinicians in other specialties often take a population approach too, especially in primary care.

Key to understanding public health is recognizing that many patients have had their health adversely affected by social, environmental or behavioural factors. The three pillars of public health intervene to address these:

- *health improvement:* implementing interventions to prevent ill-health and improve population health
- *health protection:* preventing, controlling and monitoring infectious, environmental, chemical and radiological hazards to population health
- *healthcare public health:* maximizing the benefits of healthcare interventions and reducing inequalities, using tools such as screening and health economics.

Skills required in public health can be developed by critically appraising relevant articles in journals, by undertaking local quality improvement projects, and by seeking out opportunities to work with national or local groups focusing on health or sustainability. Many public health departments in local authorities will be happy to discuss public health or arrange placements.

INTRODUCTION

When viewed on a population level, health is a broad concept. Social determinants of health are numerous and varied, stretching from climate change through to health behaviours (see **Fig. 14.4** later). The Alma Ata (World Health Organization (WHO) conference) declaration of 1978 stated that 'health, which is a state of complete physical, mental and social wellbeing, and not merely the absence of disease or infirmity, is a fundamental human right' and that 'the attainment of the highest possible level of health is a most important worldwide social goal whose realization requires the action of many other social and economic sectors in addition to the health sector'. It goes on to assert the key importance of addressing inequalities. Those working in public health strive to bring about change at a scale that will maximize benefit, while reducing inequalities in health.

The origins of public health lie in the big cities of industrialized nations in the mid-nineteenth century, where pioneers such as John Snow (**Box 14.1**) began studying patterns of transmissible disease and intervening to prevent the spread of infection. The development of germ theory, the discovery of means to prevent communicable diseases (such as vaccination and sanitation), and epidemiological insights into key causes of non-communicable diseases (such as smoking) allowed public health teams to attain a crucial position in improving the health of the whole population (**Box 14.2**). Latterly, healthcare public health has brought academic rigour to the study of aspects of healthcare delivery and to ensuring that maximum benefit is derived at a population level from healthcare services.

Public health and global health

This chapter focuses primarily on public health in higher-income countries. Public health issues more commonly associated with low- to middle-income countries, such as communicable and nutritional diseases, are covered in Chapter 13 ('Global health'). However, non-communicable diseases, such as cardiovascular disease and cancer, are now the leading cause of death globally (Global Burden of Disease 2017), meaning that the contents of this chapter are relevant for all settings.

Further reading

Institute for Health Metrics and Evaluation. *Global Burden of Disease Compare*, 2017; https://vizhub.healthdata.org/gbd-compare/.
International Conference on Primary Health Care. *Declaration of Alma-Ata*, 1978; https://www.who.int/publications/almaata_declaration_en.pdf?ua=1.

KEY CONCEPTS IN PUBLIC HEALTH

Epidemiology and causality

Epidemiology is the study of how often diseases occur in different groups of people, and why. It is central to the discipline and practice of public health medicine. Understanding the patterns of disease distribution in a population can reveal factors that may be associated with that disease. For example, the demonstration of a link between smoking and lung cancer by Sir Richard Doll and Sir Austin Bradford Hill in 1950 is a seminal piece of epidemiological research. If epidemiological associations are causal, then working to reduce or mitigate identified causes may provide an opportunity to prevent future disease. Bradford Hill laid out nine criteria to be considered when judging whether an association is likely to be causal (**Box 14.3**).

Health needs assessments

Health Needs Assessments (HNAs) are key tools used in public health medicine to drive improvement in health within a population. HNAs aim to determine healthcare needs systematically and to compare them with current service provision in order to identify gaps. A health need (whenever individuals are not completely well) and a health*care* need (if there is an ability for them to benefit from care) should be differentiated: that is, if an evidence-based intervention has been shown to improve the health of the individuals with the condition in question, as not all diseases are amenable to treatment. Real healthcare needs must be distinguished from either demand (what individuals may wish to buy or use) or supply (current provision) (**Fig. 14.1**).

Three techniques for producing HNAs have been described (Stevens and Raftery 1997):

- *epidemiological* – summarizing data on healthcare needs from a range of sources by time, place and person

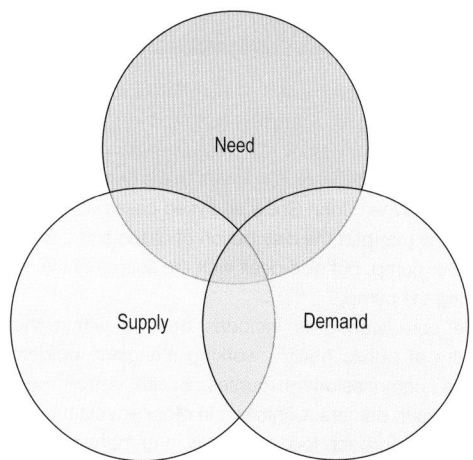

Fig. 14.1 Demand, supply and need.

- *comparative* – comparing needs, as well as service provision and service usage, between different populations
- *corporate* – consulting with stakeholders, such as healthcare professionals, commissioners and patients, to identify priorities.

Life expectancy and quality of life

Life expectancy at birth is defined as the number of years that a newborn could be expected to live if current mortality rates continue. Life expectancy has generally been rising across the world, although an Organisation for Economic Co-operation and Development (OECD) report from 2019 notes that the rate of improvement has slowed in several European countries since 2011, including France, Germany, Sweden, the Netherlands and the UK, and life expectancy has fallen in the USA in recent years.

Healthy life expectancy, defined as the number of years lived in self-assessed good health, adds a quality of life component to estimates of life expectancy. While healthy life expectancy in many countries is generally rising, it is doing so at a lower rate than life expectancy. This means that although people in most countries are living longer, they are experiencing more years in poor health. There is also a strong link to deprivation. For example, individuals living in the most deprived areas of England spend more of their life in poor health, in comparison to those in areas of lesser deprivation (**Fig. 14.2**).

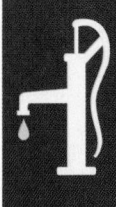

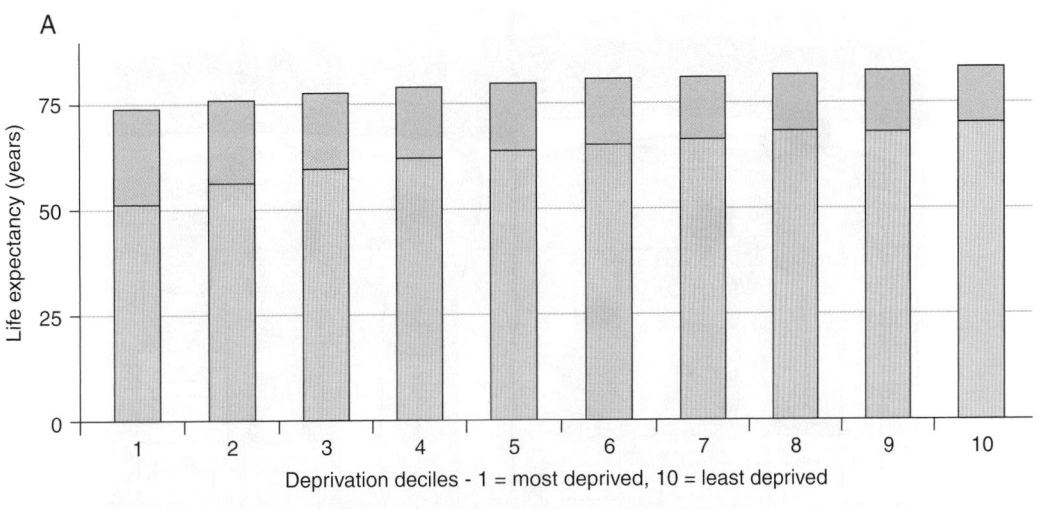

A

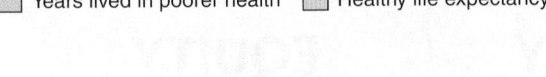

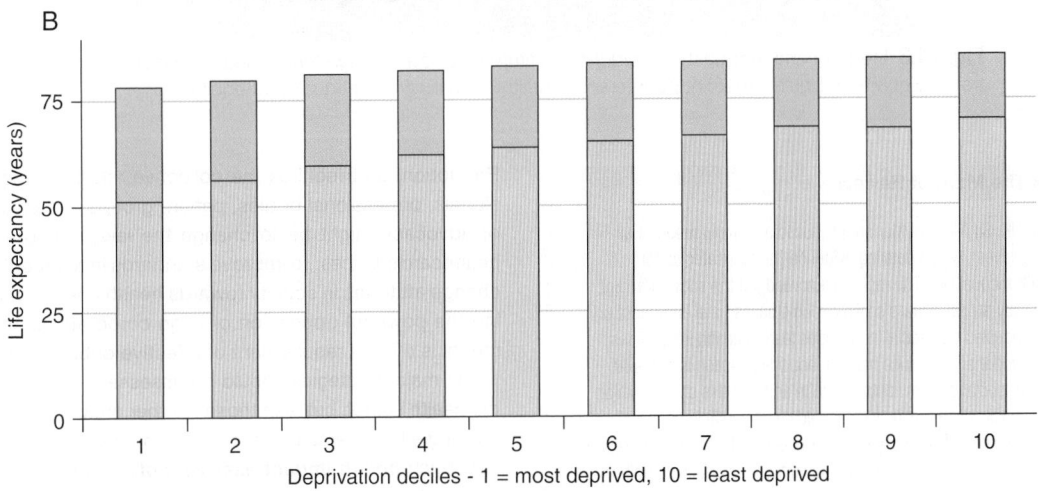

B

Fig. 14.2 Healthy life expectancy at birth and years lived in poorer states of health by national deprivation deciles (England, 2015–2017). (A) Males. (B) Females. *(Office for National Statistics. Annual Population Survey.)* (Reprint from Health state life expectancies by national deprivation deciles, England and Wales: 2015 to 2017 http://www.nationalarchives.gov.uk/doc/open-government-licence/version/3/.)

Health inequalities

Health inequalities are differences in health status between groups of individuals, which differ based on gender, ethnicity, disability, area of residence, socioeconomic status or other factors. Health differences arising from such characteristics often represent an injustice, especially if they are potentially avoidable and thus inequitable (inherently unjust and unfair). One of public health's fundamental principles is to strive to reduce such inequalities and to make health outcomes fairer for the population (**Fig. 14.3** and **Box 14.4**). However, this is often complicated by Tudor Hart's *inverse care law*, which states that the availability of good healthcare often varies inversely with need, particularly where market forces are operating.

Deprivation

Examples of health inequalities that are amenable to change are those associated with deprivation. Deprivation can be measured by a basket of indicators within defined geographical areas. One

example is the **Index of Multiple Deprivation**, which uses data across seven domains to compare relative deprivation across small areas in England. The domains encompass:
- income levels
- employment levels
- education and skills within a population
- levels of chronic ill-health and disability
- crime
- barriers to housing and local services
- the living environment.

A number of poor health outcomes have been found to correlate with deprivation. For example, it has been shown that children living in deprived areas have a higher prevalence of dental caries than those in less deprived areas. Water fluoridation is a public health intervention that improves oral health across the population but has been shown to have the most impact in those who are more deprived, thereby reducing health inequality. Other adverse outcomes associated with deprivation extend throughout the life-course, and include

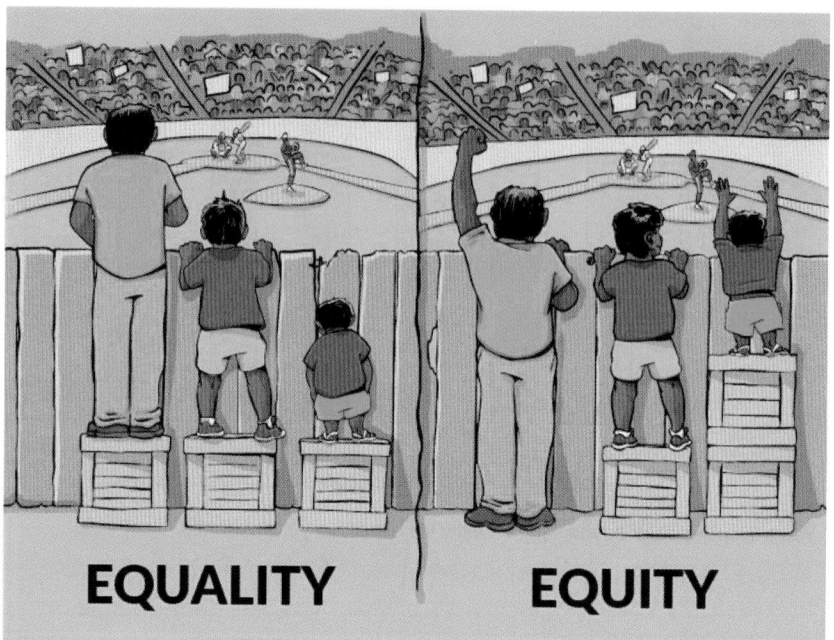

Fig. 14.3 Inequity and inequality. *(Interaction Institute for Social Change. Artist: Angus Maguire.* Illustrating Equality vs Equity, 2016; http://interactioninstitute.org/illustrating-equality-vs-equity/.)

> ⓘ **Box 14.4** The Marmot Review
>
> In 2010 in the UK, Sir Michael Marmot produced a seminal report, 'Fair Society Healthy Lives', which detailed evidence-based strategies for reducing health inequalities. The report acknowledged the social gradient in health, whereby an individual's social circumstances have an impact on health, and recognized that social inequalities lead to health inequalities. Marmot concluded that, to reduce health inequalities, action is required across the wider social determinants of health and that this should exhibit proportionate universalism (i.e. actions should be universal to all but proportionate in scale and intensity to the level of disadvantage). The report stated that actions to tackle inequalities should focus on six overlapping policy objectives:
>
> 1. Giving all children the best start in life
> 2. Enabling people of all ages to maximize their potential and acquire control over their lives
> 3. Creating fair employment and good work opportunities for all
> 4. Ensuring that everyone has a healthy standard of living
> 5. Creating and developing healthy, sustainable communities
> 6. Strengthening preventative health measures

low birth weight, higher infant mortality, increased chronic disease and premature death. Data suggest that inequalities in health due to deprivation are widening. In the UK, official statistics from 2014–16 demonstrate that life expectancy in the 10% *least* deprived areas of England and Wales was 9 years longer for males and 7 years longer for females than in the 10% *most* deprived areas, and that these gaps are widening.

Politics and advocacy

The WHO defines health advocacy as 'a combination of individual and social actions designed to gain political commitment, policy support, social acceptance and systems support for a particular health goal or programme'. It is a key component of health promotion, as detailed within the WHO's Ottawa Charter for Health Promotion, and requires the collective efforts of medical professionals, professional bodies, patient groups and charities. Targets of advocacy might be to change the law, to improve access to healthcare services, to improve standards in the food industry or to change attitudes in society towards healthy behaviours. Overcoming the powerful opposition of large corporations and/or governments is often a requirement of effective public health advocacy.

All major strategies should be assessed – not just those within the health sector, but also those in other areas such as transport or housing – to understand their impact on health and health inequalities. Such **health impact assessments** can be used to maximize the positive health consequences and minimize the adverse ones (both indirect and direct), together with reducing health inequalities.

Examples of successful health advocacy include smoking bans and reduction of salt intake.

Smoking bans

A number of countries have introduced bans on smoking in the workplace and in public spaces; a few (such as New Zealand and Finland) have announced a target to be 'tobacco-free' by a designated point in the future. International data from the USA and Europe have revealed a variety of improved health outcomes since the introduction of smoking bans, including reductions in preterm births, childhood hospital admissions for asthma, and emergency admissions for myocardial infarction. Despite unequivocal evidence of public health benefits, opponents of smoking bans have suggested they are examples of governments acting as a 'nanny state', or have expressed concern over the potential for a shift in smoking behaviour into private homes (which does not seem to have occurred). However, in general, smoking bans received public support, including among smokers, and much of the opposition came from large tobacco companies.

Reduction of daily salt intake

Regularly exceeding the maximum amount of salt recommended for daily consumption is common across the world

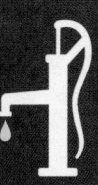

and is strongly associated with hypertension, cardiovascular disease and premature mortality. Health advocacy efforts have been based on public education campaigns, clear labelling of the salt content of foods, and salt reduction targets for the food industry. Most salt in Western diets is found in processed food, and an approach based on purely individual behaviour change is widely regarded as insufficient to tackle the problem. To make stronger gains, the food industry needs to reduce salt further within prepared food in supermarkets and food outlets. Such widespread change requires government commitment, with imposed targets and incentives for reducing salt within the food industry.

Further reading

Bradford Hill A. The environment and disease: association or causation? *Proc R Soc Med* 1965; 58:295–300.
Doll R, Bradford Hill A. Smoking and carcinoma of the lung: preliminary report. *Br Med J* 1950; 2:739–748.
Marmot M, Atkinson T, Bell J et al. *Fair Society, Healthy Lives: The Marmot Review*, 2010; http://www.instituteofhealthequity.org/resources-reports/fair-society-healthy-lives-the-marmot-review/fair-society-healthy-lives-full-report-pdf.pdf.
Office for National Statistics. *Health State Life Expectancies by National Deprivation Deciles, England and Wales: 2014 to 2016*; https://www.ons.gov.uk/peoplepopulationandcommunity/healthandsocialcare/healthinequalities/bulletins/healthstatelifeexpectanciesbyindexofmultipledeprivationimd/englandandwales2014to2016.
Stevens A, Raftery J (eds). *Health Care Needs Assessment*, 2nd series. Oxford: Radcliffe; 1997.
Tudor Hart J. The inverse care law. *Lancet* 1971; 297:405–412.

PILLARS OF PUBLIC HEALTH

Although models of public health provision vary in different countries, services are often delivered at the level of local government or regional health authorities. National bodies, such as the Centers for Disease Control and Prevention (CDC) in the USA or Public Health England (PHE), are responsible for collation of health statistics, support for national vaccination programmes and advice to government on other aspects of health policy.

The work of public health services can be described according to the three pillars of public health:
- health improvement
- health protection
- healthcare public health.

Health improvement

While it might seem self-evident that preventing a disease is better than dealing with the consequences, there is also strong economic evidence to support the case for prevention. For example, a number of studies have demonstrated that smoking cessation services both improve population health and reduce healthcare costs overall. When considering approaches to prevention, they can be classified as primary, secondary or tertiary (**Box 14.5**).

Wider determinants of health

Wider determinants of health (WDHs) are the broader social, economic, political and environmental circumstances that influence health outcomes throughout life. Dahlgren and Whitehead (1991), subsequently modified by Barton and Grant (2006), developed an influential model of the main determinants of health, in which, at the core, are constitutional factors such as sex, age and genetics; overlapping layers represent individual lifestyle factors, followed by the WDHs (**Fig. 14.4**). The core attributes are relatively fixed but, as the layers of influence extend outwards, the determinants are amenable to change:
- The first layer represents individual *lifestyle behaviours*, such as diet, physical activity, smoking and alcohol consumption.
- The second layer represents the *communities in which individuals live* – social networks that influence health and the health behaviours we exhibit.
- Next, *living and working conditions* have an impact on health, for example, the quality of an individual's employment, housing and education.
- Finally, the prevailing *socioeconomic, cultural and environmental conditions* affect the health of the whole population, and these are influenced by local, regional, national and international factors.

These overlapping layers exert an influence over each other and there is a complex interplay between them.

Air pollution

Air pollution is an example of a WDH, representing a huge environmental health risk globally. Poor air quality has a range of short- and long-term health impacts, including but not limited to cardiovascular and respiratory disease, emergency hospital admissions and death. One of the first demonstrations of these effects was during the 'great smog of London' in 1952, which contributed towards a large number of deaths. This led to the Clean Air Act of 1956, which limited the burning of solid fuel for heating in urban areas.

A range of pollutants are known to be harmful to health, including particulate matter and nitrogen dioxide. Although tackling air pollution requires individual efforts, the problem cannot be adequately addressed without local, national and international policy change. Examples of interventions for tackling air pollution include:
- setting objectives and limits for different pollutants
- encouraging use of active transport instead of cars

---

i **Box 14.5 Levels of prevention of disease**

Primary
- Involves reduction in exposure to risk factors, focusing either on the whole population or on high-risk subgroups
- Examples include healthy lifestyle interventions for the prevention of cardiovascular disease, or workplace-based interventions to reduce asbestos exposure
- Focusing on the whole population may result in Rose's *prevention paradox* – such strategies may have a relatively small impact at an individual level, despite large benefits at a population level or for those at highest risk

Secondary
- Involves detecting disease at an early stage and undertaking prompt intervention to reduce the disease's impact
- Examples include screening programmes, or prescription of statins for hypercholesterolaemia to reduce the likelihood of myocardial infarction or stroke

Tertiary
- Aims to reduce or mitigate long-term complications of a disease and maximize functioning
- Examples are HbA_{1c} monitoring in diabetes mellitus to minimize long-term micro- and macrovascular complications, or neuro-rehabilitation after head injury

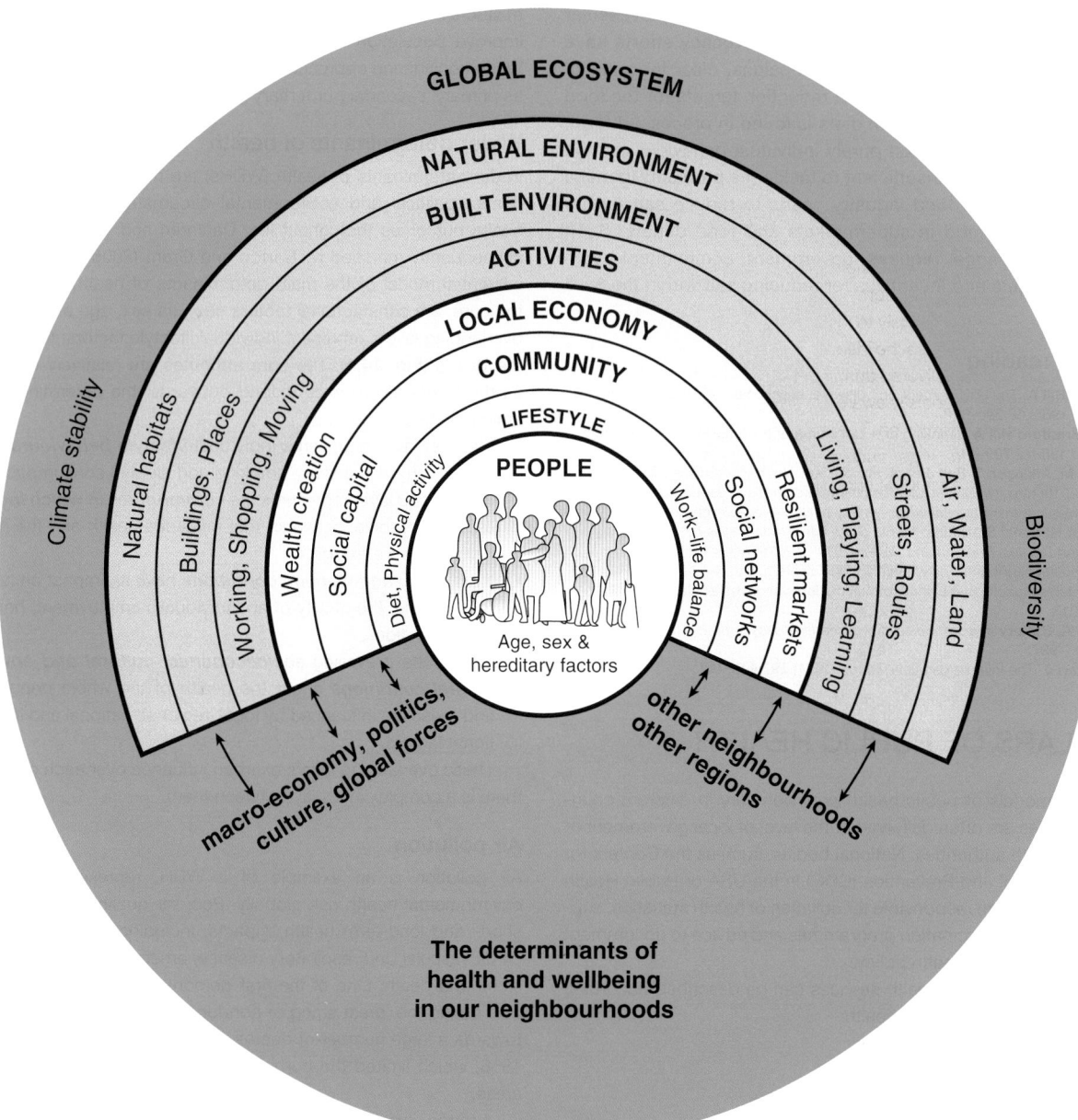

Fig. 14.4 The health map. *(Barton H, Grant M. A health map for the local human habitat.* J R Soc Promot Health *2006; 126:252–253. ISSN 1466-4240 developed from the model by Dahlgren G, Whitehead M. 'The main determinants of health' model, 1991, version accessible in: Dahlgren G, Whitehead M.* European Strategies for Tackling Social Inequities in Health: Levelling up, Part 2. *Copenhagen: WHO Regional Office for Europe, 2007; http://www.euro.who.int/__data/assets/pdf_file/0018/103824/E89384.pdf.)*

- encouraging manufacturers to produce cleaner vehicles, and industry to adopt greener technologies
- introducing ultra-low emissions zones in urban areas and 'no-idling zones' around schools.

Poor air quality affects the whole population, but also represents a significant health inequality in that more vulnerable members of society have higher exposure (for example, those living in more deprived areas) or are more susceptible to harm (such as young children or the elderly). Thus it is imperative to ensure that any interventions aimed at tackling air pollution also aim to address such inequalities.

Behaviour change

Behaviour change provides a crucial opportunity to improve health significantly. However, unhealthy behaviours are often complex and deeply ingrained. For example, the COM-B model recognizes that the interrelated components of *c*apability, *o*pportunity and *m*otivation must all be addressed before *b*ehaviour will be changed. At a population level, instigating change requires holistic and sustained interventions across a range of policy types. Interventions may be classified as individual, structural, fiscal or legal (**Fig. 14.5**), although there may be significant overlap between these: for instance, structural and fiscal approaches are often enshrined in legislation.

Individual interventions

Clinical consultations can be a prime setting in which to encourage individual-level behavioural change. The 'Making Every Contact Count' initiative seeks to encourage clinicians, and a broader range of professionals, to consider how they can build health promotion into their routine patient or client interactions. For example, professionals working in education or in the emergency services may identify issues of poor mental or physical health, isolation or violence. They may have an initial conversation about the issues they have identified, before signposting to a range of other local services that may provide further support.

While brief advice is unlikely to instigate long-term change if delivered in isolation, it may raise the idea of change higher up the patient's agenda, particularly if delivered during a 'teachable moment' when an individual becomes especially aware of their health, such as during an unexpected hospital admission. There are several models to describe individual behaviour change, such as Prochaska and DiClemente's 1983 Stages of Change model (**Fig. 14.6**). Individual-level behaviour

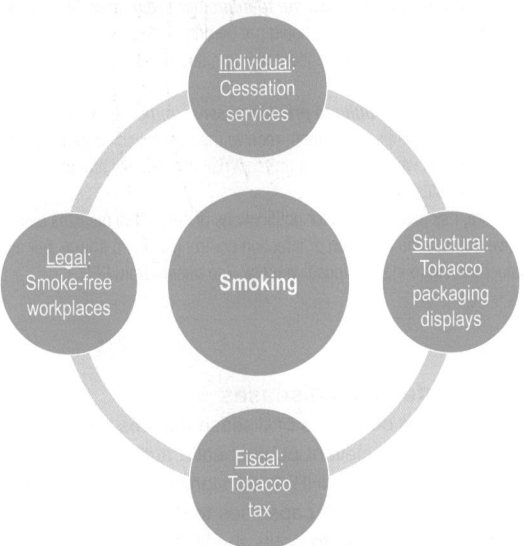

Fig. 14.5 Examples of initiatives to reduce smoking.

change therapies have been found to be highly cost-effective: for example, brief advice given to adult patients in primary care about increasing their physical activity has been shown to cost £1730 per quality-adjusted life-year (QALY) gained. A commonly used threshold for determining the cost-effectiveness of a healthcare intervention is £20 000–£30 000 per QALY gained.

Structural interventions

Structural approaches to behaviour change may be achieved through 'nudging' individuals to default to healthier choices. The nudge theory of behavioural economics rose to prominence in 2008 with the publication of 'Nudge: Improving Decisions about Health, Wealth and Happiness' by Richard Thaler and Cass Sunstein, leading to Thaler being awarded the 2017 Nobel Prize for Economics. Nudge theory proposes that small tweaks to frame a choice more favourably or render an option easier are often sufficient to increase its uptake, and that decisions are not based purely on underlying rationale. A Cochrane review in 2015 concluded that individuals consistently eat more food when offered large portions or use larger items of tableware. Promoting package and portion size reductions could be a tool to reduce weight gain.

Fiscal interventions

Fiscal measures may also encourage behaviour change, through either the taxation of potentially harmful choices to render them less attractive, or the subsidization of healthy ones to make them more favourable. The WHO encourages countries to tax sugary drinks, and many have implemented such legislation. Measures to improve healthy eating by subsidizing school dinners or offering free vitamin supplements to children and pregnant women may enhance health outcomes and also reduce inequality (**Box 14.6**). These measures often operate at a national level through the introduction of governmental policy, which may be associated with new legislation.

Legal interventions

In addition to the introduction of taxes, legislative approaches to encourage behaviour change may include the regulation or prohibition of unhealthy activities. It was estimated in 2008 in the UK that

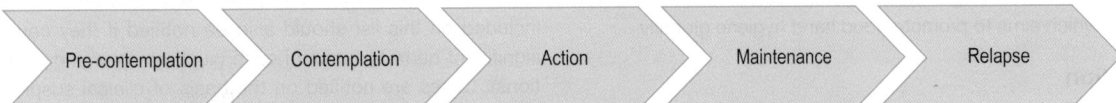

Fig. 14.6 Stages of Change model. *(Adapted from Prochaska J, DiClemente C. Stages and processes of self-change of smoking: toward an integrative model of change.* J Consult Clin Psychol *1983; 51:390–395.)*

---

i Box 14.6 Fiscal measures to improve diet and nutrition

Taxing harmful behaviours

- Poor oral health, including the presence of dental caries, is the most prevalent condition worldwide (Global Burden of Disease 2017). Reducing sugar consumption is predicted to improve oral health, as well as tackle obesity.
- An excise tax on sugar-sweetened beverages ('sugar tax') is an example of a fiscal policy that aims to encourage manufacturers to reduce the sugar content of their products, as well as dissuading individuals from consuming products with high sugar levels.
- Such a tax has been introduced in a number of jurisdictions over recent years and initial results are promising. In the UK the government introduced a Soft Drinks Industry Levy in 2018 and it is estimated that half of manufacturers reformulated their drinks to avoid it. An evaluation of a similar tax in Berkeley,

California, found that it was associated with a 21% decrease in sugar-sweetened beverages in low-income neighbourhoods, indicating that the policy has the potential not only to improve health, but also to reduce health inequalities.

Subsidizing healthy behaviours

- It has been estimated that 1 billion people globally have vitamin D deficiency, and there has been a rise in cases of rickets in some countries.
- This can be prevented by eating a diet rich in vitamin D and calcium, or by taking vitamin D supplements.
- The Healthy Start vitamins scheme was introduced in the UK in 2006 and provides free vitamin supplements (including vitamin D) for pregnant women and young children in low-income families.

over the previous 25 years since the wearing of seatbelts became compulsory, at least 60 000 lives had been saved and 600 000 severe injuries had been prevented. Legal approaches to behaviour change are often used once other methods have been tried without adequate success, since they may be perceived as paternalistic, attracting political controversy and significant lobbying from industry.

Further reading

Avineri E, Goodwin P. *Individual Behaviour Change: Evidence in Transport and Public Health*. London: Department for Transport, 2010; http://eprints.uwe.ac.uk/11211.
Falbe J, Thompson H, Becker C et al. Impact of the Berkeley excise tax on sugar-sweetened beverage consumption. *Am J Public Health* 2016; 106:1865–1871.
National Institute for Health and Care Excellence. *NICE Public Health Guideline 49: Behaviour Change: Individual Approaches*. NICE 2014; https://www.nice.org.uk/guidance/ph49.
Owen L, Pennington B, Fischer A et al. The cost-effectiveness of public health interventions examined by NICE from 2011 to 2016. *J Public Health* 2017; 40:557–566.
Rose G. Strategy of prevention: lessons from cardiovascular disease. *Br Med J* 1981; 282:1847–1851.

Health protection

Health protection involves anticipating and controlling infectious, environmental, chemical and radiological hazards to public health. There are three main areas of activity: prevention, control and monitoring (surveillance).

Prevention

Prevention within health protection is concerned with reducing the risk of transmission of infectious diseases. Two key examples of this are hand hygiene and vaccination.

Hand hygiene

This is one of the simplest yet most effective public health (prevention and control) measures. Basic hand-washing in communities minimizes the spread of infection (e.g. reducing the risk of *Escherichia coli* infection in petting zoos, or disrupting the transmission of norovirus in schools), but is also the main way of combating hospital-acquired infections and preventing the spread of antimicrobial resistance. The WHO recognizes the significant impact that such a simple measure can have in saving lives through its Clean Care is Safer Care campaign, which aims to promote good hand hygiene globally.

Vaccination

Vaccination has had a huge impact on the burden of infectious disease, second only to clean water provision. Vaccination programmes confer benefit to the individual and to the population as a whole (especially its most vulnerable members) through herd immunity, whereby a high proportion of population immunity reduces person-to-person transmission. The basic reproduction number (R_0) is the number of secondary infections produced by a typical infection in a totally susceptible population. For diseases with a high R_0 (e.g. measles), higher coverage is required to attain herd protection.

Vaccination programmes are tailored to the national prevalence of particular diseases. Selective vaccination programmes aim to protect those at highest risk of certain diseases (e.g. for travellers or healthcare workers), while mass vaccination programmes aim to contain (control), eliminate or eradicate disease (**Box 14.7**). Some vaccines provide protection *after* exposure in some cases (e.g. the measles, mumps and rubella (MMR) vaccine, which can be used to help limit the spread of a measles outbreak by immunizing previously unvaccinated contacts of a known case, **Box 14.8**).

Box 14.7 Control, elimination and eradication

- *Control* is defined as when the amount or impact of a disease within a population has reduced to a locally acceptable level.
- *Elimination* is when the disease incidence within a defined area is zero.
- *Eradication* occurs when the disease incidence is zero worldwide and no environmental reservoir exists. This has been achieved only for smallpox.

(Adapted from Dowdle WR, The principles of disease elimination and eradication. Bull World Health Org 1998; 76(Suppl 2):22–25.)

Box 14.8 Notification of suspected measles cases

Recent outbreaks of measles in Europe and the USA have been seen primarily among individuals who have not received the measles, mumps and rubella (MMR) vaccination. Post-exposure prophylaxis (PEP), if delivered promptly, can prevent contacts of known sufferers from developing measles, or may attenuate their symptoms if they go on to develop the disease.

PEP can be delivered in two ways:

- *Using a dose of MMR vaccine to induce active immunity.* However, MMR is a live vaccine and should not be administered to immunocompromised individuals or pregnant women, and is inappropriate for some infants.
- *Using immunoglobulin to provide passive immunity.* This is recommended for groups who cannot receive the MMR vaccine for the reasons listed above, who are often at greatest risk of morbidity and mortality from measles infection.

Therefore, risk assessments for notifications of suspected measles cases involve not only the provision of infection control (isolation) advice, but also contact tracing to identify those who stand to benefit from PEP.

Control

Control of infectious diseases

Rapid response to outbreaks of disease requires timely notification of new cases to the relevant public health authorities. The International Health Regulations (IHR) 2005 signify an agreement between 196 countries to build their capacities to detect, assess and report public health events, and to notify the WHO of any event that may constitute a 'public health emergency of international concern'. In England, the most recent national legislation lists 32 diseases and 60 causative organisms as notifiable, and other infections not included on this list should also be notified if they could present significant harm to human health (such as emerging or new infections). Cases are notified on the basis of clinical suspicion to the local health protection team, and notification should not be delayed while awaiting confirmation.

Health protection teams will then perform a risk assessment for each notification they receive, and will introduce control measures specific to the disease and the context to mitigate identified risks, working in conjunction with environmental health officers from the local authority. Control measures may include:

- provision of infection prevention and control advice
- isolation of infected individuals
- post-exposure prophylaxis.

Control of environmental hazards

Public health services are also notified of local environmental, chemical or radiological hazards that threaten the health of the public. These threats are wide-ranging and include air pollution, drinking water contamination and exposure to radiation. Public health professionals work with the relevant experts, emergency services, local government and industry to identify and mitigate these hazards.

Monitoring (surveillance)

'Emerging infectious diseases' (EIDs) is a term that encompasses newly emerging pathogens, pathogens whose incidence is increasing and/or that are appearing in new populations, and pathogens that are re-emerging in different forms (e.g. multidrug-resistant (MDR) and extensively drug-resistant (XDR) tuberculosis). Many of these EIDs are zoonoses (of animal origin), including, for example, human immunodeficiency virus (HIV) and Middle East respiratory syndrome coronavirus (MERS-CoV, **Box 14.9**). Other recent examples of EIDs include Zika virus associated with microcephaly, Ebola virus disease associated with outbreaks in West Africa and the Democratic Republic of Congo, and SARS-CoV2, responsible for the global COVID-19 pandemic which continues to unfold at the time of publication.

The reasons why new infections appear and old ones return are multifactorial and include:

- **population movement** to new geographical areas, e.g. displacement following war or natural disasters
- **a rise in global trade and travel**
- **ecological changes**, such as those driven by climate change or severe weather events (which can, for example, have an impact on vectors implicated in the transmission of pathogens); or changes in agricultural practices (which can, for example, alter the likelihood of coming into contact with sources of infection)
- **technologies in healthcare**, e.g. xenotransplantation or increased antibiotic use (associated with the development of antimicrobial resistance).

Well-developed surveillance mechanisms are key in the early detection of new and emerging pathogens that may represent a significant future threat to health. This monitoring facilitates outbreak investigations (**Box 14.10**), as well as informing broader infection prevention policy (**Box 14.11**).

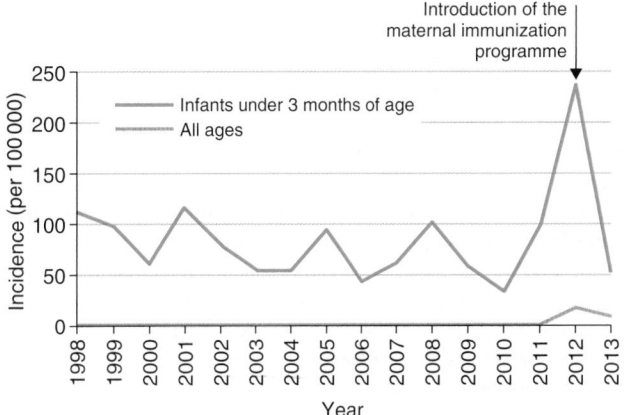

Fig. 14.7 Incidence of laboratory-confirmed cases of pertussis, England (1998–2013). *(By kind permission of Public Health England. The Green Book, Ch. 24, p. 4, Fig. 24.2. https://assets.publishing.serv ice.gov.uk/government/uploads/system/uploads/attachment_data/file/ 514363/Pertussis_Green_Book_Chapter_24_Ap2016.pdf.)*

Further reading

Andre FE, Booy R, Bock HL et al. Vaccination greatly reduces disease, disability, death and inequity worldwide. *Bull World Health Org* 2008; 86:81–160.

Dowdle WR. The principles of disease elimination and eradication. *Bull World Health Org* 1998; 76(Suppl 2):22–25.

Grant K, Byrne L. *Disease Detectives: Using Supermarket Loyalty Cards to Trace an E coli Outbreak*, 2018; https://publichealthmatters.blog.gov.uk/2018/09/26/dise ase-detectives-using-supermarket-loyalty-cards-to-trace-an-e-coli-outbreak/.

Morens DM, Fauci AS. Emerging infectious diseases: threats to human health and global stability. *PLoS Pathog* 2013; 9:e1003467.

Morse SS. Factors in the emergence of infectious diseases. *Emerg Infect Dis* 1995; 191:7–15.

Parikh SR, Andrews NJ, Beebeejaun K et al. Effectiveness and impact of a reduced infant schedule of 4CMenB vaccine against group B meningococcal disease in England: a national observational cohort study. *Lancet* 2016; 388:2775–2782.

Public Health England. *Emerging Infections: How and Why They Arise*, 2019; htt ps://www.gov.uk/government/publications/emerging-infections-characteristics-epidemiology-and-global-distribution/emerging-infections-how-and-why-they-arise.

Healthcare public health

Healthcare public health is the final of the three domains of public health, defined as being concerned with maximizing population benefits from healthcare interventions and reducing health inequalities. It involves the prioritization of limited resources, the prevention of disease and the improvement of healthcare outcomes via 'design, access, utilisation and evaluation of effective and efficient health and social care interventions, settings and pathways of care' (Faculty of Public Health 2017).

Screening

Screening aims to reduce the harm caused by a disease and its complications by detecting the disease or its risk factors at an early enough stage for it to have a beneficial impact on outcome.

Screening tests do not diagnose disease; they determine who should be investigated further for diagnosis and treatment. Screening can be:

- opportunistic, e.g. assessment of smoking status during a primary care visit
- part of a coordinated programme, with quality assurance and programme monitoring.

Although screening programmes are commissioned and delivered to improve health outcomes, screening has the potential to do harm, and so the benefits and risks need to be carefully considered, and screening should be implemented only when certain criteria are met (**Boxes 14.12** and **14.13**). In the UK, there are currently 11 population screening programmes (**Box 14.14**).

Screening for prostate cancer

An example of uncertainty around implementation of screening programmes is prostate cancer. This is a common cancer, although rates vary across countries. Some men have slow-growing asymptomatic tumours that may never require treatment, whereas others present with aggressive metastatic disease. Prostate-specific antigen (PSA) is a glycoprotein that can be detected in blood and is associated with a range of conditions affecting the prostate, including but not limited to prostate cancer. For example, elevated PSA levels are also found with benign prostatic enlargement, increasing age, inflammation and after ejaculation. Additionally, some medications may lower PSA levels.

A systematic review in 2018 demonstrated that PSA screening resulted in a possible small reduction in disease-specific mortality over 10 years but no reduction in overall mortality. The authors estimated that this equates to 1 less death from prostate cancer per 1000 men screened, but that the harms of such an approach would include 1 man hospitalized for sepsis, 3 experiencing urinary incontinence and 25 experiencing erectile dysfunction from the same 1000 screened. There is concern that population-level PSA screening would result in overdiagnosis and overtreatment, further complicated by the fact that optimum treatment is not always clear and treatment often has side-effects. As a result, many European countries have no population-wide screening programme, but in the UK asymptomatic men over 50 years who request PSA testing are given advice regarding the risks and benefits of testing so that they can make an informed choice about whether to undergo screening.

Antimicrobial resistance

This occurs when microorganisms develop resistance to commonly used antimicrobial drugs and are not suppressed by pharmacological agents that would normally inhibit their growth or kill them (see **Chapter 8**). Examples include meticillin-resistant *Staphylococcus aureus* (MRSA), XDR tuberculosis and carbapenemase-producing Enterobacteriaceae (CPE). These multiply-drug-resistant organisms are an emerging cause of hospital-acquired infections, which can result in outbreaks, are associated with high morbidity and mortality,

---

Box 14.12 Wilson and Jungner criteria for screening tests

Wilson and Jungner (1968) developed the classical screening criteria to determine whether or not a condition/disease should be subject to screening:
- The condition should represent an important health problem.
- There should be an accepted treatment.
- Diagnostic and treatment facilities should be available.
- There should be a recognizable latent or early symptomatic stage.

- There should be an appropriate test or examination.
- The test should be acceptable to the population.
- The natural history of the condition should be well understood.
- There should be agreement on who to treat.
- The cost of case-finding should be economically balanced in relation to possible expenditure on medical care as a whole.
- Case-finding should be a continuous process.

Wilson JMG, Jungner G. Principles and practice of screening for disease. Geneva: World Health Organization; 1968.

Box 14.13 Screening test performance

Negative screening tests do not necessarily confirm the absence of disease. Screening test performance can be evaluated by assessing the disease status against the test result.
- *False positives* occur when individuals with no disease test positive.
- *False negatives* occur when individuals with disease test negative.
- Sensitivity and specificity describe how well the screening test performs against a gold standard (criterion) test:
  - *Sensitivity* is the ability of the test to detect all cases of disease.
  - *Specificity* is the ability of the test to detect all disease-free cases.
- Both positive and negative predictive values are dependent on the population disease prevalence:
  - *Positive predictive value (PPV)* is the probability of having the disease, given a positive test result.
  - *Negative predictive value (NPV)* is the probability of not having the disease, given a negative test result.

	Disease present	Disease absent	
Test positive	True positive (A)	False positive (B)	A+B
Test negative	False negative (C)	True negative (D)	C+D
	A+C	B+D	TOTAL

Sensitivity = $A/(A+C) \times 100$
Specificity = $D/(D+B) \times 100$
Prevalence = $A+C/TOTAL \times 100$
PPV = $A/(A+B) \times 100$
NPV = $D/(D+C) \times 100$

Box 14.14 UK screening programmes

Antenatal and newborn
- Sickle cell and thalassaemia
- Fetal anomaly
- Infectious diseases in pregnancy
- Newborn and infant physical examination
- Newborn blood spot
- Newborn hearing

Adult
- Diabetic eye (from 12 years of age)
- Abdominal aortic aneurysm
- Breast cancer
- Cervical cancer
- Bowel cancer

and have the potential to develop into even more drug-resistant strains (**Box 14.15**).

The cornerstones of prevention of the spread of antimicrobial resistance include:

- **Early case recognition** using robust surveillance mechanisms, e.g. screening new admissions to hospital for asymptomatic carriage of some organisms.
- **Antimicrobial stewardship**:
  - ○ Antibiotics are prescribed only when clinically indicated.
  - ○ Local prescribing guidelines are adhered to.
  - ○ Use of broad-spectrum antibiotics is minimized.
  - ○ Dose, route and length of administration are monitored.
  - ○ Antibiotics are stopped or switched promptly, as appropriate (see p. 159).
- **Public education campaigns** to reduce antibiotic demand.
- **Good hand hygiene** on the part of healthcare workers.
- **Reduction of agricultural antibiotic use**.
- **Promotion of vaccination**.
- **Research** to develop new classes of antimicrobial agent.

Health economics

Demand for healthcare often exceeds the finite resources available to deliver it. These finite resources include not only money but also the availability of space and appropriately trained staff. As not all demands for healthcare can be met, the concept of **opportunity cost** arises: if resource is used for one intervention, less will be available to do something else. The benefits gained from the chosen option should be greater than the benefits foregone by not choosing the alternative. Opportunity cost may be minimized by resourcing interventions with maximal cost-effectiveness.

Measuring outcomes

A prerequisite for maximal cost-effectiveness is maximal efficiency. Efficiency describes using the minimum resource to produce the same output, or alternatively, maximizing the output gained from using the same resource. When comparing interventions that produce the same output, such as an antihypertensive that, on average, reduces blood pressure by the same extent, the intervention that is cheaper will be most efficient (this is known as cost minimization). If the interventions produce different types of output, then a common measure of health is needed to permit comparison: if both treatments are being used for the same disease, then a disease-specific measure may be used.

Comparing treatments between completely different diseases requires a generic measure of the amount of health gained (termed **'utility'**). The two most commonly used measures of utility are the **quality-adjusted life year (QALY)** and the **disability-adjusted life year (DALY)**. A QALY is 1 year of life in perfect health, whereas a DALY is the inverse: 1 year of healthy life that has been lost due to premature death. The aim is to maximize the number of QALYs gained or minimize the number of DALYs lost.

Measuring cost-effectiveness

When the interventions being compared involve both different outputs and different costs, then a measure of utility in comparison to cost is produced. These cost–utility analyses produce an **incremental cost-effectiveness ratio (ICER)**, which can then be compared by policy-makers to make funding decisions across the healthcare system (**Box 14.16**). The threshold at which interventions are deemed to be cost-effective depends on the resources available in a particular setting. For example, in England, funding recommendations are made by the National Institute for Health and Care Excellence (NICE), and a threshold of between £20 000 and £30 000 per QALY gained is currently used to determine whether an intervention should be recommended by NICE.

The ethics of funding decisions

Health economics does not only concern cost-effectiveness. The use of funds, and particularly of public funds, should be fair, as well as representing good value. The determination of 'fairness' is an ethical one, and contextual to the society in which the health system is operating. It is commonly said that the benefit of using QALYs is that they are uniform across conditions ('a QALY is a QALY is a QALY'), but whether this should be applied in all circumstances is debatable. For example:

- Is extending life by 1 month when a patient is only expected otherwise to live for 1 month the same as extending life by 1 month when a patient can be expected otherwise to live for 20 years?
- Should the amount a funder is willing to pay per QALY be the same for all diseases, when it is recognized that treatments for rare diseases are more expensive (to allow pharmaceutical companies to cover their research and development costs among a smaller sales volume)?

In the UK, specific rules have been introduced with respect to end-of-life treatments and to rare diseases in an attempt to answer these questions.

Service delivery

Research has shown that active consideration of the needs of patient groups when planning how and where interventions are to be delivered has the potential to improve patients' health at a population level. Tailoring service design to patient needs can be observed in the use of outreach services for areas with high numbers of hard-to-reach individuals, to increase accessibility. For example, homelessness is a risk factor for tuberculosis, but individuals who are homeless may be less likely to present to healthcare services with symptoms and so may remain undiagnosed; once diagnosed, they may also be less likely to complete courses of treatment. Novel outreach services run to engage homeless people in the wider community have been described that use mobile X-ray diagnostic units to provide tuberculosis screening in the community.

Centralization

Where the volumes of patients with a particular condition are low, the quality of care that patients receive may be improved by service centralization, which ensures that they are seen by teams dealing with sufficient numbers of cases to make their care routine, not unusual. Services may be delivered using a 'hub-and-spoke' model, whereby problems of lower complexity are dealt with in local

---

ℹ Box 14.15 Antimicrobial resistance

The advent of antimicrobial resistance is one of the biggest current threats to public health, as it has the potential to render individuals susceptible to a wide range of currently treatable microorganisms. As a result, 'low-risk' procedures (e.g. joint replacements) may become hazardous due to the infection risk, and treatment options for cancers or organ transplantation may become untenable if immunosuppression poses too great a threat. The O'Neill review, commissioned by the UK government, estimated that deaths from antimicrobial resistance could reach 10 million per year worldwide by 2050 unless preventative action is taken.

---

i   Box 14.16 Cost–utility calculations

Treatment A

- In comparison to current treatment, treatment A would extend patients' lives by a further 3 years, each at half the 'perfect' quality of life
- Net QALYs gained = $3 \times 0.5 = 1.5$
- Treatment A costs £45 000 per patient (one-off sum) more than the current treatment
- Cost–utility = $45\,000 / 1.5 = £30\,000$ per QALY

Treatment B

- In comparison to current treatment, treatment B would not prolong patients' lives, but it would improve their quality of life from 30% to 50% (with a life expectancy from treatment of 10 years)
- Net QALYs gained = $10 \times 0.2 = 2$
- Treatment B costs £1600 per patient per year (ongoing)
- Cost–utility = $(1600 \times 10) / 2 = £8000$ per QALY
  Therefore, treatment B is more cost-effective than treatment A.

---

hospitals and problems of higher complexity or acuity are referred to a tertiary centre. For example, in London, city-wide stroke services were reorganized in 2010 with the introduction of eight 'hyperacute' stroke units where emergency care, including thrombolysis, is delivered; these are supported by a number of other local stroke units, to which patients are subsequently 'stepped down' for rehabilitation. A 2013 evaluation concluded that this service reorganization was associated with significantly improved patient survival and reduced healthcare costs.

Centralization has a number of benefits, including:

- allowing investment in specialized healthcare professionals and equipment
- helping to ensure that clinicians remain up to date with current evidence
- reducing unwarranted variation between units.

However, any centralization is a trade-off against increased travel time for patients (which might reduce accessibility, potentially inequitably), and may be politically controversial if there is a perception that local hospitals are being undermined.

Further reading

Ilic D, Djulbegovic M, Hung Jung J et al. Prostate cancer screening with prostate-specific antigen (PSA) test: a systematic review and meta-analysis. *Br Med J* 2018; 362:k3519.

Hunter R, Davie C, Rudd A et al. Impact on clinical and cost outcomes of a centralized approach to acute stroke care in London: a comparative effectiveness before and after model. *PLOS One* 2013; 8:e70420.

O'Neill J. *Tackling Drug-Resistant Infections Globally: Final Report and Recommendations*, 2016; https://amr-review.org/sites/default/files/160518_Final%20paper_with%20cover.pdf.

Public Health England. *Prostate Cancer Risk Management Programme (PCRMP): Benefits and Risks of PSA Testing*, 2016; https://www.gov.uk/government/publications/prostate-cancer-risk-management-programme-psa-test-benefits-and-risks/prostate-cancer-risk-management-programme-pcrmp-benefits-and-risks-of-psa-testing.

World Health Organization. *Global Action Plan on Antimicrobial Resistance*, 2015; http://apps.who.int/iris/bitstream/handle/10665/193736/9789241509763_eng.pdf;jsessionid=FB427A3145FC610B10462FA952207167?sequence=1.

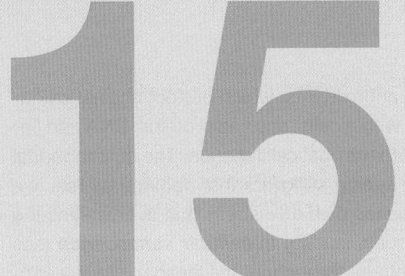

15

Geriatric medicine, frailty and multimorbidity

Adam Harper, Iain Wilkinson and Joanna Preston

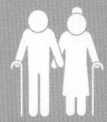

CORE SKILLS AND KNOWLEDGE

Geriatric medicine focuses on the medical care of older people. Increasingly, the criteria for specialist geriatric care are defined by the presence of multiple problems and/or frailty rather than chronological age. Medical care is provided within a multidisciplinary team.

Geriatricians cover the range of general medicine in older adults, in both acute hospital settings (the emergency department and specialist wards) and the community (rehabilitation wards or patients' homes). Geriatricians support other specialists with specific issues such as the management of multimorbidity, delirium or complex discharge planning. Subspecialty work includes falls, orthogeriatrics, stroke medicine and Parkinson's disease, along with evolving areas such as oncogeriatrics.

Key skills in geriatric medicine include:
- managing the complexity inherent in ageing physiological systems and interacting diseases and treatments
- making pragmatic and holistic decisions for individual patients in the face of uncertainty, including understanding and individualizing the evidence base
- working with allied health professionals to address patients' challenging social circumstances
- caring and advocating for the most vulnerable and frail of adult patients.

INTRODUCTION

There have been incredible changes in human life expectancy over the last 200 years, with increasing numbers of people enjoying fulfilling lives up until their nineties and beyond. These changes reflect numerous factors, ranging from improved sanitation and nutrition to the development of antibiotics. Preventative measures, such as reductions in cardiovascular disease through blood pressure control, can postpone the onset of disease. Increasingly, many diseases are treatable or even curable, including numerous cancers and chronic infections such as human immunodeficiency virus (HIV). In turn, many people are living with one or more chronic conditions, which may require ongoing treatment and intervention to reduce any negative impact on the individual's quality of life. These interventions may have their own side-effects, and ageing itself has an impact on the body and its function, requiring a specific approach.

In the 1960s, Bernard Isaacs described four *'Geriatric Giants'*, a fifth being added later as medical interventions progressed:
1. incontinence
2. immobility
3. intellectual impairment
4. instability
5. iatrogenesis.

More recently, *'5Ms'* have been proposed by Mary Tinnetti (**Box 15.1**).

Presentations of illnesses often differ in older age. For example, the physical symptoms and signs associated with depression are common, and difficult to differentiate from those of organic disease. A diagnosis of depression may be signalled by reduced social interaction and by the fact that the patient does not leave their home when this is unexplained by any co-morbidities or physical disability.

Investigation and interpretation of results must also be balanced against pragmatic considerations. For example, finding a pulmonary nodule in a frail person should prompt the questions, 'If this were malignant, what would the patient want? Are they fit for surgery or chemo- or radiotherapy? Will their present co-morbidities and disabilities allow them to tolerate further investigations?' Another common scenario is a person who is experiencing postural hypotension due to antihypertensives. It may be prudent to accept a higher blood pressure than guidelines would suggest in order to reduce the risk of falling. These decisions must be discussed with patients as part of shared decision-making, but finding a balance can prove difficult for patient and clinicians alike. At its heart, geriatric medicine is the interplay between the patient, the medical teams and the declining physiology of the ageing process.

> ℹ **Box 15.1 The 5Ms of geriatric medicine**
>
> - *Mind*: mentation, dementia, delirium, depression
> - *Mobilization*: impaired gait and balance, fall injury prevention
> - *Medications*: polypharmacy, optimal prescribing and deprescribing, adverse drug reactions
> - *Multicomplexity*: multimorbidity, complex bio-/psychosocial situations
> - *Matters most*: each individual's own meaningful health outcome goals and care preferences
>
> Tinetti M, Huang A, Molnar F. The Geriatrics 5M's: A new way of communicating what we do. *J Am Geriatr Soc* 2017; 65(9): 2115

AGEING

Ageing is a progressive physiological decline associated with living beyond roughly the age of 30. Bernhard Strehler defined ageing as:

- *Universal*: the process must happen to all members of a species.
- *Intrinsic*: it takes place via endogenous processes, i.e. it must not depend on external factors.
- *Progressive*: changes leading to ageing must occur progressively throughout a person's lifespan.
- *Deleterious*: it is bad for the individual.

Virtually all physiological functions lose efficiency with ageing, and individuals lose the capacity to maintain homeostasis when faced by external challenges. Where a younger person stumbling over a kerb would have the strength and reflexes to adjust and maintain their balance, an older person is more likely to fall.

Ageing happens at differing rates between individuals. Some aspects are easily apparent, such as the hair turning grey. Other aspects are less obvious, such as accumulation of atheroma (plaque) within blood vessels. Ageing will eventually occur in everyone, but can be influenced by a number of factors, such as genetic make-up, activity levels and environment. Some factors are associated with accelerated ageing, such as smoking and diabetes. Others are protective and slow the ageing process, such as a balanced diet and regular exercise.

Why do we age?

Theories of ageing can broadly be split into two: those concerned with the limited replication of cells and those related to evolution.

Theories related to limited cell replication

Telomere shortening

Telomeres protect the ends of chromosomes from errors in DNA during replication. With each cell replication, a small piece of the telomere is removed until it eventually becomes too short to provide this protective effect, which may lead to clinical problems associated with ageing including an increased risk of cancers.

Damage accumulation theory

Ageing is a result of fault accumulation at cellular and molecular levels due to a limitation of maintenance and repair mechanisms. The primary problems do not lie with the cells themselves, but with the regulation of mechanisms keeping the cell division process efficient and safe.

Free radical theory

Free radicals, derived from chemical reactions involving oxygen molecules (oxidation), occur more frequently in older cells. Species with high levels of free radicals have shorter life expectancies. Free radicals are balanced by antioxidants, which protect against oxidative damage to elements within cells, such as proteins, DNA and lipids – all of which are vital for normal cell function. The mitochondrial theory of free radicals in ageing suggests that damage by reactive oxygen species (ROS) causes oxidative stress that overwhelms the antioxidant cellular defences, leading to **cellular senescence** (see later). Chronic oxidative stress throughout the lifespan plays a critical role in ageing overall. There is some evidence that antioxidants can reduce this damage but no clinically relevant outcomes have been observed.

Theories related to evolution

Evolutionary theories are based on the idea that the biological processes associated with ageing provide an advantage earlier in life in terms of reproduction and survival of the species. As humans now regularly survive beyond reproductive age, individual negative biological impacts later in life may be seen as payback for this group advantage.

Disposable soma theory

This suggests that an organism must budget for the limited energy available to it and preferentially focus on reproduction rather than maintaining the mature body, leading to inefficiencies in cell replication later in life.

Mutation accumulation theory

This theory supports the disposable soma idea by asserting that DNA mutations taking place after reproductive age cannot affect future generations, meaning that there is no evolutionary imperative to correct them or develop protection against consequent defects.

Antagonistic pleiotropy theory

This theory takes the idea one step further, suggesting that genes that are protective or beneficial in early life become detrimental later in life. An example is sickle cell disease, which is protective against malaria in earlier life.

Calorie restriction

Calorie restriction is thought to prolong life expectancy, mediated through reduction of oxidative damage and anti-inflammatory benefits. This is supported by animal studies, and by the example of the population of the Japanese island of Okinawa, who, through cultural calorie restriction, boast the highest prevalence of centenarians worldwide.

Cell senescence

Cell senescence, when cells stop dividing but remain metabolically active, leads to a pro-inflammatory state. It is different from apoptosis, which is programmed cellular death followed by removal of the cell from the system in an organized way. Cells with senescent properties are seen in the tissues of those with age-related diseases, such as osteoarthritis, pulmonary fibrosis, atherosclerosis and Alzheimer's disease. Exactly what the mechanism is that leads from one to the other is unclear.

Senescence is not just seen in the context of ageing. Another example is wound healing. Once a wound is healed, the myofibroblast cells go into acute senescence to prevent excessive fibrosis at the site. Senescence also occurs when the blood supply for an embryo is being built. In these circumstances, it is a programmed process, triggered by specific stimuli and targeting specific types of cell. In ageing, the process appears unscheduled and more random. Clearance of aged cells that have undergone senescence is much less efficient. This may be due to the reduced immune function associated with ageing.

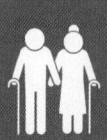

Applied anatomy and physiology of ageing

One of the key aspects of providing medical care for older people is distinguishing between normal ageing and disease. Ageing affects each organ differently. Presentations that probably arise as single-organ pathology in younger adults are likely to have more than one cause in older adults. For example, anaemia in a young woman is likely to be related to menstrual bleeding. In an older woman the anaemia might represent chronic disease, such as myelofibrotic bone marrow that is unable to respond quickly to increased demand for red cells, exacerbated by a poor nutritional state with low iron and folate levels. Older adults need to have their physical conditions assessed and managed alongside their functional and social circumstances.

What commonly differentiates people with the same apparent condition(s) is the ability of their whole system to balance these conditions in a way that keeps the person functioning. This difference is usually accounted for by the presence of frailty as an underlying physiological process.

As we age, our organs function less well, with the percentage function of each individual system reducing by the order of 0.5–1% per organ system per year from the age of 30. **Fig. 15.1** is based on a large international cohort. Similar graphs can be drawn for maximum usage of oxygen (VO_s max), cardiac output, maximum heart rate or renal function.

Further reading

Pellegrino ED, Thomasma DC. *The Virtues in Medical Practice*. Oxford, New York: Oxford University Press; 1994.
Strehler BL. *Time, Cells and Aging*, 2nd edn. New York: Academic Press; 1977.

INVESTIGATIONS IN OLDER ADULTS

Normal ranges stated by laboratories account for the values expected for the majority of the population, but older adults (like children) are outliers compared with the whole population. The altered anatomy and physiology in older adults mean that routine investigations need to be interpreted with this in mind (**Boxes 15.2** and **15.3**).

TAKING A HISTORY

When symptoms can be non-specific and many conditions present in an atypical manner, it can be difficult knowing where to start. Asking open questions like 'What is your biggest concern today?' can help. In those with confusion, timelines of presentation may not be reliable, but you can usually get a feel for immediate concerns, such as pain or breathlessness. Do not be afraid to ask about difficult issues (e.g. bladder and bowel dysfunction, death and dying); patients often want to explore these areas but are hesitant to bring them up themselves.

A key aspect of geriatric medicine is the ability to think in detail about the current issue while maintaining a longer-term, bigger picture of the person and their life. Geriatricians often manage patients with interacting multimorbidity, polypharmacy and physiological decline. They need the ability to focus on those aspects that might be troubling the patient (e.g. constipation or a dry mouth) while being aware of overall progressive decline, reservations about interventions and the potential need for advanced care-planning.

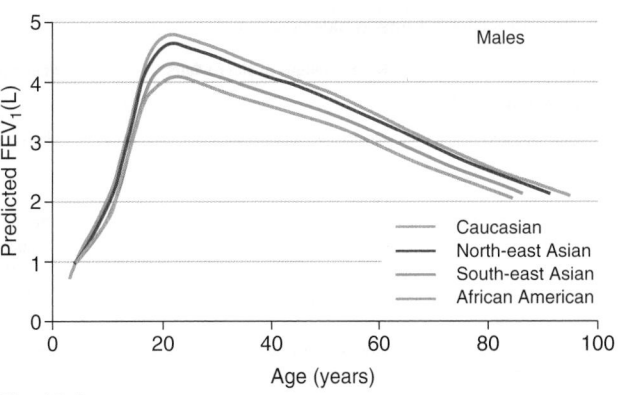

Fig. 15.1 Change in forced expiratory volume in 1 sec (FEV_1) with age. *(Stanojevic S, Quanjer P, Miller MR, et al. The Global Lung Function Initiative: dispelling some myths of lung function test interpretation.* Breathe *2013; 9:462–474.)*

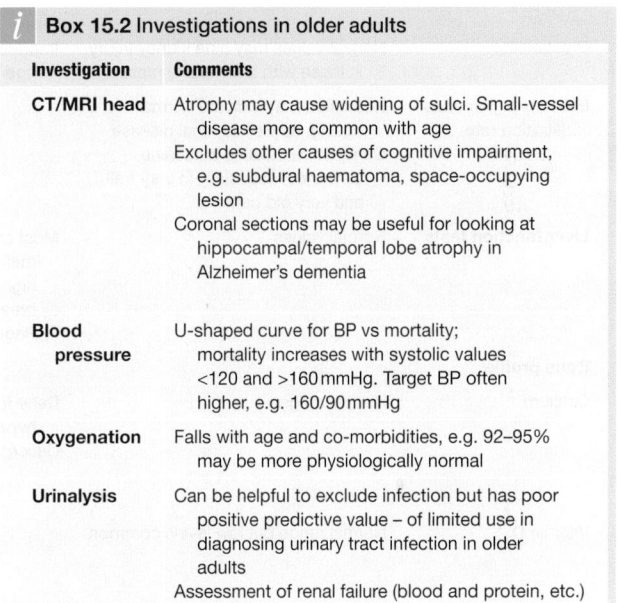

Box 15.2 Investigations in older adults

Investigation	Comments
CT/MRI head	Atrophy may cause widening of sulci. Small-vessel disease more common with age
	Excludes other causes of cognitive impairment, e.g. subdural haematoma, space-occupying lesion
	Coronal sections may be useful for looking at hippocampal/temporal lobe atrophy in Alzheimer's dementia
Blood pressure	U-shaped curve for BP vs mortality; mortality increases with systolic values <120 and >160 mmHg. Target BP often higher, e.g. 160/90 mmHg
Oxygenation	Falls with age and co-morbidities, e.g. 92–95% may be more physiologically normal
Urinalysis	Can be helpful to exclude infection but has poor positive predictive value – of limited use in diagnosing urinary tract infection in older adults
	Assessment of renal failure (blood and protein, etc.)

MULTIMORBIDITY, SARCOPENIA AND FRAILTY

Multimorbidity

Older people are more likely to have multiple medical issues. By 2035, around two-thirds of people over 65 years of age will have multimorbidity. Within the UK, for example, such patients currently account for 50% of general practitioner consultations, 55% of hospital admissions and 80% of prescriptions. Each condition often requires a number of medications, with treatments potentially interacting adversely. This can lead to *prescribing cascades*, whereby medications are given for one condition and then further medications are required to counter the side-effects (e.g. the co-prescription of aspirin with a proton-pump inhibitor).

Sarcopenia

Sarcopenia is closely related to frailty (**Box 15.4**). It is a progressive and generalized muscle disorder associated with an increased risk

i Box 15.3 Blood tests in older adults

Blood test	Normal ranges in older adults	High values	Low values
Full blood count			
Haemoglobin	Normal values lower	High in dehydration	Review medication for antiplatelets/ anticoagulation that increase bleeding risk and for gastric irritants
White cell count	Remain normal	Infection. As with any abnormal white cell count, check the differential of the cell count. CLL in particular may present as an incidental raised white cell count of lymphocytes	
Platelets	Remain normal	Temporary rise: acute-phase reactant	Often drug- or sepsis-induced May indicate bone marrow dysfunction
Serum creatinine and electrolytes			
Sodium	Normal values	Dehydration associated with reduced homeostasis of thirst axis	Commonly medication-related
Potassium	Normal values		Low values may impair muscle function
Creatinine	Normal values may hide kidney injury in those with low muscle mass	Impaired renal function due to age-related nephron loss	Low muscle mass from sarcopenia
Estimated glomerular filtration rate	Reduction may indicate normal ageing, as well as renal disease Consider calculating creatinine clearance, especially in very frail and very old patients		Less useful in the very underweight and very overweight
Liver function tests	Normal values	Most commonly gallstone disease or malignancy. Alkaline phosphatase high in bony metastases (prostate, breast), vitamin D deficiency and Paget's bone disease	Albumin: Acute: catabolic states, e.g. infection, cancer Chronic: poor nutritional state
Bone profile			
Calcium	Normal range	Dehydration, malignancy and primary hyperparathyroidism Causes confusion and constipation	Adjust for albumin level Poor dietary intake (mild) Recent parenteral treatment for osteoporosis (e.g. denosumab, zoledronic acid)
Vitamin D	Normal range but low levels common		Nutritional deficiency, reduced sunlight exposure N.B. Impact on bone health
Other			
Erythrocyte sedimentation rate	Normal values increase with age	>100 mm per Hour should prompt investigation for vasculitis or malignancy Polymyalgia rheumatica common	
Creatine kinase	Normal range	Review medication for statins, neuroleptics Rhabdomyolysis after a long period on the floor after falling	
C-reactive protein	Normal range	Sepsis, acute inflammation/ physiological stress, e.g. surgery	
Thyroid function	Normal range	May cause confusion, delusions, tremor	May cause confusion, constipation, myopathy N.B. Borderline low thyroid state can be associated with longer life expectancy
Iron/ferritin/transferrin index (TI)	Normal range	Ferritin is acute-phase reactant; consider checking TI	Low in iron-deficient anaemia (may be disproportionately normal in acute infection and iron deficiency anaemia)

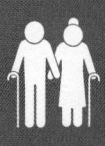

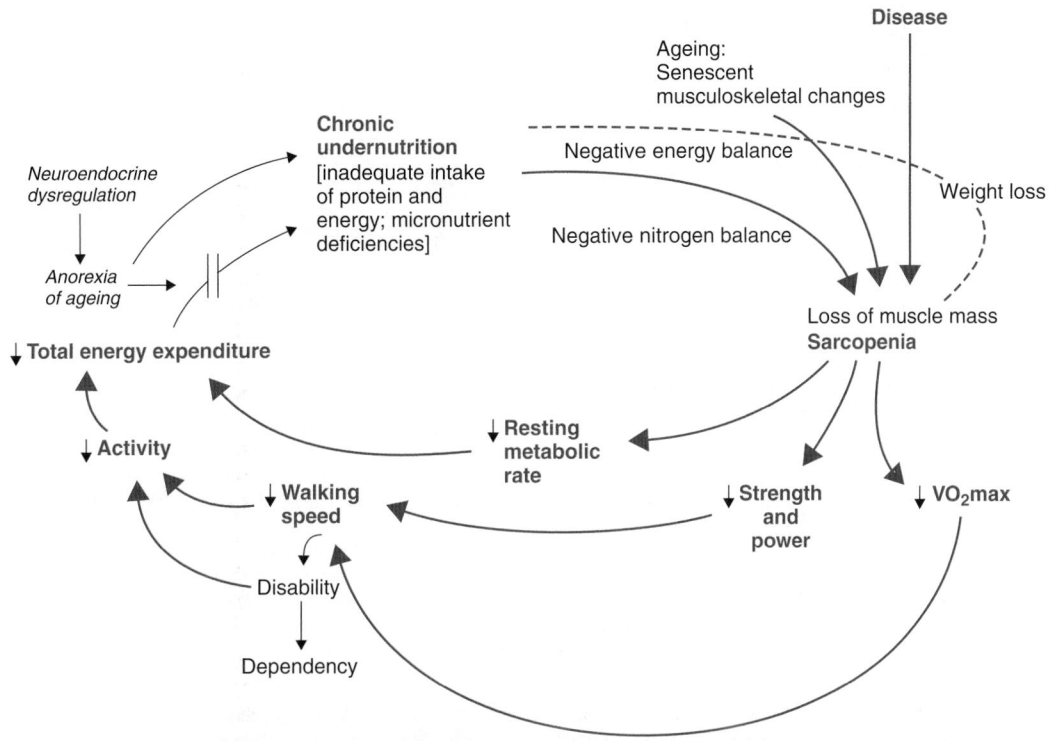

Fig. 15.2 The frailty cycle. *(Adapted from Clegg A, Young J. The frailty syndrome.* Clin Med *2011; 11:72-75.)*

Box 15.4 The European Working Group on Sarcopenia in Older People (2018)

Criterion	Definition
1. Low muscle strength	*Probable sarcopenia* is identified by criterion 1
2. Low muscle quantity or quality	*Confirmed sarcopenia* requires criteria 1 and 2
3. Low physical performance	*Severe sarcopenia* requires criteria 1, 2 and 3

---

of adverse outcomes, including falls and fractures. Muscle fibres reduce in number, the fast-twitch type II muscle fibres in particular. The result is loss of their explosive power, which is needed for functions such as sprinting, standing from a chair or even coughing.

In sarcopenia, VO₂ max within muscle reduces, as does gait speed. Reduction in physical activity leads to a reduction in energy usage; when coupled with the relative anorexia of ageing, this leads to an energy deficit. With this energy deficit, cells that are predetermined to undergo apoptosis do not have sufficient free adenosine triphosphate (ATP) to allow this process to occur. Instead, the cell undergoes necrosis, which uses more ATP and worsens the energy deficit. When this occurs in muscle tissue, it leads to worsening sarcopenia and development of the cycle of frailty (**Fig. 15.2**).

Frailty

Frailty is 'a state of increased vulnerability to stressors due to age-related declines in physiologic reserve across neuromuscular, metabolic, and immune systems'. It is the effect of systemic ageing (the underlying process) rather than chronological age. It is possible to be chronologically old and not frail, likewise to be young and very frail. As an individual organ's ability to react to a physiological stressor reduces with age, the impact of a given illness on that organ system will have a greater effect. A minor infection (e.g. an uncomplicated urinary tract infection, UTI) will have little impact on

a young and fit patient but may cause serious delirium and morbidity in the cognitively impaired, especially when combined with frailty or serious multimorbidity.

Frailty, multimorbidity and disability are distinct entities that often co-exist. The difference is important in the management of patients.

- *Frailty* is a risk of a deterioration when faced with a physiological stressor.
- *Multimorbidity* involves two or more medical conditions that may or may not interact.
- *Disability* is physical or mental impairment that has a 'substantial' and 'long-term' negative effect on a person's ability to carry out normal daily activities.

Identifying frailty

A number of models have been developed to describe frailty and the manner in which it evolves. Frailty is relatively simple to recognize when it is severe but more challenging when mild. Its recognition ensures that patients are managed according to their functional level rather than their chronological age.

Frailty recognition is an effective way of identifying people who may be at greater risk of future hospital admission, care home placement or death; those with severe frailty have more than a four times greater annual risk for these outcomes. Interventions targeted at actively managing frailty around a stressor, such as elective surgery, show better outcomes.

The key benefits to patients of a definition of frailty and an active search for it are twofold:

Box 15.5 Fried's phenotypic frailty assessment[a]

Domain	Suggested assessment
Weight loss	Loss of ≥4.5kg or ≥5% of body mass in the last year
Gait speed	6 sec or more to walk 4m (0.66m/sec)
Energy expenditure	Low levels of energy expenditure/physical activity in lowest 20% of population (men <383kcal/week; women <270kcal/week)
Subjective feeling of lethargy	Subjective feeling of exhaustion: Felt that everything they did was 'an effort' in the last week Could not 'get going' in the last week
Muscle strength	Grip strength as a score within the lowest 20%, stratified by gender

[a]Three or more define frailty.
(From Fried LP, Tangen CM, Walston J et al., Cardiovascular Health Study Collaborative Research Group. Frailty in older adults: evidence for a phenotype. Gerontol A Biol Sci Med Sci *2001; 56(3):M146–156.)*

- It prompts an objective assessment of patients (Comprehensive Geriatric Assessment, CGA; see later) to identify those who might benefit from optimization.
- It acts as a trigger for the point at which medicine stops following standardized protocols and becomes a balance between the two questions that Edmund Pellegrino termed 'prudential': 'What *can* be done for the patient?' and 'What *should* be done for the patient?'

Identification and stratification of population-level frailty could assist in planning for future demands on health and social care while allowing targeted interventions to help people age well. Upskilling of all those working with older adults is a priority. This runs in parallel with Geriatrics teams supporting specialist services, from perioperative care to specific patient populations, in areas such as oncogeriatrics and HIV medicine.

Two main theories can also be used to identify frailty: frailty as a phenotype and frailty as an accumulation of deficits.

Frailty phenotype

In 2001, Linda Fried published her model of frailty (including the frailty cycle described earlier), and demonstrated that becoming frail was associated with negative outcomes in terms of length of life and institutionalization (**Box 15.5**).

Frailty Index – accumulation of deficits

The Frailty Index (FI) defines frailty from a list of medical conditions, physiological parameters, and observations on factors that become more common with increasing age and are associated with negative health outcomes. This method has been used largely in research but now, with the development (in the UK) of the e-Frailty Index, it can be run on routinely collected data from GP records.

The Clinical Frailty Scale (CFS)

The Clinical Frailty Scale (CFS) correlates with the more in-depth FI. It uses clinical descriptors and images to stratify older adults according to level of vulnerability. It has been validated in a number of clinical settings but only after a CGA has been carried out. It is increasingly being employed for identification purposes, however, due to its ease of use (**Fig. 15.3**).

Further reading

National Institute for Health and Care Excellence. NICE Guideline 56: *Multimorbidity: Clinical Assessment and Management*. NICE 2016; https://www.nice.org.uk/guidance/ng56.

1 Very fit
People who are robust, active, energetic and motivated. These people commonly exercise regularly. They are among the fittest for their age.

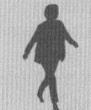
2 Well
People who have no **active disease symptoms** but are less fit than category 1. Often, they exercise or are very **active occasionally**, e.g. seasonally.

3 Managing well
People whose **medical problems are well controlled**, but are **not regularly active** beyond routine walking.

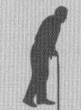
4 Vulnerable
While **not dependent** on others for daily help, often **symptoms limit activities**. A common complaint is being 'slowed up', and/or being tired during the day.

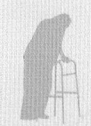
5 Mildly frail
These people often have **more evident slowing**, and need help in **high-order IADLs** (finances, transport, heavy housework, medications). Typically, mild frailty progressively impairs shopping and walking outside alone, meal preparation and housework.

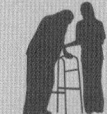
6 Moderately frail
People need help with **all outside activities** and with keeping house. Inside, they often have problems with stairs and need help with bathing and might need minimal assistance (cueing, standby) with dressing.

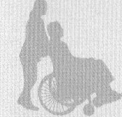
7 Severely frail
Completely dependent for personal care, from whatever cause (physical or cognitive). Even so, they seem stable and not at high risk of dying (within ~6 months).

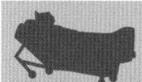
8 Very severely frail
Completely dependent, approaching the end of life. Typically, they could not recover even from a minor illness.

9 Terminally ill
Approaching the end of life. This category applies to people with **a life expectancy <6 months**, who are **not otherwise evidently frail**.

Scoring frailty in people with dementia

The degree of frailty corresponds to the degree of dementia. Common **symptoms in mild dementia** include forgetting the details of a recent event, though still remembering the event itself, repeating the same question/story and social withdrawal.

In **moderate dementia** recent memory is very impaired, even though individuals seemingly can remember their past life events well. They can do personal care with prompting.

In **severe dementia** patients cannot undertake personal care without help.

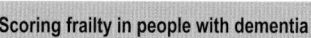
Fig. 15.3 The Clinical Frailty Scale. IADLs, instrumental activities of daily living. (© 2007–2009 Version 1.2 All rights reserved. Geriatric Medicine Research, Dalhousie University, Halifax, Canada.)

COMPREHENSIVE GERIATRIC ASSESSMENT

Once a patient is identified as being frail, what can be done to help them? There is no single treatment to cure frailty. Inaction is likely to result in worsening frailty, functional decline and disability. Therefore, a proactive assessment of each of the potential clinical and subclinical deficits is needed.

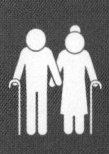

Box 15.6 Domains of the Comprehensive Geriatric Assessment

Domain	Assessment area	Assessment	Examples of assessment tools
Physical symptoms	Pain	Location, severity, impact on quality of life	Numerical scales Visual scales, e.g. Abbey Pain Scale (for patients with dementia)
	Continence	Exploration of both storage and voiding; lower urinary tract symptoms	Bladder diary *or* Post-void residual bladder volume
	Sensory impairment	Hearing assessment Check for ear wax	
		Visual assessment	Snellen chart Optician/ophthalmology review (including glaucoma, cataracts, macular degeneration)
	Musculoskeletal problems	Mobility, range of movement	Berg Balance Scale Timed Up and Go test
	Multimorbidity management	Multimorbidity management approach (e.g. NICE Guideline 56, see 'Further reading'): Identify disease vs treatment burden Discuss with patient and agree a shared management plan Review on a regular basis	Polypharmacy assessment tools, e.g. STOPP-START, Beers Ascertain patient's priorities of care: symptom relief (AF rate control) versus future prevention (AF anticoagulation)
Mental health symptoms	Mood assessment	Mental health assessment, including full mental state examination	Geriatric Depression Scale (GDS) Hospital Anxiety and Depression Scale (HADS) Cornell Depression Scale (for patients with cognitive impairment)
	Cognitive assessment	Detailed cognitive assessment, including collateral history from a relative or carer	Abbreviated Mental Test score Mini-mental state examination (MMSE) Six-item Cognitive Impairment Test (6-CIT) Montreal Cognitive Assessment (MOCA) Clock drawing task (e.g. CLOX 1) Addenbrooke's Cognitive Assessment-Revised (ACE-R)
Functional abilities	Activities of daily living (ADL) assessment	Personal ADLs: Washing/dressing Bed transfers Toileting needs Domestic ADLs: Food preparation Housework	Barthel Index (personal ADLs) Nottingham Extended ADL Scale (includes domestic ADLs and higher-level functional assessments)
Living environment	Home visit or access visit Usually led by occupational therapists	Assessment for hazards around home (e.g. lighting, flooring)	
		Assessment for safety, e.g. heating, cooker safe for patient to use, stair rails	
Social support network	Financial assessment	Often performed by social services	
	Carers' assessment	Care Act (UK)	
Future wishes	Advanced care planning	Nomination of power of attorney, CPR decisions and advance decision to refuse treatment (see p. 84)	DNACPR; ceilings of treatment (e.g. ward-based ceiling of care) ReSPECT document Locally agreed advanced care plan

AF, atrial fibrillation; CPR, cardiopulmonary resuscitation; DNACPR, do not attempt cardiopulmonary resuscitation; STOPP-START, Screening Tool of Older People's potentially inappropriate Prescriptions-Screening Tool to Alert doctors to Right Treatments.

Comprehensive Geriatric Assessment (CGA) is not something that is just delivered by doctors; it is a multidimensional, interdisciplinary diagnostic *process* focused on determining a person's medical, psychological and functional capability in order to develop a coordinated and integrated plan for treatment and long-term follow-up. As such, it is firmly rooted in the biological, psychological and sociological approach to thinking about patients and their conditions. CGA involves exploring a number of domains (**Box 15.6**). The further roles of the multidisciplinary team (MDT) are explored later.

In older adults with frailty there is often a large overlap between symptoms caused by disease, by treatment of disease, by normal ageing and by accelerated ageing. More practically, CGA can be thought of as a process of good holistic care delivered by a focused MDT, which goes above and beyond simply managing the acute problem with which the person has presented. If an older person is not managed in this way, care becomes reactive to a series of acute problems, rather than a proactive problem-solving process.

Compared to those given 'usual' care, those who undergo CGA during an acute admission have favourable outcomes. At 6 and 12 months, respectively, the number needed to treat (NNT) is 20 and 25 to prevent institutionalization and 17 for unnecessary death. By comparison, the NNT for many medications is in the hundreds to thousands range.

One area that remains to be fully explored is how best to identify patients who would benefit from a CGA who are not in an acute hospital. The proactive assessment of patient frailty is one means of doing this. Once patients are identified as frail (or becoming frailer), then a proactive CGA, in either the community or a day hospital setting, would seem to be a pragmatic approach.

Multidisciplinary team working

In order to deliver true CGA, geriatricians need to work as part of an expert MDT. Communication between the whole of the MDT is essential to ensure that patient care plans are discussed and developed together. Each team member's specialist skills are better utilized, making for a more egalitarian approach to care, rather than the traditional hierarchical one with the senior doctor as the leader (**Box 15.7**). Learning about geriatric medicine therefore requires an understanding not only of the role of the doctor in delivering CGA, but also of the roles of each member of the MDT.

ADVANCE CARE PLANNING

Advance care planning (ACP) involves discussing the approach to a patient's future care, often prior to their becoming unwell (see p. 84). ACP is a continuous process of communication between patients, their loved ones and healthcare professionals. It is not always possible or appropriate to cover everything in one conversation. Patients may want to think through often complex issues and discuss their plans with their loved ones. Plans should also be subject to regular review in case patients have changed their mind.

One of the most common decisions concerns resuscitation status. Many older people recognize that they are coming towards the end of their lives. Even though they are in good health, many would like to be allowed a natural death in the event of a cardiorespiratory arrest. Others may want to live for as long as possible and ask for all that medicine can do to prolong their lives. Events that may precede resuscitation should be planned for too, such as hospitalization for treatment of infections.

ACPs often focus on the dying phase but can be expanded to include what constitutes living well. Statements of wishes and preferences can range from where a person lives (e.g. in their own home or in a care home) to their favourite foods.

ACP discussions can be started at any time if the patient is willing and ready. They should be specifically considered in patients diagnosed with progressive conditions, such as neurodegenerative diseases, where there is the potential for capacity to be lost in the latter stages. Any agreed outcomes should be documented and available to all who need access to them, including the patient and their family, ambulance staff, GPs, community teams and hospital teams. This can also be a good time to highlight the importance of ensuring that wills and power of attorney are considered.

---

i **Box 15.7 Common members of the multidisciplinary team and their roles**

Job	Role	Clinical example
Dietician	Assessment of nutritional status and support of healthy weight during illness and health	Falls: ensuring adequate calorie intake for muscle maintenance Cognition: adaptations to meal routine to optimize nutrition, e.g. opportunistic meal times
Discharge coordinator	In-hospital coordination of complex discharges	Coordination of multiple agencies, e.g. social services, specialist equipment, funding streams, safeguarding
Doctor	Medical diagnoses and optimization, including reversible conditions and prescribing Prognostication	Falls: causes and interventions, bone health assessment and prescription Polypharmacy: medication review Inputs into most CGA domains
Nurse	Delivery of hands-on care for older patients, assessment of holistic and physical needs, including medication compliance, skin care, continence	Continence: assessment and management Skin: wound care and pressure damage Medication: delivery and compliance
Occupational therapist	Functional assessments and management (including cognition) aiming for a greater degree of independence	Falls: assessments and adaptations for maximizing independence; optimization of environment, e.g. ensuring furniture of a reasonable height to stand from easily; movement-sensitive lighting, pendant alarms, 'key safe' (small box with combination lock outside property containing house keys for carers) Cognition: cognitive assessment, activities of daily living assessments, kitchen function and safety assessments
Pharmacist	Optimization of medicine compliance Addressing polypharmacy/interactions	Falls: review of contributing medications
Physiotherapist	Optimization of physical functioning in relation to musculoskeletal function	Falls: gait analysis, exercise programmes to improve balance and strength, walking aids Continence: pelvic floor exercises
Podiatrist	Assessment and management of foot health	Falls: reduction of foot pain, suitable footwear for deformities
Psychologist	Instigation and direction of talking therapies, e.g. cognitive behavioural therapy	Falls: fear of falling counselling Mood: talking therapies, including in early dementia
Social worker	Assessment of social functioning and safety	Falls: home adaptations, provision of care Cognition: capacity assessments in relation to welfare and finances Carer strain: assessments as part of Care Act (UK) Welfare: assistance with finances
Speech and language therapist	Swallowing and communication	Communication strategies, support for capacity decisions where communication impaired Dysphagia: recommendations for minimizing risks and advance care planning
Voluntary sector	Supporting social interaction and function	Falls: exercise classes Cognition: dementia cafés, dementia friends Nutrition: assistance with shopping

CGA, Comprehensive Geriatric Assessment.

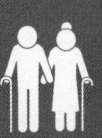

THE MOST COMMON ISSUES IN OLDER PEOPLE

Polypharmacy

Prescribing in older people

While prescribing for older people is largely the same as for younger people, there are some key differences. The approach should be based around the patient's physiological rather than chronological age. There are numerous mechanisms behind the altered pharmacokinetics in older people (**Box 15.8**) but the net result is that older patients tend to suffer increased side-effects from their medications.

Drug interactions

One-third of patients over 65 living in the UK take six or more medications, with 5% taking more than ten. Polypharmacy leads to increased drug interactions and increased potential for **drug–drug** interactions (e.g. cholinesterase inhibitors and anticholinergics) and **drug–disease** interactions (e.g. non-steroidal anti-inflammatory drugs worsening hypertension). Polypharmacy accounts in part for up to 6.5% of all iatrogenic hospital admissions.

Patient choice

Polypharmacy may leave patients unhappy with their medication burden, which can lead to poor concordance overall (**Box 15.9**). Many prefer to take fewer medicines, accepting an increased risk of further events and potentially shortened life expectancy (e.g. forgoing a statin after an acute coronary syndrome). A patient's priorities of care (what is most important to them) often rate immediate symptom control over preventative interventions. When prescribing, clarifying the goals and educating patients about the benefits of treatment are key to supporting them in making treatment choices.

Evidence base

Few clinical trials involve patients over 80 years old, and those who are included tend to be fitter than those encountered in clinical practice, especially those in secondary care. Reported levels of benefit and risk of harm from medications studied in younger, non-frail, non-co-morbid groups cannot therefore be assumed to be the same as in older, frailer cohorts with higher levels of co-morbidity. Research that includes frailer populations with multimorbidity is inherently very difficult due to the confounding issues seen in such cohorts and the practicalities of obtaining consent or attending follow-up visits. However, it would be wrong to deny patients the benefits of treatment on the grounds that there is no evidence base: *the absence of an evidence base is not the same as the absence of benefit.*

Benefits of therapy

The levels of benefit from interventions differ between age groups. For example, there is increasing evidence in older diabetic patients treated with insulin that tighter target HbA_{1c} levels of <50 mmol/mol (<6.7%) are associated with worse outcomes (increased mortality, increased weight gain) than in those patients with a more relaxed target HbA_{1c} of 47.5–57.4 mmol/mol (6.5–7.4%). In older people with diabetes, the avoidance of immediate complications (e.g. hypoglycaemic events) should be prioritized over prevention

---

 Box 15.8 Reasons for altered pharmacokinetics in older people

Drug absorption
- Gastric pH gradually increases with age (exacerbated by medications such as proton-pump inhibitors)
- Gastric emptying slows

Drug distribution
The main physiological changes that occur with ageing and lead to adverse drug reactions are probably:
- Increased body fat and decreased body water (as a proportion of total body weight)
- Increased volume of distribution for fat-soluble drugs, and so medications may accumulate due to an increased elimination half-life; this means that their effects may continue despite the drug being stopped
- Decreased volume of distribution for water-soluble drugs, and so drugs such as digoxin need a reduced loading dose

- Altered permeability of the blood–brain barrier, and so the brain of an older adult can be exposed to higher levels of medication, causing adverse effects

Drug metabolism
- Reduced hepatic blood flow and hence clearance of medications that have high hepatic excretion ratio, e.g. amitriptyline

Elimination/kidneys
- With age, there is a reduction in renal mass and renal blood flow; eGFR decreases by 0.5% per year after the age of 20
- Affects clearance of water-soluble drugs such as diuretics, NSAIDs and digoxin

  N.B. In older adults, a 'normal' creatinine may be associated with significant renal impairment.

eGFR, estimated glomerular filtration rate; NSAIDs, non-steroidal anti-inflammatory drugs.

Box 15.9 Optimizing compliance and concordance

Understand what medications are and are not being taken
- The patient may be taking certain medications only; exercise caution when increasing medications without understanding this, to avoid causing iatrogenic complications.
- Why might the patient not want particular medications?
- Review side-effects (e.g. diuretics causing incontinence).
- Review aims of treatment (see later).

Understand problems around taking the medications
- Dysphagia: is there a liquid or patch alternative?
- Dexterity: can the patient take the medication from the packaging? Aids are available for inhalers and eye drops.
- Cognition: is the patient forgetting to take the medication, or taking a second dose of one already taken? Are they managing complicated instructions, e.g.

for oral bisphosphonates, or variable-dosing medications such as insulin or warfarin?
- Visual impairment: consider large-font labelling.

Simplify regimens
- Is a particular time of day better to take the medications?
- Consider once-a-day, modified-release preparations.
- Reduce inappropriate polypharmacy.
- Agree which medications the patient wishes to take.
- Use blister packs to reduce the need to coordinate multiple medications and aid monitoring of compliance.

Review care needs
- Is supervision or prompting required?

Utility	Medications that:	Examples
More useful ↕ **Less useful**	Provide immediate relief for distressing symptoms	Analgesics, antiemetics
	Modify an acute condition that is life-threatening or will soon result in distressing symptoms if not treated	Antibiotics for severe sepsis Diuretics for acute heart failure
	Modify a chronic condition that may progress to become life-threatening or progress to cause significant symptoms if not treated	Methotrexate for rheumatoid arthritis
	Have the potential to prevent serious disease without a symptomatic benefit	Antihypertensives, antiplatelet agents
	Are unlikely to be useful in either the short or the long term	Fish oils, glucosamine
	Are used for indications where non-pharmacological therapy is equally or more effective	Physiotherapy for back pain Sleep hygiene vs long-term benzodiazepines

Fig. 15.4 Hierarchy of utility of medications. *(Adapted from Consultant Pharmacy Services, A Guide to Deprescribing. 2016; http://www.cpsedu.com.au/uploads/Documents/Deprescribing%202016%20 Version/00%20General%20Fact%20Sheet%20(SINGLE).pdf.)*

of longer-term consequences, which may take decades to develop. Similarly, while targets for blood pressure tend to be around 130/80 mmHg in younger patients, outcomes for older patients are better with a higher target: there is a U-shaped curve with an optimum of 160/90 mmHg (i.e. there is an increased risk of adverse events and mortality when blood pressure is significantly higher or lower than this). Some of these adverse events relate to the side-effects of antihypertensives, such as orthostatic hypotension, falls, and associated morbidity and mortality.

Clinical decision-making

Many tools exist to aid clinical decision-making with respect to polypharmacy. They aim to summarize the evidence for a given medication in older adults and allow a negotiated approach between patient and clinician regarding the stopping and starting of medications. Examples include the Beers Criteria, Screening Tool of Older People's potentially inappropriate Prescriptions-Screening Tool to Alert doctors to Right Treatments (STOPP-START), Anti-Cholinergic Burden (ACB) Scale and the Scottish polypharmacy app (see **Box 15.6**). **Figure 15.4** shows the potential hierarchy of utility for medications that might be considered when undertaking a polypharmacy review.

Falls (instability)

Most of us take for granted the amazing complexity of the process that maintains an upright posture. High levels of functioning are needed across multiple systems, including musculoskeletal, neurological and cardiovascular. While anyone of any age can fall, it is said that 'young people trip, old people fall'. For many older or frail adults there are numerous, cumulative risk factors for falling that, individually, would be unlikely to produce major instability (**Boxes 15.10** and **15.11**). Assessment of falls is one of the most complex areas for geriatricians and can take significant time. Asking about falls should nevertheless be part of routine practice for all professionals working with older people.

Approximately 5% of fallers over 65 years of age will sustain an injury that is serious enough to limit normal activities. Most

> **Box 15.10 Falls in the UK**
>
> - One-third of people over 65 years fall at least once per year.
> - Half of people aged over 80 years fall at least once per year.
> - Over 250 000 emergency hospital admissions each year relate to falls.
> - Falls are estimated to cost the National Health Service £2.3 billion per year.
> - Falls from 2 m or less are the most common mechanism of injury for major trauma in older people in the UK.

> **Box 15.11 Categories of risk factors for falling**
>
> | Category | Optimizable | Static |
> |---|---|---|
> | **Intrinsic** | Concurrent illness, cardiac syncope, medications | Weakness from previous stroke |
> | **Extrinsic** | Trip hazards, grab rails | Stairs into house |

falls occur during the daytime, when people are most active, and only around 20% take place overnight. Risk factors include cognitive impairment, medications, alcohol excess and a change of environment, such as being admitted to hospital or moving to new accommodation.

Breaking down the contributing risk factors helps provide some structure for assessing and developing a management plan for a person who has fallen (**Box 15.12** and **Fig. 15.5**), and for targeting those risk factors that are reversible. An approach to the assessment of falls is summarized in **Box 15.13**.

Loss of consciousness is a worrying symptom but of those patients who do actually lose consciousness, over 30% are unaware that this occurred. Often patients try to rationalize what has happened, stating 'I must have tripped.' Normally, people will put their arms out when falling to protect themselves. Be suspicious of syncopal falls where this has not happened and there are facial injuries. Items to check include lying and standing blood pressure, electrocardiogram (ECG), and medications such as antihypertensives or diuretics. Management of syncope is largely the same at all ages (see p. 1029).

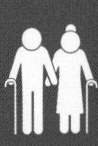

? Box 15.12 Some risk factors for falls with possible management strategies

Risk factor	Causes	Investigation and management
Unsteady gait	Varied: Gait assessment for speed, sway, hesitancy, degree of heel strike, time with both feet on the ground Balance assessment, including cerebellar examination	Physiotherapy assessment: Balance and strength exercises Review of walking aids Encouragement to keep active Appropriate and well-fitting footwear
Leg weakness	Multiple causes Spinal disease Sarcopenia Disuse/deconditioning Motor neurone disease Myopathy	Neurological assessment Clinical assessment Imaging, e.g. MRI Physiological, e.g. EMG/nerve conduction studies Targeted physiotherapy
Peripheral sensory impairment	Peripheral neuropathy, e.g. diabetes, vitamin B_{12} deficiency Reduced proprioception	Optimization of risk factors Physiotherapy and occupational therapy for adaptive measures
Joint instability	Greater likelihood of tripping and falling due to pain or reduced range of movement of hips and knees in osteoarthritis	Analgesia: topical, oral, intra-articular; consider joint replacement Walking aids to reduce stress though joint Physiotherapy to improve strength around joint
Pain	Antalgic gait Side-effects of pain medication, e.g. drowsiness from opioids	Optimization and individualization of pain control
Cerebrovascular disease	Large-vessel – causing focal visual, sensory and motor deficits Small-vessel – frequently dismissed Both associated with: Gait dyspraxia Marche à petits pas Cognitive impairment Urinary incontinence	Optimization of vascular risk factors
Cognitive impairment	Inability to pre-empt hazards, resulting in reduced safety awareness Impaired executive function – planning complex tasks Increased activity: 'wandering' Inability to use/remember walking aids	Screening for reversible causes of confusion Review of medication, e.g. opiates, sedatives, anticholinergic burden Occupational therapy for home safety
Depression	Association with reduced activity and consequent weakness, poor nutritional intake and poor sleep Impact on cognitive/executive function Interplay between depression and fear of falling	Activity can improve mood and increase interaction with social world Antidepressants may be required but can contribute further to falls Avoidance of medications most associated with postural hypotension (e.g. tricyclics) Monitoring for hyponatraemia and QTc prolongation
Visual impairment	Visual field defects: stroke, macular degeneration, glaucoma Visual neglect: stroke Reduced visual acuity: lens changes, retinopathy *Reduced hazard awareness*	Optician review, ideally annually Improvement of lighting around house; consider movement-sensitive lights for nocturia
Hearing impairment	Conductive: wax Sensorineural loss: commonly age-related plus other causes Social isolation *Reduced hazard awareness*	Audiological assessment for hearing aids Treatment for ear wax
Medication/ polypharmacy	Exacerbation of postural hypotension Dehydration Electrolyte imbalances Confusion and sedating effects	Medication review (see earlier) Over-the-counter medications Alcohol history
Postural hypotension	Frequent association with antihypertensive treatment; may be intermittent Symptoms can be vague	Ambulatory BP monitoring if associated with hypertension Review of target BP – loosening control is often a pragmatic solution Minimization of vasodilating and dehydrating medications, e.g. ACE inhibitors, diuretics, nitrates
Electrolyte imbalances	Mild–moderate derangements often dismissed, but associated with non-specific muscle weakness, malaise, constipation Severe derangements can lead to arrhythmias, seizures, myopathies presenting as a fall Often medication- or hydration-related	Blood tests Correction of abnormalities Review of medications Review of diet
Anaemia	Causes fatigue, weakness and breathlessness Increased risk of postural hypotension if volume loss-associated Pernicious anaemia causes vitamin B_{12} deficiency, which can lead to peripheral sensory neuropathy and SACD Frequent association with chronic disease and iron deficiency	Establishment of underlying cause Consideration of: Blood transfusion Iron replacement B_{12} and folate supplementation

Continued

? Box 15.12 Some risk factors for falls with possible management strategies—cont'd

Risk factor	Causes	Investigation and management
Urinary incontinence	Overactive bladder Results in rushing to toilet – especially problematic if there are also gait problems	Treatment of continence; consider specialist referral Minimization of diuretics
Diabetes mellitus	Multiple falls risk, including: Hypoglycaemic episodes Visual impairment – retinopathy/cataracts Peripheral sensory neuropathy and autonomic dysfunction	Check of FBC control – diary HbA$_{1c}$ higher target for frail older adults – higher mortality associated with HbA$_{1c}$ <50 Retinal screening Check for neuropathy/postural BP
Brady- and tachy-arrhythmia (e.g. AF or CHB)	Reduction of cerebral perfusion and increase in falls risk	If ECG is abnormal, cardiac monitoring may be required (e.g. 24-h/7-day tape)
Fear of falling	Very common, especially after major falls but can be independent of falling Association with changes in gait pattern to be less steady, further potentiating fear Physical activity may reduce, exacerbating muscle weakness Complex interplay between depression and fear of falling	Cognitive behavioural therapy Exercise (particularly tai chi) Review of walking aids to aid confidence and independence Treatment of underlying anxiety/depression
Vertigo, e.g. BPPV	Vestibular disorders in older people common and frequently unrecognized	Head impulse test: peripheral vs central cause Dix–Hallpike: BPPV Epley manoeuvres or vestibular exercises (e.g. Cooksey–Cawthorne) ENT or specialist physiotherapy input
Foot health	Foot deformities and pain contribute to falls risk and poorly fitting footwear Leg length discrepancies	Podiatry referral Trimming of toenails Well-fitting footwear; may need specialist input

ACE, angiotensin-converting enzyme; AF, atrial fibrillation; BP, blood pressure; BPPV, benign paroxysmal positional vertigo; CHB, complete heart block; ECG, electrocardiogram; EMG, electromyography; ENT, ear, nose and throat; FBC, full blood count; MRI, magnetic resonance imaging; SACD, subacute combined degeneration of the spinal cord.

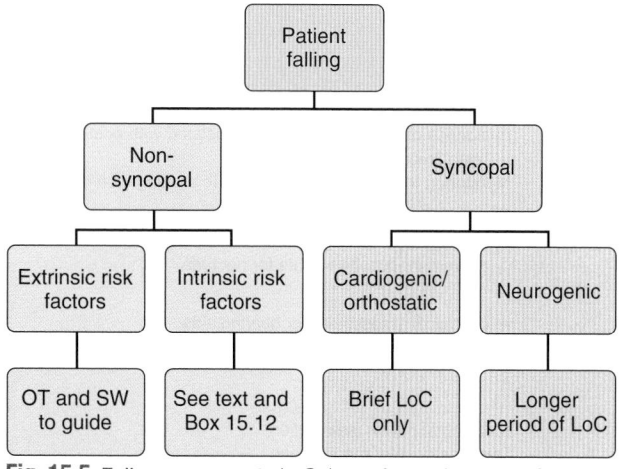

Fig. 15.5 Falls assessment. LoC, loss of consciousness; OT, occupational therapist; SW, social worker.

Consequences of falls

Most falls result in minor or no injuries. However, consequences can include fractures and trauma.

Fear of falling

Even after minor falls, patients can develop a fear of falling. This is characterized by anxiety around mobilizing and is associated with an increasing loss of confidence and hesitant gait (see **Box 15.11**). As a result, people often reduce the amount of walking they do and stop going out of the house. In turn, they develop reduced muscle strength and an increased risk of falling. There is also a danger of social isolation and depression.

Fragility fractures

Fragility fractures occur following an injury from a standing height or lower, and range from vertebral fractures (where there may even be no fall) to wrist, proximal humeral, pubic rami and neck of femur fractures. Most of these are associated with osteoporosis and enquiry should be made about:

- previous fractures, including site, history and age at the time
- age of menopause for female patients
- history of previous osteoporosis treatment.

Sometimes there is no history of trauma. These atraumatic fractures can be due to severe osteoporosis but other causes should be considered, particularly malignancy (e.g. breast, prostate, myeloma, lung), and investigated accordingly. Long-term anti-resorptive bone therapy (i.e. bisphosphonates, denosumab) can cause bones to become unnaturally brittle, especially if it is given as a parenteral treatment or at high doses for malignancy. This can result in unusual fractures, often atraumatic ones, such as fractures of the femoral shaft.

Neck of femur fractures

In England, there are approximately 60000 neck of femur fractures per year, accounting for 15% of all fragility fractures (**Fig. 15.6**). They represent a significant injury for an older person:

- They account for 1.8 million inpatient bed days per year.
- Some 20% of patients suffering a neck of femur fracture require transfer to long-term care within 1 year.
- Mortality is 5% at 30 days and 30% at 1 year.

In a number of countries there has been a drive to develop geriatric liaison services to deliver CGA for patients with hip fractures. The geriatrician's role in perioperative care covers the issues outlined in **Box 15.13** and includes:

Box 15.13 Assessment of falls

Immediate management
- Treatment of acute illness (ABC approach)
- Assessment for injuries
- Pain control: consider regional anaesthesia (fascia iliaca nerve block for hip fractures) to minimize opiate use
- Preparation for safer surgery if required, e.g. optimizing fluid balance, correcting clotting (if on anticoagulants)

History and examination (ideally including collateral information)
N.B. Cover events leading to fall, risk factors for falling, consequences of fall
- Events prior to the fall; previous falls/near-misses; baseline mobility (e.g. any aids, asking why they are needed – muscle weakness, balance, other)
- Any loss of consciousness?
- Medication review; alcohol history
- Full examination; consider risk factors, e.g. aortic stenosis, evidence of Parkinsonism, cerebellar issues, visual screen
- Postural blood pressure
- Inspect gait: even without formal training, think about how unsteady this looks, including turning, and how well a walking aid is used and whether the patient looks comfortable with it
- List risk factors for falls; address where possible

Investigations
- Bloods tests:
  - Full blood count (e.g. anaemia, evidence of sepsis)
  - Serum creatinine and electrolytes (evidence of acute kidney injury, electrolyte imbalance)
  - Glucose/HbA$_{1c}$
  - Bone profile/vitamin D
  - Thyroid function, micronutrient levels (vitamin B$_{12}$, folic acid, iron studies)

- ECG: e.g. conduction abnormalities
- Imaging:
  - Plain X-rays/cross-sectional imaging for possible fractures
  - CT head (evidence of large- or small-vessel cerebrovascular disease; exclusion of trauma, e.g. subdural haemorrhage)

Acute hospital admission
- Major trauma, including 'silver trauma' (older people with multiple injuries, often from low-impact trauma, such as falling from standing height), head injuries, fractures (e.g. hip)
- Possible/likely acute illness requiring inpatient care (e.g. intravenous antibiotics, fluids)
- Inability to mobilize safely
- Care needs that cannot be met in the community
  N.B. Not all fractures require admission, depending on mobility and social circumstances (e.g. wrist, neck of humerus, pubic rami).

Factors that should prompt further assessment
- Frequent falls without recent input from a specialist team, when the risk of further falls is felt to be high
- Possible syncope
- Polypharmacy
- Referral to relevant specialists, depending on findings from assessments (e.g. Parkinson's disease specialist)
  N.B. Usually done in the outpatient department.

Further management
- Provide oral and written information about falls
- Assess for and manage osteoporosis (e.g. DEXA scan, optimization of calcium/vitamin D levels, anti-resorptive bone medications or teriparatide)
- Advise regular optician review (e.g. screen for cataract, glaucoma)

CT, computed tomography; DEXA, dual-energy X-ray absorptiometry; ECG, electrocardiogram.

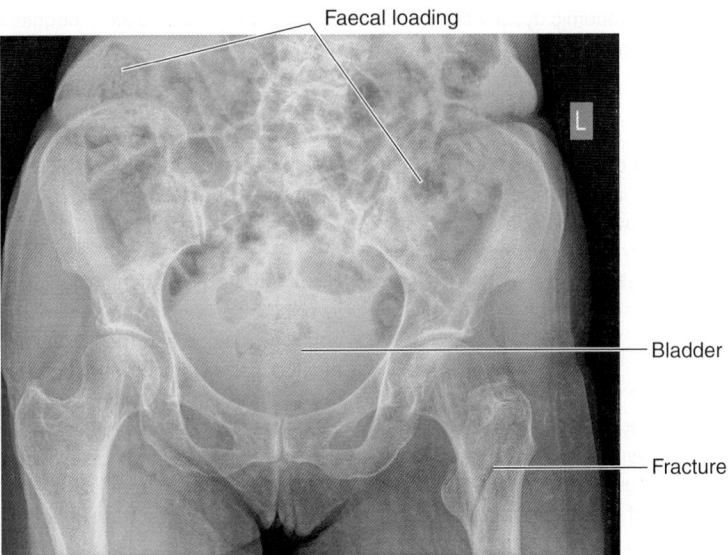

Fig. 15.6 **A left-sided intertrochanteric hip fracture.** Also of note, there is a large bladder (smooth shadowing in the lower pelvis), likely to be associated with urinary retention, for which the patient would need a catheter. Faecal loading is also visible, so laxatives should be started.

- pain management
- management of venous thrombotic risk
- recognition and management of delirium
- management of bowels and bladder
- assessment and management of bone health and osteoporosis.

In the UK the widespread establishment of orthogeriatric services has led to a halving of 1-month mortality for hip fractures (from around 10% to around 5%).

Institutionalization

Falls and their consequences contribute to approximately 40% of admissions to care homes. The fact of being in a care home does not in itself improve gait or remove the risk of falling; indeed, the risk of falling may initially increase on moving into a care home. However, it does mean that there are people on hand to help reduce the risk and to assist if someone does fall.

Postural hypotension

Cerebral autoregulation is responsible for maintaining stable blood flow through the brain. In old age, this becomes less well controlled, causing the brain to become more vulnerable to changes in systemic blood pressure and, in turn, to postural instability and falls. The prevalence of postural (orthostatic) hypotension in the community is 1 in 5 older adults.

On standing, normal physiological responses should result in maintenance of a normal blood pressure. This requires:
- normal plasma volume, i.e. the person must not be dehydrated (younger people compensate well for this)
- intact baroreceptors and reflexes
- venomotor tone, the ability of blood vessels to respond to changes in blood flow.

Symptoms of postural hypotension (**Box 15.14**) typically occur on or soon after standing; they are rare when a person is sitting or lying down, unless they have been lying for a long period and then attempt to sit upright or stand. Some definitions of 'significant drop' are provided in **Box 15.15**.

Aetiology

Acute postural hypotension is seen with a reduced intravascular volume, e.g. decreased oral intake, excessive diuresis or excessive fluid losses as in diarrhoea, vomiting or haemorrhage.

Chronic causes are principally:
- **Medications**: classically, diuretics, beta-blockers and other anti-arrhythmics, antihypertensives and vasodilators.
- **Autonomic dysfunction**: associated with diabetes mellitus, Parkinson's disease and multisystem atrophy (medications for Parkinson's disease may exacerbate this further). Some autoimmune conditions can also cause autonomic dysfunction.
- **Poor vascular compliance**: seen in ageing blood vessels due to a reduction in elasticity and increased calcification.

Management

The evidence base behind management of postural hypotension is poor and only a couple of medications are licensed for use. The goal is to minimize symptoms and improve standing time, in order to enable activities of daily living through improvement of standing blood pressure without excessive supine hypertension (**Box 15.16**).

Delirium

Delirium (sometimes called acute intellectual impairment or acute confusional state) is a common neuropsychiatric syndrome characterized by disturbed consciousness, cognitive function or perception. The characteristic feature is a lack of 'attention'. It has an acute onset (1–2 days) and fluctuating course. It is the most common psychosis seen in hospital, occurring in 20–30% of medical and 50% of orthogeriatric patients.

Delirium occurs for a large number of reasons; anything that causes a physiological stress can be a trigger. One useful way of thinking about delirium is to consider its predisposing and precipitating factors (**Box 15.17**).

As a person becomes more cognitively frail (or has significant predisposing risk factors), there is less physiological and cerebral reserve, and so smaller precipitants may trigger delirium. Delirium can be thought of as an acute brain failure. Patients admitted to hospital with delirium have:

Box 15.14 Measurement of postural blood pressure

1. Ensure that you are able to stand the patient up, getting help beforehand if necessary.
2. Use a manual sphygmomanometer, ideally.
3. Lie the patient down for 5 min.
4. Measure blood pressure.
5. Stand the patient up and measure blood pressure in the first minute.
6. Repeat at 3 min.
7. If blood pressure is still dropping, repeat and keep checking until it resolves.
8. Repeat if symptoms change at any point.

(Adapted from Royal College of Physicians: https://www.rcplondon.ac.uk/projects/outputs/measurement-lying-and-standing-blood-pressure-brief-guide-clinical-staff.)

Box 15.15 Definitions of a 'significant' drop in blood pressure

- **Classic**: reduction of 20/10 mmHg within 3 min of standing
- **Initial**: reduction of 40/20 mmHg in first 15 sec – a beat-to-beat recording is required
- **Delayed**: no agreed definition but occurring >3 min
- **In hypertensive patients**: reduction of 30 mmHg systolic – variability higher in this group

- an increased length of stay by an average of 8 days
- worse physical and cognitive recovery at 6 and 12 months
- an increased need for institutional care
- a 1.5-fold increase in mortality risk in the year following admission.

Delirium is characteristically fluctuant and may follow a hyperactive, hypoactive or mixed picture (**Box 15.18**).

Screening tools to aid recognition of delirium include the Confusion Assessment Method (CAM, **Box 15.19**) and the 4AT test (*A*lertness, *A*ttention, four-question *A*bbreviated Mental Test (AMT4) and *A*cute change). A key feature is the recognition of a change in cognitive state. This has led to the development of the *Single QUestion in Delirium* (SQUID): 'Do you think this patient has been more confused lately?'

Assessment and management

History and examination, including collateral information from family or carers, should aim to establish the duration and nature of any cognitive change and then focus on what altered for the patient in the hours or days prior to that change. There are a number of easy-to-use and swift screening tools (e.g. the 4AT test) that can aid the identification of delirium in clinical practice. Some types of dementia can have a fluctuating course, such as Lewy body disease, though the duration and pattern can help differentiate this. Patients may be worse by late afternoon or early evening; this is known as 'sundowning syndrome'. Management approaches are summarized in **Box 15.20**.

Pharmacological management

Sedatives and antipsychotics can be used to treat delirium, but only when a person is a risk to themselves or others and conservative measures have failed. There is no evidence that these interventions treat (as opposed to sedate) delirium at a physiological level. The drugs themselves are deliriogenic and so can lead to a perpetuation of delirium. When necessary, the lowest dose to control symptoms should be used (e.g. risperidone 0.25 mg, lorazepam 0.5 mg, haloperidol 0.5 mg).

i Box 15.16 Management options in postural hypotension

Recommendation	Detail	Explanation
Abdominal binders	'Corsets' beneficial in about 50%; usefulness comes down to practicalities Compression stockings (TEDs) – full-length, grade 2 and above. Logistically difficult to put on or to tolerate high pressures exerted. Below-knee TEDS unhelpful as amount of blood in calves is relatively small	Large volume of blood and baroreceptors in splanchnic and mesenteric circulation
Bolus of water	Drinking water – conflicting evidence: needs to be fluid bolus, 500 mL of water within 5 min with benefit lasting around 90 min. Useful if timing of hypotension is predictable, e.g. first thing in morning	Fluid bolus causes change in osmolality of portal blood supply and induces autonomic response in blood pressure
Bed elevation	Elevating head of bed to 30 degrees from horizontal	Lower renal perfusion pressure leading to decreased diuresis and therefore fluid retention, to maintain peripheral capillary pressure on standing up Another benefit is avoidance of supine hypertension in patient with impaired baroreceptor responsiveness lying flat
Counter-manoeuvres	Standing on toes, pelvic and abdominal clenches Crossing legs and squeezing, squeezing buttocks/thighs/calves while standing Standing slowly – education programmes with physiotherapy	Physical manoeuvres to increase blood return to heart by improving peripheral resistance Engaging venous return of mesenteric and splanchnic blood volume Unclear mechanism
Drugs (limited evidence)	Fludrocortisone Midodrine	Increases fluid retention Alpha-adrenergic agonist increasing peripheral vascular resistance
Education for self-management	STOP what you are doing when you recognize symptoms coming on SIT down: allow blood pressure to recover DRINK some water, the most modifiable factor in the immediate term THINK about triggers: recognize patterns to manage	Patient understanding that their blood pressure responses are not normal and that they need to find ways to adapt to live with this in longer term
Exercise	Moderate exercise Practising getting up and standing slowly to avoid symptoms	Improves orthostatic tolerance
Fluid intake	Keeping well hydrated	Maintains plasma volume

? Box 15.17 Predisposing and precipitating factors in delirium

Predisposing factors
- Cognitive impairment
- Older age
- Parkinson's disease
- Severe illness
- Depression
- Sensory impairment (hearing or visual loss)
- Presence of multiple co-morbidities
- Polypharmacy

Precipitant examples
- Analgesia
- Anaesthesia

- Change in location/environment
- Constipation
- Dehydration
- Electrolyte abnormalities
- Infection
- New medications/change in medication dose
- Pain
- Sleep deprivation
- Surgery
- Alcohol withdrawal

Prognosis

Usually, delirium clears within a week or two but full cognitive recovery often takes longer: up to 3 months. Rarely, it may never resolve. Those with more marked underlying cognitive impairments are less likely to regain their previous level of cognition. Delirium is both inflammatory and toxic to the cerebrum, and pathological studies show that the length of time for which delirium lasts correlates with the increased neuropathological changes commonly associated with dementia. Those who experience delirium are more likely to be diagnosed with dementia in the subsequent 1–2 years.

Urinary tract infections

UTIs are common in older adults. However, they are also commonly misdiagnosed or over-diagnosed without clear evidence. This can result in potentially dangerous overuse of antibiotics and over-looking (or missing) the actual cause of the patient's presentation. Recurrent UTIs in particular should be questioned. Often evidence is lacking and alternative diagnoses, such as vulvovaginal atrophy, should be investigated.

A diagnosis of UTI is likely with a short history of new-onset dysuria alone, or two or more of:

---

i **Box 15.18 Delirium subtypes and their features**

Delirium subtype	Characteristics	Notes
Hyperactive	Agitation Paranoia Anxiety Hallucinations (may reach out, trying to pluck things from air) Disorientation Startling easily Carphologia or floccillation (lint-picking movements) Restlessness Wandering; associated risk of falls	Patients receive medical attention as they identify themselves May need pharmacological intervention if safety at risk
Hypoactive	Quiet, sleepy Little psychomotor agitation May have paranoia and anxiety Reduced oral intake Increased pressure sore risk	Patients do not often disturb staff and so are easily missed Poorer prognosis
Mixed	A mixture of both the above subtypes May be present at same time or alternate	Most common subtype

---

i **Box 15.19 Confusion Assessment Method (CAM) screening tool for delirium[a]**

Feature	Description
1. Acute onset and fluctuating course *AND*	Often from collateral information Is there evidence of an acute change in mental status from the patient's baseline? Does the (abnormal) behaviour fluctuate during the day?
2. Inattention	Does the patient have difficulty focusing attention, e.g. distractible, difficulty following conversation?
AND **3. Disorganized thinking** *OR*	Is the patient's thinking disorganized or incoherent, e.g. rambling or irrelevant conversation, unclear or illogical flow of ideas, or unpredictable switching from subject to subject?
4. Altered level of consciousness	What is the patient's level of consciousness? Normal – alert Abnormal – vigilant (hyperalert), lethargic (drowsy, easily roused), stupor (difficult to rouse) or coma (unrousable)

[a]The diagnosis of delirium by CAM requires the presence of:
- both features 1 *and* 2
- and *either* 3 or 4.

- frequency or urgency
- incontinence
- delirium
- worsening mobility
- suprapubic discomfort
- fever
- visible haematuria.

Investigations

A midstream specimen of urine (MSU) should guide antibiotic use prior to their initiation, if there is diagnostic uncertainty. This may help reduce microbial resistance in the longer term. Urine dips are of limited value (**Box 15.21**).

---

y **Box 15.20 Management of delirium**

This is mostly centred around multifactorial interventions:
1. Identify underlying precipitant(s), e.g. constipation, new medications, pain, electrolyte imbalance, infection.
2. Address treatable causes.
3. Minimize sensory impairments, e.g. hearing aids, glasses.
4. Reduce sensory distractions, e.g. closing of some curtains, reduction of loud noises, consistent staff, gentle lighting.
5. Re-orientate (where not distressing to do so):
   - Clock/calendar
   - Radio
   - Personal objects
   - Family photos
   - 'REACH out to me'/'This is me' documents – can be used to structure background information that will help in management and care.
6. Social support and family presence – encourage and allow family members to be present. Any delusions and hallucinations should be neither endorsed nor challenged.
7. Pharmacological measures are of limited benefit.

---

i **Box 15.21 Urine dipsticks in the diagnosis of urinary tract infection**

Public Health England guidance (2018) suggests not using urine dipsticks in the over-65 population.
- In conjunction with symptoms, dipsticks have a sensitivity of around 77%.
- In the absence of symptoms (e.g. as a screen in a patient with confusion), sensitivity falls to 44%.
- The frequency of positive urine dips in institutional care is very high: up to 50% of females in nursing homes have asymptomatic bacteriuria. In non-care-home residents the figure is lower, ranging from 6% to 16% in females aged 65–90.
- The negative predictive value of dipsticks is 100% for nursing home residents.
- In the presence of long-term catheters, dipsticks will almost always be positive (colonization).

Asymptomatic bacteriuria is bacterial colonization without active infection in the urinary tract. It can cause false positives on urine dipsticks and raised white cell counts on MSU samples.

Management

- In the absence of systemic features of sepsis (see p. 156), treat with empirical antibiotics when a UTI is suspected.
- Review with MSU sensitivities when available.
- Change the catheter as soon as possible if it has been present for more than 7 days before antibiotics, if it is clinically safe to do so.

Recurrent UTIs

- Hold off antibiotics if possible and send 2–3 MSU samples.
- Consider alternative diagnoses if MSUs are repeatedly negative, including vulvovaginal atrophy in peri- and postmenopausal women, sexually transmitted infections, urethritis and prostatitis.
- Ensure that non-specific symptoms are not being inappropriately attributed to UTIs.
- In truly recurrent UTIs, specific management is often required (**Box 15.22**).

Urinary incontinence

Up to 50% of women will be incontinent at some time in their life. For men, urinary tract symptoms and difficulty passing urine are also common but less well studied. Incontinence is under-recognized and undertreated. Many people will not volunteer their symptoms; even if asked directly, not everyone will be comfortable talking about it.

Incontinence has a huge impact on a person's quality of life and often on their relationships with partners and family. Poorly controlled urinary incontinence is a common reason for admissions to residential care due to carer strain. It is independently associated with falls and is a modifiable risk factor for them. For those who are bedbound, incontinence can cause local irritation in areas prone to pressure damage, increasing the risk of breakdown of skin integrity.

There are four main types of urinary incontinence but there is often overlap between them.

Stress incontinence

Urine leaks from the bladder due to higher pressures than the pelvic muscles are able to contain. This is commonly due to weakness or damage to the pelvic floor muscles, and previous pregnancy is a risk factor. A typical history with this kind of incontinence is for it to occur on coughing, laughing or straining.

Management may be conservative or surgical. Conservative measures can cure stress incontinence and so are first-line treatment (**Box 15.23**). If they fail, surgical referral should be considered. Surgery aims to support the pelvic floor either through suspension of the bladder higher up from the external sphincter or by bulking the pelvic floor itself.

Urge incontinence (overactive bladder)

In this type, the bladder becomes irritable, causing the person to feel that they urgently need to empty it when it is not actually full. Symptoms include frequency, urgency and nocturia. If these are of new onset, the trigger may be a UTI. Chronic infection should be excluded as a cause.

When a history is taken, the questions need to be broader than in stress incontinence. Many people will have adapted their lifestyles to minimize the risk of being incontinent, so questions might include:

- Do you ever not make it to the toilet in time?
- When you feel the urge to go to the toilet, are you able to hold it or do you need to go quickly? What happens if you do not?
- If you are going out, do you plan your day around the availability of toilets?
- Do you use continence pads?

Management begins with conservative measures, as for stress incontinence (see **Box 15.23**). Additionally, it includes avoiding bladder irritants, including dehydration (concentrated urine) and caffeine. Bladder training aims for a slow increase of the amount of time from feeling the urge to pass urine to micturition. If these measures fail, some patients benefit from medications such as antimuscarinics (e.g. oxybutynin, tolterodine). Around half of patients will have stopped taking the medication by 3 months and only one-third will still be taking it at 1 year due to its anticholinergic side-effects, which include dry eyes or mouth, constipation and confusion. The latter means that these drugs are relatively contraindicated in those with cognitive impairment. Beta-3 agonists, such as mirabegron, can be used as second-line therapy but carry a risk of accelerated hypertension.

Overflow incontinence

This is due to bladder outflow tract obstruction. The most common cause is prostate enlargement, and thus this is a disorder commonly seen in older men (see p. 1480). Other precipitants include medications (e.g. anticholinergics) and constipation. Symptoms include difficulty initiating micturition, poor stream and terminal dribbling, and overflow incontinence can lead to renal failure due to obstructive uropathy. Catheterization may be required, either in the short or long term, to alleviate the obstruction.

Functional incontinence

This involves the patient being unable to reach the toilet, rather than there being a primary urogenital problem. For example, someone with poor mobility may be unable to get to the toilet in time but would otherwise be continent if their mobility improved. In states of impaired cognition, such as delirium or advanced dementia, the signals for micturition are no longer interpreted normally, resulting in the passing of urine without conscious processing and thus in incontinence. Management requires CGA to address any modifiable components, such as pain control, to allow improved mobilization. This can include environmental adaptations, which may make toileting easier. Regular toileting can be helpful for those with advanced dementia and good mobility; this involves prompting the person to go to the toilet at regular intervals, before they need to go urgently, to minimize the risk of incontinence.

Older adult abuse and safeguarding

Abuse of older adults is defined as a single or repeated act that causes harm or distress to an older person, or lack of appropriate action. It can take place within any relationship where there is an expectation of trust. There are a number of different types of abuse (**Box 15.24**) and it is quite common for a number of these to occur simultaneously.

Older people are particularly vulnerable to abuse. Worldwide, the World Health Organization (WHO) has found that approximately

ⓘ Box 15.24 Some types of abuse

Type	Features	What to look for
Physical	e.g. Hitting, scratching Misuse of medicine, both under-medicating (e.g. inadequate analgesia) and over-medicating (e.g. excessive sedation) Forcible feeding or withholding of food Restraint	Unusual pattern of injuries Absence of clear explanation Frequent injuries for which medical treatment has not been sought
Sexual	Any sexual activity the patient cannot or does not consent to	Bruising, particularly to thighs, buttocks and upper arms Bleeding, infections, pain, sexually transmitted disease or itching in genital region
Psychological or emotional	Social isolation Removal of mobility or communication aids Preventing patient from meeting their religious needs	Change in psychological state in presence of another person Low self-esteem or withdrawn appearance
Financial or material	Preventing patient from accessing their own money or assets Arranging less care than is needed to save money (e.g. to maximize an inheritance) Moving into a person's home rent-free and/or under duress	Recent changes, e.g. to property ownership Obtaining lasting power of attorney after patient is assessed as lacking mental capacity to manage their finances
Discriminatory	Unequal treatment based on age, cognition, etc.	
Organizational or institutional	Settings such as nursing and residential homes, hospitals Lack of respect for dignity and privacy, e.g. during bathing or toileting	Inappropriately prioritizing care of younger patients Precluding all patients with dementia from rehabilitation, regardless of their potential to improve
Neglect or acts of omission	Denial of access to basic needs, including food, shelter, clothing, heating, personal and medical care Failure to administer medications appropriately	Malnourished appearance Untreated medical conditions or injuries Pressure damage
Self-neglect	Failure to carry out personal hygiene, where behaviour impacts on safety Squalid or unsanitary conditions Unkempt appearance Non-compliance with care	Health risk to neighbours

❓ Box 15.25 Risk factors for abuse

Patient factors
- Frailty or any serious health condition
- Physical or sensory disability, e.g. reduced mobility, poor vision
- Memory problems or dementia; other mental health problems; learning disability
- Previous episodes of abuse
- Low income or socioeconomic status

Social factors
- Substance misuse by abuser
- Mental health problems in abuser

- Shared living situation
- Abuser's dependency on the older person (often financial)
- Difficult family relationships
- Social isolation

Care provider factors
- Poor staff training or support, e.g. in institutions
- Policies operating in the interests of the institution rather than the residents
- Poor resources, e.g. to pay for carers or provide suitable environment

1 in 10 older people experience abuse each month. They also found that two-thirds of older people with dementia have been abused. Obtaining clear data is very difficult, and there is concern that these figures are under-estimates. Some risk factors for abuse are shown in **Box 15.25**.

Older people are often afraid to talk about cases of abuse to family, friends or the authorities, with fewer than 1 in 20 cases being reported. Even where abuse is recognized, many victims are unwilling to discuss or pursue complaints, especially if family are involved.

Cognitive impairment is a major risk factor for abuse, where recall of specific issues around the abuse is patchy and unreliable, making clarification of concerns difficult. The key point is to be aware of the issue and to have a low threshold for escalating possible concerns.

While older men have the same risk of abuse as women, older females are at higher risk of neglect and financial abuse in some cultures where women have unequal social status, particularly when

they are widowed. Women may also be at higher risk of more persistent and severe forms of abuse and injury.

Management

Safeguarding is the protection of people's health and wellbeing, enabling them to live safely and free from neglect or abuse in conjunction with their own wishes and beliefs. Preventative strategies include:
- clear support, education and guidance for patients and care-givers
- education at an institutional level, and clear guidelines on the management of specific conditions, e.g. behavioural and psychological symptoms of dementia (BPSD)
- involvement of patients and advocates in the development of policies and guidelines
- external assessments, e.g. Care Quality Commission.

Recognizing abuse can be difficult. There should be a low threshold for escalating concerns to the relevant specialists, who can then investigate and act where necessary. Often, this will be led by social services.

Rehabilitation

Rehabilitation is a multidisciplinary process through which an individual's functional level is optimized, including physical, psychological and social aspects of function. It can take place anywhere, from the patient's home to acute inpatient settings; even on the intensive care unit, there are interventions to help longer-term function. Rehabilitation is dependent on working closely with the patient and the wider MDT, including (where relevant) community and hospital-based services.

While the emphasis is on returning patients to their pre-morbid level of function, a limitation of functional regain, such as after a major stroke, must be recognized. In such cases, helping the patient adjust to the new functional level is a fundamental aspect of the process.

Most commonly, we think of rehabilitation occurring after an acute illness, such as a stroke or pneumonia. However, it also plays a key part in chronic conditions, such as Parkinson's disease and reduced mobility. Increasingly, its role in preparing people for interventions such as surgery is being recognized; this is known as 'pre-habilitation' and aims to expedite recovery and improve longer-term outcomes.

A number of factors affect the likely outcome from rehabilitation:

- *Premorbid status.* A frailer patient is less likely to improve as much as those who are stronger prior to their acute illness.
- *Reasons for deterioration.* An acute injury or illness, from which full or nearly full recovery might be expected, should be compared with progressive underlying illness, such as cancer or motor neurone disease, in which it is possible to achieve short-term gains but patients will deteriorate over the longer term.
- *Co-morbidities.* Where possible, these should be addressed through CGA. Areas that bring particular benefit include pain management (e.g. in arthritis of the knee), blood pressure (too low can increase falls risk) and Parkinson's disease (timing sessions to periods of the day when control is better).
- *Cognitive impairment.* This may reduce the patient's ability to follow instructions in the intervals between sessions. However, significant improvements may occur and cognition alone should not preclude rehabilitation. The clinician should also be aware that recognizing and treating pain in patients with dementia can be difficult but that poor control will have an impact on progress.
- *Depression.* Be suspicious when patients fail to progress as expected. Trying to discriminate between depression and an adjustment reaction following an acute illness (e.g. loss of function following a stroke) can be difficult, and monitoring over a period of weeks is often necessary.
- *Motivation.* Rehabilitation takes effort on the part of the patient and there is great variability in how much individuals are willing to engage.

A distinction should be made between patients who have a realistic chance of making a meaningful improvement and those who have no realistic chance of seeing a significant change. One of the key principles of rehabilitation is goal-setting, with clear and achievable targets over appropriate timescales. For example, in a patient needing a Zimmer frame and assistance from two people to transfer between bed and chair, rather than the goal being 'To improve transferring', a better target would be 'To develop to transferring with one person and a Zimmer frame within 1 week'.

Complex discharge planning

Discharge planning can be a complex balance of managing risk, expectations and resources. It requires close multidisciplinary working across primary and secondary care to fit best with a patient's wishes. The discharge destination from an acute hospital can be directly to home or to an intermediate care facility for further rehabilitation or convalescence. A number of factors affect a patient's discharge and destination (**Box 15.26**).

Typically, when patients are preparing for discharge, assessments are carried out in hospital; however, this may involve exploring the patient's mobility in a place where distances may be significantly greater than at home, and kitchen assessments take place in an unfamiliar environment. Occupational therapy home visits evaluate a patient's ability to function within their home environment, and people often do significantly better there. Some schemes, such as Discharge to Assess (D2A), complete all assessments in the patient's home, with essential equipment and care being put in place on the same day. This can reduce time spent in hospital and often results in lower care needs than were predicted from hospital-based assessments.

Managing risk is a crucial part of discharge planning. Risk cannot be removed completely from any discharge; the aim is to recognize predictable risks, minimize them, and then make further decisions with the person involved.

Besides patients' own homes, there are alternative options for older people. The most common ones available in the UK are outlined in **Box 15.27**.

Carer strain

A widely accepted definition of a carer is someone who provides unpaid, informal support to family or friends who could not manage without this help. In the UK, there are around 5 million unpaid carers. Many may struggle with the demands of their role. They may lose their sense of self and their own wellbeing, or experience an enhanced level of anxiety and stress, particularly if they are subject to:

- increased physical or verbal abuse
- being woken during the night.

Other factors that have a major impact include depression in the patient and incontinence, with faecal incontinence being particularly difficult for carers to manage. Carers may, in addition, have medical issues of their own. Assumptions should not be made regarding a carer's capacity or willingness either to start taking responsibility or to continue to care for a person. Carers should be actively involved in decisions surrounding a patient's care.

Ways to help reduce carer strain include:

- *recognition and appreciation* of what the carer is doing
- *financial support*, e.g. a carer or attendance allowance
- *maximizing performance status*, e.g. making transfers easier
- *addressing co-morbidities*, e.g. treating depression
- *periods of respite*, e.g. day centres, where the carer can take some time off; a sitting service; rolling respite, where the patient spends 1–2 weeks every 2 months, for example, in a care home; and asking friends and family to help for periods, either regularly or on a more *ad hoc* basis
- *holidays*, provided by companies who specialize in holidays for people with health conditions, with carers on site; often, patient and carer will travel together.

ℹ Box 15.26 Factors affecting discharge planning

Patient factors

- *Patient wishes.* Some patients are desperate to remain in their own home for as long as possible, while others can feel very trapped and isolated there, preferring somewhere that has other people around, such as a care home.
- *Medical issues and prognosis.* Has the issue leading to hospital admission resolved (e.g. hip fracture, pneumonia) or is it likely to be progressive (e.g. lung cancer)? What is the likely prognosis? For those with a short prognosis, e.g. a few weeks, it may be better to take more risks and maximize time at home, as opposed to aiming for rehabilitation when there is a longer prognosis.
- *Functional status.* How much are patients able to do for themselves? At a simple level, if a patient can walk to the toilet and back, support can be put in place for most other issues. Were they struggling at home before admission? What support do they need overnight, such as with toileting or wandering? If there are issues with continence, this can make things difficult at home; faecal incontinence in particular is harder to manage there. Mobility is a major issue, with falls being one of the leading reasons for admission to a care home. N.B. Falls can occur anywhere, including at home, in hospital or in a care home, though the latter two have staff to reduce the risk or help after the event.
- *Cognition.* This affects a patient's ability to care for themselves and their safety awareness, as well as their ability to call for help appropriately, either through pendant alarms or telephones. Some may need increasing support with meals, either ready-made for oven or microwave, or delivered to the home. Some patients may forget or have poor insight into their cognitive problems, in which case options such as turning off the gas supply to the cooker can make discharge home safer. Reversal of a patient's sleep pattern (day–night reversal) can make it much harder for a spouse to offer support, as their own sleep pattern will also be affected. Patients with cognitive impairment tend to function far better in a familiar environment than elsewhere, and home visits from the occupational therapists should be considered before any permanent moves to a care home.

Home factors

- *Suitability for frailer people or those with cognitive impairment.* Some homes are more suitable than others. Cramped spaces can be difficult, although it is easier for people with reduced mobility to hold on to the walls. Some beautiful rickety cottages with little steps between each room can be a disaster! Modern purpose-built flats for older people are usually fine.
- *Stairs.* These can be a challenge, though having a toilet on each floor makes things easier.
- *Potential for adaptations.* Is there space for a hoist? Can the bathroom be adapted to house a walk-in shower? Can a stairlift be installed?

Social factors

- *Co-habitation.* This can provide physical support, such as assistance with activities of daily living (from washing and dressing to housework), as well as someone to call for help if there are any problems. Be aware of the physical and cognitive level of the spouse, who may also be frail with multiple co-morbidities. Live-in carers are another option, though expensive.
- *Financial status.* Is the patient able to pay for support and equipment?
- *Family wishes.* While patient wishes are vitally important, the family members are the ones who pick up the pieces when things do not work out. Balancing a patient's wishes with what is realistic can be tricky, as can balancing them with the family's wishes, which may not be the same as the patient's. Where a patient has capacity for decisions regarding specific issues, these should be respected wherever possible. *N.B. Beware of abuse (financial abuse and neglect) when the family agree only to an insufficient care package in their attempts to preserve their inheritance.*

Resources

- Availability of and funds for carers.
- Availability of and funds for equipment.
- Access to rehabilitation units.
- Local schemes for domiciliary care – can rehabilitation be done from the patient's own home?

ℹ Box 15.27 Non-home-based living options in the UK

- *Care home.* This can mean a residential or nursing home.
- *Residential home.* This is suitable for people who need minimal assistance with mobility, transfers and some personal care.
- *Nursing home.* This is suitable for people requiring significant support, supervision and care, with trained nurses present to support delivery.
- *Warden-assisted living/sheltered accommodation.* Residents have their own flats. A warden is accessible at certain times and is able to provide some support, though not with personal care. Often there are communal areas.
- *Extra-care sheltered accommodation.* This is sheltered accommodation that also has on-site carers who can provide additional care more flexibly.

Loneliness

As people age and experience associated disability and frailty, their personal world may progressively shrink – in some cases to a single room. This is commonly associated with an increase in social isolation and loneliness. Approximately 50% of the population over 75 years of age in the UK live alone, with around 10% of older people reporting loneliness. There are two main facets to loneliness:

- *emotional* – stemming from the absence of an intimate relationship or a close emotional attachment (e.g. a partner or a best friend)
- *social* – stemming from the absence of a broader group of contacts or an engaging social network (e.g. friends, colleagues and people in the neighbourhood).

Loneliness may be regarded as a new 'geriatric giant' and is linked with numerous negative health outcomes. The negative impact of loneliness on health equates to smoking 15 cigarettes a day, and people who suffer a high degree of loneliness are twice as likely to develop Alzheimer's disease. Conversely, people taking part in health-maintaining and independence-maintaining behaviours are less likely to feel isolated and more likely to feel that their community is a good one to grow old in. Loneliness has complex causes and the most effective schemes to deal with it take a broad view, targeting higher-risk groups including those from lower socioeconomic backgrounds, the widowed, the physically isolated, people who have given up driving and those with sensory impairment.

Further reading

Ahmed H, Farewell D, Jones HM et al. Antibiotic prophylaxis and clinical outcomes among older adults with recurrent urinary tract infection: cohort study. *Age Ageing* 2019; 48:228–234.
Anyanwagu U, Mamza J, Donnelly R et al. Relationship between HbA$_{1c}$ and all-cause mortality in older patients with insulin-treated type 2 diabetes: results of a large UK Cohort Study. *Age Ageing* 2019; 48:235–240.
Schaeffer AJ, Nicolle LE. Urinary tract infections in older men. *N Engl J Med* 2016; 374:562–571.

AGEING WELL AND ADVANTAGES OF AGEING

Amid the common negative rhetoric around the challenges that face healthcare and society at large, we should not forget that older adults are exactly that: adults who have grown to an older age, bringing their personalities, experiences and individuality with them. Modern healthcare systems were originally set up to deliver emergency and life-saving treatments for predominantly single-organ conditions. Emergency department attendances are increasingly characterized by, for example, relapses in chronic conditions, the consequences of a fall, a breakdown in social care or functional difficulties, including a decrease in mobility. These changes in the nature of emergency and acute care reflect the fact that in many ways medicine is achieving its fundamental goals: to help all members of society live their lives and participate fully in society, and to optimize their wellbeing.

Health and wellbeing

The Institute for Public Policy Research (2009) has identified five essential elements of wellbeing:

- resilience
- independence
- health
- income and wealth
- having a role and time.

Building resilience within an individual and their support network is increasingly seen as a buffer against the effects of frailty. This may be achieved by optimizing cognition, mood, social networks, mobility, physical reserves and so on.

We should be conscious not to equate the diseases we see with a lack of wellbeing or meaningful life. A study by Strawbridge et al. in 2002 looked at two different definitions of successful ageing in the prediction of wellbeing, comparing a self-rating scale with Rowe and Kahn's criteria for successful ageing (absence of disease, disability and risk factors). The proportion of individuals rating themselves as ageing successfully was 50.3%, compared with only 18.8% classified as ageing successfully according to Rowe and Kahn's criteria. Although absence of chronic conditions and maintenance of functioning were positively associated with successful ageing on both definitions, many participants with chronic conditions and functional limitations still rated themselves as ageing successfully.

There is good evidence and NICE guidance to support mid-life interventions as being beneficial in improving health and reducing frailty in later life. These include:

- smoking cessation
- promotion of physical activity
- reduction of alcohol consumption
- improvement of diet
- maintenance of a healthy weight.

Societal and economic advantages

In high-income countries, there is an increasing and active population of older people who are making major contributions to society. An Age UK study found that in 2013, older people contributed an estimated £61 billion to the economy in England (>5% of gross domestic product). This was six times the amount spent by local authorities on social care. The main financial contributions came through continued working, informal caring, providing childcare for grandchildren to enable their children to work, and volunteering. Clearly, the benefits extend far beyond the financial aspects, with older people's skills, knowledge and experience supporting many aspects of society.

Further reading

McCormick J with Clifton J, Sachrajda A et al. *Getting On: Well-being in Later Life*. Institute for Public Policy Research 2009; https://www.ippr.org/files/images/media/files/publication/2011/05/getting_on_1744.pdf.
MDTea podcasts. www.thehearingaidpodcasts.org.uk. A set of podcasts made by a multiprofessional faculty who work with older people - funded by Health Education England (KSS).
National Institute for Health and Care Excellence. NICE Guideline 16: *Dementia, Disability and Frailty in Later Life – Mid-life Approaches to Delay or Prevent Onset*. NICE 2015; https://www.nice.org.uk/guidance/ng16/chapter/1-Recommendations.
Strawbridge W, Wallhagen M, Cohen R. Successful aging and well-being: self-rated compared with Rowe and Kahn. *Gerontologist* 2002; 42:727–733.

16

Haematology

Michael F. Murphy, K. John Pasi and Noemi Roy

CORE SKILLS AND KNOWLEDGE

Haematologists treat patients with disorders of the blood. This chapter focuses on general haematology, including the investigation of anaemia and non-malignant white-cell and bleeding disorders, alongside the safe management of blood transfusion. Haematological malignancies (see Ch. 17) and thrombotic disease (Ch. 29) are dealt with elsewhere.

The skills and responsibilities of haematologists extend beyond caring for the patients with specific haematological disorders attending their wards and clinics, and include ensuring that blood results reported by the analysers in the haematology laboratory are accurate, establishing that blood used for transfusions is safe and available when and where it is needed, helping other specialties interpret results of laboratory tests and guiding the use of blood products.

Key learning objectives for general haematology at undergraduate level include:

- understanding anaemia – its causes, investigation and management
- assessing whether disorders of white blood cells and platelets are due to primary haematological disease or secondary to other causes
- understanding the way that blood transfusions are carried out and the mechanisms by which safety is ensured
- understanding the mechanisms of disorders of haemostasis and thrombosis, as well as their investigation and management.

Specific opportunities for learning haematology include attending ward rounds on inpatient haematology units, attending haematology clinics to understand the problems that cause patients to be referred from general practice, seeking out patients on a haematology day unit or medical admissions ward to understand the immediate and long-term management of haematological disorders, and attending laboratory 'morphology' meetings, where laboratory science is correlated with individual patient care.

CLINICAL SKILLS FOR HAEMATOLOGY

History

Symptoms of haemtological disease tend to be caused by the particular abnormalities seen in individual cell lines, as described in **Table 16.1**. As well as taking a full general history and examining throughly, the features identified below should be specifically sought.

Examination

The figure opposite illustrates a number of physical signs of haematological disease. Most can be attributed to the effects of over- or under-production of different cell lineages, or are features (such as splenomegaly) of underlying haematological disease processes.

Investigations

Investigation of haematological disease generally begins with examination of the peripheral blood (**Box 16.1**). Bone marrow aspiration, with or without biopsy, is a crucial investigation in the diagnosis and monitoring of many haematological disorders. These procedures allow determination of cellularity (increased or decreased?) as well as morphology (do the blood cell precursor cells look as they should?). **Fig. 16.1** (pp. 322–323) illustrates the procedure and the cell lineages present in bone marrow; see also page 328 and **Box 16.2**.

Table 16.1 Key questions from the history and clinical signs are highlighted to guide the investigation of abnormal blood counts and common haematological presentations

	Too many	Too few
Red cells	**Too many red blood cells** • Headache and blurred vision • Any hypoxia or dehydration? • Could it be secondary? • Is there associated high white count, especially basophils? • Check JAK$_2$ for primary polycythaemia	**Too few red blood cells** • Shortness of breath, fatigue • Any chest pain? • Severe anaemia can exacerbate ischaemic heart disease and need rapid treatment • Are white cells low as well? • Think about bone marrow failure • Look at trends over time – is this new or ongoing? • Ask about diet to look for haematinic deficiencies • Remember vegans have poor intake of iron and B$_{12}$
White cells	**Too many white cells** • Any recent infection? • High neutrophils are usually reactive • Is there a history of allergy, asthma, eczema? This raises eosinophil count • Remember to request a blood film so the morphology can be assessed • Immature white cells indicate malignant haematological disorders	**Too few white cells** • Any recent infection? This can be the cause or the effect of low white cells • Ask about mouth ulcers and family history • Benign neutropenia is seen in young women • Take a good drug history • Look for side effects of each drug – low white cells is common • Make sure patients with neutrophils $<1 \times 10^9$ know who to call if they have a fever • Neutropenic sepsis is fatal if not treated rapidly with i.v. antibiotics
Platelets	**Too many platelets** • Headache, itching • Any bleeding? • Very high platelets increase risk of bleeding • Is there evidence of infection or malignancy? • Secondary thrombocytosis is more common than primary • Look for splenomegaly: all myeloproliferative disorders are associated with this	**Too few platelets/abnormal clotting** • Bleeding: look for petechiae and blood blisters • Any recent infection? • Immune thrombocytopenia often follows viral infection • Ask about rheumatological disorders • Take a good drug history • Look for side-effects of each drug – low platelets is common • Understand what platelet counts are safe for procedures • Platelet transfusions are rarely needed for immune thrombocytopenia • Bleeding history: ask about previous operations, labour, dental extractions

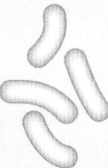

Box 16.1 Normal values for peripheral blood

	Male	Female
Haemoglobin (Hb) (g/L)	135–175	115–155
Packed cell volume (PCV) (haematocrit; L/L)	0.4–0.54	0.37–0.47
Red cell count (RCC) (10^{12}/L)	4.5–6.0	3.9–5.0
Mean corpuscular volume of red cell (MCV) (fL)		80–96
Mean corpuscular haemoglobin (MCH) (pg)		27–32
Mean corpuscular haemoglobin concentration (MCHC) (g/L)		320–360
Red blood cell distribution width (RDW) (%)		11–15
White cell count (WCC) (10^9/L)		4.0–11.0
Platelets (10^9/L)		150–400
Erythrocyte sedimentation rate (ESR) (mm/h)		<20
Reticulocytes		0.5–2.5% (50–100 × 10^9/L)

General
Colour - Pale (e.g. anaemia)
- Plethoric
(e.g. polycythaemia)
- Jaundice
Short of breath

Fundoscopy
Haemorrhage
(e.g. in thrombocytopenia)
Papilloedema
Enlarged veins

Lymph nodes
Cervical
Axillary
Inguinal
Other sites

Purpura

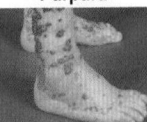

Petechiae

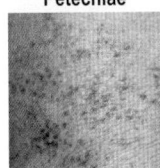

Skin
Purpura
Bruises
Petechiae
(thrombocytopenia)

Oedema

Angular stomatitis

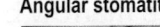
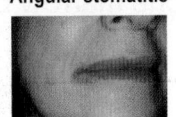

(From Epstein O 2008 Clinical Examination, 4th edn, with permission)

Mouth
Angular stomatitis
(iron deficiency)
Lips - telangiectasia
(hereditary
haemorrhagic
telangiectasia)
Tongue - Smooth/glossitis
Gum hypertrophy
(acute myeloid leukaemia)
Tonsils - enlarged

Abdomen
Hepatomegaly
Splenomegaly
Ascites
Masses
Inguinal lymph nodes

Hands
Koilonychia (iron deficiency)
Perfusion/circulation
Telangiectasia

Joints
Swelling
Deformity
Movements restricted

Check peripheral circulation
Toes - gangrene
(e.g. thrombocytosis)

Gangrene

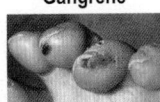

(From Epstein O 2008 Clinical Examination, 4th Edn, Elsevier, with permission)

Bone marrow biopsy

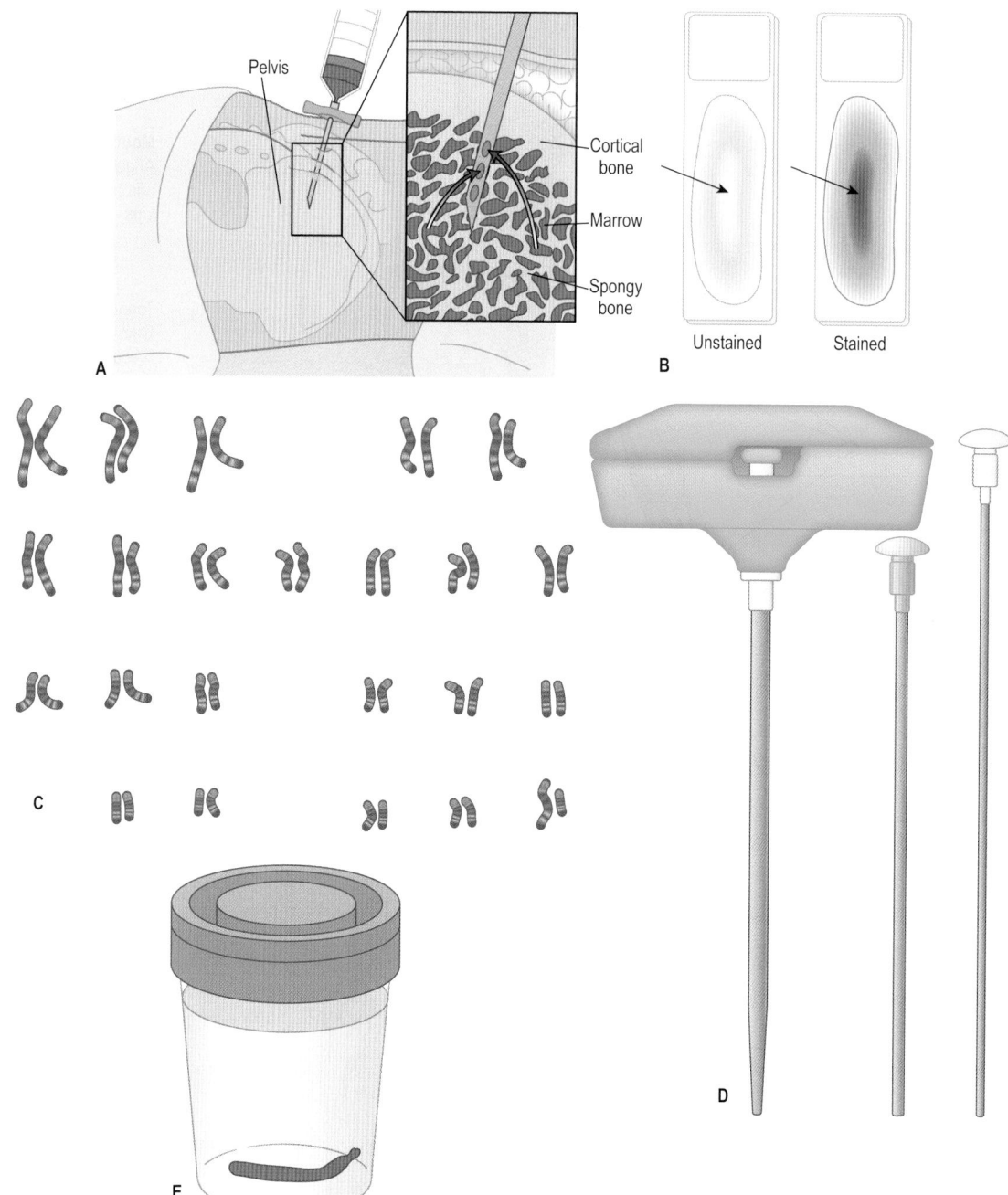

Fig. 16.1 Bone marrow aspiration and biopsy. **(A)** This is generally carried out as an outpatient procedure under local anaesthetic, using aseptic technique. Consent is obtained, and then the skin overlying the superior posterior iliac crest is cleaned and local anaesthetic injected subcutaneously and around the periosteum, which is extremely well innervated. Once the area is numb, an aspirate needle is used to obtain a liquid sample. **(B)** The sample is spread on a slide, stained and examined under the microscope for morphology. **(C)** A sample is also sent for cytogenetic analysis and a karyotype is generated, allowing identification of gross chromosomal rearrangements such as gain or loss of chromosomes or translocations. **(D)** A trephine needle is needed to obtain a bone biopsy. **(E)** The biopsy is a hard core of bone, which must be decalcified in chelating solution before being embedded in paraffin. Sections are then cut and stained, permitting the architecture of the marrow cells to be examined, and immunohistochemistry to be carried out to detect abnormal cell populations.

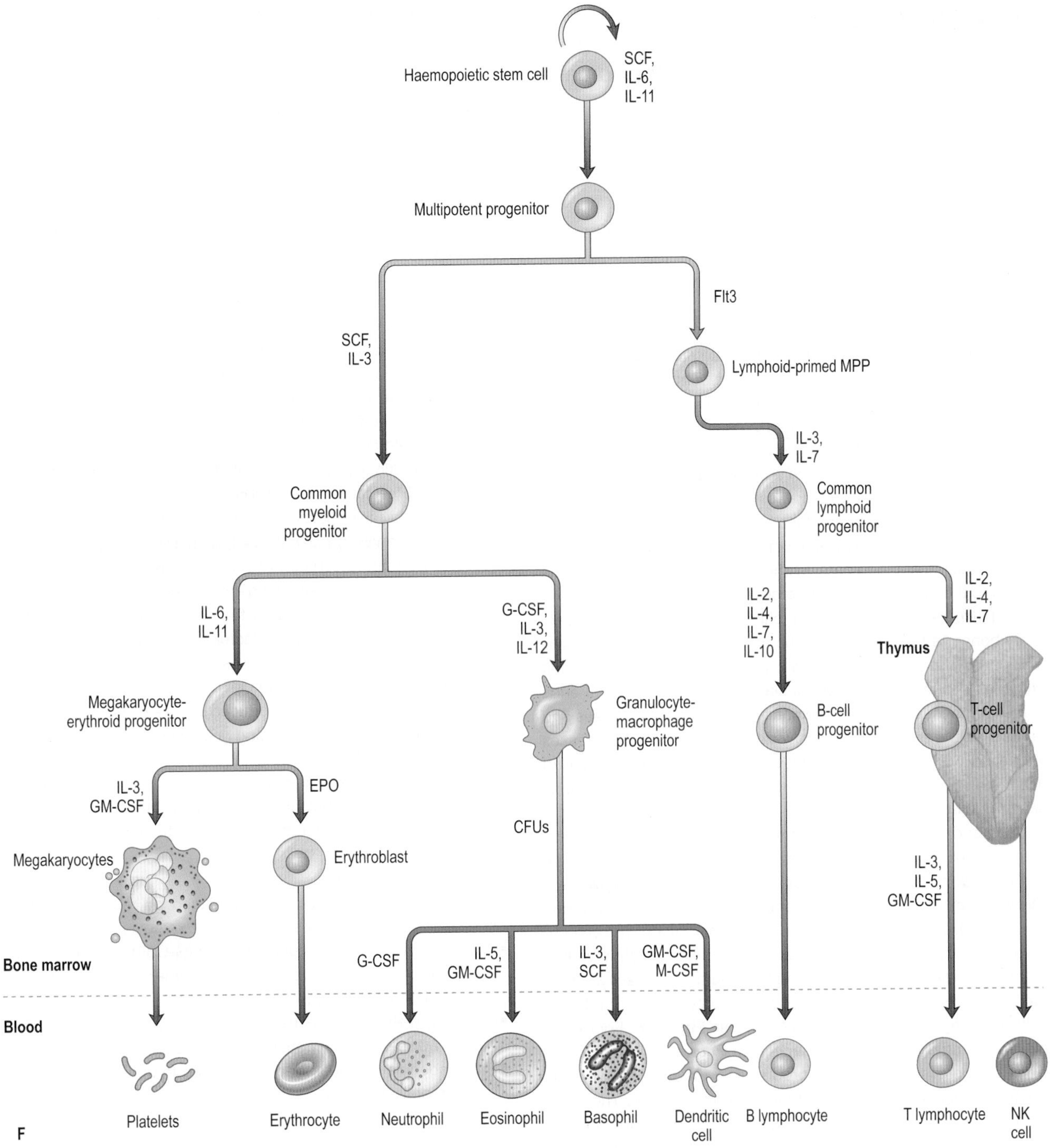

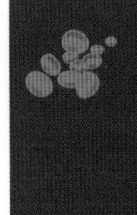

Haemopoietic stem cell — SCF, IL-6, IL-11

Multipotent progenitor

SCF, IL-3

Flt3

Lymphoid-primed MPP

IL-3, IL-7

Common myeloid progenitor

Common lymphoid progenitor

IL-6, IL-11

G-CSF, IL-3, IL-12

IL-2, IL-4, IL-7, IL-10

IL-2, IL-4, IL-7

Thymus

Megakaryocyte-erythroid progenitor

Granulocyte-macrophage progenitor

B-cell progenitor

T-cell progenitor

IL-3, GM-CSF

EPO

CFUs

IL-3, IL-5, GM-CSF

Megakaryocytes

Erythroblast

Bone marrow

G-CSF

IL-5, GM-CSF

IL-3, SCF

GM-CSF, M-CSF

Blood

Platelets   Erythrocyte   Neutrophil   Eosinophil   Basophil   Dendritic cell   B lymphocyte   T lymphocyte   NK cell

F

Fig. 16.1—cont'd **(F)** Haemopoiesis arises from multipotent stem cells, which give rise to all different blood types according to the presence of internal and external regulatory molecules, hormones and cytokines. As such, cell numbers are closely coordinated to respond rapidly to changes in requirements. EPO erythropoietin; Flt3, Fms-like tyrosine kinase 3; G-CSF, granulocyte-colony-stimulating factor; GM-CSF, granulocyte-macrophage-colony-stimulating factor; IL, interleukin; MPP, multipotent progenitor; NK, natural killer; SCF, stem cell factor; TPO, thrombopoietin.

INTRODUCTION

The formation of blood cells (haemopoiesis)

Blood consists of:
- red cells
- white cells
- platelets
- plasma, in which the above elements are suspended.

Plasma is the liquid component of unclotted blood, which contains soluble fibrinogen. Serum is what remains after formation of the fibrin clot.

The haemopoietic system includes the bone marrow, liver, spleen, lymph nodes and thymus. There is a huge turnover of cells, with red cells surviving for approximately 120 days, platelets approximately 7 days but granulocytes only 7 hours. The production of as many as 10^{13} new myeloid cells (all blood cells except for lymphocytes) per day in the normal healthy state requires tight regulation according to the needs of the body.

Blood islands are formed in the yolk sac in the third week of gestation and produce primitive blood cells, which migrate to the liver and spleen. These organs are the chief sites of haemopoiesis from 6 weeks' to 7 months' gestation, when the bone marrow becomes the main source of blood cells. In childhood and adult life, the bone marrow is the only source of blood cells in a normal person.

At birth, haemopoiesis takes place in the marrow of nearly every bone. As the child grows, the active red marrow is gradually replaced by fat (yellow marrow) so that haemopoiesis in the adult becomes confined to the central skeleton and the proximal ends of the long bones. Only if the demand for blood cells increases and persists do the areas of red marrow extend. Pathological processes interfering with normal haemopoiesis may result in resumption of haemopoietic activity in the liver and spleen, which is referred to as *extramedullary haemopoiesis*.

All blood cells are derived from pluripotent stem cells. These stem cells have two key properties: the first is *self-renewal* – that is, the production of more stem cells – and the second is *proliferation and differentiation* into progenitor cells, committed to one specific cell line. Pluripotent stem cells differentiate into mature blood cells through intermediate progenitor cells, which have lost the ability to self-renew but have high proliferative capacity. These progenitor cells can be broadly classified according to the blood cells that they are programmed to make (see **Fig. 16.1**). For example, the common lymphoid progenitor (CLP) gives rise to T and B lymphoid cells; the former are produced in the thymus, whereas B cell production primarily occurs in the bone marrow. The common myeloid progenitor (CMP) gives rise to all non-lymphoid cells in the bone marrow via a series of intermediate progenitor cells. These cells cannot be identified in bone marrow biopsies but are recognized by their ability to form colonies (reflecting their high proliferative capacity) when haemopoietic cells are immobilized in a soft gel matrix, the so-called colony-forming unit (CFU), which are named according to the type of cell they produce.

These haemopoietic stem and progenitor cells interact closely with a number of components contained within the specialized microenvironment of the bone marrow, including non-haemopoietic stromal cells, blood vessels and extracellular matrix, together creating a nurturing microenvironment for blood cell development. Central to this microenvironment are haemopoietic growth factors produced by stromal cells in the bone marrow and elsewhere, which are key regulators of blood cell production.

Haemopoietic growth factors

Haemopoietic growth factors are glycoproteins, which regulate the differentiation and proliferation of haemopoietic progenitor cells and the function of mature blood cells. Some growth factors are present in the circulation, whereas other growth factors are produced within the bone marrow microenvironment by stromal cells such as fibroblasts, osteoblasts or endothelial cells, or at sites of inflammation by activated T cells, monocytes and macrophages. Growth factors act on their respective cell surface receptors, expressed on haemopoietic cells at various stages of development, to maintain the haemopoietic progenitor cells and to stimulate increased production of one or more cell types in response to stresses such as blood loss and infection (see **Fig. 16.1**).

These haemopoietic growth factors, including erythropoietin (EPO), interleukin (IL)-3, IL-6, IL-7, IL-11, IL-12, β-catenin, stem cell factor (SCF, Steel factor or C-kit ligand) and Fms-like tyrosine kinase 3 (Flt3), act via their specific receptor on cell surfaces to stimulate downstream signalling within the cell, such as the cytoplasmic Janus kinase (JAK) pathway. This, in turn, activates signalling cascades within the cell, ultimately altering gene expression in the cell nucleus and thus influencing behaviour of the cell: for example, to promote proliferation. Colony-stimulating factors (CSFs; the prefix indicates the cell type – see **Fig. 16.1**), as well as interleukins and EPO, regulate the lineage-committed progenitor cells.

Thrombopoietin (TPO) is produced in the kidneys, liver and certain bone marrow stromal cells, and acts to control platelet production, along with IL-6 and IL-11.

In addition to these factors, which stimulate haemopoiesis, there are other factors that inhibit the process; these include tumour necrosis factor (TNF) and transforming growth factor beta (TGF-β).

Uses in treatment

Many growth factors have been produced by recombinant DNA techniques and are being used clinically. Examples include:
- granulocyte-colony-stimulating factor (G-CSF), used to accelerate haemopoietic recovery after chemotherapy and haemopoietic cell transplantation
- erythropoietin, used to treat anaemia in patients with chronic kidney disease and in patients with certain blood cancers
- thrombopoietin receptor agonists, used to treat immune thrombocytopenic purpura.

Peripheral blood

Automated cell counters are used to measure the haemoglobin (Hb) concentration and the number and size of red cells, white cells and platelets (see **Box 16.1**). Other indices can be derived from these values. A blood film examined by a haematologist or technician experienced in blood cell morphology is still an essential adjunct to the above, as definitive abnormalities of cells can be seen. This is particularly important in some haematological emergencies such as acute promyelocytic leukaemia (see p. 391) or thrombotic thrombocytopenic purpura (see p. 374), which require specific therapy within hours of diagnosis to prevent high rates of mortality.

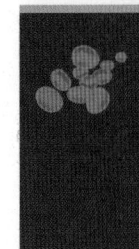

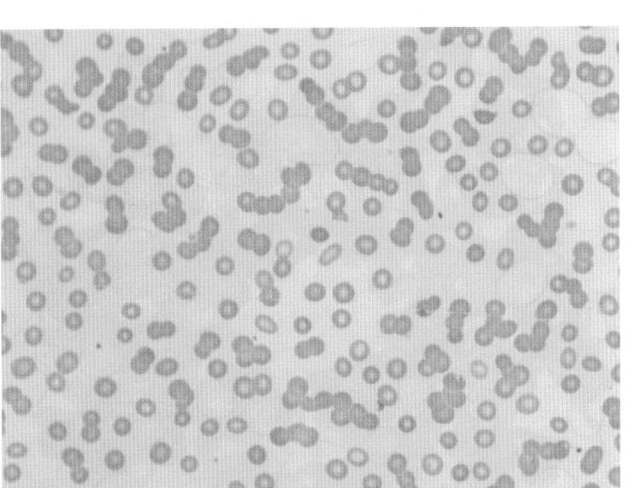

Fig. 16.2 Peripheral blood film (total magnification 400×) showing rouleaux formation in the red blood cells. In states of increased plasma protein concentration (e.g. infection, inflammation, paraprotein), the discoid red cells stack together like coins.

- **The mean corpuscular volume (MCV)** of red cells is a useful index and is used to classify anaemia (see **Fig. 16.7**).
- **The red cell distribution width (RDW)** is a measure of the variability in size of red blood cells. An elevated RDW suggests increased variation in red cell size – that is, anisocytosis – and this is seen in iron deficiency.
- **The white cell count (WCC)** (or white blood count, WBC) gives the total number of circulating leucocytes in addition to differential counts, specifically enumerating neutrophils, monocytes, lymphocytes, eosinophils and basophils.
- **Reticulocytes** are young red cells and usually comprise less than 2.5% of red cells. The reticulocyte count gives a guide to erythroid activity in the bone marrow. An increased count is seen with increased marrow activity: for example, following haemorrhage or haemolysis, and during the response to treatment with a specific haematinic. A low count in the presence of anaemia indicates an inappropriate response by the bone marrow and may be seen in bone marrow failure (from whatever cause) or a deficiency of a haematinic.
- **The erythrocyte sedimentation rate (ESR)** is the rate of fall of red cells in a column of blood and is a measure of the acute-phase response. The pathological process may be immunological, infective, ischaemic, malignant or traumatic. A raised ESR reflects an increase in the plasma concentration of large proteins, such as fibrinogen and immunoglobulins. These proteins cause rouleaux formation, with red cells clumping together and therefore falling more rapidly (**Fig. 16.2**). The ESR increases with age, and is higher in females than in males.
- **Plasma viscosity** is a measurement that is used instead of the ESR in some laboratories. It is also dependent on the concentration of large molecules such as fibrinogen and immunoglobulins. It is not affected by the level of haemoglobin.
- **C-reactive protein (CRP)** is a protein produced in the acute-phase response. It is synthesized exclusively in the liver and rises within 6 hours of an acute event. The CRP level rises with fever (possibly triggered by IL-1, IL-6, TNF-α and other cytokines), in inflammatory conditions and after trauma. It follows the clinical state of the patient much more rapidly than

the ESR and is unaffected by the level of haemoglobin, but it is less helpful than the ESR or plasma viscosity in monitoring chronic inflammatory diseases such as systemic lupus erythematosus (SLE).

THE RED CELL

Erythropoiesis

Red cell precursors pass through several stages in the bone marrow. The earliest morphologically recognizable cells are proerythroblasts. Smaller erythroblasts result from cell divisions, and precursors at each stage progressively contain less RNA and more haemoglobin in the cytoplasm. The nucleus becomes more condensed and is eventually extruded from the late normoblast in the bone marrow when the cell becomes a reticulocyte.

- **Reticulocytes** contain residual ribosomal RNA and are still able to synthesize haemoglobin. They remain in the marrow for about 1–2 days and are released into the circulation, where they lose their RNA and become mature red cells (erythrocytes) after another 1–2 days. Mature red cells are non-nucleated biconcave discs.
- Nucleated red cells (**late erythroblasts**) are not normally present in peripheral blood, but are present in extramedullary haemopoiesis and some marrow disorders (see p. 366).
- About 10% of **erythroblasts** die in the bone marrow, even during normal erythropoiesis. Survival of erythroblasts is dependent on erythropoietin cell signalling. The natural 10% excess production of erythroblasts (ineffective erythropoiesis) ensures a rapid drop in haemoglobin – e.g. with acute haemorrhage or haemolysis, resulting in a rise in EPO production – and causes a rapid increase in terminally differentiated red blood cells. Ineffective erythropoiesis is substantially increased in some anaemias, such as thalassaemia major and megaloblastic anaemia.
- **Erythropoietin** is a hormone that controls erythropoiesis. This heavily glycosylated polypeptide with a molecular weight of 30 400 Da is produced in the peritubular cells in the kidneys (90%) and in the liver (10%). Its production is regulated mainly by tissue oxygen tension, increasing production in the face of hypoxia: e.g. with anaemia or cardiac or pulmonary disease. The erythropoietin gene is one of a number of genes that is regulated by the hypoxic sensor pathway. The 3′-flanking region of these genes has a hypoxic response element, which is necessary for the induction of transcription of the gene in hypoxic cells. Hypoxia-inducible factor 1 (HIF-1) is a transcription factor, which binds to the hypoxia response element and acts as a master regulator of several genes that are responsive to hypoxia. Erythropoietin stimulates an increase in the proportion of bone marrow precursor cells committed to erythropoiesis by allowing a greater number of erythroid precursors to survive, and CFU-E are stimulated to proliferate and differentiate. Increased 'inappropriate' production of erythropoietin occurs in certain tumours, such as renal cell carcinoma, and from other causes, resulting in secondary erythrocytosis.

Haemoglobin synthesis

Haemoglobin performs the main functions of red cells, carrying oxygen to the tissues and returning carbon dioxide from the tissues to

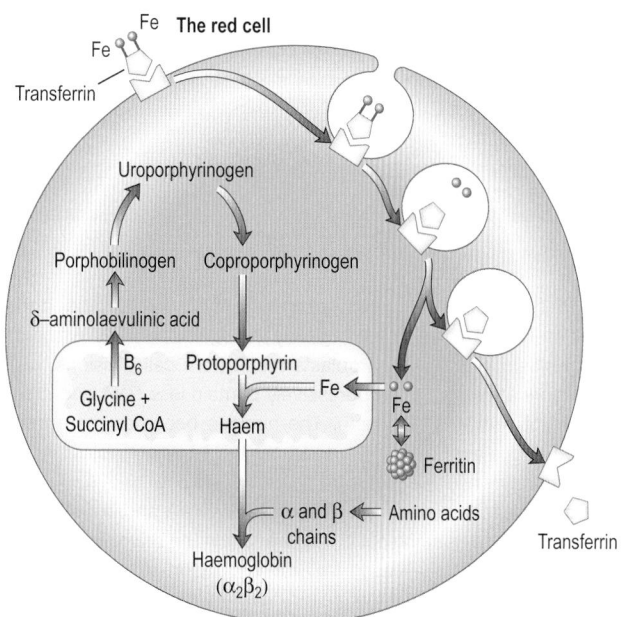

Fig. 16.3 **Haemoglobin synthesis.** Transferrin attaches to a surface receptor on developing red cells. Iron is released and transported to the mitochondria, where it combines with protoporphyrin to form haem. Protoporphyrin itself is manufactured from glycine and succinyl CoA. Haem combines with α and β chains (formed on ribosomes) to make haemoglobin.

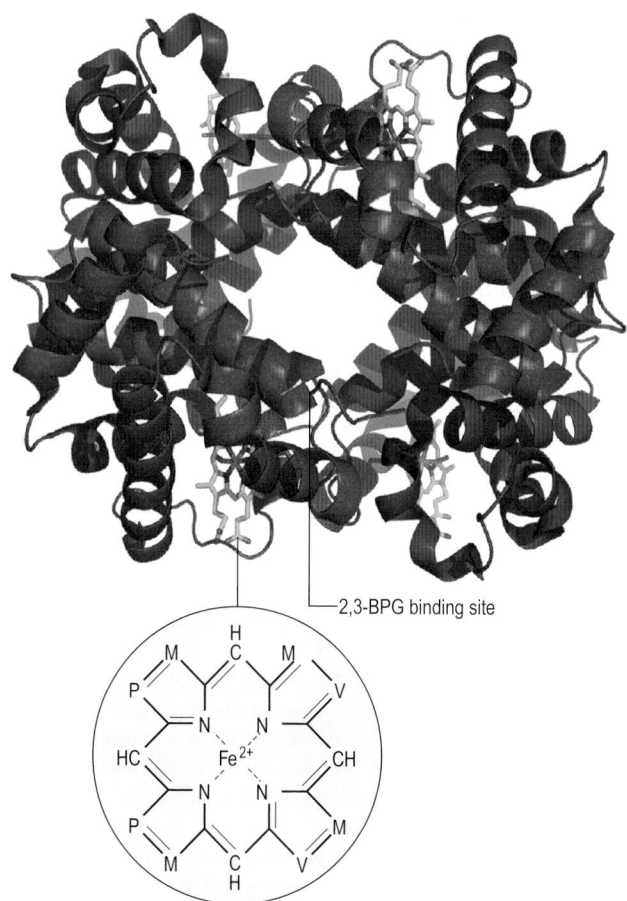

Fig. 16.4 Model of the haemoglobin molecule showing α (red) and β (blue) chains. Bisphosphoglycerate (2,3-BPG) binds in the centre of the molecule and stabilizes the deoxygenated form by cross-linking the β chains. M, methyl; P, propionic acid; V, vinyl.

the lungs. Each normal adult haemoglobin molecule (HbA) has a molecular weight of 68 kDa and consists of two α and two β globin polypeptide chains ($\alpha_2\beta_2$). HbA comprises about 97% of the haemoglobin in adults. Two other haemoglobin types, HbA_2 ($\alpha_2\delta_2$) and HbF ($\alpha_2\gamma_2$), are found in adults in small amounts (1.5–3.2% and <1%, respectively) (see p. 340).

Haem synthesis occurs in the mitochondria of the developing red cell (**Fig. 16.3**). The major rate-limiting step is the conversion of glycine and succinic acid to δ-aminolevulinic acid (ALA) by ALA synthase. Vitamin B_6 is a coenzyme for this reaction, which is inhibited by haem and stimulated by erythropoietin. Two molecules of δ-ALA condense to form a pyrrole ring (porphobilinogen). These rings are then grouped in fours to produce protoporphyrins and, with the addition of iron, haem is formed. Haem is then inserted into the globin chains to form a haemoglobin molecule. The structure of haemoglobin is shown in **Fig. 16.4**.

Haemoglobin function

The biconcave shape of red cells provides a large surface area for the uptake and release of oxygen and carbon dioxide. Haemoglobin becomes saturated with oxygen in the pulmonary capillaries, where the partial pressure of oxygen is high and haemoglobin has a high affinity for oxygen. Oxygen is released in the tissues, where the partial pressure of oxygen is low and haemoglobin has a low affinity for oxygen.

In adult haemoglobin, a haem group is bound to each of the four globin chains; the haem group has a porphyrin ring with a ferrous atom, which can reversibly bind one oxygen molecule. The haemoglobin molecule exists in two conformations, relaxed

(R) and taut (T), corresponding to oxyhaemoglobin and deoxyhaemoglobin, respectively. The binding of one oxygen molecule to deoxyhaemoglobin increases the oxygen affinity of the remaining binding sites; this property is known as 'cooperativity' and is the reason for the sigmoid shape of the oxygen dissociation curve (see **Fig. 10.3**). The binding of oxygen can also be influenced by secondary effectors, such as hydrogen ions, carbon dioxide and red cell bisphosphoglycerate (2,3-BPG). Red cell metabolism produces 2,3-BPG from glycolysis, and the binding of 2,3-BPG stabilizes the T conformation, thus reducing its affinity for oxygen and increasing release of oxygen in the tissues. The P_{50} is the partial pressure of oxygen at which the haemoglobin is 50% saturated with oxygen. When the primary limitation to oxygen transport is in the periphery – for example, during heavy exercise or in anaemia – the P_{50} is increased to enhance oxygen unloading. Furthermore, hydrogen ions and carbon dioxide added to blood cause a reduction in the oxygen-binding affinity of haemoglobin (the Bohr effect), also helping the exchange of carbon dioxide and oxygen in the tissues. When the primary limitation is in the lungs – for example, in lung disease or high-altitude exposure – the P_{50} is reduced to enhance oxygen loading. A summary of normal red cell production and destruction is given in **Fig. 16.5**.

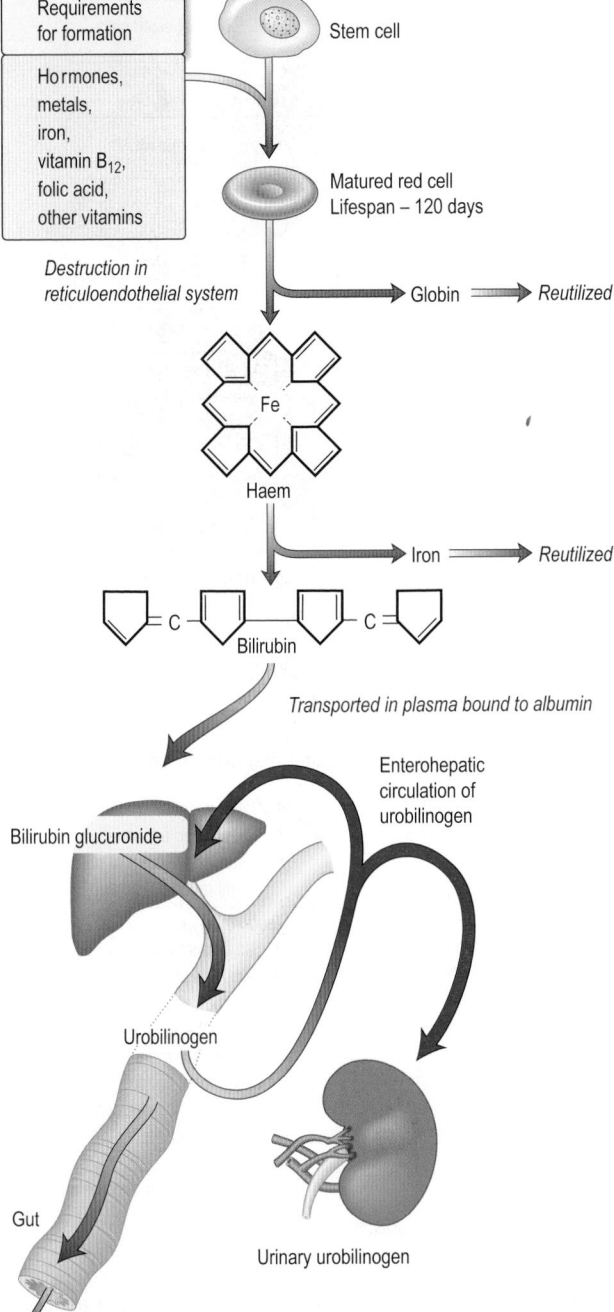

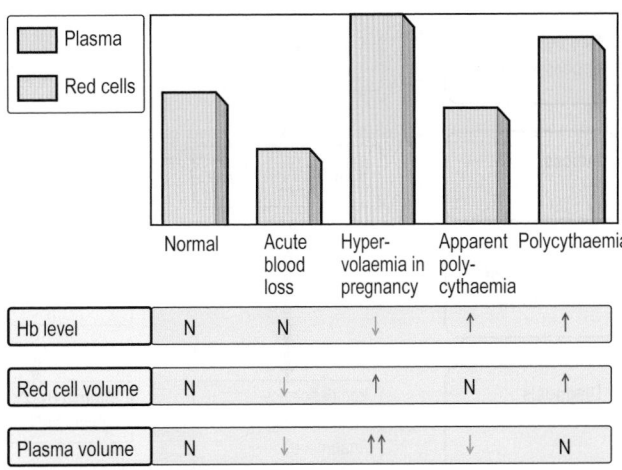

	Normal	Acute blood loss	Hyper-volaemia in pregnancy	Apparent poly-cythaemia	Polycythaemia
Hb level	N	N	↓	↑	↑
Red cell volume	N	↓	↑	N	↑
Plasma volume	N	↓	↑↑	↓	N

Fig. 16.6 Alterations of haemoglobin in relation to plasma.

combined with a small increase in red cell volume, as occurs in pregnancy.

Anaemia can be classified in a variety of ways. For example, it can be divided into that due to decreased production or increased destruction, or alternatively into inherited or acquired causes. One common way of categorizing the various types of anaemia is by the MCV, as shown in **Fig. 16.7**. Anaemias are therefore commonly described as:

- hypochromic microcytic with a low MCV
- normochromic normocytic with a normal MCV
- macrocytic with a high MCV.

While there is some biological rationale for this classification, some types of anaemia can present in more than one category.

Clinical features

Patients with anaemia may be asymptomatic. A slowly falling level of haemoglobin allows for haemodynamic compensation and enhancement of the oxygen-carrying capacity of the blood. A rise in 2,3-BPG causes a shift of the oxygen dissociation curve to the right, so that oxygen is more readily given up to the tissues. Where blood loss is rapid, more severe symptoms will occur, particularly in elderly people.

Symptoms

The symptoms of anaemia are non-specific and include breathlessness, fatigue, headaches, palpitations and faintness. Anaemia exacerbates cardiorespiratory problems, especially in the elderly. For example, angina or intermittent claudication may be precipitated by anaemia. A good way to assess the effects of anaemia is to ask about breathlessness in relation to different levels of exercise (e.g. walking on the flat or climbing one flight of stairs).

Signs

- Pallor.
- Tachycardia.
- Systolic flow murmur.
- Cardiac failure.
  Specific signs seen in the different types of anaemia include:
- koilonychia – spoon-shaped nails seen in longstanding iron deficiency anaemia
- jaundice – found in haemolytic anaemia

Fig. 16.5 Red cell production and breakdown. (See p. 1266.)

ANAEMIA: AN INTRODUCTION

Anaemia is present when there is a decrease in haemoglobin in the blood below the reference level for the age and sex of the individual (see **Box 16.1**). Alterations in haemoglobin concentration may occur as a result of changes in the plasma volume, as shown in **Fig. 16.6**. A reduction in the plasma volume will lead to a spuriously high haemoglobin; this is seen in dehydration and in the clinical condition of apparent polycythaemia (see p. 356). A raised plasma volume produces a spurious anaemia, even when

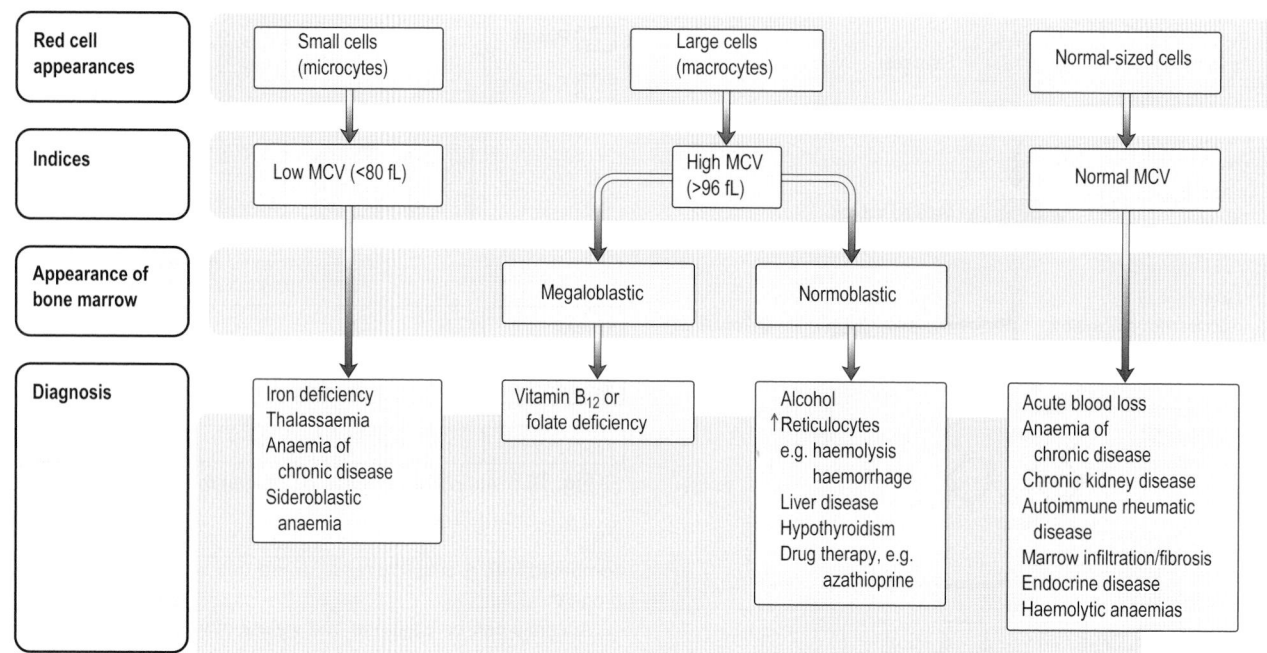

Fig. 16.7 Classification of anaemia. MCV, mean corpuscular volume.

- bone deformities – found in thalassaemia major
- leg ulcers – occur in association with sickle cell disease.
  Anaemia is not a final diagnosis and a cause should always be sought.

Investigations
Peripheral blood

A low haemoglobin should always be evaluated with the:
- red cell indices
- WCC
- platelet count
- reticulocyte count (as this indicates marrow activity)
- blood film, as abnormal red cell morphology (see **Fig. 16.9**) may indicate the diagnosis.

Where two populations of red cells are seen, the blood film is said to be dimorphic. This may, for example, be seen in patients with 'double deficiencies': for example, in combined iron and folate deficiency in coeliac disease or following treatment of anaemic patients with the appropriate haematinic where old red cells exhibit the changes associated with that deficiency and newly produced red cells have a normal morphology. Dimorphic populations are also seen after blood transfusion.

Bone marrow

Techniques for obtaining bone marrow are shown in **Box 16.2** and on page 322.

Examination of the bone marrow is performed to further investigate abnormalities found in the peripheral blood:
- **Aspiration** provides a film that can be examined by microscopy for the morphology of the developing haemopoietic cells. The liquid sample obtained at aspiration can also be used for immunophenotyping (assessment of the presence or absence of antigens on the surface of cells), cytogenetic investigations, assessment for molecular markers or microbiological culture).
- **The trephine** provides a core of bone that is processed as a histological specimen and allows an overall view of the bone mar-

Box 16.2 Techniques for obtaining bone marrow

Explain the technique to the patient and obtain consent.

Aspiration
- Site – usually iliac crest
- Give local anaesthetic injection
- Use special bone marrow needle (e.g. Salah)
- Aspirate marrow
- Make smear with glass slide
- Stain with:
  - Romanowsky technique
  - Perls' reaction (acid ferrocyanide) for iron

Trephine

Indications
- 'Dry tap' obtained with aspiration

- Better assessment of cellularity, e.g. aplastic anaemia
- Better assessment of presence of infiltration or fibrosis

Technique
- Site – usually posterior iliac crest
- Give local anaesthetic injection
- Use special needle (e.g. Jamshidi – longer and wider than for aspiration)
- Obtain core of bone
- Fix in formalin; decalcify – this takes a few days
- Stain with:
  - Haematoxylin and eosin
  - Reticulin stain

row architecture, cellularity and presence/absence of abnormal infiltrates. The specimen can be used for immunohistochemical investigations.

The following are assessed:
- cellularity of the marrow
- type of erythropoiesis (e.g. normoblastic or megaloblastic)
- morphology of all cell lineages
- cellularity of the various cell lines
- infiltration of the marrow, i.e. presence of non-haemopoietic cells such as cancer cells
- iron stores.

MICROCYTIC ANAEMIA

Microcytic anaemia most commonly results from iron deficiency, the most common cause of anaemia globally, affecting 30% of the world's population. This is because of the body's limited ability to absorb iron and the frequent loss of iron owing to bleeding. Although iron is abundant, most is in the insoluble ferric (Fe^{3+}) form, which has poor bioavailability. Ferrous (Fe^{2+}) iron is more readily absorbed.

The other causes of a microcytic hypochromic anaemia (see **Fig. 16.7**) include those due to a defect in globin production (thalassaemia, see p. 341) or a defect in haem synthesis, termed sideroblastic anaemia. When anaemia of chronic disease is long-standing, the iron restriction results in a fall in MCV and patients become microcytic.

Iron
Dietary intake
The average daily diet in the UK contains 15–20 mg of iron, although normally only 10% of this is absorbed. Absorption may be increased to 20–30% in iron deficiency and pregnancy.

Non-haem iron is mainly derived from cereals, which are commonly fortified with iron; it forms the main part of dietary iron. Haem iron is derived from haemoglobin and myoglobin in red or organ meats. Haem iron is better absorbed than non-haem iron, whose availability is more affected by other dietary constituents.

Absorption
Factors influencing iron and haem iron absorption are shown in **Fig. 16.8** and **Box 16.3**.

Dietary haem iron is more rapidly absorbed than non-haem iron derived from vegetables and grain. Most haem is absorbed in the proximal intestine, with absorptive capacity decreasing distally. The intestinal haem transporter HCP1 (haem carrier protein 1) has been identified and found to be highly expressed in the duodenum. It is upregulated by hypoxia and iron deficiency. Some haem iron may be absorbed intact into the circulation via the cell by two exporter

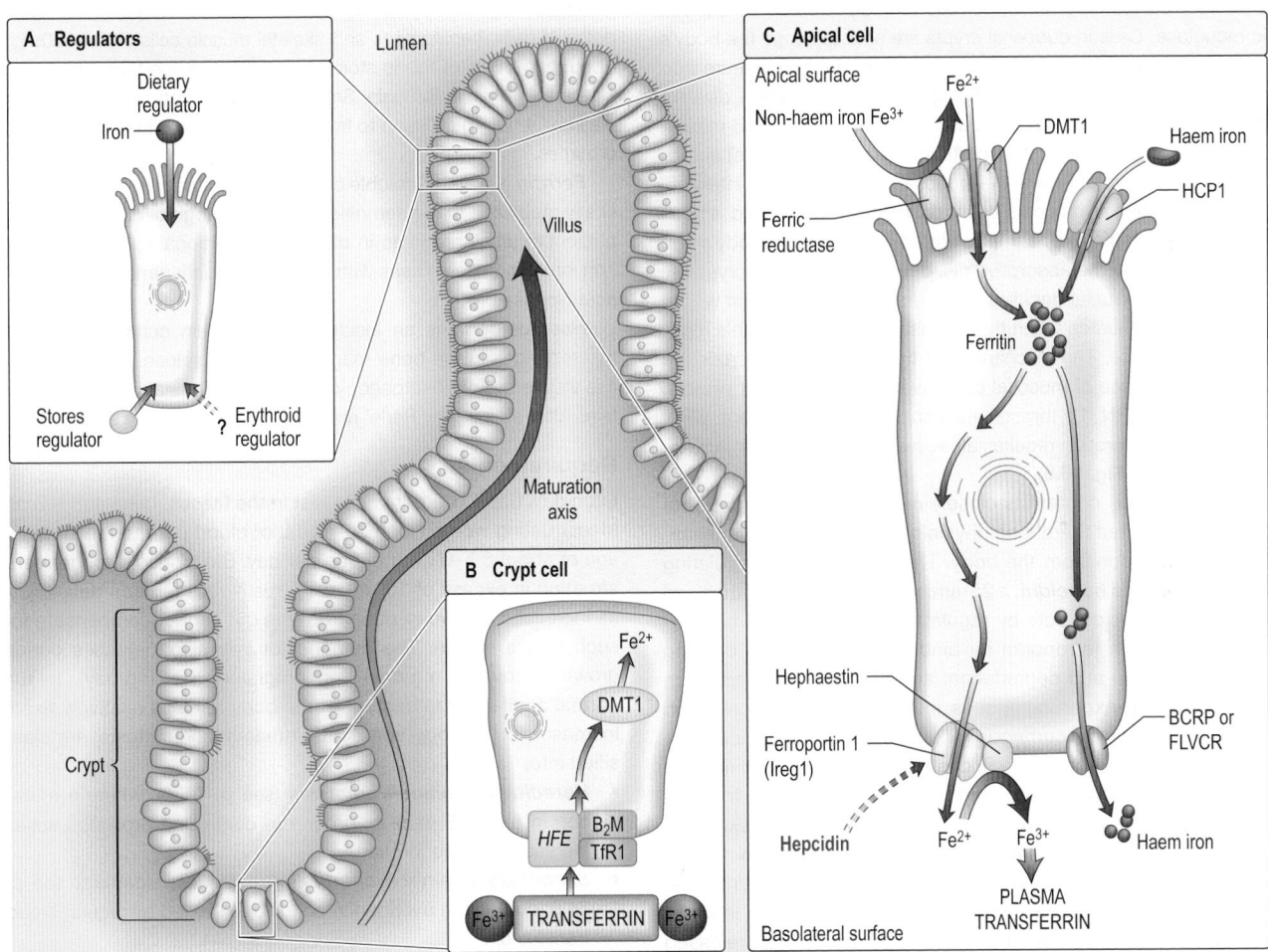

Fig. 16.8 Iron absorption. **(A)** *Regulation of the absorption of intestinal iron.* The iron-absorbing cells of the duodenal epithelium originate in the intestinal crypts and migrate towards the tip of the villus as they differentiate (maturation axis). Absorption of intestinal iron is regulated by at least three independent mechanisms, although the protein hepcidin is key. First, iron absorption is influenced by recent dietary iron intake (*dietary regulator*). After a large dietary bolus, absorptive cells are resistant to iron uptake for several days. Second, iron absorption can be modulated considerably in response to body iron stores (*stores regulator*). Third, a signal communicates the state of bone marrow erythropoiesis to the intestine (*erythroid regulator*). **(B)** *Duodenal crypt cells* sense body iron status through the binding of transferrin to the *HFE/B$_2$M/TfR1* gene complex. Cytosolic enzymes change the oxidative state of iron from ferric (Fe^{3+}) to ferrous (Fe^{2+}). A decrease in crypt cell iron concentration upregulates the divalent metal transporter (DMT1). This increases as crypt cells migrate up the villus and become mature absorptive cells. **(C)** *Apical cell*. Dietary iron is reduced from the ferric to the ferrous state by the brush border ferric reductase. **DMT1** facilitates iron absorption from the intestinal lumen. The export proteins, e.g. ferroportin 1 and hephaestin, transfer iron from the enterocyte into the circulation, depending on the hepcidin level. A second pathway absorbs intact haem iron into the circulation via BRCP and FLVCR. BCRP, breast cancer resistant protein; B$_2$M, β$_2$-microglobulin; FLVCR, feline leukaemia virus subgroup C; HCP1, haem carrier protein-1; *HFE*, hereditary haemochromatosis gene; TfR1, transferrin receptor.

Box 16.3 Factors influencing iron absorption

- Haem iron is absorbed better than non-haem iron
- Ferrous iron is absorbed better than ferric iron
- Gastric acidity helps to keep iron in the ferrous state and soluble in the upper gut
- Formation of insoluble complexes with phytate or phosphate decreases iron absorption
- Iron absorption is increased with low iron stores and increased erythropoietic activity, e.g. bleeding, haemolysis, high altitude
- Absorption is decreased in iron overload, except in hereditary haemochromatosis, where it is increased

proteins: BCRP (breast cancer resistant protein) and FLVCR (feline leukaemia virus subgroup C) (see **Fig. 16.8**).

Non-haem iron absorption occurs primarily in the duodenum. Non-haem iron is dissolved in the low pH of the stomach and reduced from the ferric to the ferrous form by a brush border ferric reductase. Cells in duodenal crypts are able to sense the body's iron requirements and retain this information as they mature into cells capable of absorbing iron at the tips of the villi. A protein, divalent metal transporter 1 (DMT1) or natural resistance-associated macrophage protein (NRAMP2), transports iron (and other metals) across the apical (luminal) surface of the mucosal cells in the small intestine.

Once inside the mucosal cell, iron may be transferred across the cell to reach the plasma, or be stored as ferritin; the body's iron status at the time the absorptive cell developed from the crypt cell is probably the crucial deciding factor. Iron stored as ferritin will be lost into the gut lumen when the mucosal cells are shed; this regulates iron balance. The mechanism of transport of iron across the basolateral surface of mucosal cells involves a transporter protein, ferroportin 1 (FPN 1), through its iron-responsive element (IRE). This transporter protein requires an accessory, multicopper protein, hephaestin (see **Fig. 16.8**).

The body iron content is closely regulated by the control of iron absorption but there is no physiological mechanism for eliminating excess iron from the body. The key molecule regulating iron absorption is **hepcidin**, a 25-amino acid peptide synthesized in the liver. Hepcidin acts by regulating the activity of the iron-exporting protein ferroportin by binding to ferroportin, causing its internalization and degradation, and thereby decreasing iron efflux from iron-exporting tissues into plasma. Therefore, high levels of hepcidin (occurring in inflammation states) via inflammatory cytokines, e.g. IL-6, will destroy ferroportin and limit iron absorption, and low levels of hepcidin (e.g. in anaemia, low iron stores, hypoxia) will encourage iron absorption. For example, in patients with haemochromatosis (see **Fig. 34.27**), mutations in the genes HFE, HJV and TfR2 interrupt hepcidin synthesis. Therefore, in the intestinal cells, a deficiency of hepcidin leads to less ferroportin being bound and thus more iron will be released into the plasma.

A longstanding mystery is why anaemias characterized by ineffective erythropoiesis, such as thalassaemia, are associated with excessive and inappropriate iron absorption. This has now been shown to be due to the downregulation of hepcidin and upregulation of ferroportin, mediated by a newly identified hormone produced by developing erythroblast-erythroferrone (Erfe).

Transport in the blood

The normal serum iron level is about 13–32 µmol/L; there is a diurnal rhythm, with higher levels in the morning. The serum iron value is of little use clinically for assessing patients' iron status. Iron is transported in the plasma bound to transferrin, a β-globulin that is synthesized in the liver. Each transferrin molecule binds two atoms of ferric iron and is normally one-third saturated. Most of the iron bound to transferrin comes from macrophages in the reticuloendothelial system and not from iron absorbed by the intestine. These recycle the iron obtained from senescent red blood cells when haemoglobin is broken down. Transferrin-bound iron becomes attached by specific receptors to erythroblasts and reticulocytes in the marrow and the iron is removed (see **Fig. 16.3**).

In an average adult male, 20 mg of iron, chiefly obtained from red cell breakdown in the macrophages of the reticuloendothelial system, is incorporated into haemoglobin every day.

Iron stores

About two-thirds of the total body iron is in the circulation as haemoglobin (2.5–3 g in a normal adult man). The rest is stored in reticuloendothelial cells, hepatocytes and skeletal muscle cells (500–1500 mg). About two-thirds of this is stored as ferritin and one-third as haemosiderin in normal individuals. Small amounts of iron are also found in plasma (about 4 mg bound to transferrin), with some in myoglobin and enzymes.

Ferritin is a water-soluble complex of iron and protein. It is more easily mobilized than haemosiderin for haemoglobin formation. It is present in small amounts in plasma, proportional to the degree of iron loading, but also rises with infection and inflammation as it is an acute-phase protein.

Haemosiderin is an insoluble iron–protein complex found in macrophages in the bone marrow, liver and spleen. Unlike ferritin, it is visible by light microscopy in tissue sections and bone marrow films after staining by Perls' reaction.

Requirements

Each day, 0.5–1.0 mg of iron is lost in the faeces, urine and sweat. Menstruating women lose 30–40 mL of blood per month, an average of about 0.5–0.7 mg of iron per day. Blood loss through menstruation in excess of 100 mL will usually result in iron deficiency, as increased iron absorption from the gut cannot compensate for such losses of iron. The demand for iron also increases during growth (about 0.6 mg/day) and pregnancy (1–2 mg/day). In the normal adult the iron content of the body remains relatively fixed. Increases in the body iron content (haemochromatosis) are classified into:

- **Hereditary haemochromatosis** (see p. 1300), where a mutation in the HFE gene or other iron-controlling proteins causes increased iron absorption.
- **Secondary haemochromatosis** (transfusion siderosis; see p. 343), due to iron overload in conditions treated by regular blood transfusion.
- **Non-transfusional iron overload**, where ineffective erythropoiesis drives uncontrolled iron absorption from the gut via erythroferrone. This occurs in thalassaemia and other inherited anaemias (e.g. sideroblastic anaemia).

Iron deficiency

Iron deficiency anaemia develops when there is inadequate iron for haemoglobin synthesis. The causes are:
- blood loss
- increased demands, e.g. growth and pregnancy
- decreased absorption (e.g. post-gastrectomy)
- poor intake

Most iron deficiency is due to blood loss, usually from the uterus or gastrointestinal tract. Premenopausal women are in a state of precarious iron balance owing to menstruation. A common cause of iron deficiency worldwide is blood loss from the gastrointestinal tract resulting from parasites such as hookworm infestation. The poor quality of the diet, predominantly containing vegetables, also contributes to the high prevalence of iron deficiency in low income countries. Even in developed countries, iron deficiency is not uncommon in infancy, when iron intake is insufficient for the demands of growth. It is more prevalent in infants born prematurely or where the introduction of mixed feeding is delayed.

Clinical features

The symptoms of anaemia are described on page 327. The following well-known clinical features of iron deficiency are generally seen only in cases of very longstanding iron deficiency:

- brittle nails
- spoon-shaped nails (koilonychia)
- atrophy of the papillae of the tongue
- angular stomatitis
- brittle hair
- a syndrome of dysphagia and glossitis (Plummer–Vinson or Paterson–Brown–Kelly syndrome, see p. 1169).

The diagnosis of iron deficiency anaemia relies on a clinical history, which should include questions about dietary intake, self-medication with non-steroidal anti-inflammatory drugs (NSAIDs; may give rise to gastrointestinal bleeding), and the presence of blood in the faeces (which may be a sign of haemorrhoids or carcinoma of the lower bowel). In women, careful enquiry should be made about the duration of periods, the occurrence of clots, and the number of sanitary towels or tampons used (3–5 per day is normal, see **Box 39.1**).

Investigations

- **Blood count and film.** A characteristic blood film is shown in **Fig. 16.9**. The red cells are microcytic (MCV <80 fL) and hypochromic (mean corpuscular haemoglobin (MCH) <27 pg). There is poikilocytosis (variation in shape) and anisocytosis (variation in size).
- **Serum iron and iron-binding capacity.** Serum iron is not helpful in the assessment of clinical iron status. The transferrin saturation is a more accurate measure and iron deficiency is regularly present when this falls below 19% (**Box 16.4**).
- **Serum ferritin.** The level of serum ferritin reflects the amount of stored iron. The normal values for serum ferritin are 30–300 µg/L (11.6–144 nmol/L) in males and 15–200 µg/L (5.8–96 nmol/L) in females. In simple iron deficiency, a low serum ferritin confirms the diagnosis. However, ferritin is an acute-phase reactant, and levels increase in the presence of inflammatory or malignant diseases and also in the presence of liver damage. This can result in a normal or mildly raised ferritin level, even in the presence of iron deficiency. Very high levels of ferritin may be observed in hepatitis and in a rare disease, haemophagocytic lymphohistiocytosis (see p. 525).
- **Serum soluble transferrin receptors.** The number of transferrin receptors released into the serum from bone marrow erythroblasts increases in iron deficiency. The results of this immunoassay compare well with results from bone marrow aspiration in terms of estimating iron stores. This assay can help to distinguish between iron deficiency and anaemia of chronic disease (see **Box 16.4**), and may avoid the need for bone marrow examination; however, it is not readily available in routine clinical practice. It may sometimes be helpful in the investigation of complicated causes of anaemia.
- **Other investigations.** These will be indicated by the clinical history and examination. Investigations of the gastrointestinal tract are often required to determine the cause of the iron deficiency (see p. 1185).

Differential diagnosis

The presence of anaemia with microcytosis and hypochromia does not necessarily indicate iron deficiency. The most common of the other causes are thalassaemia, sideroblastic anaemia and anaemia of chronic disease, and in these disorders the iron stores are normal

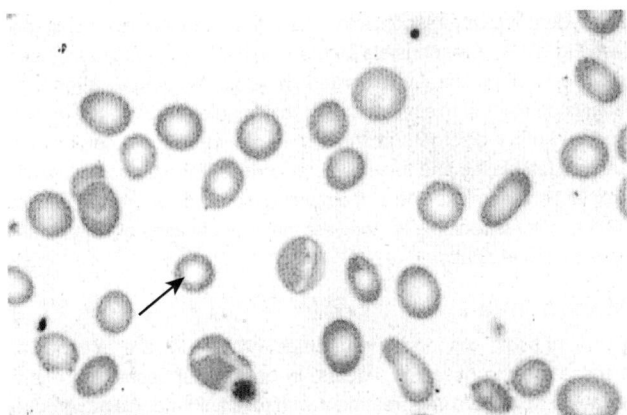

Fig. 16.9 Hypochromic microcytic cells (arrowed) on a blood film. Poikilocytosis (variation in shape) and anisocytosis (variation in size) are seen.

---

i **Box 16.4 Microcytic anaemia: differential diagnosis**

	Iron deficiency	Anaemia of chronic disease	Thalassaemia trait (α or β)	Sideroblastic anaemia
MCV	Reduced	Low normal or normal	Very low for degree of anaemia	Low in inherited type but often raised in acquired type
Serum iron	Reduced	Reduced	Normal	Raised
Serum TIBC	Raised	Reduced	Normal	Normal
Serum ferritin	Reduced	Normal or raised	Normal	Raised
Serum soluble transfer receptors	Increased	Normal	Normal or raised	Normal or raised
Iron in marrow	Absent	Present	Present	Present
Iron in erythroblasts	Absent	Absent or reduced	Present	Ring forms

MCV, mean corpuscular volume of red cells; TIBC, total iron binding capacity.

or increased. The differential diagnosis of microcytic anaemia is shown in **Box 16.4**.

Management

The correct management of iron deficiency is to find and treat the underlying cause, and to give iron to correct the anaemia and replace iron stores. Patients with iron deficiency who are taking iron will increase their haemoglobin level by approximately 10 g/L per week, unless, of course, other factors, such as bleeding, are present.

Oral iron is all that is required in most cases. The best preparation is ferrous sulphate. A 200 mg tablet provides 60 mg of elemental iron. Side-effects, such as nausea, diarrhoea or constipation, are extremely common and compliance is notoriously poor, particularly when the standard dose of 200 mg three times daily is prescribed. Emerging evidence supports the finding that after a dose of oral iron is taken, serum hepcidin levels rise quickly, suppressing the absorption of subsequent doses. Clinical trials will reveal whether optimal iron dosing would be daily, alternate day or even every 3 days. Optimizing absorption includes taking the tablets fasting with a glass of orange juice (vitamin C helps convert ferric to ferrous iron, aiding absorption). Tannins in tea inhibit iron absorption and should be avoided.

In developing countries, distribution of iron tablets and fortification of food are the main approaches for the alleviation of iron deficiency. However, iron supplementation programmes have been ineffective, mainly because of poor compliance. There are also concerns regarding the increased risk of infection in a population where malaria and other parasites are endemic.

Oral iron should be given for long enough to correct the haemoglobin level and to replenish the iron stores; this can take 6 months. The most common causes of failure to respond to oral iron are:

*   lack of compliance
*   ongoing blood loss
*   incorrect diagnosis, e.g. thalassaemia trait.

These possibilities should be considered before parenteral (injected) iron is used. However, parenteral iron is indicated, for example, for those who are intolerant to oral preparations, those with severe malabsorption and those with chronic disease (e.g. inflammatory bowel disease). Iron stores are replaced much faster with parenteral iron than with oral iron but the haematological response is no quicker. Parenteral iron can be given by slow intravenous infusion of low-molecular-weight iron dextran (a test dose is required because of the risk of anaphylactoid reactions), iron sucrose, ferric carboxymaltose or iron isomaltoside 1000; oral iron should be discontinued.

Anaemia of chronic disease

One of the most common types of anaemia, particularly in hospital patients, is the anaemia of chronic disease, occurring in individuals with chronic inflammatory disease, such as Crohn's disease, rheumatoid arthritis, SLE, polymyalgia rheumatica and malignant disease, or with chronic infections such as tuberculosis. There is decreased release of iron from the bone marrow to developing erythroblasts, an inadequate erythropoietin response to the anaemia, and decreased red cell survival.

High levels of hepcidin expression in these contexts play a key role (see earlier). As numerous pathogens are dependent on iron for multiplication, reacting to infection and inflammation by increasing hepcidin levels and sequestering iron from the circulation became evolutionarily advantageous, and IL-6 produced during infection is a potent driver of hepcidin expression. However, chronic inflammatory conditions result in raised hepcidin levels and poor delivery of iron to the marrow, and hence anaemia. Measurement of hepcidin levels is emerging as a useful test to help distinguish anaemia of chronic disease from iron deficiency anaemia.

The serum iron and the total iron binding capacity (TIBC) are low, and the serum ferritin is normal or raised because of the inflammatory process. The serum soluble transferrin receptor level is normal (see **Box 16.4**). Stainable iron is present in the bone marrow but iron is not seen in the developing erythroblasts. Patients do not respond to oral iron therapy, and treatment is, in general, that of the underlying disorder, though intravenous iron may help. Recombinant erythropoietin therapy is used in the anaemia of renal disease (see p. 1394), and occasionally in inflammatory disease (rheumatoid arthritis, inflammatory bowel disease).

Sideroblastic anaemia

Sideroblastic anaemias are inherited or acquired disorders characterized by a refractory anaemia (that does not respond to simple haematinic supplementation), a variable number of hypochromic cells in the peripheral blood, and excess iron and ring sideroblasts in the bone marrow. The presence of ring sideroblasts is the diagnostic feature of sideroblastic anaemia. There is accumulation of iron in the mitochondria of erythroblasts owing to disordered haem synthesis, forming a ring of iron granules around the nucleus that can be seen with Perls' reaction. The blood film is often dimorphic; ineffective haem synthesis is responsible for the microcytic hypochromic cells. Sideroblastic anaemias can be inherited as an X-linked disease transmitted by females or as an autosomal recessive form. A structural defect in δ-ALA synthase, the pyridoxine-dependent enzyme responsible for the first step in haem synthesis (see **Fig. 16.3**), is responsible for the X-linked form. Acquired causes include myeloproliferative disorders, myeloid leukaemia, drugs (e.g. isoniazid), alcohol misuse and lead toxicity (see p. 274). It can also occur in other disorders such as rheumatoid arthritis, carcinomas and megaloblastic and haemolytic anaemias. Primary acquired sideroblastic anaemia is one of the myelodysplastic syndromes (see p. 397) and is responsible for the vast majority of cases of sideroblastic anaemia in adults.

Management

Some patients respond when drugs or alcohol are withdrawn, if these are the causative agents. In occasional cases, there is a response to pyridoxine. Treatment with folic acid may be required to treat accompanying folate deficiency.

Further reading

Camaschella C. Iron-deficiency. *Blood* 2019; 133:30–39.
DeLoughery TG. Microcytic anaemia. *N Engl J Med* 2014; 371:1324–1331.
Fleming RE, Ponka P. Iron overload in human disease. *N Engl J Med* 2012; 366:1548–1550.
Hentze MW, Muckenthaler MU, Galy B et al. Two to tango: regulation of mammalian iron absorption. *Cell* 2010; 142:24–38.
Stoffel NU, Cercamondi CI, Brittenham G et al. Iron absorption from oral iron supplements given on consecutive versus alternate days and as single morning doses versus twice-daily split dosing in iron-depleted women: two open-label, randomised controlled trials. *Lancet Haematol* 2017; 4:e524–e533.
Weiss G, Ganz T, Goodnough LT. Anaemia of inflammation. *Blood* 2019; 133:40–50.

NORMOCYTIC ANAEMIA

Normocytic, normochromic anaemia is seen in anaemia of chronic disease, in some endocrine disorders (e.g. hypopituitarism, hypothyroidism and hypoadrenalism) and in some haematological disorders (e.g. aplastic anaemia and some haemolytic anaemias) (see **Fig. 16.7**). In addition, this type of anaemia is seen acutely following blood loss.

MACROCYTIC ANAEMIAS

These can be divided into megaloblastic and non-megaloblastic types, depending on bone marrow findings.

Megaloblastic anaemia

Megaloblastic anaemia is characterized by the presence in the bone marrow of erythroblasts with delayed nuclear maturation because of defective DNA synthesis (megaloblasts). Megaloblasts are large and have large immature nuclei. The nuclear chromatin is more finely dispersed than normal and has an open, stippled appearance (**Fig. 16.10**). In addition, giant metamyelocytes are frequently seen in megaloblastic anaemia. These cells are about twice the size of normal cells and often have twisted nuclei. Megaloblastic changes occur in:

- vitamin B_{12} deficiency or abnormal vitamin B_{12} metabolism
- folic acid deficiency or abnormal folate metabolism
- other defects of DNA synthesis, such as congenital enzyme deficiencies in DNA synthesis (e.g. orotic aciduria), or those resulting from therapy with drugs interfering with DNA synthesis (e.g. hydroxycarbamide (hydroxyurea), azathioprine)
- myelodysplasia due to dyserythropoiesis.

Haematological findings

- The MCV is characteristically over 96 fL unless there is a coexisting cause of microcytosis, in which case there may be a dimorphic picture with a normal/low average MCV.
- The peripheral blood film shows oval macrocytes with hypersegmented polymorphs with six or more lobes in the nucleus (**Fig. 16.11**).
- If severe, there may be leucopenia and thrombocytopenia.
- The lactate dehydrogenase (LDH) is typically elevated (sometimes extremely so), reflecting ineffective erythropoiesis.

Biochemical basis of megaloblastic anaemia

The key biochemical problem common to both vitamin B_{12} and folate deficiency is a block in DNA synthesis owing to an inability to methylate deoxyuridine monophosphate to deoxythymidine monophosphate, which is then used to build DNA (**Fig. 16.12**). The methyl group is supplied by the folate coenzyme, methylene tetrahydrofolate.

Deficiency of folate reduces the supply of this coenzyme; deficiency of vitamin B_{12} also reduces its supply by slowing the demethylation of methyltetrahydrofolate (methyl THF) and preventing cells from receiving tetrahydrofolate for synthesis of methylene tetrahydrofolate polyglutamate.

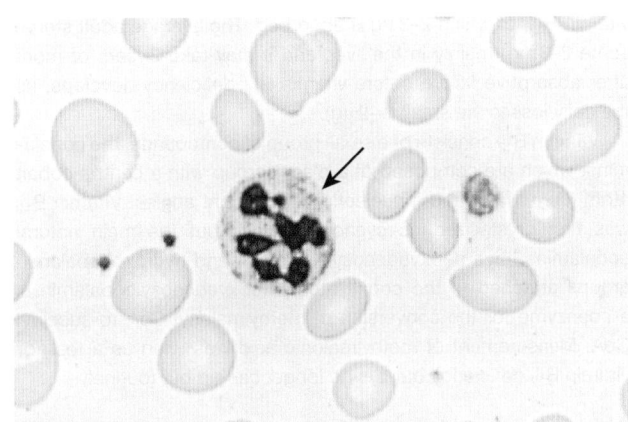

Fig. 16.11 Macrocytes and a hypersegmented neutrophil (arrowed) on a peripheral blood film.

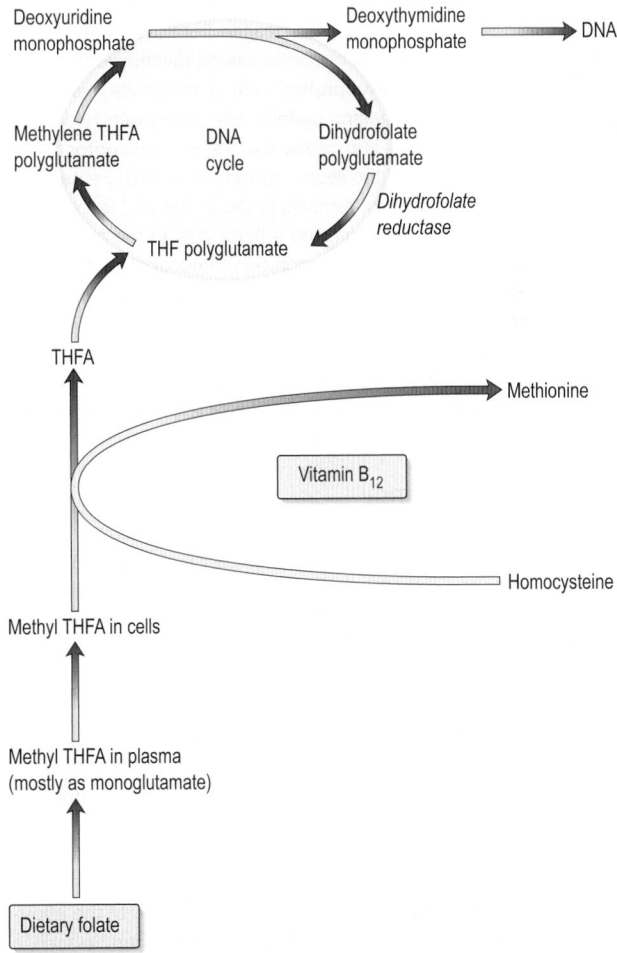

Fig. 16.12 Biochemical basis of megaloblastic anaemia. The metabolic relationship between vitamin B_{12} and folate, and their role in DNA synthesis. THFA, tetrahydrofolate.

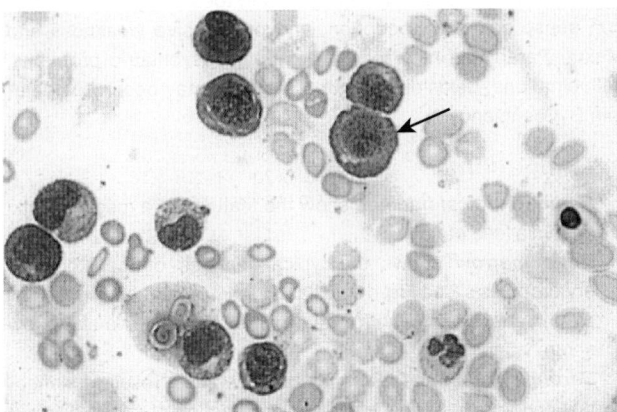

Fig. 16.10 Megaloblasts (arrowed) in the bone marrow.

Other congenital and acquired forms of megaloblastic anaemia are due to interference with purine or pyrimidine synthesis, causing an inhibition in DNA synthesis.

Vitamin B₁₂ (cobalamin)

Vitamin B_{12} is synthesized by certain microorganisms, and humans are ultimately dependent on animal sources. It is found in meat, fish, eggs and milk, but not in plants. Vitamin B_{12} is not usually destroyed by cooking. The average daily diet contains 5–30 µg of vitamin B_{12}, of which 2–3 µg is absorbed. The average adult stores some 2–3 mg, mainly in the liver, and it may take 2 years or more after absorptive failure before vitamin B_{12} deficiency develops, as the daily losses are small (1–2 µg).

Vitamin B_{12} consists of a small group of compounds, the cobalamins, which are composed of a planar group with a central cobalt atom (corrin ring) and a nucleotide set at right angles. Vitamin B_{12} was first crystallized as cyanocobalamin, but the main natural cobalamins have deoxyadenosyl-, methyl- and hydroxocobalamin groups attached to the cobalt atom. Deoxyadenosylcobalamin is a coenzyme for the conversion of methylmalonyl CoA to succinyl CoA. Measurement of methylmalonic acid was used as a test for vitamin B_{12} deficiency but it is no longer carried out routinely.

Absorption and transport

Vitamin B_{12} is liberated from protein complexes in food by gastric enzymes and then binds to a vitamin B_{12}-binding protein ('R' binder), which is related to plasma transcobalamin I (TCI) and is derived from saliva. Vitamin B_{12} is released from the 'R' binder by pancreatic enzymes and then becomes bound to intrinsic factor.

Intrinsic factor is a glycoprotein with a molecular weight of 45 kDa. It is secreted by gastric parietal cells along with H^+ ions. It combines with vitamin B_{12} and carries it to a specific receptor on the surface of the mucosa of the ileum, cubilin. Vitamin B_{12} enters the ileal cells and intrinsic factor remains in the lumen and is excreted. Vitamin B_{12} is transported from the enterocytes to the bone marrow and other tissues by the glycoprotein transcobalamin II (TCII). Vitamin B_{12} bound to TCII is known as holotranscobalamin or 'active B_{12}', as this is the form of vitamin B_{12} that is taken up by cells. Although TCII is the essential carrier protein for vitamin B_{12}, the amount of B_{12} on TCII is low. Vitamin B_{12} in plasma is mainly bound to TCI (70–90%). About 1% of an oral dose of B_{12} is absorbed 'passively' without the need for intrinsic factor.

Vitamin B₁₂ deficiency

There are a number of causes of B_{12} deficiency and abnormal B_{12} metabolism (**Box 16.5**). The most common cause of vitamin B_{12} deficiency in adults is pernicious anaemia. Malabsorption of vitamin B_{12} because of pancreatitis, coeliac disease or treatment with metformin is mild and does not usually result in significant vitamin B_{12} deficiency.

Pernicious anaemia

Pernicious anaemia (PA) is an autoimmune disorder in which there is atrophic gastritis with loss of parietal cells in the gastric mucosa and consequent failure of intrinsic factor production and vitamin B_{12} malabsorption.

Pathogenesis

This disease is common in the elderly, about 1 in 8000 of the population aged over 60 years being affected in the UK. It can be seen in all races and is more common in females than males.

There is an association with other autoimmune diseases, particularly thyroid disease, Addison's disease and vitiligo. Approximately

---

> **Box 16.5** Vitamin B_{12} deficiency and abnormal B_{12} utilization: further causes[a]
>
> **Low dietary intake**
> - Veganism
>
> **Impaired absorption**
> *Stomach*
> - Pernicious anaemia
> - Gastrectomy
> - Congenital deficiency of intrinsic factor
>
> *Small bowel*
> - Ileal disease or resection
>
> - Bacterial overgrowth
> - Tropical sprue
> - Fish tapeworm (*Diphyllobothrium latum*)
>
> **Abnormal utilization**
> - Congenital transcobalamin II deficiency
> - Nitrous oxide (inactivates B_{12})
>
> [a]See text.

50% of all patients with PA have thyroid antibodies. There is a higher incidence of gastric carcinoma with PA (1–3%) than in the general population.

Parietal cell antibodies are present in the serum in 90% of patients with PA, and also in 10% of normal individuals. Conversely, intrinsic factor antibodies, although found in only 50% of patients with PA, are specific for this diagnosis.

Pathology

Autoimmune gastritis (see p. 1173) affecting the fundus is present, with plasma cell and lymphoid infiltration. The parietal and chief cells are replaced by mucin-secreting cells. There is achlorhydria and absent secretion of intrinsic factor. The histological abnormality can be improved by corticosteroid therapy, which supports an autoimmune basis for the disease.

Clinical features

The onset of PA is insidious, with progressively increasing symptoms of anaemia. Patients are sometimes said to have a lemon-yellow colour owing to a combination of pallor and mild jaundice, caused by excess breakdown of haemoglobin. A red, sore tongue (glossitis) and angular stomatitis are sometimes present.

The neurological changes, if left untreated for a long time, can be irreversible. These neurological abnormalities occur only with very low levels of serum B_{12} (<60 ng/L or 50 pmol/L) and occasionally are seen in patients who are not clinically anaemic. The classical neurological features are those of a polyneuropathy progressively involving the peripheral nerves and the posterior and eventually the lateral columns of the spinal cord (subacute combined degeneration; see p. 891). Patients present with symmetrical paraesthesiae in the fingers and toes, early loss of vibration sense and proprioception, and progressive weakness and ataxia. Paraplegia may result. Dementia, psychiatric problems, hallucinations, delusions and optic atrophy may occur from vitamin B_{12} deficiency.

Investigations

- **Haematological findings** show the features of a megaloblastic anaemia (see p. 333).
- **Bone marrow** shows the typical features of megaloblastic erythropoiesis (see **Fig. 16.10**), although it is frequently not sampled in cases of straightforward macrocytic anaemia and a low serum vitamin B_{12}.
- **Serum bilirubin** and LDH may be raised as a result of ineffective erythropoiesis. Normally, a minor fraction of serum bilirubin results from premature breakdown of newly formed red cells in

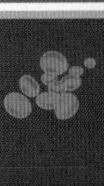

the bone marrow. In many megaloblastic anaemias, where the destruction of developing red cells is much increased, the serum bilirubin can be increased.

- **Serum vitamin B$_{12}$** is usually well below 160 ng/L, which is the lower end of the normal range. Serum vitamin B$_{12}$ can be assayed using radio-isotope dilution or immunological assays. Numerous factors can affect B$_{12}$ levels, such as pregnancy and the oral contraceptive pill, which lower it.
- **Holotranscobalamin** is the 'active' fraction of cobalamin, and its measurement may be a better marker for vitamin B$_{12}$ deficiency than serum vitamin B$_{12}$.
- **Serum methylmalonic acid (MMA) and homocysteine (HC)** are raised in B$_{12}$ deficiency but testing is recommended only in complex cases, such as those where there is a strong suspicion of vitamin B$_{12}$ deficiency but the vitamin B$_{12}$ level is normal.

Absorption tests

Vitamin B$_{12}$ absorption tests are no longer performed in the UK, as radioactive B$_{12}$ is not available.

Gastrointestinal investigations

In PA, there is achlorhydria. Intubation studies can be performed to confirm this but are rarely carried out in routine practice. Endoscopy or barium meal examination of the stomach is performed only if gastric symptoms are present.

Differential diagnosis

Vitamin B$_{12}$ deficiency must be differentiated from other causes of megaloblastic anaemia, principally folate deficiency, but usually this is quite clear from the blood levels of these two vitamins.

PA should be distinguished from other causes of vitamin B$_{12}$ deficiency by testing for intrinsic factor antibodies (see **Box 16.5**). Patients negative for intrinsic factor antibodies with no other cause of vitamin B$_{12}$ deficiency may still have PA.

Management

See later.

Folic acid

Folic acid monoglutamate is not itself present in nature but occurs as polyglutamates. Folates are present in food as polyglutamates in the reduced dihydrofolate or tetrahydrofolate (THF) forms. Polyglutamates are broken down to monoglutamates in the upper gastrointestinal tract, and during the absorptive process these are converted to methyl THF monoglutamate, which is the main form in the serum. The methylation of homocysteine to methionine requires both methylcobalamin and methyl THF as coenzymes. This reaction is the first step in which methyl THF entering cells from the plasma is converted into folate polyglutamates. Intracellular polyglutamates are the active forms of folate and act as coenzymes in the transfer of single carbon units in amino acid metabolism and DNA synthesis (see **Fig. 16.12**).

Dietary intake

Folate is found in green vegetables, such as spinach and broccoli, and offal, such as liver and kidney. Cooking causes a loss of 60–90% of the folate. The minimal daily requirement is about 100 μg.

Folate deficiency

The causes of folate deficiency are shown in **Box 16.6**. The main cause is poor intake, which may occur alone or in combination

with excessive utilization or malabsorption. The body's reserves of folate are about 10 mg. On a deficient diet, folate deficiency develops over the course of about 4 months, but folate deficiency may develop rapidly in patients who have both a poor intake and excess utilization of folate (e.g. patients in intensive care units).

Folic acid supplements at the time of conception and in the first 12 weeks of pregnancy reduce the incidence of neural tube defects. In the USA and Canada, mandatory fortification of grain products, such as bread, flour and rice, has substantially improved folate status and has been associated with a significant fall in neural tube defects. There is controversy about the role of folate supplementation in the reduction of cardiovascular and cerebrovascular disease by lowering homocysteine levels.

Clinical features

Patients with folate deficiency may be asymptomatic or may present with symptoms of anaemia or those of the underlying cause. Glossitis can occur. Unlike with B$_{12}$ deficiency, neuropathy does not occur.

Investigations

The haematological findings are those of a megaloblastic anaemia (see p. 333).

Blood measurements

Serum folate reflects recent folate status and intake. It is usually measured by immunological methods; a level below 3 μg/L (7 nmol/L) is indicative of folate deficiency. The amount of folate in the red cells is a measure of tissue folate over the lifetime of red cells; a level below 150 μg/L (340 nmol/L) is consistent with folate deficiency, but measurement of the serum folate is usually sufficient to diagnose folate deficiency.

Further investigations

In many cases of folate deficiency the cause is not obvious from the clinical picture or dietary history. Occult gastrointestinal disease should then be suspected and appropriate investigations, such as small bowel biopsy, may be performed.

Management and prevention of megaloblastic anaemia

Treatment depends on the type of deficiency. Blood transfusion is not usually indicated in chronic anaemia; indeed, it can be dangerous to transfuse elderly patients, as heart failure may be precipitated. Folic acid may produce a haematological response in vitamin B_{12} deficiency but may aggravate the neuropathy. Large doses of folic acid alone should not be used to treat megaloblastic anaemia unless the serum vitamin B_{12} level is known to be normal. In severely ill patients it may be necessary to treat with both folic acid and vitamin B_{12} while awaiting serum levels.

Management of vitamin B_{12} deficiency

Hydroxocobalamin $1000\,\mu g$ can be given intramuscularly to a total of 5–6 mg over the course of 2 weeks; $1000\,\mu g$ is then necessary every 3 months for the rest of the patient's life.

Clinical improvement may occur within 48 hours and a reticulocytosis can be seen some 2–3 days after starting therapy, peaking at 5–7 days. Improvement of the polyneuropathy may occur over 6–12 months but longstanding spinal cord damage is irreversible. Hypokalaemia can occur and, if severe, supplements should be given. Iron deficiency often develops in the first few weeks of therapy. Hyperuricaemia also occurs but clinical gout is uncommon. In patients who have had a total gastrectomy or an ileal resection, vitamin B_{12} should be monitored; if levels are low, prophylactic vitamin B_{12} should be given. Vegans may require oral B_{12} supplements.

Oral treatment with vitamin B_{12} can also be used in patients but good compliance with treatment is required.

Management of folate deficiency

Folate deficiency can be corrected by giving 5 mg of folic acid daily; the same haematological response occurs as is seen after treatment of vitamin B_{12} deficiency. Treatment should be given for about 4 months to replace body stores. Any underlying cause, such as coeliac disease, should be treated.

Prophylactic folic acid ($400\,\mu g$ daily) is recommended for all women planning a pregnancy and in early pregnancy to reduce neural tube defects.

Women who have had a child with a neural tube defect should take 5 mg folic acid daily before and during a subsequent pregnancy.

Prophylactic folic acid, in a dose of 5 mg daily or weekly, is also given to patients with chronic haematological disorders where there is rapid cell turnover and to those undergoing renal dialysis.

Macrocytosis without megaloblastic changes

A raised MCV with macrocytosis on the peripheral blood film can occur with a normoblastic rather than a megaloblastic bone marrow.

A common *physiological* cause of macrocytosis is pregnancy. Macrocytosis may also occur in the newborn. Common *pathological* causes are:

- alcohol excess
- liver disease
- reticulocytosis (e.g. due to haemolysis)
- hypothyroidism
- some haematological disorders (e.g. aplastic anaemia, myelodysplasia, pure red cell aplasia, multiple myeloma)
- drugs (e.g. hydroxycarbamide, azathioprine)

- cold agglutinins due to autoagglutination of red cells (see p. 353) (the MCV decreases to normal with warming of the sample to $37°C$).

In all these conditions, normal levels of vitamin B_{12} and folate will be found. The exact mechanisms in each case are uncertain, but in some there is increased lipid deposition in the red cell membrane.

An increased number of reticulocytes also leads to a raised MCV because they are large cells.

High alcohol consumption is a frequent cause of a raised MCV, and in such patients the MCV can be used as a surrogate marker for monitoring excessive alcohol consumption. A full-blown megaloblastic anaemia can also occur in people who use alcohol to excess; this is due to a toxic effect of alcohol on erythropoiesis and/or to dietary folate deficiency.

Further reading

British Committee for Standards in Haematology. Guidelines for the diagnosis and treatment of cobalamin and folate disorders. *Br J Haematol* 2014; 166:496–513.

ANAEMIA DUE TO MARROW FAILURE (APLASTIC ANAEMIA)

Aplastic anaemia is defined as pancytopenia with hypocellularity (aplasia) of the bone marrow; there are no leukaemic, cancerous or other abnormal cells in the peripheral blood or bone marrow. It is usually an acquired condition but may rarely be inherited.

Aplastic anaemia is due to a reduction in the number of pluripotent stem cells (see **Fig. 16.1**), together with a fault in those remaining or an immune reaction against them so that they are unable to repopulate the bone marrow. Failure of only one cell line may also occur, resulting in isolated deficiencies such as the absence of red cell precursors in pure red cell aplasia. Evolution to myelodysplasia, paroxysmal nocturnal haemoglobinuria (PNH) or acute myeloid leukaemia occurs in some cases, probably owing to the emergence of an abnormal clone of haemopoietic cells.

Aetiology

The causes of aplasia are shown in **Box 16.7**. Immune mechanisms are probably responsible for most cases of idiopathic acquired aplastic anaemia and play a part in at least the persistence of many secondary cases. Activated cytotoxic T cells in blood and bone marrow are responsible for the bone marrow failure.

Many drugs may cause marrow aplasia, including cytotoxic drugs such as busulfan and doxorubicin, which are expected to cause transient aplasia as a consequence of their therapeutic use. However, some individuals develop aplasia due to sensitivity to non-cytotoxic

---

? Box 16.7 Causes of aplastic anaemia

Primary
- Inherited, e.g. Fanconi anaemia
- Idiopathic acquired (67% of cases)

Secondary
- Chemicals, e.g. benzene, toluene, glue sniffing
- Drugs:
  - e.g. Chemotherapeutic
  - Antibiotics, e.g. chloramphenicol, gold, penicillamine, phenytoin, carbamazepine, carbimazole, azathioprine

- Insecticides
- Ionizing radiation
- Infections:
  - Viral, e.g. hepatitis, Epstein–Barr virus, human immunodeficiency virus (HIV), erythrovirus
  - Other, e.g. tuberculosis
- Paroxysmal nocturnal haemoglobinuria
- Miscellaneous, e.g. pregnancy

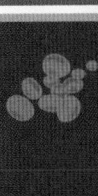

drugs such as chloramphenicol, gold, carbimazole, chlorpromazine, phenytoin, ribavirin, tolbutamide, NSAIDs, and many others that have been reported to cause aplasia as a rare side-effect.

Inherited aplastic anaemias are rare. Multiple gene mutations have been identified. Several are tumour suppressor genes and have been seen in one-third of aplastic anaemias. Fanconi anaemia is inherited as an autosomal recessive condition and is associated with skeletal, skin, eye, renal and central nervous system abnormalities. It usually presents between the ages of 5 and 10 years and is associated with an increased risk of malignancies.

Clinical features

The clinical manifestations of marrow failure from any cause are anaemia, bleeding and infection. Bleeding is often the predominant initial presentation of aplastic anaemia with bruising and minimal trauma or blood blisters in the mouth. Physical findings include ecchymoses, bleeding gums and epistaxis. Mouth infections are common. Lymphadenopathy and hepatosplenomegaly are rare in aplastic anaemia.

Investigations

- Pancytopenia.
- The virtual absence of reticulocytes.
- A hypocellular or aplastic bone marrow with increased fat spaces (**Fig. 16.13**).

Differential diagnosis

Aplastic anaemia must be differentiated from other causes of pancytopenia (**Box 16.8**). A bone marrow trephine is essential for assessment of the bone marrow cellularity.

Management and prognosis

The treatment of aplastic anaemia depends on the underlying cause and the likelihood of spontaneous recovery of blood counts. Careful attention to supportive care is essential while awaiting bone marrow recovery and, in some cases, specific treatment can be used to accelerate marrow recovery.

The main danger is infection and stringent measures should be undertaken to avoid this (see also p. 116). Any suspicion of infection in a severely neutropenic patient (neutrophil count of $<0.5 \times 10^9$/L) should lead to the immediate institution of broad-spectrum parenteral antibiotics. Supportive care, including transfusions of red cells and platelets, should be given as necessary. The cause of the aplastic anaemia must be eliminated if possible.

The course of aplastic anaemia can be variable, ranging from a rapid spontaneous remission to a persistent, increasingly severe pancytopenia, which may lead to death through haemorrhage or infection. The most reliable determinants for the prognosis are the number of neutrophils, reticulocytes and platelets, and the cellularity of the bone marrow.

A bad prognosis (i.e. severe aplastic anaemia) is associated with the presence of two of the following three features:

- neutrophil count of $<0.5 \times 10^9$/L
- platelet count of $<20 \times 10^9$/L
- reticulocyte count of $<40 \times 10^9$/L.

Haemopoietic stem cells (allogeneic bone marrow transplantation) are the treatment of choice for patients with severe aplastic anaemia under the age of 40 who have a human leucocyte antigen (HLA)-identical sibling donor, where it gives a 75–90% chance of long-term survival.

Immunosuppressive therapy is recommended for:

- patients with severe disease over the age of 40
- younger patients with severe disease who do not have an HLA-identical sibling donor
- patients who do not have severe disease but who are transfusion-dependent.

The standard immunosuppressive treatment is antithymocyte globulin (ATG) and ciclosporin, which results in response rates of 60–80% and 5-year survival rates of 75–85%.

Stem cell transplantation using matched unrelated donors is an option for patients under the age of 50 who have no matched sibling donor, and who have failed to respond to immunosuppression with ATG and ciclosporin; the results are improving (5-year survival of 65–73%). The main problems are graft rejection, graft-versus-host disease and viral infections.

Levels of haemopoietic growth factors (see **Fig. 16.1**) are normal or increased in most patients with aplastic anaemia, and so these factors are ineffective as primary treatment.

Steroids should not be used to treat severe aplastic anaemia, except for serum sickness due to ATG.

Adult pure red cell aplasia is associated with a thymoma in 5–15% of cases and thymectomy occasionally induces a remission. It may also be associated with autoimmune disease or be idiopathic. Steroids, cyclophosphamide, azathioprine and ciclosporin are effective treatments in some cases.

Further reading

British Society of Haematology. Guidelines for the diagnosis and management of adult aplastic anaemia. *Br J Haematol* 2016; 172:187-207.

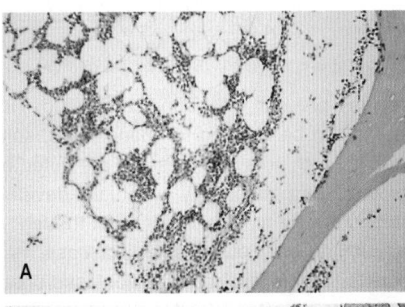

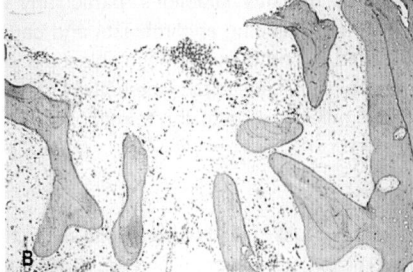

Fig. 16.13 Bone marrow trephine biopsies in low-power view. **(A)** Normal cellularity. **(B)** Hypocellularity in aplastic anaemia.

? Box 16.8 Causes of pancytopenia

- Aplastic anaemia (see Box 16.7)
- Drugs
- Megaloblastic anaemia
- Bone marrow infiltration or replacement:
  - Hodgkin and non-Hodgkin lymphoma
  - Acute leukaemia
  - Myeloma
  - Secondary carcinoma
  - Myelofibrosis
- Hypersplenism
- Systemic lupus erythematosus
- Disseminated tuberculosis
- Paroxysmal nocturnal haemoglobinuria
- Overwhelming sepsis

HAEMOLYTIC ANAEMIAS: AN INTRODUCTION

Haemolytic anaemias are caused by increased destruction of red cells. The red cell normally survives about 120 days, but in haemolytic anaemias the red cell survival times are considerably shortened.

Breakdown of normal red cells occurs in the macrophages of the bone marrow, liver and spleen (see **Fig. 16.5**).

Consequences of haemolysis

Shortening of red cell survival does not always cause anaemia, as there is a compensatory increase in red cell production by the bone marrow. If the red cell loss can be contained within the marrow's capacity for increased output, then a haemolytic state can exist without anaemia (**compensated haemolytic disease**). The bone marrow can raise its output by 6–8 times by increasing the proportion of cells committed to erythropoiesis (**erythroid hyperplasia**) and by expanding the volume of active marrow. In addition, immature red cells (**reticulocytes**) are released prematurely. These cells are larger than mature cells and stain with a light blue tinge on a peripheral blood film (the description of this appearance on the blood film is **polychromasia**) due to the presence of residual ribosomal RNA. Reticulocytes may be counted accurately as a percentage of all red cells on a blood film using a supravital stain for residual RNA (e.g. new methylene blue).

Sites of haemolysis

Extravascular haemolysis

In most haemolytic conditions, red cell destruction is extravascular. The red cells are removed from the circulation by macrophages in the reticuloendothelial system, particularly the spleen.

Intravascular haemolysis

When red cells are rapidly destroyed within the circulation, haemoglobin is liberated. This is initially bound to plasma haptoglobins but these soon become saturated.

Excess free plasma haemoglobin is filtered by the renal glomerulus and enters the urine, although small amounts are reabsorbed by the renal tubules. In the renal tubular cell, haemoglobin is broken down and becomes deposited in the cells as **haemosiderin**. This can be detected in the spun sediment of urine using Perls' reaction. Some of the free plasma haemoglobin is oxidized to **methaemoglobin**, which dissociates into **ferrihaem** and globin. **Plasma haemopexin** binds ferrihaem, but if its binding capacity is exceeded, ferrihaem becomes attached to albumin, forming **methaemalbumin**. On spectrophotometry of the plasma, methaemalbumin forms a characteristic band; this is the basis of **Schumm's test**.

The **liver** plays a major role in removing haemoglobin bound to haptoglobin and haemopexin, and also any remaining free haemoglobin. Free haemoglobin is toxic and scavenges nitric oxide, which is a critical signalling molecule for smooth muscle relaxation and the control of pulmonary pressures.

Evidence for haemolysis

Increased red cell breakdown is accompanied by increased red cell production. This is shown in **Fig. 16.14**.

Demonstration of shortened red cell lifespan

Red cell survival can be estimated from ^{51}Cr-labelled red cells given intravenously but this test is rarely performed.

Intravascular haemolysis

This is suggested by haemosiderinuria, very low or absent haptoglobins, and the presence of methaemalbumin (positive Schumm's test).

Various laboratory studies will be necessary to determine the exact type of haemolytic anaemia present. The causes of haemolytic anaemias are shown in **Box 16.9**.

INHERITED HAEMOLYTIC ANAEMIA

Red cell membrane defects

The normal red cell membrane consists of a lipid bilayer crossed by integral proteins with an underlying lattice of proteins (or cytoskeleton), including spectrin, actin, ankyrin and protein 4.1, attached to the integral proteins (**Fig. 16.15**).

Hereditary spherocytosis

Hereditary spherocytosis (HS) is the most common inherited haemolytic anaemia in Northern Europeans, affecting 1 in 5000. It can be inherited in an autosomal dominant or recessive manner, but in some patients occurs by spontaneous (*de novo*) mutation. In the absence of a family history, the most important differential diagnosis is that of autoimmune haemolytic anaemia, which can usually be excluded by a negative direct antiglobulin test. HS is caused by defects in the red cell membrane, resulting in the cells losing part of the cell membrane as they pass through the spleen, possibly because the lipid bilayer is inadequately supported by the membrane skeleton. The best-characterized defect is a deficiency in the structural protein spectrin but quantitative defects in other membrane proteins have been identified (see **Fig. 16.15**), with ankyrin defects being the most common. The abnormal red cell membrane in HS is associated functionally with an increased permeability to sodium, and this requires an increased rate of active transport of sodium out of the cells, which is dependent on adenosine triphosphate (ATP), produced by glycolysis. The surface-to-volume ratio decreases and the cells become spherocytic. Spherocytes are more rigid and less deformable than normal red cells. They are unable to pass through the splenic microcirculation so they have a shortened lifespan.

Clinical features

The condition may present with jaundice at birth. However, the onset of jaundice can be delayed for many years; some patients may go through life with no symptoms and are detected only during family studies. The patient may eventually develop anaemia, gallstones, splenomegaly or, rarely, ulcers on the leg. As in many haemolytic anaemias, the course of the disease may be interrupted by aplastic, haemolytic and megaloblastic crises. Aplastic anaemia usually occurs after infections, particularly with parvovirus, which infects developing erythroblasts and causes temporary abolition of red cell production. Megaloblastic anaemia is the result of folate depletion, caused by hyperactivity of the bone marrow. Chronic haemolysis leads to the formation of pigment gallstones (see p. 1315).

Investigations

- **Anaemia.** This is usually mild but occasionally can be severe.
- **Blood film.** This shows spherocytes (**Fig. 16.16**) and polychromasia.
- **Haemolysis.** This is evident (e.g. the serum bilirubin and urinary urobilinogen will be raised).

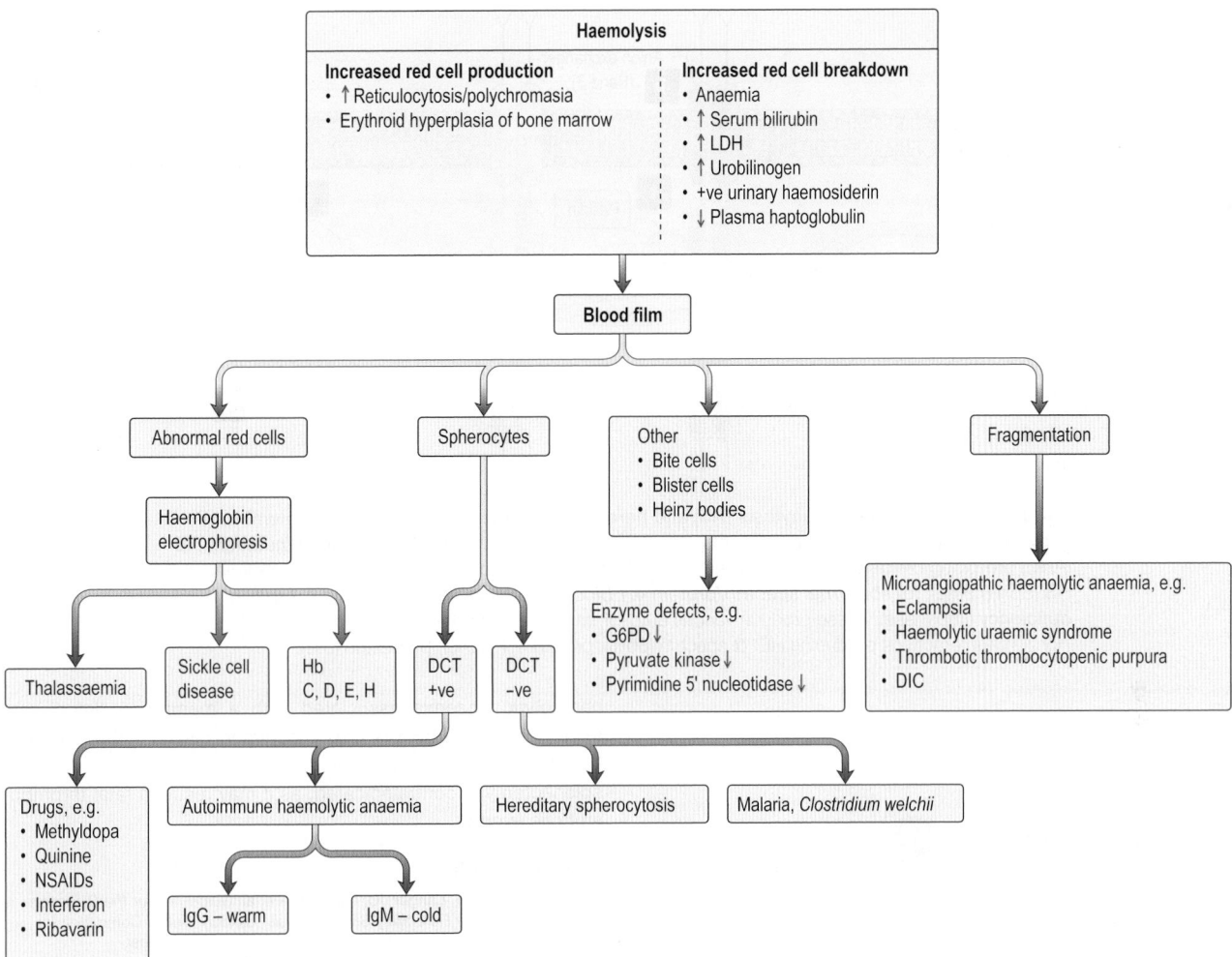

Fig. 16.14 Haemolysis: diagnostic and haematological features. DCT, direct Coombs' test; DIC, disseminated intravascular coagulation; G6PD, glucose-6-phosphate dehydrogenase; LDH, lactate dehydrogenase; NSAIDs, non-steroidal anti-inflammatory drugs.

? Box 16.9 Causes of haemolytic anaemia

Inherited

Red cell membrane defect
- Hereditary spherocytosis
- Hereditary elliptocytosis

Haemoglobin abnormalities
- Thalassaemia
- Sickle cell disease

Metabolic defects
- Glucose-6-phosphate dehydrogenase deficiency
- Pyruvate kinase deficiency
- Pyrimidine kinase deficiency

Acquired

Immune
- Autoimmune (see Box 16.16):
  - Warm
  - Cold
- Alloimmune:
  - Haemolytic transfusion reactions
  - Haemolytic disease of the newborn
  - After allogeneic bone marrow or organ transplantation

- Drug-induced

Non-immune
- Acquired membrane defects:
  - Paroxysmal nocturnal haemoglobinuria
- Mechanical:
  - Microangiopathic haemolytic anaemia
  - Valve prosthesis
  - March haemoglobinuria
- Secondary to systemic disease:
  - Renal and liver failure

Miscellaneous
- Infections, e.g. malaria, mycoplasma
- *Clostridium perfringens* (*welchii*), generalized sepsis
- Drugs and chemicals causing damage to the red cell membrane or oxidative haemolysis
- Hypersplenism
- Burns

- **Osmotic fragility.** When red cells are placed in solutions of increasing hypotonicity, they take in water, swell and eventually lyse. Spherocytes tolerate hypotonic solutions less well than do normal biconcave red cells. Osmotic fragility tests are infrequently carried out in routine practice but may be useful to confirm suspicion of spherocytosis on a blood film.
- **Direct antiglobulin (Coombs') test.** This is negative in hereditary spherocytosis, virtually ruling out autoimmune haemolytic anaemia, in which spherocytes are also commonly present.

Management

Most patients require no specific treatment or need occasional transfusions during pregnancy or intercurrent infections. Rarely, patients are transfusion-dependent. For the remainder, splenectomy is indicated to relieve symptoms due to anaemia or splenomegaly, reverse growth failure and prevent recurrent gallstones. It is best to postpone splenectomy until after childhood, as sudden overwhelming fatal infections, usually due to encapsulated organisms such as pneumococci, may occur (see p. 357). Splenectomy should be preceded by appropriate immunization and followed by life-long penicillin prophylaxis. In addition to the well-known risk of bacterial infection, there is also a significant risk of adverse arterial and venous thromboembolic events after splenectomy and this needs to be taken into account when deciding whether to proceed to splenectomy.

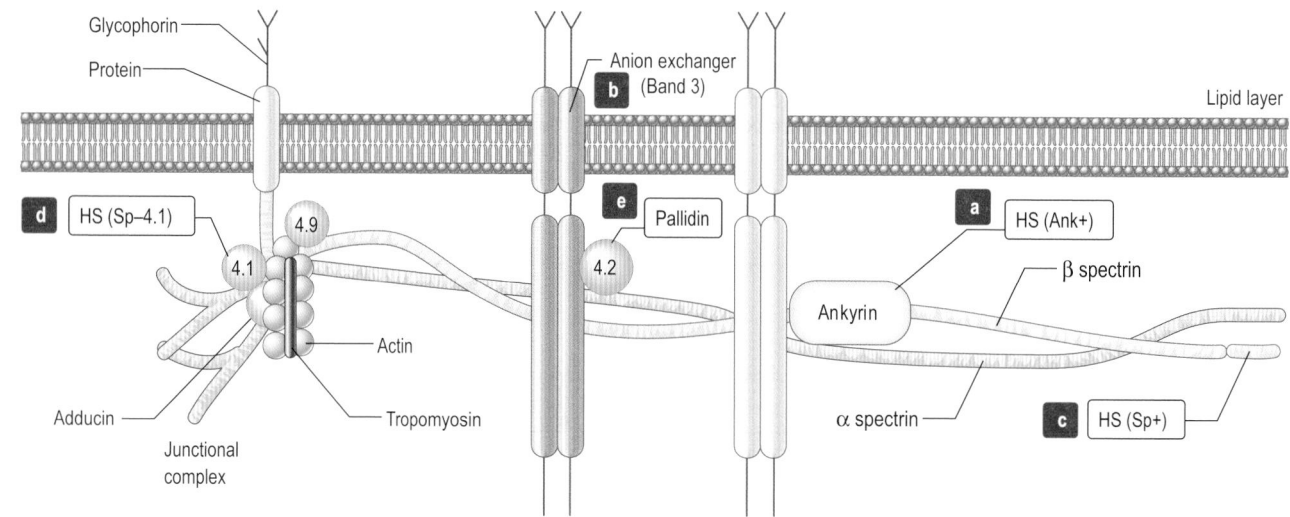

Fig. 16.15 Hereditary spherocytosis (HS) and hereditary elliptocytosis (HE): red cell membrane showing the sites of the principal defects. Vertical interactions producing HS: **(a)** *ankyrin mutation*, HS (Ank+) producing deficiency (45% of cases); **(b)** HS *band 3 deficiency* (20%); **(c)** *β spectrin deficiency*, HS (Sp+) (<20%); **(d)** *abnormal spectrin/protein 4.1 binding*, HS (Sp–4.1); **(e)** *protein 4.2 (pallidin) deficiency* (Japanese). These produce various autosomal dominant and recessive forms of the disease. Horizontal interactions producing HE: α spectrin (80%), protein 4.1 (15%), β spectrin (5%).

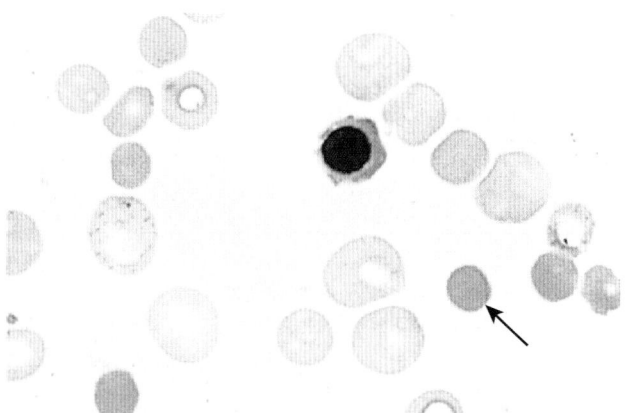

Fig. 16.16 Spherocytes (arrowed). This blood film also shows reticulocytes, polychromasia and a nucleated erythroblast.

Following splenectomy, the spherocytes persist but the haemoglobin usually returns to normal, as the red cells are no longer destroyed.

Hereditary elliptocytosis

This disorder of the red cell membrane is inherited in an autosomal dominant manner and has a prevalence of 1 in 2500 in Caucasians. The red cells are elliptical due to deficiencies of protein 4.1 or the spectrin/actin/4.1 complex, which leads to weakness of the horizontal protein interaction and to the membrane defect (see **Fig. 16.15**). Clinically, it is a similar condition to HS but milder. Only a minority of patients have anaemia and only occasional individuals require splenectomy.

Rarely, hereditary spherocytosis or elliptocytosis may be inherited in a homozygous fashion, giving rise to a severe haemolytic anaemia sometimes necessitating splenectomy in early childhood (hereditary pyropoikilocytosis).

Hereditary stomatocytosis

Stomatocytes are red cells in which the pale central area appears slit-like. Their presence in large numbers may occur in a hereditary

haemolytic anaemia associated with a membrane defect, but excess alcohol intake is also a common cause. Although these hereditary conditions are very rare, a correct diagnosis is required; splenectomy is contraindicated, as it may result in fatal thrombo-embolic events.

Further reading

Bolton-Maggs PHB, Langer JC, Iolascon A et al. *Guidelines for the Diagnosis and Management of Hereditary Spherocytosis*. London: British Committee for Standards in Haematology; 2011; https://b-s-h.org.uk/guidelines/.
Mohandas N. Inherited hemolytic anemia: a possessive beginner's guide. *Hematology* 2018; 2018:377–381.

Haemoglobin abnormalities

In early embryonic life, haemoglobins Gower 1, Gower 2 and Portland predominate. Later, fetal haemoglobin (HbF), which has two α and two γ chains, is produced (**Fig. 16.17**). There is increasing synthesis of β chains from 13 weeks' gestation and at term there is 80% HbF and 20% HbA. Completion of the haemoglobin switch from HbF to HbA occurs after birth, when the genes for γ chain production are further suppressed and there is rapid increase in the synthesis of β chains. BCL IIA, a zinc finger protein, is one of a number of proteins that suppress γ gene expression and is a key genome editing target in the effort to reactivate HbF in adults with haemoglobinopathies. There is little HbF produced (normally <1%) from 6 months after birth. The δ chain is synthesized just before birth and HbA$_2$ (α$_2$δ$_2$) remains at a level of about 2% throughout adult life (**Box 16.10**).

A normal individual has four α-globin chain genes (see **Fig. 16.17**), with two α-globin genes on each haploid genome (genes derived from one parent). These are situated close together on chromosome 16. The genes controlling the production of ε, γ, δ and β chains are close together on chromosome 11. The globin genes are arranged on chromosomes 16 and 11 in the order in which they are expressed and combine to give different haemoglobins. Normal haemoglobin synthesis is discussed on page 326.

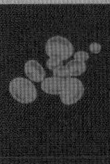

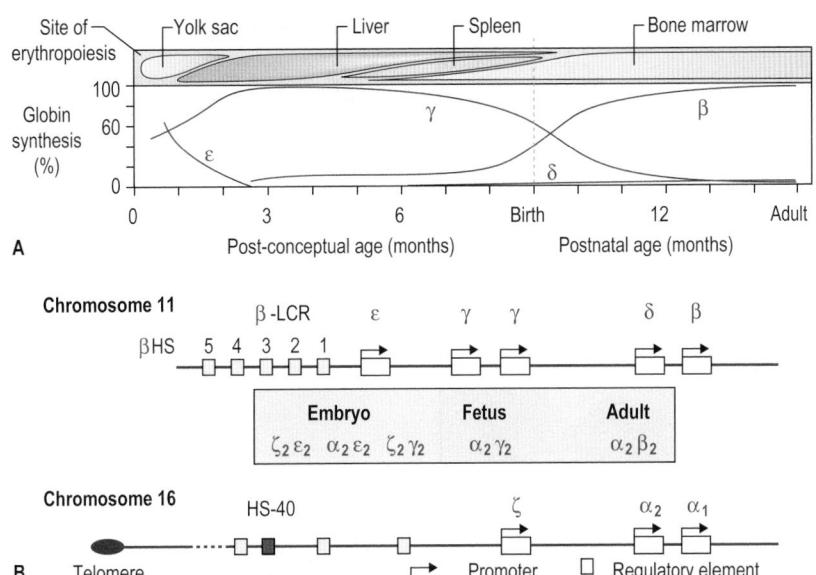

Fig. 16.17 Normal development switches in globin expression. (A) Sites of haemopoiesis and globin changes at various gestational ages. **(B)** Structure of α-like and β-like globin gene clusters. HS, major upstream regulatory element; LCR, locus control region. *(From Higgs DR, Engel JD, Stamatoyannopoulos G. Thalassaemia.* Lancet *2012; 379:373–383, with permission.)*

Box 16.10 Some types of haemoglobin (Hb)

	Hb	Structure	Comment
Normal	A	$\alpha_2\beta_2$	Comprises 97% of adult Hb
	A_2	$\alpha_2\delta_2$	Comprises 2% of adult Hb Elevated in β-thalassaemia
	F	$\alpha_2\gamma_2$	Normal Hb in fetus from third to ninth month
			Increased in β-thalassaemia
			Comprises <1% of Hb in adult
Abnormal chain production	H	β_4	Found in α-thalassaemia Biologically useless
	Barts	γ_4	Comprises 100% of Hb in homozygous α-thalassaemia Biologically useless
Abnormal chain structure	SC	$\alpha_2\beta_2{}^S\alpha_2\beta_2{}^C$	Substitution of valine for glutamine acid in position 6 of β chain Substitution of lysine for glutamic acid in position 6 of β chain

Further reading

Forget BG. Progress in understanding the hemoglobin switch. *N Engl J Med* 2011; 365:852–854.
Sankaran VG. Targeted therapeutic strategies for fetal hemoglobin induction. *Hematology* 2011; 2011:459–465.

Haemoglobinopathies

Abnormalities can occur in:

- globin chain production – quantitative defect (e.g. thalassaemia)
- structure of the globin chain – qualitative defect (e.g. sickle cell disease)
- combined defects of globin chain production and structure (e.g. sickle cell β-thalassaemia).

The thalassaemias

The thalassaemias affect people throughout the world (**Fig. 16.18**), and at least 60 000 severely affected individuals are born every year. Normally, there is balanced (1:1) production of α and β chains.

The defective synthesis of globin chains in thalassaemia leads to 'imbalanced' globin chain production, causing precipitation of the excess globin chains within the red cell precursors and resulting in ineffective erythropoiesis. Precipitation of globin chains in mature red cells leads to haemolysis. This concept of globin chain imbalance is critical in understanding the relationship between a patient's genotype and phenotype (the greater the imbalance, the worse the phenotype), as well as understanding how novel therapies are being used to ameliorate the disease.

Beta-thalassaemia

In ***homozygous*** (identical mutations on both alleles) or ***compound heterozygous*** (different damaging mutations on both alleles) β-thalassaemia, either no normal β chains are produced (β^0) or β-chain production is very reduced (β^+). This leaves an excess of α chains, which precipitate in erythroblasts and red cells, causing ineffective erythropoiesis and haemolysis. In the carrier (heterozygous) state, the excess α chains combine with δ and result in modestly increased quantities of HbA$_2$, which

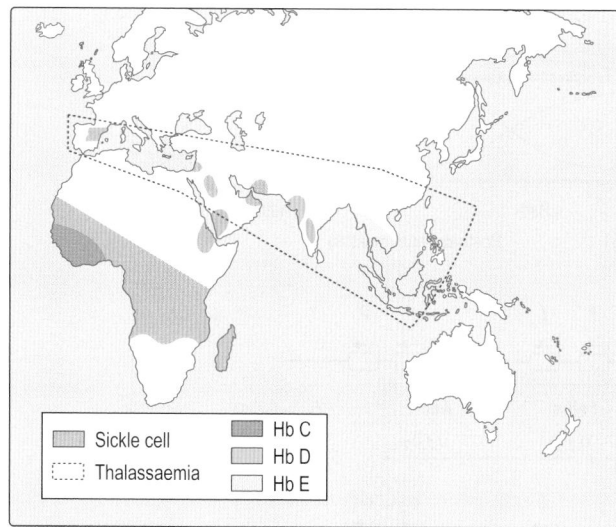

Fig. 16.18 Major haemoglobin abnormalities: geographical distribution.

Map legend:
- Sickle cell
- Thalassaemia
- Hb C
- Hb D
- Hb E

Box 16.11 Usual findings in beta thalassaemia

Type of thalassaemia	Homozygous or compound heterozygous phenotype	Heterozygous phenotype
β^+	**Transfusion dependent anaemia** *HPLC at diagnosis:* HbA (10-30%), HbF (70-90%) HbA$_2$ variable	**Mild reduction in Hb** *HPLC:* HbA (90-95%), raised HbA$_2$ (3.6-4.2%)
β^0	**Transfusion dependent anaemia** *HPLC at diagnosis:* HbF (95-98%) HbA2 variable	**Mild reduction in Hb** *HPLC:* HbA (90-95%), raised HbA$_2$ (4-5%)

is used to screen for β-thalassaemia carrier status. Heterozygous β-thalassaemia carriers exhibit asymptomatic microcytosis with or without mild anaemia. **Box 16.11** shows the findings in the homozygote and heterozygote for the common types of β-thalassaemia.

Genetics

The molecular errors accounting for over 200 genetic defects leading to β-thalassaemia have been characterized. Unlike in α-thalassaemia, the defects are mainly point mutations rather than gene deletions. The mutations result in defects in transcription, RNA splicing and modification, translation via frame shifts and nonsense codons producing highly unstable β-globin, which cannot be utilized.

Clinical syndromes

Clinical syndromes in thalassaemia have changed in recent years, moving away from the 'major' and 'minor' descriptions and focusing on whether they are 'transfusion-dependent thalassaemias' (TDTs) or 'non-transfusion-dependent thalassaemias' (NTDTs; **Fig. 16.19**). Patients who have NTDT may require occasional blood transfusions, particularly during times of infection or pregnancy. Patients with NTDT may be transferred to the TDT category if it is decided that regular transfusions would improve their growth, development and wellbeing. Thalassaemia trait is the term still used to describe the symptomless heterozygous carrier state.

Thalassaemia trait (carrier)

This common carrier state (heterozygous β-thalassaemia) is asymptomatic. Anaemia is mild or absent. The red cells are hypochromic and microcytic with a low MCV and MCH, and the condition may be confused with iron deficiency. However, the two are easily distinguished, as in thalassaemia trait the serum ferritin and the iron stores are normal (see **Box 16.4**). The RDW is usually normal (see p. 324). Haemoglobin electrophoresis usually shows a raised HbA$_2$

Thalassaemia carrier	NTDT	TDT
Thalassaemia trait	'Thalassaemia intermedia'	'Thalassaemia major'
No transfusions	Intermittent transfusions	Transfusion dependence
Heterozygous for one of: • 1 or 2 deletions of α globin • β^0-globin mutation (no β globin produced) • β$^+$-globin mutation (small amount of β globin produced)	• HbH disease (3 α gene deletions) • HbE/β-thalassaemia • β-thalassaemia trait with co-inherited multiple copies of α globin • β-thalassaemia major with co-inherited hereditary persistence of fetal haemoglobin or α-thalassaemia	Homozygous or compound heterozygous for either: • β^0-globin mutation (no β globin produced) • β$^+$-globin mutation (small amount of β globin produced)

Fig. 16.19 Clinical syndromes in thalassaemia. The terms 'thalassaemia intermedia' and 'thalassaemia major' have been replaced by 'non-transfusion-dependent thalassaemia' (NTDT) and 'transfusion-dependent thalassaemia' (TDT). Patients can fluctuate between these categories, depending on their life circumstances. In addition, the link between the genotype and the phenotype of affected individuals is influenced by modifying factors such as the reactivation of γ globin or the co-inheritance of changes in the number of α-globin genes.

and often a slightly raised HbF (see **Fig. 16.23**). Iron should not be given to these patients unless they also have proven coincidental iron deficiency.

Non-transfusion-dependent thalassaemia (NTDT)

This condition was previously referred to as thalassaemia intermedia. Patients are symptomatic with moderate anaemia (Hb 70–100 g/L) but do not require regular transfusions.

NTDT occurs in patients in whom the effects of the excess α-globin chains are attenuated. This can be due to a reduction in their production (co-inheritance of α-thalassaemia) or due to the α-chains being 'mopped up' by γ chains. While there is usually very little γ-chain production after birth, some patients may co-inherit

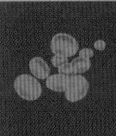

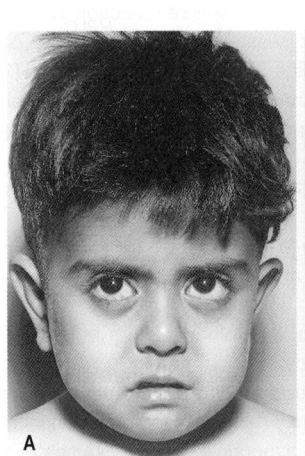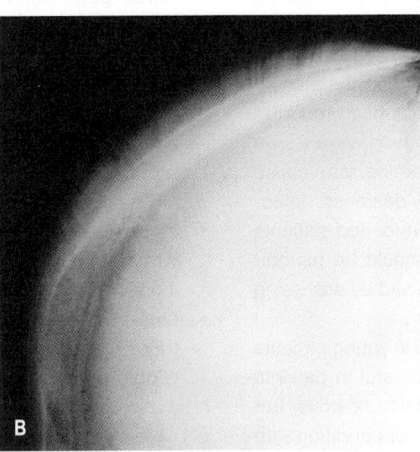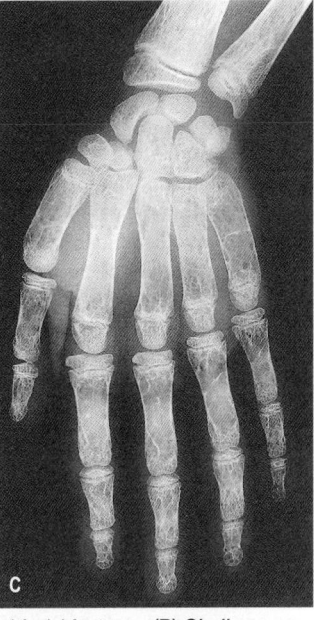

Fig. 16.20 Thalassaemia. **(A)** *Child with thalassaemia*, showing the typical facial features. **(B)** *Skull X-ray* of a child with β-thalassaemia, showing the 'hair-on-end' appearance. **(C)** *X-ray of a hand*, showing expansion of the marrow and a thinned cortex.

'hereditary persistence of fetal haemoglobin', in which γ-chain production is increased, sometimes to substantial amounts. By reducing α-chain production or increasing that of γ chains, there is less excess α-chain precipitation, thus helping to reduce the degree of globin imbalance and causing a consequent reduction in ineffective erythropoiesis and haemolysis.

Conversely, NTDT may also arise from the inheritance of a heterozygous β⁺ mutation and an excess of α-chain genes. This condition (e.g. triplicated α-chain genes) arises in the same meiotic division that results in one α-chain deletion (see **Fig. 16.23**). The more α-chain genes are inherited, the greater the imbalance and the more severe the phenotype.

Patients with NTDT may have splenomegaly and bone deformities. Recurrent leg ulcers, gallstones and infections are also seen. These patients may be iron-overloaded despite a lack of regular blood transfusions. This is caused by excessive iron absorption, which results from the underlying dyserythropoiesis that drives Erfe production, suppressing hepcidin to undetectable levels (see p. 329).

Transfusion-dependent thalassaemia (TDT)

This condition was previously referred to as thalassaemia major. Most children affected by homozygous or compound heterozygous β-thalassaemia present during the first year of life with:

- failure to thrive and recurrent bacterial infections
- severe anaemia from 3 to 6 months, when the switch from γ- to β-chain production should normally occur
- extramedullary haemopoiesis that soon leads to hepatosplenomegaly and bone expansion, giving rise to the classical thalassaemic facies (**Fig. 16.20A**).

Skull X-rays in these children show the characteristic 'hair-on-end' appearance of bony trabeculation as a result of expansion of the bone marrow into cortical bone (**Fig. 16.20B**). The expansion of the bone marrow is also shown in an X-ray of the hand (**Fig. 16.20C**).

The classic features of untreated thalassaemia major are generally observed only in patients from countries that do not have good blood transfusion support.

Management of symptomatic thalassaemia

The aims of treatment are to suppress ineffective erythropoiesis, prevent bony deformities and allow normal activity, growth and development.

- **Long-term folic acid** supplements are required.
- **Regular transfusions** should be given to keep the haemoglobin above 100 g/L. Blood transfusions may be required every 4–6 weeks.
- **Splenectomy** was previously used to reduce the transfusion requirements of patients with NTDT; these are associated with the development of pulmonary hypertension, however, and should be used only rarely. Splenectomy is usually delayed until after the age of 6 years because of the risk of infection; prophylaxis against infection is required (see p. 357).
- **Iron overload**, caused by repeated transfusions (transfusion haemosiderosis), may lead to damage to the endocrine glands, liver, pancreas and myocardium by adolescence. Among these complications of iron overload, cardiomyopathy and associated cardiac tachyarrhythmias are the leading causes of morbidity and mortality. Magnetic resonance imaging (MRI; myocardial T_2-relaxation time) is useful for monitoring iron overload in thalassaemia; both the heart and the liver can be monitored. Iron chelation using the once-daily oral iron chelator deferasirox is now standard wherever it is available and economically accessible. Elsewhere, desferrioxamine remains the standard chelator, although it has to be administered parenterally. Desferrioxamine is given

as an overnight subcutaneous infusion on 5–7 nights each week. Ascorbic acid 200 mg daily is given, as it increases the urinary excretion of iron in response to desferrioxamine. Often, young children have a very high standard of chelation, as it is organized by their parents. However, when the children become adults and take on this role themselves, chelation may become problematic. Deferiprone, an oral iron chelator, has been available for some years and is usually used for cardiac iron overload or in combination with another chelator.

- **Intensive treatment with desferrioxamine** has been reported to reverse damage to the heart in patients with severe iron overload, but excessive doses of desferrioxamine may cause cataracts, retinal damage and sensorineural deafness. Infection with *Yersinia enterocolitica* occurs in iron-loaded patients treated with desferrioxamine. Iron overload should be periodically assessed by measuring the serum ferritin and by assessing hepatic iron stores by MRI.
- **Bone marrow transplantation** has been used in young patients with HLA-matched siblings. It has been successful in patients in good clinical condition with a 3-year mortality of <5%, but there is a high mortality (>50%) in patients in poor condition with iron overload and liver dysfunction. Only 25% of patients have a sibling-matched donor.
- **Prenatal diagnosis and gene therapy** are discussed on pages 15 and 22.
- **Testing of patients' partners** should be carried out. If both partners have β-thalassaemia trait, there is a 1 in 4 chance of the pregnancy resulting in a child having β-thalassaemia major/TDT. Therefore, couples in this situation must be offered prenatal diagnosis and counselling (see p. 17).

Alpha-thalassaemia

Genetics

In contrast to β-thalassaemia, α-thalassaemia is often caused by gene deletions, although mutations of the α-globin genes may also occur. The gene for α-globin chains is duplicated on both chromosomes 16: that is, a normal person has a total of four α-globin genes. Deletion of one α-chain gene (α^+) or both α-chain genes (α^0) on each chromosome 16 may occur (**Box 16.12** and **Fig. 16.21**). The former is the most common of these abnormalities.

- **Four-gene deletion** (deletion of both genes on both chromosomes). There is no α-chain synthesis and only Hb Barts (γ4) is present. Hb Barts cannot carry oxygen and is incompatible with life (see **Boxes 16.10** and **16.12**). Infants are either stillborn at

28–40 weeks or die very shortly after birth. They are pale and oedematous, and have enormous livers and spleens – a condition called hydrops fetalis. If this is detected *in utero*, intra-uterine transfusions can be given so that the fetus can grow and survive until term, at which point the baby will have TDT.

- **Three-gene deletion.** The severe reduction in α-chain synthesis results in HbH disease, which is common in parts of Asia. HbH has four β-chains, although patients with HbH disease also have low levels of HbA and Hb Barts. HbA_2 is normal or reduced. HbH does not transport oxygen and precipitates in erythroblasts and erythrocytes. There is moderate anaemia (Hb 70–100 g/L) and splenomegaly (thalassaemia intermedia). The patients usually have NTDT.
- **Two-gene deletion** (α-thalassaemia trait). There is microcytosis with or without mild anaemia. HbH bodies may be seen on staining a blood film with brilliant cresyl blue.
- **One-gene deletion.** The blood picture is usually normal but there may be microcytosis.

Globin chain synthesis studies for the detection of a reduced ratio of α to β chains may be necessary for the definitive diagnosis of α-thalassaemia trait, although standard DNA analysis using gene sequencing can detect the most common deletions that lead to α-thalassaemia trait.

Further reading

Benz EJ, Jr. Newborn screening for α-thalassaemia – keeping up with globalization. *N Engl J Med* 2011; 364:770–771.
Brittenham GM. Iron-chelating therapy for transfusional iron overload. *N Engl J Med* 2011; 364:146–156.
Higgs DR, Engel JD, Stamatoyannopoulos G. Thalassaemia. *Lancet* 2012; 379:373–383.
Piel FB, Weatherall DJ. The α thalassaemias. *N Engl J Med* 2014; 371:1908, 1916.
Taher AT, Musallam KM, Cappellini MD et al. Optimal management of β thalassaemia intermedia. *Br J Haematol* 2011; 152:512–523.

Sickle syndromes

Sickle cell haemoglobin (HbS) results from a single-base mutation of adenine to thymine, which produces a substitution of valine for glutamic acid at the sixth codon of the β-globin chain ($\alpha_2\beta_2^{6glu \rightarrow val}$). In the homozygous state (**sickle cell anaemia**), both genes are abnormal (HbSS), whereas in the heterozygous state (**sickle cell trait**, HbAS), only one gene carries the gene. As the synthesis of HbF is normal, the disease usually does not manifest itself until the HbF decreases to adult levels at about 6 months of age.

The sickle gene is most common in Africans (up to 25% gene frequency in some populations) but is also found in India, the Middle East and Southern Europe. Its distribution mirrors that of malaria infestation.

Pathogenesis

Deoxygenated HbS molecules are insoluble and polymerize. The flexibility of the cells is decreased, and they become rigid and take up their characteristic sickle appearance (**Fig. 16.22**). This process is initially reversible but, with repeated sickling, the cells eventually lose their membrane flexibility and become irreversibly sickled. This is due to dehydration, partly caused by potassium leaving the red cells via a calcium-activated potassium channel called the Gardos channel. These irreversibly sickled cells are dehydrated and dense, and will not return to normal when oxygenated. Sickling can produce:

ⓘ Box 16.12 The α-thalassaemias

Number of α-globin genes deleted	Genotype[a]	Hb type	Clinical picture
4	--/--	Hb Barts (γ4)	Hydrops fetalis
3	--/-α	HbH (β4)	Moderately severe anaemia
			Splenomegaly
2	-α/-α	HbA	Mild anaemia
	Or	Some HbH bodies	
	--/αα		
1	αα/-α	HbA	Very mild anaemia or no anaemia

[a]The normal α-globin genotype is αα/αα (i.e. four α-globin genes present).

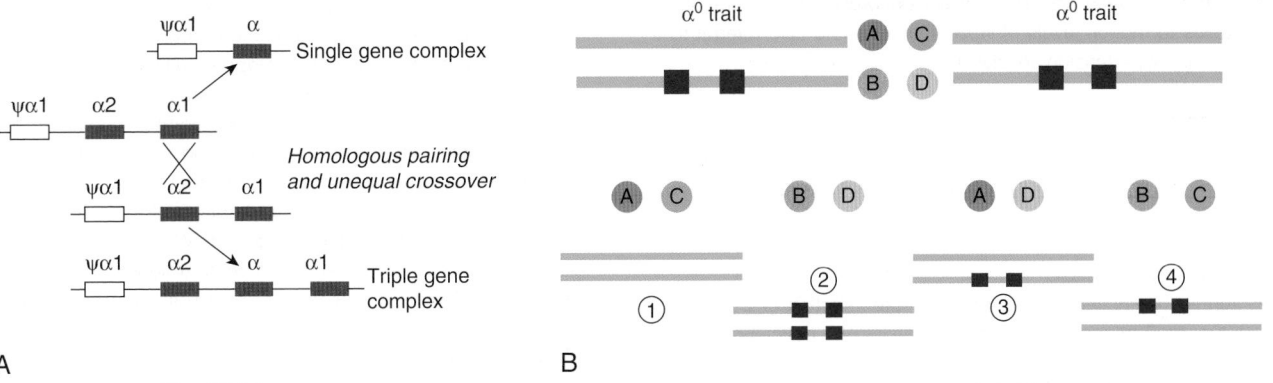

Fig. 16.21 Alpha-thalassaemia. **(A)** Deletions of α globin result from unequal crossover during the process of homologous recombination that occurs during meiosis. This also results in one allele with a triplicated α gene, which is of no clinical consequence in healthy individuals but can exacerbate the globin chain imbalance in individuals with reduced or abnormal β globin. **(B)** Possible outcomes from a pairing of two individuals with α⁰ thalassaemia. There is a 25% risk of hydrops fetalis in the fetus; hence the need for prenatal screening. There is a 25% chance that the offspring will have all four α-globin chains and a 50% chance that the offspring will be an α⁰ carrier.

- shortened red cell survival
- impaired passage of cells through the microcirculation, leading to obstruction of small vessels and tissue infarction.

Sickling is precipitated by infection, dehydration, cold, acidosis or hypoxia. In many cases, the cause is unknown, but adhesion proteins on activated endothelial cells (vascular cell adhesion molecule 1, or VCAM-1) may play a causal role, particularly in vaso-occlusion when rigid cells are trapped, facilitating polymerization. HbS releases its oxygen to the tissues more easily than does normal haemoglobin, and patients therefore feel well despite being anaemic (except, of course, during crises or complications).

Depending on the type of haemoglobin chain combinations, three clinical syndromes occur:

- **Homozygous HbSS** patients have the most severe disease. Patients with co-inheritance of HbS and β-thalassaemia can have equally severe disease.
- **Combined heterozygosity (HbSC) for HbS and C** (see later) causes patients to suffer intermediate symptoms.
- **Heterozygous HbAS (sickle cell trait)** patients have no symptoms (see p. 348).

Sickle cell anaemia
Clinical features
Vaso-occlusive crises

An early presentation may be acute pain in the hands and feet (dactylitis) owing to vaso-occlusion of the small vessels. Severe pain in other bones, such as the femur, humerus, vertebrae, ribs and pelvis, occurs in older children and adults. These attacks vary greatly in frequency from patient to patient, and sometimes in the same patient from year to year. Patients with sickle cell disease can be fairly asymptomatic or require multiple hospital admissions a year from painful vaso-occlusive crises. Overall, 25% of patients with sickle cell disease report experiencing pain on a daily basis. Fever often accompanies the pain.

Acute chest syndrome

This occurs in up to 30%, and pulmonary hypertension and chronic lung disease are the most common causes of death in adults with sickle cell disease. The acute chest syndrome is caused by infection,

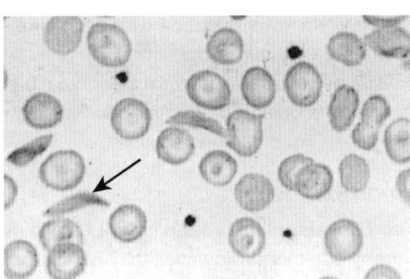

Fig. 16.22 Sickle cells (arrowed) and target cells.

fat embolism from necrotic bone marrow in a vaso-occlusive crisis or pulmonary infarction due to sequestration of sickle cells. It is comprised of shortness of breath, chest pain, pyrexia, hypoxia and new chest X-ray changes due to consolidation. The presentation may be gradual or very rapid, carrying a risk of death in a few hours. Management is with pain relief, high-flow supplemental oxygen and antibiotics (cefotaxime and clarithromycin), which should be started immediately. Exchange transfusion will reduce the amount of HbS to less than 20% if there is no improvement. Ventilation (continuous positive airways pressure, CPAP) may be necessary. Infections can be due to chlamydia and mycoplasma, as well as *Streptococcus pneumoniae*. Use of an incentive spirometer to encourage deep breathing in patients admitted with vaso-occlusive crises reduces the risk of developing the acute chest syndrome.

Pulmonary hypertension

Pulmonary hypertension (defined as a mean pulmonary artery pressure of >25 mmHg by right heart catheterization) is a known consequence of sickle cell anaemia, occurring in approximately 10% of patients. Its mechanism is not understood but contributory factors probably include sickle cell vasculopathy, damage from repeated chest crises, and repeated thromboembolism and intravascular haemolysis with consequent effects on reactive oxygen species and levels of scavenging nitric oxide. Development of pulmonary hypertension raises the risk of hypoxaemia and worsening sickle cell crises, and is an independent risk factor for mortality in patients with sickle cell anaemia. Diagnosis of pulmonary hypertension in patients with sickle cell anaemia should prompt consideration of therapies to reduce levels of HbS (see later) and also referral to a pulmonary hypertension specialist.

Anaemia

Chronic haemolysis produces a stable haemoglobin level, usually in the 60–80 g/L range, but an acute fall in haemoglobin can occur owing to:

- splenic sequestration
- bone marrow aplasia
- further haemolysis due to drugs, acute infection or associated glucose-6-phosphate dehydrogenase (G6PD) deficiency.

Splenic sequestration

Vaso-occlusion produces an acute painful enlargement of the spleen. There is splenic pooling of red cells and hypovolaemia, leading in some to circulatory collapse and death. The condition supervenes in childhood before multiple infarctions have occurred. The latter eventually lead to a fibrotic, non-functioning spleen. Liver sequestration can also occur.

Bone marrow aplasia

This most commonly follows infection with parvovirus B19, which invades proliferating erythroid progenitors. There is a rapid fall in haemoglobin with no reticulocytes in the peripheral blood because of the failure of erythropoiesis in the marrow. Patients may require transfusion until their bone marrow recovers.

Long-term problems

- **Growth and development.** Young children are short but regain their height by adulthood. However, they remain below the normal weight. Sexual maturation is often delayed and may require hormone therapy.
- **Bones.** Bones are a common site for vaso-occlusive episodes, leading to chronic infarcts. Avascular necrosis of hips and shoulders, compression of vertebrae, and shortening of bones in the hands and feet occur. These episodes are commonly the cause of the painful crisis. Osteomyelitis is more frequent in sickle cell disease and is caused by *Staphylococcus aureus*, *Streptococcus pneumoniae* and salmonella (see p. 484). Occasionally, hip joint replacement may be required.
- **Infections.** Infections are common in tissues susceptible to vaso-occlusion, such as bones, lungs and kidneys.
- **Leg ulcers.** These occur spontaneously (vaso-occlusive episodes) or follow trauma, and are usually found over the medial or lateral malleoli. They often become infected and are quite resistant to treatment; sometimes blood transfusion may facilitate ulcer healing.
- **Cardiac problems.** Cardiac problems occur, with cardiomegaly, arrhythmias and iron overload cardiomyopathy. Myocardial infarctions are caused by thrombotic episodes, which are not secondary to atheroma.
- **Neurological complications.** These occur in 25% of patients and include transient ischaemic attacks, fits, cerebral infarction, cerebral haemorrhage and coma. About 11% of patients under 20 years of age suffer strokes without a stroke prevention programme. The most common finding is obstruction of a distal intracranial internal carotid artery or a proximal middle cerebral artery. About 10% of children without neurological signs or symptoms have abnormal blood-flow velocity indicative of clinically significant arterial stenosis; such

patients have a very high risk of stroke. It has been demonstrated that if children with stenotic cranial artery lesions, as demonstrated on transcranial Doppler ultrasonography, are maintained on a regular red cell transfusion exchange programme that is designed to suppress erythropoiesis, so that no more than 30% of the circulating red cells are their own, about 90% of strokes in such children are prevented. Whether they need to remain on these transfusions for life remains to be determined. Silent infarcts, seen on MRI but not manifesting clinically, have been shown to be common in children with sickle cell disease and associated with poor educational attainment.

- **Cholelithiasis.** Pigment stones occur as a result of chronic haemolysis.
- **Liver complications.** Chronic hepatomegaly and liver dysfunction are caused by trapping of sickle cells.
- **Renal complications.** Chronic tubulointerstitial nephritis occurs (see p. 1385).
- **Priapism.** An unwanted painful erection occurs because of vaso-occlusion and can be recurrent. This requires urgent treatment, as it may result in impotence. Treatment is with an α-adrenergic blocking drug, analgesia and hydration.
- **Eye complications.** Background retinopathy, proliferative retinopathy, vitreous haemorrhages and retinal detachments all occur. Regular yearly eye checks are required.
- **Pregnancy.** Impaired placental blood flow causes spontaneous abortion, intrauterine growth retardation, pre-eclampsia and fetal death. Painful episodes, infections and severe anaemia occur in the mother.

Investigations

- **Blood count.** The level of haemoglobin is in the 60–80 g/L range, with a high reticulocyte count (10–20%).
- **Blood films.** These can show features of hyposplenism (see **Fig. 16.28**) and sickling (see **Fig. 16.22**).
- **Sickle solubility test.** A mixture of HbS in a reducing solution such as sodium dithionite gives a turbid appearance because of precipitation of HbS, whereas normal haemoglobin gives a clear solution. A number of commercial kits, such as Sickledex, are available for rapid screening for the presence of HbS, e.g. before surgery in appropriate ethnic groups and in the emergency department.
- **Haemoglobin electrophoresis** (**Fig. 16.23**). This is always needed to confirm the diagnosis. There is no HbA, 80–95% HbS and 2–20% HbF.
- **Parents.** The parents of the affected child will show features of sickle cell trait.

Management

Precipitating factors (see earlier) should be avoided or treated quickly. The complications that require inpatient management are shown in **Box 16.13**.

Acute painful attacks require supportive therapy with intravenous fluids, along with adequate analgesia. Oxygen and antibiotics are given only if specifically indicated. Crises can be extremely painful and require strong, usually narcotic, analgesia. Morphine is the drug of choice. Milder pain can sometimes be relieved by codeine, paracetamol and NSAIDs (**Box 16.14**). Use of incentive spirometry is recommended for patients hospitalized for a vaso-occlusive crisis.

Infection prophylaxis is with penicillin 500 mg daily and vaccination with polyvalent pneumococcal, meningococcal and

Haemophilus influenzae type b vaccine, as all patients are without a functioning spleen (see p. 357). Folic acid is given to all patients with haemolysis.

Anaemia

Blood transfusions should be given only when there are clear indications. Patients with steady state anaemia, those having minor surgery or those having painful episodes without complications should not be transfused. Transfusions should be given acutely for acute chest syndrome and acute anaemia associated with splenic sequestration or an aplastic crisis, aiming for a haemoglobin of 100 g/L and HbS below 30%. Before elective operations, top-up transfusions given to increase the haemoglobin to 100 g/L reduce the risk of perioperative complications. During pregnancy, repeated transfusions may be used to reduce the proportion of circulating HbS to below 30% to prevent sickling and improve placental function. Regular exchange transfusions are given to children with a history of stroke (secondary prevention) or a high risk of stroke as assessed by transcranial Doppler (primary prevention). Exchange transfusions may be necessary in patients with severe or recurrent crises, or before emergency surgery. Red cells for transfusion should be matched for Rhesus (Rh) and Kell blood groups to minimize the risk of alloimmunization, which arises from the ethnic mismatch between blood donors and recipients. Ideally, patients requiring long-term transfusion, such as those with sickle cell anaemia and thalassaemia, should undergo molecular blood group typing before their first transfusion.

Hydroxycarbamide (hydroxyurea) has been widely used as therapy for sickle cell anaemia. It acts, at least in part, by increasing HbF concentrations. Hydroxycarbamide has been shown in trials to reduce the episodes of pain, the acute chest syndrome and the need for blood transfusions. Whereas, initially, only selected patients were offered hydroxycarbamide treatment, it is now offered to almost all patients with sickle cell disease from the age of 12 months. It has been shown to be safe and effective, and probably reduces long-term complications such as renal dysfunction. Blood counts must be carefully monitored to detect the development of neutropenia, which is a side-effect of the treatment.

Stem cell transplantation has been used to treat sickle cell anaemia, although in lower numbers than for thalassaemia. Children and adolescents younger than 16 years of age, who have severe complications (strokes, recurrent chest syndrome or refractory pain) and have an HLA-matched donor, are the best candidates for transplantation.

Counselling

A multidisciplinary team should be involved, with regular clinic appointments to build up relationships. Adolescents require careful counselling over psychosocial issues and drug and birth control.

Prognosis

Some patients with HbSS die in the first few years of life from either infection or episodes of sequestration. However, there is marked individual variation in severity of disease and some

---

Box 16.13 Complications of sickle cell disease requiring inpatient management

- Pain – uncontrolled by non-opiate analgesia
- Swollen, painful joints
- Acute sickle chest syndrome or pneumonia
- Mesenteric sickling and bowel ischaemia
- Splenic or hepatic sequestration

- Central nervous system deficit
- Cholecystitis (pigment stones)
- Cardiac arrhythmias
- Renal papillary necrosis resulting in colic or severe haematuria
- Hyphaema and retinal detachment
- Priapism

Box 16.14 Management of acute painful crisis in opioid-naive adults with sickle cell disease

Morphine/diamorphine
- 0.1 mg/kg i.v./s.c. every 20 min until pain controlled
- *Then* 0.05–0.1 mg/kg i.v./s.c. (or oral morphine) every 2–4 h

Patient-controlled analgesia (PCA)
Example for adults >50 kg

Diamorphine/morphine
- Continuous infusion: 0–10 mg/h
- PCA bolus dose: 2–10 mg
- Dose duration: 1 min
- Lockout time: 20–30 min

Adjuvant oral analgesia
- Paracetamol 1 g 6-hourly
- ± Ibuprofen[a] 400 mg 8-hourly
- *Or* diclofenac[a] 50 mg 8-hourly

Laxatives (all patients)
For example:
- Lactulose 10 mL × 2 daily
- Senna 2–4 tablets daily
- Sodium docusate 100 mg × 2 daily

- Macrogol 1 sachet daily
- Lubiprostone

Other adjuvants

Antipruritics
- Hydroxyzine 25 mg × 2 as required

Antiemetics
- Prochlorperazine 5–10 mg × 3 as required
- Cyclizine 50 mg × 3 as required

Anxiolytic
- Haloperidol 1–3 mg oral/i.m. × 2 as required

[a]Caution advised with non-steroidal anti-inflammatory drugs in renal impairment.
(Adapted from Rees DC, Olujohungbe AD, Parker NE et al. Guidelines for the management of the acute painful crisis in sickle cell disease. Br J Haematol 2003; 120:744–752.)

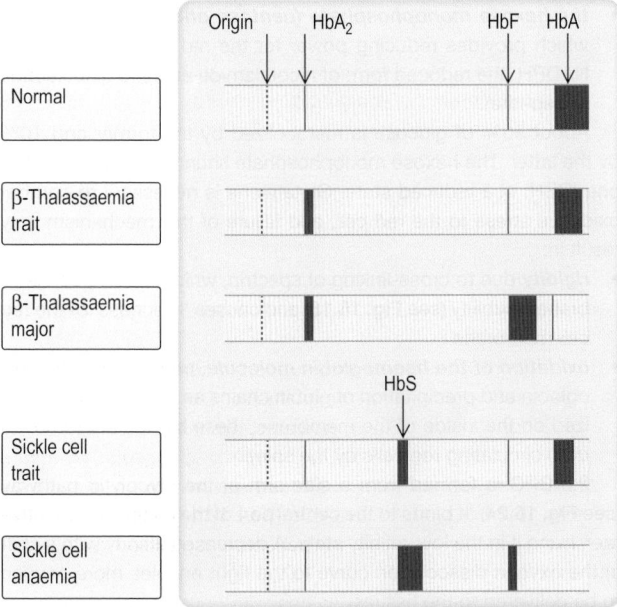

Fig. 16.23 Patterns of haemoglobin electrophoresis.

patients have a relatively normal lifespan with few complications. In most, length and quality of life are adversely affected and regular monitoring is important to prevent long-term complications.

Sickle cell trait

These individuals have no symptoms unless extreme circumstances cause anoxia, such as flying in a non-pressurized aircraft. At a population level, sickle cell trait gives some protection against *Plasmodium falciparum* malaria (see p. 564), and consequently the sickle gene has been seen as an example of a balanced polymorphism (where the advantage of the malaria protection in the heterozygote is balanced by the mortality of the homozygous condition). However, for an individual, the presence of sickle cell trait does not obviate the need for antimalarial prophylaxis. Typically, there is 60% HbA and 40% HbS. It should be emphasized that, unlike with thalassaemia trait, the blood count and film of a person with sickle cell trait are normal. The diagnosis is made by a positive sickle test or by haemoglobin electrophoresis (see **Fig. 16.23**).

Other structural globin chain defects

There are very many haemoglobin variants and most are not associated with any clinical manifestations. However, some haemoglobin variants may interact with HbS: for example, compound heterozygosity for HbC and HbS gives rise to HbSC disease. The clinical course of HbSC disease is generally somewhat milder than that of HbSS disease, but there is an increased likelihood of retinopathy and thrombosis, which may lead to thrombosis in pregnancy.

Combined defects of globin chain production and structure

Abnormalities of haemoglobin structure (e.g. HbS, C) can occur in combination with thalassaemia. The combination of β-thalassaemia trait and sickle cell trait (sickle cell β-thalassaemia) resembles sickle cell anaemia (HbSS) clinically.

HbE ($\alpha_2\beta_2^{26glu \rightarrow lys}$) is the most common haemoglobin variant in South-east Asia and the second most prevalent haemoglobin variant worldwide. HbE heterozygotes are asymptomatic; the haemoglobin level is normal but red cells are microcytic. Homozygous HbE causes a mild microcytic anaemia, but the combination of heterozygosity for HbE and β-thalassaemia produces a variable anaemia, which can be as severe as TDT (β-thalassaemia major).

Prenatal screening and diagnosis of severe haemoglobin abnormalities

Of the offspring of parents who both have either β-thalassaemia or sickle cell trait, 25% will have TDT or sickle cell anaemia, respectively. Recognition of these heterozygous states in parent and family counselling provides a basis for antenatal screening and diagnosis (see p. 17).

Pregnant women with either sickle cell trait or thalassaemia trait must be identified at antenatal booking either by selective screening of high-risk groups on the basis of ethnic origin or by universal screening of all pregnant women. Beta-thalassaemia trait can always be detected by a low MCV and MCH, and confirmed by haemoglobin electrophoresis. However, sickle cell trait is undetectable from a blood count and the laboratory needs a specific request to screen for sickle cell trait. Clearly, universal antenatal screening avoids such problems.

If a pregnant woman is found to have a haemoglobin defect, her partner should be tested. Antenatal diagnosis is offered if both are affected, as there is a risk of a severe fetal haemoglobin defect, particularly TDT. Fetal DNA analysis can be carried out using amniotic fluid, chorionic villus or fetal blood samples. Termination of pregnancy is discussed if the fetus is found to be severely affected. Chorionic villus biopsy has the advantage that it can be carried out in the first trimester, thus avoiding the need for second-trimester terminations.

Further reading

Qureshi A, Kaya B, Pancham S et al. Guideleines for the use of hydroxycarbamide in children and adults with sickle cell disease. *Br J Haematol* 2018; 181:460–475.
Rees DC, Williams TN, Gladwin MT. Sickle-cell disease. *Lancet* 2010; 376: 2018–2031.
Vichinsky E. Chronic organ failure in adult sickle cell disease. *Hematology* 2017; 2017:435–439.
Yawn BP, Buchanan GR, Afenyi-Annan AN et al. Management of sickle cell disease. *JAMA* 2014; 312:1033–1048.

Metabolic disorders of the red cell

Red cell metabolism

The mature red cell has no nucleus, mitochondria or ribosomes and is therefore unable to synthesize proteins. Red cells have only limited enzyme systems but they maintain the viability and function of the cells. In particular, energy is required in the form of ATP for maintenance of the flexibility of the membrane and the biconcave shape of the cells to allow passage through small vessels, and for regulation of the sodium and potassium pumps to ensure osmotic equilibrium. In addition, it is essential for haemoglobin to be maintained in the reduced state.

The enzyme systems responsible for producing energy and reducing power (**Fig. 16.24**) are:

- *the glycolytic (Embden–Meyerhof) pathway*, in which glucose is metabolized to pyruvate and lactic acid with production of ATP
- *the hexose monophosphate (pentose phosphate) pathway*, which provides reducing power for the red cell in the form of NADPH (the reduced form of nicotinamide adenine dinucleotide phosphate).

About 90% of glucose is metabolized by the former and 10% by the latter. The hexose monophosphate shunt maintains glutathione (GSH) in a reduced state. Glutathione is necessary to combat oxidative stress to the red cell, and failure of this mechanism may result in:

- *rigidity* due to cross-linking of spectrin, which decreases membrane flexibility (see **Fig. 16.15**) and causes 'leakiness' of the red cell membrane
- *oxidation of the haemoglobin molecule*, producing methaemoglobin and precipitation of globin chains as Heinz bodies localized on the inside of the membrane; these bodies are removed from circulating red cells by the spleen.

2,3-BPG is formed from a side-arm of the glycolytic pathway (see **Fig. 16.24**). It binds to the central part of the haemoglobin tetramer, fixing it in the low-affinity state. A decreased affinity with a shift in the oxygen dissociation curve to the right enables more oxygen to be delivered to the tissues.

In addition to the G6PD, pyruvate kinase and pyrimidine 5′ nucleotidase deficiencies described here, there are a number of rare enzyme deficiencies that need specialist investigation.

Glucose-6-phosphate dehydrogenase deficiency

The glucose-6-phosphate dehydrogenase (G6PD) enzyme occupies a vital position in the hexose monophosphate shunt (see **Fig.** 16.24), oxidizing glucose-6-phosphate to 6-phosphoglycerate with the reduction of NADP to NADPH. The reaction is necessary in red cells where it is the only source of NADPH, which is used via glutathione to protect the red cell from oxidative damage. G6PD deficiency is a common condition that presents with a haemolytic anaemia and affects millions of people throughout the world, particularly in Africa, around the Mediterranean, and in the Middle East (around 20%) and South-east Asia (up to 40% in some regions).

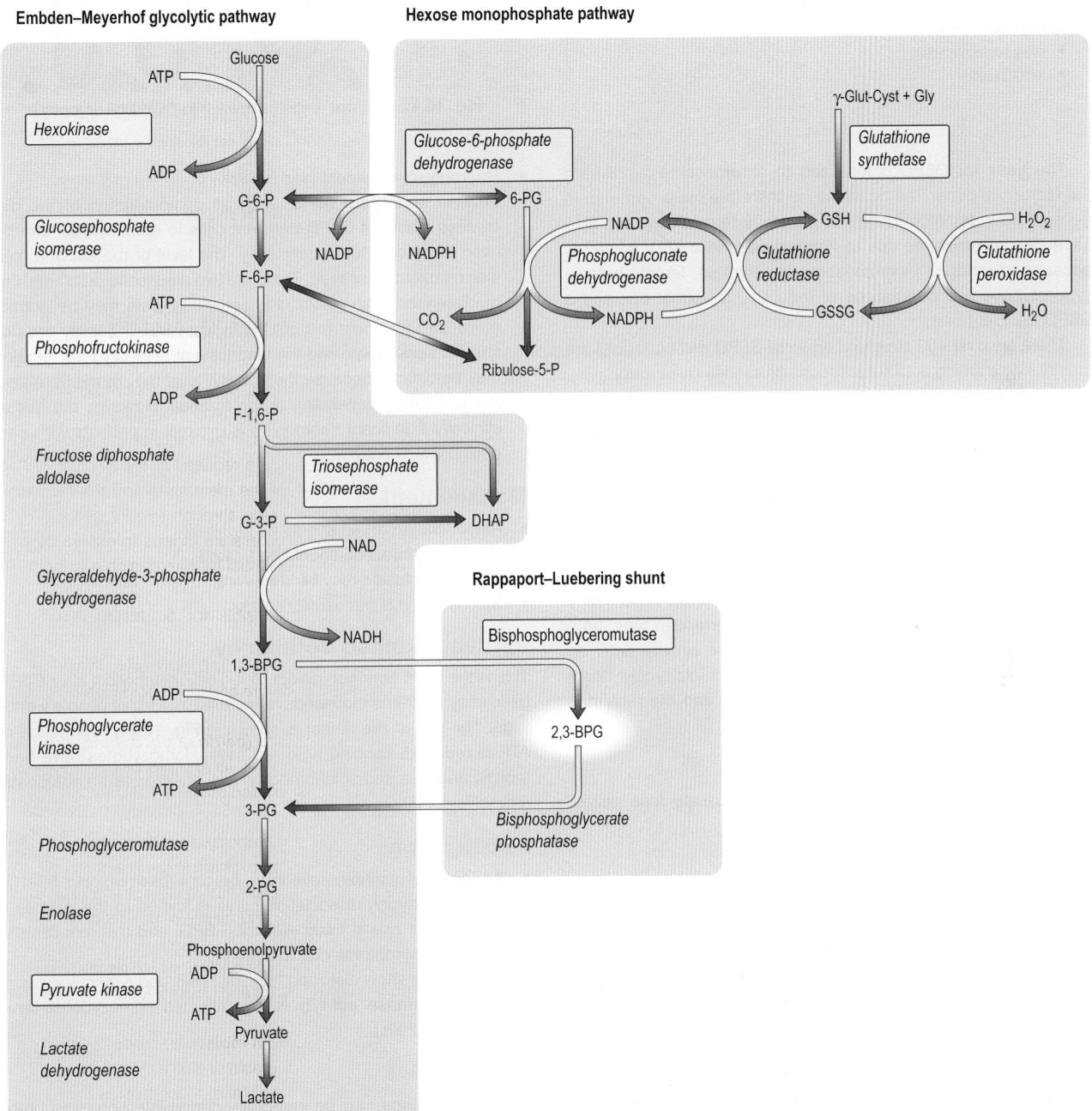

Fig. 16.24 Glucose metabolism pathways. The enzymes in green boxes indicate documented hereditary deficiency diseases. ADP, adenosine diphosphate; ATP, adenosine triphosphate; BPG, bisphosphoglycerate; DHAP, dihydroxyacetone phosphate; F, fructose; G, glucose; GSH, reduced glutathione; GSSG, oxidized glutathione; NADH, reduced nicotinamide adenine dinucleotide; NADP, nicotinamide adenine dinucleotide phosphate; NADPH, reduced NADP; P, phosphate; PG, phosphoglycerate.

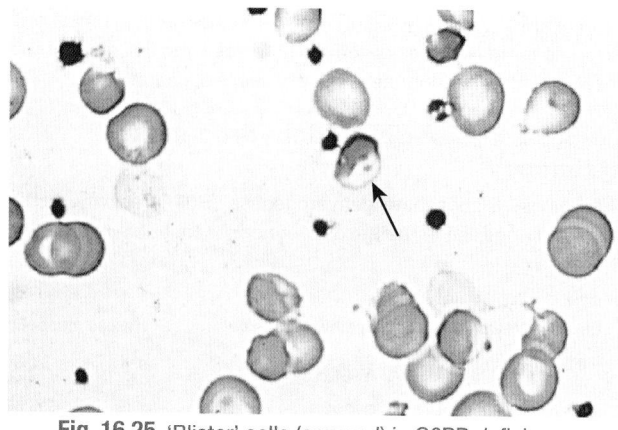

Fig. 16.25 'Blister' cells (arrowed) in G6PD deficiency.

The gene for G6PD is localized to chromosome Xq28 near the factor VIII gene. The deficiency is therefore more common in males than in females. However, female heterozygotes can also have clinical problems due to lyonization (see p. 21), whereby, because of random X-chromosome inactivation, female heterozygotes have two populations of red cells: a normal one and a G6PD-deficient one.

There are over 400 structural types of G6PD and mutations are mostly single amino acid substitutions (missense point mutations). The World Health Organization (WHO) has classified variants by the degree of enzyme deficiency and severity of haemolysis. The most common ones with normal activity are called type B+, which is present in almost all Caucasians and about 70% of black Africans, and type A+, which is present in about 20% of black Africans. There are many variants with reduced activity but only two are common. In the African or A− type, the degree of deficiency is mild and more marked in older cells. Haemolysis is self-limiting, as the young red cells newly produced by the bone marrow have nearly normal enzyme activity. However, in the Mediterranean type, both young and old red cells have very low enzyme activity. After an oxidant shock, the haemoglobin level may fall precipitously; death may follow unless the condition is recognized and the patient is transfused urgently.

Clinical syndromes

- Acute drug-induced haemolysis (**Box 16.15**) – usually dose-related.
- Favism (ingestion of fava beans).
- Chronic haemolytic anaemia.
- Neonatal jaundice.
- Infections and acute illnesses – also precipitate haemolysis in patients with G6PD deficiency.
  Mothballs containing naphthalene can also cause haemolysis.

The clinical features are due to rapid intravascular haemolysis with symptoms of anaemia, jaundice and haemoglobinuria.

Investigations

- **Blood count** is normal between attacks.
- **During an attack**, the blood film may show irregularly contracted cells, bite cells (cells with an indentation in the membrane), blister cells (cells in which the haemoglobin appears to have become partially detached from the cell membrane, **Fig. 16.25**), Heinz bodies (red cell inclusions composed of denatured haemoglobin, best seen on films stained with methyl violet) and reticulocytosis.

- **Haemolysis** is evident (see p. 338).
- **Several screening tests**, such as demonstration of the decreased ability of G6PD-deficient cells to reduce dyes, can be used to detect G6PD deficiency. The level of the enzyme may also be directly assayed. There are two diagnostic problems: immediately after an attack, the screening tests may be normal (because the oldest red cells with least 6GPD activity are destroyed selectively); and the diagnosis of heterozygous females may be difficult because the enzyme level may range from very low to normal, depending on Lyonization. However, the risk of clinically significant haemolysis is minimal in patients with borderline G6PD activity.

Management

- Any offending drugs should be stopped.
- Underlying infection should be treated.
- Blood transfusion may be life-saving.
- Splenectomy is not usually helpful.

Pyruvate kinase deficiency

This is the most common defect of red cell metabolism after G6PD deficiency; it affects thousands rather than millions of people worldwide. The site of the defect is shown in **Fig. 16.24**. Production of ATP is reduced, causing rigid red cells. Homozygotes have haemolytic anaemia and splenomegaly. It is inherited as an autosomal recessive condition.

Investigations

- **Anaemia** of variable severity is present (haemoglobin 50–100 g/L). The oxygen dissociation curve is shifted to the right as a result of the rise in intracellular 2,3-BPG, and this reduces the severity of symptoms due to anaemia.
- **Blood films** show distorted ('prickle') cells and a reticulocytosis.
- **Pyruvate kinase activity** is low (affected homozygotes have levels of 5–20%).

Management

Blood transfusions may be necessary during infections and pregnancy. Splenectomy may improve the clinical condition and is usually advised for patients requiring frequent transfusions.

Pyrimidine 5′ nucleotidase deficiency

This autosomal recessive disorder produces a haemolytic anaemia with basophilic stippling of the red cells. The enzyme degrades

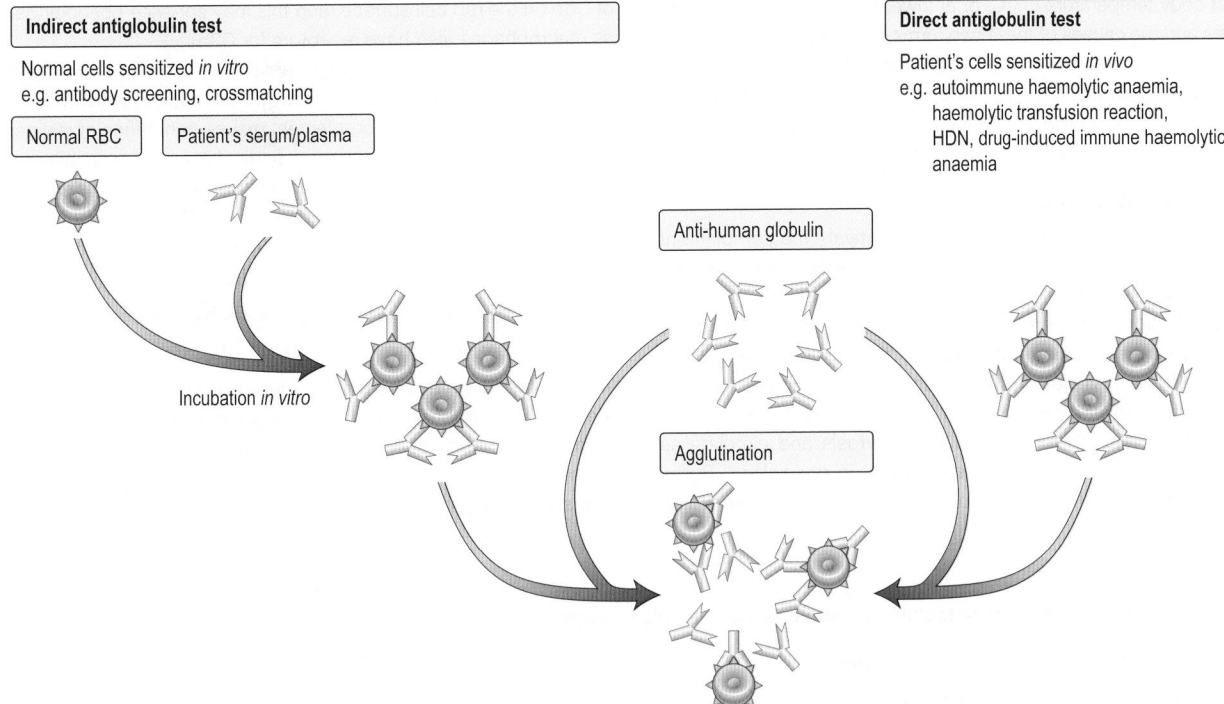

Fig. 16.26 Antiglobulin (Coombs') tests. The anti-human globulin forms bridges between the sensitized cells, causing visible agglutination. The direct test detects patients' cells sensitized *in vivo*. The indirect test detects normal cells sensitized *in vitro*. HDN, haemolytic disease of newborn; RBC, red blood cell.

pyrimidine nucleotides to cytidine and uridine (pentose phosphate shunt), which in turn leads to the degradation of RNA in the reticulocytes. Lack of the enzyme results in accumulation of partially degraded RNA, which shows as basophilic stippling in mature red cells. The enzyme is also inhibited by lead, and thus basophilic stippling is seen in lead poisoning (see p. 274). The hereditary form can be diagnosed by measuring the enzyme in erythrocytes. A screening test using the ultraviolet absorption spectrum of red cells is available.

Further reading

Grace RF, Glader B. Red blood cell enzyme disorders. *Pediatr Clin North Am* 2018; 65:579–595.

ACQUIRED HAEMOLYTIC ANAEMIA

These anaemias may be divided into those that have immune, non-immune or other causes (see **Box 16.9**).

Aetiology
Causes of immune destruction of red cells
- Autoantibodies.
- Drug-induced antibodies.
- Alloantibodies.

Causes of non-immune destruction of red cells
- Acquired membrane defects (e.g. paroxysmal nocturnal haemoglobinuria; see p. 353).
- Mechanical factors (e.g. prosthetic heart valves or microangiopathic haemolytic anaemia; see p. 355).

- Secondary to systemic disease (e.g. renal and liver disease).

Miscellaneous causes
- Various toxic substances can disrupt the red cell membrane and cause haemolysis (e.g. arsenic, and toxins produced by *Clostridium perfringens* (*welchii*)).
- Malaria frequently causes anaemia owing to the combination of a reduction in red cell survival and reduced production of red cells.
- Hypersplenism (see p. 356) results in reduced red cell survival, which may also contribute to the anaemia seen in malaria.
- Extensive burns lead to denaturation of red cell membrane proteins and reduced red cell survival.
- Some drugs (e.g. dapsone, sulfasalazine) cause oxidative haemolysis with Heinz bodies.
- Some ingested chemicals (e.g. weedkillers such as sodium chlorate) can cause severe oxidative haemolysis leading to acute kidney injury.

Autoimmune haemolytic anaemias

Autoimmune haemolytic anaemias (AIHAs) are acquired disorders resulting from increased red cell destruction due to red cell autoantibodies. These anaemias are characterized by the presence of a positive direct antiglobulin (Coombs') test, which detects the autoantibody on the surface of the patient's red cells (**Fig. 16.26**).

AIHA is divided into 'warm' (65%), 'cold' (30%) and mixed (5%) types, depending on whether the antibody attaches better to the red cells at body temperature (37°C) or at lower temperatures. The major features and the causes of these two forms of AIHA are shown in **Box 16.16**. In warm AIHA, IgG antibodies predominate and the direct antiglobulin test is positive with IgG alone, IgG and complement, or complement only. In cold AIHA, the antibodies are usually IgM. They easily elute off red cells, leaving complement, which is detected as C3d.

Immune destruction of red cells

IgM or IgG red cell antibodies, which fully activate the complement cascade, cause lysis of red cells in the circulation (intravascular haemolysis).

IgG antibodies frequently do not activate complement and the coated red cells undergo extravascular haemolysis (**Fig. 16.27**). They either are completely phagocytosed in the spleen through an interaction with Fc receptors on macrophages, or lose part of the cell membrane through partial phagocytosis and circulate as spherocytes until they become sequestered in the spleen. Some IgG antibodies partially activate complement, leading to deposition of C3b on the red cell surface, and this may enhance phagocytosis, as macrophages also have receptors for C3b.

Non-complement-binding IgM antibodies are rare and have little or no effect on red cell survival. IgM antibodies, which partially rather than fully activate complement, cause adherence of red cells to C3b receptors on macrophages, particularly in the liver, although this is an ineffective mechanism of haemolysis. Most of the red cells are released from the macrophages when C3b is cleaved to C3d, and then circulate with C3d on their surface.

'Warm' autoimmune haemolytic anaemias
Clinical features

These anaemias may occur at all ages and in both sexes, although they are most frequent in middle-aged females. They can present as a short episode of anaemia and jaundice but they often remit and relapse, and may progress to an intermittent chronic pattern. The spleen may be palpable. Infections or folate deficiency may

---

i **Box 16.16 Causes and major features of autoimmune haemolytic anaemias**

	Warm	Cold
Temperature at which antibody attaches best to red cells	37°C	Lower than 37°C
Type of antibody	IgG	IgM
Direct Coombs' test	Strongly positive	Positive
Causes of primary condition	Idiopathic	Idiopathic

Causes of secondary condition	Autoimmune
	   rheumatic disorders, e.g. systemic lupus
	   erythematosus
	Chronic lymphocytic leukaemia
	Lymphomas
	Hodgkin lymphoma
	Carcinomas
	Drugs: many, including methyldopa, penicillins,
	   cephalosporins, non-steroidal anti-inflammatory
	   drugs, quinine, interferon
		Infections, e.g. infectious mononucleosis,
		   Mycoplasma pneumoniae, other viral
		   infections (rare)
		Lymphomas
		Paroxysmal cold haemoglobinuria (IgG)

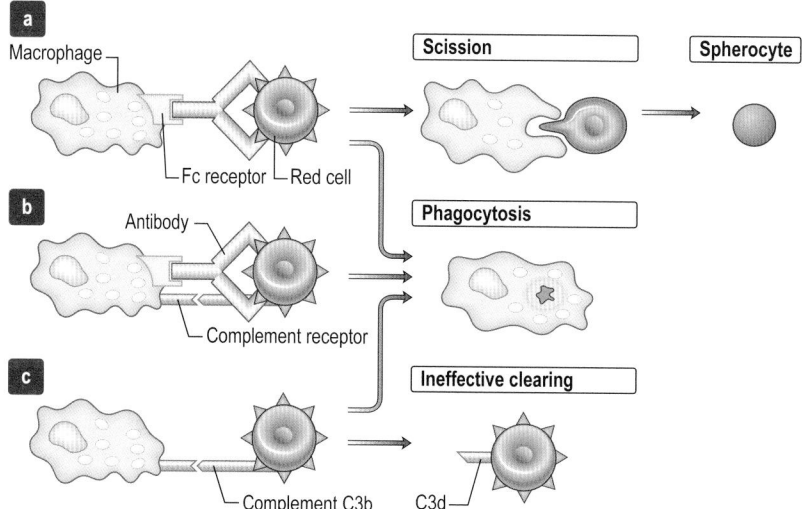

Fig. 16.27 Extravascular haemolysis. This is due to interaction of antibody-coated cells with cells in the reticuloendothelial system, predominantly in the spleen. **(a)** Spherocytosis results from partial phagocytosis. **(b)** Complete phagocytosis may occur and is enhanced if there is complement as well as antibody on the cell surface. **(c)** Cells coated with complement only are ineffectively removed and circulate with C3d or C3b on their surface.

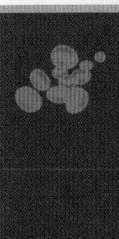

provoke a profound fall in the haemoglobin level. AIHAs are primary (50%) or secondary to an associated disorder (50%). The most common underlying cause is a lymphoproliferative disorder (see **Box 16.16**).

Investigations

- *Haemolytic anaemia* is evident (see p. 338).
- *Spherocytosis* is present as a result of red cell damage.
- *Direct antiglobulin test* is positive, with either IgG alone (35%), IgG and complement (56%), or complement alone (9%) being found on the surface of the red cells.
- *Autoantibodies* may have specificity for the Rh blood group system (e.g. for the e antigen).
- *Autoimmune thrombocytopenia* and/or neutropenia may also be present (*Evans syndrome*; see p. 373).
- *Abdominal CT scan* should be carried out to detect abdominal lymphoma.

Management and prognosis

Corticosteroids (e.g. prednisolone in a dose of 1 mg/kg daily) are effective in inducing a remission in about 80% of patients. Steroids reduce both production of the red cell autoantibodies and destruction of antibody-coated cells. Splenectomy is the most effective second-line therapy, but many patients prefer to avoid it because of the lack of a guaranteed successful outcome, its potential complications and the need to take antibiotic prophylaxis (see p. 357). Rituximab is effective in patients who fail to respond to steroids. Blood transfusion may be necessary if there is severe anaemia, although compatibility testing is complicated by the presence of red cell autoantibodies.

'Cold' autoimmune haemolytic anaemias

Low titres of IgM cold agglutinins reacting at 4°C are normally present in plasma and are harmless. At low temperatures, these antibodies can attach to red cells and cause their agglutination in the cold peripheries of the body. In addition, activation of complement may cause intravascular haemolysis when the cells return to the higher temperatures in the core of the body.

After certain infections (such as those caused by mycoplasma, cytomegalovirus or Epstein–Barr virus (EBV)), increased production of polyclonal cold agglutinins may occur, producing a mild to moderate transient haemolysis.

Chronic cold haemagglutinin disease

Chronic cold haemagglutinin disease (CHAD) usually occurs in the elderly, with a gradual onset of haemolytic anaemia owing to the production of monoclonal IgM cold agglutinins. After exposure to cold, the patient develops an acrocyanosis similar to Raynaud's as a result of red cell autoagglutination.

Investigations

- *Red cells* agglutinate in the cold or at room temperature. Agglutination is sometimes seen in the sample tube after cooling but is more easily observed on a peripheral blood film made at room temperature. The agglutination is reversible after warming the sample. The agglutination may cause a spurious increase in the MCV (see p. 324).
- *Cold agglutinin test* demonstrates a markedly elevated titre in CHAD to more than 1:512.
- *Direct antiglobulin test* is positive with complement (C3d) alone.
- *Monoclonal IgM antibodies* have specificity for the Ii blood group system, usually for the I antigen but occasionally for the i antigen.

Management

Any underlying cause should be treated, if possible. Patients should avoid exposure to cold. Steroids, alkylating agents (chemotherapy) and splenectomy are usually ineffective. Treatment with anti-CD20 (rituximab) has been successful in some cases. Blood transfusion may be necessary, and if so, the patient should be in a warm environment; compatibility testing may be difficult due to the cold agglutinin.

Paroxysmal cold haemoglobinuria

Paroxysmal cold haemoglobinuria (PCH) is a rare condition associated with common childhood infections, such as measles, mumps and chickenpox. Intravascular haemolysis is associated with polyclonal IgG complement-fixing antibodies. These antibodies are biphasic, reacting with red cells in the cold in the peripheral circulation, with lysis occurring due to complement activation when the cells return to the central circulation. The antibodies have specificity for the P red cell antigen. The lytic reaction is demonstrated *in vitro* by incubating the patient's red cells and serum at 4°C and then warming the mixture to 37°C (Donath–Landsteiner test). Haemolysis is self-limiting but red cell transfusions may be necessary.

Drug-induced immune haemolytic anaemia

Drug-induced immune haemolytic anaemias are rare, although over 100 drugs have been reported to cause immune haemolytic anaemia.

Testing for drug-dependent red cell antibodies is not routinely available, and rechallenge with the drug to confirm the diagnosis of drug-induced immune haemolytic anaemia is not advisable. Confirmation of the diagnosis requires:

- a temporal association between administration of a drug and haemolytic anaemia
- a positive direct antiglobulin test
- recovery after withdrawal of the drug.

Further reading

Hill QA, Stamps R, Massey E et al on behalf of the British Society for Haematology. The diagnosis and management of primary autoimmune haemolytic anaemia. *Br J Haem* 2017; 176:395–411.
Hill QA, Stamps R, Massey E et al on behalf of the British Society for Haematology. Guidelines on the management of drug-induced immune and secondary autoimmune haemolytic anaemia. *Br J Haem* 2017; 177:208–220.

Alloimmune haemolytic anaemia

Antibodies produced in one individual react with the red cells of another. This situation occurs in haemolytic disease of the newborn, in haemolytic transfusion reactions (see p. 360), and after allogeneic bone marrow, renal, liver, cardiac or intestinal transplantation when donor lymphocytes transferred in the allograft ('passenger lymphocytes') may produce red cell antibodies against the recipient and cause haemolytic anaemia.

Haemolytic disease of the newborn

Haemolytic disease of the newborn (HDN) is caused by fetomaternal incompatibility for red cell antigens. Maternal alloantibodies against fetal red cell antigens pass from the maternal circulation via the placenta into the fetus, where they destroy the fetal red cells. Only IgG antibodies are capable of transplacental passage from mother to fetus.

The most common type of HDN is that due to ABO incompatibility, where the mother is usually group O and the fetus group A.

HDN due to ABO incompatibility is usually mild and exchange transfusion is rarely needed. HDN due to RhD incompatibility has become much less common in developed countries following the introduction of anti-D prophylaxis (see later). HDN may be caused by antibodies against antigens in many blood group systems (e.g. other Rh antigens such as c and E, and Kell, Duffy and Kidd; see p. 357).

Sensitization occurs as a result of passage of fetal red cells into the maternal circulation (which most readily occurs at the time of delivery), so that first pregnancies are rarely affected. However, sensitization may occur at other times – for example, after a miscarriage, ectopic pregnancy or blood transfusion – or be due to episodes during pregnancy that cause transplacental bleeding, such as amniocentesis, chorionic villus sampling and threatened miscarriage.

Clinical features

These vary from a mild haemolytic anaemia of the newborn to intrauterine death from 18 weeks' gestation with the characteristic appearance of hydrops fetalis (hepatosplenomegaly, oedema and cardiac failure).

Kernicterus occurs owing to severe jaundice in the neonatal period, when the unconjugated (lipid-soluble) bilirubin exceeds 250 μmol/L and bile pigment deposition occurs in the basal ganglia. This can result in permanent brain damage, choreoathetosis and spasticity. In mild cases, it may present as deafness.

Investigations

Routine antenatal serology

All mothers should have their ABO and RhD groups determined and tested for atypical antibodies after attending the antenatal booking clinic. These tests should be repeated at 28 weeks' gestation.

If an antibody is detected, its blood group specificity should be determined and the mother should be retested at least monthly. A rising antibody titre of IgG antibodies or a history of HDN in a previous pregnancy is an indication for referral to a fetal medicine unit.

Antenatal assessment and treatment

If a clinically significant antibody capable of causing HDN, such as anti-D, anti-c or anti-K, is detected, the father's phenotype provides useful information for predicting the likelihood of the fetus carrying the relevant red cell antigen. If the father is heterozygous, the genotype of the fetus can be determined from fetal DNA from maternal plasma.

The severity of anaemia is assessed by Doppler flow velocity of the fetal middle cerebral artery; measurement of bile pigments in the amniotic fluid is no longer routinely used. If the infant appears to have severe anaemia on non-invasive monitoring, ultrasound-guided fetal blood sampling is used to confirm this directly; if necessary, an intrauterine fetal transfusion of red cells is given.

Birth of an affected infant

A sample of cord blood is obtained at birth. This shows:
- anaemia with a high reticulocyte count
- a positive direct antiglobulin test
- a raised serum bilirubin.

Postnatal management

In mild cases, phototherapy may be used to convert bilirubin to water-soluble biliverdin, which can be excreted by the kidneys. Bilirubin levels need to be monitored and phototherapy may be needed for several days. In more severely affected cases, exchange transfusion may be necessary to replace the infant's antibody-coated red cells with normal antigen-negative red cells and to remove bilirubin. Indications for exchange transfusion include severe anaemia or a high or rapidly rising bilirubin level.

The blood used for exchange transfusions should:
- be ABO-compatible with the mother and infant
- lack the antigen against which the maternal antibody is directed
- be fresh (no more than 5 days from the day of collection)
- be irradiated to prevent transfusion-associated graft-versus-host disease (TA-GvHD) and be cytomegalovirus (CMV)-seronegative to prevent transmission of CMV.

Avoidance of exchange transfusion is beneficial because of its risks. Antenatal administration of intravenous immunoglobulin to the mother significantly reduces the need for exchange transfusion.

Prevention of RhD immunization in the mother

Anti-D should be given after delivery when all of the following conditions are fulfilled:
- The mother is RhD-negative.
- The fetus is RhD-positive.
- There is no maternal anti-D detectable in the mother's serum, i.e. the mother is not already immunized.

The dose is 500 IU of IgG anti-D intramuscularly within 72 hours of delivery. The **Kleihauer test** assesses the number of fetal cells in the maternal circulation. A blood film prepared from maternal blood is treated with acid, which elutes HbA. HbF is resistant to this treatment and can be seen when the film is stained with eosin. If large numbers of fetal red cells are present in the maternal circulation, a higher or additional dose of anti-D will be necessary.

Prophylaxis may be required by RhD-negative women at other times when sensitization may occur, such as after an ectopic pregnancy, threatened miscarriage or termination of pregnancy. The dose of anti-D is 250 IU before 20 weeks' gestation and 500 IU after 20 weeks. A Kleihauer test should be carried out after 20 weeks to determine whether more anti-D is required.

Of previously non-immunized RhD-negative women carrying RhD-positive fetuses, 1–2% became immunized by the time of delivery. Antenatal prophylaxis with anti-D has been shown to reduce the incidence of immunization during pregnancy, and its routine use has been implemented in the UK. It can be given as two doses of anti-D immunoglobulin of either 500 IU or 1500 IU (one at 28 weeks' gestation and one at 34 weeks), or as a single dose of 1500 IU either at 28 weeks' gestation or between 28 and 30 weeks. In the UK in 2016, the National Institute for Care and Health Excellence (NICE) recommended fetal D typing using maternal plasma to avoid the administration of anti-D to RhD-negative women carrying RhD-negative fetuses.

Further reading

British Committee for Standards in Haematology (BCSH). Guideline for the use of anti-D immunoglobulin for the prevention of haemolytic disease of the fetus and newborn. *Transfus Med* 2014; 24:8–20.

White J, Qureshi H, Massey E et al on behalf of the British Committee for Standards in Haematology. Guideline for blood grouping and red cell antibody testing in pregnancy. *Transfus Med* 2014; 26:246–263.

Non-immune haemolytic anaemia

Paroxysmal nocturnal haemoglobinuria

Paroxysmal nocturnal haemoglobinuria (PNH) is a rare form of haemolytic anaemia that results from the clonal expression of haemopoietic stem cells that have mutations in the X-linked gene *PIG-A*. These mutations cause impaired synthesis of glycosylphosphatidylinositol (GPI), which anchors many proteins, such as decay accelerating factor (DAF; CD55), to the cell surface, and membrane inhibitor of reactive lysis (MIRL; CD59) to cell membranes. CD55, CD59 and other proteins are involved in complement degradation (at the C3 and C5 levels), and in their absence, the haemolytic action of complement continues.

Clinical features

The major clinical signs are intravascular haemolysis, venous thrombosis and haemoglobinuria. Haemolysis may be precipitated by infection, iron therapy or surgery. Characteristically, only the urine voided at night and in the morning on waking is dark in colour, although the reason for this phenomenon is not clear. In severe cases, all urine samples are dark. Urinary iron loss may be sufficient to cause iron deficiency. Some patients present insidiously with signs of anaemia and recurrent abdominal pains.

Venous thrombotic episodes may occur at atypical sites and severe thromboses may be a feature: for example, in hepatic (Budd–Chiari syndrome), mesenteric or cerebral veins. The cause of the increased predisposition to thrombosis is not known, but may be complement-mediated activation of platelets deficient in CD55 and CD59. Another suggestion is that intravascular haemolysis, which releases haemoglobin in the plasma, lowers plasma nitric oxide, causing the symptoms and venous thrombosis.

Investigations

- *Intravascular haemolysis* is evident (see p. 338).
- *Flow cytometric analysis* of red cells with anti-CD55 and anti-CD59 is undertaken.
- *Bone marrow* is sometimes hypoplastic (or even aplastic), despite haemolysis.

Management and prognosis

PNH is a chronic disorder requiring supportive measures such as blood transfusions, which are necessary for patients with severe anaemia. However, treatment with **eculizumab** has revolutionized therapy. The drug is administered intravenously every 7 days for the first 5 weeks, and then every 2 weeks thereafter. It is a recombinant humanized monoclonal antibody that prevents the cleavage of C5 (and therefore formation of the membrane attack complex). It reduces intravascular haemolysis, haemoglobinuria and the need for transfusion, and improves quality of life. Eculizumab also lowers the risk of thrombosis, the leading cause of mortality in PNH. It is now also being used in pregnancy. The most serious risk of terminal complement blockade is infection with *Neisseria meningitidis*; thus, vaccination against *N. meningitidis* is recommended 2 weeks before commencing treatment.

Long-term anticoagulation may be necessary acutely for patients with recurrent thrombotic episodes. Its long-term value is unclear with the use of eculizumab. In patients with bone marrow failure, treatment options include immunosuppression with antilymphocyte globulin, ciclosporin or bone marrow transplantation. Eculizumab does not alleviate bone marrow failure. Bone marrow transplantation has been successfully carried out using either HLA-matched sibling donors in patients under the age of 50 or matched unrelated donors in patients under the age of 25.

The course of PNH is variable. PNH may transform into aplastic anaemia or acute leukaemia, but may remain stable for many years and the PNH clone may even disappear, which must be taken into account if considering potentially dangerous treatments such as bone marrow transplantation. The median survival is 10–15 years.

Further reading

Brodsky RA. Paroxysmal nocturnal haemoglobinuria. *Blood* 2014; 124:2804–2811.

Mechanical haemolytic anaemia

Red cells may be injured by physical trauma in the circulation. Direct injury may cause immediate cell lysis or be followed by resealing of the cell membrane with the formation of distorted red cells or 'fragments'. These cells may circulate for a short period before being destroyed prematurely in the reticuloendothelial system.

The causes of mechanical haemolytic anaemia include:
- damaged artificial heart valves
- march haemoglobinuria, in which there is damage to red cells in the feet, associated with prolonged marching or running
- microangiopathic haemolytic anaemia (MAHA), in which fragmentation of red cells occurs in an abnormal microcirculation because of malignant hypertension, eclampsia, haemolytic uraemic syndrome, thrombotic thrombocytopenic purpura, vasculitis or disseminated intravascular coagulation.

POLYCYTHAEMIA

Polycythaemia (or erythrocytosis) is defined as an increase in haemoglobin or haematocrit (HCT). Haematocrit is a more reliable indicator of polycythaemia than haemoglobin, which may be disproportionately low in iron deficiency. Relative erythrocytosis is where the red cell volume is normal but there is a decrease in the plasma volume.

Polycythaemia can be classified as primary or secondary. Primary polycythaemia (polycythaemia vera) is a neoplastic process (see p. 394). Secondary polycythaemia can be congenital or acquired. The latter is due to either an appropriate increase in erythropoietin in response to hypoxia, or an inappropriate increase in erythropoietin associated with ectopic production by tumours, such as a renal carcinoma. The causes of polycythaemia are given in **Box 16.17**.

? Box 16.17 Causes of polycythaemia

Primary
- Polycythaemia vera

Congenital
- Mutations in erythropoietin receptor
- High-oxygen-affinity haemoglobins
- Mutations in hypoxia-sensing pathways, e.g. Chuvash polycythaemia mutation in von Hippel–Lindau gene

Secondary

Due to an appropriate (hypoxic) increase in erythropoietin
- High altitude
- Chronic lung disease
- Cardiovascular disease (right-to-left shunt)
- Sleep apnoea

- Morbid obesity
- Heavy smoking

Due to an inappropriate increase in erythropoietin
- Renal disease: renal cell carcinoma, Wilms' tumour
- Hepatocellular carcinoma
- Adrenal tumours
- Cerebellar haemangioblastoma
- Massive uterine leiomyoma
- Over-administration of erythropoietin
- Treatment with androgen preparations

Relative
- Stress or spurious polycythaemia
- Dehydration
- Burns

Secondary polycythaemias

Many high-oxygen affinity haemoglobin mutants (HOAHMs) have been described that lead to increased oxygen affinity but decreased oxygen delivery to the tissues, resulting in compensatory polycythaemia. A congenital autosomal recessive disorder (Chuvash polycythaemia) is due to a defect in the oxygen-sensing erythropoietin production pathway caused by a mutation of the von Hippel–Lindau (*VHL*) gene, resulting in an increased production of erythropoietin.

Serum erythropoietin (EPO) levels are normal or raised in secondary polycythaemia. Rarely, the discovery of a high EPO level may be a clue to the presence of an EPO-secreting tumour.

Management

Treatment is that of the precipitating factor; for example, renal or posterior fossa tumours need to be resected if possible. The most common cause is heavy smoking, which can produce as much as 10% carboxyhaemoglobin, and this can lead to polycythaemia because of a reduction in the oxygen-carrying capacity of the blood. Heavy smokers also often have respiratory disease.

Complications of secondary polycythaemia are distinct to those seen in polycythaemia vera, and although hyperviscosity symptoms and thromboembolic episodes can occur, management depends on the underlying cause. Complications due to myeloproliferative disease, such as progression to myelofibrosis or acute leukaemia, do not develop. Venesection may be symptomatically helpful in certain patients with secondary polycythaemia, particularly if the HCT is above 0.54.

'Relative' or 'apparent' polycythaemia (Gaisböck's syndrome)

This condition was originally thought to be stress-induced. The red cell volume is normal there is a relative polycythaemia, as a result of a decreased plasma volume. 'Relative' polycythaemia is more common than polycythaemia vera and occurs in middle-aged men, particularly in association with smoking, high alcohol intake, obesity and high blood pressure. The condition may present with cardiovascular problems, such as myocardial or cerebral ischaemia. For this reason, it may be justifiable to venesect selected patients. Management also requires modification of lifestyle factors, such as smoking and alcohol.

THE SPLEEN

The spleen is the largest lymphoid organ in the body and is situated in the left hypochondrium. There are two anatomical components:
- the red pulp, consisting of sinuses lined by endothelial macrophages and cords (spaces)
- the white pulp, which has a structure similar to that of lymphoid follicles.

Blood enters via the splenic artery and is delivered to the red and white pulp. During the flow the blood is 'skimmed', with leucocytes and plasma preferentially passing to white pulp. Some red cells pass rapidly through into the venous system while others are held up in the red pulp.

Function

Sequestration and phagocytosis

Normal red cells, which are flexible, pass through the red pulp into the venous system without difficulty. Old or abnormal cells are damaged by the hypoxia, low glucose and low pH found in the sinuses of the red pulp and are therefore removed by phagocytosis along with other circulating foreign matter. Howell–Jolly and Heinz bodies and sideroblastic granules have their particles removed by 'pitting' and are then returned to the circulation. IgG-coated red cells are removed through their Fc receptors by macrophages.

Extramedullary haemopoiesis

Pluripotential stem cells are present in the spleen and proliferate during severe erythroid stress, such as in haemolytic anaemia, thalassaemia major and myelofibrosis. This occurs due to the presence of anaemia, despite every available marrow cavity already being fully engaged in haemopoiesis. It is usually a feature of ineffective erythropoiesis.

Immunological function

About 25% of the body's T lymphocytes and 15% of B lymphocytes are present in the spleen. The spleen shares the function of production of antibodies with other lymphoid tissues.

Blood pooling

Up to one-third of the platelets are sequestrated in the spleen and can be rapidly mobilized. Enlarged spleens pool a significant percentage (up to 40%) of the red cell mass.

Splenomegaly

The spleen enlarges from under the left costal margin inferiorly and medially. It is dull to percussion and it may be possible to palpate a notch along its leading edge, which further differentiates the mass from an enlarged left kidney. The spleen typically measures 11 cm in its longest dimension. An enlarged spleen is only palpable if it is 1.5–2 times the size of a normal spleen. Ultrasound or CT scanning may be used to confirm splenomegaly and may also provide other useful information, such as the presence of abdominal lymphadenopathy.

Aetiology

A clinically palpable spleen can have many causes:
- *infection*:
  - acute, e.g. septic shock, infective endocarditis, typhoid, infectious mononucleosis
  - chronic, e.g. tuberculosis, brucellosis
  - parasitic, e.g. malaria, kala-azar and schistosomiasis
- *inflammation*: rheumatoid arthritis, sarcoidosis, SLE
- *haematological factors*: haemolytic anaemia, haemoglobinopathies, and the leukaemias, lymphomas and myeloproliferative disorders
- *portal hypertension*: liver disease
- *miscellaneous*: storage diseases (e.g. Gaucher's disease), amyloidosis, primary and secondary neoplasias, tropical splenomegaly.

Massive splenomegaly is seen in myelofibrosis, chronic myeloid leukaemia, chronic malaria, kala-azar or, rarely, Gaucher's disease.

Hypersplenism

This can result from splenomegaly of any cause. It is commonly seen with splenomegaly due to haematological disorders, portal hypertension, rheumatoid arthritis (Felty's syndrome) and lymphoma. Hypersplenism produces:
- pancytopenia
- haemolysis due to sequestration and destruction of red cells in the spleen
- increased plasma volume.

Management

This is often dependent on the underlying cause; splenectomy is sometimes required for severe anaemia or thrombocytopenia.

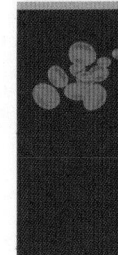

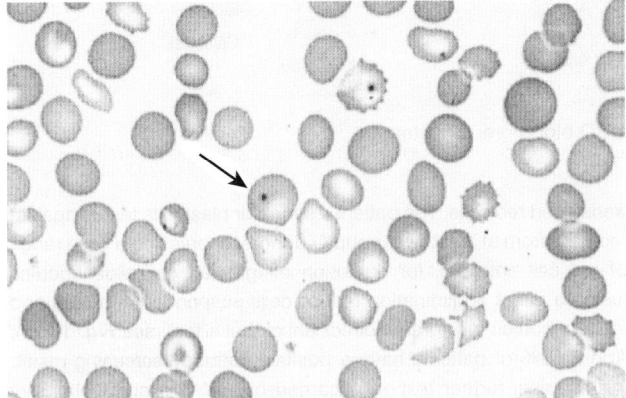

Fig. 16.28 Post-splenectomy film with Howell–Jolly bodies (arrowed). Target cells and irregularly contracted cells are also shown.

Problems after splenectomy

Splenectomy is performed mainly for:

- trauma
- immune thrombocytopenic purpura (see p.373)
- haemolytic anaemias (see p. 338)
- hypersplenism.

One immediate problem is an increased platelet count (usually 600–1000 × 10⁹/L) for 2–3 weeks. Thromboembolic phenomena may occur. In the longer term, there is an increased risk of overwhelming infections, particularly pneumococcal ones.

Prophylaxis against infection after splenectomy or splenic dysfunction

See **Box 16.18** for prophylactic measures. All patients should be educated about the risk of infection and the importance of its early recognition and treatment. They should be given an information leaflet and should carry a card or bracelet to alert health professionals to their risk of overwhelming infection.

Post-splenectomy haematological features

- **Thrombocytosis** persists in about 30% of cases.
- **WCC** is usually normal but there may be a mild lymphocytosis and monocytosis.
- **Abnormalities in red cell morphology** are the most prominent changes and include Howell–Jolly bodies (contain basophilic nuclear remnants), Pappenheimer bodies (contain sideroblastic granules), target cells and irregular contracted red cells (**Fig. 16.28**). Pitted red cells can be counted.

Splenic atrophy

This is seen in sickle cell disease due to infarction. Hyposplenism is also seen in a wide range of non-haematological diseases, including coeliac disease, dermatitis herpetiformis and, occasionally, ulcerative colitis. Post-splenectomy haematological features are seen.

Further reading

Di Sabatino A, Carsetti R, Corazza GR. Post-splenectomy and hyposlenic states. *Lancet* 2011; 378:86–97.

BLOOD TRANSFUSION

The cells and proteins in the blood express antigens that are controlled by polymorphic genes: that is, a specific antigen may be present in some individuals but not in others. A blood transfusion may immunize the recipient against donor antigens that the recipient lacks (alloimmunization), and repeated transfusions increase the risk. Similarly, the transplacental passage of fetal blood cells during pregnancy may alloimmunize the mother against fetal antigens inherited from the father. Antibodies stimulated by blood transfusion or pregnancy, such as Rh antibodies, are termed **immune antibodies** and are usually IgG, in contrast to **naturally occurring antibodies**, such as ABO antibodies, which are made in response to environmental antigens present in food and bacteria, and are usually IgM.

BLOOD GROUPS

The blood group antigens are proteins, glycoproteins or carbohydrates attached to glycoproteins on the surface of red cells; more than 300 blood groups are recognized. The ABO and Rh systems are the two major blood groups, but incompatibilities involving many other blood groups (e.g. Kell, Duffy, Kidd) may also cause haemolytic transfusion reactions and/or HDN.

ABO system

This is the most important blood group system in transfusion practice because naturally occurring IgM anti-A and anti-B antibodies are capable of producing rapid and severe intravascular haemolysis of incompatible red cells.

The ABO system is under the control of three allelic genes, *A*, *B* and *O*, producing the genotypes and phenotypes shown in **Box 16.19**.

The precursor for A and B antigens is the H antigen, which codes for an enzyme that attaches fucose to galactose on an oligosaccharide structure on the red cell membrane (**Fig. 16.29**). The *A* and *B* genes control specific enzymes responsible for the addition to H of *N*-acetylgalactosamine for group A, and ᴅ-galactose for group B. The *O* gene is amorphic and does not transform H; therefore O is

> ### Box 16.19 The ABO system: antigens and antibodies
>
> | Phenotype | Genotype | Antigens | Antibodies | Frequency UK (%) |
> |---|---|---|---|---|
> | O | OO | None | Anti-A and anti-B | 43 |
> | A | AA or AO | A | Anti-B | 45 |
> | B | BB or BO | B | Anti-A | 9 |
> | AB | AB | A and B | None | 3 |

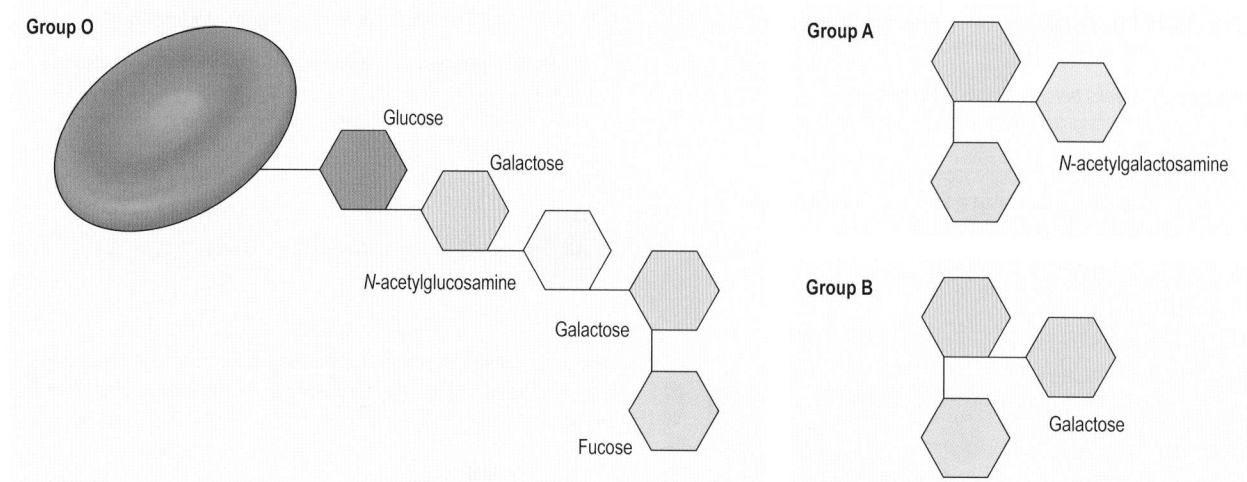

Fig. 16.29 Sugar chains in the ABO blood group system.

not antigenic. The A, B and H antigens are present on most body cells. They are also found in soluble form in tissue fluids, such as saliva and gastric juice, in the 80% of the population who possess secretor genes.

Rh system

There is a high frequency of development of IgG RhD antibodies in RhD-negative individuals after exposure to RhD-positive red cells. The antibodies formed cause HDN and haemolytic transfusion reactions.

This system is coded by allelic genes: *C* and *c*, *E* and *e*, and *D* and no *D*, signified as *d*. They are inherited as triplets on each chromosome 1, one from each pair of genes (i.e. *CDE/cde*). RhD-negative individuals have no D protein in the red cell membrane, which explains why it is so immunogenic when RhD-negative individuals are exposed to RhD antigen through transfusion or pregnancy. In Caucasians, the RhD-negative phenotype almost always results from a complete deletion of the *RhD* gene; in black Africans, it can also result from an inactive gene containing stop codons in the reading frame.

PROCEDURE FOR BLOOD TRANSFUSION IN HOSPITALS

The safety of blood transfusion in hospitals depends on meticulous attention to detail at each stage leading to and during the transfusion. Avoidance of simple errors involving patient and blood sample identification at the time of collection of the sample for compatibility testing and at the time of transfusion would avoid most serious haemolytic transfusion reactions, almost all of which involve the ABO system.

Pre-transfusion compatibility testing

Blood grouping

The ABO and RhD groups of the patient are determined.

Antibody screening

The patient's serum or plasma is screened for atypical antibodies that may cause a significant reduction in the survival of the transfused red cells. The patient's serum or plasma is tested against red cells from at least two group O donors, expressing a wide range of red cell antigens, for detection of IgM red cell alloantibodies (using a direct agglutination test of cells suspended in saline) and IgG antibodies (using an indirect antiglobulin test, see **Fig. 16.26**). About 10% of patients have a positive antibody screening result; in this case, further testing is carried out using a comprehensive panel of typed red cells to determine the blood group specificity of the antibody (clinically significant red cell antibodies are detected in about 20% of patients with positive antibody screens).

Selection of donor blood and compatibility testing

Selection procedures

Donor blood of the same ABO and RhD group as the patient is selected. Matching for additional blood groups is carried out for patients with clinically significant red cell antibodies (see later), and for patients who are likely to be multi-transfused and are at high risk of developing antibodies: for example, in sickle cell disease. Many hospitals routinely provide Kell-negative blood for women of childbearing age to minimize the risk of alloimmunization due to anti-K and subsequent HDN.

Compatibility testing procedures

Timing of sample collection

The timing of sample collection for compatibility testing must take account of pregnancy or recent transfusion, as both may stimulate antibodies that could cause a haemolytic transfusion reaction. Blood samples should be collected no more than 3 days in advance of the transfusion if the patient has been transfused or pregnant within the preceding 3 months.

Patients without atypical red cell antibodies

The full crossmatch involves testing the patient's serum or plasma against the donor red cells suspended in saline in a direct agglutination test, and also using an indirect antiglobulin test. In many hospitals this serological crossmatch is now omitted, as a negative antibody screen makes it highly unlikely that there will be any incompatibility with the donor units. Error in the collection or labelling of the patient sample or a mix-up of samples in the laboratory are much greater risks. Where the antibody screen is negative, laboratories can use their information system to check the patient records and authorize the release of ABO-compatible donor units (**computer or electronic crossmatching**).

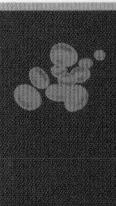

> **Box 16.20 Complications of blood transfusion**
>
> **Immunological**
>
> *Alloimmunization and incompatibility*
> - Red cells:
>   - Immediate haemolytic transfusion reactions
>   - Delayed haemolytic transfusion reactions
> - Leucocytes and platelets:
>   - Non-haemolytic (febrile) transfusion reactions
>   - Transfusion-related acute lung injury (TRALI)
>   - Poor survival of transfused platelets and granulocytes
>   - Post-transfusion purpura
>   - Transfusion-associated graft-versus-host disease (TA-GvHD)
> - Plasma proteins:
>   - Urticarial and anaphylactic reactions
>
> **Non-immunological**
>
> *Transmission of infection*
> - Viruses:
>   - HAV, HBV, HCV, HEV
>   - HIV
>   - CMV, HTLV-1, West Nile virus, Dengue, Zika
> - Parasites:
>   - Malaria, trypanosomiasis, babesia
> - Bacteria
> - Prions
>
> *Transfusion-associated circulatory overload (TACO)*
>
> *Iron overload*
> - Due to multiple transfusions (see p. 343)
>
> *Bleeding and electrolyte changes*
> - May be caused by massive transfusion of stored blood
>
> CMV, cytomegalovirus; HAV/HBV/HCV/HEV, hepatitis A/B/C/E virus; HIV, human immunodeficiency virus; HTLV-1, human T-cell leukaemia (or lymphotropic) virus 1; WNV, West Nile virus.

Electronic issue can be extended to previously unallocated blood at fridges remote from the main laboratory ('*remote blood issue*'). This is only possible using blood fridges that are electronically linked to the blood transfusion laboratory information system. The printing of compatibility labels for the blood and its collection are under electronic control, applying the same rules as electronic issue from the main laboratory. Issue of blood using this process reduces the time it takes to provide blood for patients needing it urgently, particularly at hospitals without a blood transfusion laboratory, because transport of blood from the central laboratory is not required. There are good examples of centralized transfusion services in cities such as Oxford in the UK, and Pittsburgh and Seattle in the USA, and this model is likely to be increasingly employed in the future.

Patients with atypical red cell antibodies

Donor blood should be selected that lacks the relevant red cell antigen(s), as well as being of the same ABO and RhD group as the patient. A full crossmatch should always be carried out in case new antibodies have developed.

Several other systems for blood grouping, antibody screening and crossmatching are available to hospital transfusion laboratories. They do not depend on agglutination of red cells in suspension, but rather on the differential passage of agglutinated and unagglutinated red cells through a column of dextran gel matrix (e.g. DiaMed and Ortho Biovue systems), or on the capture of antibodies by red cells immobilized on the surface of a microplate well (e.g. Capture-R solid phase system).

Blood ordering

Hospitals are increasingly relying on electronic systems for blood ordering; some include algorithms for the appropriate use of blood, with 'alerts' if there is non-compliance with agreed blood count triggers for transfusion. Electronic systems also provide the tools for feedback of comparative data on blood use to clinical teams and for the improved documentation of consent to transfusion.

Elective surgery

Many hospitals have guidelines for the ordering of blood for elective surgery (maximum surgical blood ordering schedules). These are aimed at reducing unnecessary crossmatching, which increases the risk of blood eventually becoming outdated and wasted. Many operations in which blood is required only occasionally for unexpectedly high blood loss can be classified as '*group and save*'; this means that, where the antibody screen is negative, blood is not reserved in advance but can be made available quickly if necessary – that is, in a few minutes – using the electronic crossmatch procedure described. If a patient has atypical antibodies, and is undergoing any procedure or surgery that may result in the need for transfusion, compatible blood should always be reserved in advance; this may take several days if the patient has multiple or unusual antibodies.

Emergencies

There may be insufficient time for full pre-transfusion testing. The options include:
- Blood required immediately – 2 units of O RhD-negative blood ('*emergency stock*') are used, to allow additional time for the laboratory to group the patient.
- Blood required in 10–15 min – blood of the same ABO and RhD groups as the patient is used ('*group compatible blood*').
- Blood required in 45 min – most laboratories will be able to provide fully crossmatched blood within this time.

COMPLICATIONS OF BLOOD TRANSFUSION

Reporting schemes under the term '*haemovigilance*' have been established in many countries, including the Serious Hazards of Transfusion (SHOT) scheme in the UK, which produced its first report in 1997. SHOT reported 136 deaths due to blood transfusion between 2010 and 2017, of which 54% were due to pulmonary complications: predominantly transfusion-associated circulatory overload (TACO; **Box 16.20**). Delays in transfusion were thought to be responsible for 23% of deaths, and other complications of transfusion for the remainder. **Fig. 16.30** shows data from the SHOT reports indicating that '*incorrect blood component transfused*' is the most frequent type of serious incident; it may result in mortality or serious morbidity, although it is not the most frequent cause of morbidity and mortality. Errors in clinical areas, in either the collection of the blood sample for compatibility testing, the collection of blood from the fridge and/or the administration of blood, are more frequent than laboratory errors.

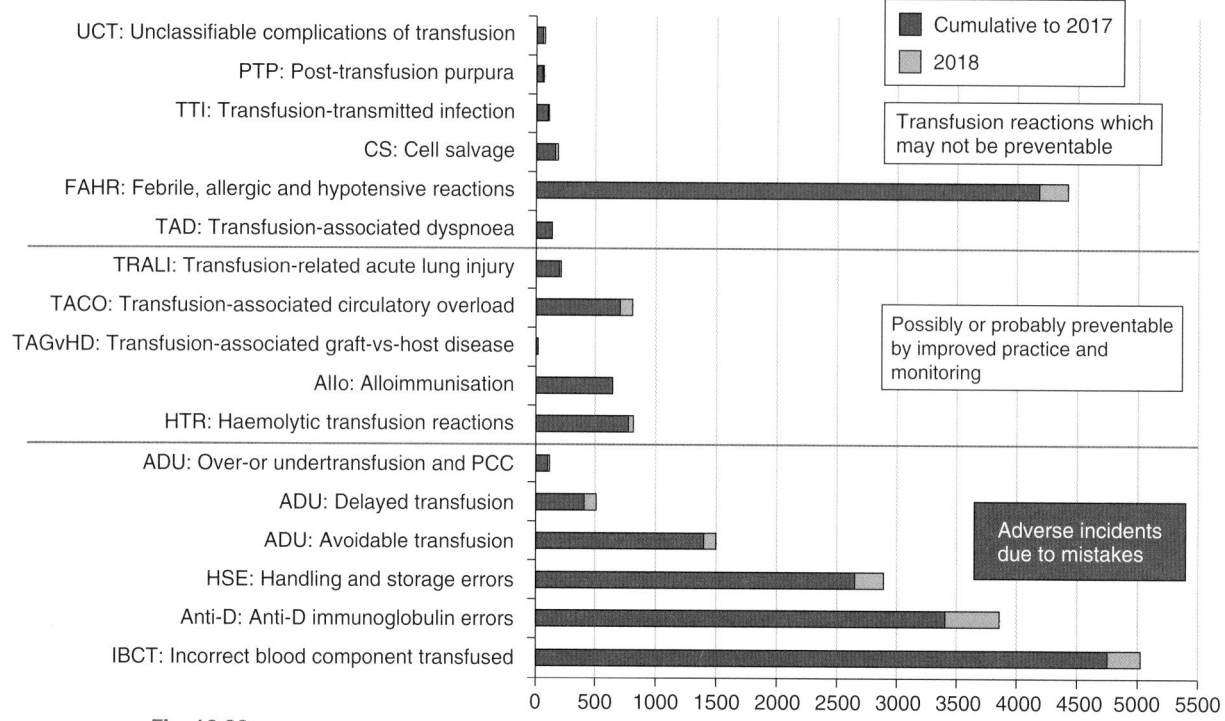

Fig. 16.30 Cumulative data for SHOT categories 1996 to 2017 n=19815. The adverse events are divided into transfusion reactions that may not be preventable, those that are probably or possibly preventable, and those caused by mistakes. Those reported in 2018 are indicated in blue at the right-hand side of each bar. PCC, Prothrombin complex concentrates. *(From S Narayan (ed.). D Poles et al. On behalf of the Serious Hazards of Transfusion (SHOT) Steering Group. The 2018 Annual SHOT Report (2019).)*

Prevention of wrong blood transfusions

The potentially serious consequences of errors in transfusion emphasize the need for meticulous procedures. Good training of staff is essential, and regular reviews of practice to ensure compliance with standard procedures are also required. New approaches include the use of barcode patient identification and new technology at the bedside. Handheld devices can prompt staff through the key steps and check that the barcode on the patient's wristband matches the barcode on the unit of blood (**Box 16.21**).

Immunological complications

Alloimmunization

Blood transfusion carries a risk of alloimmunization to the many 'foreign' antigens present on red cells, leucocytes, platelets and plasma proteins. Alloimmunization also occurs during pregnancy – to fetal antigens inherited from the father and not shared by the mother (see p. 353).

Alloimmunization does not usually cause clinical problems, such as a haemolytic transfusion reaction, with the first transfusion but these may occur with subsequent transfusions. There may also be delayed consequences of alloimmunization, such as HDN and rejection of tissue or organ transplants.

Incompatibility

Transfusion of blood cells, such as red cells and platelets, into a recipient who has antibodies against antigens on the cells may result in poor survival of the transfused cells, and also in harmful effects of the antigen–antibody reaction.

Box 16.21 Bedside checks for blood unit compatibility

- The traditional pre-transfusion bedside checking required two nurses and checks of multiple items of written documentation.
- With barcode technology, a handheld computer prompts the nurse through the key steps, including asking the patient to state their full name and date of birth, and checking that these match the details on the unit's compatibility label, attached by the transfusion laboratory.
- The nurse uses the computer to scan the barcode on the patient's wristband, which contains full patient details.
- The computer checks that the patient's details match those on the unit's compatibility label barcode after pre-transfusion testing.
- The unit's compatibility label barcode also contains the unique number of the unit, which is matched with the unit number at the top left of the bag to ensure that the blood bank has attached the right compatibility label to the bag.

Red cell complications: haemolytic transfusion reaction (immediate)

This is the most serious and life-threatening complication of blood transfusion and is usually due to ABO incompatibility. There is complement activation by the antigen–antibody reaction, usually caused by IgM anti-A and/or anti-B antibodies. The initial symptoms and signs, such as rigors, lumbar pain, dyspnoea, hypotension and haemoglobinuria, may begin a few minutes after starting the transfusion. Renal failure may develop. Activation of coagulation also occurs, and bleeding due to disseminated intravascular coagulation (DIC) is a bad prognostic sign. Emergency treatment for shock (see p. 220) is needed to maintain blood pressure and renal function.

Diagnosis

This is confirmed by finding evidence of haemolysis (e.g. haemoglobinuria), and incompatibility between donor and recipient. All documentation should be checked to detect errors such as:

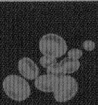

- failure to check the identity of the patient when taking the sample for compatibility testing (i.e. sample from the wrong patient)
- mislabelling of the blood sample with the wrong patient's name
- simple labelling or handling errors in the laboratory
- errors in the collection of blood, leading to delivery of the wrong blood to the ward/theatre
- failure to perform proper identity checks before the blood is transfused (i.e. blood transfused to the wrong patient).

Investigations

To confirm where the error occurred, blood grouping should be carried out on:
- the patient's original sample (used for the compatibility testing)
- a new sample taken from the patient after the reaction
- the donor units.

At the first suspicion of any serious transfusion reaction, the transfusion should always be stopped, and the donor units returned to the blood transfusion laboratory with a new blood sample from the patient to exclude a haemolytic transfusion reaction.

Red cell complications: haemolytic transfusion reaction (delayed)

This occurs in patients alloimmunized by previous transfusions or pregnancies. The antibody level is too low to be detected by pre-transfusion compatibility testing but a secondary immune response is seen after the transfusion, resulting in destruction of the transfused cells, usually by IgG antibodies.

Haemolysis is usually extravascular, as the antibodies are IgG, and the patient may develop anaemia and jaundice about a week after the transfusion, although most episodes are clinically silent. The blood film shows spherocytosis and reticulocytosis. The direct antiglobulin test is positive and detection of the antibody is usually straightforward.

Leucocyte complications: non-haemolytic (febrile) transfusion reactions

The typical cause of febrile reactions after red cell transfusions is the presence of leucocyte antibodies in patients who have previously been transfused or pregnant. Antibodies against donor leucocytes lead to the release of pyrogens. The mechanism of febrile reactions is different after platelet transfusions, where the release of cytokines from donor leucocytes is the most likely cause. Typical signs are flushing and tachycardia, fever (>38°C), chills and rigors, which are uncomfortable for the patient but not life-threatening. Aspirin may be used to reduce the fever, although it should not be given to patients with thrombocytopenia. The routine introduction of leucocyte-reduced blood in the UK to minimize the risk of transmission of variant Creutzfeldt–Jakob disease (vCJD) by blood transfusion (see later) has reduced the incidence of febrile reactions. Universal leucocyte reduction of all blood components is common in European countries, but the proportion of blood components that are leucocyte-reduced is variable across the USA.

Transfusion-related acute lung injury

Potent leucocyte antibodies in the plasma of donors, who are usually multiparous women, may cause transfusion-related acute lung injury (TRALI), characterized by dyspnoea, fever, cough, and shadowing in the perihilar and lower lung fields on the chest X-ray. Prompt respiratory support is essential and mechanical ventilation is frequently necessary. TRALI usually resolves within 48–96 hours but the mortality was 13% in the 305 cases of TRALI reported to SHOT up to 2013. The avoidance of female plasma in the preparation of fresh frozen plasma (FFP) and pooled platelets, and the testing of female plateletpheresis donors for leucocyte antibodies have been implemented in many developed countries to reduce the risk of TRALI, and the number of reported cases has reduced considerably.

Transfusion-associated graft-versus-host disease

Transfused donor lymphocytes that share an HLA haplotype with the patient are able to circulate, as they are not rejected; they may recognize the patient as 'foreign' and cause an acute GvHD reaction, including pancytopenia. It is usually fatal but no cases have occurred in the UK for many years, probably because of routine leucocyte reduction of blood components. However, certain groups of immunosuppressed patients at particular risk of TA-GvHD should receive irradiated blood to minimize the danger. Such patients include those with congenital or acquired immunodeficiencies: for example, individuals who have had treatment with purine analogue drugs, patients with Hodgkin lymphoma, those who have undergone haemopoietic stem cell transplantation, and fetuses and neonates who have received an intrauterine transfusion.

Platelet complications: post-transfusion purpura

See page 372.

Plasma protein complications: urticaria and anaphylaxis

Urticarial reactions are often attributed to plasma protein incompatibility but, in most cases, they are unexplained. They are common but rarely severe; stopping or slowing the transfusion and administering chlorphenamine 10 mg i.v. are usually sufficient treatment.

Anaphylactic reactions (see p. 64) occasionally occur; severe reactions are seen in patients lacking IgA, who produce anti-IgA that reacts with IgA in the transfused blood. The transfusion should be stopped and **adrenaline** (**epinephrine**) 0.5 mg i.m. and **chlorphenamine** 10 mg i.v. should be given immediately; endotracheal intubation may be required. Patients who have had severe urticarial or anaphylactic reactions should receive washed red cells, or blood from IgA-deficient donors for patients with IgA deficiency.

Immunosuppression

Transfusions are known to have a negative effect on the survival of subsequent renal allografts, due to transfusion-induced immunomodulation. The precise mechanism is unclear but may be associated with the transfusion of allogeneic leucocytes. Other possible clinical effects caused by transfusion-induced immunosuppression, such as an increase in postoperative infection and tumour recurrence, have been proposed but remain unproven.

Non-immunological complications

Transmission of infection

While stringent measures are being taken to minimize the risk of transfusion-transmitted infection, it may never be possible to guarantee that donor blood is absolutely 'safe'. The current approach to the safety of blood components and plasma in the UK and other developed countries is cautious but it is not an absolute guarantee of safety. Clinicians should always consider the patient's requirement for transfusion carefully, and only transfuse if clinically appropriate (see later).

Viral transmission

Donor blood in the UK is currently tested for hepatitis B virus (HBV), hepatitis C virus (HCV), hepatitis E virus (HEV), human immunodeficiency virus (HIV)-1 and human T-cell leukaemia (or lymphotropic) virus 1 (HTLV-1). CMV-seronegative blood is given to fetuses, neonates and pregnant women. Blood services continue a vigilant search for new infectious agents ('emerging' infections) that may be transmitted by blood transfusion and for methods to prevent their transmission, including donor screening, testing and pathogen inactivation. Donor questionnaires record recent travel to exclude possible risk of West Nile virus (WNV), the causal agent of meningoencephalitis, which has been transmitted by transfusion and transplantation in the USA, or Zika virus in light of the 2015-16 epidemic.

The risk of transmission of viral infections by blood transfusion varies from country to country, depending on factors such as the underlying prevalence of transfusion-transmitted infections in the population and the measures taken to minimize the risk of transmission. Viral transmission via blood transfusion is still a major issue in lower income countries. In the UK, the risk of transmission of HIV by blood transfusion is extremely low: less than 1 in 19 million units transfused. Prevention is based on self-exclusion of donors in 'high-risk' groups and testing of each donation for anti-HIV. The risk of transmission of HBV is less than 1 in 2 million units transfused. There have been no cases of transmission of HCV in the UK since 2010. Various measures, including treatment with solvents and detergents, are used for inactivating viruses in plasma products, such as coagulation factor concentrates or intravenous immunoglobulin.

Bacterial transmission

Bacterial contamination of blood components is rare but it is one of the most frequent causes of death associated with transfusion. Some organisms, such as *Yersinia enterocolitica*, can proliferate in red cell concentrates stored at 4°C, but platelet concentrates stored at 22°C are a more frequent cause of contamination. Measures to avoid bacterial contamination include strict donor arm cleansing, diversion of the initial blood collection to samples for testing rather than into the collection bag, and bacterial detection systems for platelet concentrates, which have been implemented in most developed countries. Such systems were implemented in the UK in 2011, and there have been no cases of bacterial transfusion-transmitted infections since 2017.

Transfusion-transmitted syphilis is very rare. Spirochaetes do not survive for more than 72 hours in blood stored at 4°C, and each donation is tested using the **Treponema pallidum haemagglutination assay** (TPHA).

Variant Creutzfeldt–Jakob disease

In the UK, four transmissions of vCJD occurred following a blood transfusion; the last one was reported in 2004. A number of measures were taken to minimize the risk, including universal leucocyte reduction of blood components in 1999 because the prion protein was thought to be primarily associated with lymphocytes. Blood donors are excluded if they have had a blood transfusion since 1980. UK donor plasma is not used for the manufacture of blood products; imported plasma from the USA is employed instead. For children under the age of 16 years, FFP is sourced from plasma (from unremunerated donors) imported from the USA, on the basis that exposure to bovine spongiform encephalitis (BSE) from food was eliminated by 1 January 1996. FFP for this group is treated with methylthioninium chloride (methylene blue) to inactivate viruses.

Transfusion-associated circulatory overload

See page 1077.

Iron overload

See page 343.

STRATEGIES FOR THE AVOIDANCE OF UNNECESSARY TRANSFUSION

These include:

- strict evidence-based criteria for the use of blood components and blood products, both the threshold ('trigger') for decision-making about the need for transfusion, e.g. haemoglobin concentration or platelet count, and the dose; single-unit transfusions are often sufficient to raise the patient's blood count above the threshold for transfusion ('Don't use 2 when 1 will do')
- discontinuing drug therapy such as anticoagulants and antiplatelet drugs wherever possible, as these may potentiate bleeding in surgical patients
- identification and treatment of anaemia prior to surgery and in pregnancy
- use of antifibrinolytic drugs, e.g. tranexamic acid in major surgery
- use of intraoperative cell salvage of blood in major surgery.

Artificial haemoglobin solutions and other blood substitutes suitable for routine clinical use have not yet been developed. They generally have a short intravascular half-life, and a recent meta-analysis found a significant risk of mortality and myocardial infarction.

Autologous transfusion

An alternative to using blood from volunteer donors is to use the patient's own blood. There are three types of autologous transfusion:

- **Predeposit.** The patient donates 2–5 units of blood at approximately weekly intervals before elective surgery.
- **Preoperative haemodilution.** Immediately before surgery, 1 or 2 units of blood are removed from the patient and then retransfused to replace operative losses.
- **Blood salvage.** Blood lost during or after surgery may be collected and retransfused. Several techniques of varying levels of sophistication are available. The operative site must be free of bacteria and bowel contents. Salvage was thought to be contraindicated in cancer surgery because of the risk of facilitating metastases but many centres are using it with apparent safety in this setting.

The use of predeposit autologous transfusion was largely driven by concerns about transfusion-transmitted infection, particularly in the USA. It has been abandoned in the UK and in most developed countries, except for rare cases when it is not possible to identify compatible blood because of multiple antibodies. There is little evidence that predeposit autologous transfusion reduces blood requirements, and blood is perceived as being 'safe'. Blood salvage is increasingly being employed as a way of avoiding the use of donor blood. In developing countries, autologous blood and blood from relatives are commonly chosen because of a lack of donor blood.

BLOOD, BLOOD COMPONENTS AND BLOOD PRODUCTS

Most blood collected from donors is processed as follows:

- **Blood components**, such as red cell and platelet concentrates, FFP and cryoprecipitate, are prepared from a single donation of blood by simple separation methods such as centrifugation and

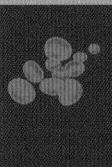

are transfused without further processing. Platelet concentrates are also prepared by plateletpheresis (see later).

- **Blood products**, such as coagulation factor concentrates, albumin and immunoglobulin solutions, are prepared by complex processes using the plasma from many donors as the starting material (UK donor plasma is not used; see earlier).

In most circumstances, it is preferable to transfuse only the blood component or product required by the patient (**'component therapy'**) rather than using whole blood. This is the most effective way of using donor blood, which is a scarce resource, and reduces the risk of complications from transfusion of unnecessary components of the blood.

Patients should be provided with information about blood transfusion wherever possible, and given the opportunity to ask questions: for example, about alternatives to transfusion. This discussion should be documented. Some patients, such as Jehovah's Witnesses, may refuse transfusion and need specialized management when they undergo surgery or receive medical treatments that usually require blood transfusion.

Whole blood

A unit of whole blood consists of 450 mL ± 10% of blood from a suitable donor plus 63 mL of anticoagulant, which is then leucocyte-depleted. Blood stored at 4°C is given a 'shelf-life' of 5 weeks in the UK (6 weeks in some other countries), when at least 70% of the transfused red cells should survive normally. Whole blood is rarely used for transfusion, as donated blood is processed into red cell concentrates and other blood components. However, there is renewed interest in considering its use in major haemorrhage.

Red cell concentrates

Virtually all the plasma is removed and is replaced by about 100 mL of an optimal additive solution, such as SAG-M, which contains sodium chloride, adenine, glucose and mannitol. The mean volume is about 330 mL. The PCV is about 0.57 L/L but the viscosity is low, as there are no plasma proteins in the additive solution; this allows fast administration, if necessary.

Red cell concentrates are used to increase the oxygen-carrying capacity of patients with major haemorrhage, and to treat non-bleeding patients with severe anaemia by maintaining the haemoglobin above 70 g/L; a higher threshold – haemoglobin of 90 g/L, say – is used in severe cardiovascular disease. Algorithms for the management of major haemorrhage highlight the need for the early transfusion of FFP and platelets to support haemostasis (**Fig. 16.31**).

Washed red cell concentrates

These are preparations of red cells suspended in saline, produced by cell separators that remove all but traces of plasma proteins. They are used in patients who have had severe recurrent urticarial or anaphylactic reactions.

Platelet concentrates

These are prepared either by centrifugation of whole blood or by plateletpheresis of blood from single donors using cell separators. They may be stored for up to 7 days at 22°C with agitation and bacterial culture to minimize the risk of bacterial transmission. They are used to treat bleeding in patients with severe thrombocytopenia, and prophylactically to prevent bleeding in patients with bone marrow failure when the platelet count is $<10 \times 10^9$/L.

Granulocyte concentrates

These are prepared from whole blood as **'buffy coats'** or from blood from single donors using cell separators, and are used for patients with severe neutropenia when there is evidence of bacterial infection. The numbers of granulocytes collected may be increased by treating donors with G-CSF and steroids. The half-life of granulocytes is of the order of a few hours only and thus granulocytes need to be collected and transfused on a daily basis, making the practicalities of this treatment challenging.

Fresh frozen plasma

FFP is prepared by freezing the plasma from 1 unit of blood to −30°C to maintain the concentration of coagulation factors. The volume is approximately 200 mL. FFP contains all the coagulation factors present in fresh plasma and is used mostly for replacement of coagulation factors in acquired coagulation factor deficiencies, such as massive haemorrhage and DIC. It may be further treated by a pathogen-inactivation process – for example, methylene blue or solvent detergent – to minimize the risk of disease transmission. For children, see page 362.

Prothrombin complex concentrates

These contain factors II, VII, IX and X, and have replaced FFP as the recommended treatment for rapid reversal of warfarin overdose in patients with an elevated international normalized ratio (INR) and bleeding because of their superior efficacy and lower risk of allergic reactions and volume overload.

Cryoprecipitate

This is obtained by allowing the frozen plasma from a single donation to thaw at 4–8°C and removing the supernatant. The typical adult dose is 2 pools each containing 5 donor units. Cryoprecipitate contains factor VIII:C, von Willebrand factor (VWF) and fibrinogen, and may be useful in DIC and other conditions where the fibrinogen level is very low. Fibrinogen concentrates are now available, and are increasingly being used for the treatment of patients with acquired disorders of haemostasis.

Specific coagulation factor concentrates

Specific factor concentrates are available for factors VII, VIII, IX, X, XI, XIII and VWF. These are freeze-dried preparations of the specific factor prepared from large pools of plasma. All products come from plasma sources at low risk of vCJD and are virus-inactivated during manufacture with either heat or chemicals. They are used for treating patients with inherited coagulation factor deficiencies, where recombinant coagulation factor concentrates are unavailable (see p. 375).

Albumin

There are two preparations:

- **Human albumin solution 4.5%** contains 45 g/L albumin and 160 mmol/L sodium. It is available in 50, 100, 250 and 500 mL bottles.
- **Human albumin solution 20%** contains approximately 200 g/L albumin and 130 mmol/L sodium. It is available in 50 and 100 mL bottles.

Human albumin solutions are considered to be inappropriate fluids for acute volume replacement or the treatment of shock. However, they are indicated for treatment of acute severe hypoalbuminaemia and as the replacement fluid for plasma exchange. The 20% albumin solution is particularly useful for patients with nephrotic syndrome or liver disease who are fluid-overloaded and resistant to diuretics.

Normal immunoglobulin

This is prepared from normal plasma. It is used to treat hypogammaglobulinaemia, prevent infections, and in high doses to treat

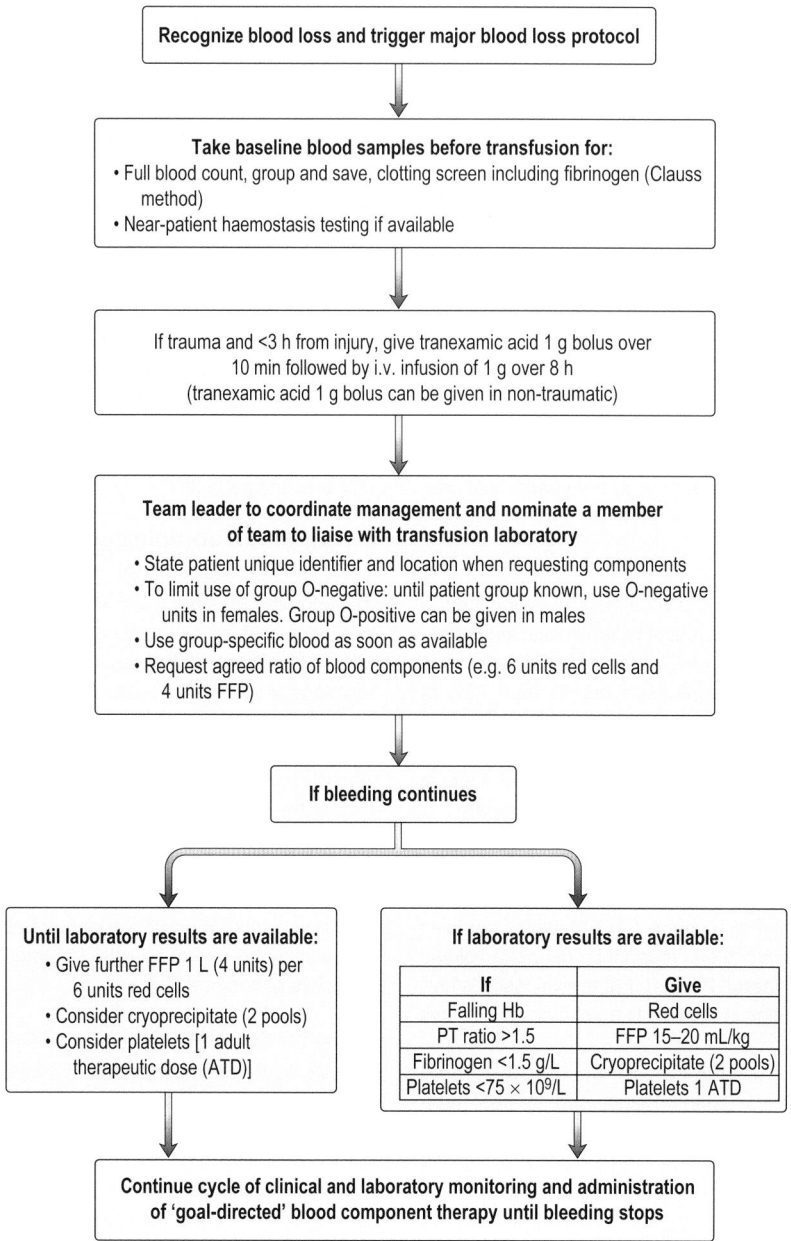

Fig. 16.31 Algorithm for the management of major haemorrhage. FFP, fresh frozen plasma; PT, prothrombin time. *(From Norfolk D 2013* Handbook of Transfusion Medicine. *The Stationery Office, with permission. Available at www.transfusionguidelines.com.)*

patients with autoimmune disorders: for example, immune thrombocytopenic purpura (see p. 374).

Specific immunoglobulins

These are obtained from donors with high titres of antibodies. Many preparations are available, such as anti-D, anti-hepatitis B and anti-varicella zoster.

Therapeutic use of haemopoietic stem cell transplantation

The use of haemopoietic stem cells to regenerate the bone marrow of patients whose own, usually diseased, marrow has been ablated by radiation and/or chemotherapy is the first and, to date, the only routine 'stem cell therapy' in clinical practice. Haemopoietic stem cell transplantation (HSCT) is used in a range of haematological

malignancies, and occasionally in other cancers and non-malignant disorders, such as sickle cell disease. It relies on the regenerative potential of transfused haemopoietic stem cells to repopulate the marrow niche that has been rendered temporarily or permanently hypoplastic by chemotherapy with or without additional radiotherapy. Such procedures vary in the source of the stem cells (**Box 16.22**) and in the type and intensity of the preparatory conditioning regimen.

Autologous stem cell transplantation

Most anticancer drugs have a sigmoid dose–response relationship, which suggests that, up to a point, a higher dose of a cytotoxic drug will induce a greater response. However, increasing a cytotoxic drug dose is often not possible owing to toxicity. For those chemotherapeutic agents with a dose-limiting toxicity of bone marrow failure, infusion of previously harvested haemopoietic stem cells is able to 'rescue' the haemopoietic system and permits the use of higher doses to overcome tumour drug resistance. Haemopoietic stem cells are collected either from the patient's bone marrow or, more commonly, from the peripheral blood by leucopheresis, following stem cell mobilization from the marrow niche by the administration of the growth factor G-CSF (see p. 324), with or without chemotherapy. These stem cells are stored by cryopreservation and then re-infused intravenously after an intensive chemotherapy regimen. This approach has been particularly effective in relapsed lymphomas, myeloma and germ cell tumours, and the large majority of HSCT procedures are carried out to treat these conditions. However, tumour contamination of the re-infused stem cells remains a reality. The infused stem cells take a period of 2–4 weeks to regenerate normal blood cell production, and therefore patients undergoing autologous HSCT experience a prolonged period of severe cytopenias and immunosuppression, with a consequent treatment-related mortality in the region of 1–5%.

Allogeneic HSCT

Conventional myeloablative allogeneic HSCT

Conventional myeloablative allogeneic HSCT combines the cytotoxic effect of high-dose chemotherapy and/or radiotherapy with a potent immunotherapy effect. Historically, the transplantation of donor haemopoietic cells has been combined with myeloablative chemotherapy with or without radiotherapy, with the dual effects of treating the malignancy and causing temporary immunosuppression that allows the graft to 'take'. Donors are usually fully matched at the major HLA antigens. Thus siblings are more likely to be found to be potential donors (25% chance for each sibling) than unrelated volunteers, who have to be carefully selected by HLA matching using large sample registries of potential donors. Allogeneic transplantation has been successfully used in a number of haemopoietic malignancies: most commonly, acute leukaemias. Engraftment of the donor immune system, with anti-tumour activity (graft-versus-tumour), is primarily responsible for the increased effectiveness of this approach. Complications include GvHD, an alloimmune reaction of the donor cells against normal host organs, which can affect 30–50% of transplant recipients and is potentially fatal. Immunosuppression, both from conditioning therapy and from the immunosuppressive drugs (ciclosporin or tacrolimus) given to prevent GvHD, results in a high incidence of opportunistic infection and viral reactivation, such as CMV. All patients receive prophylactic antibacterial, antifungal and antiviral drugs. Mortality from conventional allogeneic stem cell transplantation is therefore a major problem, with 15–40% at risk of dying from the procedure, depending on the age and status of the recipient and the degree of HLA compatibility of the donor. The use of donor lymphocyte infusions following allogeneic HSCT, while losing some of the specificity, has produced the strongest evidence for the efficacy of immunotherapy via graft-versus-tumour activity with clinical remissions observed, albeit with a risk of triggering GvHD.

Non-myeloablative allogeneic HSCT

The considerable toxicity associated with conventional myeloablative allogeneic HSCT limits use of the procedure to younger patients. This is problematic, as many haematological malignancies for which allogeneic HSCT is indicated primarily affect older patients. To address this, allogeneic HSCT approaches using 'reduced-intensity conditioning' have been developed since the turn of the century and are based on drugs such as fludarabine, which are primarily immunosuppressive rather than myeloablative. This maintains the anticancer 'graft-versus-leukaemia' effect of the transplant without the toxicity of conventional allogeneic stem cell transplantation. Treatment-related mortality is lower and the technique can be used successfully, particularly in the elderly and those with co-morbidities. GvHD remains an obstacle to success, however. Non-myeloablative allogeneic transplants are now more common than conventional myeloablative HSCT procedures.

Further reading

Ainley LI, Hewitt PE. Haematology patients and the risk of transfusion transmitted infection. *Br J Haem* 2018; 180:473–483.

Bolton-Maggs PHB (ed), Poles D, Watt A et al on behalf of the Serious Hazards of Transfusion (SHOT) Steering Group. *The 2017 Annual SHOT Report*. Manchester: SHOT; 2018; http://www.shotuk.org.

Carson JL, Triulzi DJ, Ness PM. Indications for and adverse effects of red cell transfusion. *N Engl J Med* 2017; 377:1261–1272.

Delaney M, Wendel S, Bercowitz RS et al for the Biomedical Excellence for Safer Transfusion (BEST) Collaborative. Transfusion reactions: prevention, diagnosis and treatment. *Lancet* 2016; 388:1945–1950.

Goodnough LT, Murphy MF. Do liberal transfusions cause more harm than good? *Br Med J* 2014; 350:13–15.

Murphy MF, Roberts DJ, Yazer MH (eds). *Practical Transfusion Medicine*, 5th edn. Oxford: Wiley–Blackwell; 2017.

Norfolk D (ed). *Handbook of Transfusion Medicine*, 5th edn. Norwich: UK Blood Services/The Stationery Office; 2013; http://www.transfusionguidelines.org.

Padhi S, Kemmis-Betty S, Rajesh S et al. Blood transfusion: summary of NICE guideline. *Br Med J* 2015; 351:h5832.

Seed CR, Hewitt PE, Dodd RY et al. Creutzfeldt-Jakob disease and blood transfusion safety. *Vox Sang* 2018; 113:220–231.

Shander A, Goodnough LT. From tolerating anemia to treating anemia. *Ann Intern Med* 2019; 170:125–126.

THE WHITE CELL

The five types of leucocyte found in peripheral blood are: neutrophils, eosinophils and basophils (all called granulocytes), and lymphocytes and monocytes (see also Ch. 3). The development of these cells is shown in **Fig. 16.1**.

Neutrophils

The earliest morphologically identifiable precursors of neutrophils in the bone marrow are myeloblasts, large cells constituting up to 3% of the nucleated cells in the marrow. The nucleus is large and contains 2–5 nucleoli. The cytoplasm is scanty and contains no granules. Promyelocytes are similar to myeloblasts but have some primary cytoplasmic granules, containing enzymes such as myeloperoxidase. Myelocytes are smaller cells without nucleoli but with more abundant cytoplasm and both primary and secondary granules. Indentation of the nucleus marks the change from myelocyte to metamyelocyte. The mature neutrophil is a smaller cell with a nucleus that has 2–5 lobes, with predominantly secondary granules in the cytoplasm, which contain lysozyme, collagenase and lactoferrin.

Peripheral blood neutrophils are equally distributed into a circulating pool and a marginating pool lying along the endothelium of blood vessels. In contrast to the prolonged maturation time of about 10 days for neutrophils in the bone marrow, their half-life in the peripheral blood is extremely short: only 6–8 hours. In response to stimuli (e.g. infection, corticosteroid therapy), neutrophils are released into the circulating pool from both the marginating pool and the marrow. Immature white cells are released from the marrow when a rapid response (within hours) occurs in acute infection (described as a 'shift to the left' on a blood film).

Function

The prime function of neutrophils is to ingest and kill bacteria, fungi and damaged cells. Neutrophils are attracted to sites of infection or inflammation by chemotaxins. Recognition of foreign or dead material is aided by the coating of particles with immunoglobulin and complement (opsonization), as neutrophils have Fc and C3b receptors (see p. 44). The material is ingested into vacuoles, where it is subjected to enzymic destruction; this is either oxygen-dependent, with the generation of hydrogen peroxide (myeloperoxidase), or oxygen-independent (lysosomal enzymes and lactoferrin). Leucocyte alkaline phosphatase (LAP) is an enzyme found in leucocytes. It is raised when there is a neutrophilia due to an acute illness. It is also raised in polycythaemia and myelofibrosis, and reduced in chronic myeloid leukaemia.

Neutrophil leucocytosis

A rise in the number of circulating neutrophils to more than 10×10^9/L occurs in bacterial infections or is a result of tissue damage. It may also be seen in pregnancy, during exercise, secondary to smoking and after corticosteroid administration (**Box 16.23**). With any tissue necrosis, there is a release of various soluble factors, causing a leucocytosis. Interleukin 1 is also released in tissue necrosis and causes a pyrexia. The pyrexia and leucocytosis that accompany a myocardial infarction are a good example of this and may be wrongly attributed to infection.

A ***leucoerythroblastic blood film*** (an overproduction of white cells, with many immature cells and nucleated red cells) may occur in severe infection, tuberculosis, malignant infiltration of the bone marrow, and occasionally after haemorrhage, haemolysis and severe haemolytic or megaloblastic anaemia.

Neutropenia and agranulocytosis

Neutropenia is defined as a circulatory neutrophil count of less than 1.5×10^9/L. The causes are given in **Box 16.24**. A virtual absence of neutrophils is called agranulocytosis. Note that patients from African and Caribbean backgrounds may have somewhat lower neutrophil counts, termed 'ethnic neutropenia'. This is due to a greater proportion of the neutrophils residing close to the vessel walls and not an absolute reduction in total neutrophil production or function.

Neutropenia caused by viruses is probably the most common type. Chemotherapy and radiotherapy predictably produce neutropenia; many other drugs (e.g. anti-thyroid drugs such as carbimazole, and some antibiotics) have been known to produce an idiosyncratic cytopenia and a drug cause should always be considered.

Clinical features

Infections may be frequent, are often serious, and become more likely as the neutrophil count falls. An absolute neutrophil count of less than 0.5×10^9/L is regarded as 'severe' neutropenia and may be associated with life-threatening infections, such as pneumonia and septicaemia. A characteristic glazed mucositis occurs in the mouth, and ulceration is common.

? Box 16.23 Causes of a neutrophil leucocytosis

- Bacterial infections
- Tissue necrosis, e.g. myocardial infarction, trauma
- Inflammation, e.g. gout, rheumatoid arthritis
- Drugs, e.g. corticosteroids, lithium
- Acute haemorrhage or haemolysis
- Administration of granulocyte colony-stimulating factor (G-CSF)
- Haematological:
  – Myeloproliferative disease
  – Leucoerythroblastosis (see text)
- Physiological, e.g. pregnancy, exercise
- Malignant disease, e.g. bronchial, breast, gastric
- Metabolic, e.g. renal failure, acidosis
- Congenital, e.g. leucocyte adhesion deficiency, hereditary neutrophilia
- Smoking

? Box 16.24 Causes of neutropenia

Acquired
- Viral infection
- Severe bacterial infection, e.g. typhoid
- Felty's syndrome (rheumatoid arthritis-associated)
- Autoimmune neutropenia
- Pancytopenia from any cause, including drug-induced marrow aplasia (see p. 336).
- Drug-induced agranulocytosis, e.g. carbimazole
- Pure white cell aplasia

Inherited

- Ethnic (neutropenia is common in African and Caribbean ethnicities)
- Kostmann's syndrome (severe infantile agranulocytosis) due to mutation in the elastane 2 (*ELA2*) gene
- Cyclical (genetic mutation in *ELA2* gene with neutropenia every 2–3 weeks)
- Others, e.g. Schwachman–Diamond syndrome, dyskeratosis congenita, Chédiak–Higashi syndrome

---

Investigations

The blood film shows marked neutropenia. The appearance of the bone marrow will indicate whether the neutropenia is due to depressed production or increased destruction of neutrophils. Neutrophil antibody studies are performed if an immune mechanism is suspected. Viral serology, in particular for HIV, should be undertaken.

Management

Antibiotics should be given as necessary to patients with acute severe neutropenia (see p. 116). Exposure to infections should be minimized.

If the neutropenia seems likely to have been caused by a drug, all current drug therapy should be stopped. Recovery of the neutrophil count usually occurs after about 10 days. G-CSF (see p. 324) is used to decrease the period of neutropenia after chemotherapy and haemopoietic transplantation. It is also employed successfully in the treatment of chronic neutropenia.

Steroids and high-dose intravenous immunoglobulin are used to treat patients with severe autoimmune neutropenia and recurrent infections, and G-CSF has produced responses in some cases.

Eosinophils

Eosinophils are slightly larger than neutrophils and are characterized by a nucleus, usually with two lobes, and large cytoplasmic granules that stain deep red. The eosinophil plays a part in allergic responses (see p. 45) and in the defence against infections with helminths and protozoa.

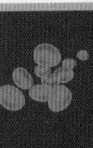

Box 16.25 Causes of eosinophilia

Parasitic infestations, e.g.:
- *Ascaris*
- Hookworm
- *Strongyloides*

Allergic disorders, e.g.:
- Hayfever (allergic rhinitis)
- Other hypersensitivity reactions, including drug reactions

Skin disorders, e.g.:
- Urticaria
- Pemphigus
- Eczema

Pulmonary disorders, e.g.:
- Bronchial asthma
- Tropical pulmonary eosinophilia
- Allergic bronchopulmonary aspergillosis
- Eosinophilic granulomatosis with polyangiitis

Malignant disorders, e.g.:
- Hodgkin lymphoma
- T-cell non-Hodgkin lymphoma
- Carcinoma
- Eosinophilic leukaemia
- Acute myeloid leukaemia
- Myeloproliferative diseases associated with platelet-derived growth factor rearrangements

Miscellaneous disorders, e.g.:
- Hypereosinophilic syndrome
- Sarcoidosis
- Hypoadrenalism
- Eosinophilic gastroenteritis

Eosinophilia is defined as more than 0.4×10^9/L eosinophils in the peripheral blood. The causes of eosinophilia are listed in **Box 16.25**.

Basophils

The nucleus of basophils is similar to that of neutrophils but the cytoplasm is filled with large, black granules. The granules contain histamine, heparin and enzymes such as myeloperoxidase. The physiological role of the basophil is not known. Binding of IgE causes the cells to degranulate and release histamine and other contents involved in acute hypersensitivity reactions (see p. 62).

Basophils are usually few in number ($<1 \times 10^9$/L) but are significantly increased in some myeloproliferative disorders, such as chronic myeloid leukaemia. Basophilia should prompt further investigations.

Monocytes

Monocytes are slightly larger than neutrophils. The nucleus has a variable shape and may be round, indented or lobulated. The cytoplasm contains fewer granules than neutrophils. Monocytes are precursors of tissue macrophages and dendritic cells; they spend only a few hours in the blood but can continue to proliferate in the tissues for many years.

A monocytosis ($>0.8 \times 10^9$/L) may be seen in chronic bacterial infections, such as tuberculosis or infective endocarditis, chronic neutropenia and myelodysplasia, particularly chronic myelomonocytic leukaemia.

Lymphocytes

Lymphocytes form nearly half of circulating white cells. They descend from pluripotent stem cells (see **Fig. 16.1**). Circulating lymphocytes are small cells, a little larger than red cells, with a dark-staining central nucleus. There are two main types: T and B lymphocytes (see p. 43).

Lymphocytosis (lymphocyte count $>5 \times 10^9$/L) occurs in response to viral infections, particularly EBV, CMV and HIV, and chronic infections such as tuberculosis and toxoplasmosis. It is also found in chronic lymphocytic leukaemia and in some lymphomas.

HAEMOSTASIS

The integrity of the circulation is maintained by blood flowing through intact vessels lined by endothelial cells. Haemostasis is the host defence mechanism that protects this integrity after injury to the vessel wall and tissue injury. It is a complex process that depends on interactions between the vessel wall, leucocytes, platelets, and coagulation and fibrinolytic mechanisms. Haemostatic systems are normally quiescent but, following tissue injury, become rapidly activated. The formation of the haemostatic plug is shown in **Fig. 16.32**.

Vessel wall

The vessel wall is lined by endothelium, which, in normal conditions, prevents platelet adhesion and thrombus formation. This property is partly due to its negative charge but also to:
- thrombomodulin and heparan sulphate expression
- synthesis of prostacyclin (prostaglandin I$_2$, PGI$_2$) and nitric oxide (NO), which cause vasodilation and inhibit platelet aggregation
- production of plasminogen activator.

Injury to vessels causes reflex vasoconstriction, while endothelial damage results in loss of antithrombotic properties, activation of platelets and coagulation, and inhibition of fibrinolysis (see **Fig. 16.32**).

Platelets

Platelet adhesion
When the vessel wall is damaged, the escaping platelets come into contact with and adhere to collagen and subendothelial bound VWF. This adherence is mediated through glycoprotein Ib (GPIb). Glycoprotein IIb/IIIa is then exposed, forming a second binding site for VWF. Within seconds of adhesion to the vessel wall, platelets begin to undergo a shape change from a disc to a sphere, spread along the subendothelium, and release the contents of their cytoplasmic granules. These are the dense bodies (containing adenosine diphosphate (ADP) and serotonin) and the α-granules (containing platelet-derived growth factor, platelet factor 4, β-thromboglobulin, fibrinogen, VWF, fibronectin, thrombospondin and other factors).

Platelet activation
The release of ADP leads to a conformational change in the fibrinogen receptor, the glycoprotein IIb/IIIa complex (GPIIb/IIIa), on the surfaces of adherent platelets, allowing it to bind to fibrinogen (**Fig. 16.33**).

Platelet aggregation
As fibrinogen is a dimer, it can form a direct bridge between platelets and so binds platelets into activated aggregates (platelet aggregation; see **Fig. 16.32B**), and further platelet release of ADP occurs. A self-perpetuating cycle of events is set up, leading to formation of a platelet plug at the site of the injury.

A

Platelet adhesion **Platelet release**

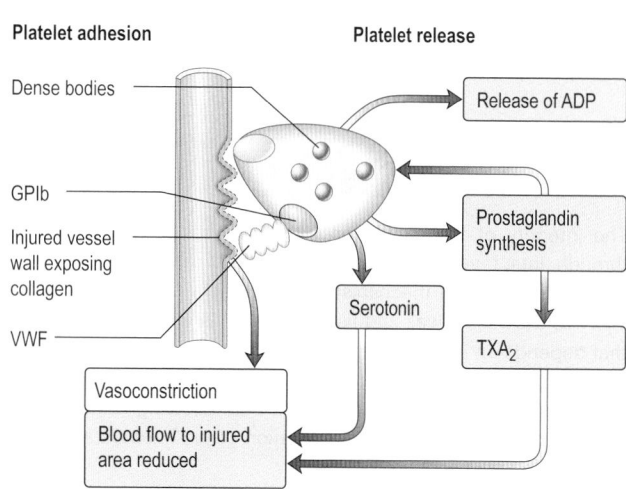

B

Platelet aggregation **Coagulation**

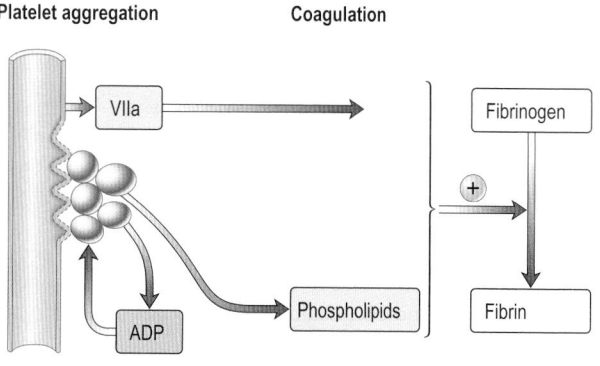

C

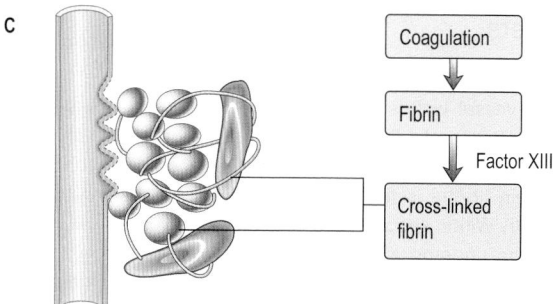

Fig. 16.32 Formation of the haemostatic plug: sequential interactions between the vessel wall, platelets and coagulation factors. **(A)** *Contact of platelets with collagen* via the platelet receptor glycoprotein Ib (GPIb) and von Willebrand factor (VWF) in plasma activates platelet prostaglandin synthesis, which stimulates release of adenosine diphosphate (ADP) from the dense bodies. Vasoconstriction of the vessel occurs as a reflex and by release of serotonin and thromboxane A$_2$ (TXA$_2$) from platelets. **(B)** *Release of ADP from platelets* induces platelet aggregation and formation of the platelet plug. The coagulation pathway is stimulated, leading to the formation of fibrin. **(C)** *Fibrin strands are cross-linked by factor XIII* and stabilize the haemostatic plug by binding platelets and red cells.

Coagulation

After platelet aggregation and release of ADP, the exposed platelet membrane phospholipids are available for the assembly of coagulation factor enzyme complexes (tenase and prothrombinase). The presence of thrombin encourages fusion of platelets, and fibrin formation reinforces the stability of the platelet plug. Central to normal platelet function is *prostaglandin synthesis*, which is induced by platelet activation and leads to the formation of thromboxane A$_2$ (TXA$_2$) in platelets (**Fig. 16.34**). TXA$_2$ is a powerful vasoconstrictor and also lowers cyclic adenosine monophosphate (AMP) levels and initiates the platelet release reaction. Prostacyclin (PGI$_2$) is synthesized in vascular endothelial cells and opposes the actions of TXA$_2$. It produces vasodilation and increases the level of cyclic AMP, preventing platelet aggregation on the normal vessel wall, as well as limiting the extent of the initial platelet plug after injury.

Coagulation and fibrinolysis

Coagulation involves a series of enzymatic reactions that lead to the conversion of soluble plasma fibrinogen to fibrin-based clot (**Fig. 16.35**). Roman numerals are used for most of the factors, but I and II are referred to as fibrinogen and prothrombin, respectively; III, IV and VI are redundant. The active forms are denoted by 'a'. The coagulation factors are primarily synthesized in the liver and are either serine protease enzyme precursors (factors IX, X and XI, and thrombin) or co-factors (V and VIII), except for fibrinogen, which is polymerized to form fibrin.

Coagulation pathway

This enzymatic amplification system was traditionally divided into 'extrinsic' and 'intrinsic' pathways. This concept is useful for the interpretation of clinical laboratory tests, such as the prothrombin time (PT) and activated partial thromboplastin time (APTT) (see **Fig. 16.39**), but is unrepresentative and oversimplifies *in vivo* coagulation. Coagulation is initiated by tissue damage (see **Fig. 16.35**):

- Tissue damage exposes tissue factor (TF), which binds to factor VII.
- The TF–factor VII complex directly converts factor X to active factor Xa, and some factor IX to factor IXa.
- In the presence of factor Xa, tissue factor pathway inhibitor (TFPI) inhibits further generation of factor Xa and factor IXa.
- Following inhibition by TFPI, the amount of factor Xa produced is insufficient to maintain coagulation. Further factor Xa, to allow haemostasis to progress to completion, can be generated only by the alternative factor IX/factor VIII pathway. However, enough thrombin exists at this point to activate factor VIII, which dramatically increases the activity of factor IXa (generated by TF–factor VIIa), so further activation of factor X can proceed. Without the amplification and consolidating action of factor VIII/factor IX, bleeding will ensue, as generation of factor Xa is insufficient to sustain haemostasis.
- Similarly, thrombin activates factor V, dramatically enhancing the conversion of prothrombin to thrombin by factor Xa.
- Thrombin hydrolyses the peptide bonds of fibrinogen, releasing fibrinopeptides A and B, and allowing polymerization between fibrinogen molecules to form fibrin. At the same time, thrombin, in the presence of calcium ions, activates factor XIII, which stabilizes the fibrin clot by cross-linking adjacent fibrin molecules.

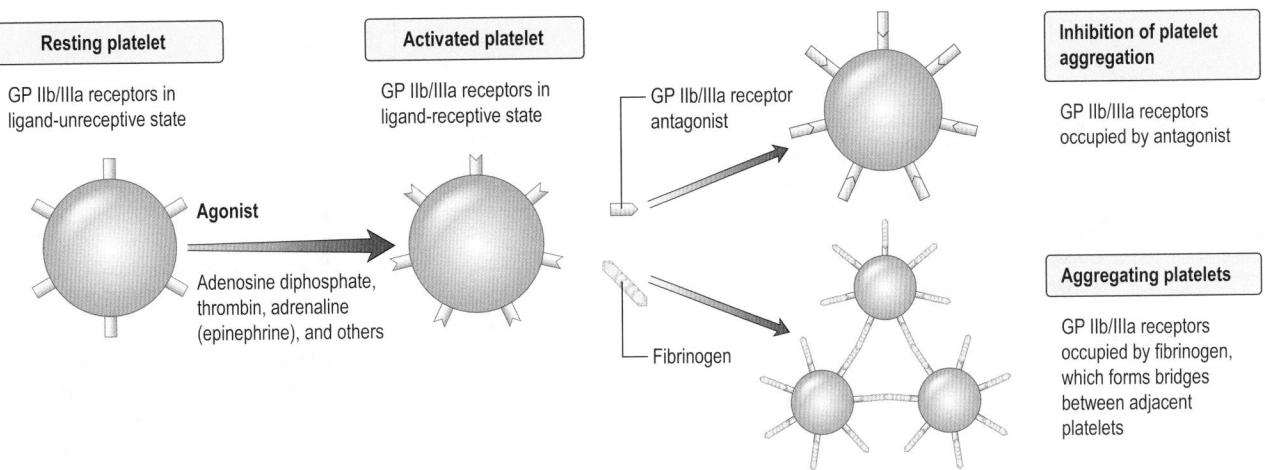

Fig. 16.33 The role of glycoprotein IIb/IIIa in platelet aggregation and the inhibition of platelet aggregation by inhibitors of glycoprotein IIb/IIIa receptors.

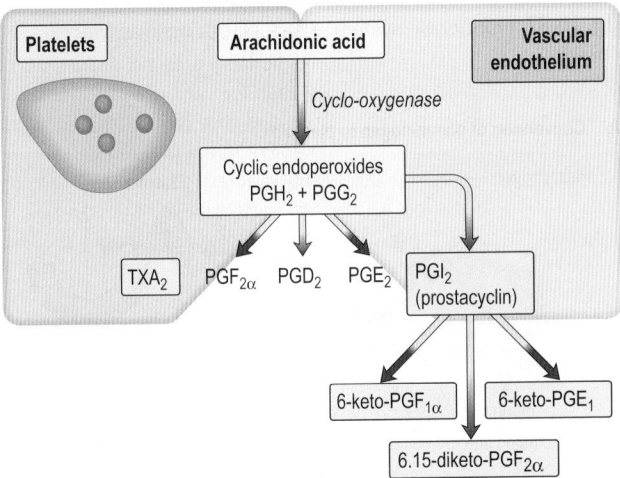

Fig. 16.34 Prostaglandin (PG) synthesis. TXA_2, thromboxane A_2.

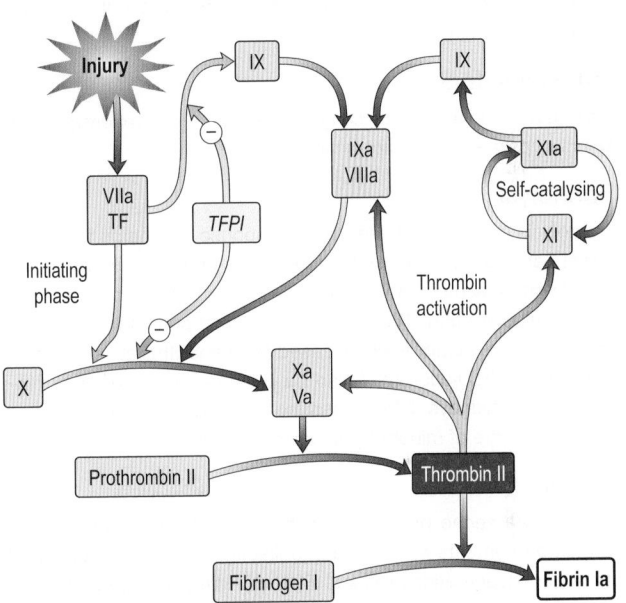

Fig. 16.35 Coagulation mechanism. The *in vivo* pathway begins with the tissue factor–factor VIIa (VIIa–TF) complex activating factor X (Xa) and amplifying factor IX (IXa). Thrombin activates factor XI (XIa), as well as factor IXa, VIIIa, and Va and Xa complexes. TFPI, tissue factor pathway inhibitor.

Factor VIII

Factor VIII is a key co-factor in the coagulation pathway. It is associated with its carrier protein VWF. When activated, factor VIII increases the conversion of factor X to Xa by factor IXa by approximately 200 000 fold. VWF functions to protect factor VIII from premature proteolytic breakdown and locates it to areas of vascular injury. Factor VIII:C has a molecular weight of about 350 kDa.

Von Willebrand factor

VWF is a glycoprotein with a monomeric molecular weight of about 250 kDa, which readily forms multimers in the circulation with molecular weights of up to 20 000 kDa. It is synthesized by endothelial cells and megakaryocytes, and stored in platelet granules as well as endothelial cells. The high-molecular-weight multimeric forms of VWF are the most biologically active (see p. 376 and **Fig. 16.40**). It has a primary role as an adhesive protein binding to platelets, surface glycoproteins and constituents of connective tissue. It also acts as a carrier protein for factor VIII.

Factor V

Factor V is similar to factor VIII in that it is a non-enzymatic co-factor. In its thrombin-activated form, factor Va, it significantly enhances the conversion of prothrombin to thrombin.

Physiological limitation of coagulation

Without a physiological system to limit blood coagulation, excessive thrombosis could ensue. The natural anticoagulant mechanism regulates and localizes thrombosis to the site of injury.

Antithrombin

Antithrombin (AT), a member of the serine protease inhibitor (serpin) superfamily, is a potent inhibitor of coagulation. It inactivates the serine proteases by forming stable complexes with them, and its action is greatly potentiated by heparin.

Activated protein C

This is generated from its vitamin K-dependent precursor, protein C, by thrombin; thrombin activation of protein C is greatly enhanced when thrombin is bound to thrombomodulin on endothelial cells (**Fig. 16.36**). Activated protein C inactivates factor Va and factor VIIIa, reducing further thrombin generation.

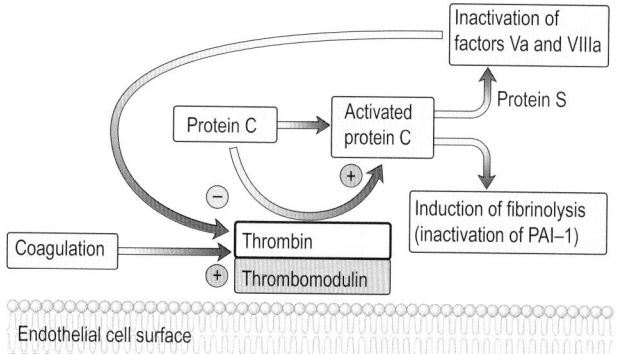

Fig. 16.36 Activation of protein C. PAI-1, plasminogen activator inhibitor 1.

Protein S

This is a co-factor for protein C, which acts by enhancing binding of activated protein C to the phospholipid surface. It circulates bound to C4b binding protein but some 30–40% remains unbound and active (free protein S).

Other inhibitors

Other natural inhibitors of coagulation include α_2-macroglobulin, α_1-antitrypsin and α_2-antiplasmin.

Fibrinolysis

Fibrinolysis is a normal haemostatic response that helps to restore vessel patency after vascular damage. The principal component is the enzyme plasmin, which is generated from its inactive precursor plasminogen (**Fig. 16.37**). This is achieved principally via tissue plasminogen activator (t-PA) released from endothelial cells. Some plasminogen activation may also be promoted by urokinase, produced in the kidneys. Other plasminogen activators (factor XII and prekallikrein) are of minor physiological importance.

Plasmin

Plasmin is a serine protease, which breaks down fibrinogen and fibrin into fragments X, Y, D and E, collectively known as fibrin (and fibrinogen) degradation products (FDPs). D-dimer is produced when cross-linked fibrin is degraded. Its presence in the plasma indicates that the coagulation mechanism has been activated.

Fibrinolytic system

This is activated by the presence of fibrin. Plasminogen is specifically adsorbed to fibrin and fibrinogen by lysine-binding sites. However, little plasminogen activation occurs in the absence of polymerized fibrin, as fibrin also has a specific binding site for plasminogen activators, whereas fibrinogen does not (**Fig. 16.38**).

Tissue plasminogen activator

This is inactivated by plasminogen activator inhibitor-1 (PAI-1). Activated protein C inactivates PAI-1 and therefore induces fibrinolysis (see **Fig. 16.36**). Inactivators of plasmin, such as α_2-antiplasmin (see **Fig. 16.38**) and thrombin-activatable fibrinolysis inhibitor (TAFI), also contribute to the regulation of fibrinolysis.

Investigation of bleeding disorders

Although the precise diagnosis of a bleeding disorder depends on laboratory tests, much information is obtained from a structured history and physical examination.

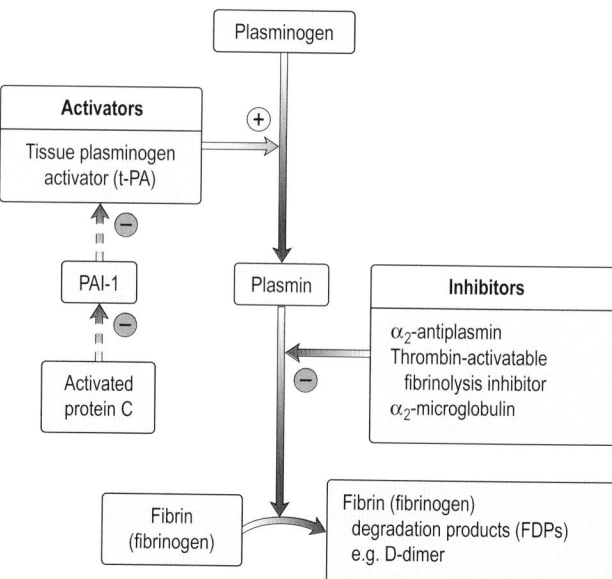

Fig. 16.37 Fibrinolytic system. PAI-1, plasminogen activator inhibitor-1.

A   Conversion of plasminogen to plasmin

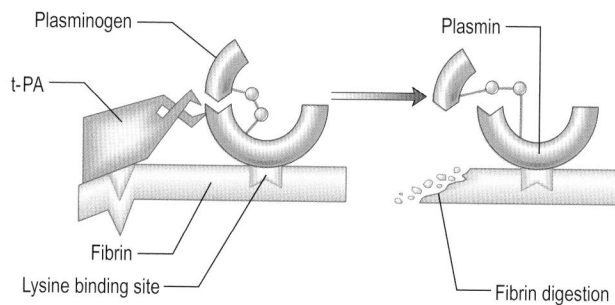

B   Plasmin α_2–antiplasmin complex

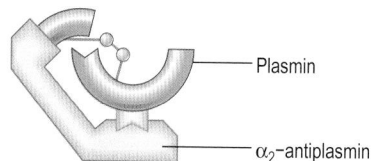

Fig. 16.38 Fibrinolysis. **(A)** *The conversion of plasminogen to plasmin* by tissue plasminogen activator (t-PA) occurs most efficiently on the surface of fibrin, which has binding sites for both plasminogen and t-PA. **(B)** *Free plasmin in the blood is rapidly inactivated by α_2-antiplasmin.* Plasmin generated on the fibrin surface is partially protected from inactivation. The lysine-binding sites on plasminogen are necessary for the interaction between plasmin(ogen) and fibrin, and between plasmin and α_2-antiplasmin.

Is there a generalized haemostatic defect?

Supportive evidence for a generalized haemostatic defect includes bleeding from multiple sites, spontaneous bleeding, and excessive bleeding after injury.

Is the defect inherited or acquired?

A family history of a bleeding disorder should be sought. Severe inherited defects usually become apparent in infancy, sometimes at the time of birth with prolonged bleeding from the umbilical cord,

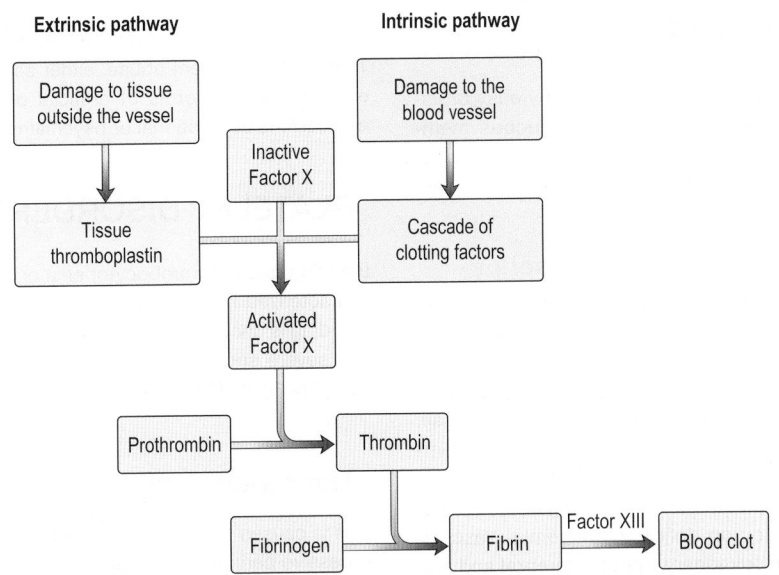

Extrinsic pathway   **Intrinsic pathway**

Fig. 16.39 The classic *in vitro* extrinsic and intrinsic coagulation cascade, as relevant to the prothrombin time (PT) and activated partial thromboplastin time (APTT). See text and Fig. 16.35. Initiation of coagulation differs significantly *in vitro* from *in vivo*.

while mild inherited defects may only come to attention later in life: for example, with excessive bleeding after surgery, childbirth, dental extractions or trauma. Some milder defects are revealed by routine coagulation screens that are performed before surgical procedures.

Is the bleeding suggestive of a vascular/platelet defect or a coagulation defect?

Vascular/platelet bleeding

This is characterized by easy bruising and spontaneous bleeding from small vessels. There is often bleeding into the skin. Purpura includes both petechiae, small skin haemorrhages varying from pinpoint size to a few millimetres in diameter that do not blanch on pressure, and ecchymoses, larger areas of bleeding into the skin. Bleeding also occurs from mucous membranes, especially the nose and mouth.

Coagulation disorders

These are typically associated with bleeding after injury or surgery and, in more severe forms, haemarthroses and muscle haematomas. There is often a short delay between the precipitating event and overt haemorrhage or haematoma formation.

Laboratory investigations

Blood count and film

These show the number and morphology of platelets and any blood disorder, such as leukaemia or lymphoma. The normal range for the platelet count is $150–400 \times 10^9/L$.

Coagulation tests

These are performed on blood collected into citrate, which neutralizes calcium ions and prevents clotting.

- ***The prothrombin time (PT)*** (also see p. 1016) is measured by adding tissue factor (thromboplastin) and calcium to the patient's plasma and establishing the length of time taken for the blood to clot. The normal PT is 11.5–13.5 sec. When used to measure warfarin-based oral anticoagulation, the PT is expressed as the international normalized ratio, or INR (see p. 1016). The PT measures factors VII, X, V, prothrombin and fibrinogen (the clas-

sic 'extrinsic' pathway, **Fig. 16.39**), and is prolonged if any of these factors is low. It may also be abnormal in liver disease, or if the patient is on oral anticoagulants, including warfarin and some direct oral anticoagulants that target factor Xa.

- ***The activated partial thromboplastin time (APTT)*** is also sometimes known as the PTT with kaolin (PTTK). It is measured by adding a surface activator (such as kaolin, micronized silica or ellagic acid), phospholipid (to mimic platelet membrane) and calcium to the patient's plasma. The normal APTT is 26–37 s and depends on the exact methodology. The APTT measures factors XII, XI, IX, VIII, X, V, prothrombin and fibrinogen (the classic 'intrinsic' pathway), and is prolonged in deficiencies of one or more of these factors. It is not dependent on factor VII.

- ***The thrombin time (TT)*** is measured by adding thrombin to the patient's plasma. The normal TT is 12–14 s; it is prolonged in fibrinogen deficiency, in qualitative defects of fibrinogen (dysfibrinogenaemia) or in the presence of inhibitors such as heparin or FDPs.

- ***Correction tests*** can be used to differentiate prolonged times in the PT, APTT and TT due to various coagulation factor deficiencies and inhibitors of coagulation. Prolonged PT, APTT or TT due to coagulation factor deficiencies can be corrected by addition of normal plasma to the patient's plasma. Failure to correct after addition of normal plasma is suggestive of the presence of an inhibitor of coagulation.

- ***Factor assays*** are used to confirm coagulation defects, especially where a single inherited disorder is suspected.

- ***Special tests of coagulation*** will often be required to confirm the precise haemostatic defect. Such tests include estimation of fibrinogen and FDPs, platelet function tests such as platelet aggregation, and platelet granule contents.

- ***Bleeding time*** measures platelet plug formation *in vivo*. Classically, a sphygmomanometer cuff is inflated to 40 mmHg and, using a template, standardized incisions are made in the forearm. The time taken for bleeding to stop is recorded. Prolonged times are seen in platelet function defects, and when the platelet count is $<100 \times 10^9/L$. Nowadays, this test is very rarely done, as it can scar and is painful.

VASCULAR DISORDERS

Vascular disorders (**Box 16.26**) are characterized by easy bruising and bleeding into the skin. Bleeding from mucous membranes sometimes occurs but the bleeding is rarely severe. Laboratory investigations, including the bleeding time, are normal.

Hereditary haemorrhagic telangiectasia

This is a rare disorder with autosomal dominant inheritance. In most cases, mutations occur in one of three genes – *ENG*, *ALK1* or *SMAD4* – that encode components of the TGF-β signalling pathway that is involved in blood vessel development. Dilation of capillaries and small arterioles produces characteristic small, red spots that blanch on pressure in the skin and mucous membranes, particularly the nose and gastrointestinal tract. Recurrent epistaxis and chronic gastrointestinal bleeding are the major problems that cause chronic iron deficiency anaemia. Vascular malformations also occur in pulmonary, hepatic cerebral and spinal vasculature.

Easy bruising syndrome

This is a common benign disorder often seen in otherwise healthy women. It is characterized by bruises on the arms, legs and trunk with minor trauma, possibly because of skin vessel fragility. It may give rise to the suspicion of a serious bleeding disorder.

Senile purpura and purpura due to steroids

These are both caused by atrophy of the vascular supporting tissue.

Purpura due to infections

This is mainly caused by damage to the vascular endothelium. The rash of meningococcal septicaemia is particularly characteristic (see **Fig. 20.21**).

Henoch–Schönlein purpura

This is mainly a disease of children (see p. 1368). It is a type III hypersensitivity (immune complex) reaction that is often preceded by an acute upper respiratory tract infection. Purpura is seen mainly on the legs and buttocks. Abdominal pain, arthritis, haematuria and glomerulonephritis also occur. Recovery is usually spontaneous but some patients develop renal failure.

Episodes of inexplicable bleeding or bruising

These may represent abuse, either self-inflicted or caused by others. The various forms of artificial or factitious purpura may be expressions of emotional or psychiatric disturbance.

PLATELET DISORDERS

Bleeding due to thrombocytopenia or abnormal platelet function is characterized by purpura and bleeding from mucous membranes. Bleeding is uncommon with platelet counts of more than 50×10^9/L, and severe spontaneous bleeding is unusual with platelet counts over 20×10^9/L (**Box 16.27**).

Thrombocytopenia

This is caused by reduced platelet production in the bone marrow, excessive peripheral destruction of platelets or sequestration in an enlarged spleen (**Box 16.28**). The underlying cause may be revealed

---

i Box 16.27 Clinical effects caused by different levels of platelet count

Platelet count ($\times 10^9$/L)	Clinical defect
>500	Haemorrhage or thrombosis
500–100	No clinical effect
100–50	Moderate haemorrhage after injury
50–20	Purpura may occur Haemorrhage after injury
<20	Purpura common Spontaneous haemorrhage from mucous membranes Intracranial haemorrhage (rare)

(From Colvin BT. Disorders of haemostasis. Medicine *2004; 32:27–33, with permission from Elsevier.)*

? Box 16.28 Causes of thrombocytopenia

Impaired production
- Selective megakaryocyte depression:
  - Rare congenital defects
  - Drugs, chemicals and viruses
- As part of a general bone marrow failure:
  - Cytotoxic drugs and chemicals
  - Radiation
  - Megaloblastic anaemia
  - Leukaemia
- Myelodysplastic syndromes
- Myeloma
- Myelofibrosis
- Solid tumour infiltration
- Aplastic anaemia
- HIV infection

Excessive destruction or increased consumption
- Autoimmune – immune thrombocytopenic purpura

- Drug-induced, e.g. glycoprotein IIb/IIIa inhibitors, penicillins, thiazides
- Secondary immune (systemic lupus erythematosus, chronic lymphocytic leukaemia, viruses, drugs, e.g. heparin, bivalirudin)
- Alloimmune neonatal thrombocytopenia
- Post-transfusion purpura
- Disseminated intravascular coagulation
- Thrombotic thrombocytopenic purpura

Sequestration
- Splenomegaly
- Hypersplenism

Dilutional
- Massive transfusion

---

i Box 16.26 Vascular disorders

Congenital
- Hereditary haemorrhagic telangiectasia (Osler–Weber–Rendu disease)
- Connective tissue disorders (Ehlers–Danlos syndrome, osteogenesis imperfecta, pseudoxanthoma elasticum, Marfan's syndrome)

Acquired

Severe infections
- Septicaemia
- Meningococcal infections
- Measles
- Typhoid

Autoimmune disorders
- Henoch–Schönlein purpura
- Systemic lupus erythematosus
- Rheumatoid arthritis

Drug-induced disorders
- Steroids
- Sulphonamides

Others
- Senile purpura
- Easy bruising syndrome
- Scurvy
- Factitious purpura

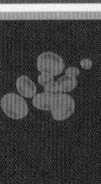

by history and examination but a bone marrow examination will show whether the numbers of megakaryocytes are reduced, normal or increased, and will provide essential information on morphology. Specific laboratory tests may be useful to confirm the presence of conditions such as PNH or SLE.

Immune thrombocytopenic purpura

In immune thrombocytopenic purpura (ITP), thrombocytopenia is due to immune destruction of platelets. The antibody-coated platelets are removed following binding to Fc receptors on macrophages.

ITP in children

This occurs most commonly in the 2–6-year age group. ITP has an acute onset with mucocutaneous bleeding and there may be a history of a recent viral infection, including varicella zoster or measles. Although bleeding may be severe, life-threatening haemorrhage is rare (approximately 1%). Bone marrow examination is not usually performed unless there are atypical clinical or laboratory features.

ITP in adults

The presentation is usually less acute than in children. ITP is characteristically seen in women and may be associated with other autoimmune disorders such as SLE, thyroid disease and autoimmune haemolytic anaemia (Evans syndrome). It is also seen in patients with chronic lymphocytic leukaemia and solid tumours, and after infections with viruses such as HIV. Platelet autoantibodies are detected in about 60–70% of patients and are presumed to be present, although not detectable, in the remaining patients; the antibodies often have specificity for platelet membrane glycoproteins IIb/IIIa and/or Ib.

Clinical features

Major haemorrhage is rare and is seen only in patients with severe thrombocytopenia. Easy bruising, purpura, epistaxis and menorrhagia are common. Physical examination is normal except for evidence of bleeding. Splenomegaly is rare.

Investigations

The only blood count abnormality is thrombocytopenia. The diagnosis is based on exclusion of other causes of thrombocytopenia using the history, clinical examination, blood count and blood film. Normal or increased numbers of megakaryocytes are found in the bone marrow, but bone marrow examination is unnecessary unless there are unusual findings clinically or on the blood film. The detection of platelet autoantibodies is not essential for confirmation of the diagnosis.

Management

Children

Children do not usually require treatment, as the thrombocytopenia is short-lived. Treatment should be reserved for serious bleeding or urgent surgery. Where treatment is necessary, corticosteroids and intravenous immunoglobulin are effective in more than 80% of children and raise the count more rapidly than steroids alone. Chronic ITP is unusual in children and requires specialist management.

Adults

Patients with platelet counts of more than 30×10^9/L generally require no treatment unless they are about to undergo a surgical procedure. Those with even lower platelet counts may not require treatment unless they have spontaneous bruising or bleeding.

First-line therapy

This consists of oral corticosteroids (1 mg/kg body weight). Approximately 66% will respond to prednisolone but relapse is common when the dose is reduced. Only 33% of patients can expect a long-term response, and long-term remission is seen in just 10–20% of patients after stopping prednisolone. Patients who fail to respond to corticosteroids or require high doses to maintain a safe platelet count should be considered for splenectomy.

Intravenous immunoglobulin is effective. It raises the platelet count in 75%, and in 50% the platelet count will normalize. Responses are only transient (3–4 weeks), with little evidence of any lasting effect. However, intravenous immunoglobulin is very useful where a rapid rise in platelet count is desired: for example, before surgery.

Second-line therapy

Therapies include:
- **Splenectomy**, to which the majority of patients respond; two-thirds will achieve a normal platelet count. About 50% of patients who do not have a complete response can still expect some improvement in the platelet count.
- **Rituximab (anti-CD20)**, to which about 60% of patients respond, although only 15–20% have long-lasting responses.
- **Thrombopoietin receptor agonists**, such as romiplostim and eltrombopag, which drive increased platelet production. They have been shown to increase platelet counts significantly in ITP on a long-term basis and are approved drugs for refractory ITP.
- **Platelet transfusions**, reserved for intracranial or other extreme haemorrhage, where emergency splenectomy may be justified.

Other immune thrombocytopenias

Drugs

Many drugs have been reported to cause immune thrombocytopenia. The same drugs can be responsible for immune haemolytic anaemia, thrombocytopenia or neutropenia in different patients.

Heparin-induced thrombocytopenia

See page 1014.

Neonatal alloimmune thrombocytopenia

This condition is due to fetomaternal incompatibility for platelet-specific antigens, usually for human platelet alloantigen 1a (HPA-1a), and is the platelet equivalent of HDN. The mother is HPA-1a-negative and produces antibodies that destroy the HPA-1a-positive fetal platelets. Thrombocytopenia is self-limiting after delivery, but platelet transfusions may be required initially to prevent or treat bleeding associated with severe thrombocytopenia; platelets are prepared from HPA-1a-negative volunteers or the mother herself. Severe bleeding, such as intracranial haemorrhage, may also occur *in utero*.

Antenatal treatment of the mother – usually with intravenous immunoglobulin and/or steroids – has been effective in preventing haemorrhage in severely affected cases.

Post-transfusion purpura

Post-transfusion purpura (PTP) is rare, occurring 7–10 days after a transfusion of platelet-containing blood components, usually red cells. PTP is associated with a platelet-specific alloantibody, usually anti-HPA-1a in an HPA-1a-negative individual. PTP always occurs in patients who have previously been immunized, either by blood transfusion or by pregnancy; hence it is more common in women. The cause of the destruction of the patient's own platelets is not well understood but they may be destroyed as 'bystanders' during the acute immune response to HPA-1a. PTP is self-limiting; intravenous immunoglobulin is the treatment of choice if there is severe thrombocytopenia and/or bleeding.

Thrombotic thrombocytopenic purpura

Thrombotic thrombocytopenic purpura (TTP) is a rare but very serious condition, in which platelet consumption leads to profound thrombocytopenia. There is a characteristic symptom complex of florid purpura, fever, fluctuating cerebral dysfunction and microangiopathic haemolytic anaemia with red cell fragmentation, often accompanied by acute kidney injury. The coagulation screen is usually normal but LDH levels are markedly raised as a result of haemolysis. TTP stems from endothelial damage and microvascular thrombosis. This occurs due to a reduction in ADAMTS-13 (*a di*sintegrin-like *and m*etalloproteinase domain with *t*hrombospondin-type motifs), a protease that is normally responsible for regulating the size of VWF. ADAMTS-13 is needed to break down ultra-large von Willebrand factor multimers (UL VWFMs) into smaller, haemostatically active fragments that interact with platelets. Reduction in ADAMTS-13 results in the adhesion and aggregation of platelets to UL VWFMs and multiorgan microthrombi. In most sporadic cases, there is a true deficiency of the ADAMTS-13, associated with antibodies to ADAMTS-13. In some congenital cases, the deficiency is due to mutations in the *ADAMTS-13* gene. Secondary causes of acute TTP include pregnancy, oral contraceptives, SLE, infection and drug treatment, including the use of ticlopidine and clopidogrel. Such cases may have a variable ADAMTS-13 activity at presentation, and may or may not have associated antibodies to ADAMTS-13.

Management

Plasma exchange is the mainstay of treatment. It provides a source of ADAMTS-13 and removes associated autoantibody in acute TTP. Cryoprecipitate and solvent-detergent FFP both contain ADAMTS-13. Pulsed intravenous methylprednisolone is given acutely; increasingly, rituximab is also a primary treatment of choice. Disease activity is monitored by measuring the platelet count and serum LDH. Platelet concentrates are contraindicated. The untreated condition has a mortality of up to 90% but modern management has reduced this figure to about 10%. Recurrent and relapsing TTP occurs, often associated with a persistent lack of ADAMTS-13. In secondary TTP cases, identifiable precipitating drugs should be stopped. Caplacizumab is a single-variable-domain immunoglobulin directed to the A1 region of the VWF. It inhibits the VWF interaction with glycoprotein Ib and has recently been shown to lead to faster normalization of the platelet count and a lower rate of recurrent TTP.

Platelet function disorders

Platelet function disorders (**Box 16.29**) are usually associated with excessive bruising and bleeding and, in some of the acquired forms, with thrombosis. The platelet count is often normal and the bleeding time is prolonged. The rare inherited defects of platelet function require more detailed investigations, such as platelet aggregation studies and factor VIII and VWF assays, as there is often a clinical overlap in symptoms with von Willebrand disease.

If there is serious bleeding or if the patient is about to undergo surgery, drugs with antiplatelet activity should be withdrawn and any underlying condition should be corrected if possible.

> *i* **Box 16.29 Inherited and acquired types of platelet dysfunction**
>
> **Inherited**
> - *Glanzmann's thrombasthenia* – lack of platelet membrane glycoprotein IIb/IIIa complex, resulting in defective fibrinogen binding and failure of platelet aggregation
> - *Bernard–Soulier syndrome* – lack of platelet membrane glycoprotein Ib/IX/V complex (the binding site for von Willebrand factor), causing failure of platelet adhesion and moderate thrombocytopenia
> - *Storage pool disease* – lack of the storage pool of platelet dense bodies, causing poor platelet function
>
> **Acquired**
> - Myeloproliferative disorders
> - Renal and liver disease
> - Paraproteinaemias
> - Drug-induced, such as with non-steroidal anti-inflammatory drugs (aspirin) or other platelet inhibitory drugs

Platelet dysfunction can be a major component of bleeding in renal disease, although other components are often also seen. The degree of the platelet-related defect is broadly proportional to the plasma urea concentration: platelet function is impaired by urea, guanidinosuccinic acid and other phenolic metabolites that accumulate in chronic kidney disease. Dialysis partially corrects platelet function. The haematocrit should be increased to over 0.30 and non-specific use of desmopressin may be helpful. Platelet transfusions may be required if these measures are unsuccessful or if the risk of bleeding is high.

Thrombocytosis

The platelet count may rise above 400×10^9/L as a result of:
- splenectomy
- malignant disease
- inflammatory disorders, such as rheumatoid arthritis and inflammatory bowel disease
- major surgery and haemorrhage
- myeloproliferative disorders
- iron deficiency.

Thus, thrombocytosis is part of the acute-phase reaction, although platelet numbers are also elevated following splenectomy because of the loss of a major site of platelet destruction.

Essential thrombocythaemia, a myeloproliferative neoplasm (see p. 394), and other myeloproliferative conditions such as polycythaemia vera, myelofibrosis and chronic myeloid leukaemia, may also be associated with a high platelet count.

A persistently elevated platelet count can lead to arterial or venous thrombosis. It is usual to treat the underlying cause of the thrombocytosis but sometimes a small dose of aspirin (75 mg) is also given. In myeloproliferative diseases, the primary risk is thrombosis and specific action is often taken to reduce the platelet count, usually with hydroxycarbamide (hydroxyurea). Paradoxically, there is also a risk of abnormal bleeding if the platelet count is very high.

Further reading

British Committee for Standards in Haematology. Guideline for the investigation and management of adults and children presenting with a thrombocytosis. *Br J Haematol* 2010; 149:352–375.

Scully M, Cataland SR, Peyvandi F et al. Caplacizumab treatment for acquired thrombotic thrombocytopenic purpura. *N Engl J Med* 2019; 380:335–346.

Veyradier A. Von Willebrand factor – a new target for TTP treatment? *N Engl J Med* 2016; 374:583–585.

A Normal

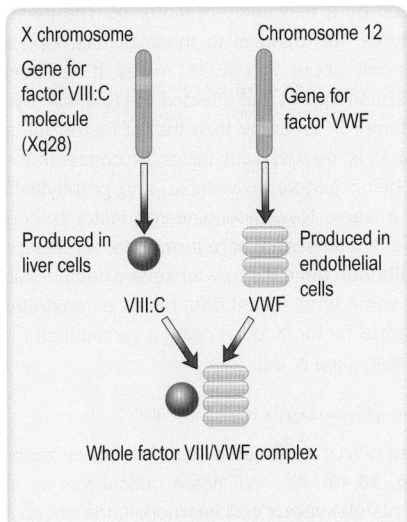

B Haemophilia A

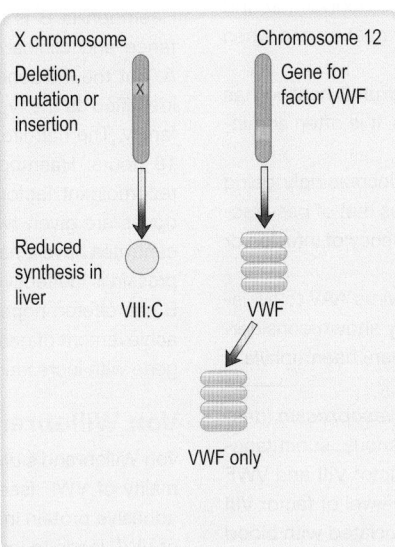

C von Willebrand's disease

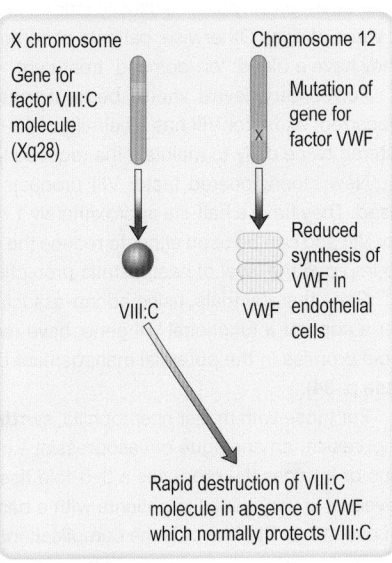

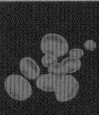

Fig. 16.40 Synthesis of factor VIII and von Willebrand factor (VWF) in inherited coagulation disorders. **(A)** Normal factor VIII synthesis. **(B)** Haemophilia A, showing defective synthesis of factor VIIIc. **(C)** Von Willebrand's disease, showing reduced synthesis of VWF.

INHERITED COAGULATION DISORDERS

Inherited coagulation disorders are uncommon and usually involve deficiency of one factor only. Acquired coagulation disorders occur more frequently and almost always involve several coagulation factors (see p. 377).

In inherited coagulation disorders, deficiencies of all factors have been described. Those leading to abnormal bleeding are rare, apart from haemophilia A (factor VIII deficiency), haemophilia B (factor IX deficiency) and von Willebrand's disease.

Haemophilia A

This is due to a lack of factor VIII. VWF is normal in haemophilia (**Fig. 16.40**). The prevalence of haemophilia A is about 1 in 5000 of the male population. It is inherited as an X-linked disorder. If a female carrier has a son, he has a 50% chance of having haemophilia; a daughter has a 50% chance of being a carrier. All daughters of men with haemophilia are carriers and the sons are normal.

Although a large number of different genetic defects have been found in the factor VIII gene, a common gene inversion in intron 22 is causative in approximately 50% of families with severe disease. There is a high mutation rate, one-third of cases being apparently sporadic with no family history of haemophilia.

Clinical features and investigations

The clinical features depend on the level of factor VIII. The normal level of factor VIII is 50–150 IU/dL.

- **Levels of <1 IU/dL (severe haemophilia)** are associated with frequent spontaneous bleeding from early life, typically into joints and muscles. Without adequate treatment, such recurrent bleeding into joints leads to crippling joint deformity.
- **Levels of 1–5 IU/dL (moderate haemophilia)** are associated with severe bleeding following injury and occasional spontaneous bleeds.

i **Box 16.30** Blood changes in haemophilia A, von Willebrand's disease and vitamin K deficiency

	Haemophilia A	von Willebrand's disease	Vitamin K deficiency
Bleeding time	Normal	↑	Normal
Prothrombin time	Normal	Normal	↑
Activated partial thromboplastin time	↑+	↑±	↑
Factor VIII:C	↓++	↓	Normal
Von Willebrand factor	Normal	↓	Normal

- **Levels of >5 IU/dL (mild haemophilia)** are usually associated with bleeding only after injury or surgery. Diagnosis in this group can often be delayed until quite late in life.

With treatment, life expectancy today is very good. The most common causes of death in people with haemophilia are cancer and heart disease, as for the general population, rather than bleeding, although cerebral haemorrhage is much more frequent than in the general population. The main laboratory features of haemophilia A are shown in **Box 16.30**. The abnormal findings are an isolated prolongation of the APTT and a reduced level of factor VIII. The PT, bleeding time and VWF level are normal.

Management

Bleeding is treated by administration of **factor VIII concentrate** by intravenous infusion to achieve normalization of levels. Factor VIII concentrate is available as a plasma-derived or recombinant product. Recombinant products are the treatment of choice but economic constraints often limit availability, particularly in developing countries.

Many patients with severe haemophilia treat themselves at home with regular factor VIII infusions three or more times per week, to prevent recurrent bleeding into joints and subsequent joint damage. Such 'prophylaxis' is usually started in early childhood (around 2 years of age). Otherwise, patients at home may treat as and when they have a bleed: 'on-demand' treatment.

For surgery, levels should be kept to normal until healing has occurred; as factor VIII has a half-life of 12 hours, it is often administered twice daily to maintain the required level.

New bioengineered factor VIII products are increasingly being used. They have a half-life approximately 1.5 times that of base factor VIII and can be used either to reduce the frequency of infusion or to improve the level of haemostatic protection.

Gene therapy trials, using adeno-associated virus AAV to transfer a copy of a functional VIII gene, have recently shown considerable promise in the potential management of severe haemophilia A (see p. 34).

For those with milder haemophilia, *synthetic vasopressin* (desmopressin, an analogue of vasopressin) – intravenous, subcutaneous or intranasal – produces a 3–5-fold rise in factor VIII and VWF levels. It is very useful in patients with a baseline level of factor VIII of over 10 IU/dL. It avoids the complications associated with blood products and is useful for treating and preventing bleeding in mild haemophilia.

People with haemophilia should be registered at a comprehensive care centre (CCC), which takes responsibility for their full medical care, including social and psychological support.

Complications

Up to 30% of people with severe haemophilia will, during their lifetime, develop antibodies to factor VIII that inhibit its action. Such inhibitors usually develop after the first few treatment doses of factor VIII. Inhibitors are relatively rare in moderate and mild haemophilia, and are often associated with specific molecular defects.

Management of inhibitor patients is very difficult, as infused factor VIII is rapidly inactivated. Acute bleeding events require treatment with agents that can bypass factor VIII, such as recombinant factor VIIa or activated prothrombin complex concentrates. Alternative non-factor replacement therapies using bispecific antibodies that can bind both factor IX and factor X, so partially mimicking factor VIII, have been shown to be highly effective alternative therapies to prevent bleeding in haemophilia A with inhibitors and are increasingly being used. Such treatments can also be effective in patients without inhibitors.

In those recently identified as having developed an inhibitor, the long-term aim is to eradicate the inhibitory antibody. This is done using immune tolerance induction strategies, sometimes with additional immunosuppression, and is successful in around 80% of cases.

Although a historical legacy of plasma-derived concentrates, the risk of *viral transmission* has been virtually eliminated (see p. 361). Many died as a consequence of HIV and HCV infection, however a considerable number of patients remain that have HIV and/or HCV infection.

Carrier detection and antenatal diagnosis

Owing to lyonization early in embryonic life (i.e. random inactivation of one chromosome; see p. 21), some female carriers may have low levels of factor VIII while others will have normal levels. Carrier detection is, therefore, definitively carried out using molecular genetic testing/mutation analysis. Antenatal diagnosis may be carried out by molecular analysis of chorionic villus biopsy at 11–12 weeks' gestation if selective termination is being considered, or by third-trimester amniocentesis if not.

Haemophilia B (Christmas disease)

Haemophilia B is caused by a deficiency of factor IX. The inheritance and clinical features are identical to those of haemophilia A, but the incidence is only about 1 in 30 000 males. It has been identified as the type of haemophilia that affected the Russian royal family. The half-life of factor IX is longer than that of factor VIII, at 18 hours. Haemophilia B is treated with factor IX concentrates, recombinant factor IX being generally available, and prophylactic doses are given twice a week. New bioengineered factor IX concentrates have a half-life 3–5 times that of regular factor IX. Desmopressin is ineffective. Although gene therapy for severe haemophilia B has offered hope for some time, recent data have demonstrated achievement of near-normal factor IX levels using a variant factor IX gene with increased activity (see p. 34).

Von Willebrand's disease

von Willebrand's disease (VWD) is caused by a deficiency or abnormality of VWF (see **Fig. 16.40**). As VWF has a critical role as an adhesive protein in the platelet vessel wall interaction, the absence of VWF leads to impaired platelet adhesion to the subendothelium. Reduced VWF levels also lead to factor VIII deficiency, as factor VIII is not protected from premature degradation. VWF reduction in VWD therefore leads to a dual haemostatic defect.

The VWF gene is located on chromosome 12 and numerous mutations have been identified. VWD has been classified into three types:

- **Type 1** is partial quantitative deficiency of VWF; significant type 1 VWD is usually inherited as an autosomal dominant.
- **Type 2** is due to a qualitative abnormality of VWF; it too is usually inherited as an autosomal dominant.
- **Type 3** is recessively inherited and patients have virtually complete deficiency of VWF. Their parents are often phenotypically normal.

Many subtypes of VWD are described, particularly type 2 variants, which reflect the specific qualitative changes in the VWF protein.

Clinical features

These are very variable. Type 1 and type 2 patients usually have relatively mild clinical features. Bleeding follows minor trauma or surgery, and epistaxis and menorrhagia often occur. Haemarthroses are rare. Type 3 patients have more severe bleeding but rarely experience the joint and muscle bleeds seen in haemophilia A.

Characteristic laboratory findings are shown in **Box 16.30**. Classically VWF activity is measured as its platelet dependent function in the presence of ristocetin.

Management

Management depends on the severity of the condition and may be similar to that of mild haemophilia, including the use of desmopressin where possible. Although recombinant VWF is becoming available, plasma-derived factor VIII concentrates that contain intact VWF are the mainstay of replacement therapy. These specific products are used to treat bleeding or to cover surgery in patients who require replacement therapy, such as those with type 3 (severe) VWD and those who do not respond adequately to desmopressin. Cryoprecipitate could be used as a source of VWF but is avoided if possible, since it is not virus-inactivated.

Further reading

Peters R, Harris T. Advances and innovations in haemophilia treatment. *Nat Rev Drug Discov* 2018; 17:493–508.
Peyvandi F, Garagiola I, Young G. The past and future of haemophilia: diagnosis, treatments, and its complications. *Lancet* 2016; 388:187–197.

ACQUIRED COAGULATION DISORDERS

Vitamin K deficiency

Vitamin K is necessary for the γ-carboxylation of glutamic acid residues on coagulation factors II, VII, IX and X, and on proteins C and S. Without it, these factors cannot bind calcium.

Deficiency of vitamin K (see also p. 1239) may be due to:

- *inadequate stores*, as in HDN and severe malnutrition, especially when combined with antibiotic treatment
- *malabsorption of vitamin K*, a fat-soluble vitamin, which occurs in cholestatic jaundice owing to the lack of intraluminal bile salts
- *oral anticoagulant drugs*, many of which are vitamin K antagonists.

The PT and APTT are prolonged (see **Box 16.30**) and there may be bruising, haematuria and gastrointestinal or cerebral bleeding. Minor bleeding is treated with phytomenadione (vitamin K_1) 10 mg intravenously. Some correction of the PT is usual within 6 hours but it may not return to normal for 2 days.

Newborn babies have low levels of vitamin K and this may cause minor bleeding in the first week of life (*classical haemorrhagic disease of the newborn*). Vitamin K deficiency also causes *late haemorrhagic disease of the newborn*, which occurs 2–26 weeks after birth and results in severe bleeding such as intracranial haemorrhage. Most infants with these syndromes have been exclusively breast-fed, and both conditions are prevented by administering 1 mg i.m. vitamin K to all neonates (see p. 1239). Concerns about the safety of this strategy are unfounded.

Liver disease

Liver disease may result in a number of defects in haemostasis:

- *Vitamin K deficiency.* This occurs owing to intrahepatic or extrahepatic cholestasis.
- *Reduced synthesis.* Reduced synthesis of coagulation factors (including natural anticoagulant proteins) may be the result of severe hepatocellular damage. The use of vitamin K does not improve the results of abnormal coagulation tests, but it is generally given to ensure that a treatable cause of failure of haemostasis has not been missed.
- *Thrombocytopenia.* This results from hypersplenism due to splenomegaly associated with portal hypertension, or from folic acid deficiency.
- *Functional abnormalities.* Functional abnormalities of platelets and fibrinogen are found in many patients with liver failure.
- *Disseminated intravascular coagulation.* DIC occurs in acute hepatic failure.

Disseminated intravascular coagulation

Disseminated intravascular coagulation (DIC) never occurs in isolation. Recognition that the patient has a clinical disorder that may result in DIC (**Box 16.31**) is the key to investigation and management. DIC arises because of systemic activation of coagulation either by release of procoagulant material, such as tissue factor, or via cytokine pathways as part of the inflammatory response. Such systemic activation leads to widespread generation of fibrin and deposition in blood vessels, leading to thrombosis and multiorgan failure. Due to the widespread coagulation activation there is consumption of platelets and coagulation factors, and secondary activation of fibrinolysis leading to production of FDPs and D-dimer. These further contribute to the coagulation defect by inhibiting fibrin polymerization (**Fig.**

> **?** **Box 16.31** Causes of disseminated intravascular coagulation
>
> - Malignant disease
> - Septicaemia (e.g. Gram-negative, including meningococcal)
> - Haemolytic transfusion reactions
> - Obstetric causes (e.g. abruptio placentae, amniotic fluid embolism, pre-eclampsia)
> - Trauma, burns, surgery
> - Other infections (e.g. *falciparum* malaria)
> - Liver disease
> - Snake bite

16.41). The consequences of these changes are a mixture of initial thrombosis, followed by a bleeding tendency due to consumption of coagulation factors and dysregulated fibrinolytic activation.

Clinical features

The underlying disorder is usually obvious. The patient is often acutely ill and shocked. The clinical presentation of DIC varies from no bleeding at all to profound haemostatic failure with widespread haemorrhage. Bleeding may occur from the mouth, nose and venepuncture sites, and there may be widespread ecchymoses.

Thrombotic events occur as a result of vessel occlusion by fibrin and platelets. Any organ may be involved but the skin, brain and kidneys are most often affected.

Investigations

The diagnosis needs to encompass both clinical and laboratory aspects. It is often suggested by the underlying condition of the patient. If the patient has an underlying disorder known to be compatible with overt DIC, the International Society on Thrombosis and Haemostasis (ISTH) scoring system is a useful diagnostic tool and provides an objective assessment (**Box 16.32**).

In severe cases with haemorrhage:

- The PT, APTT and TT are usually very prolonged and the fibrinogen level is markedly reduced.
- High levels of FDPs, including D-dimer, are found, owing to the intense fibrinolytic activity stimulated by the presence of fibrin in the circulation.
- There is severe thrombocytopenia.
- The blood film may show fragmented red blood cells.

Management

The cornerstone of management is treatment of the underlying condition and intensive support to manage hypoxia, acidosis and organ failure. In those that are not bleeding, this is often all that is necessary. Transfusions of platelet concentrates, FFP, cryoprecipitate and red cell concentrates is indicated in patients who are bleeding or to cover interventions. Transfusion of blood components on the basis of coagulation tests alone is not required. Inhibitors of fibrinolysis, such as tranexamic acid, should not be used in DIC, as dangerous fibrin deposition may result. In those cases with a dominant thrombotic component, the cautious use of unfractionated heparin should be considered. In critically ill, non-bleeding patients with DIC, thromboprophylactic doses of heparin are recommended.

Excessive fibrinolysis

Excessive fibrinolysis occurs in certain malignancies, such as acute promyelocytic leukaemia, and also during surgery involving tumours of the prostate, breast, pancreas and uterus owing to release of tissue plasminogen activators.

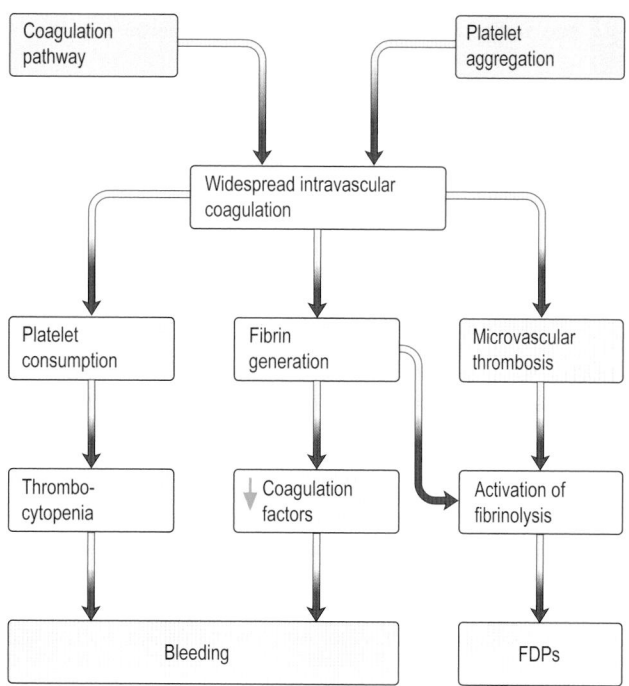

Fig. 16.41 Disseminated intravascular coagulation. FDPs, fibrin degradation products.

> **i** **Box 16.32** ISTH diagnostic scoring system for disseminated intravascular coagulation (DIC)

Parameter	Score
Platelet count	>100 × 10⁹/L = 0
	<100 × 10⁹/L = 1
	<50 × 10⁹/L = 2
Elevated fibrin marker (e.g. D-dimer, fibrin degradation products)	No increase = 0
	Moderate increase = 2
	Strong increase = 3
Prolonged prothrombin time	<3 s = 0
	>3 s but <6 s = 1
	>6 s = 2
Fibrinogen level	>1 g/L = 0
	<1 g/L = 1

Calculate score:
>5 compatible with overt DIC: repeat score daily
<5 suggestive of non-overt DIC: repeat in next 1–2 days

ISTH, International Society on Thrombosis and Haemostasis.

Primary hyperfibrinolysis is very rare but activation of fibrinolysis occurs in DIC as a secondary event in response to intravascular deposition of fibrin.

The clinical picture is similar to that of DIC, with widespread bleeding. Laboratory investigations are also similar, with a prolonged PT, APTT and TT, a low fibrinogen level and increased FDPs, although fragmented red cells and thrombocytopenia are not seen because disseminated coagulation with widespread fibrin deposition is not present.

If the diagnosis is certain, fibrinolytic inhibitors, such as tranexamic acid, can be given but evidence for their efficacy is lacking.

Massive transfusion

Few platelets and reduced levels of clotting factors are found in stored blood, although there are adequate amounts of the other coagulation factors. During massive transfusion (defined as transfusion of a volume of blood equal to the patient's own blood volume within 24 hours, e.g. >10 units in an adult), the platelet count and PT and APTT should be checked at intervals.

Transfusion of platelet concentrates, FFP and cryoprecipitate should be given if thrombocytopenia or defective coagulation is thought to be contributing to continued blood loss. Other problems of massive transfusion are described on page 221.

Inhibitors of coagulation

Factor VIII autoantibodies arise occasionally in patients without haemophilia but with autoimmune disorders such as SLE, in elderly patients, with malignant disease and sometimes after childbirth. There can be severe bleeding. Immediate bleeding problems are managed with concentrates that bypass factor VIII activity (e.g. recombinant factor VIIa or activated prothrombin complex concentrates, see p. 363). Longer-term therapy aims to eliminate the autoantibody using immunosuppression, such as steroids, cyclophosphamide or rituximab.

Lupus anticoagulant antibodies (see p. 460) are autoantibodies directed against phospholipids (antiphospholipid antibodies); they cause prolongation of phospholipid-dependent coagulation tests, particularly the APTT, but do not inhibit coagulation factor activity.

Further reading

Gando S, Levi M, Toh C-H. Disseminated intravascular coagulation. *Nat Rev Dis Primers* 2016; 2:1–16.
George JN, Nester CM. Syndromes of thrombotic microangiopathy. *N Engl J Med* 2014; 371:654–666.
Hunt BJ. Bleeding and coagulopathies in critical care. *N Engl J Med* 2014; 370:847–859.
Lillicrap D. Von Willebrand disease: advances in pathogenetic understanding, diagnosis and therapy. *Blood* 2013; 122:3735–3740.
Tripodi A, Mannucci PM. The coagulopathy of chronic liver disease. *N Engl J Med* 2011; 365:147–156.

Significant websites

https://b-s-h.org.uk/guidelines/ *British Society for Haematology guidelines*
http://www.bloodline.net *General website on haematology*
http://www.hemophilia.org *US National Hemophilia Foundation*
http://www.isth.org/ *International Society on Thrombosis and Haemostasis (ISTH)*
http://www.shotuk.org *Serious Hazards of Transfusion (SHOT) scheme, covering UK and Ireland NHS and private hospitals, affiliated to the Royal College of Pathologists (based at the Manchester Blood Transfusion Centre)*
http://www.transfusionguidelines.org.uk *UK Blood Transfusion and Tissue Transplantation Services Professional Guidelines, including* Handbook of Transfusion Medicine
http://www.transfusion.org Transfusion, *the journal of the American Association of Blood Banks*
http://www.wfh.org *World Federation of Hemophilia*

17

Haematological oncology

Jonathan Sive and Vanessa Foggo

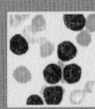

CORE SKILLS AND KNOWLEDGE

The haematological malignancies include leukaemias, myeloproliferative neoplasms, lymphomas and myeloma. They are uncommon but not rare, lymphoma being the fifth most common cancer in the UK.

Haemato-oncologists divide their time between inpatient care, outpatient clinics, chemotherapy day units and the diagnostic laboratory. In smaller centres, malignant haematology may comprise only one aspect of the work of a haematologist. In larger centres, haematologists will focus purely on the treatment of malignant disease. Here, they will often be engaged with clinical trials, medical education and research.

Inpatient wards accommodate those requiring investigation and those receiving intensive chemotherapy, in addition to patients requiring management of the acute complications caused by their disease or its treatment. More specialist units will accommodate patients undergoing autologous or allogeneic stem cell transplantation (SCT).

Key to learning objectives for haemato-oncology at undergraduate level include:

- understanding acute leukaemia and the role of SCT
- learning about the lymphomas and myeloma, and their different management strategies
- having an appreciation of the key approaches to treatment with use of cytotoxics, immunotherapy, small molecules and radiotherapy
- managing emergencies in haemato-oncology: leucostasis, hyperviscosity, tumour lysis syndrome and spinal cord compression.

Specific opportunities for learning haemato-oncology include attending ward rounds on inpatient haemato-oncology wards and transplant units, spending time at the haemato-oncology day unit and becoming familiar with how chemotherapy is delivered, meeting patients presenting with haematological malignancy and following their diagnostic work-up, and attending the haemato-oncology multidisciplinary team meeting to review diagnostic material, and to discuss management options.

CLINICAL SKILLS FOR HAEMATOLOGICAL ONCOLOGY

History

Ask about relevant symptoms (which may each arise acutely or have a chronic and insidious onset) and risk factors for malignancy, and elicit the information needed for guiding treatment (**Box 17.1**).

Assessing suitability for treatment

A patient's **performance status** is a key determinant of how well they are likely to cope with intensive anti-cancer treatment, such as chemotherapy or stem cell transplantation (SCT) (see **Box 6.13**). Asking questions about various activities of daily living (personal care, e.g. washing and dressing, and domestic tasks, e.g. shopping or preparing food) allows performance status to be assessed, and also monitored over time.

 Box 17.1 Taking a history in haemato-oncology

Symptoms of bone marrow failure
- Symptoms of anaemia – fatigue, shortness of breath, reduced exercise capacity
- Thrombocytopenia – easy bruising/bleeding
- Leucopenia – recurrent infection

Symptoms caused by mass effect of malignant tissue
- Abdominal discomfort from splenic enlargement
- Neck, jaw, axillary or groin swelling from enlarged lymph nodes

Systemic symptoms
- Malaise
- Fevers (>38°C)
- Sweats (particularly at night, drenching)
- Weight loss (should always be quantified: >10% unintentional weight loss over 6 months is considered significant)

Family history
- Haematological problems and malignancy
- Potential donors where allogeneic transplantation may be considered: ages and health of siblings

Risk factors
- Previous exposure to cytotoxins
- Previous exposure to ionizing radiation
- Viral infection

Fitness for treatment
- Medical co-morbidity that may influence treatment approach
- Social circumstances, including an assessment of performance status (see later)

Examination

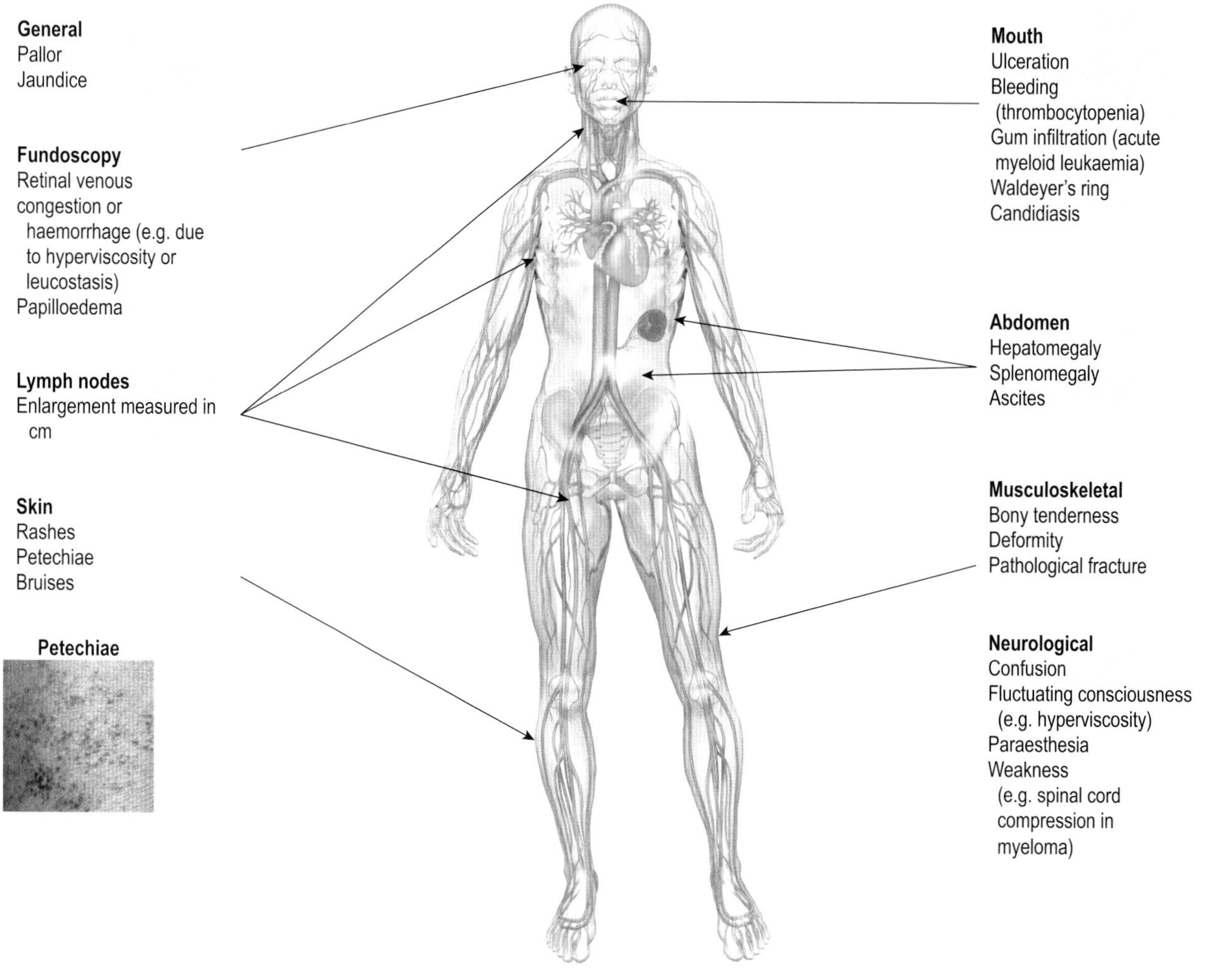

General
Pallor
Jaundice

Fundoscopy
Retinal venous congestion or haemorrhage (e.g. due to hyperviscosity or leucostasis)
Papilloedema

Lymph nodes
Enlargement measured in cm

Skin
Rashes
Petechiae
Bruises

Petechiae

Mouth
Ulceration
Bleeding (thrombocytopenia)
Gum infiltration (acute myeloid leukaemia)
Waldeyer's ring
Candidiasis

Abdomen
Hepatomegaly
Splenomegaly
Ascites

Musculoskeletal
Bony tenderness
Deformity
Pathological fracture

Neurological
Confusion
Fluctuating consciousness (e.g. hyperviscosity)
Paraesthesia
Weakness (e.g. spinal cord compression in myeloma)

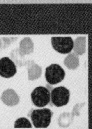

Cytotoxics
- Target rapidly growing cells and have historically formed the basis of conventional anti-cancer chemotherapy, remaining the backbone of most treatment regimens
- Classes include alkylating agents (e.g. cyclophosphamide), anthracyclines (e.g. doxorubicin), vinca alkaloids (e.g. vincristine) and purine analogues (e.g. mercaptopurine, 6-MP)

Immunotherapy
- Monoclonal antibodies target a protein on the surface of the malignant cell (rituximab, one of the most commonly used monoclonal antibodies in the treatment of haematological malignancies, targets the CD20 molecule on B lymphocytes and triggers cell death)
- Antibodies either target the tumour cell directly or can act as a vector for toxins

Corticosteroids
- Synthetic high-dose corticosteroids, e.g. dexamethasone, induce cell death in malignant lymphoid cells
- Have a prominent role alongside other forms of anti-cancer treatment in all B-cell malignancies, including myeloma

Molecular therapy
- An increased understanding of the pathophysiology of disease has allowed the development of treatments targeting specific pathways, e.g. FLT3 inhibitors such as midostaurin, which block abnormal cell signalling in acute myeloid leukaemia, or venetoclax, which blocks the mutated anti-apoptotic protein Bcl-2 in chronic lymphocytic leukaemia

Stem cell transplantation
- Involves transfer of pluripotent stem cells from either a donor (allogeneic) or the patient (autologous), following myeloablative chemo- or radiotherapy
- Generally attempted once remission has been achieved using other forms of therapy, to destroy any malignant cells
- Transplanted cells permit bone marrow recovery, and in allogeneic SCT replace the patient's own abnormal bone marrow with an alternative, normally functioning, haemopoietic system

Novel therapies
- e.g. Chimeric antigen receptor (CAR) T-cell therapy, an experimental treatment that involves collecting a patient's own T cells and modifying them to express a receptor that will bind a particular protein expressed by the tumour; the cells are expanded and re-infused, and when they meet their target malignant cell, they attack and destroy it
- Dramatic responses may be observed, even in chemotherapy-resistant cancer

Radiotherapy
- Targets solid tumour masses, e.g. groups of enlarged lymph nodes in early-stage lymphomas, plasmacytomas (see p. 410) and residual disease post treatment

Surgery
- Although of limited use in treatment of these conditions, surgery has a role in obtaining diagnostic tissue through biopsy
- Neurosurgery may relieve spinal cord compression, though steroids and radiotherapy are more frequently indicated
- Orthopaedic fixation of pathological fractures may be required in patients with myeloma

Treatments

Treatment plans (**Box 17.2**) are guided by a large volume of clinical trial evidence that exists for all haematological malignancies, and often patients can be offered enrolment into clinical trials of novel agents.

Aims of treatment

Not all treatment intent will be curative. In indolent disease, treatments are focused on slowing progression or managing symptoms and complications. Factors affecting treatment include:

- **Patient factors.** Performance status or frailty scores are helpful in estimating how well patients may tolerate a particular treatment. Open discussion with the patient is vital. Potential side-effects and complications of treatment must be balanced against the likelihood of a favourable outcome.
- **Disease factors.** Better understanding of pathophysiology has given us prognostic markers (e.g. FLT3 in acute myeloid leukaemia), and data gathered from large-cohort analyses inform increasingly accurate scoring systems.
- **Treatment factors.** The expense of newer therapies results in restricted prescribing in most healthcare systems. Enrolment in clinical trials gives some access to these drugs before their cost-effectiveness can be fully evaluated.

INTRODUCTION

Haematological malignancies cover a wide range of blood-based and solid cancers, and their diversity and nomenclature can be confusing. The updated 2016 World Health Organization (WHO) classification contains over 150 distinct entities, many of which have been added since the previous version from 2008. There is an increasing emphasis on underlying genetic abnormalities, as well as histology and immunophenotype. It is beyond the needs of generalists (and most haematologists) to be aware of all these conditions, but a few principles can hopefully provide an overview of this group of cancers and their pathogenesis, clinical behaviour and treatment.

Aetiology

(See **Box 6.4**.)

Like all cancers, haematological malignancies are caused by the **acquisition of genetic changes** within a normal cell, leading to development of a clonal population. These may be large-scale chromosomal abnormalities (translocations, deletions or duplications), which can be detected by cytogenetic analysis, or point mutations within a specific gene, which require DNA sequencing technology for analysis (**Fig. 17.1**).

Most of these events are random, although their incidence generally **increases with age**. However, not all mutations will necessarily lead to a malignancy and there is an increasing awareness of the accumulation of mutations as part of the normal ageing process. For example, mutations in genes such as *DNMT3A* and *ASXL1* are commonly found in older people's myeloid cells with no evidence of myelodysplasia (MDS) or acute myeloid leukaemia (AML); this is referred to as CHIP – clonal haemopoiesis of indeterminate potential. Similarly, the t(14;18) translocation associated with follicular lymphoma is found in around 50% of healthy individuals' circulating lymphocytes.

Previous **radiation exposure** (usually as part of radiotherapy treatment for a previous cancer) and **cytotoxic chemotherapy** can cause genetic abnormalities and subsequent malignancy. This is most commonly seen in myeloid malignancy with the development of therapy-related MDS or AML.

Viral infections are implicated as a cause of a number of haematological cancers: for example, human T-cell leukaemia (or lymphotropic) virus type 1 (HTLV-1) in adult T-cell leukaemia/lymphoma (ATLL), in which integration of viral DNA into regulatory T cells leads to malignant transformation. Epstein–Barr virus (EBV) can have a similar effect in other lymphomas, including Hodgkin lymphoma. Human immunodeficiency virus (HIV) infection predisposes to certain non-Hodgkin lymphomas, but the mechanisms appear to be primarily immunosuppression and co-infection with other viruses such as EBV and human herpesvirus 8 (HHV8), rather than direct HIV viral integration.

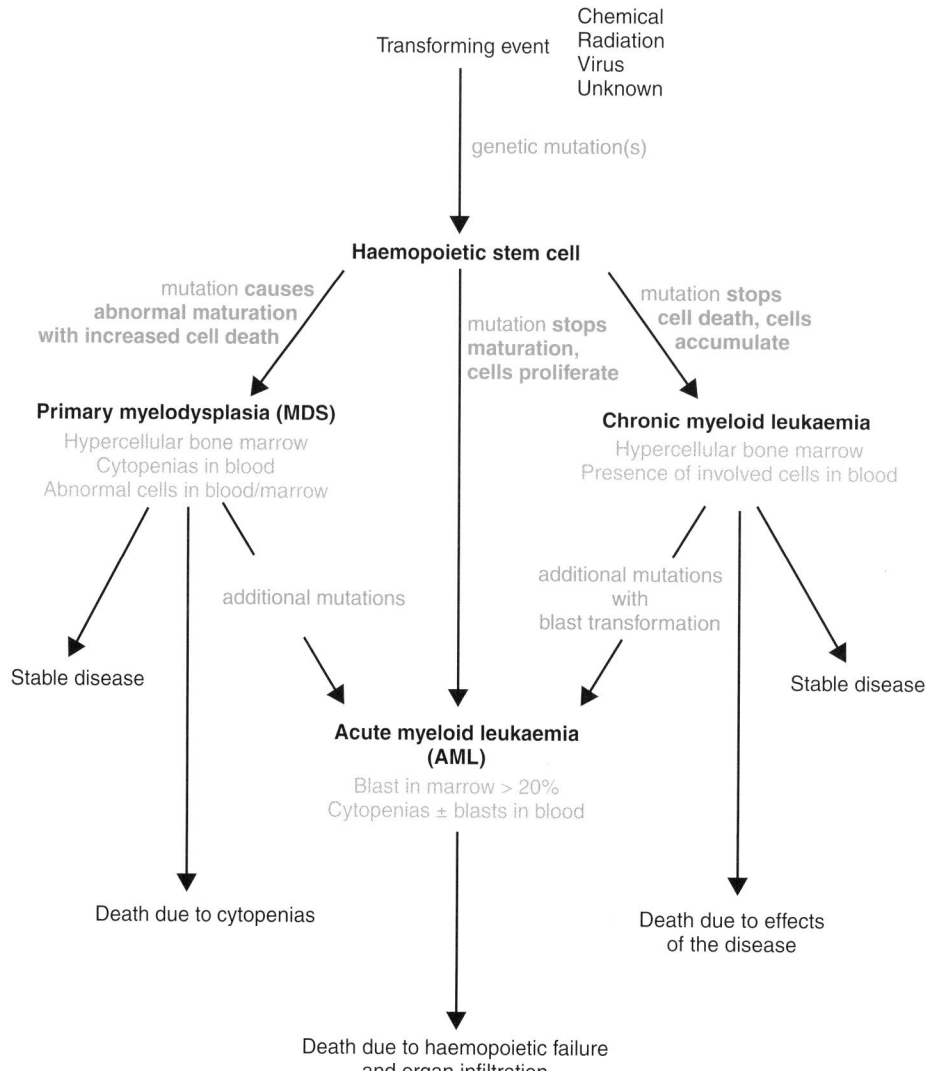

Fig. 17.1 Acquisition of clonal changes. *(Adapted from http://eclinpath.com/hematology/leukemia/ transforming-aligorithm/.)*

Immunosuppression due to long-term use of systemic therapies can increase the risk of lymphoma. This is seen most commonly in post-transplant lymphoproliferative disorder (PTLD), which can occur in patients receiving immunosuppressive therapy after renal or other transplants. Again, the majority of cases are due to EBV infection.

Congenital conditions that predispose to haematological malignancy are rare, but a small number of conditions do exist in which a germline genetic disorder increases the risk of leukaemias developing. These include Down's syndrome (trisomy 21), which can be associated with a transient myeloproliferative disorder in the neonatal period as well as an increased risk of both AML and acute lymphoblastic leukaemia (ALL), and bone marrow failure syndromes, such as Fanconi anaemia (see p. 337).

Pathogenesis

Haematological malignancies can mainly be characterized based on the ***normal counterpart cell within the haemopoietic system***. For example, AML is derived from a haemopoietic stem cell that has acquired mutations, leading to rapid proliferation of an abnormal population. These cells share some morphological and immunophenotypic appearances with normal myeloid precursor cells in the bone marrow, but their unchecked proliferation and inability to undergo differentiation lead to a neoplastic population. Myeloma, in contrast, is a cancer of plasma cells derived from a post-germinal centre B cell, whose function in producing antibodies is reflected in the abnormal monoclonal paraprotein that their malignant counterpart secretes.

Haematological cancers can be broadly divided between ***myeloid*** and ***lymphoid*** lineages (see **Fig. 16.1**). Myeloid disorders arise from those lineages within the marrow that produce granulocytes, red cells or platelets. Lymphoid disorders can arise from either B- or T-cell lineages. This classification is summarized in **Box 17.3** and the specific subdivision of the lymphoid malignancies is illustrated in **Fig. 17.2**. This division may not, however, accurately represent the cell of origin: for example, chronic myeloid leukaemia (CML) can undergo a lymphoid blast transformation into an ALL-like disease, reflecting the fact that the CML clone is derived from a haemopoietic stem cell (HSC) with both myeloid and lymphoid differentiation potential.

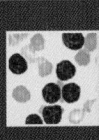

Box 17.3 Classification of leukaemia and lymphoma

Timeframe	Myeloid (bone marrow)	Lymphoid (bone marrow)	Lymphoid (node)
Acute			
Immature cells predominate	Acute myeloid leukaemia	Acute lymphoblastic leukaemia	Lymphoma: 'high-grade', 'aggressive', e.g. Burkitt lymphoma
	Myelodysplastic syndrome	Myeloma	
Chronic			
Mature cells predominate	Chronic myeloid leukaemia	Chronic lymphocytic leukaemia	Lymphoma: 'low-grade', 'indolent', e.g. follicular lymphoma
	Other myeloproliferative disorders	Others	

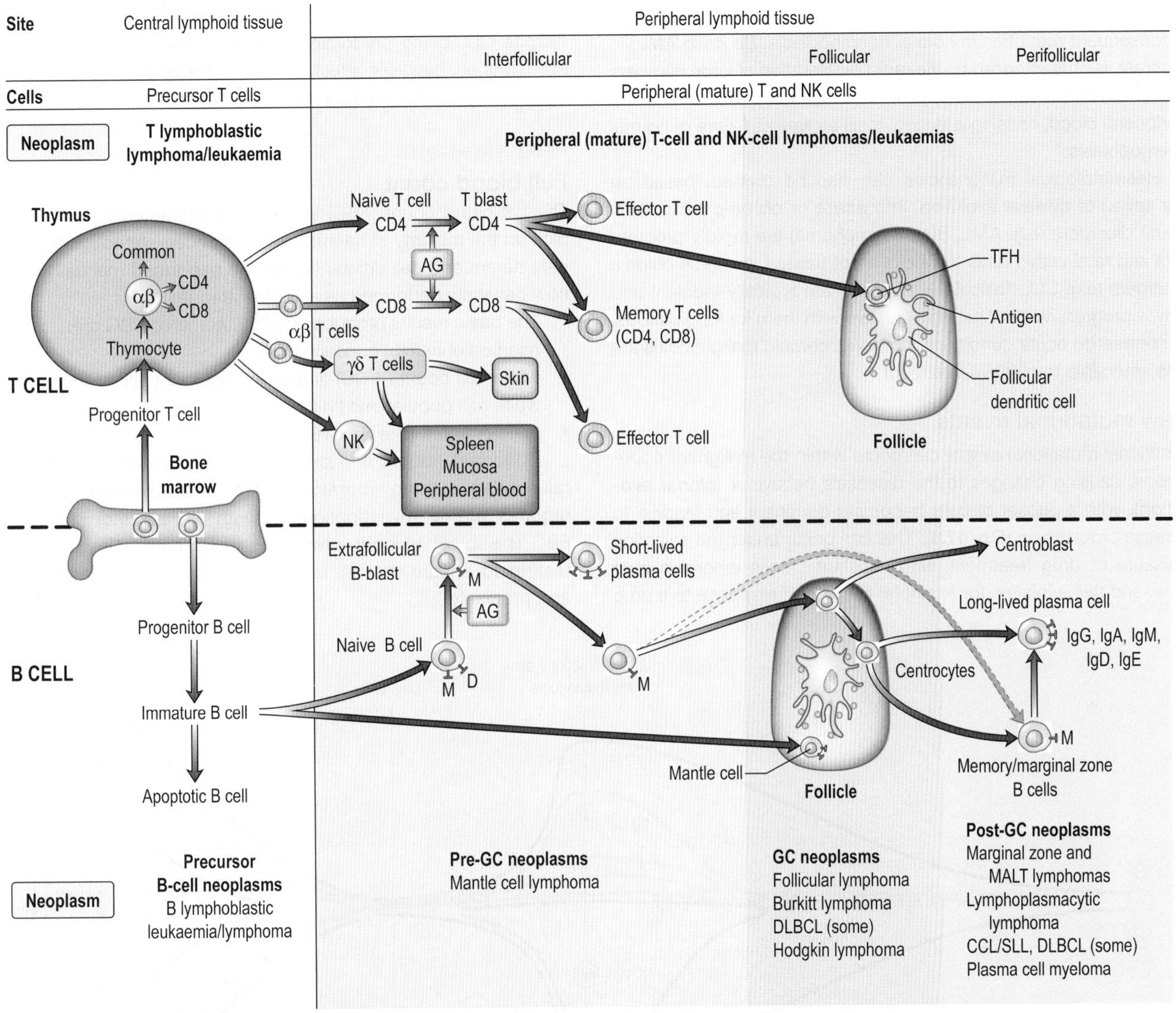

Fig. 17.2 Differentiation of T and B lymphocytes and their relationship to neoplasms. *Top (above dotted line): T-cell differentiation.* Progenitor T cells from the bone marrow enter the thymus and develop into different naive T cells. αβ T cells leave the thymus, are exposed to antigen (AG) and undergo blast transformation. They then develop into CD4+ and CD8+ effector and memory T cells. T regulatory cells are the major type of CD4+ effector cell. The other specific effector T cells are the follicular helper T cell (TFH) in the germinal centres (GC). On antigenic stimulation, T-cell responses to antigenic stimulation pathways of natural killer cells (NK) and γδ T cells are unknown.

Bottom: B-cell differentiation. Precursor B cells mature in the bone marrow and undergo apoptosis or mature to naive B cells. Following exposure to antigen and blast transformation, they develop into short-lived plasma cells or enter the GC. Somatic hypermutation and heavy chain class switching occur here (not shown). The transformed cells of the GC (centroblasts) undergo apoptosis or develop into centrocytes. Post-GC cells include long-lived plasma cells and memory/marginal cells.

DLBCL, diffuse large B-cell lymphoma; CLL/SLL, chronic lymphocytic leukaemia/small lymphocytic lymphoma; Ig, immunoglobulin; MALT, mucosa-associated lymphoid tissue. *(Redrawn from information in Swerdlow SH, Campo E, Harris NL et al. (eds). WHO Classification of Tumours of Haematopoietic and Lymphoid Tissues, 4th edn. Geneva: WHO; 2008.)*

Early genetic changes

The number, type and sequence of acquired genetic mutations determine the phenotype of the condition. CML, for example, has a clear initiating event (the Philadelphia chromosome translocation) that defines the condition and has led to effective targeted therapy. Other malignancies have a wider variety of driver mutations, producing a more heterogeneous group of conditions with variable responses to different treatments.

Cellular phenotypes

The pattern of mutations can lead to a more **dysplastic** (abnormal appearance and function) or more **proliferative** phenotype. The stem cell defect in MDS, for example, leads to dysplastic cells with a consequent reduction in normal haemopoiesis. *De novo* AML, in contrast, is characterized by the rapid proliferation of large numbers of immature cells, which can move out of the bone marrow into the peripheral blood, causing a leucocytosis as well as failure of normal haemopoiesis.

Haematological malignancies can also be divided, based on the speed of disease evolution, into **acute** or **chronic** conditions. Acute disorders (e.g. AML, Burkitt lymphoma) are rapidly progressive and fatal within days to weeks if not treated, whereas chronic disorders (e.g. CLL, follicular lymphoma) are typically indolent and slowly progressive, and patients can live with them for long periods. In contrast to acute conditions, however, chronic malignancies are less amenable to curative treatment.

New mutational events

Additional mutational events can occur within the malignant populations, causing changes to the disease's behaviour (**clonal evolution**), with a subset of cells becoming dominant and leading to disease progression (**Fig. 17.3**). This can occur under the selection pressure of drug treatment, with resistant clones emerging over time, and this explains, for example, the loss of response to a drug after a period of remission. A sudden change in behaviour from a chronic to acute condition is often called a **high-grade transformation**, with examples including Richter's transformation of CLL to a high-grade lymphoma, or blast crisis of CML.

Leukaemic and lymphomatous presentations

A final division can be made between **blood-based** or **solid** presentations, depending on whether there is primarily a marrow-based leukaemic presentation (with or without obvious circulating disease in the peripheral blood), or a nodal or extranodal lymphomatous presentation (in which soft tissue masses predominate). Again, this distinction is not hard and fast; CLL and small lymphocytic lymphoma (SLL) are considered to be essentially the same disease, despite CLL being predominantly blood-based and SLL primarily solid. It does, however, affect treatment strategies, and the need for imaging in staging and response assessment.

Investigations

Full blood count

The full blood count (FBC) is the most fundamental test used to pick up the majority of haematological cancers. Although the basic parameters and cell differential can be performed manually, this is now generally performed as an automated test.

The basic results produced by an automated FBC are:

- haemoglobin (Hb) concentration
- white cell count (WCC) and proportions of cells in the different white cell populations ('differential')
- platelet count (see **Box 16.1**).

Abnormal counts and cell populations should automatically raise a flag, alerting laboratory staff to an unexpected result that requires further investigation. As with all laboratory tests, the FBC is subject to both internal and external quality assurance testing to ensure that all laboratories report results accurately and precisely.

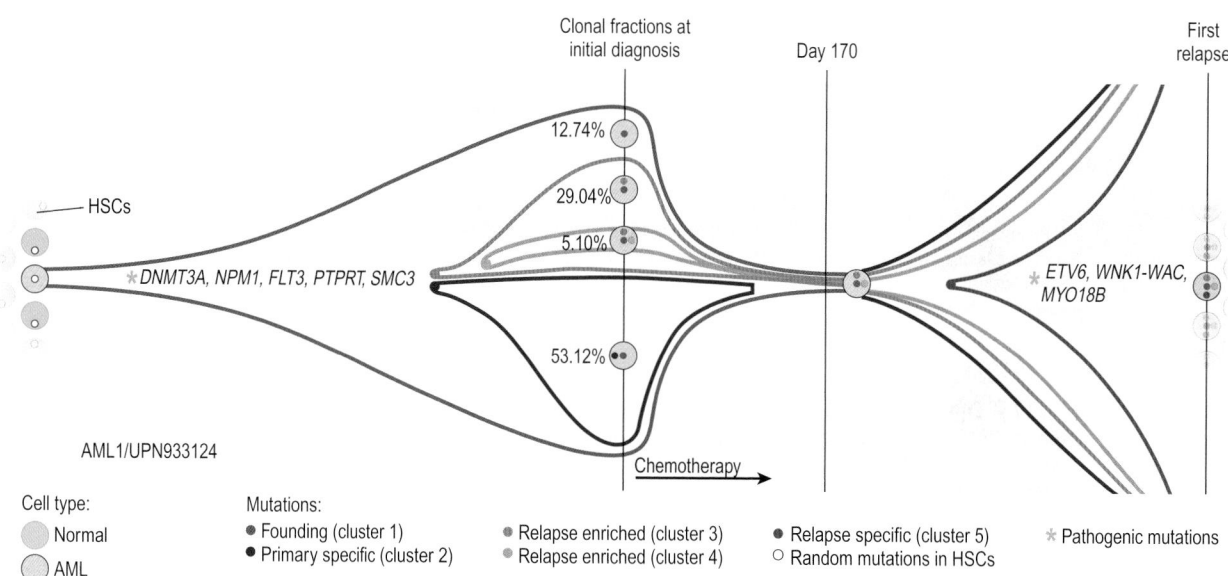

Fig. 17.3 Clonal evolution in a population of leukaemic cells from a patient with acute myeloid leukaemia (AML). The founding clone in the primary tumour contained somatic mutations in the genes *DNMT3A*, *NPM1*, *PTPRT*, *SMC3* and *FLT3* that are all recurrent in AML and probably relevant for pathogenesis; one subclone within the founding clone evolved to become the dominant clone at relapse by acquiring additional mutations, including recurrent mutations in *ETV6* and *MYO18B*, and a *WNK1-WAC* fusion gene. HSC, haemopoietic stem cell *(From Ding L, Ley TJ et al. Clonal evolution in relapsed acute myeloid leukaemia revealed by whole-genome sequencing.* Nature *2012; 481:506–510.)*

Morphology

Blood films

Blood cells can be easily viewed by spreading a droplet of blood into a film on to a microscope slide and staining it to reveal the appearance and number of the cells (**Fig. 17.4**). Certain conditions have morphological features that are characteristic (e.g. Auer rods in AML cells), and although definitive diagnosis usually requires additional tests (see later), expertise at blood film examination remains a key skill for all haematologists involved in diagnosis.

Bone marrow aspirate morphology

While many leukaemias are visible in the peripheral blood, others blood cancers require examination of the cells within the bone marrow to make a formal diagnosis. Slide preparation and staining techniques are similar, and the normal marrow aspirate shows a wide range of precursor cells at various stages of development (see **Fig. 16.1**).

Histology

Histological examination can be performed on a bone marrow biopsy (trephine), which can provide better assessment of cellularity and fibrosis, as well as an overall assessment of the tissue structure and the presence and character of any malignant population (**Fig. 17.5**). Immunohistochemical staining can provide a specific diagnosis. The same staining techniques are also used on lymph node and other biopsies, in particular for lymphomas.

Biochemistry

Routine biochemical testing is used to assess organ damage and tumour lysis. Specific tests (e.g. lactate dehydrogenase (LDH),

beta-2-microglobulin (B2M)) are used as part of a number of staging systems in myeloma and lymphoma.

Immunological assessment of paraproteins is an essential part of the diagnosis and response assessment of myeloma and some other blood cancers (see later).

Immunophenotyping

Cell surface proteins act as markers that can be used to characterize and quantify malignant cell populations. Analysis of solid samples (bone marrow trephines, lymph node biopsies etc.) is performed by *immunohistochemistry*.

On liquid samples (peripheral blood, bone marrow aspirate and so on), it is performed by *flow cytometry.* In this process, cells are stained with fluorescently labelled antibodies and analysed with specially designed analysers. The combination of cell size and appearance, together with the pattern of surface markers, identifies a profile or *immunophenotype* that is characteristic of a particular diagnosis (**Fig. 17.6**).

Immunophenotypic identification of malignant cell populations is an essential part of the diagnosis of almost all haematological malignancies. As an example, acute leukaemia cells may appear identical by morphology but have very different immunophenotype profiles:

- AML (CD13+, CD33+, CD117+)
- B-lineage ALL (CD10+, CD19+)

This information has a direct impact on treatment, different chemotherapy combinations being used for the different conditions (**Fig. 17.7**).

Cytogenetics

Cancer is characterized by genetic abnormalities within the malignant cell populations, and these abnormalities can increasingly be detected in many haematological cancers, either to confirm a diagnosis, or to act as biomarkers that can provide information on the likely timescale and behaviour of the disease (*prognostic*), and/or the likely response to a specific drug or treatment (*predictive*).

Chromosomal abnormalities (translocations, insertions, deletions, inversions) may be detected by two major cytogenetic techniques:

- *G-band karyotyping* detects large structural abnormalities in chromosomes when they are condensed during metaphase. This technique will detect the t(9;22) Philadelphia chromosome translocation in CML (see **Fig. 2.23**), and many of the major structural abnormalities associated with AML prognosis (e.g. inv16, monosomy 7).

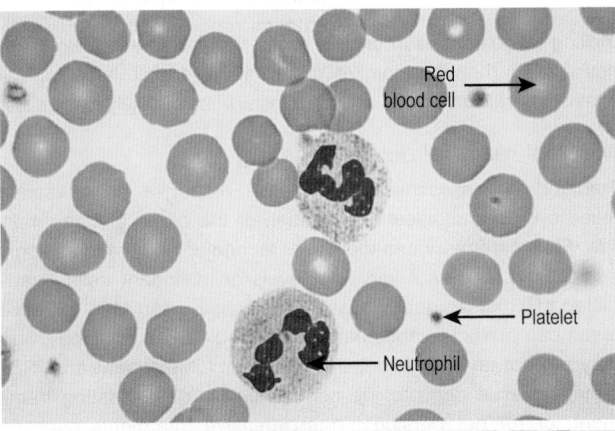

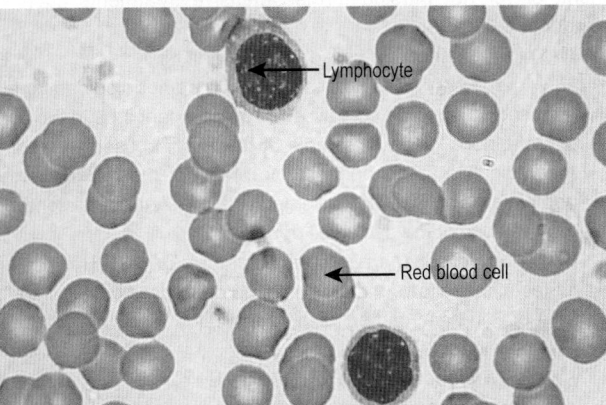

Fig. 17.4 Normal blood films.

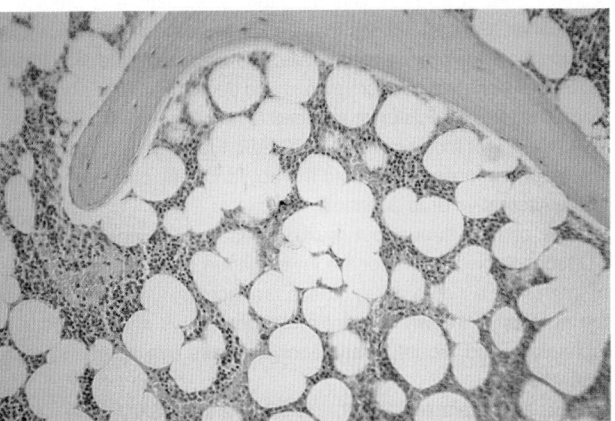

Fig. 17.5 Normal bone marrow trephine.

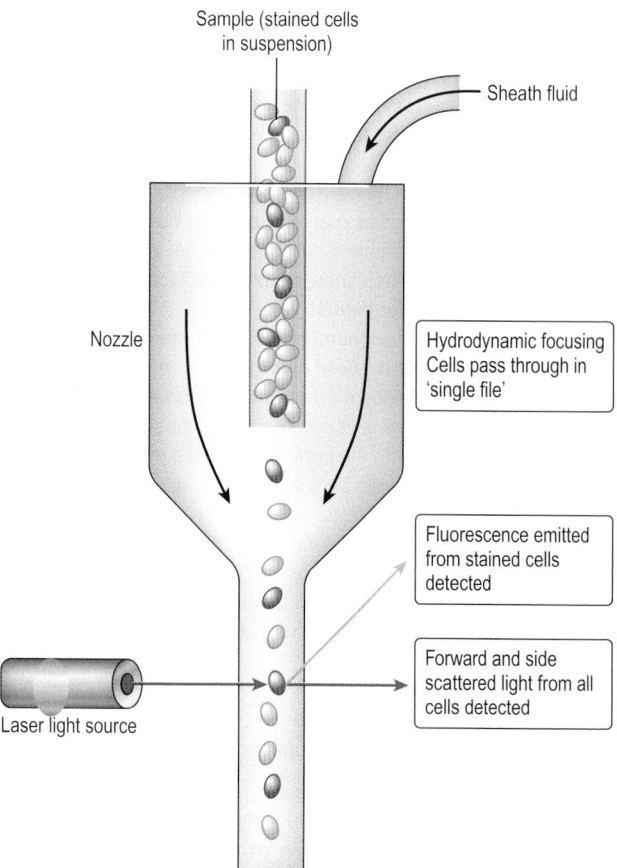

Fig. 17.6 Flow cytometer showing how cells are stained and then characterized with a laser light source and detectors. This method can produce detailed information on cell size, composition and surface markers that can be used to characterize both normal and malignant cell populations.

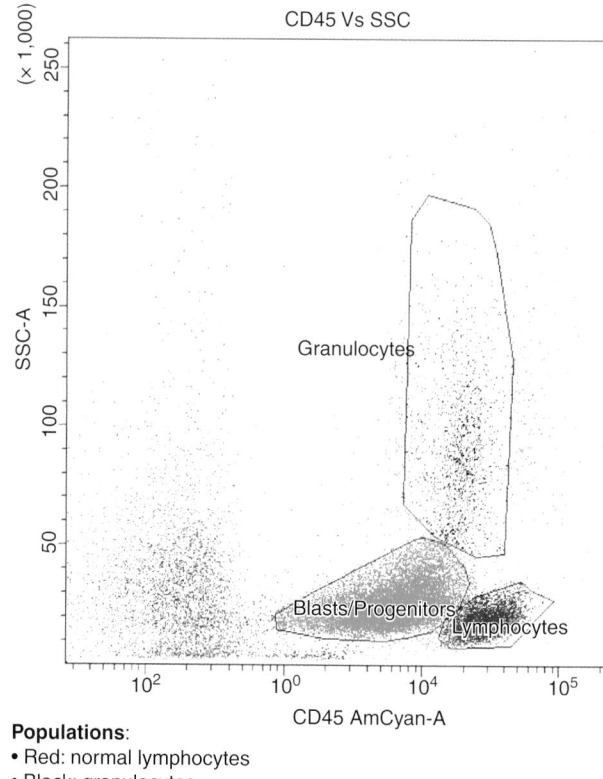

Populations:
• Red: normal lymphocytes
• Black: granulocytes
• Green: progenitors (blasts)

Fig. 17.7 Flow cytometry plot from a patient with **B-ALL (B lymphoblastic leukaemia).** *Courtesy Timothy Farren, Barts Health NHS Trust, London, UK.*

• ***Fluorescence in situ hybridization (FISH)*** assesses cells during interphase and so is useful for slower-growing cancers; however, it will only detect specific abnormalities using pre-designed fluorescently labelled probes. This technique is commonly used for detecting prognostically significant abnormalities in myeloma (e.g. t(4;14), 17p deletion) (see **Fig. 17.11**).

Molecular genetics

Abnormalities in specific genes can be detected by DNA sequencing technologies, again providing important prognostic and predictive information. Gene mutations that are known to be of relevance may be specifically screened for. In AML, for example, mutations in the *FLT3* gene denote a poor prognosis, and detection of this abnormality may lead to a decision to proceed to an allogeneic transplant. In CML, the T315I mutation in the *BCR-ABL* fusion gene is associated with poor response to standard therapy, and may prompt a change to the alternative drug ponatinib.

Use of high-throughput 'next-generation sequencing' (see p. 31) technologies allows for the investigation of a number of genes of interest in a single assay. These are increasingly being used as the number of known relevant mutations grows and advances in technology and bio-informatic analysis make this approach more cost-effective.

As an example, *TET2*, *SF3B1* and *ASXL1* are commonly mutated in MDS, and their detection can be helpful in

making this diagnosis in unclear cases, as well as informing prognosis. With the development of novel drugs that have activity against specific mutations, the use of gene panels is likely to increase.

Minimal residual disease testing

Traditionally, assessment of disease response in leukaemia relied on morphological examination of the blood or bone marrow. Flow cytometry and molecular technologies are increasingly being used to detect very low levels of malignant cells in so-called minimal residual disease (MRD) assays. An MRD-positive result can predict relapse before it is visible by morphology, and may prompt an early change in treatment. Conversely, an MRD-negative result can provide confidence for de-escalating treatment, or for not pursing further intensive treatments such as allogeneic transplant.

Two major methods are used for MRD testing:
• ***Flow cytometry.*** This utilizes the same methodology as immunophenotyping to detect low levels of malignant cells in the peripheral blood. Ideally, a sample at diagnosis is used to identify the distinctive immunophenotypic profile of the malignant cell population. This can then be employed to look for persistence or early relapse of the same cell population.
• ***Quantitative polymerase chain reaction (qPCR).*** This powerful technique allows the amplification of a specific sequence of DNA or RNA, and can be used to detect low levels of disease in a number of conditions:
  – ***gene fusions***, e.g. *BCR-ABL* in CML
  – ***immunoglobulin gene rearrangements*** in B-cell ALL
  – ***T-cell receptor gene rearrangements*** in T-cell ALL.

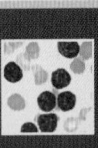

Tissue typing

For patients who may go on to allogeneic stem cell transplantation (SCT), it is important to collect a blood sample for tissue typing at diagnosis, so that potential donors may be identified. Testing identifies donors who match the patient's human leucocyte antigen (HLA) type and is done by genetic testing, ideally at the HLA-A, B, C, DP, DQ and DR loci. Testing packs can be sent out to siblings, to be returned for testing at the regional laboratory. If no related donors are identified, a search can be performed on national and international donor registries.

Radiological imaging

Although, as with all cancers, a tissue sample is required to make a diagnosis and commence treatment, radiological imaging plays a key role in the staging, response assessment and investigation of haematological cancers.

Plain films

These are rarely used for formal staging but may still be helpful in initial investigation and assessment of complications (e.g. long bone fractures as a presenting symptom of myeloma).

Ultrasound scans

These are useful for assessment of soft tissue masses: for example, in the characterization of enlarged lymph nodes. Ultrasound-guided biopsies are a common method of making an initial lymphoma diagnosis.

Computed tomography scans

These are frequently employed to gain accurate imaging to stage tumours at diagnosis and to assess response. In myeloma, where the main site of organ damage is the bones, low-dose, non-contrast computed tomography (CT) scans are sufficient, whereas assessment of soft tissue masses – for example, in lymphoma – requires a contrast scan. CT-guided biopsies are an effective method of obtaining tissue from deeper-lying areas.

Nuclear medicine scans

Nuclear medicine scans, especially fluorodeoxyglucose positron emission tomography (FGD-PET), are increasingly used in combination with CT (CT-PET) to visualize metabolically active areas of disease. This technique is helpful for assessing response after therapy, and in particular to distinguish between active residual tumour and fibrotic tissue after treatment.

Magnetic resonance imaging

Magnetic resonance imaging (MRI) can provide detailed views of particular organs and has benefits in a number of specific situations (e.g. bone marrow, brain, spinal cord). Diffusion-weighted MRI can provide functional information similar to that obtained by PET scanning and is increasingly being used in myeloma assessment.

Multidisciplinary team and specialist integrated haematological malignancy diagnostic service

As already outlined, a number of different techniques are used in making a diagnosis of a haematological cancer, as well as in providing the relevant staging and prognostic information to guide treatment. Diagnostic reports can be integrated into a single document, incorporating all relevant pathological information. This is often carried out as part of a specialist integrated haematological malignancy diagnostic service (SIHMDS), which may be run on a regional basis.

Review of pathology and radiology results at diagnosis, response assessment and disease progression should ideally be done in a multidisciplinary team (MDT) meeting, where clinical, pathological and radiological data can be discussed by an extended expert team, who can then formulate a specific management plan for the patient.

Further reading

Bain BJ. *Blood Cells: A Practical Guide*, 5th edn. Oxford: Wiley–Blackwell.
Chen X, Cherian S. Acute myeloid leukemia immunophenotyping by flow cytometric analysis. *Clin Lab Med* 2017; 37:753–769.
Kroft SH, Harrington AM. Flow cytometry of B-cell neoplasms. *Clin Lab Med* 2017; 37:697–723.
Rack KA, van den Berg E, Hafterlach C et al. European recommendations and quality assurance for cytogenomic analysis of haematological neoplasms. *Leukemia* 2019; 33:1851–1867.

LEUKAEMIAS

There are four main subtypes, as discussed earlier:
- acute myeloid leukaemia (AML)
- acute lymphoblastic leukaemia (ALL)
- chronic myeloid leukaemia (CML)
- chronic lymphocytic leukaemia (CLL).

These are relatively uncommon diseases with an incidence of about 10/100 000 per year. They can occur at any age and the type of leukaemia varies with age: ALL is mainly seen in childhood and CLL is a disease of the elderly.

Leukaemia can be diagnosed by examination of a stained slide of peripheral blood and bone marrow, but immunophenotyping, cytogenetics and molecular genetics are essential for complete subclassification and prognostication. The lineage and degree of maturity of the leukaemic clone can be assessed by morphology and immunophenotype.

Aetiology

In the majority of patients the cause is unknown but several factors have been associated:

- ***Radiation.*** This can induce genetic damage to haemopoietic precursors; ALL, AML and CML have been seen in increased incidences in survivors of Hiroshima, Nagasaki and, more recently, Chernobyl, and in patients treated with ionizing radiation.
- ***Chemicals and drugs.*** Exposure to benzene, used in industry, may lead to marrow damage. AML occurs after treatment with chemotherapy drugs such as alkylating agents (e.g. melphalan) and topoisomerase-II inhibitors (e.g. etoposide).
- ***Genetic factors.*** Leukaemia risk is highly elevated in a number of germline conditions that result in genetic instability or bone marrow failure. These include Fanconi anaemia, ataxia telangiectasia and Li–Fraumeni syndrome. The risk is elevated some 30 times in Down's syndrome (trisomy 21). There is a high degree of concordance among monozygotic twins. Several genes have also been associated with familial AML, such as *CEBPA* and *RUNX1*.
- ***Viruses.*** ATLL is a rare type of leukaemia that is associated with HTLV-1, found particularly in Japan and the Caribbean.

Acute leukaemias

The acute leukaemias increase in incidence with advancing age. ***Acute myeloid (myeloblastic, myelogenous) leukaemia*** has a median age at presentation of 65 years and may arise *de novo* or against a background of myelodysplasia or prior cytotoxic chemotherapy ('therapy-related'). *Acute lymphoid (lymphoblastic) leukaemia* has a substantially lower median age at presentation and, in addition, is the most common malignancy in childhood. The simplified WHO classification shown in **Box 17.4** also shows that a small number of acute leukaemias have an indeterminate immunophenotype between myeloid and lymphoblastic.

Clinical features

The majority of patients with acute leukaemia, regardless of subtype, present with symptoms (**Box 17.5**) reflecting inadequate haemopoiesis secondary to infiltration of the bone marrow by leukaemic cells, symptoms due to tissue infiltration by leukaemic cells, the consequences of a high white blood cell count, or substance release from the tumour cells.

Investigations

For confirming diagnosis

- **Blood count.** Haemoglobin and platelets are low. White blood cell count is usually raised, reflecting the proliferating population, but may be low if the leukaemic cells are confined to the bone marrow.
- **Blood film.** Blast cells are almost invariably seen (**Fig. 17.8A**). Lineage may be identified morphologically, e.g. the presence of Auer rods is pathognomonic for a diagnosis of AML.
- **Bone marrow aspirate.** Increased cellularity (**Fig. 17.8B**), reduced erythropoiesis and reduced megakaryocytes may be seen. Replacement by blast cells is over 20% (often approaching 100%). Lineage is confirmed by immunophenotyping, e.g. AML – CD33 or CD13; B lineage ALL – CD10 and CD19; and T lineage ALL – CD3 (see **Fig. 17.7**). Cytogenetic and FISH analysis, as well as molecular genetics, may be used for prognostication.
- **Chest X-ray.** Mediastinal widening is often present in T-lymphoblastic leukaemia.
- **Cerebrospinal fluid examination.** This is performed in all patients with ALL, as the risk of central nervous system involvement is high. It is less critical in AML.
- **Coagulation profile.** This is performed to exclude the presence of disseminated intravascular coagulation (DIC), particularly associated with acute promyelocytic leukaemia (APML): raised prothrombin time and activated partial thromboplastin time,

reduced fibrinogen, and increased fibrinogen degradation products, e.g. D-dimers.

For planning therapy

- **Biochemistry**: serum urate, renal and liver function tests.
- **Cardiac function**: electrocardiography and echocardiogram to assess cardiac function before considering intensive chemotherapy, which may include cardiotoxic anthracycline drugs.
- **HLA type**: performed for identification of potential stem cell donors for allogeneic transplantation.
- **HIV, hepatitis B virus (HBV) and hepatitis C virus (HCV) status.**

> **i** **Box 17.4 World Health Organization classification of acute leukaemia**
>
> **Acute myeloid leukaemia (AML) and related neoplasms**
> - AML with recurrent genetic abnormalities
> - AML with myelodysplasia-related changes
> - Therapy-related myeloid neoplasm
> - AML, not otherwise specified[a]
> - Myeloid sarcoma
> - Myeloid proliferation associated with Down's syndrome
>
> **Blastic plasmacytoid dendritic cell neoplasm**
> **Acute leukaemias of ambiguous lineage**
> **B-cell lymphoblastic leukaemia/lymphoma**
> **T-cell lymphoblastic leukaemia/lymphoma**
>
> [a]These entities correspond with the French–American–British classification.
> *(Adapted from Swerdlow SH, Campo E, Harris NL et al (eds). World Health Organization Classification of Tumours of Haematopoietic and Lymphoid Tissues, rev 4th edn. Lyon: IARC Press; 2017, with permission from the World Health Organization.)*

> **i** **Box 17.5 Symptoms and signs of leukaemia**
>
> | | Symptoms | Signs | Type |
> |---|---|---|---|
> | **Marrow failure** | | | |
> | Anaemia | Breathlessness Fatigue Angina Claudication | Pallor Cardiac flow murmur | ALL/AML |
> | Neutropenia | Infections | Fever Mouth ulcers Septic focus | |
> | Thrombocytopenia | Bleeding and bruising | Petechiae Gum bleeding Fundal haemorrhage | |
> | **High WCC** | | | |
> | Leucostasis | Breathlessness | Hypoxia, pulmonary infiltrates | ALL/AML |
> | | Headache | Reduced GCS | |
> | | Confusion | | |
> | | Visual problems | Retinal vein dilation, papilloedema, fundal haemorrhage | |
> | **Tissue infiltration** | | | |
> | Marrow | Bone pain | | ALL/AML |
> | Gums | | Gum hypertrophy | AML |
> | Skin | | Violaceous skin deposits | AML |
> | Liver/spleen | | Hepatosplenomegaly | ALL/AML |
> | Nodes | | Lymphadenopathy | ALL/AML |
> | CNS | Headache | Cranial nerve palsies | ALL/ (AML) |
> | Testes | | Testicular enlargement | ALL |
> | Mediastinum | | Mediastinal mass, SVCO | ALL |
> | **Substance release** | | | |
> | DIC | Bleeding and bruising | Ecchymoses Bleeding i.v. sites | AML |
> | Hyperuricaemia | Acute gout | Renal stones, tophi | ALL/AML |
> | | Tumour lysis | Acute kidney failure | |
>
> ALL, acute lymphoid leukaemia; AML, acute myeloid leukaemia; CNS, central nervous system; DIC, disseminated intravascular coagulation; GCS, Glasgow Coma Scale score; SVCO, superior vena caval obstruction; WCC, white cell count.

Management

Untreated acute leukaemia is invariably fatal, most often within weeks to months, though with judicious palliative care it may be extended, perhaps to a year. Treatment with curative intent may be successful, or may fail, either because the leukaemia does not respond (refractory), because the disease returns after an initial favourable response (relapse), or because the patient succumbs to complications of the therapy (treatment-related mortality).

At initial presentation, acute leukaemias range from being probably curable (e.g. childhood 'good-risk' ALL) through to probably incurable (e.g. AML with adverse cytogenetic features in the elderly). Since curative treatment carries considerable morbidity and potential mortality, it is essential for the risk/benefit ratio to be clearly understood by physician and patient alike.

Palliative therapy

Every attempt should be made to ensure that patients are able to stay at home as much as possible, while making available the full range of supportive care. Palliation may well include low-dose chemotherapy in addition to blood product support and antimicrobials.

Curative therapy

The decision to treat with curative intent, particularly if successful, implies severe disruption of normality for the patient and family for at least 6 months and often up to a year. In the short term, it may demand transfer to another hospital, as acute leukaemia should be treated only in units seeing a sufficient number of patients. It is highly likely to involve admission to hospital for up to a month in the first instance, with further, partly predictable, subsequent admissions of several days' to weeks' duration, requiring discussions and decisions about work or education.

The decision to treat with curative intent implies that the chance of cure justifies the risks of the therapy. It does not imply that cure is guaranteed or even expected.

Active therapy

Supportive care

This forms the basis of treatment, whether for cure or palliation:

- ***Avoidance of symptoms of anaemia*** (keeping haemoglobin <80–100 g/L). Repeated transfusion of packed red cells is needed (irradiation of cells may be required, e.g. in patients who have received purine analogue drugs such as fludarabine).
- ***Prevention or control of bleeding*** (keeping platelet count $>10 \times 10^9$/L in the stable patient, $>20 \times 10^9$/L in the septic patient, or $>50 \times 10^9$/L if a procedure is planned, e.g. lumbar puncture). The role of prophylactic platelet transfusion has been evaluated and remains superior to any alternative, certainly for patients with AML.
- ***Correction of coagulation abnormalities.*** This is achieved with fresh frozen plasma (FFP) to keep the activated partial thromboplastin time ratio and international normalized ratio (INR) <1.5 times normal, and with cryoprecipitate to keep the fibrinogen level >1.5 g/dL. This is a particular risk in APML, which is associated with activation of the coagulation system (DIC). Norethisterone is given to women of menstrual age to avoid menorrhagia during their thrombocytopenic phase.
- ***Treatment of infection*** (see **Box 6.25**):
  - ***Prophylactic.*** Education of patients, relatives and staff about diet, hand-washing and isolation facilities is necessary. Selected antibiotics, antifungals, antivirals and *Pneumocystis jirovecii* prophylaxis may be required.
  - ***Therapeutic.*** Fever is managed using a local protocol/algorithm for antibiotic and antifungal combinations.
- ***Control of hyperuricaemia (tumour lysis).*** This should be achieved with hydration, prophylactic allopurinol and occasionally rasburicase (see p. 118).

Indwelling venous devices, such as a peripherally inserted central catheter (PICC) or Hickman line, are required to allow easy access to the blood for tests and administration of therapy. Sperm banking is offered to postpubertal men and oocyte collection to women, if there is time before treatment.

Specific treatment

The initial requirement of therapy is to return the peripheral blood and bone marrow to normal (complete remission, CR). This 'induction chemotherapy' is tailored to the particular leukaemia and the individual patient's risk factors. Since this treatment is not leukaemia-specific but also impairs normal bone marrow function, it leads to a major risk of life-threatening infection, which increases the risk of early death in the short term.

Successful remission induction is always followed by further treatment (consolidation), which consists either of further cycles of chemotherapy or of allogeneic haemopoietic stem cell 'bone marrow' transplantation. The specific treatment details are determined by the type of leukaemia and by the patient's risk factors and tolerance of treatment. Without consolidation, recurrence is almost inevitable, reflecting the lack of sensitivity of a morphological 'complete remission'. Cytogenetics and molecular genetic techniques can identify residual leukaemic cells not detected morphologically (minimal residual disease, MRD), which are highly predictive of recurrence.

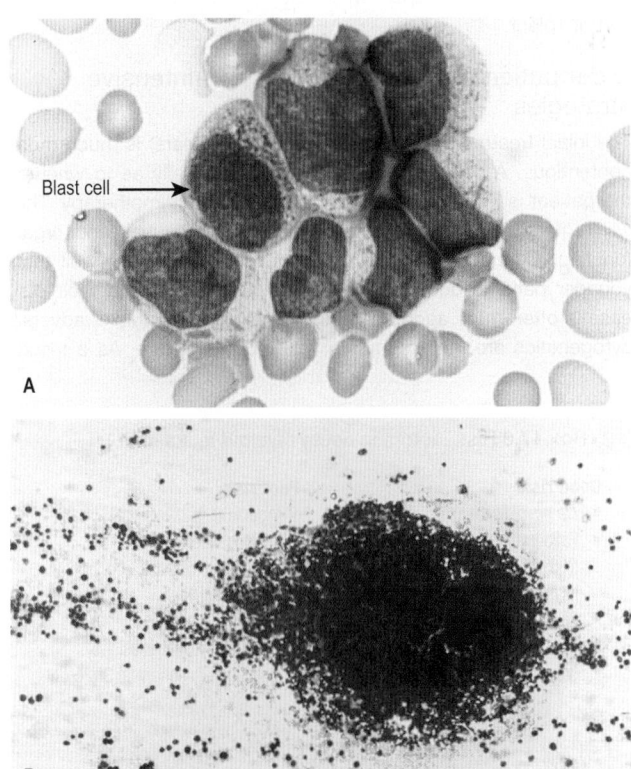

Blast cell →

A

B

Fig. 17.8 Acute leukaemia. (A) Peripheral blood film showing characteristic blast cells. The arrow points to the abnormal blast cell. **(B)** Bone marrow aspirate showing particle with increased cellularity. *(Courtesy of Dr Manzoor Mangi.)*

Refractory disease

Failure to achieve morphological CR with two cycles of therapy ('refractory') carries almost as bad a prognosis as the untreated leukaemia. If CR can be achieved – by new experimental approaches, for instance – cure may still be possible with SCT (see p. 364). A small proportion of patients with refractory disease may also be cured by myeloablative SCT.

Stem cell transplant

The decision on whether to proceed to allogeneic transplant is based on two factors:
- **Relapse risk.** This depends on cytogenetic and other risk factors at diagnosis, and response to induction therapy (morphology and MRD).
- **Transplant-related mortality (TRM).** This varies, depending on the age and fitness of the patient and the quality of the donor match.

Patients should proceed to transplantation only if the reduction in relapse risk outweighs likely TRM, leading to an improved overall survival. For example, transplantation would be appropriate for a younger, fitter patient with poor-risk disease, but not for someone with inv(16) (lower relapse risk) or an older patient with multiple co-morbidities (high predicted TRM).

Acute myeloid leukaemia
Prognosis

In AML, the prognosis is dependent on a range of key variables, the main ones being age, cytogenetics and specific gene mutations (**Fig. 17.9** and **Box 17.6**), and, increasingly, the presence of MRD after initial therapy.

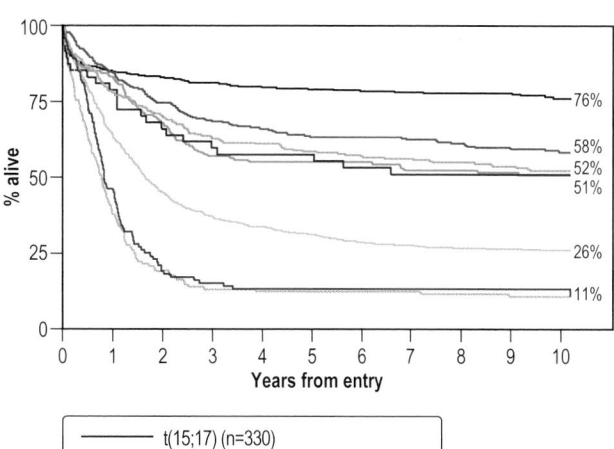

Fig. 17.9 **Prognosis related to cytogenetics and molecular data in acute myeloid leukaemia (AML).** Outcome of younger adults with AML treated in the Medical Research Council AML10 and AML12 trials, stratified according to cytogenetic and molecular abnormalities. *(Reproduced with permission from Smith ML, Hills RK, Grimwade D. Independent prognostic variables in acute myeloid leukaemia.* Blood Rev *2011; 25:39–51.)*

Management
Young patients: intensive therapy unless unfit

Treatment with curative intent is undertaken in the majority of adults below the age of 60 years, provided there is no significant co-morbidity. Treatment success reflects the cytogenetic pattern. CR will be achieved in about 80% of patients under the age of 60. Failure is due to either resistant leukaemia (10%) or treatment-related mortality (10%) – usually caused by infection or haemorrhage. Approximately 50% of those entering CR will be cured (i.e. approximately 40% overall), although this varies from 60–70% in the favourable cytogenetic group to 10–20% in the adverse cytogenetic group.

Those with 'favourable risk' disease (e.g. inv(16)) are treated with moderately intensive combination chemotherapy. This always includes an anthracycline such as daunorubicin and cytarabine, and consolidation with a minimum of a further three cycles of treatment given at 3–4-week intervals. Patients with favourable-risk disease do not benefit from allogeneic SCT during their first complete remission, as the risks outweigh the benefits.

Those with 'intermediate-risk' disease (e.g. normal karyotype, +8, +21) are a heterogeneous and increasingly complex group. Where possible, they should be given consolidation chemotherapy after an initial remission has been achieved, followed by allogeneic transplantation in most cases. The confirmation of deep remission by MRD negativity (e.g. of *NPM1* transcripts) may be sufficient to move some patients into a good risk group and remove the need for transplant.

Patients with adverse cytogenetics (e.g. 7–, 5–, complex karyotype) should proceed to SCT in first complete remission (CR1) because they respond poorly to conventional chemotherapy and have a high risk of relapse, which can be reduced to some extent by transplant.

Older patients: intensive versus non-intensive strategies

The initial treatment of the older patient (>60 years) is much more contentious. A decision needs to be taken initially as to whether the patient is 'fit' enough to tolerate intensive chemotherapy. This will require a full assessment of their co-morbidities and organ function. Older patients tolerate cytotoxic therapy less well than younger patients due to additional co-morbidities, and their disease is often more aggressive in its biology; for example, adverse cytogenetics are more common with increasing age. As a result,

---

> **i** **Box 17.6 Risk factors in acute myeloid leukaemia**
>
> **Good risk**
> - *De novo* disease
> - Favourable cytogenetics: t(15; 17) t(8; 21) or inv(16) or its variant t(16; 16)
> - CEBPA bi-allelic mutation
> - NPM1 mutation with FLT3 wild type
>
> **Poor risk**
> - Age >60
> - Male gender
> - Secondary disease, e.g. prior MDS or MPN
> - High WCC
> - Adverse cytogenetics: −5, del(5q), −7, abnormal 3q26 or a complex karyotype
> - FLT3 internal tandem duplication mutation
> - MRD positivity post induction chemotherapy
>
> CEBPA, transcription factor CCAAT/enhancer binding protein; FLT3, FMS-like tyrosine kinase 3; MDS, myelodysplasia; MPN, myeloproliferative neoplasm; MRD, minimal residual disease; NPM1, nucleophosmin; WCC, white cell count.

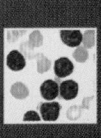

treatment-related morbidity and mortality are both higher and outcome is less successful.

Reduced-intensity allogeneic transplantation is increasingly being used for this group but is still limited by its toxicity. For those who are not fit for intensive chemotherapy, treatment will have a palliative aim to improve marrow function and to maximize quality of life. Choice of therapy will include low-dose cytarabine, azacitidine, oral cytotoxics (such as hydroxycarbamide) or enrolment into any one of a range of clinical trials of novel agents.

Relapsed AML

The management of recurrence is undertaken on an individual basis, since the overall prognosis is very poor, despite the fact that second remissions may be achieved. Long survival following recurrence is rarely achieved without allogeneic transplantation. Novel or trial therapies should be considered. The use of MRD monitoring may identify patients in CR who are in the early stages of relapse and need pre-emptive therapy before frank marrow relapse occurs.

Newer agents that target the *FLT3* mutation present in a significant proportion of cases of AML (e.g. midostaurin) may be given in conjunction with conventional chemotherapy. Other novel therapies include chemotherapy-labelled monoclonal antibodies (gemtuzumab ozogamicin) and hypomethylating agents (e.g. azacitidine).

Acute promyelocytic leukaemia

Acute promyelocytic leukaemia (APML) is a variant of AML, occurring in 10–15% of cases. It is characterized by the translocation t(15; 17), which produces a *PML-RARA* fusion gene and has particular morphological features. There is an almost invariable coagulopathy, which remains a major cause of early death. The empirical discovery that all-*trans*-retinoic acid (ATRA) causes differentiation of promyelocytes and rapid reversal of the bleeding tendency was a major breakthrough.

APML is treated with ATRA combined with several courses of chemotherapy, or in combination with arsenic trioxide, which induces apoptosis via activation of the caspase cascade (see **Fig. 3.9**). CR and molecular remission (MR) occur in at least 90% of younger adults with APML, and at least 70% will expect to be cured. Transplantation is necessary only if the leukaemia is not eliminated at the molecular level, or following recurrence and re-induction therapy.

Acute lymphoblastic leukaemia

This condition may present in leukaemic phase with significant marrow involvement (acute lymphoblastic leukaemia, ALL) or as localized bulky disease, typically a mediastinal mass (lymphoblastic lymphoma). The tumour cells in each condition are indistinguishable and similar therapies are therefore used.

Prognosis

A number of clinical and laboratory features are determinants of treatment response and survival in ALL (**Box 17.7**). Increasingly, therapeutic strategies based on prognostic risk are being used in management. MRD stratification is increasingly employed to select patients who are at high risk (for treatment intensification) or low risk (for treatment de-escalation).

The prognosis of ALL in childhood is now excellent: CR is achieved in almost all, with up to 80% being alive without recurrence at 5 years. Failure occurs most frequently in those with high presentation blast counts or an 11q23 *MLL* translocation. Current treatment strategies lessen therapy for 'good-risk' children in

order to avoid some of the long-term consequences of therapy, such as avascular necrosis of bone, infertility, neurotoxicity and cardiotoxicity.

The situation is far less satisfactory for adults, the prognosis getting worse with advancing years. Co-morbidity and t(9; 22) translocation increase in frequency with age. Between 30% and 40% of patients continue in durable first remissions, resulting in approximately 25–30% overall patient cure. Disease that is refractory to first-line therapy carries a very poor prognosis.

As with AML, most recurrences occur within the first 3 years and the outcome is extremely poor. Second remissions, though usually achieved, are rarely durable, except following allogeneic transplantation. Isolated extramedullary recurrences, however, may be cured.

Management

As with AML, the overall strategy is to achieve an initial remission with induction chemotherapy, and then consolidate the response with either further cycles of chemotherapy, or an allogeneic transplant in selected patients, depending on relapse risk and estimated TRM. The drug combinations used differ, however, with initial induction typically consisting of vincristine, a glucocorticoid, an anthracycline and asparaginase, and different agents used for consolidation cycles. Similar to AML, older and less fit patients may receive a non-intensive treatment strategy, which is not curative in intent but aims to prolong life and reduce complications.

A major difference between treatment for ALL and that for AML is the need for central nervous system-directed therapy, due to the higher risk of infiltration. Prophylaxis should be given with intrathecal chemotherapy (under platelet cover if necessary) as soon as blasts are cleared from the blood. Depending on risk, this may be continued for up to 2 years and complemented by high doses of systemic cytarabine or methotrexate. Cranial irradiation was previously given to all patients to reduce the risk of relapse within the central nervous system; risk-adapted strategies now reserve this for those patients at very high risk.

The presence of the t(9;22) Philadelphia translocation (see **Fig. 2.23**) has traditionally been associated with increased risk, but the use of imatinib and other tyrosine kinase inhibitors (TKIs) originally developed for CML have improved outcomes considerably. These agents can be used in combination with intensive or non-intensive chemotherapy.

---

i **Box 17.7 Risk factors in acute lymphoblastic leukaemia (ALL)**

Risk factor	Good	Poor
Age	Younger	Older
WCC	$<30 \times 10^9$/L for B lineage $<100 \times 10^9$/L for T lineage	$>30 \times 10^9$/L for B lineage $>100 \times 10^9$/L for T lineage
Immunophenotype	CD10+ common ALL	Pro-B ALL
Cytogenetic aberrations	t(12; 21) hyperdiploidy	t(9; 22) or t(4; 11) hypodiploidy
Time to response	Early clearance of blasts	Failure to achieve CR within 3–4 weeks
Minimal residual disease	MRD negative	MRD positive
Extramedullary disease	CSF clear	CSF positive

CR, complete remission; CSF, cerebrospinal fluid; MRD, minimal residual disease; WCC, white cell count.

After intensive induction and consolidation, maintenance therapy is used to reduce the risk of disease recurrence in those patients who did not receive a transplant. This is typically comprised of 2 years of treatment with methotrexate and mercaptopurine, although more intensive regimens are used by many groups.

Novel cytotoxic drugs, including clofarabine and nelarabine, are increasingly used for relapsed/refractory cases, as are a range of monoclonal antibodies in B-ALL, including rituximab (anti-CD20), inotuzumab (calicheamicin-labelled anti-CD22) and blinatumomab (CD19/CD3 bi-specific T-cell engager antibody). Chimeric antigen receptor T-cell (CAR-T) immunotherapy has shown significant promise in ALL and is likely to see increased use in coming years.

Further reading

Bullinger L, Döhner K, Döhner H. Genomics of acute myeloid leukemia diagnosis and pathways. *J Clin Oncol* 2017; 35:934–946.

Döhner H, Weisdorf DJ, Bloomfield CD. Acute myeloid leukemia. *N Engl J Med* 2015; 373:1136–1152.

Iacobucci I, Mullighan CG. Genetic basis of acute lymphoblastic leukemia. *J Clin Oncol* 2017; 35:975–983.

Richard-Carpentier G, Kantarjian H, Jabbour E. Recent advances in adult acute lymphoblastic leukemia. *Curr Hematol Malig Rep* 2019; 14:106–118.

Chronic leukaemias

Chronic myeloid leukaemia

Chronic myeloid leukaemia, which accounts for about 14% of all leukaemias, is a member of the family of myeloproliferative neoplasms (MPNs); it is almost exclusively a disease of adults, the peak of presentation being between 40 and 60 years. It is defined by the presence of the Philadelphia chromosome (see **Fig. 2.23**), which is demonstrated either cytogenetically (95%) or molecularly (5%). Unlike the acute leukaemias, which are either rapidly reversed or rapidly fatal, CML has a more slowly progressive course through three distinct phases: chronic phase, accelerated phase and blast crisis. If left untreated, the disease will evolve through these phases and ultimately transform to acute leukaemia (blast crisis – 75% myeloid, 25% lymphoid) or myelofibrosis, with death in a median of 3–4 years. Fortunately, targeted therapy to arrest disease progression is highly effective in the majority of patients.

Clinical features

CML usually presents in the chronic phase and some patients have no symptoms.

Symptoms

When present, symptoms include:
- symptomatic anaemia (e.g. shortness of breath)
- abdominal discomfort due to splenomegaly
- weight loss
- fever and sweats in the absence of infection
- headache (occasionally) or priapism due to hyperleucocytosis
- bruising and bleeding (uncommon).

Signs

These include:
- pallor
- splenomegaly, often massive
- lymphadenopathy (uncommon; suggests blast crisis)
- extramedullary soft tissue leukaemic deposit – 'chloroma' (indicates blast crisis)
- retinal haemorrhage due to leucostasis.

Investigations

- **Blood count.** Haemoglobin is low (normochromic and normocytic) or normal; the white blood cell count is raised (usually >100 × 10^9/L); and platelets are low, normal or raised.
- **Blood film.** There is neutrophilia with the whole spectrum of mature myeloid precursors. Basophils and eosinophils are elevated. Increased numbers of blasts are suggestive of an accelerated phase or blast crisis (**Fig. 17.10**).
- **Bone marrow aspirate.** Increased cellularity is seen, with greater numbers of myeloid precursors. Cytogenetics reveals a t(9; 22) translocation (the Philadelphia chromosome; see **Fig. 2.23B**).
- **FISH or RT-PCR.** These demonstrate the cytogenetic/molecular abnormality. They are also used to monitor response to therapy quantitatively.

Management

Treatment has been transformed by the advent of imatinib, a TKI that specifically blocks the enzymatic action of the BCR-ABL fusion protein and is still usually first-line treatment for the chronic phase, although second-generation TKIs may be used. Imatinib produces a complete cytogenetic remission (no detectable Ph+ cells in the marrow) in 70% of patients. A significant proportion will lose molecularly detectable BCR-ABL transcripts from the blood, achieving a molecular response (MR) of varying depths: MR3 (a 3 log reduction; <0.1%), MR4 (<0.01%) or MR5 (<0.001%). Side-effects of imatinib include nausea, headache, rashes and cytopenias. Imatinib can be continued indefinitely, although discontinuation can be considered in those who respond optimally and achieve a sustained deep molecular response (MR4). Patients need to be closely monitored, with around two-thirds able to remain off treatment without disease recurrence.

Resistance to imatinib as a single agent may develop as a result of secondary BCR-ABL kinase mutations beyond t(9; 22). If patients do not tolerate imatinib or respond suboptimally, mutation analysis should be performed and a second-generation TKI, such as dasatinib, nilotinib or bosutinib, should be commenced. Those who have developed a T315I mutation should be offered ponatinib.

In accelerated and blast phases the approach is to combine a second-line TKI with intensive chemotherapy, as for acute leukaemia. SCT should then be considered with the aim of achieving a durable remission.

Chronic lymphocytic leukaemia

Chronic lymphocytic leukaemia (CLL) is the most common leukaemia, occurring predominantly in later life and increasing in frequency with advancing years (the median age of presentation is around 70 years). It results from the clonal expansion of small B lymphocytes with characteristic immunophenotype. The majority of patients are asymptomatic and are identified as a chance finding on

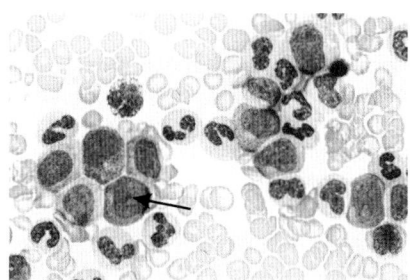

Fig. 17.10 Blood film showing blast cells (arrow) in chronic myeloid leukaemia.

a blood count performed for another indication. Others, however, present with the features of marrow failure or immunosuppression. The median survival is about 10 years and prognosis correlates with clinical stage at presentation (**Box 17.8**). A number of cytogenetic and molecular abnormalities are now recognized as being of prognostic significance (see later). This condition may present in leukaemic phase with significant marrow/blood involvement (CLL) or may present as localized disease (small lymphocytic lymphoma, SLL). The tumour cells in each condition are indistinguishable and a similar therapeutic approach is therefore used. Nearly all cases of CLL will be preceded by a monoclonal B-cell lymphocytosis (MBL) where there are fewer than 5×10^9/L circulating clonal B cells. However, this condition is also present in approximately 12% of the healthy population, and the relationship between MBL and CLL is analogous to that between monoclonal gammopathy of uncertain significance (MGUS) and myeloma (see p. 407). High-count MBL (over 0.5×10^9/L) should be distinguished from low-count MBL populations, as these patients will need review at least annually for disease evolution and infection risk.

Clinical features

The majority of patients are asymptomatic at presentation. When they are present, common symptoms are:

- recurrent infection because of (functional) leucopenia and immune failure (reduced immunoglobulins)
- anaemia due to haemolysis or marrow infiltration
- painless lymphadenopathy
- left upper quadrant discomfort (from splenomegaly).
  The most common findings on examination are:
- anaemia
- lymphadenopathy (may involve a single area or be generalized)
- hepatosplenomegaly, sometimes massive.

> ### i Box 17.8 The Rai and Binet staging systems for chronic lymphocytic leukaemia[a]
>
> | Stage | Risk | Manifestations | Recommended treatment |
> |---|---|---|---|
> | **Rai staging system** | | | |
> | 0 | Low | Lymphocytosis | Watch and wait |
> | I | Intermediate | Lymphadenopathy | Treat only with progression[b] |
> | II | Intermediate | Splenomegaly, lymphadenopathy or both | Treat only with progression[b] |
> | III | High | Anaemia, organomegaly | Treat in most cases |
> | IV | High | One or more of the following: anaemia, thrombocytopenia and organomegaly | Treat in most cases |
> | **Binet staging system** | | | |
> | A | Low | Lymphocytosis, <3 lymphoid areas enlarged[c] | Watch and wait |
> | B | Intermediate | ≥3 lymphoid areas enlarged[c] | Treat only with progression |
> | C | High | Anaemia, thrombocytopenia or both | Treat in most cases |
>
> [a]Lymphocytosis is present in all stages of the disease. [b]Progression is defined by weight loss, fatigue, fever, massive organomegaly and a rapidly increasing lymphocyte count. [c]Lymphoid areas include the cervical, axillary and inguinal lymph nodes, the spleen and the liver.

Investigations

- **Blood count** reveals a normal or low haemoglobin; a raised white blood cell count, which may be very high; lymphocytosis (criteria for diagnosis $>5 \times 10^9$/L); and normal or low platelets.
- **Blood film** demonstrates small or medium-sized mature and normal-appearing lymphocytes. Smudge cells may be seen *in vitro*. No immature blasts are evident.
- **Bone marrow** reflects peripheral blood, often very heavily infiltrated with lymphocytes.
- **Immunophenotyping** typically shows CD19+, CD5+ or CD23+ B cells with weak expression of CD22, CD79b and surface immunoglobulin (kappa and lambda light chains).
- **Cytogenetics/FISH analyses** identifying 17p deletion or p53 mutation is essential prior to treatment, as this will influence choice of therapy (**Fig. 17.11**).
- **Direct Coombs' test** may be positive if there is haemolysis.
- **Immunoglobulins** are low or normal.

Prognosis

The clinical course of CLL is variable. Prognosis is influenced by age and clinical stage, as well as pace of disease, measured by doubling time. Cytogenetic abnormalities are detected in more than 90% of cases. Patients with an isolated deletion of 13q have a better prognosis, in contrast to those with either 11q deletion or 17p deletion (sites of the tumour suppressor genes *ATM* and *TP53*, respectively), who tend to follow a rapidly evolving clinical course. Mutation within the immunoglobulin heavy chain variable region (IGHV) predicts an indolent course, and expression of ZAP70, a 70-kDa tyrosine kinase protein, correlates reasonably well with mutational status. Patients with mutated IGHV have median survival of more than 20 years in contrast to 8 years in patients with unmutated IGHV. High expression of CD38 on leukaemic cells may also indicate an adverse prognosis. Next-generation sequencing (see p. 31) has identified certain genes (*NOTCH1*, *SF3B1*) whose mutation influences prognosis.

Management

In CLL, the major consideration is when to treat; indeed, 30% of patients will never require intervention. Treatment depends on disease 'stage' (see **Box 17.8**). Early-stage disease is usually managed expectantly, advanced-stage disease is always treated immediately,

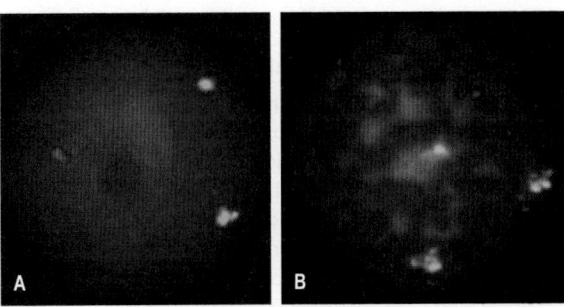

Fig. 17.11 Fluorescence *in situ* hybridization (FISH) photomicrograph of a patient with chronic lymphocytic leukaemia. **(A)** 17p (green probe) and 11q (red probe) shows two green signals (*TP53* deletion) with normal diploid complement of 11q. **(B)** 12 centromere (green probe) and 13q14 (red probe) shows three green signals (trisomy 12) with normal diploid complement of 13q. (*Courtesy of Debra Lillington, Barts and the London NHS Trust.*)

and the approach to the intermediate stage is variable. Indications for treatment are:

- marrow failure, manifest by worsening anaemia and/or thrombocytopenia that is not autoimmune
- massive or progressive splenomegaly or lymphadenopathy
- progressive disease demonstrated by doubling of the lymphocyte count in less than 6 months
- systemic symptoms (fever, night sweats or weight loss)
- presence of haemolysis or other immune-mediated cytopenias that are poorly responsive to steroids.

General/supportive treatment

Anaemia due to haemolysis is treated with steroids. Anaemia and thrombocytopenia caused by marrow infiltration are treated with chemotherapy and, when necessary, transfusion. Erythropoietin (EPO, see p. 325) may avoid the need for transfusions, particularly in patients receiving chemotherapy. Infection is treated as indicated, with prophylactic antibiotic, antiviral, anti-*Pneumocystis* and antifungal therapy potentially being given during periods of chemotherapy. Immunoglobulin replacement may be helpful, as well as pneumococcal, *Haemophilus influenzae* type B (Hib) and influenza vaccination. Live vaccines should be avoided. Allopurinol is given to prevent hyperuricaemia.

Specific treatment

Choice of therapy will depend on patient-related factors, such as age and co-morbidity, adverse prognostic features, and anticipated response to and toxicities of therapy. A range of therapies are available and these must be tailored to the patient's age, fitness, prior therapy exposure and concurrent co-morbidities.

- ***Ibrutinib***, a Bruton's tyrosine kinase (BTK) inhibitor, should be offered to those individuals with TP53 disruption, as they are poorly responsive to conventional chemo-immunotherapy. This is taken orally and is generally well tolerated, although an increased risk of atrial fibrillation is observed. Venetoclax (a BCL-2 inhibitor) is a second-line option.
- ***Fludarabine***, a purine analogue, in combination with cyclophosphamide and rituximab, is still first-line treatment for younger, fitter patients.
- ***Obinutuzumab*** or ***ofatumumab***, both novel anti-CD20 monoclonal antibodies, are preferred in the elderly or less fit to rituximab in combination with chlorambucil. Bendamustine is an alternative alkylator that may be appropriate for first-line therapy in older and less fit patients who cannot tolerate FCR (fludarabine, cyclophosphamide, rituximab).
- ***Allogeneic SCT*** with non-myeloablative conditioning regimens is occasionally considered in fit patients with high-risk disease.

Lymphomatous transformation

CLL may undergo lymphomatous (Richter's) transformation in 5–10% of cases, most typically to diffuse large B-cell lymphoma, although Hodgkin-like transformation is also recognized. In around half of cases, the high-grade lymphoma is clonally unrelated to the CLL clone and these cases respond to treatment in a similar way to *de novo* diffuse large B-cell lymphoma (DLBCL). Where lymphoma is clonally related, outcomes are poorer.

Hairy cell leukaemia

Hairy cell leukaemia (HCL) is a clonal proliferation of abnormal B (or, very rarely, T) cells, which, as in CLL, accumulate in the bone marrow and spleen. It is a rare disease; median age at presentation is 52 years and the male to female ratio is 4 : 1. The bizarre name relates to the appearance of the cells on a blood film and in the bone marrow: they have an irregular outline owing to the presence of filament-like cytoplasmic projections. *BRAF* mutations (see p. 691) are seen in almost all cases.

Clinical features

Clinical features include anaemia, fever and weight loss. Splenomegaly occurs in 80% but lymphadenopathy is uncommon. Anaemia, neutropenia, thrombocytopenia and low monocyte counts are found.

Management

The purine analogues cladribine and pentostatin have specific activity in this condition; complete remission is achieved in 90% with just one cycle of treatment. The remissions can last for many years and patients can be successfully retreated. Splenectomy or rituximab is sometimes used in cases that do not respond to these drugs.

Further reading

Baccarani M, Deininger MW, Rosti G et al. European LeukemiaNet recommendations for the management of chronic myeloid leukemia: 2013. *Blood* 2013; 122:872–884.
Etienne G, Guilhot J, Rea D et al. Long-term follow-up of the French Stop Imatinib (STIM1) study in patients with chronic myeloid leukemia. *J Clin Oncol* 2017; 35:298–305.
Schuh AH, Parry-Jones N, Appleby N et al. Guideline for the treatment of chronic lymphocytic leukaemia: a British Society for Haematology guideline. *Br J Haematol* 2018; 182:344–359.

MYELOPROLIFERATIVE NEOPLASMS

Myeloproliferative neoplasms are clonal stem cell disorders characterized by uncontrolled proliferation of one or more of the cell lines in the bone marrow, usually erythroid, myeloid and/or megakaryocyte lines. Myeloproliferative disorders include:

- polycythaemia vera (PV)
- essential thrombocythaemia (ET)
- myelofibrosis
- chronic myeloid leukaemia (CML).

The first three disorders are grouped together, as there can be transition from one disease to another: for example, PV can lead to myelofibrosis. They may also transform to AML. They are often characterized by a genetic lesion in *JAK2*, *MPL* or *CALR*. The non-leukaemic myeloproliferative neoplasms (PV, ET and myelofibrosis) will be discussed in this section, CML having been described earlier.

Polycythaemia vera

The investigation of polycythaemia is covered on page 395. While it is important to exclude secondary causes of polycythaemia, the presence of a mutation of the *JAK2* gene is strongly suggestive of primary polycythaemia (polycythaemia vera). This is a clonal stem cell disorder in which there is an excessive proliferation of erythroid, myeloid and/or megakaryocytic progenitor cells. Over 95% of patients with PV have acquired mutations of the *JAK2* gene, in the vast majority of cases a point mutation that causes the substitution of phenylalanine for valine at position 617 (JAK2V617F). *JAK2* is a cytoplasmic tyrosine kinase that transduces signals, especially those triggered by haemopoietic growth factors such as EPO, in normal and neoplastic cells. The significance of the discovery of the *JAK2* mutation in myeloproliferative neoplasms is two-fold: first, and of immediate significance, is the clinical utility of the detection of *JAK2* mutations for the diagnosis of PV, and second is the prospect of the development of new treatments for the myeloproliferative disorders based on targeting *JAK2* activity.

Clinical features

The onset is insidious. PV is more common in patients aged over 60 and may present with fatigue, itching, vertigo, headache and visual disturbance. These symptoms are common in the older population and consequently PV is easily missed. Patients may also present with complications of the disease relating to thrombosis or haemorrhage. Increasingly, PV is detected on routine blood tests conducted for other reasons. Severe itching may occur after a hot bath or when the patient is warm. Gout due to increased cell turnover may be a feature, and peptic ulceration occurs in a minority of patients. Thrombosis and haemorrhage are the major complications of PV.

The patient may be plethoric, and have a dusky cyanosis and injection of the conjunctivae. The spleen is palpable in 70% and is useful in distinguishing PV from secondary polycythaemia. The liver is enlarged in 50% of patients.

Diagnosis

JAK2 mutation screening is routine in the investigation of polycythaemia and is fully incorporated into diagnostic criteria. Although World Health Organization (WHO) criteria require a bone marrow biopsy for diagnosis in adults, current British guidelines do not mandate this in the presence of a confirmed *JAK2* mutation (**Box 17.9**). Red cell mass studies are now rarely required.

The measurement of red cell and plasma volume is not routinely required. Measurement of serum ferritin can be useful to detect cases of iron-deficient PV. There may be a raised serum uric acid, leucocyte alkaline phosphatase and raised serum vitamin B_{12} and vitamin B_{12} binding protein (transcobalamin 1).

Management
Course and treatment

Treatment is designed to maintain a normal blood count and to prevent the complications of the disease, particularly thromboses and haemorrhage. The aim is to keep the haematocrit below 0.45.

There are three types of specific treatment:
- **Venesection**. During initial phases of treatment, the removal of 400–500 mL of blood weekly will successfully relieve many of the symptoms of PV. Iron deficiency eventually limits erythropoiesis

---

and only infrequent venesection is required. Venesection is often used as the sole treatment, with the aim of maintaining a haematocrit of <0.45.
- **Chemotherapy**. Continuous or intermittent treatment with hydroxycarbamide (hydroxyurea) is used in patients who do not tolerate venesection or who have other poorly controlled features of the disease, such as thrombocytosis, symptomatic splenomegaly or thrombosis. Interferon-alfa is also effective; it is administered by subcutaneous injection but can cause unacceptable toxicity. Low-dose intermittent busulfan may be more convenient for elderly people but use must be weighed against potential long-term complications, such as the increased risk of leukaemia development.
- **Ruxolitinib**. This *JAK2* inhibitor is more widely used in myelofibrosis but may have a role in patients who have severe symptoms such as pruritus or splenomegaly.
- **Low-dose aspirin**. Aspirin 75 mg daily with the above treatments is routinely used for patients with PV in the absence of contraindications
- **Anagrelide**. This inhibits megakaryocyte differentiation and is useful for thrombocytosis.

Iron replacement should be avoided in patients with iron-deficient PV, as this can result in a dangerous rebound polycythaemia.

General measures
- **Allopurinol**. This can be given to block uric acid production. The pruritus is lessened by avoiding very hot baths.
- **Surgery**. Polycythaemia should be controlled before surgery. Patients with uncontrolled PV have a high operative risk. In an emergency, the haematocrit must be reduced by venesection and appropriate fluid replacement.

Prognosis

PV develops into myelofibrosis in 12–21% of cases and into AML in 5% as part of the natural history of the disease.

Essential thrombocythaemia

ET is a myeloproliferative neoplasm, closely related to PV, which is characterized by a persistently raised platelet count. Patients usually have normal haemoglobin levels, although mild anaemia may occur. The WCC is elevated in some patients. At diagnosis, the platelet count will usually be above 600×10^9/L and may be as high as 2000×10^9/L, or rarely even higher.

Clinical features

ET presents either symptomatically with thromboembolic or, less commonly, bleeding problems, or incidentally (e.g. at a routine medical check). Erythromelalgia, severe burning pain, erythema and warmth of the extremities (primarily the feet and, to a lesser extent, the hands) may occur.

Investigations

The diagnosis of ET is based on a sustained platelet count of 450×10^9/L or more, in the absence of a possible reactive cause of thrombocytosis (**Box 17.10**) and of other haematological malignancy associated with thrombocytosis (e.g. PV, myelofibrosis). In selected cases a bone marrow biopsy is necessary; however, the requirement for this has largely been replaced by molecular tests. The *JAK2* mutation test (see PV) is useful in that the gene is mutated in about half of all cases of ET, confirming a myeloproliferative neoplasm. For the remaining 50% of patients with a normal *JAK2* gene, testing for mutations in calreticulin (*CALR*) or the thrombopoietin

---

> **i** **Box 17.9 Recommended diagnostic criteria for polycythaemia vera (PV)**
>
> **JAK2-positive PV (requires both criteria)**
> - A1: Haematocrit >0.52 in men, >0.48 in women *or* raised red cell mass (>25% above predicted)
> - A2: Mutation in *JAK2*
>
> **JAK2-negative PV (requires A1–A4 plus another A or two B criteria)**
> - A1: Haematocrit ≥0.60 in men, ≥0.56 in women *or* raised red cell mass (>25% above predicted)
> - A2: Absence of mutation in *JAK2*
> - A3: No cause of secondary erythrocytosis
> - A4: Bone marrow histology consistent with PV
> - A5: Palpable splenomegaly
> - A6: Presence of an acquired genetic abnormality (excluding *BCR-ABL*) in the haemopoietic cells
> - B1: Thrombocytosis (platelet count >450×10^9/L)
> - B2: Neutrophil count >10×10^9/L in non-smokers, ≥12.5×10^9/L in smokers
> - B3: Radiological evidence of splenomegaly
> - B4: Low serum erythropoietin
>
> *(Adapted from BSH Guidelines: https://onlinelibrary.wiley.com/doi/full/10.1111/bjh.15648.)*

Box 17.10 Causes of thrombocythaemia

Haematological cancers
- Essential thrombocythaemia
- Polycythaemia vera
- Myelofibrosis
- CML
- Myelodysplasia with del(5q)
- MDS/MPN overlap syndromes e.g. CMML, atypical CML

Reactive
- Infection
- Inflammation
- Haemorrhage
- Postoperative
- Inflammatory conditions (e.g. inflammatory bowel disease rheumatoid arthritis)

Haemolysis
Hyposplenism
- Functional or surgical

Iron deficiency
Drugs
- Corticosteroids
- Thrombopoietin receptor agonists
Rebound post chemotherapy
Solid malignancy

CMML, chronic myelomonocytic leukaemia; MDS, myelodysplasia; MPN, myeloproliferative neoplasms.
(Adapted from British Society for Haematology Thrombocythemia guidelines, https://onlinelibrary.wiley.com/doi/full/10.1111/j.1365-2141.2010.08122.x.)

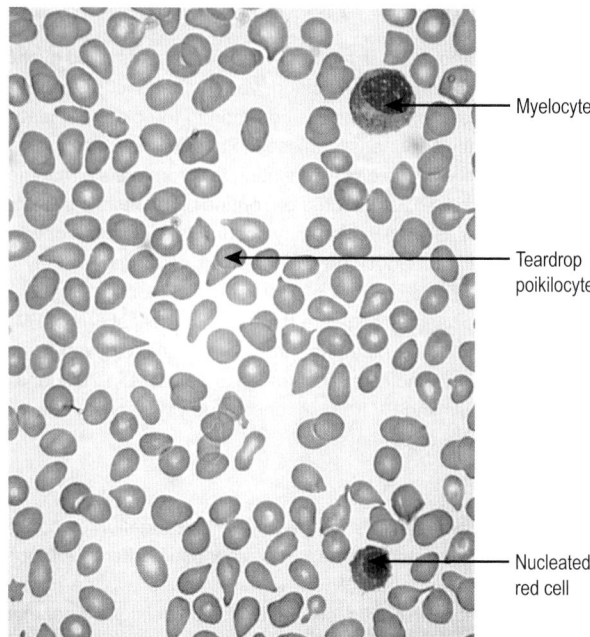

Fig. 17.12 Leucoerythroblastic blood film with teardrops in myelofibrosis.

receptor (*MPL*) will be informative in most cases, abrogating the need for a bone marrow biopsy. As a generalization, a person with a very high platelet count ($>1000 \times 10^9$/L), who is clinically normal with good health, will most likely prove to have ET. In a patient who has a lower platelet count (e.g. 600×10^9/L) and is in poor health, the diagnosis can be more difficult.

Management

Due to the thrombotic risk, aspirin should be given to all ET patients, unless contraindicated. Treatment to reduce the platelet count ('cytoreduction') is recommended for patients with any high-risk feature:
- age >60 years
- platelet count $>1500 \times 10^9$/L
- disease-related thrombosis or haemorrhage.

Treatment is usually with hydroxycarbamide (hydroxyurea), to control the platelet count to below 400×10^9/L. Alternative cytoreductive agents include anagrelide or busulfan. Interferon-alfa is also effective; it is administered by subcutaneous injection but can be difficult to tolerate due to side-effects. ET may eventually transform into PV, myelofibrosis or acute leukaemia, but the disease may not progress for many years.

Secondary thrombocytosis

Other disorders that may give rise to reactive high platelet counts include autoimmune rheumatic disorders and malignancy. Individuals who have been splenectomized (for any reason, including trauma) sometimes have high platelet counts.

Myelofibrosis

Myelofibrosis is a debilitating myeloproliferative neoplasm characterized by clonal proliferation of stem cells and abnormal myeloid cells in the bone marrow, liver, spleen and other organs. It may be

primary or develop late in the course of ET or PV. Increased fibrosis in the bone marrow is caused by hyperplasia of abnormal megakaryocytes, which release fibroblast-stimulating factors such as platelet-derived growth factor.

Clinical features

The disease presents insidiously with lethargy, weakness and weight loss. Patients often complain of a 'fullness' in the upper abdomen due to splenomegaly, which may be massive. Severe pain related to respiration may indicate perisplenitis secondary to splenic infarction, and bone pain and attacks of gout can complicate the illness. Extramedullary haemopoiesis can develop, typically in the spleen but also affecting other organs. Bruising and bleeding occur because of thrombocytopenia or abnormal platelet function.

Investigations

- **Full blood count** shows anaemia with leucoerythroblastic features. Poikilocytes and red cells with characteristic teardrop forms are seen (**Fig. 17.12**). The WCC may be $>100 \times 10^9$/L, and the differential WCC may be very similar to that seen in CML; leucopenia may also develop later. The platelet count may be very high but in later stages thrombocytopenia occurs.
- **Bone marrow aspiration** is often unsuccessful owing to the fibrotic state of the bone marrow, which may give a clue to the presence of the condition. A bone marrow trephine is necessary to show the markedly increased fibrosis. Increased numbers of megakaryocytes may be seen.
- **Cytogenetic and molecular analysis** shows the absence of the Philadelphia chromosome (*BCR-ABL* fusion gene); this helps to distinguish myelofibrosis from CML. A *JAK2* mutation is present in approximately 60% of cases and a *CALR* mutation in 25%.

Management

This consists of general supportive measures, such as blood transfusion, analgesics, antihistamines and allopurinol. Treatment for myelofibrosis is often difficult but an estimation of prognosis from a prognostic scoring system is a good basis on which to start planning a strategy for the individual patient. This may range from observation alone in those with the best prognosis to drug treatment or allogeneic SCT, offering a hope of cure for younger patients.

Historically, symptomatic splenomegaly was managed using hydroxycarbamide, radiotherapy and, in some cases, splenectomy. However, the latter is associated with very significant morbidity and mortality in patients with myelofibrosis and the former two are of limited benefit. A new and very promising development in the treatment of myelofibrosis is targeted therapy with *JAK* inhibitors. Ruxolitinib is the first such *JAK* inhibitor treatment in routine clinical use. Ruxolitinib results in substantial spleen reduction and improvement in symptoms in many patients with higher-risk myelofibrosis. Although ruxolitinib may improve life expectancy in patients with myelofibrosis, it does not eradicate the disease and underlying fibrosis remains in the vast majority of patients.

Prognosis

Patients may survive for 10 years or more, though median survival is 4–5 years with risk factors for poor prognosis, including cytopenias, presence of circulating blast cells, constitutional symptoms and the presence of poor-risk cytogenetics (e.g. monosomy 7) or molecular genetic mutations (e.g. *ASXL1* or *EZH2*). Death occurs in 10–20% of cases by transformation to AML. The other most common causes of death are progressive bone marrow failure and infection.

Other myeloproliferative neoplasms

Rare myeloproliferative neoplasms include **chronic eosinophilic leukaemia**, a disorder that is associated with gene fusions that activate tyrosine kinase activity and may be treated with imatinib, as for CML; **chronic neutrophilic leukaemia**; and a heterogeneous group described as '**myeloproliferative neoplasm, unclassifiable**'.

MYELODYSPLASIA

Myelodysplasia (MDS) describes a group of acquired bone marrow disorders caused by a defect in haemopoietic stem cells. They are characterized by progressive bone marrow failure with quantitative and qualitative abnormalities in at least one of the three myeloid cell lines (red cells, granulocyte/monocytes and platelets). MDS covers a heterogeneous group of conditions with varying presentations and prognosis, for which there is a wide spectrum of treatment approaches ranging from observation to allogeneic SCT. Although the natural history of MDS is variable, there is a high morbidity and mortality owing to bone marrow failure and transformation to AML, which occurs in about 30% of cases. The current WHO classification of MDS is shown in **Box 17.11**.

Clinical features

MDS occurs mainly in the elderly and presents with symptoms of anaemia, infection or bleeding due to pancytopenia. MDS should be suspected in patients with otherwise unexplained cytopenias or macrocytosis.

Investigations

Serial blood counts show evidence of increasing bone marrow failure with anaemia, neutropenia and thrombocytopenia, either alone or in combination.

The bone marrow cellularity can be increased, normal or reduced, irrespective of the pancytopenia. Dysplasia in one or more of the erythroid, granulocytic and megakaryocytic lineages is usually present (**Fig. 17.13**). The percentage of bone marrow blast cells is important for classification and prognostic risk stratification in MDS. If this percentage rises above 20%, the diagnosis changes from MDS to AML. Ring sideroblasts seen with a specific iron stain are present in some subtypes.

Cytogenetic abnormalities (e.g. 7–, 5–) are common and are important for prognostic stratification. Certain specific abnormalities will also change the diagnosis to AML irrespective of blast count: for example, t(8;21) and inv(16). Somatic point mutations are commonly present. A poor survival rate is seen in those carrying mutations in *TP53*, *E2H2*, *ETV6*, *RUNX1* and *ASXL1*.

Management

MDS is a heterogeneous disease and management is dependent on clinical features and predicted prognosis; the latter can be estimated using international prognostic scoring systems that incorporate blood counts, bone marrow blast percentage and cytogenetics. Treatment strategy is based on the behaviour and clinical burden of the disease and the likely prognosis, as well as the age and fitness of the patient. For example, an older patient may be managed with transfusion support alone, while a younger, fitter patient with high-risk disease may be considered for the higher-risk but potentially curative strategy of allogeneic SCT.

---

i | **Box 17.11 World Health Organization classification of myelodysplasia (MDS)**

Name	Dysplastic lineages	Cytopenias[a]	BM and PB blasts
MDS with single lineage dysplasia (MDS-SLD)	1	1 or 2	BM <5%, PB <1%, no Auer rods
MDS with multi-lineage dysplasia (MDS-MLD)	2 or 3	1–3	BM <5%, PB <1%, no Auer rods
MDS with ring sideroblasts (MDS-RS)			BM <5%, PB <1%, no Auer rods
MDS with isolated del(5q)	1–3	1–2	BM <5%, PB <1%, no Auer rods
MDS with excess blasts (MDS-EB)			
MDS-EB-1	0–3	1–3	BM 5–9% or PB 2–4%, no Auer rods
MDS-EB-2	0–3	1–3	BM 10–19% or PB 5–19%, or Auer rods
MDS, unclassifiable (MDS-U)			

[a]Cytopenias defined as: Haemoglobin <100 g/L; platelet count <100 × 10^9/L; neutrophil count <1.8 × 10^9/L. BM, bone marrow; PB, peripheral blood.
(Adapted from Swerdlow SH, Campo E, Harris NL et al (eds). WHO Classification of tumours of haematopoietic and lymphoid tissues. Blood 2016; 127:2375–2390.)

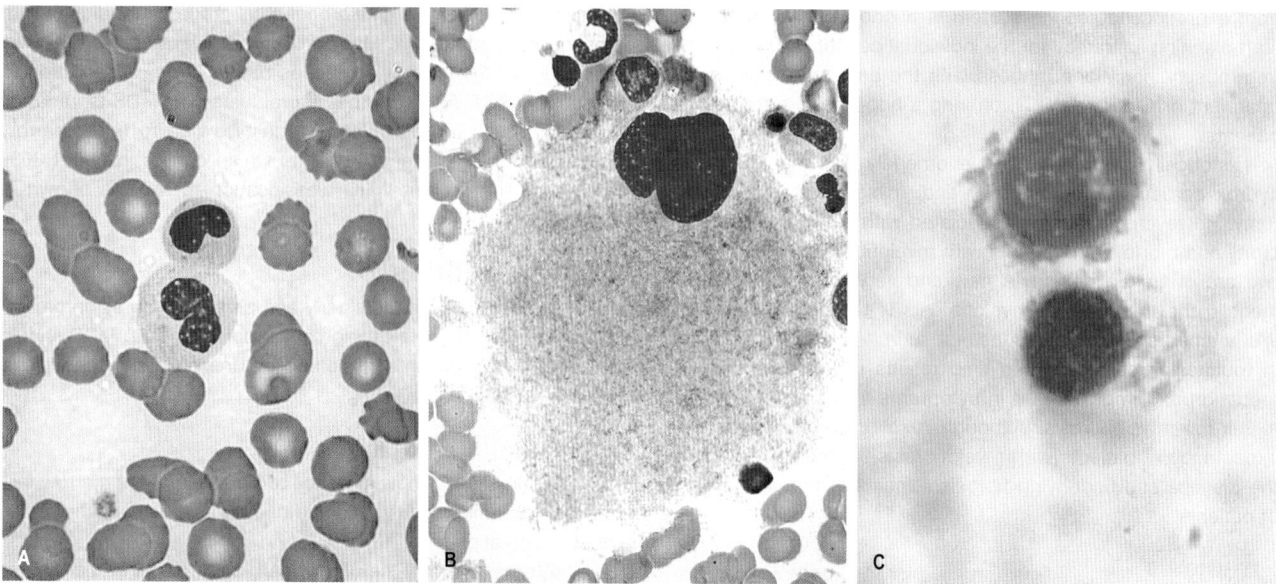

Fig. 17.13 Myelodysplastic syndrome. (A) Pseudo-Pelger neutrophil with bilobed nucleus. **(B)** Dysplastic megakaryocyte in the bone marrow. **(C)** Iron stain of the bone marrow showing 'ring sideroblasts'.

Treatment options include the following:
- ***Supportive care*** is the mainstay for all patients with MDS and symptomatic low blood counts. It includes red cell and platelet transfusion, and the prevention and treatment of MDS-associated bleeding and infection.
- ***Erythropoietin*** can be used in selected patients with low-risk MDS, symptomatic anaemia and inappropriately low endogenous EPO levels.
- ***Iron chelation*** should be considered for patients with good prognostic MDS who develop secondary iron overload (transfused with more than 20 units of red cells or serum ferritin >1000 µg/L).
- ***Hypomethylating agents*** (e.g. azacitidine, decitabine) are useful in selected patients.
- ***Immunosuppressive agents***, such as ciclosporin and antithymocyte globulin, may be used in selected patients with a hypocellular bone marrow.
- ***Intensive chemotherapy*** schedules used for AML (see p. 390) may be used in selected patients with high-risk MDS and higher numbers of bone marrow blasts, but the remission rate is less than for AML, and prolonged pancytopenia may occur owing to poor haemopoietic regeneration caused by the defect in stem cells.
- ***Lenalidomide*** (a thalidomide analogue) has been proven to be remarkably successful in the treatment of early-stage MDS with a chromosome 5q deletion (the 5q– syndrome).
- ***Allogeneic SCT*** offers the hope of cure for carefully selected MDS patients who have a matched donor. Due to the potential morbidity and mortality associated with allogeneic SCT, this procedure is usually restricted to patients without major co-morbidities who have higher-risk MDS and in whom the risk : benefit balance is clear.

MDS/MPN overlap syndromes

This is mixed group of conditions that have both dysplastic and proliferative features. It includes:
- chronic myelomonocytic leukaemia (CMML)
- atypical chronic myeloid leukaemia (aCML) (*BCR-ABL*-negative)
- juvenile myelomonocytic leukaemia (JMML)

- MDS/MPN with ring sideroblasts and thrombocytosis
- MDS/MPN, unclassifiable.

Due to the rarity of these conditions, protocols are less well established but treatment principles are similar to those for MDS (e.g. supportive care for cytopenias) and MPNs (e.g. cytoreduction for elevated blood counts). Similarly, more intensive approaches, including transplantation, may be considered for selected younger patients.

Further reading

Harrison CN, Bareford D, Butt N et al. Guideline for investigation and management of adults and children presenting with a thrombocytosis. *Br J Haematol* 2010; 149:352–375.
Harrison CN, McLornan DP. Current treatment algorithm for the management of patients with myelofibrosis, JAK inhibitors, and beyond. *Hematology Am Soc Hematol Educ Program* 2017; 2017:489–497.
Killick SB, Carter C, Culligan D et al. Guidelines for the diagnosis and management of adult myelodysplastic syndromes. *Br J Haematol* 2014; 164:503–525.
McMullin MF, Harrison CN, Ali S et al. A guideline for the diagnosis and management of polycythaemia vera: a British Society for Haematology guideline. *Br J Haematol* 2019; 184:176–191.

LYMPHOMAS

The lymphomas are malignancies of the lymphoid system and disease may arise at any site where lymphoid tissue is present. Certain subtypes have increased in frequency over the past 50 years for reasons that are not clear, the overall incidence being 15–20 per 100 000 population, which makes them the fifth most common malignancy in the Western world. Most often, patients have peripheral lymphadenopathy or symptoms due to occult lymph nodes, although approximately 20% arise at primary extranodal sites. A relatively small proportion present with lymphoma-associated 'B' symptoms of weight loss, fever and sweats. The natural history and clinical course vary widely with the subtype.

A significant proportion of patients are cured, and many others are helped, in terms of both quality and length of life.

The increasingly complex WHO classification of tumours of haemopoietic and lymphoid tissues primarily distinguishes Hodgkin lymphoma from non-Hodgkin lymphoma, an umbrella term covering a multiply subclassified spectrum of B- and T-cell malignancies.

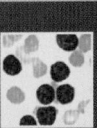

Overall management strategy common to all lymphomas

A suspected diagnosis of lymphoma should always be confirmed by an excision biopsy of the relevant tissue that is large enough to allow histological, immunological and molecular analysis. Core biopsy is an acceptable substitute for biopsy of impalpable, 'occult' disease but fine needle aspiration is inadequate. The opinion of an expert haemato-pathologist is essential.

Investigations

Once the diagnosis is established, treatment strategy will depend on the outcome of investigations that are common to all the lymphomas (**Box 17.12**). These allow prognosis to be estimated and inform treatment decisions; a 'stage' is notionally assigned to the modification of the Ann Arbor classification for all nodal lymphomas (see later), despite the fact that this was planned only for Hodgkin lymphoma.

The tests listed in **Box 17.12** are essential for planning specific therapy. Serum uric acid measurement is helpful, particularly in those lymphomas that carry a risk of tumour lysis syndrome (see p. 118); tests of cardiac function are valuable when potentially cardiotoxic chemotherapy is to be recommended, as is assessment of HIV and hepatitis B and C status.

Once treatment has begun, benefit is assessed at intervals, and re-evaluation ('restaging') performed at the end of a course of therapy. Depending on the outcome, future plans will be made. In the event of a decision to stop treatment, surveillance will initially be close, the interval between attendances being extended with the passage of time. Beyond 5 years, the focus of attention is on the possible long-term consequences of therapy rather than the disease itself. When initial therapy has been less successful than wished, management is dictated by individual circumstances. As conventional treatment options are exhausted, experimental therapy may be broached.

Hodgkin lymphoma

Hodgkin lymphoma (HL) has a stable incidence of approximately 3 per 100 000 in the Western world, and there is a male predominance of approximately 1.3:1. The majority of cases occur between the ages of 16 and 65, with a peak in the third decade.

---

i **Box 17.12 Investigation of the patient with lymphoma**

For diagnosis

- Clinical history and examination
- Performance status
- Comprehensive geriatric assessment (see p. 302)[a]
- Chest X-ray for mediastinal widening (see **Fig. 17.15**)
- CT scan of chest, abdomen, pelvis ± neck
- CT-PET scan (see **Fig. 17.16**)
- ± Bone marrow biopsy (only required if PET is not be used to assess bone marrow involvement for staging)
- Blood count, differential, film

For planning specific therapy

- Electrolytes and renal function, liver function tests and biochemistry
- Serum uric acid
- Virology: HIV, hepatitis B and C
- Cardiac function (e.g. echocardiogram)
- Respiratory function (e.g. spirometry testing)
- Referral for fertility preservation[a]

[a]Depending on circumstances.
CT, computed tomography; HIV, human immunodeficiency virus; PET, positron emission tomography.

Aetiology

There is epidemiological evidence linking previous infectious mononucleosis with HL; up to 40% of patients with HL have increased Epstein–Barr virus (EBV) antibody titres at the time of diagnosis, and EBV DNA has been demonstrated in tissue from patients with HL. These data suggest a role for EBV in pathogenesis. Other viruses have not been detected but other environmental and occupational exposures to pathogens have been postulated.

Diagnosis

HL is subclassified, according to the WHO classification (**Box 17.13**), into:

- *classic Hodgkin lymphoma* (*CHL*), the hallmark of which is the Reed–Sternberg cell (**Fig. 17.14**). CHL accounts for 90–95% of cases and is further subdivided into four distinct categories.
- *Nodular lymphocyte-predominant HL* (*NLPHL*), characterized by the lymphocyte-predominant or 'popcorn cell'.

Clinical features

The most common presentation of HL is painless cervical lymphadenopathy, commonly described in examination as 'rubbery'. A smaller proportion of patients (often young women) present with disease localized to the mediastinum, with cough due to mediastinal lymphadenopathy (**Fig. 17.15**); others present with 'generalized disease', including hepatosplenomegaly and constitutional 'B' symptoms. Other less common symptoms, undoubtedly associated with HL but not recognized in the staging classification, are pruritus and alcohol-related pain at the site of lymphadenopathy.

---

i **Box 17.13 WHO pathological classification of Hodgkin lymphoma (HL)**

Type	Histology classification	Proportion of HL
Nodular lymphocyte-predominant HL		5%
Classical HL	Nodular sclerosing	70%
	Mixed cellularity	20%
	Lymphocyte-rich	5%
	Lymphocyte-depleted	Rare

(Courtesy WHO.)

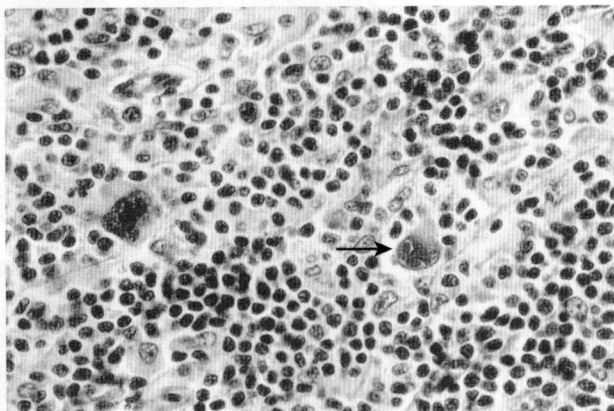

Fig. 17.14 Histological appearance of Hodgkin lymphoma. Scattered mononuclear Hodgkin cells and a classical malignant binucleate Reed–Sternberg cell (arrowed) are seen to right of centre on a background of benign small lymphocytes and histiocytes. *(Courtesy of Dr AJ Norton.)*

Investigations

These are summarized in **Box 17.12**. Baseline PET-CT is standard practice to establish extent and distribution of metabolically active sites of disease (**Fig. 17.16**). This enables 'stage' to be assigned according to the Cotswolds modification of the Ann Arbor classification (**Box 17.14**). Patients with early-stage disease should be categorized as having favourable or unfavourable disease (**Box 17.15**). The Hasenclever International Prognostic Score (IPS) is applied to patients with advanced-stage disease (**Box 17.16**). On the basis of 'stage' and other prognostic factors, patients with HL are divided into three groups (see **Box 17.15**). Criteria for unfavourable disease are defined by either Germal Hodgkin Study Group (GHSG) or European Organization for Research and Treatment of Cancer (EORTC) parameters.

Management

Principles of management

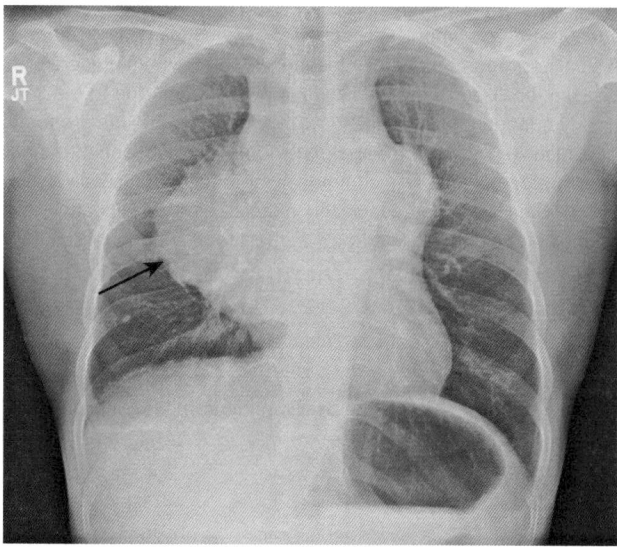

Fig. 17.15 Chest X-ray showing a mediastinal mass (arrowed) that is due to Hodgkin lymphoma.

Management is aimed towards a curative intent with expectation of success. Older patients, with or without co-morbidity, require considerable modification of therapy. Patients with HIV infection should be managed, in conjunction with their HIV clinicians, in the same way as those who are seronegative. NLPHL is a separate entity that, being strongly CD20-positive, is often treated with rituximab chemo-immunotherapy. Early-stage disease can be treated with radiotherapy alone.

> ### *i* Box 17.14 Cotswolds modification of Ann Arbor staging of Hodgkin lymphoma
>
> | Stage | Description |
> |---|---|
> | I | Involvement of a single lymph-node region or lymphoid structure (e.g. spleen, thymus, Waldeyer's ring) or involvement of a single extralymphatic site |
> | II | Involvement of two or more lymph node regions on the same side of the diaphragm; localized contiguous involvement of only one extranodal organ or site and lymph node region(s) on the same side of the diaphragm (IIE). The number of anatomical regions involved should be indicated by a subscript (e.g. II$_3$) |
> | III | Involvement of lymph node regions on both sides of the diaphragm (III), which may also be accompanied by involvement of the spleen (IIIS) or by localized involvement of only one extranodal organ site (IIIE) or both (IIISE) |
> | IV | Diffuse or disseminated involvement of one or more extranodal organs or tissues, with or without associated lymph node involvement |
>
> **Designations applicable to any disease state**
>
> | | |
> |---|---|
> | A | No symptoms |
> | B | Fever (temperature >38°C), drenching night sweats, unexplained loss of >10% of body weight within the previous 6 months |
> | X | Bulky disease (a widening of the mediastinum by more than one-third or the presence of a nodal mass with a maximal dimension >10cm) |
> | E | Involvement of a single extranodal site that is contiguous or proximal to the known nodal site |
>
> *(Adapted from Diehl V, Thomas RK, Re D et al. Hodgkin's lymphoma – diagnosis and treatment. Lancet Oncol 2004; 5:19–26, with permission from Elsevier.)*

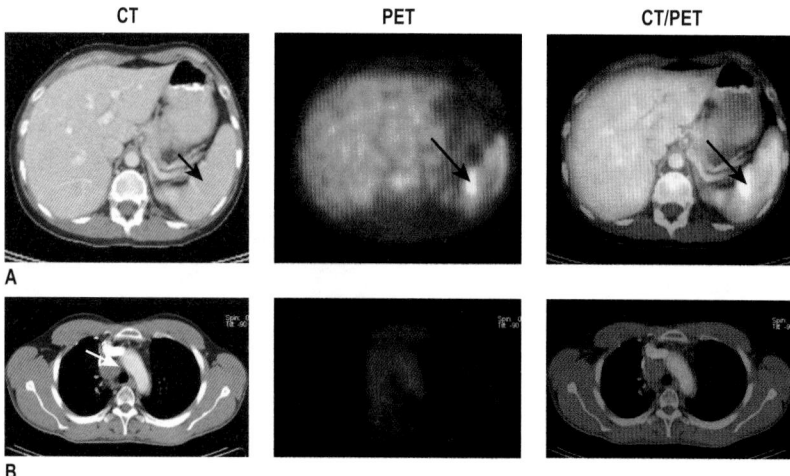

Fig. 17.16 **Positron emission tomography (PET) and computed tomography (CT) in the investigation of Hodgkin lymphoma. (A)** Lymphoma in spleen (arrowed) detected on PET (centre) and CT/PET (right), but not on CT (left). **(B)** Malignant lymphoma: mediastinal mass on CT scan (left), shown to be metabolically inactive on PET (centre) and PET/CT (right). *(Courtesy of Dr N Avril.)*

Treatment of early-stage disease

Chemotherapy, comprising 2–4 cycles of doxorubicin, bleomycin, vinblastine and dacarbazine (ABVD), which is non-sterilizing and of a low second cancer risk, followed by involved field radiotherapy (20–30 Gy), results in more than 90% experiencing sustained remission. Current trials suggest that radiotherapy should not be omitted, as doing so leads to small increases in relapse rates.

Treatment of advanced-stage disease

This is also curable for a significant proportion of patients (see **Box 17.16**). Cyclical chemotherapy starts with two cycles of ABVD before interim PET scanning determines future cycles (response-adjusted therapy). Involved field irradiation to sites that were initially bulky is considered on completion of chemotherapy.

The major short-term toxicity relates to myelosuppression and mucositis, the mortality being no more than 1% and the long-term risks being to the heart and lungs. Infertility and second malignancy are uncommon.

After two cycles of treatment, patients undergo interim scanning and response-adjusted therapy. When interim PET shows complete metabolic remission, bleomycin can be dropped from future cycles to minimize pulmonary toxicity for those with a good prognosis. If interim PET shows residual disease, therapy is escalated to BEACOPP with the addition of etoposide (E), procarbazine (P) and prednisolone (P). This regimen has a greater toxicity profile, with an impact on late effects.

Management of resistant and relapsed disease

Patients with primary refractory disease or relapsed disease are offered salvage chemotherapy with the aim of achieving a complete metabolic remission. This is followed by high-dose therapy with a BEAM autograft (carmustine, etoposide, cytarabine and melphalan).

> **Box 17.15 Hodgkin lymphoma: prognostic groups**
>
> | Prognostic group | Description |
> |---|---|
> | Early favourable | Stage I+II without unfavourable prognostic factors |
> | Early unfavourable | Stage I+II with unfavourable factors |
> | Advanced | The remainder |

> **Box 17.16 Advanced-stage Hodgkin lymphoma (Hasenclever score)**
>
> | Clinical prognostic factors | Score | |
> |---|---|---|
> | | 0 | 1 |
> | Serum albumin | Normal | <40 g/L |
> | Haemoglobin | >105 g/L | <105 g/L |
> | Age | <45 years | >45 years |
> | Sex | Female | Male |
> | Stage | <IV | IV |
> | Leucocytosis | <15 × 10⁹/L | >15 × 10⁹/L |
> | Lymphopenia | >0.6 × 10⁹/L | <0.6 × 10⁹/L |
>
> **Cumulative score**
> Score 0: 84% freedom from progression at 5 years; 89% overall survival
> Score 1: 77%; 90%
> Score 2: 67%; 81%
> Score 3: 60%; 78%
> Score 4: 51%; 61%
> Score 5 or more: 42%; 56%

Experimental approaches

With such excellent results with first- and second-line conventional therapy, the number of patients who experience treatment failure is small. However, this subset has poor outcomes and requires new treatment strategies. The antigen-targeted immunoconjugate, anti-CD-30–auristatin (SGN-35, brentuximab), can be used in patients relapsing following autologous SCT if they have had at least two previous therapies. The immune checkpoint blockers pembrolizumab and nivolumab show promising response rates. Identifying these high-risk patients at diagnosis, with the aim of incorporating these drugs upfront in more intensive regimens, is the focus of current clinical trials. Allogeneic haemopoietic stem cell transplantation (HSCT) has a role, though its timing, in the context of newer drugs, is under discussion.

Long-term follow-up

The risks of late effects of therapy, particularly second malignancy and cardiac and endocrine problems, require appropriate surveillance.

Non-Hodgkin lymphomas

As defined by the WHO classification (**Box 17.17**), approximately 80% of non-Hodgkin lymphoma (NHL) is of B-cell origin and 20% of T-cell origin, there being considerable geographical variation. The incidence has increased, not necessarily for all subtypes, from 5 to 15 per 100 000 per year in the last half-century.

Aetiology

A family history is associated with a minor increase in risk of lymphoma, and common genetic polymorphisms with only a small risk for an individual may be significant in population terms. Certain inherited immunodeficiency syndromes, such as ataxia–telangiectasia and Wiskott–Aldrich syndrome, are associated with an increased risk of lymphoma. Patients with HIV-related immunosuppression or those on immunosuppressive drugs also have an increased risk. Infective viral precipitants are known, such as HTLV-1, which is causally related to adult T-cell lymphoma/leukaemia. There is a very strong epidemiological relationship between EBV and endemic Burkitt lymphoma, and a lesser one with both sporadic Burkitt lymphoma and Hodgkin lymphoma. Bacterial infection may also cause disease: for example, *Helicobacter pylori* in gastric mucosa-associated lymphoid tissue (MALT) lymphoma, and *Chlamydia psittaci* in ocular MALT lymphoma.

Pathogenesis

Malignant clonal expansion of lymphocytes occurs at different stages of lymphocyte development, leading to the different subtypes of lymphoma (see **Fig. 17.2**). In general, neoplasms of non-dividing mature lymphocytes are 'indolent', whereas those of proliferating cells (e.g. lymphoblasts) are much more 'aggressive'. Malignant transformation is usually due to errors in gene rearrangements, which occur during the class switch, or gene recombinations for immunoglobulin and T-cell receptors. Thus, many of the errors occur within immunoglobulin loci or T-cell receptor loci.

The NHLs are subclassified according to the cell of origin (T or B lineage) and the stage of lymphocytic maturation at which they develop (precursor or mature).

> ℹ️ **Box 17.17 Modified World Health Organization classification of lymphoid neoplasms (2017)**
>
> **B-cell lymphomas**
>
> Mature B-cell lymphoma
> - Chronic lymphocytic leukaemia/small lymphocytic lymphoma
> - B-cell prolymphocytic leukaemia
> - Splenic marginal zone lymphoma
> - Hairy cell leukaemia
> - Lymphoplasmacytic lymphoma
> - Extranodal marginal zone B-cell lymphoma of mucosa-associated lymphoid tissue (MALT-lymphoma)
> - Nodal marginal zone lymphoma
> - Follicular lymphoma
> - Mantle cell lymphoma
> - Diffuse large B-cell lymphoma
> - Primary diffuse large B-cell lymphoma of the central nervous system
> - Primary mediastinal (thymic) large B-cell lymphoma
> - Intravascular large B-cell lymphoma
> - Primary effusion lymphoma
> - Burkitt lymphoma/leukaemia
>
> **T/NK cell lymphomas**
>
> Mature T/NK-cell lymphoma
> - T-cell prolymphocytic leukaemia
> - T-cell large granular lymphocytic leukaemia
> - Chronic lymphoproliferative disorder of NK cells
> - Aggressive NK-cell leukaemia
> - Adult T-cell leukaemia/lymphoma
> - Extranodal NK/T-cell lymphoma, nasal type
> - Enteropathy-type T-cell lymphoma
> - Hepatosplenic T-cell lymphoma
> - Subcutaneous panniculitis-like T-cell lymphoma
> - Mycosis fungoides
> - Sézary's syndrome
> - Primary cutaneous CD30+ peripheral T-cell lymphoproliferative disorders
> - Peripheral T-cell lymphoma, unspecified
> - Angio-immunoblastic T-cell lymphoma
> - Anaplastic large-cell lymphoma *ALK*-positive
> - Anaplastic large-cell lymphoma *ALK*-negative
>
> *ALK*, anaplastic lymphoma kinase (gene); ALL, acute lymphoblastic leukaemia; NK, natural killer.
> *(From Swerdlow SH, Campo E, Harris NL et al (eds). WHO Classification of tumours of haematopoietic and lymphoid tissues. Blood 2016; 127:2375–2390.)*

Genetic features

Burkitt lymphoma was the first tumour in which a cytogenetic change was shown to involve the translocation of a specific gene (**Box 17.18**). The most frequent change is where the *MYC* oncogene is translocated from chromosome 8 to a position near the constant region of the immunoglobulin heavy chain gene (IGH) on chromosome 14, resulting in upregulation of *MYC*. Other cytogenetic abnormalities associated with human lymphoma are the t(14; 18) in follicular lymphoma, involving upregulation of *BCL2*, or the t(11; 14) in mantle cell lymphoma, involving upregulation of the cell cycle regulator cyclin D1. Gene expression profiling and next-generation sequencing (see p. 31) have identified new molecular subclasses of lymphoma with prognostic significance.

Clinical features

The most common presentation overall is with painless lymphadenopathy or with local symptoms caused by a lymph node mass. Primary extranodal lymphomas present with soft tissue masses and related symptoms at the relevant site.

The more common subtypes of NHL are described here.

> ℹ️ **Box 17.18 Chromosome translocations in non-Hodgkin lymphoma**
>
> | Type | Translocation | Genes | Function |
> |------|---------------|-------|----------|
> | **Follicular** | t(14; 18) | *IGH/BCL2* | Suppressor of apoptosis |
> | **Mantle cell** | t(11; 14) | *CCND1/IGH* | Cell cycle regulator |
> | **Diffuse large B cell** | t(3; 4) | *BCL6* | Cell cycle regulator |
> | **Burkitt** | t(8; 14) | *MYC/IGH* | Transcription factor |
> | **Anaplastic** | t(2; 5) | *NPM1/ALK* | Tyrosine kinase |
> | **MALT** | t(11; 18) | *BIRC3/MALT1* | Suppressor of apoptosis |
>
> MALT, mucosa-associated lymphoid tissue.

B-cell lymphomas

See **Fig. 17.17**.

Follicular lymphoma

This is the second most common NHL (comprising approximately 20% of lymphomas worldwide).

Clinical features and course

Follicular lymphoma occurs in middle to late life, being rare in childhood. The majority of patients present with painless lymphadenopathy at more than one site, although a small proportion will be ill, some with 'B' symptoms. Percutaneous core biopsy or excisional biopsy establish the grade and tumour and may reveal transformation to DLBCL.

Treatment, where indicated, is with chemo-immunotherapy, targeting the CD20 antigen expressed on almost all B-cell lymphomas. The illness has been shown to regress spontaneously in some cases, which has led to an expectant policy of treatment for many patients. The clinical course following initiation of treatment is remitting–recurring. Transformation to DLBCL occurs in up to 25% of patients over 15 years. Death is due to resistant disease, transformed or not, the complications of therapy, or unrelated causes. The median survival now exceeds 10 years. Prognostic factors comprising the Follicular Lymphoma International Prognostic Index (FLIPI) are shown in **Box 17.19**.

Management

General management

The 'well' patient – asymptomatic, without organ impairment, 'bulky disease' or evidence of rapid progression or transformation – should be managed expectantly, after a careful explanation of the rationale. Around 50% of patients will progress and require therapy over the following 2.5 years, 20% will undergo spontaneous regression and 15% will require no treatment more than 10 years from diagnosis. Indications for treatment of low-grade NHL are shown in **Box 17.20**.

Initial treatment: early disease

Stage IA or 2A non-bulky disease is treated with involved field radiotherapy, which almost always induces complete remission, 50% of patients being disease-free after 10–15 years. In terms of overall survival, there are no randomized trials to show that this is better than expectant management (i.e. observing and treating if progression occurs).

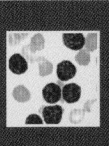

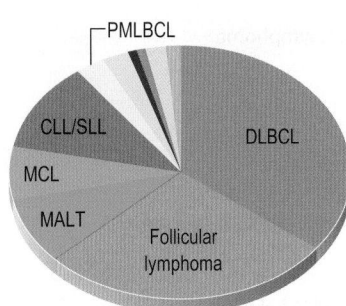

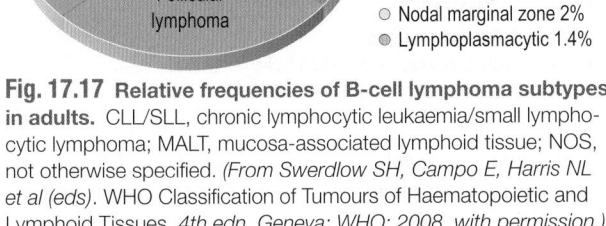

- Diffuse large B-cell 37%
- Follicular 29%
- MALT lymphoma 9%
- Mantle cell lymphoma 7%
- CLL/SLL 12%
- Primary med large B-cell 3%
- High-grade B, NOS 2.5%
- Burkitt 0.8%
- Splenic marginal zone 0.9%
- Nodal marginal zone 2%
- Lymphoplasmacytic 1.4%

Fig. 17.17 Relative frequencies of B-cell lymphoma subtypes in adults. CLL/SLL, chronic lymphocytic leukaemia/small lymphocytic lymphoma; MALT, mucosa-associated lymphoid tissue; NOS, not otherwise specified. *(From Swerdlow SH, Campo E, Harris NL et al (eds).* WHO Classification of Tumours of Haematopoietic and Lymphoid Tissues, *4th edn. Geneva: WHO; 2008, with permission.)*

 Box 17.19 Adverse prognostic factors in non-follicular lymphoma (FLIPI)

- Haemoglobin <120 g/L
- >4 nodal sites involved
- Age >60 years
- Stage III or IV disease
- Elevated serum lactate dehydrogenase

FLIPI, Follicular Lymphoma International Prognostic Index.

i **Box 17.20 Indications for treatment of low-grade non-Hodgkin lymphoma at presentation or progression**

- Stage I disease; possibly limited stage II disease
- Rapidly progressive disease
- Organ impairment (i.e. bone marrow failure, urinary tract obstruction)
- Bulky disease (i.e. lymph node mass >7 cm)
- Histological transformation
- Ascites or pleural effusion
- Philosophy of physician and patient

Initial treatment: advanced disease (stages II–IV)

Chemo-immunotherapy incorporating an anti-CD20 monoclonal antibody (either rituximab or obinutuzumab) is the treatment of choice. 'R-CHOP' (rituximab with cyclophosphamide, doxorubicin, vincristine and prednisolone) and R-bendamustine are used in patients with FLIPI scores of 0–1; O-CHOP (obinutuzumab substituted for rituximab) and O-bendamustine is used in those with FLIPI scores of 2 or more. The two antibody treatments show no overall survival difference, but progression-free survival at 3 years appears improved with the use of obinutuzumab. It has been shown that continuing rituximab or obinutuzumab 'maintenance' every 2 months for 2 years also lengthens progression-free survival, although any benefits for overall survival remain unproven.

Second therapy and beyond

Patients are managed expectantly in the first instance, provided full re-evaluation, including repeat biopsy, reveals no evidence of transformation. A number of options are available, which will be determined by the individual patient and the first-line therapy. Options include the range of chemo-immunotherapy chosen as first-line treatment and also use of purine analogues. Maintenance can again be given. When second remission is achieved, in appropriate patients, high-dose treatment and autologous SCT are used to consolidate the response. Occasionally, in fitter patients, allogeneic HSCT is considered.

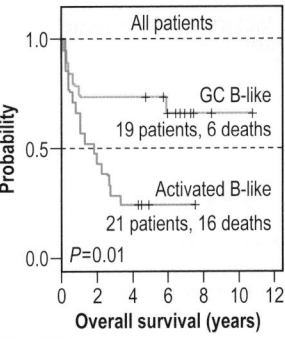

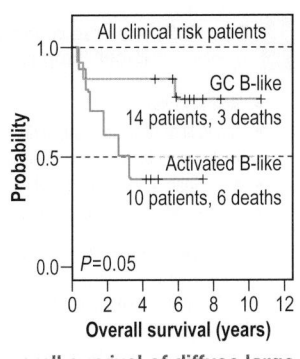

Fig. 17.18 Kaplan–Meier plot of overall survival of diffuse large B-cell lymphoma patients. Patients are grouped on the basis of gene expression profiling. GC, germinal centre cell. *(Reproduced with permission from Alizadeh AA. Distinct types of diffuse large B-cell lymphoma identified by gene expression profiling.* Nature 2000; 403:503–511.)

Prognosis

There has been a dramatic improvement in the overall survival pattern of follicular lymphoma since anti-CD20 therapy initiation. Median survival has been extended well beyond 10 years. Improvements in disease-free survival, after both initial and second-line therapy, are encouraging.

Diffuse large B-cell lymphoma

This is the most common adult lymphoma worldwide (increasing in incidence with age) and the second most common lymphoma in childhood, accounting for approximately 30% of all cases. There is a slight male preponderance. Our understanding of DLBCL's molecular and genetic features is growing, which has led to the description of subgroups. Gene expression profiling has recognized germinal centre B-cell-like (GCB) and activated B-cell like (ABC) subgroups, with the latter having an inferior clinical outcome (**Fig. 17.18**). Patients with *MYC*, *BCL2* and/or *BCL6* rearrangements represent a subtype of DLBCL that does considerably less well with conventional therapy. This increased understanding of variability within the disease may help us define groups of patients who are likely to do badly with conventional treatment, and towards whom future targeted therapies may be directed.

Clinical features

The majority of patients present with painless lymphadenopathy clinically, at one or several sites. Intra-abdominal disease presents with bowel symptoms due to compression or infiltration of the gastrointestinal tract. In a small proportion, there is a primary mediastinal presentation, with symptoms and signs akin to those of HL. There may be 'B' symptoms, which should not be confused with symptoms related to the site of involvement. Investigation will lead to the demonstration of either locally or systemically advanced disease in the majority of cases. The illness is itself rapidly progressive without intervention, death occurring within months rather than years.

Management

Initial treatment

Treatment should be initiated immediately after the diagnosis is confirmed. In younger patients without co-morbidity there is a high expectation of cure. Treatment is assigned on the basis of the revised International Prognostic Index (R-IPI; **Box 17.21** and **Fig. 17.19**).

- Age >60 years
- Stage III or IV, i.e. advanced disease
- High serum lactate dehydrogenase level
- More than one extranodal site involved
- ECOG performance status 2 or more (see **Box 6.13**)

ECOG, Eastern Cooperative Oncology Group; R-IPI, revised International Prognostic Index. 1 point is given for each prognostic marker. These classify the prognosis as very good (0 points), good (1-2 points) or poor (>2 points). See **Fig. 17.19** for the impact of these categories on survival.

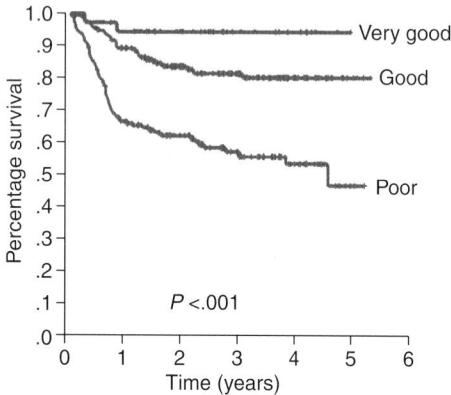

Fig. 17.19 Survival curves for the revised International Prognostic Index (R-IPI) in diffuse large B-cell lymphoma. *(Adapted from Sehn LH, Berry B, Chhanabhai M et al. The revised IPI is a better predictor of outcome than the standard IPI for patients with DLBCL treated with RCHOP. Blood 109; 1857–1861.)*

Early-stage disease

In stage IA disease, three cycles of R-CHOP, followed by involved field radiotherapy, or three further cycles of R-CHOP are used. For bulky disease, six cycles are preferred prior to radiotherapy. Interim imaging may be useful where response is not assessable clinically.

Advanced-stage disease

The age of the patient and co-morbidity are critical for both the selection of treatment and the prognosis. Six cycles of R-CHOP is standard care for the large majority of patients of all ages with DLBCL. Dose can be reduced in elderly or frail patients. In those with cardiac impairment, R-GCVP is preferred (with gemcitabine in place of the anthracycline doxorubicin). Radiotherapy to bulky disease should be considered at the end of chemotherapy.

Involvement of the central nervous system, most often meningeal, is an uncommon but devastating complication, confirming a very poor prognosis overall. Patients with a high LDH, and more than two extranodal sites or disease in breast, testis or epidural anatomical sites should receive three or four cycles of intrathecal methotrexate; alternatively, high-dose methotrexate (which crosses the blood–brain barrier) may be considered.

Second (and subsequent) therapy

Although the patient may respond initially to alternative chemotherapy, the prognosis is poor after failure of initial therapy or subsequent progression. The major issues to be addressed are whether treatment is to be undertaken with palliative or curative intent, and if the latter, what are the expectations of success. The ***palliative approach*** involves both chemotherapy and irradiation.

The ***curative approach*** involves re-evaluation, followed by second-line (salvage) chemotherapy; the response rate is approximately 50%. If at least a further partial remission is achieved, patients proceed to high-dose chemotherapy followed by an autograft. Overwhelmingly, the best results are achieved in those entering a second CR. When disease does not respond to salvage chemotherapy, clinical trials, including novel agents, may be considered.

Prognosis

The outlook for patients with DLBCL improved after the incorporation of rituximab into the initial therapy, overall survival now being between 32% and 83%, depending on risk group. The challenge of progressive disease following initial treatment is considerable, with less than 20% of patients overall staying alive in the long term.

Burkitt lymphoma

This is the most rapidly proliferating lymphoma, with a doubling time approaching 100% and a very rapid evolution. The most common childhood malignancy worldwide, it has a male to female preponderance of approximately 3:1 and occurs at all ages. There are three types (**Box 17.22**).

The most common presenting feature in the endemic type is a rapidly growing jaw tumour in a young child (**Fig. 17.20**). The next most common is an abdominal mass that is often associated with bone marrow involvement. Other common sites are the central nervous system, kidney and testis.

Investigation is along conventional lines for lymphoma and must be conducted as a matter of urgency. A different staging classification is applied to children.

Management

Burkitt lymphoma should be treated with curative intent whenever feasible, regardless of HIV status. Once investigation is completed, the patient must be haemodynamically and metabolically stable prior to initiation of specific therapy. Particular attention must be paid to the risk of the tumour lysis syndrome and so rasburicase prophylaxis should be given if available (see p. 118). Very frequent monitoring of electrolyte balance, especially potassium and phosphate levels, is essential for at least 72 hours after treatment is commenced.

Standard treatment is comprised of intensive, cyclical combination chemotherapy, if possible, to include cyclophosphamide, methotrexate and cytarabine in high doses. The details of this, and the number of cycles administered, will be determined by the number of low-risk features. Prophylactic central nervous system therapy is essential: intrathecal methotrexate or cytarabine is often given, in addition to high-dose systemic administration.

Prognosis

In the Western world, the prognosis of Burkitt lymphoma has improved markedly in recent years. The chances of cure are 90% for 'low-risk' patients and exceed 60% for 'poor-risk' patients, as well as HIV-positive cases, provided all treatment can be administered.

Patients are considered cured if they reach 2 years in remission. For those who relapse or do not achieve remission, prognosis is poor. Although there may be further chemoresponsiveness, it is rare for second-line therapy to be more than transiently beneficial, regardless of whether it is followed by consolidation with either myeloablative chemotherapy or allogeneic HSCT.

Mantle cell lymphoma

This is one of the less common B-cell lymphomas, usually presenting in later life, with a male to female preponderance of 3:1. The most frequent presentation is with painless lymphadenopathy, often generalized. There may be non-specific symptoms of tiredness, or features related to the gastrointestinal tract. 'B' symptoms occur in fewer than 50%. Examination and standard investigation usually confirm generalized lymphadenopathy with or without hepatosplenomegaly. In patients with bowel symptoms, multiple lesions are frequently found on endoscopy. The bone marrow is usually involved and there may well be lymphoma cells in the peripheral blood (**Fig. 17.21**). The t(11; 14) translocation with dysregulation of cyclin D1 is a classical feature of this lymphoma. IGHV mutation status and expression of *SOX11* can identify a subtype of indolent disease that can be monitored without the need for immediate treatment.

Management

In the majority of patients, therapy is started after investigation has been completed. It is usual for disease to regress with chemotherapy, although it is not often that CR is achieved. A prognostic index (MIPI) is used to help determine the best treatment option. Younger, fitter patients are treated with relatively intensive chemoimmunotherapy, incorporating cycles of high-dose cytarabine and cyclophosphamide with rituximab, followed by high-dose therapy and autologous SCT (e.g. BEAM or LEAM autograft (lomustine, etoposide, cytarabine and melphalan)). Allogeneic transplantation is considered in appropriate patients with high-risk disease. Older, less fit patients are treated with less intensive therapy, such as R-CHOP followed by rituximab maintenance, or bortezomib-containing regimens. Progression is inevitable and there are a range of second-line approaches, including ibrutinib (a BTK inhibitor), bortezomib and bendamustine.

Prognosis

Untreated mantle cell lymphoma has a natural history that lies between that of DLBCL and follicular lymphoma with features of high- and low-grade lymphoma. The prognosis is around 8–12 years in patients well enough to tolerate intensive therapy.

Lymphoplasmacytic lymphoma

This is an uncommon B-cell malignancy, which is known as **Waldenström's macroglobulinaemia** when associated with an immunoglobulin M (IgM) paraprotein and bone marrow infiltration. It usually occurs in later life, the incidence being approximately the same in men and women. It may be preceded by IgM monoclonal gammopathy of uncertain significance (MGUS), in which there is an IgM paraprotein but no bone marrow infiltration of symptoms relating to the paraprotein. The presentation is with lymphadenopathy or, alternatively, symptoms of anaemia or hyperviscosity caused by the paraprotein (e.g. headaches, visual disturbance). Examination

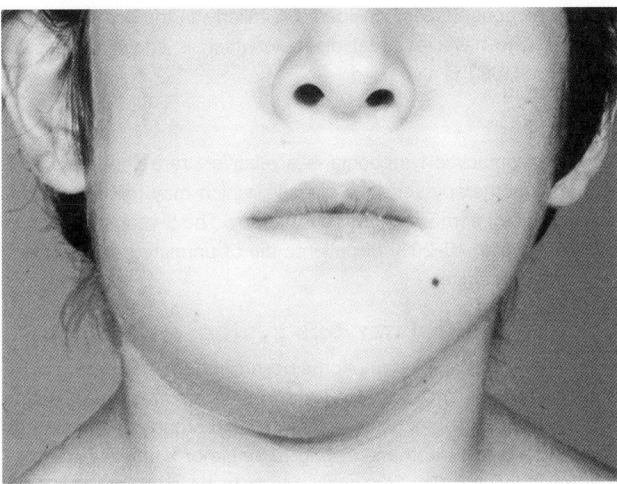

Fig. 17.20 A child with Burkitt lymphoma.

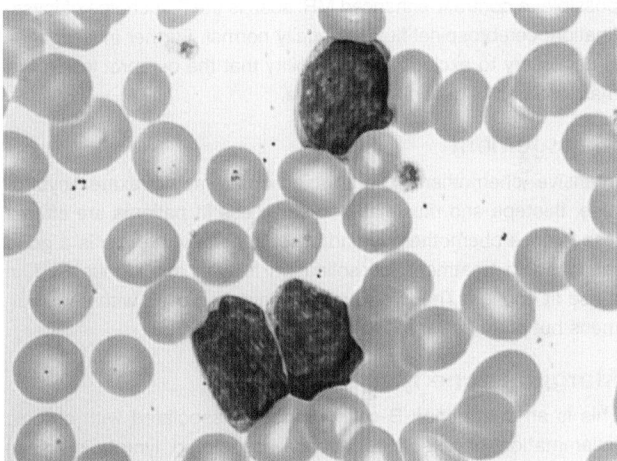

Fig. 17.21 Peripheral blood film from a patient with mantle cell lymphoma. Cells circulating in the peripheral blood can have a variable appearance. Some cases can be confused with chronic lymphoid lymphoma (CLL)/small lymphocytic lymphoma, and immunophenotyping/cytogenetic analysis is needed to differentiate. In this case the chromatin in the lymphoma cells has a more open pattern than that typically seen with CLL cells. (Wright-Giemsa stain x1000.) *(From Keohane EM, Otto CM, Walenga JM.* Rodak's Hematology: Clinical Principles and Applications, *6th edn. Elsevier Inc., 2020, Fig. 34.8.)*

and investigation usually reveal little beyond minimal adenopathy and, commonly, splenomegaly.

Management

Following completion of investigation, the critical decision is whether to initiate specific therapy or not. In an emergency, with severe symptoms of hyperviscosity, it is most appropriate to lower the paraprotein by plasmapheresis. Other symptomatic patients should receive a rituximab-containing regimen. Responses are seen in the majority of cases but with variable depth and durability. Treatment is appropriate only when symptomatic progression is clearly documented, most often by a fall in the haemoglobin or a significant rise in the IgM paraprotein. In this setting, ibrutinib can be used, and is effective particularly in patients with *MYD88* mutations (present in 90%) and wild-type *CXCR4* (mutated in 30%). In the very small proportion of younger patients in whom CR is achieved, consolidation with autologous SCT is considered. Similarly, in the same group of patients who have recurrent disease, which is again responsive, allogeneic HSCT is also used.

Prognosis

Lymphoplasmacytic lymphoma is a relatively rare chemotherapy- and immunotherapy-sensitive disease, which may follow an indolent course for some years without therapy. The 5-year survival rate is around 78%; 10–20% of patients die of unrelated causes, as it presents in later life.

Primary central nervous system lymphoma

This diffuse, large B-cell lymphoma occurs in both the immunocompetent (predominantly age 55–70) and the immunosuppressed, in the context of HIV infection or following solid organ transplantation. It presents with symptoms relating to single or multiple parenchymal mass lesions. The diagnosis needs to be made on the basis of a biopsy, particularly in the immunocompromised, in whom an infectious aetiology of the symptoms, such as toxoplasmosis, is possible. A contrast-enhanced MRI scan is the first choice of investigation; cerebrospinal fluid is usually normal. Further investigation is necessary to exclude the possibility that the cerebral lesion is a manifestation of generalized disease.

Management

Intensive chemotherapy, with high-dose methotrexate, cytarabine, thiotepa and rituximab, is used. Less fit patients are offered less intense chemotherapy and/or radiotherapy. If there is a good response to treatment, consolidation is with autologous SCT in those fit enough. The overall results have improved with new regimens but prognosis remains poor.

Marginal zone lymphoma

This is an uncommon B-cell lymphoma associated with chronic inflammation or infection. Mucosa-associated lymphoid tissue (MALT) is the commonest form of marginal zone lymphoma. MALT of the salivary glands is linked with Sjögren's syndrome. Gastric MALT lymphoma is closely associated with *Helicobacter pylori* infection and presents with symptoms of gastric ulceration or a mass, indigestion or bleeding; the diagnosis is made by endoscopic biopsy to include confirmation of both lymphoma and *H. pylori* status. Careful assessment of extranodal sites is required.

Management

Management is dependent on whether or not disease is localized and symptomatic. If only 'low-grade' gastric MALT lymphoma is present, *Helicobacter* eradication therapy is the treatment of choice

(see p. 1175). This almost invariably alleviates the symptoms. Re-evaluation is carried out after 6, 12 and 24 months with endoscopy, repeat biopsy and photography. In general, a conservative approach is followed, as responses may take many months to achieve and rapid progression is very unlikely. Failure is uncommon, but if it does occur, biopsy should be repeated. If the histology is unchanged after further *Helicobacter* eradication therapy (if necessary), either rituximab chemotherapy, single-agent rituximab or low-dose involved-field radiotherapy is likely to be effective or possibly curative. Overall, the prognosis is very good, a very large proportion of patients being alive 10 years after diagnosis.

Any evidence of transformation to DLBCL should be treated as high-grade lymphoma. *Helicobacter* eradication therapy should also be given but should not be considered definitive treatment. The potential risk of gastric perforation or haemorrhage because of therapy is not a contraindication to treatment. Surgery is rarely needed but irradiation is used for persistent disease. The prognosis is approximately the same as for nodal DLBCL of equivalent extent.

Peripheral T-cell lymphomas

T-cell lymphomas can present in nodal, extranodal, cutaneous and predominantly leukaemic forms. They describe a large group of rare diseases, less common than their B-cell counterparts and varying in their behaviour from indolent to aggressive. Many subtypes carry poor prognoses due to disappointing responses to treatment (**Fig. 17.22**).

The two most common subtypes of nodal T-cell lymphoma are 'peripheral T-cell lymphoma, not otherwise specified (NOS)' and 'angio-immunoblastic T-cell lymphoma', which together account for about 50% of T-cell lymphomas. Both occur in the middle-aged to elderly population, the primary presentation being lymphadenopathy. In contrast to the B-cell lymphomas, 'B' symptoms are common. Patients with angio-immunoblastic T-cell lymphoma also present with inflammatory symptoms of fever, rash and arthritis. Anaplastic T-cell lymphoma (ALCL), particularly when anaplastic lymphoma kinase (ALK)-positive, has a better prognosis than other subtypes.

Management

Following standard investigation, which usually reveals widespread disease, patients are treated with cyclical combination chemotherapy as for DLBCL. CD20 is not expressed on T cells and so rituximab is not used; as yet, there is no equivalent drug for T-cell lymphoma. Symptoms almost invariably resolve, although

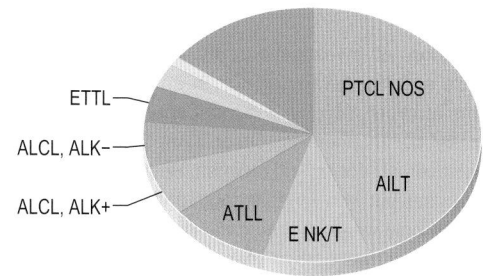

Peripheral T-cell lymphoma – NOS 25.9%
Angio-immunoblastic 18.5%
Extranodal natural killer/T-cell lymphoma 10.4%
Adult T-cell leukaemia/lymphoma 9.6%
Anaplastic large-cell lymphoma, ALK+ 6.6%
Anaplastic large-cell lymphoma, ALK– 5.5%

Enteropathy-type T-cell 4.7%
Primary cutaneous ALCL 1.7%
Hepatosplenic T-cell 1.4%
Subcutaneous panniculitis-like 0.9%
Unclassifiable PTCL 2.5%
Other disorders 12.2%

Fig. 17.22 Relative frequencies of T-cell lymphoma subtypes in adults. ALK, anaplastic lymphoma kinase; NOS, not otherwise specified. *(Reproduced with permission from WHO. Swerdlow SH, Campo E, Harris NL et al (eds). WHO Classification of Tumours of Haematopoietic and Lymphoid Tissues, 4th edn. Geneva: WHO; 2008; Fig 8.07.)*

they may recur between cycles. Overall, the outcome of treatment is worse than for DLBCL, in terms of quality of response, duration of response and overall survival. Other than in ALCL, autologous SCT or allograft should be considered in first remission. Second-line therapy is rarely satisfactory, although a small proportion of patients may benefit from allogeneic SCT to consolidate a second response.

Mycosis fungoides and Sézary's syndrome

Mycosis fungoides is the most common cutaneous lymphoma. It predominantly arises in, and is confined to, the skin, spreading to other organs only latterly in the disease. The rare leukaemic variant is known as Sézary's syndrome. It has a long natural history, presenting with multiple erythematous lesions, plaques and tumours, and multiple skin biopsies are required to establish a diagnosis. The presentation and management of skin disease are discussed on page 692. A wide range of agents can be used in advanced-stage disease, it is rare to achieve a durable response and the prognosis is poor. Early-stage disease carries a relatively good prognosis. Median survival for Sézary's syndrome is 3.1 years.

Further reading

Barrington SF, Kirkwood AA, Franceschetto A et al. PET-CT for staging and early response: results from the Response-Adapted Therapy in Advanced Hodgkin Lymphoma study. *Blood* 2016; 127:1531–1538.
Cheson BD, Fisher RI, Barrington SF et al. Recommendations for initial evaluation, staging, and response assessment of Hodgkin and non-Hodgkin lymphoma: the Lugano classification. *J Clin Oncol* 2014; 32:3059–3068.
Ferreri AJ, Cwynarski K, Pulczynski E et al. Chemoimmunotherapy with methotrexate, cytarabine, thiotepa, and rituximab (MATRix regimen) in patients with primary CNS lymphoma: results of the first randomisation of the International Extranodal Lymphoma Study Group-32 (IELSG32) phase 2 trial. *Lancet Haematol* 2016; 3:e217–227.
Sesques P, Johnson NA. Approach to the diagnosis and treatment of high-grade B-cell lymphomas with MYC and BCL2 and/or BCL6 rearrangements. *Blood* 2017; 129:280–288.
Swerdlow SH, Campo E, Harris NL et al (eds). WHO Classification of Tumours of Haematopoietic and Lymphoid Tissues. *Blood* 2016; 127:2375–2390.

MYELOMA AND OTHER PLASMA CELL DISORDERS

The classification of this group of related conditions is presented in **Box 17.23**; the most significant is myeloma.

Myeloma

Myeloma (or multiple myeloma) is a cancer of plasma cells. As with their normal counterpart, these cells usually produce immunoglobulin, but the neoplastic nature of the population means this is a non-functional monoclonal paraprotein (or 'M band'). The paraprotein is usually an intact immunoglobulin, most commonly IgG (55%) or IgA (20%), and more rarely IgM or IgD. There is normally also an imbalance in the free light chains (kappa or lambda), which can be detected in the urine (Bence Jones protein) and blood (serum free light chains, SFLC) (**Fig. 17.23**). Around 15% of cases will have no intact immunoglobulin but are light chain only, while 5% of cases are completely non-secretory.

Not all paraproteins are produced by plasma cell disorders. B-cell lymphoproliferative disorders, such as low-grade B-cell NHL and CLL can produce a paraprotein, and Waldenström's macroglobulinaemia is caused by an IgM-producing lymphoplasmacytic lymphoma. Non-malignant disorders producing a paraprotein include poorly controlled HIV infection and autoimmune conditions, although these are more likely to be transient and should resolve with treatment of the underlying condition.

The abnormal plasma cell population can be identified on bone marrow aspirate or biopsy (trephine), with the imbalance of kappa:lambda restricted plasma cells demonstrated by flow cytometry (aspirate) or immunohistochemistry (biopsy) (**Fig. 17.24**).

Myeloma is predominantly a disease of the elderly, median age at presentation being over 60 years. It is rare under 40 years of age. The annual incidence is 4 per 100 000 and disease is more common in males and in black Africans, but less common in Asians.

Clinical features

These include
- bone pain: most commonly backache, owing to vertebral involvement (60%)
- symptoms of anaemia
- recurrent infections
- symptoms of renal failure (20–30%)
- symptoms of hypercalcaemia
- rarely, symptoms of hyperviscosity and bleeding due to thrombocytopenia.

Patients can be asymptomatic, the diagnosis being suspected by abnormal 'routine' blood tests. Life-threatening complications are shown in **Box 17.24**.

The clinical features of myeloma are related to the underlying pathology:
- **Bone marrow infiltration with plasma cells.** This results in anaemia, neutropenia and thrombocytopenia.
- **Paraprotein secretion.** This may (rarely) result in symptoms of hyperviscosity. In addition, there is a reduction in the levels of normal immunoglobulin (immune paresis), contributing to the tendency to contract recurrent infections (**Fig. 17.25**).
- **Free light chain secretion.** This leads to deposition in the renal tubules, causing renal impairment by cast nephropathy. Other factors such as hypercalcaemia, use of non-steroidal anti-inflammatory drugs (NSAIDs) and, rarely, the deposition of AL amyloid can also contribute to renal injury (see p. 1357).
- **Bone disease.** Dysregulation of bone remodelling leads to the typical lytic lesions, usually seen in the spine, skull, long bones and ribs (**Fig. 17.26**). There is increased osteoclastic activity without increased osteoblast formation of bone, causing fractures of long bones, vertebral collapse and hypercalcaemia. Soft tissue plasmacytomas also occur and they are the usual cause of spinal cord compression.

> *i* **Box 17.23 World Health Organization classification of plasma cell neoplasms (2017)**
>
> - Monoclonal gammopathy of undetermined significance
> - Plasma cell myeloma
> - Plasma cell myeloma variants:
>   - Smouldering (asymptomatic) plasma cell myeloma
>   - Non-secretory myeloma
>   - Plasma cell leukaemia
> - Plasmacytoma:
>   - Solitary plasmacytoma of bone
>   - Extra-osseous plasmacytoma
> - Monoclonal immunoglobulin deposition diseases
>   - Primary amyloidosis (see p. 1357)
>   - Light chain and heavy chain deposition diseases
> - Heavy chain diseases:
>   - Gamma (γ) heavy chain disease
>   - Mu (μ) heavy chain disease
>   - Alpha (α) heavy chain disease

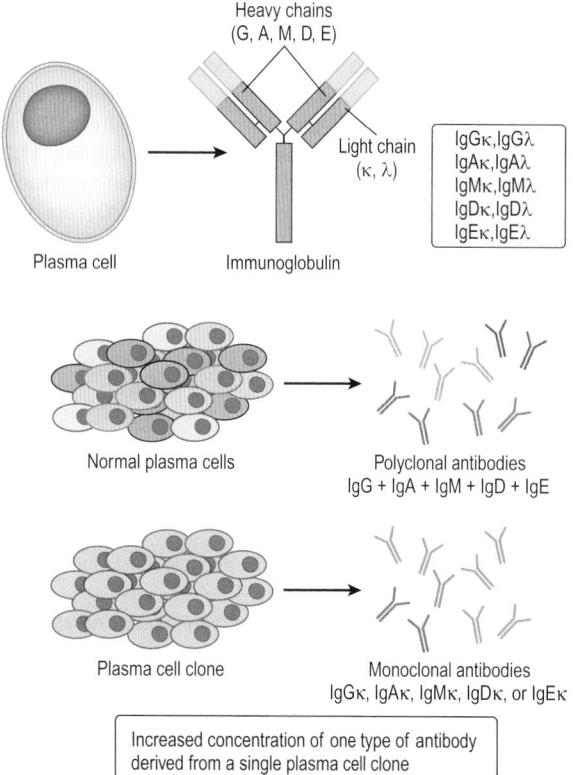

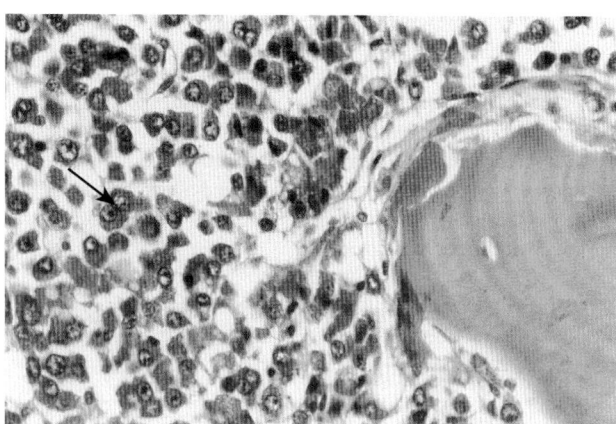

Fig. 17.23 Plasma cells produce immunoglobulins (antibodies) with different heavy and light chain combinations. Normally, a mixed population of plasma cells will produce a polyclonal mixture of different immunoglobulins. In myeloma, the malignant plasma cell population is derived from a single clone, which produces a single type of immunoglobulin that can be detected by blood or urine assays.

> **_i_** **Box 17.24 Life-threatening complications of myeloma**
>
> - **_Renal impairment_** – often a consequence of hypercalcaemia – requires urgent attention and patients may need to be referred for long-term peritoneal dialysis or haemodialysis
> - **_Hypercalcaemia_** should be treated by rehydration and use of bisphosphonates, such as pamidronate
> - **_Spinal cord compression_** due to myeloma is treated with dexamethasone, followed by radiotherapy to the lesion delineated by a magnetic resonance imaging scan
> - **_Hyperviscosity_** due to high circulating levels of paraprotein may be corrected by plasmapheresis

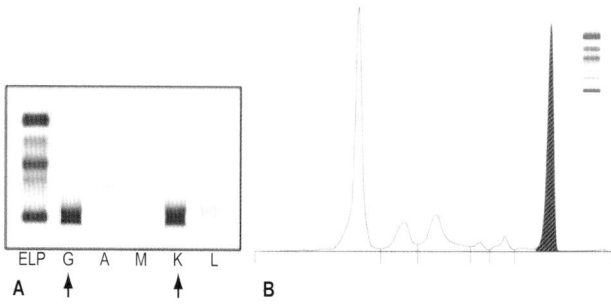

Fig. 17.25 Serum protein electrophoresis and immunofixation. (A) Immunofixation of immunoglobulin G (IgG) kappa monoclonal paraprotein in a patient with an IgG K paraprotein. The column on the far left is the total serum electrophoresis stained with anti-protein reagents. Albumin is at the top and the increased immunoglobulins at the bottom. These are shown to stain with anti-IgG and anti-kappa light chain reagents (arrows). **(B)** Quantitation and serum electrophoresis of IgG paraprotein. The paraprotein is quantified (right) by calculating the area under the paraprotein spike and comparing it with the albumin concentration. A, immunoglobulin A; ELP, electrophoresis; G, immunoglobulin G; K, kappa; L, lambda; M, immunoglobulin M.

Fig. 17.24 Multiple myeloma. Histology shows replacement of the medullary cavity by abnormal plasma cells with some binucleate forms (arrowed). A residual bony trabeculum is present towards the right. *(Courtesy of Dr AJ Norton.)*

Diagnosis

The spectrum of plasma cell disorders is classified based on the degree of plasma cell infiltration and the presence of end-organ damage (**Box 17.25**). Previously, a diagnosis of myeloma required more than 10% plasma cell infiltrate, together with at least one of the four '**CRAB**' features:

- hyper**c**alcaemia: Ca >2.75 mmol/L
- **r**enal impairment: creatinine clearance <40 mL/min or serum creatinine >177 µmol/L
- **a**naemia: haemoglobin <100 g/L or >20 g/L below normal
- **b**one involvement: one or more osteolytic lesions of ≥5 mm on X-ray, CT scan or PET scan.

The diagnostic criteria were updated in 2014 to include three additional 'biomarker' features, which are associated with a high risk of transformation to symptomatic disease:

- involved:uninvolved SFLC ratio (e.g. kappa:lambda) of ≥100
- bone marrow plasma cell infiltration of ≥60%
- ≥2 focal lesions on MRI scan.

Although they may be related, other non-CRAB manifestations of end-organ damage (e.g. hyperviscosity, recurrent bacterial infections, AL amyloidosis, peripheral neuropathy) are non-specific and not diagnostic of myeloma. The presence of a paraprotein does not in itself make a diagnosis of myeloma.

Investigations

General

- **_Full blood count._** Haemoglobin, white cell count and platelet count are normal or low.
- **_Erythrocyte sedimentation rate._** This is often high.
- **_Blood film._** There may be rouleaux formation as a consequence of the paraprotein. Circulating plasma cells are present in the aggressive plasma cell leukaemia variant of myeloma.

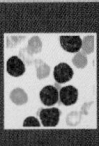

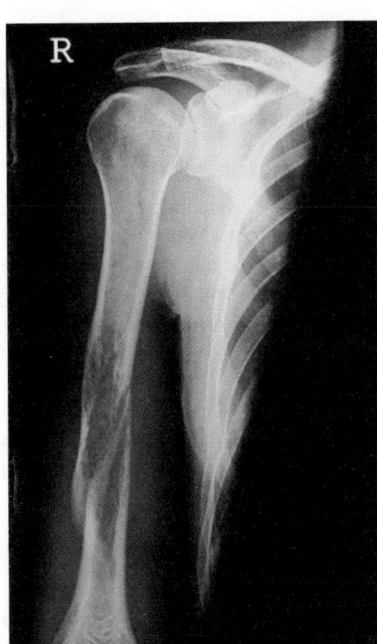

Fig. 17.26 Pathological fracture of long bone. A plain film showing a spiral fracture through the right humerus. This patient, who was previously fit and well, presented with fracture of his right arm.

> **i** | **Box 17.25 Classification and definitions of plasma cell disorders (IMWG 2016)**

	MGUS	Smouldering myeloma	Active myeloma
Clonal plasma cells in bone marrow	<10%	10–60%	>10%
Presence of myeloma-defining events	None	None	Yes
Likelihood of progression	~1% per year	~10% per year	n/a

IMWG, International Myeloma Working Group; MGUS, monoclonal gammopathy of undetermined significance.

- **Serum creatinine and electrolytes**. There may be evidence of kidney injury (see earlier).
- **Serum calcium.** This is normal or raised. Serum alkaline phosphatase is usually normal.
- **B2M and LDH**. These are measured to establish a prognostic score. B2M is a marker of renal impairment and cell turnover.

Immunology

- **Total protein** is normal or raised.
- **Serum protein electrophoresis and immunofixation** characteristically shows a monoclonal band and immune paresis (see **Fig. 17.25**). The SFLC assay may show an abnormal ratio and an increased total amount of free kappa or lambda chains.
- **Urine electrophoresis and immunofixation** can assess light-chain excretion, although this is now being superseded by the SFLC assay.

Radiology

- **Skeletal imaging.** CT, CT-PET or whole-body MRI may show characteristic lytic lesions. X-ray skeletal surveys are now outdated due to their poor sensitivity, although plain films may pick up a presenting pathological fracture.

- **MRI spine.** This is useful if there is back pain; it may show imminent compression or collapse. It can also pick up occult lesions not seen on CT (as per the updated diagnostic criteria).

Histology

Bone marrow aspirate or trephine shows characteristic infiltration by clonal plasma cells (see **Fig. 17.24**).

Staging and prognosis

Patients can be risk-stratified using the International Staging System (ISS), based on the levels of albumin and B2M:

- **ISS Stage I**: B2M <3.5 g/L and serum albumin ≥35 g/L.
- **ISS Stage II**: neither stage I nor stage III.
- **ISS Stage III**: B2M ≥5.5 g/L.

Via FISH and microarray techniques, cytogenetic abnormalities can be detected in most cases of myeloma, and have a bearing on prognosis. Hyperdiploidy is associated with a good prognosis, while some translocations affecting the IgH locus on chromosome 14 are associated with poor prognosis – for example, t(4;14), t(14;16) and t(14;20) – as are other findings such as 17p–, 1q+ and 1p–. The most important of these, together with LDH levels, have been incorporated into a revised ISS staging system (R-ISS):

- **R-ISS I**: ISS stage I *and* normal LDH *and* no del(17p), t(4;14) or t(14;16) by FISH.
- **R-ISS II**: neither stage I nor stage III.
- **R-ISS III**: ISS stage III *and* elevated LDH *and/or* del(17p), t(4;14) or t(14;16) by FISH.

This system is based on clinical trial data, and clearly divides patients into distinct groups for overall survival (10 years, 6 years and 1.3 years) for R-ISS groups I, II and III.

Management

Supportive therapy

- **Anaemia** should be corrected; blood transfusion may be required. Erythropoietin often helps. Transfusion should be undertaken slowly in patients with hyperviscosity.
- **Hypercalcaemia and kidney injury** should be treated urgently with hydration, bisphosphonates and high-dose steroids. Hyperviscosity can be managed with plasmapheresis.
- **Infection** should be treated promptly with antibiotics.
- **Bone pain** can be alleviated most rapidly by radiotherapy and systemic chemotherapy or high-dose dexamethasone. NSAIDs should be avoided because of the risk of acute kidney injury. Bisphosphonates such as zoledronate, which inhibit osteoclast activity, help ensure rapid normocalcaemia and, given long-term, reduce skeletal events such as pathological fracture, cord compression and bone pain.
- **Pathological fractures** may also be prevented by prompt orthopaedic surgery with pinning of lytic bone lesions at critical sites seen on the skeletal survey, such as the femoral shaft. Kyphoplasty and vertebroplasty may be useful in treating vertebral fractures.

Specific therapy

Although myeloma remains incurable for the vast majority of patients, there is now a large number of drugs that can be used in combination and in sequence to prolong survival and reduce complications.

- **Steroids.** Dexamethasone and prednisolone both commonly form part of combination therapies, and of initial management of acute complications.

- *Cytotoxic chemotherapy drugs*, e.g. melphalan and cyclophosphamide. Melphalan is used as high-dose therapy in autologous SCT.
- *Proteasome inhibitors.* Bortezomib was the first of these agents and is commonly given subcutaneously. Carfilzomib, an irreversible proteasome inhibitor, may have greater efficacy but can have cardiotoxic side-effects. Ixazomib is a newer oral agent.
- *'Immunomodulatory drugs'.* Thalidomide, and subsequent agents such as lenalidomide and pomalidomide, act in conjunction with the cereblon protein to alter the transcriptional profile of myeloma cells, leading to cell death. They can be given over an extended period of time.
- *Monoclonal antibodies.* Daratumumab and isatuximab (anti-CD38), as well as elotuzumab (anti-SLAMF7), have anti-myeloma activity, particularly when given in combination with other agents.
- *Others.* These include bendamustine, panobinistat and venetoclax.

Anti-myeloma agents typically work most effectively when given in combination: for example, bortezomib, thalidomide and dexamethasone are highly efficacious when used together. Combinations are selected based on efficacy, side-effect profile and previous treatment history, as well as funding availability: many are high-cost drugs.

Younger patients who are fit enough for intensive chemotherapy will typically have an autologous SCT in their first and sometimes second remission, to consolidate a good response to therapy. This typically increases the duration of remission and overall survival time. Myeloma will inevitably relapse after each initial response, and although subsequent remissions are achievable, they tend to be less sustained with each treatment course as the cancer becomes more resistant to treatment. Despite this, current treatments have transformed the prognosis of myeloma with ongoing improvement; in this fast-moving field, further improvements are expected.

Immunological therapies have the potential to cure a small subset of patients, with the use of allogeneic transplant sometimes considered for young patients with high-risk disease. CAR-T cell immunotherapy has great potential but is currently an investigational treatment.

Smouldering (asymptomatic) myeloma

In this condition there is a significant paraprotein (IgG or IgA >30 g/L, or urinary light chain excretion >0.5 g/day) and/or a marrow plasma cell infiltration of more than 10% but no end-organ damage or biomarkers of symptomatic myeloma. Most, but not all, patients will eventually progress to symptomatic myeloma, with a median time to progression of about 5 years. The risk is highest for those with an elevated SFLC ratio, high bone marrow plasma cell infiltration and paraprotein over 30 g/L. These patients can be managed with close monitoring in clinic.

Monoclonal gammopathy of undetermined significance

Monoclonal gammopathy of undetermined significance (MGUS) describes an isolated finding of a monoclonal paraprotein in the serum or urine that does not fulfil the diagnostic criteria for smouldering or symptomatic myeloma. The risk of progression to myeloma is approximately 1% per year, with risk factors including elevated SFLC ratio, paraprotein of more than 15 g/L and non-IgG subtype.

Solitary plasmacytoma

This is an isolated tumour of neoplastic plasma cells. It may be a solitary plasmacytoma of bone within the skeleton or a soft tissue extramedullary plasmacytoma outside the marrow cavity. These can be treated curatively with radiotherapy, although a high proportion (especially bone plasmacytomas) will eventually progress to systemic myeloma.

Heavy chain diseases

These rare conditions are characterized – as the name suggests – by the production of a heavy-chain-only paraprotein. They are usually caused by a B-cell lymphoproliferative condition.

Monoclonal gammopathies of clinical significance

Apart from the entities outlined above, in which the plasma cell disorder is acting in a malignant or pre-malignant manner, there are a number of other conditions in which the clonal population is relatively small but secondary clinical effects occur. These are discussed in more detail in the relevant organ-based chapters.

- *AL amyloidosis* involves organized fibrillary deposits in the kidneys, heart, gastrointestinal tract, skin and nerves. It is usually caused by a lambda-light chain isotype. Other subtypes of amyloid (e.g. hereditary ATTR amyloid and reactive AA amyloid) are not caused by a plasma cell disorder (see p. 1358).
- *Monoclonal gammopathies of renal significance* constitutes a group of renal pathologies caused by immunoglobulin deposition (see p. 1365). Like AL amyloid, all of these may be treated with myeloma-directed therapies, e.g. bortezomib, cyclophosphamide and dexamethasone.
- *POEMS syndrome* is a rare disease characterized by *p*olyneuropathy, *o*rganomegaly, *e*ndocrinopathy, *m*onoclonal plasma cell disorder and *s*kin changes (see p. 890). High levels of vascular endothelial growth factor (VEGF) are common and may be the mediating mechanism.

Further reading

Fermand JP, Bridoux F, Dispenzieri A et al. Monoclonal gammopathy of clinical significance: a novel concept with therapeutic implications. *Blood* 2018; 132:1478–1485.
Go RS, Rajkumar SV. How I manage monoclonal gammopathy of undetermined significance. *Blood* 2018; 131:163–173.
Palumbo A, Avet-Loiseau H, Oliva S et al. Revised International Staging System for multiple myeloma: a report from International Myeloma Working Group. *J Clin Oncol* 2015; 33:2863–2869.
Rajkumar SV. Multiple myeloma: 2016 update on diagnosis, risk-stratification, and management. *Am J Hematol* 2016; 91:719–734.
Tandon N, Rajkumar SV, LaPlant B et al. Clinical utility of the Revised International Staging System in unselected patients with newly diagnosed and relapsed multiple myeloma. *Blood Cancer J* 2017; 7:e528.

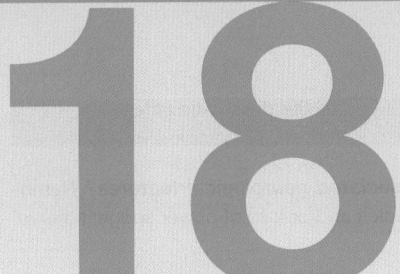

18

Rheumatology

Anisur Rahman and Ian Giles

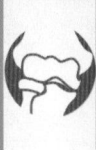

CORE SKILLS AND KNOWLEDGE

Musculoskeletal complaints are very common, comprising 25–30% of consultations in primary care. The majority of patients have soft tissue complaints or osteoarthritis, with inflammatory arthritis and autoimmune rheumatic diseases having a much lower prevalence, of between 0.01% and 1% of the population.

Rheumatology is mainly an outpatient specialty, with care being delivered by multidisciplinary teams including nurse specialists, physiotherapists and other allied health professionals. Apart from general rheumatology clinics, specialist clinics often exist (sometimes in tertiary referral centres) for patients with inflammatory conditions such as rheumatoid arthritis or systemic lupus erythematosus. Few patients require admission to hospital but many receive day case infusions of biological disease-modifying drugs.

Key learning outcomes in musculoskeletal disease include:

- learning to distinguish mechanical from inflammatory problems, and then identifing the number and pattern of joint involvement as well any extra-articular features in patients with inflammatory multisystem disease
- becoming familiar with the main drug categories, of analgesics and medication that alters the immune response
- learning how to examine joints, and when to order autoantibody tests.

Opportunities for learning include sitting in general and specialist rheumatology clinics, observing musculoskeletal and joint injection lists, talking with and examining patients attending day units for infusions of medication, and attending imaging meetings.

CLINICAL SKILLS FOR RHEUMATOLOGY

Taking a musculoskeletal history

In most rheumatological disorders (**Box 18.1**), the diagnosis is *clinical*: that is, made on the history and examination, and then supported by investigations. Taking a thorough history is therefore crucial, and the main points to consider are:

1. **Who is the patient?**
- *Age*: osteoarthritis, polymyalgia rheumatica and giant cell arteritis present mainly in patients over the age of 50. Autoimmune rheumatic diseases and inflammatory arthritis frequently present in people under 50.
- *Gender*: rheumatoid arthritis (RA), Sjögren's syndrome, systemic lupus erythematosus (SLE) and systemic sclerosis are more common in women, whereas gout and ankylosing spondylitis are more common in men.
- *Ethnicity*: SLE is more common in African–Caribbean people than in other ethnicities.
- *Occupation*: jobs that involve heavy use of one part of the body can lead to soft tissue pain and/or OA; for example, in the low back, hips and knees of people who do a lot of heavy lifting. Musculoskeletal pain may also affect people's ability to do their job, or care for children or dependents. The effects of these on quality of life should be assessed.

2. **Has something happened to the patient?**
- *Physical trauma:* trauma to a particular region of the body may cause pain there and/or in related regions.
- *Psychosocial stress and depression*: physical, psychological and social factors interact to contribute to symptoms. In musculoskeletal disorders, pain may cause distress and poor sleep, which in turn build up muscle tension and worsen the pain (see p. 429). Acute stressful events, such as bereavement, bullying, abuse and redundancy, may exacerbate these symptoms.

3. **What are the symptoms?**
- Pain:
  - *Where is it?* The pattern of joint involvement is a useful clue to the diagnosis (**Box 18.2**).
  - *Is it arising from joints, spine, muscles or bone, with local tenderness?*
  - *Could it be referred from another site?* Joint pain is localized but may radiate distally – shoulder to upper arm; hip to thigh and knee.
  - *Is it constant, intermittent or episodic?*
  - *Are there aggravating or precipitating factors?* Is it made worse by activity and eased by rest (mechanical), or worse after rest (inflammatory)?

- *Are there any associated neurological features?* Numbness, pins and needles and/or loss of power suggest 'nerve' involvement.
- Stiffness:
  - Is it generalized or localized?
  - Does it affect the limb girdles or periphery?
  - Is it worse in the morning and relieved by activity?

Joint stiffness for more than 30 minutes each morning – think of inflammatory arthritis. Morning spinal stiffness in younger adults – think of axial spondyloarthritis (e.g. ankylosing spondylitis) (see p. 448). Shoulder and pelvic girdle stiffness and pain in a patient over 55 years may be polymyalgia rheumatica (see p. 464).
- Swelling
  - *Does it affect one joint or several?* Look for symmetry or asymmetry, and/or a peripheral or proximal pattern. An acute monoarthritis may be due to trauma, gout, pseudogout or sepsis (fever or immunosuppression). A polyarthritis is more likely to be due to OA or RA.
  - *Is it constant or does it come in short-lived or longer episodes?*
  - *Is there associated inflammation* (redness and warmth)?
- Extra-articular symptoms:
  - Osteoarthritis and soft tissue problems are not usually associated with symptoms outside the joints.
  - Features such as rash, breathlessness, neurological symptoms or blood disorders suggests that the locomotor problems may be one facet of a more systemic disorder, such as RA, psoriatic arthritis or SLE.

4. **What medication is the patient taking?**
- *Could a drug be a cause?* Diuretics may precipitate gout in men and older women. Steroids can cause avascular necrosis.
- *Have the symptoms responded to medication?* A good response to a trial of oral or intramuscular corticosteroid suggests an inflammatory or autoimmune problem.

5. **What is the family history?**

ℹ Box 18.1 The 'top 10' rheumatic conditions that students should understand

- Regional musculoskeletal conditions
- Chronic pain syndromes
- Osteoarthritis
- Rheumatoid arthritis
- Spondyloarthropathies
- Crystal arthropathies
- Infection-related arthritis
- Autoimmune rheumatic diseases
- Systemic vasculitides
- Juvenile idiopathic arthritis

? Box 18.2 Distinguishing patterns of rheumatic disease

Regional	Inflammatory	Multisystem
• Localized joint pain	• Widespread joint pain	• Fever
• Increased pain with activity	• Reduced pain with activity	• Fatigue
• Short-lived stiffness	• Prolonged early morning stiffness	• Rash
• Distal radiation	• Multiple joint swelling	• Alopecia
• Joint swelling	• Functional limitation	• Raynaud's phenomenon
• Functional limitation	• Widespread joint abnormalities on examination	• Positive systems enquiry
• Localized joint abnormalities on examination		• Systems abnormalities on examination

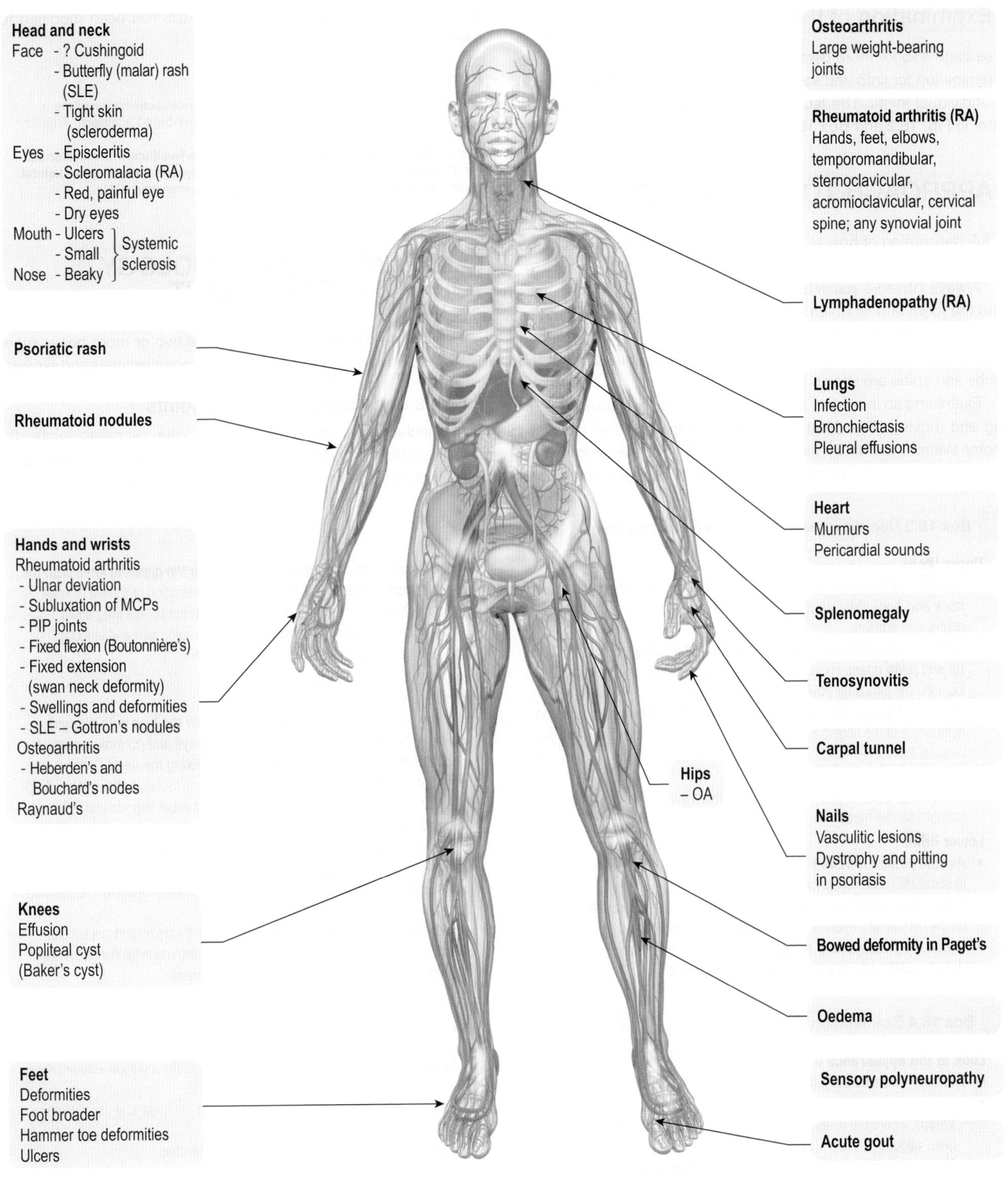

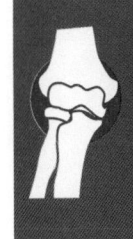

Head and neck
Face - ? Cushingoid
      - Butterfly (malar) rash
        (SLE)
      - Tight skin
        (scleroderma)
Eyes - Episcleritis
      - Scleromalacia (RA)
      - Red, painful eye
      - Dry eyes
Mouth - Ulcers ⎫ Systemic
      - Small   ⎬ sclerosis
Nose - Beaky   ⎭

Psoriatic rash

Rheumatoid nodules

Hands and wrists
Rheumatoid arthritis
 - Ulnar deviation
 - Subluxation of MCPs
 - PIP joints
 - Fixed flexion (Boutonnière's)
 - Fixed extension
   (swan neck deformity)
 - Swellings and deformities
 - SLE – Gottron's nodules
Osteoarthritis
 - Heberden's and
   Bouchard's nodes
Raynaud's

Knees
Effusion
Popliteal cyst
(Baker's cyst)

Feet
Deformities
Foot broader
Hammer toe deformities
Ulcers

Osteoarthritis
Large weight-bearing
joints

Rheumatoid arthritis (RA)
Hands, feet, elbows,
temporomandibular,
sternoclavicular,
acromioclavicular, cervical
spine; any synovial joint

Lymphadenopathy (RA)

Lungs
Infection
Bronchiectasis
Pleural effusions

Heart
Murmurs
Pericardial sounds

Splenomegaly

Tenosynovitis

Carpal tunnel

Hips
 – OA

Nails
Vasculitic lesions
Dystrophy and pitting
in psoriasis

Bowed deformity in Paget's

Oedema

Sensory polyneuropathy

Acute gout

Examination of the joints

See page 415 for more detail on how to structure both a screening examination for limb and spinal disease and a detailed examination of individual joints. The technique for joint aspiration is presented later in **Fig. 18.2** and **Box 18.7**.

APPROACH TO THE PATIENT

A full description of how to take a musculoskeletal history is found on page 412.

Always observe patients, looking for disabilities, as they walk into the room and sit down. General and neurological examinations are often necessary, and may reveal some of the signs described in the figure on page 413. Guidelines for rapid examinations of the limbs and spine are shown in **Box 18.3**.

Examining an individual joint involves three stages: looking, feeling and moving (**Box 18.4**). A screening examination of the locomotor system, known by the acronym GALS (*g*lobal *a*ssessment of the *l*ocomotor *s*ystem), has been devised. Video demonstrations

are available (see 'Further reading'). GALS has been modified for examination of children.

Further reading

Foster HE, Kay LJ, May CR et al. Pediatric regional examination of the musculoskeletal system: a practice and consensus-based approach. *Arthritis Care Res* 2011; 63:1503–1510.
https://www.versusarthritis.org/about-arthritis/healthcare-professionals/clinical-assessment-of-the-musculoskeletal-system/the-musculoskeletal-examination-gals/ *Musculoskeletal screening examination: GALS.*

ANATOMY AND PHYSIOLOGY OF THE NORMAL JOINT

A joint can be defined as a place where two or more bones meet. There are three types of joints: fibrous, fibrocartilaginous and synovial.

Fibrous and fibrocartilaginous joints

These include the intervertebral discs, the sacroiliac joints, the pubic symphysis and the costochondral joints. Skull sutures are fibrous joints. Little movement occurs at such joints.

 Box 18.3 Rapid examinations of the limbs and spine

Upper limbs
- *Raise the arms sideways to the ears* (*abduction*). *Reach behind the neck and back.* Difficulties with these movements indicate a shoulder or rotator cuff problem.
- *Hold the arms forwards, with elbows straight and fingers apart, palm up and palm down.* Fixed flexion at the elbow indicates an elbow problem. Examine the hands for swelling, wasting and deformity.
- *Place the hands in the 'prayer' position with the elbows apart.* Flexion deformities of the fingers may be due to arthritis, flexor tenosynovitis or skin disease. Painful restriction of the wrist limits the person's ability to move the elbows out with the hands held together.
- *Make a tight fist.* Difficulty with this indicates a loss of flexion or grip. Grip strength can be measured.

Lower limbs
- *Ask the patient to walk* a short distance away from and towards you, and to stand still. Look for abnormal posture or stance.
- *Ask the patient to stand on each leg.* Severe hip disease causes the pelvis on the non-weight-bearing side to sag (positive Trendelenburg test).
- *Watch the patient stand and sit*, looking for hip and/or knee problems.
- *Ask the patient to straighten and flex each knee.*

- *Ask the patient to place each foot in turn on the opposite knee with the hip externally rotated.* This tests for painful restriction of the hip or knee. Abnormal hips or knees must be examined with the patient lying down.
- *Move each ankle up and down.* Examine the ankle joint and tendons, medial arch and toes while the patient is standing.

Spine
Stand behind the patient.
- *Ask the patient to (a) bend forwards to touch the toes with straight knees, (b) extend backwards, (c) flex sideways and (d) look over each shoulder, flexing and extending and side-flexing the neck.* Observe abnormal spinal curves – scoliosis (lateral curve), kyphosis (forward bending) or lordosis (backward bending). A cervical and lumbar lordosis and a thoracic kyphosis are normal. Muscle spasm is worse while standing and bending. Leg length inequality leads to a scoliosis that decreases on sitting or lying (the lengths are measured with the patient lying down).
- *Ask the patient to lie supine.* Examine any restriction of straight-leg raising (see disc prolapse, below).
- *Ask the patient to lie prone.* Examine for anterior thigh pain during a femoral stretch test (flexing knee while prone), which indicates a high lumbar disc problem.
- *Palpate the spine and buttocks for tender areas.*

 Box 18.4 Examination of the joint

Look at the appearance of the joint
- Swelling – could be bony, fluid or synovial
- Deformity:
  - *Valgus*, where the distal bone is deviated laterally (e.g. knock-knees or genu valgum)
  - *Varus*, where the distal bone is deviated medially (bow-legs or genu varum)
  - Fixed flexion or hyperextension
- Rash – especially psoriasis
- Muscle wasting – easier to see in large muscles like the quadriceps
- Scars – from surgery or trauma
- Signs of inflammation
- Symmetry:
  - Are the right and left joints (e.g. hips, knees, any other paired joint) the same?
  - If not, which do you think is abnormal?

Feel
- Swelling:
  - *Fluid swelling* (effusion) usually represents increased synovial fluid in inflammatory arthritis, but can be due to blood or pus

  - *Synovial swelling* is rubbery or boggy and usually occurs in inflammatory arthritis
  - *Bony swelling*, such as Heberden's nodes in the fingers, is usually seen in osteoarthritis
  - Warmth – a warm joint may be inflamed or infected
  - Tenderness – may represent joint inflammation, but many people have chronic tenderness all over the body (e.g. in fibromyalgia)

Move
- Active movement:
  - Is the range full and pain-free?
  - Is the movement fluid?
  - In the hands, can the patient perform fine movements?
  - In the legs, can the patient walk properly?
- Compare movements on the right and left sides – are they symmetrical?
- Is there crepitus when the joint is moved?
- If active movement is limited, try passive movement:
  - In a joint problem both will usually be affected.
  - In a muscle or nerve problem, passive movement may remain full.

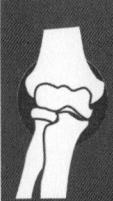

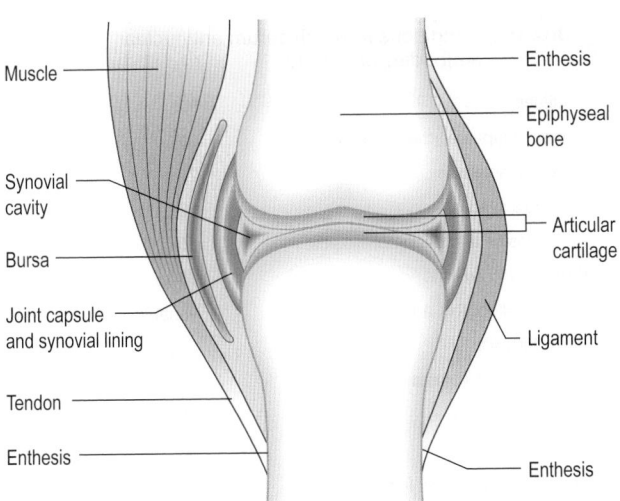

Fig. 18.1 Normal synovial joint.

Muscle

Synovial cavity

Bursa

Joint capsule and synovial lining

Tendon

Enthesis

Enthesis

Epiphyseal bone

Articular cartilage

Ligament

Enthesis

Synovial joints

Synovial joints (**Fig. 18.1**) include the ball-and-socket joints (e.g. hip) and the hinge joints (e.g. interphalangeal). They are designed to allow movement, which is restricted to a required range, and stability is maintained during use. The load is distributed across the surface, thus preventing damage by overloading or disuse. Each structural component of a synovial joint plays a key functional role, and different components are affected in different disease processes.

Juxta-articular bone

Bone structure and physiology are discussed on page 473. The bone that abuts a joint (juxta-articular bone) is highly vascular and comprises a light framework of mineralized collagen enclosed in a thin coating of tougher, cortical bone. It withstands pressure poorly if the normal intra-articular covering of hyaline cartilage is worn away, as in osteoarthritis (OA; see p. 433). This process can lead to abnormalities of bone growth and remodelling (see p. 433).

Articular cartilage

The hyaline cartilage lining the bones within a joint is called articular cartilage. It is avascular and derives nourishment from synovial fluid. It is predominantly composed of type II collagen, encoded by the *COL2A1* gene, which forms a mesh-like network. Chondrocytes secrete collagen and proteoglycans, and are embedded in the cartilage. Defects in articular cartilage and underlying bone are features of **osteoarthritis**.

Synovium and synovial fluid

The joint capsule, which is connected to the periosteum, is lined with synovium, which is a few cells thick and vascular. Its surface is smooth, non-adherent, and is permeable to proteins and crystalloids. Synovial fluid is a highly viscous fluid secreted by the synovial cells and has a similar consistency to plasma. Glycoproteins ensure a low coefficient of friction between the cartilaginous surfaces. Tendon sheaths and bursae are also lined by synovium. Inflammation of the synovium is a feature of **inflammatory arthritis**.

Ligaments and tendons

These structures stabilize joints. Ligaments are variably elastic and this contributes to the stiffness or laxity of joints (see p. 432). Tendons are inelastic and transmit muscle power to bones. The joint capsule is formed by intermeshing tendons and ligaments. The point where a tendon or ligament joins a bone is called an **enthesis** and may be the site of inflammation. Whereas most ligaments and tendons run outside the joints, some, like the supraspinatus tendon in the shoulder and the cruciate ligaments in the knee, run through the joint. Inflammation or trauma to these joints can cause severe joint symptoms.

Blood vessels and nerves

The ligaments, periosteum, synovial tissue and capsule of the joint are richly supplied by blood vessels and nerves. Pain usually derives from inflammation of these sites because the synovial membrane is relatively insensitive.

Skeletal muscle

This tissue consists of bundles of myocytes containing actin and myosin molecules. These molecules interdigitate and form myofibrils, which cause muscle contraction in a similar way to myocardial muscle (see p. 1024). Bundles of myofibrils (fasciculi) are covered by connective tissue, the perimysium, which merges with the epimysium (covering the muscle) and forms the tendon, which attaches to the bone surface (enthesis).

Though not strictly a component of the joint itself, muscles are so closely related to joints that strain and tension in muscles are commonly interpreted by patients as joint pain. Pain in muscles and ligaments (myofascial pain) is a very common cause of locomotor symptoms. Primary inflammatory disease of muscle (myositis) is far less common.

INVESTIGATION OF RHEUMATIC DISEASE

Investigations are unnecessary in many of the common musculoskeletal problems; the diagnosis is clear from the history and examination findings. Tests help to exclude another condition and to reassure the patient or their primary care physician.

Useful blood screening tests

- Full blood count:
  - *Haemoglobin.* Normochromic, normocytic anaemia suggests chronic inflammatory and autoimmune diseases. Hypochromic, microcytic anaemia indicates iron deficiency, sometimes due to non-steroidal anti-inflammatory drug (NSAID)-induced gastrointestinal bleeding.
  - *White cell count.* Neutrophilia is seen in bacterial infection (e.g. septic arthritis). It also occurs with corticosteroid treatment. Lymphopenia is found in viral illnesses or SLE. Neutropenia may reflect drug-induced bone marrow suppression. Eosinophilia is seen in eosinophilic granulomatosis with polyangiitis (EGPA) (see p. 991).
- *Platelets.* Raised platelets occur with any chronic inflammation. Thrombocytopenia is seen in drug-induced bone marrow suppression and may be a feature of SLE.
- *Erythrocyte sedimentation rate (ESR) and C-reactive protein (CRP).* An increase in these reflects inflammation. Plasma viscosity is also raised in inflammatory disease.
- *Bone and liver biochemistry.* A raised serum alkaline phosphatase may indicate liver or bone disease. A rise in liver enzymes is often seen with drug-induced toxicity. For other investigations of bone, see pages 474.

Other blood and urine tests

- Protein electrophoresis (and/or immunofixation), serum free light chain testing and urinary Bence Jones protein – to exclude myeloma as a cause of a raised ESR.

i **Box 18.5** Conditions in which rheumatoid factor (RF) is found in the serum

Condition	RF (IgM) %
Autoimmune rheumatic diseases	
Rheumatoid arthritis	70
Systemic lupus erythematosus	25
Sjögren's syndrome	90
Systemic sclerosis	30
Polymyositis/dermatomyositis	50
Juvenile idiopathic arthritis	Variable
Viral infections	**Hyperglobulinaemias**
Hepatitis	Chronic liver disease
Infectious mononucleosis	Sarcoidosis
	Cryoglobulinaemia
Chronic infections	**Normal population**
Tuberculosis	Elderly
Leprosy	Relatives of people with rheumatoid arthritis
Infective endocarditis	
Syphilis	

i **Box 18.6** Conditions in which serum antinuclear antibodies are found

Condition	%
Systemic lupus erythematosus	95
Systemic sclerosis	70
Sjögren's syndrome	80
Polymyositis and dermatomyositis	40
Rheumatoid arthritis	30
Juvenile idiopathic arthritis	Variable
Other diseases	
Autoimmune hepatitis	100
Drug-induced lupus	>95
Myasthenia gravis	50
Idiopathic pulmonary fibrosis	30
Diabetes mellitus	25
Infectious mononucleosis	5–10
Normal population	8

- Serum uric acid – for gout.
- Antistreptolysin O titre – in rheumatic fever.

Serum autoantibody studies

- *Rheumatoid factors (RFs)* (see also p. 439). RFs are detected by enzyme-linked immunosorbent assay (ELISA). RFs are antibodies (usually immunoglobulin (Ig) M, but also IgG or IgA) against the Fc portion of IgG. They are detected in 70% of people with RA, but are not diagnostic. RFs are detected in many autoimmune rheumatic disorders (e.g. SLE), in chronic infections, and in asymptomatic older people (**Box 18.5**).
- *Anti-citrullinated peptide antibodies (ACPA).* These antibodies are directed against citrullinated antigens, vimentin, fibrinogen, alpha enolase and type II collagen. They are measured by an ELISA technique and are present in up to 80% of people with RA. They have a high specificity for RA (90%, with a sensitivity of 60%). They are helpful in early disease when the RF is negative, to distinguish it from acute transient synovitis (see **Box 18.28**). Positivity for RF and/or ACPA is associated with a worse prognosis and an increase in the likelihood of bony erosions in people with RA.
- *Antinuclear antibodies (ANAs).* These are detected by indirect immunofluorescent staining of fresh frozen sections of rat liver or kidney or Hep-2 cell lines. Different patterns reflect a variety of antigenic specificities that occur with different clinical pictures. ANA is used as a screening test for SLE and systemic sclerosis – a negative ANA makes either condition highly unlikely – but low titres occur in RA and chronic infections and in normal individuals, especially the elderly (**Box 18.6**).
- *Anti-double-stranded DNA (dsDNA) antibodies.* These are usually detected by a precipitation test (Farr assay), ELISA or an immunofluorescent test using *Crithidia luciliae* (which contains dsDNA). Raised anti-dsDNA is highly specific for SLE; the levels usually rise and fall in parallel with disease activity so can be used to monitor the level of treatment required.
- *Anti-extractable nuclear antigen (ENA) antibodies* (see **Box 18.38**). These produce a speckled ANA fluorescent pattern,

and can be identified by ELISA. The most commonly measured ENAs are:

- *anti-Ro and anti-La*, which occur in Sjögren's syndrome and SLE
- *anti-Sm*, which is highly specific for SLE
- *anti-Jo-1*, which is the most common of the anti-tRNA synthetase enzymes that occur in some people with dermatomyositis or polymyositis
- *anti-topoisomerase I (anti-Scl 70)*, which is specific for systemic sclerosis
- *anti-RNA polymerase I and III*, which occur in systemic sclerosis and are associated with pulmonary fibrosis.
- *Anti-neutrophil cytoplasmic antibodies (ANCAs)* (see p. 466). These are predominantly IgG autoantibodies directed against the primary granules of neutrophil and macrophage lysosomes. They are strongly associated with small-vessel vasculitis. Two major clinically relevant ANCA patterns are recognized on *immunofluorescence*:
  - *proteinase 3 (PR3-ANCA)*, also called cytoplasmic or cANCA, producing a granular immunofluorescence and seen in granulomatosis with polyangiitis (GPA)
  - *myeloperoxidase (MPO-ANCA)*, also called perinuclear or pANCA, producing a perinuclear stain and seen in microscopic polyangiitis and EGPA.
- *Antiphospholipid antibodies* These are detected in the antiphospholipid syndrome (see p. 456).
- *Complement.* Low complement levels indicate consumption and suggest an active disease process in SLE.

Joint aspiration and examination of synovial fluid

Examination of joint (or bursa) fluid is used mainly to diagnose septic, reactive or crystal arthritis. The appearance of the fluid is an indicator of the level of inflammation. The procedure is often undertaken in combination with injection of a corticosteroid. Aspiration alone is therapeutic in crystal arthritis (**Fig. 8.2** and **Box 18.7**).

Aspiration and analysis of synovial fluid are always indicated when septic or crystal-induced arthritis is suspected, particularly a monoarthritis. Normal fluid is clear and straw-coloured, and contains fewer than 3000 white blood cells (WCC)/mm^3. Inflammatory

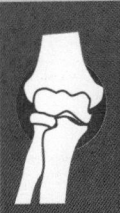

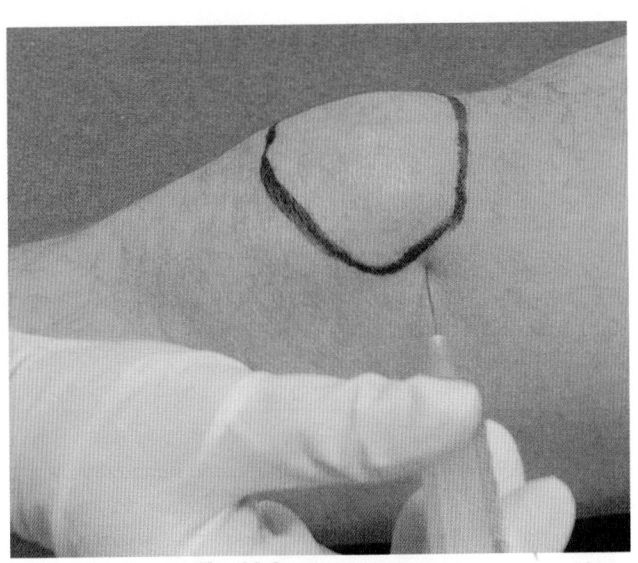

Fig. 18.2 Joint aspiration.

Box 18.7 Joint aspiration

This is a sterile procedure that should be carried out in a clean environment. Explain the procedure to the patient; obtain consent.

1. Decide on the site to insert the needle and mark it.
2. Clean the skin and your hands scrupulously.
3. Draw up local anaesthetic (and corticosteroid if it is being used).
4. Insert the needle, injecting local anaesthetic as it advances; if a joint effusion is suspected, attempt to aspirate as you advance it.
5. If fluid is obtained, change syringes and aspirate fully.
6. Examine the fluid in the syringe and decide whether or not to proceed with a corticosteroid injection (if fluid is clear or slightly cloudy) or send for microbiological tests.
7. Cover the injection site and advise the patient to rest the affected area for a few days. Warn the patient that the pain may increase initially but to report urgently if this persists beyond a few days, if the swelling worsens or if they become febrile, because this might indicate an infected joint.

Aspirated fluid is sent for microscopy, Gram-stain and culture. Different types of crystals can be identified using polarized light microscopy. Fluid from septic arthritis is often excessively turbid.

---

fluid is cloudy and contains more than 3000 WCC/mm³. Septic fluid is opaque and less viscous, and contains up to 75 000 WCC/mm³. There is much overlap.

Polarized light microscopy is performed for crystals:

- **gout**: negatively bi-refringent, needle-shaped crystals of sodium urate
- **calcium pyrophosphate deposition arthropathy**: rhomboidal, weakly positively bi-refringent crystals of calcium pyrophosphate.

Gram-staining is essential if septic arthritis is suspected and may identify the organism immediately. Joint fluid should be cultured and antibiotic sensitivities requested.

Diagnostic imaging and visualization

- **X-rays** can be diagnostic in certain conditions (e.g. established RA) and are the first investigation in many cases of trauma. X-rays can detect joint space narrowing, erosions in RA, calcification in soft tissue, new bone formation, e.g. osteophytes, and decreased bone density (osteopenia) or increased bone density (osteosclerosis):
  - In acute low back pain (see p. 421), X-rays are indicated only if the pain is persistent, recurrent, associated with neurological symptoms or signs, worse at night or associated with symptoms such as fever or weight loss.

- Radiological changes are common in older people and may not indicate symptomatic OA or spondylosis, a term that implies OA within the spine.
  - X-rays are of little diagnostic value in early inflammatory arthritis but are useful as a baseline from which to judge later change.
- **Ultrasound** is particularly useful for periarticular structures, soft tissue swellings and tendons, and for detecting active synovitis in inflammatory arthritis. It is increasingly used to examine the shoulder and other structures during movement, e.g. shoulder impingement syndrome (see p. 419). Doppler ultrasound measures blood flow and hence inflammation. Ultrasound may be used to guide local corticosteroid injections.
- **Magnetic resonance imaging (MRI)** shows bone changes and intra-articular structures in striking detail. Visualization of particular structures can be enhanced with different resonance sequences. T_1-weighted MRI is used for anatomical detail, T_2-weighted for fluid detection and short tau inversion recovery (STIR) for the presence of bone marrow oedema. MRI is more sensitive than X-rays in the early detection of articular and periarticular disease. Gadolinium injection enhances inflamed tissue. MRI is especially useful for detection of damage to non-bony tissues in or near joints, e.g. meniscal tears in the knee and torn rotator cuff muscles in the shoulder; detection of nerve root compression in the spine; detection of inflamed muscle in myositis; and early detection of synovitis in inflammatory arthritis.
- **Computerized axial tomography (CT)** is useful for detecting changes in calcified structures but the dose of radiation is high.
- **Bone scintigraphy** utilizes radionuclides, usually ⁹⁹ᵐTc, and detects abnormal bone turnover and blood circulation; although non-specific, it helps in detecting areas of inflammation, infection or malignancy. It is best used in combination with other anatomical imaging techniques.
- **Dual-energy X-ray absorptiometry (DXA) scanning** uses very low doses of X-irradiation to measure bone density and is used in the screening and monitoring of osteoporosis.
- **Positron emission tomography (PET) scanning** uses radionuclides, which decay by emission of positrons. ¹⁸F-Fluorodeoxyglucose uptake indicates areas of increased glucose metabolism. PET is used to locate tumours and demonstrate large-vessel vasculitis, e.g. Takayasu's arteritis (see p. 1132). PET scans are combined with CT to improve anatomical details.

Other tests to investigate rheumatological disease

- **Arthroscopy** is a direct means of visualizing a joint, particularly the knee or shoulder. Biopsies can be taken, surgery performed in certain conditions (e.g. repair or trimming of meniscal tears), and loose bodies removed.
- **Nerve conduction studies and electromyography** are used to diagnose nerve entrapment syndromes (such as carpal or tarsal tunnel) and to distinguish myositis from neuropathies.

CLINICAL CONDITIONS IN RHEUMATOLOGY

These can be divided into three types:

- **Pain arising from soft tissues around joints**, such as muscles and tendons. The joints themselves are normal. These are the most common locomotor problems, and are generally self-limiting or respond to simple analgesia, physiotherapy or exercise.

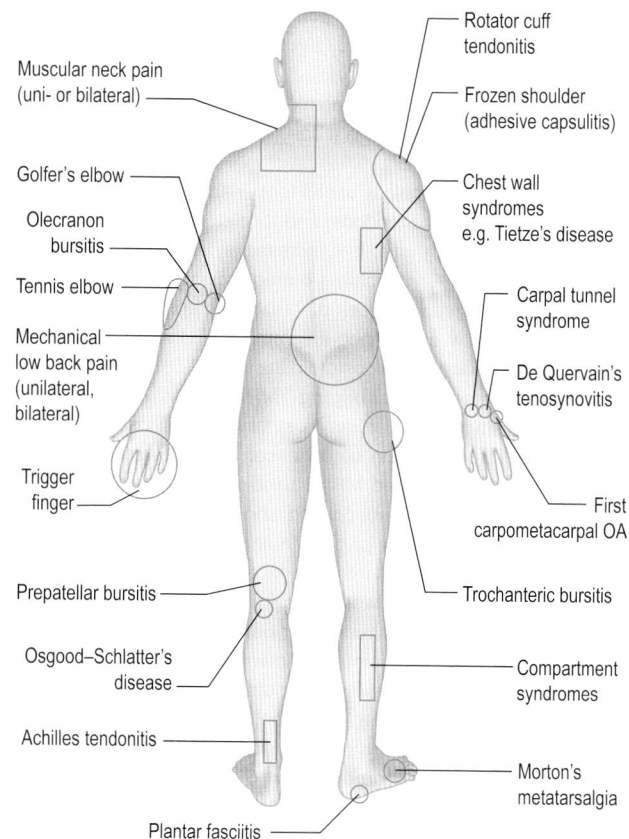

Fig. 18.3 Common regional musculoskeletal problems. OA, osteoarthritis.

- *Diseases of the joints themselves.* Osteoarthritis is more common than inflammatory arthritis, especially in the elderly.
- *Autoimmune rheumatic diseases.* These include disorders such as systemic lupus erythematosus (SLE), where the locomotor symptoms are just one manifestation of a systemic disorder.

COMMON REGIONAL MUSCULOSKELETAL PROBLEMS

See **Fig. 18.3**.

Pain in the neck and shoulder

See **Box 18.8**.

Mechanical or muscular neck pain (shoulder girdle pain)

Unilateral or bilateral muscular-pattern neck pain is common and usually self-limiting. Chronic burning neck pain occurs because of muscle tension from anxiety and stress.

Spondylosis seen on X-ray increases after the age of 40 years but it is not always related to pain. Spondylosis can, however, cause stiffness and increases the risk of mechanical or muscular neck pain. Muscle spasm is palpable and tender, and may lead to abnormal neck posture (e.g. acute torticollis). Muscular-pattern neck pain is not localized but affects the trapezius muscle, the C7 spinous process and the paracervical musculature (shoulder girdle pain). Pain often radiates upwards to the occiput and is commonly

---

? Box 18.8 Pain in the neck and shoulder

- Trauma (e.g. a fall)
- Mechanical or muscular neck pain
- Whiplash injury
- Disc prolapse – nerve root entrapment
- Ankylosing spondylitis
- Shoulder lesions:
  - Rotator cuff tendonitis
  - Calcific tendonitis or bursitis
  - Impingement syndrome or rotator cuff tear
  - Adhesive capsulitis (true 'frozen' shoulder)
  - Inflammatory arthritis or osteoarthritis
- Polymyalgia rheumatica
- Fibromyalgia (chronic widespread pain)
- Chronic (work-related) upper-limb pain syndrome
- Tumour

---

i Box 18.9 Cervical nerve root entrapment: symptoms and signs

Nerve root	Sensory changes	Reflex loss	Weakness
C5	Lateral arm	Biceps	Shoulder abduction
			Elbow flexion
C6	Lateral forearm	Biceps	Elbow flexion
	Thumb and index finger	Supinator	Wrist extension
C7	Middle finger	Triceps	Elbow extension
C8	Medial forearm	None	Finger flexion
	Little and ring fingers		
T1	Medial upper arm	None	Finger abduction and adduction

---

associated with tension headaches. These features are also seen in chronic widespread pain (see p. 429).

Management

Patients are given short courses of analgesic therapy, along with reassurance and explanation. Physiotherapists can help to relieve spasm and pain, teach exercises and relaxation techniques, and improve posture. An occupational therapist can advise about the ergonomics of the workplace if the problem is work-related (see p. 430).

Nerve root entrapment

This is caused by an acute cervical disc prolapse or pressure on the root from spondylotic osteophytes narrowing the root canal.

Acute cervical disc prolapse presents with unilateral pain in the neck, radiating to the interscapular and shoulder regions. This diffuse, aching, dural pain is followed by sharp, electric shock-like pain down the arm, in a nerve root distribution, often with pins and needles, numbness, weakness and loss of reflexes (**Box 18.9**).

Cervical spondylosis occurs in the older patient with posterolateral osteophytes compressing the nerve root and causing root pain (see **Fig. 26.64**), commonly at C5/C6 or C6/C7; it is seen on oblique radiographs of the neck. An MRI scan clearly distinguishes facet joint OA, root canal narrowing and disc prolapse.

Management

A support collar, rest, analgesia and sedation are used initially as necessary. Patients should be advised not to carry heavy items.

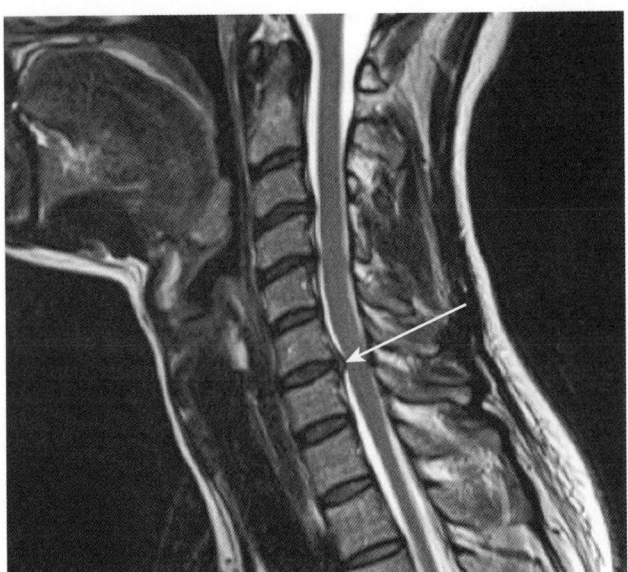

Fig. 18.4 Magnetic resonance image of the cervical spine. A large central disc prolapse (arrowed) is shown at the C6/7 level, and smaller disc bulges at C3/4 and C4/5.

They usually recover in 6–12 weeks. MRI is the investigation of choice if surgery is being considered or the diagnosis is uncertain (**Fig. 18.4**). A cervical root block, administered under direct vision by an experienced pain specialist, may relieve pain while the disc recovers. Neurosurgical referral is recommended if the pain persists or if the neurological signs of weakness or numbness are severe or bilateral. Bilateral root pain, with or without long track symptoms or signs, is a neurosurgical emergency because a central disc prolapse may compress the cervical spinal cord. Posterior osteophytes may cause spinal claudication and cervical myelopathy.

Whiplash injury

Whiplash injury results from acceleration–deceleration forces applied to the neck, usually in a road traffic accident when the car of a person wearing a seat belt is struck from behind. A simple decision plan based on clinical criteria helps to distinguish those most at risk and who warrant radiography. There is a low probability of serious bony injury if there is:
- no midline cervical tenderness
- no focal neurological deficit
- normal alertness
- no intoxication
- no other painful distracting injury.

CT scans are reserved for those with bony injury. MRI scans occasionally show severe soft tissue injury. Whiplash injuries may lead to litigation or insurance claims.

Whiplash injury is a common cause of chronic neck pain, although most people recover within a few weeks or months. Delayed recovery depends, in part, on the severity of the initial injury. The pattern of chronic neck pain is often complex, involving pain in the neck, shoulder and arm. It may be accompanied by subjective symptoms, such as headache, dizziness and poor concentration. The subjective nature of these symptoms has led to controversy about their cause.

Management

Management is with reassurance (the patient is often distressed and anxious), analgesia, a short-term support collar and physiotherapy. Pain may take a few weeks or months to settle and the patient

- Rotator cuff tendonitis pain is worse at night and radiates to the upper arm.
- Painful shoulders produce secondary muscular neck pain.
- Muscular neck pain (also known as shoulder girdle pain) does not radiate to the upper arm.
- Cervical nerve root pain is usually associated with pins and needles or neurological signs in the arm.

should be warned of this. Clinical trial evidence shows no benefit with prolonged physiotherapy.

Pain in the shoulder

The shoulder is a shallow joint with a large range of movement. The humeral head is held in place by the rotator cuff, which is part of the joint capsule. It comprises the tendons of infraspinatus and teres minor posteriorly, supraspinatus superiorly, and teres major and subscapularis anteriorly. The rotator cuff (particularly supraspinatus) prevents the humeral head from blocking against the acromion during abduction; the deltoid pulls up and the supraspinatus pulls in to produce a turning movement, and the greater tuberosity glides under the acromion without impingement. Shoulder pathology restricts or is made worse by shoulder movement. Specific diagnoses are difficult to make clinically but may be clearer on imaging.

Pain in the shoulder can sometimes be due to problems in the neck; the differential diagnosis is shown in **Box 18.10**. Early inflammatory arthritis and polymyalgia rheumatica in the elderly may present with shoulder pain.

Rotator cuff (supraspinatus) tendonosis

This condition is a common cause of shoulder pain at all ages. It follows trauma in 30% of cases and is bilateral in under 5%. The pain radiates to the upper arm and is made worse by arm abduction and elevation, which are often limited. The pain is often worse during the middle of the range of abduction, reducing as the arm is raised fully; a so-called 'painful arc syndrome'. When examined from behind, the scapula rotates earlier than usual during elevation. Passive elevation reduces impingement and is less painful. Severe pain virtually immobilizes the joint, although some rotation is retained (compare adhesive capsulitis; see below). There is also painful spasm of the trapezius. There may be an associated subacromial bursitis. Isolated subacromial bursitis occurs after direct trauma, falling on to the outstretched arm or elbow. Acromioclavicular osteophytes increase the risk of impingement and may need to be removed surgically.

X-ray is often normal but ultrasound is very useful to distinguish bursitis, tendonitis and partial or complete tendon tears. Corticosteroid injections can be guided by ultrasound.

Management

Analgesics, NSAIDs and/or physiotherapy may suffice, but severe pain responds to an injection of corticosteroid into the subacromial bursa (see **Fig. 18.5**). Patients should be warned that 10% will develop worse pain for 24–48 hours after injection. Some 70% improve over 5–20 days and mobilize the joint themselves. Physiotherapy helps persistent stiffness. If injection in the clinic is unsuccessful ultrasound-guided corticosteroid injections may be more effective.

Torn rotator cuff

This condition is caused by trauma but also occurs spontaneously in the elderly and in RA. It prevents active abduction of the arm

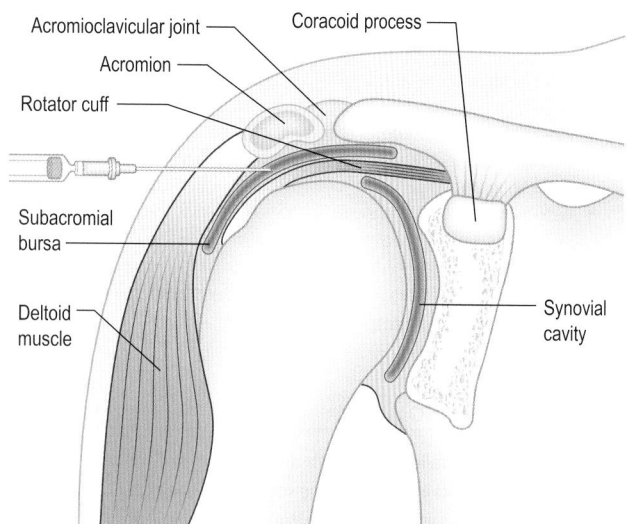

Fig. 18.5 The shoulder region, showing site of injection and subacromial space.

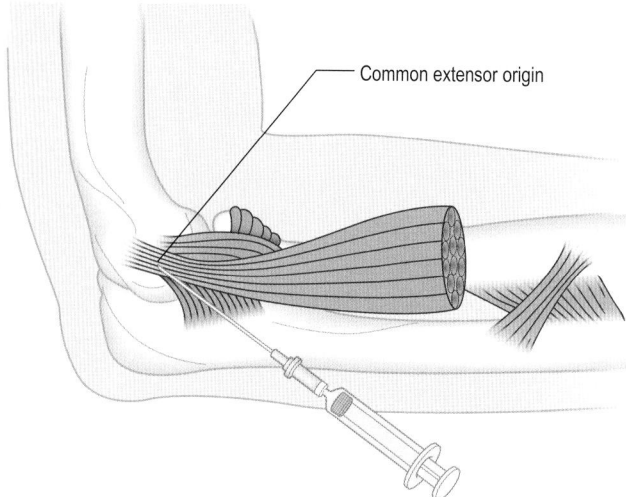

Fig. 18.6 Injection for tennis elbow.

but patients learn to initiate elevation using the unaffected arm. Once elevated, the arm can be held in place by the deltoid muscle. In younger people, the tear is repaired surgically but this is rarely possible in the elderly or in RA. Some patients require arthroscopic surgery.

Calcific tendonosis and bursitis

Calcium pyrophosphate deposits in the tendon are visible on X-ray but they are not always symptomatic. The pathogenesis is unclear, although ischaemia may play a part. The deposit is usually just proximal to the greater tuberosity. It may lead to acute or chronic recurrent shoulder pain and restriction of movement. A local corticosteroid injection may relieve the pain. The calcification may persist or resolve. Aspiration or breaking up of the deposit under ultrasound control may be required for persistent pain. Rarely, arthroscopic removal is necessary.

Shedding of crystals into the subacromial bursa causes a bursitis with severe pain and shoulder restriction. The shoulder feels hot and is swollen, and an X-ray shows a diffuse opacity in the bursa. The differential diagnosis of calcific bursitis is gout, pseudogout or septic arthritis. Aspiration and injection with corticosteroid can help.

Adhesive capsulitis (true 'frozen' shoulder)

This condition can develop with rotator cuff lesions, or following hemiplegia, chest or breast surgery, or myocardial infarction and in diabetics. Initially, it causes severe shoulder pain and a gradually reducing range of movement, leading to a 'frozen' phase where there is loss of all shoulder movements but little pain. NSAIDs and intra-articular injections of local anaesthetic and corticosteroids are helpful in the painful phase. Subsequently, there is usually a gradual improvement in function over weeks to months. Therapeutic exercises and physiotherapy help in later phases. Once the pain settles, arthroscopic release speeds functional recovery.

Pain in the elbow

Pain in the elbow can be due to epicondylitis, inflammatory arthritis or, occasionally, OA.

Epicondylitis

Two common sites where the insertions of tendons into bone become inflamed (enthesitis) are the common wrist extensor origin at the lateral humeral epicondyle ('tennis elbow') and the common wrist flexor origin at the medial epicondyle ('golfer's elbow'). Despite the names, both conditions are usually unrelated to either sport!

There is local tenderness. Pain radiates into the forearm on using the affected muscles –typically, gripping or holding a heavy bag in tennis elbow or carrying a tray in golfer's elbow. Pain at rest also occurs.

Management

Advise rest and arrange review by a physiotherapist. A local injection of corticosteroid at the point of maximum tenderness is helpful when the pain is severe (**Fig. 18.6**) but needs physiotherapy follow-up to prevent recurrences. Avoid the ulnar nerve when injecting golfer's elbow. Both conditions settle spontaneously eventually, but occasionally persist and require surgical release.

Pain in the hand and wrist

See **Box 18.11**. Hand pain is commonly caused by injury or repetitive, work-related activities. When associated with pins and needles or numbness, it suggests a neurological cause arising at the wrist, elbow or neck. Pain and stiffness that are worse in the morning are due to tenosynovitis or inflammatory arthritis. The distribution of hand pain often indicates the diagnosis.

Tenosynovitis

The finger flexor tendons run through synovial sheaths and under loops that hold them in place. Inflammation occurs with repeated or unaccustomed use, or in inflammatory arthritis. The thickened sheaths are often palpable.

Flexor tenosynovitis causes finger pain when gripping and stiffness of the fingers in the morning. Occasionally, a tendon causes a trigger finger, when the finger remains flexed in the morning or after gripping, and has to be pulled straight. A tender tendon nodule is palpable, usually in the distal palm. Trigger finger or thumb is more common in diabetic patients.

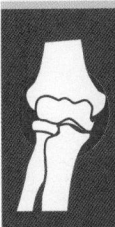

❓ Box 18.11 Causes of pain in the hand and wrist

All ages	Older patients
• Trauma/fractures	• Nodal OA:
• Tenosynovitis:	– DIPs (Heberden's nodes)
– Flexor (with/without triggering)	– PIPs (Bouchard's nodes)
– Dorsal	– First carpometacarpal joint
– De Quervain's	• Trauma – scaphoid fracture
• Carpal tunnel syndrome	• Pseudogout
• Ganglion	• Gout:
• Inflammatory arthritis	– Acute
• Raynaud's syndrome (see p. 1131)	– Tophaceous
• Complex regional pain syndrome type I (see p. 430)	

DIPs/PIPs, distal/proximal interphalangeal joints.

Dorsal tenosynovitis is less common, except in RA. The hourglass swelling extends from the back of the hand and under the extensor retinaculum.

De Quervain's tenosynovitis causes pain and swelling around the radial styloid, where the abductor pollicis longus tendon is held in place by a retaining band. There is local tenderness, and the pain at the styloid is worsened by flexing the thumb into the palm.

Management

Resting, splinting and NSAIDs may help. Local corticosteroids injected alongside the tendon under low pressure (not into the tendon itself) are helpful. Occasionally, surgery is needed if symptoms persist.

Carpal tunnel syndrome

This condition arises due to median nerve compression in the limited space of the carpal tunnel. Thickened ligaments, tendon sheaths or bone enlargement can cause it, but it is usually idiopathic. (Causes are discussed on p. 888.) The history is usually typical and diagnostic, the patient waking with numbness, tingling and pain in a median nerve distribution. The pain may radiate to the forearm. Wasting of the thenar eminence muscles develops with sensory loss in the radial three and a half fingers. The pain may be produced by tapping the nerve in the carpal tunnel (Tinel's sign) or by holding the wrist in flexion (Phalen's test).

Management

Management is with a splint to hold the wrist in dorsiflexion overnight, which relieves the symptoms and is diagnostic; used nightly for several weeks, it may produce full recovery. If it does not, a corticosteroid injection into the carpal tunnel (avoid the nerve!) helps in about 70% of cases, although it may recur. Persistent symptoms or nerve damage produce prolonged latency across the carpal tunnel on nerve conduction studies and require surgical decompression.

Other conditions causing pain
Inflammatory arthritis

This may present with pain, swelling and stiffness of the hands. In RA, the wrists, proximal interphalangeal (PIP) joints and metacarpophalangeal (MCP) joints are affected symmetrically. In psoriatic arthritis and reactive arthritis, a finger may be swollen (dactylitis), or the distal interphalangeal (DIP) joints and nails are affected asymmetrically.

Nodal osteoarthritis

This affects the DIP and, less commonly, PIP joints, which are initially swollen and red. The inflammation and pain settle but bony swellings remain (see p. 435).

First carpometacarpal osteoarthritis

This causes pain at the base of the thumb when gripping, or painless stiffness at the base of the thumb, often in people with nodal OA.

Scaphoid fractures

These cause pain in the anatomical snuffbox. They are not seen immediately on X-ray; if there is clinical suspicion, a cast is necessary. Untreated scaphoid fractures can eventually cause pain because of failed union.

Ganglion

A ganglion is a jelly-filled, often painless swelling caused by a partial tear of the joint capsule or tendon sheath. The wrist is a common site. Treatment is not essential, as many resolve or cause little trouble; otherwise, surgical excision is the best option.

Dupuytren's contracture

This condition is a painless, palpable fibrosis of the palmar aponeurosis, with fibroblasts invading the dermis. It causes puckering of the skin and gradual fixed flexion, usually of the ring and little fingers. It is more common in males, Caucasians, individuals with diabetes mellitus, and those who overuse alcohol. A similar fibrosis occurs in the feet and is often more aggressive. Intralesional steroid injections may help in early disease and some advocate transcutaneous needle aponeurotomy. Percutaneous collagenase injection into the lesion has been shown to be effective in several studies and is now first-line treatment used before surgery. Surgical release of the contracture is restricted to those with severe deformity of the fingers.

Pain in the lower back

Low back pain is a common symptom. It is often traumatic and work-related, although lifting apparatus, other mechanical devices and improved office seating help to avoid it. Episodes are generally short-lived and self-limiting, and patients attend a physiotherapist or osteopath more often than a doctor. Chronic back pain is the cause of 14% of long-term disability in the UK. The causes are listed in **Box 18.12**.

❓ Box 18.12 Causes of pain in the back (lumbar region)

Mechanical	Metabolic
• Trauma	• Osteoporotic spinal fractures (see p. 477)
• Muscular and ligamentous pain	• Osteomalacia (see p. 483)
• Lumbar spondylosis	• Paget's disease (see p. 482)
• Facet joint osteoarthritis	**Neoplastic (see p. 485)**
• Lumbar disc prolapse	• Metastases
• Spinal and root canal stenosis	• Multiple myeloma
• Spondylolisthesis	• Primary tumours of bone
• Disseminated idiopathic skeletal hyperostosis (DISH)	**Referred pain**
• Fibromyalgia, chronic widespread pain (see p. 430)	
Inflammatory	
• Infective lesions of the spine	
• Axial spondyloarthritis/sacro-iliitis (see p. 448)	

Box 18.13 Management of back pain

- Most back pain presenting to a primary care physician needs no investigation
- Pain between the ages of 20 and 55 years is likely to be mechanical and is managed with analgesia, brief rest if necessary and physiotherapy
- Patients should stay active within the limits of their pain
- Early treatment of the acute episode, advice and exercise programmes reduce long-term problems and prevent chronic pain syndromes
- Physical manipulation of uncomplicated back pain produces short-term relief and enjoys high patient satisfaction ratings
- Psychological and social factors may influence the time of presentation
- Appropriate early management reduces long-term disability

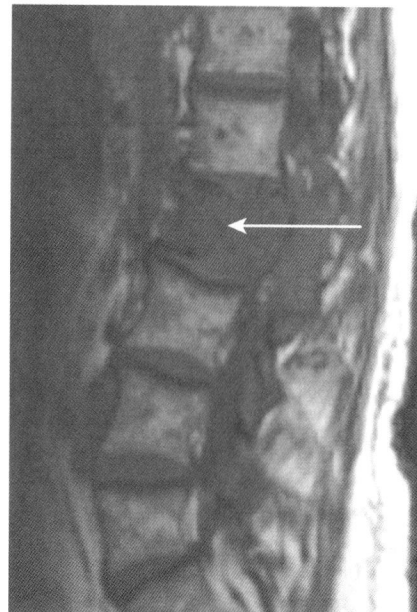

Fig. 18.8 Spinal metastasis in L2. The patient had severe back pain and weight loss, and prior carcinoma of the breast.

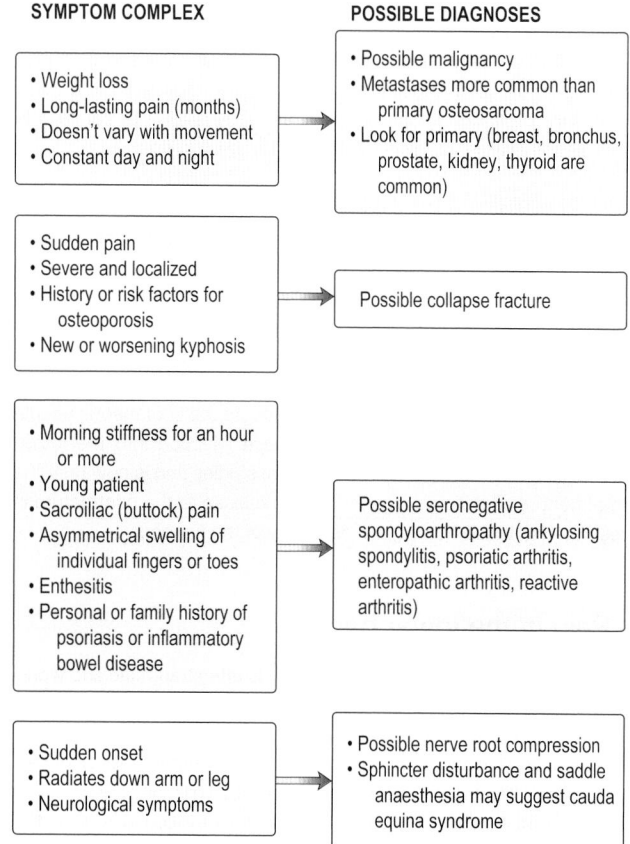

SYMPTOM COMPLEX

- Weight loss
- Long-lasting pain (months)
- Doesn't vary with movement
- Constant day and night

POSSIBLE DIAGNOSES

- Possible malignancy
- Metastases more common than primary osteosarcoma
- Look for primary (breast, bronchus, prostate, kidney, thyroid are common)

- Sudden pain
- Severe and localized
- History or risk factors for osteoporosis
- New or worsening kyphosis

- Possible collapse fracture

- Morning stiffness for an hour or more
- Young patient
- Sacroiliac (buttock) pain
- Asymmetrical swelling of individual fingers or toes
- Enthesitis
- Personal or family history of psoriasis or inflammatory bowel disease

- Possible seronegative spondyloarthropathy (ankylosing spondylitis, psoriatic arthritis, enteropathic arthritis, reactive arthritis)

- Sudden onset
- Radiates down arm or leg
- Neurological symptoms

- Possible nerve root compression
- Sphincter disturbance and saddle anaesthesia may suggest cauda equina syndrome

Fig. 18.7 Diagnoses for serious causes of back pain.

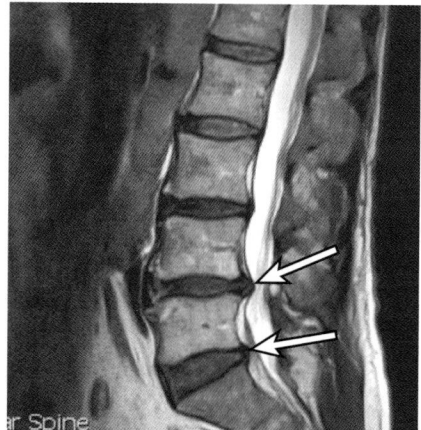

Fig. 18.9 Magnetic resonance image of the lumbar spine. A large disc prolapse is shown at the L4/L5 level and a smaller prolapse at L5/S1 (arrowed). The signal from all the lumbar discs indicates dehydration.

The majority of cases of low back pain are uncomplicated and arise from mechanical causes. Management of this type of back pain is summarized in **Box 18.13**.

One should be alert to clues in the history and examination that could suggest more serious causes of low back pain. These '**red flag**' clues (summarized in **Fig. 18.7**) include the following:

- starts before the age of 20 years or after 50
- pain has persisted for more than 6 weeks
- is worse at night or in the morning, when an inflammatory arthritis (e.g. ankylosing spondylitis), infection or a spinal tumour may be the cause
- is associated with a systemic illness, fever or weight loss
- is associated with neurological symptoms or signs, especially new onset incontinence, which may suggest cauda equina compression.

Investigations

- **Spinal X-rays** are required only if the pain is associated with 'red flag' symptoms or signs.
- **MRI** (**Figs. 18.8** and **18.9**) is preferable to CT scanning when neurological signs and symptoms are present. CT scans demonstrate bony pathology better. Interpretation of the relevance of the findings may require a specialist opinion.
- **Bone scans** are useful in infective and malignant lesions but are also positive in degenerative lesions.
- **Full blood count, ESR and biochemical tests** are required only when the pain is likely to be due to malignancy, infection or a metabolic cause. Normal ESR and CRP distinguish mechanical back pain from polymyalgia rheumatica, a likely differential in the elderly.

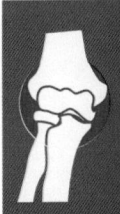

Mechanical low back pain

Mechanical low back pain starts suddenly, may be recurrent and is helped by rest. It is often precipitated by an injury and may be unilateral or bilateral. It is usually short-lived.

Examination

The back is stiff and a scoliosis may be present when the patient is standing. Muscular spasm is visible and palpable, and causes local pain and tenderness. It lessens when sitting or lying. Excessive rest should be avoided. Once a patient develops low back pain, although the episode itself is usually self-limiting, there is a significantly increased risk of further back pain episodes. Risk factors for recurrent back pain include:

- female sex
- increasing age
- pre-existing chronic widespread pain (fibromyalgia)
- psychosocial factors, such as high levels of psychological distress, poor self-rated health and dissatisfaction with employment.

Chronic low back pain is a major cause of disability and time off work and is reduced by appropriate early management.

Spinal movement occurs at the disc and the posterior facet joints, and stability is normally achieved by a complex mechanism of spinal ligaments and muscles. Any of these structures may be a source of pain. An exact anatomical diagnosis is difficult but some typical syndromes are recognized (see below). They are often associated with, but not necessarily caused by, radiological spondylosis (see p. 893).

Postural back pain develops in individuals who sit in poorly designed, unsupportive chairs.

Lumbar spondylosis

The fundamental lesion in spondylosis occurs in an intervertebral disc, a fibrous structure whose tough capsule inserts into the rim of the adjacent vertebrae. This capsule encloses a fibrous outer zone and a gel-like inner zone. The disc allows rotation and bending.

Changes in the discs occasionally start in teenage years or early twenties and often increase with age. The gel changes chemically, breaks up, shrinks and loses its compliance. The surrounding fibrous zones develop circumferential or radial fissures. In the majority, this is initially asymptomatic but visible on MRI as decreased hydration. Later, the discs become thinner and less compliant. These changes cause circumferential bulging of the intervertebral ligaments.

Reactive changes develop in adjacent vertebrae; the bone becomes sclerotic and osteophytes form around the rim of the vertebra (see **Fig. 18.9**). The most common sites of lumbar spondylosis are L5/S1 and L4/L5.

In young people, disc prolapse through an adjacent vertebral end-plate produces a Schmorl's node on X-ray. This process is painless but may accelerate disc degeneration.

Spondylosis may be symptomless but can cause:

- episodic mechanical spinal pain
- progressive spinal stiffening
- facet joint pain
- acute disc prolapse, with or without nerve root irritation
- spinal stenosis
- spondylolisthesis.

Facet joint syndrome

Lumbar spondylosis also causes secondary OA of the misaligned facet joints. Pain is typically worse on bending backwards and when straightening from flexion. It is lumbar in site, unilateral or bilateral,

and radiates to the buttock. The facet joints are well seen on MRI and may show OA, an effusion or a ganglion cyst. Direct corticosteroid injections into the joints under imaging may help but their long-term value is unclear. Physiotherapy to reduce hyperlordosis and weight reduction are helpful.

Management of mechanical back pain

Adequate analgesia to allow normal mobility and avoidance of bed rest is best, combined with physical treatments such as physiotherapy, back muscle training regimens and manipulation. Manipulation produces more rapid pain relief in some patients. Acupuncture may help. Re-education in lifting and exercises help to prevent recurrent attacks of pain. Most episodes recover, irrespective of the treatment given. A positive approach probably reduces the development of chronic pain. A comfortable sleeping position should be adopted using a mattress of medium (not hard) firmness.

Acute lumbar disc prolapse

The central disc gel may extrude into a fissure in the surrounding fibrous zone and cause acute pain and muscle spasm. These events are often self-limiting. A disc prolapse occurs when the extrusion extends beyond the limits of the fibrous zone (see **Fig. 18.9**). The weakest point is posterolateral, where the disc may impinge on emerging spinal nerve roots in the root canal.

The episode often starts dramatically during lifting, twisting or bending, and produces a typical combination of low back pain and muscle spasm, and severe, lancinating pains, paraesthesia, numbness and neurological signs in one leg (rarely both). The back pain is diffuse and usually unilateral, and radiates into the buttock. The muscle spasm leads to a scoliosis that reduces when lying down. The nerve root pain develops with, or soon after, the onset. The site of the pain and other symptoms are determined by the root affected (**Box 18.14**). A central high lumbar disc prolapse may cause spinal cord compression and long tract signs (i.e. upper motor neurone). Below L2/L3, it produces lower motor neurone lesions.

Examination

On examination, the back often shows a marked scoliosis and muscle spasm. The straight-leg-raising test, while the patient is lying, is positive in a lower lumbar disc prolapse – raising the straight leg beyond 30° produces pain radiating down the leg further than the knee. Slight limitation or pain in the back limiting this movement is seen with mechanical back pain. Pain in the affected leg produced by a straight raise of the other leg suggests a large or central disc

---

> ℹ **Box 18.14 Lumbar nerve root entrapment: symptoms and signs**

Nerve root	Sensory changes	Reflex loss	Weakness	Usual disc prolapse
L2	Front of thigh	None	Hip flexion/ adduction	L1/2
L3	Inner thigh and knee	Knee	Knee extension	L2/3
L4	Inner calf	Knee	Knee extension	L3/4
L5	Outer calf	None	Inversion of foot	L4/5
	Upper, inner foot		Dorsiflexion of toes	
S1	Posterior calf	Ankle	Plantar flexion of foot	L5/S1
	Lateral border of foot			

prolapse. Look for perianal sensory loss and urinary retention or incontinence, which indicate a cauda equina lesion – a neurosurgical emergency (see p. 893). An upper lumbar disc prolapse produces a positive femoral stretch test: pain in the anterior thigh when the knee is flexed in the prone position.

Management

Advise a short period (2–3 days) of bed rest, lying flat for a lower disc but semi-reclining for a high lumbar disc, and prescribe analgesia and muscle relaxants. Once the pain is tolerable, encourage the patient to mobilize and refer them to a physiotherapist for exercises and preventative advice. The investigation of choice is MRI, which identifies the abnormal disc and any compressed nerves. An imaging-guided epidural or nerve root canal injection reduces pain rapidly, although the evidence that it speeds resolution or prevents surgery is unclear. Caudal epidural injections are less effective than lumbar ones. Resuscitation equipment must be available for these procedures. Referral to a surgeon for possible microdiscectomy or hemi-laminectomy is necessary if the neurological signs are severe, if the pain persists and is severe for more than 6–10 weeks, or if the disc is central. If bladder or anal sphincter tone is affected, it becomes a neurosurgical emergency.

Spinal and root canal stenosis

Progressive loss of disc height, OA of the facet joints, posterolateral osteophytes and buckling of the ligamentum flavum all contribute to root canal stenosis. These changes cause nerve root pain or spinal root claudication – pain and paraesthesiae in a root distribution brought on by walking and relieved slowly by rest. The associated sensory symptoms, slower recovery when the patient rests, and presence of normal foot pulses distinguish this from peripheral arterial claudication. Severe cervical spondylosis may also produce spinal claudication, often with arm symptoms and signs.

The investigation of choice to identify the location and extent of stenosis is MRI. Spinal canal stenosis at more than one level is often associated with severe spondylosis and/or a congenitally narrow spinal canal. It causes buttock and bilateral leg pain, 'heaviness', paraesthesiae and numbness when walking. Rest helps, as does bending forwards, a manoeuvre that opens the spinal canal. Specialist surgical advice is necessary.

Spondylolisthesis

This condition occurs in adolescents and young adults when bilateral congenital pars interarticularis defects cause instability and permit a vertebra to slip, with or without preceding injury. Rarely, a cauda equina syndrome develops, with loss of bladder and anal sphincter control, and saddle-distribution anaesthesia. It is diagnosed radiologically and can be seen on plain radiographs, though MRI may be necessary if entrapment of nerve roots or cauda equina syndrome is suspected. Low back pain in adolescents warrants investigation, and spondylolisthesis requires orthopaedic assessment. It needs monitoring during the growth spurt.

A degenerative spondylolisthesis may also develop in older people with lumbar spondylosis and OA of the facet joints.

Diffuse idiopathic skeletal hyperostosis

Diffuse idiopathic skeletal hyperostosis (DISH, or Forestier's disease) affects the spine and extraspinal locations. It causes bony overgrowths and ligamentous ossification, and is characterized by flowing calcification over the anterolateral aspects of the vertebrae. The spine is stiff but not always painful, despite the dramatic changes seen on plain radiographs, which are the imaging investigation of choice. Ossification at muscle insertions around the pelvis produces radiological 'whiskering'. Similar changes occur at the patella and in the feet. It is more common in people with metabolic syndrome (high body mass index (BMI), diabetes mellitus, hypertension and dyslipidaemia; see p. 1250).

Management is with analgesics or NSAIDs for pain, and exercise to retain movement and muscle strength.

Osteoporotic crush fracture of the spine

Osteoporosis is asymptomatic but leads to an increased risk of fracture of peripheral bones, particularly neck of femur and wrist, and thoracic or lumbar vertebral crush fractures. Such vertebral fractures may develop with no or minimal trauma. They may develop painlessly or cause agonizing localized pain that radiates around the ribs and abdomen. Multiple fractures lead to an increased thoracic kyphosis. They cause disability and reduced quality of life. The diagnosis is confirmed by X-rays, showing loss of anterior vertebral body height and wedging, with sparing of the vertebral endplates and pedicles. Bone oedema on MRI indicates that a fracture is recent. An underlying tumour and pathological fracture need to be excluded.

Management

Advise bed rest and analgesia until the severe pain subsides over a few weeks, then gradual mobilization. It may warrant hospitalization, and the prescription of intravenous bisphosphonates or subcutaneous or nasal calcitonin to relieve pain. There may be some residual pain and deformity.

The role of percutaneous vertebroplasty and balloon kyphoplasty remains unclear; there are no randomized controlled trials (RCTs) showing any benefit. Both involve inserting a needle through a pedicle into the affected vertebral body under CT guidance with the aim of stabilizing the fracture. Kyphoplasty involves inflating a balloon filled with methyl methacrylate cement in order to restore vertebral shape. Vertebroplasty is the injection of cement alone, without restoring vertebral shape. Pain relief is usual with both but the risks are higher with vertebroplasty.

Bone density measurement and preventative treatment of osteoporosis are essential (see p. 477).

Septic discitis

Septic discitis may cause severe pain and rapid adjacent vertebral destruction. It is seen on MRI and requires urgent neurosurgical referral.

Ankylosing spondylitis

Buttock pain and low back stiffness in a young adult suggest axial spondyloarthritis (e.g. ankylosing spondylitis) (see p. 448), especially if they are worse at night and in the morning.

Pain in the hip

'Hip' refers to a wide area between the upper buttock, trochanter and groin. It is useful to ask the patient to point to the site of pain and its field of radiation (**Box 18.15**).

Osteoarthritis of the hip

OA (see p. 433) is the most common cause of hip joint pain in a person over the age of 50 years. It gives rise to pain in the buttock and groin on standing and walking. Stiff hip movements cause difficulty in putting on a sock and may produce a limp. Sudden-onset pain may be associated with an effusion on MRI and can be treated by an ultrasound-guided steroid injection. Severe hip OA is characterized by pain and limitation even at rest and abnormal gait. In severe cases, total hip replacement is the only successful therapy.

Lateral hip pain syndrome: trochanteric bursitis and gluteus medius tendonopathy

This syndrome may be due to trochanteric bursitis and caused by trauma or unaccustomed exercise. It also occurs in inflammatory arthritis. The pain over the trochanter is worse on going up stairs, lying on that side in bed and crossing the legs. The best management is unclear but exercises help, as may a local corticosteroid injection, although the evidence base for treatment is poor. Surgery is rarely necessary. Lateral hip pain may be referred from the upper lumbar spine. A tear of the gluteus medius tendon at its insertion into the trochanter causes a similar syndrome but does not respond to injection.

Meralgia paraesthetica

This condition causes numbness and burning dysaesthesia (increased sensitivity to light touch) over the anterolateral thigh, and may be precipitated by a sudden increase in weight, an injury or pelvic surgery. It is usually self-limiting but can be helped by amitriptyline or gabapentin at night.

Fracture of the femoral neck

This fracture usually occurs after a fall, occasionally spontaneously. There is pain in the groin and thigh, weight-bearing is painful or impossible, and the leg is shortened and externally rotated. Occasionally, a fracture is not displaced and remains undetected. X-rays are diagnostic. Anyone with a hip fracture, especially after minimal trauma, should be reviewed for osteoporosis (see p. 477).

Avascular necrosis (osteonecrosis) of the femoral head

This condition is uncommon but occurs at any age. (Risk factors are discussed on p. 482.) There is severe hip pain. X-rays are diagnostic after a few weeks, when a well-demarcated area of increased bone density is visible at the upper pole of the femoral head. The affected bone may collapse. Early, the X-ray is normal but bone scintigraphy or MRI demonstrates the lesion and shows bone marrow oedema.

Inflammatory arthritis of the hip

Inflammatory arthritis produces pain in the groin and stiffness, which is worse in the morning. RA rarely presents with hip pain, although the hip is involved eventually in severe RA. Ankylosing spondylitis and other seronegative spondyloarthropathies cause inflammatory hip arthritis in younger people.

Polymyalgia rheumatica

Bilateral hip, buttock and thigh pain and stiffness that are worse in the morning in an elderly patient may be attributable to polymyalgia rheumatica (see p. 464). Neck and shoulder pain and stiffness are usually also present.

Pain in the knee

The knee depends on ligaments and quadriceps muscle strength for stability. It is frequently injured, particularly during sports. Trauma or overuse of the knee leads to a variety of peri- and intra-articular problems. Some are self-limiting; others require physiotherapy, local corticosteroid injections or surgery.

Painful knee problems can be divided into those that arise within the joint and those that arise in the soft tissues around the joint (**Box 18.16**). Only problems arising within the joint are likely to cause accumulation of fluid (effusion). Identification and aspiration of fluid from effusions are relevant diagnostic procedures.

Knee joint effusions

An effusion of the knee causes swelling, stiffness and pain. The pain is more severe with an acute onset and with increasing inflammation because the capsule that contains the pain receptors is stretched. A full clinical history must include a past medical, family and drug history.

Examination

A large and tense effusion is easily seen and felt on each side of the patella and in the suprapatellar pouch, and is fluctuant. The effusion delays the patella tapping against the femur when it is pressed firmly and quickly with the knee held straight and relaxed (the 'patellar tap' sign). Small effusions also demonstrate the 'bulge' sign when the patient is lying with the quadriceps relaxed. For this test, apply a gentle sweeping pressure, first to the medial side of the joint and then, watching the medial dimple, to the lateral side. Slightly delayed bulging of the medial dimple indicates fluid in the joint.

? Box 18.15 Pain in the hip: causes

Hip region problems	Main sites of pain
Osteoarthritis of hip	Groin, buttock, front of thigh to knee
Trochanteric bursitis (or gluteus medius tendonopathy)	Lateral thigh to knee
Meralgia paraesthetica	Anterolateral thigh to knee
Referred from back	Buttock
Facet joint pain	Buttock and posterior thigh
Fracture of neck of femur	Groin and buttock
Inflammatory arthritis	Groin, buttock, front of thigh to knee
Sacroiliitis (ankylosing spondylitis)	Buttock(s)
Avascular necrosis	Groin and buttocks
Polymyalgia rheumatica	Lumbar spine, buttocks and thighs

? Box 18.16 Pain in the knee: causes

Problems arising within the joint
- Osteoarthritis
- Inflammatory arthritis
- Meniscal tear
- Cruciate ligament tear
- Chondromalacia
- Osteochondritis dissecans
- Spontaneous osteonecrosis of the knee

Problems arising in tissues around the joint

Medial
- Medial ligament strain
- Anserine bursitis

Anterior
- Pre-patellar bursitis
- Infrapatellar bursitis
- Quadriceps tendon enthesitis
- Osgood–Schlatter disease

Posterior
- Popliteal (Baker's) cyst

Other
- Hypermobility syndrome
- Referred from hip joint

Trauma and overuse

Investigations

These are:

- blood tests (urate, blood cultures)
- aspiration (see **Fig. 18.2**) and examination of the knee effusion.

The basic technique of aspiration is described in **Box 18.7**. If the fluid obtained is very cloudy, septic arthritis (or occasionally gout) is the likeliest diagnosis. Slightly cloudy or blood-stained fluid that does not clot is likely to indicate pseudogout. Frank blood that clots suggests a haemarthrosis. Fluid should be sent for Gram-stain and culture if sepsis is suspected. It should be sent for polarized light microscopy if looking for crystals (see p. 436).

Pain arising from within the knee

Osteoarthritis of the knee

Minor radiographic changes of OA (see **Fig. 18.16**) are very common in those aged over 50 years and do not usually cause pain, which is more likely to arise from surrounding soft tissues. X-ray appearances and the degree of pain felt in OA of the knee are not closely correlated. Marked valgus, varus or fixed flexion deformities suggest severe OA. For severe cases, surgery, usually total knee replacement, is the treatment of choice. In milder cases, pain relief, physiotherapy and, sometimes, intra-articular corticosteroid injections may help.

Inflammatory arthritis of the knee

Monoarthritis of the knee, associated with severe pain and marked redness, may be due to septic arthritis, gout or pseudogout. A cool, clear, viscous effusion is seen in elderly people with moderate or severe symptomatic OA (see p. 434). RA rarely presents with knee involvement alone, though seronegative spondyloarthritis may do so.

Haemarthrosis of the knee

This condition is caused by:

- trauma: meniscal, cruciate or synovial lining tear
- clotting or bleeding disorders, e.g. haemophilia, sickle cell disease or von Willebrand's disease.

Torn meniscus

The menisci are partially attached fibrocartilages that stabilize the rounded femoral condyles on the flat tibial plateaux. In the young, they are resilient, but this decreases with age. They can be torn by an injury, commonly in sports that involve twisting and bending. The history is usually diagnostic. There is immediate medial or lateral knee pain and swelling within a few hours. The affected side is tender. If the tear is large, the knee may lock flexed. The immediate treatment is to apply ice. MRI demonstrates the tear (**Fig. 18.10**). In most circumstances, especially in active sportspeople, early arthroscopic repair or trimming of the torn meniscus is essential. Surgical intervention reduces recurrent pain, swelling and locking but not the risk of secondary OA. In older patients with OA plus meniscal tear, surgery is no more effective than physiotherapy alone. The long-term benefit of early repair of tears is not yet known. Post-surgical quadriceps exercises aid a return to sport and other activities.

Torn cruciate ligaments

Torn cruciate ligaments account for around 70% of knee haemarthroses in young people. They often coexist with a meniscal tear. Partial cruciate tears are difficult to diagnose clinically. On flexing the knee to 90°, a torn anterior cruciate allows the tibia to be pulled forwards on the femur. MRI is the investigation of choice. Such

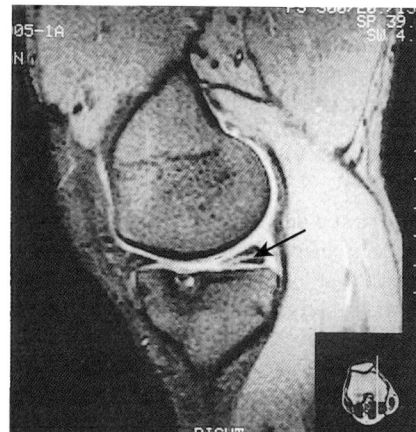

Fig. 18.10 Magnetic resonance image of a knee. A complete tear of the posterior horn of the medial meniscus is shown, extending to its lower surface (arrowed).

injuries need urgent orthopaedic referral, reconstructive surgery usually being necessary in young active adults. There is a significant incidence of secondary OA.

Chondromalacia patellae

This diagnosis is made arthroscopically. The retropatellar cartilage is fibrillated. In most cases, the pain settles eventually. When there is patellar misalignment, it may need surgery, as does recurrent patellar dislocation in adolescent girls.

Osteochondritis dissecans

This condition occasionally causes knee pain and swelling in adolescents and young adults, more commonly males. It is probably traumatic, possibly with hereditary predisposing factors. A fragment of bone and its attached cartilage detach by shearing, most commonly from the lateral aspect of the medial femoral condyle.

There is aching pain after activity and, if the fragment becomes loose, locking or 'giving way' occurs. The lesion is seen on a tunnel-view X-ray but MRI is more sensitive, especially if the fragment is undisplaced. Undisplaced lesions are treated with rest, then isometric quadriceps exercises. Loose fragments can be fixed arthroscopically or removed. A similar lesion affecting the lateral femoral condyle occurs in older people.

Spontaneous osteonecrosis of the knee

Osteonecrosis may occur spontaneously or after injury. There is local pain and there are marked bone marrow changes on MRI (**Fig. 18.11A**) or single-photon emission computed tomography (SPECT; **Fig. 18.11B**). In particular, weight-bearing must be avoided. Pamidronate by infusion is sometimes used. Spontaneous osteonecrosis of the knee (SONK) may progress to bone infarction and require replacement surgery.

Pain from structures around the knee

Medial knee pain

There may be medial or lateral ligament strain but the medial ligament is more commonly affected. There is pain at the ligament's insertion into the upper medial tibia, which is worsened by standing or stressing the affected ligament.

Anserine bursitis causes pain and localized tenderness 2–3 cm below the posteromedial joint line in the upper part of the tibia at

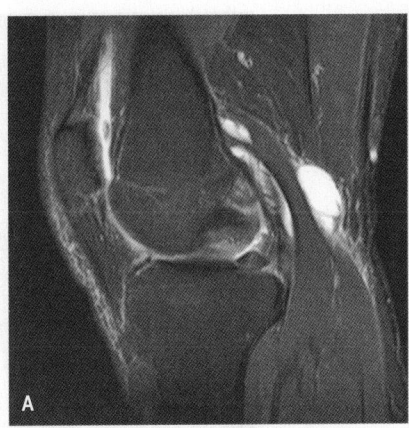 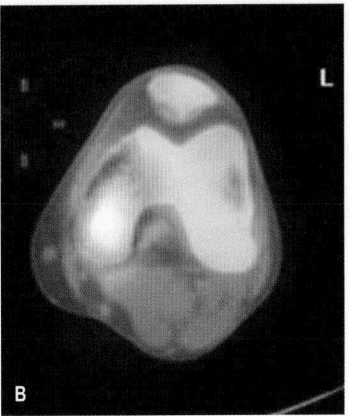

Fig. 18.11 Spontaneous osteonecrosis of the knee. **(A)** Magnetic resonance image showing a high signal in the posterior aspect of the femoral condyle, a small effusion and a popliteal cyst. **(B)** Single-photon emission computed tomography (SPECT) image showing a high signal in the posterior medial femoral condyle.

the site of the bursa. It occurs in obese women, often with valgus deformities, and in breast-stroke swimmers.

Management is with physiotherapy and a local corticosteroid injection.

Anterior knee pain

Anterior knee pain is common in adolescence. In many cases, no specific cause is found, despite investigation. This is called 'anterior knee pain syndrome' and settles with time. Isometric quadriceps exercises and avoidance of high heels both help the condition. Patients and parents often need firm reassurance. Abnormal patellar tracking may be a cause and may need surgical treatment. Hypermobility of joints causes joint pain, maltracking and, rarely, recurrent patellar dislocation (see also p. 432).

Pre- and infrapatellar bursitis

This can occur in patients whose jobs involve frequent kneeling ('housemaid's knee', 'clergyman's knee', 'carpet-layer's knee'). There is local pain, tenderness and sometimes swelling. Avoidance of kneeling and a local corticosteroid injection are helpful. Septic bursitis can occur.

Osgood–Schlatter disease

Osgood–Schlatter disease causes pain and swelling over the tibial tubercle. It is a traction apophysitis of the patellar tendon and occurs particularly in teenage sports players.

Enthesitis

This may occur at the patellar end of the quadriceps tendon (jumper's knee).

Posterior knee pain

Popliteal cyst (Baker's cyst)

In approximately 5% of people with a knee effusion, a swollen, painful popliteal cyst develops. The semi-membranosus bursa in some individuals has a valve-like connection to the knee, allowing the effusion to flow into the bursa but not back. The cyst is best seen and felt in the popliteal fossa with the patient standing.

Ruptured popliteal cyst

Fluid escapes into the soft tissue of the popliteal fossa and upper calf, causing sudden and severe pain, swelling and tenderness of the upper calf.

A history of previous knee problems and the sudden onset of pain and tenderness high in the calf suggest a ruptured cyst rather than a deep vein thrombosis (DVT). A diagnostic ultrasound examination distinguishes a ruptured cyst from a DVT (see p. 1003), which can avoid inappropriate treatment with anticoagulants. Analgesics or NSAIDs, rest with the leg elevated, and aspiration and injection with corticosteroids into the knee joint are required.

Pain in the shin, calf and ankle

Sever's disease

This is a traction apophysitis of the Achilles tendon in young people (compare Osgood–Schlatter disease, p. 427).

Pain at the insertion of the Achilles tendon into the calcaneum is an enthesitis. This is traumatic or it can complicate spondyloarthritis. Raising the shoe heel reduces pain. Occasionally, a low-pressure corticosteroid injection near the enthesis is necessary.

Achilles tendonosis

This causes a painful, tender swelling a few centimetres above the tendon's insertion. Advise against walking barefoot and jumping. Tendon damage or rupture can occur with quinolone, e.g. ciprofloxacin therapy. Therapeutic ultrasound is helpful. (*Caution*: a local injection may cause the tendon to rupture.) Autologous platelet concentrates are used but evidence of efficacy is poor. Procedures to remove or sclerose new blood vessels in the inflamed areas may help.

Achilles bursitis

This lies clearly anterior to the tendon and can be safely injected with corticosteroid.

Compartment syndromes

The muscles of the lower leg are enclosed in fascial compartments, with little room for expansion to occur. Compartment syndromes can be acute and severe, such as following exercise.

In *anterior tibial syndrome* there is severe pain in the front of the shin, occasionally with foot drop. Immediate surgical decompression to prevent muscle necrosis is sometimes required.

? Box 18.17 Pain in the foot and heel: causes

Foot pain
- Structural – flat (pronated) or high-arched (supinated)
- Hallux valgus/rigidus (± osteo-arthritis)
- Metatarsalgia
- Morton's neuroma
- Stress fracture
- Inflammatory arthritis
- Acute, monoarticular – gout
- Chronic, polyarticular – rheumatoid arthritis
- Chronic, pauciarticular – spondyloarthritis
- Tarsal tunnel syndrome

Heel pain
- Plantar fasciitis: below heel
- Plantar spur: below heel
- Achilles tendonitis/bursitis: behind heel
- Sever's disease: behind heel
- Arthritis of ankle/subtaloid joints

Chronic compartment syndrome produces pain in the lower leg that is aggravated by exercise and may therefore be mistaken for a vascular or neurological disorder.

Pain in the foot

See **Box 18.17**. The feet are subjected to extreme pressures by weight-bearing and inappropriate shoes. They are commonly painful. Broad, deep, thick-soled shoes are essential for sporting activities, prolonged walking or standing, and in people with congenitally flat or arthritic feet.

There are two common types of foot deformity:
- *Flat feet.* These stress the ankle and throw the hindfoot into a valgus (everted) position. A flat foot is rigid and inflexible.
- *High-arched feet.* These place pressure on the lateral border and ball of the foot.

The foot is affected by a variety of inflammatory arthritic conditions. After the hand, the foot joints are the most commonly affected by RA. The diagnosis depends on assessment of the distribution of the joints affected, the pattern of other joint problems or the finding of an associated condition (e.g. psoriasis; see p. 664).

Hallux valgus

The big toe migrates laterally. In the congenital form, the first metatarsal bone is displaced medially (metatarsus primus varus). The shape of modern shoes causes later onset of hallux valgus. It is a common complication of RA.

Hallux rigidus

OA of the first metatarsophalangeal (MTP) joint in a normally aligned or valgus joint causes hallux rigidus: a stiff, dorsiflexed and painful big toe. Careful choice of footwear and the help of a podiatrist suffice for most cases but some require surgery.

Metatarsalgia

This is common, especially in women who wear high heels, after trauma and in those with hammer toes. The ball of the foot is painful to walk and stand on. Callosities and pressure-induced bursae develop under the metatarsal heads. RA causes misalignment of the metatarsal bones and severe metatarsalgia.

Management is with podiatry and the wearing of appropriate shoes. Surgery is occasionally needed, particularly in the rheumatoid forefoot.

Morton's neuroma

This usually occurs between the third and fourth metatarsal heads. It causes pain, burning and numbness in the adjacent surfaces

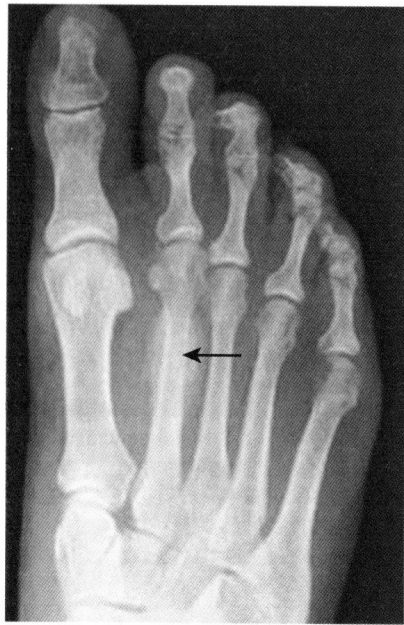

Fig. 18.12 Callus forming around a stress fracture. The image shows a stress fracture of the second metatarsal at 4 weeks. X-rays initially were normal.

of the affected toes when walking. It is helped by wearing wider, cushion-soled shoes. Occasionally, a steroid injection or excision is necessary.

Stress fractures of the metatarsals

These cause sudden, severe, weight-bearing pain in the distal shaft of the fractured metatarsal bone. They occur after unaccustomed walking or with new shoes. There is local tenderness and swelling, but initially X-rays are normal and diagnosis delayed (**Fig. 18.12**). A radioisotope bone scan or MRI reveals the fracture earlier than X-rays. Reduced weight-bearing for a few weeks usually suffices. Underlying osteoporosis may be a cause.

Tarsal tunnel syndrome

This is an entrapment neuropathy of the posterior tibial nerve at the medial malleolus. It produces burning, tingling and numbness of the toes, sole and medial arch. The nerve is tender below the malleolus and, when tapped, produces a shock-like pain (Tinel's sign). A local steroid injection under the retinaculum, between the medial malleolus and calcaneum, is helpful.

Pain under the heel

See **Box 18.17**.

Plantar fasciitis

This is an enthesitis at the insertion of the plantar fascia into the calcaneum. It produces localized pain under the heel when standing and walking, and local tenderness. It occurs alone or in spondyloarthritis. Obesity, particularly in flat-footed people who walk a lot, can predispose to plantar fasciitis.

Plantar spurs

These are traction lesions at the insertion of the plantar fascia in older people and are usually asymptomatic. They become painful after trauma.

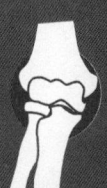

Calcaneal bursitis

This is a pressure-induced (adventitious) bursa that produces diffuse pain and tenderness under the heel. Compression of the heel pad from the sides is painful, which distinguishes it from plantar fascia pain.

Clinical features and management of heel pain

Whatever the cause, heel pain is always worse in the morning as soon as weight is placed on the foot.

All these lesions are treated with heel pads, and reduced walking; they are often self-limiting. A dorsiflexion splint at night to stretch the plantar fascia is worth trying. When an injection is necessary, a medial approach is used, rather than advancing through the heel pad, often under ultrasound guidance.

Pain in the chest

Musculoskeletal conditions are sometimes a cause of chest pain. An example is Tietze's disease. In this condition, pain arises from the costosternal junctions. It is usually unilateral and affects one, two or three ribs. There is local tenderness, which helps to make the diagnosis. The condition is benign and self-limiting. It often responds well to anti-inflammatory drugs. Other causes of chest wall pain include rib fractures due to trauma, osteoporosis or a malignant deposit. Costochondral pain occurs in ankylosing spondylitis (see p. 448). In people with heart disease, costochondral pain may cause severe anxiety but it is not like angina and the patient should be reassured.

Pain associated with sport and the performing arts

Pain in muscles and soft tissues is common after sport or associated with performing arts, such as dancing or playing musical instruments. General advice, such as warming up properly and using appropriate supportive footwear for running, can help. However, in cases of prolonged pain or where the person suffering pain is a professional sportsperson or performer, referral to a sports medicine specialist is advisable.

Further reading
Balagué F, Mannion A, Pellise F et al. Non-specific low back pain. *Lancet* 2012; 379:482–491.
Coombes BK, Bisset L, Vicenzino B. Efficacy and safety of corticosteroid injections and other injections for management of tendinopathy: a systematic review of randomised controlled trials. *Lancet* 2010; 376:1751–1767.
Ensrud KE, Schousboe JT. Clinical practice. Vertebral fractures. *N Engl J Med* 2011; 364:1634–1642.
Klazan CA, Lohle PN, de Vries J et al. Vertebroplasty versus conservative treatment in acute osteoporotic vertebral compression fractures: an open-labelled study. *Lancet* 2010; 376:1085–1092.
Lamb SE, Hansen Z, Lall R et al. Group cognitive behavioural therapy for low back pain in primary care. *Lancet* 2010; 375:916–923.
Ropper AH, Zafonte RD. Sciatica. *N Engl J Med* 2015; 372:1240–1248.

CHRONIC PAIN SYNDROMES

Chronic pain is defined as pain lasting more than 3 months (the natural tissue-healing time). Many rheumatological illnesses (e.g. RA and OA) cause pain of such duration but are not considered as chronic pain syndromes. In chronic pain syndromes, the pain generally has no clear structural cause or curative treatment and is often combined with psychological distress, poor sleep and altered use of the

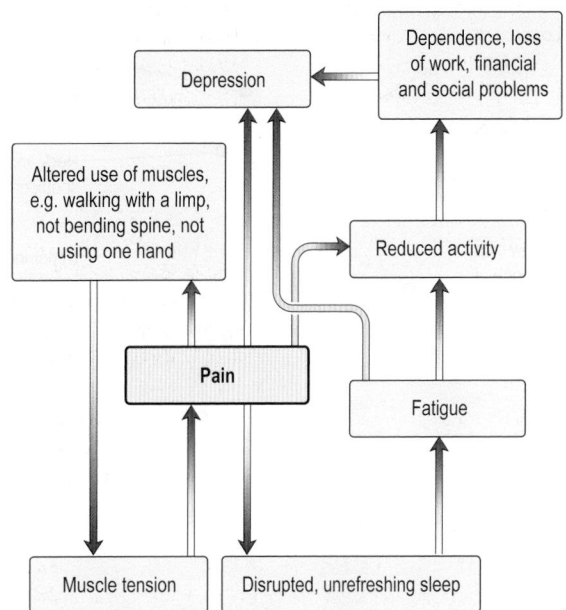

Fig. 18.13 Interaction of physical and psychological factors in chronic widespread pain.

muscles due to the pain (called fear-avoidance behaviour or abnormal pain behaviour). This altered behaviour can lead to more stress and tension in the muscles, exacerbating the pain (**Fig. 18.13**).

The pain suffered by these patients is neither imaginary nor artefactual, even though there may be no structural abnormality in the painful area. There is a problem with the pain processing system in the nervous system, leading to amplification of pain signals. Psychological factors often contribute to this amplification, and the pain can make psychological distress worse, in a vicious circle. The combination of physical pain and psychological distress makes these syndromes difficult to manage.

Living with chronic pain is difficult. Patients may become anxious, depressed or socially isolated, and their quality of life is reduced. There are often adverse effects on employment, personal relationships and dependence on others. Consultations need to address these issues, as well as the pain itself, to be effective. In chronic pain syndromes, patients need help to lead a more normal life despite their pain, and are best referred to a specialist, multidisciplinary pain service. Medications alone are not the answer.

These syndromes can be conveniently subdivided into chronic widespread pain (above and below the waist and on both sides of the body) and chronic regional pain (any other distribution). Both are very common. Epidemiological studies show that the prevalence of chronic widespread pain is 10–11% and that of chronic regional pain 20–30%.

Chronic widespread pain

Pain that starts in a single area can spread to other areas of the body, as more muscles become tense and tender. Conversely, patients with chronic widespread pain can develop new, localized causes of pain (e.g. appendicitis, OA) that can be treated successfully. It should not be assumed that every pain in these patients is always due to the same chronic problem.

Two of the main causes of chronic widespread pain are fibromyalgia and hypermobility spectrum disorders (see p. 432).

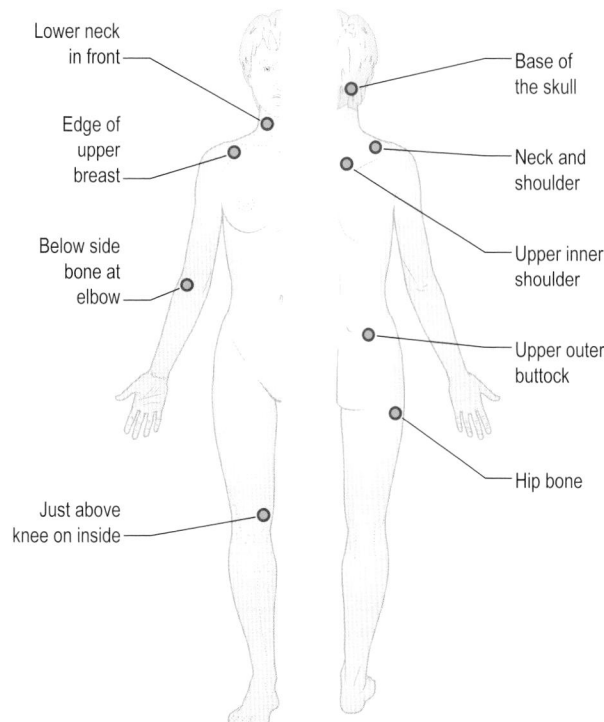

Fig. 18.14 Trigger points in fibromyalgia.

Fibromyalgia

Fibromyalgia is not a diagnosis of exclusion. It can occur in patients who have other illnesses like RA and SLE. Individuals suffer chronic widespread pain with disrupted and unrefreshing sleep, constant tiredness and tender points detectable on pressing their muscles (**Fig. 18.14**). Multiple other symptoms, such as irritable bowel syndrome (IBS), tension headaches, dysmenorrhoea, atypical facial or chest pain and forgetfulness, often coexist. It occurs in about 1 in 50 people, can develop at any age and affects women more than men (2:1). The diagnosis is clinical, and blood tests and imaging are normal. These tests may be requested to exclude other causes of pain.

Management

See p. 771. A clear explanation of the diagnosis is vital. While being honest about the fact that there is no cure for fibromyalgia, it is also necessary to reassure the patient that it is not arthritis and that the pain is not causing damage to joints or muscles. Many patients have never had an explanation of the cause of their symptoms, which leads to fear and doubt. Treatment options that can be offered to help (not cure) are described below. Management guidelines stress use of non-drug measures instead of or alongside drugs.

Drugs

There is evidence from clinical trials for use of analgesics, anticonvulsants and antidepressants. Commonly used drugs include amitriptyline (which may also improve sleep), pregabalin, paracetamol, tramadol and gabapentin. Benefits, however, are often short-term and adverse effects common.

Non-drug therapies

A sympathetic, psychosocial, multidisciplinary approach is appropriate. A graded, supervised aerobic exercise regimen over 3 months is safe and effective. When depression is present, it should be treated.

Cognitive behavioural therapy can help the person to pace their life more effectively and to cope better. Pain management programmes, combining psychology with physiotherapy, are designed to improve physical function and quality of life but do not reduce pain intensity. Acupuncture can lessen pain in some cases but the effect is usually transient.

Chronic regional pain

Chronic (work-related) upper-limb pain syndrome

This term is preferred to 'repetitive strain injury' (RSI). The predominant symptoms are pain in all or part of one or both arms. A specific lesion, such as tennis elbow or carpal tunnel syndrome, or muscular-pattern neck pain often develops first, and early recognition and treatment may prevent chronicity. After a variable period, the pain becomes more diffuse and no longer simply work-related, and there is often severe distress. It is seen in keyboard workers and in musicians. When it arises at work, it is often at a time of stress, such as changing work practices, shortage of staff or disharmony.

Management

If possible, there should be a brief period off work and a gradual return to activity as the pain settles. Use of analgesia and NSAIDs, with physiotherapy, is helpful during the initial phase to prevent a vicious circle developing. Amitriptyline or pregabalin is helpful for some patients.

A review of working practices and the positioning of screen, keyboard and chair are essential, as is support of the patient by their manager. Musicians are helped by expert advice on playing technique and should reduce playing times temporarily, but not stop completely.

Temporomandibular pain dysfunction syndrome

This pain syndrome is a disorder of the temporomandibular joint that is associated with nocturnal tooth grinding or abnormalities of bite. It occurs in anxious people. It gives rise to pain in one or both temporomandibular joints.

Dental correction of the bite helps a few, but when no dental cause is found, low-dose tricyclic antidepressant therapy is used. Many patients are made worse by unnecessary dental treatment.

Complex regional pain syndrome

Complex regional pain syndrome (CRPS) is a rare condition (prevalence 20:100000), in which regional neuropathic pain is associated with abnormal sensory, autonomic, motor and/or trophic changes. There are two types. In CRPS type I, there is no identifiable overt nerve lesion, whereas such a lesion is identifiable in CRPS type II. CRPS usually occurs after trauma but the pain is disproportionate in time or intensity to that usually caused by such an injury. It may also develop after central nervous system lesions (e.g. strokes) or without cause.

Its features are pain and other sensory abnormalities, including hyperaesthesia; and autonomic vasomotor dysfunction, leading to abnormal blood flow and sweating; and motor system abnormalities, leading to structural changes of superficial and deep tissues (trophic changes). Not all components need be present. The sensory, motor and sympathetic nerve changes are not restricted to the distribution of a single nerve and may be remote from the site of

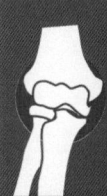

injury. The early phase, with pain, swelling and increased skin temperature, is difficult to diagnose but potentially reversible.

After a period of weeks or months, a second, still painful, dystrophic phase develops, characterized by articular stiffness, cold skin and trophic changes, often with localized osteoporosis.

A late phase involves continued pain, skin and muscle atrophy, and muscle contractures, and is extremely disabling.

Diagnosis is clinical – a high index of suspicion and recognition of the unusual distribution of the pain. There are no specific or sensitive investigations, though demineralization may be seen on X-ray. Bone scan and MRI are not required to make the diagnosis.

Management

Management is difficult and the problem often very disabling. The evidence base for treatment is poor. Early diagnosis, effective pain relief and general care of the patient are essential. NSAIDs, tricyclic antidepressants, serotonin–norepinephrine reuptake inhibitors, and pregabalin or gabapentin are used in the early phase, together with active exercise of the limb, encouraged by a physiotherapist. Intravenous bisphosphonates can also be effective. Referral to a specialist pain clinic is essential. Nerve blocks were used in the past but are less common now. Intravenous immunoglobulins have been used in clinical trials but are not yet an accepted therapy.

Further reading
Fukushima FB, Bezerra DM, Vilas Boas PJF et al. Complex regional pain syndrome. *Br Med J* 2014; 348:g3683.
Macfarlane GJ, Kronisch C, Dean LE et al. EULAR revised recommendations for the management of fibromyalgia. *Ann Rheum Dis* 2017; 76:318–328.
Rahman A, Underwood, M, Carnes D. Fibromyalgia. *Br Med J* 2014; 348:g1224.

ANALGESIC AND ANTI-INFLAMMATORY DRUGS FOR MUSCULOSKELETAL PROBLEMS

The key to using drugs, particularly in chronic disorders and the elderly, is to balance risk and benefit and to review their appropriateness constantly. **Box 18.18** shows the main drugs available.

Simple and compound analgesic agents

Simple agents, such as paracetamol, aspirin or codeine compounds (or combination preparations), used when necessary or regularly, relieve pain and improve function. Sleep may also be improved. Side-effects are relatively infrequent, although drowsiness and constipation occur with codeine preparations, especially in the elderly.

Stronger analgesics, such as dihydrocodeine, tramadol or morphine derivatives, should be used only for severe pain.

Non-steroidal anti-inflammatory drugs

Non-steroidal anti-inflammatory drugs (NSAIDs) have anti-inflammatory and centrally acting analgesic properties. They inhibit cyclo-oxygenase (COX), a key enzyme in the formation of prostaglandins, prostacyclins and thromboxanes (see p. 1176). There are two specific cyclo-oxygenase enzymes:
- **COX-1** is the constitutive form present in many normal tissues.
- **COX-2** is the form mainly induced in response to pro-inflammatory cytokines and is not found in most normal tissues

Box 18.18 Analgesics and NSAIDs

Drug	Dose	Frequency
Analgesics[a]		
To be taken only if needed. Maximum doses are indicated.		
Paracetamol	500–1000 mg	6-hourly
Paracetamol (500 mg) and codeine (8–30 mg)	1–2 tablets	6-hourly
Dihydrocodeine	30–60 mg	Every 6–8 h
Paracetamol with dihydrocodeine (e.g. 'Co-dydramol' preparations)	1–2 tablets	Every 6–8 h
Non-steroidal anti-inflammatory drugs (NSAIDs)		
Always to be taken with food. Slow-release preparations are used in inflammatory conditions or if more regular pain control is needed. Examples are shown.		
Ibuprofen	200–400 mg	Every 6–8 h
Ibuprofen slow-release	600–800 mg	12-hourly
Diclofenac	25–50 mg	8-hourly
Diclofenac slow-release	75–100 mg	×1–2 daily
Naproxen	250 mg	×3–4 daily
Naproxen slow-release	550 mg	×2 daily
Celecoxib[b]	100–200 mg	×2 daily

[a]In order of potency. [b]COX-2-specific NSAID (coxib).

(except the kidney). It is associated with oedema and the nociceptive and pyretic effects of inflammation.

Effects and side-effects

Most of the older NSAIDs are non-specific and block both enzymes but with variable specificity ('non-specific NSAIDs', or nsNSAIDs). Their therapeutic effect depends on blocking COX-2 and their side-effects mainly on blocking COX-1. COX-1 protects the gastric mucosa and blocking it accounts for the majority of upper gastrointestinal side-effects.

The most common side-effects with non-specific NSAIDs are indigestion or skin rashes. More serious upper gastrointestinal side-effects are gastric erosions and peptic ulceration with perforation and bleeding. These occur more frequently in the elderly, in whom mortality is higher, in long-term use, and in those with high-risk factors: a history of ulcers, *Helicobacter pylori*, and concurrent corticosteroid or anticoagulant therapy. Ibuprofen, in combination with low-dose aspirin, significantly increases the risk of severe gastrointestinal bleeding. Practice guidelines recommend proton pump inhibitors in high-gastrointestinal-risk patients on non-specific NSAIDs. H_2 blockers are less effective as gastroprotective agents. Prostaglandin E_2 analogues, such as misoprostol, reduce ulcer complications and are popular, but may cause nausea and diarrhoea. Lower gastrointestinal side-effects of non-specific NSAIDs are becoming more common.

COX-2 inhibitors ('coxibs') produce fewer gastrointestinal side-effects but these still occur. Coxibs are used in patients who have a high risk of gastrointestinal disease but are avoided in patients with cardiovascular risks. In fact, all NSAIDs except naproxen can cause an increase in risk of cardiovascular events, such as myocardial infarction or stroke. All these drugs, including naproxen, increase the risk of heart failure.

Coxibs and NSAIDs may reduce renal function, especially in the elderly (see **Box 36.23**).

Box 18.19 The major types of collagen

Collagen structure	Type number	Encoding gene	Associated conditions
Fibrillar	I, II, III, V, XI	*COL1A1–2, COL2A2, COL3, COL5, COL11*	Osteogenesis imperfecta, Ehlers–Danlos syndrome (subtypes)
Basement membrane	IV	*COL4A1–5*	Alport's syndrome (see p. 1362)
Fibril-associated collagen with interrupted triple helix (FACIT)	IX, XII, XIV	*COL9, 12, 14*	
Filament-producing	VI	*COL6A1–3*	
Network-forming	VIII, X	*COL8A1, 10A1*	
Anchoring fibril	VII	*COL7A1*	Epidermolysis bullosa (see p. 688)

Uses

- *In musculoskeletal pain and in OA and spondylosis*, short courses of NSAIDs or coxibs are used but simple analgesia is often more appropriate.
- *In crystal synovitis*, NSAIDs and coxibs have a true anti-inflammatory effect.
- *In chronic inflammatory synovitis*, NSAIDs and coxibs do not alter the chronic inflammatory process or decrease the risk of joint damage, but they do reduce pain and stiffness.
- *In inflammatory arthritis and situations where more constant pain control is needed*, slow-release preparations are useful.
- *In chronic arthritis*, NSAID gels have some value.

The standard advice is to use NSAID in the lowest dose possible for the shortest time necessary to control pain. Be aware of the patient's gastrointestinal and cardiac risks before prescribing NSAIDs or coxibs.

Further reading

Coxib and Traditional NSAID Trialists Collaboration. Vascular and upper gastrointestinal effects of non-steroidal anti-inflammatory drugs: meta-analyses of individual participant data from randomized trials. *Lancet* 2013; 382:769–779.
Schmidt M, Sorensen HT, Pedersen L. Diclofenac use and cardiovascular risks: series of nationwide cohort studies. *BMJ* 2018; 362:k3426.

DISORDERS OF COLLAGEN

Collagen is responsible for many of the structural, tensile and load-bearing properties in the various tissues where it is found. The structure of collagen is discussed on page 415. Thirty or more dispersed genes encode for more than 19 different types of collagen (**Box 18.19**).

Hypermobile Ehlers–Danlos syndrome and hypermobility spectrum disorders

Hypermobility is very common (15–20% of adults); it may be demonstrated by showing increased flexibility in the thumbs, little fingers, elbows, knees and lumbar spine, and quantified using the

Box 18.20 Beighton hypermobility score[a] and diagnostic criteria for joint hypermobility syndrome

Joint	Finding	Score
Little (fifth) finger	Passive dorsiflexion >90°	1 for each side
Thumb	Passive dorsiflexion to the flexor aspect of the forearm	1 for each side
Elbow	Hyperextends >10°, extends ≤10°	1 for each side
Knee	Hyperextends >10°, extends ≤10°	1 for each side
Forward flexion of trunk with the knees fully extended	Palms can rest flat on the floor	1

Diagnostic criteria for joint hypermobility syndrome: Beighton score ≥4; arthralgia for ≥3 months in ≥4 joints.

[a]In this 9-point system, the higher the score, the higher the laxity. Young adults can score 4–6.

Beighton score (**Box 18.20**). The majority of hypermobile people suffer no adverse effects from the hypermobility but in some it can cause recurrent subluxations of individual joints and/or persistent widespread musculoskeletal pains. According to the 2017 classification, these people are classified into two groups; hypermobile Ehlers–Danlos syndrome (hEDS) for those who fulfil specific classification criteria and hypermobility spectrum disorder (HSD) for those who do not. Both groups may suffer other symptoms such as bowel disturbance, easy scarring and faintness on standing (postural orthostatic tachycardia syndrome; POTS), and the combination can be very disruptive to normal life. Treatment of the musculoskeletal symptoms relies on specialist physiotherapy to advise on exercises that take the patient's hypermobility into account. Pain management programmes can be helpful in more severe cases. It is usually better to avoid surgery due to difficulties in healing.

Other forms of Ehlers–Danlos syndrome

Whereas hEDS (EDS type 5) is the most common form of EDS and has no known genetic basis, there are 12 rarer forms that have all been linked to particular genes encoding collagen or collagen modifiers. EDS types 1,4, 6 and 13 are autosomal dominant whereas the others are autosomal recessive (12 can be either). *Note:* numbering of these syndromes changed in 2017.

Marfan's syndrome

This condition is described on pages 1113–1115.

Osteogenesis imperfecta

This is a heterogeneous group of disorders inherited mainly in autosomal dominant fashion with mutations in *COL1A1* and *COL1A2* genes. There are four main types of osteogenesis imperfecta and clinical subtypes are also described (V, VI and VII). The major clinical feature is bone fragility but other collagen-containing tissues are also involved, such as tendons, skin and eyes.

- *Type I*: mild bony deformities, blue sclerae, defective dentine, early-onset deafness, hypermobility of joints and heart valve disorders
- *Type II*: death in the perinatal period
- *Type III*: severe bone deformity and blue sclerae
- *Type IV*: fewer fractures, normal sclerae, normal lifespan but can also be severe, as in type III.

Management with daily oral risedronate in children improves BMD and reduces fracture risk. Intravenous pamidronate is another option. Prognosis is variable, depending on the severity of the disease. Stem cell therapy is being used. Types I and IV are associated with normal lifespan and people with these forms continue to have increased fracture risk into adulthood.

Achondroplasia

Achondroplasia ('dwarfism') is diagnosed in the first years of life. The disease is inherited in an autosomal dominant manner and is caused by a defect in the fibroblast growth factor receptor-3 gene. The trunk is of normal length but the limbs are very short and broad due to abnormal endochondral ossification. The vault of the skull is enlarged, the face is small and the nose bridge is flat. Intelligence is normal.

Further reading

Castori M, Tinkle M, Levy H et al. A framework for the classification of joint hypermobility and related conditions. *Am J Med Genet C Semin Med Genet* 2017; 175C:148–157.
Malfait F, Francomano C, Byers P et al. The 2017 international classification of the Ehlers-Danlos syndromes. *Am J Med Genet C Semin Med Genet* 2017; 175C:8–26.

OSTEOARTHRITIS

Osteoarthritis (OA) is the most common type of arthritis. It results from damage to articular cartilage induced by an interaction of genetic, metabolic and biomechanical factors, leading to an inflammatory response affecting cartilage, subchondral bone, ligaments, menisci, synovium and capsule. Despite intense investigation, disease-modifying therapies remain elusive for this condition.

Epidemiology

Globally approximately 1 in 5 women and 1 in 10 men aged over 60 years have symptomatic OA, such that 80% have limitations in movement and 25% cannot perform major daily activities of life. Worldwide it has a variable pattern of presentation. For instance, hip OA is less common and knee OA more common in Asians than in Europeans. Beyond 55 years of age, women are affected more commonly than men by a familial pattern of inheritance in nodal and primary generalized forms of OA with variable patterns of distribution (**Fig. 18.15**). Resulting disabilities have major socioeconomic resource implications, particularly in the developed world where OA is one of the ten most disabling diseases in older adults.

Aetiology and pathogenesis

Cartilage is a matrix of water (>70%) and organic extracellular matrix components, mainly type II collagen and aggrecan or other proteoglycans (see p. 414); it has a smooth surface and shock-absorbing properties. OA is now considered a disease of the whole joint with alterations in subchondral bone, ligaments, capsule, synovial membrane as well as articular cartilage. Consequent structural changes include surface fibrillation and ulceration with loss of cartilage that exposes underlying bone to increased stress, producing microfractures and cysts leading to abnormal sclerotic subchondral bone and overgrowths at the joint margins, called osteophytes (**Fig. 18.16**). Inflammatory changes may also occur. This process produces a spectrum of OA, ranging from atrophic disease in which cartilage destruction occurs without any subchondral bone response, to hypertrophic disease with massive new bone formation at the joint margins.

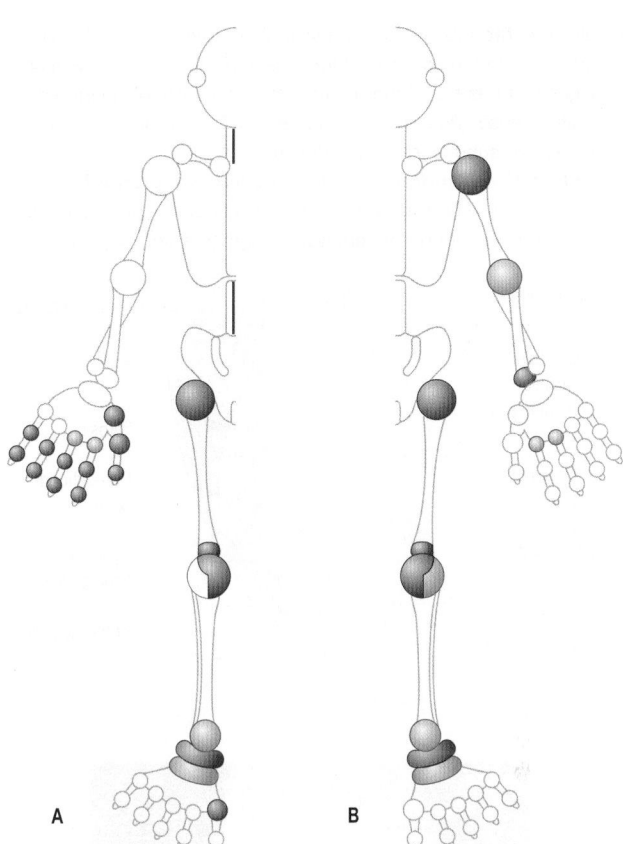

Fig. 18.15 Typical distribution of affected joints in arthritis. **(A)** Primary generalized osteoarthritis. **(B)** Pyrophosphate arthropathy. Red circles indicate the more commonly affected sites, and blue the less commonly affected sites.

Various mechanisms have been suggested:
- **Abnormal stress and loading**, leading to mechanical cartilage damage.
- **Obesity** is a risk factor for developing OA of the hand and knee and thought to trigger metabolic inflammation via adipokines, released from adipose tissue, inducing pro-inflammatory cytokines that cause cartilage and bone damage.
- **Matrix degradation** by matrix metalloproteinase (MMP)-1, MMP-2, MMP-3, MMP-9, MMP-13, which are secreted by chondrocytes in an inactive form. Extracellular activation then leads to the degradation of both collagen and proteoglycans around chondrocytes.
- **Tissue inhibitors of metalloproteinases** (TIMPs) regulate the MMPs. Disturbance of this regulation may lead to an increase in cartilage degradation over synthesis and contribute to the development of OA.
- **Osteoprotegerin (OPG), RANK and RANK ligand (RANKL)** control subchondral bone remodelling. Their levels are significantly different in OA chondrocytes.
- **Aggrecanase** production is stimulated by pro-inflammatory cytokines, and aggrecan (the major proteoglycan) levels fall.
- **Inflammatory mediator release** (including interleukin-1, IL-1 and tumour necrosis factor-alpha, TNF-α) stimulates metalloproteinase production, and IL-1 inhibits type II collagen production. IL-6 and IL-8 may also be involved. The production of cytokines by macrophages and that of MMPs by chondrocytes in OA are dependent on the transcription factor nuclear factor kappa B (NF-κB).

- **Growth factors**, including insulin-like growth factor 1 (IGF-1) and transforming growth factor beta (TGF-β), are involved in collagen synthesis, and their deficiency may play a role in impairing matrix repair. Paradoxically, increased TGF-β may also cause increased subchondral bone density.
- **Cell derived and/or cartilage breakdown products**, such as alarmins, fibronectin fragments, hyaluronic acid fragments, collagen fragments, proteoglycan fragments and high mobility

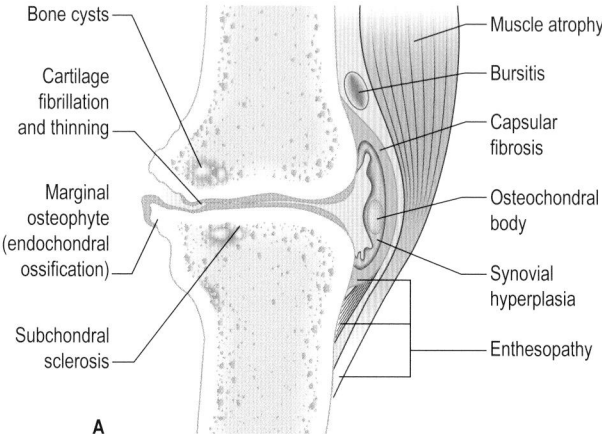

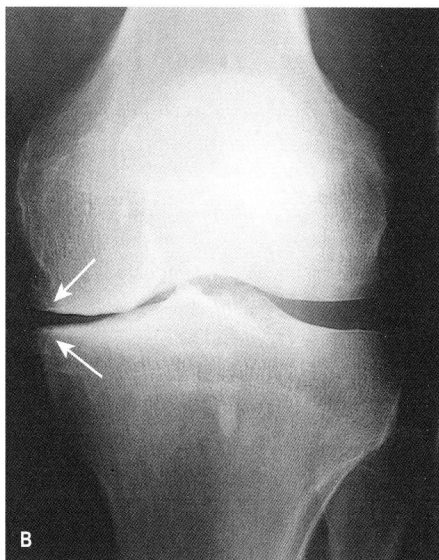

Fig. 18.16 Early osteoarthritis of a knee. **(A)** Pathology. **(B)** On the X-ray, there is medial compartment narrowing owing to cartilage thinning with subarticular sclerosis and marginal osteophyte formation (arrowed).

group box proteins, act to further deregulate chondrocyte function and contribute to cartilage degradation.

- **Vascular endothelial growth factor (VEGF)** from macrophages is a potent stimulator of angiogenesis and may contribute to inflammation and neovascularization in OA. Innervation can accompany vascularization of the articular cartilage.
- **A strong hereditary element** underlying OA is suggested by twin studies. The influence of genetic factors is estimated at 35–65%. To date, genome-wide association studies (GWAS) have identified several common variants associated with knee or hip OA, although the individual risk alleles exert only moderate to small effects. Loci that are associated with OA include genes encoding components of the TGF-β and bone morphogenetic protein signalling pathways: growth/differentiation factor 5 (GDF5); type II iodothyronine deiodinase (DIO2), which regulates synthesis of triiodothyronine that is involved in cartilage maintenance and repair; proteins involved in apoptosis and mitochondrial damage; molecules that regulate the turnover of extracellular matrix components; and proteins that are associated with inflammation and immune responses.
- **In the Caucasian population**, there is an inverse relationship between the risk of developing OA and osteoporosis.
- **Gender.** In women, weight-bearing sports produce a two- to threefold increase in risk of OA of the hip and knee. In men, there is an association between hip OA and certain occupations: farming and labouring. OA may flare after the female menopause or after cessation of hormone replacement therapy.
- **Periarticular enthesitis** is recognized in nodal generalized OA (NGOA) and may be difficult to distinguish from PsA at DIP joints.

The term **primary OA** may be used when various predisposing factors (**Box 18.21**), occur in the absence of other conditions that may cause secondary OA (**Box 18.22**).

Clinical features

OA affects many joints, in diverse clinical patterns, typically causing mechanical pain with movement and/or loss of function. Hip and knee OA are major causes of disability. Early OA is rarely symptomatic, however, unless accompanied by a joint effusion, while advanced radiological and pathological OA is not always symptomatic.

Symptoms are usually gradual in onset and progressive. Episodic disease flare-ups may be inflammatory in nature, although typically ESR and/or CRP are normal. Radiological OA is not inevitably progressive. Radiological improvement is uncommon but has been observed, suggesting that repair is possible.

---

i **Box 18.21 Factors predisposing to osteoarthritis (OA)**

- **Obesity**: This predicts a later risk of radiological and symptomatic OA of the hip and hand in population studies
- **Heredity**: There is a familial tendency to develop nodal and generalized OA
- **Gender**: Polyarticular OA is more common in women; a higher prevalence after the menopause suggests a role for sex hormones
- **Hypermobility** (see p. 432): Increased range of joint motion and reduced stability lead to OA
- **Osteoporosis**: There is a reduced risk of OA
- **Diseases**: See **Box 18.22**
- **Trauma**: A fracture through any joint predisposes. Meniscal and cruciate ligament tears cause OA of the knee

- **Congenital joint dysplasia**: This alters joint biomechanics and leads to OA. Mild acetabular dysplasia is common and leads to earlier onset of hip OA
- **Joint congruity**: Congenital dislocation of the hip or a slipped femoral epiphysis or Perthes' disease predispose; osteonecrosis of the femoral head (see p. 425) in children and adolescents causes early-onset OA
- **Occupation**: Miners develop OA of the hip, knee and shoulder, cotton workers OA of the hand, and farmers OA of the hip
- **Sport**: Repetitive use and injury in some sports cause a high incidence of lower-limb OA

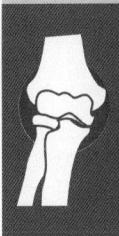

Primary OA
- No known cause

Secondary OA
Pre-existing joint damage
- Rheumatoid arthritis
- Gout
- Spondyloarthritis
- Trauma
- Overuse/abnormal use, e.g. athletes
- Septic arthritis
- Paget's disease

- Avascular necrosis, e.g. corticosteroid therapy

Metabolic disease
- Cartilage calcification
- Hereditary haemochromatosis
- Acromegaly

Systemic disease
- Haemophilia – recurrent haemarthrosis
- Haemoglobinopathies, e.g. sickle cell disease
- Neuropathies

i Box 18.23 Features of nodal osteoarthritis

- Demonstrates a familial nature
- Has a higher incidence in women
- Shows a typical pattern of polyarticular involvement of the hand joints
- Develops in late middle age and around female menopause
- Has a generally good long-term functional outcome
- Is associated with osteoarthritis of the knee, hip and spine (nodal generalized osteoarthritis)

Symptoms
- Joint pain with movement and/or weight-bearing.
- Short-lived morning joint stiffness.
- Functional limitation.

Signs
- Crepitus.
- Restricted movement.
- Bony enlargement.
- Joint effusion and variable levels of inflammation.
- Bony instability and muscle wasting.

Clinical subsets
Localized OA
Nodal OA

In nodal OA (**Box 18.23**), joints of the hand are usually affected one at a time over several years, with the DIPs more frequently involved than the PIPs. Nodal OA often begins around the female menopause, with inflammation causing painful, tender, swollen interphalangeal joints and impairment of hand function. At this stage, enthesitis can be seen on MRI. Intra-articular corticosteroid injections may be helpful at this stage. The inflammatory phase settles after some months or years, leaving painless bony swellings posterolaterally: **Heberden's nodes (DIPs)** and **Bouchard's nodes (PIPs)**, along with stiffness and deformity (**Fig. 18.17**). Functional impairment is usually limited, although PIP OA restricts grip more than DIP involvement. On X-ray, the nodes are marginal osteophytes and there is joint space loss.

Thumb-base OA coexists with nodal OA causing pain and disability, which decrease as the joint stiffens. The 'squared' hand in OA (see **Fig. 18.17**) is caused by bony swelling of the first carpometacarpal joint and fixed adduction of the thumb. Function is rarely severely compromised.

Polyarticular hand OA is associated with a slightly increased frequency of OA at other sites.

Hip OA

Hip OA affects 7–25% of adult Caucasians but is significantly less common in black African and Asian populations. There are

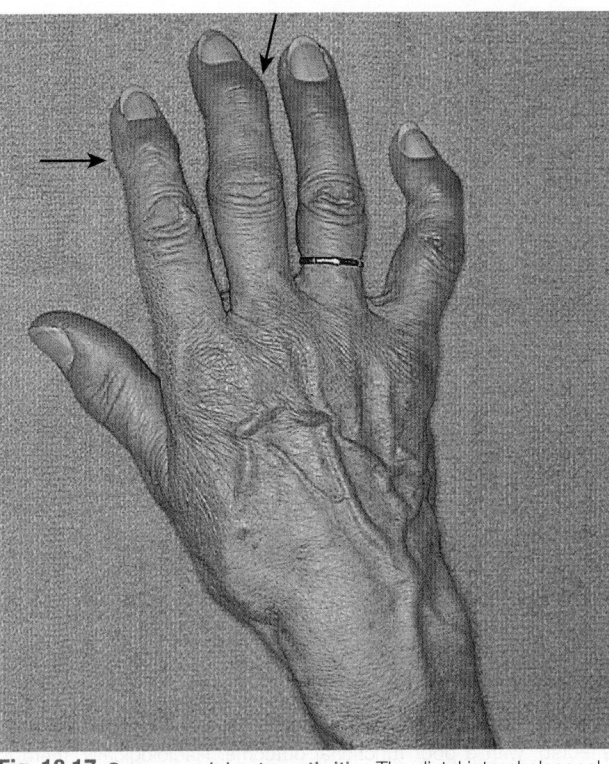

Fig. 18.17 Severe nodal osteoarthritis. The distal interphalangeal joints (DIPs) demonstrate Heberden's nodes (arrowed). The middle finger DIP joint is deformed and unstable. The thumb is adducted and the bony swelling of the first carpometacarpal joint is clearly shown – 'the squared hand of nodal osteoarthritis'.

two major subgroups defined by the radiological appearance. The most common is *superior-pole hip OA*, where joint space narrowing and sclerosis predominantly affect the weight-bearing upper surface of the femoral head and adjacent acetabulum. This finding is most common in men and unilateral at presentation, although both hips may become involved in progressive disease. Early onset of hip OA is associated with acetabular dysplasia or labral tears. Less commonly, *medial cartilage loss* occurs. This appearance is seen most commonly in women and is associated with hand involvement (NGOA), and is usually bilateral. It is more rapidly disabling.

Knee OA

The prevalence of symptomatic knee OA is 40% in individuals over 75 years of age and is more common in women. There is a strong relationship with obesity. The disease is generally bilateral and strongly associated with nodal OA of the hand in elderly women, or as part of generalized OA. The medial compartment is most commonly affected, leading to a varus (bow-legged) deformity. Often, retropatellar OA is also present. Previous trauma and meniscal and cruciate ligament tears are risk factors for developing knee OA. Bone marrow lesions seen on MRI predict disease progression and eventual joint replacement.

Primary generalized OA

This condition is rare and usually seen in combination with NGOA. Other affected areas include the knees, first MTP, hip and intervertebral (spondylosis) joints. Its onset is often sudden and severe. There is a female preponderance and a strong familial tendency. Periarticular ligamentous pathology may have an important role in the phenotypic expression of NGOA.

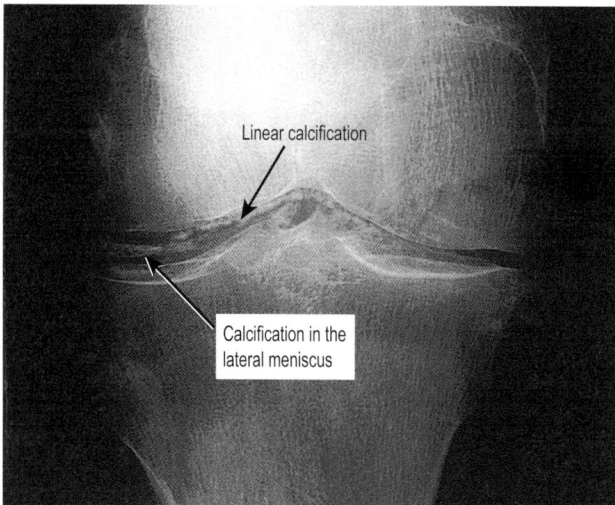

Fig. 18.18 Cartilage calcification of the knee. Note the linear calcification in the hyaline cartilage and calcification of the lateral meniscus (plus mild secondary osteoarthritis).

Erosive OA

In this rare subgroup, the DIPs and PIPs are inflamed and equally affected, with a poor functional outcome. Radiologically, there is marked osteolysis. Destructive phases are followed by phases of remodelling.

Crystal-associated OA

This condition most commonly occurs with calcium pyrophosphate deposition (CPPD) in the cartilage. It increases in frequency with age and causes cartilage calcification (CC) on over 40% of knee X-rays in the over-eighties, but is usually asymptomatic. The joints most frequently affected are the knees (hyaline cartilage and fibro-cartilage) and wrists (triangular fibrocartilage; see **Fig. 18.15**). There is patchy linear CC on X-ray (**Fig. 18.18**).

A chronic arthropathy (pseudo-OA) occurs, predominantly in elderly women with severe CC. There is a florid inflammatory component and marked osteophyte and cyst formation visible on X-rays that predominantly affects the knees, then wrists and shoulders. CC is associated with CPPD crystal-induced arthritis (see p. 451).

A rare, rapidly destructive arthritis in elderly women, affecting shoulders, hips and knees, is associated with the finding of crystals of calcium apatite in a bloody joint effusion. The outlook is poor and joints require early surgical replacement.

Investigations

- **Blood tests** lack specificity; the ESR is usually normal, although high-sensitivity CRP may be slightly raised. RFs and antinuclear antibodies are negative.
- **X-rays** are abnormal only when the damage is advanced. They are useful in preoperative assessments. For knees, a standing X-ray (stressed) is used to assess cartilage loss, and 'skyline' views in flexion are used for patello-femoral OA.
- **MRI** demonstrates meniscal tears, early cartilage injury and sub-chondral bone marrow changes (osteochondral lesions).
- **Arthroscopy** reveals early fissuring and surface erosion of the cartilage.
- **Aspiration of synovial fluid** if there is a painful effusion shows a viscous fluid with few leucocytes (see p. 416).

Management

The guiding principle is to treat the symptoms and disability, not the radiological appearances; depression and poor quadriceps strength are better predictors of pain than radiological severity in OA of the knee. Patient education about the disease and its effects reduces pain, distress and disability, and increases compliance with treatment. Psychological or social factors alter the impact of the disease.

Physical measures

Weight management is recognized to reduce the risk of development of OA and slow its progression. Women who lost an average of 5 kg decreased their risk for knee OA by 50% in the Framingham study. As little as 1% change in body weight in obese adults modifies the rate of knee cartilage loss. Overall, maintenance of muscle mass and reduction of adiposity is central to OA management. Exercises for strength and stability are useful and land-based exercise programmes for the hip and knee improve physical function and pain. Hydrotherapy helps, especially in lower-limb OA. Insoles for flat feet and a walking stick held on the contralateral side to the affected lower limb joint are useful. Transcutaneous electrical nerve stimulation, acupuncture and thermotherapy may be adjuncts for treating OA but are not universally recommended due to their limited evidence of efficacy.

Medication

Topical, oral and injectable therapies are available and potential benefit must be balanced against potential side-effects, especially in the elderly. First-line therapies include topical or oral NSAIDs. Paracetamol has limited efficacy in OA (see **Box 18.18**). NSAIDs or coxibs should be used intermittently when possible due to their toxicities. Topical rubefacients, such as capsaicin, may be used as a supplementary analgesic. Opioids are a last resort and should be used cautiously in older patients.

Intra-articular corticosteroid injections produce short-term improvement when there is a painful joint effusion. Frequent injections into the same joint should be avoided. Heterogeneity of relevant studies of intra-articular hyaluronan preparations displays limited efficacy.

Glucosamine and chondroitin (sold as food supplements) have no clinically relevant effect on joint pain or joint space narrowing.

There are no proven agents that halt or reverse OA, although they are greatly needed.

Surgery

Arthroscopy for knee OA is rarely beneficial. Replacement arthroplasty, however, has transformed the management of severe OA to reduce pain, improve function, restore quality of life and regain independence. Increasing numbers of arthroplasties, particularly hip and knee, are being performed worldwide each year with shortened recovery times, improved durability and mortality. However, an increasing trend for hip or knee arthroplasty in patients less than 60 years of age is associated with an increased lifetime risk of revision surgery. Serious complications occur in less than 1%, with venous thromboembolism and infection being the most serious. These slight but definite risks make it essential for the patient to be certain that surgery is necessary. Resurfacing hip surgery has become popular but may have higher complication rates in women, particularly with metal on metal resurfacing. Uni-compartmental knee replacement is a less major procedure and may be appropriate in some cases.

Other surgical procedures include re-alignment osteotomy of the knee or hip, excision arthroplasty of the first MTP and base of the thumb, and fusion of a first MTP joint.

1. Rheumatoid arthritis (associated with antibodies)
2. Spondyloarthritis (associated with human leucocyte antigen (HLA)-B27)
3. Metabolic arthritis (e.g. associated with crystals)

Monoarthritis
- Crystal arthritis
- Septic arthritis
- Palindromic rheumatism
- Traumatic ± haemathrosis
- Juxta-articular bone tumour
- *PsA*
- *ReA*
- *RA*

Oligoarthritis
- ReA
- Palindromic rheumatism

- Crystal arthritis
- Septic arthritis
- *PsA*
- *ReA*

Polyarthritis
- RA
- PsA, AxSpA
- ReA
- Post-viral
- Lyme arthritis
- EA
- Arthritis associated with EN

AxSpA, axial spondyloarthropathy; EA, enteropathic arthritis; EN, erythema nodosum; PsA, psoriatic arthritis; RA, rheumatoid arthritis; ReA, reactive arthritis. Italics indicate less common pattern of joint involvement.

Further reading

Hunter DJ. Viscosupplementation for osteoarthritis of the knee. *N Engl J Med* 2015; 372:1040–1047.
Martel-Pelletier J, Barr AJ et al. Osteoarthritis. *Nat Rev Dis Primers* 2016; 2:16072.
Pivec R. Hip arthroplasty. *Lancet* 2012; 380:1768–1777.

INFLAMMATORY ARTHRITIS

Inflammatory arthritis is characterized by synovial inflammation. The three main subgroups of inflammatory arthritis are rheumatoid arthritis (RA), spondyloarthritis and crystal arthritis (**Box 18.24**). The diagnosis of these conditions is helped by distinguishing:
- the number and pattern of joint involvement (symmetrical or asymmetrical, large or small) (**Box 18.25**)
- presence of any non-articular disease
- a past and family history
- periodicity of the arthritis (single acute, relapsing, chronic and progressive).

Certain non-articular diseases, such as psoriasis, iritis, IBD, nonspecific urethritis or recent dysentery, suggest spondyloarthritis. There may be evidence of recent viral illness (rubella, hepatitis B or erythrovirus), rheumatic fever, or a tick bite and skin rash (Lyme disease). In early arthritis, it may not be possible to make a specific diagnosis until the disease has evolved from an undifferentiated arthritis into a chronic form.

There is a distinct genetic separation of rheumatoid-pattern synovitis and spondyloarthritis; RA (see below) is associated with a genetic marker in the class II major histocompatibility complex (MHC) genes, while spondyloarthritis shares certain alleles in the B locus of class I MHC genes, usually B27 (see p. 448).

In general, the pain and stiffness of inflammatory arthritis are worse in the morning, often lasting for several hours and improving with activity, in contrast with the much shorter morning stiffness and mechanical pain with activity of OA. Inflammatory markers (ESR and CRP) are typically raised in inflammatory arthritis. Specific types of arthritis are discussed below.

Early inflammatory polyarthritis

Undifferentiated polyarthritis requires urgent referral to a rheumatologist for diagnosis and treatment, including the early introduction of disease-modifying agents when indicated (see p. 445). In persistent inflammatory arthritis, sustained remission depends on rapid diagnosis and intensive treatment. Poor prognostic features for undifferentiated polyarthritis are:
- polyarticular onset
- positive anti-citrullinated peptide antibodies (ACPA)
- positive rheumatoid factor
- joint erosion on X-ray at presentation
- disease for longer than 3–6 months.

RHEUMATOID ARTHRITIS

RA is a chronic inflammatory rheumatic disease. It has a multifactorial pathogenesis, with various genetic and environmental factors being implicated, giving rise to immune dysregulation with consequent joint inflammation and tissue damage. Patients typically develop a chronic symmetrical polyarthritis with systemic inflammation.

Epidemiology

RA has a worldwide distribution affecting 0.5–1% of the population (with a female preponderance of 3 : 1). The prevalence is low in black African and Chinese people. The incidence is falling. RA is the 42nd highest contributor to global disability just below malaria and just above iodine deficiency. It presents from early childhood (when it is rare) to late old age. The most common age of onset is between 30 and 50 years.

Aetiology and pathogenesis

There has been a greater understanding of genetic and environmental factors in the last two decades.
- ***Genetic factors***. There is an increased incidence in first-degree relatives and a high concordance amongst monozygotic twins of up to 15%. Over 100 loci are associated with disease risk and progression. There is a strong association between susceptibility to RA and certain human leucocyte antigen (HLA) haplotypes: HLA-DR4, which occurs in 50–75% of patients and correlates with a poor prognosis, as does possession of certain shared alleles of HLA-DRB1*04. The possession of these shared epitope alleles in HLA-DRB1 (S2 and S3P) increases susceptibility to RA and may predispose to anti-cyclic citrullinated peptide antibody (ACPA) development against citrullinated antigens. Citrullination is a process that modifies antigens, allowing them to fit into the shared epitope on HLA alleles. A genome-wide association study in ACPA-positive RA found an association with loci near HLA-DRB1 and PTPN22 in people of European descent. These genes affect the presentation of autoantigens (*HLA-DRB1*), T-cell receptor signal transduction (*PTPN22*) and targets of ACPA (*PAD14*).
- ***Environment***. Smoking and other forms of bronchial stress increase the risk of RA with HLA-DR4 and acts synergistically with HLA-DRB1 to increase the risk of having ACPA. Mucosal surfaces of the oral cavity, upper respiratory tract and gut are colonized by commensal microorganisms; a population known

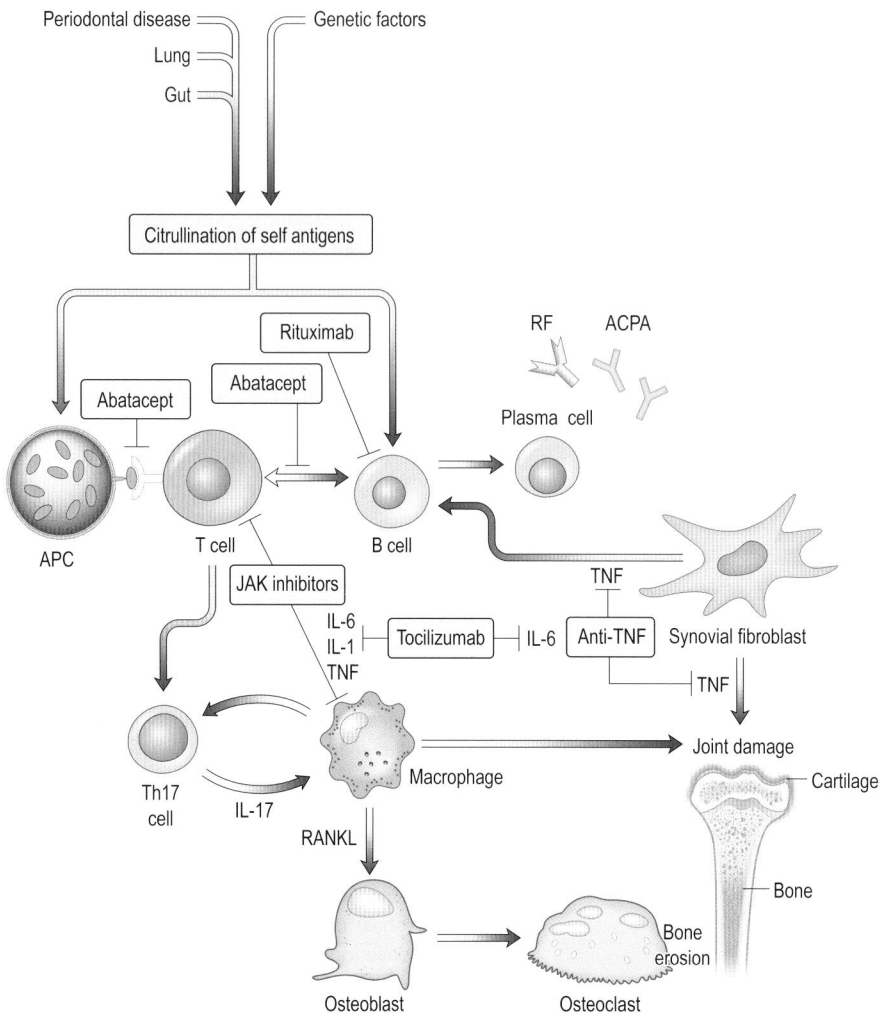

Fig. 18.19 Pathogenesis of rheumatoid arthritis. Environment–gene interactions promote citrullination of self proteins, which can then be detected by T and B cells; this leads to a loss of tolerance and promotion of the inflammatory response, resulting in joint damage. Targeted therapy is shown in yellow. ACPA, anti-citrullinated peptide antibody; APC, antigen-presenting cell; IL, interleukin; RANKL, receptor activator of nuclear factor kappa B ligand; RF, rheumatoid factor; Th, T helper; TNF, tumour necrosis factor.

as the microbiome. Alterations in the microbiome may facilitate developments in innate and adaptive immunity that predispose to RA, such as the association of periodontal disease and alterations in the gut microbiome with RA.

- **Autoantibodies.** Rheumatoid factor (RF), autoantibodies to the Fc portion of immunoglobulin G, are found in 75–80% of RA patients and are relatively specific for diagnosis of RA but have little predictive value in the general population. In contrast, ACPA are more specific and sensitive to RA.

Immunology

RA is primarily a synovial disease, and synovitis occurs when chemoattractants produced in the joint recruit circulating inflammatory cells. Over-production of tumour necrosis factor-alpha (TNF-α) leads to synovitis and joint destruction. Interaction of macrophages and T and B lymphocytes drives this over-production. TNF-α stimulates over-production of IL-6, as well as other cytokines. The increased understanding of the immunopathogenesis of this disease has informed the development of targeted biological therapies (**Fig. 18.19**).

Dysfunction of certain cell types are significant in immunopathogenesis:

- **Synovial cells** in chronic rheumatoid synovitis are predominantly fibroblast-like synoviocytes and macrophage-like synoviocytes that produce pro-inflammatory cytokines.
- **Osteoclasts** cause bone and cartilage destruction.
- **Synovial B cells**, activated by cytokine-activated macrophages and T cells, produce autoantibodies, of which IgM and IgA RF are the most typical in RA. As RFs bind the Fc portion of IgG, they have the potential for self-aggregation and immune complex formation in the synovium. These may then trigger macrophages via IgG Fc receptors to produce even more cytokines, including IL-1, IL-8, TNF-α and granulocyte–macrophage colony-stimulating factor, and fibroblasts to produce IL-6.
- **Synovial fibroblasts** have high levels of the adhesion molecule, vascular cell adhesion molecule (VCAM-1, a molecule that supports B-lymphocyte survival and differentiation), decay accelerating factor (DAF, a factor that prevents complement-induced cell lysis) and cadherin II (which mediates cell-to-cell interac-

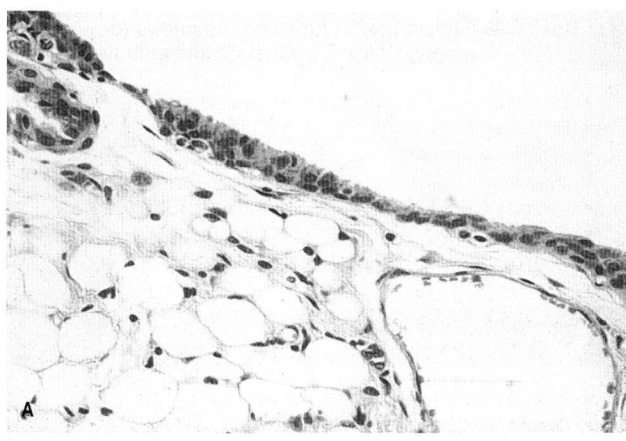

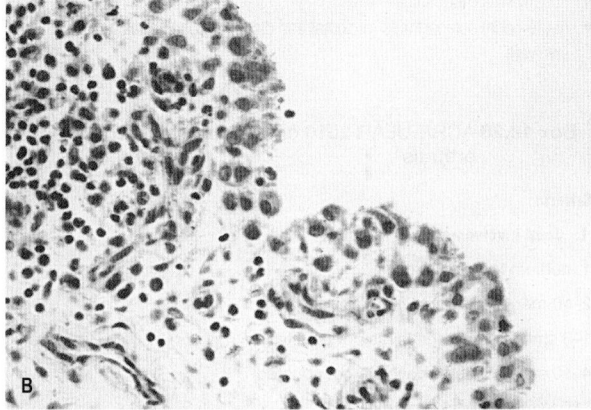

Fig. 18.20 Histological appearance of synovium in rheumatoid arthritis (RA). **(A)** Normal synovium. **(B)** Synovial appearances in established RA, showing marked hypertrophy of the tissues with infiltration by lymphocytes and plasma cells. *(From Shipley M. Colour Atlas of Rheumatology, 3rd edn. London: Mosby–Wolfe; 1993, with permission.)*

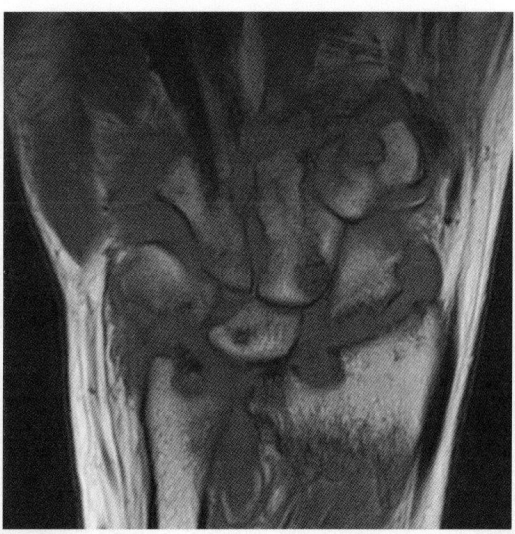

Fig. 18.21 Magnetic resonance imaging of erosions in rheumatoid arthritis. *(From Elias-Jones C. Crash Course Orthopaedics and Rheumatology, 3rd edn. Edinburgh: Elsevier, 2015.)*

tions). These molecules may facilitate the formation of ectopic lymphoid tissue in synovium.

- ***T cells*** can be a part of the destructive process. The pro-inflammatory cytokine IL-17 is produced by a specific subset, Th17 helper cells (see p. 51), which produce IL-17, 21 and 22, and TNF-α. The normal regulatory T cells are suppressed by TGF-β and interleukins (produced by macrophages and dendritic cells), allowing Th17 helper cells to increase.

The ***triggering antigen***, which leads to self-maintained inflammation in RA, remains unclear. Triggers for ACPA production include filaggrin, type II collagen and vimentin. There is little evidence that type II collagen is the triggering antigen, although it is a cause of arthritis in animal models of RA. Smoking is a potential trigger, particularly in ACPA-positive RA).

Pathology

RA is typified by widespread, persistent synovitis of joints, tendon sheaths or bursae. Normal synovium comprises a thin lining layer that contains fibroblast-like synoviocytes and macrophages overlying loose connective tissue. In RA, the synovium becomes greatly thickened, causing 'boggy' swelling around joints and tendons, with proliferation of the synovium into folds and fronds, and infiltration by a variety of inflammatory cells, including polymorphs, which transit through the tissue into the joint fluid, and lymphocytes and plasma cells. The normally sparse surface layer of lining cells becomes hyperplastic and thickened (**Fig. 18.20**). There is marked vascular proliferation. Increased permeability of blood vessels and the synovial lining layer leads to joint effusions containing lymphocytes and dying polymorphs.

The hyperplastic synovium spreads from the joint margins to the cartilage surface. This 'pannus' of inflamed synovium damages the underlying cartilage by blocking its normal route for nutrition and by the direct effects of cytokines on the chondrocytes. The cartilage becomes thinned and the underlying bone exposed. Local cytokine production and joint disuse combine to cause juxta-articular osteoporosis during active synovitis.

Fibroblasts from the proliferating synovium also grow along the course of blood vessels between the synovial margins and the epiphyseal bone cavity, and damage the bone. This process is shown by MRI (**Fig. 18.21**) to occur in the first 3–6 months following onset of the arthritis before the diagnostic, ill-defined, juxta-articular bony 'erosions' appear on X-ray (**Fig. 18.22**). This early damage justifies the use of disease-modifying anti-rheumatic drugs (DMARDs; see p. 445) within 3 months of onset of the arthritis to try to induce disease remission and prevent erosion formation. Erosions lead to a variety of deformities and contribute to long-term disability.

Rheumatoid factors and anti-citrullinated peptide antibodies (ACPA)

RFs (see p. 416) are of any immunoglobulin class (IgM, IgG or IgA), but the most common tests employed clinically detect IgM RF. The term 'seronegative RA' is used when the standard tests for IgM RF are persistently negative. These patients tend to have a more limited pattern of synovitis.

IgM RF is not diagnostic of RA and its absence does not rule the disease out; however, it is a useful predictor of prognosis. A persistently high titre in early disease implies more persistently active synovitis, more joint damage leading to greater disability, thus justifies earlier use of DMARDs.

ACPAs (see p. 416) are usually present with RF in RA. They are better predictors of a transition from early transient inflammatory arthritis to persistent synovitis and early RA. RF and ACPA together are even more specific.

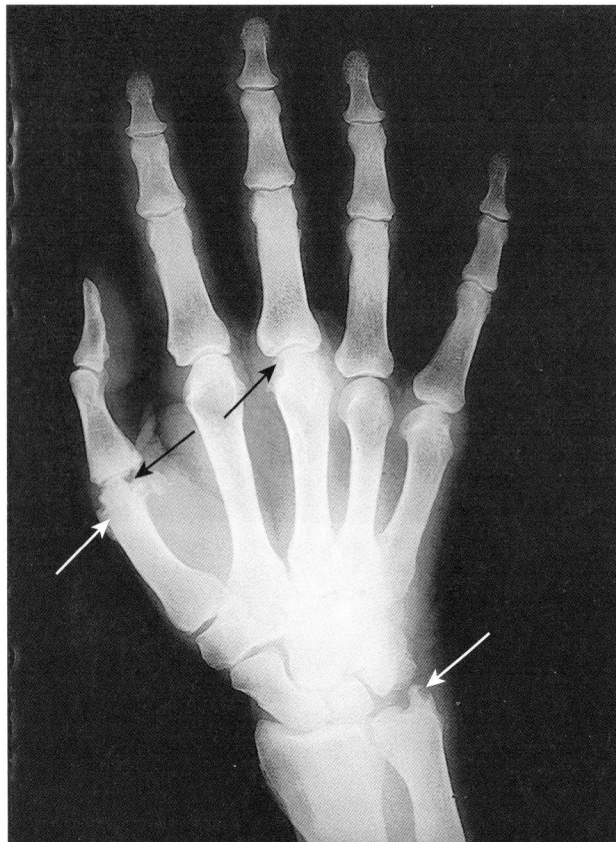

Fig. 18.22 X-ray of early rheumatoid arthritis. Typical erosions may be seen at the thumb (black and white arrows on the left), middle metacarpophalangeal joints (central black arrow) and ulnar styloid (white arrow on the right).

Clinical features

Typical presentation

RA typically presents (≈70%) as a progressive, symmetrical, periph-eral polyarthritis, evolving over a period of a few weeks or months in patients between 30 and 50 years of age, although the disease can occur at any age. Less commonly (≈15%), a rapid onset can occur over a few days (or explosively overnight), with a severe sym-metrical, polyarticular involvement, especially in the elderly. Factors indicating a poor prognosis are listed in **Box 18.26**. The differential diagnosis of early RA is shown in **Box 18.27**.

Current classification criteria from 2010 are more suitable for assessing and diagnosing early arthritis than previous versions because they do not rely on later changes, such as erosions and extra-articular disease to distinguish RA (**Box 18.28**).

In early RA, the combination of at least one swollen joint for more than 6 weeks with no prior injury, no associated history or family his-tory of spondyloarthritis or associated conditions such as psoriasis (see p. 664), and a positive ACPA test is the best way to select patients for earlier treatment to avoid joint damage. This evidence-based approach has been shown to reduce the risk of the develop-ment of damage and permanent joint deformities.

Symptoms and signs of early RA

Most patients complain of pain and stiffness of the small joints of the hands (MCPs, PIPs) and feet (MTPs). The DIPs are usually spared. Wrists, elbows, shoulders, knees and ankles are also affected. In most cases, multiple joints are involved, but 10% of patients pres-ent with a monoarthritis of the knee or shoulder or with carpal tunnel

Box 18.26 Factors predicting a poor prognosis for progression in early rheumatoid arthritis

- Older age
- Female sex
- Symmetrical small joint involvement
- Morning stiffness >30 min
- >4 swollen joints
- Cigarette smoking
- Co-morbidity
- C-reactive protein >20 g/dL
- Positive rheumatoid factor and anti-citrullinated peptide antibodies

Box 18.27 Differential diagnosis of early rheumatoid arthritis

- Postviral arthritis: rubella, hepatitis B or erythrovirus
- Seronegative spondyloarthropathies
- Polymyalgia rheumatica
- Acute nodal osteoarthritis (proximal and distal interphalangeal joints involved)

Box 18.28 ACR/EULAR 2010 criteria for rheumatoid arthritis[a]

Criteria	Points
1. Joint involvement	**0–5**
1 medium to large joint	0
2–10 medium to large joints	1
1–3 small joints (large joints not counted)	2
4–10 small joints (large joints not counted)	3
>10 joints; at least one small joint	5
2. Serology	**0–3**
Negative RF and negative ACPA	0
Low positive RF or low positive ACPA	2
High positive RF or high positive ACPA	3
3. Acute-phase reactants	**0–1**
Normal CRP and normal ESR	0
Abnormal CRP or abnormal ESR	1
4. Duration of symptoms	**0–1**
<6 weeks	0
≥6 weeks	1

[a]The cut-off point for RA is at ≥6 points. Patients can also be classified as having RA if they have both typical erosions and longstanding disease previously satisfying the classification criteria. ACPA, anticitrullinated peptide antibody; ACR, American College of Rheumatology; CRP, C-reactive protein; EULAR, European League Against Rh. (*Adapted from Scott DL, Wolfe F, Huizinga TW. Rheumatoid arthritis.* Lancet *2010; 376:1094–1108.)*

syndrome. The pain and stiffness are significantly worse in the morning. Sleep disturbance and fatigue are common complaints.

The joints are usually warm and tender with some joint swelling. There is limitation of movement and muscle wasting. Deformities and non-articular features develop if the disease cannot be con-trolled (see below).

RA in older patients may mimic polymyalgia rheumatica; the synovitis becomes apparent as the corticosteroid dose is reduced.

Other presentations

The variable presentations and progression of RA are shown in **Box 18.29**. Relapses and remissions occur either spontaneously or on drug therapy. Active disease, producing progressive joint damage, requires targeted treatment to induce remission.

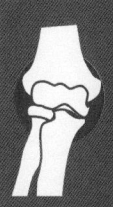

- *Palindromic.* Palindromic monoarticular attacks last 24–48 h; 50% progress to other types of RA.
- *Transient.* Disease is self-limiting, lasting <12 months and leaving no permanent joint damage. It is usually seronegative for IgM RF and ACPA. Some of these patients may have undetected postviral arthritis.
- *Remitting.* There is a period of several years during which the arthritis is active but then remits, leaving minimal damage.
- *Chronic, persistent.* This is the most typical form; it may be seropositive or seronegative for IgM RF. The disease follows a relapsing and remitting course over many years. Seropositive (plus ACPA) patients tend to develop greater joint damage and long-term disability. They warrant earlier and more aggressive treatment with disease-modifying agents.
- *Rapidly progressive.* The disease progresses remorselessly over a few years and leads rapidly to severe joint damage and disability. It is usually seropositive (plus ACPA), has a high incidence of systemic complications and is difficult to treat.

ACPA, anti-citrullinated peptide antibody; RF, rheumatoid factor.

Seronegative RA initially affects the wrists more often than the fingers and has a less symmetrical joint involvement. It has a better long-term prognosis but some cases progress to severe disability. This form can be confused with psoriatic arthropathy, which has a similar distribution (see p. 450).

Palindromic rheumatism is unusual (5%) and consists of 24–48-hour episodes of acute monoarthritis. The joint becomes acutely painful, swollen and red, but resolves completely. Further attacks occur in the same or other joints. About 50% of patients develop typical chronic rheumatoid synovitis after a delay of months or years. The rest remit or continue with acute episodic arthritis. Detection of RF or ACPA predicts conversion to chronic, destructive synovitis.

Complications
Septic arthritis
This serious complication has significant morbidity and mortality. In immunosuppressed patients, affected joints may not display the typical signs of inflammation with accompanying fever found in patients with an intact immune system. Treatment is with systemic antibiotics (see p. 455) and drainage.

Amyloidosis
Amyloidosis (see p. 1357) is found in a very small number of people with uncontrolled RA. RA is the most common cause of secondary AA amyloidosis. AL amyloidosis causes a polyarthritis that resembles RA in distribution and is also often associated with carpal tunnel syndrome and subcutaneous nodules.

Joint involvement in RA
These changes are seen in established disease or when early drug treatment has been ineffective.

Hands and wrists
In early disease, the fingers are swollen, painful and stiff. Inflamed flexor tendon sheaths increase functional impairment and may cause a carpal tunnel syndrome. Joint damage causes:

- *A combination of ulnar drift and palmar subluxation of the MCPs.* This change (**Fig. 18.23**) leads to unsightly deformity, but function may be preserved once the patient has learned to adapt and pain is controlled.
- *Fixed flexion* (buttonhole or boutonnière deformity) or *fixed hyperextension* (swan-neck deformity) of the PIP joints, which impairs hand function.

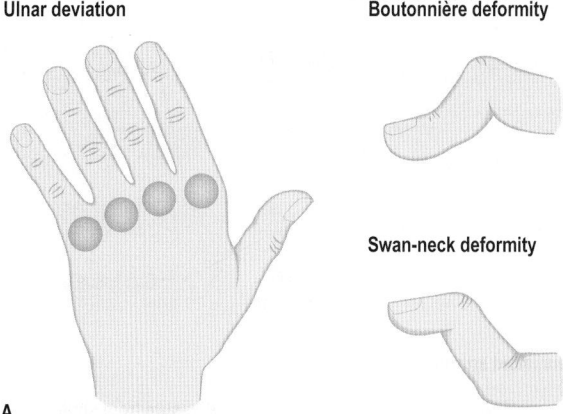

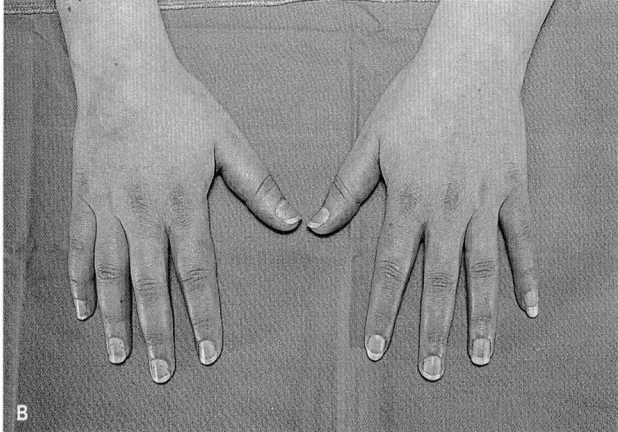

Fig. 18.23 Rheumatoid arthritis. (A) Characteristic hand deformities. **(B)** Early rheumatoid arthritis – dorsal tenosynovitis of the right wrist and small joints of both hands with spindling of the fingers.

- *Swelling and dorsal subluxation of the ulnar styloid,* which causes wrist pain. It may also cause rupture of the finger extensor tendons, leading to a sudden drop of the little and ring fingers that requires urgent surgical repair.

Shoulders
RA commonly affects the shoulders. Initially, the symptoms mimic rotator cuff tendonosis (see p. 419) with a painful arc syndrome and pain in the upper arms at night. Further joint damage leads to global stiffening; rotator cuff tears become more common and interfere with dressing, feeding and personal toilet.

Elbows
Synovitis of the elbows causes swelling and a painful fixed flexion deformity. In late disease, flexion may be lost and severe difficulties with feeding result, especially combined with shoulder, hand and wrist deformities.

Feet
One of the earliest manifestations of RA is painful swelling of the MTP joints.

- The foot becomes broader and a hammer-toe deformity develops.
- Exposure of the metatarsal heads to pressure by the forward migration of the protective fibrofatty pad (**Fig. 18.24**) causes pain.
- Ulcers or calluses may develop under the metatarsal heads and over the dorsum of the toes.

Normal

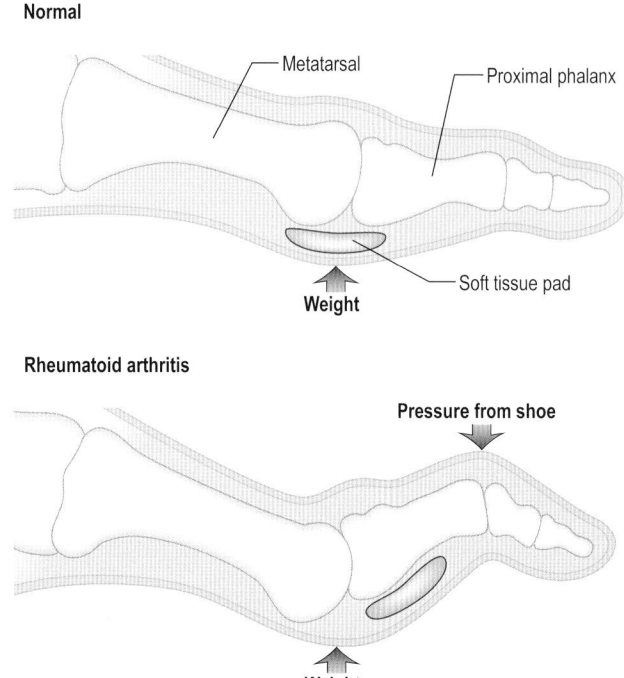

Rheumatoid arthritis

Fig. 18.24 The toes in rheumatoid arthritis. There is exposure of the metatarsal heads with forward migration of the soft tissue pad.

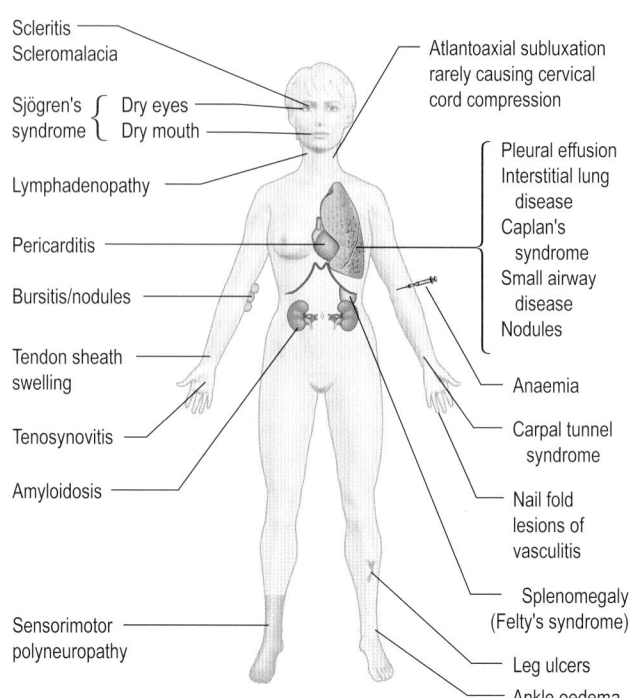

Fig. 18.25 Non-articular manifestations of rheumatoid arthritis.

- Mid- and hindfoot RA causes a flat medial arch and loss of flexibility of the foot.
- The ankle often assumes a valgus position.

Appropriate broad, deep, cushioned shoes are essential but rarely wholly adequate, and walking is often painful and limited. Podiatry helps and surgery may be required.

Knees

Massive synovitis and knee effusions occur but respond well to aspiration and steroid injection (see p. 416). A persistent effusion increases the risk of popliteal cyst formation and rupture (see p. 427). In later disease, erosion of cartilage and bone causes loss of joint space on X-ray and damage to the medial and/or lateral and/or retropatellar compartments of the knees. Depending on the pattern of involvement, the knees may develop a varus or valgus deformity. Secondary OA follows. Total knee replacement may be required to restore mobility and relieve pain.

Hips

The hips are occasionally affected in early RA but less commonly so than the knees at all stages of the disease. Pain and stiffness are accompanied by radiological loss of joint space and juxta-articular osteoporosis. The latter may permit medial migration of the acetabulum (protrusio acetabulae). Later, secondary OA develops. Hip replacement may be necessary.

Cervical spine

Painful stiffness of the neck in RA is often muscular, but it may be due to rheumatoid synovitis affecting the synovial joints of the upper cervical spine and the bursae, which separate the odontoid peg from the anterior arch of the atlas and its retaining ligaments. This synovitis leads to bone destruction, damages the ligaments and causes atlantoaxial or upper cervical vertebral instability. Subluxation and local synovial swelling may damage the spinal cord, producing

pyramidal and sensory signs. MRI is the imaging of choice, but lateral flexed and extended neck X-rays can demonstrate instability. In late RA, difficulty walking that cannot be explained by articular disease, weakness of the legs or loss of control of bowel or bladder may be due to spinal cord compression and is a neurosurgical emergency.

Imaging of the cervical spine in flexion and extension is recommended in patients with RA before surgery or upper gastrointestinal endoscopy to check for instability and reduce the risk of cord injury during intubation.

Other joints

The temporomandibular, acromioclavicular, sternoclavicular, cricoarytenoid and any other synovial joint can be affected.

Non-articular manifestations

See **Fig. 18.25**.

Soft tissue surrounding joints

Subcutaneous nodules are firm and intradermal, generally occurring over pressure points: typically, the elbows, the finger joints and the Achilles tendon in patients with seropositive erosive disease. They can be removed surgically but they tend to recur.

The olecranon and other bursae may be swollen (bursitis).

Tenosynovitis of flexor tendons in the hand can cause stiffness and occasionally a trigger finger. Swelling of the extensor tendon sheath over the dorsum of the wrist is common.

Muscle wasting around joints is common. Corticosteroid-induced myopathy occurs. Osteoporosis is more common in poorly controlled RA.

Less common non-articular manifestations

Non-articular complications are less common, probably because of more effective disease control.

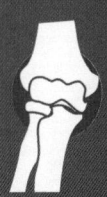

Lungs

Findings in the lungs (see p. 992) include:

- airways disease: from predominant bronchiectasis (cough and daily sputum) to predominant obliterative bronchiolitis (progressive breathlessness)
- pleural disease: pleural effusion (asymptomatic to mildly breathless) and thickening
- interstitial lung disease: a combination of inflammation and basal lung fibrosis
- peripheral, intrapulmonary nodules: asymptomatic but may cavitate, especially with pneumoconiosis (Caplan's syndrome)
- infective lesions, e.g. tuberculosis in patients on biological DMARDs.

Vasculitis

Vasculitis (see p. 464) is uncommon. Risk factors include high titres of RF and active extra-articular disease elsewhere. Findings include:

- widespread cutaneous vasculitis with necrosis of the skin
- mononeuritis multiplex (see p. 888).

Heart and peripheral vessels

Poorly controlled RA with a persistently raised CRP and high cholesterol is a cardiovascular risk factor, independent of traditional risk factors (i.e. high cholesterol and hypertension). Other cardiovascular problems include:

- pericarditis, which is rarely symptomatic
- endocarditis and myocardial disease, rarely symptomatic, found at postmortem in approximately 20% of cases.

Nervous system

- Peripheral sensory neuropathies: mononeuritis multiplex or symmetrical peripheral neuropathy – due to vasculitis of the vasa nervorum.
- Compression neuropathies: carpal or tarsal tunnel syndrome – due to synovitis.
- Cord compression: due to atlantoaxial subluxation (see earlier).

Eyes

- Sicca syndrome causes dry mouth and eyes (see Sjögren's syndrome, p. 464).
- Scleritis and episcleritis occur in severe, seropositive disease, resulting in painful red eye.
- Scleromalacia perforans is a rare feature.

Kidneys

Amyloidosis causing proteinuria, nephrotic syndrome and chronic kidney disease occurs rarely in severe, longstanding RA, due to the deposition of highly stable serum amyloid A protein (SAP) in the intercellular matrix of a variety of organs (see p. 1357).

Spleen, lymph nodes and blood

Felty's syndrome is splenomegaly and neutropenia in a patient with RA. Leg ulcers and sepsis are complications. HLA-DR4 is found in 95% of such patients, compared with 50–75% of people with RA alone.

Anaemia is almost universal and is usually normochromic and normocytic. It may be iron-deficient owing to gastrointestinal blood loss from NSAID ingestion, or rarely haemolytic (Coombs-positive). There may be a pancytopenia due to hypersplenism in Felty's syndrome or as a complication of DMARD treatment. A high platelet count occurs with active disease.

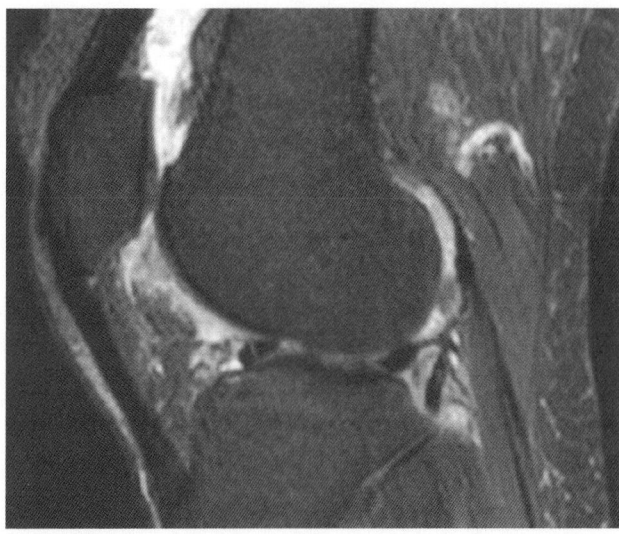

Fig. 18.26 MRI of chronic rheumatoid arthritis of the knee. There is inflamed synovium throughout joint and spreading into the popliteal bursa.

Diagnosis and investigations

Diagnosis relies on the clinical features described earlier. The predictors of poor prognosis arthritis are listed in **Box 18.26**. Initial investigations include:

- **Blood count** may show a normochromic, normocytic anaemia.
- **ESR and/or CRP** are raised in proportion to the activity of the inflammatory process and are useful in monitoring treatment.
- **Serology** reveals ACPA positivity (see p. 416) that may be present early in the disease (and even predate it by many years), and in early inflammatory arthritis indicates the likelihood of progressing to RA. RF is present in approximately 75–80% of cases and ANA at low titre in 30%.
- **X-rays** show soft tissue swelling in early disease, but ultrasound and MRI (**Fig. 18.26**) are useful to demonstrate synovitis and early erosions.
- **Aspiration of the joint** may be needed if an effusion is present. The aspirate looks cloudy owing to white cells. In a suddenly painful joint, septic arthritis should be suspected (see p. 454).
- **Musculoskeletal ultrasound** is a very effective way of demonstrating persistent synovitis when deciding on the need for DMARDs or assessing their efficacy.

Other investigations will depend on the clinical picture, as outlined above. In severe disease, extensive imaging of joints may be required.

Management

See **Box 18.30**. The diagnosis of RA inevitably causes concern and fear in the patient and requires explanation and reassurance. Anyone with persistent arthritis should be referred urgently to a rheumatologist if small joints of hands or feet are affected, more than one joint is affected, or there has already been a delay of more than 3 months from symptom onset.

The doctor should have a positive approach and remind the patient that, with the help of drugs, most people continue to lead a more or less normal life, as the aim of therapy is disease remission. Furthermore, early therapy targeted at remission within 3 months of symptom onset is more likely to achieve sustained remission with subsequent drug tapering. People should be helped and encouraged to stay at work, as 30% lose their job within 2 years of

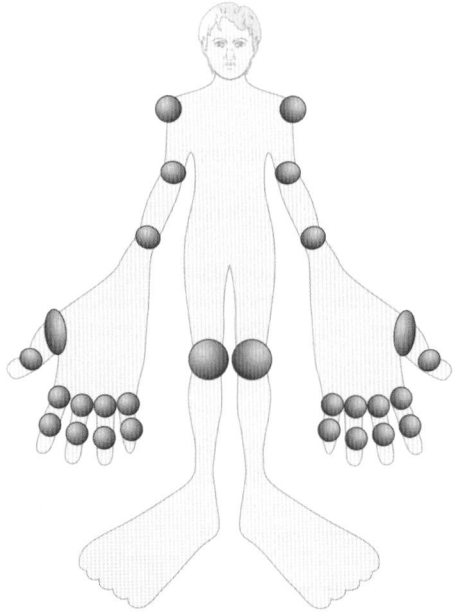

Number of tender joints = t
Number of swollen joints = sw
Erythrocyte sedimentation rate in mm/h = ESR
Visual analogue scale of overall health in mm = GH

Calculate on online calculator (www.4s-dawn.com/DAS28) or calculate on equation below:

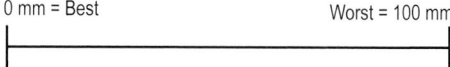

0 mm = Best   Worst = 100 mm

$$DAS28 = 0.56*\sqrt{(t)} + 0.28*\sqrt{(sw)} + 0.70*Log(ESR) + 0.014*GH$$

Fig. 18.27 Calculation of disease activity score from 28 joints (DAS28).

diagnosis. Patients adjust and cope remarkably with time and support from the specialist team in a rheumatology unit (including doctors, nurses, physiotherapists, podiatrists and psychologists) and from leaflets, websites and local patient groups.

Patients from socially deprived backgrounds and smokers have a worse prognosis. Due to the increased prevalence of cardiovascular risk in RA, aggressive management of traditional cardiac risk factors and suppression of disease are required.

Drug therapy

No curative agent exists for RA but early recognition and an intensified treat to target (T2T) regime, with regular review until remission occurs, improves outcomes. Less frequent review is then continued to assess disease activity, damage, function and co-morbidities.

The disease activity score DAS28 is widely used to measure disease activity in RA by counting the number of tender and swollen joints in 28 joints in the upper limbs and knees, combining these values with the ESR and the patient's assessment of their general health on a visual analogue scale to generate a numerical score (**Fig. 18.27**). A DAS28 score of greater than 5.1 implies active disease, less than 3.2 low disease activity and less than 2.6 remission.

For newly diagnosed patients, treatment typically begins with a combination of fast-acting corticosteroid (its dose/duration limited to give benefit with minimal side-effects) and slow-acting conventional synthetic (cs)DMARDs. With regular and frequent review the T2T approach enables optimization and intensification of therapy with effective doses of csDMARDs, often in combination to prevent the long-term irreversible damaging effects of joint inflammation.

For patients who fail to achieve low disease activity or remission with csDMARDs biological therapies (bDMARDS) are then used to achieve the desired target. If efficacy is not achieved, or subsequently lost, then switching to an alternative bDMARD is indicated. A new therapeutic class of DMARDs that inhibit intracellular Janus kinase (JAK) enzymes are now licensed in RA. These drugs, known as targeted synthetic (ts)DMARDs, have oral bioavailability, rapid onset of action and efficacy similar to bDMARDs.

Non-steroidal anti-inflammatory drugs and coxibs

Most people with RA require an NSAID to relieve night pain and morning stiffness in addition to DMARDs. The individual response to NSAIDs varies greatly, so several different drugs may have to be tried for at least a week to find the most effective (see **Box 18.18**). The major side-effects of NSAIDs and the use of coxibs are discussed on page 431. If gastrointestinal side-effects are prominent, or the patient is over 65 years of age, add a proton pump inhibitor. For additional relief, a simple analgesic is taken as required (e.g. paracetamol or a combination of codeine or dihydrocodeine and paracetamol).

Corticosteroids

The early use of corticosteroids slows down the course of the disease but intensive short courses in very early arthritis do not appear to stop progressive disease. Corticosteroids are a common cause of secondary osteoporosis; therefore, concomitant vitamin D and bisphosphonates are necessary to reduce fracture risk in patients expected to be on corticosteroid therapy for more than 3 months' duration.

Intra-articular injections with semi-crystalline steroid preparations have a powerful but sometimes only short-lived effect.

Intramuscular depot injections (40–120 mg depot methylprednisolone) are used to help induce remission while waiting for DMARDs to work and to control severe disease flares.

Oral corticosteroids are powerful disease-controlling drugs but cause a number of problems (**Box 18.31**; see also **Box 21.20**); they are best avoided in the long term because side-effects are inevitable. Early intensive short-term regimens are often used to help induce remission. Corticosteroids are invaluable to people with

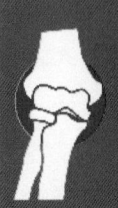

Box 18.31 Problems associated with the use of corticosteroids

- Patients are increasingly anxious about the use of corticosteroids because of adverse publicity about their potential side-effects. This must be discussed frankly and the risks of not using corticosteroids in treatment should be described and balanced against the risks posed by the drugs themselves.
- Patients must be warned to avoid sugars and saturated fats, and to eat less because of the risk of weight gain.
- The skin becomes thin and easily damaged.
- Patients should be monitored for diabetes and hypertension.
- Cataract formation may be accelerated.
- Osteoporosis develops within 3 months on doses above 7.5 mg daily. Monitor with DXA scan and treat with calcium, vitamin D and bisphosphonate (see p. 479).

DXA, dual-energy absorptiometry.

severe disease who have extra-articular manifestations such as vasculitis.

Disease-modifying anti-rheumatic drugs

Various DMARDs are listed in **Box 18.32**. Their beneficial effect is not immediate, taking 2–3 months to become apparent. As monotherapy, csDMARDs often have only a partial effect, achieving between 20% and 50% improvement by ACR criteria for disease remission (**Box 18.33**), and are frequently used in combination.

Early intervention with csDMARDs within 3 months of disease onset improves the outcome. Combinations of up to four drugs (steroids, sulfasalazine, methotrexate and hydroxychloroquine) may be used; the number of agents then reduced once remission has been achieved. Several DMARDs are contraindicated in pregnancy (see **Box 38.9**). Effective treatment with DMARDs including TNF-α blockers reduces the increased cardiovascular risk in RA.

Methotrexate

Methotrexate remains the anchor drug in RA therapy, although it should not be used in pregnancy. A screening history, chest X-ray and an interferon gamma release assay (IGRA) in high-risk patients are performed to exclude tuberculosis. Initial pneumococcal and annual influenza vaccinations are given. The starting *weekly* dose of 7.5–10 mg orally is increased up to 15–25 mg as necessary to T2T (see p. 444). It is well tolerated, although nausea or poor absorption may limit its efficacy, in which case it is given by subcutaneous injection. Oral folic acid reduces side-effects but may also lessen efficacy. Full blood counts and liver biochemistry should be monitored. Methotrexate usually works within 1–2 months. More patients remain on this agent than on most other DMARDs, indicating that it is effective and has relatively few side-effects.

Sulfasalazine

Sulfasalazine is well tolerated and can be used during pregnancy. The usual starting dose of 500 mg per day is increased to a maintenance dose of 2–3 g per day. Around 50% of patients respond in the first 3–6 months, but efficacy can be lost.

Hydroxychloroquine

A dose of 200–400 mg daily is well tolerated. It is used alone in mild disease or commonly as an adjunct to other DMARDs. Due to the risk of irreversible retinopathy with increasing dose and duration of use, baseline formal ophthalmic examination is now recommended within 1 year of commencing therapy. This initial screening is followed by annual optician review until 5 years of therapy are completed then annual ophthalmic assessment is required.

Leflunomide

This csDMARD prevents pyrimidine production in proliferating lymphocytes through blockade of the enzyme dihydro-orotate dehydrogenase, thus blocking clonal expansion of T cells. It has a long half-life of 4–28 days. A dose of 20 mg daily (10 mg if diarrhoea is a problem) is used. Diarrhoea diminishes with time. Blood monitoring is obligatory (full blood count, platelets, liver biochemistry). The onset of action is 4 weeks with some further improvement sustained at 2 years. Leflunomide works in some patients who have failed to respond to methotrexate. Its long half-life means that it is best avoided in women planning a family.

Biological therapies

These drugs are more expensive than csDMARDs. Costs, however, are being reduced by the introduction of biosimilar medicines – medicines that are highly similar to another (originator) drug and have been shown to have no clinically meaningful differences in quality, safety or efficacy from the originator compound.

TNF-α blockers

These agents are used after at least two csDMARDs (usually sulfasalazine and methotrexate) have failed. They are usually given in combination with methotrexate to reduce loss of efficacy due to anti-drug antibody formation.

- **Etanercept** is a fully humanized p75 TNF-α receptor IgG1 fusion protein given by self-administered subcutaneous injection. Around 65% of patients respond well. Some develop an injection reaction.
- **Adalimumab** is a fully human monoclonal antibody against TNF-α, given along with methotrexate.
- **Infliximab** is a monoclonal antibody against TNF-α, given intravenously and co-prescribed with methotrexate to prevent loss of efficacy because of antibody formation.
- **Certolizumab pegol** is a Fab fragment of a humanized TNF-α inhibitor monoclonal antibody that has polyethylene glycol (PEG) groups attached to reduce immunogenicity and prolong half-life. The presence of PEG and lack of Fc portion are likely responsible for its minimal transfer across the placenta and into breast milk. It is useful with or without methotrexate for severe active RA.
- **Golimumab** is a human IgG1-κ monoclonal antibody against TNF, which is given by subcutaneous injection once monthly for severe RA.

These products slow or halt erosion formation in up to 70% of people with RA and produce healing in a few. Malaise and tiredness improve in a manner that is not seen with csDMARDs. Secondary failure may occur with all in the first year; changing to another anti-TNF agent is justified and often regains control of the disease. Failure to respond to one does not predict failure to others. Currently, biosimilars exist for etanercept, infliximab and adalimumab.

Safety data. Various national registries exist to study adverse events, long-term outcomes and problems arising from biological therapies. To date, the results are reassuring. Infection rates are increased with TNF-α blockers, particularly in the first few months of treatment, but the rate then declines. There is a known association between RA and non-Hodgkin's lymphoma (NHL) but, overall, registers have not shown an increased risk of NHL in patients with RA treated with TNF-α blockers, to date. There is no convincing evidence of any increased risk of other cancers. Reactivation of

i   Box 18.32 Disease-modifying anti-rheumatic drugs (DMARDs)

Drug	Dose	Side-effects	Monitoring
Sulfasalazine (enteric coated)	500 mg daily after food, increasing to 2–3 g daily	Nausea Skin rashes and mouth ulcers Neutropenia and/or thrombocytopenia Abnormal liver biochemistry	Baseline FBC, serum creatinine and electrolytes, LFTs, then at 2, 4, 6 and 10 weeks, then 3-monthly
Methotrexate (give pneumococcal and annual influenza vaccinations)	7.5–10 mg increasing to max. 25 mg weekly, orally or s.c.	Nausea, mouth ulcers and diarrhoea Abnormal liver biochemistry Neutropenia and/or thrombocytopenia Renal impairment Rare – pulmonary fibrosis	Baseline FBC, serum creatinine and electrolytes, LFTs, then at 2, 4, 6 and 10 weeks, then 3-monthly
Leflunomide	10–20 mg daily, occasionally with initial loading dose	Diarrhoea Neutropenia and/or thrombocytopenia Abnormal liver biochemistry Alopecia Hypertension	Baseline FBC, serum creatinine and electrolytes, LFTs, then at 2, 4, 6 and 10 weeks, then 3-monthly

Cytokine modulators
TNF-α blockers

Drug	Dose	Side-effects	Monitoring
Etanercept (alone or with methotrexate)	s.c. 25 mg × 2-weekly or 50 mg weekly	Injection site reactions Heart failure Reversible lupus-like syndrome Infections Hypersensitivity reactions Rare – demyelination and autoimmune syndromes	Monitor as per concomitant DMARD; if monotherapy repeat FBC, serum creatinine and electrolytes, and LFTs 3–6 monthly
Adalimumab (with methotrexate)	s.c. 40 mg alternate weeks		
Infliximab (with methotrexate)	i.v. 3–10 mg/kg every 4–8 weeks		As per etanercept
Certolizumab pegol (alone or with methotrexate)	s.c. 400 mg in weeks 0, 2, 4, then 200 mg fortnightly		As per etanercept
Golimumab	s.c. monthly 50 mg		

Other biological agents (used with methotrexate)

Drug	Dose	Side-effects	Monitoring
Rituximab	i.v. 500–1000 mg	Hypo-/hypertension Pruritus and skin rash Back pain Rare – toxic epidermal necrolysis	
Abatacept	i.v. 10 mg/kg on days 1, 15, 30 and then monthly s.c. preparations available	Nausea, vomiting Headache Rare – hypersensitivity	Monitor as per concomitant DMARD; if monotherapy repeat FBC, serum creatinine and electrolytes and LFTs 3–6 monthly
Tocilizumab	i.v. 8 mg/kg infusion	Headache Skin eruption and stomatitis Fever Anaphylactic reactions	As per abatacept plus baseline and 3-month check of lipids with repeat at physician's discretion
Sarilumab	s.c. 200 mg alternate weeks	Dyslipidaemia, neutropenia, thrombocytopenia, skin reactions	As per tocilizumab

JAK inhibitors

Drug	Dose	Side-effects	Monitoring
Tofacitinib	5 mg oral twice daily	Anaemia, cough, neutropenia, diarrhoea, dyslipidaemia, dyspnoea, fatigue, gastritis, headache, hypertension, skin reactions	Baseline as per etanercept, then monitor FBC, serum creatinine and electrolytes, and LFTs at 4 and 8 weeks then 3-monthly. Check lipids at baseline and after 8 weeks
Baricitinib	4 mg oral once daily in adults 18–74 years; 2 mg oral once daily in adults ≥75 years	Dyslipidaemia, herpes zoster, increased risk of infection, nausea, oropharyngeal pain, thrombocytosis, acne, neutropenia, weight gain	As per tofacitinib

CD19, cluster of differentiation 19; FBC, full blood count; i.v., intravenous; JAK, Janus kinase inhibitor; LFTs, liver function tests; s.c., subcutaneous; TNF-α, tumour necrosis factor-alpha.

- Tender joint count (including feet and ankles) ≤1
- Swollen joint count (including feet and ankles) ≤1
- C-reactive protein ≤1 mg/L
- Patient global assessment ≤1 (on a 10-cm visual analogue scale)

ACR, American College of Rheumatology; EULAR, European League Against Rheumatism.

old tuberculosis may occur but is probably less common with etanercept. A pre-treatment chest X-ray is recommended, with IGRA and specialist review for high-risk groups. Tuberculosis should be treated before these agents are prescribed, and a course of prophylaxis is used in latent disease. Hepatitis B and C infection requires risk analysis and regular aminotransferase monitoring if anti-TNF agents are prescribed. They should not be used in patients who have severe cardiac failure. To date, there is no evidence of an adverse effect on pregnancy outcome but care is essential (see **Box 38.6**).

Other biological agents

- **Rituximab** is a chimeric monoclonal antibody (see p. 67), directed against the CD20 receptor expressed on pre-B and mature B cells. Rituximab produces significant improvement in RF-positive RA for 8 months to several years when used alone or in combination with corticosteroids and/or methotrexate. This clinical improvement is associated with a 6–9-month B-cell lymphopenia. A re-flare is often accompanied by a return of peripheral B lymphocytes and rise in CRP. Repeated courses, with disease flare, are well tolerated and around 80% of RF-positive patients respond, with 50–60% showing persistent disease control; however, immunoglobulin levels should be monitored, as they may fall with repeated treatments. Rituximab is mainly used in patients who have failed to respond to anti-TNF agents and a biosimilar exists.
- **Abatacept** is a recombinant fusion protein of CTLA4 and the Fc portion of IgG1, which selectively modulates T-cell activation by co-stimulation blockade. It may be used in patients who do not respond to anti-TNF regimens.
- **Tocilizumab and sarilumab** are monoclonal antibodies against the anti-IL-6 receptor that may be used with methotrexate for moderate to severe RA, usually after at least one other biologic has failed, but may also be considered as a first-line biological therapy.

Targeted synthetic DMARDS

Tofacitinib and baricitinib are oral JAK inhibitors that may be used in combination with methotrexate, or as monotherapy in patients who cannot take methotrexate, and have severe disease.

Switching between DMARDs and tapering therapy

Patients who fail to respond initially (primary failure) or subsequently lose efficacy (secondary failure) to a bDMARD over time will usually be switched to another bDMARD. In patients who lose response to a TNF-α blocker it is helpful to measure drug levels and for presence of neutralizing anti-drug antibodies (ADA), where possible. If the drug level is therapeutic then a non-TNF-α blocker is preferred. Alternatively, if the drug level is sub-therapeutic, non-adherence or the presence of ADA are likely explanations and switching to another TNF-α blocker or a different class of bDMARD are viable alternatives. If primary or secondary failure occurs to a subsequent

bDMARD the switching process may be repeated multiple times. Switching to tsDMARDs may now be considered.

In patients who achieve sustained remission (>1 year) it is now commonplace to attempt dose reduction of DMARDs by either dose reduction or prolongation of dosing interval. Potential biomarkers of responsiveness are being explored to ensure a precision medicine approach to each individual patient.

Physical measures

Input is required from the multidisciplinary team. Physiotherapists advise a combination of rest for active arthritis and exercises to maintain joint range and muscle power. Exercise in a hydrotherapy pool is popular and effective. Occupational therapists help to manage activities of daily living despite the arthritis and provide functional adaptations in the home or at work. Family and friends should be involved. Podiatry, footwear advice and psychological support should also be offered to all people with RA.

Surgery

Surgery has a useful role in the long-term approach to patient management but is less frequently needed as therapeutic disease control becomes more effective. Its main objectives are prophylactic, to prevent joint destruction and deformity, and reconstructive, to restore function.

Surgical options in RA include: surgical synovectomy; tendon repair; osteotomy to realign weightbearing surfaces; joint fusion to stabilize damaged joints that are not easily replaced; small joint implant arthroplasty, e.g. metacarpophalangeal joints; excision arthroplasties of the metatarsal heads to reduce metatarsal pain; and total joint replacement arthroplasty of the shoulder, elbow, wrist, hip, knee and ankle. The main aim of joint arthroplasty is to reduce pain and improve function, requiring careful planning with explanation of risks and outcomes to the patient.

Prognosis

A poor prognosis is indicated by:

- **a clinical picture** of an insidious rather than an explosive onset of RA, female sex, increasing number of peripheral joints involved and the level of disability at the onset
- **blood tests** showing a high CRP/ESR, normochromic normocytic anaemia, and high titres of ACPA and of RF
- **X-rays** with early erosive damage (*note*: ultrasound and MRI can show cartilage and bone damage prior to conventional X-rays).

Prognosis can be altered dramatically with early DMARD therapy and T2T regime (see p. 444) under expert supervision.

SPONDYLOARTHRITIS

The term spondyloarthritis (SpA) describes a group of conditions affecting the spine and peripheral joints with familial clustering and a link to certain type 1 HLA antigens (**Box 18.34**). These conditions share genetic factors and increasing implication of the IL-17 pathway in pathogenesis. Joint involvement differs from RA, being more

i **Box 18.34** Spondyloarthritis

- Axial spondyloarthritis, including ankylosing spondylitis
- Psoriatic arthritis
- Reactive arthritis (sexually acquired)
- Post-dysenteric reactive arthritis
- Enteropathic arthritis (ulcerative colitis/Crohn's disease)

limited with a different distribution and associated extra-articular features. These diseases occasionally present in childhood.

They may also be categorized according to their predominant clinical manifestation of axial (sacroiliac and/or spine) or peripheral (arthritis, enthesitis and/or dactylitis) disease with possible overlap. Distinct SpA conditions exist (see **Box 18.34**).

Histologically, synovitis is similar to that of RA, but there is no production of RF or ACPA. Inflammation of the enthesis (junction of ligament or tendon and bone) and joint ankylosis develop more commonly than in RA. All are associated with an increased frequency of sacroiliitis and HLA-B27.

Aetiology

These disorders have a striking association with HLA-B27, particularly ankylosing spondylitis (AS). HLA type B27 is present in more than 90% of Caucasians with AS but only 8% of controls. HLA-B27 exhibits a number of unusual characteristics, including a high tendency to misfold. The types of arthritis that follow a precipitating infection are called reactive arthritis (see p. 450).

Axial spondyloarthritis

Axial spondyloarthritis (AxSpA) occurs in 1% of the general population. It is an inflammatory disorder primarily affecting sacroiliac joints or fibrous and synovial joints of the spine that are detectable on MRI. When radiographic changes at the sacroiliac joints are present, the term ankylosing spondylitis (AS) is used.

Ankylosing spondylitis

It is now recognized that AS forms part of the spectrum of AxSpA. It presents with inflammatory back pain and sacroiliac inflammation. It is seen in 0.2–0.5% of the population in Northern Europe and approximately 0.5% in the USA, affecting mainly young adults (late teens to early thirties) and occurring worldwide, with a male to female ratio of 3 : 1. Women present later and are under-diagnosed. The frequency of AxSpA in different populations is roughly paralleled by the incidence of HLA-B27; Africans and Japanese have a low incidence of both HLA-B27 and AS, while the North American Haida Indians have a high incidence of both.

Aetiology

A combination of genetic and environmental features:
- Among white individuals with AS, 95% carry HLA-B27, in contrast to 8% of most white populations. Twin studies indicate a much higher disease concordance in HLA-B27-positive monozygotic twins (up to 70%) than in dizygotic twins (about 20–25%).
- Other genes lying within the MHC (the *IL-1* gene cluster and *CYP2D6*) also influence susceptibility to AS but the disease is polygenic and GWAS have identified significant associations with the endoplasmic reticulum aminopeptidase (*ERAP*)-1 and *IL-23* genes.
- The association of *ERAP-1* with AxSpA may support the arthritogenic peptide hypothesis, whereby disease is triggered by presentation of peptide by HLA-B27 to CD8-positive T cells. Furthermore, misfolding of HLA-B27 leads to the production of IL-23, and T cells resident in entheses promote inflammation characteristic of SpA in response to IL-23.
- The finding of increased frequency of Th17 cells and various genetic association studies have implicated the IL-23-IL-17 axis in pathogenesis and this knowledge has been translated into therapies that target this pathway.

> **Box 18.35 Back pain criteria for diagnosing axial/ ankylosing spondylitis**
>
> - *Age of onset* <45 years
> - *Insidious onset*
> - *Improvement of back pain with exercise*
> - *No improvement of back pain with rest*
> - *Pain at night* with improvement on getting up
>   The presence of **four of the five criteria suggests ankylosing spondylitis with 80% sensitivity**. All criteria have high sensitivity.

> **Box 18.36 Non-articular problems in spondyloarthritis**
>
> - Uveitis, in all types
> - Cutaneous lesions in reactive arthritis (keratoderma blennorrhagica), histologically identical to pustular psoriasis
> - Nail dystrophy, in psoriasis and reactive arthritis
> - Aortitis, occasionally in ankylosing spondylitis and reactive arthritis

---

- Reports of dysbiosis in the gut microbiome of AS patients supports previous work indicating a link between gut microbiota, intestinal inflammation and AxSpA.
- Lymphocyte and plasma cell infiltration occurs with local erosion of bone at the attachments of the intervertebral and other ligaments (enthesitis), which heals with new bone (syndesmophyte) formation.

Clinical features

Initially, the diagnosis is often missed because the patient is asymptomatic between episodes and radiological abnormalities are absent.
- *Back pain* with episodic inflammation of the sacroiliac joints in the late teenage years or early twenties is the first manifestation of AxSpA.
- *Pain in one or both buttocks* and low back pain and stiffness are typically worse in the morning and relieved by exercise.
- *Retention of the lumbar lordosis during spinal flexion* is an early sign. Later, paraspinal muscle wasting develops.

Criteria for classifying inflammatory back pain as AxSpA are shown in **Box 18.35**. These criteria encompass the whole spectrum of disease, with evidence of sacroiliitis being based on radiographic or MRI evidence of disease. Spinal stiffness can be measured by Schober's test; skin over the midline of the spine is marked 5 cm below and 10 cm above the dimples of Venus and the increase in distance between those marks during flexion is recorded. An increase of less than 5 cm implies spinal stiffness.

Non-spinal complications (uveitis or costochondritis) suggest the diagnosis of SpA (**Box 18.36**):
- *Costochondral junction inflammation* causes anterior chest pain. Measurable reduction of chest expansion is due to costovertebral joint involvement.
- *Peripheral joint involvement* is asymmetrical and affects a few, predominantly large, joints. Hip involvement leads to fixed flexion deformities of the hips and further deterioration of posture. Young teenage boys occasionally present with a lower-limb monoarthritis, which later develops into AS.
- *Acute anterior uveitis* occurs in approximately 30% of patients with AxSpA and related diseases, and is occasionally the presenting complaint. Severe eye pain, photophobia and blurred vision are an emergency (see p. 921).
- *Other extra-articular features* include:
  - cardiovascular disease – aortic incompetence occurs in up to 1% of patients with established AS and cardiac conduction abnormalities in around 5%

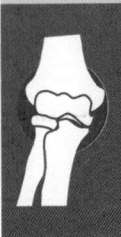

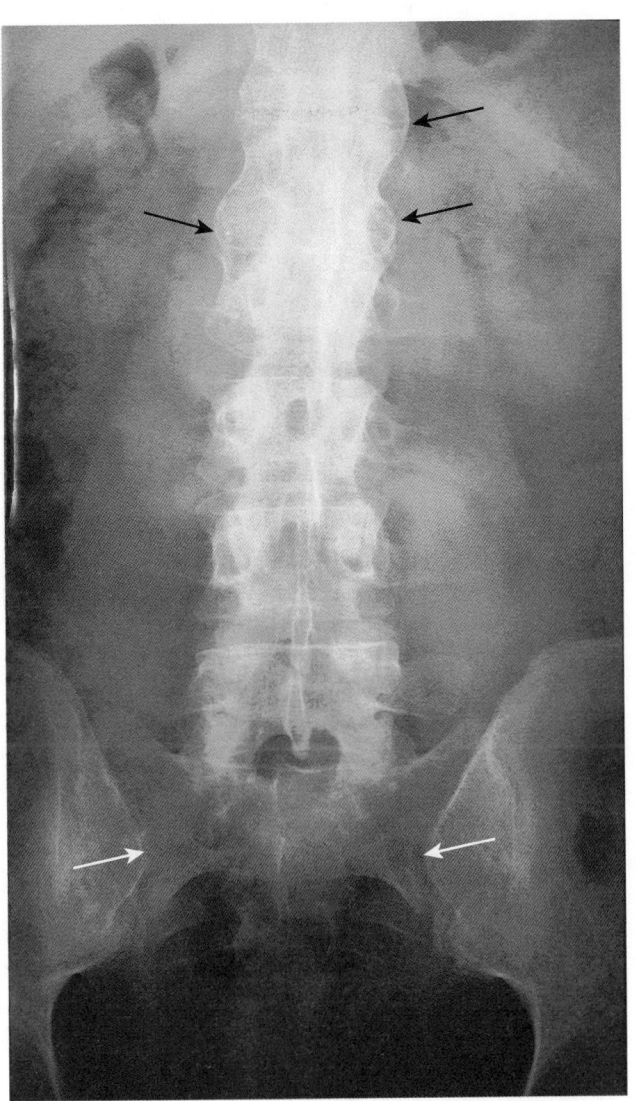

Fig. 18.28 X-ray of ankylosing spondylitis. The sacroiliac joints are eroded and show marginal sclerosis (white arrows). There is bridging syndesmophyte formation at the thoracolumbar junction (black arrows).

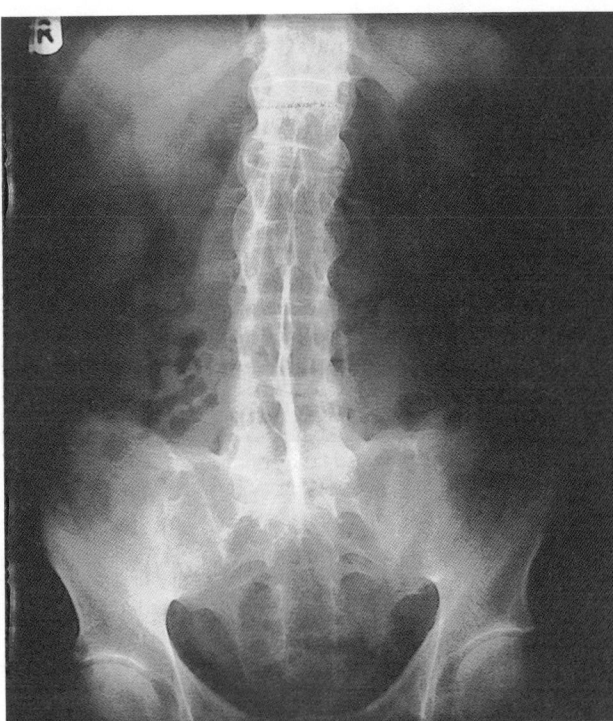

Fig. 18.29 X-ray of bamboo spine in ankylosing spondylitis. In advanced disease, there is calcification of the interspinous ligaments and fusion of the facet joints, as well as syndesmophytes at all levels. The sacroiliac joints fuse.

- respiratory disease – rarely, chest wall rigidity is associated with interstitial lung disease
- renal impairment – reported in 10–35% of patients with AS and most commonly linked to chronic NSAID use
- axial osteoporosis – occurs in approximately 25%, with vertebral fracture in 10%.

Overall clinical assessment of disease activity is based on a 1–10 score for levels of fatigue, spinal pain, arthralgia, swelling, localized tenderness, inflammation of tendons/enthesis, and duration and severity of morning stiffness. It is measured using the Bath Ankylosing Spondylitis Disease Activity Index (see Further reading).

Investigations

- **Blood.** ESR and CRP are usually raised.
- **HLA B27 testing.** This test is not definitive due to the high frequency of HLA-B27 in the population, but may strengthen or confirm suspected diagnoses.
- **X-rays.** The medial and lateral cortical margins of both sacroiliac joints lose definition owing to erosions and eventually become sclerotic (**Fig. 18.28**). Radiological appearances in the spine of

blurring of the upper or lower vertebral rims at the thoracolumbar junction are caused by an enthesitis at the insertion of the intervertebral ligaments and may eventually affect the whole spine causing bony spurs (syndesmophytes), bony ankylosis and permanent stiffening. The sacroiliac joints eventually fuse, as may the costovertebral joints, reducing chest expansion. Calcification of the intervertebral ligaments and fusion of the spinal facet joints and syndesmophytes leads to what is often called a 'bamboo' spine (**Fig. 18.29**).
- **MRI.** MRI with gadolinium demonstrates sacroiliitis before it is seen on X-rays, as well as persistent enthesitis.

Management

- The key to effective management of AS is early diagnosis so that a regimen of preventative exercises is started before syndesmophytes have formed. Morning exercises aim to maintain spinal mobility, posture and chest expansion; regular NSAIDs to improve symptoms and signs of SpA are often required to achieve this goal.
- Failure to control pain and to encourage regular spinal and chest exercises leads to an irreversible dorsal kyphosis and wasted paraspinal muscles, which, along with stiffening of the cervical spine, makes forward vision difficult.
- When the inflammation is active and the morning pain and stiffness are too severe to permit effective exercise, an evening dose of a long-acting or slow-release NSAID or an NSAID suppository improves sleep, pain control and exercise compliance.
- Sulfasalazine, methotrexate and leflunomide may help peripheral arthritis but not spinal disease.
- When NSAIDs have failed, the TNF-α-blocking drugs adalimumab, etanercept, golimumab, certolizumab and infliximab (see **Box 18.32**) have all been shown to reduce symptoms of spinal

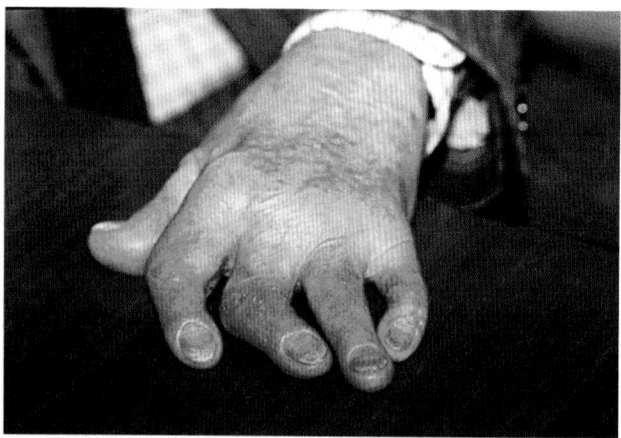

Fig. 18.30 Hand showing psoriatic arthritis mutilans. All the fingers are shortened and the joints unstable, owing to underlying osteolysis.

and peripheral joint inflammation substantially and to improve function, as well as quality of life. Evidence of reduction of bony progression, however, has not been found. Relapse occurs on stopping therapy but may be delayed by several months making intermittent treatment feasible.

- Other bDMARDs including the IL-12 and IL-23 blocker ustekinumab and the IL-17 blocker secukinumab are alternative options in SpA.

Prognosis

With exercise and pain relief, the prognosis is excellent and over 80% of patients are fully employed. The advent of bDMARD therapies has reduced the morbidity of severe disease, lowering the risk of permanent spinal stiffness and progressive peripheral joint disease.

Psoriatic arthritis

The prevalence of psoriasis is 2–3% worldwide; in this population, around 10% have arthritis, which precedes skin disease in around 15% of cases. A family history of psoriasis may be a clue to the diagnosis. The aetiology and pathogenesis are described on page 664.

Clinical features

Patterns of psoriatic arthritis include:
- **Mono- or oligoarthritis.**
- **Polyarthritis:** often begins with an asymmetrical pattern and progresses to be virtually indistinguishable from RA.
- **Spondylitis:** unilateral or bilateral sacroiliitis and early cervical spine involvement; only 50% are HLA-B27-positive.
- **Distal interphalangeal arthritis:** the most typical pattern of joint involvement in psoriasis, often with adjacent nail dystrophy (see p. 665) reflecting enthesitis extending into the nail root. Dactylitis, in which an entire finger or toe is swollen, with joint and tendon sheath involvement, is characteristic of this condition.
- **Arthritis mutilans:** affects about 5% of patients who have psoriatic arthritis and causes marked periarticular osteolysis and bone shortening ('telescopic' fingers) (**Fig. 18.30**).

Radiologically, psoriatic arthritis is erosive but the erosions are central in the joint, not juxta-articular, and produce a 'pencil in cup' appearance (**Fig. 18.31**). The skin and nail disease can be mild and may develop after the arthritis.

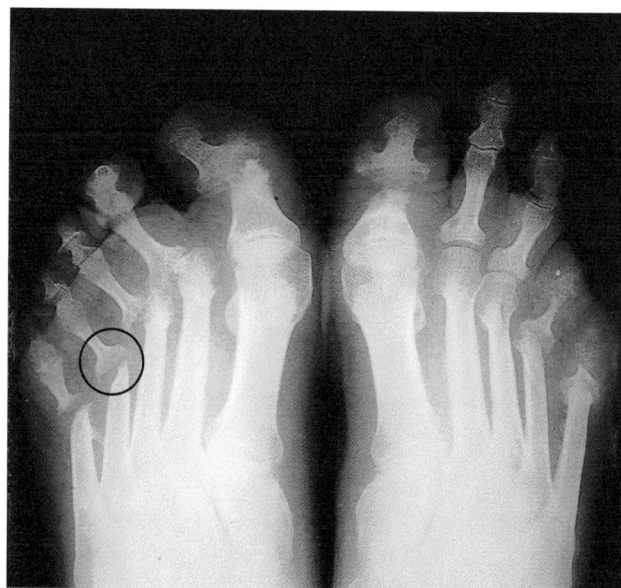

Fig. 18.31 X-ray of psoriatic arthritis. There is osteolysis of the metatarsal heads and central erosion of the proximal phalanges to produce the 'pencil in cup' appearance (circle). All the lesser toes are subluxed.

Management and prognosis

NSAIDs and/or analgesics help the pain but can occasionally worsen the skin lesions. Local synovitis responds to intra-articular corticosteroid injections. Sulfasalazine, methotrexate and leflunomide are commonly used in patients with persistent peripheral joint synovitis, although none has a proven effect on slowing the development of joint damage. Hydroxychloroquine is best avoided because it may rarely cause acute psoriatic skin reactions. Similarly, oral corticosteroids may destabilize skin disease; they are best avoided but are valuable when injected into a single inflamed joint.

Various bDMARDs and tsDMARDs are now available and highly effective for severe skin and joint disease in patients where csDMARDs, principally methotrexate, have failed. The bDMARDs include anti-TNF-α agents, such as etanercept and golimumab (see p. 445); IL-17 inhibitors, secukinumab and ixekizumab; and ustekinumab, an anti-IL-12/23 inhibitor. The tsDMARDs include apremilast, an oral PDE4 inhibitor and tofacitinib, a JAK inhibitor.

Reactive arthritis

Reactive arthritis is a sterile synovitis, which occurs following an infection. Spondyloarthritis develops in 1–2% of patients after an acute attack of dysentery, or after a sexually acquired infection – non-specific urethritis (NSU) in the male, non-specific cervicitis in the female. In males, positivity for HLA-B27 increases the risk of developing reactive arthritis after such an infection by 30–50-fold but not all patients are HLA-B27-positive. Women are less commonly affected.

Aetiology

A variety of organisms can be the trigger, including strains of *Salmonella* or *Shigella* spp. in bacillary dysentery. *Yersinia enterocolitica* causes diarrhoea and a reactive arthritis. In NSU, the organisms are *Chlamydia trachomatis* or *Ureaplasma urealyticum*.

People with reactive arthritis are not more susceptible to infection but appear to respond differently. Bacterial antigens or bacterial DNA have been found in the inflamed synovium of affected joints,

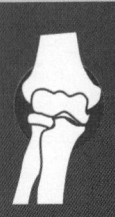

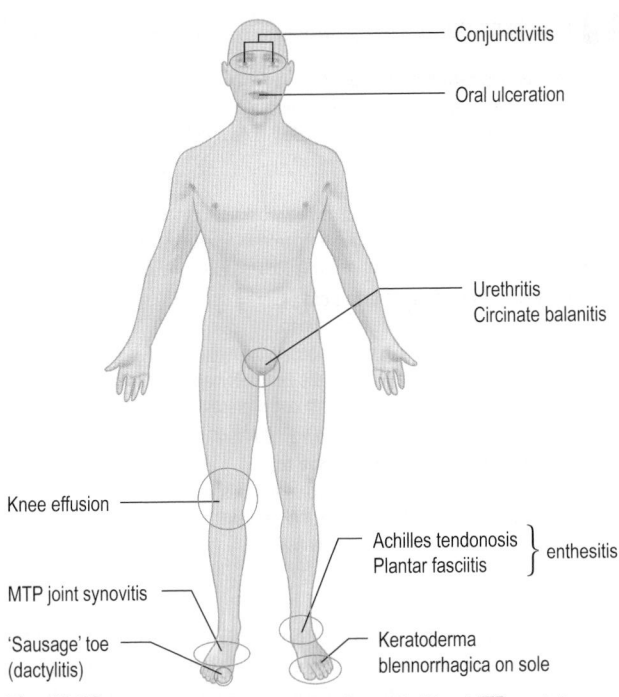

Conjunctivitis

Oral ulceration

Urethritis
Circinate balanitis

Knee effusion

Achilles tendonosis
Plantar fasciitis } enthesitis

MTP joint synovitis

'Sausage' toe
(dactylitis)

Keratoderma
blennorrhagica on sole

Fig. 18.32 Clinical features of reactive arthritis. MTP, metatarsophalangeal.

suggesting that this persistent antigenic material is driving the inflammatory process. The methods by which HLA-B27 increases susceptibility to reactive arthritis include:

- T-cell receptor repertoire selection
- molecular mimicry causing autoimmunity against HLA-B27 and/or other self antigens
- mode of presentation of bacteria-derived peptides to T lymphocytes.

There are other organisms that also trigger reactive arthritis but have a different genetic basis; see post-streptococcal arthritis (p. 544), gonococcal arthritis (p. 455) and brucellosis (p. 456). In these conditions, the line between reactive arthritis and septic arthritis is more indistinct and they can cause both.

Clinical features

Typically an acute, asymmetrical, lower-limb arthritis, this occurs days to weeks after the infection. The arthritis may be the presenting complaint if the infection is mild or asymptomatic. Enthesitis is common, causing plantar fasciitis or Achilles tendon enthesitis (see p. 428), and dactylitis may also occur (**Fig. 18.32**); 70% of patients recover fully within 6 months but many have a relapse.

In susceptible individuals with reactive arthritis, sacroiliitis and spondylitis may also develop. Sterile conjunctivitis occurs in 30%. Acute anterior uveitis complicates more severe or relapsing disease but is not synchronous with the arthritis.

The skin lesions resemble psoriasis:

- **Circinate balanitis** in the uncircumcised male causes painless superficial ulceration of the glans penis. In the circumcised male, the lesion is raised, red and scaly. Both heal without scarring.
- **Keratoderma blennorrhagica** involves the skin of the feet and hands, which develops painless, red and often confluent raised plaques and pustules that are histologically similar to pustular psoriasis.
- **Nail dystrophy** occurs.

Management

Treating persisting infection with antibiotics alters the course of the arthritis, once it has developed. Cultures should be taken and any infection treated. Sexual partners must be screened.

Pain responds well to NSAIDs and locally injected or oral corticosteroids. The majority of individuals with reactive arthritis have a single attack that settles, but a few develop a disabling relapsing and remitting arthritis. Relapsing cases are sometimes treated with sulfasalazine or methotrexate (see **Box 18.32**).

Enteropathic arthritis associated with inflammatory bowel disease

Enteropathic synovitis occurs in up to 10–15% of patients who have ulcerative colitis or Crohn's disease (see p. 1198). The link between the bowel disease and the inflammatory arthritis is not clear. The arthritis is asymmetrical and predominantly affects lower-limb joints. An HLA-B27-associated sacroiliitis or spondylitis also occurs. The joint symptoms may predate the development of bowel disease and lead to its diagnosis.

Remission of ulcerative colitis or total colectomy usually leads to remission of the joint disease, but arthritis can persist even in well-controlled Crohn's disease.

Management

Inflammatory bowel disease should be treated (see **Ch. 32**). In all cases of enteropathic arthritis, the symptoms are helped by NSAIDs, although they may make diarrhoea worse. A monoarthritis is best treated by intra-articular corticosteroids. Sulfasalazine is more frequently prescribed than mesalazine, as it may help both bowel and joint disease. The bDMARDs that are used to treat arthritis and inflammatory bowel disease are the TNF-α-blocking drugs infliximab, adalimumab and certolizumab, and ustekinumab, the IL-12/23 inhibitor.

Crystal arthritis

Aetiology

The two main types of crystal-induced arthritis are caused by sodium urate and calcium pyrophosphate crystals, which are distinguished by their different shapes and refringence properties under polarized light with a red filter (**Fig. 18.33**). Rarely, crystals of calcium apatite (see p. 436) or cholesterol cause acute synovitis.

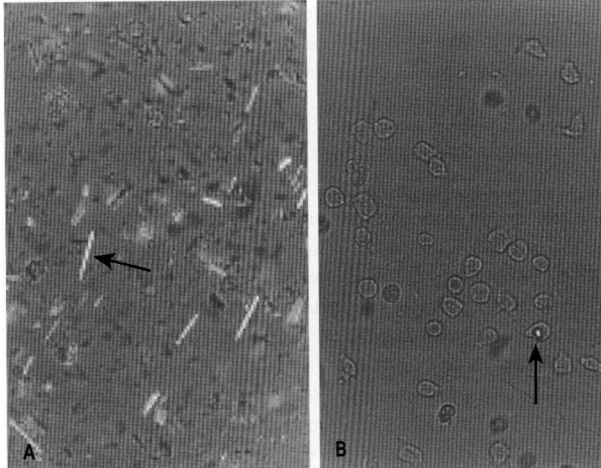

Fig. 18.33 Crystal arthritis. **(A)** Needle-shaped urate crystals (arrowed). **(B)** A small, intracellular pyrophosphate crystal (arrowed). Both are viewed under polarized light with a red filter.

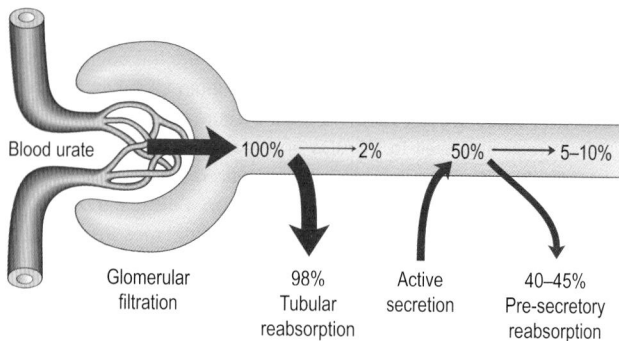

Fig. 18.34 Urate renal transport. The net result is that about 5–10% of the glomerular load is excreted in the urine under normal circumstances.

Blood urate   100% → 2%   50% → 5–10%

Glomerular filtration   98% Tubular reabsorption   Active secretion   40–45% Pre-secretory reabsorption

Gout and hyperuricaemia

Gout is an inflammatory arthritis associated with hyperuricaemia and intra-articular sodium urate crystals.

Epidemiology

The prevalence of gout has increased in recent decades to 2.5% in the UK and 3.9% in the USA. Asian populations are also increasingly at risk as their diet becomes more Western. This rising prevalence is due to changing diets with purine-rich foods, high saturated fats and fructose-containing drinks; alcohol misuse; increasing co-morbidities that promote hyperuricaemia; and suboptimal management. Gout is more common in men than women (5:1); it rarely occurs before young adulthood (when it suggests a specific genetic defect), and seldom in pre-menopausal females. Some 85–90% of cases are idiopathic. Hyperuricaemia is common in certain ethnic groups (e.g. Maoris).

The last two steps of purine metabolism in humans are the conversion of hypoxanthine to xanthine, and of xanthine to uric acid, catalysed by the enzyme xanthine oxidase. Serum uric acid (SUA) levels are higher in men than in women. Pathological hyperuricaemia is defined as a SUA level of 408 μmol/L above which monosodium urate crystal formation occurs in vitro at physiological pH and temperature, although it may occur in peripheral joints with lower tissue pH and temperature, e.g. 360 μmol/L at 35°C and 300 μmol/L at 30°C. Hyperuricaemia is mostly asymptomatic, although OA joints are more prone to attacks of gout. The range of SUA for individuals with gout is higher than in healthy controls. SUA levels increase with age, obesity, a 'Western' diet (see earlier) and combined hyperlipidaemia, diabetes mellitus, ischaemic heart disease and hypertension (metabolic syndrome; see p. 1250). Gout is often familial.

Pathogenesis of hyperuricaemia and gout

Uric acid is the final product of endogenous and dietary purine metabolism in humans, and SUA depends on the balance between purine synthesis, ingestion of dietary purines and the elimination of urate by the kidney (66%) and intestine (33%).

Some 90% of people with gout have impaired excretion of uric acid (10% have increased production due to high cell turnover and <1% due to an inborn error of metabolism). Renal excretion is coordinated by a group of secretory and reabsorptive renal tubular urate transport molecules, some of which are targets of urate-lowering drugs. These molecules can be grouped into reabsorptive urate anion exchangers (URAT1/SLC22A12, OAT4/SLC22A11 and OAT10/SLC22A3), the resorptive GLUT9/SLC2A9 urate transporter,

secretory anion-exchange transporters (OAT1, OAT2 and OAT3) and sodium-phosphate transporter proteins (NPT1/SLC17A1 and NPT4/SLC17A3), and the ATP-driven secretory pump MRP4/SLC17A3 (**Fig. 18.34**). The secretory transporter ABCG2 is significant in the gut, with reduced functioning contributing to extrarenal under-excretion. GWAS have identified prominent loci encoding urate transporters: primarily SLC2A9 and ABCG2; with a second tier dominated by genes encoding SLC22A11, SLC22A12, SLC17A1 and SLC17A3. Causes of hyperuricaemia are shown in **Box 18.37**.

Gout as an autoinflammatory disease

The involvement of the innate immune system and inflammasomes indicates that gout is an autoinflammatory disease, similar to the hereditary periodic fevers (see p. 452). This response is initiated when monosodium urate crystals interact with resident macrophages to form and activate NLRP3 inflammasome. Caspase 1 is recruited by the activated inflammasome (see p. 46) leading to activation of IL-1β and cellular activation, which triggers an IL-8-mediated influx of neutrophils. Ingestion by polymorphonuclear leucocytes of monosodium urate crystals causes the release of pro-inflammatory cytokines, particularly IL-1β and complement. Colchicine inhibits the microtubule formation that is necessary for this process to occur.

Clinical features

Hyperuricaemia may be asymptomatic or may cause:
- **Acute gout**, followed by an asymptomatic intercritical phase; a second acute attack is likely within 2 years.
- **Chronic interval gout**, with acute attacks superimposed on low-grade inflammation and potential joint damage.
- **Chronic polyarticular tophaceous gout**, which is rare and characterized by chronic joint pain, activity limitation, structural joint damage and frequent flares.
- **Urate renal stone** formation (see p. 1373).

Acute gout presents typically in a middle-aged male with a sudden onset of agonizing pain, swelling and redness of the first MTP joint. The attack may be precipitated by excess food, alcohol, dehydration or diuretic therapy. Untreated attacks last about 7 days. Recovery is typically associated with desquamation of the overlying

? Box 18.37 Causes of hyperuricaemia

Impaired excretion of uric acid
- Chronic renal disease (clinical gout unusual)
- Drug therapy, e.g. thiazide diuretics, low-dose aspirin
- Hypertension
- Lead toxicity
- Primary hyperparathyroidism or hypothyroidism
- Increased lactic acid production from alcohol, exercise, starvation
- Glucose-6-phosphatase deficiency (interferes with renal excretion)

Increased production of uric acid

Increased purine synthesis de novo due to:
- Hypoxanthine–guanine–phosphoribosyl transferase (HGPRT) reduction (an X-linked inborn error causing the Lesch–Nyhan syndrome)
- Phosphoribosyl-pyrophosphate synthase overactivity
- Glucose-6-phosphatase deficiency with glycogen storage disease type 1

Increased turnover of purines due to:
- Myeloproliferative disorders, e.g. polycythaemia vera
- Lymphoproliferative disorders, e.g. leukaemia
- Others, e.g. carcinoma, severe psoriasis

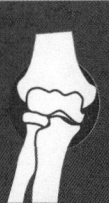

skin. In 25% of attacks, a joint other than the great toe is affected. Triggers for flares include acute medical or surgical illness, dehydration, or dietary factors such as alcohol intake or purine-rich foods.

In severe attacks, overlying crystal cellulitis makes gout difficult to distinguish clinically from infective cellulitis. A family or personal history of gout and the finding of a raised SUA suggest the diagnosis but, if in doubt, blood and joint fluid cultures should be taken to exclude sepsis.

Chronic tophaceous gout is described below.

Investigations

The clinical picture is often diagnostic, as is the rapid response to NSAIDs or colchicine.
- *Joint fluid microscopy* is the most specific and diagnostic test but is technically difficult.
- *Serum uric acid* is usually raised (>600 μmol/L). If it is not, it should be rechecked several weeks after the attack, as levels fall immediately after an acute episode. Acute gout rarely occurs with SUA in the lower half of the normal range below the saturation point of 360 μmol/L.
- *Serum urea, creatinine* and estimated glomerular filtration rate (eGFR) are monitored for signs of renal impairment.

Management

The use of NSAIDs or coxibs in high doses rapidly reduces the pain and swelling. The first dose should be taken at the first indication of an attack:
- *naproxen*: 750 mg immediately, then 500 mg every 8–12 hours
- *diclofenac*: 75–100 mg immediately, then 50 mg every 6–8 hours. After 24–48 hours, reduced doses are given for a further week.
Caution: NSAIDs may cause renal impairment. In individuals with renal impairment or a history of peptic ulceration, alternative treatments include:
- *Colchicine*: loading doses will cause diarrhoea or colicky abdominal pain, so 500 μg 2–3 times per day is usually sufficient to terminate attacks without side-effects.
- *Corticosteroids*: oral prednisolone or intramuscular or intra-articular depot methylprednisolone is used.

Dietary advice

The first attacks may be separated by up to 2 years and are managed symptomatically. Recognition and prompt treatment, including lifestyle modifications, are paramount. Advice to reduce alcohol intake, especially beer, which is high in purines and fructose, and consumption of non-diet carbonated soft drinks, also high in fructose, is essential; other dietary change include reduction of total calorie and cholesterol intake, and avoidance of purine-rich foods, such as offal, red meat, shellfish and spinach. These modifications can reduce serum urate by 15% and delay the need for drugs that reduce serum urate levels. Dietary advice is readily available on the Internet.

Treatment with agents that reduce serum uric acid levels

The aim of treatment is to reduce and maintain the uric acid level below 360 μmol/L in all patients, and in those with severe gout, such as tophi or frequent attacks, a lower level below 300 μmol/L is required to achieve clinical remission.

Allopurinol

Allopurinol should only be used when the attacks are frequent and severe (despite dietary changes), or associated with renal impairment or tophi, or when the patient finds NSAIDs or colchicine difficult to tolerate. Allopurinol is a xanthine oxidase inhibitor, which reduces SUA levels rapidly; it is relatively non-toxic but should be used at low doses (50–100 mg) in renal impairment. It should never be started within a month of an acute attack and always under cover of NSAIDs or colchicine for the first 2–4 weeks before and 4 weeks after starting allopurinol, as it may induce acute gout. The dose can be increased gradually from 100 mg every few weeks until the uric acid level is below the 360 μmol/L level. Skin rashes and gastrointestinal intolerance are the most common side-effects. A hypersensitivity reaction is the most serious but rare adverse event, as is bone marrow suppression.

Febuxostat

Febuxostat (80–120 mg) is a non-purine analogue inhibitor of xanthine oxidase that is well tolerated and as effective as allopurinol. It is safer in renal impairment, as it undergoes hepatic metabolism rather than renal excretion, and is helpful in patients who cannot tolerate allopurinol. All-cause mortality and cardiovascular mortality, however, are higher with febuxostat than with allopurinol. Allopurinol remains the drug of first choice, unless there are strong contra-indications to its use.

Pegloticase

Pegloticase, a pegylated recombinant uricase given intravenously, lowers urate levels dramatically but is typically reserved for patients with severe, refractory gout in whom target serum urate concentrations are not achieved or who cannot tolerate oral urate-lowering therapy (ULT).

Uricosuric agents

These also lower the SUA but their use is restricted throughout Europe by the very rare occurrence of serious hepatotoxicity. *Benzbromarone* acts on the URAT1 transporter and is well tolerated. *Sulfinpyrazone* and *probenecid* are best avoided in renal impairment. Availability of these drugs varies between countries – in the UK, benzbromarone and probenecid can be obtained for treating named patients.

Losartan

Losartan is an angiotensin I receptor antagonist and is uricosuric in hypertensive patients with gout. It may reduce the risk of gout in patients with the metabolic syndrome.

Targeted therapies

The IL-1 receptor inhibitor, anakinra, canakinumab (an anti-human IL-1β monoclonal antibody) and rilonacept (a dimeric fusion protein consisting of portions of IL-1R and the IL-1R accessory protein linked to the Fc portion of IgG1) have shown efficacy. The high cost of these agents, however, means they may only be considered in patients resistant to standard therapy. Lesinurad, a URAT1 inhibitor, is now licensed but its unfavourable cost-effectiveness ratio limits its availability.

Chronic tophaceous gout

Individuals with persistently high levels of uric acid can present with chronic tophaceous gout, as sodium urate forms smooth white deposits (tophi) in skin and around joints, on the ear, fingers (**Fig. 18.35**) or the Achilles tendon. Large deposits are unsightly and ulcerate. There is chronic joint pain and sometimes superimposed acute gouty attacks.

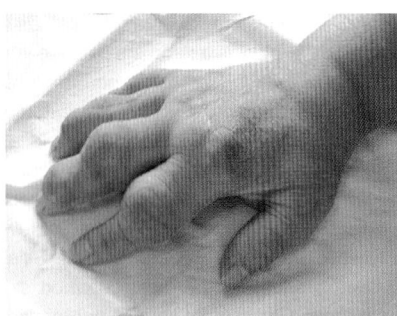

Fig. 18.35 Gout with tophi. *(Courtesy of Dr Varkey Alexander, Al-Sabah Hospital, Kuwait.)*

Periarticular deposits lead to a halo of radio-opacity and clearly defined ('punched out') bone cysts on X-ray.

Tophaceous gout is often associated with renal impairment and/or the long-term use of diuretics. There may be acute or chronic urate nephropathy or renal stone formation. Whenever possible, diuretics should be stopped or changed to less urate-retaining ones, such as bumetanide. Treatment is with allopurinol and/or uricosuric agents (see above). Pegloticase is used in people undergoing chemotherapy for malignancies (to prevent tumour lysis syndrome), and in those rare individuals who have refractory tophaceous gout.

Calcium pyrophosphate dihydrate deposition arthropathy (CPPD)

Deposition of calcium pyrophosphate dehydrate (CPP) crystals in hyaline and fibrocartilage is the most common cause of cartilage calcification. Previous terms, including pseudogout, have been unified into calcium pyrophosphate dihydrate deposition (CPPD) arthropathy. CPPD-associated arthritis is the third most common inflammatory arthritis, which increases with age, OA, joint trauma/injury and metabolic disease (hyperparathyroidism, haemochromatosis, hypomagnesaemia), and has a familial predisposition. Shedding of crystals into a joint precipitates acute synovitis that resembles gout, except that it is more common in elderly women and usually affects the knee or wrist.

Diagnosis

Diagnosis is made by detecting rhomboidal, weakly positively bi-refringent crystals in joint fluid (see **Fig. 18.33**), or is deduced from the presence of cartilage calcification on X-ray. Joint fluid looks purulent so should be sent for culture to exclude septic arthritis, as the attacks may also be associated with fever and a raised white blood cell count.

Management

There is no specific treatment to eliminate calcium pyrophosphate crystals. Therefore, management is focused on symptom control and treatments overlap with those for gout and OA. An evidence base is lacking in this condition, however, and there have been no randomized controlled clinical trials of acute management. Aspiration of the joint reduces the pain dramatically but it is usually necessary to use an NSAID or colchicine, as for gout. If infection can be excluded, an intra-articular injection of a corticosteroid helps. CPP crystals activate the NLRP3 inflammasome-IL-1 pathway (see p. 46) and although benefits have been shown with anakinra in small studies it was not superior to prednisolone.

Basic calcium phosphate deposition disease

Basic calcium phosphate (BCP) crystals, including hydroxy-apatite, tricalcium phosphate and octacalcium phosphate, can be deposited in any tissues, particularly at intra-articular and periarticular locations. Crystal formation is thought to be partly regulated by the effects of extracellular inorganic phosphate on chondrocytes and is linked with the development of OA. BCP crystals cause joint damage through induction of fibroblast proliferation, inflammatory cytokines (IL-1β and TNF-α), nitric oxide and metalloproteinases.

BCP crystal deposits in periarticular soft tissue may be asymptomatic or can cause acute calcific periarthritis (particularly in the supraspinatus tendon), tendonitis, bursitis and enthesitis. Less frequently, they can cause arthritis. In acute attacks, periarticular tissues or joints can be swollen, tender and hot. This presentation may mimic cellulitis, gout, CPPD disease and septic arthritis. Periarticular or articular BCP crystal deposits are also found in an extremely destructive chronic arthropathy of the elderly that occurs most often in shoulders (Milwaukee shoulder) or other large joints, such as the hips and knees, and in erosive OA of the fingers.

Diagnosis

The diagnosis is made clinically and septic arthritis should be excluded. A neutrophilia with elevation of ESR and CRP may occur during an acute attack. Intra- and/or periarticular calcifications, with or without erosive, destructive or hypertrophic changes, may be seen on X-ray. Alizarin red S staining is not specific for BCP crystals in synovial fluid and other calcium-containing particulates are also stained by this method.

Management

Management of acute attacks is similar to that of CPPD disease with NSAIDs, oral colchicine, aspiration of effusions and/or intra-/periarticular injection of steroids to try to shorten the duration of symptoms. In patients with underlying progressive articular changes, the response to medical therapy is usually less rewarding. Total joint replacement may be required for patients with severe destructive arthropathy in large joints.

Further reading

Andres M, Sivera F, Pascual E. Therapy for CPPD: options and evidence. *Curr Rheumatol Rep* 2018; 20:31.
Dalbeth N, Merriman TR, Stamp LK. Gout. *Lancet* 2016; 388:2039–2052.
Kiely PDW, Nikiphorou E. Management of rheumatoid arthritis. *Medicine* 2018; 46:216–221.
McInnes IB, Schett G. Pathogenetic insights from the treatment of rheumatoid arthritis. *Lancet* 2017; 389:2328–2337.
Paine A, Ritchlin. Targeting the IL23/IL-17 axis in axial spondylarthritis. *Curr Opin Rheumatol* 2016; 28:359–367.
Raine C, Keat A. Axial spondylarthritis. *Medicine* 2018; 46:231–236.
Ritchlin CT, Colbert RA, Gladman D. Psoriatic arthritis. *N Eng J Med* 2017; 376:957–970.
http://basdai.com *Bath Ankylosing Spondylitis Disease Activity Index.*

INFECTIONS OF JOINTS

Septic arthritis of native (non-prosthetic) joints occurs via direct injury or by blood-borne infection from an infected skin lesion or other site, with approximately 2 cases per 100000 people per year. It is a medical emergency that requires prompt treatment to prevent irreversible joint destruction and has a significant mortality of up to 11%, reaching 50% in polyarticular sepsis.

Risk factors for septic arthritis include age greater than 80 years, diabetes mellitus, RA, prosthetic joints, recent joint surgery, skin infection, intravenous drug use, alcoholism and prior intra-articular corticosteroid injection

Septic arthritis

The organism that most commonly causes septic arthritis is *Staphylococcus aureus*. Other organisms include streptococci, other species of staphylococcus, *Neisseria gonorrhoeae*, *Haemophilus influenzae* in children, and these and other Gram-negative organisms in the elderly or complicating RA.

Clinical features

Suspected septic arthritis is a medical emergency. In young and previously fit people, the joint is hot, red, swollen and agonizingly painful; it is held immobile by muscle spasm. In contrast, the onset may be insidious with a lack of systemic symptoms in the elderly, the immunosuppressed and patients with RA, and a high index of suspicion is needed. In 20% of patients, the sepsis affects more than one joint.

Investigations

- **Aspirate** the joint and send the fluid for urgent Gram-staining and culture. The fluid is usually frankly purulent. The culture techniques should include those for gonococci and anaerobes.
- **Blood cultures** are often positive.
- **Leucocytosis** is usual, unless the person is severely immunosuppressed.
- **X-rays** are of no value in diagnosis in acute septic arthritis.
- **Skin wound swabs, sputum and throat swab or urine** may be positive and indicate the source of infection.

Management

There are no RCTs to guide management in adults. The prognosis is similar for patients with a proven microbiological diagnosis to those with a suspected but not proven diagnosis; therefore, it is vital to treat on the basis of clinical suspicion, probability (with subsequent confirmed identity) of organism, local pattern of antibiotic sensitivity and microbiological advice.

Therapy should be started immediately before culture results are available because joint destruction may occur within weeks.

- The joint should be aspirated and then immobilized initially, followed by early physiotherapy to prevent stiffness and muscle wasting.
- Intravenous antibiotics should be given for 2 weeks and then oral antibiotics for a further 4 weeks. Response is monitored clinically and with ESR and CRP.

Empirical treatment in septic arthritis

Empirical regimens vary according to local advice and index of suspicion. For suspected Gram-positive infection first-line therapy is vancomycin, with clindamycin or cephalosporin second-line. For suspected Gram-negative infection first-line therapy is a third-generation cephalosporin with IV ciprofloxacin second-line. In confirmed methicillin-sensitive *Staphylococcus aureus* (MSSA) primary options include flucloxacillin alone or combined with fusidic acid or gentamicin, while penicillin-allergic patients should receive clindamycin or a third-generation cephalosporin. In cases of methicillin-resistant *Staphylococcus aureus* (MRSA), vancomycin is the drug of choice. Antibiotics should be altered according to sensitivities. Drainage of the joint and/or arthroscopic joint washouts are required in all cases.

Management of infected prostheses

Long-term goals of prosthetic joint infection are to eradicate the infection, reduce pain and restore function. Two-stage surgery is required to remove the prosthesis followed by treatment with appropriate IV antibiotics for 4–6 weeks before a new prosthesis is inserted. A 2–6-week course of pathogen-directed IV antibiotics followed by 3–6 months of oral antibiotics are also given.

Specific types of bacterial arthritis

Gonococcal arthritis

Disseminated gonococcal infection occurs in 0.5–3% of patients infected with *Neisseria gonorrhoeae*. It is a common cause of acute arthritis in previously fit young adults, with increasing rates in men in general and men who have sex with men.

Patients present with a fever and characteristic pustules on the distal limbs, often in association with polyarthralgia and tenosynovitis. Blood cultures are reportedly positive in up to 70% of cases, particularly those with skin lesions, tenosynovitis and polyarthralgia. Nucleic acid amplification tests may be positive even when cultures are negative. Patients should be screened for other STIs. Later, large-joint mono- or pauciarticular arthritis may follow. Culture is usually positive from the genital tract, although the joint fluid may be sterile. It is not clear whether this joint inflammation is simply a septic arthritis (which responds rapidly to antibiotics), or whether there is also a reactive element to a variety of virulence and growth factors specific to *N. gonorrhoeae*.

Management consists of initial IV ceftriaxone (or cefotaxime or ceftizoxime) repeatedly until clinical improvement occurs, plus a single oral dose of azithromycin or alternatively a week of doxycycline. In the absence of purulent arthritis after 2–3 days of improvement a 7-day course of therapy may be completed with intramuscular ceftriaxone. Purulent arthritis, however, often requires 7–14 days of IV therapy and joint drainage.

Tuberculous arthritis

Around 1% of people with tuberculosis develop joint and/or bone involvement. It occurs as the primary disease in children. In adults, it is usually due to haematogenous spread from secondary pulmonary or renal lesions. The onset is insidious and diagnosis often delayed.

The organism invades the synovium or intervertebral disc. There are caseating granulomas and rapid destruction of cartilage and adjacent bone. Some patients develop a reactive polyarthritis (Poncet's disease).

Osteoarticular TB most commonly affects the spine (50%), hip (12–15%), knee (10%) and ribs (10%). Patients become febrile with night sweats, anorexia and weight loss. The usual risk factors for tuberculosis apply – debility, excess alcohol use or immunosuppression. HIV-positive/AIDS patients are at particular risk.

Investigations should include culture of fluid, and culture and biopsy of the synovium. *Mycobacterium tuberculosis* is the usual organism but atypical mycobacteria are occasionally implicated. A chest X-ray should be performed. Initially, joint or spinal X-rays may be normal but joint-space reduction and bone destruction develop rapidly if treatment is delayed. MRI shows the abnormality earlier in the spine and CT-guided biopsy from the affected disc is often necessary to obtain cultures.

Management is as for pulmonary tuberculosis with therapy for 9 months. The joint should be rested and the spine immobilized in the acute phase.

Meningococcal arthritis

Joint inflammation may complicate meningococcal septicaemia, presenting as a migratory polyarthritis. Organisms are rarely cultured from the joint and most cases are due to immune-complex deposition. Treatment is urgent with immediate penicillin therapy.

Infective endocarditis

This condition may present with arthralgia, polymyalgia rheumatica-like symptoms or an infective arthritis (see p. 1103).

Lyme arthritis

About 25% of people with Lyme disease develop arthralgia, less commonly an acute pauciarticular arthritis (see p. 549); this usually resolves but 10% of untreated cases go on to develop a chronic arthritis. There are no positive markers of an ongoing infection in these patients).

Diagnosis is by the detection of IgM antibodies against the spirochaete *Borrelia burgdorferi*.

Treatment with antibiotics (amoxicillin or doxycycline) is highly effective in early disease.

Brucellosis

Brucellosis (see p. 548) has a worldwide distribution. The most common cause of chronic brucellosis and of arthritis is *Brucella melitensis*. There is usually a migratory large-joint mono- or oligo-articular arthritis, which is septic or reactive. Arthritis is more common in chronic infections of more than 6 months.

Leprosy

Acute or chronic symmetrical polyarthritis resembling RA, swollen hands and feet due to lepra reactions, tenosynovitis and thickened nerves with or without cutaneous manifestations are seen in leprosy (see p. 550).

Arthritis in viral disease

A transient polyarthritis or arthralgia can occur before, during or after many viral illnesses. These include infectious mononucleosis, chickenpox, mumps, adenovirus, rubella, erythrovirus B19, hepatitis B and C, arboviral infections and HIV. In most of these, it is due to a direct toxic effect or immune-complex deposition.

Rubella

In rubella (see p. 518), the virus can occasionally be isolated from the joint. This arthritis is rare in countries where rubella vaccination is routine. It occurs in up to 50% of young adult females a few days after rubella infection (6% of men). It is a symmetrical polyarthritis involving the MCP or PIP joints most commonly, but many joints can be affected. It closely resembles RA. IgM rubella antibodies are present. It resolves within a few weeks in most cases. A mild arthritis occurs rarely 2–4 weeks after rubella vaccination.

Erythrovirus B19

Erythrovirus B19 (see p. 519) causes an acute, self-limiting arthritis and is associated with erythema infectiosum ('slapped cheek disease').

Hepatitis

In hepatitis B infection (see p. 1277), a sudden, symmetrical polyarticular arthritis of the small joints of the hands occurs in approximately one-third of patients, often in the prodromal phase, and mostly resolves before the onset of jaundice. Hepatitis C infection causes type II mixed cryoglobulinaemia (see p. 1368).

Arbovirus

Arbovirus infections (see p. 522), which are endemic in many parts of the world, give rise to an arthralgia and/or arthritis. For example, the Ross River virus causes an epidemic polyarthritis in Australia and the South Pacific; it involves the small joints of the hands and clears in 2–4 weeks. Other viral infections causing epidemic arthritis include chikungunya (see p. 524) and o'nyong-nyong.

Musculoskeletal aspects of infection with HIV and AIDS

Musculoskeletal manifestations are common in these patients and are often caused by triggers such as opportunistic infections and drug therapy rather than HIV itself. Infective arthritis seen in these immunosuppressed patients often has minimal symptoms and signs. Certain of the antiviral agents cause an acute arthritis, possibly because of crystallization in the joint.

Arthralgia is common in AIDS. There is a **seronegative, predominantly lower-limb arthritis**, similar to psoriasis or Reiter's disease. **Spondylitis** also occurs but is not associated with HLA-B27. **Avascular necrosis**, possibly associated with corticosteroids or alcohol, is seen.

Non-articular diseases, such as Sjögren- and lupus-like syndromes, systemic vasculitis of the necrotizing and hypersensitivity types and myositis, also occur.

Fungal infections

Fungal infections of joints occur rarely. Bone abscesses may be seen. Destructive joint lesions can also occur with blastomycosis. A benign polyarthritis accompanied by erythema nodosum occasionally occurs in coccidioidomycosis and histoplasmosis. Culture of purulent synovial fluid and skin tests for fungi may help the diagnosis.

Further reading

Coakley G, Mathews CJ. Septic arthritis. *BMJ Best Practice* 2018; Apr 05:1–31.

AUTOIMMUNE RHEUMATIC DISEASES

Autoimmunity and autoantibodies

Autoimmune diseases are conditions in which the immune system attacks tissues of the body. The antigens can be present in multiple organs so the clinical manifestations are systemic and diverse. In some diseases, such as Graves' disease, Hashimoto's thyroiditis and type 1 diabetes mellitus, only a single organ is affected. Each individual autoimmune rheumatic disease (ARD) has a characteristic pattern of symptoms and signs, which are used to make the diagnosis. In some ARDs, there are also characteristic autoantibodies (i.e. antibodies that recognize antigens that are normal constituents of the body, such as DNA and phospholipids). Positive blood tests for autoantibodies are useful but not essential in the diagnosis of ARDs (**Box 18.38**).

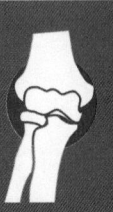

Antibody	Disease	Prevalence
ds-DNA	SLE	70%
Anti-histone	Drug-induced lupus	–
Anti-centromeric	Limited scleroderma	70%
Anti-Ro (SS-A)	SLE	40–60%
	Primary Sjögren's	60–90%
Anti-La (SS-B)	SLE	15%
	Primary Sjögren's	35–85%
Anti-Sm	SLE	10–25% (Caucasian)
		30–50% (black African)
Anti-Ul-RNP	SLE	30%
	Overlap syndrome	
Anti-Jo-1 (anti-synthetase)	Polymyositis	30%
	Dermatomyositis	
Anti-topoisomerase-1 (Scl-70)	Diffuse cutaneous SSc	30%

Box 18.38 Antinuclear autoantibodies and disease associations

ds-DNA, double-stranded DNA; RNP, ribonucleoprotein; Ro, La, first two letters of name of patients; Sm, Smith, patient's name; SS-A, SS-B, Sjögren's syndrome A and B; SSc, systemic scleroderma; SLE, systemic lupus erythematosus.

Systemic lupus erythematosus

Systemic lupus erythematosus (SLE) is an inflammatory, multisystem autoimmune disorder with arthralgia and rashes as the most common clinical features, and cerebral and renal disease as the most serious problems.

Epidemiology

SLE occurs worldwide and is about nine times as common in women as in men, with a peak age of onset between 20 and 40 years. The prevalence varies between ethnic groups, being highest (at 1:250) in African/Caribbean women. In other populations, the prevalence varies between 1:1000 and 1:10000.

Aetiology

The cause is unknown but there are several predisposing factors:
- **Heredity.** There is a higher concordance rate in monozygotic twins (up to 25%) compared with dizygotic twins (3%). First-degree relatives have a 3% chance of developing the disease but approximately 20% have autoantibodies.
- **Genetics.** Three whole-genome analyses have led to the identification of approximately 20 genes linked to the development of SLE. These include some HLA genes, as well as genes involved in T- and B-lymphocyte function and genes related to autophagy and interferon function. Homozygous deficiencies of the complement genes C1q, C2 or C4 are very rare but convey a high risk of developing SLE.
- **Sex hormone status.** Pre-menopausal women are most frequently affected.
- **Drugs.** Drugs such as hydralazine, isoniazid, procainamide and penicillamine can induce a form of SLE that is usually mild, in that the kidneys and central nervous system are not affected.
- **Ultraviolet light.** This can trigger flares of SLE, especially in the skin.
- **Exposure to Epstein–Barr virus.** This has been suggested as a trigger for SLE.

Pathogenesis

When cells die by apoptosis, the cellular remnants appear on the cell surface as small blebs that carry self antigens. These antigens include nuclear constituents (e.g. DNA and histones), which are normally hidden from the immune system. In people with SLE, removal of these blebs by phagocytes is inefficient, so that they are transferred to lymphoid tissues, where they can be taken up by antigen-presenting cells. The self antigens from these blebs can then be presented to T cells, which in turn stimulate B cells to produce autoantibodies directed against these antigens (see p. 64). It has been shown that, in some patients, the autoantibodies are present in stored blood samples that were taken years before the patient developed clinical features of SLE. The combination of availability of self antigens and failure of the immune system to inactivate B cells and T cells that recognize these self antigens (i.e. a breakdown of *tolerance*; see p. 64) leads to the following immunological consequences.
- Development of autoantibodies that either form circulating complexes or deposit by binding directly to tissues.
- Activation of complement and influx of neutrophils, causing inflammation in those tissues.
- Abnormal cytokine production: increased blood levels of IL-10 and interferon-alpha are particularly closely linked to high activity of inflammation in SLE. However, no form of anticytokine biological therapy has yet been adopted routinely in the treatment of SLE.

More recently, other cells have been implicated in the pathogenesis of SLE. These include dendritic cells, which are activated by immune complexes containing nucleic acids to produce interferon, and invariant natural killer T cells (iNKT cells), which are reduced in number and function in patients with SLE.

Pathology

SLE of the skin and kidneys is characterized by deposition of complement and IgG antibodies, and by influx of neutrophils and lymphocytes. Biopsies of other tissues are carried out less frequently but can show vasculitis affecting capillaries, arterioles and venules. The synovium of joints can be oedematous and may contain immune complexes. Haematoxylin bodies (rounded, blue, homogeneous haematoxylin-stained deposits) are seen in inflammatory infiltrates and are thought to result from the interaction of antinuclear antibodies and cell nuclei.

The pathology of lesions in other organs is described in the appropriate chapters.

Clinical features

The manifestations of SLE vary greatly between patients. Most patients suffer fatigue, arthralgia and/or skin problems. Involvement of major organs is less common but more serious (**Fig. 18.36**).

General features

Fever is common in exacerbations. Patients complain of marked malaise and tiredness, and these symptoms do not correlate with disease activity or severity of organ-based complications.

Joints and muscles

Joint involvement is the most common clinical feature (>90%). Patients often present with symptoms resembling RA with symmetrical small joint arthralgia. Joints are painful but characteristically appear clinically normal, although sometimes there is slight soft tissue swelling surrounding the joint. Deformity because of joint capsule and tendon contraction is rare, as are bony erosions. Rarely, major joint deformity resembling RA (known as **Jaccoud's arthropathy**) is seen. Avascular necrosis affecting the hip or knee is a rare complication of the disease or of treatment with corticosteroids.

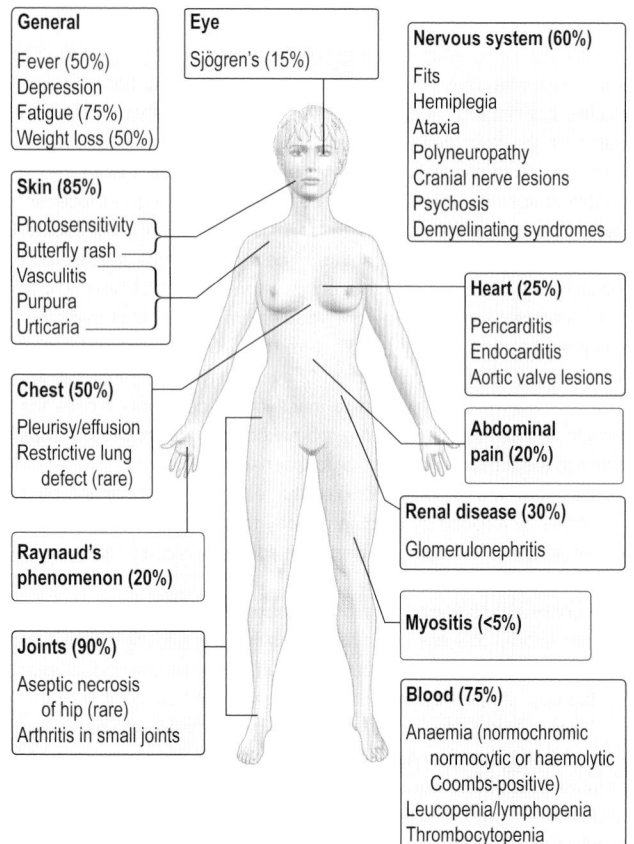

General
Fever (50%)
Depression
Fatigue (75%)
Weight loss (50%)

Eye
Sjögren's (15%)

Nervous system (60%)
Fits
Hemiplegia
Ataxia
Polyneuropathy
Cranial nerve lesions
Psychosis
Demyelinating syndromes

Skin (85%)
Photosensitivity
Butterfly rash
Vasculitis
Purpura
Urticaria

Heart (25%)
Pericarditis
Endocarditis
Aortic valve lesions

Chest (50%)
Pleurisy/effusion
Restrictive lung
    defect (rare)

**Abdominal
pain (20%)**

Renal disease (30%)
Glomerulonephritis

**Raynaud's
phenomenon (20%)**

Myositis (<5%)

Joints (90%)
Aseptic necrosis
    of hip (rare)
Arthritis in small joints

Blood (75%)
Anaemia (normochromic
    normocytic or haemolytic
    Coombs-positive)
Leucopenia/lymphopenia
Thrombocytopenia

Fig. 18.36 Clinical features of systemic lupus erythematosus.

Myalgia is present in up to 50% of patients but a true myositis is seen in only less than 5%. If myositis is prominent, the patient may well have an overlap ARD with both polymyositis and SLE.

Skin

The skin (see p. 682) is affected in 85% of cases. Erythema, in a 'butterfly' distribution on the cheeks of the face and across the bridge of the nose (see **Fig. 22.40**), is characteristic. Vasculitic lesions on the fingertips and around the nail folds, purpura and urticaria occur. In 40–50% of cases, there is photosensitivity (especially in patients positive for anti-Ro antibodies). Prolonged exposure to sunlight can lead to exacerbations of the disease. Livedo reticularis, palmar and plantar rashes, pigmentation and alopecia are seen. Scarring alopecia can lead to irreversible bald patches. Raynaud's phenomenon (see p. 1131) is common and may precede the development of other clinical problems by years.

Discoid lupus is a benign variant of lupus in which only the skin is involved. The rash is characteristic and appears on the face as well-defined erythematous plaques that progress to scarring and pigmentation (see p. 681). Subacute cutaneous lupus erythematosus, a rare variant, is described on page 682.

Lungs

Up to 50% of patients will have lung involvement at some time during the course of the disease (see p. 992). Recurrent pleurisy and pleural effusions (exudates) are the most common manifestations and are often bilateral. Pneumonitis and atelectasis are seen; in some patients a restrictive lung defect develops, with loss of lung volumes and raised hemidiaphragms. This 'shrinking

lung syndrome' is poorly understood but may have a neuromuscular basis. Rarely, pulmonary fibrosis occurs, more commonly in overlap syndromes (see p. 463). Intrapulmonary haemorrhage associated with vasculitis is a rare but potentially life-threatening complication.

Heart and cardiovascular system

The heart is involved in 25% of cases. Pericarditis, with small pericardial effusions detected by echocardiography, is common. A mild myocarditis also occurs, giving rise to arrhythmias. Aortic valve lesions and a cardiomyopathy can rarely be present. A non-infective endocarditis involving the mitral valve (Libman–Sacks syndrome) is very rare. Raynaud's, vasculitis, and arterial and venous thromboses can occur, especially in association with the antiphospholipid syndrome (see below). There is an increased frequency of ischaemic heart disease and stroke in people with SLE, which is partly due to altered levels of common risk factors such as hypertension and lipid levels, but the presence of chronic inflammation over many years may also be contributory. It is not known whether intensive treatment of cardiovascular risk factors or use of statins in SLE will alter the risk of developing coronary disease or stroke.

Kidneys

A classification of types of nephritis is given on page 1353. Post-mortem studies suggest that histological changes are very frequent, but clinical renal involvement occurs in only approximately 30% of cases. All patients should have regular screening of urine for blood and protein. An asymptomatic patient with proteinuria may be in the early stages of lupus nephritis, and treatment may prevent progression to renal impairment. Proteinuria should be quantified and haematuria should prompt examination for urinary casts or fragmented red cells that suggest glomerulonephritis. Renal biopsy is used to define the type and severity of nephritis. Renal vein thrombosis can occur in nephrotic syndrome or in association with antiphospholipid antibodies.

Nervous system

Involvement of the nervous system occurs in up to 60% of cases and symptoms often fluctuate. There may be a mild depression, but occasionally, more severe psychiatric disturbances occur. Epilepsy, migraines, cerebellar ataxia, aseptic meningitis, cranial nerve lesions, cerebrovascular disease or a polyneuropathy may be seen. The pathogenic mechanism for cerebral lupus is complex. Lesions may be due to vasculitis or immune complex deposition, thrombosis or non-inflammatory microvasculopathy. In people with cerebral lupus, infection should be excluded, or treated in parallel with administration of corticosteroids and immunosuppression.

Eyes

Retinal vasculitis can cause infarcts, which appear as hard exudates, and haemorrhages. There may be episcleritis, conjunctivitis or optic neuritis, but blindness is uncommon. Secondary Sjögren's syndrome is seen in about 15% of cases.

Gastrointestinal system

Mouth ulcers are common and may be a presenting feature. These may be painless or become secondarily infected and painful. Mesenteric vasculitis can produce inflammatory lesions involving the small bowel (infarction or perforation). Liver involvement and pancreatitis are uncommon.

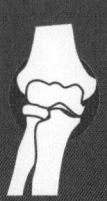

Investigations

Blood

- *A full blood count* may show a leucopenia, lymphopenia and/or thrombocytopenia. Anaemia of chronic disease or autoimmune haemolytic anaemia also occurs. The ESR is raised in proportion to the disease activity. In contrast, the CRP is usually normal but may be high when the patient has lupus pleuritis or peritonitis, arthritis or a coexistent infection.
- *Urea and creatinine* only rise when renal disease is advanced. Low serum albumin or high urine albumin/creatinine ratio are earlier indicators of lupus nephritis.
- *Autoantibodies* of many different types may be present in SLE but the most significant are ANA, anti-dsDNA, anti-Ro, anti-Sm and anti-La (see **Box 18.38**). Antiphospholipid antibodies are present in 25–40% of cases but not all of these patients develop antiphospholipid syndrome (see later).
- *Serum complement* C3 and C4 levels are often reduced during active disease. The combination of high ESR, high anti-dsDNA and low C3 may herald a flare of disease. All these markers tend to return towards normal as the flare improves, but in some patients, anti-dsDNA levels will remain high even during clinical remission.

Histology

Characteristic histological and immunofluorescent abnormalities (deposition of IgG and complement) are seen in biopsies from the kidney and skin.

Diagnostic imaging

CT scans of the brain sometimes show infarcts or haemorrhage with evidence of cerebral atrophy. MRI can detect lesions in white matter that are not seen on CT. However, it can be very difficult to distinguish true vasculitis from small thrombi.

Management

General measures

The disease and its management should be discussed with the patient, particularly the effect upon the patient's lifestyle: for example, appearance and debility due to fatigue. Patients are advised to avoid excessive exposure to sunlight and it is also necessary to reduce cardiovascular risk factors.

Symptomatic treatment

Arthralgia, arthritis, fever and serositis all respond well to standard doses of NSAIDs (see p. 431). Topical corticosteroids are effective and widely used in cutaneous lupus. Antimalarial drugs (chloroquine or hydroxychloroquine) help mild skin disease, fatigue and arthralgias that cannot be controlled with NSAIDs, but patients require regular eye checks because of potential retinal toxicity. It is now thought that retinal changes occur in up to 7.5% of patients on long-term treatment with hydroxychloroquine, with increased risk in those taking more than 5 mg/kg per day.

Corticosteroids and immunosuppressive drugs

Single intramuscular injections of long-acting corticosteroids or short courses of oral corticosteroids are useful in treating severe flares of arthritis, pleuritis or pericarditis. In some cases, these symptoms can only be kept under control using long-term oral corticosteroids.

Renal or cerebral disease and severe haemolytic anaemia or thrombocytopenia must be treated with high-dose oral corticosteroids, and the first two of these require immunosuppressive drugs in addition. Cyclophosphamide was most commonly used to achieve remission in these severe forms of lupus but has largely been replaced by mycophenolate mofetil, which has fewer side-effects. Azathioprine is also used to maintain remission. Newer agents, which specifically target cells or cytokines in the immune system, are coming into use, especially in refractory cases. These include rituximab (anti-CD20) and belimumab, which are both monoclonal antibodies acting against B lymphocytes. Other drugs, such as anti-interferon agents, are being investigated in large clinical trials.

Prognosis

An episodic course is characteristic, with exacerbations and complete remissions that may last for long periods. However, SLE can also be a chronic persistent condition. The mortality rate in SLE has fallen dramatically over the last 50 years; the 10-year survival rate is about 90%, but this is lower if major organ-based complications are present. Deaths early in the course of disease are mainly due to renal or cerebral disease or infection. Later, coronary artery disease and stroke become more prevalent. Chronic progressive destruction of joints, as seen in RA and OA, occurs rarely, but a few patients develop deformities such as ulnar deviation. People with SLE have an increased long-term risk of developing some cancers, especially lymphoma.

Pregnancy and SLE

Fertility is usually normal, except in severe disease, and there is no major contraindication to pregnancy. Recurrent miscarriages can occur, especially in women with antiphospholipid antibodies. Exacerbations can arise during pregnancy and are frequent postpartum. The patient's medications should be reviewed. Mycophenolate should be stopped, whereas azathioprine, hydroxychloroquine and low-dose oral corticosteroids are safe. Hypertension must be controlled. People with anti-Ro or anti-La antibodies have a 2% risk of giving birth to babies with neonatal lupus syndrome (rash, hepatitis and fetal heart block).

Antiphospholipid syndrome

Patients who have thrombosis (arterial or venous) and/or recurrent miscarriages (see p. 1471), and who also have persistently positive blood tests for antiphospholipid antibodies (aPL), have the antiphospholipid syndrome (APS). Antiphospholipid antibodies can be detected by several different tests:

- The *anticardiolipin test*, which detects antibodies (IgG or IgM) that bind the negatively charged phospholipid, cardiolipin.
- The *lupus anticoagulant test*, which detects changes in the ability of blood to clot in a test tube. Despite the name, it is not a test for lupus. It is a test for APS. The *anticoagulant* effect caused by aPL in the test tube causes an opposite *procoagulant* effect inside the body because the balance of factors stimulating thrombosis is different there.
- The *anti-β_2-glycoprotein I test*, which detects antibodies that bind β_2-glycoprotein I, a molecule that interacts closely with phospholipids.

A persistently positive test (i.e. positive on at least two occasions ≥12 weeks apart) in one or more of these assays is needed to diagnose APS. However, some people who test positive for aPL will never develop APS; that is, not all aPLs are harmful. APS can present in patients who already have another ARD, especially SLE. APS can also occur on its own (primary APS).

New diagnostic tests for APS are being developed and include anti-prothrombin assays, tests for IgA aPL and tests for antibodies to the N-terminal domain of β_2-glycoprotein I. Although not currently used in clinical practice, these tests may soon be helpful for assessing the overall thrombosis risk of a patient with APS, or for diagnosing patients with 'seronegative' APS who have typical clinical features but test negative for anticardiolipin, lupus anticoagulant and anti-β_2-glycoprotein I.

Pathogenesis

Negatively charged phospholipids and β-glycoprotein I are present on the outer surface of apoptotic blebs, and so aPLs are believed to arise by a similar mechanism to the lupus autoantibodies described above. Pathogenic aPLs bind to the N-terminal domain of β_2-glycoprotein I. Changes in the oxidation state of β_2-glycoprotein I in patients with APS enhance the availability of this domain to bind aPLs, and this interaction is facilitated when the protein is bound to phospholipid on the surface of cells such as endothelial cells, platelets, monocytes and trophoblasts. This change alters the functioning of those cells, leading to thrombosis and/or miscarriage.

Clinical features

Ischaemic strokes occur in about 20% of patients and deep vein thrombosis in about 40%. Unlike most causes of thrombophilia, APS can cause either arterial or venous thrombosis (though rarely both in the same patient). Some 27% of women who have had two or more spontaneous miscarriages have APS.

Large studies, however, show that people with APS can also have many other features, including:
- thrombocytopenia
- chorea, migraine and epilepsy
- valvular heart disease
- cutaneous manifestations (e.g. livedo reticularis)
- positive Coombs test
- renal impairment due to ischaemia in the small renal vessels.

Catastrophic APS is a rare variant (about 1% of cases) in which multiple infarcts in different organs of the body cause failure of multiple organs simultaneously. There is a high mortality from catastrophic APS.

Management

In people with APS who have had one thrombosis or more, the recommended treatment to prevent further thrombosis is long-term anticoagulation with warfarin. The target INR is lower in people with a history of venous compared to arterial thrombosis. Pregnant women with APS are given oral aspirin and subcutaneous low-molecular-weight heparin from early in gestation. This therapy reduces the chance of a miscarriage but pre-eclampsia and poor fetal growth remain common. There are no definite guidelines for managing people with aPL who have never had thrombosis. Aspirin or clopidogrel is sometimes given prophylactically, especially in those with high-IgG aPL. Warfarin is given much more rarely in these circumstances, but may be indicated in patients at particularly high risk; for example, those who test positive for all three of anticardiolipin, lupus anticoagulant and anti-β_2-glycoprotein I. Newer anticoagulants that act against specific clotting factors are replacing warfarin in some clinical situations and may come into use in APS. An example is the factor X inhibitor rivaroxaban, which has been the subject of two clinical trials in APS, though its place in management of APS is not yet clear.

Systemic sclerosis (scleroderma)

Systemic sclerosis (SSc, or scleroderma; see p. 681) is a multisystem disease and is distinct from localized scleroderma syndromes, such as morphea, that do not involve internal organ disease and are rarely associated with vasospasm (Raynaud's phenomenon). SSc has the highest case-specific mortality of any of the autoimmune rheumatic diseases. It occurs worldwide but there may be racial or ethnic differences in clinical features. For example, renal involvement is less frequent in Japanese cases.

The incidence of SSc is 10/million population per year with a 3 : 1 female to male ratio. The peak incidence is between 30 and 50 years of age. It is rare in children.

Environmental risk factors for scleroderma-like disorders include exposure to vinyl chloride, silica dust, adulterated rapeseed oil and trichloroethylene. Drugs such as bleomycin also produce a similar picture. Although unusual, familial cases are reported and twin cohorts suggest higher concordance in monozygotic pairs, consistent with genetic determinants of aetiology.

Pathology and pathogenesis
Vascular features

Widespread vascular damage involving small arteries, arterioles and capillaries is an early lesion. There is initial endothelial cell damage with release of cytokines, including endothelin-1, which causes vasoconstriction. There is continued intimal damage with increasing vascular permeability, leading to cellular activation and activation of adhesion molecules (E-selectin, VCAM, intercellular adhesion molecule 1 (ICAM-1)), with migration of cells into the extracellular matrix. Migrating lymphocytes are IL-2-producing cells, expressing surface antigens such as CD3, CD4 and CD5. All these factors cause release of other mediators (e.g. IL-1, 4, 6 and 8, TGF-β and platelet-derived growth factor) with activation of fibroblasts. Plasma levels of the chemokine CXCL4 are elevated in SSc and correlate with skin and lung fibrosis.

The damage to small blood vessels also produces widespread obliterative arterial lesions and subsequent chronic ischaemia.

Fibrotic features

Fibroblasts synthesize increased quantities of collagen types I and III, as well as fibronectin and glycosaminoglycans, producing fibrosis in the lower dermis of the skin as well as the internal organs. It is possible that antibodies to platelet-derived growth factor receptor, which have been found in blood of people with SSc, stimulate fibroblasts to cause fibrosis.

Clinical features

See **Fig. 18.37**.

Raynaud's phenomenon

Raynaud's phenomenon is seen in almost all cases and can precede the onset of the full-blown disease by many years.

Limited cutaneous scleroderma (LcSSc): 70% of cases

This condition usually starts with Raynaud's phenomenon many years (up to 15) before any skin changes. The skin involvement is limited to the hands, face, feet and forearms. The skin is tight over the fingers and often produces flexion deformities of the fingers. Involvement of the skin of the face produces a characteristic 'beak'-like nose and a small mouth (microstomia). Painful digital ulcers and telangiectasia with dilated nail-fold capillary loops are seen. Digital ischaemia may lead to gangrene. Gastrointestinal tract involvement is common. Pulmonary hypertension develops in 21% of people with LcSSc and pulmonary interstitial disease also occurs.

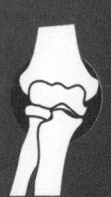

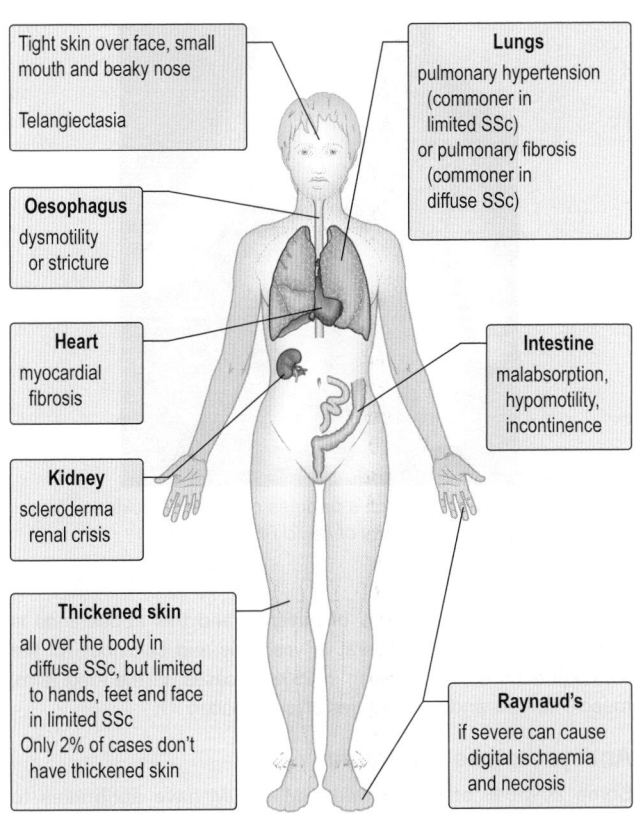

Tight skin over face, small mouth and beaky nose

Telangiectasia

Lungs
pulmonary hypertension (commoner in limited SSc) or pulmonary fibrosis (commoner in diffuse SSc)

Oesophagus
dysmotility or stricture

Heart
myocardial fibrosis

Intestine
malabsorption, hypomotility, incontinence

Kidney
scleroderma renal crisis

Thickened skin
all over the body in diffuse SSc, but limited to hands, feet and face in limited SSc Only 2% of cases don't have thickened skin

Raynaud's
if severe can cause digital ischaemia and necrosis

Fig. 18.37 Clinical features of systemic sclerosis (SSc).

Diffuse cutaneous scleroderma (DcSSc): 30% of cases

Initially oedematous in onset, skin sclerosis rapidly follows. Raynaud's phenomenon usually starts just before or concomitant with the oedema.

Diffuse swelling and stiffness of the fingers is rapidly followed by more extensive skin thickening, which can involve most of the body in the severest cases. Later, the skin becomes atrophic. Early involvement of other organs occurs with general symptoms of lethargy, anorexia and weight loss.

- **Gastrointestinal involvement** includes heartburn, reflux or dysphagia due to oesophageal involvement (see p. 1168), which is almost invariable. Anal incontinence occurs in many patients. Malabsorption from bacterial overgrowth due to dilatation and atony of the small bowel is not infrequent; more rarely, dilatation and atony of the colon occurs. Pseudo-obstruction is a known complication.
- **Renal involvement** is acute or chronic (see p. 1368). Acute hypertensive renal crisis used to be the most common cause of death in systemic sclerosis. Angiotensin-converting enzyme (ACE) inhibitors and better care, along with dialysis and renal transplantation, have changed this.
- **Lung disease**, both fibrosis (in 41% of cases) and pulmonary hypertension (17% of cases), contributes significantly to mortality in SSc. Pulmonary hypertension can be isolated or secondary to fibrosis, and high plasma levels of endothelin-1 are seen.
- **Myocardial fibrosis** leads to arrhythmias and conduction defects. Pericarditis is found occasionally.

Sometimes, these systemic features occur without skin involvement (SSc *sine* scleroderma).

Investigations

- **Full blood count.** A normochromic, normocytic anaemia occurs and a microangiopathic haemolytic anaemia is seen in some people with renal disease.
- **Serum creatinine and electrolytes.** Urea and creatinine rise in acute kidney injury.
- **Autoantibodies** (see **Box 18.38**):
  - **In LcSSc**: speckled, nucleolar or anti-centromere antibodies (ACAs) occur in 70% of cases. Anti-Th/To antibodies target small nuclear ribonucleoproteins and are found in up to 7% of cases of LcSSC.
  - **In DcSSc**: there are anti-topoisomerase-1 antibodies (called anti-Scl-70) in 30% of cases, and anti-RNA polymerase (I, II and III) antibodies in 20–25%. Anti-Scl-70 is highly specific for DcSSC. Anti-RNA polymerase positivity is associated with an increased risk of renal involvement. Anti-U3RNP antibodies bind a small nuclear ribonucleoprotein called fibrillarin and are present in up to 6% of patients with SSc – more commonly in DcSSc than LcSSc.
- **RF** is positive in 30%.
- **ANA** is positive in 95%.
- **Urine** microscopy and, if there is proteinuria, the urine albumin/creatinine ratio should be measured.
- **Imaging:**
  - **Chest X-ray:** to exclude other pathology, for changes in cardiac size and established lung disease.
  - **Hands:** deposits of calcium around the fingers (in severe cases, erosion and absorption of the tufts of the distal phalanges, termed 'acro-osteolysis').
  - **Barium swallow:** generally confirms impaired oesophageal motility. Scintigraphy, manometry, impedance and upper gastrointestinal endoscopy are also valuable.
  - **Echocardiogram and lung function tests** should be carried out annually to monitor for development of pulmonary fibrosis or pulmonary hypertension.
  - **High-resolution CT:** to demonstrate fibrotic lung involvement.
- **Other investigations** of gastrointestinal tract, lung, renal and cardiac as appropriate.

Management

Treatment should be organ-based in order to try to control the disease. Currently, there is no cure. In contrast to many other ARDs, corticosteroids and immunosuppressants are rarely used in SSc, with the exception of SSc-related pulmonary fibrosis.

- **Education**, counselling and family support are essential.
- **Regular exercises** and skin lubricants may limit contractures but no treatment has proven efficacy in reducing skin fibrosis.
- **Raynaud's phenomenon** may be improved by hand warmers and oral vasodilators (calcium-channel blockers, ACE inhibitors, angiotensin receptor blockers). In severe cases, parenteral vasodilators (prostacyclin analogues and calcitonin gene-related peptide) are used. Lumbar sympathectomy can help foot symptoms. Radical micro-arteriolysis (digital sympathectomy) can be used where individual fingers or toes are severely ischaemic, and thoracic sympathectomy under video-assisted thoracic surgery is now performed.
- **Oesophageal symptoms** can almost always be improved by proton pump inhibitors but prokinetic drugs are rarely helpful.
- **Symptomatic malabsorption** requires nutritional supplements and rotational antibiotics to treat small intestinal bacterial overgrowth.

- **Renal involvement** requires intensive control of hypertension. The first drug of choice is an ACE inhibitor. Vigilance for hypertensive scleroderma renal crisis (SRC) is critical, especially in early-stage dcSSc with rapidly progressive skin and tendon friction rubs. High-dose corticosteroids (above 10 mg prednisolone daily) may increase the risk of SRC.
- **Pulmonary hypertension** is treated with oral vasodilators, oxygen and warfarin. Advanced cases should receive prostacyclin therapy (inhaled, subcutaneous or intravenous) or the oral endothelin-receptor antagonist, bosentan. Right heart failure is treated conventionally and transplantation (heart–lung or single lung) is used in eligible cases.
- **Pulmonary fibrosis** is currently treated with immunosuppression, most often with cyclophosphamide or azathioprine combined with low-dose oral prednisolone.

Prognosis

In limited cutaneous scleroderma, the disease is often milder, with much less severe internal organ involvement and a 70% 10-year survival. Pulmonary hypertension is a significant later cause of death. Lung fibrosis and severe gut involvement also determine mortality. In diffuse disease, where organ involvement is often severe at an earlier stage, many patients die of pulmonary, cardiac or renal involvement. Overall, pulmonary involvement (vascular or interstitial) accounts for around 50% of scleroderma-related deaths.

Localized forms of scleroderma occur either in patches (morphea; see p. 681) or linear forms. These are more commonly seen in children and adolescents, and do not convert into systemic forms, although ANA may occur in localized scleroderma and, very occasionally, localized and systemic forms coexist.

Polymyositis and dermatomyositis

Polymyositis (PM) is a rare disorder of unknown cause, in which the clinical picture is dominated by inflammation of striated muscle, causing proximal muscle weakness. When the skin is involved, it is called 'dermatomyositis' (DM). The incidence is about 2–10/million population *per annum* and it occurs in all races and at all ages. The aetiology is unknown, although viruses (e.g. *Coxsackie*, rubella, influenza) have been implicated and persons with HLA-B8/DR3 appear to be genetically predisposed.

Clinical features

Adult polymyositis

Women are affected three times more commonly than men.

The onset can be insidious, over months, or acute. General malaise, weight loss and fever can develop during the acute phase, but the cardinal symptom is proximal muscle weakness. The shoulder and pelvic girdle muscles become wasted but are not usually tender. Face and distal limb muscles are not usually affected. Movements such as squatting and climbing stairs become difficult. As the disease progresses, involvement of pharyngeal, laryngeal and respiratory muscles can lead to dysphonia and respiratory failure. These severe complications are rare if the disease is treated early.

Adult dermatomyositis

This condition is also more common in women. Apart from muscle weakness, these patients often suffer from myalgia, polyarthritis and Raynaud's phenomenon, but DM is primarily distinguished from PM by the characteristic rash. This typically affects the eyelids, where heliotrope (purple) discoloration is accompanied by periorbital oedema, and the fingers, where purple–red, raised vasculitic patches are seen. These patches occur over the knuckles (Gottron's

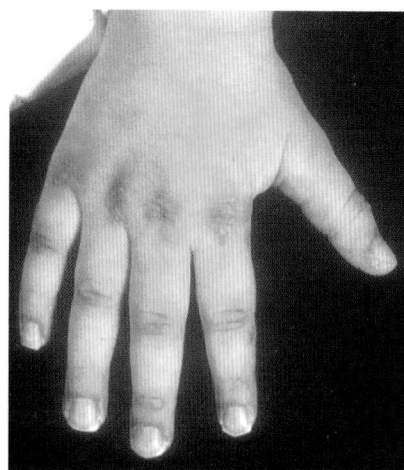

Fig. 18.38 Purplish Gottron's papules over the knuckles (dermatomyositis). *(Courtesy of David Paige, London.)*

papules; **Fig. 18.38**) in 70% of patients, and this appearance is highly specific for DM. Ulcerative vasculitis and calcinosis of the subcutaneous tissue are seen in 25% of cases. In the long term, muscle fibrosis and contractures of joints occur.

Antisynthetase syndrome

Some 20–30% of people with PM or DM have antibodies to tRNA synthetase enzymes. These people are more likely to develop pulmonary interstitial fibrosis, Raynaud's phenomenon, arthritis, and hardening and fissuring of skin over the pulp surface of the fingers (mechanic's hands). This variant of PM/DM is sometimes called antisynthetase syndrome and often has a poor outcome. Respiratory muscles are affected in PM/DM and this compounds the effects of interstitial fibrosis. Dysphagia is seen in about 50% of patients owing to oesophageal muscle involvement.

Association with other ARDs

There is an association with other ARDs (e.g. SLE, RA and SSc) and their associated clinical features, such as deforming arthritis, malar rash and skin sclerosis.

Association with malignancies

The relative risk of cancer is 2.4 for male and 3.4 for female patients, and a wide variety of cancers have been reported. The onset and clinical picture do not differ in malignancy-associated disease from those of typical DM/PM. The associated cancer may not become apparent for 2–3 years, and recurrent, refractory or ANA-negative DM should prompt a search for occult malignancy.

Malignancy (e.g. lung, ovary, breast, stomach) can also predate the onset of myositis, particularly in males with DM.

Childhood dermatomyositis

This variant most commonly affects children between the ages of 4 and 10 years. The typical rash of DM is usually accompanied by muscle weakness. Muscle atrophy, subcutaneous calcification and contractures may be widespread and severe. Ulcerative skin vasculitis is common and recurrent abdominal pain due to vasculitis is also a feature. Adults who have suffered from childhood DM may have chronic damage (e.g. contractures) or show effects of long-term corticosteroid or immunosuppressive therapy.

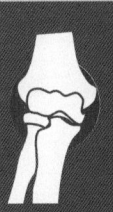

Investigations

- **Serum creatine kinase (CK)**, aminotransferases, lactate dehydrogenase (LDH) and aldolase are usually raised and are useful guides to muscle damage, but may not reflect activity.
- **ESR** and **CRP** may be raised.
- **Serum autoantibody studies** include antinuclear antibody testing, which is usually positive in people with DM. RF is present in up to 50%, and many **myositis-specific antibodies** (MSAs) have been recognized and correlate with certain subsets. Antisynthetase antibodies have been described above.
- **Electromyography (EMG)** shows a typical triad of changes with myositis: spontaneous fibrillation potentials at rest, polyphasic or short-duration potentials on voluntary contraction, and salvos of repetitive potentials on mechanical stimulation of the nerve.
- **MRI** can be used to detect abnormally inflamed muscle.
- **Needle muscle biopsy** shows fibre necrosis and regeneration in association with an inflammatory cell infiltrate with lymphocytes around the blood vessels and between muscle fibres. Open biopsy allows more thorough assessment.
- **Screening for malignancy** is usually limited to relatively non-invasive investigations such as chest X-ray, mammography, pelvic/abdominal ultrasound and CT scanning, urine microscopy and a search for circulating tumour markers.
- **PET** scanning can detect malignancy.

Management

Bed rest may be helpful but must be combined with an exercise programme. Prednisolone is the mainstay of treatment: 0.5–1.0 mg/kg body weight as initial therapy, continued until at least 1 month after myositis has become clinically and enzymatically inactive. Tapering of steroids must be slow. Early intervention with steroid-sparing agents, such as methotrexate, azathioprine, ciclosporin, cyclophosphamide and mycophenolate mofetil, is common, especially where there is clinical relapse or a rise in CK as the dose of steroids is reduced. Intravenous immunoglobulin therapy (IVIG) is helpful in some recalcitrant cases. Treatment of childhood DM tends to be more intensive, with earlier use of immunosuppressive agents. Use of biological agents such as rituximab has been described. Rituximab is more likely to be effective in autoantibody-positive cases.

Inclusion body myositis

Inclusion body myositis is an idiopathic inflammatory myopathy usually occurring in men over 50 years. Weakness of the pharyngeal muscles causes difficulty in swallowing in over 50%. It is a slowly progressive weakness of mainly distal muscles. In contrast to polymyositis, the CK is only slightly elevated; the EMG shows both myopathic and neuropathic changes. On MRI, the changes are often more distal but can be similar to those of polymyositis. A muscle biopsy shows inflammation and basophilic rimmed vacuoles with diagnostic filamentous inclusions and vacuoles on electron microscopy. A trial of corticosteroids is worthwhile but generally the response is poor.

Sjögren's syndrome

The syndrome of dry eyes (keratoconjunctivitis sicca) in the absence of RA or any of the autoimmune diseases is known as 'primary Sjögren's syndrome'. There is an association with HLA-B8/DR3. Dryness of the mouth, skin or vagina may also be a problem. Salivary and parotid gland enlargement is seen. In the majority of cases, dryness and fatigue are the only symptoms, and Sjögren's syndrome is irritating and inconvenient rather than dangerous. However, in a minority there may be systemic symptoms such as:

- arthralgia and occasional non-progressive polyarthritis, like that seen in SLE (but much less common)
- Raynaud's phenomenon
- dysphagia and abnormal oesophageal motility, as seen in systemic sclerosis (but less common)
- other organ-specific autoimmune disease, including thyroid disease, myasthenia gravis, primary biliary cirrhosis, autoimmune hepatitis and pancreatitis
- renal tubular defects (uncommon) causing nephrogenic diabetes insipidus and renal tubular acidosis
- pulmonary diffusion defects and fibrosis
- polyneuropathy, fits and depression
- vasculitis
- increased incidence of non-Hodgkin's B-cell lymphoma.

Pathology and investigations

Biopsies of the salivary gland or of the lip show a focal infiltration of lymphocytes and plasma cells.

- **Schirmer tear test.** A standard strip of filter paper is placed on the inside of the lower eyelid; wetting of less than 10 mm in 5 minutes indicates defective tear production.
- **Rose Bengal staining.** Staining of the eyes shows punctate or filamentary keratitis.
- **Laboratory abnormalities.** These include raised immunoglobulin levels, circulating immune complexes and autoantibodies. RF is usually positive. Antinuclear antibodies are found in 80% of cases and anti-mitochondrial antibodies are found in 10%. Anti-Ro (SSA) antibodies are found in 60–90%, compared with 10% of cases of RA and secondary Sjögren's syndrome.

Management

Symptomatic treatment is with artificial tears and saliva replacement solutions. Hydroxychloroquine may help fatigue and arthralgia. Corticosteroids are rarely needed but are used to treat persistent salivary gland swelling or neuropathy. A trial of rituximab in Sjögren's syndrome did not demonstrate efficacy and this drug is not used.

'Overlap' syndromes and undifferentiated autoimmune rheumatic disease

An **overlap syndrome** is one where the patient shows the characteristic clinical features of more than one ARD. Treatment of each ARD is usually the same as when they occur separately.

Undifferentiated ARD is a term used for the condition of patients who have evidence of autoimmunity (e.g. positive autoantibody test) and some clinical features of such diseases (commonly, Raynaud's phenomenon and/or arthralgia) but not enough to make a clear diagnosis of any individual ARD. These patients sometimes develop a clearer ARD over time, but some always remain undifferentiated and tend to have relatively mild disease without major organ problems.

Further reading

Bakshi J, Tejera Segura B, Wincup C et al. Unmet needs in the pathogenesis and treatment of systemic lupus erythematosus. *Clin Rev Allergy Immunol* 2018; 55:352–367.
Giannokopoulos B, Krilis S. The pathogenesis of the antiphospholipid syndrome. *N Engl J Med* 2013; 368:1033–1044.
Rahman A, Isenberg DA. Systemic lupus erythematosus. *N Engl J Med* 2008; 358:929–939.
Ruiz-Irastorza G, Crowther M, Branch W et al. Antiphospholipid syndrome. *Lancet* 2011; 376:1498–1509.
Tsokos G. Systemic lupus erythematosus. *N Engl J Med* 2011; 378:1949–1961.

i **Box 18.39 Types of systemic vasculitis**

Large vessel
- Giant cell arteritis/polymyalgia rheumatica
- Takayasu's arteritis

Medium vessel
- Classical polyarteritis nodosa (PAN)
- Kawasaki's disease

Small vessel
- Microscopic polyangiitis
- Granulomatosis with polyangiitis   ⎫
- Eosinophilic granulomatosis   ⎬ ANCA-associated
  with polyangiitis (30–50% ANCA-positive)   ⎭
- Immunoglobulin A (Henoch–Schönlein) vasculitis   ⎫
- Cutaneous leucocytoclastic vasculitis   ⎬ ANCA-negative
- Essential cryoglobulinaemia   ⎭

ANCA, anti-neutrophil cytoplasmic antibodies.

i **Box 18.40 Other conditions associated with vasculitis[a]**

Infective
- E.g. subacute infective endocarditis

Non-infective
- Vasculitis with rheumatoid arthritis
- Systemic lupus erythematosus
- Scleroderma

- Polymyositis/dermatomyositis
- Drug-induced Behçet's disease
- Goodpasture's syndrome
- Hypocomplementaemia
- Serum sickness
- Paraneoplastic syndromes
- Inflammatory bowel disease

[a]See also Box **18.39**.

SYSTEMIC INFLAMMATORY VASCULITIS

Vasculitis is a histological term describing inflammation of the vessel wall. Vasculitis can be seen in many diseases (**Boxes 18.39** and **18.40**). The group of diseases described in this section (systemic inflammatory vasculitides) is characterized by widespread vasculitis leading to systemic symptoms and signs, generally requiring treatment with corticosteroids and/or immunosuppressive drugs. Two main features are helpful in classifying these vasculitides: the *size of the blood vessels involved* and the *presence or absence of anti-neutrophil cytoplasmic antibodies (ANCA)* in the blood. Revisions in the commonly used terms for various vasculitides have been proposed to reflect increased pathophysiological understanding of these conditions (**Fig. 18.39** and see **Box 18.39**).
- *Large-vessel vasculitis* refers to the aorta and its major tributaries.
- *Medium-vessel vasculitis* refers to medium- and small-sized arteries and arterioles.
- *Small-vessel vasculitis* refers to small arteries, arterioles, venules and capillaries.

Large-vessel vasculitis

Polymyalgia rheumatica and giant cell (temporal) arteritis are systemic illnesses of the elderly. Both are associated with the finding of a giant cell arteritis on temporal artery biopsy.

Polymyalgia rheumatica

Polymyalgia rheumatica (PMR) causes a sudden onset of severe pain and stiffness of the shoulders and neck, and of the hips and lumbar spine: a limb girdle pattern. These symptoms are worse in the morning, lasting from 30 minutes to several hours. The clinical history is usually diagnostic and the patient is always over 50 years old. Up to 25% of patients may have some inflammation of peripheral joints.

Approximately one-third of patients develop systemic features of tiredness, fever, weight loss, depression and occasionally nocturnal sweats, especially if PMR is not diagnosed and treated early. A differential diagnosis is shown in **Box 18.41**.

Investigation of PMR

- *A raised ESR and/or CRP* is a hallmark of this condition. It is rare to see PMR without an acute-phase response. If it is absent, the diagnosis should be questioned and the tests repeated a few weeks later before treatment is started.
- *Serum alkaline phosphatase and γ-glutamyl-transpeptidase* may be raised as markers of the acute inflammation.
- *Anaemia* (mild normochromic, normocytic) is often present.
- *Temporal artery biopsy* shows giant cell arteritis in 10–30% of cases, but is rarely performed unless giant cell arteritis is also suspected.

Giant cell arteritis

Giant cell arteritis (GCA) is inflammatory granulomatous arteritis of large cerebral arteries, which occurs in association with PMR. The patient may have current PMR or a history of recent PMR, or may be on treatment for PMR. It is extremely rare under 50 years of age. Presenting symptoms of GCA include severe headaches, tenderness of the scalp (combing the hair may be painful) or of the temple, claudication of the jaw when eating, and tenderness and swelling of one or more temporal or occipital arteries. The most feared manifestation is sudden, painless, temporary or permanent loss of vision in one eye due to involvement of the ophthalmic artery (see p. 852). Systemic manifestations of severe malaise, tiredness and fever occur.

Investigations in GCA

- Normochromic, normocytic anaemia.
- ESR is usually raised (in the region of 50–120 mm/h) and the CRP very high.
- Liver biochemistry may be abnormal, as in PMR. The albumin may be low.
- A temporal artery biopsy from the affected side is the definitive diagnostic test. This should be taken before, or within 7 days of starting, high doses of corticosteroids. The lesions are patchy and the whole length of the biopsy (>1 cm long) must be examined; even so, negative biopsies occur.
- Ultrasound scanning of the temporal arteries is increasingly used – if diagnostic features are seen, biopsy can be avoided. The *histological features* of GCA are:
- Cellular infiltrates of CD4+ T lymphocytes, macrophages and giant cells in the vessel wall. Note that giant cells are not visible in all cases.
- Granulomatous inflammation of the intima and media.
- Breaking up of the internal elastic lamina.
- Giant cells, lymphocytes and plasma cells in the internal elastic lamina.

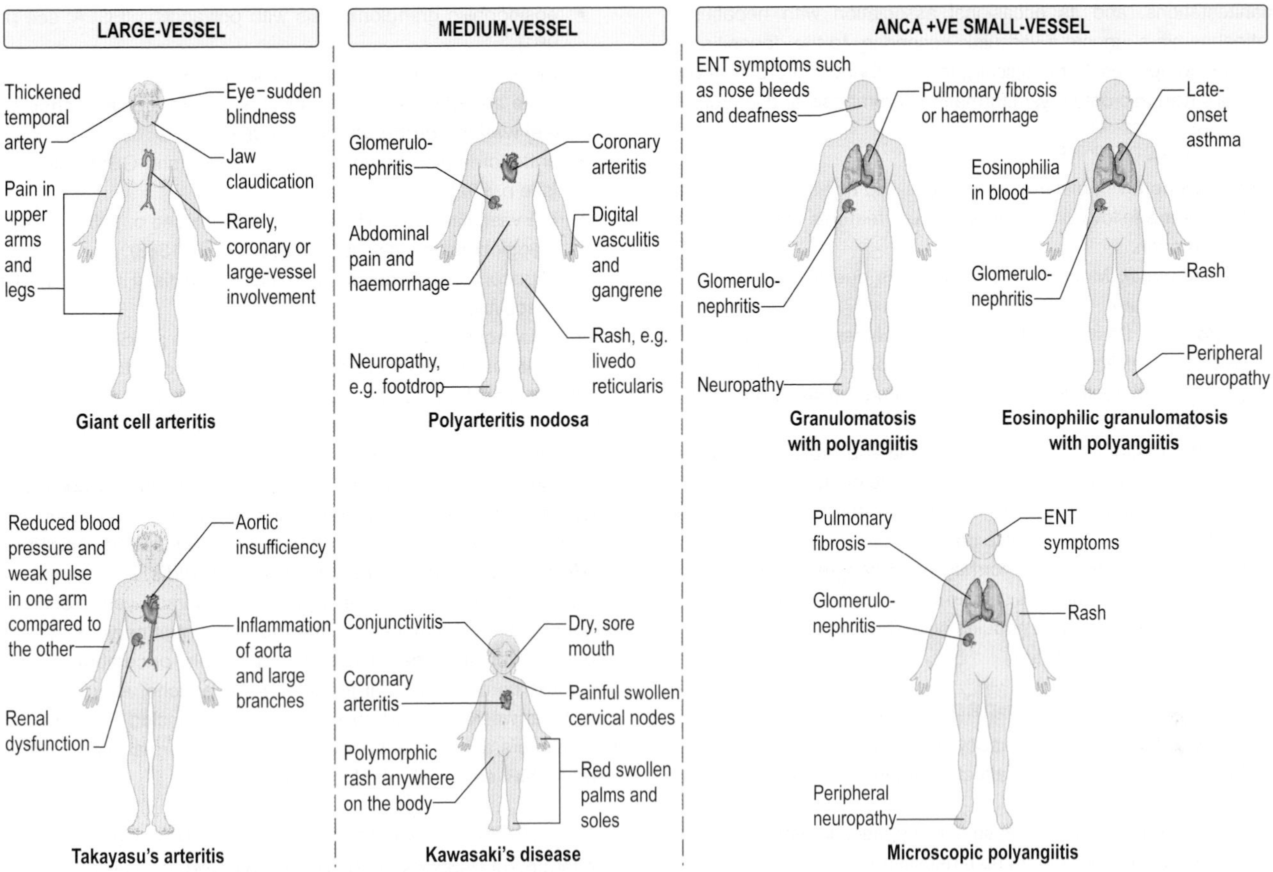

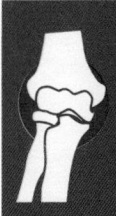

LARGE-VESSEL

Thickened temporal artery

Eye–sudden blindness

Jaw claudication

Pain in upper arms and legs

Rarely, coronary or large-vessel involvement

Giant cell arteritis

Reduced blood pressure and weak pulse in one arm compared to the other

Aortic insufficiency

Inflammation of aorta and large branches

Renal dysfunction

Takayasu's arteritis

MEDIUM-VESSEL

Glomerulo-nephritis

Coronary arteritis

Digital vasculitis and gangrene

Abdominal pain and haemorrhage

Rash, e.g. livedo reticularis

Neuropathy, e.g. footdrop

Polyarteritis nodosa

Conjunctivitis

Dry, sore mouth

Coronary arteritis

Painful swollen cervical nodes

Polymorphic rash anywhere on the body

Red swollen palms and soles

Kawasaki's disease

ANCA +VE SMALL-VESSEL

ENT symptoms such as nose bleeds and deafness

Pulmonary fibrosis or haemorrhage

Late-onset asthma

Eosinophilia in blood

Glomerulo-nephritis

Glomerulo-nephritis

Rash

Neuropathy

Peripheral neuropathy

Granulomatosis with polyangiitis

Eosinophilic granulomatosis with polyangiitis

Pulmonary fibrosis

ENT symptoms

Glomerulo-nephritis

Rash

Peripheral neuropathy

Microscopic polyangiitis

Fig. 18.39 Clinical features of systemic inflammatory vasculitides. These illnesses all frequently present with joint pain, as well as systemic symptoms such as fatigue, malaise and weight loss. The most common organ-specific manifestations are shown. Giant cell arteritis is usually seen in people over 50, whereas Takayasu's disease is seen in people under 50. Kawasaki's disease is usually seen in children under 5. ANCA, anti-neutrophil cytoplasmic antibodies; ENT, ear, nose and throat.

> **? Box 18.41 Symptom patterns in some muscle disorders**
>
> - *Polymyositis* – proximal muscle ache and weakness
> - *Polymyalgia rheumatica* – proximal morning stiffness and pain
> - *Myopathy* – weakness, but no pain or stiffness

Management of PMR or GCA

Corticosteroids produce a dramatic reduction of symptoms of PMR within 24–48 hours of starting treatment, provided the dose is adequate. If this improvement does not occur, the diagnosis should be questioned and an alternative cause sought, such as RA, vasculitis, infection or malignancy. Corticosteroid treatment should reduce the risk of patients who have PMR developing GCA. NSAIDs are less effective and should not be used.

In GCA, corticosteroids are obligatory because they significantly reduce the risk of irreversible visual loss and other focal ischaemic lesions, but much higher doses are needed than in PMR. If GCA is suspected, it may not be possible to arrange an ultrasound scan or temporal artery biopsy rapidly. In these circumstances, treatment should not be delayed, especially if there have already been episodes of visual loss or stroke.

Starting daily doses of prednisolone are:

- **PMR**: 15 mg prednisolone as a single dose in the morning
- **GCA**: 60–100 mg prednisolone, usually in divided doses.

The dose should then be reduced gradually in weekly or monthly steps. While the dose is above 20 mg, the step reductions are 5 mg, reducing the evening doses first. Between 20 mg and 10 mg, the reduction can be in 2.5-mg steps, but below 10 mg the rate should be slower and the steps of 1 mg each. Most patients will eventually be able to stop corticosteroids after 12–18 months but up to 25% may need low doses long term. Steroid-sparing immunosuppressive agents are used in refractory cases where it is hard to reduce the corticosteroid dose without causing a flare of disease or a rise in ESR or CRP. A clinical trial showed that a combination of the anti-interleukin receptor 6 receptor agent tocilizumab with corticosteroid gave higher rates of remission than corticosteroid alone.

Calcium and vitamin D supplements, and sometimes bisphosphonates, are necessary to prevent osteoporosis while high-dose steroids are being used (see p. 479).

Takayasu's arteritis

Takayasu's arteritis is a granulomatous inflammation of the aorta and its major branches (see p. 1132).

Medium-sized vessel vasculitis

Polyarteritis nodosa

Classical polyarteritis nodosa (PAN) is a rare condition that usually occurs in middle-aged men. It is accompanied by severe systemic manifestations, and its occasional association with hepatitis B antigenaemia suggests a vasculitis secondary to the deposition of immune complexes. Pathologically, there is fibrinoid necrosis of vessel walls with microaneurysm formation, thrombosis and infarction.

Clinical features

These include fever, malaise, weight loss and myalgia. These initial symptoms are followed by dramatic acute features that are due to organ infarction.

- **Neurological.** Mononeuritis multiplex is due to arteritis of the vasa nervorum.
- **Abdominal.** Pain is due to arterial involvement of the abdominal viscera, mimicking acute cholecystitis, pancreatitis or appendicitis. Gastrointestinal haemorrhage occurs because of mucosal ulceration.
- **Renal.** Presentation is with haematuria and proteinuria. Hypertension and acute/chronic kidney disease occur.
- **Cardiac.** Coronary arteritis causes myocardial infarction and heart failure. Pericarditis also occurs.
- **Skin.** Subcutaneous haemorrhage and gangrene occur. A persistent livedo reticularis is seen in chronic cases. Cutaneous and subcutaneous palpable nodules occur but are uncommon.
- **Lung.** Involvement is rare.

Investigations and management

- **Blood count.** Anaemia, leucocytosis and a raised ESR occur.
- **Biopsy.** Material from an affected organ shows features listed above.
- **Angiography.** Microaneurysms in hepatic, intestinal or renal vessels can be demonstrated if necessary.
- **Other investigations.** These are performed as appropriate (e.g. electrocardiogram and abdominal ultrasound), depending on the clinical problem. ANCA is positive only rarely in classic PAN.

Treatment is with corticosteroids, usually in combination with immunosuppressive drugs such as azathioprine.

Kawasaki's disease

Kawasaki's disease is an acute systemic vasculitis involving medium-sized vessels, affecting mainly children under 5 years of age. It is very frequent in Japan and an infective trigger is suspected. Fewer than 10% of cases occur in adults.

Clinical features and management

The characteristic clinical features are fever lasting longer than 4 days, bilateral conjunctival congestion, dry red lips and oral cavity, cervical lymphadenopathy, rash and redness of the palms and soles.

Cardiovascular changes in the acute stage include pancarditis and coronary arteritis, leading to aneurysms or dilatation visible on echocardiography, MRI or angiography.

Treatment is with a single dose of high-dose intravenous immunoglobulin (2 g/kg), which prevents the coronary artery disease, followed after the acute phase by aspirin 200–300 mg daily. There is no evidence that steroid treatment improves the outcome.

Small-vessel vasculitis

The two revised categories of small-vessel vasculitis (SVV) are:
- ANCA-associated vasculitis (AAV), characterized by a **paucity of vessel wall immunoglobulin** and presence (in many but not all patients) of ANCA, including:
  - granulomatosis with polyangiitis (GPA; see p. 991)

- eosinophilic granulomatosis with polyangiitis (EGPA; see p. 991)
  - microscopic polyangiitis (MPA; see p. 991).
- Immune complex (ANCA-negative) SVV, with a **prominence of vessel wall immunoglobulin** including:
  - anti-glomerular basement membrane (anti-GBM) disease (see p. 992)
  - IgA vasculitis (IgAV, Henoch–Schönlein) (see p. 1367)
  - cryoglobulinaemic vasculitis (CV) (see p. 1368)
  - hypocomplementaemic urticarial vasculitis (HUV, anti-C1q vasculitis)
  - cutaneous leucocytoclastic vasculitis (see p. 682).

Cutaneous leucocytoclastic vasculitis is the characteristic acute purpuric lesion that histologically involves the dermal postcapillary venules. This lesion affects only the skin and should be differentiated from similar lesions produced in systemic vasculitis. The purpura may be accompanied by arthralgia and glomerulonephritis. Hepatitis C infection is common and may be an aetiological agent. The condition can also be caused by drugs such as sulphonamides and penicillin.

Primary central nervous system vasculitis is a very rare condition (incidence 2–4 cases per million person years) characterized by clinical features confined to the central nervous system and characteristic appearances on angiography or cerebral biopsy. The most common clinical features are headache, altered cognition, focal weakness and stroke. Blood tests, including inflammatory markers and autoantibodies, are usually normal but a normal cerebral MRI essentially excludes the diagnosis.

Management of small-cell vasculitis

The treatment depends on the organs involved. Vasculitis confined to the skin may not require systemic treatment, whereas involvement of major organs (e.g. lungs or kidneys in GPA) requires high-dose corticosteroids, immunosuppression and, sometimes, plasma exchange. Clinical trials have shown that depletion of B cells with rituximab is as effective as cyclophosphamide in treating AAV and can help reduce the dose of corticosteroids required to maintain remission. In EGPA, the anti-interleukin 5 agent mepolizumab has been found to be effective in a clinical trial.

Behçet's disease

Behçet's disease is an inflammatory disorder of unknown cause. There is a striking geographical distribution, it being most common in Turkey, Iran and Japan. The prevalence per 100 000 is 10–15 in Japan and 80–300 in Turkey. There is a link to the HLA-B51 allele, with a relative risk of 5–10; this association is not seen in patients in the USA and Europe.

Clinical features

The cardinal clinical feature is recurrent oral ulceration. The **international criteria for diagnosis** require oral ulceration and any two of the following:
- genital ulcers
- defined eye lesions, including an anterior or posterior uveitis or retinal vascular lesions
- defined skin lesions – erythema nodosum, pseudofolliculitis and papulopustular lesions
- positive skin pathergy test (see below)
- oral ulcers – aphthous or herpetiform.

Other manifestations include a self-limiting peripheral mono- or oligoarthritis affecting knees, ankles, wrists and elbows; gastrointestinal symptoms of diarrhoea, abdominal pain and anorexia;

pulmonary and renal lesions; thrombophlebitis (especially in the legs); vasculitis; and a brainstem syndrome, organic confusional states and a meningoencephalitis. All the common manifestations are self-limiting except for the ocular attacks. Repeated attacks of uveitis can cause blindness.

The **pathergy reaction** is highly specific to Behçet's disease. Skin injury – by a needle prick, for example – leads to papule or pustule formation within 24–48 hours. Blood tests usually show raised ESR and CRP but not autoantibodies.

Management

Corticosteroids, immunosuppressive agents and ciclosporin are used for chronic uveitis and the rare neurological complications. Colchicine helps erythema nodosum and joint pain. Thalidomide may be useful in some cases, although side-effects of drowsiness and peripheral neuropathy are common. It should not be used in pregnant women because of phocomelia (limb abnormalities). Anti-TNF agents can be used to control severe uveitis and serious manifestations such as neurological and gastrointestinal Behçet's disease.

Further reading

Jennette JC, Falk RJ, Bacon PA et al. 2012 revised International Chapel Hill Consensus Conference nomenclature of vasculitides. *Arthritis Rheum* 2013; 65:1–11.
Kermani TA, Warrington KJ. Polymyalgia rheumatica. *Lancet* 2013; 381:63–72.
Stone JH, Tuckwell K, Dimonaco S et al. Trial of tocilizumab in giant cell arteritis. *N Engl J Med* 2017; 377:317–328.
Warrell DA, Cox TM, Firth JD (eds). *Oxford Textbook of Medicine*, 5th edn. Oxford: Oxford University Press; 2010. Section 19.11 Autoimmune rheumatic disorders and vasculitides; Section 21.10.2 The kidney in systemic vasculitis.
Wechsler ME, Akuthota P, Jayne D et al. Mepolizumab or placebo for eosinophilic granulomatosis with polyangiitis. *N Engl J Med* 2017; 376:1921–1932.

ARTHRITIS IN CHILDREN

Joint and limb pains are common in children but arthritis is, fortunately, rare. Babies and young children may present with immobility of a joint or a limp, but the diagnosis can be extremely difficult. **Fig. 18.40** summarizes the differential diagnosis.

Juvenile idiopathic arthritis

A full description of juvenile idiopathic arthritis (JIA) is beyond the scope of this textbook. A brief account is provided below.

JIA is classified according to the extent and type of joint involvement. A particularly severe form, **systemic onset JIA (Still's disease)** presents with high fever (>39°C), rash, lymphadenopathy, hepatosplenomegaly and/or serositis. Joint involvement is often not the most prominent symptom. High-dose corticosteroids and immunosuppressants such as methotrexate are used for treatment.

In contrast, patients with **oligoarticular** (<5 joints involved) and **polyarticular** (≥5 joints) JIA complain mainly of joint pain and swelling.

The oligoarticular form is more common. In childhood, these patients can develop uveitis and require regular screening by slit lamp examination. Outlook is usually good but approximately 25% develop an extended form where more joints can be involved over time leading to destructive arthritis persisting into adulthood.

Polyarticular JIA is divided into RF-positive and RF-negative subtypes, of which the RF-positive form is more aggressive.

Enthesitis-related arthritis tends to affect teenage and younger boys, mainly involves lower limb joints and entheses and is associated with HLA-B27 positivity.

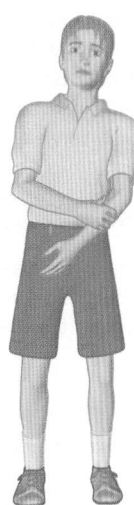

Juvenile idiopathic arthritis	Other conditions
Systemic arthritis Oligoarthritis (persistent) Oligoarthritis (extended) Polyarthritis (rheumatoid-factor positive) Polyarthritis (rheumatoid-factor negative) Enthesitis-related arthritis Psoriatic arthritis Unclassified	Henoch–Schönlein purpura Infections, e.g. tuberculosis, septic arthritis, viral arthritis Rheumatic fever Hypermobility syndrome Leukaemia Sickle cell disease SLE and other autoimmune rheumatic disease Transient synovitis of the hip Perthes' disease

Fig. 18.40 The differential diagnosis of arthritis in children. SLE, systemic lupus erythematosus.

Children with JIA are generally managed by specialist paediatric rheumatologists but come under the care of adult rheumatologists later in life. At this stage, they may be on long-term maintenance DMARDs for which management and monitoring are as for adult-onset inflammatory arthritis. However, they may also have damaged joints or side-effects of long-term medications (such as steroid-induced osteoporosis) which require close attention. Joint replacement surgery in patients who have had JIA may be required earlier in life than in other groups.

RHEUMATOLOGICAL PROBLEMS SEEN IN OTHER DISEASES

Gastrointestinal and liver disease

- Enteropathic synovitis (see p. 451).
- Autoimmune hepatitis (see p. 1286) may be accompanied by an arthralgia similar to that seen in SLE. Joint pain occurs in a bilateral, symmetrical distribution, predominantly affecting the small joints of the hands. Joints usually look normal but sometimes there is a slight soft tissue swelling. These patients often have positive tests for antinuclear antibodies.
- Primary biliary cholangitis patients occasionally have a symmetrical arthropathy.
- Hereditary haemochromatosis is associated with arthritis in 50% of cases, which is often the first sign of the disease and cartilage calcification is common.
- Whipple's disease (see p. 1194) is accompanied by fever and arthralgia.

Respiratory disease

Sarcoidosis

- Sarcoidosis (see p. 985) is a multisystem granulomatous disease associated with erythema nodosum in 20% of cases at or soon after the onset of the disease. A chest X-ray shows hilar lymphadenopathy in 80% of cases. The serum ACE may be raised.

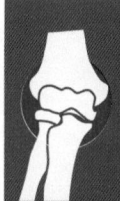

- Several patterns of arthritis occur later in the disease. These include a transient rheumatoid-like polyarthritis and an acute monoarthritis that can be mistaken for gout. Bone cysts can also develop.
- *Treatment* is with NSAIDs; if these fail to control the symptoms, corticosteroids are usually very effective.

Malignant disease

It is not uncommon for malignant diseases to present with musculoskeletal symptoms. Gout occurs in conditions such as chronic myeloid leukaemia. Neoplastic disease of bone is described on page 485.

Hypertrophic pulmonary osteoarthropathy

Hypertrophic pulmonary osteoarthropathy (HPO) is a paraneoplastic, non-metastatic complication, frequently associated with carcinoma of the bronchus. It may be the presenting feature of the disease. It rarely occurs with other conditions that also cause clubbing, presenting most often in middle-aged men with pain and swelling of the wrists and ankles. Other joints are occasionally involved. Primary HPO is a hereditary condition involving a mutation in the *HPGD* gene that degrades prostaglandin E_2 (PGE_2), thus allowing over-production of PGE_2, which may cause clubbing.

The diagnosis is made on the presence of clubbing of the fingers (usually gross in primary HPO) and periosteal new bone formation along the shafts of the distal ends of the radius, ulna, tibia and fibula on X-ray. A chest X-ray usually shows the malignancy.

Management should be directed at the underlying carcinoma; if this can be removed, the arthropathy disappears. NSAIDs relieve the symptoms.

Paraneoplastic polyarthritis

This condition is seen with carcinoma of the breast in women and of the lung in men, and also with renal cell carcinoma. The neoplasm may be occult at onset and the diagnosis is then difficult to make.

Skin disease

Psoriatic arthritis

This disease is discussed on page 450.

Erythema nodosum

Erythema nodosum (see p. 677) is accompanied by arthritis in over 50% of cases. The knees and ankles are particularly affected, being swollen, red and tender. The arthritis subsides, along with the skin lesions, within a few months. Treatment is with NSAIDs or occasionally steroids.

Neurological disease

Neuropathic (Charcot's) joints

These are damaged by trauma as a result of the loss of the protective pain sensation. The site of the neuropathic joint depends on the localization of the pain loss:

- In tabes dorsalis, the knees and ankles are most often affected.
- In diabetes mellitus, the joints of the tarsus are involved.
- In syringomyelia, the shoulder is involved.

Neuropathic joints are not painful, although there may be painful episodes associated with crystal deposition. Presentation is usually with swelling and instability. Eventually, severe deformities develop.

The characteristic finding is a swollen joint with abnormal but painless movement, in association with neurological findings that depend on the underlying disease (e.g. dissociated sensory loss in syringomyelia or polyneuropathy in diabetes). X-ray changes are characteristic, with gross joint disorganization and bony distortion.

Treatment is symptomatic. Surgery may be required in advanced cases.

Blood disease

Arthritis due to haemarthrosis is a common presenting feature of people with *haemophilia* (see p. 375). Attacks begin in early childhood in most cases and are recurrent. The knee is the most commonly affected joint but the elbows and ankles are sometimes involved. The arthritis can lead to bone destruction and disorganization of joints. Apart from replacement of factor VIII, affected joints require initial immobilization followed by physiotherapy to restore movement and measures to prevent and correct deformities.

Sickle cell crises (see p. 345) are often accompanied by joint pain that particularly affects the hands and feet in a bilateral, symmetrical distribution. Affected joints usually look normal but are occasionally swollen. This condition may also be complicated by avascular necrosis (see p. 425) and by osteomyelitis.

Arthritis can also occur in *acute leukaemia* (see p. 388); it may be the presenting feature in childhood. The knee is particularly affected and is very painful, warm and swollen. Treatment is directed at the underlying leukaemia. Arthritis may also occur in chronic leukaemia, with leukaemic deposits in and around the joints.

Individuals with *transfusion-dependent thalassaemia* (see p. 343) are living longer and are presenting with back pain due to premature disc degeneration, secondary spondylosis and crush fractures caused by osteoporosis. There is marked discal calcification.

Endocrine and metabolic disorders

Hypothyroid patients may complain of pain and stiffness of proximal muscles, resembling polymyalgia rheumatica. They may also have carpal tunnel syndrome. Less often, there is an arthritis accompanied by joint effusions, particularly in the knees, wrist and small joints of the hands and feet. These problems respond rapidly to thyroxine.

Hyperparathyroidism may be complicated by cartilage calcification and acute CPPD.

In *acromegaly*, arthralgia occurs in about 50% of patients, particularly the small joints of the hands and knees. There may be a carpal tunnel syndrome.

In *Cushing's disease*, back pain is common.

Joint disorders related to *diabetes mellitus* are described on page 735.

Familial hypercholesterolaemia is associated with oligo- or polyarthritis, usually with tendon xanthomata. Arthritis also occurs in combined hyperlipidaemia.

MISCELLANEOUS ARTHROPATHIES

Familial Mediterranean fever

Periodic fever syndromes are a group of autoinflammatory disorders that present with recurrent attacks of fever in childhood and adult life.

Familial Mediterranean fever (FMF) is the most common inherited autoinflammatory disease. It is an autosomal recessive condition recognized worldwide but most prevalent in populations originating from the eastern Mediterranean. Mutations in the *MEFV* gene on chromosome 16 that encodes for pyrin, a suppressor of the activation of caspase 1, leads to increased biosynthesis of IL-1β and inflammation in FMF.

Symptoms of FMF are recurrent episodes of fever, arthritis and serositis. Peritonitic abdominal pain occurs in 80% of attacks. Pleuritic chest pain occurs in 15% of cases and is unilateral. Arthritis is rare and usually monoarticular, lasting up to 1 week. The CRP is markedly raised during the attacks. The condition may be mistaken for palindromic rheumatism (see p. 441), but such attacks are not usually accompanied by fever.

The diagnosis can be made by PCR, if available, but is based on the clinical picture and exclusion of other conditions.

Treatment involves lifelong colchicine 1000–1500 µg daily, which can usually prevent the attacks. In resistant patients, IL-1 inhibitors (anakinra and canakinumab) are licensed. In general, the disorder is benign, but in 25% of cases, renal amyloidosis develops (see p. 1357).

Other periodic fevers are being increasingly recognized. These include tumour necrosis factor receptor-associated periodic syndrome (TRAPS), mevalonate kinase deficiency (MKD), cryopyrin-associated periodic syndrome (CAPS), and periodic fever, aphthous stomatitis, pharyngitis and adenitis (PFAPA).

SAPHO (synovitis, acne, palmoplantar pustulosis, hyperostosis, osteitis)

This rare autoinflammatory disorder, linked to various HLA associations, dysregulation of IL-1 and *Cutibacterium acnes* infection, is considered on a spectrum with SpA, autoinflammatory disorders and pustular dermatoses. It produces chronic multifocal osteitis with anterior chest wall pain and peripheral synovitis. There is inflammatory cytokine release and global neutrophil activation. NSAIDs, methotrexate or TNF inhibitors (see pp. 444–445) may help.

Osteochondromatosis

In this condition, foci of cartilage form within the synovial membrane. These foci become calcified and then ossified (osteochondromas). They may give rise to loose bodies within the joint. The condition occurs in a single joint of a young adult and X-rays are usually diagnostic.

Management involves removal of loose bodies and synovectomy.

Pigmented villonodular synovitis

This is characterized by exuberant synovial proliferation that occurs either in joints or in tendon sheaths. The main manifestation in joints is recurrent haemarthrosis. It may produce progressive local bone destruction. A malignant form is seen occasionally.

Management is synovectomy or radiotherapy for more widespread cases or those that have failed surgery.

Relapsing polychondritis

Relapsing polychondritis is a rare inflammatory condition of cartilage. It occurs equally in males and females, usually the elderly. Tenderness, inflammation and eventual destruction of cartilage occur, mainly in the ear, nose, larynx or trachea. A seronegative polyarthritis occurs, as well as episcleritis and evidence of a vasculitis (e.g. glomerulonephritis). The diagnosis is clinical with laboratory evidence of acute inflammation.

Treatment involves corticosteroids and immunosuppressive agents.

Further reading
Lachmann HJ. Periodic fever syndromes. *Best Pract Res Clin Rheumatol* 2017; 31:596–609.

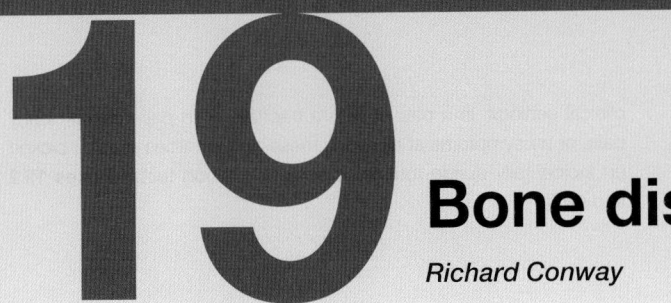

Bone disease

Richard Conway

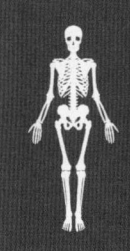

CORE SKILLS AND KNOWLEDGE

Bone disease is common in the general population, although frequently undiagnosed and often asymptomatic. Some 50% of women and 25% of men will suffer an osteoporotic fracture in their lifetime. Bone diseases are even more prevalent in those with coexisting medical conditions and the elderly. Bone disease specialists work in a variety of disciplines including general practice, rheumatology, endocrinology and medicine for the elderly, dividing their time between outpatient bone health clinics and inpatient fracture liaison services. Specialist nurses, radiographers, orthopaedic surgeons and allied health professionals all have important roles in helping to care for patients with bone disease.

Key learning objectives in bone disease include:

- understanding osteoporosis – its causes, diagnosis and treatment
- knowing when to investigate for other bone disorders, including bone infections and malignancy
- understanding 'bone profile' blood tests, dual X-ray absorptiometry (DXA) scanning and fracture risk assessment tools.

Learning opportunities in bone health include attending specialist bone health clinics, and attending fracture liaison service ward rounds where the underlying causes of fragility fractures are addressed.

CLINICAL SKILLS FOR BONE DISEASE

History

Clinical features

- Bone disease such as osteoporosis is often asymptomatic.
- *Severe, acute-onset pain* suggests a fracture (**Box 19.1**), which can occur with minimal trauma if the bone is fragile due to osteoporosis or malignancy.
- *Progressive localized bone pain* may suggest primary or secondary malignancy, or localized Paget's disease.

Risk factors for osteoporosis:

- Increased age.
- Early menopause without use of hormone replacement therapy.
- Hypogonadism in men.
- Corticosteroid use.
- Intestinal malabsorption.
- Obesity.
- Immobility.

Examination

Bone disease often presents with no physical signs, particularly in developed countries where good diet, early diagnosis and effective management of infectious disease prevent serious abnormalities. The commonest anatomical sites for various diseases of bone to occur are shown in the diagram; physical signs will vary from severe acute deformity and pain (if fracture occurs), through varying levels of tenderness, swelling and deformity in slowly progressive disease, to no observable changes in clinically silent disease.

Biochemical tests

A number of biochemical tests can be used to investigate the presence of bone disease. These are best described by their use in different clinical settings: in a patient with a fracture, or in patients with bony pain, or no symptoms at all (when these abnormalities may be picked up incidentally during routine or screening blood tests) (**Boxes 19.2** and **19.3**).

---

i **Box 19.1 Evaluation of a patient with a fracture**

Why has fracture occurred?
- Traumatic – high impact trauma
- Fragility – force equivalent to fall from less than standing height – implies osteoporosis or other bone disorder
- Pathological – consider when multiple fractures, systemic symptoms, unusual sites.

Investigations of fragility fracture
- Calcium/phosphate/magnesium
- 1,25 dihydroxyvitamin D/parathyroid hormone/alkaline phosphatase
- Myeloma screening – serum electrophoresis, serum and urine free light chains, immunoglobulins

- Dual X-ray absorptiometry (DXA) scanning.

Treatment of fragility fracture
- Fracture risk assessment
- Most patients with fragility fracture have osteoporosis and warrant treatment
- Calcium/vitamin D if required
- Oral bisphosphonate
  - Denosumab is alternative
  - Consider recombinant parathyroid hormone (PTH) if very high risk.

---

i **Box 19.2 Evaluation of a patient with a fragility fracture**

Ca	ALP	PTH	Probable diagnosis	Confirmatory test
N	N/H	N	**Osteoporosis**	DXA scanning
H	H	L	**Malignancy**	Nuclear medicine bone scan, investigation for likely site of primary (e.g. CT chest/abdomen/pelvis, mammogram)
N/H	H	H	**Primary hyperparathyroidism**	MIBI nuclear medicine parathyroid scan (see p. 645)
L	H	H	**Secondary hyperparathyroidism**	Check renal function for evidence of chronic kidney disease mineral and bone disorder (CKD-MBD, p. 1394)

ALP, alkaline phosphatase; Ca, calcium; CT, computed tomography; DXA, dual X-ray absorptiometry; H, high; L, low; MIBI, sestamibi; N, normal; PTH, parathyroid hormone.

---

i **Box 19.3 Evaluation of a patient with bone pain or no symptoms**

Ca	Phos	ALP	Probable diagnosis	Confirmatory test
L	L	H	**Osteomalacia**	Low vitamin D
N	N	H	**Paget's disease of bone**	Plain X-ray, isotope bone scan
L/N/H	H	H	**CKD-MBD**	Check renal function

ALP, alkaline phosphatase; Ca, calcium; CKD-MBD, chronic kidney disease mineral and bone disorder; H, high; L, low; N, normal; phos, phosphate.

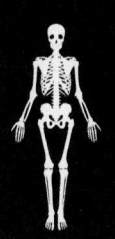

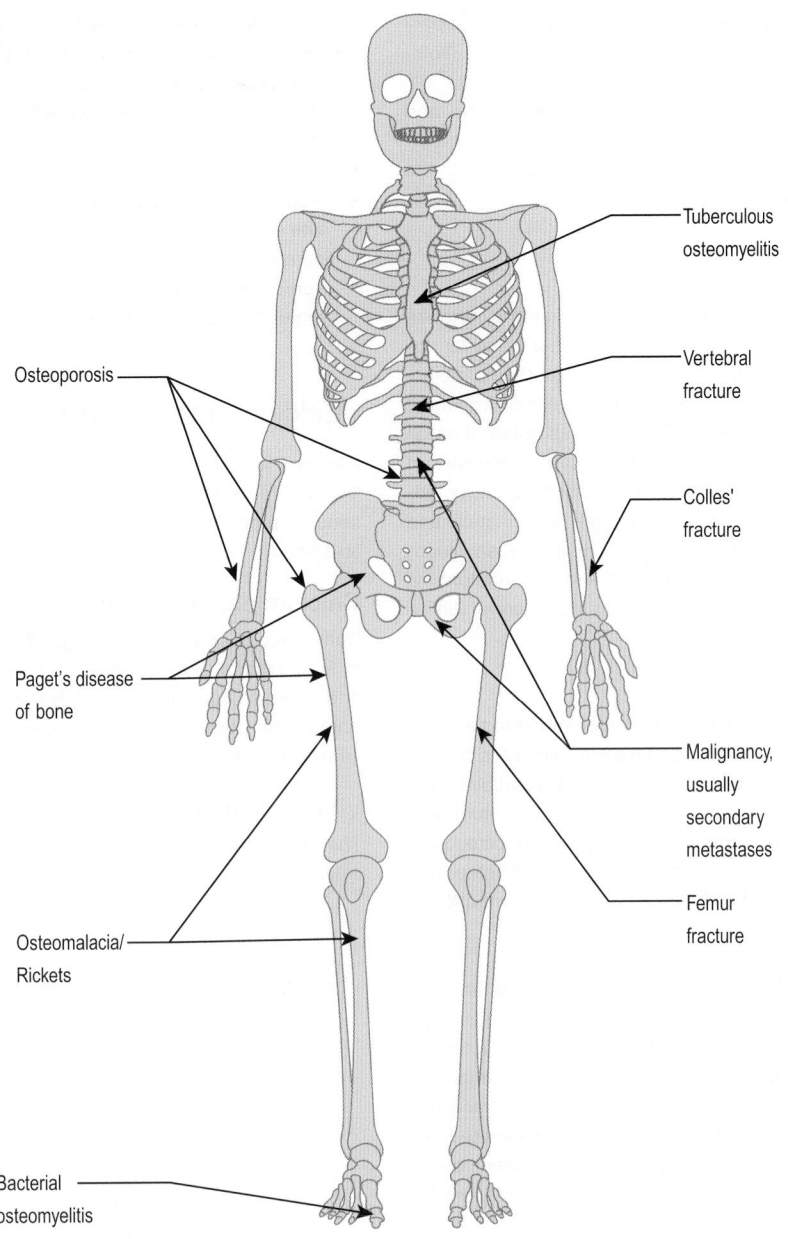

Osteoporosis

Tuberculous osteomyelitis

Vertebral fracture

Colles' fracture

Paget's disease of bone

Malignancy, usually secondary metastases

Femur fracture

Osteomalacia/ Rickets

Bacterial osteomyelitis

ANATOMY AND PHYSIOLOGY OF BONE

Bone is a specialized connective tissue serving three major functions:

- *mechanical* – supplying structure and muscle attachment for movement
- *metabolic* – providing the body's primary store of calcium and phosphate
- *protective* – enclosing the marrow and other vital organs.

This chapter covers the connective tissue functions of bone; bone marrow function is discussed in Chapter 16.

Bone structure

Bone comprises cells and a matrix of organic protein and inorganic mineral. Long bones (femur, tibia, humerus) and flat bones (skull,

scapula) have different embryological templates, with varying proportions of cortical and trabecular bone.

- *Cortical (compact or lamellar) bone* forms the shaft of long bones and the outer shell of flat bones. Formed of concentric rings of bone, it is particularly adapted to withstand bending strain.
- *Trabecular (cancellous) bone* is found at the ends of long bones and inside flat bones. Comprising a network of interconnecting rods and plates of bone, it offers resistance to compressive loads. It is also the main site of bone turnover for mineral homeostasis.
- *Woven bone* lacks an organized structure. It appears in the first few years of life, at sites of fracture repair and in high-turnover bone disorders such as Paget's disease.

Matrix components

- *Type I collagen* is the main protein, forming parallel lamellae of differing density (which impairs spreading of cracks). In cortical bone, concentric lamellae form around a central blood supply (Haversian system), which communicates via transverse (Volkmann's) canals.

- **Non-collagen proteins** include osteopontin, osteocalcin and fibronectin.
- **Bone mineral** largely consists of calcium and phosphate in the form of hydroxyapatite.

Bone cells

Osteoblasts

Derived from local mesenchymal stem cells, these cells synthesize matrix (osteoid) and regulate its mineralization. After bone formation, the majority of osteoblasts are removed by apoptosis, others remaining at the bone/marrow interface as lining cells or within the bone as osteocytes. Osteoblasts regulate bone resorption through the balance in expression of the stimulatory receptor activator of nuclear factor kappa B ligand (RANKL) and its antagonist, osteoprotegerin (OPG). Osteoblasts are rich in alkaline phosphatase and express receptors for parathyroid hormone (PTH), oestrogen, glucocorticoids, vitamin D, inflammatory cytokines and the transforming growth factor-beta (TGF-β) family, all of which may therefore influence bone remodelling.

Osteocytes

These small cells, derived from osteoblasts, are embedded in bone and interconnected with each other and with bone-lining cells through cytoplasmic processes. They respond to mechanical strain by undergoing apoptosis or through altered cell signalling, which in turn activates bone formation with or without prior resorption. As osteocytes also express RANKL and OPG, the relative importance of osteocytes and osteoblasts in bone resorption function continues to be explored.

Osteoclasts

These cells have the unique capacity to resorb bone and are derived from haemopoietic precursors of the macrophage lineage. In response to RANKL, macrophage colony stimulating factor (M-CSF) and local adhesion factors (integrins), osteoclasts attach to bone, creating a ruffled border that forms a number of extracellular lysosomal compartments. Hydrogen ions are actively secreted into these spaces and the acid environment removes the mineral phase before specialized cysteine proteases (e.g. cathepsin K) resorb the collagen matrix.

Bone growth and remodelling

Longitudinal growth occurs at the epiphyseal growth plate, a cartilage structure between the epiphysis and metaphysis (**Fig. 19.1**). Cartilage production is tightly regulated, with subsequent mineralization and growth finally arrested at 18–21 years, when the epiphysis and metaphysis fuse.

In adults, bone is regularly remodelled to ensure repair of microdamage and turnover of calcium and phosphate for homeostasis. This remodelling cycle is carried out by the basic multicellular unit (BMU; **Fig. 19.2**). Signals initiating resorption include osteocyte apoptosis and altered signalling (sclerostin, prostaglandins, RANKL and other molecules), resulting in localized retraction of bone-lining cells and binding of multinucleate osteoclasts to the bone surface, followed by bone resorption. Bone formation involves reciprocal effects of *wnt* versus *dickkopf* (*Dkk*) and sclerostin on the LRP5/6-β-catenin pathway. The switch from resorption to formation may rely on osteocyte signalling or on release of signals from the bone matrix, such as TGF-β. Bone remodelling is said to be coupled when formation follows resorption, but may be unbalanced when the amount of bone removed is not replaced with an equal amount. Examples of bone remodelling include:

- Myeloma cells have dual lytic effects, with enhanced expression of RANKL and *Dkk*
- In rheumatoid arthritis, RANKL and *Dkk* are increased
- In spondyloarthritis (characterized by new bone formation alongside erosion) *Dkk* is inhibited, with the increased *wnt* activity also increasing OPG relative to RANKL
- Corticosteroids may increase osteocyte SOST expression, and stimulate expression of *Dkk*.

Calcium homeostasis and its regulation

Calcium homeostasis is regulated by the effects of PTH and 1,25-dihydroxyvitamin D_3 on gut, kidney and bone. Calcium-sensing receptors are present in the parathyroid glands, kidney and brain.

Calcium absorption and distribution

Daily calcium consumption (**Fig. 19.3**), primarily from dairy foods, is 20–25 mmol (800–1000 mg). The combined effect of calcium and vitamin D deficiency contributes to the bone fragility seen in some older people. Intestinal absorption of calcium is reduced by vitamin D deficiency and in malabsorption states (see p. 1245).

Vitamin D metabolism

The primary source of vitamin D (**Fig. 19.4**) in humans is photoactivation in the skin of 7-dehydrocholesterol to cholecalciferol, which

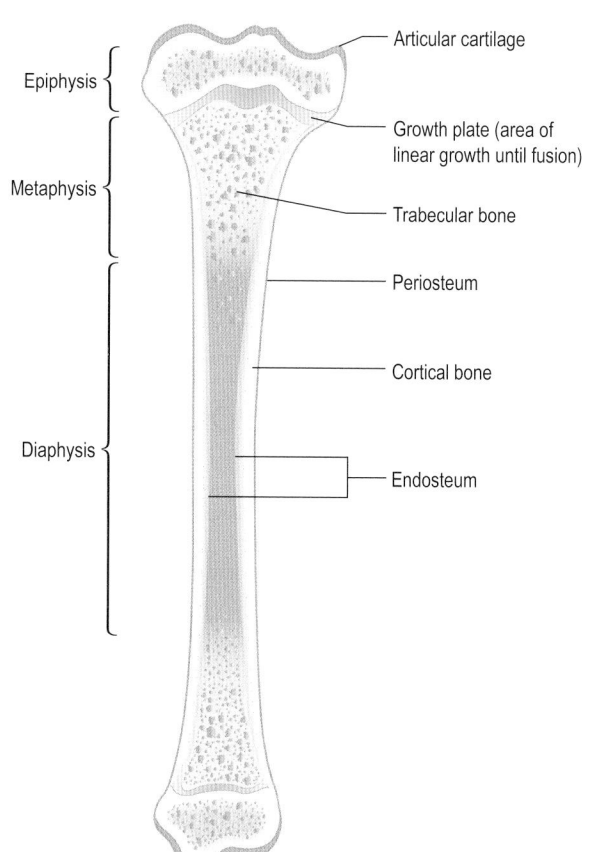

Epiphysis {

Metaphysis {

Diaphysis {

Articular cartilage

Growth plate (area of linear growth until fusion)

Trabecular bone

Periosteum

Cortical bone

Endosteum

Fig. 19.1 A longitudinal section of a growing long bone. *(From NICE guidelines: Osteoporosis – primary prevention. http://www.nice.org.uk/Guidance/TA160 (23 July 2012).)*

is then converted first in the liver to 25-hydroxyvitamin D (25(OH)D$_3$) and subsequently in the kidney (by the enzyme 1α-hydroxylase) to 1,25-dihydroxyvitamin D$_3$. (This step can occur in lymphomatous and sarcoid tissue, resulting in hypercalcaemia.) Regulation of the latter step is by PTH, phosphate and feedback inhibition by 1,25-dihydroxyvitamin D$_3$.

Parathyroid hormone

Parathyroid hormone (PTH), an 84-amino-acid hormone, is secreted from the chief cells of the parathyroid gland, which have calcium-sensing and vitamin D receptors. PTH increases renal phosphate excretion and increases plasma calcium by:

- increasing osteoclastic activity in bone (a rapid response)
- increasing intestinal absorption of calcium (a slower response)
- increasing 1α-hydroxylation of vitamin D (the rate-limiting step)
- increasing renal tubular reabsorption of calcium.

Hypomagnesaemia can suppress the normal PTH response to hypocalcaemia.

Calcitonin

Calcitonin is produced by thyroid C cells. Although calcitonin inhibits osteoclastic bone resorption and increases the renal excretion of calcium and phosphate, neither excess calcitonin (seen in medullary carcinoma of the thyroid) nor its deficiency following thyroidectomy has significant skeletal effects in humans.

Further reading

Rosen CJ. Vitamin D insufficiency. *N Engl J Med* 2011; 364:248–254.
Xiong J, Onal M, Jilka RL et al. Matrix-embedded cells control osteoclast formation. *Nat Med* 2011; 17:1235–1241.
Zebaze RM, Ghasem-Zadeh A, Bohte A et al. Intracortical remodelling and porosity in the distal radius and post-mortem femurs of women: a cross-sectional study. *Lancet* 2010; 375:1729–1736.
http://courses.washington.edu/bonephys/ *Bone physiology*.

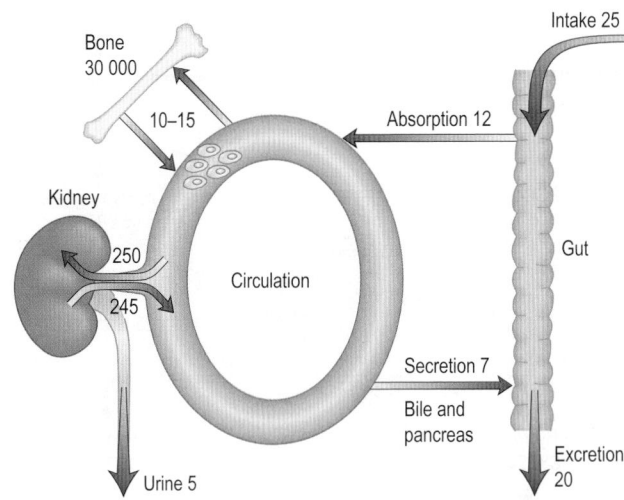

Fig. 19.3 Calcium exchange in the normal human. The amounts are shown in mmol per day.

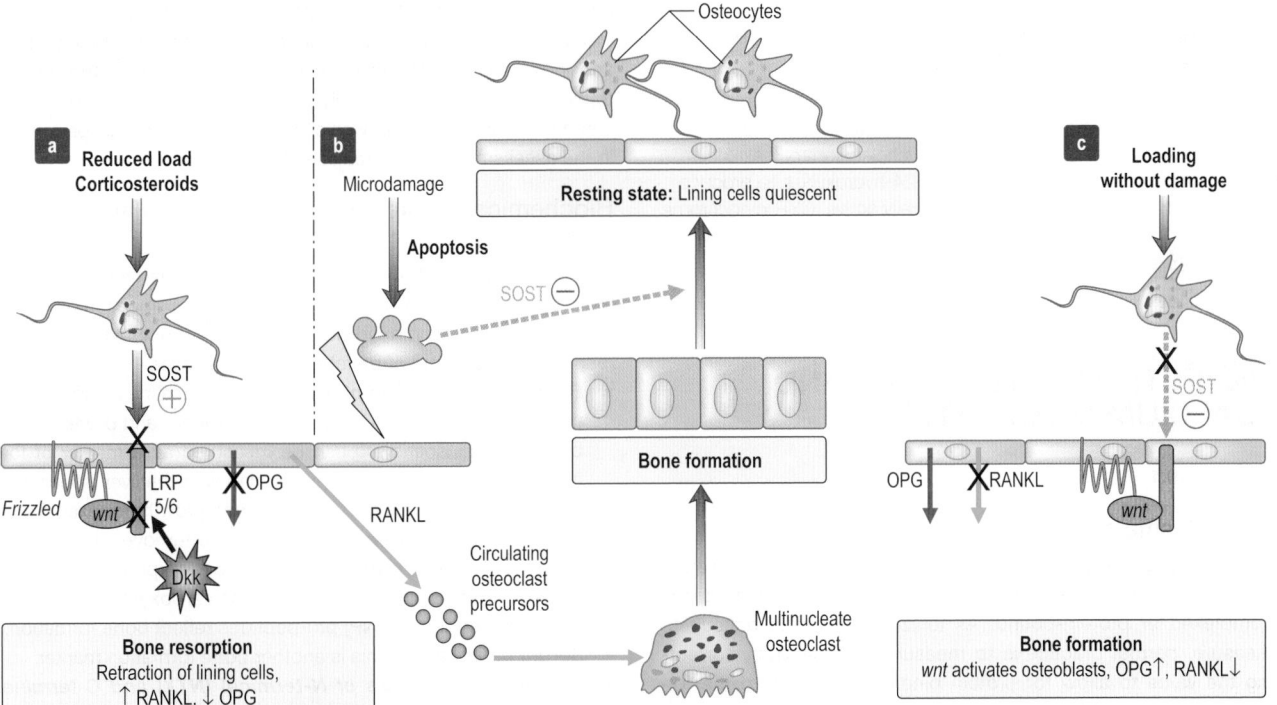

Fig. 19.2 Bone is remodelled in response to alterations in two reciprocal systems. **(a)** *Quiescent bone* may experience *reduced load,* in response the osteocyte increases expression of *sclerostin (SOST+)*, inhibiting the response to *wnt* via the **LRP5/frizzled co-receptor complex** (orange). **(b)** *Microdamage* causes osteocyte apoptosis with direct osteoclast-generating effects via receptor activator of nuclear factor kappa B ligand (RANKL), and loss of the inhibitory effect of SOST on later bone formation (dashed line, SOST–). The osteoblastic lining cells retract from an area of bone, forming a bone remodelling unit, while increased expression of RANKL and reduced osteoprotegerin (OPG) activates the formation of bone-resorbing multinucleate osteoclasts from circulating precursors; the resorbed area is then replaced by new osteoid, formed by cuboidal osteoblasts. As new osteocytes are formed, SOST levels rise and the osteoblasts cease formation, the majority undergoing apoptosis. **(c)** If bone experiences *loading without damage*, *sclerostin expression* is reduced (SOST–), increasing signal response to *wnt*, activation of osteoblast bone formation, and increased OPG expression.

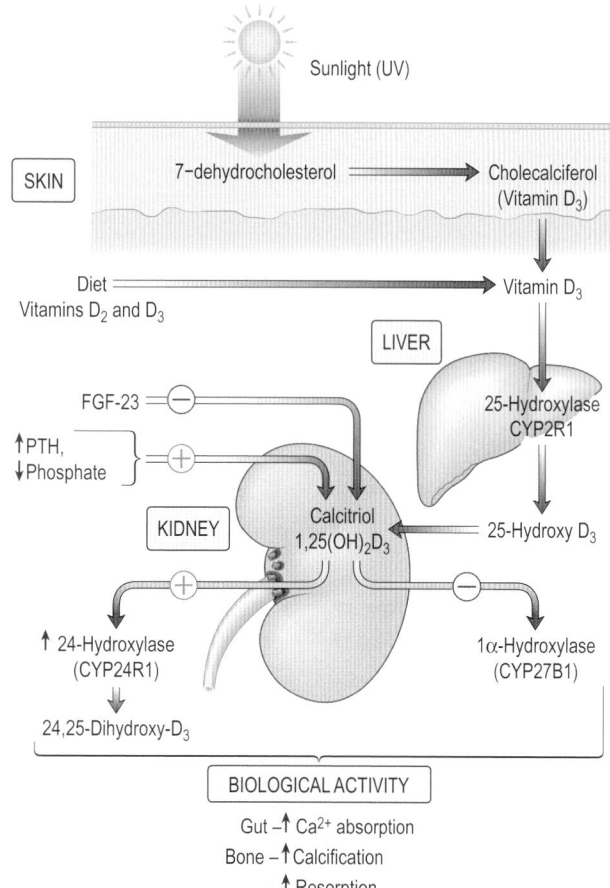

Fig. 19.4 The metabolism and actions of vitamin D. The biologically active agent is 1,25-dihydroxycholecalciferol (calcitriol). It inhibits 1α-hydroxylase and stimulates 24-hydroxylase to produce 24,25-dihydroxy-D_3, which is not biologically active. CYP, cytochrome P enzyme; FGF23, fibroblast growth factor 23 secreted mainly by osteocytes (see p. 192).

INVESTIGATION OF BONE AND CALCIUM DISORDERS

See **Box 19.1**.

Total plasma calcium

Normal range is 2.2–2.6 mmol/L. About 40% of circulating calcium is ionized and physiologically active; the remainder is complexed or protein-bound. As ionized calcium is difficult to measure, normal practice is to measure total calcium, correcting the value to allow for protein binding according to the following formula: add or subtract 0.02 mmol/L for each g/L of a simultaneous albumin level below or above 40 g/L. For critical measurements, samples should be taken in the fasting state and without a tourniquet (the latter may increase local plasma calcium concentration).

Plasma phosphate

Normal range is 0.8–1.4 mmol/L. Phosphate is essential to most biological systems. High levels are found in chronic kidney disease (CKD) and hypoparathyroidism, while low levels are associated with primary hyperparathyroidism, hypophosphataemic rickets and

osteomalacia, and other disorders associated with reduced renal tubular phosphate reabsorption.

Plasma PTH

Normal range is 10–65 ng/L (1.3–7.6 pmol/L). The PTH assay measures the intact hormone. In hypercalcaemia not due to hyperparathyroidism, serum PTH levels are suppressed. Lithium toxicity may be associated with raised PTH levels; in familial hypocalciuric hypercalcaemia (FHH), serum PTH may be normal or marginally elevated.

Serum 25-hydroxyvitamin D

Vitamin D status is best assessed using serum 25-hydroxyvitamin D_3, as 1,25-dihydroxyvitamin D_3 has a short half-life and does not accurately reflect true vitamin D status. ***Vitamin D deficiency*** is defined as <25 nmol/L (10 ng/mL) and ***vitamin D insufficiency*** as less than 75 nmol/L (30 ng/mL). Rickets and osteomalacia occur with prolonged vitamin D deficiency.

The significance of vitamin D insufficiency is uncertain but it has been linked to a wide range of conditions, including ischaemic heart disease, multiple sclerosis and a variety of cancers. Recent evidence suggests that racial differences are present in the assessment of vitamin D status. Black Americans have consistently lower levels of 25-hydroxyvitamin D_3 than white Americans but also lower levels of ***vitamin D-binding protein***, resulting in equivalent bio-available 25-hydroxyvitamin D_3.

24-hour urinary calcium

Normal range 2.5–7.5 mmol/24 h (100–300 mg/24 h). This is increased where renal tubular reabsorption of calcium is decreased, and in hypercalcaemia. One exception is FHH, where the genetic defect leads to inappropriately reduced calcium excretion. Measurement of 24-hour urinary calcium excretion should be performed in the assessment of hypercalcaemic patients.

Biochemical markers of bone formation and resorption

The clinical use of these biochemical markers is limited by large biovariability and measurement variance. Serial measurements at the same time of day in individual patients are useful in assessing response to treatment of metabolic bone diseases.

* ***Bone-specific alkaline phosphatase.*** Circulating alkaline phosphatase is derived from bone, liver, neutrophils and placenta. The bone-specific isoenzyme can be measured as a marker of formation, although there is some overlap with the liver isoenzyme. Elevated serum levels occur during bone growth: for example, in adolescents, fracture repair and high-bone-turnover states.
* ***Type 1 collagen pro-peptides.*** These are by-products of collagen synthesis. Serum levels of both the carboxyterminal (P1CP) and aminoterminal (P1NP) pro-peptides reflect bone formation.
* ***Serum osteocalcin.*** This is another bone formation marker.
* ***Serum or urine levels of N-terminal (NTX) and C-terminal (CTX) cross-linked telopeptides.*** These reflect bone resorption. They may change rapidly in response to anti-resorptive drugs or in disease states, and have been used to assess fracture risk.

Diagnostic imaging

* ***Plain radiographs.*** These identify fractures, tumours and infections. Other specific features may be seen (see following sections).
* ***Radionucleotide imaging.*** The uptake of a [99m]technetium-labelled bisphosphonate in bone reflects bone turnover and blood flow. Increased uptake is therefore seen in fractures, tu-

mour and metastatic deposits, infection and Paget's disease of bone.

- **Magnetic resonance imaging (MRI).** This is the most sensitive and specific test for the diagnosis of osteomyelitis. It is also useful in the detection of stress fractures, which may not be demonstrated on plain radiographs. A technique to suppress the high signal associated with bone marrow (such as STIR sequences; see p. 417) allows highly sensitive recognition of 'bone marrow oedema', a non-specific feature of a number of bone disorders, including osteonecrosis.
- **Bone biopsy (Fig. 19.5).** A core of bone is removed, including both cortices of the iliac crest, using a trephine. The non-decalcified specimen is examined for static and dynamic (bone turnover) indices. An oral tetracycline is given to the patient prior to the biopsy, for 2 days on two occasions 10 days apart, allowing assessment of the rate of bone turnover and mineralization. Biopsy is rarely performed but is useful in the assessment of renal bone disease and osteomalacia.
- **Bone densitometry measurements** (see p. 478).

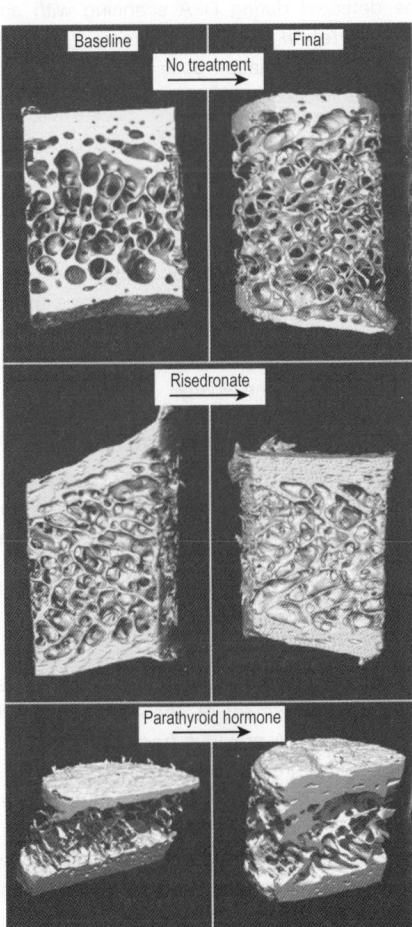

Fig. 19.5 Computerized images of bone biopsies in osteoporosis. These images demonstrate changes in bone architecture over time. **Upper pair**: Without treatment, the bone cortex becomes thinner and numerous trabecular rods and plates are lost. **Centre pair**: In response to bisphosphonate treatment, resorption is reduced, with preservation of bone mineral and structure. **Lower pair**: In response to anabolic therapy, bone is increased at both trabecular and cortical sites. *(From Jiang Y, Zhao JJ, Mitlak BH et al. Recombinant human parathyroid hormone (1–34) improves both cortical and cancellous bone structure.* J Bone Miner Res *2003; 18:1932–1941, with permission of the American Society for Bone and Mineral Research.)*

OSTEOPOROSIS

Osteoporosis is defined as 'a disease characterized by low bone mass and micro-architectural deterioration of bone tissue, leading to enhanced bone fragility and an increase in fracture risk'.

Using bone densitometry at the hip or spine measured by dual X-ray absorptiometry (DXA), the World Health Organization (WHO) also defines osteoporosis as a bone density of 2.5 standard deviations (SDs) below the young healthy adult mean value (T-score ≤−2.5) or lower. Values between −1 and −2.5 SDs below the young adult mean are termed 'osteopenia'. The rationale for this definition is the inverse relationship between bone mineral density (BMD) and fracture risk in postmenopausal women and older men. However, this definition should not be applied to younger populations.

Fractures due to osteoporosis are a major cause of morbidity and mortality in elderly populations, with osteoporotic fractures of the spine causing acute pain or deformity and postural back pain. One in two women and one in five men aged 50 years will have an osteoporotic fracture during their remaining lifetime. As the risk of fracture increases with age, changing population demographics will increase the burden of disease.

Pathogenesis

Osteoporosis results from increased bone breakdown by osteoclasts and decreased bone formation by osteoblasts, leading to loss of bone mass.

Bone mass decreases with age (**Fig. 19.6**) but will depend on the 'peak' mass attained in adult life and on the rate of loss in later life. Genetic factors are the single most significant influence on peak bone mass. Multiple genes are involved, including collagen type 1A1, vitamin D receptor and oestrogen-receptor genes. Nutritional factors, sex hormone status and physical activity also affect peak mass. Not all causes of osteoporosis affect bone remodelling and architecture in the same way.

Oestrogen deficiency results in increased numbers of remodelling units, premature arrest of osteoblastic synthetic activity and perforation of trabeculae, with a loss of resistance to fracture that is not fully reflected in the bone density measurement.

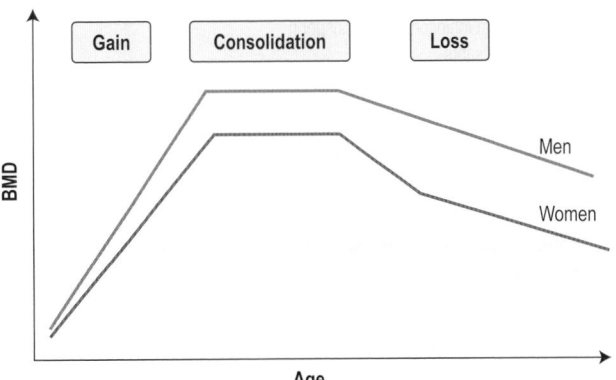

Fig. 19.6 Lifetime changes in bone mineral density (BMD). Peak bone mass is achieved between 20 and 30 years of age, and consolidated up to around the age of 40 years. Then, age-related bone loss occurs in both men and women, with an accelerated loss in women starting around the time of menopause, which lasts between 5 and 10 years.

Glucocorticoids induce a high-turnover state initially, with increased fracture risk evident within 3 months of starting therapy. More prolonged use leads to a reduced-turnover state but with a net loss due to reduced synthesis (through inhibition of the *wnt*-LRP5/6 axis).

Ageing results in increased turnover at the bone/vascular interface within cortical bone, resulting in structural weakness (trabecularization of cortical bone).

Risk factors

Risk factors for fracture may exert their effect through reducing BMD, or they may increase risk over that attributable to BMD (BMD-independent) (**Box 19.4**). Oestrogen deficiency is a major factor in the pathogenesis of accelerated bone loss due to a normal or premature menopause, or amenorrhoea in patients with anorexia nervosa and in athletes. In the elderly, vitamin D insufficiency and consequent hyperparathyroidism reduce BMD. However, previous fracture, increasing age, glucocorticoid therapy, smoking and falls increase the risk of fracture at any given BMD. For instance, 10% of women who are 65 years old and have a T-score of –2 at the hip would be expected to sustain a fracture over the next 10 years; if similar women had a Colles' fracture, smoked and had prolonged exposure to steroids, their risk would be closer to 26% in the same period.

 Box 19.4 Risk factors for fragility fractures

Bone mineral density-dependent
- Female sex
- Caucasian/Asian ethnicity
- Gastrointestinal disease
- Hypogonadism
- Immobilization
- Chronic liver disease
- Chronic kidney disease
- Low dietary calcium intake
- Vitamin D insufficiency
- Chronic obstructive pulmonary disease
- Cushing's syndrome
- Hyperthyroidism
- Hyperparathyroidism
- Diabetes mellitus
- Mastocytosis
- Multiple myeloma
- Osteogenesis imperfecta

Drugs
- Heparin
- Calcineurin inhibitors, e.g. ciclosporin
- Anticonvulsants
- Thiazolidinediones
- Aromatase inhibitors
- Anti-androgens
- Gonadotrophin-releasing hormone (GnRH) analogues
- Proton pump inhibitors
- ?Selective serotonin reuptake inhibitors

Bone mineral density-independent
- Increasing age
- Previous fragility fracture
- Family history of hip fracture
- Low body mass index
- Smoking
- Excess alcohol use
- Glucocorticoid therapy
- High bone turnover
- Increased risk of falling
- Rheumatoid arthritis

BMD-dependent risk factors respond to bone-directed treatment. BMD-independent risk factors benefit from additional targeted intervention (e.g. reduction of falls risk – see p. 306).

Clinical features

Fracture is the only cause of symptoms in osteoporosis. ***Vertebral fracture*** is suggested by the sudden onset of severe back pain. However, two in every three vertebral fractures are asymptomatic. Pain from mechanical derangement, increasing kyphosis, height loss and abdominal protuberance may follow vertebral fracture. ***Colles' fractures*** typically follow a fall on an outstretched arm. ***Fractures of the proximal femur*** usually occur in older individuals falling on their side or back.

Other causes of low-trauma fractures must not be overlooked, including metastatic disease and myeloma.

Investigations

Plain X-rays (**Fig. 19.7**) may show fractures including previously asymptomatic vertebral fractures. Such clinically silent fractures may also be detected during DXA scanning with an additional analysis (called ***vertebral fracture assessment***, **Box 19.5**) carried out with a much lower radiation dose than conventional imaging. Increased bone radiolucency suggests low BMD but requires confirmation with DXA.

Bone density

DXA measures areal bone density (mineral per surface area rather than a true volumetric density), usually of the lumbar spine and proximal femur. It is precise and accurate, uses low doses of radiation and is the 'gold standard' in diagnosis of osteoporosis (**Fig. 19.8**). Because of osteophytes, spinal deformity and vertebral fractures, spinal values may be artefactually elevated and should be interpreted with caution in the elderly.

Associated disease and risk factors

Investigations to exclude other diseases or identify contributory factors associated with osteoporosis should be performed and are particularly necessary in men, in whom secondary causes are more common (see **Box 19.4**).

Selection of individuals for treatment: risk assessment

The goal of osteoporosis treatment is to reduce fracture risk (**Box 19.6**). Thus, assessment of absolute fracture risk should be made in every case. A previous fracture is the strongest risk factor for further fractures. DXA is useful in guiding treatment decisions (**Box 19.7; Fig. 19.8**). Patients with a previous fragility fracture or a BMD T-score less than or equal to –2.5 should be considered for treatment. It is vital to recognize, however, that the majority of fragility fractures occur in women with a T-score better than –2.5 (**Fig. 19.9**). In these patients an assessment for future fracture risk should be made; this can be performed using clinical judgement by an experienced physician or using formal risk calculators, for example FRAX (**Box 19.8**). The threshold for recommending treatment in this setting will be determined by the cost-effectiveness of treatment in a particular healthcare setting and by clinical judgement. For example, in the USA, the National Osteoporosis Foundation recommends treatment if the 10-year probability of hip fracture is more than or equal to 3% or if major osteoporotic fracture is more than or equal to 20%.

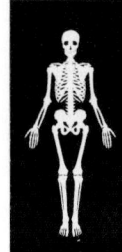

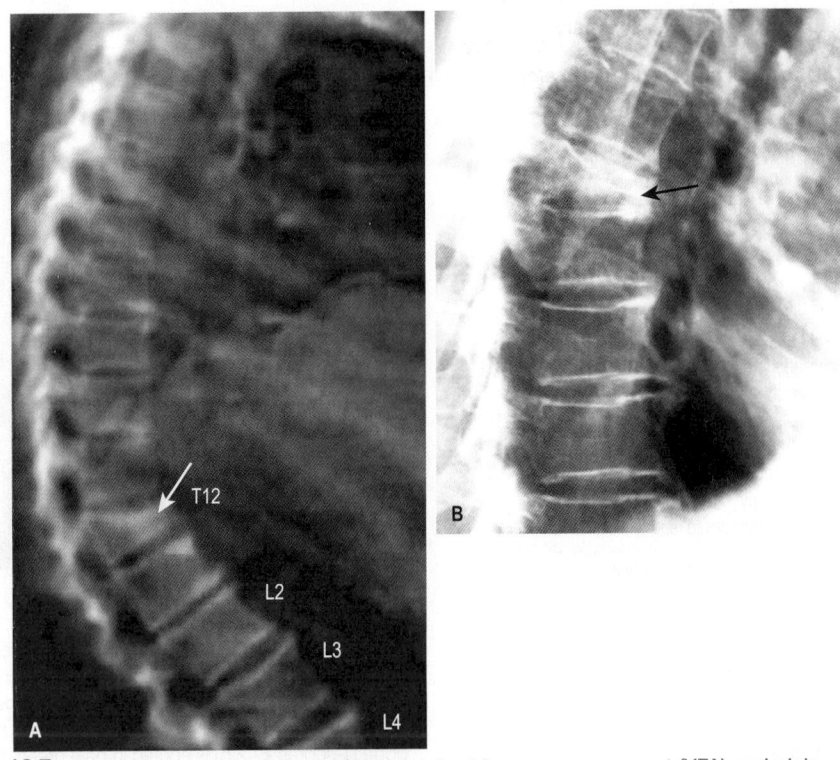

Fig. 19.7 Vertebral fracture as seen on DXA vertebral fracture assessment (VFA) and plain radiograph. **(A)** The VFA image shows a vertebra with reduced height at T12 (arrow). **(B)** The radiograph shows a typical wedge compression fracture.

| _i_ | **Box 19.5** Vertebral fracture assessment (VFA) |

- Radiographic image of lateral spine generated using DXA
- Lower radiation than formal X-ray
- Can be done at same time as DXA
- Used to identify previously unsuspected vertebral fractures
- If vertebral fragility fracture identified, treatment for osteoporosis indicated irrespective of T-score

DXA, dual-energy X-ray absorptiometry.

Prevention and management

- **_Symptomatic management._** New vertebral fractures may require bed rest for 1–2 weeks with strong analgesia and gradual physiotherapy to restore confident mobilization (see p. 424). Non-spinal fractures should be treated by conventional orthopaedic means. In fractured neck of femur, early surgical intervention, and early mobilization post-surgery, are associated with improved outcomes.
- **_Calcium and vitamin D._** Daily intakes of 800–1200 mg of calcium and 400–800 IU of vitamin D are recommended throughout life for optimum bone health. Dietary intake of calcium, and vitamin D from sunshine and diet, are preferable. For those not meeting calcium intake targets, or those with low serum 25-hydroxyvitamin D_3 levels, supplements are recommended (**Box 19.9**).
- **_Lifestyle measures._** Weight-bearing exercise for 30 minutes three times a week may increase BMD, while gentle exercise in the elderly may reduce the risk of falls and improve the protective responses to falling (see p. 306). Smoking and excess alcohol use should be avoided.

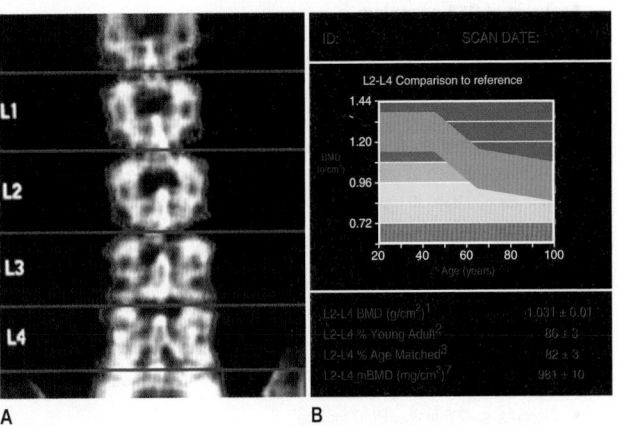

Fig. 19.8 Dual-energy X-ray absorptiometry (DXA) of the lumbar spine. **(A)** Anteroposterior image of the lumbar spine. **(B)** The patient's value is expressed in relation to the reference range.

- **_Reduction of falls._** Physiotherapy and assessment of home safety are helpful. Hip protectors do reduce fractures in the elderly in residential care when worn correctly, but compliance is poor.

Pharmacological intervention

Most interventions (see **Fig. 19.5**) act by inhibiting bone resorption (anti-resorptives), the exception being PTH peptides, which stimulate bone formation. The impression from bone turnover markers that strontium ranelate may have both anti-resorptive and stimulatory effects remains poorly understood.

The evidence base for the **_anti-fracture efficacy_** of interventions varies. Treatments with proven efficacy at all major fracture

Treatment is guided by risk of fracture, not BMD alone.
Fracture risk assessment should be performed, either using clinical judgement or a formal risk assessment calculator (e.g. http://www.shef.ac.uk/FRAX and many others; see **Box 19.8**).

Do not under-estimate the risk from steroids or previous fracture.

Oral bisphosphonates (alendronate, risedronate) are first-line treatment in many cases. Other options include:

- ***denosumab***:
  - difficulty taking bisphosphonate
  - poor adherence to treatment
  - falling BMD on bisphosphonate
  - new fracture on a bisphosphonate
  - after 5–10 years on bisphosphonate
- ***teriparatide*** if there are multiple vertebral fractures or very low BMD
- ***i.v. zoledronate*** after hip fracture.

BMD monitoring is recommended in:
- all treated patients to monitor therapy
- all untreated cases if a BMD reduction would lead to treatment.

BMD, bone mineral density; DXA, dual-energy X-ray absorptiometry.

Indications for DXA scanning
- Women aged ≥65
- Men aged ≥70
- Fragility fracture
- Women <65 with risk factors (see **Box 19.4**)
- Men <70 with risk factors (see **Box 19.4**)
- Monitoring of BMD in those on treatment

Features of DXA scanning
- Low-dose radiation X-ray
- Measures a real BMD
- Gives BMD in g/cm^2, which is difficult to interpret so translated to T or Z score
- T-score generated by comparing result with female, white, aged 20–29 years taken from the NHANES III study database.
- Z score generated by comparing result with person of same age and ethnicity and used to report to report BMD in pre-menopausal women and men aged <50

Interpretation of DXA
BMD measured at lumbar spine, total hip, femoral next (± radius)
In postmenopausal women and men aged ≥50:
- T-score ≤−2.5 = osteoporosis
- T-score ≤−1.0 to <−2.5 = osteopenia/low BMD
- T-score >−1.0 = normal BMD
- Z scores ≤−2.0 is 'low BMD for age'
  Interpretation of Z scores is complex and beyond the scope of this text

BMD, bone mineral density; DXA, dual-energy X-ray absorptiometry.

sites (particularly spine and hip) are preferable (**Box 19.10**). Hence, the bisphosphonates and denosumab are generally regarded as first-line options in the majority of postmenopausal women with osteoporosis.

Bisphosphonates

As synthetic analogues of bone pyrophosphate, bisphosphonates adhere to hydroxyapatite and inhibit osteoclasts. Alendronate and risedronate are given as once-weekly doses, zoledronate as a once-yearly infusion, and ibandronate usually as a once-monthly oral therapy (a 3-monthly intravenous injection is rarely used).

Oral bisphosphonates should be taken fasting, with a large drink of water, while standing or sitting upright. The patient should then remain upright and avoid food and drink for at least 30 minutes.

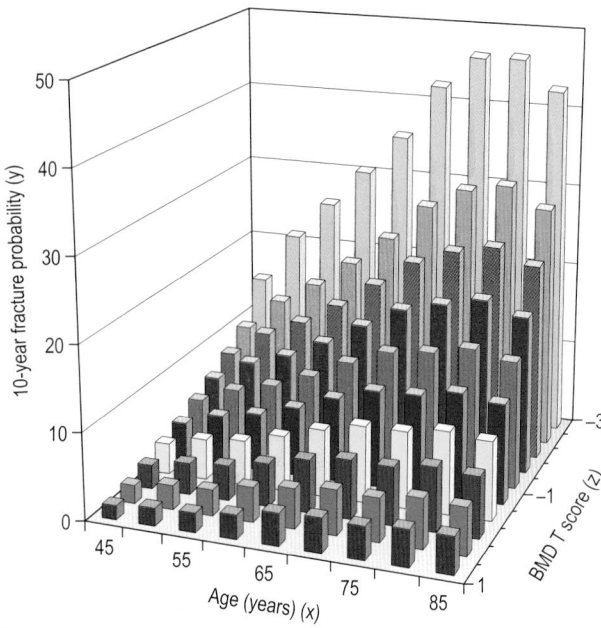

Fig. 19.9 Graph illustrating the combined effects of age (x-axis) and reduced bone mass (expressed as T-scores on the z-axis) on the 10-year probability of fracture (y-axis) in a population of women. Reduced bone mass osteopenia, T-scores between −1 and −2.5. Osteoporotic bone (T-scores <−2.5) is shown in pale green. Note that the risk of fracture may be greater in an older woman with osteopenia than in a young woman with osteoporosis. *(Data from Kanis JA. Diagnosis of osteoporosis and assessment of fracture risk. Lancet 359:1929–1936.)*

Fracture risk assessment:
- Should be performed in all patients
- Can be performed clinically or using risk assessment calculators.
FRAX is one of a number of fracture risk assessment tools available:
- Treatment is generally indicated if a 10-year major fracture risk ≥20% or hip fracture risk ≥ 3%
- These tools enable quantification of fracture risk and guide treatment decisions
- They provide estimates of fracture risk based on a set number of variables
- In certain situations they will not accurately estimate fracture risk so must be used in combination with clinical judgement

Treatment phase
- Vitamin D 50 000 iu weekly PO × 6–8 weeks **or** vitamin D 30 000 iu IM × 2 doses

Maintenance phase
- Vitamin D 800–1000 iu daily PO × lifelong

Bisphosphonates are generally well tolerated but may be associated with upper gastrointestinal side-effects such as oesophagitis, particularly if the dosing instructions are not closely followed. Bisphosphonates should be used with careful monitoring in patients who have chronic kidney disease (stage 4 or 5). Osteonecrosis of the jaw is a rare complication of high-dose intravenous bisphosphonates in patients who have malignant disease. It is associated with poor dental hygiene. As prolonged suppression of bone turnover is linked with atypical femoral fractures, it is currently advised to reassess bisphosphonate

i **Box 19.10** Evidence for fracture risk reduction of current treatment options at specific sites in postmenopausal women

Intervention	Vertebral fracture	Non-vertebral fracture	Hip fracture
Alendronate	+	+	+
Risedronate	+	+	+
Ibandronate	+	+[a]	ND
Zoledronate	+	+	+
Bazedoxifene	+	ND	ND
Raloxifene	+	ND	ND
Strontium ranelate	+	+	+[a]
Denosumab	+	+	+[a]
Teriparatide	+	+	ND

[a]Demonstrated only in high-risk subgroup. ND, not demonstrated.

treatment after 5 years. Only those with vertebral fractures and a T-score at the neck of femur below −2.5 at this 5-year scan appear to have a reduced risk of fracture with continued treatment.

Denosumab

Denosumab is a fully human monoclonal antibody to RANKL administered as a single subcutaneous injection every 6 months. It is an anti-resorptive agent that increases BMD and reduces fractures at the spine, hip and other non-vertebral sites. Fracture risk reduction is equivalent to that of bisphosphonates. Unlike bisphosphonates, the benefit of denosumab is rapidly lost on cessation, therefore if stopped it should be replaced by an alternative agent. Adverse effects are infrequent: most commonly dysuria, rarely cellulitis. Osteonecrosis of the jaw and atypical femoral fractures have also been reported

Strontium ranelate

This is rarely used due to concerns over cardiovascular and thromboembolic adverse events. It has weak anti-resorptive activity whilst maintaining bone formation. It reduces the risk of vertebral fractures in postmenopausal women with osteoporosis, and the risk of hip and other non-vertebral fractures in high-risk subgroups (women with previous fracture and T-scores at the hip of −2.4 or less).

Selective oestrogen-receptor modulators

Selective oestrogen-receptor modulators (SERMs) include raloxifene and bazedoxifene. They are rarely used to treat osteoporosis. They have no stimulatory effect on the endometrium but activate oestrogen receptors in bone. Both prevent BMD loss at the spine and hip in postmenopausal women but have been found to reduce only vertebral fracture rates. Leg cramps and flushing may occur, and the risk of thromboembolic complications is also increased to a degree similar to that seen with hormone replacement therapy (HRT; see p. 1468 and **Box 39.3**). The use of SERMs is associated with a small increase in the risk of stroke.

Recombinant human parathyroid hormone

Recombinant human PTH peptide 1–34 (teriparatide) and recombinant human PTH 1–84 are anabolic agents that stimulate bone formation. Teriparatide reduces vertebral and non-vertebral fractures in postmenopausal women with established osteoporosis, although data on hip fracture are not available. It is given by daily subcutaneous injection for 24 months. Recombinant human PTH 1–84 is also administered by once-daily subcutaneous injection but has been shown to reduce only vertebral fractures. An anti-resorptive drug should be given on completion of PTH peptide therapy to maintain the increase in BMD. Non-osteoporotic bone diseases, such as osteomalacia, should be excluded prior to treatment. PTH peptide therapy is difficult for patients to take and associated with more adverse events than other agents and therefore is mainly indicated in severe cases of vertebral osteoporosis or in those who fail to respond to other therapies. Teriparatide may cause mild transient hypercalcaemia but routine monitoring is not required. Nausea and headache may occur. Recombinant human PTH 1–84 is associated with a higher incidence of hypercalcaemia and hypercalciuria, and routine monitoring is advised. Neither agent should be used in people with skeletal metastases or osteosarcoma.

Hormone replacement therapy

Because of its adverse effects on breast cancer and cardiovascular disease risk, HRT is not indicated for osteoporosis except in early postmenopausal women who also have significant perimenopausal symptoms.

Calcitriol (1,25-dihydroxyvitamin D$_3$) and calcitonin

These may reduce vertebral fracture rate, although the data are inconsistent.

Combination therapies

Combination therapies, either with two anti-resorptive agents, or an anti-resorptive and an anabolic agent, often produce larger increases in BMD than monotherapy but have not been shown to result in greater fracture reduction.

Surgery

This is very rarely indicated in osteoporotic vertebral fractures. Percutaneous vertebroplasty and balloon kyphoplasty are discussed on page 424. Hip fractures are dealt with by hip replacements or stabilization with pins.

Treatment of specific conditions
Glucocorticoid-induced osteoporosis

Individuals requiring continuous oral glucocorticoid therapy for 3 months or more (at any dose) should be assessed for coexisting risk factors (age, previous fracture, hormone status). Postmenopausal women, men aged over 50 years and any individuals who have sustained a fragility fracture should receive treatment without waiting for DXA scanning. DXA results and fracture risk assessment guide treatment for other patients (see **Boxes 19.5, 19.7** and **19.8**). Bisphosphonates, denosumab and teriparatide are approved in this setting.

Osteoporosis in men

Alendronate, risedronate, denosumab and teriparatide are approved for use in men. In men with osteoporosis who have clinical and biochemical evidence of hypogonadism, testosterone replacement is also used.

Further reading

Coughlan T, Dockery F. Osteoporosis and fracture risk in older people. *Clin Med* 2014; 14:187–191.
Cummings SR, Martin J, McClung MR et al. Denosumab for prevention of fractures in postmenopausal women with osteoporosis. *N Engl J Med* 2009; 361:756–757.

Favus MJ. Bisphosphonates for osteoporosis. *N Engl J Med* 2010; 363:2027–2035.

Gourley ML, Fine JP, Preisser JS et al. Bone-density testing interval and transition to osteoporosis in older women. *N Engl J Med* 2012; 366:225–233.

Rachner TD, Khosla S, Hofbauer LC. Osteoporosis: now and the future. *Lancet* 2011; 377:1276–1287.

Weinstein RS. Glucocorticoid-induced bone disease. *N Engl J Med* 2011; 365:62–70.

http://www.nof.org/ *National Osteoporosis Foundation clinical guidelines.*

http://www.shef.ac.uk/FRAX *FRAX tool for 10-year probability of hip fracture and 10-year probability of major osteoporotic fracture.*

OSTEONECROSIS

This is also known as aseptic, avascular or ischaemic necrosis of bone. Over 80% of cases are attributed to glucocorticoid treatment or alcohol excess. Less frequent causes include sickle cell disease, systemic lupus erythematosus (SLE), deep-sea diving (Caisson's disease), endocrine disorders (e.g. Cushing's, diabetes mellitus), trauma, human immunodeficiency virus (HIV) infection and irradiation.

Osteonecrosis usually presents with joint pain, the shoulder or hip being most commonly affected, but can be asymptomatic, particularly on the opposite side in the same person. It may only be recognized when it results in collapse of the articular bone.

MRI best confirms the diagnosis by showing bone marrow oedema. If advanced, it can be seen on plain X-rays.

Management is mainly symptomatic. Surgical options include drilling through the bone cortex (decompression), vascularized bone grafts, or rotation of the affected bone away from the load-bearing area; however, joint replacement is often required. Bisphosphonates may reduce pain, and progression has been reduced with statin therapy in steroid-associated osteonecrosis.

PAGET'S DISEASE OF BONE

Paget's disease of bone is a focal disorder of bone remodelling. Increased osteoclastic bone resorption is followed by a compensatory increase in new bone formation, increased local bone blood flow and fibrous tissue in adjacent bone marrow. Ultimately, formation exceeds resorption but the new woven bone is weaker than normal bone, which leads to deformity and increased fracture risk. Paget's disease does not spread but can become symptomatic at previously silent sites.

Epidemiological studies are difficult because most affected individuals are asymptomatic. Paget's disease is most often seen in Europe and particularly in northern England. It affects men and women (2:3) over the age of 40 years. The incidence approximately doubles per decade thereafter, with up to 10% of individuals radiologically affected by the age of 90. For unknown reasons, the incidence and severity of Paget's disease have decreased in recent years.

Aetiology and pathogenesis

Genetic factors are implicated in Paget's disease. A positive family history is noted in about 15%. Mutations in *SQSTM1*, which encodes the osteoclast mediator protein p62, have been reported in up to 10% of cases. Intracellular inclusions in the osteoclasts in pagetic lesions are believed to be paramyxovirus nucleocapsid (e.g. canine distemper virus, measles or respiratory syncytial virus). However, similar inclusions are seen in other bone disorders, and theories of a viral aetiology in Paget's remain contentious. Altered expression of *c-fos* (an oncogene) is one suggested mechanism linking viral infection with the pathogenic changes in osteoclasts, which are more numerous and contain an increased number of nuclei (up to 100).

Clinical features

Clinical features are summarized in **Fig. 19.10A**. Between 60% and 80% of people with radiologically identified Paget's disease are asymptomatic. Diagnosis often follows the finding of an asymptomatic elevation of serum alkaline phosphatase, or a plain X-ray performed for other indications. The disease may involve one bone (monostotic, in 15%) or many (polyostotic). The most common sites, in order of frequency, are pelvis, femur, lumbar spine, skull and tibia (see **Fig. 19.10C**). Small bones of the feet and hands are rarely involved.

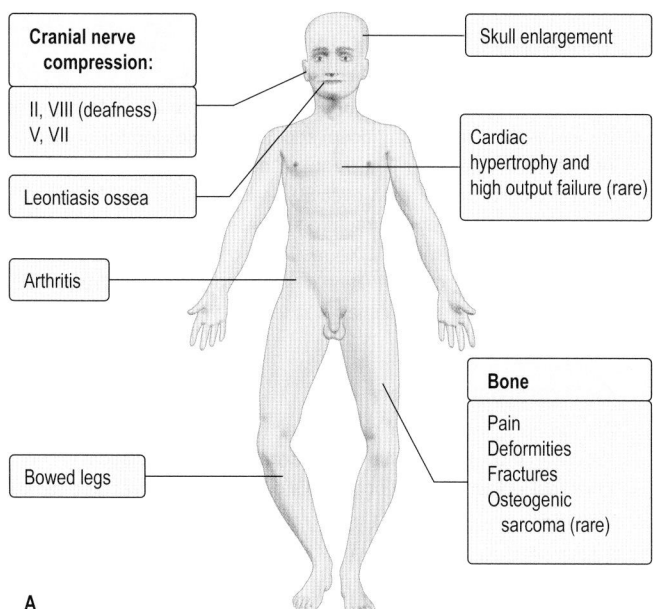

Cranial nerve compression:
II, VIII (deafness)
V, VII

Leontiasis ossea

Arthritis

Bowed legs

Skull enlargement

Cardiac hypertrophy and high output failure (rare)

Bone
Pain
Deformities
Fractures
Osteogenic sarcoma (rare)

A

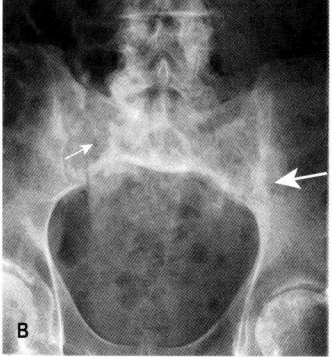

B

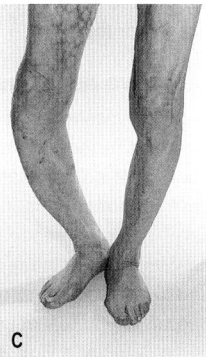

C

Fig. 19.10 Paget's disease. (A) Clinical features. **(B)** X-ray appearance of the pelvis, showing osteolytic (thin arrow) and osteosclerotic (thick arrow) lesions. **(C)** Legs showing bowing of the tibia caused by increased bone growth. Note the erythema ab igne on the medial aspect of the thigh.

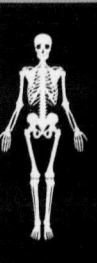

Symptoms and complications include:
- bone pain
- joint pain when an involved bone is close to a joint, leading to cartilage damage and osteoarthritis
- deformities, in particular bowed tibia and skull changes
- neurological complications – nerve compression (deafness from VIIIth cranial nerve involvement; cranial nerves II, V and VII may also be involved); spinal stenosis; hydrocephalus due to blockage of the aqueduct of Sylvius
- high-output cardiac failure and myocardial hypertrophy due to increased bone blood flow (rarely seen with modern management)
- hypercalcaemia – rarely seen outside the setting of fracture
- pathological fractures
- osteosarcoma – occurs in fewer than 1% of cases of Paget's and may be heralded by an increase in bone pain or swelling in a previous pagetic bone area.

Investigations

- **Increased serum alkaline phosphatase** with normal serum calcium and phosphate reflects increased bone turnover. Levels may be normal with limited or monostotic Paget's disease. Levels are reduced with treatment and increased during relapse.
- **Vitamin D** should be measured, as deficiency is frequent in the age group affected by Paget's disease and should be corrected (see **Box 19.9**) to avoid hypocalcaemia following bisphosphonate treatment.
- **X-ray** features (see **Fig. 19.10B**) vary from predominantly lytic lesions (osteoporosis circumscripta in the skull is characteristic), through a mixed phase, to a mainly sclerotic phase of bone expansion, cortical thickening and coarsening of the trabecular pattern.
- **Isotope bone scans** are useful to determine the extent of skeletal involvement but are unable to distinguish between Paget's disease and sclerotic metastatic carcinoma (especially breast and prostate).

Management

Bisphosphonates are the mainstay of treatment. New bone formed after treatment is lamellar, not woven (reflecting normalization of bone turnover rather than a direct effect on osteoblasts). Repeat treatment courses are guided by recurrence of symptoms and by rising alkaline phosphatase. In addition to treatment of symptomatic patients, treatment of asymptomatic lesions is appropriate if there is a significant risk of potential complications, such as fracture in weight-bearing long bones or the spine, nerve entrapment or deafness with skull involvement, and before orthopaedic procedures in involved bone (to reduce vascularity).

Intravenous bisphosphonates

Zoledronate is the most commonly used agent for Paget's disease, administered as a single infusion over 15 minutes. **Pamidronate** is an alternative but takes longer to infuse and is less potent; some patients develop drug resistance for unknown reasons. Both drugs can be associated with a first-dose reaction characterized by 'flu-like' symptoms, including transient pyrexia over 24–48 hours, which can be ameliorated with paracetamol.

Oral bisphosphonates

Oral bisphosphonates are used at doses higher than those for osteoporosis (e.g. 30 mg risedronate daily for 2 months, or 40 mg

alendronate daily for 6 months) and are less effective than intravenous zoledronic acid.

Surgery

Joint replacement or osteotomy is sometimes necessary to correct deformity or pain due to associated degenerative joint disease. Neurosurgery may be needed where there is spinal disease. Osteosarcoma usually requires amputation, though wide excision and limb salvage can be successful at distal sites.

Further reading

Ralston SH. Paget's disease of bone. *N Engl J Med* 2013; 368:644–650.

RICKETS AND OSTEOMALACIA

Osteomalacia is defective mineralization of newly formed bone matrix or osteoid. Rickets is defective mineralization at the epiphyseal growth plate and is found in association with osteomalacia in children.

Aetiology

Many factors can result in defective mineralization of the osteoid. For normal mineralization, adequate levels of vitamin D, calcium and phosphate, adequate activity of alkaline phosphatase, a normal pH at the osteoid surface and normal osteoid composition are all necessary (**Box 19.11**).

The most common cause of osteomalacia is hypophosphataemia due to hyperparathyroidism secondary to vitamin D deficiency. The most common cause of vitamin D deficiency worldwide is dietary deficiency. Bread, milk and cereals in high-income countries are now fortified with vitamin D. This has led to a much-reduced incidence of osteomalacia and rickets.

Vitamin D is produced in the skin through the action of sunlight on 7-dehydrocholesterol (see **Fig. 19.4**). Lack of sun exposure can lead to vitamin D deficiency, especially in individuals living in temperate regions who keep large parts of the skin covered throughout the year.

? Box 19.11 Causes of rickets/osteomalacia

Deficient intake or absorption of vitamin D
- Inadequate sun exposure or deficient synthesis in skin
- Low dietary intake
- Malabsorption: coeliac disease, Crohn's disease, gastrectomy, bariatric surgery, primary biliary cirrhosis

Defective 1α-hydroxylation
- Chronic kidney disease
- Vitamin D-dependent rickets type I – due to deficiency of 1α-hydroxylase

Primary renal phosphate wasting
- Renal tubular acidosis (also by causing metabolic acidosis)
- Hereditary hypophosphataemic rickets (vitamin D-resistant rickets)
- Dent's disease
- Fanconi's syndrome
- Multiple myeloma
- Tumour-induced osteomalacia

Inhibitors of mineralization
- Fluoride, aluminium, bisphosphonates
- Metabolic acidosis

Defective vitamin D receptors
- Hereditary vitamin D-resistant rickets (previously known as vitamin D-dependent rickets type II)

Vitamin D is a fat-soluble vitamin, so gastrointestinal disease can result in malabsorption. Gastrectomy, various forms of bariatric surgery, cystic fibrosis, coeliac disease, Crohn's disease and primary biliary cirrhosis are well-recognized causes.

Due to the intimate involvement of the kidney in phosphate balance, a number of causes of osteomalacia are mediated by the kidney (see p. 1394). Primary renal phosphate wasting occurs in tumour-induced osteomalacia, multiple myeloma and Fanconi's syndrome. Proximal (type 2) renal tubular acidosis can cause osteomalacia due to both renal phosphate wasting and abnormal osteoid pH secondary to metabolic acidosis.

Clinical features

Osteomalacia may be asymptomatic and identified incidentally on routine investigations following a fragility fracture. When symptomatic, it characteristically causes muscle weakness and widespread bone pain. Muscle weakness is due to a multifactorial proximal myopathy, with low vitamin D, hypophosphataemia and high PTH levels all contributing. It results in a characteristic waddling gait with difficulty climbing stairs and getting out of a chair. Generalized bone pain and tenderness are thought to be caused by hydration of the demineralized matrix, resulting in periosteal distension. The pain is typically a dull ache that is worse on weight-bearing and walking. It can be reproduced by pressure on the sternum or tibia. Insufficiency fractures can occur when the quality of the bone is insufficient to handle the stress of weight-bearing.

At birth, neonatal rickets may present as craniotabes (a thin, deformed skull). In the first few years of life, there may be widened epiphyses at the wrists and beading at the costochondral junctions, producing the 'rickety rosary', or a groove in the rib cage (Harrison's sulcus). In older children, lower limb deformities are seen. A myopathy may also occur. Hypocalcaemic tetany may occur in severe cases.

Investigations

- **Serum alkaline phosphatase** is elevated in 90% of cases.
- **Low serum calcium**, **low phosphate** and **elevated PTH** are each present in approximately half of the cases.
- **Serum** 25-hydroxyvitamin D_3 is low, usually less than 25 nmol/L (10 ng/mL).
- **Serum FGF-23** is elevated in many people with tumour-induced osteomalacia and in hypophosphataemic rickets.
- **Plain radiographs** demonstrate decreased bone mineralization. The characteristic finding in osteomalacia is Looser's pseudofractures. These are narrow radiolucent lines with sclerotic borders running perpendicular to the cortex. They can be found at any site but are most commonly seen in the femur and pelvis.
- **Tetracycline-labelled bone biopsy** is the gold standard diagnostic test. This is not practical in most clinical settings and is used mainly in research studies.

Management

Vitamin D replacement is the cornerstone of treatment. Treatment involves two stages: an initial loading stage to replenish body stores of vitamin D, and a subsequent maintenance phase to avoid repeat deficiency (see **Box 19.9**). All patients should also receive supplementary calcium of 1000–1200 mg/day. In nutritional deficiency, recommended initial replacement is with vitamin D 50 000 units per week orally. The initial replacement dose should be continued for 6–8 weeks. Vitamin D is also available as an intramuscular injection; two doses of 300 000 units are usually enough to replenish body stores. Adequacy of vitamin D replacement should be confirmed by repeat measuring of vitamin D levels. This should be followed by maintenance supplementation with 800–1000 units of vitamin D per day.

Doses for children are lower and are age-dependent. People with gastrointestinal disease and vitamin D deficiency due to malabsorption need higher doses of 10 000–50 000 units per day of vitamin D.

Tumour-induced osteomalacia is best treated by removal of the causative neoplasm, which is usually occult and frequently benign. This leads to rapid resolution of symptoms.

Further reading

Elder CJ, Bishop NJ. Rickets. *Lancet* 2014; 383:1665–1676.
Pearce SH, Cheetham TD. Diagnosis and management of vitamin D deficiency. *BMJ* 2010; 340:b5664.

BONE INFECTIONS

Acute and chronic osteomyelitis

Osteomyelitis is more common in children and arises due to haematogenous spread to the vascular metaphysis. In high-income countries, it occurs in around 8 per 100 000 children per year, but it is more common in low-income countries, with boys affected twice as often as girls. In adults it generally occurs in the setting of other medical conditions, such as type 2 diabetes mellitus and chronic skin ulceration where it infiltrates the bone through direct spreading.

Staphylococcus is the organism responsible for 90% of cases of acute osteomyelitis. Other organisms include *Haemophilus influenzae* and *Salmonella*; infection with the latter may occur as a complication of sickle cell disease. The classic presentation is with fever and localized bone pain with overlying tenderness and erythema.

Diagnosis

- Imaging:
  - Plain X-ray is not sensitive in early infection but demonstrates chronic damage.
  - MRI is highly sensitive in early disease.
  - Nuclear medicine bone scans are also helpful.
- **Blood cultures** may be positive.
- **Bone biopsy and culture** identifies the organism and sensitivities.

Management

Treatment of osteomyelitis is with intravenous antibiotics. Switching to oral antibiotics can be considered after 2 weeks with continuation for a further 4 weeks. Choice of antibiotic is determined by the causative agent and local guidelines. Surgical drainage and removal of dead bone (sequestrum) may be necessary but recurrence is common.

Delayed treatment leads to chronic osteomyelitis. In chronic osteomyelitis, sinus formation is common. Subacute osteomyelitis is associated with a chronic abscess within the bone (Brodie's abscess).

Tuberculous osteomyelitis

This is usually due to haematogenous spread from a reactivated primary focus in the lungs or gastrointestinal tract. The disease starts in intra-articular bone. The spine is commonly involved (***Pott's disease***), with damage to the bodies of two neighbouring vertebrae leading to vertebral collapse and acute angulation of the spine (gibbus). Later, an abscess forms ('cold abscess'). Pus can track along tissue planes

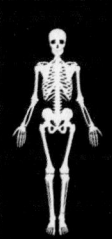

and discharge at a point far from the affected vertebrae. Symptoms consist of local pain and later swelling if pus has collected. Systemic symptoms of malaise, fever and night sweats occur.

Management is as for pulmonary tuberculosis but extended to 9 months (see p. 969), together with initial immobilization.

NEOPLASTIC DISEASE OF BONE

Bone pain may be due to multiple myeloma, lymphoma, a primary tumour of bone or secondary deposits. The pain is typically unremitting and worse at night, and there are other clinical clues such as weight loss or ill-health.

Malignant tumours of bone are shown in **Box 19.12**. The most common tumours are metastases from the bronchus, breast and prostate. Metastases from kidney and thyroid are less common. Primary bone tumours are rare and most commonly seen in children and young adults.

Symptoms are usually related to the anatomical position of the tumour, with local bone pain. Systemic symptoms (e.g. malaise and pyrexia) and aches and pains occur and may be related to hypercalcaemia. The diagnosis of metastases may be evident from the history and examination, particularly in the setting of a known primary tumour. Symptoms from bony metastases may also be the first presenting feature of a malignancy, however.

Investigations

- *Skeletal isotope scans* show bony metastases as 'hot' areas.
- *X-rays* may show metastases as osteolytic areas with bony destruction. Osteosclerotic metastases are characteristic of prostatic carcinoma.
- *MRI* is used particularly for vertebral lesions.
- *CT and computed tomography-positron emission tomography (CT-PET)* are useful.
- *Serum alkaline phosphatase* may be raised.
- *Hypercalcaemia* occurs in 10–20% of patients who have metastatic malignancies, or can be due to ectopic parathormone or PTH-related protein secretion.
- *Prostate-specific antigen* (PSA) and serum acid phosphatase are raised in the presence of prostatic metastases.

Management

Treatment is usually with analgesics and anti-inflammatory drugs. Local radiotherapy to bone metastases relieves pain and reduces

---

> *i* **Box 19.12** Malignant neoplasms of bone
>
> - Metastases (osteolytic):
>   - Lung
>   - Breast
>   - Prostate (often osteosclerotic as well)
>   - Thyroid
>   - Kidney
> - Multiple myeloma
> - Primary bone tumours (rare; seen in the young), e.g.:
>   - Osteosarcomas
>   - Fibrosarcomas
>   - Chondromas
>   - Ewing's tumour

the risk of pathological fracture. Some tumours respond to chemotherapy; others are hormone-dependent and respond to hormonal therapy. Bisphosphonates (see p. 483) can help symptomatically. Occasionally, pathological fractures require internal fixation.

SCHEUERMANN'S DISEASE

This disease predominantly occurs in adolescent boys. The main feature is a progressive dorsal kyphosis of the thoracic spine. Pain may or may not be present. The cause is unknown. A genetic predisposition, exacerbated by excessive exercise prior to epiphyseal fusion, is one suggested explanation. Older patients with kyphosis may be referred with suspected osteoporotic fractures but found to have long-standing kyphosis due to Scheuermann's. Management is focused on postural exercises and avoidance of precipitants. Surgery may be undertaken to correct kyphosis in severe cases.

Bibliography

Rosen CJ, ed. *Primer on the Metabolic Bone Diseases and Disorders of Mineral Metabolism*, 8th edn. Hoboken, New Jersey: Wiley-Blackwell, American Society for Bone and Mineral Research; 2013.

Significant websites

http://nof.org *National Osteoporosis Foundation – useful clinicians' guide.*
http://www.iscd.org *International Society for Clinical Densitometry – guidelines on DXA scanning.*
http://www.nos.org.uk/ *UK National Osteoporosis Society – useful information and reviews of ongoing research.*

Infectious disease

Gavin Barlow, William L. Irving and Peter J. Moss

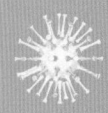

CORE SKILLS AND KNOWLEDGE

Most infections are either self-managed or cared for by community services. Hospital-based infection services manage patients with complicated or severe infections that require expertise from trained infection specialists, in settings that vary from outpatient clinics (for example, those that treat patients with chronic infections such as tuberculosis), to critical care units.

There are two main clinical infection subspecialties, although increasingly the dividing line is blurred. Clinical microbiologists and virologists predominantly provide specialist infectious diseases advice concerning patients in the care of other doctors, and also manage the microbiology laboratory. Infectious disease specialists are often trained as general physicians, and may treat patients directly under their care or provide a 'laboratory liaison service' for doctors working in other teams.

Key skills to master in infectious diseases include:

- taking a comprehensive history from patients in order to draw up a thorough account of their presentation and risk factors
- understanding the geographical distribution of different types of infectious agent and their varied clinical presentations
- being familiar with the role of laboratory-based experts in interpreting complex microbiological investigations.

The best way to learn about infectious diseases is by following patients as the story of their illness unfolds. Assess patients in the clinical environment where they present (often the emergency department), review available and subsequent investigations, and discuss them with the healthcare professionals caring for these individuals. Reflect on whether the initial assessment, investigations and management were appropriate in light of any problems that emerged (e.g. adverse drug reactions or the need to intensify therapy), and review the subsequent processes of care (e.g. de-escalation of antibiotic therapy) and the final infection diagnosis.

CORE CONTENT

Although it is necessary for doctors to be aware of a wide range of infectious diseases, it is easy for students reading chapters on the subject to lose themselves among rare and exotic diagnoses and struggle to prioritize key content. The lists in **Box 20.1** represent an attempt to identify infections, emergencies and pathogens that doctors need not just to know about, but to know well.

 Box 20.1 Key infections, emergencies, pathogens and concepts in infectious diseases

'Top 10' infections
- Respiratory infections, including pneumonia
- Diarrhoeal diseases
- Tuberculosis
- HIV infection
- Hepatitis B and C
- Malaria
- Urinary tract infection
- Skin and soft tissue infections
- Meningitis
- *Staphylococcus aureus* and *Escherichia coli* bacteraemia (see Ch. 8)

'Top 10' infection emergencies
- Sepsis
- Severe community-acquired pneumonia
- The ill returning traveller
- The severely ill HIV-positive patient
- Meningitis and encephalitis
- Endocarditis
- Necrotizing fasciitis
- Native joint septic arthritis
- Infection control for highly pathogenic transmissible diseases (e.g. Ebola, avian influenza, etc., see p. 507)
- Neutropenic sepsis (see p. 116)

'Top 10' pathogens to know about
- *Streptococcus pneumoniae*
- Influenza A virus
- *Mycobacterium tuberculosis*
- HIV
- *Plasmodium falciparum*
- *Escherichia coli*
- *Staphylococcus aureus* (including meticillin-resistant)
- Multi-resistant Gram-negative organisms (see p. 167)
- *Candida albicans*
- Hepatitis B and C viruses

'Top 10' concepts in infection care
- Sepsis
- Infection source control
- Finding the focus in bloodstream infections (bacteraemia)
- Multidisciplinary infection care
- Confidentiality in infection care
- Infection prevention and control measures
- Outbreak control
- Immunization
- Net state of immunosuppression
- Oral rehydration solution

CLINICAL SKILLS FOR INFECTIOUS DISEASE

History

Many patients with infectious diseases present with symptoms that are obviously suggestive of a particular type of infection. Others do not, and may present with non-specific symptoms (e.g. fever, malaise, vomiting or a rash). Taking a full history is critical in reaching a diagnosis (**Box 20.2**). A detailed description of how to ask about different risk factors is given later in this chapter (see p. 492), but a basic summary can be based around the crucial question *'Why has this patient, from this place, presented at this time, with these symptoms?'*

Box 20.2 Taking a history in infectious diseases

Patient
- Age:
  - Children and the very old are more susceptible than young adults to some types of infectious disease.
- Sex: remember to consider the possibilities of sex-specific diagnoses:
  - Epididymo-orchitis or prostatitis in men.
  - Pelvic inflammatory disease or tampon-related toxic shock syndrome in women.
- Occupation:
  - Contact with animals raises the possibility of zoonotic infections.
  - Healthcare workers may acquire infectious diseases from their patients.
- Co-morbidity and immunosuppression:
  - Some infectious diseases (e.g. bacterial meningitis or pneumococcal pneumonia) can affect even previously fit and healthy individuals.
  - Most infectious diseases are more common in immunosuppressed individuals, although the presentation might be blunted or less severe.
  - Certain co-morbidities raise the risk of specific types of infection, e.g. incomplete bladder emptying in neurological disease raises the risk of urinary tract infection (UTI).
  - Significant immunosuppression (e.g. in organ transplant recipients or patients with significant bone marrow disease) increases the risk of infection by a wide range of atypical (opportunistic) pathogens, including fungi, low-pathogenicity viruses and non-tuberculous mycobacteria.
- Socio-economic status
  - Malnutrition, poor sanitation, homelessness and overcrowding increase the risk of a number of 'diseases of poverty'
- Activities:
  - People who inject drugs are at risk of blood-borne viruses and bacterial bloodstream infection.
  - Unprotected sex presents the risk of developing body-fluid-borne viruses and various sexually transmitted infections (see Ch. 37).
  - Freshwater swimming is a risk factor for leptospirosis and (in certain regions) schistosomiasis.
  - Domestic pets can transmit disease, including cat-scratch fever or toxoplasmosis.
- Close contacts:
  - Diseases that occur in outbreaks (e.g. food poisoning) may also present in household or other close contacts.
- Uncommon exposures:
  - Where a diagnosis is unclear, taking time to revisit the history and ask about any unusual activities or exposures is sometimes helpful. Activities that may not be common in a particular setting, e.g. caving, cleaning aquariums, art restoration or repairing air-conditioning systems, all carry risks for developing particular infectious diseases. Unless you ask, you may never find out.

Place
- A detailed travel history is essential (see p. 492):
- Travel to tropical and subtropical countries may be a risk factor for a wide range of infectious diseases, including malaria, dengue and typhoid.
- Chronic infectious diseases, such as tuberculosis or viral hepatitis, may have been acquired during a childhood spent in endemic regions and then present in adulthood.
- Recent geographically localized epidemics, such as Middle Eastern respiratory syndrome (MERS) or Ebola (Central Africa), should be borne in mind
- Contact with healthcare settings:
  - Nursing or residential home residents are at risk of developing infectious diseases that are usually associated with hospital inpatients (such as 'hospital acquired pneumonia' or *Clostridium difficile* infection).
  - There are significant global differences in antibiotic resistance rates, so patients who have been inpatients in, or travelled to, other countries may present with multi-resistant organisms not usually seen in their country of residence.

Time
- It is often helpful to produce a timeline describing the development (and perhaps resolution) of different symptoms over time.
- Symptoms of many acute viral and bacterial infectious diseases emerge over several days.
- Symptom duration of more than 2 weeks suggests chronic infection (e.g. tuberculosis, leishmaniasis, brucellosis, human immunodeficiency virus (HIV)) or a non-infectious (e.g. autoimmune or malignant) disease process.
- Abrupt onset of severe symptoms suggests a highly virulent organism and may imply the need for urgent and empirical treatment before a diagnosis is made.
- Some diseases have characteristic time courses, e.g. the biphasic febrile response in dengue, or the initial 'Katayama fever' followed by haematuria seen in *Schistosoma haematobium* infection.

Symptoms
- Producing a clear account of the different general and organ-specific symptoms experienced by the patient is crucial.
- Sepsis is a physiological state that must not be missed, as it always requires empirical antibiotic therapy (see Ch. 8).
- Some symptoms suggest the involvement of a particular anatomical site or organ system, such as localized pain, jaundice or the bloody diarrhoea of dysentery.
- Other symptoms, such as headache, and vomiting or watery diarrhoea, often occur non-specifically in various infectious and non-infectious diseases, and should not be presumed to imply neurological or gastrointestinal disease, respectively.
- Some infectious diseases have unique pathological features that, if properly described, are highly suggestive of a particular diagnosis, e.g. the 'erythema migrans' rash of Lyme disease, or the progressive phases of typhoid.

Examination

A full examination is essential in patients presenting with fever or other signs of infectious disease. Where the site of infection is not clear from the history, signs found on examination can help form a diagnosis. The figure shows pathogens commonly affecting different organ systems, allowing a move from a clinical syndrome to a likely microbial diagnosis.

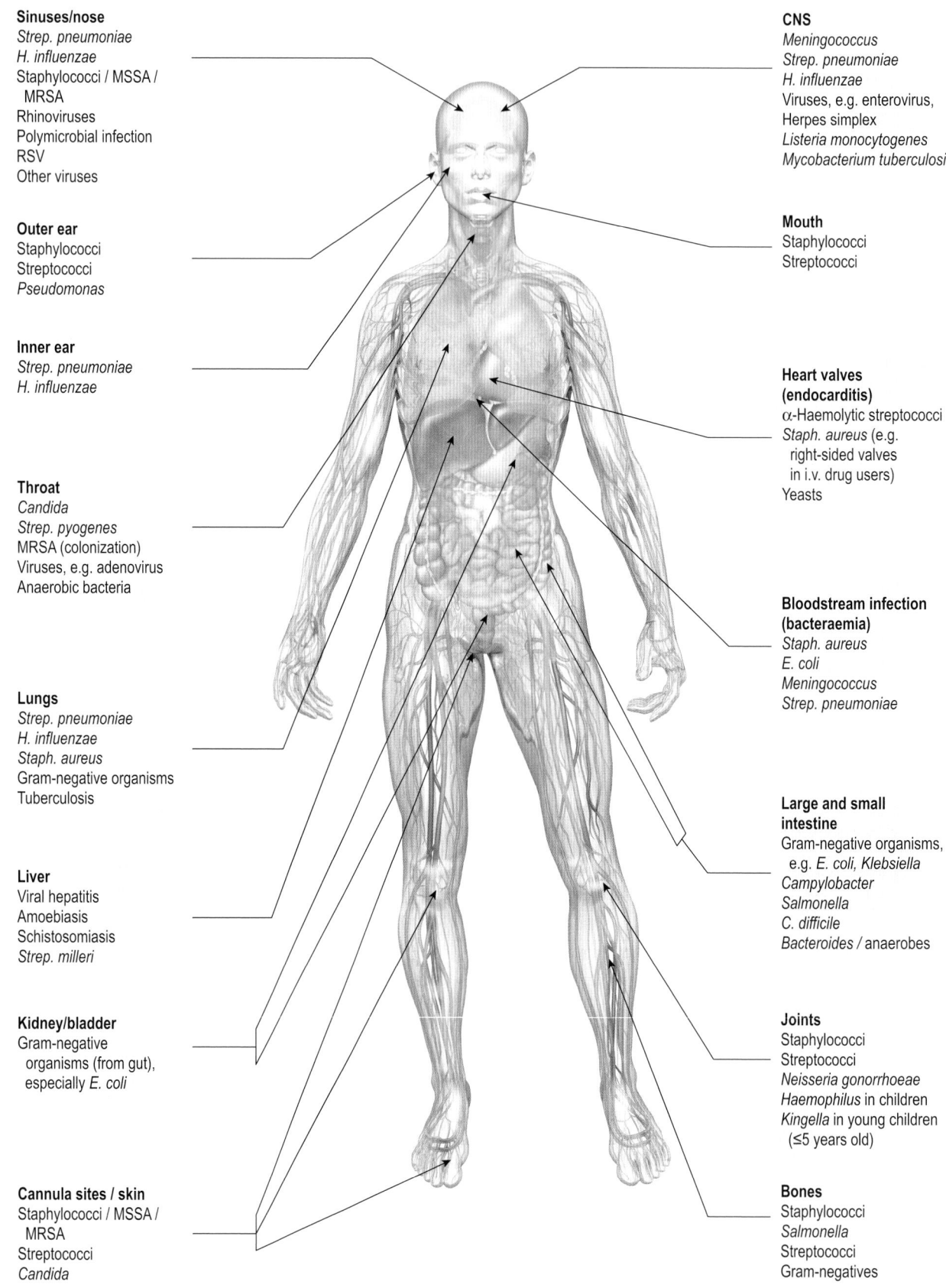

Sinuses/nose
Strep. pneumoniae
H. influenzae
Staphylococci / MSSA / MRSA
Rhinoviruses
Polymicrobial infection
RSV
Other viruses

Outer ear
Staphylococci
Streptococci
Pseudomonas

Inner ear
Strep. pneumoniae
H. influenzae

Throat
Candida
Strep. pyogenes
MRSA (colonization)
Viruses, e.g. adenovirus
Anaerobic bacteria

Lungs
Strep. pneumoniae
H. influenzae
Staph. aureus
Gram-negative organisms
Tuberculosis

Liver
Viral hepatitis
Amoebiasis
Schistosomiasis
Strep. milleri

Kidney/bladder
Gram-negative organisms (from gut), especially *E. coli*

Cannula sites / skin
Staphylococci / MSSA / MRSA
Streptococci
Candida

CNS
Meningococcus
Strep. pneumoniae
H. influenzae
Viruses, e.g. enterovirus, Herpes simplex
Listeria monocytogenes
Mycobacterium tuberculosis

Mouth
Staphylococci
Streptococci

Heart valves (endocarditis)
α-Haemolytic streptococci
Staph. aureus (e.g. right-sided valves in i.v. drug users)
Yeasts

Bloodstream infection (bacteraemia)
Staph. aureus
E. coli
Meningococcus
Strep. pneumoniae

Large and small intestine
Gram-negative organisms, e.g. *E. coli, Klebsiella*
Campylobacter
Salmonella
C. difficile
Bacteroides / anaerobes

Joints
Staphylococci
Streptococci
Neisseria gonorrhoeae
Haemophilus in children
Kingella in young children (≤5 years old)

Bones
Staphylococci
Salmonella
Streptococci
Gram-negatives

MRSA, meticillin-resistant *Staphylococcus aureus*; MSSA, meticillin-susceptible *Staphylococcus aureus*; RSV, respiratory syncytial virus.

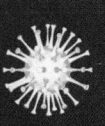
INTRODUCTION

'Infection' is defined as the process of pathogenic organisms invading and multiplying in or on a host's tissues. The term should be reserved for situations in which this results in harm, rather than when a microorganism simply colonizes the host without ill effect. The majority of microbes cause no harm. The relationship between the nature of colonizing microorganisms and human health is increasingly being recognized in studies of the human microbiome (see p. 504). Some microbes, however, including colonizing bacteria (e.g. *Staphylococcus aureus*) have the potential to cause disease in the right circumstances.

Infectious agents

The causative agents of infectious diseases can be divided into four groups:

Prions are the simplest infectious agents, consisting of a single protein molecule. They contain no nucleic acid and therefore no genetic information; their ability to propagate within a host relies on inducing the conversion of endogenous prion protein PrP^c into an abnormal protease-resistant isoform referred to as PrP^{Sc} or PrP^{Res}. Prion diseases are described on page 535.

Viruses contain both protein and nucleic acid, and so carry the genetic information for their own reproduction. However, they lack the apparatus to replicate autonomously, relying instead on 'hijacking' the cellular machinery of the host. They are small (usually <300 nanometres (nm) in diameter) and each virus possesses only one type of nucleic acid (either RNA or DNA).

Bacteria are usually larger than viruses. They are enclosed by a cell membrane and most have a cell wall, although some (e.g. *Mycoplasma* spp.) have only a cell membrane. This makes them naturally resistant to cell-wall-acting antibacterial agents (e.g. β-lactam antibiotics, including penicillin, and glycopeptide antibiotics, such as vancomycin; see Chapter 8).

Eukaryotes are the most sophisticated infectious organisms and include unicellular protozoa, fungi (which can be unicellular or filamentous) and multicellular parasitic worms. Other higher classes, such as the insects and the arachnids, also contain species that can envenom, injure or parasitize humans and cause disease; these are discussed in more detail in the topic pages online.

The figure on page 490 provides an overview of common microorganisms that cause infections. **Fig. 20.1** shows the approximate global distribution of selected human pathogens in 2019.

Further reading

http://bsac-vle.com/ *British Society for Antimicrobial Chemotherapy (BSAC) Virtual Learning Environment.*
https://apps.who.int/iris/bitstream/handle/10665/273826/EML-20-eng.pdf?ua=1 *WHO Model List of Essential Medicines.*
https://www.britishinfection.org/trainees/ *British Infection Association (BIA).*
https://www.jrcptb.org.uk/specialties/infectious-diseases-and-tropical-medicine *Joint Royal Colleges of Physicians Training BoardInfectious Diseases and Tropical Medicine.*
https://www.rcplondon.ac.uk/education-practice/advice/specialty-spotlight-infectious-diseases *Royal College of Physicians: Specialty Spotlight – Infectious Diseases.*

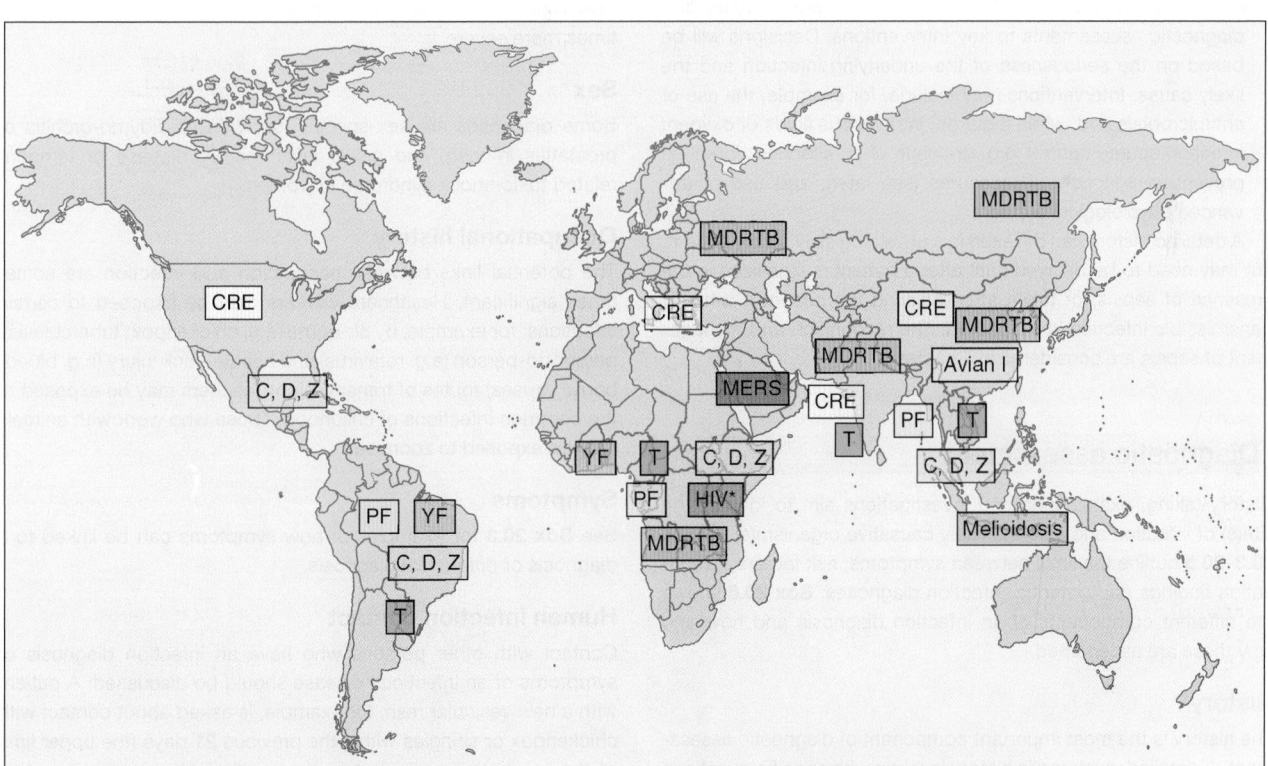

Fig. 20.1 Approximate global distribution of selected human pathogens (2019). This map is not exhaustive or geographically precise, and should not be used to guide clinical practice; a reliable travel health source (e.g. Travel Health Pro) should always be consulted. Avian I, avian influenza; C, Chikungunya virus; CRE, carbapenem-resistant Enterobacteriaceae; D, dengue virus; HIV*, human immunodeficiency virus (global distribution but highest prevalence in Africa); MDRTB, multi-drug-resistant tuberculosis; MERS, Middle East respiratory syndrome coronavirus; PF, *Plasmodium falciparum* malaria; T, typhoid fever; YF, yellow fever; Z, Zika virus.

CLINICAL APPROACH TO THE PATIENT WITH A SUSPECTED INFECTION

Fever is the cardinal feature of infection, but not all febrile illnesses are infections and not all infections present with a fever. **Fig. 20.2** provides an outline of the approach to the patient with acute (undifferentiated) fever of unclear cause. Fever is usually intermittent, so may not be present at the time of presentation, and occurs less commonly in elderly patients. Infection can also present with hypothermia (temperature <36°C), which is a poor prognostic sign. The biological behaviours of the pathogen and the consequent host responses are responsible for the clinical expression of disease, which sometimes allows clinical recognition. Knowledge of the incubation period following exposure can be helpful (e.g. up to 21 days for chickenpox), while symptoms of cough, sputum and pleuritic chest pain may suggest lobar pneumonia. Fever and neck stiffness characterize meningitis but do not inform about the microbial cause or management.

The three critical points in the assessment and management of a patient with fever, suspected infection or sepsis are:
- *Physiological assessment* (severity of illness), predominantly based on systematic examination of key physiological markers at initial presentation and subsequently.
- *Diagnostic assessment*, predominantly based on history-taking, examination and interpretation of those diagnostic tests available at presentation and subsequently performed (see later) in the context of the history and examination.
- *Management assessment*, based on linking physiological and diagnostic assessments to key interventions. Decisions will be based on the seriousness of the underlying infection and the likely cause. Interventions may include, for example, the use of antimicrobials and, when required, intravenous fluids or oxygen; infection source control (e.g. drainage of an abscess); infection prevention and control measures (see later); and use of advanced physiological support.

A detailed history can be taken in a physiologically stable patient, but may need to be delayed until after a patient is stabilized in the presence of sepsis, or taken after isolating the patient if a highly transmissible infection is suspected. The recognition and management of sepsis are considered in Chapter 8.

Diagnostic assessment

History-taking, examination and investigations aim to identify the site(s) of infection and also the likely causative organism(s). **Boxes 20.3–20.5** outline the links between symptoms, risk factors, examination findings and potential infection diagnoses. **Box 20.6** shows the different components of an infection diagnosis and how and why these are ascertained.

History

The history is the most important component of diagnostic assessment. A detailed, systematic history is taken with specific questions about the nature, timing and periodicity of symptoms (see **Box 20.1**), in particular in relation to any infection exposures and other risk factors (see **Box 20.4**). If symptoms started after the upper limit of the incubation period of any potential transmissible infection exposure identified, the diagnosis is unlikely. Consideration of the incubation period is irrelevant for many infections, however: for

example, when the invading pathogen is often a colonizer of the host, such as in *Staph. aureus* bloodstream infections, or when a specific exposure history cannot be identified, or the patient's history and examination signs are not diagnostic.

Symptoms are often non-specific (e.g. a 3-day history of lethargy, loss of appetite and shivers), but may lead to a diagnosis or differential diagnosis through careful interpretation and problem-solving (e.g. by linking the patient's symptoms to their exposures and risk factors and then to potential clinical infection diagnoses and causal pathogens; examination findings and any available test results also need to be considered). In patients with sepsis, a full history should be obtained after, or at the same time as, initiating emergency medical management (see p. 157) to avoid therapeutic delay. If the patient is confused, the history may have to be obtained from a relative or friend. With some exceptions, patients with short, acute symptom histories are more likely to have infections due to microbes that tend to cause acute presentations (e.g. *Streptococcus pneumoniae* infection in a patient with a 3-day history of shivers, cough with production of green sputum, and right-sided pleuritic chest pain). Patients with longer symptom histories are more likely to have infections due to microbes that tend to cause chronic presentations (e.g. pulmonary tuberculosis in a patient with a 2-month history of sweats, weight loss and cough productive of blood-stained sputum, and who has recently returned from living in sub-Saharan Africa).

Key diagnostic information in the patient's history includes:

Age

Older patients are more prone to some infections (e.g. *Clostridium difficile* infection or pneumonia). Some infections (e.g. glandular fever, chickenpox) are less common in older adults but are sometimes more severe.

Sex

Some diagnoses are sex-specific, such as epididymo-orchitis or prostatitis in men, and pelvic inflammatory disease or tampon-related toxic-shock syndrome in women.

Occupational history

The potential links between occupation and infection are sometimes significant. Healthcare workers may be exposed to certain infections: for example, by air-borne (e.g. chickenpox, tuberculosis), person-to-person (e.g. rotavirus) and needle-stick injury (e.g. blood-borne viruses) routes of transmission. Teachers may be exposed to the common infections of childhood. Those who work with animals may be exposed to zoonoses.

Symptoms

See **Box 20.3** for examples of how symptoms can be linked to a diagnosis or differential diagnosis.

Human infection contact

Contact with other persons who have an infection diagnosis or symptoms of an infectious disease should be discussed. A patient with a new vesicular rash, for example, is asked about contact with chickenpox or shingles within the previous 21 days (the upper limit of the incubation period). A patient with gastroenteritis is asked about contact with other people with similar symptoms, when that contact was with respect to the start of symptoms, and the social context of that contact. A patient with recurrent skin abscesses is asked about contact with other persons with recurrent skin infections (e.g. to assess the risk of transmission of Panton–Valentine–leukocidin (PVL) producing *Staph. aureus* skin infections).

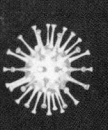

Risk factors/ Exposures

- Age
- Occupation
- Human contact
- Animal contact
- Travel
- Food and drink
- Sexual exposure
- Pregnancy
- Drug use and needle exposure
- Leisure activities

Symptom history

- Timeline / chronicity / periodicity
- Fever, sweats, shivers, rigors
- Rash / glands / masses (abscesses)
- Headache / agitation / confusion / seizures
- Ear pain/discharge; runny/congested nose; eye symptoms; sinus pain; throat; mouth; swallowing (e.g. candidiasis)
- Cough / sputum (colour/blood) / shortness of breath / pleuritic chest pain
- Abdominal pain / symptoms (nature/location/radiation) / diarrhoea
- Urinary – dysuria / frequency / urgency / haematuria, etc.
- Genital – discharge (and nature) / itching / ulceration, etc.
- Limb pain, swelling, warmth, redness
- Bone/joint/spine pain, swelling, warmth, redness

Medical history

- Previous infections
- Co-morbidities
- Immunosuppressing conditions – *net state of immunosuppression*
- Devices / prostheses
- Vaccination history
- Medications
  - recent antimicrobials
  - immunosuppression
  - acid suppression
  - HIV / hepatitis, etc.
- Allergies / intolerances

General investigations

Full blood count

Urea / electrolytes

Liver enzymes

C-reactive protein

Other biomarkers (e.g. procalcitonin) as indicated or used nationally/locally

Lactate (sepsis)

Coagulation (sepsis, hepatitis)

CD4 count / viral load in HIV patients

Other tests as appropriate (e.g. autoantibodies, thyroid tests, ferritin)

ECG (e.g. pericarditis)

Radiology

Chest X-ray

Ultrasound

Echocardiography

CT

MRI

Nuclear imaging as available/appropriate after discussion with radiologist

Examination

- Temperature (repeat regularly)
- Skin – rash, splinter haemorrhages, wounds, ulcers (remove dressings)
- Device / prosthesis / implant sites (e.g. i.v. lines, cardiac devices, urinary catheters, etc.)
- Neck stiffness
- Eyes – conjunctivitis, photophobia
- Mouth and throat, ears and nose
- Lymph nodes
- Murmurs (other signs of endocarditis)
- Focal chest signs
- Abdomen
- Genitourinary / rectal
- Lower limbs / bone / joints / spine
- Sites of inflammation – redness, warmth, swelling, pain

Infection prevention and control
Problem-solving
Differential diagnosis
Diagnosis

Management

- Multidisciplinary care
- Shared decision-making with patient
- Antimicrobials / medications, etc. (as appropriate)
- Source control (e.g. drainage of abscess)
- Foci of bloodstream infections (e.g. endocarditis)
- Re-evaluation from top if diagnosis unclear or patient does not respond / improve or deteriorates

Microbiology / Virology

Blood cultures x2 for all patients; x3 if endocarditis or other 'deep' site of infection suspected

Urine culture (if patient has symptoms or is unable to give history; only a negative urine dip test for leucocytes/ nitrites is useful)

Malaria film and/or rapid diagnostics (as indicated)

Pus; do not swab clean, uninfected wounds

Screening swabs (for MRSA and/or CRE)

Sputum (culture, rapid respiratory diagnostics; x3 if TB suspected; induced or BAL if required)

Throat / nasopharyngeal swab / sample (culture, rapid respiratory diagnostics)

Cerebrospinal fluid (microscopy, culture, protein, glucose, virology)

Aspiration / biopsy / operative tissue for histology and/or microscopy and culture; may need to be radiologically guided

Faeces (tests depend on differential diagnosis)

Nucleic acid amplification tests (e.g. PCR)

Immunodiagnostics (e.g. serology)

Fig. 20.2 Clinical approach to the patient with fever of unclear cause but without sepsis. For patients with sepsis, see Chapter 8. BAL, bronchoalveolar lavage; CRE, carbapenem-resistant Entero-bacteriaceae; CT, computed tomography; ECG, electrocardiogram; HIV, human immunodeficiency virus; MRE, magnetic resonance enterography; MRI, magnetic resonance imaging; MRSA, meticillin-resistant *Staphylococcus aureus*; PCR, polymerase chain reaction; TB, tuberculosis.

? Box 20.3 Linking symptoms elicited from the patient history to infection diagnoses

Element(s) in the symptom history of a patient with acute fever or possible infection	Example infection diagnoses
Acute headache, non-blanching rash, neck stiffness, photophobia	Meningococcal meningitis
Acute headache, neck stiffness, photophobia	Meningitis (bacterial, viral, fungal)
Acute agitation, confusion	Encephalitis
Ear pain with pus-like discharge	Otitis externa
Maxillary sinus area pain	Sinusitis
Sore throat, large neck glands (lymph nodes)	Tonsillitis, glandular fever syndromes
Sore, ulcerated mouth/throat with rash on hands/feet	Hand, foot and mouth (viral) infection, other viral infections (remember syphilis in patients with rashes on their hands/feet)
Cough, dyspnoea, pleuritic chest pain	Lower respiratory tract infection, pneumonia
Fever, shivers, rigors	Bloodstream infection (usually bacterial), malaria, viral infections (e.g. influenza), endocarditis, causes of fever/pyrexia of unknown origin (if history is ≥2 weeks); all may or may not be associated with other symptoms
Non-specific abdominal pains/cramps and diarrhoea	*Clostridium difficile* infection, gastroenteritis
Right upper quadrant pain	Biliary tract infection, liver abscess, pneumonia adjacent to diaphragm
Left iliac fossa pain	Diverticulitis, left ovarian abscess
Renal angle pain with urinary symptoms	Pyelonephritis, renal abscess
Frequency, urgency, pain on micturition	Urinary tract infection
Pelvic pain	Pelvic inflammatory disease, ovarian abscess (if pain is unilateral)
Penile or vaginal discharge	Sexually transmitted infections, retained tampon (females)
Back pain	Discitis (with or without epidural abscess)
Red, swollen, hot joint	Septic arthritis (non-infection diagnoses such as gout and reactive arthritis should be considered, see p. 455)
Red, swollen, hot, painful limb	Cellulitis, soft tissue infection
Pain, redness and discharge at the site of a prosthesis or invasive device	Prosthesis/invasive device infection

? Box 20.4 Linking risk factors elicited from the patient history to infection diagnoses

Element(s) in the risk factor history of a patient with acute fever or possible infection	Example infection diagnoses
Alcohol abuse	Spontaneous bacterial peritonitis (if ascites), invasive pneumococcal disease (*Streptococcus pneumoniae*), tuberculosis
Diverticular disease	Diverticulitis, diverticular abscess
Gallstones	Biliary tract infection, pancreatitis
Immunosuppression/HIV	Opportunistic bacterial (e.g. nocardiosis), fungal (e.g. cryptococciosis) and viral infections (e.g. cytomegalovirus)
Intravenous drug use	Bloodstream infection, especially *Staphylococcus aureus*, blood-borne infections (e.g. HIV, hepatitis B and C, malaria)
Lung disease, smoker	Respiratory tract infections/pneumonia, e.g. with *Haemophilus influenzae* (chronic obstructive pulmonary disease) and *Pseudomonas aeruginosa* (in cystic fibrosis and bronchiectasis)
Prostheses/invasive devices	Prosthesis/invasive device infection
Recent abdominal surgery	Intra-abdominal infection/peritonitis, abscess(es), wound infection
Recent influenza	Secondary bacterial infection (e.g. with Lancefield group A streptococci or meningococcus)
Recent hospitalization	Healthcare-associated infections, e.g. pneumonia and urinary tract, surgical site and bloodstream infections; at higher risk of an antimicrobial-resistant pathogen
Recent new sexual partner	Chlamydia, gonorrhoea, HIV, syphilis, other sexually transmitted infections
School or university student, military person	Meningococcal disease, mumps, other infections based on local contemporaneous epidemiology
Splenectomy	Pneumococcal, *Haemophilus* spp., and meningococcal infections (vaccination and antibiotic prophylaxis reduce but do not eliminate risk)
Travel abroad	E.g. dengue, malaria, legionnaires' disease, leptospirosis, typhoid (depends on travel history)
Urinary tract problems (e.g. renal stone, benign prostatic hypertrophy)	Urinary tract infection, pyelonephritis

Animal contact

Domestic (e.g. cats and *Toxoplasma gondii* infection), farm (e.g. sheep and *Coxiella burnetii* infection) and wild animal (e.g. bats and rabies) contact is discussed.

Travel history

Some diseases are more prevalent in certain geographical locations. A detailed travel itinerary, including any flight stopovers, should be taken from anyone who is unwell after arriving from another country. Previous travel should also be covered, as some infections may be chronic or recurrent (e.g. *Plasmodium vivax* malaria). It is necessary to find out not only which countries were visited but also the type of environment and length of stay; a prolonged stay in a remote jungle village carries much higher health risks than a short holiday in an air-conditioned coastal holiday resort, even in the same country. Food and water consumption, bathing and swimming, animal and insect contact, and contact with human illness need to be established. Enquiry should be made about sexual contacts, drug use and medical treatment (especially parenteral).

In some parts of the world, a high-proportion of professional sex workers are human immunodeficiency virus (HIV)-positive, and hepatitis B and C (HBV/HCV) are very common in some parts of Africa and

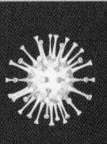

Examination finding(s) in a patient with fever or possible infection	Site of infection/diagnosis
Meningism, petechial rash	Meningitis (most likely meningococcal)
Cervical lymphadenopathy, enlarged tonsils	Tonsillitis (viral or bacterial), glandular fever syndromes (including HIV)
Tachypnoea, coarse focal crackles (can be bilateral)	Lower respiratory tract infection, pneumonia
Temperatures ≥37.8°C, new-onset regurgitant systolic murmur	Endocarditis
Right upper quadrant tenderness	Biliary tract or liver infection
Abdominal tenderness with rebound/guarding	Intra-abdominal infection (peritonitis)
Left iliac fossa tenderness	Diverticulitis/diverticular abscess, ovarian abscess in females
Right iliac fossa tenderness	Appendicitis/appendix abscess, ovarian abscess in females
Suprapubic tenderness (± catheter)	Urinary tract infection, pelvic inflammatory disease in females
Renal angle tenderness	Pyelonephritis, renal abscess
Red, hot, swollen limb	Cellulitis, soft tissue infection (consider necrotizing fasciitis if pain is out of keeping with examination appearances or if there is severe pain, rapidly progressing history and 'odd' examination appearance/findings)
Intravascular devices ± erythema, pus, etc.	Device infection, bloodstream infection, endocarditis

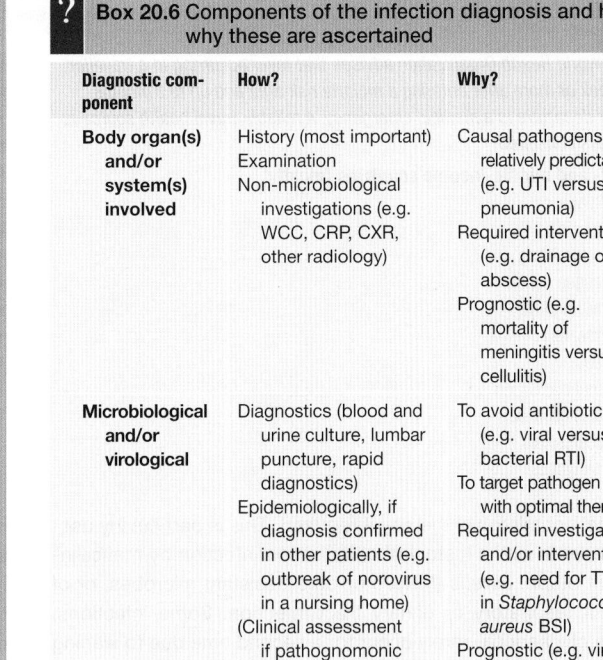

? **Box 20.6** Components of the infection diagnosis and how/why these are ascertained

Diagnostic component	How?	Why?
Body organ(s) and/or system(s) involved	History (most important) Examination Non-microbiological investigations (e.g. WCC, CRP, CXR, other radiology)	Causal pathogens are relatively predictable (e.g. UTI versus pneumonia) Required intervention (e.g. drainage of abscess) Prognostic (e.g. mortality of meningitis versus cellulitis)
Microbiological and/or virological	Diagnostics (blood and urine culture, lumbar puncture, rapid diagnostics) Epidemiologically, if diagnosis confirmed in other patients (e.g. outbreak of norovirus in a nursing home) (Clinical assessment if pathognomonic signs)	To avoid antibiotics (e.g. viral versus bacterial RTI) To target pathogen with optimal therapy Required investigation and/or intervention (e.g. need for TTE in *Staphylococcus aureus* BSI) Prognostic (e.g. viral meningitis versus bacterial) Epidemiology (for disease and resistance surveillance)
Prognostic (severity)	Physiology Age, co-morbidity, etc. Clinical and/or microbiological diagnosis (see earlier) if available	Dictates level of required intervention (i.e. sepsis versus self-limiting infection) Informs discussion with patient and relatives

BSI, bloodstream infection; CRP, C-reactive protein; CXR, chest X-ray; RTI, respiratory tract infection; TTE, transthoracic echocardiogram; UTI, urinary tract infection; WCC, white cell count.

Asia. Special tests may be needed, depending on the epidemiological risks and clinical signs, and malaria rapid antigen diagnostic tests and thick/thin blood films are mandatory in anyone who is unwell after being in a malarious area. A reliable resource such as Travel Health Pro (see Further reading) is consulted regarding current infectious disease alerts and endemic risks for the countries visited. Some of the more common causes of a febrile illness in returning travellers are listed in **Box 20.7**.

Food and drink history

Exposure to unclean water and uncooked, unpasteurized or contaminated foods or drinks (e.g. *Listeria monocytogenes* infection from soft cheeses), and illness in other people also exposed, should be asked about.

Sexual activity

The sexual history is often omitted or poorly taken, but is essential if diagnoses, such as HIV infection, are not to be missed. Sexual exposure is common in travellers. Sexually transmitted infections are discussed in Chapter 37.

Pregnancy

Pregnant women may be more susceptible to some infections (e.g. malaria, HIV infection, and listeriosis) and may be at higher risk of severe infections (e.g. disseminated herpes simplex virus (HSV) infection/hepatitis, hepatitis E, influenza, malaria and measles).

Intravenous drug use and needle exposure

As well as blood-borne viruses (mostly HIV, HBV and HCV), drug injectors are susceptible to a wide variety of bacterial and fungal infections, in particular those due to *Staph. aureus* and *Streptococcus pyogenes* (group A streptococcus), as a result of contamination of the injecting equipment or inoculation from the patient's colonized skin. Abscesses (e.g. in the psoas or other muscles) and soft tissue infections at the site of injection are common, especially in the groin, and may involve adjacent vascular structures (e.g. to form pseudoaneurysms) and bones (osteomyelitis). Bloodstream and haematogenously spread infections, including endocarditis (often right-sided), spinal infections and bone/joint infections, are also common. Other needle exposures, such as tattooing, body piercing, needle-stick injury and receipt of blood products (especially outside of developed countries), are also risk factors for blood-borne infections.

Leisure activities

Certain pastimes (e.g. open-water swimming and leptospirosis) may predispose to water-borne infections or zoonoses.

Previous infections

Previous infections are reviewed. This may provide a useful clue to both the organ/system and microbiological/virological diagnoses (see **Box 20.6**); previous microbiological results, especially for the prior 12 months, are reviewed for any pathogens isolated and associated antimicrobial susceptibilities in order to guide

> **? Box 20.7 Causes of febrile illness in travellers returning from the tropics and other countries**
>
> *The World Health Organization advises that fever occurring in a traveller 1 week or more after entering a malaria risk area and up to 3 months after departure is a medical emergency. A reliable travel health source is always consulted*
>
> **Low- and middle-income countries (mostly)**
> - Malaria
> - Typhoid
> - Leptospirosis
> - Dengue
> - Chikungunya
> - Dysentery
> - Hepatitis A
> - Amoebiasis
> - Schistosomiasis
> - Tuberculosis
> - Tick typhus
>
> **Specific geographical areas (see text)**
> - Ebola
> - Middle Eastern respiratory syndrome (MERS)
> - Zika
> - Histoplasmosis
> - Brucellosis
>
> **Worldwide**
> - Multi-drug- and extensively drug-resistant Gram-negative infections
> - Upper respiratory tract infection
> - Pneumonia
> - Influenza and other common viral infections
> - Traveller's diarrhoea
> - Other common infections

empirical antimicrobial therapy if required. This is particularly useful in patients with a history of colonization/infection by meticillin-resistant *Staph. aureus* (MRSA) or other resistant microbes, or of recurrent respiratory or urinary tract infection. Some infections, such as chickenpox, rarely occur for a second time due to waning immunity, although chickenpox may recrudesce from latency in the form of shingles (zoster). Patients who are infected with dengue virus for a second time are at higher risk of developing severe forms of the infection.

Co-morbidities

The potential association between co-morbid illnesses and infections is considered (e.g. haematological malignancy and medication-related immune suppression are risk factors for invasive pneumococcal disease, and opportunistic infections, such as *Pneumocystis jirovecii* infection).

Devices/prostheses/implants

Symptoms relating to any recently inserted or longstanding devices, prostheses or implants are discussed (e.g. increasing pain in a total hip replacement; swelling and warmth over a pacemaker insertion site).

Vaccination history

Patients who have not received certain childhood (e.g. measles, mumps) or pre-travel (e.g. typhoid) vaccines are at higher risk if exposed.

Medications

Some medications increase the risk of certain infections (e.g. proton pump inhibitors and histamine$_2$ antagonists may predispose to gastrointestinal infections, including, for example, *Salmonella* spp. gastroenteritis and *C. difficile* infection, but not norovirus, which is not acid-sensitive). The patient's recent antimicrobial exposure should also be ascertained; it is well known, for example, that individuals recently exposed to an antimicrobial are more likely subsequently to harbour microorganisms resistant to that antimicrobial (and possibly to other antimicrobials too) and this may influence prescribing decisions.

Allergies/intolerances

The detailed nature of any prior allergies and/or intolerances should be determined with respect to antimicrobials or infection-related drugs (e.g. HIV medications).

Immunosuppression

Increasing age and co-morbidity, as well as advances in medical treatment over recent decades, have led to a huge increase in the number of patients living with immunodeficiency states of varying degrees. Cancer chemotherapy, immunosuppressive drugs, including the increasing use of monoclonal antibody-based biologic therapy (e.g. infliximab), and the worldwide HIV epidemic have all contributed. Given that, in modern medicine, a patient's immunosuppression status is often multifactorial because of age, co-morbidity and therapy, for example, an assessment of the patient's **net state of immunosuppression** is an important concept in determining the nature of the infections of which a patient is at risk. For example, an otherwise well 60-year-old on low-dose maintenance prednisolone for polymyalgia rheumatica is considerably less immunosuppressed, and hence at lower risk of infections, than an 82-year-old with diabetes, rheumatoid arthritis and a past history of a renal transplantation, who is taking a variety of immunosuppressant and disease-modifying medications. The temporality of immunosuppression is also a factor: patients within 6 months of solid organ transplantation, for example, are at higher risk, as this period corresponds to the most intense time of immunosuppression. Patients who do not have a spleen (or a functional spleen) are at risk of infections caused by capsulated bacteria (i.e. pneumococci, *Haemophilus* spp. and meningococci; see p. 357).

The presentation may be atypical in the immunocompromised patient, with few, if any, localizing symptoms or signs. Infection can be due to organisms that are not usually pathogenic, including environmental bacteria and fungi (opportunistic microbes). The normal physiological responses to infection (e.g. fever, neutrophilia) may be diminished or absent. The onset of symptoms may be sudden and the course of the illness fulminant. A high index of suspicion for infections in immunosuppressed individuals is required, with early investigation (e.g. computed tomography (CT) thorax for invasive pulmonary aspergillosis in a patient receiving highly immunosuppressant cancer chemotherapy and with new chest X-ray shadowing) and rapid intervention. Common causes of infection in immunosuppressed patients are shown in **Box 20.8**. For neutropenic sepsis, see page 116 .

Clinical examination

A careful and systematic examination covering all systems is required in order to avoid missing subtle signs, such as splinter haemorrhages in endocarditis or the petechial rash of early meningococcal disease. The examination is used to support or refute likely differential diagnoses based on the history and may also help guide the approach to investigations; new differential diagnoses may also emerge based on examination findings.

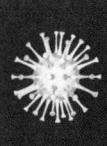

Clothes and dressings should be removed to inspect underlying skin, wounds (including historic wounds) and invasive devices (e.g. pacemaker sites). Skin rashes (**Fig. 20.3**) and lymphadenopathy are common features of infectious diseases but can occur in non-infectious conditions, such as lymphoma. The ears (e.g. necrotizing otitis externa), nose (e.g. common cold), eyes (e.g. Roth's spots in endocarditis), mouth (e.g. Koplik's spots in measles) and

throat (e.g. tonsillitis) should all be inspected carefully. Infections commonly associated with a rash are listed in **Box 20.9**. Auscultation of the heart, for murmurs, is critical in patients with fever of unknown cause, bloodstream infections and other potential signs of endocarditis. Likewise, examination of the musculoskeletal system, including palpation of the spine (i.e. discitis), is performed in patients with bloodstream infection, especially that due to *Staph. aureus*, and fever/pyrexia of unknown cause.

Abdominal examination, including the renal angles (i.e. pyelonephritis, see p. 1383), should be performed in patients with Gram-negative bloodstream infection (e.g. that due to *Escherichia coli*, *Klebsiella pneumoniae*, *Proteus mirabilis*, etc.) as the urinary tract (most commonly), intra-abdominal sites and the liver/biliary tract (liver enzymes are often elevated) are the most common underlying foci of infection. Rectal, vaginal and penile examinations are required in those at risk of sexually transmitted infections (see pp. 411–412). The fever pattern may occasionally be helpful – for example, the tertian fever of *falciparum* malaria – but in most patients fever is non-specific and not diagnostic. **Box 20.5** outlines the potential links between some examination findings and diagnoses of infection.

Investigations

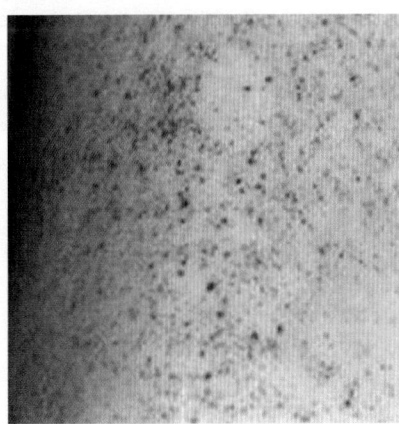

Fig. 20.3 Skin rashes and lymphadenopathy are common non-specific features of infectious diseases.

Box 20.8 Common causes of infection in immunocompromised patients

Deficiency	Causes	Organisms (examples)
Neutropenia	Chemotherapy Myeloablative therapy Immunosuppressant drugs	*Escherichia coli* *Klebsiella pneumoniae* *Staphylococcus aureus* *Staph. epidermidis* *Aspergillus* spp. *Candida* spp.
Cellular immune defects	HIV infection Lymphoma Myeloablative therapy Congenital syndromes	Respiratory syncytial virus Cytomegalovirus Epstein–Barr virus Herpes simplex and zoster *Salmonella* spp. *Mycobacterium* spp. (esp. *M. avium* complex infections) *Cryptococcus neoformans* *Candida* spp. *Cryptosporidium parvum* *Pneumocystis jirovecii* *Toxoplasma gondii*
Humoral immune deficiencies	Congenital syndromes Chronic lymphocytic leukaemia Corticosteroids	*Haemophilus influenzae* *Streptococcus pneumoniae* Enteroviruses
Terminal complement deficiencies (C5–C9)	Congenital syndromes	*Neisseria meningitidis* *N. gonorrhoeae*
Splenectomy	Surgery Trauma	*Strep. pneumoniae* *N. meningitidis* *H. influenzae* Malaria

Box 20.9 Infections commonly associated with a rash

Macular/maculopapular
- Measles
- Rubella
- Enteroviruses
- Human herpesvirus 6
- Epstein–Barr virus
- Cytomegalovirus
- Human erythrovirus (parvovirus) B19
- Human immunodeficiency virus (HIV)
- Dengue
- Typhoid
- Secondary syphilis
- Rickettsial spotted fevers

Vesicular
- Chickenpox (varicella zoster virus)
- Shingles (varicella zoster virus)
- Herpes simplex virus
- Hand, foot and mouth disease (Coxsackie virus, enterovirus 71)
- Herpangina (Coxsackie virus)

Petechial/haemorrhagic
- Meningococcal septicaemia
- Any septicaemia with disseminated intravascular coagulation (DIC)
- Rickettsiae
- Viruses (see **Box 20.37**)

Erythematous
- Scarlet fever
- Lyme disease (erythema chronicum migrans)
- Toxic shock syndrome
- Human erythrovirus (parvovirus) B19

Urticarial
- *Toxocara*
- *Strongyloides*
- *Schistosoma*
- Cutaneous larva migrans

Others
- Tick typhus (eschar)
- Primary syphilis (chancre)
- Anthrax (ulcerating papule)

The results of investigations are used to support, confirm or refute likely differential diagnoses based on the history and examination findings, and may also lead to new differential diagnoses and the need for further investigations. In some infections, such as chickenpox, the clinical presentation is so distinctive that no investigations are necessary to confirm the diagnosis. In other mild and self-limiting infections, such as those frequently managed in primary and ambulatory care settings (e.g. minor skin infections, upper respiratory tract infections, cystitis, etc.), extensive investigations will not change management and are therefore unwarranted, as the diagnosis and treatment are clear. Some patients, especially when they are being managed in secondary care or when an antibiotic prescription may be avoidable, require further tests to determine the organ/system/site of infection and microbiological cause, and thereby to guide required intervention(s). A shared decision-making approach should be taken with the patient to avoid tests, treatments or procedures that are unlikely to be of benefit (see p. 11).

General investigations

Box 20.10 shows general investigations for a patient with acute fever or suspected infection of unclear cause. It is vital to review at presentation any tests that have been performed previously, including prior microbiological tests. Treating a patient known to harbour resistant microorganisms with an antibiotic to which those organisms are resistant may be unwise, depending on clinical circumstances: for

Box 20.10 General investigations and possible causes in suspected infection

Investigation	Possible causes
Full blood count	
Neutrophilia	Bacterial infection Inflammation
Neutropenia	Viral infection Brucellosis Typhoid Typhus Severe sepsis
Lymphocytosis	Viral infection
Lymphopenia	HIV infection (not specific) Other viral infections
Atypical lymphocytes	Infectious mononucleosis
Eosinophilia	Invasive parasitic infection
Thrombocytopenia	Sepsis Malaria Some viral infections
Erythrocyte sedimentation rate or C-reactive protein	Elevated in many infections
Serum creatinine and electrolytes	Potentially deranged in severe illness from any cause
Procalcitonin	Elevated particularly in bacterial infection
Liver enzymes	
Minor elevation of transferases	Non-specific feature of many infections Mild viral hepatitis
High transferases, elevated bilirubin	Viral hepatitis (usually A, B or E)
Coagulation	May be deranged in hepatitis and sepsis
Serum lactate	Used in the assessment of sepsis

example, a patient presenting with pyelonephritis should not be treated with co-amoxiclav if *E. coli* resistant to co-amoxiclav were recently grown from a mid-stream urine specimen. The exact tests performed will vary, depending on clinical presentation and differential diagnoses, severity of illness and available resources:

General blood tests

These provide clues to the diagnosis or organ/system involved (e.g. raised liver enzymes in liver or biliary tract infection), but in general are non-specific and non-diagnostic. Helpful tests may include:

- ***The full blood count and differential white cell count.*** In adults, lymphopenia is commonly associated with various viral infections, whereas neutrophilia, particularly if marked, is more likely to be associated with bacterial infections, although such associations are far from being a precise science in clinical practice.
- ***The erythrocyte sedimentation rate (ESR), plasma viscosity and/or C-reactive protein (CRP).*** These may be raised in infection and other inflammatory states.
- ***Liver biochemistry and function.***
- ***Serum creatinine and electrolytes.*** These assess for infection-related acute kidney injury.
- ***Coagulation screen*** (in suspected sepsis and hepatitis).
- ***Serum lactate*** (in suspected sepsis).

CRP is a non-specific marker of inflammation and is raised in many different infections, and in acute and chronic non-infection conditions associated with inflammation (e.g. rheumatoid arthritis). It is more useful in monitoring response to treatment than in making a diagnosis, although it is sometimes used as a point-of-care test in primary or ambulatory care to guide the need for antibiotic therapy in acute bronchitis (using cut-offs of 100 mg/L for an antibiotic prescription, 20–100 mg/L for a delayed prescription and <20 mg/L for no antibiotic).

The exact role of procalcitonin in the diagnostic and prognostic assessment of bacterial infections is controversial; it may have a useful role in antibiotic stewardship (see p. 159) when used within algorithms, particularly for respiratory tract infections and in the critical care environment, to determine when it is safe to start or stop antibiotic therapy.

Radiological imaging

X-ray (e.g. pneumonia), ultrasound (e.g. abscess), echocardiography (endocarditis), computed tomography (CT; e.g. intra-abdominal infection) and magnetic resonance imaging (MRI; e.g. bone and spinal infections) are used to identify and localize infections. Positron emission tomography (PET) and single-photon emission computed tomography (SPECT) have also proved useful in localizing infection, especially when combined with CT scanning, when the focus of infection is unclear. Biopsy or aspiration of tissue for microbiological examination is often facilitated by ultrasound or CT guidance. Indium- or technetium-labelled white cell scans (using white cells harvested from the patient prior to the test) may also help to localize infection. When possible, cases are discussed with a radiologist before ordering tests – for example, PET or white cell scans – to ensure that patients receive the optimal investigations in the context of their individual clinical presentation and prior investigations.

Microbiological investigations

It is often helpful to discuss the clinical problem with an infection specialist to ensure that appropriate tests are performed to identify the causative organism and that specimens are collected and transported correctly. Accurate completion of the request form, including clinical information, antimicrobial history, epidemiological and risk

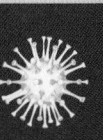

factor details (e.g. onset and duration or symptoms, recent travel, etc.) enable laboratory staff to add or delete tests appropriately.

Microscopy

The most widely utilized microscopic technique is the Gram stain, which determines the shape (cocci or bacilli) and Gram status (positive or negative) of bacteria. This allows most pathogenic bacteria to be classified into four groups: Gram-positive cocci, Gram-negative cocci, Gram-positive bacilli and Gram-negative bacilli. To some extent, this then dictates empirical antibacterial therapy, if appropriate. **Box 20.11** shows some key bacterial causes of bloodstream infections in the UK, along with their shape and Gram status, and how bacterial identity links to potential foci of infection.

Culture

Specimens for culture should, ideally, be taken prior to administration of, or a change in, antibiotic therapy. Once antibiotics are commenced, however, there will be an impact on the microbiome (see p. 504), including infecting pathogens, resulting in potentially misleading results. Culture techniques can be applied to a wide variety of bacteria, fungi, protozoa and viruses. However, some organisms are difficult to grow and may require special culture media and/or conditions. Viruses are particularly difficult (and, in many cases, impossible) to culture in the laboratory. Antimicrobial susceptibility testing is performed on isolates thought to be clinically significant. Increasingly, traditional culture techniques are combined with new technologies, such as fluorescence in situ hybridization (FISH), matrix-assisted laser desorption ionization time-of-flight (MALDI-TOF) mass spectroscopy, morphokinetic cellular analysis, polymerase chain reaction (PCR) testing of identifier genes, and whole-genome sequencing (WGS) of pathogenic organisms. This reduces the time to identification of pathogens, informs subsequent antimicrobial susceptibility testing (including whether a pathogen produces an extended-spectrum β-lactamase (ESBL) or carbapenemase – associated with multidrug resistance in Gram-negative bacteria) - and enables linkage of bacteria and patients in outbreaks. In the future, new technologies may be applied directly to blood samples, possibly replacing the current culturing process.

Specimens sent for microscopy and/or culture (**Box 20.12**) are described here.

- **Blood** is sent for bacterial culture in hospitalized patients if systemic infection is suspected, regardless of whether fever is present at the time of presentation. Additional blood cultures are taken if fever subsequently occurs. In patients with suspected endocarditis or cardiac device infection or other 'deep' foci of infection (e.g. psoas abscess, discitis, etc.), at least three sets of blood cultures are taken.
- **Urine** is sent for microscopy and culture in patients with urinary tract symptoms, and also in patients unable to provide a clear history, when urinary tract infection (UTI)/sepsis is suspected. Urine culture is not indicated in asymptomatic patients able to provide a clear history, regardless of whether they are catheterized or not.
- **Cerebrospinal fluid (CSF)** (meningitis, encephalitis)**, sputum** (e.g. pneumonia, tuberculosis)**, articular fluid** (e.g. septic arthritis, prosthetic joint infection)**, pus** (e.g. abscess) and **biopsy** (e.g. of a lymph node) specimens are sent when clinically indicated.
- **Swabs** of clean wounds, without pus or surrounding cellulitis, are avoided because of the risk of identifying colonizing

bacteria and encouraging inappropriate antibiotic prescribing. Infection doctors prefer a specimen rather than a swab of a specimen; tissues, aspirates and fluids are usually preferred. Vaginal swabs are useful, however, to identify *Candida* spp., *Trichomonas vaginalis* and other bacterial causes of vaginitis; nucleic acid amplification techniques (see next section) are more commonly used to screen for *Neisseria gonorrhoeae* and *Chlamydia* spp.

- **Special culture techniques or prolonged culture** are required for *Mycobacteria* spp., slow-growing bacteria, such as *Actinomyces* spp. and *Brucella* spp., and sometimes fungi; the laboratory must be informed of patients with suspected unusual infections or infections due to fastidious microbes.
- **Faecal culture** should be reserved for cases of suspected bacterial gastroenteritis or dysentery, especially when there may be public health implications. Faecal culture for viruses is not helpful; antigen or nucleic acid detection techniques (see next section) are more appropriate, especially in the investigation of an outbreak of diarrhoea and vomiting (e.g. norovirus). Protozoa (e.g. amoebiasis, giardiasis) may be a cause of diarrhoea in returning travellers, immunocompromised patients, toddlers, men who have sex with men, and farm workers, and in any case of prolonged unexplained diarrhoea; antigen or PCR-based tests are a useful adjunct to traditional microscopy. Detection of a specific clostridial toxin is a more reliable test for *C. difficile* infection than culture.

Nucleic acid detection

Specific genes from many pathogenic microorganisms have been cloned and sequenced. Nucleic acid probes can be designed to detect these sequences, identifying pathogen-specific nucleic acid in body fluids or tissue. The use of nucleic acid amplification techniques (NAATs), such as PCR, has increased the power of these tests to detect very small quantities of microbial material. Such techniques not only are exquisitely sensitive, but also enable quantitation (e.g. viral load testing in HIV and hepatitis B and C) and subspeciation (e.g. at genotype level). NAAT tests have been widely used for viral infections (e.g. for influenza infection), but increasingly PCR-based bacterial identification is also employed in clinical practice. This allows 'screening' of clinical samples from sterile sites for a wider range of organisms, but because of the risk of detecting contaminating, colonizing or multiple bacteria, results must be interpreted carefully in the context of clinical findings.

Immunodiagnostic tests

These can be divided into two types:

- tests that detect **microbial components** (antigens), using a polyvalent antiserum or a monoclonal antibody (e.g. hepatitis B surface antigen, galactomannan in *Aspergillus* spp. infections)
- tests that detect an **antibody response** to infection (serological tests).

These investigations are valuable in the identification of organisms that are difficult to culture, especially viruses, atypical bacteria and fungi, and can also be helpful when antibiotics have been administered before samples were obtained. Elevated antibody titres on a single occasion (especially of immunoglobulin (Ig) G) are rarely diagnostic and it may be difficult to distinguish between past and acute infection. Paired serological tests taken a few weeks apart to observe IgG seroconversion, or specific assays for IgM antibodies (indicating an acute infection), are useful retrospectively to confirm the diagnosis, but rarely change the acute management of the patient. Avidity testing may also enable recent infection (low-avidity antibodies) and historical infection (high-avidity antibodies)

? Box 20.11 Key bacterial and fungal causes of bloodstream infections in the UK

Common bacterial causes of bloodstream infection	Potential sources (foci) of bloodstream infection
Gram-negative bacilli (rods)	
Escherichia coli and other coliforms	Urinary tract (most commonly) Biliary tract (common) Other intra-abdominal Healthcare-associated pneumonia; community-acquired pneumonia if *Klebsiella pneumoniae* Other HAIs Bone/joint/spine Meningitis (especially neonates)
Pseudomonas spp.	HAIs, especially pneumonia and i.v./urinary catheters (most common) Neutropenic mucositis Urinary tract Skin/soft tissue/wounds (less common) Bone/joint/spine (less common)
Bacteroides spp.	Intra-abdominal Wounds
Gram-positive cocci	
Staphylococcus aureus (MSSA and MRSA)	Skin/soft tissue/wounds Bone/joint/spine Endocarditis I.v. drug use, including infected deep venous thrombosis and septic pulmonary emboli Vascular infections, including grafts I.v. and urinary catheters Other HAIs Abscesses, especially psoas, epidural and pyomyositis Meningitis (rare)
Group A (*Streptococcus pyogenes*), B, C and G streptococci	Skin/soft tissue/wounds/necrotizing fasciitis Bone/joint/spine Genitourinary (esp. group B streptococci) Neonatal sepsis/meningitis (group B streptococci) Tonsillitis
Viridans group streptococci (e.g. *Streptococcus mitis* and *mutans* groups)	Endocarditis Abscesses, especially liver and brain Bone/joint/spine (rare)
Streptococcus pneumoniae (pneumococcus)	Upper/lower respiratory tract Pneumonia Meningitis Endocarditis (rare)
Coagulase-negative staphylococci	Usually skin contamination, but consider prosthesis/device infection if repeat multiple blood cultures are positive for same bacteria with same antibiotic susceptibilities
Enterococcus spp.	HAIs, especially i.v. and urinary catheters (common) Urinary tract Intra-abdominal Endocarditis
Gram-negative cocci	
Neisseria meningitidis (meningococcus)	Meningitis Bloodstream infection Others, including septic arthritis and pneumonia, are rare
Fungi	
Candida spp.	HAIs, especially i.v. catheters and other devices (common) Intra-abdominal (especially patients who have had abdominal surgery and prolonged hospital stay and/or are/have been in critical care) Urinary tract I.v. drug use Endocarditis

HAI, healthcare-associated infection; MRSA, meticillin-resistant *Staphylococcus aureus*; MSSA, meticillin-susceptible *Staphylococcus aureus*.

to be distinguished. Numerous serological tests are available; they should be used only in light of the clinical presentation and exposure/risk history.

Pyrexia of unknown origin

History, clinical examination and simple investigation will reveal the cause of a fever in many patients. In a small number, no diagnosis is apparent, despite continuing symptoms. The term pyrexia of unknown origin (PUO) is sometimes used to describe this problem. Various definitions have been suggested for PUO; a useful one is 'a fever persisting for more than 2 weeks, with no clear diagnosis despite intelligent and intensive investigation'. Patients who are known to have HIV or other immunosuppressive conditions are normally excluded from the definition of PUO, as the investigation and

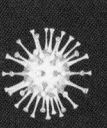

Box 20.12 Specimens and indications for microscopy, culture and other microbiological tests

Specimen	Investigation	Indication
Blood	Giemsa stain for malaria	Any symptomatic traveller returning from a malarious area
	Malaria rapid antigen detection test	
	Stains for other parasites	Specific tropical infections
	Culture	All suspected bacterial infections
Urine	Microscopy and culture	All suspected bacterial infections
	TB culture	Suspected TB Unexplained leucocytes in urine
	NAAT	STIs
Faeces	Microscopy ± iodine stain	Suspected protozoal diarrhoea; helminth infection
	Culture	All unexplained diarrhoea
	PCR/antigen detection	Suspected viral diarrhoea in children
	Clostridium difficile toxin	Diarrhoea following hospital stay or antibiotic treatment
Throat swabs	Culture	Suspected bacterial tonsillitis and pharyngitis
	PCR	Viral meningitis
	PCR/antigen detection	Viral respiratory infections where urgent diagnosis is considered necessary
Sputum	Culture	Pneumonia, respiratory tract infections
	Auramine stain/TB culture (liquid culture; see p. 968)	Suspected TB
	Other special stains/ cultures	Immunocompromised patients Suspected fungal infections
Cerebrospinal fluid	Microscopy and culture	Suspected meningitis
	Auramine stain/TB culture	Suspected TB, meningitis
	Other special stains/ cultures	Immunocompromised patients Suspected fungal infections
	PCR	Suspected encephalitis or viral or bacterial meningitis
Rash aspirate:		
Petechial	Microscopy and culture	Meningococcal disease
Vesicular	PCR/antigen detection/ viral culture	Herpes simplex/zoster

(NAAT, nuclear acid amplification test; PCR, polymerase chain reaction; STI, sexually transmitted infection; TB, tuberculosis.)

management of these patients are different. Successful diagnosis of the cause of PUO depends on knowledge of the likely and possible aetiologies; non-infection causes are common. These have been documented in a number of studies and are summarized in **Box 20.13**.

A detailed history and examination is essential, including a medication (the commencement of medications in relation to symptoms) and family history, and breast, spine and testicular examinations. Examination should be repeated on a regular basis to identify new signs as they appear. It is also worth retaking the history intermittently, as previously undisclosed important information, particularly about sexual exposures, may emerge. Investigative findings to date should be reviewed, obvious omissions amended and abnormalities followed up (e.g. raised serum liver enzymes trigger further thought about and possible investigation for liver and biliary tract pathologies; raised serum creatine kinase may suggest myositis or a medication-related adverse effect; a markedly elevated serum ferritin may suggest adult-onset Still's disease). Confirmation should be sought that the patient does have objective evidence of a raised temperature; this may require admission to hospital if the patient is not already under observation. Some people have an exaggerated circadian temperature variation (usually peaking in the evening), which is asymptomatic and not pathological.

The range of tests available has already been discussed. Investigation is guided by the history and particular abnormalities on examination or initial test results, but in some cases 'blind' investigation is necessary. Some investigations, especially blood cultures (at least three are taken), should be repeated regularly and prolonged culturing may be justified, depending on epidemiological exposure (e.g. *Brucella* spp.). Serial monitoring of inflammatory markers such as CRP allows assessment of progress. Ultrasound, echocardiography, CT, MRI, PET and labelled white-cell scanning can all help establish a diagnosis if used appropriately; the temptation to scan all patients with PUO from head to toe as a first measure should be avoided. Imaging may also be useful for identifying an appropriate site for biopsy. Biopsy of the bone marrow (and, less frequently, liver) may be useful, and temporal artery biopsy is used to confirm suspected temporal arteritis (see p. 464). Bronchoscopy is used to obtain samples for microbiological and histological examination if sputum specimens are inadequate or absent and a respiratory diagnosis is suspected. Molecular and serological tests have greatly improved the diagnosis of infectious causes of PUO, but these tests should be ordered and interpreted only in the context of the patient's presentation and exposure/risk history. Some non-infection conditions (e.g. lymphoma) can be challenging to diagnose and may, for example, require more than one lymph node biopsy.

Management

Management of a patient with a persistent fever is aimed at the underlying cause. If possible, only symptomatic treatment should be given until a clear diagnosis is made. Blind antibiotic therapy may make diagnosis of an occult infection more difficult, and empirical steroid therapy may cause deterioration of an infection or mask an inflammatory response without treating the underlying cause. In a few patients, no cause of fever is found, despite many months of investigation and follow-up. In most of these individuals, symptoms settle spontaneously, and if no definite cause has been identified after 2 years, the long-term prognosis is good.

Non-antimicrobial principles of infection care

See **Box 20.2** for other important concepts in infection and page 158 for infection source control (e.g. draining of an abscess) and finding the underlying focus in bloodstream infections.

? Box 20.13 Causes of pyrexia of unknown origin

Infection (20–40%)
- Pyogenic abscess
- Tuberculosis
- Infective endocarditis
- Toxoplasmosis
- Epstein–Barr virus infection
- Cytomegalovirus infection
- Primary HIV infection
- Brucellosis
- Lyme disease

Malignant disease (10–30%)
- Lymphoma
- Leukaemia
- Renal cell carcinoma
- Hepatocellular carcinoma
- Other malignancies

Vasculitides (15–20%)
- Adult Still's disease
- Systemic lupus erythematosus
- Granulomatosis with polyangiitis
- Giant cell arteritis
- Polymyalgia rheumatica

Miscellaneous (10–25%)
- Drug fevers
- Thyrotoxicosis
- Inflammatory bowel disease
- Sarcoidosis
- Granulomatous hepatitis
- Factitious fever
- Familial Mediterranean fever

Undiagnosed (5–25%)

Multidisciplinary infection care

It has increasingly been recognized that complex infections and infectious diseases cannot be managed singlehandedly by a lone specialist clinician, regardless of experience. Many infections require multidisciplinary teams to provide optimal care and clinical outcomes. A good example is that of orthopaedic infections. These require the expertise of multiple doctors (e.g. orthopaedic surgeons, plastic surgeons, infection doctors and radiologists), nurses (e.g. specialist outpatient parenteral antibiotic therapy (OPAT) staff), pharmacists and professionals allied to medicine, such as physiotherapists. Care plans are discussed at multidisciplinary meetings and/or clinics, which all attend. There are many other infections and situations for which the multidisciplinary team approach is necessary, such as HIV infection, tuberculosis, hepatitis, diabetic foot infection, OPAT, infection prevention and control, and antimicrobial stewardship. A weekly multidisciplinary infection meeting to discuss outpatients or inpatients with complicated infections is a standard of good departmental practice for adequately resourced infection departments.

Shared decision-making

Infection practice is often 'grey'. Patients frequently present with non-specific histories and examination findings, and tests are often not diagnostic. The degree of investigation and intervention is determined by the severity or seriousness of the clinical presentation. A clear diagnosis is not always possible, and it is therefore important to use a shared patient–healthcare professional decision-making approach to avoid tests, treatments or procedures that are unlikely to be of benefit. Discussing the following four questions with patients may be useful in determining appropriate investigation and management strategies:
- What are the benefits?
- What are the risks?
- What are the alternatives?
- What if I do nothing?

Confidentiality

Many infections (e.g. hepatitis, HIV and tuberculosis) continue to be associated with social stigma. It is important to maintain patient confidentiality about the diagnosis at all times. Case notes should not be left lying around and electronic patient records should not be visible in public areas. The patient's permission is always sought prior to discussion with spouses, partners, relatives or friends, or communication with their primary care physician, although the latter is always encouraged to facilitate high-quality integrated care. Confidentiality is broken only when there is an overwhelming individual or public health risk, although multidisciplinary discussion and legal advice are usually sought beforehand.

Re-evaluation

Patients with sepsis and other serious infections need to be evaluated regularly, sometimes several times a day. Whether as an outpatient or inpatient, those who remain symptomatic without a clear diagnosis are re-evaluated by retaking the history and performing repeat examinations and appropriate investigations using a shared decision-making approach. If the patient's clinical condition deteriorates or does not respond to therapy, or if adverse effects occur on intervention, careful re-evaluation is essential. Such patients are discussed at the hospital's multidisciplinary infection meeting.

Further reading

Bhargava A, Ralph R, Chatterjee B et al. Assessment and initial management of acute undifferentiated fever in tropical and subtropical regions. *BMJ* 2018; 363:k4766.
Drago F, Ciccarese G, Gasparini G et al. Contemporary infectious exanthems: an update. *Future Microbiol* 2017; 12:171–193.
Fishman JA. Infection in organ transplantation. *Am J Transplant* 2017; 17:856–879.
Infections parts 1 to 4. *Medicine* 2017, 45(10):587–656; 2017, 45(11):657–726; 2017, 45(12):727–806; 2018, 46(1):1–76.
Infectious Diseases Society of America. *Laboratory Diagnosis of Infectious Disease*; https://www.idsociety.org/practice-guideline/laboratory-diagnosis-of-infectious-diseases/.

EPIDEMIOLOGY AND PREVENTION OF INFECTIONS

Infectious diseases remain one of the main causes of morbidity and mortality in humans, particularly in low- and middle-income countries (LMICs), where they are associated with poverty and overcrowding. In high-income countries, increasing prosperity and hygiene (most importantly), along with universal immunization and antibiotics, have reduced the prevalence of infections. Increasingly, difficult-to-treat, antibiotic-resistant microorganisms are being isolated, however, and diseases such as HIV infection, influenza viruses, malaria, measles and Middle East respiratory syndrome (MERS) continue to be problematic. Ebola and Zika viruses have recently emerged as much greater concerns than they were historically.

Increased population mobility

There is increased global mobility, both enforced (as a result of war, civil unrest and natural disaster) and voluntary (for tourism

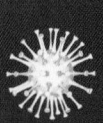

> **_i_ Box 20.14 Leading causes of mortality worldwide, 2016**
>
> | Cause of death | Mortality | |
> | --- | --- | --- |
> | | Millions (annual) | Crude mortality (/100 000) |
> | Ischaemic heart disease | 9.4 | 126 |
> | Stroke | 5.8 | 77 |
> | Chronic obstructive pulmonary disease | 3.0 | 41 |
> | Lower respiratory infections | 2.9 | 40 |
> | Alzheimer's disease and other dementias | 2.0 | 27 |
> | Trachea, bronchus and lung cancers | 1.7 | 23 |
> | Diabetes mellitus | 1.6 | 21 |
> | Road injury | 1.4 | 19 |
> | Diarrhoeal diseases | 1.4 | 19 |
> | Tuberculosis | 1.3 | 17 |
>
> _(Data from World Health Organization, www.who.int.)_

and economic benefit). This has aided the spread of infectious diseases and allowed previously localized pathogens to be imported and to establish themselves across much wider territories (e.g. New Delhi metallo-β-lactamase (NDM)-producing Gram-negative bacteria). Greater movement of livestock and animals has enabled the spread of zoonotic diseases, while changes in farming and food-processing methods have contributed to an increase in the incidence of food- and water-borne diseases. Deteriorating social conditions in the inner city areas of major conurbations have facilitated the resurgence of tuberculosis and other infections. Prisons and refugee camps, where large numbers of people are forced to live in close proximity, often in poor conditions, also continue to provide breeding grounds for devastating epidemics of infectious disease. There are ongoing concerns about the deliberate release of infectious agents, such as anthrax, by terrorist groups or national governments.

Changing patterns of disease

In LMICs, successes such as the eradication of smallpox, the near-eradication of Guinea worm infection (dracunculiasis) and reductions in leprosy have been balanced or outweighed by new problems. Communicable, maternal, neonatal and nutritional conditions, for example, were still responsible for 56% of deaths in the World Health Organization (WHO) African region in 2015. Although the leading causes of death globally are increasingly non-communicable diseases, lower respiratory tract infections, diarrhoeal diseases and tuberculosis are still the fourth, ninth and tenth most common causes of death, respectively (**Box 20.14**).

- New or relapsed cases of tuberculosis remain common at 140 per 100 000 population, with 600 000 cases of rifampicin-resistant (the most important anti-tuberculosis antibiotic) and 490 000 cases of multidrug-resistant tuberculosis diagnosed globally each year. Progress in reducing malaria has stalled, with funding being the main barrier; in 2016, there were 216 million patients with malaria globally, compared to 237 million in 2010 and 210 million in 2013.

- Some 325 million people live with hepatitis B or C, although the incidence of hepatitis B in those <5 years old has decreased from 4.7% in the pre-vaccine era to 1.3% in 2015.

- In 2016, approximately 1 million people (12% of whom were children) still died of HIV-related disease (compared to 1.9 million in 2005), despite the availability of effective therapy; globally, only half of those living with HIV receive anti-retroviral therapy. Global HIV incidence has fallen, however, from 0.4 per 1000 uninfected population in 2005 to 0.26 per 1000 uninfected population in 2016, but remains high in Africa (1.24 per 1000 population). Neglected tropical diseases, such as filariasis, onchocerciasis and trachoma, remain problematic, with 1.5 billion persons requiring mass or individual treatment in 2016 (versus 2 billion in 2010); 409 million persons were from low-income countries, which account for just 9% of the total global population.

Factors limiting control of infectious diseases in LMICs

Infections are often multiple and there is synergy between different infections (e.g. tuberculosis and HIV) and other factors such as malnutrition. Many of the infectious diseases affecting LMICs are preventable or treatable, but continue to thrive due to lack of money, infrastructure and political will. The surveillance of infectious diseases is generally poor in such countries, resulting in a slow response to emerging problems (e.g. Ebola in the West Africa region in 2013). It seems likely that the ongoing emergence of highly drug-resistant Gram-negative bacterial infections will affect the poor and vulnerable disproportionately. The impact of global warming on the spread and incidence of infections remains uncertain. Both natural climatic events and the gradual global change in weather conditions can affect the spread and transmission of infectious diseases. Changes in temperature directly influence the behaviour of insect vectors, while changes in rainfall have an effect on water-borne disease. Climate change also triggers population movement and migration, indirectly affecting infection transmission.

Goals in international development

The WHO set eight Millennium Development Goals (MDGs, see p. 278) that were meant to have been achieved by 2015, including combating HIV, malaria and other diseases; these have now evolved into 17 Sustainable Development Goals (SDGs). While a lot has been achieved by public/private partnerships and other charitable funders, it is clear that there is still much to be done, as is demonstrated by ongoing malaria transmission.

Acquisition of infection

Many infections are acquired from other people, who may be symptomatic or asymptomatic carriers. Some bacteria, like the meningococcus, are common transient commensals but cause invasive disease in a small minority of those colonized, sometimes after other infections such as influenza. Infections with other organisms, such as hepatitis B virus, can be followed in some cases by an asymptomatic but potentially infectious carrier state.

Box 20.15 Zoonotic infections

Disease	Pathogen	Animal reservoir	Mode of transmission
Prions			
vCJD	Prion protein	Cattle	Ingestion (CNS tissue)
Viruses			
Lassa fever	Arenavirus	Multimammate rats	Direct contact
Avian influenza	Influenza H5N1	Birds	Inhalation
Japanese encephalitis	Flavivirus	Pigs	Mosquito bite
Rabies	Rhabdovirus	Dogs and other mammals	Saliva, faeces (bats)
Yellow fever	Flavivirus	Primates	Mosquito bite
Monkeypox	Orthopox virus	Rodents, small mammals	Uncertain
SARS	Coronavirus	Unsure, most likely bats	Droplet
MERS	Coronavirus	Camels	Droplet
COVID-19	Coronavirus	Unsure, possible snakes or pangolin	Droplet
Bacteria			
Gastroenteritis	*Escherichia coli*	Cattle, chickens	Ingestion (contaminated food)
	Salmonella enteritidis and others	Chickens, cattle	Ingestion (meat, eggs)
	Campylobacter jejuni	Various, e.g. chickens	Ingestion (meat. milk, water)
Leptospirosis	*Leptospira interrogans*	Rodents	Ingestion (urine)
Brucellosis	*Brucella abortus*	Cattle.	Contact; ingestion of milk/cheese
	Brucella melitensis	Sheep goats	
Anthrax	*Bacillus anthracis*	Cattle, sheep	Contact; ingestion
Lyme disease	*Borrelia burgdorferi*	Deer	Tick bite
Cat-scratch disease	*Bartonella henselae*	Cats	Flea bite
Plague	*Yersinia pestis*	Rodents	Flea bite
Typhus	Various *Rickettsia* spp.	Various	Arthropod bite
Ornithosis (psittacosis)	*Chlamydia psittaci*	Psittacine and other birds	Aerosol
Others			
Toxoplasmosis	*Toxoplasma gondii*	Cats and other mammals	Ingestion (meat, faeces)
Hydatid disease	*Echinococcus granulosus*	Dogs	Ingestion (faeces)
Trichinosis	*Trichinella spiralis*	Pigs, bears	Ingestion (meat)
Toxocariasis	*Toxocara canis*	Dogs	Ingestion
Cutaneous larva migrans	*Ancylostoma caninum*	Dogs	Penetration of skin by larvae
Leishmaniasis	*Leishmania* spp.	Dogs	Ingestion

CNS, central nervous system; MERS, Middle East respiratory syndrome; SARS, severe acute respiratory syndrome; vCJD, variant Creutzfeldt–Jakob disease.

Zoonoses are infections that can be transmitted from wild or domestic animals to humans. Infection can be acquired in a number of ways:

- direct contact with the animal
- ingestion of meat or animal products
- contact with animal urine or faeces, aerosol inhalation
- via an arthropod vector
- by inoculation of saliva in a bite wound.

Many zoonoses can also be transmitted from person to person. Some zoonoses are listed in **Box 20.15**.

Most microorganisms do not have a vertebrate or arthropod host but are free-living in the environment. The vast majority of these environmental organisms are non-pathogenic but some can cause human disease (**Box 20.16**). Person-to-person transmission of these infections is rare. Some parasites may have a stage of their life cycle that is environmental (e.g. the free-living larval stage of *Strongyloides stercoralis* and the hookworms), even though the adult worm requires a vertebrate host. Other pathogens can survive for periods in water or soil and are transmitted from host to host via this route (see later); these should not be confused with true environmental organisms.

Routes of transmission

Endogenous infection

The body's own endogenous flora (often called the **microbiome**) can cause infection if the organism gains access to a usually sterile site. This can happen by simple mechanical transfer, such as when colonic bacteria enter the female urinary tract. The non-specific host defences may be breached, for example, by cutting or scratching the skin and allowing surface commensals to gain access to deeper tissues; this is frequently the aetiology of cellulitis. There may be more serious defects in host immunity owing to disease or chemotherapy, allowing normally harmless skin and bowel flora to produce invasive disease.

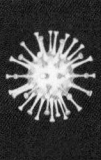

Box 20.16 Environmental organisms that can cause human infection

Organism	Disease (most common presentations)
Bacteria	
Burkholderia pseudomallei	Melioidosis
Burkholderia cepacia	Lung infection in cystic fibrosis
Pseudomonas spp.	Various
Legionella pneumophila	Legionnaires' disease (pneumonia)
Bacillus cereus	Gastroenteritis
Listeria monocytogenes	Various
Clostridium tetani	Tetanus
Clostridium perfringens	Gangrene, septicaemia
Non-tuberculous mycobacteria	Pulmonary infections
Fungi	
Candida spp.	Local and disseminated infection
Cryptococcus neoformans	Meningitis, pulmonary infection
Histoplasma capsulatum	Pulmonary infection
Coccidioides immitis	Pulmonary infection
Mucor spp.	Mucormycosis (rhinocerebral, cutaneous)
Sporothrix schenckii	Lymphocutaneous sporotrichosis
Blastomyces dermatitidis	Pulmonary infections
Aspergillus fumigatus	Pulmonary infections

Box 20.17 Infections transmitted by arthropod vectors

Vector	Disease	Microorganism
Mosquito	Malaria	*Plasmodium* spp.
	Lymphatic filariasis	*Wuchereria bancrofti, Brugia malayi*
	Yellow fever	Flavivirus
	West Nile fever	Flavivirus
	Dengue	Flavivirus
	Zika	Flavivirus
Sandfly	Leishmaniasis	*Leishmania* spp.
	Bartonellosis	*Bartonella bacilliformis*
Blackfly	Onchocerciasis	*Onchocerca volvulus*
Tsetse fly	Sleeping sickness	*Trypanosoma brucei*
Flea	Plague	*Yersinia pestis*
	Endemic typhus	*Rickettsia typhi*
Reduviid bug	Chagas' disease	*Trypanosoma cruzi*
Louse	Epidemic typhus	*Rickettsia prowazekii*
	Louse-borne relapsing fever	*Borrelia recurrentis*
Hard tick	Lyme disease	*Borrelia burgdorferi*
	Typhus (spotted fever group)	*Rickettsia* spp.
	Babesiosis	*Babesia* spp.
	Tick-borne relapsing fever	*Borrelia duttonii*
	Tick-borne encephalitis	Flavivirus
	Congo–Crimean haemorrhagic fever	Nairovirus (Bunyavirus)

Air-borne spread

Many respiratory tract pathogens are spread from person to person by aerosol or droplet transmission. Secretions containing the infectious agent are coughed, sneezed or breathed out and are then inhaled by a new host. Some enteric viral infections may also be spread by aerosols of faeces or vomit. Environmental pathogens, such as *Legionella pneumophila*, and zoonoses, such as ornithosis, are also acquired by aerosol inhalation, while rabies virus may be inhaled in the dust from bat droppings.

Faeco-oral spread

Transmission of organisms by the faeco-oral route occurs by direct transfer, by contamination of clothing or household items or, most commonly, via contaminated food or water. Human and animal faecal pathogens enter the food supply at any stage. Raw sewage is used as fertilizer in many parts of the world, contaminating growing vegetables and fruit. Poor personal hygiene can result in contamination during production, packaging, preparation or serving of food. In the Western world, centralization of the food supply and increased processing of food have allowed the potential for relatively minor episodes of contamination to cause widely disseminated outbreaks of food-borne infection.

Water-borne faeco-oral spread is usually the result of inadequate access to clean water and safe sewage disposal, and is common throughout the developing world. Worldwide, 5.2 billion people (71% of the global population) have access to clean water, but only 39% have access to safe sanitation. An estimated 870 000 deaths globally each year are due to unsafe water and sanitation and sub-optimal hygiene.

Vector-borne disease

Many tropical infections, including malaria, are spread from person to person or from animal to person by an arthropod vector. Vector-borne diseases are also found in temperate climates but are relatively uncommon, although may become more prevalent due to climate change. In most cases, part of the parasite life cycle takes place within the body of the arthropod and each parasite species requires a specific vector. Some vector-borne diseases are shown in **Box 20.17**.

Direct person-to-person spread

Organisms can be passed on directly in a number of ways. Sexually transmitted infections are dealt with in Chapter 37. Skin infections such as ringworm, and ectoparasites such as scabies and head lice, can be spread by simple skin-to-skin contact. Other organisms are passed on by transmission from blood (or, occasionally, some other body fluid) to blood. Blood-to-blood transmission can occur during sexual contact; from mother to infant, either transplacentally or in the peripartum; between intravenous drug users sharing any part of their injecting equipment; when infected medical or other (e.g. tattoo needles) equipment is reused; if contaminated blood or blood products are transfused; or in any sporting or accidental contact when blood is spilled. Ingestion of infected breast milk is another route of person-to-person spread for some infections (e.g. HIV), although in LMICs breastfeeding is still recommended when HIV-positive women are taking anti-retroviral therapy.

> **Box 20.18** Notifiable diseases in England and Wales[a]
>
> - Acute encephalitis
> - Acute infectious hepatitis
> - Acute meningitis
> - Acute poliomyelitis
> - Anthrax
> - Botulism
> - Brucellosis
> - Cholera
> - COVID-19
> - Diphtheria
> - Enteric fever (typhoid and paratyphoid)
> - Food poisoning
> - Haemolytic uraemic syndrome (HUS)
> - Infectious bloody diarrhoea
> - Invasive group A streptococcus
> - Legionnaires' disease
> - Leprosy
> - Malaria
> - Measles
> - Meningococcal septicaemia
> - Middle east respiratory syndrome (MERS)
> - Mumps
> - Plague
> - Rabies
> - Rubella
> - Scarlet fever
> - Severe acute respiratory syndrome (SARS)
> - Smallpox
> - Tetanus
> - Tuberculosis
> - Typhus
> - Viral haemorrhagic fever
> - Whooping cough
> - Yellow fever
> - Zika virus
>
> [a]Diseases are notifiable to Local Authority Proper Officers under the Health Protection (Notification) Regulations 2010. Report other diseases that may present significant risk to human health under the category 'other significant disease'.

Indirect person-to-person spread

Many organisms can be spread from person to person indirectly by contamination of fomites (e.g. door handles), which are subsequently touched by another person. Common examples include respiratory viruses, such as influenza, and healthcare-associated pathogens, such as MRSA and the spores of *C. difficile*. This is sometimes an overlooked route of transmission; minimization requires, for example, hand-washing immediately after sneezing or coughing and when moving from ward to ward in a hospital, and optimal cleaning regimens in institutions.

Direct inoculation

Infection can occur when pathogenic organisms breach the normal mechanical defences by direct inoculation (e.g. environmental contamination of bone after an open fracture, leading to subsequent osteomyelitis). Some of the circumstances in which this can occur are covered under endogenous infection and blood-to-blood transmission, described earlier. Some environmental organisms may be inoculated by accident; this is a common mode of transmission of tetanus and certain fungal infections. Rabies virus is inoculated by the bite of an infected animal.

Consumption of infected material

Although many food-related zoonotic infections are due to contamination of food with animal faeces (and are thus spread by the faeco-oral route), several diseases are transmitted directly in animal products. These include some strains of *Salmonella* (eggs, chicken meat), brucellosis (unpasteurized milk), *E. coli*, and the prion diseases kuru and variant Creutzfeldt–Jakob disease (vCJD; neural tissue).

Classification of outbreaks

The type of outbreak has a bearing on the public health measures that need to be instituted for its control.

- **Person-to-person** is where infection is passed from one infected individual to another and outbreaks of infection are separated by the incubation period. Control measures may include hand and personal hygiene (a sensible early control measure in any outbreak), immunization (e.g. influenza, measles) and antiviral agents (e.g. influenza).
- **Point source** is where there is a single source of infection, e.g. food eaten at a social function. All those infected will develop symptoms at the same time, around the expected incubation period. If the point source is temporary or removed, and provided there is no person-to-person or other mode of transmission, new cases decline after the incubation period.
- **Common source** is where there is a single source of infection but infections are spread over a period of time, e.g. a contaminated food preparation facility or restaurant. Many people may be exposed over a potentially long period of time. Once the source is identified, control measures may include cleaning and disinfecting the facility, closing the facility or restaurant, recalling food, and informing the public on how to make food safe (such as by cooking it) or to avoid or throw food away.
- **Epidemic** is when there is an increased and unusually widespread infection in the community, causing waves of infection. Epidemics spread through communities and may affect those who have no active immunity to that infection.
- **Pandemic** is an epidemic, as defined above, occurring worldwide or over a very wide geographical area and crossing international boundaries, usually affecting a large number of people.

Some infectious diseases should be notified to the public health authorities, so that they are aware of cases and outbreaks, and can respond accordingly. Diseases that are notifiable in England and Wales are listed in **Box 20.18** (see also Further reading for the *List of Notifiable Organisms (Causative Agents)* in the UK).

The prevention of and response to epidemics and pandemics is complex and depends on the underlying cause, but will be multifactorial in approach and may include:

- routine and enhanced disease surveillance
- identification and tracing of contacts, including rapid diagnostics, and epidemiological investigation
- public awareness campaigns (e.g. focused on hand and personal hygiene and/or other control measures; to provide reassurance)
- enhanced infection prevention and control procedures
- isolation or cohort nursing in healthcare facilities admitting patients and other institutions (e.g. nursing homes)
- use of mass antimicrobials (e.g. antiviral agents in influenza epidemics) and immunization as appropriate and available.

Efficient coordination of such responses by local, regional, national (e.g. Public Health England) or international organizations (e.g. WHO) is essential. The Ebola outbreak in West Africa in 2013 is a good example of how a slow initial response, in a challenging environment, can lead to grave consequences.

Infection prevention and control

Relatively few patients with infections present a serious risk to healthcare workers and other contacts or patients. The appearance of diseases such as strains of influenza with high mortality, the occasional importation of Lassa fever or Ebola (see p. 532), ongoing concerns about the bioterrorist use of microbes, and the emergence of extensively drug-resistant bacterial infections (e.g. tuberculosis and Gram-negative bacteria, especially carbapenemase-producing or carbapenemase-resistant *E. coli* and *K. pneumoniae*) mean that the potential remains for unexpected outbreaks of life-threatening or almost untreatable infections, including within healthcare settings.

During the worldwide outbreak of severe acute respiratory syndrome (SARS) in 2003, scrupulous infection control procedures reduced the spread of infection. However, in the 'inter-epidemic' period, it is difficult to maintain a high level of alert. Healthcare workers should remain vigilant because the early symptoms of many of these diseases are non-specific. Methods of preventing infection depend on the source and route of transmission.

Healthcare-associated infections

The burden of morbidity, mortality and costs attributed to healthcare-associated infection (HAI) has been highlighted in many high-income countries. Although data from LMICs are sparse, the impact of HAI is likely to be even greater. *C. difficile*, *Staph. aureus* (especially MRSA), vancomycin-resistant enterococci and the increasingly difficult-to-treat, multi- and extensively drug-resistant Gram-negative infections are all strongly associated with healthcare contact and remain a problem in hospitals worldwide. In 2011 the proportion of inpatients with an HAI in acute hospitals in England was 6.4%. In Europe, 1 in 18 inpatients have an HAI at any one time. The most frequent HAIs affect the respiratory and urinary tracts, as well as surgical sites. There has been a notable decline, however, in the incidences of, and mortality caused by, MRSA bloodstream and *C. difficile* infections in the UK. This has been due to higher standards of basic infection prevention and control, including rapid isolation of patients, hospital cleaning and universal MRSA screening (and decolonization therapy, if positive) on entry to acute hospitals and prior to surgery, and improved care of intravenous access devices.

HAI prevention and control measures

Poor infection control practice in hospitals and other healthcare environments can cause the transfer of infection from person to person. It is essential for all healthcare workers to wash or clean their hands before and after patient contact; whenever necessary, they should wear gloves, aprons and other protective equipment. This is particularly important when they are performing invasive procedures, dealing with infected wounds or manipulating indwelling devices. Care should also be taken when in contact with patients known to be colonized or infected with a resistant organism (e.g. carbapenemase-producing *K. pneumoniae*), those infected by communicable pathogens with high mortality (e.g. Ebola, for which high-security isolation and extreme care are mandatory), or those with diarrhoea (e.g. *C. difficile* infection).

Interventions that health workers should focus on to prevent and control HAIs are described here.

Care bundle approach

There is a set (typically 3–5) of simple actions – ideally, highly evidence-based – that healthcare professionals should always implement in a certain situation (e.g. inserting a urinary catheter) to minimize the risk of a negative outcome. As an example, see the *Matching Michigan* approach to reducing infections associated with central intravenous catheters (see Further reading).

Hand hygiene

The WHO's 'Five Moments for Hand Hygiene' (see Further reading) are applied before and after all patient contacts, including before and after aseptic procedures, and after contact with body fluids and the patient environment. Soap and water (rather than an alcohol-based rub) should be used after visible contamination of hands and when patients are vomiting or have diarrhoea, even if gloves are used. In low-income settings, in the absence of soap and water, alcohol-based hand rub should be used if available.

Personal protective equipment

Gloves should be worn for all invasive procedures, including venesection, and contact with sterile sites, mucous membranes, bodily fluids or non-intact skin. Disposable plastic aprons should be used when there is a risk of contamination of clothing or skin; if there is a risk of extensive contamination, surgical gowns should be worn. Respiratory protection should be worn for patients with high-consequence respiratory-spread pathogens, such as avian influenza and MERS.

Aseptic technique

This should be adopted for all invasive procedures, when using and manipulating invasive devices, and when in contact with all wounds.

Urinary catheters

These should be inserted only when it is essential to do so and then removed as soon as is possible; they must be inserted using an aseptic technique. A clear care plan should be in place for longer-term catheters. Overuse or poor care of urinary catheters increases the risk of *E. coli* bloodstream infection, a current target for HAI reduction in the UK.

Vascular access devices

Insert a vascular catheter only when there is a clear plan to use it; check the device daily and remove as soon as is possible. Use 2% chlorhexidine gluconate in 70% isopropyl alcohol for skin decontamination prior to insertion and to clean the access port or hub prior to use. Ensure that a clear care plan is in place for medium- or long-term devices.

Adequate hydration

Dehydrated patients are at higher risk of urinary tract infections. Oral hydration is preferred to intravenous if possible (there is a lower risk of infection with an intravenous device), and patients should be encouraged to drink a variety and an adequate quantity of fluids.

Communication

This is essential when transferring patients with transmissible infections (e.g. chickenpox, MERS, and infections caused by multi- and extensively drug-resistant bacteria) between admission areas, wards, hospitals and institutions, including residential and nursing homes.

Isolation

The appropriateness of isolation, if available, should be considered. Infections with a high risk to public health (e.g. Ebola and MERS) are isolated within high-security, hospital-based, negative-pressure isolation facilities using enhanced respiratory, personal protective equipment and decontamination procedures. In the UK there are only two such sites for the management of suspected Ebola infection. Patients hospitalized with highly infectious respiratory-spread pathogens, such as chickenpox and measles, are isolated in negative-pressure isolation facilities. Patients with high-consequence pathogens spread by direct or indirect person-to-person contact (colonization or infection), such as *C. difficile* and multi-drug-resistant Gram-negative bacteria, are, ideally, housed in side-rooms with *en suite* toileting facilities and appropriate contact precautions (hand hygiene and personal protective equipment). If there are few such facilities available, then risk assessment is essential (i.e. patients posing the highest risk to the health of the public, other patients and healthcare staff are housed in the available isolation facilities). If no such facilities exist, then basic precautions (hand hygiene, personal protective equipment, etc.) are still applied and cohort isolation is considered (i.e. patients with the same microbiologically confirmed infection are housed on the same ward).

Other infection prevention and control measures (non-HAI)

Although effective antimicrobial chemotherapy is available for many diseases, the ultimate aim of any infectious disease control programme is to prevent infection occurring. This is achieved either by:
* eliminating the source or mode of transmission of an infection (see p. 504), *or*
* reducing host susceptibility to environmental pathogens:

Eradication of reservoir

In a few diseases, for which humans are the only natural reservoir of infection, it may be possible to eliminate disease by an intensive programme of case-finding, treatment and immunization (as in the case of smallpox). If there is an animal or environmental reservoir, complete eradication is unlikely but local control methods may decrease the risk of human infection (e.g. killing of rodents to control plague, leptospirosis and other diseases).

For arthropod- or vector-borne infections

It may be possible to destroy the vector species and/or to take measures to avoid being bitten (e.g. insect repellent sprays, impregnated bed nets).

For food-borne infections

Improvements in food handling and preparation result in less contamination during processing, transport or preparation. Organisms that are intrinsically present in food can be killed by appropriate preparation and cooking. Improved surveillance and regulation of the food industry, as well as better health education for the public, are necessary.

For faeco-oral infections

Improvements in water supply and sanitation (recognized in the WHO's SDGs) could dramatically decrease the prevalence of faeco-oral infections.

For blood-borne infections

Blood transfer may be prevented by optimal use of medical equipment. Donated blood is routinely tested for infection in most high-income countries.

Box 20.19 Examples of passive immunization available

Infection	Antibody	Indication
Bacterial		
Tetanus	Human tetanus immune globulin	Prevention and treatment
Diphtheria	Horse serum	Prevention and treatment
Botulism	Horse serum	Treatment
Viral		
Hepatitis A Measles	Human normal immune globulin	Prevention (rarely required since vaccine introduced)
Hepatitis B	Human hepatitis B immune globulin	Prevention
Varicella zoster	Human varicella zoster immune globulin	Prevention

For infections spread by air-borne and direct contact

Some air-borne respiratory infections and some infections spread by direct contact can be controlled by isolating patients, although this is often difficult. Positive pressure isolation (in which the flow of air is from the patient's room into the ward) is useful in uninfected patients with severe immunodeficiency to protect them from infection. Neuraminidase inhibitors may reduce the transmission of influenza viruses to at-risk persons.

Immunization, immunoprophylaxis and immunotherapy

Immunization has changed the course and natural history of many infectious diseases. Passive immunization by administering preformed antibody, in the form of either immune serum or purified normal immunoglobulin, provides short-term immunity and has been effective in both the prevention (immunoprophylaxis) and the treatment (immunotherapy) of a number of bacterial and viral diseases (**Box 20.19**). The active immunization schedule currently recommended is summarized in **Box 20.20**. Long-lasting immunity is achieved only by active immunization with a live attenuated or an inactivated organism, or a subunit thereof (**Box 20.21**). Active immunization may also be performed with microbial toxin (either native or modified): that is, a toxoid. Immunization should be kept up to date, with booster doses being given throughout life according to the vaccines booster schedule. Travellers to LMICs, especially if visiting rural areas for prolonged periods, should enquire about further specific immunizations.

In 1974 the WHO introduced the Expanded Programme on Immunization (EPI). By 1994, more than 80% of the world's children had been immunized against tuberculosis, diphtheria, tetanus, pertussis, poliomyelitis and measles. It is hoped that poliomyelitis will be eradicated worldwide in the near future, matching the past success of global smallpox eradication. Introduction of conjugate vaccines against *Haemophilus influenzae* type b (Hib) and *Strep. pneumoniae* has proved highly effective in controlling invasive *H. influenzae* infection, notably meningitis, and reducing invasive pneumococcal disease, and can have a positive effect on antibiotic resistance (**Fig. 20.4**). The incidence of group C meningococcal infections in the UK is now so low that the childhood immunization schedule has been modified. A safe and immunogenic vaccine against *Neisseria meningitidis* serogroup B has now been included in the childhood

Box 20.20 Recommended childhood immunization schedules

Time of immunization	Vaccine
UK	
8 weeks old	Diphtheria, tetanus, pertussis (whooping cough), polio, Hib and hepatitis B (DTaP/IPV/Hib/HepB) Pneumococcal conjugate (PCV13) Rotavirus Meningococcal group B (MenB)
12 weeks old	Diphtheria, tetanus, pertussis, polio, Hib and hepatitis B (DTaP/IPV/Hib/HepB) Rotavirus
16 weeks old	Diphtheria, tetanus, pertussis, polio, Hib and hepatitis B (DTaP/IPV/Hib/HepB) Pneumococcal conjugate (PCV13) Meningococcal group B (MenB)
1 year old	Hib/MenC conjugate Pneumococcal conjugate (PCV13) Measles, mumps and rubella (MMR) Meningococcal group B (MenB)
Eligible paediatric age group	Influenza (live attenuated)
3 years and 4 months old, or soon after	Diphtheria, tetanus, pertussis and polio (DTaP/IPV) Measles, mumps and rubella (MMR)
12–13 years old	Human papillomavirus vaccine (HPV)
Around 14 years old	Tetanus, diphtheria and polio (Td/IPV) Meningococcus groups A, C, W and Y
WHO for all children[b]	
As soon as possible after birth	BCG + HBV
6 weeks old	DPT + PV + HBV + Hib + PCV + rotavirus
10 weeks old	DPT + PV + HBV + Hib + PCV + rotavirus
14 weeks old	DPT + PV + Hib + PCV + rotavirus
9 or 12 months old	Measles (second dose at a minimum of 4 weeks later) + rubella
As soon as possible after 9 years old	HPV (2 doses at least 6 months apart)

[a]For more detailed advice about childhood immunization, consult *The Green Book* (see Further reading). [b]Model scheme for all children; different schedules and/or additional vaccines are recommended in some locations: https://www.who.int/immunization/policy/Immunization_routine_table2.pdf?ua=1.
BCG, bacille Calmette–Guérin; DPT, diphtheria, pertussis, tetanus triple vaccine; HBV, hepatitis B vaccine; Hib, *Haemophilus influenzae* type b; HPV, human papillomavirus vaccine; PCV, pneumococcal conjugate vaccine; PV, polio vaccine. Mumps vaccine is also given in many developing countries.

Box 20.21 Examples of active immunization available

Live attenuated vaccines
- Oral polio (Sabin) (not recommended, used only for outbreaks)
- MMR (measles, mumps, rubella)[a]
- Rotavirus
- Varicella zoster
- Yellow fever
- BCG
- Typhoid

Toxoids
- Diphtheria
- Tetanus

Recombinant vaccines
- Hepatitis B

Inactivated and/or conjugate vaccines
- Hepatitis A
- Pertussis
- Typhoid – whole-cell and Vi antigen
- Polio (Salk) for routine use
- Influenza
- Human papillomavirus (HPV)
- Cholera (oral) – includes toxoid
- Meningococcus groups A, B, C, W135 and Y
- Rabies
- Anthrax
- Tick-borne encephalitis
- Japanese encephalitis
- Pneumococcal
- *Haemophilus influenzae* type b

[a] Individual vaccines for measles, mumps and rubella are not licensed in the UK. BCG, bacille Calmette–Guérin.

regularly updated) are often the best source of advice on travel health (see Further reading).

Further reading

Addisu A, Adriaensen W, Balew A et al.; Ethiopia SORT IT Neglected Tropical Diseases Group. Neglected tropical diseases and the sustainable development goals: an urgent call for action from the front line. *BMJ Glob Health* 2019; 4:e001334.
Gislason MK. Climate change, health and infectious disease. *Virulence* 2015; 6:539–542.
Pronovost P, Needham D, Berenholtz S et al. An intervention to decrease catheter-related bloodstream infections in the ICU. *N Engl J Med* 2006; 355:2725–2732.
World Health Organization. *Five Moments for Hand Hygiene*; https://www.who.int/gpsc/tools/Five_moments/en/.
World Health Organization. *Managing Epidemics: Key Facts about Major Deadly Diseases*; https://www.who.int/emergencies/diseases/managing-epidemics/en/.
https://travelhealthpro.org.uk *Travel Health Pro.*
https://www.gov.uk/government/collections/immunisation-against-infectious-disease-the-green-book *The Green Book – Immunisation Against Infectious Disease.*
https://www.gov.uk/guidance/notifiable-diseases-and-causative-organisms-how-to-report *List of Notifiable Organisms (Causative Agents)* for the UK.

vaccination schedules of some countries. Childhood immunization (e.g. tetanus) should be maintained throughout adulthood; this is often overlooked by patients and healthcare professionals alike.

Protection for travellers to developing/tropical countries

There has been a huge increase in the number of people travelling to developing countries, mainly for recreation, leisure and family visits. The risk of infection depends on the area to be visited, the type of activity and the underlying health of the traveller. Advice should always be based on an individual assessment.

Protection for travellers against infection can be divided into three categories (**Box 20.22**). Because situations and risks can change rapidly, websites such as Travel Health Pro (which are

PRINCIPLES AND MECHANISMS OF INFECTION

Host–organism interactions, including the human microbiome

Each of us is colonized by huge numbers of microorganisms (10^{14} bacteria, plus viruses, fungi, protozoa and worms), with which we coexist. Many mucosal surfaces and organs (e.g. skin, lungs, and

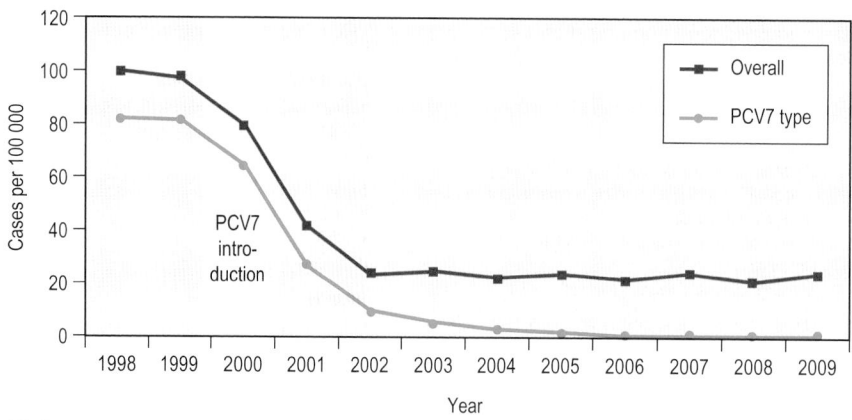

Fig. 20.4 Decline in invasive pneumococcal disease in young children following introduction of a pneumococcal conjugate vaccine (PCV) in the USA. (*From the Centers for Disease Control and Prevention, http://www.cdc.gov/pneumococcal/surveillance.html, with permission.*)

ⓘ Box 20.22 Protection for travellers against infection

Personal protection, e.g.:
- Insect repellents
- Impregnated bed netting
- Avoidance of animals
- Care with food and drink
- Condoms
- Care with travel (i.e. road traffic accidents)

Chemoprophylaxis, e.g. antimalarials

Immunization, e.g.:
- Yellow fever
- Hepatitis A and B
- Typhoid

---

gastrointestinal and genitourinary tracts) in humans have their own unique community of microbes, often called the **microbiome**. Within our gastrointestinal tract (GIT), for example, there are approximately 10^{11}–10^{12} microbes per gram of content with each person carrying at least 160 species, but often many more. A very high proportion of the GIT microbiome bacteria are anaerobic, which means that antibiotics with anti-anaerobic activity (e.g. clindamycin) can profoundly disrupt the nature of this microbial community. The human microbiome also acts as a reservoir for antimicrobial resistance, with many antimicrobials promoting the emergence of resistance through microbiome effects.

The development of the human microbiome is complex; normal vaginal delivery (or not Caesarian section), breast-feeding, diet and the living environment, for example, may have an impact on it. The effect of change in the human microbiome, particularly of the GIT, on host metabolism and immunity is increasingly associated with health states, including, for example, cancer (where it has been shown to change the patient's response to chemotherapy), diabetes and other metabolic diseases, host metabolism of medications, inflammatory bowel disease, mental health and rheumatological diseases. Early use of antibiotics, or disruption of the microbiome by other means, may therefore have a prolonged impact on microbiome community structure and, through that, on health and disease states later in life. On the other hand, it may be possible to protect and manipulate the microbiome therapeutically to the benefit of health, and not just infectious diseases; existing examples, not necessarily widely implemented in current clinical practice, include the use of probiotics and faecal transplantation to prevent and treat recurrent *C. difficile* infection, respectively, and selective decontamination of the digestive tract to prevent infections in critically ill patients.

Most microbiome microorganisms are commensal or symbiotic, living on or within humans without causing harm, but some are potentially pathogenic in the right circumstances: 'the right bug in the wrong place'. Infection and illness may be caused by microbes that are usually harmless evading the body's defences and infecting abnormal sites (e.g. *Staphylococcus epidermidis* and prosthetic joint infection). Endogenous GIT commensals may also cause disease in the host, either because they physically transfer to an inappropriate site (e.g. the bowel coliform *E. coli* causing urinary tract infection, sometimes called uropathogenic *E. coli*) or because the host immune response or the protective nature of endogenous bacteria has been reduced (e.g. oral candidiasis in an immunocompromised host and following exposure to antibiotics). Alternatively, disease may be caused by exposure to exogenous pathogenic organisms that are not part of the human microbiome (e.g. *Legionella* spp., rabies virus).

The symptoms and signs of infection are a result of the interaction between host and pathogen. In some cases, such as the early stages of influenza, symptoms are almost entirely due to killing of host cells by the invading organism. Usually, however, the harmful effects of infection are caused by a combination of direct microbial pathogenicity and the body's immune response to infection. In meningococcal bloodstream infection, for example, much of the tissue damage is caused by cytokines released in an attempt to fight bacteria.

Specificity of microorganisms

When the wrong microbes reach the right place, they are often highly specific with respect to the organ or tissue they infect (see p. 490). For example, a number of viruses are hepatotropic, such as those responsible for hepatitis A, B, C and E, and for yellow fever. This predilection for specific sites in the body relates partly to the presence of appropriate receptors on different cell types, partly to the immediate environment in which the organism finds itself, and partly to the nature of the organism. *Staph. epidermidis*, for example, is a facultative anaerobe (i.e. can live in oxygenated and non-oxygenated environments) that usually lives on the human skin, an aerobic environment, but which has a predilection to forming biofilms on medical devices (e.g. of central venous lines and hip replacements) in less aerobic environments when it reaches the right place. Other important facultative anaerobes include *E. coli*, other staphylococcal species and streptococci species. In contrast, *Mycobacterium tuberculosis* is an obligate aerobe (i.e. it needs oxygen) and *Bacteroides* spp. (found in the human GIT) and *Clostridium* spp. are obligate anaerobes (i.e. cannot live in atmospheric conditions), which partly explains the nature of the infections these bacteria cause. *Clostridium* spp. form spores, however, that enable survival in atmospheric conditions, and thereby their spread to the GIT of other human hosts.

Even within a species of bacterium there are sometimes clear differences between strains with regard to their ability to cause certain clinical presentations. There are many different strains of *Streptococcus pneumoniae*, for example, with some asymptomatically colonizing the nasopharyngeal microbiome, some more likely to invade and cause pneumococcal bloodstream infection, and certain different invasive strains more likely to cause empyema or meningitis, while other strains are more likely to cause pneumonia without bloodstream infection. Likewise, some strains of *E. coli* (enterotoxin-producing strains) are more likely to cause gastrointestinal disease (see p. 539), whereas uropathogenic *E. coli* are more likely to cause UTI.

Pathogenesis

Fig. 20.5 summarizes some of the steps that are followed during the pathogenesis of infection. Pathogens have developed a variety of mechanisms to evade host defences. For example, some produce toxins directed at phagocytes – *Staph. aureus* (α-toxin), *Strep. pyogenes* (streptolysin) and *Clostridium perfringens* (α-toxin) – while others can survive within macrophages. Several pathogens possess a capsule that protects against complement activation (e.g. *Strep. pneumoniae*). Antigenic variation can also help evasion of host defences – for example, antigenic shift and drift in influenza – which is the reason why influenza vaccines are modified from year to year.

Epithelial attachment

Many bacteria attach to epithelium cells using the adhesion molecules (called adhesins) of specific organelles called pili (or fimbriae). Enterotoxigenic and uropathogenic *E. coli* use fimbriae, for example, to attach to enterocytes and urothelial cells, respectively. Following attachment, some bacteria, such as *Staph. epidermidis* and *Pseudomonas aeruginosa*, may produce an extracellular 'slime' layer and recruit additional bacteria to form a 'protective' biofilm. Biofilms are difficult to eradicate and are frequently associated with medical devices and persistent infections. Many viruses and protozoa (e.g. *Plasmodium* spp., *Entamoeba histolytica*) attach to specific epithelial target-cell receptors, while others have attachment organs (e.g. the buccal plates of hookworms) that firmly grip the intestinal epithelium.

Colonization and invasion

Following epithelial attachment, pathogens may remain on the surface epithelium or tissue invasion may follow.

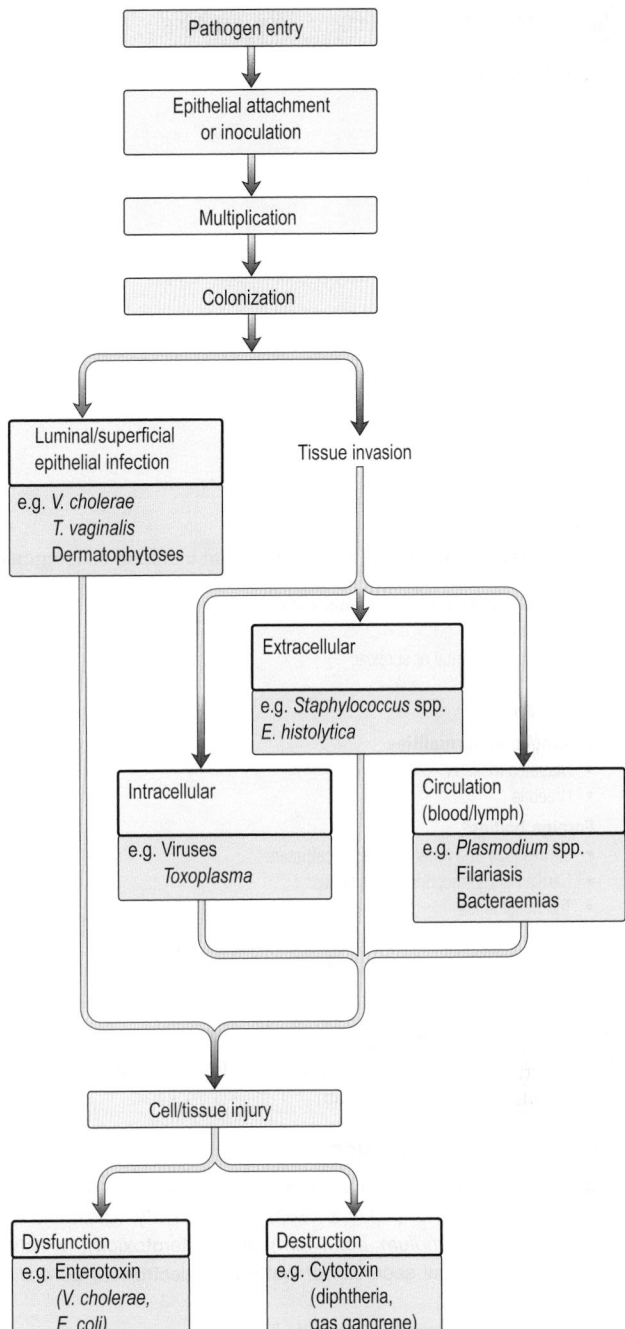

Fig. 20.5 The pathogenesis of infection.

Invasion may result in:
- an intracellular location for the pathogen (e.g. viruses, *Mycobacterium* spp., *T. gondii*, *Plasmodium* spp.)
- an extracellular location for the pathogen (e.g. pneumococci, *E. coli*, *E. histolytica*)
- invasion directly into the blood or lymph circulation (e.g. schistosome schistosomula and trypanosomes).

Tissue dysfunction or damage

Microorganisms produce disease by a number of mechanisms, as described here.

? Box 20.23 Clinical conditions produced by *Staphylococcus aureus*

Due to invasion

Skin
- Furuncles
- Cellulitis
- Impetigo
- Carbuncles

Lungs
- Pneumonia
- Lung abscesses

Heart
- Endocarditis
- Pericarditis

Central nervous system
- Meningitis
- Brain abscesses

Bones and joints
- Osteomyelitis, arthritis

Miscellaneous
- Parotitis
- Pyomyositis
- Septicaemia
- Enterocolitis

Due to toxin
- Staphylococcal food poisoning
- Scalded skin syndrome
- Bullous impetigo
- Staphylococcal scarlet fever
- Toxic shock syndrome

---

i Box 20.24 Examples of host factors that increase susceptibility to staphylococcal infections[a]

Injury to skin or mucous membranes
- Abrasions
- Trauma (accidental or surgical)
- Burns
- Insect bites

Metabolic abnormalities
- Diabetes mellitus
- Uraemia

Foreign bodies[b]
- Intravenous and other indwelling catheters
- Cardiac and orthopaedic prostheses
- Tracheostomies

Abnormal leucocyte function
- Job's syndrome
- Chédiak–Higashi syndrome
- Steroid therapy
- Drug-induced leucopenia

Postviral infections
- Influenza

Miscellaneous conditions
- Excess alcohol consumption
- Malnutrition
- Malignancies
- Old age
- Recent antibiotic therapy

[a]Predominantly *Staphylococcus aureus*. [b]Often *Staph. epidermidis*.

Cell lysis

The presence of replicating viruses may interfere with host-cell metabolism, resulting in cell death.

Exotoxins and endotoxins

- ***Exotoxins*** have many diverse actions, including inhibition of protein synthesis (diphtheria toxin), neurotoxicity (*Clostridium tetani* and *Clostridium botulinum*) and enterotoxicity, which results in intestinal secretion of water and electrolytes (*E. coli*, *Vibrio cholerae*).
- ***Endotoxin*** is a lipopolysaccharide (LPS) in the cell wall of Gram-negative bacteria. It is responsible for many of the features of sepsis (see p. 156). The effects of endotoxin are mediated predominantly by release of tumour necrosis factor (TNF).

The clinical expression of disease caused by *Staph. aureus* varies according to site, invasion and toxin production (**Box 20.23**). Furthermore, host susceptibility to infection may be linked to genetic or acquired defects in host immunity that may complicate intercurrent infection, injury, ageing and metabolic disturbances (**Box 20.24**).

Host response to infection
Natural defences

The natural host defences to infection are those of an intact surface epithelium with local production of secretions, antimicrobial enzymes (e.g. lysozyme in the eye) and, in the stomach, gastric acidity. The latter is reduced by proton pump inhibitors, increasing the risk of some gastroenteritic infections, including *C. difficile* infection. The mucociliary escalator of the large airways is destroyed by smoking.

Immunological defences

The immunological response to infection is described in Chapter 3.

Metabolic and immunological consequences of infection

Fever

Body temperature is controlled by the thermoregulatory centre in the anterior hypothalamus and is usually maintained at approximately 36.8°C in health, with diurnal and inter-individual variation of about ±1.0°C. Gram-negative bacteria contain LPS and peptidoglycan; the latter is also a component of Gram-positive bacterial cell walls. Monocytes and dendritic cells recognize these, leading to the formation of inflammatory cytokines, such as interleukin (IL)-1, IL-6, IL-12, tumour necrosis factor alpha (TNF-α) and many others. These act on the thermoregulatory centre by increasing prostaglandin (PGE$_2$) synthesis. The antipyretic effect of salicylates is brought about, at least in part, through their inhibitory effects on prostaglandin synthase.

Fever production has a positive effect on the course of infection. However, for every 1°C rise in temperature, there is a 13% increase in resting metabolic rate and oxygen consumption. Fever leads to

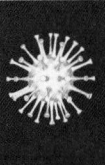

i Box 20.25 Human DNA viruses

Structure		Approximate size	Family	Viruses
Symmetry	*Envelope*			
Icosahedral	–	80 nm	Adenovirus	**Adenoviruses** (>50 serotypes)
Icosahedral	+	100 nm (160 nm with envelope)	Herpesvirus	**Herpes simplex virus types 1 and 2** **Varicella zoster virus** **Cytomegalovirus** **Epstein–Barr virus** **Human herpesvirus type 6 (HHV-6)** **Human herpesvirus type 7 (HHV-7)** **Human herpesvirus type 8 (HHV-8)**
Icosahedral	+	42 nm	Hepadnavirus	**Hepatitis B virus (HBV)**
Icosahedral	–	50 nm	Papillomavirus	**Human papillomaviruses** (>100 types)
Icosahedral	–	40–45 nm	Polyomavirus	**Polyomaviruses JC, BK, KI, WU**
Icosahedral	–	23 nm	Parvovirus	**Erythrovirus B19, bocavirus**
Complex	+	300 nm × 200 nm	Poxvirus	**Variola virus** **Vaccinia virus** **Monkeypox** **Cowpox** **Orf** **Molluscum contagiosum**

increased energy requirements, therefore, at a time when anorexia leads to decreased food intake, resulting in an increase in skeletal muscle breakdown to provide energy. Fever in non-infection conditions can be deleterious.

The inflammatory response

The inflammatory response is a fundamental biological response to a variety of stimuli, including microorganisms or their products, such as endotoxin, which acts on monocytes and macrophages. Non-phagocytic cells (lymphocytes, natural killer cells) are also involved. The release of cytokines – notably, TNF-α, IL-1, IL-6 and interferon gamma (IFN-γ) – leads to the release of a cascade of other mediators involved in inflammation and tissue remodelling, such as interleukins, prostaglandins, leukotrienes and corticotropin. See Further reading for more information about the pathogenesis of infection by some key human bacterial, viral and protozoan pathogens.

Further reading

McLellan LK, Hunstad DA. Urinary tract infection: pathogenesis and outlook. *Trends Mol Med* 2016; 22:946–957.

Musser JM, DeLeo FR. Molecular pathogenesis lessons from the world of infectious diseases research. *Am J Pathol* 2015; 185:1502–1504; https://www.ncbi.nlm.nih.gov/pmc/articles/PMC4450309/. *Editorial on four associated articles.*

Selber-Hnatiw S, Rukundo B, Ahmadi M et al. Human gut microbiota: toward an ecology of disease. *Front Microbiol* 2017; 8:1265.

Thomer L, Schneewind O, Missiakas D. Pathogenesis of Staphylococcus aureus bloodstream infections. *Annu Rev Pathol* 2016; 11:343–364.

Walter EJ, Hanna-Jumma S, Carraretto M et al. The pathophysiological basis and consequences of fever. *Crit Care* 2016; 20:200.

VIRAL INFECTIONS

Viruses are much smaller than other infectious agents and carry their genome as either DNA or RNA (but never both). Details of the structure, size and classification of human DNA and RNA viruses are shown in **Boxes 20.25** and **20.26**, respectively. Since viruses are metabolically inert, they must live intracellularly, using the host cell for synthesis of viral proteins and nucleic acid. Viruses have a central nucleic acid core (genome) surrounded by a protective protein coat (capsid) that is antigenically unique for a particular virus.

The capsid imparts a helical or icosahedral structure to the virus. Some viruses also possess an outer envelope consisting of lipid and protein.

OUTCOMES OF VIRUS INFECTION OF A CELL

Replication of viruses within a cell may result in sufficient distortion of normal cell function to result in cell death: a ***cytocidal*** or ***cytolytic*** infection. However, acute cell death is not an inevitable consequence of virus infection of a cell. In a ***chronic***, or ***persistent***, infection, virus replication continues throughout the lifespan of the cell but does not interfere with the normal cellular processes necessary for cell survival. Hepatitis B and C viruses may interact with cells in this way. Some viruses, such as those of the herpesvirus family, are able to go ***latent*** within a cell; in such a state, the virus genome is present within the cell, but there is very little, if any, production of viral proteins and no production of mature virus particles. Finally, some viruses are able to ***transform*** cells, leading to uncontrolled cell division: for example, Epstein–Barr virus infection of B lymphocytes, resulting in the generation of an immortal lymphoblastoid cell line.

VIRUS INFECTIONS OF THE SKIN AND MUCOUS MEMBRANES

Many virus infections are associated with skin rashes (exanthems) or eruptions on the mucous membranes (enanthems) (see **Box 20.9**), and so clinical syndromes based on the nature of the rash (which may be ***vesicular*** (i.e. consisting of fluid-filled vesicles) or ***maculopapular***) are often highly specific to the causative agent.

Vesicular viral rashes

Herpes simplex virus infection

Members of the *Herpesviridae* family of viruses cause a wide range of human diseases (**Box 20.27**). The hallmark of all herpesvirus

Box 20.26 Human RNA viruses

Structure		Approximate size	Family	Viruses
Symmetry	Envelope			
Icosahedral	–	30 nm	Picornaviruses	**Poliovirus** **Coxsackievirus** **Echovirus** **Enterovirus 68–71** **Hepatitis A virus** **Rhinovirus**
Icosahedral	–	80 nm	Reoviruses	**Reovirus** **Rotavirus**
Icosahedral	+	50–80 nm	Togaviruses	**Rubella virus** **Alphaviruses**
Icosahedral	+	50–80 nm	Flaviviruses	**Yellow fever virus** **Dengue virus** **Zika virus** **Japanese encephalitis virus** **West Nile virus** **Hepatitis C virus** **Tick-borne encephalitis virus**
Spherical	+	80–100 nm	Bunyaviruses	**Congo–Crimean haemorrhagic fever** **Hantavirus** **Rift Valley fever virus**
Spherical	–	35–40 nm	Caliciviruses	**Norovirus** **Sapovirus**
Spherical	–	28–30 nm	Astroviruses	**Astrovirus**
Spherical	–	30–34 nm	Hepeviruses	**Hepatitis E virus**
Helical	+	80–120 nm	Orthomyxoviruses	**Influenza viruses A, B and C**
Helical	+	100–300 nm	Paramyxoviruses	**Parainfluenza viruses 1–4** **Measles virus** **Mumps virus** **Respiratory syncytial virus** **Human metapneumovirus** **Nipah virus** **Hendra virus**
Helical	+	80–220 nm	Coronaviruses	**229E, OC43, NL63, HK1, SARS, MERS, SARS-CoV2**
Helical	+	60–175 nm	Rhabdoviruses	**Lyssavirus – rabies**
Helical	+	100 nm	Retroviruses	**Human immunodeficiency viruses 1 and 2** **Human T-cell leukaemia/lymphotropic viruses 1 and 2**
Helical	+	100–300 nm	Arenaviruses	**Lassa virus** **Lymphocytic choriomeningitis virus**
Pleomorphic	+	Filaments or circular forms; 100 × 130–2600 nm	Filoviruses	**Marburg virus** **Ebola virus**

MERS, Middle East respiratory syndrome; SARS, severe acute respiratory syndrome.

infections is the ability of the viruses to establish latent infections that persist for the life of the individual.

Two types of herpes simplex virus (HSV; **Fig. 20.6**) have been identified: HSV-1 is the major cause of herpetic stomatitis, herpes labialis ('cold sore'), keratoconjunctivitis and encephalitis, whereas HSV-2 causes genital herpes and may also be responsible for systemic infection in the immunocompromised host. These divisions are not rigid, however, for HSV-1 can give rise to genital herpes and HSV-2 can cause infections in the mouth. The site of latency for both HSV-1 and 2 is the nerve cell body.

HSV-1

The portal of entry of HSV-1 infection is usually via the mouth or, occasionally, the skin. The primary infection may go unnoticed, or may produce a severe inflammatory reaction with vesicle formation leading to painful ulcers (gingivostomatitis; **Fig. 20.7**). Latent virus may be reactivated from the trigeminal ganglion by stress, trauma, febrile illnesses and ultraviolet radiation, producing the recurrent form of the disease known as herpes labialis ('cold sore'). Approximately 70% of the population is infected with HSV-1 and recurrent infections occur in one-third of individuals. Reactivation often produces localized paraesthesiae in the lip before the appearance of a cold sore.

Complications of HSV-1 infection include transfer to the eye (dendritic ulceration, keratitis), acute encephalitis (see p. 871), nail-bed infections (herpetic whitlow) and erythema multiforme (p. 678).

HSV-2

The clinical features, diagnosis and management of genital herpes are described on page 1421. The virus remains latent in the sacral ganglia and, during recurrence, can produce a radiculomyelopathy, with pain in the groin, buttocks and upper thighs. Primary anorectal herpes infection is common in men who have sex with men.

Box 20.27 Major diseases caused by human herpesviruses

Subfamily	Virus	Children	Adults	Immunocompromised
Alphaherpesviruses	Herpes simplex type 1	Stomatitis[a] Herpes simplex encephalitis	Cold sores Herpes simplex encephalitis Keratitis Erythema multiforme	Dissemination
	Herpes simplex type 2	Neonatal herpes[a]	Primary genital herpes[a] Recurrent genital herpes	Dissemination
	Varicella zoster virus	Chickenpox[a]	Shingles	Dissemination
Betaherpesviruses	Cytomegalovirus	Congenital[a]	Infectious mononucleosis[a] Hepatitis	Pneumonitis Retinitis Hepatitis Gastrointestinal
	Human herpesvirus type 6	Roseola infantum[a]		Pneumonitis Encephalitis
	Human herpesvirus type 7	Roseola infantum[a]		?Encephalitis
Gammaherpesviruses	Epstein–Barr virus		Infectious mononucleosis[a] Burkitt's lymphoma Nasopharyngeal carcinoma	Lymphoma
	Human herpesvirus type 8		Kaposi's sarcoma	Kaposi's sarcoma

[a]Signifies primary infection.

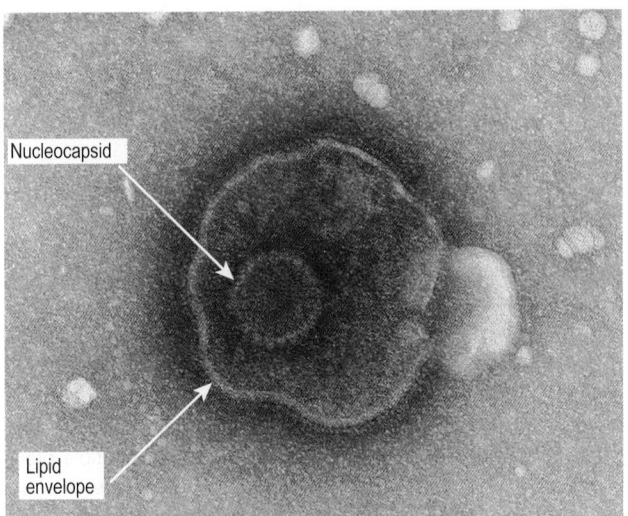

Fig. 20.6 Electron micrograph of herpes simplex virus.

Nucleocapsid

Lipid envelope

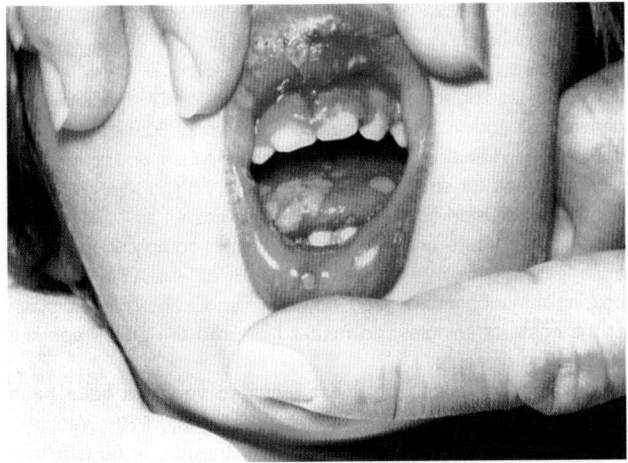

Fig. 20.7 Primary herpes simplex type 1 (gingivostomatitis).

Neonates may develop primary HSV infection following vaginal delivery in the presence of active genital HSV infection in the mother, particularly if the maternal disease is a primary, rather than a recurrent, infection. The disease in the baby varies from localized skin lesions (about 10–15%) to widespread visceral disease most often affecting the lungs, liver and brain, with a poor prognosis. Caesarean section should therefore be performed if active genital HSV infection is present during labour.

Immunocompromised patients, such as those receiving intensive cancer chemotherapy or those with acquired immunodeficiency syndrome (AIDS), may develop disseminated HSV infection involving many of the viscera. In severe cases, death may result from hepatitis and encephalitis. Eczema herpeticum is a serious complication in individuals with eczema, where the non-intact skin allows spread of lesions across large areas and bloodstream access, which may lead to herpetic involvement of internal organs.

Diagnosis and management

Confirmation of clinical diagnosis is most commonly obtained by detection of HSV DNA in vesicle fluid by genome amplification. Treatment of HSV-associated disease is with aciclovir and derivatives.

Varicella (chickenpox) and herpes zoster (shingles)

Infection with varicella zoster virus (VZV), another herpesvirus, produces two distinct diseases: varicella (chickenpox) and herpes zoster (shingles). The **primary infection**, chickenpox, usually occurs in childhood, the virus entering through the mucosa of the upper respiratory tract. In some countries (e.g. the Indian subcontinent), a different epidemiological pattern exists, with most infections occurring in adulthood. Chickenpox is rarely contracted twice by the same individual. Infectious virus is spread from the throat and from fresh skin lesions by air-borne transmission or direct contact. The period of infectivity in chickenpox extends from 2 days before the appearance of the rash until the skin lesions are all at the crusting stage. Following recovery from chickenpox, the virus remains latent in dorsal root and cranial nerve ganglia. **Reactivation** of infection results in shingles.

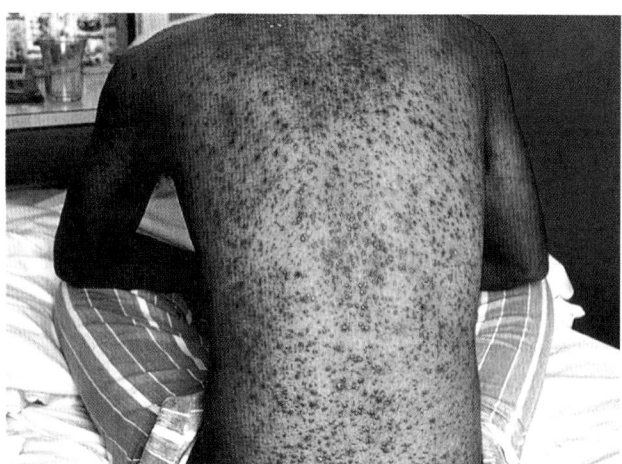

Fig. 20.8 Chickenpox in an adult. Generalized varicella zoster virus (VZV) infection.

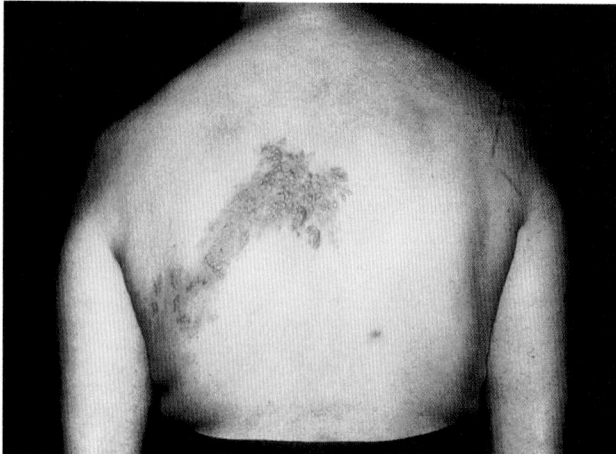

Fig. 20.9 Shingles. Varicella zoster virus (VZV) affecting a dermatome. (*Reproduced with kind permission of the Imperial College School of Medicine.*)

Clinical features of chickenpox

Some 14–21 days after exposure to VZV, a brief prodromal illness of fever, headache and malaise heralds the eruption of chickenpox, characterized by the rapid progression of macules to papules to vesicles to pustules in a matter of hours (**Fig. 20.8**). In young children the prodromal illness may be very mild or absent. The illness tends to be more severe in older children and can be debilitating in adults. The lesions occur on the face, scalp, trunk and, to a lesser extent, the extremities. It is characteristic to see lesions at all stages of development on the same area of skin. Fever subsides as soon as new lesions cease to appear. Eventually, the pustules crust and heal without scarring.

Complications include pneumonia, which generally begins 1–6 days after the skin eruption, and bacterial superinfection of skin lesions. Pneumonia is more common in adults than in children, and cigarette smokers are at particular risk. Pulmonary symptoms are usually more striking than the physical findings, although a chest X-ray usually shows diffuse changes throughout both lung fields. Central nervous system (CNS) involvement occurs in about 1 per 1000 cases and most commonly presents as an acute truncal cerebellar ataxia. The immunocompromised are susceptible to disseminated infection, with multiorgan involvement. Women in pregnancy are prone to severe chickenpox and, in addition, there is a risk of intrauterine infection with structural damage to the fetus (if maternal infection is within the first 20 weeks of pregnancy, the risk of varicella embryopathy is 1–2%).

Clinical features of shingles

Shingles (see p. 672) arises from the reactivation of VZV latent within the dorsal root or cranial nerve ganglia. It may occur at any age but is most common in the elderly, producing skin lesions similar to those of chickenpox, although classically they are unilateral and restricted to a sensory nerve (i.e. dermatomal) distribution (**Fig. 20.9**). The onset of a shingles rash is usually preceded by severe dermatomal pain, indicating the involvement of sensory nerves in its pathogenesis. Virus is disseminated from freshly formed vesicles and may cause chickenpox in susceptible contacts.

The most common complication of shingles is post-herpetic neuralgia (PHN; see p. 672). Occurrence of PHN is related to age (more likely in the elderly) and the intensity of the original shingles rash.

Diagnosis

The diseases are usually recognized clinically but can be confirmed by detection of VZV DNA within vesicular fluid, electron microscopy, immunofluorescence or culture of vesicular fluid, and serology.

Prevention and management

Chickenpox usually requires no treatment in healthy children and infection results in life-long immunity. Aciclovir and derivatives are licensed for this indication in the USA. However, the disease may be fatal in the immunocompromised, who should therefore be offered protection after exposure to the virus, with zoster-immune globulin (ZIG) and high-dose aciclovir at the first sign of development of the disease.

Antiviral therapy with aciclovir or a similar drug may be offered to patients over the age of 16 years, if they present within 72 hours of onset. Prophylactic ZIG is recommended for susceptible pregnant women exposed to VZV and, if chickenpox develops, aciclovir treatment should be given but the drug is *not* licensed for use in pregnancy. If a woman has chickenpox at term, her baby should be protected by ZIG if delivery occurs within 7 days of the onset of the mother's rash. An effective live attenuated varicella vaccine is licensed as a routine vaccination of childhood in the USA; it is available on a named patient basis in the UK and for susceptible healthcare workers.

Shingles involving motor nerves – for example, the VIIth cranial nerve, leading to facial palsy – is also treated with aciclovir (or derivatives). Antiviral therapy has been shown to reduce the burden of PHN when treatment is given in the acute phase, and is therefore recommended for shingles in the over-65s. Shingles involving the ophthalmic division of the trigeminal nerve has an associated 50% incidence of acute and chronic ophthalmic complications. Early treatment with aciclovir reduces this to 20% or less. As for chickenpox, all immunocompromised individuals should be given aciclovir at the onset of shingles, no matter how mild the attack appears when it first presents.

Both recombinant and live attenuated vaccines have been shown to reduce shingles-related morbidity and PHN. Vaccination is recommended for all adults over the age of 60 (USA) or 70 (UK).

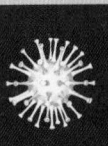

i **Box 20.28** Enteroviruses (excluding polioviruses)

Disease	Coxsackievirus		Echovirus	Enterovirus
	A (Types A1–A22, A24)	B (Types B1–B6)	(Types 1–9, 11–17, 29–33)	(Types 68–71)
Cutaneous and mucosal				
Herpangina	+++	+	+	
Hand, foot and mouth	+++	+	+	++
Erythematous rashes	+	+	+++	
Conjunctivitis	+			
Neurological				
Paralytic	+	±	+	+
Meningitis	++	++	+++	+
Encephalitis	++	++	±	+
Cardiac				
Myocarditis and peri-carditis	+	+++		
Muscular				
Myositis (Bornholm disease)	+	+++	+	

+++, often causes; ++, sometimes causes; +, rarely causes; ±, possibly causes.

Picornavirus infections

The picornaviruses (pico = small) are a large family of RNA viruses, which includes the enteroviruses, rhinoviruses, parecho-viruses and also hepatitis A virus (see p. 1276). The term entero-virus refers to their enteric means of spread: that is, via the faecal–oral route. The enteroviruses include poliovirus types 1–3, Coxsackie A and B viruses, echoviruses and enteroviruses (EV) 68–71. There are several newly described EVs yet to be officially classified. All enteroviruses are now grouped into four species, A–D, with the species letter being incorporated in the virus type name: for example, EV D68. They are responsible for a broad spectrum of disease involving the skin and mucous membranes, muscles, nerves, heart (**Box 20.28**) and, rarely, other organs, such as the liver and pancreas. They are frequently associated with pyrexial illnesses and are the most common cause of asep-tic meningitis (see later).

Herpangina

This is mainly caused by Coxsackie A viruses. It presents with a vesicular eruption on the fauces, palate and uvula, and the lesions evolve into ulcers. The illness is usually associated with fever and headache but is short-lived, recovery taking place within a few days.

Hand, foot and mouth disease

This is mainly caused by Coxsackievirus A16 or A10 (EV A16, EV A10). It is also the main feature of infection with EV A71. Oral lesions are similar to those seen in herpangina but may be more extensive in the oropharynx. Vesicles and a maculopapu-lar eruption also appear, typically on the palms of the hands and the soles of the feet, but also on other parts of the body. This infection commonly affects children. Recovery occurs within a week.

Poxvirus infections

Smallpox (variola)

This disease was eradicated in 1977 following an aggressive vac-cination policy. Its possible use in bioterrorism has resulted in the re-introduction of smallpox vaccination in some countries.

Monkeypox

This rare zoonosis occurs in small villages in tropical rainfor-ests in several countries of West and Central Africa. Its clinical effects, including a generalized vesicular rash, are indistinguish-able from those of smallpox, but person-to-person transmis-sion is unusual. Most infections occur in children who have not been vaccinated against smallpox. Disease can be severe, with mortality rates of 10–15% in unvaccinated individuals. Sero-logical surveys indicate that several species of squirrel are the likely animal reservoir. The virus was introduced into the USA in 2003 via small West African mammals illegally imported as pets. Widespread infection of prairie dogs resulted and there were 37 laboratory-confirmed cases in humans. Two imported cases were reported in the UK in 2018, with spread to a third case who was a healthcare worker.

Cowpox

Cowpox produces large vesicles that are classically found on the hands of individuals in contact with infected cows. The lesions are associated with regional lymphadenitis and fever. Cowpox virus has been found in a range of species, including domestic and wild cats, and the reservoir is thought to exist in a range of rodents.

Vaccinia virus

This laboratory virus does not occur in nature in either humans or animals. Its origins are uncertain but it has been invaluable in its use as the vaccine to prevent smallpox.

Orf

This poxvirus causes contagious pustular dermatitis in sheep and hand lesions in humans (see p. 672).

Molluscum contagiosum

This is discussed on page 672.

Human papillomavirus infections

These cause warts (see p. 672) and cervical cancer (p. 130).

Maculopapular viral rashes

Measles (rubeola)

Measles virus is a paramyxovirus (see **Box 20.26**). Measles is a highly communicable disease that occurs worldwide. With the intro-duction of aggressive immunization policies, the global incidence of and mortality from measles fell by 80% between 2000 and 2017, but there were still approximately 110000 measles-related deaths in 2017, mostly in children under the age of 5 and largely in Africa and South-east Asia. It is spread by droplet infection, and the period of infectivity is from 4 days before until 2 days after the onset of the rash.

Clinical features

The incubation period is 8–14 days. Two distinct phases of the dis-ease can be recognized.

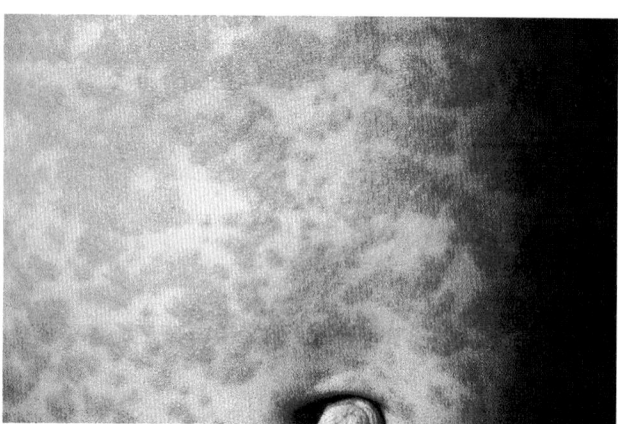

Fig. 20.10 Measles. (*Courtesy of Dr MW McKendrick, Royal Hallamshire Hospital, Sheffield.*)

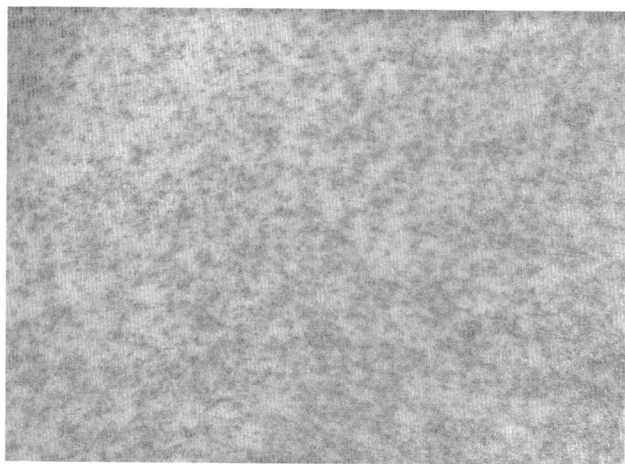

Fig. 20.11 Rubella rash.

Typical measles

- ***Pre-eruptive and catarrhal stage***, the stage of viraemia and viral dissemination. Malaise, fever, rhinorrhoea, cough, conjunctival suffusion and the pathognomonic Koplik's spots – small, greyish, irregular lesions surrounded by an erythematous base, found in greatest numbers on the buccal mucous membrane opposite the second molar tooth – are present during this stage.
- ***Eruptive or exanthematous stage***, characterized by the presence of a maculopapular rash that initially occurs on the face, chiefly the forehead, and then spreads rapidly to involve the rest of the body (**Fig. 20.10**). At first, the rash is discrete but later it may become confluent and patchy, especially on the face and neck. It fades in about 1 week and leaves behind a brownish discoloration.

The most feared complication in an immunocompetent child is post-measles encephalomyelitis, occurring within 2 weeks of the rash in 1/1000–1/5000 cases of measles. This is most likely an autoimmune disorder triggered by the measles infection, as virus is not present in the brain substance. Prognosis is poor, with a high mortality (30%), and severe residual damage in survivors.

Measles carries a high mortality in the malnourished and those who have other diseases. Complications are common in such individuals and include bacterial pneumonia, bronchitis, otitis media and severe diarrhoea. Less commonly, myocarditis, hepatitis and encephalomyelitis occur. In the malnourished or those with defective cell-mediated immunity, the classical maculopapular rash may not develop and there may be widespread desquamation. The virus also causes the rare condition subacute sclerosing panencephalitis, which may follow measles infection occurring early in life (<18 months of age). Persistence of the virus with reactivation before puberty results in accumulation of virus in the brain, progressive mental deterioration and a fatal outcome (see p. 872).

Maternal measles, unlike rubella, does not cause fetal abnormalities. It is, however, associated with spontaneous abortions and premature delivery.

Diagnosis and management

Most cases of measles are diagnosed clinically but detection of measles-specific IgM in blood or oral fluid, or genome or antigen detection from nasopharyngeal aspirates or throat swabs, should be used to confirm the diagnosis.

Management is supportive. Antibiotics are indicated only if secondary bacterial infection occurs. Vitamin A supplements lower the number of deaths from measles by 50%, and also reduce eye damage and blindness, and therefore two doses of vitamin A supplements given 24 hours apart are recommended for all children with measles.

Prevention

A previous attack of measles confers a high degree of immunity and second attacks are uncommon. Normal human immunoglobulin given within 5 days of exposure effectively aborts an attack of measles. It is indicated following exposure for previously unimmunized children below 3 years of age, for pregnant women and for those with debilitating disease.

Active immunization

Children in the UK are immunized with the combined mumps/measles/rubella (MMR) vaccine (see **Box 20.20**). In developing countries, the first measles vaccination is given at 9 months.

Rubella

Rubella ('German measles') is caused by a spherical, enveloped RNA virus of the *Rubivirus* genus belonging to the family of togaviruses. While the disease can occur sporadically, epidemics are not uncommon. It has a worldwide distribution. Spread of the virus is via droplets; maximum infectivity occurs before and during the time the rash is present.

Clinical features

The incubation period is 14–21 days, averaging 18 days. The clinical features are largely determined by age, symptoms being mild or absent in children under 5 years.

During the prodrome, the patient may develop malaise, fever, mild conjunctivitis and lymphadenopathy involving particularly the suboccipital, post-auricular and posterior cervical groups of lymph nodes. Small petechial lesions on the soft palate (Forchheimer spots) are suggestive but not diagnostic. Splenomegaly may be present.

The eruptive or exanthematous phase usually occurs within 7 days of the initial symptoms. The rash first appears on the forehead and then spreads to involve the trunk and limbs. It is pinkish red, macular and discrete, although some of these lesions may coalesce (**Fig. 20.11**). It usually fades by the second day and rarely persists beyond 3 days after its appearance.

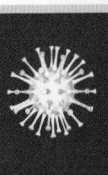

Complications

Complications are rare. They include superadded pulmonary bacterial infection, arthralgia (more common in females), haemorrhagic manifestations due to thrombocytopenia, and encephalitis. Maternal infection in pregnancy may result in the congenital rubella syndrome. Rubella affects the fetuses of up to 90% of all women who contract the infection during the first trimester of pregnancy. The incidence of congenital abnormalities diminishes in the second trimester and no ill-effects result from infection in the third trimester.

Congenital rubella syndrome is characterized by the presence of fetal cardiac malformations (especially patent ductus arteriosus and ventricular septal defect), eye lesions (especially cataracts), microcephaly, mental retardation and deafness. Hepatosplenomegaly, myocarditis, interstitial pneumonia and metaphyseal bone lesions also occur.

Diagnosis and management

Laboratory diagnosis is essential, especially in pregnancy, to distinguish the illness from other virus infections (e.g. erythrovirus B19, echovirus) and drug rashes. This is achieved by detection of rubella-specific IgM by enzyme-linked immunosorbent assay (ELISA) in an acute serum sample, preferably confirmed by demonstration of IgG seroconversion (or a rising titre of IgG) in a subsequent sample taken 14 days later. Viral genome can be detected in throat swabs (or oral fluid samples), urine and, in the case of intrauterine infection, the products of conception.

Management is supportive.

Prevention

Several live attenuated rubella vaccines have been used and have had great success in preventing this illness. They have been successfully combined with measles and mumps vaccines in the MMR vaccine. Use of the vaccine is contraindicated during pregnancy or if there is a likelihood of pregnancy within 3 months of immunization. Inadvertent use of the vaccine during pregnancy has not, however, revealed a risk of teratogenicity.

Erythrovirus infections

Human erythrovirus (also known as parvovirus) B19 causes erythema infectiosum (fifth disease), a common infection in schoolchildren. The rash is typically on the face (the *'slapped cheek'* appearance). The patient is well and the rash can recur over weeks or months. Asymptomatic infection occurs in 20% of children. Non-specific respiratory tract illness may also occur. In adults, the rash may be clinically indistinguishable from that of rubella. Moderately severe self-limiting polyarthropathy is common if infection occurs in adulthood, especially in women (this is also true of rubella). The virus infects bone marrow cells, and aplastic crisis may occur in patients with chronic haemolysis (e.g. sickle cell disease). Chronic infection with anaemia occurs in immunocompromised subjects. Hydrops fetalis (3% risk) and spontaneous abortion (9% risk) may result from maternal infection in the first and second trimesters of pregnancy.

Diagnosis of acute infection is by detection of parvovirus-specific IgM and/or DNA.

Human herpesvirus types 6 and 7 infection

These human herpesviruses occur worldwide and exist as latent infections in over 85% of the adult population. They are spread by contact with oral secretions. Human herpesvirus type 6 (HHV-6) causes roseola infantum (exanthem subitum), which presents as a high fever followed by a generalized macular rash in infants. HHV-6 is a common cause of febrile convulsions, and aseptic meningitis or encephalitis is a rare complication.

The full spectrum of disease due to HHV-7 has not yet been fully characterized but, like HHV-6, it may cause roseola infantum in infants. Both viruses have been associated with encephalitis in heavily immunosuppressed patients, such as bone marrow transplant recipients.

Management

Supportive management is recommended for the common infantile disease. Ganciclovir can be used in the immunocompromised.

Further reading

Moss WJ. Measles. *Lancet* 2017; 390:2490–2502.
Phuc L, Rothberg M. Herpes zoster infection. *BMJ* 2019; 364:k5095.

VIRUS INFECTIONS OF THE RESPIRATORY TRACT

Many viruses can cause upper respiratory tract infection (URTI): for example, in the nose (rhinitis), throat (tonsillitis, pharyngitis), sinuses (sinusitis), ear (otitis media), eye (conjunctivitis) or larynx (laryngitis) (**Box 20.29**). Infections below the larynx are referred to as lower respiratory tract infections (LRTIs). URTIs are common but relatively trivial; LRTIs are less common but may result in hospitalization and even death.

Upper respiratory tract infections

The common cold – coryza, rhinitis

Rhinovirus infection is the most common cause of the common cold (see p. 945). Peak incidence rates occur in the colder months,

Box 20.29 Virus infections of the respiratory tract

Virus	Disease
Upper respiratory tract infections	
Rhinoviruses (>100 serotypes)	Common cold, rhinitis
Parainfluenza viruses 1–4	Croup
Coronaviruses OC43, 229E	Common cold
Respiratory syncytial virus	Cough, sore throat
Human metapneumovirus	Cough, sore throat
Adenoviruses (>50 serotypes)	Pharyngitis, conjunctivitis Common cold (see p. 945)
Enteroviruses (Coxsackie, echo, EV D68)	Bronchiolitis in young babies
Lower respiratory tract infections	
Influenza A, B	Epidemics and pandemics of influenza
Respiratory syncytial virus	Bronchiolitis, pneumonia in young babies
SARS-Coronavirus 2	Coronavirus disease 2019 (COVID-19)
Rarely	
Cytomegalovirus	Pneumonitis in immuno-compromised
Varicella zoster virus	Pneumonia in adults with primary infection
Measles	Giant-cell pneumonia in immunocompromised
Coronaviruses	Pneumonia, regional or wide-spread outbreaks

especially spring and autumn. There are multiple rhinovirus serotypes (>100), which explains why infection occurs throughout life and makes vaccine control impracticable. In contrast to enteroviruses, which replicate at 37°C, rhinoviruses grow best at 33°C (the temperature of the upper respiratory tract), which explains the localized disease characteristic of common colds.

Human coronaviruses were first isolated in the mid-1960s and the majority of isolates (related to the reference strains 229E and OC43) have been associated with common colds. In 2004 and 2005, two new coronavirus infections of humans were described: NL63 and HKU1. These are also associated with coryzal symptomatology. Coronaviruses have recently become of interest owing to the discovery of three new viruses causing life-threatening LRTI (see later).

Parainfluenza

Parainfluenza is caused by the parainfluenza viruses types I–IV; these have a worldwide distribution and cause acute respiratory disease.

Parainfluenza is essentially a disease of children and presents with features similar to those of the common cold. When infection is severe, a brassy cough with inspiratory stridor and features of laryngotracheitis (croup) are present. Fever usually lasts for 2–3 days and may be more prolonged if pneumonia develops. The development of croup is due to submucosal oedema and consequent airway obstruction in the subglottic region. This may lead to cyanosis, subcostal and intercostal recession and progressive airway obstruction. Infection in the immunocompromised is usually prolonged and may be severe. Management is supportive with oxygen, humidification and sedation when required. The role of steroids and the antiviral agent ribavirin is controversial.

Adenovirus infection

Over 50 adenovirus serotypes have been identified as human pathogens, infecting a number of different cell types and therefore resulting in different clinical syndromes. Adenovirus infection commonly presents as an acute pharyngitis, and extension of infection to the larynx and trachea in infants may lead to croup. By school age, the majority of children show serological evidence of previous infection. Certain subtypes produce an acute conjunctivitis associated with pharyngitis. In adults, adenovirus causes acute follicular conjunctivitis and, rarely, pneumonia that is clinically similar to that produced by *Mycoplasma pneumoniae* (see p. 963). Adenoviruses 40 and 41 cause gastroenteritis (see p. 529) without respiratory disease, and adenovirus infection may be responsible for acute mesenteric lymphadenitis in children and young adults, which may lead to intussusception in infants. Infection in an immunocompromised host, such as a bone marrow transplant recipient, may result in multisystem failure and fatal disease.

Other viral causes of URTI

Human erythrovirus B19 infection may present as a URTI. Bocavirus is a recently identified parvovirus, which accounts for around 3–5% of respiratory tract infections in young children. Enteroviruses, such as Coxsackie and echoviruses, are occasionally found in respiratory tract secretions of young babies, and there has been much interest recently in EV D-68, which appears to infect the respiratory tract predominantly. WU and KI polyomaviruses may be associated with respiratory tract infections in young children.

Lower respiratory tract infections

Viral infections resulting in life-threatening LRTIs are influenza, respiratory syncytial virus and the Middle East respiratory syndrome and severe acute respiratory syndrome (SARS)-associated

Box 20.30 Influenza pandemics of the 20th century

Year	Virus subtype	Comments
1918–19	H1N1	'Spanish' flu, >40 million deaths
1957	H2N2	'Asian' influenza
1968	H3N2	
1976[a]	H1N1	'Russian' influenza; not thought to be a natural occurrence
2009	A(H1N1)pdm09	Derived from swine influenza

coronaviruses. However, other causes of viral pneumonia occasionally arise (see **Box 20.29**), and at the time of going to press, a novel coronavirus (SARS-CoV2) has been identified as the causative agent of an outbreak originating in Wuhan, China, which has spread throughout the world.

Influenza

Influenza viruses belong to the family of orthomyxoviruses, having a segmented negative-strand RNA genome. The influenza virus is a spherical or filamentous enveloped virus. Haemagglutinin (H), a surface glycoprotein, aids attachment of the virus to the surface of susceptible host cells at specific sialic acid receptor sites. Release of progeny viruses from the cell surface, effected by budding through the cell membrane, is facilitated by the enzyme neuraminidase (N), which is also present on the viral envelope. Three types of influenza virus are recognized – A, B and C – distinguishable by the nature of their internal proteins. In addition, 18 H subtypes (H1–H18) and 11 N subtypes (N1–N11) have been identified for influenza A viruses but only H1, H2, H3, N1 and N2 have established stable lineages in the human population since 1918.

- *Influenza A* is generally responsible for pandemics and epidemics.
- *Influenza B* often causes smaller or localized, milder outbreaks but can also result in severe disease and mortality. There are no subtypes of influenza B.
- *Influenza C* rarely produces disease in humans.

Antigenic shift generates new influenza A subtypes carrying different H and/or N proteins on their surface, which emerge at irregular intervals and give rise to influenza pandemics. Possible mechanisms include:

- Genetic reassortment of the eight RNA segments of the virus with that of an avian influenza virus. This requires co-infection of a host with both human and avian viruses. Pigs are thought to be the likely mixing vessel, although this could theoretically also occur in humans.
- Trans-species transmission of an avian influenza virus to humans. Viruses transmitted in this way are usually not well adapted to growth in their new host but adaptation may occur as a result of spontaneous mutations, leading to the emergence of a pandemic strain.

Antigenic drift (minor changes in influenza A and B viruses) results from Darwinian evolution, with randomly occurring point mutations leading to amino acid changes in the two surface glycoproteins, haemagglutinin and neuraminidase, against the selection pressure of previously existing humoral immunity. This enables the virus to evade previously induced immune responses and is the process whereby annual influenza epidemics arise.

Thus, changes due to antigenic shift or drift render the individual's immune response less able to combat the new variant.

Incidence increases during the winter months. Spread is mainly by droplet infection but fomites and direct contact have also been implicated. Influenza pandemics of the 20th century are listed in **Box 20.30**.

In 1997, avian influenza A/H5N1 viruses were first isolated from humans in Hong Kong, raising the spectre of another pandemic. Since then, the virus has spread across Asia, Europe and Africa. There have been several hundred human cases, with a mortality approaching 50%. While this virus is highly pathogenic to humans, due to the induction of a cytokine storm within the lungs, it still has not evolved to replicate well in human cells and human-to-human spread is unusual. However, anxieties remain that either genetic reassortment will occur in a human co-infected with human A(H1N1) pdm09 or A(H3N2) virus, or adaptive mutations will occur within infected human hosts, such that a truly pandemic strain will emerge.

In April 2009, a novel influenza A virus, now referred to as A(H1N1) pdm09, was identified in patients with severe respiratory illness in Mexico and North America. The virus quickly spread across the world, with the WHO declaring an official pandemic in June 2009. The virus was the end-product of several reassortments between pre-existing swine, avian and human virus lineages, with the swine H1 protein showing around 20% amino acid sequence divergence from previously circulating human seasonal H1N1 influenza viruses. Although unquestionably highly transmissible (with estimates of millions of infections worldwide within 1 year), this pandemic virus was, perhaps fortunately, not especially virulent. Most infections occurred in children; adults over 50 years of age had evidence of pre-existing protective immunity. A minority of infections resulted in serious disease, with an estimated 200 000 deaths worldwide. Risk factors for serious disease included pre-existing underlying medical conditions, age below 5 years, obesity and pregnancy. The pandemic was declared officially over by the WHO in August 2010, the virus now behaving as a normal seasonal influenza virus and replacing the previously circulating A(H1N1) virus.

Novel influenza viruses may continue to infect humans sporadically, raising the possibility of a new pandemic. In 2013, over 100 cases of infection with an H7N9 virus were reported from China. As of December 2018, there had been 1567 confirmed cases, with 615 deaths. Most cases gave a history of exposure to live animals, including chickens.

Purified haemagglutinin and neuraminidase from recently circulating strains of influenza A and B viruses are incorporated in current vaccines.

The clinical features, diagnosis, treatment and prophylaxis of influenza are discussed on page 947.

Respiratory syncytial virus infection

Respiratory syncytial virus (RSV) is a paramyxovirus that causes many respiratory infections in epidemics each winter. It is a common cause of bronchiolitis in infants, complicated by pneumonia in approximately 10% of cases. The infection normally starts with upper respiratory symptoms. After an interval of 1–3 days, a cough and low-grade fever may develop. The onset of bronchiolitis is characterized by dyspnoea and hyperexpansion of the chest with subcostal and intercostal recession. The disease may be severe and potentially fatal in babies with underlying cardiac, respiratory (including prematurity) or immunodeficiency disease. The virus undergoes antigenic drift and, consequently, re-infection occurs throughout life. RSV is occasionally the cause of outbreaks of influenza-like illness or pneumonia in the elderly (in residential homes) and the immunocompromised.

Transfer of infection between children in hospital (hospital-acquired infection) commonly occurs unless infected patients are isolated or cohorted. Meticulous attention to hand-washing and other infection control measures reduces the risk of transmission by staff members (see p. 292).

Diagnosis and management

Genome detection or immunofluorescence on nasopharyngeal aspirates is the usual way of confirming the diagnosis.

Management is generally supportive but aerosolized ribavirin can be given to severe cases, particularly those with underlying cardiac or respiratory disease.

Prevention

No vaccine is currently available for RSV but high-risk children (including those with bronchopulmonary dysplasia and congenital heart disease) can be protected against severe disease by monthly administration of either a hyperimmune globulin against RSV, or a humanized monoclonal antibody (palivizumab) during the winter months.

Metapneumovirus

Human metapneumovirus (hMPV) belongs to the same virus family as RSV and causes approximately 10% of LRTIs in infants and young children. Infection is clinically indistinguishable from that caused by RSV.

Coronavirus infection – severe acute respiratory and Middle East respiratory syndromes

In November 2002, an apparently new viral LRTI occurred in China and spread rapidly in other parts of the Far East and, from there, across the world. This disease, of which bronchopneumonia is a major feature, is known as 'severe acute respiratory syndrome' (SARS); it is caused by a previously unknown coronavirus (SARS-CoV). Similarity of this virus to coronaviruses isolated from civet cats, raccoons and ferret badgers indicates that SARS is a zoonotic disease. Bats are the likely host species. The epidemic was finally brought under control in the summer of 2003, by which time there had been more than 8000 cases with approximately 800 deaths. Naturally acquired infection has not been reported since.

In 2012, a new coronavirus, Middle East respiratory syndrome coronavirus (MERS-CoV), was identified in a patient who died of acute respiratory failure in Saudi Arabia. There have been over 2200 cases since, across 27 countries, although mostly in the Middle East; mortality is around 35%. The most likely source is from dromedary camels. Person-to-person spread within healthcare settings is another major source, with the largest outbreaks in Saudi Arabia, United Arab Emirates and the Republic of Korea.

In December 2019, yet another coronavirus was identified in an outbreak of severe respiratory disease in Wuhan, China. This virus is now known as SARS Coronavirus 2 (SARS-CoV-2), and the associated disease is Coronavirus Disease 2019 (COVID 19). Whilst mortality is not as high as with SARS-CoV (current estimates are of the order of 1-5%), this virus is clearly more transmissible and has spread explosively around the world. As of May 2020, there are approaching 5 million cases and 300,000 deaths recorded globally. It is feared that many more people will become infected over the next year or so, with millions of deaths.

Further reading

Arabi YM, Balkhy HH, Hayden FG et al. Middle East respiratory syndrome. *N Engl J Med* 2017; 376:584–594.
Florin TA, Plint AC, Zorc JJ. Viral bronchiolitis. *Lancet* 2017; 389:211–224.
Paules C, Subbarao K. Influenza. *Lancet* 2017; 390:697–708.
Shi T, McAllister DA, O'Brien KL et al. Global, regional, and national disease burden estimates of acute lower respiratory infections due to respiratory syncytial virus in young children in 2015: a systematic review and modelling study. *Lancet* 2017; 390:946–958.

SYSTEMIC VIRAL INFECTIONS

Dengue

This is the most common arthropod-borne viral infection in humans, whose global incidence has increased dramatically in recent years; over 100 million cases occur every year in the tropics, with over 10 000 deaths from severe dengue (previously known as haemorrhagic fever)

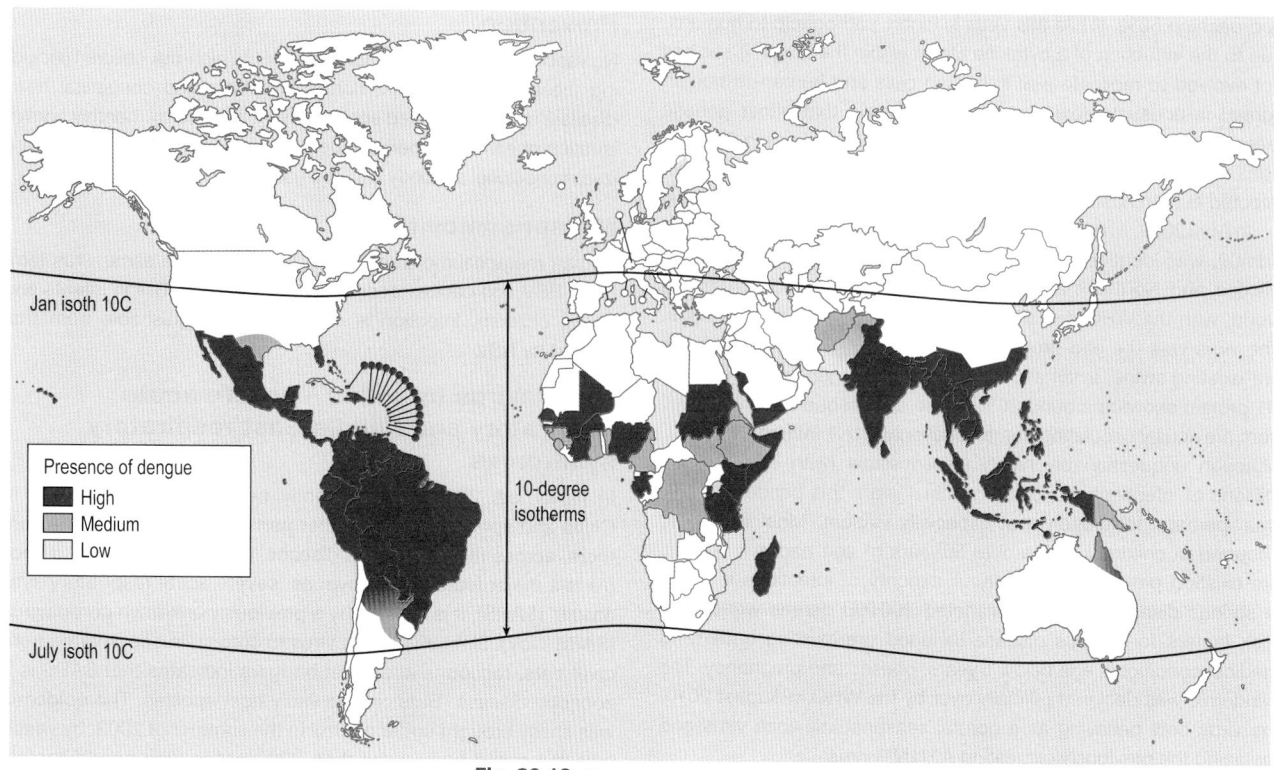

Fig. 20.12 Global dengue burden.

ℹ **Box 20.31** Arbovirus (arthropod-borne) infection

Defining features of arboviruses
- Arboviruses are zoonotic viruses, transmitted through the bites of insects, especially mosquitoes and ticks
- >385 viruses are classified as arboviruses
- Most are members of the families of togaviruses, flaviviruses and bunyaviruses (see **Box 20.32**)
- *Culex, Aedes* and *Anopheles* mosquitoes account for transmission of the majority of these viruses

Clinical features of arbovirus infection
- Most arbovirus diseases are generally mild; epidemics are frequent, and when these occur, the mortality is high

- In general, the incubation period is short (<10 days). Common features include a biphasic illness, pyrexia, conjunctival suffusion, a rash, retro-orbital pain, myalgia and arthralgia. Lymphadenopathy is seen in dengue
- *Haemorrhage* (from increased vascular permeability, capillary fragility, consumptive coagulopathy) is a feature of some arbovirus infections (see **Box 20.37**)
- *Encephalitis* resulting from cerebral invasion may be prominent in some arbovirus fevers

---

(**Fig. 20.12**). Dengue is caused by a flavivirus. The disease is endemic in all tropical regions, including northern Australia, most South-east Asian countries, tropical Africa and the Middle East, and Caribbean countries. Cases of dengue are also imported into the continental USA and Europe (e.g. Italy) via tourists returning from endemic countries.

Viruses spread by insects are collectively referred to as arthropod-borne viruses, or arboviruses (**Boxes 20.31** and **20.32**). Four different antigenic serotypes of dengue virus are recognized and all are transmitted by the daytime-biting mosquito *Aedes aegypti*, which breeds in standing water in refuse dumps in inner cities. *A. albopictus* is a less common transmitter. Humans are infective during the first 3 days of the illness (viraemic stage; **Fig. 20.13**). Mosquitoes become infective about 2 weeks after feeding on an infected individual and remain so for life. The disease is usually endemic. Heterotypic immunity between serotypes after the illness is partial and lasts only a few months, although homotype immunity is life-long.

Clinical features

The incubation period is 5–6 days following the mosquito bite. Asymptomatic or mild infections are common. Two clinical forms are recognized (see **Fig. 20.14**).

Classic dengue fever

Classic dengue fever is characterized by the abrupt onset of fever, malaise, headache, facial flushing, retrobulbar pain that worsens on eye movements, conjunctival suffusion and severe backache, which is a prominent symptom. Lymphadenopathy, petechiae on the soft palate and transient, morbilliform skin rashes may also appear on the limbs with subsequent spread to involve the trunk. Desquamation occurs subsequently. Cough is uncommon. The fever subsides after 3–4 days, the temperature returning to normal for a couple of days, after which the fever returns, together with the features already mentioned, but milder. This biphasic or 'saddleback' pattern is considered characteristic. Severe fatigue, a feeling of being unwell and depression are common for several weeks after the fever has subsided.

Severe dengue

Severe dengue is potentially deadly and is believed to arise from two or more sequential infections with different dengue serotypes. It is characterized by the capillary leak syndrome, thrombocytopenia, haemorrhage, hypotension and shock. It is characteristically a disease of children, occurring most commonly in South-east Asia. The disease has a mild start, often with symptoms of an URTI. This

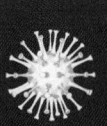
Box 20.32 Some arboviruses

Family	Genus	Viruses	Transmission	Predominant clinical syndrome
Togaviridae	Alphaviruses	Eastern, Western, Venezuelan equine encephalitis	Mosquito-borne	E
				F
		Chikungunya		F
		Ross River		F
Flaviviiridae	Flaviviruses	St Louis encephalitis	Mosquito-borne	E
		Japanese encephalitis		E
		Murray Valley encephalitis		E
		Yellow fever (see p. 531)		H
		Dengue (see pp. 521–524)		H
		Zika		F
		West Nile		E
		Louping ill	Tick-borne	E
		Tick-tome encephalitis		E
		Kyasanur Forest virus		H
		Omsk haemorrhagic fever		H
Bunyaviridae	Orthobunyaviruses	La Crosse	Mosquito-borne	E
	Phleboviruses	Rift Valley fever	Mosquito-borne	F
	Nairoviruses	Congo-Crimean haemorrhagic fever	Tick-borne	H

E, encephalitis or aseptic meningitis; F, tropical fever, often with headache, myalgia, rash, arthralgia; H, haemorrhagic fever.

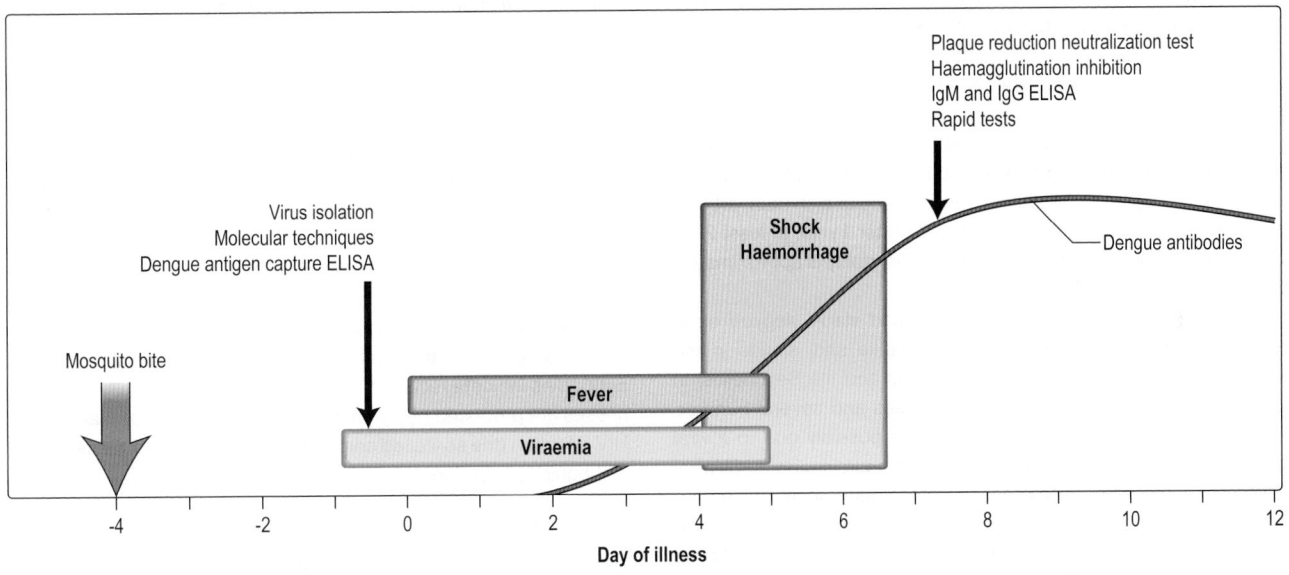

Fig. 20.13 Dengue infection – course and timing of diagnosis. ELISA, enzyme-linked immunosorbent assay; Ig, immunoglobulin. (*From Halstead SB. Dengue. Lancet 2007; 370:1644–1652, with permission.*)

is followed by the abrupt onset of shock and haemorrhage into the skin and ear, epistaxis, haematemesis and melaena, known as the **dengue shock syndrome**, which has a mortality of up to 44%. Serum complement levels are depressed and there is laboratory evidence of disseminated intravascular coagulation (DIC, see p. 377).

Diagnosis and management

- Isolation of dengue virus by tissue culture, or detection of viral RNA by genome amplification in sera obtained during the first few days of illness, is diagnostic.
- Detection of virus-specific IgM antibodies, or of rising IgG titres in sequential serum samples, confirms the diagnosis.
- Blood tests show leucopenia and thrombocytopenia.

Management is supportive, with analgesics and adequate fluid replacement. Corticosteroids are of no benefit and convalescence can be slow. In dengue haemorrhagic fever blood transfusion may be necessary, as well as intensive care support.

Prevention

Travellers should be advised to sleep under impregnated nets but this is not very effective, as the mosquito bites in the daytime. Topical insect repellents should be used. Adult mosquitoes should be destroyed by sprays, and breeding sites, such as small pools of stagnant water, should be eradicated. A live recombinant tetravalent dengue vaccine has been licensed, although concerns have arisen that vaccination of seronegative individuals may paradoxically increase the risk of severe dengue. Several other vaccines are in clinical trials.

Zika virus infection

Zika virus, a flavivirus closely related to dengue viruses, came to prominence in 2016 following an explosive pandemic throughout South and Central America, and the Caribbean. Like dengue, Zika is an arbovirus, transmitted to humans by *Aedes* mosquitoes. Illness, when it arises, is usually unremarkable, with fever, myalgia, eye pain, prostration and maculopapular rash, with spontaneous resolution. However, the epidemiological association of Zika virus outbreaks with subsequent dramatic increases in the number of cases of microcephaly in infants (e.g. Brazil reported a 20-fold increase in incidence from 2014 to 2015) led the WHO to declare Zika a public health emergency of international concern. Precise data on the magnitude of the risk of congenital brain abnormalities in a Zika-affected pregnancy are not yet available. The WHO has also concluded that Zika virus is a trigger of the Guillain–Barré syndrome. Accurate diagnosis of infection is complicated by serological cross-reactivity with dengue viruses. Further research on the consequences of infection with Zika virus is urgently needed.

Chikungunya

Chikungunya virus is an alphavirus, a genus within the family of togaviruses. There are eight alphaviruses that result in human disease and all are arboviruses, transmitted by mosquitoes. They are globally distributed and tend to acquire their names from the location where they were first isolated (such as Ross River, Eastern, Venezuelan and Western equine encephalitis viruses) or from the local expression for a major symptom caused by the virus (such as chikungunya, meaning 'doubled up'). Chikungunya infection is characterized by fever, headache, maculopapular skin rash, arthralgia, myalgia and sometimes encephalitis. After 1 year, at least 20% of patients still suffer recurrent joint pains. Mortality is approximately 0.1%, mostly in the elderly or very young.

Major epidemics of chikungunya, spread via *A. aegypti* or *A. albopictus*, were reported in India, Sri Lanka and islands in the Indian Ocean (including Reunion, Mauritius and the Seychelles) in 2005 and 2006, with at least 1 million cases and several hundred deaths. The severity of these epidemics is possibly due to a viral strain, with mutations resulting in a higher neurovirulence. Several European countries reported cases of chikungunya in returning travellers, including 133 cases in the UK in 2006. The increased numbers of infected returning travellers may result in the local *Aedes* mosquito population becoming infected, giving rise to outbreaks in countries where it has not previously been described: for example, in Italy (2007) and the French mainland (2010). In 2013, an outbreak in the Caribbean islands spread to contiguous Central and South American countries, and over 200 cases were reported in 2014 in the USA.

A number of chikungunya vaccines are currently undergoing clinical trials.

Infectious mononucleosis: Epstein–Barr virus infection

Globally, most individuals are infected with the herpesvirus Epstein–Barr virus (EBV) at an early age (0–5 years), at which time clinical symptoms are unusual. Infection at an older age is associated with an acute febrile illness known as infectious mononucleosis (glandular fever), which occurs worldwide in adolescents and young adults. EBV is probably transmitted in saliva and by aerosol.

Clinical features

The predominant symptoms of infectious mononucleosis are fever, headache, malaise and sore throat. Palatal petechiae and a transient macular rash are common, the latter occurring in 90% of patients who have received ampicillin (inappropriately) for the sore throat. Cervical lymphadenopathy, particularly of the posterior cervical nodes, and splenomegaly are characteristic. Mild hepatitis is common, resulting in clinical jaundice in 10% of young adults, but other complications such as myocarditis, meningitis, encephalitis, mononeuritis multiplex, cerebellar ataxia and mesenteric adenitis are rare. Splenic rupture may occur in the first 3 weeks of illness and contact sport should be avoided during this period. Some young adults may remain debilitated and depressed for some months after infection.

The site of EBV latency is resting memory B lymphocytes. Evidence for reactivation of latent virus in healthy individuals is controversial, although this is thought to occur in immunocompromised patients. Severe, often fatal, infectious mononucleosis may result from a rare X-linked lymphoproliferative syndrome affecting young boys. Those who survive have an increased risk of hypogammaglobulinaemia and/or lymphoma. EBV is the cause of oral hairy leucoplakia in AIDS patients and is intimately linked to the generation of a number of malignancies (see later). EBV is a cause of haemophagocytic lymphohistiocytosis (HLH), a rare condition presenting with fever, rash, jaundice, hepatosplenomegaly and enlarged lymph nodes. Blood tests show cytopenia and a high ferritin, and the bone marrow shows haemophagocytosis. HLH can be primary (inherited) or secondary (e.g. to EBV), and has a high mortality.

Diagnosis

EBV infection should be strongly suspected if atypical mononuclear cells (activated CD8-positive T lymphocytes) are found in the peripheral blood in large numbers. It can be confirmed during the second week of infection by a positive Paul–Bunnell reaction, which detects heterophile antibodies (IgM) that agglutinate sheep erythrocytes, in around 90% of cases. False-positives can occur in other conditions, such as viral hepatitis, Hodgkin lymphoma and acute leukaemia. The Monospot test is a sensitive and easily performed screening test for heterophile antibodies. Specific EBV IgM antibodies indicate recent infection by the virus. Clinically similar illnesses are produced by cytomegalovirus, toxoplasmosis and acute HIV infection (the so-called seroconversion illness) but these can be distinguished serologically.

Management

The majority of cases require no specific treatment and recovery is rapid. Corticosteroid therapy is advised when there is neurological involvement (e.g. encephalitis, meningitis, Guillain–Barré syndrome), marked thrombocytopenia or haemolysis, or tonsillar enlargement that is so marked as to cause respiratory obstruction.

Cytomegalovirus infection

Clinically significant cytomegalovirus (CMV) infection arises in two patient groups in particular:

- fetuses who acquire the infection transplacentally and are born congenitally infected
- patients who are immunocompromised, such as transplant recipients or people with HIV infection.

As with all herpesviruses, CMV persists for life, usually as a latent infection in cells of the monocyte/macrophage lineage, and so may become reactivated, especially in immunocompromised patients. Over 50% of the adult population has serological evidence of latent CMV infection.

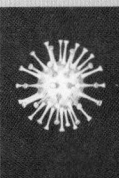

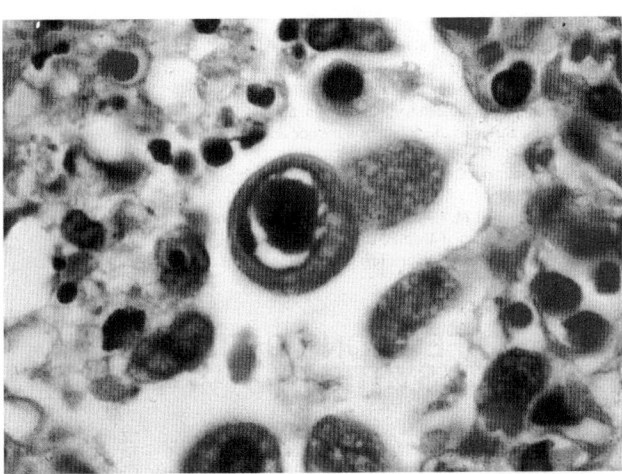

Fig. 20.14 Typical 'owl's eye' inclusion-bearing cell infected with cytomegalovirus.

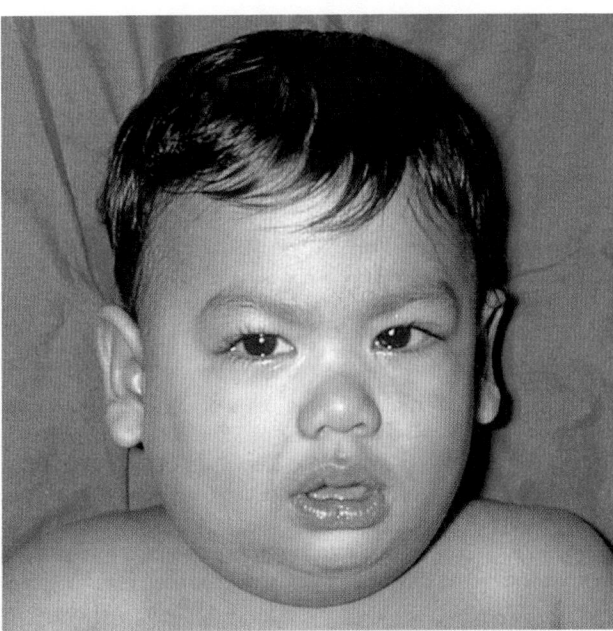

Fig. 20.15 Mumps: a child with a swollen face. (*From Chaudhry B, Harvey DR*. Mosby's Color Atlas and Text of Paediatrics and Child Health. *Edinburgh: Mosby; 2001. © Elsevier 2001.*)

Clinical features

In healthy children and adults, CMV infection is usually asymptomatic but occasionally may result in a glandular fever-like illness, with fever, lymphocytosis with atypical lymphocytes, and hepatitis with or without jaundice. The Paul–Bunnell test for heterophile antibody is negative. Infection may be spread in saliva (accounting for extensive person-to-person spread in childcare units), sexual intercourse or blood transfusion, and transplacentally to the fetus. In an immunocompromised patient (see Ch. 40), CMV infection may involve multiple organ systems, common manifestations being retinitis, pneumonitis, diffuse involvement of the gastrointestinal tract and encephalitis.

Intrauterine infection may arise from either primary or reactivated maternal infection. CMV is, by far, the most common congenital infection; in developed countries, 0.3–1% of all babies are born congenitally infected with CMV. Around 5–10% of such babies have severe disease evident at birth, with a poor prognosis (cytomegalic inclusion disease). CNS involvement may cause microcephaly and motor disorders. Jaundice and hepatosplenomegaly are common and thrombocytopenia and haemolytic anaemia also occur. Periventricular calcification is seen on skull X-ray. A further 5–10% of infected babies are normal at birth but developmental abnormalities become apparent later: for example, sensorineural nerve deafness. The remaining 80–85% of infected babies are normal at birth and develop normally.

Diagnosis

Serological tests can identify latent (IgG) or primary (IgM) infection. However, most infections are now diagnosed by detection and quantification of CMV DNA or RNA using molecular amplification techniques, in blood or other body fluid samples. The virus can also be identified in tissues by the presence of characteristic intranuclear 'owl's eye' inclusions (**Fig. 20.14**) on histological staining and by direct immunofluorescence.

Management

In the immunocompetent, infection is usually self-limiting and no specific treatment is required. In the immunosuppressed, ganciclovir reduces retinitis and gastrointestinal damage, and can eliminate CMV from blood, urine and respiratory secretions. It is less effective against pneumonitis. In patients who are continually immunocompromised, maintenance therapy may be necessary. Drug resistance may arise during long-term therapy, such as in transplant recipients.

Bone marrow toxicity is common. Valganciclovir, foscarnet and cidofovir are also available, and there are promising new drugs undergoing clinical trial including brincidofovir, maribavir and letermovir (see p. 533). Treatment of CMV in neonates is difficult, but therapy of infected babies with evident CNS involvement has been shown to improve long-term hearing outcome, and 6 months of valganciclovir therapy is now recommended for symptomatic neonates.

Mumps

Mumps virus is a paramyxovirus. It is spread by droplet infection, by direct contact or through fomites. Humans are the only known natural hosts. The peak period of infectivity is 2–3 days before the onset of the parotitis and for 3 days afterwards.

Clinical features

The incubation period averages 18 days. Although no age is exempt, this is primarily a disease of school-age children and young adults; it is uncommon before the age of 2 years. The prodromal symptoms are non-specific and include fever, malaise, headache and anorexia. This is usually followed by severe pain over the parotid glands, with either unilateral or bilateral parotid swelling (**Fig. 20.15**). The enlarged glands obscure the angle of the mandible and may elevate the ear lobe, which does not occur in cervical lymph node enlargement. Trismus due to pain is common at this stage. Submandibular gland involvement occurs less frequently.

Complications

CNS involvement is the most common extra-salivary gland manifestation of mumps. Clinical meningitis occurs in 5% of all infected patients, and 30% of patients with CNS involvement have no evidence of parotid gland involvement.

Epididymo-orchitis develops in about one-third of patients who develop mumps after puberty. Bilateral testicular involvement results in sterility in only a small percentage of these patients. Pancreatitis, oophoritis, myocarditis, mastitis, hepatitis and polyarthritis may also occur.

Box 20.33 Human lymphotropic retroviruses

Subfamily	Virus	Disease
Lentiviruses	HIV-1	AIDS
	HIV-2	AIDS
Oncoviruses	HTLV-1	Adult T-cell leukaemia/lymphoma Tropical spastic paraparesis
	HTLV-2	Myelopathy

AIDS, acquired immunodeficiency syndrome; HIV, human immunodeficiency virus; HTLV, human T-cell leukaemia/lymphotropic virus.

Diagnosis and management

The diagnosis of mumps is on the basis of the clinical features. Viral RNA can be demonstrated by genome detection assays in saliva, throat swabs, urine and CSF. Serological demonstration of a mumps-specific IgM response in an acute blood or oral fluid sample is also diagnostic.

Treatment is supportive. Attention should be paid to adequate nutrition and mouth care. Analgesics should be used to relieve pain.

Prevention

Children in the UK are immunized with the live attenuated MMR vaccine (see **Box 20.20**) and the mumps vaccine is given in most developing countries. Vaccination is contraindicated in immunosuppressed individuals, pregnant women or those with severe febrile illnesses.

HIV infections

The human immunodeficiency viruses (HIV) belong to the family of retroviruses (**Box 20.33**), and are characterized by their ability to replicate through a DNA intermediate using the enzyme reverse transcriptase.

HIV-1 and the related virus, HIV-2, are further classified as lentiviruses ('slow' viruses) because of their slowly progressive clinical effects. They give rise to the acquired immunodeficiency syndrome (AIDS) and are discussed in Chapter 37.

Human T-cell leukaemia/lymphotropic virus infection

Human T-cell leukaemia/lymphotropic virus type 1 (HTLV-1) causes adult T-cell leukaemia/lymphoma and tropical spastic paraparesis.

Myocarditis and skeletal muscle infection

Enterovirus infection is a cause of acute myocarditis and pericarditis (see **Box 20.28**), from which, in general, there is complete recovery. However, these viruses can also cause chronic congestive cardiomyopathy and, rarely, constrictive pericarditis. Skeletal muscle involvement, particularly of the intercostal muscles, is a feature of Bornholm disease, a febrile illness usually due to Coxsackie B viruses. The pain may be of such intensity as to mimic pleurisy or an acute abdomen. The infection affects both children and adults, and may be complicated by meningitis or cardiac involvement. Myocarditis and pericarditis are also discussed on pages 1118 and 1125.

Postviral/chronic fatigue syndrome

Many viral infections have been implicated aetiologically, including EBV, Coxsackie B viruses, echoviruses, CMV and hepatitis A virus. Non-viral causes, such as allergy to *Candida* spp., have also been proposed. Only a minority of patients have an identifiable precipitating infectious illness (see also p. 770).

Further reading

Honein M. Recognising the global impact of Zika virus infection during pregnancy. *N Engl J Med* 2018; 378:1055–1056.
Hviid A, Rubin S, Muhlemann K. Mumps. *Lancet* 2008; 371:932–944.
Luzuriaga K, Sullivan JL. Infectious mononucleosis. *N Engl J Med* 2010; 362:1993–2000.
Massad E, Bezerra Coutinho FA. The cost of dengue control. *Lancet* 2011; 377:1630–1631.
Weaver SC, Lecuit M. Chikungunya virus and the global spread of a mosquito-borne disease. *N Engl J Med* 2015; 372:1231–1239.
Wilder-Smith A, Ooi EE, Horstick O et al. Dengue. *Lancet* 2019; 393:350–363.

VIRUS INFECTIONS OF THE NERVOUS SYSTEM

Acute flaccid paralysis, including poliomyelitis

A number of enteroviruses may infect the nervous system (see **Box 20.25**), with different clinical outcomes. Infection with polioviruses 1, 2 and 3, classified within enterovirus species C, may result in acute flaccid paralysis (AFP). Polioviruses are excreted in faeces and spread via the faecal–oral route. They have a propensity for the nervous system, especially the anterior horn cells of the spinal cord and cranial motor neurones.

Clinical features

The incubation period is 7–14 days. Although polio is essentially a disease of childhood, no age is exempt. The clinical manifestations vary considerably. The most common outcome (95% of individuals) is asymptomatic seroconversion. AFP, also known as *paralytic poliomyelitis*, arises in only approximately 0.1% and 1% of infected children and adults, respectively. It follows about 4–5 days after an initial illness of fever, sore throat and myalgia. Meningeal irritation and muscle pain occur and are followed by the onset of asymmetric flaccid paralysis without sensory involvement. Factors predisposing to the development of paralysis include male sex, exercise early in the illness, trauma, surgery or intramuscular injection, which localize the paralysis, and recent tonsillectomy (bulbar poliomyelitis).

Aspiration pneumonia, myocarditis, paralytic ileus and urinary calculi are late complications of poliomyelitis.

AFP may also arise from infection with a number of other enteroviruses, and indeed, AFP is now more commonly caused by these viruses than by polioviruses. EV A71, more usually associated with hand, foot and mouth disease, has a particular predilection for neuroinvasion. Epidemics of EV A71 are not infrequent; an estimated 6 million cases have occurred globally since 2009, with over 2000 deaths from a variety of serious neuromotor syndromes. Inactivated EV A71 vaccines have been approved for clinical use in China. Acute flaccid myelitis has also been associated recently with outbreaks of EV D68 infection in the USA and UK.

Diagnosis

All cases of AFP must be investigated to exclude poliovirus infection. Diagnosis is by detection of EV RNA in a throat swab, faecal sample or CSF, followed by sequencing to identify precisely which EV is present. Sequencing also enables a distinction to be made between wild poliovirus and vaccine strains.

Management

Management is supportive. Bed rest is essential during the early course of the illness. Respiratory support with intermittent positive-pressure respiration is required if the muscles of respiration are involved.

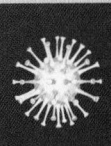

Prevention and control of poliomyelitis

In 1988, the World Health Assembly adopted the goal of eliminating poliomyelitis worldwide. Since then, the estimated 350 000 cases arising annually in 125 countries have been reduced by over 99%, with only Pakistan, Nigeria and Afghanistan never having terminated indigenous transmission. Only 33 cases of wild-type poliomyelitis were documented in 2018. The eradication campaign has relied on improvements in sanitation, hygiene and the widespread use of polio vaccines. However, spread of infection via travel from endemic countries has led to the disease reappearing in a number of states, including China, Cameroon, Syria and Somalia, and in 2014 the WHO declared the spread of poliomyelitis to be a global public health emergency. The creation of a poliomyelitis-free world remains the goal, and there is a revised strategic plan to achieve this by 2023. Vaccination remains the bedrock of the campaign. New preparations of inactivated intramuscular poliovirus vaccine (IPV) have greater potency than the original Salk IPV. The greater reliability of IPV in hot climates and the scientific and ethical problems of continuing to use oral polio vaccine (OPV) in countries free from poliomyelitis mean that IPV has replaced OPV in the routine immunization schedules in many countries.

Meningitis

Enteroviruses are the most common viral cause of aseptic meningitis, although a number of other viruses may also result in this syndrome (**Box 20.34**).

Encephalitis

Encephalitis may arise by direct virus invasion of nervous tissue, or by induction of an aberrant cross-reactive immune response (post-infectious encephalitis). While HSV is the most common cause of sporadic encephalitis worldwide (see p. 871), a number of other virus infections may also present with an encephalitic illness.

Japanese encephalitis

Japanese encephalitis is a mosquito-borne encephalitis caused by a flavivirus. It has been reported most frequently in the rice-growing countries of South-east Asia and the Far East. *Culex tritaeniorhynchus* is the usual vector and this feeds mainly on pigs, as well as birds such as herons and sparrows. Humans are accidental hosts.

The incubation period is 5–15 days. Most infections are asymptomatic. When disease arises, the onset is heralded by severe rigors. Fever, headache and malaise last 1–6 days. Weight loss is prominent. In the acute encephalitic stage the fever is high (38–41°C), neck rigidity occurs and neurological signs, such as altered consciousness, hemiparesis and convulsions, develop. Mental deterioration occurs over a period of 3–4 days and culminates in coma. Mortality varies from 7% to 40% and is higher in children. Residual neurological defects, such as deafness, emotional lability and hemiparesis, occur in about 70% of patients who have had CNS involvement. Convalescence is prolonged. Antibody detection in serum and CSF by IgM capture ELISA is a useful rapid diagnostic test. Vaccines containing formalin-inactivated viruses derived from mouse brain are available and effective. Management is supportive.

West Nile encephalitis

West Nile virus was first recognized in the Western hemisphere (New York, USA) in 1999, having been previously reported in Africa, Asia and parts of Europe. By the end of 2009, the US outbreak had resulted in over 25 000 human cases and over 1100 deaths. The vast majority of infections are asymptomatic. In a minority of cases, infection presents as a febrile illness with a maculopapular rash, 1% resulting in severe encephalitis. Disease severity and mortality are age-related, being greatest in the elderly. The primary hosts of infection are birds. It is spread by mosquitoes (*Culex* spp.) and may also infect humans and horses. It can also be transmitted by blood transfusions, breast-feeding and organ donation from an infected individual. Diagnosis is by genome detection in appropriate samples, or specialized serology for the detection of IgM virus-specific antibodies.

? Box 20.34 Viral causes of meningitis and encephalitis

Virus	Comments	Outcome
Meningitis		
Enteroviruses, esp. Coxsackie B and echoviruses		
Mumps virus		
Herpes simplex viruses		
Encephalitis, direct invasion		
Herpes simplex viruses	Most common cause of sporadic encephalitis. Any age	High morbidity and mortality
Mumps virus	Spread from meninges, resulting in meningoencephalitis	Most patients recover
Measles virus	Subacute sclerosing encephalitis	Rare, high mortality
Varicella zoster virus	May cause vasculitis	May arise with reactivation (shingles)
Cytomegalovirus	Only in immunocompromised	Poor prognosis
Enteroviruses	EV 71; otherwise, usually in immunocompromised only	
HIV	Dementia is main feature	
Japanese encephalitis virus	Flavivirus, mosquitoborne	
West Nile encephalitis virus	Flavivirus, mosquitoborne	Birds are primary host. Higher mortality in elderly
Tick-borne encephalitis viruses	Flaviviruses, tick-borne	
Lymphocytic choriomeningitis virus	Arenavirus	House mouse is primary host
Hendra, Nipah viruses	Paramyxoviruses	Zoonotic infections from horses, pigs
Rabies virus	Acquired from animal or bat bite	Almost always fatal
JC virus	Only in immunocompromised	Results in progressive multifocal leucoencephalopathy
Eastern, Venezuelan encephalitis viruses	Alphaviruses, mosquito-borne	Geographically restricted to the Americas
Encephalitis, post-infectious		

May arise from a number of different virus infections, including measles (1 in 1000–5000 cases of measles), influenza, varicella zoster

Tick-borne encephalitis

This arises from infection with a flavivirus (actually a series of closely related viruses) transmitted by *Ixodes* spp. ticks. It occurs in an area extending from Western Europe to Japan. The tick is the main reservoir for the virus, which is transmitted when it feeds on mice and other rodents.

The disease starts 4–28 days after a bite from an infected tick and is biphasic in 80% of patients. After a symptom-free period of about 7 days, fever, malaise, headache and fatigue are followed by encephalitis. There may be associated limb paralysis, which is due to anterior horn cell involvement, mainly of the cervical region. Cranial nerve involvement also occurs. Tick-borne encephalitis virus (TBEV) IgM and IgG antibodies are present and the virus can be detected in blood by genome detection assays. Overall mortality is about 1% (but can be considerably higher for certain strains); 30% of cases have impairment in neurological function with persistent paralysis in 6%. A preventative vaccine is available.

Lymphocytic choriomeningitis

This infection is a zoonosis, the natural reservoir of lymphocytic choriomeningitis (LCM) virus (an arenavirus; see **Box 20.26**) being the house mouse. Infection is by inhalation from urine-contaminated rubbish and is characterized by:

- non-nervous-system illness, with fever, malaise, myalgia, headache, arthralgia and vomiting
- *meningitis* in addition to the above symptoms.

Occasionally, a more severe form occurs, with encephalitis leading to disturbance of consciousness.

This illness is generally self-limiting and requires no specific treatment.

Hendra and Nipah virus infection

Hendra and Nipah viruses cause zoonotic infections in humans who have been in contact with infected animals (horses and pigs, respectively). The viruses are named after the locations where they were first isolated: Hendra in Australia and Nipah in Malaysia. Both are classified as paramyxoviruses, and fruit bats are their natural hosts. Hendra virus has caused severe respiratory distress in horses and humans, and Nipah virus caused a major outbreak of viral encephalitis (265 cases and 105 deaths) in Malaysia between September 1998 and April 1999; subsequent outbreaks have been reported in India and Bangladesh. Management of these conditions is supportive and no vaccines are currently available.

Rabies

Rabies is a major problem in some countries, with an estimated 55 000 deaths per year worldwide. Established infection is almost invariably fatal; there are only a handful of recorded cases of survival from clinical rabies. It is caused by the rabies virus, a single-stranded RNA virus of the lyssavirus genus within the family of rhabdoviruses. The virus is bullet-shaped and has spike-like structures arising from its surface containing glycoproteins that cause the host to produce neutralizing, haemagglutination-inhibiting antibodies. The virus has a marked affinity for nervous tissue and the salivary glands. It exists in two major epidemiological settings:

- *Urban rabies* is most frequently transmitted to humans through rabid dogs and, less frequently, cats.
- *Sylvan (wild) rabies* is maintained in the wild by a host of animal reservoirs such as foxes, skunks, jackals, mongooses and bats.

With the exception of Australia, New Zealand and the Antarctic, human rabies has been reported from all continents. Transmission is usually through the bite of an infected animal. However, the percentage of rabid bites leading to clinical disease ranges from 10% (on the legs) to 80% (on the head). Other forms of transmission, if they occur, are rare.

The virus replicates in the muscle cells near the entry wound. It penetrates the nerve endings and travels in the axoplasm to the spinal cord and brain. In the CNS, the virus again proliferates before spreading to the salivary glands, lungs, kidneys and other organs via the autonomic nerves.

Clinical features

The incubation period is variable, ranging from a few weeks to several years; on average, it is 1–3 months. In general, bites on the head, face and neck have a shorter incubation period than those elsewhere. In humans, two distinct clinical varieties of rabies are recognized:

- *Furious rabies* – the classic variety. The only characteristic feature in the prodromal period is the presence of pain and tingling at the site of the initial wound. Fever, malaise and headache are also present. About 10 days later, marked anxiety and agitation or depressive features develop. Hallucinations, bizarre behaviour and paralysis may also occur. Hyperexcitability, the hallmark of this form of rabies, is precipitated by auditory or visual stimuli. Hydrophobia (fear of water) is present in 50% of patients and is due to severe pharyngeal spasms on attempting to eat or drink. Aerophobia (fear of air) is considered pathognomonic of rabies. Examination reveals hyper-reflexia, spasticity and evidence of sympathetic overactivity indicated by pupillary dilation and diaphoresis. The patient goes on to develop convulsions, respiratory paralysis and cardiac arrhythmias. Death usually occurs in 10–14 days.
- *Dumb rabies* – the paralytic variety. This presents with a symmetrical ascending paralysis that resembles the Guillain–Barré syndrome.

Diagnosis

The diagnosis of rabies is generally made clinically. Skin-punch biopsies are used to detect antigen with an immunofluorescent antibody test on frozen section. Viral RNA can be detected by genome amplification. Isolation of virus from saliva or the presence of antibodies in blood or CSF may establish the diagnosis. Negri bodies are detected at postmortem in 90% of all patients with rabies: these are eosinophilic, cytoplasmic, ovoid bodies, 2–10 nm in diameter, seen in greatest numbers in the neurones of the hippocampus and the cerebellum. The diagnosis should be made pathologically on the biting animal using genome amplification, immunofluorescence on brain tissue using fluorescently labelled anti-rabies antibody or tissue culture of the brain.

Management

Once CNS disease is established, therapy is symptomatic, as death is virtually inevitable. The patient should be nursed in a quiet, darkened room. Nutritional, respiratory and cardiovascular support may be necessary.

Drugs such as morphine, diazepam and chlorpromazine should be used liberally in patients who are excitable.

Prevention and control
Pre-exposure prophylaxis

This is given to individuals with a high risk of contracting rabies, such as laboratory workers, animal handlers and veterinarians. Three doses of human diploid (HDCV) or purified chick embryo cell vaccine (PCEV), given by deep subcutaneous or intramuscular injection on days 0, 7 and 28, provide effective immunity. A reinforcing dose is given after 12 months and additional reinforcing doses are given every 3–5 years, depending on the risk of exposure. Vaccines of nervous tissue origin are still used in some parts of the world. These, however, are associated with significant side-effects and should not be used if HDCV is available.

Post-exposure prophylaxis

The wound should be cleaned carefully and thoroughly with soap and water, and left open. Human rabies immunoglobulin should be given immediately (20 IU/kg); half should be injected around the area of the wound and the other half should be given intramuscularly. Five 1.0 mL doses of HDCV should be given intramuscularly: the first dose is given on day 0 and is followed by injections on days 3, 7, 14 and 28. Reaction to the vaccine is uncommon. Protection mediated by this protocol is almost 100%.

Control

Domestic animals should be vaccinated if there is any risk of rabies in the country. In the UK, control has been by quarantine of imported animals for 6 months and no indigenous case of rabies has been reported for many years. The Pet Travel Scheme (PETS) enables certain pet animals to enter or re-enter Great Britain without quarantine if they come from qualifying countries via designated routes, are carried by authorized transport companies and meet the conditions of the scheme. Wild animals in 'at-risk' countries must be handled with great care.

Progressive multifocal leucoencephalopathy

JC virus, a polyomavirus, is the cause of progressive multifocal leucoencephalopathy (PML), which presents as dementia in the immunocompromised and is due to multiple foci of demyelination in cerebral white matter. Virus replicates in the nucleus of oligodendrocytes, resulting in cell lysis and breakdown of the myelin sheath. The virus is usually acquired in childhood, and may reactivate if the host immune system becomes compromised in later life (see p. 1446). Reactivation of JC virus and development of PML have recently been described in multiple sclerosis patients treated with the monoclonal antibody, natalizumab, directed against the cell adhesion molecule, α4 integrin.

Further reading

Hemachuda T, Ugolini G, Wacharapluesadee S. Human rabies: neuropathogenesis, diagnosis and treatment. *Lancet Neurol* 2013; 12:498–513.
Tyler KL. Acute viral encephalitis. *N Engl J Med* 2018; 379:557–566.
Zaffran M, McGovern M, Hossaini R et al. The polio endgame: securing a world free of all polioviruses. *Lancet* 2018; 391:11–12.

VIRUS INFECTIONS OF THE GASTROINTESTINAL TRACT

Virus infections that commonly result in acute gastroenteritis (diarrhoea and vomiting) are listed in **Box 20.35**.

Rotavirus infection

Rotaviruses are a major cause of infantile gastroenteritis worldwide. The virus (Latin *rota* = wheel) is so named because of its electron microscopic appearance with a characteristic circular outline and radiating spokes (**Fig. 20.16**). It belongs to the reoviruses family, which have double-stranded RNA segmented genomes. More than 200 000 infected children under the age of 5 years are estimated to die annually in resource-deprived countries. The prevalence is higher during the winter months in non-tropical areas. Asymptomatic infections are common and bottle-fed babies are more likely to be symptomatic than those that are breast-fed.

Adults may become infected with rotavirus but symptoms are usually mild or absent. The virus may, however, cause diarrhoea in immunosuppressed adults, or outbreaks in patients on care of the elderly wards.

Clinical features

The illness is characterized by vomiting, fever, diarrhoea and the metabolic consequences of water and electrolyte loss.

Diagnosis and differential diagnosis

The diagnosis can be established by genome amplification, or ELISA for the detection of rotavirus antigen in faeces and by electron microscopy of faeces. Histology of the jejunal mucosa in children shows shortening of the villi, with crypt hyperplasia and mononuclear cell infiltration of the lamina propria.

Management and prevention

Management is directed at overcoming the effects of water and electrolyte imbalance with adequate oral rehydration therapy and, when indicated, intravenous fluids (**Box 20.36**). Antibiotics should not be prescribed.

Rotavirus vaccines

Despite a major setback when the first licensed rotavirus vaccine was rapidly withdrawn from the market in 1999 following reports of increased rates of intussusception, two live vaccines have been developed and are now used in many countries. One (Rotarix) contains an attenuated human strain, the relevant antigens being P[8] and G1; the other (Rotateq) is based on a bovine parent strain and comprises five single-gene reassortants, each containing a human-strain outer capsid gene encoding the most common human antigenic

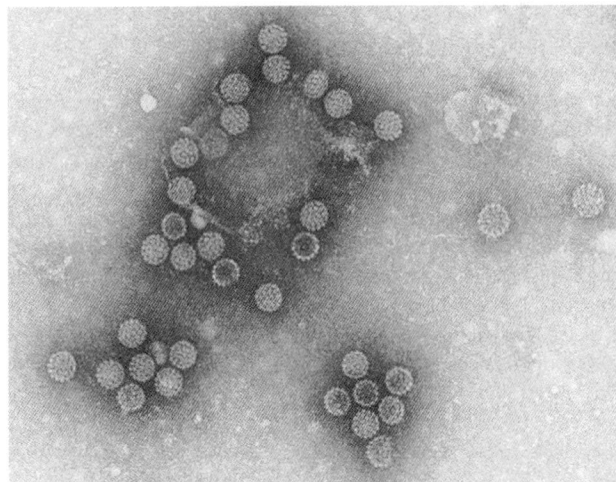

Fig. 20.16 Electron micrograph of human rotavirus.

Box 20.35 Viruses associated with gastroenteritis

- Rotaviruses (groups A, B and C)
- Enteric adenoviruses (types 40 and 41)
- Caliciviruses (includes noroviruses and sapoviruses)
- Astroviruses

> **Box 20.36** Oral rehydration solutions (ORS) and intravenous solutions used in moderate and severe diarrhoea[a]

Solution	Salts (mmol/L)				Substance added (per L of water)	
	Na+	K+	Cl-	Glucose	Substance	Quantity
Oral[b]						
World Health Organization (hypo-osmolar formulation)	75	20	65	75	NaCl	2.6 g
					Na citrate	2.9 g
					KCl	1.5 g
					Glucose	13.5 g
Cereal-based	85	–	80	–	Cooked rice	80 g
					Salt (NaCl)	5 g
Household	85	–	80	111	Glucose	20 g
					Salt (NaCl)	5 g
UK/Europe	35–60	20	37	90–200	Pre-prepared solutions	
Intravenous						
Ringer's lactate[b]	131	5	111	0	Pre-prepared	

[a]In children under 5, zinc supplements (10 mg daily under 6 months, 20 mg daily over 6 months) should ideally be given along with ORS.
[b]ORS should be administered by encouraging the patient to take small, regular sips of fluid. If vomiting occurs, administration should be paused for 10 min and then cautiously restarted. ORS can be administered via a nasogastric tube if swallowing is impaired. If patients are severely dehydrated, intravenous fluids are preferred. [b]Contains Ca^{2+} 2 mmol/L and HCO_3^- (as lactate).

types (P[8] and G1–4). Routine rotavirus vaccination (2 doses at 8 and 12 weeks of age) was introduced in the UK in 2012. Vaccine efficacy against severe rotavirus gastroenteritis is around 90%.

Calicivirus infection

The caliciviruses are an extensive virus family, named after the cup-shaped (Latin *calyx* = cup) indentations on their viral surface seen by electron microscopy. The family contains four genera, two of which, the noroviruses and sapoviruses, infect humans and cause gastroenteritis.

Norovirus is the major cause of acute non-bacterial gastro-enteritis, causing outbreaks in nursing homes, hospitals, schools, leisure centres and restaurants, and on cruise ships. In countries that have adopted routine rotavirus vaccination of infants, noro-virus has become the leading cause of clinically significant acute gastroenteritis in children. Transmission is mostly faecal–oral, with outbreaks suggesting a common source, such as food and water, and fomites. Aerosol transmission also occurs and noroviruses can be detected in vomit. Illness is usually self-limiting (12–48 h) and mild, consisting of nausea, headache and abdominal cramps, fol-lowed by diarrhoea and vomiting, which may be the only feature (winter vomiting). Diagnosis is by demonstration of viral nucleic acid or antigen in diarrhoeal faeces. Treatment is with oral rehydration solutions. Prevention can be difficult but hand-washing and good hygienic food preparation are required.

Sapovirus causes gastroenteritis, mainly in children.

Further reading

Banyai K, Estes MK, Martella V et al. Viral gastroenteritis. *Lancet* 2018; 392:175–186.
Santosham M. Rotavirus vaccines – a new hope. *N Engl J Med* 2017; 376: 1170–1171.

VIRAL HEPATITIS

A number of distinct virus infections may result in inflammation of the liver (hepatitis). The viruses belong to different virus fami-lies, are spread by different routes, and may have differing clinical consequences (see **Box 34.7**). Viral hepatitis is discussed further in Chapter 34.

VIRUSES AND MALIGNANT DISEASE

Around 15–20% of all human malignant disease arises from infec-tion. Recognition of the infectious cause of a particular cancer raises the possibility of developing an anti-cancer vaccine, as has now happened for both hepatitis B virus and human papillomavirus.

Hepatitis viruses and primary hepatocellular carcinoma

Globally, hepatocellular carcinoma is the second most common cause of death due to malignant disease. A high percentage arises in patients infected with either hepatitis B or C viruses (see pp. 126 and 1308).

Human papillomaviruses and cancer of the uterine cervix

Papillomaviruses tend to produce chronic infections (see also p. 672). Human papillomaviruses (HPVs), of which there are at least 100 types, are responsible for the common skin and genital warts, and certain types (mainly 16 and 18) are the cause of carcinoma of the cervix, cancers in other genital areas (vagina, vulva, penis, anus) and some oral cancers (type 16). Vaccines against HPV types 16 and 18 are available. The current recommendations in many coun-tries are for vaccination of all girls at age 9–14 years, although some countries (including the UK) are increasingly opting to vaccinate both boys and girls. (For *anogenital warts*, see p. 1420.)

Epstein–Barr virus and malignant disease

EBV infection has been associated with a number of malignant diseases, including Burkitt lymphoma, undifferentiated nasopha-ryngeal carcinoma, post-transplant lymphoma, the immunoblastic lymphoma of AIDS patients, some forms of Hodgkin lymphoma and gastric cancer. Different levels of expression of EBV latency genes occur in these proliferative conditions, and various co-factors are

Flavivirus
- Yellow fever (urban and sylvan)
- Dengue haemorrhagic fever
- Kyasanur Forest disease
- Omsk haemorrhagic fever

Bunyavirus
- Rift Valley fever
- Congo–Crimean haemorrhagic fever
- Hantavirus infections

Arenavirus
- Argentinian haemorrhagic fever
- Bolivian haemorrhagic fever
- Lassa fever
- Epidemic haemorrhagic fever

Filovirus
- Marburg
- Ebola

[a]Most of these are arboviruses. Some (e.g. Hantavirus, Lassa fever) have a rodent vector. The source and transmission route of filoviruses are not known.

also involved in their pathogenesis; for example, in Burkitt lymphoma, the most common tumour of childhood in sub-Saharan Africa, epidemiological evidence points to an interplay between EBV infection and the presence of hyperendemic (i.e. present all year round) malaria.

Kaposi's sarcoma and human herpesvirus type 8

HHV-8 is strongly associated with the aetiology of all forms of Kaposi's sarcoma. Antibody prevalence is high in those with tumours but relatively low in the general population of most industrialized countries. High rates of infection (>50% population) have been described in Central and Southern Africa, and this matches the geographical distribution of classical Kaposi's sarcoma before the era of AIDS. HHV-8 is transmitted sexually and through exposure to blood from needle-sharing. It is thought that salivary transmission may be the predominant route in Africa. HHV-8 RNA transcripts have been detected in Kaposi's sarcoma cells and in circulating mononuclear cells from patients with the tumour. This virus also has an aetiological role in two rare lymphoproliferative diseases: multicentric **Castleman's disease** (a disorder of the plasma cell type) and **primary effusion lymphoma** (body-cavity-based lymphoma), which is characterized by pleural, pericardial or peritoneal lymphomatous effusions in the absence of a solid tumour mass.

Other rare malignancies due to virus infection

HTLV-1, a lentivirus belonging to the same virus family as HIV, is the aetiological agent of adult T-cell leukaemia/lymphoma. Merkel cell polyomavirus has been identified in the malignant tissue of the rare Merkel cell carcinoma of the skin.

Further reading

Huh WK, Joura EA, Giuliano AR et al. Final efficacy, immunogenicity, and safety analyses of a nine-valent human papillomavirus vaccine in women aged 16–26 years: a randomised, double-blind trial. *Lancet* 2017; 390:2143–2159.

VIRAL HAEMORRHAGIC FEVERS

These comprise infection with a range of different viruses (**Box 20.37**), which have in common the clinical feature of haemorrhagic manifestations.

Yellow fever

Yellow fever, caused by a flavivirus, is an illness of widely varying severity. It is confined to Africa (90% of cases) and South America between latitudes 15°N and 15°S. For poorly understood reasons, yellow fever has not been reported from Asia, despite the fact that climatic conditions are suitable and the vector, *Aedes aegypti*, is common. The infection is transmitted in the wild by *A. africanus* in Africa and the *Haemagogus* species in South and Central America. Extension of infection to humans (via the mosquito from monkeys) leads to the occurrence of 'jungle' yellow fever. *A. aegypti*, a domestic mosquito that lives in close relationship to humans, is responsible for human-to-human transmission in urban areas (urban yellow fever). Once infected, a mosquito remains so for life.

Clinical features

The incubation period is 3–6 days. Mild infection is indistinguishable from other viral fevers such as influenza or dengue.

Three phases are recognized in the severe (classical) illness. Initially, the patient presents with a high fever of acute onset, usually 39–40°C, which then returns to normal in 4–5 days. During this time, headache is prominent. Retrobulbar pain, myalgia, arthralgia, a flushed face and suffused conjunctivae are common. Epigastric discomfort and vomiting are present when the illness is severe. Relative bradycardia (Faget's sign) is present from the second day of illness. The patient then makes an apparent recovery and feels well for several days. Following this 'phase of calm', the patient again develops increasing fever, deepening jaundice and hepatomegaly. Ecchymosis, bleeding from the gums, haematemesis and melaena may occur. Coma, which is usually a result of uraemia or haemorrhagic shock, occurs for a few hours preceding death. The mortality rate is up to 40% in severe cases. Liver pathology shows mid-zone necrosis and eosinophilic degeneration of hepatocytes (Councilman bodies; see p. 1275).

Diagnosis and management

The diagnosis is established by a history of travel and vaccination status, and by isolation of the virus (when possible) from blood during the first 3 days of illness. Serodiagnosis is possible but in endemic areas cross-reactivity with other flaviviruses is a problem.

Management is supportive. Bed rest (under mosquito nets), analgesics and maintenance of fluid and electrolyte balance are required.

Prevention and control

Yellow fever is an internationally notifiable disease. It is easily prevented by using the attenuated 17D chick embryo vaccine. Vaccination is not recommended for children under 9 months, pregnant women or immunosuppressed patients, unless there are compelling reasons. For the purposes of international certification, immunization is valid for 10 years, but protection lasts much longer than this and probably for life. The WHO Expanded Programme of Immunization includes yellow fever vaccination in endemic areas.

Congo–Crimean haemorrhagic fever

Congo–Crimean haemorrhagic fever (CCHF) virus belongs to the *Nairovirus* genus of the family *Bunyaviridae*. This family contains more than 200 viruses, grouped into a number of genera, most of which are arthropod-borne.

CCHF disease is found mainly in Asia and Africa. The primary hosts are cattle and hares, and the vectors are *Hyalomma* ticks. Following an incubation period of 3–6 days, there is an influenza-like illness with fever and haemorrhagic manifestations. The mortality is 10–50%.

Hantavirus infection

Hantaviruses belong to the Hantavirus genus of the Bunyaviridae and are enzootic viruses of wild rodents, which are spread by aerosolized excreta and not by insect vectors. The most severe form of this infection is Korean haemorrhagic fever (also known as haemorrhagic fever with renal syndrome, HFRS). This condition has a mortality of 5–10% and is characterized by fever, shock and haemorrhage followed by an oliguric phase. Milder forms of the disease are associated with related viruses (e.g. Puumala virus) and may present as nephropathia epidemica, an acute fever with renal involvement, seen in Scandinavia and other European countries in people who have been in contact with bank voles. In the USA a hantavirus (transmitted by the deer mouse) termed Sin Nombre was identified as the cause of outbreaks of acute respiratory disease (hantavirus pulmonary syndrome, HPS) in adults. Other hantavirus types and rodent vector systems have been associated with this syndrome.

Diagnosis of hantavirus infection is made by ELISA detection of specific antibodies.

Rift Valley fever

Rift Valley fever, caused by a virus from the *Phlebovirus* genus of the *Bunyaviridae,* is primarily an acute febrile illness of livestock: sheep, goats and camels. It is found in southern and eastern Africa. The vector is *Culex pipiens* in East Africa and *Aedes caballus* in southern Africa, but disease can be transmitted by the bite of an infected animal. Following an incubation period of 3–6 days, the patient has an acute febrile illness that is difficult to distinguish clinically from other viral fevers. The temperature pattern is usually biphasic. The initial febrile illness lasts 2–4 days and is followed by a remission and a second febrile episode. Complications are indicative of severe infection and include retinopathy, meningoencephalitis, haemorrhagic manifestations and hepatic necrosis. Mortality approaches 50% in severe forms. Management is supportive. Animals can be vaccinated.

Lassa fever

Lassa fever virus belongs to the family *Arenaviridae.* Arenaviruses are pleomorphic, round or oval viruses with diameters ranging from 50 to 300 nm. The virion surface has club-shaped projections and the virus itself contains a variable number of characteristic electron-dense granules that represent residual, non-functional host ribosomes. Lassa fever illness was first documented in the town of Lassa, Nigeria, in 1969 and is confined to sub-Saharan West Africa (Nigeria, Liberia and Sierra Leone). The multimammate rat, *Mastomys natalensis*, is known to be the reservoir. Humans are infected by ingesting foods contaminated by rat urine or saliva containing the virus. Person-to-person spread by body fluids also occurs. Only 10–30% of infections are symptomatic. Related arenaviruses are the causative agents of Argentinian and Bolivian haemorrhagic fevers.

Clinical features

The incubation period is 7–18 days. The disease is insidious in onset and characterized by fever, myalgia, severe backache, malaise and headache. A transient maculopapular rash may be present. A sore throat, pharyngitis and lymphadenopathy occur in over 50% of patients. In severe cases, there may be epistaxis and gastrointestinal bleeding: hence the classification of Lassa fever as a viral haemorrhagic fever. The fever usually lasts 1–3 weeks, and recovery within 1 month of the onset of illness is usual. However, death occurs in 15–20% of hospitalized patients, usually from irreversible hypovolaemic shock.

Diagnosis

The diagnosis is established by serial serological tests (including the Lassa virus-specific IgM titre) or by genome detection in throat swab, serum or urine.

Management

Management is supportive. In addition, clinical benefit and a reduction in mortality can be achieved with ribavirin therapy, if given in the first week.

In non-endemic countries, strict isolation procedures should be used, the patient ideally being nursed in a flexible-film isolator. Specialized units for the management of Lassa fever and other haemorrhagic fevers have been established in the UK. As Lassa fever virus and other causes of haemorrhagic fever (Marburg/Ebola and Congo–Crimean haemorrhagic fever viruses; see **Box 20.37**) have been transmitted from patients to staff in healthcare situations, great care should be taken in handling specimens and clinical material from these patients.

Marburg virus disease and Ebola virus disease

These severe, haemorrhagic, febrile illnesses are discussed together because their clinical manifestations are similar, and the causative negative-strand RNA viruses belong to the same virus family, the *Filoviridae*, so called because the viruses have a filamentous appearance on electron microscopy. The diseases are named after Marburg in Germany and the Ebola river region in the Sudan and Zaire, where these viruses first appeared. Their natural reservoir has not been identified and the precise mode of spread from one individual to another has not been elucidated. The genus *Ebolavirus* contains five defined species, which vary in terms of case fatality rates: less than 40% for Bundibugyo, 50% for Sudan and 40–90% for Ebola viruses. There has been only one (non-fatal) case of Tai Forest virus infection. Reston virus, the only Asian species, has not been associated with human mortality.

Epidemics have occurred periodically in recent years, mainly in sub-Saharan Africa. Filoviruses are zoonotic pathogens, with fruit bats thought to be the natural host. The illness is characterized by the acute onset of severe headache, myalgia, vomiting and high fever, followed by prostration. On about the fifth day of illness a non-pruritic maculopapular rash develops on the face and then spreads to the rest of the body. Diarrhoea is profuse and associated with abdominal cramps and vomiting. Haematemesis, melaena or haemoptysis may occur between days 7 and 16. Hepatosplenomegaly and facial oedema are usually present. In Ebola virus disease, chest pain and a dry cough are prominent symptoms.

In August 2014 the WHO declared the ongoing outbreak of Ebola virus infection in West Africa a public health emergency of international concern, with an estimated several thousand

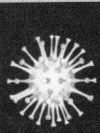

deaths. Guinea, Sierra Leone and Liberia were the worst affected countries. As of early 2020, an outbreak in the Democratic Republic of Congo has involved over 3000 cases, with over 2000 deaths.

Treatment is symptomatic, although a number of experimental therapies, including monoclonal antibodies (e.g. Mab114) and the antivirals remdesivir and favipiravir, are being tried. Experimental vaccines are also being developed. In the absence of effective therapy, accurate diagnosis and infection control precautions are the only intervention strategies. Lack of infrastructure to support rapid molecular diagnostic techniques, and to allow institution of the meticulous patient isolation necessary to interrupt human-to-human transmission of infection, has contributed to generating the recent large outbreaks. Asymptomatic people may be infected but have a low viral count, making transmission unlikely.

Further reading

Houlihan C, Behrens R. Lassa fever. *Br Med J* 2017; 358:j2986.
Lewnard JA. Ebola virus disease: 11323 deaths later, how far have we come? *Lancet* 2018; 392:189–190.

ANTIVIRAL DRUGS

Drugs for HIV infection are discussed on page 1435, and the treatment of hepatitis C and B virus infections on page 1281.

Anti-herpesvirus drugs

Nucleoside analogues

Aciclovir. Aciclovir (**Fig. 20.17A**; also known as acycloguanosine) is an acyclic nucleoside analogue that acts as a chain terminator of herpesvirus DNA synthesis. This drug is converted to aciclovir monophosphate by a virus-encoded thymidine kinase produced by the alpha herpesviruses, herpes simplex types 1 and 2, and varicella zoster virus (**Box 20.38**). Conversion to the triphosphate is then achieved by cellular enzymes. Aciclovir triphosphate acts as a potent inhibitor of viral (but not cellular) DNA polymerase and also competes with deoxyguanine triphosphate for incorporation into the growing chains of herpesvirus DNA, thereby resulting

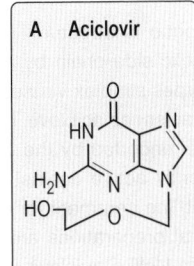
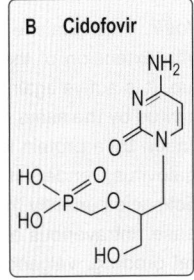

Fig. 20.17 The structure of antiviral drugs. **(A)** Aciclovir. **(B)** Cidofovir.

---

i **Box 20.38 Antiviral agents[a]**

Virus	Structure/mode of action	Drug	Route of administration	Notes
Anti-herpesvirus	Nucleoside analogue	Aciclovir	Oral, i.v., topical	HSV, VZV
		Valaciclovir	Oral	HSV, VZV
		Famciclovir	Oral	HSV, VZV
		Ganciclovir	i.v.	CMV
		Valganciclovir	Oral	CMV
	Nucleotide analogue	Cidofovir	i.v.	CMV
		Brincidofovir	Oral	CMV
	Pyrophosphate analogue	Foscarnet	i.v.	CMV
	Helicase primase inhibitor	Pritelivir	Oral	HSV
	UL97 inhibitor	Maribavir	Oral	CMV
	Terminase inhibitor	Letermovir	Oral	CMV
Anti-influenza	Neuraminidase inhibitor	Zanamivir	Inhaled	Influenza A, B
		Oseltamivir	Oral	Influenza A, B
		Peramivir	i.v.	Influenza A, B
	Endonuclease inhibitor	Baloxavir	Oral	Influenza A, B
Anti-hepatitis B virus	Nucleoside analogue	Lamivudine	Oral	Rapid resistance
		Telbivudine	Oral	Rapid resistance
		Entecavir	Oral	High barrier to resistance
	Nucleotide analogue	Adefovir	Oral	
		Tenofovir	Oral	High barrier to resistance
Other	Nucleoside analogue	Ribavirin	Oral, i.v.	Broad spectrum; RSV, HCV
	Interferons		i.m.	Pegylated
	Monoclonal antibody	Palivizumab	i.m.	RSV

[a]For drugs used in HIV, see p. 1435; for drugs used in the treatment of hepatitis C virus infection, see p. 1283). CMV, cytomegalovirus; HCV, hepatitis C virus; HSV, herpes simplex virus; i.m., intramuscular; i.v., intravenous; RSV, respiratory syncytial virus; VZV, varicella zoster virus.

in chain synthesis termination due to its acyclic structure. This highly specific mode of activity, targeted only to virus-infected cells, means that aciclovir has very low toxicity. Crystallization in the renal tubules is a well-recognized adverse effect and patients should be well hydrated, particularly when high-dose intravenous therapy is being used. Intravenous, oral and topical preparations are available for the treatment of herpes simplex and varicella zoster virus infections. Treatment does not eliminate latent virus and so relapses do occur.

Valaciclovir. This is an oral prodrug of aciclovir. Coupling of valine to the acyclic side-chain of aciclovir allows better intestinal absorption. The valine is removed by enzymic action and aciclovir is released into the circulation. A similar prodrug of a related nucleoside analogue (penciclovir) is the antiherpes drug famciclovir. The mode of action and efficacy of famciclovir are similar to those of aciclovir.

Ganciclovir. This guanine analogue is structurally similar to aciclovir, with extension of the acyclic side-chain by a carboxymethyl group. It is active against herpes simplex viruses and varicella zoster virus by the same mechanism as aciclovir. In addition, phosphorylation by a protein kinase, encoded by the *UL97* gene of cytomegalovirus, renders it potently active against this virus. Thus, ganciclovir is currently the first-line treatment for cytomegalovirus disease. Intravenous and oral preparations are available, as is an oral prodrug, valganciclovir. Unlike aciclovir, ganciclovir has a significant toxicity profile, including neutropenia, thrombocytopenia and, rarely, sterilization by inhibition of spermatogenesis. It is therefore reserved for the treatment or prevention of life- or sight-threatening cytomegalovirus infection in immunocompromised patients.

Nucleotide analogues

Cidofovir. This is a phosphonate derivative of an acyclic nucleoside that acts as a viral DNA polymerase inhibitor (**Fig. 20.17B**). Phosphorylation to the active triphosphate moiety is entirely by host cell enzymes. It is administered intravenously for the treatment of severe cytomegalovirus infections when other drugs are inappropriate. It is given with probenecid and, as it is nephrotoxic, particular attention should be paid to hydration and monitoring of renal function.

Brincidofovir. This drug consists of cidofovir bound to a lipid moiety, enabling an oral route of administration and avoiding renal toxicity; it has shown great promise in clinical trials.

Pyrophosphate analogues

Foscarnet (sodium phosphonoformate). This is a simple pyrophosphate analogue that inhibits viral DNA polymerases. It is active against herpesviruses and its main roles are as a second-line treatment for severe cytomegalovirus disease and in the treatment of aciclovir-resistant herpes simplex infection. It is given intravenously but the potential for severe side-effects, particularly renal damage, limits its use.

Novel anti-herpesvirus agents

New drugs undergoing clinical trials include pritelivir, an inhibitor of the herpes simplex viral helicase–primase enzyme complex; maribavir, an inhibitor of the product of the *UL97* gene of cytomegalovirus, which plays a key role in allowing viral egress from an infected cell; and letermovir, an inhibitor of the cytomegalovirus terminase enzyme complex, which cuts the string of cytomegalovirus genomes synthesized in an infected cell into unit-length genomes for packaging in the capsid.

Anti-influenza drugs

Adamantanes

Amantadine. The use of amantadine and derivatives in the treatment and prophylaxis of influenza has largely been superseded by the neuraminidase inhibitors. Amantadine is active prophylactically and therapeutically against influenza A (but not B) virus. CNS side-effects, such as insomnia, dizziness and headache, may occur and the drug is poorly tolerated, especially in the elderly.

Neuraminidase inhibitors

Zanamivir (administered by inhalation) and *oseltamivir* (an oral preparation). These drugs inhibit the action of the neuraminidase of influenza A and B. Both have been shown to be effective in reducing the duration of illness in influenza if given within the first 48 hours. Oseltamivir is also available for the prophylaxis of influenza among contacts of an index case. Intravenous peramivir and zanamivir were both reported to be effective in treating patients during the 2010 influenza pandemic, but neither is currently licensed for routine use in this way.

Novel anti-influenza drugs

Baloxavir inhibits the cap-dependent endonuclease activity of the influenza polymerase. Clinical trials have shown efficacy similar to that of oseltamivir, and this drug achieved Food and Drug Administration approval in October 2018.

Anti-hepatitis B drugs

A number of nucleoside and nucleotide analogues have been shown to inhibit the reverse transcriptase function of hepatitis B virus and thereby suppress viral replication (see p. 1281). The first such agents, *lamivudine* and *adefovir*, have largely been superseded by the more potent drugs *entecavir* and *tenofovir*, both of which also have a considerably higher barrier to resistance.

Telbivudine is also a nucleoside analogue inhibitor of HBV DNA polymerase activity.

Other drugs

Ribavirin. This synthetic purine nucleoside derivative, which interferes with 5′-capping of messenger RNA, is active against several RNA and DNA viruses, at least *in vitro*. Its major use is in the treatment of chronic hepatitis C infection in combination with other agents, although it has no effect when given alone. It is administered orally. Haemolytic anaemia is the most frequent adverse reaction. It is also administered by a small-particle aerosol generator (SPAG) to infants with acute respiratory syncytial virus (RSV) infection. Another indication is in the treatment of Lassa fever virus infection.

Palivizumab. This monoclonal antibody is specifically indicated to prevent seasonal RSV infection in infants at high risk of this infection. It is administered by intramuscular injection.

Interferons

These are naturally occurring proteins with a multiplicity of actions, including antiviral, immunomodulatory and antiproliferative effects. Interferons are produced by virus-infected cells, macrophages and lymphocytes. They induce an antiviral state in uninfected cells, through

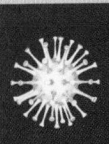

activation of a complex set of biochemical pathways. They have been synthesized commercially and are licensed for therapeutic use.

The potency of INF-α has been enhanced by coupling the protein with polyethylene glycol. The resulting pegylated (PEG) interferon, given once weekly, has been shown to improve the response to, and reduce the side-effects from, treatment for hepatitis B and C (see p. 1281).

Further reading

Poole CL, James SH. Antiviral therapies for herpesviruses: current agents and new directions. *Clin Ther* 2018; 40:1282–1298.

TRANSMISSIBLE SPONGIFORM ENCEPHALOPATHIES (PRION DISEASES)

Transmissible spongiform encephalopathies (TSEs) are caused by the accumulation in the nervous system of a protein, termed a 'prion', which is an abnormal isoform (PrP^{Sc}) of a normal host protein (PrP^{c}).

Although familial forms of prion disease are known to exist, these conditions can be transmissible, particularly if brain tissue enters another host. There is no convincing evidence for the presence of nucleic acid in association with prions, and it is the abnormal prion protein itself that is infectious and can trigger a conversion of the normal protein into the atypical isoform. After infection, a long incubation period is followed by CNS degeneration associated with dementia or ataxia, which invariably leads to death. Histology of the brain reveals spongiform change with an accumulation of the abnormal prion protein in the form of amyloid plaques.

The human prion diseases are Creutzfeldt–Jakob disease, including the sporadic, familial, iatrogenic and variant forms of the disease, Gerstmann–Straussler–Scheinker syndrome, fatal familial insomnia and kuru.

- *Creutzfeldt–Jakob disease (CJD)*. CJD occurs sporadically worldwide with an annual incidence of 1 per million of the population. Although, in most cases, the epidemiology remains obscure, iatrogenic transmission to others has occurred as a result of administration of human cadaveric growth hormone or gonadotrophin, from dura mater and corneal grafting and in neurosurgery from reuse of contaminated instruments and electrodes (iatrogenic CJD).
- *Variant CJD (vCJD)*. In the UK, knowledge that large numbers of cattle with the prion disease, bovine spongiform encephalopathy (BSE), had gone into the human food chain, led to enhanced surveillance for emergence of the disease in humans. Based on transmission studies in mice and on glycosylation patterns of prion proteins, the evidence is convincing that this has occurred and, to date, there have been approximately 180 confirmed and suspected cases of vCJD (human BSE) in the UK and 50 in the rest of the world. In contrast to sporadic CJD, which presents with dementia at a mean age of onset of 60 years, vCJD presents with ataxia, dementia, myoclonus and chorea at a mean age of onset of 29 years.
- *Gerstmann–Straussler–Scheinker syndrome and fatal familial insomnia*. These are rare prion diseases, usually occurring in families with a positive history. The pattern of inheritance is autosomal dominant with some degree of variable penetrance. The gene encoding PrP^{c} in these families often contains mutations.
- *Kuru*. This disease was described and characterized in the Fore highlanders in north-east New Guinea. Transmission was associated with ritualistic cannibalism of deceased relatives. With

the cessation of cannibalism by 1960, the disease has gradually diminished and recent cases had all been exposed to the agent before 1960.

The infectious agents of prion disease have remarkable characteristics. In the infected host there is no evidence of inflammatory, cytokine or immune reactions. The agent is highly resistant to decontamination, and infectivity is not reliably destroyed by autoclaving or by treatment with formaldehyde and most other gas or liquid disinfectants. It is very resistant to γ-irradiation. Autoclaving at a high temperature (134–137°C for 18 min) is used for decontamination of instruments and hypochlorite (20 000 p.p.m. available chlorine) or 1 molar sodium hydroxide is used for liquid disinfection. Uncertainty about the reliability of any methods for safe decontamination of surgical instruments has necessitated the introduction of guidelines for patient management.

Further reading

Mackenzie G, Will R. Creutzfeldt-Jakob disease: recent developments. *F1000Res* 2017; 6:2053.

BACTERIAL INFECTIONS

UBIQUITOUS BACTERIAL INFECTIONS

Bacteria are ubiquitous single-celled organisms that form the major part of the normal human microbiome. Bacterial infection is caused by commensal bacteria invading normally sterile parts of the body, or by pathogenic bacteria that are not normal commensal organisms. Infection can be the result of translocation of bacteria from non-sterile to sterile areas (e.g. from the gut to the urinary tract), acquisition from other people or animals, or transmission on fomites or in the environment.

In some cases, bacterial infection may be localized to a specific site, with few or no systemic symptoms. In other circumstances a localized infection may be accompanied by systemic illness or sepsis syndrome (see Ch. 8). Sometimes there is no obvious localized infection and the presentation is undifferentiated sepsis. In a few cases, bacteria cause illness through release of a specific toxin, which produces symptoms distant from the actual site of infection (**Box 20.39**).

Some bacterial infections are found worldwide, while others are particularly common in tropical/subtropical countries or in areas that have poorer access to fresh water, good hygiene and medical care. These factors are often interdependent, and many of the conditions that are traditionally labelled as 'tropical' are, in fact, related to socioeconomic conditions rather than climate.

Many of the common organ-specific bacterial conditions are covered in the relevant system chapters and the sepsis syndrome is described in Chapter 8. This section deals with those bacterial infections that do not fit readily into an organ-specific model, and those that are more defined by geographical and economic constraints than by body site.

BACTERIAL INFECTIONS OF THE SKIN AND SOFT TISSUES

Most common bacterial infections of skin and soft tissue are covered in Chapter 22, although some of the more unusual causes are described here and listed in **Box 20.40**. The majority of soft tissue infections are caused by *Staphylococcus aureus*, and while most *Staph. aureus* infections remain superficial, this organism can spread from the skin to cause a variety of more serious infections (see **Box 20.23**). Staphylococci are part of the normal microflora of the human skin and nasopharynx; up to 25% of people are carriers of *Staph. aureus*, the species responsible for the majority of staphylococcal infections. Other species of staphylococci are only rarely pathogenic.

Box 20.39 Classification of more common bacteria affecting humans

Bacteria	Cocci	Bacilli	Others
Aerobic			
Gram-positive	Staphylococcus aureus Staph. epidermidis Streptococcus pneumoniae Strep. pyogenes (group A) Strep. agalactiae (group B) Enterococci Viridans streptococci	Listeria monocytogenes Corynebacterium diphtheriae Bacillus anthracis B. cereus	
Gram-negative	Neisseria gonorrhoeae N. meningitidis Moraxella catarrhalis Bordetella pertussis	Escherichia coli Klebsiella spp. Proteus spp. Haemophilus influenzae Legionella spp. Salmonella spp. Shigella spp. Campylobacter jejuni Helicobacter pylori Pseudomonas spp. Brucella spp. Acinetobacter spp. Burkholderia spp. Vibrio cholerae Yersinia pestis	
Anaerobic			
Gram-positive	Peptococci Peptostreptococci	Actinomyces spp. Clostridium perfringens C. difficile C. botulinum C. tetani	
Gram-negative		Bacteroides fragilis group Fusobacterium spp.	
Spirochaetes			Treponema pallidum Leptospira spp. Borrelia spp.
Others			Mycobacterium spp. Mycoplasma pneumoniae Ureaplasma spp. Chlamydia spp. Rickettsia spp.

Invasive staphylococcal infection

Invasive staphylococcal infection is often associated with breaches in the skin: for example, those due to injecting drug use, iatrogenic cannulation, surgery or trauma. Other predisposing factors are listed in **Box 20.24**. In clinical situations, scrupulous attention to disinfection and hygiene when performing invasive procedures can minimize the risk of infection. Although *Staph. aureus* is the most common species of staphylococcus implicated in intravenous catheter-related infections, other normally non-pathogenic species, such as *Staph. epidermidis* (which is often intrinsically resistant to flucloxacillin), may be found. Flucloxacillin remains the first-choice antibiotic in staphylococcal infection when the organism is known to be sensitive (see p. 163 and **Box 8.8**), but with the increasing prevalence of meticillin-resistant *Staph. aureus* (MRSA), alternative anti-staphylococcal agents are being used more widely.

Staphylococcal virulence factors

Staph. aureus can produce a variety of toxins and virulence factors that affect the type and severity of infection. These include staphylococcal enterotoxin A, superantigenic staphylococcal exotoxins, toxic shock toxin 1 and Panton Valentine–leukocidin (PVL). The last of these has been found mainly in community-associated strains of *Staph. aureus* (both MRSA and meticillin-sensitive *Staph. aureus*, MSSA), rather than in hospital-acquired or epidemic strains. PVL-producing MRSA and MSSA are becoming an increasingly common cause of invasive soft tissue and lung infections in some countries (notably the USA), although it is unclear whether PVL itself is directly responsible for the increased virulence.

Meticillin-resistant *Staphylococcus aureus*

Staph. aureus is commonly resistant to penicillin, and isolated resistance to other β-lactam antibiotics, such as meticillin (now rarely used) and flucloxacillin, has been recognized since the development of the first semi-synthetic penicillins in the early 1960s. However, in the last 40 years, strains of meticillin-resistant *Staphylococcus aureus* (MRSA) with resistance to a much wider range of antibiotics have emerged.

MRSA is usually found as a skin commensal, especially in hospitalized patients or nursing home residents. However, it can cause a variety of infections in soft tissues and elsewhere, and can lead to death. It is particularly associated with surgical wound infections. Eradication of the organism is difficult and people who are known

---

Box 20.40 Bacterial causes of superficial skin and soft tissue infection

Specific risk factors	Likely organisms
None	Staphylococcus aureus Streptococcus pyogenes
Diabetes, peripheral vascular disease	Group B streptococci
Animal bite	Pasteurella multocida, Capnocytophaga canimorsus
Freshwater exposure	Aeromonas hydrophila
Seawater exposure	Vibrio vulnificans
Lymphoedema, stasis dermatitis	Groups A, C and G streptococci
Hot tub exposure	Pseudomonas aeruginosa
Malignant otitis externa	Pseudomonas aeruginosa
Human bite	Fusobacterium spp.

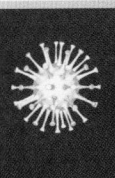

to be colonized should be isolated from those at risk of significant infection. Topical decolonization is often used to decrease bacterial load prior to invasive procedures but is of limited efficacy in clearing carriage completely. Careful attention to hand-washing and hygiene is the main method of controlling spread (see p. 292).

Although MRSA is generally regarded as a hospital-associated organism, it is commonly seen in people away from this setting, both as a colonizer and as a cause of disease. Often the organisms are the typical 'hospital' strains of MRSA and have been acquired directly or indirectly from a healthcare setting (e.g. in workers in care homes). However, there is an increasing prevalence in some countries of true community-associated MRSA (CA-MRSA), with no discernible links to hospital or residential care. These CA-MRSA strains have different resistance profiles to those of typical hospital strains (often retaining sensitivity to tetracyclines, clindamycin and co-trimoxazole) and are more likely to produce PVL.

Pasteurellosis

Pasteurella multocida is found in the oropharynx of up to 90% of cats and 70% of dogs. It can cause soft tissue infections following animal bites. Although the infection initially resembles other forms of cellulitis, there is a greater tendency to spread to deeper tissues, resulting in osteomyelitis, tenosynovitis or septic arthritis. It can also spread haematogenously to other organs, including the lungs and heart. The organism is sensitive to penicillin, but as infections following animal bites are often polymicrobial, co-amoxiclav is a better choice.

Cat-scratch disease

Cat-scratch disease is a zoonosis caused by *Bartonella henselae*. Asymptomatic bacteraemia is relatively common in domestic and especially feral cats, and human infection is probably due to direct inoculation from the claws or via cat flea bites. Regional lymphadenopathy appears 1–2 weeks after infection; the nodes become tender and may suppurate. Histology of the nodes shows granuloma formation and the illness may be mistaken for mycobacterial infection or lymphoma. There are usually few systemic symptoms in immunocompetent patients, although more severe disease may be seen in the immunocompromised. In these patients, tender cutaneous or subcutaneous nodules are seen (**bacillary angiomatosis**), which may ulcerate. The lymphadenopathy resolves spontaneously over weeks or months, although surgical drainage of very large suppurating nodes may be necessary. *B. henselae* is sensitive to azithromycin, doxycycline and ciprofloxacin, but drug selection and clinical benefit of treatment vary according to the primary site of the infection and the immune status of the patient.

Toxin-mediated skin disease

A number of skin conditions, although caused by bacteria, are mediated by exotoxins rather than direct local tissue damage.

Staphylococcal scalded skin syndrome

The scalded skin syndrome is caused by a toxin-secreting strain of *Staph. aureus* (see p. 669). It principally affects children under the age of 5. The toxin, exfoliatin, causes intra-epidermal cleavage at the level of the stratum corneum, leading to the formation of large, flaccid blisters that shear readily. It is a relatively benign condition and responds to treatment with flucloxacillin.

Toxic shock syndrome

Toxic shock syndrome (TSS) is usually due to toxin-secreting staphylococci but toxin-secreting streptococci have also been implicated. Although historically associated with vaginal colonization and tampon use in women, this is not always the case. The exotoxin (normally toxic shock syndrome toxin 1, TSST-1) induces cytokine release, causing abrupt onset of fever and shock, with a diffuse macular rash and desquamation of the palms and soles. Many patients are severely ill and mortality is about 5%. Management is mainly supportive, although the organism should be eradicated.

BACTERIAL INFECTIONS OF THE RESPIRATORY TRACT

Infections of the respiratory tract are divided into those affecting the upper respiratory tract and those affecting the lower respiratory tract, which are separated by the larynx. The majority of common respiratory infections are covered elsewhere.

Upper respiratory tract infections

Scarlet fever

Scarlet fever occurs when the infectious organism (usually *Streptococcus* group A but occasionally group C or G) produces erythrogenic toxin in an individual who does not possess neutralizing antitoxin antibodies. Infections may be sporadic or epidemic, occurring in residential institutions such as schools, prisons and military establishments.

Clinical features

The onset of this relatively mild disease, which mainly affects children, is 2–4 days following a streptococcal infection (usually in the pharynx). Common features include regional lymphadenopathy, fever, rigors, headache and vomiting. The rash, which blanches on pressure, usually appears on the second day of illness. It is generalized but typically absent from the face, palms and soles. It usually lasts about 5 days and is followed by extensive desquamation of the skin (**Fig. 20.18**). The face is flushed, with characteristic circumoral pallor. Early in the disease the tongue has a white coating, through which

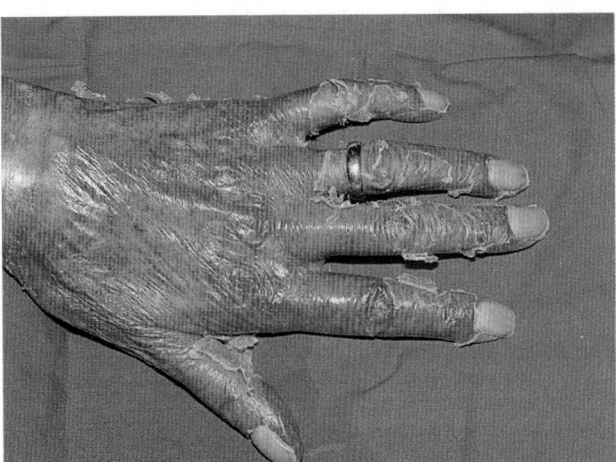

Fig. 20.18 Scarlet fever rash, showing desquamation.

prominent bright red papillae can be seen ('strawberry tongue'). Later the white coating disappears, leaving a raw-looking, bright red colour ('raspberry tongue'). The patient is infective for 10–21 days after the onset of the rash, unless treated with antibiotics.

Scarlet fever may be complicated by peritonsillar or retropharyngeal abscesses and otitis media.

The diagnosis is established by the typical clinical features, and culture of a throat swab. Scarlet fever should be treated with penicillin, to which group A streptococcus is invariably sensitive.

Diphtheria

Diphtheria (caused by *Corynebacterium diphtheriae* or *C. ulcerans*) occurs worldwide. Its incidence in the West has fallen dramatically following widespread active immunization, but the disease has re-emerged in Eastern Europe. Transmission is mainly through airborne droplet infection. *C. diphtheriae* is a Gram-positive bacillus; only strains that carry the *tox*+ gene are capable of toxin production.

Clinical features

Diphtheria was formerly a disease of childhood but may affect adults in countries where childhood immunization has been interrupted or uptake is poor. The incubation period is 2–7 days. The manifestations are local (due to the membrane) or systemic (due to exotoxin). The presence of a membrane, however, is not essential to the diagnosis.

Nasal diphtheria is characterized by the presence of a unilateral, serosanguineous nasal discharge that crusts around the external nares.

Pharyngeal diphtheria is associated with the greatest toxicity and is characterized by marked tonsillar and pharyngeal inflammation and, usually, the presence of a membrane. The tough, greyish-yellow membrane is formed by fibrin, bacteria, epithelial cells, mononuclear cells and polymorphs, and is firmly adherent to the underlying tissue. Regional lymphadenopathy, often tender, is prominent and produces the so-called 'bull-neck'.

Laryngeal diphtheria is usually a result of extension of the membrane from the pharynx. A husky voice, a brassy cough and, later, dyspnoea and cyanosis due to respiratory obstruction are common features.

Diphtheria toxin principally affects the heart and the nervous system. Clinically evident myocarditis occurs, sometimes weeks after initial infection, in a proportion of patients with pharyngeal or laryngeal diphtheria. Acute circulatory failure due to myocarditis may occur in convalescent individuals around the tenth day of illness and can often be fatal. Neurological manifestations occur either early in the disease (palatal and pharyngeal wall paralysis) or several weeks after its onset (cranial nerve palsies, paraesthesiae, polyneuropathy or, rarely, encephalitis).

Cutaneous diphtheria (caused by *C. ulcerans*) is uncommon but seen in association with burns and in individuals with poor personal hygiene. Typically, the ulcer is punched-out with undermined edges and is covered with a greyish-white to brownish adherent membrane. Constitutional symptoms are uncommon.

Diagnosis

This must be made on clinical grounds since therapy is usually urgent; the mortality rate is about 10%. It is confirmed by bacterial culture and toxin studies.

Management

Antitoxin therapy is the only specific treatment. It must be given promptly to prevent further fixation of toxin to tissue receptors, since fixed toxin is not neutralized by antitoxin. Depending on the severity, 20 000–100 000 units of horse-serum antitoxin should be administered intramuscularly, after an initial test dose to exclude any allergic reaction. Intravenous therapy may be required in a very severe case. There is a risk of acute anaphylaxis after antitoxin administration, and of serum sickness 2–3 weeks later (**Box 20.41**). However, the risk of death outweighs the problems of anaphylaxis. Antibiotics (penicillin, amoxicillin or a macrolide) should be administered concurrently to eliminate the organisms and thereby remove the source of toxin production.

The cardiac and neurological complications need intensive supportive therapy. Recovery and rehabilitation can take many weeks.

Prevention

Patients with suspected diphtheria must be isolated and the local public health authorities should be informed. Staff caring for the patient should have documented immunization status. All contacts of the patient should have throat swabs sent for culture; those with a positive result should be treated with antibiotic, and be given active immunization or a booster dose of diphtheria toxoid. Diphtheria is prevented by active immunization in childhood (see p. 508). Travellers to high-risk countries may require a booster dose, even if they have had childhood immunization (although monovalent diphtheria vaccine is no longer available).

Acute epiglottitis

Acute epiglottitis has been virtually eliminated among children in countries that have introduced *Haemophilus influenzae* vaccine, as in the UK. Occasionally, infections are seen in adults. The clinical features are described on page 947.

Lower respiratory tract infections

Pneumonia, lung abscess and tuberculosis

For community-acquired pneumonia, see page 963; hospital-acquired pneumonia, page 965; and pneumonia in immunocompromised persons, page 967.

Lung abscess is described on page 965.

Tuberculosis is described on page 967.

Further reading

Barlow RS, Reynolds RE, Cieslak PR et al. Vaccinated children and adolescents with pertussis infections experience reduced illness severity and duration. *Clin Infect Dis* 2014; 58:1523–1529.

Murhekar M. Epidemiology of diphtheria in India, 1996–2016: implications for prevention and control. *Am J Trop Med Hyg* 2017; 97:313–318.

Box 20.41 Antitoxin administration

- Many antitoxins are heterologous and therefore dangerous
- Hypersensitivity reactions are common
  Prior to treatment
- Question the patient about:
  - allergic conditions (e.g. asthma, hay fever)
  - previous antitoxin administration

- Read the instructions on the antitoxin package carefully
- Always give a subcutaneous test dose
- Have adrenaline (epinephrine) available

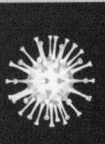

BACTERIAL INFECTIONS OF THE GASTROINTESTINAL TRACT

Gastroenteritis

The most common form of acute gastrointestinal infection is gastroenteritis, causing diarrhoea with or without vomiting. Children in the developing world can expect, on average, 3–6 bouts of severe diarrhoea annually. Although oral rehydration programmes have cut the death toll significantly, more than half a million children die every year as a direct result of diarrhoeal disease. In the Western world, diarrhoea is both less common and less likely to cause death, but remains a major cause of morbidity, especially in the elderly. Other groups at increased risk of infectious diarrhoea include travellers to developing countries, people in residential care and infants in daycare facilities.

Viral gastroenteritis (see p. 529) is a common cause of diarrhoea and vomiting in young children but is less commonly seen in adults, other than in the context of common source outbreaks (usually due to norovirus). It is a major cause of morbidity and mortality among infants in low-income countries. Protozoal and helminthic gut infections (see pp. 563 and 573) are rare in the West but relatively common in developing countries. However, the most common cause of significant adult gastroenteritis worldwide is bacterial infection.

Bacteria can cause diarrhoea in three different ways (**Box 20.42**). Some species may employ more than one of these methods. In addition to these direct mechanisms, a proportion of people develop post-infectious irritable bowel syndrome, a functional bowel disorder triggered by infection but persisting after resolution of the inflammation (see p. 1187).

Mucosal adherence

Most bacteria causing diarrhoea must first adhere to specific receptors on the gut mucosa: a number of different molecular adhesion mechanisms have been elaborated. For some pathogens this is merely the prelude to invasion or toxin production but others, such as enteropathogenic *Escherichia coli* (EPEC), cause mucosal lesions and produce a secretory diarrhoea as a direct result of adherence. Enteroaggregative *E. coli* (EAggEC) adhere in an aggregative pattern, with the bacteria clumping on the cell surface, and their toxin causes persistent diarrhoea. Diffusely adhering *E. coli* (DAEC) adheres in a uniform manner and may also cause diarrhoea. Both are seen mainly in low-income countries with poor hygiene and inadequate clean water supply.

E. coli O104:H4, which has caused huge outbreaks of gastroenteritis in Germany and other developed countries, has two different diarrhoea-causing *E. coli* pathotypes: typical enteroaggregative *E. coli* and Shiga-toxin-producing *E. coli*.

Mucosal invasion

Invasive pathogens, such as *Shigella* spp., enteroinvasive *E. coli* (EIEC) and *Campylobacter* spp., penetrate the intestinal mucosa. Initial entry into the mucosal cells is facilitated by the production of 'invasins', which disrupt the host-cell cytoskeleton. Subsequent destruction of the epithelial cells allows further bacterial entry, which also causes the typical symptoms of dysentery: low-volume bloody diarrhoea with abdominal pain.

Toxin production

Gastroenteritis can be caused by different types of bacterial toxin. **Enterotoxins** produced by bacteria adhering to the intestinal epithelium induce excessive fluid secretion into the bowel lumen, leading to watery diarrhoea without physically damaging the mucosa (e.g. cholera, enterotoxigenic *E. coli*, ETEC). Some enterotoxins that are pre-formed in food primarily cause vomiting (e.g. enterotoxigenic *Staph. aureus* and *Bacillus cereus*). **Cytotoxins** damage the intestinal mucosa and, in some cases, vascular endothelium as well (e.g. *E. coli* O157).

Clinical syndromes

Bacterial gastroenteritis can be divided on clinical grounds into two broad syndromes: **watery diarrhoea** (usually due to enterotoxins or adherence) and **dysentery** (usually due to mucosal invasion and damage) (**Box 20.43**). With some pathogens, such as *Campylobacter jejuni*, there may be overlap between the two syndromes. A third clinical type of infective gastroenteritis, **chronic diarrhoea**, is rarely bacterial in origin.

---

i | **Box 20.42** Pathogenic mechanisms of bacterial gastroenteritis

Pathogenesis	Mode of action	Clinical presentation	Examples
Mucosal adherence	Effacement of intestinal mucosa	Moderate watery diarrhoea	Enteropathogenic *Escherichia coli* (EPEC) Enteroaggregative *E. coli* (EAggEC) *E. coli* O14:H4 Diffusely adhering *E. coli* (DAEC)
Mucosal invasion	Penetration and destruction of mucosa	Dysentery	*Shigella* spp. *Campylobacter* spp. Enteroinvasive *E. coli* (EIEC)
Toxin production:			
Enterotoxin	Fluid secretion without mucosal damage	Profuse watery diarrhoea	*Vibrio cholerae* *Salmonella* spp. *Campylobacter* spp. Enterotoxigenic *E. coli* (ETEC) *Bacillus cereus* *Staphylococcus aureus* producing enterotoxin B *Clostridium perfringens* type A
Cytotoxin	Damage to mucosa	Dysentery	*Salmonella* spp. *Campylobacter* spp. Enterohaemorrhagic *E. coli* O157 (EHEC) *E. coli* O104:H4

Management of infective diarrhoea is usually syndromic (see later), as, except during outbreaks, the causative organism is rarely known at presentation. Bacterial gastroenteritis is usually self-limiting and in otherwise healthy individuals does not require anti-bacterials, unless the infection is particularly severe or prolonged. An exception is dysentery in children, where antibiotic therapy is proven to reduce mortality (**Box 20.44**).

Salmonella

Gastroenteritis can be caused by many of the numerous sero-types of non-typhoidal *Salmonella* (all of which are members of a single species of Gram-negative bacillus, *S. choleraesuis*), but the most commonly implicated are *S. enteritidis* and *S. typhimurium* (*S. typhi* and *S. paratyphi*, the causes of enteric fever, which are covered on p. 554). These organisms, which are found all over the world, are commensals in the bowels of livestock (especially poultry) and oviducts of chicken (where the eggs can become infected). They are usually transmitted to humans in contaminated foodstuffs and water.

Salmonellae can affect both the large and the small bowel, and induce diarrhoea both by production of enterotoxins and by invasion. The typical symptoms commence abruptly, 12–48 hours after infection, and consist of nausea, cramping abdominal pain, diarrhoea and sometimes fever. The diarrhoea can vary from pro-fuse and watery to a bloody dysentery syndrome. Spontaneous resolution usually occurs in 3–6 days, although the organism may persist in the faeces for several weeks. Bloodstream infec-tion occurs in 1–4% of cases and is more common in the elderly and the immunosuppressed; some serotypes are more prone to cause bacteraemia than others. Occasionally, this is complicated by metastatic infection, especially of atheroma on vascular endo-thelium, with potentially devastating consequences. In healthy adults, *Salmonella* gastroenteritis is usually a relatively minor ill-ness, but young children and the elderly are at risk of significant dehydration.

Specific diagnosis is made by culturing the organism from blood or faeces, but management is usually empirical and includes oral rehydration. Antibiotic resistance in salmonellae is increasing, with 13% of European human isolates now resistant to ciprofloxacin. Resistance to azithromycin or third-generation cephalosporins remains rare.

Campylobacter jejuni

The Gram-negative bacillus *C. jejuni* is a zoonotic organism, exist-ing as a bowel commensal in many species of livestock, includ-ing poultry and cattle. It is found worldwide and is an important cause of childhood gastroenteritis in developing countries. Adults in these countries may be tolerant of the organism, excreting it asymptomatically. In the West, it is a common cause of sporadic food-borne outbreaks of gastroenteritis. About 50 000 cases are confirmed annually in England and Wales, but the actual incidence is much higher. The most common sources are undercooked meat

---

? Box 20.43 Bacterial causes of watery diarrhoea and dysentery

Watery diarrhoea	Dysentery
• *Bacillus cereus* ⎱ plus profuse vomiting • *Staphylococcus aureus* ⎰ • *Vibrio cholerae* • Enterotoxigenic *Escherichia coli* (ETEC) • Enteropathogenic *Escherichia coli* (EPEC) • *Salmonella* spp. • *Campylobacter jejuni* • *Clostridium perfringens* • *Clostridium difficile*	• *Shigella* spp. • *Salmonella* spp. • *Campylobacter* spp. • Enteroinvasive *Escherichia coli* (EIEC) • Enterohaemorrhagic *Escherichia coli* (EHEC) • *Yersinia enterocolitica* • *Vibrio parahaemolyticus* • *Clostridium difficile*

---

i Box 20.44 Antibiotics in adult acute bacterial gastroenteritis

Condition	Indications	Drug of choice	Other drugs	Benefits
Dysentery Suspected or confirmed shigellosis	Most patients	Ciprofloxacin 500 mg twice daily	Azithromycin 500 mg once daily Ceftriaxone 2 g daily (i.v. or i.m.)	Relieve symptoms Shorten illness Reduce mortality in children Decrease transmission
Cholera	Severely dehydrated patients only (World Health Organization guidance)	Ciprofloxacin 500 mg twice daily	Tetracycline 250 mg four times daily Azithromycin 1 g single dose Doxycycline 300 mg single dose	Relieve symptoms Shorten illness
Empirical therapy of watery diarrhoea[a]	Severe symptoms Prolonged illness Elderly patients Immunosuppressed	Ciprofloxacin 500 mg twice daily	Azithromycin 500 mg once daily Co-trimoxazole 960 mg twice daily	Relieve symptoms Shorten illness May decrease complications
Travellers' diarrhoea[a]	Rarely used	Ciprofloxacin 500 mg twice daily	Co-trimoxazole 960 mg twice daily	Relieve symptoms Shorten illness
Treatment of confirmed *Salmonella*[a]	Symptoms not improving (rarely needed)	Ciprofloxacin 500 mg twice daily	Azithromycin 500 mg once daily	May shorten illness
Treatment of confirmed *Campylobacter*[a]	Symptoms not improving (rarely needed)	Azithromycin 500 mg once daily	Co-trimoxazole 960 mg twice daily	May shorten illness
Clostridium difficile	Most cases (unless symptoms resolved)	Vancomycin 125–250 mg four times daily	Metronidazole 400 mg three times daily Fidaxomicin 200 mg twice daily	Relieve symptoms Shorten illness May reduce relapse rate

[a]Antibiotics are not needed for the majority of adult cases in developed countries.

(especially beefburgers and chicken), and contaminated milk products and water. In many developed countries there is significant seasonal variation, with peaks associated with warm weather and barbecues.

Like *Salmonella*, *Campylobacter* can affect the large and small bowel and can cause a wide variety of symptoms. The incubation period is usually 2–4 days, after which there is an abrupt onset of nausea, diarrhoea and severe abdominal cramps. The diarrhoea is usually profuse and watery, but an invasive haemorrhagic colitis is sometimes seen. Bacteraemia is very rare, and infection is usually self-limiting in 3–5 days. Diagnosis is made from stool cultures. Quinolone resistance is now widespread in developed countries (45% in the UK and nearly 90% in Spain); this is due in part to the use of antibiotics in intensive livestock farming. Antibiotics are not usually indicated, but if symptoms are severe, azithromycin is the drug of choice.

Shigella

Shigellae are enteroinvasive Gram-negative bacteria, which cause classical bacillary dysentery. The principal species causing gastroenteritis are *S. dysenteriae*, *S. flexneri* and *S. sonnei*, which are found with varying prevalence in different parts of the world. All cause a similar syndrome, as a result of damage to the intestinal mucosa. Some strains of *S. dysenteriae* also secrete a cytotoxin affecting vascular endothelium. Although shigellae are found worldwide, transmission is strongly associated with poor hygiene, and of the 165 million episodes of shigella dysentery estimated by the WHO to occur every year, 99% are in economically less developed countries. The main burden falls on children: shigella dysentery kills nearly 50 000 children under 5 years old every year.

The organism is spread from person to person (either directly, or via contaminated food or water) and only a small number of bacteria need to be ingested to cause illness (<200, compared with 10^4 for *Campylobacter* and >10^5 for *Salmonella*). Symptoms start 24–48 hours after ingestion and typically consist of frequent, small-volume stools containing blood and mucus. Dehydration is not as significant as in the secretory diarrhoeas but systemic symptoms

and intestinal complications are worse. The illness is usually self-limiting in 7–10 days, but in children in developing countries it can carry a significant mortality.

Antibiotic treatment decreases the severity and duration of diarrhoea, reduces mortality in children, and possibly lowers the risk of further transmission. Resistance to antibiotics is widespread and, wherever possible, treatment should be based on known local sensitivity patterns. Antibiotics such as nalidixic acid and co-trimoxazole, which were widely used in the past, are no longer recommended by the WHO, due to extensive resistance. Most guidelines recommend ciprofloxacin as the first-choice antibiotic but resistance to this antibiotic is also increasing rapidly in some parts of the world. Other options include azithromycin, cefixime and ceftriaxone, but these all have disadvantages compared to the cheap and safe ciprofloxacin.

Enteroinvasive *Escherichia coli*

Enteroinvasive *E. coli* (EIEC) causes an illness that is indistinguishable from shigellosis. Definitive diagnosis is made by stool culture but most cases are probably treated empirically as shigellosis.

Enterohaemorrhagic *Escherichia coli*

Enterohaemorrhagic *E. coli* (EHEC; usually serotype O157:H7 and also known as verotoxin-producing *E. coli*, VTEC) is a well-recognized cause of gastroenteritis in humans. It is a zoonosis that is usually associated with cattle, and there have been a number of major outbreaks (notably in Scotland, Japan and the USA) linked to contaminated food. A variety of modes of transmission have been reported and the epidemiology of EHEC infection is a paradigm for all enteric livestock-associated zoonoses (**Fig. 20.19**). EHEC secretes a toxin (Shiga-like toxin 1) that affects vascular endothelial cells in the gut and in the kidney. After an incubation period of 12–48 hours, it causes diarrhoea (frequently bloody), associated with abdominal pain and nausea. Some days after the onset of symptoms the patient may develop thrombotic thrombocytopenic purpura (see p. 374) or haemolytic uraemic syndrome (see p. 1368). These are more

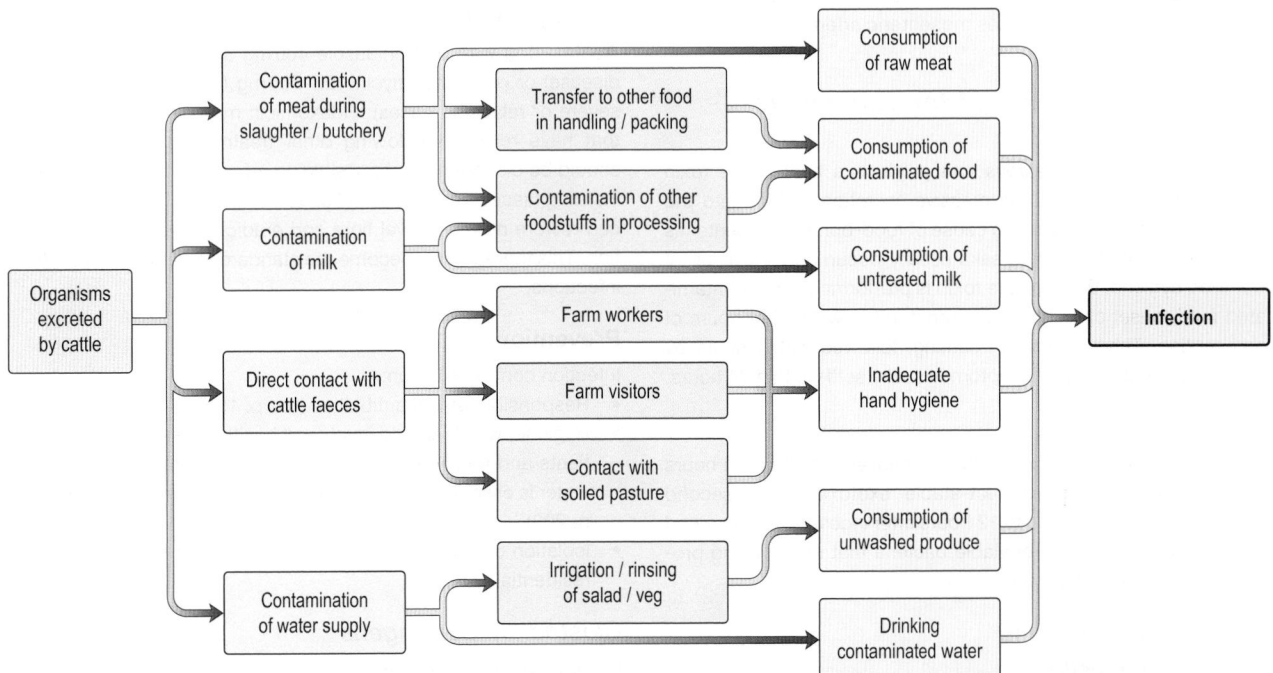

Fig. 20.19 Routes of human infection with *Escherichia coli* O157.

common in children and may lead to permanent renal damage or death. Non-O157 serotypes are of increasing concern.

Between May and June 2011, the largest ever recorded outbreak of Shiga toxin-producing *E. coli* (STEC) causing HUS was recorded in Germany. The outbreak was caused by the O104 serotype and over 2000 people were affected. High rates of HUS were observed in adults not in the typical 'at-risk' age range. The increased virulence of this strain is possibly due to it having two different pathotypes (see p. 539).

Treatment is mainly supportive; there is evidence that antibiotic therapy might precipitate HUS by causing increased toxin release, although this remains controversial.

Enterotoxigenic *Escherichia coli*

Enterotoxigenic *E. coli* (ETEC) produce both heat-labile and heat-stable enterotoxins, which stimulate secretion of fluid into the intestinal lumen. The result is watery diarrhoea of varying intensity, which usually resolves within a few days. Transmission is normally from person to person via contaminated food and water. The organism is common in developing countries and is a major cause of travellers' diarrhoea (see later).

Vibrio

Cholera, due to *Vibrio cholerae*, is the prototypic pure enterotoxigenic diarrhoea; it is described on page 553.

V. parahaemolyticus can cause acute watery diarrhoea after consumption of contaminated raw fish or shellfish. Explosive diarrhoea, abdominal cramps and vomiting occur, with fever in 50%. The infection is self-limiting but can last for up to 10 days.

Yersiniosis

Yersinia enterocolitica infection is a zoonosis of a variety of domestic and wild mammals. Human disease can arise via either contaminated food products, such as pork, or direct animal contact. *Y. enterocolitica* can cause a range of gastroenteric symptoms, including watery diarrhoea, dysentery and mesenteric adenitis. The illness is usually self-limiting but ciprofloxacin may shorten the duration. *Y. pseudotuberculosis* is a much less common human pathogen; it causes mesenteric adenitis and terminal ileitis.

Enterotoxin-producing *Staphylococcus aureus*

Some strains of *Staph. aureus* can produce a heat-stable toxin (enterotoxin B), which causes massive secretion of fluid into the intestinal lumen. It is a common cause of food-borne gastroenteritis in Europe and the USA, outbreaks usually occurring as a result of poor food hygiene. Because the toxin is pre-formed in the contaminated food, onset of symptoms is rapid, often within 2–4 hours of consumption. There is violent vomiting, followed within hours by profuse watery diarrhoea. Symptoms usually settle within 24 hours.

Bacillus cereus

B. cereus produces two toxins. The first causes vomiting 2–4 hours after ingesting pre-formed heat-stable exotoxins. The second causes watery diarrhoea up to 12 hours after ingestion of uncooked food that contains spores or viable bacteria that multiply and produce a toxin within the bowel.

Clostridial infections
Clostridium difficile

C. difficile can cause watery diarrhoea, colitis and pseudomembranous colitis. It is a Gram-positive, anaerobic, spore-forming bacillus that is found in the bowel flora of 3–5% of the asymptomatic population (increasing to up to 20% in hospitalized people).

Pathogenesis

C. difficile produces two toxins: toxin A is an enterotoxin, while toxin B is cytotoxic and causes bloody diarrhoea. It usually causes illness either in patients who have been given antibiotic therapy that has eliminated other bowel commensals, or in those who are debilitated for other reasons. Almost all antibiotics have been implicated but an increase in cases has been attributed in part to greater use of quinolones. Hospital-acquired infections remain common, partly due to increased spread from person to person and via fomites, and partly to high rates of antibiotic use in hospitalized people. Strains of *C. difficile* with greater capacity for toxin production have been reported (e.g. ribotype 027) in a number of hospital outbreaks, with a high mortality.

Clinical features

C. difficile-associated diarrhoea (CDAD) can begin anything from 2 days to some months after taking antibiotics. Elderly hospitalized patients are most frequently affected. It is unclear why some carriers remain asymptomatic. Symptoms can range from mild diarrhoea to profuse, watery, haemorrhagic colitis, along with lower abdominal pain. The colonic mucosa is inflamed and ulcerated, and can be covered by an adherent membrane-like material (pseudomembranous colitis). The disease is usually more severe in the elderly and can cause intractable diarrhoea; occasionally, it can cause toxic megacolon. Markers of severity include:

- temperature >38.5°C
- white cell count >15×10^9
- serum creatinine >50% above baseline
- raised serum lactate
- severe abdominal pain.

Diagnosis

Diagnosis is made by detecting A or B toxins in the stools using ELISA, or PCR for C. *difficile* nucleic acid.

Management

Treatment is with metronidazole 400 mg three times daily (in mild disease) or oral vancomycin 125–500 mg four times daily (in more severe or relapsing cases). Fidaxomicin may be effective in cases that have relapsed following other treatments. Other antibiotics should be discontinued if possible. In refractory or relapsing cases, instilling faeces from the bowel of a healthy donor (faecal transplant) can restore normal bowel flora and eradicate the *C. difficile* infection. This therapy may become the standard for refractory *C. difficile* infections.

Prevention

Infection control relies on:

- Responsible use of antibiotics (see p. 159).
- Hygiene, which should involve all health workers, as well as patients and relatives. Washing hands thoroughly using soap and water is essential, as alcohol disinfectants do not kill spores (see p. 292).
- Isolation of patients with symptomatic *C. difficile* in hospitals or residential care.

Clostridium perfringens

C. perfringens infection is due to inadequately cooked food, usually meat or poultry allowed to cool for a long time, during which period the spores germinate. The ingested organism produces an enterotoxin that causes watery diarrhoea with severe abdominal pain, usually without vomiting.

Travellers' diarrhoea

Travellers' diarrhoea is defined as the passage of three or more unformed stools per day in a resident of an industrialized country travelling in a developing nation. Infection is usually food- or water-borne and younger travellers are most often affected (probably reflecting behaviour patterns). Reported attack rates vary from country to country but approach 50% for a 2-week stay in some nations. The disease is usually benign and self-limiting; treatment with quinolone antibiotics may hasten recovery but is not normally necessary. Prophylactic antibiotic therapy may also be effective for short stays but should not be used routinely. The common causative organisms are listed in **Box 20.45**.

Management of acute gastroenteritis

In children in low-income countries, untreated diarrhoea has a high mortality due to dehydration, often on a background of malnutrition and other chronic infection. Death and serious morbidity are less common in adults but still occur, particularly in developing countries and in the elderly.

The mainstay of treatment for all types of gastroenteritis is oral rehydration solutions (ORS) (**Fig. 20.20**; see **Box 20.36**). The use and formulation of ORS are discussed on page 553. Antibiotics may

sometimes have a role, especially in children in developing countries. It is also important to remember that other diseases, notably UTIs and chest infections in the elderly, and malaria at any age, can present with acute diarrhoea. Most cases of acute gastroenteritis (especially in developed countries) resolve within 10 days; if symptoms persist, other causes, such as colitis, are more likely.

Food poisoning

Food poisoning is a legally notifiable condition in England and Wales. There is some overlap between food poisoning (defined as 'any disease of an infective or toxic nature caused by or thought to be caused by the consumption of food and water') and gastroenteritis. However, not all cases of gastroenteritis are due to food poisoning, as the pathogens are not always food- or water-borne. Conversely, some types of food poisoning (e.g. botulism) do not primarily cause gastroenteritis. Common bacterial causes of food poisoning are listed in **Box 20.46**. Food poisoning may also be caused by a number of non-infectious organic and inorganic toxins (**Box 20.47**).

The increase in reported food poisoning in developed countries is due, at least in part, to changes in the production and distribution of food. Livestock raised and slaughtered under modern intensive farming conditions is frequently contaminated with *Salmonella* or *Campylobacter*. However, the main problem is not at this stage. Only 0.02–0.1% of the eggs from a flock of chickens infected with *S. enteritidis* will be affected and then only at a level of less than 20 cells per egg – harmless to most healthy individuals. It is flaws in the processing, storage and distribution of food products that allow massive amplification of the infection, resulting in extensive contamination. The internationalization of the food supply encourages widespread and distant transmission of the resulting infections.

Enteric fever, *Helicobacter pylori*, Whipple's disease and bacterial peritonitis

Enteric fever: see page 554.
H. pylori: see page 1173.
Whipple's disease: see page 1194.
Bacterial peritonitis: see page 1222.

? Box 20.45 Commonly identified causes of travellers' diarrhoea[a]

Organism	Frequency (varies from country to country)
Enterotoxigenic *Escherichia coli*	30–70%
Shigella spp.	0–15%
Campylobacter spp.	0–15%
Salmonella spp.	0–10%
Viral pathogens	0–10%
Giardia intestinalis	0–3%

[a] In most cases, no microbiological diagnosis is made.

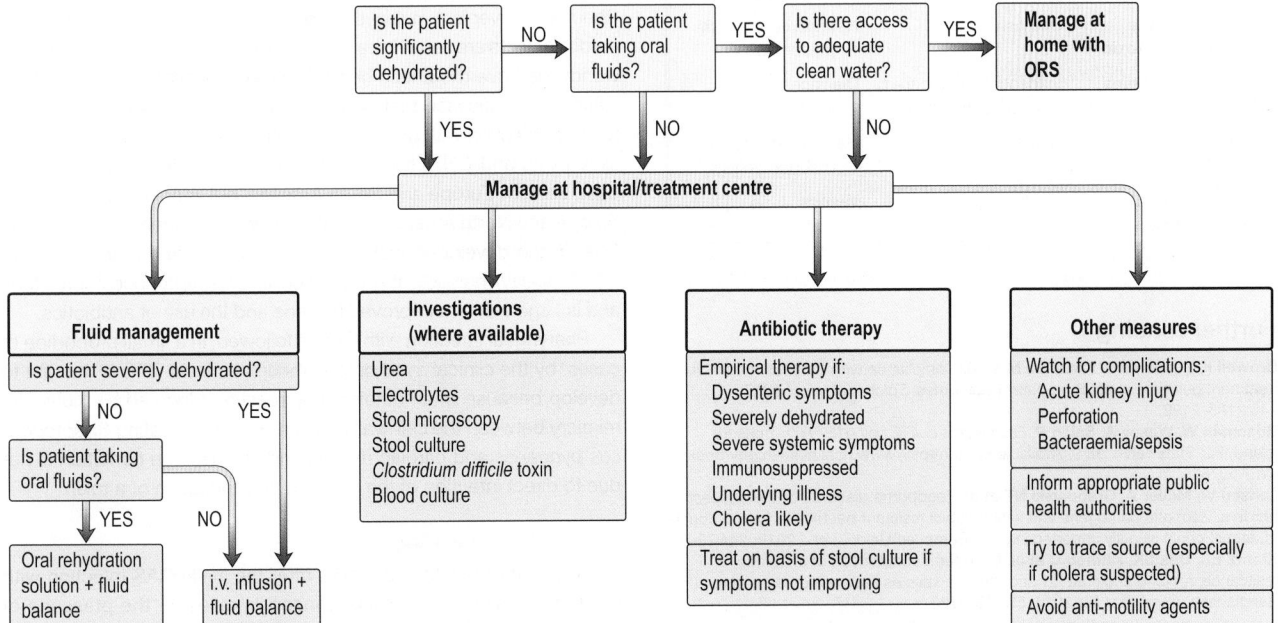

Fig. 20.20 Gastroenteritis: management plan. ORS, oral rehydration solution.

? Box 20.46 Bacterial causes of food poisoning

Organism	Source/vehicles	Incubation period	Symptoms	Diagnosis	Recovery
Staphylococcus aureus	Humans – contaminated food and water	2–4 h	Diarrhoea, vomiting, dehydration	Culture of organism in vomitus or remaining food	<24 h
Escherichia coli (ETEC)	Salads, water, ice	24 h	Watery diarrhoea	Stool culture	1–4 days
E. coli O157:H7	Cattle – contaminated foodstuffs	12–48 h	Watery diarrhoea ± haemorrhagic colitis, HUS	Stool culture	10–12 days
Yersinia enterocolitica	Milk, pork	2–14 h	Abdominal pain, vomiting, diarrhoea	Stool culture	2–30 days
Bacillus cereus	Environment – rice, ice cream, chicken	1–6 h 6–14 h	Vomiting Diarrhoea	Culture of organism in faeces and food	Rapid
Clostridium perfringens	Environment – contaminated food	8–22 h	Watery diarrhoea, cramping pain	Culture of organism in faeces and food	2–3 days
Listeria monocytogenes	Environment – milk, raw vegetables, dairy products, unpasteurized cheese	Variable	Colic, diarrhoea, vomiting	Stool culture	Variable
Vibrio parahaemolyticus	Seafood	2–48 h	Diarrhoea, vomiting	Stool, food	2–10 days
Clostridium botulinum	Environment – bottled or canned food	18–24 h	Brief diarrhoea and paralysis due to neuromuscular blockade	Demonstration of toxin in food or faeces	10–14 days
Salmonella spp.	Cattle and poultry – eggs, meat	12–48 h	Abrupt diarrhoea, fever, vomiting	Stool culture	Usually 3–6 days but may be up to 2 weeks
Campylobacter jejuni	Cattle and poultry – meat, milk	48–96 h	Diarrhoea ± blood, fever, malaise, abdominal pain	Stool culture	3–5 days
Shigella spp.	Humans – contaminated food and water	24–48 h	Acute watery, bloody diarrhoea	Stool culture	7–10 days

ETEC, enterotoxigenic *Escherichia coli*; HUS, haemolytic uraemic syndrome.

? Box 20.47 Organic toxins causing food poisoning[a]

Toxin	Source	Illness
Scombrotoxin	Tuna, mackerel	Histamine fish poisoning
Ciguatoxin	Barracuda, snapper	Ciguatera (diarrhoea and paraesthesia)
Dinoflagellate plankton toxin	Shellfish	Neurotoxic shellfish poisoning
Haemagglutinins	Inadequately prepared dried kidney beans	Diarrhoea and vomiting
Unknown	Buffalo fish	Haff disease (toxic rhabdomyolysis)
Phallotoxins, amatoxins	Mushrooms	Various

[a]See online topics.

Further reading

Crowell KT, Julian KG, Katzman M et al. Compliance with Clostridium difficile treatment guidelines: effect on patient outcomes. *Epidemiol Infect* 2017; 145:2185–2192.

Gossman W, Wasey A, Salen P. *Escherichia coli (E coli 0157 H7)*. Treasure Island, FL: StatPearls; 2019. Available from: https://www.ncbi.nlm.nih.gov/books /NBK507845/.

Jansen W, Müller A, Grabowski NT et al. Foodborne diseases do not respect borders: Zoonotic pathogens and antimicrobial resistant bacteria in food products of animal origin illegally imported into the European Union. *Vet J* 2019; 244:75–82.

Klontz ES, Das SK, Ahmed D et al. Long term comparison of antibiotic resistance in Vibrio cholerae O1 and Shigella species between urban and rural Bangladesh. *Clin Infect Dis* 2014; 58:e133–136.

BACTERIAL INFECTIONS OF THE CARDIOVASCULAR SYSTEM

Infective endocarditis is discussed on page 1103.

Rheumatic fever

Rheumatic fever is a multisystem disorder but is included here as the cardiac effects are usually the most significant (about 35 million people worldwide have rheumatic heart disease). It is an immune-mediated inflammatory disease that occurs in children and young adults as a result of infection with group A streptococci (GAS). It affects the heart, skin, joints and CNS. It is relatively common in the Middle and Far East, Eastern Europe and South America, but is now rare in Western Europe and North America. This decline in the incidence of rheumatic fever in the developed world (from 10% of children in the 1920s to 0.01% today) parallels the reduction in all streptococcal infections and is largely due to improved hygiene and the use of antibiotics.

Pharyngeal infection with GAS is followed, in a small proportion of cases, by the clinical syndrome of rheumatic fever. This is thought to develop because of an autoimmune reaction triggered by molecular mimicry between the cell-wall M proteins of the infecting *Streptococcus pyogenes* and cardiac myosin and laminin. The condition is not due to direct infection of the heart or the production of a toxin.

Clinical features

The disease presents 2–3 weeks after the initial GAS infection with fever, joint pains and malaise. Diagnosis relies on the presence of

i **Box 20.48 Modified Jones criteria for the diagnosis of rheumatic fever**

Evidence of antecedent streptococcal infection
- Positive throat culture for group A streptococcus
- Good clinical history (e.g. of scarlet fever)
- Elevated antistreptolysin O titre (or other serological assay for streptococci)

Major criteria
- Carditis
- Polyarthritis
- Chorea
- Erythema marginatum
- Subcutaneous nodules

Minor criteria
- Fever
- Arthralgia (unless arthritis counted as major criterion)
- Previous rheumatic fever
- Raised erythrocyte sedimentation rate/C-reactive protein
- Leucocytosis
- Prolonged PR interval on electrocardiogram (unless carditis counted as major criterion)

two or more major clinical manifestations, or one major manifestation plus two or more minor features, in addition to evidence of current or recent streptococcal infection. These are known as the modified Jones criteria (**Box 20.48**).

Carditis manifests as new or changed heart murmurs, development of cardiac enlargement or cardiac failure, appearance of a pericardial effusion, or electrocardiographic (ECG) changes of pericarditis, myocarditis or cardiac arrhythmias.

Non-cardiac features include fever, arthritis, Sydenham's chorea (see p. 862) and skin lesions. The arthritis is typically a fleeting migratory polyarthritis affecting large joints such as the knees, elbows, ankles and wrists. Once the acute inflammation disappears, the rheumatic process leaves the joints normal. Skin manifestations include erythema marginatum, a transient pink rash with slightly raised edges, which occurs in 20% of cases, and small painless subcutaneous nodules.

Management

The streptococcal infection should be eradicated with penicillin. If the diagnosis is suspected clinically, antibiotics should be administered, even if nasal or pharyngeal swabs do not culture the streptococci.

The arthritis of rheumatic fever usually responds to non-steroidal anti-inflammatory drugs (NSAIDs), although these have no impact on long-term cardiac sequelae. There is no good evidence that steroids are of benefit, although some experts give high-dose prednisolone if there is severe carditis. In areas of high prevalence, recurrence is common and persistent cardiac damage more likely. Further infection can largely be prevented by prophylaxis with daily oral or monthly intramuscular benzathine penicillin until the age of 20 years or for 10 years after the latest attack. Erythromycin or clarithromycin is used if the patient is allergic to penicillin. Any streptococcal infection that does develop should be treated promptly.

Prognosis

More than 50% of those who suffer acute rheumatic fever with carditis will later (after 10–20 years) develop chronic rheumatic valvular disease, predominantly affecting the mitral and aortic valves.

BACTERIAL INFECTIONS OF THE NERVOUS SYSTEM

The central and peripheral nervous systems can be affected by a variety of microorganisms, including bacteria, viruses (see p. 868) and protozoa (p. 563), which cause disease by direct invasion or via toxins. The nervous system is also vulnerable to prion disease (pp. 535 and 884).

Bacterial meningitis

The most common bacterial disease affecting the CNS is acute meningitis (see p. 869), which causes about 175 000 deaths per year, predominantly in the developing world. The most common causes are *Neisseria meningitidis* (or meningococcus) and *Streptococcus pneumoniae*, while tuberculous meningitis (see p. 870) is common in sub-Saharan Africa and parts of Asia.

Haemophilus influenzae type b (Hib) was once a common cause of meningitis in children, but since an effective vaccine has been available serious *H. influenzae* infections have become rare in countries that have also instituted immunization programmes; however, invasive *H. influenzae* infection remains common in some parts of the world.

Other less common causes of meningitis in adults include group B streptococci, *Listeria monocytogenes* (see p. 548), *Staph. aureus* and Gram-negative bacilli. These organisms are usually associated with an underlying illness or immunocompromising condition, or with a CSF leak.

N. meningitidis is also an important cause of bloodstream infection and sepsis. There is a spectrum of presentation ranging from pure meningitis with few systemic features to a typical sepsis syndrome without clinical evidence of meningitis.

Meningococcal sepsis

Neisseria meningitidis is found worldwide. Twelve serogroups have been identified, of which six (A, B, C, W, X and Y) cause significant outbreaks of infection. In sub-Saharan Africa and parts of Asia, where group A meningococcus is prevalent, it usually causes epidemic disease. The main burden falls on the so-called 'meningitis belt', which includes 25 countries across Africa stretching from Senegal in the west to Ethiopia in the east. Groups X, Y and W can also cause epidemic infection, while groups B and C (the predominant strains in Europe and North America) tend to be sporadic.

Humans are the only known reservoir for the organism, which is carried asymptomatically in the nasopharynx of 5–20% of the general population. Meningococcal disease occurs when the bacteria invade the nasal mucosa and enter the bloodstream; this happens only in a small percentage of those colonized. Invasion depends on both host and bacterial factors. It is more likely to take place soon after colonization has occurred, and following viral upper respiratory infections.

Clinical features

Invasive meningococcal infection may cause meningitis, the meningococcal sepsis syndrome or both. Meningitic disease (see p. 868) usually presents with the classical triad of headache, fever and neck stiffness. Vomiting, diminished consciousness and focal neurological signs sometimes occur, although many patients, especially in the early stages, have only mild symptoms. Meningococcal blood stream infection causes the typical features of septic shock, such as fever, myalgia and hypotension (see p. 218), and may be accompanied by a petechial or haemorrhagic rash (**Fig. 20.21**). In some cases the patient can deteriorate rapidly, with shock, DIC and multiorgan failure.

Diagnosis

The presence of meningitis and sepsis syndrome with a typical rash is strongly suggestive of meningococcal disease. The rash is not always present, however, and its absence does not rule out the diagnosis. Gram-negative diplococci may be seen on Gram stain of CSF or of aspirate from petechiae; meningococci can also be cultured from CSF or blood, or detected by PCR. PCR can also be used to identify the serogroup, which may be important for public health management.

Management

N. meningitidis is sensitive to benzylpenicillin (in most cases), third-generation cephalosporins, and chloramphenicol; cefotaxime or ceftriaxone is the recommended treatment in the UK (see **Box 26.57**). Meningococcal sepsis should be managed in the same way as any other form of bacterial sepsis (see p. 157). The mortality from meningococcal sepsis in developed countries is currently approximately 10%, while that from meningococcal meningitis alone is less than 5% (see later). Mild neurological sequelae (especially vestibular nerve damage) are common but serious brain damage is relatively unusual.

The meningococcal C conjugate vaccine has contributed to an overall reduction of invasive meningococcal disease in the UK: only 755 cases were reported in England and Wales in 2017, compared with 2784 in 1999 (when the group C meningococcal immunization programme began). Group B vaccines were licensed and approved for use in the UK in 2014, and were introduced into the routine childhood/young adult immunization programme in 2017. A combined A/C/W135/Y vaccine is available for control of outbreaks caused by these strains and for travellers to endemic areas: it gives relatively short-term protection. A cheap and effective conjugate meningococcal A vaccine, giving long-term immunity, has been distributed widely in the African meningitis belt, with more than 280 million people in 21 countries receiving the vaccine so far.

In an outbreak, close contacts of a case of meningococcal disease should be given prophylaxis with oral rifampicin or ciprofloxacin to eradicate the bacteria from the nasopharynx and reduce the risk of onward spread (this has little impact in epidemic areas). In some outbreak situations, contacts should be offered immunization.

Cerebral abscess

This is covered on page 873.

Toxin-mediated infections

Botulism

Clostridium botulinum is a common environmental organism that produces spores that can survive heating to 100°C. It can cause illness through a number of routes:

- contamination of canned or bottled foodstuffs, in which the anaerobic organism can multiply and elaborate a neurotoxin
- infection of wounds
- contamination of injectable drugs (especially heroin).

In botulism (food poisoning), the toxin is ingested and causes profound neuromuscular blockade, leading to autonomic and motor paralysis. The first symptoms, occurring 18–24 hours after ingestion, are nausea and diarrhoea. These are followed by cranial nerve palsies and then progressive symmetrical paralysis, leading to respiratory failure.

The diagnosis is usually clinical and is confirmed by detection of toxin in faeces or in contaminated food. Management is mainly supportive, with mechanical ventilation if necessary. Antitoxin is available in some countries (including the UK); the risk of anaphylaxis is relatively high and antitoxin should be used only in severe cases. A subcutaneous test dose should be given before intravenous or intramuscular injection. Antibiotics have no proven role. The overall mortality from botulism is high, but patients who survive the acute paralysis can make a full recovery.

A similar clinical picture can follow the contamination of wounds, or injection of street heroin contaminated with *C. botulinum*; in infants, botulism may be related to bowel colonization by the organism.

Tetanus

Tetanus is also due to a toxin-secreting clostridium: *C. tetani*. The organism is found in soil, and illness usually results from a contaminated wound. The injury itself may be trivial and disregarded by the individual. Tetanus can also complicate injecting drug use, if the drug (usually heroin) is contaminated with *C. tetani*. In developing countries, neonatal tetanus follows contamination of the umbilical stump, often after the area is dressed with dung. The overall incidence of tetanus across the world has fallen significantly in the past 20 years, due mainly to active immunization.

The organism is not invasive and clinical manifestations of the disease are due to the potent neurotoxin, tetanospasmin. Tetanospasmin causes disinhibition at synapses, neuromuscular blockade and skeletal muscle spasm, and acts on the sympathetic nervous system. The end result is marked flexor muscle spasm and autonomic dysfunction.

Clinical features

The incubation period varies from a few days to several weeks. The most common form of the disease is generalized tetanus. General malaise is rapidly followed by trismus (lockjaw) due to masseter muscle spasm. Spasm of the facial muscles produces the characteristic grinning expression known as *risus sardonicus*. If the disease is severe, painful reflex spasms develop, usually within 24–72 hours of the initial symptoms. The interval between the first

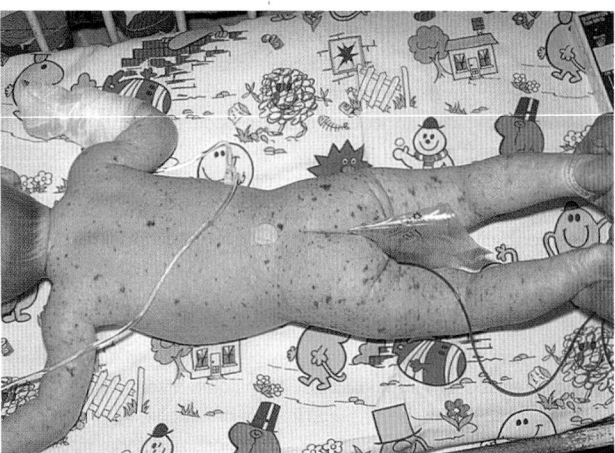

Fig. 20.21 Meningococcal infection, showing a purpuric rash.

symptom and the first spasm is referred to as the 'onset time'. The spasms may occur spontaneously but are easily precipitated by noise, handling of the patient or light. Respiration may be impaired because of laryngeal spasm; oesophageal and urethral spasm lead to dysphagia and urinary retention, respectively, and there is arching of the neck and back muscles (opisthotonus). Autonomic dysfunction produces tachycardia, a labile blood pressure, sweating and cardiac arrhythmias. Patients with tetanus are mentally alert.

Death results from aspiration, hypoxia, respiratory failure, cardiac arrest or exhaustion. Mild cases with rigidity usually recover. Poor prognostic indicators include a short incubation period, short onset time and extremes of age.

Localized tetanus is a milder form of the disease. Pain and stiffness are confined to the site of the wound, with increased tone in the surrounding muscles. Recovery is usual.

Cephalic tetanus is uncommon but invariably fatal. It usually occurs when the portal of entry of *C. tetani* is the middle ear. Cranial nerve abnormalities, particularly of the VIIth nerve, are usual. Generalized tetanus may or may not develop.

Neonatal tetanus is characterized by failure to thrive, poor sucking, grimacing and irritability, followed by the rapid development of intense rigidity and spasms. Mortality approaches 100%. One aim of the WHO's EPI is to eliminate this condition by immunizing all women of child-bearing age, providing clean delivery facilities, and strengthening surveillance in high-risk areas.

Diagnosis

Few diseases resemble tetanus in its fully developed form and the diagnosis is therefore usually clinical. Rarely, *C. tetani* is isolated from wounds. Phenothiazine overdosage, strychnine poisoning, meningitis and tetany can occasionally mimic tetanus.

Management

If tetanus is suspected, any wound must be cleaned and debrided to remove the source of toxin. Human tetanus immunoglobulin 250 units should be given, along with an intramuscular injection of tetanus toxoid. If the patient is already protected, a single booster dose of the toxoid is given; otherwise, the full three-dose course of adsorbed vaccine is required (see later).

In established disease, management consists of supportive medical and nursing care. Improvement in this area has contributed, more than any other single measure, to the decrease in the mortality rate from 60% to nearer 20%. Patients are nursed in a quiet, isolated, well-ventilated, darkened room. Benzodiazepines are used to control spasms and sedate the patient; if the airway is compromised, intubation and mechanical ventilation may be necessary. Magnesium sulphate infusion may decrease the need for antispasmodics.

Antibiotics and antitoxin should be administered, even in the absence of an obvious wound. Intravenous metronidazole for 7–10 days is the drug of choice, although penicillin is also effective. Human tetanus immunoglobulin (HTIG) should be given as soon as possible, by either intravenous infusion or intramuscular injection, to neutralize any circulating toxin. If HTIG is not available, human normal immunoglobulin (HNIG) can be used. If the patient recovers, active immunization should be instituted, as immunity following tetanus is incomplete.

Prevention

An effective, safe and relatively cheap vaccine means that tetanus is an eminently preventable disease. After initial active immunization, boosters are recommended at 10-year intervals for all adults. Infant immunization schedules in all countries include tetanus. Protection by passive immunization with HTIG or HNIG is short-lived, lasting only about 2 weeks.

Further reading

Rodrigo C, Fernando D, Rajapakse S. Pharmacological management of tetanus: an evidence-based review. *Crit Care* 2014; 18:217.
Webb RH, Grant C, Harnden A. Acute rheumatic fever. *Br Med J* 2015; 351:h3443.

BACTERIAL BONE AND JOINT INFECTIONS

See pages 454 and 484.

BACTERIAL INFECTIONS OF THE URINARY TRACT

See page 1381.

SYSTEMIC/MULTISYSTEM BACTERIAL INFECTIONS

Many infections are confined to a particular body organ or system, owing to the metabolic requirements of the organism, the route of infection or the response of host defences. Other infections can potentially affect several systems or the entire body. Under unusual circumstances, such as altered host immunity, infections that are normally circumscribed may become systemic. The general principles of systemic infections, bacteraemia and the sepsis syndrome are described in Chapter 8, as are the common causes of sepsis. This section describes some specific and less common bacterial infections that cause multisystem disease in an immunocompetent host.

Leptospirosis

Leptospirosis is a zoonosis caused by the spirochaete *Leptospira interrogans*. There are over 200 serotypes. The main types affecting humans are:

- *L. i. icterohaemorrhagiae* (normal host: rodents)
- *L. i. canicola* (dogs and pigs)
- *L. i. hardjo* (cattle)
- *L. i. pomona* (pigs and cattle).

Leptospires are excreted in the animals' urine and enter the host through a skin abrasion or intact mucous membranes. Leptospirosis can also be caught by ingestion of contaminated water. The organism can survive for many days in warm freshwater and for up to 24 hours in seawater.

In England and Wales, between 50 and 100 cases of leptospirosis are reported every year, although many mild infections probably go undiagnosed. It is traditionally an occupational disease of farmers, vets and others who work with animals, but is increasingly associated with recreational activities that bring people into closer contact with rodents or contaminated water. Outbreaks of leptospirosis have also been associated with flooding.

Clinical features

In 1896, Weil described a severe illness consisting of jaundice, haemorrhage and renal impairment caused by *L. i. icterohaemorrhagiae*, but fortunately 90–95% of infections are subclinical or cause only a mild fever. The incubation period of leptospirosis is usually 7–14 days and the illness typically has two phases. A leptospiraemic phase, which lasts for up to a week, is followed after a couple of days' interval by an immunological phase. The first phase is characterized by severe headache, malaise, fever, anorexia and myalgia. Most patients have conjunctival suffusion. Hepatosplenomegaly, lymphadenopathy and various skin rashes are sometimes seen. The second phase is usually mild. Meningism is common; if lumbar puncture is performed, there is often CSF lymphocytosis. The majority of patients recover uneventfully at this stage.

In severe disease, there may not be a clear distinction between phases. Following the initial symptoms, patients progressively develop hepatic and kidney injury, haemolytic anaemia and circulatory collapse. Cardiac failure and pulmonary haemorrhage may also occur. Even with full supportive care, the mortality is around 10%, rising to 15–20% in the elderly.

Diagnosis

The diagnosis is usually a clinical one. Leptospires can be cultured from blood or CSF during the first week of illness, but culture requires special media and may take several weeks. Leptospiral DNA can be detected by PCR in the blood and urine. A minority of patients may also excrete the organism in their urine from the second week onwards. Confirmation is usually serological. Specific IgM antibodies start to appear from the end of the first week and the diagnosis is often made retrospectively with a microscopic agglutination test (MAT) showing a fourfold rise. There is typically a leucocytosis and, in severe infection, thrombocytopenia and an elevated creatine phosphokinase.

Management

Early antibiotic therapy may limit progress of the disease, and penicillin or ceftriaxone should be given in severe cases. The efficacy of antibiotics in mild disease is debated; if they are used, oral doxycycline is the best choice. Intensive supportive care is needed for those patients who develop hepatorenal failure.

Brucellosis

Brucellosis (Malta fever, undulant fever) is caused by various species of *Brucella*, a Gram-negative intracellular coccobacillus. It is a zoonosis, especially of goats, sheep and cattle, and has a worldwide distribution (although the UK is officially 'brucellosis-free'). A handful of imported human cases are diagnosed in England each year. The highest incidence is in the Mediterranean countries, the Middle East and the tropics; there are about 500 000 new cases diagnosed per year worldwide.

The organisms usually gain entry into the human body via the mouth; less frequently, they may enter via the respiratory tract, genital tract or abraded skin. The bacilli travel in the lymphatics and infect lymph nodes. This is followed by haematogenous spread with ultimate localization in the reticulo-endothelial system. Acquisition is usually by the ingestion of raw milk from infected cattle or goats, although occupational exposure is also common. Person-to-person transmission is rare.

Clinical features

The incubation period of acute brucellosis is 1–3 weeks. The onset is insidious, with malaise, headache, weakness, generalized myalgia and night sweats. The fever pattern is classically undulant, although continuous and intermittent patterns are also seen. Lymphadenopathy and hepatosplenomegaly are common; sacroiliitis, arthritis,

osteomyelitis, epididymo-orchitis, meningoencephalitis and endocarditis have all been described.

Untreated brucellosis can give rise to chronic infection, lasting a year or more. This is characterized by easy fatigability, myalgia and occasional bouts of fever and depression. Splenomegaly is usually present. Occasionally, infection can lead to localized brucellosis, which may not be associated with systemic symptoms. Bones and joints, spleen, endocardium, lungs, urinary tract and nervous system may be involved.

Diagnosis

Blood (or bone marrow) cultures are positive during the acute phase of illness in 50% of patients (higher in *B. melitensis*) but prolonged culture is needed. In chronic disease, serological tests are of greater value. The *Brucella* agglutination test, which demonstrates a fourfold or greater rise in titre (>1 in 160) over a 4-week period, is highly suggestive of brucellosis. An elevated serum IgG level is evidence of current or recent infection; a negative test excludes chronic (non-localized) brucellosis. In localized brucellosis, antibody titres are low and the diagnosis is usually established by culturing the organisms from the involved site. Species-specific PCR tests are also available.

Management and prevention

Brucellosis should be treated with a combination of doxycycline, rifampicin and an aminoglycoside (usually gentamicin). Prevention and control involve careful attention to hygiene when handling infected animals, eradication of infection in animals through vaccination, and the pasteurization of milk. No vaccine is available for use in humans.

Listeriosis

Listeria monocytogenes is an environmental organism that is widely disseminated in soil and decayed matter. It affects both animals and humans; the most common route of human infection is in contaminated foodstuffs. The organism can grow at temperatures as low as 4°C and the most commonly implicated foods are unpasteurized soft cheeses, raw vegetables and chicken pâtés. Listeriosis is a rare but serious infection affecting mainly neonates, pregnant women, the elderly and the immunocompromised. *L. monocytogenes* has also been recognized as a cause of self-limiting, food-borne gastroenteritis in healthy adults, but the incidence of this is unknown.

In pregnant women, *Listeria* causes an influenza-like illness, but infection of the fetus can lead to septic abortion, premature labour and stillbirth. Early treatment of *Listeria* in pregnancy may prevent this but the overall fetal loss rate is about 50%. In the elderly and the immunocompromised, *Listeria* can cause bacteraemia, meningoencephalitis and a variety of focal infections.

The diagnosis is established by culture of blood, CSF or other body fluids. The treatment of choice for adult listeriosis is ampicillin plus gentamicin. Co-trimoxazole and meropenem are also effective but the organism is resistant to cephalosporins.

Q fever

Q fever is a zoonosis caused by *Coxiella burnetii*, a Gram-negative intracellular bacterium. Infection is widespread in domestic, farm and other animals, birds and arthropods; spread is mainly by ticks. Modes of transmission to humans are by dust, aerosol and unpasteurized milk from infected cows. The formation of spores means that *C. burnetii* can survive in extreme environmental conditions for long periods. The infective dose is very small, so that minimal animal contact is required. One reported outbreak occurred among inhabitants of a village through which infected sheep had passed.

A large outbreak in the Netherlands (with 4000 human cases) was linked to goat farming, with the main risk factor being residence within 5 km of an affected farm. Infection in the UK is rare and usually associated with farm and abattoir workers.

Clinical features

Symptoms begin insidiously 2–4 weeks after infection. Fever is accompanied by influenza-like symptoms with myalgia and headache. The acute illness usually resolves spontaneously but pneumonia or hepatitis may develop. In pregnant women, Q fever can cause severe fetal damage. Occasionally, infection can become chronic, with endocarditis, myocarditis, uveitis, osteomyelitis or other focal infections.

C. burnetii is an obligate intracellular organism and does not grow on standard culture media. Diagnosis is made serologically using an immunofluorescent assay. Antibody tests for two different bacterial antigens allow distinction between acute and chronic infection. A PCR assay is available but the sensitivity is low.

Management

Treatment with doxycycline or azithromycin shortens the duration of the acute illness and there is emerging evidence that it may reduce the incidence of chronic sequelae. For chronic Q fever, including endocarditis, doxycycline is often combined with rifampicin or hydroxychloroquine. Even prolonged courses of treatment may not clear the infection. A vaccine is available for those at high risk.

Lyme disease

Lyme disease is caused by spirochaetes of the genus *Borrelia*. *B. burgdorferi* is the sole cause of Lyme disease in the USA. In Europe, *B. afzelii* and *B. garinii* are also implicated. Lyme disease is a zoonosis of deer and other wild mammals. It has increased in both incidence and detection; it is now known to be widespread in the USA, Europe, Russia and the Far East. About 1000 autochthonous laboratory-confirmed infections are reported in England and Wales each year, but many other cases may be diagnosed clinically or are subclinical. Infection is transmitted from animal to human by ixodid ticks and is most likely to occur in rural wooded areas in spring and early summer. In places where other tick-borne infections such as ehrlichia are endemic, simultaneous co-infection may occur.

Clinical features

Early localized disease presents about a week after the tick bite with erythema migrans (a macular rash; **Fig. 20.22**), lymphadenopathy,

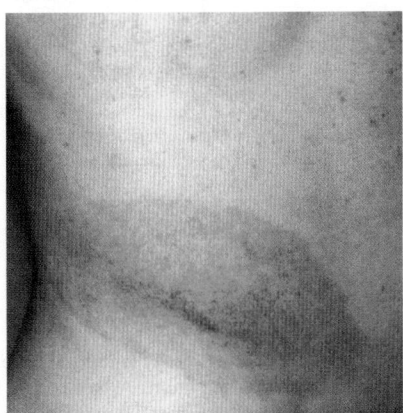

Fig. 20.22 The skin lesion erythema migrans, at the site of a tick bite.

and associated fever and headache. Most people recover spontaneously at this stage, with no further symptoms or signs. A small number may develop early disseminated disease, which occurs days to weeks after the appearance of erythema migrans. There can be a more widespread rash, and a small proportion of untreated cases may develop neurological complications such as meningitis, encephalitis, cranial or peripheral neuritis, or radiculopathies. Cardiac involvement is seen in the USA but is rare elsewhere. Myalgia and arthritis may also occur at this stage. Late Lyme disease, which is rare, can cause chronic arthritis, encephalomyelitis and other neurological disorders, and acrodermatitis chronica atrophicans. Much of the damage in late Lyme disease is likely to be immune-mediated, and although antibiotics should be given to eradicate any persistent infection, there is no evidence to support a role for prolonged antibiotic treatment.

Diagnosis

The clinical features and epidemiological considerations are usually strongly suggestive. The presence of a typical rash after potential risk exposure requires antibiotic treatment without further diagnostic tests (which may well be negative at this stage anyway). The diagnosis can be confirmed only rarely by isolation of the organisms from blood, skin lesions or CSF. IgM antibodies are detectable in the first month and IgG antibodies are invariably present late in the disease. Sensitive antibody detection tests are available but false-positive results occur and an initial positive test should always be followed by a confirmatory immunoblot assay. Even a genuine positive IgG result may be a marker of previous exposure rather than of ongoing infection.

Management

Amoxicillin or doxycycline given early in the course of the disease shortens the duration of the illness in approximately 50% of patients. Disseminated or late disease should be treated with 2–4 weeks of intravenous ceftriaxone. However, treatment is unsatisfactory and preventative measures are recommended. In tick-infested areas, repellents and protective clothing should be worn. Prompt removal of any tick is essential, as infection is unlikely to take place unless the tick has been attached for more than 48 hours. Ticks should be grasped with forceps near to the point of attachment to the skin and then withdrawn by gentle traction. Antibiotic prophylaxis following a tick bite is not usually justified, even in areas where Lyme disease is common. There is currently no effective vaccine.

Tularaemia

Tularaemia is due to infection with *Francisella tularensis*, a Gram-negative coccobacillus. It is primarily a zoonosis, usually acquired from rodents. Infection can be transmitted by arthropod vectors or by the handling of infected animals, when the microorganisms enter through minor abrasions or mucous membranes. Occasionally, infection occurs from contaminated water or from uncooked meat. The disease is widely distributed in North America, Northern Europe and Asia, but the particularly virulent type A subspecies is seen only in the USA. It is relatively rare, occurring mainly in hunters, trappers and others in close contact with animals; about 800 cases per year are recorded in Europe, mainly in Scandinavia.

The incubation period of 2–7 days is followed by a generalized illness. The most common presentation is ulceroglandular tularaemia. A papule occurs at the site of inoculation. This ulcerates and is followed by tender, suppurative lymphadenopathy. Rarely, this can be followed by bacteraemia, leading to septicaemia, pneumonia or meningitis. These forms of the disease carry a high mortality if untreated.

Routine cultures are often negative, and diagnosis has traditionally been made serologically. PCR is now becoming the standard diagnostic test.

Doxyxcycline can be used in mild disease but the most effective antibiotics are aminoglycosides and quinolones.

Further reading

Hu LT. Lyme disease. *Ann Intern Med* 2016; 164:ITC65–ITC80.
Kampschreur LM, Delsing CE, Groenwold RHH et al. Chronic Q fever in the Netherlands 5 years after the start of the Q fever epidemic: results from the Dutch Chronic Q Fever Database. *J Clin Microbiol* 2014; 52:1637–1643.
Maurin M, Gyuranecz M. Tularaemia: clinical aspects in Europe. *Lancet Infect Dis* 2016; 16:113–124.

BACTERIAL INFECTIONS SEEN IN DEVELOPING AND TROPICAL COUNTRIES

Skin, soft tissue and eye disease

Leprosy (Hansen's disease)

Leprosy is caused by the acid-fast bacillus *Mycobacterium leprae*. Unlike other mycobacteria, this does not grow in artificial media or even in tissue culture. Apart from the nine-banded armadillo, humans are the only natural host of *M. leprae*, although it can be grown in the footpads of mice.

The WHO has provided free drug treatment for leprosy since 1995. The campaign to control the disease has been hugely successful, with more than 16 million people having been cured of the disease since the year 2000. The number of people with active leprosy has fallen from 5.4 million in 1985 to about 175 000 at the end of 2015, largely as the result of supervised multidrug treatment regimens. The majority of the remaining cases are in India and Brazil; despite the successes, many new infections are occurring in these countries. The WHO has published a Global Leprosy Strategy, with the aim of eradicating the disease completely.

The precise mode of transmission of leprosy is still uncertain but it is likely that nasal secretions play a role. Infection is related to poverty and overcrowding. Once an individual has been infected, subsequent progression to clinical disease appears to be dependent on several factors. Males appear to be more susceptible than females and there is evidence from twin studies of a genetic susceptibility. The main factor, however, is the response of the host's cell-mediated immune system.

Two **polar types** of leprosy are recognized, with most patients falling on a spectrum between (**Fig. 20.23**):

- **Tuberculoid leprosy** is a localized disease that occurs in individuals with a high degree of cell-mediated immunity (CMI). The T-cell response to the antigen releases interferon, which activates macrophages to destroy the bacilli (Th1 response), but with associated destruction of the tissue.
- **Lepromatous leprosy** is a generalized disease that occurs in individuals with impaired CMI. Here the tissue macrophages fail to be activated and the bacilli multiply intracellularly. Th2 cytokines are produced.

In the 1960s the spectrum was divided into five clinico-pathological groups (**Fig. 20.24**). This remains the 'gold standard' classification, but for the purposes of treatment the WHO has defined two main patterns of disease:

- **Paucibacillary leprosy** has five or fewer skin lesions with no bacilli
- **Multibacillary leprosy** has six or more lesions that may have bacilli.

Skin smears are not always available in practice and the distinction must be made on clinical grounds alone. Concern has been raised that this may lead to undertreatment of some people incorrectly identified as having paucibacillary leprosy, but overall the WHO regimen has been remarkably successful.

Clinical features

The incubation period is typically from 2 to 6 years, although it may be as short as a few months or as long as 20 years. The onset of leprosy is generally insidious (although acute onset is known to occur). Patients may present with a transient rash, features of an acute febrile illness, evidence of nerve involvement, or with any combination of these.

Diagnosis

The diagnosis of leprosy is essentially clinical, with hypopigmented/reddish patches with loss of sensation, and thickening of peripheral nerves. Acid-fast bacilli (AFB) may be seen on skin-slit smears. Occasionally, nerve biopsies are helpful. Detection of *M. leprae* DNA is possible in all forms of leprosy using PCR and can be employed to assess the efficacy of treatment.

Management

Multidrug therapy (MDT) is essential because of developing drug resistance (up to 40% of bacilli in some areas are resistant to dapsone). Much shorter courses of treatment are now being used; the current WHO-recommended drug regimens for leprosy are shown in **Box 20.49** but longer therapy is required in severe cases. Follow-up, including skin smears where possible, is obligatory. Immunological reactions ('lepra reactions') can occasionally occur after treatment is started, especially in borderline and lepromatous disease (**Box 20.50**).

Patients should be taught self-care of their anaesthetic hands and feet to prevent ulcers. Cheap canvas shoes with cushioned insoles are protective.

Leprosy should be treated in specialist centres with adequate physiotherapy and occupational therapy support. Surgery and physiotherapy also play a role in the management of trophic ulcers and deformities of the hands, feet and face.

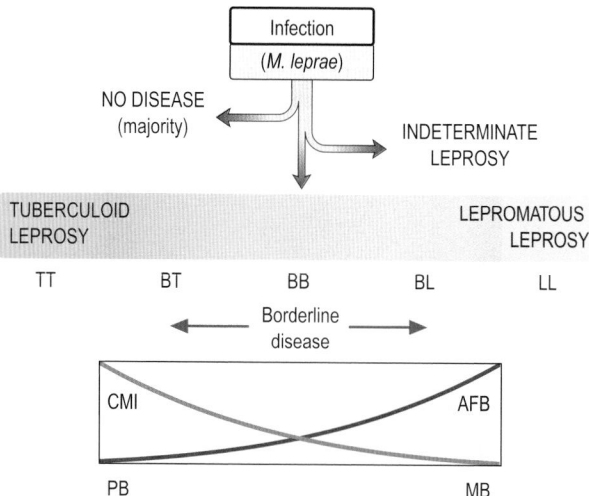

Fig. 20.23 Clinical spectrum of leprosy with the combined Ridley–Jopling and WHO classification. AFB, acid-fast bacilli; BB, borderline; BL, borderline lepromatous; BT, borderline tuberculoid; CMI, cell-mediated immunity; LL, lepromatous leprosy; MB, multibacillary; PB, paucibacillary; TT, tuberculoid leprosy.

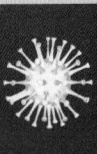

Prognosis in tuberculoid leprosy is good, even if untreated; lepromatous leprosy is progressive if untreated.

Prevention

The prevention and control of leprosy depend on rapid treatment of infected patients, particularly those with lepromatous and borderline lepromatous types, to decrease the bacterial reservoir.

Anthrax

Anthrax is caused by *Bacillus anthracis*. The spores of these Gram-positive bacilli are extremely hardy and withstand extremes of temperature and humidity. The organism is capable of toxin production and this property correlates most closely with its virulence. The disease occurs worldwide but is most common in Africa and Southern Asia. Surveillance data are limited but the likely global annual incidence is in the tens of thousands. In Europe and the USA there are only very occasional cases. Transmission is through direct contact with an infected animal; infection is most frequently seen in farmers, butchers, and dealers in wool and animal hides. Spores can also be ingested or inhaled. Cases in the USA have been caused by the deliberate release of anthrax spores as a bioterrorist weapon.

Clinical features

The incubation period is 1–10 days.

Cutaneous anthrax is the most common form. The small, erythematous, maculopapular lesion is initially painless. It may subsequently vesiculate and ulcerate, with formation of a central black eschar. The illness is self-limiting in the majority of patients, but occasionally perivesicular oedema and regional lymphadenopathy may be marked and toxaemia can occur.

Inhalational anthrax (wool-sorter's disease) follows inhalation of spores. A febrile illness is accompanied by a non-productive cough and retrosternal discomfort; pleural effusions are common. If the disease is untreated, mortality is about 90%; in the bioterrorism cases in the USA, it was 45%, despite treatment.

Gastrointestinal anthrax is due to consumption of undercooked, contaminated meat. It presents as severe gastroenteritis, sometimes with haematemesis and bloody diarrhoea. In some cases, systemic toxin spread may lead to shock and death.

Diagnosis

The diagnosis is established by demonstration of the organism in smears from cutaneous lesions or by culture of blood and other body fluids. Serological confirmation can be obtained using ELISAs that detect antibodies to both the organism and a toxin. PCR tests are available.

Management

Ciprofloxacin is considered the best treatment. In mild cutaneous infections, oral therapy for 2 weeks is adequate. In more severe infections, high doses of intravenous antibiotics are needed, along with appropriate supportive care. The monoclonal antibody raxibacumab has been shown in animal studies to improve survival in

---

 Box 20.49 Recommended treatment regimens for leprosy in adults (modified WHO guidelines

Multibacillary leprosy (LL, BL, BB)	Paucibacillary leprosy (BT, TT)
• Rifampicin 600 mg once monthly, supervised	• Rifampicin 600mg once monthly, supervised
• Clofazimine 300mg once monthly, supervised	• Dapsone 100 mg daily, self-administered
• Clofazimine 50mg daily, self-administered	• Treatment continued for 6 months
• Dapsone 100 mg daily, self-administered	**Single-lesion paucibacillary leprosy**
• Treatment continued for 12 months	• Rifampicin 600 mg ⎤ (as a single dose) • Ofloxacin 400 mg ⎥ • Minocycline 100 mg ⎦

BB, borderline; BL, borderline lepromatous; BT, borderline tuberculoid; LL, lepromatous; TT, tuberculoid.

A **Tuberculoid (TT)**	B **Borderline tuberculoid (BT)**	C **Borderline (BB)**	D **Borderline lepromatous (BL)**	E **Lepromatous (LL)**
Skin lesion (usually single) - hypopigmented - anaesthetic - clearly defined edges - thickened local nerve(s) May heal spontaneously	Several skin lesions - similar to TT Thickened peripheral nerves - deformities of hands/feet	Numerous skin lesions - varying size Widespread nerve involvement and deformity	Numerous florid skin lesions - variable size and form - contain many AFB Variable nerve involvement Neurotrophic atrophy of digits	Extensive skin infiltration Mucous membrane involvement Nasal septal perforation - 'Leonine facies' Glove and stocking anaesthesia Multiple nerve palsies Neurotrophic atrophy of digits

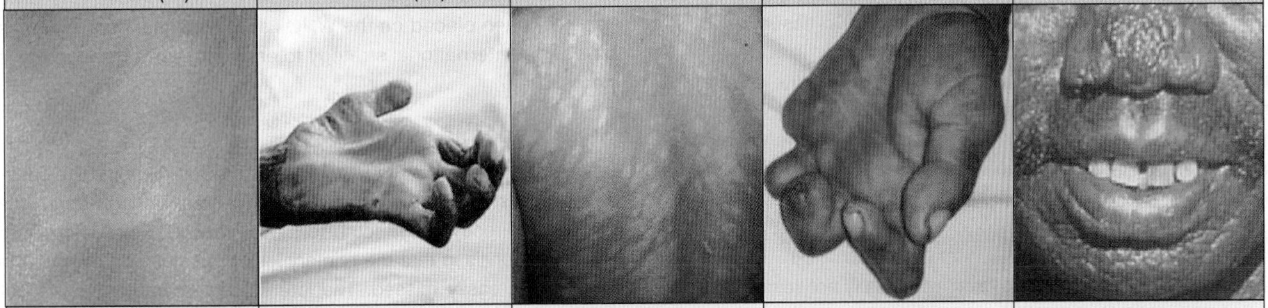

Fig. 20.24 The spectrum of disease in leprosy. AFB, acid-fast bacilli. (*C, From Cohen J, Powderly JG. Infectious Diseases, 3rd edn. London: Mosby; 2010, with permission. E, From Goering R et al. Mims' Medical Microbiology, 5th edn. London: Mosby; 2013, courtesy of DA Lewis, with permission.*)

> **Box 20.50** Lepra reactions following commencement of anti-mycobacterial treatment
>
> **Type 1**
> - Occurs in borderline disease
> - Type IV hypersensitivity reaction
> - Lasts for many months
> - Upgrading (→TT) or downgrading (→BB)
> - Abrupt onset of nerve palsies in upgrading
> - Treatment:
>   - Prednisolone
>
> **Type 2 (erythema nodosum leprosum)**
> - Occurs in lepromatous disease
> - Type III (immune complex) hypersensitivity reaction
> - Lasts days to weeks:
>
> - Fever
> - Arthralgia
> - Subcutaneous nodules
> - Iridocyclitis
> - Rare since clofazimine included in treatment
> - Treatment:[a]
>   - Analgesia
>   - Clofazimine (if not already started)
>   - Prednisolone if eye involvement
>   - Continuation of anti-mycobacterial treatment
>
> [a]Thalidomide no longer has any role in the management of lepra reactions. BB, borderline; TT, tuberculoid.

inhalational anthrax. Any suspected case should be reported to the relevant authority.

Control

Any infected animal that dies should be burned and the area in which it was housed disinfected. Where animal husbandry is poor, mass vaccination of animals may prevent widespread contamination but needs to be repeated annually. A human vaccine is available for those at high risk and prophylactic ciprofloxacin is used following exposure. Some countries are establishing public health policies to deal with the deliberate release of anthrax spores.

Mycobacterial ulcer (buruli ulcer)

Buruli ulcer, caused by *Mycobacterium ulcerans*, is seen in humid rural areas of the tropics, especially in Africa. About 2000 cases per year are reported to the WHO but this does not reflect the true prevalence (which is much higher). The mode of transmission remains unknown. A small subcutaneous nodule at the site of infection gradually ulcerates, involving subcutaneous tissue, muscle and fascial planes, and occasionally bone. The ulcers are usually large with undermined edges and markedly necrotic bases due to mycolactone (a toxin produced by the mycobacterium). Smears taken from necrotic tissue generally reveal numerous acid-fast bacilli; a PCR assay is widely available. Combination therapy with rifampicin plus one of streptomycin, clarithromycin or moxifloxacin, given for 8 weeks, will heal ulcers in many cases. However, in more severe cases, surgical debridement and, where possible, skin grafting may be needed as well.

Tropical ulcer

Tropical ulcer is a non-specific infection, usually polymicrobial, seen in damp, hot climates. A wide variety of organisms have been implicated but there is no characteristic bacterium associated with the condition. Good wound hygiene is the mainstay of management, with antibiotic therapy used (either empirically or based on culture) as needed.

Endemic treponematoses
Yaws

Yaws (caused by *Treponema pallidum* subspecies *pertenue*) is the most widespread and common of the endemic treponemal diseases, although it has been eradicated from a number of areas. Most cases are now reported from West Africa and the South Pacific. After an incubation period of weeks or months, a primary inflammatory reaction occurs at the inoculation site, from which organisms can be isolated. Dissemination of the organism leads to multiple papular lesions containing treponemes; these skin lesions usually involve the palms and soles. There may also be bone involvement, particularly affecting the long bones and those of the hand.

Approximately 10% of those infected go on to develop late yaws. Bony gummatous lesions may progress to cause gross destruction and disfigurement, particularly of the skull and facial bones, interphalangeal joints and long bones. Plantar hyperkeratosis is characteristic. As in syphilis, there may be a latent period between the early and late phases of the disease but visceral, neurological and cardiovascular problems do not occur.

In endemic areas the diagnosis is usually clinical. The causative organism can be identified from the exudative lesions under darkground microscopy. Serological tests for syphilis are positive and do not differentiate between the conditions. Rapid point-of-care, species-specific tests are used but do not distinguish between past and current infection. PCR diagnosis is not widely available but may become important in the yaws eradication campaign, as it is necessary to distinguish active from treated infection.

Single-dose oral azithromycin has now replaced intramuscular benzathine penicillin as the treatment of choice. This drug has now been placed on the WHO list of essential medicines, as part of the international strategy to eradicate yaws through mass treatment.

Bejel (endemic syphilis)

Bejel is seen in Africa, the Middle East and Central Asia. The causative organism (*Treponema endemicum*) enters through abrasions in the skin directly or by mouth-to-mouth contact. Bejel differs from venereal syphilis in that the primary lesion is small and often in the mouth; it is easily missed. The late stages resemble syphilis but cardiological and neurological manifestations are rare.

Pinta

Pinta (caused by *Treponema carateum*) is restricted mainly to Central and South America. There is no effective surveillance and the current prevalence is unknown. It is milder than the other treponematoses and confined to the skin. The primary lesion is a pruritic red papule, usually on the hand or foot. It may become scaly but never ulcerates, and is generally associated with regional lymphadenopathy. In the later stages, similar lesions can continue to occur for up to 1 year, associated with generalized lymphadenopathy. Eventually, the lesions heal, leaving hyperpigmented or depigmented patches.

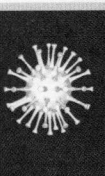

The diagnosis of bejel and pinta is largely clinical. Treatment is still with benzathine penicillin usually, although it is likely that azithromycin will prove to be effective. Surveillance, diagnosis and treatment are much less well coordinated than for yaws.

Trachoma

Trachoma is caused by the intracellular bacterium *Chlamydia trachomatis* (which can also cause a number of sexually transmitted infections, see p. 1416). It is the most common infectious cause of blindness in the world. It is estimated that there are 21 million active infections and 2 million people who have been blinded by trachoma. It is a disease of poverty, found mainly in the tropics and the Middle East, and is entirely preventable. Trachoma commonly occurs in children and is spread by direct transmission or by flies. Isolated infection is probably self-limiting and it is repeated infection that leads to chronic eye disease.

Clinical features

Infection is bilateral and begins in the conjunctiva, with marked follicular inflammation and subsequent scarring. Damage to the upper eyelid causes entropion, leaving the cornea exposed to further abrasion from the eyelashes rubbing against it (trichiasis). The corneal scarring that eventually occurs leads to blindness.

Trachoma may also occur as an acute ophthalmic infection in the neonate.

Diagnosis and management

The diagnosis is generally made clinically.

Systemic therapy with a single dose of azithromycin is the treatment of choice, but re-infection is common and repeated treatments are often needed. In some endemic areas, routine mass drug administration is used in children. Once infection has been controlled, surgery may be required for eyelid reconstruction and for treatment of corneal opacities.

Prevention

Community health education, improvements in water supply and sanitation (pit latrines), and earlier case reporting could have a substantial impact on disease prevalence. This is reflected in the 'SAFE' approach to trachoma:

- surgery
- antibiotics
- facial cleanliness
- environmental improvement.

The WHO Global Partnership for Trachoma Eradication is working with numerous countries throughout the world: Iran, Nepal and Ghana are the latest previously endemic countries to be declared trachoma-free.

Further reading

Mitjà O, Marks M, Konan DJ. Global epidemiology of yaws: a systematic review. *Lancet Glob Health* 2015; 3:e324–331.
Stamm LV. Pinta: Latin America's forgotten disease? *Am J Trop Med Hyg* 2015; 93:901–903.
https://www.who.int/lep/epidemiology/en/. Leprosy.

Gastrointestinal infections

Cholera

Cholera is caused by the curved, flagellated, Gram-negative bacillus *Vibrio cholerae*. The organism is killed by temperatures of 100°C in a few seconds but can survive in ice for up to 6 weeks.

The fertile, humid plains of the River Ganges in West Bengal have traditionally been regarded as the home of cholera. However, a series of pandemics have spread the disease across the world, usually following trade routes. The seventh pandemic currently affects large areas of Asia, sub-Saharan Africa and the Americas. Until recently, all outbreaks of cholera were caused by *V. cholerae* O1, which is responsible for the current pandemic. In the 1990s a new serogroup (O139 Bengal) caused outbreaks of an illness indistinguishable from O1 cholera, but it has not been reported outside Bangladesh, India and South-east Asia. Outbreaks of cholera are common when there is disruption of water supplies and sanitation: for example, that due to natural disasters or to conflict. More than a million cases of cholera have been reported in Yemen during the last 2 years of the civil war in that country.

Transmission is by the faeco-oral route. Contaminated water plays a major role in the dissemination of cholera, although contaminated foodstuffs and contact carriers may contribute in epidemics. Achlorhydria or hypochlorhydria facilitates passage of the cholera bacilli into the small intestine. Here they proliferate, elaborating an exotoxin that produces massive secretion of isotonic fluid into the intestinal lumen. Cholera toxin also releases serotonin (5-hydroxytryptamine, 5-HT) from enterochromaffin cells in the gut, which activates a neural secretory reflex in the enteric nervous system. This may account for at least 50% of cholera toxin's secretory activity. *V. cholerae* also produces other toxins (zona occludens toxin (ZOT) and accessory cholera toxin (ACT)), which contribute to its pathogenic effect.

Clinical features

The incubation period varies from a few hours to 6 days. The majority of patients with cholera have a mild illness that cannot be distinguished clinically from diarrhoea due to other infective causes. In severe cases, there is abrupt onset of profuse painless diarrhoea, followed by vomiting. As the illness progresses, the typical 'rice water' stool, flecked with mucus, may be seen. There is massive fluid loss, and if this is not replaced, the features of hypovolaemic shock (cold clammy skin, tachycardia, hypotension and peripheral cyanosis) and dehydration (sunken eyes, hollow cheeks and a diminished urine output) can develop within hours. Muscle cramps may be severe. Children may present with convulsions owing to hypoglycaemia.

As long as the patient can be adequately rehydrated the prognosis is good, with a gradual return to normal clinical and biochemical parameters in 1–3 days.

Diagnosis

This is largely clinical. Examination of freshly passed stools may demonstrate rapidly motile organisms (although this is not diagnostic, as *Campylobacter jejuni* may give a similar appearance). A rapid dipstick test is also available. Stool and rectal swabs should be taken for culture to confirm the diagnosis and establish antibiotic sensitivity. Cholera should always be reported to the appropriate public health authority.

Management

The mainstay of treatment is rehydration, and with appropriate and effective rehydration therapy, mortality has decreased to less than 1%. Oral rehydration is usually adequate, but intravenous therapy is sometimes required (**Fig. 20.25**). Antibiotics may shorten the duration and severity of diarrhoea but should be given only to patients with severe dehydration.

Oral rehydration solutions (**ORS**) are based on the observation that glucose (and other carbohydrates) enhance sodium and water absorption in the small intestine, even in the presence of secretory

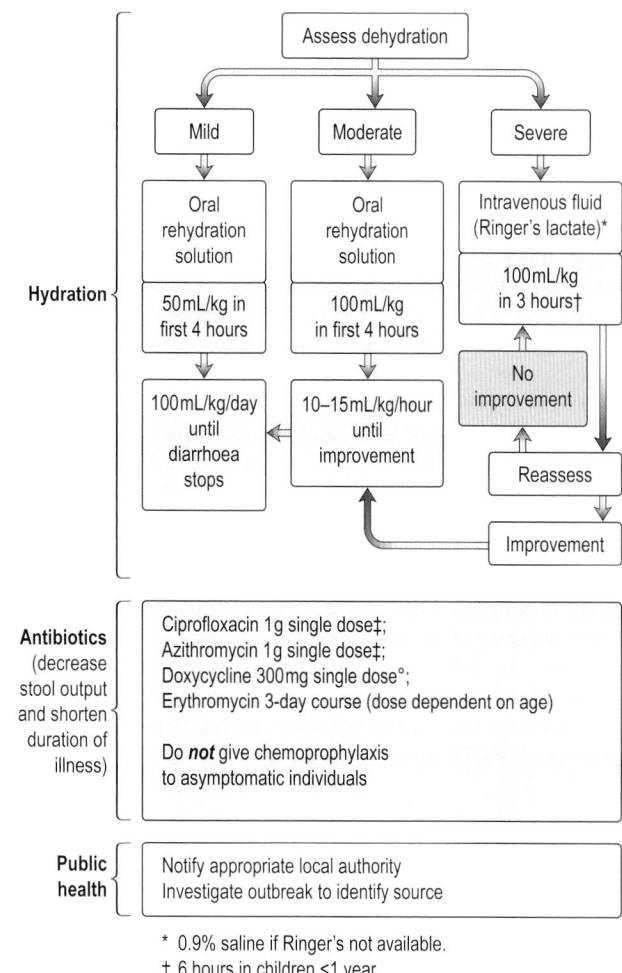

* 0.9% saline if Ringer's not available.
† 6 hours in children <1 year.
‡ Adult doses: adjust for age.
° Not in children/adolescents.

Fig. 20.25 The management of cholera.

loss due to toxins. Additions such as amylase-resistant starch to glucose-based ORS have been shown to increase the absorption of fluid. Cereal-based electrolyte solutions have been found to be as effective as sugar/salt ORS and actually reduce stool volume, as well as rehydrating. The WHO and UNICEF recommend the use of reduced-osmolarity ORS (with zinc supplementation) for all types of diarrhoea: the small risk of hyponatraemia with this formulation is far outweighed by the improved efficacy. Suitable solutions for rehydration are listed in **Box 20.36**.

Immunization is now recommended by the WHO in potential or actual outbreak situations. Two killed oral vaccines are available. The best preventative measures, however, are good hygiene and improved sanitation. In 2017, the WHO announced a new strategy: 'Ending Cholera: a Roadmap to 2030'. It has three elements:
* early detection and quick response to contain outbreaks
* prevention of cholera recurrence in cholera 'hotspots'
* coordination of technical support, advocacy, resource mobilization, and partnership at local and global levels.

Enteric fever

Over 17 million new cases of enteric fever occur annually worldwide, mainly in India and Africa, causing 150 000 deaths per year. Enteric fever is an acute systemic illness characterized by fever, headache and abdominal discomfort. *Typhoid*, the typical form of

enteric fever, is caused by *Salmonella typhi*. A similar but generally less severe illness known as *paratyphoid* is due to infection with *S. paratyphi* A, B or C. Humans are the only natural host for *S. typhi*, which is transmitted in contaminated food or water. The incubation period is 10–14 days.

Clinical features

After ingestion, the bacteria invade the small bowel wall via Peyer's patches, from where they spread to the regional lymph nodes and then to the blood. The onset of illness is insidious and non-specific, with intermittent fever, headache and abdominal pain. Physical findings in the early stages include abdominal tenderness, hepatosplenomegaly, lymphadenopathy and a scanty maculopapular rash ('rose spots'). Without treatment (and occasionally even after treatment), serious complications can arise, usually in the third week of illness. These include meningitis, lobar pneumonia, osteomyelitis, intestinal perforation and intestinal haemorrhage. The fourth week is characterized by gradual improvement but in areas with limited healthcare up to 30% of those infected will die and 10% of untreated survivors will relapse. This compares with a mortality rate of 1–2% in the USA.

After clinical recovery, up to 10% of patients will continue to excrete *S. typhi* for several months: these are termed **convalescent carriers**. Between 1% and 4% will continue to carry the organism for more than a year: this is **chronic carriage**. The usual site of carriage is the gall bladder, and chronic carriage is associated with the presence of gallstones. However, in parts of the Middle East and Africa where urinary schistosomiasis is prevalent, chronic carriage of *S. typhi* in the urinary bladder is also common.

Paratyphoid fever is associated with a milder and shorter illness, and complications are uncommon.

Diagnosis

The definitive diagnosis of enteric fever requires the culture of *S. typhi* or *S. paratyphi* from the patient. Blood culture is positive in most cases in the first 2 weeks. Culture of intestinal secretions, faeces and urine is also used, although care must be taken to distinguish acute infection from chronic carriage. Bone marrow culture is more sensitive than blood culture but is rarely required, except in patients who have already received antibiotics. Leucopenia is common but non-specific. Serological investigations, such as the Widal antigen test, are of little practical value, are easily misinterpreted and should not be used.

Management

Increasing antibiotic resistance is seen in isolates of *S. typhi*, especially in the Indian subcontinent. Chloramphenicol, cotrimoxazole and amoxicillin may still be effective in some cases, but resistance to all of these drugs (known as multidrug-resistant (MDR) typhoid) is spreading rapidly. For example, the proportion of *S. typhi* isolates with MDR typhoid in Malawi rose from 7% in 2010 to 97% in 2014. In most areas the treatment of choice is now a quinolone (e.g. ciprofloxacin 500 mg twice daily), but resistance is starting to appear to these agents as well, and ideally treatment should be based on known local resistance patterns. In a few countries (notably Pakistan), so-called extensively drug-resistant (XDR) typhoid is becoming common; this is resistant to quinolones and to third-generation cephalosporins, and only azithromycin and carbapenems are still effective.

The patient's temperature may remain elevated for several days after antibiotics are started and this alone is not a sign of treatment failure. Prolonged antibiotic therapy may eliminate the carrier

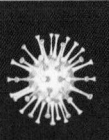

state, but in the presence of gall bladder disease it is rarely effective. Cholecystectomy is not usually justified on clinical or public health grounds.

Prevention

This is mainly through improved sanitation and clean water. Travellers should avoid drinking untreated water, taking ice in drinks or eating ice creams. Vaccination with either injectable inactivated or oral live attenuated vaccines gives partial protection and should be used for travellers to high-risk areas. A new conjugate vaccine that provides more effective and longer-lasting immunity has recently become available; with funding from the Global Alliance for Vaccines and Immunization (GAVI), this new vaccine is to be rolled out to children in endemic countries from 2019.

Further reading

Dyson ZA, Klemm EJ, Palmer S et al. Antibiotic resistance and typhoid. *Clin Inf Dis* 2019; 58:S165–170.
https://www.gavi.org/about/mission/. *Immunization*.

Systemic infections

Tuberculosis

See page 967.

Non-tuberculous mycobacterial infections

Environmental mycobacteria can cause a wide variety of infections in susceptible hosts (**Box 20.51**). These are discussed in more detail on page 972.

Plague

Plague is caused by *Yersinia pestis*, a Gram-negative bacillus. Sporadic cases of plague (as well as occasional epidemics) occur worldwide but it is relatively uncommon: about 1000 cases per year are reported to the WHO, with a 10% mortality. The majority are in Madagascar and Central Africa, although the disease is occasionally seen in developed countries (usually associated with hunting). The main reservoirs are woodland rodents, which transmit infection to domestic rats (*Rattus rattus*). The usual vector is the rat flea, *Xenopsylla cheopis*. These fleas bite humans when there is a sudden decline in the rat population. Occasionally, spread of the

organisms may be through infected faeces being rubbed into skin wounds, or through inhalation of droplets.

Clinical features

Four clinical forms are recognized: bubonic, pneumonic, septicaemic and cutaneous.

- **Bubonic plague** is the most common form, accounting for about 90% of cases. The incubation period is 2–7 days. The onset of illness is acute, with high fever, chills, headache, myalgia, nausea, vomiting and, when severe, prostration. This is rapidly followed by the development of lymphadenopathy (buboes), most commonly involving the inguinal region. Characteristically, these are matted and tender, and suppurate in 1–2 weeks.
- **Pneumonic plague** is characterized by the abrupt onset of features of a fulminant pneumonia with bloody sputum, marked respiratory distress, cyanosis, and death in almost all affected patients.
- **Septicaemic plague** presents as an acute fulminant infection with evidence of shock and DIC. If it is left untreated, death usually occurs in 2–5 days.
- **Cutaneous plague** can present as a pustule, eschar or papule, or as extensive purpura, which can become necrotic and gangrenous.

Diagnosis

This is based on clinical, epidemiological and laboratory findings. Microscopy (on blood or lymph node aspirate) or a rapid dipstick antigen detection test can provide a presumptive diagnosis in an appropriate clinical setting. Confirmation is by blood or lymph node culture, or paired serological tests.

Management

Treatment is urgent and should be instituted before the results of culture studies are available. *Y. pestis* remains sensitive to most antibiotics for Gram-negative bacteria. Gentamicin is the most widely used agent: doxycycline, ciprofloxacin and chloramphenicol are also effective.

Prevention

Prevention of plague is largely dependent on control of the flea population. Outhouses or huts should be sprayed with insecticides that are effective against the local flea. During epidemics, rodents should not be killed until the fleas are under control, as the fleas will leave dead rodents to bite humans. Tetracycline is an effective chemoprophylactic agent for those at risk during an outbreak. Both killed and attenuated vaccines have been available for many years but have limited efficacy and are not widely used.

Relapsing fevers

These conditions are so named because, after apparent recovery from the initial infection, recurrences may occur after a week or more without fever. They are caused by spirochaetes of the genus *Borrelia*.

Louse-borne relapsing fever

This condition (caused by *B. recurrentis*) is spread by body lice and only humans are affected. Classically, it is an epidemic disease of armies and refugees, although it is also endemic in the highlands of Ethiopia and Yemen, and in the Andes. Lice are spread from person to person when humans live in close contact in impoverished conditions. The spirochaete penetrates through the skin or mucosa when infected lice are crushed by scratching or by biting (a traditional

Box 20.51 Examples of non-tuberculous mycobacteria causing disease in humans

Clinical	Common cause	Rare cause
Chronic lung disease	*Mycobacterium avium-intracellulare* *M. kansasii*	*M. malmoense* *M. xenopi*
Local lymph-adenitis	*M. avium-intracellulare* *M. scrofulaceum*	*M. malmoense* *M. fortuitum*
Skin and soft tissue infection		
Fish tank granuloma	*M. marinum*	
Abscesses, ulcers, sinuses	*M. fortuitum* *M. chelonae*	*M. haemophilum*
Bone and joint infection	*M. kansasii* *M. avium-intracellulare*	*M. scrofulaceum*
Disseminated infection (in HIV)	*M. avium-intracellulare*	

means of killing the insect, hence the adage 'man bites louse is more dangerous than louse bites man'). Symptoms begin 3–10 days after infection and consist of abrupt high fever, generalized myalgia and headache. A petechial or ecchymotic rash may be seen. In severe cases the condition then deteriorates, with delirium, hepatospleno-megaly, jaundice, bleeding and circulatory collapse. A proportion of those who recover have no further symptoms but the majority experience one or more relapses of diminishing intensity over the weeks following the initial illness. Severity varies enormously, with many people experiencing only mild symptoms, and some develop-ing antibodies with no history of clinical illness. In some epidemics, however, mortality in untreated people has exceeded 50%.

Tick-borne relapsing fever

This is caused by *B. duttoni* and other *Borrelia* species, spread by soft (argasid) ticks of the genus *Ornithodoros*. Rodents are the main reservoir of infection and humans are incidental hosts, acquiring the spirochaete from the saliva of the infected tick. The disease is found worldwide and is endemic in parts of North America and Europe, but the clinical burden falls mainly in Africa. It is particularly com-mon where traditional mud huts are the principal form of human shelter, as the ticks live in the walls and feed on inhabitants at night. The illness is generally similar to the louse-borne disease, with the same variability in presentation and severity.

Diagnosis and management

Spirochaetes can be demonstrated microscopically in the blood during febrile episodes; organisms are more numerous in louse-borne relapsing fever. Treatment is usually with tetracycline or doxy-cycline. A severe Jarisch–Herxheimer reaction (see p. 1424) occurs in many patients, especially those who have the louse-borne form.

Prevention

Control of infection relies on elimination of the vector. Ticks live for years and remain infected, passing the infection to their prog-eny. These reservoirs of infection should be controlled by spraying houses with insecticides and reducing the number of rodents. Post-exposure prophylaxis has been shown to be effective in areas where tick-borne disease is highly endemic. Infested patients should be deloused by washing with a suitable insecticide. All clothes must be thoroughly disinfected.

Rickettsiae and rickettsia-like infections

Rickettsiae (and the closely related orientiae) are small, intracellular bacteria that are spread to humans by arthropod vectors, including body lice, fleas, hard ticks and larval mites. Rickettsiae inhabit the alimentary tract of these arthropods and infection is spread to the human host by inoculation of their faeces through broken human skin, generally produced by scratching. Rickettsiae multiply intra-cellularly and can enter most mammalian cells, although the main lesion produced is a vasculitis caused by invasion of endothelial cells of small blood vessels. Multisystem involvement is usual.

Typhus is the collective name given to a group of diseases caused by *Rickettsia* species. **Box 20.52** provides a list of some of the more important rickettsial diseases; with the advent of molecu-lar techniques, many new species of *Rickettsia* causing human dis-ease have been identified and more than 30 pathogenic species are now recognized. Various ways of classifying rickettsial disease have been proposed, based on genetic typing, clinical presentation and geography. None of these is ideal, as species that are geneti-cally very similar can occur in different parts of the world and there is considerable overlap between the various rickettsial syndromes.

? Box 20.52 Infections caused by rickettsiae

Disease	Organism	Reservoir	Vector
Typhus fever group			
Epidemic typhus	*Rickettsia prowazekii*	Human	Human body louse
Endemic (murine) typhus	*R. typhi*	Rodent	Rat flea
Spotted fever group			
African tick typhus	*R. africae*	Various mammals	Hard tick
Mediterrane-an spotted fever	*R. conorii*	Rodent, dog	Hard tick
Rocky Mountain spotted fever	*R. rickettsii*	Rodent, dog	Hard tick
Rickettsial pox	*R. akari*	Rodent	Mite
Flea-borne spotted fever	*R. felis*	Various mammals	Flea
Scrub typhus	*Orientia tsut-sugamushi*	Trombiculid mite	Trombiculid mite

A useful clinical approach is to divide rickettsial infections into three groups: typhus, spotted fever and scrub typhus (although the organisms causing the last of these are now strictly classified as orientiae and not rickettsiae).

Typhus group

Epidemic typhus

The vector of epidemic typhus is the human body louse and, as with louse-borne relapsing fever, epidemics are associated with war and refugees.

The incubation period of 1–3 weeks is followed by an abrupt febrile illness associated with profound malaise and generalized myalgia. Headache is severe and there may be conjunctivitis with orbital pain. A measles-like eruption appears around the fifth day. At the end of the first week, signs of meningoencephalitis appear and CNS involvement may progress to coma. At the height of the illness, splenomegaly, pneumonia, myocarditis and gangrene at the peripher-ies may be evident. Oliguric acute kidney injury occurs in fulminating disease, which is usually fatal. Recovery begins in the third week but is generally slow. If untreated, the disease may recur many years after the initial attack, owing to rickettsiae that lie dormant in lymph nodes. The recrudescence, which is now rarely seen due to appropriate use of antibiotics in the primary phase, is known as Brill–Zinsser disease.

Endemic (murine) typhus

This is an infection of rodents that is inadvertently spread to humans by rat fleas. The disease closely resembles epidemic typhus but is much milder and rarely fatal.

Spotted fever group

A variety of *Rickettsia* species, collectively known as the spot-ted fever group rickettsiae, cause the illnesses known as spotted fevers. In most cases the vector is a hard tick. Although the caus-ative organism and the name of the illness vary from place to place, the clinical course is common to all.

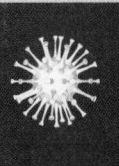

The typical feature of the spotted fevers is a widespread petechial rash (**Fig. 20.26**), although a variety of other types of skin lesion are seen, especially in Rocky Mountain spotted fever. An exception is the form of African tick typhus caused by *R. africae*, which often presents without a rash.

After an incubation period of 4–10 days, an eschar (a black, crusted, necrotic papule) may develop at the site of the bite in association with regional lymphadenopathy (**Fig. 20.27**). There is abrupt onset of fever, myalgia and headache, accompanied by a maculopapular rash that may become petechial. Neurological, haematological and cardiovascular complications can occur, as in epidemic typhus, although these are uncommon.

Scrub typhus

Found throughout Asia and the Western Pacific (and also reported occasionally from Africa), this disease is spread by larval trombiculid mites (chiggers). An eschar can often be found at the site of the bite. The clinical illness is very variable, ranging from a mild illness to fulminant and potentially fatal disease. The more severe cases resemble epidemic typhus. Unlike in other types of typhus, the organism is passed on to subsequent generations of mites, which consequently act as both reservoir and vector.

Diagnosis

The diagnosis of all types of rickettsial infection is generally made on the basis of the history and clinical course. It can be confirmed serologically or by PCR.

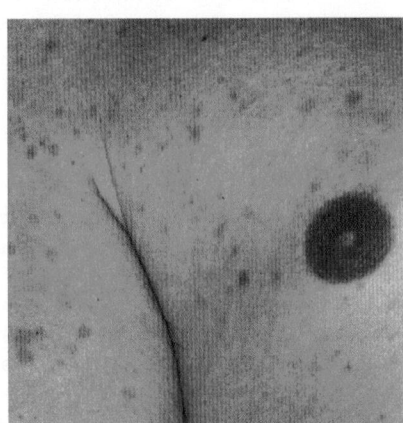

Fig. 20.26 The petechial rash of rickettsial spotted fever.

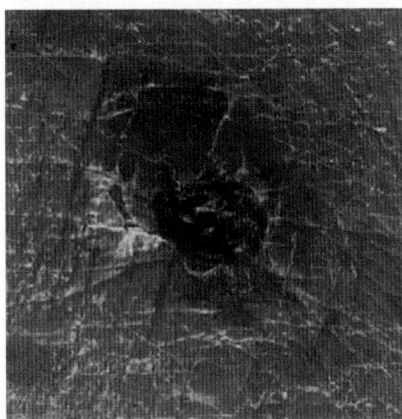

Fig. 20.27 An eschar developing at the site of the bite in rickettsial disease.

Management and prevention

Doxycycline or tetracycline given for 5–7 days is the treatment of choice. Ciprofloxacin is also effective. Prophylactic doxycycline 200 mg weekly protects against scrub typhus; it is reserved for highly endemic areas. Rifampicin is also used when resistance to tetracycline is present. Seriously ill patients need intensive care. Control of typhus is achieved by eradication of the arthropod vectors: lice and fleas can be eradicated from clothing with insecticides (0.5% malathion or DDT). Control of rodents is necessary in endemic typhus and some of the spotted fevers. Areas of vegetation infested with trombiculid mites can be cleared by chemical spraying from the air. Bites from ticks and mites should be avoided by wearing protective clothing on exposed areas of the body. The likelihood of infection from ticks is related to the duration of feeding; in high-risk areas the body should be inspected twice a day, as the bites are painless, and any ticks should be removed.

Bartonellosis

Bartonella spp. are intracellular bacteria closely related to the rickettsiae. A number of human diseases can be caused by these organisms; as in rickettsial disease, infection is usually spread from animals via an arthropod vector (**Box 20.53**).

Carrion's disease (*Bartonella bacilliformis*)

This disease is largely restricted to the habitat of its main vector, the sandfly, in the river valleys of the Andes mountains at an altitude of 500–3000 m. Two clinical presentations are seen, which may occur alone or consecutively. ***Oroya fever*** is an acute febrile illness causing myalgia, arthralgia, severe headache and confusion, followed by a haemolytic anaemia. ***Verruga peruana*** consists of eruptions of reddish-purple haemangiomatous nodules, resembling bacillary angiomatosis. It may follow 4–6 weeks after Oroya fever or be the presenting feature of infection. Spontaneous resolution may occur over a period of months or years. Carrion's disease is frequently complicated by superinfection, especially with *Salmonella* spp.

? Box 20.53 Human infections caused by *Bartonella* spp. and *Ehrlichia* spp.

Disease	Organism	Reservoir	Vector
Bartonella			
Carrion's disease	*Bartonella bacilliformis*	Unknown	Sandfly
Cat-scratch disease	*B. henselae*	Cat	Cat flea
Bacillary angiomatosis	*B. henselae*	Cat	Cat flea
Trench fever	*B. quintana*	Human	Body louse
Ehrlichia			
Human monocytic ehrlichiosis (HME)	*Ehrlichia chaffeensis*	Deer	Hard tick
Human granulocytic ehrlichiosis (HGE)[a]	*Ehrlichia ewingii Anaplasma phagocytophilum*[b]	Small mammals and deer	Hard tick

[a]Also known as human granulocytic anaplasmosis. [b]Formerly known as *Ehrlichia phagocytophilia*.

The diagnosis is made by culturing bacilli from blood or peripheral lesions. Serological tests have been developed but are not widely available.

Treatment with chloramphenicol or tetracycline is effective in acute disease but less so in verruga peruana. Carrion's disease is a paradigm for eradicable but neglected diseases of poverty. It is readily treatable, geographically constrained and has no known hosts other than humans. However, because of the areas in which it is found, there is almost no surveillance or organized treatment programme.

Cat-scratch disease and bacillary angiomatosis (*Bartonella henselae*)

These are described on page 537.

Trench fever

Trench fever is caused by *Bartonella quintana* and transmitted by human body lice. It is mainly seen in refugees and the homeless. It is characterized by cyclical fever, chills and headaches, accompanied by myalgia and pretibial pain. The disease is usually self-limiting but it can be treated with erythromycin or doxycycline if symptoms are severe.

Ehrlichiosis

Ehrlichiosis and anaplasmosis are infections caused by tick-borne, rickettsia-like bacteria. At least three species have been implicated: *Ehrlichia chaffeensis*, which causes human monocytic ehrlichiosis (HME), and *E. ewingii* and *Anaplasma phagocytophilum* (formerly known as *E. phagocytophilum*), which cause human granulocytic ehrlichiosis (HGE, also known as human granulocytic anaplasmosis). All cause a rather non-specific febrile illness with fever, myalgia and headache. Treatment is with doxycycline. The vectors are hard ticks and the main reservoir hosts are deer. As with most tick-borne zoonoses, the avoidance of tick bites and the prompt removal of feeding ticks are the best forms of prevention.

Other bacterial infections

Melioidosis

This term refers to infections caused by the Gram-negative bacterium *Burkholderia pseudomallei*. This environmental organism, which is found in soil and surface water, is distributed widely in the tropics and subtropics. The majority of clinical cases of melioidosis occur in South-east Asia. Infection follows inhalation or direct inoculation. More than half of all patients with melioidosis have predisposing underlying disease; it is particularly common in people with diabetes.

B. pseudomallei causes a wide spectrum of disease and the majority of infections are probably subclinical. Illness may be acute or chronic, and localized or disseminated, but one form may progress to another and individual patients may be difficult to categorize. The most serious form is septicaemic melioidosis, which is often complicated by multiple metastatic abscesses; it is frequently fatal. Serological tests are available but definitive diagnosis depends on isolating the organism from blood or appropriate tissue. *B. pseudomallei* has extensive intrinsic antibiotic resistance. The most effective agent is ceftazidime, given intravenously for 2–4 weeks; this should be followed by several months of co-amoxiclav or co-trimoxazole to prevent relapses.

Actinomycosis

Actinomyces spp. are branching, Gram-positive higher bacteria, which are normal mouth and intestine commensals; they are particularly associated with poor mouth hygiene. *Actinomyces* have a worldwide distribution but are a rare cause of disease in the West.

Cervicofacial actinomycosis, the most common form, usually occurs following dental infection or extraction. It is often indolent and slowly progressive, is associated with little pain, and results in induration and localized swelling of the lower part of the mandible. Sinuses and tracts develop, with discharge of 'sulphur' granules. **Thoracic actinomycosis** follows inhalation of organisms, usually into a previously damaged lung. The clinical picture is not distinctive and is often mistaken for malignancy or tuberculosis. Symptoms such as fever, malaise, chest pain and haemoptysis are present. Empyema occurs in 25% of patients and local extension produces chest-wall sinuses with discharge of 'sulphur' granules.

Abdominal and pelvic actinomycosis most frequently affects the caecum. Characteristically, an indurated mass is felt in the right iliac fossa. Later, sinuses develop. The differential diagnosis includes malignancy, tuberculosis, Crohn's disease and amoeboma. The incidence of pelvic actinomycosis appears to be increasing with wider use of intrauterine contraceptive devices. Occasionally, actinomycosis becomes disseminated to involve any site.

Diagnosis is by microscopy and culture of the organism. Treatment often involves surgery, as well as antibiotics. Penicillin is the drug of choice and should usually be given for 4–6 weeks, followed by oral amoxicillin for at least 3–4 months after clinical resolution (longer courses may be required if source control is not feasible). Tetracyclines are also effective.

Nocardia infections

Nocardia spp. are Gram-positive branching bacteria, found in soil and decomposing organic matter. *N. asteroides* and, less often, *N. brasiliensis* are the main human pathogens.

Mycetoma is the most common illness. It is a result of local invasion by *Nocardia* spp. and presents as a painless swelling, usually on the sole of the foot (Madura foot). The swelling of the affected part of the body continues inexorably. Nodules gradually appear, which eventually rupture and discharge characteristic 'grains', which are colonies of organisms. Systemic symptoms and regional lymphadenopathy are rare. Sinuses may occur several years after the onset of the first symptom. A similar syndrome may be produced by other branching bacteria and also by species of eumycete fungi, such as *Madurella mycetomi* (see p. 561).

Pulmonary disease, which follows inhalation of the organism, presents with cough, fever and haemoptysis; it is usually seen in the immunocompromised. Pleural involvement and empyema occur. In severely immunosuppressed patients, initial pulmonary infection may be followed by disseminated disease.

The diagnosis is often delayed, partly because of inadequate specimens and partly because *Nocardia* requires prolonged culture on standard media. Severe pulmonary or disseminated infection may require parenteral treatment. Co-trimoxazole, linezolid, ceftriaxone and amikacin have all been used successfully, but *in vitro* sensitivities are variable and there is no consensus on the best treatment.

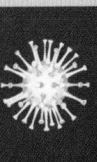

ANTIBIOTIC THERAPIES

Drugs used to combat bacterial infections are described on page 161.

Further reading

Bonell A, Lubell Y, Newton PN et al. Estimating the burden of scrub typhus: a systematic review. *PLoS Negl Trop Dis* 2017; 11:e0005838.
Dworkin MS, Schwan TG, Anderson DE et al. Tick-borne relapsing fever. *Infect Dis Clin North Am* 2008; 22:449–viii.
Gomes C, Pons MJ, del Valle Mendoza J et al. Carrion's disease: an eradicable illness? *Infect Dis Poverty* 2016; 5:105.
Parola P, Paddock CD, Dance D. Treatment and prophylaxis of melioidosis. *Int J Antimicrob Agents* 2014; 43:310–318.
Valour F, Sénéchal A, Dupieux C et al. Actinomycosis: etiology, clinical features, diagnosis, treatment, and management. *Infect Drug Resist* 2014; 7:183–197.
https://wwwnc.cdc.gov/travel/yellowbook/2018/infectious-diseases-related-to-travel/rickettsial-spotted-and-typhus-fevers-and-related-infections-including-anaplasmosis-and-ehrlichiosis. *Rickettsia*.

FUNGAL INFECTIONS

Morphologically, fungi can be grouped into three major categories:
- yeasts and yeast-like fungi, which reproduce by budding
- moulds, which grow by branching and longitudinal extension of hyphae
- dimorphic fungi, which behave as yeasts in the host but as moulds *in vitro*.

Despite the fact that fungi are ubiquitous, systemic fungal infections are relatively rare (in contrast to superficial fungal infections of the skin, nails and orogenital mucosae). Systemic mycoses are usually seen in immunocompromised patients and in critical care settings, and are becoming more prevalent as this population increases.

Fungal infections are transmitted by inhalation of spores, contact with the skin or direct inoculation. This last can occur through penetrating injuries, injecting drug use or iatrogenic procedures. Fungi may also produce allergic pulmonary disease. Some fungi, such as *Candida albicans*, are human commensals. Fungal infections are usually divided into systemic, subcutaneous or superficial (**Box 20.54**). However, these divisions can be misleading, as many fungi that cause superficial infection in the healthy host can cause invasive or disseminated infection in immunocompromised patients, while 'deep' subcutaneous infections can invade other organs to cause systemic disease.

SYSTEMIC FUNGAL INFECTIONS

Candidiasis

Candidiasis is the most common fungal infection in humans and is predominantly caused by *Candida albicans*, although other species of *Candida* are increasingly seen. *Candida* are small asexual yeasts. They are found worldwide, and most species that cause serious invasive disease are also normal oropharyngeal and gastrointestinal commensals.

Clinical features

Most human candidiasis is superficial. Vaginal thrush and oral thrush are the most common forms, typically seen in the very young, the elderly, patients on antibiotic therapy and those who are immunosuppressed. Candidal oesophagitis presents with painful dysphagia. Cutaneous candidiasis typically occurs in intertriginous areas. It is also a cause of paronychia.

Invasive candidiasis is usually associated with intravascular devices (especially in intensive care units) and with profound immunosuppression (e.g. due to treatment of haematological malignancy). Dissemination can lead to meningitis, visceral and pulmonary abscesses, endophthalmitis and osteomyelitis.

Diagnosis and management

The fungi can be demonstrated in scrapings from infected lesions, tissue secretions or, in invasive disease, from blood cultures. Serological tests for beta D glucan, a fungal cell wall component, can be used to look for systemic fungal infection, but are common to many pathogenic fungi and the test does not distinguish different infections.

Treatment varies, depending on the site and severity of infection, and on the sensitivity of the organism. Superficial lesions may respond to topical nystatin or amphotericin B, although systemic agents may be needed for more extensive infection. For invasive infection, parenteral therapy with amphotericin B, fluconazole, voriconazole or echinocandins is necessary. Many non-*albicans* species are intrinsically resistant to many antifungals and even *C. albicans* can develop extensive resistance (especially to azoles).

Candida auris

Since 2010 there has been an increase in human colonization and infection with *C. auris*, a species first identified in Japan in 2009 and which has no known environmental niche. *C. auris* is particularly worrying as it is intrinsically resistant to many antifungals, and sometimes to all three major classes of drug. It is also spread readily from person to person (especially in healthcare settings), and can survive for extended periods on hard surfaces despite normal cleaning and disinfection processes. Laboratory diagnosis is difficult and it can easily be mistaken for other species. Healthcare-associated outbreaks have been reported from a number of countries across all continents.

Histoplasmosis

Histoplasmosis is caused by *Histoplasma capsulatum*. Spores can survive in moist soil for several years, particularly when the soil is

---

i **Box 20.54 Important fungal infections**

Systemic
- Histoplasmosis
- Cryptococcosis
- Coccidioidomycosis
- Blastomycosis
- Zygomycosis (mucormycosis)
- Candidiasis
- Aspergillosis
- *Pneumocystis jirovecii* (formerly *P. carinii*)

Subcutaneous
- Sporotrichosis
- Subcutaneous zygomycosis
- Chromoblastomycosis
- Mycetoma

Superficial
- Dermatophytosis
- Superficial candidiasis
- *Malassezia* infections

enriched by bird and bat droppings. Histoplasmosis occurs world-wide but is most commonly seen in the Ohio and Mississippi river valleys, where over 80% of the population have been subclinically exposed. An increasing number of cases are being reported from parts of Asia (especially China). Transmission is mainly by inhalation of the spores, particularly when clearing out attics, barns and bird roosts, or exploring caves.

Clinical features

Primary pulmonary histoplasmosis is usually asymptomatic. Calcification in the lungs, spleen and liver occurs in patients from areas of high endemicity. When symptomatic, primary pulmonary histoplasmosis generally presents as a mild influenza-like illness, although symptoms can be more severe. Occasionally, there can be complications such as secondary bacterial pneumonia, pleural effusions, erythema nodosum and erythema multiforme.

Chronic pulmonary histoplasmosis is clinically similar to pulmonary tuberculosis (see p. 967). It is usually seen in white American males over the age of 50 years. Disseminated histoplasmosis resembles disseminated tuberculosis, with fever, lymphadenopathy, hepatosplenomegaly, weight loss, leucopenia and thrombocytopenia. Rarely, features of meningitis, hepatitis, hypoadrenalism, endocarditis and peritonitis may dominate the clinical picture.

Diagnosis

Definitive diagnosis is possible by culturing the fungi (e.g. from sputum) or by demonstrating them on histological sections. *H. capsulatum* glycoprotein can be detected in the urine and serum of those with acute pulmonary and disseminated infection. Antibodies usually develop within 3 weeks of the onset of illness and are best detected by complement fixation or immunodiffusion (sensitivity of 95% and 90%, respectively). Although molecular detection tests are available, they are not in widespread use.

Management

Only symptomatic acute pulmonary histoplasmosis, chronic histoplasmosis and acute disseminated histoplasmosis require therapy. Itraconazole is effective in mild to moderate disease. Severe infection is treated with intravenous amphotericin B for 1–2 weeks, followed by itraconazole for a total of 12 weeks, or with voriconazole. Surgical excision of histoplasmomas (granulomatous pulmonary nodules caused by *H. capsulatum*) or chronic cavitatory lung lesions, and release of adhesions following mediastinitis may be required.

African histoplasmosis

This is caused by a specific subspecies: *Histoplasma capsulatum* var. *duboisii*, the spores of which are larger than those of *H. capsulatum*. Skin lesions (e.g. abscesses and nodules), lymph node involvement and lytic bone lesions are prominent. Pulmonary lesions do not occur. Treatment is similar to that for *H. capsulatum* infection.

Aspergillosis

Aspergillosis is caused by one of several species of dimorphic fungi of the genus *Aspergillus*. Of these, *A. fumigatus* is the most common, although *A. flavus* and *A. niger* are also recognized. These fungi are ubiquitous in the environment and are commonly found on decaying leaves and trees. Humans are infected by inhalation of the spores. Disease manifestation depends on the dose of the spores inhaled, as well as the immune response of the host. Three major forms of the disease are recognized: bronchopulmonary allergic aspergillosis, aspergilloma and invasive aspergillosis.

Diagnosis and treatment are described on page 993.

Cryptococcosis

Cryptococcosis is caused by the yeast-like fungus *Cryptococcus neoformans*. It has a worldwide distribution, with bird droppings being an important mode of spread. The spores gain entry into the body through the respiratory tract, where they elicit a granulomatous reaction. Pulmonary symptoms are, however, uncommon. Meningitis, which usually occurs in those with HIV infection or lymphoma, is a common mode of presentation and often develops subacutely. Less commonly, lung cavitation, hilar lymphadenopathy, pleural effusions and pulmonary fibrosis occur. Skin and bone involvement are rare.

Diagnosis and management

Diagnosis is established by demonstrating the organisms in appropriately stained tissue sections. A positive latex cryptococcal agglutinin test performed on the CSF is diagnostic of cryptococcosis.

Liposomal amphotericin B alone or in combination with flucytosine for 2 weeks is followed by oral fluconazole. Therapy should be continued for 8 weeks if meningitis is present. Fluconazole has greater CSF penetration and is used when toxicity is encountered with amphotericin B and flucytosine, and as maintenance therapy in immunocompromised patients, especially those with HIV infection (see p. 1443).

Coccidioidomycosis

Coccidioidomycosis is caused by the non-budding spherical form (spherule) of *Coccidioides immitis*. This is a soil saprophyte and is found in the southern USA, Central America and parts of South America. Humans are infected by inhalation of the thick-walled, barrel-shaped spores called arthrospores. Occasionally, epidemics of coccidioidomycosis have been documented following dust storms.

Clinical features

The majority of patients are asymptomatic and the infection is detected only by the conversion of a skin test using coccidioidin (extract from a culture of mycelial growth of *C. immitis*) from negative to positive. Acute pulmonary coccidioidomycosis presents after an incubation period of about 10 days with fever, malaise and cough. Erythema nodosum, erythema multiforme, phlyctenular conjunctivitis and, less commonly, pleural effusions may occur. Complete recovery is usual.

Pulmonary cavitation with haemoptysis, pulmonary fibrosis, meningitis, lytic bone lesions, hepatosplenomegaly, skin ulcers and abscesses may occur in severe disease.

Diagnosis

The organism can be identified in respiratory secretions and cultured in specialist laboratories. Serological tests are also widely used for diagnosis. These include the highly specific latex agglutination and precipitin tests (IgM), which are positive within 2 weeks of infection and decline thereafter. Other tests include complement fixation, ELISA and radioimmunoassay.

A complement fixation test (IgG) performed on the CSF is diagnostic of coccidioidomycosis meningitis; it becomes positive within 4–6 weeks and remains so for many years.

Management

Mild pulmonary infections are self-limiting and require no treatment, but progressive and disseminated disease mandates urgent therapy. Itraconazole or fluconazole for 6 months is the treatment of choice for primary pulmonary disease, with more prolonged courses for cavitating or fibronodular disease. Fluconazole in high dose (600–1000 mg

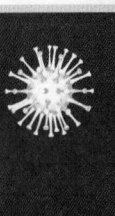

daily) is given for meningitis. Voriconazole or posaconazole is used for poor responders. Surgical excision of cavitatory pulmonary lesions or localized bone lesions may be necessary.

Blastomycosis

Blastomycosis is a systemic infection caused by the biphasic fungus *Blastomyces dermatitidis*. Although previously believed to be confined to certain parts of North America, it has now been reported from South America, India and the Middle East.

Clinical features

Blastomycosis primarily involves the skin, causing non-itchy papular lesions that later develop into ulcers with red verrucous margins. The ulcers are initially confined to the exposed parts of the body but later involve the unexposed parts as well. Atrophy and scarring may occur. Pulmonary involvement presents as a solitary lesion resembling a malignancy or gives rise to radiological features similar to the primary complex of tuberculosis. Systemic symptoms, such as fever, malaise, cough and weight loss, are usually present. Bone lesions are common and present as painful swellings.

Diagnosis and management

The diagnosis is confirmed by demonstrating the organism in histological sections or by culture, although results can be negative in 30–50% of cases. Enzyme immunoassay may be helpful, although there is some cross-reactivity of antibodies to *Blastomyces* with *Histoplasma*.

Itraconazole is preferred for treating mild to moderate disease in the immunocompetent for periods of up to 6 months. In severe or unresponsive disease and in the immunocompromised, amphotericin B is usually used.

Paracoccidioidomycosis

Sometimes known as 'South American blastomycosis', paracoccidioidomycosis is caused by dimorphic fungi of the genus *Paracoccioides*. It is confined to localized areas of Brazil and neighbouring countries. Like the other pathogenic dimorphic fungi it is usually acquired by inhalation. It can cause a wide variety of systemic and local manifestations, although skin lesions are particularly common. Itraconazole is generally the best treatment, although amphotericin B can be used in severe cases.

Mucormycosis

The terminology relating to mucormycosis and zygomycosis is confusing. **Invasive zygomycosis** (also known as **mucormycosis**) is rare and is caused by several fungi, including *Mucor* spp., *Rhizopus* spp. and *Absidia* spp. It usually occurs in immunocompromised or severely ill patients and has a high mortality. The hallmark of the disease is vascular invasion with marked haemorrhagic necrosis.

Rhinocerebral mucormycosis is a specific, locally invasive form of the condition. Nasal stuffiness, facial pain and oedema, and necrotic, black nasal turbinates are characteristic. It is rare and is mainly seen in people with diabetes.

Other forms of invasive zygomycosis include pulmonary and disseminated infection (in immunosuppressed patients) and gastrointestinal infection (in malnutrition).

Subcutaneous zygomycosis is described later.

Management of locally invasive and systemic disease is with amphotericin B and surgical debridement, but even with the best care mortality exceeds 50%. The newer triazoles, posaconazole and isavuconazole, have been shown to be effective in mucormycosis but their role in therapy remains unclear.

Further reading

Kullberg BJ, Arendrup MC. Invasive candidiasis. *N Engl J Med* 2015; 373:1445–1456.

Pappas PG, Kauffman CA, Andes DR et al. Clinical practice guideline for the management of candidiasis: 2016 update by the Infectious Diseases Society of America. *Clin Inf Dis* 2016; 62:e1–e50.

Skiada A, Lass-Floerl C, Klimko N et al. Challenges in the diagnosis and treatment of mucormycosis. *Med Mycol* 2018; 56:S93–S101.

Theel ES, Doern CD. β-D-glucan testing is important for diagnosis of invasive fungal infections. *J Clin Microbiol* 2013; 51:3478–3483.

SUBCUTANEOUS FUNGAL INFECTIONS

Sporotrichosis

Sporotrichosis is caused by the saprophytic fungus *Sporothrix schenckii*, which is found worldwide. It is common in soil and on plants, and infection classically follows cutaneous inoculation from thorns ('rose handler's disease). A reddish, non-tender, maculopapular lesion develops at the site of inoculation; this is referred to as 'plaque sporotrichosis'. Satellite lesions may develop over time. Pulmonary involvement and disseminated disease occur very rarely.

Treatment with itraconazole 100–200 mg/day for 3–6 months is usually curative.

Subcutaneous zygomycosis

Subcutaneous zygomycosis can be a form of mucormycosis in immunocompromised patients, as described earlier. However, the term is also used to describe a largely tropical condition caused by filamentous fungi of the *Basidiobolus* genus, and typically associated with inoculation injuries and trauma. The disease usually remains confined to the subcutaneous tissues and muscle fascia. It presents as a brawny, woody infiltration involving the limbs, neck and trunk. Amphotericin B is the drug of choice, usually in combination with surgical debridement. Even the cutaneous/subcutaneous form of the infection carries a significant mortality.

Chromoblastomycosis

Chromoblastomycosis (chromomycosis) is caused by fungi of various genera, including *Phialophora*, *Wangella* and *Fonsecaea*. These are found mainly in tropical and subtropical countries. Chromoblastomycosis presents initially as a small papule, usually at the site of a previous injury, which persists for several months before ulcerating. The lesion later becomes warty and encrusted, and gradually spreads. Satellite lesions may be present. Itching is common. The drug of choice is amphotericin B in combination with itraconazole or voriconazole. Cryosurgery is used to remove local lesions.

Mycetoma (Madura foot)

Mycetoma may be due to subcutaneous infection with fungi (*Eumycetes* spp.) or bacteria (see p. 558). It is largely confined to the tropics. Infection results in local swelling, which may discharge through sinuses. Bone involvement may follow.

Management consists of surgical debridement, combined with antimicrobials chosen according to the aetiological agent.

Pneumocystis jirovecii infection

Genetic analysis has shown *Pneumocystis jirovecii* to be homologous with fungi. *P. jirovecii* disease is almost invariably associated with immunodeficiency states, particularly AIDS (see p. 1443).

SUPERFICIAL FUNGAL INFECTIONS

Dermatophytosis

Dermatophytoses are chronic fungal infections of keratinous structures, such as the skin, hair or nails. The main causative organisms are species of the genera *Trichophyton*, *Microsporum* and *Epidermophyton*.

Malassezia infection

Malassezia spp. are found on the scalp and greasy skin, and are responsible for seborrhoeic dermatitis, pityriasis versicolor (hypo- or hyperpigmented rash on the trunk) and *Malassezia* folliculitis (itchy rash on the back) (see p. 674).

Treatment of any superficial fungal infection is with topical antifungals, or oral triazole drugs if infection is refractory or more extensive.

ANTIFUNGAL DRUGS

Fungal infections range from trivial superficial skin and nail infections to life-threatening systemic conditions. The antifungal armoury is relatively limited, and because fungal cells share more enzymes and other pathways with human cells than do bacteria, targeting the pathogen without harming host metabolism is more difficult. There are three main groups of parenteral drugs for treating severe fungal infections: amphotericin, triazoles and echinocandins (**Box 20.55**). Although each has specific licence indications, antifungal drugs often have to be given empirically in severely ill patients. The best choice from among the available agents depends on a number of factors, including local resistance patterns and availability, potential for toxicity, and cost, and many countries have specific national guidelines.

Polyenes

Polyenes react with the sterols in fungal membranes, increasing permeability and thus damaging the organism. The most potent is **amphotericin**, which is used intravenously in severe systemic fungal infections. Nephrotoxicity is a major problem and dosage levels must take background renal function into account. Liposomal formulations of amphotericin are less toxic and are used in preference where cost is not prohibitive. **Nystatin** is not absorbed through mucous membranes and is therefore useful for the treatment of oral and enteric candidiasis and for vaginal infection. It can only be given orally or as pessaries.

Azoles

Imidazoles

Imidazoles are broad-spectrum antifungal drugs. They act by inhibiting fungal sterol synthesis, resulting in damage to the cell wall.

Ketoconazole is active orally but can produce liver damage, and is now rarely used systemically. It continues to be used topically, along with **clotrimazole** and **miconazole**, for the treatment of ringworm, and cutaneous and genital candidiasis. **Econazole** is used for the topical treatment of cutaneous and vaginal candidiasis and dermatophyte infections, while **tioconazole** is indicated for fungal nail infections.

Triazoles

These drugs also act by interfering with fungal sterol synthesis. **Itraconazole** was the first triazole to be used widely in clinical practice, but its relatively poor absorption and failure to penetrate CSF mean that it has largely been superseded (except for a few specific conditions such as histoplasmosis and blastomycosis). **Fluconazole** is well absorbed and has excellent CNS penetration; it is used for mucosal and invasive candidiasis and for the treatment of CNS infection with *Cryptococcus neoformans*. Some non-*albicans Candida* species are intrinsically resistant to fluconazole, and resistance can develop in *C. albicans*. **Voriconazole** has broad-spectrum activity that includes most *Candida*, *Cryptococcus* and *Aspergillus* species and other filamentous fungi. It is available for oral and intravenous use. Adverse effects include visual disturbance, abnormalities of liver enzymes and a variety of dermatological problems (including a possible link with squamous cell carcinoma). It also has significant drug–drug interactions with drugs metabolized by the CYP450 enzymes and, like all the triazoles, can cause QTc prolongation. It is indicated for invasive aspergillosis and severe *Candida* infections unresponsive to amphotericin and fluconazole, respectively, and also for empirical treatment of suspected or confirmed severe fungal infection. **Posaconazole** has a similar range of activity and is also associated with hepatotoxicity and CYP450 interactions. **Isavuconazole** is the newest triazole: it is licensed for use in invasive mould disease and mucormycosis but (largely due to cost) is generally a second- or third-line agent.

Echinocandins

These act by inhibiting the cell-wall polysaccharide glucan. **Caspofungin**, which is administered intravenously, is active against *Candida* spp. and *Aspergillus* spp., and is indicated for invasive candidiasis and invasive aspergillosis unresponsive to other drugs, as well as for empirical therapy in seriously ill patients. Other echinocandins include **micafungin** and **anidulafungin**, approved for the treatment of disseminated candidiasis. Severe hepatotoxicity has been reported with micafungin and liver biochemistry must be monitored.

Flucytosine

The fluorinated pyridine derivative flucytosine is used in combination with amphotericin B for cryptococcal meningitis. Side-effects

---

 Box 20.55 Antifungal agents

Polyenes
- Amphotericin, nystatin

Echinocandins
- Caspofungin
- Anidulafungin
- Micafungin

Azoles
- Miconazole, ketoconazole, fluconazole, itraconazole, voriconazole, posaconazole, isavuconazole

- Topical clotrimazole, sulconazole, tolnaftate, econazole, tioconazole

Allylamines
- Terbinafine

Other antifungals
- Amorolfine (topical only)
- 5-Flucytosine
- Griseofulvin

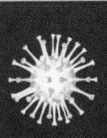

are uncommon, although it may cause bone marrow suppression. It is active when given orally or parenterally, but there is very limited availability in resource-poor settings.

Allylamines

Terbinafine has broad-spectrum antifungal and also anti-inflammatory activity. It is well absorbed orally and accumulates in keratin. It is useful for the treatment of superficial mycoses, such as dermatophyte infections, onychomycosis and cutaneous candidiasis. A topical formulation is also available to treat fungal skin infections.

PROTOZOAL INFECTIONS

Protozoa are unicellular eukaryotic organisms. They are more complex than bacteria and belong to the animal kingdom. Although many protozoa are free-living in the environment, some have become parasites of vertebrates, including humans, often developing complex life cycles involving more than one host species. In order to be transmitted to a new host, some protozoa transform into hardy cyst forms, which can survive harsh external conditions. Others are transmitted by an arthropod vector, in which a further replication cycle takes place before infection of a new vertebrate host.

BLOOD AND TISSUE PROTOZOA

Malaria

Human malaria is usually caused by one of four species of the genus *Plasmodium*: *P. falciparum*, *P. vivax*, *P. ovale* or *P. malariae*. Occasionally, other species of malaria more commonly found in primates (e.g. *P. knowlesi*) can affect humans. Human malaria probably originated from animal malarias in Central Africa but was spread around the globe by human migration. Public health measures and changes in land use have eradicated malaria in most developed countries, although the potential for malaria transmission still exists in many areas. Some 220 million people were infected in 2017, with 415 000 deaths (mainly in African children). Over 25 000 infections per year occur in travellers from non-malarious countries.

Epidemiology

Malaria is transmitted by the bite of female anopheline mosquitoes. The parasite undergoes a temperature-dependent cycle of development in the gut of the insect, and its geographical range therefore depends on the presence of the appropriate mosquito species and an adequate temperature. The disease occurs in endemic or epidemic form throughout the tropics and subtropics, except for some areas above 2000 m (**Fig. 20.28**).

In areas of so-called **stable transmission** (including much of sub-Saharan Africa), transmission occurs consistently year round. The bulk of the mortality is seen in children, while those who survive

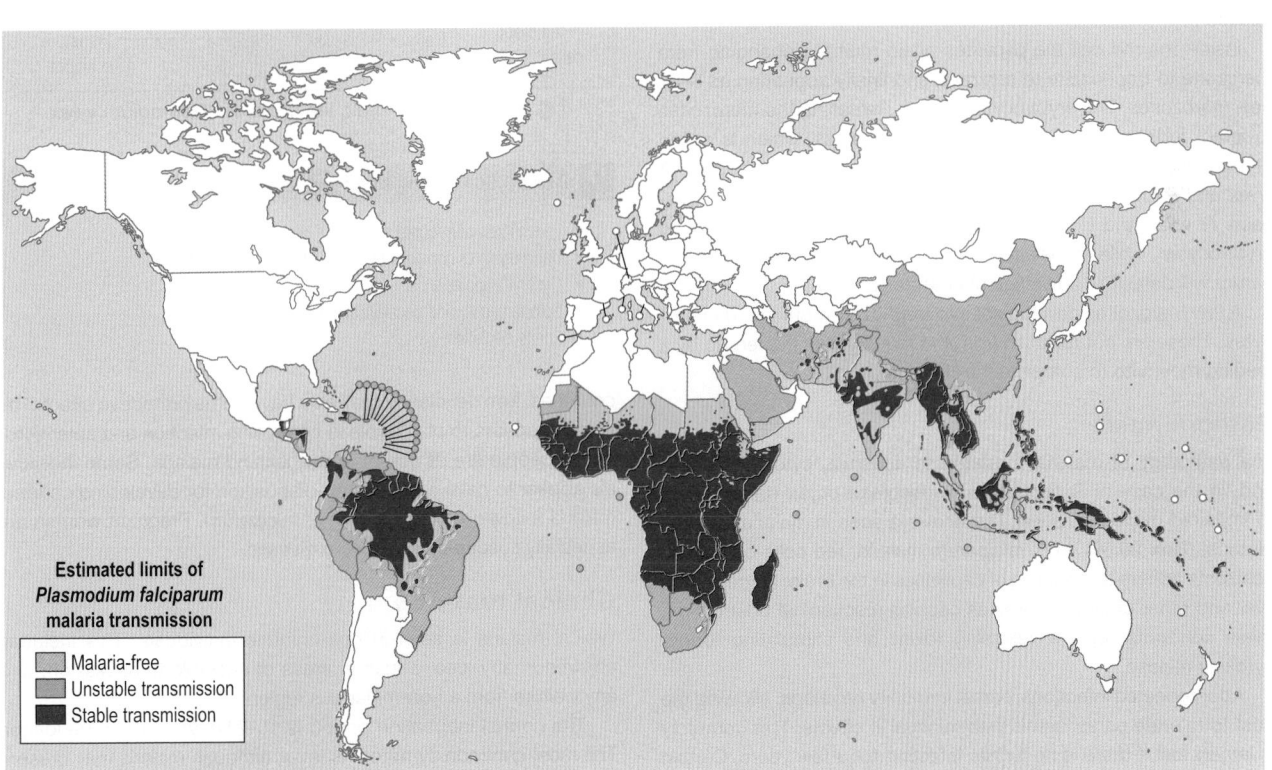

Estimated limits of *Plasmodium falciparum* malaria transmission

☐ Malaria-free
☐ Unstable transmission
■ Stable transmission

Fig. 20.28 *Plasmodium falciparum* malaria transmission: geographical distribution. *Grey areas* are likely to be risk-free, either because health surveillance reports 0 cases for 3 years, because low temperatures or high aridity are likely to preclude transmission, or because specific medical intelligence exists defining the area as risk-free. *Pink areas* are where local transmission cannot be ruled out but levels of risk are extremely low, with annual case incidence reported at less than 1 per 10 000. *Red areas* are at risk of stable malaria transmission. This is a very broad classification of risk, including any regions where the annual case incidence is likely to exceed 1 per 10 000. (*From Malaria Atlas Project, with permission; http://www.map.ox.ac.uk/browse-resources/transmission-limits/Pf_limits/world/.*)

to adulthood acquire significant immunity; low-grade parasitaemia is still present but causes few symptoms. **Unstable transmission** occurs when there is erratic, seasonal or low-level transmission (e.g. in the Sahel belt, where mosquitoes feed only in the rainy season). In these circumstances, little protective immunity develops and symptomatic malaria occurs at all ages. Changes in environmental or social conditions in such areas can lead to epidemics with substantial mortality in all age groups.

Malaria can also be transmitted in contaminated blood transfusions. It has occasionally been seen in injecting drug users who share needles, and in patients with a hospital-acquired infection related to contaminated equipment. Rare cases are acquired outside the tropics when mosquitoes are transported from endemic areas ('airport malaria'), or when the local mosquito population becomes infected by a returning traveller.

Parasitology

The female mosquito becomes infected after taking a blood meal containing gametocytes, the sexual form of the malarial parasite (**Fig. 20.29**). The developmental cycle in the mosquito usually takes 7–20 days (depending on temperature), culminating in the migration of infective sporozoites to the insect's salivary glands. The sporozoites are inoculated into a new human host and those not destroyed by the immune response are rapidly taken up by the liver. Here they multiply inside hepatocytes as merozoites: this is pre-erythrocytic (or hepatic) sporogeny. After a few days the infected hepatocytes rupture, releasing merozoites into the blood, from where they are rapidly taken up by erythrocytes. In the case of *P. vivax* and *P. ovale*, a few parasites remain dormant in the liver as hypnozoites. These may reactivate at any time subsequently, causing relapsing infection.

Inside the red cell the parasites again multiply, changing from merozoite to trophozoite to schizont, and finally appearing as 8–24 new merozoites. The erythrocyte ruptures, releasing the merozoites to infect further cells. Each cycle of this process, which is called erythrocytic schizogony, takes about 48 hours in *P. falciparum*, *P. vivax* and *P. ovale* disease, and about 72 hours in *P. malariae* disease. *P. vivax* and *P. ovale* mainly attack reticulocytes and young erythrocytes, while *P. malariae* tends to attack older cells; *P. falciparum* will parasitize any stage of erythrocyte.

A few merozoites develop not into trophozoites but into gametocytes. These are not released from the red cells until taken up by a feeding mosquito to complete the life cycle.

Pathogenesis

The pathology of malaria is related to anaemia, cytokine release and, in the case of *P. falciparum*, widespread organ damage due to impaired microcirculation. The anaemia seen in malaria is multifactorial (**Box 20.56**). In *P. falciparum* malaria, red cells containing schizonts adhere to the lining of capillaries in the brain, kidneys, gut, liver and other organs. As well as causing mechanical obstruction, these schizonts rupture, releasing toxins and stimulating further cytokine release.

After repeated infections, partial immunity develops, allowing the host to tolerate parasitaemia with minimal ill effects. This immunity is largely lost if there is no further infection for a few years. Certain genetic traits also confer some immunity to malaria. People who lack the Duffy antigen on the red cell membrane (a common finding in West Africa) are not susceptible to infection with *P. vivax*. Certain haemoglobinopathies (including sickle cell trait) also give some protection against the severe effects of malaria; this may account for the persistence of these otherwise harmful mutations in tropical

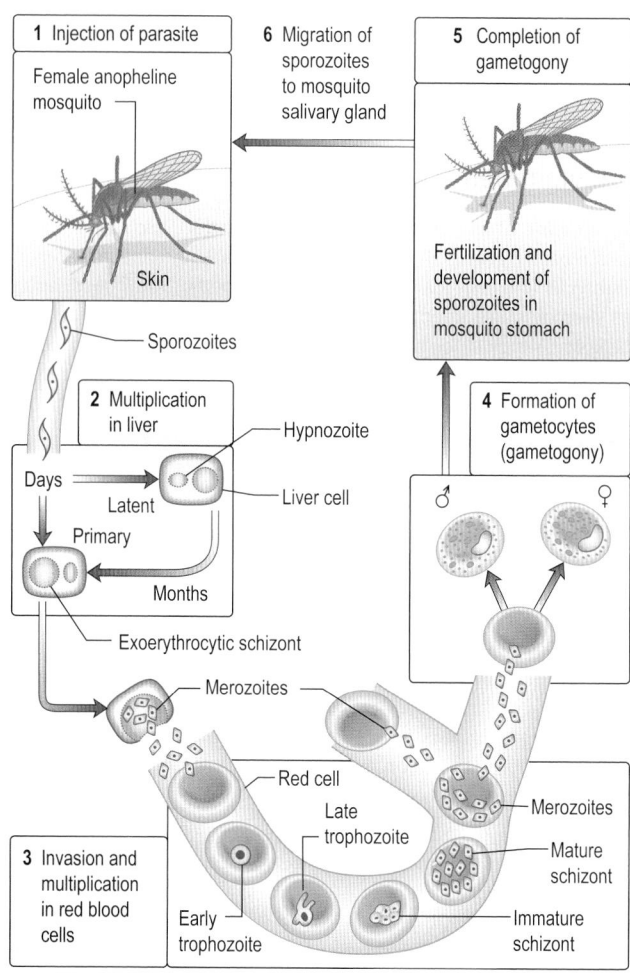

Fig. 20.29 A schematic life cycle of *Plasmodium vivax*.

1 Injection of parasite
Female anopheline mosquito
Skin
Sporozoites

2 Multiplication in liver
Hypnozoite
Days
Latent
Primary
Months
Liver cell
Exoerythrocytic schizont

3 Invasion and multiplication in red blood cells
Merozoites
Early trophozoite
Red cell
Late trophozoite
Merozoites
Mature schizont
Immature schizont

4 Formation of gametocytes (gametogony)
♂   ♀

5 Completion of gametogony
Fertilization and development of sporozoites in mosquito stomach

6 Migration of sporozoites to mosquito salivary gland

❓ Box 20.56 Causes of anaemia in malaria infection

- Haemolysis of infected red cells
- Haemolysis of non-infected red cells (blackwater fever)
- Dyserythropoiesis
- Splenomegaly and sequestration
- Folate depletion

---

countries. Iron deficiency may also have some protective effect. The spleen appears to play a role in controlling infection and splenectomized people are at risk of overwhelming malaria. Some individuals appear to have a genetic predisposition for developing cerebral malaria following infection with *P. falciparum*. Pregnant women are especially susceptible to severe disease.

Clinical features

Typical malaria is seen in non-immune individuals. This includes children in any area, adults in areas of unstable transmission, and any visitors from a non-malarious region.

The normal incubation period is 10–21 days but can be longer. The most common symptom is fever, although malaria may present initially with general malaise, headache, vomiting or diarrhoea. At first the fever may be continual or erratic; the classical tertian or quartan fever appears only after some days. The temperature often reaches 41°C and is accompanied by rigors and drenching sweats.

The illness caused by *P. vivax* or *P. ovale* infection is usually relatively mild (although *P. vivax* can occasionally cause severe

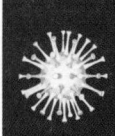

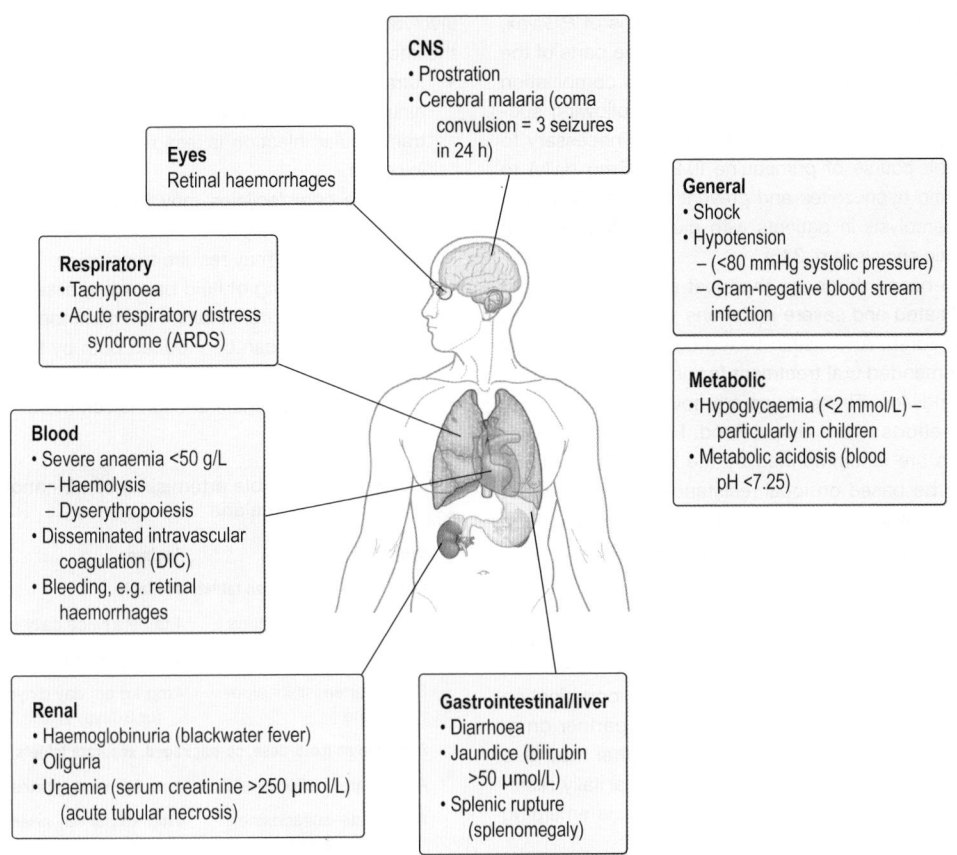

Fig. 20.30 Features of severe *falciparum* malaria.

disease). Anaemia develops slowly and there may be tender hepatosplenomegaly. Spontaneous recovery usually occurs within 2–6 weeks but hypnozoites in the liver can cause relapses for many years after infection. Repeated infections often cause chronic ill health due to anaemia and hyper-reactive splenomegaly.

P. malariae infection also causes a relatively mild illness but tends to run a more chronic course. Parasitaemia may persist for years, with or without symptoms. In children, *P. malariae* infection is associated with glomerulonephritis and nephrotic syndrome.

P. knowlesi is primarily a parasite of macaque monkeys but causes human malaria in certain areas of South-east Asia. The clinical picture is very variable, ranging from a chronic relatively mild illness similar to *P. malariae*, through to fulminant and fatal disease.

P. falciparum infection causes, in many cases, a self-limiting illness similar to the other types of malaria, although the paroxysms of fever are usually less marked. However, it may also cause serious complications (**Fig. 20.30**) and the vast majority of malaria deaths are due to *P. falciparum*. Patients can deteriorate rapidly, and children in particular progress from reasonable health to coma and death within hours. A high parasitaemia (>1% of red cells infected) is an indicator of severe disease, although patients with apparently low parasite levels may also develop complications (peripheral parasite counts can be misleading, as many parasitized cells are sequestered in the microcirculation). Cerebral malaria is marked by diminished consciousness, confusion and convulsions, often progressing to coma and death. Untreated, it is universally fatal. Blackwater fever is due to widespread intravascular haemolysis, affecting both parasitized and unparasitized red cells, giving rise to dark urine.

Hyper-reactive malarial splenomegaly (tropical splenomegaly syndrome) is seen in older children and adults in areas where malaria is hyperendemic. It is associated with an exaggerated immune response to repeated malaria infections and is characterized by anaemia, massive splenomegaly and elevated IgM levels. Malaria parasites are scanty or absent. Tropical splenomegaly syndrome usually responds to prolonged treatment with prophylactic antimalarial drugs.

Diagnosis

Malaria should be in the differential diagnosis of anyone who presents with a febrile illness in, or having recently left, a malarious area. *Falciparum* malaria is unlikely to present more than 3 months after exposure, even if the patient has been taking prophylaxis, but *vivax* malaria may cause symptoms for the first time up to a year after leaving a malarious area.

Diagnosis is usually made by identifying parasites on a Giemsa-stained thick or thin blood film (thick films are more difficult to interpret and it may be difficult to speciate the parasite, but they have a higher yield). At least three films should be examined before malaria is declared unlikely. Rapid antigen detection tests are available for near-patient use. In many endemic areas, malaria is over-diagnosed on clinical grounds and a definite diagnosis should be made wherever possible. Serological tests are of no diagnostic value.

Parasitaemia is common in endemic areas and the presence of parasites does not necessarily mean that malaria is the cause of the patient's symptoms. Further investigation, including a lumbar puncture, may be needed to exclude bacterial infection.

Management
Uncomplicated malaria

Chloroquine is still widely used to treat non-*falciparum* malaria (**Box 20.57**) and in many areas it remains effective. However, there is increasing resistance to chloroquine in some strains of *P. vivax*, and co-infection with *P. falciparum* is common in some parts of the world. It is therefore sensible to use oral artemisinin combination therapy, where available, for all cases of malaria. Following successful treatment of *P. vivax* or *P. ovale* malaria, it is necessary to give a 2- to 3-week course of primaquine (0.25–0.5 mg daily) to eradicate the hepatic hypnozoites and prevent relapse. This drug can precipitate haemolysis in patients with glucose-6-phosphate dehydrogenase deficiency (see p. 346).

The artemisinin-based drugs are the most effective treatment for both uncomplicated and severe infections with *P. falciparum*, in adults and in children. Artemisinin-based combination therapy (ACT) is the recommended oral treatment for uncomplicated *falciparum* malaria worldwide. These drugs are now widely available, partly through the efforts of the Global Fund. Five different fixed-dose combinations are recommended by the WHO (**Box 20.58**); the choice should be based on local resistance to the 'partner'. A sixth combination, artesunate–pyronaridine, has recently been approved by the European Medicines Agency, and may be useful in areas where there is resistance to current partner drugs. In order to limit the development of resistance, artemisinin derivatives should never be given as monotherapy. Partial resistance to artemether has already been reported in parts of South-east Asia, and also in South and Central America. As long as combination therapy is used and the parasite is sensitive to the partner drug, ACT will still be effective. Longer courses of artemether may also overcome the partial resistance. However malaria partially resistant to artemether, and resistant to all partner drugs, is emerging along the Mekong river.

In addition to treating the acute infection, the WHO recommends that a single dose of primaquine should be given as a gametocide, to decrease onward transmission.

Severe falciparum malaria

Severe malaria, indicated by the presence of any of the complications discussed earlier or a parasite count of more than 1% in a non-immune patient, is a medical emergency (**Box 20.59**). Anyone involved in managing patients with malaria should be familiar with the latest WHO guidelines.

- Intravenous artesunate is more effective than intravenous quinine and should be used where available. Absorption from intramuscular injection is less reliable than that from intravenous injection.
- Intensive care facilities may be needed, including mechanical ventilation and dialysis.
- Severe anaemia may require transfusion.
- Careful monitoring of fluid balance is essential; both pulmonary oedema and pre-renal failure are common.
- Hypoglycaemia can be induced both by the infection itself and by quinine treatment.
- Superadded bacterial infection is common.

i **Box 20.58 Suitable artemisinin combination therapies (ACT) for malaria**

Drugs	Regimen
Fixed-dose combination tablets available	
Artemether–lumefantrine	4 tablets twice daily for 3 days[a]
Artesunate–amodiaquine	4 mg/kg per day artesunate for 3 days
Dihydroartemisinin–piperaquine	4 mg/kg per day dihydroartemisinin for 3 days
Available as fixed-dose, co-packaged, separate tablets	
Artesunate–mefloquine[b]	4 mg/kg per day artesunate for 3 days
Artesunate–sulfadoxine–pyrimethamine[c]	4 mg/kg per day artesunate for 3 days
Alternatives where no combination packages are available	
Artesunate + clindamycin	2 mg/kg per day + 10 mg/kg twice daily for 7 days
Artesunate + doxycycline	2 mg/kg per day + 3.5 mg/kg per day for 7 days

[a]Adult dose: reduce dose by body weight for children. [b]Combination tablet manufactured but not widely available. [c]Not suitable for *P. vivax* or mixed infections. Different fixed-dose combinations available.

i **Box 20.57 Drug treatment of uncomplicated malaria**

Parasite	Drugs	Regimen	Plus	Regimen
Plasmodium vivax *P. ovale* *P. malariae*	Chloroquine	600 mg[a] 300 mg[b] 6 h later 300 mg 24 h later 300 mg 24 h later	Primaquine	0.25–0.5 mg/kg per day for 2–3 weeks
	or (if known resistance to chloroquine, or dual infection with P. falciparum)			
	ACT (not artesunate + SP)	3 days	Primaquine	0.25–0.5 mg/kg per day for 2–3 weeks
P. falciparum (adults, endemic zone)	ACT	3 days	Primaquine	0.75 mg/kg single dose
	or (if not available)			
	Quinine + doxycycline	7 days	Primaquine	0.75 mg/kg single dose
P. falciparum (pregnant women)	First trimester: quinine + doxycycline[c]	7 days		
	Second/third trimesters: ACT	3 days		
P. falciparum (infants)	ACT	3 days; appropriate dose for body weight	Primaquine	0.75 mg/kg single dose
P. falciparum (returning travellers)	Atovaquone–proguanil *or* quinine + doxycycline	7 days		

[a]10 mg/kg in children. [b]5 mg/kg in children. [c]Use ACT only if quinine is not available. ACT, artemisinin-based combination therapy; SP, sulfadoxine–pyrimethamine.

Box 20.59 Drug treatment of severe *falciparum* malaria in adults and children

Drug/route	Immediate dose	Subsequent doses
Severe malaria is an emergency: after rapid assessment and confirmation of diagnosis, if possible, treatment should be started with whatever parenteral treatment is available. The options, in order of preference, are:		
1. Intravenous artesunate	2.4 mg/kg	2.4 mg/kg at 12 and 24 h, then daily (up to 7 days)
2. Intravenous quinine	20 mg/kg[a]	10 mg/kg 8-hourly (up to 7 days)
3. Intramuscular artesunate	2.4 mg/kg	2.4 mg/kg at 12 and 24 h, then daily (up to 7 days)
4. Intramuscular artemether	3.2 mg/kg	1.6 mg/kg daily
5. Rectal artesunate	10 mg/kg	Transfer to centre where parenteral therapy available
Continue parenteral treatment for at least 24 h, regardless of improvement in condition. After this, if the patient is improving, switch to oral therapy to complete 7 days with:		
ACT		
Or	Plus	Primaquine 0.75 mg/kg single dose
Quinine + doxy-cycline		

[a]10 mg/kg if patient has already received oral quinine or mefloquine.
ACT, artemisinin-based combination therapy.

Box 20.60 Strategy for controlling malaria

1. Aggressive control in highly endemic countries, to reduce mortality and decrease transmission
2. Progressive eradication at the endemic margins, to shrink the 'malaria map'
3. Research into new vaccines, new drugs, new diagnostics and better ways of delivering malaria care

Prevention and control

Malaria is a priority for the WHO, which announced its 'Roll Back Malaria' campaign in 1998. This has had considerable success, and global malaria-specific mortality decreased by 25% between 2000 and 2010. However, the latest WHO Global Malaria Report (2018) shows that, following an unprecedented period of success in reducing malaria incidence and mortality, progress has stalled, with no significant improvement between 2015 and 2017. Although some countries either have eradicated malaria or plan to do so soon, for much of Africa the aim remains control rather than eradication. A three-part strategy is now widely endorsed and supported by governments and non-governmental organizations (**Box 20.60**).

As with many vector-borne diseases, control of malaria relies on a combination of case treatment, vector eradication and personal protection from vector bites, such as that provided by insecticide (permethrin)-treated nets. Mosquito eradication is usually achieved by a combination of insecticide use (e.g. house spraying with DDT) and manipulation of the habitat (e.g. marsh drainage). Alongside these elements, there has been renewed interest in chemoprevention, in which children in endemic areas are given monthly doses of antimalarials during the rainy season. This has been shown to reduce the incidence of malaria but may lead to an increased risk of drug resistance. Pregnant women, who are at greater risk of complications from

Box 20.61 Malaria prophylaxis for adult travellers

Area visited	Prophylactic regimen	Alternative
No chloroquine resistance	Chloroquine 300 mg weekly	Proguanil 200 mg daily
Limited chloroquine resistance	Chloroquine 300 mg weekly	Doxycycline 100 mg daily
	Plus	*Or*
	Proguanil 200 mg daily	Malarone 1 tablet daily
		or
		Mefloquine 250 mg weekly
Significant chloroquine resistance	Mefloquine 250 mg weekly	Doxycycline 100 mg daily
		or
		Malarone 1 tablet daily

malaria, may also be offered chemoprevention (although drug options are limited). Enormous effort (and resource) has been devoted to the search for a malaria vaccine, and some progress has been made. The first vaccine to go through large-scale phase 3 clinical trials, RTS,S/AS01, prevented approximately 39% of predicted cases of malaria, with an associated reduction in mortality and need for transfusion. Pilot implementation programmes are now being developed, although there are currently no plans for widespread use of the vaccine.

Non-immune travellers to malarious areas should take measures to avoid insect bites, such as using a repellent (diethyltoluamide (DEET) 20–50% in lotions and sprays) and sleeping under a mosquito net. Antimalarial prophylaxis should also be taken in most cases, although this is never 100% effective (**Box 20.61**). The precise choice of prophylactic regimen depends both on the individual traveller and on the specific itinerary; further details can be found in national formularies or travel advice centres.

Trypanosomiasis

African trypanosomiasis (sleeping sickness)

Sleeping sickness is caused by trypanosomes transmitted to humans by the bite of the tsetse fly (genus *Glossina*) (although mother to child transmission has also occasionally been reported). It is endemic in a belt across sub-Saharan Africa, extending to about 14 degrees north and 20 degrees south: this marks the natural range of the tsetse fly. Two subspecies of trypanosome cause human sleeping sickness: *Trypanosoma brucei gambiense* ('Gambian sleeping sickness') and *T. b. rhodesiense* ('Rhodesian sleeping sickness').

Epidemiology

Sleeping sickness due to *T. b. gambiense* accounts for 97% of reported new cases. It is currently found in 24 countries in an area stretching from Uganda in Central Africa, west to Cameroon and south as far as Angola, but Democratic Republic of Congo (DRC) and Central African Republic are the only countries still reporting significant numbers. Humans are the major reservoir and infection is transmitted by riverine *Glossina* species (e.g. *G. palpalis*).

Sleeping sickness due to *T. b. rhodesiense* occurs in 13 countries in East and Central Africa but cases are rare and sporadic. It is a zoonosis of both wild and domestic animals. In endemic situations, it is maintained in game animals and transmitted by savannah flies such as *G. morsitans*. Previous epidemics have been related to cattle and the vectors were riverine flies.

Political upheavals during the 1990s disrupted established treatment and control programmes, resulting in major epidemics in Angola, DRC and Uganda. By 1997, as many as 500 000 people were affected by sleeping sickness. A concerted control programme has gradually brought this number under control: by 2009 there were fewer than 10 000 cases reported, and in 2017 fewer than 1500. The WHO believes that it is on course to eliminate African trypanosomiasis as a public health problem by 2020.

Parasitology

Tsetse flies bite during the day and, unlike most arthropod vectors, both males and females take blood meals. An infected insect may deposit metacyclic trypomastigotes (the infective form of the parasite) into the subcutaneous tissue. These cause local inflammation ('trypanosomal chancre') and regional lymphadenopathy. Within 2–3 weeks the organisms invade the bloodstream, subsequently spreading to all parts of the body, including the brain.

Clinical features

T. b. gambiense causes a chronic, slowly progressive illness. Episodes of fever and lymphadenopathy occur over months or years and hepatosplenomegaly may develop. Eventually, infection reaches the CNS, causing headache, behavioural changes, confusion and daytime somnolence. As the disease progresses, patients may develop tremors, ataxia, convulsions and hemiplegias; eventually, coma and death supervene. Histologically, there is a lymphocytic meningoencephalitis, with scattered trypanosomes visible in the brain substance.

T. b. rhodesiense sleeping sickness is a much more acute disease. Early systemic features may include myocarditis, hepatitis and serous effusions, and patients can die before the onset of CNS disease. If they survive, cerebral involvement occurs within weeks of infection and is rapidly progressive.

Diagnosis

Diagnosis involves three stages:
- screening using serological tests (only available for *T. b. gambiense*) and clinical signs
- confirmation of the presence of parasites in body fluids
- assessment of stage of disease.

The card agglutination test for trypanosomiasis (CATT) is a robust and easy-to-use field assay for screening. If this is positive (or there are clinical signs of disease), Giemsa-stained smears of thick or thin blood films, or of lymph node aspirate, should be examined for parasites. Blood films are usually positive in *T. b. rhodesiense* infection but may be negative in *T. b. gambiense* disease; concentration techniques may increase the yield. The main investigation for staging disease is lumbar puncture: examination of CSF is essential in patients with evidence of trypanosomal infection. CNS involvement causes lymphocytosis and elevated protein in the CSF, and parasites may be seen in concentrated specimens. A single dose of suramin should be given to patients with parasitaemia prior to lumbar puncture, to avoid inoculation into the CSF.

Management

The treatment of sleeping sickness remained largely unchanged for more than 40 years but better drugs are now available for *T. b. gambiense* infection and further new agents are undergoing clinical trials. In both forms of disease, treatment is usually effective if

given in the first stage (i.e. before the onset of CNS involvement) (**Box 20.62**). The treatment of choice for second-stage (CNS) disease in *T. b. gambiense* is a combination of eflornithine and nifurtimox, a therapy introduced in 2009 and provided free of charge via the WHO. Melarsoprol remains the only treatment for CNS infection with *T. b. rhodesiense*. It is extremely toxic: 2–10% of patients develop an acute encephalopathy, with a 50–75% mortality; peripheral neuropathy and hepatorenal toxicity are also common. Between 3% and 6% of patients relapse following melarsoprol treatment.

Control

Control programmes coordinated by the WHO have been effective in many areas. As in many vector-borne diseases, prevention depends largely on elimination, control or avoidance of the vector.

South American trypanosomiasis (Chagas' disease)

Chagas' disease is widely distributed in rural areas of South and Central America, where up to 7 million people are infected. Since 2009, more cases have been detected in other parts of the world, due to increased migration from Latin America. The disease is caused by *Trypanosoma cruzi*, which is transmitted to humans in the faeces of blood-sucking reduviid bugs (also called cone-nose or assassin bugs). Faeces infected with *T. cruzi* trypomastigotes are rubbed in through skin abrasions, mucosa or conjunctiva. The bugs, which live in mud or thatch buildings, feed on a variety of vertebrate hosts (e.g. rats, opossums) at night, defecating as they do so.

The parasites spread in the bloodstream before entering host cells and multiplying. Cell rupture releases them back into the circulation, where they can be taken up by a feeding bug. Further multiplication takes place in the insect gut, completing the trypanosome life cycle. Human infection can also occur via contaminated blood transfusion or, occasionally, by transplacental spread.

Clinical features

Acute infection usually occurs in children and often passes unnoticed. A firm, reddish papule is sometimes seen at the site of entry, associated with regional lymphadenopathy. In the case of conjunctival infection, there is swelling of the eyelid, which may close the eye (Romaña's sign). There may be fever, lymphadenopathy, hepatosplenomegaly and, rarely, meningoencephalitis. Acute Chagas' disease is occasionally fatal in infants but normally there is full recovery within a few weeks or months.

Some 10–30% of people go on to develop chronic Chagas' disease after a latent period of many years. The pathogenesis remains controversial, although the most likely explanation is an autoimmune response to persistent parasite DNA integrated into

---

Box 20.62 Drugs used in the treatment of African trypanosomiasis

Disease stage	*Trypanosoma brucei gambiense*	*Trypanosoma brucei rhodesiense*
1	Pentamidine	Suramin[a]
2 (central nervous system)	Eflornithine + nifurtimox Eflornithine Monotherapy (melarsoprol)	Melarsoprol

[a]Severe allergic reactions common: give test dose.

the host genome. The heart is commonly affected, with conduction abnormalities, arrhythmias, aneurysm formation and cardiac dilation. Gastrointestinal involvement leads to progressive dilation of parts of the gastrointestinal tract; this commonly results in mega-oesophagus (causing dysphagia and aspiration pneumonia) and megacolon (causing severe constipation).

Diagnosis

Trypanosomes may be seen on a stained blood film during the acute illness. PCR is also sensitive in the acute phase. In chronic disease, serological tests are the most useful method, although they need to be interpreted in the clinical context.

Management and control

Nifurtimox and benznidazole are the main drugs used. Both are highly effective in acute infection, with a cure rate of over 90%, but much less so in chronic disease. They are relatively toxic, with adverse reactions in up to 40% of patients, and new drugs are urgently needed. Anti-arrhythmic drugs and pacemakers may be needed in cardiac disease and surgical treatment is sometimes required for gastrointestinal complications.

In the long term, prevention of Chagas' disease relies on improved housing and living conditions, and eradication of vectors. Several coordinated multinational vector control programmes have been implemented, with some success in reducing transmission. Screening of blood donors and pregnant women in high-risk areas can reduce transmission through non-vector routes.

Leishmaniasis

This group of diseases is caused by protozoa of the genus *Leishmania*, which are transmitted by the bite of the female phlebotomine sandfly (**Box 20.63**). Leishmaniasis is seen in localized areas of Africa, Asia (particularly India and Bangladesh), Europe, the Middle East and South and Central America. It is strongly linked to poverty and poor hygiene. Certain parasite species are specific to each geographical area. The clinical picture is dependent on the species of parasite and on the host's cell-mediated immune response. Asymptomatic infection, in which the parasite is suppressed or eradicated by a strong immune response, is common in endemic areas, as demonstrated by a high incidence of positive leishmanin skin tests. Symptomatic infection may be confined to the skin (sometimes with spread to the mucous membranes) or widely disseminated throughout the body (visceral leishmaniasis). Relapse of previously asymptomatic infection is seen in patients who become immunocompromised, especially those with HIV infection.

In some areas, leishmania is primarily zoonotic, whereas in others humans are the main reservoir of infection. In the vertebrate host the parasites are found as oval amastigotes (Leishman–Donovan bodies). These multiply inside the macrophages and cells of the reticuloendothelial system and are then released into the circulation as the cells rupture. Parasites are taken into the gut of a feeding sandfly (genus *Phlebotomus* in the Old World, genus *Lutzomyia* in the New World), where they develop into the flagellate promastigote form. These migrate to the salivary glands of the insect, where they can be inoculated into a new host.

Visceral leishmaniasis

Clinical features

Visceral leishmaniasis (kala azar) is caused by *L. donovani*, *L. infantum* or *L. chagasi*, and is prevalent in localized areas of Asia, Africa, the Mediterranean littoral and South America. In parts of India, where humans are the main host, the disease occurs in epidemics. In most other areas, it is endemic, and it is mainly children and visitors to the area who are at risk. The main animal reservoirs in Europe and Asia are dogs and foxes, while in Africa it is carried by various rodents. Between 50 000 and 100 000 new cases occur each year, the vast majority in Brazil, East Africa and the Indian subcontinent. Mortality rates have fallen in Asia due to improved treatment programmes, but not in Africa, where conflicts have disrupted management initiatives.

The incubation period is usually 1–2 months but may be several years. The onset of symptoms is insidious and the patient may feel quite well, despite markedly abnormal physical findings. Fever is common and may be high and intermittent, although usually low-grade. The liver and especially the spleen become enlarged; lymphadenopathy is common in African kala azar. The skin becomes rough and pigmented. If the disease is not treated, profound pancytopenia develops and the patient becomes wasted and immunosuppressed. Death usually occurs within a year and is normally due to bacterial infection or uncontrolled bleeding.

Diagnosis

Specific diagnosis is made by demonstrating the parasite in stained smears of aspirates of bone marrow, lymph node, spleen or liver. The organism can also be cultured from these specimens. Specific serological tests are positive in 95% of cases. Pancytopenia, hypoalbuminaemia and hypergammaglobulinaemia are common. The leishmanin skin test is usually negative, indicating a poor cell-mediated immune response.

Management

The most widely used drugs for visceral leishmaniasis remain the pentavalent antimony salts (e.g. sodium stibogluconate and meglumine antimoniate), despite toxicity and increasing resistance. Intravenous amphotericin B (preferably liposomal, which may be curative as a single-dose treatment) is effective but expensive; intramuscular

? Box 20.63 *Leishmania* species causing visceral and cutaneous disease

Disease type	Species complex	Species
Visceral leishmaniasis	*L. donovani*	*L. donovani* *L. infantum* *L. chagasi*
Cutaneous leishmaniasis	*L. tropica*	*L. tropica*
	L. major	*L. major*
	L. aethiopica	*L. aethiopica*
	L. mexicana	*L. mexicana* *L. amazonensis* *L. garnhami* *L. pifanoi* *L. venezuelensis*
	L. braziliensis	*L. braziliensis* *L. guyanensis* *L. panamanensis* *L. peruviana*
Mucocutaneous leishmaniasis		*L. braziliensis*

paromomycin is cheaper and also has a good cure rate. The oral drug miltefosine has been shown in India to be highly effective, especially in combination with liposomal amphotericin; this and other combination therapies are increasingly being used to shorten treatment courses and limit resistance. The recommended treatment regimens vary from region to region and are available from the WHO (see Further reading).

Successful treatment may be followed in a small proportion of patients by a skin eruption called **post-kala azar dermal leishmaniasis** (PKDL). It starts as a macular or maculopapular nodular rash, which spreads over the body. It is most often seen in Sudan and India, and is difficult to treat, although it may improve with miltefosine.

HIV co-infection

Visceral leishmaniasis is strongly associated with HIV-related immunosuppression (see p. 1444), and the two infections may be passed on together through injecting drug use. In Southern Europe, antiretroviral therapy has largely controlled the problem, but increasing numbers of cases are being seen in Brazil and India.

Cutaneous leishmaniasis

Cutaneous leishmaniasis is caused by a number of geographically localized species, which may be zoonotic or anthroponotic. It is by far the most common form of the disease, with up to a million new cases worldwide every year. Some 95% of these occur in just seven countries: Iran, Iraq, Syria, Algeria, Afghanistan, Brazil and Colombia.

Following a sandfly bite, *Leishmania* amastigotes multiply in dermal macrophages. The local response depends on the species of *Leishmania*, the size of the inoculum, and the host immune response. Single or multiple painless nodules appear 1 week to 3 months after the bite (**Fig. 20.31**). These enlarge and ulcerate with a characteristic erythematous raised border. An overlying crust may develop. The lesions heal slowly over months or years, sometimes leaving a disfiguring scar.

L. major and *L. tropica* are found in Russia and Eastern Europe, the Middle East, Central Asia, the Mediterranean littoral and sub-Saharan Africa. The reservoir for *L. major* is desert rodents, while *L. tropica* has a mainly urban distribution with dogs and humans as reservoirs. *L. aethiopica* is found in the highlands of Ethiopia and Kenya, where the animal reservoir is the hyrax. The skin lesions caused by these species usually heal spontaneously with scarring; this may take a year or more in the case of *L. tropica*. Leishmaniasis recidivans is a rare chronic relapsing form caused by *L. tropica*.

L. mexicana is found predominantly in Mexico, Guatemala, Brazil, Venezuela and Panama; infection usually runs a benign course with spontaneous healing within 6 months. *L. braziliensis* infections (which are seen throughout tropical South America) also usually heal spontaneously but may take longer.

L. mexicana amazonensis and *L. aethiopica* may occasionally cause diffuse cutaneous leishmaniasis. This is rare and is characterized by diffuse infiltration of the skin by Leishman–Donovan bodies. Visceral lesions are absent.

Diagnosis and management

The diagnosis can often be made clinically in a patient who has been in an endemic area. Giemsa stain on a split-skin smear will demonstrate *Leishmania* parasites in 80% of cases. Biopsy tissue from the edge of the lesion can be examined histologically and parasites identified by PCR; culture is less often successful. The leishmanin skin test is positive in over 90% of cases but does not distinguish between active and resolved infection. Serology is unhelpful.

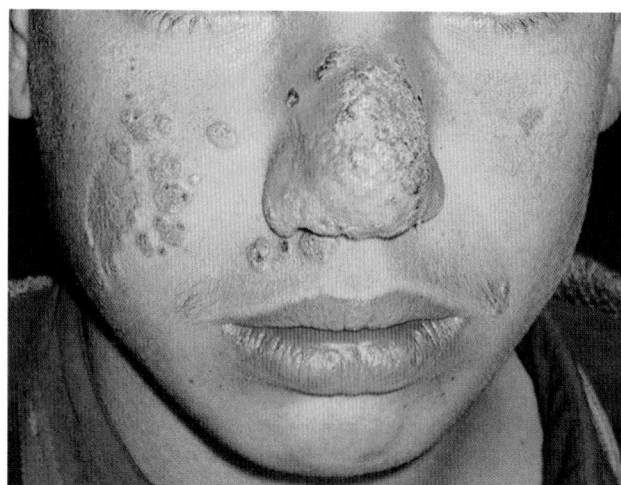

Fig. 20.31 Hyperkeratotic nodular cutaneous leishmaniasis lesions and leishmaniasis recidivans (on the right cheek) due to *Leishmania tropica*. (*From Bailey MS, Lockwood DNJ. Cutaneous leishmaniasis. Clin Dermatol 2007; 25:203–211.*)

Small lesions usually require no treatment. Large lesions or those in cosmetically sensitive sites can sometimes be treated locally by curettage, cryotherapy or topical antiparasitic agents. In other cases, systemic treatment with pentavalent antimonials, amphotericin or triazole antifungal drugs may be needed.

Mucocutaneous leishmaniasis

Mucocutaneous leishmaniasis occurs in 3–10% of infections with *L. b. braziliensis* and is most common in Bolivia and Peru. It can also follow infection with *L. aethiopica*. The cutaneous sores are followed months or years later by indurated or ulcerating lesions affecting mucosa or cartilage, typically on the lips or nose ('espundia'). The condition can remain static, or there may be progression over months or years affecting the nasopharynx, uvula, palate and upper airways.

Diagnosis and management

Biopsies usually show only very scanty organisms, although parasites can be detected by PCR; serological tests are frequently positive.

Amphotericin B is the treatment of choice, if available, although systemic antimonial compounds are widely used; miltefosine may also be effective. Relapses are common following treatment. Patients may die because of secondary bacterial infection or, occasionally, laryngeal obstruction.

Prevention of leishmaniasis relies on control of vectors and/or reservoirs of infection. Insecticide spraying, control of host animals and treatment of infected humans may all be helpful. Personal protection against sandfly bites is also important, especially in travellers visiting endemic areas. Sandflies are poor fliers and sleeping off the ground helps prevent bites.

Other protozoal diseases of the blood and tissues

Toxoplasmosis

Toxoplasmosis is caused by the intracellular protozoan parasite *Toxoplasma gondii*. The sexual form of the parasite lives in the gut of the definitive host, the cat, where it produces oocysts. After a period of maturing in the environment, these oocysts become the source

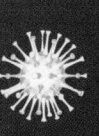

> **_i_ Box 20.64 Pathogenic human intestinal protozoa**
>
> **Amoebae**
> - _Entamoeba histolytica_
>
> **Flagellates**
> - _Giardia intestinalis_
>
> **Ciliates**
> - _Balantidium coli_
>
> **Coccidia**
> - _Cryptosporidium parvum_
> - _Isospora belli_
> - _Sarcocystis_ spp.
> - _Cyclospora cayetanensis_
>
> **Microspora**
> - _Enterocytozoon bieneusi_
> - _Encephalitozoon_ spp.

of infection for secondary hosts, which may ingest them. In the secondary hosts (which include humans, cattle, sheep, pigs, rodents and birds) there is disseminated infection. Following a successful immune response, the infection is controlled but dormant parasites remain encysted in host tissue for many years. The life cycle is completed when carnivorous felines eat infected animal tissue. Humans are infected either from contaminated cat faeces or undercooked infected meat; transplacental infection may also occur.

Clinical features

Toxoplasmosis is common: seroprevalence in adults in the UK is about 25%, rising to 90% in some parts of Europe. Most infections are asymptomatic or trivial. Symptomatic patients usually present with lymphadenopathy, mainly in the head and neck. There may be fever, myalgia and general malaise; occasionally, there are more severe manifestations, including hepatitis, pneumonia, myocarditis, and choroidoretinitis. Lymphadenopathy and fatigue can sometimes persist for months after the initial infection.

Congenital toxoplasmosis may also be asymptomatic but can produce serious disease. Clinical manifestations include microcephaly, hydrocephalus, encephalitis, convulsions and mental retardation. Choroidoretinitis is common; occasionally, this may be the only feature.

Immunocompromised patients, especially those with HIV infection, are at risk of serious infections with _T. gondii_. In acquired immunodeficiency states, this is usually due to reactivation of latent disease (see p. 1444).

Diagnosis

Diagnosis is usually made serologically. IgG antibodies detectable by the Sabin–Feldman dye test remain positive for years; acute infection can be confirmed by demonstrating a rising titre of specific IgM.

Management

Acquired toxoplasmosis in an immunocompetent host rarely requires treatment. In those with severe disease (especially eye involvement), sulfadiazine and pyrimethamine are given for 4 weeks, along with folinic acid. The management of pregnant women with toxoplasmosis aims to decrease the risk of fetal complications. However, there is only weak evidence that giving spiramycin, either alone or in combination with sulfadiazine (which is the recommended treatment), has any significant effect on the frequency or severity of fetal damage. Infected infants should be treated from birth. The treatment of toxoplasmosis in HIV-positive patients is covered on page 1444.

Babesiosis

Babesiosis is a tick-borne parasitic disease, diagnosed most commonly in North America and Europe. It is a zoonosis of rodents and cattle, and is occasionally transmitted to humans; infection is more common and more severe in those who are immunocompromised following splenectomy. The causative organisms are the _Plasmodium_-like _Babesia microti_ (rodents) and _B. divergens_ (cattle).

The incubation period averages 10 days. In patients with normal splenic function the illness is usually mild. In splenectomized individuals, systemic symptoms are more pronounced and haemolysis is associated with haemoglobinuria, jaundice and acute kidney injury. Examination of a peripheral blood smear may reveal the characteristic _Plasmodium_-like organisms.

The standard treatment of severe babesiosis is a combination of quinine 650 mg and clindamycin 600 mg orally three times daily for 7 days. Atovaquone and azithromycin is an alternative combination therapy.

Further reading

Burza S, Croft SL, Boelaert M. Leishmaniasis. _Lancet_ 2018; 392:951–970.
Draper SJ, Sack BK, King CR et al. Malaria vaccines: recent advances and new horizons. _Cell Host Microbe_ 2018; 24:43–56.
Liu Q, Zhou XN. Preventing the transmission of American trypanosomiasis and its spread in non-endemic countries. _Infect Dis Poverty_ 2015; 4:60.
Maldonado YA, Read JS, AAP Committee on Infectious Diseases. Diagnosis, treatment, and prevention of congenital toxoplasmosis in the United States. _Pediatrics_ 2017; 139:e20163860.
Singh B, Daneshvar C. Human infections and detection of Plasmodium knowlesi. _Clin Microbiol Rev_ 2013; 26:165–184.
World Health Organization. _Control of the Leishmaniases_. Geneva: WHO; 2010.
http://www.theglobalfund.org. _The Global Fund_.
http://www.who.int/leishmaniasis/resources/en/. _WHO Technical Report 949 Control of the Leishmaniases_.
http://www.who.int/malaria/publications/. _WHO guidelines for the treatment of malaria_.
http://www.wwarn.org. _Up-to-date information on resistance to all antimalarials_.

GASTROINTESTINAL PROTOZOA

The major gastrointestinal protozoal parasites of humans are shown in **Box 20.64**.

Amoebiasis

Amoebiasis is caused by _Entamoeba histolytica_. There are three morphologically identical species of amoeba, which can be distinguished by molecular techniques after culture of the trophozoite:
- **_E. histolytica_**, which is pathogenic
- **_E. dispar_**, which is non-pathogenic
- **_E. moshkovskii_**, which is of uncertain significance.

Amoebiasis occurs worldwide, although much higher incidence rates are found in the tropics and subtropics.

The organism exists both as a motile trophozoite and as a cyst that can survive outside the body. Cysts are transmitted by ingestion of contaminated food or water, or they can be spread directly by person-to-person contact. Trophozoites emerge from the cysts in the small intestine and then pass on in to the colon, where they multiply.

Clinical features

It is believed that many individuals can carry the pathogen without obvious evidence of clinical disease (asymptomatic cyst passers). However, this may be due, in some cases, to the misidentification of non-pathogenic *E. dispar* as *E. histolytica*, and it is not clear how often true *E. histolytica* infection is symptomless. In affected people, *E. histolytica* trophozoites invade the colonic epithelium, probably with the aid of their own cytotoxins and proteolytic enzymes. The parasites continue to multiply and eventually cause frank ulceration of the mucosa. If penetration continues, trophozoites may enter the portal vein, via which they reach the liver and cause intrahepatic abscesses. This invasive form is serious and may even be fatal.

The incubation period of intestinal amoebiasis is highly variable and may be as short as a few days or as long as several months. The usual course is chronic, with mild intermittent diarrhoea and abdominal discomfort. This may progress to bloody diarrhoea with mucus, sometimes accompanied by systemic symptoms such as headache, nausea and anorexia. Less commonly, infection presents as acute amoebic dysentery, resembling bacillary dysentery or acute ulcerative colitis.

Complications are unusual but include toxic dilation of the colon, chronic infection with stricture formation, severe haemorrhage, amoeboma and amoebic liver abscess. Amoebic liver abscesses often develop in the absence of a recent episode of colitis. Tender hepatomegaly, a high swinging fever and profound malaise are characteristic, although early in the course of the disease both symptoms and signs may be minimal. The clinical features are described in more detail on page 1306.

Diagnosis

Microscopic examination of fresh stool or colonic exudate obtained at sigmoidoscopy has been the standard means of diagnosing colonic amoebic infection. To confirm the diagnosis, motile trophozoites containing red blood cells must be identified; the presence of amoebic cysts alone does not imply disease. However, it is impossible to distinguish with certainty between the pathogenic and non-pathogenic species of *Entamoeba* using microscopy, and it is recommended that, wherever possible, species-specific molecular methods should be used. Sigmoidoscopy and barium enema examination may show colonic ulceration but are rarely diagnostic.

The amoebic fluorescent antibody test is positive in at least 90% of patients with liver abscess and in 60–70% with active colitis. Seropositivity is low in asymptomatic cyst passers.

Management

Metronidazole 800 mg three times daily for 5 days is given in amoebic colitis; a lower dose (400 mg three times daily for 5 days) is usually adequate in liver abscess. Tinidazole is also effective. After treatment of the invasive disease, the bowel should be cleared of parasites with a luminal amoebicide such as diloxanide furoate.

Prevention

Amoebiasis is difficult to eradicate because of the substantial human reservoir of infection. Progress will only be through improved standards of hygiene and sanitation, and better access to clean water. Cysts are destroyed by boiling but chlorine and iodine sterilizing tablets are not always effective.

Giardiasis

Giardia intestinalis is a flagellate (**Fig. 20.32**) that is found worldwide. It causes small intestinal disease, with diarrhoea and malabsorption. Prevalence is high in many developing countries and it is the most common parasitic infection in travellers returning to the UK. In certain parts of Europe and in some rural areas of North America, large water-borne epidemics have been reported. Person-to-person spread may occur in day nurseries and residential institutions. The organism exists as both a trophozoite and a cyst, the latter being the form in which it is transmitted.

The organism sometimes colonizes the small intestine and may remain there without causing detriment to the host. In other cases, severe malabsorption may occur, which is thought to be related to morphological damage to the small intestine. The changes in architecture are usually mild partial villous atrophy; subtotal villous atrophy is rare. The mechanism by which the parasite causes alteration in mucosal architecture and produces diarrhoea and intestinal malabsorption is unknown, though there is evidence that the morphological damage is immune-mediated. Bacterial overgrowth has also been found in association with giardiasis and may contribute to fat malabsorption.

Clinical features

Many individuals excreting *Giardia* cysts have no symptoms. Others become ill within 1–3 weeks of ingesting cysts; symptoms include diarrhoea, often watery in the early stage of the illness, nausea, anorexia, and abdominal discomfort and bloating. In most these symptoms resolve after a few days, but in some they persist. Stools may then become paler, with the characteristic features of steatorrhoea. If the illness is prolonged, weight loss occurs and can be marked. Chronic giardiasis, frequently seen in developing countries, can result in growth retardation in children.

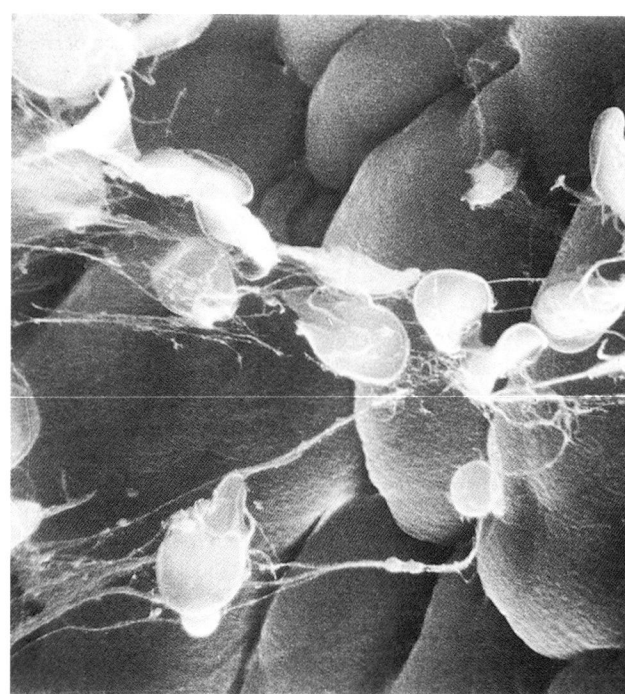

Fig. 20.32 *Giardia intestinalis* on small intestinal mucosa. (*Courtesy of Dr A Phillips*)

Diagnosis

Both cysts and trophozoites can be found in the stool, but negative stool examination does not exclude the diagnosis since the parasite may be excreted at irregular intervals. The parasite can also be seen in duodenal aspirates (obtained with either an endoscope or a luminal capsule) and in histological sections of jejunal mucosa.

Management

Metronidazole 2 g as a single dose on three successive days will cure the majority of infections, although sometimes a second or third course is necessary. Alternative drugs include tinidazole, nitazoxanide and albendazole. Preventative measures are similar to those outlined earlier for *E. histolytica*.

Cryptosporidiosis

This organism is found worldwide, cattle being the major natural reservoir. It has also been demonstrated in supplies of drinking water in the UK. The parasite is able to reproduce both sexually and asexually; it is transmitted by oocysts excreted in the faeces.

In healthy individuals, cryptosporidiosis is a self-limiting illness. Acute watery diarrhoea is associated with fever and general malaise lasting for 7–10 days. In immunocompromised patients, especially those with HIV, diarrhoea is severe and intractable (see p. 1444). Cryptosporidium may also be an important cause of childhood diarrhoea in resource-poor countries, contributing to overall morbidity and mortality.

Diagnosis is usually made by faecal microscopy, although the parasite can also be detected in intestinal biopsies. There is no reliable treatment but nitazoxanide may be of benefit.

Balantidiasis

Balantidium coli is the only ciliate that produces clinically significant infection in humans. It is found throughout the tropics, particularly in Central and South America, Iran, Papua New Guinea and the Philippines. It is usually carried by pigs, and infection is most common in those communities that live in close association with swine. Its life cycle is identical to that of *E. histolytica*. *B. coli* causes diarrhoea and sometimes a dysenteric illness, with invasion of the distal ileal and colonic mucosa. Trophozoites rather than cysts are found in the stool. Treatment is with tetracycline or metronidazole.

Blastocystis hominis infection

B. hominis is a strictly anaerobic protozoal pathogen that inhabits the colon. The pathogenicity for humans remains controversial. Many people appear to excrete the organism with no symptoms at all, but there are numerous reports of people with diarrhoea whose symptoms improve after eradication of the parasite. Whether this is due to pathogenic and non-pathogenic subspecies or individual host variation is unclear.

Cyclospora cayetanensis infection

C. cayetanensis, a coccidian protozoal parasite, was originally recognized as a cause of diarrhoea in travellers to Nepal. It has been detected in stool specimens from immunocompetent and immunodeficient people worldwide. Infection is usually self-limiting but can be treated with co-trimoxazole.

Microsporidiosis

Protozoa of the phylum Microsporea can cause diarrhoea in patients with HIV/AIDS (see p. 1444).

Further reading

Sparks H, Nair G, Castellanos-Gonzalez A et al. Treatment of cryptosporidium: what we know, gaps, and the way forward. *Curr Trop Med Rep* 2015; 2:181–187.

HELMINTHIC INFECTIONS

Worm infections are very common in developing countries, causing much disease in both humans and domestic animals. Worms are frequently imported into industrialized countries. The most common human helminth infections are listed in **Box 20.65**. Eight of the 17 'neglected tropical diseases' identified by the WHO as causing major morbidity in the poorest areas are caused by helminths. Even those parasites that, in developed countries, are regarded as little more than an inconvenience (e.g. roundworm or whipworm) cause huge morbidity in resource-poor settings due to the very high worm burden in children.

> **Box 20.65 Helminths commonly infecting humans**

	Helminth	Common name/disease caused
Nematodes (roundworms)		
Tissue-dwelling worms	*Wuchereria bancrofti*	Filariasis
	Brugia malayi/timori	Filariasis
	Loa loa	Loiasis
	Onchocerca volvulus	River blindness
	Dracunculus medinensis	Dracunculiasis
	Mansonella perstans	Mansonellosis
Intestinal human nematodes	*Enterobius vermicularis*	Threadworm
	Ascaris lumbricoides	Roundworm
	Trichuris trichiura	Whipworm
	Necator americanus	Hookworm
	Ancylostoma duodenale	Hookworm
	Strongyloides stercoralis	Strongyloidosis
Zoonotic nematodes	*Toxocara canis*	Toxocariasis
	Trichinella spiralis	Trichinellosis
Trematodes (flukes)		
Blood flukes	*Schistosoma* spp.	Schistosomiasis
Lung flukes	*Paragonimus* spp.	Paragonimiasis
Intestinal/hepatic flukes	*Fasciolopsis buski*	
	Fasciola hepatica	
	Clonorchis sinensis	
	Opisthorchis felineus	
Cestodes (tapeworms)		
Intestinal adult worms	*Taenia saginata*	Beef tapeworm
	Taenia solium	Pork tapeworm
	Diphyllobothrium latum	Fish tapeworm
	Hymenolepis nana	Dwarf tapeworm
Larval tissue cysts	*Taenia solium*	Cysticercosis
	Echinococcus granulosus	Hydatid disease
	Echinococcus multilocularis	Hydatid disease
	Spirometra mansoni	Sparganosis

Helminths are the largest internal human parasite. They reproduce sexually, generating millions of eggs or larvae. **Nematodes** and **trematodes** have a mouth and intestinal tract, while **cestodes** absorb nutrients directly through the outer tegument. All worms are motile, although once the adults are established in their definitive site, they rarely migrate further. Adult helminths may be very long-lived: up to 30 years in the case of the schistosomes.

Many helminths have developed complex life cycles, involving more than one host. Both primary and intermediate hosts are often highly specific to a particular species of worm. In some cases of human infection, humans are the primary host, while in others, humans are a non-specific intermediary or are coincidentally infected. Multiple infections with different helminths are common in endemic areas. Mass treatment programmes, in which one or more antihelminthic drugs are given on a regular (usually annual) basis, are used to keep the total worm load down, and the WHO recommends treating all schoolchildren at regular intervals in areas where helminth infections are common (**Box 20.66**).

NEMATODES

Tissue-dwelling worms

Filariasis

Several nematodes belonging to the superfamily Filarioidea can infect humans (**Box 20.67**). The adult worms are long and thread-like, ranging from 2 cm to 50 cm in length; females are generally much larger than males. Larval stages are inoculated into humans by various species of biting flies (each specific to a particular parasite). The adult worms that develop from these larvae mate, producing millions of offspring (microfilariae), which migrate in the blood or skin. These are ingested by feeding flies, in which the remainder of the life cycle takes place. Disease, which may be caused either by the adult worms or by microfilariae, stems from the host immune response to the parasite and is characterized by massive eosinophilia. Adult worms are long-lived (10–15 years) and re-infection is common, so that disease tends to be chronic and progressive.

Lymphatic filariasis

Lymphatic filariasis, which may be caused by different species of filarial worm, has a scattered distribution in the tropics and subtropics. Almost 1 billion people in developing countries are at risk. *Wuchereria bancrofti* is transmitted to humans by a number of mosquito species, mainly *Culex fatigans*. Adult female worms (5–10 cm long) live in the lymphatics, releasing large numbers of microfilariae into the blood. Generally, this occurs at night, coinciding with the nocturnal feeding pattern of *C. fatigans*. Non-periodic forms of *W. bancrofti*, transmitted by day-biting species of mosquito, are found in the South Pacific. *Brugia malayi* (and the closely related *B. timori*) is very similar to *W. bancrofti*, exhibiting the same nocturnal periodicity. The usual vectors are mosquitoes of the genus *Mansonia*, although other mosquitoes have been implicated.

Many filarial worms coexist with symbiotic *Wolbachia* bacteria, which are, in themselves, a cause of inflammation in the human host.

Clinical features

Following the bite of an infected mosquito, the larvae enter the lymphatics and are carried to regional lymph nodes. Here, they grow and mature for 6–18 months.

Adult worms produce allergic lymphangitis. The clinical picture depends on the individual immune response, which in turn may depend on factors such as age at first exposure. In endemic areas, many people have asymptomatic infection. Sometimes early infection is marked by bouts of fever accompanied by pain, tenderness and erythema along the course of affected lymphatics. Involvement of the spermatic cord and epididymis is common in Bancroftian filariasis. These acute attacks subside spontaneously in a few days but usually recur. Recurrent episodes cause intermittent lymphatic obstruction, which in time can become fibrotic and irreversible. Obstructed lymphatics may rupture, causing cellulitis and further fibrosis; there may also be chylous pleural effusions and ascites. Over time, there is progressive enlargement, coarsening

---

ⓘ Box 20.66 Drugs used in mass treatment of helminth infections

Drug	Infection
Diethylcarbamazine (DEC)	Loiaisis Filariasis
Ivermectin	Loiaisis Filariasis Onchocerciasis Strongyloidiasis
Albendazole	Filariasis (with DEC) Intestinal helminths
Praziquantel	Schistosomiasis

? Box 20.67 Diseases caused by the filarial worms

Organism	Adult worm	Microfilariae	Major vector	Clinical signs	Distribution
Wuchereria bancrofti	Lymphatics	Blood	*Culex* spp.	Fever Lymphangitis Elephantiasis	Tropics
Brugia timori/malayi	Lymphatics	Blood	*Mansonia* spp.	Fever Lymphangitis Elephantiasis	East and South-east Asia, South India, Sri Lanka
Loa loa	Subcutaneous	Blood	*Chrysops* spp.	'Calabar' swellings Urticaria	West and Central Africa
Onchocerca	Subcutaneous	Skin, eye	*Simulium* spp.	Subcutaneous nodules Eye disease	Africa, South America
Mansonella perstans	Retroperitoneal	Blood	*Culicoides* spp.	Allergic eosinophilia	Sub-Saharan Africa, South America

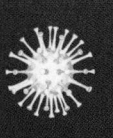

and fissuring of the skin, leading to the classical appearances of elephantiasis. The limbs or scrotum may become hugely swollen. Eventually, the adult worms will die, but the lymphatic obstruction remains and tissue damage continues. Elephantiasis takes many years to develop and is seen only in association with recurrent infection in endemic areas.

Occasionally, the predominant features of filarial infection are pulmonary. Microfilariae become trapped in the pulmonary capillaries, generating an intense local allergic response. The resulting pneumonitis causes cough, fever, weight loss and shifting radiological changes, associated with a high peripheral eosinophil count. This is known as **tropical pulmonary eosinophilia**.

Diagnosis

The clinical picture in established disease is usually diagnostic, although similar lymphatic damage may occasionally be caused by silicates absorbed through the feet from volcanic soil (podoconiosis). Parasitological diagnosis has traditionally relied on detecting microfilariae in blood films or skin snips, but rapid and sensitive near-patient antigen detection tests are now available.

Management

Diethylcarbamazine (DEC) kills both adult worms and microfilariae. Serious allergic responses may occur as the parasites are killed, and particular care is needed when using DEC in areas endemic for loiasis. Mass treatment programmes, using combinations of DEC, ivermectin and albendazole to target various helminthic infections, are deployed in many parts of the world; the exact regimens depend on local situations. The WHO reported in 2017 that over 7 billion courses of treatment had been given to 850 million people since 2000, and several countries have eliminated filariasis as a significant public health problem. There is currently much interest in using new agents to kill the symbiotic *Wolbachia* bacteria, without which the adult worm will eventually die. However, the best way of incorporating this tactic into the overall management strategy remains unclear. Vector control with insecticide bed nets is helpful in certain areas.

Loiasis

Loiasis is found in the humid forests of West and Central Africa. The causative parasite, *Loa loa*, is a small (3–7 cm) filarial worm, found in the subcutaneous tissues. The microfilariae circulate in the blood during the day but cause no direct symptoms. The vectors are day-biting flies of the genus *Chrysops*.

Adult worms migrate around the body in subcutaneous tissue planes. Worms may be present for years, frequently without causing symptoms. From time to time, localized, tender, hot, soft tissue swellings (Calabar swellings) occur due to hypersensitivity, often near a joint. These are produced in response to the passage of a worm and usually subside over a few days or weeks. There may also be more generalized urticaria and pruritus. Occasionally, a worm may be seen crossing the eye under the conjunctiva; it may also enter retro-orbital tissue, causing severe pain. Short-term residents of endemic areas often have more severe manifestations of the disease.

Microfilariae may be seen on stained blood films, although these are often negative. Serological tests are relatively insensitive and cross-react with other microfilariae. There is usually massive eosinophilia. DEC, which was used in early treatment campaigns, can cause severe allergic reactions associated with parasite killing and is being replaced by newer agents. Ivermectin in single doses of 200–400 µg/kg is effective but may also cause severe reactions occasionally. Albendazole, which brings about a more

gradual reduction in microfilarial load, may be preferable in heavily infected patients. Mass treatment with either DEC or ivermectin can decrease the transmission of infection but the mainstay of prevention is vector avoidance and control.

Onchocerciasis

Onchocerciasis (river blindness) affects 37 million people worldwide, of whom 250 000 are blind and 500 000 visually impaired; most of these are in West and Central Africa, with small foci in Yemen and in Central and South America. It is the result of infection with *Onchocerca volvulus*. Infection is transmitted by day-biting flies of the genus *Simulium*.

Pathogenesis

Infection occurs when larvae are inoculated into humans by the bite of an infected fly. The worms mature in 2–4 months and can live for more than 15 years. Adult worms, which can reach lengths of 50 cm (although they are <0.5 mm in diameter), live in the subcutaneous tissues. They may form fibrotic nodules, especially over bony prominences and sites of trauma. Huge numbers of microfilariae are distributed in the skin and may invade the eyes. Live microfilariae cause relatively little harm but dead parasites may cause severe allergic reactions, with hyaline necrosis and loss of tissue collagen and elastin. In the eye a similar process causes conjunctivitis, sclerosing keratitis, uveitis and secondary glaucoma. Choroidoretinitis is also seen occasionally.

Clinical features

Symptoms usually start about a year after infection. Initially, there is generalized pruritus, with urticaria and fleeting oedema. Subcutaneous nodules (which can be detected by ultrasound) start to appear, and in dark-skinned individuals there is hypo- and hyperpigmentation from excoriation and inflammatory changes. Over time, more chronic inflammatory changes appear, with roughened, inelastic skin. Superficial lymph nodes become enlarged and, in the groin, may hang down in loose folds of skin ('hanging groin'). Eye disease, which is associated with chronic heavy infection, usually first manifests as itching and conjunctival irritation. This gradually progresses to more extensive eye disease and eventually to blindness.

Diagnosis

In endemic areas the diagnosis can often be made clinically, especially if supported by finding eosinophilia on a blood film. In order to identify parasites, skin snips taken from the iliac crest or shoulder are placed in saline under a cover slip. After 4 hours, microscopy will show microfilariae wriggling free on the slide. If this is negative, DEC can be applied topically under an occlusive dressing and will provoke an allergic rash in the majority of infected people (modified Mazzotti reaction). Slit-lamp examination of the eyes may reveal the microfilariae. However, skin snip tests are less reliable in lower worm loads and are therefore of limited value in assessing success of treatment. Rapid near-patient serological card tests are under evaluation, and PCR tests are being developed.

Management and prevention

A single dose of ivermectin kills microfilariae and prevents their return for 6–12 months. There is little effect on adult worms and so annual (or more frequent) retreatment is needed. In patients co-infected with *Loa loa*, ivermectin may occasionally induce severe allergic reactions, including a toxic encephalopathy. An alternative agent, moxidectin, is currently under investigation.

The WHO Onchocerciasis Control Programme (OCP), which started in 1974, had a considerable impact on the disease in West Africa. A combination of vector control measures and, more recently, mass treatment with ivermectin led to a decrease in both infection rates and progression to serious disease. The control programme has been handed over to local governments by the WHO, and local mass treatment programmes are still running in most endemic countries. Eradication may eventually be possible, as humans are the only host, but measures are required over a long period because of the longevity of the worm (10–15 years).

Mansonellosis

Mansonella perstans is a filarial worm transmitted by biting midges of the genus *Culicoides*. Small numbers of microfilariae are found in the blood, and although they do not cause serious disease, there may be minor allergic reactions and an eosinophilia.

Dracunculiasis

Infection with the Guinea worm, *Dracunculus medinensis*, occurs when water fleas (copepods) containing the parasite larvae are swallowed in contaminated drinking water. Ingested larvae mature and the female worm, which can reach over 1 metre in length, migrates through connective and subcutaneous tissue for 9–18 months before surfacing on the skin. The uterus of the worm ruptures, releasing larvae that are ingested by the small crustacean water fleas, and the cycle is completed.

The diagnosis is clinical. The traditional management, extracting the worm over several days by winding it round a stick, is probably still the most effective. The worm should not be damaged. Antibiotics may be needed to control secondary infection.

Prevention and control of dracunculiasis has been one of the success stories in tropical medicine. Large-scale eradication programmes (involving removal of water fleas, and thus infective larvae, by chemical treatment or simple filtration) have been in place for several years. In 1989, active surveillance in Africa identified nearly a million cases of dracunculiasis; similar (though probably more robust) surveillance in 2018 found only 28 cases. The disease is now confined to a handful of small areas of Africa, notably in South Sudan, Chad and Angola.

Human intestinal nematodes

Adult intestinal nematodes (also referred to sometimes as soil-transmitted helminths, or geohelminths) live in the human gut. There are two main types of life cycle, both usually including a soil-based stage. In some species, infection is spread by ingestion of eggs (which often require a period of maturation in the environment); in others, the eggs hatch in the soil and larvae penetrate directly through the skin of a new host. *Strongyloides* (see p. 577) is unusual in that it is the only nematode that is able to complete its life cycle entirely within the human host without requiring a stage in the environment or an insect vector. Larvae may hatch before leaving the colon and so are able to re-infect the host by penetrating the intestinal wall and entering the venous system.

Although light infestations with intestinal worms cause few symptoms, heavy worm loads cause significant morbidity, especially in children. Cheap, effective and safe treatments are available and the WHO promotes mass treatment programmes for those at risk (without individual diagnosis): 600 million children in endemic areas received albendazole or mebendazole in 2017 (**Box 20.68**).

Ascariasis (roundworm infection)

Ascaris lumbricoides is a pale yellow worm, 20–35 cm in length (**Fig. 20.33**). It is found worldwide but is particularly common in poor rural communities, where there is heavy faecal contamination of the immediate environment. Larvae hatch and penetrate the duodenum, migrating through the tissues to the lungs before being expectorated and swallowed. The adult worms live in the small intestine. Ova are deposited in faeces and require a 2–4-month maturation in the soil before they are infective.

Infection is usually asymptomatic, although heavy infections are associated with nausea, vomiting, abdominal discomfort and anorexia. Worms can sometimes obstruct the small intestine, the most common site being the ileocaecal valve. They may also occasionally invade the appendix, causing acute appendicitis, or the bile

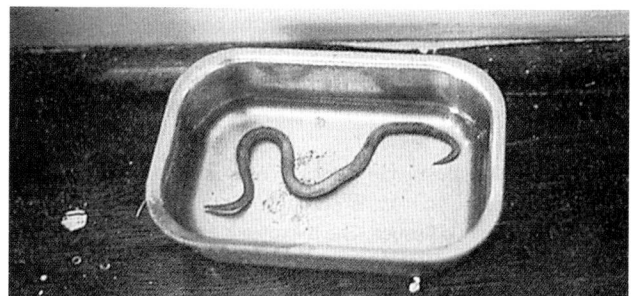

Fig. 20.33 *Ascaris lumbricoides.* The worm is approximately 20 cm long.

> **Box 20.68 Drugs used for treating human intestinal nematodes**[a]

Drug	Dosage	Ascaris	Hookworm	Enterobius	Trichuris	Strongyloides
Piperazine	75 mg/kg	++	+	++	–	–
Pyrantel pamoate	10 mg/kg	++	+	++	–	–
Oxantel pamoate	10 mg/kg	++	+	n/a	++	–
Albendazole	400 mg[b]	++	++	++	+	+
Mebendazole	500 mg[c]	++	++	++	+	+
Tiabendazole	25 mg/kg[b]	n/a	n/a	n/a	n/a	++
Levamisole	2.5 mg/kg	++	+	n/a	n/a	–
Ivermectin	200 μg/kg[d]	n/a	n/a	n/a	n/a	++

++, highly effective; +, moderately effective; –, ineffective; n/a, drug not used for this indication/no data available. [a]Single dose unless otherwise stated. [b]Twice daily for 3 days in strongyloidiasis. [c]WHO-recommended dose for developing countries; in the UK, commonly given as 100 mg single dose for threadworm or 100 mg twice daily for 3 days for whipworm. [d]Once daily for 2 days.

duct, resulting in biliary obstruction and suppurative cholangitis. Larvae in the lung may produce pulmonary eosinophilia. Heavy infection in children, especially those who are already malnourished, may have significant effects on nutrition and development. Serious morbidity and mortality are relatively rare in ascariasis, but the huge number of people infected means that on a global basis roundworm infection causes a significant burden of disease, especially in children.

Ascaris eggs can be identified in the stool and, occasionally, adult worms emerge from the mouth or the anus. They may also be seen on barium enema studies. Appropriate drug treatments are shown in **Box 20.68**. Very rarely, surgical or endoscopic intervention may be required for intestinal or biliary obstruction.

Threadworm (*Enterobius vermicularis*)

E. vermicularis is a small (2–12 mm) worm, which is common throughout the world. Larval development takes place mainly in the small intestine and adult worms are normally found in the colon. The gravid female deposits eggs around the anus, causing intense itching, especially at night. Unlike those of *A. lumbricoides*, the eggs do not require a maturation period in soil, and infection is often directly transmitted from anus to mouth via the hands. Eggs may also be deposited on clothing and bed linen, and are subsequently either ingested or inhaled. Apart from discomfort and local excoriation, infection is usually harmless.

Ova can be collected either by using a moistened perianal swab or by applying adhesive cellophane tape to the perianal skin. They can then be identified by microscopy.

The most commonly used drugs are mebendazole and piperazine (see **Box 20.68**). However, isolated treatment of an affected person is often ineffective. Other family members (especially small children) may also need to be treated and the whole family should be given advice about personal hygiene. Two courses of treatment 2 weeks apart may break the cycle of autoinfection.

Whipworm (*Trichuris trichiura*)

Infections with whipworm are common worldwide, especially in poor communities with inadequate sanitation. Adult worms, which are 3–5 cm long, inhabit the terminal ileum and caecum, although in heavy infection they are found throughout the large bowel. The head of the worm is embedded in the intestinal mucosa. Ova are deposited in the faeces and require a maturation period of 3–4 weeks in the soil before becoming infective.

Infection is usually asymptomatic, but mucosal damage can occasionally be so severe that there is colonic ulceration, dysentery, or rectal prolapse.

Diagnosis is made by finding ova on stool microscopy, or occasionally by seeing adult worms on sigmoidoscopy. Drug treatment is shown in **Box 20.68**.

Hookworm

Hookworm infections, caused by the human hookworms *Ancylostoma duodenale* and *Necator americanus*, are found worldwide. They are relatively rare in developed countries but very common in areas with poor sanitation and hygiene; overall, about 25% of the world's population is affected. Hookworm infection is a major contributing factor to anaemia in the tropics. *A. duodenale* is found mainly in East Asia, North Africa and the Mediterranean, while *N. americanus* is the predominant species in South and Central America, South-east Asia and sub-Saharan Africa.

Adult worms (which are about 1 cm long) live in the duodenum and upper jejunum, where they are often found in large numbers. They attach firmly to the mucosa using the buccal plate, feeding on blood. Eggs passed in the faeces develop in warm, moist soil, producing infective filariform larvae. These penetrate directly through the skin of a new host and are carried in the bloodstream to the lungs. Having crossed into the alveoli, the parasites are expectorated and then swallowed, thus arriving at their definitive home.

Clinical features

Local irritation as the larvae penetrate the skin ('ground itch') may be followed by transient pulmonary signs and symptoms, often accompanied by eosinophilia. Light infections, especially in a well-nourished person, are often asymptomatic. Heavier worm loads may be associated with epigastric pain and nausea, resembling peptic ulcer disease. Chronic heavy infection, particularly on a background of malnourishment, may cause iron deficiency anaemia and hypoproteinaemia. Heavy infection in children is associated with delays in physical and mental development.

Diagnosis and management

The diagnosis is made by finding eggs on faecal microscopy. In infections heavy enough to cause anaemia, these will be present in large numbers. The aim of treatment in endemic areas is reduction of worm burden rather than complete eradication; albendazole given as a single dose is the best drug (see **Box 20.68**).

Strongyloidiasis

Strongyloides stercoralis is a small (2 mm long) worm that lives in the small intestine. It is found in many parts of the tropics and subtropics, and is especially common in Asia. Eggs hatch in the bowel, and larvae are found in the stool. Usually, these are non-infective rhabditiform larvae, which require a further period of maturation in the soil before they can infect a new host, but sometimes this maturation can occur in the large bowel. Infective filariform larvae can therefore penetrate directly through the perianal skin, re-infecting the host. In this way, autoinfection may continue for years or even decades. Some war veterans who were imprisoned in the Far East during the Second World War were found to have active strongyloidiasis over 50 years later. After skin penetration, the life cycle is similar to that of the hookworm, except that the adult worms may burrow into the intestinal mucosa, causing a local inflammatory response.

Clinical features

Following skin penetration, *S. stercoralis* causes a similar local dermatitis to hookworm. In autoinfection, this manifests as a migratory linear weal around the buttocks and lower abdomen (**cutaneous larva currens**). In heavy infections, damage to the small intestinal mucosa can cause malabsorption, diarrhoea and even perforation. There is usually a persistent eosinophilia.

In patients who are immunosuppressed (e.g. by corticosteroid therapy or intercurrent illness), filariform larvae may penetrate directly through the bowel wall in huge numbers, causing an overwhelming and usually fatal generalized infection (the strongyloidiasis hyperinfestation syndrome). This condition is often complicated by Gram-negative bacteraemia due to bowel organisms.

Diagnosis and management

Motile larvae may be seen on stool microscopy, especially after a period of incubation. Serological tests are also useful. The best drug for treating strongyloidiasis is ivermectin (200 μg/kg daily for 2 days); albendazole and tiabendazole are also effective. In hyperinfection, antibiotics against Gram-negative organisms should be given.

Zoonotic nematodes

A number of nematodes that are principally parasites of animals may also affect humans. The most common are described here.

Trichinosis

The normal hosts of *Trichinella spiralis*, the cause of trichinosis, include pigs, bears and warthogs. Humans are infected by eating undercooked meat from these animals. Ingested larvae mature in the small intestine, where adults release new larvae that penetrate the bowel wall and migrate through the tissues. Eventually, these larvae encyst in striated muscle.

Light infections are usually asymptomatic. Heavier loads of worms produce gastrointestinal symptoms as the adults establish themselves in the small intestine, followed by systemic symptoms as the larvae invade. The latter include fever, oedema and myalgia. Massive infection may occasionally be fatal but usually the symptoms subside once the larvae encyst.

The diagnosis can usually be made from the clinical picture, associated eosinophilia and serological tests. If necessary, it can be confirmed by muscle biopsy a few weeks after infection. Longstanding infection may be revealed by the presence of numerous calcified cysts on X-ray. Albendazole (20 mg/kg for 7 days), given early in the course of the illness, will kill the adult worms and decrease the load of larvae reaching the tissues. Analgesia and steroids may be needed for symptomatic relief.

Toxocariasis (visceral larva migrans)

Eggs of the dog roundworm, *Toxocara canis*, are occasionally ingested by humans, especially children. The eggs hatch and the larvae penetrate the small intestinal wall and enter the mesenteric circulation, but are then unable to complete their life cycle in a 'foreign' host. Many are held up in the capillaries of the liver, where they generate a granulomatous response, but some may migrate into other tissues, including lungs, striated muscle, heart, brain and eye. In most cases, infection is asymptomatic and the larvae die without causing serious problems. In heavy infections, there may be generalized symptoms (fever and urticaria) and eosinophilia, as well as focal signs related to the migration of the parasites. Pulmonary involvement may cause bronchospasm and chest X-ray changes. Ocular infection may produce a granulomatous swelling mimicking a retinoblastoma, while cardiac or neurological involvement is occasionally fatal. Rarely, larvae survive in the tissues for many years, causing symptoms long after infection.

Isolation of the larvae is difficult and the diagnosis is usually made serologically. Albendazole 400 mg daily (5–10 mg/kg in children) for a week is the most effective treatment.

Cutaneous larva migrans

Cutaneous larva migrans is caused by the larvae of the non-human hookworms, *Ancylostoma braziliense* and *A. caninum*. Like human hookworms, these hatch in warm, moist soil and then penetrate the skin. In humans, they are unable to complete a normal life cycle and instead migrate under the skin for days or weeks until they eventually die. The wandering of the larva is accompanied by a clearly defined, serpiginous, itchy rash, which progresses at the rate of about 1 cm per day. There are usually no systemic symptoms. The diagnosis is purely clinical. Single larvae may be treated with a 15% solution of topical tiabendazole; multiple lesions require systemic therapy with a single dose of albendazole 400 mg or ivermectin 150–200 µg/kg.

TREMATODES

Trematodes (flukes) are flat, leaf-shaped worms. They have complex life cycles, often involving freshwater snails and intermediate mammalian hosts. Disease is caused by the inflammatory response to eggs or to the adult worms.

Water-borne flukes

Schistosomiasis

Schistosomiasis affects over 200 million people in the tropics and subtropics, mostly in sub-Saharan Africa. Chronic infection causes significant morbidity and, after malaria, it has the greatest socioeconomic impact of any parasitic disease. Schistosomiasis is largely a disease of the rural poor but has also been associated with major development projects, such as dams and irrigation schemes.

Parasitology and pathogenesis

There are three species of schistosome that commonly cause disease in humans: *Schistosoma mansoni*, *S. haematobium* and *S. japonicum*. *S. mekongi* and *S. intercalatum* also affect humans but have a very restricted distribution (**Fig. 20.34**). Eggs are passed in the urine or faeces of an infected person and hatch in freshwater to release the miracidia. These ciliated organisms penetrate the tissue of the intermediate host, a species of water snail specific to each species of schistosome. After multiplying in the snail, large numbers of fork-tailed cercariae are released back into the water, where they can survive for 2–3 days. During this time the cercariae can penetrate the skin or mucous membranes of the definitive host, humans. Transforming into schistosomulae, they pass through the lungs before reaching the portal vein, where they mature into adult worms (the male is about 20 mm long and the female a little larger). Worms pair in the portal vein before migrating to their final destination: mesenteric veins in the case of *S. mansoni* and *S. japonicum*, and the vesicular plexus for *S. haematobium*. Here they may remain for many years, producing vast numbers of eggs. The majority of these are released in urine or faeces, but a small number become embedded in the bladder or bowel wall and a few are carried in the circulation to the liver or other distant sites.

The pathology of schistosome infection varies with species and stage of infection. In the early stages, there may be local and systemic allergic reactions to the migrating parasites. As eggs start to be deposited, there is a local inflammatory response in the bowel or bladder, while ectopic eggs may produce granulomatous lesions anywhere in the body. Chronic heavy infection, in which large numbers of eggs accumulate in the tissues, leads to fibrosis, calcification and, in some cases, dysplasia and malignant change. Morbidity and mortality are related to duration of infection and worm load, as well as to the species of parasite. Children in endemic areas tend to have the heaviest worm load because of both increased exposure to infection and differences in the immune response between adults and children.

Clinical features

Cercarial penetration of the skin may cause local dermatitis ('swimmer's itch'). After a symptom-free period of 3–4 weeks, systemic allergic features may develop, including fever, rash, myalgia and pneumonitis (Katayama fever). These allergic phenomena are common in non-immune travellers but are rarely seen in local populations, who are usually exposed to infection from early childhood

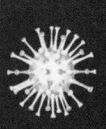

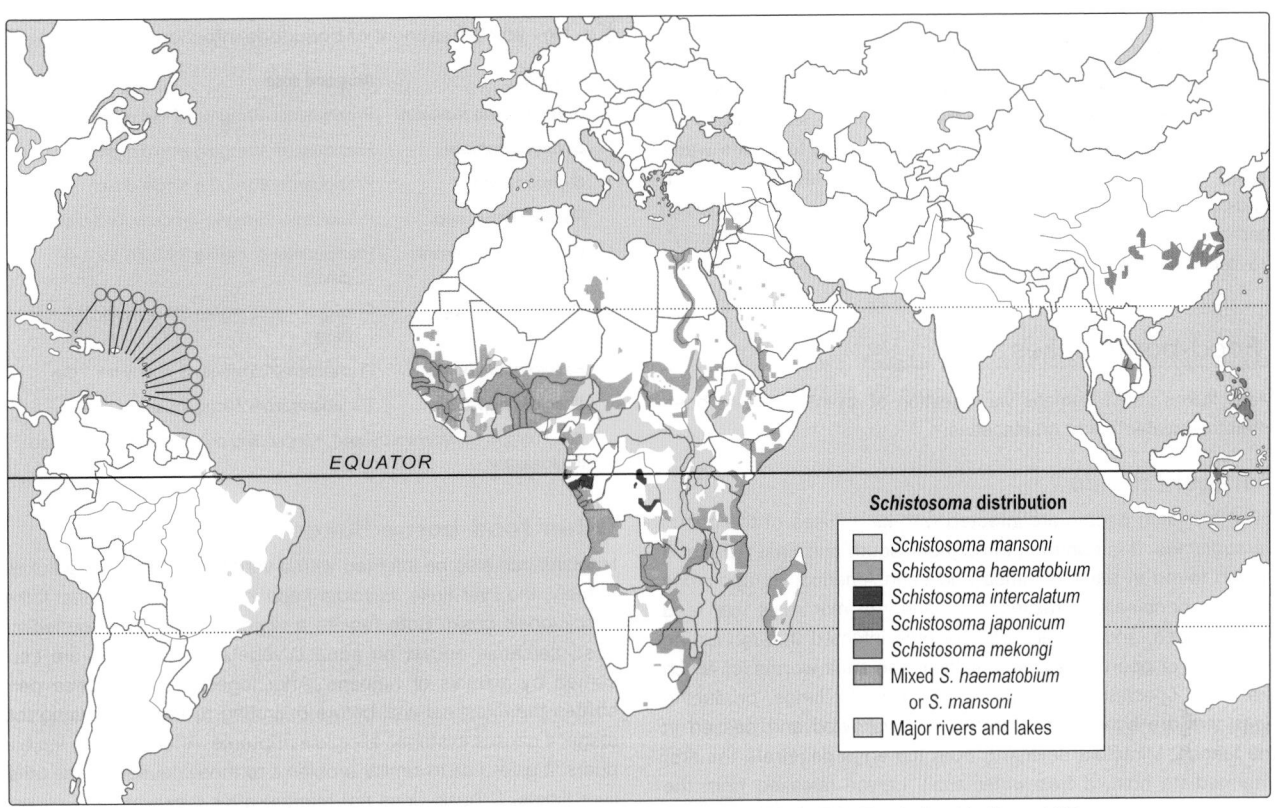

Fig. 20.34 Schistosomiasis: geographical distribution. *(From Colley DG, Bustinduy AL, Secor WE, King CH. Human schistosomiasis. Lancet 2014; 383:2253–22264, with permission.)*

onwards. If infection is sufficiently heavy, symptoms from egg deposition may start to appear 2–3 months after infection.

S. haematobium infection (bilharzia)

The earliest symptom is usually painless terminal haematuria. As bladder inflammation progresses, there is increased urinary frequency and groin pain. Obstructive uropathy develops, leading to hydronephrosis, chronic kidney disease and recurrent urinary infection. There is a strong association between chronic urinary schistosomiasis and squamous cell bladder carcinoma. The genitalia may also be affected and ectopic eggs may cause pulmonary or neurological disease.

S. mansoni

This usually affects the large bowel. Early disease produces superficial mucosal changes, accompanied by blood-stained diarrhoea. Later, the mucosal damage becomes more marked, with the formation of rectal polyps, deeper ulceration and, eventually, fibrosis and stricture formation. Ectopic eggs are carried to the liver, where they cause an intense granulomatous response. Hepatitis is followed by progressive periportal fibrosis, leading to portal hypertension, oesophageal varices and splenomegaly (see p. 1306). Hepatocellular function is usually well preserved.

S. japonicum

Unlike the other species, S. japonicum infects numerous other mammals apart from humans. It is similar to S. mansoni but infects both large and small bowel and produces a greater number of eggs. Disease therefore tends to be more severe and rapidly progressive. Hepatic involvement is more common and neurological involvement is seen in about 5% of cases.

Diagnosis

Schistosomiasis is suggested by relevant symptoms following freshwater exposure in an endemic area. In the early allergic stages the diagnosis can only be made clinically. When egg deposition has started, the characteristic eggs (with a terminal spine in the case of *S. haematobium* and a lateral spine in the other species) can be detected on microscopy. In *S. haematobium* infection the best specimen for examination is a filtered midday urine sample; parasites may also be found in semen. *S. mansoni* and *S. japonicum* eggs can usually be found in faeces or in a rectal snip. Serological tests are available and may be useful in the diagnosis of travellers returning from endemic areas, although the test may not become positive for 12 weeks after infection; a direct parasitological diagnosis should always be made if possible. In chronic disease X-rays, ultrasound examinations and endoscopy may show abnormalities of the bowel or urinary tract, although these are non-specific. Liver biopsy may show the characteristic periportal fibrosis.

Management

The aim of treatment in endemic areas is to decrease the worm load and therefore minimize the chronic effects of egg deposition. It may not always be possible (or even desirable) to eradicate adult worms completely, and re-infection is common. However, a 90% reduction in egg output has been achieved in mass treatment programmes, and in light infections, where there is no risk of re-exposure, the drugs are usually curative. The most widely used is praziquantel (**Box 20.69**), which is effective against all species of schistosome, well tolerated and reasonably cheap. Nearly 90 million people in sub-Saharan Africa received praziquantel through coordinated treatment programmes in 2016.

Prevention

Prevention of schistosomiasis is difficult and relies on a combination of approaches. Mass treatment of the population (especially children) will decrease the egg load in the community. Health education programmes, the provision of latrines and access to a safe water supply should decrease contact with infected water. Attempts to eradicate the snail host have generally been unsuccessful, although man-made bodies of water can often be made less 'snail-friendly'. Travellers should be advised to avoid potentially infected water.

Food-borne flukes

Many flukes infect humans via ingestion of an intermediate host, often freshwater fish or crustaceans.

Paragonimiasis

Over 20 million people are infected with lung flukes of the genus *Paragonimus*. It is common throughout South and East Asia, and is also found in parts of Africa and Latin America. *Paragonimus* spp. are principally parasites of a variety of mammals that feed on crustacea, and humans can become infected through eating uncooked or poorly prepared shellfish. The adult worms (of which the major species is *P. westermani*) live in the lungs, producing eggs that are either expectorated, or swallowed and passed in the faeces. Miracidia emerging from the eggs penetrate the first intermediate host, a freshwater snail. Larvae released from the snail seek out the second intermediate host, freshwater crustacea, in which they encyst as metacercariae. After consumption by mammalian hosts, cercariae penetrate the small intestinal wall and migrate directly from the peritoneum to the lungs across the diaphragm. Having established themselves in the lung, the adult worms may survive for 20 years.

The common clinical features are fever, cough and mild haemoptysis. In heavy infections the disease may progress, sometimes mimicking pneumonia or pulmonary tuberculosis. Ectopic worms may cause signs in the abdomen or the brain.

The diagnosis is made by detection of ova on sputum or stool microscopy. Radiological appearances are variable and non-specific. Treatment is with praziquantel or triclabendazole: the latter, which has a simpler regimen and is supplied free through the WHO, is generally preferred. Prevention involves avoidance of inadequately cooked shellfish.

Liver flukes

Humans can become infected with a variety of liver flukes. Terminology is confused: three parasite species, *Clonorchis sinensis*, *Opisthorchis felineus* and *O. viverrini*, are commonly referred to as the human liver flukes, although feline and other mammals are the principal hosts. *C. sinensis* and *O. viverrini* are almost entirely confined to East and South-east Asia, while the distribution of *O. felineus* extends across Central Asia as far as Eastern Europe. Adult worms live in the bile ducts, releasing eggs into the faeces. The parasite requires two intermediate hosts, a freshwater snail and a fish, and humans are infected by consumption of raw fish. The cycle is completed when excysted worms migrate from the small intestine into the bile ducts.

Infection is often asymptomatic but may be associated with cholangitis and biliary carcinoma. The diagnosis is made by identifying eggs on stool microscopy. Treatment is with praziquantel, and infection can be avoided by preparing and cooking fish adequately.

> **Box 20.69 Treatment of trematode infections**

Parasite	Drug and dose
Schistosoma mansoni	Praziquantel 40 mg/kg single dose[a]
S. haematobium	Praziquantel 40 mg/kg single dose[a]
S. japonicum	Praziquantel 60 mg/kg single dose[a]
Paragonimus spp.	Praziquantel 25 mg/kg 8-hourly for 3 days
Clonorchis sinensis	Praziquantel 25 mg/kg 8-hourly for 1–3 days[b]
Opisthorchis spp.	Praziquantel 25 mg/kg 8-hourly for 1–3 days[b]
Fasciolopsis buski	Praziquantel 25 mg/kg 8-hourly for 1 day
Fasciola hepatica	Triclabendazole 10 mg/kg single dose[c]

[a]May be split to minimize nausea. [b]Depending on worm load. [c]Repeated if necessary.

Other food-borne flukes

Humans can also be infected with a variety of other animal flukes: notably, the liver fluke, *Fasciola hepatica*, and the intestinal fluke, *Fasciolopsis buski*. Both require a water snail as an intermediate host; cercariae encyst on aquatic vegetation and then are consumed by animals or humans. After ingestion, *F. hepatica* penetrates the intestinal wall before migrating to the liver: during this stage, it causes systemic allergic symptoms. After reaching the bile ducts, it gives rise to similar problems to those caused by the other liver flukes. *F. buski* does not migrate after it excysts and causes mainly bowel symptoms.

Management of trematode infections

For drug treatment, see **Box 20.69**.

CESTODES

Cestodes (tapeworms) are ribbon-shaped worms, which vary from a few millimetres to several metres in length. Adult worms live in the human intestine, where they attach to the epithelium using suckers on the anterior portion (scolex). From the scolex arises a series of progressively developing segments, called proglottids. The mature distal segments contain eggs, which either may be released directly into the faeces, or are carried out with an intact detached proglottid. The eggs are consumed by intermediate hosts, after which they hatch into larvae (oncospheres). These penetrate the intestinal wall of the host (pigs, cattle or other animals) and encyst in the tissues. Humans ingest the cysts in undercooked meat and the cycle is completed when the parasites excyst in the stomach and develop into adult worms in the small intestine. Infections are usually solitary but several adult tapeworms may coexist. The exceptions to this life cycle are the dwarf tapeworm, *Hymenolepis nana*, which has no intermediate host and is transmitted from person to person by the faeco-oral route; and *Taenia solium*, which can cause either normal tapeworm infection (when humans are the definitive host) or cysticercosis (when humans are the intermediate host).

Taenia saginata

T. saginata, the beef tapeworm, may reach a length of several metres. It is found in all countries where undercooked beef is eaten, although human infection can largely be eradicated by good abattoir hygiene and inspection regimes, and the main burden of disease falls on economically less developed countries. The adult worm causes few,

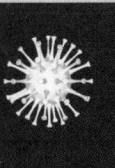

if any, symptoms, and is not a significant cause of chronic health problems. Infection is usually discovered when proglottids are found in faeces or on underclothing, often causing considerable anxiety. Ova may also be seen on stool microscopy. Infection can be cleared with a single dose of praziquantel (10 mg/kg).

Taenia solium and cysticercosis

T. solium, the pork tapeworm, is generally smaller than *T. saginata*, although it can still reach 6 metres in length. It is particularly common in South America, South Africa, China and parts of South-east Asia. As with *T. saginata*, infection is usually asymptomatic. The ova of the two species are identical but the proglottids can be distinguished on inspection.

Pork tapeworm infection is acquired by eating uncooked pork. Treatment is with praziquantel or niclosamide. Drug treatment should not be accompanied by a purgative, as was previously believed.

Cysticercosis occurs when humans become the intermediate host of the parasite, and is caused by cysts rather than the adult worm. It follows the ingestion of eggs from contaminated food and water. Faeco-oral autoinfection can occur but is rare. Patients with tapeworms do not usually develop cysticercosis, and individuals with cysticercosis do not usually harbour tapeworms. Following the ingestion of eggs the larvae are liberated, penetrate the intestinal wall and are carried to various parts of the body, where they develop into cysticerci. These are cysts, 0.5–1 cm in diameter, containing the scolex of a new adult worm. Common sites for cysticerci include subcutaneous tissue, skeletal muscle and brain.

Superficial cysts may be felt under the skin but usually cause no significant symptoms. Cysts in the brain can give rise to a variety of problems, including epilepsy, personality change, hydrocephalus and focal neurological signs (see p. 872). These may only appear many years after infection.

Muscle cysts tend to calcify and are often visible on X-rays. Cutaneous cysts can be excised and examined. Brain cysts are less prone to calcification and are often seen only on CT or MRI scan. Serological tests may support the diagnosis.

Management of cysticercosis

Following years of controversy, recent studies suggest that antihelminthic drugs are of benefit in most cases of neurocysticercosis, although their role in other forms of cysticercosis remains unproven. Albendazole 15 mg/kg daily for 8–20 days is the drug of choice; the alternative is praziquantel 50 mg/kg daily (in divided doses) for 15 days.

Successful treatment is accompanied by increased local inflammation, and corticosteroids should be given during and after the course of antihelminthic. Prevention of cysticercosis depends mainly on good hygiene.

Cerebral cysticercosis

Anticonvulsants should be given for epilepsy, and surgery may be indicated if there is hydrocephalus (see p. 876).

Diphyllobothrium latum

Infection with the fish tapeworm, *D. latum*, is common in Northern Europe and Japan, owing to the consumption of raw fish. The adult worm reaches a length of several metres but, like the other tapeworms, usually causes no symptoms. A megaloblastic anaemia (due to competitive utilization of vitamin B_{12} by the parasite) may occur. Diagnosis and treatment are the same as for *Taenia* species.

Hydatid disease

Hydatid disease occurs when humans become an intermediate host of the dog tapeworm, *Echinococcus granulosus*. The adult worm lives in the gut of domestic and wild canines and the larval stages are usually found in sheep, cattle and camels. Humans may become infected either from direct contact with dogs, or from food or water contaminated with dog faeces. After ingestion, the parasites excyst, penetrate the small intestine wall, and are carried to the liver and other organs in the bloodstream. A slow-growing, thick-walled cyst is formed, inside which further larval stages of the parasite develop. The life cycle cannot be completed unless the cyst is eaten by a dog. Hydatid disease is prevalent in areas where dogs are used in the control of livestock, especially sheep. It is common in Argentina, Peru, Central Asia, China and parts of East Africa, and about 1 million people are infected worldwide.

Symptoms depend mainly on the site of the cyst. The liver is the most common organ affected (60%), followed by the lung (20%), kidneys (3%), brain (1%) and bone (1%). The symptoms are those of a slowly growing benign tumour. Pressure on the bile ducts may cause jaundice. Rupture into the abdominal cavity, pleural cavity or biliary tree may occur. A cyst rupturing into a bronchus may result in its expectoration and spontaneous cure, but if secondary infection supervenes, a chronic pulmonary abscess will form. Focal seizures can occur if cysts are present in the brain. Renal involvement produces lumbar pain and haematuria. Calcification of the cyst occurs in about 40% of cases. The diagnosis and treatment of hydatid liver disease are described on page 1307.

A related parasite of foxes, *E. multilocularis*, causes a similar but more severe infection, alveolar hydatid disease. These cysts are invasive and metastases may occur; if untreated, the disease is usually fatal. Treatment requires radical surgery as well as antihelminthic treatment.

Further reading

Colley DG, Bustinduy AL, Secor WE et al. Human schistosomiasis. *Lancet* 2014; 383:2253–2264.
Hong WD, Benayoud F, Nixon GL et al. AWZ1066S, a highly specific anti-Wolbachia drug candidate for a short-course treatment of filariasis. *Proc Nat Acad Sci* 2019; 116:1414–1419.
Okello AL, Thomas LF. Human taeniasis: current insights into prevention and management strategies in endemic countries. *Risk Manag Healthc Policy* 2017; 10:107–116.
Papier K, Williams GM, Luceres-Catubig R et al. Childhood nutrition and parasitic helminth infections. *Clin Infect Dis* 2014; 59:234–243.
Qian MB, Utzinger J, Keiser J et al. Clonorchiasis. *Lancet* 2016; 387:800–810.

ARTHROPOD ECTOPARASITES

Arthropods, which include the arachnid ticks and mites as well as insects, may be responsible for human disease in several ways.

LOCAL HYPERSENSITIVITY REACTIONS

Local lesions may be caused by hypersensitivity to allergens in arthropod saliva. This common reaction, known as papular urticaria, is nonspecific and is seen in the majority of people in response to the bite of a variety of blood-sucking arthropods, including mosquitoes, bugs, ticks, lice and mites (**Fig. 20.35**). Occasionally, tick bites may cause a more severe systemic allergic response, especially in previously sensitized individuals. The saliva of some tick species contains a neurotoxin, which causes flaccid paralysis in the victim following a bite; this condition is rare but occurs worldwide, most commonly in children.

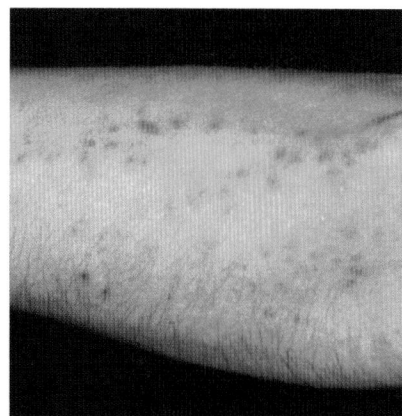

Fig. 20.35 Papular urticaria due to bedbug bites.

RESIDENT ECTOPARASITE INFECTIONS

Most ectoparasites alight on humans only to feed (although some species of lice live in very close proximity to the skin: body lice in clothing, and head and pubic lice on human hairs, see p. 675). However some types of parasite are actually resident within the skin, causing more specific local lesions.

Scabies

See page 674.

Jiggers

Jiggers is due to infection with the jigger flea, *Tunga penetrans*, and is common throughout South America and Africa. The pregnant female flea burrows into the sole of the foot, often between the toes. The egg sac grows to about 0.5 cm in size, before the eggs are discharged on to the ground. The main danger is bacterial infection or tetanus. The flea should be removed with a needle or scalpel and the area kept clean until it heals.

Myiasis

Myiasis is caused by invasion of human tissue by the larva of certain flies, principally the Tumbu fly, *Cordylobia anthropophaga* (found in sub-Saharan Africa) and the human botfly, *Dermatobia hominis* (Central and South America). The larvae, which hatch from eggs laid on laundry and linen, burrow into the skin to form boil-like lesions; a central breathing orifice may be visible. Again, the main risk is secondary infection. It is not always easy to extract the larva; covering it with petroleum jelly may bring it up in search of air.

SYSTEMIC ENVENOMING

Many arthropods can cause local or systemic illness through envenoming: that is, injection of venom. A detailed discussion of spider, scorpion and other bites is beyond the scope of this chapter (see Further reading and online topics).

VECTORS OF INFECTION

By far the most important role of arthropods in causing human disease is as vectors of parasitic and viral infections. Some of these infections are shown in **Box 20.17** and discussed in detail elsewhere.

Further reading

Erickson TB, Cheema N. Arthropod envenomation in North America. *Emerg Med Clin North Am* 2017; 35:355–375.

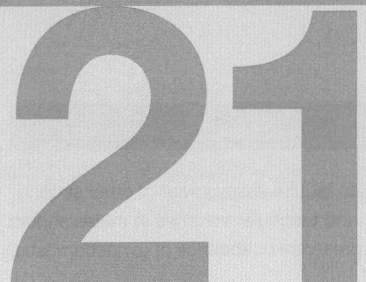

21

Endocrinology

Helena Gleeson, Narendra Reddy and Miles J. Levy

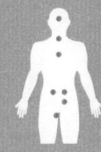

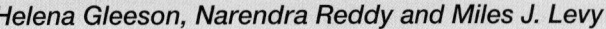

CORE SKILLS AND KNOWLEDGE

Many endocrine conditions are common and seen outside the hospital setting. They often affect young people and can usually be cured or completely controlled with appropriate therapy. For example, the UK prevalence of hypothyroidism is 2%, and it is usually managed in primary care. Excluding obesity (Ch. 33) and diabetes mellitus (Ch. 23), the commonest endocrine disorders are thyroid disorders; menstrual disorders; disorders affecting reproduction; hyperparathyroidism; and increasingly incidental findings in endocrine organs found on scans being done for other reasons – termed 'incidentalomas'.

Most endocrinologists specialize in both diabetes and endocrinology, seeing patients in outpatient clinics and often looking after general medical inpatients. Joint clinics that include specialist endocrine surgeons, endocrine oncologists, obstetricians, gynaecologists and paediatricians combine the expertise patients require in one clinical environment. Specialist nurses oversee dynamic testing of endocrine function, and coordinate education and management of patients with endocrine conditions.

Key skills required in endocrinology include:
- Mastering key principles of hormone action (such as negative feedback) in order to distinguish primary from secondary gland failure.
- Understanding the concept of dynamic endocrine tests and interpreting their results.
- Becoming familiar with the hormones most commonly used in endocrine replacement including levothyroxine, hydrocortisone and testosterone (in men) and oestrogen/progestogen (in women).

The best way to learn about endocrinology is to attend specialist and general outpatient clinics, where patients presenting with endocrine syndromes are evaluated and complex dynamic tests are planned and interpreted. Attend specialist multidisciplinary team meetings (MDTs) to learn about the radiology, histology and different management approaches to endocrine disease.

CLINICAL SKILLS FOR ENDOCRINOLOGY

History and examination

Specific features of the history relevant in endocrine disease are described in **Box 21.1**. On examination, weight, height, body mass index (BMI), blood pressure and general habitus should be documented, together with the presence or absence of specific signs of deficiency or excess of individual hormone axes indicated in the diagram opposite. Emergency presentations are listed in **Box 21.2**. In addition:

- In people with suspected pituitary disease, visual fields and adjacent cranial nerves should be assessed.
- In thyroid disease, the presence of goitre or orbitopathy should be documented.

- In hypogonadism both sexes require assessment of other secondary sexual characteristics, and testicular volumes in males should be documented as well as presence or absence of gynaecomastia.

Dynamic endocrine tests

Because of intra-individual and diurnal variations in the levels of many clinically relevant hormones, a single blood test often does not provide the information necessary to make a diagnosis (see p. 590). Dynamic endocrine tests assess the response of an endocrine axis to a specific challenge and are performed according to detailed protocols, which must be followed precisely. There are two types of dynamic tests – stimulation and suppression tests (**Box 21.3**).

 Box 21.1 Taking a history in endocrine assessment

General symptoms of a variety of endocrine disorders
- Tiredness, weakness, lack of energy or drive

Other common 'hormonal' symptoms
- Changes in body size and shape
- Changes in appetite or thirst
- Problems with libido and sexual function
- Changes in menstrual cycle
- Changes in the skin (dryness, greasiness, acne, bruising, thinning or thickening)
- Abnormal hair distribution (loss or excess)
- Subfertility or pregnancy loss

Role of hormones in physical development
- Growth and development in childhood
- Age of menarche
- Age of puberty
- Problems of sexual development

Risk factors common to a range of endocrine disorders
- Previous surgery or radiation involving endocrine glands
- Current or previous medication with endocrine side-effects
- A previous or family history of autoimmune disease
- A previous or family history of atypical tumours
- A family history of obesity, early-onset cardiovascular disease or any symptoms similar to those the patient is experiencing

---

Box 21.2 The 'top 10' endocrine emergencies

Diagnosis	Presentation	Page number
Severe hyponatraemia	Non-specific neurological symptoms and signs including confusion, drowsiness, coma and seizures if severe	183
Severe hypercalcaemia	Thirst, dehydration, polyuria	645
Hypoadrenal crisis	Collapse, postural hypotension, hypoglycaemia, history of chronic steroid use	603
Rapid dehydration in diabetes insipidus	Severe dehydration with ongoing polyuria; thirst; drowsiness, coma or seizures; history of diabetes insipidus or chronic lithium use	603
Pituitary apoplexy	Sudden severe headache (may be mistaken for subarachnoid haemorrhage) in a patient with known or undiagnosed pituitary tumour	596
Thyrotoxicosis	Fever, tachycardia, anxiety, tremor, dysrhythmia, e.g. fast atrial fibrillation	614
Severe hypothyroidism	Bradycardia, hypotension, drowsiness or coma	613
Hypoglycaemia	Sweating, confusion, drowsiness or coma. Regular user of insulin or sulphonylurea	716
Diabetic ketoacidosis	Vomiting, fever, dehydration, acidosis with Kussmaul respiration, hyperglycaemia. History of type 1 diabetes	722
Hyperglycaemic hyperosmolar state	Drowsiness or coma. Severe dehydration and hyperglycaemia. Signs of intercurrent illness. History of type 2 diabetes	725

Box 21.3 Dynamic endocrine tests

	Stimulation test	Suppression test
Assess for	Hormone deficiency	Hormone excess
Abnormal result	Inadequate rise in hormone level after stimulation, suggesting damage to target gland limiting maximum secretory output	Inadequate suppression of hormone level, indicating failure of negative feedback control and likely autonomous hormone secretion
Example	Short ACTH (synacthen) test for adrenal insufficiency	Dexamethasone suppression test for Cushing's disease

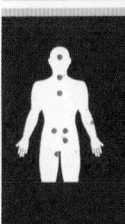

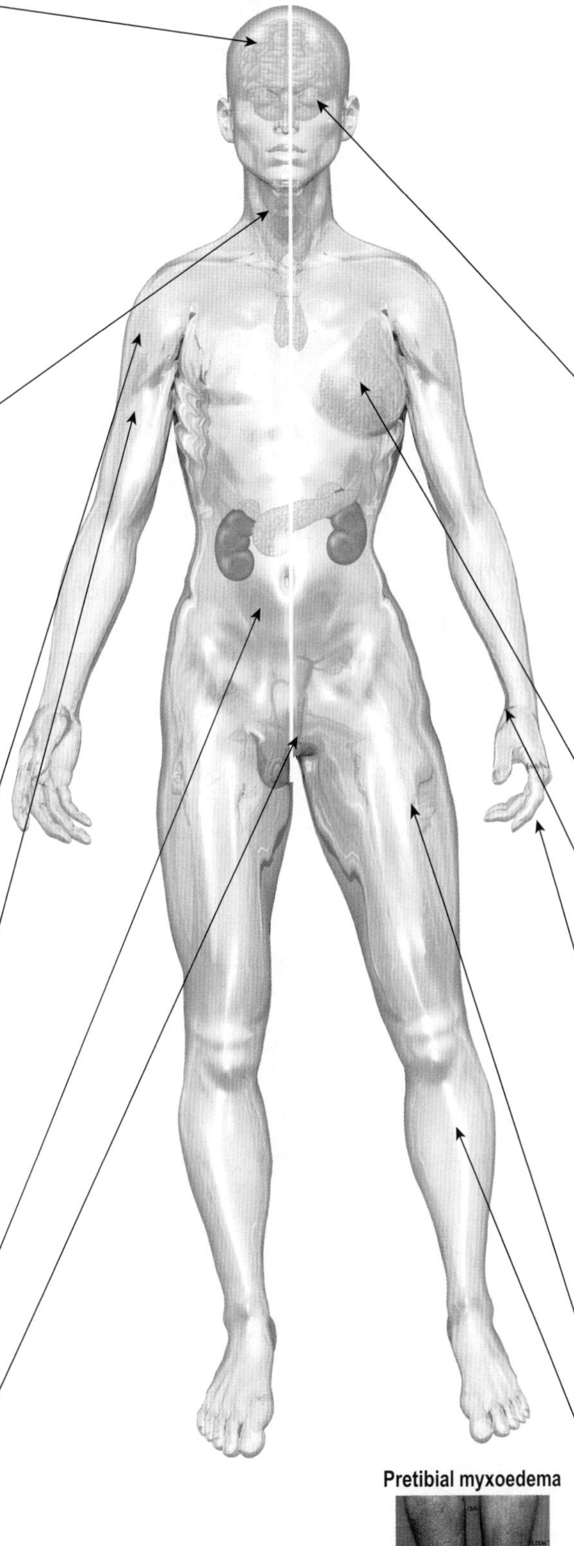

Hair
Alopecia
Coarse hair
Frontal balding

Facial features
Hypothyroid
- coarse features
- 'peaches and cream' complexion
- puffy eyes
- dry skin
Hyperthyroid
- eye problems

Neck
Goitre
Thyroid nodules

Goitre

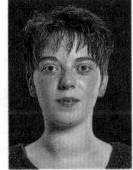

Vitiligo

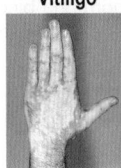

Skin
Vitiligo (autoimmune disease)
Pigmentation
Hair distribution

Blood pressure
↑ Cushing's
   Conn's
   Phaeochromocytoma
   Hypertension
   Acromegaly
   Thyroid disease
↓ Adrenal insufficiency

Central
Obesity
Striae (Cushing's)

Genitalia
Testicular volume
Pubertal development
Virilization

General
Look for features of:
 Hypothyroidism
 Hyperthyroid
 Acromegaly
 Mood
 - depressed/lethargic
 - restlessness
 - memory
 Voice – hoarse
 Weight – loss or gain
 Sweating
 Hirsutism

Eyes
- Signs of Graves' orbitopathy - proptosis, erythema, swelling
- Diplopia
- Visual fields defects
- Ophthalmoscopy
  - Papilloedema
  - Pale optic discs

Exophthalmos

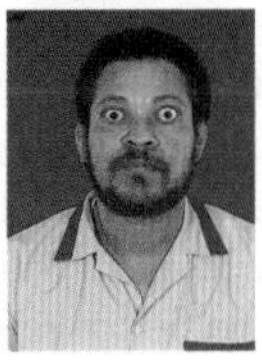

Breasts
Gynaecomastia
Galactorrhoea

Pulse
Atrial fibrillation

Hands
Sweating, tremor, palmar erythema
Carpal tunnel
Large, spade-like hands (acromegaly)
Pigmentation of creases (Addison's)

Acromegaly

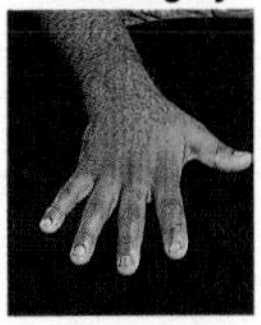

Proximal myopathy

Pretibial myxoedema

Pretibial myxoedema

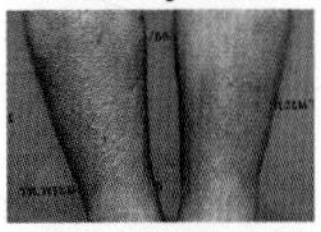

(From Rojanametin K, Masaru T. J Am Coll Dermatol 2015; 73:e195-e196, with permission)

INTRODUCTION

The endocrine system consists of glands that exert their actions at distant parts of the body via the production of biologically active hormones secreted into the bloodstream. Unlike the neurological system, which produces an immediate response, the endocrine system typically has a slower and longer-lasting effect on the body. The main endocrine glands are the pituitary, thyroid, adrenals, gonads, parathyroids and pancreas, and the common endocrine problems seen in clinical practice are shown in **Fig. 21.1**. The pituitary gland, a pea-sized structure situated at the base of the brain, plays a key role in the control and feedback mechanisms of the endocrine system and has been termed the 'conductor of the endocrine orchestra'

Hormonal activity

Synthesis, storage and release of hormones

Hormones have several chemical structures: polypeptide, glycoprotein, steroid or amine. Hormone release is the end-product of a cascade of intracellular events. In the case of polypeptide hormones, neural or endocrine stimulation of the cell causes increased transcription from DNA to a specific messenger RNA (mRNA), which is, in turn, translated to the peptide product. This is often a precursor molecule that may itself be biologically inactive. This 'prohormone' is further processed before being packaged into granules, in the Golgi apparatus. These granules are transported to the plasma membrane before release, which is itself regulated by a complex combination of intracellular regulators. Hormone release may be in a brief spurt caused by the sudden stimulation of granules, often induced by an intracellular Ca^{2+}-dependent process, or 'constitutive' (immediate and continuous secretion).

Plasma transport

Most classical hormones are secreted into the systemic circulation. In contrast, hypothalamic releasing hormones are released into the pituitary portal system so that higher concentrations of the releasing hormones reach the pituitary than occur in the systemic circulation.

Many hormones are bound to proteins within the circulation. In most cases, only the free (unbound) hormone is available and thus biologically active. This binding serves to buffer against rapid changes in plasma levels of the hormone, and some binding protein interactions are also involved in the active regulation of hormone action. Many tests of endocrine function measure total rather than free hormone, which can give rise to difficulties in interpretation when binding proteins are altered in disease states or by drugs.

Binding proteins comprise both specific, high-affinity proteins of limited capacity, such as thyroxine-binding globulin (TBG), cortisol-binding globulin (CBG), sex-hormone-binding globulin (SHBG) and insulin-like growth factor (IGF)-binding proteins (e.g. IGF-BP3), and other less specific, low-affinity ones, such as prealbumin and albumin.

Hormone action and receptors

Hormones act by binding to specific receptors in the target cell. Most hormone receptors are proteins with complex tertiary structures. The structure of the hormone-binding domain of the receptor complements the tertiary structure of the hormone, while changes in other parts of the receptor in response to hormone binding are responsible for the effects of the activated receptor within the cell. The structure of common hormones and their receptors is described under individual hormone axes.

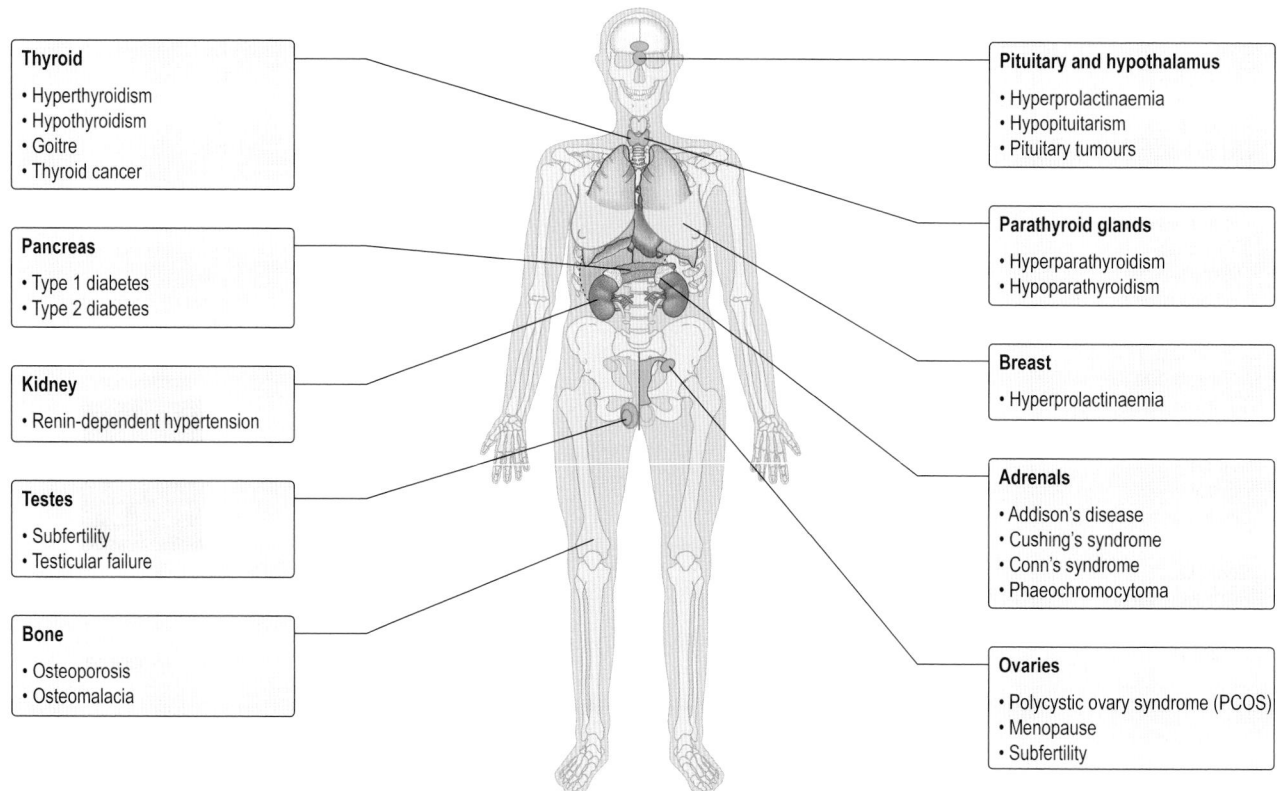

Thyroid
- Hyperthyroidism
- Hypothyroidism
- Goitre
- Thyroid cancer

Pancreas
- Type 1 diabetes
- Type 2 diabetes

Kidney
- Renin-dependent hypertension

Testes
- Subfertility
- Testicular failure

Bone
- Osteoporosis
- Osteomalacia

Pituitary and hypothalamus
- Hyperprolactinaemia
- Hypopituitarism
- Pituitary tumours

Parathyroid glands
- Hyperparathyroidism
- Hypoparathyroidism

Breast
- Hyperprolactinaemia

Adrenals
- Addison's disease
- Cushing's syndrome
- Conn's syndrome
- Phaeochromocytoma

Ovaries
- Polycystic ovary syndrome (PCOS)
- Menopause
- Subfertility

Fig. 21.1 The major endocrine organs and common endocrine problems.

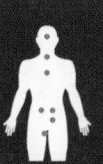

Hormone receptors are broadly divided into:

- *cell surface or membrane receptors*: transmembrane receptors that contain hydrophobic sections spanning the lipid-rich plasma membrane and trigger internal cellular messengers
- *nuclear receptors*: bind hormones and translocate them to the nucleus, where they bind hormone response elements of nuclear DNA via characteristic amino-acid sequences (e.g. so-called 'zinc fingers').

Abnormal receptors are an occasional cause of endocrine disease.

Mechanisms of hormone–receptor action

Common structural mechanisms of hormone–receptor action include:

- *G-protein coupled receptors (7-transmembrane or serpentine receptors).* These bind hormones on their extracellular domain and activate the membrane G-protein complex with their intracellular domain. The activated complex may then:
  - stimulate cyclic AMP (cAMP) generation by adenylate cyclase – activating further intracellular kinases and leading to phosphorylation
  - activate phospholipase C (PLC), leading to generation of inositol 1,4,5-triphosphate (IP_3) and release of intracellular calcium – in turn, leading to calmodulin-dependent kinase activity and phosphorylation
  - lead to diacylglycerol (DAG) activation of C-kinase and subsequent protein phosphorylation.

Most peptide hormones act via G-protein coupled receptors.

- *Dimeric transmembrane receptors.* These receptors, from several receptor superfamilies, bind hormone in their extracellular components (sometimes causing dimerization of the receptor monomer) and directly phosphorylate intracellular messengers via intracellular components, leading to a variety of intracellular activation cascades. Growth hormone, prolactin and IGF-1 act via this type of receptor.
- *Lipid-soluble molecules.* These pass through the cell membrane and bind with their *nuclear receptors* in the cell cytoplasm before translocation of the activated hormone–receptor complex to the nucleus; here, it binds to nuclear DNA, often in combination with a multi-component complex of promoters, inhibitors and transcription factors. This interaction leads to increased transcription of the relevant gene product. Steroid and thyroid hormones act via this type of receptor.

Hormone release and binding to receptors

The activation of intracellular kinases, phosphorylation, release of intracellular calcium and other 'second messenger' pathways, and the direct stimulation of DNA transcription may result in the following:

- stimulation/release of pre-formed hormone from storage granules
- stimulation/synthesis of hormone and other cellular components
- opening/closing of ion or water channels in the cell membrane (e.g. calcium channels or aquaporin water channels)
- activation/deactivation of other DNA binding proteins, leading to stimulation or inhibition of DNA transcription.

In each case, binding of the hormone to its receptor is the first step in a cascade of intracellular events, which eventually lead to the overall effects of that hormone on cellular function.

The sensitivity and/or number of receptors for a hormone are often decreased after prolonged exposure to a high hormone

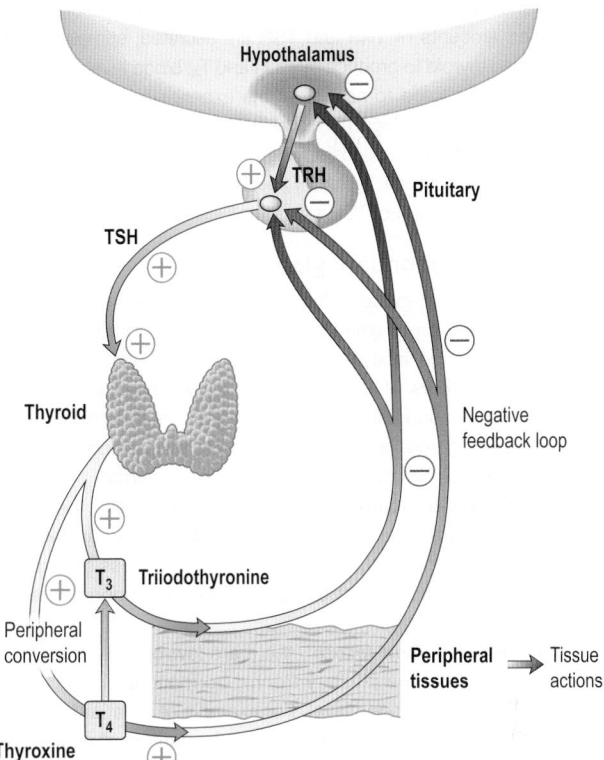

Fig. 21.2 The hypothalamic–pituitary–thyroid axis. Pituitary thyroid-stimulating hormone (TSH) is secreted in response to hypothalamic thyrotrophin-releasing hormone (TRH) and stimulates secretion of T_4 and T_3 from the thyroid. T_4 and T_3 have actions in peripheral tissues and exert negative feedback on the pituitary and hypothalamus.

concentration, the receptors thus becoming less sensitive ('down-regulation', e.g. angiotensin II receptors, β-adrenoceptors). The reverse is true when stimulation is absent or minimal, the receptors showing increased numbers or sensitivity ('upregulation').

Control and feedback

Most hormone systems are under tight regulatory control (typically by the hypothalamic–pituitary (HP) axis) by a system known as negative feedback. An example of the negative feedback system in the hypothalamic–pituitary–thyroid axis is demonstrated in **Fig. 21.2** and described here:

- Thyrotrophin-releasing hormone (TRH) is secreted in the hypothalamus and travels via the portal system to the pituitary, where it stimulates the thyrotrophs to produce thyroid-stimulating hormone (TSH).
- TSH is secreted into the systemic circulation, where it stimulates increased iodine uptake by the thyroid, and synthesis and release of thyroxine (T_4) and triiodothyronine (T_3).
- Serum levels of T_3 and T_4 are increased by TSH; in addition, the conversion of T_4 to T_3 (the more active hormone) in peripheral tissues is stimulated by TSH.
- T_3 and T_4 enter cells, where they bind to nuclear receptors and promote increased metabolic and cellular activity.
- Levels of T_3, from the blood and from local conversion of T_4, are sensed by receptors in the pituitary and the hypothalamus. If they rise above normal, TRH and TSH production is suppressed, leading to reduced T_3 and T_4 secretion.
- Peripheral T_3 and T_4 levels fall to normal.

- If T_3 and T_4 levels are low – for example, after thyroidectomy, increased amounts of TRH and TSH are secreted, stimulating the remaining thyroid to produce more T_3 and T_4; blood levels of T_3 and T_4 may be restored to normal, at the expense of increased TSH drive, reflected by a high TSH level: 'compensated euthyroidism'.
- Conversely, in thyrotoxicosis, when factors other than TSH itself are maintaining high T_3 and T_4 levels, the same mechanisms lead to suppression of TSH secretion.

Primary and secondary gland failure

It is useful in clinical endocrinology to distinguish between 'primary' disease of the end-organ gland (e.g. that due to autoimmune destruction, atrophic change, infiltration or surgical removal of the gland) and 'secondary' disorders of the same axis, caused by disease of the pituitary gland. An understanding of the negative feedback system is key to interpreting endocrine blood results and diagnosing the site of the disease process in clinical practice. In general terms:

- **'Primary' gland failure** due to a disease process in the endocrine end-organ (thyroid, adrenal or gonad) will lead to deficiency of the hormone produced by that gland and a loss of negative feedback and subsequent elevation in the corresponding anterior pituitary hormone.
- In **'secondary gland failure'**, there are low or 'inappropriately normal' levels of the pituitary trophic hormone in the face of a low end-organ hormone level. For example, if a patient has low circulating free T_3 (fT_3) and T_4 levels in the context of a low TSH, pituitary disease should be suspected.

Hormone excess

Abnormal hormone excess due to a disease process in the primary endocrine gland, or excess amount of exogenous hormone, will lead to increased negative feedback and suppression of the corresponding pituitary hormones. For example, in autoimmune hyperthyroidism, free T_3 and T_4 levels are elevated in the context of a suppressed TSH. Equally, the presence of a non-suppressed plasma pituitary hormone in the context of excess primary hormone implies that the pituitary, rather than the primary gland itself, is the cause. For example, in pituitary-driven Cushing's disease, cortisol levels are elevated but ACTH is not suppressed.

Hormone resistance

In certain situations, receptor abnormalities can give rise to abnormal negative feedback due to hormone resistance, which can lead to an unusual pattern of blood results. For example, thyroid hormone resistance, due to mutations in the thyroid hormone receptor, is characterized by an elevation in thyroid hormones with a non-suppressed TSH. With this pattern of thyroid results, the clinician should also consider the rare diagnosis of a TSH-secreting pituitary tumour, as well as the possibility of assay issues.

Measurement of hormones

Hormones are routinely measured by biochemical assays in the laboratory. It is possible to measure pituitary trophic hormones and the hormones produced by the end-organ glands, but hypothalamic hormones are not measured in practice because of their low concentration and local action within the HP axis. Circulating levels of most hormones are very low (10^{-9}–10^{-12} mol/L) and cannot be measured by simple chemical techniques. Hormones are therefore usually measured by immunoassays, which rely on highly specific polyclonal or monoclonal antibodies, which bind to the hormone being measured. This hormone–antibody interaction is measured by use of labelled hormone after separation of bound and free fractions (**Fig. 21.3**).

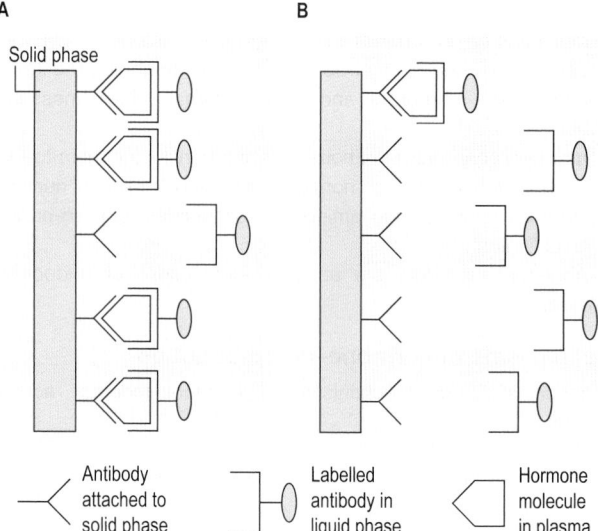

Fig. 21.3 Principles of measurement of hormone levels in plasma by immunoassay. (Precise details vary with different assays and manufacturers.) Immunoassays use two antibodies specific to the hormone being measured: one typically attached to a solid phase and one labelled antibody in the liquid phase. **(A)** High hormone levels in plasma: a large amount of hormone binds to antibody in solid phase; a large amount of labelled antibody is linked to solid phase via molecules of the hormone. **(B)** Low hormone levels in plasma: less hormone, and therefore less labelled antibody, is linked to the solid phase. Label (radioactive, chemiluminescent, enzymatic or fluorescent) can be measured in either solid or liquid phase after separation of phases; levels of label will be proportional to the amount of hormone in the sample.

Immunoassays are sensitive but have limitations. In particular, the immunological activity of a hormone, as used in developing the antibody, may not necessarily correspond to biological activity and there may be false-positive and negative results. The patient's blood may also contain heterophile antibodies, which interact with the animal antibodies used in the assay and produce falsely low or high values. When there is a discrepancy between endocrine blood results and the clinical presentation, the clinician must question the validity of an endocrine result, and liaise with chemical pathology. It may be necessary for the sample to be measured in a different laboratory using an alternative antibody, or to measure hormones in ways other than immunoassay. Examples of alternative techniques include equilibrium dialysis, high-pressure liquid chromatography (HPLC) and mass spectroscopy.

Hormone-binding proteins

Many hormones are transported in the bloodstream by a specific binding protein (see p. 586). It is more helpful to measure the free hormone rather than total bound hormone level, as this is the part that is biologically active. Some modern assays attempt to measure the free hormone level directly (e.g. free T_4) and are a more accurate reflection of biological activity, although many assays still measure total hormone level.

Cortisol, which is bound to cortisol-binding globulin (CBG), and testosterone, which is bound to sex-hormone-binding globulin (SHBG), are still usually measured in their total form and can be affected by alterations in binding protein levels. In women who are pregnant or on the combined oral contraceptive pill, high oestrogen levels may lead to an elevation in CBG, which can overestimate cortisol and give the false impression of

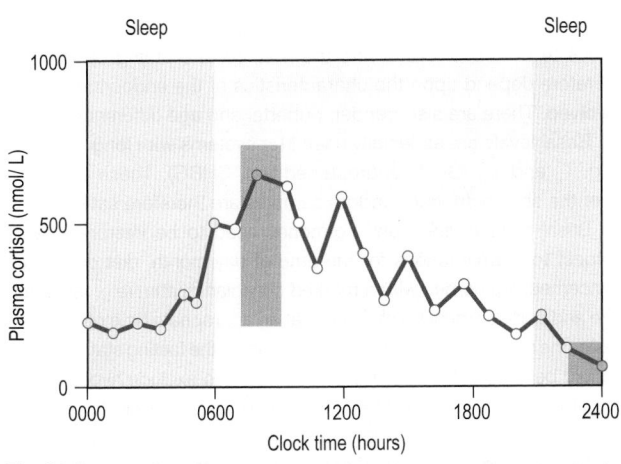

Fig. 21.4 Plasma cortisol levels during a 24-hour period. Note both the pulsatility and the shifting baseline. Normal ranges for 09:00 hours (180–700 nmol/L) and 24:00 hours (<100 nmol/L; must be taken when asleep) are shown in the red boxes. Grey shading shows sleep.

hypercortisolaemia. In people with diabetes mellitus or other insulin-resistant states that may lower SHBG levels, low total testosterone levels may give the false impression of androgen deficiency. Conversely, hyperthyroidism or oestrogen excess can cause an elevation in SHBG, leading to apparently high total testosterone levels.

Patterns of hormonal secretion

Hormone secretion can be continuous or intermittent, for example:

- **Continuous secretion** is shown by the thyroid hormones, with a half-life of 7–10 days for T_4 and 6–10 hours for T_3, and with little variation in levels over the day, month and year.
- **Pulsatile secretion** is the normal pattern for the gonadotrophins, luteinizing hormone (LH) and follicle-stimulating hormone (FSH), with major pulses released every 1–2 hours, depending on the phase of the menstrual cycle. Growth hormone (GH) is also secreted in a pulsatile fashion, with undetectable levels in between pulses. A single measurement is therefore not helpful to diagnose GH deficiency or excess.

Biological rhythms

Circadian means changes over the 24 hours of the day–night cycle and is best shown for the pituitary–adrenal axis. **Fig. 21.4** shows plasma cortisol measured over 24 hours; levels are highest in the early morning and lowest overnight. Additionally, cortisol release is pulsatile, following the pulsatility of pituitary ACTH. Thus, 'normal' cortisol levels vary during the day and great variations can be seen in samples taken only 30 minutes apart.

The menstrual cycle is an example of a longer and more complex (28-day) biological rhythm (see p. 1467).

Other regulatory factors

- **Stress.** Physiological 'stress' and acute illness produce rapid increases in ACTH and cortisol, GH, prolactin, adrenaline (epinephrine) and noradrenaline (norepinephrine). These can occur within seconds or minutes.
- **Sleep.** Secretion of GH and prolactin is increased during sleep, especially the rapid eye movement (REM) phase.
- **Feeding and fasting.** Many hormones regulate the body's control of energy intake and expenditure, and are therefore influenced by feeding and fasting. Secretion of insulin increases, while testosterone and GH decrease after ingestion of food, and

secretion of a number of hormones is altered during prolonged food deprivation.

i **Box 21.4** Types of autoimmune disease affecting endocrine organs

Organ and frequency, if known[a]	Antibody	Antigen, if known	Clinical syndrome
Stimulating			
Thyroid (1 in 100)	Thyroid-stimulating immuno-globulin (TSI, TSAb)	Thyroid-stimulating hormone (TSH) receptor	Graves' disease, neonatal thyrotoxicosis
Destructive			
Thyroid (1 in 100)	Thyroid microsomal	Thyroid peroxidase enzyme (TPO)	Primary hypothyroidism (myxoedema)
	Thyroglobulin	Thyroglobulin	
	Immunoglobulin (Ig) G4		Riedel's thyroiditis
Adrenal (1 in 20 000)	Adrenal cortex	21-Hydroxylase enzyme	Primary hypoadrenalism (Addison's disease)
Pancreas (1 in 500)	Islet cell	Glutamic acid decarboxylase (GAD; see p. 706)	Type 1 diabetes
Stomach	Gastric parietal cell	Gastric parietal cell	Pernicious anaemia
	Intrinsic factor	Intrinsic factor	
Skin	Melanocyte		Vitiligo
Ovary (1 in 500)	Ovary		Primary ovarian failure
Testis	Testis		Primary testicular failure
Parathyroid	Parathyroid chief cell		Primary hypoparathyroidism
Pituitary	Pituitary-specific cells		Autoimmune hypophysitis
			Selective hypopituitarism (e.g. growth hormone (GH) deficiency, diabetes insipidus)

[a]Frequencies are approximate and refer to the population in Northern Europe.
Note: Other related diseases include myasthenia gravis and autoimmune liver diseases.

Aetiology and pathology

Aetiological mechanisms common to many endocrine disorders are described as follows.

Autoimmune disease

Organ-specific autoimmune diseases can affect every major endocrine organ (**Box 21.4**). They are characterized by the presence of specific antibodies in the serum, often present years before clinical symptoms are evident, usually more common in women and have a strong genetic component, often with an identical-twin concordance rate of 50% and with human leucocyte antigen (HLA) associations (see individual diseases).

Endocrine tumours

Most endocrine tumours are benign, although a cytological or histological diagnosis may be needed if there is suspicion of malignancy. Clinical presentation depends on whether the tumour is functional or non-functional, the latter presenting only as a mass clinically or on imaging. Palpable thyroid nodules are common, and mass effects are a frequent presentation of pituitary adenomas, but the increased use of high-resolution ultrasound and detailed cross-sectional imaging has revealed a very high prevalence of asymptomatic, incidentally discovered thyroid, adrenal and pituitary lesions, commonly termed 'incidentalomas'.

Functional tumours cause their effects via excess secretion of the relevant hormone. While often considered to be 'autonomous' – that is, independent of the physiological control mechanisms – many functional tumours do show evidence of feedback occurring at a higher 'set-point' than normal (e.g. adrenocorticotrophic hormone (ACTH) secretion from a corticotroph adenoma). This is relevant in the dynamic assessment of endocrine diseases, such as in the differential diagnosis of Cushing's syndrome.

Endocrine adenomas typically present in a single gland, although rarer multiple endocrine neoplasia (MEN) syndromes exist that are due to very specific mutations of a single gene, such as the mutations of the *RET* proto-oncogene in MEN 2 or the *MEN1* gene mutation in MEN 1 (see p. 649). The diagnosis of some endocrine tumours, particularly at a young age, or the identification of a family history should prompt genetic screening.

Enzyme defects

The biosynthesis of most hormones involves many stages. Deficient or abnormal enzymes can lead to absent or reduced production of the secreted hormone. In general, severe deficiencies present early in life with obvious signs; partial deficiencies usually present later with mild signs or are only evident under stress. An example of an enzyme deficiency is congenital adrenal hyperplasia (CAH), whose molecular basis has also been identified as mutations or deletions of the gene encoding the relevant enzymes (see p. 604).

Receptor abnormalities

There are rare conditions in which hormone secretion and control are normal but the receptors are defective; thus, if androgen receptors are defective, normal levels of androgen will not produce masculinization (e.g. androgen insensitivity syndrome). There are also a number of rare syndromes of diabetes and insulin resistance from receptor abnormalities (see **Box 23.4**); other examples include nephrogenic diabetes insipidus, pseudohypoparathyroidism and thyroid hormone resistance.

Endocrine investigations

Endocrine function is assessed by measurement of hormone levels in blood (or, more precisely, in plasma or serum) and sometimes in other body fluids on samples obtained basally and in response to stimulation and suppression tests.

Basal blood levels

Assays for all clinically relevant pituitary and end-organ hormones are available.

The time, day and conditions of measurement make great differences to hormone levels, and the method and timing of samples therefore depend upon the characteristics of the endocrine system involved. There are also gender, pubertal and age differences.

Basal levels are especially useful for systems with long half-lives (e.g. T_4 and T_3, IGF-1, androstenedione, SHBG). These vary little over the short term and random samples are therefore satisfactory.

Basal samples for many hormones need to be interpreted with respect to normal ranges for the time of day/month, diet or posture concerned. Hormones with a marked circadian rhythm (e.g. testosterone and cortisol) must be measured at an appropriate time of day. Testosterone should be measured before 11am in the fasting state; cortisol should be checked between 8am and 10am to exclude hypoadrenalism, but at midnight to demonstrate normal low levels (to exclude Cushing's). LH/FSH, oestrogen and progesterone vary with time of menstrual cycle, and renin/aldosterone may vary with sodium intake, posture and age. For these hormones, all relevant details must be recorded or the results may prove uninterpretable.

Stress-related hormones

Measurement of stress-related hormones may be problematic either because the patient is stressed by hospital attendance or venepuncture, leading to falsely high levels (e.g. catecholamines, prolactin; sampling via an indwelling needle may be required, some time after initial venepuncture), or because low levels in a non-stressed individual are unable to confirm an adequate reserve required for normal physiological stress (cortisol and GH).

Urine collections

Collections over 24 hours have the advantage of providing an 'integrated mean' of a day's secretion but, in practice, are often incomplete or wrongly timed. They also vary with sex and body size or age. Written instructions should be provided for the patient to ensure accurate collection. Examples of hormones measured in this way are catecholamines and urinary free cortisol levels.

Saliva

Saliva is sometimes used for steroid estimations, especially in children or for samples taken at home. Midnight salivary cortisol levels are increasingly used for the diagnosis of Cushing's syndrome due to the practical difficulties in obtaining a midnight blood sample.

Stimulation and suppression tests

These tests are used when basal levels give equivocal information. In general, stimulation tests are used to confirm suspected deficiency of hormone secretion, and suppression tests to confirm suspected excess (see **Box 21.3**). These tests are valuable in many instances. For example, where the secretory capacity of a gland is damaged, maximal stimulation by the trophic hormone will give a diminished output. Thus, in the short ACTH stimulation test for adrenal reserve (**Box 21.5**; **Fig. 21.5A**), the healthy subject shows a normal response while the subject with primary hypoadrenalism (Addison's disease) demonstrates an impaired cortisol response to tetracosactide (an ACTH analogue).

A patient with a hormone-producing tumour usually fails to show normal negative feedback. A patient with Cushing's disease (excess pituitary ACTH) will thus fail to suppress ACTH and cortisol production when given a dose of synthetic steroid, in contrast to normal subjects. **Fig. 21.5B** shows the response of a normal subject given dexamethasone 1 mg at midnight; cortisol is suppressed the following morning. The subject with Cushing's disease shows inadequate suppression.

Indications
- Diagnosis of Addison's disease
- Screening test for ACTH deficiency

Procedure
- I.v. cannula for sampling
- Any time of day, but best at 09:00 hours; non-fasting and may indicate deficiency)

- Tetracosactide 250 µg, i.v. or i.m. at time 0
- Measure serum cortisol at time 0 and time +30 min

Normal response
- 30 min cortisol >600 nmol/L[a]
  – (400–600 nmol/L borderline

[a]Precise cortisol normal ranges are variable between laboratories and assays; appropriate local reference ranges must be used.

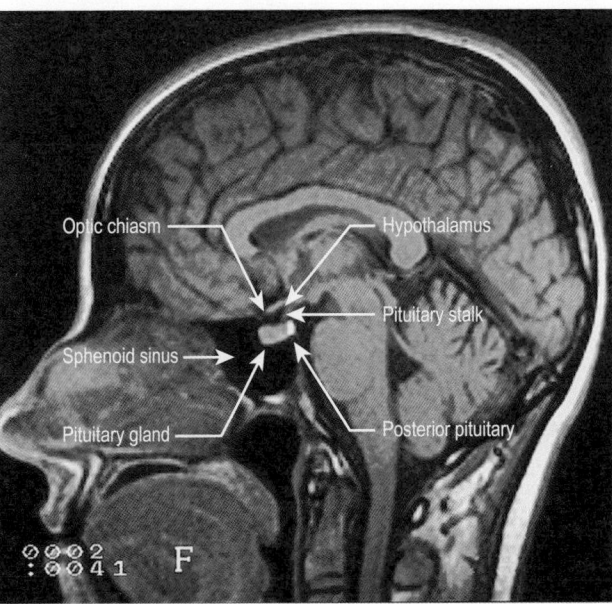

Fig. 21.6 Magnetic resonance imaging (MRI) of a sagittal section of the brain, showing the pituitary fossa and adjacent structures. *(By kind permission of Dr Martin Jeffree.)*

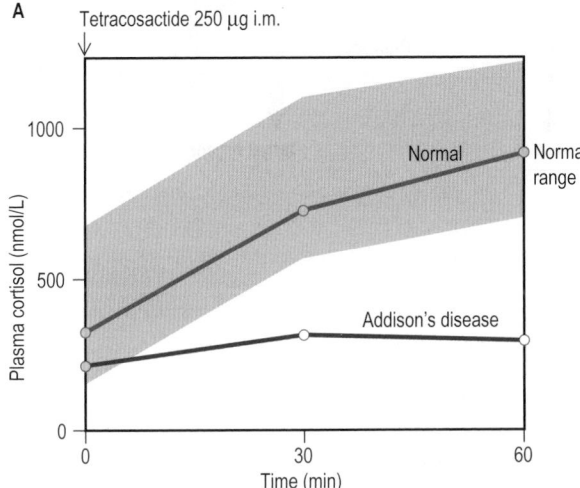

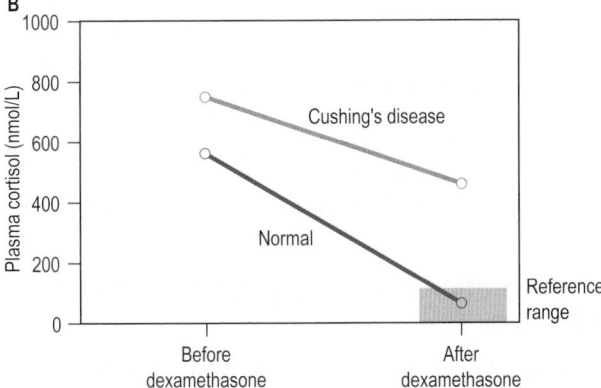

Fig. 21.5 Short ACTH stimulation and dexamethasone suppression tests. **(A)** The short ACTH stimulation test shows a normal response in a healthy subject and a decreased response in a patient with Addison's disease. **(B)** Dexamethasone suppression tests in a normal subject and in a patient with Cushing's disease, showing inadequate suppression.

The detailed protocol for each test must be followed exactly, since differences in technique will produce variations in results.

Radiological investigations

Magnetic resonance imaging (MRI), computed tomography (CT) and ultrasound give detailed images of endocrine glands but should be interpreted in clinical and biochemical context. Incidental endocrine tumours are common ('incidentalomas') and may have no clinical significance. Conversely, functional endocrine tumours may be too small to visualize on routine imaging. There is an increasing role for functional imaging e.g. positron emission tomography (PET) to detect endocrine tumours. Selective venous sampling is a useful interventional technique to localize hormone excess and is discussed in the relevant section.

THE PITUITARY GLAND AND HYPOTHALAMUS

Anatomy

Most peripheral hormone systems are controlled by the hypothalamus and pituitary. The hypothalamus is sited at the base of the brain around the third ventricle and above the pituitary stalk, which leads down to the pituitary itself, carrying the hypophyseal–pituitary portal blood supply.

The anatomical relations of the hypothalamus and pituitary (**Fig. 21.6**) include the optic chiasm above the pituitary fossa; any expanding lesion from the pituitary or hypothalamus can thus produce visual field defects by pressure on the chiasm. Such upward expansion of the gland through the diaphragma sellae is termed 'suprasellar extension'. Lateral extension of pituitary lesions may involve the vascular and nervous structures in the cavernous sinus and may rarely reach the temporal lobe of the brain. The pituitary is itself encased in a bony box; therefore, any lateral, anterior or posterior expansion must cause bony erosion.

Embryologically, the anterior pituitary is formed from an upgrowth of Rathke's pouch (ectoderm); this meets an outpouching of the third ventricular floor, which becomes the posterior pituitary. This combination of primitive gut and neural tissue provides an essential link between the rapidly responsive central nervous system and the longer-acting endocrine system. Several transcription factors – LHX3, HESX1, PROP1, POU1F1 – are responsible for the

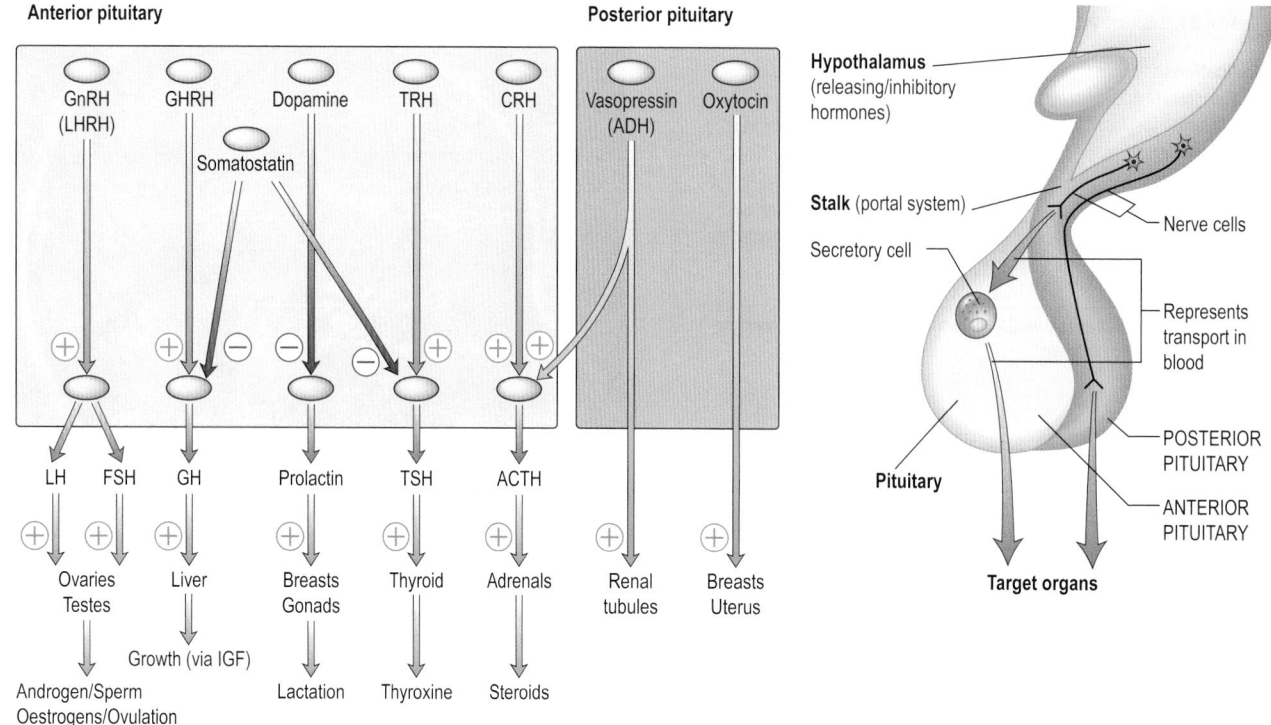

Fig. 21.7 Hypothalamic releasing hormones and the pituitary trophic hormones. ADH, anti-diuretic hormone; CRH, corticotrophin-releasing hormone; FSH, follicle-stimulating hormone; GH, growth hormone; GHRH, growth hormone-releasing hormone; GnRH, gonadotrophin-releasing hormone; IGF, insulin-like growth factor; LH, luteinizing hormone; TRH, thyrotrophin-releasing hormone.

differentiation and development of the pituitary cells. Mutation of these produces pituitary disease.

Physiology

Hypothalamus

This contains many vital centres for such functions as appetite, thirst, thermal regulation and sleeping/waking. It acts as an integrator of many neural and endocrine inputs to control the release of pituitary hormone-releasing factors. It plays a role in circadian rhythm, menstrual cyclicity, and responses to stress, exercise and mood.

Hypothalamic neurones secrete pituitary hormone-releasing and inhibiting factors and hormones into the portal system; these run down the stalk to the pituitary. As well as the classical hormones (**Fig. 21.7**), the hypothalamus also contains large amounts of other neuropeptides and neurotransmitters such as neuropeptide Y, vasoactive intestinal peptide (VIP) and nitric oxide, which can also alter pituitary hormone secretion.

Synthetic hypothalamic hormones and their antagonists are available for the testing of many aspects of endocrine function and for treatment.

Anterior pituitary

The majority of anterior pituitary hormones are under predominantly positive control by the hypothalamic releasing hormones; the exception is prolactin, which is under tonic inhibition by dopamine. Pathological conditions interrupt the flow of hormones between the hypothalamus and pituitary gland, and therefore cause deficiency of most hormones but oversecretion of prolactin. There are five major anterior pituitary axes: the gonadotrophin axis, the growth axis, prolactin, the thyroid axis and the adrenal axis.

Posterior pituitary

The posterior pituitary is neuroanatomically connected to specific hypothalamic nuclei and acts merely as a storage organ. Antidiuretic hormone (ADH, also called vasopressin) and oxytocin, both nonapeptides, are synthesized in the supraoptic and paraventricular nuclei in the anterior hypothalamus. They are then transported along the axon and stored in the posterior pituitary (see **Fig. 21.7**). This means that damage to the stalk or pituitary alone does not prevent synthesis and release of ADH and oxytocin. ADH is discussed on pages 641–643; oxytocin produces milk ejection and uterine myometrial contraction.

Presentation of pituitary and hypothalamic disease

Diseases of the pituitary can cause under- or overactivity of each hypothalamic–pituitary–end-organ axis. The clinical features of the syndromes associated with such altered pituitary function, such as Cushing's syndrome, can be the presenting symptom of pituitary disease or of end-organ disease and are discussed later. First, however, we look at the clinical features of pituitary disease that are common to all hormonal axes.

Pituitary space-occupying lesions and tumours

Pituitary tumours (**Box 21.6**) are the most common cause of pituitary disease, and the great majority are benign pituitary adenomas, usually monoclonal in origin. Problems are caused by:

- local effects of a tumour
- excess hormone secretion
- inadequate production of hormone by the remaining normal pituitary, i.e. hypopituitarism.

Approach for a possible or proven mass

Is there a tumour?

If there is, how big is it and what **local anatomical effects** is it exerting? Pituitary and hypothalamic space-occupying lesions, hormonally active or not, can cause symptoms by pressure on, or infiltration of:

- the visual pathways, with field defects and visual loss (most common)
- the cavernous sinus, with III, IV and VI cranial nerve lesions
- bony structures and the meninges surrounding the fossa, causing headache
- hypothalamic centres: altered appetite, obesity, thirst, somnolence/wakefulness or precocious puberty

Box 21.6 Characteristics of common pituitary and related tumours

Tumour or condition	Usual size	Most common clinical presentation
Prolactinoma	Most <10 mm (micro-prolactinoma)	Galactorrhoea, amenorrhoea, hypogonadism, erectile dysfunction
	Some >10 mm (macroprolactinoma)	As above plus headaches, visual field defects and hypopituitarism
Acromegaly	Few mm to several cm	Change in appearance, visual field defects and hypopituitarism
Cushing's disease	Most small: few mm (some cases are hyperplasia)	Central obesity, cushingoid appearance (local symptoms rare)
Nelson's syndrome	Often large: >10 mm	Post-adrenalectomy, pigmentation, sometimes local symptoms
Non-functioning tumours	Usually large: >10 mm	Visual field defects; hypopituitarism (microadenomas may be incidental finding)
Craniopharyngioma	Often very large and cystic (skull X-ray abnormal in >50%; calcification common)	Headaches, visual field defects, growth failure (50% occur below age 20; about 15% arise from within sella)

- the ventricles, causing interruption of cerebrospinal fluid (CSF) flow and hydrocephalus
- the sphenoid sinus, causing CSF rhinorrhoea.

Investigations

- **MRI of the pituitary.** MRI is superior to CT (**Fig. 21.8**) and readily shows any significant pituitary mass. Small lesions within the pituitary fossa, 'microadenomas', are very common on MRI (10% of normal individuals in some studies). Such small lesions are sometimes detected during MRI of the head for other reasons – so-called 'pituitary incidentalomas'.
- **Visual fields.** These should be plotted formally by automated computer perimetry or Goldmann perimetry, but clinical assessment by confrontation using a small red pin as the target is also sensitive and valuable. Common defects are upper temporal quadrantanopia and bitemporal hemianopia (see p. 810).

Is there a hormonal excess?

There are three major conditions that are usually caused by excess secretion from pituitary adenomas and which will show positive immunostaining for the relevant hormone:

- prolactin excess (**prolactinoma or hyperprolactinaemia**): histologically, prolactinomas are 'chromophobe' adenomas (a description of their appearance on classical histological staining)
- GH excess (**acromegaly or gigantism**): somatotroph adenomas, usually 'acidophil', and sometimes due to specific G-protein mutations (see p. 633)
- excess ACTH secretion (**Cushing's disease and Nelson's syndrome**): corticotroph adenomas, usually 'basophil'.

Many tumours are able to synthesize several pituitary hormones, and occasionally more than one hormone is secreted in clinically significant excess (e.g. both GH and prolactin).

The clinical features of acromegaly, Cushing's disease or hyperprolactinaemia are usually (but not always) obvious (see pp. 602 and 639). Tumours producing LH, FSH or TSH are well described but very rare.

Some common pituitary tumours cause no clinically apparent hormone excess and are referred to as 'non-functioning' tumours. Laboratory studies such as immunocytochemistry or *in situ* hybridization show that these tumours may often produce small amounts of LH and FSH or the α-subunit of LH, FSH and TSH, and occasionally ACTH.

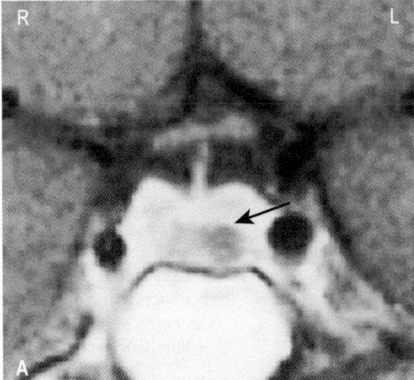
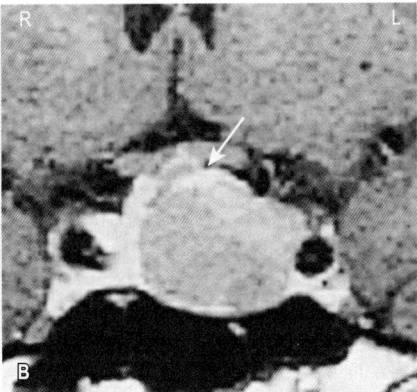
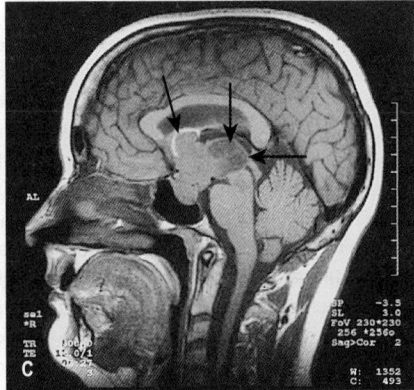

Fig. 21.8 Investigation of the pituitary gland. (A) Left-sided lucent intrasellar microadenoma (arrowed) (coronal MRI). The pituitary stalk is deviated slightly to the right. **(B)** Macroadenoma with moderate suprasellar extension, and lateral extension compressing the left cavernous sinus (coronal MRI). The top of the adenoma is compressing the optic chiasm (arrowed). **(C)** Pituitary macroadenoma with massive suprasellar extension (arrowed) (sagittal MRI).

Box 21.7 Tests of hypothalamic–pituitary (HP) function

All hormone levels are measured in plasma unless otherwise stated.
Tests **shown in bold** are those normally measured on a single basal 09:00 hours sample in the initial assessment of pituitary function.

Axis	Basal investigations		Common dynamic tests	Other tests
	Pituitary hormone	**End-organ product/function**		
Anterior pituitary				
HP–ovarian	**LH**	**Oestradiol**		Ovarian ultrasound
	FSH	Progesterone (day 21 of cycle)		LHRH test[a]
HP–testicular	**LH**	**Testosterone**		Sperm count
	FSH			LHRH test[a]
Growth	GH	**IGF-1**	Insulin tolerance test	GH response to sleep, exercise or arginine infusion
		IGF-BP3	Glucagon test	GHRH test[a]
Prolactin	**Prolactin**		–	–
HP–thyroid	**TSH**	**Free T$_4$, T$_3$**		TRH test[a]
HP–adrenal	ACTH	**Cortisol**	Insulin tolerance test	Glucagon test
			Short ACTH (tetracosactide) stimulation test	CRH test[a]
				Metyrapone test
Posterior pituitary				
Thirst and osmoregulation		**Plasma/urine osmolality**	Water deprivation test	Hypertonic saline infusion

[a]Releasing hormone tests were a traditional part of pituitary function testing but have been largely replaced by the advent of more reliable assays for basal hormones. They test only the 'readily releasable pool' of pituitary hormones, and normal responses may be seen in hypopituitarism. Bold text indicates commonly performed investigations.
ACTH, adrenocorticotrophic hormone; CRH, corticotrophin-releasing hormone; FSH, follicle-stimulating hormone; GH, growth hormone; GHRH, growth hormone-releasing hormone; IGF, insulin-like growth factor; LH, luteinizing hormone; LHRH, luteinizing hormone-releasing hormone; TRH, thyroid-releasing hormone; TSH, thyroid-stimulating hormone.

Is there a deficiency of any hormone?

Clinical examination may give clues; thus, short stature in a child with a hypothalamic pituitary mass is likely to be due to GH deficiency. An adult complaining of lethargy with pale skin is likely to be deficient in TSH and/or ACTH. Milder deficiencies may not be obvious and require specific testing (**Box 21.7**).

Management

Management depends on the type and size of tumour (**Box 21.8**). Decisions about pituitary tumour management are made in an MDT setting, which typically comprises an endocrinologist, pituitary surgeon and radiologist. In general, therapy has three aims: removal/control of the tumour, reduction of excess hormone secretion and replacement of hormone deficiencies.

Removal/control of tumour

This is only required if the tumour is large enough to cause, or is likely to cause, anatomical effects or if it is secreting excess hormones. Small tumours producing no significant symptoms, pressure or endocrine effects may be observed with appropriate clinical, visual field, imaging and endocrine assessments.

- *Surgery* via the trans-sphenoidal route is usually the treatment of choice. Very large tumours are occasionally removed via the open transcranial (usually transfrontal) route.
- *Radiotherapy* – by conventional linear accelerator or newer stereotactic techniques – is usually employed when surgery is impracticable or incomplete, as it controls but rarely abolishes tumour mass. The conventional regimen involves a dose of 45 Gy, given as 20–25 fractions via three fields. Stereotactic techniques use either a linear accelerator or multiple cobalt sources ('gamma-knife').
- *Medical therapy* with somatostatin analogues and/or dopamine agonists sometimes causes shrinkage of specific tumour types (see p. 638) and, if successful, can be used as primary therapy, particularly in the case of prolactinomas.

Box 21.8 Comparisons of primary treatments for pituitary tumours

Treatment method	Advantages	Disadvantages
Surgical		
Trans-sphenoidal adenomectomy or hypophysectomy	Relatively minor procedure Potentially curative for microadenomas and smaller macroadenomas	Some extrasellar extensions may not be accessible Risk of CSF leakage and meningitis
Transcranial (usually transfrontal) route	Good access to suprasellar region	Major procedure; danger of frontal lobe damage High chance of subsequent hypopituitarism
Radiotherapy		
External (40–50 Gy)	Non-invasive Reduces recurrence rate after surgery	Slow action, often over many years Not always effective Possible late risk of tumour induction
Stereotactic	Precise administration of high dose to lesion	Long-term follow-up data limited
Medical		
Dopamine agonist therapy (e.g. bromocriptine, cabergoline)	Non-invasive; reversible	Usually not curative; significant side-effects in minority Concerns about fibrotic reactions
Somatostatin analogue therapy (octreotide, lanreotide)	Non-invasive; reversible	Usually not curative; causes gallstones; expensive
Growth hormone receptor antagonist (pegvisomant)	Highly selective	Usually not curative; very expensive

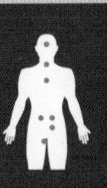

Axis	Usual replacement therapies
Adrenal	Hydrocortisone 15–25 mg daily (starting dose 10 mg on rising/5 mg lunchtime/5 mg evening) (Normally no need for mineralocorticoid replacement)
Thyroid	Levothyroxine 100–150 µg daily
Gonadal	
Male	Testosterone intramuscularly, orally, transdermally or implant
Female	Cyclical oestrogen/progestogen orally or as patch
Fertility	HCG plus FSH (purified or recombinant) or pulsatile GnRH to produce testicular development, spermatogenesis or ovulation
Growth	Recombinant human GH used routinely to achieve normal growth in children
	Also advocated for replacement therapy in adults, where GH has effects on muscle mass and wellbeing
Thirst	Desmopressin 10–20 µg 1–3 times daily by nasal spray or orally 100–200 µg 3 times daily. Carbamazepine, thiazides and chlorpropamide are very occasionally used in mild diabetes insipidus
Breast (prolactin inhibition)	Dopamine agonist (e.g. cabergoline 500 µg weekly)

FSH, follicle-stimulating hormone; GH, growth hormone; HCG, human chorionic gonadotrophin.

Reduction of excess hormone secretion

Reduction is usually obtained by surgical removal but sometimes by medical treatment. Useful control can be achieved with dopamine agonists for prolactinomas or somatostatin analogues for acromegaly, but ACTH secretion usually cannot be controlled by medical means. GH antagonists are also available for acromegaly (see p. 638).

Replacement of hormone deficiencies

See **Box 21.9**. Replacement of hormone deficiencies, i.e. hypopituitarism, is discussed further on page 597.

Differential diagnosis of pituitary or hypothalamic masses

Although pituitary adenomas are the most common mass lesion of the pituitary (90%), a variety of other conditions may also present as a pituitary or hypothalamic mass and form part of the differential diagnosis.

Other tumours

- **Craniopharyngioma** (1–2%), a usually cystic hypothalamic tumour that is often calcified and arises from Rathke's pouch. It is the most common pituitary tumour in children but may present at any age (**Fig. 21.9**).
- **Uncommon tumours** include meningiomas (**Fig. 21.10**), gliomas, chondromas, germinomas and pinealomas. Primary pituitary carcinomas are very rare, but occasionally prolactin- and ACTH-secreting tumours present in an aggressive manner, which may require chemotherapy in addition to conventional treatment. Metastases occasionally present as apparent pituitary tumours, typically accompanied by headache and diabetes insipidus.

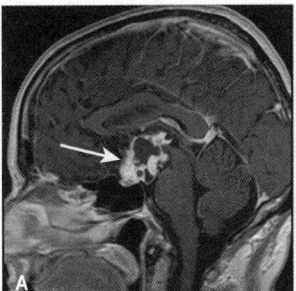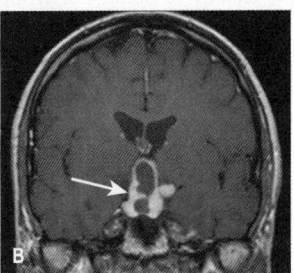

Fig. 21.9 Craniopharyngioma (arrowed): a partially cystic pituitary and suprasellar mass. **(A)** Sagittal MRI. **(B)** Coronal MRI.

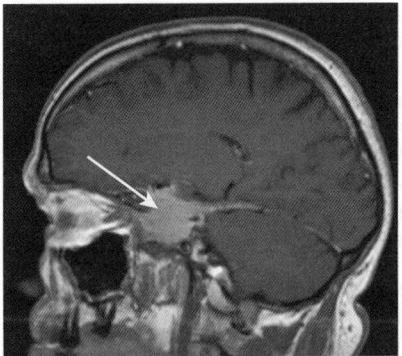

Fig. 21.10 Meningioma (arrowed) involving the pituitary fossa. Note the typical 'dural tail'.

Hypophysitis and other inflammatory masses

A variety of inflammatory masses occur in the pituitary or hypothalamus. These include rare pituitary-specific conditions (e.g. autoimmune (lymphocytic) hypophysitis, giant cell hypophysitis, postpartum hypophysitis), or pituitary manifestations of more generalized disease processes (sarcoidosis, Langerhans' cell histiocytosis, granulomatosis with polyangiitis). These lesions may be associated with diabetes insipidus and/or an unusual pattern of hypopituitarism.

Other lesions

Carotid artery aneurysms may masquerade as pituitary tumours and must be diagnosed before surgery. Cystic lesions may also present as a pituitary mass, including arachnoid and Rathke cleft cysts.

Hypopituitarism
Pathophysiology

Deficiency of hypothalamic releasing hormones or of pituitary trophic hormones can be selective or multiple. Thus isolated deficiencies of GH, LH/FSH, ACTH, TSH and vasopressin (ADH) are all seen, some cases of which are genetic and congenital, and others sporadic and autoimmune or idiopathic in nature.

Multiple deficiencies usually result from tumour growth or other destructive lesions. There is generally a progressive loss of anterior pituitary function. GH and gonadotrophins are usually first affected. Hyperprolactinaemia, rather than prolactin deficiency, occurs relatively early because of loss of tonic inhibitory control by dopamine. TSH and ACTH are usually last to be affected.

Panhypopituitarism refers to deficiency of all anterior pituitary hormones; it is most commonly caused by pituitary tumours, surgery or radiotherapy. Vasopressin (ADH) will only be significantly

Congenital
- Isolated deficiency of pituitary hormones (e.g. Kallmann's syndrome)
- *POU1F1* (Pit-1), Prop1, HESX1 mutations

Infective
- Basal meningitis (e.g. tuberculosis)
- Encephalitis
- Syphilis

Vascular
- Pituitary apoplexy
- Sheehan's syndrome (postpartum necrosis)
- Carotid artery aneurysm

Immunological
- Autoimmune (lymphocytic) hypophysitis
- Pituitary antibodies

Neoplastic
- Pituitary or hypothalamic tumour
- Craniopharyngioma
- Meningioma
- Gliomas
- Pinealoma
- Secondary deposits, especially breast
- Lymphoma

Traumatic
- Skull fracture through base
- Surgery, especially transfrontal
- Perinatal trauma

Infiltrations
- Sarcoidosis
- Langerhans' cell histiocytosis
- Hereditary haemochromatosis
- Hypophysitis:
  – Postpartum
  – Giant cell

Others
- Radiation damage
- Fibrosis
- Chemotherapy
- Immunotherapy (ipilimumab, pembrolizumab, nivolumab)
- Empty sella syndrome

'Functional'
- Anorexia nervosa
- Starvation
- Emotional deprivation

affected if the hypothalamus is involved by a hypothalamic tumour or major suprasellar extension of a pituitary lesion, or if there is an infiltrative/inflammatory process. Posterior pituitary deficiency with diabetes insipidus is rare in an uncomplicated pituitary adenoma.

Genetics

Specific genes are responsible for the development of the anterior pituitary, involving interaction between signalling molecules and transcription factors. For example, mutations in *PROP1* and *POU1F1* (previously *PIT-1*) prevent the differentiation of anterior pituitary cells (precursors to somatotroph, lactotroph, thyrotroph and gonadotroph cells), leading to deficiencies of GH, prolactin, TSH and gonadotrophin-releasing hormone (GnRH). In addition, novel mutations within GH and growth hormone-releasing hormone (GHRH) receptor genes have been identified, which explain the pathogenesis of isolated GH deficiency in some children. Despite these advances, most cases of hypopituitarism do not have specific identifiable genetic causes.

Aetiology

Disorders that cause hypopituitarism are listed in **Box 21.10**. Pituitary and hypothalamic tumours, and surgical or radiotherapy treatment, are the most common.

Clinical features

Symptoms and signs depend upon the extent of hypothalamic and/or pituitary deficiencies, and mild deficiencies may not lead to any complaint. In general, symptoms of deficiency of a pituitary-stimulating hormone are the same as those of primary deficiency of the peripheral endocrine gland (e.g. TSH deficiency and primary hypothyroidism cause similar symptoms due to lack of thyroid hormone secretion).

- *Secondary hypothyroidism, hypoadrenalism, hypogonadism* and *GH deficiency* lead to tiredness and general malaise and reduced quality of life.
- *Hypothyroidism* causes weight gain, slowness of thought and action, dry skin, cold intolerance, constipation and potentially bradycardia and hypothermia.
- *Hypoadrenalism* causes mild hypotension, hyponatraemia and, ultimately, cardiovascular collapse during severe intercurrent stressful illness.
- *Hypogonadism* leads to loss of libido, loss of secondary sexual hair, amenorrhoea and erectile dysfunction and, eventually, osteoporosis.
- *Hyperprolactinaemia* may cause galactorrhoea and hypogonadism, including amenorrhoea.
- *GH deficiency* causes growth failure in children, and impaired wellbeing in some adults.
- *Weight gain* (due to hypothyroidism; see above), or *weight loss* in severe combined deficiency.
- Longstanding *panhypopituitarism* gives the classic picture of pallor with hairlessness ('alabaster skin').

Particular syndromes related to hypopituitarism are described below.

Kallmann's syndrome

This is isolated gonadotrophin (GnRH) deficiency (see p. 626) caused by mutations in the *KAL1* gene, which is located on the short (p) arm of the X chromosome. Kallmann's classically causes anosmia because the *KAL1* gene provides instructions to make anosmin, which has a role both in development of the olfactory system and in migration of GnRH-secreting neurones.

Septo-optic dysplasia

This rare congenital syndrome (rarely associated with mutations in the *HESX1* gene), presents in childhood with two out of the clinical triad of midline forebrain abnormalities, optic nerve hypoplasia and hypopituitarism.

Sheehan's syndrome

This is due to pituitary infarction following postpartum haemorrhage and is rare in developed countries but not uncommon in countries where there are not established obstetric services.

Pituitary apoplexy

A pituitary tumour occasionally enlarges rapidly owing to infarction or haemorrhage. This may produce severe headache, double vision and sudden severe visual loss, sometimes followed by acute life-threatening hypopituitarism. Often, pituitary apoplexy can be managed conservatively with replacement of hormones and close monitoring of vision, although if there is a rapid deterioration in visual acuity and fields, surgical decompression of the optic chiasm may be necessary (**Fig. 21.11**).

'Empty sella' syndrome

An 'empty sella' is sometimes reported on pituitary imaging. This is sometimes due to a defect in the diaphragma and extension of the subarachnoid space (cisternal herniation), or may follow

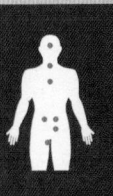

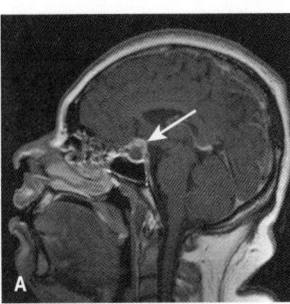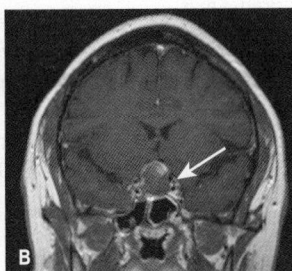

Fig. 21.11 Pituitary apoplexy. A bright area of haemorrhage at the top of a pituitary adenoma (arrowed) is shown. **(A)** Sagittal MRI. **(B)** Coronal MRI.

Box 21.11 Insulin tolerance test

Indications
- Diagnosis or exclusion of ACTH and GH deficiency

Procedure
- Test explained to patient and consent obtained
- Should only be performed in experienced, specialist units
- Exclude cardiovascular disease (ECG), epilepsy or unexplained blackouts; exclude severe untreated hypopituitarism (basal cortisol must be >100 nmol/L; normal free T_4)
- I.v. hydrocortisone and glucose available for emergency
- Overnight fast, begin at 08:00–09:00 hours
- Soluble insulin, 0.15 U/kg, i.v. at time 0
- Glucose, cortisol and GH levels at 0, 30, 45, 60, 90, 120 min

Normal response
- Cortisol rises above 550 nmol/L[a]
- GH rises above 7 ng/L (severe deficiency = <3 ng/L (<9 mU/L))
- Glucose must be <2.2 mmol/L to achieve adequate stress response

[a]Precise cortisol normal ranges are variable between laboratories and assays; appropriate local reference ranges must be used.
ACTH, adrenocorticotrophic hormone; ECG, electrocardiogram; GH, growth hormone.

---

spontaneous infarction or regression of a pituitary tumour. All or most of the sella turcica is devoid of apparent pituitary tissue but, despite this, pituitary function is usually normal, the pituitary being eccentrically placed and flattened against the floor or roof of the fossa.

Investigations

Each axis of the hypothalamic–pituitary system requires separate investigation. However, the presence of normal gonadal function in women as evidenced by the menstrual cycle obviates the need for investigation.

Investigations range from measurement of simple basal levels (e.g. TSH and free T_4 for the thyroid axis) to stimulatory tests for the pituitary and tests of feedback for the hypothalamus (see **Box 21.7**). Assessment of the hypothalamic–pituitary–adrenal (HPA) axis is complex: depending on the assay basal 9am cortisol levels above 400 nmol/L usually indicate adequate reserve, while levels below 100 nmol/L predict an inadequate stress response. In many cases, basal levels are equivocal and a dynamic test is essential. The insulin tolerance test (**Box 21.11**) is widely regarded as the 'gold standard' but the short ACTH stimulation test (see **Box 21.5**), though an indirect measure, is used by many as a routine test of HPA status as long as it is performed 6 weeks after any pituitary insult. Occasionally, the difference between ACTH deficiency and normal HPA axis can be subtle, and interpretation requires experience.

Management

- Glucocorticoid and thyroid hormones are essential for life. Both are given as oral replacement drugs, hydrocortisone and levothyroxine respectively, as in primary thyroid and adrenal failure, with the aim of restoring the patient to clinical and biochemical normality (see **Box 21.9**); for levothyroxine replacement, levels are monitored by routine hormone assays, whereas for hydrocortisone replacement monitoring is more limited to symptoms. ***Note:*** Thyroid replacement therapy should not commence until normal adrenal axis function has been demonstrated or glucocorticoid replacement therapy initiated, as an adrenal 'crisis' may otherwise be precipitated.
- Sex hormone replacement is with testosterone in males and a combination of oestrogen and progestogen in females, both for symptomatic control and for prevention of long-term problems related to deficiency (e.g. osteoporosis).

- When fertility is desired, gonadal function is stimulated directly by human chorionic gonadotrophin (HCG, mainly acting as LH) or by purified or biosynthetic gonadotrophins, or indirectly by pulsatile gonadotrophin-releasing hormone (GnRH – also known as luteinizing hormone-releasing hormone, LHRH) if gonadotrophs are undamaged; their use should be restricted to specialist units.
- GH replacement therapy is given for growth in a child, under the care of a paediatric endocrinologist. If the adolescent remains deficient at the achievement of adult height, GH replacement therapy can be offered until patients reach their mid-twenties to maximize muscle and bone mass. In adult GH deficiency, GH replacement therapy also produces improvements in body composition, work capacity and psychological wellbeing, together with reversal of lipid abnormalities associated with high cardiovascular risk, and often results in significant symptomatic benefit. The National Institute for Health and Care Excellence (NICE) recommends GH replacement for children and adolescents with GH deficiency, and in adults with severe GH deficiency and significant quality-of-life impairment. It is expensive and in the UK costs £2500–6000 per annum.
- Glucocorticoid deficiency may mask impaired urine concentrating ability, with diabetes insipidus only becoming apparent after glucocorticoid replacement therapy because glucocorticoids are required for excretion of free water.

Further reading

Dattani MT. Growth hormone deficiency and combined pituitary deficiency: does the genotype matter? *Clin Endocrinol* 2005; 63:121–130.
National Institute for Health and Clinical Excellence. *NICE Technology Appraisal 64: Human Growth Hormone (Somatotropin) in Adults with Growth Hormone Deficiency.* NICE 2003; http://www.nice.org.uk/guidance/ta64.
Rajasekaran S, Vanderpump M, Baldeweg S et al. UK guidelines for the management of pituitary apoplexy. *Clin Endocrinol* 2011; 74:9–20.
Schneider HJ, Aimaretti G, Kreitschmann-Andermahr I et al. Hypopituitarism. *Lancet* 2007; 369:1151–1470.

---

i **Box 21.12** Hormones and receptors of the hypothalamic–pituitary–adrenal axis

Hormone	Source	Site of action	Hormone structure	Receptor	Post-receptor activity
Corticotrophin-releasing hormone (CRH)	Hypothalamus	Pituitary	Peptide – 41 AA	Membrane – 7TM CRF1	G-proteins cAMP
Adrenocorticotrophic hormone (ACTH)	Pituitary	Adrenal	Peptide – 39 AA	Membrane – 7TM ACTHR (MCR2)	G-proteins cAMP
Cortisol	Adrenal	All tissues	Steroid ring	Nuclear GRα	Transcription GRE

7TM, 7 transmembrane (G-protein coupled receptor); AA, amino acids; GRE, glucocorticoid response element.

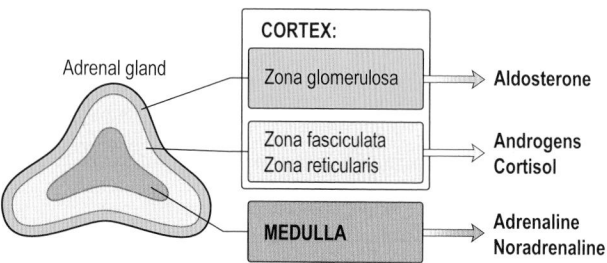

Fig. 21.12 The adrenal gland and its hormones.

i **Box 21.13** The major actions of glucocorticoids

Increased or stimulated:
- Gluconeogenesis
- Glycogen deposition
- Protein catabolism
- Fat deposition
- Sodium retention
- Potassium loss
- Free water clearance
- Uric acid production
- Circulating neutrophils

Decreased or inhibited:
- Protein synthesis
- Host response to infection
- Lymphocyte transformation
- Delayed hypersensitivity
- Circulating lymphocytes
- Circulating eosinophils

i **Box 21.14** The relative potency of equal amounts of common natural and synthetic steroids

Steroid	Glucocorticoid effect	Mineralocorticoid effect
Cortisol (hydrocortisone)[a]	1	1
Prednisolone	4	0.7
Dexamethasone	40	2
Aldosterone	0.1	400
Fludrocortisone	10	400

[a]Cortisol is arbitrarily defined as 1.

HYPOTHALAMO–PITUITARY–ADRENAL AXIS

Anatomy and physiology

The human adrenals (**Box 21.12**) together weigh 8–10 g and comprise an outer cortex and inner medulla. The cortex has three zones: the zona glomerulosa, which secretes aldosterone under the control of the renin–angiotensin system, and the zona fasciculata and zona reticularis, which produce glucocorticoids, cortisol, and sex steroids and androgens under feedback control of the hypothalamic–pituitary–adrenal (HPA) axis. The inner medulla synthesizes, stores and secretes catecholamines (see later and **Fig. 21.12**).

The adrenal cortex

The steroids produced by the adrenal cortex are grouped into three classes, based on their predominant physiological effects: glucocorticoids, mineralocorticoids and androgens.

Glucocorticoids

These are named after their effects on carbohydrate metabolism. Major actions are listed in **Box 21.13**. They act on intracellular corticosteroid receptors and combine with coactivating proteins to bind the 'glucocorticoid response element' (GRE) in specific regions of DNA to cause gene transcription. Glucocorticoid action is modified locally by the action of 11β-hydroxysteroid dehydrogenase (11βHSD). 11βHSD type 1 converts inactive cortisone into active cortisol, hence amplifying the hormone signal, while 11βHSD type 2 does the opposite.

The relative potency of common steroids is shown in **Box 21.14**.

Mineralocorticoids

The predominant effect of mineralocorticoids is on the extracellular balance of sodium and potassium in the distal tubule of the kidney. Aldosterone, produced solely in the zona glomerulosa, is the predominant mineralocorticoid in humans (about 50%); corticosterone makes a small contribution to overall mineralocorticoid activity. Mineralocorticoids act on type 1 corticosteroid receptors, while glucocorticoids act on type 2 receptors, both having a very similar structure. The mineralocorticoid activity of cortisol is weak but cortisol is present in considerable excess. The mineralocorticoid receptor in the kidney is protected from this excess by the intrarenal conversion ('shuttle') of cortisol to cortisone by 11βHSD type 2.

Androgens

Although secreted in considerable quantities, most androgens have relatively weak intrinsic androgenic activity until metabolized peripherally to testosterone or dihydrotestosterone. Dihydrotestosterone is metabolized from testosterone by 5α-reductase and is a potent androgen receptor agonist. The androgen receptor has been well characterized and mutations within this gene may cause androgen insensitivity syndromes.

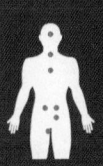

A

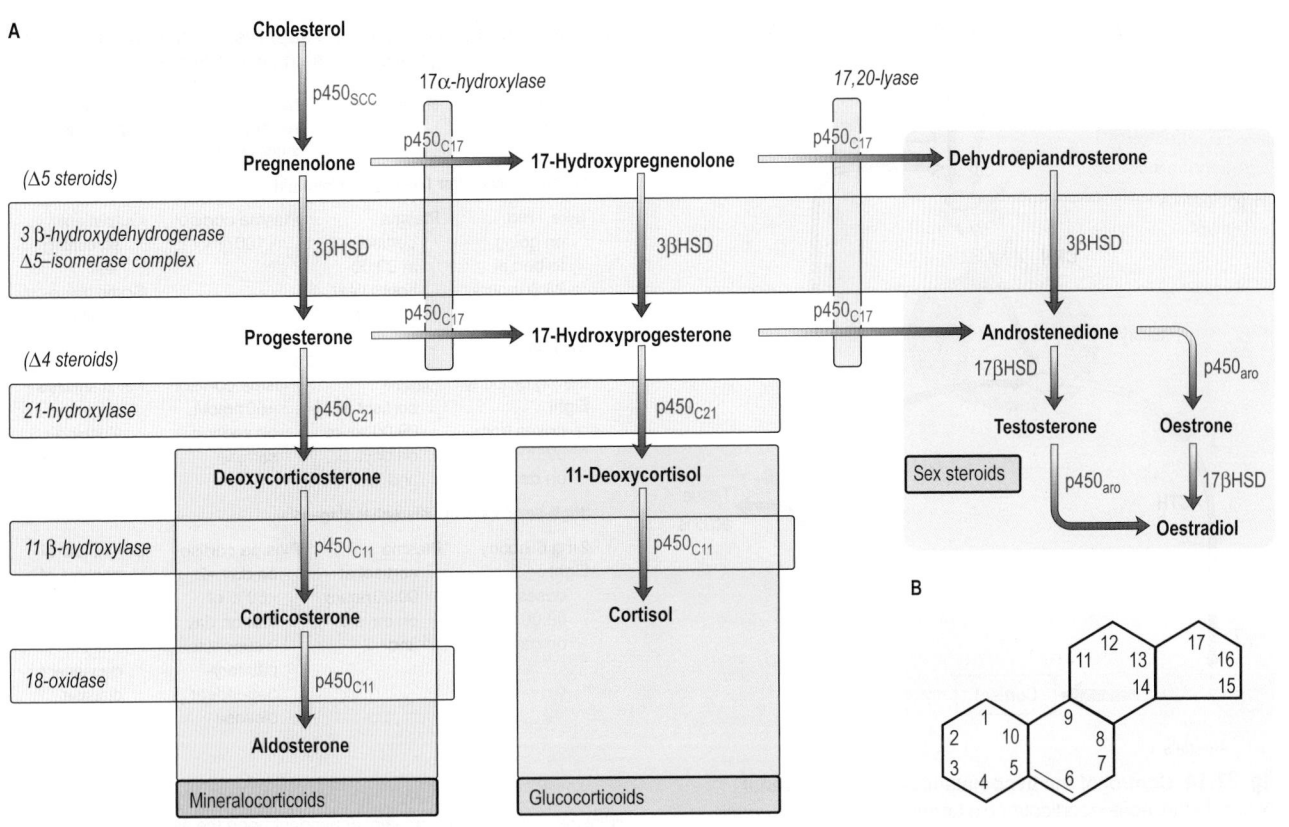

Fig. 21.13 Steroid pathways and molecule. (A) The major steroid biosynthetic pathways. Steroid hormones are synthesized in the adrenal glands and gonads from the initial substrate via a series of interconnected enzymatic steps. The reactions catalysed are shown by shaded boxes with italic labels. The molecular identity of the enzymes is shown in red; some catalyse more than one reaction. The p450 enzymes are in mitochondria, 3β-hydroxysteroid dehydrogenase (3βHSD) in cytoplasm; 17βHSD and p450aro (aromatase) are found mainly in gonads. **(B)** The steroid molecule.

Biochemistry

All steroids have the same basic skeleton (**Fig. 21.13B**) and the chemical differences between them are slight. The major biosynthetic pathways are shown in **Fig. 21.13A**.

Physiology

Glucocorticoid production by the adrenal is under hypothalamic–pituitary control (**Fig. 21.14**).

Corticotrophin-releasing hormone (CRH) is secreted in the hypothalamus in response to circadian rhythm, stress and other stimuli. CRH travels down the portal system to stimulate *adrenocorticotrophin (ACTH)* release from the anterior pituitary. Hypothalamic vasopressin (antidiuretic hormone, ADH) also stimulates ACTH secretion and acts synergistically. ACTH is derived from the prohormone pro-opiomelanocortin (POMC), which undergoes processing within the pituitary to produce ACTH and a number of other peptides, including beta-lipotrophin and beta-endorphin. Many of these peptides, including ACTH, contain melanocyte-stimulating hormone (MSH)-like sequences, which cause pigmentation when levels of ACTH are markedly raised as in Addison's disease.

Circulating ACTH stimulates cortisol production in the adrenal. The secreted cortisol (or any other synthetic corticosteroid administered to the patient) causes negative feedback on the hypothalamus and pituitary to inhibit further CRH/ACTH release. The set-point of this system varies through the day according to the circadian rhythm, and is usually overridden by severe stress. Unlike cortisol, mineralocorticoids and sex steroids do not cause negative feedback on the CRH/ACTH axis.

Following adrenalectomy or other adrenal damage (e.g. Addison's disease), cortisol secretion is absent or reduced; ACTH levels will therefore rise.

Mineralocorticoid secretion is mainly controlled by the renin–angiotensin system (see p. 1346).

Investigation of glucocorticoid abnormalities
Basal levels

Cortisol has a circadian rhythm and increases in response to stress. When taking a blood sample, remember:

- Sampling time should be recorded.
- Basal cortisol levels should be taken between 8am and 10am, near the peak of the circadian variation, if investigating for deficiency
- Stress should be minimized
- Appropriate reference ranges (for time and assay method) should be used.

The measurement of ACTH levels are only really required once an abnormality in cortisol levels has been identified. A plasma sample is required and has to be transported on ice to the lab immediately.

Suppression tests are used if excess cortisol is suspected, and stimulation tests are used if cortisol deficiency is suspected.

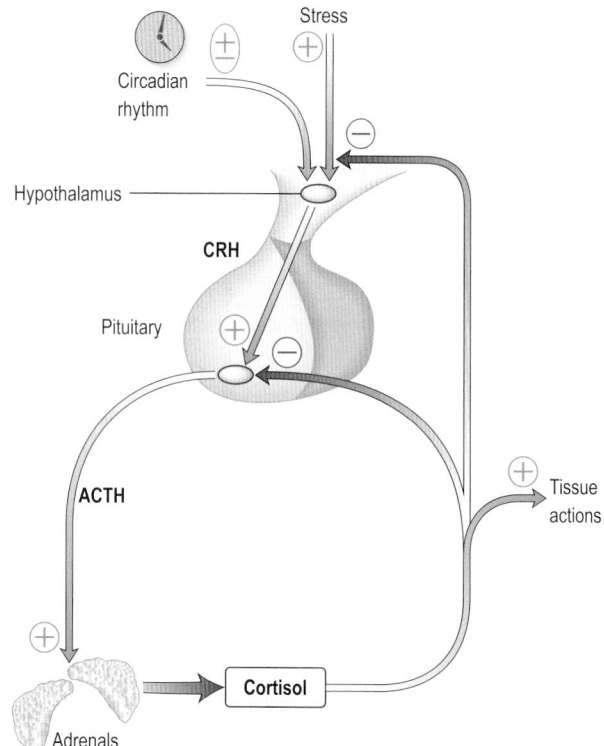

Fig. 21.14 Control of the hypothalamic–pituitary–adrenal axis. Pituitary adrenocorticotrophic hormone (ACTH) is secreted in response to hypothalamic corticotrophin-releasing hormone (CRH), triggered by circadian rhythm, stress and other factors, and stimulates secretion of cortisol from the adrenal. Cortisol has multiple actions in peripheral tissues and exerts negative feedback on the pituitary and hypothalamus.

Dexamethasone suppression tests

Administration of a synthetic glucocorticoid (dexamethasone) to a normal subject produces suppression of CRH and ACTH levels, and thus of endogenous cortisol secretion (dexamethasone is not measured by most cortisol assays). Three forms of the test, used in the diagnosis and differential diagnosis of Cushing's syndrome, are available (**Box 21.15**).

ACTH stimulation tests

Synthetic ACTH (tetracosactide, which consists of the first 24 amino acids of human ACTH) is given to stimulate adrenal cortisol production (see **Box 21.5** and **Fig. 21.5**).

Cushing's syndrome

Cushing's syndrome describes the clinical state of increased free circulating glucocorticoid. It is most often iatrogenic following the therapeutic administration of synthetic steroids. The next most common cause is excess endogenous secretion of ACTH from a pituitary adenoma, when it is called Cushing's disease (see below).

Pathophysiology and aetiology

Spontaneous Cushing's syndrome is rare, with an incidence of fewer than 5/million per year.

Causes of Cushing's syndrome are usually subdivided into two groups (**Box 21.16**):

- Increased circulating ACTH from the pituitary (65% of cases), known as Cushing's disease, or from an 'ectopic', non-pituitary,

---

Box 21.15 Dexamethasone suppression test in the diagnosis of Cushing's syndrome

Test and protocol	Measurement[a]	Normal test result or positive suppression	Use and explanation
Dexamethasone (for Cushing's): overnight			
Take 1 mg on going to bed at 23:00 hours	Plasma cortisol at 09:00 hours next morning	Plasma cortisol <100 nmol/L	Outpatient screening test Some 'false-positives'
'Low-dose'			
0.5 mg 6-hourly Eight doses from 09:00 hours on day 0	Plasma cortisol at 09:00 hours on days 0 and +2	Plasma cortisol <50 nmol/L on second sample	For diagnosis of Cushing's syndrome
'High-dose' used in differential diagnosis			
2 mg 6-hourly Eight doses from 09:00 hours on day 0	Plasma cortisol at 09:00 hours on days 0 and +2	Plasma cortisol on day +2 <50% of that on day 0 suggests pituitary-dependent disease	Differential diagnosis of Cushing's syndrome Pituitary-dependent disease suppresses in about 90% of cases

[a]Plasma cortisol values are very dependent upon the assay used; local reference ranges must be consulted.

Box 21.16 Causes of Cushing's syndrome

ACTH-dependent disease
- Pituitary-dependent (Cushing's disease)
- Ectopic ACTH-producing tumours

Non-ACTH-dependent disease
- Adrenal adenomas
- Adrenal carcinomas
- Exogenous steroids

ACTH, adrenocorticotrophic hormone.

ACTH-producing tumour elsewhere in the body (10%) with consequent glucocorticoid excess ('ACTH-dependent' Cushing's).
- A primary excess of endogenous cortisol secretion (25%) by an adrenal tumour or, more rarely, by bilateral primary pigmented nodular hyperplasia (PPNH) with suppression of ACTH ('non-ACTH-dependent' Cushing's). Rare cases are due to aberrant expression of receptors for other hormones (e.g. glucose-dependent insulinotrophic peptide (GIP), LH or catecholamines) in adrenal cortical cells. Germline changes in protein kinase A (PKA) can also result in adrenal hyperplasia and adenomas.

History and examination

The clinical features of Cushing's syndrome are illustrated in **Fig. 21.15**.
- **Pigmentation** occurs only with ACTH-dependent causes (most frequently in ectopic ACTH syndrome).
- **A cushingoid appearance** can also be caused by excess alcohol consumption (pseudo-Cushing's syndrome); the pathophysiology is poorly understood.

Symptoms	
General	
Change of appearance	
Weight gain (central)	
Hair growth/acne	
Thin skin/easy bruising	
Mental changes	
Depression	
Psychosis	
Insomnia	
Muscular weakness	
Back pain	
Amenorrhoea/oligomenorrhoea	
Poor libido	
Growth arrest in children	
Polyuria/polydipsia	
Old photographs may be useful	

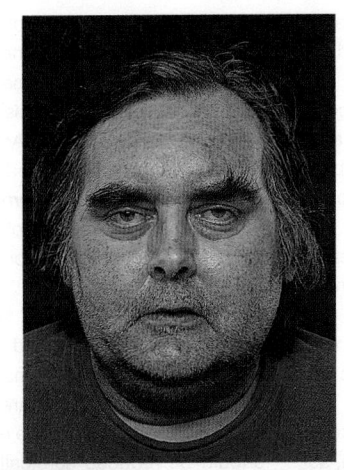
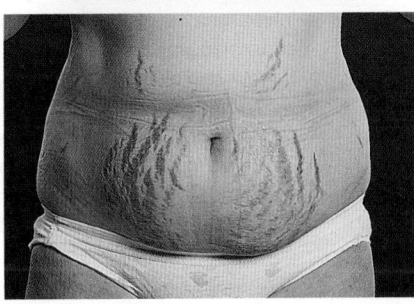

Signs	
General	**Proximal myopathy**
Plethora	Proximal muscle wasting
Moon face	
Hypertension	
'Buffalo hump'	
Central obesity	
Depression/psychosis	
Glycosuria	
Oedema	
Skin	
Thin skin	
Hirsutism	
Acne	
Bruising	
Poor wound healing	
Skin infections	
Striae (purple or red)	
Pigmentation	
Musculoskeletal	
Osteoporosis	
Pathological fractures (esp. vertebrae and ribs)	
Kyphosis	
Rib fractures	

Fig. 21.15 Cushing's syndrome: symptoms and signs. *Bold italic* type indicates signs of most value in discriminating Cushing's syndrome from simple obesity and hirsutism.

- *Impaired glucose tolerance* or frank diabetes is common, especially with ectopic ACTH.
- *Hypokalaemia* due to the mineralocorticoid activity of cortisol is common with ectopic ACTH secretion.
- *Hypertension* is common in all causes of Cushing's syndrome.

Investigations

There are two phases to investigation.

Confirmation

Most patients with obesity and hypertension or women with obesity and hirsutism do not have Cushing's syndrome, but some cases of genuine Cushing's can also relatively subtle clinical signs. Confirmation rests on demonstrating inappropriate cortisol secretion that is not suppressed by exogenous glucocorticoids; difficulties occur with obesity and depression, where cortisol dynamics are often abnormal. Random cortisol measurements are of no value. Occasional patients are seen with 'cyclical Cushing's', in which the abnormalities come and go.

Investigations to confirm the diagnosis include:

- *48-h low-dose dexamethasone test* (see **Box 21.15**). Normal individuals suppress plasma cortisol to less than 50 nmol/L. People with Cushing's syndrome fail to show complete suppression of plasma cortisol levels (although levels may fall substantially in a few cases). This test is highly sensitive (>97%). The overnight dexamethasone test is simpler but has a higher false-positive rate so often used as an initial screening test, before progressing to the longer test.
- *24-hour urinary free cortisol measurements.* This is another screening test. It is simple but less reliable; repeatedly normal values render the diagnosis unlikely, but some people with Cushing's syndrome have normal values on some collections (approximately 10%).

- *Circadian rhythm.* After 48 h in hospital, cortisol samples are taken at 09:00 hours and 24:00 hours (without warning the patient and ideally when they are asleep). Normal subjects show a pronounced circadian variation (see Fig. 21.4); those with Cushing's syndrome have high midnight cortisol levels (>100 nmol/L), though the 09:00 hours value may be normal. Increasingly, loss of circadian rhythm recorded using *midnight or late-night salivary cortisol* collected at home can be used for the diagnosis and surveillance of Cushing's, removing the need for a hospital stay.
- *Other tests.* There are frequent exceptions to the classic responses to diagnostic tests in Cushing's syndrome. If any clinical suspicion of Cushing's remains after preliminary tests, then specialist investigations are still indicated. These *may include the insulin stress test, desmopressin stimulation test* (see **Box 21.53**) *and corticotrophin releasing hormone (CRH)* tests.

Differential diagnosis of the cause

This can be extremely difficult on symptoms and signs alone since all causes can result in clinically identical Cushing's syndrome. The classical ectopic ACTH syndrome is distinguished by a short history, pigmentation, weight loss, hypokalaemia, diabetes and plasma ACTH levels above 200 ng/L, but many ectopic tumours are benign and mimic pituitary disease closely, both clinically and biochemically. Severe hirsutism/virilization suggests an adrenal tumour.

Biochemical and radiological procedures for diagnosis include:

- If *plasma ACTH levels* are low or undetectable (<10 ng/L) on two or more occasions, this is a reliable indicator of non-ACTH-dependent disease and adrenal imaging should be planned, using *adrenal CT or MRI scan*. Adrenal adenomas and carcinomas causing Cushing's syndrome are relatively large and always detectable by CT. Carcinomas are distinguished by their large size and irregular outline, and signs of infiltration or metastases. Bilateral adrenal hyperplasia may be seen in ACTH-dependent causes or in ACTH-independent nodular hyperplasia.

- If **plasma ACTH levels** are normal or high on two or more occasions, this is a reliable indicator of ACTH-dependent disease and pituitary imaging should be planned in the first instance and biochemical tests to distinguish between pituitary and ectopic sources of ACTH.
- **Pituitary MRI.** A pituitary adenoma may be seen but the adenoma is often small and not visible in a significant proportion of cases.
- **High-dose dexamethasone suppression test** (see **Box 21.15**). Failure of significant plasma cortisol suppression suggests an ectopic source of ACTH (or an adrenal tumour).
- **CRH test.** An exaggerated ACTH and cortisol response to exogenous CRH suggests pituitary-dependent Cushing's disease, as ectopic sources rarely respond.
- **Chest X-ray.** A carcinoma of the bronchus or a bronchial carcinoid is sought. Carcinoid lesions may be very small; if ectopic ACTH is suspected, whole-lung, mediastinal and abdominal **CT scanning** should be performed.
  Further investigations may involve:
- **Selective catheterization** of the inferior petrosal sinus to measure ACTH for pituitary lesions, or blood samples taken throughout the body to look for ectopic sources.
- **Radiolabelled octreotide** (^{111}In octreotide) is occasionally helpful in locating ectopic ACTH sites.

Management
Cushing's syndrome

Successful treatment with a normal biochemical profile should lead to reversal of clinical features. However, untreated Cushing's syndrome has a very poor prognosis, with death from venous thromboembolism, hypertension, myocardial infarction, infection and heart failure. Whatever the underlying cause, cortisol hypersecretion should be controlled prior to surgery or radiotherapy. Considerable morbidity and mortality are otherwise associated with operating on unprepared patients, especially when abdominal surgery is required.

The usual drug is **metyrapone**, an 11β-hydroxylase blocker, which is given in doses of 750 mg to 4 g daily in 3–4 divided doses. **Ketoconazole** (200 mg three times daily) is also used and is synergistic with metyrapone. Plasma cortisol should be monitored, aiming to reduce the mean level during the day to 150–300 nmol/L, equivalent to normal production rates. **Aminoglutethimide**, **trilostane** (which reversibly inhibits 3-hydroxysteroid dehydrogenase/5–5,4 isomers) and **etomidate** infusion (in severe cases) are occasionally used.

Choice of further treatment depends upon the cause.

Cushing's disease (pituitary-dependent hypercortisolism)

- **Trans-sphenoidal removal of the tumour** is the treatment of choice. Selective adenomectomy nearly always leaves the patient ACTH-deficient immediately postoperatively, and this is a good prognostic sign. Overall, pituitary surgery results in remission in 75–80% of cases, but results vary considerably and an experienced surgeon is essential.
- **External pituitary irradiation** alone is slow-acting, only effective in 50–60% even after prolonged follow-up, and mainly used after failed pituitary surgery. Children respond much better to radiotherapy, 80% being cured. Stereotactic radiotherapy can be useful in selected cases.

- **Medical therapy** to reduce ACTH (e.g. bromocriptine, cabergoline and cyproheptadine) is rarely effective. The somatostatin analogue pasireotide may provide medical control of Cushing's in some patients, but is associated with hyperglycaemia as a common side-effect. Aggressive corticotroph adenomas may respond to temozolomide chemotherapy.
- **Bilateral adrenalectomy** is an effective last resort if other measures fail to control the disease (see 'Nelson's syndrome' later). This can be performed laparoscopically.

Cushing's syndrome due to other causes

Adrenal adenomas should be resected laparoscopically. Contralateral adrenal suppression may last for a year or more.

Adrenal carcinomas are highly aggressive and the prognosis is poor. In general, if there are no widespread metastases, tumour bulk should be reduced surgically. The adrenolytic drug mitotane may inhibit growth of the tumour and prolong survival, though it can cause nausea and ataxia. Some would also give radiotherapy to the tumour bed after surgery.

Tumours secreting ACTH ectopically should be removed if possible. Otherwise chemotherapy/radiotherapy may be used, depending on the tumour. Control of the Cushing's syndrome with metyrapone or ketoconazole is beneficial for symptoms, and bilateral adrenalectomy may be appropriate to give complete control of Cushing's syndrome if prognosis from the tumour itself is reasonable.

If the source of ACTH is not clear, cortisol hypersecretion should be controlled with medical therapy until a diagnosis can be made.

Nelson's syndrome

Nelson's syndrome occurs in about 20% of cases after bilateral adrenalectomy for Cushing's disease and is characterized by increased pigmentation (because of high levels of ACTH), associated with an enlarging pituitary tumour. The syndrome is rare now that adrenalectomy is an uncommon primary treatment, and its incidence may be reduced by pituitary radiotherapy soon after adrenalectomy. The Nelson's adenoma may be treated by pituitary surgery and/or radiotherapy (unless given previously).

Further reading

Colao A, Petersenn S, Newell-Price J et al. A 12-month phase 3 study of pasireotide in Cushing's disease. *N Engl J Med* 2012; 366:914–924.

Drake WM, Stiles CE, Howlett TA et al. A cross-sectional study of the prevalence of cardiac valvular abnormalities in hyperprolactinemic patients treated with ergot-derived dopamine agonists. *J Clin Endocrinol Metab* 2014; 99:90–6.

Feelders RA, Hofland LJ. Medical treatment of Cushing's disease. *J Clin Endocrinol Metab* 2013; 98:425–438.

Howlett TA, Willis D, Walker G et al. Control of growth hormone and IGF1 in patients with acromegaly in the UK: responses to medical treatment with somatostatin analogues and dopamine agonists. *Clin Endocrinol* 2013; 79: 689–699.

Klibanski A. Prolactinomas. *N Engl J Med* 2010; 362:1219–1226.

Addison's disease
Pathophysiology and aetiology

In this condition, there is destruction of the entire adrenal cortex. Glucocorticoid, mineralocorticoid and sex steroid production are therefore all reduced. This differs from hypothalamic–pituitary disease, in which mineralocorticoid secretion remains largely intact, being predominantly stimulated by angiotensin II. Adrenal sex steroid production is also largely independent of pituitary action. In Addison's disease, reduced cortisol levels lead, through feedback, to increased CRH and ACTH production, the latter being directly responsible for the hyperpigmentation.

Addison's disease is rare, with an incidence of 3–4/million per year and prevalence of 40–60/million. Primary adrenal insufficiency shows a marked female preponderance and is usually caused by autoimmune disease (>90% in the UK), but in countries with a high prevalence of HIV/AIDS, tuberculosis is an increasing cause. Autoimmune adrenalitis results from the destruction of the adrenal cortex by organ-specific autoantibodies, with 21-hydroxylase as the common antigen. There are associations with other autoimmune conditions in polyglandular autoimmune syndromes types I and II (e.g. type 1 diabetes mellitus, pernicious anaemia, thyroiditis, hypoparathyroidism, premature ovarian insufficiency; see p. 648).

All other causes are rare (**Box 21.17**). In patients with degenerative neurological symptoms, a diagnosis of adrenoleukodystrophy should be excluded. In childhood the most common cause of primary adrenal insufficiency is congenital adrenal hyperplasia (CAH).

History and examination

See **Fig. 21.16**. The symptomatology of Addison's disease is often non-specific. These symptoms may be the prelude to an addisonian crisis with severe hypotension and dehydration precipitated by intercurrent illness, accident or operation.

Pigmentation (dull, slaty, grey–brown) is the predominant sign in over 90% of cases.

Postural systolic hypotension, due to hypovolaemia and sodium loss, is present in 80–90% of cases, even if supine blood pressure is normal. Mineralocorticoid deficiency is the cause of the hypotension.

? Box 21.17 Causes of primary hypoadrenalism

- Autoimmune disease
- Tuberculosis (<10% in UK)
- Surgical removal
- Haemorrhage/infarction:
  – Meningococcal septicaemia
  – Venography
- Infiltration:
  – Malignant destruction
  – Amyloid
- Schilder's disease (adrenal leukodystrophy)

Investigations

Once Addison's disease is suspected, investigation is urgent. If the patient is seriously ill or hypotensive, hydrocortisone 100 mg should be given intravenously or intramuscularly, together with intravenous 0.9% saline. Ideally, this should be done immediately after a blood sample is taken for later measurement of plasma cortisol. Full investigation should be delayed until emergency treatment (see below) has improved the patient's condition. Otherwise, tests are as follows:

- **Single cortisol measurements** are of little value, although a random cortisol below 100 nmol/L during the day is highly suggestive, and a random cortisol higher than 550 nmol/L makes the diagnosis unlikely.
- **The short ACTH stimulation test** should be performed (see Box 21.5 and Fig. 21.5). Note that an absent or impaired cortisol response confirms the presence of hypoadrenalism but does not differentiate Addison's disease from ACTH deficiency or iatrogenic suppression by steroid medication. The long ACTH test is no longer used because of the availability of accurate ACTH assays.
- **A 09:00-hours plasma ACTH level** is measured, a high level (>80 ng/L) with low cortisol confirming primary adrenal insufficiency.
- **Adrenal antibodies** are present in approximately 90% of cases of autoimmune adrenalitis.
- **Chest and abdominal X-rays** or cross-sectional imaging of the abdomen (CT or MRI) may show evidence of tuberculosis and/or calcified adrenals (**Fig. 21.17**).
- **Plasma renin activity** is high due to low serum aldosterone.
- **Serum creatinine and electrolytes** classically show hyponatraemia, hyperkalaemia and a high urea, but they can be normal.
- **Blood glucose** may be low, with hypoglycaemia.
- **Hypercalcaemia and anaemia** (after rehydration) are sometimes seen.

Management

Acute hypoadrenalism needs urgent treatment (**Box 21.18**).

Symptoms
Weight loss
Malaise
Weakness
Fever
Anorexia
Nausea/vomiting
Diarrhoea
Abdominal pain
Constipation
Depression
Confusion
Myalgia
Joint or back pain
Impotence/amenorrhoea
Syncope from postural hypotension

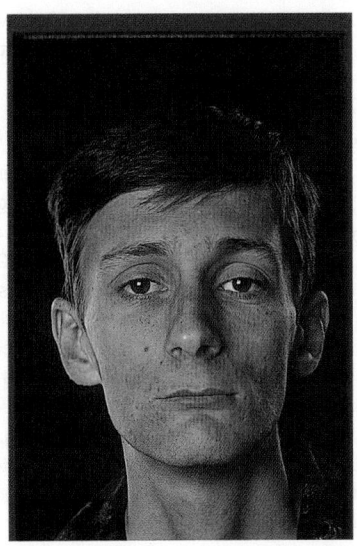

Signs
General
Loss of weight
General wasting
Pigmentation, especially of new scars and palmar creases
Buccal pigmentation
Postural hypotension
Loss of body hair (vitiligo)
Dehydration

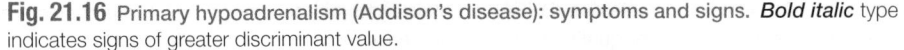

Fig. 21.16 Primary hypoadrenalism (Addison's disease): symptoms and signs. *Bold italic* type indicates signs of greater discriminant value.

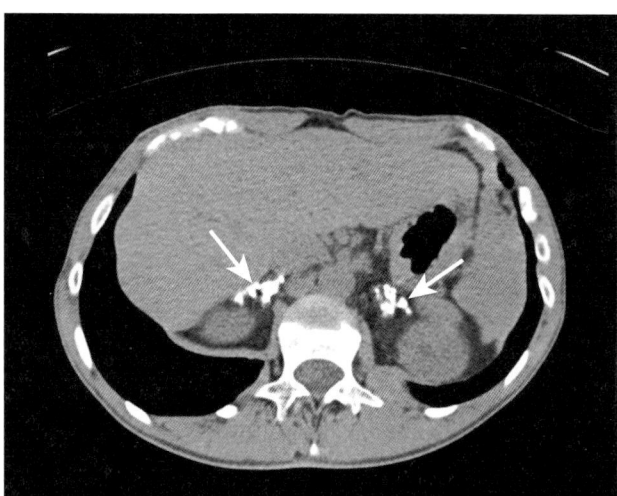

Fig. 21.17 CT scan showing bilateral adrenal calcification.

Box 21.18 Management of acute hypoadrenalism

Clinical context
Hypotension, hyponatraemia, hyperkalaemia, hypoglycaemia, dehydration, pigmentation often with precipitating infection, infarction, trauma or operation. The major deficiencies are of salt, steroid and glucose.

Requirements
Assuming normal cardiovascular function, the following are required:
• 1 L of 0.9% saline should be given over 30–60 min with 100 mg of i.v. bolus hydrocortisone
• Subsequent requirements are several litres of saline within 24 h (assessing with central venous pressure line if necessary) plus hydrocortisone, 100 mg i.m., 6-hourly, until the patient is clinically stable
• Glucose should be infused if there is hypoglycaemia
• Oral replacement medication is then started, unless the patient is unable to take oral medication: initially, hydrocortisone 20 mg, 8-hourly, reducing to 20–30 mg in divided doses over a few days (see **Box 21.19**)
• Fludrocortisone is unnecessary acutely, as the high cortisol doses provide sufficient mineralocorticoid activity – it should be introduced before discharge

i **Box 21.19 Average replacement steroid dosages for adults with primary hypoadrenalism**

Drug	Dose
Glucocorticoid	
Hydrocortisone	20–30 mg daily (e.g. 10 mg on waking, 5 mg at 12:00 hours, 5 mg at 18:00 hours)
rarely	
Prednisolone	7.5 mg daily (5 mg on waking, 2.5 mg at 18:00 hours)
very rarely	
Dexamethasone	0.75 mg daily (0.5 mg on waking, 0.25 mg at 18:00 hours)
Mineralocorticoid	
Fludrocortisone	50–300 µg daily

Long-term treatment is with replacement glucocorticoid and mineralocorticoid; tuberculosis must be treated if present or suspected. Replacement dosage details are shown in **Box 21.19**. Dual-release, oral, once-daily hydrocortisone preparations are becoming increasingly available. Dehydroepiandrosterone (DHEA) replacement has also been advocated by some for quality of life;

some studies suggest that this may cause symptomatic improvements, although others show no clear benefit and acne and hirsutism occur.

Adequacy of glucocorticoid dose is judged by:
• clinical wellbeing and restoration of normal, but not excessive, weight; ideally aiming for a low dose, for example, total dose of hydrocortisone between 15 and 25 mg split in two or three divided doses throughout the day
• measuring cortisol levels during the day while on replacement hydrocortisone (cortisol levels cannot be used for synthetic steroids) is not recommended as an assessment of dose adequacy.

Adequacy of fludrocortisone replacement is assessed by:
• restoration of serum electrolytes to normal
• no evidence of hypertension or postural hypotension (it should not fall >10 mmHg systolic after 2 minutes' standing)
• suppression of plasma renin activity to high normal.

Patient advice
All patients requiring replacement steroids should:
• know how to increase steroid replacement by doubling the dose for intercurrent illness
• carry a 'steroid card'
• wear a MedicAlert bracelet (or similar), which gives details of their condition so that emergency replacement therapy can be given if found unconscious
• keep an (up-to-date) ampoule of hydrocortisone at home in case oral therapy is impossible, for administration by self, family, ambulance or doctor.

Secondary hypoadrenalism
This may arise from:
• hypothalamic–pituitary disease (inadequate ACTH production) *or*
• long-term steroid therapy leading to ACTH suppression.

Most people with hypothalamic–pituitary disease have panhypopituitarism (see p. 595) and need T_4 replacement, as well as cortisol; in this case, hydrocortisone must be started before T_4.

Long-term corticosteroid medication for non-endocrine disease is the most common cause of secondary hypoadrenalism. The hypothalamic–pituitary axis and the adrenal may both be suppressed and the patient may have vague symptoms of feeling unwell. ACTH levels are low in secondary hypoadrenalism. Weaning off steroids is often a long and difficult process.

Congenital adrenal hyperplasia
Pathophysiology
Congenital adrenal hyperplasia (CAH) is an autosomal recessive disorder resulting in deficiency of an enzyme in the cortisol synthetic pathways. There are six major types; most common is 21-hydroxylase deficiency (CYP21A2), which occurs in about 1 in 15 000 births and is due to defects on chromosome 6 near the HLA region, affecting one of the cytochrome p450 enzymes (p450C21).

As a result, cortisol secretion is reduced and feedback leads to increased ACTH secretion, causing adrenal hyperplasia. Diversion of the steroid precursors into the androgenic steroid pathways occurs (see **Fig. 21.13A**). Thus, 17-hydroxyprogesterone, androstenedione and testosterone levels are increased, leading to virilization. Aldosterone synthesis may be impaired with resultant salt wasting.

The other forms affect 11β-hydroxylase, 17α-hydroxylase, 3β-hydroxysteroid dehydrogenase and a cholesterol side-chain cleavage enzyme (p450scc) (see **Fig. 21.13A**).

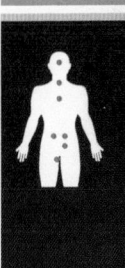
History and examination

Classical CAH presents at birth with:

- Ambiguous genitalia in females (clitoral hypertrophy, urogenital abnormalities and labioscrotal fusion are common) *or*
- Adrenal failure (collapse, hypotension, hypoglycaemia), sometimes with a salt-losing state (hypotension, hyponatraemia). The syndrome may be unrecognized in the male until a salt-losing crisis occurs, usually within 10 days of birth.

Non-classical disease presents later as precocious puberty with hirsutism; rare, milder cases present in adult life, usually accompanied by primary amenorrhoea. Hirsutism developing before puberty is suggestive of CAH.

Investigations

In many developed countries neonatal screening for CAH takes place by assessing 17OHP in dried blood spots soon after birth. This approach would prevent undiagnosed children presenting with adrenal failure and identify those that may present later with precocious puberty.

Expert advice is essential in the confirmation and differential diagnosis of 21-hydroxylase deficiency; with ambiguous genitalia, advice must be sought urgently before any assignment of gender is made.

Unless 17 OHP levels are very elevated (>30 nmol/L) a synacthen test should be performed with measurement of 17OHP and cortisol at 0 and 60 minutes. If 17OHP levels at baseline or after synacthen are above 30 nmol/L 21 hydroxylase deficiency is confirmed.

Assessment of mineralocorticoid activity is also required.

Management

Glucocorticoid activity must be replaced, as must mineralocorticoid activity if deficient. The practice in CAH of giving the larger dose of glucocorticoid at night to suppress the morning ACTH peak, with a smaller dose in the morning, is largely outdated. Correct dosage is often difficult to establish in the **child** but should ensure normal androstenedione and mildly elevated 17OHP levels while allowing normal growth; excessive replacement leads to stunting of growth. In **adults**, clinical features and biochemistry (plasma renin, androstenedione and 17-hydroxyprogesterone) are used to modify treatment. The use of modified-release hydrocortisone may have a role in the management of CAH.

Prenatal diagnosis

Prenatal genetic counselling is essential (see **Ch. 2**). There is a 1 : 4 chance of an affected child if one child in the family is already affected. In a parent with CAH, genetic testing of the partner provides important information about the risk of having an affected child. Dexamethasone can be offered to the mother as it may prevent virilization of an affected female fetus by suppressing ACTH levels. There are, however, concerns about the potential adverse consequences of this practice.

Problems of therapeutic steroid therapy

Apart from their use as therapeutic replacement for endocrine deficiency states, synthetic glucocorticoids are widely used for many non-endocrine conditions. Short-term use (e.g. for acute asthma) carries only small risks of significant side-effects, except for the simultaneous suppression of immune responses. The danger lies in their continuance, often through medical oversight or patient default. In general, therapy for 3 weeks or less, or a dose of

---

> **i** **Box 21.20** Major adverse effects of corticosteroid therapy

Physiological
- Adrenal suppression (secondary)

Pathological

Cardiovascular
- Increased blood pressure

Gastrointestinal
- Pancreatitis

Renal
- Polyuria
- Nocturia

Central nervous
- Depression
- Euphoria
- Psychosis
- Insomnia

Endocrine
- Weight gain
- Glycosuria/hyperglycaemia/diabetes

- Impaired growth
- Amenorrhoea

Bone and muscle
- Osteoporosis
- Proximal myopathy and wasting
- Avascular necrosis of the hip
- Pathological fractures

Skin
- Thinning
- Easy bruising

Eyes
- Cataracts

Increased susceptibility to infection
(Signs and fever are frequently masked)
- Septicaemia
- Fungal infections
- Reactivation of tuberculosis
- Skin infections (e.g. fungi)

---

prednisolone of less than 5 mg per day, will not result in significant long-term suppression of the normal adrenal axis.

Long-term therapy with synthetic or natural steroids will, in most respects, mimic endogenous Cushing's syndrome. Exceptions are the relative absence of hirsutism, acne, hypertension and severe sodium retention, as the common synthetic steroids have low androgenic and mineralocorticoid activity.

Excessive doses of steroids may also be absorbed from skin when strong dermatological preparations are used, and along with inhaled steroids may rarely cause Cushing's syndrome; they may, however, quite commonly cause adrenal suppression.

The major hazards are detailed in **Box 21.20**. In the long term, many are of such severity that the clinical need for high-dose steroids should be continually and critically assessed. Steroid-sparing agents should always be considered, and screening and prophylactic therapy for osteoporosis introduced (see p. 477). New targeted biological therapies for inflammatory conditions may reduce the incidence of steroid-induced adrenal suppression.

Supervision of steroid therapy

All patients receiving steroids should carry a 'steroid card'. They should be made aware of the following points:

- Long-term steroid therapy must never be stopped suddenly.
- Doses should be reduced very gradually, with most being given in the morning at the time of withdrawal; this minimizes adrenal suppression. Many believe that 'alternate-day therapy' produces less suppression.
- Depending on current dose, doses need to be increased at times of serious intercurrent illness, accident and stress. Double doses should be taken during these periods.
- Other physicians, anaesthetists and dentists must be told about steroid therapy.

Patients should also be informed of potential side-effects, and all this information should be documented in the clinical record. If prophylactic use of bisphosphonate therapy is required to prevent

Box 21.21 Steroid cover for operative procedures[a]

Procedure	Premedication	Intra- and postoperative	Resumption of normal maintenance
Simple procedures (e.g. gastroscopy, simple dental extractions)	Hydrocortisone 100 mg i.m.	–	Immediately if no complications and eating normally
Minor surgery (e.g. laparoscopic surgery, veins, hernias)	Hydrocortisone 100 mg i.m.	Hydrocortisone 20 mg orally 6-hourly or 50 mg i.m. 6-hourly for 24 h if not eating	After 24 h if no complications
Major surgery (e.g. hip replacement, vascular surgery)	Hydrocortisone 100 mg i.m.	Hydrocortisone 50–100 mg i.m. 6-hourly for 72 h	After 72 h if normal progress and no complications Perhaps double normal dose for 2–3 days
GI tract surgery or major thoracic surgery (not eating or ventilated)	Hydrocortisone 100 mg i.m.	Hydrocortisone 100 mg i.m. 6-hourly for 72 h or longer if still unwell	When patient eating normally again Until then, higher doses (to 50 mg 6-hourly) may be needed

[a]A useful summary of surgical steroid guidelines can be found at: http://www.addisons.org.uk/.

the development of osteoporosis (following NICE guidance), patients should be informed of the rationale.

Steroids and surgery

Any patient receiving steroids, or who has recently received a 4 week course of steroids (within the last 6 months) and may still have adrenal suppression, requires steroid cover around the time of surgery (**Box 21.21**).

Incidental adrenal tumours ('incidentalomas')

With the advent of abdominal CT, MRI and high-resolution ultrasound scanning, unsuspected adrenal masses have been discovered in 3–10% of scans (increasing with age). The two issues with an incidental adrenal mass are:
* whether the lesion is functional or non-functional
* whether it is benign or malignant.

Most incidentalomas are asymptomatic and benign, but direct questioning may reveal symptoms of endocrine hypersecretion such as cushingoid features, catecholamine excess, virilization in women, or evidence of endocrine hypertension (see **Box 31.2**).

Box 21.22 Endocrine causes of hypertension

Excessive renin, and thus angiotensin II, production
* Renal artery stenosis
* Other local renal disease
* Renin-secreting tumours

Excessive production of catecholamines
* Phaeochromocytoma

Excessive growth hormone (GH) production
* Acromegaly

Excessive aldosterone production
* Adrenal adenoma (Conn's syndrome)
* Idiopathic adrenal hyperplasia
* Dexamethasone-suppressible hyperaldosteronism

Excessive production of other mineralocorticoids
* Cushing's syndrome (massive excess of cortisol, a weak mineralocorticoid)
* Congenital adrenal hyperplasia (in rare cases)
* Tumours producing other mineralocorticoids, e.g. corticosterone

Exogenous 'mineralocorticoids' or enzyme inhibitors
* Liquorice ingestion (inhibits 11β-hydroxylase)
* Misuse of mineralocorticoid preparations

Even in the absence of symptoms, biochemical tests to exclude secretory activity should be performed, as adrenal adenomas often secrete cortisol at a low level – 'autonomous cortisol secretion', which may confer increased cardiovascular risk. If no endocrine activity is found, then most authorities recommend removal only of large adrenal tumours (>4–5 cm) because of the risk of malignancy. Smaller, hormonally inactive lesions are usually left alone.

Phaeochromocytoma must be excluded before surgery due to the risk of perioperative hypertensive or hypotensive crises (see p. 608).

Primary hyperaldosteronism

Increased mineralocorticoid secretion from the adrenal cortex, termed primary hyperaldosteronism, accounts for 5–10% of all hypertension. Other endocrine causes of hypertension should also be considered if there is clinical suspicion (**Box 21.22**). It is impracticable to screen all hypertensive patients for secondary endocrine causes. The highest chances of detecting such causes are in patients:
* under 35 years, especially those without a family history of hypertension
* with accelerated (malignant) hypertension
* with hypokalaemia
* resistant to conventional antihypertensive therapy (e.g. more than three drugs) *or*
* with unusual symptoms (e.g. sweating attacks or weakness).

Pathophysiology

Primary hyperaldosteronism is characterized by excess aldosterone production leading to sodium retention, potassium loss and the combination of hypokalaemia and hypertension. This must be distinguished from secondary hyperaldosteronism, which arises when there is excess renin (and hence angiotensin II) stimulation of the zona glomerulosa. Common causes of secondary hyperaldosteronism are accelerated hypertension and renal artery stenosis, when the patient will also be hypertensive. Causes associated with normotension include congestive cardiac failure and cirrhosis, where excess aldosterone production contributes to sodium retention.

Aetiology

Adrenal adenomas (Conn's syndrome; see **Box 21.22**) originally accounted for 60% of cases of primary hyperaldosteronism but represented a rare cause of hypertension. The use of the aldosterone:renin ratio in the routine investigation of hypertension now suggests that hyperaldosteronism due to bilateral adrenal hyperplasia (idiopathic hyperaldosteronism) is much more common than the classical Conn's adenoma.

History and examination

The usual presentation is simply hypertension; hypokalaemia (<3.5 mmol/L) is frequently not present. The few symptoms are non-specific; rarely, muscle weakness, nocturia and tetany are seen. Hypertension may be severe and associated with renal, cardiac and retinal damage.

Adenomas, often very small, are more common in young females, while bilateral hyperplasia rarely occurs before the age of 40 years and is more common in males.

Investigations

Beta-blockers and other drugs may interfere with renin activity, and spironolactone, angiotensin-converting enzyme (ACE) inhibitors and angiotensin II receptor antagonists will all affect results; all should be discontinued, if possible. The characteristic features of investigation are as follows:

- **Plasma aldosterone:renin ratio (ARR)** is now most frequently used as a screening test for the condition, but raised ARR alone does not confirm the diagnosis (if the renin is low enough, ARR will always be high). Note that normal ranges are highly assay-dependent.
- **Elevated plasma aldosterone levels** are not suppressed with 0.9% saline infusion (2 L over 4 h) or fludrocortisone administration. Between 30% and 50% of people with a raised ARR on screening will suppress normally, excluding the diagnosis.
- **Suppressed plasma renin activity** or immunoreactivity is seen.
- **Hypokalaemia** is often present but a normal potassium does not exclude the diagnosis.
- **Urinary potassium loss** greater than 30 mmol daily during hypokalaemia is inappropriate.

Once a diagnosis of hyperaldosteronism is established, differentiation of adenoma from hyperplasia involves adrenal CT or MRI, but small adenomas may be missed and non-functioning incidentalomas also occur. Further information is obtained from diurnal/postural changes in plasma aldosterone levels (which tend to rise with adenomas between 09:00 hours supine and 13:00 hours erect samples; in contrast, they fall with hyperplasia), measurement of 18-OH cortisol levels (raised in adenoma), and venous catheterization for aldosterone levels. All of these tests have pitfalls and exceptions.

Management

An adenoma can be removed surgically, usually laparoscopically; blood pressure falls in 70% of patients. Those with hyperplasia should be treated with the aldosterone antagonist, spironolactone (100–400 mg daily); frequent side-effects include nausea, rashes and gynaecomastia. The pure aldosterone receptor antagonist, eplerenone, is a useful alternative if side-effects preclude the use of spironolactone (see p. 179) Spironolactone metabolites have been linked with tumour development in animals but not in humans. Amiloride and calcium-channel blockers are moderately effective in controlling hypertension but do not correct the hyperaldosteronism.

Glucocorticoid (or dexamethasone)-suppressible hyperaldosteronism

This rare condition is caused by a chimeric gene on chromosome 8. A fusion gene resulting from an unusual crossover at meiosis between the genes encoding aldosterone synthase and adrenal 11β-hydroxylase produces aldosterone, which is under ACTH control. Treatment with glucocorticoid resolves the problem.

Syndrome of apparent mineralocorticoid excess

This causes the clinical syndrome of primary hyperaldosteronism but with low renin and aldosterone levels. Reduced activity of the enzyme 11β-hydroxysteroid dehydrogenase type 2 (11βHSD2) prevents the normal conversion in the kidney of cortisol (which is active at the mineralocorticoid receptor) to cortisone (which is not), and therefore 'exposes' the mineralocorticoid receptor in the kidney to the usual molar excess of cortisol over aldosterone in the blood. While the inherited syndrome is rare, the same clinical syndrome can occur with excessive ingestion of liquorice, which inhibits the 11βHSD2 enzyme.

The adrenal medulla

The adrenal medulla is the innermost part of the adrenal gland, consisting of cells that secrete the major catecholamines, noradrenaline (norepinephrine) and adrenaline (epinephrine), which produce the sympathetic nervous response. The catecholamines are interconverted in the adrenal medulla, and an increase in levels of their metabolites in the urine is a marker of abnormal hypersecretion (**Fig. 21.18**).

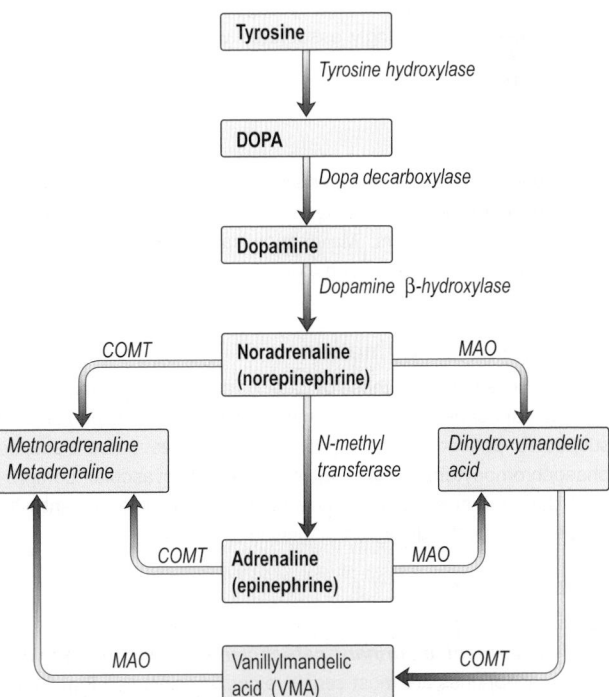

Fig. 21.18 The synthesis and metabolism of catecholamines. COMT, catechol-O-methyl transferase; MAO, monoamine oxidase.

Symptoms
- Anxiety or panic attacks
- Palpitations
- Tremor
- Sweating
- Headache
- Flushing
- Nausea and/or vomiting
- Weight loss
- Constipation or diarrhoea
- Raynaud's phenomenon
- Chest pain
- Polyuria/nocturia

Signs
- Hypertension
- Tachycardia/arrhythmias
- Bradycardia
- Orthostatic hypotension
- Pallor or flushing
- Glycosuria
- Fever
- (Signs of hypertensive damage)

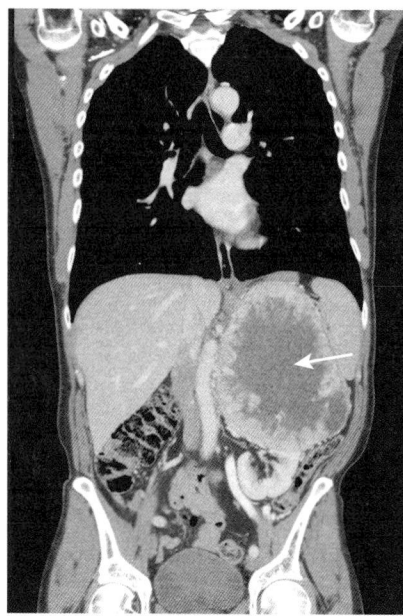

Fig. 21.19 MRI scan showing a massive left-sided phaeochromocytoma.

Phaeochromocytoma and paraganglioma

These are very rare tumours of the sympathetic nervous system (less than 1 in 1000 cases of hypertension) that secrete catecholamines, noradrenaline (norepinephrine), adrenaline (epinephrine) and their metabolites (see **Fig. 21.18**):

- 90% arise in the adrenal medulla (*phaeochromocytomas*)
- 10% occur elsewhere in the sympathetic chain (*paragangliomas*).

Some are associated with MEN 2 (see below), von Hippel–Lindau's (VHL) syndrome (see p. 887) and neurofibromatosis. Most tumours release both noradrenaline (norepinephrine) and adrenaline (epinephrine), but large tumours and extra-adrenal tumours produce almost entirely noradrenaline.

Paragangliomas typically occur in the head and neck but are also found in the thorax, pelvis and bladder. They are more closely associated with other genetic associations than phaeochromocytoma. The association of paraganglioma, bilateral adrenal phaeochromocytomas, positive family history or young age at presentation is seen in multiple endocrine neoplasms (see p. 650). Mutations in the succinate dehydrogenase (*SDHD*) gene have been shown to be strongly associated with the development of paraganglioma.

Pathology

Oval groups of cells occur in clusters and stain for chromogranin A; 25% are multiple and 10% malignant, the latter being more frequent in extra-adrenal tumours. Malignancy cannot be determined on simple histological examination alone.

History and examination

The clinical features are those of catecholamine excess and are frequently, but not necessarily, intermittent (**Box 21.23**). All people with suspected phaeochromocytomas must be investigated because phaeochromocytomas may cause acute cardiovascular compromise during routine medical procedures and can also present with sudden death if the diagnosis is missed.

Investigations

Specific tests are:

- **Measurement of urinary catecholamines and metabolites** (metanephrines are most sensitive and specific; see **Fig. 21.18**) is a useful screening test; normal levels on three 24-hour collections of metanephrines virtually exclude the diagnosis. Many drugs, e.g. tricyclics, and dietary vanilla interfere with these tests.
- **Resting plasma metanephrines** are raised.
- **Plasma chromogranin A** (a storage vesicle protein) is raised.
- **Clonidine suppression test** may be appropriate but should only be performed in specialist centres.
- **CT/MRI scans**, initially of the abdomen, are helpful to localize the tumours, which are often large (**Fig. 21.19**).
- **Scanning with [131I]meta-iodobenzylguanidine (MIBG)** produces specific uptake in sites of sympathetic activity with about 90% success. It is particularly useful with extra-adrenal tumours. ^{18}F-deoxyglucose positron emission tomography (PET) is also used by some centres (**Fig. 21.20**).
- **Genetic testing** for *MEN2*, *VHL*, *SDHB* and *SDHD* mutations should be performed in all people with confirmed phaeochromocytoma or paraganglioma.

Management

Tumours should be removed if possible; 5-year survival is about 95% for non-malignant tumours. Medical preoperative and perioperative treatment is vital and includes complete alpha- and beta-blockade with phenoxybenzamine (20–80 mg daily in divided doses), then propranolol (120–240 mg daily), plus intravenous hydration to re-expand the contracted plasma volume. Alpha-blockade must precede the beta-blockade, as worsened hypertension may otherwise result. Labetalol is not recommended. Surgery in the unprepared patient is fraught with dangers of both hypertension and hypotension; expert anaesthesia and an experienced surgeon are vital, and sodium nitroprusside, phentolamine (a rapid-acting α-blocker) and magnesium should be available in case sudden severe hypertension develops.

When operation is not possible, combined alpha- and beta-blockade can be used long term. Radionucleotide treatment with MIBG has been employed but has had limited success in malignant phaeochromocytoma.

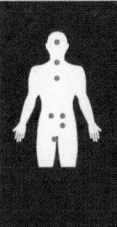

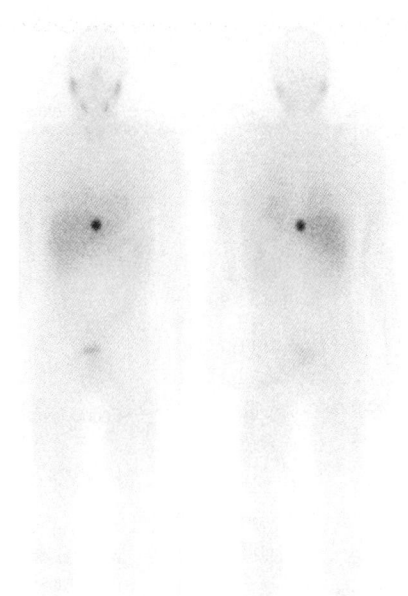

Fig. 21.20 MIBG scan showing a solitary area of increased uptake in the liver consistent with metastasis from a phaeochromocytoma. MIBG, meta-iodobenzylguanidine.

Patients should be kept under clinical and biochemical review after tumour resection, as over 10% of tumours recur or a further tumour develops. Catecholamine excretion measurements should be performed at least annually.

Further reading

Auchus RJ, Arlt W. Approach to the patient: the adult with congenital adrenal hyperplasia. *J Clin Endocrinol Metab* 2013; 98:2645–2655.
Lenders JW, Duh QY, Eisenhofer G et al and the Endocrine Society. Pheochromocytoma and paraganglioma: an Endocrine Society clinical practice guideline. *J Clin Endocrinol Metab* 2014; 99:1915–1942.
Merke DP, Bornstein SR. Congenital adrenal hyperplasia. *Lancet* 2005; 365:2125–2136.
Van Nederveen FH, Korpershoek E, Lenders JW et al. Somatic SDHB mutation in an extraadrenal phaeochromocytoma. *N Engl J Med* 2007; 357:306–308.
Young WF. The incidentally discovered adrenal mass. *N Engl J Med* 2007; 356:601–610.

THE THYROID AXIS

The metabolism of virtually all nucleated cells of many tissues is controlled by the thyroid hormones. Overactivity or underactivity of the gland is the most common of all endocrine problems.

Anatomy and physiology

Anatomy

The thyroid gland consists of two lateral lobes connected by an isthmus. It is closely attached to the thyroid cartilage and to the upper end of the trachea, and thus moves on swallowing. It is often palpable in healthy women.

Embryologically, it originates from the base of the tongue and descends to the middle of the neck. Remnants of thyroid tissue can sometimes be found at the base of the tongue (lingual thyroid) and along the line of descent. The gland has a rich blood supply from superior and inferior thyroid arteries.

The thyroid gland consists of follicles lined by cuboidal epithelioid cells. Inside is the colloid (the iodinated glycoprotein thyroglobulin), which is synthesized by the follicular cells. Each follicle is surrounded by basement membrane, and between them are parafollicular cells containing calcitonin-secreting C cells.

Physiology
Synthesis

The thyroid synthesizes two hormones:
- triiodothyronine (T_3), which acts at the cellular level
- L-thyroxine (T_4), which is the prohormone.

Inorganic iodide is trapped by the gland via an enzyme-dependent system, oxidized and incorporated into the glycoprotein thyroglobulin to form mono- and diiodotyrosine, and then T_4 and T_3 (**Fig. 21.21**).

More T_4 than T_3 is produced, but T_4 is converted in some peripheral tissues (liver, kidney and muscle) to the more active T_3 by 5′-monodeiodination; an alternative 3′-monodeiodination yields the inactive reverse T_3 (rT_3). The latter step occurs particularly in severe non-thyroidal illness (see later).

In plasma, more than 99% of all T_4 and T_3 is bound to hormone-binding proteins (thyroxine-binding globulin, TBG; thyroid-binding prealbumin, TBPA; and albumin). Only free hormone is available for action in the target tissues, where T_3 binds to specific nuclear receptors within target cells. Many drugs and other factors affect TBG; all may result in confusing total T_4 levels in blood, and most laboratories therefore now measure free T_4 levels.

Control of the hypothalamic–pituitary–thyroid axis

Thyrotrophin-releasing hormone (TRH), a peptide produced in the hypothalamus, stimulates the pituitary to secrete thyroid-stimulating hormone (TSH) (see Fig. 21.2). TSH, in turn, stimulates growth and activity of the thyroid follicular cells via the G-protein-coupled TSH membrane receptor (**Box 21.24**). The T_3 and T_4 subsequently secreted into the circulation by follicular cells exert negative feedback on the hypothalamus, as described on page 587.

Circulating T_4 is peripherally deiodinated to T_3, which binds to the thyroid hormone nuclear receptor (TR) on target organ cells to cause modified gene transcription. There are two TR receptors (TR-α and TR-β) and the tissue-specific effects of T_3 are dependent upon the local expression of these TR receptors. TR-α knockout mice show poor growth, bradycardia and hypothermia, while TR-β knockout mice show thyroid hyperplasia and high T_4 levels in the presence of inappropriately normal circulating TSH, suggesting a role for the latter receptors in thyroid hormone resistance (see p. 618).

Physiological effects of thyroid hormones

The physiological effects of thyroid hormones are summarized in **Box 21.25**.

Dietary iodine requirement

Globally, dietary iodine deficiency is a major cause of thyroid disease, as iodine is an essential requirement for thyroid hormone synthesis. The recommended daily intake of iodine should be at least 140 µg, and dietary supplementation of salt and bread has reduced the number of areas where 'endemic goitre' still occurs (see later).

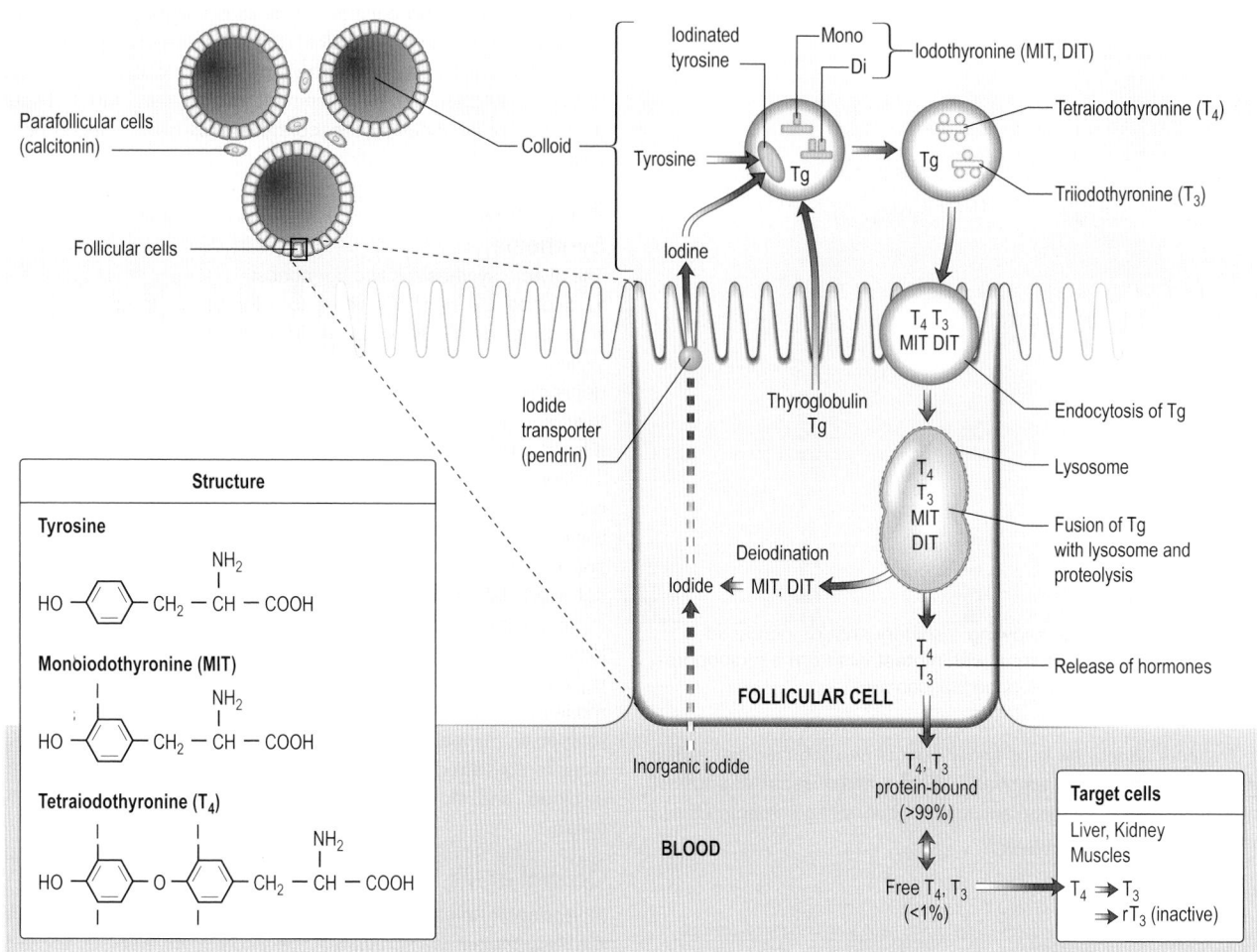

Fig. 21.21 Synthesis and metabolism of the thyroid hormones. Tg, thyroglobulin.

ⓘ Box 21.24 Hormones and receptors of the hypothalamic–pituitary–thyroid axis

Hormone	Source	Site of action	Hormone structure	Receptor	Post-receptor activity
Thyrotrophin-releasing hormone (TRH)	Hypothalamus	Pituitary	Peptide – 3 AA	Membrane – 7TM TRHR	G-proteins PLC/IP$_3$
Thyroid-stimulating hormone (TSH)	Pituitary	Thyroid	Glycoprotein: α and β subunits	Membrane – 7TM TSHR	G-proteins cAMP/ PLC/IP$_3$
Thyroxine and triiodothyronine (T$_4$ and T$_3$)	Thyroid	All tissues	Thyronines – 4/3 iodine atoms	Nuclear TR-α and β	Transcription TRE/RXR

7TM, 7 transmembrane (G-protein coupled receptor); AA, amino acids; TRE/RXR, thyroid hormone response element/response silencing region.

Investigations: thyroid function tests

Immunoassays for free T$_4$, free T$_3$ and TSH are widely available. There are only minor circadian rhythms and measurements may be made at any time. Particular uses of the tests are summarized in **Box 21.26**, with typical findings in common disorders.

TSH measurement

In most circumstances, TSH levels can discriminate between hyperthyroidism, hypothyroidism and euthyroidism (normal thyroid gland function). Exceptions are hypopituitarism, and the 'sick euthyroid' syndrome where low levels (which normally imply hyperthyroidism) occur in the presence of low or normal T$_4$ and T$_3$ levels. As a single test of thyroid function, TSH measurement is the most sensitive in most circumstances, but accurate diagnosis requires at least two

tests: for example, TSH plus free T$_4$ or free T$_3$ where hyperthyroidism is suspected; TSH plus serum free T$_4$ where hypothyroidism is likely.

TRH test

This has been rendered almost obsolete by modern sensitive TSH assays, except for investigation of hypothalamic–pituitary dysfunction. TRH (protirelin) is occasionally used to differentiate between thyroid hormone resistance and TSHoma in the context of raised fT$_4$ and TSH levels. Typically, after TRH administration, there is a rise in TSH in thyroid hormone resistance, while in TSHoma there is a flat response due to continued autonomous TSH secretion, which does not respond to TRH.

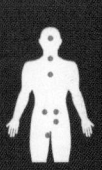

> **Box 21.25 Physiological effects of thyroid hormone**

Target	Effect
Cardiovascular system	Increases heart rate and cardiac output
Bone	Increases bone turnover and resorption
Respiratory system	Maintains normal hypoxic and hypercapnic drive in respiratory centre
Gastrointestinal system	Increases gut motility
Blood	Increases red blood cell 2,3-BPG[a], facilitating oxygen release to tissues
Neuromuscular function	Increases speed of muscle contraction/relaxation and muscle protein turnover
Carbohydrate metabolism	Increases hepatic gluconeogenesis/glycolysis and intestinal glucose absorption
Lipid metabolism	Increases lipolysis and cholesterol synthesis and degradation
Sympathetic nervous system	Increases catecholamine sensitivity and β-adrenergic receptor numbers in heart, skeletal muscle, adipose cells and lymphocytes. Decreases cardiac α-adrenergic receptors

[a]2,3-BPG, 2,3-bisphosphoglyceric acid.

> **Box 21.26 Characteristics of blood thyroid function tests in common thyroid disorders[a]**

	TSH (0.3–3.5 mU/L)	Free T$_4$ (10–25 pmol/L)	Free T$_3$ (3.5–7.5 pmol/L)
Thyrotoxicosis	**Suppressed (<0.05 mU/L)**	**Increased**	**Increased**
Primary hypothyroidism	Increased (>10 mU/L)	Low/low-normal	Normal or low
TSH deficiency	Low-normal or subnormal	**Low/low-normal**	Normal or low
T$_3$ toxicosis	Suppressed (<0.05 mU/L)	Normal	**Increased**
Compensated euthyroidism	**Slightly increased (5–10 mU/L)**	**Normal**	Normal

[a]The clinically most informative tests in each situation are shown in **bold**. TSH, thyroid-stimulating hormone.

Problems in interpretation of thyroid function tests

There are three major areas of difficulty: serious acute or chronic illness, pregnancy and use of oral contraceptives, and certain drugs.

Serious acute or chronic illness

Thyroid function is affected in several ways:
- reduced concentration and affinity of binding proteins
- decreased peripheral conversion of T$_4$ to T$_3$ with more rT$_3$
- reduced hypothalamic–pituitary TSH production.

Systemically ill patients can therefore have an apparently low total and free T$_4$ and T$_3$ with a normal or low basal TSH (the 'sick euthyroid' syndrome). Levels are usually only mildly below normal and are thought to be mediated by interleukins IL-1 and IL-6; the tests should be repeated after resolution of the underlying illness.

> **Box 21.27 Causes of hypothyroidism**

Primary disease of thyroid

Congenital
- Agenesis
- Ectopic thyroid remnants

Defects of hormone synthesis
- Iodine deficiency
- Dyshormonogenesis
- Anti-thyroid drugs
- Other drugs (e.g. lithium, amiodarone, interferon)

Autoimmune
- Atrophic thyroiditis
- Hashimoto's thyroiditis
- Postpartum thyroiditis

Infective
- Post-subacute thyroiditis

Post-surgery

Post-irradiation
- Radioactive iodine therapy
- External neck irradiation

Infiltration
- Tumour

Secondary (to hypothalamic–pituitary disease)

Hypopituitarism
- Isolated TSH deficiency

Peripheral resistance to thyroid hormone

TSH, thyroid-stimulating hormone.

Pregnancy and oral contraceptives

These lead to greatly increased TBG levels and thus to high or high-normal total T$_4$. Free T$_4$ is usually normal. Normal ranges for free T$_4$ and TSH alter with the normal physiological changes during pregnancy and TSH is often slightly suppressed in the first trimester, but this rarely causes clinical problems.

Drugs

Amiodarone decreases T$_4$ to T$_3$ conversion and free T$_4$ levels may therefore be above normal in a euthyroid patient; conversely, amiodarone may induce both hyper- and hypothyroidism – the TSH level is usually reliable.

Many drugs affect thyroid function tests by interfering with protein binding but this now rarely causes a problem with free T$_4$ assays.

Anti-thyroid antibodies

Serum antibodies to the thyroid are common.
- ***Destructive antibodies*** are directed against the microsomes or against thyroglobulin; the antigen for thyroid microsomal antibodies is the thyroid peroxidase (TPO) enzyme. TPO antibodies are found in up to 20% of the normal population, especially older women, but only 10–20% of these develop overt hypothyroidism.
- ***TSH receptor IgG antibodies*** (***TRAb***) typically stimulate, but occasionally block, the receptor. They are specific for Graves' disease (see p. 614).

Hypothyroidism

Pathophysiology

Underactivity of the thyroid is usually primary, caused by disease of the thyroid, but may be secondary to hypothalamic–pituitary disease (reduced TSH drive) (**Box 21.27**). Primary hypothyroidism is one of the most common endocrine conditions, with an overall UK prevalence of over 2% in women but under 0.1% in men; lifetime prevalence for an individual is higher – perhaps as high as 9% for women and 1% for men, with mean age at diagnosis around 60 years. The worldwide prevalence of subclinical hypothyroidism varies from 1% to 10%.

Aetiology of primary hypothyroidism

See **Box 21.27**.

Autoimmune

Atrophic (autoimmune) hypothyroidism

This is the most common cause of hypothyroidism and is associated with anti-thyroid autoantibodies, leading to lymphoid infiltration of the gland and eventual atrophy and fibrosis. It is six times more common in females and the incidence increases with age. The condition is associated with other autoimmune diseases, such as pernicious anaemia, vitiligo and other endocrine deficiencies. Occasionally, intermittent hypothyroidism occurs with subsequent recovery; antibodies that block the TSH receptor may sometimes be involved in the aetiology.

Hashimoto's thyroiditis

This form of autoimmune thyroiditis, again more common in women and most common in late middle age, produces atrophic changes with regeneration, leading to goitre formation. The gland is usually firm and rubbery but may range from soft to hard. TPO antibodies are present, often in very high titres (>1000 IU/L). Patients may be hypothyroid or euthyroid, though they may go through an initial toxic phase, 'Hashi-toxicity'. Levothyroxine therapy may shrink the goitre, even when the patient is not hypothyroid.

Postpartum thyroiditis

This is usually a transient phenomenon observed following pregnancy. It may cause hyperthyroidism, hypothyroidism or the two sequentially. It is believed to result from the modifications to the immune system necessary in pregnancy, and histologically is a lymphocytic thyroiditis. The process is normally self-limiting, but when conventional antibodies are found there is a high chance of this proceeding to permanent hypothyroidism. Postpartum thyroiditis may be misdiagnosed as postnatal depression, emphasizing the need for thyroid function tests in this situation.

Defects of hormone synthesis

Iodine deficiency

Dietary iodine deficiency still exists (see p. 1245) as 'endemic goitre' in some areas where goitre, occasionally massive, is common. The patients may be euthyroid or hypothyroid, depending on the severity of iodine deficiency. The mechanism is thought to be borderline hypothyroidism leading to TSH stimulation and thyroid enlargement in the face of continuing iodine deficiency. Iodine deficiency is still a problem in the Netherlands, Western Pacific, India, South-east Asia, Russia and parts of Africa. Efforts to prevent deficiency by providing iodine in salt continue worldwide but often with incomplete success. Even in the late 20th century, of the 500 million with iodine deficiency in India, about 2 million had cretinism (see later).

Dyshormonogenesis

This rare condition is due to genetic defects in the synthesis of thyroid hormones; patients develop hypothyroidism with goitre. One particular familial form is associated with sensorineural deafness due to a deletion mutation in chromosome 7, causing a defect of the transporter pendrin (Pendred's syndrome) (see **Fig. 21.21**).

History and examination

Hypothyroidism produces many symptoms (**Fig. 21.22**). The alternative term 'myxoedema' refers to the accumulation of mucopolysaccharide in subcutaneous tissues. The classic picture of the slow, dry-haired, thick-skinned, deep-voiced patient with weight gain,

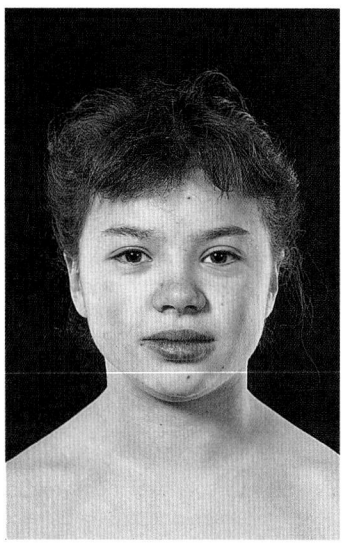

Symptoms	Signs	
General	**Mental slowness**	
Tiredness/malaise	Psychosis/dementia	Periorbital oedema
Weight gain	Ataxia	Deep voice
Cold intolerance	Poverty of movement	(Goitre)
Change in appearance	Deafness	
Goitre		
	'Peaches and cream'	**Dry skin**
Depression	complexion	Mild obesity
Psychosis	**Dry thin hair**	
Coma	Loss of eyebrows	
Poor memory		
	Hypertension	Myotonia
Hair – dry, brittle, unmanageable	Hypothermia	Muscular hypertrophy
Skin – dry, coarse	Heart failure	Proximal myopathy
	Bradycardia	**Slow-relaxing reflexes**
Arthralgia	Pericardial effusion	
Myalgia		
Muscle weakness/stiffness		
Poor libido		
Puffy eyes	Cold peripheries	Anaemia
Deafness	Carpal tunnel syndrome	
Constipation	Oedema	
Anorexia		

Fig. 21.22 Hypothyroidism: symptoms and signs. *Bold italic* type indicates symptoms or signs of greater discriminant value. A history from a relative is often revealing. Symptoms of other autoimmune disease may be present.

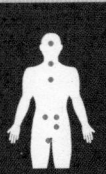

cold intolerance, bradycardia and constipation makes the diagnosis easy. Milder symptoms are, however, more common and hard to distinguish from other causes of non-specific tiredness. Many cases are detected on biochemical screening.

Special difficulties in diagnosis may arise in certain circumstances:

- **Children with hypothyroidism** may not show classic features but often have a slow growth velocity, poor school performance and sometimes arrest of pubertal development.
- **Young women with hypothyroidism** may not show obvious signs. Hypothyroidism should be excluded in all people with oligomenorrhoea/amenorrhoea, menorrhagia, infertility or hyperprolactinaemia.
- **The elderly** show many clinical features that are difficult to differentiate from normal ageing. Hypothyroidism should be excluded in elderly patients with cognitive impairment.

Investigation of primary hypothyroidism

Serum TSH is the investigation of choice; a high TSH level confirms primary hypothyroidism. A low free T_4 level confirms the hypothyroid state (and is also essential to exclude TSH deficiency if clinical hypothyroidism is strongly suspected and TSH is normal or low).

Thyroid and other organ-specific antibodies may be present. Other abnormalities include the following:

- **anaemia**, which is usually normochromic and normocytic in type but may be macrocytic (sometimes this is due to associated pernicious anaemia) or microcytic (in women, due to menorrhagia or undiagnosed coeliac disease)
- **increased serum aspartate transferase levels**, from muscle and/or liver
- **increased serum creatine kinase levels**, with associated myopathy
- **hypercholesterolaemia** and hypertriglyceridaemia
- **hyponatraemia** due to an increase in ADH and impaired free water clearance.

Management
Replacement therapy

Replacement therapy with levothyroxine (thyroxine, i.e. T_4) is given for life. The starting dose will depend upon the severity of the deficiency and on the age and fitness of the patient, especially their cardiac performance: 100 μg daily for the young and fit, 50 μg (increasing to 100 μg after 2–4 weeks) for the small, old or frail. People with ischaemic heart disease require even lower initial doses, especially if the hypothyroidism is severe and longstanding. Most physicians would then begin with 25 μg daily and perform serial electrocardiograms (ECGs), increasing the dose at 3- to 4-week intervals if angina does not occur or worsen, and the ECG does not deteriorate. Occasional patients develop 'thyrotoxic' (hyperthyroid) symptoms despite normal fT4 levels if the dose is increased too rapidly.

Monitoring

The aim is to restore T_4 and TSH to well within the normal range. Adequacy of replacement is assessed clinically and by thyroid function tests after at least 6 weeks on a steady dose. If serum TSH remains high, the dose of T_4 should be increased in increments of 25–50 μg, and the tests repeated at 6–8-week intervals until TSH becomes normal, ideally in the lower third of the normal range. Complete suppression of TSH should be avoided because of the risk of atrial fibrillation and osteoporosis. The usual maintenance dose is 100–150 μg given as a single daily dose. An annual thyroid function test is recommended – this is usually performed in the primary care setting, often assisted and prompted by district 'thyroid registers'.

Clinical improvement on T_4 may not begin for 2 weeks or more, and full resolution of symptoms may take 6 months. The necessity for lifelong therapy must be emphasized and the possibility of other autoimmune endocrine disease developing, especially Addison's disease or pernicious anaemia, should be considered. During pregnancy, an increase in T_4 dosage of about 25–50 μg is often needed to maintain relatively stricter TSH range of 0.3–2.5 mU/L, and the necessity for optimal replacement during pregnancy is emphasized by the finding of reductions in cognitive function in children of mothers with elevated TSH during pregnancy.

In cases where there is difficulty normalizing the TSH, compliance issues, concurrent medication that can interfere with thyroxine absorption (such as iron, calcium compounds and proton pump inhibitors) and undiagnosed coeliac disease should be considered.

A few people with primary hypothyroidism complain of incomplete symptomatic response to T_4 replacement. Combination T_4 and T_3 replacement has been advocated in this context, but randomized clinical trials show no consistent benefit in quality-of-life symptoms.

Borderline hypothyroidism or 'compensated euthyroidism'

Patients are frequently seen with low-normal serum T_4 levels and slightly raised TSH levels. Treatment with levothyroxine is normally recommended where the TSH is consistently above 10 mU/L, or when possible symptoms, high-titre thyroid antibodies, or lipid abnormalities are present. Where the TSH is only marginally raised, the tests should be repeated 3–6 months later, as a significant proportion will be normal on repeat testing. Conversion to overt hypothyroidism is more common in men or when TPO antibodies are present. In practice, vague symptoms in people with marginally elevated TSH (below 10 mU/L) rarely respond to treatment, but a 'therapeutic trial' of replacement may be needed to confirm that symptoms are unrelated to the thyroid. It is also considered best to normalize TSH during (and ideally before) pregnancy to avoid potential fetal adverse effects.

Myxoedema coma

Severe hypothyroidism, especially in the elderly, may present with confusion or even coma. Myxoedema coma is very rare; hypothermia is often present and the patient may have severe cardiac failure, pericardial effusions, hypoventilation, hypoglycaemia and hyponatraemia. The mortality was previously at least 50% and patients require full intensive care. Optimal treatment is controversial and data are lacking; most physicians would advise T_3 orally or intravenously in doses of 2.5–5 μg every 8 hours, then increasing as above. Large intravenous doses should not be used. Additional measures, though unproven, should include:

- oxygen (by ventilation if necessary)
- monitoring of cardiac output and pressures
- gradual rewarming
- hydrocortisone 100 mg i.v. 8-hourly
- glucose infusion to prevent hypoglycaemia.

Myxoedema madness

Depression is common in hypothyroidism. Rarely, with severe hypothyroidism in the elderly, the patient may become frankly demented or psychotic, sometimes with striking delusions. This may occur shortly after starting T_4 replacement.

? Box 21.28 Causes of hyperthyroidism

Common
- Graves' disease (autoimmune)
- Toxic multinodular goitre
- Solitary toxic nodule/adenoma

Uncommon
- Acute thyroiditis
  - Viral (e.g. de Quervain's)
  - Autoimmune
  - Post-irradiation
  - Postpartum
- Gestational thyrotoxicosis (HCG-stimulated)
- Neonatal thyrotoxicosis (maternal thyroid antibodies)
- Exogenous iodine

- Drugs – amiodarone, immunotherapy (ipilimumab, pembrolizumab, nivolumab)
- Thyrotoxicosis factitia (secret T_4 consumption)

Rare
- TSH-secreting pituitary tumours
- Metastatic differentiated thyroid carcinoma
- HCG-producing tumours
- Hyperfunctioning ovarian teratoma (struma ovarii)

HCG, human chorionic gonadotrophin; TSH, thyroid-stimulating hormone.

? Box 21.29 Differential diagnosis of thyrotoxicosis

	Graves' disease	Solitary or multinodular thyrotoxicosis	Thyroiditis
History	Symptoms of thyrotoxicosis	Symptoms of thyrotoxicosis	Symptoms of thyrotoxicosis Recent viral infection Recent delivery of child Painful neck swelling
Clinical examination	Signs of thyrotoxicosis Diffuse goitre Extrathyroidal manifestations including ophthalmopathy	Signs of thyrotoxicosis Palpable solitary nodule or multinodular goitre	Signs of thyrotoxicosis Diffuse goitre Tender on palpation
Biochemical tests	TSH suppressed FT4 and FT3 elevated	TSH suppressed FT4 and FT3 elevated (only FT3 elevated in T3 toxicosis)	TSH suppressed FT4 and FT3 elevated Raised inflammatory markers (ESR, CRP)
Immunological tests	TSH receptor antibodies raised TPO antibodies raised		TPO antibodies may be raised
Thyroid isotope uptake scan (Scintiscan ^{99}Tm)	Diffuse uptake of tracer	Focal uptake of tracer in nodules with reduced uptake in rest of thyroid gland	Minimal uptake of tracer

Screening for hypothyroidism

The incidence of *congenital* hypothyroidism is approximately 1 in 3500 births. Untreated, severe hypothyroidism produces permanent neurological and intellectual damage ('cretinism'). Routine screening of the newborn using a blood spot, as in the Guthrie test, to detect a high TSH level as an indicator of primary hypothyroidism is efficient and cost-effective; cretinism is prevented if T_4 is started within the first few months of life.

Screening of *elderly* patients for thyroid dysfunction has a low pick-up rate, is controversial and is not currently recommended unless as part of a confusion screen. However, patients who have undergone thyroid surgery or received radio-iodine should have regular thyroid function tests, as should those receiving lithium or amiodarone therapy.

Hyperthyroidism

Hyperthyroidism (thyroid overactivity, thyrotoxicosis) is common, affecting perhaps 2–5% of all females at some time and having a sex ratio of 5:1; it most often occurs between the ages of 20 and 40 years. Nearly all cases (>99%) are caused by intrinsic thyroid disease; a pituitary cause is extremely rare (**Box 21.28**). Most common patterns of hyperthyroidism and their distinctive features are outlined in **Box 21.29**.

Graves' disease

This is the most common cause of hyperthyroidism and is due to an autoimmune process. Serum IgG antibodies bind to TSH receptors in the thyroid, stimulating thyroid hormone production; that is, they behave like TSH. These TSH receptor antibodies (TSHR-Ab) are specific for Graves' disease. Persistent high levels predict a relapse when drug treatment is stopped. There is an association with HLA-B8, DR3 and DR2; the concordance rate amongst monozygotic twins is 50% and that in dizygotic twins is 5%. There is an association with cytotoxic T lymphocyte-associated antigen 4 (CTLA-4), HLA-DRBP*08 and DRB3*0202 on chromosome 6. The mechanism of immune damage is illustrated in **Fig. 3.16**.

Yersinia enterocolitica, *Escherichia coli* and other Gram-negative organisms contain TSH-binding sites. This raises the possibility that the initiating event in the pathogenesis may be an infection with possible 'molecular mimicry' in a genetically susceptible individual, but the precise initiating mechanisms remain unproven in most cases.

Thyroid eye disease is a feature of Graves' disease. It may accompany the hyperthyroidism in many cases but patients may also be euthyroid or hypothyroid. Other components of Graves' disease, such as Graves' dermopathy, are very uncommon. Rarely, lymphadenopathy and splenomegaly may occur. Graves' disease is also associated with other autoimmune disorders such as pernicious anaemia, vitiligo and myasthenia gravis.

The natural history is one of fluctuation, many patients showing a pattern of alternating relapse and remission; perhaps only 40% of subjects have a single episode. Many patients eventually become hypothyroid.

Other causes of hyperthyroidism/thyrotoxicosis
Solitary toxic adenoma/nodule

This is the cause of about 5% of cases of hyperthyroidism. While the hyperthyroidism will be controlled by the anti-thyroid drugs, it does not usually remit after a course of anti-thyroid drugs.

Symptoms		Signs	
General		*Tremor*	Proximal myopathy
Weight loss		*Hyperkinesis*	Proximal muscle wasting
Irritability/behaviour change		Psychosis	Onycholysis
Restlessness			Palmar erythema
Malaise			
Itching			
Sweating		*Tachycardia or atrial*	Graves' dermopathy*
Tall stature (in children)		*fibrillation*	Thyroid acropachy
Breathlessness		*Full pulse*	Pretibial myxoedema
Palpitations		*Warm vasodilated*	
Heat intolerance		*peripheries*	
Stiffness		Systolic hypertension	
Muscle weakness		Cardiac failure	
Tremor		*Exophthalmos**	
Choreoathetosis		*Lid lag and 'stare'*	
		Conjunctival oedema	
Thirst		Ophthalmoplegia*	
Vomiting		Periorbital oedema	
Diarrhoea		*Goitre, bruit*	
		Weight loss	
Eye complaints*			
Oligomenorrhoea			
Loss of libido			
Gynaecomastia			
Onycholysis			
Goitre			
*Only in Graves' disease		*Only in Graves' disease	

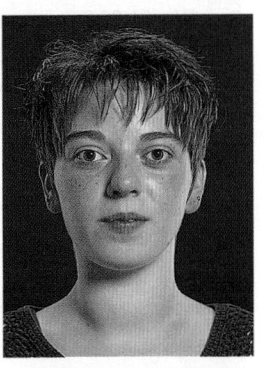
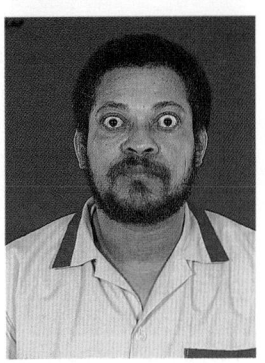

Fig. 21.23 Hyperthyroidism: symptoms and signs. *Bold italic* type indicates symptoms or signs of greater discriminant value.

Toxic multinodular goitre

This commonly occurs in older women. Again, anti-thyroid drugs are rarely successful in inducing a remission, although they can control the hyperthyroidism.

De Quervain's thyroiditis

This is transient hyperthyroidism from an acute inflammatory process, probably viral in origin. Apart from the toxicosis, there is usually fever, malaise and pain in the neck with tachycardia and local thyroid tenderness. Thyroid function tests show initial hyperthyroidism, the erythrocyte sedimentation rate (ESR) and plasma viscosity are raised, and thyroid uptake scans show suppression of uptake in the acute phase. Hypothyroidism, usually transient, may then follow after a few weeks. Treatment of the acute phase is with aspirin, using short-term prednisolone in severely symptomatic cases.

Postpartum thyroiditis

This is described on page 612.

Amiodarone-induced thyrotoxicosis

Amiodarone, a class III antiarrhythmic drug (see p. 1067), causes two types of hyperthyroidism.

- *Type I amiodarone-induced thyrotoxicosis (AIT)* is associated with pre-existing Graves' disease or multinodular goitre. In this situation, hyperthyroidism is probably triggered by the high iodine content of amiodarone.

- *Type II AIT* is not associated with previous thyroid disease and is thought to be due to a direct effect of the drug on thyroid follicular cells, leading to a destructive thyroiditis with release of T_4 and T_3. Type II AIT may be associated with a hypothyroid phase several months after presentation. Because amiodarone inhibits the deiodination of T_4 to T_3, biochemical presentation of both types of AIT may be associated with higher $T_4:T_3$ ratios than usual.

Immunotherapy-induced thyrotoxicosis

Cancer immunotherapy drugs that block negative regulators on T cell, called immune checkpoint inhibitors (ipilimumab, pembrolizumab, nivolumab) have been found to be effective in wide range cancers. These drugs cause immune-related adverse events (irAEs) in various organs, including in endocrine glands, resulting in thyroiditis (15%), hypophysitis (9%), adrenalitis (1%) and type 1 diabetes mellitus (<1%). Thyroiditis is the most common of endocrine irAEs and occurs between 3 and 12 weeks after initiation of the drug. Treatment is with beta-blockers, analgesia and, rarely, with anti-thyroid medication if thyrotoxicosis persists, especially with symptoms.

History and examination

The symptoms and signs of hyperthyroidism affect many systems (**Fig. 21.23**). Symptomatology and signs vary with age and with the underlying aetiology.

- *The eye signs – lid lag and 'stare'* – may occur with hyperthyroidism of any cause but other features of thyroid eye disease (see below) occur only in Graves' disease.

- **Graves' dermopathy** is rare and can occur on any extensor surface. **Pretibial myxoedema** is the most commonly described and is an infiltration of the skin on the shin. **Thyroid acropachy** is very rare and consists of clubbing, swollen fingers and periosteal new bone formation.
- **In the elderly**, a frequent presentation is with atrial fibrillation, other tachycardias and/or heart failure, often with few other signs. Thyroid function tests are mandatory in any patient with atrial fibrillation.
- **Children** frequently present with excessive height or excessive growth rate, or with behavioural problems such as hyperactivity. They may also show weight gain rather than loss.
- **So-called 'apathetic thyrotoxicosis'** in some elderly patients presents with a clinical picture more like that of hypothyroidism. There may be very few signs and a high degree of clinical suspicion is essential.

Differential diagnosis

Hyperthyroidism is often clinically obvious but treatment should never be instituted without biochemical confirmation.

Differentiation of the mild case from anxiety states may be difficult; useful positive clinical markers are eye signs, a diffuse goitre, proximal myopathy and wasting. Weight loss, despite a normal or increased appetite, is a very useful clinical symptom of hyperthyroidism. The hyperdynamic circulation with warm peripheries seen with hyperthyroidism can be contrasted with the clammy hands of anxiety.

Investigations

- **Serum TSH** is suppressed in hyperthyroidism (<0.05 mU/L), except for the very rare instances of TSH hypersecretion.
- **A raised free T_4 or T_3** confirms the diagnosis; T_4 is almost always raised but T_3 is more sensitive, as there are occasional cases of isolated 'T_3 toxicosis'.
- **TSH receptor stimulating antibodies (TSHR-Ab)** are now measured routinely and the third-generation tests are 97–99% specific for Graves' disease.
- **Thyroid peroxidase (TPO)** and thyroglobulin antibodies are present in 80% of cases of Graves' disease, but are also found in normal individuals.
- **Scintiscan ^{99}Tm** is used in patients who are antibody negative to look for toxic nodular disease.

Management

Three possibilities are available: anti-thyroid drugs, radio-iodine and surgery. Practices and beliefs differ widely within and between countries.

Anti-thyroid drugs

Carbimazole is most often used in the UK, and propylthiouracil (PTU) is also an option. **Thiamazole** (methimazole), the active metabolite of carbimazole, is used in the USA. These drugs inhibit the formation of thyroid hormones and also have other minor actions; carbimazole/thiamazole is also an immunosuppressive agent. Initial doses and side-effects are detailed in **Box 21.30**.

Although thyroid hormone synthesis is reduced very quickly, the long half-life of T_4 (7 days) means that clinical benefit is not apparent for 10–20 days. As many of the manifestations of hyperthyroidism are mediated via the sympathetic system, beta-blockers are used to provide rapid partial symptomatic control; they also decrease peripheral conversion of T_4 to T_3. Preferred drugs are those without intrinsic sympathomimetic activity, e.g. propranolol (see **Box 21.30**).

Box 21.30 Drugs used in the treatment of hyperthyroidism

Drug	Usual starting dose	Side-effects	Remarks
Anti-thyroid drugs			
Carbimazole	20–40 mg daily, 8-hourly or in single dose	Rash, nausea, vomiting, arthralgia, agranulocytosis (0.1%), jaundice	Active metabolite is thiamazole (methimazole) Mild immunosuppressive activity
Propylthiouracil (PTU)	100–200 mg 8-hourly	Rash, nausea, vomiting, agranulocytosis, hepatotoxicity	Additionally blocks conversion of T_4 to T_3
Beta-blocker for symptomatic control			
May need higher doses than normal			
Propranolol	40–80 mg every 6–8 h		Avoid in asthma Use agents without intrinsic sympathomimetic activity as receptors are highly sensitive

They should not be used alone for hyperthyroidism except when the condition is self-limiting, as in subacute thyroiditis.

Subsequent management is either by gradual dose titration or by a 'block and replace' regimen. Neither regimen has been shown to be unequivocally superior. TSH often remains suppressed for many months after clinical improvement and normalization of T_4 and T_3.

Dosage regimen

Gradual dose titration

1. Start carbimazole 20–40 mg daily.
2. Review after 4–6 weeks and reduce the dose of carbimazole, depending on clinical state and fT_4/fT_3 levels. TSH levels may remain suppressed for several months and are unhelpful at this stage.
3. When the patient is clinically and biochemically euthyroid, stop beta-blockers.
4. Review thyroid function regularly during the planned course of treatment (typically 18 months – but some use courses between 6 and 24 months).
5. Reduce carbimazole if fT_4 falls below or TSH rises above normal, and when approaching the end of the planned course.
6. Increase carbimazole if fT_4 or fT_3 is above normal (and consider if TSH remains suppressed after several months with a normal fT_4).
7. Stop treatment at the end of the course if the patient is euthyroid on 5 mg daily carbimazole. PTU is used in similar fashion (see **Box 21.30**).

'Block and replace' regimen

With this policy, full doses of anti-thyroid drugs, usually carbimazole 40 mg daily, are given to suppress the thyroid completely while replacing thyroid activity with 100 µg of levothyroxine daily once euthyroidism has been achieved. This is continued usually for 18 months, the claimed advantages being the avoidance of over- or undertreatment and the better use of the immunosuppressive action of carbimazole. This regimen is contraindicated in pregnancy, as T_4 crosses the placenta less well than carbimazole.

Relapse

About 50% of patients will relapse after a course of carbimazole or PTU, mostly within the following 2 years but occasionally much later. Long-term anti-thyroid therapy is then used, or surgery or radiotherapy is considered (see below). Most patients (90%) with hyperthyroidism have a diffuse goitre but those with large single or multinodular goitres are unlikely to remit after a course of anti-thyroid drugs and will usually require definitive treatment. Severe biochemical hyperthyroidism is also less likely to remain in remission.

Toxicity

The major side-effect of drug therapy is agranulocytosis, which occurs in approximately 1 in 1000 patients, usually within 3 months of treatment. All patients must be warned to seek immediate medical attention and to have a check of their white blood cell count if they develop unexplained fever or sore throat; written information is essential. Rashes are more frequent and usually require a change of drug. If toxicity occurs on carbimazole, PTU may be used, and vice versa; side-effects are only occasionally repeated on the other drug.

Radioactive iodine

Radioactive iodine (RAI) is given to patients of all ages, although it is contraindicated in pregnancy and while breast-feeding. RAI is the most common treatment modality in the USA, whereas anti-thyroid drugs tend to be favoured in Europe.

^{131}*Iodine* is given in an empirical dose (usually 400–550 MBq) because of variable uptake and radiosensitivity of the gland. It accumulates in the thyroid and destroys the gland by local radiation, although it takes several months to be fully effective.

Patients must be rendered euthyroid before treatment. They should stop anti-thyroid drugs at least 4 days before radio-iodine, and not recommence until 3 days after radio-iodine. Patients on PTU should stop anti-thyroid medication before RAI earlier than those on carbimazole because it has a radioprotective action. Many patients do not need to restart anti-thyroid medication after treatment.

Early discomfort in the neck and immediate worsening of hyperthyroidism are sometimes seen. If worsening occurs, the patient should receive propranolol (see **Box 21.30**); if necessary, carbimazole can be restarted. Euthyroidism normally returns in 2–3 months. People with dysthyroid eye disease are more likely to show worsening of eye problems after radio-iodine than after anti-thyroid drugs; this represents a partial contraindication to RAI, although worsening can usually be prevented by steroid administration.

Long-term surveillance

Hypothyroidism affects the majority of subjects over the following 20 years. Some 75% of patients are rendered euthyroid in the short term, but a small proportion remain hyperthyroid and may require a second dose of radio-iodine. Long-term surveillance of thyroid function is necessary, with frequent tests in the first year after therapy and at least annually thereafter.

There is no increased risk of malignancy after RAI.

Surgery

Thyroidectomy should be performed only in patients who have previously been rendered euthyroid. Conventional practice is to stop the anti-thyroid drug 10–14 days before operation and to give potassium iodide (60 mg three times daily), which reduces the vascularity of the gland and reduces thyroid hormone synthesis by inhibiting organification of iodine (Wolff–Chaikoff effect).

The operation should be performed only by experienced surgeons to reduce the chance of complications:

> **i** | **Box 21.31 Choice of surgery or radio-iodine therapy for hyperthyroidism**
>
> **Indications for surgery or radio-iodine**
> - Patient choice
> - Persistent drug side-effects
> - Poor compliance with drug therapy
> - Recurrent hyperthyroidism after drugs
>
> **Indications for surgery**
> - A large goitre, which is unlikely to remit after anti-thyroid medication

- Early postoperative bleeding causing tracheal compression and asphyxia is a rare emergency that mandates immediate removal of all clips/sutures to allow escape of the blood/haematoma.
- Laryngeal nerve palsy occurs in 1%. Vocal cord movement should be checked preoperatively. Mild hoarseness is more common and thyroidectomy is best avoided in professional singers!
- Transient hypocalcaemia occurs in up to 10% but with permanent hypoparathyroidism in fewer than 1%.
- Ongoing thyroid function depends on the operation performed. With a single toxic nodule, excision of the lesion is curative. With Graves' disease or multinodular goitre, the traditional 'subtotal' thyroidectomy, aiming for euthyroidism on no treatment, results in recurrent hyperthyroidism in 1–3% within 1 year, then 1% per year and hypothyroidism in about 10% of patients within 1 year, and then increasing with time. 'Near-total' thyroidectomy is therefore now preferred, with inevitable hypothyroidism but a much-reduced risk of recurrence.

Indications for either surgery or radio-iodine are given in **Box 21.31**.

Special situations in hyperthyroidism
Thyroid crisis or 'thyroid storm'

This rare condition, with a mortality of 10%, is a rapid deterioration of hyperthyroidism with hyperpyrexia, severe tachycardia, extreme restlessness, cardiac failure and liver dysfunction. It is usually precipitated by stress, infection or surgery in an unprepared patient, or by radio-iodine therapy. With careful management, it should no longer occur and most cases referred to as a 'crisis' are simply severe but uncomplicated thyrotoxicosis.

Treatment is urgent. Propranolol in full doses is started immediately together with potassium iodide, anti-thyroid drugs, corticosteroids (which suppress many of the manifestations of hyperthyroidism) and full supportive measures. Control of cardiac failure and tachycardia is also necessary.

Occasionally, hyperthyroidism can lead to a thyrotoxic cardiomyopathy, which causes ischaemic changes on a 12-lead ECG; these reverse after euthyroidism is achieved (**Fig. 21.24**).

Hyperthyroidism in pregnancy and neonatal life

Since hyperthyroidism typically affects young women, pregnancies, both planned and unplanned, inevitably occur during anti-thyroid treatment. PTU is usually the preferred anti-thyroid drug at conception and in the first trimester of pregnancy or in any woman planning pregnancy, due to rare reports of congenital abnormalities with carbimazole, which have not been described with PTU (p. 1459). However, carbimazole is recommended in the second and third trimesters, as liver problems are more frequently described on PTU.

The high level of HCG found in normal pregnancy is a weak stimulator of the TSH receptor, commonly causing suppressed TSH with slightly elevated fT$_4$/fT$_3$ in the first trimester, which may be

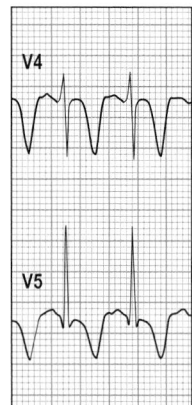

Fig. 21.24 Thyrotoxic cardiomyopathies. ECG showing marked lateral T-wave inversion.

associated with hyperemesis gravidarum. True maternal hyperthyroidism occurring *de novo* during pregnancy is, however, uncommon and usually mild. Diagnosis can be difficult because of the overlap with symptoms of normal pregnancy and misleading thyroid function tests, although TSH is largely reliable. The pathogenesis is almost always Graves' disease.

Thyroid-stimulating immunoglobulin (TSI) crosses the placenta to stimulate the fetal thyroid. Carbimazole and PTU (see below) also cross the placenta but T_4 does so poorly, so a 'block and replace' regimen is contraindicated. The smallest dose necessary of PTU or carbimazole (see earlier) is used and the fetus must be monitored. If necessary (when high doses are needed, or there is poor patient compliance or drug side-effects), surgery can be performed, preferably in the second trimester. RAI is absolutely contraindicated.

The fetus and maternal Graves' disease

Any mother with a history of Graves' disease may have circulating TSI. Even if she is euthyroid after surgery or RAI, the immunoglobulin may still be present to stimulate the fetal thyroid, and the fetus can thus become hyperthyroid.

Any such patient should therefore be monitored during pregnancy. Fetal heart rate provides a direct biological assay of fetal thyroid status, and monitoring should be performed at least monthly. Rates above 160/minute are strongly suggestive of fetal hyperthyroidism, and maternal treatment with PTU and/or propranolol is used. Direct measurement of TSHR-Ab may be helpful to predict neonatal thyrotoxicosis in this situation. To prevent a euthyroid mother becoming hypothyroid, T_4 may be given, as this does not easily cross the placenta. Sympathomimetics, used to prevent premature labour, are contraindicated, as they may provoke fatal tachycardia in the fetus. The paediatrician should be informed and the infant checked immediately after birth, as overtreatment with PTU or carbimazole can cause fetal goitre. Breast-feeding while on the usual doses of carbimazole or PTU appears to be safe.

Hyperthyroidism may also develop in the neonatal period, as TSI has a half-life of approximately 3 weeks. Manifestations in the newborn include irritability, failure to thrive and persisting weight loss, diarrhoea and eye signs. Thyroid function tests are difficult to interpret, as neonatal normal ranges vary with age.

Untreated neonatal hyperthyroidism is probably associated with hyperactivity in later childhood.

Thyroid hormone resistance

Thyroid hormone resistance is an inherited condition, caused by an abnormality of the thyroid hormone receptor. Mutations to the receptor (TR β) result in the need for higher levels of thyroid hormones to achieve the same intracellular effect. As a result, the normal feedback control mechanisms (see Fig. 21.2) result in high blood levels of T_4 with a normal TSH in order to maintain a euthyroid state. This has two consequences:

• Thyroid function tests appear abnormal, even when the patient is euthyroid and requires no treatment. Specialist review is needed to differentiate this condition from hyperthyroidism due to inappropriate TSH secretion.

• Different tissues contain different thyroid hormone receptors and, in some families, receptors in certain tissues may have normal activity. In this case, the level of thyroid hormones to maintain euthyroidism at pituitary and hypothalamic levels (which controls secretion of TSH) may be higher than that required in other tissues such as heart and bone, so that these tissues may exhibit 'thyrotoxic' effects in spite of a normal serum TSH. This 'partial thyroid hormone resistance' can be very difficult to manage effectively.

Thyroid hormone resistance is diagnosed on the basis of a raised T_4/T_3 in the context of a non-elevated TSH. The differential diagnosis of this pattern of blood results includes TSHoma and laboratory assay interference.

Long-term consequences of hyperthyroidism

Long-term follow-up studies of hyperthyroidism show a slight increase in overall mortality, which affects all age groups, is not fully explained and tends to occur in the first year after diagnosis. Thereafter, the only long-term risk of adequately treated hyperthyroidism appears to be an increased risk of osteoporosis. People with persistently suppressed TSH levels have an increased likelihood of developing atrial fibrillation, which may predispose to thromboembolic disease.

Graves' orbitopathy (ophthalmopathy)

Pathophysiology

Graves' orbitopathy is due to a specific immune response that causes retro-orbital inflammation (**Fig. 21.25**). Swelling and oedema of the extraocular muscles lead to limitation of movement and to proptosis, which is usually bilateral but can sometimes be unilateral. Ultimately, increased pressure on the optic nerve may cause optic atrophy. Histology of the extraocular muscles shows focal oedema and glycosaminoglycan deposition followed by fibrosis. The precise autoantigen that leads to the immune response remains to be identified, but it appears to be an antigen in retro-orbital tissue with similar immunoreactivity to the TSH receptor.

Eye disease is a manifestation of Graves' disease and can occur in patients who may be hyperthyroid, euthyroid or hypothyroid. Thyroid dysfunction and orbitopathy usually occur within 2 years of each other, although sometimes a gap of many years is seen. TSH receptor antibodies are almost invariably found in the serum; their role in the pathogenesis is becoming clearer (see **Fig. 21.25**). Orbitopathy is more common and more severe in smokers.

Clinical features

The clinical appearances are characteristic (see **Fig. 21.23**) but thyroid eye disease demonstrates a wide range of severity. A high proportion of people with Graves' disease notice some soreness, painful watering or prominence of the eyes, and the 'stare' of lid retraction is relatively common. More severe proptosis occurs in a minority of cases, and limitation and discomfort of eye movement

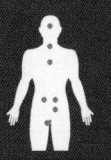

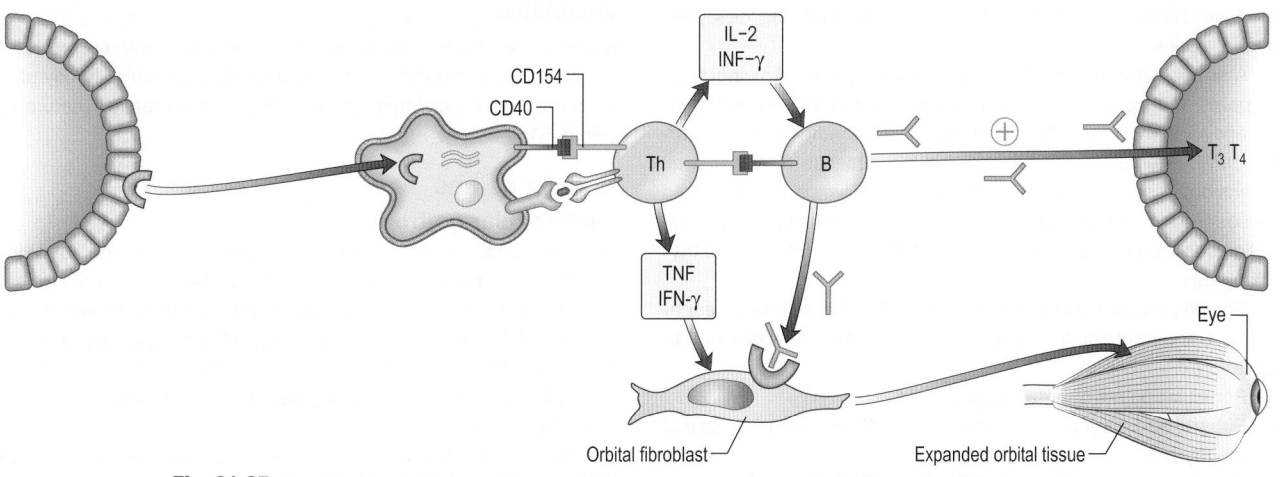

Fig. 21.25 Model of the initiation of thyrotrophin-receptor autoimmunity in Graves' ophthalmopathy and its consequences. Thyrotrophin receptor is internalized and degraded by antigen-presenting cells that present thyrotrophin-receptor peptides, in association with major histocompatibility complex (MHC) class II antigens, to helper T (Th) cells. These cells become activated, interact with autoreactive B cells through CD154–CD40 bridges, and secrete interleukin 2 (IL-2) and interferon-gamma (IFN-γ). These cytokines induce the differentiation of B cells into plasma cells that secrete anti-thyrotrophin-receptor antibodies. Anti-thyrotrophin-receptor antibodies (green) recognize the thyrotrophin receptor on orbital fibroblasts and, in conjunction with the secreted type 1 helper T cytokines, IFN-γ and tumour necrosis factor (TNF), initiate the tissue changes characteristic of Graves' ophthalmopathy. These antibodies stimulate the thyrotrophin receptor on thyroid follicular epithelial cells, leading to hyperplasia and increased production of the thyroid hormones triiodothyronine (T$_3$) and thyroxine (T$_4$). *(Adapted from Bahn RS. Graves' ophthalmology. N Engl J Med 2010; 362:726–738.)*

and visual impairment due to optic nerve compression are relatively uncommon. Proptosis and lid retraction may limit the ability to close the eyes completely so that corneal damage may occur. There is periorbital oedema, and conjunctival oedema and inflammation.

Eye manifestations do not parallel the degree of biochemical thyrotoxicosis or the need for anti-thyroid therapy, but exacerbation of eye disease is more common after radio-iodine treatment (15% versus 3% on anti-thyroid drugs). Sight is threatened in only 5–10% of cases, but the discomfort and cosmetic problems cause great patient anxiety.

Investigations

If the appearance is characteristic, consideration is needed as to whether the patient requires review by an ophthalmologist. Investigation would include:

- TSH, fT$_3$ and fT$_4$ measurement.
- MRI or CT of the orbits to exclude retro-orbital space-occupying lesions. In Graves' orbitopathy, there may be enlarged muscles and oedema, with a taut optic nerve due to raised intra-orbital pressure.
- Assessment of vision, particularly optic nerve function.

Management

If the patient is thyrotoxic, this should be treated, but treatment will not directly result in an improvement of the ophthalmopathy; hypothyroidism must be avoided, as it may exacerbate the eye problem. Smoking should be stopped. Treatment of the eyes may be either local or systemic, and always requires close liaison between specialist endocrinologist and ophthalmologist:

- *Methylcellulose or hypromellose eyedrops* or ointment are given to aid lubrication and improve comfort.
- *Sleeping upright* affords some patients relief.
- *Taping the eyelids* ensures closure at night.

- *Systemic steroids* (prednisolone 30–120 mg daily) usually reduce inflammation if more severe symptoms are present. Pulse intravenous methylprednisolone may be used initially and is more rapidly effective in severe cases.
- *Surgical decompression of the orbit(s)* may be required, particularly if pressure of orbital contents on the optic nerve threatens vision (often called a 'hot' decompression), and at a later, stable stage for cosmetic reasons ('cold' decompression).
- *Lid surgery* will protect the cornea if lids cannot be closed, and can be useful later for cosmetic reasons.
- *Corrective eye muscle surgery* may improve diplopia due to muscle changes; it should be deferred until the situation has been stable for 6 months and should follow any orbital decompression.
- *Irradiation of the orbits* (20 Gy in divided doses) is used in some centres. This reduces inflammation and ocular motility but has little effect on proptosis; its precise role is debated.
- *Immunomodulatory agents* may produce a response in some patients when conventional treatments fail, although clinical trial evidence is inconsistent.
- *Selenium* may have a beneficial effect on mild orbitopathy in some patients.

Goitre (thyroid enlargement)

Goitre is more common in women than in men and may be either physiological or pathological.

Clinical features

Goitres are present on examination in up to 9% of the population. Most commonly, a goitre is noticed as a cosmetic defect by the patient or by friends or relatives. The majority are painless, but pain or discomfort can occur in acute varieties. Large goitres can produce dysphagia and difficulty in breathing, implying oesophageal or tracheal compression.

A small goitre may be more easily visible (on swallowing) than palpable. Clinical examination should record the size, shape, consistency and mobility of the gland, as well as whether its lower margin can be demarcated (thus implying the absence of retrosternal extension). A bruit may be present. Associated lymph nodes should be sought and the tracheal position determined if possible. Examination should never omit an assessment of the patient's clinical thyroid status.

Specific enquiry should be made about any medication, especially iodine-containing preparations, and possible exposure to radiation.

Particular points of note are as follows:

- Puberty and pregnancy may produce a diffuse increase in size of the thyroid.
- Pain in a goitre may be caused by thyroiditis, bleeding into a cyst or (rarely) a thyroid tumour.
- Excessive doses of carbimazole or PTU will induce goitre.
- Iodine deficiency and dyshormonogenesis (see earlier) can also cause goitre.

Diagnosis

There are four major aspects to any goitre: its pathological nature, whether it is causing any compressive symptoms, the patient's thyroid status and whether it is of cosmetic concern. The nature can often be judged clinically. Goitres (**Box 21.32**) are usually separable into diffuse and nodular types, the causes of which differ.

Diffuse goitre

Simple goitre

In this instance, no clear cause is found for enlargement of the thyroid, which is usually smooth and soft. It may be associated with thyroid growth-stimulating antibodies.

Autoimmune thyroid disease

Hashimoto's thyroiditis and Grave's disease thyrotoxicosis are both associated with firm diffuse goitre of variable size. A bruit is often present in thyrotoxicosis.

Thyroiditis

Acute tenderness in a diffuse swelling, sometimes with severe pain, is suggestive of an acute viral thyroiditis (de Quervain's). It may produce transient clinical hyperthyroidism with an increase in serum T_4 (see p. 615).

Nodular goitres

Multinodular goitre

Most common is the multinodular goitre, especially in older patients. The patient is usually euthyroid but may have clinical hyperthyroidism or subclinical hyperthyroidism (suppressed or low TSH levels but normal free T_4 and T_3). Multinodular goitre is the most common cause of tracheal and/or oesophageal compression and can lead to laryngeal nerve palsy. It may also extend retrosternally (**Fig. 21.26**).

The classical 'multinodular goitre' is usually readily apparent clinically, but it should be noted that modern, high-resolution ultrasound frequently reports multiple small nodules in glands, which are clinically diffusely enlarged and associated with autoimmune thyroid disease. These nodules are also found in up to 40% of the normal population.

? Box 21.32 Goitre: causes and types

Diffuse
- Simple:
  - Physiological (puberty, pregnancy)
- Autoimmune:
  - Graves' disease
  - Hashimoto's disease
- Thyroiditis:
  - Acute (de Quervain's thyroiditis)
- Iodine deficiency (endemic goitre)
- Dyshormonogenesis
- Goitrogens (e.g. sulphonylureas)

Nodular
- Multinodular goitre
- Solitary nodular
- Fibrotic (Riedel's thyroiditis)
- Cysts

Tumours
- Adenomas
- Carcinoma
- Lymphomas

Miscellaneous
- Sarcoidosis
- Tuberculosis

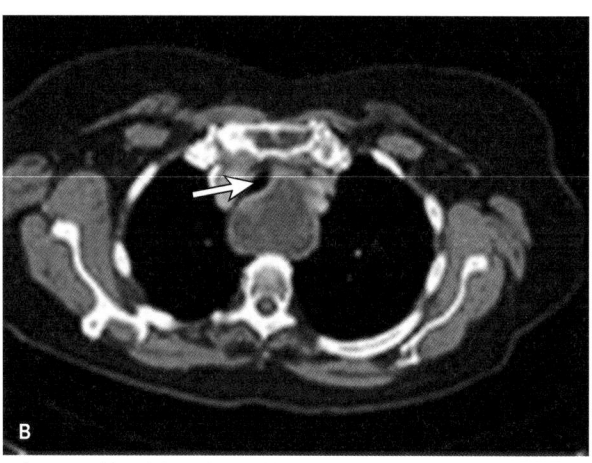

Fig. 21.26 Imaging of goitre. (A) Tc scan showing a multinodular goitre, with predominant involvement of the left lobe of the thyroid (anterior view with arrowed anatomical marker at the sternal notch). **(B)** Retrosternal goitre showing deviation and compression of the trachea (arrowed) on CT.

Solitary nodular goitre

Such a goitre presents a difficult problem of diagnosis. Malignancy should be of concern in any solitary nodule; however, the majority of such nodules are cystic or benign and, indeed, may simply be the largest nodule of a multinodular goitre. The diagnostic challenge is to differentiate the small minority of malignant nodules, which require surgery, from the majority of benign nodules, which do not. Sometimes a history of rapid enlargement, associated lymph nodes or pain may suggest an aggressive malignancy, but most thyroid cancers are painless and slow-growing so that investigations are paramount. Risk factors for malignancy include previous irradiation, longstanding iodine deficiency and occasional familial cases.

Solitary toxic nodules are quite uncommon and may be associated with T₃ toxicosis.

Fibrotic goitre (Riedel's thyroiditis)

Fibrotic goitre is a rare condition, usually producing a 'woody' gland. It is associated with other midline fibrosis and is often difficult to distinguish from carcinoma, being irregular and hard. Clinical clues include systemic symptoms of inflammation and elevation in inflammatory markers; it has been shown to be an IgG₄-related disease.

Malignancy

In addition to thyroid carcinomas (see later), the thyroid is rarely the site of a metastatic deposit or the site of origin of a lymphoma.

Investigations

Clinical findings will dictate the appropriate initial tests:

- **Thyroid function tests** should include measurement of TSH plus free T₄ or T₃ (see **Box 21.7**).
- **Thyroid antibodies** are assessed to exclude an autoimmune aetiology.
- **Ultrasound** with high resolution is a sensitive method for delineating nodules and can demonstrate whether they are cystic or solid. In addition, a multinodular goitre may be demonstrated when only a single nodule is palpable. Unfortunately, even cystic lesions can be malignant and thyroid tumours may arise within a multinodular goitre; therefore fine-needle aspiration (see below) is often required and is performed under ultrasound control at the same time as the scan.
- **Chest and thoracic inlet X-rays or CT scan** may detect tracheal compression and large retrosternal extensions in people with a very large goitre or clinical symptoms.
- **Fine-needle aspiration (FNA)** should be performed in the outpatient clinic or during ultrasound if the appearance is suggestive of potential malignancy, based on defined ultrasound criteria, as in people with a solitary nodule or a dominant nodule in a multinodular goitre, there is a 5% chance of malignancy. Cytology in expert hands can usually differentiate the suspicious or definitely malignant nodule. FNA reduces the necessity for surgery but there is a 5% false-negative rate, which must be borne in mind (and the patient appropriately counselled). Continued observation is required when an isolated thyroid nodule is assumed to be benign without excision.
- **Thyroid scan** (⁹⁹ᵐTc) can be useful to distinguish between functioning (hot) or non-functioning (cold) nodules. A hot nodule is only rarely malignant; however, a cold nodule is malignant in 10% of cases and FNA has largely replaced isotope scans in the diagnosis of thyroid nodules.

Management
Euthyroid goitre

Many goitres are small, cause no symptoms and can be observed (including self-monitoring by the patient in the long term). In particular, during puberty and pregnancy, a goitre associated with euthyroidism rarely requires intervention and the patient can be reassured that spontaneous resolution is likely. Indications for surgical intervention are:

- **The possibility of malignancy.** A positive or suspicious FNA makes surgery mandatory, and surgery may be necessary if doubt persists, even in the presence of a negative FNA (especially if the patient is concerned by the false-negative rate).
- **Pressure symptoms on the trachea or, more rarely, the oesophagus.** The possibility of retrosternal extension should be excluded.
- **Cosmetic reasons.** A large goitre often causes considerable anxiety to the patient, even though it is functionally and anatomically benign.

RAI has also been advocated for the treatment of euthyroid goitre, particularly when surgery is an unattractive option.

Toxic nodule

This is initially treated with anti-thyroid drugs but surgery or radioiodine is often required.

Thyroid carcinoma

Types of thyroid carcinoma, with their characteristics and treatment, are listed in **Box 21.33**. While not common, these tumours are responsible for 400 deaths annually in the UK and there is an annual incidence of 30 000 cases in the USA. Over 75% occur in women. They present in 90% of cases as thyroid nodules (see above), but occasionally with cervical lymphadenopathy (about 5%), or with lung, cerebral, hepatic or bone metastases.

Carcinomas derived from thyroid epithelium may be papillary or follicular (differentiated), or anaplastic (undifferentiated). Medullary carcinomas (about 5% of all thyroid cancers) arise from the calcitonin-producing C cells. The pathogenesis of thyroid

Box 21.33 Types of thyroid malignancy

Cell type	Frequency	Behaviour	Spread	Prognosis
Papillary	70%	Occurs in young people	Local, sometimes lung/bone secondaries	Good, especially in young
Follicular	20%	More common in females	Metastases to lung/bone	Good if resectable
Medullary cell	5%	Often familial	Local and metastases	Poor, but indolent course
Anaplastic	<5%	Aggressive	Locally invasive	Very poor
Lymphoma	2%	Variable		Sometimes responsive to radiotherapy

epithelial carcinomas is not understood, except for occasional familial papillary carcinoma, and those cases related to previous head and neck irradiation or ingestion of RAI (e.g. post-Chernobyl). These tumours are minimally active hormonally and are extremely rarely associated with hyperthyroidism; over 90%, however, secrete thyroglobulin, which can therefore act as a tumour marker after thyroid ablation.

Papillary and follicular carcinomas

The primary treatment is surgical: normally total or near-total thyroidectomy for local disease. Regional or more extensive neck dissection is needed where there is local nodal spread or involvement of local structures.

Most tumours will take up iodine, and UK and other guidelines currently recommend RAI ablation of residual thyroid tissue postoperatively for most people with differentiated thyroid cancer. After ablation of normal thyroid in this way, RAI may be used to localize residual disease (scanning using low doses) or to treat it (using high doses: 5.5–7.5 GBq). When disease does recur, local invasion and lymph node involvement is most common, and lungs and bone are the most common sites of distant metastases.

To minimize risk of recurrence patients are treated with suppressive doses of levothyroxine (sufficient to suppress TSH levels below the normal range). Patient progress is monitored, both clinically and biochemically, using serum thyroglobulin levels as a tumour marker. The measurement of thyroglobulin is most sensitive when TSH is high but this requires the withdrawal of levothyroxine therapy. Recombinant TSH (thyrotropin alpha, rhTSH) 900 µg (2 doses over 48 h) is used to stimulate thyroglobulin without stopping levothyroxine therapy. Detectable thyroglobulin suggests recurrence, in which case whole-body ^{131}I scanning is required. Unfortunately, the presence of anti-thyroglobulin antibodies can make the assay unreliable.

The ***prognosis*** is extremely good when differentiated thyroid cancer is excised while confined to the thyroid gland, and the specific therapies available lead to a relatively good prognosis even in the presence of metastases at diagnosis. Accepted markers of high risk include greater age (>40 years), larger primary tumour size (>4 cm) and macroscopic invasion of capsule and surrounding tissues. Recently, oral sorafenib has shown a good short-term response in locally advanced and metastatic differentiated thyroid cancers that were refractory to RAI.

Medullary carcinoma

Medullary thyroid carcinoma (MTC) is a neuroendocrine tumour of the calcitonin-producing C cells of the thyroid. This condition is often associated with MEN 2 (see p. 650). Approximately 25% of patients diagnosed with MTC have a mutation of the *RET* proto-oncogene, although the other manifestations of MEN 2 may be absent; hence the importance of genetic counselling and family screening. People with MEN 2 mutations are advised to have a prophylactic thyroidectomy as early as 5 years of age to prevent the development of MTC.

Total thyroidectomy and wide lymph node clearance are usually indicated in MTC. Local invasion or metastasis is frequent, and the tumour responds poorly to treatment, although progression is often slow. Recent biological therapy with vandetanib and cabozantinib has shown benefit in advanced medullary thyroid carcinoma.

Anaplastic carcinomas and lymphoma

These do not respond to RAI, and external radiotherapy produces only a brief respite.

Further reading

Abraham P, Bevan JS. Antithyroid drug regimen for treating Graves' hyperthyroidism. *Cochrane Database Syst Rev* 2010; 1:CD003420.
Bahn RS. Graves ophthalmopathy. *N Engl J Med* 2010; 362:726–738.
Brent GA. Thyroid function and screening in pregnancy. *N Engl J Med* 2012; 366:562–568.
Burman KD, Wartofsky L. Thyroid nodules. *N Engl J Med* 2015; 373: 2347–2356.
Franklyn JA, Boelaert K. Subclinical thyroid disease: where is the evidence? *Lancet Diabetes Endocrinol* 2013; 1:172–173.
Franklyn JA, Boelaert K. Thyrotoxicosis. *Lancet* 2012; 379:1155–1166.
Haugen BR, Wartofsky L. American Thyroid Association management guidelines for adult patients with thyroid nodules and differentiated thyroid cancer. *Thyroid* 2016; 26:1–133.
Perros P, Boelaert K, Colley S et al and the British Thyroid Association. Guidelines for the management of thyroid cancer. *Clin Endocrinol* 2014; 81(S1):1–22.
Ross DS. Radioiodine therapy for hyperthyroidism. *N Engl J Med* 2011; 364:542–550.

HYPOTHALAMO–PITUITARY–GONADAL AXIS

The hypothalamo–pituitary–gonadal axis controls progress through puberty (p. 633) and the capacity for reproduction. Terminology in reproductive medicine is shown in **Box 21.34**.

Anatomy and physiology

Embryology

Up to 8 weeks of gestation, the sexes share a common development, with a primitive genital tract including the Wolffian and

---

Box 21.34 Definitions in reproductive medicine

Term	Definition
Erectile dysfunction	Inability of the male to achieve or sustain an erection adequate for satisfactory intercourse
Azoospermia	Absence of sperm in the ejaculate
Oligospermia	Reduced numbers of sperm in the ejaculate
Libido	Sexual interest or desire; often difficult to assess and greatly affected by stress, tiredness and psychological factors
Menarche	Age at first period
Primary amenorrhoea	Failure to begin spontaneous menstruation by age 16
Secondary amenorrhoea	Absence of menstruation for 3 months in a woman who has previously had cycles
Oligomenorrhoea	Irregular long cycles; often used for any length of cycle above 35 days
Dyspareunia	Pain or discomfort in the female during intercourse
Menstruation	Onset of spontaneous (usually regular) uterine bleeding in the female
Virilization	Occurrence of male secondary sexual characteristics in the female

Müllerian ducts. Additionally, there are a primitive perineum and primitive gonads.

- In the presence of a Y chromosome, the potential testis develops while the ovary regresses.
- In the absence of a Y chromosome, the potential ovary develops and related ducts form a uterus and the upper vagina.

Production of Müllerian inhibitory factor from the early 'testis' produces atrophy of the Müllerian duct, while, under the influence of testosterone and dihydrotestosterone, the Wolffian duct differentiates into an epididymis, vas deferens, seminal vesicles and prostate. Androgens induce transformation of the perineum to include a penis, penile urethra and scrotum containing the testes, which descend in response to androgenic stimulation. At birth, testicular volume is 0.5–1 mL. The number of oocytes in the ovaries of a female fetus has reached a maximum by the end of the second trimester of *in utero* development. At birth, the ovaries contain about 3 million oocytes, of which only 400 000 will remain by the time puberty occurs. With the onset of menarche, these oocytes will activate and grow, leading to ovulation and then menstruation.

Physiology

An outline of the hypothalamic–pituitary–gonadal axis is shown in **Fig. 21.27**.

Pulses of gonadotrophin-releasing hormone (GnRH) are released from the hypothalamus and stimulate luteinizing hormone (LH) and follicle-stimulating hormone (FSH) release from the pituitary. LH and FSH are composed of two glycoprotein chains (α and β subunits). The α subunits are identical and are shared with TSH, while the β subunit confers specific biological activity (**Box 21.35**)

The male

1. LH stimulates testosterone production from Leydig cells of the testis.
2. Testosterone acts via nuclear androgen receptors, which interact with co-regulatory proteins to produce the appropriate tissue responses: progress through puberty, anabolism and the maintenance of libido. It also acts locally within the testis to aid spermatogenesis. Testosterone circulates largely bound to sex hormone-binding globulin (SHBG) (see p. 588). Testosterone feeds back on the hypothalamus/pituitary to inhibit GnRH secretion.
3. FSH stimulates the Sertoli cells in the seminiferous tubules to produce mature sperm and the inhibins A and B.
4. Inhibin feeds back to the pituitary to decrease FSH secretion. Activin, a related peptide, counteracts inhibin.

The female

Female physiology is more complex (see **Figs 21.27** and **21.28**).

1. During puberty in response to pulses of hypothalamic GnRH, pituitary secretes LH and FSH, which stimulate androgen and oestrogen production from the ovaries resulting in progress through puberty followed by menarche and the establishment of the menstrual cycle.
2. The menstrual cycle depends upon the activity of hypothalamic GnRH. Pulses of GnRH, at about 2-hour intervals, stimulate release of pituitary LH and FSH.
3. Menstrual cycles are often irregular during adolescence, particularly the interval from the first cycle to the second cycle as immaturity of the hypothalamic–pituitary–ovarian axis during the early years after menarche often results in anovulation and cycles may be somewhat long (90% of cycles: 21–45 days). By

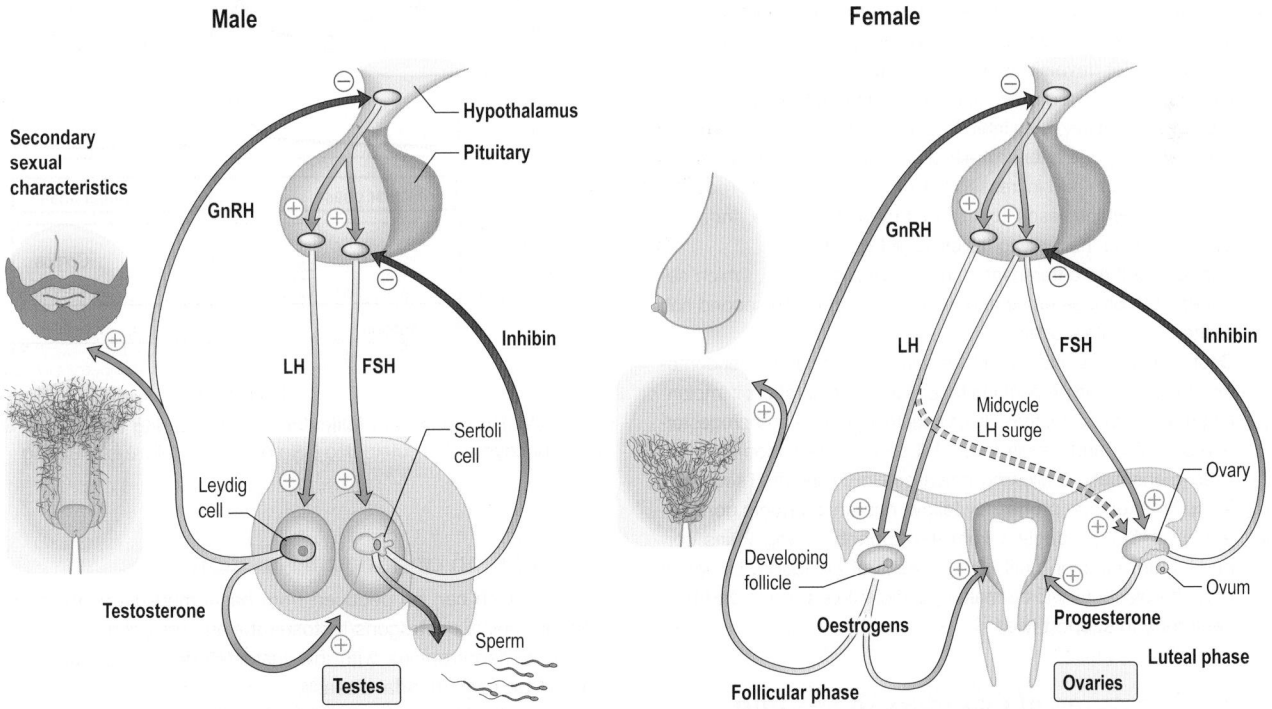

Fig. 21.27 Male and female hypothalamic–pituitary–gonadal axes. Luteinizing hormone (LH) and follicle-stimulating hormone (FSH) are secreted in pulses in response to hypothalamic gonadotrophin-releasing hormone (GnRH) and have different effects on the gonads (see text). Testosterone and oestrogens have multiple peripheral effects and exert negative feedback on LH secretion. Inhibin exerts negative feedback on FSH secretion.

> ℹ **Box 21.35 Hormones and receptors of the hypothalamic–pituitary–gonadal axis**

Hormone	Source	Site of action	Hormone structure	Receptor	Post-receptor activity
Gonadotrophin-releasing hormone (GnRH; LHRH)	Hypothalamus	Pituitary	Peptide – 10 AA	Membrane – 7TM GnRH-R1	G-proteins PLC/IP₃
Luteinizing hormone (LH)	Pituitary	Gonad	Glycoprotein: α and β subunits	Membrane – 7TM LHhCGR	G-proteins cAMP
Follicle-stimulating hormone (FSH)	Pituitary	Gonad	Glycoprotein: α and β subunits	Membrane –7TM FSHR	G-proteins cAMP
Oestradiol	Ovary	Uterus, breast bone, vascular	Steroid ring	Nuclear ER α and β (ESR1/ESR2)	Homo-/heterodimer ERE Transcription
Testosterone	Testis	Many tissues	Steroid ring	Nuclear AR (NR3C4)	Dimer ARE Transcription
Inhibin and activin	Gonad	Pituitary–hypothalamus	Peptide dimers α and β subunits	Transmembrane dimerized	Phosphorylation by receptor

7TM, 7 transmembrane (G-protein coupled receptor); AA, amino acids; ARE, androgen response element; cAMP, adenylate cyclase → cyclic adenosine monophosphate; ERE, oestrogen response element; LHhCGR, luteinizing hormone human chorionic gonadotrophin receptor; LHRH, luteinizing hormone-releasing hormone; PLC/IP₃, phospholipase C/inositol triphosphate.

the third year after menarche, 60–80% of menstrual cycles are 21–34 days long, as is typical of adults.

4. LH stimulates ovarian androgen production by the ovarian theca cells.

5. FSH stimulates follicular development and activity of aromatase (an enzyme required to convert ovarian androgens to oestrogens) in the ovarian granulosa cells. FSH also stimulates release of inhibin from ovarian stromal cells, which inhibits FSH release. Activin counteracts inhibin (see **Fig. 21.27**).

6. Although many follicles are 'recruited' for development in early folliculogenesis, by day 8–10 a 'leading' (or 'dominant') follicle is selected for development into a mature Graafian follicle.

7. Oestrogens have a double feedback action on the pituitary (see **Fig. 21.27**). Initially, they inhibit gonadotrophin secretion (negative feedback) but, later, high-level exposure results in increased GnRH secretion and increased LH sensitivity to GnRH (positive feedback), which leads to the mid-cycle LH surge, inducing ovulation from the leading follicle (see **Fig. 21.28**).

8. The follicle then differentiates into a corpus luteum, which secretes both progesterone and oestradiol during the second half of the cycle (luteal phase).

9. Oestrogen initially and then progesterone cause uterine endometrial proliferation in preparation for possible implantation; if implantation does not occur, the corpus luteum regresses and progesterone secretion and inhibin levels fall so that the endometrium is shed (menstruation), allowing increased GnRH and FSH secretion.

10. If implantation and pregnancy follow, human chorionic gonadotrophin (HCG) production from the trophoblast maintains corpus luteum function until 10–12 weeks of gestation, by which time the placenta will be making sufficient oestrogen and progesterone to support itself.

Clinical features of disorders of sex and reproduction

A detailed history and examination of all systems are required (**Box 21.36**). A man having regular satisfactory intercourse or a woman with regular ovulatory periods is most unlikely to have significant endocrine disease, assuming the history is accurate.

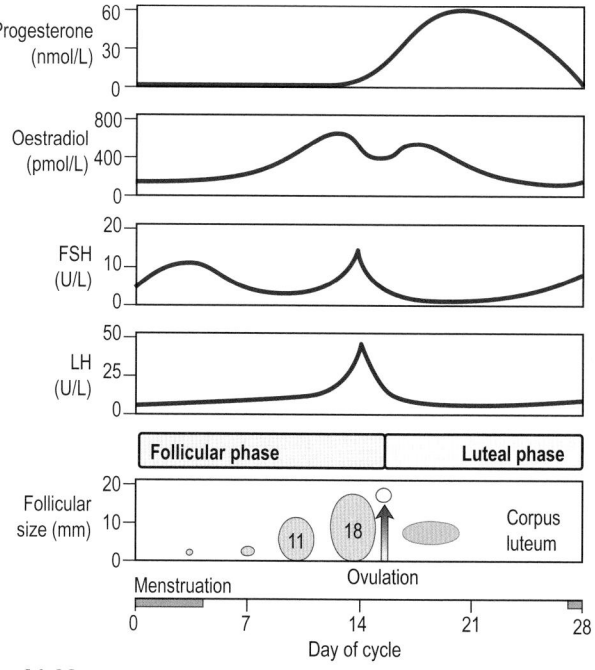

Fig. 21.28 Hormonal and follicular changes during the normal menstrual cycle. LH, luteinizing hormone; FSH, follicle-stimulating hormone.

Investigation of gonadal function

In adults much can be deduced from basal measurements of the gonadotrophins, oestrogens/testosterone and prolactin:

- High gonadotrophins with low testosterone or oestradiol indicates primary gonadal disease.
- Low levels of testosterone/oestradiol with low or normal LH/FSH imply hypothalamic–pituitary disease.
- Demonstration of ovulation (by measurement of luteal phase serum progesterone and/or by serial ovarian ultrasound in the follicular phase) or a healthy sperm count (20–200 million/mL, >60% grade I motility and <20% abnormal forms) provides

Box 21.36 Sexual and menstrual disorders

History
- Menstruation – timing of bleeding and cycle
- Relationship of symptoms to cycle
- Breasts (tenderness/galactorrhoea)
- Hirsutism and acne
- Libido and potency
- Problems with intercourse
- Past fertility and future plans

Physical signs
- Evidence of systemic disease
- Secondary sexual characteristics
- Extent/distribution of hair
- Genital size (testes, ovaries, uterus)
- Clitoromegaly
- Breast development, gynaecomastia
- Galactorrhoea

Box 21.37 Tests of gonadal function

Test	Uses/comments
Male	
Basal testosterone	Normal levels exclude hypogonadism
Sperm count	Normal count excludes deficiency Motility and abnormal sperm forms should be noted
Female	
Basal oestradiol	Normal levels exclude hypogonadism
Luteal phase progesterone (days 18–24 of cycle)	If >30 nmol/L, suggests ovulation
Ultrasound of ovaries	To confirm ovulation
Both sexes	
Basal LH/FSH	Demonstrates state of feedback system for hormone production (LH) and germ cell production (FSH)
HCG test (testosterone or oestradiol measured)	Response shows potential of ovary or testis; failure demonstrates primary gonadal problem
Clomifene test (LH and FSH measured)	Tests hypothalamic negative feedback system; clomifene is an oestrogen antagonist and causes LH/FSH to rise
LHRH test (rarely used)	Shows adequacy (or otherwise) of LH and FSH stores in pituitary

FSH, follicle-stimulating hormone; HCG, human chorionic gonadotrophin; LH, luteinizing hormone; LHRH, luteinizing hormone-releasing hormone.

absolute confirmation of normal female or male reproductive endocrinology, but these tests are not always essential.
- Pregnancy provides complete demonstration of normal male and female function.
- Hyperprolactinaemia can be confirmed or excluded by direct measurement. Levels may increase with stress; if this is suspected, a cannula should be inserted and samples taken through it 30 minutes later.

More detailed tests are indicated in **Box 21.37**.

Disorders in the male

Hypogonadism
History and examination

How a male presents depends on age. Hypogonadism in an adolescent would present with delayed puberty and/or growth, whereas an

Box 21.38 Effects of androgens and consequences of androgen deficiency in the male

Physiological effect	Consequences of deficiency
General	
Maintenance of libido	Loss of libido
Deepening of voice	High-pitched voice (if prepubertal)
Frontotemporal balding	No temporal recession
Facial, axillary and limb hair	Decreased hair
Maintenance of erectile and ejaculatory function	Loss of erections/ejaculation
Pubic hair	
Maintenance of male pattern	Thinning and loss of pubic hair
Testes and scrotum	
Maintenance of testicular size/consistency (needs gonadotrophins as well)	Small, soft testes
Rugosity of scrotum	Poorly developed penis/scrotum
Stimulation of spermatogenesis	Subfertility
Musculoskeletal	
Epiphyseal fusion	Eunuchoidism (if prepubertal)
Maintenance of muscle bulk and power	Decreased muscle bulk
Maintenance of bone mass	Osteoporosis

adult may present with poor libido, erectile dysfunction and loss of secondary sexual hair (**Box 21.38**). Hypogonadism may also be an incidental finding, such as one that emerges during investigation for subfertility. Semen volume is usually maintained as sperm makes up for only a very small proportion of seminal fluid volume; most is prostatic fluid. The testes may be small and soft, and there may be gynaecomastia. Except with subfertility, the symptoms are usually those of androgen deficiency.

Causes of male hypogonadism are shown in **Box 21.39**.

Investigations

Hypogonadism may be immediately apparent but basal levels of testosterone, LH and FSH should be measured. These will allow the distinction to be made between primary gonadal (testicular) failure and hypothalamic–pituitary disease.

If primary gonadal failure is identified, chromosomal analysis (e.g. to exclude Klinefelter's syndrome) is required. In secondary gonadal failure, gonadotrophin deficiency, pituitary MRI scan, prolactin levels and other pituitary function tests are needed.

A frequent cause of referral is men with poor libido or erectile dysfunction with equivocal lowering of serum testosterone (7–10 nmol/L) without elevation of gonadotrophins. If the testosterone was taken in the morning, such test results can be interpreted as mild gonadotrophin deficiency or lower end of the normal, but may also be seen in people with obesity and diabetes mellitus, who commonly have low circulating SHBG levels associated with insulin resistance and therefore low total testosterone levels but normal free testosterone levels. Regular use of opiate analgesia may lead to gonadotrophin deficiency and should be considered. 'Anabolic' steroid (i.e. androgen) abuse causes similar biochemical findings and is likely if the patient appears well virilized. A therapeutic trial of testosterone replacement is often justified and forms part of the

- Reduced gonadotrophins (hypothalamic–pituitary disease):
  - Hypopituitarism
  - Selective gonadotrophic deficiency, Kallmann's syndrome, normosmic idiopathic hypogonadotropic hypogonadism
  - Severe systemic illness
  - Severe underweight
- Hyperprolactinaemia
- Primary gonadal disease (congenital):
  - Anorchia/Leydig cell agenesis
  - Cryptorchidism (testicular maldescent)
  - Chromosome abnormality
- (e.g. Klinefelter's syndrome)
  - Enzyme defects: 5α-reductase deficiency
- Primary gonadal disease (acquired):
  - Testicular torsion
  - Orchidectomy
  - Local testicular disease
  - Chemotherapy/radiation toxicity
  - Orchitis (e.g. mumps)
  - Chronic kidney disease
  - Cirrhosis/alcohol
  - Sickle cell disease
- Androgen receptor deficiency/ abnormality

i **Box 21.40 Androgen replacement therapy**

Route	Preparation	Dose	Remarks
Dermal	Testosterone gel	50–100 mg	Rubs on shoulders
	Testosterone patch	300 μg/24 h	Self-adhesive
Intra-muscular	Testosterone enanthate	250 mg every 3 weeks	Frequent injections
	Testosterone unde-canoate	1 g every 3 months	Painful Large-volume injection
	Testosterone propionate	50–100 mg every 2–3 weeks	Very frequent injections Short half-life
Oral	Testosterone unde-canoate	120–160 mg daily, in divided doses	Variable dose, irregular absorption
Implant	Testosterone implant	600 mg every 4–5 months	Requires implant procedure Scarring, infection

investigation in some patients; full pituitary evaluation may be required in such cases to exclude other pituitary disease.

Management

The cause of hypogonadism can rarely be reversed and testosterone replacement therapy should be commenced to control current symptoms and prevent osteoporosis in the long term. Replacement is usually given by transdermal gel or by intramuscular injection (**Box 21.40**). In gonadotrophin deficiency, LH and FSH (purified or synthetic) or pulsatile GnRH may be used when fertility is required.

Special instances of hypogonadism
Cryptorchidism

Cryptorchidism (or undescended testes) is usually treated by surgical exploration and orchidopexy in early childhood. After that age, the germinal epithelium is increasingly at risk, and lack of descent by puberty is associated with subfertility. A short trial of HCG occasionally induces descent; an HCG test with a testosterone response

72 hours later excludes anorchia. Intra-abdominal testes have an increased risk of developing malignancy; if presentation is after puberty, orchidectomy is advised. Patients may present in adulthood with a history of cryptorchidism with primary testicular failure (due to the testicular damage before or during surgery) or gonadotrophin deficiency (presumably the initial cause of maldescent).

Klinefelter's syndrome

Klinefelter's syndrome is a common chromosomal abnormality, affecting 1 in 1000 males (47XXY and variants, e.g. 46XY/47XXY mosaicism), i.e. a male with an extra X chromosome. There is both a loss of Leydig cells and seminiferous tubular dysgenesis. If not identified on amniocentesis, only 10% are diagnosed prepuberty; early indications of the condition include cryptorchidism, behavioural problems, and learning disabilities as well as tall stature. In adolescence, gynaecomastia and micro-orchidism (mostly from the age of 14 years), as well as a poor muscular bulk with excessive long legs (due to lack of epiphyseal closure), small shoulders and broad hips should raise suspicion. Most patients have a normal puberty; while in adulthood, infertility is one of the most common presentations. There is also a predisposition to diabetes mellitus, breast cancer, emphysema and bronchiectasis; these are all unrelated to the testosterone deficiency.

Clinical examination shows a wide spectrum of features with small, pea-sized but firm testes, usually gynaecomastia and other signs of *androgen deficiency*. Confirmation is by chromosomal analysis.

Treatment is androgen replacement therapy if deficient in testosterone. The majority of men with Klinefelter's syndrome have relative testosterone deficiency (low-normal levels). The evidence that testosterone replacement in these men has positive benefits is lacking but should be discussed and trialled. No treatment is possible for the abnormal seminiferous tubules and infertility, although advances in fertility techniques and microdissection testicular sperm extraction (*microTESE*), offers some hope to men wanting to father their own child.

Kallmann's syndrome

This is isolated GnRH deficiency. It is associated with decreased or absent sense of smell (anosmia), and sometimes with other bony (cleft palate), renal and cerebral abnormalities (e.g. colour blindness). It is often familial and is usually X-linked, resulting from a mutation in the *KAL1* gene, which encodes anosmin-1 (producing loss of smell); one sex-linked form is due to an abnormality of a cell adhesion molecule. Management is that of secondary hypogonadism (see p. 626). Fertility is possible with gonadotrophin therapy.

Normosmic idiopathic hypogonadotropic hypogonadism

This refers to isolated GnRH deficiency in the absence of anosmia. Known mutations account for less than 15% of normosmic idiopathic hypogonadotropic hypogonadism (nIHH). Mutations include the *KISS1* gene, which codes for kisspeptin, the protein that acts on the GPR54 receptor, and the *FGFR1* gene.

Oligospermia and azoospermia

These may be secondary to gonadotrophin deficiency and can be corrected by gonadotrophin therapy. More often, they result from primary testicular diseases, in which case they are rarely treatable, although advances in fertility techniques and microdissection testicular sperm extraction (microTESE), offers some hope to men with primary hypogonadism wanting to father their own child.

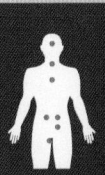

- Physiological:
  - Neonatal
  - Pubertal
  - Old age
- Hyperthyroidism
- Hyperprolactinaemia
- Renal disease
- Liver disease
- Hypogonadism (see **Box 21.39**)
- Oestrogen-producing tumours (testis, adrenal)

- HCG-producing tumours (testis, lung)
- Starvation/refeeding
- Carcinoma of breast
- Drugs:
  - Oestrogenic: oestrogens, cannabis, digoxin, diamorphine
  - Antiandrogens: spironolactone, cimetidine, cyproterone
  - Others: gonadotrophins, cytotoxics

HCG, human chorionic gonadotrophin.

Azoospermia with normal testicular size and low FSH levels suggests a vas deferens block, which is sometimes reversible by surgical intervention.

Gynaecomastia

Gynaecomastia is development of breast tissue in the male. Causes are shown in **Box 21.41**. It is due to an imbalance between free oestrogen and free androgen effects on breast tissue.

Pubertal gynaecomastia

This occurs in perhaps 50% of normal boys, often asymmetrically. It usually resolves spontaneously within 6–18 months, but after this duration may require surgical removal, as fibrous tissue will have been laid down. The cause is thought to be relative oestrogen excess, and the oestrogen antagonist tamoxifen is occasionally helpful.

Gynaecomastia in the older male

This requires a full assessment to exclude potentially serious underlying disease, such as bronchial carcinoma and testicular tumours (e.g. Leydig cell tumour). However, aromatase activity (see p. 624) increases with age and may be the cause of gynaecomastia in this group. Aromatase is an enzyme of the cytochrome P450 family and converts androgens to produce oestrogens. Drug effects are common (especially digoxin and spironolactone), and once these and significant liver disease are excluded, most cases have no definable cause. Painful gynaecomastia may be treated with a 3–6-month trial of tamoxifen, and surgery is occasionally necessary if the symptoms or cosmetic appearance are unacceptable.

The ageing male

In the male, there is no sudden 'change of life'. However, there is a progressive loss of sexual function with reduction in morning erections and frequency of intercourse.

The age of onset varies widely. Typically, overall testicular volume diminishes and SHBG and gonadotrophin levels gradually rise, but other men present with low or borderline testosterone without elevation of LH/FSH. Low testosterone certainly increases the risk of osteoporosis and, in some studies, is associated with increased cardiovascular risk. It remains unclear to what extent general symptoms of lack of energy, drive, muscle strength and general wellbeing may relate to these hormonal changes, but a recent trial of testosterone replacement showed no benefit in general symptoms although there was an improvement in sexual

Physiological effect	Consequences of deficiency
Breast	
Development of connective and duct tissue	Small, atrophic breast
Nipple enlargement and areolar pigmentation	
Pubic hair	
Maintenance of female pattern	Thinning and loss of pubic hair
Vulva and vagina	
Vulval growth	Atrophic vulva
Vaginal glandular and epithelial proliferation	Atrophic vagina
Vaginal lubrication	Dry vagina and dyspareunia
Uterus and tubes	
Myometrial and tubal hypertrophy	Small, atrophic uterus and tubes
Endometrial proliferation	Amenorrhoea
Skeletal	
Epiphyseal fusion	Eunuchoidism (if prepubertal)
Maintenance of bone mass	Osteoporosis

function. Loss of libido and erectile dysfunction are, however, common symptoms, even when hormones are normal, and long-term outcome studies of testosterone replacement are still awaited. Therefore, the decision to offer testosterone replacement to an ageing male is currently based on full clinical and biochemical assessment and full discussion of potential risks (including prostate disease) as well as benefits. If testosterone is unequivocally low (<7 pmol/L) and there are symptoms specific to androgen deficiency (low libido, erectile dysfunction and loss of early morning erections), most authorities would recommend replacement. However, few would treat if testosterone is higher than 12 pmol/L with normal LH/FSH. Clinically, a large proportion of cases are in the borderline range (7–12 pmol/L), which can lead to difficulties in reaching a firm diagnosis. There is an increasing move towards measuring fasting testosterone levels, as food intake may decrease testosterone, leading to an incorrect diagnosis of androgen deficiency.

Disorders in the female

Hypogonadism

Impaired ovarian function, whether primary or secondary, will lead to both oestrogen deficiency and abnormalities of the menstrual cycle. The latter is very sensitive to disruption, cycles becoming anovulatory and irregular before disappearing altogether. Symptoms will depend on the age at which failure develops. Thus, before puberty, primary amenorrhoea will occur, possibly with delayed puberty; after puberty, secondary amenorrhoea and symptoms of oestrogen deficiency.

Oestrogen deficiency

The physiological effects of oestrogens and symptoms/signs of deficiency are shown in **Box 21.42**.

ℹ️ **Box 21.43 Clinical assessment of amenorrhoea**

History
- ? Pregnant
- Date of onset
- Age of menarche, if any
- Sudden or gradual onset
- General health
- Weight – absolute and changes in recent past
- Stress (job, lifestyle, examinations, relationships)
- Excessive exercise
- Drugs
- Hirsutism, acne, virilization
- Headaches/visual symptoms
- Sense of smell
- Past history of pregnancies
- Past history of gynaecological surgery

Examination
- General health
- Body shape and skeletal abnormalities
- Weight and height
- Hirsutism and acne
- Evidence of virilization
- Maturity of secondary sexual characteristics
- Galactorrhoea
- Normality of vagina, cervix and uterus

Amenorrhoea

Absence of periods or markedly irregular infrequent periods (oligomenorrhoea) is the most common presentation of female gonadal disease. The clinical assessment of such patients is shown in **Box 21.43**, and common causes are listed in **Box 21.44**. Causes can be divided into whether amenorrhoea is primary or secondary, whether associated with oestrogen deficiency or not, whether oestrogen deficiency is due to gonadotrophin deficiency or ovarian insufficiency, whether it is associated with another condition, and whether amenorrhoea is due to structural problems.

Polycystic ovary syndrome

Polycystic ovary syndrome is an example of amenorrhoea that could either be primary or secondary and is not associated with oestrogen deficiency. It is the most common cause of oligomenorrhoea and amenorrhoea (see below).

Hypothalamic and weight-related amenorrhoea

Amenorrhoea with low oestrogen and gonadotrophins in the absence of organic pituitary disease is described as hypothalamic amenorrhoea. This may be related to 'stress'; low body weight, excessive exercise or previous weight loss; stopping the contraceptive pill; or severe illness. However, some patients appear to have defective cycling mechanisms without apparent explanation.

A minimum body weight is necessary for regular menstruation. While anorexia nervosa is the extreme form of weight loss (see p. 797), amenorrhoea is common and may be seen at weights within the 'normal' range. It is possible that alterations in leptin levels are responsible for the hypothalamic dysfunction seen in this situation. Restoration of body weight to above the 50th centile for height is usually effective in restoring menstruation, but in the many cases where this cannot be achieved then oestrogen replacement is necessary.

Premature ovarian insufficiency

Premature ovarian insufficiency is the preferred term to describe premature menopause or ovarian failure of onset before the age of 40. The cause may be autoimmune, and is rarely caused by identifiable genetic causes such as the fragile X pre-mutation or Turner's syndrome; most commonly, however, it is of unknown aetiology, although often familial. Repeat measurements of LH/FSH levels are necessary before a diagnosis of premature ovarian insufficiency is given because of the psychological impact of this diagnosis and the possibility that a single elevation of LH/FSH might simply be the mid-cycle ovulatory surge. Iatrogenic causes, such as bilateral oophorectomy and following cancer therapy with radiotherapy and some chemotherapy agents also cause premature ovarian insufficiency. In some scenarios, ovarian function can fluctuate; therefore, in younger women, consideration needs to be given as to whether contraception is required, and the combined oral contraceptive pill is the best option for hormone replacement therapy (HRT).

Turner's syndrome is a cause of premature ovarian insufficiency, frequently with delayed puberty and primary amenorrhoea, although some girls do undergo menarche and establish a menstrual cycle but remain at risk of premature ovarian insufficiency. The phenotype is female with female external genitalia. There is gonadal dysgenesis with streak ovaries. Features include short stature, webbing of the neck (up to 40%), a wide carrying angle of the elbows, high-arched palate and low-set ears. These patients also have an increased incidence of autoimmune disease (2%), bicuspid aortic valves, aortic coarctation and dissection, coronary artery disease, hypertension, type 2 diabetes, horseshoe kidneys, lymphoedema, reduced bone density, hearing problems and inflammatory bowel disease (0.3%).

Investigation of oligo-amenorrhoea

Basal levels of FSH, LH, oestrogen and prolactin allow initial distinction between primary gonadal and hypothalamic–pituitary causes (**see Box 21.44**). Elevation of LH and FSH to menopausal levels usually confirms the diagnosis. Subsequent investigations are also shown in **Box 21.44**.

Anti-Müllerian hormone (AMH) released from granulosa cells of preantral and small antral follicles in the ovary, a marker of '*ovarian reserve*', is being increasingly used in context of secondary amenorrhoea, especially in infertility centres: PCOS (usually high level), premature ovarian insufficiency (low), hypogonadotropic hypogonadism (normal or low), and menopause (low). It is shown to be helpful in deciding the type of infertility treatment strategy to be adopted, specifically in premature ovarian insufficiency or hypogonadotropic hypogonadism cases where low AMH level indicates poor follicular reserve, therefore oocyte donation is recommended. Whereas adequate AMH level means there is hope for oocyte retrieval following gonadotrophin stimulation protocols to facilitate *in vitro* fertilization (IVF).

Management

Treatment is that of the cause wherever possible (e.g. hypothyroidism, low weight, stress, excessive exercise). Hyperprolactinaemia should be corrected (see below). Polycystic ovary syndrome is discussed in detail below.

When oestrogen deficiency is not reversed, HRT should almost always be given, as the risk of osteoporosis and other conditions related to oestrogen deficiency almost always outweighs the risks of HRT at this younger age. HRT may still also be actively recommended when normal menopause occurs relatively early (e.g. before the age of 50).

In younger and older women with premature ovarian insufficiency ovarian function may recover or fluctuate, and therefore consideration should be given to using the combined oral contraceptive pill if fertility is not desired.

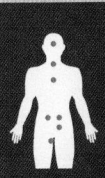

? Box 21.44 Differential diagnosis and investigation of amenorrhoea

Hormone results					Possible diagnoses	Secondary tests
LH	FSH	E2	PRL	T		
↑	↑	↓	N	N	Ovarian failure	
					Ovarian dysgenesis[a]	Karyotype
					Premature ovarian failure[a]	Ultrasound of ovary/uterus
					Steroid biosynthetic defect[a]	Laparoscopy/biopsy of ovary
					(Oophorectomy)	HCG stimulation
					(Chemotherapy)	
					Resistant ovary syndrome	
↓	↓	↓	N	N	Gonadotrophin failure	
					Hypothalamic–pituitary disease[a]	Pituitary MRI if diagnosis unclear
					Kallmann's syndrome/nIHH[a]	Possibly LHRH test
					Possible hypothalamic causes:	Serum free T$_4$
					Hypothalamic amenorrhoea[a]	Possibly full assessment of pituitary function
					Weight-related amenorrhoea[a]	
					Exercise-induced amenorrhoea and anorexia[a]	
					Post-pill amenorrhoea	
					General illness[a]	
↓	↓	↓	↑/↑↑	N	Hyperprolactinaemia	
					Prolactinoma[a]	See pages 639–641
					Idiopathic hyperprolactinaemia[a]	Serum free T$_4$/TSH
					Hypothyroidism[a]	Pituitary MRI
					Polycystic ovarian disease[a]	Other tests for PCOS
					Physiological in lactation	
					Dopamine-antagonist drugs	
↑/N	N	N	N/↑	N/↑	Polycystic ovary syndrome[a]	
					Rarely, Cushing's syndrome	Androstenedione, DHEAS
						SHBG
						Ultrasound of ovary
						Progesterone challenge
						See page 601 (Cushing's syndrome)
N/↓	N/↓	N/↓	N	↑↑	Androgen excess	
					Gonadal or adrenal tumour	Imaging ovary/adrenal
					Congenital adrenal hyperplasia[a]	17a-OH-progesterone
N	N	↑	↑	N	Pregnancy	Pregnancy test
N	N	N	N	N	Uterine/vaginal abnormality	
					Imperforate hymen[a]	Examination findings (?EUA)
					Absent uterus[a]	Ultrasound of pelvis
					Lack of endometrium	Progesterone challenge
						Hysteroscopy

[a]These conditions may present as primary amenorrhoea.
DHEAS, dehydroepiandrosterone sulphate; E2, oestradiol; EUA, examination under anaesthesia; FSH, follicle-stimulating hormone; HCG, human chorionic gonadotrophin; LH, luteinizing hormone; LHRH, luteinizing hormone-releasing hormone; nIHH, normosmic idiopathic hypogonadotropic hypogonadism; PCOS, polycystic ovary syndrome; PRL, prolactin; SHBG, sex hormone-binding globulin; T, testosterone.

When fertility is desired, in gonadotrophin deficiency, gonadotrophins can be given to achieve ovulation. Ovarian insufficiency is rarely treatable and often the option for pregnancy is donor eggs. There is a rare condition called 'resistant' ovary, where high-dose gonadotrophin therapy can occasionally lead to folliculogenesis.

Hirsutism

Normal hair versus hirsutism

The extent of normal hair growth varies between individuals, families and races, being more extensive in the Mediterranean and some Asian subcontinent populations. These normal variations in body hair, and the more extensive hair growth seen in patients complaining of hirsutism, represent a continuum from no visible hair to extensive cover with thick, dark hair. It is therefore impossible to draw an absolute dividing line between 'normal' and 'abnormal' degrees of facial and body hair in the female. Soft vellus hair is normally present all over the body; this type of hair on the face and elsewhere is 'normal' and is not sex hormone-dependent. Hair in the beard, moustache, breast, chest, axilla, abdominal midline, pubic and thigh areas is sex hormone-dependent. Any excess in the latter regions is thus a marker of increased ovarian or adrenal androgen production: most commonly, polycystic ovary syndrome (PCOS) but occasionally other rarer causes.

Aetiology

- **Idiopathic hirsutism**. People with hirsutism, no elevation of serum androgen levels and no other clinical features are sometimes labelled as having 'idiopathic hirsutism'. However, studies suggest that most people with 'idiopathic hirsutism' have some radiological or biochemical evidence of PCOS on more detailed investigation, and several studies have demonstrated evidence of mild PCOS in up to 20% of the normal female population. Familial or idiopathic hirsutism does occur, but usually involves a distribution of hair growth that is not typically androgenic.
- **Ovarian hyperthecosis**. This is a non-malignant ovarian disorder characterized by luteinized thecal cells in the ovarian stroma, which secrete testosterone. The clinical features are similar to those of PCOS but tend to present in perimenopausal women, and serum testosterone levels are higher than typically seen in PCOS.
- **Iatrogenic hirsutism**. This occurs after treatment with androgens, or more weakly androgenic drugs such as progestogens or danazol.
- **Non-androgen-dependent hair growth (hypertrichosis)**. This occurs with drugs such as phenytoin, diazoxide, minoxidil and ciclosporin.
- **Other causes**. Rarer and more serious endocrine causes of hirsutism and virilization include congenital adrenal hyperplasia (CAH; see p. 604), Cushing's syndrome (p. 600), and androgen-secreting (virilizing) tumours of the ovary and adrenal.

Management

See page 631.

Polycystic ovary syndrome

Polycystic ovary syndrome (PCOS) is the most common cause of hirsutism in clinical practice, affecting about 1 in 5 women worldwide. It is characterized by multiple small cysts within the ovary (**Fig. 21.29**) (which represent arrested follicular development) and by excess androgen production from the ovaries (and to a lesser extent from the adrenals).

Measured levels of androgens in blood vary widely from patient to patient and may remain within the normal range, but SHBG levels are often low (due to insulin resistance and high insulin levels), leading to high free androgen levels. In PCOS, there is thought to be an increased frequency of the GnRH pulse generator, causing an increase in LH pulses and androgen secretion. The response of the hair follicle to circulating androgens also seems to vary between individuals with otherwise identical clinical and biochemical features, and the reason for this variation in end-organ response remains poorly understood.

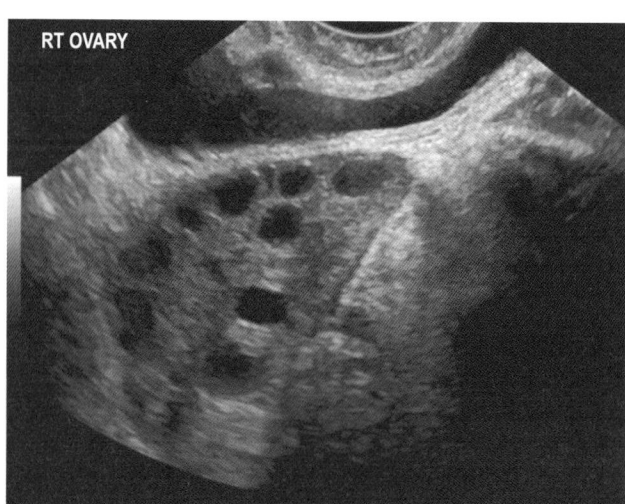

Fig. 21.29 Polycystic ovary syndrome. Ultrasound of the ovary, revealing multiple cysts with central ovarian stroma showing increased echo texture.

PCOS is frequently associated with:
- **hyperinsulinaemia and insulin resistance**, the prevalence of type 2 diabetes being 10 times higher than in normal women
- **hypertension, hyperlipidaemia and increased cardiovascular risk** (the metabolic syndrome; see p. 1250), which is 2–3 times higher in PCOS, and studies suggest that PCOS per se confers an absolute increase in cardiovascular end-points.

Obesity with PCOS is an additional risk factor for insulin resistance. The precise mechanisms that link the aetiology of polycystic ovaries, hyperandrogenism, anovulation and insulin resistance are still to be elucidated, and whether the basic defect is in the ovary, adrenal or pituitary, or is a more generalized metabolic defect, remains unknown. Frequently, there is a family history of either PCOS or type 2 diabetes, suggesting a genetic component.

In routine clinical practice, the majority of people with objective signs of androgen-dependent hirsutism will have PCOS, and investigation is mainly required to exclude rarer and more serious causes of virilization.

History and examination

Most patients with PCOS present with amenorrhoea/oligomenorrhoea and/or hirsutism and acne, shortly after menarche. Frequently, patients are also obese with evidence of insulin resistance. Clinical, biochemical and radiological features of PCOS merge imperceptibly into those of the normal populations.
- **Hirsutism.** This should be recorded objectively, ideally using a scoring system, both to document the problem and to monitor treatment. The method and frequency of physical removal (e.g. shaving, plucking) should also be recorded. The development of hirsutism commonly provokes severe distress in young women and may lead to avoidance of normal social activities. Most patients who complain of hirsutism will have an objective excess of hair on examination, but occasionally very little will be found (and appropriate counselling is then indicated).
- **Age and speed of onset.** Hirsutism related to PCOS usually begins around the time of the menarche and increases slowly and steadily in the teens and twenties. Rapid progression and prepubertal or late onset suggest a more serious cause.
- **Accompanying virilization.** Hirsutism due to PCOS may be severe and affect all androgen-dependent areas on the face and body. However, more severe virilization (clitoromegaly, recent-onset

frontal balding, male phenotype) implies substantial androgen excess, and usually indicates a rarer cause rather than PCOS. Thinning of head hair in a male pattern – androgenic alopecia – occurs in a proportion of women with uncomplicated PCOS, typically with a familial tendency for premature androgen-related hair loss in both sexes.

- **Menstruation.** Most people with PCOS will have some disturbance of menstruation, typically oligo-/amenorrhoea, although more frequent erratic bleeding can also occur. However, PCOS can present as hirsutism with regular periods or as irregular periods, with no evidence of hirsutism or acne.
- **Weight.** Many people with PCOS are also overweight or obese. The obesity worsens the underlying androgen excess and insulin resistance, and inhibits the response to treatment; it is an indication for appropriate advice on diet and exercise. In severe cases, the insulin resistance may have a visible manifestation as acanthosis nigricans on the neck and in the axillae. In addition to worsening the symptoms of PCOS, central obesity in PCOS significantly increases the likelihood of developing diabetes and cardiovascular disease.

Investigations and differential diagnosis

- **Serum total testosterone.** This is often elevated in PCOS and is invariably substantially raised in virilizing tumours (usually >5 nmol/L). People with hirsutism and normal testosterone levels frequently have low levels of SHBG, leading to high free androgen levels. The **free androgen index** ([testosterone/SHBG] *100) is often used and is high; free testosterone is difficult to measure directly.
- **Other androgens.** Androstenedione and dehydroepiandrosterone sulphate are frequently elevated in PCOS, and even higher in congenital adrenal hyperplasia (CAH) and virilizing tumours.
- **17α-Hydroxyprogesterone.** This is elevated in classical CAH, but may be apparent in late-onset CAH only after stimulation tests.
- **Gonadotrophin levels.** LH hypersecretion is a frequent feature of PCOS, but the pulsatile nature of secretion of this hormone means that a 'classic' increased LH/FSH ratio is not always observed on a random sample.
- **Oestrogen levels.** Oestradiol is usually normal in PCOS, but oestrone levels (which are rarely measured) are elevated because of peripheral conversion. Levels are variable in other causes.
- **Ovarian ultrasound.** This is a useful investigation (see **Fig. 21.28**). Typical features are those of a thickened capsule, multiple 3–5 mm cysts and a hyperechogenic stroma. Prolonged hyperandrogenization from any cause may lead to polycystic changes in the ovary. Ultrasound may also reveal virilizing ovarian tumours, although these are often small.
- **Serum prolactin.** Mild hyperprolactinaemia is common in PCOS but rarely exceeds 1500 mU/L.

If an androgen-secreting tumour is suspected clinically or after investigation, then more complex investigations include dexamethasone suppression tests, CT or MRI of adrenals, and selective venous sampling.

Diagnosis

Most patients presenting with a combination of hirsutism and menstrual disturbance will be shown to have PCOS, but the rarer alternative diagnoses should be excluded; the latter include late-onset CAH (early onset, raised serum 17α-hydroxyprogesterone), Cushing's syndrome (look for other clinical features), and virilizing

tumours of the ovary or adrenals (severe virilization, markedly elevated serum testosterone).

The consensus **(Rotterdam) criteria 2003** for diagnosis of PCOS are at least two of the following:

- clinical and/or biochemical evidence of hyperandrogenism
- oligo-ovulation and/or anovulation
- polycystic ovaries on ultrasound.

Management
Local therapy for hirsutism

Regular plucking, bleaching, use of depilatory cream, waxing or shaving is used. Such removal neither worsens nor improves the underlying severity of hirsutism. More 'permanent' solutions include electrolysis and a variety of 'laser' hair removal systems; all appear effective but have not been evaluated in long-term studies, are expensive, and still often require repeated long-term treatment. **Eflornithine cream** (an antiprotozoal) inhibits hair growth by inhibiting ornithine decarboxylase, but is effective in only a minority of cases and should be discontinued if there is no improvement after 4 months.

Systemic therapy for hirsutism

This always requires a year or more of treatment for maximal benefit, and long-term therapy is frequently required as the problem tends to recur when treatment is stopped. The patient must therefore always be an active participant in the decision to use systemic therapy and must understand the rare risks as well as the benefits. Weight loss (at least 5%) should also be encouraged, as many patients have improvement in symptoms.

- **Oestrogens** (e.g. oral contraceptives) suppress ovarian androgen production and reduce free androgens by increasing SHBG levels. Combined hormone pills will produce a slow improvement in hirsutism in a majority of cases and should normally be used first unless there is a contraindication, such as a history of thrombosis. After the menopause, HRT preparations that contain medroxyprogesterone (rather than more androgenic progestogens) may be helpful.
- **Cyproterone acetate** (50–100 mg daily) is an antiandrogen but is also a progestogen, teratogen and a weak glucocorticoid. Given continuously, it produces amenorrhoea, and so is normally given for days 1–14 of each cycle. In women of childbearing age, contraception is essential.
- **Spironolactone** (200 mg daily) also has antiandrogen activity and can cause useful improvements in hirsutism. In women of childbearing age, contraception is essential.
- **Finasteride** (5 mg daily), a 5α-reductase inhibitor that prevents the formation of dihydrotestosterone in the skin, has also been shown to be effective but long-term experience is limited. In women of childbearing age, contraception is essential.
- **Flutamide**, another antiandrogen, is less commonly used owing to the high incidence of hepatic side-effects. In women of childbearing age, contraception is essential.

Treatment of menstrual disturbance

- **Cyclical oestrogen/progestogen** administration will regulate the menstrual cycle and remove the symptom of oligo- or amenorrhoea. This is most frequently an additional benefit of the treatment of hirsutism, but may also be used when menstrual disturbance is the only symptom.
- **Metformin** (500 mg three times daily) is commonly used in this condition because of the recognized association between PCOS and insulin resistance. It may improve menstrual cyclicity and ovulation; some patients also report improvement in hirsutism and ease of weight loss, but gastrointestinal upset may limit use.

Box 21.45 Disorders of sexual differentiation

Condition	Chromosomes	Gonads	Phenotype	Remarks
Turner's syndrome	45X (50%) 46,X,i (Xq) (5–10%) 45,X, mosaicism (remainder)	Streak	Female	Often morphological features (e.g. short stature, web neck, coarctation of aorta)
Gonadal dysgenesis	46XY	Streak or minimal testes[a]	Immature female	
Congenital adrenal hyperplasia	46XX	Ovary	Female with variable virilization	Obvious androgen excess
Virilizing tumour	46XX	Ovary	Female with variable virilization	Obvious androgen excess
True hermaphroditism	46XX/XY or mosaic	Testis and ovary	Male or ambiguous	
Klinefelter's syndrome	47XXY	Small testes	Male, often with gynaecomastia	Many are hypogonadal
Testicular feminization	46XY	Testes[a]	Ambiguous or infantile female	Androgen receptor defective
Testicular synthetic defects	46XY	Testes[a]	Cryptorchid, ambiguous	
5α-Reductase deficiency	46XY	Testes	Cryptorchid, ambiguous	Impaired conversion of testosterone to dihydro-testosterone
Anorchia	46XY	Absent	Immature female	

[a]Gonadectomy advised because of high risk of malignancy.
i, isochromosome.

Treatment for fertility in PCOS

- **Clomifene or letrozole** is given daily on days 2–6 of the cycle and is effective in 75% of women in achieving ovulation. It can occasionally cause the **ovarian hyperstimulation syndrome**, an iatrogenic complication of ovulation induction therapy, consisting of ovarian enlargement, oedema, hypovolaemia, acute kidney injury and possibly shock; specialist supervision is essential. It is recommended that clomifene and letrozole should not normally be used for more than six cycles (owing to a possible increased risk of ovarian cancer in patients treated for longer than recommended).
- **Low-dose FSH** is used for non-responders to clomifene.
- **Metformin** alone may improve ovulation and achieve conception.

Wedge resection of the ovary was a traditional therapy but is now rarely required, although laparoscopic ovarian electrodiathermy may be helpful.

Disorders of sex development

Disorders of sex development (DSD) are a rare group of conditions that can be divided into 46XY and 46XX DSD and encompass conditions of abnormalities in androgen synthesis, action and excess and gonadal development and persistent Müllerian duct syndrome or sex chromosomal DSD (**Box 21.45**). Such cases always require extensive, multidisciplinary clinical management. An individual's sex can be defined in several ways:

- **Chromosomal sex.** The normal female is 46XX, the normal male 46XY. The Y chromosome confers male sex; if it is not present, development follows female lines.
- **Gonadal sex.** This is determined predominantly by chromosomal sex but requires normal embryological development.
- **Phenotypic sex.** This describes the normal physical appearance and characteristics of male and female body shape. This, in turn, is a manifestation of gonadal sex and subsequent sex hormone production.

- **Social sex (gender).** This is heavily dependent on phenotypic sex and normally assigned on appearance of the external genitalia at birth.
- **Sexual orientation** – heterosexual, homosexual or bisexual.

Further reading

Basaria S. Male hypogonadism. *Lancet* 2014; 383:1250–1263.
Carel JC, Léger J. Precocious puberty. *N Engl J Med* 2008; 358:2366–2377.
Caronia LM, Martin C, Welt CK et al. A genetic basis for functional hypothalamic amenorrhea. *N Engl J Med* 2011; 364:215–225.
Gordon CM. Functional hypothalamic amenorrhea. *N Engl J Med* 2010; 363:365–371.
Mani H, Levy MJ, Davies MJ et al. Diabetes and cardiovascular events in women with polycystic ovary syndrome: a 20-year retrospective cohort study. *Clin Endocrinol* 2013; 78:926–934.
Rotterdam ESHRE/ASRM-Sponsored PCOS Consensus Workshop Group. Revised 2003 consensus on diagnostic criteria and long-term health risks related to polycystic ovary syndrome. *Fertil Steril* 2004; 81:19–25.
Snyder PJ, Bhasin S, Cunningham AM et al. Effects of testosterone treatment in older men. *N Engl J Med* 2016; 374:611–624.
Webber L, Vermeulen N. ESHRE Guideline: Management of women with premature ovarian insufficiency. *Hum Reprod* 2016; 31:926–937.

GROWTH AND PUBERTY

Normal growth and puberty

There are factors other than GH axis and the hypothalamo–pituitary–gonadal axis that influence linear growth and adult height and timing of puberty in the human:

- **Genetic factors.** Children of two short parents will probably be short and similarly for tall parents. Timing of parental puberty is a strong determinant of timing of puberty in the child.
- **Nutritional factors.** Adequate nutrients must be available. Impaired growth can result from inadequate dietary intake or small bowel disease (e.g. coeliac disease). Puberty is affected by whether a child is undernourished or obese.
- **General health.** Any serious systemic disease in childhood is likely to reduce growth and/or delay puberty (e.g. chronic kidney disease or chronic infection).

- *Small for gestational age*; 15% of these infants do not catch up and can also have an earlier and more rapidly progressive puberty. There is some evidence that low birth weight may predispose to hypertension, diabetes and other health problems in later adult life (see p. 1246).
- *Emotional deprivation and psychological factors.* These can impair growth by complex, poorly understood mechanisms, probably involving temporarily decreased GH secretion.

In general, there are three overlapping phases of growth: infantile (0–2 years), which appears to be largely dependent on substrates (food); childhood (age 2 years to puberty), which is largely GH-dependent; and the adolescent 'growth spurt', dependent on GH and adequate sex hormone production during puberty.

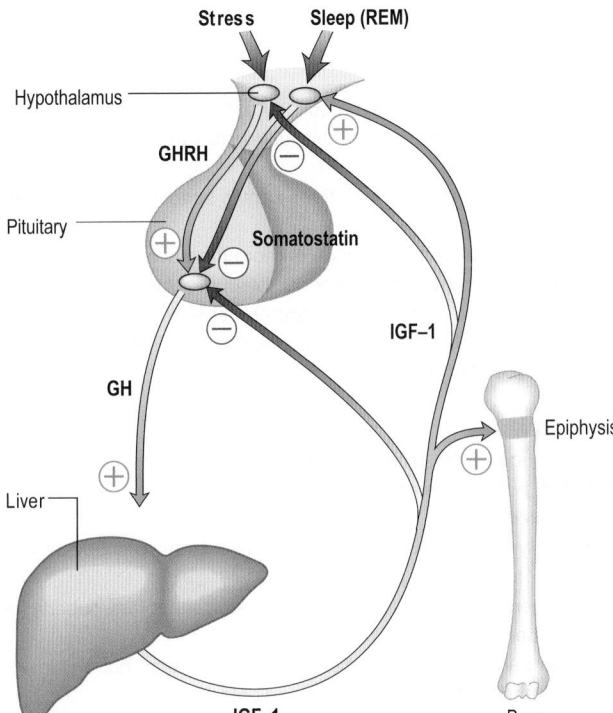

Fig. 21.30 The control of growth hormone (GH) and insulin-like growth factor-1 (IGF-1). Pituitary GH is secreted under dual control of growth hormone-releasing hormone (GHRH) and somatostatin, and stimulates release of IGF-1 in the liver and elsewhere. IGF-1 has peripheral actions, including bone growth, and exerts negative feedback to the hypothalamus and pituitary. REM, rapid eye movement.

Physiology

Growth hormone (GH) is the pituitary factor responsible for stimulation of body growth in humans. Its secretion is stimulated by GHRH, released into the portal system from the hypothalamus; it is also under inhibitory control exerted by somatostatin (**Fig. 21.30**). A separate GH-stimulating system involves a distinct receptor (GH secretagogue receptor), which interacts with ghrelin. It is not known how these two systems interact but, because ghrelin is synthesized in the stomach, a nutritional role is suggested for GH.

- *GH* acts by binding to a specific (single transmembrane) receptor located mainly in the liver (**Box 21.46**). This induces an intracellular phosphorylation cascade involving the Janus kinase/ signal transducing activators of transcription (JAK/STAT) pathway (see p. 68). STAT proteins are translocated from the cytoplasm into the cell nucleus and cause GH-specific effects by binding to nuclear DNA.
- *Insulin-like growth factor-1 (IGF-1)*, a somatomedin, stimulates growth. Its hepatic secretion is stimulated by a tissue-specific effect of GH on the liver. There are multiple IGF-binding proteins (IGF-BP) in plasma; IGF-BP3 can be measured clinically to improve assessment of GH status, particularly in children.

The metabolic actions of the system are:
- increasing collagen and protein synthesis
- promoting retention of calcium, phosphorus and nitrogen, necessary substrates for anabolism
- opposing the action of insulin (a 'counter-regulatory' hormone effect).

GH release is intermittent and mainly nocturnal, especially during REM sleep. The frequency and size of GH pulses increase during the growth spurt of adolescence and decline thereafter. Acute stress and exercise both stimulate GH release, while, in the normal subject, hyperglycaemia suppresses it.

IGF-1 may, in addition, play a major role in maintaining neoplastic growth. A relationship has been shown between circulating IGF-1 concentrations and breast cancer in premenopausal women and prostate cancer in men.

Puberty

The mechanisms initiating puberty are thought to result from withdrawal of central inhibition of GnRH release and involve a complex interplay between hypothalamic peptides, as well as external factors. Environmental and physical factors (including body fat changes and physical exercise) are involved in the timing of puberty, as well as the genetic factors required for pubertal maturation. Kisspeptin is the endogenous ligand for kisspeptin receptor *KISS1R*, formerly known as *GPR54* (a G-protein-coupled receptor gene), and this

Box 21.46 Hormones and receptors of the hypothalamic–pituitary–GH axis

Hormone	Source	Site of action	Hormone structure	Receptor	Post-receptor activity
Growth hormone-releasing hormone (GHRH)	Hypothalamus	Pituitary	Peptide – 44 AA	Membrane – 7TM	G-proteins cAMP
Somatostatin (inhibitory GHRIH)	Hypothalamus	Pituitary	Cyclic peptide – 14 or 28 AA	Membrane – 7TM SST2 + SST5	G-proteins Inhibit cAMP
Growth hormone	Pituitary	Liver and other tissues	Peptide – 191 AA	Transmembrane Dimerized GHR	JAK2 STAT
Insulin-like growth factor 1 (IGF-1)	Liver and locally elsewhere	Many tissues	Peptide – 70 AA 3 S=S bridges	Transmembrane – IGFR 2α + 2β subunits	Receptor tyrosine kinase

7TM, 7 transmembrane (G-protein coupled receptor); AA, amino acids; cAMP, adenylate cyclase → cyclic adenosine monophosphate; GHRIH, growth hormone-releasing inhibitory hormone; JAK, Janus kinase; STAT, signal transducers and activators of transcriptions; SST, somatostatin receptor subtypes.

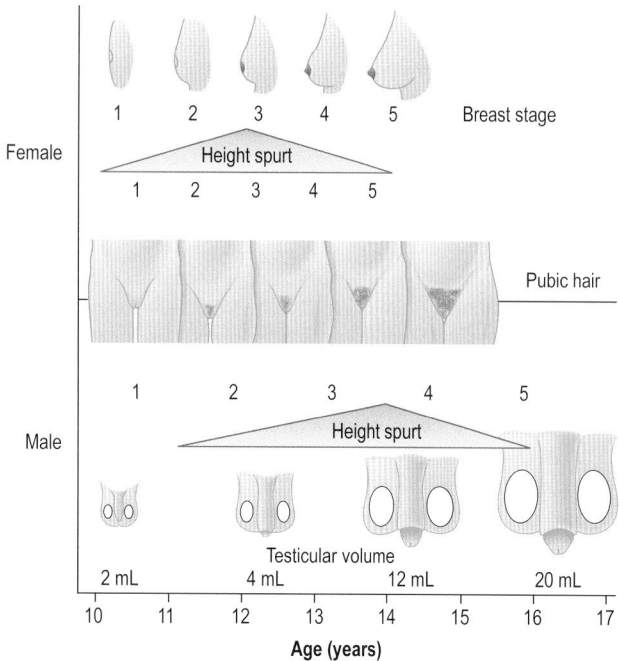

Fig. 21.31 The age of development of features of puberty. Stages and testicular size show mean ages, and all vary considerably between individuals. The same is true of the height spurt, shown here in relation to other data. Numbers 2–5 indicate stages of development.

peptide is believed to play a crucial role in the regulation of GnRH production and the timing of puberty.

LH and FSH are both low in the prepubertal child. In early puberty, FSH begins to rise first, initially in nocturnal pulses; this is followed by a rise in LH with a subsequent increase in testosterone/oestrogen levels. The milestones of puberty in the two sexes are shown in **Fig. 21.31**.

The relevant aspects of history and examination in the assessment of problems are shown in **Box 21.47**.

Assessment of growth and puberty

Growth

Charts showing normal centiles of height and weight are essential to monitor growth; they are available for normal British children (**Fig. 21.31**) and many other national and ethnic groups. Height must be measured, ideally at the same time of day on the same instrument by the same trained observer.

Height velocity is more helpful than current height. It requires at least two measurements some months apart and, ideally, multiple serial measurements. Height velocity is the rate of current growth (centimetres per year), while the current attained height is largely dependent upon previous growth. Standard deviation scores (SDS) based on the degree of deviation from age–sex norms are widely used.

The approximate target centile range for height of a child can be predicted by calculating 'mid-parental height' from parental heights:
1. add parental heights
2. divide by 2
3. add 7 cm for a boy *or* subtract 7 cm for a girl.

Target centile range is two centile spaces (around 9 cm) more or less of the mid-parental height.

Thus, with a father of 180 cm and mother of 154 cm, the mid-parental height would be 174 cm for a son and 160 cm for a daughter; and the target centile range for the son between 165 and 181 cm would be considered normal, and for the daughter between 151 and 169 cm.

Box 21.47 Assessment of problems of growth and development

History
- Pregnancy records
- Rate of growth (home/school records, e.g. heights on kitchen door)
- Comparison with peers at school and siblings
- Change in appearance (old photographs)
- Change in shoe/glove/hat size or frequency of 'growing out' of these
- Age of appearance of pubic hair, breasts, menarche
- History of headaches or visual problems

Physical signs
- Evidence of systemic disease
- Body habitus, size, relative weight, proportions (span versus height)
- Skin thickness, interdental separation
- Facial features
- Spade hands/feet
- Grading of secondary sexual characteristics
- Evidence of visual field defect and/or papilloedema or optic atrophy on fundoscopy

Further investigations are required if:
- height is below the 0.4th centile, unless already fully investigated at an earlier age
- height centile is more than three centile spaces below the mid-parental centile
- drop in height centile position of more than two centile spaces, as long as measurement error has been excluded
- smaller centile falls or discrepancies between child's and mid-parental centile, if seen in combination, or if associated with possible underlying disease.

Puberty

A knowledge of the timing and tempo of normal puberty and the stages of puberty are essential.

In males:
- Puberty before 9 years in boys is likely to be precocious and further assessment is necessary.
- Between 9 and 14 years most boys will be either 'pre-puberty' or 'in puberty'.
- If there are no signs of puberty by 14 years, then puberty is delayed and further assessment is indicated.
- From 14 to 17 years most boys will be either 'in puberty' or 'completing puberty'
- After 17 years boys will usually be 'completing puberty'. If this is not the case, maturation is delayed and further assessment may be needed.

In females:
- Puberty before 8 years in girls is likely to be precocious and further assessment is necessary.
- Between 8 and 13 years most girls will be either 'prepuberty' or 'in puberty'.
- If there are no signs of puberty by 13 years, then puberty is delayed and further assessment is indicated.
- From 13 to 16 years most girls will be either 'in puberty' or 'completing puberty'.
- After 16 years girls will usually be 'completing puberty' when menarche will have occurred. If this is not the case, maturation is delayed and further assessment may be needed.

Tanner staging

In males the first sign of puberty is testicular volumes reaching 4 mL; testicular volumes continue to increase until adult sizes are reached (15–25 mL). Other aspects that are staged from 1 to 5, with stage 1

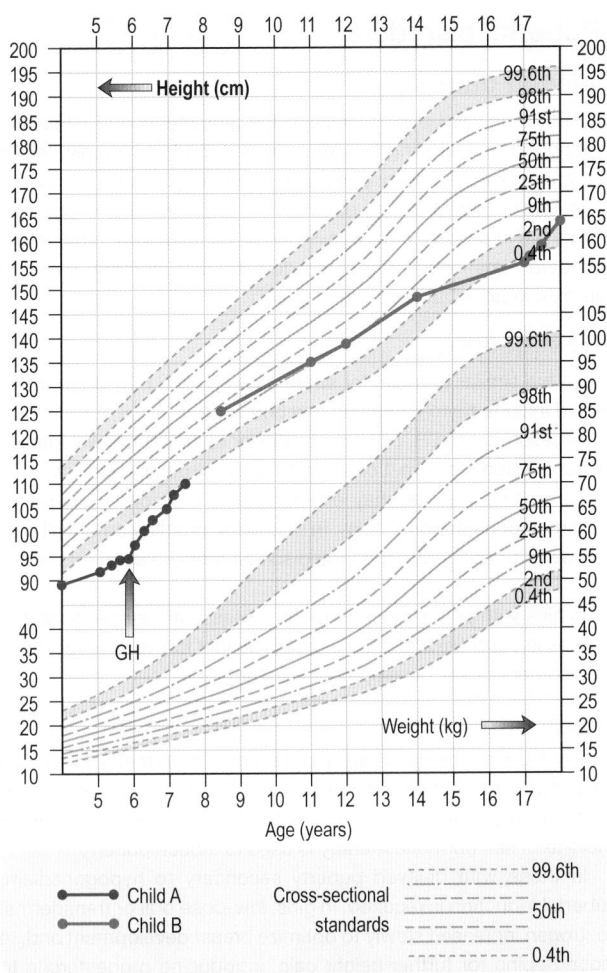

Fig. 21.32 A height chart for boys. **Child A** (red) illustrates the course of a child with hypopituitarism, initially treated with cortisol and thyroxine, but showing growth only after growth hormone (GH) treatment. **Child B** (blue) shows the course of a child with constitutional growth delay without treatment.

prepubertal (no signs of puberty) and stage 5 adult appearance, are genitalia (changes in the scrotum and penis) and pubic hair (5 stages). Axillary hair has two stages. Spermarche happens around stage 4.

In girls the development of breast buds signals the start of puberty (Tanner stage 2), and continue to develop until adult shape of breasts and nipples (stage 5). As in boys, pubic hair and axillary hair are also staged, with menarche happening around stage 4.

During puberty is also a period of rapid growth, which happens earlier in girls than boys.

Disorders of stature

Short stature

When children or their parents complain of short stature, particular attention should focus on:

- small for gestational age
- possible systemic disorders – any system but especially small bowel disease
- evidence of skeletal, chromosomal or other congenital abnormalities
- possible symptoms and signs of a hypothalamic or pituitary tumour
- endocrine status – particularly thyroid
- dietary intake and use of drugs, especially steroids for asthma
- emotional, psychological, family and school problems.

School, general practitioner, clinic and home records of height and weight should be obtained, if possible, to allow growth-velocity calculation. If unavailable, such data must be obtained prospectively.

A child with normal growth velocity is unlikely to have significant endocrine disease and the most common cause of short stature in this situation is familial short stature or constitutional delay. However, low growth velocity without an apparent systemic cause requires further investigation. Sudden cessation of growth suggests major physical disease; if no gastrointestinal, respiratory, renal or skeletal abnormality is apparent, then a cerebral tumour or hypothyroidism is most likely.

Consistently slow-growing children require full endocrine assessment. Features of the more common causes of growth failure are given in **Box 21.48**.

i	**Box 21.48** Clinical features of common causes of short stature				
Cause	**Family history**	**Growth pattern, clinical features and puberty**	**Bone age**	**Remarks**	
Constitutional delay	Often present	Slow from birth, immature but appropriate with late but spontaneous puberty	Moderate delay	Often difficult to differentiate from GH deficiency Growth velocity measurement vital	
Familial short stature	Positive	Slow from birth, clinically normal with normal puberty	Normal	Need heights of family members Growth velocity normal	
GH insufficiency	Rare	Slow growth, immature, often overweight, delayed puberty	Moderate delay, increasing with time	Early investigation and treatment vital Increased suspicion if child is plump	
Primary hypothyroidism	Rare	Slow growth, immature and delayed puberty	Marked delay	Measure TSH, T_4 in all cases of short stature Clear clinical signs not obvious	
Small bowel disease	Sometimes	Slow, immature, usually thin for height, delayed puberty	Delayed	Diarrhoea and/or macrocytosis/anaemia Occasionally no gastrointestinal symptoms	

GH, growth hormone; TSH, thyroid-stimulating hormone.

Around the time of puberty, if constitutional delay is clearly shown and symptoms require intervention, then very-low-dose sex steroids in 3- to 6-month courses will usually induce acceleration of growth.

Investigations

- **Thyroid function tests.** Serum TSH and free T_4 should be measured to exclude hypothyroidism.
- **Assessment of bone age.** Non-dominant hand and wrist X-rays allow assessment of bone age by comparison with standard charts. Bone age will be delayed in constitutional delay, endocrinopathies and chronic disease
- **Karyotyping in females.** Turner's syndrome (see p. 628) is associated with short stature. It is thought that this is due to a defect in the short stature homeobox (*SHOX*) gene, which has a role in non-GH-mediated growth.
- **GH status.** Not all children with short stature require this assessment, particularly as the test has a high false-positive rate, and therefore it should be considered only in ongoing growth failure with no other explanation. Basal levels of GH are of little value, therefore dynamic tests include the GH response to insulin (the 'gold standard'; see **Box 21.11**), arginine + GHRH and glucagon are used. Tests should only be performed in centres experienced in their use and interpretation. Normal responses depend on test and GH assay used.
- **Blood levels of IGF-1 and IGF-BP3.** These may provide evidence of GH undersecretion.
- **MRI pituitary/brain.** If symptoms are suggestive of cerebral tumour or there is evidence of GH insufficiency this will be required to investigate for hypothalamic pituitary tumour.

Management of short stature

Systemic illness should be treated and primary hypothyroidism managed with levothyroxine.

A watch and wait approach to those with constitutional delay, potentially with a very-low-dose sex steroids in 3- to 6-month courses to kick-start puberty and induce acceleration of growth.

For GH insufficiency, recombinant GH (somatropin) is given as nightly injections in doses of 0.17–0.35 mg/kg per week, with dose adjustments made according to clinical response and IGF-1 levels. Treatment is expensive and should be supervised in expert centres.

Other indications for growth hormone are in conditions without GH insufficiency, such as Turner's syndrome and *SHOX* gene haploinsufficiency (skeletal dysplasia), chronic renal failure on dialysis (resistance to GH-dependent IGFs), Prader–Willi syndrome (partial GH insufficiency), small for gestational age without catch-up. In some countries it is also offered to children with idiopathic short stature.

Familial cases of resistance to GH that is caused by an abnormal GH receptor (Laron-type dwarfism) are well described. They are very rare but may respond to therapy with synthetic IGF-1 (mecasermin).

Tall stature

The most common causes are hereditary (two tall parents), idiopathic (constitutional) or early developmental factors (eventually resulting in short stature). Tall stature can occasionally be due to hyperthyroidism. Other causes include chromosomal abnormalities (e.g. Klinefelter's syndrome, Marfan's syndrome) or metabolic abnormalities. GH excess secondary to a GH-secreting pituitary adenoma causing gigantism is a very rare cause and is usually clinically obvious.

Pubertal disorders

Delayed puberty

Causes of delayed puberty include the aforementioned causes of hypogonadism including hypogonadism as part of hypopituitarism but many cases represent constitutional delay, particularly in boys.

In constitutional delay, pubertal development, bone age and stature are in parallel. A family history may confirm that other family members experienced the same delayed development, which is common in boys but very rare in girls.

Investigations

These are similar to those for short stature which may coexist and should include thyroid function and bone age.

Assessment of LH, FSH, oestradiol or testosterone will identify primary hypogonadism. Low normal gonadotrophins with low oestradiol or testosterone may either represent secondary hypogonadism or constitutional delay. In paediatric practice an LHRH may also be performed, although the discriminatory value of this test is low.

In girls with primary amenorrhoea, assessment for pelvic abnormalities is essential and if the uterus is absent further investigations for disorders of sex development are warranted.

Management

In constitutional delay, if any progression into puberty is evident clinically, investigations are not required. When delay is great and problems are serious (e.g. severe teasing at school), low-dose, short-term sex hormone therapy is used to induce puberty.

In those with delayed puberty secondary to hypogonadism, pubertal induction is required. In girls, low-dose oral or transdermal oestrogen increased slowly to optimize breast development and, in those hoping for further height gain, introducing progesterone to induce withdrawal bleed when bleeding occurs, or after 2 years of unopposed oestrogen. In boys, pubertal induction is with testosterone. The dose is less critical unless optimizing height.

Precocious puberty

True precocious puberty can be divided into gonadotrophin-dependent and gonadotrophin-independent (secondary to exposure to either endogenous or sometimes exogenous sex steroids) types. Gonadotrophin-independent causes can also initiate gonadotrophin-dependent precocious puberty, as is the case in congenital adrenal hyperplasia. All cases require assessment by a paediatric endocrinologist.

True precocious puberty must be distinguished from normal variants:

- **Premature thelarche.** This is early breast development alone and is usually transient, at age 2–4 years. It may regress or persist until puberty. There is no evidence of follicular development.
- **Premature adrenarche.** This is early development of pubic hair without significant other changes, usually after the age of 5 years and more commonly in girls. It is also more common in obese children due to reduced SHBG levels, leading to higher free circulating androgens.

Gonadotrophin-dependent precocious puberty

- **Idiopathic precocity** is most common in girls and very rare in boys. This is a diagnosis of exclusion. With no apparent cause for premature breast or pubic hair development, and an early growth spurt, it may be normal and may run in families.

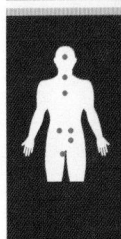

Symptoms		Signs

Symptoms

Head and neck
Change in facial appearance
Headaches
Visual deterioration
Deep voice
Goitre

General
Tiredness
Weight gain
Breathlessness
Excessive sweating
Muscular weakness
Joint pain

Hormonal
Amenorrhoea or oligomenorrhoea
  in women
Galactorrhoea
Impotence or poor libido

Increased glove or hat size

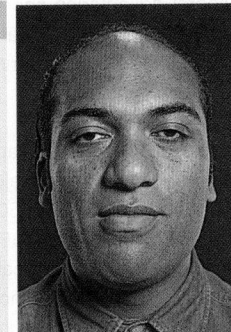
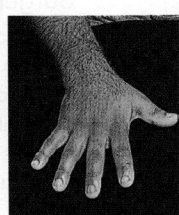
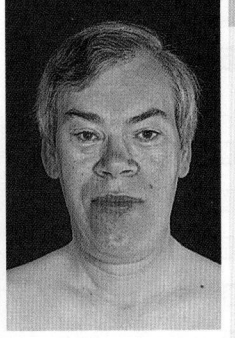
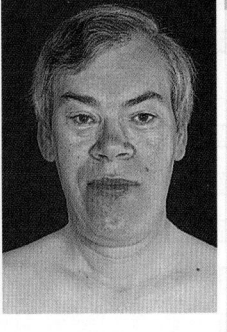
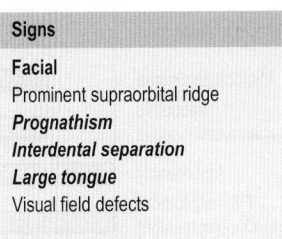
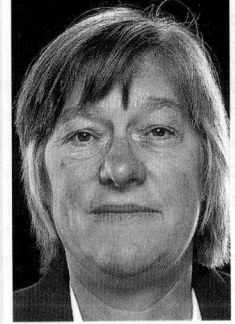
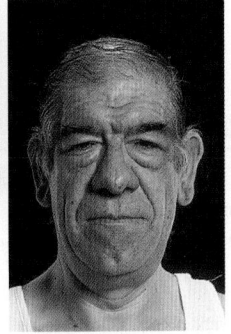

Signs

Facial
Prominent supraorbital ridge
Prognathism
Interdental separation
Large tongue
Visual field defects

General
Hirsutism
Thick greasy skin

Hands
Spade-like hands and feet
Tight rings on fingers
Carpal tunnel syndrome

Other
Galactorrhoea
Hypertension
Heart failure
Oedema
Arthopathy
Proximal myopathy
Glycosuria (plus possible signs of
  hypopituitarism)

Fig. 21.33 Acromegaly: symptoms and signs. *Bold italic* type indicates signs of greater discriminant value.

- *Cerebral precocity* is when precocious puberty is associated with a cerebral abnormality, acquired or otherwise, such as a tumour, previously acquired brain injury, for example, radiotherapy. In boys, tumours must be rigorously excluded and MRI scan is almost always indicated to exclude this diagnosis. The most common finding is a hypothalamic hamartoma, a benign tumour that can be associated with seizures.

Gonadotrophin-independent precocious puberty

The most common cause is congenital adrenal hyperplasia. Other causes include testicular or ovarian disorders, such as testotoxicosis or McCune–Albright's syndrome (MAS; see also p. 650). MAS usually occurs in girls, with precocity, polyostotic fibrous dysplasia and skin pigmentation (café-au-lait patches). HCG-secreting tumours, androgen- and oestrogen-secreting tumours, including teratomas, are important conditions to exclude.

Management

Treatment is often required to maximize adult height, reduce psychosocial impact, and delay menarche. Treatment depends on whether the cause is gonadotrophin-dependent or independent. If the cause is gonadotrophin-dependent, treatment with long-acting GnRH analogues (given by nasal spray, by subcutaneous injection or by implant) causes suppression of gonadotrophin release via downregulation of the receptor – and therefore reduced sex hormone production – and is moderately effective. If the cause is gonadotrophin-independent, inhibitors of steroidogenesis, antiandrogens, and aromatase inhibitors are also used.

Further reading

Allen DB, Cuttler L. Clinical practice. Short stature in childhood – challenges and choices. *N Engl J Med* 2013; 368:1220–1228.
Savage MO, Burren CP, Rosenfeld RG. The continuum of growth hormone–IGF-I axis defects causing short stature: diagnostic and therapeutic challenges. *Clin Endocrinol* 2010; 72:721–728.

Acromegaly and gigantism

Growth hormone stimulates skeletal and soft tissue growth. GH excess therefore produces gigantism in children (if acquired before epiphyseal fusion) and acromegaly in adults. Both are due to a GH-secreting pituitary tumour (somatotroph adenoma) in almost all cases. Hyperplasia due to ectopic GHRH excess is very rare. Overall incidence is approximately 3–4/million per year and the prevalence is 50–80/million worldwide. Acromegaly usually occurs sporadically, although gene mutations can rarely give rise to familial acromegaly: typically, the *AIP* gene in familial isolated pituitary adenoma. In familial acromegaly, there is an increased onset before puberty compared with sporadic cases, leading to a higher prevalence of gigantism.

History and examination

Symptoms and signs of acromegaly are shown in **Fig. 21.33**. One-third of patients present with changes in appearance, and one-quarter with visual field defects or headaches; in the remainder, the diagnosis is made by an alert observer in another clinic: for example, in general practice, or in the diabetes, hypertension, dental, dermatology departments. Sleep apnoea is common and requires investigation and treatment if there are suggestive symptoms (see p. 960). Sweating, headaches and soft tissue swelling are particularly useful symptoms of persistent GH secretion. Headache is very common in acromegaly and may be severe, even with small tumours; it is often improved after surgical cure or with somatostatin analogues.

Investigations

- *GH levels* may exclude acromegaly if they are undetectable, but a detectable value is non-diagnostic taken alone. Normal adult levels are below 0.5 µg/L for most of the day, except during stress or a 'GH pulse'.
- *A glucose tolerance test* is diagnostic if there is no suppression of GH. Acromegalics fail to suppress GH below 0.3 µg/L and

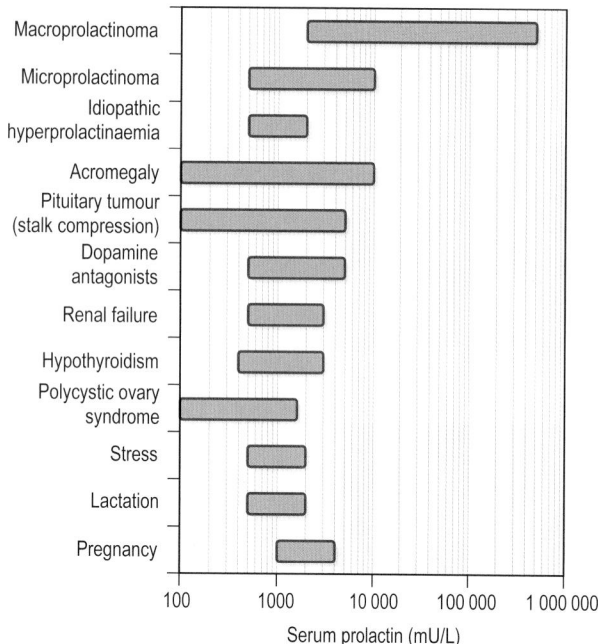

Fig. 21.34 Range of serum prolactin seen in common causes of hyperprolactinaemia.

some show a paradoxical rise; about 25% of acromegalics have a positive diabetic glucose tolerance test.

- **IGF-1 levels** are almost always raised in acromegaly; a single plasma level of IGF-1 reflects mean 24-hour GH levels and is useful in diagnosis. A normal IGF-1, together with random GH of less than 1 µg/L, may be taken to exclude acromegaly if the diagnosis is clinically unlikely.
- **Visual field examination** commonly reveals defects, such as bitemporal hemianopia.
- **MRI scan** of the pituitary is carried out if the above tests are abnormal. This will almost always reveal the pituitary adenoma. In cases where no clear lesion is present, or in postoperative cases where residual disease is being sought, there is increasing interest in the use of functional imaging such as positron emission tomography (PET).
- **Pituitary function** commonly demonstrates partial or complete anterior hypopituitarism.
- **Prolactin** levels show mild to moderate hyperprolactinaemia in 30% of patients (**Fig. 21.34**). In some, the adenoma secretes both GH and prolactin.

Management

Untreated acromegaly results in markedly reduced survival. Most deaths occur from heart failure, coronary artery disease and hypertension-related causes. In addition, there is an increase in deaths due to neoplasia, particularly large bowel tumours; guidance advocates regular colonoscopy to detect and remove colonic polyps in order to reduce the risk of colonic cancer, although the evidence is inconclusive. Treatment is therefore indicated in all except the elderly or those with minimal abnormalities. The aim of therapy is to achieve a mean GH level below 2.5 µg/L; this is not always 'normal' but has been shown to reduce mortality to normal levels and is therefore considered a 'safe' GH level. A normal IGF-1 is also a goal of therapy. Occasionally, there can be discordance between GH and IGF-1 levels, which can create management dilemmas.

When present, hypopituitarism should be corrected and concurrent diabetes and/or hypertension should be treated conventionally; both usually improve with treatment of the acromegaly.

The general advantages and disadvantages of surgery, radiotherapy and medical treatment are discussed on page 597. Progress can be assessed by monitoring GH and IGF-1 levels.

Surgery

Trans-sphenoidal surgery is the appropriate first-line therapy. It will result in clinical remission in a majority of cases (60–90%) with pituitary microadenoma, but in only 50% of those with macroadenoma. Very high preoperative GH and IGF-1 levels are also poor prognostic markers of surgical cure. Surgical success rates are variable and highly dependent upon experience, and a specialist pituitary surgeon is essential. Transfrontal surgery is rarely required except for massive macroadenomas. There is a recurrence rate of approximately 10%.

Pituitary radiotherapy

External radiotherapy is normally used after pituitary surgery fails to normalize GH levels rather than as primary therapy. It is often combined with medium-term treatment using a somatostatin analogue, dopamine agonist or GH antagonist because of the slow biochemical response to radiotherapy, which may take 10 years or more; it is also often associated with hypopituitarism, which makes it unattractive in patients of reproductive age. Stereotactic (gamma-knife) radiotherapy is used in some centres, as it delivers a more concentrated field of radiation.

Medical therapy

There are three receptor targets for the treatment of acromegaly: pituitary somatostatin receptors and dopamine (D₂) receptors, and GH receptors in the periphery.

Somatostatin receptor agonists

Octreotide and **lanreotide** are synthetic analogues of somatostatin, which act selectively on somatostatin receptor subtypes (SSTR2 and SSTR5) and are highly expressed in GH-secreting tumours. These drugs were used as a short-term treatment while other modalities become effective, but now are sometimes used as primary therapy. They reduce GH and IGF levels in most patients but do not all achieve treatment targets. Both drugs are typically administered as monthly depot injections and are generally well tolerated; they are, however, associated with an increased incidence of gallstones and are expensive. Pasireotide (acting on SSTR 1, 2, 3 and 5) is a newer agent but its role in acromegaly is still being evaluated.

Dopamine agonists

Dopamine agonists act on D₂ receptors (see pp. 222–223) and can be given to shrink tumours prior to definitive therapy or to control symptoms and persisting GH secretion; they are probably most effective in mixed GH-producing (somatotroph) and prolactin-producing (mammotroph) tumours. Typical doses are bromocriptine 10–60 mg daily or cabergoline 0.5 mg daily (higher than for prolactinomas). Given alone, they reduce GH to 'safe' levels in only a minority of cases, but are useful for mild residual disease or in combination with somatostatin analogues. Drugs with combined somatostatin and dopamine receptor activity are under development.

Growth hormone antagonists

Pegvisomant (a genetically modified analogue of GH) is a GH receptor antagonist that exerts its effect by binding to and preventing dimerization of the GH receptor. It does not lower GH levels or reduce tumour size but has been shown to normalize IGF-1 levels in 90% of patients. It is given by daily injection and its main role at the present time is treatment of patients in whom GH and IGF levels

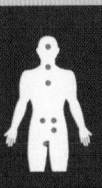

Hormone	Source	Site of action	Hormone structure	Receptor	Post-receptor activity
Dopamine	Hypothalamus	Pituitary	Amine	Membrane – 7TM D2 receptor	G-proteins Inhibit cAMP
Prolactin	Pituitary	Breast Other tissues	Peptide – 199 AA	Transmembrane PRLR Class 1 cytokine	JAK2 and other pathways

7TM, 7 transmembrane (G-protein coupled receptor); AA, amino acids; cAMP, adenylate cyclase → cyclic adenosine monophosphate; JAK, Janus kinase.

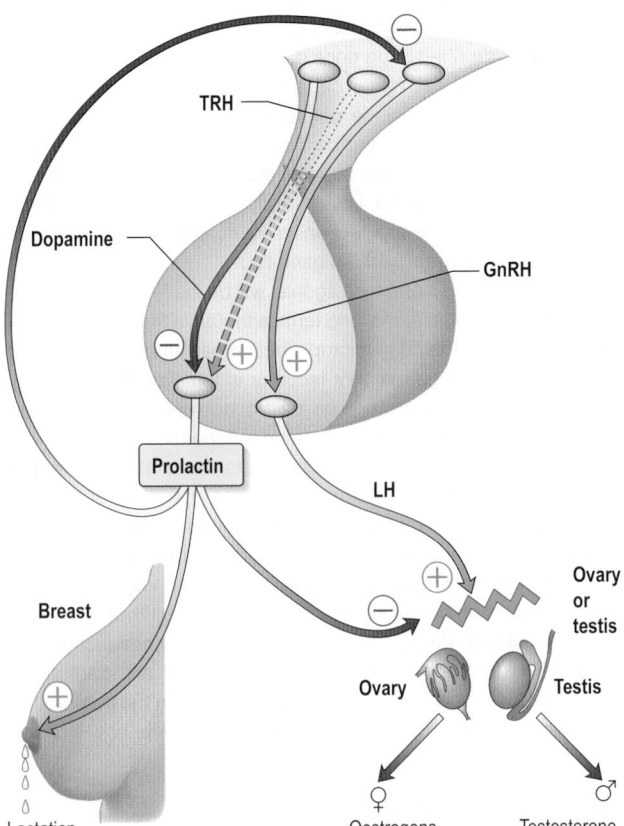

Fig. 21.35 **The control and actions of prolactin.** Prolactin is mainly controlled by tonic inhibition by hypothalamic dopamine. Prolactin stimulates lactation but also inhibits both hypothalamic gonadotrophin-releasing hormone (GnRH) secretion and the gonadal actions of luteinizing hormone (LH). TRH, thyrotrophin-releasing hormone.

cannot be reduced to safe levels with somatostatin analogues alone, or by surgery or radiotherapy.

Hyperprolactinaemia

The hypothalamic–pituitary control of prolactin secretion is illustrated in **Fig. 21.35**. Prolactin is a large peptide secreted in the pituitary and acts via a transmembrane receptor stimulating JAK2 and other pathways (**Box 21.49**).

Prolactin is under tonic dopamine inhibition; factors known to increase prolactin secretion (e.g. TRH) are probably of less relevance unless the patient has primary hypothyroidism. Prolactin stimulates milk secretion (but not breast tissue development) but also inhibits gonadal activity. It decreases GnRH pulsatility at the hypothalamic level and, to a lesser extent, blocks the action of LH on the ovary or testis, producing hypogonadism even when the pituitary–gonadal axis itself is intact.

The role of prolactin outside pregnancy and lactation is not well defined, although there is some epidemiological evidence of a link between high prolactin levels and breast cancer, which has led to an interest in the development of prolactin receptor antagonists.

Physiological hyperprolactinaemia occurs in pregnancy, lactation and severe stress, as well as during sleep and coitus. The range of serum prolactin seen in common causes of hyperprolactinaemia is illustrated in **Fig. 21.34**. Mildly increased prolactin levels (400–600 mU/L) may be physiological and asymptomatic but higher levels require a diagnosis. Levels above 5000 mU/L always imply a prolactin-secreting pituitary tumour.

Aetiology

Hyperprolactinaemia has many causes:

- **Physiological.** These include pregnancy, lactation, stress, sleep, exercise and coitus.
- **Pathological.** These include prolactinoma, co-secretion of prolactin in tumours causing acromegaly, stalk compression due to pituitary adenomas and other pituitary masses, polycystic ovarian syndrome, primary hypothyroidism and idiopathic hyperprolactinaemia. Rarer causes include renal failure, liver failure, postictal state and chest wall injury (e.g. following herpes zoster).
- **Drug-induced.** Drug causes include **oestrogens** (e.g. contraceptive pill), **dopamine antagonists** (e.g. antipsychotics such as phenothiazines), **antidepressants** (e.g. tricyclics, selective serotonin reuptake inhibitors (SSRIs)), **antiemetics** (e.g. metoclopramide, domperidone) and **others** (e.g. verapamil, cimetidine, methyldopa).

History and examination

Patients may present with features of hyperprolactinaemia or structural symptoms from a pituitary tumour with headaches and visual loss. This latter presentation is more common in males.

It usually presents with:

- Galactorrhoea, spontaneous or expressible (60% of cases). Note that many people with galactorrhoea do not have hyperprolactinaemia – 'normoprolactinaemic galactorrhoea' – and the causes are poorly understood.
- Oligomenorrhoea or amenorrhoea.
- Decreased libido in both sexes.
- Decreased potency in men.
- Subfertility.
- Symptoms or signs of oestrogen or androgen deficiency – in the long term osteoporosis may result, especially in women.
- Delayed or arrested puberty in the peripubertal patient.
- Mild gynaecomastia – often seen in men due to the associated hypogonadism rather than being a direct effect of prolactin.

Additionally, headaches and/or visual field defects occur if there is a pituitary macroadenoma (more common in men).

Investigations

Hyperprolactinaemia should be confirmed by repeat measurement. If there are no clinical features of hyperprolactinaemia, the possibility of ***macroprolactinaemia*** should be considered. This is a higher-molecular-weight complex of prolactin bound to IgG, which is physiologically inactive but occurs in a small proportion of normal people and can therefore lead to unnecessary treatment. Macroprolactinaemia can be diagnosed in the laboratory by precipitation of immunoglobulin G (IgG) with polyethylene glycol, after which prolactin levels will be normal on testing; most laboratories will do this routinely. Hyperprolactinaemia should be excluded in all patients presenting with a pituitary mass.

Further tests are appropriate after physiological and drug causes have been excluded:

* ***Visual fields*** should be checked.
* ***Primary hypothyroidism*** must be excluded since this is a cause of hyperprolactinaemia.
* ***Anterior pituitary function*** should be assessed if there is any clinical evidence of hypopituitarism or radiological evidence of a pituitary tumour (see **Boxes 21.5, 21.7** and **21.11**).
* ***MRI of the pituitary*** is necessary if there are any clinical features suggestive of a pituitary tumour, and desirable in all cases when prolactin is significantly elevated (>1000 mU/L).

In the presence of a pituitary mass on MRI, the level of prolactin helps determine whether the mass is a prolactinoma or a non-functioning pituitary tumour causing stalk-disconnection hyperprolactinaemia: levels of above 5000 mU/L in the presence of a macroadenoma, or above 2000 mU/L in the presence of a microadenoma (or with no radiological abnormality) strongly suggest a prolactinoma (see p. 593). Macroprolactinoma refers to tumours above 10 mm in diameter, microprolactinoma to smaller ones. Tumours that are approximately 10 mm are termed mesoadenomas.

Occasionally, very large prolactinomas can be associated with such high serum prolactin levels that some assays give an artefactual falsely low result (known as the 'hook effect'). If suspected, this can be excluded by serial dilutions of the serum sample.

Management

In all patients with a macroprolactinoma treatment is recommended to reduce the size of the tumour. It is also recommended in those with troublesome galactorrhoea. In those with sex steroid deficiency lowering prolactin levels should reverse hypogonadism and avoid the long-term effects, although for those intolerant of the medication sex steroid replacement is an alternative approach. Therefore some patients, for example, women postmenopause with microprolactinomas, may not require any treatment.

Medical treatment

Hyperprolactinaemia is controlled with a dopamine agonist.

* ***Cabergoline*** (500 µg once or twice a week, judged on clinical response and prolactin levels) is the best-tolerated and longest-acting drug, and is the drug of choice.
* ***Bromocriptine*** is the longest-established therapy and is therefore preferred if pregnancy is planned; initial doses should be small (e.g. 1 mg), taken with food and gradually increased to 2.5 mg two or three times daily. Side-effects, which prevent effective therapy in a minority of cases, include nausea and vomiting, dizziness and syncope, constipation and cold peripheries.
* ***Quinagolide*** (75–150 µg once daily) is an alternative.

Complications, seen when cabergoline is used in higher doses in Parkinson's disease, include pulmonary, retroperitoneal and pericardial fibrotic reactions, and cardiac valve lesions. Patients need monitoring, although studies suggest that adverse effects appear to be very rare in those on lower, 'endocrine' doses. In addition, patients can also develop neuropsychiatric side-effects, including compulsive behaviours such as gambling.

In most cases, a dopamine agonist will be the first and only therapy, and can be used in the long term, although a trial of discontinuation can be considered in microprolactinomas after 2–3 years, as a significant percentage may not recur, or in females at the onset of the menopause who are not on oestrogen replacement therapy. Prolactinomas usually shrink in size on a dopamine agonist, and in macroadenomas any pituitary mass effects commonly resolve (**Fig. 21.36**). Macroprolactinomas may not recur after several years of dopamine agonist therapy in a minority of cases, but in the majority, hyperprolactinaemia will return if treatment is stopped.

In patients planning ***pregnancy***, it is useful to know the size of the pituitary lesion before starting dopamine agonist therapy. Rarely, tumours enlarge during pregnancy to produce headaches and visual field defects. Dopamine agonists, which are traditionally stopped after conception, particularly when used in the treatment of microprolactinomas, can be restarted if there are any signs of tumour growth during pregnancy.

Trans-sphenoidal surgery

Surgery may rarely be needed in patients who are intolerant of or unresponsive to dopamine agonists. Surgery may restore normoprolactinaemia in people with microadenoma, but is rarely completely successful in those with macroadenomas and risks damage to normal pituitary function. Therefore, most patients and

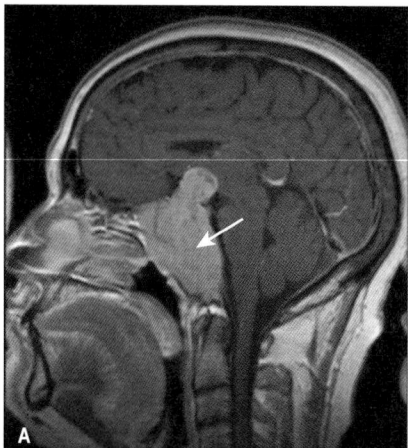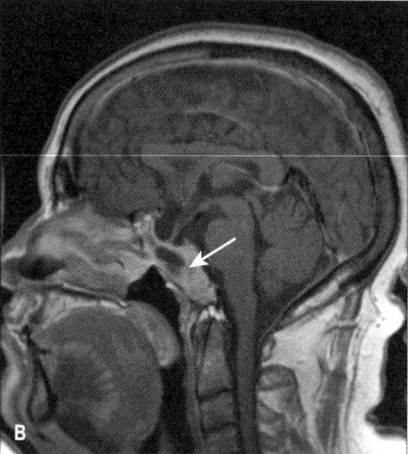

Fig. 21.36 Macroprolactinoma (arrowed). **(A)** Before treatment. **(B)** After 2 years' treatment with the dopamine agonist cabergoline, showing marked adenoma shrinkage.

physicians elect to continue medical therapy rather than proceed to surgery. Prolactin should therefore always be measured before surgery on any mass in the pituitary region. Some surgeons believe that long-term bromocriptine increases the hardness of the adenoma and makes resection more difficult, but others dissent from this view.

Radiotherapy

Also rarely needed, radiotherapy usually controls adenoma growth and is slowly effective in lowering prolactin, but causes progressive hypopituitarism. It may be advocated after medical tumour shrinkage or after surgery in larger tumours, especially where families are complete or if the drug treatment is poorly tolerated, but most workers simply advocate continuation of dopamine agonist therapy in responsive cases.

THE THIRST AXIS

Thirst and water regulation are largely controlled by vasopressin, also known as ADH, which is synthesized in the hypothalamus (see p. 591) and then migrates in neurosecretory granules along axonal pathways to the posterior pituitary. Pituitary disease alone without hypothalamic involvement therefore does not lead to ADH deficiency, as the hormone can still 'leak' from the damaged end of the intact axon.

At normal concentrations, the kidney is the predominant site of action of vasopressin. Vasopressin stimulation of the V_2 receptors (**Box 21.50**) allows the collecting ducts to become permeable to water via the migration of aquaporin-2 water channels, thus permitting reabsorption of hypotonic luminal fluid (see p. 175). Vasopressin therefore reduces diuresis and results in overall retention of water. At high concentrations, vasopressin also causes vasoconstriction via the V_1 receptors in vascular tissue.

Changes in plasma osmolality are sensed by osmoreceptors in the anterior hypothalamus. Vasopressin secretion is suppressed at levels below 280 mOsm/kg, thus allowing maximal water diuresis. Above this level, plasma vasopressin increases in direct proportion to plasma osmolality. At the upper limit of normal (295 mOsm/kg), maximum antidiuresis is achieved and thirst is experienced at about 298 mOsm/kg (**Fig. 21.37**).

Other factors affecting vasopressin release are shown in **Box 21.51**.

Disorders of vasopressin secretion or activity include:
- cranial diabetes insipidus with deficiency as a result of hypothalamic disease

- 'nephrogenic' diabetes insipidus – a rare condition in which the renal tubules are insensitive to vasopressin, and an example of a receptor abnormality
- inappropriate excess of the hormone, also called syndrome of inappropriate antidiuretic hormone (SIADH), a common cause of hyponatraemia in hospital patients.

While diabetes insipidus is uncommon, they need to be distinguished from the occasional patient with 'primary polydipsia', and those whose renal tubular function has been impaired by electrolyte abnormalities, such as hypokalaemia or hypercalcaemia. Similarly other causes of hyponatraemia need to be excluded prior to diagnosing and investigating SIADH.

Diabetes insipidus
History and examination

Deficiency of vasopressin (ADH) or insensitivity to its action leads to excess excretion of dilute urine with a compensatory increase

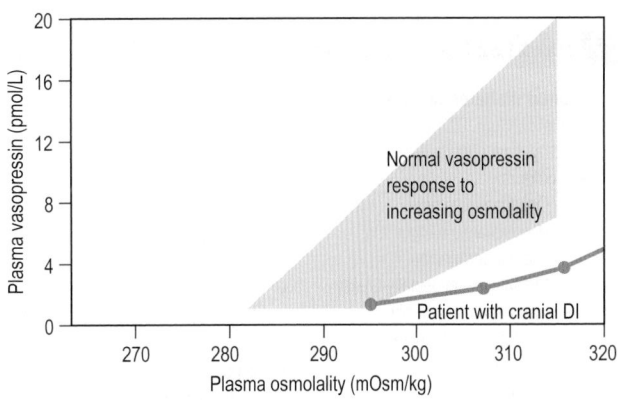

Fig. 21.37 Plasma vasopressin response to increasing osmolality in normal subjects and in a patient with diabetes insipidus (DI).

Box 21.51 Factors affecting vasopressin (ADH) release

Increased by
- Increased osmolality
- Hypovolaemia
- Hypotension
- Nausea
- Hypothyroidism
- Angiotensin II
- Adrenaline (epinephrine)
- Cortisol
- Nicotine
- Antidepressants

Decreased by
- Decreased osmolality
- Hypervolaemia
- Hypertension
- Ethanol
- α-Adrenergic stimulation

Box 21.50 Hormones and receptors of the posterior pituitary axes

Hormone	Source	Site of action	Hormone structure	Receptor	Post-receptor activity
Vasopressin (antidiuretic hormone, ADH)	Hypothalamus → pituitary	Kidney	Peptide – 9 AA	Membrane – 7TM AVPR2	G-proteins cAMP Aquaporin-2
	Hypothalamus → pituitary	Vascular	Peptide – 9 AA	Membrane – 7TM AVPR1A	G-proteins PLC/IP$_3$
	Hypothalamus → portal veins	Pituitary (ACTH secretion)	Peptide – 9 AA	Membrane – 7TM AVPR1B	G-proteins PLC/IP$_3$
Oxytocin	Hypothalamus → pituitary	Uterus and breast	Peptide – 9 AA	Membrane – 7TM OXTR	G-proteins

7TM, 7 transmembrane (G-protein coupled receptor); AA, amino acids; ARE, androgen response element; AVPR, arginine vasopressin receptor; cAMP, adenylate cyclase → cyclic adenosine monophosphate; OXTR, oxytocin receptor.

in thirst (polydipsia). Daily urine output may reach as much as 10–15 L, leading to dehydration that may be very severe if the thirst mechanism or consciousness is impaired or the patient is denied fluid.

Diabetes insipidus (DI) may be masked by simultaneous cortisol deficiency; cortisol replacement allows a water diuresis and DI then becomes apparent.

Aetiology

Causes of DI are listed in **Box 21.52**. The most common is hypothalamic–pituitary surgery, following which transient DI is common, frequently remitting after a few days or weeks. Typically, inflammatory lesions of the pituitary stalk are associated with DI (**Fig. 21.38**).

Familial isolated vasopressin deficiency causes DI from early childhood and is dominantly inherited, caused by a mutation in the *AVP-NPII* gene. **DIDMOAD (Wolfram's) syndrome** is a rare autosomal recessive disorder comprising diabetes insipidus, diabetes mellitus, optic atrophy and deafness, and is caused by mutations in the

WFS1 gene on chromosome 4. MRI may show an absent or poorly developed posterior pituitary.

Biochemistry

- High or high-normal plasma osmolality with low urine osmolality (in primary polydipsia, plasma osmolality tends to be low).
- Resultant high or high-normal plasma sodium (hypernatraemia).
- High 24-hour urine volumes (<2 L excludes the need for further investigation).
- Failure of urinary concentration with fluid deprivation.
- Restoration of urinary concentration with vasopressin or an analogue.

The latter two points are studied with a formal water deprivation test (**Box 21.53**). In normal subjects, plasma osmolality remains normal while urine osmolality rises above 600 mOsm/kg. In DI, plasma osmolality rises while the urine remains dilute, only concentrating after exogenous vasopressin is given (in 'cranial' DI), or not concentrating after vasopressin if nephrogenic DI is present. An alternative is measurement of plasma vasopressin during hypertonic saline infusion, but these measurements are not widely available.

Management

The synthetic vasopressin (ADH) analogue, desmopressin, is the treatment of choice in cranial DI. It has a longer duration of action

---

❓ Box 21.52 Causes of diabetes insipidus

Cranial diabetes insipidus
- Familial (e.g. DIDMOAD)
- Idiopathic (often autoimmune)
- Tumours:
  - Craniopharyngioma
  - Hypothalamic tumour, e.g. glioma, germinoma
  - Metastases, especially breast
  - Lymphoma/leukaemia
  - Pituitary with suprasellar extension (rare)
- Infections:
  - Tuberculosis
  - Meningitis
  - Cerebral abscess
- Infiltrations:
  - Sarcoidosis
  - Langerhans' cell histiocytosis
- Inflammatory:
  - Hypophysitis
- Post-surgical:
  - Transfrontal
  - Trans-sphenoidal

- Vascular:
  - Haemorrhage/thrombosis
  - Sheehan's syndrome
  - Aneurysm
- Trauma (e.g. head injury)

Nephrogenic diabetes insipidus
- Familial (e.g. vasopressin receptor gene, aquaporin-2 gene defect)
- Idiopathic
- Renal disease (e.g. renal tubular acidosis)
- Hypokalaemia
- Hypercalcaemia
- Drugs (e.g. lithium, demeclocycline, glibenclamide)
- Sickle cell disease
- Prolonged polyuria due to any cause, including cranial DI and primary polydipsia – can cause mild temporary nephrogenic DI

DI, diabetes insipidus; DIDMOAD, diabetes insipidus, diabetes mellitus, optic atrophy and deafness.

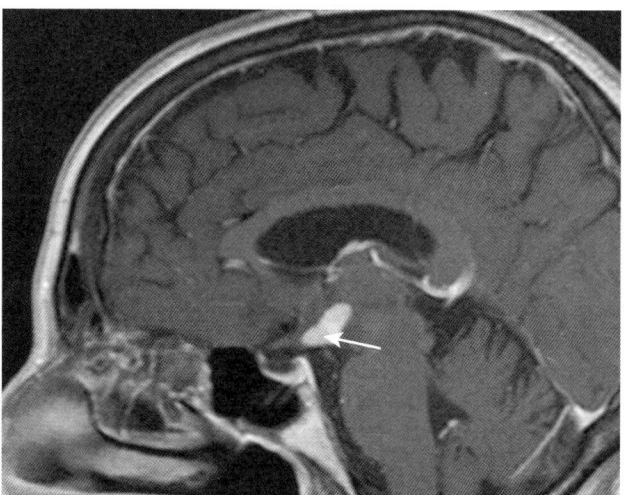

Fig. 21.38 MRI showing a thickened pituitary stalk in hypophysitis.

🩺 Box 21.53 Water deprivation test

Indications
- Diagnosis or exclusion of diabetes insipidus (DI).

Procedure
- Fasting and no fluids from 07:30 h (or overnight if only mild DI is expected and polyuria is only modest).
- Monitor serum and urine osmolality, urine volume and weight hourly for up to 8 h.
- Abandon fluid deprivation if weight loss >3% occurs.
- If serum osmolality is >300 mOsm/kg and/or urine osmolality <600 mOsm/kg, give desmopressin 2 μg i.m. at end of test. Allow free fluid but measure urine osmolality for 2–4 h.

Interpretation
- *Normal response* – serum osmolality remains within normal range (275–295 mOsm/kg). Urine osmolality rises to >600 mOsm/kg.
- *Diabetes insipidus (DI)* – serum osmolality rises above normal without adequate concentration of urine osmolality (i.e. serum osmolality >300 mOsm/kg; urine osmolality <600 mOsm/kg).
- *Nephrogenic DI* – if desmopressin does not concentrate urine.
- *Cranial DI* – if urine osmolality rises by >50% after desmopressin.

than vasopressin and has no vasoconstrictive effects. It can be given intranasally as a spray 10–40 µg once or twice daily, and orally as 100–200 µg three times daily, or intramuscularly 2–4 µg daily. Response is variable and must be monitored carefully with enquiry about fluid input/output and plasma osmolality measurements. The main problem is avoiding water overload and consequent hyponatraemia (see p. 183). Where there is an underlying cause (e.g. a hypothalamic tumour), this should be investigated and treated.

Alternative agents in mild DI, probably working by sensitizing the renal tubules to endogenous vasopressin, include thiazide diuretics, carbamazepine (200–400 mg daily) or chlorpropamide (200–350 mg daily) but these are rarely used.

Nephrogenic diabetes insipidus

In this condition, renal tubules are resistant to normal or high levels of plasma vasopressin (ADH). Nephrogenic diabetes insipidus may be inherited as a rare sex-linked recessive, with an abnormality in the vasopressin-2 receptor, or as an autosomal post-receptor defect in an ADH-sensitive water channel, aquaporin-2. More commonly, it can be acquired as a result of renal disease, sickle cell disease, drug ingestion (e.g. lithium), hypercalcaemia or hypokalaemia. Wherever possible, the cause should be reversed (see **Box 21.52**). Polyuria is helped by thiazide diuretics.

Other causes of polyuria and polydipsia

Diabetes mellitus, hypokalaemia and hypercalcaemia should be excluded. In the case of diabetes mellitus, the cause is an osmotic diuresis secondary to glycosuria, which leads to dehydration and an increased perception of thirst owing to hypertonicity of the extracellular fluid.

Primary polydipsia

This is a relatively common cause of thirst and polyuria. It is a psychiatric disturbance characterized by the excessive intake of water. Plasma sodium and osmolality fall as a result and the urine produced is appropriately dilute. Vasopressin levels become virtually undetectable. Prolonged primary polydipsia may lead to the phenomenon of 'renal medullary washout', with a fall in the concentrating ability of the kidney.

Characteristically, the diagnosis is made by a water deprivation test. A low plasma osmolality is usual at the start of the test, and since vasopressin secretion and action can be stimulated, the patient's urine becomes concentrated (although 'maximum' concentrating ability may be impaired); the initially low urine osmolality gradually increases with the duration of the water deprivation.

Syndrome of inappropriate antidiuretic hormone secretion
History and examination

Inappropriate secretion of ADH (also called vasopressin) leads to retention of water and hyponatraemia. The presentation of the syndrome of inappropriate antidiuretic hormone secretion (SIADH) is usually vague, with confusion, nausea, irritability and, later, fits and coma. There is no oedema. Mild symptoms usually occur with plasma sodium levels below 125 mmol/L and serious manifestations are likely below 115 mmol/L. The elderly may show symptoms with milder abnormalities.

The syndrome must be distinguished from dilutional hyponatraemia due to excess infusion of glucose/water solutions or diuretic administration (thiazides or amiloride; see p. 183).

Investigations

The usual features are:
- dilutional hyponatraemia due to excessive water retention
- euvolaemia (in contrast to hypovolaemia of sodium and water depletion states)
- low plasma osmolality with 'inappropriate' urine osmolality >100 mOsm/kg (and typically higher than plasma osmolality)
- continued urinary sodium excretion >30 mmol/L (lower levels suggest sodium depletion or 'hypovolaemic hyponatraemia', and should respond to 0.9% saline infusion)
- absence of hypokalaemia (or hypotension)
- normal renal and adrenal and thyroid function.
  The causes are listed in **Box 21.54**.

Hyponatraemia is very common during illness in frail elderly patients and it may sometimes be clinically difficult to distinguish SIADH from salt and water depletion, particularly when mixed clinical features are present. Under these circumstances, a trial infusion of 1–2 L 0.9% saline is given. SIADH will not respond (but will excrete the sodium and water load effectively); sodium depletion will respond. ACTH deficiency can give a very similar biochemical picture to SIADH; therefore it is necessary to ensure that the hypothalamic–pituitary–adrenal axis is intact, particularly in neurosurgical patients, in whom ACTH deficiency may be relatively common.

Management

The underlying cause should be corrected where possible. Symptomatic relief can be obtained by the following measures:
- ***Fluid intake*** should be restricted to 500–1000 mL daily. If tolerated and complied with, this will correct the biochemical abnormalities in almost every case.
- ***Frequent measurement*** of plasma osmolality, serum sodium and body weight is needed.
- ***Demeclocycline*** (600–1200 mg daily) is given if water restriction is poorly tolerated or ineffective; this inhibits the action of vasopressin on the kidney, causing a reversible form of nephrogenic diabetes insipidus. However, it often causes photosensitive rashes.
- ***Hypertonic saline*** may be indicated when the syndrome is very severe (i.e. acute and symptomatic), but this is potentially dangerous and should only be used with extreme caution (see p. 185).

> **? Box 21.54 Common causes of the syndrome of inappropriate antidiuretic hormone secretion (SIADH)**
>
> **Tumours**
> - Small-cell carcinoma of lung
> - Prostate
> - Thymus
> - Pancreas
> - Lymphomas
>
> **Pulmonary lesions**
> - Pneumonia
> - Tuberculosis
> - Lung abscess
>
> **Central nervous system causes**
> - Meningitis
> - Tumours
>
> - Head injury
> - Subdural haematoma
> - Cerebral abscess
> - Systemic lupus erythematosus
> - Vasculitis
>
> **Metabolic causes**
> - Alcohol withdrawal
> - Porphyria
>
> **Drugs**
> - Chlorpropamide
> - Carbamazepine
> - Cyclophosphamide
> - Vincristine
> - Phenothiazines

- **Vasopressin V$_2$ antagonists**, e.g. tolvaptan 15 mg daily, are being used with good results.

Further reading

Spasovski G, Vanholder R, Allolio B et al. Clinical practice guideline on diagnosis and treatment of hyponatraemia. *Eur J Endocrinol* 2014; 170:G1–G47.

DISORDERS OF CALCIUM METABOLISM

Serum calcium levels are mainly controlled by parathyroid hormone (PTH) and vitamin D. Hypercalcaemia is much more common than hypocalcaemia and is frequently detected incidentally with multichannel biochemical analysers. Mild asymptomatic hypercalcaemia occurs in about 1 in 1000 of the population, with an incidence of 25–30 per 100 000 population. It occurs mainly in elderly females and is usually due to primary hyperparathyroidism.

Parathyroid hormone

There are normally four parathyroid glands, which are situated posterior to the thyroid; occasionally, additional glands exist or they may be found elsewhere in the neck or mediastinum. PTH, an 84-amino-acid hormone derived from a 115-residue pre-prohormone, is secreted from the chief cells of the parathyroid glands. PTH levels rise as serum ionized calcium falls. The latter is detected by specific G-protein-coupled, calcium-sensing receptors on the plasma membrane of the parathyroid cells. PTH has several major actions, all serving to increase plasma calcium by:

- increasing osteoclastic resorption of bone (occurring rapidly)
- increasing intestinal absorption of calcium (a slow response)
- increasing synthesis of 1,25-dihydroxyvitamin D$_3$
- increasing renal tubular reabsorption of calcium
- increasing excretion of phosphate.

  PTH effects are mediated at specific membrane receptors on the target cells, resulting in an increase of adenyl cyclase messenger activity.

  Vitamin D metabolism is discussed on page 474.

  PTH measurements use two-site immunometric assays that measure only the intact PTH molecule; interpretation requires a simultaneous calcium measurement in order to differentiate most causes of hyper- and hypocalcaemia.

Hypercalcaemia

Pathophysiology and aetiology

The major causes of hypercalcaemia are listed in **Box 21.55**; primary hyperparathyroidism and malignancies are by far the most common (>90% of cases). Hyperparathyroidism itself may be primary, secondary or tertiary. Primary hyperparathyroidism is caused by single (>80%) parathyroid adenomas or by diffuse hyperplasia of all the glands (15–20%); multiple parathyroid adenomas are rare. Involvement of multiple parathyroid glands may be part of a familial syndrome (e.g. MEN type 1 or 2a). Parathyroid carcinoma is rare (<1%), though it usually produces severe and intractable hypercalcaemia. Hyperparathyroidism–jaw tumour syndrome is a rare familial cause of hyperparathyroidism that may be associated with parathyroid carcinoma and maxillary or mandibular tumours.

Primary hyperparathyroidism

Primary hyperparathyroidism is of unknown cause, though it appears that adenomas are monoclonal. Hyperplasia may also be monoclonal. Chromosomal rearrangements in the 5′ regulatory region of the parathyroid hormone gene have been identified, and inactivation of some tumour suppressor genes at a variety of sites may also be involved.

Secondary hyperparathyroidism

Secondary hyperparathyroidism (see p. 1394) is physiological compensatory hypertrophy of all parathyroids because of hypocalcaemia, such as occurs in chronic kidney disease or vitamin D deficiency. PTH levels are raised but calcium levels are low or normal, and PTH falls to normal after correction of the cause of hypocalcaemia where this is possible.

Tertiary hyperparathyroidism

Tertiary hyperparathyroidism is the development of apparently autonomous parathyroid hyperplasia after longstanding secondary hyperparathyroidism, most often in renal failure. Plasma calcium and phosphate are both raised, the latter often grossly so. Parathyroidectomy is necessary at this stage.

Clinical features

Mild hypercalcaemia

Mild hypercalcaemia (e.g. adjusted calcium <3 mmol/L) is frequently asymptomatic, but more severe hypercalcaemia can produce a number of symptoms:

? Box 21.55 Causes of hypercalcaemia

Excessive parathyroid hormone (PTH) secretion
- Primary hyperparathyroidism (most common by far), adenoma (common), hyperplasia or carcinoma (rare)
- Tertiary hyperparathyroidism
- Ectopic PTH secretion (very rare indeed)

Malignant disease – low PTH levels (second most common cause)
- Myeloma
- Secondary deposits in bone
- Production of osteoclastic factors by tumours
- PTH-related protein secretion

Excess action of vitamin D
- Iatrogenic or self-administered excess
- Granulomatous diseases, e.g. sarcoidosis, tuberculosis
- Lymphoma

Excessive calcium intake
- 'Milk-alkali' syndrome

Other endocrine disease (mild hypercalcaemia only)
- Thyrotoxicosis
- Addison's disease

Drugs
- Thiazide diuretics
- Vitamin D analogues
- Lithium administration (chronic)
- Vitamin A

Miscellaneous
- Long-term immobility
- Familial hypocalciuric hypercalcaemia

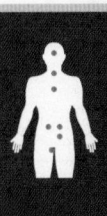

- **General.** There may be tiredness, malaise, dehydration and depression.
- **Renal.** Renal colic occurs from stones. Polyuria or nocturia, haematuria and hypertension are seen. The polyuria results from the effect of hypercalcaemia on renal tubules, reducing their concentrating ability – a form of mild nephrogenic diabetes insipidus. Primary hyperparathyroidism is present in about 5% of patients who present with renal calculi.
- **Bones.** There may be bone pain. Hyperparathyroidism mainly affects cortical bone, and bone cysts and locally destructive 'brown tumours' occur but only in advanced disease. Only 5–10% of all cases have definite bony lesions even when sought. Bone disease may be more apparent when there is coexisting vitamin D deficiency.
- **Abdomen.** There may be abdominal pain.
- **Chondrocalcinosis** and ectopic calcification. These are occasional features.
- **Corneal calcification.** This is a marker of longstanding hypercalcaemia but causes no symptoms.

There may also be symptoms from the underlying cause. Malignant disease is usually advanced by the time hypercalcaemia occurs, typically with bony metastases. The common primary tumours are bronchus, breast, myeloma, oesophagus, thyroid, prostate, lymphoma and renal cell carcinoma. True 'ectopic PTH secretion' by the tumour is very rare, and most cases are associated with raised levels of PTH-related protein. This is a 144-amino-acid polypeptide, the initial sequence of which shows an approximate homology with the biologically active part of PTH, which is necessary in fetal development but does not have a clearly defined role in the adult. Bone-resorbing cytokines and prostaglandins may be involved locally where there are metastatic skeletal lesions, leading to local mobilization of calcium by osteolysis with subsequent hypercalcaemia.

Severe hypercalcaemia

Severe hypercalcaemia (>3 mmol/L) is usually associated with malignant disease, hyperparathyroidism, chronic kidney disease or vitamin D therapy.

Investigations and differential diagnosis
Biochemistry

Several fasting serum calcium and phosphate samples should be taken.
- **Serum PTH.** The hallmark of primary hyperparathyroidism is hypercalcaemia and hypophosphataemia with detectable or elevated intact PTH levels during hypercalcaemia. When this combination is present in an asymptomatic patient, then further investigation is usually unnecessary. However, an undetectable PTH level in the context of hypercalcaemia always requires further investigation to exclude malignancy or other pathology (see **Box 21.54**).
- **Hyperchloraemic acidosis.** This is often mild.
- **Renal function.** This is usually normal but should be measured as a baseline.
- **24-h urinary calcium** or single calcium creatinine ratio. This should be measured in a young patient with modest elevation in calcium and PTH to exclude familial hypocalciuric hypercalcaemia (see p. 646).
- **Elevated serum alkaline phosphatase.** This is found in severe parathyroid bone disease, but otherwise it suggests an alternative cause for hypercalcaemia.

Where PTH is undetectable or equivocal, a number of other tests may lead to the diagnosis:
- Protein electrophoresis/immunofixation: to exclude myeloma.
- Serum TSH: to exclude hyperthyroidism.
- 9am cortisol and/or ACTH test: to exclude Addison's disease.
- Serum ACE: helpful in the diagnosis of sarcoidosis.

Imaging

The success of parathyroid imaging is highly operator-dependent and choice therefore depends on local skills and experience. Imaging is frequently far less accurate than parathyroid exploration by an expert surgeon, where the success rate is at least 90%. Methods include:
- Radioisotope scanning using ^{99m}Tc-sestamibi, which is approximately 90% sensitive in detecting adenomas; it is enhanced with single-photon emission computed tomography (SPECT).
- Ultrasound, which is simple and safe, although insensitive for small tumours.
- High-resolution CT scan or MRI (more sensitive). A CT scan of the thorax, abdomen and pelvis will often show malignancy or granulomatous disease in patients with hypercalcaemia and a suppressed PTH level.

Dual energy X-ray absorptiometry (DXA) bone density scanning is useful to detect bone effects in asymptomatic people with hyperparathyroidism in whom conservative management is planned.

Abdominal X-rays may show renal calculi or nephrocalcinosis. High-definition hand X-rays can show subperiosteal erosions in the middle or terminal phalanges. Neither is required as part of diagnosis unless symptoms of renal calculi are present or there is evidence of renal failure.

Management of hypercalcaemia

Details of emergency treatment for severe hypercalcaemia are given in **Box 21.56**. This should be followed by oral therapy unless the underlying disease can be treated.

Management of primary hyperparathyroidism
Medical management

There are no effective medical therapies at present for primary hyperparathyroidism, but a high fluid intake should be maintained and replacement of vitamin D in those that are deficient appears to have no detrimental effect on calcium levels. New therapeutic agents that target the calcium-sensing receptors (e.g. cinacalcet) are of proven value in parathyroid carcinoma and in dialysis patients (see p. 1396), and are used in primary hyperparathyroidism where surgical intervention is contraindicated.

Surgery

There is agreement that surgery is indicated in primary hyperparathyroidism for:
- symptoms of hypercalcaemia such as thirst, frequent or excessive urination, or constipation or
- end-organ disease (renal stones, fragility fractures or osteoporosis) or
- an albumin-adjusted serum calcium level of 2.85 mmol/L or above.

The situation where plasma calcium is mildly raised (2.65–2.85 mmol/L) is more controversial. Most authorities feel that young patients should be operated on, as should those who have reduced cortical bone density or significant hypercalciuria, as this is associated with stone formation.

In older patients without these problems, or in those unfit for or unwilling to have surgery, conservative management is indicated. Regular measurement of serum calcium and of renal function is necessary. Bone density of cortical bone should be monitored if conservative management is used. Hyperparathyroidism can cause non-specific symptoms of weakness, fatigue and depression, and it can be difficult to determine whether these symptoms are related to hypercalcaemia or coincidental.

Surgical technique and complications

Parathyroid surgery should be performed only by experienced surgeons, as the minute glands may be very difficult to define, and it is difficult to distinguish between an adenoma and normal parathyroid. In expert centres, over 90% of operations are successful, involving removal of the adenoma or removal of all four hyperplastic parathyroids. Minimal access surgery is used, and some centres measure PTH levels intraoperatively to ensure that the adenoma has been removed.

Other than postoperative hypocalcaemia (see below), the other rare complications are those of thyroid surgery: bleeding and recurrent laryngeal nerve palsies (<1%). Vocal cord function should be checked preoperatively.

⊕   Box 21.56 Management of acute severe hypercalcaemia

Acute hypercalcaemia often presents with dehydration, nausea and vomiting, nocturia and polyuria, drowsiness and altered consciousness. The serum Ca^{2+} is >3 mmol/L and sometimes as high as 5 mmol/L. While investigation of the cause is under way, immediate treatment is mandatory if the patient is seriously ill or if the Ca^{2+} is >3.5 mmol/L.

- *Rehydrate* using at least 4–6 L of 0.9% saline on day 1, and 3–4 L for several days thereafter. Central venous pressure (CVP) may need to be monitored to control the hydration rate.
- *Intravenous bisphosphonates* are the treatment of choice for the hypercalcaemia of malignancy or of undiagnosed cause. Pamidronate is preferred (60–90 mg as an intravenous infusion in 0.9% saline or glucose over 2–4 h or, if less urgent, over 2–4 days). Levels fall after 24–72 h, lasting for approximately 2 weeks. Zoledronic acid is an alternative.
- *Prednisolone* (30–60 mg daily) is effective in some instances (e.g. in myeloma, sarcoidosis and vitamin D excess) but in most cases is ineffective.
- *Calcitonin* (200 units i.v. 6-hourly) has a short-lived action and is little used.
- *Oral phosphate* (sodium cellulose phosphate 5 g three times daily) produces diarrhoea.

If initial exploration is unsuccessful, a full work-up, including venous catheterization and scanning, is essential, remembering that parathyroid tissue can be ectopic.

Postoperative care

The major danger after operation is hypocalcaemia, which is more common in patients who have significant bone disease and/or vitamin D deficiency – the 'hungry bone' syndrome. Some authorities pre-treat such patients with alfacalcidol 2 µg daily from 2 days pre-operatively for 10–14 days, and routine vitamin D replacement (preferably without calcium) is always indicated if deficiency is diagnosed. Chvostek's and Trousseau's signs (see below) are monitored, as well as biochemistry. Plasma calcium measurements are performed at least daily until stable, with or without replacement; a mild transient hypoparathyroidism often continues for 1–2 weeks. Depending on its severity, oral or intravenous calcium should be given temporarily, as only a few patients (<1%) will develop longstanding surgical hypoparathyroidism.

Familial hypocalciuric hypercalcaemia

This uncommon autosomal dominant, and usually asymptomatic, condition demonstrates increased renal reabsorption of calcium despite hypercalcaemia. PTH levels are normal or slightly raised and urinary calcium is low. Familial hypocalciuric hypercalcaemia is caused by loss-of-function mutations in the gene on the long arm of chromosome 3 encoding for the calcium-ion-sensing G-protein-coupled receptor in the kidney and parathyroid gland. Family members are often affected and this is detected by genetic analysis. Parathyroid surgery is not indicated, as the course appears benign. This diagnosis can be differentiated from hyperparathyroidism in an isolated case by the calcium : creatinine ratio in blood and urine.

Hypocalcaemia
Pathophysiology

Hypocalcaemia may be due to deficiencies of calcium homeostatic mechanisms, or secondary to high phosphate levels or other causes of hypocalcaemia (**Box 21.57**). All forms of hypoparathyroidism, except transient surgical effects, are uncommon.

Aetiology

- *Chronic kidney disease* is the most common cause of hypocalcaemia.
- *Severe vitamin D deficiency* may cause mild, and occasionally severe, hypocalcaemia.

? Box 21.57 Causes of hypocalcaemia

Increased phosphate levels
- Chronic kidney disease (common)
- Phosphate therapy

Hypoparathyroidism
- Surgical – after neck exploration (thyroidectomy, parathyroidectomy – common)
- Congenital deficiency (DiGeorge's syndrome)
- Idiopathic hypoparathyroidism (rare)
- Severe hypomagnesaemia

Vitamin D deficiency
- Osteomalacia/rickets
- Vitamin D resistance

Resistance to PTH
- Pseudohypoparathyroidism

Drugs
- Calcitonin
- Bisphosphonates
- Other
  - Acute pancreatitis (quite common)
  - Citrated blood in massive transfusion (not uncommon)
  - Low plasma albumin, e.g. malnutrition, chronic liver disease
  - Malabsorption, e.g. coeliac disease

PTH, parathyroid hormone.

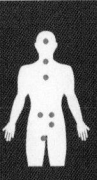

- ***Hypocalcaemia after thyroid or parathyroid surgery*** is common but usually transient; fewer than 1% of thyroidectomies leave permanent damage (see above).
- ***Idiopathic hypoparathyroidism*** is one of the rarer autoimmune disorders, and is often accompanied by vitiligo, cutaneous candidiasis and other autoimmune disease.
- ***DiGeorge's syndrome*** (see p. 60) is a familial condition in which the hypoparathyroidism is associated with intellectual impairment, cataracts and calcified basal ganglia, and occasionally with specific autoimmune disease.
- ***Pseudohypoparathyroidism*** is a syndrome of end-organ resistance to PTH owing to a mutation in the $G_S\alpha$-protein (GNAS1), which is coupled to the PTH receptor. It is associated with short stature, short metacarpals, subcutaneous calcification and sometimes intellectual impairment. Variable degrees of resistance involving other G-protein-linked hormone receptors may also be seen (TSH, LH, FSH).
- ***Pseudo-pseudohypoparathyroidism*** describes the phenotypic defects but without any abnormalities of calcium metabolism. Individuals with this condition may share the same gene defect as those with pseudohypoparathyroidism and be members of the same families.

Clinical features

Hypoparathyroidism presents as neuromuscular irritability and neuropsychiatric manifestations. Paraesthesiae, circumoral numbness, cramps, anxiety and tetany (**Box 21.58**) are followed by convulsions, laryngeal stridor, dystonia and psychosis. Two signs of hypocalcaemia are Chvostek's sign (gentle tapping over the facial nerve causes twitching of the ipsilateral facial muscles) and Trousseau's sign (inflation of the sphygmomanometer cuff above systolic pressure for 3 min induces tetanic spasm of the fingers and wrist). Severe hypocalcaemia may cause papilloedema and, frequently, a prolonged QT interval on the ECG.

Investigations

The clinical history and picture is usually diagnostic and is confirmed by a low serum calcium (after correction for any albumin abnormality). Additional tests include:
- ***Serum and urine creatinine.*** These test for renal disease.
- ***PTH levels*** in the serum. These are absent or inappropriately low in hypoparathyroidism, high in other causes of hypocalcaemia.
- ***Parathyroid antibodies.*** These are present in idiopathic hypoparathyroidism.
- ***25-hydroxyvitamin D serum level.*** This is low in vitamin D deficiency.
- ***Magnesium level.*** Severe hypomagnesaemia results in functional hypoparathyroidism, which is reversed by magnesium replacement.
- ***X-rays of metacarpals.*** Short fourth metacarpals occur in pseudohypoparathyroidism.

Box 21.58 Causes of tetany

In the presence of alkalosis
- Hyperventilation
- Excess antacid therapy
- Persistent vomiting
- Hypochloraemic alkalosis, e.g. primary hyperaldosteronism

In the presence of hypocalcaemia
See **Box 21.56**

Management

In vitamin D deficiency, colecalciferol is the most appropriate treatment. In other cases, alpha-hydroxylated derivatives of vitamin D are preferred for their shorter half-life, and especially in renal disease, as the others require renal hydroxylation. Usual daily maintenance doses are 0.25–2 μg for alfacalcidol (1α-OH-D$_3$). During treatment, plasma calcium must be monitored frequently to detect hypercalcaemia. Oral calcium supplements may be used in the early stages of treatment, and severe hypocalcaemia presenting as an emergency may occasionally require replacement with intravenous calcium gluconate. In hypoparathyroidism, PTH therapy is being used in clinical trials.

Further reading

Fraser WD. Hyperparathyroidism. *Lancet* 2009; 374:145–158.
Marcocci C, Cetani F. Primary hyperparathyroidism. *N Engl J Med* 2011; 365:2389–2397.
Shoback D. Hypoparathyroidism. *N Engl J Med* 2008; 359:391–403.
Society for Endocrinology. *Emergency Endocrine Guidance: Acute Hypercalcaemia*; Society for Endocrinology 2013; https://www.endocrinology.org/clinical-practice/clinical-guidance/emergency-guidelines/.
Society for Endocrinology. *Emergency Endocrine Guidance: Acute Hypocalcaemia*; Society for Endocrinology 2013; https://www.endocrinology.org/clinical-practice/clinical-guidance/emergency-guidelines/.

HYPOGLYCAEMIA IN THE NON-DIABETIC PATIENT

Hypoglycaemia develops when hepatic glucose output falls below the rate of glucose uptake by peripheral tissues. Hepatic glucose output may be reduced by:
- inhibition of hepatic glycogenolysis and gluconeogenesis by insulin
- depletion of hepatic glycogen reserves by malnutrition, fasting, exercise or advanced liver disease
- impaired gluconeogenesis (e.g. following alcohol ingestion).

In the first of these categories, insulin levels are raised, the liver contains adequate glycogen stores and the hypoglycaemia can be reversed by injection of glucagon. In the other two situations, insulin levels are low and glucagon is ineffective. Peripheral glucose uptake is accelerated by high insulin levels and by exercise, but these conditions are normally balanced by increased hepatic glucose output.

The most common symptoms and signs of hypoglycaemia are neurological. The brain consumes about 50% of the total glucose produced by the liver. This high energy requirement is needed to generate ATP, used to maintain the potential difference across axonal membranes.

Insulinomas

Insulinomas are pancreatic islet cell tumours that secrete insulin. Most are sporadic but some patients have multiple tumours arising from neural crest tissue (multiple endocrine neoplasia). Some 95% of these tumours are benign. The classic presentation is with fasting hypoglycaemia, but early symptoms may also develop in the late morning or afternoon. Recurrent hypoglycaemia is often present for months or years before the diagnosis is made, and the symptoms may be atypical or even bizarre; the presenting features in one series are given in **Box 21.59**. Common misdiagnoses include

---

Box 21.59 Presenting features of insulinoma

- Diplopia
- Sweating, palpitations, weakness
- Confusion or abnormal behaviour
- Loss of consciousness
- Grand mal seizures

psychiatric disorders, particularly pseudodementia in elderly people, epilepsy and cerebrovascular disease. Whipple's triad remains the basis of clinical diagnosis. This is satisfied when:

- symptoms are associated with fasting or exercise
- hypoglycaemia is confirmed during these episodes
- glucose relieves the symptoms.

A fourth criterion – demonstration of inappropriately high insulin levels during hypoglycaemia – may usefully be added.

The diagnosis is confirmed by the demonstration of hypoglycaemia in association with inappropriate and excessive insulin secretion. Hypoglycaemia is demonstrated by:

- Measurement of overnight fasting (16 h) glucose and insulin levels on three occasions. About 90% of patients with insulinomas will have low glucose and non-suppressed (normal or elevated) insulin levels.
- A prolonged 72-hour supervised fast if overnight testing is inconclusive and symptoms persist.

Autonomous insulin secretion is demonstrated by lack of the normal feedback suppression during hypoglycaemia. This may be shown by measuring insulin, C-peptide or proinsulin during a spontaneous episode of hypoglycaemia.

Management

The most effective therapy is surgical excision of the tumour but insulinomas are often very small and difficult to localize. Many techniques can be used to attempt to localize insulinomas. Sensitivity and specificity vary between centres and between operators. These include highly selective angiography, contrast-enhanced high-resolution computed tomography scanning, scanning with radiolabelled somatostatin (some insulinomas express somatostatin receptors), and endoscopic and intraoperative ultrasound scanning. Venous sampling for the detection of 'hot spots' of high insulin concentration in the various intra-abdominal veins is still used occasionally.

Medical treatment with diazoxide is useful when the insulinoma is malignant, when a tumour cannot be located and when elderly patients have mild symptoms. Symptoms may also remit on treatment with a somatostatin analogue (octreotide or lanreotide).

Hypoglycaemia with other tumours

Hypoglycaemia may develop in the course of advanced neoplasia and cachexia, and has been described in association with many tumour types. Certain massive tumours, especially sarcomas, may produce hypoglycaemia owing to the secretion of insulin-like growth factor-1. True ectopic insulin secretion is extremely rare.

Postprandial hypoglycaemia

If frequent venous blood glucose samples are taken following a prolonged glucose tolerance test, about 1 in 4 subjects will have at least one value below 3 mmol/L. The arteriovenous glucose difference is quite marked during this phase, so that very few are truly hypoglycaemic in terms of arterial (or capillary) blood glucose content. Failure to appreciate this simple fact led some authorities to believe that postprandial (or reactive) hypoglycaemia was a potential 'organic' explanation for a variety of complaints that might otherwise have been considered psychosomatic. An epidemic of false 'hypoglycaemia' followed, particularly in the USA. Later work showed a poor correlation between symptoms and biochemical hypoglycaemia. Even so, a number of otherwise normal people occasionally become pale, weak and sweaty at times when meals are due, and report benefit from advice to take regular snacks between meals.

True postprandial hypoglycaemia may develop in the presence of alcohol, which 'primes' the cells to produce an exaggerated insulin response to carbohydrate. The person who substitutes alcoholic beverages for lunch is particularly at risk. Postprandial hypoglycaemia sometimes occurs after gastric surgery, owing to rapid gastric emptying and mismatching of nutrient absorption and insulin secretion. This is referred to as 'dumping' but it is now rarely encountered (see p. 1176).

Hepatic and renal causes of hypoglycaemia

The liver can maintain a normal glucose output despite extensive damage, and hepatic hypoglycaemia is uncommon. It is, however, a particular problem with acute hepatic failure.

The kidney has a subsidiary role in glucose production (via gluconeogenesis in the renal cortex), and hypoglycaemia is sometimes a problem in terminal renal failure.

Hereditary fructose intolerance occurs in 1 in 20 000 live births and can cause hypoglycaemia.

Endocrine causes of hypoglycaemia

Deficiencies of hormones antagonistic to insulin are rare but well-recognized causes of hypoglycaemia. These include hypopituitarism, isolated adrenocorticotrophic hormone (ACTH) deficiency and Addison's disease.

Drug-induced hypoglycaemia

Many drugs have been reported to produce isolated cases of hypoglycaemia, but usually only when other predisposing factors are present:

- Sulphonylureas may be used in the treatment of diabetes or may be taken by people without diabetes in suicide attempts.
- Quinine may produce severe hypoglycaemia in the course of treatment for *falciparum* malaria.
- Salicylates may cause hypoglycaemia, usually after accidental ingestion by children.
- Propranolol can induce hypoglycaemia in the presence of strenuous exercise or starvation.
- Pentamidine, used in the treatment of resistant *Pneumocystis* pneumonia (see p. 1443), may produce hypoglycaemia .

Alcohol-induced hypoglycaemia

Alcohol inhibits gluconeogenesis. Alcohol-induced hypoglycaemia occurs in poorly nourished chronic alcohol users, binge drinkers, and children who have taken relatively small amounts of alcohol, since they have a diminished hepatic glycogen reserve. They present with coma and hypothermia (hypothermia is a feature of hypoglycaemia, due to the suppression of central thermoregulation, particularly the shivering response; children manifest hypothermia more frequently due to their high ratio of surface area to body mass).

Factitious hypoglycaemia

This is a relatively common variant of self-induced disease and is more common than an insulinoma. Hypoglycaemia is produced by surreptitious self-administration of insulin or sulphonylureas. Many patients in this category have been extensively investigated for an insulinoma. Measurement of C-peptide levels during hypoglycaemia should identify patients who are injecting insulin; sulphonylurea abuse can be detected by chromatography of plasma or urine.

OTHER ENDOCRINE DISORDERS

Diseases of many glands

Polyglandular autoimmune syndromes

Primary endocrine gland failure is commonly caused by autoantibodies (see **Box 21.4**) and there may be multiple gland deficiencies. Most common are the associations of primary hypothyroidism and

ℹ Box 21.60 Multiple endocrine neoplasia (MEN) syndromes

Organ	Frequency	Tumours/manifestations
Type 1		
Parathyroid	95%	Adenomas/hyperplasia
Pituitary	70%	Adenomas – prolactinoma, ACTH- or GH-secreting (acromegaly)
Pancreas	50%	Islet cell tumours (secreting insulin, glucagon, somato-statin, VIP, pancreatic poly-peptide, GH-releasing factor) Zollinger–Ellison syndrome (gastrinoma) Non-functional tumour
Adrenal	40%	Non-functional adenoma
Thyroid	20%	Adenomas – multiple or single
Type 2a		
Adrenal	Most	Phaeochromocytoma (70% bilateral) Cushing's syndrome
Thyroid	Most	Medullary carcinoma (calcitonin-producing)
Parathyroid	60%	Hyperplasia
Type 2b		
Type 2a with marfanoid phenotype and intestinal and visceral ganglioneuromas but not hyperparathyroidism. Neuromas also present around lips and tongue		

ACTH, adrenocorticotrophic hormone; GH, growth hormone; VIP, vasoactive intestinal peptide.

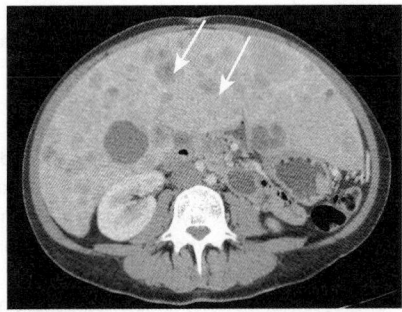

Fig. 21.39 Multiple liver metastases (arrowed) from a pancreatic endocrine tumour in multiple endocrine neoplasia type 1.

mutation must also occur, such as deletion or loss of a normal homologous chromosome.

MEN 1

The defect in MEN 1 is in a novel gene (*menin*) on the long arm of chromosome 11, which encodes for a 610-amino-acid protein. *Menin* represses a transcription factor (*JunD*), and lack of *JunD* suppression leads to decreased apoptosis and oncogenesis. People with the *MEN1* gene carry one mutant gene and a wild-type gene (i.e. are heterozygous). When the wild-type gene undergoes a random somatic mutation during life, this leads to loss of heterozygosity and explains the late onset of tumours at any stage (the 'two hit' hypothesis). MEN 1 is classically associated with pancreatic, parathyroid and pituitary tumours, although other glands may be affected (**see Box 21.60; Fig. 21.39**).

MEN 2a and 2b

MEN 2a and 2b are caused by mutations of the *RET* proto-oncogene on chromosome 10 (see medullary thyroid cancer, p. 622). This gene encodes for a transmembrane glycoprotein receptor. For MEN 2a, the mutation is in the extracellular domain; for 2b, it is in the intracellular domain. MEN 2 is classically associated with parathyroid tumours, phaeochromocytoma and medullary thyroid carcinoma (see **Box 21.60**). Unlike MEN 2a, MEN 2b is associated with a marfanoid phenotype and intestinal and visceral ganglioneuromas, as well as neuromas around the lips and tongue.

Management

Management of established tumours in MEN is largely the same as treatment for similar tumours occurring sporadically. In MEN 1, four-gland parathyroidectomy is usually recommended when surgery is needed since all glands are typically involved. However, the essence of management in MEN is annual screening to detect tumours at an early, treatable stage.

Screening

A careful family history is essential. If the precise gene mutation has been identified in a particular family, then family members at risk can be offered genetic screening for the presence of the mutation, ideally in childhood. In affected individuals, biochemical screening and periodic imaging are then required.

Screening for MEN 1

Hyperparathyroidism is usually the first manifestation, and serum calcium is the simplest screening test in families with no identified mutation. In an established case (or gene-positive family member), other screening bloods include prolactin, GH/IGF-1 and 'gut hormones' (see **Box 32.4**). Periodic imaging of pancreas, adrenals and pituitary is usually performed. People with MEN 1 can develop

type 1 diabetes, and either of these with Addison's disease or pernicious anaemia.

Autoimmune polyendocrinopathy type 1

Autoimmune polyendocrinopathy type 1 (APS-1) is an autosomal recessive disorder and is caused by *AIRE* gene mutations. This condition is also associated with non-endocrine manifestations. The *AIRE* gene is present in the epithelium of the thymus and is involved in the presentation of self-antigens to thymocytes. Mutations will allow persistence of thymic lymphocytes, which react against self antigens and cause development of autoimmune disorders. Mucocutaneous candidiasis often develops before the onset of endocrine deficiencies, such as hypothyroidism, Addison's disease, type 1 diabetes, hypoparathyroidism, primary hypogonadism, nail dystrophy, vitiligo and dental enamel hypoplasia.

Autoimmune polyendocrinopathy type 2

Autoimmune polyendocrinopathy type 2 (APS-2) is not associated with candidiasis and is also known as Schmidt's syndrome, typically when hypothyroidism, Addison's disease, type 1 diabetes, myasthenia gravis and primary hypogonadism are present in combination; coeliac disease is also an association.

Multiple endocrine neoplasias

Multiple endocrine neoplasia (MEN) is the name given to the simultaneous or metachronous occurrence of tumours involving a number of endocrine glands (**Box 21.60**). The condition is inherited in an autosomal dominant manner and arises from the expression of recessive oncogenic mutations, most of which have been isolated. Affected persons may pass on the mutation to their offspring in the germ cell, but for the disease to become evident, a somatic

metastases to the liver from non-functional pancreatic tumours that are clinically silent; this emphasizes the need for regular screening imaging.

Screening for MEN 2

Serum calcium levels will easily detect hyperparathyroidism.

- *Medullary carcinoma of thyroid (MCT).* With the known presence of the gene defect, total thyroidectomy is recommended in early childhood or as soon as the gene defect is identified. Calcitonin is a useful tumour marker.
- *Phaeochromocytoma.* Metanephrine or catecholamine estimations are required.

McCune–Albright syndrome

This condition is associated with autonomous hypersecretion of a number of endocrine glands at a young age. Gonadotrophin-independent puberty occurs, with Leydig cell hyperplasia in males and ovarian oestrogen production in girls. Pituitary hypersecretion may lead to hyperprolactinaemia, acromegaly or gigantism. Cushing's syndrome due to nodular hyperplasia of the adrenal cortex is observed, as well as autonomous functioning thyroid nodules. Non-endocrine manifestations include café-au-lait patches and increased bone deformity and fractures due to polyostotic fibrous dysplasia. The pathological basis is a point mutation of the *GNAS1* gene that inhibits GTPase activity, leading to persistent activation of cAMP-mediated endocrine secretion.

Ectopic hormone secretion

This term refers to hormone synthesis, and normally secretion, from a neoplastic non-endocrine cell, most usually seen in tumours that have some degree of embryological resemblance to specialist endocrine cells. The clinical effects are those of the hormone produced, with or without manifestations of systemic malignancy. The most common situations seen are the following:

- *Hypercalcaemia of malignant disease*, often from squamous cell tumours of lung and breast, often with bone metastases. Where metastases are not present, most cases are mediated by secretion of PTH-related protein (PTHrP), which has considerable sequence homology to PTH; a variety of other factors may sometimes be involved but very rarely PTH itself. Treatment is discussed on page 645.
- *SIADH* (see p. 643). Again, this is most commonly caused by a primary lung tumour.
- *Ectopic ACTH syndrome* (see p. 601). Small-cell carcinoma of the lung, carcinoid tumours and medullary thyroid carcinomas are the most common causes, though many other tumours rarely cause it.
- *Production of insulin-like activity.* This may result in hypoglycaemia (see p. 716).
- *Carcinoid syndrome.* This is the collection of symptoms (diarrhoea, abdominal pain and loss of appetite; flushing of the skin, particularly the face; tachycardia; breathlessness and wheezing) when a neuroendocrine tumour, usually one that has spread to the liver, releases hormones such as serotonin into the bloodstream. Measurement of 24 hour urinary 5HIAAs is required for diagnosis.

Endocrine treatment of other malignancies

See Chapter 6.

Bibliography

Jameson JL, DeGroot L. *Endocrinology*, 7th edn. Philadelphia: WB Saunders; 2015.
Wass JA, Stewart P (eds). *Oxford Textbook of Endocrinology and Diabetes*, 2nd edn. Oxford: Oxford University Press; 2011.

Significant websites

http://www.addisons.org.uk/ *Addison's Self Help Group (UK): information and guidelines on Addison's and steroid replacement.*
http://www.endocrine.niddk.nih.gov/ *US National Institutes of Health, National Institute of Diabetes and Digestive and Kidney Diseases.*
http://www.endocrineweb.com *Endocrine web resources.*
http://www.endocrinology.org *UK Society for Endocrinology.*
http://www.endo-society.org *Endocrine Society.*
http://www.endotext.org/ *Online endocrinology textbook.*
http://www.medicalert.org.uk *Emergency identification system for people with hidden medical conditions.*
http://www.pituitary.org.uk *Pituitary Foundation (UK charity): comprehensive information for patients and GPs.*
http://www.thyroidmanager.org/ *Online thyroid disease textbook.*
http://www.tss.org.uk *UK Turner Syndrome Support Society.*

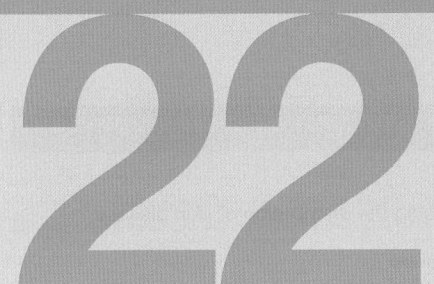

22

Dermatology

Sarah H. Wakelin

CORE SKILLS AND KNOWLEDGE

Skin diseases are common and their burden on a population level is significant. They cause considerable distress to patients and a few are life-threatening, including pemphigus, severe drug reactions and melanoma, the fifth most common cancer in the UK.

Dermatology is primarily an outpatient specialty, although admission is sometimes needed for severe inflammatory or infectious skin disease when associated with systemic symptoms. The demand for specialist care exceeds supply and teledermatology is evolving as a means of triaging referrals and offering remote access to specialist advice. Suspected malignant melanoma and squamous cell carcinoma require rapid access to specialist assessment. Dermatologists work in multidisciplinary teams with oncologists, pathologists, radiotherapists and plastic or maxillofacial surgeons to provide diagnosis and treatment.

Key skills include:

- examining the skin and describing common skin lesions and rashes accurately

- understanding the management of common skin complaints, including acne, eczema, psoriasis, skin infections and malignancies
- recognizing life-threatening skin conditions, including melanoma, severe drug reactions and aggressive skin and soft tissue infection
- understanding the role of topical therapies, oral immunosuppressants, phototherapy and biological drugs in the treatment of skin disease.

Dermatology is best learned by practical experience gained through interviewing and examining patients in outpatient clinics. Attending a skin cancer multidisciplinary team meeting gives insight into the expanding range of anti-cancer therapy available. Talking with patients who are receiving day treatment and phototherapy sheds light on the importance of improving chronic skin disease and its impact on quality of life.

CLINICAL SKILLS FOR DERMATOLOGY

History and examination

Skin complaints generally consist of **lesions** ('lumps and bumps') and **rashes**. Diagnosis is by taking a detailed history (**Box 22.1**) and examining the whole skin surface, as well as the hair, nails and oral cavity. Diagnostic accuracy can be increased by palpation (to assess depth of lesions) and by use of a **dermatoscope** (a handheld magnifying device with strong and sometimes polarized light).)

The **distribution** (**Box 22.2** and **Fig. 22.1**), **pattern** (**Fig. 22.2**) and **appearance** (**Fig. 22.3**) of disease should be described.

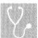 **Box 22.1** Taking a history in dermatology

History of the presenting complaint
- Time course: duration, changes in distribution/appearance over time
- Local symptoms: itching, pain and tenderness, bleeding
- Involvement of mouth, nails, hair or genitalia
- Provoking factors: temperature, sunlight, medication
- Features of systemic inflammatory disease, e.g. malaise, fever
- Symptoms in other systems: eyes, joints, internal organs

Risk factors
- History of autoinflammatory or autoimmune disease
- Current and recent medications, previous history of drug allergy
- Family history of skin disease (e.g. psoriasis, skin cancer) and atopy
- Skin type, cumulative sunlight exposure, use of sunbeds
- Time spent in tropical countries

Psychological factors[a]
- Depression and anxiety
- Disturbed body image, effect on relationships and self-confidence

[a]Screening tools for psychological distress, e.g. patient health questionnaire (PHQ)-9 and generalized anxiety disorder (GAD)-7, may be useful in assessment.

i **Box 22.2** Describing the distribution of skin disease

- **Generalized** or **localized**
- **Unilateral** or **bilateral**
- **Symmetrical** or **asymmetrical**
- **Acral** (primarily affecting the extremities – fingers, toes, nose, ears and penis) or **truncal** (primarily affecting the torso)

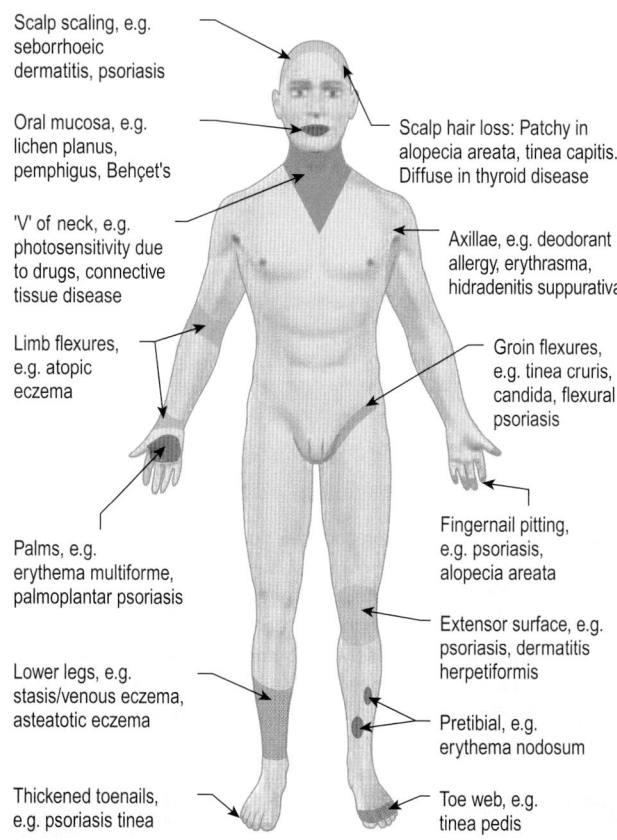

Scalp scaling, e.g. seborrhoeic dermatitis, psoriasis

Oral mucosa, e.g. lichen planus, pemphigus, Behçet's

'V' of neck, e.g. photosensitivity due to drugs, connective tissue disease

Limb flexures, e.g. atopic eczema

Palms, e.g. erythema multiforme, palmoplantar psoriasis

Lower legs, e.g. stasis/venous eczema, asteatotic eczema

Thickened toenails, e.g. psoriasis tinea

Scalp hair loss: Patchy in alopecia areata, tinea capitis. Diffuse in thyroid disease

Axillae, e.g. deodorant allergy, erythrasma, hidradenitis suppurativa

Groin flexures, e.g. tinea cruris, candida, flexural psoriasis

Fingernail pitting, e.g. psoriasis, alopecia areata

Extensor surface, e.g. psoriasis, dermatitis herpetiformis

Pretibial, e.g. erythema nodosum

Toe web, e.g. tinea pedis

Fig. 22.1 Examination of the skin surface.

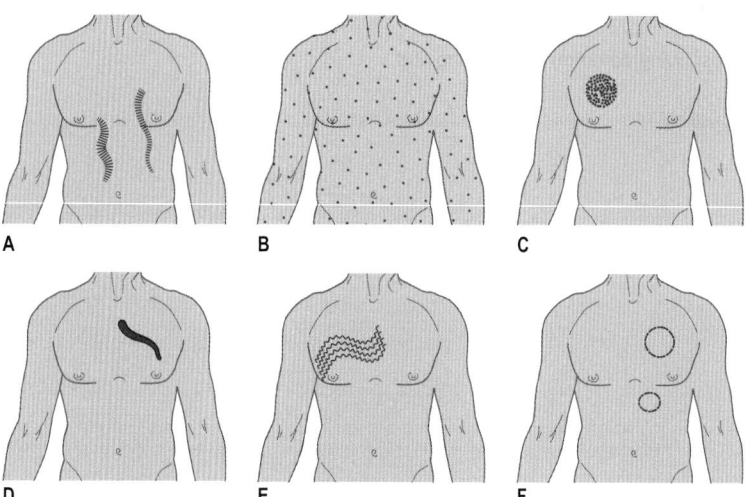

Fig. 22.2 Describing patterns in skin disease. **(A)** Serpiginous. **(B)** Scattered. **(C)** Grouped. **(D)** Linear. **(E)** Whorled. **(F)** Annular.

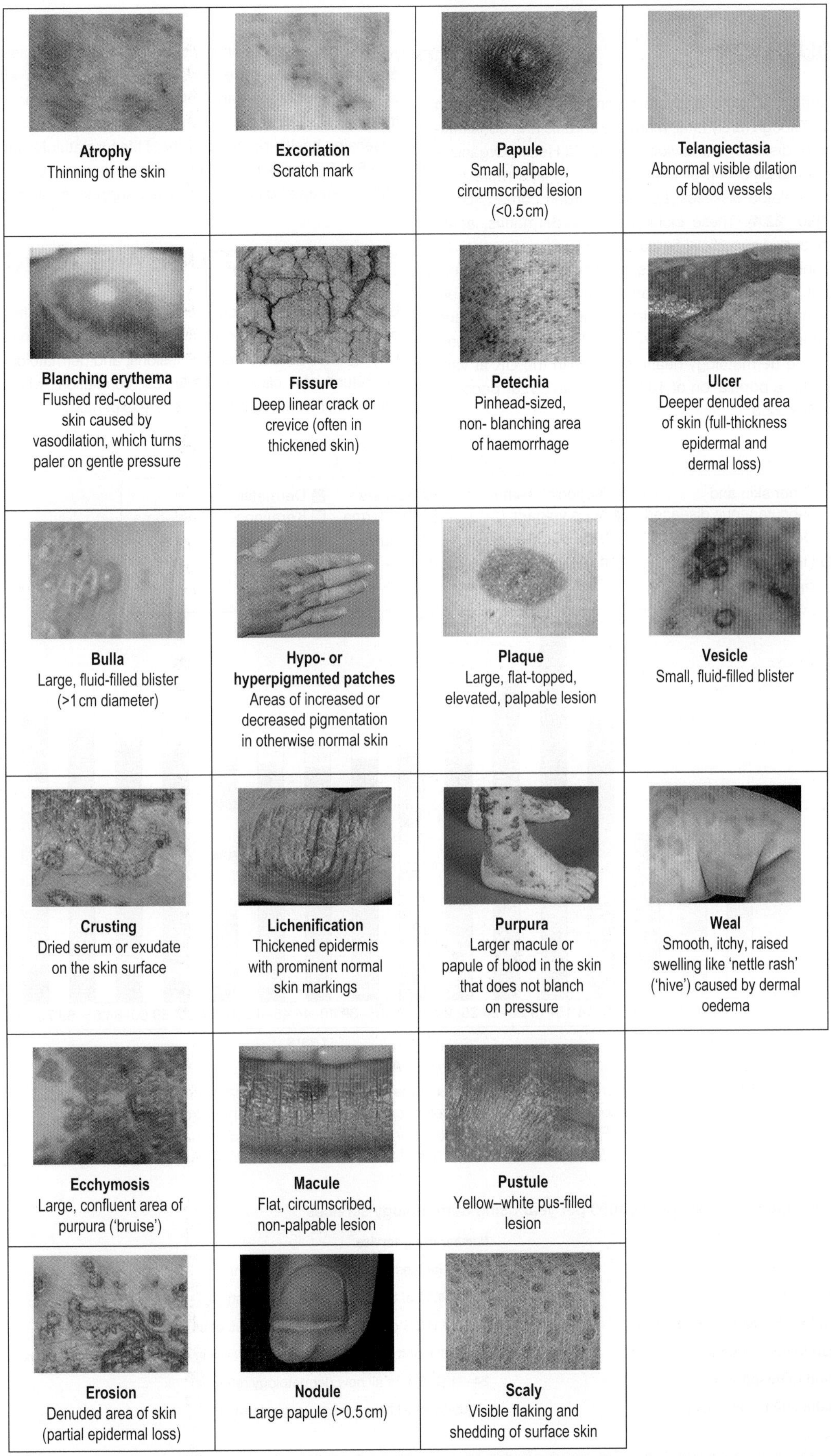

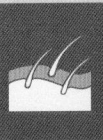

Atrophy
Thinning of the skin

Excoriation
Scratch mark

Papule
Small, palpable,
circumscribed lesion
(<0.5 cm)

Telangiectasia
Abnormal visible dilation
of blood vessels

Blanching erythema
Flushed red-coloured
skin caused by
vasodilation, which turns
paler on gentle pressure

Fissure
Deep linear crack or
crevice (often in
thickened skin)

Petechia
Pinhead-sized,
non- blanching area
of haemorrhage

Ulcer
Deeper denuded area
of skin (full-thickness
epidermal and
dermal loss)

Bulla
Large, fluid-filled blister
(>1 cm diameter)

**Hypo- or
hyperpigmented patches**
Areas of increased or
decreased pigmentation
in otherwise normal skin

Plaque
Large, flat-topped,
elevated, palpable lesion

Vesicle
Small, fluid-filled blister

Crusting
Dried serum or exudate
on the skin surface

Lichenification
Thickened epidermis
with prominent normal
skin markings

Purpura
Larger macule or
papule of blood in the skin
that does not blanch
on pressure

Weal
Smooth, itchy, raised
swelling like 'nettle rash'
('hive') caused by dermal
oedema

Ecchymosis
Large, confluent area of
purpura ('bruise')

Macule
Flat, circumscribed,
non-palpable lesion

Pustule
Yellow–white pus-filled
lesion

Erosion
Denuded area of skin
(partial epidermal loss)

Nodule
Large papule (>0.5 cm)

Scaly
Visible flaking and
shedding of surface skin

Fig. 22.3 Terminology describing types of lesion. *(Petechia image reproduced with permission from W Piette. Purpura and coagulation. In: Bolognia JL, Jorizzo JL (eds). Dermatology, 2nd edn. London: Elsevier; 2003. Blanching erythema image from Astle BJ, Duggleby W, Potter PA et al. Canadian Fundamentals of Nursing, 6th edn. Elsevier Canada, a division of Reed Elsevier Canada, Ltd; 2019. Hypopigmentation image from Douglas G, Nicol F, Robertson C. Macleod's Clinical Examination, 13th edn. Edinburgh: Churchill Livingstone/Elsevier; 2013.)*

INTRODUCTION

Skin diseases affect all ages and are among the most common human ailments. Though rarely fatal, many are chronic and constitute a leading cause of disability worldwide. The World Health Organization International Classification of Disease (ICD) 10 lists more than 1000 skin or skin-related diseases, but most burden comes from a few diseases (**Fig. 22.4**). These include eczema/dermatitis, acne, psoriasis, urticaria, and superficial fungal, bacterial (impetigo, cellulitis, abscesses) and viral infections (warts, molluscum contagiosum).

People with a skin complaint seek advice from various sources, including the Internet, pharmacists, primary care practitioners and specialists in intermediate or secondary care. The estimated number of people using dermatology health services in the UK at various entry points for a population of 100 000 over a 1-year period is summarized in **Box 22.3**.

The psychosocial impact of chronic skin disease can be great and should always be considered, including its effect on work, schooling, recreation and relationships. The dermatology life quality index (DLQI) and children's DLQI are simple validated tools for assessing health-related quality of life for patients with skin disease. The SWIFT check-up tool (see Further reading) can also be used to identify areas of difficulty and what support is needed.

SKIN STRUCTURE AND FUNCTION

Understanding the structure and function of the skin helps make sense of the signs and symptoms of skin disease. The skin can be biopsied to diagnose rashes or remove lesions, and dermatology offers a great opportunity for clinico-pathological correlation, where clinician and pathologist work together and share expertise.

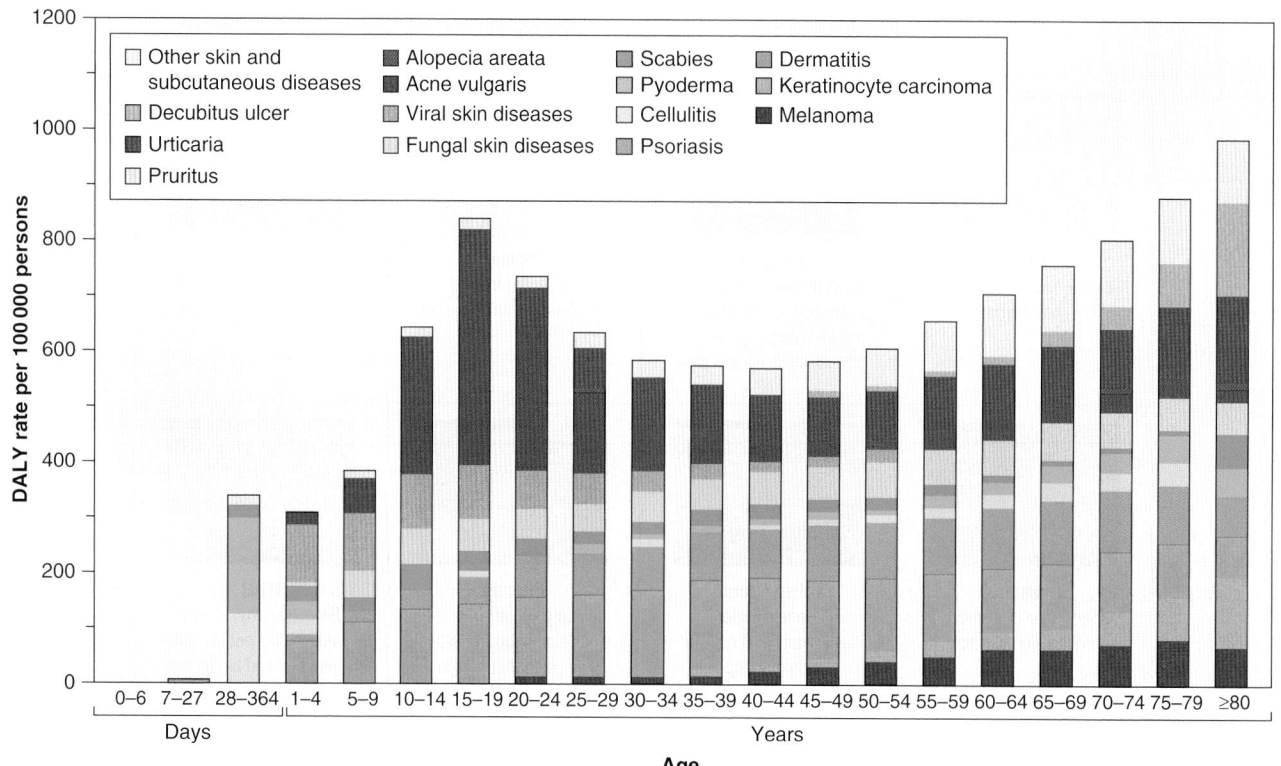

Fig. 22.4 Age distribution of skin and subcutaneous disease burden. Disability-adjusted life year (DALY) rate per 100 000 persons from 15 skin disease categories throughout the human lifespan. *(From Karimkhani C, Dellavalle RP, Coffeng LE et al. Global skin disease morbidity and mortality: an update from the Global Burden of Disease Study 2013. JAMA Dermatol 2017; 153:406-412, Fig. 1.)*

i **Box 22.3 Number of persons per 100 000 per year using dermatology services**

Group	Number using service
Number with a skin complaint	25 000 (at least 25% of total population)
Number who will self-treat	7500 (30% of those with skin complaint)
Number who will seek advice from their GP	14 550[a] (15% of total population or 19% of all GP consultations)
Number referred to dermatologist	1162 (8% of those attending their GP for skin problems or 1.2% of total population)
Number admitted to hospital	24–31 (2–3% of all new dermatology referrals)
Number of deaths due to skin disease	5[b] (0.4% of all new dermatology referrals)

[a]Excludes skin neoplasms, viral warts, herpes simplex and scabies.
[b]Includes people dying from cellulitis, chronic ulcer of the skin and severe drug reactions who might not have been admitted under a dermatologist's care.
(UK data. From Williams HC. Dermatology. In: Stevens A, Raftery J (eds). Health Care Needs Assessment, Series II. Oxford: Radcliffe Medical Press; 1997, pp. 261–348. Reproduced with kind permission of Rook's Textbook of Dermatology, 9th edn; http://www.rooksdermatology.com.)

Whole skin

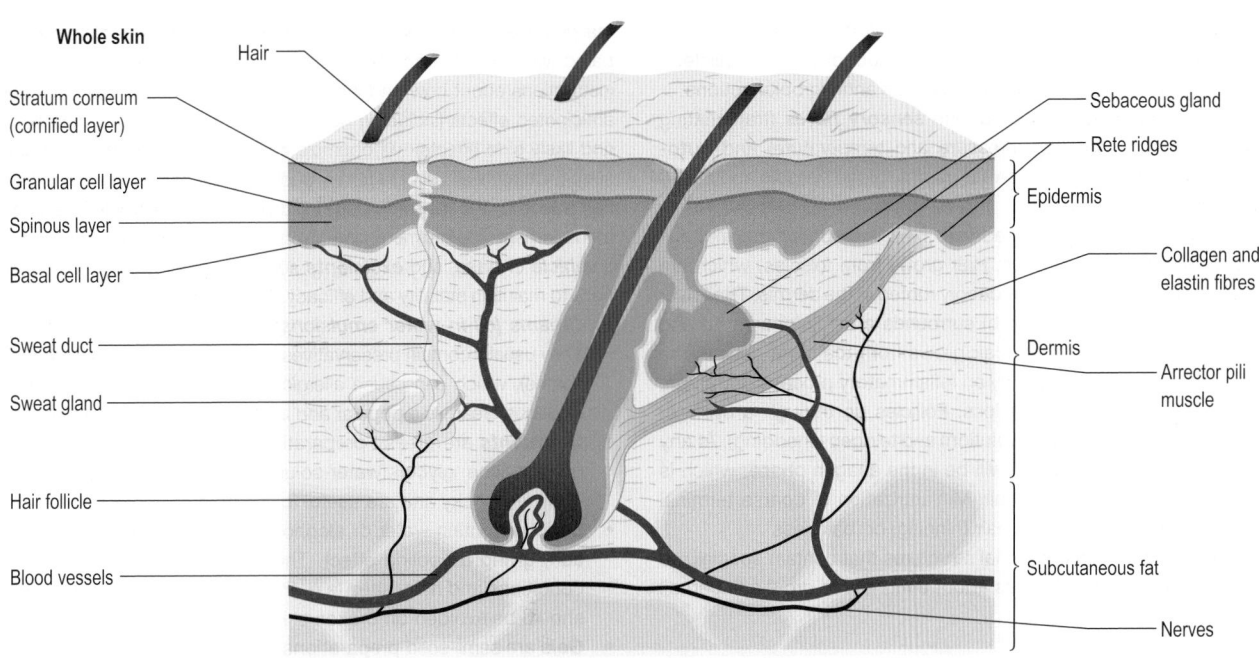

Hair

Stratum corneum
(cornified layer)

Granular cell layer

Spinous layer

Basal cell layer

Sweat duct

Sweat gland

Hair follicle

Blood vessels

Sebaceous gland

Rete ridges

Epidermis

Collagen and
elastin fibres

Dermis

Arrector pili
muscle

Subcutaneous fat

Nerves

Fig. 22.5 The structure of the skin.

> **i** **Box 22.4 Functions of the skin**
>
> - Physical barrier against friction and shearing forces
> - Protection against chemicals and ultraviolet radiation
> - Protection against infection (innate and acquired immunity)
> - Prevention of excessive water loss or absorption
> - Temperature regulation
> - Ultraviolet-induced synthesis of vitamin D
> - Wound healing

The skin is comprised of three distinct layers: the epidermis, dermis and subcutis (**Fig. 22.5**).

An overview of the functions of the skin is provided in **Box 22.4**.

Epidermis

The epidermis functions as a renewable dynamic barrier again the environment and pathogens, and plays an essential role in homeostasis. Its thickness ranges from 0.05 to 1.5 mm, depending on body site, and it is tethered to the underlying dermis by the dense protein network of the basement membrane zone (BMZ, see **Fig. 22.43**). Inherited or autoimmune-induced deficiencies of BMZ proteins lead to fragility and blistering of the skin and mucous membranes (see p. 686).

The epidermis is a **stratified squamous epithelium**, composed mostly of **keratinocytes** (keratin-synthesizing cells) that originate from a proliferating **basal layer**. They differentiate and migrate out to the surface to be shed as dead, flattened **squames**. Epidermal differentiation is a highly complex process involving 'switching on' and 'off' genes that regulate protein and lipid synthesis. Basal keratinocytes synthesize the **keratin** filaments of the cytoskeleton and desmosomal proteins (desmoplakin, desmoglein) for cell-to-cell cohesion. **Lipids** are synthesized in the granular layer and secreted to form a watertight intercellular layer. **Filaggrin** is expressed in the outer stratum corneum, where it acts as a 'natural moisturizing factor', keeping the skin hydrated and pliable. The stratum corneum provides most of the skin's barrier function, and deficiency in filaggrin leads to 'leaky',

dry skin that cracks, allowing entry of allergens and pathogens. Filaggrin gene mutations are common and have been identified as a major risk factor for atopic eczema and other atopic diseases. Changes in lipid and protease activity in the outermost epidermis lead to shedding (desquamation). The keratinocyte's journey from basal cell to skin surface normally takes about 30 days but is considerably faster in psoriasis (see p. 664), leading to thickened, scaly skin.

Keratinocytes also secrete cytokines, such as interleukins, interferon-gamma (IFN-γ) and tumour necrosis factor-alpha (TNF-α), in response to injury; these stimulate wound healing and protect against microbial invasion. They also produce antimicrobial peptides that form part of the innate immune system. Deficiency of these peptides may increase susceptibility to staphylococcal and viral infection in people with atopic eczema. The epidermis contains a network of **Langerhans cells** (dendritic cells) that capture and process antigens for presentation to T lymphocytes. Melanin-synthesizing **melanocytes** reside in the basal layer and transfer ultraviolet (UV)-protecting pigment to adjacent keratinocytes. The epidermis also contains nerve endings and sensory cells (**Merkel cells**).

Dermis

The dermis is a tough matrix of **collagen** and **elastin fibres**, surrounded by a gel-like ground substance. These fibres give skin its strength and elasticity. It also contains cells (fibroblasts, mast cells, lymphocytes and dendritic cells), blood and lymphatic vessels, nerves, muscle and **appendages** (sweat glands, sebaceous glands and hair follicles). The upper **papillary dermis** has finger-like projections that contain terminal capillary networks. The lower **reticular dermis** is thicker and denser. **Eccrine sweat glands** are found throughout the skin, except for the mucosal surfaces, and carry out thermoregulatory sweating. **Apocrine sweat glands** are found in the axillae and anogenital area, and do not function until puberty. **Sebaceous glands** are also inactive until puberty, when they excrete the oily substance sebum, under the influence of androgens. They are most numerous on the 'greasy' (seborrhoeic) sites of the central face, scalp and upper torso. Sebum flows on to the skin surface via the pilosebaceous duct of the hair follicle. It contributes to skin barrier function and has antimicrobial actions.

The skin is richly innervated with **sensory fibres** (transmitting touch, pain/itch, vibration, pressure and temperature) and **autonomic fibres** that innervate sweat glands, blood vessels and arrector pili for thermoregulation.

The skin surface is covered with **hair**, except for the mucous membranes, palms and soles. Hair grows from follicles, which are modified epidermal structures deeply rooted in the dermis. The lower portion of the hair follicle (bulb) surrounds a richly innervated and vascularized dermal papilla. Hair grows from the stem cells in the bulb. If this area is damaged by an inflammatory process or trauma, this leads to permanent hair loss. Follicles go through a cycle of anagen (growth), catagen (involution) and telogen (shedding). At any one time, most hairs (>90%) will be in the anagen phase, which is usually 3–5 years for scalp hair. Miniaturization of coarse terminal scalp hairs with age leads to hair thinning, or 'baldness'.

Nails are modified epidermal structures that contain specialized tough keratin proteins. It takes about 6 months to grow a fingernail and 1 year to grow a toenail.

Subcutis

The subcutaneous layer consists of lobules of adipose tissue separated by fibrous septa with sparse blood vessels and nerves. This layer provides insulation and cushioning against trauma.

INVESTIGATION OF SKIN DISEASE

The most common dermatological investigations are microscopy and culture of microbial swabs and fungal tests (mycology) of skin, hair or nail clippings (**Box 22.5**). Skin lesions may be removed by shaving, curetting or excision, depending on their depth and the suspected diagnosis. This can be done under local anaesthetic as an outpatient procedure. All skin specimens should be sent for histology. Immunofluorescence tests on skin and serum are indicated in suspected immunobullous diseases (see p. 686).

PRINCIPLES OF DERMATOLOGICAL THERAPY

Topical therapy

The skin is easily accessible to topical therapy and this is an effective and generally safe way of treating many rashes and some low-grade

---

> **i**　**Box 22.5 Common dermatological investigations**
>
> - Microbial swab (impetigo, folliculitis, candida); viral swab (herpes simplex virus, varicella zoster virus)
> - Mycology (fungal studies) of plucked hair/scalp brushings (tinea capitis)
> - Mycology of nail clippings (onychomycosis)
> - Mycology of skin scrapings (tinea, pityriasis versicolor)
> - Skin biopsy (histology, immunohistochemistry, direct immunofluorescence)
> - Blood tests (routine bloods, inflammatory markers, autoantibodies, indirect immunofluorescence)
> - Urinalysis (glucose, red cells) and urine microscopy (red cells, casts)
> - Patch tests for allergic contact dermatitis

---

malignancies with a reduced risk of systemic adverse effects compared with oral therapy. Attention to cosmetic acceptability, clear instructions about how and when to apply, duration of treatment and anticipated effects (including how quickly the complaint should settle and likely side-effects) will optimize patient adherence. It is helpful to specify quantities in simple terms, such as a 'pea-sized' portion to treat half a face or the 'fingertip unit' for topical corticosteroids in eczema management. Topical medicaments consist of an **active ingredient**, in a **vehicle** or **base**, and **excipients** such as **preservatives** or **emulsifiers** to maintain stability and efficacy. The following formulations exist:

- **Creams (oil-in-water emulsions)** are light and easily absorbed. They usually contain preservatives, such as parabens (hydroxybenzoates), which can cause allergic contact dermatitis (see below). Aqueous cream is a popular and inexpensive soap substitute.
- **Ointments** are greasy preparations based in vehicles such as polyethylene glycol (water-soluble) or petrolatum (insoluble). They feel sticky and are useful for treating dry, flaky rashes.
- **Lotions** contain water or alcohol that evaporates after application, giving a cooling effect. They are useful for weeping skin conditions and hairy sites (e.g. the scalp). Alcohol based-lotions should be avoided on broken skin, as they sting.
- **Gels** are semi-solid preparations of high-molecular-weight polymers. They are non-greasy and liquefy on contact with the skin. They are used to treat oily or hairy areas (e.g. scalp).
- **Pastes** are thick, adherent ointments containing a powder, e.g. Lassar's paste. They are rarely used now due to poor cosmetic acceptability.

Adverse effects of topical therapies

- **Systemic absorption** may occur when large areas of inflamed skin are treated, especially with occlusive bandages or dressings. Neonates are particularly susceptible due to their relatively high body surface area and immature skin barrier.
- **Contact allergy** may develop to the drug (e.g. hydrocortisone, neomycin), vehicle (e.g. lanolin, cetearyl alcohol) or excipients (e.g. chlorocresol, parabens). It should be considered in any patient with an unresponsive dermatitis or new dermatitis following topical treatment. Ointments contain fewer excipients and so are less likely to cause contact allergy.
- **Folliculitis** can occur due to blockage of hair follicles, especially with ointments in hot weather and on sweaty, occluded skin (bandages, tight clothing).

Corticosteroids can cause a range of adverse effects (see p. 661) but have a very good safety profile when used correctly.

Phototherapy

Phototherapy with sunlight has been used to treat skin diseases since ancient times. Modern phototherapy uses specific wavelengths in the UV spectrum for anti-inflammatory or pigment-inducing effects. The conditions most commonly treated with phototherapy are psoriasis, eczema, polymorphic light eruption, cutaneous T-cell lymphoma and vitiligo. Narrow-band UVB (311 nm /TL01) was developed specifically to treat psoriasis and is the treatment of choice in most cases. UVA therapy is given with systemic or topical psoralens (psoralen + UVA = PUVA) to enhance its photobiological effects. Commercial tanning beds predominantly deliver low doses of UVA and have limited effectiveness in treating skin disease.

Narrow-band UVB therapy is given two or three times a week for 6–10 weeks. It has superseded broad-band UVB, as it is more effective. PUVA is usually given twice a week. If the psoralen is taken orally, UV-protective glasses must be worn for the day of treatment

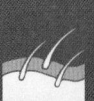

to protect the retina. PUVA is used less widely nowadays because it is associated with an increased risk of skin cancer, especially squamous cell carcinoma. The maximum recommended lifetime dose of UVA is 1000 joules (approximately 200 treatments).

Unaffected regions of skin or high-risk areas like the scrotum should be covered during phototherapy. To avoid adverse effects, patients should be carefully selected and their skin cancer risk assessed. People with very fair skin and freckles are at increased risk of burning and the UV dosage has to be carefully adjusted and escalated according to skin type.

Systemic therapy

A wide range of systemic drugs are used to treat skin disease. Some are used off-licence, especially for uncommon diseases where no licensed option exists. The risks and benefits should be carefully considered and discussed with the patient, so they can share in treatment decisions. Drugs include:

- antibiotics (antibacterial, antiviral and antifungal therapy)
- antiandrogens
- anti-inflammatories (antihistamines, antimalarials, colchicine, corticosteroids, dapsone, phosphodiesterase inhibitors, thalidomide)
- immunosuppressants (azathioprine, ciclosporin, cyclophosphamide, methotrexate, mycophenolate mofetil)
- retinoids (acitretin, alitretinoin, isotretinoin)
- biologics (for psoriasis, eczema, urticaria).

ERYTHRODERMA AND LOSS OF SKIN FUNCTION ('SKIN FAILURE')

Erythroderma ('red skin') is a term used to describe widespread inflammation affecting 90% or more of the body surface. There are several causes (**Box 22.6**), of which underlying skin disease and drug hypersensitivity are the most common. Extensive skin inflammation causes pain, soreness and irritation, and leads to loss of normal skin function, especially fluid and temperature regulation. Symptoms include thirst, fever and chills, malaise and dizziness. Erythroderma requires urgent medical treatment to avoid life-threatening complications (see next section). Examination should seek features of an underlying dermatosis, such as scalp or nail psoriasis. There may be associated generalized lymphadenopathy and a skin biopsy may be indicated, especially in suspected cutaneous lymphoma. In non-malignant disease, lymph nodes are often mildly enlarged and histology shows non-specific, reactive changes.

Complications

These include:

- high-output cardiac failure from increased blood flow
- hypothermia from heat loss
- pre-renal acute kidney injury from fluid depletion
- hypoalbuminaemia
- catabolism and increased basal metabolic rate
- secondary bacterial infection
- ***capillary leak syndrome***: the most severe complication and potentially fatal, though rare. Release of inflammatory mediators from the skin causes extensive vascular leakage with oedema, hypovolaemic shock and acute respiratory distress syndrome (ARDS) (see p. 232).

Management

Intensive supportive treatment includes maintaining body temperature (with space blankets and heaters) and close monitoring of vital signs and fluid and electrolyte balance. Skin swabs should be taken if secondary infection is suspected. All non-essential medication should be stopped. Topical therapy with a bland emollient or mild topical steroid can be initiated while the underlying cause is identified, at which point systemic therapy may be indicated: for example, ciclosporin for psoriasis (see p. 666).

COMMON RASHES

Acne and related disorders

Acne

Acne is one of the most common skin complaints globally, affecting over 85% of adolescents and often persisting into adulthood. In women, a late-onset chronic variant starting in the twenties is increasingly recognized. Acne can have a profound effect on self-esteem and mood, leading to anxiety, depression and even suicidal ideation. This may have little correlation with apparent disease severity. Lesions arise in the pilosebaceous follicle, which becomes blocked due to abnormal keratinization and increased production of altered sebum, leading to comedones. Microcomedones (microscopic comedones) can be found in biopsies of normal-looking acne-prone skin. Blockage of the pilosebaceous duct is followed by alteration in its microbiome, especially involving *Cutibacterium acnes* (formerly *Propionibacterium acnes*), leading to activation of innate immunity (**Fig. 22.6A**). This causes an inflammatory response with influx of neutrophils that release elastase, causing connective tissue damage. Scarring may follow with profound long-term psychological consequences. Post-inflammatory hyperpigmentation (see p. 693) is also a common sequela in dark-skinned people.

Clinical features

Acne affects the face and upper torso, where the sebaceous glands are dense and affected skin is usually greasy (seborrhoea). Lesions are classified as:

- ***non-inflammatory*** – open comedones (blackheads) or closed comedones (whiteheads)
- ***inflammatory*** – papules, pustules (**Fig. 22.6B**), nodules and cysts
- ***scars*** – raised (hypertrophic) or depressed/pitted (box, rolling and ice-pick).

Uncommon acne variants are shown in **Box 22.7**.

Severe acne may be associated with various autoinflammatory syndromes characterized by fever and aseptic inflammation (**Box 22.8**).

? Box 22.6 Causes of erythroderma

Common
- Atopic eczema
- Psoriasis
- Drugs (e.g. sulphonamides, gold, sulphonylureas, penicillin, allopurinol, captopril)
- Seborrhoeic eczema
- Idiopathic

Rare
- Chronic actinic dermatitis

- Cutaneous T-cell lymphoma (Sézary's syndrome)
- Malignancy (especially leukaemias)
- Pemphigus foliaceus
- Pityriasis rubra pilaris (a hereditary disorder of keratinization)
- HIV infection
- Toxic shock syndrome

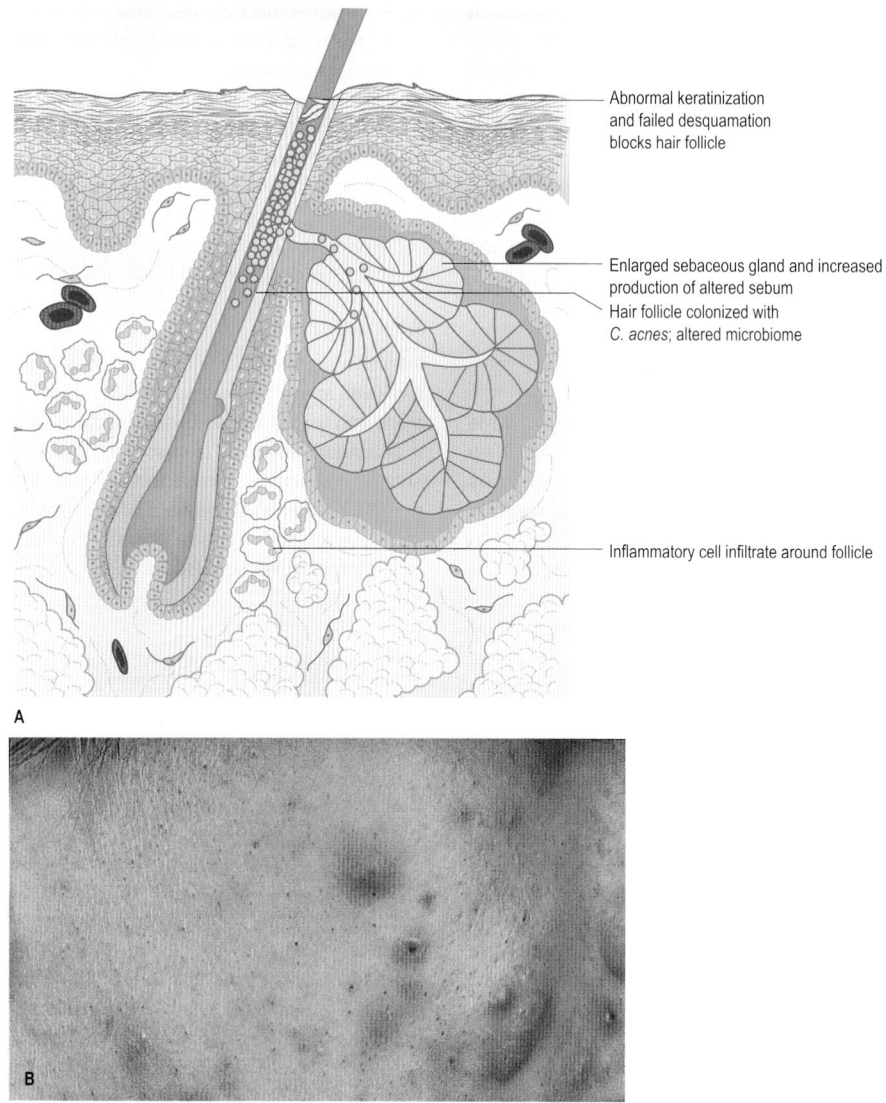

Fig. 22.6 Acne. (A) Pilosebaceous unit, which becomes blocked in acne. **(B)** Comedones and inflammatory lesions in facial acne. *(A, From Eichenfield LF, Frieden IJ, Mathes EF et al.* Neonatal and Infant Dermatology, *3rd edn. Elsevier Inc.; 2015; Fig. 2.1. Courtesy of Randall Hayes.)*

In figure A labels: Abnormal keratinization and failed desquamation blocks hair follicle; Enlarged sebaceous gland and increased production of altered sebum; Hair follicle colonized with *C. acnes*; altered microbiome; Inflammatory cell infiltrate around follicle.

Management

The diagnosis of acne is usually straightforward. Treatment should target the primary pathogenic lesion: the *microcomedone* and associated inflammatory response. The choice depends on whether lesions are predominantly non-inflamed or inflamed, disease severity or scarring, response to previous treatment and degree of psychological upset (**Box 22.9**).

Topical retinoids, azelaic acid, salicylic acid and benzoyl peroxide (BPO) are **keratolytic** and help unblock pores but also cause dry, flaky skin. This can be managed with a non-comedogenic/oil-free moisturizer. **Tetracyclines** and **erythromycin** are licensed for oral use in acne but their prolonged use may encourage the emergence of resistant bacteria. They should not be prescribed long term or without non-antibiotic topical therapy, as the latter reduce the emergence of resistant bacteria (**Box 22.10**). In females, the *combined oral contraceptive pill* and a formulation containing additional *cyproterone acetate* (a mild antiandrogen) may be of benefit due to a reduction in sebum excretion. Low-dose spironolactone is another useful option. Progesterone-only pills ('mini-pills') may aggravate acne.

Oral isotretinoin is a highly effective treatment licensed for severe inflammatory acne, especially with scarring. It is also used in milder recalcitrant cases associated with severe psychological upset. It causes dryness of the mucous membranes and has a range of other potential adverse effects. A major concern is its potent teratogenicity, so females of childbearing age must use highly effective contraception and follow a specific pregnancy prevention programme. Oral isotretinoin has been associated with depression and rare cases of suicide, so mood should be carefully monitored. However, for most acne sufferers, emotional wellbeing improves as their acne clears. High-intensity light treatment (blue light, intense pulsed light) has also been reported to lessen inflammatory lesions, and ablative laser therapy and physical treatment, such as dermabrasion, may improve the appearance of scars. However, these are not 'magic wands' and a key goal of acne treatment is to *prevent* scar formation.

Hidradenitis suppurativa ('acne inversa')

Hidradenitis suppurativa (HS) is a chronic inflammatory disorder that affects the apocrine pilosebaceous follicles of the axillae, the inguinal

Box 22.7 Clinical variants of acne

Infantile acne
- Typically starts between 3 and 12 months of age
- Triggered by maternal androgens

Acne excoriée
- Mainly affects young women who pick mild acne spots, leaving prominent excoriations
- There is usually underlying psychological upset

Drug-induced acneiform eruptions
- May be caused by corticosteroids, vitamin B_{12}, isoniazid and epidermal growth factor receptor (EGFR) inhibitors
- Comedones are absent

Pomade acne
- Caused by oily scalp cosmetics
- Typically affects the forehead

Oil acne
- Caused by prolonged (e.g. occupational) contact with oils

- Usually affects the legs

Chloracne
- Caused by exposure to toxins (e.g. dioxin)
- Widespread comedones and large, straw-coloured, non-inflamed cysts

Acne conglobata
- A severe form of cystic acne with abscesses and interconnecting sinuses
- Usually affects young men

Acne fulminans
- There is associated fever, weight loss and musculoskeletal pain
- Systemic steroids and oral isotretinoin are required

Follicular occlusion triad
- Severe cystic acne with cellulitis of the scalp (see p. 695) and hidradenitis suppurativa (see p. 658)

---

i **Box 22.8 Acne-associated autoinflammatory syndromes**

- SAPHO syndrome: synovitis, acne, pustulosis, hyperostosis, osteitis
- PAPA: PG, acne, pyogenic arthritis
- PASH: PG, acne, suppurative hidradenitis (hidradenitis suppurativa)
- PAPASH: PG, psoriatic arthritis, suppurative hidradenitis (hidradenitis suppurativa)
- PASS: PG, acne, seronegative spondyloarthritis

PG, pyoderma gangrenosum (see p. 678).

Box 22.9 Treatment of acne

Mild/physiological acne
- Step 1: Provide acne-friendly/oil-free skin care: salicylic acid washes (keratolytic)

Comedonal acne
- Step 2: Add topical retinoid or azelaic acid (keratolytic)

Inflammatory acne
- Step 3: Give topical retinoid + BPO
  - BPO ± topical or oral antibiotic (antimicrobial)

Severe acne
- Step 4: Consider oral isotretinoin
  - Antiandrogen therapy (cyproterone acetate, spironolactone) may be useful in females with moderate acne and seborrhoea

BPO, benzoyl peroxide.

Box 22.10 Prescribing antibiotics for acne

- Avoid long-term prescription (>6 months) of oral antibiotics
- Do not use topical antibiotic monotherapy (co-prescribe with retinoid or benzoyl peroxide)
- Avoid prescribing dissimilar oral and topical antibiotics

area and around the breasts ('apocrine acne'). It is characterized by recurrent abscesses, draining sinuses and scarring, and is associated with the metabolic syndrome, obesity and smoking. Patients are often disabled by pain and malodorous discharging lesions; there is no definitive treatment. Bacterial biofilms within the occluded follicles may explain the disappointing results of antibiotic therapy. Treatment options include oral tetracycline, combined rifampicin and clindamycin, acitretin and adalimumab (anti-TNF). Surgery may be required to drain abscesses and to excise the affected areas of skin.

Rosacea

Rosacea (**Fig. 22.7**) is a common inflammatory rash predominantly affecting the central face. It usually starts in mid-adult life and it is more common in fair-skinned people. The cause is unknown but pathogenesis may involve chronic sun damage, and an increased innate immune response triggered by the commensal mite *Demodex folliculorum* and leading to synthesis of pro-angiogenic and pro-inflammatory mediators.

Clinical features

The main features are diffuse erythema and inflammatory papules and pustules. Flushing and telangiectasia may be early features and can be aggravated by hot drinks, alcohol, sunlight and changes in temperature (erythemato-telangiectatic rosacea). This may be followed by papules and pustules (papulopustular rosacea) but, unlike acne, there are no comedones. Ocular involvement can lead to blepharitis, keratitis and conjunctivitis. Later complications include sebaceous gland and soft tissue overgrowth (phymatous rosacea), especially of the nose in men, causing rhinophyma and facial lymphoedema. Use of topical steroids can exacerbate or trigger rosacea.

Management

Treatment is suppressive rather than curative. Topical metronidazole, azelaic acid or ivermectin may be used for long-term control, with intermittent courses of oral tetracyclines. Subantimicrobial doses of doxycycline are effective due to an anti-inflammatory effect. Flushing and erythema do not respond to antibacterial drugs and treatment options include cosmetic concealers, topical brimonidine and vascular laser therapy. Rhinophyma can be debulked surgically or with an ablative laser (e.g. CO_2 laser).

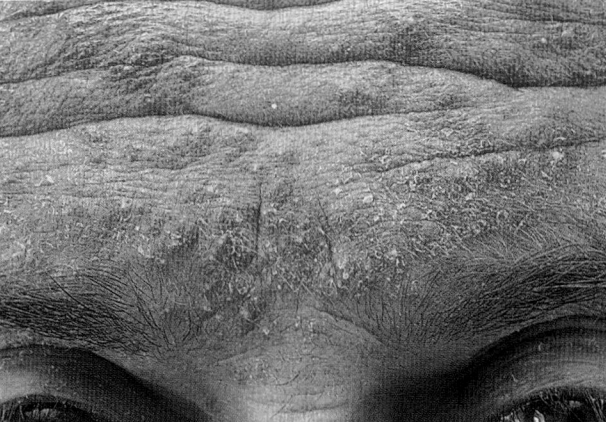

Fig. 22.7 Rosacea. Papules and pustules on background erythema. There are no comedones.

Perioral dermatitis

Perioral dermatitis is a distinctive rosacea-like rash that typically affects the nasolabial fold and area around the mouth in young women in a 'diamond' distribution. It is characterized by small inflammatory papules and pustules with overlying scaling. Topical steroids may trigger the complaint in susceptible individuals and are often continued inadvertently as the rash flares when they are discontinued. Treatment is with an oral tetracycline, as for rosacea, and with weaning off topical steroids.

Other rarer causes of facial rashes

These include autoimmune rheumatic diseases, lymphocytic and granulomatous infiltrates.

Further reading

Ingram JR, Collier F, Brown D et al. British Association of Dermatologists guidelines for the management of hidradenitis suppurativa (acne inversa) 2018; *Br J Dermatol* 2018; 180:1009–1017.
Nast A, Dréno B, Bettoli V et al. European evidence based (S3) guidelines for the treatment of acne. *J Eur Acad Dermatol Venereol* 2012; 26(Suppl 1):1–29.
Zaenglein AL. Acne vulgaris. *N Engl J Med* 2018; 379:1343–1352.

Eczema/dermatitis

The terms 'eczema' and 'dermatitis' are used interchangeably to describe an extremely common type of inflammatory rash. In the developed world, eczema may affect about 10% of the population at any one time, with up to 40% experiencing an episode of eczema during their lifetime. Eczema is classified as **constitutional** or **endogenous**, and **contact** or **exogenous** (**Box 22.11**). It can also be classified according to duration (acute, subacute or chronic).

The cardinal features of inflammation are manifest in eczema as erythema, swelling, itch/soreness and loss of normal (skin barrier) function. In acute eczema, oedema is prominent and tiny vesicles or larger bullae may be seen within inflamed skin. Skin swelling subsides to leave dry, flaky skin. Scratching leads to excoriations with serosanguinous exudate. Repeated scratching or rubbing causes thickened skin with the prominent lines (lichenification) of chronic eczema. The thickened skin is not supple and cracks easily, predisposing to fissures, especially on hands and feet. Secondary bacterial infection may occur and cause crusts, papules and pustules. The histology of eczema correlates with the clinical features: in acute eczema the keratinocytes are swollen with increased intercellular fluid ('spongiosis'), while in chronic disease there is little oedema but prominent thickening of the epidermis (acanthosis) and scaling (hyperkeratosis). Inflammatory cells are present around the upper dermal vessels in all patterns.

Atopic eczema

This type of constitutional eczema is extremely common, affecting up to 20% of children. It usually starts under the age of 2 years and is often associated with other atopic diseases, which present in a sequence described as the 'atopic march'. The majority (80–90%) of children with early-onset atopic eczema will spontaneously improve and 'clear' before the teenage years, 50% being free of the condition by the age of 6. Recurrence may occur in adulthood, especially as a localized hand eczema. Onset in later childhood or adulthood is often associated with a more chronic relapsing course.

Aetiology

Atopic eczema is a highly prevalent chronic inflammatory skin disease that arises from a combination of genetic, immunological and environmental factors that lead to skin barrier dysfunction and an altered skin microbiome. A positive family history of atopic disease is often present: there is 90% concordance in monozygotic twins but only 20% in dizygotic twins. If one parent has atopic disease, the risk of a child developing eczema is about 20–30%. If both parents have atopic eczema, the risk is more than 50%.

Genetic studies have identified a primary abnormality in skin barrier function: in particular, loss-of-function mutations in the filaggrin gene, which are associated not only with atopic eczema but with other atopic diseases and food allergy. Filaggrin deficiency leads to impaired skin barrier function and dry skin, allowing antigens and microbes to penetrate the epidermis. There is an initial activation of Th2 CD4 lymphocytes in the skin, with increased interleukin (IL)-4, IL-5 and IL-13 levels that lead to raised levels of immunoglobulin E (IgE) and IL-31, a key mediator of itch. Scratching leads to further epidermal damage. The later chronic inflammatory phase is more complex and also involves Th1, Th17/IL-23, Th22 cells and the Janus kinase (JAK)/STAT pathway (see p. 68).

Defects in the innate immune system have also been identified in atopic eczema, including epidermal antimicrobial peptides, Toll-like receptor 2 expression and epidermal tight junctions. This may explain the predisposition to cutaneous infection, particularly with *Staphylococcus* spp. and herpes simplex virus. Paradoxically, a lack of infection (in infancy) may skew the immune system towards a Th2 axis, favouring development of eczema ('hygiene hypothesis').

Blockade of the IL-4/IL-13 pathway is being used therapeutically in the management of eczema and asthma, and anti-IL-31 therapy shows promise in the treatment of itch.

Exacerbating factors

Exposure to soap and detergent skin cleansers dries and damages the epidermis and promotes inflammation. In some patients, repeated infections with *Staph. aureus* induce flares, which may be mediated by superantigen exotoxins that cause widespread T-cell activation. Teething, dribbling and lip licking may trigger facial eczema in infancy and childhood. Severe anxiety or stress may exacerbate eczema in some individuals. Pet dander can aggravate eczema. The role of house dust mites and diet is less clear-cut. Immediate/type 1 hypersensitivity to food allergens (cow's milk, egg, soya, wheat, fish and nuts) is common in young children with severe atopic eczema. Ingestion of food causes perioral and sometimes generalized urticaria (hives) and gastrointestinal symptoms (reflux, vomiting and diarrhoea). Rarely, there may be a delayed hypersensitivity to foods such as cow's milk that manifests with an eczema flare after 12–24 hours. This cannot be investigated with prick tests or blood tests and the mechanism is unclear. The diagnosis is made by taking a careful dietary history, followed by oral food challenge tests. There is some evidence that food allergens may play a role in triggering atopic eczema and that dairy products or eggs can worsen eczema in a minority of infants under 12 months of age.

Clinical features

Atopic eczema has a variable clinical presentation. The characteristic sites involved are the flexures of the elbows, knees, ankles and

---

i **Box 22.11 Classification of eczema**

Endogenous
- Atopic eczema
- Seborrhoeic eczema
- Venous ('gravitational') eczema
- Discoid eczema
- Asteatotic eczema
- Chronic hand/foot eczema
- Lichen simplex/nodular prurigo

Exogenous
- Irritant contact eczema
- Allergic contact eczema

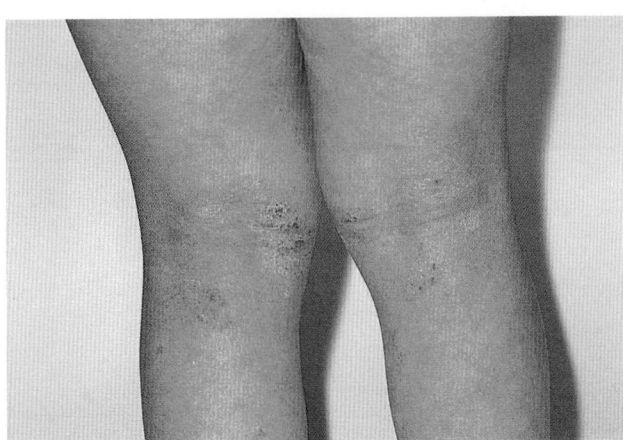

Fig. 22.8 Atopic eczema behind the knees.

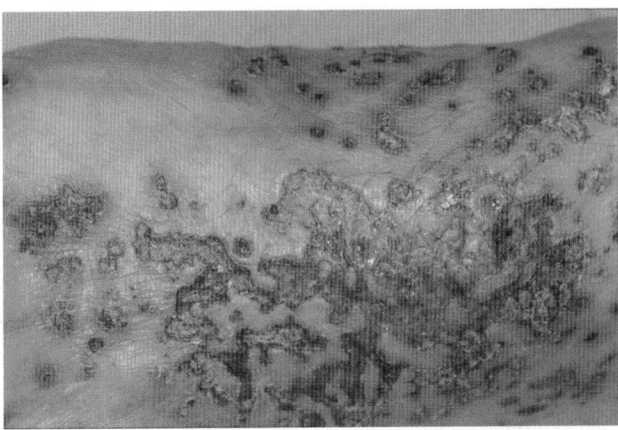

Fig. 22.9 Eczema herpeticum. Multiple punched-out crusted erosions.

wrists (**Fig. 22.8**), and around the neck. In infants, eczema often starts on the cheeks before spreading to the body. Clinical features of acute or chronic eczema (see earlier) may predominate and the pattern can change with time. Pruritus is usually severe, leading to excoriations and lichenification. In dark skin types the distribution may be different, with an 'inverse pattern' predominantly affecting the extensor surfaces, and follicles can be prominent. Pigmentary changes – hyper- and hypopigmentation – may follow the inflammatory phase of eczema and are often slow to resolve.

In some atopic individuals the skin of the upper arms and thighs feel rough due to follicular hyperkeratosis ('keratosis pilaris'). Prominent skin creases on the palms ('hyperlinear palms') and dry, 'fish-like' scaling of the skin of the lower legs (ichthyosis vulgaris) point to underlying deficiencies in filaggrin.

Secondary infection

Secondary bacterial infection with *Staph. aureus* and/or streptococci is common, especially in moist flexural areas such as the neck and groin. Pustules, oedema and golden-crusted inflamed papules strongly suggest secondary infection.

Cutaneous viral infections (e.g. viral warts and molluscum) may be more widespread in atopic eczema. Herpes simplex virus (HSV) can cause widespread infection of the skin, ***'eczema herpeticum'***. This appears as multiple small blisters or painful, punched-out crusted papules (**Fig. 22.9**) that are associated with malaise and pyrexia. Urgent systemic antiviral therapy is indicated to reduce the risk of disseminated life-threatening infection. An extensive form of hand, foot and mouth disease may also occur in children with eczema, with blisters and crusted lesions extending over large areas of the limbs and face ('eczema coxsackium'). Ocular complications of atopic eczema include conjunctival irritation and, less commonly, keratoconjunctivitis and cataract.

Investigations

Atopic eczema is diagnosed on the history and clinical features. About 80% of patients also have laboratory features of atopy (raised total IgE and allergen-specific IgE and mild eosinophilia).

Management

General measures include avoiding irritants (especially bar and liquid soap). Clothing should be made of soft, 'breathable' fabric such as cotton (see **Box 22.12**). Manipulating the diet (e.g. following a dairy-free or egg-free diet) may help a minority of infants with moderate to severe eczema. However, this should be done only under the expert guidance of a dietician, to ensure adequate intake of nutrients such as calcium.

---

i **Box 22.12** Management of atopic eczema

- Education and explanation
- Avoidance of irritants/allergens
- Emollients
- Bath oils/soap substitutes
- Topical therapies:
  - Steroids
  - Immunomodulators
- Adjunct therapies:
- Oral antibiotics
- Sedating antihistamines
- Bandaging
- Phototherapy
- Systemic therapy, e.g. oral prednisolone, ciclosporin

---

i **Box 22.13** Classification of topical corticosteroids by potency

Very potent
- 0.05% clobetasol propionate
- 0.3% diflucortolone valerate

Potent
- 0.1% betamethasone valerate
- 0.025% fluocinolone acetonide

Moderately potent
- 0.05% clobetasone butyrate
- 0.05% alclometasone dipropionate

Mild
- 2.5% hydrocortisone
- 1% hydrocortisone

Topical therapies

Topical therapies (see p. 656) are sufficient to control atopic eczema in most people. The key components are moisturizers/emollients and topical corticosteroids. Fragrance-free moisturizers should be used liberally on all dry skin areas and reapplied as often as needed. Some can also be used as soap substitutes. Dermatology nurse-led education of eczema sufferers and their families provides psychological support and improves adherence to treatment.

Topical corticosteroids remain the bedrock of eczema treatment and for most patients they provide reasonable disease control. They are usually applied once or twice a day to inflamed skin. Topical corticosteroids are classified into four groups, according to potency (**Box 22.13**). Select an appropriate potency, according to the body site, surface area and patient age, to minimize the risk of adverse effects (**Box 22.14**) and allow safe, intermittent long-term treatment. Unfortunately, 'steroid phobia' is common among patients or their carers, and leads to under-use of an otherwise effective treatment. Potent steroids should be used for short periods only and weaned down to milder steroids, or used intermittently as the eczema settles. Regular use of emollients may reduce steroid usage.

Mild steroids rarely cause skin atrophy but this is a significant risk with potent and superpotent steroids, especially if applied under occlusion or with a keratolytic such as salicylic acid. Mild steroids are used to treat eczema on the face and flexures, especially in the periocular area and in young children. Potent steroids are usually required to treat palmoplantar eczema due to the thick stratum corneum at this site. The 'fingertip unit' can be used to guide topical steroid dosage.

Moisturizers with or without topical steroids can be applied under occlusive damp tubular gauze bandages ('wet wraps'). These can improve efficacy but are time-consuming to apply. Paste bandages containing ichthammol can also be useful for resistant or lichenified eczema of the limbs.

Topical calcineurin inhibitors (TCIs) (tacrolimus ointment and pimecrolimus cream) are licensed for the treatment of atopic eczema in adults and children over the age of 2 years. They do not cause skin atrophy and are therefore useful for delicate areas such as the face and eyelids. They are less effective on thick skin due to poor penetration. The main adverse effect is a burning or prickling sensation that usually improves with continued treatment. Initial concerns that the immunosuppressant effects of TCIs would increase the risk of skin cancer have not proved to be founded, but patients are advised to avoid sun exposure and vaccinations. Tacrolimus ointment can also be used prophylactically twice a week to prevent eczema flares.

Antibiotics and antiseptics

Antibiotics are indicated if there are clinical signs of infection and are usually given orally for 7–10 days. Flucloxacillin is the treatment of choice for staphylococcal infection and phenoxymethylpenicillin for streptococcal disease. Erythromycin is an alternative for those with penicillin allergy. Topical antiseptics are often used as emollient washes or bath additives, or in the form of 'bleach baths'. They may cause irritation.

Sedating antihistamines

These may be useful at bedtime, but as histamine is not a key mediator in the itch of eczema they are often of limited benefit.

Second-line therapy and new drugs

These are used in severe, unresponsive eczema, especially if it is interfering with an individual's life (e.g. growth, sleeping, schoolwork or job). Ultraviolet phototherapy (see p. 656) and systemic immunosuppressants (ciclosporin, azathioprine and methotrexate) can be helpful. Short, tapering courses of oral prednisolone usually provide rapid disease control but relapse is common on withdrawal. The risks and benefits of long-term systemic therapy require careful evaluation and should be discussed with the patient or their carer.

The anti-IL-4/IL-13 monoclonal antibody dupilumab, given by subcutaneous injection every 2 weeks, has been shown to be a highly effective and safe treatment for adult atopic eczema and is now licensed in the UK to treat moderately severe disease. Various other biological drugs and small-molecule drugs are under investigation, and include phosphodiesterase-4 inhibitors and JAK inhibitors.

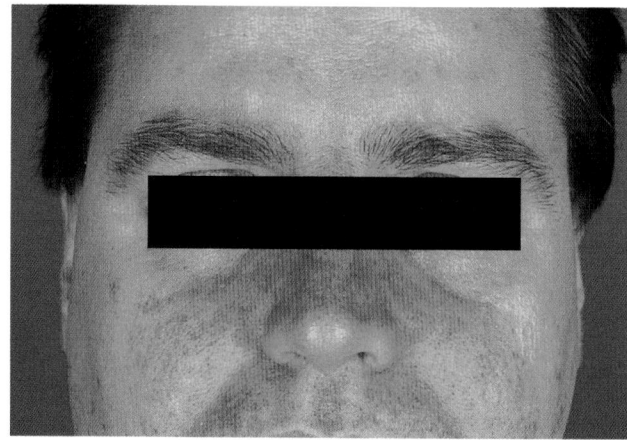

Fig. 22.10 Seborrhoeic eczema affecting the sides of the nose.

Seborrhoeic eczema

Clinical features

Seborrhoeic eczema is extremely common in adults of all ages and in its mildest form is often overlooked. As the name implies, it affects greasy areas. On the face, it presents with scaling and erythema around the nose (**Fig. 22.10**), medial eyebrows, hairline and ear canals. Itch is variable. Dandruff is thought to be a mild variant of scalp seborrhoeic dermatitis. More severe scalp involvement can look like psoriasis (sebo-psoriasis). The presternal area may be affected in men and other sites include the large flexures and anogenital area. A generalized form of seborrhoeic eczema presents as erythroderma in the elderly (see p. 657). Children are not affected until puberty. Cradle cap and a non-itchy napkin dermatitis may represent infantile variants of seborrhoeic eczema.

Aetiology

It is thought that a lipophilic commensal yeast, *Malassezia* (see p. 674), triggers the inflammatory skin changes of seborrhoeic dermatitis in susceptible individuals. Host immunity is also involved, and seborrhoeic dermatitis is one of the earliest skin manifestations of HIV infection (see p. 676). Its prevalence is also increased in Parkinson's disease.

Management

Seborrhoeic dermatitis usually runs a chronic relapsing course and treatment is suppressive rather than curative. Topical azole antifungal creams, with short-term use of mild- to moderate-potency steroids according to body site, are usually helpful. TCIs are an effective option but are unlicensed for this form of dermatitis. Ketoconazole-containing shampoo is useful to treat scalp involvement and as maintenance therapy.

Venous eczema (varicose eczema, stasis, gravitational eczema)

Venous eczema usually affects the elderly and those with varicose veins or a history of venous thrombosis. The inner calf is involved and there are usually coexistent signs of venous hypertension, including haemosiderin deposition, lipodermatosclerosis and varicose ulceration. The eczematous changes range from mild erythema and scaling to an acute exudative inflammatory rash. It may be complicated by allergic contact dermatitis to medicated creams or bandages, and patch tests should be done if there is an inadequate response to treatment.

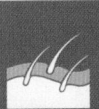

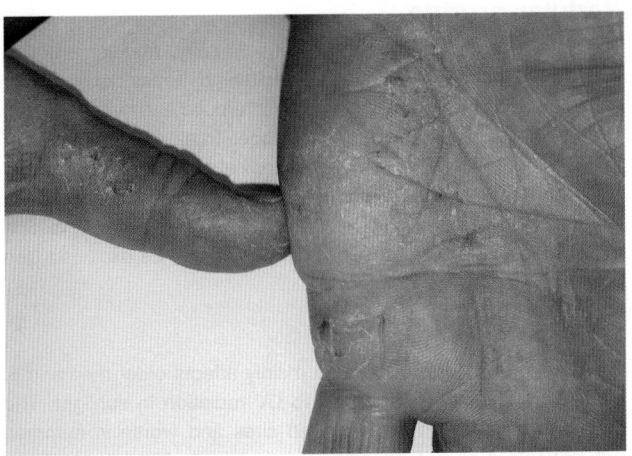

Fig. 22.11 Hand eczema.

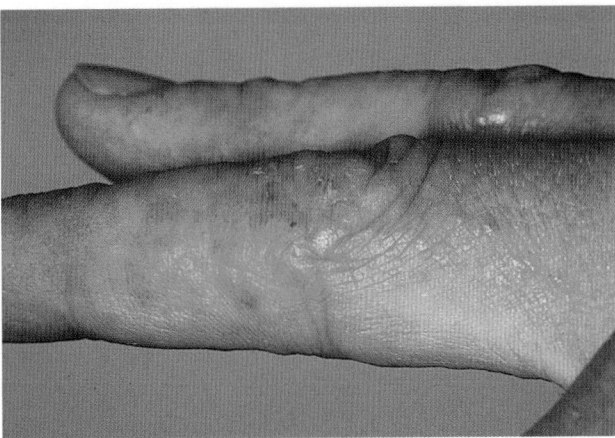

Fig. 22.12 Pompholyx eczema. *(Courtesy of Dr A Bewley, London.)*

Management

This includes use of bland (perfume-free) emollients such as a 50:50 liquid paraffin:white soft paraffin mix, and short-term prescription of a moderately potent topical steroid. Underlying venous hypertension should be managed with compression hosiery or vascular surgery. Paraffin-containing emollients are a fire hazard as they impregnate clothes and bedding, making them highly flammable.

Discoid eczema (nummular eczema)

Discoid eczema is characterized by well-demarcated, inflamed scaly patches, sometimes with tiny vesicles. It usually affects the limbs and torso, and is intensely itchy, which helps differentiate it from psoriasis. Lesions may be secondarily infected with *Staph. aureus*. The cause is unknown. Potent topical steroids are usually required to clear individual lesions.

Asteatotic eczema (winter eczema, eczema craquelé)

This form of eczema often affects older people in wintertime and can be intensely pruritic. It involves the lower legs, lower back and other areas that have few sebaceous glands. These areas are particularly vulnerable to the drying effects of soap and water. The rash resembles crazy paving with dry scales and inflamed cracks. Frequent use of a bland moisturizer and soap substitute is usually all that is needed.

Hand eczema

Hand eczema (**Fig. 22.11**) is a common problem that has a significant impact on quality of life. It often runs a chronic relapsing course for many years, with a reported lifetime prevalence of up to 15%. Different clinical patterns are recognized, and the morphology may be mixed and can vary with time in an affected individual.

The underlying causes are:
- **Contact dermatitis/eczema** – due to an external harsh substance (**irritant**) or allergy-provoking substance (**allergen**).
- **Endogenous dermatitis/eczema** – where no external factors can be identified. There may also be involvement of the feet.

In reality, hand eczema often has a complex and mixed aetiology due to an inherent endogenous eczema tendency and an additional irritant and/or allergic component.

Mild **irritant hand eczema** typically causes dry, sore, chapped skin on the dorsal hands and the finger webs. It is extremely common in cold, dry weather and in people who wash their hands

Box 22.15 Common contact allergens

- **Fragrance** ('parfum') – in fine fragrances, toiletries, moisturizers, household products
- **Rubber chemicals** – in household and examination gloves and footwear
- **Metals** – in jewellery, buckles, spectacle frames and gadgets, including mobile phones
- **Chemical hair dye** – in permanent and semi-permanent colorants
- **Preservative chemicals** – in cosmetics, toiletries, and household and industrial products
- **Topical antibiotics and antiseptics** – prescribed and over-the-counter
- **Other ingredients in medicated creams** – e.g. lanolin, hydrocortisone
- **Adhesives** – in footwear, acrylic nails, superglue
- **Leather and textile dyes**

frequently, either at home (especially when caring for young children) and/or in occupations such as catering, healthcare and hairdressing. Hand eczema is a common finding in people with **atopic eczema** and the hand may be the only site involved in adulthood. **Vesicular** hand eczema or 'pompholyx' is characterized by multiple intensely itchy blisters, especially on the sides of the fingers and palms (**Fig. 22.12**). A **hyperkeratotic** form of eczema is characterized by dry, scaly plaques and cracks on the palms and soles, and shares similarities with psoriasis at these sites. Localized eczema of the finger pulps is called '**pulpitis**'.

Severe chronic hand eczema often leads to sick leave and job loss. It is a considerable financial and societal burden, as it impairs the ability to work and to carry out the tasks of daily living. **Patch testing** should be considered in all patients with chronic hand eczema to identify contact allergies, as it is not possible to distinguish which patients have an allergic contact dermatitis from the clinical appearance. A careful history of occupation and recreational activities may indicate the need to test with extra allergens: for example, plants in a gardener or rubber glove chemicals in a surgeon.

Management of chronic hand eczema includes use of emollients and moderate to potent topical corticosteroids (see p. 660), minimizing contact with irritants and avoiding exposure to allergens (**Box 22.15**). This may involve wearing protective gloves and sometimes a change of occupation. The oral retinoid alitretinoin is an effective treatment for topical steroid-refractory severe chronic hand eczema. It leads to clearance or significant improvement in over half of all patients over a 6-month course. Like all oral retinoids, it is a teratogen, and a pregnancy prevention programme must be followed.

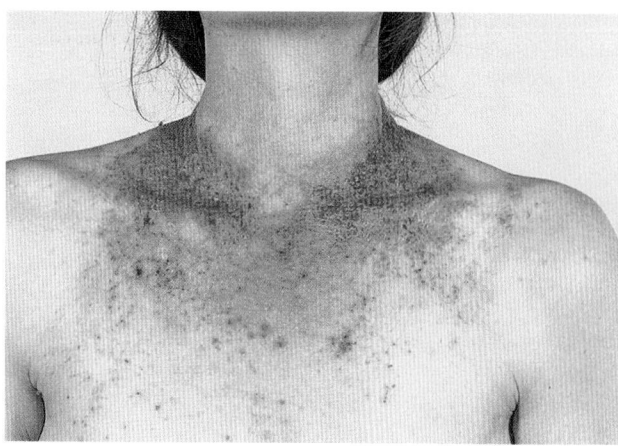

Fig. 22.13 Contact eczema secondary to perfume allergy.

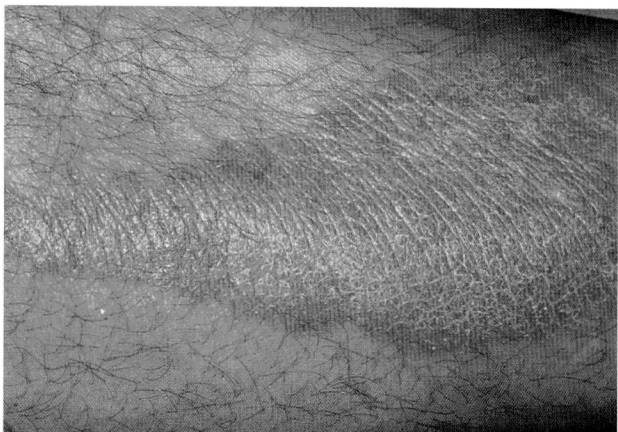

Fig. 22.14 Lichen simplex from chronic rubbing.

Allergic and irritant contact eczema

Allergic contact eczema is an example of a delayed-type hypersensitivity. The rash does not usually appear until at least 12–24 hours after skin contact and may even be delayed by several days, so the cause is often unsuspected. The hands, face and neck (**Fig. 22.13**) are commonly involved due to their frequent contact with allergens. Other body sites that are often affected by allergic contact dermatitis include the lower leg, ear canal and anogenital area (due to medicaments) and the feet (from footwear). Patch testing should be considered in all patients with suspected allergic contact eczema or where this cannot be excluded.

Irritant contact eczema is a common complaint and mainly affects the hands. People with a history of atopic eczema are at significantly increased risk. The most common cause is frequent contact with soap or detergents and water at work ('wet work'). Occupations with increased risk include hairdressing, catering and healthcare.

Lichen simplex

This is a chronic form of eczema in which the skin is thickened and lined (lichenified) in response to repeated rubbing and scratching (**Fig. 22.14**). Common sites are the nape of the neck, outer calves and anogenital area. Short-term use of a potent or superpotent topical steroid and topical antipruritics (e.g. menthol) often helps to break the itch–scratch cycle, along with habit reversal techniques. There may be underlying emotional stress: hence the alternative name, 'neurodermatitis'.

Nodular prurigo

This is a chronic, widespread, intensely itchy, nodular eruption that is perpetuated by picking and scratching. It may develop on a background of atopic eczema. Scattered eroded and hyperkeratotic nodules are typically found on the upper trunk and the extensor surfaces of the limbs. Unfortunately, topical corticosteroids, sedating antihistamines and antipruritics have limited effectiveness. The diagnosis is made by exclusion of other pathologies and may require a skin biopsy. Medical causes of pruritus should be excluded (see Box 22.20).

Chronic actinic dermatitis

This uncommon form of eczema mainly affects older men and is caused by excessive sensitivity to UV radiation in sunlight. The rash is prominent on sun-exposed sites and worse in summer, but patients may not be aware of their underlying photosensitivity. A clear cut-off line can usually be found between clothed (unaffected) and exposed (affected) sites. Specialist assessment is needed. Monochromator phototesting across the solar spectrum can be done to confirm UVB sensitivity and other causative wavelengths.

Further reading

Li R, Hadi S, Guttman-Yassky E. Current and emerging biologic and small molecule therapies for atopic dermatitis. *Expert Opin Biol Ther* 2019; 19:367–380.
Tsianakas A. Dupilumab: a milestone in the treatment of atopic dermatitis. *Lancet* 2016; 386:4–5.

Psoriasis

Psoriasis is a common chronic inflammatory skin disease that affects 2% of the population. It is characterized by well-demarcated, red plaques with a thick, silver scale. Various clinical patterns are recognized and severity is highly variable. There are two peak ages of onset: early (age 16–22) is more common and is often associated with a positive family history, while late-onset disease peaks around 55–60 years. Moderate to severe psoriasis is often associated with an inflammatory arthritis, metabolic syndrome and increased risk of cardiovascular disease. Depression and impaired body image are common co-morbidities.

Aetiology

The condition appears to be polygenic, with epigenetic and environmental triggers. Twin studies show 73% concordance in monozygotic twins, compared with 20% in dizygotic pairs. Multiple genetic psoriasis susceptibility loci have been identified, including *PSORS1* (which accounts for 35–50% of the heritable component).

The pathogenesis of psoriasis is complex and incompletely understood, but there have been considerable advances in recent years. Abnormalities of T-cell homeostasis – in particular, the pro-inflammatory T17 axis – are believed to be involved in creating an inflammatory loop with dendritic cells and keratinocytes. This causes overproduction of antimicrobial peptides, inflammatory cytokines and chemokines, amplifying the immune response and driving abnormally rapid keratinocyte proliferation. The end result is thickened, inflamed skin (plaques) with thick overlying scale.

Clinical features

Different patterns of psoriasis are recognized and can occur together. Certain drugs can aggravate psoriasis, particularly lithium, antimalarials and beta-blockers.

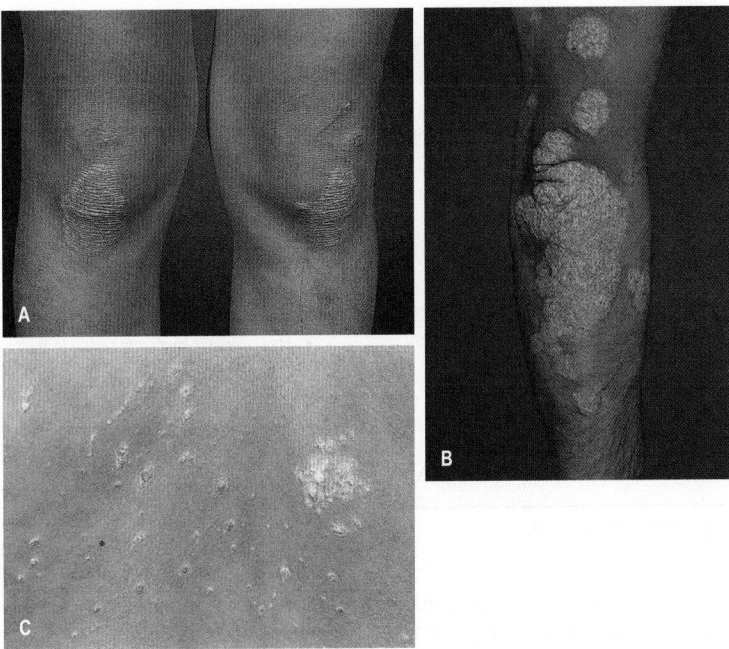

Fig. 22.15 Psoriasis. **(A)** Chronic plaque psoriasis of the knees. **(B)** Chronic plaque psoriasis on the elbows of an Indian patient. **(C)** Guttate psoriasis in an African patient. *(Courtesy of Dr P Matondo, Lusaka, Zambia.)*

- **Chronic plaque psoriasis** is the most common variant and is characterized by pink–red, well-demarcated plaques with silver–white scales, seen especially on extensor surfaces of the knees (**Fig. 22.15A**) and elbows (**Fig. 22.15B**). The lower back, ears and scalp are often also involved. New plaques of psoriasis occur at sites of skin trauma (Köbner phenomenon). The lesions can become itchy or sore, and bleed easily when scales are removed.

- **Flexural psoriasis** tends to affect older adults with a raised body mass index. It is characterized by well-demarcated, shiny plaques with little, if any, scaling affecting the large flexures of the groin, natal cleft, axillae and submammary area. The rash is often misdiagnosed as candida intertrigo (see p. 674) but has a sharp margin and lacks satellite lesions. Anogenital involvement is common and can cause considerable psychosexual upset.

- **Guttate psoriasis** is the term given to a 'raindrop-like' pattern of psoriasis, most commonly seen in children and young adults (**Fig. 22.15C**). The rash develops over days and consists of very small circular or oval plaques on the torso. It is usually triggered by a streptococcal throat infection. Guttate psoriasis resolves spontaneously and in up to one-third of individuals does not recur. However, the remainder experience recurrent guttate attacks or develop chronic plaque psoriasis.

- **Erythrodermic and pustular psoriasis** are the most severe variants and are manifestations of extensive inflammatory skin disease. They may occur together and may be preceded by unstable widespread chronic plaque disease. There is often associated systemic upset with malaise, fever and circulatory disturbance (see p. 657). The pustules are sterile and can be triggered by sudden withdrawal of potent topical or systemic corticosteroids. A more common localized, pustular rash on the palms and soles (palmoplantar pustulosis) is considered to be a variant of psoriasis. It occurs almost exclusively in heavy cigarette smokers.

Nail changes affect up to 50% of people with psoriasis (**Fig. 22.16**). Features include:
- pitting of the nail plate

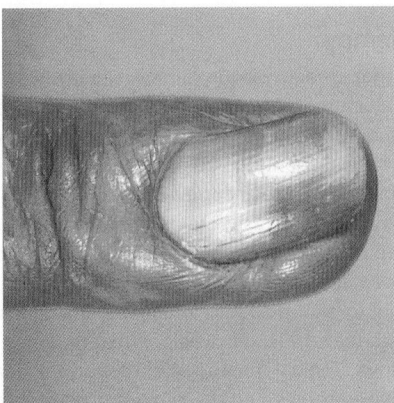

Fig. 22.16 Psoriasis of the nail. Yellowish brown discoloration and distal nail plate separation (onycholysis).

- distal separation of the nail plate (onycholysis) and, rarely, loss of the nail plate
- pink- (salmon patch) to yellow–brown (oil-drop) discoloration
- subungual hyperkeratosis.

Topical therapy is usually ineffective but systemic medication and biologics can improve nail dystrophy. Toenail psoriasis can be difficult to distinguish from nail tinea (see p. 673) and the two diseases may coexist.

Psoriatic arthritis and enthesitis (see p. 450) may affect up to 40% of individuals with moderate to more severe psoriasis. Joint symptoms can present before skin disease but most individuals have scalp or nail psoriasis. People with psoriasis should be asked specifically about joint symptoms and the Psoriasis Epidemiology Screening Tool (PEST) score can be used as a guide for rheumatological referral.

Management

There is no curative treatment and the choice of therapy is determined on an individual basis, according to the site and severity of

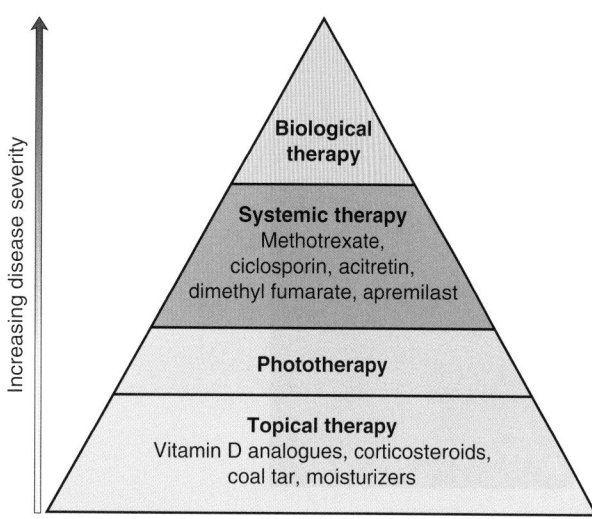

Fig. 22.17 Management of psoriasis.

disease, its psychological impact, co-morbidities such as cardio-vascular or liver disease, and the individual's wishes (**Fig. 22.17**). Most people with chronic plaque psoriasis will have the condition for life, though it may fluctuate in severity. A supportive and empathic approach is needed, as people with psoriasis often feel stigmatized by their skin disease.

Topical therapy

This is given for chronic plaque psoriasis, usually as a vitamin D analogue (calcipotriol, calcitriol, tacalcitol) and an emollient to reduce scaling. Moderate or potent corticosteroids may also be used. Other topical agents include coal tar and tazarotene (a retinoid), though these are less popular due to irritancy. Dithranol is seldom used nowadays, as it stains the skin and clothing. Salicylic acid can help remove scales but increases steroid potency when used concurrently. Topical therapy is usually applied once or twice daily to skin plaques. Vitamin D analogues should be limited to less than 100 g per week as higher doses may cause hypercalcaemia. Topical therapy is often not practical for widespread plaque psoriasis and the next option is usually narrow-band UVB phototherapy. Traditional regimes combining tar or dithranol and UVB were once common but newer therapies have taken their place. Treatment of difficult-to-treat sites is outlined in **Box 22.16**.

Phototherapy

Guttate psoriasis is usually treated with topical therapies and/or UVB phototherapy (see p. 656). Chronic plaque psoriasis may also respond to phototherapy with UVB or PUVA. Topical PUVA can be helpful for palmoplantar psoriasis, including palmoplantar pustulosis.

Systemic therapy

Systemic therapy is usually indicated for widespread disease that has failed to respond to topical agents and phototherapy. It may also be needed to manage associated psoriatic arthritis and milder disease with psychological upset. All medication has potential adverse effects and toxicities and patients should be provided with user-friendly information, such as the British Association of Dermatologists patient leaflets.

Methotrexate is given orally or by subcutaneous injection in low dose (up to 25 mg) once a week, with folic acid on other days to reduce gastrointestinal upset. It is a teratogen, so pregnancy

- The scalp is considered a 'difficult to treat' site, as thick scales build up, hindering penetration of topical drugs. Scaling needs removal with keratolytic agents, e.g. silicone lotion or coconut oil and salicylic acid ointment. These can be applied overnight and washed out with a coal tar shampoo.
- Flexural and genital psoriasis requires special consideration, as the skin is easily irritated and prone to secondary infection and steroid atrophy. Treatment usually consists of intermittent mild to moderate steroids used alone or in combination with antimicrobial agents. Calcitriol and 0.1% tacrolimus ointment can also be effective.
- Nail psoriasis responds poorly to topical therapy and usually requires systemic drugs.

must be avoided. Regular blood tests are needed to check liver function and monitor for bone marrow suppression. Measurement of serum procollagen 3 peptide levels and liver fibroelastography (see p. 1270) have evolved as routine non-invasive alternatives to liver biopsy to monitor for hepatotoxicity. Non-steroidal anti-inflammatory drugs (NSAIDs) should be avoided, especially in the elderly, as they reduce renal excretion of methotrexate metabolites and may cause toxicity.

Ciclosporin is a selective immunosuppressant that inhibits T lymphocytes. It has been widely used in the treatment of severe psoriasis and is a useful drug in unstable or erythrodermic disease due to its rapid onset of action. However, long-term use is often complicated by nephrotoxicity and hypertension.

Acitretin is an oral retinoid used to treat psoriasis and rarer inherited scaly skin diseases (Darier disease, congenital ichthyosis). It is less effective than ciclosporin or methotrexate but lacks immunosuppressant effects and may be used in combination with UVB and PUVA. All oral retinoids are potent teratogens. Acitretin's metabolites have an extremely long half-life and pregnancy must be avoided for 3 years after completing treatment, so this drug is not suitable for women of childbearing age. New immunomodulator drugs licensed for use in psoriasis include the phosphodiesterase-4 inhibitor ***apremilast*** and ***dimethyl fumarate***. Other drugs in clinical trials include the JAK pathway inhibitor tofacitinib.

Biological therapy

Advances in understanding the immunopathogenesis of psoriasis have led to development of an expanding and increasingly effective group of targeted biological drugs that block pro-inflammatory cytokines or their receptors. The UK's National Institute for Health and Care Excellence (NICE) restricts use of these drugs to patients with severe psoriasis (defined by a Psoriasis Area Severity Index (PASI) of >10 and DLQI of >10), in whom phototherapy and conventional systemic drug therapy have failed, are contraindicated or are not tolerated. Anti-TNF-α drugs (infliximab, etanercept, adalimumab) were the first group of biologics licensed for use in psoriasis. These have been followed by IL-12/23, IL-17 and selective IL-23 inhibitors. The latest allow the majority of patients to achieve a 90% reduction in PASI score ('PASI 90'). However, all biologic drugs remain expensive and have potential toxicity, as the long-term safety of the newer agents remains unknown.

Further reading

Boehncke W-H, Schön MP. Psoriasis. *Lancet* 2015; 386:983–994.
https://pathways.nice.org.uk/pathways/psoriasis. *NICE pathway for management of psoriasis.*
Ruzicka T, Hanifin JM, Furue M et al. Anti–interleukin-31 receptor A antibody for atopic dermatitis. *N Engl J Med* 2017; 376:826–835.
Sonja Stände M, Yosipovitch G, Legat FJ et al. Trial of nemolizumab in moderate-to-severe prurigo nodularis. *N Engl J Med* 2020; 382:706–716.

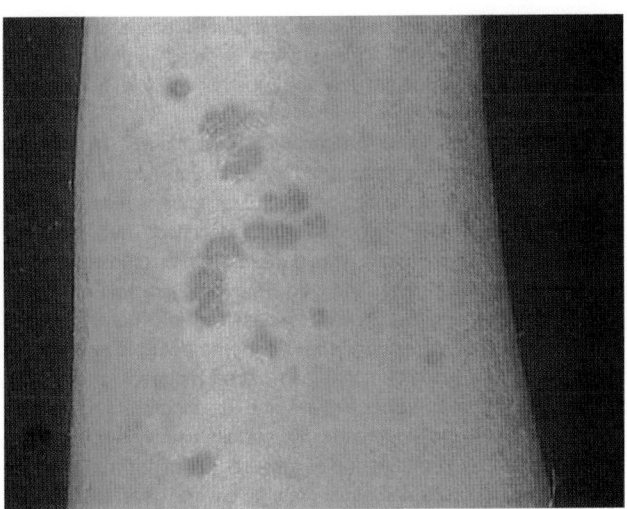

Fig. 22.18 Lichen planus.

Other common papulosquamous rashes

Pityriasis rosea

Pityriasis rosea is an acute, self-limiting exanthem, which is thought to be caused by a viral infection, possibly human herpesvirus (HHV)-6 and HHV-7. It usually affects older children or young adults and there is an increased incidence in spring and autumn. The rash is most prominent on the torso and proximal limbs, and consists of circular or oval pink macules with a collarette of fine scale. It is usually preceded by a larger solitary 'herald patch'. Lesions tend to run along dermatomal lines of the back, giving a 'Christmas tree' pattern. The rash is usually asymptomatic or mildly itchy and resolves within 4–8 weeks. Treatment is not usually required but emollients and a mild steroid cream may be used for pruritus. Severe pityriasis rosea in the first trimester of pregnancy has been associated with fetal loss, and off-label use of aciclovir may be considered.

Polymorphic light eruption ('prickly heat')

This sun-induced rash is common in young women and is usually triggered by unusually intense exposure to strong sunshine on holiday. In most cases it is mild and wrongly attributed to heat ('prickly heat'). Typically, an itchy papular rash develops on sun-exposed areas, particularly the 'V' of the neck, shoulders and arms, several hours after sun exposure. Vesicles or plaques may occur: hence 'polymorphic'. A minority of people with polymorphic light eruption (PLE) are severely affected and develop the rash in temperate zones, starting in spring or early summer. It is thought to be caused by a delayed-type hypersensitivity to an endogenous antigen that occurs in the skin after UV exposure (photoantigen). Mild cases can be managed by avoiding the sun (with high sun protection factor (SPF) sunscreens and clothing) and gradually building up tolerance to sunlight. Short courses of prednisolone can be given for prophylaxis or treatment. People who are troubled by severe PLE can be 'desensitized' with a short course of UVB phototherapy in early spring, which enables them to tolerate subsequent sun exposure.

Lichen planus

Lichen planus (LP) is a chronic inflammatory skin disease affecting the skin and mucosal membranes. It is thought to be a cytotoxic T-cell-mediated autoimmune disease and potential triggers include hepatitis B virus and hepatitis C virus. However, in most cases there is no identifiable cause. Mucosal involvement is seen in about 50% of patients with cutaneous LP and the oral mucosa may also be affected in isolation. LP-like (lichenoid) rashes may be caused by drugs (e.g. antihypertensives, antimalarials, NSAIDs) and contact allergens.

LP appears as clusters of intensely pruritic, purple–pink, polygonal papules (**Fig. 22.18**) that usually affect the flexural aspect of wrists, forearms and lower legs. The rash may be widespread and lead to scarring hair loss and nail damage.

Close inspection of the papules shows fine white streaks (Wickham's striae). Lesions can fuse into plaques, especially on the lower legs, where they turn warty and hyperkeratotic. After resolution, post-inflammatory hyperpigmentation is common, especially in people with darker skin. LP may köbnerize: that is, localize to areas of superficial trauma.

Mucosal involvement ranges from asymptomatic, reticulate white streaks on the buccal mucosa and lateral tongue to a severe, painful, erosive gingivitis and glossitis (erosive LP). Delayed-contact allergy to metals in amalgam fillings may cause localized LP-like changes on the oral mucosa. The anogenital mucosa may be affected by LP and lesions on the penis are often annular. A severe erosive variant can affect the vulva and vagina in women.

Histology of LP is usually diagnostic and shows a dense infiltrate of lymphocytes along the dermo-epidermal junction, which becomes damaged with degenerate (apoptotic) basal keratinocytes.

Cutaneous LP usually resolves within 1–2 years, though it may relapse. Hypertrophic disease and mucosal disease are usually more persistent. Malignant change and development of squamous cell carcinoma may rarely complicate chronic ulcerated LP. Skin and mucosal lesions usually respond to potent or superpotent topical corticosteroids and topical tacrolimus (see p. 656). Widespread skin disease may require tapering courses of oral steroids, phototherapy, oral retinoids or systemic immunosuppressants.

Granuloma annulare

Granuloma annulare usually affects children and young adults. It is usually asymptomatic and characterized by clusters of small flesh-coloured or slightly erythematous papules (with no scaling) in a ring shape with a dusky centre. These typically affect the dorsal hands and/or feet. The cause is unknown; several systemic associations have been proposed but not proven, including diabetes mellitus and thyroid disease. Localized granuloma annulare is usually self-limiting and resolves after a few years. Potent topical or intralesional steroids can be tried if needed.

Lichen sclerosus

Lichen sclerosus (LS) is a common inflammatory dermatosis of the genital area. The cause is unknown but may be autoimmune, and preceding infection or trauma and an occluded, moist environment may act as triggers. In females, the usual age of onset is before puberty or after the menopause. Males may develop LS at any age. Lesions are intensely pruritic or sore, and appear as shiny, ivory–white, fissured patches on the vulva, or on the glans penis and distal foreskin or penile shaft. Additional perianal involvement is common in females, leading to a 'figure-of-eight' distribution. Telangiectasia may be evident, and early lesions in girls can present with haemorrhagic blisters that are occasionally mistaken for signs of sexual abuse.

The scarring and atrophy that accompany longstanding LS cause changes in the vulval structure, with loss and fusion of the labia minora and scarring of the clitoral hood. Involvement of the foreskin can cause phimosis, and urethral disease may cause strictures and impaired micturition. Profound sexual dysfunction can result from LS in both men and women.

The diagnosis is usually made by the clinical appearance. Histology shows thickened ('hyalinized') dermal collagen and a thin, flat (atrophic) epidermis.

Short-term courses of potent or superpotent topical corticosteroids improve the signs and symptoms of LS. TCIs may also be helpful. The condition may remit spontaneously after several years, especially in children. Unresponsive phimosis may necessitate circumcision. Longstanding anogenital LS is associated with an increased risk of squamous cell carcinoma in affected sites.

Further reading

Lewis FM, Tatnall FM, Velangi SS et al. British Association of Dermatologists' guidelines for the management of lichen sclerosus 2018. *Br J Dermatol* 2018; 178:839–853.

Urticaria and angio-oedema

Urticaria (hives, 'nettle rash') is a common skin condition characterized by short-lived, itchy swellings or 'weals' that clear within minutes to hours without residual dryness or skin flaking (**Fig. 22.19**). The short-lived nature of individual swellings and lack of skin surface changes help distinguish urticaria from other inflammatory rashes, especially eczema. *Angio-oedema* is a similar disorder involving deeper tissues and usually affecting the lips, tongue and eyelids. Urticaria and angio-oedema may occur together or separately, and have a range of causes.

Aetiology and clinical features

Urticaria and angio-oedema with weals are caused by dermal mast cell degranulation and release of a range of pro-inflammatory mediators (including histamine) that cause vasodilation and increased capillary permeability. Mast cell degranulation may be triggered by various stimuli, including *drugs* (opiates, aspirin), *physical triggers* (friction, pressure, sweating), *allergens* and *autoantibodies*. Urticaria is classified as acute or chronic (>6 weeks' duration). Chronic urticaria is divided into spontaneous (or idiopathic) and inducible types (**Fig. 22.20**).

Acute urticaria is often triggered by infections. It may also be the presenting feature of immediate (type 1) allergy, especially in young children with atopic eczema (see p. 64). Common causes include food (nuts, egg, milk), drugs (penicillin) and natural rubber latex. Allergic urticaria may be localized to an area of skin (contact urticaria) – for example, due to latex gloves, or take the form of a more widespread reaction that can evolve to anaphylaxis (see p. 69). Measurement of allergen-specific IgE and/or skin prick tests and allergen challenge tests can be done to confirm an allergic cause.

Chronic inducible urticaria has a range of causes, including friction (symptomatic dermographism), pressure (delayed pressure urticaria), cold (cold urticaria), sunshine (solar urticaria) and sweating (cholinergic urticaria). Physical tests, such as lightly scratching the skin for dermographism or an ice cube test for cold urticaria, are helpful in demonstrating the cause.

Chronic spontaneous urticaria (*CSU*) is thought to have an underlying autoimmune basis, and in some individuals functional autoantibodies against the high-affinity IgE receptor on mast cells and basophils or against IgE antibodies can be identified. There is also an association with autoimmune thyroid disease. Chronic urticaria is seldom caused by food allergy, and food allergy tests are not indicated.

Angio-oedema without weals is classified into hereditary and acquired variants. *Hereditary angio-oedema* (*HAE*) is a rare autosomal dominant condition that can cause recurrent and severe swellings of the skin, upper airways and intestinal tract. Laryngeal involvement may be life-threatening. Attacks usually start in childhood and can be spontaneous or triggered by minor trauma. Skin swellings are not itchy and usually last for several days. HAE types I and II are caused by mutations in the *SERPING1* gene that result in decreased plasma levels of functional C1 esterase inhibitor (C1NH). This allows unchecked activation of the complement cascade. Serum complement C4 can be measured as a screening test. C1NH activity is normal in type III HAE. All forms of HAE are caused by increased levels of bradykinin.

Acquired angio-oedema may be idiopathic or associated with lymphoproliferative or autoimmune disorders. Drugs can also cause angio-oedema, especially angiotensin-converting enzyme (ACE) inhibitors and angiotensin II receptor antagonists. The rate is up to four times higher in Afro-Caribbean patients and onset may be delayed by months or years after starting therapy, so a careful drug history is essential.

Management

Acute urticaria is usually self-resolving. Allergic urticaria and angio-oedema may require emergency treatment with intramuscular adrenaline (epinephrine) and intravenous steroids (see **Box 3.22**). *Chronic urticaria* is managed with non-sedating antihistamines such as loratadine 10 mg daily; the dose may be increased fourfold if needed for symptom control. Montelukast may also be helpful in those with aspirin sensitivity. NSAIDs and opiate analgesics should be avoided, as they can aggravate urticaria. The biological anti-IgE drug omalizumab is licensed for antihistamine-refractory CSU.

Management of *HAE* used to be limited to prophylaxis with attenuated androgens (stanozolol, danazol), which were poorly tolerated, and treatment of acute attacks was with fresh frozen plasma. Newer selective therapies include plasma-derived and recombinant C1NH, a kallikrein inhibitor (ecallantide) and a bradykinin B2 receptor

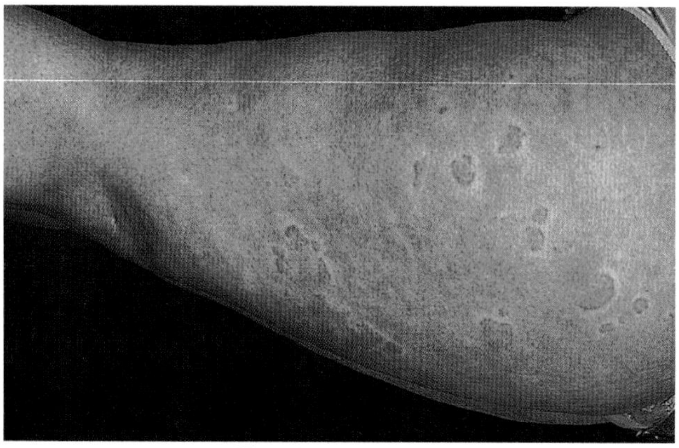

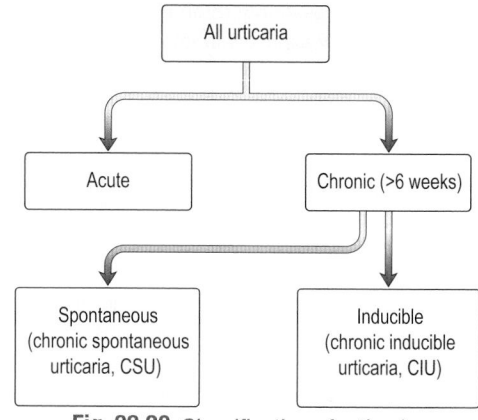

Fig. 22.19 Urticaria.

Fig. 22.20 Classification of urticaria.

antagonist (icatibant). These newer products can be used for treatment of acute attacks of HAE, and C1NH is also used for prophylaxis.

Urticarial vasculitis

If urticarial weals are painful and last for more than 24 hours, leaving bruising or a blemish, this may indicate an underlying vasculitis rather than ordinary urticaria. The patient should be thoroughly assessed with a vasculitis screen of blood tests, skin biopsy and urinalysis.

Further reading

Buss PJ, Christiansen SC. Hereditary angioedema. *N Engl J Med* 2020;382:1136–1148.

SKIN INFECTIONS

The skin is home to a diverse population of microbes (microbiome), most of which are commensals (permanent non-pathogenic residents) or transients (temporary residents). Many skin pathogens can also be found on living skin as commensals, and microbial dysregulation, altered environmental factors, trauma, host immunity and host genetic variation may drive the transition from commensal to pathogen and subsequent skin disease. The microbiome of the skin varies greatly, according to body site and between individuals, and its role in health and disease is the subject of considerable interest.

Bacterial infections

(See also Chapter 20.)

Impetigo

Impetigo is a highly contagious infection that usually affects children (**Fig. 22.21**) and is spread by direct contact. Infected areas appear as inflamed plaques with a golden, crusted surface, typically around the mouth and nose. It is caused by *Staphylococcus aureus* or *Streptococcus pyogenes*. Toxin-producing strains of staphylococcus can also cause blisters (bullous impetigo; see later). Skin and nasal swabs should be taken if the complaint is extensive or recurrent, or constitutes a suspected outbreak.

Management

Localized impetigo may be treated with topical fusidic acid. Mupirocin should be reserved for cases caused by meticillin-resistant *Staphylococcus aureus* (MRSA). The new topical antibiotic retapamulin is effective but expensive, and is used as second-line treatment. Widespread infection or bullous impetigo should be treated with oral antibiotics for 7 days (flucloxacillin or erythromycin or clarithromycin if the patient is penicillin-allergic). Affected individuals should avoid school or work until the lesions are dry or for 48 hours after starting antibiotics.

Toxin-mediated skin disease

Staphylococcal scalded skin syndrome (SSSS) and toxic shock syndrome (TSS) are diseases caused by bacterial secretion of toxins, the latter representing a life-threatening illness requiring urgent medical treatment. Blistering lesions seen in SSSS can resemble toxic epidermal necrolysis (TEN, see p. 697) but the mucous membranes are not involved in SSSS and blistering occurs higher in the epidermis. The intra-epidermal split of SSSS can be demonstrated by histology of a frozen section of skin. Further details of management and prognosis are given on page 537.

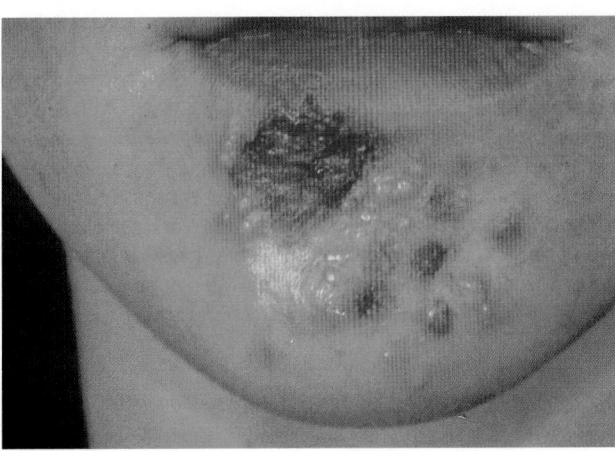

Fig. 22.21 Impetigo. Crusted, blistering lesions on the chin.

Cellulitis and erysipelas

Cellulitis and erysipelas are caused by superficial and deeper infection of the dermis and subcutaneous tissues, respectively. It is not always possible to make a clear distinction. Both complaints present with tender confluent areas of inflamed skin and are often associated with fever and malaise. Cellulitis typically affects the lower leg or arm and may spread proximally. Other sites that may be affected include the abdomen and perianal and periorbital areas. Erysipelas is more common on the face and is more sharply demarcated. Localized blistering (clear or blood-stained), necrosis, abscess formation, lymphangitis and lymphadenopathy may occur. The most common infective organisms are β-haemolytic streptococcus and *Staph. aureus*. Gram-negative or anaerobic bacteria may cause infection in immunocompromised people and those with diabetes.

Lymphoedema, obesity, venous stasis and toe-web fungal infection are risk factors for lower limb cellulitis. The skin should be carefully examined to look for fissures or erosions that can allow entry of pathogens. Skin swabs are usually negative unless taken from broken skin. Serological tests can confirm a streptococcal infection (antistreptolysin O titre (ASOT) and anti-DNAse B titre).

Management

Systemic antibiotics (flucloxacillin or erythromycin) are indicated; they may be given as high-dose oral therapy, or intravenously via ambulatory care or as an inpatient, depending on the patient's age, disease severity and co-morbidities. Single-dose dalbavancin may be an alternative to conventional antibiotics in the treatment of acute bacterial skin infections in adults, avoiding the need for hospitalization or repeat attendance.

Up to 50% of people with cellulitis experience repeat episodes. Prophylactic antibiotic therapy reduces the risk of further attacks during treatment but the effect wears off after discontinuation.

Necrotizing fasciitis

This fulminant, rapidly spreading, life-threatening bacterial infection of the subcutaneous and deep soft tissues causes severe tissue destruction and is associated with a high mortality. A number of organisms can cause necrotizing fasciitis: spontaneous disease that arises in previously health people is often caused by group A streptococcus (GAS), while disease related to abdominal surgery or immunosuppression is often caused by mixed aerobic and anaerobic populations.

Necrotizing fasciitis is characterized by severe pain that is out of proportion to the apparent signs of skin inflammation. Infection tracks rapidly along tissue planes, causing spreading erythema, swelling, pain and sometimes tissue crepitus. Patients are typically febrile and severely unwell, and urgent surgical intervention (with extensive debridement or amputation) and intravenous antibiotic therapy are required. High-dose benzylpenicillin and clindamycin are used in confirmed GAS infection, and a broad-spectrum antibiotic combination with additional metronidazole is used where the pathogen is unknown. Typically, the C-reactive protein (CRP) and white cell count are significantly raised. Imaging is sometimes helpful (e.g. by revealing gas in deep tissues) but should not delay urgent surgical intervention. Multiorgan failure is common and mortality is high.

Gas gangrene

Gas gangrene is caused by deep tissue infection with *Clostridium* spp. (especially *C. perfringens*), following contaminated penetrating injuries – historically, battlefield wounds but now commonly found in intravenous drug users and patients who have undergone gastrointestinal tract surgery. Initial infection develops in damaged, necrotic tissue; toxins secreted by the bacteria destroy surrounding tissue and permit rapid spread of infection, contributing to severe systemic effects. Treatment is by surgical debridement of necrotic tissue and intravenous benzylpenicillin and clindamycin.

Folliculitis

Folliculitis is a common superficial inflammatory disorder of the hair follicle, which presents as itchy or tender small papules and pustules (pimples). It may be caused by trauma, chemical irritation and infection with a range of pathogens, most commonly *Staph. aureus*. Predisposing factors include friction, occlusion, sweating, obesity and diabetes. A deeper variant affecting beard follicles ('sycosis barbae') causes multiple swollen papules that may coalesce to form pustule-studded plaques. The main differential diagnosis is pseudo-folliculitis barbae, which is caused by ingrowth of curly hairs.

Extensive, itchy folliculitis may be a manifestation of human immunodeficiency virus (HIV) infection (see p. 1431). The Gram-negative bacterium *Pseudomonas aeruginosa* may cause outbreaks of folliculitis stemming from inadequately disinfected hot tubs and pools.

Treatment is with topical antiseptics, topical antibiotics or oral antibiotics; management should address the underlying predisposing factors.

Boils (furuncles) and carbuncles

Boils or furuncles are deeper infections of hair follicles and surrounding tissue, and appear as painful, red, pus-filled swellings. They are usually caused by *Staph. aureus*. Boils may coalesce to form carbuncles, which are larger swellings with multiple pus-discharging openings and systemic upset. They may spread from person to person due to poor hygiene or overcrowding, and are more common in people with diabetes, malnutrition and immunosuppression. A recent increase in UK hospital admissions for boils and other acute skin conditions may be due to the increased virulence of community-onset MRSA, which secretes a cytotoxin called **Panton–Valentine leukocidin (PVL)** (see p. 536). This is associated with outbreaks of severe recurrent boils and skin abscesses in healthy adults. Skin swabs should be taken from all patients with severe or recurrent folliculitis to determine antibiotic sensitivities and screen specifically for PVL toxin-producing strains of staphylococci.

Management

Isolated boils can be treated with hot bathing alone. Anti-staphylococcal oral antibiotics for 10–14 days are required for widespread infection or facial involvement. PVL-positive strains

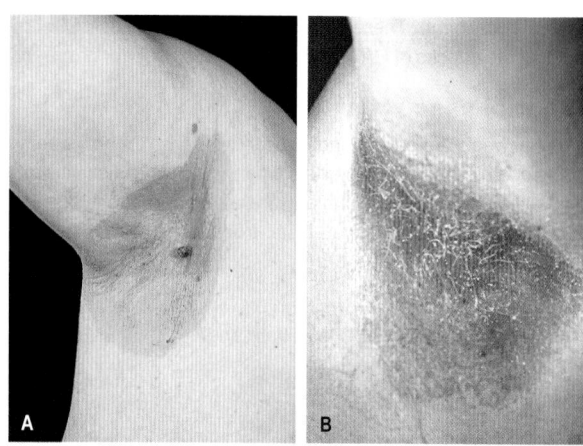

Fig. 22.22 Erythrasma. **(A)** Erythrasma of the axilla. **(B)** Pink fluorescence under a Wood's lamp.

mandate prolonged therapy with a combination of antibiotics such as rifampicin and clindamycin. Larger boils and abscesses may need incision and drainage. Screening of family contacts, nasal decolonization and use of antiseptic washes (e.g. chlorhexidine) are recommended.

Ecthyma

Ecthyma is also caused by streptococci (group A β-haemolytic), *Staph. aureus* or occasionally both. It presents as chronic, well-demarcated, deep ulcers with a necrotic crust and exudate. It is associated with malnutrition and poor hygiene: for example, in intravenous drug users.

Management is with topical antiseptics, systemic antibiotics and improved nutrition.

Ecthyma gangrenosum presents with distinctive necrotic skin ulcers with a central thick, dark brown or black eschar. It is typically caused by *Pseudomonas septicaemia* in an immunocompromised or neutropenic patient. Invasion of a microbe through the subcutaneous vasculature leads to a haemorrhagic occlusive vasculitis. Intensive parenteral antibiotic therapy is imperative to reduce the associated high mortality.

Erythrasma and pitted keratolysis

Erythrasma is a superficial skin infection caused by *Corynebacterium minutissimum*. It presents as orange–beige scaly plaques in the large flexures (axillae and groin) or maceration in the toe webs (**Fig. 22.22**) and is often misdiagnosed as a fungal infection. Corynebacteria are part of the normal skin microbiome but can also act as pathogens. They show a characteristic coral-pink fluorescence when examined with Wood's light (UVA). Corynebacteria are also implicated in **pitted keratolysis**, which appears as multiple punched-out areas and maceration of the skin on weight-bearing plantar surfaces. There is usually associated hyperhidrosis and malodour.

Management of erythrasma is with topical or oral macrolides. Pitted keratolysis responds to astringents such as potassium permanganate soaks, antiperspirants and topical imidazoles or fusidic acid.

Further reading

Dalal A, Eskin-Schwartz M, Mimouni D et al. Interventions for the prevention of recurrent erysipelas and cellulitis. *Cochrane Database Syst Rev* 2017; 6:CD009758.

Lin HS, Lin PT, Tsai YS et al. Interventions for bacterial folliculitis and boils (furuncles and carbuncles). *Cochrane Database Syst Rev* 2018; 8:CD013099.

National Institute for Health and Care Excellence. *Impetigo – Summary*. NICE 2015; http://cks.nice.org.uk/impetigo#!topicsummary.

Mycobacterial infections

Leprosy (Hansen's disease)

Leprosy (see p. 550) typically involves the skin and peripheral nerves. The clinical features depend on the host's immune response to the infecting organism, *Mycobacterium leprae*.

Tuberculoid leprosy presents with a few larger, hypopigmented (see **Fig. 20.24**) or erythematous plaques with an inflamed border. Sensation is absent within lesions, which are dry and hairless due to nerve damage. Nerves may be enlarged and palpable. Biopsy shows a granulomatous infiltrate around nerves but no organisms.

Indeterminate leprosy presents with small, hypopigmented or erythematous, circular, scaly macules with reduced sensation. It may resolve spontaneously or progress to one of the other types. Biopsy reveals a perineural granulomatous infiltrate and scant acid-fast bacilli.

Lepromatous leprosy presents with multiple inflammatory papules, plaques and nodules. Loss of the eyebrows ('madarosis') and nasal stuffiness are common. Skin thickening and severe disfigurement may follow. Biopsy shows numerous acid-fast bacilli.

Diagnosis and management are discussed on page 551.

Skin manifestations of tuberculosis

Tuberculosis (see p. 967) can occasionally cause skin manifestations:

* **Lupus vulgaris** usually arises as a post-primary infection. It commonly presents on the head or neck with red–brown nodules that look like apple jelly when pressed with a glass slide ('diascopy'). They heal with scarring, and new lesions slowly spread out to form a chronic solitary, erythematous plaque. Chronic lesions are at high risk of developing into squamous cell carcinoma.
* **Tuberculosis verrucosa cutis** arises in people who are partially immune to the organism but suffer further skin inoculation. It presents as warty lesions on a 'cold' erythematous base.
* **Scrofuloderma** occurs due to discharge from an affected lymph node into the skin with ulceration and scarring.
* **The tuberculides** are a group of rashes caused by a hypersensitivity response to underlying *Mycobacterium tuberculosis* infection. Erythema nodosum is the most common (see p. 677). Erythema induratum (Bazin's disease) is a similar rash with deep inflammatory nodules on the calves rather than the shin that may ulcerate.

Mycobacterium marinum infection (fish tank/ swimming pool granuloma)

This atypical/non-tuberculous mycobacterial infection presents with one or more painless inflammatory nodule on a hand or upper limb. Infection is usually acquired by coming into contact with non-chlorinated water or by cleaning out a fish tank without gloves. The diagnosis is usually made from the occupational or recreational history and clinical features. A skin biopsy shows granulomatous inflammation, and *Mycobacterium marinum* may be identified by prolonged culture at low temperature or polymerase chain reaction (PCR) of skin lesions.

Treatment is with combination oral antibiotics (e.g. clarithromycin and ciprofloxacin) for 8–12 weeks, according to microbiological guidance.

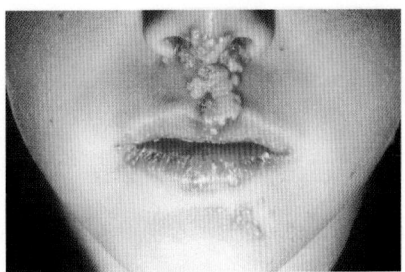

Fig. 22.23 Primary herpes simplex infection.

Viral infections

Viral exanthem

The most common cutaneous manifestation of viral infections is a widespread maculopapular rash or exanthem that predominantly affects the torso and proximal limbs. It is probably caused by deposition of immune complexes of antibody and viral antigen within dermal blood vessels. Many different viruses can cause exanthems, e.g. echovirus (see p. 517), measles (see p. 517) human herpesvirus 6 (see p. 519) and Epstein–Barr virus (see p. 524). The rash resolves spontaneously in 7–10 days.

Slapped cheek syndrome (erythema infectiosum, fifth disease)

See page 519.

Herpes simplex virus

Most people are infected with herpes simplex virus (HSV) type 1 in childhood, and infection is often subclinical. Overt primary infection causes clusters of painful blisters on the face (**Fig. 22.23**) or a painful ulcerative gingivostomatitis. HSV infection can also affect other sites, such as the neck in people who play contact sports or the fingers of healthcare workers ('herpetic whitlow'). Some individuals experience recurrent attacks of HSV ('cold sores') around the lips. HSV 2 infection (see p. 1421) is usually sexually acquired and associated with anogenital ulceration. Recurrence may cause skin lesions at non-genital sites such as the buttock and lower back. Immunosuppression and UV exposure can trigger a recurrence of HSV.

Complications of HSV infection include corneal ulceration, eczema herpeticum (see p. 661), chronic severe anogenital ulceration in HIV infection, and erythema multiforme.

Management

Oral antiviral therapy (aciclovir, valaciclovir) may be given for severe primary HSV and painful genital HSV. Eczema herpeticum, neonatal infection and infection in immunocompromised patients require parenteral antiviral therapy. Cold sores may be treated with aciclovir cream, used early to shorten an attack. Frequent recurrences can be treated with prophylactic oral therapy.

Varicella zoster virus

Varicella zoster virus (VZV) causes the common childhood infection chickenpox and also herpes zoster (see p. 515).

Herpes zoster (shingles)

'Shingles' results from reactivation of latent VZV infection. It may be preceded by a prodromal phase of itch, tingling or pain, followed by a painful, unilateral, blistering eruption in a dermatomal distribution

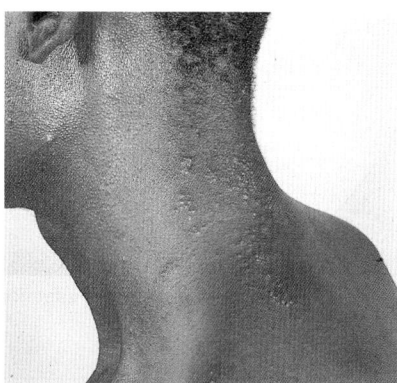

Fig. 22.24 Herpes zoster in an African male. *(Courtesy of Dr P Matondo, Lusaka, Zambia.)*

(**Fig. 22.24**; see also **Fig. 20.9**). The blisters occur in crops and may become purulent before crusting. The rash lasts 2–4 weeks and is usually more severe in the elderly or immunocompromised with involvement of more than one dermatome.

Complications of shingles include severe, persistent pain (post-herpetic neuralgia), ocular disease (if the ophthalmic nerve is involved) and, rarely, a motor neuropathy.

Management

Herpes zoster requires adequate analgesia and antibiotics (if secondary bacterial infection is present). Oral antiviral therapy should be started within 72 hours of the onset of the rash and continued for 7–10 days to reduce pain, severity and viral shedding. Parenteral therapy is indicated in immunocompromised patients. A live-attenuated shingles vaccine is available to boost immunity against VZV in the elderly and reduce the risk of developing herpes zoster.

Human papillomavirus

Human papillomavirus (HPV) infection causes skin and anogenital 'viral' warts.

Common warts are papules with a keratotic rough surface, often seen on the hands and feet but also at other sites. Small black dots (thrombosed vessels) may be visible on close examination (**Fig. 22.25**). Warts on the face may become elongated ('filiform'). Children and adolescents are usually affected. Spread is by direct contact and is facilitated by trauma. They may also affect the beard area in men and spread due to shaving.

Plantar warts (**verrucae**) affect the soles of the feet. They are flattened due to pressure but still have a characteristic warty (papillomatous) surface. Black dots can be seen if the skin is pared down (unlike callosities). Warts may be tender if they affect pressure points or are sited around nail folds.

Plane warts are much less common and are caused by certain HPV subtypes. They are smaller and flatter than common warts and often flesh-coloured or lightly pigmented; they are best seen with side-on lighting. They are usually multiple and are frequently found on the face or the backs of the hands.

Anogenital warts (see p. 1420).

Management

There is no definitive cure and warts may persist for months or years before spontaneously clearing. They are often recalcitrant in people with impaired immunity (e.g. transplant recipients). Regular

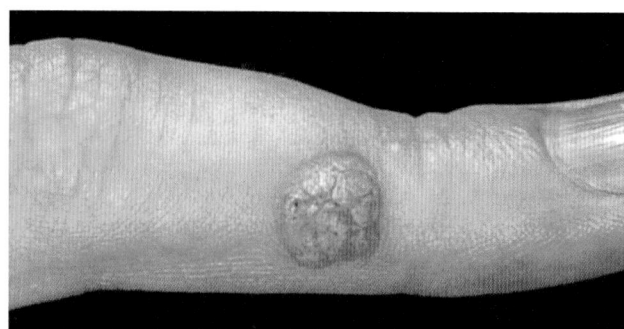

Fig. 22.25 Viral wart.

use of a topical keratolytic agent (e.g. 10–26% salicylic acid) after removal of hyperkeratotic skin may hasten resolution and is the mainstay of treatment. Liquid nitrogen cryotherapy can also be effective. Other destructive treatments include curettage and cautery, and laser therapy, but these may cause considerable pain and scarring.

Molluscum contagiosum

Molluscum contagiosum is a common childhood skin infection and is caused by a pox virus. Lesions are multiple small (1–3 mm), translucent, firm papules with a central dimple ('umbilicated') containing soft, white, keratinous matter that can be extruded by squeezing. Mollusca may exhibit the Köbner phenomenon (see p. 665) and can affect any body site. Occasionally, larger ('giant') lesions of up to a centimetre in diameter may occur.

Lesions usually appear in crops over 6–12 months before resolving spontaneously. Treatment is not required, but destructive therapies such as cryotherapy or curettage may be helpful in older children. Potassium hydroxide 5% lotion can be used in younger children. Genital mollusca are usually sexually transmitted in adults. Widespread infection should raise the possibility of immunosuppression, especially HIV infection (see Chapter 37).

Orf

Orf is a pox virus infection of young sheep and goats. People who handle the infected animal may become infected themselves. Orf has long been recognized in farm workers but may also affect children, who catch the infection at 'petting stations' in city farms. Lesions appear as 1–2 cm red papules on the hands with an inflamed border that blisters; alternatively, they turn into pustules and resolve spontaneously after 4–6 weeks, conferring life-long immunity. Occasionally, orf is complicated by erythema multiforme (see p. 677).

Further reading

Sterling JC, Gibbs S, Haque Hussain SS. British Association of Dermatologists' guidelines for the management of cutaneous warts 2014. *Br J Dermatol* 2014; 171:696–712.
van der Wouden JC, van der Sande R, Kruithof EJ et al. Interventions for cutaneous molluscum contagiosum. *Cochrane Database Syst Rev* 2017; 5:CD004767.

Fungal infections

Fungal skin diseases have a high prevalence in humans, 'thrush' and 'athlete's foot' being two extremely common examples. In most cases, infection is superficial and limited to the stratum corneum, which elicits no inflammation, or the deeper layers of the epidermis, including hair and nails, where inflammation may be triggered by the fungus or its products. Subcutaneous mycoses include a range of

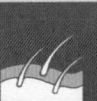

infections of the subcutaneous tissues, usually following traumatic inoculation. The inflammatory response may extend upwards to the epidermis.

There are three groups of pathogenic fungi that commonly affect the outer layer of skin or keratinizing epithelium: dermatophytes, *Candida albicans* and *Malassezia* (formerly *Pityrosporum*).

Dermatophyte infection

Dermatophyte (tinea) fungi invade and grow in dead keratin. The three main genera that affect humans are *Trichophyton*, *Microsporum* and *Epidermophyton*. They tend to form an expanding annular lesion due to lateral growth: hence the name 'ringworm'. Tinea may be transmitted to humans by other people (anthropophilic), animals (zoophilic) or soil (geophilic). The clinical appearance depends on the infecting organism, the site affected and the host reaction.

Tinea of the body usually presents with asymmetrical, scaly, inflamed patches with clearer centres and a scaly, raised border. Occasionally, vesicles or pustules may be seen. Treatment with topical steroids reduces inflammation and masks clinical signs, while allowing spread of the infection – **'tinea incognito'**. The rash typically flares when steroids are stopped, which often prompts further use of steroids and leads to widespread infection. Tinea infections are classified according to body site: tinea corporis (body), tinea facei (face), tinea barbae (beard), tinea cruris (groin), tinea manuum (hand), tinea pedis (foot), tinea capitis (scalp) and tinea unguium (nails). Multiple sites may be affected and skin, hair and nails should be examined.

Asymmetrical scaly rashes should be investigated for fungal infection by mycology of skin scrapings.

Tinea cruris is more common in men than women and presents with an intensely itchy rash in the groin, with a scaly border that extends on to the thighs (**Fig. 22.26**).

Tinea pedis (athlete's foot) is extremely common in adults and is often confined to the toe webs, where the skin looks white, macerated and fissured. It may extend more widely on to the soles and sides of the feet, causing dryness, scaling and erythema, and the toenails are also often affected. Tinea pedis frequently flares in hot weather, causing pustules or blisters, and this can be misdiagnosed as eczema. Infection may also spread to the palm (**tinea manuum**), especially in manual workers. Annular lesions are rarely seen on palmoplantar skin.

Tinea capitis is the most common dermatophyte infection in young children, especially those of black African origin, whose hair and scalp seem more susceptible to fungal invasion. Adults and the elderly are rarely affected. Fungus may confine itself to the hair shaft (endothrix) or spread out over the hair surface (ectothrix). The latter may fluoresce under a Wood's lamp (UV light). Scalp ringworm is spread by close contact (especially in schools and households) and by sharing of brushes or clippers. Migration has led to changing patterns of fungal infections in Europe (e.g. *Trichophyton tonsurans* from Central America, *Trichophyton violaceum* from India and Pakistan). The majority of UK cases are due to *T. tonsurans* (which does not fluoresce).

The clinical appearance of scalp ringworm varies from mild diffuse scaling with no hair loss (similar to dandruff) to the more typical appearance of bald, scaly patches with broken hairs. An increased host response causes pustules and an inflammatory exudate, and certain types of tinea can trigger a severe inflammatory reaction with a swollen purulent mass or 'kerion'. This may be mistaken for a bacterial infection and inappropriately treated with an antibiotic. Extensive infection is occasionally accompanied by a widespread

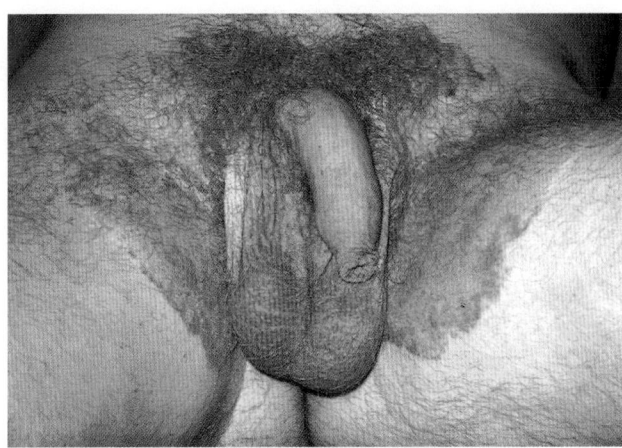

Fig. 22.26 **Tinea cruris.** Ringworm of the groin.

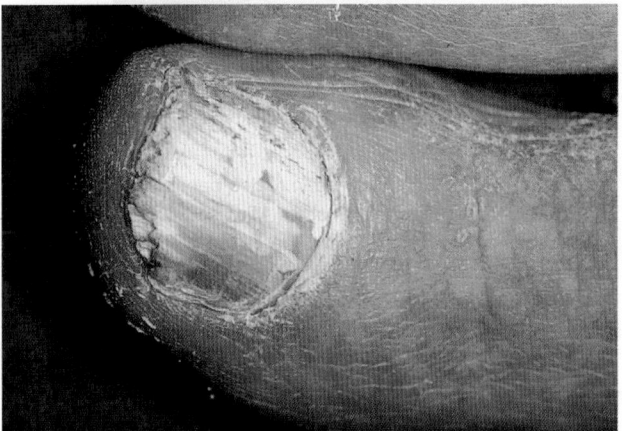

Fig. 22.27 Dermatophyte infection of the nail. White, crumbling dystrophy.

papulopustular rash on the trunk. This so-called 'id reaction' probably relates to the host immune response to the fungus. It resolves when the infection is treated.

Tinea unguium and onychomycosis

Onychomycosis is a broad term for fungal nail infection. Tinea unguium refers to a dermatophyte infection of the fingernails or toenails (**Fig. 22.27**). *Trichophyton rubrum* is the most common pathogen.

Tinea toenail infection is a common finding in the elderly and is usually asymptomatic. Fingernail infection is less common. Affected nails are dystrophic, thick (subungual hyperkeratosis) and discoloured (white–yellow–beige). Infection usually starts at the distal or lateral nail edges and then spreads proximally. The whole nail plate may be destroyed in advanced disease. The **differential diagnoses** include nail psoriasis and traumatic nail dystrophy (which may coexist with fungal infection).

Management

Localized tinea of the body or flexures is treated with an antifungal cream (clotrimazole, miconazole or terbinafine for 1–2 weeks). Nystatin is ineffective. More widespread infection, tinea pedis, tinea manuum and tinea capitis require oral antifungal therapy with itraconazole or terbinafine for 1–2 months. The diagnosis should be confirmed with skin scrapings taken from the active margin or across the affected area. Clippings should be taken from the proximal crumbly, white area of affected nails and plucked hairs or scrapings for diagnosis of scalp

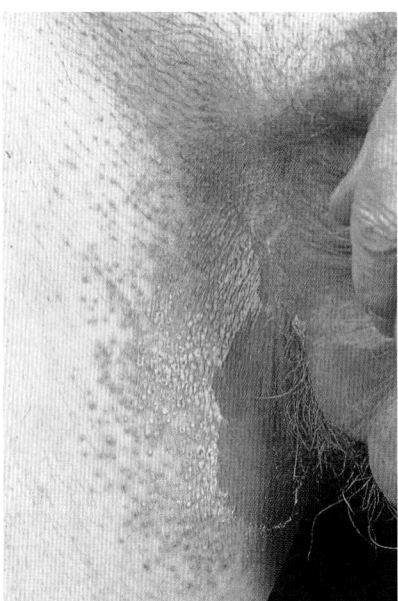

Fig. 22.28 Intertrigo with satellite lesions typical of candidiasis.

tinea. Specimens are transported in folded paper to keep them dry and prevent bacterial contamination. Microscopy and mycological culture confirm the diagnosis and identify the organism. Molecular diagnostic techniques, including PCR, analysis are gaining in popularity as they can offer high sensitivity and rapid results.

Toenail tinea infection requires prolonged oral antifungal therapy. Oral terbinafine for 3–6 months can clear up to 80% of cases but relapses are common. Itraconazole may be given as a continuous or pulsed regimen. Griseofulvin is a less effective drug but is still used for childhood tinea capitis.

Candidosis

Candida is a common species of yeast that causes a variety of skin infections. *Candida albicans* (see also p. 559) is a commensal in the gastrointestinal tract and vagina. It can overgrow on occluded moist skin, causing nappy rash, intertrigo of the large flexures in obese people (**Fig. 22.28**), and vulvovaginal candidiasis or 'thrush'. The glans penis may be affected in uncircumcised males (candidal balanitis). Other species of *Candida* may be isolated from vaginal infections and immunocompromised hosts.

Candidal intertrigo causes irritation and soreness; affected areas are glazed and inflamed, with a ragged, peeling edge that may contain a few small pustules. Spotty erythema may extend beyond the affected border (satellite lesions).

Candida may also affect the moist interdigital clefts of the toes and mimic tinea pedis. In people who frequently immerse their hands in water (e.g. cleaners, caterers), *Candida* may cause chronic infection of the nail folds ('paronychia') and nail infection (candida onychomycosis). *Candida* can also infect the oral mucosa, especially after broad-spectrum antibiotics and in the immunocompromised and older denture wearers. Affected mucosal surfaces are inflamed with superficial white or creamy pseudomembranous plaques, which can easily be scraped away. The diagnosis can be confirmed with microscopy and culture of a specimen taken with a routine microbial swab.

Management

Predisposing factors should be treated. Diabetes should be excluded. Topical therapy (azoles or nystatin) is usually adequate, except for nail infection, and may take the form of creams, pessaries,

lozenges or powder, depending on body site. Recurrent vulvovaginal candidiasis (see p. 1444) is a common complaint in women and may require oral azole antifungal therapy.

Malassezia

This lipophilic yeast family (formerly called *Pityrosporum*, see p. 562) is part of the normal skin microbiome. Colonization is prominent at areas rich in sebaceous glands: the scalp, large flexures and upper trunk. Over a dozen different species of *Malassezia* have been identified and there is increasing evidence of their causal role in three common dermatoses:
*   pityriasis versicolor
*   seborrhoeic eczema (see p. 662)
*   *Pityrosporum* (*Malassezia*) folliculitis.

Pityriasis versicolor is a common complaint in young adults, especially in warm climates. It causes widespread pink–beige scaly macules on the torso. Variable pigmentation is characteristic, with pale areas developing after tanning and in darker-skinned individuals as the yeast impairs melanin synthesis. The diagnosis is usually made clinically but can be confirmed by microscopy of skin scrapings, which shows spherical yeast and short pseudohyphae ('meatballs and spaghetti'). Treatment is with topical azoles or oral itraconazole for resistant cases. Anti-dandruff shampoos containing selenium sulphide or ketoconazole may also be used as a body wash. The pigment changes take months to resolve and recurrences are common.

Pityrosporum folliculitis is also common in young men and causes small, itchy, monomorphic papules and pustules on the upper back, shoulders and face. It may be confused with acne. Topical and oral azole antifungals can be effective but the complaint often relapses quickly.

Subcutaneous mycoses

Subcutaneous mycoses (see p. 561) are a rare group of localized infections of the skin and subcutaneous tissues that follow traumatic implantation of the fungal agent, a soil saprophyte. The causative organisms vary geographically and disease examples include sporotrichosis (worldwide), chromoblastomycosis and mycotic mycetoma (tropical and subtropical). Sporotrichosis, or 'rose gardener's disease', usually causes a slowly growing, inflamed nodule at the site of skin inoculation, with new lesions developing along lymphatics and blood vessels – 'sporotrichoid spread'. Treatment is with oral itraconazole.

Further reading

Ahmeen M, Lear JT, Madan V et al. British Association of Dermatologists' guidelines for the management of onychomycosis 2014. *Br J Dermatol* 2014; 171:937–958.

Infestations

Scabies

Scabies is an ectoparasite infestation with the mite *Sarcoptes scabiei*. It can affect all races and people of any social class, and is most common in children and young adults but can affect any age group. There are 300 million cases of scabies in the world each year. It is more common in poorer countries with social overcrowding, especially sub-Saharan Africa, and at any time there are approximately 130 million untreated cases. Although scabies is considered a trivial complaint, infectious complications include neonatal septicaemia, post-streptococcal nephritis and rheumatic fever. These cause

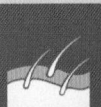

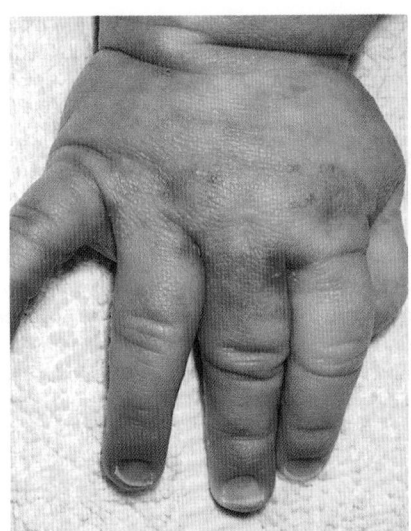

Fig. 22.29 Scabies. Itchy papules and pustules centred on the web spaces of the hand.

Box 22.17 Treatment of scabies

- Treat all skin below the neck, including the genitalia, palms and soles, and under the nails. Treat the head and neck regions in infants (up to 2 years of age).
- Treat all close contacts at the same time, *even if asymptomatic.*
- Reapply scabicide to the hands if they are washed during the treatment period.
- Wash or clean recently worn clothes (preferably at 60°C) to avoid re-infection.
- Repeat the application after 1 week.

considerable morbidity. Scabies is spread by close or prolonged contact, such as within households or care homes, and by sexual contact. It presents with a widespread, intensely itchy, excoriated, eczematous rash that is triggered by a hypersensitivity ('allergy') response to mite antigens. Pruritus is usually worse at night and disturbs sleep. Small, red papules, vesicles and occasionally pustules occur anywhere on the body but rarely on the face, except in neonates. The distribution of lesions is helpful in making a diagnosis (**Fig. 22.29**). Sites of predilection are the finger webs, palms, soles, wrists, axillae, male genitalia, and around the nipples and umbilicus. The rash may be complicated by secondary bacterial infection.

The diagnostic sign is fine linear or curved burrows a few millimetres long, but these are not always visible and dermoscopy may help. Scabies can be confirmed by demonstrating the mite and/or eggs on microscopy of potassium hydroxide-treated skin scrapings from the tip of a burrow, but this is time-consuming and treatment is usually based on clinical features and risk factors.

Management

A topical scabicide (e.g. 5% permethrin) is applied overnight. For the treatment to be successful, the measures listed in **Box 22.17** should be followed.

Malathion can be used if permethrin is unavailable; benzyl benzoate is employed occasionally but is irritant and should not be used in children. Oral ivermectin, as 2 doses 2 weeks apart, is effective, especially for use in communal settings (e.g. residential homes), but is unlicensed for this indication. Pruritus takes a few weeks to settle and can be managed with antihistamines and cooling creams such as 2% menthol.

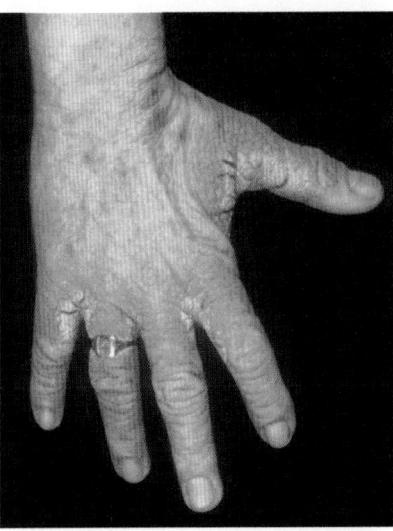

Fig. 22.30 Crusted scabies in a patient with chronic myeloid leukaemia.

Crusted scabies (Norwegian scabies)

Crusted scabies is a variant that affects elderly or immunocompromised people who are infested with a large number of mites (**Fig. 22.30**). Pruritus may be mild or absent. Individuals are highly infectious and may be the source of outbreaks if the diagnosis is delayed – which it often is, due to lack of symptoms. Hyperkeratotic crusted lesions characteristically affect the hands and feet. There may be a widespread inflammatory rash with scaly, crusted plaques resembling infected eczema or psoriasis. Meticulous barrier nursing is needed to protect staff against infestation. Hyperkeratotic scales should be removed with a keratolytic agent before application of a scabicide. Oral ivermectin is often required for effective eradication of all mites.

Lice

Lice are blood-sucking ectoparasites that cause three patterns of infection in humans.

Head lice (pediculosis capitis) infestation is an extremely common problem in schoolchildren, especially girls. Lice spread by close contact and cause pruritus, leading to excoriations and papules around the hairline of the neck and ears. The diagnosis is made by identifying eggs ('nits'), which are firmly stuck to the hair shaft, or the adult lice, which can be caught between the teeth of a fine comb. **Management** aims at eradication but this is difficult because treatment is time-consuming and re-infestations are common. Lotions containing traditional topical insecticides, such as malathion, carbaryl and phenothrin, are used less widely because of resistance and are being replaced by physical treatments such as dimeticone and isopropyl myristate. Fine combing of wet hair after applying conditioner can also be done repeatedly to remove young lice before they mature. Treatment needs to be repeated meticulously until all eggs have hatched.

Body lice (pediculosis corporis) are associated with poverty and neglect, and are seldom seen in developed countries except in long-term homeless people. They are spread by direct contact or by sharing of infested clothing. The lice and eggs are not usually seen on the patient's skin but can be found on close inspection of clothing. Infestation presents with itchy papules and excoriations. **Management** consists of malathion or permethrin for the patient and high-temperature washing and drying of clothing.

Pubic lice (crabs, phthiriasis pubis) are transmitted by direct contact, usually sexual (see p. 1425). Infestation presents with itching, especially at night. Lice can be seen near the base of the hair with eggs somewhat further up the shaft. Occasionally, eyebrows, eyelashes and the beard area are affected. *Management* is as for head lice, but all sexual contacts should be treated and the patient screened for other sexually transmitted diseases.

Arthropod-borne diseases ('insect bites' or papular urticaria)

These stem from contact with an animal (e.g. dog, cat, bird) that is infested with fleas (*Cheyletiella*) or from bites from flying insects (e.g. midges, mosquitoes). Animals infested with fleas usually scratch vigorously, leading to scaly, thickened skin. Flea eggs can lie dormant in soft furnishings (e.g. carpets) for many months, hatching when disturbed by vibrations. Bites present as itchy, urticated lesions, which are often grouped in clusters or lines. The legs are most commonly affected and lesions can blister in hot weather. Some individuals react more vigorously to bites while others appear unaffected. Anti-flea treatment of the animal and furnishings is required. Repellents and appropriate clothing help reduce bites from flying insects.

Bed bug infestation is a common problem worldwide and is caused by bites from small, brown/black, apple seed-sized insects that emerge from the seams of bedding at night when attracted to the warmth and carbon dioxide emissions of a sleeping human body. Their bites occur in groups or lines as intensely itchy papules on exposed areas, including the face and neck. Infestations usually require expert pest control for eradication. Further advice may be obtained in the UK from the National Pest Technicians Association, a professional trade body (see Further reading).

Further reading

Fuller LC. Epidemiology of scabies. *Curr Opin Inf Dis* 2013; 26:123–126.
National Institute for Health and Care Excellence. *Head Lice – Management*. NICE 2016; https://cks.nice.org.uk/head-lice.
http://www.npta.org.uk. *UK National Pest Technicians Association*.

Tropical dermatoses

Skin diseases that feature among the 'neglected tropical diseases' defined by the World Health Organization (WHO) include scabies, leprosy, leishmaniasis, dracunculiasis (guinea worm), lymphatic filariasis and onchocerciasis. These are endemic in poor countries and constitute a huge physical and financial burden on their societies. Travellers who have visited tropical or subtropical countries may also be affected by skin diseases, especially cutaneous leishmaniasis, cutaneous larva migrans and myiasis. Rashes may also be a feature of systemic tropical infections such as dengue, schistosomiasis and rickettsial diseases.

Leishmaniasis (see p. 569) is caused by a protozoon, *Leishmania*, and is acquired from the bite of a sandfly vector. Cutaneous, mucocutaneous and visceral disease (kala azar) may occur, depending on the infecting organism and host response. *Cutaneous leishmaniasis* (see p. 570) is the most common form and presents as a chronic ulcer (oriental sore), which heals slowly over many months with scarring.

Cutaneous larva migrans is caused by direct contact with the larvae of hookworm from animal faeces, usually acquired by walking or lying on sandy beaches. Larvae penetrate the skin and cause an intensely itchy serpiginous lesion, which migrates as the larva burrows within the epidermis.

Myiasis is an infestation of the skin with developing fly larvae (maggots). Species that can penetrate intact skin to cause boil-like lesions include botfly and tumbu fly.

HUMAN IMMUNODEFICIENCY VIRUS AND THE SKIN

HIV infection is associated with a range of infective, inflammatory and malignant skin diseases that may be severe, atypical, difficult to diagnose and recalcitrant (see p. 1431). Advances in highly active anti-retroviral therapy (ART, see p. 1435) have dramatically reduced the prevalence of these diseases in recent years in countries with early access to therapy. However, awareness must be maintained, as they may be a presenting feature of undiagnosed HIV infection.

Seroconversion rash

This non-specific maculopapular exanthem affects up to 75% of individuals a few weeks after contracting HIV. There may be associated fever, malaise, myalgia, lymphadenopathy and mouth ulceration (or oral candidiasis). Symptoms usually resolve within a few weeks. This episode is often dismissed as 'flu' and the diagnosis missed. Patients are highly infectious at this time due to very high viral loads.

Cutaneous infection and opportunistic infection

These are increased due to HIV-induced immune deficiency. Molluscum contagiosum is common, especially on the face, and lesions may be large (>1 cm in diameter) and extensive (a pattern rarely seen in immunocompetent adults). Other viral infections that are typically more severe or widespread include herpes simplex, shingles and viral warts. Bacterial infections (e.g. staphylococcal boils) and fungal infections (tinea and *Candida*) are also common. Recalcitrant and recurrent oropharyngeal candidiasis is a particular problem.

Opportunistic infections that may affect the skin include cytomegalovirus (pustules or necrotic ulcers) or *Cryptococcus* (red papules, psoriasiform or molluscum-like lesions). Diagnosis can be difficult and depends on skin biopsies and culture.

Inflammatory dermatoses

Severe, extensive seborrhoeic eczema (see p. 662) is common and may be the presenting sign of HIV. Psoriasis is typically more severe in patients with HIV and close liaison between dermatologist and HIV physicians is needed, especially with low CD4 counts (<200/ mm^3), due to the risk of further immunosuppression with systemic therapy (e.g. ciclosporin) and drug interactions.

Drug rashes

These are much more common in HIV patients. Reactions (maculopapular rash) to co-trimoxazole, dapsone (used in *Pneumocystis* prophylaxis) and anti-retroviral drugs appear to be particularly frequent. Drug rashes may be severe (especially with nevirapine and efavirenz), resulting in erythroderma (see p. 656) or toxic epidermal necrolysis (see p. 697). Other unusual conditions include nail or mucosal pigmentation from zidovudine, paronychia from indinavir and lipodystrophy (of the face and abdomen/buttocks) from protease inhibitors. As protease inhibitors and zidovudine are now used much less often in first-line drug combinations, the latter side-effects are rare today.

Cutaneous malignancy

HIV infection is associated with an increased risk of several malignancies. Cutaneous malignancy (Kaposi's sarcoma, see p. 692) was one of the earliest recognized manifestations of HIV infection that led to the description of the acquired immune deficiency syndrome (AIDS). Most HIV-related cancers are associated with co-infection with oncogenic viruses; Kaposi's sarcoma (HHV-8), lymphoma (Epstein–Barr virus) and epithelial squamous cell carcinoma (HPV). Pre-malignant conditions, such as the intraepithelial dysplasias (cervix – CIN, penis – PIN, anal – AIN), are also increased in HIV infection. The risk of malignant transformation at all three sites is high and should be assessed by screening. Kaposi's sarcoma is much more common in men who have sex with men who have HIV than in other groups, but is infrequently seen nowadays in patients on ART.

'Specific' HIV dermatoses

'Itchy folliculitis' / HIV folliculitis (also called papular pruritic eruption or eosinophilic folliculitis) is commonly found in association with declining CD4 counts. It presents with intensely itchy papules and excoriations around hair follicles and occurs most commonly over the upper trunk and upper arms (**Fig. 22.31**).

Oral hairy leucoplakia presents with fixed white plaques with vertical ridges on the sides of the tongue. Unlike candidiasis, the lesions cannot be scraped off. It was first recognized in HIV disease but can rarely occur in other forms of immunosuppression and is thought to be due to co-infection with Epstein–Barr virus.

Immune reconstitution inflammatory syndrome

Several infections can be unmasked or can paradoxically worsen 2–4 months after commencing ART as the CD4 lymphocyte count recovers – the so-called immune reconstitution inflammatory syndrome (IRIS). Most commonly described are ano-genital HSV infection, viral warts, tinea folliculitis, molluscum and genital warts. IRIS affects up to 25% of patients on ART and is thought to reflect the response of a recovering immune system against pathogens that were already present. IRIS may also be responsible for an increase in inflammatory rashes, such as folliculitis and subacute lupus erythematosus.

Further reading

Chang CC, Sheikh V, Sereti I et al. Immune reconstitution disorders in patients with HIV infection: from pathogenesis to prevention and treatment. *Curr HIV/AIDS Rep* 2014; 11:223–232.
Vangipuram R, Tyring SK. AIDS-associated malignancies. *Cancer Treat Res* 2019; 177:1–21.

SKIN SIGNS OF SYSTEMIC DISEASE

Most skin diseases are isolated complaints but a few are associated with underlying systemic disease, of which they may be the presenting feature.

Erythema nodosum

Erythema nodosum (see also p. 677) has a number of disease associations (**Box 22.18**). It presents as painful or tender, dusky bruise-like swellings over the shins, which fade over several weeks (**Fig. 22.32**). It is most common in young women. There may be associated arthralgia, malaise and fever. Inflammation occurs in the deeper dermis and the subcutaneous fat (panniculitis), and can be confirmed with a skin biopsy.

Management includes symptomatic relief with NSAIDs, light compression socks and rest. Any underlying cause should be treated. It usually resolves spontaneously but persistent cases can be treated with anti-inflammatory drugs (dapsone, colchicine) or prednisolone.

Erythema multiforme

Erythema multiforme is an acute self-limiting rash characterized by distinctive 'target lesions' on the distal limbs, palms and soles

> **Box 22.18** Causes of erythema nodosum

- Streptococcal infection[a]
- Drugs (e.g. sulphonamides, oral contraceptive pill)
- Sarcoidosis[a]
- Idiopathic[a]
- Bacterial gastroenteritis, e.g. *Salmonella, Shigella, Yersinia*
- Fungal infection (histoplasmosis, blastomycosis)
- Tuberculosis
- Leprosy
- Inflammatory bowel disease
- *Chlamydia* infection

[a]Common causes.

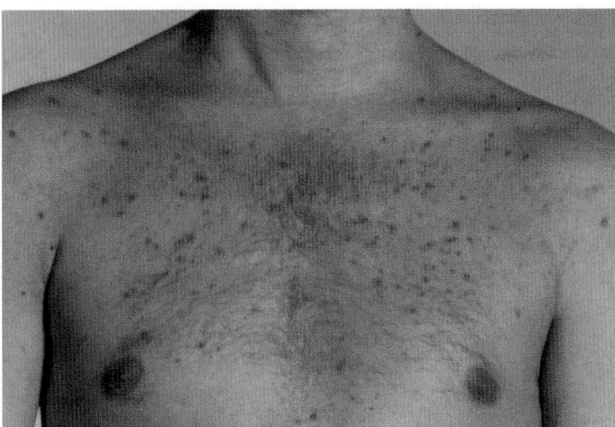

Fig. 22.31 Itchy folliculitis of HIV infection on the upper trunk and proximal limbs.

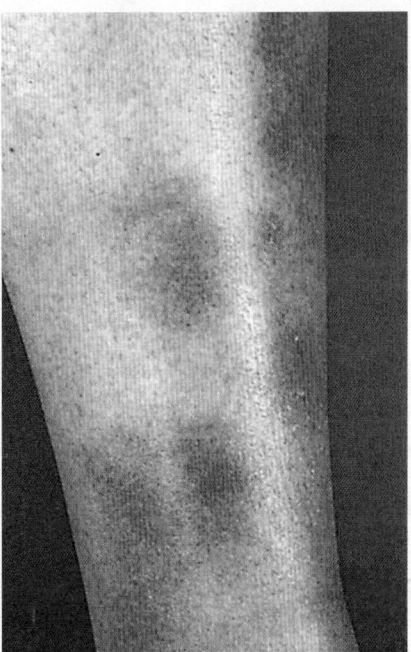

Fig. 22.32 Erythema nodosum in a patient with HIV on co-trimoxazole.

(acral sites). These are concentric rings of erythema with a dusky centre, which can blister. There is variable inflammation/ulceration of the mouth, lips and other mucosal sites. In erythema multiforme major, mucosal ulceration is severe and there may be fever and systemic upset (**Fig. 22.33**). The most common trigger is herpes simplex virus. Other causes include orf (see p. 672) and drugs (e.g. anticonvulsants). In 50% of cases there is no identifiable cause. *Mycoplasma pneumoniae* infection may trigger severe erythema multiforme-like mucosal ulceration with minimal skin changes: *M. pneumoniae*-associated mucositis (MPAM).

Management is supportive, with analgesia and parenteral fluids until dysphagia has resolved. MPAM requires antimicrobial therapy. Infection can be confirmed by *M. pneumoniae* PCR.

The clinical features of erythema multiforme major – Stevens–Johnson syndrome – are shown in **Box 22.19**. The role of systemic steroids in this condition remains controversial.

Pyoderma gangrenosum

Pyoderma gangrenosum (PG) is a rare ulcerating skin disease of unknown cause, often associated with systemic inflammatory conditions, especially inflammatory bowel disease. It may also be associated with inflammatory arthritis and haematological malignancies. It is classified as a 'neutrophilic' disease and shares clinicopathological similarities with autoinflammatory diseases in which there is an infection-like host response in the absence of a microbial trigger. The most common presentation is with painful inflammatory nodules that rapidly turn into enlarging purulent ulcers ('pyoderma') with a purple undermined edge. PG may occur spontaneously or postoperatively in a surgical wound or stoma, when it can be misdiagnosed as a wound infection.

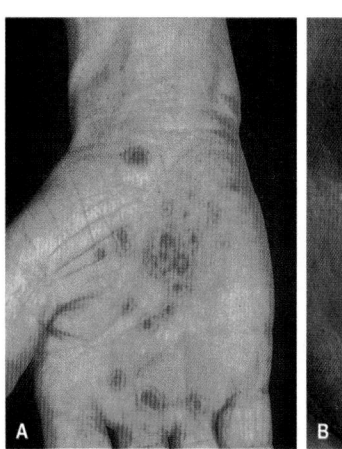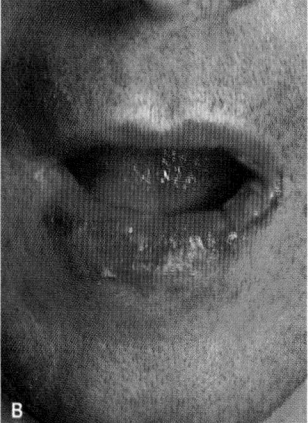

Fig. 22.33 Erythema multiforme major. **(A)** Target lesions of the palm. **(B)** Mucosal involvement around the mouth.

Skin lesions are rich in neutrophils but histological features are non-specific and so the diagnosis is made on clinical features. Superpotent topical corticosteroids may help in very mild cases. Systemic therapy with moderate to high-dose systemic corticosteroids and/or ciclosporin is usually needed. Anti-TNF therapy, such as infliximab, may be used for refractory cases. The clinical course is unpredictable and unrelated to underlying inflammatory bowel disease activity. PG ulcers heal with mesh-like (cribriform) scars (**Fig. 22.34**).

Sweet's syndrome (acute febrile neutrophilic dermatosis)

Sweet's syndrome is a rare disorder characterized by fever, malaise and an acute eruption of tender, red–purple lumps on the head, neck and upper body (**Fig. 22.35**). As in PG, the skin lesions contain abundant neutrophils (neutrophilic dermatosis). There is usually no underlying illness, but the syndrome may be associated with haematological malignancy and can be induced by drugs, including granulocyte colony stimulating factor. It is usually treated with systemic corticosteroids or anti-neutrophil drugs (dapsone, colchicine).

Behçet's syndrome

Behçet's syndrome (see p. 466) is an inflammatory disorder characterized by recurrent oral ulcers and eye lesions, genital ulcers or skin lesions. Skin changes include erythema nodosum, papulopustular acne-like lesions, thrombophlebitis and skin pathergy (prolonged inflammation or pustulation at the site of needle-prick or other minor skin injuries). The syndrome is probably a vasculitis and many organs can be involved. Milder disease and skin lesions may respond well to colchicine or dapsone.

Sarcoidosis

Sarcoidosis (see also p. 985) is a multisystem granulomatous disorder of unknown aetiology. Skin involvement occurs in 20–30% of cases and usually presents with red–brown papules, nodules and plaques. The nose may be extensively involved (lupus pernio). Lesions may hypo- or hyperpigmented, especially in dark skin. Erythema nodosum (see p. 677) is sometimes seen in acute sarcoidosis. Although sarcoidosis may be localized to the skin, all patients should be investigated for systemic involvement (see p. 987). Cutaneous sarcoid responds poorly to topical therapy but superpotent or intralesional corticosteroids or topical tacrolimus may occasionally help.

Further reading

Marzano AV, Borghi A, Wallach D et al. A comprehensive review of neutrophilic diseases. *Clin Rev Allergy Immunol* 2018; 54:114–130.

_i_ Box 22.19 Clinical spectra of erythema multiforme, Stevens–Johnson syndrome and toxic epidermal necrolysis

Diagnosis	Skin lesions	Mucosal lesions	Other signs/symptoms
Erythema multiforme (EM)	Three-ring target lesions, often hands and feet	EM major only	Recent infection (herpes simplex virus, *Mycoplasma*)
Stevens–Johnson syndrome (SJS)	Scattered macules/blisters scattered over face, trunk, proximal limbs (<10% body surface area) Occasional two-ring target lesion	Always	Fever Skin tenderness Recent drug exposure
Toxic epidermal necrolysis (TEN)	As for SJS but >30% body surface area involved	Always	As for SJS Respiratory and gastrointestinal lesions Hypotension Decreased consciousness
SJS/TEN overlap	As for SJS (10–30% body surface area involved)	Always	

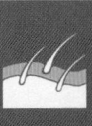

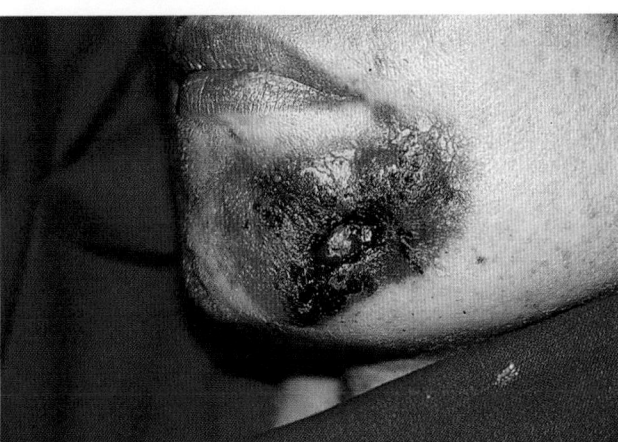

Fig. 22.34 Pyoderma gangrenosum.

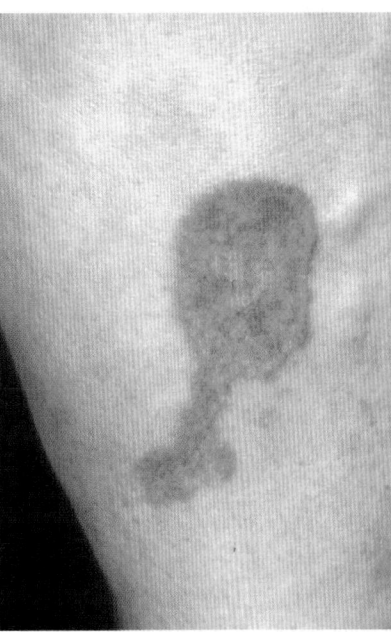

Fig. 22.36 Necrobiosis lipoidica on the shin in type 1 diabetes mellitus.

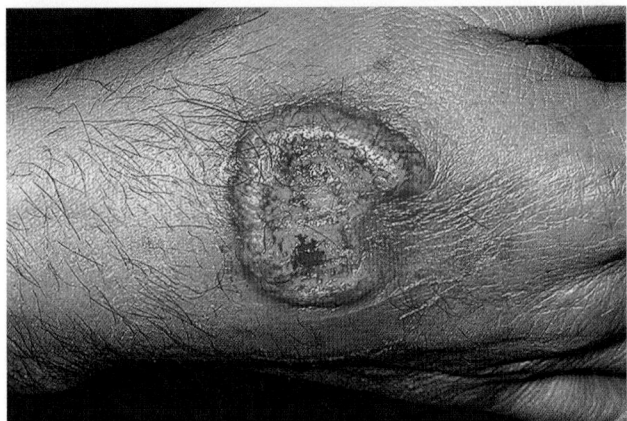

Fig. 22.35 Sweet's syndrome. Lesions are tender erythematous papules and plaques that can also be pseudovesicular or pustular. Lesions tend to be multiple but isolated lesions are seen. *(From Habif TP, Dinulos JGH, Chapman MS et al. Skin Disease: Diagnosis and Treatment. Elsevier Inc.; 2018; Fig. 11.33.)*

Endocrine disease

Thyroid disease

(See also Ch. 21.) Individuals with **hypothyroidism** have cold, dry skin and brittle hair with diffuse thinning and loss of the outer third of the eyebrows. There may be a jaundice-like appearance due to carotene excess with firm, gelatinous (myxoedematous) skin.

Hyperthyroidism may be associated with hyperhidrosis, onycholysis and diffuse alopecia. The extrathyroid manifestations of Graves' disease include dermopathy (pretibial myxoedema), which classically presents with non-pitting infiltration, plaques on the shins and, in severe cases, thyroid acropachy, characterized by clubbing and soft tissue swelling of the fingers and toes with periosteal reaction of the bones.

Diabetes mellitus

Diabetes mellitus (see also p. 735) can have a number of skin manifestations and complications, mediated mainly by hyperglycaemia and hyperinsulinaemia. They include:

- fungal infection (e.g. candidiasis, see p. 674)
- bacterial infections (e.g. recurrent boils, see p. 670)
- arterial and neuropathic ulcers

- poor or delayed healing
- xanthomas
  Specific dermatoses of diabetes include:
- necrobiosis lipoidica (a patch of spreading erythema over the shin, which becomes yellowish and atrophic in the centre and may ulcerate, **Fig. 22.36**)
- diffuse granuloma annulare (see p. 667)
- diabetic stiff skin/cheiroarthropathy (tight, waxy skin over the fingers with limitation of joint movement owing to thickened collagen).

Cushing's syndrome

Skin manifestations due to high cortisol include hirsutism, central obesity, moon face and buffalo hump. Florid purple striae distensae, or 'stretch marks', skin atrophy, telangiectasia and increased susceptibility to folliculitis and candidiasis may occur (see pp. 670 and 674). Hyperpigmentation also occurs in cases with increased circulating adrenocorticotropic hormone (ACTH; ectopic ACTH syndromes or Cushing's disease, see p. 602).

Striae distensae are caused by ruptures in dermal collagen and elastic tissue. They are a common finding over the abdomen, hips and breasts in normal female puberty and pregnancy, and in obesity, and over the lumbosacral area in adolescent males. The cause is unclear but they are associated with rapid growth. There is no effective treatment but they fade from pink/purple to pale silvery lines with time. Striae are also seen in Marfan's syndrome.

Addison's disease

Generalized hyperpigmentation occurs secondary to raised circulating ACTH levels (see also p. 599). This may be prominent in the palmar creases, oral mucosa, lips, large flexures, genitals and nail beds.

Acanthosis nigricans

Acanthosis nigricans presents with thickened, hyperpigmented, velvet-textured skin around the large flexures (**Fig. 22.37**). It can appear warty when advanced. The most common and mildest

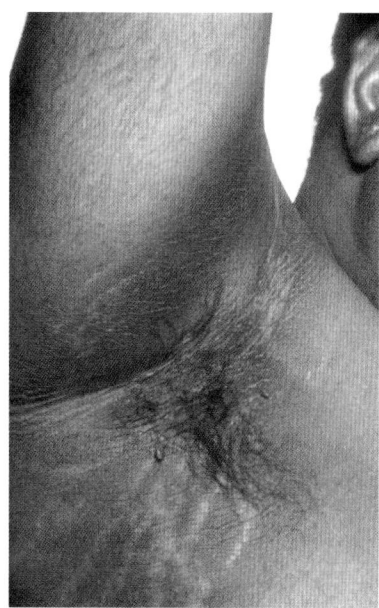

Fig. 22.37 Acanthosis nigricans in the axilla of an obese individual.

form is associated with obesity and insulin resistance). Late-onset, severe disease with mucosal involvement is usually a paraneoplastic phenomenon caused by underlying malignancy, especially gastrointestinal tumours. Acanthosis nigricans may also be triggered by niacin therapy.

Flushing

Facial flushing in response to emotional stimuli (blushing) is a normal physiological response that can cause embarrassment and may be associated with social phobia. Pathological causes include carcinoid syndrome, other neuroendocrine tumours and drugs. Treatment of idiopathic flushing includes cosmetic camouflage, beta-blockers and clonidine. Cognitive therapy and selective serotonin reuptake inhibitors may help with associated depression and anxiety.

Metabolic disease

Hyperlipidaemias

Hyperlipidaemia (see also p. 746) may present with xanthomas, which are abnormal lipid deposits in the skin. A fasting lipid profile should be checked in all patients, though it may be normal in the most common type, **xanthelasma**, which presents with asymptomatic yellow plaques around the eyes. There are a number of other clinical variants of **xanthoma**, including:

- **tuberous xanthoma** (firm orange–yellow nodules and plaques on extensor surfaces)
- **tendon xanthoma** (firm subcutaneous swellings attached to tendons)
- **plane xanthoma** (orange–yellow macules often affecting palmar creases)
- **eruptive xanthoma** (numerous small, yellowish papules, commonly on the buttocks).

Porphyria cutanea tarda

Porphyria cutanea tarda (PCT, see p. 755) is a rare metabolic disorder associated with liver disease; it is usually precipitated by alcohol excess or hepatitis C virus (HCV) infection, and 20% of cases have underlying haemochromatosis (see p. 1300). PCT presents with

sun-induced blisters, fragile skin, scarring and milia, especially on the dorsal hands, and hypertrichosis.

Management is with repeated venesection to reduce iron overload, alcohol avoidance and low-dose antimalarial drugs. Antiviral therapy is indicated for underlying HCV infection.

Pruritus

The pathophysiology of pruritus (itch) is complex and incompletely understood. It may be caused by peripheral mechanisms (as in skin disease), central or neuropathic mechanisms (as in multiple sclerosis), neurogenic mechanisms (as in cholestasis/μ-opioid receptor stimulation) or psychogenic mechanisms (e.g. parasitophobia). Evidence suggests that low stimulation of unmyelinated C-fibres in the skin is associated with the sensation of itch; high stimulation produces pain. Histamine, tachykinins (e.g. substance P) and cytokines (e.g. IL-31) may also play a role. In the central nervous system μ-opioid receptors may regulate the perception and intensity of itch.

Pruritus is a characteristic feature of many inflammatory rashes, especially atopic eczema, scabies and lichen planus. It also occurs with asteatotic eczema (see p. 663) and cholinergic urticaria, where the rash may be subtle and overlooked. Pruritus is common in the elderly and usually due to skin dryness (xerosis). Generalized pruritus without a rash can be caused by a number of medical problems (**Box 22.20**).

Management involves use of soap substitutes and symptomatic measures (as for asteatotic eczema). Phototherapy, low-dose amitriptyline or gabapentin may help in intractable cases. If a pruritic skin disease is not evident, patients should be fully investigated for underlying systemic disease.

Haematological disease

Anaemia (especially iron-deficient), iron overload, polycythaemia vera and lymphoproliferative diseases such as lymphoma can present with generalized pruritus. Iron deficiency can also present with hair shedding (see p. 331), glossitis, angular cheilitis and brittle or spoon-shaped nails (koilonychia).

Amyloidosis

Amyloid may be deposited in the skin in localized cutaneous forms due to repeated scratching (macular amyloid) or in association with underlying systemic disease. About 50% of patients with systemic amyloid will have skin involvement. Amyloid deposits in the oral cavity present with macroglossia and mucosal papules. Deposition in and around blood vessels causes fragility with petechiae and purpura, especially in the periocular skin and large flexures. In primary systemic amyloid, there is usually an underlying monoclonal plasma cell proliferation. Multidisciplinary treatment of the underlying disease is required.

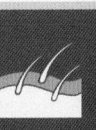

Chronic liver disease

Chronic liver disease may present with jaundice, palmar erythema, spider naevi, white nails and hyperpigmentation. Pruritus is common in cholestatic disease, including cholestasis of pregnancy (see p. 1455).

Chronic renal disease

End-stage renal disease (ESRD, see also p. 1397) is commonly associated with intractable pruritus. Pallor, hyperpigmentation and ecchymoses also occur. ESRD may rarely be associated with non-inflammatory, PCT-like blistering and fragility (pseudo-porphyria). Longstanding renal transplant recipients are at high risk of recurrent viral warts and squamous cell carcinomas (see p. 690) due to immunosuppression. *Calciphylaxis* is a rare life-threatening disorder caused by vascular calcification and occlusion, and characterized by extremely painful, ulcerating plaques (see p. 1396). *Nephrogenic fibrosing dermopathy/nephrogenic systemic fibrosis* is a severe scleroderma-like skin disease that affects people with severe renal impairment. The disease can develop rapidly, with swelling and woody thickening of the skin, and internal organs may be affected. Exposure to gadolinium-containing contrast agents used in magnetic resonance imaging (MRI) has been identified as a trigger.

Further reading

Millington GW, Collins A, Lovell CR et al. British Association of Dermatologists' guidelines for the investigation and management of generalized pruritus in adults without an underlying dermatosis 2018. *Br J Dermatol* 2018; 178:34–60.

Autoimmune rheumatic disease

Dermatomyositis

The rash of dermatomyositis (see also p. 462) has a lilac colour, likened to that of a heliotrope, and is often in a photosensitive, cape-like distribution. It can itch and there may be prominent oedema around the eyes and poikiloderma (reticulate pigmentation, atrophy and telangiectasia). Purple nodules or plaques appear over the knuckles (Gottron's papules, see **Fig. 18.38**) and extensor surfaces. The nail folds and cuticles are ragged with dilated capillaries. Investigations include serum muscle enzymes, myositis-specific antibodies, MRI scan, muscle biopsy and electromyography. Skin biopsy changes are non-specific. Myositis-specific antibody tests include anti-Mi-2 (highly specific for dermatomyositis), anti-MDA-5 (interstitial lung disease) and anti-TIF1-gamma (malignancy-associated disease, see p. 463).

Juvenile dermatomyositis usually starts before the age of 10. It is associated with cutaneous calcinosis and muscle contractures. The adult form usually occurs after the age of 40. Some cases are associated with malignancy, especially gynaecological, and this requires thorough investigation. Other cases are associated with connective tissue diseases, including scleroderma and lupus erythematosus (see p. 456).

Skin disease may respond to sunscreens and the antimalarial drug hydroxychloroquine. Myositis usually requires high-dose corticosteroids and immunosuppressant drugs.

Scleroderma

The term scleroderma refers to a thickening or hardening of the skin due to abnormal dermal collagen. It is not a diagnostic entity in itself. Systemic sclerosis and morphea both show sclerodermatous changes but are distinct conditions:

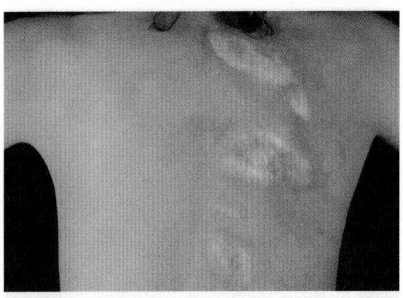

Fig. 22.38 Morphea. Hyperpigmentation and scarring on the trunk.

- *Systemic sclerosis* (often called scleroderma) has cutaneous and systemic features, and is discussed on page 460. Skin changes may be the presenting feature in the localized CREST variant.
- *Morphea* (localized cutaneous scleroderma) is confined to the skin or subcutis and usually presents in children or young adults. It is more common in females and the cause is unknown. Lesions usually appear on the trunk as bluish-red thickened plaques with a shiny white indurated or atrophic centre (**Fig. 22.38**). A severe linear variant in childhood is associated with atrophy of underlying deep tissues and can lead to unequal limb growth or scarring alopecia.

Rarely, scleroderma-like skin changes may occur in chronic *Borrelia* infection (acrodermatitis chronica atrophicans), chronic graft-versus-host disease and eosinophilic myalgia syndrome (due to tryptophan therapy).

Potent topical steroids, oral (or pulsed intravenous) steroids, methotrexate or phototherapy can be helpful. Systemic treatment is indicated for subcutaneous disease to minimize scarring.

Lupus erythematosus

Lupus is a chronic multisystem autoimmune inflammatory disease (see p. 461). Skin involvement falls into three broad categories:
- chronic discoid lupus erythematosus (CDLE)
- subacute cutaneous lupus erythematosus (SCLE)
- systemic lupus erythematosus (SLE).

The cause is unknown but inherited factors, UV exposure and drugs may be relevant. All forms of lupus are more common in women.

Chronic discoid lupus erythematosus

Chronic discoid lupus erythematosus (CDLE) is characterized by chronic erythematous, scaly, atrophic plaques with telangiectasia, especially on the face or other sun-exposed sites (**Fig. 22.39**). Lesions are often hypopigmented and close examination may show plugged follicles. Scalp involvement leads to patchy scarring alopecia. Oral involvement (erythematous patches or ulcers) occurs in 25% of cases. A minority of patients also suffer with Raynaud's phenomenon or chilblain-like lesions (chilblain lupus). About 30% of patients have positive antinuclear antibodies and about 5% develop overt systemic disease.

Skin biopsy shows a dense infiltration of lymphocytes around the hair follicles and damage to the basal layer of the epidermis. Direct immunofluorescence may demonstrate granular deposits of IgM and C3 at the dermo-epidermal junction ('lupus band'). CDLE usually lasts for many years, with fluctuations in severity before 'burning out'.

Treatment is with high-factor sunscreens and potent topical steroids. Widespread or unresponsive disease and associated arthritis may require antimalarial therapy (hydroxychloroquine),

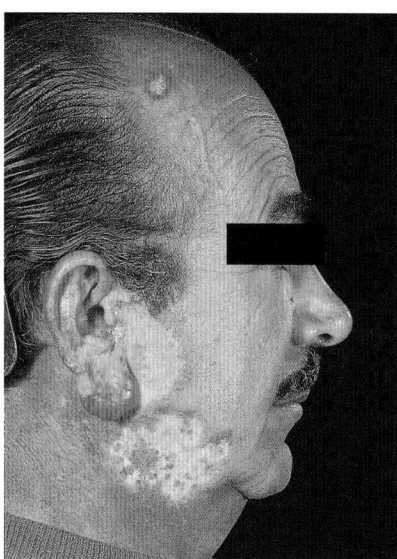

Fig. 22.39 Chronic discoid lupus erythematosus. Scaling, atrophy and hypopigmentation.

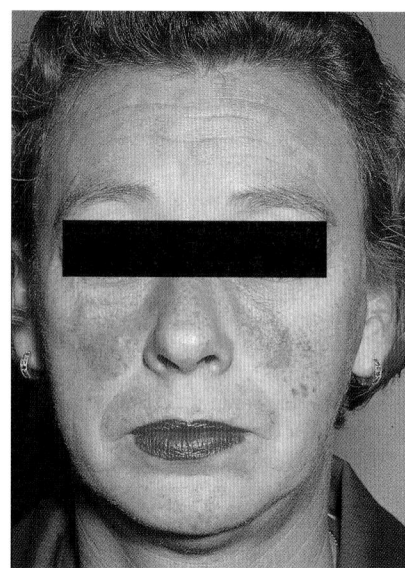

Fig. 22.40 Systemic lupus erythematosus. Macular erythema on the cheeks ('butterfly rash').

systemic steroids or immunosuppressants. Thalidomide has been used for recalcitrant CDLE.

Subacute cutaneous lupus erythematosus

Subacute cutaneous lupus erythematosus (SCLE) is an uncommon variant that presents with widespread annular, papulosquamous lesions and plaques on the upper torso and upper limbs. It typically flares a few weeks after sun exposure. Systemic symptoms, such as arthralgia and mouth ulceration, are seen but significant organ involvement is rare. It may be drug-induced. Anti-Ro and anti-La antinuclear antibodies are usually positive (see p. 459).

Treatment is with antimalarials, dapsone or systemic steroids.

Systemic lupus erythematosus

Systemic lupus erythematosus (SLE; see also p. 457) seldom presents with skin features, as other organ involvement (arthritis, nephritis) usually predominates. The classical 'butterfly' rash affects the central face in a rosacea-like distribution (**Fig. 22.40**). Palmar erythema, dilated nail-fold capillaries, splinter haemorrhages, digital infarcts, purpura and livedo reticularis (see later) may be evident due to vascular inflammation or occlusion.

Treatment is described on page 459.

Disorders of blood vessels and lymphatics

Vasculitis

Vasculitis (see also p. 464) is an inflammatory disorder of blood vessels that causes endothelial damage. Cutaneous vasculitis may be an isolated problem or part of a multisystem disease with involvement of other organs. The most commonly used classification is based on the size of blood vessel involved (see **Boxes 18.39** and **18.40**) and the presence or absence of antineutrophil cytoplasmic antibody (ANCA).

The features of cutaneous vasculitis are haemorrhagic papules, pustules, nodules or plaques, which may erode and ulcerate. Lesions are purpuric and do not blanch with pressure. Blotchy erythema in a broken livedo/reticulate pattern (see next section) may be seen, with areas of infarction and necrosis. Pyrexia and arthralgia are common associated features. Other clinical features depend on the underlying cause. A thorough clinical evaluation will determine

the likely causes and guide further investigations. Routine bloods and urinalysis should be carried out to exclude renal involvement.

Leucocytoclastic vasculitis is the most common cutaneous vasculitis and involves small vessels. It usually affects the lower legs as a symmetrical palpable purpura and is rarely associated with systemic involvement. It can be caused by drugs (15%), infection (15%), inflammatory disease (10%) or malignant disease (<5%) but often no cause is found (55–60%). Histology of an early lesion confirms blood vessel inflammation (rather than primary occlusion) and indicates the size of the blood vessel involved, as well as the presence of additional diagnostic features such as granulomas. Treatment is with analgesia, support stockings, and dapsone or prednisolone to control inflammation and heal ulceration.

Livedo reticularis

The term livedo reticularis describes a mesh-like (reticulate), blotchy, purple–red discoloration of the skin. It usually affects the lower limbs and is more noticeable in the cold but does not disappear on rewarming (unlike physiological livedo). The colour change is due to sluggish blood flow in dermal venules. This may be caused by blood abnormalities of the blood (high viscosity, coagulopathy, cryoglobulinaemia) or vessel wall (vasculitis, e.g. polyarteritis nodosa, calcification). If the network or mesh pattern is broken and irregular ('livedo racemosa'), underlying systemic disease is likely. *Livedoid vasculopathy* is characterized by broken livedo, painful leg ulcers and *atrophie blanche* (see later). It may be associated with antiphospholipid syndrome and SLE.

Leg ulcers

Leg ulcers are common and can have many causes (**Box 22.21**). Venous ulcers are the most common type in developed countries (**Fig. 22.41**).

Venous ulcers

Venous ulcers are the result of sustained venous hypertension in the superficial veins, due to incompetent valves in the deep or perforating veins or to previous deep vein thrombosis. The increased pressure causes extravasation of fibrinogen through the capillary

- Venous hypertension
- Arterial disease (e.g. atherosclerosis)
- Neuropathic disease (e.g. diabetes, leprosy)
- Neoplastic disease (e.g. squamous or basal cell carcinoma)
- Vasculitis (e.g. rheumatoid arthritis, systemic lupus erythematosus, pyoderma gangrenosum)
- Infection (e.g. ecthyma, tuberculosis, deep mycoses, Buruli ulcer, syphilis, yaws)
- Haematological disease (e.g. sickle cell disease, spherocytosis)
- Drug (e.g. hydroxycarbamide)
- Other (e.g. necrobiosis lipoidica, trauma, artefact)

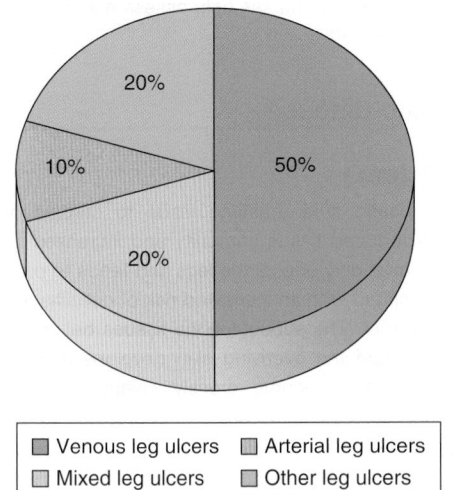

Venous leg ulcers **Arterial leg ulcers**
Mixed leg ulcers **Other leg ulcers**

Fig. 22.41 Types of leg ulcer. *(From Griffiths C, Barker J, Bleiker T et al. (eds).* Rook's Textbook of Dermatology, *9th edn.* Chichester: John Wiley & Sons; 2016.)

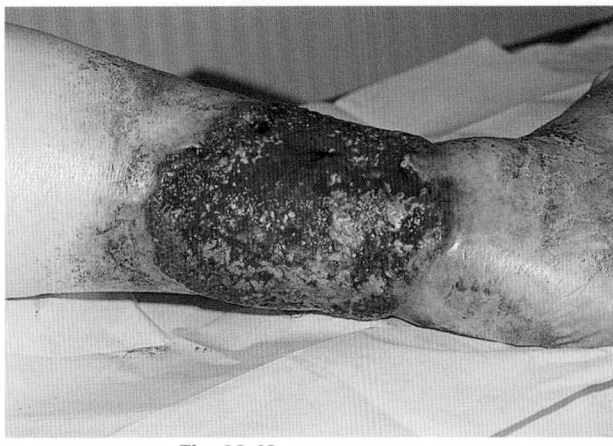

Fig. 22.42 Venous leg ulcer.

walls, giving rise to perivascular fibrin deposition, which leads to poor oxygenation of the surrounding skin.

Venous ulcers are common in later life, affecting 1% of the population over the age of 70. They are often chronic or recurrent and create a significant burden on healthcare resources. Ulceration is most common on the lower leg above the medial malleolus (**Fig. 22.42**). Dilated foot, leg and thigh veins are usually evident. Other signs include:

- oedema of the lower legs
- venous/stasis/gravitational eczema (see p. 662)
- brown pigmentation from haemosiderin
- lipodermatosclerosis (the combination of induration, reddish-brown pigmentation and inflammation) – a fibrosing panniculitis of the subcutaneous tissue
- scarring white atrophy with telangiectasia (*atrophie blanche*).

Management is with graduated multilayer compression bandaging and leg elevation to improve venous return. Three- or four-layer bandaging is suitable for people who are immobile, and two-layer bandaging for those who are mobile. Doppler studies (ankle:brachial pressure index) should be performed before compression to exclude significant arterial disease. Treatment can be delivered effectively in the community by appropriately trained nurses. Non-adherent dressings are used to keep the ulcer moist. Alternative dressings (alginate, hydrogel, hydrocolloid) may be helpful for heavy exudate and slough. With adequate compression, up to 80% of ulcers can be healed within 6 months. Slower healing rates occur in patients with poor mobility, bilateral disease

and very large ulcers that have been present for over 6 months. Diuretics are sometimes indicated to reduce oedema, and pentoxifylline may be a useful adjunct. Microbial swabs and antibiotics are indicated only when there are clinical signs of infection or cellulitis.

Painful venous leg ulcers require adequate analgesia. Split-thickness skin grafting can aid healing in resistant cases. Support stockings (individually fitted) should be worn for life after healing, to lessen recurrence. Underlying venous disease should be assessed. Modern vascular surgical interventions may accelerate healing and reduce the risk of ulcer recurrence.

Arterial ulcers

Arterial ulcers present as punched-out, painful lesions higher up the leg or on the feet in people with underlying peripheral vascular disease, particularly smokers. The affected leg is cold and pale with loss of hair. Peripheral pulses are absent or weak and Doppler ultrasound studies can confirm underlying arterial disease.

Management depends on keeping the ulcer clean and covered, adequate analgesia and vascular surgical intervention if appropriate. Compression bandaging must be avoided.

Neuropathic ulcers

Neuropathic ulcers usually occur over pressure areas of the feet, such as the metatarsal heads, owing to repeated trauma. They are usually associated with diabetes and peripheral neuropathy. In some developing countries, leprosy is a common cause.

Management involves keeping the ulcer clean and reducing pressure or trauma to the affected area. People with diabetes need meticulous foot care and correctly fitting shoes (see p. 733).

Pressure ulcers (decubitus ulcers, bedsores)

Pressure ulcers or sores are a severe manifestation of pressure-induced skin and soft tissue injury. They affect elderly, immobile, unconscious or paralysed patients and are due to skin and soft tissue ischaemia from sustained pressure over a bony prominence: most commonly, the heel and sacrum. Healthy individuals feel the discomfort of continued pressure, even during sleep, and relieve pressure by changing body position. Pressure injuries may be graded and range from non-blanchable erythema of intact skin (stage 1) to deep ulcers extending to the bone (stage IV).

There are numerous risk factors for the development of pressure ulcers (**Box 22.22**). The majority of ulcers arise in hospital, with approximately 70% appearing in the first 2 weeks of hospitalization and 70% occurring in orthopaedic patients, especially those on

Prolonged immobility
- Paraplegia
- Arthritis
- Severe physical disease
- Apathy
- Operation and postoperative states
- Plaster casts
- Intensive care

Decreased sensation
- Coma
- Neurological disease

- Diabetes mellitus
- Drug-induced sleep

Vascular disease
- Atherosclerosis
- Diabetes mellitus
- Scleroderma
- Vasculitis

Poor nutrition
- Anaemia
- Hypoalbuminaemia
- Vitamin C or zinc deficiency

traction. Deep ulcers are associated with a high mortality rate. The early sign of red/blue skin discoloration can lead rapidly to ulcers within hours. Leaving patients on hard emergency room trolleys or sitting them in chairs for prolonged periods must be avoided.

Management

See **Box 22.23**.

Prevention

Prevention is better than cure and a risk assessment should be undertaken on newly admitted patients. The best-known risk assessment tools are the Norton Scale and Waterlow Pressure Ulcer Risk Assessment, which yield a numerical score (**Box 22.24**). Specialist tissue viability nurses help assess risk, deliver care and train other clinical staff.

Box 22.23 Management of pressure ulcers

- Ensure bed rest with pillows and fleeces to keep pressure off bony areas (e.g. sacrum and heels) and prevent friction
- Provide air-filled cushions for patients in wheelchairs
- Provide special pressure-relieving mattresses and beds
- Maintain regular turning but avoid pressure on hips
- Give adequate nutrition
- Apply non-irritant occlusive moist dressings (e.g. hydrocolloid)
- Prescribe adequate analgesia (may need opiates)
- Consider plastic surgery (debridement and grafting in selected cases)
- Treat the underlying condition

Lymphatic disease

Lymphoedema

Impaired lymphatic fluid drainage leads to chronic non-pitting oedema with reduced tissue immunity and increased fat deposition. It most commonly affects the legs and tends to progress with age. It is associated with an increased risk of cellulitis, which often becomes recurrent. The subcutaneous tissues become thickened and indurated, and the overlying skin develops a warty texture. Affected limbs may become grossly enlarged. Lymphoedema can be primary (and present early in life) and due to an inherited

i **Box 22.24 Pressure ulcer risk assessment tools**

Norton Scale for pressure ulcers[a]

Physical			Neurology			Activity			Mobility			Incontinence	
4			Good	4		Alert	4		Ambulant	4		Full	4	None
3			Fair	3		Apathetic	3		Walks with help	3		Slightly	3	Occasionally incontinent
2			Poor	2		Confused	2		Not bound	2		Limited	2	Usually incontinent
1			Very poor	1		Stupor	1		Bedfast	1		Very limited; immobile	1	Doubly incontinent

Waterlow Pressure Ulcer Risk Assessment[b]

Build/weight for height		Visual skin type		Continence		Mobility		Sex/Age		Appetite	
Average	0	Healthy	0	Complete	0	Fully mobile	0	Male	1	Average	0
Above average	2	Tissue paper	1	Occasionally incontinent	1	Restricted/difficult	1	Female	2	Poor	1
Below average	3	Dry	1	Catheter/incontinent of faeces	2	Restless/fidgety	2	14–18	1	Anorectic	2
		Oedematous	1	Doubly incontinent	3	Apathetic	3	50–64	2		
		Clammy	1			Inert/traction	4	65–75	3		
		Discoloured	2					75–80	4		
		Broken/spot	3					81+	5		

Special risk factors

1. Poor nutrition, e.g. terminal cachexia	8	
2. Sensory deprivation, e.g. diabetes, paraplegia, cerebrovascular disease	6	
3. High-dose anti-inflammatory or steroid in use	3	
4. Smoking 10+ per day	1	
5. Orthopaedic surgery/fracture below waist	3	

Assessment value

At risk	10
High risk	15
Very high risk	20

[a]Low scores carry a high risk.
[b]See assessment value, bottom right of table.

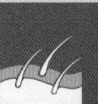

abnormality of lymphatic vessels (e.g. Milroy's disease), or can be secondary and due to obstruction of lymphatic vessels (e.g. filarial infection or malignant disease).

Management is with compression stockings and physical massage. Causes of high central venous pressure, low albumin and local inflammation should be treated. Long-term antibiotics are indicated for recurrent cellulitis (see p. 669), as each episode of cellulitis causes further damage to the lymph vessels. Surgery should be avoided.

Further reading

Gohel MS, Heatly F, Liu X et al. A randomized trial of early endovenous ablation in venous ulceration. *N Engl J Med* 2018: 378:2105–2114.
National Institute for Health and Care Excellence. *Clinical Knowledge Summary: Leg Ulcer – Venous*. NICE 2019; https://cks.nice.org.uk/leg-ulcer-venous.
National Institute for Health and Care Excellence. *NICE Clinical Guideline 179: Pressure Ulcers: Prevention and Management*. NICE 2014; https://www.nice.org.uk/guidance/CG179.

Systemic malignant disease

Certain rashes may be a non-metastatic manifestation of an underlying malignancy: these are the ***paraneoplastic dermatoses*** (**Box 22.25**). Rarely, internal malignancies can metastasize to the skin, where they usually present as papules or nodules that may ulcerate.

Genetic disease

Neurofibromatosis type 1

Type 1 neurofibromatosis (von Recklinghausen's disease) is an autosomal dominant condition caused by mutations in the *NF1* gene. It often presents in childhood with multiple *café-au-lait* spots (brown macules, >5mm in diameter, and more than five lesions) and axillary freckling. Learning difficulties and skeletal dysplasia can occur. Iris Lisch nodules may be seen on slit-lamp examination. Neurofibromas appear in adulthood as fleshy skin polyps and smooth soft dermal tumours, and can be extensive. A number of endocrine disorders are rarely associated, including phaeochromocytoma, acromegaly and Addison's disease.

Tuberous sclerosis

The tuberous sclerosis complex (TSC) is an autosomal dominant condition of variable severity, characterized by a range of benign or hamartomatous tumours. The main clinical features are learning and behavioural difficulties, epilepsy and skin lesions:

- adenoma sebaceum (reddish papules or fibromas around the nose)
- periungual fibroma (nodules arising from the nail bed)
- shagreen patches (firm, flesh-coloured plaques on the trunk)
- ash-leaf hypopigmentation (pale macules best seen with Wood's UV lamp)
- forehead plaque (indurated, flesh-coloured patch)
- *café-au-lait* patches.

Internal hamartomas can arise in the heart, lung, kidney, retina and central nervous system. Inhibition of the mammalian target of rapamycin (mTOR) signalling pathway with drugs such as rapamycin may help to shrink TSC-associated tumours.

Ehlers–Danlos syndrome

Ehlers–Danlos syndrome (see also p. 432) refers to a group of inherited disorders of connective tissue that affect the structure and function of the skin, eyes, ligament, joints, blood vessels and internal organs. The underlying defects are varied and involve abnormalities of collagen fibril synthesis and extracellular matrix molecules. They are characterized by joint hypermobility, easy bruising and lax skin that heals with tissue paper scars.

Pseudoxanthoma elasticum

Pseudoxanthoma elasticum is a rare autosomal recessive disease involving fragmentation and calcification of elastic tissue in the dermis, blood vessels and eye. The skin changes of slackness, wrinkling and yellowing (resembling plucked chicken skin) are most evident in the flexures, especially the sides of the neck. Non-cutaneous features include recurrent gastrointestinal bleeding, vascular occlusion and aneurysms, and angioid streaks on the retina.

PHOTOSENSITIVITY

Photosensitivity disorders are characterized by abnormal sensitivity to the UV and sometimes the visible range of the solar spectrum. Several rare skin diseases are primarily caused by sunlight (primary photodermatoses) and a larger number are aggravated by sun exposure (photoaggravated photodermatoses), including connective tissue diseases (dermatomyositis and cutaneous lupus). The rashes of pellagra (see p. 1241) and the porphyrias (see p. 755), and certain drug hypersensitivities, are also triggered by UV exposure (see p. 697) (**Box 22.26**).

ℹ Box 22.25 Non-metastatic cutaneous manifestations of underlying malignancy

Dermatosis	Tumour
Dermatomyositis	Lung, gastrointestinal tract, genitourinary tract
Acanthosis nigricans	Gastrointestinal tract, lung, liver
Paget's disease of the nipple (localized eczema-like changes on nipple and areola)	Ductal breast carcinoma
Erythroderma	Lymphoma/leukaemia
Tylosis (thickened palms/soles)	Oesophageal carcinoma
Tripe palms (velvet palms)	Pulmonary, gastric
Ichthyosis (dry flaking of skin)	Lymphoma
Erythema gyratum repens (concentric rings of erythema, which change rapidly)	Lung, breast
Necrolytic migratory erythema (burning, geographic and spreading annular areas of erythema)	Glucagonoma
Paraneoplastic pemphigus	Lymphoproliferative

❓ Box 22.26 Differential diagnosis of photosensitive rashes

Photoexacerbated/provoked rashes

Autoimmune rheumatic disorders
- Lupus erythematosus
- Dermatomyositis

Metabolic disease
- Porphyrias (see p. 755)
- Pellagra (see p. 1241)

Drugs
- Thiazides
- Phenothiazines
- Tetracyclines
- Amiodarone

Plant phototoxins
- Phytophotodermatitis (photosensitivity induced by contact of the skin with certain plants, e.g. celery, hogweed, rue, lime, fig tree)

Skin disease
- Rarely, atopic eczema, psoriasis, lichen planus (these usually improve in sunlight)

Idiopathic photodermatoses
- Polymorphic light eruption
- Chronic actinic dermatitis
- Solar urticaria

BLISTERING AND BULLOUS SKIN DISEASE

There are many causes of skin blisters, the most common being **infection** (HSV, chickenpox, impetigo, cellulitis), **insect bites** – especially on the lower legs – and **trauma** (burns and friction). Blistering may also be a feature of eczema, especially on the hands and feet (pompholyx, see p. 663).

Very rarely, blistering is due to skin fragility caused by genetically determined abnormalities in the structural proteins of the dermo-epidermal junction and basal keratinocytes (**mechanobullous diseases**) or their destruction by antibodies in autoimmune (**immunobullous**) disease. The level at which fragility and blistering occur varies according to disease and affects the clinical presentation (see **Fig. 22.43**). It can be demonstrated by light and electron microscopy and immunofluorescence (IMF) studies. Autoantibody deposits (at the BMZ or between keratinocytes) can be identified by direct IMF of affected (perilesional) skin, and indirect IMF identifies autoantibodies in serum.

Immunobullous diseases

Pemphigus

Pemphigus vulgaris is a rare and potentially life-threatening blistering disease. It is more common in Ashkenazi Jews and people from the Indian subcontinent. It may affect all ages but usually starts in adulthood. Pathogenic IgG4 antibodies against desmosomal proteins (desmoglein 1 and 3) lead to loss of keratinocyte adhesion in the skin and mucous membranes, causing superficial (intraepidermal) blisters, erosions and mucosal ulcers.

Oral involvement is common and is the presenting sign in up to 50% of patients. Skin lesions appear as flaccid blisters that rupture easily, leaving weeping and crusted erosions. Blisters can be extended with gentle lateral pressure (Nikolsky's sign).

Pemphigus foliaceus is a rarer variant, in which the target antigen is desmoglein 1. This antigen is not expressed in the oral mucosa, which is therefore unaffected. Desmoglein 1 is predominantly expressed in the upper epidermis, which detaches, leaving crusts and erosions rather than blisters. It usually affects the seborrhoeic areas before becoming more widespread. Endemic pemphigus foliaceus occurs in the Limão Verde area of Brazil and is thought to be triggered by an infectious agent carried by biting insects. A pemphigus foliaceus-like rash can be induced by drugs (e.g. captopril, penicillamine).

Paraneoplastic pemphigus is a very rare malignancy-associated disorder characterized by painful oral erosions and a polymorphic inflammatory ash. It is usually associated with a lymphoproliferative neoplasm.

Direct IMF of perilesional skin in pemphigus shows intercellular IgG deposition. Circulating anti-epidermal antibodies can also be detected and their titre correlates with disease activity. Histology of affected skin shows intraepidermal cleavage above the basal cell layer with separation of individual keratinocytes (acantholysis) in pemphigus vulgaris. The split occurs higher in the epidermis in pemphigus foliaceus.

Management

High-dose systemic corticosteroids are usually effective in controlling pemphigus, followed by longer-term, steroid-sparing immunosuppressive drugs including azathioprine, cyclophosphamide, methotrexate and rituximab (an anti-CD20 monoclonal antibody).

Bullous pemphigoid

Bullous pemphigoid is more common than pemphigus in Western Europe and usually affects adults over 60. Pemphigoid gestationis is a rare variant that occurs in pregnancy and post-partum. Autoantibodies against a 230 kDa or 180 kDa hemidesmosomal protein ('bullous pemphigoid antigen 1' and 'type XVII collagen')

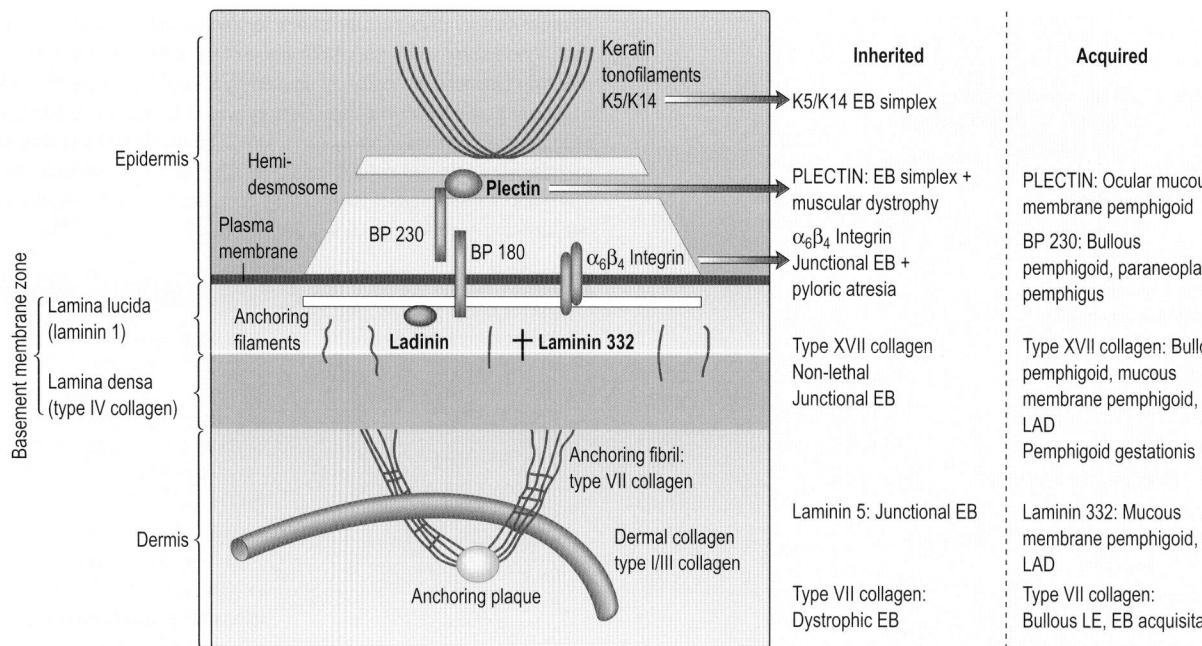

Fig. 22.43 Section of the basement membrane zone. The structural sites of damage in bullous disorders. EB, epidermolysis bullosa; K, keratin; LAD, linear IgA disease; LE, lupus erythematosus.

play a pathogenic role and cause a split through the epidermal BMZ (see p. 654). This can be seen on routine histology as a subepidermal split. Direct IMF shows deposition of IgG and complement at the dermo-epidermal junction. Lesions are often itchy and present as large, tense, serous or haemorrhagic blisters (bullae) with an inflamed ('urticated') base. Blistering may be widespread, affecting the torso and limbs, especially the lower abdomen and thighs (**Fig. 22.44**). Mucosal ulceration is not prominent, except in a rare variant of pemphigoid, mucous membrane pemphigoid (formerly called cicatricial pemphigoid). This presents with erosions and ulceration of the mucosal surfaces and scarring eye disease, with fusion of the eyelids, corneal damage and visual loss.

Management

Oral corticosteroids (prednisolone 0.5 mg/kg per day) are usually initiated for disease control, with a steroid-sparing drug such as azathioprine or mycophenolate mofetil for long-term management. These drugs require careful monitoring in the elderly due to their increased risk of adverse drug effects, which contributes to the increased mortality associated with pemphigoid. Oral tetracyclines are also used for their anti-inflammatory actions and may be safer drugs. Mild localized pemphigoid can be managed by daily application of a very potent topical steroid to drained (popped) blisters. Treatment can usually be withdrawn after a few years but the disease often relapses.

Linear IgA disease

Linear IgA disease (LAD) is a rare pemphigoid-like disorder of adults and children caused by pathogenic IgA autoantibodies that target various BMZ proteins, including type XVII collagen and laminin-332 (see **Fig. 22.43**). The cause is unknown but LAD may be induced by drugs, especially vancomycin. Direct IMF of skin shows linear IgA deposition along the dermo-epidermal junction. LAD characteristically presents with circular clusters of golden blisters, described as a 'string of jewels' (**Fig. 22.45**). It usually responds to treatment with dapsone (see below).

Dermatitis herpetiformis

Dermatitis herpetiformis (DH) is a cutaneous manifestation of coeliac disease (see p. 1189). Both conditions are genetically determined and triggered by dietary gluten. DH presents with an intensely itchy, eczematous rash that predominantly affects the elbows, knees, scalp and buttocks. Small blisters may be visible but are often scratched away, leaving excoriations and crusted erosions. DH is more common in males (whereas coeliac disease has a female predominance); it can present at any age but usually appears in early adulthood. Nearly all patients with DH have small intestinal changes of coeliac disease (villous atrophy/inflammation) but lack gastrointestinal symptoms. Autoantibodies against tissue transglutaminase (TG) 2 occur in the serum and bowel in DH and coeliac disease, with additional IgA antibodies against TG3 occurring in DH. The latter can be demonstrated in the skin by direct IMF, which reveals granular IgA deposits in the dermal papillae and along the BMZ. Histology of DH shows subepidermal blistering and a florid infiltrate of neutrophils causing micro-abscesses in the dermal papillae.

Management

Patients should avoid all dietary gluten (see p. 1191). Treatment with dapsone or sulphonamides, sometimes at low dose, usually gives rapid relief from itch. If a strict gluten-free diet is followed, oral medication can usually be withdrawn after 2 years. Dapsone causes mild dose-related haemolysis, which is usually well tolerated except in cardiorespiratory disease. It is contraindicated in people with glucose-6-phosphate dehydrogenase deficiency, as they are at risk of severe drug-induced haemolysis. Other rare adverse effects of dapsone include hepatitis, drug hypersensitivity syndrome (including DRESS, see p. 698) and peripheral neuropathy.

Further reading

Collin P, Salmi TT, Hervonen K et al. Dermatitis herpetiformis: a cutaneous manifestation of coeliac disease. *Ann Med* 2017; 49:23–31.

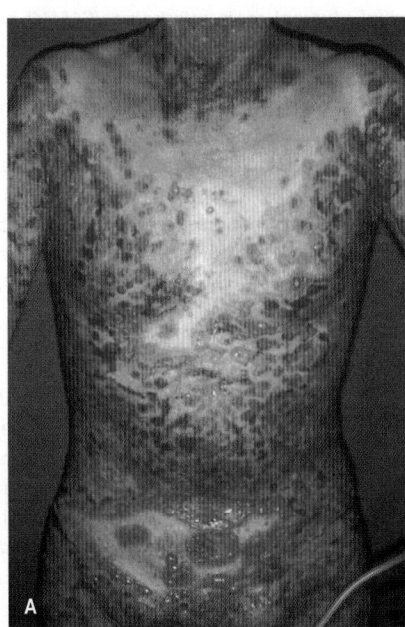

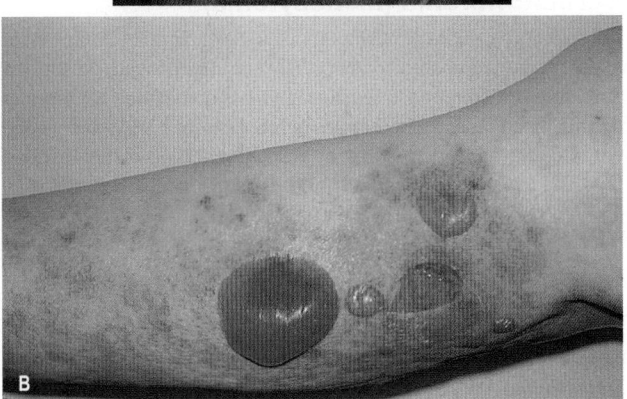

Fig. 22.44 Bullous pemphigoid. (A) Widespread blistering. **(B)** Large, tense bullae.

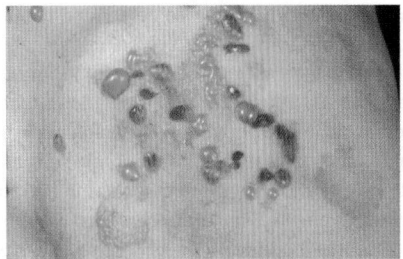

Fig. 22.45 Linear IgA disease. Typical circular clustering of blisters.

Mechanobullous diseases (epidermolysis bullosa)

This rare group of inherited skin diseases is caused by defective or absent structural skin proteins, leading to fragile skin that blisters with minimal trauma. Blisters and erosions usually appear at or shortly after birth. The degree of skin fragility is highly variable, ranging from mild friction blisters to severe, extensive and life-limiting skin loss ('butterfly babies'). There are three broad groups of disorders:

- **Epidermolysis bullosa simplex** is the mildest form and causes localized blisters on the hands and feet that heal without scarring. It is inherited as an autosomal dominant trait and caused by synthesis of abnormal cytoskeleton proteins (e.g. keratins 5 and 14) in the basal epidermis.
- **Dystrophic epidermolysis bullosa** is a debilitating, life-limiting disease characterized by deep erosions, blisters and scarring. The underlying abnormality is mutations in the type VII collagen gene that cause impaired or absent synthesis of anchoring fibrils in the deep part of the BMZ. Mucosal involvement can affect the larynx and oesophagus, causing voice loss and dysphagia. Nails are absent and the digits may become fused by the scarring, causing mitten-like deformities. Affected individuals have a high risk of developing aggressive squamous cell carcinomas within chronically inflamed skin. There is no curative therapy at present and management is supportive.
- **Junctional epidermolysis bullosa** is the most severe form and is characterized by a split in the lamina lucida of the BMZ due to mutations in genes controlling synthesis of various structural proteins (laminin-332, $\alpha_6\beta_4$ integrin, type XVII collagen). It presents at birth with widespread blistering and areas of absent skin, and is usually fatal in early childhood.

Investigations and management

Investigation and treatment of epidermolysis bullosa should be carried out in a specialist centre. Ultrastructural skin tests and genetic testing provide a precise diagnosis and prognosis, and are required for genetic counselling. Prenatal diagnosis and pre-implantation diagnosis are available for severe forms of epidermolysis bullosa. Treatment options are limited to pain management and skin grafting with cultured keratinocytes. Gene therapy and bone marrow transplantation are two new approaches that are undergoing clinical trials.

SKIN TUMOURS

Benign skin tumours

Melanocytic naevi

Melanocytic naevi are the most common benign neoplasm in humans. **Congenital melanocytic naevi** are present at birth in 1–2% of newborns. Small solitary lesions are common and harmless, but larger lesions (>20 cm diameter) and multiple smaller naevi may be associated with neurological complications, including epilepsy and an increased risk of melanoma. **Acquired melanocytic naevi (moles)** appear in childhood, adolescence and early adult life, increasing in size and number. Benign naevi usually have even pigmentation and regular borders. They start as flat brown macules with proliferation of melanocytes at the dermo-epidermal junction (junctional naevi). With later downward growth of melanocytes into the dermis (compound naevi), the mole becomes raised and palpable, eventually maturing into an intradermal naevus with

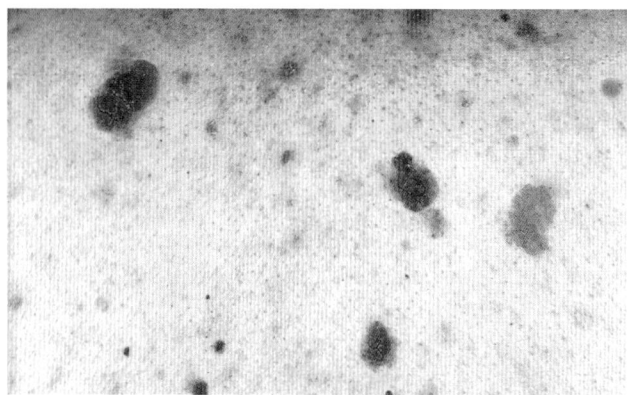

Fig. 22.46 Seborrhoeic warts (basal cell papillomas).

loss of pigment. Although the risk of malignant transformation of a benign mole is extremely low, the presence of more than 100 common naevi is associated with a sevenfold increase in the risk of melanoma.

Atypical naevi are acquired moles that have irregular pigment and are larger (>5 mm) than common naevi, often with ill-defined, 'fuzzy' borders. They may show dysplastic features on histology but the clinical and microscopic features do not always tally. Atypical naevi are associated with an increased risk of melanoma. Individuals with **familial atypical mole syndrome (FAMM)** have a large number of atypical naevi and a high lifetime risk of melanoma. They require long-term follow-up with serial photography and dermoscopy of atypical lesions. Atypical naevi that lack features of melanoma and do not warrant excision on presentation can be reviewed and rephotographed at 3-monthly intervals to detect early features of malignant change.

Blue naevus is an acquired blue–grey mole caused by a deeper proliferation of melanocytes in the mid-dermis.

Basal cell papilloma (seborrhoeic keratosis/wart)

This is an extremely common, harmless growth that affects older adults and is caused by overgrowth of the basal keratinocytes. Lesions range from flesh-coloured to very dark brown, and have a greasy, 'stuck-on' appearance (**Fig. 22.46**). The surface is rough and warty, and may contain tiny keratin cysts. They can be removed under local anaesthetic with curettage, or treated with cryotherapy or electrodesiccation.

Dermatofibroma (histiocytoma)

Dermatofibromas are firm, smooth, pink–beige nodules, which have a peripheral pigmented margin. They are often found on the leg and are more common in females. There is sometimes a history of trauma or an insect bite. The lesion consists of histiocytes, blood vessels and varying degrees of fibrosis. Excision is not needed unless lesions are symptomatic or there is diagnostic uncertainty.

Epidermoid cyst ('sebaceous cyst') and pilar cyst

Epidermoid cysts are cystic swellings derived from an occluded follicle. They have a central punctum and contain 'cheesy' keratinous matter. Cysts may enlarge and can become secondarily infected and inflamed. Pilar cysts are similar lesions that occur on the scalp. They may be multiple and familial. Symptomatic cysts can be excised under local anaesthetic.

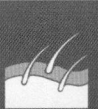

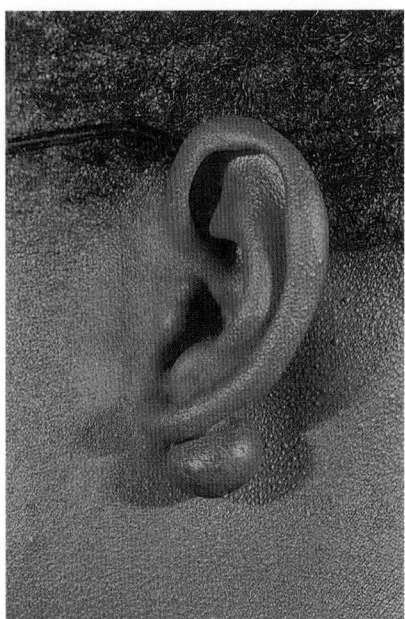

Fig. 22.47 Keloid scar of the lobe of the ear.

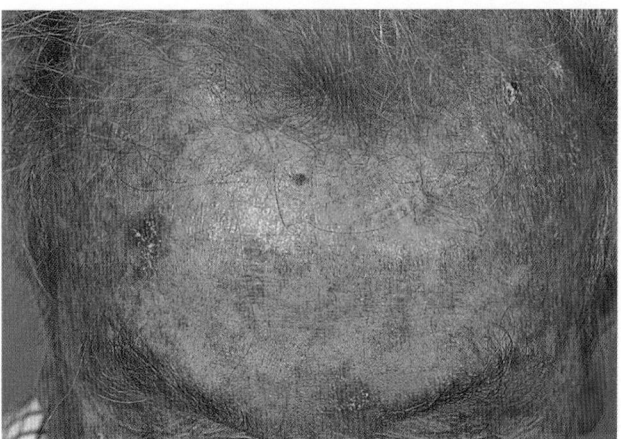

Fig. 22.48 Solar keratoses with background actinic damage.

Pyogenic granuloma

Pyogenic granulomas are benign vascular proliferations that present as rapidly growing, friable, red nodules that bleed easily. They may follow minor trauma and often occur on the face or fingers. Excision is advisable and lesions should always be sent for histology to exclude amelanotic malignant melanoma.

Cherry angioma (Campbell de Morgan spots)

Cherry angiomas are benign angiokeratomas that appear as tiny, pinpoint, red papules, especially on the trunk, and increase with age. No treatment is required.

Keloids and hypertrophic scars

Abnormal wound healing with excessive dermal fibrosis leads to hypertrophic scars and keloid formation. Hypertrophic scars remain confined to the borders of the original wound and usually regress spontaneously. Keloids (**Fig. 22.47**) can arise spontaneously or after minimal trauma, and proliferate and enlarge beyond the wound margins. They are often itchy and tend to affect young, dark-skinned adults. Sites of predilection include the shoulders, upper back and chest, earlobes and chin. Treatment options include silicone gel or dressings, pressure garments, cryotherapy and intralesional corticosteroids. Non-essential surgery should be avoided.

Dysplastic/pre-malignant skin lesions

Actinic (solar) keratoses

These are common on the sun-exposed areas of fair-skinned individuals in later life, especially bald scalps. They appear as scaly, erythematous papules or patches and feel gritty and rough. The surrounding skin usually shows signs of chronic sun damage (**Fig. 22.48**), with wrinkles and solar lentigines. A small minority (<1%) of actinic keratoses undergo malignant transformation into squamous cell carcinoma. Lesion-based treatments include cryotherapy and curettage and cautery. Field treatments, aimed at clearing visible and subclinical lesions over a larger area, include topical 5-fluorouracil, imiquimod and diclofenac.

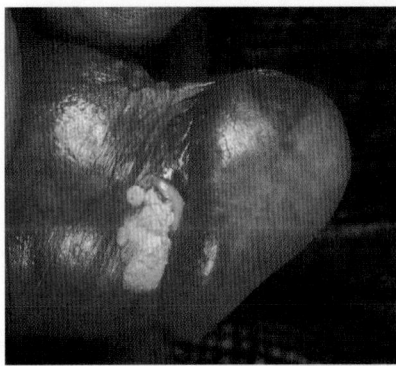

Fig. 22.49 Erythroplasia of glans penis (penile intraepithelial neoplasia).

Topical photodynamic therapy (PDT) using 5-aminolaevulinic acid or its methyl ester is another option, but is expensive and may be painful.

Bowen's disease (intraepithelial carcinoma)

This is an indolent form of intraepidermal (*in situ*) squamous cell carcinoma that rarely progresses to invasive disease. It typically affects the lower legs in fair-skinned women or the torso in men, and is thought to be caused by chronic UV exposure. Lesions appear as a slowly enlarging, well-demarcated, scaly red patch or plaque resembling psoriasis but lacking thick silvery scale. A variant of Bowen's disease can affect the genital mucosa and is referred to as vulval, penile or anal intraepithelial neoplasia. This presents with non-specific erythematous patches ('erythroplasia', **Fig. 22.49**) or warty papules (Bowenoid papulosis). There is a strong link with HPV-16 and 18 infection. Genital Bowen's disease is more common in immunosuppressed individuals, including those with HIV, and perianal disease may extend into the rectum. Treatment options are similar to those for actinic keratosis.

Keratoacanthoma

Keratoacanthomas are rapidly growing epidermal tumours that develop as a red papule with a central crater-like, crusty keratinous plug (**Fig. 22.50**). They occur on sun-exposed skin in later life and often reach 2–3 cm in diameter. Although they regress spontaneously after about 3 months, leaving a pitted scar, they are usually excised, as it can be extremely difficult to distinguish them from squamous cell carcinoma.

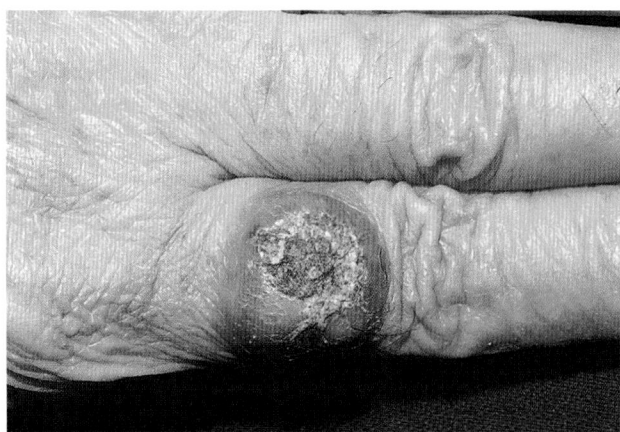

Fig. 22.50 Keratoacanthoma.

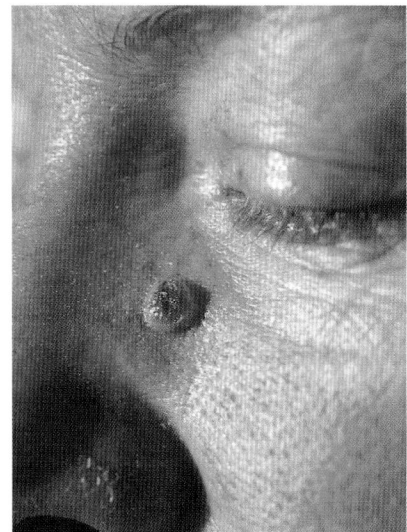

Fig. 22.51 Ulcerating basal cell carcinoma.

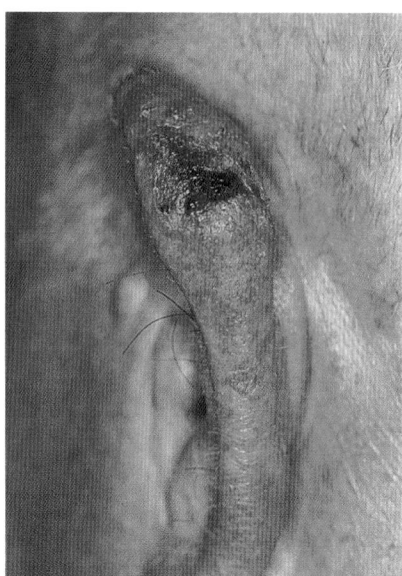

Fig. 22.52 Squamous cell carcinoma.

Malignant skin tumours

Basal cell carcinoma

Basal cell carcinomas (BCCs) are the most common form of skin cancer and their incidence is increasing by 10% a year worldwide. Fair-skinned elderly individuals in sunny climates are at greatest risk but other genetic factors are also involved. The exact aetiology of BCCs is unknown but they are thought to arise from pluripotential cells in the basal epidermis or follicular structures. Mutations in *PTCH1*, the human homologue of the 'Patched' gene that regulates the Hedgehog intracellular signalling pathway, have been detected in sporadic BCCs and Gorlin's syndrome (hereditary BCC syndrome). BCCs typically appear as a slowly enlarging, pearly or shiny nodule on the head and neck area, which bleeds easily with minor trauma and fails to heal (nodulocystic BCC). The border of ulcerated lesions is raised, with a pearly appearance (**Fig. 22.51**) and overlying, branch-like (arborizing) telangiectasia. Pigmented, superficial and morpheic (scar-like) variants exist. Although BCCs have minimal metastatic potential, they cause significant morbidity by local invasion into adjacent tissues: hence the common term 'rodent ulcer'.

Management

The treatment of choice for most BCCs is a wide excision with histology to ensure complete removal of the tumour with adequate margins. Mohs micrographic surgery is preferred for morpheic BCCs and tumours involving the nasal creases, as these are more likely to recur. Superficial BCCs can be managed with non-surgical treatment, including cryotherapy, photodynamic therapy and topical imiquimod. Radiotherapy remains an option in those who are unable to tolerate surgery. Vismodegib inhibits the Hedgehog signalling pathway and normalizes keratinocyte proliferation. It can halt or even clear advanced or inoperable BCC, but is very expensive and may be poorly tolerated due to its adverse effects.

Squamous cell carcinoma

Squamous cell carcinoma (SCC) is the second most common skin cancer. Like BCC, it is derived from keratinocytes. It has a higher metastatic potential than BCC and a clearer correlation with chronic cumulative UV-induced skin damage. SCC mainly affects the exposed sites of fair-skinned older people. It can arise in pre-existing solar keratoses or Bowen's disease, and can also complicate areas of chronic inflammation, as in lupus vulgaris. Rarely, multiple tumours may arise due to arsenic ingestion in early life. Multiple aggressive tumours also occur in people who are immunosuppressed, such as transplant recipients.

Clinically, SCCs are enlarging, ill-defined, keratotic or warty, inflamed plaques or nodules that may ulcerate and bleed easily (**Fig. 22.52**). The risk of metastasis to lymph nodes increases in SCC with 'high-risk' features, which guides the need for long-term follow-up (**Box 22.27**).

Management

In the UK, patients with suspected SCC should be referred urgently for specialist assessment by the local hospital's multidisciplinary skin cancer team. Treatment is complete surgical excision with a wide margin (≥5 mm). Radiotherapy is also used. Education about sun avoidance is key to reducing the risk of further SCC development.

Lentigo maligna

This pigmented macule occurs on sun-damaged skin, usually of the face, in elderly people ('Hutchinson's melanotic freckle'). At first it resembles a solar lentigo (see p. 693) but it enlarges considerably

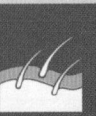

over several years and has an asymmetrical border and irregular pigmentation. Lentigo maligna represents a slow-growing intraepidermal form of melanoma, similar to a melanoma *in situ*, where malignant cells grow radially without dermal invasion. However, invasive disease, lentigo maligna melanoma (see next section), may occur, especially in larger lesions. Treatment is by excision if possible but tumour margins are difficult to define clinically. Confocal microscopy or excision by Mohs' technique can help improve margin control. Complete removal with wide margins may involve disfiguring surgery, and although its cure rate is low, topical imiquimod may be an alternative when surgery is contraindicated.

Malignant melanoma

Malignant melanoma (or just 'melanoma') is the most serious form of skin cancer, as although it represents only 4% of cases of skin cancer, it causes 80% of skin cancer deaths. The incidence increases with age but it may also affect young people. The increasing incidence in recent years is thought to be due to more extensive recreational sun exposure, especially intermittent intense exposure (sunbathing in particular) and sunburn in childhood. Other risk factors include fair skin, multiple melanocytic naevi, a family history of melanoma and immunosuppression. About 75% of cutaneous melanomas arise *de novo* from normal skin, the remainder arising from a pre-existing naevus. A number of oncogenes and tumour suppressor proteins have been implicated in the pathogenesis. About 60% of human melanomas have an activating mutation in the BRAF V600 protein kinase, which is now a target for 'personalized' chemotherapy (see later).

Diagnosis of melanoma is not always easy but the clinical signs listed in **Box 22.28** help distinguish malignant from benign moles. Examination with a dermatoscope (a hand-held polarized light source with magnification) aids clinical diagnosis and is an essential skill for clinicians who assess pigmented lesions.

Four clinical types exist:
- **Lentigo maligna melanoma** is invasive tumour that develops within pre-existing lentigo maligna. It is usually apparent as a new nodule.
- **Superficial spreading malignant melanoma** is a large, flat, irregularly pigmented lesion that grows laterally before vertical invasion develops.
- **Nodular malignant melanoma** (**Fig. 22.53**) is the most aggressive type. It presents as a rapidly growing pigmented nodule, which bleeds or ulcerates. Rarely, it is amelanotic (non-pigmented) and can mimic pyogenic granuloma.
- **Acral lentiginous malignant melanomas** arise as pigmented lesions on the palm or sole or under the nail, and usually present late. They may not be related to sun exposure.

Management

In the UK, all people with suspected melanoma should be referred urgently (2-week wait pathway) to the local hospital's multidisciplinary skin cancer team. Surgery remains the definitive treatment

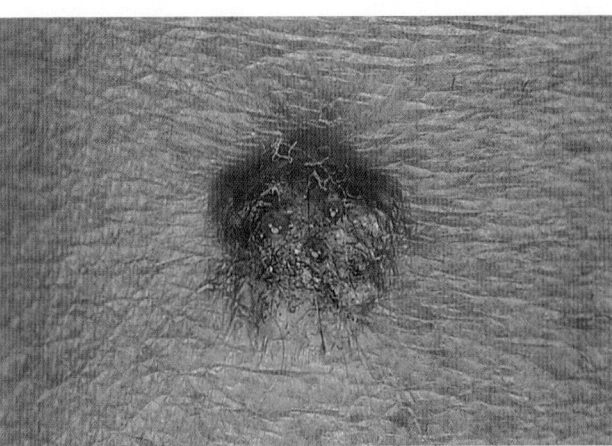

Fig. 22.53 Nodular malignant melanoma.

for primary melanoma and early wide excision of thin tumours is usually curative. Suspicious lesions should be completely and promptly excised with a narrow (2 mm) margin for review by a dermatopathologist experienced in melanoma diagnosis. The pathological staging of the primary melanoma depends on the Breslow thickness of the melanoma – that is, the depth of dermal invasion – and whether the tumour is ulcerated. The 8th *American Joint Committee on Cancer (AJCC) melanoma staging system*, published in 2017, defines four broad categories of tumour, T1–4, ranging from T1a (<0.8 mm thickness without ulceration) to T4b (>4.0 mm with ulceration). These categories guide the margins of the subsequent wide local excision and the likely benefit from a sentinel lymph node biopsy (SLNB) to detect occult metastases in the adjacent lymph nodes. The latest NICE guidelines recommend that SLNB should be offered to patients with stage 1B–2C melanoma with a Breslow thickness of more than 1 mm. Patients with clinically evident lymphadenopathy or positive SLNB are further evaluated with positron emission tomography–computed tomography (PET-CT) to detect distant metastases.

Treatment for metastatic melanoma (stages 3 and 4) has been revolutionized in the last few years with the advent of targeted therapy. This includes the oral tyrosine kinase inhibitors vemurafenib and dabrafenib, and the MEK inhibitor trametinib for patients whose melanomas demonstrate the *BRAF V600* mutation. They are more effective than conventional chemotherapy when given in combination, but toxicity and tumour resistance are limitations. Immunotherapy with immune checkpoint-blocking agents, including CTLA4 antibody (ipilimumab) and programmed death 1 protein antibody (PD-1 antibody – pembrolizumab, nivolumab), has led to significant improvements in survival for patients with advanced melanoma with tolerable toxicity.

Type	Wavelength	Properties
Visible radiation (visible light)	400–700 nm	Visible light
Ultraviolet A (UVA)	400–315 nm	Long wave, black light, not absorbed by the ozone layer
Ultraviolet B (UVB)	315–280 nm	Medium wave, mostly absorbed by the ozone layer
Ultraviolet C (UVC)	280–100 nm	Short wave, germicidal, completely absorbed by the ozone layer and atmosphere

UV exposure and photoprotection

The solar spectrum at the earth's surface includes visible light and medium- and long-wave ultraviolet (UV): that is, UVB and UVA. Short-wavelength UVC is filtered out by the atmosphere (**Box 22.29**). UVB and UVA are potentially mutagenic and carcinogenic, especially in fair-skinned people. They cause sunburn (predominantly UVB), premature ageing or photodamage (predominantly UVA). UV radiation has immunosuppressive effects that enhance skin cancer development. Systemic medication may lead to abnormal sensitivity to UV and phototoxic or photoallergic rashes. This is thought to be the underlying mechanism behind the recently identified increase in risk of non-melanoma skin cancer among patients on long-term thiazide therapy.

Sunscreens protect against UVA and UVB irradiation but are no substitute for protective clothing and restriction of exposure, especially in young children. They work by absorbing or filtering UV radiation (e.g. benzophenones, cinnamates, salicylates) or reflecting it (zinc/titanium dioxide). New sunscreen chemicals have been developed to give better protection, and the particle size of reflective sunscreens can be reduced (micronized) to improve their cosmetic acceptability. Modern creams are formulated to provide broad-spectrum protection against UVA and UVB. The sun protection factor (SPF) is a measure of UVB protection and the degree to which exposure can be prolonged before burning. However, in many cases, sunscreens are not applied in adequate amounts and so do not provide the SPF as labelled. UV-absorbing chemicals may occasionally cause allergic contact dermatitis and, in rare instances, photoallergic contact dermatitis (where the sunscreen becomes allergenic with UV exposure).

Sunlight is the main source of vitamin D and individuals who do not have photosensitivity benefit from short-term sun exposure (without burning) to maintain levels. This is particularly necessary for people with darker skins living in temperate climates, who are at risk of vitamin D deficiency. Advice about sun protection therefore needs to take into account the individual's skin type.

Further reading

http://www.bad.org.uk/for-the-public/skin-cancer/. *British Association of Dermatologists Sunscreen fact sheet.*
http://www.sunsmart.org.uk/. *Information from Cancer Research UK on sun, UV and cancer.*

Primary cutaneous T-cell lymphoma (mycosis fungoides)

Mycosis fungoides is a rare lymphoproliferative disease that usually follows an indolent course. It presents with pruritic, scaly patches, which typically start on the buttocks and can resemble eczema, psoriasis or fungal infection; asymmetry and atrophy are useful

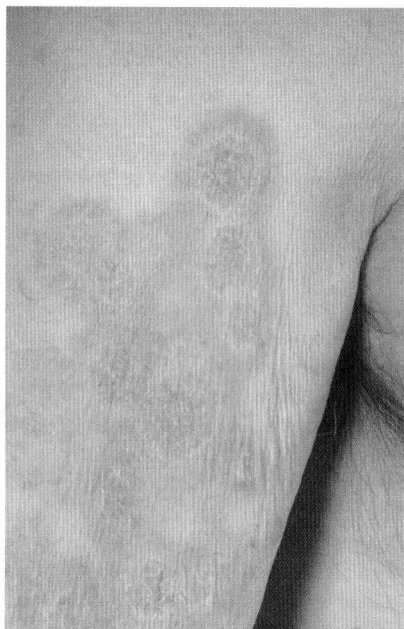

Fig. 22.54 Patch-stage mycosis fungoides.

clues (**Fig. 22.54**). Skin biopsy shows invasion of the epidermis by atypical T lymphocytes (exocytosis), and T-cell receptor gene rearrangement studies show that the infiltrate is clonal.

Occasionally, patches evolve into nodules or tumours, which may metastasize to lymph nodes and internal organs. ***Sézary's syndrome*** (see p. 407) is a rare erythrodermic variant of cutaneous T-cell lymphoma with peripheral lymphadenopathy and peripheral blood involvement; it is seen mostly in elderly men. Mycosis fungoides and Sézary's syndrome usually run chronic relapsing courses. Treatment choices depend on disease stage and extent. Patch and plaque-stage mycosis fungoides usually responds to potent topical corticosteroids and UV phototherapy. Advanced disease treatment options include radiotherapy, oral retinoids (bexarotene) and chemotherapy. Sézary's syndrome is treated with extracorporeal photopheresis, in which the patient's leucocytes are mixed with psoralen and irradiated with UVA *ex vivo*.

Kaposi's sarcoma

This tumour of vascular and lymphatic endothelium presents as purplish nodules and plaques. There are three types:

- ***The 'classic' or 'sporadic' form*** occurs in elderly males, especially Jewish people from Eastern Europe. It presents as slow-growing macules, plaques or nodules on the foot and lower limb.
- ***The 'endemic' form*** occurs in males from Central Africa and has more widespread skin and lymph node involvement. Oedema is a prominent feature.
- ***The immunosuppression-related form*** is more severe and is most common in HIV-positive men who have sex with men. Lesions are widespread with additional involvement of the oral cavity, bowel and lungs.

All three types have a strong association with human herpesvirus-8 (HHV-8) but other factors must be involved, as HHV-8 seroprevalence is up to 10% in the USA and 50% in some African countries. ART (see p. 1435) significantly reduces the incidence of Kaposi's sarcoma in people with HIV infection.

Treatment of advanced Kaposi's sarcoma is with radiotherapy, immunotherapy or chemotherapy.

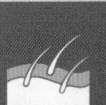

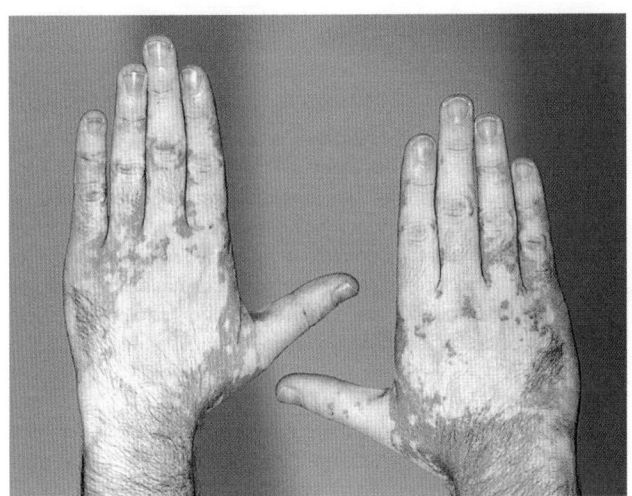

Fig. 22.55 Vitiligo of the hands. Areas of depigmentation.

Further reading

Gershenwald JE, Scolyer RA. Melanoma staging: American Joint Committee on Cancer (AJCC) 8th Edition and beyond. *Ann Surg Oncol* 2018; 25:2015–2110.
Luke JJ, Flaherty KT, Ribas A et al. Targeted agents and immunotherapies: optimizing outcomes in melanoma. *Nat Rev Clin Oncol* 2017; 14:463–482.

DISORDERS OF PIGMENTATION

Hypopigmentation

Vitiligo

Vitiligo is a chronic depigmenting skin disorder that affects 1–2% of the world population; about a third of all cases start in childhood. It is thought be due to autoimmune T cell-mediated destruction of melanocytes and is associated with other autoimmune disease, especially that of the thyroid. Vitiligo presents with asymptomatic, symmetrical, well-demarcated macules of complete pigment loss and typically affects the face, genitalia and bony prominences (**Fig. 22.55**). Pigment may be lost from overlying hair. Lesions are not inflamed. Treatment is often unsatisfactory and has no impact on the long-term outcome. Potent topical corticosteroids, topical tacrolimus and UV phototherapy may stimulate repigmentation, and this usually starts around hair follicles, giving a speckled appearance. Repigmentation is less likely in established lesions and acral sites. Sunblocks should be used to prevent burning. Patients may benefit from psychological support and skin camouflage advice.

Post-inflammatory hypopigmentation

Pale patches may be left after resolution of an inflammatory complaint, especially eczema and psoriasis. They are more noticeable in people with a dark skin or a tan and can be mistaken for vitiligo, but lesions are *hypo*pigmented rather than *de*pigmented. Pigmentation recovers over several months as long as the underlying condition has been treated. Pityriasis alba is a common hypopigmented variant of atopic eczema seen on the cheeks and arms of dark-skinned children, where there is little inflammation but prominent pallor. Hypopigmented patches are also common in pityriasis versicolor (see p. 674) and may occur in mycosis fungoides (see p. 692).

Leprosy

Tuberculoid leprosy and indeterminate leprosy (see also p. 550) can present with anaesthetic hypopigmented patches and should always be considered in people from endemic regions. Lesions may also show hair loss and decreased sweating.

Oculocutaneous albinism

This rare group of autosomal recessive disorders is caused by reduced or absent pigment synthesis in the skin, hair and eyes. It can affect all races. Individuals have pale skin, white or yellow hair, and a pink iris. Ocular manifestations include photophobia, nystagmus and a squint. Meticulous UV protection is required to prevent sunburn and reduce the risk of skin cancer.

Hyperpigmentation

Freckles (ephelides)

These extremely common pigmented macules appear in childhood after sun exposure. They fade in the winter.

Lentigines

These persistent pigmented macules look similar to freckles. They may rarely be associated with systemic syndromes (e.g. Peutz–Jeghers, see p. 1197; LEOPARD/Noonan's (*l*entigines, *E*CG abnormalities, *o*cular hypertension, *p*ulmonary stenosis, *a*bnormalities of genitalia, *r*etardation of growth and *d*eafness). Solar lentigines ('age spots', 'liver spots') are common on the dorsal hands and face and on bald scalps in older, fair-skinned people.

Café-au-lait macules

These may occur as an isolated abnormality. Multiple lesions are also a feature of neurofibromatosis types 1 and 2, tuberous sclerosis, ataxia telangiectasia, multiple endocrine neoplasia type 1 and McCune–Albright syndrome.

Melasma (chloasma)

This is a common complaint in pregnant women and in women taking hormonal contraception. Asymptomatic beige–brown patches develop on the forehead, temples and cheeks. Topical azelaic acid, retinoic acid or 2–5% hydroquinone may help reduce pigmentation. Meticulous sun protection with high SPF sunscreens is needed to prevent relapse.

Post-inflammatory hyperpigmentation

This phenomenon occurs in dark-skinned individuals at the sites of skin trauma or inflammatory rashes, such as acne, lichen planus and eczema. It improves slowly over many months.

Metabolic/endocrine effects

Generalized skin darkening can occur with chronic liver disease, especially haemochromatosis (see p. 1300), and endocrine disease.

Urticaria pigmentosa (cutaneous mastocytosis)

This disorder is caused by a benign proliferation of cutaneous mast cells. It presents most commonly in childhood as multiple pigmented macules that become red, itchy and urticated if they are rubbed (Darier's sign), and occasionally blister. Extensive mast cell degranulation can lead to systemic symptoms, such as wheeze, flushing, syncope, diarrhoea and, very rarely, anaphylaxis. This may be triggered by drugs, including aspirin and opiates, and allergens. Childhood urticaria pigmentosa usually resolves spontaneously but adult-onset disease is often persistent. Histology of skin lesions shows increased numbers of mast cells. Most cases are due to somatically acquired activating mutations of the *KIT* receptor that controls mast cell proliferation and apoptosis. Rarely, in adult and neonatal disease, mast cell infiltration may involve internal organs (bone, gastrointestinal tract, liver, spleen – *systemic mastocytosis*). There is a small risk of developing mast cell leukaemia. Treatment of cutaneous mastocytosis is aimed at controlling the symptoms of mast cell mediator release with antihistamines and cromoglicate, and minimizing the risk of anaphylaxis.

Further reading

Ezzedine K, Eleftheriadou V, Whitton M et al. Vitiligo. *Lancet* 2015; 386:74–84.
JP Hill, JM Batchelor. An approach to hypopigmentation. *BMJ* 2016; 355:i6534.

NAIL DISORDERS

- *Psoriasis* (see p. 664), *fungal infection* (p. 672) and *trauma* are the most common causes of abnormal nail growth (dystrophy).
- *Pitting* can be caused by psoriasis, alopecia areata, atopic eczema and trauma.
- *Onycholysis* (distal nail plate separation) is caused by psoriasis, thyrotoxicosis, trauma and, rarely, a phototoxic drug reaction (e.g. with tetracyclines).
- *Koilonychia* (thin, spoon-shaped nails) can be caused by iron deficiency anaemia.
- *Leuconychia* (white nails) is seen in hypoalbuminaemia.
- *Beau's lines* (transverse lines) are horizontal grooves in the nail due to a temporary growth arrest associated with an acute severe illness.
- *Yellow-nail syndrome* is a rare disorder based on the triad of thickened, slow-growing, yellow nails, pulmonary manifestations (cough, bronchiectasis, pleural effusion) and lower limb lymphoedema.
- *Subungual hyperkeratosis* is thickening of the nail plate, usually due to tinea infection (see p. 673), psoriasis, trauma or a combination of these.
- *Onychogryphosis* is severe nail thickening and curvature (ram's horn), which is common in the elderly, especially in the big toenail, where trauma from ill-fitting footwear may be relevant.
- *Longitudinal melanonychia* (brown streaks) of multiple nails is a common finding in dark-skinned people. An acquired solitary pigmented streak may be caused by a melanocytic naevus and needs to be differentiated from subungual melanoma (see p. 688), especially if the pigmentation spreads on to the adjacent nail fold ('Hutchinson's sign').
- *Subungual haemorrhage* is common in the great toe-nails after trauma (football, running downhill). The red–brown pigmentation grows out with the nail over several months with clear proximal growth.
- *Clubbing* is discussed on page 937.

Nail dystrophy is also a feature of various genodermatoses including *nail patellar syndrome, ectodermal dysplasias* (abnormal hair, teeth and nail) and *pachyonychia congenita*.

Further reading

Iorizzo M. Tips to treat the 5 most common nail disorders: brittle nails, onycholysis, paronychia, psoriasis, onychomycosis. *Dermatol Clin* 2015; 33:175–307.

HAIR DISORDERS

Hair loss (alopecia)

There are many causes of hair loss, or alopecia (**Box 22.30**). They are broadly divided into localized and diffuse patterns, and non-scarring alopecia (where follicles are preserved) and scarring alopecia (where an inflammatory process causes permanent destruction of follicles). Patients may complain of increased hair shedding and/or thinning. Dermoscopic (trichoscopic) examination can help to identify whether follicles are still present and histology of scalp biopsies is helpful when there is diagnostic uncertainty.

Androgenic alopecia

Androgenic alopecia (male-pattern baldness) is the most common cause of non-scarring hair loss and a feature of normal human ageing. It is thought to be caused by a genetically determined increased sensitivity to androgens and there is often a positive family history. It may present in adolescence with a receding frontal hairline, followed by thinning over the vertex. Women may be similarly affected, but usually later in life, with milder loss and preservation of the frontal hair margin (female-pattern alopecia). If acne, hirsutism and menstrual disturbance are also present, there may be underlying polycystic ovary syndrome or an androgenic disorder.

Treatment options include topical minoxidil or oral 5-alpha-reductase inhibitors (finasteride or dutasteride). These can halt progression and may induce modest regrowth, if used early in disease and continued indefinitely. Approximately one-third of patients will not respond to either therapy. Finasteride is well tolerated but may cause sexual adverse effects, such as loss of libido in about 1% of men; it should not be taken or handled by pregnant women, as it can cause feminization of a male fetus. Oral antiandrogen therapy (e.g. cyproterone acetate or spironolactone) may help some women.

Alopecia areata

Alopecia areata is a non-scarring hair loss disorder with a lifetime prevalence of about 2%. It is thought to be an organ-specific autoimmune disease of the hair follicle that occurs due to loss of hair follicle immune privilege. It is associated with other organ-specific autoimmune diseases and runs an unpredictable course ranging in severity from a temporary small, solitary patch of scalp hair loss (alopecia areata) to total loss of scalp hair (*alopecia totalis*) and, rarely, scalp and body hair (*alopecia universalis*). Hair loss can have a major impact on body image and quality of life, with associated depression and social isolation.

Alopecia areata usually presents in children or young adults with patches of baldness (**Fig. 22.56**). These may regrow spontaneously, to be followed by new areas of hair loss. The presence of broken hairs and 'exclamation mark' hairs (narrow at the scalp and wider

---

? Box 22.30 Causes of alopecia

Scarring alopecia
- Discoid lupus erythematosus
- Kerion (tinea capitis)
- Lichen planus
- Dissecting cellulitis
- X-irradiation
- Idiopathic ('pseudopelade')

Non-scarring alopecia
- Androgenic alopecia
- Telogen effluvium
- Alopecia areata
- Trichotillomania (self-induced hair-pulling)
- Tinea capitis
- Traction alopecia
- Metabolic (iron deficiency, hypothyroidism)
- Drugs (e.g. heparin, isotretinoin, chemotherapy)

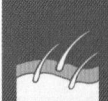

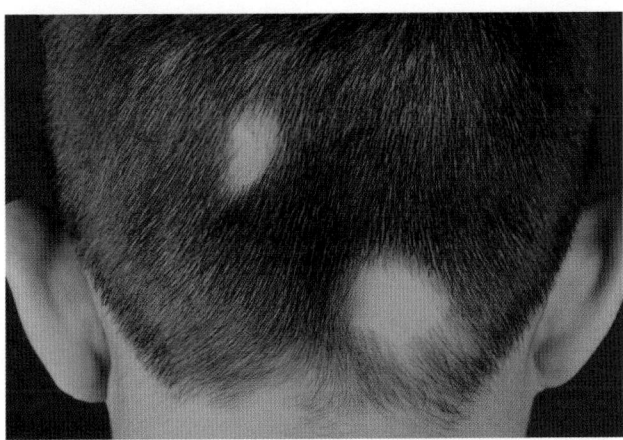

Fig. 22.56 Alopecia areata.

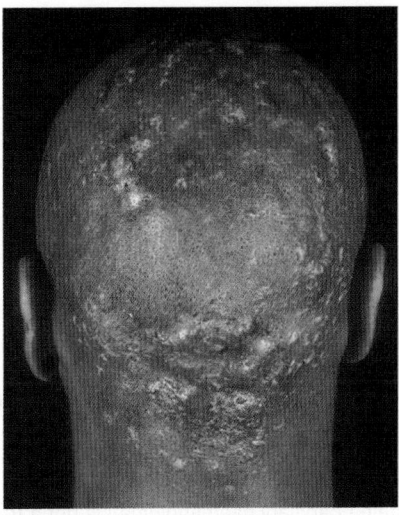

Fig. 22.57 Dissecting cellulitis of the scalp in an African–Caribbean male.

and more pigmented at the tip) at the edge of a bald area is diagnostic. The nails may be pitted or roughened.

Management has no effect on the long-term disease course. Potent topical or injected steroids may trigger regrowth of localized patchy hair loss. Repeated application of a contact sensitizer (contact immunotherapy) such as diphencyprone can be helpful in more extensive disease. Oral JAK inhibitors have recently been shown to reverse hair loss in moderate to severe alopecia areata. In the UK, patients with extensive hair loss are eligible for prescribed wigs and may benefit from joining patient support groups.

Traction alopecia

This form of scarring hair loss is caused by mechanical damage to the hair follicle from pulling the hair back into a bun or tight plaits. It is more common in black Africans.

Telogen effluvium

This type of diffuse, non-scarring hair loss is associated with increased hair shedding and usually presents 2 or 3 months after pregnancy or a severe illness. It occurs when a larger percentage of scalp hairs enters the telogen phase of hair shedding at the same time. Spontaneous recovery is usual after a few months, though a chronic variant is recognized.

Metabolic causes of hair loss

Iron deficiency may be associated with increased hair shedding and hair thinning, and is a common finding in menstruating women who do not eat red meat. The exact relationship between serum iron or ferritin levels and optimum hair growth is unclear.

Dissecting cellulitis

This is a chronic scarring folliculitis of the scalp that predominantly affects black men and may be associated with severe acne and hidradenitis suppurativa. Crusted papules and pustules occur with underlying diffuse swelling (**Fig. 22.57**). Prolonged courses of anti-staphylococcal oral antibiotics such as rifampicin and clindamycin may be helpful.

Increased hair growth

Hirsutism

Hirsutism (see p. 629) refers to a male pattern of hair growth in females. Racial variation in hair growth must be considered, as certain races (e.g. Mediterranean and Asian) normally have more male-pattern hair growth than Northern European females. If virilizing

features (deep voice, clitoromegaly, dysmenorrhoea, acne) are present, a full endocrine assessment is necessary. Hirsutism can cause severe psychological distress in some individuals.

Management involves physical methods, such as bleaching, waxing, electrolysis, intense pulsed light (IPL) and laser therapy. Oral anti-androgen therapy is occasionally helpful.

Hypertrichosis

Hypertrichosis refers to excessive hair growth at any site and occurs in both sexes. It can be seen in anorexia nervosa, porphyria cutanea tarda and underlying malignancy, and is caused by certain drugs (e.g. ciclosporin, minoxidil).

Further reading

Mella JM, Perret MC, Manzotti M et al. Efficacy and safety of finasteride therapy for androgenetic alopecia: a systematic review. *Arch Dermatol* 2010; 146:1141–1150.
Rajab F, Drake LA, Senna MM et al. Alopecia areata: a review of disease pathogenesis. *Br J Dermatol* 2018; 179:1033–1048.

BIRTH MARKS AND NEONATAL RASHES

Infantile haemangiomas (strawberry naevus, cavernous haemangioma)

Infantile haemangiomas are the most common benign tumour of infancy with a prevalence of 4.5% (**Fig. 22.58**). They present shortly after birth as a single red, lumpy nodule that grows rapidly for the first few months. Multiple lesions can also occur. They resolve spontaneously over several years. Parental reassurance is usually all that is required.

Treatment is indicated for lesions associated with:

- visual obstruction or feeding difficulties
- ulceration or bleeding
- life-threatening lesions associated with high-output cardiac failure from vascular shunting or consumptive coagulopathy (Kasabach–Merritt syndrome).

Treatment has been revolutionized by the use of oral propranolol to shrink infantile haemangiomas rapidly. Topical timolol may also be effective. The mechanism of action is unclear. Treatment needs to be continued for at least 6 months.

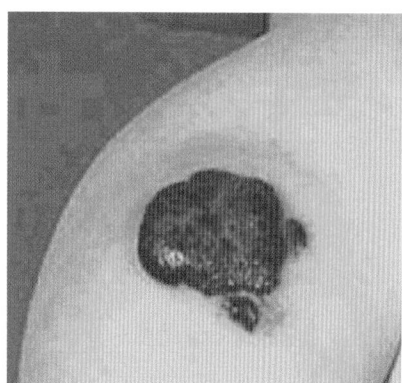

Fig. 22.58 Strawberry naevus (cavernous haemangioma).

Port-wine stain (naevus flammeus)

Port-wine stain ('capillary haemangioma') is not a true haemangioma but an abnormal dilation of dermal capillaries. It presents at birth as a flat, red area and is commonly found on the face. It does not improve and may become thickened with age. If the lesion occurs in the distribution of the first division of the trigeminal nerve, it may be associated with ipsilateral meningeal vascular anomalies that can cause epilepsy and even hemiplegia (Sturge–Weber syndrome). Periocular lesions may be associated with glaucoma and so ophthalmological follow-up is required.

Treatment of port-wine stains is with a vascular laser: for example, a pulsed dye laser. Facial lesions respond best but lesions can darken after several years and require retreatment.

Congenital melanocytic naevi

See page 688.

Mongolian blue spot

This appears in infants as a deep blue–grey, bruise-like area, usually over the sacrum or back (**Fig. 22.59**); it is occasionally mistaken for a sign of child abuse. Mongolian blue spot is due to the presence of melanocytes in the deeper dermis. It is very common in Oriental children, less common in black Africans and rare in Caucasians. It usually disappears by the age of 7 years.

Toxic erythema of the newborn (erythema neonatorum)

Toxic erythema of the newborn describes a common transient, blotchy, maculopapular rash in newborns. The rash is occasionally pustular and the child is not well, but the complaint resolves spontaneously within a few days.

Milia

'Milk spots' are small follicular epidermal cysts. These pinhead white papules are commonly found on the face of infants. They resolve spontaneously.

Nappy rash ('diaper dermatitis')

This is an irritant contact dermatitis caused by prolonged skin contact with faeces and urine. It is much less common nowadays due to the high absorbency of disposable nappies. The flexures are usually spared, which is a useful differentiating feature from atopic eczema. Satellite lesions around the edge may indicate secondary infection with *Candida*. A recalcitrant purpuric nappy rash in the

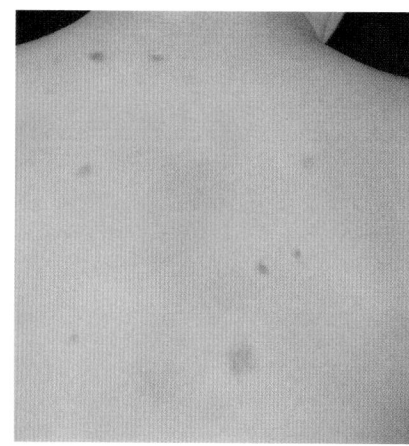

Fig. 22.59 Urticaria pigmentosa (mastocytosis) and Mongolian blue spot in a baby.

groins and axillae should be biopsied to exclude rarer pathology such as Langerhans cell histiocytosis.

Management involves frequent changing of the nappy and regular application of a barrier cream.

Acrodermatitis enteropathica

This rare but distinctive rash (see p. 1244) is a manifestation of zinc deficiency, which can occur in three settings:

- an inherited defect in zinc transporter protein in the gastrointestinal tract (presents after breast-feeding finishes)
- low levels in breast milk in breast-fed infants (presents during breast-feeding)
- patients on total parenteral nutrition without adequate zinc replacement.

There is an erythematous, sometimes blistering, rash around the perineum, mouth, hands and feet. It may be associated with photophobia, diarrhoea and alopecia.

In the inherited form the rash presents when breast-feeding finishes, as breast milk usually has high levels of zinc that override the poor absorption. These patients will need life-long oral zinc replacement therapy to improve the skin and ensure normal neurological development. The second type needs replacement only until breast-feeding finishes. The response to zinc is rapid and dramatic.

Further reading

Leaute-Labreze C, Harper JI, Hoeger PH. Infantile hemangioma. *Lancet* 2017; 390:85–94.

DRUG ERUPTIONS

Cutaneous adverse drug reactions are common and range from mild, and predictable, dose-related effects such as phototoxicity from doxycycline or mucocutaneous dryness from oral isotretinoin, to idiosyncratic, severe and life-threatening eruptions (severe cutaneous adverse drug reactions, SCAR). The diagnosis of drug eruptions can be challenging because individual drugs can cause different rashes and these sometimes mimic constitutional inflammatory rashes or viral rashes. The clinical features can also be mixed. A high index of suspicion and a detailed drug history are essential. Underlying viral infection, especially HIV, and systemic disease, such as systemic lupus and leukaemia, may also increase the risk of drug rashes (see **Fig. 22.32**). Allergy

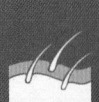

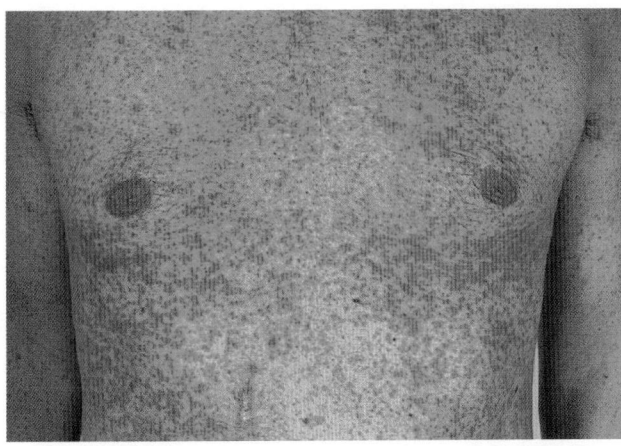

Fig. 22.60 Morbilliform drug rash due to penicillin allergy.

tests (prick tests and patch tests) have a limited role, especially in the acute setting, and drug challenge tests are time-consuming and potentially risky.

Maculopapular (morbilliform) exanthems

These are the most common type of hypersensitivity rash (**Fig. 22.60**). They start on the torso and spread to the face and limbs, but spare the mucosae. They are self-limiting and usually clear within 1–2 weeks.

Fixed drug eruptions

These inflamed patches recur at the same site each time a drug is taken. They may blister, and often resolve with hyperpigmentation.

Drug-induced and drug-exacerbated dermatoses

Drugs may exacerbate pre-existing skin disease and can also trigger or induce skin disease that resembles a constitutional dermatosis (**Box 22.31**).

Severe cutaneous adverse drug reactions

Severe drug rashes are listed in **Box 22.32**. Common causes include antibiotics, NSAIDs, anticonvulsants, allopurinol, dapsone and nevirapine. Early recognition and drug withdrawal can minimize morbidity and mortality. Recent advances in pharmacogenetics have identified human leucocyte antigen (HLA) associations, and cytochrome P450 polymorphisms that are associated with an increased risk of reaction to certain drugs.

Stevens–Johnson syndrome and toxic epidermal necrolysis

Stevens–Johnson syndrome (SJS) and toxic epidermal necrolysis (TEN) are severe mucocutaneous disorders that are considered variants of a disease spectrum. They are characterized by varying extents of blistering/epidermal detachment and mucosal ulceration (see **Box 22.19**):

_i_ Box 22.31 Dermatoses induced or aggravated by drugs

Dermatosis	Drugs
Acne	Androgens (danazol)
Acneiform	Corticosteroids, EGFR inhibitors
Angio-oedema	ACE inhibitors
Urticaria	Penicillin, aspirin, NSAIDs, iodine contrast media
Vasculitis	Gold, hydralazine, NSAIDs, proton pump inhibitors
Fixed drug eruption	Phenolphthalein in laxatives, tetracyclines, paracetamol
Pigmentation	Minocycline (black), amiodarone (slate-grey)
Lupus erythematosus	Minocycline, anti-TNF biologics, isoniazid, interferons
Photosensitivity	Thiazides, quinolones, tetracyclines, diuretics, amiodarone
Pseudoporphyria	Naproxen, diuretics
Leg ulcers	Hydroxyurea
Anogenital ulcers	Nicorandil
Erythema nodosum	Sulphonamides, oral contraceptive
Erythema multiforme	Barbiturates, etravirine
Lichen planus-like (lichenoid)	Antimalarials, thiazides, statins, diuretics
Psoriasiform	Methyldopa, gold, lithium, beta-blockers
Toxic epidermal necrolysis	Penicillin, co-trimoxazole, carbamazepine, NSAIDs, nevirapine, efavirenz
Pemphigus	Penicillamine, ACE inhibitors
Erythroderma	Gold, sulphonylureas, allopurinol, nevirapine, efavirenz

ACE, angiotensin-converting enzyme; EGFR, epidermal growth factor receptor; NSAIDs, nonsteroidal anti-inflammatory drugs; TNF, tumour necrosis factor.

_i_ Box 22.32 Severe cutaneous adverse drug reactions

- Stevens–Johnson syndrome (SJS) and toxic epidermal necrolysis (TEN)
- Drug reaction with eosinophilia and systemic symptoms (DRESS)
- Acute generalized exanthematous pustulosis (AGEP)
- Erythroderma/exfoliative dermatitis
- Serum sickness-like reactions

- **_SJS_**: <10% skin detachment; one or two mucosal sites involved (oral, genital, ocular)
- **_SJS–TEN_** overlap: 10–30% skin detachment
- **_TEN_**: >30% skin detachment; all mucosal sites involved in most cases.

The onset is usually 1–2 weeks after drug exposure. Initial symptoms are non-specific (malaise, myalgia, fever and cough). These are followed by tender maculopapular erythematous lesions on the torso and inflamed mucosal surfaces. Target lesions usually affect the hands and feet in SJS. In TEN there is widespread flaccid blistering with skin that wrinkles like wet wallpaper on gentle pressure (Nikolsky's sign). Features of skin failure can ensue (see p. 657). Respiratory mucosal and pulmonary involvement may require ventilation, and upper gastrointestinal involvement can cause haemorrhage. Patients are at high risk of sepsis and require expert intensive supportive care, as for extensive burns. Multiorgan failure may occur and the mortality for TEN ranges from 30% to 50%. 'SCORTEN' is

i **Box 22.33** SCORTEN prognostic score in toxic epidermal necrolysis

Risk factor	0	1
Age	<40 years	>40 years
Associated malignancy	No	Yes
Heart rate (b.p.m.)	<120	>120
Serum urea (mmol/L)	<9.6	>9.6
Detached or compromised body surface	<10%	>10%
Serum bicarbonate (mmol/L)	>20	<20
Serum glucose (mmol/L)	<13.9	>13.9

The more risk factors present, the higher the SCORTEN score, and the higher the mortality rate:
0–1 risk factors: 3.2% mortality
2: 12.1%
3: 35.3%
4: 58.3%
≥5: >90%

(From Bastuji-Garin S, Fouchard N, Bertocchi M et al. SCORTEN: a severity-of-illness score for toxic epidermal necrolysis. J Invest Dermatol *2000; 115:149–153.)*

a clinical severity score that can help assess prognosis (**Box 22.33**). All potential causative drugs should be stopped.

Treatment with high-dose steroids, ciclosporin and intravenous immunoglobulin therapy remains controversial, as high-quality clinical trials are lacking.

Drug reaction with eosinophilia and systemic symptoms/drug hypersensitivity syndrome

Drug reaction with eosinophilia and systemic symptoms (DRESS)/drug hypersensitivity syndrome usually starts 2–6 weeks after initial exposure and is characterized by widespread erythema, facial oedema, fever, lymphadenopathy and hepatosplenomegaly. Blood eosinophilia is usual with elevated hepatic transferases. Pneumonia and nephritis can develop and a mortality rate of 10% has been reported. Treatment is with systemic steroids tapered over at least 3 months. Aromatic anticonvulsants are one of the most common causes of DRESS and, as they cross-react, all drugs of this group must be avoided in the future. Sodium valproate is a suitable alternative.

Acute generalized exanthematous pustulosis/toxic pustuloderma

Acute generalized exanthematous pustulosis (AGEP)/toxic pustuloderma is an exanthem with numerous small, non-follicular, sterile pustules around the neck, axillae and groin. It usually starts a few days after drug exposure and resolves with peeling. There may be mild systemic upset but internal organs are not involved. Localized forms can occur. Florid cases can resemble pustular psoriasis. Topical steroids and emollients can be used to relieve symptoms.

Further reading

Creamer D, Walsh SA, Dziewulski P. UK guidelines for the management of Stevens Johnson syndrome/toxic epidermal necrolysis in adults 2016. *Br J Dermatol* 2016; 174:1194–1227.

Bibliography

Griffiths C, Barker J, Bleiker T et al (eds). *Rook's Textbook of Dermatology*, 9th edn. Chichester: John Wiley & Sons; 2016.

Websites

http://dermnetnz.org/ Dermatology information and images.
http://hardinmd.lib.uiowa.edu/dermpictures.html Dermatology images (atlas).
http://www.aad.org American Academy of Dermatology.
http://www.bad.org.uk British Association of Dermatologists.
http://www.debra.org.uk Dystrophic Epidermolysis Bullosa Association.
http://www.eczema.org National Eczema Society.
http://www.evidence.nhs.uk/ National Institute for Health and Care Excellence (NICE): clinical guidelines, systematic reviews, evidence-based synopses, image database.
http://www.pcds.org.uk Primary Care Dermatology Society.
http://www.psoriasis-association.org.uk Psoriasis Association.
http://www.skin-camouflage.net British Association of Skin Camouflage.
http://www.thecochranelibrary.com Cochrane Library: systematic reviews of treatment.
http://www.vitiligosociety.org.uk Vitiligo Society.
https://www.nice.org.uk/guidance Dermatology treatment guidelines in the UK.

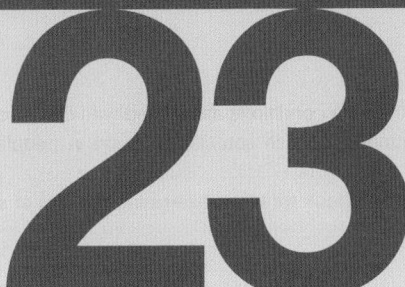

Diabetes mellitus

Richard I.G. Holt

CORE SKILLS AND KNOWLEDGE

Diabetes is the most prevalent and clinically important endocrine disorder, affecting around 10% of the adult population in most countries. Many go on to develop life-limiting complications including cardiovascular, renal, eye and neurological disease. Most consultant diabetologists will be trained in both diabetes and endocrinology as well as general internal medicine; although many diabetes specialists focus solely on diabetes. Some sub-specialize in areas including inpatient care, diabetes in pregnancy, technology (insulin pumps and continuous glucose monitoring), and pancreas or islet-cell transplantation.

Most people with diabetes will be seen in outpatient clinics either in primary or secondary care, although approximately 15% of all inpatients have diabetes. Many are admitted for other reasons but diabetes may complicate their hospital stay.

Key skills within diabetes include:

- listening to people with diabetes (as with any patient with a long-term condition), and involving them actively in the management of their illness, and understanding the role of the multidisciplinary team in preventing and managing long-term diabetic complications
- learning about the acute management of diabetic emergencies (hypoglycaemia, diabetic ketoacidosis and hyperosmolar, hyperglycaemic state)
- developing confidence in prescribing insulin therapy and the wide range of oral hypoglycaemic agents

Diabetes is best learned in outpatient settings by listening to people with diabetes. As diabetes is a long-term condition, there is an opportunity to build up long-term patient relationships. Diabetic emergencies are common reasons for admission to hospital and people presenting with these may be found in the hospital emergency department or acute admissions unit.

CLINICAL SKILLS FOR DIABETES MELLITUS

Diabetes mellitus is a chronic condition and people with diabetes may present to healthcare services for routine monitoring of their condition, or for a host of reasons related or unrelated to their diabetes. Treatment for diabetic emergencies, which may be the presentation when diabetes is first diagnosed, is covered on page 722. This section outlines an approach to people with diabetes in non-emergency settings (**Box 23.1**).

Routine checks in people with diabetes

All people with diabetes should be screened regularly to assess for their level of glycaemic control and the emergence of any complications. **Box 23.2** shows the checks (covering history, examination and selected investigations) that should form part of the annual screening process.

Examination

The physical examination carried out in people with diabetes will be determined by the clinical context and any presenting complications. The figure presents a range of physical signs seen in people with diabetes: some are a direct result of complications of hyperglycaemia, and some are conditions associated with diabetes (e.g. vitiligo, an autoimmune disease sometimes found in people with type 1 diabetes).

Box 23.3 lists features to look for when examining the feet of a person with diabetes.

 Box 23.1 Taking a history in diabetes mellitus (see also Box 1.7)

Presenting complaint
- Why has the patient attended?
- Could their presenting complaints be related to a complication of diabetes?

Diagnosis of diabetes
- When were they diagnosed?
- Did they present as an emergency, or with symptomatic hyperglycaemia, or was diabetes picked up without symptoms through routine screening?
- What type of diabetes do they have?
  - Might it be secondary to another disease process (p. 704)?
  - Is there any reason to suspect monogenic diabetes (p. 709)?

Management of the disease
- What do they understand about the role of self-management in diabetes?
- Do they monitor their capillary or interstitial glucose?
  - Do they keep a diary of the results?
  - What are the usual readings?
  - Is there evidence of hypoglycaemia or hyperglycaemia?
- Have they ever required hospital (or intensive care) admission for diabetic emergencies?
- Do they ever suffer from hypoglycaemic episodes?
  - Are they aware if they are becoming hypoglycaemic?
  - Have they needed external help to manage an episode of hypoglycaemia?
- Do they drive, or engage in any other activities that may raise safety concerns in the context of hypoglycaemia?

Medications
- Do they see a primary care clinician or hospital specialist to manage their diabetes?
  - Are they in contact with a specialist nurse or dietitian?

- What medication do they use to control their blood glucose?
- If they inject insulin, do they rotate injection sites?
  - What size needles do they use?
- Are they able to adjust doses of insulin or other medications according to blood glucose levels and carbohydrate intake?
- What other medications are they taking?

Complications
- Have they suffered any cardiovascular events?
  - What is their cardiovascular risk, and is this being appropriately managed?
- Are they undergoing regular retinal screening?
  - Have they required any retinal intervention?
- Do they supply regular urine samples to screen for diabetic nephropathy?
  - Are they taking ACE inhibitors or angiotensin receptor blockers?
- Have they had any problems with neuropathy or vascular disease affecting their feet?
  - Have they experienced a foot ulcer?
  - Have they needed an amputation?

Social history
- Do they smoke? If so, have they tried to quit?
- Are they aware of key lifestyle interventions around healthy eating, weight reduction and exercise?

 Box 23.2 Annual screening checks in people with diabetes

General health
- Level of knowledge about diabetes
- Weight and BMI
- Diet and eating habits
- Exercise

Glycaemic control
- Glycated haemoglobin (HbA$_{1c}$)
- Glucose monitoring
- Medication
- Review of insulin injection sites

Development of complications
- Retinal screening, ideally by retinal photography

- Visual acuity
- Urine albumin : creatinine ratio (ACR)
- Serum urea and electrolytes; estimated glomerular filtration rate (eGFR)
- Examination of feet for vascular disease and neuropathy
- Full blood count
- Thyroid function
- Liver function

Cardiovascular risk
- Smoking status
- Blood pressure
- Lipid profile
- Overall cardiovascular risk using validated risk model, e.g. QRISK

 Box 23.3 Examination of feet

Features of vascular disease
- Pale discoloration
- Loss of hair
- Cool temperature
- Absent pulses (begin in foot and proceed up legs)
- Reduced capillary refill time
- Evidence of gangrene or infection

Features of neuropathy
- Clawing of toes, loss of plantar arch
- Neuropathic ulcers
- Joint deformity (Charcot's joint)
- Glove and stocking sensory loss (check with monofilament)
- Loss of vibration sense, proprioception and pain
- Loss of ankle jerk

General observation
Does patient look well/
unwell?
Weight loss (T1DM)
Weight gain (T2DM)
Dehydrated?
Breathing (air hunger,
Kussmaul breathing)

Face
Cranial nerve palsy,
particularly CNIII
Eye movements
Ptosis

Neck
Carotid pulses/bruits
Check thyroid gland for
goitre (autoimmune)

Hands
Carpal tunnel
Dupuytren's contracture
Muscle wasting
Limited joint movement

Dupuytren's contracture

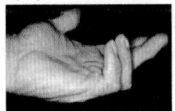

*(From Palastanga N. Anatomy and
Human Movement, 6th edn, with
permission.)*

Abdomen
Hepatomegaly (fatty liver)

Skin
Vitiligo (autoimmune)
Pigmentation (e.g. axillary
acanthosis nigricans in
insulin resistance)
Granuloma annulare
Bullosis

Vitiligo

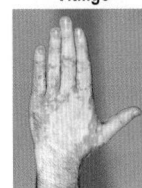

Eyes
Fundoscopy
- Cataracts, against red
reflex
- Retinopathy (p. 726)
- Visual acuity
Eyelids – xanthelasma

Cataracts

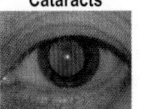

Retinopathy

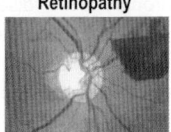

Mouth
Candidiasis

Insulin injection sites
Bruising
Lipohypertrophy
Lipoatrophy (rare)

Legs
Muscle wasting
Hair loss
Sensory neuropathy (glove
and stocking)
Reflexes (lost in
sensorimotor neuropathy)
Necrobiosis lipoidica

Feet
• Feel for peripheral pulses
• Skin – colour, ulcers,
gangrene
• Look between toes for
infection
• Sensory loss
- Neuropathic foot ulcer
- Charcot neuroarthropathy

Neuropathic ulcer

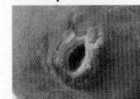

Charcot joints

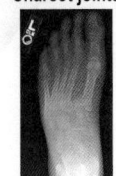

*(From Miller MD. Presentation,
Imaging and Treatment of Common
Musculoskeletal Conditions,
Saunders 2011, with permission.)*

Aims of physical examination in diabetic patients:

* Assessing for diabetic emergencies - diabetic ketoacidosis, hypoglycaemia.
* Establishing the presence of complications - neuropathy, eyes and
retinopathy, kidney disease, skin changes including ulceration, cardiovascular
disease including peripheral vascular disease, foot complications, soft tissue
infection.
* Assessment of cardiovascular risk factors — blood pressure, stigmata of
hyperlipidaemia, weight and Body Mass Index
* Revealing signs of auto-immune disease — vitiligo, thyroid disease
* Assessment of injection sites

INTRODUCTION

Diabetes mellitus is a complex metabolic disorder characterized by chronic hyperglycaemia due to relative insulin deficiency, resistance or both. In 2017, the International Diabetes Federation estimated that 425 million people (1 in 11 of the global population) had diabetes, and estimates an increase to 693 million by 2045 (**Fig. 23.1**).

Diabetes is associated with a number of short- and long-term complications that reduce quality of life and life expectancy, and are associated with major health costs. These include acute metabolic disturbance, macrovascular disease (leading to an increased prevalence of coronary artery disease, peripheral vascular disease and stroke), and microvascular damage causing retinopathy, nephropathy and neuropathy.

Diabetes was responsible for approximately 4 million deaths or 10.7% of all deaths in 2017, outnumbering the combined number of global deaths from human immunodeficiency virus (HIV)/acquired immune deficiency syndrome (AIDS), tuberculosis and malaria. A diagnosis of diabetes in a man or woman at the age of 55 years reduces life expectancy by 5 and 6 years, respectively. By contrast, type 2 diabetes diagnosed after the age of 80 years has a limited effect on life expectancy. Heart disease is the most common cause of death and accounts for two-thirds of all deaths in people with diabetes aged 65 years or older.

PHYSIOLOGY OF INSULIN STRUCTURE, SECRETION AND ACTION

Insulin is the key hormone involved in the regulation of cellular energy supply and macronutrient balance derived from food. It is a 51-amino acid peptide hormone comprising two polypeptide chains, the A and B chains (**Fig. 23.2**), and is synthesized in the β cells of the pancreatic islets of Langerhans (**Fig. 23.3**). The synthesis, intracellular processing and secretion of insulin by the β cell is typical of the way that the body produces and manipulates many peptide hormones. **Fig. 23.4** illustrates the cellular events triggering the release of insulin-containing granules. After secretion, insulin enters the portal circulation and is carried to the liver, its prime target organ. About 50% of secreted insulin is extracted and degraded in the liver; the remainder is broken down by the kidneys. C-peptide is only partially extracted by the liver (and hence provides a useful index of the rate of insulin secretion) but is mainly degraded by the kidneys.

Insulin is secreted at a slow background rate throughout the day, resulting in a low plasma insulin concentration between meals and overnight. In response to eating, there is a rapid rise in circulating insulin concentration, which falls back to baseline within 2 hours (**Fig. 23.5**).

The insulin receptor

Insulin exerts its actions through binding to a receptor, which straddles the cell membrane of many cells (**Fig. 23.6**). The receptor comprises a dimer with two α-subunits, which include the binding sites for insulin, and two β-subunits, which traverse the cell membrane. When insulin binds to the α-subunits, it induces a conformational change in the β-subunits, resulting in activation of tyrosine kinase and initiation of a cascade response involving a host of other intracellular substrates. The insulin-receptor complex is then internalized by the cell, insulin is degraded, and the receptor is recycled to the cell surface.

Glucose metabolism

Blood glucose levels are tightly regulated in health and rarely stray outside the range of 3.5–8.0 mmol/L (63–144 mg/dL),

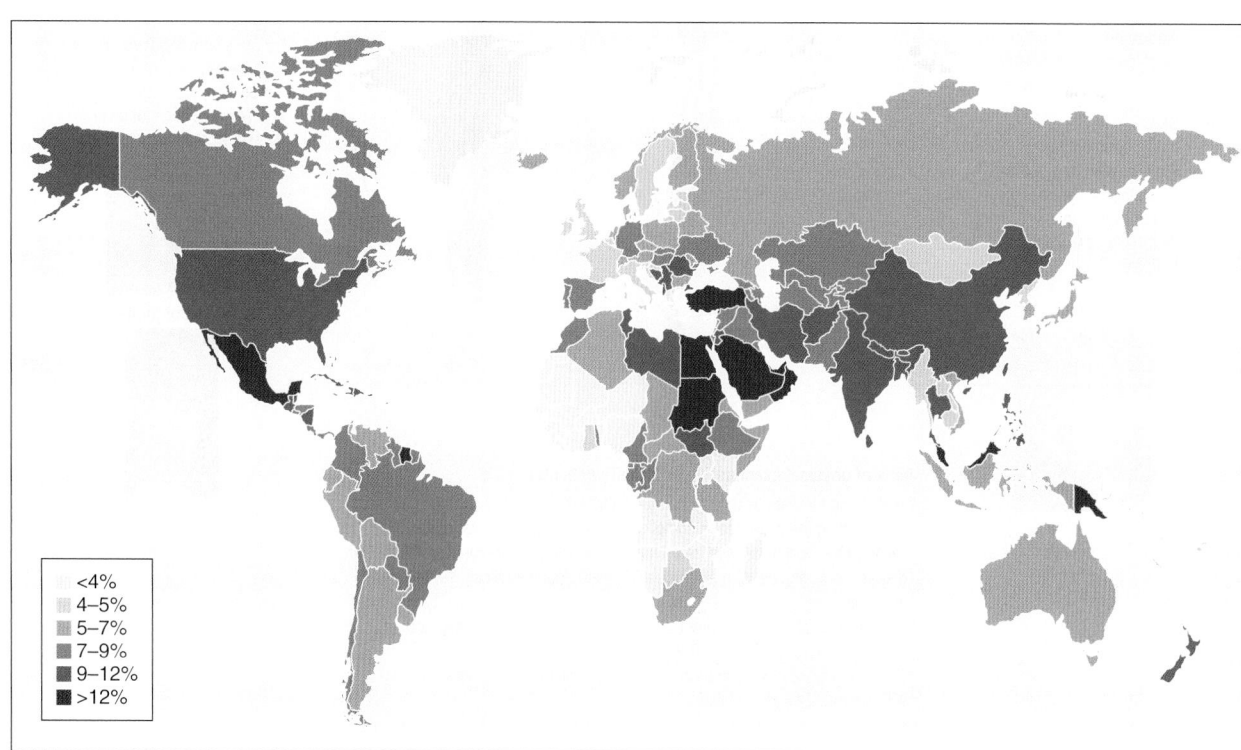

Fig. 23.1 Estimated age-adjusted prevalence of diabetes in adults aged 20–79 years in 2017. (From IDF Diabetes Atlas, 8th edition.)

<4%
4–5%
5–7%
7–9%
9–12%
>12%

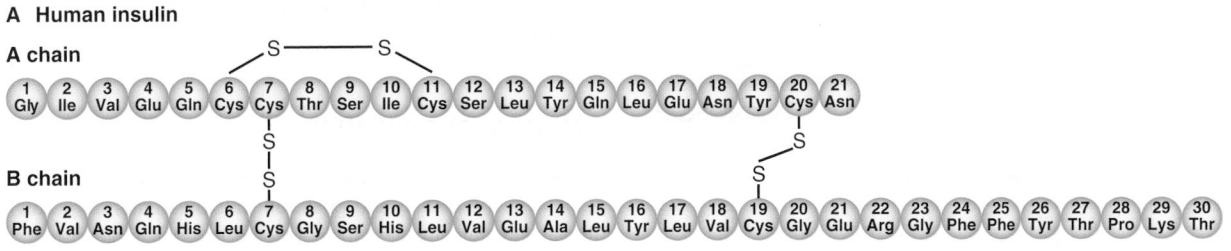

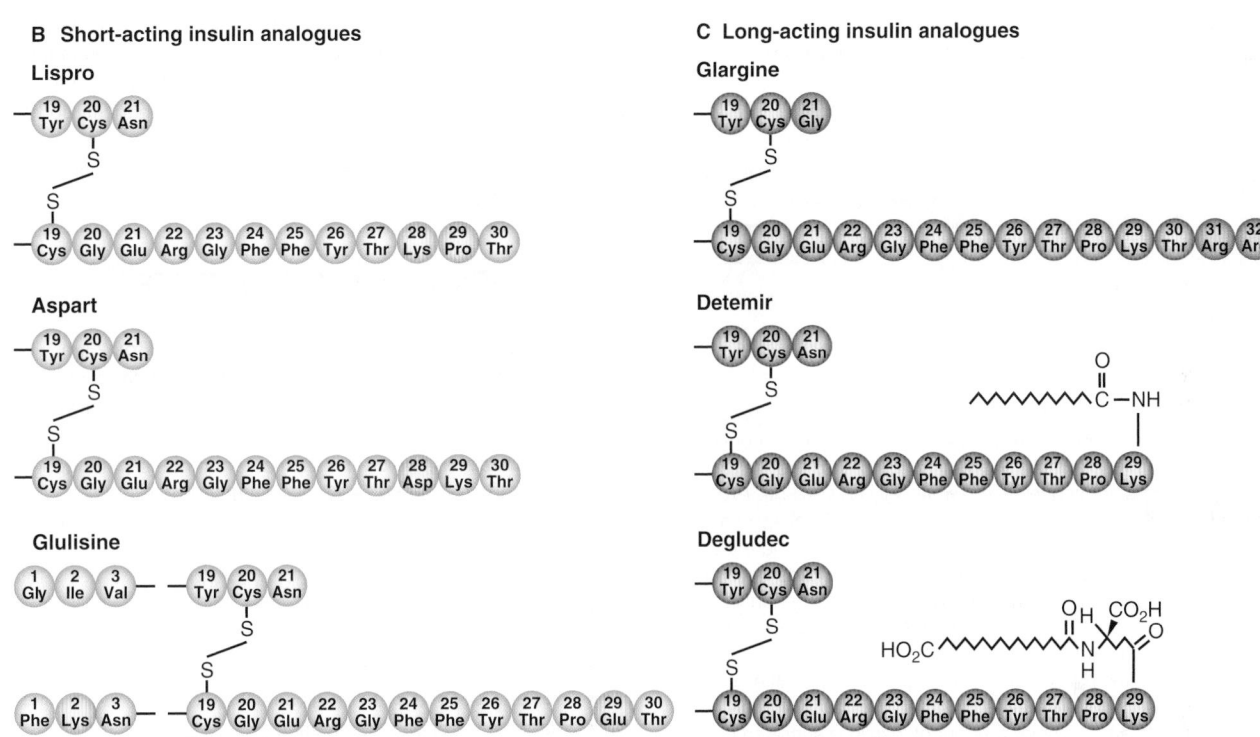

Fig. 23.2 Amino acid structure of insulin. **(A)** Human insulin. **(B)** Modification of human insulin produces rapid-acting insulin analogues. *Lispro* is created by reversing the order of the amino acids proline and lysine in positions 28 and 29 of the B chain. *Aspart* is a similar analogue created by replacing proline at position 28 of the B chain with an aspartic acid residue. *Glulisine* is a similar analogue created by replacing asparagine at position B3 with lysine and the lysine in position B29 is replaced by glutamic acid. **(C)** Modification of human insulin produces long-acting insulin analogues. *Insulin glargine* is created by replacing asparagine in position 21 of the A chain with a glycine residue and adding two arginines to the end of the B chain. *Detemir* discards threonine in position 30 of the B chain and adds a fatty acyl chain to lysine in position B29. *Degludec* is created by removing the threonine at position 30 of the B chain and the attachment, via a glutamic acid linker of a 16-carbon fatty diacid to the lysine at position 29 of the B chain.

despite the widely varying effects of food, fasting and exercise. Tight control of glucose is necessary because some tissues, particularly the brain, are highly dependent on glucose as an energy source while high glucose concentration irreversibly damages cellular proteins.

The principal organ of glucose homeostasis is the liver, which absorbs and stores glucose (as glycogen) in the post-absorptive state and releases it into the circulation between meals to match the rate of glucose utilization by peripheral tissues. The liver also combines three-carbon molecules derived from breakdown of fat (glycerol), muscle glycogen (lactate) and protein (e.g.

alanine) into the six-carbon glucose molecule by the process of gluconeogenesis.

Glucose production

More than 90% of the approximately 200 g of glucose utilized daily is derived from liver glycogen and hepatic gluconeogenesis, with the remainder coming from renal gluconeogenesis.

Glucose utilization

The major consumer of glucose is the brain, whose function depends on an uninterrupted supply of this substrate. Its

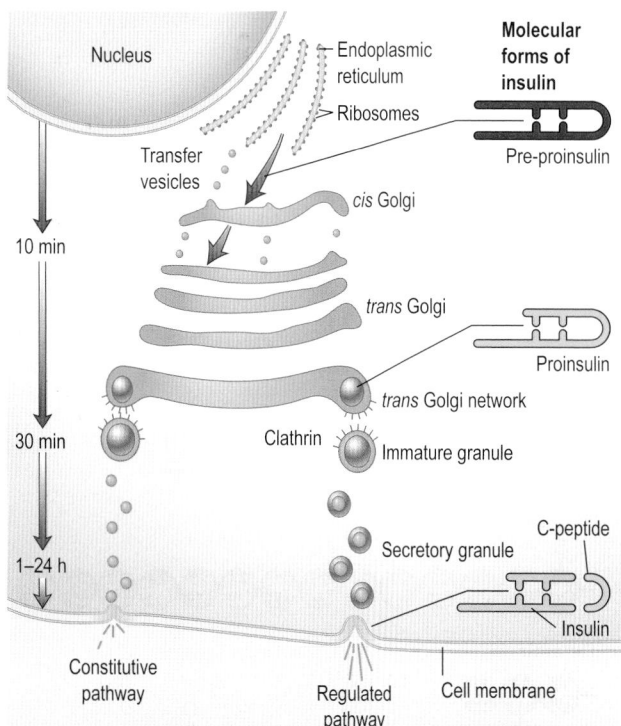

Fig. 23.3 Part of a β cell. The ribosomes manufacture **pre-proinsulin** from insulin messenger RNA (mRNA). The hydrophobic 'pre' portion of pre-proinsulin allows it to transfer to the Golgi apparatus, and is subsequently enzymatically cleaved off. **Pro-insulin** is parceled into secretory granules in the Golgi apparatus. These mature and pass towards the cell membrane, where they are stored before release. The proinsulin molecule folds back on itself and is stabilized by disulphide bonds. The biochemically inert peptide fragment known as **connecting (C-)peptide** splits off from proinsulin in the secretory process, leaving insulin as a complex of two linked peptide chains. Equimolar quantities of insulin and C-peptide are released into the circulation via the **'regulated pathway'**. A small amount of insulin is secreted by the β cell directly via the **'constitutive pathway'**, which bypasses the secretory granules.

requirement is 1 mg/kg body weight per minute, or approximately 100 g daily in a 70 kg person. Glucose uptake by the brain is obligatory and is not dependent on insulin, and the glucose used is oxidized to carbon dioxide and water. Tissues such as muscle and fat have insulin-responsive glucose transporters and absorb glucose in response to postprandial peaks in glucose and insulin. At other times, energy requirements are largely met by fatty acid oxidation. Glucose taken up by muscle is stored as glycogen or metabolized to lactate or carbon dioxide and water. Fat uses glucose as a substrate for triglyceride synthesis; lipolysis releases fatty acids from triglyceride together with glycerol, a substrate for hepatic gluconeogenesis.

Glucose transport

Cell membranes are not inherently permeable to glucose. A family of specialized glucose-transporter (GLUT) proteins carry glucose through the membrane into cells. The function of GLUT-1 to -3 is insulin-independent but insulin stimulates glucose uptake into muscle and adipose tissue through GLUT-4. GLUT-4 is normally present in the cytoplasm, but after insulin binds to its receptor, GLUT-4

moves to the cell surface where it creates a pore for glucose entry (see **Fig. 23.6**).

Hormonal regulation

Insulin is a major regulator of intermediary metabolism but its actions in the fasting and postprandial states differ (**Fig. 23.7**). In the fasting state, insulin's main action is to regulate glucose release by the liver, while in the postprandial state, it additionally promotes glucose uptake by fat and muscle.

A number of 'counter-regulatory hormones' that antagonize the action of insulin are also important in maintaining normoglycaemia. As glucose concentration falls below the normal range, glucagon is secreted from the pancreatic α-cells. At the same time, a number of other hormones, including noradrenaline (norepinephrine), cortisol and growth hormone, are released. These counter-regulatory hormones increase hepatic glucose production and reduce its utilization in fat and muscle for any given insulin concentration.

CLASSIFICATION OF DIABETES

Diabetes may be primary (idiopathic) or secondary (**Box 23.4**). Gestational diabetes refers to glucose intolerance appearing for the first time in pregnancy and is described in more detail on page 740. Primary diabetes is classified into:

- **Type 1 diabetes**, which usually has an immune pathogenesis and is characterized by severe insulin deficiency.
- **Type 2 diabetes**, which results from a combination of insulin resistance and less severe insulin deficiency.
  Secondary diabetes can be subdivided into:
  - diabetes secondary to genetic defects
  - diabetes secondary to exocrine pancreatic disease
  - diabetes secondary to endocrine disease
  - diabetes secondary to drugs and chemicals
  - diabetes secondary to infection
  - uncommon forms of immune-mediated diabetes
  - other genetic syndromes sometimes associated with diabetes.

  Box 23.5 lists the key features of the different types of diabetes. Type 1 diabetes and type 2 diabetes represent two distinct diseases from the epidemiological point of view, but from a clinical perspective, the two conditions appear as a spectrum – distinct at the two ends but overlapping in the middle.

Approximately 1–3% of cases of diabetes diagnosed under the age of 30 years are caused by mutations in a single gene (monogenic mutation). Although uncommon, it is important to recognize because the treatments and implications are different from type 1 diabetes or type 2 diabetes.

All forms of diabetes result from inadequate insulin secretion relative to the body's needs, and progressive insulin secretory failure is characteristic of both common forms of diabetes. Thus, some people with immune-mediated type 1 diabetes may not require insulin at the point of diagnosis, whereas many with type 2 diabetes will eventually do so.

Type 1 diabetes mellitus
Epidemiology

Type 1 diabetes is a disease of insulin deficiency and accounts for 5–10% of all cases of diabetes. It typically presents in

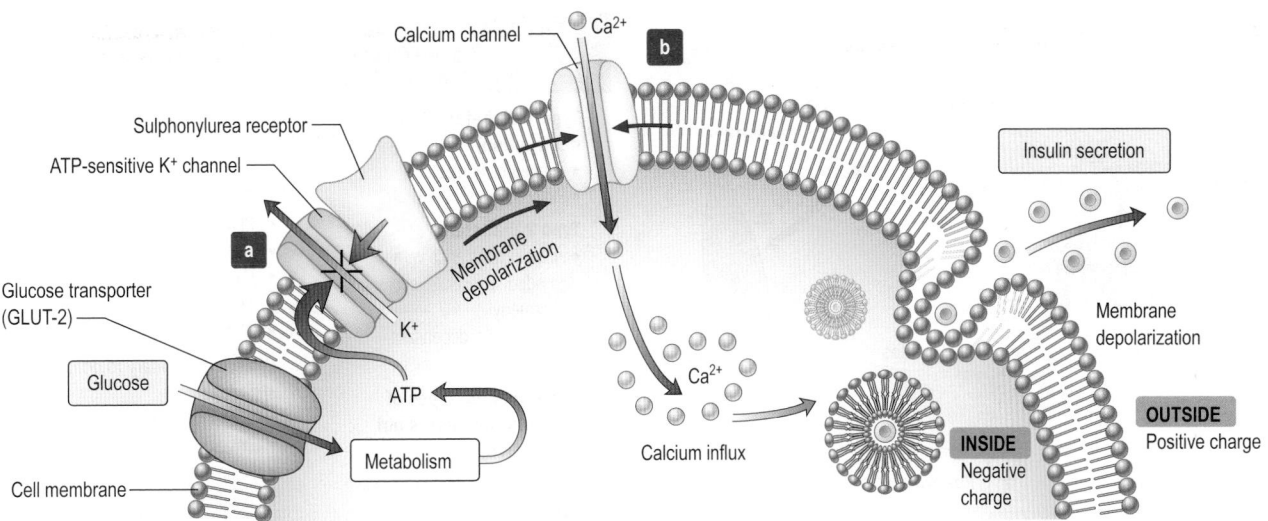

Fig. 23.4 The local regulation of insulin secretion from β cells. Glucose (on the left) enters the β cell via the GLUT-2 transporter protein, which is closely associated with the glycolytic enzyme glucokinase. Metabolism of glucose within the β cell generates adenosine triphosphate (ATP). ATP closes potassium channels in the cell membrane **(a)**. If a sulphonylurea binds to its receptor, this also closes potassium channels. Closure of potassium channels predisposes to cell membrane depolarization, allowing calcium ions to enter the cell via calcium channels in the cell membrane **(b)**. The rise in intracellular calcium triggers activation of calcium-dependent phospholipid protein kinase which, via intermediary phosphorylation steps, leads to fusion of the insulin-containing granules with the cell membrane and exocytosis of the insulin-rich granule contents. Similar mechanisms produce hormone-granule secretion in many other endocrine cells.

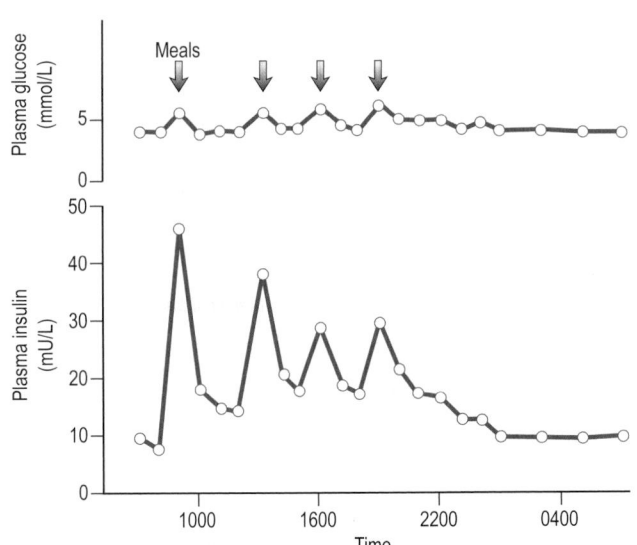

Fig. 23.5 Glucose and insulin profiles in people without diabetes.

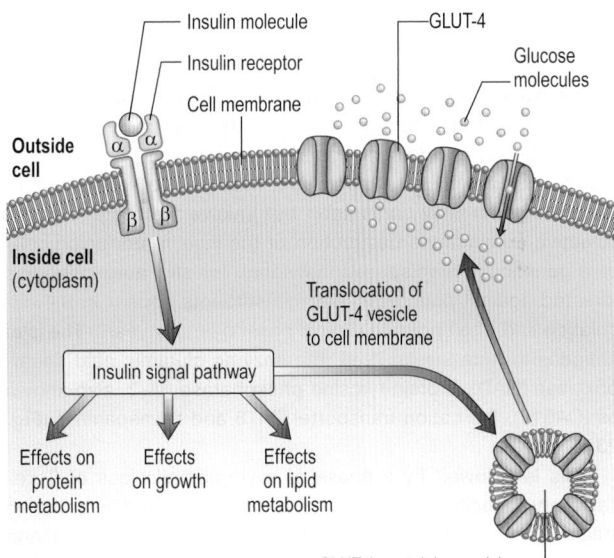

Fig. 23.6 Insulin signalling in peripheral cells (e.g. muscle and adipose tissue). The insulin receptor consists of α- and β-subunits linked by disulphide bridges (top left). The β-subunits straddle the cell membrane. The transporter protein GLUT-4 (bottom right) is stored in intracellular vesicles. The binding of insulin to its receptor initiates many intracellular actions, including translocation of these vesicles to the cell membrane, carrying GLUT-4 with them; this allows glucose transport into the cell.

childhood and young adulthood, reaching a peak incidence around the time of puberty, but can present at any age. In 2017, globally over a million children and adolescents had type 1 diabetes with approximately 132 600 new cases every year. The incidence of type 1 diabetes varies dramatically throughout the world, with the highest rates being in northern Europe and the Middle East.

Type 1 diabetes is subdivided into type 1A (immune-mediated) and type 1B (non-immune-mediated). The vast majority of those affected, especially in Western countries, have type 1A disease. A 'slow-burning' variant with slower progression to insulin deficiency occurs in later life and is termed latent autoimmune diabetes in adults (LADA).

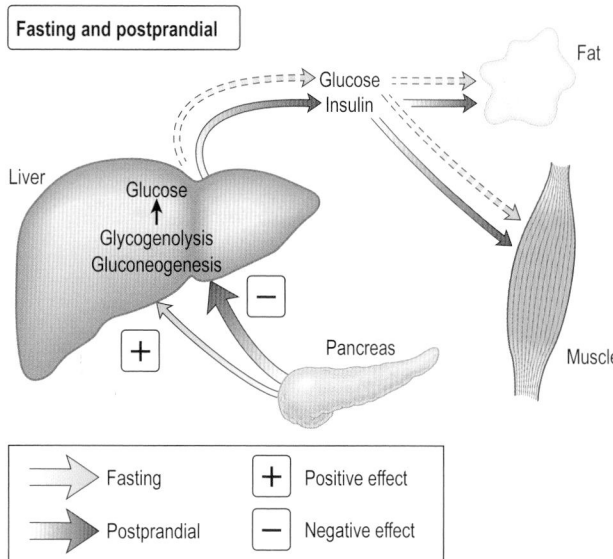

Fasting and postprandial

Fig. 23.7 **Fasting and postprandial effects of insulin.** In the *fasting state*, insulin concentrations are low and it acts mainly as a hepatic hormone, modulating glucose production (via glycogenolysis and gluconeogenesis) from the liver. Hepatic glucose production rises as insulin levels fall. In the *postprandial state*, insulin concentrations are high and it then suppresses glucose production from the liver and promotes the entry of glucose into peripheral tissues, particularly skeletal muscle and fat (increased glucose utilization).

Aetiology

Type 1 diabetes belongs to a family of immune-mediated organ-specific diseases, which include autoimmune thyroid disease, coeliac disease, Addison's disease and pernicious anaemia. The precise molecular mechanisms that lead to type 1 diabetes are incompletely understood but involve the triggering of a selective autoimmune destruction of the insulin producing cells of a genetically predisposed individual. Initially, autoantibodies directed against pancreatic islet constituents appear in the circulation and often predate clinical onset by many years. The islet antigens include insulin itself, the enzyme glutamic acid decarboxylase (GAD), protein tyrosine phosphatase (IA-2, also known as ICA512), the cation transporter ZnT8 and tetraspanin 7 (**Fig. 23.8**).

This is followed by a phase of asymptomatic loss of β cell secretory capacity; histologically, this is characterized by a chronic inflammatory mononuclear cell infiltrate of T lymphocytes and macrophages in the islets, known as insulitis (**Fig. 23.9**). Eventually, when the remaining β cells are no longer able to produce enough insulin to meet the body's needs, diabetes symptoms start to develop.

Some recovery of endogenous insulin secretion may occur over the first few months after diagnosis and treatment initiation (the 'honeymoon period'). During this time, the insulin dose may need to be reduced or even stopped. Recent studies have shown that some people with type 1 diabetes continue to produce small amounts of insulin for many decades after diagnosis. It is unclear why this occurs but it seems that strict glucose control from diagnosis can prolong β cell function.

The ability to detect autoantibodies in children prior to the development of type 1 diabetes is paving the way for trials to prevent the

---

Box 23.4 Aetiological classification of diabetes mellitus, based on classification by the American Diabetes Association[a]

Type 1 diabetes (β-cell destruction)
- Immune-mediated
- Idiopathic

Type 2 diabetes
- Insulin resistance with inadequate insulin secretion
- Formerly non-insulin-dependent diabetes

Other specific types of diabetes (this list is not exhaustive)

Diabetes secondary to genetic defects
- Genetic defects of β-cell function
  - MODY (maturity-onset diabetes of the young)
    - Glucokinase mutations
    - Hepatic nuclear factor mutations
  - Neonatal diabetes
  - Mitochondrial diabetes
- Genetic defects of insulin action
  - Leprechaunism
  - Type A insulin resistance
  - Rabson–Mendenhall syndrome
  - Lipoatrophic diabetes

Diabetes secondary to exocrine pancreatic disease
- Chronic pancreatitis
- Haemochromatosis
- Pancreatic surgery or trauma
- Cystic fibrosis
- Neoplasia
- Fibrocalculous pancreatopathy

Diabetes secondary to endocrine disease
- Acromegaly
- Cushing's syndrome
- Phaeochromocytoma
- Glucagonoma
- Hyperthyroidism
- Somatostatinoma
- Aldosteronoma

Diabetes secondary to drugs and chemicals
- Glucocorticoids
- Thiazide diuretics
- Antipsychotics
- β-adrenergic receptor blockers

Infections
- Congenital rubella
- Cytomegalovirus
- Mumps

Uncommon forms of immune-mediated diabetes
- Stiff man syndrome
- Anti-insulin receptor antibodies

Other genetic syndromes sometimes associated with diabetes:
- Down's syndrome
- Klinefelter's syndrome
- Turner's syndrome
- Prader–Willi syndrome
- DIDMOAD (Wolfram's) syndrome
- Friedreich's ataxia
- Huntington's chorea
- Laurence–Moon–Biedl syndrome
- Myotonic dystrophy
- Porphyria

Gestational diabetes

[a]People with any form of diabetes may require insulin treatment at some stage of their disease. Such use of insulin does not, of itself, classify an individual's diabetes. DIDMOAD, diabetes insipidus, diabetes mellitus, optic atrophy and deafness.
(Adapted from American Diabetes Association. Diagnosis and classification of diabetes mellitus. Diabetes Care 4;37(Suppl. 1):S81–S90.)

---

disease by immune modulation, but these interventions are still in early development.

Genetic susceptibility and inheritance

Increased susceptibility to type 1 diabetes is inherited but the disease is not genetically predetermined. The identical twin of a person with type 1 diabetes has a 30–50% chance of developing the disease, which implies that non-genetic factors must also be involved. The risk of developing diabetes by age 20 years is greater with a father with diabetes (5–7%) than with a mother with diabetes (2–5%). If one child in a family has type 1 diabetes, each sibling has a 4–6% risk of developing diabetes. This risk rises to about 20% in siblings with the same human leucocyte antigen (HLA) genotype as the proband.

Box 23.5 Spectrum of diabetes: a comparison of the different types of diabetes mellitus

Features	Type 1	Type 2	Monogenic	Secondary
Age	Younger (usually <30 years)	Older (usually >30 years)	Neonates to early adulthood	Usually middle or older age
Weight loss	Usually present	Usually no	No	Depends on underlying cause
Symptom duration	Weeks	Months/years	Months	Weeks or months
Seasonal onset	Yes	No	No	No
Heredity	HLA-DR3 or DR4 in >90%	No HLA links	Present in almost all with on-set in early adulthood or (more commonly) earlier	Unusual unless diabetes secondary to genetic conditions such as haemochromatosis
Pathogenesis	Autoimmune disease	No immune disturbance	No immune disturbance	No immune disturbance
Ketonuria	Yes	No or minimal	No or minimal	May be present
Severity of symptoms	Can be marked	Variable but usually mild	Not usually severe	Depends on underlying cause
Biochemical	C-peptide disappears	C-peptide persists	C-peptide persists	C-peptide persists

HLA, human leucocyte antigen.

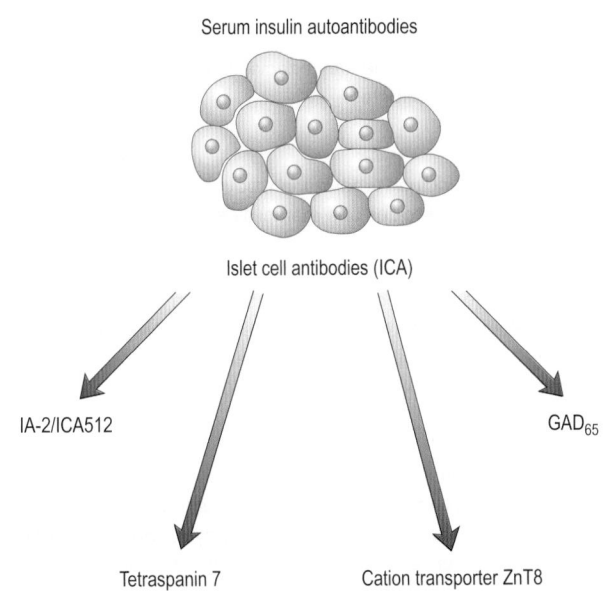

Fig. 23.8 **Islet autoantibodies.** Islet cell antibodies (ICA) are detected by a fluorescent antibody technique that detects binding of autoantibodies to islet cells. Much of this staining reaction is due to antibodies specific for **glutamic acid decarboxylase** (GAD) and **protein tyrosine phosphatase** (IA-2, also known as ICA512). Other islet autoantibodies involved are the cation transporter ZnT8 and the recently identified tetraspanin 7. Insulin autoantibodies also appear in the circulation but do not contribute to the ICA reaction.

Human leucocyte antigen system

Genetic susceptibility is polygenic but the greatest contribution comes from polymorphisms in the HLA region. HLA genes are highly polymorphic and modulate the body's immune defence system. More than 90% of people with type 1 diabetes carry HLA-DR3-DQ2, HLA-DR4-DQ8 or both, as compared with some 35–40% of the background population. By contrast, certain HLA alleles confer protective effects, for example DQB1*0602.

Other genes or gene regions

Genome-wide association studies have greatly broadened our understanding of the genetic background to type 1 diabetes and

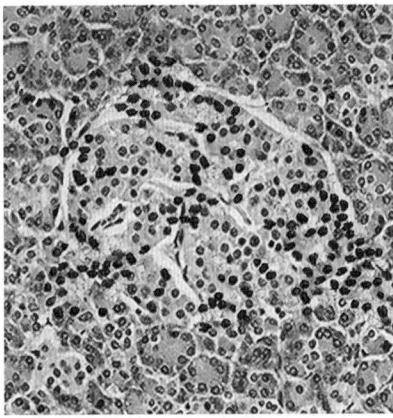

Fig. 23.9 Pancreatic islet showing infiltration by chronic inflammatory cells (insulitis).

have identified more than 50 non-HLA genes or gene regions that influence risk to a minor extent. These include the gene encoding insulin and other genes involved in immune responses.

Environmental factors

Despite the genetic susceptibility to type 1 diabetes, 80–90% of people with newly diagnosed type 1 diabetes do not have a close family history of diabetes and only 10% of individuals with HLA-susceptible genes develop type 1 diabetes. This implies that genetic factors do not account entirely for the development of type 1 diabetes, and environmental triggers are also important.

A large number of putative environmental factors have been identified but none of these is either necessary or sufficient to cause type 1 diabetes. These include:

- **maternal factors**, such as gestational infection and older age
- **viral infections**, including enteroviruses such as Coxsackie B4
- **exposures to dietary constituents**, such as early introduction of cow's milk and relative deficiency of vitamin D
- **environmental toxins**, e.g. alloxan, Vacor
- **childhood obesity**
- **psychological stress.**

How these environment factors interact with the immune system is uncertain and there are several theories to explain this:

- The environmental factor damages the β cells leading to presentation of self-antigens to the T-helper cells, which trigger the autoimmune response against the remaining healthy β cells.
- The self-antigens may be modified and become antigenic.
- An immune response against the environment factor may cross-react with self-antigens, so-called 'molecular mimicry'.
- The 'hygiene hypothesis' proposes that a cleaner environment with less early stimulation of the immune system in childhood may lead to a relatively immature immune system prone to auto-immunity.

Type 2 diabetes mellitus

Epidemiology

Type 2 diabetes is the most common form of diabetes, accounting for around 90% of all cases; it is also one of the most common non-communicable diseases. The prevalence of type 2 diabetes is rising rapidly because of a combination of population growth, an ageing population and longer survival with type 2 diabetes, earlier age at onset and better diagnosis. Type 2 diabetes is a disease of nutrient excess and the incidence has increased with the obesity epidemic, poor quality diet and reduced physical activity.

The prevalence of type 2 diabetes varies markedly across the world with the highest rates being in the Middle East and Pacific Islands, and lowest in Africa and Europe. Although often viewed as a disease of affluence, around three-quarters of those with type 2 diabetes live in low- and middle-income countries and the most rapid rise in incidence is occurring in countries with rapidly growing economies, such as India and China. Two-thirds of people with diabetes live in urban areas.

Aetiology

Genetic susceptibility and inheritance

Identical twins of people with type 2 diabetes have more than a 50% chance of developing diabetes; the risk to non-identical twins or siblings is approximately 25%, confirming a strong inherited component to the disease. Type 2 diabetes is a polygenic disorder and, as with type 1 diabetes, genome-wide studies of association between common DNA variants and disease have allowed identification of numerous susceptibility loci. Several of these loci define β cell development or function, and there is no overlap with the immune function genes identified for type 1 diabetes. Transcription factor-7-like 2 (TCF7-L2) is the most common variant observed in type 2 diabetes in Europeans, and KCNQ1 (a potassium voltage-gated channel) in Asians. Most of the identified genetic markers exert very modest risk and together explain less than 20% of the heritability of type 2 diabetes.

Ageing

Pancreatic β-cell function declines with age and so the incidence of type 2 diabetes increases with age; most people are diagnosed after the age of 40 and one-third of those living with type 2 diabetes are older than 65. However, type 2 diabetes is becoming increasingly common in children and young adults.

Fetal origins of diabetes

There is a J-shaped relationship between low weight at birth and at 12 months of age and glucose intolerance later in life, particularly in those who gain excessive weight in adulthood. The concept is that poor nutrition early in life impairs β-cell development and function, predisposing to diabetes later on. Low birth weight also predisposes to a number of other chronic diseases in adulthood including heart disease, hypertension and osteoporosis.

Obesity

Obesity increases the risk of type 2 diabetes up to 80–100-fold and accounts for 80–85% of the overall risk of developing type 2 diabetes. In Western Europe and North America, 80–90% of adults with type 2 diabetes are overweight and nearly a half are obese. A central distribution of fat increases the risk of type 2 diabetes, and so for any given level of obesity, the more visceral fat an individual has, the higher the risk of type 2 diabetes.

Diet

Although diet can affect the risk of diabetes through changes in body weight, certain dietary patterns are associated with higher or lower risks of type 2 diabetes. Components that increase the risk include: dietary fat, particularly saturated fat, red and processed meat, consumption of fried food, including French fries, increased intake of white rice and sugar-sweetened beverages. Wholegrains, increased fruit and vegetable intake, fermented dairy products, oily fish and a Mediterranean dietary pattern are associated with lower rates of type 2 diabetes.

Physical inactivity

Physical inactivity and sedentary behaviour are also associated with an increased risk of diabetes.

Other factors

Other risk factors include urbanization, poverty, abnormal sleep patterns, environmental toxins and mental illness.

Pathogenesis

The relative role of defects in insulin secretion and action in the pathogenesis of type 2 diabetes has been much debated and likely differs between different people. However, both defects are necessary to develop diabetes.

Abnormalities of insulin action

Insulin action is diminished in type 2 diabetes through the development of insulin resistance, which is defined as the inability of insulin to produce its usual biological effects at physiological concentrations. It is characterized by an impaired ability of insulin to:

- inhibit hepatic glucose output
- stimulate glucose uptake into skeletal muscle, and
- suppress lipolysis in adipose tissue.

The underlying mechanisms of insulin resistance are not fully understood but result from nutrient excess. Intracellular triglyceride accumulates in the liver and skeletal muscle and impedes the phosphorylation of the post-receptor insulin receptor substrate, IRS-1. Although this defect reduces insulin action with regards to glucose and lipid metabolism, insulin is still able to activate the mitogen-activated protein (MAP) kinase pathway, which regulates a number of intracellular pathways involved in inflammation, cellular proliferation and atherosclerosis.

Abnormalities of insulin secretion

Insulin resistance alone does explain the development of diabetes as only one-fifth of those with the degree of insulin resistance characteristic of diabetes develop the condition. As insulin resistance develops, the body's response is to increase insulin secretion and so early diabetes is often associated with insulin hypersecretion. This observation led some to question the role of β-cell function in the aetiology of diabetes. Nevertheless, insulin secretory abnormalities manifest early in the course of type 2 diabetes and progress with time; an early sign is loss of the first phase of the normal biphasic insulin secretion. Even though circulating insulin concentrations are higher than in people without diabetes, they are still inadequate to restore glucose homeostasis. By the time of diagnosis, at least 50% of β-cell mass and function has been lost. Relative insulin lack is associated with increased glucose production from the liver (owing to inadequate suppression of gluconeogenesis) and reduced insulin-mediated glucose uptake by peripheral tissues. Hyperglycaemia and lipid excess are toxic to β cells, at least *in vitro*, a phenomenon known as glucotoxicity, which is thought to cause further β-cell loss and further deterioration of glucose homeostasis. With time, insulin secretion declines, an observation referred to as the 'Starling curve' of the pancreas. This time course varies widely between individuals.

Type 2 diabetes is thus a condition in which insulin deficiency relative to increased demand leads to insulin hypersecretion by a depleted β-cell mass and progression towards absolute insulin deficiency, requiring insulin therapy.

Other hormonal abnormalities

Glucagon secretion is increased in type 2 diabetes, likely because of diminished intra-islet insulin, and leads to increased hepatic glucose output.

The insulin response to oral glucose is greater than the response to intravenous glucose, a phenomenon known as the incretin effect. The effect is mediated by two hormones, glucagon like peptide-1 (GLP-1) and glucose-dependent insulinotrophic polypeptide (GIP), which are released by the gastrointestinal tract following eating. Their major action is to increase glucose-induced β-cell insulin secretion, while suppressing glucagon secretion, but they also slow gastric emptying and induce satiety. Both hormones have short half-lives in the circulation, being degraded within minutes predominantly by the enzyme dipeptidyl peptidase-4 (DPP4). The incretin effect is impaired in type 2 diabetes.

Glucose reabsorption in the kidney

The sodium-glucose transporter 2 (SGLT2) is a sodium-dependent glucose transport protein located in the proximal renal tubules, whose function is to reabsorb glucose from the renal filtrate and restore it to the circulation. Its activity thus determines the renal threshold for glucose, which normally averages approximately 10–11 mmol/L (180–200 mg/dL). This prevents urinary glucose loss but is maladaptive in type 2 diabetes as this process is upregulated and serves to maintain hyperglycaemia.

Monogenic diabetes mellitus

Approximately 1–3% of people with diabetes diagnosed under the age of 30 years have monogenic diabetes, previously called 'maturity-onset diabetes of the young' (MODY) (**Box 23.6**). Monogenic diabetes is caused by a single gene mutation, which is dominantly inherited and predominantly affects β-cell function. Extra-pancreatic features may also be present. Many people with monogenic diabetes are misdiagnosed with either type 1 or type 2 diabetes and so monogenic diabetes should be considered in people presenting with early-onset diabetes in association with an affected parent, and early-onset diabetes in approximately 50% of relatives. It is likely that as awareness improves, the diagnosis rate will increase.

Type 1 diabetes does not present in children before 6 months of age and so infants who develop diabetes at this age are likely to have a monogenic defect. Transient neonatal diabetes mellitus occurs soon after birth and resolves at a median of 12 weeks; around 50% of people ultimately relapse later in life. Most have an abnormality of imprinting of the *ZAC* and *HYMAI* genes on chromosome 6q. The most common cause of permanent neonatal diabetes mellitus is mutations in the *KCNJ11* gene encoding the Kir6.2 subunit of the β-cell potassium–adenosine triphosphate (ATP) channel.

Neurological features are seen in 20% of children. Diabetes results from defective insulin release rather than β-cell destruction, and can be treated successfully with sulphonylureas, even after many years of insulin therapy.

Further reading

Chatterjee S, Khunti K, Davies MJ. Type 2 diabetes. *Lancet* 2017; 389:2239–2251.
Defronzo RA. Banting Lecture. From the triumvirate to the ominous octet: a new paradigm for the treatment of type 2 diabetes mellitus. *Diabetes* 2009; 58:773–795.
DiMeglio LA, Evans-Molina C, Oram RA. Type 1 diabetes. *Lancet* 2018; 391:2449–2462.
International Diabetes Federation. *IDF Diabetes Atlas*, 9th edn; https://www.diabetesatlas.org/.
Kahn SE, Cooper ME, Del Prato S. Pathophysiology and treatment of type 2 diabetes: perspectives on the past, present and future. *Lancet* 2014; 383:1068–1083.
Katsarou A, Gudbjörnsdottir S, Rawshani A et al. Type 1 diabetes. *Nat Rev Dis Primers* 2017; 3:17016.
McCarthy MI. Genetics of T2DM in 2016: biological and translational insights from T2DM genetic. *Nat Rev Endocrinol* 2017; 13:71–72.
Nolan CJ, Damm P, Prentki M. Type 2 diabetes across generations: from pathophysiology to prevention and management. *Lancet* 2011; 378:169–181.

Box 23.6 Monogenic causes of diabetes[a]

Features	Glucokinase	*HNF-1a*	*HNF-1b*	*HNF-4a*	*IPF-1*
Chromosomal location	7p	12q	17q	20q	13q
Proportion of all cases	15%	70%	2%	5%	<1%
Onset	Present from birth	Teens/twenties	Teens/twenties	Teens/thirties	Teens/thirties
Progression	Little deterioration with age	Progressive hyperglycaemia	Progression unclear	Progressive hyperglycaemia	Progression unclear
Microvascular complications		Frequent	Frequent	Frequent	
Other features	None	Low renal glucose threshold (glycosuria) Raised HDL cholesterol	Renal cysts, proteinuria, chronic kidney disease	Increased birth weight Neonatal hypoglycaemia Low HDL and raised LDL cholesterol	

[a]The glucokinase gene is intimately involved in the glucose-sensing mechanism within the pancreatic β cell. The hepatic nuclear factor (HNF) genes and the insulin promoter factor-1 (IPF-1) gene control nuclear transcription in the β cell, where they regulate its development and function. Abnormal nuclear transcription genes may cause pancreatic agenesis or more subtle progressive pancreatic damage. A handful of families with autosomal dominant diabetes have been described with mutations in neurogenic differentiation factor-1 (NeuroD1).

CLINICAL APPROACH TO THE PATIENT WITH DIABETES

Presentation

Presentation may be acute, subacute or asymptomatic, or an individual may present with a complication of diabetes.

Acute presentation

Children and young adults often present with a 2–6-week history of the classic triad of symptoms:
- **polyuria** due to the osmotic diuresis that results when blood glucose levels exceed the renal threshold
- **thirst and polydipsia** due to the resulting loss of fluid and electrolytes
- **weight loss** due to fluid depletion and accelerated breakdown of fat and muscle secondary to insulin deficiency.

Ketonuria is often present in young people and may progress to ketoacidosis if these early symptoms are not recognized and treated.

Subacute presentation

The clinical onset may be prolonged over several months or years, particularly in older people. Thirst, polyuria and weight loss are usually present, but the individual may complain of other symptoms such as lack of energy, visual blurring (owing to glucose-induced changes in refraction), or pruritus vulvae or balanitis due to *Candida* infection.

Complications as the presenting feature

These include:
- staphylococcal skin infections
- retinopathy noted during a visit to the optician
- a polyneuropathy causing tingling and numbness in the feet
- erectile dysfunction
- arterial disease, resulting in myocardial infarction or peripheral gangrene.

Asymptomatic diabetes

It is estimated that approximately half of people with diabetes are unaware of their condition. This proportion varies across the world, from about a third in high-income countries to three-quarters in some low-income countries. Consequently, up to one-third of diagnoses are made as an incidental finding and several countries have introduced screening programmes to identify those with asymptomatic undiagnosed diabetes.

Physical examination at diagnosis

Evidence of weight loss and dehydration may be present, and the breath may smell of ketones. Older people may present with established complications. Occasionally, there will be physical signs of an illness causing secondary diabetes (see **Boxes 23.4** and **23.5**). People with severe insulin resistance may have acanthosis nigricans, which is characterized by blackish pigmentation at the nape of the neck and in the axillae (see **Fig. 22.37**). Hypertension is present in 50% of people with type 2 diabetes and in a higher proportion of people of African and Caribbean ethnicity.

 Box 23.7 World Health Organization diagnostic criteria for diabetes[a]

- Fasting plasma glucose >7.0 mmol/L (126 mg/dL)
- Random plasma glucose >11.1 mmol/L (200 mg/dL)
- HbA$_{1c}$ >6.5% (48 mmol/mol)

One abnormal laboratory value is diagnostic in symptomatic individuals; two values are needed in asymptomatic people. The glucose tolerance test (see **Box 23.8**) is only required where there is diagnostic uncertainty and for diagnosis of cystic fibrosis-related diabetes and gestational diabetes.

[a]There is no such thing as mild diabetes. All people who meet the criteria for diabetes are liable to develop disabling long-term complications.

Box 23.8 The 75 g oral glucose tolerance test: World Health Organization criteria[a]

Timing of test	Normal	Impaired glucose tolerance	Diabetes mellitus
Fasting	<6.0 mmol/L <106 mg/dL	<7.0 mmol/L <126 mg/dL	≥7.0 mmol/L ≥126 mmol/L
2 h after glucose[b]	<7.8 mmol/L <140 mg/dL	7.8–11.0 mmol/L 140–200 mg/dL	≥11.1 mmol/L ≥200 mg/dL

[a]Only a fasting and a 120-min sample are needed. Results are for venous plasma; whole-blood values are lower.
[b]Adult 75 g glucose in 300 mL water; child 1.75 g glucose/kg body weight.

Diagnosis and investigations

Once considered, diabetes is easy to diagnose. This may be by a laboratory measurement of fasting plasma glucose (FPG), random glucose or a 2-hour plasma glucose after a 75-g oral glucose tolerance test (OGTT). The use of glycated haemoglobin (HbA$_{1c}$; also called A$_{1c}$ in the USA) was introduced as an alternative method in 2011. HbA$_{1c}$ is an integrated measure of an individual's prevailing blood glucose concentration over several weeks and is also used to guide treatment decisions.

Diabetes can be diagnosed if the fasting plasma glucose is higher than or equal to 7.0 mmol/L (126 mg/dL) or the random or 2-hour glucose tolerance test plasma glucose is more than or equal to 11.1 mmol/L (200 mg/dL) or the HbA$_{1c}$ is higher than or equal to 48 mmol/mol (6.5%).

When overt symptoms are present, only one biochemical test is needed but in the absence of clear symptoms, two abnormal glucose or HbA$_{1c}$ tests are required (**Boxes 23.7** and **23.8**). Fasting, 2-hour glucose and HbA$_{1c}$ identify slightly different populations of people with diabetes; that is, someone may be diagnosed by one criteria but not another. However, with time, people will eventually cross the diagnostic threshold for the other tests.

The diagnostic criteria recognize two further categories of abnormal glucose concentrations: impaired fasting glycaemia (IFG) and impaired glucose tolerance (IGT). Collectively these have been described as 'pre-diabetes' but this is not strictly accurate because the majority will never develop diabetes. Neither IFG nor IGT are clinical entities in their own right but they identify people who are at high risk of diabetes and cardiovascular disease. Individuals with IGT have a similar risk of cardiovascular disease as those with frank diabetes, but do not develop microvascular complications. Impaired fasting glucose (IFG) only overlaps with IGT to a limited extent, and the associated risks of cardiovascular disease and future diabetes are not directly comparable.

Impaired glucose tolerance can only be diagnosed with a glucose tolerance test (see **Box 23.8**) and is complicated by poor reproducibility of the key 2-hour value in this test. Impaired fasting glucose is defined as a fasting plasma glucose between 6.1 and 6.9 mmol/L (110–126 mg/dL) and has the practical advantage that it avoids the need for a glucose tolerance test. The ADA definition of IFG differs slightly from the WHO criteria in that the ADA threshold is 100 mg/dL (5.6 mmol/L).

Glycosuria cannot be used to diagnose diabetes, but requires further investigation. It is commoner in older people, who have an altered renal threshold for glucose. It may also occur in familial renal glycosuria, which is a monogenic disorder affecting function of the sodium–glucose co-transporter (*SGLT2*) and found in about 1 : 400 of the population.

Other investigations

No further tests are needed to diagnose diabetes, but measurement of C-peptide and islet auto-antibodies can help determine the type of diabetes. C-peptide can be measured in blood or urine; it is often present when type 1 diabetes is diagnosed but disappears with time and is a more useful investigation in people with a duration of diabetes longer than 5 years. Other routine investigations include urine testing for protein, a full blood count, urea and electrolytes, liver biochemistry and random lipids. The latter test is useful to exclude associated hyperlipidaemia and, if elevated, should be repeated as a fasting measurement after diabetes has been brought under control. Investigations of secondary causes of diabetes or associated autoimmune disease may be appropriate (see **Box 23.4**).

Further reading

American Diabetes Association. Diagnosis and classification of diabetes mellitus. *Diabetes Care* 2018; 41(Suppl 1):S13–S27.

PREVENTION OF TYPE 2 DIABETES

A dramatic reduction in the incidence of adult-onset diabetes was documented during the Second World War when food was scarce. More recently, clinical trials in individuals with IGT have shown that it is possible to prevent or at least delay the development of type 2 diabetes by lifestyle and/or pharmacological interventions. The lifestyle interventions aim to reduce body weight, reduce dietary fat intake, in particular saturated fat, while increasing dietary fibre and moderate physical activity to approximately 30 minutes a day. Several drugs, including metformin and orlistat, reduce incident diabetes but these are less effective than lifestyle change and should be reserved for those who cannot change their lifestyle or whose glucose concentration continues to rise despite lifestyle change. Bariatric surgery to treat morbid obesity can normalize elevated blood glucose; the effect on glucose precedes weight loss, suggesting a direct metabolic effect of surgery, possibly mediated by gut hormones, as well as an effect of long-term weight loss.

Given limited healthcare resources, interventions are targeted at those at highest risk and who will benefit most. Several risk assessment algorithms are available to identify those at highest risk of diabetes. Measurement of blood glucose will identify people with IFG or IGT.

Further reading

Diab M, Barhoosh HA, Daoudi B et al. Prevention and screening recommendations in type 2 diabetes: review and critical appraisal of clinical practice guidelines. *Prim Care Diabetes* 2019; 13:197–203.

National Institute of Diabetes and Digestive and Kidney Diseases. *Preventing Type 2 Diabetes*; https://www.niddk.nih.gov/health-information/diabetes/overview/preventing-type-2-diabetes.
National Institute for Health and Care Excellence. *NICE Public Health Guideline 38: Type 2 Diabetes: Prevention in People at High Risk.* NICE 2012; https://www.nice.org.uk/guidance/ph38.

MANAGEMENT OF DIABETES

Aims of diabetes care

For most people, diabetes is a life-long condition. Except for a few hours a year spent in contact with healthcare professionals, the majority of people with diabetes will look after their condition themselves for most of the time. It is therefore vital that people develop the skills to manage their condition effectively. The aims of diabetes care and management are fourfold:

- Prevention of life-threatening diabetes emergencies, such as diabetic ketoacidosis and hypoglycaemia with effective management when they do occur
- Treatment of hyperglycaemic symptoms
- Minimization of long-term complications through screening and effective control of hyperglycaemia and other cardiovascular risk factors
- Avoidance of iatrogenic side-effects, such as hypoglycaemia.

Fortunately, individuals with diabetes usually do not experience life-threatening diabetes emergencies frequently (the incidence of diabetic ketoacidosis is roughly two episodes per 100 person-years while the rate of severe hypoglycaemia is ≈2.5 events per person-year) and hyperglycaemic symptoms are easily treated. Therefore, most of the discussions regarding diabetes management revolve around maintaining good diabetes control to prevent long-term complications whilst balancing the short-term adverse events associated with treatment. Hyperglycaemia drives microvascular complications and it is unsurprising that the impact of improved glucose control on small-vessel complications, such as retinopathy and nephropathy, has been compellingly demonstrated.

The Diabetes Control and Complications Trial (DCCT) compared standard and intensive insulin therapy in a large trial of young people with type 1 diabetes, some of whom had no evidence of retinopathy or microalbuminuria (primary prevention group) at the beginning of the trial and others who already had evidence of these complications (secondary prevention group). Despite intensive therapy, mean blood glucose levels were still 40% above the non-diabetic range, but even at this level of control, the risk of primary progression to retinopathy was reduced by 60%, nephropathy by 30% and neuropathy by 20% over 7 years with intensive insulin therapy. These benefits persisted beyond the end of the trial despite equivalent levels of glucose control in the post-trial period.

The UK Prospective Diabetes Study (UKPDS) compared standard and intensive treatment in a large trial in people with recently diagnosed type 2 diabetes. Intensive treatment was associated with a 25% overall reduction in microvascular disease end-points, a 33% reduction in albuminuria and a 30% reduction in the need for laser treatment for retinopathy in the more intensively treated people. Similar to the DCCT, these benefits persisted for many years after conclusion of the trial (the 'legacy effect'). This study also showed blood pressure control to be equally necessary in the prevention of retinopathy, but there is no legacy effect and good blood pressure control needs to be maintained.

Although there is an association between glucose and large-vessel disease, which extends well into the glucose range of the general population, with no clear cut-off for risk, the benefits of reducing hyperglycaemia are less certain for macrovascular disease. In this context, we should remember that diabetes affects not only carbohydrate metabolism, but also lipid and protein metabolism. People with diabetes often have other cardiovascular risk factors, such as dyslipidaemia, hypertension and obesity, and these risk factors may play a more important role than hyperglycaemia. Both the DCCT and UKPDS studies showed a reduction in cardiovascular events in the post-trial follow-up period in the intensive treatment groups, suggesting that early control of hyperglycaemia may improve the long-term risk of cardiovascular disease.

In both the DCCT and UKPDS, the achieved levels of glycaemic control were above those of people without diabetes and so further trials were undertaken in people with type 2 diabetes to assess whether further lowering of glucose to normoglycaemia would yield greater benefits. These trials confirmed the benefits for microvascular disease but did not improve cardiovascular outcomes and in the Action to Control Cardiovascular Risk in Diabetes (ACCORD) study, more people died in the intensively treated group than the standard arm. Exactly why this occurred is uncertain, but it seems likely that any benefit of improved glucose control was outweighed by iatrogenic side-effects, such as hypoglycaemia and weight gain.

Most guidelines advocate HbA$_{1c}$ targets between 48 mmol/mol and 58 mmol/mol (6.5–7.5%) but as the benefits and risks of improved glycaemic control differ between people with diabetes, the actual glycaemic targets should be determined for each individual taking into account the factors shown in **Box 23.9**. Realistic goals should be agreed with each person, considering what is likely to be achievable. This applies particularly to older people and those with a limited prognosis.

> **Box 23.9 Factors to consider with individualizing glycaemic targets for people with diabetes**
>
> **Stringent glycaemic control**
> - No hypoglycaemia
> - Less complexity/polypharmacy
> - Lifestyle or metformin only
> - Short disease duration
> - Long life expectancy
> - No cardiovascular disease
>
> **Less stringent control**
> - History of severe hypoglycaemia
> - High burden of therapy
> - Longer disease duration
> - Limited life expectancy
> - Extensive co-morbidity
> - Cardiovascular disease

Role of self-management education

As the onus of diabetes management lies with the individual with diabetes, it is essential that the individual is equipped with the skills for this task. People with diabetes need to understand the risks of diabetes and the potential benefits of glycaemic control and other measures such as maintaining a lean weight, stopping smoking and taking care of their feet. If healthcare professionals do not provide accurate information, misinformation from others will take its place. In order to address this need, diabetes self-management education has become an important cornerstone of diabetes care, delivered by all members of the diabetes multidisciplinary team (**Fig. 23.10**). The education needs to be tailored to the individual by embracing a 'patient-centred approach'.

Structured educational programmes with a clear philosophy, such as 'Dose Adjustment for Normal Eating' (DAFNE), that employ trained facilitators using a written curriculum are seen as the gold standard. These programmes improve diabetes knowledge and quality of life, glycaemic control and reduce mortality. Education should not be viewed as a once-off inoculation and regular ongoing support and updates will be needed.

Diet

Diet plays a key role in the management and clinical care of all people with diabetes. However, there has been a lot of controversy about what constitutes an ideal or optimal diet for a person with, or at risk of, diabetes. Previous guidance focused on the ideal macronutrient composition of the diet, but the latest guidance highlights the role of certain foods and dietary patterns. In common with the general population, people should be encouraged to eat more vegetables, fruits, wholegrains, fish, nuts and pulses while reducing the consumption of red and processed meat, refined carbohydrates and sugar-sweetened beverages. As no one diet is effective in managing diabetes, it is important to adopt an individualized approach taking into consideration the person's personal and cultural preferences. **Box 23.10** summarizes the latest Diabetes UK dietary recommendations for people with diabetes.

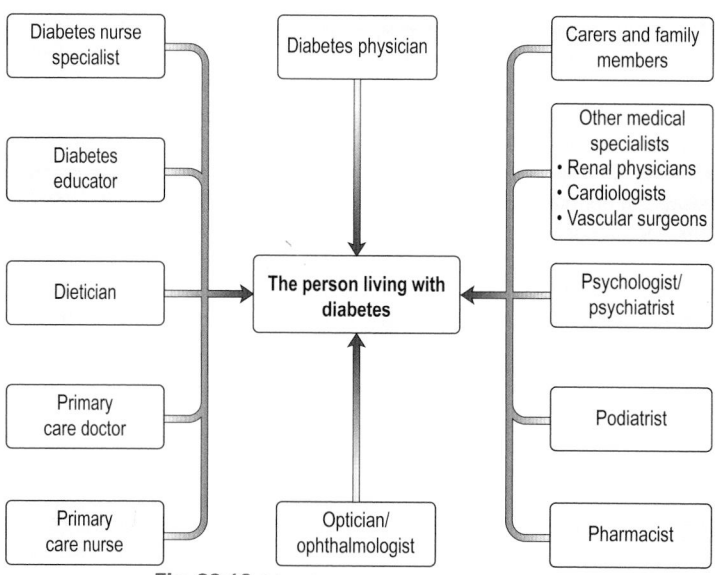

Fig. 23.10 Members of the diabetes team.

Box 23.10 Abbreviated summary of the evidence-based nutrition guidelines for the management of diabetes, hyperlipidaemia and hypertension

- Nutrition advice should be offered to all people with diabetes, hyperlipidaemia and hypertension and those at risk of developing type 2 diabetes as part of an integrated package of education and clinical care.
- Dietary advice should be individualized and culturally sensitive.
- People with type 1 diabetes should be supported to identify and quantify their dietary carbohydrate intake in order to support the adjustment of insulin dose to carbohydrate intake.
- People with type 2 diabetes, hyperlipidaemia, hypertension or at risk of developing type 2 diabetes who are overweight should be supported to lose at least 5% of their weight by reducing calorie intake and increasing energy expenditure.
- Low glycaemic index foods are encouraged.
- A Mediterranean-style diet or equivalent healthy eating pattern should be encouraged. Key features of these diets include:
  - Decreasing salt intake to <6 g/day
  - Eating two portions of oily fish each week
  - Eating more wholegrains, fruit and vegetables, fish, nuts and legumes (pulses)
  - Consuming less red and processed meat, refined carbohydrates and sugar-sweetened beverages
  - Replacing saturated fats with unsaturated fats, and limiting intake of trans-fatty acids
  - Limiting alcohol intake to ≤14 units/week

(Based on the Diabetes UK evidence-based nutrition guidelines for the management of diabetes.)

One exception to the food-based recommendations concerns carbohydrate intake, which is important for people using intensive insulin regimens, particularly those with type 1 diabetes. In people without diabetes, the amount of insulin produced after eating is dependent on the carbohydrate consumed. In order to optimize glycaemic control, people need to match their insulin dose to the carbohydrate in the meal and so it is important to teach people how to 'carbohydrate count'. Several books and apps are available to help with this process.

The peak blood glucose after a meal varies with the type of carbohydrate. For example, the glucose profile after eating pasta is much flatter than that seen after eating the same amount of carbohydrate as a sugary drink because pasta has a lower 'glycaemic index'. Foods with a low glycaemic index are encouraged to prevent rapid swings in plasma glucose.

Importance of weight loss in type 2 diabetes

For many years, it was thought that type 2 diabetes was an incurable progressive condition; however, the latest evidence challenges this view. People who can be supported to lose 10–15 kg of body weight through lifestyle, pharmacological or surgical treatment can enter remission.

Bariatric or metabolic surgery (see p. 1252) is a treatment option for people with severe obesity. The National Institute for Health and Care Excellence (NICE) recommends consideration of surgery in those with a body mass index (BMI) higher than 40 kg/m², or in those with a BMI of more than 35 kg/m² and co-morbidities, such as diabetes. In the USA, the Food and Drug Administration (FDA)-recommended BMI thresholds are lower. The most common operations are gastric bypass and sleeve gastrectomy. These operations lead to a mean weight loss of approximately 30% and diabetes remission in up to 70% of people, depending on the duration of diabetes. Surgery also improves quality of life and reduces cardiovascular disease and mortality. The operative mortality is low (1 in 1000) but there are long-term consequences for nutrition, bone health and suicide.

Physical activity

No treatment for diabetes is complete without exercise as physical activity has profound benefits, including improved fitness, reduced insulin requirement and better glycaemic control, lower cardiovascular risk and greater life expectancy. The maxim that *some exercise is better than no exercise and more exercise is better than some exercise* applies. People with diabetes should be advised to take at least 150 minutes of aerobic exercise and resistance training per week spread over a minimum of 3 days. Prior to exercise, however, it is important to ascertain whether the individual has either macrovascular or microvascular complications as these may be exacerbated by unaccustomed activity.

People with type 1 diabetes should be advised that physical activity can reduce the insulin requirement and lead to unstable glucose levels during and immediately after exercise and a later risk of severe hypoglycaemia.

Tobacco smoking

Smoking can adversely affect glucose management as well as increasing the risk of a number of medical conditions and so healthcare professionals should support people who smoke to quit.

Insulin

Prior to discovery of insulin in 1921, the life expectancy of people with type 1 diabetes was only 3–4 months. Many people died from diabetic ketoacidosis but it was possible to survive for several years on diets of around 500–700 calories/day; these individuals had a wretched existence until either the person broke their diet or died from starvation. The discovery of insulin is rightly considered one of the greatest medical advances of the 20th century as the lives of millions of people with diabetes have been transformed by its discovery. Insulin is always indicated in people with type 1 diabetes and is often needed in those with type 2 diabetes as the condition progresses.

The philosophy of insulin therapy is to mimic the normal physiological secretion of insulin as closely as possible (see **Fig. 23.5**). This involves the use of both long-acting insulin to replicate the basal secretion of insulin and short-acting insulin to cover mealtimes.

Insulin was historically derived from beef or pig pancreas but this has been replaced by highly purified biosynthetic insulin, which is produced by adding a DNA sequence coding for insulin or proinsulin into cultured yeast or bacterial cells.

Short-acting insulins

Soluble human insulin is absorbed slowly, reaching a peak 60–90 minutes after subcutaneous injection. Its action tends to persist after meals, predisposing to hypoglycaemia. Absorption is delayed because soluble insulin forms stable hexamers (six insulin molecules around a zinc core), which need to dissociate to monomers or dimers before it can enter the circulation.

This delay is inconvenient for people with diabetes because the insulin should be injected 20–30 minutes prior to a meal, which often is not feasible. ***Short-acting insulin analogues*** (***insulin lispro***, ***insulin aspart*** and ***insulin glulisine***) have been engineered that dissociate more rapidly following injection without altering the biological effect (see **Fig. 23.2**). These ***insulin analogues*** enter and disappear from the circulation more rapidly than soluble insulin. A newer formulation of insulin aspart has been developed that dissociates and enters the circulation even more rapidly.

The use of short-acting insulin analogues in people with type 1 diabetes reduces total and nocturnal hypoglycaemic episodes and improves glycaemic control as judged by postprandial glucose concentrations and HbA$_{1c}$. The benefits in people with type 2 diabetes are more modest but short-acting insulin analogues seem to provide better control of HbA$_{1c}$ and postprandial glucose than soluble human insulin.

Intermediate and longer-acting insulins

The action of human insulin can be prolonged by the addition of zinc or protamine. The most widely used form is NPH (neutral protamine Hagedorn) or isophane insulin but its use is hampered by variability from one injection to another, the need to re-suspend the insulin prior to injection and a peak action, which generally occurs in the middle of the night. Long-acting analogues have been developed to delay absorption and prolong the duration of action (see **Fig. 23.2**). Insulin glargine is soluble in the vial as a slightly acidic (pH 4) solution but precipitates at subcutaneous pH, thus prolonging its duration of action. A concentrated formulation of insulin glargine is now available with a longer and flatter duration of action than the standard preparation. ***Insulin detemir*** and ***insulin degludec*** have a fatty acid 'tail' that binds to serum albumin; the slow dissociation from the bound state prolongs the duration of action. In the case of insulin degludec, it forms long multihexamer chains at the site of injection, which only dissociate very slowly. Long-acting insulin analogues reduce hypoglycaemia for people with both type 1 diabetes and type 2 diabetes, particularly at night.

As insulin analogues are more expensive than NPH insulin, in the case of type 2 diabetes NICE recommends that insulin analogues are reserved for people who do not respond well to NPH insulin. The European Association of the Study of Diabetes and American Diabetes Association consensus report on the management of type 2 diabetes notes the benefits of insulin analogues but highlights that the way in which insulin is used has a greater impact on the effectiveness and adverse effects of insulin than differences between insulin formulations.

Strengths of insulin

Most insulin is formulated as 100 units/mL but more concentrated forms are available, for example insulin glargine is available as U300 (300 units/mL) as described above. Insulin degludec is available in two concentrations: 100 and 200 units/mL. The pen devices for these insulins indicate how many units of insulin are given but there is a significant danger of overdose if the insulin is withdrawn from the pen and administered using an insulin syringe. A number of warnings have been issued to prevent this practice.

Some people with diabetes experience severe insulin resistance and require massive insulin doses. U500-strength insulin is available for these individuals allowing them to inject the same dose of insulin in one-fifth of the usual volume. Rare syndromes of insulin resistance exist, but most cases are unexplained (see **Box 23.4**). Insulin resistance associated with antibodies directed against the insulin receptor has been reported in people with acanthosis nigricans.

Twice-daily mixed soluble and intermediate insulins

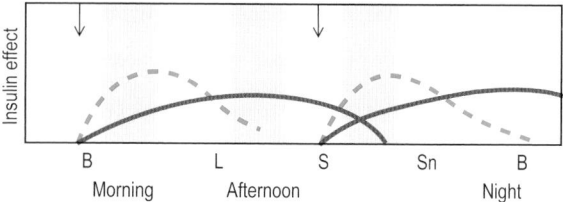

Three-times-daily soluble with intermediate- or long-acting insulin given before bedtime

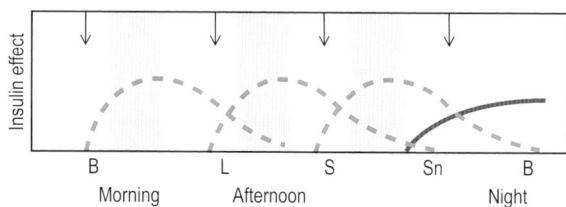

Three-times-daily rapid-acting analogue with long-acting analogue insulin given before bedtime

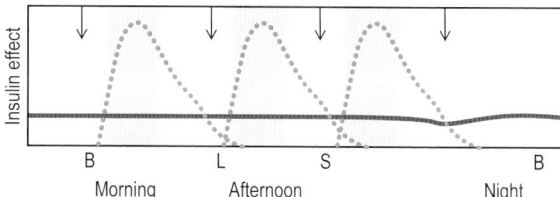

Fig. 23.11 Insulin regimens. Profiles of soluble insulins are shown as dashed lines; intermediate- or long-acting insulin as solid lines (purple); and rapid-acting insulin as dotted lines (blue). The arrows indicate when the injections are given. B, breakfast; L, lunch; S, supper; Sn, snack (bedtime).

Insulin regimens

Many different combinations of insulin are used to treat people with diabetes but there are several regimens that are more commonly used. The possible treatment options should be discussed with the individual to find the one that is most suitable to their needs and lifestyle.

Basal-bolus regimen

The basal-bolus regimen involves the administration of both short- and long-acting insulin. Long-acting insulin is injected 1–2 times per day to provide the background (basal) insulin to keep the glucose concentration consistent during periods of fasting (**Fig. 23.11**). Short-acting insulin is given shortly before eating as a bolus to control glucose concentration following a meal. This regimen most closely mimics normal insulin physiology and is more flexible than other regimens as each injection can be adjusted individually.

This regimen is the treatment of choice for people with type 1 diabetes but is increasingly used in younger people with type 2 diabetes. The flexibility is of great value to people who have busy jobs, work shifts and travel regularly. The main disadvantage of a basal-bolus regimen is the number of injections.

Twice-daily mixed insulin regimen

A mixture of short- and long-acting insulin is injected before breakfast and the evening meal (see **Fig. 23.11**). There are a number of insulin preparations with premixed insulin but it is also possible to self-mix the insulin. This regimen is used more commonly for people with type 2 diabetes but may be used by people with type 1 diabetes when it is not possible inject four times a day. The main disadvantage of this regimen is the lack of a lunch-time bolus and higher basal levels between meals, which increase the risk of hypoglycaemia.

Basal-only and basal-plus insulin regimens

As people with type 2 diabetes are able to produce insulin, it may be possible to use a less intensive insulin regimen. Basal long-acting insulin at night, together with other non-insulin treatments during the day, is initially as effective as multidose insulin regimens and is less likely to promote weight gain. Addition of mealtime insulin may become necessary to control postprandial hyperglycaemia.

Insulin administration

Insulin is administered subcutaneously by intermittent injection or by insulin pumps (continuous subcutaneous insulin infusion, CSII). The usual injection sites are the front and upper outer side of the thigh, the abdominal wall, buttocks and upper outer arms. Injection technology has improved dramatically since insulin was first discovered; although insulin may be drawn up from a vial into special plastic insulin syringes, an increasing number of people now use insulin pens, which may be disposable with pre-filled insulin or re-usable by changing the insulin cartridge when empty. The pens are portable, use a fine 4–5 mm needle and have a simplified procedure for dialing the insulin dose. Compared with needles and syringes, pens are more convenient, more accurate, easier to use and produce a less painful injection. Even though most injections are virtually painless, people are understandably apprehensive and must learn how to give insulin safely and effectively.

Introduced over 35 years ago, insulin pumps are small devices that continuously infuse insulin into the subcutaneous tissue. The technology has progressively improved and allows the user to give varying amounts of basal insulin throughout the day with mealtime boluses, guided by the pump software. The latest pumps connect with continuous glucose monitors that allow the pump to suspend the insulin infusion if the glucose levels are low or predicted to become low. The long-term goal is to develop a completely 'closed loop' system or 'artificial pancreas' where the glucose monitor and pump automatically control the insulin infusion rate to maintain normal glucose concentrations without input from the wearer. Pump therapy in people with type 1 diabetes improves glycaemic control, reduces hypoglycaemia and leads to better quality of life compared with multiple daily injections. These benefits have led to an increasing number of pump users although the uptake of CSII varies across the world; up to 40% of people with type 1 diabetes use pumps in the USA compared with 12.2% in the UK.

The disadvantages of pump therapy include the nuisance of being attached to a gadget, skin infections, the risk of ketoacidosis if the flow of insulin is interrupted (since there is no protective reservoir of injected basal insulin) and cost.

Lipohypertrophy and lipoatrophy

Fatty lumps, known as lipohypertrophy, may occur following the overuse of a single injection site with any type of insulin.

Local allergic responses sometimes occur early in therapy but usually resolve spontaneously. As modern insulin is highly purified, insulin allergy is rare. However, immunoglobulin G immune complexes against the insulin can be formed that can produce local atrophy of fat tissue (lipoatrophy).

As well as being unsightly, lipohypertrophy and lipoatrophy interfere with insulin absorption thereby compromising insulin action. Generalized allergic responses and injection site abscesses are exceptionally rare.

Inhaled insulin

The first inhaled insulin was withdrawn from the market in 2007 on the grounds of limited clinical demand, although lung cancer was also observed. The FDA approved a new formulation (Afrezza) in July 2014.

Challenges of insulin therapy

Although insulin and the means of administering insulin continue to improve, achieving optimal glycaemic control is extremely challenging for people living with diabetes for a number of reasons:

- The therapeutic index of insulin is low, meaning that when too little insulin is administered, glucose concentrations rise outside the normal range while if too much insulin is administered, glucose concentrations fall in the hypoglycaemic range.
- Insulin requirements are highly variable from one person to another and vary within the same individual within a day and between days.
- In people without diabetes, insulin is secreted directly into the portal circulation and reaches the liver in high concentration where 50% is cleared on first passage. By contrast, insulin injected subcutaneously passes into the systemic circulation. People treated with insulin therefore have lower portal insulin levels and higher systemic levels relative to normal physiology.
- Subcutaneous insulin takes longer to enter and achieve peak plasma levels and it is slower to leave the circulation.
- The absorption of subcutaneous insulin into the circulation from one injection to the next is variable.
- Basal insulin levels adapt to the metabolic needs of people without diabetes but injected insulin peaks and declines, with resulting swings in metabolic control in those with diabetes.
- Bolus insulin doses should ideally be adjusted to the carbohydrate content of the meal.
- Carbohydrate counting is difficult because many foods do not list the carbohydrate content.
- It is not always possible to determine how much will be eaten, as appetite may change.
- The rate of absorption of glucose is affected by the glycaemic index and amount of protein and fat in the meal.
- Calculating the appropriate dose of insulin requires advanced mathematical skills.
- There are no holidays from diabetes; an individual using a basal bolus regimen will need to inject approximately 1500 times a year.
- The price of giving too much insulin is hypoglycaemia, which is unpleasant and often embarrassing.
- The pens or devices can fail.

It is critically important that people are trained to use their insulin effectively and safely and this forms a central component of diabetes self-management education for people with diabetes. As their insulin requirement changes, people should be encouraged to adjust their insulin doses with a view to maintaining blood glucose values between 4 mmol/L and 7 mmol/L (70–126 mg/dL) before meals and between 4 mmol/L and 10 mmol/L (70–180 mg/dL) after meals, assuming that this can be achieved without troublesome hypoglycaemia (**Box 23.11**).

Professional advice should be available to support people with diabetes who experience problems; alongside this is a responsibility

Box 23.11 Guide to adjusting insulin dosage according to blood glucose test results

Time	Blood glucose persistently too high	Blood glucose persistently too low
Before breakfast	Increase evening long-acting or pre-mixed insulin	Reduce evening long-acting or pre-mixed insulin
Before lunch	Increase morning short-acting or pre-mixed insulin	Reduce morning short-acting or pre-mixed insulin, or take a mid-morning snack
Before evening meal	Increase morning long-acting or pre-mixed insulin or lunch short-acting insulin	Reduce morning long-acting or pre-mixed insulin or lunch short-acting insulin, or increase mid-afternoon snack
Before bed	Increase evening short-acting or pre-mixed insulin	Reduce evening short-acting or pre-mixed insulin

Adjustment should be approximately 10% of the current dose.

Box 23.12 The six steps to insulin safety

- The right person
- The right insulin
- The right dose
- The right device
- The right way
- The right time

for healthcare professionals to prescribe insulin safely (**Box 23.12**). Insulin prescribing errors, with potentially fatal consequences, are one of the most common causes of iatrogenic harm. There are many different types of insulin, often with similar sounding names, that are used in different ways and contribute to the confusion surrounding prescription.

Hypoglycaemia

Hypoglycaemia (low blood glucose) is the most common side-effect of insulin therapy and is the major limitation to what can be achieved with insulin treatment. A recent consensus report defined a glucose concentration below 3.0 mmol/L (54 mg/dL) as 'clinically significant hypoglycaemia' but recognized that any value below 4.0 mmol/L (70 mg/dL) represented an 'alert value' that required treatment. 'Severe hypoglycaemia' is defined as hypoglycaemia requiring external help for recovery. Most people treated with insulin will experience several episodes of symptomatic hypoglycaemia per week and one to two severe episodes per year. Despite the advances in insulin therapy, the incidence of hypoglycaemia has not changed over the last 25 years. Interestingly with the advent of continuous glucose monitoring, it is apparent that asymptomatic hypoglycaemia occurs much more frequently than previously thought. Hypoglycaemia is more common in people with type 1 diabetes, where there is absolute insulin deficiency, and with longer duration of diabetes. It occurs more frequently in young children and those trying to achieve tight glycaemic control.

Hypoglycaemia greatly impairs quality of life and induces fear and anxiety in the person with diabetes, their family and carers. In an older study, the fear of severe hypoglycaemia was worse than the fear of developing blindness or end-stage renal disease. Nocturnal hypoglycaemia can be particularly disruptive. In addition to

Box 23.13 Some of the consequences of hypoglycaemia

Acute symptoms
- Autonomic
  - Sweating, paraesthesiae, feeling hot, shakiness, anxiety, palpitations and pallor
- Neuroglycopenia
  - Slurring of speech, altered behaviour, loss of concentration, drowsiness, low mood, dizziness, hemiplegia, fits, coma and, rarely, death
  - Loss of warning with recurrent hypoglycaemia and long duration of diabetes

Medical
- Increased risk of falls
- Increased risk of myocardial infarction
  - Increased thrombosis
- Atherosclerotic plaque instability
- Cardiac arrhythmias
- Increased risk of hospitalization
- Increased risk of sudden death

Psychological
- Poor quality of life
- Embarrassment
- Fear of hypoglycaemia
  - Reduced medication taking to avoid future episodes
  - Higher HbA$_{1c}$

Financial
- Inability to work effectively
- Increased out-of-pocket expenses
- Increased medical costs
  - Extra visits
  - More glucose testing

the psychological effects, hypoglycaemia is associated with a number of long-term medical consequences, including cardiovascular events and falls (**Box 23.13**).

Hypoglycaemia is caused when more insulin is injected than is needed. Irregular eating habits, unusual exertion and alcohol excess may all precipitate hypoglycaemic episodes but insulin errors and variation in insulin absorption, for example as a result of lipohypertrophy, are also important. The times of greatest risk are before meals, during the night, and during and after exercise.

The mechanisms that protect against hypoglycaemia in people without diabetes are compromised because of abnormal islet cell function or defective counter-regulatory hormone secretion. The delivery of insulin after injection cannot be halted and glucagon secretion is impaired because its main regulator is a fall of intra-islet insulin. Even the third line defence of counter-regulatory hormones and other sympathetic nervous system responses to hypoglycaemia may become diminished in people with long-standing diabetes or recurrent hypoglycaemia.

Symptoms and signs

The symptoms of hypoglycaemia can be divided into two main categories, autonomic and neuroglycopenic, although non-specific symptoms may also be experienced (see **Box 23.13**). Autonomic symptoms and signs occur because of activation of the adrenergic and cholinergic parts of the autonomic nervous system. As the brain is dependent on glucose as its primary fuel source, neuroglycopenic symptoms arise from inadequate glucose supply to the brain.

Usually, autonomic symptoms develop before cognitive impairment. This is clinically important as these symptoms alert the individual to hypoglycaemia and prompt them to take corrective action. In longstanding diabetes or after repeated episodes of hypoglycaemia, the autonomic symptoms may only develop at glucose levels below the threshold for neuroglycopenic symptoms. When this occurs, hypoglycaemia awareness becomes impaired and the person is at increased risk of severe hypoglycaemia. Awareness improves if hypoglycaemia is scrupulously avoided.

The symptoms and signs of hypoglycaemia resolve once the hypoglycaemia is treated and the glucose returns to within the normal range.

Management of hypoglycaemia

Hypoglycaemia is an acute medical emergency that requires immediate treatment with 15–20g of oral glucose. This should be repeated after 15 minutes if the glucose concentration has not risen above 4.0mmol/L (70mg/dL). The glucose can be taken either as a liquid or solid food containing fast acting carbohydrate, such as glucose tablets or sugary sweets, e.g. Jelly Babies. More carbohydrate than necessary should not be taken in order to prevent rebound hyperglycaemia.

The diagnosis of severe hypoglycaemia resulting in confusion or coma is simple and usually made on clinical grounds, backed by a bedside blood test. Many people with diabetes carry a card or wear a bracelet or necklace saying that they have diabetes, and these should be sought in unconscious patients. The treatment is either intramuscular glucagon or intravenous glucose. Glucagon acts by mobilizing hepatic glycogen and works almost as rapidly as glucose. It is simple to administer and can be given at home by relatives. It does not work when liver glycogen levels are low, for example, after a prolonged fast. Once the individual revives, they should eat some longer-acting carbohydrate to replenish glycogen reserves.

After the acute event has been treated, it is important to ascertain why the hypoglycaemia occurred to try to prevent future episodes.

Weight gain

As insulin is an anabolic hormone and the absence of insulin leads to profound weight loss, it is unsurprising that many people gain weight whilst treated with insulin. Restoration of normal weight is a therapeutic effect, but some individuals experience excessive weight gain, especially if the insulin dose is increased inappropriately. Excessive weight gain may be the consequence of frequent hypoglycaemia if an individual takes excess carbohydrate to treat or prevent hypoglycaemia (so called 'defensive eating'). Weight gain can be offset, to some extent, by dietary measures and exercise.

Oral non-insulin treatments for type 2 diabetes

Unlike type 1 diabetes, there are alternative pharmacological treatments for type 2 diabetes when dietary and other lifestyle changes do not adequately bring the glucose into the target range. These treatments are adjuncts rather than alternatives to dietary and lifestyle management.

Biguanides: metformin

Metformin is currently the only available biguanide. It was introduced into clinical practice in the 1950s alongside two other biguanides, phenformin and buformin, but these latter two agents were withdrawn because of a high risk of lactic acidosis.

Mode of action

The precise mechanism of action of metformin remains unclear but may involve the activation of the enzyme adenosine monophosphate (AMP) kinase, which regulates cellular energy metabolism. Metformin reduces the rate of gluconeogenesis, and hence hepatic glucose output, and increases insulin sensitivity. It does not affect insulin secretion, does not induce hypoglycaemia and does not predispose to weight gain. In addition to its effects on glucose, it may also suppress appetite and stabilize weight.

Clinical use

Metformin is the best-validated treatment for type 2 diabetes and appears as the first-line pharmacological agent in all type 2 diabetes guidelines. Metformin may be given in combination with all other oral diabetes treatments as well as GLP-1 receptor agonists or insulin. It lowers fasting plasma glucose by 2–4mmol/L (36–72mg/dL), corresponding to a fall in HbA_{1c} of 11–22mmol/mol (1–2%). In UKPDS, metformin treatment led to an unexpected reduction in cardiovascular events. Metformin has been used alongside insulin in people with type 1 diabetes but only with limited efficacy.

Adverse effects

Unwanted effects include gastrointestinal side-effects (10–20%), such as anorexia, nausea, abdominal discomfort and diarrhoea. The effects can be mitigated by starting at low dose and gradually increasing until the desired therapeutic effect is achieved. A slow-release preparation of metformin appears to be better tolerated.

Metformin is contraindicated in renal impairment, cardiac failure and hepatic failure because of the risk of lactic acidosis. Metformin should not be started in someone whose estimated glomerular filtration rate (eGFR) is less than 45mL/min per 1.73m^2 and should be stopped if the eGFR falls below 30mL/min per 1.73m^2.

Metformin must be stopped prior to intravascular administration of iodinated contrast agent because of the risk of renal failure and subsequent lactic acidosis. Treatment can be restarted 48 hours after the test if there has been no deterioration in renal function. Similarly, metformin should be stopped temporarily around surgery or during other intercurrent illnesses that may affect lactate clearance. Metformin should be avoided in people with a history of alcohol misuse.

Metformin reduces gastrointestinal vitamin B_{12} absorption, but only rarely causes anaemia.

Sulphonylureas

Sulphonylureas were originally derived from sulfonamide antibiotics after it was recognized that the latter caused hypoglycaemia during a typhoid epidemic in Marseilles, France in 1942 (**Box 23.14**).

Mode of action

Sulphonylureas act on the β cell to induce insulin secretion. They are ineffective in people without a functional β-cell mass and therefore have no effect in people with type 1 diabetes. Sulphonylureas bind to the sulphonylurea receptor on the β-cell membrane, which closes ATP-sensitive potassium channels and blocks potassium efflux. The resulting depolarization promotes calcium influx and stimulates insulin release (see **Fig. 23.4**).

Clinical use

Most clinical guidelines recommend that sulphonylureas can be used as an alternative first-line agent where metformin is contraindicated or not tolerated. As monotherapy, sulphonylureas typically reduce fasting plasma glucose by 2–4mmol/L (36–72mg/dL), corresponding to a fall in HbA_{1c} of 11–22mmol/mol (1–2%). Although this is more effective than many other oral agents in the short term (1–3 years), the sulphonylurea effect wears off as the β-cell mass declines. Sulphonylureas can also be used in combination with other oral antidiabetes agents or basal insulin, although it is usually stopped when the individual requires short-acting insulin at mealtimes.

Adverse effects

Weight gain, typically 1–4kg, and hypoglycaemia are the most common side effects. Hypoglycaemia affects about one-fifth of those taking the drug but severe hypoglycaemia is uncommon.

i   **Box 23.14** Examples of non-insulin drugs used to treat diabetes[a]

Drug class	Examples
Biguanides	Metformin
Sulphonylureas	Gliclazide
	Glimepiride
	Glibenclamide
	Glipizide
	Tolbutamide
Meglitinides	Repaglinide
	Nateglinide
Thiazolidinediones	Pioglitazone
DPP-4 inhibitors	Sitagliptin
	Linagliptin
	Vlidagliptin
	Alogliptin
	Saxagliptin
SGLT2 inhibitors	Dapagliflozin
	Empagliflozin
	Canagliflozin
Alpha-glucosidase inhibitors	Acarbose
	Miglitol
	Voglibose
GLP-1 receptor agonists	Exenatide
	Liraglutide
	Lixisenatide
	Dulaglutide
	Semaglutide
	Albiglutide

[a]This list is not exhaustive and other drugs are in development in many of these classes.

The risk of hypoglycaemia is increased with longer acting sulphonylureas, excessive alcohol intake, older age and during intercurrent infection. Severe sulphonylurea-induced hypoglycaemia should be managed in hospital for up to 48 hours with glucose support until the drug has cleared from the circulation. Sulphonylureas should be used with care in people with liver or renal disease.

Meglitinides or post-prandial insulin releasers

Meglitinides are short-acting agents that promote insulin secretion in response to meals.

Mode of action

Like sulphonylureas, meglitinides act by closing the K^+-ATP channel in the β cells (see **Fig. 23.4**). They are rapidly metabolized and have a short duration of action of less than 3 hours. They were designed to restore early-phase post-prandial insulin release without prolonged stimulation during subsequent periods of fasting.

Clinical use

Meglitinides may be used to treat people with post-prandial hyperglycaemia with normal fasting glucose levels. They may be useful in older frail people where there is an imperative to avoid hypoglycaemia. However, meglitinides are less effective than other drugs and their role in diabetes management is not well established.

Adverse effects

Hypoglycaemia and weight gain are the most common adverse effects but these are generally less severe than with sulphonylureas.

Thiazolidinediones or 'glitazones'

Three thiazolidinediones have been launched but troglitazone was withdrawn because of liver toxicity and rosiglitazone has been withdrawn or restricted because of concerns about cardiovascular safety. In many countries, pioglitazone is the only available thiazolidinedione.

Mode of action

Thiazolidinediones reduce insulin resistance by interaction with peroxisome proliferator-activated receptor-gamma (PPAR-γ), a nuclear receptor that regulates large numbers of genes, including those involved in lipid metabolism and insulin action. The paradox that glucose metabolism should respond to a drug that binds to nuclear receptors mainly found in fat cells is still not fully understood. One suggestion is that these drugs act indirectly via the glucose–fatty acid cycle, lowering free fatty acid levels and thus promoting glucose consumption by muscle. They reduce hepatic glucose production, an effect that is synergistic with that of metformin, and also enhance peripheral glucose uptake. Like metformin, the glitazones potentiate the effect of endogenous or injected insulin.

Clinical use

Thiazolidinediones can be used as monotherapy or in combination with other antidiabetes drugs, including insulin. Thiazolidinediones do not cause hypoglycaemia as monotherapy and pioglitazone may specifically benefit people with non-alcoholic fatty liver disease, a frequent co-morbidity of type 2 diabetes. As the effect on plasma glucose is indirect, thiazolidinediones may take up to 3 months to reach their maximal effect.

Adverse effects

The most common adverse effect is weight gain of 5–6 kg, but pioglitazone may cause fluid retention precipitating heart failure. Mild anaemia and osteoporosis resulting in peripheral bone fractures have been reported.

Dipeptidyl peptidase-4 inhibitors or 'gliptins'

Dipeptidyl peptidase-4 (DPP4) inhibitors have been used since 2006 and are one of two classes of drug that improve glycaemic control by enhancing the incretin effect (see p. 709).

Mode of action

These drugs inhibit the enzyme DPP4, which prevents the rapid inactivation of glucagon-like peptide-1 (GLP-1), which in turn increases insulin secretion and reduces glucagon secretion.

Clinical use

DPP-4 inhibitors are most effective in the early stages of type 2 diabetes, when insulin secretion is relatively preserved, and are currently recommended for second-line use in combination with metformin or a sulphonylurea. Although they only have relatively modest effects on glucose lowering, they are included in most type 2 diabetes treatment algorithms because they are well tolerated. DPP-4 inhibitors do not promote weight gain, have a low risk of hypoglycaemia and can be used safely in people with renal impairment.

Adverse effects

Nausea may occur and there have been occasional reports of acute pancreatitis. DPP-4 inhibitors do not alter the incidence of myocardial infarction, but saxagliptin may increase the risk of heart failure.

Sodium-glucose transporter 2 inhibitors ('flozins')

SGLT2 inhibitors have been available since 2011 (see **Box 23.14**). In addition to their effects on blood glucose, they lower body weight, improve renal dysfunction and reduce the risk of atherosclerotic cardiovascular events and heart failure.

Mode of action

SGLT2 inhibitors lower the renal threshold for glucose, consequently increasing urinary glucose excretion. This has the effect of removing both glucose and calories from the circulation, thus lowering blood glucose by 7–13 mmol/mol (0.6–1.2%) and facilitating weight loss (≈2–4 kg over 6–12 months). They alter glomerular haemodynamics, which may underlie the observed benefits on renal function.

Exactly how SGLT2 inhibitors reduce the risk of myocardial infarction, stroke, cardiovascular death and heart failure is uncertain; however, several hypotheses have been suggested including:

- increased natriuresis leading to fluid loss and small reductions in systolic blood pressure
- increased production of ketones acting as a 'superfuel' for the heart
- vasodilation through blockade of the renin–angiotensin system
- direct effects on the heart.

Clinical use

SGLT2 inhibitors can be used as monotherapy but are used more typically in combination with all other antidiabetes drugs. This class has become rapidly established in clinical practice and in type 2 diabetes guidelines because of their cardiovascular benefits, weight loss and low risk of hypoglycaemia. The glucose lowering effect is dependent on good renal function but the renoprotective benefits are seen in people with lower eGFR. This is leading to an expansion of their use in people with reduced eGFR.

SGLT2 inhibitors are licensed as adjunctive therapy to insulin in type 1 diabetes. In this context, SGLT2 inhibitors confer additional benefits by lower HbA_{1c} by 5–6 mmol/mol (0.4–0.5%) despite lower total daily insulin doses and weight loss. The reduction in HbA_{1c} does not increase the risk of hypoglycaemia but does carry a higher risk of diabetic ketoacidosis and fungal infections.

Adverse effects

The most common adverse effects are genital candidiasis and dehydration. Rarer side effects include diabetic ketoacidosis, Fournier's gangrene and lower limb amputation. Diabetic ketoacidosis may occur in people with diagnosed type 2 diabetes. In general, these people are insulin deficient and may have unrecognized type 1 diabetes. A diagnostic trap is that glucose concentrations may be normal or minimally raised in this situation.

Alpha-glucosidase inhibitors

Alpha-glucosidase inhibitors, such as acarbose, are designer drugs that reduce carbohydrate absorption after a meal.

Mode of action

Alpha-glucosidase inhibitors prevent α-glucosidase, the last enzyme involved in carbohydrate digestion, from breaking down disaccharides to monosaccharides. This slows the absorption of glucose after a meal and lowers post-prandial glucose.

Clinical use

Although α-glucosidase inhibitors can be used as monotherapy or in combination with all other antidiabetes drugs, they are not widely used because of their limited efficacy and gastrointestinal side-effects.

Adverse effects

The major side-effects are gastrointestinal and include flatulence, abdominal distension and diarrhoea, as unabsorbed carbohydrate is fermented in the bowel.

Other oral therapies
Quick-release bromocriptine

Abnormal circadian rhythm is associated with the development of insulin resistance, obesity and diabetes. When administered at daybreak, quick-release bromocriptine appears to reset hypothalamic dopamine circadian rhythms. It lowers HbA_{1c} by 5–8 mmol/mol (0.5–0.7%) either as monotherapy or in combination with other antidiabetes medications. The drug is well tolerated.

Colesevelam

Colesevelam is a bile acid-binding resin that lowers cholesterol, and can reduce blood glucose concentrations by an unknown gastrointestinal mechanism.

Non-insulin injectable therapies for type 2 diabetes

GLP-1 receptor agonists

GLP-1 receptors are a heterogeneous class of drugs that act by enhancing the incretin effect. The class is divided into two main groups; the first are drugs that are derived from the protein exendin, which is found in the saliva of an Arizonian desert lizard. Exendin has 53% sequence homology with human GLP-1 and is resistant to cleavage by DPP-4. The second group are analogues of human GLP-1.

The pharmacokinetics has been modified to prolong the duration of action. The first GLP-1 receptor agonists were given twice daily but now there are once-weekly preparations. At present GLP-1 receptor agonists require injection but oral formulations are in late development.

Clinical trials have demonstrated that human GLP-1 analogues, but not exendin-based GLP-1 receptor agonists, reduce the risk of myocardial infarction, stroke, cardiovascular death and heart failure.

Mode of action

GLP-1 receptor agonists enhance the incretin effect by activating the GLP-1 receptor. Unlike DPP-4 inhibitors that restore physiological GLP-1 levels, GLP-1 receptor agonists achieve pharmacological levels and are therefore more potent that DPP-4 inhibitors. In addition to their effects on the pancreas to increase insulin secretion and decrease glucagon, they also act on the hypothalamus to reduce appetite and food intake leading to weight loss. The size of effect has led to the licensing of liraglutide as an anti-obesity treatment. Short acting GLP-1 receptors agonists also slow gastric emptying.

GLP-1 receptors are widely expressed in the cardiovascular system and GLP-1 analogues appears to protect the heart against ischaemic damage, both through direct effects on the heart as well as indirect effects, such as lowered blood pressure and free fatty acids.

Clinical use

Despite the need for injection, clinical guidelines endorse their use and GLP-1 receptor agonists are now widely used in combination with other antidiabetes agents, as second- or third-line therapies. They should not be combined with DPP-4 inhibitors as the DPP-4 inhibitor does not confer any additional benefit. There are differences in efficacy between GLP-1 receptor agonist and head-to-head clinical trials have shown reductions of HbA_{1c} in the ranges 9–19 mmol/mol (0.8–1.8%) and reduction of weight from −0.6–4.3 kg. As GLP-1 receptor agonists cause weight loss, they are particularly suitable for people with obesity.

Adverse effects

The most common side-effects of GLP-1 receptor agonists are gastrointestinal and include nausea and vomiting, bloating and diarrhoea. These tend to diminish with time and occur less frequently with longer-lasting GLP-1 receptor agonists. There is a low risk of hypoglycaemia but this may occur if GLP-1 receptor agonists are combined with insulin or sulphonylureas. GLP-1 receptor agonists should not be used in people with a history of pancreatitis because of a risk of acute pancreatitis. Recent studies have not confirmed earlier concerns about links with pancreatic and thyroid cancer.

Amylin analogues

Pramlintide is an analogue of amylin and is approved in the USA for use in people with either type 1 or insulin-treated type 2 diabetes. Amylin is co-secreted with insulin and delays gastric emptying, suppresses post-prandial glucagon secretion and increases satiety. It is not widely used.

Which drug and when?

With the introduction of increasing numbers of drugs to treat type 2 diabetes, the choice of which drug and when becomes more and more relevant. As type 2 diabetes is characterized by progressive β-cell failure and glucose control deteriorates over time, this requires a progressive and pre-emptive escalation of diabetes therapy. There is strong evidence of delays in treatment escalation, which exposes the individual with diabetes to prolonged periods of hyperglycaemia and the inherent risks of complications.

All guidelines currently recommend metformin as the first-line treatment for most people with type 2 diabetes whose glucose levels remain above target despite optimal lifestyle management. However, what comes next is more contentious. As new treatments and new evidence of the effectiveness of these treatments, guidance about how to use these is continually updated. The European Association for the Study of Diabetes and American Diabetes Association have recently produced a comprehensive consensus report about the management of hyperglycaemia in diabetes.

Decisions about treatment should be individualized and shared with the person with diabetes. The importance of diabetes self-management education is highlighted to enable the person with diabetes to make an informed choice. Clinicians are advised to consider specific patient characteristics and factors that will inform the discussion (**Box 23.15**).

Where the individual has established atherosclerotic cardiovascular disease, a GLP-1 receptor agonist or SGLT2 inhibitor with proven cardiovascular benefit is recommended. Where heart failure or chronic kidney disease is present, an SGLT2 inhibitor is the treatment of choice. Approximately a quarter of individuals with diabetes will fall into this category. For the remaining three-quarters, if there

---

> *i* **Box 23.15 Considerations when choosing treatment for type 2 diabetes**
>
> **Characteristics of the person with diabetes**
> - Current lifestyle
> - Co-morbidities
>   - Atherosclerotic vascular disease
>   - Heart failure
>   - Chronic kidney disease
> - Clinical characteristics
>   - Age
>   - Weight
>   - Current HbA_{1c}
> - Psychosocial issues such as motivation and depression
> - Cultural and socioeconomic context
>
> **Specific factor**
> - Individualized HbA_{1c} target
>
> - Impact on weight and hypoglycaemia
> - Medication side-effects
> - Treatment complexity
> - Choose regimen to optimize medication taking
> - Access, cost and medication availability
>
> **Shared decision-making**
> - Involves an educated and informed person with diabetes (and their family/caregiver)
> - Seeks patient preferences
> - Ensures effective consultation
> - Empowers the person with diabetes
> - Ensures access to diabetes self-management education
>
> *(Adapted from Davies MJ, D'Alessio DA, Fradkin J et al. Management of hyperglycemia in type 2 diabetes, 2018. A consensus report by the American Diabetes Association (ADA) and the European Association for the Study of Diabetes (EASD). Diabetes Care 2018; 41:2669–2701.)*

is a pressing need to minimize weight gain or promote loss, again GLP-1 receptor agonists or SGLT2 inhibitors are recommended. In addition to GLP-1 receptor agonists and SGLT2 inhibitors, DPP4 inhibitor and thiazolidinediones may be used if there is a need to avoid hypoglycaemia. Sulphonylureas or thiazolidinediones are preferred when cost is a major issue.

When triple therapy is needed, other recommended drugs can be added. For example, if a GLP-1 receptor agonist is first added to metformin in someone with established atherosclerotic cardiovascular disease, an SGLT2 inhibitor would be an appropriate third-line choice. Beyond triple therapy, insulin is required as further additional treatments have only a minimal effect, if any.

Several fixed dose oral combinations and fixed ratio injectable combinations of insulin and GLP-1 receptor agonists are available and reduce the pill or injection burden for the person with diabetes as treatment is escalated.

Measuring the metabolic control of diabetes

Measures of glycaemic control are needed to help people with diabetes and their healthcare professionals make rational choices about therapy. There have been considerable advances in methods for monitoring over the last 30 years. Blood testing has now superseded the original urinary testing and it is possible to measure interstitial glucose continuously. Measurements of metabolic control can be divided into short-term measures that provide an almost instantaneous record of the current glucose concentration and long-term measures that provide an assessment of average glucose concentration over the preceding weeks or months.

Short-term measures of metabolic control
Self-monitoring of capillary blood glucose

The availability of hand-held meters has allowed people with diabetes to measure their capillary blood glucose concentration regularly throughout the day wherever they are. Blood is taken from the side of a fingertip (not from the top, which is densely innervated) using a special lancet. Single blood glucose concentrations are of limited value because of their wide variability, but repeated glucose measurements offer invaluable feedback that permits appropriate adjustment of treatment to be made. Some meters include bolus calculators that advise the individual on the appropriate dose of mealtime insulin based on the current glucose and estimated carbohydrate of the meal. The parameters of the automated bolus calculator (the ratio of insulin dose to carbohydrate intake and the amount that one unit of insulin will reduce glucose by) need to be programmed into the meter, usually during a consultation.

Self-monitoring of capillary blood glucose is recommended for everyone treated with insulin but some people with diet- or tablet-treated type 2 diabetes may also find testing a useful guide to therapy. Like any investigation, measuring capillary blood glucose should inform future management and so if individuals are unable or unwilling to adjust their treatment then 'testing for testing's sake' should be discouraged. Blood glucose monitoring does not, in itself, result in better control but is essential to those wishing to achieve it.

Continuous glucose monitoring

Continuous glucose monitoring (CGM) systems measure interstitial glucose every few minutes allowing the user to see trends in glucose levels throughout the day, in particular at times when testing is not usually done, for example at night. By tracking the glucose, the user can act earlier if the glucose starts to rise or fall. These devices have three parts, a sensor that sits just underneath the skin, a transmitter attached to the sensor and a display device that shows the glucose level. The sensors need to be changed frequently but with some devices can be worn for up to 14 days.

There are two types of continuous glucose monitoring:

- Real time, which allows the user to check the glucose levels at any time, as well as being able to download the results
- Retrospective, which does not allow the user to check the glucose levels in real time but the user can look back at results by downloading them.

The technology is developing extremely rapidly; some systems have alarms that alert the user to either high or low glucose levels while the latest CGM devices can be linked to pumps allowing the insulin infusion to be suspended if the glucose levels are low or predicted to become low. Clinical studies have shown that the use of CGM improves HbA_{1c} while reducing glucose variability and thereby lowering the risk of hypoglycaemia in type 1 diabetes.

The main disadvantage of CGM is the lag of 15–20 minutes between changes in blood glucose and interstitial glucose. Caution is needed if the glucose levels are changing rapidly and, if an individual experiences hypoglycaemic symptoms, they should test their capillary glucose even if the CGM reading is normal. Although many people with type 1 diabetes find CGM incredibly helpful, the wealth of data and alarms can overburden others.

Continuous glucose monitoring is recommended for people with type 1 diabetes who have problematic hypoglycaemia, including recurrent severe hypoglycaemia, impaired awareness of hypoglycaemia, or extreme fear of hypoglycaemia. CGM is also recommended for those who suffer persistent hyperglycaemia despite very frequent capillary glucose monitoring.

Long-term measures of metabolic control
Glycated haemoglobin (HbA_{1c})

As discussed on page 710, glycated haemoglobin (HbA_{1c}) is a measure of an individual's average blood glucose concentration over the previous 6–8 weeks. The glycation occurs as a two-step reaction,

---

> **_i_ Box 23.16** Limitations of HbA_{1c}

Analytical variability
- Different methods for measuring HbA_{1c} may give different results:
  - Largely addressed by standardization of the reference method
- Molecular variants of haemoglobin:
  - Fetal haemoglobin

Biological variability
- Inter-individual variability:
  - An individual with a mean glucose of 10 mmol/L (180 mg/dL) may have an HbA_{1c} value that ranges from 6.0% to 9.0% (42–75 mmol/mol), probably reflecting differences in rates of protein glycation

  - Ageing
  - Ethnicity
  - Variation in erythrocyte lifespan:
- Shortened lifespan can give spuriously low results:
  - Haemolytic anaemia
  - Acute or chronic blood loss
  - Pregnancy
- Longer lifespan can give spuriously high results:
  - Iron deficiency
- Renal failure
- HIV infection

Clinical variability
- Predictive link between HbA_{1c} and clinical outcomes is not clear-cut

---

resulting in the formation of a covalent bond between the glucose molecule and the terminal valine of the β chain of the haemoglobin molecule. The rate at which this reaction occurs is related to the prevailing glucose concentration. HbA_{1c} is expressed as a percentage of the normal haemoglobin or as the mmol concentration of HbA_{1c} per mol of normal haemoglobin (standardized range 4–6%; 20–42 mmol/mol).

As HbA_{1c} provides an integrated measure of blood glucose concentration over the life of the haemoglobin molecule (≈6 weeks), the result may be misleading if the lifespan of the red cell is altered (**Box 23.16**).

Fructosamine

Glycation albumin measured as fructosamine relates to glycaemic control over the preceding 2–3 weeks. It may be useful in people with anaemia or haemoglobinopathy but is only rarely used.

Whole-pancreas and pancreatic islet transplantation

Islet transplantation

Since 2000, there has been remarkable progress regarding the technical aspects of islet cell processing and the outcomes of islet cell transplantation. The process involves harvesting pancreatic islets from cadavers (two or three pancreata are usually needed), which are then injected into the portal vein and seed themselves into the liver. It is one of the safest and least invasive transplant procedures. Islet cell transplantation is indicated for people with type 1 diabetes who have hypoglycaemia unawareness, severe hypoglycaemic episodes and marked glucose variability. The goal of treatment is to prevent severe hypoglycaemia but about 50–70% of people receiving islet cell transplants also achieve insulin independence after 5 years.

Whole-pancreas transplantation

Worldwide, over 42 000 whole-pancreas transplantations have been performed. They are most often undertaken in people with type 1 diabetes and end-stage kidney disease at the same time as kidney transplantation. Pancreas transplant may be performed less frequently after a kidney transplant or alone. Pancreatic transplantation can establish normoglycaemia and greatly improve quality of life. There is some evidence of protection against or reversal of some diabetes complications, but this comes at the cost of long-term immunosuppression.

Further reading

American Diabetes Association. Standards of medical care in diabetes – 2019. *Diabetes Care* 2019; 42(Suppl 1): S1–S183.

Davies MJ, D'Alessio DA, Fradkin J et al. Management of hyperglycaemia in type 2 diabetes, 2018. A consensus report by the American Diabetes Association (ADA) and the European Association for the Study of Diabetes (EASD). *Diabetologia* 2018; 61:2461–2498 and *Diabetes Care* 2018; 41:2669–2701.

DCCT/Epidemiology of Diabetes Interventions and Complications Research Group. Retinopathy and nephropathy in patients with type 1 diabetes four years after a trial of intensive insulin therapy. *N Engl J Med* 2000; 342:381–389.

Dyson PA, Twenefour D, Breen C et al. Diabetes UK evidence-based nutrition guidelines for the prevention and management of diabetes. *Diabet Med* 2018; 35:541–547.

Holman RR, Paul SK, Bethel MA et al. 10 year follow-up of intensive glucose control in type 2 diabetes. *N Engl J Med* 2008; 359:1577–1589.

Kilpatrick ES, Atkin SL. Using haemoglobin A(1c) to diagnose type 2 diabetes or to identify people at high risk of diabetes. *BMJ* 2014; 348:g2867.

Lean MEJ, Leslie WS, Barnes AC et al. Durability of a primary care-led weight-management intervention for remission of type 2 diabetes: 2-year results of the DiRECT open-label, cluster-randomised trial. *Lancet Diabetes Endocrinol* 2019; 7:344–355.

Leelarathna L, Wilmot EG. Flash forward: a review of flash glucose monitoring. *Diabet Med* 2018; 35:472–482.

National Institute for Health and Care Excellence. *NICE Guideline 28: Type 2 Diabetes in Adults: Management.* NICE 2019; https://www.nice.org.uk/guidance/ng28.

National Institute for Health and Care Excellence. *NICE Guideline 17: Type 1 Diabetes in Adults: Diagnosis and Management.* NICE 2016; https://www.nice.org.uk/guidance/ng17.

Nguyen NT, Varela JE. Bariatric surgery for obesity and metabolic disorders: state of the art. *Nat Rev Gastroenterol Hepatol* 2017; 14:160–169.

Pickup JC. Is insulin pump therapy effective in type 1 diabetes? *Diabet Med* 2019; 36:269–278.

Slattery D, Choudhary P. Clinical use of continuous glucose monitoring in adults with type 1 diabetes. *Diabetes Technol Ther* 2017; 19:S55–S61.

DIABETIC METABOLIC EMERGENCIES

The main terms used are defined in **Box 23.17**.

Diabetic ketoacidosis

Diabetic ketoacidosis (DKA) remains a frequent and life-threatening complication of diabetes, with a mortality rate of approximately 1%. Population studies suggest that there are 5–8 episodes annually per 1000 people with diabetes. It occurs more frequently in younger people but the mortality is higher in older people. Although treatment has improved with better outcomes, the incidence is rising. As DKA results from marked insulin deficiency, it mostly occurs in people with type 1 diabetes but may occasionally present in people with type 2 diabetes. It is usually seen in the following circumstances:

- previously undiagnosed diabetes (10–20% of cases)
- interruption of insulin therapy (15–30% of cases)
- the stress of intercurrent illness and infection (30–40%).

The majority of cases could have been prevented by earlier diagnosis, better communication between the person with diabetes and their healthcare professional, and better self-management education. The most common error is to reduce or omit insulin because the individual feels unable to eat, owing to nausea or vomiting. This is a factor in at least 25% of all hospital admissions. Although insulin adjustment is necessary, it should never be stopped. The UK National Diabetes Inpatient Audit found that a large number of people developed DKA whilst in hospital, suggesting that healthcare professionals also make the same mistakes.

Box 23.17 Terms used in uncontrolled diabetes

Term	Definition
Ketonuria	Detectable ketone levels in the urine; it should be appreciated that ketonuria occurs after fasting in people without diabetes and may be found in people with relatively well-controlled type 1 diabetes
Ketosis	Elevated plasma ketone levels in the absence of acidosis
Diabetic ketoacidosis	A metabolic emergency in which hyperglycaemia is associated with a metabolic acidosis due to greatly raised (>3 mmol/L) ketone levels
Hyperosmolar hyperglycaemic state	A metabolic emergency in which uncontrolled hyperglycaemia induces a hyperosmolar state in the absence of significant ketosis
Lactic acidosis	A metabolic emergency in which elevated lactic acid levels induce a metabolic acidosis. In people with diabetes, it is rare and associated with biguanide therapy

Pathogenesis

Ketoacidosis is a state of uncontrolled catabolism associated with marked insulin deficiency and elevated counter-regulatory hormones, which accelerate the effects of insulin deficiency (**Fig. 23.12**). The insulin deficiency leads to hyperglycaemia secondary to increased hepatic glucose output and diminished insulin-mediated peripheral glucose uptake, which in turn causes an osmotic diuresis and profound dehydration and loss of electrolytes (**Fig. 23.13**). However, the most important biochemical abnormality in DKA is not the hyperglycaemia but the uncontrolled lipolysis in adipose tissue and uncontrolled ketogenesis in the liver. Marked insulin deficiency is a necessary precondition for DKA since very little insulin is needed to inhibit hepatic ketogenesis and the breakdown of adipose triglycerides to non-esterified fatty acids (NEFAs). NEFAs are transported to the liver where they are partially oxidized to acidic ketones bodies, such as acetoacetic acid and 3-hydroxybutyric acid, and acetone. This occurs because the absence of insulin impairs hepatic re-esterification of NEFA to triglyceride. The liver exports the ketone bodies as an alternative fuel supply, but these build up in the circulation because of impaired uptake into peripheral tissues, such as muscle. The excess ketones are excreted in the urine but also appear in the breath, producing a distinctive smell similar to that of acetone. Ketone bodies are strong organic acids that rapidly exceed the body's buffering capacity and cause severe metabolic acidosis. Ketone bodies are nauseating and many people will vomit, worsening the dehydration and electrolyte loss further. Plasma osmolality rises and renal perfusion falls, which impairs renal excretion of hydrogen ions and ketones, aggravating the acidosis. Respiratory compensation for the acidosis leads to hyperventilation, graphically described as 'air hunger'.

As the pH falls below 7.0 ([H⁺] >100 nmol/L), pH-dependent enzyme systems in many cells function less effectively and, untreated, severe ketoacidosis is invariably fatal.

Clinical features

The features of ketoacidosis are those of uncontrolled diabetes with acidosis, and include prostration, dehydration, nausea, vomiting and, occasionally, abdominal pain. The latter is sometimes so severe that it can be confused with a surgical acute abdomen. Although some people are mentally alert at presentation, others

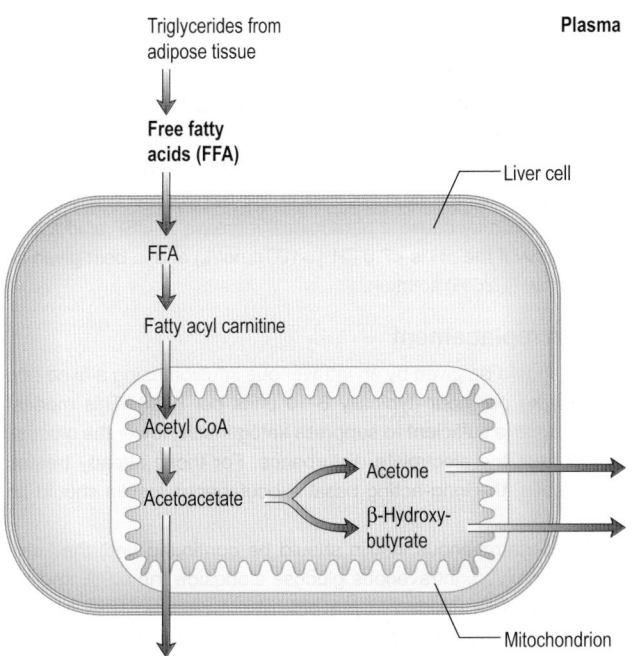

Fig. 23.12 Ketogenesis. During insulin deficiency, lipolysis accelerates and free fatty acids taken up by liver cells form the substrate for ketone formation (acetoacetate, acetone and β-hydroxybutyrate) within the mitochondrion. These ketones pass into the blood, producing acidosis. CoA, coenzyme A.

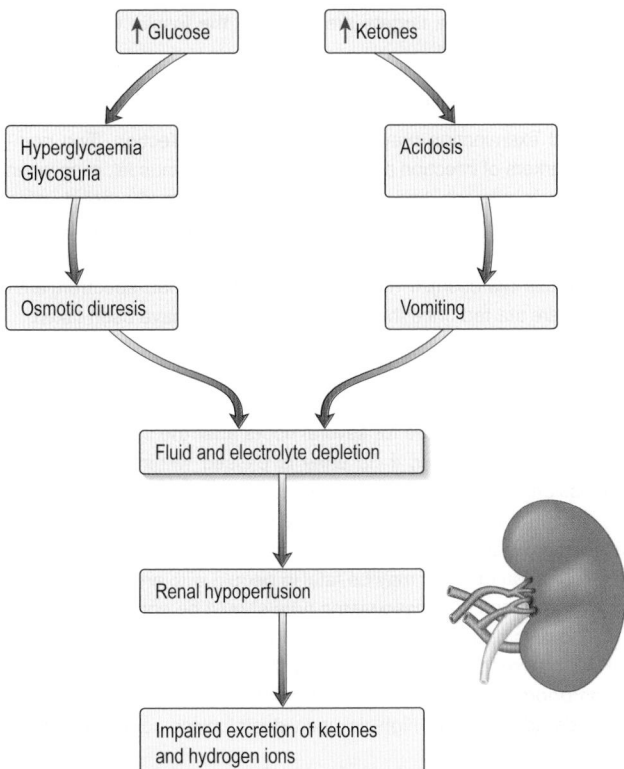

Fig. 23.13 Dehydration occurs during ketoacidosis as a consequence of two parallel processes. Hyperglycaemia results in osmotic diuresis, and hyperketonaemia results in acidosis and vomiting. Renal hypoperfusion then occurs and a vicious circle is established as the kidney becomes less able to compensate for the acidosis.

Box 23.18 Indicators of severe diabetic ketoacidosis

- Blood ketones over 6 mmol/L
- Bicarbonate level below 5 mmol/L
- Venous/arterial pH below 7.0
- Hypokalaemia on admission (under 3.5 mmol/L)
- Glasgow Coma Scale less than 12 or abnormal AVPU scale
- Oxygen saturation below 92% on air (assuming normal baseline respiratory function)
- Systolic BP below 90 mmHg
- Pulse over 100 or below 60 beats/min
- Anion gap above 16 [anion gap = $(Na^+ + K^+) - (Cl^- + HCO3^-)$]

may be confused and up to 5% present in coma. Although hyperventilation (Kussmaul respiration) may be present, it becomes less marked in very severe acidosis, owing to respiratory depression. The smell of ketones on the breath allows an instant diagnosis to be made by those able to detect the odour.

Diagnosis

This is confirmed by demonstrating hyperglycaemia with ketonaemia or heavy ketonuria, and acidosis as follows:

- Ketonaemia ≥3 mmol/L (31 mg/dL) *or* significant ketonuria (≥2 on standard urine sticks)
- Blood glucose >11 mmol/L (200 mg/dL) *or* known diabetes mellitus
- ***Bicarbonate (HCO_3^-) below 15 mmol/L (15 mEq/L)*** and/or ***venous pH <7.3.***

Blood glucose and ketones can be checked urgently at the bedside using portable meters. Blood electrolytes should be assessed as potassium abnormalities occur frequently; metabolic acidosis causes hyperkalaemia as potassium is exchanged for hydrogen ions moving into the cell. As insulin promotes the co-transport of potassium along with glucose into cells, this further exacerbates hyperkalaemia. Although serum potassium may be elevated, there is a severe whole-body potassium deficiency as significant quantities of potassium are lost in vomit and urine. The indicators of severe DKA are shown in **Box 23.18**.

Management

See **Box 23.19**; these measures should be carried out with the involvement of a specialist diabetes team. If the patient has severe DKA, they should be managed in a high dependency unit environment.

Replacement of the fluid losses

Individuals with DKA have a typical water deficit of 100 mL/kg, equivalent to 7.5 litres in a 75 kg adult. The replacement fluid of choice is 0.9% sodium chloride but Hartmann's solution is an acceptable alternative provided there are local policies to ensure the safe administration of additional potassium chloride (potassium cannot be added to Hartmann's solution). The aim of the first few litres of fluid is to correct any hypotension, replenish the intravascular deficit, and counteract the effects of the osmotic diuresis with correction of the electrolyte disturbance. Over-rapid fluid replacement may lead to cerebral oedema in children and young adults and so the remainder of the fluid should be replaced more cautiously over the next 2 days. The rate and volume of fluid replacement need to be modified in older people and in those with renal or heart failure.

Replacement of the electrolyte losses

Typical electrolytes deficits are sodium 7–10 mmol/kg, chloride 3–5 mmol/kg and potassium 3–5 mmol/kg. After the initiation of treatment with insulin, potassium levels can fall rapidly as

Box 23.19 Guidelines for the management of diabetic ketoacidosis (DKA)

Immediate measures (0–60 min after diagnosis and initiation of intravenous fluids)

1. Carry out clinical assessment to determine the severity of the DKA episode
2. Perform initial investigations, including blood ketones, capillary and venous glucose, serum creatinine and electrolytes, venous blood gases, full blood count, cultures, ECG, chest X-ray if indicated and cardiac monitoring
3. Initiate the intravenous infusion with 0.9% sodium chloride.
   a. Give 1 L over the first hour unless there is hypotension requiring more rapid correction of fluid deficit
   b. Add 40 mmol/L if the potassium is <5.5 mmol/L. Senior review is needed if the potassium is below 3.5 mmol/L
4. Commence a fixed-rate intravenous insulin infusion at a rate of 0.1 unit/kg per hour using soluble human insulin. Estimate the weight if necessary
5. Continue the long-acting basal insulin at the usual dose and time

Management from 60 min to 6 h

1. Reassess the patient
   a. Consider urinary catheterization if the patient is incontinent or anuric after 2–4 h
   b. Consider nasogastric tube insertion if the patient is obtunded or persistently vomiting
2. Continue intravenous fluids
   a. 0.9% sodium chloride 1L with potassium chloride over 2 h
   b. 0.9% sodium chloride 1L with potassium chloride over 2 h
   c. 0.9% sodium chloride 1L with potassium chloride over 4 h
   d. 0.9% sodium chloride 1L with potassium chloride over 4 h
   e. 0.9% sodium chloride 1L with potassium chloride over 6 h
3. Measure blood ketones and capillary glucose hourly
   a. If blood ketones are not falling by at least 0.5 mmol/L per hour, increase the insulin infusion rate by 1.0 unit per hour increments hourly until the ketones are falling at target rates. Seek senior review
   b. An alternative to blood ketones is venous bicarbonate which should rise by at least 3.0 mmol/L per hour
   c. A further alternative is glucose that should fall by at least 3.0mmol/L per hour (50 mg/dL)
   d. If the glucose falls below 14.0 mmol/L (250 mg/dL), commence 10% glucose given at 125 mL per hour alongside the 0.9% sodium chloride solution
4. Measure venous blood gas for pH, bicarbonate and potassium at 60 min and hourly thereafter
   a. Adjust the potassium replacement accordingly
5. Identify and treat precipitating factors

Management from 6 to 12 h

1. Reassess the patient and review biochemical and metabolic measurement to check for resolution of DKA

Conversion to subcutaneous insulin

1. Convert the patient to an appropriate subcutaneous regimen when biochemically stable (blood ketones less than 0.6 mmol/L, pH over 7.3) and ready and able to eat.

insulin promotes potassium uptake by the cells. Commercially, 0.9% sodium chloride is available with premixed potassium chloride (40 mmol/L (0.3%)) allowing the potassium to be replaced safely. Hypokalaemia and hyperkalaemia are potentially life-threatening conditions during the management of DKA and so potassium levels should be monitored frequently. There is a risk of acute pre-renal kidney injury associated with severe dehydration and so potassium should not be prescribed with the initial fluid resuscitation or if the serum potassium level remains above 5.5 mmol/L.

Hyperchloraemic acidosis may develop during treatment since a large variety of negatively charged electrolytes are lost in DKA,

which are replaced with chloride. The kidneys usually correct this spontaneously within a few days.

Restoration of the acid–base balance

In most cases, once the circulating volume is restored, the metabolic acidosis will rapidly compensate. Bicarbonate is seldom indicated because it is implicated in the development of cerebral oedema and may cause a paradoxical increase in CSF acidosis. It is used only if the pH is <7.0 ([H⁺] >100nmol/L) and is best given as an isotonic (1.26%) solution.

Insulin replacement

Insulin should be given by an intravenous infusion using a fixed rate 0.1 units/kg per hour (typically 6–10 units per hour). This modest insulin dose is sufficient to suppress ketogenesis, lower the glucose and correct the electrolyte disturbance. For those already treated with insulin, the long-acting basal subcutaneous insulin should be continued.

As the intravenous insulin should be continued until the ketosis has resolved, intravenous glucose alongside the 0.9% sodium chloride is often needed to prevent hypoglycaemia; 10% glucose is recommended once the blood glucose falls below 14.0 mmol/L (250 mg/dL) and should be continued until the person is eating and drinking normally.

Monitoring progress

The aim of treatment is lower the blood ketone concentration by 0.5 mmol/L per hour, increase the venous bicarbonate by 3.0 mmol/L per hour and reduce capillary blood glucose by 3.0 mmol/L per hour (50 mg/dL per hour) while maintaining potassium between 4.0 and 5.5 mmol/L. If these targets are not met, the insulin infusion rate should be increased.

Seeking the underlying cause

Physical examination may reveal a source of infection. Two common markers of infection are misleading: fever is unusual, even when infection is present; and polymorpholeucocytosis is present, even in the absence of infection. Relevant investigations include a chest X-ray, urine and blood cultures, and an electrocardiogram (to exclude myocardial infarction). If infection is suspected, broad-spectrum antibiotics are started once the appropriate cultures have been taken.

Other measures

As patients are significantly dehydrated on admission, it is unlikely that they will pass urine for several hours after the initiation of fluid replacement. However, if no urine is passed within 2–4 hours of admission, the insertion of a urinary catheter should be considered.

A central venous cannula may be required to monitor fluid balance in older people and those with cardiac disease.

Aspiration of vomit may be fatal in people with an impaired conscious level and so a nasogastric tube should be considered.

The dehydration, increased blood viscosity and coagulability of DKA increase the risk of a potentially fatal thromboembolism and so thromboprophylaxis with low-molecular-weight heparin should be considered in older or high-risk individuals unless contraindicated.

Complications of diabetic ketoacidosis

Cerebral oedema is a rare but serious complication with high mortality and mostly happens in children or young adults. Severe hypothermia with a core temperature of more than 33°C may occur and can be overlooked unless a rectal temperature is taken with a low-reading thermometer.

On-going management

Once the person is able to eat and keep food down, subcutaneous insulin treatment should be resumed or initiated. A subcutaneous bolus insulin is given with the meal and for those whose long-acting basal insulin was continued during the DKA episode, the insulin infusion and fluids can be discontinued 30 minutes after the meal. If the long-acting insulin was stopped, the intravenous insulin infusion and fluids should be continued until some form of background insulin has been given. The inpatient stay provides an educational opportunity to assess why the DKA occurred and what steps are needed to prevent it from happening again.

Hyperosmolar hyperglycaemic state

Hyperosmolar hyperglycaemic state, in which severe hyperglycaemia develops without significant ketosis, is the characteristic metabolic emergency of uncontrolled type 2 diabetes. People present in middle or later life, often with previously undiagnosed diabetes. Common precipitating factors include consumption of glucose-rich fluids, concurrent medication such as thiazide diuretics or steroids, and intercurrent illness. The hyperosmolar hyperglycaemic state and ketoacidosis represent two ends of a spectrum rather than two distinct disorders (**Box 23.20**). The biochemical differences may partly be explained as follows:

- **Age.** Old people experience thirst less acutely and become dehydrated more readily. In addition, the mild renal impairment associated with age results in increased urinary losses of fluid and electrolytes.
- **The degree of insulin deficiency.** This is less severe in the hyperosmolar hyperglycaemic state. Endogenous insulin levels are sufficient to inhibit hepatic ketogenesis but insufficient to inhibit hepatic glucose production.

> **i** **Box 23.20 Comparison of the electrolyte changes in diabetic ketoacidosis and the hyperosmolar hyperglycaemic state**

Examples of blood values	Severe ketoacidosis	Hyperosmolar hyperglycaemic state
Na$^+$ (mmol/L)	140	155
K$^+$ (mmol/L)	5	5
Cl$^-$ (mmol/L)	100	110
HCO$_3^-$ (mmol/L)	5	25
Urea (mmol/L)	8	15
Glucose (mmol/L)	30	50
Arterial pH	7.0[a]	7.35

The normal range of osmolality is 285–300 mOsm/kg. It can be measured directly, or can be calculated approximately from the formula:

$$Osmolality = 2(Na^+ + K^+) + glucose + urea.$$

For instance, in the example of severe ketoacidosis given above:

$$Osmolality = 2(140 + 5) + 30 + 8 = 328 \, mOsm/kg$$

and in the example of the hyperosmolar hyperglycaemic state:

$$Osmolality = 2(155 + 5) + 50 + 15 = 385 \, mOsm/kg$$

The normal anion gap is <17. It is calculated as

$$(Na^+ + K^+) - (Cl^- + HCO_3^-)$$

In the example of ketoacidosis, the anion gap is 40, and in the example of the hyperosmolar hyperglycaemic state, the anion gap is 25. Mild hyperchloraemic acidosis may develop in the course of therapy. This will be shown by a rising plasma chloride and persistence of a low bicarbonate, even though the anion gap has returned to normal.

[a][H$^+$] >100 nmol/L.

Clinical features

The characteristic clinical features are dehydration, and stupor or coma. Impaired consciousness is directly related to the degree of hyperosmolality. Evidence of underlying illness, such as pneumonia or pyelonephritis, may be present, and the hyperosmolar state may predispose to stroke, myocardial infarction or lower limb arterial insufficiency.

Investigations and management

These are (with some exceptions) similar to the guidelines for ketoacidosis. The plasma osmolality is usually extremely high. It can be measured directly or calculated as $(2(Na^+ + K^+) + glucose + urea)$, all in mmol/L. Again, the most important aspect of management is fluid replacement; 0.9% sodium chloride is the treatment of choice, but 0.45% sodium chloride may be considered if the osmolality is not declining despite adequate fluid balance. The rate of fall of plasma sodium should not exceed 10 mmol/L in 24 hours because the resultant change in osmolality may cause cerebral damage.

Fluid replacement is often enough to lower the glucose but insulin (0.05 units/kg per hour) should be used if the glucose is no longer falling with fluids alone or if the patient develops significant ketonaemia, when the diagnosis should be reconsidered. Many patients are extremely sensitive to insulin and the glucose concentration may fall rapidly with the initiation of insulin. In order to prevent cerebral damage, the fall in blood glucose should be no more than 5 mmol/L per hour (90 mg/dL per hour).

Prophylactic low-molecular-weight heparin should be given.

Prognosis

The reported mortality ranges as high as 15–20%, mainly because of the more advanced age of the patients and the frequency of intercurrent illness. Unlike ketoacidosis, the hyperosmolar hyperglycaemia state is not an absolute indication for subsequent insulin therapy, and survivors may do well on diet and oral agents.

Lactic acidosis

The risk of lactic acidosis in people taking metformin is extremely low, provided that the therapeutic dose is not exceeded and the drug is withheld in people with advanced hepatic or renal dysfunction. Patients present in severe metabolic acidosis with a large anion gap (an anion gap is <17 mmol/L in health), usually without significant hyperglycaemia or ketosis. Treatment is by rehydration and infusion of isotonic 1.26% bicarbonate. The mortality is in excess of 50%.

Further reading

Joint British Diabetes Societies Inpatient Care Group. *The Management of Diabetic Ketoacidosis in Adults*, 2nd edn. London: Diabetes UK; 2013; https://www.diabetes.org.uk/resources-s3/2017-09/Management-of-DKA-241013.pdf.
Joint British Diabetes Societies Inpatient Care Group. The management of hyperosmolar hyperglycaemic state (HHS) in adults with diabetes. *Diabet Med* 2015; 32:714–724.
Kamel KS, Halperin ML. Acid–base problems in diabetic ketoacidosis. *N Engl J Med* 2015; 372:546–554.

COMPLICATIONS OF DIABETES

Once effective treatment allowed people to survive the acute metabolic consequences of diabetes, it became apparent that long-term diabetes was associated with the development of a number of complications. These can be broadly divided into two groups: the microvascular complications that affect the capillaries and arterioles throughout the body but particularly involve the eyes (retinopathy), kidneys (nephropathy) and nerve (neuropathy), and macrovascular complications, which increase the risk of myocardial infarction, stroke and peripheral vascular disease. With improved treatment of diabetes, the incidence of diabetes complications has fallen for each individual but overall the prevalence has gone up as the number of people with diabetes has increased.

Microvascular complications

Microvascular complications are specific to diabetes and affect over 80% of individuals with diabetes. They are unusual in the first 10 years after the diagnosis of type 1 diabetes but are found in 20–50% of people with newly diagnosed type 2 diabetes as a result of the preceding undiagnosed hyperglycaemia. With the advent of screening for type 2 diabetes, the numbers with complications at presentation are falling.

Pathology of microvascular complications

Thickening of the capillary and arteriole basement membrane is the cardinal feature of microvascular complications. Although basement membrane thickening is seen in most people with diabetes, organ damage occurs much less frequently; however, with time, the small vessels become progressively narrower and eventually become blocked leading to ischaemia and tissue dysfunction. The tissues damaged by hyperglycaemia are those that have high blood flow and cannot downregulate glucose uptake in the presence of hyperglycaemia.

The mechanisms leading to damage are ill-defined but likely to be multifactorial. There is no doubt that the duration and degree of hyperglycaemia play a major role in the production of complications. However, other factors also seem to play a role as some people are relatively protected against microvascular complications despite longstanding diabetes. Twin studies suggest that genetic polymorphisms may affect the risk of developing complications. There are also racial differences in the overall rates of nephropathy; in the USA, the prevalence is highest in Pima Native American people followed by Hispanic/Mexican-Americans then black Americans with the lowest rates in people of white Northern European ancestry.

The following are consequences of hyperglycaemia and likely contribute to the development of microvascular complications. The common feature of each stems from a single hyperglycaemia-induced process of overproduction of superoxide by the mitochondrial electron chain.

Formation of advanced glycation end products (AGE)

When a wide variety of proteins are exposed to increased glucose concentrations, glucose binds irreversibly to the protein to form advanced glycation end-products (AGE). These accumulate in proportion to hyperglycaemia and time; one example of this is HbA_{1c}, which is used to diagnose diabetes and monitor treatment. AGEs cause tissue injury and inflammation via stimulation of pro-inflammatory factors, such as complement and cytokines.

Increased flux of glucose through the sorbitol–polyol pathway

When hyperglycaemia occurs, excess glucose is metabolized to sorbitol via the polyol pathway. This leads to accumulation of sorbitol and fructose, which cause changes in vascular permeability, cell proliferation and capillary structure via stimulation of protein kinase C and transforming growth factor-beta (TGF-β).

Abnormal microvascular blood flow

Hyperglycaemia swamps the normal autoregulatory mechanisms that limit tissue blood flow and the high flow rates damage the tissue, particularly when hypertension is present. Endothelial damage

occurs and vasoconstrictors, such as endothelins and thrombogenesis, are released that can lead to microvascular occlusion. Nutrients and oxygen supply are impeded.

Blockage of the renin–angiotensin system slows the progression of microvascular complications to a greater extent than other blood pressure-lowering agents, suggesting the renin–angiotensin system may have a role in the development of microvascular complications.

Growth factors and cytokines

Through increased expression of protein kinase C β (PKCβ), a number of mitogenic cytokines and growth factors, including TGF-β, tumour necrosis factor and vascular endothelial growth factor (VEGF), are upregulated.

Growth hormone–insulin-like growth factor axis

The reduction in portal insulin concentrations impairs the ability of growth hormone to generate IGF-I in the liver, which in turn leads to growth hormone hypersecretion by the pituitary gland. Growth hormone excess has been implicated in the development of microvascular complications and, indeed, pituitary ablation was used to treat retinopathy before laser therapy became available.

Diabetic retinopathy

Diabetic retinopathy (damage to the retina) is the most commonly diagnosed diabetes-related complication (**Fig. 23.14**). Its prevalence increases with the duration of diabetes and affects around one-third of all people with diabetes (**Fig. 23.15**). Approximately 20% of people with type 1 diabetes will have retinal changes after 10 years, rising to 90% after 20 years (**Box 23.21**); 20–30% of people with type 2 diabetes have retinopathy at diagnosis, 10% of people with diabetes develop sight-threatening retinopathy, and worldwide diabetic retinopathy is the most common cause of blindness in people of working age. Approximately 30% of people with diabetes will require laser photocoagulation to prevent or limit progression to proliferative retinopathy.

Early changes without vision loss

The earliest changes in the retina are known as non-proliferative or background retinopathy (see **Box 23.21**). Damage to the wall of small vessels causes microaneurysms (small red dots) within the retina. When vessel walls are breached, superficial (blot) haemorrhages occur in the ganglion cell and outer plexiform layers. Damaged blood vessels leak fluid into the retina. The fluid is cleared into the retinal veins, leaving behind protein and lipid deposits, which are seen as hard exudates. These are eventually cleared by macrophages. Micro-infarcts within the retina due to occluded vessels cause cotton wool spots. The spot is swelling of the retinal nerve fibers because normal axoplasmic transport is disrupted leading to the accumulation of axoplasmic debris. This debris is removed by macrophages. As this occurs, there may be white dots at the site of the previous cotton wool spot (cytoid bodies).

Sequential retinal photographs have demonstrated that all these lesions can heal, and it is not uncommon for changes to be seen on one occasion but not the next.

Transition to sight-threatening retinopathy

The next stage of retinopathy is known as pre-proliferative retinopathy (see **Box 23.21**). Damage to the walls of veins causes their calibre to vary (venous beading) and elongation to occur, causing venous loops.

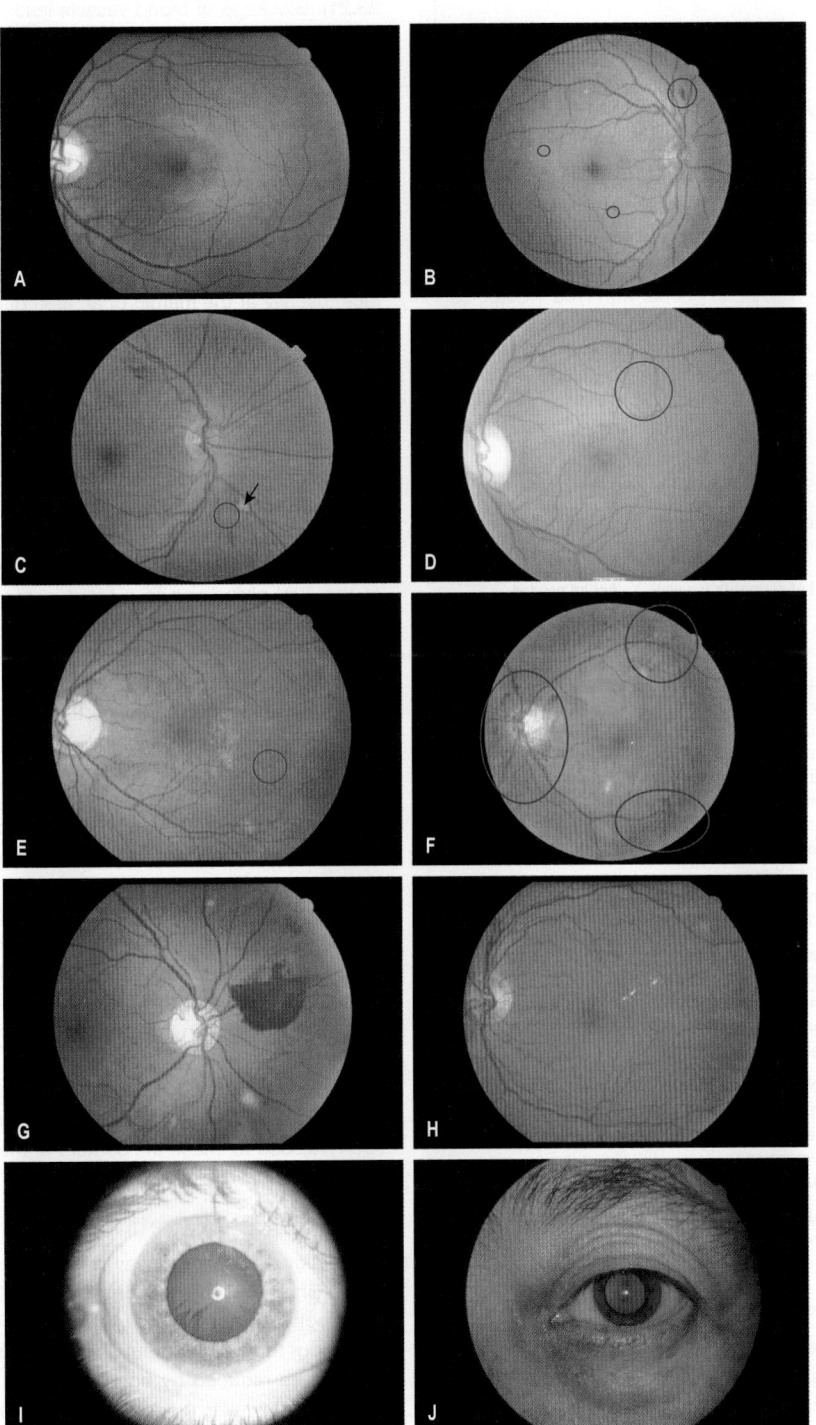

Fig. 23.14 Features of diabetic eye disease. (A) The normal macula (centre) and optic disc (to left).
(B) Microaneurysms (small circles) and blot haemorrhage (larger circle) – early non-proliferative retinopathy.
(C) Hard exudates (circled) and single cotton wool spot (arrowed) in addition to multiple blot haemorrhages in non-proliferative retinopathy. **(D)** Intraretinal microvascular abnormalities (IRMA) –
pre-proliferative retinopathy (circled). **(E)** Venous loop (circled) also indicates pre-proliferative change.
(F) Fronds of new vessels on the disc and elsewhere (proliferative; circled). **(G)** Pre-retinal haemorrhage
in proliferative disease. **(H)** Hard exudates within a disc-width of the macula (maculopathy). **(I)** Cortical
cataracts and **(J)** central cataracts can be seen against the red reflex with the ophthalmoscope.

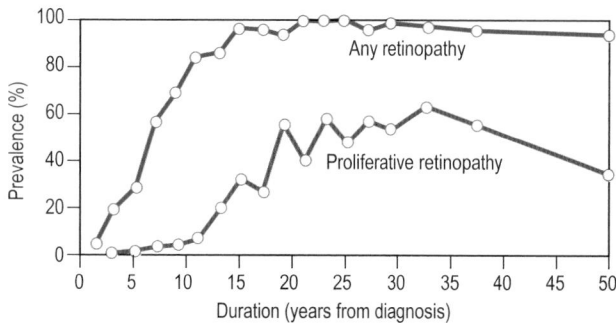

Fig. 23.15 Prevalence of retinopathy. Prevalence is shown in relation to duration of the disease in people with type 1 diabetes mellitus diagnosed under the age of 33 years. Almost all eventually develop background change and 60% progress to proliferative retinopathy. *(Data from Archives of Ophthalmology 1984; 102:520.)*

Box 23.21 Grading and management of pathological changes in diabetic retinopathy

Retinopathy grade	Retinal abnormality (cause)	Action needed
Peripheral retina		
Non-proliferative (R1)	Dot haemorrhages (capillary microaneurysms) (usually appear first) Blot haemorrhages (leakage of blood into deeper retinal layers) Hard exudates (exudation of plasma rich in lipids and protein)[a] Cotton wool spots/cytoid bodies[b]	Annual screening only
Pre-proliferative (R2)	Venous beading/loops Intraretinal microvascular abnormalities (IRMAs) Multiple deep, round haemorrhages	Non-urgent referral to an ophthalmologist
Proliferative (R3)	New blood-vessel formation/neovascularization Preretinal or subhyaloid haemorrhage Vitreous haemorrhage	Urgent referral to an ophthalmologist
Advanced retinopathy	Retinal fibrosis Traction retinal detachment	Urgent referral to an ophthalmologist – but much vision already lost
Central retina		
Maculopathy (M1)	Hard exudates within 1 disc-width of macula Lines or circles of hard exudates within 2 disc-widths of macula Microaneurysms or retinal haemorrhages within 1 disc-width of macula if associated with an unexplained visual acuity 6/12 or worse	Prompt referral to an ophthalmologist

[a]Hard exudates have a bright yellowish-white colour and are often irregular in outline with a sharply defined margin.
[b]Cotton-wool spots are greyish-white and have indistinct margins and a dull matt surface, unlike the glossy appearance of hard exudates.

Sight-threatening retinopathy

With further progression proliferative retinopathy develops (see **Box 23.21**). Blockage of blood vessels leads to areas of capillary non-perfusion. Ischaemia in these areas causes the release of vascular growth factors such as VEGF. These factors cause new blood vessels to grow in the retina (neovascularization).

Some of these new blood vessels are inside the retina and are helpful. These new intraretinal vessels, and other vessels whose walls are damaged and dilated, give the appearance of intraretinal microvascular abnormalities (IRMAs). IRMAs are a feature of pre-proliferative retinopathy.

Other new vessels emerge through the retina and lie on its surface, usually at the margin of an area of capillary closure. The normal shearing stresses that occur within the eye can cause these poorly supported new vessels to bleed. Small haemorrhages give rise to pre-retinal haemorrhages (boat-shaped haemorrhages). With further bleeding, vitreous haemorrhage may occur with sudden loss of vision. Later, collagen tissue grows along the margins of the new vessels and gives rise to fibrotic bands. These bands may contract and pull on the retina, causing further haemorrhage and *retinal detachment*. Sometimes, vessels may be induced to grow on the pupil margin (*rubeosis*) and in the angle of the anterior chamber of the eye, giving rise to a rapid increase in intraocular pressure (*rubeotic glaucoma*).

Fluorescein angiography (a fluorescent dye is injected into an arm vein and photographed in transit through the retinal vessels) may be needed to define the extent of the potentially sight-threatening diabetic retinopathy.

Maculopathy

Non-proliferative retinopathy may affect vision if it is situated within the macular area, which is responsible for fine vision (see **Box 23.21**). Fluid from leaking vessels is cleared poorly in this area because its anatomy differs from that of the rest of the retina. Above a certain rate of formation, clearance fails and macular oedema occurs. This distorts and thickens the retina at the macula. If sustained, this distortion causes loss of central vision. Capillary occlusion in the macular area will also cause loss of central vision.

Macular oedema is not visible with the ophthalmoscope or with retinal photography. For this reason, ocular coherence tomography (OCT) is used to image the content of the layers of the macula and measure retinal thickness.

Management of retinopathy

Prevention is the best way of managing retinopathy; the Diabetes Chronic Complications Trial (DCCT) and United Kingdom Prospective Diabetes Study (UKPDS) showed conclusively that the risk of the development and progression of diabetic retinopathy can be reduced by tight control of both glucose and blood pressure. However, a short-term deterioration of retinopathy may occur following rapid improvement in glycaemic control and during pregnancy and by nephropathy. The lipid-lowering drug, fenofibrate, has been shown to slow the progression of retinopathy including macular oedema. Smoking cessation is recommended.

Intravitreal injection

Repeated injections of anti-VEGF drugs, such as bevacizumab, aflibercept and ranibizumab, can control proliferative diabetic retinopathy and sight-threatening maculopathy. Studies have shown benefit over laser phototherapy for this type of maculopathy, but side-effects include infection, glaucoma, cataract and retinal detachment. The corticosteroid, triamcinolone, reduces macular oedema in the short term but may be useful while other treatments exert a more permanent effect.

Laser photocoagulation

Laser photocoagulation therapy is used to treat the new vessels of proliferative retinopathy. New vessels on the disc carry the worst prognosis and warrant urgent laser therapy. The laser should be directed at the new vessels and, in addition, at the associated areas of capillary non-perfusion (ischaemia). If the proliferative retinopathy has progressed to development of new vessels on the optic disc, then a technique known as panretinal photocoagulation is carried out. Rubeosis is also treated with panretinal photocoagulation. This involves multiple laser burns to the peripheral retina, especially in the areas of capillary non-perfusion. The principle is that by destroying the peripheral retina, the ischaemic stimulus for new vessel formation is diminished. Maculopathy may also be treated with localized laser photocoagulation.

Although laser treatment prevents blindness, the main adverse effects result from the destruction of retinal tissue. The visual field becomes permanently smaller and there is reduced dark adaptation. In essence, peripheral vision is sacrificed to maintain central vision.

Vitreoretinal surgery

Vitreoretinal surgery is used if bleeding is recurrent and preventing laser therapy. It is also employed to try to salvage some vision if an intravitreal haemorrhage fails to clear and to treat fibrotic traction retinal detachment in advanced retinopathy.

Other ways in which diabetes can affect the eye

Cataract

Cataracts are caused by the denaturation of the protein and other components of the lens of the eye, which renders it opaque. Cataracts develop earlier in people with diabetes than in the general population. Sustained very poor diabetes control with a degree of ketosis can cause an acute cataract (snowflake cataract) to develop rapidly.

Extraction and intraocular lens implantation are indicated if the cataract is causing visual disability or an inability to view the retina adequately. Cataract extraction is straightforward if there is no retinopathy present. Pre-existing retinopathy may worsen after cataract extraction.

Refractory defects

The lens can also be affected by fluctuations in blood glucose concentration, which cause refractive variability, as a result of osmotic changes within the lens (the absorption of water into the lens causes temporary hypermetropia). This presents as fluctuating difficulty in reading but people should be reassured that this resolves with better metabolic control of the diabetes.

External ocular palsies

These most commonly affect the sixth and the third nerves and are described in the section on neuropathies (see p. 731). These nerve palsies usually recover spontaneously within a period of 3–6 months.

Glaucoma

The prevalence of open-angle glaucoma is increased in people with diabetes.

Blindness

If sight loss occurs, individuals should be advised to register as blind and may require additional aids to help them to manage their diabetes. Less severe visual impairment is a bar to driving.

Clinical examination of the eye

Visual acuity should be checked using both a pinhole and distance spectacles if worn. The ocular movements are assessed to detect any ocular motor palsies. The iris is examined for rubeosis and then the pupils dilated with 1% tropicamide. About 5–10 minutes later, the eye is examined for the presence of a cataract by looking at the lens with a +10.00 lens in the ophthalmoscope and viewing the lens against the red reflex. All four quadrants of the retina and finally the macula are systematically examined. The macula is examined last because this induces the greatest discomfort, and pupillary constriction.

Eye screening

In the UK, the National Screening Committee has established universal digital photography-based screening across the country, based on a national set of standards. As a result of the early detection of retinopathy, diabetes is no longer the most common cause of blindness in those under 65 years of age in the UK. All people with diabetes over the age of 12 years are offered annual measurement of their acuity and retinal photographs. There are on-going discussions about whether the screening interval might be extended in those with no retinopathy while more frequent screening is required in some groups, for example pregnant women. **Box 23.22** shows standardized criteria for screening schemes; these are regularly inspected.

Diabetic nephropathy

Diabetic nephropathy is characterized by gradually increasing urinary albumin excretion and blood pressure as the glomerular filtration rate falls insidiously towards end-stage renal disease. It is slowly progressive and diabetic nephropathy usually manifests 15–25 years after the diagnosis of diabetes but affects 25–35% of people diagnosed under the age of 30 years. It is the leading cause of premature death in young people with diabetes.

The incidence of end-stage kidney disease has fallen in recent decades (2.5–7.8% after 30 years of type 1 diabetes), probably due to better control of blood glucose and blood pressure, but overall there are now more people with end-stage kidney disease because of the rising prevalence of both types of diabetes. Although the proportion of people with type 2 diabetes affected by end-stage kidney disease is lower, most people commencing renal replacement therapy have type 2 diabetes, because type 2 diabetes is so much commoner than type 1 diabetes. Diabetic nephropathy increases the risk of cardiovascular risk and most people with nephropathy die from cardiovascular disease before progressing to end-stage renal disease.

Pathophysiology

The earliest functional abnormality in the diabetic kidney is renal hypertrophy associated with a raised glomerular filtration rate. This appears soon after diagnosis and is related to hyperglycaemia. As the kidney becomes damaged by diabetes, the afferent arteriole (leading to the glomerulus) becomes vasodilated to a greater extent than the efferent glomerular arteriole. This increases the intraglomerular filtration pressure, further damaging the glomerular capillaries. This raised intraglomerular pressure also leads to increased local shearing forces, which likely contribute to mesangial cell hypertrophy and increased secretion of extracellular mesangial matrix material. This process eventually leads to glomerular sclerosis. The initial structural lesion in the glomerulus is thickening of the basement membrane. Associated changes result in disruption of the protein cross-linkages that normally make the membrane an effective filter. In consequence, there is a progressive leak of large molecules (particularly protein) into the urine.

Light-microscopic changes of both diffuse and nodular glomerulosclerosis become manifest; the latter is known as the Kimmelstiel–Wilson lesion. At the later stage of glomerulosclerosis, the glomerulus is replaced by hyaline material.

Albuminuria

Gradually increasing urinary albumin excretion is the hallmark of classical diabetic nephropathy. The earliest evidence of this is 'microalbuminuria', so called because the amounts of urinary albumin are too small as to be undetectable by standard dipsticks (see p. 1349). Microalbuminuria may, after some years, progress to intermittent albuminuria followed by persistent proteinuria (**Fig. 23.16**).

At the stage of persistent proteinuria, the plasma creatinine is normal but once this stage is reached, end-stage kidney disease ensues within 5–10 years, although the rate of progression varies widely between individuals. Rising plasma creatinine is a late feature.

The proteinuria may become so heavy as to induce a transient nephrotic syndrome, with peripheral oedema and hypoalbuminaemia.

A small proportion of individuals with type 1 diabetes and up to 50% of those with type 2 diabetes have non-classical diabetic nephropathy. In this situation, the glomerular filtration rates falls progressively but with little or no albuminuria.

Other features of diabetic nephropathy

Diabetic nephropathy is typically associated with a normochromic normocytic anaemia and raised erythrocyte sedimentation rate and C-reactive protein. Hypertension is a common development and may itself damage the kidney still further.

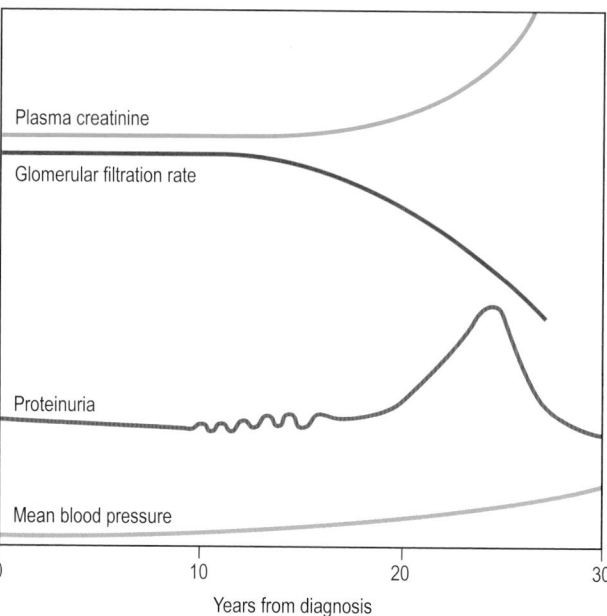

Fig. 23.16 Schematic representation of the natural history of nephropathy. The typical onset is 15 years after diagnosis. Intermittent proteinuria leads to persistent proteinuria. In time, the plasma creatinine rises as the glomerular filtration rate falls.

Screening for diabetic nephropathy

The urine of all people with diabetes should be checked regularly (at least annually) for the presence of microalbuminuria. The albumin:creatinine ratio (ACR, tested on a midstream first morning urine sample) is less than 2.5 mg/mmol in healthy men and less than 3.5 mg/mmol in healthy women. If microalbuminuria is detected, the test should be repeated twice because false-positive readings are common.

Investigation of microalbuminuria and proteinuria

Once proteinuria is present, other possible causes should be considered, but once these are excluded, a presumptive diagnosis of diabetic nephropathy can be made. Clinical suspicion of a non-diabetic cause of nephropathy may be provoked by an atypical history, the absence of diabetic retinopathy (usually, but not invariably, present with diabetic nephropathy) and the presence of red-cell casts in the urine. Renal biopsy should be considered in such cases but is rarely necessary or helpful. Plasma creatinine level and eGFR should be measured regularly.

Management of nephropathy

The management of diabetic nephropathy is similar to that of other causes of chronic kidney disease, with a number of provisos. Although diabetic nephropathy is progressive, the time course can be markedly slowed by early aggressive antihypertensive therapy, particularly with ACE inhibitors and angiotensin receptor blockers, and meticulous glycaemic control. The target blood pressure should be <130/80 mmHg but renin–angiotensin system blockers should also be used in people with normal blood pressure and persistent microalbuminuria.

The development of nephropathy also has implications for glycaemic management. Oral antidiabetes agents, partially excreted via the kidney (e.g. glibenclamide and metformin), should be avoided. As insulin clearance is reduced in advanced renal disease, insulin dosage is usually reduced. Recent trials have demonstrated

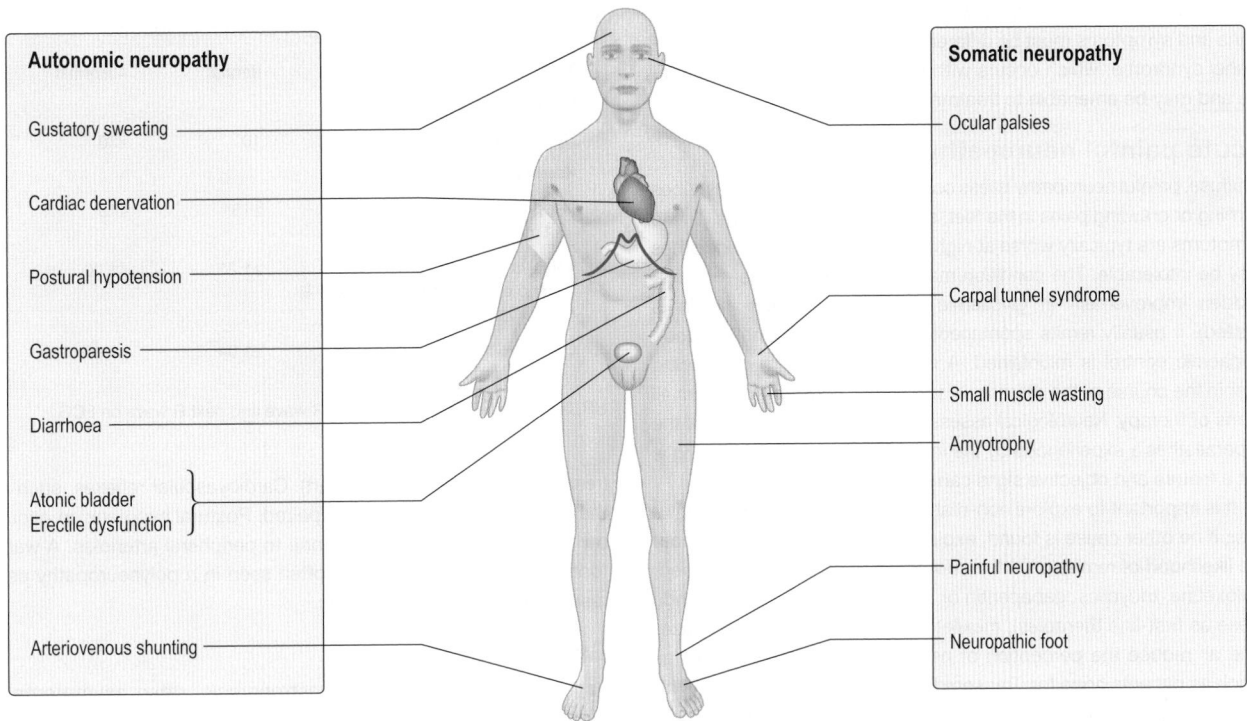

Fig. 23.17 The effects of neuropathy in people with diabetes.

that SGLT2 inhibitors slow the progression of diabetic nephropathy and preserve renal function. Attention should also be paid to the management of cardiovascular risk factors (p. 734).

Management of end-stage renal disease

Managing end-stage renal disease is made more difficult by the fact that patients often have other complications of diabetes, such as blindness, autonomic neuropathy or peripheral vascular disease. Vascular shunts tend to calcify rapidly; hence, chronic ambulatory peritoneal dialysis may be preferable to haemodialysis. The failure rate of renal transplants is somewhat higher than in people without diabetes.

Other ways that diabetes can damage the kidney

Ischaemic lesions

Arteriolar lesions, with hypertrophy and hyalinization of the vessels, can occur in people with diabetes. The appearances are similar to those of hypertensive disease and lead to ischaemic damage to the kidneys.

Urinary tract Infection

Urinary tract infections are relatively more common in women with diabetes, but not in men. Ascending infection may occur because of bladder stasis resulting from autonomic neuropathy, and infections more easily become established in damaged renal tissue. Autopsy material frequently reveals interstitial changes suggestive of infection, but ischaemia may produce similar changes and the true frequency of pyelonephritis in diabetes is uncertain. Untreated infections in people with diabetes can result in renal papillary necrosis, in which renal papillae are shed in the urine, but this complication is now very rare.

Diabetic neuropathy

Diabetes can damage peripheral nervous tissue in several ways. The vascular hypothesis postulates occlusion of the vasa nervorum as the prime cause. This seems likely in isolated mononeuropathies but the diffuse symmetrical nature of the common forms of neuropathy implies a metabolic cause. Since hyperglycaemia leads to increased formation of sorbitol and fructose in Schwann cells, accumulation of these sugars may disrupt function and structure.

The earliest functional change in nerves of people with diabetes is delayed nerve conduction velocity; the earliest histological change is segmental demyelination, caused by damage to Schwann cells. In the early stages, axons are preserved, implying prospects of recovery; at a later stage, irreversible axonal degeneration develops. Diabetic neuropathy can manifest in a number of different ways **(Fig. 23.17)**.

Symmetrical distal polyneuropathy

Peripheral neuropathy is often unrecognized by the person with diabetes in its early stages. Early clinical signs are mainly sensory and include loss of vibration sense, pain sensation (deep before superficial) and temperature sensation in the feet. At later stages, people may complain of a feeling of 'walking on cotton wool' and can lose their balance when washing the face or walking in the dark owing to impaired proprioception. Early involvement of the hands is less common and should prompt a search for non-diabetic causes. Complications include unrecognized trauma because of the loss of pain sensation.

Involvement of motor nerves to the small muscles of the feet gives rise to interosseous wasting. Unbalanced traction by the long flexor muscles leads to a characteristic shape of the foot, with a high arch and clawing of the toes, which in turn causes abnormal distribution of pressure on walking, resulting in callus formation under the first metatarsal head or on the tips of the toes. The hands show small-muscle wasting, as well as sensory changes, but these signs and symptoms must be differentiated from those of the carpal tunnel syndrome, which occurs with increased frequency in diabetes and may be amenable to treatment (p. 421).

Acute painful neuropathy

A diffuse, painful neuropathy is less common. The individual describes burning or crawling pains in the feet, shins and anterior thighs. These symptoms are typically worse at night and pressure from bedclothes may be intolerable. The condition may present at diagnosis or after sudden improvement in glycaemic control (e.g. when insulin is started). It usually remits spontaneously after 3–12 months if good glycaemic control is maintained. A more chronic form, developing later in the course of the disease, is sometimes resistant to almost all forms of therapy. Neurological assessment is difficult because of the hyperaesthesia experienced by the individual, but muscle wasting is not a feature and objective signs can be minimal.

It is important to explore non-diabetic causes (see p. 889). However, if no other cause is found, explanation and reassurance about the likelihood of remission within months may be all that is needed. Duloxetine, tricyclics, gabapentin or pregabalin (NICE recommends these as first-line therapies), mexiletine, valproate and carbamazepine all reduce the perception of neuritic pain, but usually not as much as patients hope for. Transepidermal nerve stimulation (TENS) benefits some people. Topical capsaicin-containing creams help occasionally. A few report that acupuncture has been of value.

Mononeuritis and mononeuritis multiplex (multiple mononeuropathy)

Any nerve in the body can be involved in diabetic mononeuritis; the onset is typically abrupt and sometimes painful. Radiculopathy (i.e. involvement of a spinal root) may also occur.

Isolated palsies of nerves to the external eye muscles, especially the third and sixth nerves, are more common in diabetes. A characteristic feature of diabetic third nerve lesions is that they are painless and the pupillary reflexes are retained owing to sparing of pupillomotor fibres. Full spontaneous recovery is the rule for most episodes of mononeuritis over 3–6 months. Lesions are more likely to occur at common sites for external pressure palsies or nerve entrapment (e.g. the median nerve in the carpal tunnel).

Diabetic amyotrophy

This condition is usually seen in older men with diabetes. Presentation is with painful wasting, usually asymmetrical, of the quadriceps muscles. The wasting may be very marked and knee reflexes are diminished or absent. The affected area is often extremely tender. Extensor plantar responses sometimes develop and cerebrospinal fluid (CSF) protein content is elevated. Diabetic amyotrophy is usually associated with periods of more severe hyperglycaemia and may be present at diagnosis. It often resolves over time with improved glycaemic control.

Autonomic neuropathy

Asymptomatic autonomic disturbances can be demonstrated on testing in many people with diabetes (**Box 23.23**) but symptomatic autonomic neuropathy is rare. It affects both the sympathetic and parasympathetic nervous systems and can cause disabling postural hypotension.

The cardiovascular system

Vagal neuropathy results in tachycardia at rest and loss of sinus arrhythmia. At a later stage, the heart may become denervated

Box 23.23 Bedside testing of autonomic function

Test	Normal	Abnormal
Supine to erect blood pressure		
Systolic BP fall (mmHg)	10	≥30
Heart rate responses to:		
Deep breathing (6 breaths over 1 min) max. to min. HR	≥15	≤10
Valsalva manoeuvre (15 sec): ratio of longest to shortest R–R interval	≥1.21	≤1.20
Lying to standing ratio of R–R interval of 30th to 15th beats	≥1.04	≤1.00

HR, heart rate; R–R, time between R wave and next R wave on ECG.

(resembling a transplanted heart). Cardiovascular reflexes, such as the Valsalva manoeuvre, are impaired. Postural hypotension occurs owing to loss of sympathetic tone to peripheral arterioles. A warm foot with a bounding pulse is often seen in a polyneuropathy as a result of peripheral vasodilation.

Gastrointestinal tract

Vagal damage can lead to gastroparesis, often asymptomatic but sometimes leading to intractable vomiting. Implantable devices that stimulate gastric emptying, and injections of botulinum toxin into the pylorus (to paralyse the sphincter partly), have each shown benefit in cases of this previously intractable problem.

Other symptoms resulting from altered gastrointestinal motility include dysphagia, dyspepsia, abdominal pain, constipation, diarrhoea and faecal incontinence. Autonomic diarrhoea characteristically occurs at night, accompanied by urgency and incontinence.

Small intestinal dysmotility predisposes to bacterial overgrowth, which can cause bile salt deconjugation, fat malabsorption and diarrhoea. Bacterial overgrowth may also lead to features such as anaemia and macrocytosis; treatment is with antibiotics such as tetracycline.

Bladder involvement

Loss of tone, incomplete emptying and stasis (predisposing to infection) can occur and may ultimately result in an atonic, painless, distended bladder. Treatment is with intermittent self-catheterization, permanent catheterization if that fails, and prophylactic antibiotic therapy for those prone to recurrent infection.

Sexual dysfunction

Sexual dysfunction is common in both men and women with diabetes. The overall prevalence in men is 35–40% but increases with age. Approximately 60% of men with diabetes aged 60 years or over are affected. The first manifestation is incomplete erection, which may, in time, progress to total failure; retrograde ejaculation also occurs in people with autonomic neuropathy.

The mechanisms involved in erectile dysfunction in diabetes are multifactorial and include inadequate vascular supply owing to atheroma in pudendal arteries, primary or secondary gonadal failure, hypothyroidism, anxiety, depression, alcohol excess and drugs (e.g. thiazides and beta-blockers).

When a man presents with erectile dysfunction, a detailed history and examination is needed to search for these causes. Blood is taken for luteinizing hormone, follicle stimulating hormone, testosterone, prolactin and thyroid function.

Treatment should ideally include sympathetic counselling of both partners. Phosphodiesterase type 5 inhibitors (sildenafil, tadalafil, vardenafil, avanafil), which enhance the effects of nitric oxide on smooth muscle and increase penile blood flow, are the first line treatment in those who do not take nitrates for angina. Although less effective in people with diabetes, approximately 60% of men benefit from this therapy.

Alternative treatments include:
- Apomorphine 2 mg or 3 mg sublingually 20 min before sexual activity.
- Alprostadil (prostaglandin E1 preparation), given as a small pellet inserted with a device into the urethra (125 μg initially to a maximum of 500 μg). If the partner is pregnant, barrier contraception must be used to prevent fetal exposure to the prostaglandin.
- Intracavernosal injection of alprostadil (2.5 μg initially to a maximum of 40 μg). Side-effects include priapism, which needs urgent treatment should erection last longer than 3 h.
- Vacuum devices.
- Penile prostheses.

Women with diabetes may complain of vaginal dryness and impaired sexual arousal.

The diabetic foot

Up to 50% of older people with type 2 diabetes have risk factors for foot problems and 10–15% of people with diabetes develop foot ulcers at some stage in their lives. Diabetic foot problems (**Fig. 23.18**) are responsible for nearly 50% of all diabetes-related hospital admissions. Diabetes is the most common cause of non-traumatic lower limb amputation but many diabetic amputations could be delayed or prevented by more effective self-management education and medical supervision.

Ischaemia, resulting from peripheral vascular disease, neuropathy and infection, combine to produce tissue necrosis and ulceration. Peripheral vascular disease tends to affect more distal vessels and occurs at a younger age in people with diabetes. Ischaemia compromises the ability to heal after minor trauma or infection.

Pain is a protective mechanism and the diminished sensation that results from peripheral neuropathy means that the individual is less able to perceive trauma and may continue to walk on a wounded foot thereby worsening the injury. Autonomic neuropathy reduces sweating and alters blood flow resulting in dry skin that is prone to crack and fissure.

Although ischaemia and neuropathy may coexist, certain features allow an ischaemic to be distinguished from a predominantly neuropathic aetiology (**Box 23.24**).

Charcot neuroarthropathy

Charcot arthropathy is a complication of severe neuropathy. It occurs in a well-perfused foot and can be divided into three phases:
- acute onset
- bony destruction
- radiological consolidation and stabilization.

Individuals present with an acutely swollen hot foot and about a third have pain. At this stage, it may be difficult to differentiate between Charcot arthropathy and cellulitis; if in doubt, both conditions should be treated. Acute gout and deep vein thrombosis may also masquerade as Charcot arthropathy. If treatment is delayed, the foot can become deformed as bone is destroyed, often very rapidly over a few weeks. After 6–12 months, the destructive process stabilizes. Rehabilitation is always necessary after a long period in a cast and reconstructive surgery may be needed.

The aim of treatment is to prevent or minimize bony destruction and deformity. Any resulting deformity can alter the pressure distribution across the foot and predisposes the foot to future ulceration. Immobilization in a non-weight bearing cast is the treatment of choice and should be continued until the swelling and temperature in the foot has resolved.

Management of the diabetic foot

The key to managing diabetic foot problems is prevention. Learning about the principles of foot care is essential (**Box 23.25**). Healthcare professionals should screen for foot problems at least once a year; this process should include questions about past or present ulceration, an examination of the foot to detect structural abnormalities or callus formation and an assessment of neuropathy and peripheral vascular disease. Although a clinical examination may

Box 23.24 Distinguishing features between ischaemia and neuropathy in the diabetic foot		
Feature	**Ischaemia**	**Neuropathy**
Symptoms	Claudication	Usually painless
	Rest pain	Sometimes painful neuropathy
Inspection	Dependent rubor	High arch
	Trophic changes	Clawing of toes
		No trophic changes
Palpation	Cold	Warm
	Pulseless	Bounding pulses
Ulceration	Painful	Painless
	Heels and toes	Plantar

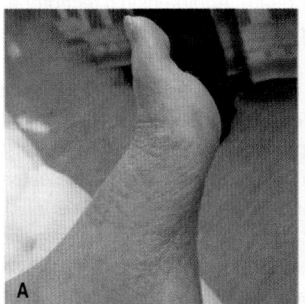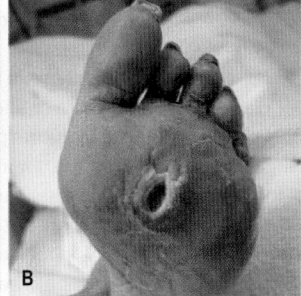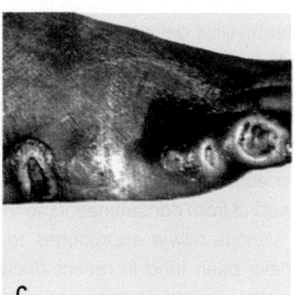

Fig. 23.18 Diabetic foot. (A) High arch and clawing of toes. **(B)** Typical neuropathic plantar ulceration. **(C)** Vascular pattern of ulceration.

23

Box 23.25 Principles of diabetic foot care

- Inspect feet daily
- Moisturize dry skin
- Seek early advice for any damage
- Take care if walking barefoot
- Check shoes inside and out for sharp bodies/areas before wearing
- Ensure shoes fit well with plenty of room for the toes
- Keep feet away from sources of heat (hot sand, hot-water bottles, radiators, fires)
- Check the bath temperature before stepping in
- Do not treat corns/callosities without professional help
- Attend a podiatrist regularly:
  – Older people with diabetes may require help to cut their toenails

reveal a distal loss of sensation, the use of monofilament, applied perpendicular to the foot and which buckles at a force of 10 g, has allowed reproducible assessments. Ability to feel that level of pressure provides protective sensation against foot ulceration. Doppler ultrasound is a useful addition to a clinical examination of the lower limb pulses. If neuropathy or impaired blood supply is detected, the individual can be warned that their foot is at increased risk of ulceration.

Foot ulceration

The key to healing an ulcer is to ensure that the foot is non-weight-bearing. Resting the affected leg may need to be supplemented with special shoes and insoles to move pressure away from critical sites, or by removable or non-removable leg casts. After healing, special shoes and insoles are likely to be needed in the long-term to protect the feet and prevent abnormal pressure repeating damage to a healed area. In neuropathic feet, particularly, sharp surgical debridement by a chiropodist is necessary to prevent callus distorting the local wound architecture and causing damage through abnormal pressure on normal skin nearby.

Ischaemia

Clinical signs of ischaemia may be confirmed by femoral angiography, which is used to localize areas of occlusion that may be amenable to bypass surgery or angioplasty.

Infection

Foot infections can take hold rapidly and should be treated as medical emergencies. Some people have termed this a 'foot attack' akin to heart attacks to emphasize the seriousness of this condition. Clinical signs may include purulent discharge, erythema, local warmth and swelling.

Early broad-spectrum antibiotics are essential, with therapy adjusted in the light of culture results. The organism grown from the skin surface may not be the organism causing deeper infection. Collections of pus are drained and excision of infected bone may be needed if osteomyelitis develops and does not respond to appropriate antibiotic therapy. Regular X-rays of the foot are needed to check on progress.

Wound environment

Dressings are used to absorb or remove exudate, maintain moisture, and protect the wound from contaminating agents; they should be easily removable. Various newer approaches to aid healing of diabetic foot ulcers have been tried in recent decades, including new dressings containing growth factors and other biologically active agents, hyperbaric oxygen, negative pressure wound therapy and bioengineered skin substitutes.

Multidisciplinary diabetic foot team

A multidisciplinary diabetic foot team, involving diabetologists working with podiatrists, orthopaedic and vascular surgeons, specialist nurses, orthotists and other healthcare professionals improves the outcome for people with diabetic foot ulcers. Rapid access to services is needed and people with diabetes should know how to contact the foot team if they develop problems.

Macrovascular complications

Atherosclerotic vascular disease

Diabetes is a risk factor for the development of atherosclerosis. Myocardial infarction, stroke, peripheral vascular disease and cardiovascular death are increased two- or threefold compared with the background population. This risk is increased up to tenfold in premenopausal women, who lose their normal protection against cardiovascular disease.

Pathogenesis

Atherosclerotic vascular disease in people with diabetes tends to occur at an earlier age, progress more rapidly and is more distal and diffuse than in people without diabetes. Although hyperglycaemia contributes to the development of macrovascular disease, unlike microvascular disease, other more important haemodynamic and metabolic mechanisms are involved. The relationship between glycaemic control and cardiovascular disease is less strong than microvascular disease but continues across the normal glucose range. The other factors include hypertension, dyslipidaemia, which is characterized by low HDL cholesterol and high triglyceride concentrations, obesity, hyperinsulinaemia and proteinuria including microalbuminuria.

Management of atherosclerotic cardiovascular risk

Addressing cardiovascular risk involves the aggressive and systematic management of each of the predisposing factors (**Box 23.26**). As discussed earlier, early tight glycaemic control reduces the long-term risk of cardiovascular disease. In people with type 2 diabetes with established cardiovascular disease, the use of SGLT2 inhibitors and GLP-1 receptor agonists is recommended because of their protective effect. Anti-hypertensive treatment produces a marked reduction in adverse cardiovascular outcomes as well as microvascular events. To achieve the target for blood pressure, most people with diabetes will need combination drug therapy. The use of ACE inhibitors or angiotensin receptor blockers may confer additional benefit. Treating people with diabetes and at least one other major cardiovascular risk factor with an ACE inhibitor produces a 25–35% lowering of the risk of heart attack, stroke, overt nephropathy or cardiovascular death. Angiotensin II receptor antagonists are sometimes preferred initially and are also used for those intolerant to ACE inhibitors.

Statins are recommended for those with diabetes over the age of 40 years or after a 10-year history of diabetes if microvascular complications are present as cardiovascular events are reduced by 20% for every 1 mmol/L reduction in LDL cholesterol. Other lipid lowering agents, such as ezetimibe or PCSK9 inhibitors, are indicated if statins are not tolerated or do not bring the cholesterol to target.

As in the general population, smoking cessation is important and help should be offered to those wishing to quit.

Low-dose aspirin reduces macrovascular risk but is associated with a morbidity and mortality from bleeding. The benefits of aspirin

Box 23.26 Target goals for cardiovascular risk factor management of people with diabetes

Parameter	Ideal	Reasonable but not ideal
HbA$_{1c}$	<7% (53 mmol/mol)	<8% (64 mmol/mol)
Blood pressure (mmHg)	<130/80	<140/85
Total cholesterol (mmol/L)	<4.0	<5.0
Low-density lipoprotein	<2.0	<3.0
High-density lipoprotein[a]	>1.1	>0.8
Triglycerides	<1.7	<2.0

[a]In women, >1.3 mmol/L. Standards from American Diabetes Association (2016).

outweigh the bleeding risk when used for secondary prevention, but in Europe it is not recommended for primary prevention.

The management of established cardiovascular disease by angioplasty or surgery is discussed in Chapter 30.

Heart failure

Heart failure is more common than atherosclerotic cardiovascular disease in people with diabetes and both heart failure with preserved ejection volume and heart failure with reduced ejection volume occur more frequently. Around two-thirds of people with type 2 diabetes have evidence of left ventricular dysfunction 5 years after the diagnosis of diabetes. The prognosis after the development of heart failure is poor, with only 10% alive after 5 years.

Despite this, heart failure has received less attention than atherosclerotic cardiovascular disease and is frequently underdiagnosed. The prevalence of undiagnosed heart failure is higher in those with increasing age, with obesity, hypertension dyspnoea or fatigue and in women.

The diagnosis and management of heart failure is similar to the general population but it is important to consider the effects of diabetes medications on the heart failure. Pioglitazone and saxagliptin, a DPP4 inhibitor, increased the risk of heart failure in clinical trials while epidemiological studies show an association between the use of insulin and sulphonylureas with heart failure. GLP-1 receptor agonists have no effect on heart failure while SGLT2 inhibitors reduce the risk.

OTHER COMPLICATIONS OF DIABETES

Non-alcoholic liver disease and other gastrointestinal manifestations of diabetes

Non-alcoholic fatty liver disease (NAFLD) is characterized by intrahepatic fat accumulation with varying degrees of hepatic inflammation and fibrosis. A small proportion of people progress to cirrhosis. NAFLD is present in up to one-fifth of the general population but the prevalence is increased in people with type 2 diabetes. Over a third of people with NAFLD have diabetes and NAFLD is an independent predictor of the development of diabetes and cardiovascular disease. It is associated with central obesity and insulin resistance (see p. 708). Management is

through weight loss and exercise. Pioglitazone may also reduce intrahepatic fat.

Malabsorption secondary to gastrointestinal dysmotility is described earlier but people with diabetes may also develop malabsorption through chronic exocrine pancreatic insufficiency. This is unusual because only 10% of pancreatic function is sufficient for normal digestion. Treatment is with pancreatic enzymes. People with type 1 diabetes have a higher prevalence of coeliac disease.

Infections

Although people with well-controlled diabetes are not more prone to infection, hyperglycaemia leads to more frequent infection through multiple disturbances in innate immunity; by contrast, humoral immunity appears relatively unaffected. Microvascular disease may further impede the immune system and likely contributes to the severity of certain infections, including malignant otitis externa, emphysematous pyelonephritis and necrotizing fasciitis. Some microorganisms, such as *Klebsiella* serotypes and *Burkholderia pseudomallei*, are more virulent in hyperglycaemic environments.

Urinary tract infections and asymptomatic bacteriuria are more common in people with diabetes, with autonomic neuropathy a common and important underlying factor. Mycotic genital infections are more common, particularly in women. Skin and soft tissue infections are more common. The risk of tuberculosis is increased in people with diabetes. Certain viral infections, such as hepatitis C, and treatment for HIV/AIDS increase the risk of diabetes.

Cancer

Certain types of cancer are more common in type 2 diabetes. The risk of carcinoma of the uterus and of the pancreas is approximately doubled, and there is a 20–50% increase in the risk of colorectal and breast cancer. These associations appear to be mediated, at least in part, by obesity, which confers similar levels of risk in the absence of hyperglycaemia, although there is also an element of reverse causation with carcinoma of the pancreas, which can precipitate or cause diabetes. People treated with metformin have been reported to have a lower cancer risk than those on other therapies, and this agent is under investigation for possible anti-tumour properties.

Skin and joints

Diabetic cheiroarthropathy refers to joint contractures in the hands as a result of long-standing diabetes. This may be diagnosed by asking the individual to join the hands as if in prayer; the metacarpophalangeal and interphalangeal joints cannot be opposed. Thickened, waxy skin can be noted on the backs of the fingers. These features may be due to glycation of collagen and are not progressive (p. 679). Frozen shoulder, Dupuytren's contracture, trigger finger, and carpal tunnel syndrome all occur more commonly in diabetes.

Fracture risk is increased in both type 1 and type 2 diabetes. Although bone mineral density is decreased in type 1 diabetes, it is increased in type 2 diabetes and so other mechanisms are at play. Thiazolidinediones decrease bone formation and bone mineral density, and increase fracture risk in type 2 diabetes. Following a fracture, healing may be delayed in people with diabetes. The risk of gout is increased in people with type 2 diabetes.

Further reading

Antonetti DA, Klein R, Gardner TW. Diabetic retinopathy. *N Engl J Med* 2012; 366:1227–1239.

DCCT/EDIC Research Group, de Boer IH, Sun W et al. Intensive diabetes therapy and glomerular filtration rate in type 1 diabetes mellitus. *N Engl J Med* 2011; 365:2366–2376.

Diabetes UK. *How to Spot a Foot Attack*; https://www.diabetes.org.uk/get_invol ved/volunteer/involve-newsletter/new-booklet-for-people-at-increased-risk-of-a-foot-attack.

Jude EB, Eleftheriadou I, Tentolouris N. Peripheral arterial disease in diabetes – a review. *Diabetes Med* 2010; 27:4–14.

Martin DF, Maguire MG. Treatment choice for diabetic macular edema. *N Engl J Med* 2015; 372:1260–1261.

National Institute for Health and Care Excellence. *NICE Guideline 19: Diabetic Foot Problems: Prevention and Management*. NICE 2019; https://www.nice.org.u k/guidance/ng19.

Pernicova I, Korbonits M. Metformin – mode of action and clinical implications for diabetes and cancer. *Nat Rev Endocrinol* 2014; 10:143–156.

White NH, Sun W, Cleary PA. Prolonged effect of intensive therapy on the risk of retinopathy complications in patients with type 1 diabetes mellitus: 10 years after the Diabetes Control and Complications Trial. *Arch Ophthalmol* 2008; 126:1707–1715.

PSYCHOSOCIAL IMPLICATIONS OF DIABETES

The interaction between mind and body is central to the management and outcome of all chronic diseases, but is particularly fascinating in the case of diabetes. People with diabetes have an increased risk of developing a number of psychological conditions, while a range of psychiatric disorders are associated with an increased risk of diabetes (**Box 23.27**). People who report chronic stress, low stress resilience, sleeping problems or depression are at increased risk of developing type 2 diabetes. Diabetes affects the quality of many aspects of life including emotional wellbeing, financial situation, leisure and work activities and relationships with friends and families.

Psychological problems associated with diagnosis

Most people show remarkable psychological resilience to a diagnosis of diabetes, despite the implications for self-management and long-term health. However, in some people, the diagnosis may lead to symptoms of anxiety and depression while others develop an 'adjustment disorder'. Transient psychological symptoms begin within 3 months of the diagnosis of the diabetes but usually resolve within 6 months. These symptoms are seen as part of the normal 'grieving process' that often accompanies the development of any chronic illness and may also develop in the parents of children with newly diagnosed diabetes.

Diabetes-related distress

Living with diabetes is demanding; it is estimated that people with type 1 diabetes need to devote up to 2 hours a day to self-management while around half of people with diabetes report that taking medication interferes with their ability to live a normal life. There are no holidays from diabetes! Diabetes self-management is often frustrating when blood glucose levels remain stubbornly out-of-target despite the individual's best efforts. More than 50% of people develop psychological symptoms, which are collectively known as diabetes distress, in response to living with the constant burden of diabetes. These include:

- experiencing worries about the future and the possibility of serious complications
- feeling guilty or anxious when the diabetes management goes awry
- feeling scared or depressed when thinking about living with diabetes
- feeling discouraged with diabetes regimen.

 Box 23.27 Bidirectional relationship between diabetes and psychiatric and psychological conditions

Psychiatric and psychological conditions that occur more frequently in people with diabetes	Psychiatric and psychological conditions that increase the risk of diabetes
• Adjustment disorders • Diabetes-related distress • Fear of hypoglycaemia • Stigma and discrimination • Anxiety • Depression • Phobia • Eating disorders	• Chronic stress • Low resilience • Sleeping problems • Anxiety • Depression • Bipolar disorder • Schizophrenia • Other psychotic conditions treated with antipsychotics

Fear of hypoglycaemia

Episodes of hypoglycaemia are frequently unpredictable and are associated with unpleasant, embarrassing symptoms associated with activation of the nervous system. It is perhaps unsurprising that many people worry about future occurrences of hypoglycaemia and some people develop significant fear of hypoglycaemia. This fear may also be experienced by other family members. Significant fear of hypoglycaemia is more common in people who have experienced loss of consciousness during a previous episode.

Depression

The prevalence of depression is increased two-fold in diabetes. Significant depressive symptoms affect approximately one in four adults with diabetes while a formal diagnosis of depressive disorders is made in 10–15% of people with diabetes. Depression is more common in women, those who are divorced and those who have experienced childhood adversity and social deprivation. In addition, there are a number of diabetes-specific risk factors associated with depression, including the development of complications and after initiation of insulin in type 2 diabetes.

Eating disorders

Eating disorders, such as anorexia nervosa and bulimia, are more common in people with diabetes. The drive to lose weight may lead to intentional insulin omission, which is reported by a third of young women aged 16–30.

Consequences of psychological and psychiatric disorders of diabetes

As well as affecting quality of life, the psychological sequelae of diabetes also impair the individual's ability to manage their diabetes. They are less likely to follow a healthy diet and exercise, less likely to take medication as prescribed and it is therefore no wonder that psychological problems are associated with higher HbA_{1c}, more frequent admissions with hypoglycaemia and diabetic ketoacidosis, a higher incidence of complications and shortened life expectancy.

Management of psychological issues

The key step to managing the psychological sequelae of diabetes is identifying the problem. It is important to ask the person with diabetes how they feel about their diabetes and whether they are experiencing difficulties with it. The diabetes specialist team will undertake much of the psychological management, but this should

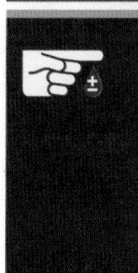

include liaison with the mental health teams to ensure appropriate referral of those with more complex problems. Some diabetes teams now include a psychologist.

A range of psychological interventions, including cognitive behavioural therapy and problem solving, have been used successfully to improve the psychological wellbeing of people with diabetes.

For people with depression, antidepressants are effective as long as they are used in adequate doses.

Social aspects of diabetes

Diabetes affects many aspects of the daily lives of people with the condition but here we will consider driving and employment.

The main issues for drivers with diabetes are hypoglycaemia and visual impairment from either retinopathy or cataract. Disability from leg amputation or neuropathy may also affect the ability to drive safely. As hypoglycaemia is the most common cause of accidents in people with insulin-treated diabetes, drivers with diabetes must take precautions to avoid hypoglycaemia while driving. In most countries, a driver with diabetes will need to inform the relevant authorities and insurance companies of their diagnosis.

Diabetes should not prevent access to most occupations but certain occupations including the armed forces, emergency services, commercial pilots, prison and security services, and jobs in potentially dangerous areas (e.g. at heights, underwater and offshore) are barred or require special precautions. Shift work can make insulin management more complex but modern long-acting insulin analogues with duration of action longer than 24 hours have made life easier.

Further reading

Fisher L, Polonsky WH, Hessler D. Addressing diabetes distress in clinical care: a practical guide. *Diabet Med* 2019; 36; https://doi.org/10.1111/dme.13967.
Holt RI, de Groot M, Golden SH. Diabetes and depression. *Curr Diab Rep* 2014; 14:491.
Holt RI, Nicolucci A, Kovacs Burns K et al. Diabetes Attitudes, Wishes and Needs second study (DAWN2™): cross-national comparisons on barriers and resources for optimal care –healthcare professional perspective. *Diabet Med* 2013; 30:789–798.
Kovacs Burns K, Nicolucci A, Holt RI et al. Diabetes Attitudes, Wishes and Needs second study (DAWN2™): cross-national benchmarking indicators for family members living with people with diabetes. *Diabet Med* 2013; 30:778–788.
http://dwed.org.uk/. *Diabetics with eating disorders*.

DIABETES IN SPECIAL SITUATIONS

Diabetes in childhood, adolescence and early adulthood

More than 1 million children have diabetes worldwide with approximately 132 600 new cases diagnosed annually. The incidence has been steadily rising over the last 50 years. Most children with diabetes have type 1 diabetes, although type 2 diabetes is becoming more common in older children.

After diagnosis, the child should be managed as an outpatient by a team comprising a paediatrician specializing in diabetes, diabetes specialist nurse, dietitian, social worker and a psychologist trained in childhood diabetes. Support and education is needed for the parents and extended families as the diagnosis of diabetes can be devastating

Insulin pump is the treatment of choice for children with type 1 diabetes although basal-bolus multiple daily injections are an acceptable alternative. As the doses of insulin are much smaller in children, even a one-unit change in dose can amount to a large percentage change. The insulin pump allows finer adjustment than multiple daily injections. Half unit pens are also available.

As the child grows up, the responsibility for managing the diabetes will shift from parent to child. Adolescence and young adulthood is characterized by complex biological, social and psychological changes, which poses unique challenges to those with diabetes. The pubertal increase in sex steroids and growth hormone increase insulin resistance by 25–30% and coupled with the increase in body size, insulin requirements can increase substantially. Insulin adjustment often lags behind these changes resulting in hyperglycaemia.

During adolescence, individuals develop a sense of self and identity and begin to establish control, autonomy and independence. This is often accompanied by anxiety as the adolescent seeks peer acceptance. Diabetes often singles out the adolescent and can leave them feeling isolated and different. Adolescents may prioritize their social network over diabetes management and studies have shown that HbA_{1c} and admissions for diabetic ketoacidosis tend to rise during the teenage years. The diabetes team needs to support the adolescent and parents through this period; success relies on empowering the individual with the skills and confidence that they can manage their diabetes.

The period of transition between paediatric and adult services is challenging and many young adults with diabetes lose contact with healthcare professionals if this process is not managed effectively. The physical transfer between paediatric and adult services is only a small component of transition and the process can take a number of years as the paediatric team, working with the adult team, provides the young adult with the information and skills needs to negotiate an adult health service independently. Although many young adults move to adult services around the age of 18–19 years, the decision to transfer should be based on skills and competencies rather than chronological age.

Emerging adulthood is a new concept that describes the early years of adulthood when an individual may be entering the world of work and moving away from home for the first time, including going to university. As well as providing many new opportunities, it is often a time for risk-taking. Many centres have now developed young adult clinics to care for the specific needs of this age group.

Diabetes in older people and at the end of life

The prevalence of diabetes in older people is increasing dramatically because of an ageing population and age-related challenges in body composition and insulin resistance. The lifetime risk of developing diabetes is 22% for women and 19% for men from the age of 60 years. More than half of those with diabetes are aged over 65 years. Approximately 25% of older people living in care homes or nursing homes have diabetes.

Diabetes places an additional burden on older people, who frequently have other chronic conditions, with up to 40% having three or more other co-morbidities. Diabetes increases the risk of dementia and the cognitive decline compromises diabetes management. Frailty, which is characterized by weight loss, weakness, decreased physical activity, exhaustion and slow gait speed, is more common in older people.

The management of diabetes in the older individual should consider the health status and needs of the person with diabetes. A thorough assessment should identify co-morbidities. Older people with diabetes are a highly heterogeneous population ranging from someone living independently in the community to a frail individual

---

Box 23.28 Glycaemic targets for older people[a]

Independent or robust	Dependent	Dependent dementia or frail	End of life
7.0–7.5%	7.0–8.0%	<8.5%	Avoid symptomatic hypoglycaemia
53–59 mmol/mol	53–64 mmol/mol	<70 mmol/mol	

[a]Glycaemic control targets should be individualized taking into account functional status, co-morbidities, especially the presence of established CVD, history and risk of hypoglycaemia, and presence of microvascular complications.
(*Available at: https://www.idf.org/e-library/guidelines/78-global-guideline-for-managing-older-people-with-type-2-diabetes.html*)

Box 23.29 Use of insulin in older people[a]

Insulin regimen	Independent or robust	Dependent frail	Dependent dementia	End of life
Basal insulin + oral anti-diabetes agents	First choice	First choice	First choice	First choice but consider withdrawal
Pre-mix insulin	Alternative first choice			
Basal-bolus insulin	Second-line	Avoid	Avoid	Avoid

[a]Choose appropriate device, usually pre-filled pen.
(*Available at: https://www.idf.org/e-library/guidelines/78-global-guideline-for-managing-older-people-with-type-2-diabetes.html*)

---

with multiple co-morbidities in a care home. Glycaemic targets should therefore be individualized taking into consideration overall health, life expectancy, cognitive decline and co-morbidities (**Box 23.28**). Maximizing quality of life should always be the focus of care.

Where possible, drugs that avoid hypoglycaemia are preferred because the associated co-morbidities, geriatric syndromes, polypharmacy, long duration of diabetes and the increased prevalence of hepatic and renal dysfunction increase the risk of hypoglycaemia. Insulin regimens should be simplified (**Box 23.29**). Furthermore, hypoglycaemia can be less easily recognized and is often misdiagnosed because of reduced autonomic symptoms.

As people approach the end of life, the goals of treatment shift from the prevention of long-term complications to the avoidance of symptomatic hyper- and hypoglycaemia, acute metabolic decompensation and drug-related adverse events. Glycaemic targets should be relaxed with the aim of keeping the glucose between 6 mmol/L and 15 mmol/L (110–270 mg/dL) to minimize the risk of hypoglycaemia and other drug-related adverse events. Insulin should usually be continued. It is important to take care to avoid foot ulceration in bedbound individuals.

Inpatient diabetes

In 2015 the UK National Diabetes Inpatient Audit showed that 4–35% of hospital inpatients had diabetes. In the majority, diabetes was not the cause for their admission but poor management of diabetes lengthens hospital stay and increases the risk of developing complications, such as hospital-acquired infection, or dying. This applies equally to medical and surgical inpatients.

While the stress of acute illness can worsen hyperglycaemia, it is hypoglycaemia that is associated with increased morbidity and mortality. As there is a lack of robust evidence demonstrating that intensive glucose management improves outcomes, the general

---

Box 23.30 Indications for intravenous insulin in hospital

Variable rates intravenous insulin infusion
- Critical care illness
- Acute coronary syndromes
- Stroke
- 'Nil by mouth' status when more than one meal will be missed (type 1 diabetes)
- General preoperative, intraoperative and postoperative care
- Stroke
- Hyperglycaemia during high-dose corticosteroid therapy
- Labour and delivery
- Other acute illness for which prompt glycaemic control is judged important for recovery

Fixed rates intravenous insulin infusion
- Diabetes emergencies:
  – Diabetic ketoacidosis
  – Hyperosmolar hyperglycaemic syndrome

---

consensus is that the main priority is to avoid hypoglycaemia and diabetes treatments need to be adjusted accordingly.

As people with diabetes may be less able to self-manage their diabetes while in hospital, it is important the diagnosis of diabetes is clearly identified in the medical records and glucose and HbA$_{1c}$ measured on admission. Errors in insulin prescribing are common and one-third of all fatal inpatient medical errors that cause death within 48 hours of the error involve insulin administration. An emphasis on insulin safety, particularly when an intravenous insulin is being used, is essential. There is an increasing move for people with insulin-treated diabetes to self-manage once they are able to so themselves on the grounds that they know how to do so much better than many hospital staff.

Many hospitals have specialized diabetes inpatient teams who take responsibility for diabetes management but all staff caring for people with diabetes should be appropriately trained and competent in the management of inpatient diabetes (see **Box 23.12**).

Intravenous insulin is required for a number of specific conditions as this mode of administration provides the greatest flexibility to meet rapidly changing insulin requirements (**Box 23.30**). Intravenous insulin is usually administered as a variable rate infusion, but the insulin rate is fixed when treating diabetic ketoacidosis. Variable-rate or fixed-rate intravenous insulin infusion is preferred to the old but more ambiguous terminology 'sliding scale'. In order to maintain patient safety, the glucose should be monitored frequently.

Management of diabetes during an admission for surgery

Both hyperglycaemia and hypoglycaemia in the postoperative period worsen surgical outcomes by increasing the risk of infection, myocardial infarction and death, and are associated with an increased duration of stay on the intensive care unit and in hospital.

The patient journey begins in primary care and general practitioners should help optimize glucose management in the preoperative period. This will reduce the likelihood of the surgery being cancelled or postponed owing to poor glycaemic control. The preoperative assessment provides a further opportunity to improve diabetes management and will allow the patient to be placed at the beginning of a morning list where possible to minimize the period of fasting and subsequent metabolic disturbance.

For people treated with insulin, unless the period of fasting is less than one missed meal, a variable-rate intravenous insulin infusion will be needed to control the glucose perioperatively. The long-acting insulin should be continued as this will prevent rebound hyperglycaemia when the intravenous insulin is stopped. Oral drugs that can cause hypoglycaemia should also be stopped for the dose immediately prior to surgery but can be resumed once the patient is eating and drinking normally. Metformin should be stopped if intravenous contrast is used.

Prior to discharge, a clear follow-up plan is needed, which should be communicated to the person with diabetes and their primary care team.

Diabetes in pregnancy

Diabetes is one of the most common medical conditions in pregnancy, affecting 2–5% of pregnant women. Approximately 85% of women with diabetes in pregnancy have gestational diabetes with the remainder having pre-existing diabetes. The epidemiology of pre-existing diabetes in pregnancy is changing as women are delaying pregnancy to an older age and the prevalence of obesity and type 2 diabetes is increasing in women of childbearing age. Whereas 25 years ago, type 2 diabetes was rare in pregnant women, the latest UK national audit has indicated that there are equal numbers of women with type 2 diabetes as type 1 diabetes.

Adverse effects of diabetes in pregnancy

Prior to the discovery of insulin, pregnancy was invariably fatal for both mother and fetus. Even in the era up to the 1960s, pregnancy remained a risky enterprise, with perinatal mortality rates of up to 40%. However, with an understanding that maternal hyperglycaemia was the major cause of fetal loss, management changed to ensure as near normoglycaemia as possible and outcomes began to improve. However, pregnancy outcomes in women with diabetes still remain worse than women without diabetes.

Diabetes in pregnancy is associated with risks to both the woman and to the developing fetus. Women with pre-existing diabetes may find it harder to conceive and in the first trimester have higher rates of miscarriage and congenital anomalies. The frequency of many developmental abnormalities, including cardiac and skeletal malformations, is increased. Although rare, the risk of caudal regression syndrome appears to be specifically increased in women with diabetes. Towards the end of pregnancy, women with either pre-existing diabetes or gestational diabetes have a higher risk of pre-term labour, hypertension and pre-eclampsia.

The risks to the fetus include higher rates of macrosomia and associated shoulder dystocia and birth injury, polyhydramnios, stillbirth and perinatal mortality, and impaired postnatal metabolic adaptation leading to higher rates of neonatal hypoglycaemia, jaundice and respiratory distress. After birth, neonatal hypoglycaemia may occur. Maternal glucose crosses the placenta but insulin does not; this leads the fetal islets to hypersecrete insulin in order to combat the rising hyperglycaemia, and rebound hypoglycaemia may occur when the umbilical cord is cut. In the longer term, offspring of mothers with diabetes have a higher risk of obesity and diabetes in adulthood.

Obesity itself adversely affects maternal and fetal outcomes. For the mother, obesity independently increases the risk of hypertension and pre-eclampsia, infections and venous thromboembolism. Through fetal overnutrition, obesity may also drive macrosomia and associated birth trauma.

Management of diabetes during pregnancy

As the adverse effects of diabetes are largely mediated by hyperglycaemia, the major aim of management in diabetic pregnancies is to maintain normoglycaemia by avoiding pre- and post-prandial hyperglycaemia without causing severe hypoglycaemia. This is a demanding process and so pregnant women with diabetes should be in contact with a specialist multidisciplinary team jointly led by a physician and obstetrician at least every 2 weeks.

Pre-conception care

Pregnancy management should begin well before conception; as pregnancy can only be diagnosed a minimum of 2 weeks after conception, it is important that optimal glycaemic control is achieved prior to conception. This requires planning on the part of both the woman with diabetes and the diabetes team. From puberty, girls with diabetes need to know about the importance of pregnancy planning and contraception until they are ready to start a family.

Once a woman expresses a desire for pregnancy, referral to a specialist diabetes preconception clinic improves the pregnancy outcomes. This provides an opportunity to review the diabetes management, discuss the need for high dose folic acid (5 mg daily) to reduce the risk of neural tube defects, ensure that microvascular screening is up-to-date and check that the woman has been immunized against rubella.

The optimal target pre-conception HbA_{1c} is below 48 mmol/mol (6.5%) when this can be achieved safely but women should be advised not to become pregnant if their HbA_{1c} is above 86 mmol/mol (10%). Target fasting plasma glucose levels 5–7 mmol/L (90–126 mg/dL) and 4–7 mmol/L (70–126 mg/dL) before meals at other times of the day are needed to achieve this level of glycaemic control. This is challenging for the women and they should be offered the opportunity to attend structured education if they have not done so already. Where necessary, insulin analogues should be used as these appear to convey advantages over human insulin. Metformin may be used while preparing for pregnancy but other oral antidiabetes drugs and GLP-1 receptor agonists should be stopped. ACE inhibitors, angiotensin II receptor antagonists and statins should be stopped prior to conception.

Antenatal management

The need for tight glycaemic control continues once a woman becomes pregnant; the target glucose levels are less than 5.3 mmol/L fasting (95 mg/dL), less than 7.8 mmol/L (140 mg/dL) 1 hour after meals and less than 6.4 mmol/L (115 mg/dL) 2 hours after meals. Women need to monitor their glucose levels by capillary blood testing; where available, continuous glucose monitoring is preferred as this increases the time that women spend in the target glucose range and is associated with improved fetal outcomes.

These stringent glycaemic targets are made harder to achieve because pregnancy changes the insulin requirement; this tends to fall in the first trimester, partly as a result of the hormonal changes in pregnancy but also because pregnancy-associated nausea and vomiting can reduce appetite. This increases the risk and severity of hypoglycaemia; for reasons that are not entirely clear, early pregnancy is associated with impaired awareness of hypoglycaemia, further increasing the likelihood of hypoglycaemia. Women and their partners need to know about the risk and how to manage it. Interestingly, the fetus tolerates maternal hypoglycaemia relatively well.

During the second and third trimesters, pregnancy induces a state of insulin resistance, which typically increases insulin requirements by 50–100% in the latter half of pregnancy. Towards the end of pregnancy, insulin absorption is delayed and so women may need to increase the length of time between the short-acting insulin injection and eating in the third trimester.

? Box 23.31 Comparison of the NICE and IADPSG diagnostic criteria for gestational diabetes

Association	Glucose load	No. of high readings needed	Fasting glucose	1-h glucose	2-h glucose
IADPSG	75 g	≥1	5.1 mmol/L 90 mg/dL	10.0 mmol/L 180 mg/dL	8.5 mmol/L 153 mg/dL
NICE	75 g	≥1	5.6 mmol/L 100 mg/dL		7.8 mmol/L 140 mg/dL

IADPSG, International Association of Diabetes and Pregnancy Study Groups; NICE, National Institute for Health and Care Excellence.

Ketoacidosis in pregnancy carries a 50% fetal mortality and therefore if it occurs in pregnancy it should be diagnosed and managed rapidly. In order to expedite the diagnosis, women should be taught to monitor blood ketones at the outset of pregnancy.

As pregnancy can accelerate the progression of retinopathy, pregnant women should be screened in the first and third trimester and in the second trimester if any retinopathy is present at the outset.

Low-dose aspirin (150 mg daily) from the 12th week of pregnancy lowers the risk of hypertension and pre-eclampsia.

Enhanced fetal surveillance is needed and a detailed ultrasound scan for fetal anomalies including a four-chamber view of the fetal heart and outflow tracts should be offered at 18–20 weeks. Growth scans and other tests of fetal wellbeing should be performed during the third trimester.

Birth

Most babies of women with diabetes are born before term following an induction of labour or elective caesarean section to reduce the risk of stillbirth. Glycaemic control during labour is usually maintained by a variable rate intravenous insulin infusion but pumps are being increasingly used as an alternative in some centres.

Postnatal care

Following birth, maternal insulin requirements drop rapidly to pre-conception levels within hours of the birth and may even be lower if a woman chooses to breast-feed. As the neonate is at increased risk of hypoglycaemia, early feeding should be encouraged with breast-feeding being the preferred option and glucose checked regularly until it is clear that the pre-feeding glucose levels are being maintained in the normal range.

Gestational diabetes

Gestational diabetes is defined as diabetes occurring for the first time in pregnancy that is clearly not overt diabetes prior to pregnancy. It is usually diagnosed in the second and third trimester of pregnancy following a 75 g oral glucose tolerance. Gestational diabetes occurs in women whose pancreatic β cells are unable to secrete sufficient insulin to meet the pregnancy-induced insulin resistance. The risk factors for gestational diabetes are the same as for type 2 diabetes and so gestational diabetes can be regarded as an early revelation of the metabolic abnormality brought on by the demands of pregnancy. Not all diabetes presenting in pregnancy is gestational. Screening may identify women with previously undiagnosed type 2 diabetes and, in a few cases, gestational diabetes may unmask pre-clinical type 1 diabetes.

Diagnosis of gestational diabetes

There is a lack of international agreement regarding the diagnosis with varying diagnostic cut-off values and number of abnormal values needed between recommendations (**Box 23.31**). Universal screening for diabetes is recommended in many countries but in

i Box 23.32 Risk factors for gestational diabetes: NICE recommendations for 75 g oral glucose tolerance test

NICE recommends undertaking a 75 g oral glucose tolerance test at 24–28 weeks gestation in women with the following risk factors:
- BMI >30 kg/m²
- Previous macrosomic baby weighing ≥4.5 kg
- Previous gestational diabetes[a]
- First-degree relative with diabetes
- Family origin with a high prevalence of diabetes:
  – South Asian, black Caribbean and Middle Eastern

[a]Women with a previous history of gestational diabetes should be offered a 75 g 2-h oral glucose tolerance test (OGTT) as soon as possible after booking (whether in the first or second trimester), and a further 75 g 2-h OGTT at 24–28 weeks if the results of the first OGTT are normal.
NICE, National Institute for Health and Care Excellence.

the UK, NICE recommends screening only women with risk factors for gestational diabetes; the advantage of the latter approach is that many low-risk women do not need the screening test and it costs less but it risks missing gestational diabetes in a significant proportion of women (**Box 23.32**).

Management of gestational diabetes

The glucose targets are the same as for pre-existing diabetes but management begins with lifestyle modification, similar to the management of type 2 diabetes (pp. 712–713). If lifestyle modification does not achieve adequate maternal glycaemia within 1–2 weeks, pharmacological therapy is indicated. Although insulin is still widely used, studies have suggested that metformin or glibenclamide (a sulphonylurea) are acceptable alternatives.

Women with gestational diabetes have a 50% chance of developing diabetes within 10 years of the pregnancy. The diabetes antenatal team should discuss this risk and the measures needed to reduce the likelihood of developing diabetes prior to discharge after the birth. An annual HbA$_{1c}$ or glucose test is recommended to diagnose asymptomatic diabetes. At present, the uptake of postnatal interventions and screening is low, and more research is needed to find out how to manage this risk more effectively.

Further reading

International Association of Diabetes in Pregnancy Study Groups Consensus Panel. International Association of Diabetes in Pregnancy Study Groups recommendations on the diagnosis and classification of hyperglycemia in pregnancy. *Diabetes Care* 2010; 33:676–682.
International Diabetes Federation. Managing older people with type 2 diabetes. Global guideline; https://www.idf.org/e-library/guidelines/78-global-guideline-for-managing-older-people-with-type-2-diabetes.html.
Joint British Diabetes Societies. Management of adults with diabetes undergoing surgery and elective procedures: improving standards; https://www.diabetes.org.uk/resources-s3/2017-09/Use%20of%20variable%20rate%20intravenous%20insulin%20infusion%20in%20medical%20inpatients_0.pdf.
Joint British Diabetes Societies. The use of variable rate intravenous insulin infusion (VRIII) in medical inpatients; https://www.diabetes.org.uk/resources-s3/2017-09/Use%20of%20variable%20rate%20intravenous%20insulin%20infusion%20in%20medical%20inpatients_0.pdf

ORGANIZATION OF DIABETES CARE

The diabetes care team involves a multidisciplinary group of healthcare professionals who are available to support the person with diabetes (see **Fig. 23.10**). As the amount of time that each person with diabetes spends with a healthcare professional is small, on average less than 6 hours a year, it is important that every contact counts and provides appropriate medical and psychosocial support. To ensure that the person with diabetes derives the maximum benefit from the time spent with their diabetes team, whether in a hospital or community setting, the consultation should be collaborative, patient-centred, goal-focused and with clear aims. As well as traditional clinic visits, people with diabetes may access diabetes care virtually through phone, email or internet contact or through educational sessions.

Much of care is focused towards minimizing the long-term complications while avoiding adverse effects from treatment. Diabetes UK has described the 15 essentials of diabetes care (**Box 23.33**) that should be assessed and discussed at least once a year.

The majority of diabetes care takes place in a primary care setting but people with diabetes with complex medical or psychological needs will require management and support in a specialist setting for some or all of their care. A close collaboration between primary and secondary healthcare professionals and among specialists is essential to ensure that care is integrated and coordinated across the wide range of disciplines involved.

People with diabetes need to be involved in decisions about their care as this improves outcomes and the likelihood that a specific management plan will be followed. It is good practice to provide the person with diabetes with copies of any letters written about them

---

i | Box 23.33 Diabetes UK 15 essentials of diabetes care

1. Blood glucose test (HbA_{1c} test)
2. Blood pressure check
3. Cholesterol and lipid check
4. Eye screening
5. Foot and leg check
6. Kidney tests
7. Advice on diet
8. Emotional and psychological support
9. Diabetes education course
10. Care from diabetes specialists
11. Free flu jab
12. Good care if in hospital
13. Support with any sexual problems
14. Help to stop smoking
15. Specialist care while planning a pregnancy

---

so that all decisions are clear, and it is easier to review the management plans at subsequent contacts.

Significant websites

http://www.diabetes.ca. *Canadian Diabetes Association site – well-designed, practical site with many links to other diabetes-related sites; a good starting point.*
http://www.diabetes.org. *American Diabetes Association – heavyweight and authoritative, with an American flavour.*
http://www.diabetes.org.uk. *Diabetes UK charity – information for patients, researchers and health professionals.*
http://www.diapedia.org. The Living Textbook of Diabetes, *sponsored by the European Association for the Study of Diabetes (EASD).*
http://www.dtu.ox.ac.uk. *Diabetes Trials Unit (University of Oxford) – research information, particularly the UK Prospective Diabetes Study results.*
http://www.idf.org. *International Diabetes Federation.*
http://www.sign.ac.uk. *Scottish Intercollegiate Guidelines Network – guidelines on a range of subjects including diabetes.*

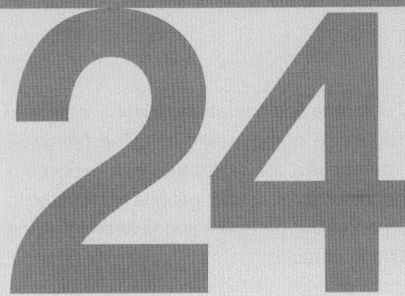

24 Lipid and metabolic disorders

Anthony S. Wierzbicki and Radha Ramachandran

CORE SKILLS AND KNOWLEDGE

Lipid disorders are common, and of great public health importance. All doctors need to be comfortable with managing such patients in the context of their overall cardiovascular risk. Inherited metabolic diseases (IMDs) are individually much rarer, although as a group not altogether uncommon.

Many patients with IMDs, including severe phenotypes of inherited lipid disorders, are diagnosed in childhood, and transition to the care of metabolic medicine specialists in tertiary referral centres in adulthood, supported by dieticians and other healthcare professionals. However, they may initially present as adults to general services, or require general or emergency management in non-specialist settings, meaning that all doctors need a basic awareness of these conditions.

Key skills in this area include:
- becoming familiar with the different drugs for lowering lipids and their role in reducing cardiovascular risk
- knowing when to suspect an inherited metabolic disease and understanding the principles of tailored therapy for rare diseases
- recognizing the acute presentations of such conditions and knowing core steps in management of these emergencies.

Opportunities for learning in this specialty include observing clinics in specialist metabolic medicine centres, and shadowing a dietician giving advice to patients on reducing cardiovascular risk.

INTRODUCTION

Lipid disorders are common, with 95% of Western populations having raised cholesterol levels compared with aboriginal/undeveloped societies. Cholesterol contributes up to half of population cardiovascular disease risk worldwide. A single genetic disorder of cholesterol metabolism – familial hypercholesterolaemia – is one of the commonest autosomal dominant disorders globally. Other disorders are less common but defects of the lipoprotein lipase pathway constitute a medical emergency as they can present as gross hypertriglyceridaemia associated with pancreatitis.

Inherited disorders of metabolism present in a variety of ways, often in childhood but sometimes in adults, as described in the second half of this chapter. Often disease will present with multi-system involvement, or in response to specific metabolic triggers such as starvation or dehydration. There may be a family history of similar symptoms or early death, or of consanguinity. It is important not to miss the diagnosis of an IMD because early institution of therapy or dietary modultation often significantly improves prognosis.

Approach to the patient

History

Significant factors relevant to lipid disorders include:
- demographics, including ethnicity.
- a cardiovascular risk factor history, including current and previous smoking, diabetes or pre-diabetes, family history of cardiovascular disease prior to age 60 (to second generation if available) and family history of hyperlipidaemia.
- a history of unexplained pancreatitis.

An IMD should be considered:
- in patients presenting with syndromes associated with particular IMDs, including encephalitis, rhabdomyolysis, acidosis, hypoglycaemia or stroke (see p. 752).
- where there is multisystem involvement.
- where there is a history of metabolic triggers (see p. 752).
- where there is a family history of similar symptoms, early death or of consanguinity.
- where an alternative more common diagnosis is not forthcoming.

It is important not to miss a diagnosis, as prognosis is often good following early institution of simply therapy or diet modulation. A confirmed diagnosis also has implications for the extended family who may benefit from early intervention and reproductive options.

Examination

Examination of a patient with a lipid disorder includes:
- noting signs of soft tissue lipid accumulation, such as tendon lumps (xanthomata), eyelid xanthelasma, and eruptive or planar xanthomata.
- measuring waist circumference and calculating body mass index (BMI).
- measuring blood pressure.

Patients with IMD may have signs relating to their clinical presentation, eg stroke or encephalitis. In some of the storage diseases, hepatosplenomegaly (sometimes massive) can be demonstrated.

Investigations

Patients with lipid disorders require a random or fasting lipid profile (see p. 745), and (at their first clinic visit) exclusion of secondary causes of proteinuria such as nephrotic syndrome (by measuring urine protein).

IMDs may require measurement of metabolites including ammonium, lactate, glucose, organic acids and amino acids in serum, urine and cerebrospinal fluid. Basic and additional tests, including the role of genetic testing, is described in Box 24.6.

DISORDERS OF LIPID METABOLISM

Physiology

Lipids are essential as fuel sources, structural components of membranes and as the basis for paracrine mediators. Lipid components can be synthesized from acetyl CoA derived from the tricarboxylic acid (Krebs) cycle pathway. Thus acetyl CoA can be made into linear chain fatty acids used mostly as fuel or the ring structures of cholesterol essential for membrane structure. The cholesterol synthesis pathway is regulated by its end-product through its rate-limiting initial enzyme, hydroxy-methyl-glutaryl coenzyme A reductase (HMG-CoAR), which is inhibited by 'statins', explaining their importance in the control of lipid disorders.

Lipids are insoluble in water and are transported in the bloodstream as macromolecular complexes. These complexes comprise a core of hydrophobic triglyceride, cholesterol and cholesterol esters surrounded by a phospholipid coat. Proteins (called apolipoproteins (apos)) on the surface of these 'lipoprotein' particles act as modulators of metabolism (e.g. enzyme cofactors) and ligands for receptors in the liver and the peripheral tissues. The structure of a chylomicron (one type of lipoprotein particle) is illustrated in **Fig. 24.1**.

Five principal types of lipoprotein particles are found in the blood (**Fig. 24.2**). They are structurally different and can be separated in the laboratory by their composition, density and electrophoretic mobility. The larger particles give postprandial plasma its cloudy appearance (lipaemia). The major apolipoproteins and most receptors have been isolated and sequenced, but the functions of some remains unclear. Plasma lipid levels are dependent on nutritional and environmental factors as well as genetic variants and contribute 55% of population-attributable risk for atherosclerotic disease. Genetic disorders of lipid metabolism are relatively common and contribute to highly increased risk of cardiovascular disease in some individuals. The pathways involved in lipid particle metabolism are concerned with exogenous lipid uptake and transport (chylomicrons), endogenous lipid synthesis and transport (apo B100-containing-particles) and reverse transport to the liver (apo A1-containing particles)

Chylomicrons

Chylomicrons (see **Fig. 24.1**) are synthesized in the small intestine post-prandially in response to the presence of gut fats (triglycerides) and cholesterol. They are secreted into the intestinal lymphatic drainage, and then pass along the thoracic duct into the bloodstream to be cleared eventually by the liver. They contain large quantities of triglycerides, some cholesterol and cholesterol esters. They are the main mechanism for transporting dietary fat, cholesterol and dietary-derived fat-soluble vitamins. Chylomicrons contain a ligand protein – apo B48 (one molecule), components of some future high-density lipoprotein (HDL) particles (apo A1 and apo A2), and acquire apoproteins C1-3 and apo-E by transfer from other particles in the bloodstream. Apo C2 binds to specific vascular surface (endothelial) receptors in adipose tissue, skeletal muscle and the liver, where the endothelial enzyme, lipoprotein lipase (LPL), hydrolyzes triglyceride into fatty acids for local uptake. The chylomicron remnant particle, containing most of the cholesterol, is taken up by the liver by a specific receptor and also by

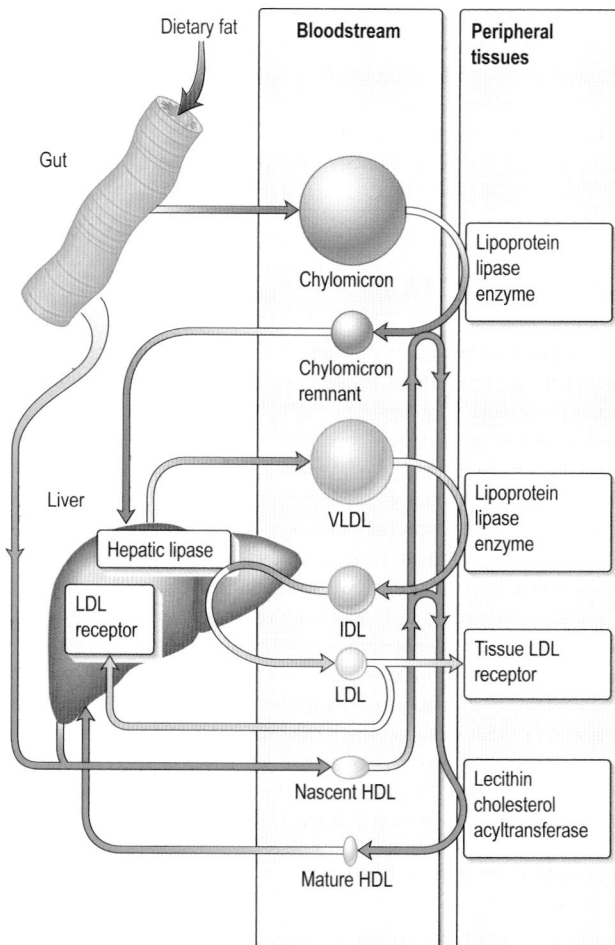

Fig. 24.2 The sites of origin of the major lipoprotein particles, showing their interaction and fate. HDL, high-density lipoprotein; IDL, intermediate-density lipoprotein; LDL, low-density lipoprotein; VLDL, very-low-density lipoprotein.

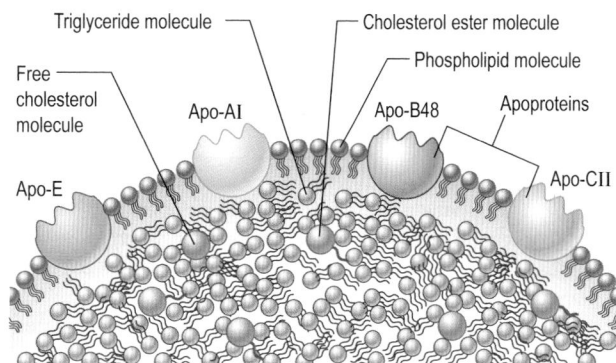

Fig. 24.1 A chylomicron particle (75–1200 nm) showing apoproteins lying in the surface membrane.

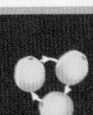

the apo-E/B-100 receptor. Clearance is determined by the balance of apo-E promoting clearance and apo C3 delaying it.

Very-low-density lipoprotein particles

Very-low-density lipoprotein (VLDL) particles are synthesized continuously in the liver. They transport the body's endogenously synthesized triglyceride and cholesterol. Apo B-100 is the signature protein component of VLDL and its metabolic derivatives, and present at one per particle. A small proportion of VLDL may complex with liver synthesized apo(a). As with chylomicrons, apo C1-3 and -E are incorporated later into VLDL by transfer from HDL particles and triglycerides are removed by LPL. This leaves a denser particle, due to partial depletion of triglyceride called an intermediate-density lipoprotein (IDL) particle.

Intermediate-density lipoprotein particles

IDL particles contain apo B-100 and apo C1-3 and apo-E molecules on the particle surface. Most IDL particles bind to liver low-density lipoprotein (LDL) (apo-E/B-100) receptors through the apo-E molecule and are catabolized. Further triglyceride removal leads to a denser remnant called LDL particles.

Low-density lipoprotein particles

LDL particles are the main carrier of cholesterol in fasting plasma, and deliver it both to the liver and to peripheral cells. The surface of the LDL particle contains apo B-100 and varying quantities of apo C-3 and apo-E. Apo B-100 is the principal ligand for the LDL (apo-E/B-100) receptor (LDLR). The LDLR binds LDL, forms coated pits on the surface of the hepatocyte, which invaginate and fuse with lysosomes and proteasomes, which destroy the LDL particle releasing its components (**Fig. 24.3**). This process is, in part, regulated by a serine protease, proprotein convertase subtilisin/kexin type 9 (PCSK9). PCSK9 binds to LDL–LDLR complexes increasing the rate of clearance of the complexes. If no PCSK9 is bound, then the LDLR can be recycled to the cell surface. The number of hepatic LDLR regulates the circulating LDL particle number and LDL cholesterol. LDL particles can deposit lipid into the walls of the peripheral vasculature through binding to elastin and other hyaline components, causing macrophage entry and atherosclerosis.

Lipoprotein(a)

The particles that comprise lipoprotein(a) are derived from VLDL by addition and covalent binding of apo(a). This protein contains multiple domain repeats (which control its plasma concentration) and an inactive plasminogen domain. Apo(a) binds in such a way to impede clearance of Lp(a) by the LDLR. High levels of Lp(a) are genetically co-dominantly inherited. Most Caucasians have little Lp(a) unlike West African populations. Lp(a) binds avidly to arterial glycans and acts to promote atherosclerosis. Patients with high levels of Lp(a) show increased rates of CVD even if they have only moderate levels of LDL-C.

High-density lipoprotein particles

Nascent high-density lipoprotein (HDL) particles are produced in both the liver and the intestine. They are initially disc-shaped and contain their signature protein apoprotein A1 (4 molecules), other apoprotein components and some phospholipid. The apoA1 molecules are arranged in an overlapping belt and can be replaced by the inflammation-associated protein serum amyloid A. HDL particles take up cholesterol from cells through the ATP-binding cassette transporter-A1 (ABC-A1). A concentration gradient for export is maintained by esterifying this cholesterol through the action of lecithin-cholesterol acyltransferase (LCAT). The particles acquire further cholesterol through ABC-G1 and also phospholipids, apo C1-3 and apo-E by transfer from chylomicrons and VLDL particles. The HDL particle transports excess cholesterol from the periphery and may transfer it to other particles, such as VLDL through the action of cholesterol ester transfer protein (CETP), or deliver cholesterol directly to the liver (reverse cholesterol transport) or to steroid-synthetic tissues (ovaries, testes, adrenal cortex). HDL particles are taken up by the liver scavenger-receptor B1 (SRB1). In contrast to apo B-100 particles, the apo A1 core is recycled and re-secreted. Highly depleted or modified HDL particles are eventually cleared by the kidney through megalin and cubilin receptors. Cholesterol in the liver can be oxidized to bile acids, which are secreted into the bile to promote cholesterol and triglyceride uptake in the gut. Excess bile salts are resorbed in the terminal ileum and recirculate in the enterohepatic circulation (see p. 1266). HDL particles also have multiple other actions including reducing inflammation, being anti-parasitic, modulating clotting factor activity, affecting bone marrow function and promoting endothelial health.

Measurement of serum lipids

In a fasting serum lipid profile, the majority of the total cholesterol concentration is present in LDL particles with about 20–30% in HDL particles. The triglyceride concentration largely reflects VLDL particles, as chylomicrons have normally been completely cleared by 8–12 hours of fasting. In non-fasting samples, the total triglyceride concentration will be raised, due to presence of triglyceride-rich chylomicrons. The laboratory will usually supply the non-HDL-cholesterol (difference of total and HDL-cholesterol) concentration as this is the strongest index of CVD risk. In patients with triglycerides below 4.5 mmol/L, and ideally fasting, the laboratory can calculate the LDL cholesterol (LDL-C) using the Friedewald formula: $LDL\text{-}C = TC - HDL\text{-}C - (TG/2.2)$. Some laboratories measure concentrations of LDL-C directly, and also of lipoprotein(a), apo B-100 and apo A1.

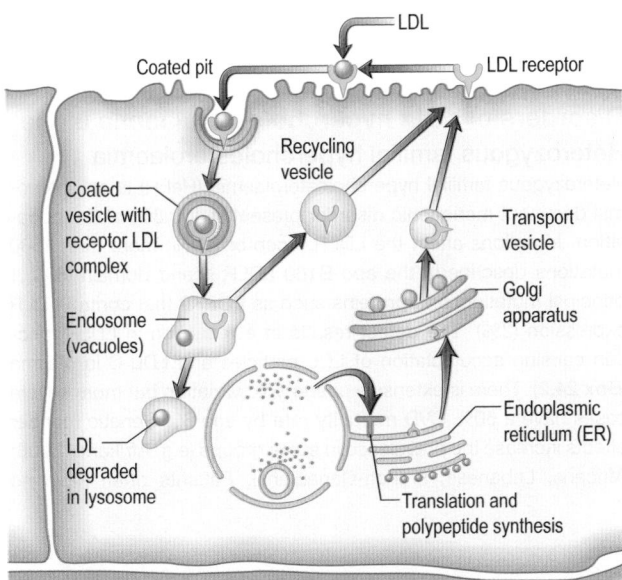

Fig. 24.3 Receptor-mediated endocytosis. Low-density lipoprotein (LDL) receptors are formed in the endoplasmic reticulum and transported via the Golgi apparatus to the surface of a hepatocyte. LDLs bind to these receptors, and are internalized and taken up by the endosome. The receptor is recycled back to the surface, while the LDL is broken down by the lysosomes, freeing the cholesterol needed for membrane synthesis.

Plasma lipids and cardiovascular risk

Population studies have repeatedly demonstrated a strong association between total, non-HDL cholesterol (the difference between total and HDL cholesterol; a surrogate for apo B-100-containing particles) and also LDL-cholesterol concentration, and CVD risk; the strongest association is with coronary heart disease. CVD risk rises progressively with total cholesterol, and with total cholesterol:HDL-C ratio (**Fig. 24.4**). Higher HDL concentrations (up to 1.8 mmol/L) protect against CVD. Triglycerides often move in opposition to HDL-C levels. There is a weak additional risk associated with triglyceride-rich VLDL or IDL particles and CVD risk. Chylomicrons do not confer an excess CVD risk but do raise the total plasma triglyceride concentrations. Raised triglyceride levels (>10 mmol/L), and especially those associated with continuing plasma persistence of chylomicrons, are associated with an increased risk of pancreatitis.

Hyperlipidaemia

Hyperlipidaemia results from genetic predispositions interacting with the environment, including nutritional factors.

Secondary hyperlipidaemia

Glucose and liver metabolism influence lipid levels. A clinical history, examination and simple investigations need to be performed to detect the causes of secondary hyperlipidaemia (**Box 24.1**), which

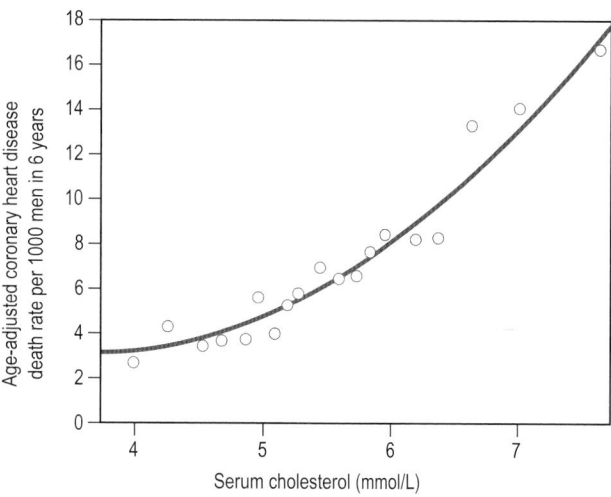

Fig. 24.4 The Multiple Risk Factor Intervention Trial. Relationship between levels of serum cholesterol and risks of fatal coronary artery disease in a longitudinal study of more than 361 000 men screened for entry into the trial. (*Data from Stamler J, Wentworth D, Neaton JD. Is relationship between serum cholesterol and risk of death from coronary heart disease continuous and graded? Findings in 356 222 primary screenees of the Multiple Risk Factor Intervention Trial (MRFIT). JAMA 1986; 256:2823.*)

may need specific treatment in their own right. Hypothyroidism, untreated diabetes, renal disease (especially nephrotic syndrome) and abnormal liver function can all raise plasma lipid levels.

Primary hyperlipidaemia

Lipid disorders can be grouped as follows:

- disorders of VLDL and chylomicrons – hypertriglyceridaemia
- disorders of LDL – hypercholesterolaemia alone
- disorders of HDL (rare)
- combined hyperlipidaemia.

Disorders of VLDL and chylomicrons: moderate and severe hypertriglyceridaemia

Most cases are caused by multiple gene variants acting together to produce a modest excess of circulating concentration of VLDL particles, such cases being termed polygenic hypertriglyceridaemia.

Lipoprotein lipase pathway deficiencies

These are rare orphan diseases that produce greatly elevated triglyceride concentrations (>20 mmol/L) owing to the persistence of chylomicrons (not VLDL particles), because their triglyceride cannot be metabolized. This may occur if the enzyme lipoprotein lipase (LPL) is defective (95% of cases), or sometimes because the normal enzyme cannot function, due to deficiencies of its apoprotein C2 co-factor (1%), a control protein affecting LPL secretion (apo-A5) (1%), a protein involved in particle maturation (lipid-maturation factor-1; LMF-1) or the cell surface receptor for LPL (glycerophosphoinositol-HDL-like binding-protein-1(GPI-HBP1). Patients with homozygous or dual deficiency present in childhood with eruptive xanthomas, lipaemia retinalis (yellow lipid particles visible in retinal arteries), pancreatitis and hepatosplenomegaly. Heterozygotes can present as adults with gross hypertriglyceridaemia. Some cases are caused by severe polygenic hypertriglyceridaemia. The presence of chylomicrons floating like cream on top of fasting lipaemic plasma suggests this diagnosis. The aetiology can be implied by measurement of the triglyceride:apoB-100 ratio or ultracentrifugation but the diagnosis is confirmed by DNA sequencing.

Disorders of LDL: hypercholesterolaemia alone
Heterozygous familial hypercholesterolaemia

Heterozygous familial hypercholesterolaemia (HeFH) is an autosomal dominant monogenic disorder present in 1 in 350 of the population. Mutations affect the LDLR receptor (90%; more than 1500 mutations described), the apo-B100 LDLR ligand domain (5%; 1 principal mutation) and proteins such as PCSK9 that control LDLR expression (2%). The defect results in a reduction in LDLR function causing accumulation of LDL particles and LDL-C in plasma (**Box 24.2**). There is extensive phenotypic variation but more severe cases have a 50% CVD mortality rate by age 65. Genetic founder effects increase the prevalence in some groups (e.g. Afrikaner South Africans, Lebanese, French-Canadians). Patients often have no

---

? Box 24.1 Causes of secondary hyperlipidaemia

- Hypothyroidism
- Diabetes mellitus (when poorly controlled)
- Obesity
- Chronic kidney disease
- Nephrotic syndrome
- Dysglobulinaemia
- Hepatic dysfunction and cholestasis

- Alcohol
- Anorexia nervosa
- Drugs:
  - Oral contraceptives in susceptible individuals
  - Retinoids, thiazide diuretics, corticosteroids, beta-blockers, sirolimus (and other immunosuppressive agents), anti-retroviral drugs

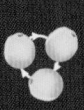

physical signs, in which case, the diagnosis is made on the presence of very high plasma cholesterol concentrations that are unresponsive to dietary modification and are usually associated with a family history of early CVD before age 60. Diagnosis is easier if pathognomonic clinical features are present but these only occur in 10%. These signs include cholesterol deposition in extensor tendons such as the Achilles or those of the fingers. Lipid deposition in the skin around the eyes (xanthelasma) may be present but is not diagnostic of FH and is more typical of high triglyceride-low HDL disorders. The diagnosis of FH is confirmed by DNA sequencing. Given its autosomal dominant inheritance, mutation screening is simple to apply and children of affected individuals have a 50% chance of inheriting the defect.

Homozygous familial hypercholesterolaemia

Homozygous familial hypercholesterolaemia (HoFH) is an ultra-orphan disorder (affecting 1 in 250 000). Affected children have minimal LDLR function in the liver. They have a hugely elevated LDL-C (greater than 13 mmol/L), and massive deposition of lipid in arterial walls, the proximal aorta and in skin on extensor surfaces (tuberose xanthomata). Most die from ischaemic heart disease by age 35 if untreated. They have a limited response to drugs such as statins but PCSK9 inhibitors have been used with some success especially in patients with point mutations. Repeated fortnightly lipid-specific plasma extraction (apheresis) can be used to remove LDL-C in patients with null mutations. LDLR function can be restored by partial lobe liver transplantation which normalizes LDL-C levels and causes regression of xanthomata. Some orphan drug therapies are licensed for use in HoFH (**Box 24.3**).

> ℹ **Box 24.2 Genetic defects underlying some lipoprotein disorders**

Disorder	Affected gene	Chromosome	Frequency
Common disorders			
Heterozygous familial hyper-cholesterolaemia	*LDLR, PCSK9* (activating)	19, 1	1:350
Familial defective apolipoprotein B	*Apo-B100* (exon 26 mostly)	2	1:5000
Hypobetalipo-proteinaemia	*Apo-B100* (various exons), MTP	2, 4	1:10 000
Familial combined hyperlipidaemia	Complex	Multiple	1:250
Familial hyper-triglyceridaemia	Mostly polygenic	Multiple	1:1000
Some rarer disorders			
'Homozygous' familial hyper-cholesterolaemia	*LDLR>PCSK9, Apo-B* (exon 26)	19	1:350 000
Lipoprotein lipase pathway deficiencies	*LPL, >apoC2, apoA5, LMF-1, GPIHBP-1*	8, 19,11, 16, 8	1:1 000 000 (homozygous)
Tangier disease	*ABC-A1*	9	Very rare
Lecithin-cholesterol acyltransferase deficiency	*LCAT*	16	Very rare
Apolipoprotein A1 deficiency	*Apo-A1*	1	Very rare

Mutations in the *apoB* and *PCSK9* genes

Mutations in the terminal part of *apoB* affect binding to the LDLR and cause another relatively common single-gene disorder resembling FH. The clinical picture resembles classical HeFH but is milder, with lower LDL-C levels as some LDLR functions are preserved. Activating mutations in *PCSK9* cause downregulation of LDLR. In contrast, inactivating mutations in PCSK9 are associated with enhanced LDLR function and lower cholesterol levels. The two disorders can be distinguished clearly only by genetic tests. The approach to treatment is the same.

Polygenic hypercholesterolaemia

This is a term used to lump together the large group of patients without evidence of monogenic cholesterol disorders above, but with cholesterol in the upper part of the normal distribution. Panels for diagnosis of polygenic variants have been devised and include genes known to significantly affect cholesterol levels and CVD disease risk such as LDLR, apo5, apo(a), apo-E and PCSK9.

Disorders of HDL

Genetic disorders of HDL metabolism are rare and recessively inherited. They include those causing low HDL-C levels including mutations in apo-A1, ABC-A1 and LCAT. Apo-A1 mutations cause low HDL-C, which are associated with amyloid deposition, and either atherosclerosis or protection from atherosclerosis depending on the exact site affected. Very high HDL-C levels are caused by mutations in cholesterol ester transfer protein (CETP) or endothelial lipase, which affect metabolism of HDL particles.

Tangier disease

Macrophages are involved in uptake of excess cholesterol in arterial walls, and donate this to HDL particles. If a defect occurs in cholesterol transport, e.g. the ABC-A1 transporter, then they accumulate cholesterol (see **Box 24.2**). In Tangier disease, cholesterol accumulates in reticuloendothelial tissue and arteries, causing enlarged, orange-coloured tonsils and hepatosplenomegaly, corneal opacities and polyneuropathy, as well as CVD.

Combined hyperlipidaemia (hypercholesterolaemia and hypertriglyceridaemia)

The most common patient group with abnormalities of serum lipid concentrations have a polygenic combined hyperlipidaemia. Patients have an increased CVD risk due to high non-HDL-C concentrations, abundant pro-atherogenic triglyceride-rich particles, high LDL-C and suppression of HDL concentrations by the hypertriglyceridaemia (low LPL, excess CETP activity).

Familial combined hyperlipidaemia (FCHL)

This is relatively common, affecting 1 in 200 of the general population. Its lipid phenotype includes hypertriglyceridaemia, hypercholesterolaemia or both, associated with premature CVD. The genetic basis for the disorder is not clear though current studies suggest the primary defect lies in excess adipose tissue fatty acid release. It is diagnosed by finding raised cholesterol and triglyceride concentrations in association with a typical family history. There are no typical physical signs.

Remnant hyperlipidaemia

This is a rare (1 in 5000) cause of combined hyperlipidaemia. It is due to accumulation of IDL remnant particles and is associated with an extremely high risk of CVD. It may be suspected in a patient with

Box 24.3 Drugs used in the treatment of hyperlipidaemia

Drug/ examples[a]	Mechanism of action	Contraindications	Adverse effects	Expected therapeutic effect	Safety
Statins					
Pravastatin Atorvastatin Rosuvastatin (Simvastatin) (Fluvastatin)	Inhibit the rate-limiting step in cholesterol synthesis (HMG-CoA reductase)	Active liver disease, pregnancy, breast feeding	Constant aches/muscle stiffness, myopathy, rhabdomyolysis; derangement of liver biochemistry Gastrointestinal upset Some statins have CYP3A4 interactions (e.g. simvastatin)	Reduce LDL cholesterol (LDL-C) by 30–60% Have modest lowering effect on triglycerides Little effect on HDL cholesterol (HDL-C) Atorvastatin and rosuvastatin are the most potent	Atorvastatin and rosuvastatin have good long-term safety and extensive outcomes evidence Avoid if possible in women of childbearing age
Cholesterol absorption inhibitors					
Ezetimibe	Inhibits gut absorption of cholesterol from food and bile; inhibits activity of NPC1L1, a lipid transporter found in the duodenum	Breast feeding	Occasional abdominal discomfort, skin rash	Reduce LDL-C by 20% Reduce triglyceride concentrations by <10% Minimal effect on HDL-C	Mostly act in gut, and recirculate in enterohepatic circulation Some safety and some outcome evidence
Bile acid sequestrants					
Colesevelam (Colestyramine) (Colestipol)	Bind bile acids in the gut, preventing enterohepatic circulation; the liver makes more bile acids from cholesterol, depleting the cholesterol pool	Biliary obstruction	Gastrointestinal side-effects are very common e.g. constipation, diarrhoea, bloating, flatulence; may reduce fat-soluble vitamin and drug absorption Other drugs bind to resins and should be taken 1 hour before or 4 hour afterwards	Reduce LDL-C by 15–25% Increase triglyceride concentration by 5–15% Have little or no effect on HDL-C	Not systemically absorbed Safety profile is good Appear safe in women of childbearing age Fat-soluble vitamin supplements may be required in children, and pregnant and breast-feeding women
Fibric acid derivatives					
Bezafibrate Fenofibrate (Ciprofibrate) (Gemfibrozil)	Activate peroxisome proliferator-activated nuclear receptors (esp. PPAR-α), producing protean effects on lipid metabolism	Severe hepatic or renal impairment, gall bladder disease, pregnancy	Reversible myositis, nausea, predisposition to gallstones, non-specific malaise, impotence Reversibly increase creatinine by 15% Drug interactions (e.g. statins) an issue with gemfibrozil	Reduce LDL-C by 0–15% Reduce triglycerides by 25–70% depending on baseline Increase HDL-C by 10–30% depending on baseline	No knowledge of effect on developing fetus, however avoid in women of childbearing age Long-term safety good and moderate beneficial CVD outcomes effects
Nicotinic acid/niacin (NA) derivatives					
Modified-release niacin (Acipimox)	Unclear: probably inhibit lipid synthesis in the liver by effect on DGAT-2	Pregnancy, breast-feeding	Value limited by frequent side-effects: painful prostaglandin D2- and E2-induced flushing, nausea, malaise, itching, abnormal liver biochemistry Glucose intolerance, hyperuricaemia, dyspepsia; hyperpigmentation may occur	Reduce LDL-C by 15–20% Reduce triglycerides by 20–40% Increase HDL-C by 10–20%	Medium-term safety good but marred by adverse effects Some monotherapy outcomes evidence Modified-release preparations better but still need high-dose aspirin to reduce flushing
Fatty acid compounds					
Omega-3 fatty acids Omega-3 fatty acid ethyl esters	Reduce hepatic VLDL secretion and inflammation via FFAR-4	Avoid with anticoagulants since bleeding time is prolonged	Occasional nausea and belching	Reduce triglycerides in severe hypertriglyceridaemia No effect on other lipids	Long-term safety is good. High-dose CVD outcomes evidence
MTP inhibitors					
Lomitapide	Inhibits MTP, which is necessary for VLDL assembly and secretion in the liver	Unclear	Abnormal liver biochemistry	Lowers LDL-C by 50% Orphan drug licensed only for homozygous familial hypercholesterolaemia	Long-term safety data very limited

Box 24.3 Drugs used in the treatment of hyperlipidaemia—cont'd

Drug/ examples[a]	Mechanism of action	Contraindications	Adverse effects	Expected therapeutic effect	Safety
Proprotein convertase subtilisin kexin (PCSK)-9 inhibitors					
Alirocumab Evolocumab	Inhibit the action of PCSK-9 to upregulate liver LDL receptor expression	Needle phobia (injectable agents)	Myalgia (flu-like illness), injection site reactions	Reduce LDL-C by 45–60% Have modest lowering effect on triglycerides Little effect on HDL-C	Good safety and CVD outcomes evidence

[a]Drugs now rarely used in brackets.

HMG-CoA, hydroxymethylglutaryl coenzyme A; CVD, cardiovascular disease; LDL, low-density lipoprotein; MTP, microsomal triglyceride transfer protein; VLDL, very-low-density lipoprotein.

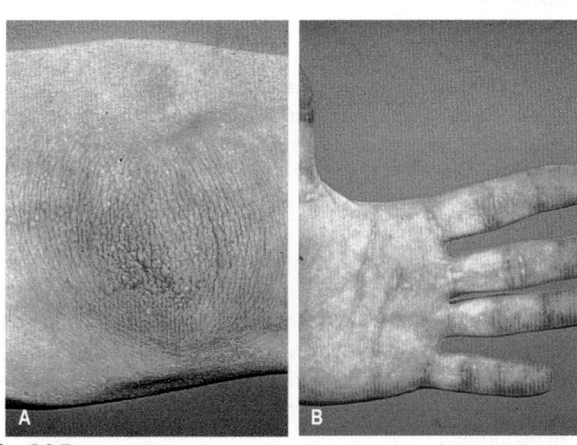

Fig. 24.5 Remnant hyperlipidaemia. **(A)** Tuberous xanthomas behind the elbow. **(B)** Lipid deposits in the hand creases.

almost equal cholesterol and triglyceride concentrations and by finding lipid deposition in the dermis visible at palmar creases (planar xanthomata, which is diagnostic) and in the skin over the knees and elbows (tuberose xanthomata) (**Fig. 24.5**). Remnant hyperlipidaemia is commonly associated with inheritance of apo-E variant alleles (e.g. homozygosity for apoprotein E2 that has reduced LDLR binding), together with aggravating factor such as another primary hyperlipidaemia. The diagnosis can be confirmed using the triglyceride:apoB-100 ratio, by genotyping apo-E or by ultracentrifugation.

Management of hyperlipidaemia

Lipid-lowering diet

The main elements of a lipid-lowering diet are similar to those for people with diabetes or hypertension (see **Box 23.10**). Additional specific measures are to:

- reduce alcohol consumption, since this may worsen primary lipid disorders at doses that would not affect normal individuals
- include foods capable of binding cholesterol such as bran or soya protein.

Aboriginal or undeveloped societies typically have a total cholesterol 3.5–4.0 mmol/L with LDL-C 1.5–2.0 mmol/L. A vegan diet can reduce cholesterol and LDL-C by 2 mmol/L and a vegetarian diet by 1 mmol/L compared to the usual western diet. Several 'nutraceutical' or alternative health products are available that can reduce LDL-cholesterol levels. Plant stanols are analogues of cholesterol that bind to gut cholesterol transporters and reduce the absorption of cholesterol. Products containing sitostanol or sitosterol reduce cholesterol by approximately 0.35–0.5 mmol/L, but with wide inter-individual variation. Red yeast rice is a Chinese medicine that contains a homologue of a statin (monacolin A) capable of reducing LDL-C by 10–20%.

Box 24.4 Drug therapy for hyperlipidaemia

Hypertriglyc-eridaemia (predominantly)	Combined hyperlipidaemia	Hypercholesterolaemia (predominantly)
First-line agents		
Fibrate	Fibrate	Statin: atorvastatin 20 mg initially; atorvastatin 80 mg for greater cholesterol lowering or patients with CVD
Additional/alternative agents		
Fish oil capsules (Niacin derivatives)	Statin may be required in addition to lower cholesterol adequately (monitor carefully for muscle aches, creatine kinase rise or worsening liver function). Avoid gemfibrozil in combination therapy Ezetimibe (to lower cholesterol further) (Niacin derivative to lower cholesterol and triglycerides further)	Ezetimibe if statin not tolerated or greater LDL-C lowering needed PCSK-9 inhibitor (Cholesterol-binding resin) (Nicotinic acid derivative)

LDL-C, low-density lipoprotein cholesterol.

Exercise, weight loss and smoking

Regular exercise, weight loss and stopping smoking all reduce CVD risk, irrespective of lipid levels.

Drugs

See **Box 24.3** for the classes of drugs used to treat hyperlipidaemia and **Box 24.4 for** principles of use.

Statins

Statins block HMG-CoA reductase, the rate-limiting step in cholesterol synthesis, leading to compensating effects that increase the expression of LDL receptors and hence a reduction in plasma cholesterol concentrations of 20–50%. Statins reduce CVD events by 21% per 1 mmol/L LDL-C reduction. Their adverse effects are uncommon, reversible and occur in 1–2% of individuals, generally within weeks of starting the drug. Generalized muscular aches (myalgia) are the most common, occasionally representing myositis if creatine kinase (CK) is raised and extending rarely to rhabdomyolysis in severe cases (CK >5000 IU/L). A pharmacogenetic effect exists for some statins due to

> ℹ **Box 24.5 Classes of drugs in clinical trials for the potential treatment of hyperlipidaemia**
>
> | Drug class | Mechanism of action |
> |---|---|
> | **Adenosine triphosphate (ATP) citrate lyase inhibitors** e.g. bempedoic acid | Inhibit activity of ATP-citrate lyase, a liver enzyme preceding HMG-CoA reductase in cholesterol synthesis pathway. Now in phase 2b/3 trials |
> | **Proprotein convertase subtilisin/kexin type 9 (PCSK9) inhibitors** e.g. inclisiran | Small interfering RNA drug that blocks PCSK9 and lowers LDL-C by 50%. 3–6-monthly dosing. Phase 3 clinical trial on CVD outcomes (ORION-4) in progress |
> | **Anti-lipoprotein(a) antisense therapy** e.g. Apo(a)Lrx | Inhibits formation of lipoprotein(a) in the liver. Reduces Lp(a) by 80%. Phase 3 clinical trials in progress |
>
> HDL, high-density lipoprotein; LDL, low-density lipoprotein; Lp(a), lipoprotein(a); RNA, ribonucleic acid.

variants in the *SLCO1B1* transporter, which increase gut uptake of the statin resulting in higher levels in plasma and increased toxicity.

Gut-acting cholesterol-lowering drugs

Ezetimibe is a gut-acting drug binding to the Niemann–Pick C1-Like protein 1 (NPC1L1) duodenal cholesterol transporter. This molecule is also the binding site for sitosterol. It reduces plasma cholesterol by 20% and has been shown to reduce CVD events when added to statin therapy.

Bile acid sequestrants (e.g. colesevelam) are drugs that bind bile acids preventing micelle formation and thus reducing gut cholesterol uptake. They reduce cholesterol by 15–20% and have some CVD outcome evidence from previous trials with monotherapy, but lack data on CVD outcomes in the era of statins. They are commonly associated with excess gastrointestinal side-effects and are now rarely used outside the context of liver disorders associated with raised cholesterol.

PCSK9 inhibitors

PCSK9 is involved in downregulating LDLR expression. Antibodies to PCSK9 (e.g. alirocumab) reduce LDL-C by 40–60% and have been shown to reduce CVD events. These drugs are used as third-line agents in familial hypercholesterolaemia, severe progressing CVD or in patients intolerant to multiple statins.

Fibrates

Fibrates are gene regulators affecting peroxisomal-proliferator activating receptors-alpha subtype (PPAR-α). They reduce triglycerides by increasing synthesis of LPL, reducing synthesis of apoC3 to promote clearance of triglyceride-rich particles (e.g. VLDL), and can increase apo-A1. They have a moderate effect in reducing CVD events.

Omega-3 fatty acids

These preparations (often termed fish oils) include the essential fatty acids docosahexaenoic acid (DHA) and eicosapentaenoic acid (EPA). They bind to specific free fatty acid receptors (FFAR-4) to affect lipid and inflammation pathways. They exert dose-proportional effects in reducing triglycerides by 20–50%. Their effects in prevention of CVD are controversial with conflicting results. Low doses in low-risk patients seem to do little but high doses of EPA in high-risk patients seem to reduce CVD events.

New classes of lipid-lowering drugs in development are listed in **Box 28.5**.

Screening

Cardiovascular disease (CVD) secondary to atherosclerosis is common. Most patients with hyperlipidaemia are asymptomatic and have no clinical signs. Screening practices for CVD vary between countries ranging from opportunistic measurements to systematic programmes targeting individuals aged greater than 40 years. Opportunistic measurement of lipids is justified for:

- a family history of coronary heart disease (especially below 60 years of age)
- a family history of lipid disorders
- the presence of physical signs, e.g. xanthoma or xanthelasma at any age; or corneal arcus before the age of 40 years
- diabetes mellitus
- hypertension
- obesity
- acute pancreatitis
- patients undergoing renal replacement therapy.

Where one family member is known to have a monogenic disorder, such as FH, siblings and children must have their plasma lipid concentrations measured.

Acute severe illnesses, such as myocardial infarction, reduce plasma lipid concentrations for up to 3 months. Lipid profiles should be measured either within 48 hours of an acute myocardial infarction (before derangement has had time to occur) or 3 months later. Cholesterol and HDL-C concentrations do not change significantly after a meal so screening is performed using random blood samples for cholesterol, triglycerides and HDL-C. Patients with moderate hypertriglyceridemia should have a repeat fasting profile performed.

Management of hypertriglyceridaemia

A serum triglyceride concentration below 2.0 mmol/L is normal. In the range 2.0–6.0 mmol/L, no specific intervention will be needed unless there are coincident CVD risk factors, and in particular a strong family history of early CVD or an increased calculated CVD risk. Patients should be told they have a minor lipid problem; and offered advice on lifestyle improvement including weight reduction if obese. The commonest causes are associated with a fatty liver (moderately raised transaminases, raised gamma-glutamyl transferase (GGT) and high triglyceride : HDL-C ratio). Some individuals have livers that respond to even moderate degrees of alcohol intake by increased production of VLDL, so a trial of abstinence is advised. Other drugs, including high-dose thiazides, oestrogens and glucocorticoids, can have a similar effects in susceptible patients.

If the triglyceride concentration remains above 6.0 mmol/L despite lifestyle measures, drug therapy is warranted (see **Boxs 28.3** and **28.4**). The severe hypertriglyceridaemia associated with disorders of the LPL pathway may require restriction of dietary fat to 10–20% of total energy intake, the use of orphan disease drugs, and the use of special preparations of medium-chain triglycerides in cooking in place of oil or fat as these are not absorbed via chylomicrons (see p. 744).

Management of hypercholesterolaemia (without hypertriglyceridaemia)

Familial hypercholesterolaemia

Individuals often require treatment with dietary measures and more than one cholesterol-lowering drug from teenage years. Ezetimibe is often added to a statin therapy **Boxs 28.3** and **28.4**) and PCSK9 inhibitors are used in severe refractory cases.

Primary prevention for people with type 2 diabetes

Lipid-lowering therapy with a moderate dose statin, or alternatives as above, is used routinely in asymptomatic individuals with type 2 diabetes alone aged over 40 years, unless the LDL-C is particularly low (<1.8 mmol/L). Calculated CVD risk usually exceeds 10% per decade in these individuals.

Primary prevention for people without diabetes

Lipid-lowering with a moderate dose statin in the first instance is offered to people after an unsuccessful trial of lifestyle intervention whose calculated CVD risk exceeds 10% over the next decade.

Secondary prevention

Statin treatment with high-dose high potency agents is warranted for any patient with known macrovascular disease (coronary artery disease, transient ischaemic attack or stroke, peripheral arterial disease), irrespective of the total or LDL-C level. The treatment target is total cholesterol below 4.0 mmol/L and LDL-C below 2 mmol/L; or alternatively, the maximum tolerated statin dose can be used. If a statin is not tolerated, combinations of other agents are tried (see **Box 28.4**).

Risk prediction tables

CVD risk is typically multifactorial. An isolated high level of a risk factor may not justify treatment unless levels are extreme (e.g. 95th centile). Epidemiological studies consistently identify age, gender, smoking, presence of type 2 diabetes, hypertension and the ratio of total cholesterol:HDL cholesterol as primary risk factors. Ancillary risk factors such as family history of premature CVD may add to predictive efficiency in some cases. CVD risk calculators rely on population studies to predict risk in individuals (see p. 1080). This is always an approximate process. The commonest tools calculate either CVD mortality (Europe) or events (USA ASCVD, UK NICE), based on 10-year, 30-year or lifetime horizons. They are unreliable in populations aged less than 40 years or greater than 75 years as CVD risk is driven principally by age. Generally, a 20% risk is considered mandatory for drug treatment while discussion should be had with patients above 10% risk on lifestyle intervention and then risks and benefits of drug treatment if no significant improvement is observed. In young individuals, treatment decisions are often based on excess relative risk driven by family history while in older patients, co-morbidities and life expectancy are significant factors to consider. In some countries imaging techniques such as coronary artery calcium scores are used to refine CVD risk predictions in borderline cases.

Management of combined hyperlipidaemia

Hypertriglyceridaemia increases CVD risk for any cholesterol concentration. Therapy is with diet in the first instance and then with drugs if required. Statins are first-line in patients with triglycerides less than 8 mmol/L while fibrates are used first-line for higher levels. Combination therapy is often required (see **Box 28.4**).

Other lipid disorders

Hypolipidaemia

Low lipid levels can be found in severe protein–energy malnutrition. They are also seen occasionally with severe malabsorption and in intestinal lymphangiectasia.

Hypobetalipoproteinaemia (see **Box 28.2**) is a benign familial condition with cholesterol levels in the range 1–3.5 mmol/L. Rare causes includes mutations in apo-B, PCSK9 and apo3.

Abetalipoproteinaemia

This is described on page 1196.

Further reading

Cholesterol Treatment Trialists' (CTT) Collaboration. Efficacy and safety of LDL-lowering therapy among men and women: meta-analysis of individual data from 174 000 participants in 27 randomised trials. *Lancet* 2015; 385:1397–1405.
Defesche JC, Gidding SS, Harada-Shiba M et al. Familial hypercholesterolaemia. *Nat Rev Dis Primers* 2017; 3:17093.
Emerging Risk Factors Collaboration. Major lipids, apolipoproteins, and risk of vascular disease. JAMA 2009; 302:1993–2000.
Grundy SM, Stone NJ, Bailey AL et al. 2018 AHA/ACC/AACVPR/AAPA/ABC/ACPM/ADA/AGS/APhA/ASPC/NLA/PCNA Guideline on the management of blood cholesterol: Executive summary: a report of the American College of Cardiology/American Heart Association Task Force on Clinical Practice Guidelines. *Circulation* 2018:139:e1046-e1081.
Mach F, Baigent C, Catapano AL et al. 2019. ESC/EAS Guidelines for the management of dyslipidaemias: lipid modification to reduce cardiovascular risk. Eur Heart J. 2020; 41:111–188.
Rabar S, Harker M, O'Flynn N, Wierzbicki AS. Lipid modification and cardiovascular risk assessment for the primary and secondary prevention of cardiovascular disease: summary of updated NICE guidance. *BMJ* 2014; 349:g4356.
Van Horn L, Carson JA, Appel LJ et al. Recommended dietary pattern to achieve adherence to the American Heart Association/American College of Cardiology (AHA/ACC) guidelines: a scientific statement from the American Heart Association. *Circulation* 2016; 134:e505–e529.

INHERITED METABOLIC DISEASES

IMDs, previously known as inborn errors of metabolism, are a heterogeneous group of complex monogenic disorders that occur due to an impairment in the activity of an enzyme involved in one or more metabolic pathways. Hundreds of disorders exist, with the number of known disorders increasing yearly. Although individually rare, collectively they are not that uncommon, with reported prevalence ranging from 1 in 800 to 1/2500 live births. IMDs are commoner in populations where consanguinity occurs. Specific founder mutations are found in societies derived from small original ancestral populations, where inter-marriage and genetic drift further increase the prevalence of specific IMDs, especially in geographically or culturally isolated populations.

Clinical signs and symptoms occur due to accumulation of substrate precursors or due to deficiencies of enzyme products. The majority of IMDs present in childhood but there is increasing recognition of adult presentations that may differ from those seen in paediatric cases. Patients may present to the emergency department with acute metabolic decompensation, or to any specialist outpatient clinic with problems related either to a previously diagnosed IMD or an as-yet undiagnosed IMD.

Patients in IMD services include those who:

- transition into adult services, having been diagnosed in childhood (newborn screening, early diagnosis and specific therapies have improved prognosis and life spans, albeit with sequelae needing ongoing medical attention; their risk of more common age-related conditions is at least as high as in the general population)
- present for the first time in adulthood (up to 40% of patients managed in dedicated Adult IMD centres as per survey in 2006).

This section will discuss acute presentations where an IMD should form part of the differential diagnosis. A few common, mostly treatable, IMDs will also be discussed separately in more detail. Wherever possible the estimated incidence is given (as lifespans improve, the prevalence of these conditions will be significantly higher than the incidence).

Special considerations

Patients with IMDs may have specific risks related to pregnancy, surgery or anaesthesia. Hence any pregnancy or surgery should be discussed with a specialist metabolic physician well in advance, to enable a personalized birth/surgical treatment plan to be drawn up.

Genetic testing, including multigene panels, whole exome and whole genome sequencing are becoming almost first-line diagnostic tools, and are likely to widen the spectrum of IMDs both in terms of phenotypic presentations and new diseases.

Acute presentations of IMDs

Patients with known IMDs or undiagnosed IMDs can present acutely to the emergency department as a result of metabolic decompensation precipitated by some metabolic triggers, including:

- catabolic states such as inter-current illness or an inability to tolerate oral food and drinks
- labour and the postpartum period
- non-compliance with IMD treatment
- drugs (therapeutic or recreational), including alcohol
- change in diet.

Management of acute presentations of inborn errors

Known IMD

Patients at risk of decompensation will often carry with them an emergency management plan provided by their specialist metabolic centre. They would, if appropriate for their condition, have been prescribed a basic oral emergency regime (ER) to use when unwell. The advice on the oral ER is usually to take 200 mL of 25% glucose polymer drink every 2 hours, with instructions to attend hospital for i.v. treatment and further management if unable to tolerate oral ER, if getting worse despite oral ER or if they fail to improve. Intravenous ER is usually an infusion of 10% glucose i.v. at 2 mL/kg per hour.

Emergency departments should ensure these patients are triaged at least as 'very urgent' and treatment and investigations instituted without delay as per plan. While prompt treatment is often associated with good prognosis, a delay can lead to permanent neurological damage or death. Patients should also be investigated and treated for metabolic triggers of acute decompensation. ERs for common metabolic conditions are available online, for example, on the British Inherited Metabolic Disease Group (BIMDG) website (see Further reading and Significant websites). Every effort should be made to contact the patient's metabolic centre for advice as soon as possible, ideally within the first hour (many metabolic centres, including in the UK, offer 24/7 on-call advice).

Suspected IMD

A diagnosis of IMD should be considered in patients presenting with encephalopathy, psychiatric presentations, acid–base disturbance, rhabdomyolysis, atypical seizure or stroke if a more common alternative diagnosis is not forthcoming. A suggestive personal and/or family history, the presence of one or more metabolic triggers, a history of aversion to certain food groups such as proteins or recent history of exclusion diets (low carbohydrate/high fat and protein diets) should alert physicians to an IMD aetiology. A basic metabolic screen should be sent off. Abnormalities in biochemistry may only be apparent during an acute episode. Therefore, samples for a basic acute metabolic screen (**Box 24.6**) should be taken at presentation. Specialist advice sought and treatment initiated as soon as possible if an IMD is suspected.

Clinical presentations where an IMD should be suspected include the disorders described here.

Encephalopathy

IMDs should be considered in all adults presenting with encephalopathy.

Both patients with known IMD and those with an as-yet undiagnosed IMD can present for the first time in adulthood with encephalopathy. Metabolic encephalopathy most commonly occurs secondary to hyperammonaemia. This must therefore be excluded urgently.

Disorders of ammonia metabolism

Ammonia is a by-product of protein catabolism. It is detoxified by conversion to urea via the urea cycle in the liver, and subsequently excreted by the kidneys. A diagnosis of IMD, most often a urea cycle defect, should be sought in patients where other more common causes of hyperammonaemia such as decompensated liver disease and drugs have been excluded. Prolonged hyperammonaemia is associated with permanent neurological deficit and death. Since prompt diagnosis and treatment can reverse progression, ammonia should be included in the first-line screening investigations for any patient presenting with encephalopathic symptoms. Ammonia samples are unstable and should be collected on ice and despatched promptly to the laboratory. If hyperammonaemia is confirmed, treatment can and should be started before the precise IMD causing hyperammonaemia is known.

The main principles of treatment are to:

- prevent catabolism by giving i.v. ER (this can be done before ammonia levels are known if index of suspicion high)
- lower plasma ammonia levels as quickly as possible – most effectively done using haemofiltration/haemodialysis in symptomatic patients
- decrease protein load by temporarily stopping all external natural protein intake (this can be done before ammonia levels are known if index of suspicion high); total protein restriction should not continue beyond 48 hours
- use ammonia scavengers like sodium benzoate/phenylbutyrate as soon as available.

Published guidelines 'Urea cycle defects – acute emergency management' are available on the BIMDG website (see Significant websites). Advice from a specialist IMD centre should be sought for ongoing management and further investigations.

Rhabdomyolysis

While trauma and drugs are the commonest causes of rhabdomyolysis, IMDs such as glycogen storage disease type 5 (see **Box 24.11**) or disorders of fatty acid metabolism (see **Box 24.12**) should be considered in patients with recurrent episodes or a suggestive history. Send samples for an acute metabolic screen including creatine kinase. In addition to standard treatment for rhabdomyolysis, patients with IMD related rhabdomyolysis will benefit from i.v. ER

Stroke

Thrombotic strokes in younger adults or a cerebral sinus thrombosis should prompt measurement of plasma homocysteine levels to exclude homocysteine/folate metabolism disorders, particularly as they are treatable.

IMDs such as mitochondrial disorders and Fabry's disease should also be considered in patients with strokes where symptoms or imaging is inconsistent with a defined vascular territory.

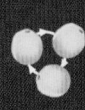

? Box 24.6 Basic and additional tests in known or suspected inherited metabolic diseases

Investigation	Timing of investigation and clinical significance
Basic metabolic screen	
FBC, renal, liver and bone profiles, CRP, ammonia, lactate, glucose, ketones (beta-hydroxybutyrate and free fatty acids), venous blood gases, CK, urate	At presentation Laboratories servicing emergency departments should return results for these tests within the hour, at any time of day or night, to enable prompt treatment
Tests of vitamin B_{12} metabolism (preferably including active vitamin B_{12} (transcobalamin and methylmalonic acid), homocysteine, and folate)	At presentation Abnormalities may be suggestive of IMDs in cobalamin and folate metabolism that are eminently treatable
2 bottles of 5 mL of lithium heparin preservative samples for plasma amino acids and acyl-carnitines	At presentation
Urine collected in a 15 mL universal container for urine organic acids (OA)	At presentation
Additional tests to consider	

If patient is undergoing a lumbar puncture and IMD is suspected send:
  one aliquot of CSF in a fluoride-oxalate tube for lactate and glucose
  one aliquot of CSF in a plain tube to the laboratory to be saved for further investigations if needed
Paired plasma fluoride-oxalate and lithium heparin samples should be sent along with the CSF samples.
CSF results can only be interpreted by comparison with serum/plasma levels
	Preferably discuss with a metabolic centre prior to taking samples. If unable to contact centre, take and send to laboratory to be saved. Ensure prior consent taken as per local guidelines

Consider sending two 5 mL EDTA preservative whole-blood samples for DNA analysis and white cell extraction	Preferably discuss with a metabolic centre prior to taking samples. If unable to contact centre or if patient perimortem, take and send to laboratory to be saved. Ensure prior consent taken as per local guidelines
Skin biopsy – DNA can be extracted from fibroblasts grown from a skin biopsy (even taken up to 24 h postmortem if sterile.) A postmortem diagnosis of individuals dying of a suspected IMD may allow screening of other family members, as well as confirming the cause of death	Preferably discuss with a metabolic centre prior to taking samples. If unable to contact centre or if patient perimortem/ immediate postmortem take and send to laboratory to be saved. Ensure prior consent taken as per local guidelines
Tissue biopsy – muscle/liver/renal and cardiac – if indicated	Preferably discuss with a metabolic centre prior to taking samples. If unable to contact centre or if patient perimortem/immediate postmortem, take and send to laboratory to be saved. Ensure prior consent taken as per local guidelines

CK, creatine kinase; CRP, c-reactive protein test; CSF, cerebrospinal fluid; EDTA, ethylene-diamine-tetra-acetic acid; FBC, full blood count.

Hypoglycaemia

While hypoglycaemia is a common neonatal/childhood presentation of glycogen storage disorders (GSDs) (see **Box 24.11**) and fatty acid oxidation disorders (FAOD) (see **Box 24.12**), presentations among adults are rare. Nevertheless, there are isolated reports of patients with IMDs such as glucokinase-activating mutations presenting for the first time in adulthood with hypoglycaemia. As it is eminently treatable, diagnosis should be considered and excluded. Insulin/C--peptide measurements and an acute metabolic screen at the time of hypoglycaemia will provide important diagnostic clues.

Acidosis

A raised unexplained anion gap may be suggestive of an IMD. Hyperlactatemia, hyperammonaemia, or ketosis without hyperglycaemia may all be diagnostic clues. Clinicians should send samples for an acute metabolic screen, including blood gases, bicarbonate, glucose and lactate at presentation if an IMD is suspected.

Mitochondrial diseases

Mitochondrial function is regulated by the interplay between nuclear genes that code for nearly 1500 mitochondrial proteins and the 37 mitochondrial genes (see p. 19). Thus, mitochondrial diseases can be caused by maternally inherited defects in the mitochondrial genome or by Mendelian inherited nuclear genome defects. *De novo* mutations are also known to occur.

Every nucleated cell in the body contains between 100 and 10 000 mitochondria that are responsible for ATP generation through oxidative phosphorylation. Hence mitochondrial dysfunction leads to clinical manifestations secondary to cellular dysfunction and premature cell death as a result of energy deficit. MDs are not that uncommon, with a reported incidence of 1 in 4300 in the UK. MDs presenting in adulthood were traditionally thought to be caused by mutations in the mitochondrial genome; however, it is now increasingly apparent that roughly 25% of mitochondrial diseases presenting for the first time in adulthood may be secondary to mutations in the nuclear genome.

Patients can present with a variable phenotype with one or more clinical features associated with mitochondrial disease, varying in severity and chronology (**Box 24.7**). Patients may sometimes present with well-defined clinical syndromes that are associated with a particular nuclear or mitochondrial mutation (**Box 24.8**). General physicians should be aware of and consider mitochondrial disease in patients with a suggestive family history, and multisystem disease where more common causes have been excluded. Investigation profiles should include glucose, lactate, acyl-carnitines and creatine kinase.

Diagnosis

While biochemistry may be indicative, confirmatory diagnosis requires specialist investigations including tissue (most often muscle) biopsy and genetic testing.

Box 24.7 Clinical features that should prompt consideration of a mitochondrial disease[a]

System	Clinical feature
Neurological	Ataxia/stroke-like episodes (predominantly occipital)/seizures/myoclonus/neuropathy/ myopathy/migraines/encephalopathic symptoms/MRI changes suggestive of mitochondrial disease
Cardiac symptoms	Cardiomyopathy/conduction defects/ Wolff–Parkinson–White syndrome
Endocrine	Diabetes, particularly in patients with a strong maternal history of diabetes, sensorineural hearing loss or a phenotype/biochemistry not typical of insulin resistance
Eyes	Non-fatigable ptosis/ophthalmoplegia/ pigmented retinopathy/cataracts/optic atrophy
Sensorineural hearing loss	Early onset, bilateral, with strong maternal family history
Gastrointestinal	Dysmotility presenting as vomiting/constipation
Other biochemistry	May have raised plasma lactate/creatine kinase

[a]Unless otherwise explained.

i **Box 24.8** Some well-described mitochondrial disease syndromes

Syndrome	Inheritance	Key feature	Additional features
Spastic paraplegia type 7 (SPG7) (6 in 100 000)	AR	Spastic paraparesis	Dysarthria/ dysphagia/ nystagmus
Progressive external ophthalmoplegia (PEO)	AD/AR Mitochondrial Sporadic	Ophthalmoplegia/ptosis	Dysphagia/ myopathy/ exercise intolerance
Optic atrophy type 1 (OPA1)	AD	Optic atrophy/ ophthalmoplegia	Sensory neural hearing loss/ ataxia/ neuropathy
Mitochondrial encephalopathy, lactic acidosis and stroke-like episodes (MELAS)	Mitochondrial	Diabetes Sensory neural hearing impairment Lactic acidosis Encephalopathy	
Leber's hereditary optic neuropathy (LHON)	Mitochondrial	Optic atrophy in early adulthood	Movement disorders, tremors, cardiac conduction defects

AD, autosomal dominant; AR, autosomal recessive.

Management

Although clinical trials are ongoing, specific therapies for mitochondrial disease are currently not available in the clinical setting. Management is largely supportive, including surveillance for and treatment of MD-associated co-morbidities such as diabetes and cardiac disease. Patients should be offered genetic counselling and a detailed pedigree history should be taken to ensure appropriate cascade testing of at-risk relatives. With the option of mitochondrial donation now becoming available, reproductive options should also be discussed.

Disorders of protein metabolism

Phenylketonuria

Phenylketonuria (PKU; incidence 1 : 20 000 globally) is an autosomal recessive amino acid metabolism disorder caused by a bi-allelic mutation in the phenylalanine hydroxylase gene. It is the most common IMD encountered in specialist metabolic centres in Europe, where the incidence is highest (1 in 5000 to 15 000 in white babies of European descent). It is characterized by elevated levels of phenylalanine in the blood, and if treatment is delayed, can result in severe intellectual disability. Early treatment within the first few days of life results in normal development. Many countries including the UK offer newborn screening for PKU, with an aim to start therapy within the first 2 weeks of life. The aim of treatment is to maintain phenylalanine levels below therapeutic targets which may vary slightly between countries. The therapeutic targets in the UK are broadly aligned to European consensus guidelines, which also advocate phenylalanine restriction for life. The mainstay of treatment is a diet restricted in natural proteins, combined with supplements (phenylalanine-free protein, vitamins and minerals) and specialist low-protein foods available on prescription. High phenylalanine levels during pregnancy can result in microcephaly, significant intellectual disability, cardiac defects and growth retardation in the baby. Women are therefore advised against unplanned pregnancy. Therapeutic targets for preconception and pregnancy are significantly lower than baseline adult targets and require close monitoring/management by specialist centres. Unplanned pregnancy in a woman with PKU is a medical emergency and should be referred to a metabolic centre to enable treatment to be started/options discussed within 24 hours. GP practices across the UK can expect to have one or more patients with PKU on their register. The oldest patients diagnosed on newborn screening in the UK are nearing 50 years of age. Clinicians can therefore expect to occasionally encounter them in their routine practice, presenting with other common age-related illness not directly linked to PKU.

Some other common protein metabolism IMDs are listed in **Box 24.9**.

Lysosomal storage disorders

Lysosomes play an important role in cell turnover. Their main function is to break down complex macromolecules to simple monomers, and to transport these monomers out of the lysosome into the cytosol for recycling. Any disruption to this process results in lysosomal storage disease (LSD). Genetically inherited LSDs are one of the commonest IMDs encountered in metabolic centres treating adult patients, with Gaucher's and Fabry's disease being the most common amongst these. A number of these conditions can present for the first time in adulthood. Prognosis is variable, dependent on residual enzyme activity. Specific therapies are now available for a number of LSDs, and hence it is important that clinicians consider LSDs in patients presenting with suggestive symptoms. A few common LSDs with specific therapies are listed in **Box 24.10**.

Disorders of carbohydrate metabolism

Glycogen storage disorders

Glycogen storage disorders (GSDs) refers to a group of IMDs where either glucose utilization (glycolysis) or glycogen mobilization (glycogenolysis or glycogen transport) is impaired. Glycogen is a glucose polymer stored most abundantly in the muscle and liver. Patients present with symptoms related to decreased availability of glucose for ATP generation and/or abnormal glycogen accumulation and impairment in other linked metabolic pathways. Effective treatments for a number of GSDs exist, and early treatment significantly improves prognosis. GSDs can be classified broadly based on the most affected organs. Some of the principal GSDs are listed in **Box 24.11**. A few other treatable IMDs of carbohydrate metabolism are listed in **Box 24.12**.

Disorders of fatty acid oxidation defects

The fatty acid oxidation pathway provides important an alternative fuel source, by using fats in situations such as fasting, exercise or illness where glucose supply may be inadequate. A detailed description of the process is beyond the scope of this book. Briefly, it involves:

- conversion of fatty acids to fatty acetyl CoA on entry through the plasma membrane
- entry of fatty acetyl CoAs into the mitochondria via the carnitine shuttle
- beta-oxidation of fatty acetyl CoAs to acetyl CoA by dehydrogenases in the mitochondria
- transfer of electrons by dehydrogenases to the respiratory chain via electron carriers.

Acetyl CoA is used either to generate ketone bodies (an alternate fuel for the brain), or for direct ATP production via Krebs cycle (e.g. in skeletal muscle). Defects in any step in the pathway results in a fatty acid oxidation disorder. Characteristic features of FAODs include hypoketotic hypoglycaemia, cardiomyopathy and myopathy with/without rhabdomyolysis. While most present in childhood, some can present for the first time in adulthood (**Box 24.13**) with myopathy and/or rhabdomyolysis. Unlike in GSD5, symptoms usually occur after prolonged exercise, a prolonged fast or during an inter-current illness, that results in a catabolic state. Once diagnosis is known, management to avoid crisis is relatively simple (see **Box 24.13**). As with all other IMDs, symptoms may be unmasked (with catastrophic consequences) by a recent change in diet, for example a ketogenic diet, in addition to all the other metabolic triggers described above. Baseline investigations to exclude these conditions and close monitoring on initiation of a therapeutic ketogenic diet for conditions such as epilepsy is mandatory.

Porphyrias

Porphyrias are a group of disorders caused by defects in the haem synthesis pathway. Detailed descriptions of the different porphyrias is beyond the scope of this book. Briefly, symptoms occur due to accumulation of toxic metabolites. A block in the early stages of synthesis leads to accumulation of porphyrin precursors including porphobilinogen (PBG) and α-aminolaevulinic acid (ALA), while a block in the late stages results mainly in accumulation of porphyrins. Porphyrin precursors are neurotoxic while porphyrins themselves induce a photosensitive blistering rash. Thus, presentations may be acute neurovisceral crisis (block in the early stages of haem synthesis – acute intermittent porphyria) or non-acute cutaneous

(block in the late stages – porphyria cutanea tarda; commonest, incidence 1:5000 to 1:70000, erythropoietic protoporphyria and congenital erythropoietic porphyria). A block in the intermediate stages cause cutaneous and neurovisceral symptoms (variegate porphyria and hereditary coproporphyria).

Acute porphyrias have an autosomal dominant inheritance and almost always present in late childhood/adulthood. Prevalence is 5:1000000 in Europe, with a much higher prevalence in South Africa (3:1000). Clinical features include abdominal pain, vomiting, neuropsychiatric symptoms, hypertension, seizures, hyponatraemia and fever. In addition to the usual triggers for metabolic decompensation in IMDs, anaesthesia and drugs (including cytochrome P450 enzyme inducers), can precipitate an acute attack. Porphyria occurs more often in women, particularly in the luteal phase of the menstrual cycle and pregnancy. Symptoms may mimic an acute abdomen, and anaesthesia during an acute attack can be catastrophic. It is treatable and hence a diagnosis of porphyria should be considered and sought early in the emergency department if symptoms are suggestive. Diagnosis is made by measuring ALA and PBG in a fresh urine sample (plain bottle, with no preservatives and always protected from light). Normal levels exclude acute porphyria and an alternative diagnosis for symptoms should be sought.

If porphyria is confirmed/likely, management should be initiated immediately.

- Remove all precipitating causes, including any triggering drugs (www.drugs-porphyria.org).
- Give supportive therapy for symptoms, and an i.v. infusion for hydration and correction of electrolyte imbalance.
- Ensure a high carbohydrate intake of at least 600 mg per day.
- Administer heme arginate (i.v.).
- Contact a porphyria reference centre for further advice. Published emergency management guidelines are available on the BIMDG website. Recurrent severe attacks may merit consideration for liver transplantation.

For details confirmatory tests of diagnosis, pathophysiology and presentations of other porphyrias see Further reading.

Peroxisomal diseases

X-Adrenoleukodystrophy

Being X-linked, presentation is more severe in males who present with the cerebral form. Symptoms usually begin between 4 and 10 years with behavioural/neuropsychiatric problems, cognitive decline and variable progressive neurological decline, which is fatal. Presentation may be delayed into adulthood, and even into the third or fourth decade. Patients also often develop adrenal insufficiency, which may precede development neurological symptoms. While no treatment exists for symptomatic patients, pre-symptomatic patients may be amenable to treatment with bone marrow transplant (BMT) or a clinical trial of gene therapy. Therefore, X-adrenoleukodystrophy (ALD) should be excluded in all patients with adrenal insufficiency where no other cause is found. Female carriers and adult males may also present with adrenomyeloneuropathy, resulting in spastic paraparesis of the lower limbs and bladder disturbances. Cerebral ALD and adrenal insufficiency almost never occur in female carriers. Adult physicians should exclude ALD in patients with suggestive symptoms, as a positive diagnosis will initiate cascade testing to find any pre-symptomatic relatives, who may be eligible for BMT, and female carriers who may benefit from prenatal counselling.

Adult Refsum's disease

Adult Refsum's (AR) is a recessive disease that results in phytanic acid accumulation in tissues and plasma secondary to mutations in the *PHYH* or *PEX7* gene. Diagnosis should be excluded in patients presenting with retinitis pigmentosa, which along with anosmia is present in almost all patients with AR. These two features often precede development of other features like ataxia, peripheral neuropathy and cataract by several years. A third of patients may have bony abnormalities such as shortened fourth metatarsals. Cardiac arrhythmias may occur, particularly when phytanic acid levels are high. Treatment includes a phytanic acid restricted diet and avoidance of fasting or rapid weight loss. Plasmapheresis may be needed. Without treatment there is gradual progressive deterioration. Elevated plasma phytanic acid levels with low pristanic acid levels is diagnostic.

Further reading

Bellettato CM, Hubert L, Scarpa M et al. Inborn errors of metabolism involving complex molecules: lysosomal and peroxisomal storage diseases. *Pediatr Clin North Am* 2018; 65:353–373.

Gorman GS, Chinnery PF, DiMauro S et al. Mitochondrial diseases. *Nat Rev Dis Primers* 2016; 2:16080.

Häberle J, Boddaert N, Alberto Burlina A et al. Suggested guidelines for the diagnosis and management of urea cycle disorders. *Orphanet J Rare Dis* 2012; 7:32.

Hollack CEM, Lachmann RH. *Inherited Metabolic Dsease in Adults: A Clinical Guide*. Oxford: Oxford University Press; 2016.

Lee B, Scaglia F. *Inborn Errors of Metabolism – From Neonatal Screening to Metabolic Pathways*. (Oxford Monographs on Medical Genetics). Oxford: Oxford University Press; 2014.

Platt FM, d'Azzo A, Davidson BL et al. Lysosomal storage diseases. *Nat Rev Dis Primers* 2018; 4:27.

Prietsch V, Lindner EM, Zschocke J et al. Emergency management of inherited metabolic disease. *J Inherit Metab Dis* 2002; 25:531–546.

Sadubray JM, Baumgartner MR, Walter J. *Inborn Metabolic Diseases: Diagnosis and Treatment*. 6th ed. Cham: Springer; 2016.

van Wegberg AMJ, MacDonald A, Ahring K et al. The complete European guidelines on phenylketonuria: diagnosis and treatment. *Orphanet J Rare Dis* 2017; 12:162.

Significant websites

www.bimdg.org.uk *British Inherited Metabolic Diseases Group*.
www.ssiem.org *Society for the Study of Inborn Errors of Metabolism*.

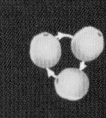

Box 24.9 Common inherited metabolic diseases of protein metabolism

Disease	Enzyme defect	Inheritance	Reported incidence	Acute decompensation/first presentation in adulthood	Common clinical features	Biochemical features	Management	Prognosis
Urea cycle defects	Mutations in one of six cycle enzymes, most commonly OTC deficiency	AR OTC is X-linked	1:8000–1:45000	Yes, including as first presentation in adulthood. May be unmasked in adulthood by a change in diet for e.g. low-carbohydrate, high-protein diets	Progressive encephalopathy. Cyclical vomiting/non-specific neuropsychiatric symptoms	When unwell: hyperammonaemia, characteristic abnormalities in AA/OA. May also have: alkalosis consistently very low urea	As for hyperammonaemia in acute setting. Life-long protein restriction, ammonia scavengers, arginine, citrulline	Good if treated promptly. Fatal if diagnosis/treatment delayed
Tyrosinaemia Type 1	Fumaryl-acetoacetate hydroxylase deficiency	AR	1:100000. More common in Quebec, Canada, due to founder mutations	Yes, first presentation in adulthood reported	Liver failure. Gastrointestinal bleeding. Fanconi's syndrome, tubulopathy, Renal rickets, acute porphyria. Guillain–Barré syndrome-like acute neurogenic crisis. Hepatocellular carcinoma	Raised tyrosine in serum AA and raised succinylacetone in urine OA	Nitisinone (NTBC). Tyrosine restriction. Tyrosine-free amino acid supplementation. Liver transplantation may be considered	Good if treated early. If patient not compliant with medication or untreated, can present in adulthood with any of clinical features described
Alkaptonuria	Homogentisate 1,2-dioxygenase deficiency	AR	1:250000 AR	Presents more often in adulthood (3rd–5th decades)	Large joint arthritis. Ochronotic pigmentation (sclera/ears). Valvular heart disease. Urine turns black on standing. Black nappies in children	Raised homogentisic acid on urine OA	Nitisinone (NTBC) improves biochemical profile	Chronic progressive disease with variable prognosis
Classical homocystinuria	Cystathionine β synthase deficiency	AR	1:40000 to 250000	Yes, including first presentation in adulthood	Thromboembolic events (stroke/arterial or venous occlusive disease). Acute lens dislocation/visual loss. Neuropsychiatric symptoms. Developmental delay. Seizures. Acute/subacute/chronic neurological deterioration. Marfanoid habitus. Osteoporosis	Raised plasma homocysteine (particularly if >50 µmol/L). Raised plasma methionine. Reduced plasma cysteine. Genetic analysis may be useful in predicting response to pyridoxine in addition to confirming diagnosis Note: folate/vitamin B_{12} deficiencies and metabolism defects can also cause mild to moderate rise in homocysteine levels – these must be excluded	Pyridoxine. Betaine. Vitamin B_{12}. Folate. Methionine-restricted diet in pyridoxine-non-responsive homocystinuria with added vitamin supplements	Variable depending on severity. Early treatment (in neonatal/early childhood) results in normal IQ and decreased risk of long-term morbidity
Defects in metabolism of branched chain amino acids **Maple syrup urine disease (MSUD)** **Propionic aciduria (PA)** **Methylmalonic aciduria (MMA)**	MSUD – branch chain α-ketoacid dehydrogenase deficiency. PA – propionyl coA carboxylase deficiency. MMA – genetically heterogenous disorder	AR	MSUD 1:185000. 1:380 in Old Order Mennonite population (PA) 1:100000, more common in Saudi Arabians 1:100000	Yes, first presentation in adults very unusual	Acute decompensation: encephalopathy, acidosis, hyperammonaemia. Developmental delay. Abnormal neurology. Cardiomyopathy (PA). Pancreatitis (MMA/PA). Renal failure (occasionally adults with milder forms of MMA may present with just renal impairment)	Metabolic acidosis with high anion gap. Hyperammonaemia during acute decompensation. Characteristic abnormalities on AA/OA and AC profiles	Natural protein restriction. Avoid catabolism. Liver transplantation (MSUD, PA). Renal/combined liver and renal transplantation (MMA). Carnitine supplementation (PA/MMA). BCAA free supplements (MSUD)	Variable depending on severity. Acute decompensations can be fatal

AA amino acids; AC, acylcarnitine profile; AR, autosomal recessive; OA organic acids; OTC, ornithine transcarbamylase.

Box 24.10 Lysosomal storage disorders

Disease	Enzyme defect	Inheritance	Reported incidence	Common clinical features	Biochemistry/diagnostic test	Management
Gaucher	Beta-glucocerebrosidase (GBA) deficiency	AR	Panethnic, 1:75 000, 1:850 in AJ population	94% of patients have non-neuronal disease (type 1) characterized by hepatosplenomegaly, bone marrow involvement, cytopaenia and skeletal symptoms such as severe bone pain and avascular necrosis Presentation can occur in adulthood Neuronopathic form is much rarer (6% of patients) Acute (1%) (type 2) – presentation almost always at <1 year of age – severe progressive neurological deficit leading to early death Chronic (5%) (type 3) – mild to severe neurological and skeletal symptoms and organomegaly Intermediate forms occur, as can late neurological presentations in adulthood with neurological symptoms including a supranuclear horizontal gaze palsy Acute complications: avascular necrosis of bone and splenic infarcts Heterozygous mutations may increase risk of Parkinson's syndrome	Deficient GBA activity in leukocytes or fibroblasts 'Gaucher cells' on biopsy Genetics	Supportive Enzyme replacement therapy (ERT) using recombinant GBA
Fabry	Alpha-galactosidase A (α-GLA) deficiency	X-linked	1:40 000. Late onset milder forms much more common	Acroparesthaesia, cornea verticillata, angiokeratomas Gastrointestinal symptoms (classical phenotype, most common presenting symptoms in paediatric population) Adults more often present with end organ disease Arrhythmia, cardiac fibrosis, hypertrophic cardiomyopathy Proteinuria, renal impairment Stroke Decreased exercise tolerance, fatigue, depression Females can also be symptomatic due to lyonization of X chromosome. End organ symptoms usually a decade later than men Wide phenotypic spectrum in both males and females based on residual enzyme activity levels	Deficient (α-GLA) activity in white cells. Activity can be normal in 60% of affected females – genetic confirmation therefore needed	Supportive ERT Cascade testing for family members at risk
Niemann–Pick B	Acid sphingo-myelinase deficiency	AR	1:250 000, 1:40 000 in AJ	Age of presentation and severity variable. Can present for the first time in adulthood Splenomegaly, hypersplenism Hepatomegaly, hepatic fibrosis, cirrhosis Dyslipidaemia (high LDL–C and triglycerides) Osteoporosis Storage facies Cherry-red macular spot (25%) Lung fibrosis causing restrictive lung disease	Deficient enzyme activity in leukocytes Genetic confirmation	Supportive Clinical trial for ERT ongoing
Tay–Sachs	Beta-hexosaminidase (isoform A) deficiency	AR	1:250 000. However, 1:25 (versus 1:250 in the general population) carrier frequency in AJ Actual incidence in Jewish populations now significantly decreased in many countries due to effective counselling	Childhood disease is fatal with rapidly progressive neurology, visceromegaly, dysmorphia and increased startle response Late onset adult disease – age of onset and severity varies Cerebellar and motor neurone dysfunction causing tremor, dysarthria, chorea, dystonia	Deficient enzyme activity in leukocytes Genetic confirmation	Supportive
Pompe's (GSD type 2)	Acid alpha-glucosidase (acid maltase) deficiency	AR	1:40 000	Adult with Pompe's usually symptomatic in 3rd–4th decade with: limb girdle muscle weakness respiratory insufficiency secondary to diaphragm weakness, which is often major cause of death acute decompensation related to respiratory failure Classical infantile form – more severe presentation in the first few months of life	Deficient enzyme activity in leukocytes Genetics Vacuolated lymphocytes Vacuolar myopathy on muscle biopsy Pulmonary function test (>20% change in VC between sitting and supine position)	Supportive ERT

AJ, Ashkenazi Jewish population; AR, autosomal recessive; VC, vital capacity.

Box 24.11 Common glycogen storage disorders (GSDs)

GSD group	Common sub-types and the specific enzyme deficiency	Incidence	Inheritance	Common clinical features	Biochemistry/diagnostic test	Principles of management
GSDs affecting mainly muscle	GSD 2 (Pompe's) see **Box 24.10**	See **Box 24.10**	See **Box 24.10**	See **Box 24.10**	See **Box 24.10**	See **Box 24.10**
	GSD 5 (McArdle's) secondary to myophosphorylase deficiency	1: 100 000	AR	First presentation in adults not unusual Exercise intolerance. Pain within 5–10 min of starting exercise; 'second wind' phenomenon, i.e. symptoms improve within a few minutes if able to continue with exercise Rhabdomyolysis	Raised creatine kinase Flat lactate with an exaggerated rise in ammonia on non-ischaemic exercise test Genetic testing PAS staining vacuolar myopathy (although muscle biopsy should not normally be needed for diagnosis)	Diagnosis and treatment prevents rhabdomyolysis Aerobic conditioning exercise programmes to improve exercise tolerance Oral glucose (for e.g. glucose polymer drink with 25% glucose) 5 min before exercise Avoid unaccustomed strenuous exercise
GSDs affecting mainly liver	GSD1 (glucose-6-phosphatase deficiency)	1:100 000	AR	Hypoglycaemia, ketosis and lactic acidosis in infancy Growth retardation Massive hepatomegaly Renal impairment Hepatic adenomas and hepatocellular carcinoma (one subtype GSD1b can present with neutropenia) No cognitive impairment if hypoglycaemia avoided. With improved treatment most transition into adulthood. Isolated case reports of first presentation in adults	Enzymology and genetic testing for diagnosis Secondary abnormalities Hyperuricemia Ketosis, lactic acidosis, hypertriglyceridaemia	Principles of management for this group of diseases includes: dietary therapy with regular doses of slow release corn-starch to maintain normoglycaemia ER Most severe cases may need continuous feed through gastrostomy Surveillance for co-morbidities as above
	GSD III (debrancher enzyme deficiency)	1:100 000, 1:5400 in North African Jewish ancestry	AR	Adults are much more likely to present with complications related to cardiac/liver involvement rather than hypoglycaemia Less severe than GSD1 Fasting hypoglycaemia less severe Ketosis, but no lactic acidosis Mild hyperlipidaemia Childhood presentation with hypoglycaemia and hepatomegaly Kidneys not involved Hepatic adenomas less common Muscle weakness with raised CK may occur Cardiac complications including ventricular hypertrophy		

AR, autosomal recessive; CK, creatine kinase; ER, emergency regimen; PAS, Periodic acid schiff staining.

Box 24.12 Other inherited metabolic diseases affecting carbohydrate metabolism

Disease	Enzyme defect	Incidence	Inheritance	Common clinical features	Biochemistry/diagnostic test	Principles of management
Galactosaemia	Most commonly galactose-1-phophate uridyltransferase deficiency	1:40000	AR	Neonatal presentation on ingestion of galactose (milk/formula) with failure to thrive, liver disease, cataract and renal tubular dysfunction. Treated adults can have: developmental delay, neurological deficits, premature ovarian failure. Adult presentation rare, however, exclude diagnosis in patients with premature ovarian failure ± cataracts ± neurological disease	Elevated levels of galactose-1-phosphate in RBCs	Immediate removal of galactose from diet as soon as suspected without awaiting diagnostic confirmation. Restriction for life. Supportive therapy including options to freeze eggs before onset of premature ovarian failure
Glucose transporter 1 (GLUT1)	GLUT1 deficiency	1:90 000	AD	Symptoms secondary to decreased facilitated glucose transport into brain via GLUT1. Symptoms include seizures, developmental delay, complex movement disorder. Symptoms worse a few hours post-prandial	Lumbar puncture after a 4-6-hour fast. Paired CSF/blood glucose ratio <0.45 suggestive. Confirmation with genetics/RBC glucose uptake studies	Ketogenic diet imitates metabolic state of fasting so brain uses ketones as alternative fuel. Ketogenic diet for life
Hereditary fructose intolerance	Aldolase B deficiency	1:20000	AR	Ingestion of fructose/sucrose/sorbitol causes acute illness (within minutes) of abdominal pain, vomiting, diarrhoea. More severe symptoms including hypoglycaemia/seizures/coma can occur. Persistent exposure leads to liver steatosis/fibrosis/failure and renal tubular disease/Fanconi's syndrome. Patients may go undiagnosed or have diagnosed delayed until adulthood due to self-restricted fructose intake and thus symptom prevention	Enzymology now replaced by genetic testing	Withdrawal of all enteral and parenteral sources of fructose. Medications/infusions/supplements should be checked for fructose. Supplementation with vitamin C and other vitamins. Prognosis good if all fructose avoided

AD, autosomal recessive; AR, autosomal recessive; RBC, red blood cell.

i **Box 24.13** Fatty acid oxidation disorders (FAODs)

Disease	Enzyme defect	Incidence	Inheritance	Common clinical features	Biochemistry/ diagnostic test	Principles of management
Medium-chain acyl-CoA dehydro-genase deficiency (MCADD)	Medium-chain acyl-CoA dehydrogenase enzyme deficiency	1:17 000, more common in people of north European descent Newborn screening in the UK and a number of other countries	AR	In adults first presentation with rhabdomyolysis, most often triggered by excess alcohol intake Paediatric presentation: hypoketotic hypoglycaemia, encephalopathy, liver dysfunction, cot death	Characteristic profile on AC/OA Genetics	Avoid fasting Regular meals No specific dietary modifications needed ER
Carnitine palmi-toyltrans-ferase 2 (CPT2) deficiency	CPT2 enzyme deficiency	Exact frequency not known >300 cases reported in the literature	AR	As above + myopathy in paediatric presentation	Characteristic profile on AC/OA Genetics	As above
Very long-chain acyl-CoA dehydro-genase (VLCAD) deficiency	VLCAD enzyme deficiency	1:40 000	AR	As in CPT2 + neuromuscular weakness, cardiomyopathy in paediatric presentation	Characteristic profile on AC/OA Genetics	As above May need cardiac surveillance and restriction of long-chain fatty acids depending on severity

AC, acylcarnitine profile; AR, autosomal recessive; ER, emergency regime; OA, organic acid profile.

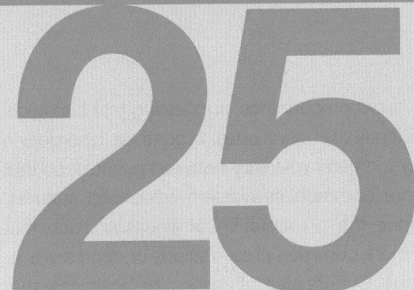

25

Liaison psychiatry

Julius Bourke

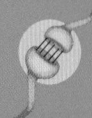

CORE SKILLS AND KNOWLEDGE

Liaison psychiatry is a subspecialty within psychiatry that primarily concerns itself with the interface between psychiatry and other medical specialties. It is a vital component of hospital medicine, supporting every medical specialty to some degree, from the most acute of presentations to more chronic problems.

Inpatient medical teams may seek the advice of a liaison psychiatrist when a patient with known psychiatric co-morbidity is admitted to hospital; when patients that develop new onset psychopathology, often in the absence of a past history; or where psychopathology arises as a clinical sign within a given medical diagnosis – for example in neurological or some endocrine disorders.

Key skills in psychological medicine include:
- performing mental state and cognitive examinations, and recognizing common psychiatric presentations encountered in general medicine

- assessing risk in the potentially suicidal patient
- understanding functional somatic syndromes found in different medical specialties
- assessing mental capacity: a vital requirement for informed consent
- understanding the roles of psychoactive medications including antidepressants, antipsychotics and sedatives in patient care; and their patterns of toxicity.

Acute aspects of psychological medicine can be learned by shadowing a liaison psychiatrist or liaison psychiatry mental health nurse in assessing psychiatric morbidity and on-going risk in patients presenting to the emergency department, including after instances of self-harm or suicide attempts. On an outpatient basis, important experience will be gained by assessing patients with functional disorders. Developing skills in psychiatric history-taking and mental state examination allows the complex biopsychosocial understanding of any condition to be unpicked.

INTRODUCTION

Psychiatry is concerned with the study and management of disorders of mental function: primarily, thoughts, perceptions, emotions and purposeful behaviours. Liaison psychiatry, or psychological medicine, is concerned primarily with psychiatric disorders in patients who have physical complaints or conditions. This chapter will mainly address this branch of psychiatry.

The long-held belief that diseases are either physical or mental has been replaced by accumulated evidence that the brain is functionally or anatomically abnormal in psychiatric disorders. Physical, psychological and social factors, and their interactions, must be looked into, in order to understand psychiatric conditions – replacing the mind/body *biomedical model* with an integrated *biopsychosocial* one.

Provision of psychiatric care in the general hospital

The structure of psychiatric services varies between countries but in broad terms, they tend to be located in three settings: in the community, in psychiatric hospitals and in general hospitals. General hospital psychiatry is referred to as liaison psychiatry. This subspecialty is increasingly recognized as an essential component of effective care in acute hospitals, reducing length of hospital stay and improving outcome measures. In the UK, 79% of hospitals now have a liaison psychiatry service; the provision may be limited to the emergency department, or in other places extend to the general wards and even the outpatient department.

Epidemiology and vulnerable patient groups

The point prevalence of psychiatric disorders in adults in the UK is about 20%, mostly composed of depressive and anxiety disorders and substance misuse (mainly alcohol) (**Box 25.1**). The prevalence is about twice as high in patients attending the general hospital, with the highest rates in the emergency department and medical wards. The most prevalent disorders among general hospital inpatients are organic brain disorders (e.g. delirium), depressive illnesses and alcohol dependence or harmful use. In more than half of such cases, a psychiatric intervention is required. Particularly vulnerable groups include those admitted to the wards with neurological disorder, including acquired brain injury, patients on the intensive care unit (where post-traumatic stress disorder (PTSD) is especially common) and older patients, who are at greater risk of organic brain disorders such as delirium. A further patient group of importance is those with a pre-existing psychiatric diagnosis.

Culture and ethnicity

These can alter the presentation and prevalence of psychiatric ill-health. Biological factors in mental illness are similar across cultures but may vary between ethnicities, whereas psychological and social factors will vary across culture. For example, the prevalence and presentation of schizophrenia vary little between countries, suggesting that biological factors operate independently of cultural ones. In contrast, disorders in which social factors play a greater role vary between cultures, so that anorexia nervosa is more common in Western-influenced cultures. Culture can also influence the presentation of illnesses, such that physical symptoms are more common presentations of depressive illness in Asia than in Europe. Culture also influences the healthcare that is sought and provided for the same condition.

CLINICAL APPROACH TO THE PATIENT WITH A PSYCHIATRIC DISORDER

Psychiatric history

The history is essential in making a diagnosis and is similar to that used in all specialties, but tailored to help to make a psychiatric diagnosis, determine possible aetiology and estimate prognosis. The interview also enables a doctor to establish a therapeutic relationship with the patient. **Box 25.2** gives essential guidance on how to conduct such an interview safely, although it is rare for a patient to harm a healthcare professional.

Components of the history are summarized in **Box 25.3**.

Box 25.1 Approximate prevalence of psychiatric disorders in different UK populations

Population/disorder	Approximate percentage
General population	20[a]
Neuroses	16
Psychoses	0.5
Alcohol misuse	5
Drug misuse	2[b]
Primary care	25
General hospital outpatients	30
General hospital inpatients	40

[a]Total in the community (general population) is 20% due to co-morbidity.
[b]An underestimate.

Box 25.2 Essentials of a safe psychiatric interview

- *Beforehand*: Ask someone with experience who knows the patient whether it is safe to interview the patient alone.
- *Access to others*: If in doubt, interview in the view or hearing of others, or accompanied by another member of staff.
- *Setting*: If safe, conduct the interview in a quiet room alone for confidentiality, not by the bed.
- *Seating*: Place yourself between the door and the patient.
- *Alarm*: If one is available, find out where the alarm is and how to use it.

Box 25.3 Summary of the components of the psychiatric history

Component	Description
Reason for referral	Why and how the patient came to the attention of the doctor
Present illness	How the illness progressed, from the earliest time at which a change was noted until the patient came to the attention of the doctor
Past psychiatric history	Prior episodes of illness, and where and how they were treated. Prior self-harm
Past medical history	This should include emotional reactions to illness and procedures
Family history	History of psychiatric illnesses and relationships within the family
Personal (biographical) history	*Childhood*: mother's pregnancy and patient's birth (complications, nature of delivery), early development and attainment of developmental milestones (e.g. learning to crawl, walk, talk). School history: age started and finished; truancy, bullying, reprimands; qualifications *Adulthood*: employment (age at first job, total number of jobs, reasons for leaving, problems at work), relationships (sexual orientation, age at first relationship, total number of relationships, reasons for ending them), children and dependants
Reproductive history	*Women*: menstrual problems, pregnancies, terminations, miscarriages, contraception and menopause
Social history	Current employment, benefits, housing, current stressors
Personality	This may help to determine prognosis. How do they normally cope with stress? Do they trust others and make friends easily? Irritable? Moody? A loner? This list is not exhaustive
Drug history	Prescribed and over-the-counter medication, units and type of alcohol/week, tobacco, caffeine and illicit drugs
Forensic history	Explain that you need to ask about this, since ill-health can sometimes lead to problems with the law. Note any violent or sexual offences. This is part of a *risk assessment*. Worst harm they have ever inflicted on someone else? Under what circumstances? Would they do the same again, were the situation to recur?
Systematic review	Psychiatric illness is not exclusive of physical illness! The two may not only coexist but also have a common aetiology

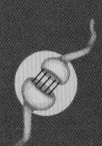
Mental state examination

The history will already have assessed several aspects of the mental state examination (MSE), but several of these will need to be expanded on and specific areas, such as cognition, tested. The MSE is typically followed by a physical examination, and concluded with an assessment of insight and risk, and a formulation that takes into account a differential diagnosis and aetiology. Each domain of the MSE is given below; abnormalities that might be detected are summarized in **Box 25.4**.

Aspects of the MSE

Appearance and general behaviour

The clothes (state, colour, style), facial appearance, eye contact, posture and movement provide information about a patient's affect. Agitation and anxiety cause an easy startle response, sweating, tremor, restlessness, fidgeting and visual scanning (for perceived danger).

Speech

The rate, rhythm, volume and content of the patient's speech should be examined for abnormalities. Speech is the only way that you can examine thought form and so this is typically observed in this section. The content of the patient's thoughts is dealt with separately (see below). Neurological abnormalities (e.g. dysarthria, dysphasia) should also be assessed.

Mood and affect

Precise terminology is used in psychiatry: the patient has an **emotion** or **feeling**, tells you about their **mood**, and what you observe is the patient's **affect**. Mood can demonstrate persistent change, fluctuations and incongruity.

Thoughts

Abnormalities of thought content and thought possession are recorded here. Delusions (see **Box 25.4**) can be further categorized as primary or secondary, depending on whether they arise *de novo* or secondary to other abnormalities of the mental state.

Abnormal perceptions

Assessing perceptions involves observation and questioning of the patient. Patients experiencing auditory hallucinations may appear startled by voices that you cannot hear, or may interact with them, for example by engaging in conversation when nobody else is in the room. Hallucinations can affect any sensory modality and specific types of hallucination and the disorders in which they are seen will be addressed later in the chapter.

Cognitive state

A cognitive examination is necessary to diagnose organic brain disorders, such as delirium and dementia. Poor concentration, confusion and memory problems are the most common subjective complaints. Screening of cognitive functions may suggest the need for more formal psychometry. Simple questioning detects about 90% of people with cognitive impairment, with about 10% false positives. Testing can be divided into tests of diffuse and focal brain functions, summarized in **Box 25.5**.

Insight and illness beliefs

Insight is the degree to which a person recognizes that they are unwell, and is minimal in people with a psychosis. **Illness beliefs** are the patient's own explanations of their ill-health, including diagnosis and causes. These beliefs may be important in determining prognosis and adherence to treatment.

Defence mechanisms

Defence mechanisms are unconscious mental processes. Although not part of the MSE examination, they help understand aspects of behaviour. Common defence mechanisms are described in **Box 25.6**.

Risk assessment

Risk assessment may sound daunting but is common to all clinical practice: for instance, when determining whether a patient with chest pain should be reviewed in the resuscitation room of the emergency department rather than a normal cubicle. Risk must be assessed in people with a psychiatric diagnosis, although the nature of 'risk' is different, comprising the risk that the patient poses to themselves and that which they pose to others (**Box 25.7**). An appraisal of risk will have started with the initial preparations for seeing a patient (see **Box 25.2**) and in checking 'forensic history' (see **Box 25.3**). Additional information from family, friends or professionals who know the patient may prove invaluable.

Severe behavioural disturbance

Patients who are aggressive or violent cause understandable apprehension in all staff, and are most commonly seen in the accident and emergency department. Information from anyone accompanying the patient, including police or carers, can help considerably. **Box 25.8** lists the main causes of disturbed behaviour.

Management of the severely disturbed patient

The primary aims of management are the control of dangerous behaviour and the establishment of a provisional diagnosis. Four specific strategies may be necessary when dealing with the violent patient (**Box 25.9**):

- reassurance and explanation
- medication
- physical restraint
- monitoring.

Remember that the behaviour exhibited is normally a reflection of an underlying disorder and so portrays suffering and often fear. The approach to the agitated or violent patient must take this into account and the steps listed intend to alleviate this suffering while maintaining the safety of the individual, other patients and staff.

Relevant physical examination

This should be guided by the history and mental state examination. Particular attention should be paid to the neurological and endocrinological examinations when organic brain syndromes and affective illnesses are suspected.

Summary or formulation

When the full history and mental state have been assessed, you should make a concise assessment or 'formulation' of the case.

Box 25.4 Mental state examination and the psychopathology it is used to detect

Type of disorder	Abnormality	Description	Typical of which disorder(s)?
Appearance and behaviour	–	Colour and state of clothes, facial appearance, eye contact, posture, movement, agitation. Startle response, sweating, tremor, restlessness, fidgeting, visual scanning (for danger), distractibility	–
Speech			
Disorders of stream of thought	Pressured speech	Rapid rate, increased volume, difficult to interrupt	Mania
	Poverty of speech	Lengthy pauses between brief utterances	Depressive illness Schizophrenia
	Thought block	A sentence is suddenly stopped for no obvious reason	Schizophrenia
Disorders of thought form	Flight of ideas	Thoughts rapidly jump from one topic to another	Mania
	Word salad or schizophasia	The connection between themes, sentences and even words is lost, resulting in unintelligible speech, although words are still identifiable	Schizophrenia Receptive (Wernicke's) aphasia
	Perseveration	Persistent, inappropriate repetition of the same thought or action	Schizophrenia, Obsessive–compulsive disorder Frontal lobe lesions
Mood			
Persistent change	Depression	Low mood, tearfulness, low spirits	Depression
	Anxiety	Constant, inappropriate or excessive worry, fear, apprehension, tension or inner restlessness	Anxiety disorders (± depressive illnesses) Drug intoxication and withdrawal
	Elation	A feeling of high spirits, exuberant happiness, vitality	Mania, drug intoxication
	Irritability	Either expressed (as in a temper or impatience) or an internal feeling of exasperation or anger	Depression (especially men) Mania
	Blunted affect	A total absence of emotion	Schizophrenia (in chronic illness)
Fluctuating change		Different emotions rapidly follow one another. Alternatively, excessive emotion over events	Mixed affective states Pseudobulbar palsy
Incongruity		Mood and context do not reflect one another, e.g. laughing while describing the death of a loved one	Schizophrenia Mania
Thoughts			
Disorders of content	Delusions	A false belief held with absolute conviction, and out of keeping with the patient's cultural, social and religious beliefs	Psychosis
	Overvalued ideas	Deeply held personal convictions that are understandable when the individual's background is known	–
	Obsessions	Recurrent, persistent thought, impulse, image or musical theme occurring despite the patient's effort to resist it. May be accompanied by compulsions (repetitive, seemingly purposeful action performed stereotypically)	Obsessive–compulsive disorder
Disorders of thought possession	Thought broadcast	The patient experiences their thoughts as being understood by others without talking	Schizophrenia
	Thought insertion	The patient's thought is perceived as being planted in their mind by someone else	Schizophrenia
	Thought withdrawal	The patient experiences their thoughts being taken away from them, without their control	Schizophrenia
Perceptions			
	Hallucinations	Perception in the absence of a stimulus, perceived in objective space with the qualities of normal perceptions	Psychosis Organic brain states, e.g. delirium
	Pseudo-hallucinations	Usually auditory: true externally sited hallucinations, but with insight into their imaginary nature, or internally sited (e.g. 'I heard a voice in my head speaking to me')	Depressive illness Personality disorders Not indicative of psychotic disorder
	Illusions	Misperceptions of external stimuli, most likely when the general level of sensory stimulation is reduced	Normal experience Some neurological disorders
	Depersonalization	A change in self-awareness such that the patient feels unreal or detached from their body. The patient is aware, however, of the subjective nature of this alteration	Anxiety disorders Schizophrenia Temporal lobe epilepsy, in healthy people when tired
	Derealization	The unpleasant feeling that the external environment has become unreal and/or remote; patients may describe themselves as though they are in a dream-like state	As in depersonalization
	Heightened sensitivity	Photosensitivity and phonosensitivity	Anxiety disorders Drug intoxication and withdrawal Migraine Epilepsy

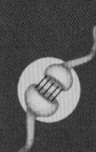

Box 25.5 Cognitive examination[a]

Cognitive domain	Assessment
Diffuse functions	
Pre-morbid intelligence	An estimate is helpful in assessing changes in cognitive abilities: ask the patient about the final year and level of their education, and the highest qualifications or skills they achieved
Orientation	Assess orientation to time, place and person. Consciousness can be defined as the awareness of the self and the environment. Clouding of consciousness is more accurately a fluctuating level of awareness and is commonly seen in delirium
Attention	Ask the patient to say the months of the year or days of the week backwards
Verbal memory	*Immediate recall or registration*: ask the patient to repeat a name and address with ten or so items, noting how many times it takes to recall it with 100% accuracy (normal is 1 or 2). *Short-term memory*: ask the patient to try to remember the address and then ask it of them again after 5 min (0 or 1 error is normal).
Long-term memory	Ask the patient to recall the news from that morning or recently. If they are not interested in the news, find out their interests (football team, favourite soap opera) and ask relevant questions. *Amnesia* is literally an absence of memory; *dysmnesia* indicates a dysfunctioning memory
Focal functions	
Frontal, temporal and parietal lobe function	These are covered in detail on pages 806–808
Behaviour	Disinhibited behaviour that cannot be explained by a psychiatric illness is suggestive of frontal lobe lesions
Sequential tasks	Ask the patient to alternate making a fist with one hand at the same time as a flat hand with the other Ask the patient to tap a table once if you tap twice, and vice versa Note any motor perseveration whereby the patient cannot change the movement once established Observe for verbal perseveration, in which the patient repeats the same answer as given previously for a different question
Abstract thinking	Ask the patient the meaning of common proverbs: a literal meaning may suggest frontal lobe dysfunction, assuming reasonable pre-morbid intelligence

[a]This correlates well with more time-consuming intelligence quotient (IQ) tests, but it will not pick up cognitive problems caused by focal brain lesions as easily.

Box 25.6 Common defence mechanisms

Defence mechanism	Description
Repression	Avoiding thinking about memories, emotions and/or impulses that would cause anxiety or distress if allowed to enter consciousness
Denial	Similar to repression and occurs when patients behave as though unaware of something that they might be expected to know, e.g. a patient who, despite being told that a close relative has died, continues to behave as though the relative were still alive
Displacement	Transferring of emotion from a situation or object with which it is properly associated to another that gives less distress
Identification	Unconscious process of taking on some of the characteristics or behaviours of another person, often to reduce the pain of separation or loss
Projection	Attribution to another person of thoughts or feelings that are in fact one's own
Regression	Adoption of primitive patterns of behaviour appropriate to an earlier stage of development. It can be seen in ill people who become child-like and highly dependent
Sublimation	Unconscious diversion of unacceptable behaviours into acceptable ones

Box 25.7 Assessment of risk

	Risk to self	Risk to others
Active	Acts of self-harm or suicide attempts Look for prior history of self-harm and what may have precipitated or prevented it	Aggression towards others – this may be actual violence or threatening behaviour A past history of aggression is a good predictor of its recurrence. Look at the severity and quality of, and remorse for, prior violent acts, as well as identifiable precipitants that might be avoided in the future (e.g. alcohol)
Passive	Self-neglect Manipulation by others	Neglect of others – always find out whether there are children or other dependants at home

Box 25.8 Main causes of disturbed behaviour

- Drug intoxication (especially alcohol)
- Delirium (acute confusional state)
- Acute psychosis
- Personality disorder

This should include a summary of the essential features of the history and examination, a differential diagnosis, possible causal factors and any further investigations or interviews that are needed. It concludes with a concise plan of treatment and a statement of the likely prognosis.

Further reading

Dudas RB, Berrios GE, Hodges JR. The Addenbrooke's Cognitive Examination (ACE) in the differential diagnosis of early dementias versus affective disorder. *Am J Geriatr Psychiatry* 2005; 13:218–226.

McAllister-Williams RH, Cousins D, Lunn B. Clinical assessment and investigation in psychiatry. *Medicine* 2012; 40:568–573.

i **Box 25.9 Management of the severely disturbed patient**

Method	Description
'Verbal de-escalation'	First step – try to defuse the situation by talking to the patient. The disturbed behaviour may be simple to correct, e.g. if staff explain their intentions on approaching the patient
Medication	Where possible, use oral medication first. Start with a short-acting benzodiazepine unless the patient is elderly or delirious (can worsen confusion and agitation). Give medications sequentially, rather than together, allowing 30 min to 1 h for them to take effect: Lorazepam (oral/i.m.) 0.5–1 mg Haloperidol (oral) 2.5–5 mg Promethazine (i.m.) 50 mg Haloperidol (i.m.) 5–10 mg Olanzapine (i.m.) 10 mg
Physical restraint	Use only to maintain safety and to administer i.m. medications. It should be performed by adequately trained psychiatric nurses and security staff. In the UK, doctors will never be involved in restraining the patient. Restraint is a potentially dangerous intervention, even more so when mixed with psychotropic medication, and deaths have occurred as a direct consequence
Monitoring	Where medications are used, monitor blood pressure, pulse, respiratory rate and oxygen saturation frequently, dictated by the level of on-going agitation and consciousness

i.m., intramuscular.

CLASSIFICATION OF PSYCHIATRIC DISORDERS

The classification of psychiatric disorders into categories is mainly based on symptoms and behaviours, since there are few diagnostic tests for psychiatric disorders. An unhelpful dualistic division of psychiatric disorders from neurological diseases exists in the main classification systems. Since the brain or nervous system is the organ affected in both psychiatric and neurological conditions, some have argued that they should all simply be classified as disorders of the nervous system.

Psychiatric classifications have traditionally divided up disorders into neuroses and psychoses:

- **Neuroses** are illnesses in which symptoms vary only in severity from normal experiences, such as depressive illness.
- **Psychoses** are illnesses in which symptoms are qualitatively different from normal experience, with little insight into their nature, such as schizophrenia.

There are several problems with this dichotomy. First, neuroses may be as severe in their effects as psychoses. Second, neuroses may cause symptoms that fulfil the definition of psychotic symptoms. For instance, someone with anorexia nervosa may be convinced that they are fat when they are thin, and this belief would meet all the criteria for a delusional belief, yet we would traditionally classify the illness as a neurosis.

The ***ICD-10 Classification of Mental and Behavioural Disorders***, published by the World Health Organization, has largely

i **Box 25.10 International Classification of Psychiatric Disorders (ICD-10)**

- Organic disorders
- Mental and behavioural disorders due to psychoactive substance use
- Schizophrenia and delusional disorders
- Mood (affective) disorders
- Neurotic, stress-related and somatoform disorders
- Behavioural syndromes
- Disorders of adult personality and behaviour
- Mental retardation

abandoned the traditional division between neurosis and psychosis, although the terms are still used. The disorders are now arranged in groups according to major common themes (e.g. mood disorders and delusional disorders). A classification of psychiatric disorders derived from ICD-10 is shown in **Box 25.10**, and this is the classification mainly used in this chapter (ICD-11 will come into effect in 2022).

The Diagnostic and Statistical Manual of the American Psychiatric Association (DSM-5) is an alternative classification system.

Further reading

American Psychiatric Association. *Diagnostic and Statistical Manual of Mental Disorders*, 5th edn. Text revision (DSM-5). Washington, DC: APA; 2013.
Jacob KS, Patel V. Classification of mental disorders: a global mental health perspective. *Lancet* 2014; 383:1433–1435.
White PD, Rickards H, Zeman AZJ. Time to end the distinction between mental and neurological illnesses. *BMJ* 2012; 344:e3454.
World Health Organization. *The ICD-10 Classification of Mental and Behavioural Disorders: Clinical Descriptions and Diagnostic Guidelines*. Geneva: World Health Organization; 1992.

AETIOLOGY OF PSYCHIATRIC DISORDERS

A psychiatric disorder may result from several causes, which may interact. It can be helpful to divide causes into the three 'Ps'– predisposing, precipitating and perpetuating factors:

- ***Predisposing factors*** often stem from early life and include genetic factors, pregnancy- and delivery-related factors, previous emotional traumas and personality factors.
- ***Precipitating factors*** are 'triggers' that may be physical, psychological or social. Whether or not they produce a disorder depends on their nature and severity, and the presence of predisposing factors.
- ***Perpetuating factors*** maintain the disorder once it has been triggered and may be physical, psychological or social. There may be more than one and these may interact.

PSYCHIATRIC ASPECTS OF PHYSICAL DISEASES

People with non-psychiatric, 'physical' diseases are more likely to suffer from psychiatric disorders than those who are well. The most common examples are mood and acute organic brain disorders (delirium). The relationship between mental and physical conditions may be understood in one of four ways:

- Psychological distress and disorders can precipitate physical diseases (e.g. the cardiac risk associated with depressive disorders, or hypokalaemia causing arrhythmias in anorexia nervosa).
- Physical diseases and their treatments can cause mental symptoms or ill-health (**Box 25.11**).

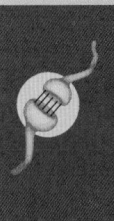

_i_ **Box 25.11 Psychiatric conditions sometimes caused by physical diseases**

Depressive illness
- Hypothyroidism
- Cushing's syndrome
- Steroid treatment
- Brain tumour

Anxiety disorder
- Thyrotoxicosis
- Hypoglycaemia (transient)
- Phaeochromocytoma
- Complex partial seizures (transient)
- Alcohol withdrawal

Irritability
- Post-concussion syndrome
- Frontal lobe syndrome
- Hypoglycaemia (transient)

Memory problem
- Brain tumour
- Hypothyroidism

Altered behaviour
- Acute drug intoxication
- Post-ictal state
- Acute delirium
- Dementia
- Brain tumour

_i_ **Box 25.12 Factors increasing the risk of psychiatric disorders in the general hospital**

Patient factors
- Previous psychiatric history
- Current social or interpersonal stresses
- Homelessness
- Recent alcohol misuse

Setting
- Accident and emergency department
- Neurology, oncology and endocrinology wards
- Intensive care unit
- Renal dialysis unit

Physical conditions
- Chronic ill-health
- Chronic pain
- Life-threatening illness
- Recent bad prognostic news
- Disabling condition
- Brain disease
- Recent live birth, stillbirth or miscarriage
- Functional illness

Treatment
- Certain drugs (e.g. dopamine agonists)
- Second postoperative day
- Surgery affecting body image (e.g. emergency stomata)

- Both the mental and physical symptoms are caused by a common disease process (e.g. Huntington's chorea, Parkinson's disease).
- Physical and mental symptoms and disorders may be independently co-morbid, particularly in the elderly.

Factors that increase the risk of a psychiatric disorder in someone with a physical disease are shown in **Box 25.12**.

Differences in management

Although the basic principles are the same as in treating psychiatric illnesses in the physically healthy, there are some differences:

- *A physical disease or treatment* may be exacerbating the psychiatric condition and may be revealed in the history (see **Box 25.11**); this should then be addressed. For example, dopamine agonists may precipitate a psychosis.
- *Disorders affecting pharmacokinetics* entail a reduction in dosage when psychotropic drugs are prescribed, e.g. fluoxetine in acute kidney injury or hepatic failure.
- *Drug interactions* should be of particular concern, e.g. lithium and non-steroidal anti-inflammatory drugs (NSAIDs).
- *Women who might become pregnant* need to avoid certain drugs, such as sodium valproate, which can cause fetal malformations.
- *A planned physical treatment* may sometimes exacerbate the psychiatric condition. An example would be high-dose steroids

---

_i_ **Box 25.13 'Functional' somatic syndromes**

- 'Tension' headaches
- Atypical facial pain
- Atypical chest pain
- Fibromyalgia (chronic widespread pain)
- Other chronic regional pain syndromes
- Chronic fatigue syndrome
- Multiple chemical sensitivity
- Premenstrual syndrome
- Irritable or functional bowel syndrome
- Irritable bladder

---

as part of chemotherapy in a patient with leukaemia and depressive illness.
- *The risk of suicide* should always be remembered in an inpatient with a mood disorder and steps should be taken to reduce that risk, such as by having a registered mental health nurse attend the patient while at risk.

Further reading

Becker AE, Kleinman A. Mental health and the global agenda. _N Engl J Med_ 2013; 369:66–73.

SICK ROLE AND ILLNESS BEHAVIOUR

The *sick role* describes the behaviour usually adopted by ill people. Such people are not expected to fulfil their normal social obligations. They are treated with sympathy by others and are only obliged to see their doctor and take medical advice or treatments.

Illness behaviour is the way in which given symptoms may be differentially perceived, evaluated and acted (or not acted) upon. We all have illness behaviour when we choose what to do about a symptom. Going to see a doctor is generally more likely with more severe, disabling and numerous symptoms and in introspective individuals who focus on their health.

Abnormal illness behaviour occurs when there is a discrepancy between the objective pathology present and the patient's response to it, in spite of adequate medical investigation and explanation.

FUNCTIONAL SOMATIC SYNDROMES

So-called *functional* (in contrast to 'organic') somatic syndromes are illnesses in which no obvious pathology is found and there is an assumed dysfunction of an organ or system. Examples are given in **Box 25.13**. The psychiatric classification of these disorders might be *somatoform disorders* but they do not fit easily within either medical or psychiatric classification systems, since they occupy the borderland between them. This classification also implies a dualistic 'mind or body' dichotomy, which is not supported by evidence. Since current classifications still support this outmoded understanding, this chapter will address these conditions in this way.

The word *psychosomatic* has had several colloquial meanings, including 'all in the mind', but the modern concept is that psychosomatic disorders are syndromes in which both physical and psychological factors are likely to be causative. So-called medically unexplained symptoms and syndromes are very common in both primary care and the general hospital. Because orthodox medicine has not been particularly effective in treating or understanding these disorders, many patients perceive their doctors as unsympathetic and seek out complementary or even alternative treatments of uncertain efficacy.

Because epidemiological studies suggest that having one of these syndromes significantly increases the risk of having another, some doctors believe that these conditions represent different manifestations of a single 'functional syndrome', indicating a global somatization process, particularly since they are also associated with depressive and anxiety disorders. However, the majority of primary care patients with one of these disorders do not have a mood or other functional disorder. It also seems that it requires a major stress or the development of a co-morbid psychiatric disorder in order for such sufferers to see their doctor, which might explain why doctors are overly impressed with the associations with both stress and psychiatric disorders. Doctors have historically tended to diagnose 'stress' or 'psychosomatic disorders' in people with symptoms that they cannot explain. History is full of such disorders being reclassified as research clarifies the pathology. An example is writer's cramp (see p. 863), which most neurologists agree is a dystonia rather than a neurosis.

The likelihood is that these functional disorders will be reclassified as their causes and pathophysiology are revealed. Functional brain scans and peripheral sensory testing suggest that central nervous system sensitization is found in a number of these disorders, which might help to explain their clustering together.

Chronic fatigue syndrome

There has probably been more controversy over the existence and causes of chronic fatigue syndrome (CFS) than any other functional somatic syndrome in recent decades. There is good evidence for the independent existence of this syndrome, although the diagnosis is made clinically and by exclusion of other fatiguing disorders. Its prevalence is 0.5–2.5% worldwide, mainly depending on how it is defined. It occurs most commonly in women between the ages of 20 and 50 years.

Clinical features

The cardinal symptom is chronic fatigue made worse by minimal exertion. The fatigue is usually both physical and mental, and is most commonly associated with:

- poor concentration
- impaired registration of memory
- alteration in sleep pattern (either insomnia or hypersomnia)
- muscular pain.

Mood disorders are present in a significant minority of patients, and can cause problems in diagnosis because of the overlap in symptoms. These mood disorders may be secondary, independent (co-morbid) or primary (with a misdiagnosis of CFS).

Aetiology

Functional disorders often have some aetiological factors in common with each other (**Box 25.14**), as well as more specific aetiologies. For instance, CFS can be triggered by certain infections, such as infectious mononucleosis and viral hepatitis. About 12% of patients who have infectious mononucleosis have CFS 6 months after the onset of infection, yet there is no evidence of persistent infection in these patients. Those fatigue states that clearly do follow on from a viral infection can also be classified as *post-viral fatigue syndromes*.

Other aetiological factors are uncertain. Immune and endocrine abnormalities noted in CFS may be secondary to the inactivity or

> **? Box 25.14 Aetiological factors commonly seen in 'functional' disorders**
>
> **Predisposing**
> - Perfectionist and introspective personality traits
> - Childhood traumas (physical and sexual abuse)
> - Similar illnesses in first-degree relatives
>
> **Precipitating (triggering)**
> - Infections (CFS, irritable bowel syndrome)
> - Traumatic events (especially accidents)
> - Acute painful conditions ('fibromyalgia' and other chronic pain syndromes)
> - Life events that precipitate changed behaviours (e.g. taking time off sick)
> - Incidents where the patient believes others are responsible
>
> **Perpetuating (maintaining)**
> - Inactivity with consequent physiological adaptation (CFS, 'fibromyalgia')
> - Avoidant behaviours (MCS, CFS)
> - Maladaptive illness beliefs (that maintain maladaptive behaviours) (CFS, MCS)
> - Excessive dietary restrictions ('food allergies')
> - Stimulant drugs (e.g. caffeine)
> - Sleep disturbance
> - Mood disorders
> - Somatization disorder
> - Unresolved anger or guilt
> - Disputed compensation claim
>
> CFS, chronic fatigue syndrome; MCS, multiple chemical sensitivities.

> **ℹ Box 25.15 Management of functional somatic syndromes**
>
> - The first principle is the identification and treatment of maintaining factors (e.g. dysfunctional beliefs and behaviours, mood and sleep disorders)
>
> **Communication**
> - Explanation of ill-health, including diagnosis and causes
> - Education about management (including self-help leaflets)
>
> **Stopping drugs**
> - E.g. caffeine causing insomnia, analgesics causing dependence
>
> **Rehabilitative therapies**
> - Cognitive behaviour therapy (to challenge unhelpful beliefs and change coping strategies)
> - Supervised and graded exercise therapy for approximately 3 months (to reduce inactivity and improve fitness)
>
> **Pharmacotherapies**
> - Specific antidepressants for mood disorders, analgesia and sleep disturbance (e.g. 10–50 mg of amitriptyline at night for sleep and pain)
> - Symptomatic medicines (e.g. appropriate analgesia, taken only when necessary)

sleep disturbance commonly seen. The role of stress is uncertain, with some indication that the influence of stress is mediated through consequent psychiatric disorders exacerbating fatigue, rather than any direct effect.

Management

The general principles of the management of functional disorders are given in **Box 25.15**. Specific management of CFS should include a mutually agreed and supervised programme of gradually increasing activity. However, only about a quarter of patients recover after treatment. It is sometimes difficult to persuade a patient to accept what are inappropriately perceived as 'psychological therapies' for such a physically manifested condition.

Antidepressants do not work in the absence of a mood disorder, pain or insomnia.

Prognosis

Prognosis is poor without treatment, with less than 10% of hospital attenders recovered after 1 year. Outcomes are worse with greater severity, increasing age, co-morbid mood disorders, and the conviction that the illness is entirely physical. A large trial showed that about 60% improve with active rehabilitative treatments, such as graded exercise therapy and cognitive behaviour therapy, when added to specialist medical care.

Fibromyalgia (chronic widespread pain)

Fibromyalgia is characterized by widespread muscle and joint pain but is also associated with chronic fatigue and sleep disturbance. The 'tender points', previously used diagnostically (see p. 430), are no longer used but their importance is still argued by some. It is commonest in women aged 40–65 years, and has a prevalence in the community of 1–11%, varying by definition. There are associations with depressive and anxiety disorders, other functional disorders, physical deconditioning and a possibly characteristic sleep disturbance (see **Box 25.14**). Functional brain scans and peripheral sensory testing support the idea of an underlying abnormal sensory processing that may be related to abnormal regulation of central opioidergic mechanisms.

Management

Apart from the general principles set out in **Box 25.15**, management consists of:

- centrally acting analgesia
- reversal of the sleep disturbance
- a physically orientated rehabilitation programme.

A meta-analysis suggests that tricyclic antidepressants such as amitriptyline and dosulepin that inhibit reuptake of both serotonin (5-hydroxytryptamine, 5-HT) and noradrenaline (norepinephrine) have the greatest effect on sleep and pain. The doses used are too low to exert an antidepressant effect and the drugs may work primarily through their hypnotic effects. Other centrally acting anti-nociceptive agents that are also antidepressants include duloxetine and milnacipran (not available in the UK), used at full doses and the gabapentinoids, pregabalin and gabapentin.

Other chronic pain syndromes

A chronic pain syndrome is a condition of chronic disabling pain for which no medical cause can be found. The psychiatric classification would be a persistent **somatoform pain disorder**; this is unsatisfactory since the criteria stipulate that emotional factors must be the main cause, of which it is difficult to be clinically certain.

The most commonly affected sites are the lower back, abdomen, genitalia, head, face, neck or all over (fibromyalgia). 'Functional' low back pain is the most common 'physical' reason for being off sick long term in the UK (see p. 421). Quite often, minor abnormalities are found on investigation but are not severe enough to explain the severity of the pain and resultant disability. These pains are often unremitting and respond poorly to analgesics. Sleep disturbance is almost universal and co-morbid psychiatric disorders are commonly found.

Aetiology

The perception of pain involves sensory (nociceptive), emotional and cognitive processing in the brain. Functional brain scans suggest that the brain responds abnormally to pain in these conditions, with increased activation in response to chronic pain. Alongside this, the brain's ability to inhibit pain through descending mechanisms in the spinal cord is impaired. The brain may then adapt to the prolonged stimulus of the pain by changing its central processing. The insula, striatum, thalamus and cingulate gyrus seem to be particularly affected, all of which are involved in the experience of pain in general. Thus, it is possible to start to understand how interactions between physiology, cognitions, emotions and behaviour might influence the perception of chronic pain.

Management

Management involves the same principles as are applied in other functional syndromes (see **Box 25.15**). Since analgesics are rarely effective and can cause long-term harm, patients should be encouraged to reduce their use gradually. It is often helpful to involve the patient's immediate family or partner, to ensure that the partner is also supported and not unconsciously discouraging progress.

Specific drug treatments are few:

- **Nerve blocks** are not usually effective.
- **Gabapentinoids:** gabapentin and pregabalin (see p. 825).
- **Dual-acting antidepressants** (serotonin and noradrenaline reuptake inhibitors, SNRIs, e.g. duloxetine) affect both serotonin and noradrenaline (norepinephrine) reuptake; these demonstrate the greatest efficacy. Low-dose tricyclic antidepressants that affect both of these neurotransmitters (e.g. amitriptyline, dosulepin) are also effective, although this may be primarily through an improvement in sleep. Selective serotonin reuptake inhibitors, SSRIs, are less effective, except in the presence of co-morbid anxiety and depressive disorders.

Irritable bowel syndrome

This is one of the most common functional somatic syndromes, affecting some 10–30% of the population worldwide. The clinical features and management of irritable bowel syndrome (IBS) and related functional bowel disorders are described in more detail in on page 1187. Although the majority of people with IBS do not have a psychiatric disorder, depressive illness should be excluded in those with constipation and a poor appetite. Anxiety disorders should be excluded in individuals with nausea and diarrhoea. Persistent abdominal pain or a feeling of emptiness may occasionally be the presenting symptom of a severe depressive illness, particularly in the elderly, with a **nihilistic delusion** that the body is empty or dead inside (see p. 776).

Management

This is dealt with in more detail in **Box 25.15**. Seeing a physician who provides specific education addressing individual illness beliefs and concerns can provide lasting benefit.

Antidepressants are frequently indicated in moderate to severe cases and the choice of agent will depend on the presence of pain, sleep disturbance and psychiatric co-morbidity, as well as the effect of drug families on bowel transit times (e.g. this is reduced with SSRIs). Milder cases will often respond well to low doses of amitriptyline, although this may be poorly tolerated. Non-pharmacological treatments are also important considerations, most commonly cognitive behaviour therapy.

Multiple chemical sensitivity, *Candida* hypersensitivity and food allergies

Some complementary health practitioners, doctors and patients themselves make diagnoses of multiple chemical sensitivities (MCS) (e.g. to foods, smoking, perfumes, petrol), *Candida* hypersensitivity and allergies (to food, tap water and even electricity). Symptoms and syndromes attributed to these putative disorders are numerous and variable, and include all the functional disorders, **mood disorders** and **arthritis**. Scientific support for the existence of these disorders is weak, particularly when double-blind methodologies have been used.

Type 1 hypersensitivities to foods such as nuts certainly exist, although they are fortunately uncommon (approximately 3/1000) (see p. 62). Direct **specific food intolerances** also occur (e.g. chocolate with migraine, caffeine with IBS).

Candidiasis can occur in the gastrointestinal tract in immunocompromised individuals, such as those with the acquired immunodeficiency syndrome (AIDS). Vaginal candidiasis can follow antibiotic treatment in otherwise healthy women. A double-blind and controlled study of nystatin in women diagnosed as having candidiasis hypersensitivity syndrome showed that vaginitis was the only condition relieved more by nystatin than placebo. There is little evidence of *Candida* having a systemic role in other symptoms. In spite of this evidence, the patient is often convinced of the legitimacy and usefulness of these diagnoses and their treatments.

Aetiology

Surveys of patients diagnosed with MCS or food allergies have shown high rates of current and previous mood and anxiety disorders (see **Box 25.14**). Eating disorders (see p. 797) should be excluded in people with food intolerances. Some patients taking very-low-carbohydrate diets as putative treatments may develop reactive hypoglycaemia after a high carbohydrate meal, which they then interpret as a food allergy.

Classical conditioning can produce intolerance to foods and smells in healthy people and this may be a causative mechanism in some individuals with intolerances. This supports the existence of these intolerance conditions, but suggests they may be conditioned responses with attendant physiological consequences. This might explain why double-blinding sometimes abolishes the reaction to the stimulus.

Management

The general principles in **Box 25.15** apply. If one assumes a phobic or conditioned response is responsible, graded exposure (systematic desensitization) to the conditioned stimulus may be worthwhile. Preliminary studies do suggest that this approach may successfully treat such intolerances, in the context of cognitive behaviour therapy.

Premenstrual syndrome

The premenstrual syndrome (PMS) consists of both physical and psychological symptoms that regularly occur during the premenstrual phase and substantially diminish or disappear soon after the period starts.

- **Physical symptoms**: headache, fatigue, breast tenderness, abdominal distension and fluid retention.
- **Psychological symptoms**: irritability, emotional lability or low mood, and tension.

The **premenstrual (late luteal) dysphoric disorder (PMDD)** is a severe form of PMS with marked mood swings, irritability,

depression and anxiety accompanying the physical symptoms. Women who suffer from mood disorders may be more prone to experience this. The prevalence of PMS does not vary between cultures and is reported by the majority (75%) of women at some time in their lives. PMDD occurs in 3–8% of women.

The cause of PMS remains unclear, although exacerbating factors include some of those outlined in **Box 25.14**. Sex hormone receptor abnormalities may play a role.

Management

The general principles in **Box 25.15** apply. Treatments with vitamin B_6 (see p. 1241), diuretics, progesterone, oral contraceptives, oil of evening primrose, and oestrogen implants or patches (balanced by cyclical norethisterone) remain empirical. Psychotherapies aimed at enhancing the patient's coping skills can reduce disability. Two trials suggest that graded exercise therapy improves symptoms. Several studies have demonstrated that SSRIs (see p. 780) are effective treatments for PMDD.

Menopause

The clinical features and management of the menopause are described on page 1468. A prospective study has shown that there is no increased incidence of depressive disorders at this time. Menopausal vasomotor symptoms are associated with sleep disturbance that may give rise to mood disturbance. Such a significant bodily change, sometimes occurring at the same time as children leave home, is naturally accompanied by an emotional adjustment that does not normally amount to a pathological state.

Further reading

Bass C, Hallingan P. Factitious disorders and malingering: challenges for clinical assessment and management. *Lancet* 2014; 383:1422–1432.
Bourke JH, Langford RM, White PD. The common link between functional somatic syndromes may be central sensitisation. *J Psychosomatic Research* 2015; 78:228–236
Ford AC, Talley NJ, Schoenfeld PS et al. Efficacy of antidepressants and psychological therapies in irritable bowel syndrome: systematic review and meta-analysis. *Gut* 2009; 58:367–378.
White PD, Goldsmith KA, Johnson AL et al. Comparison of adaptive pacing therapy, cognitive behaviour therapy, graded exercise therapy, and specialist medical care for chronic fatigue syndrome (PACE): a randomised trial. *Lancet* 2011; 377:823–836.
Yonkers KA, O'Brien PM, Eriksson E. Premenstrual syndrome. *Lancet* 2008; 371:1200–1210.

SOMATOFORM DISORDERS

As explained in the section on functional disorders (see p. 769), the classification of somatoform disorders is unsatisfactory because of their uncertain nature and aetiology. However, there are certain disorders, beyond those described above, that present frequently and coherently enough to be usefully recognized.

Somatization disorder

One in ten patients presenting with a functional disorder will fulfil the criteria of a chronic somatization disorder. The condition is composed of multiple, recurrent, medically unexplained physical symptoms, usually starting early in adult life. Symptoms may be referred to almost any part or bodily system. The patient has often had multiple medical opinions and repeated negative investigations. Medical reassurance fails to reassure the patient, who will continue to 'doctor-shop' and is usually reluctant to accept that psychological and/or social factors may play a role. Abnormal illness behaviour is evident and patients may become increasingly dependent on doctors.

The aetiology is unknown, but both mood and personality disorders are often also present. Somatization disorder is frequently associated with dependence upon or overuse of prescribed medication, usually sedatives and analgesics. There is often a history of significant childhood traumas, or chronic ill-health in the child or parent, which may play an aetiological role or help to explain difficult therapeutic relationships. The condition is probably the somatic presentation of psychological distress, although iatrogenic damage (from postoperative and drug-related problems) soon complicates the clinical picture. It is a chronic and disabling disorder, with longstanding family, relationship and/or occupational problems.

Hypochondriasis

The conspicuous feature is a preoccupation with an assumed serious disease and its consequences. Patients commonly believe that they suffer from cancer or some other serious condition. Characteristically, such patients repeatedly request investigations either to prove they are ill or to reassure themselves that they are well. Such reassurance rarely lasts long before another cycle of worry and requests begins. The symptom of hypochondriasis may be secondary to or associated with a variety of psychiatric disorders, particularly depressive and anxiety disorders. Occasionally, the hypochondriasis is delusional, secondary to schizophrenia or a depressive psychosis. Hypochondriasis may coexist with physical disease but the diagnostic point is that the patient's concern is disproportionate and unjustified.

Management of somatoform disorders

The principles outlined in **Box 25.15** apply to these disorders. Given their poor prognosis, the aim is to minimize disability. It is vital that all members of staff and close family members adopt the same approach to the patient's problems as the patient will often, consciously or unconsciously, split both medical staff and family members into 'good' and 'bad' (or caring and uncaring) people, as a way of projecting their distress.

Patients appreciate a discussion and explanation of their symptoms. You should sensitively explore possible psychological and social difficulties, if possible by asking about or demonstrating links between symptoms and stresses. Such discussion usually gives information that can be used to formulate an agreed plan of management. A contract of mutually agreed care, involving the appropriate professionals (general practitioner, and a choice of psychotherapist, physician or psychiatrist), with agreed frequency of visits and a review date, can be helpful in managing the condition. Management also includes cessation of reassurance that no serious disease has been uncovered, since this simply reinforces dependence on the doctor. Repeated investigations should be discouraged. Cognitive behaviour therapy has been shown to provide effective rehabilitation in significant numbers of patients suffering from a somatoform disorder.

DISSOCIATIVE/CONVERSION DISORDERS

Increasingly, these disorders are referred to as 'functional neurological disorders'.

A **dissociative disorder** is a condition in which there is a profound loss of awareness or cognitive ability without medical explanation. The term dissociative indicates the disintegration of different mental activities, and covers such phenomena as amnesia, fugues and non-epileptic attacks.

Conversion disorder occurs when an unresolved conflict is converted into, usually symbolic, physical symptoms as a defence against it. Such symptoms commonly include paralysis, abnormal movements, sensory loss, aphonia, disorders of gait and pseudocyesis (false pregnancy). The lifetime prevalence has been estimated at 3–6 per 1000 in women, with a lower prevalence in men. Most cases begin before the age of 35 years and are unusual in the elderly.

Clinical features

The various symptoms are usually divided into dissociative and conversion categories (**Box 25.16**). Dissociative disorders have the following three characteristics that are necessary in order to make the diagnosis:

- They occur in the absence of physical pathology that would fully explain the symptoms.
- They are produced unconsciously.
- Symptoms are not caused by overactivity of the sympathetic nervous system.
  Other characteristics include:
- Symptoms and signs often reflect a patient's ideas about illness.
- There is usually abnormal illness behaviour, with exaggeration of disability.
- There may have been significant childhood traumas.
- **Primary gain** is the immediate relief from the emotional conflict.
- **Secondary gain** refers to the social advantage gained by the patient by being ill and disabled (sympathy of family and friends, time off work, disability pension).
- Physical disease is, not uncommonly, also present (e.g. pseudoseizures are more common in someone with epilepsy).

Dissociative amnesia commences suddenly. Patients are unable to recall long periods of their lives and may even deny any knowledge of their previous life or personal identity. In a **dissociative fugue**, patients not only lose their memory but also wander away from their usual surroundings; when found, they have no memory of their whereabouts during this wandering. The differential diagnosis of a fugue state includes post-epileptic automatism, depressive illness and alcohol misuse.

Multiple personality disorder is rare but dramatic, and may be triggered by suggestion on the part of a psychotherapist. There are rapid alterations between two or more 'personalities' in the same

---

> *i* **Box 25.16 Common dissociative/conversion symptoms**
>
> **Dissociative (mental)**
> - Amnesia
> - Fugue
> - Pseudodementia
> - Dissociative identity disorder
>
> **Conversion (physical)**
> - Paralysis
> - Disorders of gait
> - Tremor
> - Aphonia
> - Mutism
> - Sensory symptoms
> - Globus
> - Pseudoseizures
> - Blindness

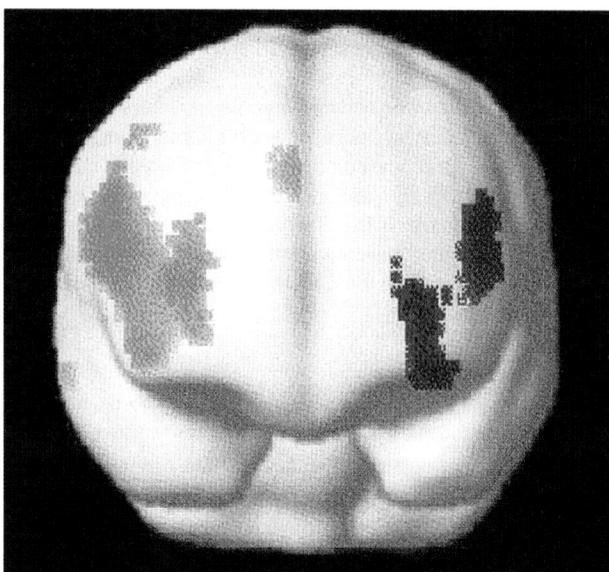

Fig. 25.1 Statistical parametric maps superimposed on a magnetic resonance imaging scan of the anterior surface of the brain, orientated as though looking at a person head on. The red region shows hypofunction of people with conversion motor symptoms. The green region shows hypofunction of healthy controls feigning the same motor abnormality. (*From Spence SA, Crimlisk HL, Cope H et al. Discrete neurophysiological correlates in prefrontal cortex during hysterical and feigned disorders of movement. Lancet 2000; 355:1243–1244, with permission.*)

person, each of which is repressed and dissociated from the other 'personalities'. A differential diagnosis is rapid-cycling bipolar affective disorder, which would explain sudden apparent changes in personality.

Differential diagnosis

Dissociation is usually a stable and reliable diagnosis over time, although high rates of co-morbid mood and personality disorders are found in chronic sufferers. Particular care should be taken to make the diagnosis on positive grounds, and not simply on the basis of an absence of a medical diagnosis. Care should also be taken to exclude or treat co-morbid psychiatric disorders.

Aetiology

Functional brain scans differ between healthy controls feigning a motor abnormality and people with a similar conversion motor symptom, which suggests that dissociation involves different areas of the brain from simulation (**Fig. 25.1**). Functional brain scanning of a patient with conversion paralysis has shown that recalling a past trauma not only activated the emotional areas, such as the amygdala, but also reduced motor cortex activity. This would suggest that conversion involves a disinhibition of voluntary will at an unconscious level, so that the patient can no longer *will* something to happen.

The psychoanalytical theory of dissociation is that it is the result of emotionally charged memories that are repressed into the unconscious at some point in the past. Symptoms are explained as the combined effects of repression and the symbolic conversion of this emotional energy into physical symptoms. This hypothesis is

 Box 25.17 Example of an explanation that might be given for a dissociative disorder

'You told me about the tremendous shock you felt when your mother suddenly died. This was particularly the case since you hadn't spoken to her for so long beforehand, after that big disagreement with her over your wedding to John. You weren't able to say goodbye before she died. Your brain was overloaded with grief, guilt and anger all at once. I wonder whether that is why you aren't able to speak now. I wonder whether it's difficult to think of anything to say that would make things right, particularly since you can't speak with your mother now.'

difficult to test, although there is some evidence that people with dissociative disorders are more likely to have suffered childhood abuse. Caution should be taken when such a history is obtained by therapies that recover childhood memories previously completely unknown to the patient.

Management

The treatment of dissociation is similar to the treatment of somatoform disorders (see **Box 25.15**). The first task is to engage the patient and their family with an acceptable explanation of the illness that makes sense to them and leads to the appropriate management (**Box 25.17**). Such an explanation would be modified by mutual discussion until an agreed understanding was achieved, which would serve as a working model for the illness. Provision of a rehabilitation programme that addresses both the physical and the psychological needs of the patient would then be planned.

- *A graded and mutually agreed plan for a return to normal function* can usually be led by the appropriate therapist (e.g. speech therapist for dysphonia, physiotherapist for paralysis).
- *A psychotherapeutic assessment* should be made at the same time, in order to determine the most appropriate psychotherapy. For instance, couple therapy will address a significant relationship difficulty; individual psychotherapy could ease an unresolved conflict from childhood (see p. 788).

Abreaction brought about by *hypnosis* or by intravenous injections of small amounts of midazolam may produce a dramatic, if sometimes short-lived, recovery. In the abreactive state, the patient is encouraged to relive the stressful events that provoked the disorder and to express the accompanying emotions: that is, to abreact. It should only be contemplated in the presence of an anaesthetist with suitable resuscitation equipment to hand.

Hypnotherapy is psychotherapy applied while the patient is in a hypnotic trance, the idea being that therapy is more easily possible because the patient is relaxed and not using repression. This may allow the therapist access to the previously unconscious emotional conflicts or memories. There are no published trials of this technique in dissociation. Care should be taken to avoid a catastrophic emotional reaction when the patient is suddenly faced with the previously repressed memories.

Prognosis

Most cases of recent onset recover quickly with treatment, while chronicity predicts a worse outcome (with the exception of non-epileptic attack disorder where it has no impact), emphasizing the importance of early diagnosis. One study found that 83% were still unwell at 12 years' follow-up.

SLEEP DIFFICULTIES

Sleep is divided into rapid eye movement (REM) and non-REM sleep:

- As drowsiness begins, the alpha rhythm on an electroencephalogram (EEG) disappears and is replaced by deepening **slow-wave** activity **(non-REM).**
- After 60–90 minutes, this slow-wave pattern is replaced by low-amplitude waves, on which are superimposed **rapid eye movements** lasting a few minutes.
- This cycle is repeated during the duration of sleep, with the REM periods becoming longer and the slow-wave periods shorter and less deep **(Fig. 25.2).**

REM sleep is accompanied by dreaming and physiological arousal. **Slow-wave sleep** is associated with release of anabolic hormones and cytokines, with an increased cellular mitotic rate. It helps to maintain host defences, metabolism and repair of cells. For this reason, slow-wave sleep is increased in those conditions where growth or conservation is required (e.g. adolescence, pregnancy, thyrotoxicosis).

Insomnia

Insomnia is difficulty in sleeping; a third of adults complain of insomnia, and in a third of these it can be severe.

Sleep disorders secondary to another medical diagnosis will not be discussed here.

Primary sleep disorders

These include sleep apnoea (see p. 960), narcolepsy (p. 858), the **restless legs syndrome** (Wittmaack–Ekbom's syndrome, also known as Willis–Ekbom disease; see p. 858) and the related **periodic leg movement disorder**, in which the legs (and sometimes the arms) jerk while asleep.

Delayed sleep phase syndrome

This occurs when the circadian pattern of sleep is delayed, so that the patient sleeps from the early hours until midday or later; it is most common in young people.

Parasomnias

Night terrors, **sleep-walking** and **sleep-talking** are non-REM phenomena, called parasomnias; they are most commonly found in children, but can recur in adults when under stress or suffering from a mood disorder.

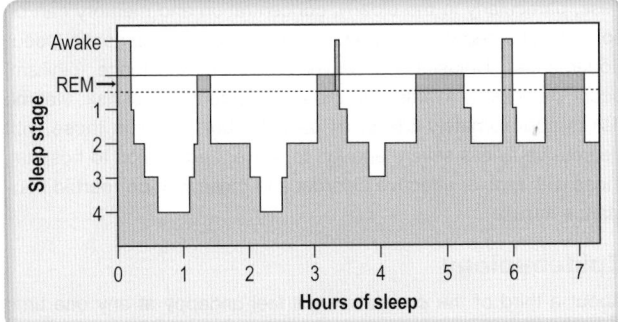

Fig. 25.2 Sleep architecture. Cycles of slow-wave sleep are interspersed with rapid eye movement (REM) sleep. Sleep is 'staged' by the electroencephalogram (EEG). Deeper sleep (stages 3 and 4) is demonstrated by slow waves on the EEG. Sleep occurs in cycles, light sleep (accompanied by REM sleep and dreaming) to deep sleep and back again, and these cycles last about 90 minutes.

Psychophysiological insomnia

This is commonly secondary to functional, mood and substance misuse disorders, and is frequently present in individuals under stress. It can often be triggered by one of these factors before becoming a habit on its own, driven by anticipation of insomnia and daytime naps.

Clinical Features

Insomnia causes daytime sleepiness and fatigue, with consequences such as road traffic accidents. Assessment should focus on mood, life difficulties and drug intake (especially alcohol, nicotine and caffeine). The timing of the insomnia should be ascertained:

- **Initial insomnia** (trouble going off to sleep) is common in mania, anxiety, depressive disorders and substance misuse.
- **Middle insomnia** (waking up in the middle of the night) occurs with medical conditions such as sleep apnoea and prostatism.
- **Late insomnia** (early morning wakening) is caused by depressive illness and malnutrition (anorexia nervosa).

Habitual **alcohol** consumption should be estimated, since even a small excess can be a potent cause of insomnia, as well as recent withdrawal. The effects of **caffeine** are easily under-estimated. Six cups of coffee a day are likely to cause insomnia in the average healthy adult. Caffeine is found not only in tea and coffee, but also in chocolate, cola drinks and some analgesics. Prescription drugs that can either disturb sleep or cause vivid dreams include appetite suppressants, glucocorticoids, dopamine agonists, lipid-soluble beta-blockers (e.g. propranolol) and certain psychotropic drugs (especially on initiation, e.g. fluoxetine, risperidone).

Hypersomnia

This is not uncommon in adolescents with depressive illness. It occurs in narcolepsy, and may temporarily follow infections such as infectious mononucleosis.

Management of insomnia

This is determined by diagnosis. Where none is immediately apparent, it is worth educating the patient about sleep hygiene. In addition:

- **Simple measures**, such as decreasing alcohol intake, having supper earlier, exercising daily, having a hot bath prior to going to bed and establishing a routine of going to bed at a consistent time, should all be tried.
- **Relaxation techniques and cognitive behaviour therapy** have a role in those with intractable insomnia.
- **Short-half-life benzodiazepines** can be useful for acute insomnia, but should not be used for more than 2 weeks continuously to avoid dependence.

> **?** **Box 25.18 Common causes of insomnia**
>
> **Primary sleep disorders**
> - Periodic leg movements
> - Restless legs syndrome
>
> **Secondary sleep disorders**
> - Psychiatric disorders:
>   - Mood disorders (mania, depressive and anxiety disorders)
>   - Delirium and dementia
> - Drug use or misuse:
>   - Addictive drug withdrawal (alcohol, benzodiazepines)
>   - Stimulant drugs (caffeine, amfetamines)
>   - Prescribed drugs (steroids, dopamine agonists)
> - Physical conditions:
>   - Pain (classically with carpal tunnel syndrome)
>   - Nocturia (e.g. from prostatism)
>   - Malnutrition

- ***Non-benzodiazepine hypnotics*** (zaleplon, zopiclone, zolpidem) act at γ-aminobutyric acid type A (GABA-A) receptors and occasional dependence has been reported.
- ***Certain antihistamines*** (e.g. diphenhydramine and promethazine) and ***antidepressants*** (e.g. amitriptyline, trazodone, mirtazapine) are not addictive and can be used as hypnotics in low dose, with the added advantage of improving slow-wave sleep. The most common adverse effects are morning sedation and weight gain.

Further reading

Falloon K, Arroll B, Elley CR et al. The assessment and management of insomnia in primary care. *BMJ* 2011; 342:d2899.
Morin CM, Benca R. Chronic insomnia. *Lancet* 2012; 379:1129–1141.
van Straten A et al. Cognitive and behavioral therapies in the treatment of insomnia: a meta-analysis. *Sleep Med Rev* 2018; 38:3–1.

MOOD (AFFECTIVE) DISORDERS

The central feature of these disorders is an abnormality of mood. Mood is best described in terms of a continuum ranging from severe depression at one extreme to severe mania at the other, with normal, stable mood in the middle. Mood disorders are divided into unipolar and bipolar affective disorders.

Unipolar affective disorders

Patients suffer from depressive episodes alone, which are commonly recurrent.

Bipolar affective disorder

Patients suffer bouts of both depression and mania. Although mania can occur by itself without depressive episodes, it is far more commonly found in association with them, although it can take several years for the first depressive illness to appear.
- ***Bipolar I*** disorder is defined as one or more manic or mixed (signs of mania and depression) episodes.
- ***Bipolar II*** is defined as a depressive episode with at least one episode of hypomania (this is shorter-lived than mania and is not accompanied by psychotic symptoms). Hypomania is noticeably abnormal but does not result in functional impairment or hospitalization.
- ***Bipolar III*** disorder is less well established and describes depressive episodes, with hypomania occurring only when taking an antidepressant.

About 10% of patients who have depressive illness are eventually found to have a bipolar illness.

Depressive disorders

Depressive disorders or 'episodes' are classified by the ICD-10 as mild, moderate or severe, with or without somatic symptoms. Severe depressive episodes are divided according to the presence or absence of psychotic symptoms.

Clinical features of depressive disorder

Whereas everyone will, at some time or other, feel 'fed up' or 'down in the dumps', it is when such symptoms become qualitatively different and pervasive or interfere with normal functioning that a depressive illness has occurred. Depressive disorder, clinical or 'major' depression, is characterized by disturbances of mood, speech, energy and ideas (**Box 25.19**). Patients often describe their

---

> ℹ️ **Box 25.19 Characteristic features of depressive illness**

Characteristic	Clinical features
Mood	Depressed, miserable or irritable
Speech	Impoverished, slow, monotonous
Energy	Reduced, lethargic, lacking motivation
Ideas	Feelings of futility, guilt, self-reproach, unworthiness, hypochondriacal preoccupations, worrying, suicidal thoughts, delusions of guilt, nihilism and persecution
Cognition	Impaired learning, pseudodementia in elderly patients
Physical	Insomnia (especially early waking), poor appetite and weight loss, constipation, loss of libido, erectile dysfunction, bodily pains
Behaviour	Retardation or agitation, poverty of movement and expression
Hallucinations	Auditory – often hostile, critical

> ℹ️ **Box 25.20 Screening questions for depressive illness**

- During the last month, have you often been bothered by feeling down, depressed or hopeless?
- During the last month, have you often been bothered by having little interest or pleasure in doing things?
- If the answer to one or both of these questions is 'yes', assess further for depressive illness

---

symptoms in physical terms. Marked fatigue and headache are the two most common physical symptoms in depressive illness and may be the first symptoms to appear. Patients describe the world as looking grey, and themselves as lacking a zest for living, and being devoid of pleasure and interest in life (anhedonia). Anxiety and panic attacks are common; secondary obsessional and phobic symptoms may emerge. Symptoms should last for at least 2 weeks and cause significant incapacity (e.g. trouble working or relating to others) in order to be considered an illness.

In the more severe forms, diurnal variation in mood can occur, patients feeling worse in the morning, after waking in the early hours with apprehension. Suicidal ideas are more frequent, intrusive and prolonged. Delusions of guilt, persecution and bodily disease are not uncommon, along with second-person auditory hallucinations insulting the patient or suggesting suicide. In severe depressive illness, particularly in the elderly, concentration and memory can be so badly affected that the patient appears to have dementia (pseudodementia). Delusions of poverty and non-existence (nihilism) occur particularly in this age group. Suicide is a real risk; lifetime risk is approximately 6% in all patients, but higher in those with depressive illness severe enough to warrant admission to hospital, those with bipolar affective disorder and those with co-morbid substance misuse.

Epidemiology

About a third of the population will feel unhappy at any one time but this is not the same as depressive illness; the middle-aged feel least happy compared with the young and elderly. The point prevalence of depressive illness is 5% in the community, with a further 3% having dysthymia (see below). It is more common in women, but there is no increase with age, and no difference by ethnic or socioeconomic group (apart from a clear association with unemployment). Married and never-married people have similar prevalence rates, with separated and divorced people having two to three times the prevalence. Depressive illnesses are becoming more common and are more frequently found in the presence of:

- physical diseases, particularly if chronic, stigmatizing or painful
- excessive and chronic alcohol use
- social stresses, particularly loss events, such as separation, redundancy and bereavement
- interpersonal difficulties with those close to the patient, especially when socially humiliated
- lack of social support, with no confiding relationship

Depressed people with another physical disorder view themselves as more sick and disabled, visit their doctors almost four times as often, stay in hospital longer, adhere less to medical advice and medication, and undergo more medical and surgical procedures. Depressive illness may be associated with increased mortality (excluding suicide) in people with physical illness, such as myocardial infarct.

Dysthymia

Dysthymia is a mild or moderate depressive illness that lasts intermittently for 2 years or more and is characterized by tiredness and low mood, lack of pleasure and low self-esteem. The mood relapses and remits, with several weeks of feeling well, soon followed by longer periods of being unwell. It can be punctuated by depressive episodes of greater severity, so-called 'double depression'.

Seasonal affective disorder

Seasonal affective disorder is characterized by recurrent episodes of depressive illness occurring during the winter months in the northern hemisphere. Symptoms are similar to an atypical depressive illness, with hypersomnia, increased appetite (with carbohydrate craving) and weight gain, and profound fatigue. Such patients have a higher prevalence of bipolar affective disorder, and some doctors are uncertain whether the condition is different from normal depressive illness, with the accentuation of mood that naturally occurs by season. However, there is evidence that seasonal depressive illness can be successfully treated with bright light therapy given in the early morning, which causes a phase advance in the circadian rhythm of melatonin. By contrast, the same treatment given in the evening has less antidepressant effect. Selective serotonin reuptake inhibitors (SSRIs) are alternative treatments.

Puerperal affective disorders

Affective illnesses and distress are common in women soon after they have given birth.

'Baby blues' describe the brief episodes of emotional lability, irritability and tearfulness arising in about 50% of women 2–3 days postpartum and resolving spontaneously in a few days.

Postpartum psychosis occurs once in every 500–1000 births. Over 80% of cases are an affective psychosis and the onset is usually within the first 2 weeks following delivery. Disorientation and confusion are often noted. Severely depressed patients may have delusional ideas that the child is deformed, evil or otherwise affected in some way, and such false ideas may lead to either attempts to kill the child or attempts at suicide. The response to speedy treatment is generally good. The recurrence rate for a psychosis in a subsequent puerperium is 20–30%.

Non-psychotic postnatal depressive disorders occur during the first postpartum year in 10% of mothers, especially in the first 3 months, with a higher prevalence in developing countries. Risk factors are first pregnancy, poor relationship with the partner, ambivalence about the pregnancy, and emotional personality traits.

A lack of emotional bonding with the baby is a common consequence. The Edinburgh Postnatal Depression Scale (EPDS) is a ten-item questionnaire that can be used as an effective screening tool.

Differential diagnosis of depressive disorders

See **Box 25.21**. Other psychiatric disorders are the most common misdiagnoses. Some 90% of patients presenting with a depressive illness while misusing alcohol will no longer be depressed 2 weeks after their last drink.

Pathological (abnormal) grief and normal grief are described on page 788. Pathological grief is closely associated with depressive illness.

Investigation of depressive disorders

A corroborative history can be valuable in helping to exclude differential diagnoses such as alcohol misuse, and in elucidating perpetuating factors such as a poor relationship with a partner. Investigations should be guided by the history and examination, but those commonly performed are:

- full blood count, urea and electrolytes, serum creatinine, estimated glomerular filtration rate (eGFR)
- liver biochemistry (including glutamyl transpeptidase)
- serum calcium
- erythrocyte sedimentation rate/C-reactive protein (ESR/CRP)
- thyroid function tests (free T_4, thyroid-stimulating hormone (TSH))
  Other tests include:
- serum cortisol (morning and evening)
- antinuclear antibody
- chest X-ray
- EEG or brain scan, as indicated.

Aetiology of unipolar depressive disorders

The aetiology of unipolar depressive disorders is multifactorial and is composed of a mixture of genetic and environmental factors.

Genetic factors

Unipolar depression is probably polygenic but no linkage has been firmly identified. The risk of unipolar depression in a first-degree relative of a patient is approximately three times that in the non-affected. The concordance of unipolar depression in monozygotic twins is between 30% and 60%, increasing with more recurrent illnesses.

Box 25.21 Common differential diagnoses of depressive illness

Other psychiatric disorders

- Alcohol misuse
- Amfetamine (and derivatives) misuse and withdrawal
- Borderline personality disorder
- Dementia
- Delirium
- Schizophrenia
- Normal and pathological grief

Organic (secondary) affective illness

Physical causes that are both necessary and sufficient as a cause

- Cushing syndrome
- Thyroid disease (although sometimes depression persists after treatment)
- Hyperparathyroidism
- Corticosteroid treatment
- Brain tumour (rarely without other neurological signs)

Polymorphisms that increase the risk of depression involve mono-amines and their receptors, but studies are inconclusive. Recent research suggests a possible role for epigenetic changes. The issue is complicated by genetic influences on sleep, emotional personality and even life events, which are all involved in the genesis of depressive illness.

Biochemical changes

Monoamines

The monoamine deficiency theory of depressive illness is supported by the efficacy of monoamine reuptake inhibitors and the depressive effect of dietary tryptophan depletion. There is, however a discrepancy between the timing of changes in neurotransmitter metabolism and clinical improvement.

Neuroimaging studies have revealed a raised density of mono-amine oxidase A (MAO-A) receptors. Depression is proposed to be related to a chronic and on-going depletion of these neurotrans-mitters as a result of increased MAO-A activity and its interaction with region-specific monoamine transporter densities. Together, these are then thought to determine the particular expression of the depressive illness and the predominance of particular symptoms.

Neuroendocrine tests suggest that the serotonin neurotransmit-ter system is downregulated. 5-HT$_{1a}$ and 5-HT$_2$ receptor subtypes are thought most likely to be involved. Receptor-labelled functional brain scans suggest that dopamine underactivity relates to anhedo-nia and psychomotor retardation.

Hypothalamo–pituitary–adrenal axis

Exogenous steroids are associated with the onset of depres-sive symptoms and people with Cushing's syndrome often dem-onstrate depressive episodes. Acute stress, whether physical or psychological, is associated with a rise in serum glucocorticoids. Severe depressive episodes have been linked with hypercortisolae-mia (although cortisol is low in 'atypical' depression), but whether this is aetiological or secondary to sleep disturbance and weight loss is unknown. This cortisol dysregulation has been associated with impaired glucocorticoid negative feedback, adrenal hyper-responsiveness to adrenocorticotrophic hormone (ACTH) and hypersecretion of cortisol-releasing hormone (CRH).

Exposure to the high levels of cortisol is thought to have a direct effect on neuronal plasticity and to lower resistance to neu-ronal damage. The hippocampus seems especially susceptible, resulting in atrophic changes. This, in turn, has further deleteri-ous effects on wider neuroendocrine function, leading to a self-perpetuating dysregulation that may serve to maintain and/or worsen the illness.

The interplay at this level becomes more complicated, with reduced central and peripheral glucocorticoid receptor sensitivity, hypothalamo–pituitary–adrenal (HPA) axis upregulation, and the release of pro-inflammatory cytokines that may, in turn, explain changes in mood, fatigue, appetite, sensitivity to pain and reduced libido (note that depression is a side-effect of interferon treatment). At the cellular level, this affects monoamine transport and causes neuronal apoptosis and dysfunction of glial cells, normally respon-sible for maintaining neuronal homeostasis.

Brain-derived neurotrophic factor

Healthy interactions between neurones and glial cells are maintained by brain-derived neurotrophic factor (BDNF), which is found in its greatest concentration in the hippocampus and cerebral cortex. It promotes cell growth and long-term potentiation (the enhancement of synchronous firing between two neurones). Pro-BDNF, its precursor,

promotes the reduction of dendritic spines and apoptosis. BDNF is then involved in the growth and activity of neural networks.

- Animal studies suggest that BDNF is reduced by stress.
- Adult humans with untreated depressive illness have lower se-rum concentrations of BDNF when compared with both healthy controls and those that have received antidepressant treatment.
- Low levels normalize with antidepressant treatment.

BDNF therefore has potential as an objective marker of depres-sion and its response to treatment, and as a pharmacological target for drug development.

Neuroimaging changes

The use of functional magnetic resonance imaging (fMRI) and positron emission tomography (PET) has revealed a number of abnormalities in the brains of people with major depression. These changes are non-specific but involve regions that are associated with both the emotional and the cognitive abnormalities seen in depression. Increased brain ventricle volume, and orbitofrontal, dor-solateral frontal and anterior cingulate cortex altered activation have been implicated. The hippocampus is smaller in several stress-related neuropsychiatric disorders, including recurrent depression.

Sleep

A reduced time between onset of sleep and REM sleep (shortened REM latency), and reduced slow-wave sleep both occur in depres-sive illness. These abnormalities persist in some patients when they are not depressed. Families with several sufferers of depressive ill-ness can share these traits, suggesting that sleep patterns may be inherited and may predispose to depression.

Childhood traumas and personality

Physical, sexual and emotional abuse and neglect in childhood pre-dispose adults to depressive illness but the effect is non-specific. Both 'neurotic' (emotional) and perfectionist personality traits are risks for depressive illness, and these may be determined as much by genetic factors as childhood environment.

Social factors

Some 30% of women will develop a depressive illness after a severe life event or difficulty, such as a divorce, and this is compounded by low self-esteem and a lack of a confiding relationship. Unemploy-ment is a significant risk factor in men.

An integrated model of aetiology

Stress is more likely to trigger depressive illness in a person pre-disposed by lack of social support and/or certain personality traits. Stress triggers various changes in both neurohormones (e.g. CRH) and neurotransmitters (e.g. serotonin) known to be altered in depres-sive illness. This suggests an integrated biopsychosocial model of depressive illness and challenges dualistic ideas that depressive ill-nesses are either psychological or physical rather than being both.

Management of depressive illness

The patient needs to know the diagnosis to provide understanding and rationalization of the overwhelming distress inherent in depres-sive illness and this in itself may have an 'antidepressant' effect. The treatment of depressive disorders involves physical, psychological and social interventions (**Box 25.22**).

Patients who are actively suicidal or severely depressed (with or without psychotic symptoms) should be admitted to hospi-tal. Admission is necessary for perhaps 1 in 1000 people with clinical depression in primary care. This allows support, listening,

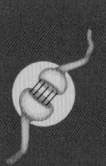

> **Box 25.22 Management of depressive illness**
>
> **Physical**
> - Cessation of depressing drugs (alcohol, steroids)
> - Regular exercise (good for mild to moderate depression)
> - Antidepressants (choice determined by adverse effects, co-morbid illnesses and interactions)
> - Adjunctive drugs (e.g. lithium; if no response to two different antidepressants)
> - Electroconvulsive therapy (ECT; if depression is life-threatening or non-responsive)
>
> **Psychological**
> - Education and regular follow-up by same professional
> - Cognitive behaviour therapy (CBT)
> - Other indicated psychotherapies (couple, family, interpersonal)
>
> **Social**
> - Financial: eligible benefits, debt counselling
> - Employment: acquiring or changing a job or career
> - Housing: adequate, secure tenancy, safe, social neighbours
> - Young children: child-care support
>
> **Treatments combined**
> - The most effective treatment is a mixture of CBT and an antidepressant

observation, the close monitoring of treatments and the prevention of suicide. The pitfall of not treating a depressive illness just because it seems an 'understandable' reaction to serious illness or difficult circumstances should be avoided. This is particularly likely to happen if the patient is elderly, or severely or terminally ill.

Psychological treatments

There is good evidence that mild to moderate depressive episodes respond well to 'talking therapies'.

Cognitive behaviour therapy

Beck developed cognitive behaviour therapy (CBT) to reverse the negative cognitive triad with which patients regard themselves, their situation and their futures. It involves the identification of the negative automatic thoughts that maintain the negative perceptions that feed depression. These commonly include catastrophizing (e.g. making a 'mountain out of a mole-hill'), over-generalizing (e.g. 'I failed an exam; therefore I am a failure as a person') and categorical ('all-or-none') thinking (e.g. 'My work is either perfect or abysmal'). CBT then involves identifying the links between these thoughts, consequent behaviour and feeling low, and then testing their logic. This is done by looking at the evidence either in the therapy sessions (e.g. Q: 'Did you pass the other exams you took?'; A: 'Yes; I guess I did') or in behavioural 'experiments' (e.g. showing the 'abysmal' work to a colleague and asking their opinion).

There is good evidence that individual CBT is as effective as antidepressant drugs for mild and moderate depressive illness, and should be offered as first-choice treatment. It is also effective in preventing a relapse of clinical depression after therapy has ceased. Individual CBT is more effective than group-delivered therapy, and computer-delivered CBT programmes are also helpful when used to supplement therapist involvement. Third-wave CBT therapies, such as mindfulness-based CBT, centred on the use of meditation, can prevent recurrence. Acceptance and commitment therapy (accepting the things that cannot be changed, and committing oneself to things that can be) shows promise.

Interpersonal psychotherapy

This psychotherapy is probably as effective as CBT in mild and moderate clinical depression. The therapist focuses on those interpersonal relationships involved in, or affected by, the patient's illness, using problem-solving techniques to help the individual to find solutions.

Other psychotherapies

Couple therapy is effective when a patient is in a problematic relationship that may be contributing to the depressive illness; both the patient and partner attend therapy.

Family therapy is effective not only to treat a family with problems, but also to assist the family to help a patient get better. It may involve understanding one family member's 'depression' as a systemic 'solution' for a wider problem within the family.

Physical treatments

Exercise and other self-help

There is good evidence that regular exercise, particularly involving other people, can help relieve depressive illness of mild severity. The benefit is independent of a physical training effect. The role of exercise is unclear but recent evidence suggests that kynurenine is prevented from crossing the blood–brain barrier, thereby reducing neuroactive metabolites. Other self-help and psycho-educational advice (e.g. reduction of alcohol consumption, regular meals and sleep–wake cycle) may be helpful, particularly if supported by bibliotherapy.

Use of drugs in the treatment of clinical depression

Moderate and severe depressive episodes can be effectively treated using medication. Antidepressants are designed to provide an acute increase in monoamine activity. They do this through either prevention of reuptake or enzymatic degradation. This occurs acutely and, although an equally rapid **depletion** of monoamines has an acute mood-lowering effect, the mood-elevating benefits of these drugs require weeks of continuous administration. The benefits are therefore unlikely to be due to this mechanism alone.

The effects of chronic administration of monoamine reuptake inhibitors are various. Examples include an increase in the synthesis of binding proteins necessary for serotonin receptor activity and increases in cyclic adenine monophosphate activation, in turn increasing BDNF synthesis, enhancing glucocorticoid receptor sensitivity and inhibiting cytokine signalling. These effects may be secondary to the acute restoration of monoamine levels but rely upon transcriptional and translational changes that alter neuronal plasticity. It is this protein synthesis-dependent process that is thought to be the final pathway responsible for the clinical effect of the drugs.

As the neurobiology for depressive illness becomes clearer, so too are novel approaches to its treatment; some of the novel targets under active investigation are listed in **Box 25.23**. A general approach to the prescription of antidepressants is outlined in **Box 25.24**.

Drug choices in specific circumstances

- *Recurrent episodes.* Maintenance treatment with the antidepressant at the dose that obtained remission should be continued for at least 2 years. Maintenance treatment beyond this point should be re-evaluated, considering age, co-morbidities and risk factors.
- *Refractory depressive illness.* While 50% may show a response, as few as 30% of individuals (outpatients) experience complete remission with the first choice of drug. Strategies available at this point are switching drug classes or augmenting with other agents. This should be overseen by a specialist.

Box 25.23 Potential targets for novel antidepressant agents

- Brain-derived neurotrophic factor (BDNF)
- Tumour necrosis factor-alpha (TNF-α)
- Interleukin-1 beta (IL-1β)
- Glucocorticoid receptors
- Corticotrophin-releasing hormone
- Melatonin-concentrating hormone
- Alpha-melanocyte stimulating hormone
- Ghrelin
- Leptin
- Orexins
- Neuropeptide Y
- Nesfatin-1

Box 25.24 A general approach to the prescription of antidepressants

- Any drugs that may contribute to or exacerbate depression, e.g. corticosteroids, should be stopped
- An ECG should be performed prior to institution of antidepressants
- Patient education should be provided (e.g. 80% of the UK public wrongly believe that antidepressants are addictive)
- Regular follow-up (especially weeks 1–6) should accompany the prescription of antidepressants to increase adherence
- All antidepressants have similar efficacy and speed of onset
- Selective serotonin reuptake inhibitors (SSRIs) are considered first-line agents
- Choice of agent will depend on safety and adverse effects, which can be used to positive effect (sedating drugs given at night to enhance sleep)
- The rate of improvement is greatest in weeks 1–2
- An alternative agent should be considered at week 4 in the absence of any response
- With resolution of symptoms, antidepressants should be continued for 6–9 months after a single episode but for at least 2 years in the case of multiple prior episodes
- Some 50% of patients who stop antidepressants immediately on recovery relapse in the next 6 months

- ***Psychotic depression.*** This needs either a combination of an antidepressant and an antipsychotic drug, or electroconvulsive therapy.
- ***Depressive episodes in bipolar affective disorder.*** Monotherapy with quetiapine has been proposed as the treatment of choice. Other drugs include mood stabilizers or olanzapine, either alone or in combination with an SSRI antidepressant (see p. 783).

Selective serotonin reuptake inhibitors

Selective serotonin reuptake inhibitors (SSRIs) selectively inhibit the reuptake of the monoamine serotonin (5-HT) within the synapse (**Fig. 25.3**). Citalopram and its levo-isomer escitalopram, as well as fluoxetine, paroxetine and sertraline have the advantage of causing less serious adverse effects than tricyclic antidepressants and do not usually cause significant weight gain. Because of their long half-lives, they can also be given just once daily, normally in the morning after breakfast. For these reasons, patients adhere better to treatment and therefore SSRIs are first-line treatments for depressive disorders.

The most common adverse effects of SSRIs resemble a 'hang-over' and include nausea, vomiting, headache, diarrhoea and dry mouth. Insomnia and paradoxical agitation can occur when first starting the drugs. Adolescents, in particular, may develop suicidal thoughts with SSRIs and only fluoxetine is licensed in the UK for adolescents. Further studies suggest that this risk is small, if present,

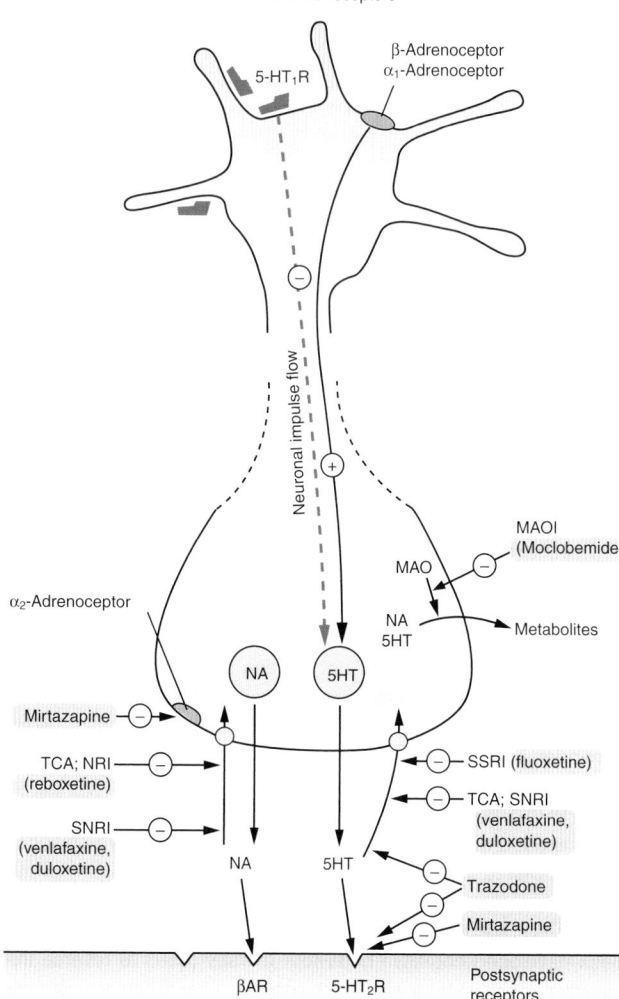

Fig. 25.3 The effect of drugs used in the treatment of depression on central nervous system serotonergic and adrenergic functioning. **(a)** The majority of released serotonin 5-HT and noradrenaline (NA; norepinephrine) is rapidly removed from the synapse by reuptake into the neurone (yellow circles). **(b)** There is a range of antidepressants, which vary in their abilities to inhibit the reuptake of serotonin or noradrenaline, thus enhancing the synapse concentrations of these transmitters. **(c)** Stimulation of presynaptic α2-adrenoceptors reduces monoamine release; mirtazapine blocks these presynaptic autoreceptors, and increases the release and transmission of noradrenaline and serotonin. **(d)** Other drugs act by significantly blocking postsynaptic receptors that are upregulated in depression. βAR, β-adrenoceptor; MAO, monoamine oxidase; MAOI, monoamine oxidase inhibitor; NA, noradrenaline; NRI, (selective) noradrenaline reuptake inhibitor; SNRI, serotonin and noradrenaline reuptake inhibitor; SSRI, selective serotonin reuptake inhibitor; TCA, 'classic' tricyclic antidepressant. (*From Waller DG, Sampson AP. Medical Pharmacoland Therapeutics, 5th edn. Elsevier; 2017, with permission.*)

and no study has shown a significant increased risk of suicide itself. One in five patients also has sexual adverse effects, including erectile dysfunction and loss of libido. Uncommon adverse effects include restless legs syndrome (see p. 858) and hyponatraemia.

A ***risk of bleeding*** is associated with SSRIs and is thought to be due to the inhibition of serotonin uptake by platelets as part of normal aggregation in response to vascular injury. To date, much of the reported incidence relates to gastrointestinal bleeding, and any patient with one or more risk factors for upper gastrointestinal bleeding, such as taking an NSAID, should be given gastro-protection with a proton pump inhibitor or advised to stop the NSAID. A risk of intra- and postoperative bleeding has also been reported. While antidepressants are certainly not a reason to withhold a surgical intervention, there is certainly an added risk, of which the surgeon and anaesthetist should be aware.

'Serotonin syndrome' is a toxic hyper-serotonergic state, which can be caused by the ingestion of two or more drugs that increase serotonin levels, e.g. an SSRI combined with a monoamine oxidase inhibitor, a dopaminergic drug (e.g. selegiline) or a tricyclic antidepressant. Symptoms include hyperthermia, agitation, confusion, tremor, diarrhoea, tachycardia and hypertension. This is a medical emergency and requires admission to hospital.

Discontinuation syndrome, a specific withdrawal syndrome, has been reported with *some* SSRIs, and may occur with any antidepressant if stopped suddenly. The syndrome is characterized by shivering, anxiety, dizziness, 'electric shocks', headache and nausea. Patients should be warned not to omit a dose and to reduce SSRIs gradually when stopping them.

A *prolonged QTc interval* has been noted, particularly with high doses of citalopram and escitalopram.

Tricyclic antidepressants

Tricyclic antidepressants (TCAs) potentiate the action of the monoamines, noradrenaline (norepinephrine) and serotonin, by inhibiting their reuptake into nerve terminals (see **Fig. 25.3**). Dosulepin, imipramine, nortriptyline and amitriptyline are the most commonly used TCAs in the UK, but with the exception of modern compounds that are safer in overdose (e.g. lofepramine), their use as antidepressants is unusual and they are more commonly prescribed in low dose as hypnotics and in the management of chronic pain. They are toxic in overdose and should be avoided in the actively suicidal patient (**Box 25.25**).

Serotonergic and noradrenergic antidepressants

These antidepressants block a number of different neurotransmitter receptors both at the synapse and elsewhere. Their different receptor profiles cause different adverse effects.

- *Dual-acting agents* (*serotonin and noradrenaline reuptake inhibitors, SNRIs*). Duloxetine is the most potent blocker of both serotonin and noradrenaline (norepinephrine) reuptake and at higher doses is equipotent for both neurotransmitters.

> **i** | **Box 25.25 Adverse effects of tricyclic antidepressants**
>
> **Antimuscarinic effects**
> - Dry mouth
> - Constipation
> - Tremor
> - Blurred vision
> - Urinary retention
>
> **Cardiovascular effects**
> - QT prolongation
> - Arrhythmias
> - Postural hypotension
>
> **Convulsant activity**
> - Lowered seizure threshold
>
> **Other effects**
> - Weight gain
> - Sedation
> - Mania (rarely)

Venlafaxine is a less potent SNRI but at higher doses it also augments dopamine transmission, although its effects remain greatest for serotonin. Nausea is the most common side-effect of both drugs. Patients on venlafaxine should be monitored for hypertension and it should not be prescribed in those with uncontrolled hypertension or cardiac arrhythmias.

- *Tetracyclics*. Trazodone is a tetracyclic compound that acts as a serotonin antagonist (except at $5\text{-}HT_1A$ receptors, where it acts as a partial agonist) and reuptake inhibitor. It is used in the treatment of anxiety and depressive disorders. It is an effective nocturnal sedative due to postsynaptic $\alpha 1$-antagonism but this may also give rise to postural hypotension and the rare side-effect of priapism.
- *Mirtazapine* is a $5\text{-}HT_{2a}$ and $5\text{-}HT_3$ receptor antagonist and a potent α_2-adrenergic blocker: a noradrenaline and selective serotonin antagonist or NSSA. It can be given at night to aid sleep and rarely causes sexual adverse effects. Sedation and weight gain are common side-effects, while agranulocytosis is uncommon.
- *Noradrenaline (norepinephrine) reuptake inhibitors* (*NRIs*). Reboxetine is an NRI that is an effective antidepressant but has also demonstrated benefit in the treatment of panic disorder and attention deficit disorder. It can cause insomnia in some patients in addition to antimuscarinic adverse effects.

Monoamine oxidase inhibitors

Monoamine oxidase inhibitors (MAOIs) act by irreversibly inhibiting the intracellular enzymes monoamine oxidase A and B, leading to an increase of noradrenaline (norepinephrine), dopamine and 5-HT in the brain (see **Fig. 25.3**). MAOIs produce a dangerous hypertensive reaction with foods containing tyramine or dopamine and therefore a restricted diet is prescribed. Tyramine is present in cheese, pickled herrings, yeast extracts, certain red wines, and any food, such as game, that has undergone partial decomposition. Dopamine is present in broad beans. MAOIs interact with drugs such as pethidine and can also cause liver damage occasionally. They are less frequently prescribed because of these restrictions.

Reversible inhibitors of monoamine oxidase A

An example of a reversible inhibitor of monoamine oxidase A (RIMA) is moclobemide. These drugs appear to have fewer adverse effects than the MAOIs (insomnia and headache, but some sexual problems) and constitute a low risk in overdose. Patients prescribed such antidepressants can eat a normal diet, but should be careful to avoid excessive amounts of food rich in tyramine (see above).

Selective irreversible inhibitors of monoamine oxidase B

Selegiline is a selective irreversible inhibitor of MAO-B. At higher doses it loses its specificity and also inhibits MAO-A. It is more frequently used in the treatment of Parkinson's disease (see p. 861) than in depression, as it prolongs the activity of levodopa because dopamine is a substrate of MAO-B.

Melatonin receptor agonist and serotonin receptor antagonist

Agomelatine is the only class member. It is an agonist at melatonin MT_1 and MT_2 receptors and a weak antagonist at $5\text{-}HT_{2C}$ receptors but does not affect the uptake of serotonin, noradrenaline (norepinephrine) or dopamine. Agomelatine has the same antidepressant efficacy as the SSRIs. It is contraindicated in hepatic impairment.

Antidepressant augmentation

If two trials of antidepressants have failed, adding a second antidepressant or drugs such as lithium or an atypical antipsychotic can be helpful.

Antidepressant use in general medicine

- **Cardiac disease.** In people with cardiac disease, SSRIs, lofepramine and trazodone are preferred over more quinidine-like compounds which may have arrhythmogenic effects.
- **Epilepsy.** SSRIs are typically first-line. Interactions with anticonvulsants should be checked.
- **Drug interactions.** Most antidepressants are metabolized by the cytochrome P450 system but relatively few inhibit cytochrome enzymes, with paroxetine and the TCAs being the exception.
- **Herbal medicine.** Antidepressants should be avoided in patients taking the herbal antidepressant St John's wort, which interacts with serotonergic drugs in particular.
- **Elderly.** Doses of antidepressants should initially be halved in the elderly and in people with renal or hepatic failure.
- **Pregnancy.** Antidepressants should be avoided if possible in pregnancy and breast-feeding. If other treatments are ineffective, the risks of drug therapy should be balanced against those of taking no treatment, since depression can affect fetal progress and future mother–child bonding. TCAs are generally believed to be safe in pregnancy, with no significant increase in congenital malformations in fetuses exposed to them. However, occasionally, their antimuscarinic adverse effects produce jitteriness, sucking problems and hyperexcitability in the newborn. Postpartum plasma levels of babies breast-fed by treated mothers are negligible. SSRIs do not seem to be teratogenic but manufacturers advise against their use in pregnancy until more data are available. Pulmonary hypertension in the newborn is a rare complication. MAOIs should be avoided during pregnancy.

Combining antidepressants with psychotherapy

Historically, the understanding has been that combining psychotherapy with antidepressants provided no additive benefit. Recently, however, a well-designed randomized controlled trial has suggested that an additive effect can be achieved with this approach (specifically, with CBT). However, this is both a modest and a specific effect. Patients with more severe and non-chronic episodes attain this benefit, while those with milder forms of the disorder, chronic depression and co-morbid personality disorders do not, when compared with antidepressants alone. Individuals who obtained benefit from the combined treatment also experienced fewer adverse effects from the antidepressants prescribed.

Electroconvulsive therapy

Electroconvulsive therapy (ECT) is the treatment of choice in severe, life-threatening depressive illness, particularly when psychotic symptoms are present. It is sometimes essential treatment when the patient is dangerously suicidal or refusing to eat and drink, and when a rapid resolution is required, such as in postpartum depressive illness, when returning baby to mother as soon as it is safe to do so forms part of the treatment.

ECT is performed under general anaesthetic and involves the passage of an electric current across two electrodes applied to the anterior temporal areas of the scalp, in order to induce a seizure. The motoric seizure is less significant than its electrophysiological evidence (spike-and-wave activity on an EEG). Treatments are normally given twice a week for 3–6 weeks.

ECT is a controversial treatment, yet it is free of serious adverse effects. Most adverse effects are due to the general anaesthetic. Post-ictal confusion and headache are not uncommon, while transient and short-term retrograde amnesia and a temporary defect in new learning can occur during the weeks of treatment, but these are typically short-lived. Autobiographical memory loss is a more common adverse effect than previously thought. This is often discrete and, in most instances, not recognized by the patient, unless the particular memory is actively sought. Patients should be forewarned of this during the consenting process.

Uncommonly used physical treatments

Transcranial magnetic stimulation (TMS) shows moderate efficacy, but is uncommonly used. **Psychosurgery** is very occasionally considered in people with severe intractable depressive illness, when all other treatments have failed (see p. 789). A third improve remarkably, while a further third improve somewhat.

Deep brain stimulation may represent major advances in the management of chronic and treatment-refractory depressive disorders, but definitive trials are not available.

Social treatments

Many people with clinical depression have associated social problems (see **Box 25.22**). Assistance with these can make a significant contribution to clinical recovery. Interventions include the provision of group support, social clubs, occupational therapy and referral to a social worker. Educational programmes, self-help groups and informed and supportive family members can help improve outcome.

Prognosis

Depression is one of the leading causes of disease burden worldwide. People with major depressive illness are between 1.5 and 2 times more likely to die than non-depressed people in the next 16 years, and the risks encompass not only suicide, but also cardiovascular disorders. Depression produces greater disability than angina, arthritis, asthma and diabetes, which makes effective treatment and prevention imperative.

Most patients have recovered by 6 months in primary care and 12 months in secondary care. About a quarter of patients attending hospital with depressive illnesses will have a recurrence within 1 year, and three-quarters will have a recurrence within 10 years. People with recurrent depressive illnesses should be offered prevention. This may involve CBT that concentrates on relapse prevention, other forms of psychotherapy, prolonged antidepressant use, and advice on lifestyle activities such as regular exercise. Full-dose antidepressants are the most effective prophylaxis in recurrent depressive disorders.

Mania, hypomania and bipolar disorder

Mania and hypomania almost always occur as part of a bipolar disorder. The clinical features of mania include a marked elevation of mood, characterized by euphoria, overactivity and disinhibition (**Box 25.26**). Hypomania lasts a shorter time and is less severe, with no psychotic features and less disability. Hypomania can be distinguished from normal happiness by its persistence, non-reactivity (not provoked by good news and not affected by bad news) and social disability.

The social disability of mania can be severe, with disinhibited behaviour leading to significant debts (from overspending), lost

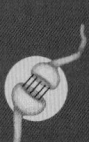

> **Box 25.26 Clinical features of mania**
>
> | Characteristic | Clinical feature |
> |---|---|
> | Mood | Elevated or irritable |
> | Speech | Fast, pressurized, flight of ideas |
> | Energy | Excessive |
> | Ideas | Grandiose, self-confident, delusions of wealth, power, influence or of religious significance, sometimes persecutory |
> | Cognition | Disturbance of registration of memories |
> | Physical | Insomnia, mild to moderate weight loss, increased libido |
> | Behaviour | Disinhibition, increased sexual activity, excessive drinking or spending |
> | Hallucinations | Fleeting auditory |

> **Box 25.27 Treatment options in acute mania or hypomania**
>
> Choice of agent is determined largely by clinical judgement, contraindications and prior response
> - Stop antidepressant medication
>
> **If the patient is NOT on antimanic medication, then start**
> - Antipsychotic, e.g. aripiprazole 15 mg daily
> - *Or* valproate 750 mg daily
> - *Or* lithium 0.4 mg daily to serum lithium of 0.4–1.0 mmol/L
>   If response is inadequate:
> - Antipsychotic + valproate or lithium
>
> **If the patient is already ON antimanic medication**
> - If taking an antipsychotic: check dose and compliance; increase if possible, or add valproate or lithium
> - If taking valproate: check plasma levels and increase dose, aiming for a serum concentration of 125 mg/L as tolerated and/or add an antipsychotic (this should be done if mania is severe)
> - If taking lithium: check plasma levels and increase dose to gain a level of 1.0–1.2 mmol/L if necessary (*Note*: higher than usual reference range) or add an antipsychotic (this should be done if mania is severe)
> - If taking carbamazepine: add an antipsychotic if appropriate
>   A short-acting benzodiazepine may be added to assist with agitation in all patients

relationships (from promiscuity or irritability), social ostracism and lost employment (from reckless or disinhibited behaviour).

Some patients have a ***rapid-cycling*** illness, with frequent swings from one mood state to another. A ***mixed affective state*** occurs when features of mania and depressive illness are seen in the same episode. ***Cyclothymia*** is a personality trait with spontaneous swings in mood that are not sufficiently severe or persistent to warrant another diagnosis.

Differential diagnosis

Acute intoxication with recreational drugs such as amfetamines, amfetamine derivatives (MDMA: Ecstasy) and cocaine can mimic mania. Up to a quarter of people with Cushing's syndrome develop mania. Similarly, corticosteroids can induce mania less commonly than depressive illness. Dopamine agonists (e.g. bromocriptine) are also known to induce mania sometimes.

Epidemiology

The lifetime prevalence of bipolar affective disorder is 1% across the world. Unlike unipolar depressive illness, it is equally common in men and women, supporting its different aetiology. There is no variation by socioeconomic class or race. The mean age of onset is 21, earlier than unipolar depression. The higher prevalence found in divorced people is probably a consequence of the condition.

Aetiology

Genetic factors

There is strong evidence for a genetic aetiology in this disorder, with a 60–80% concordance rate in monozygotic twins, compared to 15% in dizygotic twins, suggesting a high rate of heritability. Studies in adoptive twins show similar rates, so this high rate is probably genetic and not due to the family environment. Linkage studies have so far proved disappointing, with several polymorphism associations being found, similar to polymorphisms associated with schizophrenia.

Biochemical changes

Brain monoamines, such as serotonin, are increased in mania. Dexamethasone tends not to suppress cortisol levels in people with mania, suggesting a similar pattern of non-suppression to that seen in severe depressive illness.

Psychological factors

The effect of life events is weaker in bipolar compared with unipolar illnesses, most effects being apparent at first onset. Similarly,

personality does not seem to be a major influence, in contrast to unipolar depression, although there is some evidence of a link with creativity and divergent thinking that may be an advantage in the right occupation.

Management

Acute mania or hypomania

Treatment is summarized in **Box 25.27**. Acute mania is treated with an atypical antipsychotic, sodium valproate or lithium.

- The atypical antipsychotics olanzapine, quetiapine, risperidone and aripiprazole are recommended, especially with behavioural disturbance. The behavioural excitement and overactivity are usually reduced within days, but elation, grandiosity and associated delusions often take longer to respond.
- Lithium may be used in instances where compliance is likely to be good; however, the screening necessary prior to its prescription (see below) may prohibit its use in these circumstances as a first-line agent.
- Valproic acid is also helpful in hypomania or in rapid-cycling illnesses (see below).

Prevention of relapses

Since bipolar illnesses tend to be relapsing and remitting, prevention of recurrence is the major therapeutic challenge. A patient who has experienced more than two episodes of affective disorder within a 5-year period is likely to benefit from preventive treatments. Recommendations include lithium, olanzapine and valproic acid (avoided in women of childbearing age).

Lithium

Lithium (carbonate or citrate) is one of the two main agents used for prophylaxis in people with repeated episodes of bipolar illness (the other being valproic acid). It is rapidly absorbed from the gastrointestinal tract and more than 95% is excreted by the kidneys; small amounts are found in the saliva, sweat and breast milk. Renal clearance of lithium correlates with renal creatinine clearance. Lithium is a mood-stabilizing drug that prevents mania and depression. It lowers the frequency and severity of relapses by half and significantly reduces the likelihood of suicide. Its mode of action is

> **ℹ Box 25.28 Lithium**
>
> **Adverse effects**
> - Nausea
> - Diarrhoea
> - Fine tremor
> - Weight gain, mainly through increased appetite
> - Polyuria ⎫
> - Polydipsia ⎭ due to nephrogenic diabetes insipidus
>
> **Toxicity (>1.5 mmol/L, more likely with dehydration and drug interactions)**
> - Drowsiness
> - Nausea
> - Vomiting
> - Blurred vision
> - Coarse tremor
> - Ataxia
> - Dysarthria
> - Delirium
> - Convulsions
> - Coma
> - Death

unknown, but lithium is known to act on the serotonergic system. Poor response to lithium is associated with a negative family history, an unstable pre-morbid personality and a rapid-cycling illness. Pharmacogenetic work suggests that certain polymorphisms may predict response.

Plasma levels

These should be monitored weekly, with blood drawn 12 h after the last dose (a 'trough' level) until a steady state is reached and at 3-monthly intervals thereafter. The minimum level for prophylaxis is 0.4 mmol/L, with an optimum range of between 0.6 and 0.75 mmol/L. Levels higher than this may afford further protection against manic episodes but the relationship with depression is less clear. For this reason, the therapeutic range is typically quoted as 0.5–1.0 mmol/L. Fluctuations in plasma levels increase the risk of relapse.

Screening prior to starting lithium and at 6-monthly intervals thereafter includes:
- *Thyroid function* (free T_4, TSH and thyroid autoantibodies). Lithium interferes with thyroid function and can produce frank hypothyroidism. The presence of thyroid autoantibodies increases the risk.
- *Parathyroid function.* Serum calcium and parathyroid hormone levels are higher in 10% of patients.
- *Renal function* (serum urea and creatinine, eGFR and 24-h urinary volume). Long-term treatment with lithium causes two renal problems: nephrogenic diabetes insipidus (p. 643) and reduced glomerular function. The best screen for diabetes insipidus is to ask the patient about polyuria and polydipsia.

Toxicity

Patients should always carry a lithium card with them, be advised to avoid dehydration, and be warned of drug interactions, such as with NSAIDs and diuretics. As with all medications, it is vital to discuss adverse effects and signs of toxicity (**Box. 25.28**).

Pregnancy

As a rule, lithium is not advised during pregnancy, particularly in the first trimester, because of an increased risk of fetal malformation (Ebstein's anomaly). About 25% of women with a history of bipolar disorder relapse within 2 weeks of delivery. Restarting lithium within 24 h of delivery (if the mother is prepared to forgo breast-feeding) markedly reduces the risk of relapse.

Other mood stabilizers

Valproic acid (as the semisodium salt) is recommended in both prophylaxis and treatment of manic states. Second-line treatments include *lamotrigine*. *Carbamazepine* is less frequently used and more effective in mania than depressive states. Some patients who do not respond to lithium may respond to these anticonvulsants or a combination of both. People with rapid-cycling illnesses show a better response to anticonvulsants than to lithium.

Other drugs that appear to exert a prophylactic mood-stabilizing effect include *olanzapine* and *risperidone*.

Both valproate and carbamazepine are associated with neural tube defects and should be avoided in all women of childbearing age. See page 857 for other adverse effects of these drugs.

Prognosis

The mean duration of a manic episode is 2 months, with 95% making a full recovery in time. Recurrence is the rule in bipolar disorders, up to 90% relapsing within 10 years.

Further reading

BALANCE Investigators. Lithium plus valproate combination versus monotherapy for relapse prevention in bipolar disorders (BALANCE). *Lancet* 2010; 375:365–375.

Cipriani A, Barbui C, Salanti G et al. Comparative efficacy and acceptability of antimanic drugs in acute mania. *Lancet* 2011; 378:1306–1315.

Craddock N, Sklar P. Genetics of bipolar disorder. *Lancet* 2013; 381:1654–1662.

Geddes JR, Miklowitz DJ. Treatment of bipolar disorder. *Lancet* 2013; 381:1672–1682.

Grande I, Berk M, Birmaher B et al. Bipolar disorders. *Lancet* 2016; 387:1561–1572.

Krishnan V, Nestler EJ. The molecular neurobiology of depression. *Nature* 2008; 455:894–902.

Malhi G, Mann JJ. Depression. *Lancet* 2018; 392:2299–2312.

McKnight RF, Adida M, Budge K et al. Lithium toxicity profile: a systematic review and meta-analysis. *Lancet* 2012; 379:721–728.

Phillips ML, Kupfer DJ. Bipolar disorder diagnosis: challenges and future directions. *Lancet* 2013; 381:1663–1671.

Patorno E, Huybrechts KF, Bateman BT et al. Lithium use in pregnancy and the risk of cardiac malformations. *N Engl J Med* 2017; 376: 2245–2254.

Stewart DE. Depression during pregnancy. *N Engl J Med* 2011; 365:1605–1611.

SUICIDE AND SELF-HARM

(See also p. 260.) There are 800 000 suicide deaths worldwide per year. Suicide accounts for 2% of male and 1% of female deaths in England and Wales each year, equivalent to a rate of 10 per 100 000. The rate increases with age, peaking for women in their sixties and for men in their seventies. Suicide is the second most common cause of mortality in 15- to 34-year-olds. Meta-analyses of relevant studies suggest that the lifetime risk of suicide is 7% in alcohol dependence, 6% in affective disorders and 4% in schizophrenia.

The highest rates of suicide have been reported in Guyana, Lesotho and Russia, while the lowest are found in the Caribbean. Such variations may reflect differences in reporting, which may be related to religion, as much as genuine differences. The provision of mental health care to suicidal individuals varies greatly around the world; a World Health Organization (WHO) study suggests that most receive no treatment at all. Factors that increase the risk of suicide are indicated in **Box 25.29**.

A distinction must be drawn between those who attempt suicide – self-harm (SH) – and those who succeed (suicide):

Box 25.29 Factors that increase the risk of suicide

- Male sex
- Older age
- Living alone
- Immigrant status
- Recent bereavement, separation or divorce
- Unemployment or retirement
- Living in a socially disorganized area
- Family history of affective disorder, suicide or alcohol misuse
- Previous history of affective disorder, alcohol or drug misuse
- Previous suicide attempt
- Addiction to alcohol or drugs
- Severe depression or early dementia
- Incapacitating painful physical illness

Box 25.30 Guidelines for the assessment of patients who harm themselves

Questions to ask: of concern if positive answer
- Was there a clear precipitant/cause for the attempt?
- Did the patient leave a suicide note?
- Had the patient taken pains not to be discovered?
- Did the patient make the attempt in strange surroundings (i.e. away from home)?
- Would the patient do it again?

Other relevant factors
- Has the precipitant or crisis resolved?
- Was the act premeditated or impulsive?
- Is there a continuing suicidal intent?
- Does the patient have any psychiatric symptoms?
- What is the patient's social support system?
- Has the patient inflicted self-harm before?
- Has anyone in the family ever taken their life?
- Does the patient have a physical illness?

Indications for referral to a psychiatrist

Absolute indications
- Clinical depression
- Psychotic illness of any kind
- Clearly pre-planned suicidal attempt that was not intended to be discovered
- Persistent suicidal intent (the more detailed the plans, the more serious the risk)
- A violent method used

Other common indications
- Alcohol and drug misuse
- Patients over 45 years, especially if male, and young adolescents
- Those with a family history of suicide in first-degree relatives
- Those with serious (especially incurable) physical disease
- Those living alone or otherwise unsupported
- Those in whom there is a major unresolved crisis
- Persistent suicide attempts
- Any patients who give you cause for concern

- The majority of cases of SH occur in people under 35 years of age.
- The majority of suicides occur in people aged over 60.
- Suicides are more common in men, while SH is more common in women.
- Suicides are more common in older men, although rates are falling. Rates in young men are rising fast throughout the UK and Europe.
- Suicides in women are slowly falling in the UK.
- Approximately 90% of cases of SH involve self-poisoning.
- A formal psychiatric diagnosis can be made retrospectively in 90% of suicides but is unusual in SH.

There is, however, an overlap between SH and suicide. Between 1% and 2% of people who attempt suicide will kill themselves in the year following SH. The risk of suicide stays elevated in those with SH, with 0.5% *per annum* committing suicide in the following 20 years. Following the guidelines for the assessment of such patients (**Box 25.30**) will help in the identification of risk factors and the need for a psychiatric referral.

In general, it is worth trying to interview a family member or close friend and checking these points with them. Requests for immediate re-prescription on discharge should be denied, only 3 days' supply of essential medication should be given, and the patient should be requested to report to their general practitioner or to their psychiatric outpatient clinic for further supplies. Occasionally, involuntary admission to hospital may be required (see p. 800).

Further reading

Brooks SE et al. Suicide in the elderly: a multidisciplinary approach to prevention. *Clin Geriatr Med* 2019; 35:133–145.
Bruffaerts R, Demyttenaere K, Hwang I et al. Treatment of suicidal people around the world. *Br J Psychiatry* 2011; 199:64–70.
Moran P, Coffey C, Romaniuk H et al. The natural history of self-harm from adolescence to young adulthood. *Lancet* 2012; 379:236–243.
Turecki G. The molecular bases of the suicidal brain. *Nat Neurosci Rev* 2014; 15:802–816.
van Heeringen K, Mann JJ. The neurobiology of suicide. *Lancet Psychiatry* 2014; 1:63–72.
https://www.who.int/gho/mental_health/suicide_rates_crude/en/. *World Health Organization suicide rates.*

ANXIETY DISORDERS

These are conditions in which anxiety dominates the clinical symptoms. They are classified according to whether the anxiety is persistent (general anxiety) or episodic, with the episodic conditions classified according to whether the episodes are regularly triggered by a cue (phobia) or not (panic disorder). The differential diagnoses of anxiety disorders are given in **Box 25.31**. A patient with one anxiety disorder may develop others in time.

Box 25.31 Anxiety disorders: differential diagnosis

Psychiatric disorders
- Depressive illness
- Obsessive–compulsive disorder
- Pre-senile dementia
- Alcohol dependence
- Drug dependence
- Benzodiazepine withdrawal

Endocrine disorders
- Hyperthyroidism
- Hypoglycaemia
- Phaeochromocytoma

Generalized anxiety disorder

Generalized anxiety disorder (GAD) occurs in 4–6% of the population and is more common in women. Symptoms are persistent and often chronic. GAD and the related panic disorder are differential diagnoses for functional somatic syndromes, owing to the many physical symptoms that are caused by these conditions.

Clinical features

See **Box 25.32** for physical and psychological symptoms. The patient looks worried, and has a tense posture, restless behaviour, a pale and sweaty skin, or intermittent flushing. The patient takes time to go to sleep and wakes intermittently with worry dreams.

Box 25.32 Physical and psychological symptoms of anxiety

Physical symptoms

Gastrointestinal
- Dry mouth
- Difficulty in swallowing
- Epigastric discomfort
- Aerophagy (swallowing air)
- Diarrhoea (usually frequency)

Respiratory
- Feeling of chest constriction
- Difficulty in inhaling
- Over-breathing
- Choking

Cardiovascular
- Palpitations
- Awareness of missed beats
- Chest pain

Genitourinary
- Increased frequency
- Failure of erection
- Lack of libido

Nervous system
- Fatigue
- Blurred vision
- Dizziness
- Sensitivity to noise and/or light
- Headache
- Sleep disturbance
- Trembling

Psychological symptoms
- Apprehension and fear
- Irritability
- Difficulty in concentrating
- Distractibility
- Restlessness
- Depersonalization
- Derealization

Box 25.33 Hyperventilation syndrome

Clinical features
- Panic attacks – fear, terror and impending doom – accompanied by some or all of the following:
  - Dyspnoea (trouble getting a good breath in)
  - Palpitations
  - Chest pain or discomfort
  - Suffocating sensation
  - Dizziness
  - Paraesthesiae in hands and feet
  - Perioral paraesthesiae
  - Sweating
  - Carpopedal spasms

Aetiology
- Over-breathing leading to a decrease in P_aCO_2 and an increase in arterial pH, causing relative hypocalcaemia

Diagnosis
- A provocation test – voluntary over-breathing for 1 minute – provokes similar symptoms; rebreathing from a large paper bag relieves them

Management
- Explanation and reassurance is given
- The patient is trained in relaxation techniques and slow, controlled breathing
- The patient is asked to breathe into a closed paper bag

Box 25.34 Phobias

- A phobia is an abnormal fear and avoidance of an object or situation
- Phobias are common (the incidence varies from 3.5% to 12.8% worldwide), disabling and treatable with behaviour therapy

Associated conditions include hyperventilation, which is even more common in panic disorders (**Box 25.33**). The patient will either breathe rapidly and shallowly or sigh deeply, particularly when talking about the stresses in their life.

Mixed anxiety and depressive disorder

This disorder is the most common mood disorder in primary care (7% point prevalence). There are equal elements of anxiety and depression, showing how closely associated these two abnormal mood states are.

Panic disorder

Panic disorder is diagnosed when the patient has repeated, sudden attacks of overwhelming anxiety, accompanied by severe physical symptoms, usually related to both hyperventilation (see **Box 25.33**) and sympathetic nervous system overactivity (palpitations, tremor, restlessness and sweating). The lifetime prevalence is 5%. People with a panic disorder often have catastrophic illness beliefs during the panic attack, such as the conviction that they are about to die from a stroke or heart attack. The fear of a stroke is related to dizziness and headache. Fear of a heart attack accompanies chest pain (atypical chest pain). The occasional patient with longstanding attacks may no longer feel anxious and simply notices the physical symptoms.

Aetiology

Generalized anxiety and panic disorders occur four times more commonly in first-degree relatives of affected patients. Sympathetic nervous system overactivity, increased muscle tension and hyperventilation are the common pathophysiological associations. Anxiety is the emotional response to the threat of a loss, whereas depression is the response to the loss itself. There is some evidence that being bullied leads to anxiety disorders in adolescents.

Phobic (anxiety) disorders

Phobias are common conditions in which intense fear is triggered by a stimulus, or group of stimuli, that are predictable and normally cause no particular concern to others (e.g. agoraphobia, claustrophobia, social phobia). This leads to avoidance of the stimulus (**Box 25.34**). The patient knows that the fear is irrational but cannot control it. The prevalence of all phobias is 8%, with many patients having more than one. Phobias of 'medical' stimuli exist (e.g. of doctors, dentists, hospitals, blood and injections), which affect the patient's ability to receive adequate healthcare.

Aetiology

Phobias may be caused by classical conditioning, in which a response (fear and avoidance) becomes conditioned to a previously benign stimulus (e.g. a lift), often after an initiating emotional shock (e.g. being stuck in a lift). In children, phobias can arise through imagined threats (e.g. ghost stories). Women have twice the prevalence of phobias than men. Phobias aggregate in families, indicating the importance of genetic factors.

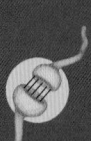

Agoraphobia

Translated as 'fear of the marketplace', this common phobia (4% prevalence) presents as a fear of being away from home, with travelling, walking down a road and going to supermarkets being common cues. At its most disabling, the patient avoids leaving home, particularly when unaccompanied. It is often associated with **claustrophobia**, a fear of enclosed spaces.

Social phobia

This is the fear and avoidance of social situations: crowds, strangers, parties and meetings. Public speaking would be the sufferer's worst nightmare. It is suffered by 2% of the population.

Simple phobias

The phobia of spiders (arachnophobia) is the most common, particularly in women. The prevalence of simple phobias is 7% in the general population. Other common phobias include insects, bats, dogs, snakes, heights, thunderstorms and the dark. Children are particularly phobic about the dark, ghosts and burglars, but the large majority grow out of these fears.

Management of anxiety disorders

Psychological management

For many people with brief episodes, discussion with a doctor concerning the nature of anxiety and its precipitants is sufficient.

- **Relaxation techniques** can be effective in mild/moderate anxiety. Relaxation can be achieved in many ways, including complementary techniques such as meditation and yoga. Conventional relaxation training involves a slowing down of the rate of breathing, muscle relaxation and mental imagery.
- **Anxiety management** training involves two stages. In the first stage, verbal cues and mental imagery are used to arouse anxiety to demonstrate the link with symptoms. In the second stage, the patient is trained to reduce this anxiety by relaxation, distraction and reassuring self-statements.
- **Biofeedback** is useful for showing patients that they are not relaxed, even when they fail to recognize it, having become so used to anxiety. Biofeedback involves feeding back to the patient a physiological measure that is abnormal in anxiety. These measures may include electrical resistance of the skin of the palm, heart rate, muscle electromyography or breathing pattern. The effect tends not to generalize to everyday life away from the feedback.
- **Behaviour therapies** are treatments that are intended to change behaviour and thus symptoms. The most common and successful behaviour therapy (with 80% success in some phobias) is graded exposure or 'systematic desensitization'. First, the patient rates the phobia into a hierarchy of worsening fears (e.g. in agoraphobia: walking to the front door with a coat on; walking out into the garden; walking to the end of the road). Second, the patient practises exposure to the least fearful stimulus until no fear is felt. Each sequentially greater fear is then addressed in order, in the same manner.
- **Cognitive behaviour therapy** (CBT; see p. 779) is the treatment of choice for panic disorder and generalized anxiety disorder because the therapist and patient need to identify the mental cues (thoughts and memories) that may subtly provoke exacerbations of anxiety or panic attacks. CBT also allows identification and alteration of the patient's 'schema', or way of looking at themselves and their situation, which feeds anxiety.

> **_i_ Box 25.35 Withdrawal syndrome with benzodiazepines**
>
> - Insomnia
> - Anxiety
> - Tremulousness
> - Muscle twitching
> - Perceptual distortions
> - Hallucinations (which may be visual)
> - Hypersensitivities (light, sound, touch)
> - Convulsions

Drug treatments

Initial 'drug' treatment should involve advice for gradual cessation of anxiogenic substances such as caffeine and alcohol (which can cause a rebound anxiety). Prescribed drugs used in the treatment of anxiety can be divided into two groups: those that act primarily on the central nervous system, and those that block peripheral autonomic receptors.

- **Benzodiazepines** are centrally acting anxiolytic drugs. They are agonists of the inhibitory transmitter γ-aminobutyric acid (GABA). Diazepam and chlordiazepoxide have relatively long half-lives (20–40 h) and are used as anti-anxiety drugs in the short term. Adverse effects include sedation and memory problems, and patients should be advised not to drive while on treatment. They can cause dependence and tolerance within 4–6 weeks, particularly in those with dependent personalities. A withdrawal syndrome (**Box 25.35**) can occur after only 3 weeks of continuous use and is particularly severe when high doses have been given for a longer time. Thus, if a benzodiazepine drug is prescribed for anxiety, it should be given in as low a dose as possible and for not more than 2–4 weeks.
- **Most SSRIs** (e.g. fluoxetine, paroxetine, sertraline, escitalopram, citalopram) are useful symptomatic treatments for generalized anxiety and panic disorders, as well as some phobias (social phobia), although doses higher than those used in depression are often required. Duloxetine, mirtazapine, venlafaxine and pregabalin are alternative treatments for GADs, with the added benefit of possibly preventing the subsequent development of depression. Treatment response is often delayed several weeks; a trial of treatment should last 3 months.
- **Antipsychotics**, such as quetiapine or olanzapine, can be effective for more severe or refractory cases.
- **Beta-blockers** are effective in reducing peripheral symptoms, as many of the symptoms of anxiety are due to an increased or sustained release of adrenaline (epinephrine) and noradrenaline (norepinephrine) from the adrenal medulla and sympathetic nerves. Beta-blockers, such as propranolol (20–40 mg two or three times daily), can reduce peripheral symptoms such as palpitations, tremor and tachycardia, but they do not help central symptoms such as anxiety.

Acute stress reactions and adjustment disorders

Acute stress reaction

This occurs in response to exceptional physical and/or psychological stress. While severe, such a reaction usually subsides within days. The stress may be an overwhelming traumatic experience (e.g. accident, battle, physical assault, rape) or a sudden change in the social circumstances, such as a bereavement. Individual vulnerability and coping capacity play a role in the occurrence and severity of an acute stress reaction, as evidenced by the fact that not all people exposed to exceptional stress develop symptoms.

Symptoms usually include an initial state of feeling 'dazed' or numb, with inability to comprehend the situation. This may be followed either by further withdrawal from the situation, or by anxiety and overactivity. No treatments beyond reassurance and support are normally necessary.

Adjustment disorder

This disorder can follow an acute stress reaction and is common in the general hospital. It is a more prolonged (up to 6 months) emotional reaction to a significant life event, with low mood joining the initial shock and consequent anxiety, but not of sufficient severity or persistence to fulfil a diagnosis of a depressive or anxiety disorder. Supportive counselling is usually a successful treatment, allowing facilitation of unexpressed feelings and fears, and education about the likely future.

Normal grief

Normal grief immediately follows bereavement, is expressed openly, and allows a person to go through the social ceremonies and personal processes of bereavement. The three stages are, first, shock and disbelief; second, the emotional phase (anger, guilt and sadness); and, third, acceptance and resolution. This normal adjustment process may take up to a year, with movement between all three stages occurring in a sometimes haphazard fashion.

Pathological (abnormal) grief

This is a particular kind of adjustment disorder. It can be characterized as excessive and/or prolonged grief, or even absent grieving with abnormal denial of the bereavement. Usually, a relative will be stuck in grief, with insomnia and repeated dreams of the dead person, anger at doctors or even the patient for dying, consequent guilt in equal measure, and an inability to 'say goodbye' to the loved person by dealing with their effects. *Guided mourning* uses cognitive and behavioural techniques to allow the relative to stop grieving and move on in life.

Post-traumatic stress disorder

PTSD is a protracted response to a stressful event or situation of an exceptionally threatening nature, likely to cause pervasive distress in almost anyone. Causes include natural or human disasters, war, serious accidents, witnessing the violent death of others, and being the victim of sexual abuse, rape, torture or terrorism. Predisposing factors, such as personality, previously unresolved traumas or a history of psychiatric illness, may prolong the course of the syndrome. These factors are neither necessary nor sufficient to explain its occurrence, which is mostly related to the intensity of the trauma, proximity to the traumatic event, and its prolonged or repeated nature.

Clinical features

The typical symptoms of PTSD include:

- *'flashbacks'*, repeated vivid reliving of the trauma in the form of intrusive memories, often triggered by a reminder of the trauma
- *insomnia*, usually accompanied by nightmares, the nocturnal equivalent of flashbacks
- *emotional blunting*, emptiness or 'numbness', alternating with *intense anxiety* on exposure to events that resemble an aspect of the traumatic event, including anniversaries of the trauma
- *avoidance* of activities and situations reminiscent of the trauma
- *emotional detachment* from other people
- *hypervigilance*, with autonomic hyperarousal and an enhanced startle reaction.

This clinical picture represents the severe end of a spectrum of emotional reactions to trauma, which might alternatively take the form of an adjustment or mood disorder. The course is often fluctuating but recovery can be expected in two-thirds of cases at the end of the first year. Complications include depressive illness and alcohol misuse. In a small proportion of cases, the condition may follow a chronic course over many years and a transition to an enduring personality change.

Management and prevention

Compulsory **psychological debriefing** immediately after a trauma does not prevent PTSD and may be harmful. Prevention is better achieved by the support offered by others who were also involved. Trauma-focused CBT and *eye movement desensitization and reprocessing (EMDR)* are the evidence-based treatments of choice. SSRIs have a place in the management of chronic PTSD but dropout from pharmacotherapy is common.

The adult consequences of childhood abuse

Estimates of the prevalence of childhood sexual abuse vary, depending on definition, but there is reasonable evidence that 20% of women and 10% of men suffered significant, coercive and inappropriate sexual activity in childhood. The abuser is usually a member of the family or known to the child in social care homes.

Adverse childhood experiences (ACEs) have a dose–response relationship with a variety of lifetime health, social and behavioural problems. Consequent adult psychiatric disorders include depressive illness, substance misuse, eating disorders, borderline personality disorder and self-harm. Adverse effects on emotional and personality development will also predispose to psychiatric disorders.

There is increasing evidence to support the impact of such early experiences on the structural and physiological development of the nervous system, with hippocampal atrophy and downregulation of the neuroendocrine axis. This is a growing area of longitudinal neurobiological research, but early findings suggest that the long-term effects of ACEs may be to adversely affect the immune system with a variety of consequences.

Management
Psychodynamic psychotherapy

Psychodynamic psychotherapy is derived from psychoanalysis and is based on several key analytical concepts. These include Freud's ideas about psychosexual development, defence mechanisms, free association as the method of recall, and the therapeutic techniques of interpretation, including that of transference, defences and dreams. Such therapy usually involves once-weekly sessions, the length of treatment varying between 3 months and 2 years. The long-term aim is symptom relief and personality change. Psychodynamic psychotherapy is classically indicated in the treatment of unresolved conflicts in early life, as might be found in non-psychotic and personality disorders. There is no convincing evidence concerning its superiority over alternative forms of treatment.

Cognitive analytical therapy

Cognitive analytical therapy is an integration of CBT and psychodynamic therapy. It is a short-term therapy involving the patient and therapist recognizing the origins of a recurrent problem, reformulating how it continues to occur, and revising other ways of coping and internalizing it, using both the transference of the patient–therapist relationship and behavioural experiments.

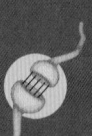

Obsessive–compulsive disorder

Obsessive–compulsive disorder (OCD) is characterized by obsessional ruminations and compulsive rituals. It is particularly associated with both depressive illness and **Tourette's syndrome** (see p. 863). The prevalence is between 1% and 2% in the general population, and patients uncommonly seek help. There is an equal distribution by gender, and the mean age of onset ranges from 20 to 40 years.

Clinical features

The obsessions and compulsions are time-consuming and intrusive, so that they affect functioning and cause considerable distress. Obsessions are often unpleasant repetitive thoughts, out of character, such as being dirty or violent. This can lead to a compulsive need to check that everything and everyone is all right and that things have been done correctly, and reassurance cannot remove the doubt that persists. Some rituals are derived from superstitions, such as actions repeated a fixed number of times, with the need to start again if interrupted. When severe and primary, OCD can last for many years and may be resistant to treatment. However, obsessional symptoms commonly occur in other disorders, most notably depressive illness, and remit with the resolution of the primary disorder.

Minor degrees of obsessional symptoms and compulsive rituals or superstitions are common in the healthy population and do not require treatment, particularly in times of stress and in children, who usually grow out of it. The mildest grade is that of obsessional personality traits, such as over-conscientiousness, tidiness, punctuality, and other indicators of a strong tendency towards conformity and inflexibility. Such individuals are *perfectionists* who are intolerant of shortcomings in themselves and others, and take pride in their high standards. When such traits are so marked that they dominate other aspects of personality, in the absence of clear-cut OCD, the diagnosis is obsessional (anankastic) personality (see p. 799).

Aetiology

Genetic factors

OCD is found in 5–7% of the first-degree relatives. Twin studies showed 80–90% concordance in monozygotic twins and about 50% in dizygotic twins. Genetic factors account for more of the variance in childhood-onset versus adult-onset cases.

Biological model

Neuroimaging studies suggest dysfunction in the orbito-striatal area (including the caudate nucleus) and dorsolateral prefrontal cortex, combined with abnormalities in serotonergic (underactive) and glutamatergic (overactive) neurotransmission. Further support for this model comes from an association with neurological disorders involving dysfunction of the striatum, including Parkinson's disease, Huntington's disease, Tourette's syndrome and Sydenham's chorea. The latter has also been associated with OCD and tic disorders in the *p*aediatric *a*utoimmune *n*europsychiatric *d*isorder *a*ssociated with *s*treptococcal infection (PANDAS). This is a rare condition in children that follows group A haemolytic streptococcal infection. OCD also can follow brain injury.

Cognitive behavioural model

Most people have occasional intrusive thoughts, but would ordinarily dismiss these as meaningless and not focus upon them further. These develop into an obsession when they assume great significance to the individual, causing greater anxiety. This anxiety motivates suppression of these thoughts, and ritual behaviours are developed to reduce anxiety further.

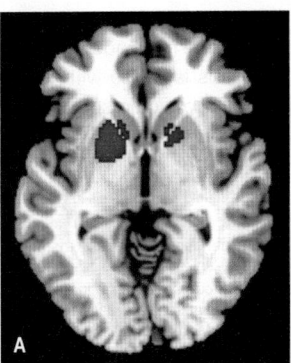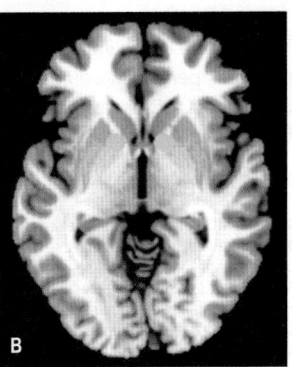

Fig. 25.4 Grey matter increase and deep brain stimulation targets in obsessive–compulsive disorder. **(A)** Main areas of increased grey matter regions (lenticular nuclei and caudate) in individuals with obsessive–compulsive disorder (red). **(B)** The usual targets for deep brain stimulation in the treatment of obsessive–compulsive disorder (green). (*From Radua J, Mataix-Cols D. Voxel-wise meta-analysis of grey matter changes in obsessive compulsive disorder.* Br J Psychiatr *2009; 195:393–402, with permission.*)

Management

Psychological management

CBT focusing on exposure and response prevention is reasonably effective. This involves confronting the anxiety-provoking stimulus in a controlled environment and not performing the associated ritual. The aim is for the individual to habituate to the stimulus, thus reducing anxiety. Since it provokes anxiety, the dropout rate is often high.

Physical management

Tricyclic antidepressants (TCAs) and serotonin reuptake inhibitors (SSRIs)

Clomipramine (a TCA) and the SSRIs are the mainstay of drug treatment. Their efficacy is independent of their antidepressant action but the doses required are usually some 50–100% higher than those effective in depression. Although many sufferers respond, relapse rates on discontinuation are high. Three months' treatment with maximum tolerated doses may be necessary for a positive response; in those who fail to respond, the addition of an antipsychotic significantly improves outcome, especially when tics occur co-morbidly. Positive correlations between reduced severity of OCD and decreased orbitofrontal and caudate metabolism following behavioural and SSRI treatments have been demonstrated in a number of studies.

Deep brain stimulation

This is a non-ablative, and therefore potentially reversible, surgical technique that involves the electrical stimulation of the basal ganglia by implanted electrodes, creating a 'functional lesion' (**Fig. 25.4**). Although this has had success, often impressively so in intractable cases, issues still remain regarding subject selection and the optimum anatomical targets.

Psychosurgery

This is very occasionally recommended in cases of chronic and severe OCD refractory to other treatments. The development of stereotactic techniques has led to the replacement of the earlier, crude leucotomies with more precise surgical interventions such as subcaudate tractotomy and cingulotomy, with small yttrium radioactive implants, which induce lesions in the cingulate area or the ventromedial quadrant of the frontal lobe.

Prognosis

Two-thirds of cases improve within a year; the remainder run a fluctuating or persistent course. The prognosis is worse with primary and severe OCD or with an anankastic pre-morbid personality when the personality is obsessional or anankastic.

Further reading

Craske, MG, Stein, MB. Anxiety. *Lancet* 2016; 388:3048–3059.
Danese A, McEwen BS. Adverse childhood experiences, allostasis, allostatic load, and age-related disease. *Physiol Behav* 2012; 106:29–39.
Fenster RJ, Lebois LAM, Ressler KJ et al. Brain circuit dysfunction in post-traumatic stress disorder: from mouse to man. *Nat Neurosci Rev* 2018; 19:535–551.
Grant JE. Obsessive-compulsive disorder. *N Engl J Med* 2014; 371:646–653.
National Institute for Health and Clinical Excellence. *NICE Guideline 116:Post-traumatic Stress Disorder*. NICE 2018; https://www.nice.org.uk/guidance/ng116/chapter/Recommendations#management-of-ptsd-in-children-young-people-and-adults.
National Institute for Health and Clinical Excellence. *NICE Clinical Guideline 113: Generalised Anxiety Disorder and Panic Disorder (with or without Agoraphobia) in Adults: Management in Primary, Secondary and Community Care*. NICE 2011; http://www.nice.org.uk/CG113/.
Shear MK. Complicated grief. *N Engl J Med* 2015; 372:153–160.

ALCOHOL MISUSE AND DEPENDENCE

A wide range of physical, social and psychiatric problems are associated with excessive drinking. Alcohol misuse occurs when a patient is drinking in a way that regularly causes problems to the patient or others.

- **The problem drinker** is one who causes or experiences physical, psychological and/or social harm as a consequence of drinking alcohol. Many problem drinkers, while heavy drinkers, are not physically addicted to alcohol.
- **Heavy drinkers** are those who drink significantly more in terms of quantity and/or frequency than is safe in the long term.
- **Binge drinkers** are those who drink excessively in short bouts, separated by often lengthy periods of abstinence. Their overall monthly or weekly alcohol intake may be relatively modest.
- **Alcohol dependence** is defined by a physical dependence on or addiction to alcohol. The term 'alcoholism' is a confusing one and has off-putting connotations of vagrancy, 'meths' drinking and social disintegration. It has been replaced by the term 'alcohol dependence syndrome'.

Epidemiology

A total of 20% of men and 10% of women drink more than double the recommended limit of 14 units per week in the UK. The amount of alcohol consumed in the UK has doubled over the last 50 years. Some 4% of men and 2% of women report alcohol withdrawal symptoms, suggesting dependence. Approximately 1 in 5 male admissions to acute medical wards is directly or indirectly due to alcohol. People with serious drinking problems have a 2–3 times increased risk of dying compared with the general population of the same age and sex.

Box 25.36 provides an estimate of what behavioural impairment can be expected in an average individual with a particular blood alcohol level. The amount of alcohol is measured for convenience in units that contain about 8 g of absolute alcohol and raise the blood alcohol concentration by 15–20 mg/dL, the amount that is metabolized in 1 h. One unit of alcohol is found in half a pint of ordinary beer (3.5% alcohol by volume, ABV) and in 125 mL of 9% wine. Note that most lagers are 5% ABV (3 units per pint) and wine is often 13% ABV and sold in 175 mL glasses (2–3 units per glass).

Box 25.36 Behavioural effects of alcohol

Blood alcohol concentration (BAC) (mg/dL)	Expected effect
20–99	Impaired coordination, euphoria
100–199	Ataxia, poor judgement, labile mood
200–299	Marked ataxia and slurred speech; poor judgement, labile mood, nausea and vomiting
300–399	Stage 1 anaesthesia, memory lapse, labile mood
400+	Respiratory failure, coma, death

Box 25.37 Common alcohol-related psychological and social problems

Psychological
- Depression
- Anxiety
- Memory problems
- Delirium tremens
- Attempted suicide
- Suicide
- Pathological jealousy

Social
- Domestic violence
- Marital and sexual difficulties
- Child abuse
- Employment problems
- Financial difficulties
- Accidents at home, on the roads, at work
- Delinquency and crime
- Homelessness

Diagnosis

Alcohol misuse should be suspected in any patient presenting with one or more of the physical problems commonly associated with excessive drinking (see p. 1258). Alcohol misuse may also be associated with a number of psychiatric symptoms/disorders and social problems (**Box 25.37**).

Guidelines

The patient's frequency of drinking and the quantity drunk during a typical week should be established. Although previous guidelines proposed different weekly limits for men and women as representing 'safe drinking', this has now been abandoned.

- 14 units per week has now been set for both sexes as 'low risk' rather than 'safe', with the declaration that there is no safe drinking level.
- 10–20 years of regularly drinking more than 14 units per week is associated with adverse health consequences, including malignancies and diseases of the cardiovascular, gastrointestinal and nervous systems.

Diagnostic markers of alcohol misuse

Laboratory parameters indicating alcohol misuse in recent weeks include elevated γ-glutamyl transpeptidase (γ-GT) and mean corpuscular volume (MCV). Blood or breath alcohol tests are useful in anyone suspected of very recent drinking.

Alcohol dependence syndrome

Dependence is a pattern of repeated self-administration that causes tolerance, withdrawal and compulsive substance use, the essential

> **Box 25.38 Symptoms of alcohol dependence**
>
> - Inability to keep to a drink limit
> - Difficulty in avoiding getting drunk
> - Spending a considerable amount of time drinking
> - Missing meals
> - Memory lapses, blackouts
> - Restlessness without drink
> - Organizing the day around drink
> - Trembling after drinking the day before
> - Morning retching and vomiting
> - Sweating excessively at night
> - Withdrawal fits
> - Morning drinking
> - Increased tolerance
> - Hallucinations, frank delirium tremens

> **Box 25.39 Diagnostic criteria for alcohol withdrawal syndrome**
>
> ***Any three of the following:***
> - Tremor of outstretched hands, tongue or eyelids
> - Sweating
> - Nausea, retching or vomiting
> - Tachycardia or hypertension
> - Anxiety
> - Psychomotor agitation
> - Headache
> - Insomnia
> - Malaise or weakness
> - Transient visual, tactile or auditory hallucinations or illusions
> - Grand mal convulsions

element of which is the continued use of the substance despite significant substance-related problems. Symptoms of alcohol dependence in a typical order of occurrence are shown in **Box 25.38**. Diagnostic criteria for alcohol withdrawal syndrome are shown in **Box 25.39**.

Course

About 25% of all cases of alcohol misuse will lead to chronic alcohol dependence. This most commonly ends in social incapacity, death or abstinence. Alcohol dependence syndrome usually develops after 10 years of heavy drinking (3–4 years in women). In some individuals who use alcohol to alter consciousness, obliterate conscience and defy social mores, dependence and loss of control may appear in only a few months or years.

Delirium tremens

Delirium tremens (DTs) is the most serious withdrawal state and occurs 1–3 days after alcohol cessation, so is commonly seen 1–2 days after admission to hospital. Patients are disorientated and agitated and have a marked tremor and visual hallucinations (e.g. insects or small animals). Signs include sweating, tachycardia, tachypnoea and pyrexia. Complications include dehydration, infection, hepatic disease or the Wernicke–Korsakoff's syndrome (see p. 891).

Aetiology of alcohol dependence

Genetic factors

Sons of alcohol-dependent people who are adopted by other families are four times more likely to develop drinking problems than are the adopted sons of non-alcohol misusers. Genetic markers include the serotonin transporter gene, dopamine-2 receptor allele A1, alcohol dehydrogenase subtypes and monoamine oxidase B activity, but they are not specific.

Environmental factors

Adverse childhood experience increases the risk of subsequent alcohol dependence and this rises if there is also a history of parental alcohol dependence or other substance misuse.

Neurobiological factors

Similar to many drugs of addiction, there is substantial empirical evidence for the involvement of dopaminergic and opioidergic neural circuitry within the striatum and ventral tegmentum. Sites where these converge, 'hedonic hotspots', underpin 'motivational salience': what we are most likely to respond to in our environment and the likelihood of the same response recurring under the same circumstances in the future. Corticotrophin-releasing hormone may have a bearing on what is potentially addictive to one individual and not to another by altering the valency of the given stimulus (good versus bad), which potentially ties continued abuse to dysregulation of the stress axis. This is not specific to alcohol and may imply that addictive behaviour is a consequence of stress but also a cause of it. Specific neurobiological causal factors have not been reliably identified.

Psychiatric illness

Psychotic, depressed, anxious and phobic patients frequently self-medicate with alcohol but this is an uncommon cause of dependency.

Excess consumption in society

The prevalence of alcohol dependence correlates with the general level of alcohol use in a society. This, in turn, is determined by price, licensing laws, availability and the societal norms concerning alcohol consumption.

Management

Psychological management of problem drinking

Successful identification at an early stage can be a helpful intervention in its own right. It should lead to:

- the provision of information concerning low-risk drinking levels
- a recommendation to cut down where indicated
- simple support and advice concerning associated problems.

This alone may prove effective. Successful alcohol misuse treatment involves ***motivational enhancement*** (***motivational therapy***), feedback, education about the adverse effects of alcohol, and agreed drinking goals. A motivational approach is based on five stages of change: pre-contemplation, contemplation, determination, action and maintenance. The therapist uses motivational interviewing and reflective listening to allow the patient to persuade himself along the five stages to change.

This technique, CBT and 12-step facilitation (as used by Alcoholics Anonymous, AA) have all been shown to reduce harmful drinking. With addictive drinking, self-help group therapy, involving long-term support by fellow members of the group (e.g. AA), is helpful in maintaining abstinence. Family and marital therapy involving both the alcohol misuser and partner may also help. Families of drinkers find meeting others in a similar situation helpful (Al-Anon).

Drug treatments for problem drinking

Alcohol withdrawal and delirium tremens

Addicted drinkers often experience considerable difficulty when they attempt to reduce or stop drinking. Withdrawal symptoms are a particular problem and delirium tremens (DTs) needs urgent treatment (**Box 25.40**). In the absence of DTs, alcohol withdrawal can be treated on an outpatient basis (see **Box 25.40**), so long as the patient attends daily for medication and monitoring, and has good

---

Box 25.40 Management of delirium tremens (DTs)

General measures
- Admit the patient to a medical bed
- Correct electrolyte abnormalities and dehydration
- Treat any co-morbid disorder (e.g. infection)
- Give parenteral thiamine slowly (250 mg daily for 3–5 days) in the absence of Wernicke–Korsakoff's syndrome
- Give parenteral thiamine slowly (500 mg daily for 3–5 days) with Wernicke–Korsakoff's encephalopathy. *Note*: Beware anaphylaxis
- Give prophylactic phenytoin or carbamazepine, if there is a previous history of withdrawal fits

Specific drug treatment
- Give one of the following orally:
  - Diazepam 10–20 mg
  - Chlordiazepoxide 30–60 mg
- Repeat 1 h after the last dose, depending on response

Fixed-schedule regimens
- Diazepam 10 mg every 6 h for 4 doses, then 5 mg 6-hourly for 8 doses *OR*
- Chlordiazepoxide 30 mg every 6 h for 4 doses, then 15 mg 6-hourly for 8 doses
- Provide additional benzodiazepine when symptoms and signs are not controlled

---

Box 25.41 Commonly used drugs of misuse and dependence

Stimulants
- Methylphenidate
- Phenmetrazine
- Phencyclidine ('angel dust')
- Cocaine
- Amfetamine derivatives
- Ecstasy (MDMA)

Hallucinogens
- Cannabis preparations
- Solvents
- Lysergic acid diethylamide (LSD)
- Mescaline

Narcotics
- Morphine
- Heroin
- Codeine
- Pethidine
- Methadone
- Tranquillizers
- Barbiturates
- Benzodiazepines

---

social support. Outpatient schedules are sometimes given over 5 days. Long-term treatment with benzodiazepines should not be prescribed in those patients who continue to misuse alcohol.

Drugs for prevention of alcohol dependence

Naltrexone, the opioid antagonist (50 mg per day), reduces the risk of relapse into heavy drinking and the frequency of drinking. *Acamprosate* (1–2 g/day) acts on several receptors, including those for GABA, noradrenaline (norepinephrine) and serotonin and reduces drinking frequency. Neither drug seems particularly helpful in maintaining abstinence. The effects of both are enhanced by combining them with counselling, but their moderate efficacy precludes regular use.

Disulfiram reacts with alcohol to cause unpleasant acetaldehyde intoxication and histamine release. There is mixed evidence of efficacy.

Oral thiamine (300 mg/day) can prevent Wernicke–Korsakoff's syndrome (see p. 891) in heavy drinkers and should *always* be prescribed.

Prognosis

Research suggests that 30–50% of alcohol-dependent drinkers are abstinent or drinking very much less up to 2 years following traditional intervention. The long-term outcome of patients treated with the latest psychological and pharmacological therapies remains uncertain.

Further reading

Friedmann PD. Alcohol use in adults. *N Engl J Med* 2013; 368:365–373.
Schuckit MA. Recognition and management of withdrawal delirium (delirium tremens). *N Engl J Med* 2014; 371:2100–2113.

DRUG MISUSE AND DEPENDENCE

In addition to alcohol and nicotine, there are a number of psychotropic substances that are taken for their effects on mood and other mental functions (**Box 25.41**).

Aetiology of drug misuse

There is no single cause of drug misuse and/or dependence. Three factors appear commonly, in a similar way to alcohol problems:
- the availability of drugs
- a vulnerable personality
- social pressures, particularly from peers.

Once regular drug-taking is established, pharmacological factors determine dependence.

Drugs of misuse and their effects

Inhaled substances

Some 1% of adolescents in the UK sniff solvents such as glue for their intoxicating effects. Tolerance develops over weeks or months. Intoxication is characterized by euphoria, excitement, a floating sensation, dizziness, slurred speech and ataxia. Acute intoxication can cause amnesia and visual hallucinations.

Nitrous oxide (laughing gas) is increasingly popular in the UK and is associated with the functional deactivation of vitamin B_{12} and potentially disabling neurological sequelae.

Amfetamines and related substances

These have temporary stimulant and euphoriant effects that are followed by fatigue and depression, the latter sometimes prolonged for weeks. Psychological rather than true physical dependence occurs with amfetamine sulphate ('speed'). Methyl amfetamine, also known as 'crystal meth', is another amfetamine psychostimulant. The high potential for abuse is associated with the activation of neural reward mechanisms involving nucleus accumbens dopamine release.

In addition to a manic-like presentation, amfetamines can produce a schizophrenia-like paranoid psychosis .

'Ecstasy' is the street name for 3,4-methylenedioxymetamphetamine(MDMA), a psychoactive phenylisopropylamine, synthesized as an amfetamine derivative. It has a brief duration of action (4–6 h). Deaths have been reported from malignant hyperpyrexia and dehydration. Acute renal and liver failure can occur.

Cocaine

Cocaine (see p. 267) is a central nervous system stimulant (with similar effects to amfetamines), derived from *Erythroxylon coca* trees grown in the Andes. In purified form, it may be taken orally, snorted or injected. If cocaine hydrochloride is converted to its base ('crack'), it can be smoked. Dependent users take large doses and alternate between withdrawal phenomena of depression, tremor and muscle pains, and the hyperarousal produced by increasing doses. Prolonged use of high doses produces irritability, restlessness, paranoid ideation and, occasionally, convulsions. Persistent sniffing of the drug can cause perforation of the nasal septum. Overdoses cause death through myocardial infarction, cerebrovascular disease, hyperthermia and arrhythmias (see p. 268).

Hallucinogenic drugs

Hallucinogenic drugs, such as lysergic acid diethylamide (LSD) and mescaline, produce distortions and intensifications of sensory perceptions, as well as frank hallucinations in acute intoxication. Psychosis is a long-term complication.

Cannabis

Cannabis is a widely used drug in some subcultures. It is derived from the dried leaves and flowers of the plant *Cannabis sativa*. It can cause tolerance and dependence. Hashish is the dried resin from the flower tops, while marijuana refers to any part of the plant. The drug, when smoked, seems to exaggerate the pre-existing mood, be it depression, euphoria or anxiety. It has specific analgesic properties. Cannabis use, especially of the more potent 'skunk', has increased in the UK. An amotivational syndrome with apathy and memory problems has been reported with chronic daily use. Cannabis may, of itself, sometimes cause psychosis in the right circumstances (see later).

Tranquillizers

Drugs that cause dependence include barbiturates and benzodiazepines. Benzodiazepine dependence is common and may be iatrogenic, when the drugs are prescribed and not discontinued. Discontinuing treatment with benzodiazepines may cause withdrawal symptoms (see **Box 25.35**). For this reason, withdrawal should be supervised and gradual.

Opiates

Physical dependence occurs with morphine, heroin and codeine, as well as with synthetic and semi-synthetic opiates such as methadone, pethidine and fentanyl. These substances display cross-tolerance – the withdrawal effects of one are reduced by administration of another. The psychological effects of opiates are a calm, slightly euphoric mood associated with freedom from physical discomfort and a flattening of emotional response. This is believed to be due to the attachment of morphine and its analogues to endorphin receptors in the central nervous system. Tolerance to this group of drugs is rapidly developed and marked, but is quickly lost following abstinence. The *opiate withdrawal syndrome* consists of a constellation of signs and symptoms (**Box 25.42**) that reaches peak intensity on the second or third day after the last dose of the opiate. These rapidly subside over the next 7 days. Withdrawal is dangerous in people with heart disease or other chronic debilitating conditions.

Opiate addicts have a relatively high mortality rate, owing to both the ease of accidental overdose and the blood-borne infections associated with shared needles. Heart disease (including infective endocarditis), tuberculosis and AIDS are common causes of death, while the complications of hepatitis B and C are also common. Some illegal supplies of heroin used by addicts contain fentanyl which increases the toxicity, leading to a high mortality, particularly in the United States.

Management of chronic misuse

Blood and urine screening for drugs is required in circumstances where drug misuse is suspected. When a patient with an opiate addiction is admitted to hospital for another health problem, advice should be sought from a psychiatrist or drug misuse clinic regarding management of their addiction while an inpatient.

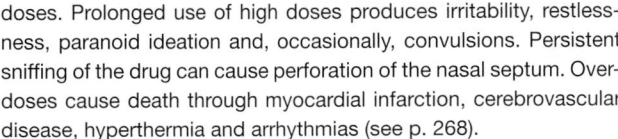

> **Box 25.42** Opiate withdrawal syndrome

12–16 h after last dose of opiate
- Yawning
- Rhinorrhoea
- Lacrimation
- Pupillary dilation
- Sweating
- Piloerection
- Restlessness

24–72 h after last dose of opiate
- Muscular twitches
- Aches and pains
- Abdominal cramps
- Vomiting
- Diarrhoea
- Hypertension
- Insomnia
- Anorexia
- Agitation
- Profuse sweating

The treatment of chronic dependence aims to help the patient either to live without drugs, or to regularize and control use, and to prevent secondary ill-health. Patients need help and advice in order to avoid a withdrawal syndrome. An overdose should be treated immediately with the opioid antagonist naloxone.

Drug-induced psychosis

Drug-induced psychosis has been reported with amfetamine and its derivatives, and with cocaine and hallucinogens. It can occur acutely after drug use but is more usually associated with chronic misuse. Psychoses are characterized by vivid hallucinations (usually auditory, but often occurring in more than one sensory modality), misidentifications, delusions and/or ideas of reference (often of a persecutory nature), psychomotor disturbances (excitement or stupor) and an abnormal affect. For diagnosis, ICD-10 requires the condition to occur within 2 weeks and usually within 48 hours of drug use, and to persist for more than 48 hours but not more than 6 months.

Cannabis use can result in anxiety, depression or hallucinations. Manic-like psychoses occurring after long-term cannabis use have been described but seem more likely to be related to the toxic effects of heavy ingestion. Evidence suggests that the risk of psychosis is significantly raised in those using cannabis at an early age (before, as compared to after, 15 years) and on a daily basis. High-potency cannabis ('skunk') is associated with an increased risk. A meta-analysis suggests that daily cannabis use doubles the risk of psychosis, and that 14% of schizophrenia in the UK would be prevented if cannabis use ceased.

Further reading

Degenhardt L, Hall W. Extent of illicit drug use and dependence, and their contribution to the global burden of disease. *Lancet* 2012; 379:55–70.
Kuepper R, van Os J, Lieb R et al. Continued cannabis use and risk of incidence and persistence of psychotic symptoms: 10-year follow-up cohort study. *BMJ* 2011; 342:d738.
Room R, Reuter P. How well do international drug conventions protect public health? *Lancet* 2012; 379:84–91.
Strang J, Babor T, Caulkins J et al. Drug policy and the public good: evidence for effective interventions. *Lancet* 2012; 379:71–83.
Strang J, Metrebian N, Lintzeris N et al. Supervised injectable heroin or injectable methadone versus optimised oral methadone as treatment for chronic heroin addicts in England after persistent failure in orthodox treatment (RIOTT): a randomised trial. *Lancet* 2010; 375:1885–1895.
Volkow ND, Baler RD, Compton WM et al. Adverse health effects of marijuana use. *N Engl J Med* 2014; 370:2219–2227.
Volkow ND, Koob GF, McLellan AT. Neurobiologic advances from the brain disease model of addiction. *N Engl J Med* 2016; 374:363–371.

SCHIZOPHRENIA

The group of illnesses conventionally referred to as 'schizophrenia' is diverse in nature and covers a broad range of perceptual, cognitive and behavioural disturbances. The point prevalence of the condition is 0.5% throughout the world, with equal gender distribution. A non-psychiatrist primarily needs to know how to recognize schizophrenia, what problems it might present with in the general hospital and how it is treated.

Aetiology

No single cause has been identified. Schizophrenia is likely to be a disease of neurodevelopmental disconnection caused by an interaction of genetic and environmental factors that affect brain development. The genetic aetiology is likely to be polygenic and non-mendelian; a recent very large study suggests there are about 100 single nucleotide polymorphisms that are associated. Schizophrenia has a heritability of about 60%. Functional neuroimaging studies and histology point towards alterations in prefrontal and, less consistently, temporal lobe function, with enlarged lateral ventricles and disorganized cytoarchitecture in the hippocampus, supporting neurodevelopmental models. Dopamine excess (D_2) is the oldest and most widely accepted neurochemical hypothesis, although this may explain only one group of symptoms (the positive ones). The cognitive impairments in schizophrenia may be related to dopamine D_1 abnormalities. The interaction between serotonergic and dopaminergic systems is likely to play a role. Glutamate and glycine have been recent pharmacological targets with promising preclinical data that has not been realized in subsequent trials.

Clinical features

The peak age of onset is the early twenties but it may start at any time. The characteristic symptoms of the condition have been termed *first-rank symptoms*. They consist of:
- *auditory hallucinations* in the third person and/or voices commenting on the patient's behaviour
- *thought withdrawal*, insertion and broadcast
- *primary delusion* (arising out of nothing)
- *delusional perception*
- *somatic passivity and feelings* – patients believe that their thoughts, feelings or acts are controlled by others.

The more of these symptoms a patient has, the more likely it is that the diagnosis is schizophrenia, but they also occur in other psychoses.

Other symptoms of *acute schizophrenia* include behavioural disturbances, other hallucinations, secondary (usually persecutory) delusions and blunting of mood. Schizophrenia is sometimes divided into 'positive' and 'negative' symptom clusters:
- *Positive schizophrenia* is characterized by acute onset, prominent delusions and hallucinations, normal brain structure, a biochemical disorder involving dopaminergic transmission, a good response to neuroleptics, and a better outcome.
- *Negative schizophrenia* is characterized by a slow, insidious onset, a relative absence of acute symptoms, the presence of apathy, social withdrawal, lack of motivation, underlying brain structure abnormalities and poor antipsychotic response.

Chronic schizophrenia is characterized by its long duration and by the 'negative' symptoms of underactivity, lack of drive, social withdrawal and emotional emptiness.

Differential diagnosis

Schizophrenia should be distinguished from:
- organic mental disorders (e.g. partial complex epilepsy)

Motor
- Acute dystonia
- Parkinsonism
- Akathisia (motor restlessness)
- Tardive dyskinesia

Autonomic
- Hypotension
- Failure of ejaculation

Antimuscarinic
- Dry mouth
- Urinary retention
- Constipation
- Blurred vision

Metabolic
- Weight gain

Others
- Precipitation of glaucoma
- Galactorrhoea (due to hyperprolactinaemia)
- Amenorrhoea
- Cardiac arrhythmias
- QTc interval prolongation
- Seizures
- Leucopenia
- Cholestatic jaundice
- Skin reactions
- Hypersensitivity

[a]The frequency and type of side-effects will depend upon the choice of antipsychotic agent and its dose.

- mood (affective) disorders (e.g. mania)
- drug psychoses (e.g. amfetamine psychosis)
- personality disorders (schizotypal).

In older patients, any acute or chronic brain syndrome can present in a schizophrenia-like manner. A helpful diagnostic point is the fact that altered consciousness and disturbances of memory do not occur in schizophrenia, and visual hallucinations are unusual.

A *schizoaffective psychosis* describes a clinical presentation in which clear-cut affective and schizophrenic symptoms coexist in the same episode.

Management

The best results are obtained by combining drug and social treatments.

Antipsychotic drugs

These act by blocking the D_1 and D_2 groups of dopamine receptors and are most effective against acute, positive symptoms and are least effective in the management of chronic, negative symptoms. Complete control of positive symptoms can take up to 3 months, and premature discontinuation of treatment can result in relapse.

As antipsychotic drugs block both D_1 and D_2 dopamine receptors, they usually produce extrapyramidal adverse effects. This limits their use in the maintenance therapy of many patients. They also block adrenergic and muscarinic receptors and thereby cause a number of other unwanted effects (**Box 25.43**).

Neuroleptic malignant syndrome

This is an infrequent but potentially dangerous adverse effect. Neuroleptic malignant syndrome is a medical emergency and should be managed by medical admission. It occurs in 0.2% of patients on antipsychotic drugs, particularly the potent dopaminergic antagonists,

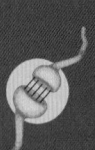

such as haloperidol. Symptoms occur a few days to a few weeks after starting treatment and consist of hyperthermia, muscle rigidity, autonomic instability (tachycardia, labile blood pressure, pallor) and a fluctuating level of consciousness. Investigations show a raised creatine kinase, raised white cell count and abnormal liver biochemistry. The more severe consequences include acute renal injury, pulmonary embolus and death. Treatment consists of stopping the drug and general resuscitation measures, such as temperature reduction. Bromocriptine enhances dopaminergic activity and dantrolene will reduce muscle tone but no treatment has proven benefit.

Pregnancy

Data on the potential teratogenicity of antipsychotic medications are still limited. The disadvantages of not treating during pregnancy have to be balanced against possible developmental risks to the fetus. The butyrophenones (e.g. haloperidol) are probably safer than the phenothiazines, such as chlorpromazine. Subsequent management decisions relating to dosage will depend primarily on the ability to avoid adverse effects, since the antiparkinsonian agents are still believed to be teratogenic and should be avoided.

Typical or first-generation antipsychotics

Phenothiazines were the first group of antipsychotics to be developed but are used less frequently now. Chlorpromazine (100–1000 mg daily) is the drug of choice when a more sedating drug is required. Trifluoperazine is used when sedation is undesirable. Fluphenazine decanoate is used as a long-term prophylactic to prevent relapse, as a depot injection (25–100 mg i.m. every 1–4 weeks). **Butyrophenones** (e.g. haloperidol 2–15 mg daily) are also powerful antipsychotics, and are used in the treatment of acute schizophrenia and mania. They are likely to cause a dystonia and/or extrapyramidal adverse effects, but are much less sedating than the phenothiazines.

Atypical antipsychotics or serotonin dopamine antagonists

Atypical, second-generation antipsychotics or serotonin dopamine antagonists (SDAs), are 'atypical' in that they block D_2 receptors less than D_1, and thus cause fewer extrapyramidal adverse effects and less tardive dyskinesia. They are now recommended as first-line drugs for newly diagnosed schizophrenia.

Risperidone is a benzisoxazole derivative with combined dopamine D_2 receptor and 5-HT_{2A}-receptor blocking properties. The drug is not markedly sedative and the overall incidence and severity of extrapyramidal adverse effects is lower than with more conventional antipsychotics. Hyperprolactinaemia can be problematic and prolactin levels should be monitored. Paliperidone is an active metabolite of risperidone. Both are available in oral and depot preparations.

Olanzapine has affinity for 5-HT_2, D_1, D_2, D_4 and muscarinic receptor sites. Clinical studies indicate that it has a lower incidence of extrapyramidal adverse effects. The apparent better compliance with the drug may be related to its lower side-effect profile and its once-daily dosage. Weight gain is a problem with long-term treatment and there is an increased risk of type 2 diabetes mellitus with this and other atypical drugs.

Other atypical antipsychotics include amisulpride, lurasidone, sulpiride, zotepine, ziprasidone and quetiapine, the latter causing less hyperprolactinaemia. Those taking atypical antipsychotics should have regular monitoring of their body mass index, cholesterol levels, blood sugar and QTc interval on ECG. No more than one antipsychotic should be prescribed routinely.

Clozapine is used in patients who have intractable schizophrenia refractory to at least two conventional antipsychotic drugs; alternatively, it may be used as first-line therapy. This drug is a dibenzodiazepine with a relative high affinity for D_4 dopamine receptors, as compared with D_1, D_2, D_3 and D_5, in addition to muscarinic and α-adrenergic receptors. It acts additionally as a partial agonist at 5-HT_{1A} receptors, which may be of benefit in treating the 'negative' symptoms of psychosis. Functional brain scans have shown that clozapine selectively blocks limbic dopamine receptors more than striatal ones, which is probably why it causes considerably fewer extrapyramidal adverse effects. Clozapine exercises a strong therapeutic effect on both intractable positive and negative symptoms. However, it is expensive and produces severe agranulocytosis in 1–2% of patients. Therefore, in the UK, for example, it can only be prescribed to registered patients by doctors and pharmacists registered with a patient-monitoring service. White cell counts should be monitored weekly for 18 weeks and then 2-weekly for the length of treatment. In addition to its antipsychotic actions, clozapine may also help reduce aggressive and hostile behaviour and the risk of suicide. It can cause considerable weight gain and sialorrhoea. There is an increased risk of diabetes mellitus, and gastrointestinal hypomotility resulting in a functional obstruction has also been reported.

Psychological management

This consists of reassurance, support and a good doctor–patient relationship. Psychotherapy of an intensive or exploratory kind is contraindicated. In contrast, individual CBT may have some efficacy, particularly in those who decline drug treatment.

Social management

Social treatment involves attention being paid to the patient's environment and social functioning. Family education can help relatives and partners to provide the optimal amount of emotional and social stimulation, so that not too much emotion is expressed (a risk for relapse). Over 90% of patients are unemployed but sheltered employment can be helpful. Assertive outreach mental health teams will follow up those adhering poorly to treatment.

Medical presentations related to treatment

The motor adverse effects of neuroleptics are the most common reason for a patient with schizophrenia to present to a physician, followed by self-harm. **Acute dystonia** normally arises in patients newly started on neuroleptics, causing torticollis. **Extrapyramidal adverse effects** are common and present in the same way as Parkinson's disease. They remit once the drug is stopped and on use of antimuscarinic drugs, such as procyclidine. **Akathisia** is motor restlessness, most commonly affecting the legs. It is similar to the restless legs syndrome but is apparent during the day. **Amenorrhoea** and **galactorrhoea** can be caused by dopamine antagonists. Postural hypotension can affect the elderly, and neuroleptics can be the cause of delirium in this age group, if their antimuscarinic effects are prominent.

Long-term benefits outweigh the risks in most cases, and long-term treatment is associated with a lower mortality rate when compared with no treatment. In this respect, the atypical antipsychotics are preferable to the typical antipsychotics and clozapine is the class leader.

Prognosis

The prognosis of schizophrenia is variable: 15–25% of people with schizophrenia recover completely, about 70% will have relapses and may develop mild to moderate negative symptoms, and about 20% will remain seriously disabled. There is some evidence that early drug treatment improves prognosis.

Further reading

Birnbaum R, Weinberger DR. Genetic insights into the neurodevelopmental origins of schizophrenia. *Nat Rev Neurosci* 2017; 18:727–740.
Howes OD, Murray RM. Schizophrenia: an integrated sociodevelopmental-cognitive model. *Lancet* 2014; 383:1677–1687.
Leucht S, Cipriani A, Spineli L et al. Comparative efficacy and tolerability of 15 antipsychotic drugs in schizophrenia: a multiple-treatments meta-analysis. *Lancet* 2013; 382:951–962.

ORGANIC MENTAL DISORDERS

Organic brain disorders result from structural pathology, as in dementia (see p. 880), or from disturbed central nervous system function, as in fever-induced delirium.

Delirium

Delirium, also termed **toxic confusional state** and **acute organic psychosis**, is an acute or subacute brain failure in which impairment of attention is accompanied by abnormalities of perception and mood. It is the most common psychosis seen in the general hospital setting, where it occurs in 14–24% of patients. This figure rises in specialist populations such as intensive care patients. Agitation is usually worse at night, with consequent sleep reversal, so that the patient is asleep in the day and awake all night. In addition to an agitated, 'hyperactive' presentation, a hypoactive variant is also recognized and is thought to represent a worse prognosis in the elderly. Most cases will demonstrate a fluctuation between these two psychomotor forms. During the acute phase, thought and speech are incoherent, memory is impaired and misperceptions occur. Episodic visual hallucinations (or illusions) and persecutory delusions occur. As a consequence, the patient may be frightened, suspicious, restless and uncooperative.

A developing, deteriorating or damaged brain predisposes a patient to develop delirium (**Box 25.44**). A large number of diseases may cause delirium, particularly in elderly patients, such that it is wise to assess for delirium in patients over 65 years who are admitted to hospital. Some causes of delirium are listed in **Box 25.45**. Delirium tremens should be considered in the differential diagnosis (see p. 791), as well as Lewy body dementia (p. 883). Diagnostic criteria are given in **Box 25.46**.

Management

History should be taken from a witness. Examination may reveal the cause. Investigation and treatment of the underlying physical disease should be undertaken (see **Box 25.45**). The patient should be carefully nursed and rehydrated in a quiet single room with a window that does not allow exits. If a high fever is present, the patient's temperature should be reduced. All current drug therapy should be reviewed and, where possible, stopped. If they are needed, ensure that patients have hearing aids, glasses and dentures. Psychoactive drugs should be avoided if possible (because of their own risk of exacerbating delirium). In severe delirium, haloperidol is an effective choice, the daily dose usually ranging between 1.5 mg (in the elderly) and 20 mg per day. Benzodiazepines should not be used as first-line medication and may prolong confusion. If necessary, the first dose can be administered intramuscularly. Olanzapine is an effective alternative, especially if given at night for insomnia.

Prognosis

Delirium usually clears within a week or two, but brain recovery usually lags behind recovery from the causative physical illness. The prognosis depends not only on the successful treatment of the causative disease, but also on the underlying state of the brain. Some 25% of the elderly with delirium will have an underlying dementia; 15% of patients do not survive their underlying illness; 40% are in institutional care at 6 months. Mortality rates are raised in patients with delirium in the 18 months after admission and this is greatest in those who present to emergency departments with the diagnosis.

? Box 25.45 Some common causes of delirium

- Systemic infection:
  - Any infection, particularly with high fever (e.g. malaria, septicaemia)
- Metabolic disturbance:
  - Hepatic failure
  - Chronic kidney disease
  - Disorders of electrolyte balance, dehydration
  - Hypoxia
- Vitamin deficiency:
  - Thiamine (Wernicke–Korsakoff's syndrome, beriberi)
  - Nicotinic acid (pellagra)
  - Vitamin B_{12}
- Endocrine disease:
  - Hypothyroidism
  - Cushing's syndrome
- Intracranial causes:
  - Trauma
  - Tumour
  - Abscess
  - Subarachnoid haemorrhage
  - Epilepsy
- Drug intoxication:
  - Anticonvulsants
  - Antimuscarinics
  - Anxiolytics/hypnotics
  - Tricyclic antidepressants
  - Dopamine agonists
  - Digoxin
- Drug/alcohol withdrawal
- Postoperative states

---

i Box 25.44 Predisposing factors in delirium

- Extremes of age (developing or deteriorating brain)
- Damaged brain:
  - Any dementia (most common predisposition)
  - Previous head injury
  - Alcohol brain damage
  - Previous stroke
- Dislocation to an unfamiliar environment (e.g. hospital admission)
- Sleep deprivation
- Sensory extremes (overload or deprivation)
- Immobilization
- Visual or hearing impairment

---

i Box 25.46 Delirium: diagnostic criteria

- Disturbance of consciousness:
  - ↓ Clarity of awareness of environment
  - ↓ Ability to focus, sustain or shift attention
- Change in cognition:
  - Memory deficit, disorientation, language disturbance, perceptual disturbance
- Disturbance develops over a short period (hours or days)
- Fluctuation over the course of a day

(Derived from American Psychiatric Association. Diagnostic and Statistical Manual of Mental Disorders, 5th edn. Text revision (DSM-5). Washington, DC: APA; 2013.)

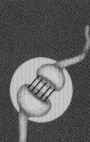

Further reading

Inouye SK, Westendorp RGJ, Saczynski JS. Delirium in elderly people. *Lancet* 2014; 383:911–922.

Marcantonio ER. Delirium in hospitalized older adults. *N Engl J Med* 2017; 377:1456–1466.

National Institute for Health and Care Excellence. *NICE Clinical Guideline 103: Delirium: Prevention, Diagnosis and Management*. NICE 2019; https://www.nice.org.uk/guidance/cg103.

van Munster BC, de Rooij S. Delirium: a synthesis of current knowledge. *Clin Med* 2014; 14:192–195.

Witlox J, Eurelings LS, de Jonghe JF et al. Delirium in elderly patients and the risk of postdischarge mortality, institutionalization, and dementia: a meta-analysis. *JAMA* 2010; 304:443–451.

EATING DISORDERS

Obesity

Obesity is the most common eating disorder (see p. 1247) and has become epidemic in many developed countries. It is usually caused by a combination of constitutional and social factors, but a binge-eating disorder and psychological determinants of 'comfort eating' should be excluded.

Anorexia nervosa

Case register data suggest an incidence rate of 19/100000 females aged between 15 and 34 years. Surveys have suggested a prevalence rate of approximately 1% among schoolgirls and university students. However, many more young women have amenorrhoea accompanied by less weight loss than the 15% required for the diagnosis of anorexia nervosa. The condition is much less common among men (ratio of 1:10).

Clinical features

The main clinical criteria for diagnosis are shown in **Box 25.47**. Clinical features include the following:

- Onset is usually in adolescence.
- There is a previous history of faddish eating.
- The patient generally eats little, yet is obsessed by food.
- Exercising is excessive.

The physical consequences of anorexia include sensitivity to cold, constipation, hypotension and bradycardia. In most cases, amenorrhoea is secondary to the weight loss. In those who also binge and vomit or abuse purgatives, there may be hypokalaemia and alkalosis.

Aetiology

Biological factors

Genetic

Some 6–10% of female siblings of affected women suffer from anorexia nervosa. There is an increased concordance amongst monozygotic twins, suggesting a genetic predisposition.

> ℹ **Box 25.47 Clinical criteria for anorexia nervosa**
>
> - Body weight >15% below the standard weight or a body mass index <17.5 kg/m² (ICD-10)
> - Self-induced weight loss: avoidance of fattening foods, vomiting, purging, exercise or appetite suppressants
> - Distortion of body image, i.e. patients regard themselves as fat when they are thin
> - Morbid fear of fatness
> - Amenorrhoea in women
>
> *(From World Health Organization. The ICD-10 Classification of Mental and Behavioural Disorders, 10th edn. Geneva: WHO; 2016.)*

Hormonal

The reductions in sex hormones and downregulation of the hypothalamic–pituitary–adrenal axis are secondary to malnutrition and usually reversed by refeeding.

Psychological factors

Individual

Anorexia nervosa has often been seen as an escape from the emotional problems of adolescence and a regression into childhood. Patients commonly have had dietary problems in early life. Perfectionism and low self-esteem are common antecedents. Studies suggest that survivors of abuse are at greater risk of developing an eating disorder, usually anorexia nervosa, in adolescence.

Family

Family problems are most commonly secondary to the stress of coping with a family member with the illness.

Social and cultural factors

There is a higher prevalence in higher social classes, Westernized families, certain occupational groups (e.g. ballet dancers and nurses) and societies where cultural value is placed on thinness.

Management

Treatment can be conducted on an outpatient basis, unless the weight loss is severe and accompanied by marked cardiovascular signs and/or electrolyte and vitamin disturbances. Hospital admission may then be unavoidable and may need to be on a medical ward initially. Uncommonly, the patient's weight loss may be so severe as to be life-threatening. If the patient cannot be persuaded to enter hospital, compulsory admission may have to be used. Inpatient treatment goals include:

- establishing a therapeutic relationship with both the patient and their family
- restoring the weight to a level between the ideal body weight and the patient's ideal weight
- providing a balanced diet, aimed at gaining 0.5–1 kg weight per week
- eliminating purgative and/or laxative use and vomiting.

Outpatient treatment should include cognitive behavioural or interpersonal psychotherapies. Family therapy is more effective than individual psychotherapy in adolescents and those still at home, and less effective in those who have left home. Motivational enhancement techniques are used with some success.

Drug treatment has met with limited success, and those drugs that increase the QTc interval should be avoided. Vitamins and minerals may need replacement.

Prognosis

The condition runs a fluctuating course, with exacerbations and partial remissions. Long-term follow-up suggests that about two-thirds of patients maintain normal weight and that the remaining one-third are split between those who are moderately underweight and those who are seriously underweight. Indicators of a poor outcome include:

- a long initial illness
- severe weight loss
- older age at onset
- bingeing and purging
- personality difficulties
- difficulties in relationships

Suicide has been reported in 2–5% of people with chronic anorexia nervosa. The mortality rate per year is 0.5% from all causes. The illness can quickly cause osteopenia, and later osteoporosis. More than one-third have recurrent affective illness, and various family, genetic and endocrine studies have found associations between eating disorders and depression.

Bulimia nervosa

This refers to episodes of uncontrolled excessive eating, which are also termed 'binges', accompanied by means to lose weight. There is a preoccupation with food and habitual behaviours to avoid the fattening effects of periodic binges. These behaviours include:

- self-induced vomiting
- misuse of drugs – laxatives, diuretics, thyroid extract or anorectics. Additional clinical features are shown in **Box 25.48**.

The lifetime prevalence of bulimia ranges between 3% and 7% for women. Bulimia is sometimes associated with anorexia nervosa. A pre-morbid history of dieting is common. The prognosis for bulimia nervosa is better than that for anorexia nervosa.

Management

Individual CBT is more effective than both interpersonal psychotherapy and drug treatments. SSRIs (e.g. fluoxetine) are also an effective treatment, even in the absence of a depressive illness, but may require high doses.

Atypical eating disorders

These include eating disorders that do not conform clinically to the diagnostic criteria for anorexia nervosa or bulimia nervosa. ***Binge-eating disorders*** (BEDs) consist of bulimia without the vomiting and other weight-reducing strategies. The new DSM-5 considers binge-eating disorder as a separate diagnosis, characterized by discrete episodes of significant overeating combined with a sense of having no control over eating during these episodes. Periods of bingeing need to be present at least once a week over a period of 3 months or more. ICD-10 continues to consider the diagnosis as an otherwise undefined eating disorder. Management strategies include self-help programmes and CBT, which are often combined with an SSRI.

Further reading

Bulik CM. The challenges of treating anorexia nervosa. *Lancet* 2014; 383:105–106.
National Institute for Health and Care Excellence. *NICE Guideline 69: Eating Disorders: Recognition and Treatment*. NICE 2017; https://www.nice.org.uk/guidance/ng69.
Royal College of Psychiatrists. *Anorexia and Bulimia*. Royal College of Psychiatrists 2015; https://www.rcpsych.ac.uk/mental-health/problems-disorders/anorexia-and-bulimia.
Treasure J, Claudino AM, Zucker N. Eating disorders. *Lancet* 2010; 375:583–593.

> *i* **Box 25.48 Clinical features of bulimia nervosa**
>
> - Physical complications of vomiting:
>   - Cardiac arrhythmias
>   - Renal impairment
>   - Muscular paralysis
>   - Tetany – from hypokalaemic alkalosis
>   - Swollen salivary glands – from vomiting
>   - Eroded dental enamel
> - Associated psychiatric disorders:
>   - Depressive illness
>   - Alcohol misuse
>   - Fluctuations in body weight within normal limits
>   - Menstrual function – periods irregular but amenorrhoea is rare
>   - Personality – perfectionism and/or low self-esteem present pre-morbidly

SEXUAL DISORDERS

Sexual disorders can be divided into sexual dysfunctions and deviations, and gender role disorders (**Box 25.49**).

Sexual dysfunction

Sexual dysfunction in men refers to the repeated inability to achieve normal sexual intercourse, whereas in women it refers to a repeatedly unsatisfactory quality of sexual satisfaction. Problems of sexual dysfunction can usefully be classified into those affecting sexual desire, arousal and orgasm.

Among men presenting for treatment of sexual dysfunction, erectile dysfunction is the most frequent complaint. The prevalence of premature ejaculation is low, except in young men, while ejaculatory failure is rare. Common female problems include reduced libido, vaginismus and anorgasmia.

Sexual drive is affected by constitutional factors, ignorance of sexual technique, anxiety about sexual performance, medical and psychiatric conditions, and certain drugs (**Boxes 25.50** and **25.51**).

The treatment of sexual dysfunction involves careful assessment of both physical and psychosocial factors, the participation (where appropriate) of the patient's partner, sex education, and specific therapeutic techniques, including relaxation, behavioural therapy and couple therapy. The introduction of phosphodiesterase type 5 inhibitors (e.g. sildenafil) has provided an effective therapy for the treatment of erectile dysfunction (see p. 1485).

Sexual deviation

Sexual deviations are regarded as unusual forms of behaviour rather than as an illness. Doctors are only likely to be involved when the behaviour involves breaking the law (e.g. paedophilia) and when there is a question of an associated mental or physical disorder. Men are more likely than women to have sexual deviations.

> *i* **Box 25.49 Classification of sexual disorders**
>
> **Sexual dysfunction**
>
> *Affecting sexual desire*
> - Low libido
>
> *Impaired sexual arousal*
> - Erectile dysfunction
> - Failure of arousal in women
>
> *Affecting orgasm*
> - Premature ejaculation
> - Retarded ejaculation
> - Orgasmic dysfunction in women
>
> **Sexual deviations**
>
> *Variations of the sexual 'object'*
> - Fetishism
> - Transvestism
> - Paedophilia
> - Bestiality
> - Necrophilia
>
> *Variations of the sexual act*
> - Exhibitionism
> - Voyeurism
> - Sadism
> - Masochism
> - Frotteurism
>
> **Disorders of the gender role**
> - Transsexualism

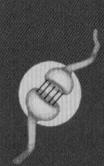

> ℹ️ **Box 25.50** Medical conditions affecting sexual performance

Endocrine
- Diabetes mellitus
- Hyperthyroidism
- Hypothyroidism

Cardiovascular
- Angina pectoris
- Previous myocardial infarction
- Disorders of peripheral circulation

Hepatic
- Cirrhosis, particularly alcohol-related

Renal
- Chronic kidney disease

Neurological
- Neuropathy
- Spinal cord lesions

Respiratory
- Asthma
- Chronic obstructive pulmonary disease

Psychiatric
- Depressive illness
- Substance misuse

> ℹ️ **Box 25.51** Drugs affecting sexual arousal

Male arousal
- Alcohol
- Benzodiazepines
- Neuroleptics
- Cimetidine
- Opiate analgesics
- Methyldopa
- Clonidine
- Spironolactone
- Antihistamines
- Metoclopramide
- Diuretics
- Beta-blockers
- Cannabis

Female arousal
- Alcohol[a]
- Central nervous system depressants
- Antidepressants (SSRIs)
- Oral combined contraceptives
- Methyldopa
- Clonidine

[a]Alcohol increases the desire but diminishes the performance. SSRIs, selective serotonin reuptake inhibitors.

Gender role disorders

Transsexualism involves a disturbance in gender identity in which the patient is convinced that their body is the wrong gender. A person's gender identity refers to the individual's sense of masculinity or femininity, as distinct from sex. There is increasing evidence that transsexualism is biologically determined, perhaps by prenatal endocrine influences, and functional brain imaging shows specific differences from normal controls.

For males, treatment includes oestrogen administration and, if surgery is to be recommended, a period of living as a woman as a trial beforehand. In the case of female transsexuals, treatment involves surgery and the use of methyltestosterone.

> ℹ️ **Box 25.52** Main categories of personality disorder

Category	Description
Borderline (emotionally unstable)	Impulsive actions Intense, short-lived emotional attachments Chronic internal emptiness Frequent self-harm Transient 'pseudo'-psychotic features Strong family history of mood disorders
Paranoid	Extreme sensitivity Suspicion Litigiousness Self-importance Preoccupation with conspiracy theories
Schizoid	Emotional coldness and detachment Limited capacity to express emotions Indifference to praise or criticism Preference for solitary activities Lack of close friendships Marked insensitivity to social norms
Antisocial	Callous unconcern for the feelings of others Incapacity to maintain enduring relationships Very low tolerance of frustration Incapacity to experience guilt and to learn from experience Tendency to blame others
Histrionic	Self-dramatization, theatricality, suggestibility Shallow and labile emotions Continual seeking for excitement and appreciation Inappropriately seductive appearance and behaviour
Narcissistic	Inflated sense of self-importance Need to be admired Self-referential nature Arrogance
Anankastic (obsessional)	Feelings of excessive doubt and caution Preoccupation with details, rules and order Perfectionism Excessive conscientiousness, scrupulousness, pedantry and rigidity
Dependent	Encouragement of others to make their personal decisions Subordination of their needs to others Unwillingness to make demands on others Feelings of inability to care for themselves Preoccupation with fears of being abandoned

---

PERSONALITY DISORDERS

These disorders comprise enduring patterns of behaviour that manifest themselves as inflexible responses to a broad range of personal and social situations. Personality disorders are developmental conditions that appear in childhood or adolescence and continue into adult life. Their prevalence is about 15% in the population. They are not secondary to another psychiatric disorder or brain disease, although they may precede or coexist with other disorders. In contrast, personality change is acquired, usually in adult life, following severe or prolonged stress, extreme environmental deprivation, serious psychiatric disorder or brain injury or disease.

Personality disorders are usually subdivided according to clusters of traits that correspond to the most frequent or obvious behavioural manifestations, but many will show the characteristics of more than one category. The main categories of personality disorder are described in **Box 25.52**.

Further reading

Bateman AW, Gunderson J, Mulder R. Treatment of personality disorder. *Lancet* 2015; 385:735–743.

Gunderson JG. Borderline personality disorder. *N Engl J Med* 2011; 364:2037–2042.

Leichsenring F, Leibing E, Kruse J et al. Borderline personality disorder. *Lancet* 2011; 377:74–84.

Newton-Howes G, Clark LA, Chanen A. Personality disorder across the life course. *Lancet* 2015; 385:727–734.

Tyrer P, Reed GM, Crawford MJ. Classification, assessment, prevalence, and effect of personality disorder. *Lancet* 2015; 385:717–726.

INVOLUNTARY DETENTION

(See also Chapter 5). Involuntary detention in hospital is typically used as a last resort and treatment on an outpatient basis is preferable in most cases. The term describes the practice of ***admitting or keeping a patient in hospital against their will***. This is done in compliance with the mental health legislation relevant to a particular country. Application for such a course of action may be made by a doctor (typically, but not always, a psychiatrist), social worker, psychologist or, in some instances, a police officer.

Mental health laws differ between countries and, in the case of the USA, also between states. However, in broad terms, the principles remain the same and are summarized in **Box 25.53**.

The potential for abuse of such 'powers' is a constant focal point for the review of such legislation. Although this is thankfully uncommon, the detention of individuals as a means to suppress dissent against regimes is well known.

> **i** **Box 25.53 The basis of mental health laws for detention**
>
> 1. The individual to be detained must be suffering from a defined mental disorder.
> 2. Detention is for the purposes of observation and refinement of the diagnosis and/or to actively treat the disorder (i.e. detention is a means to an end).
> 3. Attempts to treat the individual on an outpatient basis have failed.
> 4. The offer of a voluntary admission to hospital has been refused or is impractical.
> 5. Treatment in hospital is necessary:
>   - because it will benefit the outcome of the illness
>   - to protect the patient from harm (in terms of physical health, mental health, and abuse or manipulation at the hands of others)
>   - to protect others from harm that the patient might cause them either passively (neglect) or actively

MENTAL CAPACITY ACT

Mental capacity is the ability to make decisions about all aspects of one's life, including, but not exclusively, healthcare. All doctors need to be able to assess mental capacity. In England and Wales, a new act was passed in 2005, which, for the first time, formally protects patients who lack capacity. Some 3% of people in the UK are thought to lack capacity due to conditions affecting brain function, such as dementia. However, the assessment of capacity is specific to an individual decision, so it is possible to have capacity to make one decision but not another. The assessment of capacity is outlined in **Box 25.54**. Capacity is assumed unless there is evidence to the contrary. In the absence of capacity, it is best to act in the best interests of the patient and provide the least restrictive management, after consulting the nearest relative or an independent advocate.

> **Box 25.54 Assessment of mental capacity to make a decision**
>
> The patient lacks decision-making capacity if they have a demonstrated impairment or disturbance of their mind/brain, alongside a demonstrated inability to do any one of the following:
> - Understand relevant information
> - Retain that information for sufficient time to make the decision
> - Use or weigh that information
> - Communicate their decision

Further reading

Department for Constitutional Affairs. *Mental Capacity* Act 2005. *Code of Practice*. The Stationery Office 2007; https://assets.publishing.service.gov.uk/government/uploads/system/uploads/attachment_data/file/497253/Mental-capacity-act-code-of-practice.pdf.

National Institute for Health and Care Excellence. *NICE Guideline 108: Decision-making and Mental Capacity*. NICE 2018; https://www.nice.org.uk/guidance/NG108.

Nicholson TR, Cutter W, Hotopf M. Assessing mental capacity: the Mental Capacity Act. *BMJ* 2008; 336:322–325.

Significant websites

http://psych.org *American Psychiatric Association*.

http://www.b-eat.co.uk *Beating Eating Disorders (formerly the Eating Disorders Association)*.

http://www.cebmh.com *Centre for Evidence-Based Mental Health*.

http://www.mentalhealth.org.uk *Mental Health Foundation – charity*.

http://www.rcpsych.ac.uk *UK Royal College of Psychiatrists*.

http://www.sleepfoundation.org *National Sleep Foundation*.

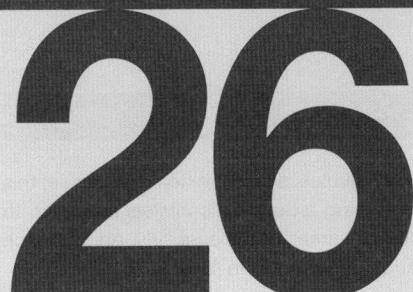

26

Neurology

Paul Jarman and Umesh Vivekananda

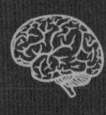

CORE SKILLS AND KNOWLEDGE

Neurology is a large and diverse subject that covers many conditions requiring long-term coordinated care and having serious effects on the daily lives of patients and their families. Neurology includes conditions as diverse as cognitive disorders involving higher-level mental functioning, and disorders of peripheral nerve and skeletal muscle.

In recent years a focus on 'acute neurology' has seen many hospitals employ neurologists supporting general medical admissions units to deal with neurological emergencies that present via the hospital emergency department (for instance meningoencephalitis or Guillain–Barré syndrome). Other neurological conditions are managed primarily in outpatients (such as epilepsy and migraine), and those causing significant disability require close cooperation with allied health professionals, primary care and community services. Neurological subspecialties include stroke, movement disorders, muscle disease and epilepsy.

Key skills in neurology include:

- distilling information gathered during a careful history and physical examination into a well-defined clinical syndrome, suggesting likely diagnoses and a rational approach to investigation
- managing neurological emergencies including stroke, coma, central nervous system infection, spinal cord compression and myasthenic crisis
- managing disability, working with other health professionals to help patients achieve a maximum level of functional independence despite advanced or progressive disease.

Opportunities for learning neurology include attending ward rounds on a stroke unit or with acute neurology teams, practising neurological examination with consenting patients, attending a range of general and specialist neurology clinics, and observing specialist neurologist investigations such as electrophysiology or lumbar puncture.

CLINICAL SKILLS FOR NEUROLOGY

History

There are many different clinical presentations of neurological disease, and specific diagnostic approaches are covered in greater depth in relevant sections of this chapter. However, patterns emerge from a properly conducted history and examination that can suggest the likely causes, site and extent of disease; this section focuses on developing a diagnostic clinical approach to patients that is relevant in all areas of the specialty. An approach to history-taking in neurology is shown in (**Box 26.1**).

 Box 26.1 Taking a history in neurology

Presenting symptoms

- Duration of symptoms, and any previous episodes
- Pattern – constant, intermittent, progressive
- Onset – sequence of events when symptoms first began, or each time they recur
- Triggers – warm baths may worsen symptoms caused by demyelination; sensory stimuli can trigger epilepsy; dietary stimuli, tiredness or stress can trigger migraines

Screening questions for other relevant features

- Systemic symptoms – fever (may suggest infection), weight loss and anorexia (may suggest malignancy with paraneoplastic neurological phenomena)
- Raised intracranial pressure symptoms – headaches worse on waking and on lying flat, vomiting, diplopia
- Visual symptoms – blurring, diplopia, flashing lights
- Bulbar symptoms – changes in speech and difficulties swallowing
- Motor symptoms – weakness, stiffness, abnormal gait
- Sensory symptoms – loss of sensation, neuropathic ('tingling' or 'electric') pain
- Loss of coordination – dizziness, staggering gait, loss of fine motor control, altered speech
- Autonomic symptoms – postural dizziness, faecal incontinence, urinary retention
- Loss of consciousness – features suggesting a neurological cause include aura, muscle jerking, tongue biting, incontinence and a drowsy post-ictal phase.
- Disturbance of higher functions – personality change, cognitive decline, loss of executive control, disinhibition, psychiatric symptoms

Past medical history

- Atherosclerotic risk factors – hypertension, diabetes, other cardiovascular disease
- Risk factors for embolic disease – atrial fibrillation, patent foramen ovale
- Diabetes – time since diagnosis, degree of glycaemic control, presence of other complications
- Malignancies, systemic inflammatory disorders, immunosuppressive conditions, e.g. HIV

Medication history

- Use of neuroactive medications, for instance antipsychotics

Family history

- History of inherited neurological disorders such as Huntington's chorea, myotonic dystrophy and Charcot–Marie–Tooth disease in close relatives

Risk factors for functional disease

- Employment status, job security, stress at work, relationships with colleagues
- Family circumstances, relationship status, conflict, bereavements

Disability and effect on lifestyle

- Mobility
- Ability to perform activities of daily living
- Current provision of carers

Lifestyle factors

- Smoking, alcohol consumption, use of illegal drugs

Safety

- Do they drive?
- What is their employment? Might their illness pose a risk to themselves or others?
- Do they take baths or go swimming alone? Any other potentially risky leisure activities?

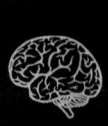

1. General examination
Level of consciousness
Orientation in time/place/person
Gait
Speech
Cognitive function
Abnormal posture of limbs
Facial expression
Blood pressure
Temperature

2. Face
Eyes
- acuity
- fields
- movements
- pupils
- fundoscopy
Facial motor control
- asymmetry
- lifting eyebrows, showing teeth
Facial sensation
- dermatomal sensory loss
Speech
Swallowing assessment
Neck stiffness

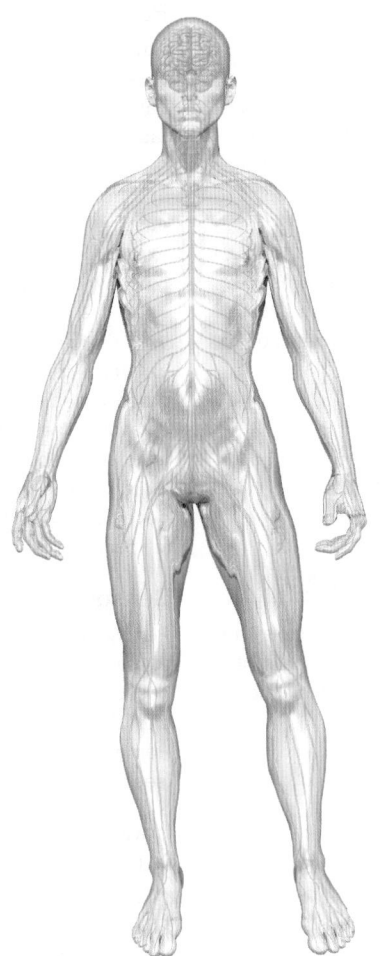

3. Limbs – motor assessment
Wasting
Fasciculation
Abnormal posture
Tone
Power
Reflexes
Plantar reflexes
Coordination

4. Limbs – sensory assessment
Ask about numbness
Light touch – cotton wool
Pain – pin prick
Joint position sense
Vibration sensation
2-point discrimination
Temperature sensation

Examination

If the neurological history focuses primarily on the likely *cause* of the neurological disease, the examination focuses on the likely *anatomical location* of the lesion. The diagram above illustrates key a basic approach to focused examination of the nervous system with key signs to elicit or exclude.

Putting it all together

Information from the history and examination should be used together in order to answer the questions in **Box 26.2**, which will direct likely diagnoses and investigations that are likely to be helpful.

? **Box 26.2 Formulating a diagnosis in neurology**

Is the lesion global or focal?
- Global lesions affect all (or most) brain functions, and typically affect cognition and consciousness
- Focal lesions affect one region of the body and resultant signs may be asymmetric

What is the timescale?
- Immediate onset symptoms are usually vascular (ischaemia or haemorrhage), or electrical (epilepsy) in aetiology
- Rapidly progressive symptoms (over days) may represent infective (e.g. meningitis) or inflammatory (e.g. demyelinating) disease
- Slowly progressive symptoms tend to be caused by degenerative diseases

Do motor lesions affect the upper or the lower motor neurone?
- Upper motor neurone (UMN) signs include increased tone (spasticity), weakness, increased reflexes and upgoing plantars – a 'pyramidal' pattern of weakness where stronger muscles (upper limb flexors, lower limb extensors) overwhelm weaker ones
- Lower motor neurone (LMN) signs include flaccid weakness, decreased or absent reflexes, wasting and fasciculations

Where is the lesion?
- Cerebral cortex/internal capsule: contralateral UMN signs
- Cerebellum: nystagmus, impaired balance/coordination
- Brainstem: impaired consciousness, global signs, cranial nerve abnormalities
- Spinal cord: UMN paraplegia/quadriplegia with sensory level
- Nerve root: LMN myotomal signs; dermatomal sensory loss
- Single peripheral nerve: LMN signs and sensory loss according to distribution of nerve
- All peripheral nerves: 'length dependent' LMN signs (worst in hands/feet), 'glove and stocking' sensory loss
- Neuromuscular junction/muscle: Only motor signs present. Fatiguability common, wasting and fasciculations

Is there a functional component?
- Are there elements that don't fit within standard neuroanatomical patterns of disease?
- Are there risk factors for functional disease (see history section opposite)?
- Functional elements commonly exist alongside organic disease

INTRODUCTION

Neurology is a broad clinical specialty that requires good clinical skills and a rational diagnostic approach to link underlying pathophysiological processes with a diverse range of clinical syndromes that affect patients' lives. The skills required cannot be replaced with investigations or imaging alone.

Some 17% of general practitioner consultations and 10% of emergency department visits are for neurological symptoms; 19% of all hospital admissions are for neurological disorders and 25% of chronic disability in adults below the age of 64 is due to neurological disease (**Box 26.3**).

CLINICAL APPROACH TO THE PATIENT WITH NEUROLOGICAL DISEASE

Clinical features of neurological disease

Pattern recognition in neurology – interpretation of history, symptoms and examination – is very reliable. Practical experience is vital. There are three critical questions in formulating a clinical diagnosis:
- What is/are the site(s) of the lesion(s)?
- What is the likely pathology?
- Does a recognizable disease fit this pattern?

Difficulty walking and falls

Change in walking pattern is a common complaint (**Box 26.4**). Arthritis and muscle pain make walking painful and slow (antalgic gait). The *pattern* of gait is valuable diagnostically.

Spasticity and hemiparesis

Spasticity (see p. 819), more pronounced in extensor muscles and with or without weakness, causes stiff, effortful and slow walking. Toes of shoes become scuffed, catching level ground. Pace shortens; a narrow base is maintained. Clonus – involuntary extensor rhythmic leg jerking – may occur.

In a hemiparesis, when spasticity is unilateral and weakness marked, the stiff, weak leg is circumducted and drags.

Parkinson's disease: shuffling gait

Stride length shortens and, in advanced forms, the gait slows to a shuffle. Posture is stooped and arm swing reduced (initially, unilaterally). Gait becomes festinant (hurried) with short, rapid steps. There is difficulty turning quickly (count the number of steps to turn around). Eventually, gait initiation difficulty and freezing episodes (sudden involuntary halts, such as when passing through a doorway) may develop. Falls are uncommon, except in late-stage disease, and may indicate a 'Parkinson's plus' syndrome.

Cerebellar ataxia: broad-based gait

In lateral cerebellar lobe disease (see p. 820), stance becomes broad-based, unstable and tremulous. Ataxia describes this incoordination. When walking, the person tends to veer to the side of the affected cerebellar lobe.

In disease of midline structures (cerebellar vermis), the trunk becomes unsteady without limb ataxia, and there is a tendency to fall backwards or sideways – truncal ataxia.

Sensory ataxia: stamping gait

Peripheral sensory loss (e.g. polyneuropathy; see p. 889) causes ataxia because of loss of *proprioception* (position sense). A broad-based, high-stepping, 'stamping' gait develops as feet are placed clumsily, relying in part on vision, so balance is worse in the dark. Romberg's test, first described in sensory ataxia of tabes dorsalis (see p. 872), becomes positive.

Lower limb weakness: high-stepping and waddling gaits

When weakness is distal, affecting ankle dorsiflexors, such as in a common peroneal nerve palsy (see p. 889), gait becomes high-stepping to avoid tripping. The sole returns to the ground with an audible *slap*.

Weakness of proximal leg muscles (e.g. polymyositis, muscular dystrophy) causes difficulty rising from sitting. Walking becomes a *waddle*, the pelvis being poorly supported by each leg.

Gait apraxia

With frontal lobe disease (e.g. diffuse cerebrovascular disease, normal-pressure hydrocephalus), *walking skills* become disorganized, despite normal motor and sensory function when examined on the couch. The gait is shuffling with small steps

---

i **Box 26.3 UK incidence of common neurological conditions**

Conditions	Events per 100 000/year
Migraine	400
Stroke	240
Dementia over age of 85	68
Epilepsy	50
Parkinson's disease	19
Severe brain injury and subdural haematoma	13
All central nervous system tumours	9
Trigeminal neuralgia	8
Meningitis	7
Multiple sclerosis	7
Myasthenia, all muscle and motor neurone disease	5

---

i **Box 26.4 Common gait abnormalities**

Cause	Gait abnormality
Stroke	Spastic/hemiparetic
Parkinson's disease	Shuffling/festinant
Cerebellar ataxia	Broad-based
Sensory neuropathy	Stamping
Position sensory loss	High-stepping
Distal weakness/foot drop	Slapping
Proximal weakness, e.g. myopathy	Waddling
Apraxia of gait, e.g. diffuse cerebrovascular disease	Incoordinated/gait initiation failure; *marche à petits pas*
Normal-pressure hydrocephalus	Hesitant
Arthritis and muscle pain	Antalgic

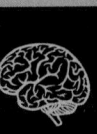

(*marche à petits pas*), gait ignition failure and hesitancy with fear of falling. Unlike in the gait of Parkinson's disease, arm swing and posture are normal. Urinary incontinence and dementia are often present.

Falls

Falls are a major health problem in elderly people, often leading to hospital admission; they are frequently a reason for requiring residential care. A third of people over the age of 65 will fall each year and 10% sustain serious injury, such as hip fracture or head injury. Falls are the leading cause of injury-related death in elderly people.

The cause of falls is usually multifactorial and a multidisciplinary approach to assessment and prevention is essential, considering both intrinsic medical risk factors and external environmental factors, such as rugs, stairs, footwear, poor lighting and so on. Medical risk factors for falls (**Box 26.5**) are additive, with multiple factors substantially increasing the risk of falling. A fuller discussion of falls prevention and risk factor modification is given in chapter 15.

Dizziness, vertigo and blackouts

Dizziness covers many complaints, from a vague feeling of unsteadiness to severe, acute vertigo. It is frequently used to describe light-headedness (e.g. due to hypotension), panic, anxiety, palpitations and chronic ill-health. The real nature of this symptom must be determined.

Vertigo (see p. 816) means the illusion of movement, a sensation of rotation or tipping. The patient feels the surroundings are spinning or moving. This is distressing and often accompanied by nausea or vomiting.

Blackout, like dizziness, is simply descriptive, implying either altered consciousness (see epilepsy, p. 852, and syncope, p. 857), transient visual disturbance as part of pre-syncope or falling, or hypoglycaemia in a diabetic patient. A good history is essential.

Collapse is a vague term but often used. It should be avoided.

Fatigue is common. When it is an isolated symptom, it rarely indicates neurological disease, although it may be a symptom of many neurological disorders. General medical causes, such as anaemia and endocrine disorders, should be excluded. No serious disease is found in many (>20%) patients referred with symptoms suggestive of possible neurological conditions.

Examination and formulation

Following a short or detailed examination, relevant findings are summarized in a brief formulation, which becomes the basis for investigation, transfer of information and management (**Boxes 26.6–26.8**).

ℹ Box 26.5 Medical risk factors for falls in the elderly

- Cognitive impairment (dementia and delirium)
- Arthritis, muscle weakness
- Disorders of balance and gait, e.g. parkinsonism, ataxia, stroke
- Visual impairment
- Postural hypotension and syncope
- Vestibular disorders

- Polypharmacy, especially with sedative drugs, neuroleptics, antihypertensives and anticonvulsants
- Alcohol excess
- Peripheral neuropathy
- Effects of ageing on strength (sarcopenia), postural stability and reaction time
- Use of walking aid

Further reading

Clarke C. The language of neurology – symptoms, signs and basic investigations. In: Clarke C, Howard R, Rossor M et al (eds). *Neurology: A Queen Square Textbook*. Oxford: Blackwell; 2009.

Box 26.6 Five-part short neurological examination

1. **Look at patient**
   - General demeanour
   - Speech
   - Gait
   - Arm swinging
2. **Head**
   - Fundi
   - Pupils
   - Eye movements
   - Facial movements
   - Tongue
3. **Upper limbs**
   - Posture of outstretched arms
   - Wasting, fasciculation
   - Power, tone
   - Coordination
   - Reflexes
4. **Lower limbs**
   - Wasting, fasciculation
   - Power, tone
   - Reflexes
   - Plantar responses
5. **Sensation**
   - Ask the patient

Box 26.7 Ten-part neurological examination

1. *State of consciousness, arousal, appearance*
2. *Mental state, attitude, insight*
3. *Cognitive function* – orientation, recall, level of intellect, language, other cortical problems, e.g. apraxia
4. *Gait and balance tests*, including tandem walking and Romberg's test
5. *Neck* – stiffness, palpation and auscultation of carotids
6. *Cranial nerves* (see Box 26.10)
7. *Motor system*
   Upper limbs:
   – Wasting and fasciculation
   – Posture of arms: drift, rebound, tremor
   – Tone: spasticity, clonus, extrapyramidal rigidity
   – Power: 0–5 scale (see **Box 26.8**)
   – Tendon reflexes: + or ++ normal; +++ pathological; 0 = absent with reinforcement
   Thorax and abdomen:
   – Respiration
   – Thoracic and abdominal muscles
   – Abdominal reflexes
   Lower limbs:
   – Wasting and fasciculation
   – Tone, power and tendon reflexes
   – Plantar responses
8. *Coordination and fine movements*
9. *Sensory system*
   – Chart area of sensory loss; start in area with abnormal sensation and move stimulus towards normal area to demarcate boundaries
   Posterior columns:
   – Vibration (128 Hz tuning fork)
   – Joint position – small movements of distal interphalangeal joints in toes and fingers
   – Light touch – use cotton wool
   – Two-point discrimination (normal: 2–4 mm fingertips, 2 cm soles)
   Spinothalamic tracts:
   – Pain: use a split orange-stick or a sterile pin (never a hypodermic needle)
   Temperature: warm and cold objects
   Cortical sensory loss – dysgraphaesthesia and astereognosis
10. *Specialized tests* as required e.g. Hallpike for vertigo, Phalen's test and so on

> **i** **Box 26.8 Muscle power: the Medical Research Council (MRC) scale**
>
> | Grade | Definition |
> |---|---|
> | 5 | Normal power |
> | 4 | Active movement against gravity and resistance |
> | 3 | Active movement against gravity only |
> | 2 | Active movement with gravity eliminated |
> | 1 | Flicker of contraction |
> | 0 | No contraction |

Dykes PC, Carroll DL, Hurley A et al. Fall prevention in acute care hospitals. *JAMA* 2010; 304:1912–1918.
Keall MD, Pierse N, Howeden-Chapman P et al. Home modifications to reduce injuries from falls in the home injury prevention (HIPI) study: a cluster-randomised controlled trial. *Lancet* 2015; 385:231–238.

FUNCTIONAL NEUROANATOMY

Neurone and synapse

The neurone is the functional unit of the entire nervous system (**Fig. 26.1**). Its cell body and axon terminate in a synapse. The size and type of each group of neurones vary. A thoracic spinal cord α-motor neurone has an axonal length of more than 1 metre and innervates between several hundred and 2000 muscle fibres in one leg – a motor unit. By contrast, some spinal or intracerebral interneurones have axons shorter than 100 μm, terminating on one neuronal cell body.

Neurotransmitters

Neurotransmitters are excitatory (acetylcholine, noradrenaline (norepinephrine), adrenaline (epinephrine), 5-hydroxytryptamine (5-HT, serotonin), dopamine, glutamate and aspartate) or inhibitory (γ-aminobutyric acid (GABA), histamine and glycine). Neuropeptides, such as vasopressin, adrenocorticotrophic hormone (ACTH), substance P and opioid peptides, as well as the purines adenosine triphosphate (ATP) and adenosine monophosphate (AMP) are both excitatory and inhibitory.

Synaptic transmission is mediated by neurotransmitters released by action potentials passing down an axon. Neurotransmitters activate postsynaptic receptors and are removed by transporter proteins. The neurotransmitter–receptor reaction increases ionic permeability and propagates a further action potential. Axonal electrical activity and synaptic chemical release are the basis of neurological function.

Clinical features of focal brain lesions: general mechanisms

The symptoms and signs suggest the area of the brain that is malfunctioning (e.g. aphasia – dominant frontal lobe, hemiparesis – the internal capsule, or a Bell's palsy – VIIth cranial (facial) nerve).

Focal lesions of the cortex, and lesions throughout the nervous system, cause symptoms and signs by two processes:

- **Suppression or destruction of neurones** and surrounding structures (**Fig. 26.2**). This is the most common process: part of the system simply fails to work.

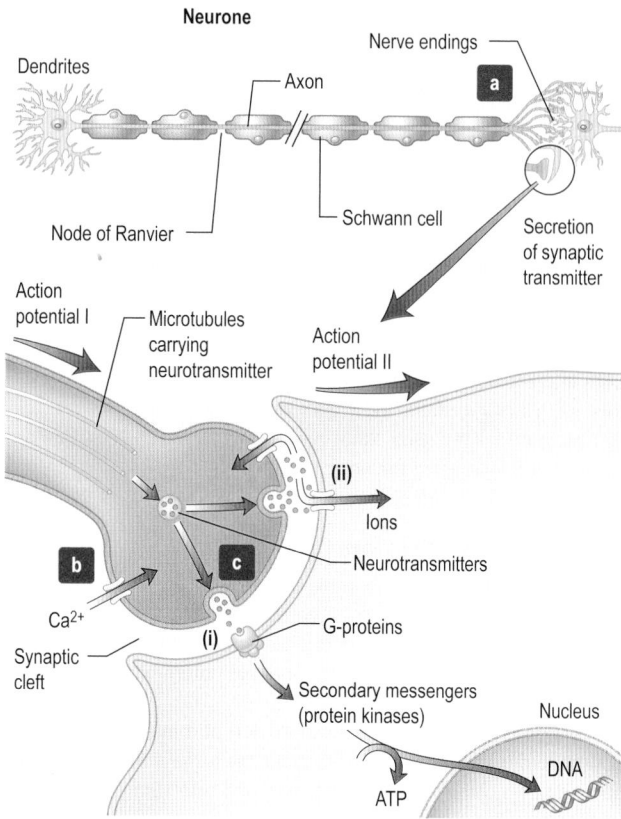

Fig. 26.1 The functional unit: neurone and neurotransmitters. (a) *The action potential* – that is, the nerve impulse – travels down the axon. Microtubules carry neurotransmitters to nerve endings. **(b) *Action potential I*** depolarizes the synaptic membrane, opening voltage-gated calcium channels. **(c)** Influx of calcium ions causes vesicles to fuse with the membrane, allowing neurotransmitter binding to receptors **(i)** and activation of secondary messengers that modulate gene transcription and also open ligand-gated channels **(ii)**. This allows ions to enter, depolarize the membrane and ***initiate action potential II.***

- ***Synchronous discharge of neurones*** by *irritative* lesions (**Fig. 26.3**), e.g. cortical lesions, causes epilepsy, either focal or generalized.

Localization within the cerebral cortex

Work on neuronal networks, functional imaging and plasticity questions the traditional views of highly specific localization of cortical function. The following paragraphs summarize areas of clinical relevance.

Dominant hemisphere (usually left)

The concept of cerebral dominance arose from a simple observation: right-handed stroke patients with acquired language disorders had destructive lesions within the left hemisphere. Right-handed (and 70% of left-handed) people have language function on the left.

More specifically, destructive lesions within the left frontotemporoparietal region cause disorders of communication:

- spoken language – **aphasia**, also called **dysphasia**
- writing – **agraphia**
- reading – acquired **alexia**.

Site of lesion	Disorder	R	L
Frontal, either	Intellectual impairment Personality change Urinary incontinence Monoparesis or hemiparesis		
Frontal, left	Broca's aphasia		
Temporo- parietal, left	Acalculia Alexia Agraphia Wernicke's aphasia Right-left disorientation Homonymous field defect		
Temporal, right	Confusional states Failure to recognize faces Homonymous field defect		
Parietal, either	Contralateral sensory loss or neglect Agraphaesthesia Homonymous field defect		
Parietal, right	Dressing apraxia Failure to recognize faces		
Parietal, left	Limb apraxia		
Occipital/ occipitoparietal	Visual field defects Visuospatial defects Disturbances of visual recognition		

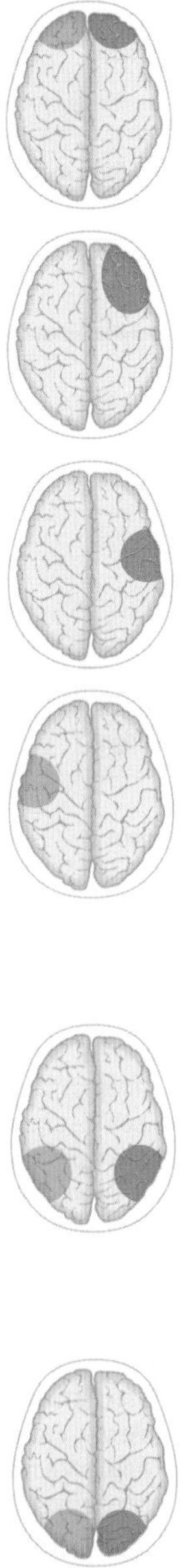

Fig. 26.2 Principal features of destructive cortical lesions in a right-handed individual.

Site of lesion	Effects	R	L

Frontal	Partial seizures–focal motor
	  seizures of contralateral limbs
	Conjugate deviation of head
	  and eyes away from the lesion		

Temporal	Formed visual hallucinations Complex partial seizures Memory disturbances (e.g. *déjà vu*)		

Parietal
 	
Parieto-occipital
	Partial seizures–focal sensory
	  seizures of contralateral limbs
	Crude visual hallucinations (e.g.
	  shapes in one part of the field)		

Occipital	Visual disturbances (e.g. flashes)		

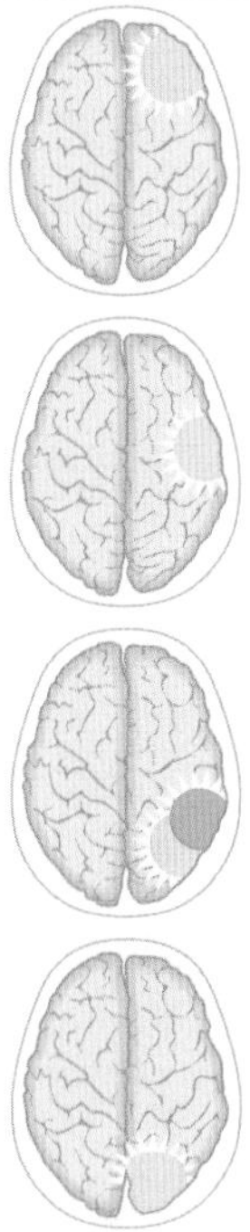

Fig. 26.3 Effects of irritative cortical lesions.

words with failure to construct sentences (sometimes described as ***telegrammatic***). Patients who recover say they knew what they wanted to say but could not get the words out.

Wernicke's (receptive, posterior) aphasia

Left temporo-parietal damage leaves fluency of language unaffected but words are muddled. This varies from insertion of a few incorrect or unnecessary words into speech to a profuse outpouring of jargon (non-existent words). Severe jargon aphasia is bizarre and often mistaken for psychotic behaviour.

Patients who recover from Wernicke's aphasia say that they found speech, both their own and others', like an unintelligible foreign language – that is, incomprehensible – but they could neither stop speaking nor understand speech.

Nominal (anomic) aphasia

This means difficulty in naming objects. Naming difficulty is an early feature in all types of aphasia. This is often tested in practice by asking patient to name parts of a watch; a more sensitive test utilizes pictures to test low-frequency words, such as rhinoceros, violin, tricycle or ladybird.

Global (central) aphasia

This means the combination of the expressive problems of Broca's aphasia and the loss of comprehension of Wernicke's, with loss of both language production and understanding. It is due to widespread damage to speech areas and is the most common aphasia after a severe left hemisphere infarct. Writing and reading are also affected.

Dysarthria

Dysarthria is disordered articulation – slurred speech. Language is intact. Paralysis, slowing or incoordination of the muscles of

Developmental dyslexia describes delayed, disorganized reading and writing ability in children, usually with normal intelligence.

Aphasia

Aphasia is loss of, or defective language from damage to, the speech centres within the left hemisphere. Numerous varieties have been described.

Broca's (expressive, anterior) aphasia

Damage in the left frontal lobe causes reduced speech fluency with relatively preserved comprehension. The patient makes great efforts to initiate language, which becomes reduced to a few disjointed

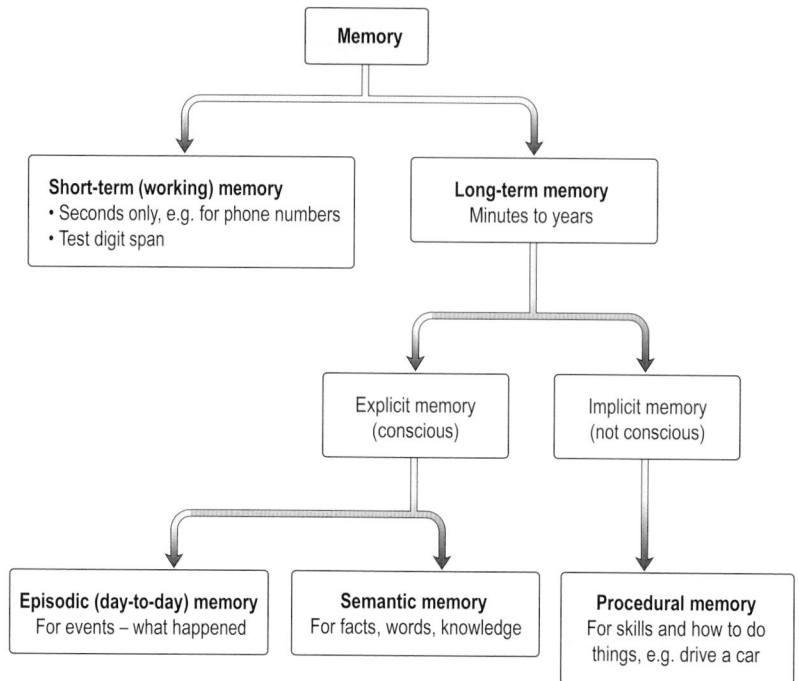

Fig. 26.4 Types of memory.

articulation, causes various patterns of dysarthria. Examples are the ***gravelly*** speech of pseudobulbar palsy (see p. 817), the ***jerky***, ataxic speech of cerebellar lesions, the hypophonic ***monotone*** of Parkinson's, and speech in myasthenia that ***fatigues*** and dies away. Many aphasic patients are also dysarthric.

Non-dominant hemisphere

Disorders in right-handed patients with right hemisphere lesions are often difficult to recognize. There are abnormalities of perception of internal and external space. Examples are loss of the way in familiar surroundings, failure to put on clothing correctly (dressing apraxia), or inability to draw simple shapes – constructional apraxia.

Memory and its disorders

Like most brain functions, memory has a modular organization, with different aspects of memory dependent on functionally and anatomically distinct brain networks. Three distinct processes are required: learning, storage and subsequent retrieval of learned information. There is a fundamental distinction between ***explicit*** memory, which can be consciously accessed, such as long-term memory for events (***episodic*** memory) and knowledge of word meaning (***semantic*** memory) on the one hand, and ***implicit*** memory, which is not conscious: for example, how to ride a bike (**Fig. 26.4**). Short-term memory is frequently misunderstood and refers to ***working*** memory lasting seconds only: for example, phone numbers.

Disorders of memory can result from damage to the medial structures of the temporal lobes and their brainstem connections – the hippocampi, fornices and mammillary bodies, as well as from damage to the thalamus and frontal lobe. The distributed anatomical basis of memory means that bilateral lesions are necessary to cause ***amnesia***. Impairment of episodic memory usually results in a temporal memory gradient: recent and new memories are mainly affected, with relative preservation of distant memories.

? Box 26.9 Causes of an amnestic syndrome[a]

- Dementia (note: multiple cognitive domains affected, not memory in isolation)
- Amnestic mild cognitive impairment (see p. 881)
- Alcohol – thiamine deficiency (Wernicke–Korsakoff's syndrome)
- Head injury (severe)
- Anoxic brain damage and that following carbon monoxide poisoning
- Stroke, including bilateral thalamic infarction, subarachnoid haemorrhage, diffuse small-vessel disease, and post cardiac surgery
- Viral, paraneoplastic and autoimmune encephalitis
- Drugs – psychotropics, anticholinergics and solvent abuse
- Bilateral invasive tumours
- Temporal lobe epilepsy and temporal lobectomy
- Following hypoglycaemia
- Temporary amnesia: transient global amnesia, transient epileptic amnesia, post-traumatic amnesia
- Dissociative (functional/psychogenic)

[a]Amnesia must be distinguished from delirium.

Memory loss (the amnestic syndrome) is frequently a symptom of dementia, especially Alzheimer's disease (see p. 881), but also occurs as an isolated entity (**Box 26.9**).

Essential elements of neuroanatomy

For clinical purposes, the complexity of neuroanatomy must be reduced to its core elements:

- cranial nerves
- three systems of motor control:
  - corticospinal or pyramidal system
  - extrapyramidal system
  - cerebellum
- motor unit
- reflex arc

- sensory pathways and pain
- control of the bladder and sexual function.

CRANIAL NERVES

See **Box 26.10**.

I: Olfactory nerve

This sensory nerve arises from olfactory (smell) receptors within nasal mucosa. Branches pierce the cribriform plate and synapse in the olfactory bulb. The olfactory tract passes to the olfactory cortex.

Anosmia (loss of the sense of smell) is caused by head injury (shearing of olfactory neurones as they pass through the cribriform plate at the skull base) or tumours of the olfactory groove (e.g. meningioma). Olfaction is temporarily (or permanently, on occasion) lost or diminished after upper respiratory infections and with local disorders of the nose. Many patients with gradual-onset anosmia over many years may be unaware of the deficit: for example, in Parkinson's disease, where anosmia precedes motor symptoms by many years but is often not noticed by the patient.

Detailed smell testing is difficult in routine clinical practice and rarely performed. Adequate testing requires use of commercially available kits, such as scratch and sniff cards or odour-filled pens with forced multiple-choice identification.

II: Optic nerve and visual system

Light regulated by the pupillary aperture is converted into action potentials by retinal rod, cone and ganglion cells (see p. 912). The lens, under control of the ciliary muscle, produces the image (inverted) on the retina. Axons in the optic nerve (1 on **Fig. 26.5**) decussate at the optic chiasm (2), and fibres from the nasal retina cross and join with uncrossed fibres originating in the temporal retina to form the optic tract (3). Each optic tract thus carries information from the contralateral visual hemifield.

From the lateral geniculate body, fibres pass in the optic radiation through the parietal and temporal lobes (4 and 5) to reach the visual cortex of the occipital lobe (6 and 7), which is somatotopically organized with macular vision located at the occipital pole.

Beyond the visual cortex, visual information is further processed by neighbouring visual association areas to detect lines, orientation, shapes, movement, colour and depth; there is even a distinct area responsible for face recognition.

Visual acuity

Visual acuity (see p. 914) is assessed in each eye with a Snellen chart and/or Near Vision Reading Types, corrected for refractive errors with lenses or a pinhole. The patient should stand 6 metres from a well-lit chart. Acuity is recorded as distance in metres from the chart over distance at which the line should be legible, e.g. 6/6 indicates 'normal' acuity and 6/60 very poor acuity.

Visual field defects

Visual fields are assessed at the bedside by confrontation – comparing the examiner's and patient's fields, one eye at a time and quadrant by quadrant. Patience and good technique are required to produce reliable results. White and red targets (traditionally, hatpins) are used to assess peripheral and central fields, respectively, although in practice a fingertip is often substituted as a cruder screening test. More detailed quantification of fields may

Number	Name	Main clinical action
I	Olfactory	Smell
II	Optic	Vision, fields, afferent light reflex
III	Oculomotor	Eyelid elevation, eye elevation, adduction, depression in abduction, efferent pupil – light reflex
IV	Trochlear	Eye intorsion, depression in adduction
V	Trigeminal	Facial (and corneal) sensation, mastication muscles
VI	Abducens	Eye abduction
VII	Facial	Facial movement, taste fibres
VIII	Vestibulocochlear	Balance and hearing
IX	Glossopharyngeal	Sensation – soft palate, taste fibres
X	Vagus	Cough, palatal and vocal cord movements
XI	Accessory	Head turning, shoulder shrugging
XII	Hypoglossal	Tongue movement

Box 26.10 Cranial nerves

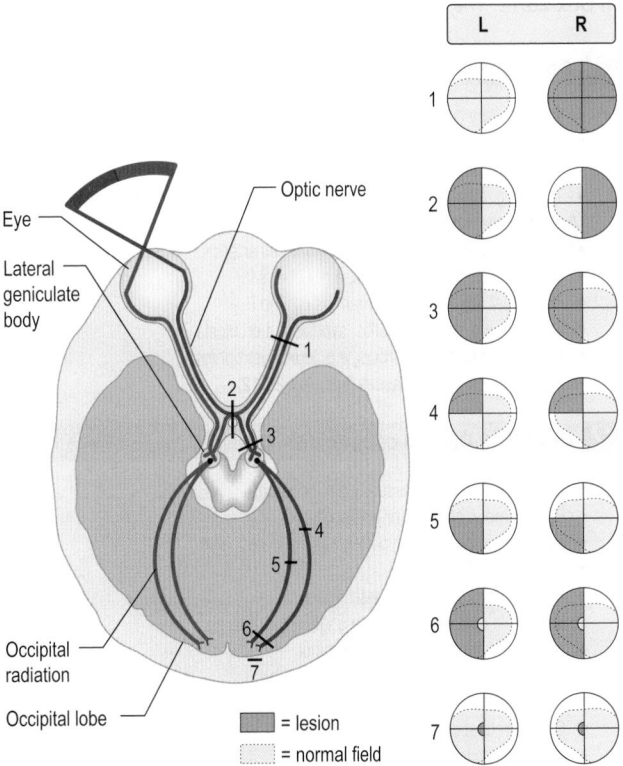

Fig. 26.5 The visual pathway. (1) Mononuclear field loss – complete optic nerve lesion. **(2)** Bitemporal hemianopia – chiasmal lesion. **(3)** Homonymous hemianopia – optic tract lesion. **(4)** Homonymous quadrantanopia – temporal lesion. **(5)** Homonymous quadrantanopia – parietal lesion. **(6)** Homonymous hemianopia with macular sparing – occipital cortex or optic radiation. **(7)** Homonymous hemianopia (hemiscotoma) – occipital pole lesion.

be obtained using Goldmann (manual) or Humphrey (automated) perimetry testing.

Field defects are described as hemianopic when half the field is affected and quadrantanopic when a quadrant is affected. Lesions posterior to the optic chiasm produce **homonymous** field defects, indicating involvement of the same part of the visual field in both eyes, as information from the two visual hemifields is separated beyond this point. Lesions damaging decussating nasal fibres at the optic chiasm cause bitemporal defects.

Retinal and local eye lesions

See pages 923–924.

Optic nerve lesions

Unilateral visual loss, commencing with a central or paracentral (off-centre) scotoma, is the hallmark of an optic nerve lesion. Because most fibres in the optic nerve subserve macular vision, lesions within the nerve disproportionately affect central vision and colour vision. A total optic nerve lesion causes unilateral blindness with loss of pupillary light reflex. Examination findings in optic neuropathy are:

* reduced acuity in the affected eye
* a scotoma (usually central)
* impaired colour vision (assess with Ishihara plates)
* an afferent pupillary defect (see below)
* optic atrophy – pale disc (develops late).
  Causes are listed in **Box 26.11**.

Papilloedema

Papilloedema means swelling of the optic disc. Causes are shown in **Box 26.12**. The earliest signs of swelling are disc pinkness, with

---

> **? Box 26.11 Causes of optic neuropathy**
>
> * Inflammatory (optic neuritis), e.g. demyelination, sarcoidosis, vasculitis
> * Optic nerve trauma or compression, e.g. glioma, meningioma, aneurysm, bone disorders affecting orbit
> * Toxic, e.g. tobacco/alcohol, ethambutol, methyl alcohol, quinine, hydroxychloroquine, radiation
> * Ischaemic optic neuropathy, e.g. giant cell arteritis
> * Hereditary optic neuropathies, e.g. Leber's
> * Nutritional deficiency, e.g. vitamins B_1 and B_{12}
> * Infection, e.g. orbital cellulitis, syphilis, tuberculosis
> * Neurodegenerative disorders, e.g. leukodystrophies
> * Papilloedema and its causes (see **Box 26.12**)

> **? Box 26.12 Causes of optic disc swelling**
>
> * Raised intracranial pressure (papilloedema)
> * Brain tumour, abscess or haemorrhage
> * Idiopathic intracranial hypertension, hydrocephalus
> * Optic nerve disease
> * Optic neuritis, e.g. multiple sclerosis
> * Ischaemic optic neuropathy, e.g. giant cell arteritis
> * Toxic optic neuropathy, e.g. methanol
> * Venous occlusion
> * Venous sinus thrombosis
> * Central retinal vein thrombosis
> * Orbital mass lesions
> * Retinal vascular disease
> * Malignant hypertension
> * Vasculitis, e.g. systemic lupus erythematosus
> * Metabolic causes
> * Hypercapnia, chronic hypoxia, hypocalcaemia
> * Disc infiltration
> * Leukaemia, sarcoidosis, optic nerve glioma

---

blurring and heaping up of disc margins, nasal first. There is loss of spontaneous pulsation of retinal veins within the disc. The physiological cup becomes obliterated, and the disc is engorged with dilated vessels. Small haemorrhages often surround the disc.

Various conditions simulate true disc swelling. Marked hypermetropic (long-sighted) refractive errors make a disc appear pink, distant and ill defined. Myelinated nerve fibres at disc margins and hyaline bodies (drusen; see p. 923) can be mistaken for disc swelling.

Disc infiltration also causes a swollen disc with raised margins (e.g. in leukaemia).

When there is doubt about disc oedema, intravenous fluorescein angiography is diagnostic; retinal leakage is seen with papilloedema.

Papilloedema produces few, if any, visual symptoms other than momentary visual obscurations with changes in posture. The underlying disease is the source of the patient's symptoms. The blind spot is enlarged but this is not noticed by the patient. However, over time, progressive and permanent constriction of visual fields occurs, ultimately culminating in optic atrophy.

Inflammatory optic neuropathy (optic neuritis)

Optic neuritis is one of the most common causes of subacute visual loss. Symptoms may vary from a mild fogging of central vision with colour desaturation to a dense central scotoma, but very rarely complete blindness. Pain on eye movements is almost universal. The optic disc usually appears normal, despite severe visual loss (unless the inflammation is at the optic nerve head, in which case the disc may appear swollen in the acute phase).

A plaque of demyelination within the optic nerve is the most common cause in Western populations. Dedicated magnetic resonance imaging (MRI) of the optic nerves may show the inflammatory plaque, and imaging of the brain may show additional inflammatory lesions, which confer a higher risk of developing multiple sclerosis (MS). Approximately 50% of patients go on to develop MS with prolonged follow-up (see p. 864). Recovery of visual acuity to 6/9 or better occurs in 95% of cases over months; recovery time is improved by high-dose intravenous or oral steroids given acutely.

Optic neuritis may be caused by infective or other inflammatory disorders, such as sarcoidosis or vasculitides (see **Box 26.11**).

Anterior ischaemic optic neuropathy

The anterior part of the optic nerve is supplied by the posterior ciliary arteries, occlusion or hypoperfusion of which leads to infarction of all or part of the optic nerve head. There is sudden or stuttering altitudinal visual loss (typically, the lower half of the visual field) with disc swelling, later replaced by optic atrophy. The other eye is affected later in one-third of cases.

Individuals with small hypermetropic discs seem to be predisposed, and often there are relatively few vascular risk factors. Less commonly, arteritis is the cause (see p. 985).

Optic atrophy

Optic atrophy means disc pallor, from loss of axons, glial proliferation and decreased vascularity. This may eventually develop following any type of optic neuropathy of sufficient severity to damage axons extensively within the nerve, including chronic papilloedema.

Optic chiasm

Bitemporal hemianopia or quadrantanopia occurs with compression of the chiasm from above or below. Common causes are:

* pituitary tumours (see p. 591)
* meningioma
* craniopharyngioma

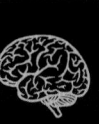

Optic tract and optic radiation

Optic tract lesions (rare) cause a homonymous hemianopia (loss of the contralateral visual field in both eyes). Optic radiation lesions cause homonymous quadrantanopic defects. Temporal lobe lesions (e.g. tumour, infarction) cause upper quadrantic defects, and parietal lobe lesions cause lower quadrantic defects.

Occipital cortex

Homonymous hemianopic defects are produced by unilateral posterior cerebral artery infarction (see p. 840). The macular cortex (at each occipital pole) supplied by the middle cerebral artery may be spared.

Widespread bilateral occipital lobe damage by infarction (**'top of the basilar'** syndrome, occlusion of the rostral basilar artery), trauma or coning causes **cortical blindness** (Anton syndrome). The patient cannot see but characteristically lacks insight into this; he or she may even deny it. Pupillary responses remain normal (see p. 840).

Pupils

A slight difference between the size of each pupil (up to 1 mm) is common (**physiological anisocoria**) and does not vary with differing light levels. The pupil tends to become smaller and irregular in old age (senile miosis); anisocoria is more pronounced. **Convergence** becomes sluggish with ageing.

Pupillary reactions to light and accommodation may be tested (**Fig. 26.6**). A bright torch (not an ophthalmoscope light!) should be used to test the pupillary light reaction.

Afferent pupillary defect (APD). A complete optic nerve lesion causes a dilated pupil and an APD. For a left APD:

- The pupil is unreactive to light (i.e. the direct reflex is absent).
- The consensual reflex (constriction of the right pupil when the left is illuminated) is absent. Conversely, the left pupil constricts

when light is shone in the intact right eye: that is, the consensual reflex of the right eye remains intact.

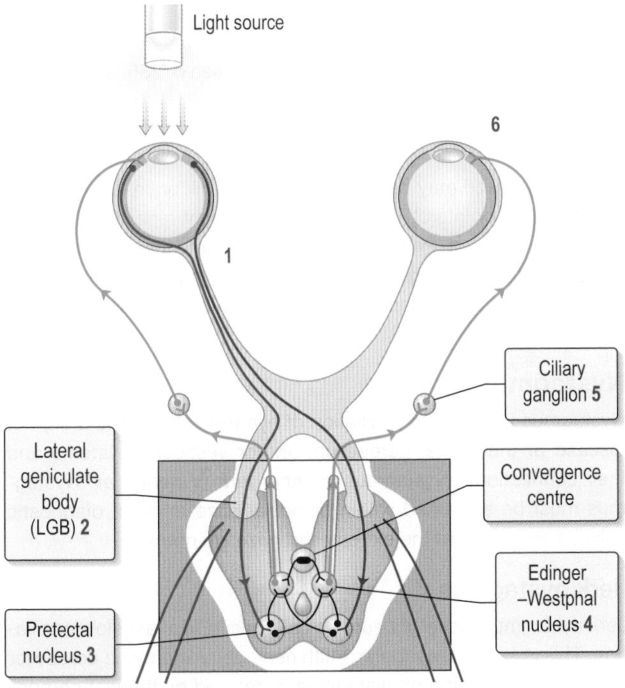

Relative afferent pupillary defect (RAPD). This occurs with incomplete damage to one optic nerve relative to the other. An RAPD is a sensitive sign of optic nerve pathology and can provide evidence of an optic nerve lesion, even after recovery of vision. For a left RAPD:

- Direct and indirect reflexes are intact in each eye but differ in relative strength.
- When the light is swung from one eye to the other, the left pupil **dilates** slightly when illuminated and **constricts** slightly when the right eye is illuminated (the consensual reflex is stronger than the direct).

Horner's syndrome

The sympathetic nervous supply to the eye is a three-neurone pathway originating in the hypothalamus and descending by way of the brainstem and cervical cord to the T1 nerve root, paravertebral sympathetic chain and, on via the carotid artery wall, to the eye. Damage to any part of the pathway results in Horner syndrome (**Box 26.13**). This is significant not only because it affects vision but also because it may indicate serious underlying pathology.

The clinical features of Horner's syndrome are:

- unilateral miosis (constricted pupil)
- partial ptosis
- loss of sweating on the same side (extent depending on the level of the lesion)
- possible subtle conjunctival injection and enophthalmos.

The miosis is most easily seen in low light, as the pupil cannot dilate, and may not be apparent in bright light.

Myotonic pupil (Holmes–Adie pupil)

This is a dilated, often irregular, pupil, and is more frequent in women; it is common and usually unilateral. There is no (or very slow) reaction to bright light and also incomplete constriction to convergence. This is due to denervation in the ciliary ganglion, of unknown cause, and has no other pathological significance. A myotonic pupil is sometimes associated with diminished or absent tendon reflexes.

Argyll Robertson pupil

Now rarely seen in clinical practice, an Argyll Robertson pupil is small and irregular; it is fixed to light but constricts on convergence. The lesion is in the brainstem surrounding the aqueduct of Sylvius. Once considered diagnostic of neurosyphilis, it is now only occasionally seen in diabetes or MS.

Fig. 26.6 Pupillary light reflex. Afferent pathway: (1) Light activates optic nerve axons. (2) Axons (some decussating at the chiasm) pass through each lateral geniculate body, and (3) synapse at pretectal nuclei. **Efferent pathway:** (4) Action potentials pass to Edinger–Westphal nuclei of the IIIrd nerve, then, (5) via parasympathetic neurones in IIIrd nerves to cause (6) pupil constriction.

Light source

6

1

Ciliary ganglion **5**

Lateral geniculate body (LGB) **2**

Convergence centre

Edinger–Westphal nucleus **4**

Pretectal nucleus **3**

? Box 26.13 Causes of Horner's syndrome

Hypothalamic, hemisphere and brainstem lesions
- Massive cerebral infarction
- Brainstem demyelination or lateral medullary infarction

Cervical cord
- Syringomyelia and cord tumours

T1 root
- Apical lung tumour or tuberculosis
- Cervical rib
- Brachial plexus trauma

Sympathetic chain and carotid artery in neck
- Following thyroid/laryngeal/carotid surgery
- Carotid artery dissection
- Neoplastic infiltration
- Cervical sympathectomy

Miscellaneous
- Congenital
- Cluster headache, usually transient
- Idiopathic

III, IV, VI: Oculomotor, trochlear and abducens nerves

These cranial nerves supply the extraocular muscles and disorders commonly result in abnormal eye movements and diplopia (double vision) due to breakdown of conjugate eye movements. Diplopia may also occur with local orbital lesions or myasthenia gravis.

Examination of eye movements

Pursuit (slow) eye movements and saccadic (fast) eye movements are tested separately. The examiner assesses the range of eye movements in all directions and asks the patient to report double vision. Jerky pursuit movements with saccadic intrusion (i.e. brief, fast saccades interspersed with slower pursuit movements), overshoot on saccadic movements, and nystagmus may indicate cerebellar or brainstem pathology.

Control of eye movements

Fast voluntary eye movements originate in the frontal lobes. Fibres descend and cross in the pons to end in the centre for lateral gaze (paramedian pontine reticular formation, PPRF), close to the VIth nerve nucleus. Each PPRF also receives input from:
- the ipsilateral occipital cortex – pathway concerned with tracking objects
- the vestibular nuclei – pathways linking eye movements with position of the head and neck (vestibulo-ocular reflex).

Conjugate lateral eye movements are coordinated from each PPRF via the medial longitudinal fasciculus (MLF; **Fig. 26.7**). Fibres

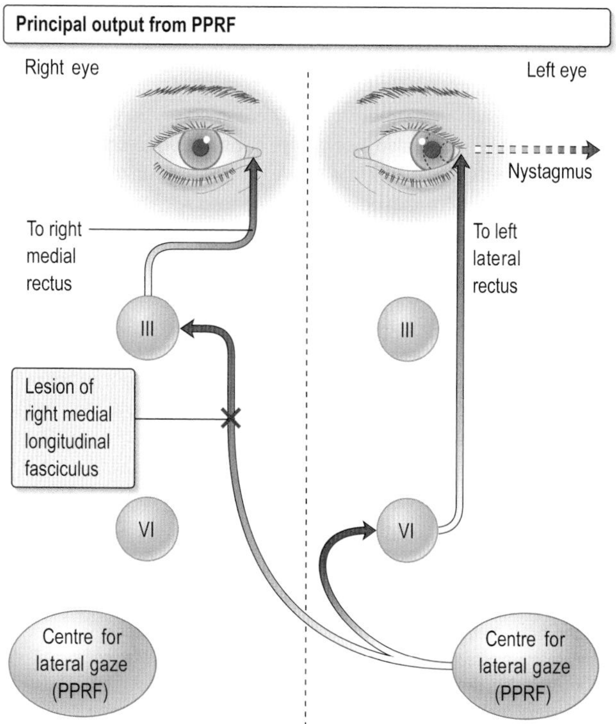

Fig. 26.7 Paramedian pontine reticular formation (PPRF) and internuclear ophthalmoplegia. Impulses from the PPRF pass via the ipsilateral VIth nerve nucleus to the lateral rectus muscle (**ab**duction), and via the medial longitudinal fasciculus to the opposite third nerve nucleus and thus to the opposite medial rectus muscle (**ad**duction). A lesion of the medial longitudinal fasciculus (X) causes failure of or slow **ad**duction in the right eye, and nystagmus in the left eye with left lateral gaze.

from the PPRF pass both to the ipsilateral VIth nerve nucleus (lateral rectus) and, having crossed the midline, to the opposite IIIrd nerve nucleus (medial rectus and other muscles) via the MLF, thus linking the eyes for lateral gaze.

Abnormalities of conjugate lateral gaze

A destructive lesion on one side allows the eyes to be driven by the intact opposite pathway. A left frontal destructive lesion (e.g. an infarct) leads to failure of conjugate lateral gaze to the right. In an acute lesion, the eyes are often deviated to the side of the lesion, past the midline, and therefore look towards the left (normal) limbs; there is usually a contralateral (i.e. right) hemiparesis.

In the brainstem, a unilateral destructive lesion involving the PPRF leads to failure of conjugate lateral gaze *towards* that side. There is usually a contralateral hemiparesis, and lateral gaze is deviated towards the side of the paralysed limbs.

Internuclear ophthalmoplegia

Damage to one MLF causes internuclear ophthalmoplegia (INO), a common complex brainstem eye movement disorder seen frequently in MS. In a right INO, there is a lesion of the right MLF (see **Fig. 26.7**). On attempted left lateral gaze, the right eye fails to **ad**duct or does so slowly in comparison to the **ab**ducting eye. The left eye develops nystagmus in **ab**duction. The side of the lesion is on the side of impaired **ad**duction, not on the side of the (obvious, unilateral) nystagmus. Bilateral INO is almost pathognomonic of MS.

One and a half syndrome

Pontine infarction involving the PPRF, VIth nerve nucleus and MLF on one side results in an ipsilateral horizontal gaze palsy and an INO, so that abduction of the opposite eye (with nystagmus) is the only horizontal eye movement possible. Vertical gaze and convergence are preserved, as they have distinct neural control mechanisms.

Vestibulo-ocular (doll's eye) reflexes

Examination is of diagnostic value in coma (see p. 236) and assessment of vertigo (see p. 816).

Abnormalities of vertical gaze

Failure of upgaze may be caused by dorsal midbrain lesions, such as pinealoma or infarct. When the pupillary light reflex fails in addition, this is called Parinaud's syndrome. Defective upgaze also develops in certain degenerative disorders (e.g. progressive supranuclear palsy). Some impairment of upgaze occurs as part of normal ageing.

Nystagmus

Nystagmus is rhythmic oscillation of eye movement; it is a sign of disease of the retina, cerebellum and/or vestibular systems and their connections. Nystagmus is either *jerk* or *pendular*. Nystagmus must be sustained within binocular gaze to be of diagnostic value; a few beats at the extremes of gaze are normal.

Jerk nystagmus

Jerk nystagmus (usual in neurological disease) is a fast/slow oscillation. This is seen in vestibular, VIIIth nerve, brainstem and cerebellar lesions. The direction of nystagmus is decided by the fast component, a reflex attempt to correct the slower, primary movement.
- *Horizontal or rotary jerk nystagmus* may be either of peripheral (vestibular) or central origin (VIIIth nerve, brainstem, cerebellum and connections).

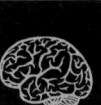

- In peripheral lesions, nystagmus is usually acute and transient (minutes or hours) and associated with severe prostrating vertigo.
- In central lesions, nystagmus tends to be long-lasting (weeks, months or more). Vertigo caused by central lesions tends to wane after days or weeks, the nystagmus outlasting it.
- **Vertical jerk nystagmus** is typically caused by central lesions.
- **Down-beat jerk nystagmus** is a rarity caused by lesions around the foramen magnum (e.g. meningioma, cerebellar ectopia).

Pendular nystagmus

Pendular describes movements to and fro, similar in velocity and amplitude. Pendular nystagmus is usually vertical and present in all directions of gaze. The causes are generally ocular (e.g. poor visual fixation from longstanding, severe visual impairment) or congenital.

III: Oculomotor nerve lesions

The nucleus of the IIIrd nerve lies ventral to the aqueduct in the midbrain. It supplies four external ocular muscles (superior, inferior and medial recti, and inferior oblique) and levator palpebrae superioris (which lifts the eyelid), and effects parasympathetic constriction of the pupil. Causes of a IIIrd nerve lesion are listed in **Box 26.14**.

Signs of a complete IIIrd nerve palsy include:
- unilateral complete ptosis (levator weakness)
- deviation of the eye down and out (unopposed lateral rectus and superior oblique)
- a fixed and dilated pupil.

Patients do not complain of diplopia as the ptosis effectively covers the eye. **Sparing of the pupil** indicates that parasympathetic fibres are undamaged; these run in a discrete bundle on the surface of the nerve, and so the pupil is of normal size and reacts normally. Diabetic IIIrd nerve infarction is usually painless and pupil-sparing, unlike compression by a posterior communicating artery aneurysm.

IV: Trochlear nerve lesions

The trochlear nerve supplies the superior oblique muscle. The patient complains of torsional diplopia (two objects at an angle) when attempting to look down (e.g. descending stairs); the head is tilted away from that side. The most common cause is head injury, often with bilateral trochlear nerve palsies occurring.

VI: Abducens nerve lesions

The abducens nerve supplies the lateral rectus muscle (**ab**duction). Lesions cause horizontal diplopia when looking into the distance, which is maximal when looking to the side of the lesion. The eye cannot be fully abducted and an esotropia (inward eye deviation) may be visible in the primary position.

The VIth nerve has a long intracranial course. It can be damaged in the brainstem (e.g. by MS or infarction). In raised intracranial pressure, it is compressed against the tip of the petrous temporal bone (this may be bilateral). The nerve sheath may be infiltrated by tumours, particularly nasopharyngeal carcinoma. Microvascular ischaemia of the nerve may occur in diabetes with acute onset, followed by recovery within 3 months in most cases.

> **? Box 26.14 Some causes of a IIIrd nerve lesion**
>
> - Aneurysm of the posterior communicating artery
> - Infarction of IIIrd nerve, e.g. diabetes, atheroma
> - Coning of the temporal lobe
> - Midbrain infarction
> - Midbrain tumour (primary or secondary)

Complete external ophthalmoplegia

Complete external ophthalmoplegia describes an immobile eye when IIIrd, IVth and VIth nerves are paralysed at the orbital apex (e.g. by metastasis) or within the cavernous sinus (e.g. by sinus thrombosis or meningioma).

Wernicke's encephalopathy due to thiamine deficiency (see p. 891) may cause a complex eye movement disorder or complete ophthalmoplegia, as may neuromuscular junction disorders such as myasthenia, botulism and some myopathies or metabolic disorders.

V: Trigeminal nerve

The trigeminal is the largest cranial nerve; it is mainly sensory with a motor component to the muscles of mastication.

Sensory fibres (**Fig. 26.8**; see also **Figs 26.13** and **26.14**) of the three divisions – ophthalmic (V_1), maxillary (V_2) and mandibular (V_3) – pass to the trigeminal (Gasserian) ganglion at the apex of the petrous temporal bone. Ascending fibres transmitting light touch enter the fifth nucleus in the pons. Descending central fibres carrying pain and temperature form the spinal tract of V, to end in the spinal fifth nucleus that extends from the medulla into the cervical cord.

Clinical features of a Vth nerve lesion

A complete Vth nerve lesion causes unilateral sensory loss on the face, scalp anterior to the vertex, and the anterior two-thirds of the tongue and buccal mucosa; the jaw deviates to that side as the mouth opens (motor fibres). Diminution of the corneal reflex is an early and sometimes isolated sign of a Vth nerve lesion.

Aetiology

- **Brainstem pathology** (infarction, demyelination or tumour) may damage the nucleus, with light touch and spinothalamic pathways sometimes being differentially involved.

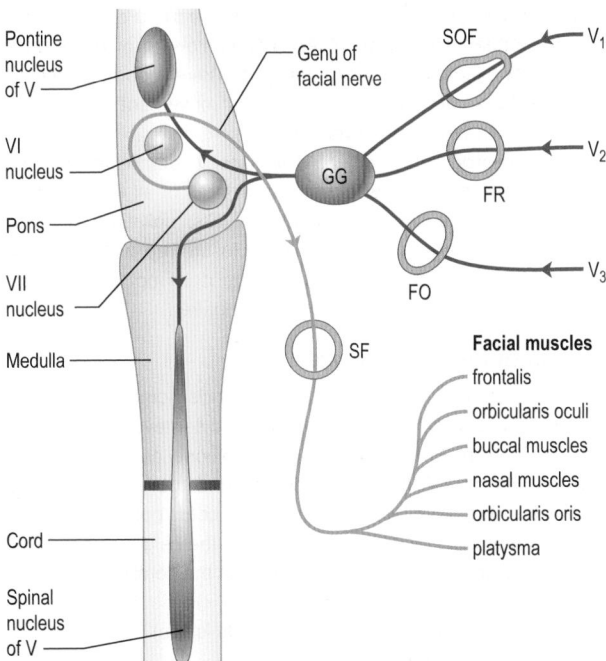

Fig. 26.8 Sensory input of fifth nerve (red) and motor output of the VIIth nerve (blue). FO, foramen ovale; FR, foramen rotundum; GG, Gasserian ganglion; SF, stylomastoid foramen; SOF, superior orbital fissure.

- *Cerebellopontine angle tumours* (acoustic neuroma or meningioma) may compress the nerve and also affect the VIIth and VIIIth nerves, producing facial weakness and deafness.
- *Cavernous sinus and skull base pathology* (tumour or infection) may affect the ganglion and proximal branches.
- *Peripheral branches* may be picked off individually, e.g. the 'numb chin syndrome' seen with a breast cancer metastasis in the mandible.

Trigeminal neuralgia

Trigeminal neuralgia is discussed with facial pain (see p. 852).

Trigeminal sensory neuropathy

This causes gradually progressive, unilateral, facial sensory loss and tingling with normal imaging. The condition is probably heterogeneous in aetiology but may have an autoimmune basis, with inflammation of the trigeminal ganglion, occurring mainly in association with mixed and undifferentiated connective tissue disease and primary Sjögren's syndrome.

VII: Facial nerve

The VIIth nerve is largely motor, supplying muscles of facial expression. It carries sensory taste fibres from the anterior two-thirds of the tongue via the chorda tympani and supplies motor fibres to the stapedius muscle. The VIIth nerve (see **Fig. 26.8**) arises from its nucleus in the pons and leaves the skull through the stylomastoid foramen. Neurones in each VIIth nucleus supplying the upper face (principally frontalis) receive bilateral supranuclear innervation.

Unilateral facial weakness

Upper motor neurone (UMN) lesions. These cause weakness of the lower part of the face on the opposite side. Frontalis is spared: normal furrowing of the brow is preserved; eye closure and blinking are largely unaffected. The earliest sign is slowing of one side of the face: for example, on baring the teeth. There is sometimes relative preservation of spontaneous emotional movement (e.g. smiling) compared with voluntary movement.

Lower motor neurone (LMN) lesions. A complete unilateral LMN VIIth lesion causes weakness (ipsilateral) of all facial expression muscles. The angle of the mouth falls; unilateral dribbling develops. Frowning (frontalis) and eye closure are weak. Corneal exposure and ulceration occur if the eye does not close during sleep. Taste sensation is frequently also impaired.

Causes of facial weakness

The most common cause of a UMN lesion is hemispheric stroke with hemiparesis on the opposite side. At lower levels, lesion sites are recognized by LMN weakness with additional signs.

Pons. Here the VIIth nerve loops around the VIth (abducens) nucleus (see **Fig. 26.8**), leading to a lateral rectus palsy (see p. 813) with unilateral LMN facial weakness. When the neighbouring PPRF and corticospinal tract are involved, there is the combination of:
- LMN facial weakness
- failure of conjugate lateral gaze (towards lesion)
- contralateral hemiparesis.

Causes include pontine tumours (e.g. glioma), MS and infarction.

Cerebellopontine angle (CPA). The neighbouring Vth, VIth and VIIIth nerves are compressed with VII in the CPA; for example, by acoustic neuroma, meningioma or metastasis.

Petrous temporal bone. The nerve may be damaged within the bony facial canal, within which lies the sensory geniculate ganglion (receiving taste fibres from the anterior two-thirds of the tongue via the chorda tympani). As well as LMN facial weakness, lesions in this region cause:
- loss of taste on the anterior two-thirds of the tongue
- hyperacusis (loud noise distortion – paralysis of stapedius).

Causes include:
- Bell's palsy
- trauma
- middle ear infection
- herpes zoster (Ramsay Hunt syndrome; see p. 815).

Skull base, parotid gland and within the face. The facial nerve can be compressed by skull base tumours and in Paget's disease of bone. Branches of VII may be damaged by parotid gland tumours as the nerve traverses the parotid, and by sarcoidosis (see p. 985) and trauma.

Bell's palsy

This common (37 per 100 000 incidence), acute facial palsy is thought to be due to viral infection/reactivation (often herpes simplex) causing swelling of nerve within the tight petrous bone facial canal. Unilateral LMN facial weakness develops over 24–48 hours, sometimes with lost or altered taste on the tongue, and hyperacusis. Pain behind the ear is common at onset. Patients often suspect a stroke and may be very distressed. Vague altered facial sensation is often reported, although examination of facial sensation is normal.

Diagnosis is made on clinical grounds and tests are usually not required. The ear (and palate) should be examined for vesicles (see Ramsay Hunt syndrome later), hearing loss or evidence of local pathology such as cholesteatoma or malignant otitis externa; parotid tumours should be excluded. Involvement of other cranial nerves means facial weakness is not due to Bell's palsy. Lyme disease may account for one-quarter of cases of facial palsy in endemic areas and HIV seroconversion is the most common cause in parts of Africa.

(*Bell's phenomenon* is the upward conjugate eye movement that occurs normally when the eyes are closed but is accentuated when the orbicularis oculi muscle is weak.)

Management and prognosis

Complete, or almost complete, recovery over 4–12 weeks occurs in at least 85% of patients, even without specific treatment. Patients should be reassured that the prognosis is good and that the condition is unlikely to recur.

Inability to blink in severe facial weakness may lead to exposure keratitis. Use of lubricating eye ointment is often required and patients should be advised to tape the eye closed carefully at night. For more severe facial weakness with complete inability to close the eye, early ophthalmological assessment is necessary and lateral tarsorrhaphy and/or insertion of a gold weight into the upper lid may be required until recovery occurs.

Early treatment with corticosteroids (prednisolone 50 mg for 10 days) improves outcome if started within 72 hours of onset. The latest evidence does not support use of antiviral agents.

Recovery sometimes takes up to a year if axons have to regrow rather than just remyelinate, in which case aberrant re-innervation of facial muscles (e.g. mouth twitching with blinking) is a frequent late complication. Plastic surgery may be helpful where recovery is not complete. Bell's palsy rarely recurs; if it does, this should prompt a search for an alternative cause.

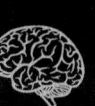

Ramsay Hunt syndrome

This is herpes zoster (shingles) of the geniculate ganglion. There is a facial palsy (identical to Bell's) with vesicles around the external auditory meatus and/or the soft palate (sensory twigs from VII). Deafness and vertigo/unsteadiness may occur. Complete recovery is less likely than in Bell's. Antiviral treatment (aciclovir/valaciclovir) is usually given with steroids.

Bilateral facial weakness

Bilateral facial palsy is rare, accounting for less than 1% of cases of facial palsy, but is more likely than unilateral palsies to have an identifiable underlying cause. Paradoxically, bilateral weakness is often less obviously apparent than unilateral weakness, as there is no facial asymmetry.

Causes include:
- infections:
  - Lyme disease (bilateral in 25% – Bannwarth's syndrome)
  - viral: human immunodeficiency virus (HIV) seroconversion, Epstein–Barr virus
  - mastoiditis (bilateral)
  - diphtheria and botulism (rare)
- sarcoidosis
- skull-base trauma and tumours
- pontine lesions, e.g. gliomas
- neuromuscular disorders as part of more generalized weakness:
  - Guillain–Barré syndrome
  - myasthenia
  - myotonic dystrophy and facioscapulohumeral dystrophy
- congenital and genetic causes (Gelsolin gene mutations).

Hemifacial spasm

Hemifacial spasm (HFS) is an irregular, painless unilateral spasm of facial muscles, usually occurring after middle age. It starts in the orbicularis oculi and usually progresses gradually over the years to involve other facial muscles on the same side. It varies from a mild to a severe, disfiguring spasm.

HFS is usually caused by compression of the root entry zone of the facial nerve, generally by vascular structures such as the vertebral or basilar arteries or their branches (a mechanism similar to that of trigeminal neuralgia; see p. 852). Other mass lesions in the cerebellopontine angle, including tumours, are the cause in approximately 1% of cases.

Occasionally, HFS may occur with ipsilateral trigeminal neuralgia, one symptom usually preceding the other: a combination called *tic convulsif*. The paroxysms of pain and spasm occur independently. A compressive cause, such as a vascular loop or other structural lesion, is usually identified.

Management

Mild cases require no treatment. Botulinum toxin injection into affected muscles every 3–4 months is now the standard treatment. Drugs (e.g. carbamazepine) are of little value. Decompression of the VIIth nerve in the CPA is sometimes helpful. Surgical decompression of the facial nerve in the posterior fossa involves interposing a non-resorbable sponge between the nerve and any adjacent vascular loop identified at operation. The procedure results in complete resolution of symptoms in up to 90% of cases but is associated with a risk of facial weakness or deafness.

Other involuntary facial movements

Myokymia of orbicularis oculi is an irritating twitch, usually of the lower eyelid. It is a normal phenomenon but sometimes a cause of anxiety. More extensive facial myokymia may result from intrinsic brainstem pathology.

Tics and tardive dyskinesia frequently involve facial or perioral muscles (see p. 863).

Blepharospasm is a form of focal dystonia affecting orbicularis oculi (see p. 863).

VIII: Vestibulocochlear nerve

Auditory fibres from the spiral organ of Corti within the cochlea pass to the cochlear nuclei in the pons. Fibres from these nuclei cross the midline and pass upwards via the medial lemnisci to the medial geniculate bodies and then to the temporal cortex.

Symptoms of a cochlear nerve lesion are deafness and tinnitus (see p. 907). Sensorineural and conductive deafness can be distinguished with tuning fork tests, e.g. Rinne's and Weber's (using a 256 Hz, not 128 Hz, tuning fork; see p. 903).

Basic investigations of cochlear lesions

- Pure tone audiometry and auditory thresholds.
- Auditory evoked potentials (recording responses from repetitive clicks via scalp electrodes; lesion levels are determined from the response pattern).

Causes of deafness

These are listed in **Box 26.15** and **Box 27.2**.

Vertigo and the vestibular system

The vestibular system of the inner ear detects head movements and has three primary functions:
- to stabilize gaze during head movements, e.g. looking ahead while running (the vestibulo-ocular reflex)
- to control posture and balance
- to facilitate perception of orientation and motion.

? Box 26.15 Some causes of vertigo and hearing loss

Conditions	Symptom(s)
Benign paroxysmal positional vertigo	V
Vestibular neuritis	V
Ménière's disease	V, D
Alcohol, antiepileptic drug intoxication	V
Cerebellar lesions	V
Partial (temporal lobe) seizures	V
Migraine	V+ phonophobia
Brainstem ischaemia	V, occasionally D
Multiple sclerosis	V, occasionally D
Mumps, intrauterine rubella and congenital syphilis	D
Advancing age (presbycusis) and otosclerosis	D
Acoustic trauma	D
Congenital, e.g. Pendred's syndrome	D
Gentamicin, furosemide	V, D
Middle and external ear disease	V, D
Cerebellopontine angle lesions, e.g. acoustic neuroma	V, D
Carcinomatous meningitis, sarcoidosis and tuberculous meningitis	V, D

D, hearing loss; V, vertigo.

Nerve impulses generated by movement of hair cells within the three semicircular canals detect head motion in the three planes (yaw/pitch/roll). Balance is maintained by integrating information from:

- the vestibular system
- the visual system
- the somatosensory system – proprioception from limbs, trunk and neck.

The **main symptoms** of vestibular lesions are vertigo and loss of balance.

Vertigo

Vertigo is the illusion of movement of the subject or surroundings, typically rotatory, and should be distinguished from other causes of non-specific dizziness. It can be described to patients as being similar to the sensation one feels after getting off a child's roundabout or after spinning on the spot and suddenly stopping.

Vomiting frequently accompanies acute vertigo of any cause. Vertigo is always made worse by head movements and patients prefer to remain still and maintain visual fixation. Walking is unsteady. Nystagmus (see p. 812) is the principal sign.

The dizzy patient

Complaints of 'dizziness' require careful history-taking and may be caused by:

- vertigo
- pre-syncopal sensations due to transient cerebral hypoperfusion, e.g. orthostatic light-headedness
- unsteadiness or disequilibrium, e.g. cerebellar or postural stability disorders
- non-specific 'dizziness', e.g. due to medication or anxiety and hyperventilation.

Causes of vertigo

Vertigo indicates a disturbance of the vestibular apparatus or brainstem and associated neural pathways (see **Box 26.15**). Causes:

- **Peripheral causes** (vestibular system) are common. Deafness and tinnitus accompanying vertigo indicate involvement of the ear or cochlear nerve (see p. 903).
- **Central causes** (brainstem and connections) are rarer. Other clinical features, such as diplopia, weakness, cerebellar signs or cranial nerve palsies, may help localize the lesion.

Peripheral (vestibular) disorders

Vestibular disorders are fully discussed elsewhere (see p. 907). Attack duration and frequency, as well as trigger factors, help the clinician distinguish on history between different pathological causes. The ability to perform a Hallpike test, head impulse test and Epley particle repositioning manoeuvre are invaluable skills for all clinicians (see p. 906; **Fig. 26.9** and see **Fig. 27.9**).

The most commonly encountered vestibular disorders presenting with vertigo are:

- **benign paroxysmal positional vertigo** (BPPV) – frequent attacks lasting seconds only (see p. 906).
- **vestibular neuronitis** – acute onset lasting days or weeks; non-recurrent
- **Ménière's disease** – recurrent attacks lasting minutes or hours, usually accompanied by hearing loss, tinnitus and a feeling of fullness in the ear
- **trauma** – vestibular disruption following head injury.

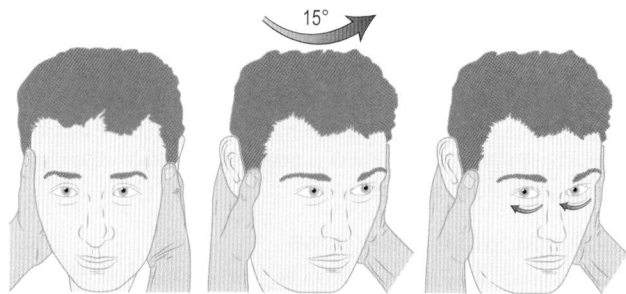

Fig. 26.9 The head impulse test. When tested on the normal side, a patient can maintain fixation on a distant object as the examiner rapidly turns the patient's head sideways through about 15°. If there is unilateral vestibulopathy, the patient cannot maintain fixation on the target and can be observed to make a voluntary eye movement (a saccade) back to the target after the head impulse, as shown on the right. It is essential for the head to be turned as rapidly as possible; otherwise, smooth pursuit eye movements will compensate for the head turn.

Central causes of vertigo

Vertigo may be a manifestation of brainstem pathology, including:

- **infarcts involving the vestibular nuclei** in the medulla (e.g. the lateral medullary syndrome)
- **demyelination** involving the brainstem
- **posterior fossa mass lesions** – e.g. tumours, haemorrhage or vascular malformations
- **migrainous vertigo** (see p. 850) – lasts hours, occurring every few weeks or months
- **CPA mass lesions** and tumours compressing the vestibular nerve (technically, these should be classified as 'peripheral' disorders, but are distinct from disorders of the vestibular apparatus)
- **drugs** – e.g. anticonvulsant toxicity and alcohol.

Although vertigo occasionally occurs in isolation with brainstem pathology, it is more typically a single component of a more complex clinical picture, associated with other symptoms or examination findings. The brainstem nuclei and tracts are tightly packed into a small space and most pathological processes affect multiple contiguous neural pathways, resulting, for example, in diplopia, eye movement disorders, cranial nerve palsies, cerebellar signs or hemiparesis.

Slowly growing CPA tumours, such as vestibular nerve schwannomas, may cause vertigo but rarely do so in the absence of unilateral deafness and tinnitus.

Basic investigations for vestibular problems

Bedside assessment is usually sufficient to make a diagnosis in the majority of patients:

- examination of eye movements for nystagmus (see p. 812)
- assessment of hearing and otoscopic examination of the ear (see p. 815)
- head impulse (thrust) test – to assess the vestibulo-ocular reflex (VOR) and identify a unilateral vestibulopathy
- Hallpike manoeuvre – a positioning test to stimulate the posterior semicircular canal and trigger an attack in BPPV (see **Fig. 27.9**).

Specialist testing is occasionally required to assess vestibular function and hearing. This includes:

- caloric testing – irrigation of the external auditory meatus with cold and then warm water to stimulate the horizontal semicircular canal and induce nystagmus; labyrinthine function is tested in each ear separately

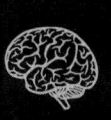

- electro-nystagmography – to quantify and characterize nystagmus under different conditions, e.g. in a rotating chair
- posturography – assesses body sway on a moving platform
- pure-tone audiograms
- high-definition MRI – provides the best structural imaging of the brainstem and CPA, and is useful where a central cause of vertigo is suspected.

Vestibular neuronitis

Vestibular neuronitis is a common but poorly understood problem. It is an acute attack of isolated vertigo with nystagmus, often with vomiting, and is believed to follow viral infections. The disturbance lasts for several days or weeks, is self-limiting and rarely recurs. Vestibular neuronitis is sometimes followed by BPPV (see p. 906). Deafness is absent. Acute treatment is with vestibular sedatives. Similar symptoms can be caused by MS or brainstem vascular lesions. Other signs are usually apparent.

Lower cranial nerves IX, X, XI, XII

The glossopharyngeal (IX), vagus (X) and accessory (XI) nerves arise in the medulla and leave the skull through the jugular foramen. The hypoglossal (XII) arises in the medulla, to leave the skull base via the hypoglossal foramen. Outside the skull, the four cranial nerves lie together, close to the carotid artery and sympathetic trunk.

Glossopharyngeal (IX)

This nerve is largely sensory, supplying sensation and taste from the posterior third of the tongue and the pharynx (afferent pathway of gag reflex). Motor fibres supply some pharyngeal muscles, and parasympathetic fibres supply the parotid.

Vagus (X)

The vagus is a mixed nerve, largely motor, which supplies striated muscle of the pharynx (efferent gag reflex pathway), larynx (including vocal cords via recurrent laryngeal nerves) and upper oesophagus. There are sensory fibres from the larynx. Parasympathetic fibres supply the heart and abdominal viscera.

Accessory (XI)

The accessory nerve, a complex motor nerve, supplies the trapezius and sternomastoid muscles.

Hypoglossal (XII)

The hypoglossal nerve is a motor nerve to tongue muscles.

IXth and Xth nerve lesions

Principal causes of IXth, Xth, XIth and XIIth nerve lesions are listed in **Box 26.16**.

Isolated lesions of IXth and Xth nerves are unusual, since disease at the jugular foramen affects both nerves and sometimes XI.

A unilateral IXth nerve lesion causes diminished sensation on the same side of the pharynx and is hard to recognize in isolation. A Xth nerve palsy produces ipsilateral failure of voluntary and reflex elevation of the soft palate (which is drawn to the opposite side) and ipsilateral vocal cords.

Bilateral lesions of IXth and Xth nerves cause palatal weakness, reduced palatal sensation, an absent gag reflex, dysphonia and choking with nasal regurgitation. **Bulbar palsy** is a general term describing palatal, pharyngeal and tongue weakness of LMN or muscle origin.

> ### Box 26.16 Principal causes of IXth, Xth, XIth and XIIth nerve lesions
>
> **Within brainstem**
> - Infarction
> - Syringobulbia
> - Motor neurone disease (motor fibres)
>
> **Around skull base**
> - Nasopharyngeal carcinoma
> - Glomus tumour
> - Neurofibroma
> - Jugular venous thrombosis
> - Trauma
>
> **Within neck and nasopharynx**
> - Nasopharyngeal carcinoma
> - Metastases
> - Carotid artery dissection (XII)
> - Trauma
> - Lymph node biopsy in posterior triangle (XI)

Recurrent laryngeal nerve lesions. Paralysis of this branch of each vagus causes hoarseness (dysphonia) and failure of the forceful, explosive part of coughing ('bovine cough'). There is no visible palatal weakness; vocal cord paralysis is seen endoscopically. Bilateral acute lesions (e.g. postoperatively) cause respiratory obstruction – an emergency.

The left recurrent laryngeal nerve (looping beneath the aorta) is damaged more commonly than the right.

Causes of recurrent laryngeal nerve lesions include:
- mediastinal primary tumours (e.g. thymoma)
- secondary spread from bronchial carcinoma
- aortic aneurysm
- trauma or surgery of neck or thorax.

XIth nerve lesions

XIth nerve lesions cause weakness of sternomastoid (rotation of the head and neck to the opposite side) and trapezius (shoulder shrugging). Nerve section (e.g. following lymph node biopsy in the neck posterior triangle) is followed by persistent neuralgic pain.

XIIth nerve lesions

LMN lesions of XII lead to unilateral tongue weakness, wasting and fasciculation. The protruded tongue deviates towards the weaker side. Bilateral supranuclear (UMN) lesions produce slow, limited tongue movements and a stiff tongue that cannot be protruded far. Fasciculation is absent.

Bulbar and pseudobulbar palsy
Bulbar palsy

This is LMN weakness of muscles whose cranial nerve nuclei lie in the medulla (the bulb). Paralysis of bulbar muscles is caused by disease of lower cranial nerve nuclei, lesions of IXth, Xth and XIIth nerves (see **Box 26.16**), malfunction of their neuromuscular junctions (e.g. myasthenia gravis, botulism) or disease of muscles themselves (e.g. dystrophies).

Pseudobulbar palsy

Describes bilateral supranuclear (UMN) lesions of lower cranial nerves producing weakness of the tongue and pharyngeal muscles. This resembles, superficially, a bulbar palsy: hence pseudobulbar. Findings are a stiff, slow, spastic tongue (not wasted), dysarthria and dysphagia. Gag and palatal reflexes are preserved and the jaw jerk exaggerated. Emotional lability (inappropriate laughing or crying) often accompanies pseudobulbar palsy. Principal causes are:
- motor neurone disease, often both UMN and LMN lesions (i.e. elements of both pseudobulbar and bulbar palsy)
- cerebrovascular disease, typically following multiple infarcts
- neurodegenerative disorders such as progressive supranuclear palsy (see p. 861)

- severe traumatic brain injury
- MS, mainly as a late event.

Difficulty swallowing, dysarthria and drooling also develop in later stages of Parkinson's disease.

Dropped head syndrome

As the name suggests, weakness of neck extensors causes neck flexion and inability to hold the head up. Seen mainly in the elderly, it is often due to isolated neck extensor myopathy of uncertain cause but may be a presenting feature of motor neurone disease, myasthenia or various myopathic disorders.

Further reading

Biousse V, Newman NJ. Ischemic optic neuropathies. *N Engl J Med* 2015; 372:2428–2436.

MOTOR CONTROL SYSTEMS

There are three systems, each of which interacts by feedback loops with the other two, with sensory input from the reticular formation:

- **The corticospinal** (or **pyramidal**) **system** enables purposive, skilled, intricate, strong and organized movements. Defective function is recognized by a distinct pattern of signs – loss of skilled voluntary movement, spasticity and reflex change – seen, for example, in a hemiparesis, hemiplegia or paraparesis.
- **The extrapyramidal system** facilitates fast, fluid movements that the corticospinal system has generated. Defective function produces slowness (bradykinesia), stiffness (rigidity) and/or disorders of movement (rest tremor, chorea and other dyskinesias). One feature (e.g. stiffness, tremor or chorea) will often predominate.
- **The cerebellum** and its connections have a role coordinating smooth and learned movement, initiated by the pyramidal system, and in posture and balance control. Cerebellar disease leads to unsteady and jerky movements (ataxia), with characteristic limb signs of past-pointing, action tremor and incoordination, gait ataxia and/or truncal ataxia.

Corticospinal (pyramidal) system

The corticospinal tracts originate in neurones of the cortex and terminate at motor nuclei of cranial nerves and spinal cord anterior horn cells. The pathways of particular clinical significance (**Fig. 26.10**) congregate in the internal capsule and cross in the medulla (decussation of the pyramids), passing to the contralateral cord as the lateral corticospinal tracts. This is the pyramidal system, disease of which causes UMN lesions. 'Pyramidal' is simply a descriptive term that draws together anatomy and characteristic physical signs; it is used interchangeably with the term UMN.

A proportion of the corticospinal outflow is uncrossed (anterior corticospinal tracts). This is of no relevance in practice.

Characteristics of pyramidal lesions

Signs of an early pyramidal lesion may be minimal (**Box 26.17**). Weakness, spasticity or changes in reflexes can predominate, or be present in isolation.

Pyramidal drift of an upper limb

Normally, the outstretched upper limbs are held symmetrically, when the eyes are closed. With a pyramidal lesion, when both upper limbs are held outstretched, palms uppermost, the affected limb

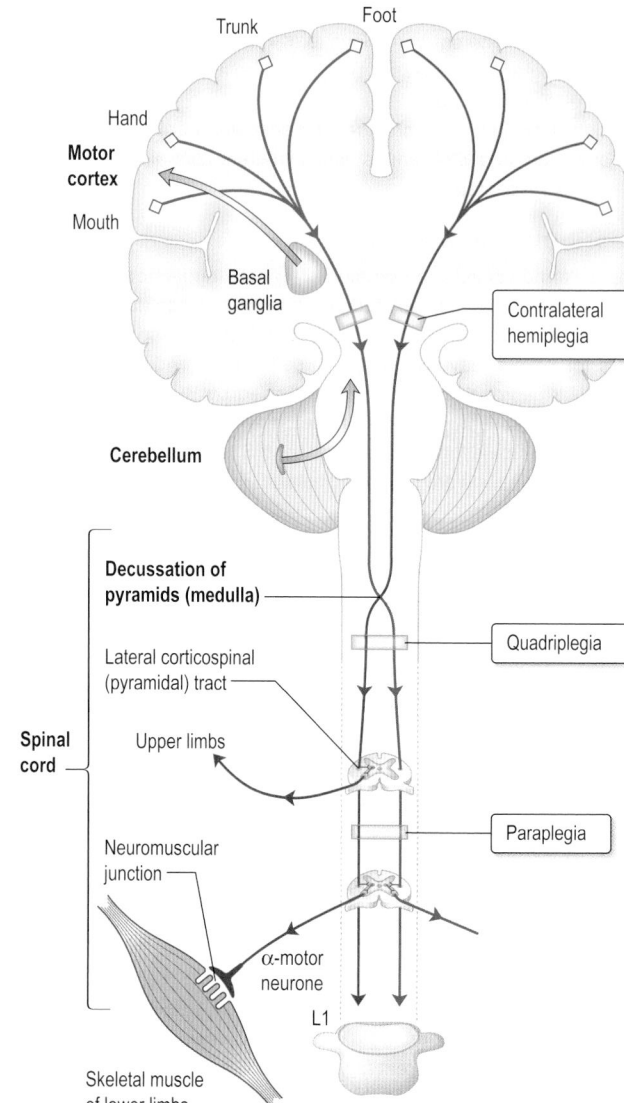

Fig. 26.10 The motor (corticospinal, pyramidal) system.

> **ℹ Box 26.17 Features of upper motor neurone lesions**
>
> - Drift of upper limb
> - Weakness with characteristic distribution
> - Changes in tone: flaccid–spastic
> - Exaggerated tendon reflexes
> - Extensor plantar response
>
> - Loss of skilled finger/toe movements
> - Loss of abdominal reflexes
> - No muscle wasting
> - Normal electrical excitability of muscle

---

drifts downwards and pronates. This sign, with slowing of fast finger movements, is an early one, sometimes occurring before weakness and/or reflex changes become apparent.

Weakness and loss of skilled movement

A unilateral pyramidal lesion above the decussation in the medulla causes weakness of the opposite limbs. When acute and complete, this weakness will be immediate and total: a hemiplegia – for example, following an internal capsule infarct. With slowly progressive lesions (e.g. a hemisphere glioma), a characteristic pattern of weakness emerges: a hemiparesis.

In the upper limb, flexors are stronger than extensors, whereas in the lower limb, extensors are stronger than flexors. In the upper arm, weaker movements are thus shoulder abduction and elbow extension; in the forearm and hand, wrist and finger extensors and abductors are weaker than their antagonists. In the lower limb, weaker movements are hip flexion, knee flexion, ankle dorsiflexion and eversion. There is also loss of skilled movement; fine finger and toe control diminishes. Wasting (except from disuse) is not a feature. When a UMN lesion is below the decussation of the pyramids – in the cervical cord, for example – hemiparesis is on the same side as the lesion; this is an unusual situation.

Changes in tone and tendon reflexes

An acute lesion of one pyramidal tract (e.g. internal capsule stroke) causes initially flaccid paralysis with loss of tendon reflexes. Increase in tone follows, usually within several days, due to loss of inhibitory effects of the corticospinal pathways and an increase in spinal reflex activity. This increase in tone (spasticity) is most easily detectable in stronger muscles. Spasticity is characterized by sudden **changing resistance** to rapid passive movement – the clasp-knife effect. Relevant tendon reflexes become exaggerated; clonus may emerge.

Changes in superficial reflexes

The normal flexor plantar response becomes extensor. In a severe acute lesion, this extensor response can be elicited from a wide area of the foot. As recovery progresses, the receptive area diminishes until the lateral posterior third of the sole remains receptive to an orange-stick stimulus (the appropriate instrument). An extensor plantar response is certain when great toe dorsiflexion is accompanied by abduction of adjacent toes. Abdominal reflexes are abolished on the affected side.

Patterns of UMN disorders

There are three main patterns:
- **Hemiparesis** means weakness of the limbs on one side; it is usually caused by a lesion in the brain and occasionally in the cord.
- **Paraparesis** means weakness of both lower limbs and is usually diagnostic of a cord lesion; bilateral medial brain lesions (e.g. parasagittal meningioma) occasionally cause paraparesis.
- **Tetraparesis** (also called **quadriparesis**) means weakness of four limbs.

Hemiplegia, paraplegia and tetraplegia (strictly) indicate *total* paralysis but are often used to describe severe weakness.

Hemiparesis

The level within the corticospinal system is recognized from particular features.

Motor cortex. Weakness and/or loss of skilled movement confined to one contralateral limb (an arm or a leg – monoparesis) or part of a limb (e.g. a clumsy hand) is typical of an isolated motor cortex lesion (e.g. an infarct or secondary neoplasm). A defect in cognitive function (e.g. aphasia) and focal epilepsy may occur.

Internal capsule. Corticospinal fibres are tightly packed in the internal capsule (about 1 cm^2); thus a small lesion causes a large deficit. A middle cerebral artery branch infarction (see p. 840) produces a sudden, dense, contralateral hemiplegia.

Pons. A pontine lesion (e.g. an MS plaque) is rarely confined to the corticospinal tract. Adjacent structures, e.g. VIth and VIIth

nuclei, MLF and PPRF (see p. 812) are involved. Diplopia, facial weakness, internuclear ophthalmoplegia (INO) and/or a lateral gaze palsy occur with contralateral hemiparesis.

Spinal cord. An isolated lesion of one lateral corticospinal tract (e.g. a cervical cord injury) causes an ipsilateral UMN lesion, the level being indicated by changes in reflexes (e.g. absent biceps, C5/6), features of a Brown–Séquard syndrome (see p. 865) and muscle wasting at the level of the lesion (p. 824).

Spastic paraparesis

Paraparesis indicates bilateral damage to corticospinal pathways, causing weakness and spasticity (or flaccid weakness in the initial phase of spinal shock after an acute cord insult). Cord compression (see p. 878) or cord diseases are the usual causes; cerebral lesions occasionally produce paraparesis. Paraparesis is a feature of many neurological conditions; finding the cause is crucial (see p. 879).

Extrapyramidal system

The extrapyramidal system is a general term for basal ganglia motor systems: that is, corpus striatum (caudate nucleus + globus pallidus + putamen), subthalamic nucleus, substantia nigra and parts of the thalamus. In basal ganglia/extrapyramidal disorders, two features (either or both) become apparent, in limbs and axial muscles:
- reduction in speed of movement (**bradykinesia**) or akinesia (no movement), with muscle rigidity
- involuntary **hyperkinetic** movements (tremor, chorea, dystonia, tics, myoclonus).

Extrapyramidal disorders are classified broadly into **akinetic–rigid syndromes** (see p. 861) where poverty of movement predominates, and **hyperkinetic** movement disorders where there are abnormal involuntary movements (see p. 862).

The most common extrapyramidal disorder is Parkinson's disease.

Essential anatomy

The corpus striatum lies close to the substantia nigra, thalami and subthalamic nuclei, lateral to the internal capsule (**Fig. 26.11**; see **Fig. 26.10**).

Function and dysfunction

Overall function of this system is modulation of cortical motor activity by a series of loops between cortex and basal ganglia (see **Fig. 26.11**). In involuntary movement disorders, there are specific changes in neurotransmitters (**Box 26.18**) rather than focal lesions seen on imaging or at postmortem.

Proposed model of principal pathways

1. Direct pathway from striatum to medial globus pallidus (GP*m*) and substantia nigra pars reticulata (SN*r*). Inhibitory **synapse F**, GABA and substance P.
2. Indirect pathway from striatum to globus pallidus, via lateral globus pallidus (GP*l*; inhibitory **synapse C**, GABA, enkephalin) and subthalamic nucleus (inhibitory **synapse D**, GABA). Terminates in GP*m*–SN*r* (in excitatory **synapse E**, glutamate).
3. Direct pathways, both inhibitory and excitatory, from substantia nigra pars compacta (SN*c*) to striatum. **Synapse A**, dopamine, D$_1$, excitatory; and **synapse B**, D$_2$, inhibitory.
4. GP*m* and SN*r* to thalamus. Inhibitory **synapse G**, GABA.
5. Thalamus to cortex. Excitatory, **synapse H.**
6. Cortex to striatum. Excitatory, glutamate.

The model helps explain how basal ganglia disease can either reduce excitatory thalamo-cortical activity at synapse H – that is, movement – causing bradykinesia, or increase it, causing hyperkinetic disorders.

Parkinson's disease (PD). This is characterized by slowness, stiffness and rest tremor (see p. 859). Degeneration in SNc causes loss of dopamine activity in the striatum. Dopamine is excitatory for synapse A and inhibitory for synapse B. Through the direct pathway there is reduced activity at synapse F, leading to increased inhibitory output (G) and decreased cortical activity (H).

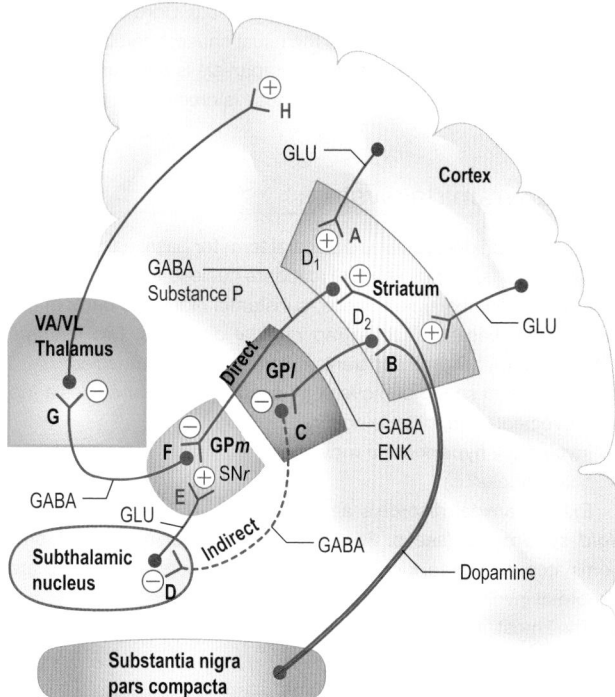

Fig. 26.11 Extrapyramidal system: connections and neurotransmitters. The *inhibitory pathways* are in blue (B, C, D, F, G) and the *excitatory pathways* are in red (A, E, H). ENK, enkephalin; GABA, γ-aminobutyric acid; GLU, glutamate; GP*l*, lateral globus pallidus; GP*m*, medial globus pallidus; SN*r*, substantia nigra pars reticulate; VA/VL, ventral anterior and ventrolateral thalamic nuclei.

---

i Box 26.18 Changes in neurotransmitters in Parkinson's and Huntington's diseases

Site	Neurotransmitter
Parkinson's	
Putamen	Dopamine ↓ 90% Noradrenaline (norepinephrine) ↓ 60% 5-HT ↓ 60%
Substantia nigra	Dopamine ↓ 90% GAD + GABA ↓↓
Cerebral cortex	GAD + GABA ↓↓
Huntington's	
Corpus striatum	Acetylcholine ↓↓ GABA ↓↓ Dopamine: normal GAD + GABA ↓↓

5-HT, 5-hydroxytryptamine; GABA, γ-aminobutyric acid; GAD, glutamic acid decarboxylase, the enzyme responsible for synthesizing GABA.

Also in PD, in the indirect pathway, dopamine deficiency results in disinhibition of neurones synapsing at C. This leads to reduced activity at D, and to increased activity of neurones in the subthalamic nucleus. There is excess stimulation at synapse E, enhancing further inhibitory output of GP*m*–SN*r*.

The net effect via both pathways is to inhibit the ventral anterior (VA) and ventrolateral (VL) nuclei of the thalamus at synapse G. Cortical (motor) activity at H is thus reduced.

Levodopa helps slowness and tremor in PD (see p. 860) but induces unwanted dyskinesias by increasing dopamine activity at synapses A and B; it is thought to do this by reversing sequences in both direct and indirect pathways.

Hemiballismus (see p. 862). Wild, flinging (ballistic) limb movements are caused by a lesion in the subthalamic nucleus, typically an infarct. This reduces excitatory activity at synapse E, reduces inhibition at G, with increased thalamo-cortical neuronal activity, and increases activity at H.

Cerebellum

The third system of motor control modulates coordination and learned movement patterns, rather than speed. Ataxia, i.e. unsteadiness, is characteristic.

The cerebellum receives afferents from:
- proprioceptive receptors (joints and muscles)
- vestibular nuclei
- basal ganglia
- the corticospinal system
- olivary nuclei.

Efferents pass from the cerebellum to:
- each red nucleus
- vestibular nuclei
- basal ganglia
- the corticospinal system.

Each lateral cerebellar lobe coordinates movement of the ipsilateral limbs. The vermis (a midline structure) is concerned with maintenance of axial (midline) posture and balance.

Cerebellar lesions

Box 26.19 summarizes the main causes of cerebellar disease. Expanding lesions obstruct the aqueduct to cause hydrocephalus, with severe pressure headaches, vomiting and papilloedema. Coning of the cerebellar tonsils (see p. 875) through the foramen magnum leads to respiratory arrest, sometimes within minutes/hours. Rarely, tonic seizures (attacks of limb stiffness) occur.

Lateral cerebellar hemisphere lesions

A lesion within one cerebellar lobe (e.g. tumour or infarction) causes disruption of the normal sequence of movements (dyssynergia) on the same side.

Posture and gait. The outstretched arm is held still in the early stages of a cerebellar lobar lesion (cf. the drift of pyramidal lesions) but there is rebound upward overshoot when the limb is pressed downwards and released. Gait becomes broad and ataxic, faltering towards the side of the lesion.

Tremor and ataxia. Movement is imprecise in direction, force and distance (dysmetria). Rapid alternating movements (tapping, clapping or rotary hand movements) become disorganized (dysdiadochokinesia). Intention tremor (action tremor with past-pointing) is seen, but speed of fine movement is preserved (cf. extrapyramidal and pyramidal lesions).

Nystagmus. Coarse horizontal nystagmus (see p. 812) develops with a lateral cerebellar lobe lesion. The fast component is always towards the side of the lesion.

Dysarthria. Halting, jerking speech (scanning speech) develops.

Other signs. Titubation – rhythmic head tremor as either forward and back (yes–yes) movements or rotary (no–no) movements – can occur, mainly when cerebellar connections are involved (e.g. in essential tremor and MS; see p. 862). Hypotonia (floppy limbs) and depression of reflexes (with slow, pendular reflexes) are also sometimes seen.

Midline cerebellar lesions

Cerebellar vermis lesions have dramatic effects on trunk and axial muscles. There is difficulty standing and sitting unsupported (truncal ataxia), with a broad-based, ataxic gait. Lesions of the flocculonodular region cause vertigo and vomiting with gait ataxia if they extend to the roof of the IVth ventricle.

Tremor

Tremor means a regular and sinusoidal oscillation of the limbs, head or trunk.

Postural tremor

Everyone has a physiological tremor (often barely perceptible) of the outstretched hands at 8–12 Hz. This is increased with anxiety, caffeine, hyperthyroidism and drugs (e.g. sympathomimetics, sodium valproate, lamotrigine, lithium) and occurs in mercury poisoning. A higher-amplitude, postural tremor is seen in benign essential tremor (usually quite fast at 5–12 Hz).

Intention tremor

Tremor exacerbated by action, with past-pointing and accompanying incoordination of rapid alternating movement (dysdiadochokinesia), occurs in cerebellar lobe disease and with lesions of cerebellar connections. Titubation (head tremor) and nystagmus may be present.

Rest tremor

Seen typically in Parkinson's disease, this tremor is noticeably worse at rest, usually 4–7 Hz (often pill-rolling, between thumb and forefinger). Unlike essential tremor, parkinsonian tremor is generally unilateral for the first few years.

Other tremors

Dystonic tremor occurs after the age of 50 and is a manifestation of dystonia that is often seen without dystonic posturing. It is generally unilateral (or asymmetric), affecting hand/arm or head, and worse with posture and certain tasks such as drinking, pouring liquids, or using cutlery or a pen. It is often mistaken for parkinsonian tremor. Holmes tremor (present at rest, action and posture) is seen following lesions of the red nucleus (e.g. infarction, multiple sclerosis).

LOWER MOTOR NEURONE LESIONS

The lower motor neurone (LMN) is the pathway from anterior horn cell (or cranial nerve nucleus) via a peripheral nerve to muscle motor end-plates. The motor unit consists of one anterior horn cell, its single fast-conducting axon that leaves the cord via the anterior root, and the group of muscle fibres (100–2000) supplied via the nerve. Anterior horn cell activity is modulated by impulses from:
- corticospinal tracts
- the extrapyramidal system
- the cerebellum
- afferents via posterior roots.

Clinical features of lower motor neurone lesions

These are seen in voluntary muscles that depend on an intact nerve supply for both contraction and metabolic integrity. Signs follow rapidly if the LMN is interrupted (**Box 26.20**).

Aetiology

Examples of LMN lesions at various levels include:
- cranial nerve nuclei (Bell's palsy) and anterior horn cell (motor neurone disease)
- spinal root – *radiculopathy*, e.g. cervical and lumbar disc protrusion (see p. 892)
- peripheral (or cranial) nerve – trauma, entrapment (see p. 888) and polyneuropathy (p. 889).

Spinal reflex arc

Components are illustrated in **Fig. 26.12**. The stretch reflex is the physiological basis for all tendon reflexes. In the knee jerk, a tap on the patellar tendon activates stretch receptors in the quadriceps. Impulses in first-order sensory neurones pass directly to LMNs (L3 and L4) that contract quadriceps. Loss of a tendon reflex is caused by a lesion anywhere along the spinal reflex path. The reflex lost indicates its level (**Box 26.21**).

Reinforcement. Distraction of the patient's attention, clenching teeth or pulling interlocked fingers enhances reflex activity

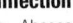 **Box 26.19 Principal causes of cerebellar syndromes**

Tumours
- Haemangioblastoma
- Medulloblastoma
- Secondary neoplasm
- Compression by acoustic neuroma

Vascular
- Haemorrhage
- Infarction
- Arteriovenous malformation

Infection
- Abscess
- HIV
- Prion diseases
- Encephalitis

Developmental
- Arnold–Chiari malformation
- Cerebral palsy

Toxic and metabolic
- Antiepileptic drugs
- Chronic alcohol use
- Carbon monoxide poisoning
- Lead poisoning
- Solvent misuse

Inherited
- Friedreich's and other spinocerebellar ataxias
- Ataxia telangiectasia

Miscellaneous
- Multiple sclerosis (common in MS)
- Hydrocephalus
- Hypothyroidism
- Paraneoplastic syndromes (rapidly progressive)
- Multiple system atrophy
- Superficial siderosis

Box 26.20 Features of lower motor neurone lesions

- Weakness
- Wasting
- Hypotonia
- Reflex loss
- Fasciculation
- Fibrillation potentials (electromyography)
- Muscle contractures
- Trophic changes in skin and nails

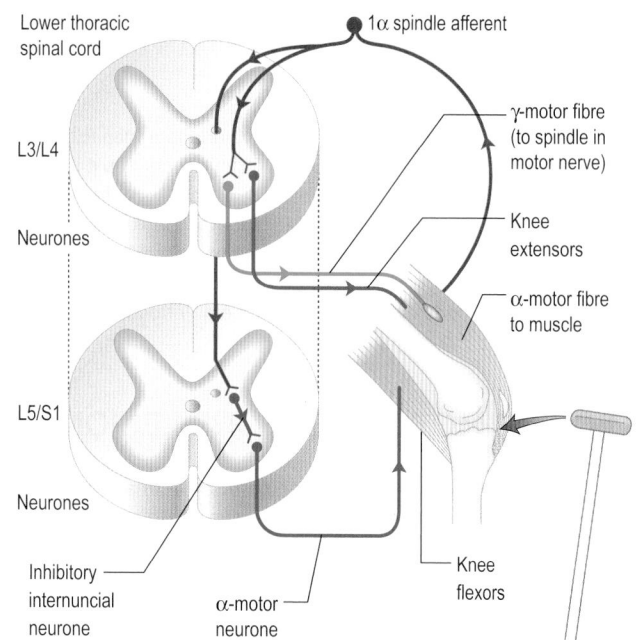

Fig. 26.12 Knee jerk: a spinal reflex arc. Sudden patellar tendon stretching generates sensory action potentials in 1α-muscle spindle afferents that synapse with γ-motor fibres to spindles and α-motor fibres. Motor action potentials cause brisk extensor muscle contraction; there is also inhibition of knee flexors.

i | **Box 26.21 Spinal levels: recording/interpretation of tendon reflexes**

Level	Reflex	Symbol	Meaning
C5–6	Supinator	0	Absent
C5–6	Biceps	±	Present with reinforcement
C7	Triceps	+	Normal
L3–4	Knee	++	Brisk, normal
S1	Ankle	+++	Exaggerated (abnormal)
		CL	Clonus

(Jendrassik manoeuvre). Such reinforcement manoeuvres should be done before a reflex is recorded as absent.

SENSORY PATHWAYS AND PAIN

Peripheral nerves and spinal roots

Peripheral nerves carry all modalities of sensation from either free or specialized nerve endings to dorsal roots and thence to the cord. Sensory distribution of spinal roots (dermatomes) is shown in **Fig. 26.13**.

Spinal cord

Posterior columns

Axons in the posterior columns whose cell bodies are in the ipsilateral gracile and cuneate nuclei in the medulla carry sensory modalities of vibration, joint position (proprioception), light touch and two-point discrimination. Axons from second-order neurones then cross in the brainstem to form the medial lemniscus, passing to the thalamus (**Fig. 26.14**).

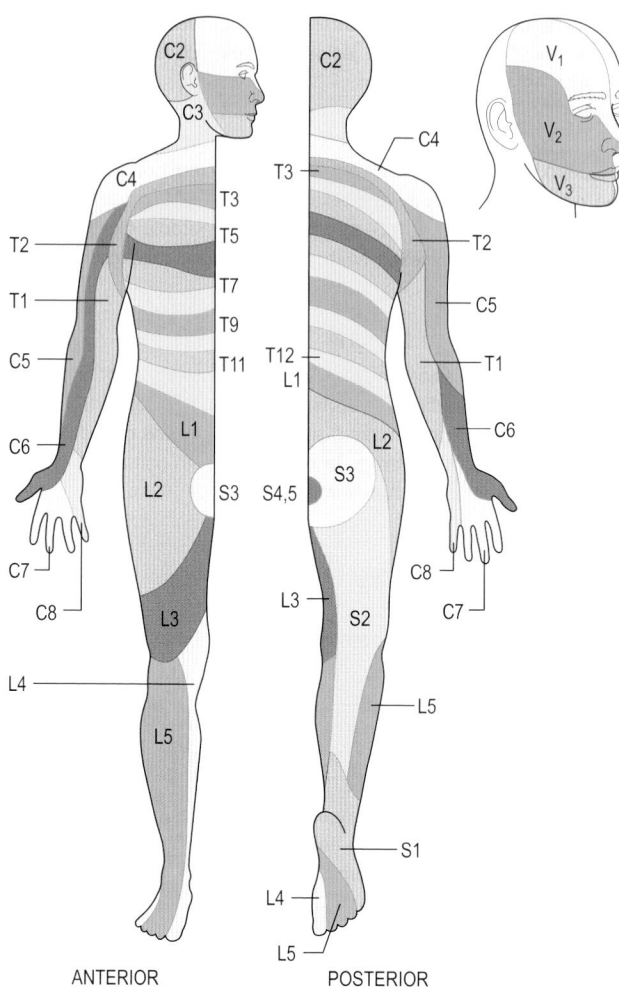

Fig. 26.13 Dermatomes of spinal roots and Vth nerve.

Spinothalamic tracts

Axons carrying pain and temperature sensation synapse in the dorsal horn of the cord, cross within the cord, and pass in the spinothalamic tracts to the thalamus and reticular formation.

Sensory cortex

Fibres from the thalamus pass to the parietal region sensory cortex (see **Fig. 26.14**). Connections exist between the thalamus, sensory cortex and motor cortex.

Lesions of the sensory pathways

Altered sensation, tingling (paraesthesia), clumsiness, numbness and pain are the principal symptoms of sensory lesions. The pattern and distribution point to the site of pathology (**Fig. 26.15**).

Peripheral nerve lesions

Symptoms are felt within the distribution of a peripheral nerve. Section of a sensory nerve is followed by complete sensory loss. Nerve entrapment (see p. 888) causes numbness, pain and tingling. Tapping the site of compression sometimes causes a sharp, electric shock-like pain in the distribution of the nerve, known as Tinel's sign, such as in carpal tunnel syndrome (see p. 888).

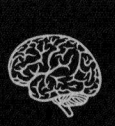

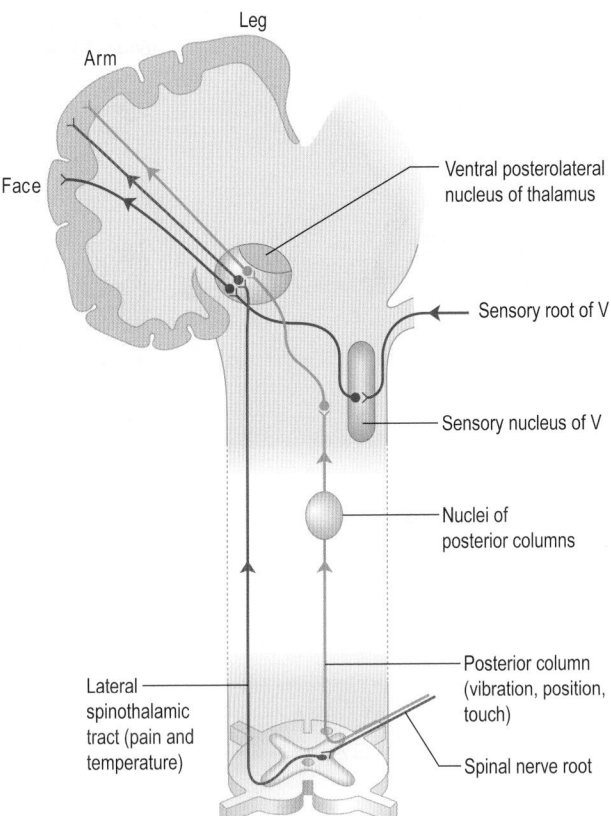

Fig. 26.14 Principal sensory pathways. Posterior columns remain uncrossed until the medulla. Spinothalamic tracts cross close to their entry into the cord.

Neuralgia

Neuralgia refers to pain, usually of great severity, in the distribution of a damaged nerve. Examples are:
- trigeminal neuralgia (see p. 852)
- postherpetic neuralgia (see p. 872)
- complex regional pain syndrome type II (causalgia) – chronic burning pain that occasionally follows peripheral nerve damage.

Spinal root lesions
Root pain

Pain of root compression is felt in the myotome supplied by the root, and there is also a tingling discomfort in the dermatome. The pain is worsened by manoeuvres that either stretch the root (e.g. straight-leg raising in lumbar disc prolapse) or increase pressure in the spinal subarachnoid space (coughing and straining). Cervical and lumbar disc protrusions (see p. 892) are common causes of root lesions.

Dorsal spinal root lesions

Section of a dorsal root causes loss of all modalities of sensation within a dermatome (see **Fig. 26.13**). However, overlap between adjacent dermatomes makes it difficult to detect anaesthesia when a single root is destroyed.

Spinal cord lesions
Posterior column lesions

These cause:
- tingling
- electric shock-like sensations
- clumsiness

- numbness
- tight band-like sensations.

These symptoms, though lateralized, are often felt vaguely without a clear sensory level. Position sense, vibration sense, light touch and two-point discrimination are diminished below the lesion. Position sense loss produces a stamping gait (sensory ataxia; see p. 804).

Lhermitte's phenomenon

Electric shock-like sensations radiate down the trunk and limbs on neck flexion. This points to a cervical cord lesion. Lhermitte's is common in acute exacerbations of MS (see p. 865), and also occurs in cervical myelopathy (p. 892), subacute combined degeneration of the cord (p. 891), radiation myelopathy (p. 893) and cord compression.

Spinothalamic tract lesions

Pure spinothalamic spinal lesions cause contralateral loss of pain and temperature sensation with a clear level below the lesion. This is called **_dissociated_** sensory loss – pain and temperature are dissociated from light touch, which remains preserved. This is seen typically in syringomyelia where a cavity occupies the central cord (see p. 879).

The spinal level is modified by lamination of fibres within the spinothalamic tracts. Fibres from lower spinal roots lie superficially and are damaged first by compressive lesions from outside the cord. As an external compressive lesion (e.g. a mid-thoracic extradural meningioma; **Fig. 26.16**) enlarges, the spinal sensory level ascends as deeper fibres become involved. Conversely, a central cord lesion (e.g. a syrinx; see p. 879) affects deeper fibres first. Spinothalamic tract lesions cause loss of pain and temperature perception (e.g. painless burns). Perforating ulcers and neuropathic (Charcot) joints develop.

Spinal cord compression

Cord compression (see **Fig. 26.16**) causes progressive spastic paraparesis (or tetraparesis/quadriparesis) with sensory loss below the level of compression. Sphincter disturbance is common. Root pain is frequent but not invariable, felt characteristically at the level of compression. With thoracic cord compression (e.g. an extradural meningioma), pain radiates around the chest and is exacerbated by coughing and straining, as meningeal root sheaths are stretched.

Damage to one spinothalamic tract (contralateral loss of pain and temperature) with the ipsilateral corticospinal tract is known as the **_Brown–Séquard syndrome_** (originally, cord hemisection). The patient complains of numbness on one side and weakness on the other. Paraparesis/spinal cord lesions are discussed on page 865.

Pontine lesions

Since lesions (e.g. an MS plaque) lie above the decussation of the posterior columns, and both medial lemniscus and spinothalamic tracts are close together, there is loss of all forms of sensation on the side opposite the lesion. Combinations of IIIrd, IVth, Vth, VIth and VIIth cranial nerve nuclei are seen, and may indicate a level (see **Fig. 26.14**).

Thalamic lesions

Thalamic pain (also called **_central post-stroke pain_** or **_thalamic syndrome_**) follows a small thalamic infarct. The patient has a stroke (hemiparesis and sensory loss). Weakness improves but deep-seated constant pain in the paretic limbs develops. Choreoathetotic movements occur. Secondary depression may lead to

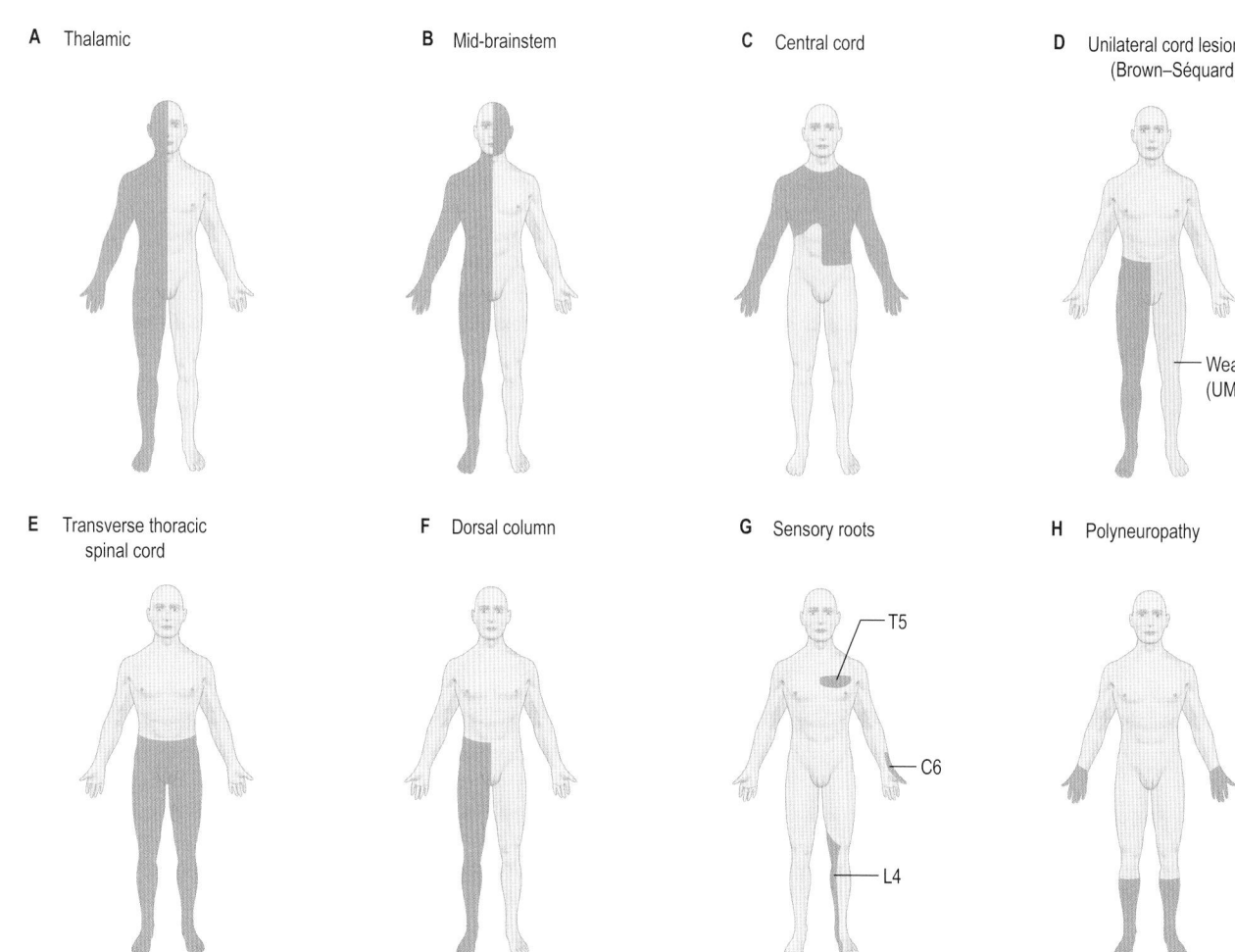

Fig. 26.15 Principal patterns of loss of sensation. (A) *Thalamic lesion:* sensory loss throughout opposite side (rare). **(B) *Brainstem lesion:*** contralateral sensory loss below face and ipsilateral loss on face. **(C) *Central cord lesion,*** e.g. syrinx: 'suspended' areas of loss, often asymmetrical and 'dissociated': i.e. pain and temperature lost but light touch intact. **(D) *Hemisection of cord/unilateral cord lesion*** – Brown–Séquard syndrome: contralateral spinothalamic (pain and temperature) loss with ipsilateral weakness and dorsal column loss below lesion. **(E) *Transverse cord lesion:*** loss of all modalities, including motor, below lesion. **(F) *Dorsal column lesion,*** e.g. multiple sclerosis: loss of proprioception, vibration and light touch. **(G) *Individual sensory root lesions,*** e.g. C6, T5, L4. **(H) *Polyneuropathy:*** distal sensory loss. UMN, upper motor neurone.

self-harm. Thalamic lesions can also cause diminished sensation alone, on the opposite side; this is less usual.

Parietal cortex lesions

Sensory loss, neglect of one side, apraxia (see p. 804) and subtle disorders of sensation occur. Pain is not a feature of destructive cortical lesions. Irritative phenomena (e.g. focal sensory seizures from a parietal cortex glioma) cause tingling sensations in a limb or elsewhere.

Pain

Pain is an unpleasant, complex sensory and emotional experience. Acute pain serves a biological purpose (e.g. withdrawal) and is typically self-limiting, ceasing as healing ensues. Some forms of chronic pain (e.g. causalgia) outlast the period required for healing and may be permanent.

Essential physiology of pain

Pain perception is mediated by small-diameter myelinated A-delta and non-myelinated C fibres. Chemicals released following injury produce pain either by direct stimulation or by sensitization of nerve endings. A-delta fibres give rise to perception of sharp, immediate pain; slower-onset, more diffuse and prolonged pain is mediated by slower-conducting C fibres.

Nociceptive (pain) impulses enter the cord via dorsal spinal roots forming synapses in the spinal cord dorsal horn (substance P and glutamate neurotransmitters). Second-order neurones then decussate to the contralateral side and ascend in the spinal cord via two main pathways: the spinothalamic tract (for pain localization) and the spinoreticular tract (mediation of the emotional component of pain; **Fig. 26.17**). Both pathways project via synapses in the thalamus to the sensory cortex and limbic system. There are projections to brainstem structures: the reticular formation (spinoreticular tract) and periaqueductal grey matter (spinothalamic tract), which modulates pain transmission via descending

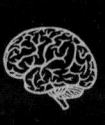

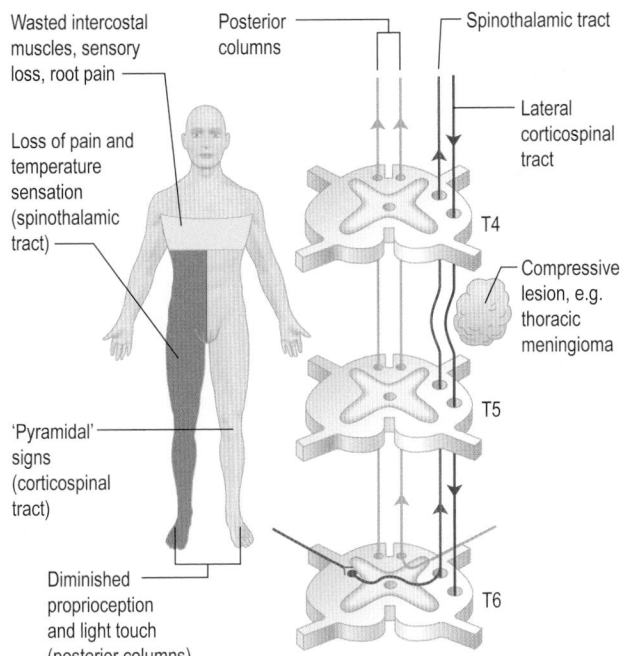

Fig. 26.16 **Spinal cord compression: features and anatomy.**

Labels on figure:
- Wasted intercostal muscles, sensory loss, root pain
- Posterior columns
- Spinothalamic tract
- Lateral corticospinal tract
- Loss of pain and temperature sensation (spinothalamic tract)
- T4
- Compressive lesion, e.g. thoracic meningioma
- T5
- 'Pyramidal' signs (corticospinal tract)
- Diminished proprioception and light touch (posterior columns)
- T6

monoaminergic pathways to the spinal cord dorsal horn. The emotional and affective components of pain, mediated through cortical and limbic networks, are now recognized to be fundamental to pain perception.

Gate theory of pain

Gate theory proposes that transmission of afferent nociceptive (pain) impulses is regulated ('gated') in the spinal cord dorsal horn synapses by afferent impulses from non-nociceptive, large-diameter sensory fibres and descending pathways from the peri-aqueductal grey (PAG) and other brainstem structures. It explains the phenomenon of rubbing a painful area to ease the pain and is also the basis of transcutaneous electrical nerve stimulation (TENS) therapy. Similar gating and modulation of afferent pain signals occur in the brainstem under the influence of connections from the thalamus and limbic system.

Peripheral and central sensitization

Sensitization is an increase in the excitability of peripheral nociceptors and central pain pathways, causing normal sensory inputs such as light touch to produce abnormal responses: that is, pain (termed *allodynia*). For example, warm water in a shower feels painfully burning on sunburnt skin and touching the scalp is painful during a migraine. This is an adaptive protective response to ensure that contact with an injured area is minimized. However, maladaptive responses to pain via this mechanism at the central or peripheral level may be the basis for chronic pain when it becomes permanent and out of proportion to the initial painful stimulus.

Plasticity and receptor changes

Pain results in neural plasticity changes and reorganization in pain pathways at spinal cord and cortical/brainstem level. These modulate pain and may be maladaptive in some cases, leading to maintenance of chronic pain. Molecular changes also occur in response to painful stimuli, including upregulation of sodium channels and receptor changes.

Neuropathic pain

Pain results directly from damage to, or dysfunction of, the pain/sensory pathways, such as in peripheral nerve damage, radiculopathy, post-stroke pain and post-herpetic neuralgia (**Box 26.22**). It is common, affecting 6–8% of people. Clinically, the pain usually has an unpleasant burning, electrical or stabbing quality, with allodynia being a frequent feature. It often becomes chronic due to peripheral and central sensitization processes.

Neurotransmitters and receptors involved in pain

These are involved in pain processing, explaining why a wide range of drug classes are helpful in treating pain.

- ***Excitatory neurotransmitters*** include substance P, glutamate and calcitonin gene-related peptide (CGRP) in the dorsal horn of the spinal cord and peripherally.
- ***Gamma-aminobutyric acid*** (**GABA**) is a key inhibitory neurotransmitter.
- ***Opioid receptors***, activated by endogenous endorphins or opiate medications, are widely distributed in pain pathways, including in the spinal cord, peri-aqueductal grey matter and other brainstem structures.
- ***Noradrenaline*** (***norepinephrine***) and 5-HT (serotonin) are distributed in descending regulatory pathways.
- ***The vanilloid receptor*** (TRPV1 – transient receptor potential cation channel VI) on peripheral nociceptors is activated by capsaicin, the active constituent of chilli peppers.

Management of chronic pain

Chronic pain is gravely disabling, distressing and difficult to treat (see p. 429). Multidisciplinary pain clinics provide the best setting for long-term management.

Management plans for intractable pain have a number of components.

Diagnostic

Rigorous attention must be paid to the diagnosis, reviewing the entire history and investigations. A specific surgical approach may become apparent (e.g. nerve root or peripheral nerve compression or trigeminal neuralgia).

Psychological

Chronic pain influences quality of life. Depression (see p. 776) is commonly associated with pain; antidepressants can help. Psychology-based pain management programmes and cognitive behavioural therapy are now a cornerstone of chronic pain management, helping people to control symptoms and the response to pain.

Analgesics

These include aspirin, paracetamol, non-steroidal anti-inflammatory drugs (NSAIDs) and opiates. Some opiates, such as tramadol and tapentadol, also have a monoamine reuptake inhibition mechanism of action. The World Health Organization (WHO) analgesic ladder (see p. 140) is useful.

Co-analgesics

Co-analgesics have a primary use other than for pain, and help when used alone or added to analgesics. They may have a synergistic effect when used in combination. Examples are:

- tricyclic antidepressants, e.g. amitriptyline
- duloxetine – a serotonin (5-HT)–noradrenaline (norepinephrine) reuptake blocker (SNRI)
- anticonvulsants, e.g. carbamazepine, gabapentin, pregabalin and lamotrigine (see **Box 7.9**)

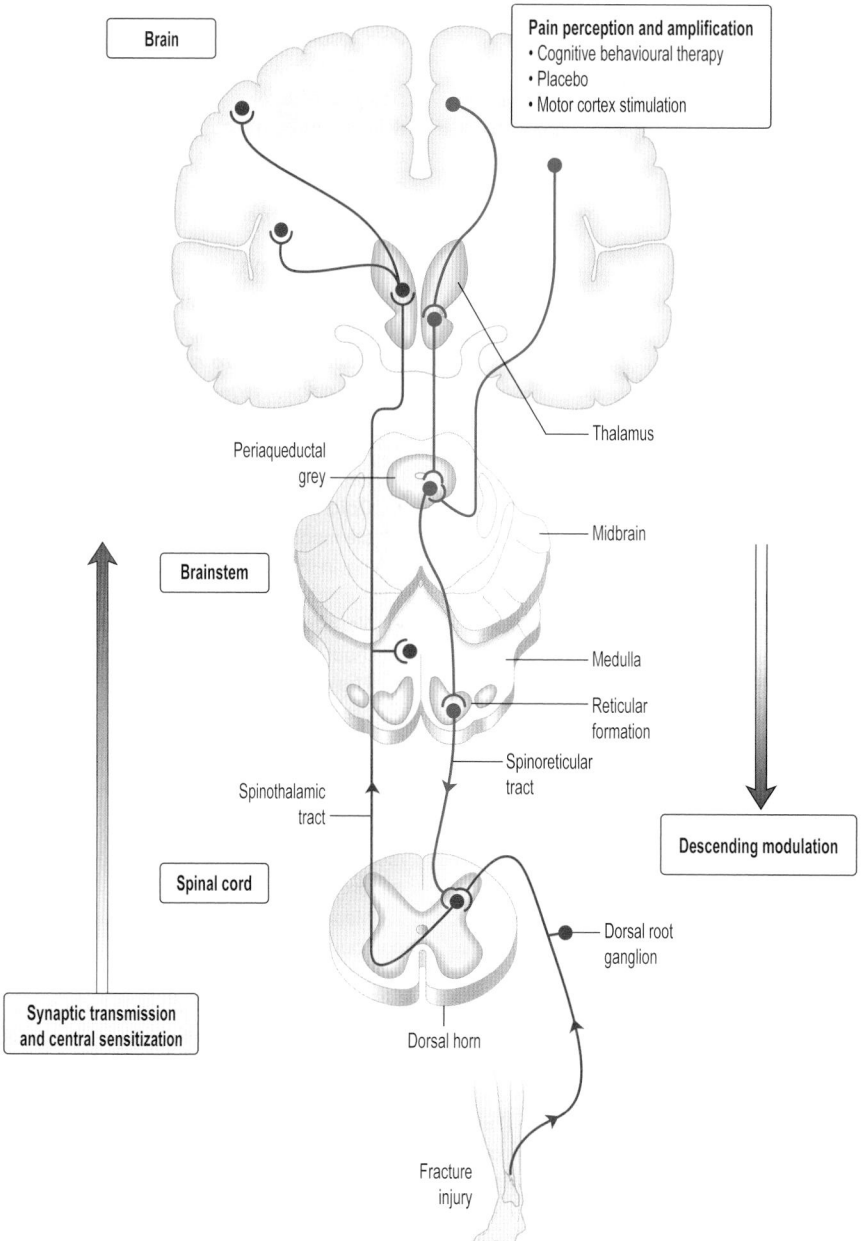

Fig. 26.17 The spinothalamic and spinoreticular tracts in pain perception.

- calcium-channel blockers, e.g. ziconotide used intrathecally
- muscle relaxants, e.g. baclofen
- *capsaicin* topical preparations – extracts from capsicum plants (chilli peppers), which bind to vanilloid receptors (see above)
- *N*-*methyl*-*D*-*aspartate (NMDA)* antagonists, e.g. ketamine
- *cannabinoids* – administered via oral spray in MS and resistant cancer pain
- *botulinum* toxin – licensed for chronic migraine; increasing evidence supports a role in modulating pain neurotransmitters.

Stimulation

Acupuncture, ice, heat, ultrasound, massage, TENS and spinal cord stimulation all achieve analgesia by gating effects on large myelinated nerve fibres.

Nerve blocks

Pain pathways can be blocked, either temporarily by local anaesthetic (by injection or with topical patches) or permanently with phenol or with radiofrequency lesions:

- somatic blocks:
  - peripheral nerve and plexus injections
  - epidural and spinal analgesia
- sympathetic blocks:
  - sympathetic ganglia injections
  - central epidural and spinal sympathetic blockade.

Neurosurgery

Highly specialized techniques have a place alongside drugs. Examples are dorsal rhizotomy, sympathectomy, cordotomy and neurostimulation.

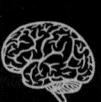

Box 26.22 Causes of neuropathic pain

Peripheral nerve injury

- Peripheral neuropathy – especially if small (pain) fibres are affected, e.g. diabetes, AL amyloid, HIV, chemotherapy (e.g. carboplatin neuropathy), vitamin deficiency, alcohol, Fabry's
- Vasculitic nerve lesions – e.g. diabetic femoral neuropathy (neuralgic amyotrophy)
- Nerve compression – carpal tunnel syndrome, meralgia paraesthetica
- Postherpetic neuralgia
- Nerve trauma or section – e.g. phantom limb pain
- Trigeminal neuralgia

Nerve root and plexus

- Radiculopathy due to intervertebral disc prolapse
- Plexopathy – e.g. inflammatory (brachial neuritis) or neoplastic infiltrative (e.g. breast cancer)

Central nervous system disorders

- Multiple sclerosis (pain is common in progressive forms)
- Post-stroke pain – e.g. thalamic strokes
- Spinal cord lesions – intrinsic cord lesions, inflammatory or vascular (infarcts) especially
- Parkinson's disease

Further reading

Caulley L, Caplan B, Ross E. Medical marijuana for chronic pain. *N Engl J Med* 2018; 379:1575–1577.
Cohen SP, Mao J. Neuropathic pain: mechanisms and their clinical implications. *BMJ* 2014; 348:f7656.
Magrinelli R, Zanette G, Tamburin S. Neuropathic pain: diagnosis and treatment. *Pract Neurol* 2013; 13:292–307.
Turk DC, Wilson HD, Cahana A. Treatment of chronic non-cancer pain. *Lancet* 2011; 377:2226–2235.

BLADDER CONTROL AND SEXUAL DYSFUNCTION

Changes in micturition and failure of normal sexual activity due to neurological conditions are seen in sacral, spinal cord and cortical disease.

Essential functions and anatomy

The bladder has two functions: storage and voiding. Afferent pathways (T12–S4) respond to pressure within the bladder and sensation from the genitalia. As the bladder distends, continence is maintained by suppression of parasympathetic outflow and reciprocal activation of sympathetic outflow. Both are under some voluntary control. Voiding takes place by parasympathetic activation of the detrusor, and relaxation of the internal sphincter (**Box 26.23**).

Cortical awareness of bladder fullness is located in the postcentral gyrus, parasagittally, while initiation of micturition is in the pre-central gyrus. Voluntary control of micturition is located in the frontal cortex, parasagittally.

Neurological disorders of micturition

Urogenital tract disease is dealt with largely by urologists. Incontinence is common and easy to recognize; neurological causes are sometimes not obvious. These are:

Cortical:
- Post-central lesions cause loss of the sense of bladder fullness.
- Pre-central lesions cause difficulty in initiating micturition.
- Frontal lesions cause socially inappropriate micturition.

Spinal cord. Bilateral UMN lesions (pyramidal tracts) cause urinary frequency and incontinence. The bladder is small and hypertonic: that is, sensitive to small changes in intravesical pressure. Frontal lesions can also cause a hypertonic bladder.

Box 26.23 Efferents to the bladder and genitalia

Nerve supply	Function
Parasympathetic S2–4	Bladder wall: contraction Internal sphincter: relaxation Penis/clitoris: engorgement
Sympathetic T12–L2	Bladder wall: relaxation Internal sphincter: contraction Orgasm, ejaculation
Pudendal nerves	External sphincter (skeletal muscle)

LMN. Sacral lesions (conus medullaris, sacral root and pelvic nerve – *bilateral*) cause a flaccid, atonic bladder that overflows (cauda equina; see p. 893), often unexpectedly.

Management. Assessment of both urological causes (e.g. calculi, prostatism, gynaecological problems) and potential neurological causes of incontinence is necessary. Intermittent self-catheterization is used by many patients who have, for example, spinal cord lesions.

Male erectile dysfunction

Failure of penile erection often has mixed organic and psychological causes. Depression is common. Erectile dysfunction is described on page 1485.

INVESTIGATION OF NEUROLOGICAL DISEASE

Neurological investigations, such as brain scans, should not be a substitute for clinical evaluation through history-taking and examination. An experienced clinician will be able to make an accurate diagnosis in most patients without recourse to investigations: for example, in most individuals presenting with headache. However, cross-sectional imaging will allow confirmation of the anatomical localization of lesions and may reveal the presence of other clinically 'silent' lesions. Imaging does not always indicate the pathological nature of a visualized lesion (careful history-taking is essential in this regard) and therefore needs to be carefully interpreted in the clinical context. Neurophysiological investigations provide information about nervous system *function* and are more diagnostically helpful than imaging in some situations: for example, in patients with primary generalized epilepsies or peripheral nerve disorders.

Unnecessary or inappropriate use of investigations, particularly brain imaging, exposes patients to risk, such as radiation; is an inefficient use of resources; and may lead to identification of incidental findings that cause considerable anxiety (there is a 3% incidental abnormality rate for brain MRI scans). Clinicians should also be familiar with the range of normal in the population; for example, the high prevalence of white-matter hyperintensities on brain MRI in older people and the range of common non-specific electroencephalogram (EEG) changes.

Neuroimaging

Skull and spinal X-rays

Skull X-rays have now been largely superseded by computed tomography (CT) and MRI. They show fractures, bone metastases, osteomyelitis, Paget's disease, sinus disease and intracranial calcification.

Spinal X-rays show fractures, congenital and destructive lesions (bone cysts, infection, metastases), and degenerative spondylosis.

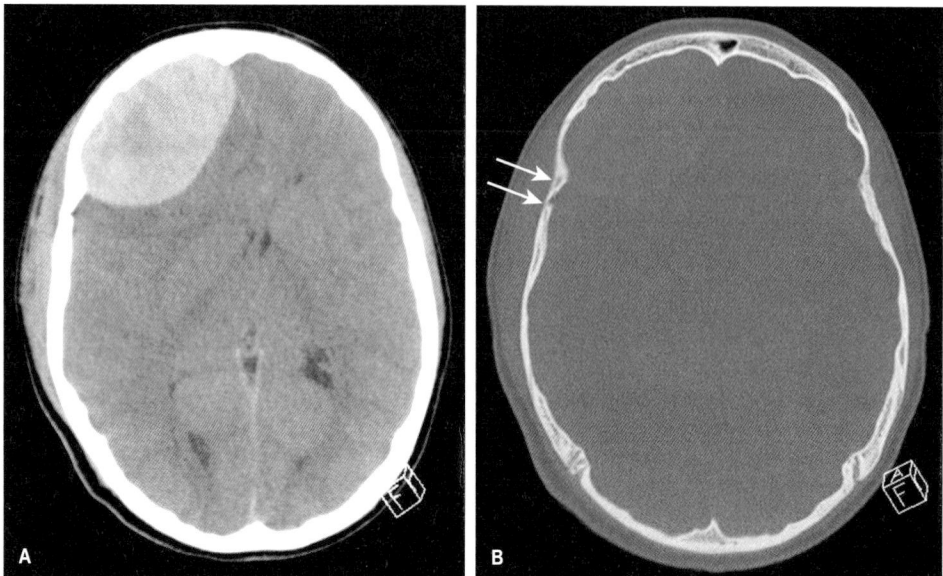

Fig. 26.18 Extradural haematoma. (A) shown by hyperintensity on CT brain window **(B)** Note the subtle linear non-depressed fracture of the right frontal bone (arrows). This extended adjacent to the middle meningeal artery.

Brain computed tomography

In brain CT, an X-ray beam and detectors revolve rapidly as the patient is moved slowly through the scanner, producing a spiral set of 'slices'. The digital data are converted to cross-sectional images.

Differences in attenuation (density, expressed as Hounsfield units) between different tissues allow accurate recognition of, for example, fresh blood, bone or calcification (**Fig. 26.18**). Enhancement with intravenous iodinated contrast delineates areas of vascular leak, such as with tumours and inflammation (**Box 26.24**).

CT angiography

Spiral CT after intravenous injection of contrast produces high-quality arterial angiograms (or venograms), which are now considered the gold standard for non-invasive angiography.

Spinal CT and CT myelography

Spinal CT is useful for assessing the bone architecture of the spine but provides little information about soft tissues, such as nerve roots, and for this purpose spinal cord MRI is required. CT myelography (spinal CT after intrathecal injection of contrast) is used for identification of spinal fluid leaks/blockage or for situations where MRI is contraindicated.

Magnetic resonance imaging

A hydrogen nucleus is a proton whose electrical charge creates a local electrical field. In MRI, protons are aligned by sudden, strong magnetic impulses and then imaged with radiofrequency waves at right angles to their alignment. The protons resonate and spin, then revert to their normal alignment. As they do so, images are made at different phases of relaxation, known as T_1, T_2, T_2 STIR, FLAIR, diffusion-weighted imaging (DWI) and other sequences. The combination of these sequences increases the diagnostic sensitivity and specificity of MRI. Gadolinium is used as intravenous contrast to show areas of increased vascularity.

The superior spatial resolution and soft tissue contrast of MRI, as compared to CT, makes MRI of the brain and spine generally preferable in the non-emergency situation. It can image pathology not easily visualized on CT, such as small lesions, white-matter disease such as MS plaques and spinal cord lesions or compression, and demonstrate anatomy more accurately.

Box 26.24 Comparison of magnetic resonance imaging and computed tomography

Advantages of CT over MRI
- Speed – brain imaging takes seconds, an advantage in restless or critically ill patients; CT is also less sensitive to artefact due to patient motion
- Patient access – critically ill patients can be monitored more easily than in an MRI scanner
- Method of choice to detect acute haemorrhage
- Detailed evaluation of bone, e.g. spinal vertebrae and fractures
- Easier identification of calcification and metal foreign bodies
- Toleration by claustrophobic patients
- Safety with implanted devices, e.g. pacemakers
- Wider availability than MRI
- Imaging modality of choice in trauma and acute stroke for these reasons

Advantages of MRI over CT
- Superior spatial resolution and soft tissue contrast for imaging of brain parenchyma, spinal cord and nerve roots, e.g. white-matter disease such as multiple sclerosis plaques and spinal cord, which are not visible on CT
- No bone artefact, so superior visualization of posterior fossa and spinal cord
- Availability of numerous special sequences, e.g. diffusion-weighted sequence sensitive to early infarction; multiple sequences increase diagnostic utility
- No ionizing radiation
- MR angiography may be performed without contrast

Doppler studies

Ultrasound is a safe, low-cost and rapid method for detecting and quantifying carotid stenosis and assessing carotid plaque burden. It is operator-dependent and less reproducible than other imaging modalities.

Catheter angiography

Contrast is injected intra-arterially in selected vessels via a catheter inserted in the femoral artery. Angiography carries a mortality and stroke risk (<1%). Images of aorta, carotid, vertebral and brain arteries demonstrate occlusion, stenoses, aneurysms and arteriovenous

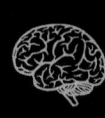

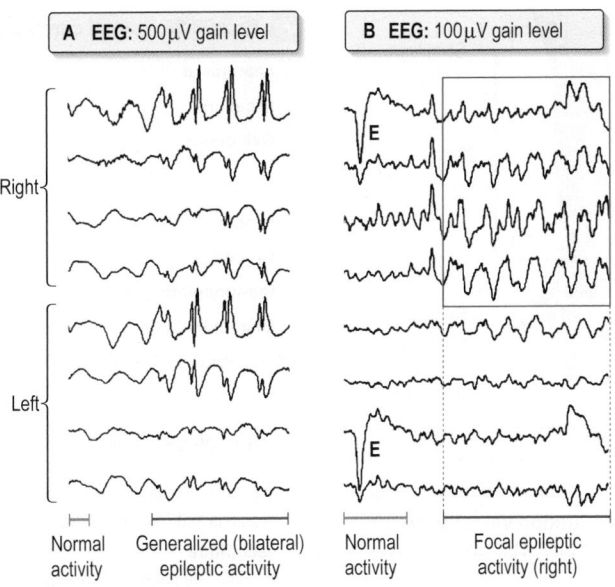

| A EEG: 500 μV gain level | B EEG: 100 μV gain level |

Right

Left

Normal activity | Generalized (bilateral) epileptic activity

E

Normal activity | Focal epileptic activity (right)

E

Fig. 26.19 Examples of EEG traces. **(A)** Normal activity followed by generalized epileptic spikes in all leads. **(B)** Normal activity followed by focal spikes in right leads. E, eye-movement artefact.

malformations (AVMs). Spinal angiography is complex and is used to identify spinal AVMs and dural fistulas. Aneurysms and AVMs may be treated by endovascular means (embolization with glue or platinum coils) during the procedure.

Positron emission tomography, single proton emission computed tomography, dopamine transporter imaging and functional MRI

These functional imaging techniques track uptake of radio-isotopes and/or metabolites. Fluorodeoxyglucose positron emission tomography (FDG-PET) is used principally to detect occult neoplasms or tumour recurrence, outside the central nervous system (CNS), or to identify large-vessel vasculitis. Dopamine transporter imaging (DAT) is used to identify reduced nigrostriatal dopaminergic terminals in parkinsonian disorders, mainly in patients with atypical tremor where the clinical diagnosis is uncertain. Functional MRI (fMRI) is largely a research tool for mapping brain function, in health and disease. New techniques using radionuclide tracers to image brain amyloid deposits in Alzheimer's disease are currently available in the research domain and limited clinical centres.

Isotope bone scanning

The radio-isotope [⁹⁹ᵐTc]-pertechnetate is given intravenously. The technique is used principally in detection of vertebral, skull and bone metastases.

Neurophysiological investigations

Electroencephalography

Brain electrical activity (**Fig. 26.19**) is recorded from scalp electrodes (20 channels simultaneously). Its main use is to characterize epilepsy syndromes. Recordings are usually made between seizures (inter-ictal). Sleep-deprived EEG and 24-hour ambulatory EEG increase diagnostic sensitivity. Videotelemetry (VT) combines continuous EEG with video over several days to record the semiology and electrical characteristics of seizures. VT is invaluable diagnostically to identify seizure type where there is clinical uncertainty, and to pinpoint the seizure focus in focal epilepsies.

Epilepsy

Spikes, or spike-and-wave abnormalities, are hallmarks of epilepsy, but it is important to emphasize that patients with epilepsy often have a normal EEG between seizures (see p. 855).

Diffuse brain disorders

Slow-wave EEG abnormalities appear in encephalopathy (e.g. hepatic coma), encephalitis and prion (Creutzfeldt–Jakob) diseases.

Brain death

The EEG is isoelectric (flat); EEG is not necessary to confirm brain death in many countries (see p. 833).

Electromyography and nerve conduction studies

Electromyography (EMG) and nerve conduction studies (NCS) are skilled investigations of nerve function that are essential for investigation of peripheral nerve, anterior horn cell, neuromuscular junction (NMJ) and, to a lesser extent, muscle disorders. NCS are highly sensitive in identification of peripheral neuropathy, and assessment of the nerves affected and the type of pathology (axonal loss versus demyelinating). In mononeuropathies, the anatomical site of the lesion may be identified with considerable accuracy and prognostic information obtained.

Electromyography

A concentric needle electrode is inserted into voluntary muscle. Amplified recordings, on an oscilloscope, are also heard through a speaker. The main EMG features include:

- normal interference pattern
- denervation and re-innervation changes
- myopathic and myotonic features (see p. 893).
  Single-fibre EMG is used for disorders of NMJ transmission.

Peripheral nerve conduction

Electrical stimulation of a peripheral nerve generates a nerve impulse that may be recorded (**Fig. 26.20**). Four measurements are of principal value in neuropathies and nerve entrapment:

- nerve conduction velocity
- distal motor latency

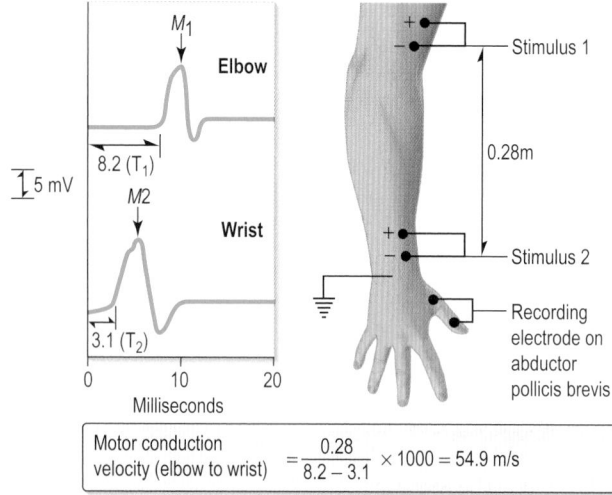

Motor conduction velocity (elbow to wrist) $= \dfrac{0.28}{8.2 - 3.1} \times 1000 = 54.9$ m/s

Fig. 26.20 Measurement of motor conduction velocity (MCV) in ulnar nerve. The recording electrode on abductor pollicis brevis measures the muscle action potential (M) from ulnar nerve stimulation at the elbow (stimulus 1) and wrist (stimulus 2). MCV calculation:
$M_1 =$ muscle action potential (MAP) from stimulus 1
$M_2 =$ MAP from stimulus 2
$T_1 =$ time from elbow to recording electrode
$T_2 =$ time from wrist to recording electrode

$$MCV = \frac{\text{distance (metres)}}{T_1 - T_2} \times 1000 = \text{m/s}$$

- sensory action potentials (SAPs)
- compound muscle action potentials (CMAPs).

Small action potential size (SAP and CMAP) indicates loss of axons. Conduction block and slowing of conduction velocity indicate demyelinating neuropathy, as saltatory conduction is lost with damage to the myelin sheath. Repetitive nerve stimulation is used to identify NMJ conduction disorders (myasthenia).

Cerebral-evoked potentials

Visual-evoked potentials (VEPs) record the interval visual stimuli take to reach the occipital cortex, and the amplitude of response. VEPs are used to confirm previous optic neuritis (see p. 810); this leaves a delayed latency despite clinical recovery.

Similar techniques for auditory and somatosensory potentials (from a limb) are also used.

Lumbar puncture and cerebrospinal fluid examination

See **Boxes 26.25** and **26.26**. Indications for lumbar puncture (LP) include:

- diagnosis of meningitis and encephalitis
- diagnosis of subarachnoid haemorrhage (in a patient with a normal CT)
- measurement of CSF pressure, e.g. idiopathic intracranial hypertension (see p. 851)
- removal of CSF therapeutically, e.g. idiopathic intracranial hypertension
- diagnosis of various conditions, e.g. MS, neurosyphilis, sarcoidosis, Behçet's, malignant meningitis, polyneuropathies
- intrathecal injection/drugs.

In suspected CNS infection, close liaison between clinician and microbiologist is essential. Specific techniques (e.g. polymerase chain reaction to identify specific pathogens) are invaluable.

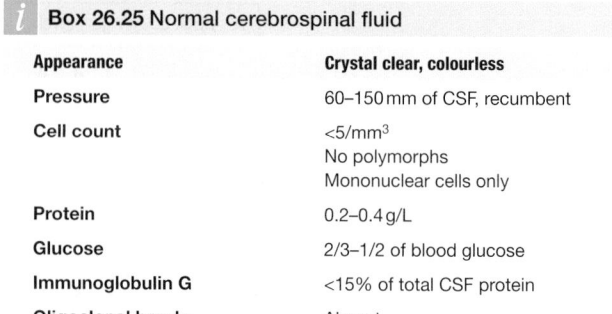

Box 26.25 Normal cerebrospinal fluid

Appearance	Crystal clear, colourless
Pressure	60–150 mm of CSF, recumbent
Cell count	$<5/\text{mm}^3$ No polymorphs Mononuclear cells only
Protein	0.2–0.4 g/L
Glucose	2/3–1/2 of blood glucose
Immunoglobulin G	<15% of total CSF protein
Oligoclonal bands	Absent

CSF, cerebrospinal fluid.

Box 26.26 Lumbar puncture

Explain the procedure to the patient and obtain consent. See list of contraindications and cautions below.

Technique
- Place the patient on the edge of the bed in the left lateral position, with knees and chin as close together as possible
- Mark the third and fourth lumbar spines. The fourth lumbar spine usually lies on a line joining the iliac crests
- Using sterile precautions, inject 2% lidocaine into the dermis by raising a bleb in either the third or fourth lumbar interspace
- Push the LP needle through the skin in the midline, steadily forwards and slightly towards the head, with the head and spine bolstered horizontally with pillows
- When you feel the needle penetrate the dura, withdraw the stylet and allow a few drops of CSF to escape
- You can then measure CSF pressure with a manometer connected to the needle. The patient's head must be on the same level as the sacrum. Normal CSF pressure is 60–150 mm of CSF. The level rises and falls with respiration and heartbeat, and rises on coughing
- Collect CSF specimens in three sterile bottles and take a sample for CSF glucose, together with a simultaneous blood glucose sample
- Record CSF naked-eye appearance: clear, cloudy, yellow (xanthochromic) or red
- Ask the patient to lie flat after the procedure to avoid subsequent headaches; this manoeuvre is probably of little value, however
- Analgesics may be required for post-LP headaches

Contraindications
- Suspicion of a mass lesion in the brain or cord. Caudal herniation of the cerebellar tonsils (coning) may occur if an intracranial mass is present and the pressure below is reduced by removal of CSF
- Any cause of raised intracranial pressure
- Local infection near the LP site
- Congenital lesions in the lumbosacral region (e.g. meningomyelocele)
- Platelet count $<40 \times 10^9/\text{L}$ and other clotting abnormalities, including anticoagulant drugs
- Unconscious patients and those with papilloedema must have a CT scan before LP

Notes
- Contraindications are relative; there are circumstances when LP is carried out despite them, for instance in the treatment of idiopathic intracranial hypertension
- Composition of normal CSF is shown in **Box 26.25**

Repeated CSF examination is often necessary in chronic infection such as tuberculosis. Post-LP headaches, worse on standing, are a common complaint for several days (or more). Prolonged headaches can be treated with caffeine or by an 'autologous intrathecal blood patch': injection of 20 mL of the patient's venous blood into the lumbar epidural space.

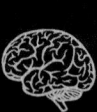

Biopsy

Interpretation of brain, tonsillar, muscle and nerve histology requires specialist neuropathology services.

Brain and meninges

Brain biopsy (e.g. of a non-dominant frontal lobe) is rarely used to diagnose inflammatory and degenerative brain diseases. CT and MR stereotactic biopsies of intracranial lesions are standard procedures.

Muscle

Muscle biopsy (usually quadriceps), with light/electron microscopy and immunohistochemical analysis, is performed routinely for diagnosis of inflammatory, metabolic and dystrophic disorders (see p. 894).

Peripheral nerve

Nerve biopsy, usually of the (sensory) sural nerve or superficial sensory branch of the radial nerve, can be of value in the diagnosis of peripheral neuropathy: for example, if vasculitis, amyloid deposition or malignant infiltration is suspected. There may be significant complications (wound healing and pain), so it should be undertaken only where all other investigations are non-diagnostic and where there is clinical evidence of a severe or progressive neuropathy.

Psychometric assessment

Psychometric testing, performed by neuropsychologists, assesses cognitive function in more detail than bedside testing during clinical examination. Decline in intellectual function, as compared with estimated pre-morbid IQ, is seen following brain injury or in dementia, for example. Individual cognitive domains, such as various types of memory, language, visuospatial function and frontal executive function, are tested separately, as they may be differentially involved in different disorders, the pattern of involvement often being of considerable diagnostic value. Serial testing at intervals of 6–12 months may be needed to show clear evidence of progression in neurodegenerative disorders such as dementias.

Routine tests

Standard blood tests, such as full blood count, erythrocyte sedimentation rate (ESR), biochemistry, glucose/HbA$_{1c}$, C-reactive protein, creatine kinase and protein electrophoresis, are helpful to identify underlying disorders such as diabetes, metabolic disorders and other systemic disorders that may underlie neurological presentations (e.g. coma or peripheral neuropathy). Relevant tests are covered in disease-specific sub-sections.

Specialized tests in specific diseases

An increasing number of highly specialized tests are employed to diagnose individual (sometimes rare) diseases (**Box 26.27**).

Genetic tests

Several hundred neurogenetic disorders are now recognized and, for many of these, specific molecular genetic investigations are available for diagnostic and predictive testing (see p. 886). As genetic testing is complex and expensive, it should only be undertaken after

---

i Box 26.27 Neurological autoantibody tests

Clinical disorder	Antibody (Ab) test
Paraneoplastic disorders: cerebellar ataxia, limbic encephalitis, opsoclonus–myoclonus, progressive encephalomyelitis with rigidity and myoclonus	Anti-Hu, Yo, Ma2/Ma1, CV2, Ri, Tr, amphiphysin
Teratoma-associated limbic encephalitis	NMDA Abs
Limbic encephalitis (non-paraneoplastic)	Anti-potassium channel, glycine Abs
Myasthenia gravis[a]	Acetylcholine receptor, MUSK Abs
Lambert–Eaton's myasthenic syndrome[a]	Voltage-gated calcium channel Abs
Neuromyelitis optica	Aquaporin 4 Abs
Stiff person syndrome	Anti-GAD Abs
Transverse myelitis	Anti-MOG Abs
Peripheral neuropathy	Anti-ganglioside and MAG Abs
Hashimoto's encephalopathy	Anti-TPO Abs
Dermatomyositis/polymyositis[a]	Anti-Jo-1 and other tRNA synthetases, SRP, Mi-2 and other Abs

[a]May also be paraneoplastic. *Abs*, antibodies.

---

senior specialist advice. Testing of panels of disease genes (e.g. for dementias or muscular dystrophies) is now available. Informed patient consent is required, as a positive test may have implications for other family members. Predictive testing in non-affected, at-risk individuals should only be undertaken after detailed genetic counselling by a specialist.

Immunological tests

An increasing number of autoimmune neurological disorders are recognized, many of which are associated with specific antibody tests (see **Box 26.27**). Many of these are paraneoplastic syndromes but an increasing number of non-cancer-related autoimmune syndromes have been identified, such as forms of encephalitis or myasthenia gravis. In addition, monoclonal paraproteins associated with plasma cell dyscrasias may cause immune-mediated peripheral neuropathy.

Further reading

Morris Z, Whiteley WM, Longstreth Jr WT et al. Incidental findings on brain magnetic resonance imaging: systematic review and meta-analysis. *BMJ* 2009; 339:b3016.
Whittaker RG. SNAPs, CMAPs and F-waves: nerve conduction studies for the uninitiated. *Pract Neurol* 2012; 12:108–115.

UNCONSCIOUSNESS AND COMA

Consciousness is dependent on the functioning of two separate anatomical and physiological systems:

- The ascending reticular activating system (ARAS), projecting from brainstem to thalamus. This determines arousal (the level of consciousness).
- The cerebral cortex, which determines the content of consciousness.

Impaired functioning of either anatomical system may cause coma.

i   **Box 26.28** Glasgow Coma Scale (GCS)[a]

Parameter	Score
Eye opening (*E*)	
Spontaneous	4
To speech	3
To pain	2
No response	1
Motor response (*M*)	
Obeys	6
Localizes	5
Withdraws	4
Flexion	3
Extension	2
No response	1
Verbal response (*V*)	
Orientated	5
Confused conversation	4
Inappropriate words	3
Incomprehensible sounds	2
No response	1

[a]GCS score = $E + M + V$ (GCS minimum = 3; maximum = 15).

Disturbed consciousness: definitions

- ***Coma***: a state of unrousable unresponsiveness. Level of consciousness represents a continuum between being alert and deeply comatose. It may be quantified using the Glasgow Coma Scale (GCS) with a score between 3 and 15 (**Box 26.28**). Coma may be conveniently defined as a GCS score of 8 or lower. Terms such as stupor and obtundation have been superseded by the GCS score and are no longer used.
- ***Delirium***: a confusional state in which reduced attention is a cardinal feature, usually with altered behaviour, cognition, orientation and a fluctuating level of consciousness (from agitation to hypoarousal; see p. 796).

Mechanisms and causes of coma

Altered consciousness is produced by four mechanisms affecting the ARAS in the brainstem or thalamus, and/or widespread impairment of cortical function (**Box 26.29** and **Fig. 26.21**).
- ***Brainstem lesion.*** A discrete brainstem or thalamic lesion, e.g. stroke, may damage the ARAS.
- ***Brainstem compression.*** A supratentorial mass lesion within the brain compresses the brainstem, inhibiting the ARAS, e.g. 'coning' from a brain tumour or haemorrhage. Mass lesions within the posterior fossa are particularly prone to causing brainstem compression and hydrocephalus.
- ***Diffuse brain dysfunction.*** Generalized severe metabolic or toxic disorders (e.g. alcohol, sedatives, uraemia, hypercapnia) depress cortical and ARAS function.
- ***Massive cortical damage.*** Unlike brainstem lesions, extensive damage of the cerebral cortex and cortical connections is required to cause coma, e.g. meningitis or hypoxic–ischaemic damage after cardiac arrest (**Fig. 26.22**).

A single focal hemisphere (or cerebellar) lesion does not produce coma, unless it compresses the brainstem. Cerebral oedema frequently surrounds masses, increasing their pressure effects.

?   **Box 26.29** Principal causes of coma: examples of mechanisms

Diffuse brain dysfunction
- Drug overdose (accidental or deliberate), including alcohol
- CO poisoning
- Traumatic brain injury
- Hypoglycaemia, hyperglycaemia
- Severe uraemia (see p. 1390)
- Hepatic encephalopathy (see p. 1297)
- Respiratory failure with CO_2 retention (see p. 956)
- Hypercalcaemia, hypocalcaemia
- Hypoadrenalism, hypopituitarism and hypothyroidism
- Hyponatraemia, hypernatraemia
- Metabolic acidosis
- Hypothermia, hyperpyrexia
- Seizures – post-ictal state and non-convulsive status
- Metabolic rarities, e.g. porphyria
- Extensive cortical damage
- Hypoxic–ischaemic brain injury, e.g. cardiac arrest
- Encephalitis, meningitis, cerebral malaria
- Subarachnoid haemorrhage

Direct effect within brainstem
- Brainstem haemorrhage, infarction or demyelination
- Brainstem neoplasm, e.g. glioma
- Wernicke–Korsakoff's syndrome

Pressure effect on brainstem
- Tumour, massive hemisphere infarction with oedema, haematoma, abscess
- Cerebellar mass

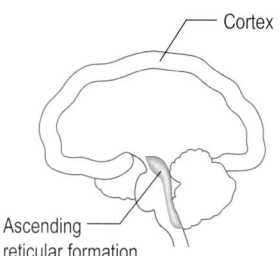

Normal

Cortex

Ascending reticular formation

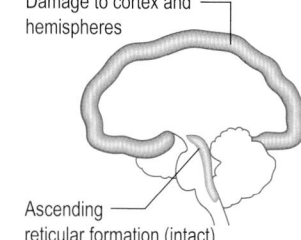

Persistent vegetative state

Damage to cortex and hemispheres

Ascending reticular formation (intact)

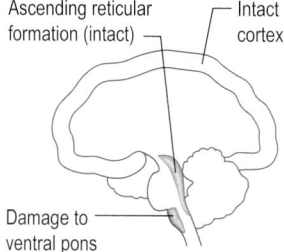

Locked-in syndrome

Ascending reticular formation (intact)

Intact cortex

Damage to ventral pons

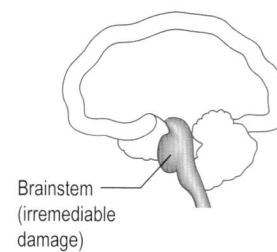

Brainstem death

Brainstem (irremediable damage)

Fig. 26.21 **Anatomy of vegetative state, locked-in syndrome and brainstem death.** *(Adapted from Bates D. Coma and brainstem death. Medicine 2004; 32.)*

The most common causes of coma are:
- metabolic disorders – 35%
- drugs and toxins – 25%
- mass lesions – 20%
- other – including trauma, stroke and CNS infections.

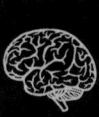

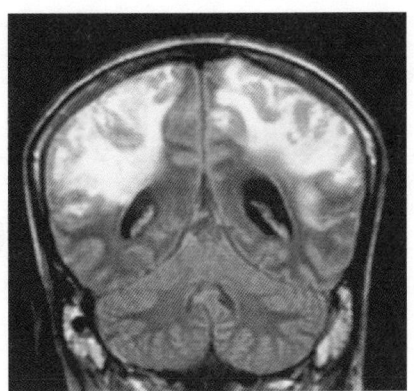

Fig. 26.22 Magnetic resonance image showing extensive cortical damage following meningitis. A permanent vegetative state resulted.

The unconscious patient

Immediate assessment and management

- Check the *a*irway, *b*reathing, *c*irculation, *d*isability and *e*xposure/*e*xamination.
- Use a point of care testing device to measure blood glucose; if the patient is hypoglycaemic, give glucose (25 mL 50%).
- Treat seizures with buccal midazolam; if not terminated, use intravenous phenytoin.
- If there is fever and meningism, give intravenous antibiotics.
- Give intravenous naloxone or flumazenil (for overdose) and thiamine (in Wernicke's encephalopathy) in people who use excess alcohol.
  Obtain as much history as possible. A limited history is one of the problems in assessing the unconscious patient. What were the circumstances? Ask paramedics, police and witnesses. Contact the patient's relatives, friends and GP, and obtain past hospital notes. Look for drug details/bottles and identification data.

General and neurological examination

General examination

(See **Fig. 26.23**.)

- Measure the patient's temperature (with a low-reading rectal thermometer if hypothermic). Check for meningism.
- Sniff the patient's breath for ketones, alcohol and hepatic fetor.
- Survey the skin for signs of trauma or spinal injury, rash (meningococcal sepsis), jaundice or stigmata of chronic liver disease, cyanosis and injection marks.
- Assess the respiratory pattern, e.g. Cheyne–Stokes (alternating hyperpnoea and periods of apnoea indicating bilateral cerebral or upper brainstem dysfunction) or acidotic (Kussmaul) respiration (deep, sighing hyperventilation seen in diabetic ketoacidosis and uraemia).

Neurological examination

Neurological examination aims to determine:

- depth of coma (GCS)
- brainstem function
- lateralization of pathology.

Depth of coma

GCS. Assessment of the GCS score is repeated regularly to determine whether the patient's level of consciousness is progressively declining. Use a painful stimulus (e.g. nail-bed pressure) to each limb and central area (sternal rub or pressure over the supraorbital nerve), and record the *best* response. Shout commands.

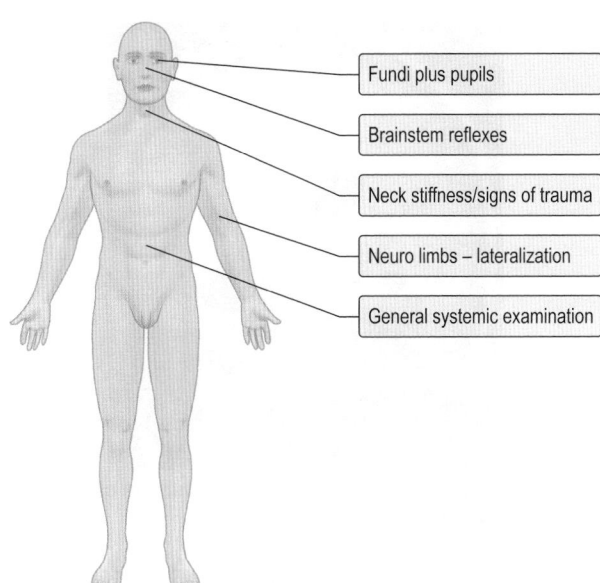

Fig. 26.23 Assessing the unconscious patient.

| Fundi plus pupils |
| Brainstem reflexes |
| Neck stiffness/signs of trauma |
| Neuro limbs – lateralization |
| General systemic examination |

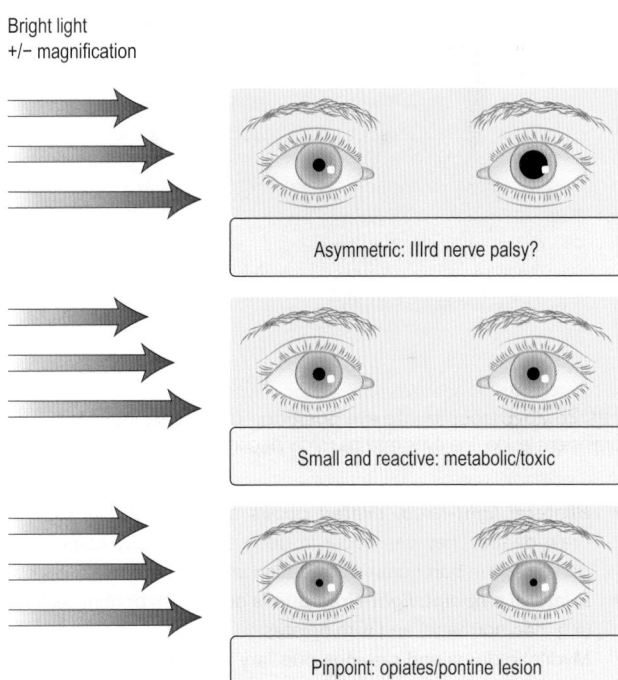

Bright light
+/– magnification

Asymmetric: IIIrd nerve palsy?

Small and reactive: metabolic/toxic

Pinpoint: opiates/pontine lesion

Fig. 26.24 Examination of the pupils.

Fundi. Look for papilloedema and subhyaloid retinal haemorrhage (seen in subarachnoid haemorrhage).

Brainstem function

Pupils

Record their size and reaction to light (**Fig. 26.24**):

- ***Dilation of one pupil*** that then becomes fixed to light indicates compression of the IIIrd nerve. This may indicate a potential neurosurgical emergency (**Fig. 26.25**).
- ***Bilateral mid-point reactive pupils*** (i.e. normal pupils) are characteristic of metabolic comas and secondary coma due to sedative drugs (except opiates).

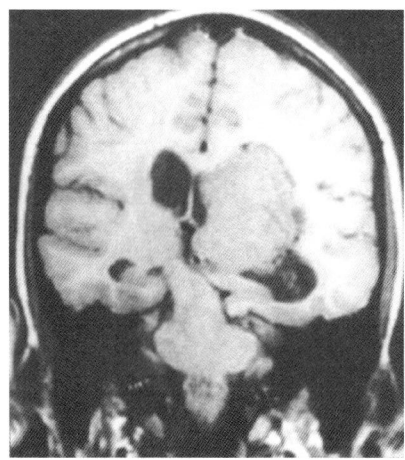

Fig. 26.25 Medial temporal lobe (uncal) herniation causing third nerve compression.

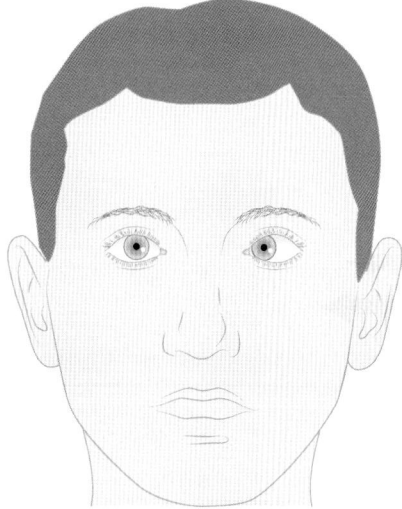

Fig. 26.26 Disconjugate eye position. This usually indicates brainstem lesion (the eyes may be mildly disconjugate in metabolic coma).

- **Bilateral light-fixed, dilated pupils** are one cardinal sign of brain death. They can occur in deep coma of any cause, but particularly in barbiturate intoxication and hypothermia.
- **Bilateral pinpoint, light-fixed pupils** occur with pontine lesions (e.g. haemorrhage) and with opiates.
  Mydriatic drugs and previous pupillary surgery can cause diagnostic difficulty.

Eye movements and position

- Disconjugate eyes (divergent ocular axes) indicate a brainstem lesion, e.g. **skew deviation** (one eye up, one eye down; **Fig. 26.26**).
- Conjugate gaze deviation means the eyes deviate towards the lesion in the frontal lobe and the normal limbs (unopposed activity of the intact frontal eye fields drives eyes to the opposite side); and away from the lesion in the brainstem and towards the weak limbs (the PPRF in the pons controls lateral gaze to the ipsilateral side; see p. 812) (**Fig. 26.27**).
- Vestibulo-ocular reflex means that passive head-turning produces conjugate ocular deviation away from the direction of rotation (doll's eye reflex). This reflex disappears in deep coma, brainstem lesions and brain death (**Fig. 26.28**).

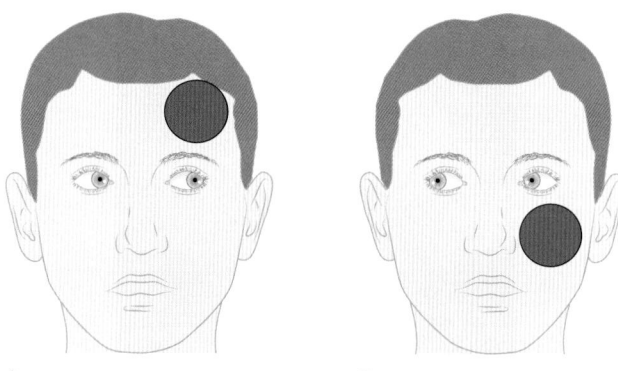

A   **B**

Fig. 26.27 Conjugate gaze deviation. (A) Frontal lesion. **(B)** Brainstem lesion.

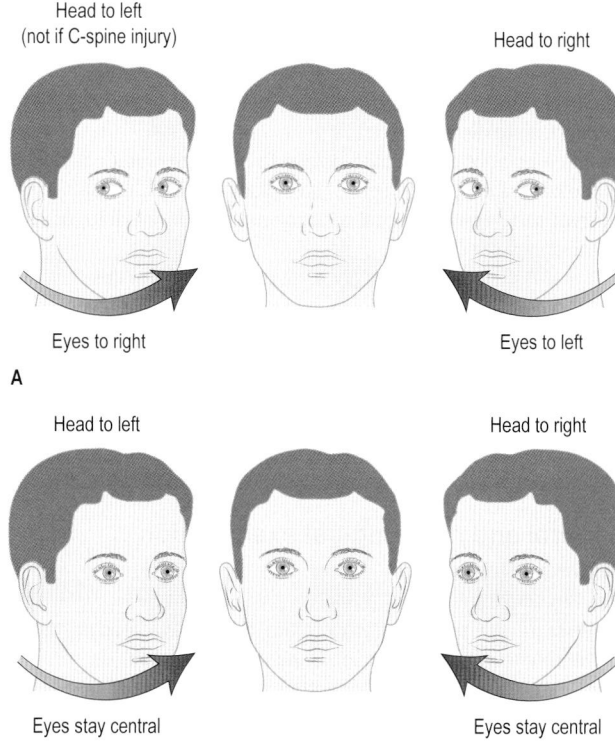

Fig. 26.28 Doll's eye movements. (A) Normal. **(B)** Abnormal.

- In light coma, slow, side-to-side eye movements are seen ('windscreen wiper' eyes; **Fig. 26.29**). This is also seen with extensive cortical damage in deep coma.

Other brainstem reflexes

- Corneal reflex.
- Gag/cough reflex (via endotracheal tube if intubated).
- Respiratory drive (see p. 932).

Lateralizing signs

Coma makes it difficult to recognize lateralizing signs. These are helpful:

- **Asymmetry of response to visual threat** in a stuporose patient: suggests hemianopia.
- **Asymmetry of face**: drooping or dribbling on one side; blowing in and out of mouth when the paralysed cheek does not move.

- **Asymmetry of tone**: unilateral flaccidity or spasticity – may be the only sign of hemiparesis.
- **Asymmetry of decerebrate and decorticate posturing.**
- **Asymmetrical response** to painful stimuli.
- **Asymmetry of tendon reflexes and plantar responses**: both plantars are often extensor in deep coma.

Coma 'look-alikes'

- Psychogenic coma.
- 'Locked-in' syndrome – complete paralysis, except for vertical eye movements/blinking in ventral pontine infarction. Patients have a functioning cerebral cortex and are fully aware but unable to communicate, except through eye movements (**Box 26.30**).
- Severe paralysis, e.g. myasthenic crisis or severe Guillain–Barré syndrome.

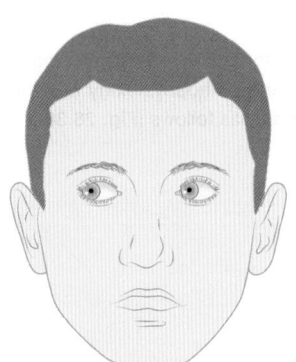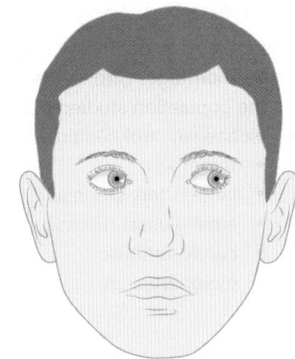

Fig. 26.29 'Windscreen wiper' eyes ('ping pong' eyes). Slow, side-to-side movements demonstrate diffuse cortical dysfunction. This is common in light coma and implies normal brainstem function. In deep coma it indicates extensive cortical damage.

Diagnosis and investigations in coma

Often the cause is evident (e.g. head injury, metabolic disorder, overdose). Where lateralizing signs or brainstem pathology are found on examination, a mass lesion or infarction/haemorrhage is likely (note that hypoglycaemia may also cause focal signs). If no cause is obvious after clinical assessment, further investigations are essential.

Blood and urine

- **Drug screen** – blood alcohol and salicylates, urine toxicology including screening for benzodiazepines, narcotics, amfetamine.
- **Biochemistry** – urea, electrolytes, glucose, calcium, liver biochemistry.
- **Metabolic and endocrine studies** – thyroid stimulating hormone, cortisol.
- **Arterial blood gases** – for acidosis or high CO_2 levels.
- **Other** – e.g. cerebral malaria (request *thick* blood film; see p. 563) and porphyria (p. 755).

Brain imaging

CT brain imaging is the most readily available and safest modality in the unconscious patient (MRI is useful where CT is normal but presents greater monitoring challenges in the unconscious patient). CT is quick and effective in demonstrating all types of brain haemorrhage and most mass lesions; infarcts may be missed in the early stages and where only the brainstem is affected.

CSF examination

LP should be performed in coma only after careful risk assessment. It is contraindicated when an intracranial mass lesion is a possibility; CT is essential to exclude this. CSF examination is likely to alter therapy only if undiagnosed meningoencephalitis or other infection is present, or in subarachnoid haemorrhage where CT may give a false-negative result, particularly after 24 hours.

? Box 26.30 Differential diagnosis of prolonged disorders of consciousness

Condition	VS	MCS	Locked-in syndrome	Coma	Death confirmed by brainstem tests
Awareness	Absent	Present	Present	Absent	Absent
Sleep–wake cycles	Present	Present	Present	Absent	Absent
Response to noxious stimuli	±	Present	Present (in eyes only)	±	Absent
Glasgow Coma Scale	E4, M1–4, V1–2	E4, M1–5, V1–4	E4, M1, V1	E1–2, M1–4, V1–2	E1, M1–3, V1
Motor function	No purposeful movement	Some consistent verbal or purposeful motor behaviour	Volitional vertical eye movements or eye blink typically preserved	No purposeful movement	None or only reflex spinal movement
Respiratory function	Typically preserved	Typically preserved	Typically preserved	Variable	Absent
EEG activity	Typically slow-wave activity	Insufficient data	Typically normal	Typically slow wave activity	Typically absent
Cerebral metabolism (PET)	Severely reduced	Intermediate reduction	Mildly reduced	Moderately to severely reduced	Severely reduced or absent
Prognosis	Variable: if permanent, continued VS or death	Variable: (if permanent, continued MCS or death)	Depends on cause but full recovery unlikely	Recovery, VS or death usually within weeks	Organ function can be sustained only temporarily with life support

EEG = electroencephalography; MCS = minimally conscious state; PET = positron emission tomography; VS = vegetative state.
(*Reproduced from Royal College of Physicians.* Prolonged Disorders of Consciousness: National Clinical Guidelines. *London: RCP, 2013; with permission.*)

Electroencephalography

EEG is of some value in the diagnosis of metabolic coma, encephalitis and non-convulsive status epilepticus.

General management

Comatose patients need careful nursing, meticulous attention to the airway, and frequent monitoring of vital functions.

Longer-term essentials are:

- skin care – turning (to avoid pressure ulcers and pressure palsies)
- oral hygiene – mouthwashes, suction
- eye care – prevention of corneal damage (lid taping, irrigation)
- fluids – nasogastric or intravenous
- feeding – via a fine-bore nasogastric tube or via PEG
- sphincters – catheterization when essential (use a penile urinary sheath if possible in men); rectal evacuation.

Prognosis in coma and the vegetative state

Prognosis depends on the cause of coma and the extent of brain damage sustained. Metabolic and toxic causes of coma have the best prognosis when the underlying problem can be corrected. Following hypoxic–ischaemic brain injury, such as after cardiac arrest, only 11% make a good recovery; after stroke, the prognosis is worse still, with only 7% recovering. Of those patients who do not recover consciousness, a substantial proportion will remain in a vegetative or minimally responsive state.

- **Vegetative state** (VS) is usually a consequence of extensive cortical damage. Brainstem function is intact and so breathing is normal without the need for mechanical ventilation, and the patient appears awake with eye-opening and sleep–wake cycles. However, there is no sign of awareness or response to environmental stimuli, except reflex movements. Feeding is via gastrostomy. Patients may remain in this state for years. It is considered permanent (PVS) if there is no recovery after 12 months where trauma is the cause, and after 6 months for all other causes. Prolonged support of patients after this time presents a number of ethical issues; families may apply to the courts for withdrawal of feeding in PVS.
- **Minimally conscious state** (MCS) describes patients with some, often fluctuating, limited awareness, with inconsistent but reproducible responses, e.g. movements in response to voice; crying or laughing in response to emotional stimuli; and vocalization in response to questions. A patient may emerge from VS into MCS. Distinguishing VS from MCS requires careful specialist assessment over a long period. Functional brain imaging has recently been used for this purpose.
- **Brainstem death** is discussed on page 236.

Distinction between these states is essential before addressing issues of prognosis and cessation of supportive care.

Further reading

Royal College of Physicians of London. *Prolonged Disorders of Consciousness: National Clinical Guidelines.* London: RCP; 2013.

STROKE

Stroke is the third most common cause of death in high-income countries (11% of all deaths in the UK) and the leading cause of adult disability worldwide. Approximately two-thirds of the global burden of stroke is in middle- and low-income countries. Stroke rates are higher in Asian and black African populations than in Caucasians. Stroke risk increases with age but one-quarter of all strokes occur before the age of 65. The death rate following stroke is 20–25%, and 40% of surviving patients are dependent at 6 months.

Definitions

- **Stroke.** To the public, stroke means weakness, usually permanent on one side, often with loss of speech. Stroke is *defined* as a syndrome of rapid onset neurological deficit caused by focal cerebral, spinal or retinal infarction or haemorrhage. Tissue injury is confirmed by neuroimaging. Hemiplegia following middle cerebral artery thromboembolism is the typical example.
- **Transient ischaemic attack (TIA)** means a brief episode of neurological dysfunction due to temporary focal cerebral or retinal ischaemia without infarction, e.g. a weak limb, aphasia or loss of vision, usually lasting seconds or minutes with complete recovery. TIAs may herald a stroke. The arbitrary time of less than 24 hours is no longer used.

Pathophysiology

The underlying pathology responsible for stroke is either infarction or haemorrhage. Stroke mechanism and pathophysiology depend on the population studied but are broadly as follows (**Fig. 26.30**):

- ischaemic stroke/infarction (85%)
  - thrombotic
  - large-artery stenosis
  - small-vessel disease
  - cardio-embolic
  - hypoperfusion

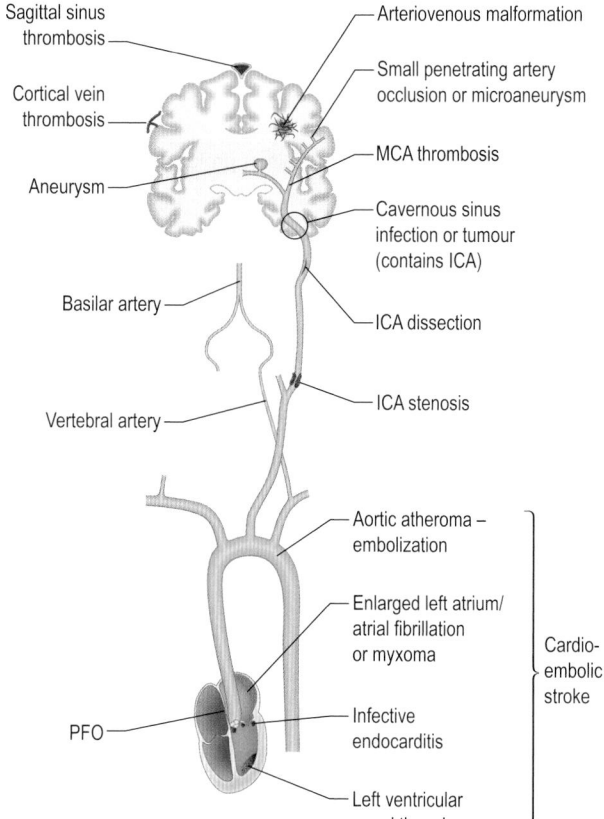

Fig. 26.30 **Pathophysiology of ischaemic stroke.** ICA, internal carotid artery; MCA, middle cerebral artery; PFO, patent foramen ovale.

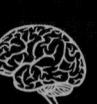

- haemorrhagic stroke (10%) (see p. 845)
  - intracerebral haemorrhage (see p. 846)
  - subarachnoid haemorrhage (see p. 848)
- other (5%), e.g. arterial dissection, venous sinus thrombosis, vasculitis (see p. 464).

Ischaemic stroke

Arterial disease and atherosclerosis are the main pathological processes causing stroke. Arterial branch points, such as the origin of the great vessels arising from the aorta, the proximal internal carotid artery and its distal intracranial branches, are particularly affected (**Fig. 26.31**). Non-Caucasian populations tend to have more intracranial narrowing and white populations more extracranial disease (which is strongly correlated with co-morbid coronary artery and peripheral vascular disease).

Thrombosis. Thrombosis at the site of ruptured mural plaque leads to artery-to-artery embolism or vessel occlusion.

Large-artery stenosis. This usually causes stroke by acting as an embolic source rather than by occluding the vessel (which may not in itself cause stroke if it occurs gradually and collateral circulation is adequate).

Small-vessel disease. Small penetrating arterial branches supply the deep brain parenchyma and are affected by a different pathological process: an occlusive vasculopathy – lipohyalinosis – that is a consequence of hypertension. This leads to small infarcts called 'lacunes' and/or gradual accumulation of diffuse ischaemic change in deep white matter.

Cardio-embolic stroke. The heart is a common source of embolic material. Atrial fibrillation (and other arrhythmias) leading to thrombosis in a dilated left atrium is the most common cause. Cardiac valve disease, including congenital valve disorders, infective vegetations, and rheumatic and degenerative calcific changes, may cause embolization. Mural thrombosis may occur in a damaged or akinetic segment of the ventricle. A patent foramen ovale (PFO), which is a common variant, may occasionally allow passage of fragments of thrombus (e.g. from a lower limb deep vein thrombosis) from the right atrium to the left when Valsalva causes shunting of blood across the PFO. Pulmonary arteriovenous fistulas may also act as a conduit for paradoxical embolization. Rarer causes include fat emboli after long bone fracture, atrial myxomas and iatrogenic causes, such as cardiac bypass and air embolism. Simultaneous infarcts in different vascular territories are very suggestive of a proximal source of emboli in the heart or aorta.

Hypoperfusion. Severe hypotension, such as in cardiac arrest, may lead to border-zone infarction in the watershed areas between vascular territories, particularly if there is severe stenosis of proximal carotid vessels. The parieto-occipital area between the middle and posterior cerebral artery territories is particularly vulnerable.

Carotid and vertebral artery dissection

Dissection accounts for around 1 in 5 strokes below the age of 40 and is sometimes a sequel of trivial neck trauma or hyperextension; for example, after whiplash, osteopathic manipulation, hairwashing in a salon or exercise. Subtle collagen disorders, such as partial forms of Marfan's syndrome, may be a predisposing factor.

Most dissections are in large extracranial neck vessels. Blood penetrates the subintimal vessel wall, forming a false lumen, but it is thrombosis within the true lumen due to tissue thromboplastin release that leads to embolization from the site of dissection and stroke, sometimes days after the initial event.

Pain in the neck or face is often the clue leading to diagnosis. Horner's syndrome or lower cranial nerve palsies may occur with carotid dissection, as these structures are intimately associated with the carotid artery in the neck.

Venous stroke

Only 1% of strokes are venous. Thrombosis within intracranial venous sinuses, such as the superior sagittal sinus, or in cortical veins, may occur in pregnancy, hypercoagulable states and thrombotic disorders, or with dehydration or malignancy. Cortical infarction, seizures and raised intracranial pressure result.

Haemorrhagic stroke

See page 846.

Transient ischaemic attacks

TIAs are usually the result of microemboli but different mechanisms produce similar clinical events. For example, TIAs may be caused by a fall in cerebral perfusion (e.g. a cardiac dysrhythmia, postural hypotension or decreased flow through atheromatous arteries). Infarction is usually averted by autoregulation. Rarely, tumours and subdural haematomas cause episodes that are indistinguishable from thromboembolic TIAs. Principal sources of emboli to the brain are cardiac thrombus and atheromatous plaques/thrombus within the aortic arch and carotid and vertebral systems. Cardiac thrombus often results from atrial fibrillation (which can be paroxysmal) or myocardial infarction. Cardiac valve disease may be a source of emboli: for example, calcific material or vegetations in infective endocarditis. Polycythaemia is also a cause.

Risk factors for stroke

The principal risk factors are those for atherosclerosis: age, smoking, dyslipidaemia, diabetes, obesity, inactivity and genetic/ethnic factors.

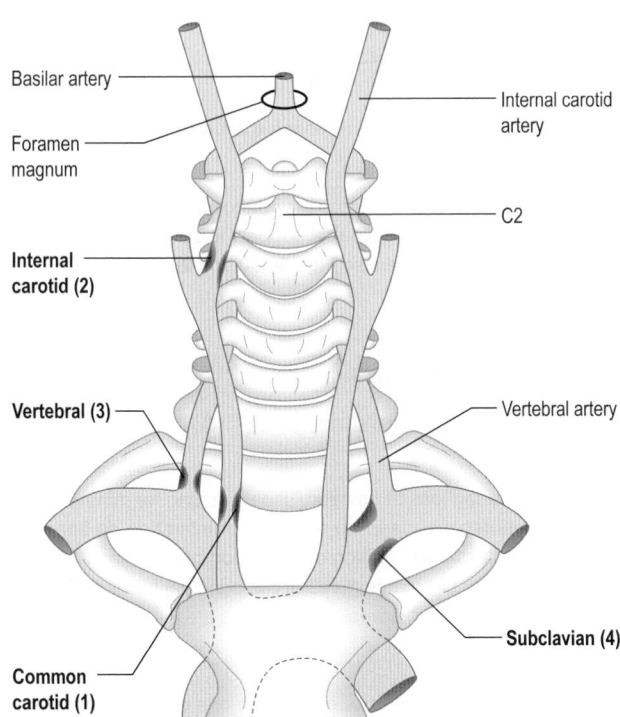

Fig. 26.31 Principal sites of stenoses in extracerebral arteries. (These are shown in bold, 1–4.)

Labels: Basilar artery, Foramen magnum, Internal carotid (2), Vertebral (3), Common carotid (1), Internal carotid artery, C2, Vertebral artery, Subclavian (4)

Box 26.31 Factors reducing stroke risk

Risk factor	Action	Reduction in stroke risk		
		Infarction	Haemorrhage	Relative risk reduction in secondary prevention
Hypertension	Treatment and monitoring	++	++	28%
Smoking	Cessation	++	+	33%
Lifestyle	Greater activity	+	0	
Alcohol	Moderate intake	+	+	
High cholesterol	Statins, diet	+	0	24%
Atrial fibrillation	Anticoagulation	++	*Increases* risk slightly	67%
Obesity	Weight reduction	Probable	Probable	
Diabetes	Good control	+	0	
Severe carotid stenosis	Surgery	++	0	44%
Sleep apnoea	Treatment	+	0	

++, major correlation with reduced stroke risk; +, moderate correlation; SAH, subarachnoid haemorrhage.

Hypertension is overall the most modifiable stroke risk factor in the population; stroke is decreasing in the 40–60 age group partly because hypertension is now more effectively identified and treated (**Box 26.31**). There is a linear relationship between blood pressure and stroke risk (see **Fig. 31.3**).

On an individual rather than population basis, anticoagulation for atrial fibrillation is the intervention resulting in the greatest stroke risk reduction.

Other risk factors and rarer causes of stroke

- Thrombocythaemia, polycythaemia and hyperviscosity states – thrombophilia (e.g. protein C deficiency, factor V Leiden) is weakly associated with arterial stroke but predisposes to cerebral venous thrombosis.
- Anticardiolipin and lupus anticoagulant antibodies (antiphospholipid syndrome; see p. 459) predispose to arterial thrombotic strokes in young patients.
- Low-dose, oestrogen-containing oral contraceptives do not increase stroke risk significantly in healthy women but probably do so in combination with other risk factors, e.g. uncontrolled hypertension or smoking.
- Migraine is a rare cause of cerebral infarction.
- Vasculitis (systemic lupus erythematosus (SLE), polyarteritis, giant cell arteritis, granulomatous CNS angiitis) is a rare cause of stroke.
- Amyloidosis can present as recurrent cerebral haemorrhage (see p. 1357).
- Hyperhomocysteinaemia predisposes to thrombotic strokes. Folic acid therapy does not reduce the incidence.
- HIV, neurosyphilis, mitochondrial disease, Fabry's disease (see p. 1367).
- Sympathomimetic drugs such as cocaine, and possibly over-the-counter cold remedies containing vasoconstrictors; neuroleptics in older patients.
- CADASIL (cerebral dominant arteriopathy with subcortical infarcts and leukoencephalopathy) is a rare inherited cause of stroke/vascular dementia.

Vascular anatomy

Knowledge of normal arterial anatomy and likely sites of atheromatous plaques and stenoses helps understanding of the main stroke syndromes.

The circle of Willis is supplied by the two internal carotid arteries (the anterior cerebral circulation) and by the vertebrobasilar

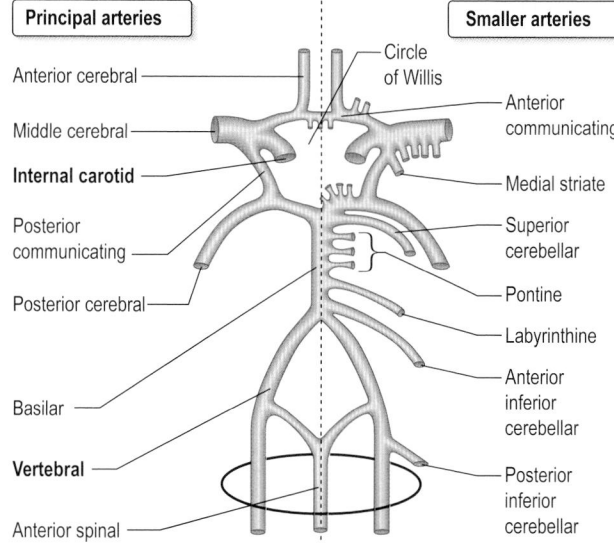

Fig. 26.32 Arteries supplying the brain and cord.

posterior cerebral circulation. The distribution of the anterior, middle and posterior cerebral arteries that supply the cerebrum is shown in **Figs 26.32** and **26.33** (see also **Figs 26.30** and **26.31**).

Clinical syndromes

Transient ischaemic attack (TIA)
Clinical features

TIAs cause sudden loss of function, usually lasting for minutes only, with complete recovery and no evidence of infarction on imaging. The previous classical definition of a duration of less than 24 hours is no longer used. Clinical features of the principal forms of TIA are given in **Box 26.32**. Hemiparesis and aphasia are the most common.

Amaurosis fugax

This is a sudden transient loss of vision in one eye. When it is due to the passage of emboli through the retinal arteries, the embolus is sometimes visible through an ophthalmoscope during an attack (Hollenhorst plaque). A TIA causing an episode of amaurosis fugax

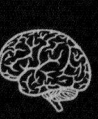

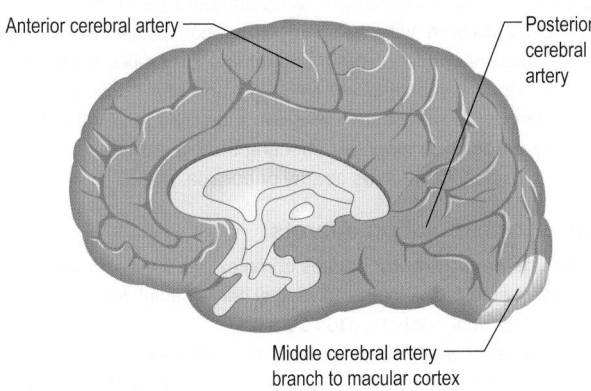

A **Medial view of right hemisphere**

Anterior cerebral artery

Posterior cerebral artery

Middle cerebral artery branch to macular cortex

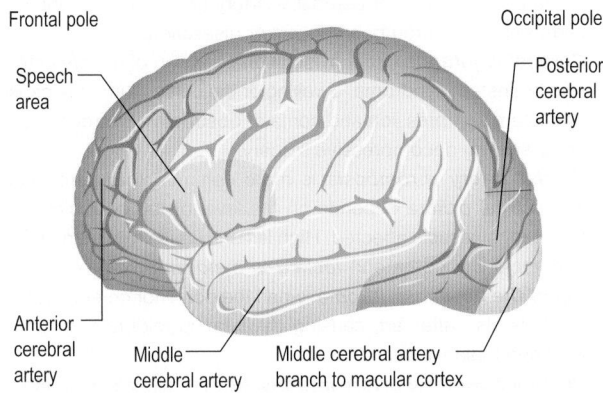

B **Lateral view of left hemisphere**

Frontal pole

Occipital pole

Speech area

Posterior cerebral artery

Anterior cerebral artery

Middle cerebral artery

Middle cerebral artery branch to macular cortex

Fig. 26.33 The three major cerebral arteries. (A) Medial view of right hemisphere. **(B)** Lateral view of left hemisphere.

is often the first clinical evidence of internal carotid artery (ICA) stenosis – a warning sign of incipient ICA territory stroke.

Diagnosis

Diagnosis of TIA is often based solely on its description. It is unusual to witness an attack, as they are so brief. Consciousness is usually preserved in TIA. There may be clinical evidence of a source of embolus, such as:

- carotid arterial bruit (stenosis)
- atrial fibrillation or other dysrhythmia
- valvular heart disease/endocarditis
- recent myocardial infarction.
  An underlying condition may be evident:
- atheroma
- hypertension
- postural hypotension
- bradycardia or low cardiac output
- diabetes mellitus
- rarely, arteritis, polycythaemia, neurosyphilis, HIV
- antiphospholipid syndrome (see p. 459).

Differential diagnosis

TIAs can be distinguished, usually on clinical grounds, from other transient episodes (see p. 857). Occasionally, events identical to TIAs are produced by mass lesions. Focal epilepsy is usually recognized by its positive features (e.g. limb jerking and loss of consciousness) and progression over minutes. In a TIA, involuntary limb movements do occur occasionally – **limb-shaking TIA** – and are

Box 26.32 Features of transient ischaemic attacks

Anterior circulation	**Posterior circulation**
Carotid system	*Vertebrobasilar system*
• Amaurosis fugax	• Diplopia, vertigo, vomiting
• Aphasia	• Choking and dysarthria
• Hemiparesis	• Ataxia
• Hemisensory loss	• Hemisensory loss
• Hemianopic visual loss	• Hemianopic visual loss
	• Bilateral visual loss
	• Tetraparesis
	• Loss of consciousness (rare)
	• Transient global amnesia (possibly)

i **Box 26.33** ABCD² score in the stratification of stroke risk

Parameter	Score
Age >60 years	1
BP >140 mmHg systolic and/or diastolic >90 mmHg	1
Clinical features	
Unilateral weakness	2
Isolated speech disturbance	1
Other	0
Duration of symptoms (min)	
>60	2
10–59	1
<10	0
Diabetes	1

A score of <4 is associated with a low risk whereas >6 is high-risk for a stroke within 7 days of a TIA. This scoring system is now no longer used to guide management, but may still inform prognosis (see text).

pathognomonic of severe carotid stenosis causing transient focal cerebral hypoperfusion. Cerebral amyloid angiopathy can cause TIA-like events; identification on imaging is necessary, as antiplatelet therapy is contraindicated.

Migraine aura causing visual loss or dysphasia, particularly when it occurs without subsequent headache in elderly people, often causes diagnostic difficulty. Headache, common but not invariable in migraine, is rare in TIA. Positive visual phenomena such as shimmering, which are typical of migraine, are not seen in TIA. The onset and evolution of symptoms is usually slower with migraine aura than TIA (minutes rather than seconds). Limb weakness is rarely due to migraine.

Prognosis

Prospective studies show that 5 years after a single thromboembolic TIA:

- 30% have had a stroke, a third of these in the first year
- 15% have suffered a myocardial infarct.

TIAs in the anterior cerebral circulation carry a more serious prognosis than those in the posterior circulation (see **Box 26.32**).

The **ABCD² score** (**Box 26.33**) was until recently used to stratify stroke risk in the first 2 days. Now *all* patients with a suspected TIA event should be referred to a TIA clinic and be seen, investigated and managed within 24 hours.

Investigations should include Doppler ultrasound of the internal carotid arteries, cardiac echo, ECG and 24-hour tape, MRI brain and MR or CT angiography. Treat with medical therapy (see p. 843) and surgery if appropriate (p. 844). Surgery or stenting of high-grade symptomatic carotid stenosis should take place within 1 week of TIA (p. 838).

Cerebral infarction

Major thromboembolic cerebral infarction usually causes an obvious stroke. The clinical picture is thus very variable, depending on the infarct site and extent.

Following vessel occlusion, brain ischaemia occurs, with electrical neuronal failure causing symptoms, followed by infarction and cell death. The infarcted region is surrounded by a swollen ischaemic area that does not function but is structurally intact. This is the *ischaemic penumbra*, which is detected on MRI and can regain function following revascularization.

Within the ischaemic area, hypoxia leads to neuronal damage. There is a fall in ATP with release of glutamate, which opens calcium channels with release of free radicals. These alterations lead to inflammatory damage, necrosis and apoptotic cell death.

Clinical features

An acute onset (over minutes) of 'negative' symptoms indicating focal deficits in brain function, such as weakness, sensory loss, dysphasia and visual loss, are the characteristic defining features of ischaemic stroke. The exact clinical picture depends on the vascular territory affected.

Anterior circulation infarcts

This includes infarcts in the territory of the internal carotid, middle cerebral (MCA), anterior cerebral (ACA) and ophthalmic arteries. Complete MCA occlusion results in devastating stroke with contralateral hemiplegia and facial weakness, hemisensory loss and neglect syndromes (parietal lobe – severe if the non-dominant side is affected), eye deviation towards the affected side (frontal eye fields), aphasia (dominant hemisphere lesions) and hemianopia. Brain swelling of infarcted tissue leads to a high risk of death due to coning – *malignant MCA infarction*. Decompressive craniectomy (**Fig. 26.34**) within the first 48 hours has been shown to reduce mortality and slightly improve the long-term severe disability.

A similar picture to MCA stroke is caused by **internal carotid occlusion**, although collateral circulation may reduce the infarct size (see **Fig. 26.31**). MCA branch occlusions produce fragments of the picture described above, such as hemiparesis, monoparesis and aphasia. Occlusion of lenticulostriate perforating arteries (or MCA occlusion with collateral circulation protecting the cortex) causes infarction of deep subcortical structures such as the internal capsule, resulting in hemiplegia and hemisensory deficits. ACA infarcts are significantly less common than MCA infarcts and typically produce hemiparesis affecting the leg more than arm, and frontal lobe deficits such as apathy or apraxia.

Posterior circulation infarcts

*   ***Brainstem infarction*** causes complex signs, depending on the relationship of the infarct to cranial nerve nuclei, long tracts and brainstem connections (**Box 26.34**).
*   ***The lateral medullary syndrome*** (Wallenberg's syndrome) is a common brainstem vascular syndrome presenting as acute vertigo with cerebellar and other signs, including Horner's syndrome (**Box 26.35** and **Fig. 26.35**). It follows thromboembolism in the posterior inferior cerebellar artery (PICA) or its branches, vertebral artery thromboembolism or dissection.
*   ***Cerebellar infarcts*** occur in isolation or as part of a more extensive brainstem syndrome. Swelling of the cerebellum may cause brainstem compression and coma or obstructive hydrocephalus necessitating decompressive surgery.
*   ***Basilar artery thrombosis*** is more common than embolism. The clinical picture depends on the level of the occlusion and the branch vessels affected. High lesions cause midbrain infarction, including coma and ***locked-in syndrome*** (see p. 832) or ***top of the basilar syndrome***, when the posterior cerebral artery (PCA) is also affected, causing devastating midbrain, occipital lobe and thalamic infarction.

Posterior cerebral artery infarcts are typically embolic. Homonymous hemianopia results from unilateral lesions, cortical blindness (***Anton's syndrome***) from bilateral lesions (see **Fig. 26.33** and p. 807). Neglect syndromes and visual agnosias are associated with involvement of more anterior visual association areas. The PCA supplies the thalamus, and posteromedial temporal lobe and infarction of these structures causes confusion or memory impairment.

Lacunar infarction

Lacunes are small (<1.5 cm³) infarcts seen on MRI or at postmortem. Hypertension is the major risk factor. Strokes without cortical features, such as pure motor stroke, pure sensory stroke, sudden

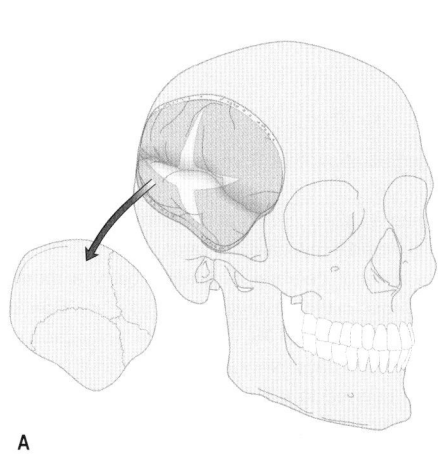

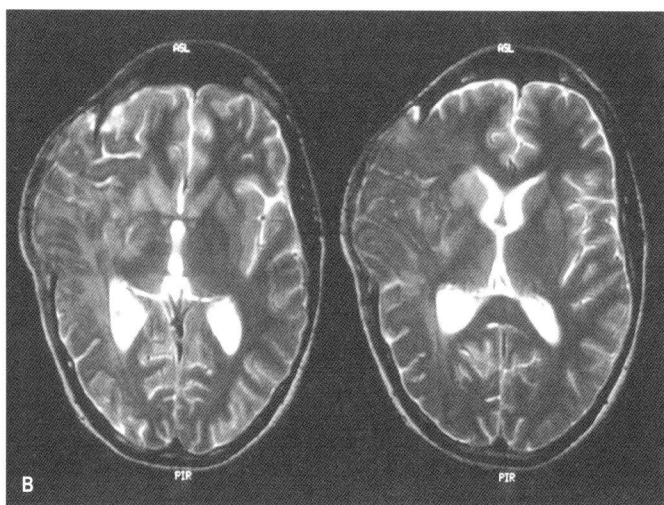

A **B**

Fig. 26.34 Decompressive craniectomy for stroke.

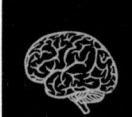

Box 26.34 Features of brainstem infarction	
Clinical feature	**Structure involved**
Hemiparesis or tetraparesis	Corticospinal tracts
Sensory loss	Medial lemniscus and spinothalamic tracts
Diplopia	Oculomotor system
Facial numbness	Vth nerve nuclei
Facial weakness	VIIth nerve nucleus
Nystagmus, vertigo	Vestibular connections
Dysphagia, dysarthria	IXth and Xth nerve nuclei
Dysarthria, ataxia, hiccups, vomiting	Brainstem and cerebellar connections
Horner's syndrome	Sympathetic fibres
Coma, altered consciousness	Reticular formation

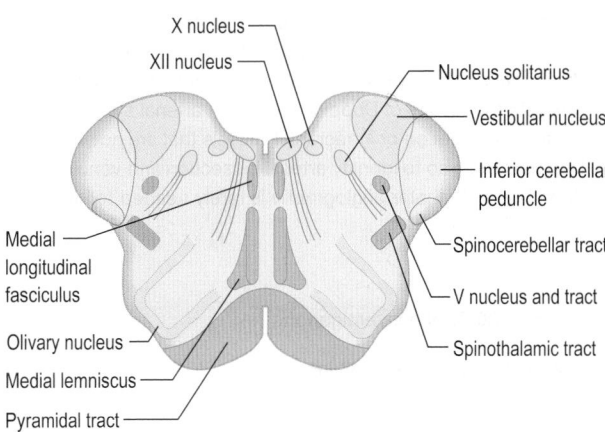

Fig. 26.35 Medulla (cross-section). Structures at risk after brainstem infarction.

Box 26.35 Some clinical stroke syndromes	
Vascular supply/region affected	**Neurological deficits**
Left middle cerebral artery	Right-sided weakness involving face and arm > leg Dysphasia
Right middle cerebral artery	Left-sided weakness involving face and arm > leg Visual and/or sensory neglect Denial of disability
Lateral medulla (posterior inferior cerebellar artery or vertebral artery)	Ipsilateral Horner's syndrome Xth nerve palsy Facial sensory loss Limb ataxia with contralateral spinothalamic sensory loss Vertigo Dysphagia
Posterior cerebral artery	Homonymous hemianopia Varied deficits due to thalamic, occipitoparietal and/or temporal lobe involvement
Internal capsule	Motor, sensory or sensorimotor loss Face = arm = leg Possible profound dysarthria from involvement of corticobulbar fibres No dysphasia or other cortical deficits
Bilateral paramedian thalamus and midbrain	Coma or reduced alertness Ophthalmoplegia Ataxia Memory impairment Thalamic pain
Carotid artery dissection	Neck/face pain Ipsilateral Horner's syndrome from compression of sympathetic plexus around the carotid artery Lower cranial nerves (Xth and XIIth most clinically obvious) Embolic infarcts in anterior circulation territory

unilateral ataxia and sudden dysarthria with a clumsy hand, are typical lacunar syndromes. Lacunar infarction is often symptomless.

Multi-infarct dementia (vascular dementia)

Multiple lacunes or larger infarcts cause generalized intellectual loss seen with advanced cerebrovascular disease. In the late stages, there is dementia (see p. 883), pseudobulbar palsy and a shuffling gait – *marche à petits pas* (small steps), sometimes called atherosclerotic parkinsonism. **Binswanger's disease** is a term for widespread low attenuation in cerebral white matter, usually with dementia, TIAs and stroke episodes in hypertensive patients (the changes being seen on imaging/autopsy).

Watershed (border-zone) infarction

Severe cerebral hypoperfusion, such as hypotension after cardiac arrest or bypass surgery, causes ischaemia in the border zones between areas supplied by the anterior, middle and posterior cerebral arteries (affecting the occipitoparietal cortex, hippocampi and motor pathways). Complex patterns of visual loss (e.g. **Balint's syndrome**), memory loss, intellectual impairment and sometimes motor deficits are typical. A vegetative state or minimally conscious state may result from severe hypoxic–ischaemic encephalopathy after prolonged cerebral hypoperfusion (see p. 836).

Investigations in stroke

The purpose of investigations in stroke is to:
- confirm the clinical diagnosis, distinguish between haemorrhage and thromboembolic infarction, and exclude stroke mimics, e.g. tumour
- identify an underlying cause for the purposes of secondary prevention and identification of stroke mimics.

Investigations in thromboembolic stroke and TIA are listed in **Box 26.36**.

Neuroimaging

- **CT** will demonstrate haemorrhage immediately but cerebral infarction is often not detected in the acute phase or only subtle changes are seen (**Fig. 26.36A**). Repeat CT at 24–48 hours may be helpful.
- **MRI** is more sensitive than CT for early changes of infarction (diffusion-weighted sequences, DWI; **Fig. 26.36B**) and for small infarcts (**Fig. 26.37**). MRI also clearly demonstrates the extent and anatomy of an infarct and shows evidence of clinically silent simultaneous infarcts that indicate an embolic cause. MRI can also help identify the underlying cause, e.g. arterial dissection using specific sequences to show the false lumen (**crescent sign**) or venous cortical infarcts. Many stroke mimics, such as demyelination, are shown with MRI but not CT. For these reasons, MRI is increasingly used in routine assessment of stroke and is essential in younger patients or in those where the cause is uncertain.

- **Vascular imaging** by carotid Doppler within 24 hours is essential to identify high-grade symptomatic carotid stenosis requiring surgery. CT or MR angiography is now widely used to corroborate the results of Doppler, to identify arterial stenosis in the posterior circulation or intracranial vessels that are not visible on Doppler, and also to identify arterial dissection and venous sinus thrombosis. Catheter angiography is rarely needed following ischaemic stroke.

ℹ️ Box 26.36 Stroke investigations

Immediate urgent investigations
Ideally within 1 hour of presentation
- CT brain scan
- Blood count and glucose (and clotting studies if anticoagulated)

Further investigations
(Within 24 h)
- Routine blood tests – blood count, erythrocyte sedimentation rate, glucose, clotting studies, lipids
- Electrocardiography (ECG) and later 24-h ECG for atrial fibrillation
- Carotid Doppler studies (in patients with anterior circulation stroke fit for surgery)

In addition
In selected patients, e.g. young stroke or no cause identified
- CT or MR angiography
- MRI brain scan with dissection protocol
- Echocardiogram (consider transoesophageal echocardiography)
- Prolonged cardiac monitoring for paroxysmal atrial fibrillation in cryptogenic stroke, e.g. implantable loop recorder
- Vasculitis screen
- Antiphospholipid antibodies
- Thrombophilia screen
- Other: genetics for CADASIL and mitochondrial disorders; alpha-galactosidase for Fabry's disease; drugs of abuse screen, e.g. cocaine

---

CADASIL, cerebral dominant arteriopathy with subcortical infarcts and leukoencephalopathy

Cardiac investigations

Identification of a cardio-embolic source of stroke, principally atrial fibrillation, is achieved with electrocardiography (ECG) or 24-hour ECG. Other causes, such as valve disease, patent foramen ovale or mural thrombus, require transthoracic echocardiography, or trans-oesophageal echo in selected patients. Recent research has shown that prolonged cardiac monitoring (e.g. with an implantable loop recorder) demonstrates paroxysmal atrial fibrillation in a significant minority of people with stroke of unknown cause.

Other investigations

In young patients with stroke or in those individuals where there is no evidence of atherosclerosis or an embolic source, more specialist investigations may be required to look for an underlying vasculitic, inflammatory, infective, metabolic or genetic cause (see **Box 26.36**).

Acute stroke: immediate care and thrombolysis

(See **Box 26.37**.) Stroke is a medical emergency. Paramedics and members of the public are encouraged to make the diagnosis of stroke on a simple history and examination – **FAST**:
Face – sudden weakness of the face
Arm – sudden weakness of one or both arms
Speech – difficulty speaking, slurred speech
Time – the sooner treatment can be started, the better.

During initial assessment, immediate, continued and meticulous attention to the airway, blood pressure and swallowing is essential. Management of unconscious or stuporose patients is outlined on page 832.

Thrombolysis

Thrombolysis significantly increases the chances of having no or minimal disability after stroke, by reducing infarct size (**Figs 26.38** and **26.39**; **Box 26.38**). Earlier treatment within the 4.5-hour time window significantly improves outcome, *so every minute counts*.

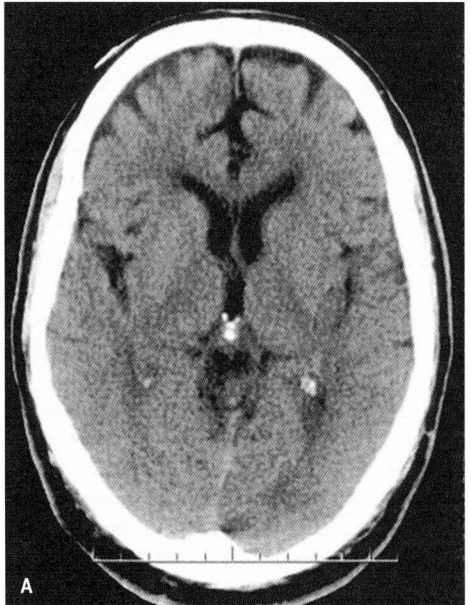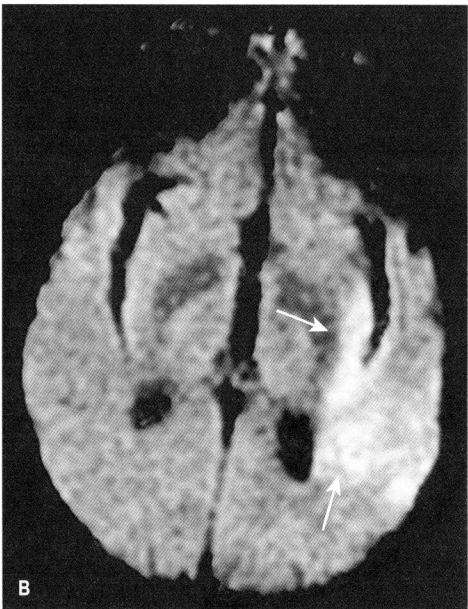

Fig. 26.36 Acute stroke seen on computed tomography (CT) scan with corresponding magnetic resonance imaging (MRI) appearance. **(A)** CT may show no evidence of early infarction. **(B)** A corresponding image seen on MRI diffusion-weighted imaging (DWI) with changes of infarction in the middle cerebral artery (MCA) territory (arrows). *(Reproduced from Ralston SH, Penman ID, Strachan MWJ et al. Davidson's Principles and Practice of Medicine, 23rd edn. Edinburgh: Elsevier; 2018. Fig. 26.4.)*

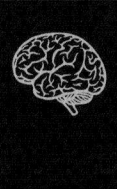

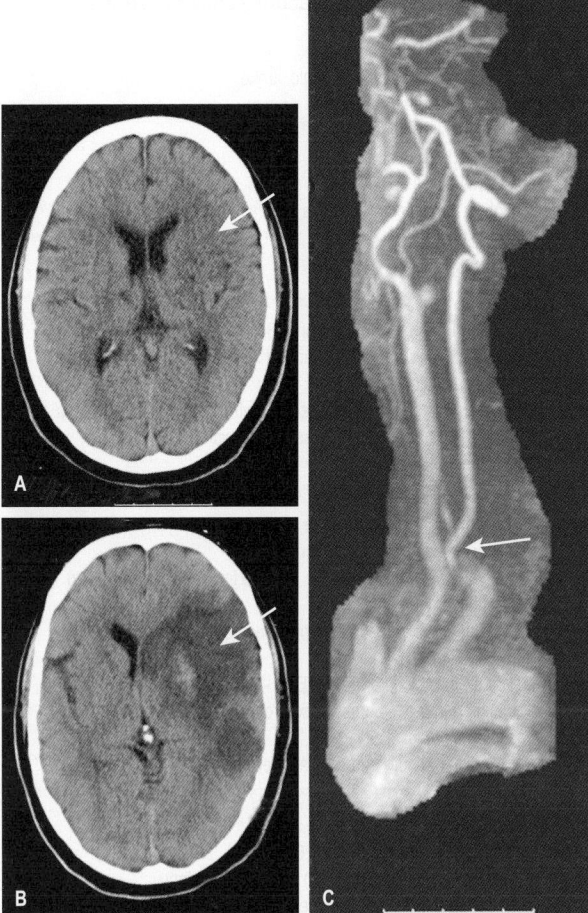

Fig. 26.37 CT imaging of cerebral infarction and subsequent magnetic resonance angiography performed in the same patient. (A) Early changes (arrowed). **(B)** Changes after 5 days (arrowed). **(C)** Magnetic resonance angiography showing internal carotid artery occlusion (arrowed). *(Courtesy of Dr Paul Jarman.)*

Approximately 10% of patients are potential candidates for thrombolysis, most being excluded due to late presentation outside the time window for treatment. Two recent studies have shown benefit, with a low complication rate, from endovascular therapy (usually performed with retrievable stents) following alteplase therapy. In both studies, patients with proximal vessel occlusion and salvageable brain tissue were selected, with improved function and reduced mortality after treatment.

In a recent meta-analysis of five trials, endovascular thrombectomy has been shown to benefit most patients with an acute stroke caused by occlusion of the proximal anterior circulation. Currently thrombectomy is performed routinely for selected cases in a number of centres.

Antiplatelet therapy and anticoagulation

High-dose aspirin (300 mg) is started 24 hours after thrombolysis, or as soon as haemorrhage is excluded if thrombolysis is contraindicated, and continued for 2 weeks before switching to clopidogrel. The number needed to treat (NNT) to prevent one stroke is 100.

Anticoagulants are started for atrial fibrillation-associated cardio-embolic stroke usually after 2 weeks to reduce the risk of acute haemorrhagic transformation of infarcts (NNT = 12). For arterial dissection, the risk of recurrent embolic stroke from the site of dissection is considered to be high enough to justify immediate

---

Box 26.37 Stroke management outline

1. Immediate general medical measures:
   - Airway: confirm patency and monitor
   - Continue care of the unconscious or stuporose patient
   - Give oxygen by mask
   - Monitor blood pressure
2. Is thrombolysis appropriate?
   - If so (see **Box 26.38**), *immediate* brain imaging is essential
3. Brain imaging:
   - CT should always be available; this will indicate haemorrhage, other pathology and sometimes infarction
4. Cerebral infarction
   - If CT excludes haemorrhage, give immediate thrombolytic therapy.
   - Give aspirin 300 mg/day if thrombolytic therapy is contraindicated
5. Cerebral haemorrhage:
   - If CT shows haemorrhage, give no drugs that could interfere with clotting; neurosurgery may occasionally be needed
6. Admit to multidisciplinary stroke unit:
   - Assess swallowing
   - Start thromboembolism prophylaxis
   - Treat medical complications, e.g. infection, hyperglycaemia, atrial fibrillation
   - Investigate for cause and risk factors (see **Box 26.36**)
   - Arrange early therapy input (physiotherapy, occupational therapy, speech and language therapy)
   - Initiate secondary prevention measures
   - Give lifestyle advice – smoking cessation, weight reduction
7. Rehabilitation – specialized unit or community

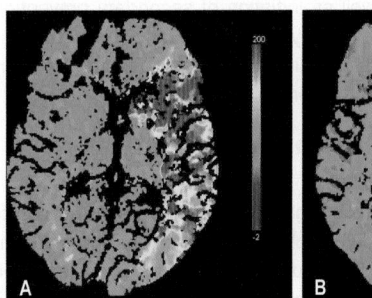
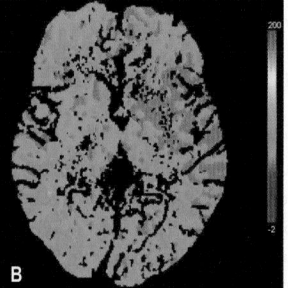

Fig. 26.38 CT perfusion scans. (A) Pre-thrombolysis. **(B)** Post-thrombolysis showing reperfusion of the ischaemic site. *(Courtesy of Professor Adrian Dixon, Cambridge Radiology Department, UK.)*

anticoagulation or antiplatelet therapy, although controlled trial evidence is lacking. Venous sinus or cortical vein thrombosis causing stroke is also treated with anticoagulation. In addition to warfarin for oral anticoagulation, direct oral anticoagulants (DOACs; see p. 1061) that inhibit factor Xa or thrombin are now available. They have the advantage over warfarin of a wider therapeutic index with a lower rate of haemorrhage, no need for monitoring and few drug interactions.

Decompressive craniectomy

This should be performed within 48 hours in MCA strokes causing infarction of more than 50% of the MCA territory to prevent coning and improve long-term outcome (see p. 840).

Stroke units

Direct admission to a stroke unit has been demonstrated to be one of the most effective interventions in acute stroke, saving lives and reducing long-term disability. Specialized multidisciplinary

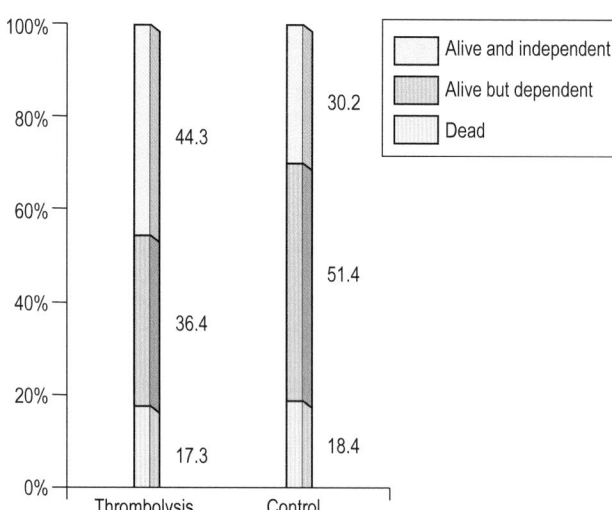

Fig. 26.39 Risk of death, dependency and good functional outcome in randomized trials of tissue plasminogen activator rt-PA given within 3 hours of acute stroke. *(Data from Stroke Module,* Cochrane Database of Systematic Reviews. *Cochrane Collaboration issue 4, 1999.)*

teams and clear protocols for aspects of care, such as swallowing assessment, thromboembolism prevention, treatment of infections, management of hyperglycaemia and other medical complications, improve quality and consistency of care, and thus outcomes. Early mobilization and access to physiotherapy, occupational therapy and speech therapy, as well as initiation of secondary prevention and patient education, are equally necessary. Early supported discharge and assessment of rehabilitation needs are also better coordinated on a stroke unit than a general ward.

Secondary prevention interventions

Antihypertensive therapy

Recognition and good control of high blood pressure are the major factors in primary and secondary stroke prevention. Transient hypertension, often seen following stroke, usually does not require treatment, provided diastolic pressure does not rise above 100 mmHg. Sustained severe hypertension needs treatment after 72 hours (see p. 1144); blood pressure should be lowered slowly to avoid any sudden fall in perfusion.

Lipid-lowering therapy

Statins, typically atorvastatin 40 mg, should be offered to all patients unless there is a contraindication, aiming for a target total cholesterol below 4 mmol/L (low-density lipoprotein <2 mmol/L).

Lifestyle modification and education

Education of patient and family is an essential aspect of secondary prevention. Smoking cessation and advice about diet, exercise, weight reduction and alcohol consumption should be started on the stroke unit and continued after discharge.

Surgery and stenting for carotid stenosis

High-grade symptomatic carotid stenosis is associated with a significant risk of recurrent stroke during the weeks after TIA or stroke. Carotid endarterectomy should be performed within 2 weeks in patients with 70–99% stenosis on the affected side, provided the initial stroke was not severely disabling. A second imaging modality, such as CT angiography, should be performed to confirm the results of Doppler studies. For patients with moderate symptomatic

Box 26.38 Thrombolysis in acute ischaemic stroke

Eligibility
- Clinical diagnosis of acute ischaemic stroke
- Assessment by experienced team
- Persisting neurological deficit
- Imaging excludes haemorrhage
- Timing of onset well established
- Thrombolysis should commence as soon as possible and up to 4.5 h after acute stroke

Exclusion criteria

Historical
- Stroke or head trauma within the prior 3 months
- Any prior history of intracranial haemorrhage
- Major surgery within 14 days
- Gastrointestinal or genitourinary bleeding within the previous 21 days
- Arterial puncture at a non-compressible site within 7 days
- Lumbar puncture within 7 days

Clinical
- Rapidly improving stroke syndrome
- Minor and isolated neurological signs
- Seizure at the onset of stroke if the residual impairments are due to post-ictal phenomena
- Symptoms suggestive of subarachnoid haemorrhage, even if the CT is normal
- Persistent systolic blood pressure (BP) >185, diastolic BP >110 mmHg, or requiring aggressive therapy to control BP
- Pregnancy
- Active bleeding or acute trauma (fracture)

Laboratory
- Platelets <100 000/mm³
- Serum glucose <2.8 mmol/L or >26.2 mmol/L
- International Normalized Ratio (INR) >1.7 if on warfarin
- Elevated partial thromboplastin time if on heparin

Dose of i.v. alteplase (tissue plasminogen activator)
- Total dose 0.9 mg/kg (max. 90 mg)
- 10% of total dose by initial i.v. bolus over 1 min
- Remainder infused intravenously over 60 min

ªSee Figure 21.38.

stenosis (50–69%), there is a modest benefit with intervention over the 3% stroke risk associated with the procedure itself. Carotid stenting is an alternative to surgery in some patients (major stroke risk is the same for surgery and stenting, but the chance of minor non-disabling stroke is higher for stenting).

The case for intervention in asymptomatic stenosis is debatable. Patients with 70–99% stenosis may have a modest stroke risk reduction at 5 years, but moderate stenosis should be treated conservatively. Screening asymptomatic individuals for carotid stenosis is not helpful. Carotid occlusion is always treated conservatively (there is no risk of distal embolization).

Stroke in the elderly

Thrombolysis is not contraindicated. Age is no barrier to recovery; elderly patients benefit from good rehabilitation. Consider social isolation, pre-existing cognitive impairment, nutrition, and skin and sphincter care, and reassess swallowing. Carotid endarterectomy over 75 years of age confers greater risk reduction than in younger patients.

Rehabilitation: multidisciplinary approach

Physiotherapy has particular value in the first few weeks after stroke to relieve spasticity, prevent contractures and teach patients to use walking aids. The benefits of physiotherapy for longer-term outcome

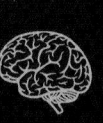

are still inadequately researched. Baclofen and/or botulinum toxin are sometimes helpful in the management of severe spasticity.

Speech and language therapists have a vital understanding of aphasic patients' problems and frustration. Return of speech is hastened by conversation generally. If swallowing is unsafe because of the risk of aspiration, either nasogastric feeding or percutaneous gastrostomy will be needed. Video-fluoroscopy while attempting to swallow is helpful.

Physiotherapy, occupational and speech therapy have a vital role in assessing and facilitating the future care pathway. Stroke is frequently devastating and, particularly during working life, radically alters the patient's remaining years. Many become unemployable, lose independence and are financially embarrassed. Loss of self-esteem makes depression common.

At home, aids and alterations may be needed: stair and bath rails, portable lavatories, hoists, sliding boards, wheelchairs, tripods, stair lifts, electric blinds and modified sleeping arrangements, kitchen, steps, flooring and doorways. Liaison between hospital-based and community care teams, and primary care physician, is essential.

Prognosis

About 25% of patients die within 2 years of a stroke, nearly 10% within the first month (see **Fig. 26.39**). This early mortality is higher following intracranial haemorrhage than ischaemic stroke. Poor outcome is likely when there is coma, a defect in conjugate gaze and hemiplegia. Many complications, such as aspiration or pressure ulcers, are preventable, particularly in the elderly. Coordinated care reduces deaths.

Recurrent strokes are, however, common (10% in the first year) and many patients die subsequently from myocardial infarction. Of initial stroke survivors, some 30–40% remain alive at 3 years.

Gradual improvement usually follows stroke, with a plateau in recovery after 12 months. One-third of survivors return to independent mobility and one-third have disability requiring institutional care.

Further reading

Bonati LH, Dobson J, Featherstone RL et al. Long-term outcomes after stenting versus endarterectomy for treatment of symptomatic carotid stenosis: the International Carotid Stenting Study (ICSS) randomised trial. *Lancet* 2015; 385:529–538.
Campbell BCV. Endovascular therapy for ischaemic stroke with perfusion imaging selection. *N Engl J Med* 2015; 372:1009–1018.
Furlan AJ. Endovascular therapy for stroke – it's about time. *N Engl J Med* 2015; 372:2347–2349.
Goyal M, Demchuk AM, Menon BK et al. Randomised assessment of rapid endovascular treatment of ischaemic stroke. *N Engl J Med* 2015; 372:1019–1030.
Goyal M, Menon BK, van Zwam WH et al. Endovascular thrombectomy of large vessel ischaemic stroke: a meta-analysis of individual patient data from five randomised trials. *Lancet* 2016; 387:1723–31.
IST-3 Collaborative Group. The benefits and harms of intravenous thrombolysis with recombinant tissue plasminogen activator within 6 h of acute ischaemic stroke (the third International Stroke Trial [IST-3]): a randomised controlled trial. *Lancet* 2012; 379:2352–2363.
Jüttler E, Unterberg A, Woitzik J et al. Hemicraniectomy in older patients with extensive middle-cerebral-artery stroke. *N Engl J Med* 2014; 370:1091–1100.
Langhorne P, Bernhardt J, Kwakkel G. Stroke rehabilitation. *Lancet* 2011; 377:1693–1702.
Qureshi AI, Caplan LR. Intracranial atherosclerosis. *Lancet* 2014; 383:984–998.
Rothwell PM, Algra A, Amarenco P. Medical treatment in acute and long-term secondary prevention after transient ischaemic attack and ischaemic stroke. *Lancet* 2011; 377:1681–1692.
Wechsler LR. Intravenous thrombolytic therapy for acute ischemic stroke. *N Engl J Med* 2011; 364:2138–2146.

INTRACRANIAL HAEMORRHAGE

This comprises:

- intracerebral and cerebellar haemorrhage
- subarachnoid haemorrhage
- subdural and extradural haemorrhage/haematoma.

Intracerebral haemorrhage
Aetiology

Intracerebral haemorrhage causes approximately 10% of strokes. It is associated with a higher mortality than ischaemic stroke (up to 50%). A large haematoma may act as a space-occupying lesion, causing raised intracranial pressure with brain displacement and herniation. Aetiology includes:

- **Hypertension.** Rupture of microaneurysms (Charcot–Bouchard aneurysms, 0.8–1.0 mm in diameter) and degeneration of small, deep, penetrating arteries are the principal pathologies. Such haemorrhage is usually massive, often fatal, and occurs in chronic hypertension and at well-defined sites: basal ganglia, pons, cerebellum and subcortical white matter. Vasopressor drugs, such as cocaine, may cause haemorrhage. Alcohol is also a risk factor (probably as a result of impaired coagulation/platelet function).
- **Cerebral amyloid angiopathy (CAA).** Deposition of amyloid-β in the walls of small and medium-sized arteries in normotensive patients, particularly over 60 years, causes *lobar* intracerebral haemorrhage (especially posterior, i.e. occipital/parietal lobes), which is often recurrent. CAA is associated with particular apolipoprotein E genotypes (E2) and is more common in patients with Alzheimer's disease. Cerebral microbleeds are usually seen on MRI sequences sensitive to haemosiderin deposition. CAA may occasionally cause TIA-like, transient neurological symptoms.
- **Secondary.** Arteriovenous malformations, cavernomas, aneurysms and dural venous thrombosis cause around 20% of intracerebral haemorrhages. Coagulopathies, anticoagulants and thrombolysis may cause haemorrhage. Haemorrhagic transformation of a large ischaemic infarct may sometimes present as a haemorrhage.

Clinical features and investigations

At the bedside, there is no entirely reliable way of distinguishing between haemorrhage and ischaemic infarcts. Intracerebral haemorrhage is more often associated with severe headache or coma. Patients on oral anticoagulants should be assumed to have had a haemorrhage unless it is proved otherwise.

Brain haemorrhage is seen on CT imaging immediately (compare infarction; see p. 843) as intraparenchymal, intraventricular or subarachnoid blood. Routine MRI may not identify an acute small haemorrhage reliably in the first few hours. MRI and MR angiography are necessary to identify underlying vascular malformations such as AVMs or aneurysms. Catheter angiography may be required in selected patients with no obvious risk factors or no underlying cause identified on imaging.

Management of haemorrhagic stroke
Medical

Treatment should be on a stroke unit or a neurological intensive care unit. Frequent monitoring of GCS and neurological signs is essential, as neurosurgery may be required. Antiplatelet drugs are, of course, contraindicated. Anticoagulation should be rapidly reversed where possible (for patients on warfarin give intravenous vitamin K and clotting factor concentrates). Control of hypertension is vital with intravenous drugs in an intensive care unit setting for systolic blood pressure higher than 180 mmHg. Measures to reduce intracranial pressure may be required, including mechanical ventilation and mannitol. Recombinant activated factor VII administration may prevent haematoma expansion but has not yet been shown to improve outcome.

Surgical

Cerebellar haematomas may cause obstructive hydrocephalus or coma due to brainstem compression; urgent neurosurgical clot

Box 26.39 Underlying causes of subarachnoid haemorrhage

Cause	(%)
Saccular (berry) aneurysms	70%
Arteriovenous malformation (AVM)	10%
No arterial lesion found	15%
Rare associations	<5%
Bleeding disorders	
Mycotic aneurysms – endocarditis	
Acute bacterial meningitis	
Tumours, e.g. metastatic melanoma, oligodendroglioma	
Arteritis (e.g. systemic lupus erythematosus)	
Spinal AVM → spinal subarachnoid haemorrhage	
Coarctation of the aorta	
Marfan or Ehlers–Danlos syndromes	
Adult polycystic kidney disease	

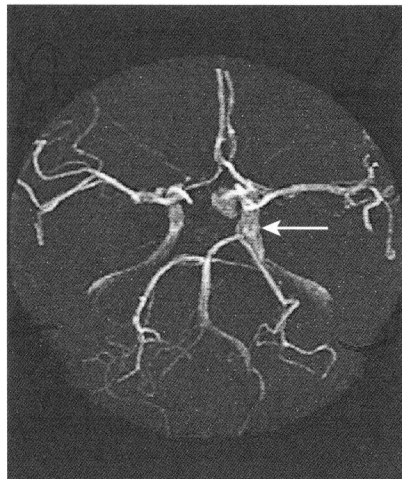

Fig. 26.40 Digital subtraction angiogram: posterior communicating artery aneurysm.

evacuation is lifesaving (and is required where the haematoma is >3 cm or the patient is drowsy or deteriorating). The role of surgical decompression for non-cerebellar bleeds is less clear-cut and liaison with neurosurgeons is vital. Use of minimally invasive surgical techniques to evacuate haematomas is an area of active research. Placement of an external ventricular drain is needed if obstructive hydrocephalus develops; for example, with extension of the haemorrhage into the ventricular system.

Subarachnoid haemorrhage

Subarachnoid haemorrhage (SAH) means spontaneous arterial bleeding into the subarachnoid space, and is usually clearly recognizable clinically from its dramatic onset. SAH accounts for some 5% of strokes and has an annual incidence of 6 per 100000.

Aetiology

The causes of SAH are shown in **Box 26.39**; it is unusual to find any contributing disease.

Saccular (berry) aneurysms

Saccular aneurysms (**Fig. 26.40**) develop within the circle of Willis and adjacent arteries. Common sites are at arterial junctions:

- between posterior communicating and internal carotid artery – posterior communicating artery aneurysm
- between anterior communicating and anterior cerebral artery – anterior communicating and anterior cerebral artery aneurysm
- at the trifurcation or a bifurcation of the middle cerebral artery – middle cerebral artery aneurysm.

Other aneurysm sites are on the basilar, posterior inferior cerebellar, intracavernous internal carotid and ophthalmic arteries. Saccular aneurysms are an incidental finding in 1% of autopsies and can be multiple.

Aneurysms cause symptoms either by spontaneous rupture, when there is usually no preceding history, or by direct pressure on surrounding structures; for example, an enlarging unruptured posterior communicating artery aneurysm is the most common cause of a painful IIIrd nerve palsy (see p. 813).

Arteriovenous malformation

Arteriovenous malformation (AVM) is a vascular developmental malformation, often with a fistula between arterial and venous systems, causing high flow through the AVM and high-pressure arterialization of draining veins. An AVM usually presents following a spontaneous intracerebral haemorrhage or with a seizure, often focal in

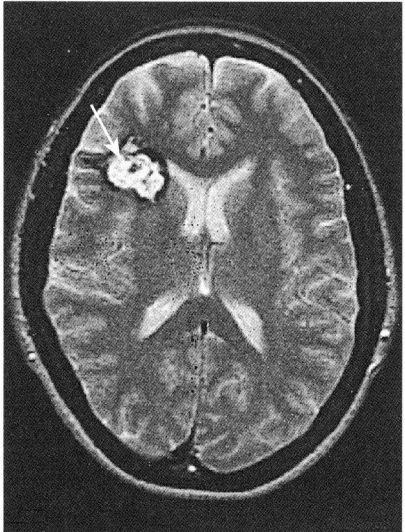

Fig. 26.41 Magnetic resonance T2-weighted image: symptomless frontal cavernoma (arrowed).

onset. The risk of a first haemorrhage in unruptured AVMs (20% fatal and 30% resulting in permanent disability) is approximately 2–3% per year. Once an AVM has caused a haemorrhage, the risk of rebleeds is increased to approximately 10% per year. AVMs may be ablated with endovascular treatment (catheter injection of glue into the nidus, usually), microsurgery or stereotactic radiotherapy. A multidisciplinary team approach with neurologist, interventional neuroradiologist and neurosurgeon is required in deciding on treatment options. There is no clear consensus on the best treatment modality or, indeed, whether the considerable risk of intervention is lower than with a conservative approach.

Cavernous haemangiomas (cavernomas) are common (0.1–0.5% prevalence) and consist of a tangle of low-pressure dilated vessels without a major feeding artery; they are frequently symptomless (**Fig. 26.41**) and seen incidentally on imaging. Multiple cavernomas often have a genetic basis. Cavernomas may cause seizures. Small haemorrhages may occur but are usually low-pressure bleeds and rarely cause severe deficits. Surgical resection is rarely needed, except where the cavernoma is gradually enlarging or causing significant neurological symptoms.

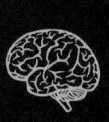

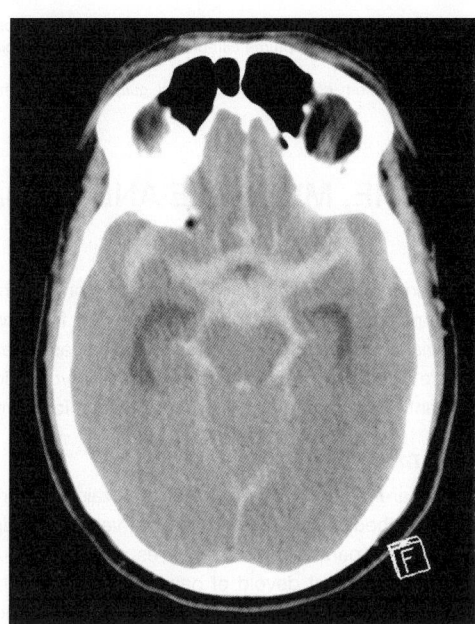

Fig. 26.42 Subarachnoid haemorrhage. Axial, non-contrast CT showing blood filling the basal cisterns around the brainstem.

Clinical features of subarachnoid haemorrhage

There is a sudden, very severe headache, often occipital (mean time to peak headache 3 min). Headache is usually followed by vomiting and often by coma and death. Survivors of SAH may remain comatose or drowsy for hours, days or longer. SAH is a *possible* diagnosis in any sudden headache.

Following major SAH, there is neck stiffness and a positive Kernig's sign. Papilloedema is sometimes present, with retinal and/or subhyaloid haemorrhage (tracking beneath the retinal hyaloid membrane). Minor bleeds cause few signs but almost invariably do cause headache (approximately 17% of patients have small 'sentinel bleeds' in the weeks before presenting with SAH).

Investigations

CT imaging is the immediate investigation (**Fig. 26.42**). Subarachnoid and/or intraventricular blood is usually seen (sensitivity of CT to detect subarachnoid blood is 95% within 24 hours of onset but much lower over subsequent days). Lumbar puncture is not necessary if SAH is confirmed by CT, but should be performed if doubt remains. CSF becomes yellow (xanthochromic) within 12 hours of SAH and remains detectable for 2 weeks. Visual inspection of supernatant CSF is usually sufficiently reliable for diagnosis. Spectrophotometry to estimate bilirubin in the CSF released from lysed cells is used to define SAH with certainty. CT angiography or catheter angiography to identify the aneurysm or other source of bleeding is performed in patients potentially fit for surgery. In some, no aneurysm or source of bleeding is found, despite a definite SAH.

Differential diagnosis

SAH must be differentiated from migraine. This is sometimes difficult but a short time to maximal headache intensity and the presence of neck stiffness usually indicate SAH. **Thunderclap headache** is used (confusingly) to describe either SAH or a sudden (benign) headache for which no cause is ever found. The syndrome of reversible cerebral vasoconstriction (Call–Fleming's syndrome) presents with thunderclap headache. Acute bacterial meningitis occasionally causes a very

abrupt headache, when a meningeal microabscess ruptures; SAH also occasionally occurs at the onset of acute bacterial meningitis. Cervical arterial dissection can present with a sudden headache.

Complications

Blood in the subarachnoid space can lead to obstructive hydrocephalus, seen on CT. Hydrocephalus can be asymptomatic but may cause deteriorating consciousness following SAH. Shunting may be necessary. Arterial spasm (visible on angiography and a cause of coma or hemiparesis) is a serious complication of SAH and a poor prognostic feature.

Management

Immediate treatment of SAH involves bed rest and supportive measures. Hypertension should be controlled. Nimodipine, a calcium-channel blocker given for 3 weeks, reduces mortality.

All SAH cases should be discussed urgently with a neurosurgical centre. Nearly half of SAH cases are either dead or moribund before reaching hospital. Of the remainder, a further 10–20% rebleed and die within weeks. Failure to diagnose SAH – for example, mistaking SAH for migraine – contributes to this mortality.

Where angiography demonstrates an aneurysm (the cause of the vast majority of SAHs), endovascular treatment by placing platinum coils via a catheter in the aneurysm sac, to promote thrombosis and ablation of the aneurysm, is now the first-line treatment. Endovascular coiling has a lower complication rate than surgery but direct surgical clipping of the aneurysm neck is still required in some selected cases. For asymptomatic (unruptured) aneurysms over 8 mm in diameter, the risk of treatment is less than the risk of haemorrhage if not treated. Patients who remain comatose or who have persistent severe deficits after SAH have a poor outlook.

Subdural and extradural bleeding

These conditions can cause death following head injuries unless treated promptly.

Subdural haematoma

Subdural haematoma (SDH) means accumulation of blood in the subdural space following rupture of a vein. This usually follows a head injury, sometimes a trivial one. The interval between injury and symptoms can be days, or may extend to weeks or months. Chronic, apparently spontaneous, SDH is common in the elderly, and also occurs with anticoagulants.

Headache, drowsiness and confusion are common; symptoms are indolent and can fluctuate. Focal deficits, such as hemiparesis or sensory loss, develop. Epilepsy occasionally occurs. Stupor, coma and coning may follow.

Extradural haemorrhage

Extradural haemorrhage (EDH) typically follows a linear skull vault fracture tearing a branch of the middle meningeal artery. Extradural blood accumulates rapidly over minutes or hours. A characteristic picture is that of a head injury with a brief duration of unconsciousness, followed by improvement (the lucid interval). The patient then becomes stuporose; there is an ipsilateral dilated pupil and contralateral hemiparesis, with rapid transtentorial coning. Bilateral fixed, dilated pupils, tetraplegia and respiratory arrest follow. An acute progressive SDH presents similarly.

Management

Possible extradural or subdural bleeding needs immediate imaging. CT (**Fig. 26.43A**) is the most widely used investigation because of

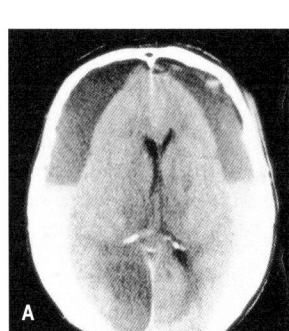
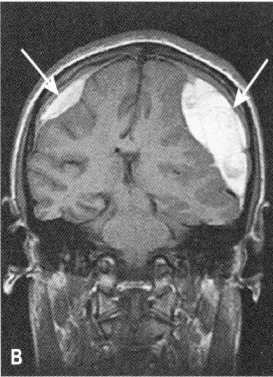

Fig. 26.43 **Bilateral subdural haematomas. (A)** CT scan. **(B)** Magnetic resonance T1-weighted image.

its immediate availability. MRI is more sensitive for the detection of small haematomas. T1-weighted MRI (**Fig. 26.43B**) shows bright images due to the presence of methaemoglobin.

EDHs *require urgent neurosurgery*; if it is performed early, the outlook is excellent. When the patient is far from a neurosurgeon, such as in wartime or at sea, drainage through skull burr holes has been lifesaving when an EDH has been diagnosed clinically.

Subdural bleeding usually needs less immediate attention but close neurosurgical liaison is necessary. Even large collections can resolve spontaneously without drainage. Serial imaging is required to assess progress.

Cortical venous thrombosis and dural venous sinus thrombosis

Intracranial venous thromboses are usually (>50%) associated with a prothrombotic risk factor, such as oral contraceptives, pregnancy, genetic or acquired prothrombotic states, and dehydration. Head injury is also a cause. Infection, such as from a paranasal sinus, may be present. Venous thromboses can also arise spontaneously.

Cortical venous thrombosis

The venous infarct leads to headache, focal signs (e.g. hemiparesis) and/or seizures. Cortical haemorrhagic infarction is shown on MRI.

Dural venous sinus thromboses

Cavernous sinus thrombosis causes eye pain, fever, proptosis and chemosis. External and internal ophthalmoplegia with papilloedema develops.

Thrombosis of the dural venous sinuses, such as when the sagittal sinus causes raised intracranial pressure with headache, papilloedema and frequently seizures, may progress to coma.

Management

MRI and MR venography (MRV) show occluded sinuses and/or veins. Treatment is with heparin initially, followed by warfarin or other oral anticoagulants for 6 months. Anticonvulsants are given if necessary.

Further reading

Knopman J, Stieg PE. Management of unruptured brain arteriovenous malformations. *Lancet* 2014; 383:581–583.
Mendelow AD, Gregson BA, Rowan EN et al; STICH II Investigators. Early surgery versus initial conservative treatment in patients with spontaneous supratentorial lobar intracerebral haematomas (STICH II): a randomised trial. *Lancet* 2013; 382:397–408.

Molyneaux AJ, Birks J, Clarke A et al. The durability of endovascular coiling versus neurosurgical clipping of ruptured cerebral aneurysms: 18-year follow-up. *Lancet* 2015; 385:691–697.
http://www.bestpractice.bmj.com. *BMJ best practice guidelines for haemorrhagic stroke.*

HEADACHE, MIGRAINE AND FACIAL PAIN

Headache is an almost universal experience and one of the most common symptoms in medical practice. It varies from an infrequent and trivial nuisance to a pointer to serious disease. Headache symptoms are unpleasant, disabling and common worldwide, and have a substantial economic impact because of time lost from work.

Mechanisms

Pain receptors are located at the base of the brain in arteries and veins, and throughout meninges, extracranial vessels, scalp, neck and facial muscles, paranasal sinuses, eyes and teeth. Curiously, brain substance is almost devoid of pain receptors. Head pain is mediated by the Vth and IXth cranial nerves and upper cervical sensory roots.

Clinical approach to the patient with headache

In assessing patients with headache, the aim should be to make a confident diagnosis based on the history. Examination is helpful in excluding underlying medical disorders as a cause of headache but will not distinguish between different types of primary headache.

There is an internationally agreed classification for headaches that defines all headache patterns. Headache is divided into primary headache disorders such as migraine, and secondary headaches due to underlying pathology such as raised intracranial pressure or meningitis (**Box 26.40**). It is also useful to distinguish between episodic (recurrent) headache, single first headache episodes and patients with chronic headache.

In an outpatient clinic setting, most headaches will be benign. Fewer than 1% of outpatients with non-acute headache have a serious underlying cause but in the emergency department there will be a much higher prevalence of serious underlying pathology presenting with headache. New-onset severe headache in those without a previous headache history, especially in older patients (>50), requires exclusion of underlying pathology causing secondary headache.

There are some widely believed 'headache myths'. Headaches are not caused by hypertension, except rarely with malignant hypertension (see p. 1138). Eye strain from refractive error does not cause headache and sinusitis is rarely the explanation for recurrent or chronic headache.

Taking a history for 'headaches'

Ask about:
- Headache location (e.g. hemicranial), severity and character (e.g. throbbing versus non-throbbing).
- Associated symptoms, e.g. nausea, photophobia, phonophobia and motion sensitivity.
- Presence of autonomic symptoms, e.g. tearing or ptosis.
- Relieving or exacerbating features, e.g. effect of posture.
- Headache pattern: is headache episodic and part of a pattern of previous similar headaches? Age at onset and headache frequency.
- Duration of headache episodes (helpful in distinguishing between different primary headache types).

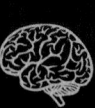

? Box 26.40 Some causes of secondary headache

- Raised intracranial pressure, e.g. idiopathic intracranial hypertension
- Infections, e.g. meningitis, sinusitis
- Giant cell arteritis
- Intracranial haemorrhage, esp. subarachnoid haemorrhage or subdural haematoma
- Low cerebrospinal fluid volume (low-pressure) headache
- Post-traumatic headache
- Cervicogenic headache
- Acute glaucoma

- Triggers.
- Pattern of analgesic use.
- Family history of headache.
- 'Red flag' symptoms: fever (meningitis, sinusitis).
- Sudden onset in less than 1 minute (SAH).
- Features of raised intracranial pressure.
- Jaw claudication (giant cell arteritis).

Examination

Examination should include fundoscopy to look for papilloedema. In older patients, temporal arteries should be palpated for loss of pulsatility and tenderness that may be features of giant cell arteritis (GCA). Fever and neck stiffness suggest meningitis. Examination is generally normal in patients with primary headache disorders.

Investigations

Investigations, including brain imaging, do not contribute to the diagnosis of primary headache disorders. Neuroimaging is indicated only where history or examination suggests an underlying secondary cause. Older patients with new-onset headache and those with 'red flag' symptoms should have brain CT. In patients over 50 with new headache, the ESR should be checked to exclude GCA.

Primary headache disorders

Migraine

Migraine is the most common cause of episodic headache (15–20% of women and 5–10% of men); in 90%, onset is before 40 years of age. Episodes of headache are associated with sensory sensitivity such as to light, sound or movement, and sometimes with nausea and vomiting. There is a spectrum of severity between individuals and from one attack to another. Migraine is usually high-impact, with inability to function normally during episodes. Headache frequency in migraine varies from an occasional inconvenience to frequent headaches severely impacting on quality of life, and may transform into chronic daily headache.

Mechanisms

Genetic factors play a part in causing the neuronal hyperexcitability that is probably the biological basis of migraine. Migraine is polygenic but a rare form of familial migraine is associated with mutations in the α-1 subunit of the P/Q-type voltage-gated calcium channel or neuronal sodium channel (*SCN1A*), and a dominant loss-of-function mutation in a potassium channel gene (*TRESK*) has been identified in some patients with migraine with aura.

The pathophysiology of migraine is now thought to have a primarily neurogenic rather than vascular basis. Spreading cortical depression – a wave of neuronal depolarization followed by depressed activity slowly spreading anteriorly across the cerebral

i Box 26.41 Migraine: simplified diagnostic criteria

Headache lasting 4 hours to 3 days (untreated)

At least two of:
- Unilateral pain (may become holocranial later in attack)
- Throbbing-type pain
- Moderate to severe intensity
- Motion sensitivity (headache made worse with head movement or physical activity)

At least one of:
- Nausea/vomiting
- Photophobia/phonophobia
- Normal examination and no other cause of headache

cortex from the occipital region – is thought to be the basis of the migraine aura. Activation of trigeminal pain neurones is the basis of the headache. The innervation of the large intracranial vessels and dura by the first division of the trigeminal nerve is known as the trigeminovascular system. Release of calcitonin gene-related peptide (CGRP), substance P and other vasoactive peptides, including 5-HT, by activated trigeminovascular neurones causes painful meningeal inflammation and vasodilation. Peripheral and central sensitization of trigeminal neurones and brainstem pain pathways makes otherwise innocuous sensory stimuli (such as CSF pulsation and head movement) painful, and light and sound are perceived as uncomfortable.

Clinical features

Migraine without aura

Migraine typically starts around puberty with increasing prevalence into the fourth decade. There is a spectrum of severity and associated features, but attacks have recognizable core features (**Box 26.41**). Most migraine attacks are usually of sufficient severity to prevent sufferers continuing with normal activities; sleep usually helps. A 'washed-out' feeling follows the attack. The scalp may be tender to touch during episodes (allodynia) and the preference is to be still in a dark, quiet environment.

Some patients recognize changes in routine as trigger factors:
- Sleep (too little or too much).
- Stress (including letdown after a period of stress).
- Hormonal factors for women – changes in oestrogen levels, e.g. menstrual migraine (usually just before menses) and worsening with the oral contraceptive pill and menopause.
- Eating – skipping meals and alcohol. Contrary to popular belief, individual foods are rarely a trigger.
- Other – sensory stimuli, such as bright lights or loud sounds; physical exertion; and changes in weather patterns, e.g. stormy weather. Minor head injuries may trigger a worsening of migraine frequency and severity.

Migraine with aura

Approximately 25% of migraine sufferers experience focal neurological symptoms immediately preceding the headache phase in some or all attacks; this is termed migraine aura. Most never experience aura, and the presence of aura is therefore not required for a diagnosis of migraine. Aura usually evolves over 5–20 minutes, with symptoms changing as the wave of spreading neuronal depression moves across the surface of the cortex. It rarely lasts longer than 60 minutes and is followed immediately by the headache phase.

Visual aura is the most common type, with positive visual symptoms such as shimmering, teichopsia (zigzag lines, also called fortification spectra) and fragmentation of the image (like looking through a pane of broken glass) often accompanied by patches of loss of vision, which may move across the visual field (scotomas) and even evolve into hemianopia or tunnel vision. Positive sensory symptoms (mainly tingling), dysphasia and, rarely, loss of motor function may also occur, and may occur successively within the same episode of aura following the visual symptoms.

Migraine aura usually presents no diagnostic difficulty, but problems with diagnosis may sometimes arise in men over the age of 50 who develop migraine aura for the first time without subsequent headache (sometimes referred to as acephalic migrainous aura). This is frequently misdiagnosed as a TIA (see p. 839). Distinguishing the two conditions is often difficult and relies on the characteristic evolution of symptoms over minutes and the presence of positive symptoms in aura, in contrast to TIA where symptom onset is acute and negative symptoms (visual loss as opposed to visual distortion and teichopsia) are the norm. There may also be a history of previous typical migraine aura in early adult life to help distinguish the conditions.

Migraine-related dizziness

Vertigo is now recognized as being a migrainous symptom in some individuals, with attacks lasting for hours in the context of migraine attacks. There is an overlap with what is sometimes described as basilar migraine, a poorly defined migraine subtype associated with brainstem aura-type symptoms before or during attacks, including perioral paraesthesiae, diplopia, unsteadiness and, rarely, reduced level of consciousness.

Hemiplegic migraine

This rare autosomal dominant disorder causes a hemiparesis and/or coma and headache, with recovery within 24 hours. Some patients have permanent cerebellar signs, as it is allelic with episodic ataxia. It is distinct from more common forms of migraine.

Management

General measures include:
- explanation
- avoidance of trigger factors and lifestyle modification where possible.

Acute treatment of attacks

Analgesics, such as high-dose dispersible aspirin (900 mg), paracetamol 1 g or an NSAID (e.g. naproxen 250–500 mg), are often effective, with an antiemetic such as metoclopramide if necessary. Acute treatment should be taken as soon as possible after onset of headache. Patients should be aware that repeated use of analgesics leads to further headaches (see medication overuse headache, p. 851).

Triptans (5-HT$_{1B/1D}$ agonists) are specific for migraine and may be effective where simple analgesics are insufficient. Sumatriptan was the first marketed; almotriptan, eletriptan, frovatriptan, naratriptan, rizatriptan and zolmitriptan are now available, with various routes of administration. Subcutaneous sumatriptan injection may be effective where vomiting prevents absorption of oral medication (note that nasal triptan sprays rely on gastrointestinal rather than nasal absorption). Triptans should be avoided when there is vascular disease, and like analgesics, they should not be overused. CGRP antagonists, e.g. telcagepant, are likely to be future effective therapy for migraine.

Migraine suppression medication

When migraine episodes are frequent (>1–2 per month, for example) and impacting on quality of life, migraine suppression medication should be offered. The key principles are that a period of 3–6 months' treatment is usually sufficient to reduce headache frequency and severity by approximately 50%, with the effect of 'resetting' migraine frequency beyond the treatment period. However, these medications will not be effective where ongoing analgesic overuse is an issue. Treatment options include:

- *Anticonvulsants.* Valproate (800 mg) or topiramate (100–200 mg daily) are generally the most effective options.
- *Beta-blockers*, e.g. propranolol slow-release 80–160 mg daily.
- *Tricyclics*, e.g. amitriptyline 10 mg, increasing weekly in 10 mg steps to 50–60 mg.
- *Candesartan.* Up to 16 mg daily.
- *Antidepressants*, e.g. venlafaxine up to 150 mg daily.
- *Botulinum toxin.* This was recommended as a treatment for chronic migraine (see p. 851). The technique involves 31 injections over the scalp and neck repeated every 3 months. Its effect is inconsistent.
- *Pizotifen.* This is rarely used. Flunarizine (a calcium antagonist) and methysergide are used in refractory patients.

Tension-type headache

The exact pathogenesis of tension-type headache (TTH) remains unclear. There is overlap with migraine, and many headaches traditionally subsumed under this category probably, in fact, represent mild migraine. Since there are no diagnostic tests to separate TTH from mild migraine it is difficult to know if the conditions are biologically distinct. In contrast to migraine, pain is usually of mild to moderate severity, bilateral and relatively featureless, with tight band sensations, pressure behind the eyes, and bursting sensations being described.

Depression is also a frequent co-morbid feature. TTH is often attributed to cervical spondylosis, refractive errors or high blood pressure; evidence for such associations is poor.

Simple analgesics are often effective but overuse should be avoided. Physical treatments, such as massage, ice packs and relaxation, are often recommended. Frequent or chronic TTH may respond to migraine suppression medications as above, with tricyclics often being used first-line.

Trigeminal autonomic cephalalgias

The trigeminal autonomic cephalalgias are a group of primary headache disorders characterized by unilateral trigeminal distribution pain (usually in the ophthalmic division of the nerve) and prominent ipsilateral autonomic features.

Cluster headache

Cluster headache is distinct from migraine and much rarer (1 per 1000). It affects adults, mostly males aged between 20 and 40. Patients describe recurrent bouts (clusters) of excruciating unilateral retro-orbital pain with parasympathetic autonomic activation in the same eye, causing redness or tearing of the eye, nasal congestion or even a transient Horner's syndrome. The pain is reputed to be the worst known to humans, and patients often contemplate, and sometimes commit, suicide, such is the severity of the pain. Unlike with migraine attacks, patients prefer to move about or rock rather than remain still.

Attacks are shorter than migraine, usually 30–90 minutes, and may occur several times per day, especially during sleep. Clusters last 1–2 months, with attacks most nights, before stopping completely and typically recurring a year or more later, often at the same time of year. Although the cause is not known, hypothalamic activation is seen on functional imaging studies during an attack.

Management. Analgesics are unhelpful. Subcutaneous suma-triptan is the drug of choice for acute treatment, as no other drug works quickly enough. High-flow oxygen is also used. Most prophylactic migraine drugs are unhelpful. Verapamil, lithium and/or a short course of steroids help terminate a bout of cluster headaches.

Paroxysmal hemicrania and SUNCT

Paroxysmal hemicrania is a rare condition with similarities to cluster headache, differing mainly in that attacks are briefer (10–30 min) and more frequent (>5 per day, at any time of day) and do not occur in clusters. Women are more often affected than men. There is a rapid and complete response to indometacin.

Short-lasting unilateral neuralgiform headache with conjunctival injection and tearing (SUNCT) is very rare. Attacks are short, 5 seconds to 2 minutes, and very frequently occur in bouts. Distinguishing SUNCT from trigeminal neuralgia can be difficult.

Other primary headache disorders

- *Primary stabbing headache* (*'ice pick headache'*) involves momentary jabs or stabs of localized pain occurring either in the same spot or moving about the head. Symptoms wax and wane, and are more common in patients with other primary headache disorders, particularly migraine. Treatment is usually not needed but this type of headache responds well to indometacin.
- *Primary cough headache* is a sudden, sharp head pain on coughing. No underlying cause is found but intracranial pathology should be excluded. The problem often resolves spontaneously. Indometacin is the treatment of choice; LP with removal of CSF can help.
- *Primary sex headache* is characterized by explosive headache at or before orgasm. It often resolves spontaneously after several attacks. Investigation to exclude SAH is required after the first episode.
- *Other varieties* of primary headache include hemicrania continua, primary exertional headache, hypnic headache (headache triggered by sleep) and primary thunderclap headache.

Chronic daily headache

This is defined as headache on 15 or more days per month for at least 3 months. Up to 4% of the population are affected by daily or near-daily headache. Although there are many possible causes, including secondary headache disorders, in practice, primary headache disorders, particularly migraine, are responsible for the majority. Where migraine is the cause, the term chronic migraine is now preferred.

Overuse of analgesic medication or triptans (termed *medication overuse headache*) is often a major factor leading to and maintaining chronicity, particularly in those with migrainous biology. Use of ten or more doses per month of any analgesic or triptan, particularly codeine or opiate-containing drugs such as co-codamol, or numerous over-the-counter analgesics, may eventually lead to transformation of episodic headache into chronic daily headache.

Explanation that medication overuse is part of the problem is essential to help patients withdraw from or substantially reduce analgesic intake. This is a difficult process for many patients, especially as there may be a period of transient rebound worsening of headache after withdrawal. Concurrent introduction of migraine suppression medication (see above) may help withdrawal but will not be effective if patients cannot withdraw from frequent analgesic use. Occasionally, hospital admission for analgesic withdrawal with parenteral administration of dihydroergotamine is required.

Secondary headache disorders

Raised intracranial pressure headache

Any headache present on waking and made worse by coughing, straining or sneezing may be due to raised intracranial pressure (ICP) caused by a mass lesion. Vomiting often accompanies pressure headaches. Visual obscurations (momentary bilateral visual loss with bending or coughing) are characteristic and seen in the presence of papilloedema. Occasionally, where ICP rises quickly, papilloedema may not be present.

Neuroimaging is mandatory if raised ICP is suspected. Where no mass lesion, venous sinus thrombosis or hydrocephalus is detected on imaging in the presence of papilloedema, idiopathic intracranial hypertension may be the cause and LP is performed to measure CSF opening pressure.

Idiopathic intracranial hypertension

Idiopathic intracranial hypertension (IIH) probably results from reduced CSF resorption. IIH typically develops in younger, overweight female patients, many of whom have polycystic ovaries. Headaches and transient visual obscurations due to the florid papilloedema are the presenting features. A VIth nerve palsy may develop – a false localizing sign (see p. 813). CSF pressure is very elevated, with normal constituents. Brain imaging is normal, although ventricles may be small and appear 'slit-like'.

Various drugs, such as tetracyclines, and vitamin A supplements have been implicated. Other causes of papilloedema should be excluded. Sagittal sinus thrombosis can cause a similar picture and should always be looked for on MR venography.

IIH is usually self-limiting. However, optic nerve damage can result from longstanding severe papilloedema with progressive loss of peripheral visual fields. Regular monitoring of visual fields with perimetry is essential. Repeated LP, acetazolamide and thiazide diuretics are used to reduce CSF production. Weight reduction is helpful. Ventriculoperitoneal shunt insertion or optic nerve sheath fenestration to protect vision is sometimes necessary.

Low-CSF-volume (low-pressure) headache

Although most often seen following LP, CSF leaks may occur spontaneously, leading to postural headache, worse on standing or sitting and relieved completely by lying flat. The patient may give a history of vigorous Valsalva, straining or coughing just prior to onset. Leptomeningeal enhancement may be seen on MRI but is not reliably present. LP is generally avoided for obvious reasons but may reveal low opening pressure. The site of the leak is usually within the spine; thus treatment consists of injection of autologous blood into the spinal epidural space to seal the leak (a 'blood patch'), or occasionally surgical repair of the dural tear. Intravenous caffeine infusion and bed rest are sometimes effective.

Post-traumatic headache

Pre-existing migraine may worsen following head injury. *De novo* headache sometimes follows a minor head injury but post-traumatic headache is an ill-defined entity. Improvement over a few weeks is the norm, but where litigation is ongoing, symptoms can persist for long periods. Subdural haematoma and low-pressure headache need to be considered as a possible cause.

Facial pain

The face has many pain-sensitive structures: teeth, gums, sinuses, temporomandibular joints, jaw and eyes. Dental causes are common and should always be considered. Facial pain is also caused by specific neurological conditions.

Trigeminal neuralgia

Trigeminal neuralgia typically starts in the sixth and seventh decades; hypertension is the main risk factor. Compression of the trigeminal nerve at or near the pons by an ectatic vascular loop is the usual cause. High-resolution MRI studies may demonstrate the vascular loop in contact with the nerve in a high proportion of cases. In younger patients, multiple sclerosis or a cerebellopontine angle tumour (acoustic schwannomas, meningiomas, epidermoids) is more likely to be the cause.

Clinical features

Paroxysms of knife-like or electric shock-like pain, lasting seconds, occur in the distribution of the Vth nerve. Pain tends to commence in the mandibular division (V_3) but may spread over time to involve the maxillary (V_2) and, occasionally, the ophthalmic divisions (V_1). Bilateral trigeminal neuralgia is rare (3%) and usually due to intrinsic brainstem pathology, such as demyelination. Episodes occur many times a day with a refractory period after each. They may be brought on by stimulation of one or more trigger zones in the face. Washing, shaving, a cold wind and chewing are examples of trivial stimuli that provoke pain. The face may be screwed up in agony. Spontaneous remissions last months or years before (almost invariable) recurrence. There are no signs of Vth nerve dysfunction on examination.

Management

Carbamazepine (600–1200 mg daily) reduces the severity of attacks in the majority. Oxcarbazepine, lamotrigine and gabapentin are also used. If drugs fail or are not tolerated, a number of surgical options are available that, in general, are more effective than medical treatments. Percutaneous radiofrequency selective ablation of the trigeminal ganglion is performed as a day-case procedure; recurrence may occur after an average of 2 years. Microvascular decompression of the nerve in the posterior fossa has a high long-term success rate (approximately 90%).

Atypical facial pain

Facial pain differs from trigeminal neuralgia in quality and distribution, and trigger points are absent. The condition is probably heterogeneous in aetiology but is believed by some (on little evidence) to be a somatic manifestation of depression. Tricyclic antidepressants and drugs used in neuropathic pain are sometimes helpful.

Other causes of facial pain

Facial pain occurs in the trigeminal autonomic cephalgias (see above), occasionally in migraine and in carotid dissection.

Giant cell arteritis (temporal arteritis)

A granulomatous large-vessel arteritis is seen almost exclusively in people over 50 (see p. 464).

Clinical features

- **Headache.** This is almost invariable in giant cell arteritis (GCA). Pain develops over inflamed superficial temporal and/or occipital arteries. Touching the skin over an inflamed vessel (e.g. when combing the hair) causes pain. Arterial pulsation is soon lost; the artery becomes hard, tortuous and thickened. The scalp over inflamed vessels may become red. Rarely, gangrenous patches appear.
- **Facial pain.** Pain in the face, jaw and mouth is caused by inflammation of facial, maxillary and lingual branches of the external carotid artery in GCA. Pain is characteristically worse on eating (jaw claudication). Mouth opening and protruding the tongue become difficult. A painful, ischaemic tongue occurs rarely.
- **Visual problems.** Visual loss from arterial inflammation and occlusion occurs in 25% of untreated cases. Posterior ciliary artery occlusion causes anterior ischaemic optic neuropathy in three-quarters of these. Other mechanisms are central retinal artery occlusion, cilioretinal artery occlusion and posterior ischaemic optic neuropathy. There is sudden monocular visual loss (partial or complete), usually painless. Amaurosis fugax (see p. 838) may precede permanent blindness.

When the posterior ciliary vessels are affected, ischaemic optic neuropathy causes the disc to become swollen and pale; retinal branch vessels usually remain normal. When the central retinal artery is occluded, there is sudden permanent unilateral blindness, disc pallor and visible retinal ischaemia. Bilateral blindness may develop, with the second eye being affected 1–2 weeks after the first.

Diagnosis and management

See page 465.

Further reading

Headache Classification Committee of the International Headache Society. The International Classification of Headache Disorders, 3rd edn (beta version). *Cephalgia* 2013; 33:629–808.
http://www.bash.org.uk *British Association for the Study of Headache guidelines on headache diagnosis and management.*

EPILEPSY AND LOSS OF CONSCIOUSNESS

Epilepsy

An epileptic seizure can be defined as a sudden synchronous discharge of cerebral neurones causing symptoms or signs that are apparent either to the patient or to an observer. For example, a limited discharge affecting only part of the cortex may cause a subjective aura apparent only to the patient, or a generalized seizure may cause a convulsion witnessed by an observer of which the patient may be unaware. This definition excludes disorders such as migrainous aura that are more gradual in onset and usually more prolonged, and EEG discharges that do not have a clinical correlate. Epilepsy is an ongoing liability to recurrent epileptic seizures.

Epidemiology

Epilepsy is common. Its population prevalence is 0.7–0.8% (higher in developing countries). Approximately 440 000 people in the UK have epilepsy. The incidence of epilepsy is age-dependent; it is highest at the extremes of life, most cases starting before the age of 20 or after the age of 60. The cumulative incidence (lifetime risk) of epilepsy is over 3% and the lifetime risk of having a single seizure is 5%. The fact that the prevalence is much lower than the cumulative incidence in part reflects the fact that epilepsy often goes into remission.

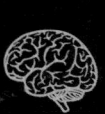

Box 26.42 Classification of seizures

1. Generalized seizures
   A. Tonic–clonic seizures (grand mal)
   B. Absence seizures with 3 Hz spike-and-wave discharge (petit mal)
   C. Myoclonic seizures
   D. Tonic, clonic and atonic seizures
2. Focal seizures (originating within one hemisphere). Characterized according to one or more features:
   A. Aura
   B. Motor (without impaired awareness, e.g. Jacksonian seizures)
   C. Awareness and responsiveness altered or retained (e.g. with impaired awareness, in temporal lobe seizures)
   A focal seizure can evolve into bilateral convulsive seizure – secondary generalization
3. Unknown (insufficient evidence to characterize as focal, generalized or both)

(Abridged from algorithm in Berg AT, Berkovic SF, Brodie MJ et al. Revised terminology and concepts for organization of seizures and epilepsies: report of the ILAE Commission on Classification and Terminology 2005–2009. Epilepsia 2010; 51:676–685.)

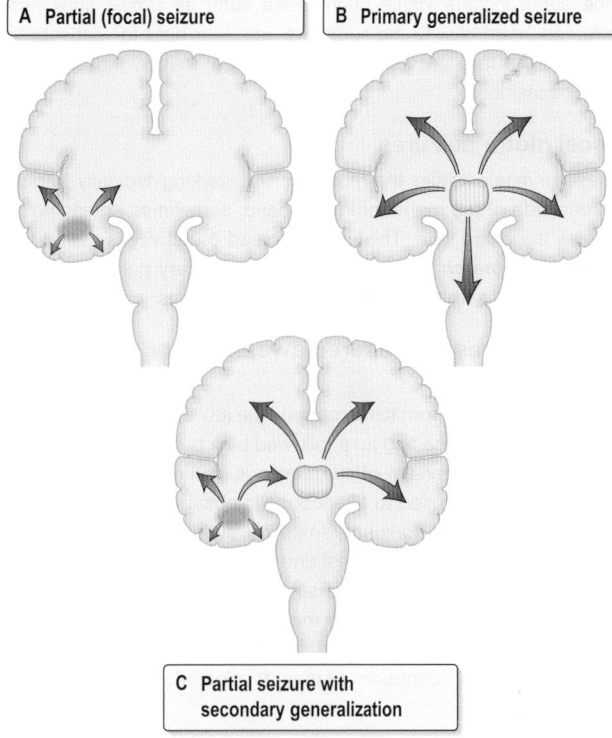

Fig. 26.44 Seizure types.

Classification

Seizures are divided by clinical pattern into two main groups (**Box 26.42** and **Fig. 26.44**): *focal* seizures and *generalized* seizures.

- *A focal seizure* is caused by electrical discharge restricted to a limited part of the cortex of one cerebral hemisphere. Focal seizures are further characterized according to whether or not there is:
  - aura, e.g. smell or auditory hallucination, déjà vu, fear, visual distortion, sensory symptoms such as tingling, abdominal rising sensation
  - motor features, e.g. one limb jerking (a Jacksonian seizure)
  - loss of awareness or responsiveness, e.g. in many temporal lobe seizures.
- *In a generalized seizure*, there is simultaneous involvement of both hemispheres, always associated with loss of consciousness or awareness.

Focal seizures with electrical activity confined to one part of the brain may spread after a few seconds, due to failure of inhibitory mechanisms, to involve the whole of both hemispheres, causing a *bilateral tonic–clonic seizure*. The patient may remember the initial focal seizure before losing consciousness, in which case this is called an *aura*; sometimes, however, the spread of electrical activity is so rapid that the patient does not experience any warning before a *bilateral tonic–clonic* seizure.

Generalized seizure types

Typical absence seizures (petit mal)

This generalized epilepsy almost invariably begins in childhood. Each attack is accompanied by 3 Hz spike-and-wave EEG activity (see **Fig. 26.19**). There is loss of awareness and a vacant expression for less than 10 seconds before returning abruptly to normal and continuing as though nothing had happened. Apart from slight fluttering of the eyelids, there are no motor manifestations. Patients often do not realize they have had an attack but may have many per day. Typical absence attacks are never due to acquired lesions such as tumours; they are a manifestation of primary generalized epilepsy. Children with absence seizures may go on to develop generalized convulsive seizures. Absence seizures are often confused with temporal lobe seizures causing transient alteration of awareness.

Generalized tonic–clonic seizures (grand mal seizures)

Prodrome. There is often no warning before generalized tonic–clonic seizures (GTCS), or there may be an aura prior to a *bilateral tonic–clonic* seizure.

Tonic–clonic phase. An initial tonic stiffening is followed by the clonic phase with synchronous jerking of the limbs, reducing in frequency over about 2 minutes until the convulsion stops. The patient may utter an initial cry and then falls, sometimes suffering serious injury. The eyes remain open and the tongue is often bitten. There may be incontinence of urine or faeces.

Post-ictal phase. A period of flaccid unresponsiveness is followed by gradual return of awareness with confusion and drowsiness lasting 15 minutes to an hour or longer. Headache is common after a GTCS.

Myoclonic, tonic and atonic seizures

Myoclonic seizures or 'jerks' take the form of momentary brief contractions of a muscle or muscle groups: for example, causing a sudden involuntary twitch of a finger or hand. They are common in primary generalized epilepsies. *Tonic seizures* consist of stiffening of the body, not followed by jerking. *Atonic seizures* involve a sudden collapse with loss of muscle tone and consciousness.

Focal seizure types

Focal seizures with aura

The nature of the aura helps to localize the seizure focus. Temporal lobe auras include déjà vu or jamais vu; fear (may be mistaken for panic attacks); olfactory, gustatory or auditory hallucinations; altered perception, such as macropsia or micropsia; an abdominal rising sensation; nausea; and vertigo. With some frontal seizures, conjugate gaze (see p. 807) deviates away from the epileptic focus and the head turns; this is known as an adversive seizure. Occipital lobe auras include visual phenomena such as zigzag lines and coloured scotomas. Some auras are vague or hard for patients to describe but they are generally stereotyped: that is, the same on each occasion.

Focal motor seizures

These originate within the motor cortex. Jerking typically begins on one side of the mouth or in one hand, sometimes spreading to involve the entire side. This visible spread of activity is called the *Jacksonian march* of a seizure. Local temporary paralysis of the limbs affected sometimes follows: Todd's paralysis.

Focal seizures with altered awareness or responsiveness

These usually arise from the temporal lobe (60%) or the frontal lobe. There is often a preceding aura followed by a period of complete or partial loss of awareness of surroundings, lasting for 1–2 minutes on average (as opposed to 10 seconds in absence seizures), which the patient generally does not remember subsequently. This stage is accompanied by speech arrest and often by *automatisms*: semi-purposeful stereotyped motions such as lip smacking or dystonic limb posturing, or more complex motor behaviours such as walking in a circle or undressing. The attacks may be followed by a short period of post-ictal confusion or may develop into a *bilateral tonic–clonic* seizure.

Epilepsy syndromes and aetiology of epilepsy

The range of causes of epilepsy (**Box 26.43**) is different at different ages and in different countries.
- *Children and teenagers*: genetic, perinatal and congenital disorders predominate.
- *Younger adults*: trauma, drugs and alcohol are common.
- *Older ages (>60 years)*: vascular disease and mass lesions such as neoplasms are important.

Primary generalized epilepsies

Presenting in childhood and early adult life, primary generalized epilepsies (PGEs) account for up to 20% of all patients with epilepsy. The cause is thought to be polygenic with complex inheritance. The brain is structurally normal but abnormalities of ion channels influencing neuronal firing, abnormalities of neurotransmitter release and synaptic connections are probably the underlying molecular pathological substrates. They include:

Box 26.43 Causes of epilepsy

- Primary generalized epilepsy, e.g. juvenile myoclonic epilepsy
- Developmental, e.g. neuronal migration abnormalities, cortical dysplasia
- Hippocampal sclerosis
- Brain trauma and surgery
- Intracranial mass lesions, e.g. tumour
- Vascular, e.g. cerebral infarction, arteriovenous malformation, venous sinus thrombosis
- Infectious, e.g. viral encephalitis, meningitis, cerebral tuberculosis, HIV, cerebral toxoplasmosis, neurocysticercosis
- Immune, e.g. NMDA receptor antibody and potassium channel antibody encephalitis
- Genetic, e.g. channelopathies
- Metabolic abnormalities, e.g. hyponatraemia, hypocalcaemia
- Neurodegenerative disorders, e.g. Alzheimer's
- Drugs, e.g. ciclosporin, lidocaine, quinolones, tricyclic antidepressants, antipsychotics, lithium, stimulant drugs such as cocaine
- Alcohol withdrawal

- *Childhood absence epilepsy*: absence seizures. Spontaneous remission by age 18 is usual.
- *Juvenile myoclonic epilepsy* (JME; **Box 26.44**): this accounts for 10% of all epilepsy patients. Typically, myoclonic jerks start in the teenage years (and are usually ignored by the patient; ask about jerks when taking an epilepsy history – see **Box 26.44**), followed by generalized tonic–clonic seizures that bring the patient to medical attention. One-third of patients also have absences. Seizures and jerks often occur in the morning after waking. Lack of sleep, alcohol and strobe or flickering lights are seizure triggers in JME. JME usually responds well to treatment, is usually associated with EEG abnormalities and requires life-long treatment.
- *Monogenic disorders*: research has identified a number of single-gene epilepsy disorders, e.g. autosomal dominant nocturnal frontal lobe epilepsy (caused by mutations in the nicotinic acetylcholine receptor gene). Many are due to mutations of neuronal voltage-gated channels, e.g. potassium and sodium channels, or ligand-gated channels and receptors (channelopathies).

Focal epilepsy

Almost any process disrupting the cortical grey matter can cause epilepsy. Seizures arise from the affected area of cortex, with or without *bilateral tonic–clonic* seizures (these may obscure the focal onset). A focal seizure onset often indicates a structural cause and detailed imaging is required to identify this. In general, the response to treatment is less good than with PGE.

Hippocampal sclerosis

This is a major cause of epilepsy. Hippocampal sclerosis (damage with scarring and atrophy of the hippocampus and surrounding cortex) is the main pathological substrate causing temporal lobe epilepsy and the leading cause of localization-related epilepsy. Childhood febrile convulsions are the main risk factor. Hippocampal sclerosis is usually visible on MRI. It is one of the more common causes of refractory epilepsy, in which case it may be amenable to surgical resection of the damaged temporal lobe.

Genetic and developmental disorders

Over 200 genetic disorders, such as tuberous sclerosis, include epilepsy among their features. These account for less than 2% of epilepsy cases. Neuronal migration defects during brain development, dysplastic areas of cerebral cortex and hamartomas contribute to seizures in both infancy and adult life.

Trauma, hypoxia and neurosurgery

Traumatic brain injury. This may cause epilepsy, sometimes years after the event. The risk is not increased after mild injury (loss of consciousness or post-traumatic amnesia <30 min). Depressed

---

Box 26.44 Juvenile myoclonic epilepsy

- 10% of all epilepsy patients
- Starts in teenage years
- Clinical features:
  - Myoclonic jerks
  - Generalized tonic–clonic seizures
  - Absence in one-third
  - Triggers: sleep deprivation, alcohol, strobe lighting
- Abnormal EEG
- Good response to treatment
- Requires life-long treatment

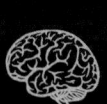

skull fracture, penetrating injury and intracranial haemorrhage increase risk significantly.

Perinatal brain injury and cerebral palsy. Periventricular leukomalacia and brain haemorrhage associated with prematurity and fetal hypoxia, may cause early-onset epilepsy. One-third of children with cerebral palsy have epilepsy.

Brain surgery. This is followed by seizures in up to 17% of cases. Prophylactic anticonvulsant use after surgery is not recommended.

Brain tumours and other mass lesions

Mass lesions involving the cortex cause epilepsy. Seizures are one of the most common presenting features of brain tumours. Brain tumours cause 6% of cases of adult-onset epilepsy.

Vascular disorders

Stroke and small-vessel cerebrovascular disease is the most common cause of epilepsy after the age of 60.

Cortical venous thrombosis or venous sinus thrombosis

Arteriovenous malformations commonly cause epilepsy.

Cavernous haemangiomas (cavernomas) usually present with epilepsy (see **Fig. 26.41**).

Neurodegenerative disorders

Neurodegenerative disorders involving the cerebral cortex, such as Alzheimer's disease, are associated with an increased risk of epilepsy.

Infection

Seizures are often the presenting feature of encephalitis, cerebral abscess and tuberculomas. They also occur in chronic meningitis (e.g. tuberculosis) and may rarely be the first sign of acute bacterial meningitis. Neurocysticercosis is a major cause of seizures in countries where the pork tapeworm is endemic, such as India and South America. HIV and complications of immunosuppression, such as cerebral toxoplasmosis, may also lead to seizures.

Immunological disorders

Autoimmune antibody-mediated encephalitis, such as that due to antibodies against potassium channels or NMDA or glycine receptors, typically present with seizures, as may autoimmune limbic encephalitis.

Alcohol and drugs

Chronic alcohol use is a common cause of seizures. These occur either during heavy drinking bouts or during periods of withdrawal. Alcohol-induced hypoglycaemia and head injury also lead to seizures.

Several drugs, including antipsychotics, tricyclic antidepressants, selective serotonin reuptake inhibitors (SSRIs), lithium, class Ib anti-arrhythmics such as lidocaine, ciclosporin and mefloquine, sometimes provoke fits, either in overdose or at therapeutic doses in individuals with a low seizure threshold. Stimulant drugs such as cocaine also cause seizures.

Withdrawal of antiepileptic drugs (especially barbiturates) and benzodiazepines may provoke seizures.

Metabolic abnormalities

Seizures can be caused by:

- hypocalcaemia, hypoglycaemia, hyponatraemia
- acute hypoxia
- uraemia, hepatic encephalopathy
- porphyria.

Diagnosis of the first fit and investigations

The diagnosis of a seizure is essentially a clinical one, based on taking a history from the patient and any witnesses (**Boxes 26.45** and **26.46**). Investigations have a limited role in distinguishing between a seizure and other causes of a blackout or attack (see p. 857).

The majority of patients referred to a first fit clinic have not had a seizure. The most common error is to misdiagnose a syncopal blackout for a seizure.

Which investigations are needed?

Blood tests, including serum calcium, and an ECG (rhythm, conduction abnormalities, QT interval) are necessary in most patients following an episode of loss of consciousness (**Box 26.47**).

Electroencephalography

EEG is most useful to categorize epilepsy and understand its cause, rather than as a means of confirming a doubtful diagnosis of epilepsy. EEG has a high false-negative rate in epilepsy (>20% even

---

Box 26.45 Diagnosis of a seizure: taking a history after an episode of loss of consciousness

Witness account is crucial.
- What happened:
  - Before: aura versus pre-syncopal prodrome
  - During: convulsion, automatisms versus brief syncopal blackout and pallor
  - After: post-ictal confusion and headache versus rapid recovery in syncope
- Circumstances:
  - Seizure triggers? Sleep deprivation, alcohol binge or drugs
  - Syncope triggers? Pain, heat, prolonged standing
- Epilepsy risk factors?
  - Childhood febrile convulsions
  - Significant head injury
  - Meningitis or encephalitis
  - Family history of epilepsy
- Previous unrecognized seizures?
  - Myoclonic jerks
  - Absences
  - Auras (focal seizures)
- Alcohol excess?
- Medication lowering seizure threshold?
- Hold a driving licence?

Box 26.46 Useful points when diagnosing epilepsy

Diagnosis is a clinical one. Tests such as EEG have little role in distinguishing between epilepsy and other attack types:
- Poor clinical discriminators between types of blackout:
  - Urinary incontinence – may occur in both seizure and syncope
  - Presence of injury
- Good discriminators between types of blackout:
  - Prolonged recovery period (seizure)
  - Bitten tongue – side of tongue usually (seizure)
  - Colour change – pallor (syncope), cyanosis (seizure)
- Stereotyped attacks are usually due to epilepsy

If in doubt, do not diagnose epilepsy – best to wait and see rather than label and treat as epilepsy. There is no role for a 'trial of anticonvulsant treatment' in uncertain cases.

i **Box 26.47** Checklist after a first seizure

- Perform tests:
  - Blood tests and ECG
  - EEG
  - MRI brain (most patients – see text)
- Avoid or remove precipitants: drugs, alcohol, sleep deprivation
- Give advice on safety: e.g. avoid swimming, baths, working at heights
- Stop driving and ask the patient to inform the Driver and Vehicle Licensing Authority (DVLA; in the UK)
- Discuss recurrence risk and treatment

with awake and sleep recordings) and a low false-positive rate (1% of people without epilepsy have epileptiform changes on EEG).

- **EEG abnormalities in epilepsy**: focal cortical spikes (e.g. over a temporal lobe) or generalized spike-and-wave activity (in PGE). Epileptic activity is continuous in status epilepticus.
- **Sleep recordings or 24-hour ambulatory EEG** increase sensitivity when routine EEG is normal.
- **Inpatient EEG videotelemetry** is helpful for diagnosis in attacks of uncertain cause.

Brain imaging

MRI is indicated in most patients after a first seizure, particularly in focal-onset seizures and in older patients where the chance of a focal brain lesion is greatest. In patients below the age of 30 with a definite electroclinical diagnosis of PGE, brain imaging is not essential.

Recurrence risk after a first fit

Some 70–80% of people will have a second seizure, the risk being highest in the first 6 months after the initial seizure. The vast majority of those who have a second seizure will have further seizures if not started on treatment. The risk of seizure recurrence is significantly increased by features of PGE on EEG, focal seizures and the presence of structural brain lesions.

Management

Emergency measures

Most seizures last only minutes and end spontaneously. A prolonged seizure (>5 min) or repeated seizures may be terminated with rectal diazepam, intravenous lorazepam or buccal midazolam. Oxygen should be given and the airway monitored in the post-ictal phase.

Status epilepticus

This medical emergency (**Box 26.48**) means continuous seizures for 30 minutes or longer (or two or more seizures without recovery of consciousness between them over a similar period). Status epilepticus has a mortality of 10–15%. The longer the duration of status, the greater the risk of permanent cerebral damage. Rhabdomyolysis may lead to acute kidney injury in convulsive status epilepticus.

Over 50% of cases occur without a previous history of epilepsy. Some 25% with apparent refractory status have **pseudostatus** (non-epileptic attack disorder).

Not all status is convulsive. In **absence status**, for example, status is non-convulsive; the patient is in a continuous, distant, stuporose state. **Focal status** also occurs. **Epilepsia partialis continua** is continuous seizure activity in one part of the body, such as a finger or a limb, without loss of consciousness. This is often due to a cortical neoplasm or, in the elderly, a cortical infarct.

 Box 26.48 Status epilepticus: management

Early status (up to 30 min)
- Administer oxygen, monitor ECG and blood pressure, perform routine blood tests (include glucose, calcium, drug screen, anticonvulsant levels urgently)
- Give lorazepam i.v. 4 mg bolus. Repeat once if necessary. Buccal midazolam is an alternative

Established status (30–90 min)
- Phenytoin: give 15 mg/kg i.v. diluted to 10 mg/mL in saline into a large vein at 50 mg/min (ECG monitoring required)

or

- Fosphenytoin: this is a prodrug of phenytoin and can be given faster than phenytoin. Doses are expressed in phenytoin equivalents (PE): fosphenytoin 1.5 mg = 1 mg phenytoin. Give 15 mg/kg (PE) fosphenytoin (15 mg × 1.5 = 26.5 mg) diluted to 10 mg/mL in saline at 50–100 mg (PE)/min

If ongoing seizures
- Phenobarbital 10 mg/kg i.v. diluted 1 in 10 in water for injection at <100 mg/min
- Valproate i.v. (25 mg/kg) is an alternative

Refractory status (>90 min) – general anaesthesia
- Only in intensive care setting; intubation and ventilation usually required
- Propofol bolus 2 mg/kg, repeat, followed by continuous infusion of 5–10 mg/kg per hour
- Thiopental and midazolam infusions may also be used
- Use continuous EEG monitoring to assess efficacy of treatment – aim for EEG burst suppression pattern
- Reinstate previous AED medication via nasogastric tube
- Establish diagnosis: CT or MRI may reveal an underlying cause
- Remember: 25% of apparent status cases turn out to be pseudostatus

i **Box 26.49** Antiepileptic drugs and common seizure types

	Generalized tonic–clonic seizures (grand mal)	Focal seizures with or without secondary generalization	Myoclonic seizures
First-line	Sodium valproate Levetiracetam Lamotrigine Carbamazepine Oxcarbazepine Topiramate	Carbamazepine Lamotrigine Levetiracetam Sodium valproate Oxcarbazepine Topiramate	Sodium valproate Levetiracetam Topiramate
Second-line and/or add-ons	Phenobarbital Clobazam Clonazepam Phenytoin	Clobazam Gabapentin Pregabalin Zonisamide Lacosamide Tiagabine	Clonazepam Clobazam Lamotrigine Piracetam
May worsen attacks			Carbamazepine Oxcarbazepine

Antiepileptic drugs

Antiepileptic drugs (AEDs; **Box 26.49**) are indicated when there is a firm clinical diagnosis of epilepsy and a substantial risk of recurrent seizures. Some general principles apply:

- Introduce AEDs at low dose and slowly titrate upwards until the seizures are controlled or side-effects become unacceptable.
- Aim for monotherapy; 70% of patients will have good seizure control with a single AED.
- If seizures are not controlled with the first AED, gradually introduce a second agent and then slowly withdraw the first AED. If the patient is still not seizure-free, then combination therapy is required.

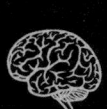

- Epilepsy is one of the few disorders where non-generic ('brand name') prescribing is justified to ensure consistent drug levels.
- Routine monitoring of AED levels is not needed and should be reserved for assessing compliance and toxicity. Measuring sodium valproate levels is rarely useful, as levels fluctuate widely.
- There are interactions between AEDs (and with other medications), e.g. between sodium valproate and lamotrigine. New-generation AEDs have fewer interactions.
- Phenytoin is no longer considered a first-line AED; it is now principally used in emergency control of seizures (see status epilepticus above). Levetiracetam is increasingly used in most types of epilepsy.

Unwanted effects of drugs

Intoxication with most AEDs causes unsteadiness, nystagmus and drowsiness. Side-effects are more common with multiple AED usage. Skin rashes are seen particularly with lamotrigine, carbamazepine and phenytoin. A wide variety of idiosyncratic drug reactions may occur, such as blood dyscrasias with carbamazepine.

Epilepsy in women

See page 1458.

Epilepsy and driving

Patients should be asked to stop driving after a seizure and to inform the regulatory authorities if they hold a driving licence. After a seizure, a temporary driving ban until seizure-free is usual but regulations vary from country to country. Many driving regulatory bodies also suggest refraining from driving while withdrawing from AEDs.

Lifestyle and safety

People with epilepsy (the term 'epileptic' is no longer used) should be encouraged to lead lives as unrestricted as reasonably possible, though observing simple safety measures such as avoiding swimming and dangerous sports like rock-climbing. Advice at home includes leaving bathroom and lavatory doors unlocked and taking showers rather than baths. Epilepsy triggers, such as sleep deprivation, excess alcohol and drugs, should be avoided, as should strobe lighting where there is EEG evidence of a photo-paroxysmal response.

Drug withdrawal

Withdrawal of AEDs should be considered after a seizure-free period of at least 2–3 years. There is a 50% seizure recurrence rate after withdrawal so detailed discussion and explanation are essential.

Refractory epilepsy

- Seizures may persist despite treatment, especially with temporal lobe epilepsy.
- Re-evaluate the diagnosis.
- Consider concordance (compliance).
- Combine AEDs and use the maximum tolerated dose.
- Refer to a specialist unit for consideration of epilepsy surgery.
- Other non-pharmacological treatments, such as vagal nerve stimulation and the ketogenic low-carbohydrate diet, may sometimes be useful.

Epilepsy surgery

Temporal lobectomy will result in seizure freedom in 50–70% of selected patients with uncontrolled seizures caused by hippocampal sclerosis (defined by imaging and confirmed by EEG).

> **?** **Box 26.50** Causes of blackouts and 'funny turns'

- Epilepsy
- Syncope:
  - Neurocardiogenic syncope (vasovagal)
  - Cardiac syncope (Stokes–Adams attacks)
  - Micturition syncope
  - Cough syncope
  - Postural hypotension
  - Carotid sinus syncope
- Non-epileptic attacks (pseudoseizures)
- Panic attacks and hyperventilation
- Hypoglycaemia
- Drop attacks
- Hydrocephalic attacks
- Basilar migraine
- Severe vertigo
- Cataplexy, narcolepsy, sleep paralysis

Other causes of blackouts

The distinction between a fit (seizure), a faint (syncope) or another type of attack is primarily a clinical one, dependent on the history and an eyewitness account (**Box 26.50**). Mistaking a syncopal loss of consciousness for a seizure is the most frequent error made in differential diagnosis.

Syncope or faints

The simple faint that over half the population experiences at some time (particularly in childhood, youth or pregnancy) is due to sudden reflex bradycardia with vasodilation of both peripheral and splanchnic vasculature (***neurocardiogenic or vasovagal syncope***).

- ***Precipitants***: a common response to prolonged standing, fear, venesection or pain. Syncope almost never occurs in the recumbent posture.
- ***Prodrome***: usually brief. There is dizziness and a light-headed feeling, often with nausea, sweating, a feeling of heat and visual grey-out.
- ***Blackout***: patients usually lie still but jerking and twitching movements can occur and are sometimes mistaken for a convulsion. Their appearance is pale. Incontinence of urine or faeces can occur and is not a good discriminator between seizure and syncope.
- ***Recovery***: rapid, usually taking place over seconds, but may be followed by a feeling of general fatigue (as opposed to post-ictal drowsiness and confusion following a seizure).

Other types of syncope

Cardiac syncope (Stokes–Adams attacks) is potentially serious and often treatable. Typically, there is little or no warning. Cardiac arrhythmias, such as those due to heart block, or left ventricular outflow tract obstruction may be the cause. Syncope during exercise is often cardiac in origin.

- ***Micturition syncope*** occurs during micturition in men, particularly at night.
- ***Cough syncope*** occurs when venous return to the heart is obstructed by bouts of severe coughing; it is also seen with laughter occasionally.
- ***Postural hypotension*** (see p. 1029) can cause syncope and occurs in the elderly, in autonomic neuropathy, and with some drugs, such as antihypertensives.
- ***Carotid sinus syncope*** (see p. 1029) is due to a vagal response caused by pressure over the carotid sinus baroreceptors in the neck: for example, due to a tight collar.
- ***Convulsive syncope*** is when collapsing in a propped-up position following a syncope results in delayed restoration of cerebral blood flow and may lead to a secondary anoxic seizure following syncope.

Investigations

A 12-lead ECG should always be performed after a syncope to identify heart block, pre-excitation or long QT syndrome. Cardiac ECG holter monitoring and echocardiography are required where cardiac syncope is suspected. An implantable loop recorder is occasionally needed for infrequent events with a possible cardiac origin. Tilt-table testing (see p. 1038) is sometimes diagnostic but has low sensitivity.

Other conditions

Non-epileptic attack disorder (pseudoseizures) regularly causes difficulty in diagnosis. Attacks may look like generalized fits. Usually, there are bizarre thrashing, non-synchronous limb movements, but there can be extreme difficulty in separating these attacks from seizures. EEG videotelemetry is valuable. Apparent status epilepticus can occur. The serum prolactin level is of some value; this rises during a grand mal seizure but not during a pseudoseizure (or a partial seizure).

Panic attacks (see p. 786) trigger sudden sympathetic activation and often hyperventilation, leading to respiratory alkalosis. They cause some or all of the following symptoms: dizziness, chest pains or tightness, a feeling of choking or shortness of breath, tingling in face and extremities, palpitations, trembling and a feeling of dissociation or of impending doom. Consciousness is usually preserved and attacks are easily recognized. Blood gases should be measured.

Hypoglycaemia (see p. 716) causes confusion followed by loss of consciousness, sometimes with a convulsion, dysphasia or hemiparesis. There is often a warning, with hunger, malaise, shaking and sweating. Prompt recovery occurs with intravenous (or oral) glucose. Prolonged hypoglycaemia causes widespread cerebral damage. Hypoglycaemic attacks unrelated to diabetes are rare (see p. 647). Feeling faint after fasting does not indicate anything serious.

Vertigo, when acute, can be sufficiently severe as to cause prostration; a few seconds' unresponsiveness sometimes follows.

Migraine, in the form of severe basilar migraine and familial hemiplegic migraine, may occasionally lead to loss of consciousness.

Drop attacks are instant, unexpected episodes of lower limb weakness with falling, largely in women over 60 years. Awareness is preserved. They are due to sudden change in lower limb tone, presumably of brainstem origin. Sudden attacks of leg weakness also occur in hydrocephalus.

TIAs are almost never a cause of loss of consciousness.

Sleep disorders

Sleep architecture and insomnia are discussed on page 775. Myoclonic jerks when falling asleep are a normal phenomenon (see p. 862). Seizures may occur predominantly or solely during sleep.

Narcolepsy and cataplexy

Narcolepsy is caused by abnormalities of the brain neurotransmitter hypocretin (orexin), which is a regulator of sleep. CSF levels are usually low, thought in most cases to be due to autoimmune damage to the hypothalamic cells secreting the neurotransmitter. Narcolepsy is strongly associated with human leucocyte antigen (HLA)-DR2 and HLA-DQBl*0602 antigens. The prevalence is estimated at 30–50/100 000.

There are four main clinical features but not all patients have the full tetrad:

- **Excessive daytime sleepiness (EDS)**. This is the usual presenting symptom and the main cause of disability. Patients have frequent irresistible sleep attacks during the day, often in inappropriate circumstances, e.g. during meals or conversations or while driving. EDS may be quantified with the Epworth Sleepiness Scale. Night-time sleep may be disrupted and, paradoxically, insomnia may occur.
- **Cataplexy.** This is sudden loss of muscle tone leading to head droop or even falling with intact awareness. Attacks are often set off by sudden surprise or emotion, e.g. laughter.
- **Hypnagogic/hypnopompic hallucinations.** These terms refer to dream-like hallucinations occurring while falling asleep or waking from sleep; these are often frightening.
- **Sleep paralysis.** A brief paralysis on waking or while falling asleep is due to intrusion of rapid eye movement (REM) atonia into wakefulness. This occasionally occurs in people without narcolepsy.

Diagnosis and management

Multiple sleep latency testing demonstrating a rapid transition from wakefulness to sleep and a short time to onset of REM sleep confirms the diagnosis. HLA testing may also be useful.

Good sleep hygiene advice is necessary. Modafinil dexamfetamine and methylphenidate are used to treat EDS, often with only partial response. Tricyclic antidepressants, particularly clomipramine, or SSRIs can improve cataplexy. Sodium oxybate is also used.

Parasomnias

Disruptive motor or verbal behaviours occurring during sleep are divided into REM and non-REM parasomnias, depending on which stage of sleep they arise in. They include sleepwalking, night terrors, confusional arousals and REM sleep behaviour disorder (which may be an early feature of Parkinson's disease).

Obstructive sleep apnoea

See page 960.

Restless leg syndrome (Willis–Ekbom disease)

Also known as Wittmaack–Ekbom's syndrome, this affects about 10% of adults, both women and men, and is also seen in children. Most people do not seek medical advice but it can be quite severe in 2–3%. The syndrome is characterized by an unpleasant sensation of 'wanting to move' the legs with throbbing or pulling, and usually occurs when the person is resting, sitting or lying; it can be totally or partially relieved by stretching or walking. It often occurs in the evenings or night-time and appears to be more frequent in the elderly. The condition is usually idiopathic and there is a familial tendency. It has been associated with pregnancy, Parkinson's disease, uraemia or a haematinic deficiency. Some drugs have been implicated.

There is no specific treatment. Dopamine agonist drugs and benzodiazepines may help. Some suggest a decreased use of alcohol or caffeine.

Further reading

Kwan P, Schachter SC, Brodie MJ. Drug resistant epilepsy. *N Engl J Med* 2011; 365:919–926.

Leach JP, Abassi H. Modern management of epilepsy. *Clin Med* 2013; 13:84–86.

Moshé SL, Perucca E, Ryvlin P et al. Epilepsy: new advances. *Lancet* 2015; 385:884–898.

Scammell TE. Narcolepsy. *N Engl J Med* 2015; 373:2054–2662.

Shorvon SD. Epilepsy and related disorders. In: Clarke C, Howard R, Rossor M et al (eds). *Neurology: A Queen Square Textbook*. Oxford: Blackwell; 2009.

http://www.epilepsysociety.org.uk. *National Society for Epilepsy, UK patient support group.*

http://www.narcolepsy.org.uk. *Narcolepsy UK.*

MOVEMENT DISORDERS

Disorders of movement divide broadly into two categories:
- *hypokinesias* – characterized by slowed movements with increased tone (parkinsonism)
- *hyperkinesias* – excessive involuntary movements.

Both types may coexist; for example, in Parkinson's disease, where there are both slowed movements and tremor. Many of these disorders (not all) relate to dysfunction of the basal ganglia.

Parkinsonian disorders

Idiopathic Parkinson's disease

In 1817, James Parkinson, a physician in Hoxton, London, published *The Shaking Palsy*, describing this common worldwide condition that has a prevalence of 150/100000. Parkinson's disease (PD) is clinically and pathologically distinct from other parkinsonian syndromes.

Aetiology

The causes of idiopathic PD are still not fully understood. The relatively uniform worldwide prevalence suggests that a single environmental agent is not responsible. There may be multiple interacting risk factors, including genetic susceptibility.

Age and gender

Prevalence increases sharply with age, particularly over 70 years, with prevalence of 1 in 200 over age 80. Ageing changes are likely to be a factor in causation. Prevalence is higher in men (1.5:1 male to female).

Environmental factors

Epidemiological studies consistently show a small increased risk with rural living and drinking well water. Pesticide exposure has been implicated and pesticide-induced rodent models of PD exist, which increases biological plausibility of a link. The chemical compound methyl-phenyl tetrahydropyridine (MPTP), a potent mitochondrial toxin, causes severe parkinsonism, leading to suggestions that oxidative stress may be a factor leading to neuronal cell death in idiopathic PD. Studies consistently show that non-smokers have a higher risk of PD than smokers (even after controlling for shorter life expectancy in smokers), an observation that is difficult to explain.

Genetic factors

Idiopathic PD is not usually familial but twin studies show there is a significant genetic component in early-onset PD (onset before 40). Several genetic loci for Mendelian inherited monogenic forms of PD have now been identified (**Box 26.51**), designated *PARK* 1–11. Most of these are rare but together they account for a large proportion of early-onset and familial PD, and a small proportion (perhaps 1–2%), of sporadic late-onset cases. The main significance of the *PARK* genes is that they provide insights into the pathophysiological mechanisms underlying PD that may be relevant to sporadic cases. Polymorphisms in these and other genes may, in combination, constitute a susceptibility to PD that can be triggered by environmental factors or the ageing process.

Pathology

The pathological hallmarks of PD are the presence of neuronal inclusions called Lewy bodies (see p. 883) and loss of the dopaminergic

i **Box 26.51 Selected Parkinson's disease (PD) genes**

Locus	Protein	Inheritance	Comments
PARK1	α-Synuclein	AD	Rare but a major protein in Lewy bodies
PARK2	Parkin	AR	Responsible for most cases of juvenile PD and 20% of early-onset PD cases
PARK6	Pink-1	AR	Rare. Protein involved in mitochondrial function
PARK8	LRRK2 (a kinase of unknown function)	AD	Phenotype almost identical to sporadic PD. Found in 1% of apparently sporadic PD patients. High frequency in Jewish and North African Arab patients

AD, autosomal dominant; AR, autosomal recessive.

neurones from the pars compacta of the substantia nigra in the midbrain that project to the striatum of the basal ganglia (see **Fig. 26.11**). Lewy bodies contain tangles of α-synuclein and ubiquitin, and become gradually more widespread as the condition progresses, spreading from the lower brainstem to the midbrain and then into the cortex. Degeneration also occurs in other basal ganglia nuclei. The extent of nigrostriatal dopaminergic cell loss correlates with the degree of akinesia.

Clinical features

PD almost always presents with the typical motor symptoms of tremor and slowness of movement but it is likely that the pathological process starts many years before these symptoms develop. By the time of first presentation, on average 70% of dopaminergic nigrostriatal cells have already been lost.

Prodromal pre-motor symptoms

Patients develop a variety of non-specific non-motor symptoms during the approximately 7 years, sometimes longer, before the motor symptoms become manifest. These include:
- anosmia (present in 90%) – the olfactory bulb is one of the first structures to be affected
- depression/anxiety (50%)
- aches and pains
- REM sleep behaviour disorder
- autonomic features – urinary urgency, hypotension
- constipation
- restless legs syndrome.

Motor symptoms

These develop slowly and insidiously, and are often initially attributed to 'old age' by patients. The core motor features of PD are:
- akinesia
- tremor
- rigidity
- postural and gait disturbance.

Slowness causes difficulty rising from a chair or getting into or out of bed. Writing becomes small (micrographia) and spidery, tending to tail off. Relatives often notice other features: slowness and an impassive face. Idiopathic PD is almost always more prominent initially on one side. The diagnosis is usually evident from the overall appearance.

Akinesia

Poverty/slowing of movement (also called bradykinesia) is the cardinal clinical feature of parkinsonism and the main cause of disability. What distinguishes it from slowness of movement from other causes is a progressive **fatiguing** and **decrement** in amplitude and speed of repetitive movements, such as opening and closing the hand or finger tapping.

There is difficulty initiating movement. The upper limb is usually affected first and is almost always unilateral for the first years. Rapid dexterous movements are impaired, causing difficulty writing (micrographia) and doing up buttons and zips, for example. Facial immobility gives a mask-like semblance of depression. Frequency of spontaneous blinking diminishes, producing a **serpentine stare**.

Tremor

Tremor is the presenting symptom in 70% of patients. It typically starts in the fingers or hand (3–6 Hz) and is unilateral initially, spreading later to the leg on the same side and, after some years, to the opposite side. The tremor is present at rest, and reduces or stops completely when the hand is in motion. It is often described as **pill-rolling** because the patient appears to be rolling something between thumb and forefinger. As with most tremors, it is made worse by emotion or stress.

Rigidity

This is a sign rather than a symptom. Stiffness on passive limb movement is described as 'lead pipe', as it is present throughout the range of movement and, unlike spasticity, is not dependent on speed of movement. When stiffness occurs with tremor (not always visible), a ratchet-like jerkiness is felt, described as 'cogwheel' rigidity.

Postural and gait changes

A stooped posture is characteristic. Gait gradually becomes shuffling with small stride length, slow turns, freezing and reduced arm swing. Postural stability eventually deteriorates, leading to falls, but this is a late-stage feature that should arouse suspicion of an alternative diagnosis if present during the first 5 years.

Speech and swallowing

Speech becomes quiet, indistinct and flat. Drooling may be an embarrassing problem and swallowing difficulty is a late feature that may eventually lead to aspiration pneumonia as a terminal event.

Cognitive and psychiatric changes

Cognitive impairment is now recognized to be common in late-stage PD (80%) and may develop into dementia. Visual hallucinations on treatment, and psychosis are not uncommon, and may herald evolving cognitive decline. Cholinesterase inhibitors (see p. 884) may be helpful.

Depression is common, probably due to involvement of serotonergic and adrenergic systems, and is a cause of reduced quality of life in PD. Anxiety is also co-morbid with PD.

Clinical evolution of PD

Most patients respond well to treatment and there is generally a period of several years in which symptoms are well controlled with relatively little disability. Response to dopaminergic drugs is never lost but treatment-related fluctuations may develop (see below), which can be limiting, especially for patients with early age at onset. Eventually, usually by the mid-seventies, late-stage, treatment-unresponsive

features, such as cognitive impairment, swallowing difficulty, loss of postural stability and falls, start to emerge.

The rate of progression is very variable, with a benign form running over several decades. Usually, the course is over 10–20 years, death resulting from bronchopneumonia and immobility.

Diagnosis

There is no laboratory test; diagnosis is made by recognizing physical signs and distinguishing idiopathic PD from other parkinsonian syndromes. Patients with suspected PD should be referred to a specialist without initiation of treatment.

MRI is normal and not necessary in typical cases. Dopamine transporter (DAT) imaging using SPECT or PET makes use of a radiolabelled ligand binding to dopaminergic terminals to assess the extent of nigrostriatal cell loss. It may occasionally be needed to distinguish PD from other causes of tremor or from drug-induced parkinsonism, but it cannot discriminate between PD and other akinetic–rigid syndromes.

Management

Education about the condition is necessary and physical activity is beneficial and should be encouraged. Dopamine replacement with levodopa or a dopamine agonist improves motor symptoms and is the basis of pharmacological therapy. Treatment of non-motor symptoms, such as depression, constipation, pain and sleep disorders, is also necessary and significantly improves quality of life.

Dopamine replacement may not always be needed in early-stage PD and is only started when symptoms begin to cause disability. The mechanism of action of drugs in PD is shown in **Fig. 26.45**.

Levodopa

Levodopa remains the most effective form of treatment and all patients with PD will eventually need it. It is combined with a dopa

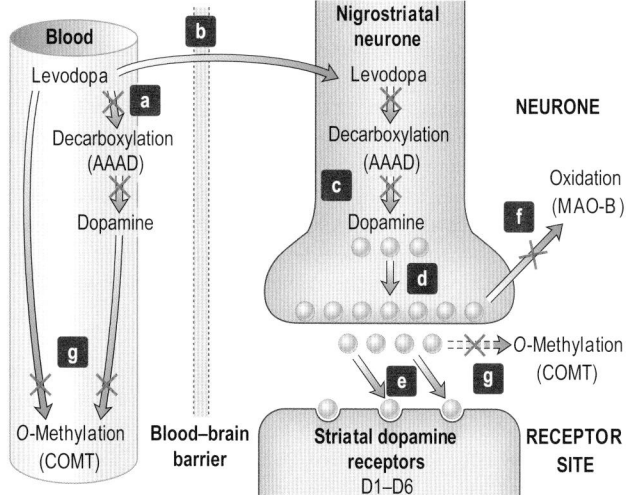

Fig. 26.45 Drugs in Parkinson's disease. Levodopa crosses the blood–brain barrier, enters the nigrostriatal neurone and is converted to dopamine. **(a)** Carbidopa and benserazide reduce peripheral conversion of levodopa to dopamine, thus reducing the side-effects of circulating dopamine. **(b)** Dietary amino acids from high-protein meals can inhibit active transport across the blood–brain barrier by competing with levodopa. **(c)** Levodopa is converted (aromatic amino acid decarboxylase, AAAD) to dopamine. **(d)** Amantadine enhances dopamine release. **(e)** Dopamine agonists react with dopamine receptors. **(f)** Monoamine oxidase (MAO)-B inhibitors block dopamine breakdown. **(g)** Catechol-O-methyl transferase (COMT) inhibitors prolong dopamine activity by blocking breakdown.

decarboxylase inhibitor – benserazide (co-beneldopa) or carbidopa (co-careldopa) – to reduce the peripheral adverse effects (e.g. nausea and hypotension); 50 mg of levodopa (e.g. co-careldopa 62.5 mg) three times daily, increasing after 1 week to 100 mg three times daily, is a typical starting dose. The response is often dramatic.

Dopamine agonists

Dopamine agonists (DAs) may be used in combination with levodopa or as initial monotherapy in younger patients (below age 65–70) with mild to moderate impairment. Although less efficacious in symptom control than levodopa and generally less well tolerated, DAs are associated with fewer motor complications over a 5-year period. Non-ergot DAs (pramipexole and ropinirole or rotigotine via transdermal patch) are used in preference to ergot-derived drugs, which may be associated with fibrotic reactions, including cardiac valvular fibrosis. Domperidone is used as an antiemetic when initiating DA therapy (other antiemetics should not be used, as they may worsen symptoms by blocking central dopamine receptors).

Other drugs used in PD

- *Selegiline* 5–10 mg once daily (a monoamine oxidase (MAO)-B inhibitor) reduces catabolism of dopamine in brain. It has a mild symptomatic effect. *Rasagiline* is another MAO-B inhibitor.
- *Amantadine* has a modest anti-parkinsonian effect but is used mainly to improve dyskinesias in advanced disease.
- *Antimuscarinics* (e.g. *orphenadrine*, *procyclidine*, *trihexyphenidyl*) may help tremor but are rarely used in PD except in younger patients. They have a high propensity to cause confusion and cognitive impairment in older patients.
- *Apomorphine* is a potent, short-acting DA administered subcutaneously by an autoinjector pen as intermittent 'rescue' injection for off periods or by continuous infusion pump. It is used in advanced PD.

Long-term response to treatment

As the disease progresses, medical therapy for PD becomes more difficult as higher doses of dopamine replacement therapy are required and response becomes more unpredictable with the development of motor fluctuations and dyskinesias; response to dopaminergic drugs is never lost, however.

Approximately 10% of patients per year develop motor complications in the form of 'wearing off' (the duration of effect of individual doses of levodopa becomes progressively shorter), dyskinesias (involuntary choreiform movements) and, eventually, 'on/off' phenomena (sudden, unpredictable transitions from mobile to immobile). Eventually, patients may alternate between the 'on' state with dopamine-induced dyskinesias and periods of complete immobility ('off').

Management of the motor complications of treatment represents one of the greatest challenges in the management of PD. Strategies include:

- dose fractionation of levodopa – increasing dose frequency
- addition of the catechol-O-methyl transferase (COMT) inhibitor *entacapone* (200 mg with each levodopa dose) to prolong duration of action; this is also available as a combined preparation with levodopa and carbidopa
- slow-release levodopa – mostly used for overnight symptoms, as absorption is erratic and difficult to predict, so limiting effectiveness in control of daytime symptoms
- avoidance of protein-rich meals (which impair levodopa absorption) and taking doses at least 40 minutes prior to meals
- apomorphine continuous subcutaneous infusion (see above)
- deep brain stimulation and levodopa intestinal gel (see below).

Deep brain stimulation

Stereotactic insertion of electrodes into the brain has proved to be a major therapeutic advance in selected patients (usually under age 70) with disabling dyskinesias and motor fluctuations not adequately controlled with medical therapy. Targets include:

- the subthalamic nucleus – response similar to levodopa with reduction in dyskinesia
- the globus pallidus – improves dyskinesia but levodopa is still required for motor symptoms
- the thalamus – for tremor only.

Dopaminergic drugs can be reduced (but not withdrawn) after deep brain stimulation (DBS). Approximately 10% of patients will be candidates at some point, usually patients with younger onset, as they have a higher rate of motor complications such as dyskinesia. There is a trend towards earlier use of DBS before motor complications become severe.

Levodopa intestinal gel infusion

Continuous infusion of this gel into the small intestine via a jejunostomy using a patient-operated pump is effective for selected patients with severe motor complications. At present, it is used only where apomorphine and DBS are contraindicated, partly because of high costs.

Tissue transplantation

Transplantation of embryonic mesencephalic dopaminergic cells directly into the putamen has produced mixed results but is potentially promising; research is ongoing to refine the technique. Stem cells and gene therapy approaches are in development.

Physiotherapy, occupational therapy and physical aids

Physiotherapy, occupational therapy and speech therapy all have a role to play in managing PD and reducing disability, speech and swallowing problems, and falls. Walking aids are often a hindrance early on, but later a frame or a tripod may help. A variety of external cueing techniques may help with freezing.

Other akinetic–rigid syndromes

Drug-induced parkinsonism

Dopamine-blocking or depleting drugs, particularly neuroleptics (with the exception of clozapine), induce parkinsonism or worsen symptoms in affected patients, and may precipitate symptoms in elderly patients in the presymptomatic phase. Antimuscarinic drugs reduce these symptoms, although tardive dyskinesia may be made worse.

Atypical parkinsonism

A number of neurodegenerative disorders affect the basal ganglia, causing prominent parkinsonism as part of the clinical picture; they may be mistaken for idiopathic PD in the early stages. These include:

- *Progressive supranuclear palsy* (Steele–Richardson–Olszewski's syndrome). This causes parkinsonism, postural instability with early falls, vertical supranuclear gaze palsy, pseudobulbar palsy and dementia. Tau deposition is seen pathologically in the substantia nigra, subthalamic nucleus and midbrain.
- *Multiple system atrophy (MSA)*. Autonomic and cerebellar symptoms occur in addition to parkinsonism. Either parkinsonism or cerebellar symptoms predominate. Pathologically, α-synuclein-positive glial cytoplasmic inclusions are found in

the basal ganglion, cerebellum and motor cortex. Patients do not respond to levodopa therapy. Management is symptomatic and they have a poorer prognosis than patients with Parkinson's disease.

- **Corticobasal degeneration.** Alien limb phenomena, myoclonus and dementia occur.

These disorders are relentlessly progressive; although they sometimes respond to levodopa, they usually cause death within a decade. 'Red flag' symptoms suggesting one of these disorders include:

- symmetrical presentation and absence of tremor
- levodopa unresponsiveness (or poor response)
- early falls (within first year)
- additional neurological features.

Wilson's disease

This rare and treatable disorder of copper metabolism is inherited as an autosomal recessive trait. Copper deposition occurs in the basal ganglia, cornea and liver (see p. 1301), where it can cause cirrhosis. All young patients (below age 50) with any hyperkinetic movement disorder or with liver cirrhosis should be screened for Wilson's disease (serum copper and caeruloplasmin should be checked). Intellectual impairment develops. Neurological damage is reversible with early treatment. Diagnosis and treatment with the chelating agent penicillamine are discussed on page 1302.

Hyperkinetic movement disorders

There are five hyperkinetic movement disorders, which can sometimes be difficult to separate from one another and may occur in combination.

- **tremor** – rhythmic sinusoidal oscillation of a body part
- **chorea** – excessive, irregular movements flitting from one body part to another ('dance-like')
- **myoclonus** – brief, electric shock-like jerks
- **tics** – stereotyped movements or vocalizations (may be temporarily suppressed)
- **dystonia** – sustained muscle spasms causing twisting movements and abnormal postures.

Essential tremor

This common condition, often inherited as an autosomal dominant trait, causes a bilateral, fast, low-amplitude tremor, mainly in the upper limbs. The head and voice are occasionally involved. Tremor is postural, such as when holding a glass or cutlery. Essential tremor occurs at any age but usually starts in early life. Tremor is slowly progressive but rarely produces severe disability. There may be a cerebellar-type action tremor component. Anxiety exacerbates the tremor.

Treatment is often unnecessary or unsatisfactory. Many patients are reassured to find they do not have PD, with which essential tremor is often confused. Small amounts of alcohol, beta-blockers (propranolol), primidone or gabapentin may help. Sympathomimetics (e.g. salbutamol) make all tremors worse. Stereotactic thalamotomy and thalamic DBS are used in severe cases.

Chorea

There are a wide variety of possible causes of chorea. These include:

- systemic disease – thyrotoxicosis, SLE, antiphospholipid syndrome, polycythaemia vera
- genetic disorders – Huntington's disease and genetic phenocopies, neuroacanthocytosis, benign hereditary chorea

- structural and vascular disorders affecting the basal ganglia
- drugs (e.g. levodopa and the oral contraceptive pill)
- post-infectious (Sydenham's chorea) – following months after streptococcal infection or as part of acute rheumatic fever
- pregnancy.

Treatment is of the underlying cause but dopamine-blocking drugs, such as phenothiazines (e.g. sulpiride) and dopamine-depleting drugs (tetrabenazine), reduce chorea (as the prototypical *excessive* movement condition the treatment is the *opposite* of PD).

Huntington's disease

Huntington's disease is a cause of chorea, usually presenting in middle life, initially with subtle 'fidgetiness' followed by development of progressive psychiatric and cognitive symptoms.

Prevalence worldwide is about 5/100 000. HD is due to a CAG trinucleotide repeat expansion, which forms the basis of the diagnostic test (see p. 30). This results in translation of an expanded polyglutamine repeat sequence in huntingtin, the protein gene product, the function of which is unclear. The expansion is thought to be a toxic 'gain-of-function' mutation. Most adult-onset patients have 36–55 repeats and there is an inverse relationship between repeat length and age at onset, with juvenile-onset patients having over 60 repeats. Expansion of the unstable CAG repeat during meiosis, particularly spermatogenesis, is the molecular basis for the phenomenon of anticipation (a tendency for successive generations to have earlier onset and more severe disease), particularly when inherited from the father.

HD is inherited in an autosomal dominant manner with complete penetrance (all gene carriers will develop the disease eventually). Previous family history is often not known. There is no disease-modifying treatment at present, although chorea can improve with treatment, such as risperidone or sulpiride, but progressive neurodegeneration leads to dementia and ultimately death after 10–20 years. Patients with small or intermediate-range expansions may present in old age with isolated chorea.

Absence of treatment results in a low take-up rate for presymptomatic testing in at-risk individuals. Test centres have protocols for counselling families and addressing ethical issues.

Hemiballismus

Hemiballismus (see **Fig. 26.11**) describes violent swinging movements of one side, usually caused by infarction or haemorrhage in the contralateral subthalamic nucleus.

Acute chorea–hemiballismus also occurs after diabetic hyperosmolar hyperglycaemia, with signal change seen in the basal ganglia on CT or MRI; it is thought to be due to osmotic shifts causing myelinolysis.

Myoclonus

Cortical myoclonus is usually distal (hands and fingers especially) and stimulus-sensitive (spontaneous but also triggered by touch or loud noises). It is caused by a wide variety of pathologies affecting the cerebral cortex; spinal and brainstem myoclonus are caused by localized lesions affecting these structures.

Primary myoclonus

Physiological myoclonus. Nocturnal myoclonus consisting of sudden jerks (often with a feeling of falling) on dropping off to sleep or waking; it is common and not pathological. The startle response is also a form of brainstem myoclonus.

Myoclonic dystonia (DYT11). Myoclonic 'lightning jerks', often with dystonia, are inherited as a rare autosomal dominant disorder due to mutations in the ε-sarcoglycan gene. The condition is thought to be allelic with benign essential myoclonus (caused by disruption of the same gene).

Myoclonus in epilepsy

Myoclonic jerks occurs in several forms of epilepsy (see p. 853). An antiepileptic drug, such as valproate, may be helpful.

Progressive myoclonic epilepsy–ataxia syndromes

These rare conditions include genetic and metabolic disorders in which myoclonus accompanies progressive epilepsy, cognitive decline and/or ataxia. **Lafora body disease**, **neuronal ceroid lipofuscinosis** and **Unverricht–Lundborg** disease are examples.

Secondary myoclonus

Myoclonus may be seen in a wide variety of metabolic disorders, including hepatic and renal failure (asterixis), as part of several dementias and neurodegenerative disorders (e.g. Alzheimer's disease) and encephalitis.

Post-anoxic myoclonus sometimes follows severe cerebral anoxia.

Tics

Tics are common (15% lifetime prevalence), brief, stereotyped movements usually affecting the face or neck but which may involve any body part; they include vocal tics. Unlike other movement disorders, they may be transiently suppressed, leading to a build-up of anxiety and overflow after release.

Simple transient tics (e.g. blinking, sniffing or facial grimacing) are common in childhood but may persist. Adult-onset tics are rare and usually have a secondary cause. The borderland between normal and pathological is vague.

Tourette's syndrome

The most common cause of tics, characterized by multiple motor tics and at least one vocal tic, starts in childhood and persists longer than a year. Boys are affected more often than girls in a 3:1 ratio. Behavioural problems, including attention deficit hyperactivity disorder (ADHD) and obsessive–compulsive disorder (OCD), are common and may sometimes be the major cause of disability. There is sometimes explosive barking and grunting of obscenities (coprolalia) and gestures (copropraxia) or echolalia (copying what other people say). Many affected individuals never come to medical attention. The cause is not known but it may be a complex problem with histaminergic neurotransmission.

Dystonias

Dystonia (**Box 26.52**) is most usefully classified by aetiology into:

- **primary dystonias** – where dystonia is the only, or main, clinical manifestation (usually genetic)

- **secondary dystonia** – due to brain injury, cerebral palsy or drugs, for example
- **hereditary degenerative dystonia** – part of a wider neurodegenerative disorder
- **paroxysmal dystonias** – rare, mostly genetic, attacks of sudden involuntary movements with elements of dystonia and chorea.

Primary dystonias

Young onset. Mutations in the *DYT1* gene locus, seen particularly in the Ashkenazi Jewish population, cause limb-onset dystonia (usually foot), before the age of 28. Most patients have a three base-pair GAG deletion in the torsinA endoplasmic reticulum ATPase protein encoded by the *DYT1* gene. Penetrance is low (autosomal dominant) and phenotype very variable, but the disorder often spreads over years to become generalized dystonia, and can result in severe disability. Cognitive function remains normal. The condition is rare and the definitive form of treatment for severe cases is DBS (electrodes inserted into the globus pallidus).

Adult onset. This is much the most common type of primary dystonia. Onset is usually around 55 and dystonia is usually focal (restricted to one body part), particularly affecting the head and neck, unlike *DYT1* dystonia. Various patterns are recognized.

Torticollis

Dystonic spasms gradually develop in neck muscles, causing the head to turn (torticollis) or to be drawn backwards (retrocollis). There may also be a jerky head tremor. A gentle touch with a fingertip at a specific site may relieve the spasm temporarily (sensory trick or 'geste').

Writer's cramp and task-specific dystonias

There is a specific inability to perform a previously highly developed, repetitive, skilled movement, such as writing. The movement provokes dystonic posturing. Other functions of the hand remain normal. Overuse may lead to task-specific dystonias in certain occupations, such as musicians, typists and even golfers.

Blepharospasm and oromandibular dystonia

These consist of spasms of forced blinking or involuntary movement of the mouth and tongue (e.g. lip-smacking and protrusion of the tongue and jaw). Speech may be affected.

Dopa-responsive dystonia

In this rare disorder, dystonia is completely abolished by small doses of levodopa. Typically, dystonic walking begins in childhood and may resemble a spastic paraparesis or even present as cerebral palsy. Dominantly inherited mutations in the *GTP* cyclohydrolase gene on chromosome 14q26.3 (necessary for synthesis of a co-factor – tetrahydrobiopterin – needed for dopamine synthesis) lead to brain dopamine deficiency. Patients with dystonic gaits are sometimes given test doses of levodopa.

Neuroleptics and movement disorders

Neuroleptics (antipsychotic drugs used to treat schizophrenia) and related drugs used as antiemetics (e.g. metoclopramide) can cause a variety of movement disorders:

- **Akathisia**. This is a restless, repetitive and irresistible need to move.
- **Parkinsonism**. This is due to D_1 and D_2 dopamine receptor blockade (see earlier).
- **Acute dystonic reactions**. Spasmodic torticollis, trismus and oculogyric crises (episodes of sustained upward gaze) develop, dramatically and unpredictably, after single doses.

ℹ️ Box 26.52 A classification of dystonias

- Generalized dystonia
- Primary torsion dystonia (PTD)
- Dopamine-responsive dystonia (DRD)
- Drug-induced dystonia (e.g. metoclopramide)
- Symptomatic dystonia (e.g. after encephalitis lethargica or in Wilson's disease)

- Paroxysmal dystonia (very rare, familial, with marked fluctuation)
- Focal dystonia
- Spasmodic torticollis
- Writer's cramp
- Oromandibular dystonia
- Blepharospasm
- Hemiplegic dystonia, e.g. following stroke
- Multiple sclerosis – rare

- **Tardive dyskinesia**. These mouthing and lip-smacking grimaces occur after several years of neuroleptic use. They often become temporarily worse when the drug is stopped or the dose reduced. Even if treatment ceases, resolution seldom follows. Atypical neuroleptics are less prone to cause this complication.

Management

Targeted injection of botulinum toxin into affected muscles is now the principal form of treatment for all focal dystonias. Antimuscarinics (e.g. trihexyphenidyl) are sometimes helpful.

Further reading

Kalia LV, Lang AE. Parkinson's disease. *Lancet* 2015; 386:896–912.
Obeso JA, Rodriguez-Oroz MC, Stamelou M et al. Expanding the universe of disorders of basal ganglion. *Lancet* 2014; 384:523–531.
Schapira AH, Olanow CW, Greenamyre JT et al. Slowing of neurodegeneration in Parkinson's disease and Huntington's disease: future therapeutic perspectives. *Lancet* 2014; 384:545–555.
Stoessi AJ, Leherly S, Strafella AD. Imaging insights into basal ganglion function, Parkinson's disease and dystonia. *Lancet* 2014; 384:532–544.

NEUROINFLAMMATORY DISORDERS

Multiple sclerosis is by far the most common neuroinflammatory disorder in Western populations. Other CNS inflammatory conditions include post-infectious disorders such as acute disseminated encephalomyelitis (ADEM) and transverse myelitis, distinct autoimmune disorders such as neuromyelitis optica (NMO) and multisystem inflammatory disorders such as sarcoidosis and Behçet's disease.

Multiple sclerosis

Multiple sclerosis (MS) is a chronic autoimmune, T-cell-mediated, inflammatory disorder of the CNS. Multiple plaques of demyelination are found throughout the brain and spinal cord, occurring sporadically over years (dissemination in space and time is crucial for diagnosis).

MS is a major cause of disability in young adults but several disease-modifying therapies are now available.

Epidemiology

- **Prevalence**. MS is a common neurological disorder with over 2 500 000 cases worldwide. In the UK, the prevalence is 1.2/1000. Approximately 80 000 people in the UK have MS.
- **Gender**. Women outnumber men by 2 : 1. There is evidence that this ratio is widening, with an increasing proportion of women being affected.
- **Age**. Presentation is typically between 20 and 40 years of age. Presentation after age 60 is rare, although diagnosis may sometimes be much delayed, occurring years after the initial symptoms.

Prevalence varies widely in different geographical regions and ethnic groups. This probably reflects both genetic (see below) and environmental influences in pathogenesis. MS is much more common in white populations and with increasing distance from the equator. Even within the UK, there is a north–south divide, prevalence being higher in Scotland than southern England. Migration studies show that children moving from a low-risk to a high-risk area (e.g. the UK) develop a higher risk of MS, similar to the population of the country to which they migrate, indicating that environmental factors are a factor in pathogenesis.

Other autoimmune disorders occur with increased frequency in patients with MS and their relatives, indicating a genetic predisposition to autoimmunity.

Aetiology and pathogenesis

MS is a T-cell-mediated autoimmune disease that causes an inflammatory process mainly within the white matter of the brain and spinal cord. The aetiology of MS is complex and not yet fully understood.

Genetic susceptibility

Multiple genes interact to confer an increased risk of MS, giving a complex polygenic inheritance pattern. Genetic differences between different populations probably account for part of the observed variation in MS incidence around the world.

Family studies show that there is a much-increased risk of MS in first-degree relatives of affected patients (approximately 5% lifetime risk of developing MS). Twin studies confirm a major genetic component to susceptibility, with 30% of monozygotic twins being concordant for MS versus 5% of dizygotic twins.

Genes. Variations in some 60 different genes have been identified as conferring an increased risk of MS; 80% of these are genes relating to immune system function and regulation, including HLA and major histocompatibility complex (MHC) polymorphisms. HLA-associated genes include haplotypes HLA-DRB1*1501, DQA1*102 and DQB1*0602. HLA-DR15 appears to be associated with an earlier disease onset.

Environmental factors

Migration studies (see above) and twin studies indicate that environmental factors play a role in the development of MS but these factors are still largely unknown. Viral infections can precipitate MS relapses, and exposure to infectious agents at critical times in development may trigger MS in genetically susceptible individuals. There is evidence that exposure to Epstein–Barr virus (EBV) may be linked to MS; EBV seropositivity is higher in patients with MS than in the general population. Human herpesvirus 6 (HHV-6) has also been implicated. Exposure to infectious agents in childhood may reduce the risk of developing MS and other autoimmune disorders (the 'hygiene hypothesis'). There is also some evidence that low levels of vitamin D and lack of sunlight exposure may be a risk factor for MS.

Pathology

Plaques of demyelination, 2–10 mm in size, are the cardinal features (**Fig. 26.46**). Plaques occur anywhere in CNS white matter but have a predilection for distinct CNS sites: optic nerves, the periventricular

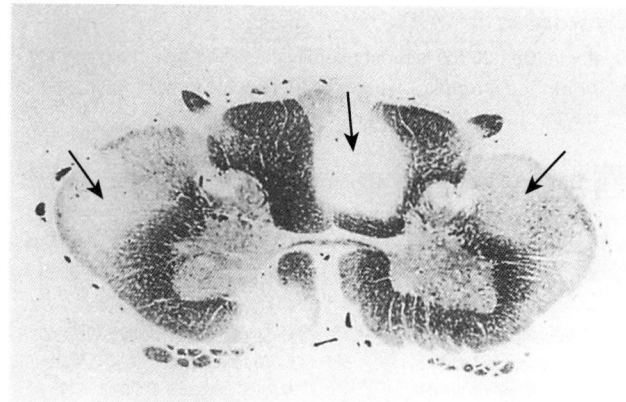

Fig. 26.46 Multiple sclerosis (MS). Cross-section of spinal cord showing MS plaques in posterior column and lateral corticospinal tracts (arrowed). *(Courtesy of the late Professor Ian Macdonald.)*

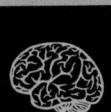

region, the corpus callosum, the brainstem and its cerebellar connections, and the cervical cord (corticospinal tracts and posterior columns). MRI studies show that most inflammatory plaques are asymptomatic. Recent advances in pathology and MRI techniques show that the grey matter of the cortex and the sub-pial meninges is also affected from an early stage in MS. Peripheral myelinated nerves are not directly affected in MS.

Acute relapses are caused by focal inflammation causing myelin damage and conduction block. Recovery follows as inflammation subsides and remyelination occurs. When damage is severe, secondary permanent axonal destruction occurs. Progressive axonal damage is the pathological basis of the progressive disability seen in progressive forms of MS. The extent of grey matter damage correlates with the severity of disability and cognitive involvement. The exact relationship between the inflammatory lesions seen in early relapsing–remitting forms of MS and the progressive axonal loss of chronic forms of MS is disputed.

Clinical features

No single group of signs or symptoms is diagnostic. A wide variety of possible symptoms may occur, depending on the anatomical site of the lesions; MS has been described as the modern 'great imitator'. The clinical time course of attacks and tempo of evolution of symptoms are as helpful as the symptoms themselves in making the diagnosis of MS.

Types of MS

There are four main clinical patterns (**Fig. 26.47**):

- **Relapsing–remitting MS** (**RRMS**) (85–90%). This is the most common pattern of MS. Symptoms occur in attacks (relapses) with a characteristic time course: onset over days and typically recovery, either partial or complete, over weeks. On average, patients have one relapse per year but occasionally many years may separate relapses (benign MS – 10% of patients). Patients may accumulate disability over time if they do not recover fully after relapses.
- **Secondary progressive MS.** This late stage of MS consists of gradually worsening disability progressing slowly over years. Some 75% of patients with relapsing–remitting MS will eventually evolve into a secondary progressive phase by 35 years after onset. Relapses may sometimes occur in this progressive phase (relapsing–progressive MS).

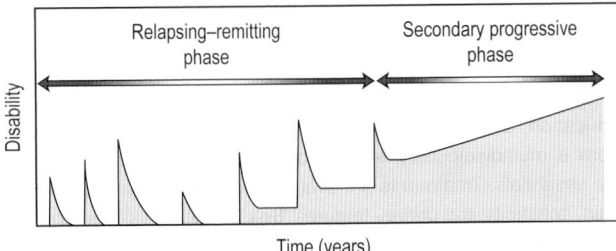

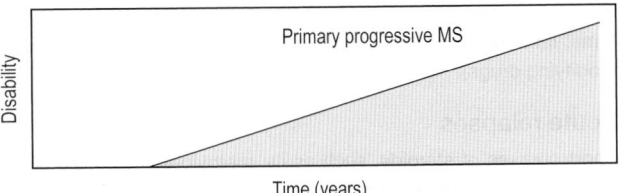

Fig. 26.47 Clinical patterns of multiple sclerosis.

- **Primary progressive MS** (**PPMS**) (10–15%). This pattern is characterized by gradually worsening disability without relapses or remissions. It typically presents later and is associated with fewer inflammatory changes on MRI.
- **Relapsing–progressive MS** (<5%). This is the least common form of MS. It is similar to PPMS but with occasional supra-added relapses on a background of progressive disability from the outset.

Clinical presentations

Three characteristic common presentations of MS are optic neuropathy (neuritis), brainstem demyelination and spinal cord lesions.

Optic neuritis

See page 810.

Brainstem demyelination

A relapse affecting the brainstem causes combinations of diplopia, vertigo, facial numbness/weakness, dysarthria or dysphagia. Pyramidal signs in the limbs occur when the corticospinal tracts are involved. A typical picture is sudden diplopia, and vertigo with nystagmus, but without tinnitus or deafness. Bilateral internuclear ophthalmoplegia (see p. 812) is pathognomonic of MS.

Spinal cord lesions

Paraparesis developing over days or weeks (see **Box 26.62**) is a typical result of a plaque in the cervical or thoracic cord, causing difficulty in walking and limb numbness with tingling, often asymmetric. Lhermitte's sign may be present (see p. 823). Sometimes the arms are also involved in high cervical cord lesions. A tight band sensation around the abdomen or chest is common with thoracic cord lesions.

Common symptoms in MS

Disability and neurological impairments accumulate gradually over the years. Several symptoms are common and many can be improved with symptomatic treatments.

- Visual changes (see p. 810).
- Sensory symptoms – often unusual, e.g. a sensation of water trickling down the skin. Sensory symptoms are the presenting feature in 40% of patients. Reduced vibration sensation and proprioception in the feet are among the most common abnormalities on examination, but examination may be normal despite significant sensory symptoms.
- Clumsy/useless hand or limb – due to loss of proprioception (often a dorsal column spinal plaque).
- Unsteadiness or ataxia.
- Urinary symptoms – bladder hyper-reflexia causing urinary urgency and frequency. Treatment is with antimuscarinics or intravesical botulinum toxin injections.
- Pain – neuropathic pain is common.
- Fatigue – a common and often debilitating symptom, which can occur in patients with otherwise mild disease. This sometimes responds to amantadine or a fatigue management programme.
- Spasticity – may require baclofen or other muscle relaxants. Occasionally, botulinum toxin injections are used for focal spasticity.
- Depression.
- Sexual dysfunction.
- Temperature sensitivity – temporary worsening of pre-existing symptoms with increases in body temperature, e.g. after exercise or a hot bath, is known as Uhthoff's phenomenon.

Unusual presentations

Epilepsy and trigeminal neuralgia (see p. 852) occur more commonly in MS patients than in the general population. Tonic spasms (frequent brief spasms of one limb) are rare but pathognomonic of MS.

Late-stage MS

Late MS causes severe disability with spastic tetraparesis, ataxia, optic atrophy, nystagmus, brainstem signs (e.g. bilateral internuclear ophthalmoplegia), pseudobulbar palsy and urinary incontinence. Cognitive impairment, often with frontal lobe features, may occur in late-stage disease. In a proportion of patients, disability eventually becomes severe, with median time to requiring walking aids of 15 years and time to wheelchair use 25 years from onset.

Diagnosis

Few other neurological diseases have a similar relapsing and remitting course. The diagnosis of MS requires two or more attacks affecting different parts of the CNS: that is, dissemination in time and space, and exclusion of other possible causes. History and support from investigations, particularly MRI, make the diagnosis. The McDonald criteria formalize the diagnostic features but are designed mainly for research purposes and rarely used in clinical practice.

When taking a history at the time of initial presentation, it is essential to ask about previous episodes of neurological symptoms, often years previously, that may represent episodes of unrecognized demyelination: for example, a severe episode of vertigo lasting weeks or loss of vision in one eye that gradually recovered.

Investigations

The purpose of investigations is to provide supportive evidence of dissemination in time and space (i.e. to show scattered demyelinating lesions that evolve over time), to exclude other diseases and to provide evidence of immunological disturbance.

- MRI of brain and cord is the definitive investigation, as it demonstrates areas of demyelination with high sensitivity. Multiple scattered plaques are usually seen (**Fig. 26.48A**), demonstrating dissemination in space. Typical lesions are oval in shape, up to 2 cm in diameter, and often orientated perpendicular to the lateral ventricles. Occasionally, large 'tumefactive' (swelling) lesions are seen (**Fig. 26.48B**). Acute lesions show gadolinium

enhancement for 6–8 weeks. Although a sensitive technique to demonstrate plaques (normal MRI in MS is possible but distinctly rare), it is limited by lower specificity. Over the age of 50, small ischaemic lesions may be difficult to distinguish from demyelination, and in younger patients other neuroinflammatory disorders such as sarcoidosis, Behçet syndrome and vasculitis may produce similar imaging appearances. The presence of spinal cord lesions is quite specific for inflammatory disorders such as MS rather than ischaemic lesions, so cord imaging is often useful where there is diagnostic difficulty.

- Plaques are rarely visible on CT.
- CSF examination is often unnecessary with suggestive MRI and a compatible clinical picture. CSF analysis shows oligoclonal IgG bands in over 90% of cases but these are not specific for MS. The CSF cell count may be raised (5–60 mononuclear cells/mm^3).
- Evoked responses, e.g. visual-evoked responses in optic nerve lesions, may demonstrate clinically silent lesions. However, since the advent of MRI, they are less used in diagnosis.
- Blood tests are used to exclude other inflammatory disorders such as sarcoidosis or SLE, or other causes of paraparesis, e.g. adrenoleukodystrophy, HIV, human T-cell lymphotropic virus 1 (HTLV-1) and vitamin B$_{12}$ deficiency.

The clinically isolated syndrome

In patients presenting with a first ever episode of neurological symptoms suggestive of neuroinflammation, termed a 'clinically isolated syndrome' (CIS), a diagnosis of MS cannot be made by definition. In up to 70% of such patients, MRI shows multiple clinically silent lesions. An abnormal brain MRI at presentation, with multiple inflammatory-type lesions, confers an 85% chance of developing MS over subsequent years (50% if presenting with optic neuritis). Patients need to be made aware of this possibility.

A second clinical event indicative of a new lesion in a different anatomical location allows the diagnosis of MS to be confirmed. Alternatively, a repeat MRI brain scan at least 1 month later showing either a new lesion or a gadolinium-enhancing lesion is sufficient to demonstrate dissemination in time and space and confirm the diagnosis, even in the absence of new symptoms.

Management

There is no cure for MS but, in recent years, several immunomodulatory treatments have been introduced that have dramatically altered the ability to modify the course of the inflammatory relapsing–remitting phase of MS. It is hoped that these will translate into reduced long-term disability but this has yet to be proved.

General measures

Education, provision of appropriate written materials and support from a multidisciplinary team, including an MS nurse specialist, are essentials. Treatments are available for various symptoms, e.g. pain, spasticity and urinary features (**Box 26.53**). Physiotherapy and occupational therapy are helpful where there is persisting impairment between relapses. Infections should be treated early, as they may precipitate relapses or lead to worsening of existing symptoms. Immunizations are safe (but not live vaccines if on disease-modifying drugs).

Acute relapses

Short courses of steroids, such as i.v. methylprednisolone 1 g/day for 3 days or high-dose oral steroids, are used for severe relapses. They speed recovery but do not influence long-term outcome.

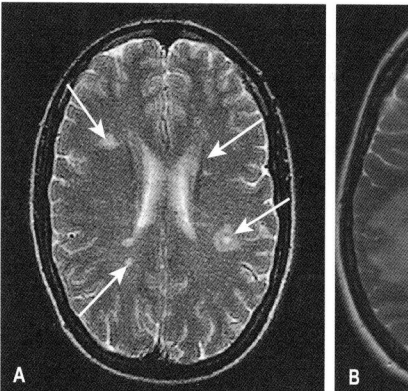
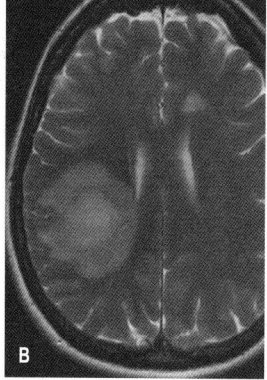

Fig. 26.48 Multiple sclerosis. (A) T2-weighted magnetic resonance image. Brain plaques are shown (arrowed). Typical lesions are oval in shape, up to 2 cm in diameter, and often orientated perpendicular to the lateral ventricles. **(B)** Tumefactive multiple sclerosis lesion.

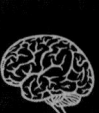

Disease-modifying drugs

Immunomodulatory disease-modifying drugs (DMDs; **Box 26.54**), such as β-interferon (both IFN-β1b and 1a, and pegylated β1a) and glatiramer acetate, reduce relapse rate by one-third and serious relapses by up to half in RRMS. They also significantly reduce development of new MRI lesions and may reduce accumulation of disability over the short term. They are self-administered by subcutaneous or intramuscular injection and are generally well tolerated, apart from influenza-like side-effects and injection site irritation. From a health economics point of view, cost is an issue, as these drugs are very expensive. IFN-β and glatiramer acetate are considered first-line DMDs. **Current recommendations** in the UK are that DMDs are offered to ambulant patients with RRMS where there have been two or more *significant* relapses over a 2-year period or after one major disabling relapse. When used after CIS, the conversion rate to definite MS is reduced from 50% to 30% over 3 years, but in the UK treatment with DMDs after CIS is rarely recommended. DMDs are not effective in primary progressive or secondary progressive MS.

Oral DMDs

Three oral agents, *fingolimod*, *teriflunomide* and *dimethyl fumarate*, have been licensed for treatment of RRMS. They all reduce relapse rate significantly and, in the case of fingolimod and dimethyl fumarate, are superior to interferons. In general, they seem well tolerated but have more serious adverse events than interferons. Their exact place in MS treatment is not yet established (cost is an issue); in some countries, they are used as first-line DMDs but in the UK are likely to be used where first-line drugs are not tolerated or not sufficiently effective.

Treatment of aggressive RRMS

Immunomodulatory drugs and biological agents (monoclonal antibodies), such as *natalizumab* and *alemtuzumab*, have shown high efficacy in preventing relapses and may reduce accumulation of disability significantly (see **Box 26.54**). They have the potential to cause serious adverse effects and are generally used only in very aggressive disease or where relapses are not reduced by β-IFN or glatiramer acetate.

Haemopoietic stem cell transplantation (AHSCT) may be used to treat aggressive MS, working in part by 'resetting' the immune system.

Other drugs and symptomatic therapies

- *Vitamin D.* There is some evidence that vitamin D supplementation may be beneficial in MS but this is still controversial. Some specialists advocate treatment with up to 2000 IU daily.
- *Fampridine* (4-aminopyridine, an oral potassium-channel blocker). This has been shown to improve walking significantly in selected patients with significant MS-related disability.
- *Other symptomatic treatments.* Symptomatic treatments are available for most complications of MS and significantly improve quality of life (see **Box 26.53**). Urinary urgency and frequency, pain, spasticity and depression are all common and treatable.

> *i* **Box 26.53 Symptomatic treatments in multiple sclerosis**

Urinary symptoms
- Antimuscarinics, e.g. oxybutynin, tolterodine, solifenacin, trospium
- Desmopressin spray ± antimuscarinic
- Intermittent self-catheterization (ISC)
- Botulinum toxin type A intravesical injections (usually also require ISC)
- Bladder training exercises
- Indwelling catheter

Spasticity
- Self-management, including stretching, physiotherapy, splinting
- Skeletal muscle relaxants: baclofen, tizanidine, clonazepam
- Gabapentin
- Botulinum toxin type A (electromyelography-guided injections) for focal spasticity
- Cannabis: oromucosal spray
- Intrathecal baclofen pump
- Intrathecal phenol – destructive procedure in advanced disease with paraplegia

Pain
- As for treatment of neuropathic pain (see p. 825)
- Trigeminal neuralgia – carbamazepine, lamotrigine
- Lhermitte's – carbamazepine

Depression
- Cognitive behavioural therapy
- Antidepressants (see p. 771)

Impaired mobility
- Physiotherapy ± walking aids
- Treat spasticity
- Fampridine – selected patients

Erectile dysfunction
- Sildenafil, tadalafil or vardenafil

Tremor
- Beta-adrenoceptor-blocking drugs
- Botulinum toxin type A injections (head or arms)
- Deep brain stimulation for severe Holmes tremor

Fatigue
- Fatigue management programme, treat depression
- Amantadine (often ineffective)

> *i* **Box 26.54 Disease-modifying drugs used in relapsing–remitting multiple sclerosis**

Drug	Mode of action	Administration	Reduction in relapse rate	Effect on disability	Adverse effects/comments
β-interferon (IFN-β1b and 1a)	Immunomodulatory	s.c. alternate days or i.m. weekly	33%	?	Few
Glatiramer acetate	Unknown	s.c. daily	33%	?	Few
Natalizumab	MCA blocks α-4 integrin vascular adhesion molecule. Prevents T cells entering CNS	i.v. monthly	68%	+	Rarely, PML (fatal) Hypersensitivity reactions
Alemtuzumab	MCA. Anti-CD52. Depletes T >B cells	i.v. once and repeat at 1 year	65% relapse-free at 4 years	++	Autoimmune disorders: Graves' disease and ITP
Fingolimod	Sphingosine-1-phosphate receptor (S1-PR) ligand. Prevents T cells leaving lymph nodes	Oral daily	60%	?+	Bradycardia and increased infection rate
Dimethyl fumarate	Unknown	Oral twice daily	50–60%	?	Good safety record in psoriasis; well tolerated but one case of PML
Teriflunomide	Blocks proliferation of activated lymphocytes	Oral daily	30%	+	Abnormal liver enzymes

ITP, immune thrombocytopenic purpura; MCA, monoclonal antibody; PML, progressive multifocal leukoencephalopathy.

Prognosis

The clinical course of MS is unpredictable; a high MR lesion load at initial presentation, high relapse rate, male gender and late presentation are poor prognostic features but not invariably so. There is wide variation in severity. Many patients continue to live independent, productive lives; a minority become severely disabled. Life expectancy is reduced by 7 years on average.

Transverse myelitis

Transverse myelitis is an acute inflammatory disorder affecting the spinal cord with cord swelling and loss of function. Typically, one or two spinal segments are affected with part or all of the cord area at that level involved (*transverse* indicates involvement of the whole cross-section of the cord at the affected level). Clinically, a myelopathy evolves over days, and recovery (often partial) follows over weeks or months. MRI is sensitive and shows cord swelling and oedema with gadolinium enhancement at the affected level(s). Usually, images are also taken of the brain to look for evidence of demyelination. CSF may be inflammatory with an excess of lymphocytes. Causes include:

- *Para-infectious autoimmune inflammatory response.* This is the most common cause and may follow viral infection or immunization, for example.
- *Systemic inflammatory disorders*, e.g. SLE, Sjögren's, sarcoidosis.
- *Infection.* This may be caused by viruses – e.g. herpesviruses, such as varicella zoster or EBV, HIV, HTLV-1 and 2 (tropical spastic paraparesis); mycobacteria, e.g. tuberculosis; bacteria – e.g. syphilis and Lyme disease; or flatworms – e.g. schistosomiasis.
- *Multiple sclerosis.* Transverse myelitis may occur as part of a relapse or be a presenting feature of MS. If the brain MRI is normal, the risk of later development of MS is around 20%; in those that do develop MS with a normal brain MRI, prognosis is better than average.
- *Neuromyelitis optica* – see below.

   Treatment is usually with high-dose steroids or other immunosuppression, or antimicrobial therapy in the case of specific infections.

Neuromyelitis optica

This is a distinct inflammatory relapsing demyelinating disorder, previously thought to be a variant of MS. It is characterized by longitudinally extensive transverse myelitis (>3 segments) and bilateral or recurrent optic neuritis. Limited forms occur, such as recurrent myelitis only. Serum antibodies to aquaporin-4 water channels on astrocytes are diagnostic. It is rarer than MS but there is a higher incidence in Asian and African Caribbean people.

   Treatment with steroids and immunosuppressive drugs is essential from the time of diagnosis, as the relapse rate is high and relapses are much more disabling than in MS. A similar syndrome that follows a monophasic course occurs with myelin oligodendrocyte (MOG) antibodies.

Acute disseminated encephalomyelitis

Acute disseminated encephalomyelitis (ADEM) is usually post-infectious, following infections such as measles, mycoplasma, mumps and rubella, and occasionally following 1–2 weeks after immunization. There is a monophasic illness with multifocal brain, brainstem and often spinal cord inflammatory lesions in white matter, with demyelination. ADEM is caused by an immune-mediated host response to infection and occurs principally in children and young adults. Mild cases recover completely. Survivors often have permanent brain damage. Treatment is supportive, with steroids and anticonvulsants.

Other neuroinflammatory conditions
Neurosarcoidosis

Neurosarcoid, with or without systemic sarcoid, causes chronic meningoencephalitis, cord lesions, cranial nerve palsies – particularly bilateral VIIth nerve lesions, polyneuropathy and myopathy (see p. 985). Diagnosis can be difficult if disease is confined to the CNS.

Behçet's disease

Behçet's principal features (see p. 466) are recurrent oral and/or genital ulceration, inflammatory ocular disease (uveitis; see p. 921) and neurological syndromes. Brainstem and cord lesions, aseptic meningitis, encephalitis and cerebral venous thrombosis occur. There is a predilection for ethnic groups along the ancient 'Silk Road' – Turkey, the Middle East and Asia. Behçet's is associated with the HLA-B51 allele.

Further reading

Frohman EM, Wingerchuk DM. Clinical practice. Transverse myelitis. *N Engl J Med* 2010; 363:564–572.
Perry M, Swain S, Kemmis-Betty S et al. Multiple sclerosis: summary of NICE guidance. *BMJ* 2014; 349:g5701.
Polman CH, Reingold SC, Banwell B et al. Diagnostic criteria for multiple sclerosis: 2010 revisions to the McDonald criteria. *Ann Neurol* 2011; 69:292–302.
Scolding N, Barnes D, Cader S et al. Association of British Neurologists: revised (2015) guidelines for prescribing disease-modifying treatments in multiple sclerosis. *Pract Neurol* 2015; 15:273–279.
http://www.mssociety.org.uk. *MS Society (UK national charity).*

NERVOUS SYSTEM INFECTION

Meningitis

Meningitis usually implies serious *infection* of the meninges (**Box 26.55**). Bacterial meningitis is fatal unless treated. Microorganisms reach the meninges either by direct extension from the ears, nasopharynx, cranial injury or congenital meningeal defect, or by bloodstream spread. Immunocompromised patients are at risk of infection with unusual organisms. Non-infective causes of meningeal inflammation include malignant meningitis, intrathecal drugs and blood following subarachnoid haemorrhage.

Pathology

In acute bacterial meningitis, the pia-arachnoid is congested with polymorphs. A layer of pus forms. This may organize to form adhesions, causing cranial nerve palsies and hydrocephalus.

   In chronic infection (e.g. tuberculosis), the brain is covered in a viscous grey–green exudate with numerous meningeal tubercles. Adhesions are invariable. Cerebral oedema occurs in any bacterial meningitis.

   In viral meningitis there is a predominantly lymphocytic inflammatory CSF reaction without pus formation, polymorphs or adhesions; there is little or no cerebral oedema unless encephalitis develops.

Clinical features
Meningitic syndrome

This is a simple triad: headache, neck stiffness and fever. Photophobia and vomiting are often present. In acute bacterial infection, there is usually intense malaise, fever, rigors, severe headache, photophobia and vomiting, developing within hours or minutes.

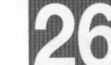

Bacteria
- *Neisseria meningitidis*
- *Streptococcus pneumoniae*[a]
- *Staphylococcus aureus*
- *Streptococcus* group B
- *Listeria monocytogenes*
- Gram-negative bacilli, e.g. *Escherichia coli*
- *Mycobacterium tuberculosis*
- *Treponema pallidum*

Viruses
- Enteroviruses:
  - ECHO
  - Coxsackie
- (Poliomyelitis – mainly eradicated worldwide)
- Mumps
- Herpes simplex
- HIV
- Epstein–Barr

Fungi
- *Cryptococcus neoformans*
- *Candida albicans*
- *Coccidioides immitis*, *Histoplasma capsulatum*, *Blastomyces dermatitidis* (USA)

[a]These organisms account for 70% of acute bacterial meningitis outside the neonatal period. A wide variety of infective agents are responsible for the remaining 30% of cases. *Haemophilus influenzae b* (Hib) has been eliminated as a cause in many countries by immunization. Malaria often presents with cerebral symptoms and a fever.

? **Box 26.56** Clinical clues in meningitis

Clinical feature	Possible cause
Petechial rash	Meningococcal infection
Skull fracture Ear disease Congenital CNS lesion	Pneumococcal infection
Immunocompromised patients	HIV with opportunistic infection
Rash or pleuritic pain	Enterovirus infection
International travel	Malaria
Occupational: work in drains, canals, polluted water, recreational swimming Clinical: myalgia, conjunctivitis, jaundice	Leptospirosis

The patient is irritable and often prefers to lie still. Neck stiffness and a positive Kernig's sign usually appear within hours.

In less severe cases (e.g. many viral meningitides), there are less prominent meningitic signs. However, bacterial infection may also be indolent, with a deceptively mild onset.

In uncomplicated meningitis, consciousness remains intact, although anyone with a high fever may be delirious. Progressive drowsiness, lateralizing signs and cranial nerve lesions indicate complications such as venous sinus thrombosis (see p. 837), severe cerebral oedema or hydrocephalus, or an alternative diagnosis such as cerebral abscess (see p. 873) or encephalitis (see p. 871).

Specific varieties of meningitis

Clinical clues point to the diagnosis (**Box 26.56**). If there is access to the subarachnoid space via skull fracture (recent or old) or occult spina bifida, bacterial meningitis can be recurrent, and the infecting organism is usually pneumococcus.

Acute bacterial meningitis

Onset is typically sudden, with rigors and high fever. Meningococcal septicaemia is associated with a petechial rash, sometimes sparse (**Box 26.57** and **Fig. 26.49**). The meningitis may be part of a generalized meningococcal septicaemia with septic shock and peripheral vascular infarcts (see p. 545). Acute septicaemic shock may develop in any bacterial meningitis.

⊕ **Box 26.57** Meningococcal meningitis and meningococcaemia: emergency treatment

Suspicion of meningococcal infection is a medical emergency requiring treatment immediately.

Clinical features
- Petechial or non-specific blotchy, red rash
- Fever, headache, neck stiffness.
  All these features may not be present – and meningococcal infection may sometimes begin like any apparently non-serious infection.

Immediate treatment for suspected meningococcal meningitis at first contact before investigation
- Third-generation cephalosporin, e.g. cefotaxime, as empirical therapy (increasing rates of penicillin resistance)
- Switch to benzylpenicillin if sensitivity confirmed
- Dexamethasone 0.6 mg/kg i.v. with or before first dose of antibiotic
  In meningitis, minutes count – delay is unacceptable.

On arrival in hospital
- Blood tests, including blood cultures, immediately
- Monitoring for septic shock.
  For further management and prophylaxis, see text.

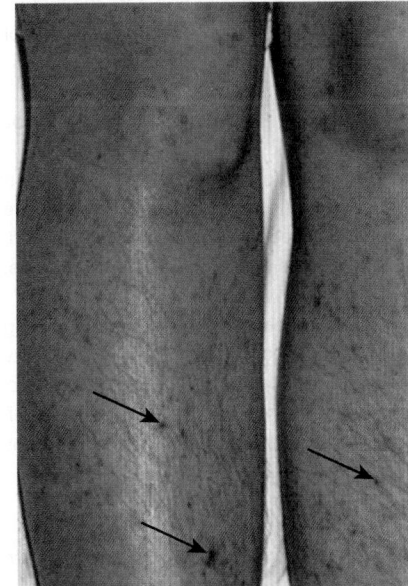

Fig. 26.49 Rash of meningococcal septicaemia with meningitis. Purpuric lesions are indicated with arrows.

Viral meningitis

This is almost always a benign, self-limiting condition lasting 4–10 days. Headache may follow for some months. There are no serious sequelae, unless an encephalitis is present (see p. 871).

Chronic meningitis (see below)

For further discussion on chronic meningitis, see later.

Differential diagnosis

It may be difficult to distinguish between the sudden headache of subarachnoid haemorrhage, migraine and acute meningitis. Meningitis should be considered seriously in anyone with headache and fever, and in any sudden headache. Neck stiffness should be looked for; it may not be obvious.

Chronic meningitis sometimes resembles an intracranial mass lesion, with headache, epilepsy and focal signs. Cerebral malaria can mimic bacterial meningitis.

Management

Recognition and immediate treatment of acute bacterial meningitis (see **Box 26.57**) are vital. Minutes save lives. Bacterial meningitis has a high mortality and morbidity. Even with optimal care, mortality is around 15%. The following applies to adult patients; management is similar in children.

When meningococcal meningitis is diagnosed clinically by the petechial rash, immediate intravenous antibiotics should be given and blood cultures taken; lumbar puncture is unnecessary. In other causes of meningitis, an LP is performed if there is no clinical suspicion of a mass lesion (see p. 830). If the latter is suspected, an immediate CT scan must be performed because coning of the cerebellar tonsils may follow LP, but normal brain imaging does not exclude raised intracranial pressure and clinical features of raised pressure contraindicate LP. Typical CSF changes are shown in **Box 26.58**. CSF pressure is characteristically elevated.

Immediate *antibiotic* treatment in acute bacterial meningitis is shown in **Box 26.59**. Treatment with antibiotics should be continued for at least 5 days.

Adjunctive immediate high-dose **steroid** (dexamethasone 0.6 mg/kg i.v. for 4 days), given with or before the first dose of antibiotics, has been shown to reduce neurological complications in bacterial meningitis (e.g. deafness), and some studies also show reduced mortality in Western populations.

Blood should be taken for cultures, glucose and routine tests. Chest and skull films should be obtained if appropriate.

CSF stains demonstrate organisms (e.g. Gram-positive intracellular diplococci – pneumococcus; Gram-negative cocci – meningococcus). Ziehl–Neelsen stain demonstrates acid-fast bacilli (tuberculosis), though TB organisms are rarely numerous. Indian ink stains fungi.

Meticulous attention should focus on microbiological studies in suspected CNS infection with close liaison between clinician and microbiologist. Specific techniques, such as polymerase chain reaction for meningococci and viruses, or CSF bacterial antigen testing, are invaluable. Syphilis serology should always be carried out.

Local infection (e.g. paranasal sinus) should be treated surgically if necessary. Repair of a depressed skull fracture or meningeal tear may be required.

Prophylaxis

Meningococcal infection should be notified to the public health authorities, and advice sought about immunization and prophylaxis of contacts. Chemoprophylaxis with rifampicin or ciprofloxacin should be offered to all close contacts. MenC vaccine is given in the UK and MenB, a meningococcal B vaccine, is now available for population immunization of infants and for use in outbreaks. A combined A and C meningococcal vaccine is sometimes used prior to travel from the UK to endemic regions, such as Africa or Asia, and there is a quadrivalent ACWY vaccine for specific events, such as the Hajj and Umrah in Mecca.

Pneumococcal conjugated vaccine is now given to infants in many countries and pneumococcal polysaccharide vaccine is offered to older adults and those with, for example, immunodeficiency or splenectomy. Pneumococcal immunization has reduced the incidence of pneumococcal meningitis.

Hib (*Haemophilus influenzae*) vaccine is given routinely in childhood in the UK and many other countries, virtually eliminating a common cause of fatal meningitis.

Chronic meningitis

Tuberculous meningitis (TBM) and *cryptococcal meningitis* typically commence with vague headache, lassitude, anorexia and vomiting. Acute meningitis can occur but is unusual. Meningitic signs often take some weeks to develop. Drowsiness, focal signs (e.g. diplopia, papilloedema, hemiparesis) and seizures are common. Syphilis, sarcoidosis and Behçet's also cause chronic meningitis. In some cases of chronic meningitis, an organism is never identified.

Investigation and management of tuberculous meningitis

TBM is a common and serious disease worldwide. Brain imaging, usually with MRI, may show meningeal enhancement, hydrocephalus and tuberculomas (see p. 876), although it may remain

---

i **Box 26.58 Typical changes in cerebrospinal fluid in viral, pyogenic and tuberculous meningitis**

	Normal	Viral	Pyogenic	Tuberculous
Appearance	Crystal clear	Clear/turbid	Turbid/purulent	Turbid/viscous
Mononuclear cells	<5/mm^3	10–100/mm^3	<50/mm^3	100–300/mm^3
Polymorph cells	Nil	Nil[a]	200–300/mm^3	0–200/mm^3
Protein	0.2–0.4 g/L	0.4–0.8 g/L	0.5–2.0 g/L	0.5–3.0 g/L
Glucose	⅔–½ blood glucose	>½ blood glucose	<½ blood glucose	<½ blood glucose

[a]Some CSF polymorphs may be seen in the early stages of viral meningitis and encephalitis.

---

i **Box 26.59 Antibiotics in acute bacterial meningitis**

Organism	Antibiotic	Alternative (e.g. allergy)
Unknown pyogenic	Third-generation cephalosporin, e.g. cefotaxime (+ vancomycin in areas of high pneumococcal penicillin/cephalosporin resistance)	Benzylpenicillin and chloramphenicol
Age >50 or immunocompromised	As above but add ampicillin to cover *Listeria*	Co-trimoxazole for *Listeria*
Meningococcus	Third-generation cephalosporin initially Switch to benzylpenicillin if confirmed sensitive	Cefotaxime
Pneumococcus	Third-generation cephalosporin, e.g. cefotaxime	Penicillin
Haemophilus	Third-generation cephalosporin, e.g. cefotaxime	Chloramphenicol

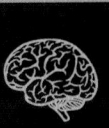

normal (see **Box 26.58** for CSF changes). In many cases, the sparse tuberculous organisms cannot be seen on staining and PCR testing should be performed, although results may be negative. Repeated CSF examination is often necessary and it will be some weeks before cultures are confirmatory. Treatment with anti-tuberculosis drugs (see p. 971) – rifampicin, isoniazid and pyrazinamide – must commence on a presumptive basis and continue for at least 9 months. Ethambutol should be avoided because of its eye complications. Adjuvant corticosteroids, such as prednisolone 60 mg for 3 weeks, are now recommended (often tapered off). Relapses and complications (e.g. seizures, hydrocephalus) are common in TBM. The mortality remains over 60%, even with early treatment.

Malignant meningitis

Malignant cells can cause a subacute or chronic, non-infective, meningitic process. A meningitic syndrome, cranial nerve lesions, paraparesis and root lesions are seen, often in confusing and fluctuating patterns. CSF cytology may demonstrate malignant cells but yield is low so multiple LPs may be required to confirm the diagnosis. Treatment with intrathecal cytotoxic agents is sometimes helpful.

Cells in a sterile CSF (pleocytosis)

A raised CSF cell count is present without an evident infecting organism. CSF pleocytosis, i.e. a mixture of lymphocytes and polymorphs, is the usual situation (**Box 26.60**).

Encephalitis

Encephalitis means acute inflammation of brain parenchyma, usually viral. In viral encephalitis, fever (90%) and meningism are usual; in contrast to meningitis, however, the clinical picture is dominated by brain parenchyma inflammation. Personality and behavioural change is a common early manifestation, which progresses to a reduced level of consciousness and even coma. Seizures (focal and generalized) are very common and focal neurological deficits, such as speech disturbance, often occur (especially in herpes simplex encephalitis).

Viral encephalitis

(See p. 527.) The viruses isolated from adult UK cases are usually herpes simplex (HSV), varicella zoster (VZV) and other herpes group viruses, HHV-6, 7, enteroviruses and adenovirus. HSV encephalitis typically affects the temporal lobes initially, and is often asymmetric. Frequently, the virus is never identified. Outside the UK, in endemic regions, different pathogens cause encephalitis, including flaviviruses (Japanese encephalitis, West Nile virus, tick-borne encephalitis) and rabies.

Local epidemics can occur. For example, in New York in the 1990s, West Nile virus caused an epidemic and Venezuelan equine virus was isolated from encephalitis cases in South America.

> **? Box 26.60 Causes of sterile CSF pleocytosis**
>
> - Partially treated bacterial meningitis
> - Viral meningitis
> - Tuberculous or fungal meningitis
> - Intracranial abscess
> - Neoplastic meningitis
> - Parameningeal foci, e.g. paranasal sinus
> - Syphilis
> - Cerebral venous thrombosis
> - Cerebral malaria
> - Cerebral infarction
> - Following subarachnoid haemorrhage
> - Encephalitis, including HIV
> - Rarities, e.g. cerebral malaria, sarcoidosis, Behçet's syndrome, Lyme disease, endocarditis, cerebral vasculitis

Investigations

- MRI shows areas of inflammation and swelling, generally in the temporal lobes in HSV encephalitis. Raised intracranial pressure and midline shift may occur, leading to coning.
- EEG shows periodic sharp and slow-wave complexes.
- CSF shows an elevated lymphocyte count (95%).
- Viral detection by CSF PCR is highly sensitive for several viruses, such as HSV and VZV. However, a false-negative result may occur within the first 48 hours of symptom onset. Serology (blood and CSF) is also helpful.
- Brain biopsy is rarely required since the advent of MRI and PCR.

Management

Suspected HSV and VZV encephalitis is treated immediately with intravenous aciclovir (10 mg/kg 3 times a day for 14–21 days), even before investigation results are available. Early treatment significantly reduces both mortality and long-term neurological damage in survivors. Seizures are treated with anticonvulsants. Occasionally, decompressive craniectomy is required to prevent coning but coma confers a poor prognosis.

Long-term complications are common and include memory impairment, personality change and epilepsy.

Autoimmune encephalitis

This group of disorders are increasingly being recognized. Auto-antibodies directed against neuronal epitopes cause a subacute encephalitic illness: limbic encephalitis or panencephalitis. Limbic encephalitis presents over weeks or months with memory impairment, confusion, psychiatric disturbance, and seizures – usually temporal lobe seizures, reflecting involvement of the hippocampus and mesial temporal lobes.

Paraneoplastic limbic encephalitis (PLE). PLE is seen particularly with small-cell lung cancer and testicular tumours, and is associated with a variety of antibodies, including anti-Hu and anti-Ma2. Antibodies can be detected in 60% of cases. MRI usually shows a hippocampal high signal. PLE precedes the diagnosis of cancer in most cases and should prompt investigation to identify the tumour.

Voltage-gated potassium channel (VGKC) limbic encephalitis. VGKC antibodies (which can be tested for) produce a variety of disorders, including limbic encephalitis with characteristic faciobrachial dystonic seizures, in combination with confusion, agitation and hyponatraemia. This usually occurs in patients over 50 years of age but is rarely associated with cancer (thymoma). Treatment is with high-dose steroids. Neuromyotonia and peripheral nerve hyperexcitability syndromes may also be seen with antibodies to VGKC.

Anti-NMDA receptor antibody encephalitis. This presents as limbic encephalitis followed by coma and often status epilepticus. Orofacial dyskinesias are characteristic. Patients are usually younger, and most have teratomas, such as ovarian.

Patients may respond to immunotherapy: intravenous immunoglobulin or plasma exchange initially, followed by steroids, rituximab or cyclophosphamide. PLE responds less well to treatment.

HIV and neurology

HIV-infected individuals frequently present with or develop neurological conditions. The human immunodeficiency virus itself is directly neuroinvasive and neurovirulent. Immunosuppression leads to indolent, atypical clinical patterns (see p. 1430). HIV patients also have a high incidence of stroke. The pattern of disease is changing with anti-retroviral (ART) therapy.

CNS and peripheral nerve disease in HIV

HIV seroconversion can cause meningitis, encephalitis, Guillain–Barré syndrome and Bell's palsy (the most common cause of Bell's palsy in South Africa).

Chronic meningitis occurs with fungi (e.g. *Cryptococcus neoformans* or *Aspergillus*), tuberculosis, *Listeria*, coliforms or other organisms. Raised CSF pressure is common in cryptococcal meningitis.

AIDS–dementia complex (ADC). A progressive, HIV-related dementia, sometimes with cerebellar signs, is still seen where ART is unavailable.

Encephalitis and brain abscess. *Toxoplasma*, cytomegalovirus, herpes simplex and other organisms cause severe encephalitis. Multiple brain abscesses develop in HIV infection, usually due to toxoplasmosis.

CNS lymphoma. This is typically fatal (see p. 406).

Progressive multifocal leukoencephalopathy (PML) is due to JC virus and occurs with very low CD4 counts (see p. 529).

Spinal vacuolar myelopathy. This occurs in advanced disease.

Peripheral nerve disease. HIV-related peripheral neuropathy is common (70%) and can be difficult to distinguish from the effects of certain ART toxic to peripheral nerves.

Other infections and post-infectious inflammatory conditions

Many other infections involve the CNS and are discussed in Chapter 20: for example, rabies, tetanus, botulism, Lyme disease and leprosy.

Herpes zoster (shingles)

This is caused by reactivation of varicella zoster virus (VZV), usually within dorsal root ganglia. Primary infection with VZV causes chickenpox, following which the virus remains latent in sensory ganglia. Development of shingles may indicate a decline in cell-mediated immunity, such as that due to age or malignancy.

Clinical patterns and complications

Dermatomal shingles. See pages 515 and 671.

Postherpetic neuralgia. This is defined as pain lasting for more than 4 months after developing shingles; it occurs in 10% of patients (often elderly). Burning, intractable pain responds poorly to analgesics. Response to treatment is unsatisfactory but there is a trend towards gradual recovery over 2 years. Amitriptyline or gabapentin is commonly used, and topical lidocaine patches may help.

Cranial nerve involvement. Only cranial nerves with sensory fibres are affected, particularly the trigeminal and facial nerves. Ophthalmic herpes is due to involvement of V_1. This can lead to corneal scarring and secondary panophthalmitis. Involvement of the geniculate ganglion of the facial nerve is also called Ramsay Hunt syndrome (see p. 815).

Myelitis. This may occur in the context of shingles, when the inflammatory process spreads from the dorsal root ganglion to the adjacent spinal cord.

Immunization. Older adults (p. 516) can be vaccinated against herpes zoster (even those who have had shingles previously), as it boosts immunity against VZV and reduces the incidence of shingles by about 50%.

Neurosyphilis

Many neurological symptoms occur, sometimes mixed (see also syphilis; p. 1422).

Asymptomatic neurosyphilis

This means positive CSF serology without signs.

Meningovascular syphilis

This causes:
- subacute meningitis with cranial nerve palsies and papilloedema
- a gumma – a chronic expanding intracranial mass
- paraparesis – a spinal meningovasculitis.

Tabes dorsalis

Demyelination in dorsal roots causes a complex deafferentation syndrome. The elements of tabes are:
- lightning pains
- ataxia, stamping gait, reflex/sensory loss, wasting
- neuropathic (Charcot) joints
- Argyll Robertson pupils (see p. 811)
- ptosis and optic atrophy.

General paralysis of the insane

The grandiose title describes dementia and weakness. The dementia of general paralysis of the insane (GPI) is typically similar to that of Alzheimer's (see p. 882). Progressive cognitive decline, seizures, brisk reflexes, extensor plantar reflexes and tremor develop. Death follows within 3 years. Argyll Robertson pupils are a usual finding. GPI and tabes are rarities in the UK.

Other forms of neurosyphilis

In *congenital* neurosyphilis (acquired *in utero*), features of combined tabes and GPI develop in childhood: taboparesis.

Secondary syphilis can be symptomless or may cause a self-limiting subacute meningitis.

Management

Benzylpenicillin 1 g daily i.m. for 10 days in primary infection eliminates any risk of neurosyphilis. Allergic (Jarisch–Herxheimer) reactions can occur; steroid cover is usually given with penicillin. Established neurological disease is arrested but not reversed by penicillin.

Neurocysticercosis

The pork tapeworm, *Taenia solium*, is endemic in Latin America, Africa, India and much of South-east Asia (see p. 581). Epilepsy is the most common clinical manifestation of neurocysticercosis and one of the most common causes of epilepsy in endemic countries. Most infected people remain asymptomatic.

Brain CT and MRI show ring-enhancing lesions with surrounding oedema when the cyst dies, and later calcification. Multiple cysts are often seen in both brain and skeletal muscle. Serological tests indicate infection but not activity. Biopsy of a lesion is rarely necessary. Management is primarily the control of seizures, and the anthelmintic agent, albendazole, is often given too (usually with steroid cover).

Subacute sclerosing panencephalitis

Persistence of measles antigen in the CNS is associated with this rare late sequel of measles. Progressive mental deterioration, fits, myoclonus and pyramidal signs develop, typically in a child. Diagnosis is made by high measles antibody titre in blood and CSF. Measles immunization protects against subacute sclerosing panencephalitis (SSPE), which has now been almost eliminated in the UK.

Progressive rubella encephalitis

Some 10 years after primary rubella infection, this causes progressive cognitive impairment, fits, optic atrophy, cerebellar and pyramidal signs. Antibody to rubella viral antigen is produced locally within the CNS. It is even rarer than SSPE.

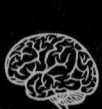

Mollaret's meningitis

Recurrent, self-limiting episodes of aseptic meningitis (i.e. no bacterial cause is found) occur over many years. Herpes simplex has been shown to be the cause in most cases.

Whipple's disease

CNS Whipple's disease, due to *Tropheryma whipplei* infection, is characterized by neurological symptoms, e.g. myoclonus, dementia and supranuclear ophthalmoplegia (see p. 1194). Diagnosis of CNS involvement is made by CSF PCR (only 50% sensitivity) or brain biopsy.

Brain and spinal abscesses

Brain abscess

Focal bacterial infection behaves as any expanding mass. The typical bacteria found are *Streptococcus anginosus* and *Bacteroides* species (from the paranasal sinuses and teeth), and staphylococci (associated with penetrating trauma). Mixed infections are common. Multiple abscesses may develop, particularly in HIV infection. Fungi also cause brain abscesses. A parameningeal infective focus (e.g. ear, nose, paranasal sinus, skull fracture) or a distant source of infection (e.g. lung, heart, abdomen) may be present. Frequently, no underlying cause is found. An abscess is more than ten times rarer than a brain tumour in the UK.

Clinical features and management

Headache, focal signs (e.g. hemiparesis, aphasia, hemianopia), epilepsy and raised intracranial pressure develop. Fever, leucocytosis and raised ESR are usual, although not invariable.

Urgent imaging is essential. MRI shows a ring-enhancing mass, usually with considerable surrounding oedema (**Fig. 26.50**). The search for a focus of infection should include a detailed examination of the skull, ears, paranasal sinuses and teeth, and distant sites

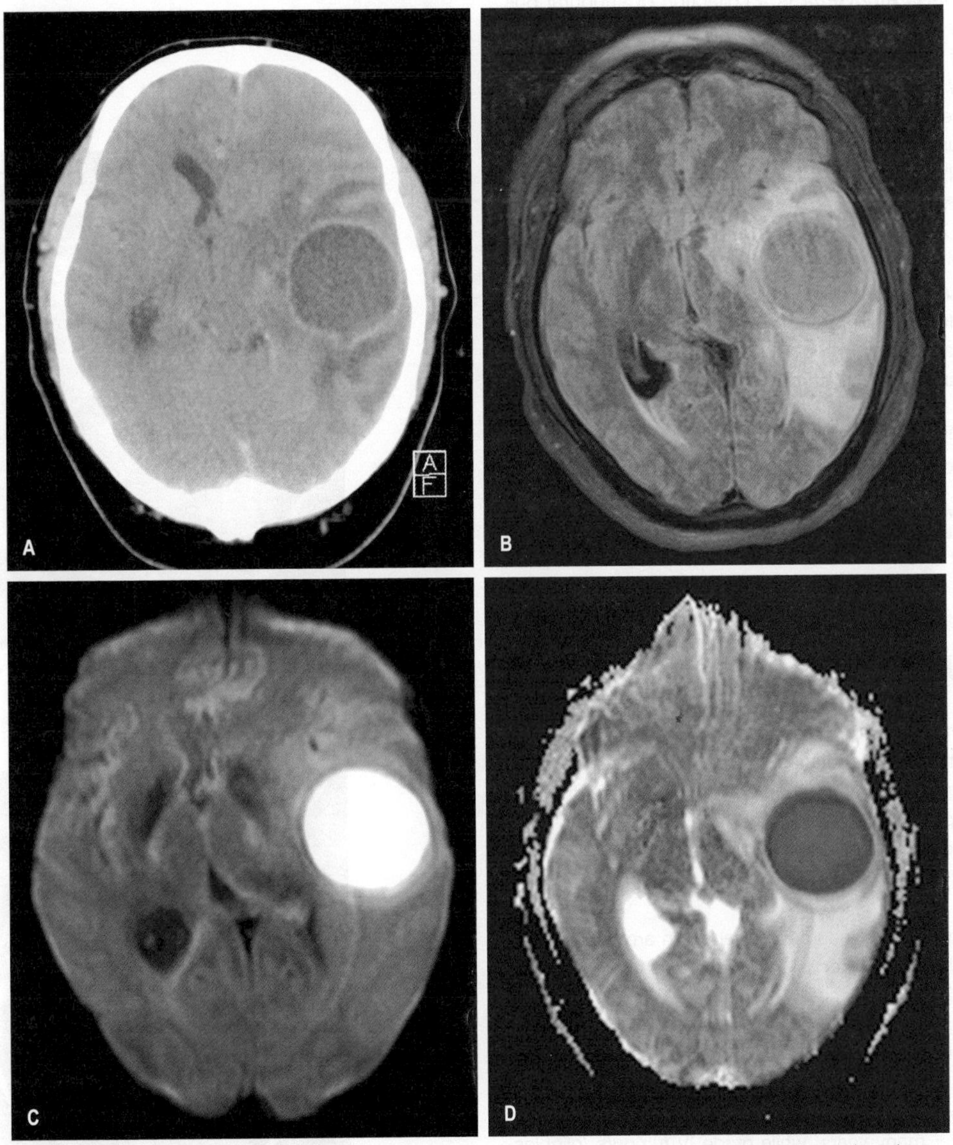

Fig. 26.50 Pyogenic cerebral abscess. (A) Axial post-contrast CT demonstrating a ring-enhancing lesion in the left temporoparietal region. **(B)** Subsequent T2-weighted fluid suppressed (FLAIR) images show the extent of surrounding oedema. MRI is also useful to characterize the lesion further. **(C)** Here, diffusion-weighted and **(D)** ADC map confirm restricted diffusion within the lesion, which is characteristic of intracranial pyogenic abscess.

such as heart and abdomen. LP is dangerous and should not be performed. Neurosurgical aspiration with stereotactic guidance allows the infective organism to be identified. Treatment is with high-dose antibiotics and, sometimes, surgical resection/decompression. Despite treatment, mortality remains high at approximately 25%. Epilepsy is common in survivors.

Brain tuberculoma

Tuberculosis causes chronic caseating intracranial granulomatous masses: tuberculomas. These are the most common intracranial masses in countries where tuberculosis is common, such as India. Brain tuberculomas either present as mass lesions *de novo* or develop during tuberculous meningitis; they are also found as symptomless intracranial calcification on imaging. Spinal cord tuberculomas also occur. Treatment is described on page 969.

Subdural empyema and intracranial epidural abscess

Intracranial subdural empyema is a collection of subdural pus, usually secondary to local skull or middle ear infection. Features are similar to those of a cerebral abscess. Imaging is diagnostic.

In **intracranial epidural abscess**, a layer of pus, 1–3 mm thick, tracks along the epidural space, causing sequential cranial nerve palsies. There is usually local infection: in the middle ear, for example. MRI shows the collection; CT is typically normal. Drainage is required, as are antibiotics.

Spinal epidural abscess

Staphylococcus aureus is the usual organism, reaching the spine via the bloodstream: for example, from a boil. Fever and back pain are followed by paraparesis and/or root lesions. Emergency imaging and antibiotics are essential and surgical decompression is often necessary.

Further reading

Brouwer MC, Tunkel GM, McKhann HGM. Brain abscess. *N Engl J Med* 2014; 371:447–456.
van de Beek D, Brouwer MC, Thwaites GE et al. Advances in treatment of bacterial meningitis. *Lancet* 2012; 380:1693–1702.
http://www.meningitisnow.org/. *Formed in 2013 by merger of Meningitis UK and the Meningitis Trust.*

BRAIN TUMOURS

Primary intracranial tumours account for 3% of all cancers. The most common tumours are outlined in **Box 26.61**, with **cerebral metastases** being more common than primary intracranial tumours (**Fig. 26.51**). Symptomless meningiomas (benign) are found quite commonly on imaging or at autopsy.

Gliomas

These malignant tumours of neuroepithelial origin are usually seen within the hemispheres, but occasionally in the cerebellum, brainstem or cord (**Fig. 26.52**). Their cause is unknown. Gliomas are occasionally associated with neurofibromatosis. They tend to spread by direct extension, virtually never metastasizing outside the CNS.

- **Astrocytomas** are gliomas that arise from astrocytes. They are classified histologically into grades I–IV. Grade I astrocytomas grow slowly over many years, while grade IV tumours (glioblastoma multiforme) cause death within several months. Cystic astrocytomas of childhood are relatively benign and usually cerebellar.
- **Oligodendrogliomas** arise from oligodendrocytes. They grow slowly, usually over several decades. Calcification is common.

Box 26.61 Common brain tumours

Tumour	Approximate frequency
Metastases	50%
Bronchus	
Breast	
Stomach	
Prostate	
Thyroid	
Kidney	
Primary malignant tumours of neuroepithelial tissues	35%
Astrocytoma	
Oligodendroglioma	
Mixed (oligoastrocytoma) glioma	
Ependymoma	
Primary cerebral	
Lymphoma	
Medulloblastoma	
Benign tumours	15%
Meningioma	
Neurofibroma	

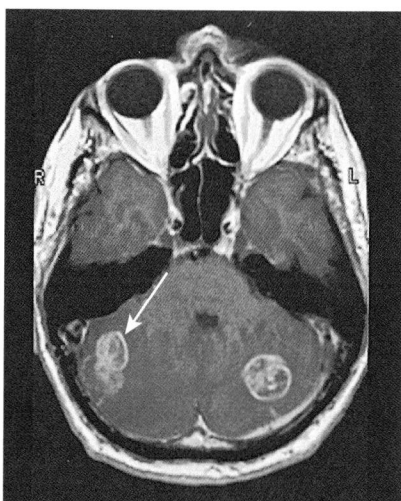

Fig. 26.51 Bilateral cerebellar metastases (arrowed): T1-weighted MRI.

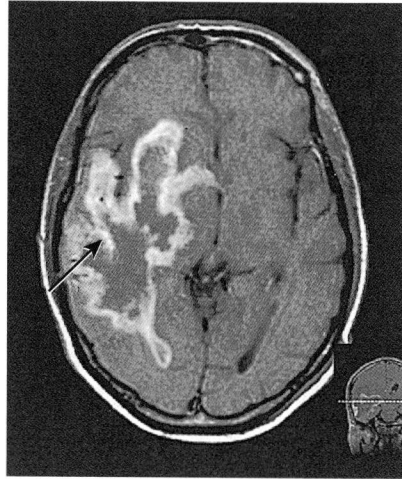

Fig. 26.52 Cerebral glioblastoma multiforme: T1-weighted MRI.

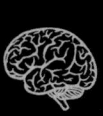

Meningiomas

These benign tumours (**Fig. 26.53**) arise from the arachnoid and may grow to a large size, usually over years. Those close to the skull erode bone or cause local hyperostosis. They often occur along the intracranial venous sinuses, which they may invade. They are unusual below the tentorium. Common sites are the parasagittal region, sphenoidal ridge, subfrontal region, pituitary fossa and skull base.

Neurofibromas (schwannomas)

These solid benign tumours arise from Schwann cells and occur principally in the cerebellopontine angle, where they arise from the VIIIth nerve sheath (acoustic neuroma; see p. 814). They may be bilateral in neurofibromatosis type 2 (see p. 886).

Other neoplasms

Other less common neoplasms include cerebellar haemangioblastomas, ependymomas of the IVth ventricle, colloid cysts of the IIIrd ventricle, pinealomas, chordomas of the skull base, glomus tumours of the jugular bulb, medulloblastomas (a cerebellar childhood tumour), craniopharyngiomas (see p. 595) and primary CNS lymphomas (p. 406). For pituitary tumours, see page 592.

Clinical features

Mass lesions within the brain produce symptoms and signs by three mechanisms:

- direct effect – the brain is infiltrated and local function is impaired, producing focal neurological signs
- secondary effects of raised intracranial pressure and shift of intracranial contents (e.g. papilloedema, vomiting, headache)
- provocation of generalized and/or focal seizures.

Although neoplasms, either secondary or primary, are the most common mass lesions in the UK, cerebral abscess, tuberculoma, neurocysticercosis, and subdural and intracranial haematomas can also produce features that are clinically similar.

Direct effects of mass lesions

The hallmark of a direct effect of a mass is local progressive deterioration of function. Tumours can occur anywhere within the brain. Three examples are given:

- **A left frontal meningioma** caused a frontal lobe syndrome over several years with vague disturbance of personality, apathy and impaired intellect. Expressive aphasia developed, followed by progressive right hemiparesis as the corticospinal pathways became involved. As the mass enlarged further, pressure headaches and papilloedema occurred.
- **A right parietal lobe glioma** caused a left homonymous field defect (optic radiation). Cortical sensory loss in the left limbs and left hemiparesis followed over 3 months. Partial seizures (episodes of tingling of the left limbs) developed.
- **A left VIIIth nerve sheath neurofibroma (acoustic neuroma, schwannoma)** in the cerebellopontine angle caused, over 3 years, progressive deafness (VIII), left facial numbness (V) and weakness (VII), followed by cerebellar ataxia on the same side.

With a hemisphere tumour, epilepsy and the direct effects commonly draw attention to the problem. The rate of progression varies greatly, from a few days or weeks in a highly malignant glioma, to several years with a slowly enlarging mass such as a meningioma. Cerebral oedema surrounds mass lesions; its effect is difficult to distinguish from that of the tumour itself.

Raised intracranial pressure

Raised intracranial pressure causing headache, vomiting and papilloedema is a relatively unusual presentation of a mass lesion in the brain. These symptoms often imply hydrocephalus: obstruction to CSF pathways. Typically, this is produced early by posterior fossa masses that obstruct the aqueduct and IVth ventricle, but only later by lesions above the tentorium. Shift of the intracranial contents produces features that coexist with the direct effects of any expanding mass:

- **Distortion of the upper brainstem** as midline structures are displaced either caudally or laterally by a hemisphere mass (see **Fig. 26.52**). This causes impairment of consciousness, progressing to coning and death as the medulla and cerebellar tonsils are forced into the foramen magnum.
- **False localizing signs**, termed false only because they do not point *directly* to the site of the mass.

  Three examples of false localizing signs are:
  - **A VIth nerve lesion**, first on the side of a mass and later bilaterally as the VIth nerve is compressed or stretched during its long intracranial course.
  - **A IIIrd nerve lesion** developing as the temporal lobe uncus herniates caudally, compressing the IIIrd nerve against the petroclinoid ligament. The first sign is ipsilateral pupil dilation as parasympathetic fibres are compressed.

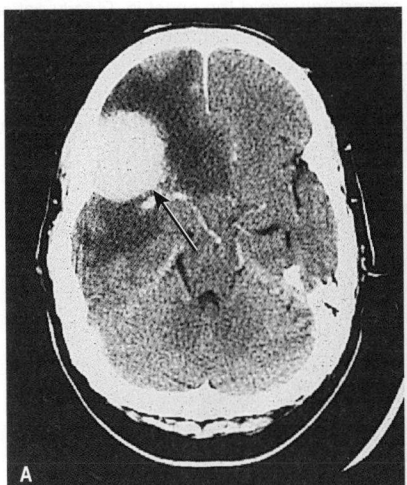
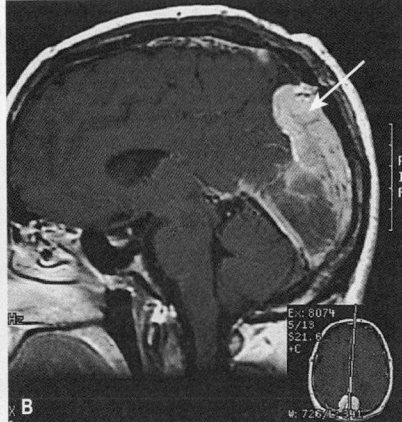
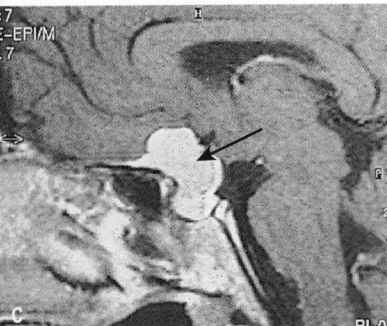

Fig. 26.53 Meningiomas (arrowed). (A) Frontal: CT. **(B)** Falx meningioma (occipital): T1-weighted MRI. **(C)** Within sella and suprasellar extension: T1-weighted MRI.

- *Hemiparesis* on the same side as a hemisphere tumour – that is, the side that might not be expected – from compression of the contralateral cerebral peduncle on the edge of the tentorium.

Seizures

Seizures are a common presenting feature of malignant brain tumours. Focal seizures, with or without altered awareness, that may evolve into bilateral tonic–clonic seizures, are characteristic of many hemisphere masses, whether malignant or benign. The pattern of focal seizure is of localizing value (see p. 853).

Investigations

Imaging

Both CT and MRI are useful in detecting brain tumours; MRI is superior for posterior fossa lesions. Benign and malignant tumours, brain abscess, tuberculosis, neurocysticercosis and infarction have characteristic, but not entirely reliable, appearances, and refined imaging techniques and biopsy are often necessary. MR angiography is used occasionally to define blood supply and MR spectroscopy to identify patterns typical of certain gliomas. PET is sometimes helpful to locate an occult primary tumour with brain metastases.

Routine tests

Since metastases are more common than primary tumours, routine tests, such as chest X-ray, should be performed.

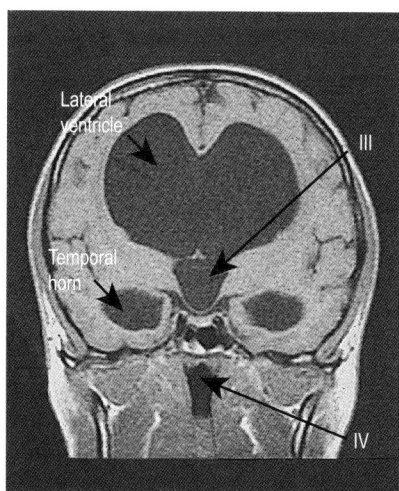

Fig. 26.54 Hydrocephalus with gross IIIrd, IVth and lateral ventricle enlargement (arrowed): T1-weighted MRI.

Lumbar puncture

This is contraindicated when there is any possibility of a mass lesion, as withdrawing CSF may provoke immediate coning. CSF examination is rarely helpful and has been superseded by imaging.

Biopsy and tumour removal

Stereotactic biopsy via a skull burr hole is carried out to ascertain the histology of most suspected malignancies. With a benign tumour, such as a symptomatic, accessible meningioma, craniotomy and removal are usual.

Management

This is discussed on page 132.

Further reading

Bredel M, Scholtens DM, Yadav AK et al. NFKBIA deletion in glioblastomas. *N Engl J Med* 2011; 364:627–637.

HYDROCEPHALUS

Hydrocephalus is an excessive accumulation of CSF within the head, caused by a disturbance of formation, flow or absorption. High pressure and ventricular dilation result (**Fig. 26.54**).

Infantile hydrocephalus

Head enlargement in infancy occurs in 1 in 2000 live births. There are several causes:

- *Arnold–Chiari malformations.* The cerebellar tonsils descend into the cervical canal (**Fig. 26.55**). Associated spina bifida is common. Syringomyelia may develop (see p. 879).
- *Stenosis of the aqueduct of Sylvius.* Aqueduct stenosis is either congenital (genetic), or acquired following neonatal meningitis/haemorrhage.
- *Dandy–Walker syndrome.* There is cerebellar hypoplasia and obstruction to IVth ventricle outflow foramina.

Hydrocephalus in adults

Hydrocephalus is sometimes an unsuspected finding on imaging. Stable childhood hydrocephalus can become apparent in adult life ('arrested hydrocephalus') but can suddenly decompensate. Combinations of headache, cognitive impairment, features of raised intracranial pressure and ataxia develop, depending on how high the CSF pressure rises and how rapid the onset is. Elderly patients with more compliant brains may present with gradual-onset gait apraxia and subtle cognitive slowing.

Hydrocephalus may be caused by:

- *posterior fossa and brainstem tumours* obstructing the aqueduct or IVth ventricular outflow

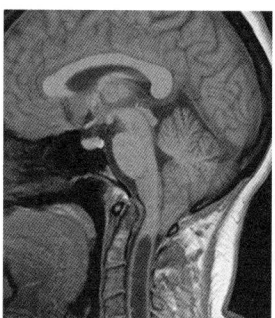
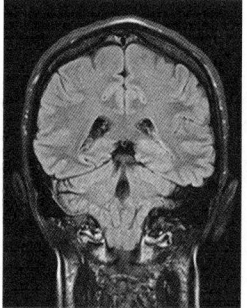
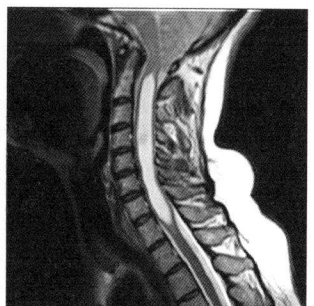

Fig. 26.55 Arnold–Chiari malformation with spinal cord syrinx.

- *subarachnoid haemorrhage*, head injury or meningitis (particularly tuberculous), causing obstruction of CSF flow and reabsorption
- *a IIIrd ventricle colloid cyst* causing intermittent hydrocephalus – recurrent prostrating headaches with episodes of lower limb weakness
- *choroid plexus papilloma* (rare) secreting CSF.

Frequently, the underlying cause of hydrocephalus remains obscure.

Management

Ventriculoperitoneal shunting is necessary when progressive hydrocephalus causes symptoms. Removal of tumours is carried out when appropriate. Endoscopic IIIrd ventriculostomy may be performed.

Normal pressure hydrocephalus

This describes a syndrome of enlarged lateral ventricles in elderly patients with the clinical triad of:

- a gait disorder – gait apraxia
- dementia
- urinary incontinence.

The term is a misnomer, as it is a low-grade hydrocephalus with intermittently raised ICP. Ventriculoperitoneal shunting may be required. A trial of prolonged drainage of lumbar CSF over several days predicts response to shunt insertion.

TRAUMATIC BRAIN INJURY

In most Western countries, head injury accounts for about 250 hospital admissions per 100 000 population annually. Traumatic brain injury (TBI) describes injuries with potentially permanent consequences. For each 100 000 people, 10 die annually following TBI; 10–15 are transferred to a neurosurgical unit, the majority of these requiring rehabilitation for a prolonged period of 1–9 months. The prevalence of survivors with a major persisting handicap is around 100/100 000. Road traffic accidents and excessive alcohol use are the principal aetiological factors in this major cause of morbidity and mortality, in many countries.

Skull fractures

Linear skull fracture of the vault or base is one indication of the severity of a blow, but in itself is not necessarily associated with any brain injury. Healing of linear fractures takes place spontaneously. *Depressed* skull fracture is followed by a high incidence of post-traumatic epilepsy. Surgical elevation and debridement are usually necessary.

Principal local complications of skull fracture are:

- *meningeal artery rupture* causing extradural haematoma (see p. 847)
- *dural vein tears* causing subdural haematoma (see p. 847)
- *CSF rhinorrhoea/otorrhoea* and consequent meningitis.

Mechanisms of brain damage

Older classifications attempted to separate *concussion*, transient coma for hours followed by apparent complete clinical recovery, from brain *contusion* – that is, bruising – with prolonged coma, focal signs and lasting damage. Pathological support for this division is poor. Mechanisms of TBI are complex and interrelated:

- diffuse axonal injury – shearing and rotational stresses on decelerating brain, sometimes at the site opposite impact (the *contrecoup* effect)

- neuronal and axonal damage from direct trauma
- brain oedema and raised intracranial pressure
- brain hypoxia
- brain ischaemia.

Clinical course

In a mild TBI, a patient is stunned or dazed for a few seconds or minutes. Following this, the patient remains alert without post-traumatic amnesia. Headache can follow; complete recovery is usual. In more serious injuries, duration of unconsciousness, and particularly of post-traumatic amnesia (PTA), helps grade severity. PTA lasting more than 24 hours defines severe TBI. The Glasgow Coma Scale (GCS; see p. 832) is used to record the degree of coma; this has prognostic value. A GCS below 5/15 at 24 hours implies a serious injury; 50% of such patients die or remain in a vegetative or minimal conscious state (see p. 836). However, prolonged coma of up to some weeks is occasionally followed by good recovery.

Recovery after severe TBI takes many weeks or months. During the first few weeks, patients are often intermittently restless or lethargic, and have focal deficits such as hemiparesis or aphasia. Gradually, they become more aware, though they may remain in PTA, being unable to lay down any continuous memory despite being awake. This amnesia may last some weeks or more, and may not be obvious clinically. PTA is one predictor of outcome. PTA of over a week implies that persistent organic cognitive deficit is almost inevitable, although return to unsupported paid work may be possible.

Late sequelae

Sequelae of TBI are major causes of morbidity and can have serious social and medicolegal consequences. They include:

- *Incomplete recovery*, e.g. cognitive impairment, hemiparesis.
- *Post-traumatic epilepsy* (see p. 854).
- *The post-traumatic (post-concussional) syndrome.* This describes the vague complaints of headache, dizziness and malaise that follow even minor head injuries. Litigation is frequently an issue. Depression is prominent. Symptoms may be prolonged.
- *Benign paroxysmal positional vertigo* (see p. 906).
- *Chronic subdural haematoma* (see p. 847).
- *Hydrocephalus* (see p. 876).
- *Chronic traumatic encephalopathy.* This follows repeated and often minor injuries. It is known as the *'punch-drunk syndrome'* and consists of cognitive impairment and extrapyramidal and pyramidal signs, seen typically in professional boxers.

Management

Immediate management

Attention to the airway is vital. If there is coma, depressed fracture or suspicion of intracranial haematoma, CT imaging and discussion with a neurosurgical unit are essential. Indications for CT vary from imaging all minor head injuries in some centres to more stringent criteria elsewhere.

In many severe TBI cases, assisted ventilation will be needed. Intracranial pressure monitoring is valuable. Hypothermia lowers intracranial pressure when used early after a TBI; an effect on outcome has been seen only in specialized neurotrauma centres. Care of the unconscious patient is described on page 833. Prophylactic antiepileptic drugs have been shown to be of no value in prevention of late post-traumatic epilepsy. Trials using progesterone have shown no benefit.

Rehabilitation

TBI cases require skilled, prolonged and energetic support. Survivors with severe physical and cognitive deficits require rehabilitation in specialized units. Rehabilitation includes care from a multidisciplinary team, including prominent physiotherapists, occupation therapists, speech and language therapists, and clinical psychologists. Many survivors are left with cognitive problems (amnesia, neglect, disordered attention and motivation) and behavioural/emotional problems (temper dyscontrol, depression and grief reactions). Long-term support for both patients and families is necessary.

Further reading

Stocchetti N, Maas AI. Traumatic intracranial hypertension. *N Engl J Med* 2014; 370:2121–2130.

SPINAL CORD DISEASE

The cord extends from C1, the junction with the medulla, to the lower vertebral body of L1, where it becomes the conus medullaris. Blood supply is from the anterior spinal artery and a plexus on the posterior cord. This network is supplied by the vertebral arteries and by several branches from lumbar and intercostal vessels, including the artery of Adamkiewicz.

Spinal cord compression

The principal features of chronic and subacute cord compression are spastic paraparesis or tetraparesis, radicular pain at the level of compression, and sensory loss below the compression (**Box 26.62**).

For example, in compression at T4 (see **Fig. 21.16**), a band of pain radiates around the thorax, characteristically worse on coughing or straining. Spastic paraparesis develops over months, days or hours, depending on underlying pathology. Numbness commencing in the feet rises to the level of compression. This is called the **sensory level** and is usually 2–3 dermatome levels below the level of anatomical compression. Retention of urine and constipation develop.

Aetiology

Disc and vertebral lesions. Central cervical disc and thoracic disc protrusion causes cord compression (see p. 892). Chronic compression due to cervical spondylotic myelopathy is frequently seen in clinical practice and is the most common cause of a spastic paraparesis in an elderly person.

Trauma. Any trauma to the back is potentially serious and the patient should be immobilized until the extent of the injury can be determined.

Spinal cord tumours. Extramedullary tumours, such as meningiomas and neurofibromas, cause cord compression (**Fig. 26.56** and **Box 26.63**) gradually over weeks to months, often with root pain and a sensory level (see p. 892). Vertebral body destruction by bony metastases, such as in prostate or breast cancer, is a common cause of spinal cord compression.

Intramedullary tumours (e.g. ependymomas) are less common and typically progress slowly, sometimes over many years. Sensory disturbances similar to syringomyelia may develop (see p. 879).

Tuberculosis. Spinal tuberculosis is the most common cause of cord compression in countries where the disease is common. There is destruction of vertebral bodies and disc spaces, with local spread of infection. Cord compression and paraparesis follow, culminating in paralysis: Pott's paraplegia.

Spinal epidural abscess. This is described on page 874.

Epidural haemorrhage and haematoma. These are rare sequelae of anticoagulant therapy, bleeding disorders or trauma, and can follow LP when clotting is abnormal. A rapidly progressive cord or cauda equina lesion develops.

Management

Acute spinal cord compression is a medical emergency. Early diagnosis and treatment are vital. MRI is the imaging technique of choice.

Routine tests (e.g. chest X-ray) may indicate a primary neoplasm or infection. Surgical exploration is frequently necessary; if decompression is not performed promptly, irreversible cord damage ensues. Results are excellent if benign tumours and haematomas are removed early. Radiotherapy is used to treat cord malignancies, or compression due to inoperable malignant vertebral body disease causing cord compression.

Other spinal cord disorders

Inflammatory cord lesions (transverse myelitis)

See page 868.

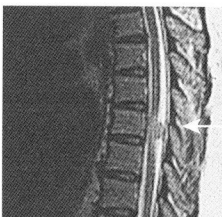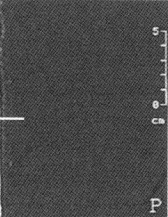

Fig. 26.56 Thoracic meningioma (arrowed) compressing the spinal cord: T2-weighted MRI.

? Box 26.62 Causes of spinal cord compression

- Spinal cord tumours
  - Extramedullary, e.g. meningioma or neurofibroma
  - Intramedullary, e.g. ependymoma or glioma
- Vertebral body destruction by bone metastases, e.g. prostate primary
- Disc and vertebral lesions:
  - Chronic degenerative and acute central disc prolapse
  - Trauma
- Inflammatory:
  - Epidural abscess
  - Tuberculosis
  - Granulomatous
- Epidural haemorrhage/haematoma

---

i Box 26.63 Principal spinal cord neoplasms

Extradural
- Metastases:
  - Bronchus
  - Breast
  - Prostate
  - Lymphoma
  - Thyroid
  - Melanoma

Extramedullary
- Meningioma
- Neurofibroma
- Ependymoma

Intramedullary
- Glioma
- Ependymoma
- Haemangioblastoma
- Lipoma
- Teratoma

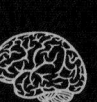

Anterior spinal artery occlusion

There is acute paraplegia and loss of spinothalamic (pain and temperature) sensation, with infarction of the anterior two-thirds of the spinal cord. This may result from aortic atherosclerosis, dissection, trauma or cross-clamping in surgery. Vasculitis, emboli, haematological disorders causing thrombosis and severe hypotension are other causes. Occlusion of the artery of Adamkiewicz, which supplies the thoracic anterior spinal artery, causes watershed infarction of the cord, typically at the T8 level where perfusion is relatively poor.

Arteriovenous malformations of the cord

Although rare, spinal arteriovenous malformations (AVMs) may be difficult to diagnose but are potentially curable. The two main types seen are dural arteriovenous fistulas (acquired) and true intramedullary AVMs (probably congenital but gradually enlarging). Dural arteriovenous fistulas occur mainly in middle-aged men due to formation of a direct connection between an artery and vein in a dural nerve root sleeve. This causes arterialization of veins with venous hypertension, and thus oedema and congestion of the spinal cord at and below the affected level. Presentation is with a gradually progressive myelopathy over months or a few years, often with thoracic back pain. MRI usually shows cord swelling (**Fig. 26.57**) and may show the enlarged arterialized veins over the surface of the cord. Spinal angiography demonstrates the fistula and allows endovascular ablation with glue, often with complete resolution of symptoms if permanent neuronal damage has not already occurred.

Genetic disorders – hereditary spastic paraparesis (HSP)

Several genetic disorders may present with a gradually evolving upper motor neurone syndrome resembling a myelopathy. Typically, spasticity and stiffness dominate the clinical picture rather than weakness, especially in hereditary spastic paraparesis (HSP). Muscle relaxants, such as baclofen, improve gait. There are 28 known genes associated with HSP, some causing 'pure' spasticity and others with associated neurological features, such as thinning of the corpus callosum.

Other genetic disorders such as adrenoleukodystrophy may cause a slowly progressive spastic paraparesis (including in manifesting female carriers), as can the spinocerebellar ataxias (see p. 887) or presenilin-1 mutations (see p. 883).

Vitamin B$_{12}$ deficiency

Subacute combined degeneration of the cord resulting from vitamin B$_{12}$ deficiency (see p. 891) is the most common example of metabolic disease causing spinal cord damage. Abuse of nitrous oxide may precipitate functional B$_{12}$ deficiency with normal serum B$_{12}$ levels.

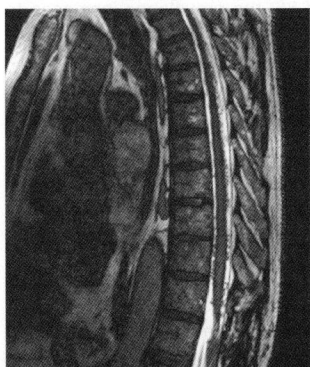
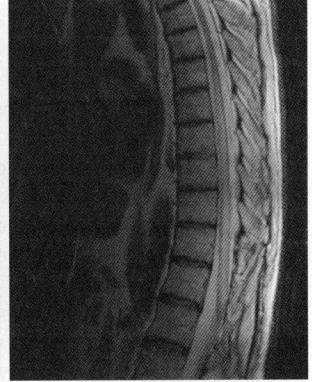

Fig. 26.57 Dural arteriovenous fistulas.

Other causes of a spastic paraparesis

Motor neurone disease may present initially with a spastic paraparesis before lower motor neurone features develop (see p. 885). Paraneoplastic disorders, radiotherapy, copper deficiency, liver failure and rare toxins (e.g. lathyrism) may cause spinal cord damage. Not all causes of paraparesis relate to spinal cord pathology; beware a parasagittal cerebral meningioma presenting with a paraparesis due to bilateral compression of the leg area of the motor cortex.

Care of the patient with paraplegia

Where patients are left with a severe paraplegia, there are several issues in long-term care, and specialist nursing is vital.

Bladder management. The bladder does not empty and urinary retention results. Patients self-catheterize or develop reflex bladder emptying, helped by abdominal pressure. Early treatment of urine infections is essential. Chronic kidney disease may develop from chronic obstruction or repeated urinary tract infection.

Bowel function. Constipation and impaction must be avoided. Following acute paraplegia, manual evacuation is necessary; reflex emptying develops later.

Skin care. Risks of pressure ulcers and their sequelae are serious. Meticulous attention must be paid to cleanliness and regular turning. The sacrum, iliac crests, greater trochanters, heels and malleoli should be inspected frequently (see p. 683). Pressure-relieving mattresses are useful initially until patients can turn themselves. If pressure ulcers develop, plastic surgery may be required. Pressure palsies, such as those of ulnar nerves, can occur.

Lower limbs. Passive physiotherapy helps to prevent contractures. Severe spasticity, with flexor or extensor spasms, may be helped by muscle relaxants such as baclofen or by botulinum toxin injections.

Rehabilitation. Many patients with traumatic paraplegia or tetraplegia return to self-sufficiency (especially if the level is at C7 or below). A specialist spinal rehabilitation unit is necessary. Lightweight, specially adapted wheelchairs provide independence. Tendon transfer operations may allow functional grip if hands are weak. Autonomic dysreflexia may be a problem. Patients with paraplegia have substantial practical, psychological and sexual needs.

Syringomyelia and syringobulbia

A syrinx is a fluid-filled cavity within the spinal cord. Syringobulbia means a cavity in the brainstem. Syringomyelia is frequently associated with the Arnold–Chiari malformation (see p. 876). The abnormality at the foramen magnum probably allows normal pulsatile CSF pressure waves to be transmitted to fragile tissues of the cervical cord and brainstem, causing secondary cavity formation. The syrinx is in continuity with the central canal of the cord. Syrinx formation may also follow spinal cord trauma and lead to secondary damage years later, and can also be caused by intrinsic cord tumours.

Pathophysiology

The expanding cavity in the cord gradually destroys spinothalamic neurones, anterior horn cells and lateral corticospinal tracts. In the medulla (syringobulbia), lower cranial nerve nuclei are affected.

Clinical features

Cases associated with the Arnold–Chiari malformation usually develop symptoms around the age of 20–30. Upper limb pain

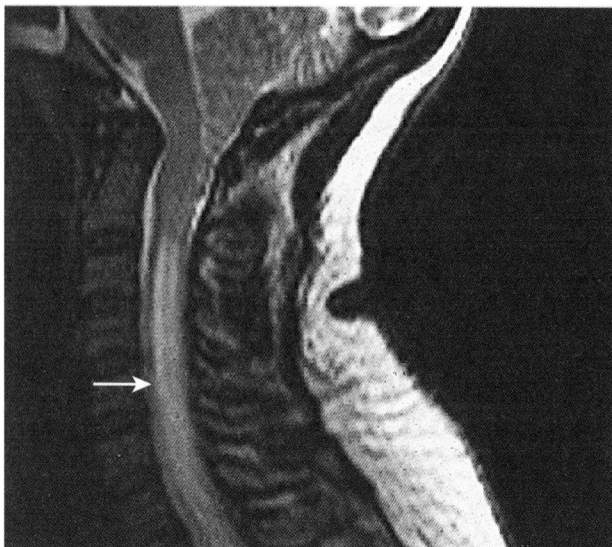

Fig. 26.58 Cervical syrinx – cavity within cord (arrowed): T2-weighted MRI.

exacerbated by exertion or coughing is typical. Spinothalamic sensory loss – pain and temperature – leads to painless upper limb burns and trophic changes. Paraparesis develops. The following are typical signs of a substantial cervical syrinx (**Fig. 26.58**):

- *a 'suspended' area of dissociated sensory loss* – i.e. spinothalamic loss in the arms and hands without loss of light touch
- *loss of upper limb reflexes*
- *muscle wasting* in the hand and forearm
- *spastic paraparesis* – initially mild
- *brainstem signs* – as the syrinx extends into the brainstem (syringobulbia) there may be tongue atrophy and fasciculation, bulbar palsy, a Horner's syndrome and impairment of facial sensation.

Investigations and management

MRI demonstrates the cavity and herniation of cerebellar tonsils. Syringomyelia is gradually progressive over several decades. Sudden deterioration sometimes follows minor trauma or occurs spontaneously. Surgical decompression of the foramen magnum often causes the syrinx to collapse.

Further reading

Ginsberg L. Disorders of the spinal cord and roots. *Pract Neurol* 2011; 11:259–267.

NEURODEGENERATIVE DISEASES

Neurodegenerative disease is an umbrella term for disorders characterized by progressive neuronal cell loss with distinct patterns in different disorders. These disorders are increasing in an ageing population.

Dementia

Dementia is a clinical syndrome with multiple causes, defined by:

- an acquired loss of higher mental function, affecting two or more cognitive domains, including:
  - episodic memory (acquisition of new information) – usually (but not always) involved
  - language function

Box 26.64 Taking a dementia history

- Memory:
  - Is the patient repetitive, e.g. with questions?
  - Is there a temporal gradient of amnesia – preservation of more distant memories with amnesia for recent events?
  - Is there difficulty learning to use new devices, e.g. computer, mobile phone?
- Functional ability:
  - Has work performance or ability to cook and do domestic tasks declined?
  - Has responsibility for finances and administration shifted to the spouse?
  - Does the patient get easily muddled?
- Personality and frontal lobe function:
  - Has personality altered?
  - More aggressive/apathetic/lacking initiative
  - Disinhibition
  - Change in food preference or religiosity
- Language:
  - Difficulty with word finding or remembering names
- Visuospatial ability:
  - Does the patient get lost in familiar places?
  - Difficulty dressing, e.g. putting jacket on the wrong way round
- Psychiatric features:
  - Features of depression
- Tempo of progression
- Family history of dementia
- Alcohol and drug use
- Medication
- Any other neurological problems, e.g. parkinsonism, gait disorder, strokes

- frontal executive function
  - visuospatial function
  - apraxia
- being of sufficient severity to cause significant social or occupational impairment
- being chronic and stable (which distinguishes it from delirium, which is acute and fluctuating).

Although dementia is usually progressive, it is not invariably so, and may even be reversible in some cases. Dementia robs patients of their independence, and is a serious burden on carers and a major socioeconomic challenge for society as a whole.

Epidemiology

Dementia is common and becoming even more so as a result of an ageing population and better case ascertainment. Age is the main risk factor, followed by family history. Over the age of 65, there is a 6% prevalence; over the age of 85, the prevalence increases to 20%.

Clinical assessment

There are two main considerations:

- Does the patient have dementia?
- Are the pattern of cognitive deficits, tempo of progression or associated features suggestive of a distinct cause? Cognitive problems need to be interpreted in the context of estimated pre-morbid abilities (e.g. based on educational attainments or occupation).

Taking a history from a spouse or relative is essential. Patients may tend to downplay or deny symptoms (anosognosia) or constantly look to the relative for answers (the 'head-turning sign'). See **Box 26.64** for the key elements in history-taking.

Examination

Conversation with the patient during history-taking may be as revealing as formal cognitive assessment but many patients hide deficits well behind an intact social façade.

Bedside cognitive assessment

The mini-mental state examination (MMSE; see p. 805) is commonly used to assess cognitive function but has its limitations, such as relative insensitivity to milder cognitive impairment and to frontal lobe dysfunction, especially in those with pre-morbid abilities. The Addenbrooke's Cognitive Examination (ACE) is a tool developed to address the deficiencies of the MMSE but is short enough to use in clinical practice.

It is useful to ask patients to give an account of recent news events to assess episodic memory.

Individual cognitive domains can be tested separately in detail: for example, clock drawing for visuospatial (parietal lobe) function, naming and reading tasks for language function, verbal fluency, conceptual similarity to test abstract thinking, and stop–go tasks, which are components of the Frontal Assessment Battery (FAB).

Check for primitive reflexes (frontal release signs), such as grasp, palmo-mental and pout reflexes, and perseveration or utilization behaviour with frontal lobe involvement.

Test:

- limb praxis – copying hand gestures and miming tasks, e.g. 'Show me how you brush your teeth'.
- oro-buccal praxis, e.g. 'Show me how you would blow out a candle'.

Complete neurological examination to look for evidence of papilloedema, parkinsonism, myoclonus and gait disorders, for example, is also necessary, in addition to is general examination and assessment of mental state.

Investigations

Investigations (**Box 26.65**) are aimed at identifying treatable causes and helping support a clinical diagnosis of dementia type. For most patients, this should include the elements listed below.

Blood tests. These should include a full blood count and measurement of vitamin B_{12}, thyroid function, urea and electrolytes, liver function, glucose and ESR.

Brain imaging. CT is adequate to exclude structural lesions (**Fig. 26.59**), such as tumours or hydrocephalus. The superior anatomical resolution of MRI helps identify patterns of regional brain atrophy and so distinguish between different types of degenerative dementia (e.g. hippocampal atrophy in Alzheimer's disease (AD) versus temporal lobe and frontal atrophy in frontotemporal dementia). Imaging also allows assessment of brain 'vascular load'. MRI is always preferable to CT in patients with cognitive disorders.

Detailed neuropsychometric assessment (see p. 831). Appropriate in most patients, this allows quantification of the relative involvement of different cognitive domains and may be helpful if performed serially over time to assess progression.

Younger patients (<65 years). More intensive investigation may be necessary. This may include EEG, genetic tests (e.g. for Huntington's, familial AD and FTD genes), voltage-gated potassium channel antibodies, anti-neuronal antibodies (for paraneoplastic limbic encephalitis), HIV serology and metabolic tests; on rare occasions, brain biopsy may be appropriate.

CSF examination. Measurement of CSF protein biomarkers has been shown to be useful in distinguishing between different types of dementia; for example, in AD, CSF tau is raised and Aβ42 reduced. In Creutzfeldt–Jakob disease (CJD) and other rapidly progressive

---

> *i* **Box 26.65** Tests in dementia

Blood tests
- Full blood count, erythrocyte sedimentation rate, vitamin B_{12}
- Urea and electrolytes
- Glucose
- Liver biochemistry
- Serum calcium
- Thyroid stimulating hormone, T_3, T_4
- HIV serology
- Syphilis serology

Imaging
- CT or MRI brain scan

Other – selected patients only
- Cerebrospinal fluid – including tau and Aβ42 measurement
- Genetic studies, e.g. for AD and FTD genes, HD, prion mutations
- Electroencephalography
- Brain biopsy

AD, Alzheimer's disease; FTD, frontotemporal dementia; HD, Huntington's disease.

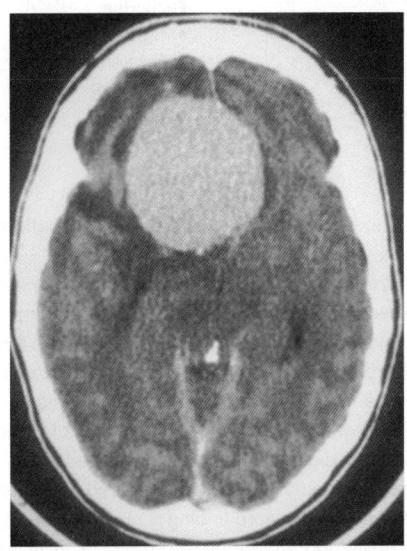

Fig. 26.59 CT scan showing a large frontal meningioma presenting with apathy and frontal dementia.

---

dementias, protein 14–3–3 is increased. A new CSF assay for abnormal prion protein, real-time quaking induced conversion (rt-QUIC), has proved to be highly sensitive and specific for CJD.

New imaging modalities. Radionuclide scans using radioactively labelled ligands that bind directly to amyloid allow amyloid deposition in the brain to be directly visualized and have great potential for earlier and more accurate diagnosis of AD. Amyloid imaging is now beginning to enter clinical practice in some specialist centres.

Mild cognitive impairment

Mild cognitive impairment (MCI) is an intermediate state between normal cognition and dementia. Often mild memory impairment, greater than expected for age but not sufficient to classify as dementia, is the only symptom ('amnestic MCI'). MCI may be a pre-dementia state, with 10–15% of patients per year developing overt AD.

Causes of dementia

There are many causes of dementia (**Box 26.66**), by far the most common being AD. Cause varies according to age (**Fig. 26.60**).

Alzheimer's disease

Although technically a definitive diagnosis can only be made by histopathology, in practice the clinical features are sufficiently characteristic that a diagnosis can usually be made with considerable

? Box 26.66 Causes of dementia

Degenerative
- Alzheimer's disease
- Dementia with Lewy bodies
- Frontotemporal dementia
- Huntington's disease
- Parkinson's disease
- Prion diseases, e.g. Creutzfeldt–Jakob

Vascular
- Vascular dementia
- Cerebral vasculitis (rare)

Metabolic
- Uraemia
- Liver failure

Toxic
- Alcohol
- Solvent misuse
- Heavy metals

Vitamin deficiency
- B_{12} and thiamine

Traumatic
- Severe or repeated brain injury

Intracranial lesions
- Subdural haematoma
- Tumours
- Hydrocephalus

Infections
- HIV
- Neurosyphilis
- Whipple's disease
- Tuberculosis

Endocrine
- Hypothyroidism
- Hypoparathyroidism

Psychiatric
- Depression causing 'pseudodementia'

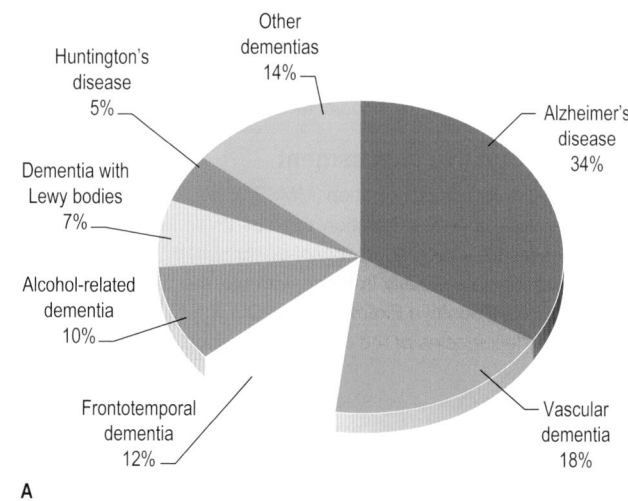

A

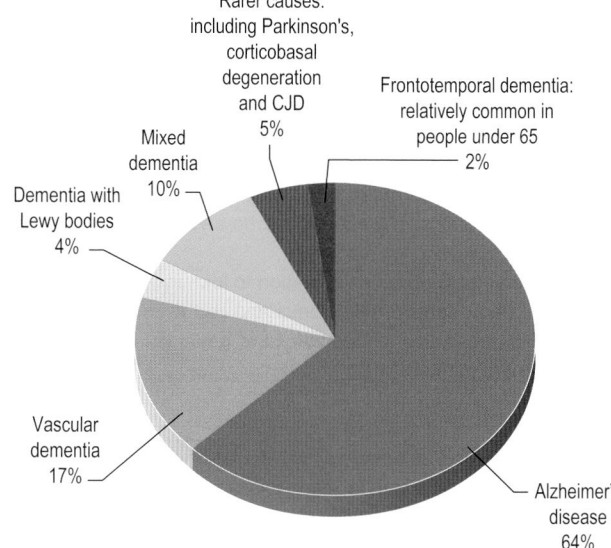

B

Fig. 26.60 Causes of dementia at different ages. (A) Under 65 years. **(B)** At 65 years or more. CJD, Creutzfeldt–Jakob disease. *(Data from Prince M, Knapp M, Guerchet M et al.* Alzheimer's Society Dementia UK Update. *London: Alzheimer's Society; 2014.)*

accuracy in life, supported by diagnostic investigations. The key clinical features are:

- **Memory impairment.** Episodic (day-to-day) memory is affected. There is progressive loss of ability to learn, retain and process new information. There is a characteristic temporal gradient, with relative preservation of distant memory and amnesia for more recent events. Patients often refer to this as 'short-term memory loss', which technically refers to loss of working memory: for example, digit span, which is preserved in AD.
- **Language.** This usually becomes impaired as the disease advances. Difficulty with word finding is characteristic.
- **Apraxia.** Ability to carry out skilled motor activities is impaired (see p. 804).
- **Agnosia.** There is a failure to recognize objects such as clothing, and places or people.
- **Frontal executive function.** Organizing, planning and sequencing are impaired.
- **Parietal presentation.** Presentation with visuospatial difficulties and difficulty with orientation in space and navigation may occur. Parietal lobe involvement is also seen as a later feature in more typical presentations.
- **Posterior cortical atrophy (PCA).** This is the least common presentation of AD with visual disorientation due to initial involvement of the occipital lobes and occipitoparietal regions. Patients have complex visual symptoms that may be difficult to describe; they often say that it is easier to see distant than close-up objects. Memory is initially well preserved.
- **Personality.** In contrast to other dementias such as frontotemporal dementia, basic personality and social behaviour remain intact until late AD.
- **Anosognosia.** Lack of insight by the patient into their difficulties is common; they may be reluctant to seek medical attention but be brought to clinic by a family member.
- **Tempo.** Onset is insidious and often not noticed by family members initially. Progression is gradual but inexorable over a decade or longer, with eventual severe deficits in multiple cognitive domains.
- **Late non-cognitive features.** Myoclonus may develop, sometimes followed by seizures (the cortex is the main site of pathology). Sleep–wake cycle reversal and incontinence may place a

great strain on carers. Motor function is usually strikingly preserved so patients are capable of wandering and getting lost. Swallowing may become impaired, leading to aspiration pneumonia – often a terminal event.

Investigations

MRI typically shows characteristic atrophy of mesial temporal lobe structures, including hippocampi, progressing eventually to generalized cerebral atrophy. Imaging may be normal in the early stages and selective regional atrophy is seen in AD variants such as 'posterior presentations', for example posterior cortical atrophy (PCA) with occipital lobe atrophy. Characteristic MRI and psychometric testing abnormalities are sufficient to make a diagnosis if the clinical picture is suggestive (a progressive amnestic cognitive disorder in an older person). CSF tau and β-amyloid measurement is helpful in cases of diagnostic difficulty but not yet widely available (see above).

Molecular pathology and aetiology

Although the cause of AD is still not known, a great deal is now understood about the molecular pathology. The pathological hallmarks are:

- The deposition of β-amyloid (Aβ) in amyloid plaques in the cortex.
- Structural and conformational changes in tau protein, i.e. hyperphosphorylation and formation of paired helical filaments, which are the binding blocks of neurofibrillary tangles. These protein aggregates damage synapses and ultimately lead to neuronal death. Early pathological changes in the brain, including Aβ deposition, pre-date clinical symptoms and diagnosis by up to 25 years.

Amyloid may also be laid down in cerebral blood vessels, leading to amyloid angiopathy.

The amyloid precursor protein (APP) is processed by secretase enzymes to form pathogenic $A\beta_{1-42}$ monomers, which polymerize into amyloid plaques (**Fig. 26.61**).

A basal forebrain cholinergic deficit occurs and may explain the therapeutic response to cholinesterase inhibitor drugs.

Genetics of AD

A first-degree relative with AD confers a doubled lifetime risk of AD. There are rare autosomal dominant monogenic early-onset forms of familial AD with high penetrance, caused by mutations in specific genes; taken together, these account for only 1% of cases of AD.

Other genes. The E4 allele of the apolipoprotein E gene confers an increased risk of AD (2–3 times lifetime risk), especially if two copies of the E4 allele are inherited (6–8 times risk). Several other candidate genes have been identified as risk factors for AD in large genome-wide association studies.

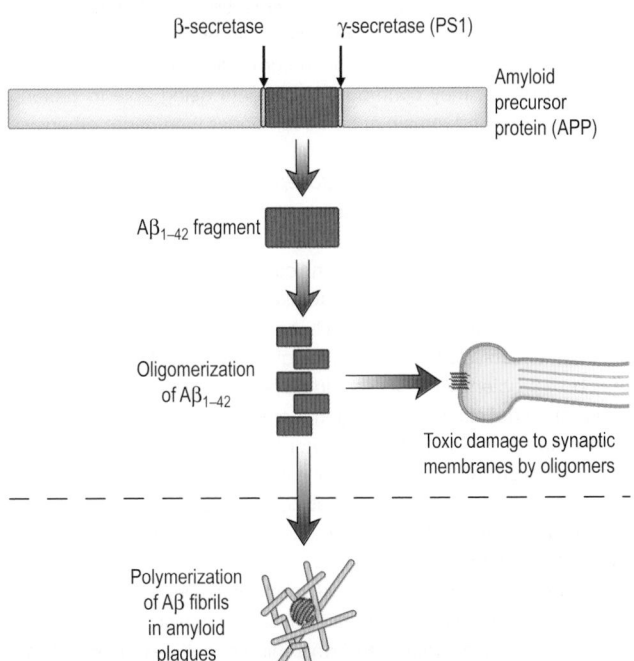

Fig. 26.61 Molecular pathogenesis of Alzheimer's disease. Processing of the amyloid precursor protein (APP) molecule by secretase enzymes releases $A\beta_{1-42}$ monomers, which are the building blocks of amyloid plaques. Aβ oligomers may damage synaptic membranes. Mutations in APP or γ-secretase (presenilin-1) cause genetic forms of Alzheimer's. Disruption of the balance between formation and degradation of $A\beta_{1-42}$ is thought to be a major problem.

Amyloid precursor protein (APP). Point mutations in the *APP* gene can cause AD, and the presence of three copies of the *APP* gene on chromosome 21 in Down's syndrome patients is responsible for the high incidence of AD in that condition.

Presenilin (PS)-1 and 2. Mutations in these genes affect the γ-secretase enzyme function (see **Fig. 26.61**). *PS1* mutations account for 50% of monogenic forms of AD. The *PS1/2* and *APP* genes may be sequenced for mutations in selected early-onset cases with a family history.

Environmental risk factors

Age is the main risk factor for AD, as incidence increases exponentially with age. Head trauma and vascular risk factors also increase AD risk. Epidemiological studies show that taking anti-inflammatory drugs over a long period may confer some protection.

Dementia with Lewy bodies and Parkinson's disease dementia

Dementia with Lewy bodies (DLB) is characterized by the early feature of visual hallucinations, fluctuating cognition with variation in attention and alertness, sleep disorders (especially REM sleep behaviour disorder), dysautonomia and parkinsonism. The visual hallucinations often take the form of people or animals, or the sense of a presence ('extracampine hallucinations'). Memory loss may be absent in the early stages. Delusions and transient loss of consciousness occur. Lewy bodies, inclusions containing aggregates of the protein α-synuclein first described in Parkinson's disease, are found in the cortex.

In DLB, the cognitive features dominate; parkinsonism may evolve later and is typically mild. In Parkinson's disease dementia (PDD), cognitive problems are a late feature, occurring at least 1 year after onset and usually after the age of 75. Both conditions may respond to cholinesterase inhibitors. Patients with DLB may be very sensitive to neuroleptic drugs with dramatic worsening.

Vascular dementia

This common cause of dementia is due to different mechanisms, including multi-infarct dementia, cerebral small-vessel disease and post-stroke dementia. Most vascular dementias are of mixed cause. Vascular dementia is distinguished from AD by its clinical features and imaging. Dementia can be progressive and similar to AD. There is sometimes a history of TIAs, or the dementia follows a succession of cerebrovascular events, or has a stepwise course. Apraxic gait disorder, pyramidal signs and urinary incontinence are common additional features. Widespread small-vessel disease seen on MRI is the typical finding and may produce a variety of cognitive deficits, reflecting the site of ischaemic damage.

Frontotemporal dementia

Frontotemporal dementia (FTD) is the term used to describe a group of neurodegenerative disorders characterized by asymmetric frontal lobe and temporal lobe atrophy on MRI and at postmortem (also called *Pick's disease*). Onset is usually below the age of 65 and there is often a family history. FTD is considerably less common than AD, prevalence being approximately 10 per 100 000 before the age of 65. There are three distinct presentations, depending on which anatomical region is affected first.

Frontal presentation. This *behavioural variant* is characterized by personality change, emotional blunting, apathy, disinhibition, carelessness and behavioural change with striking preservation of episodic memory.

Temporal presentations. *Primary progressive aphasia* is characterized by progressive impairment of language function.

Involvement of the left temporal lobe produces 'semantic dementia', with fluent speech relatively lacking in meaningful content and progressive difficulty with comprehension of the meaning of words (e.g. a patient may respond to the MMSE question 'What season is it?' by asking 'What is a season?'). The second temporal lobe presentation is **progressive non-fluent aphasia** due to peri-Sylvian atrophy, with loss of verbal fluency and increasingly telegrammatic speech.

The frontal and temporal presentations eventually merge as cognitive decline becomes more widespread.

Pathology

About 25% of cases are familial, associated with mutations in the tau and progranulin genes or hexanucleotide repeat expansion in the *C9ORF72* gene. The characteristic pathology consists of deposition of abnormally aggregated proteins: phosphorylated tau, transactive response DNA-binding protein 43 (TDP-43) or fused in sarcoma (FUS). Ten per cent of patients have overlap syndromes with motor neurone disease or parkinsonian disorders such as progressive supranuclear palsy. There is no cure or specific treatment at present.

Prion diseases, including Creutzfeldt–Jakob disease

Prion diseases (see p. 535) are transmissible neurodegenerative disorders with a long incubation period, caused by accumulation of misfolded native prion protein (PrP^c). Misfolding and conformational change in PrP^c is caused either by exposure to the abnormal misfolded isoform of the protein (PrP^{sc}) or by mutations in the PrP gene (*PRNP*), leading to toxic accumulation of PrP^{sc} as amyloid in beta-pleated sheets. Neuronal cell damage and 'spongiform' change in the brain result (see p. 535), the clinical correlate being a rapidly progressive dementia in most cases.

Creutzfeldt–Jakob disease

Creutzfeldt–Jakob disease (CJD) is the most common prion disease in humans, the animal equivalents being bovine spongiform encephalopathy (BSE) in cattle and scrapie in sheep. CJD may be sporadic, iatrogenic or familial.

Sporadic CJD is the most common form, occurring over the age of 50, with an incidence of approximately 1 per million. It is thought to be due to spontaneous somatic mutations in the *PRNP* gene or stochastic conformational change in PrP^c to PrP^{sc} with a subsequent 'domino effect' inducing misfolding in other PrP molecules. A rapidly progressive dementia leads to death within 6 months of onset. Rapidly progressive cognitive decline should always lead to suspicion of CJD. The presence of myoclonus is also a clinical clue (present in 90%). New forms of monoclonal antibody treatment are being studied.

Iatrogenic CJD is transmitted from neurosurgical instruments (prions are resistant to sterilization), transplant material (e.g. corneal grafts) and cadaveric pituitary-derived growth hormone taken from patients with CJD or presymptomatic CJD. Iatrogenic CJD has a long incubation period of several years.

Familial CJD (rare) is associated with *PRNP* gene mutations. Other clinical phenotypes, such as **familial fatal insomnia**, also occur.

Variant CJD

Variant CJD (vCJD) was first seen in the UK in 1995. vCJD patients are younger than sporadic cases, with a mean age of 29. Early symptoms are neuropsychiatric, followed by ataxia and dementia with myoclonus or chorea. The diagnosis can be confirmed by tonsillar biopsy but a sensitive blood test has been developed. vCJD

has a longer course than sporadic CJD – up to several years. vCJD and BSE are caused by the same prion strain, giving rise to speculation that transmission from animal to human food chain took place: that is, infection from BSE-infected cattle to humans (see p. 535). Transmission via blood transfusion may also occur. Most patients with vCJD and sporadic CJD have a specific polymorphism at codon 129 of the *PRNP* gene that leads to susceptibility.

Other dementias

Other neurodegenerative disorders may include dementia as one of their clinical manifestations. For example, corticobasal degeneration (CBD), progressive supranuclear palsy (PSP) and dementia may be a feature of a number of genetic and metabolic disorders, such as Huntington's disease (see p. 862) and the leukodystrophies.

Management of dementia

It is rare for a reversible cause for dementia to be found, such as normal pressure hydrocephalus or frontal meningioma. Other disorders, such as limbic encephalitis or severe depression, may present as dementia mimics and every effort should be made to distinguish these treatable conditions from degenerative dementias.

Management is supportive, to preserve dignity and to provide care for as long as possible in the familiar home environment. The burden of illness frequently falls on relatives. Dementia clinical nurse specialists form a central part of the multidisciplinary team.

General measures. Some evidence suggests that participation in cognitively demanding activities in later life may protect against or delay the onset of dementia. High-dose B vitamins may possibly slow conversion from MCI to AD in patients with above-average levels of the amino acid homocysteine. There is some recent evidence supporting use of vitamin E to slow progression.

Cognitive enhancing drugs. These have a modest symptomatic benefit in AD, equivalent to an increase in 1–2 points on the MMSE. They are not disease-modifying, so do not slow or prevent progression. Whilst there has been some dispute about the place for these drugs, they contribute to patients being able to prolong independence and remain at home for longer than might otherwise be the case.

Cholinesterase inhibitors (donepezil, rivastigmine and galantamine) increase brain acetylcholine levels by inhibiting CNS acetylcholinesterase. Patients with AD have a central cholinergic deficit. There is usually a small but significant improvement in memory, cognition and function. Cholinesterase inhibitors are also effective in DLB and Parkinson's dementia but not in FTD or vascular dementia. Side-effects, particularly cholinergic gastrointestinal symptoms, may be a problem. An ECG should be performed to exclude cardiac conduction deficits before starting therapy.

Memantine is an NMDA receptor antagonist. It is used in moderate or severe AD or where cholinesterase inhibitors are not tolerated. There is some evidence that combination of memantine and cholinesterase inhibitors is better than either used alone. It is generally well tolerated.

Psychiatric and behavioural problems. Depression is common in dementia and may be difficult to distinguish from dementia symptoms, such as apathy and worsening cognitive function. A trial of an antidepressant is appropriate where depression is suspected. Distinguishing depressive pseudodementia from organic dementia can be difficult but is crucial. Behavioural disturbance (e.g. due to agitation or delusions) and hallucinations may occur in late-stage disease. Use of antipsychotic medications is associated with significantly increased stroke risk in patients with dementia and should be used only as a last resort.

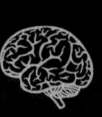

Drugs in development. The greatest need is for disease-modifying therapies that halt or slow progression in early-stage disease before significant irreversible neuronal damage has accumulated. Potential treatments in development include anti-amyloid therapies, such as monoclonal antibodies directed against Aβ and inhibitors of secretase enzymes that process APP into Aβ fragments.

Financial and legal issues. Patients may want to set up a Lasting Power of Attorney (if they retain mental capacity to do so in legal terms) to allow a spouse or relative to deal with their financial affairs on their behalf when they lose the capacity to do so. Patients and carers may be entitled to state financial benefits.

Driving. After a diagnosis of dementia, patients in the UK have a duty to inform the Driver and Vehicle Licensing Authority (DVLA), who may request a driving safety assessment.

Further reading

Bang J, Spina S, Miller BL. Frontotemporal dementia. *Lancet* 2015; 386: 1672–1682.
Mitchell SL. Advanced dementia. *N Engl J Med* 2015; 372:2533–2540.
O'Brien JT, Thomas A. Vascular dementia. *Lancet* 2015; 386:1698–1706.
Walker Z, Possin KL, Boeve BF et al. Lewy body dementias. *Lancet* 2015; 386:1683–1697.

Motor neurone disease

Motor neurone disease (MND) is a devastating condition causing progressive weakness and eventually death, usually as a result of respiratory failure or aspiration. It is relatively uncommon, with an annual incidence of 2/100 000. Presentation is usually between the ages of 50 and 75. Below age 70, men are affected more often than women. Amyotrophic lateral sclerosis (ALS) is the term more commonly used for MND in some countries.

Pathogenesis

MND predominantly affects upper and lower motor neurones in the spinal cord, cranial nerve motor nuclei and cortex. However, other neuronal systems may also be affected; 5% of patients also develop FTD (see p. 883) and up to 40% have some measurable frontal lobe cognitive impairment. MND is usually sporadic and of unknown cause, with no established environmental risk factors. Ubiquitinated cytoplasmic inclusions containing the RNA processing proteins TDP-43 and FUS are the pathological hallmarks found in axons, indicating that protein aggregation may be involved in pathogenesis, as with other neurodegenerative disorders. Oxidative neuronal damage and glutamate-mediated excitotoxicity have also been implicated in pathogenesis.

Between 5% and 10% of cases of MND are familial, and mutations in the free radical scavenging enzyme superoxide dismutase (SOD-1) and in a number of other genes, including *TDP-43* and *FUS*, have been identified. A hexanucleotide GGGGCC repeat expansion in the *C9ORF72* gene on chromosome 9 accounts for a significant proportion of familial cases of MND–FTD overlap.

Clinical features

Four main clinical patterns are seen. These different presentations usually merge as MND progresses. The sensory system is not involved and so sensory symptoms such as numbness, tingling and pain do not occur.

- *Amyotrophic lateral sclerosis* (**ALS**). This is the classic paraneoplastic presentation with simultaneous involvement of upper and lower motor neurones, usually in one limb, spreading gradually to other limbs and trunk muscles. The typical picture is one of progressive focal muscle weakness and wasting (e.g. in one hand), with muscle fasciculations due to spontaneous firing of abnormally large motor units formed by surviving axons branching to innervate muscle fibres that have lost their nerve supply. Cramps are a common but non-specific symptom. Examination often reveals upper motor neurone signs, such as brisk reflexes (a brisk reflex in a wasted muscle is a classic sign), extensor plantar responses and spasticity. Sometimes, an asymmetric spastic paraparesis is the presenting feature, with lower motor neurone features developing months later. Relentless progression of signs and symptoms over months allows confirmation of a diagnosis that may initially be suspected.
- *Progressive muscular atrophy.* This is a pure lower motor neurone presentation with weakness, muscle wasting and fasciculations, usually starting in one limb and gradually spreading to involve other adjacent spinal segments.
- *Progressive bulbar and pseudobulbar palsy* (20%). The lower cranial nerve nuclei and their supranuclear connections are initially involved. Dysarthria, dysphagia, nasal regurgitation of fluids and choking are the presenting symptoms. A fasciculating tongue with slow, stiff tongue movements is the classic finding in a mixed bulbar palsy. Emotional incontinence with pathological laughter and crying may occur in pseudobulbar palsy.
- *Primary lateral sclerosis* (rare, 1–2%). This is the least common form of MND and is confined to upper motor neurones, causing a slowly progressive tetraparesis and pseudobulbar palsy.

Diagnosis

Diagnosis is largely clinical. There are no diagnostic tests but investigations allow exclusion of other disorders and may confirm subclinical involvement of muscle groups, such as paraspinal muscles. Denervation of muscles due to degeneration of lower motor neurones is confirmed by EMG.

Cervical spondylosis causing radiculopathy with myelopathy (upper and lower motor neurone signs) can cause diagnostic difficulty. Motor neuropathies, such as multifocal motor neuropathy, can also appear like MND (see p. 889).

Prognosis and management

Survival for more than 3 years is unusual, although there are rare MND cases who survive for a decade or longer.

No treatment has been shown to influence outcome substantially. Riluzole, a sodium-channel blocker that inhibits glutamate release, slows progression slightly, increasing life expectancy by 3–4 months on average. Non-invasive ventilatory support and feeding via a gastrostomy help prolong survival. Patients should be supported by a specialist multidisciplinary team with access to palliative care and a clinical nurse specialist.

Further reading

Atarashi R, Satoh K, Sano K et al. Ultrasensitive human prion detection in cerebrospinal fluid by real-time quaking-induced conversion. *Nat Med* 2011; 17:175–178.
Howard R, McShane R, Lindesay J et al. Donepezil and memantine for moderate-to-severe Alzheimer's disease. *N Engl J Med* 2012; 366:893–903.
National Institute for Health and Care Excellence. Dementia: assessment, management and support for people living with dementia and their carers. NG97; NICE 2011; http://www.nice.org.uk.
Petersen RC. Mild cognitive impairment. *N Engl J Med* 2011; 364:2227–2234.
Prince M, Knapp M, Guerchet M et al. *Dementia UK: Update*. London: Alzheimer's Society; 2014.
Querfurth HW, LaFerla FM. Alzheimer's disease. *N Engl J Med* 2010; 362:329–344.
Warren JD, Rohrer JD, Rossor MN. Frontotemporal dementia. *BMJ* 2013; 347:f4827.

CONGENITAL DISORDERS

Cerebral palsy

Cerebral palsy (CP) is an umbrella term encompassing disparate disorders that are apparent at birth or in childhood and are characterized by non-progressive motor deficits. It is the most common form of physical disability in childhood and most affected children survive into adulthood. A variety of intrauterine and neonatal cerebral insults may cause CP, including prematurity and its complications, hypoxia, intrauterine infections and kernicterus. In many cases, no specific cause can be identified.

Clinical features

Failure to achieve normal milestones is usually the earliest feature. Specific motor syndromes become apparent later in childhood or, rarely, in adult life.
- **Spastic diplegia** – lower limb spasticity, with scissoring of gait.
- **Athetoid cerebral palsy** (see p. 862).
- **Infantile hemiparesis** – may be noted at birth or later. One hemisphere is hypotrophic and the contralateral, hemiparetic limbs small (hemiatrophy).
- **Ataxic and dystonic CP.**
- **Co-morbidity** – particularly epilepsy and learning difficulty, which are common and at least as disabling as the motor deficit.

Dysraphism

Failure of normal fusion of the fetal neural tube leads to a group of congenital anomalies. Folate deficiency during pregnancy is contributory and supplements should always be given (see p. 1242). Antiepileptic drugs, such as valproate, are also implicated (see p. 856). If there is access from the skin, such as from a sinus connecting to the subarachnoid space, bacterial meningitis may follow.
- **Meningoencephalocele** involves extrusion of brain and meninges through a midline skull defect; protrusion can be minor or massive.
- **Spina bifida** is failure of lumbosacral neural tube fusion. Several varieties occur.
- **Spina bifida occulta** is isolated failure of vertebral arch fusion (usually lumbar), often seen incidentally on X-rays (3% of the population). A dimple or a tuft of hair may overlie the anomaly; clinical abnormalities are unusual.
- **Meningomyelocele** may occur with spina bifida.

Meningomyelocele consists of elements of spinal cord and lumbosacral roots within a meningeal sac. This herniates through a vertebral defect. In severe cases, both lower limbs and sphincters are paralysed. Meningocele is a meningeal defect alone. The defect should be closed in the first 24 hours after birth.

Further reading

Colver A, Fairhurst C, Pharoah POD. Cerebral palsy. *Lancet* 2014; 383:1240–1249.
Kiernan MC, Vucic S, Cheah BC et al. Amyotrophic lateral sclerosis. *Lancet* 2011; 377:942–955.
Renton AE, Majounie E, Waite A et al. A hexanucleotide repeat expansion in C9ORF72 is the cause of chromosome 9p21-linked ALS-FTD. *Neuron* 2011; 72:257–268.

NEUROGENETIC DISORDERS

Approximately 80% of the 20000–30000 human genes are expressed in the brain. It is therefore not surprising that of the 5000 or so Mendelian disorders of humans, a high proportion are neurological disorders. Several hundred neurological disease genes have

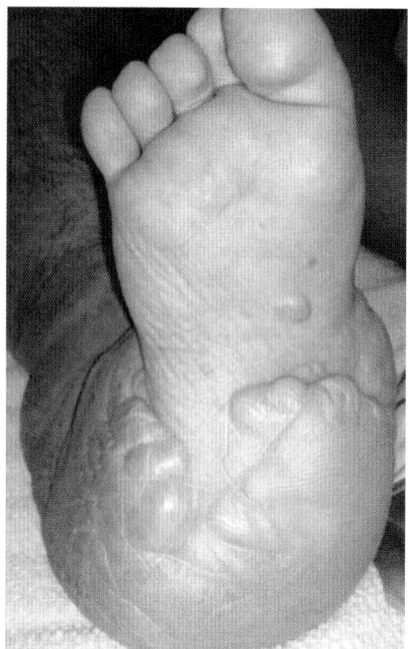

Fig. 26.62 Plexiform neurofibroma.

been identified and molecular genetic testing is now part of the neurological diagnostic process. Many of these disorders are covered in largely individual disease sections of this chapter.

Neurocutaneous syndromes

Neurofibromatosis type 1 (von Recklinghausen's disease)

One of the most common neurogenetic disorders, neurofibromatosis type 1 (NF-1) has a prevalence of 1 in 3000. Inheritance is autosomal dominant but 50% of cases are due to new mutations with no family history. The protein is called neurofibromin 1. NF-1 is characterized by multiple skin neurofibromas and pigmentation (café-au-lait patches – see p. 685, axillary freckling and Lisch nodules of the iris). The neurofibromas arise from the neurilemmal sheath.

Skin neurofibromas present as soft subcutaneous, sometimes pedunculated, lumps (see p. 685). They increase in number throughout life. Plexiform neurofibromas (**Fig. 26.62**) may develop on major nerves and proximal nerve roots, sometimes involving the spinal cord. Treatment is surgical removal if pressure symptoms develop. Associated features include learning difficulties, malignant transformation of neurofibromas, and bone abnormalities including scoliosis and fibrous dysplasia.

Neurofibromatosis type 2

Neurofibromatosis type 2 (NF-2) is much less common than NF-1. It is also autosomal dominant; the gene product, merlin or schwannomin, is a cytoskeletal protein. Many neural tumours occur:
- acoustic neuromas (usually bilateral) in 90%
- meningiomas
- gliomas (including optic nerve glioma)
- cutaneous neurofibromas (30%).

Tuberous sclerosis (epiloia)

Features of this rare multisystem, autosomal dominant condition include adenoma sebaceum, renal tumours and glial overgrowth

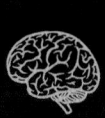

in the brain (cortical tubers and subependymal nodules). Epilepsy (70%) and learning difficulties (50%) are common complications.

Von Hippel–Lindau disease

This rare condition is dominantly inherited. Cerebellar, spinal and retinal haemangioblastomas develop and can be surgically removed. Tumours – renal cell carcinoma and phaeochromocytomas – may also occur. Polycythaemia sometimes develops.

Spinocerebellar ataxias

A wide variety of genetic disorders cause cerebellar ataxia as the sole or predominant clinical feature. Many are due to trinucleotide repeat insertions (see p. 29).

Early-onset ataxia

Most early (<20 years of age) childhood-onset inherited ataxias are autosomal recessive. Friedreich's ataxia is by far the most common, caused by a GAA trinucleotide repeat expansion in the frataxin gene (involved in mitochondrial iron metabolism). Onset is in the early teens with progressive difficulty in walking due to cerebellar ataxia and sensory neuropathy. Associated features include scoliosis, cardiomyopathy, optic atrophy, areflexia and diabetes.

Ataxia telangiectasia and ataxia with vitamin E deficiency are other rarer forms of autosomal recessive inherited ataxia.

Late-onset ataxia

Adult-onset (>20 years of age) inherited ataxias are usually dominantly inherited and there are some 30 different genetic forms, many caused by CAG trinucleotide repeats. There are three main categories of autosomal dominant cerebellar ataxia (ADCA):

- **ADCA-1**: progressive ataxia with variable additional features, including peripheral neuropathy, pyramidal and extrapyramidal signs, and cognitive impairment. ADCA-1 is caused by mutations in loci *SCA1–3*.
- **ADCA-2**: progressive ataxia with macular dystrophy. ADCA-2 is rare and involves the *SCA7* gene.
- **ADCA-3**: late adult-onset 'pure' ataxia. ADCA-3 is associated with the *SCA6* gene in 50%. Non-genetic phenocopies must be excluded.

PARANEOPLASTIC SYNDROMES

Neurological disease may accompany malignancy in the absence of metastases. These paraneoplastic syndromes are associated with anti-neuronal antibodies, believed to be involved in the generation of signs and symptoms. Numerous anti-neuronal antibodies have been described.

Clinical pictures include:

- sensorimotor neuropathy (see p. 895)
- Lambert–Eaton myasthenic–myopathic syndrome (LEMS; see p. 889) and myasthenia gravis with thymoma
- motor neurone disease variants (see p. 885)
- spastic paraparesis (see p. 879)
- cerebellar syndrome (see p. 820)
- limbic encephalitis (see p. 871)
- paraneoplastic stiff person syndrome (see p. 897).

The neurological syndrome usually precedes evidence of the neoplasm: often a small-cell bronchial carcinoma, or breast or ovarian cancer. Diagnosis is based on the clinical pattern and antibody profile. Neuroimaging is typically normal. Treatment is often unsatisfactory.

PERIPHERAL NERVE DISEASE

Mechanisms of damage to peripheral nerves

Peripheral nerves consist of two principal cellular structures: the nerve nucleus with its axon, and the myelin sheath, which is produced by Schwann cells between each node of Ranvier (see **Fig. 26.1**). Blood supply is via vasa nervorum. Several mechanisms, some coexisting, cause nerve damage.

Demyelination

Schwann cell damage leads to myelin sheath disruption. This causes a marked slowing of conduction, seen, for example, in Guillain–Barré syndrome and many genetic neuropathies.

Axonal degeneration

Axon damage causes the nerve fibre to die back from the periphery. Conduction velocity initially remains normal (compare demyelination) because axonal continuity is maintained in surviving fibres. Axonal degeneration typically occurs in toxic neuropathies. A wide range of toxic and metabolic disorders damage peripheral nerves, as their long axons (requiring cellular transport of proteins from cell body to nerve terminals) make them uniquely vulnerable. This explains the concept of length-dependent neuropathy with the longest, most vulnerable axons (to the toes) being affected first.

Compression

Focal demyelination at the point of compression causes disruption of conduction. This typically occurs in entrapment neuropathies, such as carpal tunnel syndrome.

Infarction

Microinfarction of vasa nervorum occurs in diabetes and arteritis, such as polyarteritis nodosa and eosinophilic granulomatosis with polyangiitis (see p. 991). Wallerian degeneration occurs distal to the infarct.

Infiltration

Infiltration of peripheral nerves occurs by inflammatory cells in leprosy and granulomas, such as sarcoid, and by neoplastic cells.

Nerve regeneration

Regeneration occurs either by remyelination – Schwann cells produce new myelin sheaths around an axon – or by axonal growth down the nerve sheath with sprouting from the axonal stump. Axonal growth takes place at up to 1 mm/day.

Types of peripheral nerve disease

(See **Fig. 26.63**.)

- **Neuropathy** simply means a pathological process affecting a peripheral nerve or nerves.
- **Mononeuropathy** means a process affecting a single nerve.
- **Mononeuritis multiplex** means that several individual nerves are affected.
- **Polyneuropathy** describes diffuse, symmetrical disease, usually commencing peripherally. The course may be acute, chronic, static, progressive, relapsing or towards recovery. Polyneuropathies are motor, sensory, sensorimotor and autonomic. They are classified broadly into demyelinating and

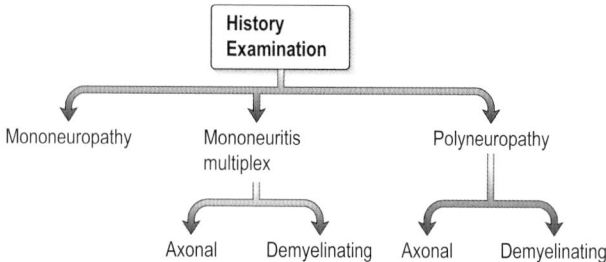

Fig. 26.63 Peripheral neuropathies. The type of neuropathy (axonal or demyelinating) can be assessed by electrical nerve studies (see p. 829).

axonal types, depending on which principal pathological process predominates. It is often impossible to separate these clinically. Many systemic diseases cause neuropathies. Widespread loss of tendon reflexes is typical, with distal weakness and distal sensory loss.

- **Radiculopathy** means disease affecting nerve roots and **plexopathy**, the brachial or lumbosacral plexus.

Diagnosis is made by clinical pattern, nerve conduction studies/ EMG, nerve biopsy, usually sural or radial, and identification of systemic or genetic disease.

Mononeuropathies

Peripheral nerve compression and entrapment

Nerves are vulnerable to mechanical compression at a few key sites (**Box 26.67**), such as the common peroneal nerve at the head of the fibula, or the ulnar nerve at the elbow. Entrapment develops in relatively tight anatomical passages, such as the carpal tunnel. Focal demyelination predominates at the compression site, and some distal axonal degeneration occurs.

These neuropathies are recognized largely by their clinical features. Diagnosis is confirmed by nerve conduction studies.

The most common are mentioned here. All are seen more frequently in people with diabetes.

Carpal tunnel syndrome

This common mononeuropathy, median nerve entrapment at the wrist, is usually known as carpal tunnel syndrome (CTS). CTS is typically not associated with any underlying disease. It is, however, seen in:

- hypothyroidism
- pregnancy (third trimester)
- rheumatoid disease
- acromegaly
- amyloidosis, including in dialysis patients.

Symptoms, signs and management are discussed on page 421.

Ulnar nerve compression

The nerve is compressed in the cubital tunnel at the elbow. This follows prolonged or recurrent pressure and elbow fracture ('tardy ulnar palsy', as onset is very delayed).

There is clawing of the hand, wasting of interossei and hypothenar muscles, and weakness of interossei and medial two lumbricals with sensory loss in the little finger and splitting of the ring finger. Decompression and transposition of the nerve at the elbow is sometimes helpful but often disappointing.

Box 26.67 Nerve compression and entrapment

Nerve	Entrapment/compression site
Median	Carpal tunnel (wrist)
Ulnar	Cubital tunnel (elbow)
Radial	Spiral groove (of humerus)
Posterior interosseous	Supinator muscle (forearm)
Lateral cutaneous of thigh	Inguinal ligament
Common peroneal	Neck of fibula
Posterior tibial	Tarsal tunnel (flexor retinaculum – foot)

The deep, solely motor branch of the ulnar nerve can be damaged in the palm by repeated trauma, such as from a crutch, screwdriver handle or cycle handlebars.

Radial nerve compression

The radial nerve is compressed acutely against the humerus: for example, when the arm is draped over a hard chair for several hours, known as Saturday night palsy. Wrist drop and weakness of brachioradialis and finger extension follow. Recovery is usual, though not invariable, within 1–3 months. Posterior interosseous nerve compression in the forearm also leads to wrist drop, without weakness of brachioradialis.

Lateral cutaneous nerve of the thigh compression

This is also known as meralgia paraesthetica and is described on page 425.

Common peroneal nerve palsy

The common peroneal nerve is compressed against the head of the fibula following prolonged squatting, yoga, pressure from a cast, prolonged bed rest or coma, or for no apparent reason. There is foot drop and weakness of ankle eversion. The ankle jerk (S1) is preserved. A patch of numbness develops on the anterolateral border of the dorsum of the foot and/or lateral calf. Confusion with an L5 motor radiculopathy may occur. Recovery is usual, though not invariable, within several months.

Hereditary neuropathy with pressure palsies

The genetic converse of Charcot–Marie–Tooth disease 1A (see p. 891), this dominantly inherited disorder is due to deletion (as opposed to duplication) of the *PMP-22* gene. Patients are susceptible to pressure palsies after minor compression episodes; even the brachial plexus may be involved. There is also a mild background neuropathy that develops gradually. Genetic testing can be performed.

Mononeuritis multiplex

This occurs in:

- diabetes mellitus
- leprosy
- vasculitis, including eosinophilic granulomatosis with polyangiitis amyloidosis
- malignancy
- neurofibromatosis
- HIV and hepatitis C infection
- multifocal motor neuropathy with conduction block.

Several nerves, such as the ulnar, median, radial and lateral popliteal, become affected sequentially or simultaneously. When multifocal neuropathy is symmetrical, there is difficulty distinguishing it from polyneuropathy.

Polyneuropathies (peripheral neuropathy)

Many diseases cause polyneuropathy. The diagnosis should not stop with identification of the polyneuropathy, but should involve a full diagnostic work-up to identify the underlying cause (**Box 26.68**). However, despite thorough investigation, the aetiology remains unknown in 50% of cases.

Clinical features. Duration, distribution and pattern of the different types of polyneuropathy vary considerably.

Neurophysiological features. Nerve conduction studies allow separation into axonal and demyelinating forms.

Diagnostic investigations (in addition to neurophysiology). A stepped approach can be taken (**Box 26.69**).

Immune-mediated neuropathies
Guillain–Barré syndrome (GBS)
Clinical features

Guillain–Barré syndrome (GBS) is also called acute inflammatory demyelinating polyradiculoneuropathy (AIDP). GBS is the most common acute polyneuropathy (3/100 000 per year); it is usually demyelinating or occasionally axonal, and has an immune-mediated, often post-infectious, basis. GBS is monophasic – it does not recur. The clinical spectrum of GBS extends to an acute motor axonal neuropathy (AMAN) and the Miller–Fisher syndrome – a rare proximal form causing ocular muscle palsies and ataxia.

Paralysis follows 1–3 weeks after an infection that is often trivial and seldom identified. *Campylobacter jejuni* and cytomegalovirus infections are well-recognized causes of severe GBS. Infecting organisms induce antibody responses against peripheral nerves. Molecular mimicry – that is, sharing of homologous epitopes between microorganism liposaccharides and nerve gangliosides (e.g. GM1) – is the possible mechanism.

The patient complains of weakness of the distal limb muscles and/or distal numbness. Low back pain is a frequent early feature. The weakness and sensory loss progress proximally, over several days to 6 weeks. Predominant proximal muscle involvement may occur and, rarely, pure sensory forms. Loss of tendon reflexes is almost invariable. In mild cases, there is mild disability before spontaneous recovery begins, but in some 20% respiratory and facial muscles become weak, sometimes progressing to complete paralysis. Autonomic features sometimes develop.

Diagnosis

This is established on clinical grounds and confirmed by nerve conduction studies; these show slowing of conduction in the common demyelinating form, prolonged distal motor latency and/or conduction block. CSF protein is often raised to 1–3 g/L; cell count and glucose level remain normal.

In the Miller–Fisher syndrome, antibodies against GQ1b (ganglioside) have a sensitivity of 90%.

The differential diagnosis includes other acute paralytic illnesses, such as botulism, cord compression, muscle disease and myasthenia.

Course and management

Paralysis may progress rapidly (hours/days) to require ventilatory support. It is essential for ventilation (vital capacity) to be monitored repeatedly to recognize emerging respiratory muscle weakness. Low-molecular-weight heparin (see p. 1014) and compression stockings should be used to reduce the risk of venous thrombosis.

Immunoglobulin given intravenously within the first 2 weeks reduces duration and severity of paralysis. Patients should be

> **Box 26.68** Varieties of polyneuropathy
>
> - Guillain–Barré syndrome
> - Chronic inflammatory demyelinating polyradiculoneuropathy
> - Idiopathic sensorimotor neuropathy
> - Metabolic, toxic and vitamin deficiency neuropathies (see **Box 26.70**)

> **Box 26.69** Investigations in peripheral neuropathy
>
> **Initial investigations**
> - Blood tests:
>   – Full blood count, erythrocyte sedimentation rate, vitamin B_{12}
>   – Renal, liver, thyroid function
>   – Glucose
>   – Protein electrophoresis, immunoglobulins/ immunofixation
>   – Antinuclear antibody
> - Chest X-ray
> - Urine: Bence Jones proteins, casts
>
> **Selected patients**
> - Nerve biopsy
> - Blood tests:
>   – Anti-ganglioside antibodies
>   – Anti-myelin-associated glycoprotein (anti-MAG) antibodies
>   – HIV, Lyme disease, hepatitis C
>   – Cryoglobulins, vasculitis screen
>   – Anti-Ro and anti-La
>   – Porphyrins
>   – Genetic tests (e.g. Friedreich's ataxia)
>   – Angiotensin-converting enzyme
>   – Serum free light chains
>   – Anti-neuronal antibodies
> - Search for malignancy
> - CSF analysis for protein
> - Labial salivary gland biopsy for Sjögren's
> - Slit-skin smear for leprosy
> - Nerve conduction studies: to differentiate axonal from demyelinating forms

screened for IgA deficiency before immunoglobulin is given, as severe allergic reactions due to IgG antibodies may occur when congenital IgA deficiency is present. Plasma exchange is an alternative. Prolonged ventilation may be necessary. Improvement towards independent mobility is gradual over many months or even years but may be incomplete. Some 5–8% die and 30% are left disabled.

Chronic inflammatory demyelinating polyradiculoneuropathy

Chronic inflammatory demyelinating polyradiculoneuropathy (CIDP) develops over months, causing progressive or relapsing proximal and distal limb weakness with sensory loss. Variants, such as the sensory ataxic form and multifocal motor neuropathy, occur. In some cases, cranial nerves may be involved.

There is no single diagnostic test but CSF protein is raised and patchy demyelination is usually seen on nerve conduction studies. Some cases are associated with a serum paraprotein. Nerve biopsy is sometimes required. CIDP responds to long-term immunosuppression with steroids or to intravenous immunoglobulin in the acute stages.

Multifocal motor neuropathy with conduction block

A distal immune-mediated focal demyelinating motor neuropathy (often asymmetrical and predominantly in the hands) develops gradually over months with profuse fasciculation; hence there is confusion with motor neurone disease (see p. 885). Conduction block and denervation are seen electrically. Antibodies to the ganglioside GM_1

are found in over 50% of cases; this is non-specific, as antibodies are sometimes seen in other neuropathies, such as GBS.

Treatment is usually with regular intravenous immunoglobulin infusions that produce immediate improvement. Steroids may cause the condition to worsen and should be avoided.

Paraproteinaemic neuropathies

Up to 70% of patients with a serum paraprotein have a neuropathy and some 10% of patients with no other identifiable cause for their neuropathy have a paraprotein. Most are associated with monoclonal gammopathy of unknown signification (MGUS; see p. 410) but they are also seen in myeloma (see p. 407). The antibody may be pathogenic for the neuropathy (e.g. anti-MAG) or coincidental in some cases.

IgM paraproteins: usually a demyelinating neuropathy. The paraproteins are often directed against myelin-associated glycoprotein (anti-MAG). The anti-MAG phenotype is a slowly progressive distal neuropathy with ataxia and prominent tremor.

POEMS syndrome (**P**olyneuropathy (demyelinating), **O**rganomegaly (hepatomegaly 50%), **E**ndocrinopathy (reduced testosterone usually), an **M** (para)protein band, and **S**kin changes): probably caused by vascular endothelial growth factor (VEGF) release from a plasmacytoma. Treatment is of the plasmacytoma/plasma cell dyscrasia.

Chronic sensorimotor neuropathy: no cause found

This situation is common. Progressive symmetrical numbness and tingling occur in hands and feet, spreading proximally in a glove and stocking distribution. Distal weakness also ascends. Tendon reflexes are lost. Symptoms may progress, remain static or occasionally remit. Autonomic features are sometimes seen.

Nerve conduction studies usually show axonal degeneration. Nerve biopsy helps to classify some cases: for example, diagnosing CIDP or unsuspected vasculitis.

Metabolic, toxic and vitamin deficiency neuropathies

Causes of the most common neuropathies are shown in **Box 26.70**.

Metabolic neuropathies

Diabetes mellitus

This is the most common cause of neuropathy in developed countries; 50% of patients with diabetes have neuropathy after 25 years. Good glycaemic control is protective against this microvascular complication of diabetes. Several varieties of neuropathy occur (see p. 731):

- **distal symmetrical sensory neuropathy**: usually mild and asymptomatic; related to diabetes duration and glycaemic control
- **acute painful sensory neuropathy** (reversible with improved glycaemic control)
- **mononeuropathy and multiple mononeuropathy (mononeuritis multiplex)**:
  - cranial nerve lesions
  - individual mononeuropathies (e.g. carpal tunnel syndrome) or mononeuritis multiplex
- **diabetic amyotrophy**: a reversible vasculitic plexopathy or femoral neuropathy
- **autonomic neuropathy.**

Uraemia

Progressive sensorimotor neuropathy develops in chronic uraemia. Response to dialysis is variable; the neuropathy usually improves after transplantation.

Thyroid disease

A mild chronic sensorimotor neuropathy is sometimes seen in both hyperthyroidism and hypothyroidism. Myopathy also occurs in hyperthyroidism (see p. 614).

Porphyria

In acute intermittent porphyria (see p. 755), there are episodes of a severe, mainly proximal neuropathy in the limbs, sometimes with abdominal pain, confusion and coma. Alcohol, barbiturates and intercurrent infection can precipitate attacks.

Amyloidosis

Polyneuropathy or multifocal neuropathy develops (see p. 1357).

Toxic neuropathies

Alcohol

Polyneuropathy, mainly in the lower limbs, occurs with chronic alcohol use. It is a common cause of neuropathy. A myopathy may accompany it. For other neurological consequences of alcohol, see **Box 26.71**.

Drugs and industrial toxins

Many drugs (**Box 26.72**) and a wide variety of industrial toxins cause polyneuropathy. Toxins include:

- lead – motor neuropathy
- acrylamide (plastics industry), trichlorethylene, hexane, fat-soluble hydrocarbons, e.g. solvent abuse; see p. 792
- arsenic, thallium and heavy metals.

 Box 26.70 Metabolic, toxic and vitamin deficiency neuropathies

Metabolic
- Diabetes mellitus
- Uraemia
- Hepatic disease
- Thyroid disease
- Porphyria
- Amyloid disease
- Malignancy
- Refsum's disease
- Critical illness

Toxic
- Drugs (see **Box 26.72**)
- Alcohol
- Industrial toxins, e.g. lead, organophosphates

Vitamin deficiency
- B_1 (thiamine)
- B_6 (pyridoxine)
- Nicotinic acid
- B_{12}

Other
- Hereditary sensorimotor neuropathies, e.g. Charcot–Marie–Tooth
- Other polyneuropathies:
  - Neuropathy in cancer
  - Neuropathy in systemic diseases
  - Autonomic neuropathy
  - HIV-associated neuropathy
  - Critical illness neuropathy

Box 26.71 Neurological effects of ethyl alcohol

- Acute intoxication:
  - Disturbance of balance, gait and speech
  - Coma
  - Head injury and sequelae
- Alcohol withdrawal:
  - Morning shakes
  - Tremor
  - Delirium tremens
- Thiamine deficiency:
  - Polyneuropathy
  - Wernicke–Korsakoff syndrome

- Epilepsy
- Acute intoxication
- Alcohol withdrawal
- Hypoglycaemia
- Cerebellar degeneration
- Cerebral infarction
- Cerebral atrophy, dementia
- Osmotic demyelination syndrome (ODS)
- Marchiafava–Bignami's syndrome (corpus callosum degeneration, rare)

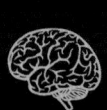

Box 26.72 Drug-related neuropathies

Drug	Neuropathy	Mode/site of action
Phenytoin	M	A
Chloramphenicol	S, M	A
Metronidazole	S, S/M	A
Isoniazid	S, S/M	A
Dapsone	M	A
Anti-retroviral drugs	S > M	A
Nitrofurantoin	S/M	A
Vincristine	S > M	A
Paclitaxel	S > M	A
Disulfiram	S, M	A
Cisplatin	S	A
Amiodarone	S, M	D, A
Chloroquine	S, M	A, D
Suramin	M > S	D, A

Vitamin deficiency neuropathies

Vitamin deficiencies cause nervous system damage that is potentially reversible if treated early, and progressive if not. Deficiencies, often of multiple vitamins, develop in malnutrition.

Thiamine (vitamin B$_1$)

Dietary deficiency causes *beriberi* (see p. 1240). Its principal features are polyneuropathy and cardiac failure. Thiamine deficiency also leads to Wernicke's encephalopathy and Korsakoff psychosis. Alcohol is the most common cause in Western countries and, rarely, anorexia nervosa or vomiting of pregnancy.

Wernicke–Korsakoff's syndrome. This thiamine-responsive encephalopathy is due to damage in the brainstem and its connections. It consists of:

- *eye signs* – nystagmus, bilateral lateral rectus palsies, conjugate gaze palsies
- *ataxia* – broad-based gait, cerebellar signs and vestibular paralysis
- *cognitive change* – acutely, stupor and coma; later, an amnestic syndrome with confabulation.

Wernicke–Korsakoff's syndrome is under-diagnosed. Thiamine should be given parenterally if the diagnosis is a possibility. Untreated Wernicke–Korsakoff's syndrome commonly leads to an irreversible amnestic state. Erythrocyte transketolase activity is reduced but the test is rarely available.

Pyridoxine (vitamin B$_6$)

Deficiency causes a mainly sensory neuropathy. In practical terms, this is seen as limb numbness developing during anti-tuberculosis therapy in slow isoniazid acetylators (see p. 971). Prophylactic pyridoxine 10 mg daily is given with isoniazid.

Vitamin B$_{12}$ (cobalamin)

Deficiency causes damage to the spinal cord, peripheral nerves and brain.

Subacute combined degeneration of the cord (*SACD*). Combined cord and peripheral nerve damage is a sequel of addisonian pernicious anaemia and, rarely, other causes of vitamin B$_{12}$ deficiency (see p. 334). Initially, there is numbness and tingling of fingers and toes; distal sensory loss, particularly of the posterior column; absent ankle jerks; and, with cord involvement, exaggerated knee jerks and extensor plantars. Optic atrophy and retinal haemorrhage may occur. In later stages, sphincter disturbance, severe generalized weakness and dementia develop. Exceptionally, dementia develops in the early stages.

Activated vitamin B$_{12}$, methylmalonic acid and homocysteine levels should be checked. Macrocytosis with megaloblastic marrow is usual, though not invariable, in SACD. Parenteral B$_{12}$ reverses nerve damage but has little effect on the cord and brain. Copper deficiency is a very rare cause of a similar picture. Nitrous oxide abuse may cause functional B$_{12}$ deficiency.

Genetic neuropathies

Inherited neuropathy may occur as 'pure' neuropathy disorders (e.g. Charcot–Marie–Tooth disease) or as part of a neurological multisystem disorder (e.g. spinocerebellar ataxias; see p. 887).

Charcot–Marie–Tooth disease

Charcot–Marie–Tooth (CMT) disease is a complex group of heterogeneous hereditary motor and sensory neuropathies (HMSNs) with multiple causative genes. Distal limb wasting and weakness typically progress slowly over many years, mostly in the legs, with variable loss of sensation and reflexes. In advanced disease, severe foot drop results but patients usually remain ambulant. Mild cases have pes cavus and toe clawing that can pass unnoticed.

- *HSMN Ia (CMT 1A)* – the most common (70% of CMT; 1:2500 births) autosomal dominant demyelinating neuropathy, caused by duplication (or point mutation) of a 1.5 megabase portion p11.2 of chromosome 17 encompassing the peripheral myelin protein 22 gene (*PMP-22*, 17p11.2).
- *HSMN Ib (CMT 1B)* – the second most common autosomal dominant demyelinating neuropathy due to mutations in the myelin protein zero gene (*MPZ*) on chromosome 1 (1q22).
- *HSMN II (CMT 2)* – rare axonal polyneuropathies also caused by *MFN2* or *KIFIB* on chromosome 1p36 and other mutations; there is prominent sensory involvement with pain and paraesthesias.
- *Distal spinal muscular atrophy* – a rare cause of the CMT phenotype.
- *CMT with optic atrophy*, deafness, retinitis pigmentosa and spastic paraparesis.
- *CMTX* – an X-linked dominant HSMN on chromosome Xq13.1; the gene product is a gap junction B1 protein (GJB1) or connexin 32.

Hereditary motor and sensory neuropathy type III

HSMN III is a rare childhood demyelinating sensory neuropathy (Déjérine–Sottas disease) leading to severe incapacity during adolescence. Nerve roots become hypertrophied. CSF protein is greatly elevated to 10 g/L or more. Point mutations, either of *PMP-22* gene or of *P0*, can generate this phenotype.

Other polyneuropathies
Neuropathy in cancer

Polyneuropathy is seen as a paraneoplastic syndrome (non-metastatic manifestation of malignancy). Polyneuropathy occurs in myeloma and other plasma cell dyscrasias via several mechanisms, including direct effects of paraproteins, amyloidosis and nerve infiltration, POEMS and effects of chemotherapy. Individual nerves may be infiltrated with malignant cells, such as lymphoma.

Neuropathies in systemic diseases

Vasculitic neuropathy occurs in SLE (see p. 457), polyarteritis nodosa (p. 465), granulomatosis with eosinophilia (p. 991) and rheumatoid disease (p. 442). Both multifocal neuropathy and symmetrical sensorimotor polyneuropathy occur.

Autonomic neuropathy

Autonomic neuropathy causes postural hypotension, urinary retention, erectile dysfunction, nocturnal diarrhoea, diminished sweating, impaired pupillary responses and cardiac arrhythmias. This can develop in diabetes and amyloidosis, and may complicate GBS and Parkinson's disease. Many varieties of neuropathy cause autonomic problems in a mild form. Occasionally, such as with amyloidosis, a severe autonomic neuropathy may occur.

Neuromuscular weakness complicating critical illness

Some 50% of critically ill intensive care unit patients with multiple organ failure and/or sepsis develop an axonal polyneuropathy (see p. 231). Typically, distal weakness and absent reflexes are seen during recovery from critical illness. Resolution is usual.

Plexus and nerve root lesions

The common conditions that cause these are summarized in **Box 26.73**.

Cervical and lumbar degeneration

Spondylosis (see p. 892) describes vertebral and ligamentous degenerative changes occurring during ageing or following trauma. Several factors produce neurological signs and symptoms:

- osteophytes – local overgrowth of bony spurs or bars
- thickening of spinal ligaments
- congenital narrowing of the spinal canal
- disc degeneration and protrusion (posterior and lateral protrusion: cord and root compression)
- vertebral collapse (osteoporosis, infection)
- rheumatoid synovitis (see p. 442)
- ischaemic changes within cord and nerve roots.

Narrowing of disc spaces, osteophytes, narrowing of exit foramina and narrowing of the spinal canal are also seen on X-rays and MRI in the *symptomless* population, commonly in the mid- and lower cervical and lower lumbar region, and so imaging must not be over-interpreted.

Lateral cervical disc protrusion

The patient complains of pain in the arm. A C7 protrusion is the most common problem (**Fig. 26.64**). There is root pain that radiates to the C7 myotome (triceps, deep to scapula and extensor aspect of forearm), with a sensory disturbance, tingling and numbness in the C7 dermatome.

In an established C7 root lesion there is:

- weakness/wasting – triceps, wrist and finger extensors
- loss of the triceps jerk (C7 reflex arc)
- C7 dermatome sensory loss.

Although the initial pain can be very severe, most cases recover with rest and analgesics. It is usual to immobilize the neck. Disc protrusion with root compression is seen on MRI. Root decompression is sometimes helpful.

Lateral lumbar disc protrusion

The L5 and S1 roots are commonly compressed by lateral prolapse of L4–L5 and L5–S1 discs; the root number below a disc interspace is compressed. There is low back pain and *sciatica*: pain radiating from the back to buttock and leg. Onset is typically acute. This can follow lifting, bending or minor injury. When pain follows such an event, it is tempting to ascribe the disc protrusion to it. However, commonly, lateral lumbar disc protrusion is apparently spontaneous; lifting or injury is usually only bringing forward an inevitable disc prolapse.

Straight-leg raising is limited. There is reflex loss, such as ankle jerk in an S1 root lesion, and weakness of plantar flexion (S1) or great toe extension (L5). Sensory loss is found in the affected dermatome.

Most sciatica resolves with initial rest and analgesia, followed by early mobilization. MRI is sometimes appropriate. Surgery is indicated when a substantial persistent symptomatic disc lesion is shown.

Acute low back pain

Acute low back pain is extremely common. Often, pain is of disc or facet joint origin. Significant nerve root compression is unusual. Maintenance of activity and a trial of gentle manipulation are recommended (see also p. 423).

Cervical spondylotic myelopathy

This is a relatively common disorder of older adults. Posterior disc protrusion (**Fig. 26.65**), common at C4–5, C5–6 and C6–7 levels, causes spinal cord compression. Congenital spinal canal narrowing, osteophytic bars, ligamentous thickening and ischaemia are contributory. Usually, there are no or few neck symptoms. The patient complains of slowly progressive difficulty walking as a spastic paraparesis develops. A reflex level in the upper limbs and evidence of

---

> ### i Box 26.73 Common root and plexus problems
>
> **Nerve root**
> - Cervical and lumbar spondylosis
> - Trauma
> - Herpes zoster
> - Tumours, e.g. neurofibroma, metastases
> - Meningeal inflammation, e.g. syphilis, arachnoiditis
>
> **Plexus**
> - Trauma
> - Malignant infiltration
> - Neuralgic amyotrophy
> - Thoracic outlet syndrome (cervical rib)

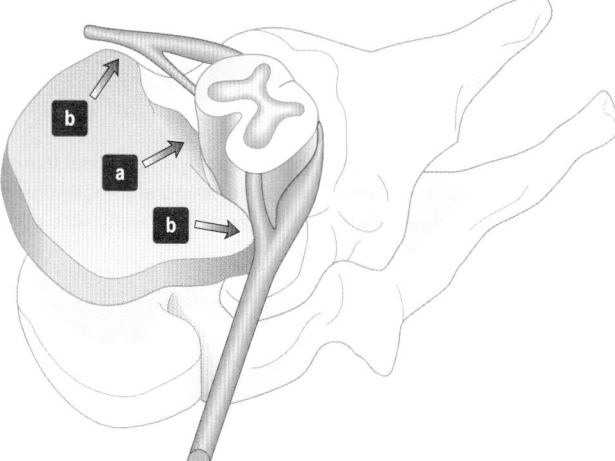

Fig. 26.64 Central and lateral disc protrusions. (a) Central disc protrusion compressing the cord. (b) Lateral disc protrusion compressing nerve roots.

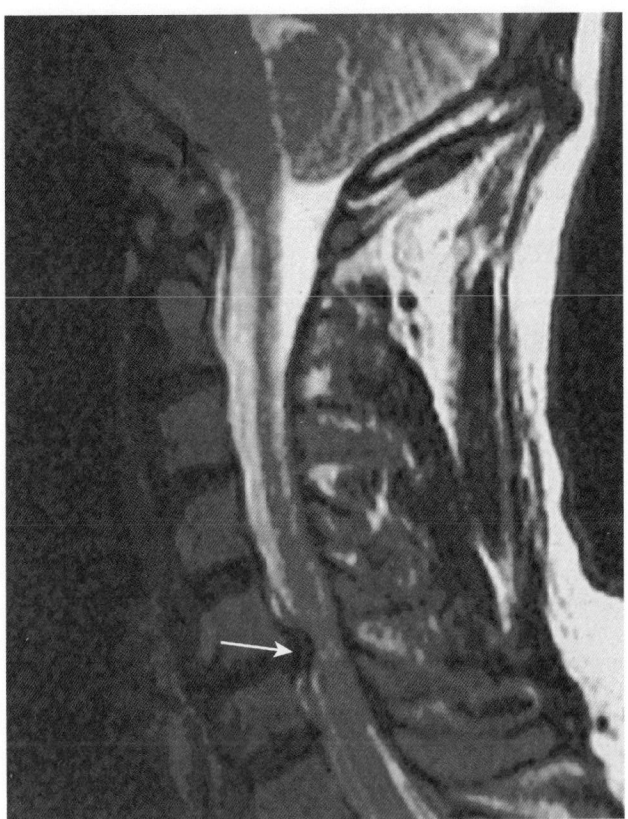

Fig. 26.65 C5/6 disc (arrowed) compressing the cord: T2-weighted MRI.

cervical radiculopathy may coexist. MRI demonstrates the level and extent of cord compression and T2 signal change is usually evident in the cervical cord at the point of maximal compression. Neck manipulation should be avoided.

Decompression by anterior cervical discectomy may be necessary when cord compression is severe or progressive. Complete recovery of the pyramidal signs may occur; progression is generally halted.

Central thoracic disc protrusion

Central protrusion of a thoracic disc is an unusual cause of paraparesis, as the thoracic spine is relatively non-mobile and disc degeneration and protrusion, other than that due to trauma, is rare.

The cauda equina syndrome

A central lumbosacral disc protrusion causes a cauda equina syndrome: that is, bilateral flaccid (compare spasticity in higher lesions) lower limb weakness, sacral numbness, retention of urine, erectile dysfunction and areflexia, usually with back pain. Multiple lumbosacral nerve roots are involved. Onset is either acute – an acute flaccid paraparesis – or chronic, sometimes with intermittent claudication. A central lumbosacral protrusion should be suspected if a patient with back pain develops retention of urine or sacral numbness. Urgent imaging and surgical decompression are indicated for this emergency. Neoplasms in the lumbosacral region can present with similar features.

Spinal stenosis

A narrow spinal canal is developmental and frequently symptomless, but a congenital narrowing of the cervical canal predisposes the cervical cord to damage from minor disc protrusion later.

In the lumbosacral region, further narrowing of the canal by disc protrusion causes root pain and/or buttock and lower limb

claudication. As the patient walks, nerve roots become hyperaemic and swell, producing buttock and lower limb pain with numbness (claudication). Surgical decompression is required.

Neuralgic amyotrophy

Severe pain in the muscles around one shoulder is followed by wasting, usually of infraspinatus, supraspinatus, deltoid and serratus anterior. A demyelinating brachial plexopathy develops over several days. The cause is unknown; an allergic or viral basis is postulated. Rarely, a similar condition develops in distal upper limb muscles or in a lower limb. Recovery of wasted muscles is usual, but not invariable, over several months.

Thoracic outlet syndrome

A fibrous band or cervical rib extending from the tip of the C7 transverse process towards the first rib compresses the lower brachial plexus roots, C8 and T1. There is forearm pain (ulnar border), T1 sensory loss and thenar muscle wasting, principally of abductor pollicis brevis. A Horner's syndrome may develop. The rib or band can be excised. Frequency of this diagnosis varies widely; thoracic outlet problems are sometimes invoked to explain ill-defined arm symptoms, typically on poor evidence.

A rib or band can also produce subclavian artery or venous occlusion. Neurological and vascular problems rarely occur together.

Malignant infiltration and radiation plexopathy

Metastatic disease of nerve roots or the brachial or lumbosacral plexus causes a painful radiculopathy and/or plexopathy. An example is apical bronchial carcinoma (Pancoast's tumour) causing a T1 and sympathetic outflow lesion: wasting of small hand muscles, pain and T1 sensory loss with an ipsilateral Horner's syndrome. This also occurs in apical tuberculosis. In the upper limb, radiotherapy following breast cancer can produce a plexopathy.

MUSCLE DISEASES

Definitions

- **Myopathy** means a disease of voluntary muscle.
- **Myositis** indicates inflammation.
- **Muscular dystrophies** are inherited disorders of muscle cells.
- **Myasthenia** means fatiguable (worse on exercise) weakness – seen in neuromuscular junction diseases.
- **Myotonia** is sustained contraction/slow relaxation.
- **Channelopathies** are ion channel disorders of muscle cells.
  Weakness is the predominant feature of muscle disease. A selection of these conditions is given in **Box 26.74**.

Pathophysiology

Muscle fibres are affected by:

- acute inflammation and fibre necrosis (e.g. polymyositis, infection)
- genetically determined metabolic failure (e.g. Duchenne muscular dystrophy)
- infiltration by inflammatory tissue (e.g. sarcoidosis)
- fibre hypertrophy and regeneration
- mitochondrial diseases
- immunological damage, e.g. myasthenia gravis and Lambert–Eaton myasthenic syndrome
- ion channel disorders, e.g. chloride channel mutations in hereditary myotonias.

ℹ **Box 26.74 Muscle disease: classification**

- Acquired
  - Inflammatory
  - Polymyositis
  - Dermatomyositis
- Inclusion body myositis
  - Viral, bacterial and parasitic infection
  - Sarcoidosis
- Endocrine and toxic
  - Corticosteroids/Cushing's
  - Thyroid disease
  - Calcium disorders
  - Alcohol misuse
  - Drugs, e.g. statins
- Myasthenic
  - Myasthenia gravis
  - Lambert–Eaton myasthenic–myopathic syndrome (LEMS)
- Genetic dystrophies
  - Duchenne
  - Facioscapulohumeral
  - Limb girdle and others
- Myotonic
  - Myotonic dystrophy
  - Myotonia congenita
- Channelopathies
  - Hypokalaemic periodic paralysis
  - Hyperkalaemic periodic paralysis
- Metabolic
  - Myophosphorylase deficiency (McArdle's syndrome)
  - Other defects of glycogen and fatty acid metabolism
- Mitochondrial disease

Diagnosis

Clinical features, including the distribution of weakness, wasting or hypertrophy, and the tempo of progression and presence of family history contribute to a clinical diagnosis. Several investigations help make a definitive diagnosis.

Serum muscle enzymes

Serum creatine kinase (CK) is a marker of muscle fibre damage and is greatly elevated in many dystrophies, such as Duchenne, and in inflammatory muscle disorders, such as polymyositis.

Neurogenetic tests

These are essential in muscular dystrophies and mitochondrial disease.

Electromyography

Characteristic EMG patterns are as follows:
- **Myopathy.** Short-duration spiky polyphasic muscle action potentials are seen. Spontaneous fibrillation is occasionally recorded.
- **Myotonic discharges.** A characteristic high-frequency whine is heard.
- **Decrement and increment.** In myasthenia gravis, a characteristic decrement in evoked muscle action potential follows repetitive motor nerve stimulation. The reverse occurs, i.e. increment, following repetitive stimulation in LEMS (see p. 895).
- In **denervation**, profuse fibrillation potentials are seen.

Muscle biopsy

Unlike neural tissue, skeletal muscle can be easily biopsied to provide a definitive diagnosis using powerful molecular immunohistochemical techniques. Histology and muscle histochemistry of fibre types demonstrate denervation, inflammation and dystrophic changes. Electron microscopy is often valuable. In dystrophies, immunohistochemistry in specialist laboratories allows identification of the abnormal muscle protein and a precise molecular diagnosis.

Imaging

MRI shows **signal changes** within muscles in some cases of myositis, and fatty replacement of muscle in chronically damaged muscles.

Inflammatory myopathies

Inflammatory myopathies, including polymyositis, dermatomyositis and inclusion body myositis, are described on pages 462 and 463. Granulomatous muscle infiltration and inflammation may occur in sarcoidosis and other disorders such as rheumatoid arthritis, causing a mild myopathy. Viral myositis may also occur, and muscles may be involved in other infections such as neurocysticercosis (see p. 872).

Metabolic and endocrine myopathies

Corticosteroids and Cushing's syndrome

Proximal weakness occurs with prolonged high-dose steroid therapy and in Cushing's syndrome (see p. 600). Selective type-2 fibre atrophy is seen on biopsy.

Thyroid disease

Several myopathies occur (see also p. 617). Thyrotoxicosis can be accompanied by severe proximal myopathy. There is also an association between thyrotoxicosis and myasthenia gravis, and between thyrotoxicosis and hypokalaemic periodic paralysis (see p. 896). Both associations are seen more frequently in South-east Asia. In ophthalmic Graves' disease, there is swelling and lymphocytic infiltration of extraocular muscles (see p. 618).

Hypothyroidism is sometimes associated with muscle pain and stiffness, resembling myotonia. a proximal myopathy also occurs.

Disorders of calcium and vitamin D metabolism

Proximal myopathy develops in hypocalcaemia, rickets and osteomalacia (see p. 483).

Hypokalaemia

Acute hypokalaemia (e.g. with diuretics) causes flaccid paralysis reversed by potassium, given slowly (see p. 188). Chronic hypokalaemia leads to mild, mainly proximal, weakness. (See also periodic paralysis; p. 896).

Alcohol and drugs

Severe myopathy with muscle pain, necrosis and myoglobinuria occurs in acute excess. A subacute proximal myopathy occurs with chronic alcohol use. A similar syndrome occurs in diamorphine and amfetamine addicts.

Drugs

Drug-induced muscle disorders include proximal myopathy (steroids), muscle weakness (lithium), painful muscles (fibrates), rhabdomyolysis (a fibrate combined with a statin, or interaction between statins and other drugs such as certain antibiotics) and malignant hyperpyrexia. Most respond to drug withdrawal.

Myophosphorylase deficiency (McArdle's syndrome)

McArdle's syndrome is a muscle-only glycogenosis where there is a deficiency of muscle glycogen phosphorylase (PYGM). It presents with muscle cramps, fatigue, anaesthetic problems and myoglobinuria after exercise in adults. Diagnosis is made on a muscle biopsy with analysis of PYGM at 11q13. Patients have a normal life span. Sucrose should be given before exercise.

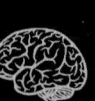

Malignant hyperpyrexia

Widespread skeletal muscle rigidity with hyperpyrexia as a sequel of general anaesthesia or neuroleptic drugs, such as haloperidol, is due to a genetic defect in the sarcoplasmic reticulum calcium-release channel of the muscle ryanodine receptor, RyR1. Death during or following anaesthesia can occur in this rarity, sometimes inherited as an autosomal dominant trait. Dantrolene is of some help for rigidity.

Neuromuscular junction disorders

Myasthenia gravis

Myasthenia gravis (MG) is an autoimmune disorder of neuromuscular junction (NMJ) transmission, characterized by weakness and fatiguability of proximal limb, bulbar and ocular muscles, the latter sometimes in isolation. The prevalence is about 4 in 100 000. MG is twice as common in women as in men, with a peak age incidence around 30 and a second smaller peak in incidence in older men.

Antibodies to acetylcholine receptor protein (anti-AChR antibodies) are pathogenic. Immune complexes of anti-AChR IgG and complement are deposited at the postsynaptic membranes, causing destruction of AChRs. Antibodies against muscle-specific receptor tyrosine kinase (anti-MuSK antibodies) have been identified in anti-AChR antibody-negative cases.

Thymic hyperplasia is found in 70% of MG patients below the age of 40. In some 10%, a thymic tumour is found (paraneoplastic myasthenia), the incidence increasing with age; antibodies to striated muscle can be demonstrated in some of these patients.

There is an association between MG and other autoimmune disorders: thyroid disease, rheumatoid disease, pernicious anaemia and SLE. Transient MG is sometimes caused by D-penicillamine treatment.

Clinical features

Weakness and fatiguability are typical. Limb muscles (proximal), extraocular muscles, speech, facial expression and mastication muscles are commonly affected. Symptoms are worse towards the end of the day. Fluctuating diplopia and ptosis (often asymmetric) are frequently early symptoms and symptoms may be confined to the eyes: ocular myasthenia. Respiratory difficulties can occur in generalized myasthenia. Early complaints of fatigue are frequently dismissed.

Complex extraocular palsies, ptosis and fatiguable proximal weakness are found on examination (prolonged upgaze should be checked and limb power tested after repetitive contractions). The reflexes are initially preserved but may be fatiguable: that is, they disappear following repetitive activity. Wasting is sometimes seen after many years.

Investigations

- **Serum anti-AChR and anti-MuSK antibodies.** Anti-AChR antibodies are present in some 80–90% of cases of generalized MG. In pure ocular MG, anti-AChR antibodies are detectable in less than 30% of cases. These antibodies are highly specific for MG and confirm the diagnosis. Anti-MuSK antibodies define a subgroup of MG patients characterized by weakness predominantly in bulbar, facial and neck muscles.
- **Repetitive nerve stimulation and single-fibre EMG.** A characteristic decrement occurs in the evoked muscle action potential during repetitive stimulation. Single-fibre EMG of orbicularis oculi is more sensitive than repetitive stimulation and shows block and jitter.
- **Imaging and other tests.** Mediastinal MRI or CT is needed to look for thymoma in all cases. Antibodies to striated muscle suggest a thymoma.

- **Tensilon (edrophonium) test.** This is seldom required and the drug is not available worldwide. Edrophonium 10 mg is given intravenously following a 1–2 mg test dose from the 10 mg vial. When the test is positive, there is substantial improvement in weakness within seconds and this lasts for up to 5 minutes. A control test using saline is performed. The sensitivity of the test is 80% but there are false-negative and false-positive tests. Occasionally, edrophonium (an anticholinesterase) causes bronchospasm and syncope. Resuscitation facilities must be available.

Course and management

MG fluctuates in severity; most cases have a protracted, life-long course. Respiratory impairment, nasal regurgitation and dysphagia occur; emergency ventilation may be required. Simple monitoring tests, such as the duration for which an arm can be held outstretched, and the vital capacity are useful.

Exacerbations are usually unpredictable and unprovoked but may be brought on by infections and by aminoglycosides and other drugs.

Drug treatment
Oral anticholinesterases

Pyridostigmine (60 mg tablet) is widely used. The duration of action is 3–4 hours, the dose (usually 3–16 tablets daily) determined by response. Pyridostigmine prolongs acetylcholine action by inhibiting cholinesterase. Overdose of anticholinesterases causes severe weakness (cholinergic crisis). Muscarinic side-effects, such as colic and diarrhoea, are common; oral propantheline (antimuscarinic) helps to reduce this. Anticholinesterases help weakness but do not alter the natural history of myasthenia.

Immunosuppressant drugs

These drugs are used in patients who do not respond to pyridostigmine or who have severe weakness. Steroids are usually used. There is improvement in 70%, although this may be preceded by an initial relapse; steroid dose should be increased slowly. Azathioprine, mycophenolate and other immunosuppressants are also used as steroid-sparing agents.

Thymectomy

Thymectomy improves myasthenia in patients with thymic hyperplasia and positive AChR antibodies (approximately one-third improve, one-third enter remission and one-third do not benefit). When a thymoma is present, the potential for malignancy makes surgery necessary but the myasthenia may not improve.

Plasmapheresis and intravenous immunoglobulin

These produce a rapid dramatic response and are used in exacerbations and severe myasthenic crisis.

Other rare myasthenic syndromes exist, such as congenital myasthenia.

Lambert–Eaton myasthenic–myopathic syndrome

Lambert–Eaton myasthenic–myopathic syndrome (LEMS) is a paraneoplastic manifestation of small-cell bronchial carcinoma due to defective acetylcholine release at the neuromuscular junction. A smaller proportion of cases are autoimmune without underlying malignancy. Proximal limb muscle weakness, sometimes with ocular/bulbar muscles, develops, with some absent tendon reflexes: a cardinal sign. Weakness tends to improve after a few minutes of muscular contraction, and absent reflexes return (compare myasthenia). Diagnosis is confirmed by repetitive nerve stimulation (increment;

see above). Antibodies to voltage-gated calcium channels are found in most cases (90%). Treatment with 3,4-diaminopyridine (DAP) is reasonably safe and effective.

Muscular dystrophies

These progressive, genetically determined disorders of skeletal and sometimes cardiac muscle have a complex clinical and neurogenetic classification.

Duchenne muscular dystrophy and Becker's muscular dystrophy

These are inherited as X-linked recessive disorders, though one-third of cases are spontaneous mutations. Duchenne muscular dystrophy (DMD) occurs in 1 in 3000 male infants. There is absence of the gene product *dystrophin*, a rod-shaped cytoskeletal muscle protein in DMD. In Becker's dystrophy, dystrophin is present but levels are low. DMD is usually obvious by the fourth year, and often causes death by the age of 20.

Dystrophin is essential for cell membrane stability. Deficiency leads to reduction in three glycoproteins (α-, β- and γ-sarcoglycans) in the dystrophin-associated protein complex (DAP complex) that links dystrophin to laminin within cell membranes.

Becker's muscular dystrophy is less severe than Duchenne and weakness only becomes apparent in young adults.

Clinical features

A boy with DMD is noticed to have difficulty running and rising to his feet; he uses his hands to climb up his legs (Gowers' sign). There is initially a proximal limb weakness with calf pseudohypertrophy. The myocardium is affected. Severe disability is typical by the age of 10.

Investigations

The diagnosis is often suspected clinically. CK is grossly elevated (100–200 times normal). Biopsy shows variation in muscle fibre size, necrosis, regeneration and replacement by fat, and on immunochemical staining, absence of dystrophin.

Management

There is no curative treatment but new gene-editing therapies are in development. Steroids may delay progression. Physiotherapy helps prevent contractures in the later stages. Non-invasive respiratory support and multidisciplinary care improve life expectancy.

Carrier detection. Females with an affected brother have a 50% chance of carrying the *DMD* gene. In carriers, 70% have a raised CK, and usually EMG abnormalities and/or changes on biopsy. Carrier and prenatal diagnosis is available with genetic counselling.

Limb-girdle and facioscapulohumeral dystrophy

These less severe but disabling dystrophies are summarized in **Box 26.75**. There are many other varieties of dystrophy; facioscapulohumeral dystrophy is one of the most common. Genes for numerous forms of limb-girdle muscular dystrophy have been identified. CK is usually moderately elevated.

Myotonias

Myotonias are characterized by continued, involuntary muscle contraction after cessation of voluntary effort: that is, failure of muscle

i **Box 26.75 Limb-girdle and facioscapulohumeral dystrophies**

	Limb-girdle	Facioscapulohumeral
Inheritance	Recessive, dominant or X-linked	Dominant, new mutations common
Onset	10–20 years	10–40 years
Muscles affected	Proximal: shoulders, pelvic girdle	Face, shoulders, scapular winging, upper arms, foot drop. Typically asymmetric
Progression	Severe disability <25 years	Life expectancy normal, slow progression
Associated features	Very variable. Contractures in Emery Dreifuss dystrophy	Occasionally, deafness and retinal abnormalities
Diagnosis	Multiple genetic types Diagnosis on muscle biopsy immunohistochemistry and genetic testing	Genetic testing (muscle biopsy usually not required but may show inflammatory changes)

relaxation. EMG is characteristic (see p. 829). The two most common myotonias are described below. Patients with myotonia tolerate general anaesthetics poorly.

Myotonic dystrophy

This autosomal dominant condition is a genetic disorder with two different triple repeat mutations: most commonly, an expanded CTG repeat in a protein-kinase (*DMPK*) gene (DM1). The less common variety (DM2) is caused by an expanded CCTG repeat in a zinc finger protein gene. There is a correlation between disease severity, age at onset and approximate size of triplet repeat mutations. There is progressive distal muscle weakness, with ptosis, weakness and thinning of the face and sternomastoids. Myotonia is typically present. Muscle disease is part of a syndrome comprising:

- cataracts
- frontal baldness
- cognitive impairment (mild)
- oesophageal dysfunction (and aspiration)
- cardiomyopathy and conduction defects (sudden death can occur in type 1)
- small pituitary fossa and hypogonadism
- glucose intolerance
- low serum IgG.

This gradually progressive condition usually becomes evident between 20 and 50 years.

Myotonia congenita

Autosomal dominant myotonia, usually mild, becomes evident in childhood. The gene, *CLC1*, codes for a muscle chloride channel. The myotonia, which persists, is accentuated by rest and by cold. Diffuse muscle hypertrophy occurs, meaning that although physically weak, the patient will have bulky muscles.

Channelopathies

Hypokalaemic periodic paralysis

This disorder is characterized by generalized weakness, including that of bulbar muscles, which often starts after a heavy carbohydrate meal or following exertion. Attacks last for several hours. The disorder often first comes to light in the teenage years and tends

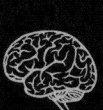

to remit after the age of 35. Serum potassium is usually below 3.0 mmol/L in an attack. The weakness responds to (slow) intravenous potassium chloride. It is usually inherited as an autosomal dominant trait caused by mutation in a muscle voltage-gated calcium channel gene (*CACLN1A3*). Other mutations in the sodium channels (*SCNA4*) and potassium channels (*KCNE3*) also occur. Acetazolamide sometimes helps prevent attacks. Weakness can be caused by diuretics. A similar condition can also occur with thyrotoxicosis.

Hyperkalaemic periodic paralysis

This condition, also autosomal dominant, is characterized by attacks of weakness, sometimes with exercise. Attacks start in childhood and tend to remit after the age of 20; they last about 30–120 minutes. Myotonia may occur. Serum potassium is elevated. An attack can be terminated by intravenous calcium gluconate or chloride. There are point mutations in a muscle voltage-gated sodium-channel gene (*SCN4A*). Acetazolamide or a thiazide diuretic can be helpful.

A very rare normokalaemic, sodium-responsive periodic paralysis also occurs.

Stiff person syndrome

Stiff person syndrome (SPS) is a rare autoimmune disease, more common in females, causing axial muscle stiffness with abnormal posture, spasms and falls. Attacks of stiffness are sometimes provoked by noise or emotion, but sometimes occur spontaneously. Between attacks, which last from hours to days or even weeks, the patient may appear normal.

Widespread muscle stiffness is typical during an attack; there are no other neurological signs. SPS has been mistaken for Parkinson's, dystonia and non-organic conditions. Anti-glutamic acid decarboxylase antibodies (anti-GAD) are found in very high titre in more than 50% of cases and are believed to be involved in the generation of muscle stiffness. Continuous motor activity in paraspinal muscles is seen on EMG.

Treatment with diazepam, other muscle relaxants and intravenous immunoglobulin can be helpful during attacks.

A form of SPS is also seen occasionally as a paraneoplastic condition associated with antibodies to the synaptic protein amphiphysin (see **Box 6.10**).

Mitochondrial diseases

These comprise a complex group of rare disorders involving muscle, peripheral nerves and CNS, characterized by morphological and biochemical abnormalities in mitochondria. Mitochondrial DNA is inherited maternally (see p. 18). The spectrum is wide, ranging from optic atrophy (see Leber's; p. 26) to myopathies, neuropathies and encephalopathy.

- *MELAS* (*m*itochondrial *e*ncephalomyopathy, *l*actic *a*cidosis, *s*troke-like episodes) is one well-recognized form.
- Chronic progressive ophthalmoplegia (CPEO) is another.
- *MERRF* describes *m*yoclonic *e*pilepsy with abnormal muscle histology, the muscle appearance being described as *r*agged *r*ed *f*ibres.

Further reading

Ryan A, Matthews E, Hanna MG. Skeletal muscle channelopathies. *Curr Opin Neurol* 2007; 20:558–563.
Shapira AHV. Mitochondrial disease. *Lancet* 2006; 368:70–82.

Bibliography

Clarke C, Howard R, Rossor M et al (eds). *Neurology: A Queen Square Textbook.* Oxford: Blackwell; 2009.

Significant websites

http://jnnp.bmjjournals.com Journal of Neurology, Neurosurgery and Psychiatry.
http://www.patient.co.uk/selfhelp.asp *UK Patient Support Group.*
http://www.theabn.org *Association of British Neurologists information service.*

Ear, nose and throat and eye disease

Francis Vaz, Nishchay Mehta and Robin D. Hamilton

CORE SKILLS AND KNOWLEDGE

Disorders of the special sense organs are common reasons for patients to present to primary or emergency care. Although many diseases are minor and self-limiting, destructive disease of these organs can lead to serious disability, and may be caused by a range of systemic inflammatory disorders.

All doctors, and especially those working in primary care, require a basic understanding of the way to approach common symptoms arising from the special sense organs. They must be able to exclude serious pathology that may result in sensory loss and treat minor problems such as uncomplicated otitis media or conjunctivitis. Care for more serious conditions relating to the ears, nose, throat (ENT) and eyes is generally carried out in specialist ENT or ophthalmology surgical outpatient services. Medical ophthalmology and clinical audiology services led by physicians are often present in specialist centres that address pathology in these organs caused by systemic diseases.

Key skills in these areas include:

- developing an appropriate diagnostic approach to the four key symptoms of ear disease: pain, discharge, hearing loss and dizziness
- recognizing life-threatening disorders of the throat, including retropharyngeal abscesses and airway compromise
- appropriately identifying sight-threatening eye emergencies and understanding their urgent management.

Learning opportunities include attending ENT and ophthalmology outpatient clinics and practising clinical skills including physical examination, otoscopy and fundoscopy.

INTRODUCTION TO ENT

ENT is a broad specialty that, in addition to covering diseases of the ears, nose and throat, is also concerned with diseases of the trachea and the skull base and is responsible for head and neck cancer, facial plastic surgery, sleep-disordered breathing as well as congenital head and neck anomalies.

One-fifth of general practice relates to ENT conditions and whilst only 3% of emergency department visits are related to ENT diagnoses, they are often the most life-threatening (e.g. acute airway obstructions and major upper airway haemorrhage). Common emergency presentations include severe and complicated upper respiratory tract infections, epistaxis, upper airway compromise, ingested or inhaled foreign bodies and penetrating neck injuries. An ENT surgeon typically begins medical treatment and if this fails can manage these emergencies using surgical intervention.

Surgical treatments for ENT conditions often involve technological aids such as endoscopes, microscopes, powered instruments, lasers and more recently robotics. In ENT, technology is not only used as an aid for surgery but can also be used as the treatment (e.g. cochlear and brain stem auditory implants). The head and neck are generally complicated anatomical regions with multiple vital structures in close proximity to each other. Whilst being mindful of this complicated anatomy, surgery varies from the fine (e.g. stapedotomy) to expansive (e.g. laryngopharyngectomy). Nearly three-quarters of the operative load has moved to day case, reducing the inpatient burden.

Multidisciplinary working is central to ENT as many conditions are managed in collaboration with other specialists (e.g. oncologists and plastic surgeons for head and neck cancer,

899

endocrinologists for thyroid disease, respiratory physicians for tracheal disease, sleep-disordered breathing and allergies, neurosurgeons for skull base disease, etc.) and allied health professionals (e.g. speech and language therapists for speech and swallowing problems, electrophysiologists for voice assessment, audiologists for hearing and balance issues, teachers of the deaf for cochlear implant patients and psychologists for body dysmorphic disorders).

CLINICAL APPROACH TO THE PATIENT WITH AN ENT COMPLAINT

When a patient presents with a location-specific symptom, it is wise to ask about other symptoms that are specific to that site. **Box 27.1** and **Fig. 27.1** list symptoms that frequently present depending on the anatomical location of the lesion. Keep in mind that the nose communicates with the ear through the Eustachian tube and with the throat through the nasopharynx, so symptoms of a disease can cross from one location to another (e.g. patients with chronic rhinosinusitis often complain of pressure in their ears).

The nature, character and chronological features of each symptom should be systematically explored. Concomitant medical problems, medication use, occupation and environmental factors are not only frequently the cause of many ENT complaints but can also be impacted by ENT treatments and so it is essential to get a full history. Whilst a comprehensive history is essential, there are certain high-yield pointers that can sometimes help make common ENT diagnoses.

Ear symptoms
Hearing loss

Upper respiratory tract infections can precede hearing loss caused by acute otitis media (painful) or otitis media with effusion (painless). Trauma can cause conductive hearing loss secondary to haemotympanum (blood in the middle ear) or disruption to the ossicular chain; additionally it can relate to trauma of the otic capsule (bony covering of inner ear) causing sensorineural hearing loss. Chemotherapy, aspirin, aminoglycoside antibiotics and loop diuretics can all cause sensorineural hearing loss. Fluctuating hearing loss

---

> ### *i* Box 27.1 Symptoms correlating with lesion location
>
> **Ear**
> - Hearing loss
> - Otalgia (ear pain)
> - Otorrhoea (ear discharge)
> - Vertigo (false perception of movement)
> - Tinnitus (false perception of external sound)
>
> **Nose**
> - Nasal blockage
> - Rhinorrhoea (anterior nasal discharge)
> - Postnasal drip
> - Dysosmia (change in sense of smell)
> - Facial pressure
>
> **Throat**
> - Odynophagia (pain on swallowing)
> - Dysphagia (difficulty swallowing)
> - Dysphonia (difficulty with voice)
> - Dyspnoea (difficulty breathing)

---

in children normally signifies otitis media with effusion, whereas in adults it signifies cochlear hydrops, autoimmune conditions and Ménière's (if associated with vertigo and tinnitus). Many types of hearing loss run in families and occupational exposure to loud noise is a common cause of hearing loss.

Vertigo

Duration of vertigo is a key feature that helps distinguish the different pathologies. Vertigo, defined as rotatory sensation, when lasting for seconds is typically benign paroxysmal positional vertigo (BPPV), when lasting for hours is typically Ménière's and when lasting for days is often caused by labyrinthitis/vestibular neuronitis. Vertigo that is triggered by loud noises suggests a breach in the otic capsule.

Tinnitus

Unilateral tinnitus may signify retrocochlear pathology (e.g. vestibular schwannoma). The nature of tinnitus can help identify causes: ringing, buzzing, humming and blowing tinnitus tends to be idiopathic and requires very little investigation beyond examination and a hearing test. However, tinnitus that is unilateral, pulsatile, related to body sounds (voice echoing in ears, sound of eyeballs moving), or objective (i.e., third party can also hear sound) needs further investigations. Loud noise exposure is the commonest cause of tinnitus and so occupational history is important.

Nose symptoms
Nasal blockage

If unilateral, this usually represents a fixed anatomical obstruction such as a nasal septal fracture-deviation or nasal polyps. If in a child, consider a foreign body. Alternating nasal blockage suggests an exaggerated nasal cycle and is a sign of nasal mucosa disease such as allergic or chronic rhinosinusitis. Chronic use of topical decongestants can lead to fixed nasal blockage and so previous medication history is important. A history of asthma and aspirin sensitivity may suggest rhinitis or nasal polyps. Knowledge about pets and seasonal variations can sometimes help with the diagnosis.

Rhinorrhoea

Unilateral clear rhinorrhoea that increases with positions of raised intracranial pressure may signify a cerebrospinal fluid (CSF) leak. Rhinorrhoea associated with nasal itch and frequent sneezing is normally allergy driven. Blood-stained rhinorrhoea may signify malignant disease. Offensive rhinorrhoea usually signifies sinus infections. Rhinorrhoea that initiates in response to changes in ambient or food temperature usually represents vasomotor rhinitis.

Dysosmia

A sudden history of anosmia following an upper respiratory infection can signify permanent and irreversible damage to the olfactory sensory lining. Gradual anosmia, especially related to other sinus symptoms (e.g. nasal blockage), may represent a failure of odorants penetrating the olfactory niche. Cacosmia (offensive smell in absence of offensive external stimulus) may represent a localized sinus infection or neurological condition. Many medications can lead to anosmia and so a full medication history is essential. Heavy metal exposure and nutritional deficiencies can also lead to anosmia and need to be explored in the history.

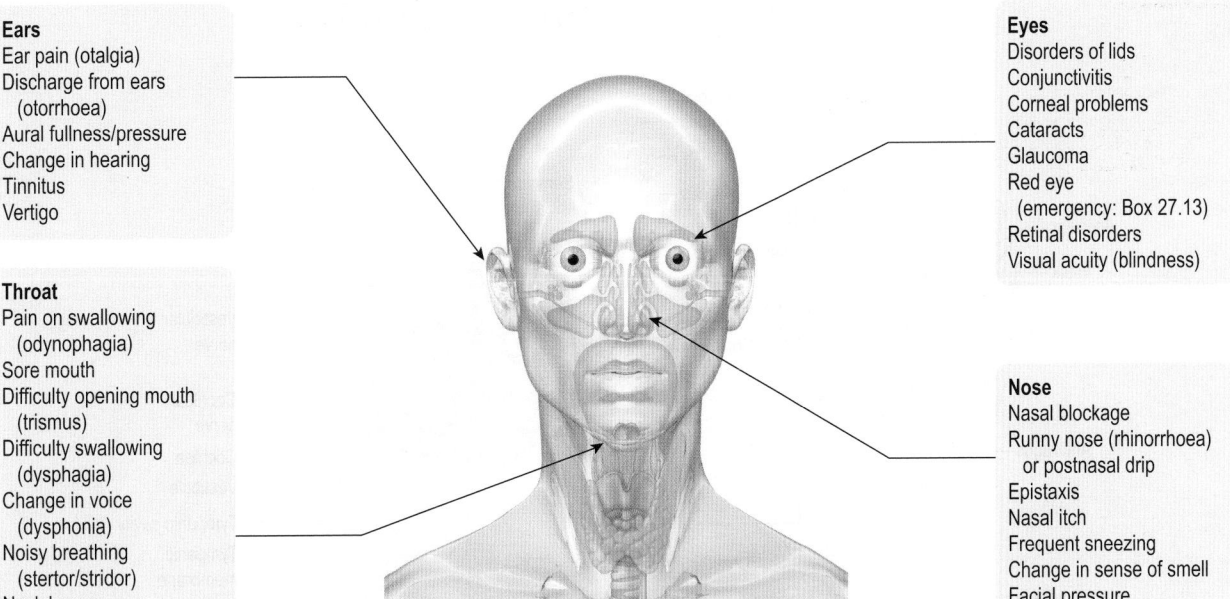

Ears
Ear pain (otalgia)
Discharge from ears (otorrhoea)
Aural fullness/pressure
Change in hearing
Tinnitus
Vertigo

Throat
Pain on swallowing (odynophagia)
Sore mouth
Difficulty opening mouth (trismus)
Difficulty swallowing (dysphagia)
Change in voice (dysphonia)
Noisy breathing (stertor/stridor)
Neck lumps

Eyes
Disorders of lids
Conjunctivitis
Corneal problems
Cataracts
Glaucoma
Red eye (emergency: Box 27.13)
Retinal disorders
Visual acuity (blindness)

Nose
Nasal blockage
Runny nose (rhinorrhoea) or postnasal drip
Epistaxis
Nasal itch
Frequent sneezing
Change in sense of smell
Facial pressure

Fig. 27.1 Symptoms of ear, nose and throat and eye disorders.

Throat symptoms

Odynophagia/dysphagia

Acute odynophagia with dysphagia is invariably related to throat infections. Chronic odynophagia is frequently related to acid reflux into the throat, but may be a sign of underlying malignancy, especially if the patient has risk factors and has suffered weight loss. Acute dysphagia usually relates to a vascular event (e.g. bulbar stroke) or impacted foreign bodies (e.g. food bolus). Chronic dysphagia to liquids more than solids may signify neurological pathology (e.g. bulbar palsy), whilst dysphagia to solids more than liquids may signify anatomical obstruction (e.g. oesophageal stricture, malignancy, pharyngeal pouch). Chronic dysphagia associated with regurgitation of undigested foods relates to pharyngeal pouch, while chronic dysphagia on the background of longstanding gastro-oesophageal reflux disease is more likely to represent a stricture.

Dyspnoea

Acute dyspnoea associated with sore throat usually signifies an infection of the upper airway and is usually preceded with coryzal symptoms. Dyspnoea resulting from upper airway disease usually presents with noisy breathing (e.g. stridor). The timing of breathing noises helps identify the location of the pathology. Inspiratory stridor signifies partial obstruction anywhere from the epiglottis to the voicebox, expiratory stridor usually signifies partial obstruction of the tracheobronchial tree, while stridor present during inspiration and expiration usually denotes disease of the area around the vocal cords.

Dysphonia

Acute dysphonia, especially with preceding symptoms of an upper respiratory tract infection, usually represents acute laryngitis. Chronic dysphonia that is worse in the morning may be related to gastro-oesophageal reflux, whereas dysphonia that gets worse throughout the day signifies voice abuse. Chronic dysphonia that does not fluctuate may suggest anatomical lesions such as a vocal cord cyst or polyp. A strained high pitch voice may suggest adductor spasmodic dysphonia, a breathy voice suggests vocal cord palsy or abductor spasmodic dysphonia, and a whispering voice suggests laryngitis. Malignancy should be considered in all patients with chronic dysphonia and a history of smoking and heavy drinking. Professional voice users are more prone to several laryngeal conditions from muscle tension dysphonia to vocal cord nodules and so an occupational history is vital.

DISORDERS OF THE EAR

ANATOMY AND PHYSIOLOGY

The ear can be divided into three parts: outer, middle and inner (**Fig. 27.2**).

The **outer ear** has a skin-lined tube 2.5 cm long leading down to the tympanic membrane (the ear drum). Its outer third is cartilaginous and contains hair and sebaceous and ceruminous glands, but the walls of the inner two-thirds are bony. The outer ear is self-cleaning, as the skin is migratory so there are no indications to use cotton wool buds. Wax should only be seen in the outer third.

The **middle ear** is an air-containing cavity derived from the branchial clefts. It communicates with the mastoid air cells superiorly, and the Eustachian tube connects it to the nasopharynx medially. The Eustachian tube ventilates the middle ear and maintains equal air pressure across the tympanic membrane. It is normally closed but opens via the action of the palatal muscles to allow air entry when swallowing or yawning. A defect in this mechanism, such as with a cleft palate, will prevent air entering the middle ear cleft, which may then fill with fluid. Lying within the middle ear cavity are the three ossicles (malleus, incus and stapes), which transmit sound from the tympanic membrane (**Fig. 27.3**) to the inner ear. On the medial wall of the

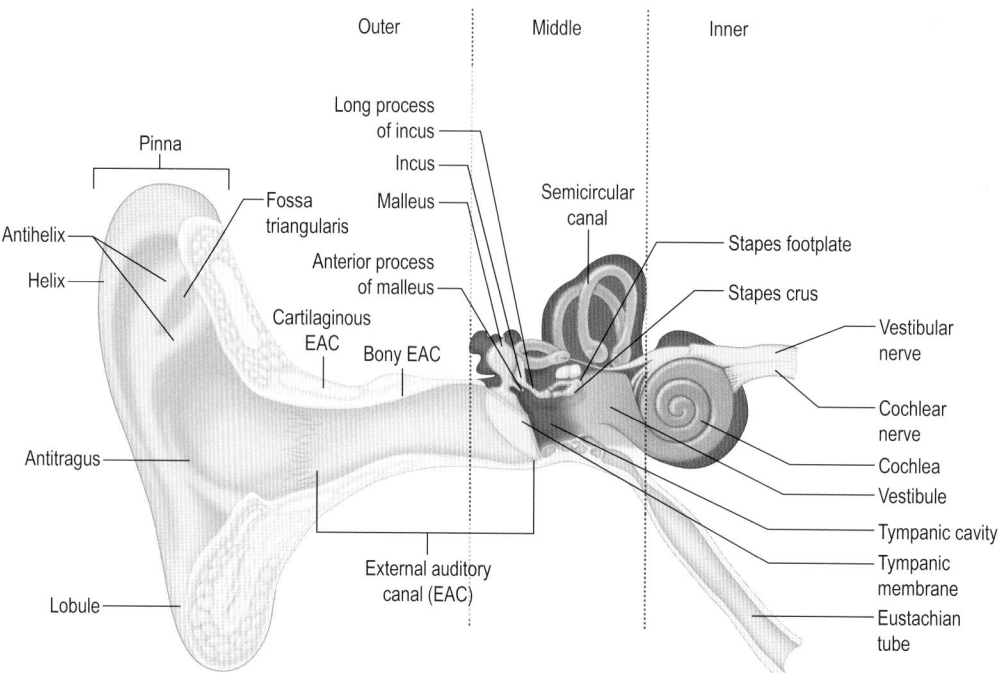

Fig. 27.2 The anatomy of the ear. The ear is anatomically divided into outer, middle and inner ear, as indicated at the top. The **outer ear** consists of the pinna and external auditory meatus, and funnels sound energy to the middle ear, selectively amplifying sounds in the 2–4 kHz range by 15 decibels (dB, speech sounds). When sound energy passes from air in the outer ear to fluid in the inner ear, it loses 30 dB due to energy that is reflected at the interface of the two mediums. The **middle ear** acts as a transformer, increasing the pressure of the acoustic wave to account for the energy lost at this air–fluid interface. As the acoustic wave moves across the tunnel of the **inner ear**, passing from the oval window to the round window, it causes maximal vibration of the basilar membrane in a location that is specific to its resonant frequency. This vibration causes the hair cell to open its ion gates and an action potential to be propagated along a fibre of the cochlear nerve. The location of the nerve fibre and the strength of its action potential allow the central nervous system to construct meaning from the sound we hear.

cavity is the horizontal segment of the facial nerve, which can be damaged during surgery or by direct extension of infection in the middle ear.

The **inner ear** contains the cochlea for hearing and the vestibule and semicircular canals for balance. There is a semicircular canal arranged in each body plane and these canals are stimulated by rotatory movement. The facial, cochlear and vestibular nerves emerge from the inner ear and run through the internal acoustic meatus to the brainstem (see **Fig. 26.8**).

Physiology of hearing

The ossicles, in the middle ear, transmit sound waves from the tympanic membrane to the cochlea. They amplify the waves by about eighteen-fold to compensate for the loss of sound waves moving from the air-filled middle ear to the fluid-filled cochlea. Hair cells in the basilar membrane of the cochlea detect the vibrations and transduce these into nerve impulses, which pass to the cochlear nucleus and then eventually to the superior olivary nuclei of both sides; thus lesions central to the cochlear nucleus do not cause unilateral hearing loss.

If the ossicles are diseased, sound can also reach the cochlea by vibration of the temporal bone (bone conduction).

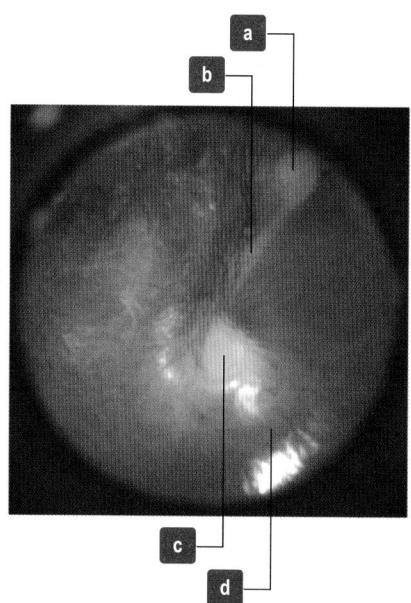

Fig. 27.3 Normal tympanic membrane. (a) Lateral process of malleus. **(b)** Handle of malleus. **(c)** Umbo. **(d)** Light reflex.

CLINICAL APPROACH TO THE PATIENT WITH A DISORDER OF THE EAR

Examination

The pinna and post-auricular region should first be examined for erythema, scars or swellings. An auroscope is used to examine the external ear canal whilst the pinna is retracted backwards and upwards to straighten the canal. Look for wax, discharge or foreign bodies. The tympanic membrane should always be seen with a light reflex anteroinferiorly. Previous repeated infections may cause a thickened, whitish drum but fluid in the middle ear may show as dullness of the drum. Perforations can be described as marginal if they involve the annulus, subtotal if the pars tensa is absent, and total if both pars tensa and the annulus are absent.

Rinne test

(See **Fig. 27.4**.)

- Normally, a tuning fork, 512 Hz, will be heard as louder if held next to the ear (i.e. air conduction) than it will if placed on the mastoid bone (***Rinne-positive***).
- If the tuning fork is perceived louder when placed on the mastoid (i.e. via bone conduction), then a defect in the conducting mechanism of the external or middle ear is present (true ***Rinne-negative***).

Weber test

(See **Fig. 27.5**.) A tuning fork placed on the forehead or vertex of a patient with normal hearing (or with symmetrical hearing loss) should be perceived centrally by the patient. A patient with unilateral conductive hearing loss will hear the sound loudest in the affected ear, whereas a patient with unilateral sensorineural hearing loss will report the sound to be loudest in the unaffected ear.

Pure-tone audiometry

The patient is asked to respond when they hear sounds presented as pure tones at varying sound intensities and frequencies. Sounds are presented to each ear (representing air conduction) and then to each mastoid in turn (representing bone conduction). An audiogram is produced by the lowest sound intensity that is reliably perceptible at each frequency tested at both ears and mastoids (**Fig. 27.6**).

COMMON DISORDERS OF THE EAR

There are four main symptoms related to ear pathology: pain (otalgia), discharge (otorrhoea), hearing loss and dizziness (vertigo). The sequence and combination of symptoms can differentiate between most conditions and therefore history is often the most useful diagnostic tool.

The painful ear (otalgia)

A painful ear is a common complaint but, due to the complex innervation, may be referred from distant sites and can thus on occasion have an obscure aetiology.

Otitis externa

When the natural barriers to infection are overcome, the skin of the ear canal can become infected. Discharge and itch are the initial presenting symptoms, followed by pain and then reduction in hearing as the ear canal closes off. Infection can spread to the pinna, causing cellulitis. Although the causative organism is most commonly bacterial (pseudomonal species, followed by staphylococcal species), it can also be fungal. There may be swelling of the pre-auricular or post-auricular lymph nodes that can be mistaken for mastoiditis.

Examination often reveals debris in the canal, which needs to be removed either by gentle mopping or preferably by suction, viewed directly under a microscope. The tympanic membrane is normal, when visible. In severe cases, the canal may be swollen

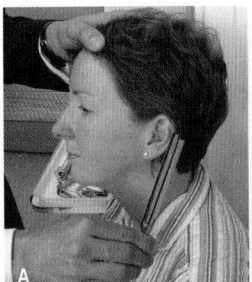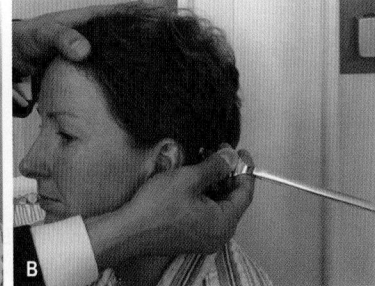

Fig. 27.4 Rinne test. Comparing conduction of sound. **(A)** Air conduction. **(B)** Bone conduction.

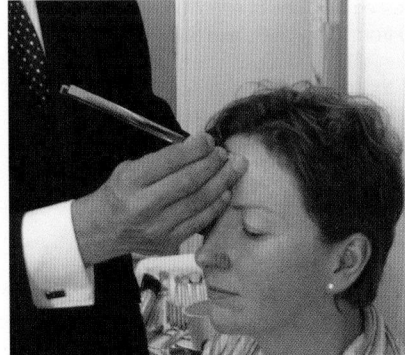

Fig. 27.5 Weber test.

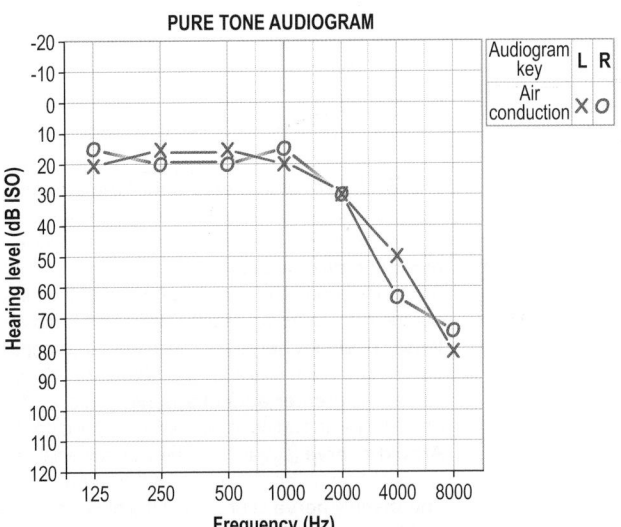

Fig. 27.6 Audiogram showing presbycusis (high-frequency loss).

and a view of the tympanic membrane impossible. Any foreign body seen should be removed with great care by trained personnel.

Treatment is with topical combination antibiotic and steroid drops in the first instance: for example dexamethasone 0.05%, framycetin sulfate 0.5% and gramicidin 0.005% drops, or hydrocortisone acetate 1% and gentamicin 0.3% drops, or a spray such as dexamethasone 0.1% with neomycin sulfate 3250 units. If symptoms do not resolve in 3–4 days, then microsuction in an ENT department is necessary.

Finafloxacin ear drops are used if there is a perforation, to reduce ototoxicity.

Otitis media

Otitis media is an infection of the middle ear seeded from the upper respiratory tract through the Eustachian tube. Therefore, the most commonly encountered pathogens are similar to those that cause upper respiratory tract infections: respiratory syncytial virus (RSV), *Streptococcus pneumoniae*, *Haemophilus influenzae* and *Moraxella catarrhalis*. Otitis media most commonly affects children under the age of 10. Infection causes inflammation of the middle ear mucosa and inflammatory exudate in the middle ear space. Due to the middle ear fluid, otitis media presents with otalgia and hearing disturbance. If it does not resolve, it can lead to tympanic membrane perforation and discharge. There are no mucous glands in the external ear canal. If the discharge is serous, then middle ear pathology is unlikely. Otitis media classically presents with otalgia followed by discharge, whereas otitis externa presents with discharge followed by otalgia. Rare complications of otitis media include mastoiditis

as the middle ear inflammatory fluid escapes from the middle ear into the mastoid, or meningitis as the infection spreads through the tegmen into the intracranial cavity. Examination shows a healthy ear canal with an erythematous and occasionally bulging tympanic membrane.

Treatment of the acute case is initially with non-steroidal anti-inflammatory drugs. Otitis media is often viral in origin – for example, following a cold – and will settle within 72 hours without antibacterial treatment. In people with systemic features or after 72 hours, a systemic antibiotic, such as amoxicillin, should be given, particularly in children under 2 years old. Topical therapy is of no value. If there is tenderness and swelling over the mastoid, then an urgent ENT opinion should be obtained.

Referred otalgia

Pain may be referred from:

- the teeth and temporomandibular joint from the auriculotemporal nerve (a branch of the mandibular (Vth cranial) nerve)
- cervical spinal problems from C1 to C3
- tonsil and tongue base problems from the glossopharyngeal (Jacobson's) nerve
- the larynx and pharynx from the vagus (Arnold's) nerve
- Ramsay Hunt syndrome, causing vesicles along the distribution of the VIIth cranial nerve.

The innervation of the pinna is from the auriculotemporal branch of the trigeminal and the first two cervical nerves (**Fig. 27.7**). Therefore, dental pain, temporomandibular joint dysfunction and upper

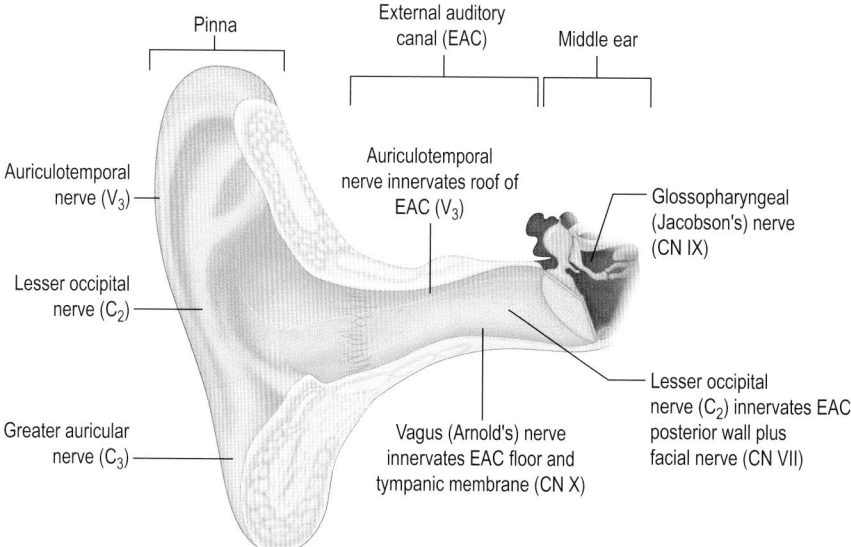

Fig. 27.7 Sensory innervation of the ear. Due to the sophisticated embryology of ear structures, the sensory innervation is complicated. Therefore otalgia can be referred from many sites, and knowledge of aural sensory innervation is a good guide for a comprehensive examination in idiopathic ear pain. The **auriculotemporal nerve** (a branch of the mandibular division of the trigeminal nerve) supplies innervation to the superolateral pinna and roof of the external auditory canal (EAC). Pathology related to the upper teeth, temporomandibular joint and parotid gland can cause referred otalgia through this nerve. The **lesser occipital nerve** (a branch from the second cervical nerve) supplies most of the medial surface of the pinna and the posterior wall of the EAC. Cervical osteoarthritis can cause referred otalgia through this nerve. The **greater auricular nerve** (a branch from the third cervical nerve) supplies the inferior portion of the pinna, including the lobule. Cervical osteoarthritis can cause referred otalgia through this nerve. **Arnold's nerve** (a branch of the vagus cranial nerve) supplies the EAC floor and lateral surface of the tympanic membrane. Tumours of the larynx and pharynx can cause referred otalgia through this nerve. **Jacobson's nerve** (a branch of the glossopharyngeal nerve) supplies innervation to the mucosa of the middle ear, including the medial surface of the tympanic membrane. Tonsillitis and pharyngitis can cause referred otalgia through this nerve. CN, cranial nerve.

cervical osteoarthritis can all present as otalgia. The ear canal is innervated by the above-mentioned nerves, and also by the facial and vagus nerves (see **Fig. 27.7**). Hence Ramsay Hunt syndrome (varicella reactivation along the sensory division of the facial nerve) causes otalgia with ear canal vesicles, whereas cancer of the larynx and pharynx can occasionally present as otalgia due to referred pain along the vagus nerve. The middle ear is innervated by the glossopharyngeal nerve and therefore infections of the pharynx are associated with otalgia.

The discharging ear (otorrhoea)

Discharge from the ear is usually due to infection of the outer or middle ear. The most common cause is otitis externa, followed by otitis media with a perforated tympanic membrane (see earlier).

Cholesteatoma

Although cholesteatoma is a rarer cause of the otorrhoea, it has severe implications if missed and should be considered in any non-resolving or recurrent case of otorrhoea. Cholesteatoma is defined as keratinizing squamous epithelium within the middle ear cleft and can present with foul-smelling otorrhoea. Examination shows a defect in the tympanic membrane full of white, cheesy material. Mastoid surgery is required to remove this sac of squamous debris, as it can erode local structures such as the ossicles or facial nerve, or even extend intracranially to cause meningitis or an intracranial abscess.

Hearing loss

Deafness can be conductive or sensorineural and these can be differentiated at the bedside by the Rinne and the Weber tests (**Box 27.2**) or with pure-tone audiometry. **Conductive hearing loss** has many causes (**Box 27.3**) but wax is the most common.

Perforated tympanic membrane

This arises from trauma or chronic middle ear disease when recurrent infection results in a permanent defect. Surgical repair is indicated only if the patient is symptomatic with recurrent discharge. The larger the perforation, the greater the impact on hearing.

Otitis media and otitis externa

As discussed above, both of these infections lead to hearing loss but the sequence of events will help differentiate the conditions: hearing loss is common and early in otitis media, but rare and late in otitis externa.

Secretory otitis media with effusion ('serous otitis media' or 'glue ear')

This is common in children because Eustachian tube dysfunction may lead to poorly ventilated middle ears. The vacuum created by poor ventilation leads to a non-inflammatory effusion. The effusion resolves naturally in the majority of cases but can persist or recur, causing a hearing loss that impacts on speech and language skills and on educational progress. The presenting complaint is hearing loss or speech delay but little association with otalgia.

Examination shows a dull tympanic membrane with loss of light reflex (**Fig. 27.8**) and occasionally fluid with air bubbles visible in the middle ear. Children with glue ear frequently have adenoidal hypertrophy and nasal blockage.

Management involves insertion of a grommet (tympanostomy tube) into the tympanic membrane, which ventilates the middle ear cavity, if the symptoms are persistent and troublesome. Antibiotic–glucocorticoid ear drops are more effective than oral antibiotics. Adenoidectomy can be added to the procedure if there is a strong history of complete nasal blockage or recurrent upper respiratory tract infections. Grommets are extruded from the tympanic membrane as it heals (over 6 months to 2 years). Developmental outcomes are not improved by grommet insertions. In most children,

---

? **Box 27.3 Causes of deafness**

Conductive	**Sensorineural**
External meatus	*Congenital*
• Wax	• Pendred's syndrome (see p. 1202)
• Foreign body	• Long QT syndrome
• Otitis externa	• Björnstad's syndrome (pili torti)
• Chronic suppuration	
	End-organ
Drum	• Advancing age
• Perforation/trauma	• Occupational acoustic trauma
	• Ménière's disease
Middle ear	• Drugs (e.g. gentamicin, furosemide)
• Otosclerosis	
• Ossicular bone problems	*VIIIth nerve lesions*
• Suppuration (otitis media)	• Acoustic neuroma
	• Cranial trauma
	• Inflammatory lesions:
	– Tuberculous meningitis
	– Sarcoidosis
	– Neurosyphilis
	– Carcinomatous meningitis
	Brainstem lesions (rare)
	• Multiple sclerosis
	• Infarction

---

i **Box 27.2 Testing hearing loss**

Type	Defect	Rinne test	Weber test
Conductive	Outer or middle ear	Negative	Sound heard louder on the affected side
Sensorineural	Inner ear or more centrally	Positive	Sound heard louder in the normal ear

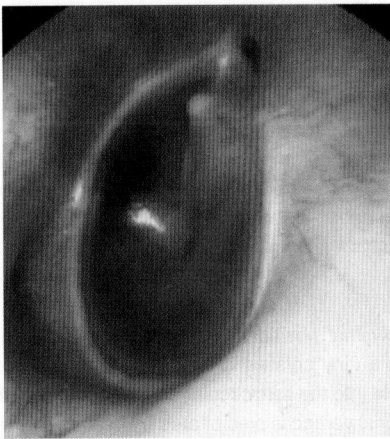

Fig. 27.8 Secretory otitis media (glue ear). Auroscopic view of the tympanic membrane, which is dull with loss of light reflex.

the middle third of the face grows around the age of 7–14 years and Eustachian tube dysfunction is rare after this.

Otosclerosis

This is usually a hereditary disorder, in which new bony deposits occur within the stapes footplate and the cochlea. Characteristically seen in the second and third decades, it is more common in females and can become worse during pregnancy. The hearing loss may be mixed, and management includes a hearing aid or replacement of the fixed stapes with a prosthesis (stapedectomy). The choice of treatment is dependent on the patient. Surgery is an excellent option, with very good success rates in the hands of a regular stapedectomist, but it always carries a small risk of complete hearing loss. Hearing aids, while safe, require the patient's compliance if they are to afford benefit.

Presbycusis

This is the most common cause of deafness. It is a degenerative disorder of the cochlea and is typically seen in old age. It can be due to the loss of outer hair cells (sensory), loss of the ganglion cells (neural) or strial atrophy (metabolic), or there can be a mixed picture. Ageing itself does not cause outer hair cell loss but environmental noise toxicity over the years is a major factor. The onset is gradual and the higher frequencies are affected most (see **Fig. 27.6**). Speech has two components: low frequencies (vowels) and high frequencies (consonants). When the consonants are lost, speech loses its intelligibility. Increasing the volume merely increases the low frequencies and the characteristic response of 'Don't shout. I'm not deaf!'

A high-frequency-specific hearing aid will do much to ease the frustrations of both the patients and their close contacts.

Noise trauma

Cochlear damage can occur, for example, from shooting without ear protectors or from industrial noise and characteristically has a loss at 4 kHz.

Acoustic neuroma

This is a slow-growing benign schwannoma of the vestibular nerve (see p. 875), which can present with progressive sensorineural hearing loss. Any patient with an asymmetric sensorineural hearing loss or sudden sensorineural hearing loss should be investigated: for example, with a magnetic resonance imaging (MRI) scan.

Dizziness/vertigo

Vertigo is usually rotatory when it arises from the ear. The presence of otalgia, otorrhoea, tinnitus or hearing loss suggests an otologic aetiology. Vestibular causes can be classified according to the duration of the vertigo. Common causes are summarized as follows:
- seconds (<1 min) – benign paroxysmal positional vertigo
- minutes to hours – Ménière's disease
- hours to days – labyrinthine or central pathology.

Benign paroxysmal positional vertigo

Benign paroxysmal positional vertigo (BPPV) is thought to occur when otoconia (tiny crystals of calcium carbonate) are dislodged from the utricle into the semicircular canals, commonly the posterior canal. Positional vertigo is precipitated by head movements, usually to a particular position, and often occurs when turning in bed or on sitting up. The onset is typically sudden and distressing. The vertigo

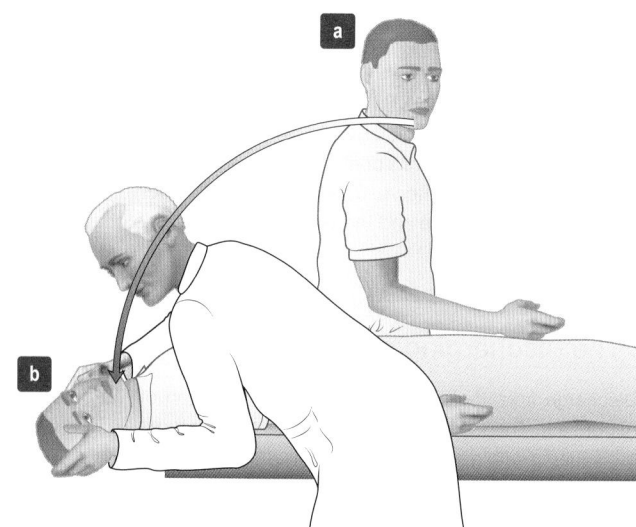

Fig. 27.9 Hallpike manoeuvre for diagnosis of benign paroxysmal positional vertigo. This can be done in the outpatient department. **(a)** The patient sits on a couch, their head turned towards one ear. **(b)** The head is supported by the examiner while the patient lies down so that their head is just below the horizontal. Nystagmus (following a latent interval of a few seconds) is commonly noted when the head has been turned towards the affected ear. This can be repeated with the patient's head turned towards the other ear.

lasts seconds (<1 min) and the phenomenon becomes less severe on repeated movements (fatigue). There is no serious underlying cause but it sometimes follows vestibular neuronitis (see p. 817), head injury or ear infection. It occurs in 50% of older people and is the most common cause of head injury in those under 50 years of age.

Diagnosis

Diagnosis is made on the basis of the history and by the *Hallpike manoeuvre* (**Fig. 27.9**). A positive Hallpike test confirms BPPV, which can be cured in over 90% of cases by the Epley manoeuvre. This involves gentle but specific manipulation and rotation of the patient's head to shift the loose otoliths from the semicircular canals.

The differential diagnosis includes a cerebellar mass, but in that case positional nystagmus (and vertigo) is immediately apparent (no latent interval) and does not fatigue.

Ménière's disease

This is a rare condition characterized by recurring, episodic, rotatory vertigo lasting 30 minutes to a few hours; attacks are recurrent over months or years. Classically, it is associated with a low-frequency sensorineural hearing loss, a feeling of fullness in the affected ear, loss of balance, tinnitus and vomiting. There is a build-up of endolymphatic fluid in the inner ear, although its precise aetiology is still unclear.

Management

Vestibular sedatives, such as cinnarizine, are used in the acute phase. Preventative measures, such as a low-salt diet, betahistine and avoidance of caffeine, are useful. If the disease cannot be controlled, then a chemical labyrinthectomy, perfusing the round window orifice with ototoxic drugs such as gentamicin, is used. Gentamicin destroys the vestibular epithelium; therefore, the patient has severe vertigo for around 2 weeks until the body compensates for the lack of vestibular input on that side. The patient will happily trade occasional mild vertigo when the balance system is challenged against the unpredictable, severe and disabling attacks of vertigo involved in Ménière's disease. There is a risk of sensorineural hearing loss and complete vestibular failure if Ménière's starts in the previously unaffected side. The final option is surgical decompression of the endolymphatic compartment of the inner ear to relieve the endolymphatic hydrops.

Labyrinthine or central causes of vertigo

(See **Box 26.15**.) These are managed with vestibular sedatives in the acute phase. Most patients will settle over a few days but continuous true vertigo with nystagmus suggests a central lesion. A patient with a deficit of vestibular function due to viral labyrinthitis or neuronitis should be able to cease vestibular sedatives within 2 weeks; long-term use can give parkinsonian side-effects, delay central compensation and thus prolong the vertigo. Vestibular rehabilitation by a physiotherapist or audiological scientist can speed up the compensation process, although most patients will be able to do this themselves with time.

Tinnitus

This is a sensation of a sound when there is no auditory stimulus. It can occur without hearing loss and results from heightened awareness of neural activity in the auditory pathways. Patients describe a hissing or ringing in their ears and this can cause much distress. It usually does not have a serious cause but vascular malformation, such as aneurysms, or vascular tumours can be associated. In these cases, the tinnitus is pulsatile and most commonly unilateral.

Management

This is difficult. A tinnitus masker (a mechanically produced, continuous soft sound) can help. Cognitive behavioural therapy through audiological services are of use and rehabilitate patients well.

Further reading

Kim J, Zee DS. Benign paroxysmal positional vertigo. *N Engl J Med* 2014; 370:1138–1147.
Kral A. Profound deafness in children. *N Engl J Med* 2010; 363:1438–1450.
Schreiber BE, Agrup C, Haskard DO et al. Sudden sensorineural hearing loss. *Lancet* 2010; 375:1203–1211.

DISORDERS OF THE NOSE

ANATOMY AND PHYSIOLOGY

(See **Fig. 27.10**.) The function of the nose is to facilitate smell and respiration:

- Smell is a sensation conveyed by the olfactory epithelium in the roof of the nose. The olfactory epithelium is supplied by the Ist cranial nerve (see p. 809).
- The nose also filters, moistens and warms inspired air and, in doing so, assists the normal process of respiration.

The external portion of the nose consists of two nasal bones attached to the rest of the facial skeleton and to the upper and lower lateral cartilages. The internal nose is divided by a midline septum that comprises both cartilage and bone. This divides the internal nose in two, from the external nostril to the posterior choanae. The posterior choanae are in continuity with the nasopharynx posteriorly.

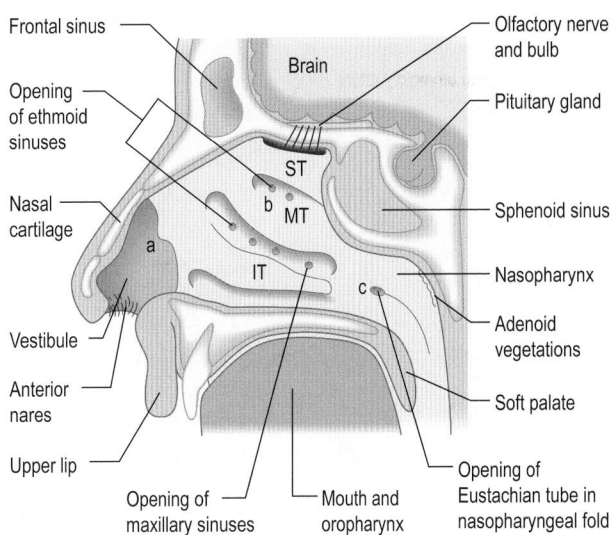

Fig. 27.10 The anatomy of the nose in longitudinal section. IT, inferior turbinate; MT, middle turbinate; ST, superior turbinate; a, internal ostium; b, respiratory region; c, choanae.

The paranasal sinuses open into the lateral wall of the nose and form a system of aerated chambers within the facial skeleton.

The blood supply of the nose is derived from branches of both the internal and external carotid arteries. The internal carotid artery supplies the upper nose via the anterior and posterior ethmoidal arteries. The external carotid artery supplies the posterior and inferior portion of the nose via the superior labial artery, greater palatine artery and sphenopalatine artery. On the anterior nasal septum there is an area of confluence of these vessels (Little's area; **Fig. 27.11A**).

CLINICAL APPROACH TO THE PATIENT WITH A DISORDER OF THE NOSE

Examination

The anterior part of the nose can be examined using a nasal speculum and light source. Endoscopes are required to examine the nasal cavity and postnasal space.

COMMON DISORDERS OF THE NOSE

Epistaxis

Nose bleeds vary in severity from minor to life-threatening. Little's area (see **Fig. 27.11A**) is a frequent site of nasal haemorrhage. First aid measures should be administered immediately, including external digital compression of the anterior lower portion of the external nose, ice packs and leaning forward. The patient should be asked to avoid swallowing any blood running posteriorly, as this causes nausea.

Not infrequently, small, recurrent epistaxes occur and these may require a visit to the emergency department for an examination and simple local anaesthetic cautery with a silver nitrate stick. If the bleeding continues profusely, then resuscitation in the form of intravenous access, fluid replacement or blood, and oxygen can be administered. If further intervention is necessary, consideration should be given to intranasal cautery of the bleeding vessel, or

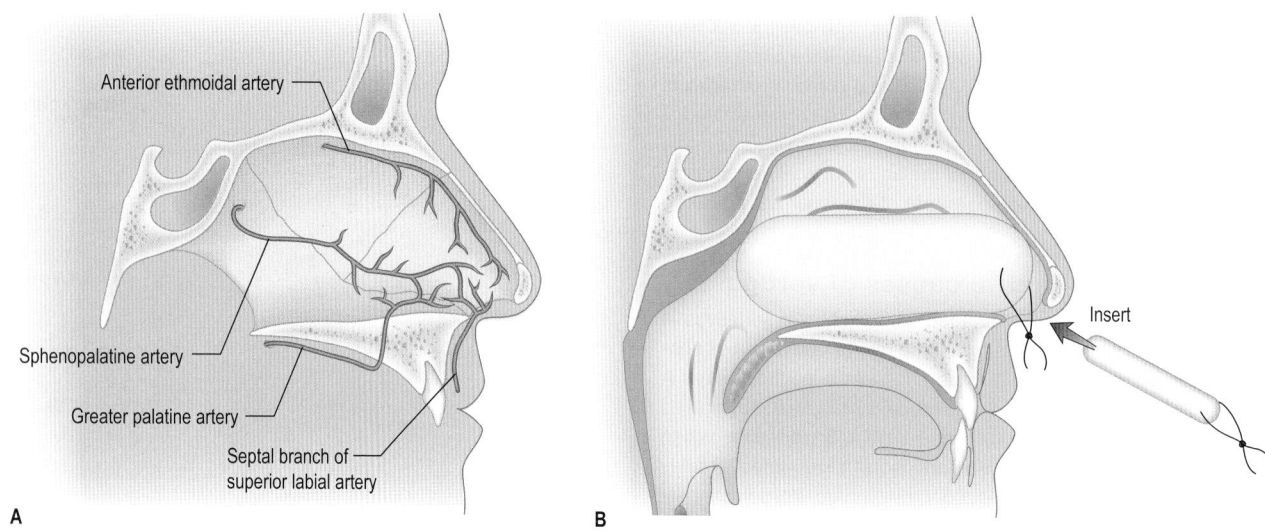

Fig. 27.11 Little's area and nasal packing. (A) Blood supply of Little's area on the septum of the nose. **(B)** Nasal pack.

intranasal packing using a variety of commercially available nasal packs (see **Fig. 27.11B**). In addition to direct treatment of the epistaxis, a cause should be sought and treated appropriately (**Box 27.4**). If the above treatments fail, surgical ligation of the sphenopalatine artery can be undertaken endoscopically or an interventional arterial embolization can be performed for the problematic vessel.

Rhinitis

See page 945.

Nasal obstruction

Nasal obstruction is a symptom and not a diagnosis. It can significantly affect a patient's quality of life. Causes include:
- **Rhinitis** (see p. 945). The most common aetiology is allergy-based. Rhinitis results in erythema of the nasal mucosa and hypertrophy of inferior turbinates. If an allergen is identified, then allergen avoidance is the mainstay of treatment. Topical steroids and/or antihistamines can be tried. If rhinitis is severe, then referral to an allergy clinic for immunotherapy is warranted. Short-term benefit can be gained in severe nasal blockage by surgically reducing the inferior turbinate.
- **Septal deviation.** Correction can be undertaken surgically.
- **Nasal polyps.** This condition occurs with inflammation and oedema of the sinus nasal mucosa. This oedematous mucosa prolapses into the nasal cavity and can cause significant nasal obstruction. In allergic rhinitis (see p. 945), the mucosa lining the nasal septum and inferior turbinates are swollen and a dark-red

or plum colour. Nasal polyps can be identified as glistening swellings, which are insensate. Treatment with intranasal steroids helps, but if polyps are large or unresponsive to medical treatment, then surgery is necessary.
- **Foreign bodies.** These are usually seen in children who present with unilateral nasal discharge. Clinical examination of the nose with a light source often reveals the foreign body, which requires removal, either in clinic or in theatre, with a general anaesthetic.
- **Sinonasal malignancy.** This is extremely rare. The diagnosis must be considered if unusual unilateral symptoms are seen, including nasal obstruction, epistaxis, pain, epiphora (watery eye), cheek swelling, paraesthesia of the cheek, unilateral serous otitis media and proptosis of the orbit.

Sinusitis

Sinusitis is an infection of the paranasal sinuses that is bacterial (mainly *Streptococcus pneumoniae* and *Haemophilus influenzae*) or occasionally fungal. It is most commonly associated with an upper respiratory tract infection and can occur with asthma. Symptoms include frontal headache, purulent rhinorrhoea, facial pain with tenderness, and fever. Sinusitis can be confused with a variety of other conditions, such as migraine, trigeminal neuralgia and cranial arteritis.

Management

Treatment for a bacterial sinusitis includes nasal decongestants, such as xylometazoline; broad-spectrum antibiotics, such as co-amoxiclav because *H. influenzae* can be resistant to amoxicillin; anti-inflammatory therapy with topical corticosteroids, such as fluticasone propionate (nasal spray) to reduce mucosal swelling; and steam inhalations.

If the symptoms of sinusitis are recurrent (**Box 27.5**) or complications such as orbital cellulitis arise, then an ENT opinion is appropriate and a computed tomography (CT) scan of the paranasal sinuses is undertaken. Plain sinus X-rays are now rarely used to image the sinuses.

CT scan of the sinuses (**Fig. 27.12**) or an MRI scan can demonstrate bony landmarks and soft tissue planes.

Functional endoscopic sinus surgery (FESS) is used for ventilation and drainage of the sinuses.

Box 27.5 Types of sinusitis

Type	Duration of symptoms
Acute	1 week to 1 month
Recurrent acute	>4 episodes of acute sinusitis per year
Subacute	1–3 months
Chronic	>3 months

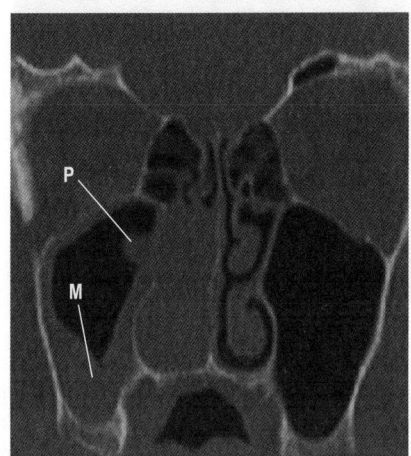

Fig. 27.12 CT of the sinuses. An inverting papilloma (P) can be seen obstructing the right nostril, and there is mucosal thickening (M) of the right maxillary sinus.

Anosmia

Olfaction is mainly under the control of cranial nerve I, although irritant, unpleasant nasal sensations are carried by cranial nerves V, IX and X. Anosmia is a complete loss of the sense of smell and *hyposmia* is a decreased sense of smell:

- A *conductive deficit* of smell occurs if odorant molecules do not reach the olfactory epithelium high in the nose.
- A *sensorineural loss* of smell is incurred if the neural transmission of smell is affected.
- Some conditions predispose to a mixed (conductive and sensorineural) loss of smell.

The main cause of a loss of smell is nasal obstruction due to upper respiratory infection or nasal polyps. Other causes include sinonasal disease, old age, drug therapy and head injury/trauma. It is difficult to predict the speed and extent of recovery in the latter causes. In many, anosmia is idiopathic, but before this diagnosis is accepted, an assessment of the patient for the possibility of an intranasal tumour or intracranial mass should be undertaken.

Fractured nose

People with a fractured nose present with epistaxis, bruising of the eyes and nasal bridge swelling. Initially, it is often difficult to assess whether the bones are deviated, particularly if there is significant swelling. Reduction of the fracture should be undertaken in the first 2 weeks after injury and can be achieved by manipulation. However, if the fracture sets, a more formal rhinoplasty may have to be undertaken at a later stage. The patient should be examined for a head injury and the nose should also be checked for a septal haematoma (**Fig. 27.13**). This is painful, can cause nasal obstruction, is fluctuant to touch on the nasal septum, and requires immediate drainage to prevent destruction of the septal cartilage.

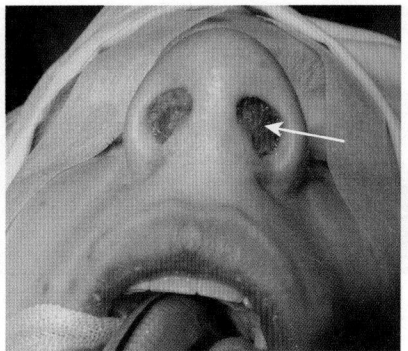

Fig. 27.13 Septal haematoma.

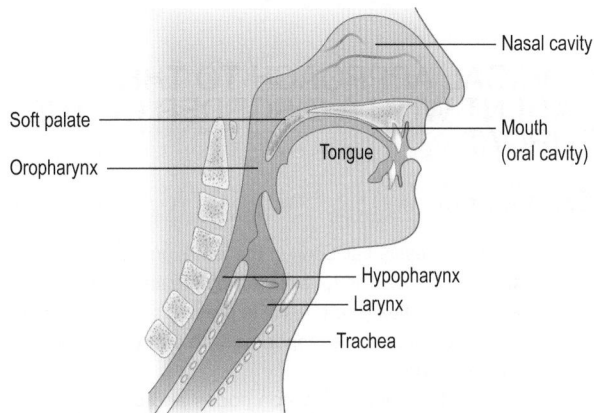

Fig. 27.14 Normal anatomy of the throat.

DISORDERS OF THE THROAT

ANATOMY AND PHYSIOLOGY

The throat can be considered as the oral cavity, the pharynx and the larynx (**Fig. 27.14**). The oral cavity extends from the lips to the tonsils. The pharynx can be divided into three areas:

- *the nasopharynx* extends from the posterior nasal openings to the soft palate
- *the oropharynx* extends from the soft palate to the tip of the epiglottis
- *the hypopharynx* extends from the tip of the epiglottis to just below the level of the cricoid cartilage, where it is continuous with the oesophagus.

Lying within the hypopharynx is the larynx. This consists of cartilaginous, ligamentous and muscular tissue that has the primary function of protecting the distal airway. The pharynx is innervated from the pharyngeal plexus.

In the larynx, there are two vocal cords that abduct (open) during inspiration and adduct (close) to protect the airway and for voice production (phonation). The main nerve supply of the vocal cords comes from the recurrent laryngeal nerves (branches of the vagus nerve), which arise in the neck, but on the left side pass down around the aortic arch and then ascend in the tracheo-oesophageal groove to the larynx.

Normal vocal cords in phonation vibrate between 90 (male) and 180 (female) times per second, giving the voice its pitch or frequency. A healthy voice requires full closure of the vocal cords with a smooth, regular pattern of vibration, and any pathology that

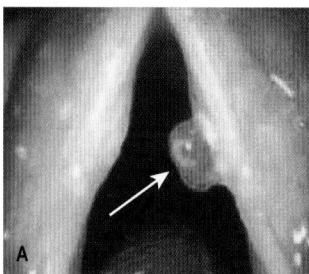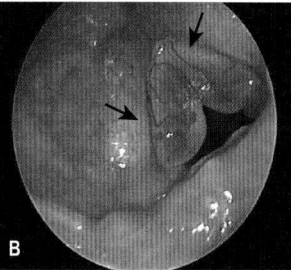

Fig. 27.15 **Disorders of the vocal cords.** **(A)** Vocal cord polyp. **(B)** Reinke's oedema of the vocal cords.

prevents full closure will result in air escaping between the vocal cords during phonation and a 'breathy' voice.

CLINICAL APPROACH TO THE PATIENT WITH A DISORDER OF THE THROAT

Examination

Good illumination is essential. Look at the teeth, gums, tongue, floor of mouth and oral cavity. The tonsils, soft palate and uvula are easily seen, and a gag reflex (see p. 817) is present. The remainder of the pharynx and larynx can be inspected with a laryngeal mirror or flexible nasendoscope.

Examination of the neck for lymph nodes and other masses is also performed.

COMMON DISORDERS OF THE THROAT

Hoarseness (dysphonia)

There are three essential components for voice production: an air source (the lungs); a vibratory source (the vocal cords); and a resonating chamber (the pharynx and nasal and oral cavities). Although chest and nasal disorders can affect the voice, the majority of hoarseness is due to laryngeal pathology.

Inflammation that increases the 'mass' of the vocal cords will cause the vocal cord frequency to fall, giving a much deeper voice. Thus listening to a patient's voice can often give a diagnosis before the vocal cords are examined.

Nodules

Nodules (always bilateral and more common in females) and polyps (**Fig. 27.15A**) are found on the free edge of the vocal cord, preventing full closure and giving a 'breathy, harsh' voice. They are commonly found in professionals who rely on their voice for their livelihood, such as teachers, singers and lawyers. They are usually related to poor technique of voice production and can usually be cured with speech therapy. If surgery is needed, great care must be taken to remain in the superficial layers of the vocal cord in order to prevent deep scarring, which leaves the voice permanently hoarse.

Reinke's oedema

This is due to a collection of tissue fluid in the subepithelial layer of the vocal cord (see **Fig. 27.15B**). The vocal cord has poor lymphatic drainage, predisposing it to oedema. Reinke's oedema is associated with irritation of the vocal cords by smoking, voice abuse, acid

+ **Box 27.6 Red flags for hoarseness requiring urgent laryngoscopy**

- Heavy smoking
- High alcohol intake
- Haemoptysis
- Dysphagia
- Pain, including otalgia
- Increasing dyspnoea

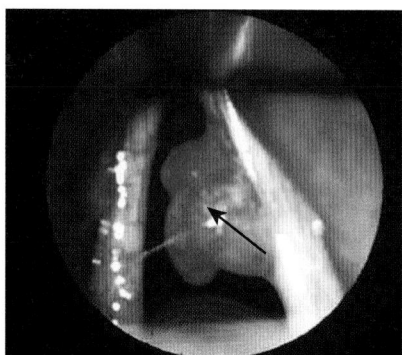

Fig. 27.16 Carcinoma of the right cord.

reflux and, very rarely, hypothyroidism. Treatment is to remove the irritation in most cases, but surgery to incise the cords and reduce the oedema will also allow the voice to return to its normal pitch.

Acute-onset hoarseness

Hoarseness, in a smoker, is a danger sign. Any patient with a hoarse voice for over 6 weeks should be seen by an ENT surgeon. Other red flag symptoms will require urgent laryngoscopy (**Box 27.6**). The voice may be deep, harsh and breathy, indicating a mass on the vocal cord (**Fig. 27.16**), or it can be weak, suggesting a paralysed left vocal cord secondary to mediastinal disease, such as bronchial carcinoma.

Early squamous cell carcinoma of the larynx has a good prognosis. Treatment is with carbon dioxide laser resection or radiotherapy. Spread and growth of the tumour can lead to referred otalgia, and, if the tumour is significant in its size, requires a laryngectomy (removal of the voicebox), with a neck dissection to remove the affected glands in the neck. A patient with a paralysed left vocal cord must have a CT of the neck and chest. Medialization of the paralysed cord to allow contact with the opposite cord can return the voice and give a competent larynx. This can be done under local or general anaesthesia, producing an immediate result whatever the long-term prognosis of the chest pathology.

Stridor

Stridor, or noisy breathing, can be divided into the following types:
- *Inspiratory*: obstruction is at the level of the vocal cords or above.
- *Mixed* (both inspiratory and expiratory): obstruction is in the subglottis or extrathoracic trachea.
- *Expiratory*: obstruction is in the intrathoracic trachea or distal airways.

All people with stridor, both paediatric and adult, are potentially at risk of asphyxiation and should be investigated fully. Severe stridor may be an indication for either intubation or a tracheostomy (**Box 27.7**).

Management
Tracheostomy

Tracheostomy tubes (**Fig. 27.17**) are:
- *Cuffed or uncuffed.* A high-volume, low-pressure cuff is used to prevent aspiration and to allow positive-pressure ventilation.

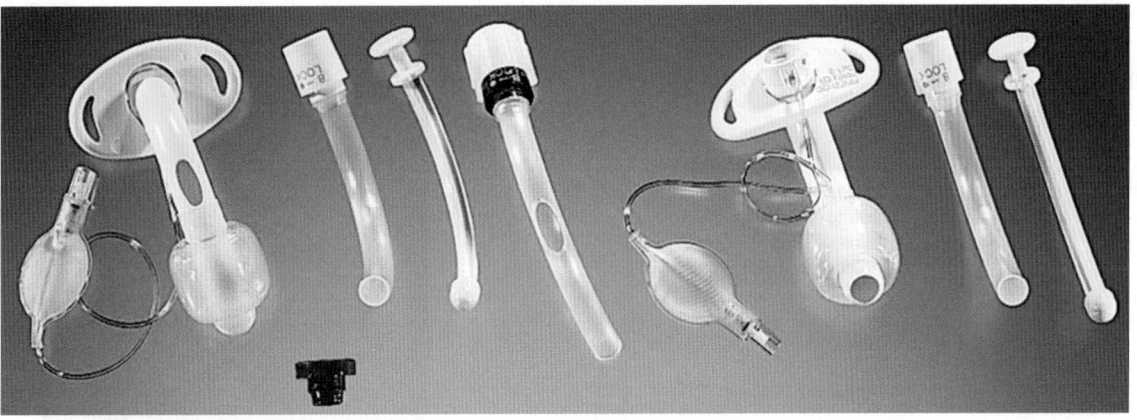

Fig. 27.17 Tracheostomy tubes and their accompanying components.

---

i **Box 27.7** Indications for tracheostomy

- Upper airway obstruction (real or anticipated)
- Long-term ventilation
- Bronchial lavage
- Incompetent larynx with aspiration

i **Box 27.8** Indications for tonsillectomy

- Suspected malignancy
- Obstructive sleep apnoea due to tonsillar hypertrophy
- Recurrent tonsillitis: five attacks a year for at least 2 years
- Quinsy in a patient with a history of recurrent tonsillitis

---

- ***Fenestrated or unfenestrated.*** A fenestrated cuff has a small hole on the greater curvature of the tube (both outer and inner), allowing air to escape upwards to the vocal cords; the patient can therefore speak. This tube often has a valve that allows air to enter from the stoma but closes on expiration, directing the air through the fenestration.

Most long-term tracheostomy tubes have an inner and an outer tube. The inner tube fits inside the outer tube and projects beyond its lower end. A major problem with a tracheostomy tube is crusting of its distal end with dried secretions, and this arrangement allows the inner tube to be removed, cleaned and replaced as frequently as required, without disrupting the outer tube.

When to decannulate a patient is often a difficult issue if laryngeal competence is unclear. Movement of the vocal cords requires an ENT examination and a speech therapist's involvement. The tracheostomy tube itself can also produce problems due to compression of the oesophagus with a cuffed tube and prevention of the larynx from rising during normal swallowing.

Tonsillitis and pharyngitis

Viral infections of the throat are common and, although many practitioners may be under pressure from the patient to give antibiotics, they should not be used. The vast majority of infections are self-limiting, settling with rest, analgesia and encouragement of fluid intake. Fungal infections, usually candidiasis, are uncommon and may indicate an immunocompromised patient or undiagnosed diabetes.

Tonsillitis

Tonsillitis, with a good history of pyrexia, dysphagia, lymphadenopathy and severe malaise, is usually bacterial; β-haemolytic streptococcus is the most common organism, which responds to penicillin V.

Glandular fever

Glandular fever (see p. 524) can also present with tonsillitis. Although, clinically, the tonsils have a confluent white exudate, there is often a petechial rash on the soft palate and an accompanying lymphadenopathy.

Quinsy (peritonsillar abscess)

Quinsy is a collection of pus outside the capsule of the tonsil, usually located adjacent to its superior pole. The patient often has trismus, making examination difficult, but the pus pushes the uvula across the midline to the opposite side. The area is usually hyperaemic and smooth but unilateral tonsil ulceration is more likely to be a malignancy. In either case, urgent referral to an ENT specialist is essential.

Indications for a ***tonsillectomy*** are shown in **Box 27.8**. This is carried out under a general anaesthetic and current surgical techniques include diathermy dissection, laser excision and coblation (using an ultrasonic dissecting probe). There are strong advocates for each technique and much will depend on the individual surgeon's preference. Some departments carry out tonsillectomy as a day-case procedure, as most reactionary bleeding will occur within the first 8 hours postoperatively.

Snoring

Snoring is caused by high-pressure airflow, resulting in vibration of soft tissue above the level of the larynx. It is a common symptom (50% of 50-year-old males will snore to some extent) and can be considered to be related to obstruction of three potential areas: the nose, the palate or/and the hypopharynx (see **Fig. 28.27**). There is a strong association between snoring and sleep-disordered breathing, such as in obstructive sleep apnoea (see p. 960).

The Epworth questionnaire (see **Box 28.29**) can assist in identification of sleep apnoea. People with a history of habitual, non-positional, heroic snoring (can be heard through a wall) require a full ENT examination and can be investigated by sleep nasendoscopy, in which a sedated, snoring patient has a flexible nasendoscope inserted to identify the source of vibration.

Nasal pathology, such as polyps, can be removed surgically with good results and most patients will benefit from lifestyle changes, such as weight loss. Stiffening or shortening the soft palate via surgery, often using a laser, can help for palatal snorers but hypopharyngeal snorers require either a dental prosthesis at night to hold the mandible forwards or continuous positive airway pressure (CPAP) via a mask (see p. 962).

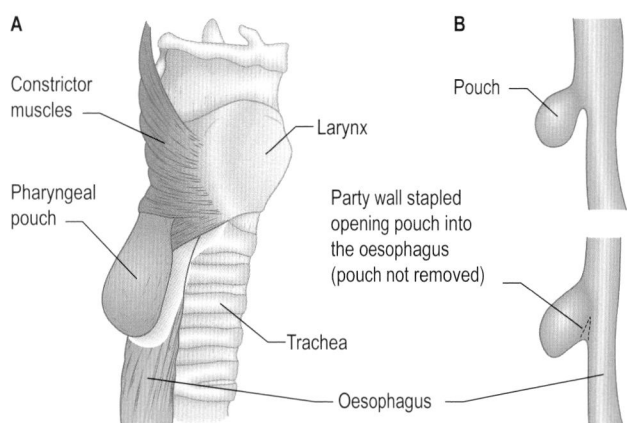

Fig. 27.18 Pharyngeal pouch. (A) Position of pharyngeal pouch. **(B)** Stapling of the party wall between oesophagus and pouch.

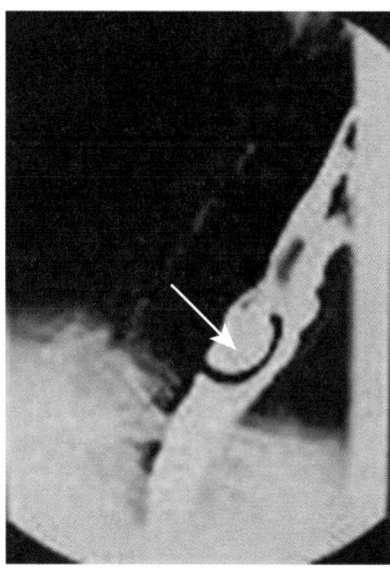

Fig. 27.19 Pharyngeal pouch shown on barium swallow.

Dysphagia

Dysphagia occurs because of any lesion between the throat and stomach. The two conditions described here are the ones usually dealt with by ENT departments. Gastroenterology departments see causes further down the gullet.

Pharyngeal pouch

A pharyngeal pouch is a herniation of mucosa through the fibres of the inferior pharyngeal constrictor muscle (cricopharyngeus) (**Fig. 27.18A**). An area of weakness known as Killian's dehiscence allows a pulsion diverticulum to form. Patients present with a neck swelling following a failed swallow attempt. They can occasionally compress the swelling to allow food particles to be pushed back into the oesophagus. They may also complain that a gurgling sound is heard in the neck following a swallow as liquid and food collect in the pouch. Occasionally, patients present with recurrent pneumonia following aspiration of food into the trachea. Diagnosis is made with a barium swallow (**Fig. 27.19**) and treatment is surgical, either via an external approach through the neck where the pouch is excised or, more commonly, via endoscopy with stapling of the party wall (see **Fig. 27.18B**).

Foreign bodies

Foreign bodies in the pharynx can be divided into three general categories: soft food bolus, coins (smooth) and bones (sharp). Soft food bolus can be initially treated conservatively with muscle relaxants for 24 hours. Impacted coins should be removed at the earliest opportunity but sharp objects require emergency removal to avoid perforation of the muscle wall.

If the patient perceives the foreign body to be to one side, then it should be above the cricopharyngeus and an ENT examination will locate it; common areas are the tonsillar fossae, base of tongue, posterior pharyngeal wall and valleculae. Radiology will identify coins, and a clinical decision can be made to see whether a coin will pass down to the stomach; in this case no further treatment is required as it will exit naturally. Some departments advocate the use of a metal detector to monitor the position of the coin in the patient, who is usually a child or has a mental disorder. Fish can be divided into those with a bony skeleton (teleosts) and those with a cartilaginous skeleton (elasmobranchs), and therefore radiology is useful only in some cases. Radiology can also identify air in the cervical oesophagus, indicating a radiolucent foreign body lying distally. A soft tissue lateral neck radiograph is the investigation of choice to delineate some of the features above.

Globus pharyngeus

This is a functional disorder and is not a true dysphagia. It is a condition with classic symptoms of an intermittent sensation of a lump in the throat. This is perceived to be in the midline at the level of the cricoid cartilage and is worse when swallowing saliva; indeed, it often disappears when ingesting food or liquids. ENT examination is clear and normal laryngeal mobility can be felt when gently rocking the larynx across the postcricoid tissues. A contrast swallow will not only show the structures below the pharynx but also assess the swallowing dynamically. Treatment is with explanation and reassurance. Antidepressants may be tried. Any suspicious area will require an endoscopy with biopsy.

Further reading

Dhillon RS, East CA. *Ear, Nose and Throat and Head and Neck Surgery*, 4th edn. Edinburgh: Churchill Livingstone; 2013.
Warner G, Burgess A, Patel S et al. *Otolaryngology and Head and Neck Surgery*. Oxford: Oxford University Press; 2009.
http://www.britishsnoring.co.uk *Interactive version of the Epworth Sleepiness Scale.*

DISORDERS OF THE EYE

Most of the major and common types of eye disease are covered below. However, diabetic eye disease (p. 726) and hypertensive eye disease (p. 1138) are discussed elsewhere.

APPLIED ANATOMY AND PHYSIOLOGY

The average length of the human eye is 24 mm. It is essentially made up of two segments:
- The smaller anterior segment is transparent and coated by the cornea; its radius is approximately 8 mm.
- The larger posterior segment is coated by the opaque sclera; its radius is approximately 12 mm.

It is the cornea and the sclera that give the mechanical strength and shape to the exposed surface of the eye.

The cornea occupies the central aspect of the globe and is one of the most richly innervated tissues in the body. This clear, transparent, avascular structure, measuring 12 mm horizontally and 11 mm vertically, provides 78% of the focusing power of the eye. The eyelids prevent the cornea from drying and becoming an irregular surface by distributing the tear film over the surface of the globe with each blink.

Anatomically, the cornea is made up of five layers:

- epithelium
- Bowman's layer (membrane)
- stroma
- Descemet's membrane
- endothelium.

The endothelial cells lining the inner surface of the cornea are responsible for maintaining the clarity of the cornea by continuously pumping fluid out of the tissue. Any factor that alters the function of these cells will result in corneal oedema and cause blurred vision.

The sclera is an opaque white structure covering four-fifths of the globe and is continuous with the cornea at the limbus. The six extraocular muscles responsible for eye movements are attached to the sclera, and the optic nerve perforates it posteriorly.

The conjunctiva covers the anterior surface of the sclera. This richly vascularized and innervated mucous membrane stretches from the limbus over the anterior sclera (where it is called the bulbar conjunctiva) and is then reflected on to the undersurface of the upper and lower lids (the tarsal conjunctiva). The area of conjunctival reflection under the lids makes up the upper and lower fornix.

The anterior chamber is the space between the cornea and the iris, and is filled with aqueous humour (**Fig. 27.20**). This fluid is produced by the ciliary body (2 µL/min) and provides nutrients and oxygen to the avascular cornea. The outflow of aqueous humour is through the trabecular meshwork and canal of Schlemm adjacent to the limbus. Any factor that impedes its outflow will increase the intraocular pressure. The upper range of normal for intraocular pressure is 21 mmHg.

The uveal tract is made up of the iris anteriorly, the ciliary body and the choroid. The **iris** is the coloured part of the eye under the transparent cornea. The muscles of the iris diaphragm regulate the size of the pupil, thereby controlling the amount of light entering the eye. The muscles of the **ciliary body** control the accommodation of the lens, and the secretory epithelium produces the aqueous humour (see above). The highly vascular **choroid** lines the inner aspect of the sclera and upon this lies the retina.

The lens lies immediately posterior to the pupil and anterior to the vitreous humour. It is a transparent biconvex structure and is responsible for 22% of the refractive power of the eye. By changing its shape, it can alter its refractive power and help to focus objects at different distances from the eye. By the fourth decade of life, this ability to change shape starts to decline and, with time, the lens starts to become less transparent and cataracts begin to develop.

The vitreous humour fills the cavity between the retina and the lens.

The retina is a multilayered structure. The metabolically active region of the retina is represented in **Fig. 27.21**. There are two types of photoreceptors in the retina: rods and cones. There are approximately 6 million cones, mainly confined to the **macula**, and these are responsible for detailed central vision and colour vision. The peripheral retina has around 125 million rods that are responsible for peripheral vision. The axons of the ganglion cells form the optic nerve (or disc) of the eye (**Fig. 27.22**).

The blood supply to the eye is via the ophthalmic artery; in particular, the central retinal artery is responsible for supplying the inner retinal layers. Venous return is through the central retinal and ophthalmic veins. Local lymphatic drainage is to the pre-auricular and submental nodes.

The sensory innervation of the eye is through the trigeminal (Vth) nerve. The six extraocular muscles are supplied by different nerves (see p. 812):

- oculomotor (IIIrd) nerve: medial, superior, inferior rectus and inferior oblique
- trochlear (IVth) nerve: superior oblique
- abducens (VIth) nerve: lateral rectus.

The oculomotor (IIIrd) nerve also supplies the upper lid and, indirectly, the pupil (parasympathetic fibres are attached to it). The facial (VIIth) nerve supplies the orbicularis and other muscles of facial expression.

Fig. 27.20 Cross-section of the eyeball.

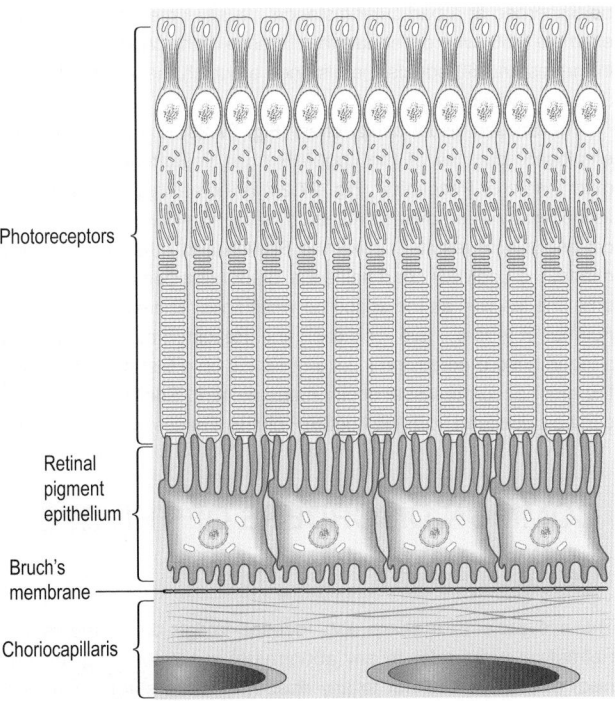

Fig. 27.21 Schematic diagram of the retina.

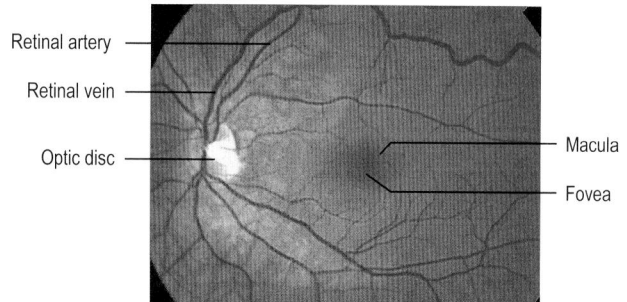
Fig. 27.22 Fundus photograph of the left eye.

CLINICAL APPROACH TO THE PATIENT WITH A DISORDER OF THE EYE

History and examination

A detailed history gives most of the facts needed to make a working diagnosis. The eye has limited mechanisms by which it can convey a diseased state. Common symptoms include alteration in visual acuity, redness, pain, discharge and photophobia.

It is essential to adopt a systematic approach to the examination of the eye. Different approaches and instruments (including direct ophthalmoscope, slit lamp with or without Goldman or Volk lens) are necessary for examination of the lids and anterior and posterior segments, as well as extraocular movements.

Visual acuity

It is vital for an accurate assessment of visual acuity to be recorded in all people with an eye problem. The visual acuity of each eye is recorded in two ways: distance visual acuity and near visual acuity. Distance vision is measured in Snellen letters or, ever more commonly, in LogMAR letters or figures of different sizes (see below). The recording is given as an expression of the line of letters that can be discerned at a particular distance, usually 6 metres (20 feet): for example 6/60, where 6 equals the distance of the chart from the eye in metres and 60 equals the distance at which the letter subtends 5′ at the nodal point.

The Snellen visual acuity chart (**Fig. 27.23**) is most commonly employed, but use of the LogMAR chart (*log*arithm of the *Mini*mum *A*ngle of *R*esolution; **Fig. 27.24**) is increasing, largely due to its necessity in studies or research, since it allows better statistical analysis of results. Unlike the Snellen and other visual acuity charts, the LogMAR chart has equal graduation between the letters on a line, as well as the space between lines. There is also a fixed number of letters – five – on each line. Research conducted using a logarithmic progression in size of letters on a test chart provides the most accurate visual acuity measurement. Snellen equivalents can be calculated from the LogMAR charts if necessary (**Fig. 27.25**).

COMMON DISORDERS OF THE EYE

Refractive errors

The eye projects a sharp and focused image on to the retina. Refractive errors refer to any abnormality in the focusing mechanism of the eye and not to any opacity in the system, such as a corneal or retinal scar.

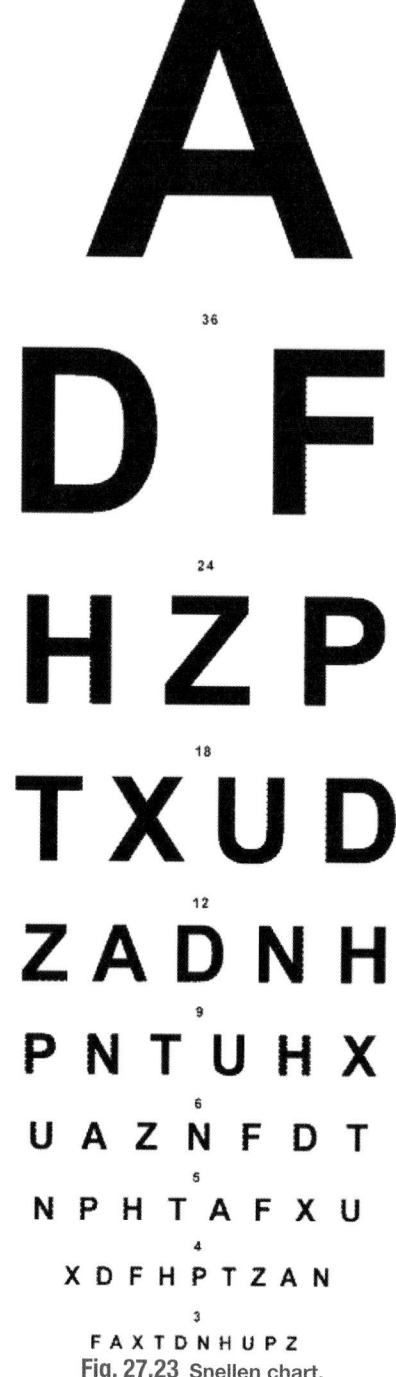
Fig. 27.23 Snellen chart.

The refraction of light in emmetropic (normal), myopic (shortsighted; negative lenses will correct) and hypermetropic (longsighted; positive lenses will correct) eyes is shown in **Fig. 27.26**.

Astigmatism is a refractive error of the eye in which there is a different degree of refraction in the different meridians of curvature. It may be myopic in one plane and hypermetropic or emmetropic in the other plane. In this situation, the front surface of the eye is shaped more like a rugby ball than a football.

Presbyopia is the term used to describe the normal ageing of the lens, which leads to a change in the refractive state of the eye. As the lens ages, it becomes less able to alter its curvature and this causes difficulty with near vision, especially reading.

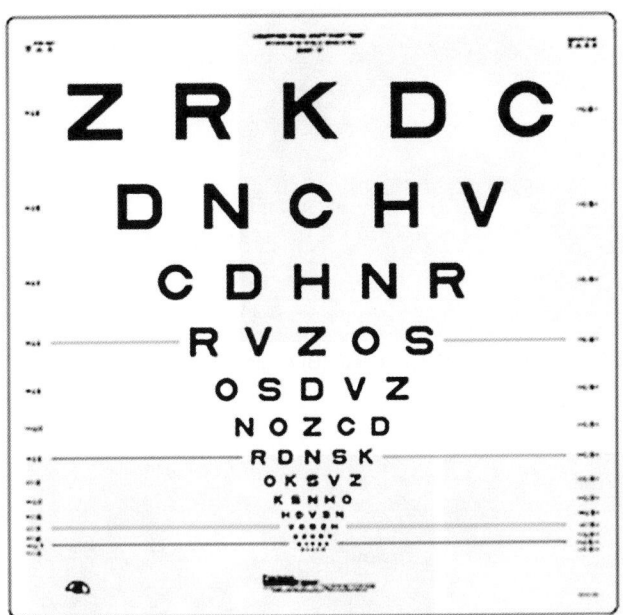

Fig. 27.24 LogMAR chart (*logarithm of the Minimum Angle of Resolution*).

20 feet (Snellen)	6 metres (Snellen)	Decimal	4 metres	log MAR
20/200	6/60	0.1	4/40	+1.0
20/160	6/48	0.125	4/32	+0.9
20/125	6/38	0.16	4/25	+0.8
20/100	6/30	0.2	4/20	+0.7
20/80	6/24	0.25	4/16	+0.6
20/63	6/19	0.32	4/12.5	+0.5
20/50	6/15	0.4	4/10	+0.4
20/40	6/12	0.5	4/8	+0.3
20/32	6/9.5	0.63	4/6.3	+0.2
20/25	6/7.5	0.8	4/5	+0.1
20/20	6/6	1.0	4/4	+0.0
20/16	6/4.8	1.25	4/3.2	−0.1
20/12.5	6/3.8	1.60	4/2.5	−0.2
20/10	6/3	2.0	4/2	−0.3

Fig. 27.25 Snellen equivalents can be calculated from the LogMAR charts if necessary. Vision is often recorded at 4 metres in studies, and logMAR equivalents or decimals are used in statistics.

Management

Errors of refraction can be corrected by using spectacles or contact lenses. The latter often result in better-quality vision but carry the risk of infection. They may be the only option in some refractive states such as keratoconus, a degenerative disorder of the eye in which structural changes within the cornea cause it to thin and to take on a more conical shape than its normal gradual curve. A number of surgical techniques can correct these errors of refraction, with varying degrees of accuracy. Phakic intraocular lenses may be used to treat high degrees of myopia but the most popular method remains the excimer laser to re-profile the corneal curvature (using PRK, LASIK and LASEK techniques). The laser either removes corneal tissue centrally to flatten the cornea in myopia or it removes tissue from the peripheral cornea to steepen it in hypermetropia.

Disorders of the lids

The lids afford protection to the eyes and help to distribute the tear film over the front surface of the globe. Excess tears are drained via

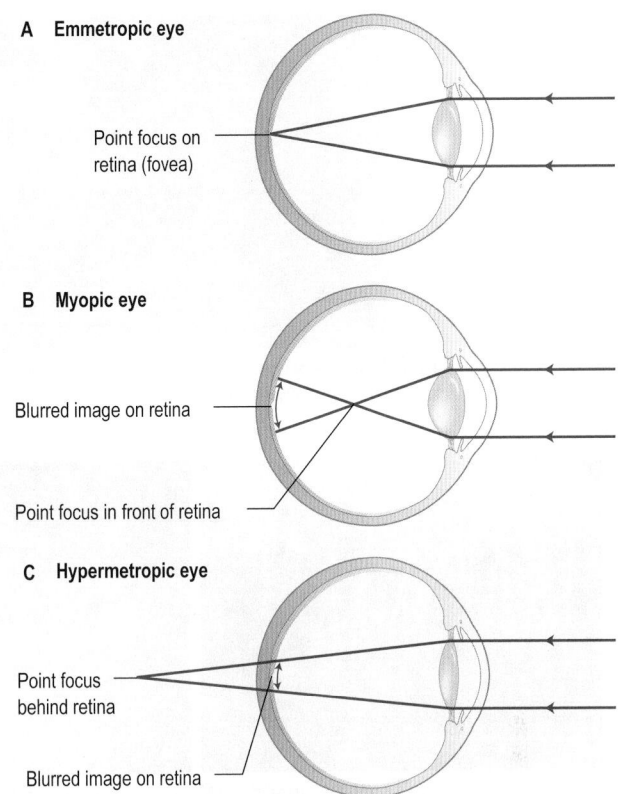

Fig. 27.26 Refraction. (A) Emmetropic (normal). **(B)** Myopic (short-sighted). **(C)** Hypermetropic (long-sighted).

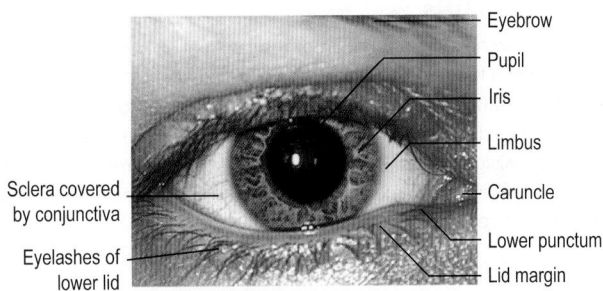

Fig. 27.27 The right eye.

the puncta and lacrimal system to the nose (**Fig. 27.27**). Malposition of the lids, factors that affect blinking and lacrimal drainage can all cause problems.

Entropion

The lid margin rolls inwards so that the lashes are against the globe (**Fig. 27.28A**). The lashes act as a foreign body and cause irritation, leading to a red eye that can mimic conjunctivitis. Occasionally, the constant rubbing of lashes against the cornea causes an abrasion. The most common cause is ageing and surgery is usually required.

Ectropion

The lid margin rolls outwards and is not apposed to the globe. As a result, the lacrimal punctum is not in the correct anatomical position to drain tears and patients usually complain of a watery eye. Underlying factors include age, VIIth nerve palsy and cicatricial skin conditions. Surgery is usually required.

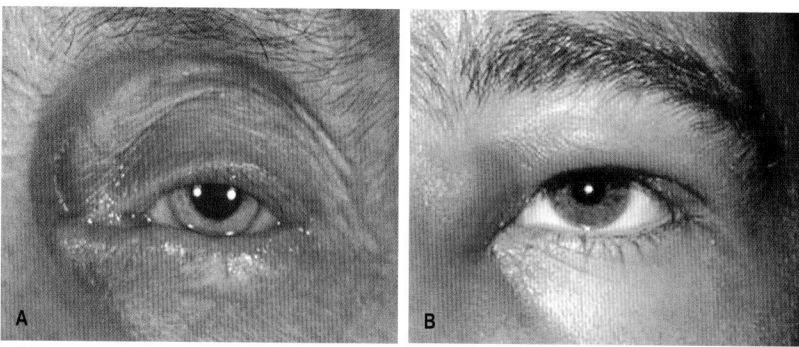

Fig. 27.28 Disorders of the eyelid. (A) Lid entropion. The lower lid appears inverted. **(B)** Acute dacryocystitis, showing a lump on the side of the nose.

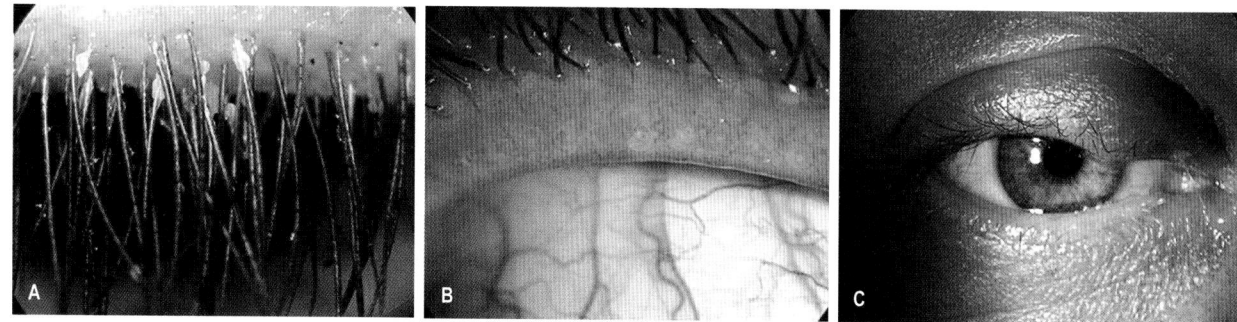

Fig. 27.29 Blepharitis. (A) Crusty and scaly deposits on the lashes and lash bases. **(B)** Upper lid showing meibomian glands plugged with oily secretions. **(C)** Blockage of the meibomian glands leads to swelling of the lid (chalazion).

Dacryocystitis

Patients who have inflammation of the lacrimal sac usually present with a painful lump at the side of the nose adjacent to the lower lid (see **Fig. 27.28B**). This should be treated with oral broad-spectrum antibiotics such as a cephalosporin, and patients should be watched carefully for signs of cellulitis. All patients should be referred to the ophthalmologist, as some have an underlying mucocele or dilated sac, and will require surgery.

Blepharitis

This is an extremely common condition in which inflammation of the lid margins may involve the lashes and lash follicles (**Fig. 27.29A**), resulting in styes, or inflammation and blockage of meibomian glands (see **Fig. 27.29B**) leading to chalazion (see **Fig. 27.29C**). Common underlying causes of blepharitis include meibomian gland dysfunction, seborrhoea and *Staphylococcus aureus* infection. Patients can be asymptomatic or complain of itchy, burning eyes because of tear film instability resulting from meibomian gland dysfunction. *Staph. aureus* is frequently responsible for chronic blepharoconjunctivitis and some patients may develop keratitis in the cornea (**Fig. 27.30**).

Management

Lid hygiene is the mainstay of treatment for blepharitis, as it helps to reduce the bacterial load and unblock meibomian glands. A short course of topical chloramphenicol or fusidic acid is useful in chronic cases, but in severe cases or cases where acne rosacea is suspected, oral doxycycline is used. Some patients are left with a lump once the acute inflammatory phase has subsided. Most of these patients find the lump, or chalazion, cosmetically unacceptable and require incision and curettage. People with keratitis should be referred to the ophthalmologist for topical steroids.

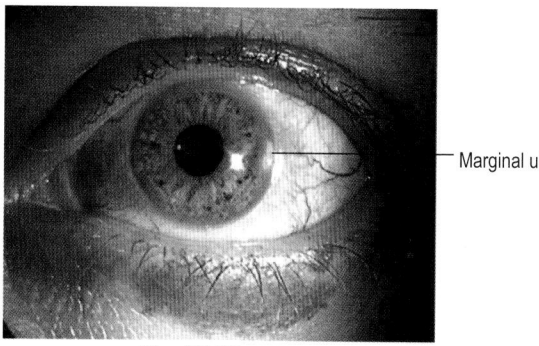

Marginal ulcer

Fig. 27.30 Marginal keratitis.

Conjunctivitis

The most common cause of a red eye, inflammation of the conjunctiva can arise from a number of causes, viral, bacterial and allergic being the most frequently encountered. Common features in all types include soreness, redness and discharge; in general, the visual acuity is good. History should include the speed of onset of the inflammation, the colour and consistency of the discharge, whether the eye is itchy, and if there has been a recent history of a cold or sore throat. In the neonate, it is vital to exclude gonococcal or chlamydial conjunctivitis associated with maternal sexually transmitted infection. The differential diagnosis of conjunctivitis is shown in **Box 27.9**.

Bacterial conjunctivitis

Bacterial conjunctivitis is uncommon, making up 5% of all cases of conjunctivitis. In the vast majority of patients, it causes a sore

? Box 27.9 Conjunctivitis

Type	Discharge	Pre-auricular node	Corneal involvement	Comment
Bacterial	Mucopurulent	–ve (except gonococci)	+ve Gonococcus	Rapid onset
Viral	Watery	+ve	+ve Adenovirus	Cold and/or sore throat
Chlamydial	Watery	+ve	+ve	Genitourinary discharge
Allergic	Stringy	–ve	+ve	Itchiness

or gritty eye in the presence of good vision. Bacterial conjunctivitis is invariably bilateral and should be suspected when conjunctival inflammation is associated with a purulent discharge.

Clinical features

Gonococcal conjunctivitis should be suspected when the onset of symptoms is rapid, the discharge is copious, and ocular inflammation includes chemosis (conjunctival oedema) and lid oedema. Gonococci are a cause of conjunctivitis, giving rise to a palpable pre-auricular node. Less acute or subacute purulent conjunctivitis with moderate discharge can be attributed to organisms such as *Haemophilus influenzae* and *Streptococcus pneumoniae*. Chronic conjunctivitis is usually associated with mild conjunctival injection and scant purulent discharge. Common organisms include *Staphylococcus aureus* and *Moraxella lacunata*.

Management

Prompt treatment with oral and topical penicillin is given in gonococcal conjunctivitis to ensure a reduced rate of corneal perforation. A Gram-stain of the conjunctival swab can quickly confirm the presence of diplococci. Gonococcal conjunctivitis is a notifiable disease in the UK. Empirical treatment for both subacute and chronic conjunctivitis involves a topical broad-spectrum antibiotic, such as chloramphenicol. Swabs should be taken if these cases do not respond to this initial treatment. Antibiotic resistance is increasing.

Chlamydial conjunctivitis

Chlamydia trachomatis (see p. 1416) in developed countries causes a sexually transmitted infection that is most prevalent in sexually active adolescents and young adults. Direct or indirect contact with genital secretions is the usual route of infections but shared eye cosmetics can also be involved. Neonatal chlamydial conjunctivitis is a notifiable disease in the UK and should be suspected in newborns with a red eye. Mothers should be asked about sexually transmitted infections.

Clinical features

The onset of symptoms is slow, and patients may complain of mild discomfort for weeks. In these cases, the red eye is associated with a scanty mucopurulent discharge and a palpable pre-auricular lymph node. In chronic cases, it is not unusual to see superior corneal vascularization. In neonates, the onset of the red eye is typically around 2 weeks after birth, whereas gonococcal conjunctivitis occurs within days of birth. Conjunctival swabs should be taken and a nucleic acid amplification test (NAAT; see p. 1416) performed prior to commencement of treatment.

Management

Topical erythromycin twice daily is commenced and patients referred to the sexual health clinic. Neonates should be started on topical erythromycin and referred to the paediatrician, as there may be associated otitis media or pneumonitis.

i Box 27.10 Trachoma

- A very common cause of blindness worldwide (see p. 553)
- Found mainly in the tropics and the Middle East
- Caused by *Chlamydia trachomatis* but not usually sexually transmitted
- Chronic conjunctival inflammation causes progressive scarring, trichiasis, entropion and subsequent corneal scarring
- The result may be severe visual impairment or blindness from corneal opacification or ulceration

Trachoma

See **Box 27.10**.

Viral conjunctivitis

Adenoviral conjunctivitis

This is highly contagious and can cause epidemics in communities. Transmission is through direct or indirect contact with infected individuals. The onset of symptoms may be preceded by a cold or influenza-like symptoms. Inflammation is commonly associated with chemosis, lid oedema and a palpable pre-auricular lymph node. Some patients develop a membrane on the tarsal conjunctiva (**Fig. 27.31**) and haemorrhage on the bulbar conjunctiva. Viral conjunctivitis can cause deterioration in visual acuity owing to corneal involvement (focal areas of inflammation). In 50% of these patients, the conjunctivitis is unilateral.

The condition is largely self-limiting in the majority of cases. Lubricants, together with a cold compress, can be a soothing element of **management** for patients. Adhering to strict hygiene and keeping towels separate from those of the rest of the household go a long way towards reducing the spread of the infection. In people with corneal involvement or intense conjunctival inflammation, topical steroids are indicated.

Herpes simplex conjunctivitis

Primary ocular herpes simplex conjunctivitis is typically unilateral. It usually causes a palpable pre-auricular lymph node, and cutaneous vesicles develop on the eyelids and the skin around the eyes in the majority. Over 50% of these patients develop a dendritic corneal ulcer (**Fig. 27.32**). The organism responsible for this condition is the herpes simplex virus (HSV), usually HSV-1, although HSV-2 can give rise to ocular infection.

Primary ocular HSV infection is self-limiting but most clinicians choose **treatment** with topical aciclovir in order to limit the risk of corneal epithelial involvement.

Molluscum contagiosum conjunctivitis

This is typically unilateral; it produces a red eye that generally goes unrecognized and comes to the forefront because patients fail to improve and the cornea starts to become involved. On close inspection, pearly, umbilicated nodules, filled with the DNA poxvirus, can be seen on the lid margin.

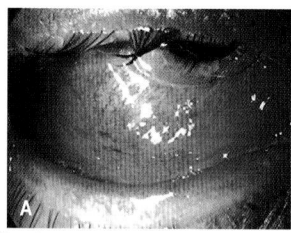
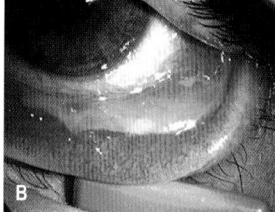

Fig. 27.31 Viral conjunctivitis. (A) Conjunctival chemosis. **(B)** Pseudomembrane on lower lid.

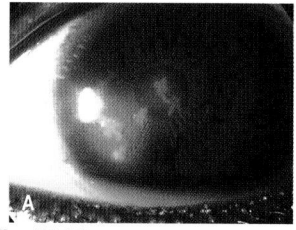
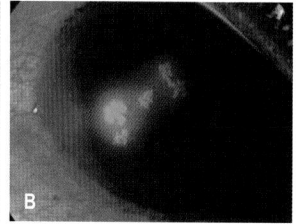

Fig. 27.32 Dendritic ulcers on the cornea. **(A)** Stained with fluorescein. **(B)** Stained with fluorescein and viewed with blue light.

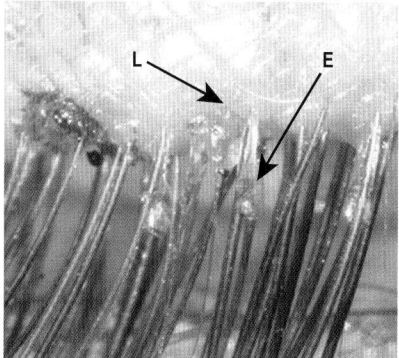

Fig. 27.33 Phthiriasis palpebrarum. The lice (L) and the nits (eggs) can be seen on the lid margins. E, empty egg.

Management includes curetting the central portion of the lesion, freezing the centre or completely excising the lesion. If the corneal involvement is severe or the eye is very inflamed, a short course of topical steroids, such as prednisolone 0.5% or dexamethasone 0.1%, is helpful.

Phthiriasis palpebrarum

Phthiriasis palpebrarum (**Fig. 27.33**) is an eyelid infestation caused by *Phthirus pubis*, or the crab louse. Infestation of the cilia and eyelid is rare. It leads to blepharitis with marked conjunctival inflammation, pre-auricular lymphadenopathy and, rarely, secondary infection at the site of louse bite.

Management

Mechanical removal of the lice with fine forceps, physostigmine 1.25% and pilocarpine gel 4% are all effective treatments.

Allergic conjunctivitis

There are five main types of allergic conjunctivitis: seasonal, perennial, vernal, atopic and giant papillary. Both seasonal and perennial allergic conjunctivitis are acute allergic conjunctival disorders. Symptoms include itching and pink to reddish eyes. These two eye conditions are mediated by mast cells and can be treated easily with cold compresses, eye washes with tear substitutes, and avoidance of allergens. The last three are difficult to treat; they are chronic and can be sight-threatening, so should be referred to an ophthalmologist.

Seasonal/perennial conjunctivitis

Seasonal allergic conjunctivitis and perennial conjunctivitis, affecting 20% of the general population in the UK, are allergic reactions to grass and tree pollen and fungal spores. Seasonal allergic conjunctivitis occurs mainly in spring and summer. Perennial allergic conjunctivitis occurs all year round but peaks in the autumn; causes include allergens, such as house-dust mites.

The main symptoms include itching, redness, soreness, watering and a stringy discharge. Occasionally, the conjunctiva may become so hyperaemic that chemosis results. This is usually associated with swollen lids.

Lowering the allergen load (reducing dust; see p. 946) is helpful. Medical *treatment* includes the use of antihistamine drops such as azelastine and emedastine, together with topical mast-cell-stabilizing agents such as sodium cromoglicate and nedocromil. Olopatadine (twice daily) has dual action and is very effective. Corticosteroid drops should be avoided. Oral antihistamines help the itching.

Corneal disorders

Trauma

Corneal abrasions

Trauma resulting in the removal of a focal area of epithelium on the cornea is very common. Abrasions usually occur when the eye is accidentally poked with a finger, a foreign body flies into the eye or something brushes against the eye.

Symptoms include severe pain, due to exposure of the corneal nerve endings, lacrimation and inability to open the eye (blepharospasm). Blinking and eye movement can aggravate the pain and foreign body sensation. The visual acuity is usually reduced. Most cases will need topical anaesthetic drops such as oxybuprocaine or tetracaine to be administered before it is possible to examine the eye. The cornea should be inspected with a blue light after instillation of fluorescein drops. The orange dye will stain the area of the abrasion. Under blue light, the abrasion lights up as green. Occasionally, foreign bodies can lodge on the undersurface of the upper lid and give rise to linear vertical abrasions. Eversion of the upper lid is necessary in all cases of abrasions (**Fig. 27.34**).

Treatment consists of a broad-spectrum topical antibiotic, such as chloramphenicol drops or ointment four times a day for 5 days. The role of padding is controversial but common practice is to pad the affected eye for 24 hours once chloramphenicol ointment has been applied to the eye.

Corneal foreign body

Occasionally, when something flies into the eye, it sticks on the cornea (**Fig. 27.35A**). It may be associated with lacrimation and photophobia. Examination is best attempted following instillation of a topical anaesthetic and should include eversion of the upper lid (see **Fig. 27.35B**). Corneal foreign bodies can usually be seen directly with a white light.

The corneal foreign body should be removed. *Treatment* involves a topical antibiotic, such as chloramphenicol four times a day for 5 days, or fusidic acid twice a day for 5 days.

High-velocity trauma

In cases of high-velocity trauma, corneal perforation or an intraocular foreign body should be suspected. Examination may show

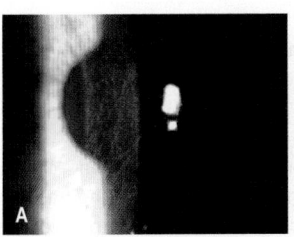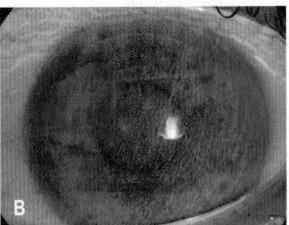

Fig. 27.34 Linear corneal abrasion. (A) Stained with fluorescein. **(B)** Stained with fluorescein and viewed with blue light.

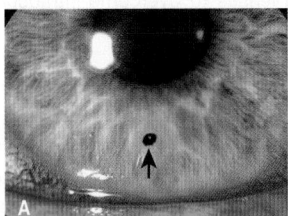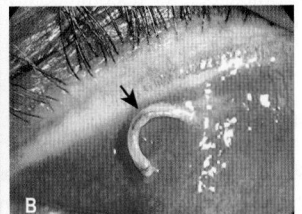

Fig. 27.35 Foreign bodies (arrowed). (A) Corneal. **(B)** Subtarsal.

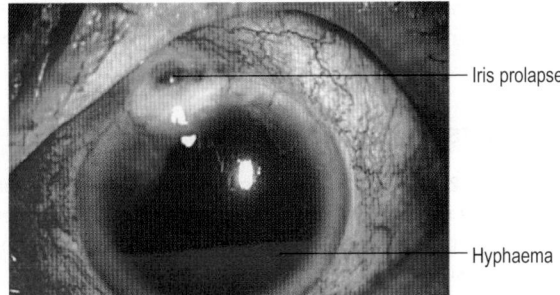

Iris prolapse

Hyphaema

Fig. 27.36 Blunt trauma. Hyphaema and globe rupture with iris prolapse.

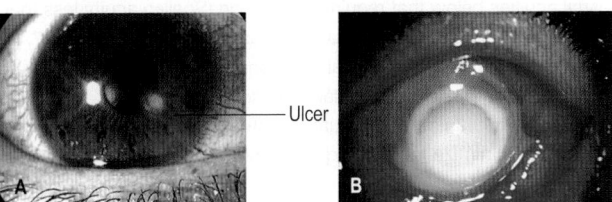

Ulcer

Fig. 27.37 Contact lens-related keratitis. (A) Corneal ulcer. **(B)** Severe keratitis with a corneal abscess and a hypopyon.

a corneal laceration and a foreign body may also be embedded in the cornea. The foreign body may be present on the iris or in the lens or vitreous. Other clues pointing towards a penetrating injury include a large subconjunctival haemorrhage, a flat anterior chamber with low intraocular pressure, and the presence of blood in the anterior chamber (hyphaema). Urgent referral to the ophthalmologist is mandatory, ensuring that no drops are instilled into the eye and that a plastic shield is placed over the eye to minimize further risk of trauma.

Blunt trauma usually results in periorbital bruising and gross lid oedema, which can make examination to exclude perforating injury difficult. These patients should be referred to the ophthalmologist for a detailed ocular examination to exclude a perforation, retinal detachment or a traumatic hyphaema (**Fig. 27.36**).

Keratitis

This is a general term used to describe corneal inflammation. Common causes include herpes simplex virus, contact lens-associated infection and blepharitis. Symptoms include the sensation of a foreign body or pain (depending on the size and depth of the ulcer), photophobia and lacrimation. Vision is reduced if the ulcer affects the visual axis.

Herpes simplex keratitis

Corneal epithelial cells infected with the virus eventually undergo lysis and form an ulcer, which is typically dendritic in shape (see **Fig. 27.32**). The ulcer stains with fluorescein and can be observed easily with a blue light. Topical immunosuppression, such as with steroid drops, or systemic immunosuppression, such as in AIDS, can lead to the centrifugal spread of the virus, such that the ulcer increases in area and is referred to as a geographic ulcer. Recurrent attacks of HSV keratitis can be triggered by ultraviolet light, stress and menstruation. All these factors are responsible for activating the virus, which normally lies dormant in the ganglion of the Vth nerve.

Treatment consists of aciclovir ointment five times a day for 2 weeks; this is usually very effective.

Contact lens-related keratitis

A small number of contact lens wearers develop infective corneal ulcers, which are potentially sight-threatening (**Fig. 27.37**). The organisms usually responsible include Gram-positive and Gram-negative bacteria. Patients should be referred to an ophthalmologist for scraping of the ulcer and commencement of antibiotic treatment.

Keratoconus

Keratoconus is an eye condition in which the normally round, dome-shaped cornea progressively thins and causes a cone-shaped bulge to develop. Aetiology is uncertain but genetic factors play a role, and the condition is more common in people with allergic diseases such as asthma, in Down's syndrome and in some disorders of collagen such as Marfan's disease. Keratoconus affects up to 1 in 1000 people and is more common in individuals of Asian heritage. It is usually diagnosed in teenagers and young people.

Management

In the early stages, spectacles or soft contact lenses may be used to correct vision. As the cornea becomes thinner and steeper, rigid gas-permeable contact lenses may be necessary.

Corneal cross-linking is a new treatment that can stop keratoconus becoming worse. It is effective in more than 9 out of 10 patients, with a single 30-minute day-case procedure, but is only suitable when the corneal shape is continuing to deteriorate. In very advanced cases, where contact lenses fail to improve vision, a corneal transplant may be needed.

Corneal dystrophy

Corneal dystrophies may be classified anatomically as comprising:
- epithelial and subepithelial dystrophies
- epithelial–stromal *TGFBI* corneal dystrophies
- stromal dystrophies
- endothelial dystrophies.

The most common endothelial dystrophy, Fuchs' corneal dystrophy, is a genetically associated degenerative disorder leading to corneal oedema and vision loss. The gene involved is *TCF4*. The condition affects both eyes; it is more common in females and is of gradual onset, leading to blindness in the 40–60 age group. There is an accumulation of deposits (guttae) in the cornea with thickening of Descemet's membrane. Treatment is by corneal transplantation.

Cataracts

Cataract (**Fig. 27.38**) is by far the most common cause of preventable blindness in the world, having an effective surgical treatment. In the UK, approximately 250 000 cataract operations are performed each year, making it the most common surgical procedure.

Aetiology

Age-related opacification of the lens (cataract) is the commonest cause of visual impairment, with 30% of people over 65 years having visual acuities below that required for driving (Snellen acuity less than 6/12). The common causes of cataracts are summarized in **Box 27.11**.

In young patients, familial or congenital causes should be excluded. Any history of ocular inflammation is noted. Cataracts diagnosed in infants demand urgent referral to the ophthalmologist in order to minimize the subsequent development of amblyopia.

Clinical features

Gradual painless deterioration of vision is the most common symptom. Other symptoms are dependent on the type of cataract: for example, a posterior capsular type would lead to glare and problems with night driving. Early changes in the lens are correctable by spectacles but eventually the opacification needs surgical intervention.

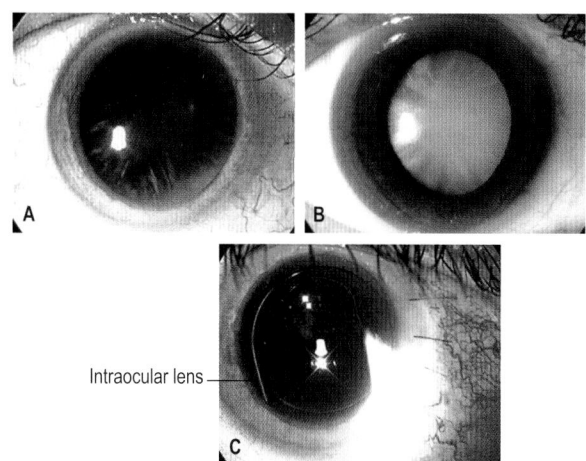

Fig. 27.38 **Cataracts.** (A) Early cataract. (B) White mature cataract. (C) Artificial intraocular lens following phacoemulsification.

Intraocular lens

Box 27.11 Cataracts: aetiology

Congenital
- Maternal infection
- Familial

Age
- Elderly

Metabolic
- Diabetes
- Galactosaemia
- Hypocalcaemia
- Wilson's disease

Drug-induced
- Corticosteroids
- Phenothiazines
- Miotics
- Amiodarone

Traumatic
- Post-intraocular surgery

Inflammatory
- Uveitis

Disorder-associated
- Down syndrome
- Dystrophia myotonica
- Lowe's syndrome

Investigations

Blood glucose, serum calcium and liver biochemistry should be measured to diagnose metabolic disorders.

Management

Small-incision extracapsular or phacoemulsification cataract extraction with the insertion of an intraocular lens is the treatment of choice (see **Fig. 27.37C**). Recent advances have enabled surgeons to perform multiple steps in the surgical process with the excimer laser to enhance visual outcomes. Lens technology has also improved and toric lenses are available to treat astigmatism, and multifocal or accommodative lenses to overcome intraocular lens-induced presbyopia.

Glaucoma

Glaucoma is due to increased pressure inside the eye, which is sufficiently elevated to cause optic nerve damage and result in visual field defects, with loss of sight (**Fig. 27.39**). Normal intraocular pressure (IOP) is 10–21 mmHg. Some types of glaucoma can result in an IOP exceeding 70 mmHg. Glaucoma is the second most common cause of blindness worldwide and the third most common cause of blind registration in the UK.

Primary open-angle glaucoma

Primary open-angle glaucoma (POAG) is the most common form of glaucoma. High intraocular pressures result from reduced outflow of aqueous humour through the trabecular meshwork (**Fig. 27.40A**). Common risk factors include age (0.02% of 40-year-olds versus 10% of 80-year-olds), race (black Africans are at five times greater risk than whites), positive family history and myopia.

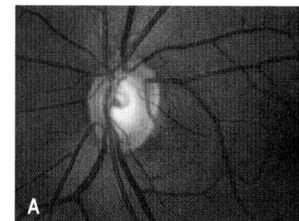
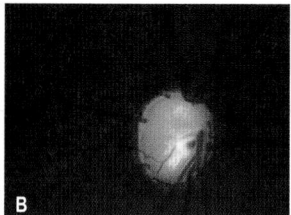

Fig. 27.39 **The optic disc.** (A) Normal optic disc. (B) Glaucomatous optic disc. The central cup is enlarged and deepened.

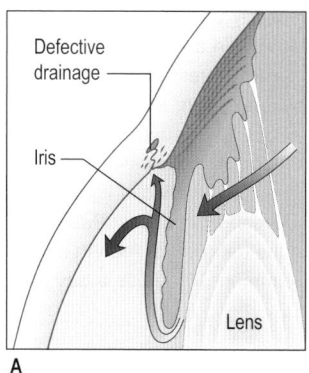
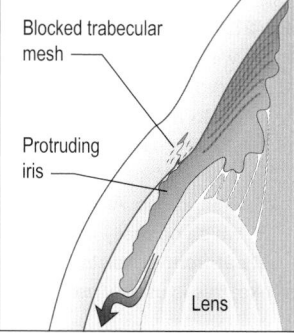

Defective drainage

Iris

Lens

Blocked trabecular mesh

Protruding iris

Lens

A   B

Fig. 27.40 **Glaucoma.** (A) Primary open-angle glaucoma. (B) Angle-closure glaucoma.

Clinical features

POAG causes a gradual, insidious, painless loss of peripheral visual field, causing loss of vision. It is initially asymptomatic and the central vision remains good until the end-stage of the disease. Usually, glaucoma is identified during a routine ophthalmic examination. Diagnosis is only made if the IOP is measured. The optic disc is inspected and shows an enlarged cup with a thin neuroretinal rim. Visual fields are assessed and show a normal blind spot with scotomas.

Management

Treatment aims to reduce the IOP, either by reducing aqueous production or by increasing aqueous drainage:

- **Beta-blockers**, such as timolol, carteolol and levobunolol, reduce aqueous production and are the most commonly prescribed topical agents. These drugs are contraindicated in people with chronic obstructive pulmonary disease, asthma or heart block.
- **Prostaglandin analogues**, such as latanoprost, bimatoprost and travoprost, increase aqueous outflow and are also used (alone or in combination with beta-blockers) for POAG, as they can reduce IOP by 30%.
- **Carbonic anhydrase inhibitors**, such as dorzolamide and acetazolamide, reduce aqueous production and are available in topical preparations. Acetazolamide is also available orally and, in this form, is the most potent drug for reducing IOP. It should not be used in patients who have a sulphonamide allergy.
- **Selective laser trabeculoplasty (SLT)** is a form of laser surgery that can lower the IOP by about 30% when used as initial therapy. It is useful when eye-drop medications are not lowering the eye pressure enough or are causing significant side-effects. It may sometimes be used as initial treatment in glaucoma, although effects commonly last 1–5 years only.

Acute angle-closure glaucoma

Acute angle-closure glaucoma (AACG) is an ophthalmic emergency. There is a sudden rise in intraocular pressure to levels over 50 mmHg. This occurs due to reduced aqueous drainage when the ageing lens pushes the iris forwards against the trabecular meshwork (see **Fig. 27.40B**). People most at risk of developing AACG are those with shallow anterior chambers, such as hypermetropes and women. The attack is more likely to occur under reduced light conditions when the pupil is dilated.

Clinical features

AACG causes sudden onset of a red, painful eye and blurred vision. Patients become unwell, with nausea and vomiting, and complain of headache and severe ocular pain. The eye is injected and tender, and feels hard. The cornea is hazy and the pupil is semi-dilated (**Fig. 27.41**). **Box 27.12** shows the differential diagnosis of the acute red eye. **Box 27.13** shows features that require **urgent referral** to an ophthalmologist.

Management

Prompt treatment is required to preserve sight and includes:

- i.v. acetazolamide 500 mg (provided there are no contraindications) to reduce IOP, *and*
- instillation of pilocarpine 4% drops to constrict the pupil to improve aqueous outflow and prevent iris adhesion to the trabecular meshwork.

Other topical drops, such as beta-blockers and prostaglandin analogues, can also be instilled if available, provided there are no contraindications. Analgesia and antiemetics are given as required.

Patients must be referred to an ophthalmologist immediately so that reduction in IOP can be monitored and other agents, such as oral glycerol or i.v. mannitol, can be administered to non-responding patients. Definitive treatment involves making a hole in the periphery of the iris of both eyes either by laser or by surgical means.

Uveitis

Uveitis is inflammation of the uveal tract, which includes the iris, ciliary body and choroid. It is classified according to the part of the uveal tract that the inflammation affects:

- **Anterior uveitis** is inflammation that affects the anterior part of the uveal tract. This can include the iris (iritis), or both the iris and the ciliary body (iridocyclitis). It is the most common type of uveitis.
- **Intermediate uveitis** is inflammation that affects the middle part of the uveal tract or eye, mainly the vitreous. It can also affect the underlying retina.
- **Posterior uveitis** is inflammation that affects the posterior part of the eye. It can affect the choroid, optic nerve head and the retina (or any combination of these structures). It includes chorioretinitis, retinitis and neuroretinitis.
- **Panuveitis** is inflammation affecting the whole of the uveal tract.

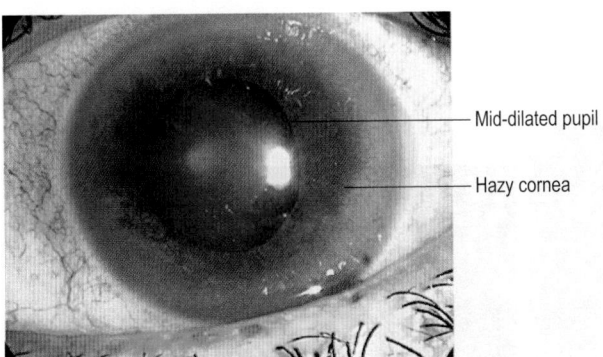

Mid-dilated pupil

Hazy cornea

Fig. 27.41 Acute angle-closure glaucoma.

? Box 27.12 Differential diagnosis of the acute red eye							
Cause	**Conjunctival injection**	**Unilateral or bilateral**	**Pain**	**Photophobia**	**Vision**	**Pupil**	**Intraocular pressure**
Conjunctivitis	Diffuse	Bilateral (often unilateral initially)	Gritty	Occasionally with adenovirus	Normal	Normal	Normal
Keratitis	Diffuse	Unilateral	Gritty	Yes	Reduced	Normal	Normal
Anterior uveitis	Circumcorneal	Unilateral	Painful	Yes	Reduced	Constricted	Normal or raised
Acute glaucoma	Diffuse	Unilateral	Severe pain	Mild	Reduced	Mid-dilated	Raised

The most common symptoms of uveitis are blurred vision, pain, redness, photophobia and floaters. Each symptom is determined by the location of the inflammation, such that photophobia and pain are common features of iritis while floaters are commonly seen with posterior uveitis.

Anterior uveitis (iritis)

The classic presentation entails a triad of eye symptoms: redness, pain and photophobia. Vision can be normal or blurred, depending on the degree of inflammation. The eye can be generally red or the injection can be localized to the limbus. The anterior chamber shows features consistent with inflammation, including cells, keratic precipitates on the corneal endothelium, fibrin or hypopyon (pus), and the pupil may have adhered to the lens (posterior synechiae) (**Fig. 27.42**). The IOP may be normal or raised, either due to cells clogging up the trabecular meshwork, or due to posterior synechiae causing aqueous humour to build up behind the iris and force the iris against the trabecular meshwork and so reduce aqueous drainage.

Management

This consists of reducing inflammation with the use of topical steroids such as dexamethasone 0.1% and dilating the pupil with

> ⊕ **Box 27.13 Red flags for a red eye**
>
> The following symptoms require **urgent** referral:
> - Severe pain
> - Photophobia
> - Reduced vision, particularly if sudden
> - Coloured halos around point of light in a patient's vision
> - Proptosis
> - Smaller pupil in affected eye
>   *Plus* on medical assessment:
> - High intraocular pressure
> - Corneal epithelial disruption
> - Shallow anterior chamber depth
> - Ciliary flush

cyclopentolate 1% to prevent formation of posterior synechiae. Dilation also allows fundoscopy to exclude posterior segment involvement. If the IOP is raised, this is treated with topical beta-blockers, prostaglandin analogues, or oral or i.v. acetazolamide. Referral should be made to the ophthalmologist.

Intermediate uveitis

This usually causes painless blurred vision, most commonly associated with floaters. It is unusual to experience photophobia and redness. Both eyes are commonly affected in intermediate uveitis.

Management

This consists of a combination of treatment for anterior and posterior uveitis depending on the degree of anterior and posterior involvement.

Posterior uveitis

This commonly causes painless, blurred vision and can progress to severe visual loss. It is commonly associated with floaters and scotomata, or blind spots in the visual field.

Posterior uveitis is often found with systemic autoimmune diseases or infections; appropriate investigations should be performed and treatment given that is aimed at the cause.

Autoimmune diseases associated with uveitis include rheumatoid arthritis and Behçet's disease, ankylosing spondylitis and positive HLA-B27 (see p. 448), reactive arthritis, sarcoidosis, psoriasis and inflammatory bowel disease (Crohn's disease and ulcerative colitis; see p. 1202). Infections, a rare cause of uveitis, include herpes simplex, herpes zoster, toxoplasmosis, cytomegalovirus, syphilis, tuberculosis, HIV infection and Lyme disease. In a number of patients, no cause is found (idiopathic uveitis).

Management

Steroids are commonly given orally, or more locally by injection into or around the eye. If steroid treatment is needed to treat uveitis in the longer term, second-line immunosuppressive drugs, such as mycophenolate mofetil, ciclosporin or azathioprine, are used.

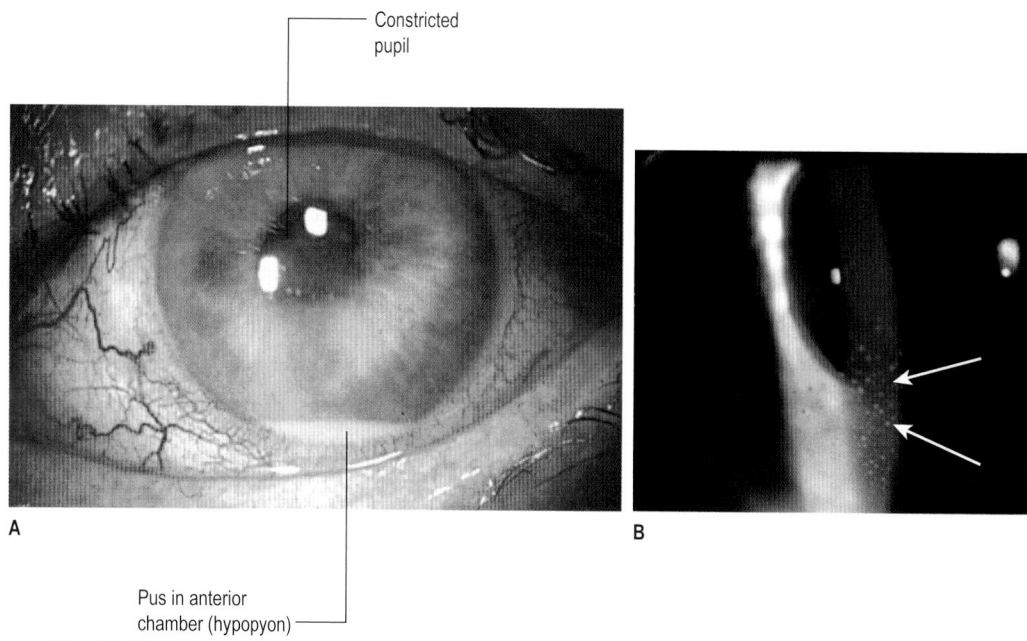

Constricted pupil

Pus in anterior chamber (hypopyon)

Fig. 27.42 Anterior uveitis. (A) Acute uveitis with hypopyon. **(B)** Keratic precipitates (arrowed) on the corneal endothelium.

Biological agents, such as rituximab or adalimumab, are showing increasing promise in more severe cases.

Disorders of the retina

Central retinal vein occlusion

Central retinal vein occlusion (CRVO) usually leads to profound, sudden, painless loss of vision with thrombosis of the central retinal vein at or posterior to the lamina cribrosa, where the optic nerve exits the globe. The thrombus causes obstruction to the outflow of blood, leading to a rise in intravascular pressure. This results in dilated veins, retinal haemorrhage, cotton wool spots and abnormal leakage of fluid from vessels, causing retinal oedema (**Fig. 27.43**). In severe cases, an afferent papillary defect (p. 811) is present and this suggests the ischaemic variant.

Predisposing factors include increasing age, hypertension and cardiovascular disease, diabetes, glaucoma and, in the younger age group, blood dyscrasias and vasculitis.

Management

Treatment of any underlying medical condition is mandatory. Referral to an ophthalmologist is essential to monitor the eye, as some patients can develop retinal ischaemia with resulting neovascularization of the retina and iris. Panretinal photocoagulation should be commenced if there is neovascularization, and intravitreal steroid or anti-vascular endothelial growth factor (anti-VEGF) therapy is also used if there is macular oedema. Patients who develop iris neovascularization – rubeosis – where these new blood vessels block the drainage angle are at risk of developing rubeotic glaucoma.

Central retinal artery occlusion

Central retinal artery occlusion (CRAO) results in sudden, painless severe loss of vision. Retinal arterial occlusion results in infarction of the inner two-thirds of the retina. The arteries become narrow and the retina becomes opaque and oedematous. A cherry-red spot

is seen at the fovea because the choroidal vasculature shows up through the thinnest part of the retina (**Fig. 27.44**). An afferent papillary defect is usually present.

Arteriosclerosis-related thrombosis is the most common cause of CRAO. Emboli from atheromas and diseased heart valves are other causes. Giant cell arteritis (see p. 464) must be excluded.

Management

CRAO is an ophthalmic emergency since studies have shown that irreversible retinal damage occurs *within 90 minutes of onset*. Ocular massage and 500 mg i.v. acetazolamide help to reduce ocular pressure and may assist in dislodging the emboli. Breathing into a paper bag allows a build-up of carbon dioxide, which acts as a vasodilator and so helps dislodge the emboli. Other options include making a corneal paracentesis to drain off some aqueous humour, thereby reducing the IOP.

People with CRAO should have a thorough medical evaluation to determine the aetiology of the emboli or thrombus. Some patients may present with transient loss of vision or amaurosis fugax (see p. 838). All people with CRAO and amaurosis fugax should be started on oral aspirin if it is not medically contraindicated.

Retinal detachment

This causes a painless, progressive visual field loss. The shadow corresponds to the area of detached retina. If the detachment affects the macula, central vision will be lost. Following a tear in the retina, fluid collects in the potential space between the sensory retina and the pigment epithelium (**Fig. 27.45**). Patients usually report a sudden onset of floaters, often associated with flashes of light (photopsia) prior to the detachment. These individuals should be referred to an ophthalmologist for a detailed fundal examination.

Retinitis pigmentosa

This is a common chronic, inherited, degenerative disease of the retina, which can be primary or part of a syndrome, and leads to blindness. There is constriction of the peripheral vision, leading to tunnel vision and progressive loss of night vision.

Ophthalmoscopy shows bone spicule deposits and attenuated retinal vessels. Several genes are implicated.

There is no treatment but high-dose vitamin A supplementation may slow progression. Gene therapy is being investigated.

Age-related macular degeneration

Age-related macular degeneration (AMD) is the most common cause of visual impairment in patients over 50 years in the Western world, and the most common cause of blind registration in this age group. It affects 10% of people over 65 years and 30% over

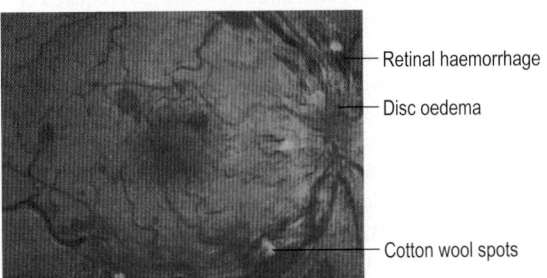

Fig. 27.43 Central retinal vein occlusion.

Retinal haemorrhage
Disc oedema
Cotton wool spots

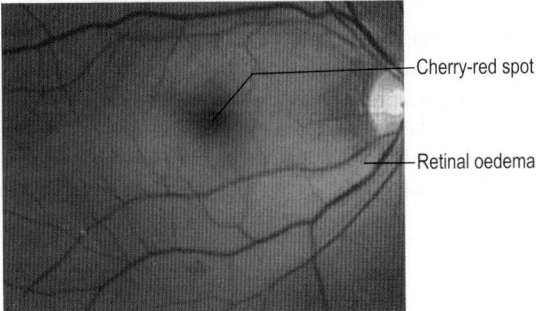

Fig. 27.44 Central retinal artery occlusion.

Cherry-red spot
Retinal oedema

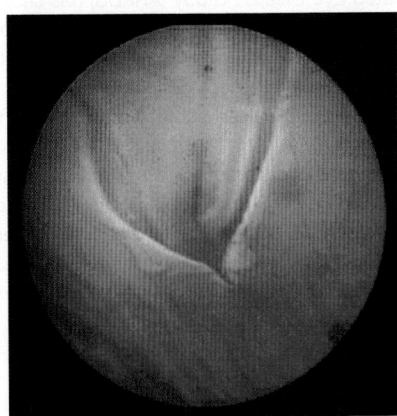

Fig. 27.45 Retinal tear leading to detachment.

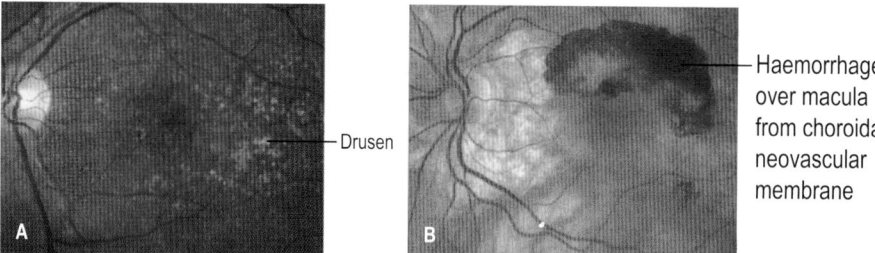

Fig. 27.46 **Age-related macular degeneration.** **(A)** With deposition of material (drusen) over the macula. **(B)** With choroidal neovascularization.

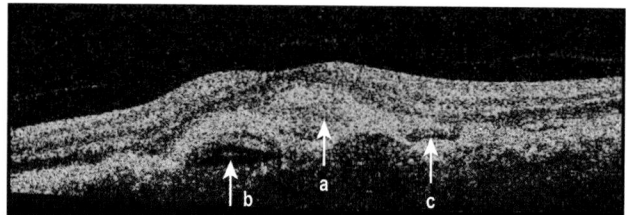

Fig. 27.47 **Age-related macular degeneration seen by optical coherence tomography.** **(a)** Area of thickened retina. **(b)** Pigment epithelial detachment. **(c)** Subretinal fluid.

80 years. Mutations in various genes have been reported: fibulin 5, complement factor H, and the Arg 80 Gly variant of complement C3.

The cause is unknown but suggested risk factors include increasing age, smoking, hypertension, hypercholesterolaemia and ultraviolet exposure.

There are two types:

- **Non-exudative (dry) macular degeneration** describes a painless and progressive loss of central vision. With age, lipofuscin deposits (drusen) are found between the retinal pigment epithelium (RPE) and Bruch's membrane (**Fig. 27.46A**; see **Fig. 27.21**). Drusen may be hard or soft, and there may be focal RPE detachment. Not all people with these changes will be affected visually but some develop distortion and blurring of their central vision. Extensive atrophy of RPE can occur (geographic atrophy).
- **Exudative (wet) AMD** (10% of cases) occurs with the development of abnormal subfoveal choroidal neovascularization in the region of the macula and causes severe central visual loss (see **Fig. 27.46B**).

Management

The Age-Related Eye Disease Study (AREDS) has shown that vitamins C and E, β-carotene, zinc and copper slow progression of the disease. The subsequent study, AREDS 2, suggests that adding lutein, zeaxanthin and omega 3 does not improve the original AREDS formula overall, unless subjects had little of the supplements in their diets.

People with central distortion or with frank macular pathology should be referred *urgently* to the ophthalmologist for assessment of treatment. Anti-VEGF, such as ranibizumab, aflibercept and bevacizumab, are given by intravitreal injections with great success; the last of these is unlicensed yet less expensive. The treatment course should be commenced *as a matter of urgency*, as vision is maintained in up to 95% of patients and improves in approximately one-third. Initial monthly monitoring with optical coherence tomography (OCT) is recommended (**Fig. 27.47**). Laser treatment and photodynamic therapy with verteporfin constituted the treatment of choice in the past for wet AMD but now have limited roles.

Severe visual loss is possible and low-vision aids, such as magnifying glasses, may help to improve a patient's independence.

Visual loss

Every patient with unexplained sudden visual loss requires ophthalmic referral (see **Box 27.14** for initial history and examination).

The common causes of blindness are similar across the world (**Box 27.15**). In developing countries, trachoma due to *Chlamydia trachomatis* (see p. 553) is also a major cause, accounting for 10% of global blindness; onchocerciasis (river blindness, due to *Onchocerca volvulus*; see p. 575) accounts for blindness in about 1 million people, although this figure is decreasing with community treatment programmes. In leprosy, 70% of patients have ocular involvement, and blindness occurs in 5–10% of these. Ocular involvement is common in cerebral malaria (see p. 565), although loss of vision is rare.

HIV infection can produce uveitis but the major problem is severe opportunistic infection of the eye when the CD4 count falls (see p. 1432) and anti-retroviral therapy is not available.

Vitamin A deficiency and xerophthalmia affect millions each year; the World Health Organization (WHO) classification of xerophthalmia by ocular signs is shown in **Box 33.15**.

The WHO lists the most common causes of blindness across the world as cataract, glaucoma, acute macular degeneration, corneal opacity, diabetic retinopathy and infections from bacteria or parasites.

⊕ **Box 27.14 Initial history and examination in sudden loss of vision**

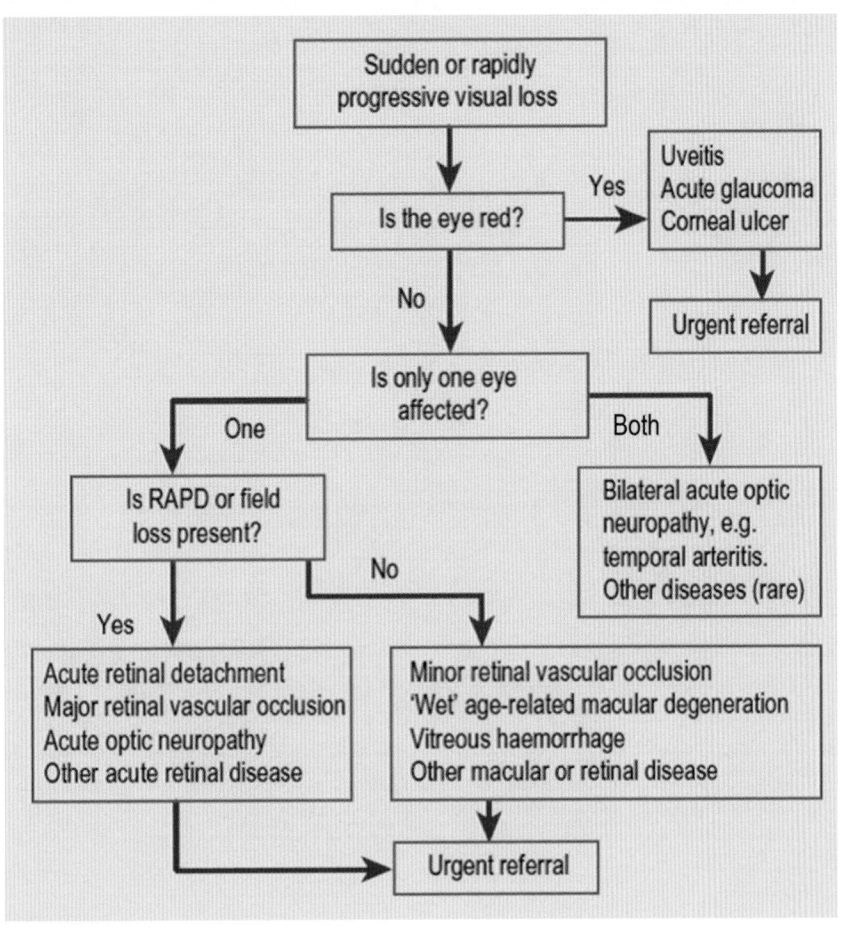

RAPD, relative afferent papillary defect.
(After Pane A, Simcock P. Practical Ophthalmology. Edinburgh: Churchill Livingstone; 2005.)

? **Box 27.15 Causes of loss of vision**

Painless loss of vision
- Cataract
- Open-angle glaucoma
- Retinal detachment
- Central retinal vein occlusion
- Central retinal artery occlusion
- Diabetic retinopathy
- Vitreous haemorrhage
- Posterior uveitis
- Age-related macular degeneration
- Optic nerve compression
- Cerebral vascular disease

Painful loss of vision
- Acute angle-closure glaucoma
- Giant cell arteritis
- Optic neuritis
- Uveitis
- Scleritis
- Keratitis
- Shingles
- Orbital cellulitis
- Trauma

Further reading

Lynn WA, Lightman S. The eye in systemic infection. *Lancet* 2004; 364:
1439–1450.
Quigley MA. Glaucoma. *Lancet* 2011; 377:1367–1377.
Rosenfeld PJ. Bevacizumab versus ranibizumab for AMD. *N Engl J Med* 2011;
364:1966–1967.
Sakimoto E, Roseblatt MI, Azar DT. Laser eye surgery for refractive errors.
Lancet 2006; 367:1432–1447.
Sheffield VC, Stone EM. Genomics and the eye. *N Engl J Med* 2011; 364:
1932–1942.
Weiss JS, Møller HU, Aldave AJ et al. IC3D classification of corneal dystrophies
– edition 2. *Cornea* 2015; 34:117–159.
Wong TY, Scott IU. Retinal vein occlusion. *N Engl J Med* 2010; 363:2135–3144.
Wright AF, Dhillon B. Major progress in Fuchs's corneal dystrophy. *N Engl J Med*
2010; 363:1072–1075.

28

Respiratory disease

Veronica White and Prina Ruparelia

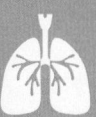

CORE SKILLS AND KNOWLEDGE

Respiratory medicine is an exciting and varied specialty caring for patients with a range of acute and chronic conditions. One-third of visits to primary care are due to a respiratory complaint, and respiratory conditions are the reason for one-quarter of medical admissions to hospital.

Respiratory physicians provide a large amount of inpatient care, for acute problems such as pneumonia or exacerbations of chronic obstructive pulmonary disease and other chronic respiratory conditions. Outpatient care is given in general clinics (for the initial investigation and diagnosis of patients with respiratory symptoms) and in more specialist ones (for long-term follow-up of individual conditions). In specialist clinics, care is shared with community teams and nurse specialists to promote the health and quality of life of patients, through education, self-management and admission-avoidance strategies. Practical procedures performed by respiratory physicians

include bronchoscopy, endobronchial ultrasound scanning and pleural interventions.

Key skills in respiratory medicine include:

- managing respiratory emergencies, including type 1 and type 2 respiratory failure, massive pleural effusion, pneumothorax and large-volume haemoptysis
- interpreting basic examination findings and respiratory investigations, i.e. chest X-rays (**Fig. 28.1**), arterial blood gas analysis and spirometry, with confidence
- understanding common treatments for respiratory conditions, including inhaled and nebulized medications, home oxygen therapy and non-invasive ventilation.

Respiratory medicine can be learned through attending general and subspecialty respiratory clinics (e.g. lung cancer, tuberculosis or sleep clinics), observing specialist investigations such as lung function measurement or bronchoscopy, attending clinics and home visits with specialist nurses, and at every opportunity interpreting arterial blood gases and using the results to alter oxygen delivery or assisted ventilation systems.

CLINICAL SKILLS FOR RESPIRATORY MEDICINE

History

The following features of the medical history are especially relevant in respiratory disease:

- **Respiratory symptoms:** cough, sputum production, breathlessness, chest pain, haemoptysis, wheeze. Specify acuity of onset, change over time, change in symptoms with location.
- **Systemic symptoms:** weight loss, malaise, night sweats.
- **Occupational exposure:** all previous occupations, with a specific focus on exposure to asbestos, to organic materials such as hay, mushrooms or cotton, or to animals. Establish any relationship of symptoms to work.

- **Smoking:** smoking history (duration of smoking and number of cigarettes smoked per day), and also attempts made to give up, including use of nicotine replacement substances such as e-cigarettes.
- **Recreational drug use:** especially smoked cannabis.
- **Family history:** respiratory conditions such as emphysema, bronchiectasis or cystic fibrosis.
- **Childhood history:** prematurity, childhood infections such as whooping cough or measles.
- **Travel history:** may be relevant in assessing risk factors for tuberculosis.

Examination

End of the bed:
- Posture – lying flat or raised
- Colour – cyanosed?
- Respiratory rate
- Pain on breathing (pleuritic)?
- Fever
- Cachexia

Anaemia
Horner's syndrome
Pursed lips
Nose – beaky

Central cyanosis

Jugular venous pressure
- Raised
- Pulsatile

Use of accessory muscles
Intercostal indrawing

CO_2 retention flap
Bounding pulse

Clubbing
Tar staining
Peripheral cyanosis

Deep vein thrombosis

Oedema (leg or sacral if
  lying down)
- Right heart failure
- Secondary to pulmonary
  hypertension

Sputum
Volume ($\uparrow\uparrow$ bronchiectasis)
Mucopurulent (infection)
Purulent (green = infection)
Blood-stained (cancer,
  pulmonary embolism,
  tuberculosis, bronchiectasis)

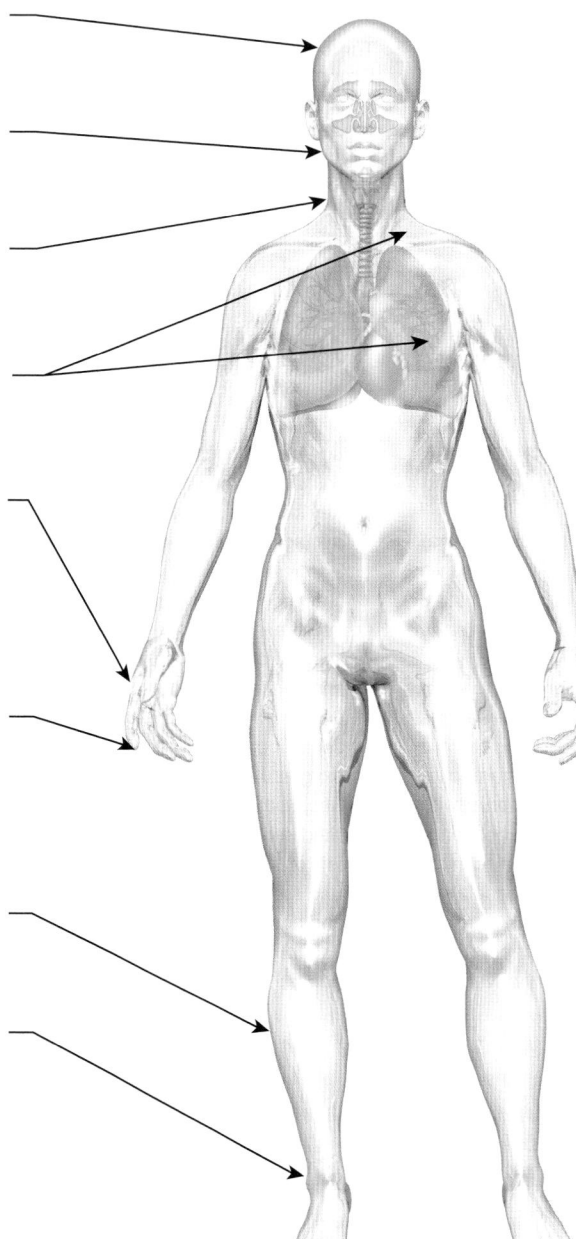

Examining the chest

Inspection
- Colour
- Breathlessness
- Deformity
- Scars
- Symmetry of movement
- Abdominal paradox
  (diaphragm weakening)
- Hyperinflation
- Prominent veins
  (SVC obstruction)
- Intercostal indrawing
- Scoliosis

Palpation
- Tracheal position
- Cricosternal distance
- Supraclavicular fossa nodes
- Apex beat
- Tenderness
  - Costochdritis
  - Rib fracture
- Liver
  - Position (low lying)
  - Enlargement

Percussion
- Dull
  - Consolidation
  - Collapse
- 'Stony dull'
  - Fluid (effusion)
- Hyperresonant
  - Pneumothorax

Auscultation
- Normal or 'vesicular'
- Bronchial breathing
- Wheeze
  - Monophonic (single large airwar obstruction)
  - Polyphonic (narrowing of small airways)
- Crackles
  - Coarse (consolidation, bronchiectasis)
  - Fine, late inspiratory (pulmonary oedema, lung fibrosis)
- Pleural rub
- Vocal resonance

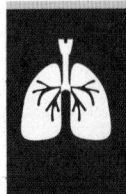

1. Preliminaries		• **Patient details:**
		  - Which patient, how old, when was this image taken?
		• **X-ray details:**
		  - Is it a posteroanterior or anteroposterior projection?
		  - Is the patient rotated?
		  - Is there adequate penetration?
		  - Has the patient taken an adequate breath?
			• Compare where available to previous X-ray images

2. Trachea		• The trachea should be widely patent and should be central in the chest	• The trachea may be pulled towards areas of fibrosis or collapse • It may be pushed away by masses, a goitre, lymphadenopathy, large pleural effusion or a tension pneumothorax
3. Mediastinum		• The aortic notch should be just visible • The left hilum should be slightly higher than the right • The hila should be symmetrical in size	• The mediastinum is widened by lymphadenopathy, masses such as thymoma, and aortic aneurysm • The hila may be pulled up or down by collapsed lobes, or enlarged by the presence of a tumour
4. Heart size		• Heart size should be less than 50% of the thoracic width on a PA chest film • Assess heart borders	• Cardiomegaly may be caused by hypertension, valvular disease, heart failure or cardiomyopathy • Loss of right heart border may suggest right middle lobe pathology • Loss of left heart border suggests lingular pathology
5. Diaphragm		• The right hemidiaphragm is usually higher than the left • Look for air/gas under the diaphragm and for elevation of the diaphragm on either side	• Air or gas under the diaphragm indicates a perforated abdominal viscus • A hemidiaphragm may be pulled up from above by lobar collapse, or pushed up from below by a large mass
6. Pleura		• The costophrenic angles should be clearly visible • Look for lung markings extending to the chest wall • Look for evidence of a lung edge	• Loss of the costophrenic angle is usually due to the presence of pleural effusions • Larger pleural effusions may cause a 'white out' on one side • Loss of lung markings or a visible lung edge suggests a pneumothorax
7. Lungs		• Is there consolidation of the upper lobe (stops at horizontal fissure), middle lobe/lingula (heart edge unclear) or lower lobe (diaphragm unclear)? • Inspect each part of the lung looking for round shadows • Inspect the lung parenchyma for interstitial changes	• Areas of consolidation may often be restricted to a lobe and are usually caused by pneumonia. An air bronchogram (airways outlined) or evidence of cavitation may be seen • Rounded shadows may be caused by cancer, inflammatory lesions, such as tuberculosis or fungal disease • Interstitial changes may be caused by pulmonary oedema or fibrosis

8. Bones		• Inspect all ribs for evidence of fractures
		• Faint bones imply osteopenia
		• Are there lytic lesions?
			• Think of systemic diseases:
			  - Osteoporosis may cause osteopenia or fractures
			  - Solid organ cancers or myeloma can cause lytic lesions

9. Soft tissue		• Observe the soft tissue around the rib cage	• Air within the skin suggests surgical emphysema
10. Miscellaneous		• Look for any externally applied devices	• Nasogastric tubes should bisect the carina and cross the diaphragm • Chest drains should terminate in the pleural space • Central venous catheters should end just above the right atrium • Pacemaker wires, and sternotomy wires imply cardiac disease

Fig. 28.1 A systematic ten-step approach to chest X-ray interpretation.

The 'top 10' respiratory conditions
- Acute and chronic cough
- Asthma
- Chronic obstructive pulmonary disease (COPD)
- Pneumonia
- Pulmonary tuberculosis
- Pneumothorax
- Pleural effusions
- Lung cancer
- Bronchiectasis
- Interstitial lung disease

The 'top 10' concepts in respiratory medicine
- Smoking cessation
- Self-management of chronic conditions
- Admission avoidance
- Home oxygen therapy
- Multidisciplinary cancer care

- Respiratory failure
- Atopy
- The 'treatment ladder' approach to asthma and COPD
- Management of chest drains
- Diagnosis and staging of lung cancer

The 'top 10' respiratory medications
- Oxygen
- β_2 agonists
- Antimuscarinics
- Oral and inhaled corticosteroids
- Combination inhalers
- Antihistamines
- Leukotriene receptor antagonists
- Mucolytics
- Monoclonal antibodies
- Antifibrotics

FUNCTION OF THE RESPIRATORY SYSTEM

The respiratory system has several key functions, the principal ones being to extract oxygen from the external environment and to dispose of carbon dioxide. This requires the lungs to function as efficient bellows, bringing in fresh air and delivering it to the alveoli, and expelling used air at an appropriate rate. Gas exchange is achieved by exposing thin-walled capillaries to the alveolar gas and matching ventilation to blood flow through the pulmonary capillary bed. The excretion of carbon dioxide by the lungs is involved in acid–base homeostasis.

The lungs expose a large surface area of body tissue to the external environment in order to achieve gas exchange, and hence they can be damaged by dusts, gases and infective agents. Host defence is therefore a key priority for the lung and is achieved by a combination of structural and immunological defences.

The pulmonary circulation also acts as a blood pool reservoir that can allow the body to respond readily to increased oxygen demands in exercise. The lungs act as a filtration system for small pulmonary emboli. The pulmonary circulation also plays a role in innate immunity: for example, in de-priming neutrophils.

Finally, the lungs have a role in speech, as the passage of air through the vocal cords is necessary for phonation.

Anatomy

Nose, pharynx and larynx

See pages 907 and 909.

Trachea, bronchi and bronchioles

The trachea is 10–12 cm in length. It lies slightly to the right of the midline and divides at the carina into right and left main bronchi. The carina lies under the junction of the manubrium sterni and the second right costal cartilage. The right main bronchus is more vertical than the left and inhaled material is therefore more likely to end up in the right lung.

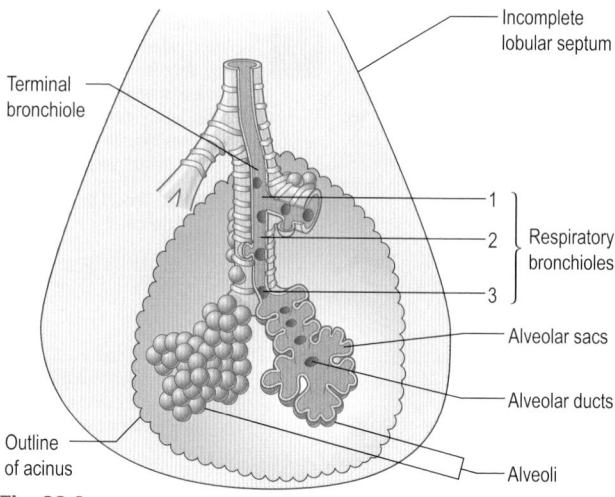

Fig. 28.2 Branches of a terminal bronchiole ending in the alveolar sacs.

The right main bronchus divides into the upper lobe bronchus and the intermediate bronchus, which further subdivides into the middle and lower lobe bronchi. On the left the main bronchus divides into upper and lower lobe bronchi only. Each lobar bronchus further divides into segmental and subsegmental bronchi. There are about 25 divisions in all between the trachea and the alveoli.

The first seven divisions are bronchi that have:
- walls consisting of cartilage and smooth muscle
- an epithelial lining with cilia and goblet cells
- submucosal mucus-secreting glands
- endocrine cells.

The next 16–18 divisions are bronchioles that have:
- no cartilage and a muscular layer that progressively becomes thinner
- a single layer of ciliated cells but very few goblet cells
- granulated Clara cells that produce a surfactant-like substance.

The ciliated epithelium is a key defence mechanism. Each cell bears approximately 200 cilia beating at 1000 beats per minute (b.p.m.) in organized waves of contraction. Mucus, which contains macrophages, cell debris, inhaled particles and bacteria, is moved by the cilia towards the larynx at about 1.5 cm/min (the 'mucociliary escalator'; see later).

The bronchioles finally divide within the acinus into smaller respiratory bronchioles that have alveoli arising from the surface (**Fig. 28.2**). Each respiratory bronchiole supplies approximately 200 alveoli via alveolar ducts. The term 'small airways' refers to bronchioles of less than 2 mm; the average lung contains about 30 000 of these.

Alveoli

There are approximately 300 million alveoli in each lung. Their total surface area is 40–80 m². The epithelial lining consists mainly of **type I pneumocytes** (**Fig. 28.3**). These cells have an extremely thin layer of cytoplasm, which only offers a thin barrier to gas exchange. Type I cells are connected to each other by tight junctions that limit the movements of fluid in and out of the alveoli. Alveoli are not completely airtight; many have holes in the alveolar wall, allowing communication between alveoli of adjoining lobules (pores of Kohn).

Type II pneumocytes are slightly more numerous than type I cells but cover less of the epithelial lining. They are found generally in the borders of the alveolus and contain distinctive lamellar vacuoles, which are the source of surfactant. Type I pneumocytes are derived from type II cells. Large alveolar macrophages are present within the alveoli and assist in defending the lung.

Lungs

The lungs are separated into lobes by invaginations of the pleura, which are often incomplete. The right lung has three lobes, whereas the left lung has two. The positions of the oblique fissures and the right horizontal fissure are shown in **Fig. 28.4**. The upper lobe lies mainly in front of the lower lobe and therefore physical signs on the right side in the front of the chest are due to lesions of the upper lobe or the middle lobe.

Pleura

The pleura is a layer of connective tissue covered by a simple squamous epithelium. The visceral pleura covers the surface of the lung, lines the interlobar fissures, and is continuous at the hilum with the parietal pleura, which lines the inside of the hemithorax. At the hilum, the visceral pleura continues alongside the branching

bronchial tree for some distance before reflecting back to join the parietal pleura. In health, the pleurae are in apposition, apart from a small quantity of lubricating fluid.

Diaphragm

The diaphragm is covered by parietal pleura above and peritoneum below. The diaphragmatic muscle fibres arise from the lower ribs and insert into the central tendon. Motor and sensory nerve fibres go separately to each half of the diaphragm via the phrenic nerves. Fifty per cent of the muscle fibres are of the slow-twitch type with a low glycolytic capacity; they are relatively resistant to fatigue.

Pulmonary vasculature and lymphatics

The lung has a dual blood supply, receiving deoxygenated blood from the right ventricle via the pulmonary artery and oxygenated blood via the bronchial circulation.

The pulmonary artery divides to accompany the bronchi. The arterioles accompanying the respiratory bronchioles are thin-walled and contain little smooth muscle. The pulmonary venules drain laterally to the periphery of the lobules, pass centrally in the interlobular and intersegmental septa, and eventually join to form the four main pulmonary veins.

The bronchial circulation arises from the descending aorta. These bronchial arteries supply tissues down to the level of the respiratory bronchiole. The bronchial veins drain into the pulmonary veins, forming part of the normal physiological shunt.

Lymphatic channels lie in the interstitial space between the alveolar cells and the capillary endothelium of the pulmonary arterioles.

The tracheobronchial lymph nodes are arranged in five main groups: pulmonary, bronchopulmonary, subcarinal, superior tracheobronchial and paratracheal. For practical purposes, these form a continuous network of nodes from the lung substance up to the trachea.

Nerve supply to the lung

The innervation of the lung remains incompletely understood. Parasympathetic and sympathetic fibres (from the vagus and sympathetic chain, respectively) accompany the pulmonary arteries and the airways. Airway smooth muscle is innervated by vagal afferents, postganglionic muscarinic vagal efferents and vagally derived nonadrenergic non-cholinergic (NANC) fibres, which use a range of neurotransmitters. Three muscarinic receptor subtypes have been

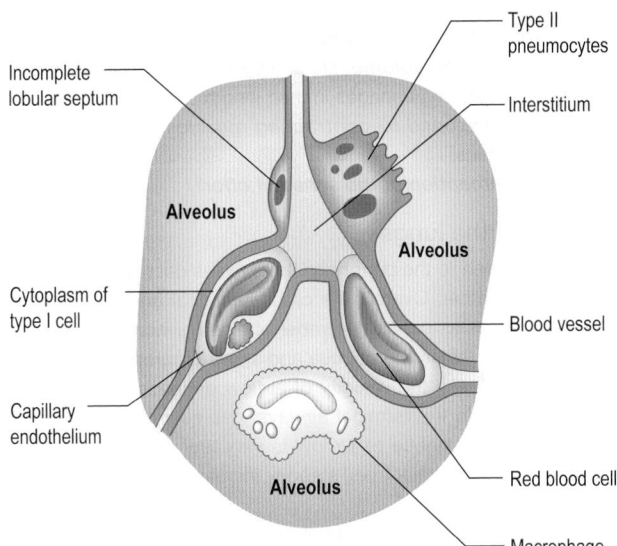

Fig. 28.3 The structure of alveoli, showing the pneumocytes and capillaries.

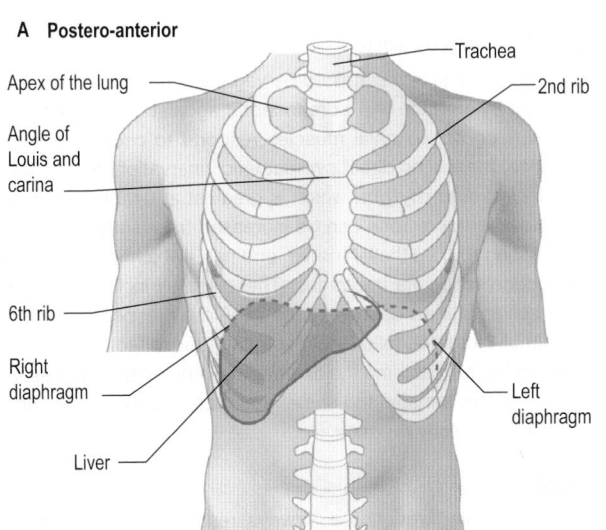

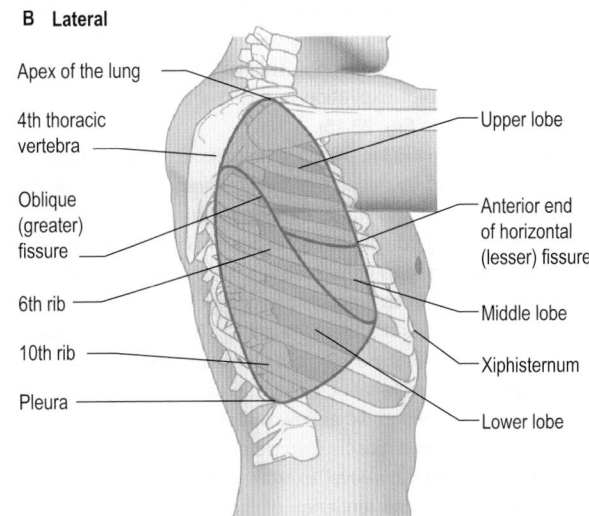

Fig. 28.4 Surface anatomy of the chest. **(A)** Anterior. **(B)** Lateral.

identified: M_1 receptors on parasympathetic ganglia, a smaller number of M_2 receptors on muscarinic nerve terminals, and M_3 receptors on airway smooth muscle. The parietal pleura is innervated from intercostal and phrenic nerves but the visceral pleura has no innervation.

Further reading

Albert RK, Spiro SG, Jett JR. *Clinical Respiratory Medicine*, 4th edn. Chicago: Mosby; 2012.

Physiology

Nose

The major functions of nasal breathing are:
- to heat and moisten the air
- to remove particulate matter.

Nasal secretions contain immunoglobulin A (IgA) antibodies, lysozyme and interferons. In addition, the cilia of the nasal epithelium move the mucous gel layer rapidly back to the oropharynx, where it is swallowed. Bacteria have little chance of settling in the nose. Mucociliary protection is less effective against viral infections because viruses bind to receptors on epithelial cells. The majority of rhinoviruses bind to an adhesion molecule, intercellular adhesion molecule 1 (ICAM-1), which is shared by neutrophils and eosinophils. Many noxious gases, such as sulphur dioxide, are almost completely removed by nasal breathing.

Breathing

Lung ventilation can be considered in two parts:
- the mechanical process of inspiration and expiration
- the control of respiration to a level appropriate for metabolic needs.

Mechanical process

The lungs have an inherent elastic property that causes them to tend to collapse away from the thoracic wall, generating a negative pressure within the pleural space. The strength of this retractive force relates to the volume of the lung: at higher lung volumes the lung is stretched more, and a greater negative intrapleural pressure is generated. **Lung compliance** is a measure of the relationship between this retractive force and lung volume. At the end of a quiet expiration the retractive force exerted by the lungs is balanced by the tendency of the thoracic wall to spring outwards. At this point, respiratory muscles are resting. The volume of air remaining in the lung after a quiet expiration is called the **functional residual capacity (FRC**; see **Fig. 28.15**).

Inspiration from FRC is an active process: a negative intrapleural pressure is created by descent of the diaphragm and movement of the ribs upwards and outwards through contraction of the intercostal muscles. During tidal breathing in healthy individuals, inspiration is almost entirely due to contraction of the diaphragm. More vigorous inspiration requires the use of accessory muscles of ventilation (sternomastoid and scalene muscles). Respiratory muscles are similar to other skeletal muscles but are less prone to fatigue. However, inspiratory muscle fatigue contributes to respiratory failure in patients with severe chronic airflow limitation and in those with primary neurological and muscle disorders.

At rest or during low-level exercise, expiration is passive and results from the natural tendency of the lung to collapse. Forced expiration involves activation of accessory muscles, chiefly those of the abdominal wall, which help to push up the diaphragm.

Control of respiration

Coordinated respiratory movements result from rhythmical discharges arising in an anatomically ill-defined group of interconnected neurones in the reticular substance of the brainstem, known as the respiratory centre. Motor discharges from the respiratory centre travel via the phrenic and intercostal nerves to the respiratory musculature.

Ventilation is controlled by a combination of neurogenic and chemical factors (**Fig. 28.5**). In healthy individuals the main driver for respiration is the arterial pH, which is closely related to the partial pressure of carbon dioxide in arterial blood. Oxygen levels in arterial blood are usually above the level that triggers respiratory drive. Typical normal values are shown in **Box 28.2**.

Breathlessness on physical exertion is normal and not considered a symptom unless the level of exertion is very light, such as when walking slowly. Surveys of healthy Western populations reveal that over 20% of the general population report themselves as breathless on relatively minor exertion. Although breathlessness is a very common symptom, the sensory and neural mechanisms underlying it remain obscure. The sensation of breathlessness is derived from at least three sources:
- *changes in lung volume*, sensed by receptors in thoracic wall muscles signalling changes in their length
- *tension developed by contracting muscles*, sensed by Golgi tendon organs
- *central perception of the sense of effort*.

Airways of the lungs

From the trachea to the periphery, the airways decrease in size but increase in number. Overall, the cross-sectional area available for airflow increases as the total number of airways increases. The airflow rate is greatest in the trachea and slows progressively towards the periphery (since the velocity of airflow depends on the cross-sectional area). In the terminal airways, gas flow occurs solely by diffusion. The resistance to airflow is very low (0.1–0.2 kPa/L in a normal tracheobronchial tree), steadily increasing from the small to the large airways.

Airways expand as the lung volume increases. At full inspiration (***total lung capacity***, TLC) they are 30–40% larger in calibre than at full expiration (***residual volume***, RV). In chronic obstructive pulmonary disease (COPD) the small airways are narrowed but this can be partially compensated by breathing closer to TLC.

Control of airway tone

Bronchomotor tone is maintained by vagal efferent nerves and can be reduced by atropine or β-adrenoceptor agonists. Adrenoceptors on the surface of bronchial muscles respond to circulating catecholamines; there is no direct sympathetic innervation. Airway tone shows a ***circadian rhythm***, which is greatest at 04.00 and lowest in the mid-afternoon. Tone can be increased transiently by inhaled stimuli acting on epithelial nerve endings, which trigger reflex bronchoconstriction via the vagus. These stimuli include cigarette smoke, solvents, inert dust and cold air. Airway responsiveness to these stimuli increases following respiratory tract infections, even in healthy subjects. In asthma the airways are very irritable, and as the circadian rhythm remains the same, asthmatic symptoms are usually worse in the early morning.

Airflow

Movement of air through the airways results from a difference between atmospheric pressure and the pressure in the alveoli; alveolar pressure is negative in inspiration and positive in expiration.

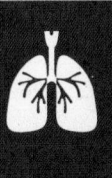

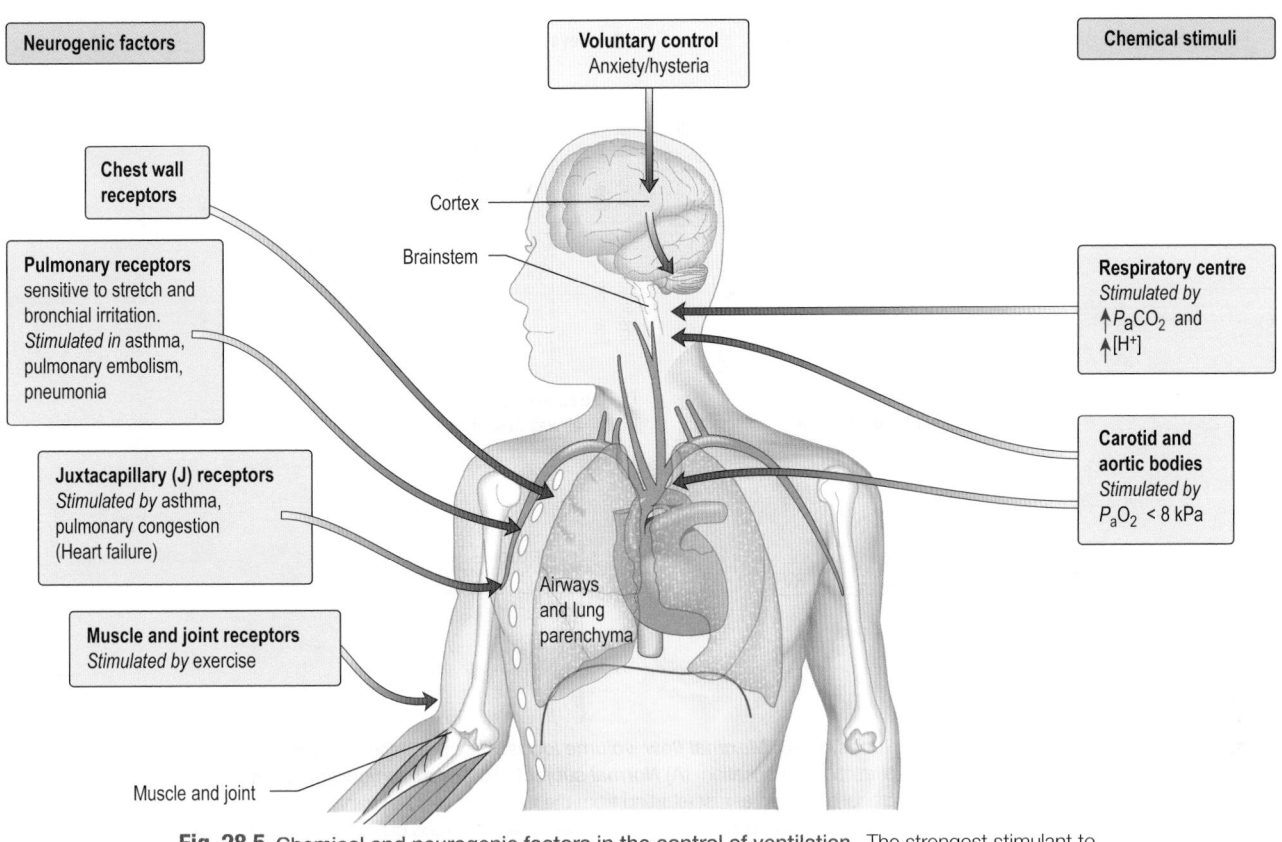

Fig. 28.5 Chemical and neurogenic factors in the control of ventilation. The strongest stimulant to ventilation is a rise in P_aCO_2, which increases [H⁺] in cerebrospinal fluid. *Sensitivity* to this may be lost in *chronic obstructive pulmonary disease*. In these patients, hypoxaemia is the chief stimulus to respiratory drive; oxygen treatment may therefore reduce respiratory drive and lead to a further rise in P_aCO_2. An increase in [H⁺] due to metabolic acidosis, as in diabetic ketoacidosis, will increase ventilation with a fall in P_aCO_2, causing deep sighing (Kussmaul) respiration. The respiratory centre is depressed by severe hypoxaemia and sedatives (e.g. opiates).

ⓘ Box 28.2 Normal values for respiratory physiology

In a typical normal adult at rest:
- Pulmonary blood flow is about 5 L/min
- This carries 11 mmol/min (250 mL/min) of O_2 to tissues
- Ventilation is about 6 L/min
- This removes 9 mmol/min (200 mL/min) of CO_2 from the body
- Normal pressure of oxygen in arterial blood (P_aO_2) is 11–13 kPa
- Normal pressure of carbon dioxide in arterial blood (P_aCO_2) is 4.8–6.0 kPa

During quiet breathing the pleural pressure is negative throughout the breathing cycle. With vigorous expiratory efforts (e.g. cough) the pleural pressure becomes positive (up to 10 kPa). This compresses the central airways, but the smaller airways do not close off because the driving pressure for expiratory flow (alveolar pressure) is also increased.

Flow–volume loops

The relationship between maximal flow rates and lung volume is demonstrated by the maximal flow–volume (MFV) loop (**Fig. 28.6A**).

In subjects with healthy lungs, maximal flow rates are rarely achieved even during vigorous exercise. However, in patients with severe COPD, limitation of expiratory flow occurs even during tidal breathing at rest (**Fig. 28.6B**). To increase ventilation, these patients have to breathe at higher lung volumes and allow more time for

expiration, both of which reduce the tendency for airway collapse. To compensate, they increase flow rates during inspiration, where there is relatively less flow limitation.

The volume that can be forced in from the residual volume in 1 second (FIV₁) will always be greater than that which can be forced out from TLC in 1 second (FEV₁). Thus, the ratio of FEV₁ to FIV₁ is less than 1. The only exception to this is when there is significant obstruction to the airways outside the thorax, such as tracheal tumour or retrosternal goitre. Expiratory airway narrowing is prevented by tracheal resistance, and expiratory airflow becomes more effort-dependent. During forced inspiration, this same resistance causes such negative intraluminal pressure that the trachea is compressed by the surrounding atmospheric pressure. Inspiratory flow thus becomes less effort-dependent, and the ratio of FEV₁ to FIV₁ is greater than 1. This phenomenon, and the characteristic flow–volume loop, are diagnostic of extrathoracic airways obstruction (**Fig. 28.6C**).

Ventilation and perfusion relationships

For optimum gas exchange there must be a match between ventilation of the alveoli ($\dot{V}$) and their perfusion ($\dot{Q}$). However, in reality there is variation in the ($\dot{V}_A/\dot{Q}$) ratio in both normal and diseased lungs (**Fig. 28.7**). In the normal lung, both ventilation and perfusion are greater at the bases than at the apices but the gradient for perfusion is steeper, so the net effect is that ventilation exceeds perfusion towards the apices while perfusion exceeds ventilation at the bases. Other

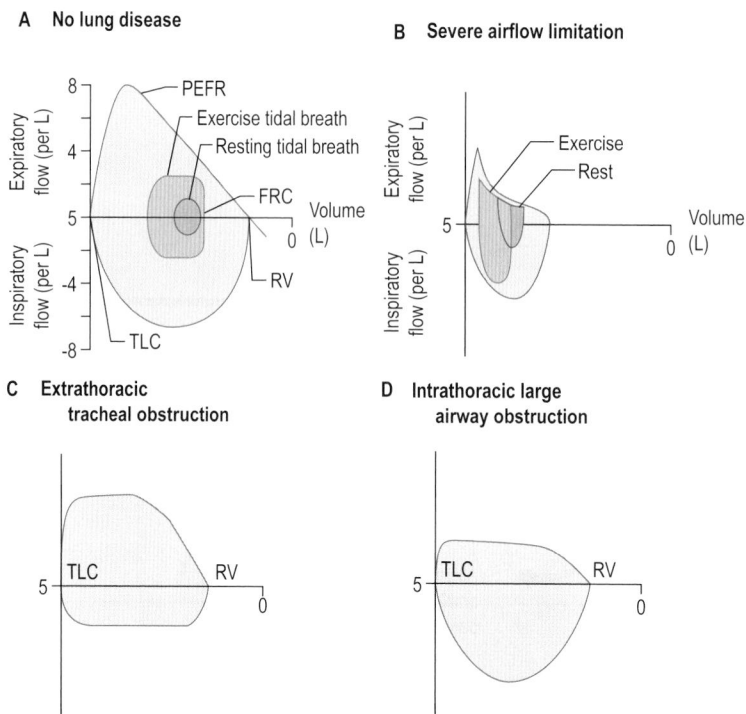

Fig. 28.6 Flow–volume loops. **(A–B)** *Maximal flow–volume loops*, showing the relationship between maximal flow rates on expiration and inspiration. **(A)** *Normal subject*. **(B)** *Severe airflow limitation*. Flow–volume loops during tidal breathing at rest (starting from the functional residual capacity, FRC) and during exercise are also shown. The highest flow rates are achieved when forced expiration begins at total lung capacity (TLC) and represent the peak expiratory flow rate (PEFR). As air is blown out of the lung, so the flow rate decreases until no more air can be forced out, a point known as the residual volume (RV). Because inspiratory airflow is dependent only on effort, the shape of the maximal inspiratory flow–volume loop is quite different, and inspiratory flow remains at a high rate throughout the manoeuvre. **(C–D)** *Flow–volume loops in large airway (tracheal) obstruction*, showing plateauing of maximal expiratory flow. **(C)** *Extrathoracic tracheal obstruction* with a proportionally greater reduction of maximal inspiratory (as opposed to expiratory) flow rate. **(D)** *Intrathoracic large airway obstruction*; the expiratory plateau is more pronounced and inspiratory flow rate is less reduced than in **(C)**. In *severe airflow limitation*, the ventilatory demands of exercise cannot be met (compare A, B), greatly reducing effort tolerance.

causes of mismatch include direct shunting of deoxygenated blood through the lung without passing through alveoli (e.g. the bronchial circulation) and areas of lung that receive no blood (e.g. anatomical deadspace, bullae and areas of under-perfusion during acceleration and deceleration, e.g. in aircraft and high-performance cars).

An increased physiological shunt results in arterial hypoxaemia since it is not possible to compensate for some of the blood being under-oxygenated by increasing ventilation of the well-perfused areas. An increased physiological deadspace just increases the work of breathing and has less impact on blood gases since the normally perfused alveoli are well ventilated. In more advanced disease this compensation cannot occur, leading to increased alveolar and arterial PCO_2 (P_aCO_2), together with hypoxaemia, which cannot be compensated for by increasing ventilation.

Hypoxaemia occurs more readily than hypercapnia because of the different ways in which oxygen and carbon dioxide are carried in the blood. Carbon dioxide is carried in three forms (in bicarbonate, in carbamino compounds and in simple solution) but the volume carried is proportional to the partial pressure of CO_2. Oxygen is carried in chemical combination with haemoglobin in the red blood cells, with a non-linear relationship between the volume carried and the partial pressure. Alveolar hyperventilation reduces the alveolar PCO_2 (P_ACO_2) and diffusion leads to a proportional fall in the carbon dioxide content of the blood (P_aCO_2). However, as the haemoglobin is already saturated with oxygen, increasing the alveolar PO_2 through hyperventilation will not increase blood oxygen content. This means that hypoxaemia due to physiological shunting cannot be compensated for by hyperventilation.

In individuals who have mild degrees of mismatch the P_aO_2 and P_aCO_2 will still be normal at rest. Increasing the requirements for gas exchange by exercise will widen the mismatch and the P_aO_2 will fall. Mismatch is by far the most common cause of arterial hypoxaemia.

Alveolar stability

Pulmonary alveoli are polygonal spaces within a sponge-like matrix. Surface tension acting at the curved internal surface tends to cause the alveoli to decrease in size. The surface tension within the alveoli would make the lungs extremely difficult to distend, were it not for the presence of surfactant, which reduces surface tension so that alveoli remain stable.

Defence mechanisms of the respiratory tract

Pulmonary disease often results from a failure of the normal host defence mechanisms of the healthy lung (**Fig. 28.8**). These can be divided into physical, physiological, humoral and cellular mechanisms.

Physical and physiological mechanisms
Humidification

This prevents dehydration of the epithelium.

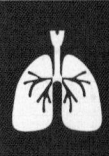

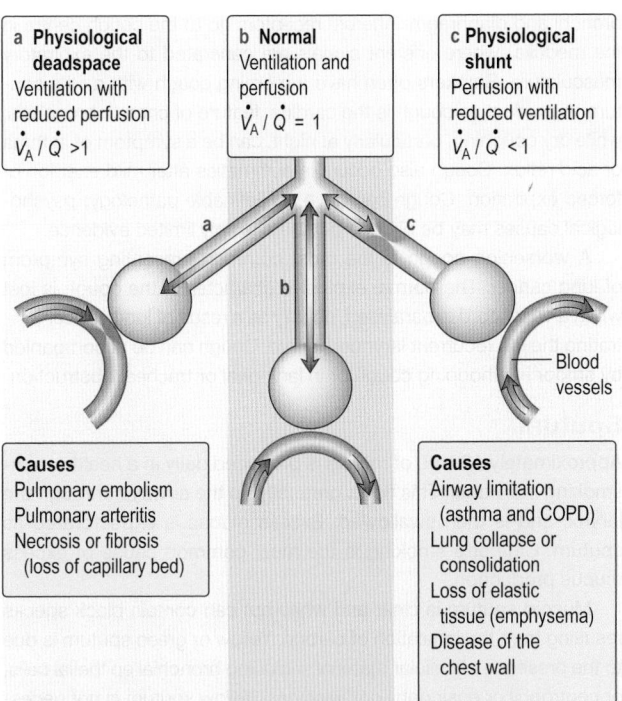

Fig. 28.7 Relationships between ventilation and perfusion: the alveolar–capillary interface. The *centre* **(b)** shows *normal ventilation* and perfusion. On the left **(a)** there is a *block in perfusion (physiological deadspace)*, while on the right **(c)** there is *reduced ventilation (physiological shunting)*. COPD, chronic obstructive pulmonary disease.

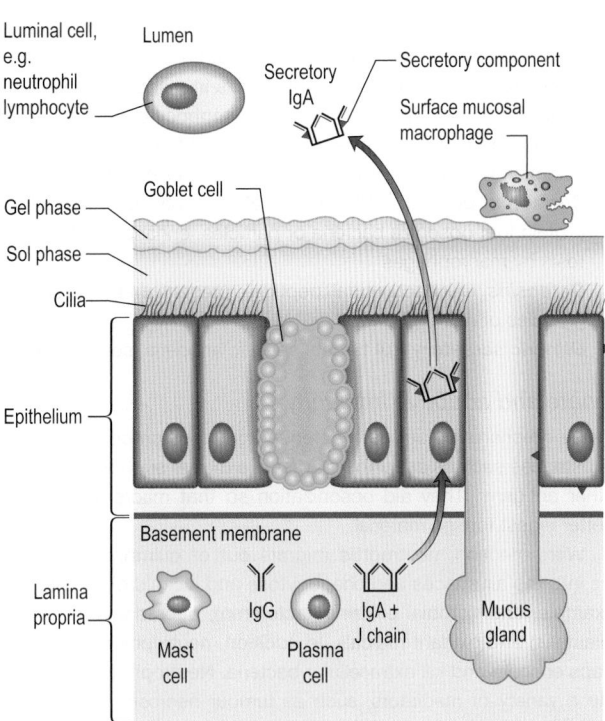

Fig. 28.8 Defence mechanisms present at the epithelial surface.

Particle removal

Over 90% of particles of more than 10 μm in diameter are removed in the nostril or nasopharynx. This includes most pollen grains, which are typically greater than 20 μm in diameter. Particles between 5 and 10 μm become impacted at the carina. Particles of less than 1 μm tend to remain airborne: thus the particles capable of reaching the deep lung are those in the 1–5 μm range.

Particle expulsion

This is facilitated by coughing, sneezing or gagging.

Respiratory tract secretions

The mucus of the respiratory tract is a gelatinous substance consisting of water and highly glycosylated proteins (mucins). The mucus forms a thick gel that is relatively impermeable to water and floats on a liquid or sol layer found around the cilia of the epithelial cells (see **Fig. 28.8**). The gel layer is secreted from goblet cells and mucus glands as distinct globules that coalesce increasingly in the central airways to form a more or less continuous mucus blanket. In addition to the mucins, the gel contains various antimicrobial molecules (lysozyme, defensins), specific antibodies (IgA) and cytokines, which are secreted by cells in airways and are incorporated into the mucus gel. Bacteria, viruses and other particles become trapped in the mucus and are either inactivated or simply expelled before they can do any damage. Under normal conditions the tips of the cilia engage with the undersurface of the gel phase and by coordinated movement they push the mucus blanket upwards and outwards to the pharynx, where it is either swallowed or coughed up. One of the major long-term effects of cigarette smoking is a reduction in mucociliary transport. This contributes to recurrent infection and prolongs contact with carcinogenic material. Air pollutants, local and general anaesthetics, and products of bacterial and viral infection also reduce mucociliary clearance.

Congenital defects in mucociliary transport (cystic fibrosis and immotile cilia syndrome) lead to recurrent infections and eventually to bronchiectasis.

The respiratory microbiome

It has always been thought that the lower respiratory tract is sterile. Recent evidence has shown that there is a resident bacterial flora that is very similar to that of the mouth. The composition of the respiratory microbiome is determined by three factors:

- *microbial immigration*, e.g. by inhalation, or microaspiration from the gastrointestinal tract
- *local growth conditions* for the bacteria, e.g. temperature, pH, nutrients, concentration and activation of local inflammatory cells, and epithelial cell interactions
- *microbial elimination* by the usual mechanisms, i.e. the mucociliary escalator, coughing and the innate and adaptive humoral mechanisms.

All of these factors will change in both acute and chronic lung conditions when there is an increase in pathological bacteria. This respiratory tract dysbiosis causes a dysregulation of the local immune response and favours the growth of bacteria: for example, in the exacerbation of chronic diseases in which inflammation is perpetuated. The background composition of the bacterial microbiome in different conditions might favour exacerbations.

Humoral and cellular mechanisms
Non-specific soluble factors

- *Alpha-antitrypsin* (α_1-antiprotease, see p. 1302) in lung secretions is derived from plasma. It inhibits chymotrypsin and trypsin, and neutralizes proteases, including neutrophil elastase.
- *Antioxidant defences* include enzymes such as superoxide dismutase and low-molecular-weight antioxidant molecules (ascorbate, urate) in the epithelial lining fluid.
- *Lysozyme* is an enzyme found in granulocytes that has bactericidal properties.

- *Lactoferrin* is synthesized from epithelial cells and neutrophil granulocytes, and has bactericidal properties.
- *Interferons* are produced by most cells in response to viral infection and are potent modulators of lymphocyte function.
- *Complement* in secretions is also derived from plasma. In association with antibodies, it plays a major role in cytotoxicity.
- *Surfactant protein A* (SPA) is one of four species of surfactant protein that opsonize bacteria or particles, enhancing phagocytosis by macrophages.
- *Defensins* are bactericidal peptides present in the azurophil granules of neutrophils.
- *Dimeric secretory IgA* targets specific antigens (see p. 1155).

Innate and adaptive immunity

These mechanisms act as a defence against microbes, inorganic substances such as asbestos, particulate matter such as dust, and other antigens. They aid opsonization so that macrophages can better ingest foreign material.

With infection, neutrophils migrate out of pulmonary capillaries into the air spaces and phagocytose and kill microbes with, for example, antimicrobial proteins (lactoferrin), degradative enzymes (elastase) and oxidant radicals. In addition, neutrophil extracellular traps ensnare and kill extracellular bacteria. Neutrophils also generate a variety of mediators, such as tumour necrosis factor alpha (TNF-α), interleukin 1 (IL-1), and chemokines that attract further inflammatory cells that assist with adaptive immunity.

Microbes are detected by host cells by pattern recognition receptors, such as toll-like receptors. These act via nuclear factor kappa B (NF-κB) transcription factors in the epithelial cells to produce adhesion molecules, chemokines and colony stimulating factors to initiate inflammation. Inflammation is necessary for innate immunity and host defence but can lead to lung damage; there is a fine line between defence and injury.

Further reading

Fahy JV, Dickey BF. Airway mucus function and dysfunction. *N Engl J Med* 2010; 363:2233–2247.
Kiley JP, Caler EV. The lung microbiome: a new frontier in pulmonary medicine. *Ann Am Thorac Soc* 2014; 11(Suppl 1):S66–S70.

CLINICAL APPROACH TO THE PATIENT WITH RESPIRATORY DISEASE

Clinical features of respiratory disease

Runny, blocked nose and sneezing

Nasal symptoms are extremely common; 'runny nose' (rhinorrhoea), nasal blockage and attacks of sneezing can be caused by allergic rhinitis (see p. 945) and by common colds (p. 945). Nasal secretions are usually thin and runny in allergic rhinitis but thicker and discoloured with viral infections. Nose bleeds and blood-stained nasal discharge are common and rarely indicate serious pathology. However, a blood-stained nasal discharge associated with nasal obstruction and pain may be the presenting feature of a nasal tumour (see p. 908). Nasal polyps typically present with nasal blockage and loss of smell.

Cough

Cough (see also p. 908) is the most common symptom of lower respiratory tract disease. It is caused by mechanical or chemical stimulation of cough receptors in the epithelium of the pharynx, larynx, trachea,

bronchi and diaphragm. Afferent receptors go to the cough centre in the medulla, where efferent signals are generated to the expiratory musculature. Smokers often have a morning cough with a little sputum. A productive cough is the cardinal feature of chronic bronchitis, while dry coughing, particularly at night, can be a symptom of asthma or acid reflux. Cough also occurs in asthmatics after mild exertion or forced expiration. Cough can have no definable pathology; psychological causes may be blamed but there is only limited evidence.

A worsening cough is the most common presenting symptom of lung cancer. The normal explosive character of the cough is lost when a vocal cord is paralysed, usually as a result of lung cancer infiltrating the left recurrent laryngeal nerve. Cough can be accompanied by stridor in whooping cough or in laryngeal or tracheal obstruction.

Sputum

Approximately 100 mL of mucus is produced daily in a healthy, non-smoking individual. This flows gradually up the airways, through the larynx, and is then swallowed. Excess mucus is expectorated as sputum. Cigarette smoking is the most common cause of excess mucus production.

Mucoid sputum is clear and white but can contain black specks resulting from the inhalation of carbon. Yellow or green sputum is due to the presence of cellular material, including bronchial epithelial cells, or neutrophil or eosinophil granulocytes. Yellow sputum is not necessarily due to infection, since granulocytes in the sputum, as seen in asthma, can give the same appearance. The production of large quantities of yellow or green sputum is characteristic of bronchiectasis.

Haemoptysis

Haemoptysis (blood-stained sputum) varies from small streaks of blood to massive bleeding. The most common cause of mild haemoptysis is acute infection (**Box 28.3**), particularly in exacerbations of COPD, but this should not be assumed without investigation. Other common causes are pulmonary infarction (e.g. secondary to pulmonary embolism), bronchial carcinoma and tuberculosis. Pink, frothy sputum is seen in pulmonary oedema, while in bronchiectasis the blood is often mixed with purulent sputum. Massive haemoptysis (>200 mL of blood in 24 h) is usually due to bronchiectasis or tuberculosis, but can also be caused in later stages of lung cancer.

Although a diagnosis can often be made from a chest X-ray (e.g. bronchiectasis, tuberculosis), a normal chest X-ray does not exclude serious disease. However, if the chest X-ray is normal, CT scanning and bronchoscopy are diagnostic in only about 5% of patients with haemoptysis.

> **? Box 28.3 Causes of haemoptysis**
>
> - Malignancy and benign lung tumours, including lung metastasis
> - Pulmonary infection, including bacterial pneumonia, tuberculosis, lung abscesses and fungal infection
> - Bronchiectasis, including cystic fibrosis
> - Pulmonary emboli
> - Congestive heart failure
> - Pulmonary fibrosis
> - Pulmonary vasculitis, e.g. Goodpasture's syndrome, microscopic polyangiitis
> - Severe pulmonary hypertension
> - Arteriovenous malformation
> - Chest trauma and foreign bodies
> - Endometriosis
> - Anticoagulation, coagulopathy
> - Drugs, e.g. cocaine, thrombolytics

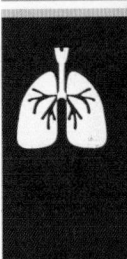

? Box 28.4 Causes of breathlessness

Acute
- Airways obstruction
- Anaphylaxis
- Asthma
- Pneumothorax
- Pulmonary embolus
- Myocardial infarction
- Pulmonary oedema
- Arrhythmias
- Anxiety

Subacute
- Pneumonia
- Exacerbation of COPD
- Angina
- Cardiac tamponade

- Metabolic acidosis
- Pain
- Pontine haemorrhage

Chronic
- COPD
- Pleural effusion
- Malignancy
- Chronic pulmonary emboli
- Restrictive lung disorders
- Congestive cardiac failure
- Valvular dysfunction
- Cardiomyopathy
- Anaemia
- Neuromuscular disorders
- Deconditioning

COPD, chronic obstructive pulmonary disease.

i Box 28.5 Medical Research Council grading of dyspnoea (breathlessness scale)

1. Not troubled by breathlessness, except on strenuous exercise
2. Short of breath when hurrying or walking up a slight hill
3. Walks slower than contemporaries on the level because of breathlessness, or has to stop for breath when walking at own pace
4. Stops for breath after about 100 m or after a few minutes on the level
5. Too breathless to leave the house, or breathless when dressing or undressing

Breathlessness

Dyspnoea (breathlessness) is a sense of awareness of increased respiratory effort that is unpleasant and recognized by the patient as inappropriate. Patients often complain of tightness in the chest; this must be differentiated from angina (**Box 28.4**). The degree of breathlessness should be assessed in relation to the patient's lifestyle. For example, a moderate degree of breathlessness will be totally disabling if the patient has to climb many flights of stairs to reach home. Breathlessness can be graded using the Medical Research Council grading of dyspnoea (**Box 28.5**).

Orthopnoea (see p. 1028) is breathlessness on lying down. While it is classically linked to heart failure, it is partly due to the weight of the abdominal contents pushing the diaphragm up into the thorax. Such patients may also become breathless on bending over.

Tachypnoea and *hyperpnoea* are, respectively, an increased rate of breathing and an increased level of ventilation. These may be appropriate responses (e.g. during exercise).

Hyperventilation is inappropriate overbreathing. This may occur at rest or on exertion, and results in a lowering of the alveolar and arterial PCO_2 (see **Box 25.33**).

Paroxysmal nocturnal dyspnoea (see p. 1028) describes acute episodes of breathlessness at night, typically due to heart failure.

Wheezing

Wheezing is a common complaint and results from airflow limitation due to any cause. The symptom of wheezing is not diagnostic of asthma; other causes include vocal cord dysfunction, bronchiolitis and COPD. Conversely, wheeze may be absent in the early stages of asthma.

Chest pain

The most common type of chest pain reported in respiratory disease is a localized sharp pain, often termed pleuritic. It is made worse by deep breathing or coughing and the patient can usually

i Box 28.6 Signs to look for in the hands

- Clubbing
- Pallor
- Warm, well-perfused palms (CO_2 retention)
- Cyanosis
- Flap
- Tremor
- Tobacco staining
- Bruising and/or thin skin
- Pulse rate and character

localize it. Localized anterior chest pain with tenderness of a costochondral junction is caused by costochondritis. Shoulder tip pain suggests irritation of the diaphragmatic pleura, while central chest pain radiating to the neck and arms is likely to be cardiac. Retrosternal soreness is associated with tracheitis, and malignant invasion of the chest wall causes a constant, severe, dull pain.

Examination of the respiratory system

Nose

See page 907.

Chest

Inspection

Observe the patient as they enter the room or move around the bed. Are they simply breathless at rest? Do they have a cough or are they wheezy? Assessment should be made of mental alertness, cyanosis, breathlessness at rest, use of accessory muscles, shape of the chest wall, any deformity or scars on the chest and movement on both sides. Kyphosis and scoliosis of the spine can cause asymmetry of the chest. CO_2 intoxication causes coarse tremor or flap of the outstretched hands. Prominent veins on the chest may imply obstruction of the superior vena cava. The patient's face may reveal signs of anaemia, or there may be a Horner's syndrome due to a Pancoast tumour.

Respiratory rate and rhythm may be altered; the normal respiratory rate is 14–16 breaths per minute. Tachypnoea is an increased respiratory rate. Apnoea is the absence of breathing; some patients have episodes of apnoea during sleep.

Hands should be inspected for evidence of tobacco staining on the fingers, clubbing or a fine tremor (**Box 28.6**).

Cyanosis (see p. 1030) is a dusky discoloration of the skin and mucous membranes, due to the presence of more than 50 g/L of desaturated haemoglobin. When it has a central cause, cyanosis is visible on the tongue (especially the underside) and lips. Patients with central cyanosis will also be cyanosed peripherally. Peripheral cyanosis without central cyanosis is caused by a reduced peripheral circulation and is noted on the fingernails and skin of the extremities, with associated coolness of the skin.

Finger clubbing is present when the normal angle between the base of the nail and the nail fold is lost (**Fig. 28.9**). The base of the nail is fluctuant owing to increased vascularity, and there is an increased curvature of the nail in all directions, with expansion of the end of the digit. Some causes of clubbing are given in **Box 28.7**. Clubbing is not a feature of uncomplicated COPD.

Palpation and percussion

The position of the trachea and apex beat should be checked. The supraclavicular fossa, cervical chains and axilla are examined for enlarged lymph nodes. The distance between the sternal notch and the cricoid cartilage (3–4 finger-breadths in full expiration) is reduced in patients with severe airflow limitation. Chest expansion should be checked; a tape measure may be used if precise or serial measurements are needed, such as in **ankylosing spondylitis**. Local discomfort over the sternochondral joints suggests costochondritis.

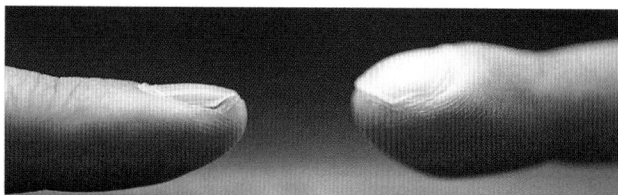

Fig. 28.9 Clubbing deformity. The finger on the right is clubbed compared with the normal-shaped finger on the left. *(From Hochberg MC, Gravallese EM, Silman AJ et al. Rheumatology, 7th edn. Elsevier Inc.; 2019; Fig. 213.2.)*

? Box 28.7 Some causes of finger clubbing

Respiratory
- Bronchial carcinoma, including hypertrophic pulmonary osteoarthropathy
- Chronic suppurative lung disease:
  - Bronchiectasis
  - Lung abscess
  - Empyema
- Idiopathic lung fibrosis
- Pleural and mediastinal tumours (e.g. mesothelioma)
- Cryptogenic organizing pneumonia

Cardiovascular
- Cyanotic heart disease
- Subacute infective endocarditis
- Atrial myxoma

Miscellaneous
- Congenital – no disease
- Cirrhosis
- Inflammatory bowel disease
- Thyroid acropachy

In rib fractures, compression of the chest laterally and anteroposteriorly produces localized pain. On percussion, liver dullness is usually detected anteriorly at the level of the sixth rib. Liver and cardiac dullness disappear when the lungs are over-inflated (**Box 28.8**).

Auscultation

The patient is asked to take deep breaths through the mouth. Inspiration should be more prolonged than expiration. Normal breath sounds are caused by turbulent flow in the larynx and sound harsher anteriorly over the upper lobes (particularly on the right). Healthy lungs filter out most of the high-frequency component, and the resulting sounds are called vesicular.

If the lung is consolidated or collapsed, the high-frequency hissing components of breath are not attenuated and can be heard as 'bronchial breathing'. Similar sounds may be heard over areas of localized fibrosis or bronchiectasis. Bronchial breathing is accompanied by whispering pectoriloquy (whispered, high-pitched sounds can be heard distinctly through a stethoscope).

Added sounds

Wheeze. Wheeze results from vibrations in the collapsible part of the airways when the large and medium-sized bronchi become constricted. It is usually heard during expiration and is commonly, but not invariably, present in asthma and COPD. In acute severe asthma, wheeze may not be heard, as airflow may be insufficient to generate the sound. Wheezes may be monophonic (single large airway obstruction) or polyphonic (narrowing of many small airways). An end-inspiratory wheeze or 'squeak' may be heard in obliterative bronchiolitis.

Crackles. These brief crackling sounds are probably produced by opening of previously closed bronchioles; early inspiratory crackles are associated with diffuse airflow limitation, while late inspiratory crackles are characteristically heard in pulmonary oedema, lung fibrosis and bronchiectasis.

Pleural rub. This creaking or groaning sound is usually well localized (said to sound like a foot crunching through fresh-fallen snow). It indicates inflammation and roughening of the pleural surfaces, which normally glide silently over one another, and is heard in association with lung infections and consolidation.

i Box 28.8 Physical signs of respiratory disease

Pathological process	Mediastinal displacement	Percussion note	Breath sounds	Vocal resonance	Added sounds
Consolidation (i.e. lobar pneumonia)	None	Dull	Bronchial	Increased	Fine crackles
Collapse					
Major bronchus	Towards lesion	Dull	Diminished or absent	Reduced or absent	None
Peripheral bronchus	Towards lesion	Dull	Bronchial	Increased	Fine crackles
Fibrosis					
Localized	Towards lesion	Dull	Bronchial	Increased	Coarse crackles
Generalized (e.g. idiopathic lung fibrosis)	None	Normal	Vesicular	Increased	Fine crackles
Pleural effusion (>500 mL)	Away from lesion (in massive effusion)	Stony dull	Vesicular reduced or absent	Reduced or absent	None
Large pneumothorax	Away from lesion	Normal or hyper-resonant	Reduced or absent	Reduced or absent	None
Asthma	None	Normal	Vesicular Prolonged expiration	Normal	Expiratory polyphonic wheeze
Chronic obstructive pulmonary disease	None	Normal	Vesicular Prolonged expiration	Normal	Expiratory polyphonic wheeze and coarse crackles
Bronchiectasis	None	Normal	Vesicular	Normal	Coarse crackles

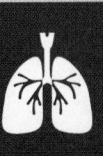

Check

- *Centring of the image.* The distance between each clavicular head and the spinal processes should be equal.
- *Penetration.* Make sure the image is not too dark and adjust the contrast.
- *View:*
  - *Postero-anterior (PA) views* are used for routine images; the X-ray source is behind the patient.
  - *Anteroposterior (AP) views* are used only in patients who are unable to stand or cannot be taken to the radiology department; the cardiac outline appears bigger and the scapulae cannot be moved out of the way.
  - *Lateral views* were used to localize pathology but have been replaced by CT scans.

Look at

- Shape and bony structure of the chest wall
- Centrality of the trachea
- Elevation/flatness of the diaphragm
- Shape, size and position of the heart
- Shape and size of the hilar shadows
- Shape and size of any lung abnormalities
- Vascular shadowing

Vocal resonance. Healthy lung attenuates high-frequency notes, as compared to the lower-pitched components of speech. Consolidated lung has the reverse effect, transmitting high frequencies well; the spoken word then takes on a bleating quality. Whispered (and therefore high-pitched) speech can be clearly heard over consolidated areas, as compared to healthy lung. Low-frequency sounds such as 'ninety-nine' are well transmitted across healthy lung to produce vibration that can be felt over the chest wall. Consolidated lung transmits these low-frequency noises less well, and pleural fluid severely dampens or obliterates the vibrations altogether. Tactile vocal fremitus is the palpation of this vibration, usually by placing the edge of the hand on the chest wall. For all practical purposes, this duplicates the assessment of vocal resonance and is not routinely performed as part of the chest examination.

Cardiovascular system examination

This gives additional information about the lungs (see p. 1029).

Additional bedside tests

Review the patient's observation chart, particularly oxygen saturations and the concentration of additional oxygen that the patient may be receiving. Inspect any sputum pots. Since so many patients with respiratory disease have airflow limitation, airflow should be routinely measured using a peak flow meter or spirometer. This is a much more useful assessment of airflow limitation than any physical sign.

Investigation of respiratory disease

Imaging

Imaging is essential in the investigation of most chest symptoms. Some diseases, such as tuberculosis or lung cancer, may be undetectable on clinical examination but may be obvious on the chest X-ray. Conversely, asthma or chronic bronchitis may be associated with a normal chest X-ray. Always try to obtain previous images for comparison.

Chest X-ray

See **Box 28.9** and **Fig. 28.1**.

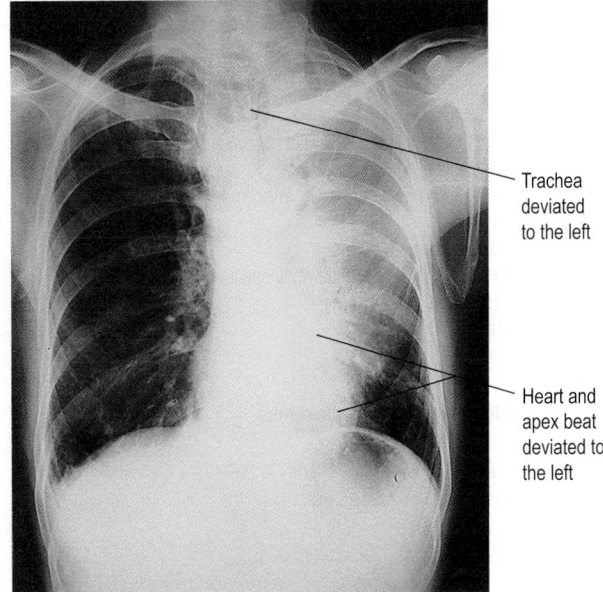

Trachea deviated to the left

Heart and apex beat deviated to the left

Fig. 28.10 Collapse of the left upper lobe. Chest X-ray showing increased opacification in the left upper and mid zone with evidence of left-sided volume loss.

- Enlarged tracheobronchial lymph nodes due to malignant disease or tuberculosis
- Inhaled foreign bodies (e.g. peanuts) in children, usually in the right main bronchus
- Bronchial casts or plugs (e.g. allergic bronchopulmonary aspergillosis)
- Retained secretions postoperatively and in debilitated patients

Collapse and consolidation

Simple pneumonia is easy to recognize (see **Fig. 28.28**) but a careful search should be made for any evidence of collapse (**Fig. 28.10** and **Box 28.10**). Loss of volume or crowding of the ribs is the best indicator of lobar collapse. The lung lobes collapse in characteristic directions:

- The lower lobes collapse downwards and towards the mediastinum.
- The left upper lobe collapses forwards against the anterior chest wall.
- The right upper lobe collapses upwards and inwards, giving the appearance of an arch over the remaining lung.
- The right middle lobe collapses anteriorly and inwards, obscuring the right heart border.
- If a whole lung collapses, the mediastinum will shift towards the side of the collapse.

  Uncomplicated consolidation does not cause mediastinal shift or loss of lung volume, and so any of these features should raise the suspicion of an endobronchial obstruction.

Pleural effusion

Pleural effusions (see **Fig. 28.31**) need to be larger than 500 mL to cause much more than blunting of the costophrenic angle. On an erect film, they produce a characteristic shadow with a curved upper edge rising into the axilla. If they are very large, the whole of one hemithorax may be opaque, with mediastinal shift away from the effusion.

? **Box 28.11** Causes of round shadows (>3 cm) in the lung

- Carcinoma
- Metastatic tumours (usually multiple shadows)
- Lung abscess (usually with fluid level)
- Encysted interlobar effusion (usually in horizontal fissure)
- Hydatid cysts (often with a fluid level)
- Arteriovenous malformations (usually adjacent to a vascular shadow)
- Aspergilloma
- Rheumatoid nodules
- Tuberculoma (may be calcification within the lesion)
- Bronchial carcinoid
- Cylindroma
- Chondroma
- Lipoma

Other shadows related to mediastinum
- Pericardium ⎤
- Oesophagus ⎬ Can be characterised by performing a lateral chest X-ray
- Spinal cord ⎦

Fibrosis

Localized fibrosis produces streaky shadowing, and the accompanying loss of lung volume causes mediastinal structures to move to the same side. More generalized fibrosis can lead to a honeycomb appearance (see p. 988), seen as diffuse shadows containing multiple circular translucencies a few millimetres in diameter.

Round shadows

Lung cancer is the most common cause of large round shadows but many other aetiologies are recognized (**Box 28.11**).

Miliary mottling

This term, derived from the Latin for millet, describes numerous minute opacities, 1–3 mm in size. The most common causes are tuberculosis, pneumoconiosis, sarcoidosis, idiopathic pulmonary fibrosis and pulmonary oedema (see **Fig. 30.15**), although pulmonary oedema is usually perihilar and accompanied by larger, fluffy shadows. Pulmonary microlithiasis is a rare but striking cause of miliary mottling.

Computed tomography

Computed tomography (CT) provides excellent images of the lungs and mediastinal structures (**Fig. 28.11**). It is essential in staging bronchial carcinoma by demonstrating tumour size, nodal involvement, metastases and invasion of mediastinum, pleura or chest wall. CT-guided needle biopsy allows samples to be obtained from peripheral masses. Staging scans should assess liver and adrenals, which are common sites for metastatic disease. Mediastinal structures are shown more clearly after injecting intravenous contrast medium.

High-resolution CT (HRCT) samples lung parenchyma with 1–2 mm thickness scans at 10–20 mm intervals and is used to assess diffuse inflammatory and infective parenchymal processes. HRCT scanning does not require any intravenous contrast. It is valuable in:

- evaluation of diffuse disease of the lung parenchyma, including sarcoidosis, hypersensitivity pneumonitis, occupational lung disease and any other form of interstitial pulmonary fibrosis
- diagnosis of bronchiectasis, having a sensitivity and specificity of >90%
- distinction of emphysema from diffuse parenchymal lung disease or pulmonary vascular disease as a cause of a low gas transfer factor with otherwise normal lung function
- suspected opportunist lung infection in immunocompromised patients
- diagnosis of lymphangitis carcinomatosa.

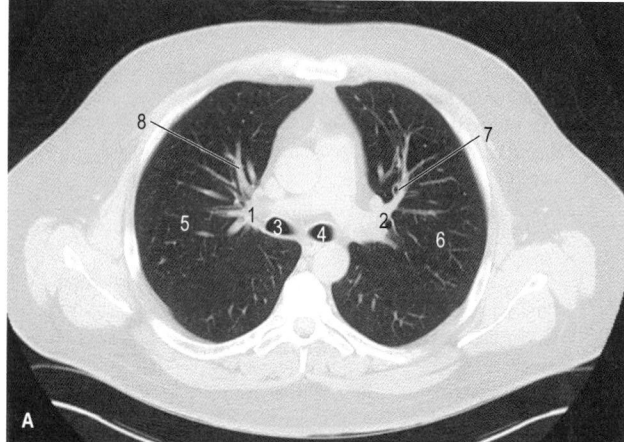
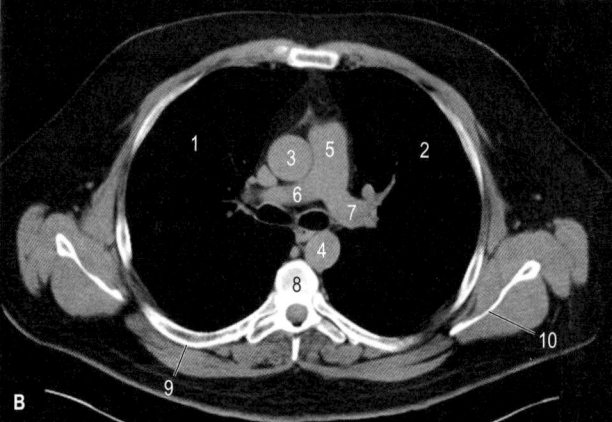
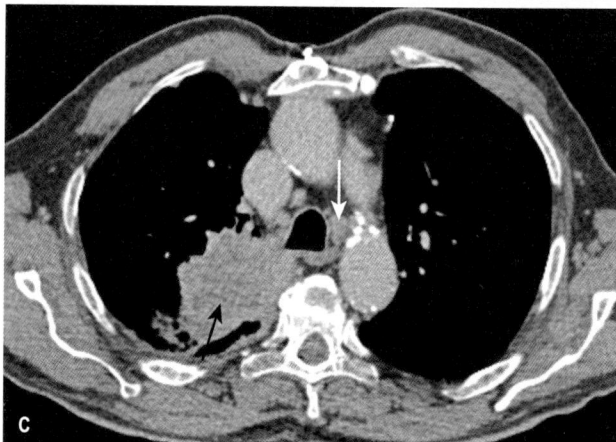

Fig. 28.11 Computed tomography scans of the lung. **(A)** Axial CT image of the thorax on lung settings. (1) Right hilum; (2) left hilum; (3) right main bronchus; (4) left main bronchus; (5) right lung; (6) left lung; (7) bronchus; (8) blood vessel. **(B)** Axial CT image of the thorax on soft tissue settings. (1) Right lung; (2) left lung; (3) ascending aorta; (4) descending aorta; (5) pulmonary trunk; (6) right pulmonary artery; (7) left pulmonary artery; (8) vertebra; (9) rib; (10) scapula. **(C)** CT chest demonstrates a right upper lobe carcinoma that is invading the mediastinum (black arrow) and prominent mediastinal lymph nodes (white arrow).

Multi-slice CT scanners can produce detailed images in two or three dimensions in any plane. This detail is particularly useful for the detection of pulmonary emboli. Pulmonary nodules and airway disease are more easily defined, reducing the need for HRCT.

CT pulmonary angiography (CTPA) is used to investigate for pulmonary embolism and enables visualization of the pulmonary

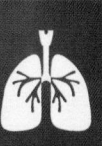

arteries. Contrast is injected and images are taken in timed fashion, so that the contrast agent is in the pulmonary circulation.

Magnetic resonance imaging

Magnetic resonance imaging (MRI) with electrocardiography (ECG) gating allows accurate imaging of the heart and aortic aneurysms. MRI has been used in staging lung cancer and assessing tumour invasion in the mediastinum and chest wall and at the lung apex because it produces good images in the sagittal and coronal planes. Vascular structures can be clearly differentiated, as flowing blood produces a signal void on MRI. Traditionally, MRI has been less useful than CT in parenchymal lung disease; however, it may have a place in interstitial lung disease assessment in the future.

Positron emission tomography–computed tomography

PET-CT combines a CT scan and positron emission tomography. Positron-emitting isotopes such as ^{18}fluorodeoxyglucose (^{18}FDG) are used as contrast and are taken up rapidly by metabolically active tissue such as lung cancers. PET imaging is used for lung cancer staging prior to curative treatment such as surgery or radiotherapy. FDG-PET can also be useful in determining an appropriate site for a biopsy and can often assist with differentiating benign from malignant tumours; however, inflammatory lesions may also be FDG-avid.

Scintigraphic imaging

Isotopic lung scans were widely used for the detection of pulmonary emboli but are now performed less often, owing to the widespread use of CTPA. They are discussed in more detail on page 1005.

Ultrasound

Two-dimensional transthoracic ultrasound is a technique used for assessing a pleural effusion. Ultrasound confirms the presence of pleural fluid and provides details about the nature of the effusion, such as whether it is a simple pleural effusion (single collection), heavily loculated with adhesions or organized (more gelatinous). Ultrasound assists in determining the best site for aspiration and it is recommended that any invasive pleural procedure, such as pleural aspiration and intercostal chest drain placement, is performed with ultrasound screening. Ultrasound-guided biopsy is used for lung masses that abut the pleura or pleural masses, if appropriate. It is also used in bronchoscopy (endobronchial ultrasound, EBUS) to stage and sample mediastinal lymph nodes (see p. 944).

Respiratory function tests

In clinical practice, airflow limitation can be assessed by relatively simple tests that have good intra-subject repeatability (**Box 28.12**). Results must be compared with predicted values for healthy subjects, as normal ranges vary with sex, age, height and ethnic group. Moreover, there is considerable variation between healthy individuals of the same size and age; the standard deviation for the PEFR is approximately 50 L/min, and for the FEV_1 approximately 0.4 L. Repeated measurements of lung function are useful for assessing the progression of disease in individual patients.

Tests of ventilatory function

These tests are used mainly to assess the degree of airflow limitation during expiration.

Spirometry

The patient takes a maximum inspiration followed by a forced expiration (for as long as possible) into the spirometer. The spirometer measures the 1-second forced expiratory volume (FEV_1) and the total volume of exhaled gas (forced vital capacity, FVC). Both FEV_1 and FVC are related to height, age, sex and ethnicity, and help to differentiate between an obstructive and a restrictive pattern of respiratory compromise (**Fig. 28.12**; **Box 28.13**).

In chronic airflow limitation (particularly COPD and asthma), the total lung capacity (TLC) is usually increased, yet there is nearly always some reduction in the FVC. This is because collapse of small

Box 28.12 Respiratory function and exercise tests			
Test	**Use**	**Advantages**	**Disadvantages**
PEFR	Monitoring changes in airflow limitation in asthma	Portable Can be used at the bedside	Effort-dependent Poor measure of chronic airflow limitation
FEV, FVC, FEV₁/FVC	Assessment of airflow limitation (the best single test)	Reproducible Relatively effort-independent	Bulky equipment but smaller portable machines available
Flow–volume curves	Assessment of flow at lower lung volumes Detection of large-airway obstruction, both intra- and extrathoracic (e.g. tracheal stenosis, tumour)	Recognizes patterns of flow–volume curves for different diseases	Sophisticated equipment needed for full test but expiratory loop possible with compact spirometry
Airways resistance	Assessment of airflow limitation	Sensitive	Technique difficult to perform
Lung volumes	Differentiation between restrictive and obstructive lung disease	Effort-independent, complements FEV_1	Sophisticated equipment needed
Gas transfer	Assessment and monitoring of extent of interstitial lung disease and emphysema	Non-invasive (compared with lung biopsy or radiation from repeated chest X-rays and CT)	Sophisticated equipment needed
Blood gases	Assessment of respiratory failure	Can detect early lung disease when measured during exercise	Invasive
Pulse oximetry	Postoperative, sleep studies and respiratory failure	Continuous monitoring Non-invasive	Measures saturation only
Exercise tests (6-min walk)	Practical assessment for disability and effects of therapy	No equipment required	Time-consuming Learning effect At least two walks required
Cardiorespiratory assessment	Early detection of lung/heart disease Fitness assessment	Differentiates breathlessness due to lung or heart disease	Expensive and complicated equipment required

CT, computed tomography; FEV, forced expiratory volume; FEV_1, forced expiratory volume in 1 sec; FVC, forced vital capacity; PEFR, peak expiratory flow rate.

A   Normal

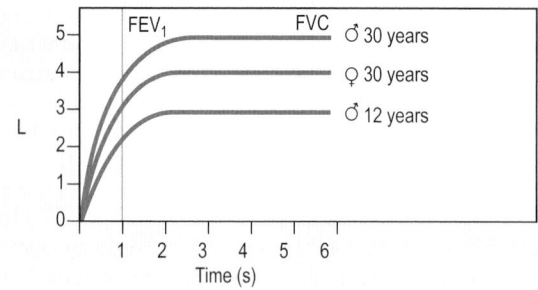

B   Restrictive pattern

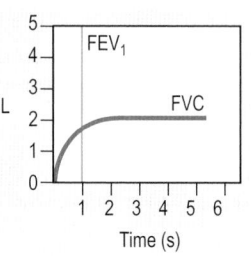

C   Airflow limitation

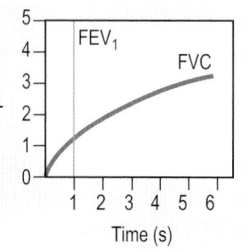

Fig. 28.12 Spirometry: volume–time curves. **(A)** Normal patterns for age and sex. **(B)** Restrictive pattern (FEV_1 and FVC reduced). **(C)** Airflow limitation (FEV_1 only reduced). FEV_1, forced expiratory volume in 1 sec; FVC, forced vital capacity.

> **ℹ   Box 28.13 FEV_1/FVC ratio**
>
> - **Normal**: approximately 75%
> - **Airflow obstruction**: reduced
> - **Restriction**: normal or increased
>
> FEV_1, forced expiratory volume in 1 second; FVC, forced vital capacity.

---

airways causes obstruction to airflow before the normal residual volume (RV) is reached. This trapping of air within the lung is a characteristic feature of these diseases.

Peak expiratory flow rate

Peak expiratory flow rate (PEFR) is an extremely simple and cheap test. Subjects take a full inspiration to total lung capacity and then blow out forcefully into the peak flow meter (**Fig. 28.13**). The best of three attempts is recorded.

Although reproducible, PEFR is mainly dependent on the flow rate in larger airways and it may be falsely reassuring in patients with moderate airflow limitation. PEFR is mainly used to diagnose asthma, and to monitor exacerbations of asthma and response to treatment. Regular measurements of peak flow rates on waking, during the afternoon and before going to bed demonstrate the wide diurnal variations in airflow limitation that characterize asthma and allow objective assessment of response to treatment (**Fig. 28.14**).

Other ventilatory function tests

Measurement of airways resistance in a body box (plethysmograph) is more sensitive but the equipment is expensive and the necessary manoeuvres are too exhausting for many patients with chronic airflow limitation.

Flow–volume loops

Plotting flow rates against expired volume (flow–volume loops, see **Fig. 28.6**) shows the site of airflow limitation within the lung. At the start of expiration from TLC, maximum resistance is from the large airways, and this affects the flow rate for the first 25% of the curve. As air is exhaled, lung volume reduces and the flow rate becomes dependent on the resistance of smaller airways. In COPD, which mainly affects the smaller airways, expiratory flow rates at 50% or 25% of the vital capacity are disproportionately reduced when compared with flow rates at larger lung volumes. Flow–volume loops also show obstruction of large airways: for example, tracheal narrowing due to tumour or retrosternal goitre.

A   Peak flow meter

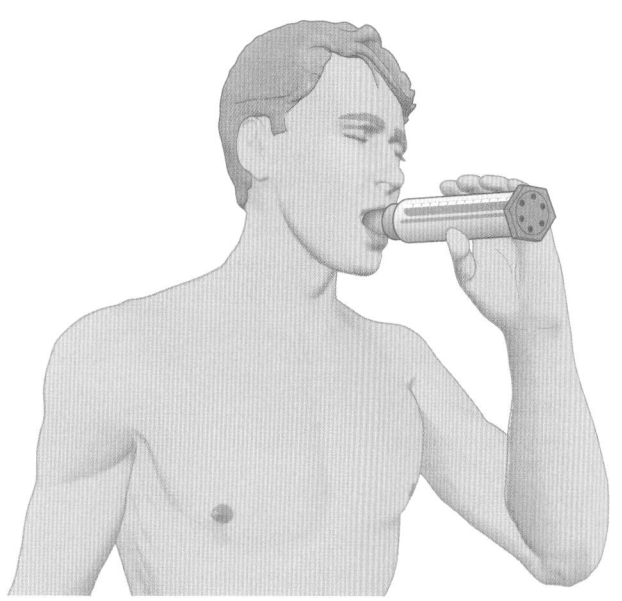

B   Graph of normal readings

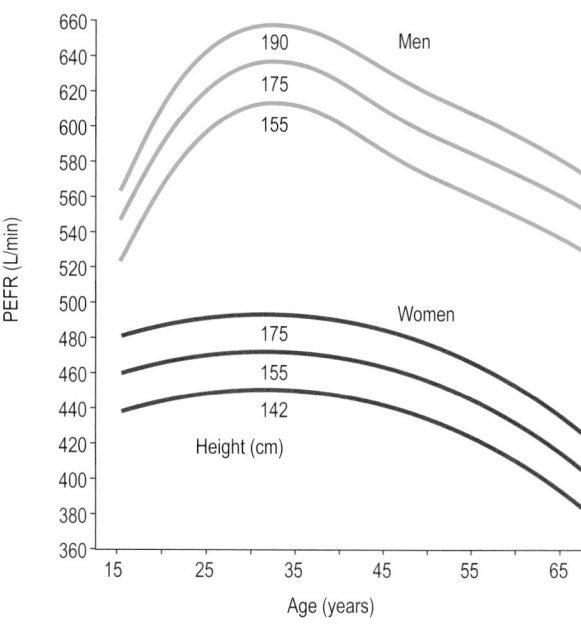

Fig. 28.13 Peak flow measurements. **(A)** Peak flow meter; the lips should be tight around the mouthpiece. **(B)** Normal readings. PEFR, peak expiratory flow rate.

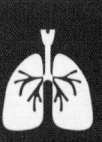

Lung volumes

The subdivisions of lung volume are shown in **Fig. 28.15**. Tidal volume and vital capacity can be measured using a simple spirometer but alternative techniques are needed to measure TLC and RV. TLC is measured by inhaling air containing a known concentration of helium and measuring its dilution in the exhaled air. RV can be calculated by subtracting the vital capacity from the TLC.

TLC measurements using this technique are inaccurate if there are large cystic spaces in the lung because helium cannot diffuse into them. Under these circumstances the thoracic gas volume can be measured more accurately using a body plethysmograph (see earlier). The difference between measurements made by these two methods shows the extent of non-communicating air space within the lungs.

Transfer factor

In normal lungs the transfer factor accurately reflects how efficiently oxygen diffuses from alveolar air into blood, and depends on the thickness of the alveolar–capillary membrane. In lung disease the diffusing capacity (D_{CO}) is also affected by the ventilation–perfusion relationship. Carbon monoxide is used as a surrogate marker to measure this, as it has a similar diffusion rate to oxygen. A low concentration of carbon monoxide is inhaled and the rate of absorption calculated. To control for differences in lung volume, the uptake of carbon monoxide is expressed relative to lung volume as a transfer coefficient (K_{CO}).

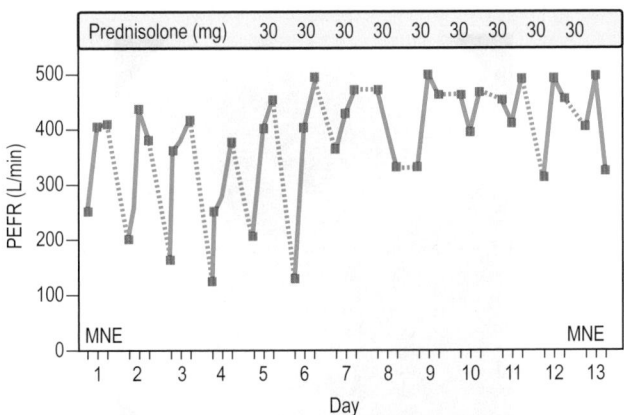

Fig. 28.14 Diurnal variability in peak expiratory flow rate (PEFR) in asthma, showing the effect of steroids. MNE, morning, noon, evening.

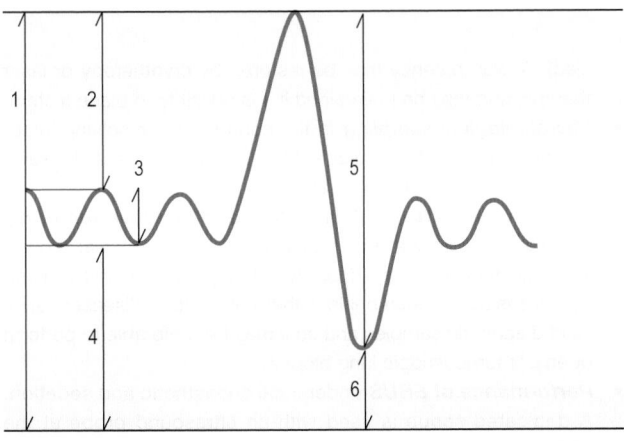

1	Total lung capacity	4	Functional residual capacity
2	Inspiratory reserve volume	5	Vital capacity
3	Tidal volume	6	Residual volume

Fig. 28.15 The subdivisions of the lung volume.

Gas transfer is reduced in patients with severe degrees of emphysema and fibrosis, but also in heart failure and anaemia. Although relatively non-specific, gas transfer is particularly useful in the detection and monitoring of diseases affecting the lung parenchyma (e.g. idiopathic pulmonary fibrosis, sarcoidosis and asbestosis). The K_{CO} is raised in pulmonary haemorrhage.

Peripheral oxygen saturation (S_pO_2) can be continuously measured using an oximeter with either ear or finger probes. Pulse oximetry has become an essential part of the routine monitoring of patients in hospital and clinics. It is also useful in exercise testing and reduces the need to measure arterial blood gases.

Measurement of blood gases

This technique is described on page 225, where a guide to interpreting blood gas analyses is provided.

Measurement of the partial pressures of oxygen and carbon dioxide in arterial blood is essential in managing respiratory failure, when repeated measurements are often the best guide to therapy.

Exhaled nitric oxide

Nitric oxide (NO) is produced by the bronchial epithelium and increases in asthma and other forms of airway inflammation. Measuring exhaled NO can guide therapy in asthma that is difficult to control (see p. 951).

Six-minute walk test

In this validated test the distance walked in metres is recorded over a period of 6 minutes. The oxygen saturations, pulse rate and distance are measured.

Cardiopulmonary exercise testing

This provides a functional assessment of cardiopulmonary reserve and provides information about cardiorespiratory and metabolic muscle function. It is usually performed on a treadmill or a cycle ergometer. Oxygen consumption, carbon dioxide production and ventilation can be calculated.

Indications include the investigation of unexplained breathlessness, establishing prognosis in respiratory illnesses and predicting risk in perioperative assessment.

Nocturnal polygraphy

This multichannel sleep study records pulse, oxygen saturation, nasal flow, body position, and thoracic and abdominal wall movements. It is useful in the investigation of sleep-disordered breathing.

Haematological and biochemical tests

It is useful to measure:
- **haemoglobin**: to detect anaemia or polycythaemia
- **packed cell volume**: as secondary polycythaemia occurs with chronic hypoxia
- **routine biochemistry**: often disturbed in lung cancer and infection
- **D-dimer**: to detect intravascular coagulation; a negative test makes pulmonary embolism very unlikely.

Other blood investigations sometimes required include α_1-antitrypsin levels, *Aspergillus* antibodies, viral and mycoplasma serology, autoantibody profiles and specific IgE measurements.

Sputum

Sputum should be inspected for colour:
- Yellowish green indicates inflammation (infection or allergy).
- Blood suggests bronchiectasis, lung cancer (see p. 976) or pulmonary infarction.

Microbiological studies (e.g. Gram stain and culture) are rarely helpful in upper respiratory tract infections or in acute or chronic bronchitis. Conversely, they are of value in:

- pneumonia
- tuberculosis (a specific request to test for acid-fast bacilli (AFB) is required)
- bronchiectasis.

Sputum cytology

This may be an adjunct in the management of asthma but is more often used in research studies. Its advantages are its speed, cheapness and non-invasive nature. A reliable cytologist is needed. Sputum can be induced by inhalation of nebulized hypertonic saline (5%). Better samples can be obtained by bronchoscopy and bronchial washings (see later).

Pleural aspiration

Diagnostic aspiration may be necessary to determine the aetiology of a pleural effusion, especially if unilateral. This is usually done under ultrasound guidance, using full aseptic precautions. A needle is inserted under local anaesthesia through an intercostal space towards the top of the area identified on ultrasound. Fluid is withdrawn and the presence of any blood is noted. Samples are sent for cytology and biochemical analysis (protein estimation, lactate dehydrogenase (LDH) and bacteriological examination, including culture and Ziehl–Neelsen/auramine staining for tuberculosis). A therapeutic aspiration can be performed in the context of a large pleural effusion to help relieve extreme breathlessness.

Pleural biopsy

A pleural biopsy may be a necessary part of the investigation of a unilateral exudative pleural effusion or suspicious pleural thickening. Pleural biopsies may be obtained with CT or ultrasound guidance. An alternative means by which to obtain a pleural biopsy is video-assisted thoracoscopy (VATS). A scope is introduced into the pleural space, allowing direct visualization and biopsy of the parietal pleura. A pleural effusion can be drained during this procedure.

Intercostal drain placement

An intercostal chest drain is an indwelling drain that is placed in the pleural space using ultrasound guidance (**Box 28.14**). It is connected to an underwater seal bottle. Circumstances in which a chest drain is placed include:

- pneumothorax
- large pleural effusion
- empyema.

Occasionally, a **long-term pleural drain** may be needed for recurrent effusions.

Fibreoptic bronchoscopy

This endoscopic procedure allows direct visualization of the endobronchial tree down to the subsegmental level (**Fig. 28.16**). The procedure is performed under local anaesthesia and sedation.

Indications for bronchoscopy (**Box 28.15**) are:

- **Visualization and biopsy of an endobronchial lesion** (suspected malignancy). An endobronchial biopsy may be taken.
- **Collapsed lung or lobe.** Bronchoscopy is performed to determine the nature of the obstruction. Possible causes include an aspirated foreign body, a mucus plug (these may be removed during the bronchoscopy by suction, or by using forceps or a dormier basket) or endobronchial tumour (which may be biop-

Box 28.14 Intercostal drainage

Explain the nature of the procedure to the patient and obtain written consent.

Technique

1. Identify the site for aspiration (using ultrasound in most cases).
2. Carefully sterilize the skin over the aspiration site.
3. Anaesthetize the skin, muscle and pleura with 2% lidocaine.
4. Make a small incision and insert an 8–12 French gauge drain, using the Seldinger technique. A needle is used to enter the pleural space and then withdrawn over a guidewire, over which the catheter is inserted. (A larger-calibre catheter is needed for drainage of empyema, or a 28 French gauge Argyle catheter.)
5. Attach to a three-way tap and 50 mL syringe, and aspirate up to 1000 mL. Stop aspiration if the patient becomes uncomfortable; shock may ensue if too much fluid is withdrawn too quickly.
6. If the drain is to stay in, secure it to skin with suture and sterile dressing.
7. Attach the drain to an underwater seal drainage bottle and allow fluid to drain. Clamp the drain and release periodically, especially if patient becomes uncomfortable (usually up to 1000 mL at a time before clamping for a few hours).
8. Perform a chest X-ray to check the position of the drain.

Pleurodesis

1. Instil lidocaine 3 mg/kg and then talc 4–5 g in 50 mL sodium chloride 0.9% solution into the pleural cavity to achieve pleurodesis in recurrent/malignant effusion.

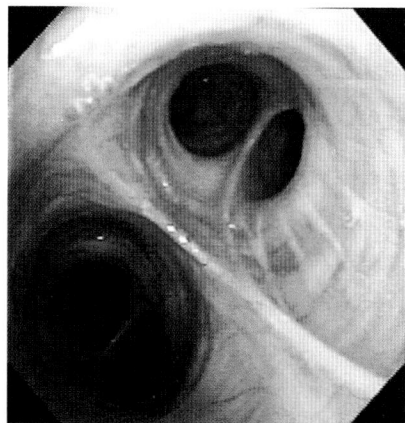

Fig. 28.16 Normal endobronchial appearances as seen at fibreoptic bronchoscopy.

sied). Airway patency may be restored by cryotherapy or laser therapy, and may be maintained if it is possible to place a stent.

- **Microbiological sampling** in the context of unresolving infection or suspected tuberculosis. More distal lesions may be sampled by washing or blind brushing.
- **Diagnosis of diffuse inflammatory and infective lung processes** by bronchoalveolar lavage and transbronchial biopsy. The yield is best in sarcoidosis, lymphangitis carcinomatosa and hypersensitivity pneumonitis. Other fibrotic lung diseases rarely yield diagnostic samples and so it may be preferable to perform open or thoracoscopic lung biopsy.
- **Performance of EBUS** under local anaesthetic and sedation. A dedicated scope is used with an ultrasound probe at the distal end, which allows detailed visualization of the mediastinal nodes. The lymph nodes can be aspirated and samples sent for cytological and microbiological examination. EBUS is performed when CT imaging shows enlarged mediastinal lymph nodes, for which the differential diagnosis includes

Informed written consent is obtained after the nature of the procedure is explained.

Indications
- Lesions requiring biopsy seen on chest X-ray
- Haemoptysis
- Stridor
- Positive sputum cytology for malignant cells with no chest X-ray abnormality
- Collection of bronchial secretions for bacteriology, especially tuberculosis
- Recurrent laryngeal nerve paralysis of unknown aetiology
- Infiltrative lung disease (to obtain a transbronchial biopsy)
- Investigation of collapsed lobes or segments and aspiration of mucus plugs

Disadvantages
- All patients require sedation to tolerate the procedure
- Minor and transient cardiac dysrhythmias occur in up to 40% of patients on passage of the bronchoscope through the larynx. Monitoring is required
- Oxygen supplementation is required in patients with P_aO_2 <8 kPa
- Fibreoptic bronchoscopy should be performed with care in the very sick, and transbronchial biopsies avoided in ventilated patients owing to the increased risk of pneumothorax
- Massive bleeding may occur after biopsy of vascular lesions or carcinoid tumours. Rigid bronchoscopy may be required to allow adequate access to the bleeding point for haemostasis

sarcoid, tuberculosis, lung cancer, lymphoma and metastatic diseases from other primary malignancies.

Mediastinoscopy

This surgical procedure is performed under general anaesthetic. A rigid scope is passed from just above the sternum into the anterior mediastinum. Mediastinoscopy is used in the diagnosis of mediastinal masses and in the staging of nodal disease in carcinoma of the bronchus. It is needed much less often since the introduction of EBUS.

Video-assisted thoracoscopic lung biopsy

VATS lung biopsy has largely replaced open thoracotomy when a lung biopsy is required (see p. 988).

Skin-prick tests

Allergen solutions are placed on the skin (usually the volar surface of the forearm) and the epidermis is broken using a 1 mm tipped lancet. A separate lancet should be used for each allergen. If the patient is sensitive to the allergen, a weal develops. The weal diameter is measured after 10 minutes. A weal of at least 3 mm diameter is regarded as positive, provided that the control test is negative. The results should always be interpreted in light of the history. Skin tests are not affected by bronchodilators or corticosteroids but antihistamines should be discontinued at least 48 hours before testing.

Bronchial provocation testing

This is performed in a lung function laboratory and may be useful in the diagnosis of asthma. Airway hyper-responsiveness (AHR) is a characteristic feature of asthma and can be demonstrated by asking patients to inhale gradually increasing concentrations of histamine or methacholine (**bronchial provocation tests**). This induces transient airflow limitation in susceptible individuals (approximately 20% of the population); the severity of AHR can be graded according to the provocation dose (PD) or concentration (PC) of the agonist that produces a 20% fall in FEV_1. Patients with clinical symptoms of asthma respond to very low doses of methacholine. AHR can also be assessed by exercise testing or inhalation of cold, dry air, mannitol or hypertonic saline.

Further reading

Bohadana A, Izbicki G, Kraman SS. Fundamentals of lung auscultation. *N Engl J Med* 2014; 370:744–751.
Ellis S. *Interpreting Chest X-rays*. Banbury: Scion; 2010.
Hansell DM, Lynch DA, Page McAdams H et al. *Imaging of Diseases of the Chest*, 5th edn. Chicago: Elsevier Mosby; 2010.

DISEASES OF THE UPPER RESPIRATORY TRACT

Rhinitis

Rhinitis is defined clinically as sneezing attacks, nasal discharge or blockage occurring for more than an hour on most days.

The common cold (acute coryza)

This highly infectious illness (see p. 519) is caused by a variety of respiratory viruses: for example, the rhinoviruses (most common), coronaviruses and adenoviruses. Infectivity from close personal contact (nasal mucus on hands) or droplets is high in the early stages of the infection. There are at least 100 different antigenic strains of rhinovirus, making it difficult for the immune system to confer protection. The incubation period varies from 12 hours to 5 days.

The clinical features are tiredness, slight pyrexia, malaise, and a sore nose and pharynx. Sneezing and profuse, watery nasal discharge are followed by thick mucopurulent secretions that may persist for up to a week. Secondary bacterial infection occurs in only a minority of cases.

Other forms of rhinitis

Rhinitis can be subdivided by the frequency with which symptoms occur:
- for a limited period of the year (seasonal or intermittent rhinitis)
- throughout the whole year (perennial or persistent rhinitis).

Seasonal rhinitis (intermittent)

This is the most common allergic disorder. It is often called 'hayfever', but as this implies that only grass pollen is responsible it is better described as seasonal (or intermittent) allergic rhinitis. Worldwide prevalence varies from 2% to 20%. Prevalence is maximal in the second decade, and up to 30% of UK teenagers and young adults are affected each June and July.

Nasal irritation, sneezing and watery rhinorrhoea occur, but many also suffer from itching of the eyes and soft palate, and occasionally even itching of the ears because of the common innervation of the pharyngeal mucosa and the ear. In addition, approximately 20% suffer from seasonal wheezing. Common seasonal allergens include tree and grass pollens and mould spores.

Since the pollination patterns of plants that give rise to high pollen counts vary from country to country, seasonal rhinoconjunctivitis and accompanying wheeze may occur at different times of year in different regions.

Perennial rhinitis (persistent)

In about 50% of patients with perennial rhinitis, symptoms of sneezing and watery rhinorrhoea predominate, while the other

50% complain mostly of nasal blockage. The patient may lose the senses of smell and taste but rarely has eye or throat symptoms. Sinusitis occurs in about 50% of cases, due to mucosal swelling that obstructs drainage from the sinuses. Perennial rhinitis is most frequent in the second and third decades, decreasing with age, and can be divided into four main types.

Perennial allergic rhinitis

The most common cause is allergy to the faecal particles of the house-dust mite, *Dermatophagoides pteronyssinus* or *D. farinae*, which may be found in dust throughout the house (**Fig. 28.17**). Mites live off desquamated human skin scales and the highest concentrations (4000 mites/g of surface dust) are found in human bedding. The next most common allergens come from domestic pets (especially cats) and are proteins derived from urine or saliva spread over the surface of the animal, as well as skin protein. Allergy to urinary protein from small mammals is a major cause of morbidity among laboratory workers. Industrial dust, vapours and fumes cause occupationally related perennial rhinitis more often than asthma.

The presence of perennial rhinitis makes the nose more reactive to non-specific stimuli, such as cigarette smoke, washing powders, household detergents, strong perfumes and traffic fumes. Although patients often think they are allergic to these stimuli, these are irritant responses and do not involve antibodies.

Perennial non-allergic rhinitis with eosinophilia

No extrinsic allergic cause can be identified, either on taking a history or testing the skin, but eosinophilic granulocytes are present in nasal secretions. Most of these patients are intolerant of aspirin/non-steroidal anti-inflammatory drugs (NSAIDs).

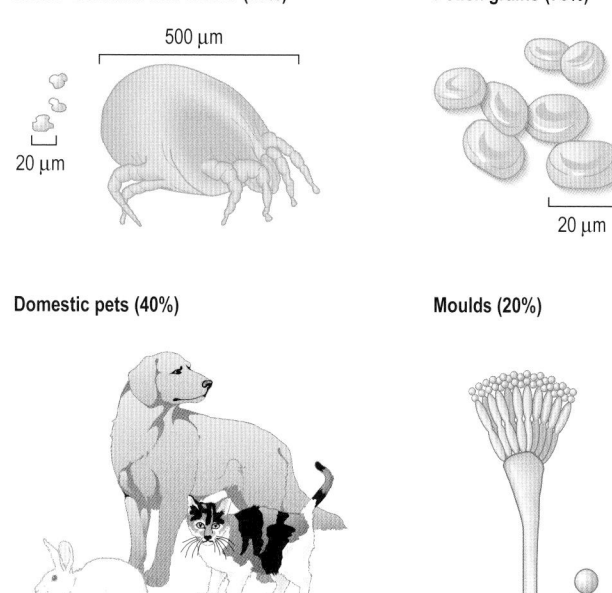

House-dust mite and faeces (80%)
500 μm
20 μm

Pollen grains (70%)
20 μm

Domestic pets (40%)

Moulds (20%)
5 μm

Fig. 28.17 Common allergens causing allergic rhinitis and asthma. These include the house-dust mite, faeces of house-dust mites, pollen grains, domestic pets and moulds. Percentages indicate the proportion of positive skin-prick tests to these allergens in patients with allergic rhinitis.

Vasomotor rhinitis

Patients with this type of perennial rhinitis have no demonstrable allergy or nasal eosinophilia. Watery secretions and nasal congestion are triggered by, for example, cold air, smoke, perfume or newsprint, possibly because of an imbalance of the autonomic nerves controlling the erectile tissue (sinusoids) in the nasal mucosa.

Nasal polyps

These are round, smooth, soft, semitranslucent, pale or yellow, glistening structures attached to the sinus mucosa by a relatively narrow stalk or pedicle, occurring in patients with allergic or vasomotor rhinitis. The mechanism(s) of their formation is not known. They contain mast cells, eosinophils and mononuclear cells in large numbers and cause nasal obstruction, loss of smell and taste, and mouth breathing, but rarely sneezing, since the mucosa of the polyp is largely denervated.

Investigations and diagnosis

The allergic factors causing rhinitis can usually be identified from the history. Skin-prick testing is used to support the history. A positive test does not necessarily mean that an allergen causes the respiratory disease. However, if there is a compatible clinical history, it is more likely to be relevant. Allergen-specific IgE antibodies can be measured in blood but such tests are much more expensive than skin tests and should be used only in patients who cannot be skin-tested for some reason (e.g. dermatographism, active eczema or inability to stop antihistamines for 3 days before skin tests).

Management
Allergen avoidance

Removal of a household pet or total enclosure of industrial processes releasing sensitizing agents can lead to cure of rhinitis and, indeed, asthma. However, pollen avoidance is impossible. Contact may be diminished by wearing sunglasses, driving with the car windows shut, avoiding walks in the countryside (particularly in the late afternoon, when the number of pollen grains is highest at ground level) and keeping bedroom windows shut at night. These measures are rarely sufficient in themselves to control symptoms. Exposure to pollen is generally lower in coastal regions, where sea breezes carry pollen grains inland.

Exposure to mite allergen can be reduced by enclosing bedding in fabric specifically designed to prevent its passage, while allowing water vapour through. This is comfortable and also reduces symptoms. Acaricides (substances toxic to mites) are less effective and cannot be recommended. Increased room ventilation and reduced soft furnishings, including carpets, curtains and soft toys, can all help to reduce the mite load.

H₁ antihistamines

Antihistamines remain the most common therapy for rhinitis; in the UK most can be purchased directly over the counter. They are particularly effective against sneezing and itching of the eyes and palate, but are less effective against rhinorrhoea and have little influence on nasal blockage. First-generation antihistamines (chlorphenamine, hydroxyzine) cause sedation and loss of concentration in all patients (including those who are not aware of the problem) and should no longer be used. Second-generation drugs, such as loratadine (10 mg once daily), desloratadine (5 mg daily), cetirizine (10 mg daily) and fexofenadine (120 mg daily), are at least as potent and do not cause sedation.

Decongestants

Drugs with sympathomimetic activity (α-adrenergic agents) are widely used to treat nasal obstruction. They may be taken orally or, more commonly, as nasal drops or sprays (e.g. ephedrine nasal drops). Xylometazoline and oxymetazoline are widely used because they have a prolonged action and tachyphylaxis does not develop. Secondary nasal hyperaemia can occur some hours later as a rebound effect and *rhinitis medicamentosa* can develop if patients take increasing quantities of decongestant to overcome this phenomenon. Although local decongestants are an effective treatment for vasomotor rhinitis, patients must be warned about rebound nasal obstruction and should use the drugs carefully. Ideally, such preparations should be prescribed for only a limited period to open the nasal airways and allow better access for other local therapy, such as topical corticosteroids.

Anti-inflammatory drugs

Sodium cromoglicate and nedocromil sodium act by blocking an intracellular chloride channel and influence mast cell and eosinophil activation and nerve function. Topical sodium cromoglicate and nedocromil sodium can be very effective in allergic conjunctivitis but are of limited value in allergic rhinitis.

Corticosteroids

The most effective treatment for rhinitis is a topical corticosteroid preparation (e.g. beclometasone, fluticasone propionate, fluticasone furoate or mometasone furoate spray). Topical steroids should be started before the beginning of seasonal symptoms. The combination of a topical corticosteroid with a non-sedating antihistamine taken regularly is particularly effective. Patients should be carefully instructed in how to use the nasal steroid device to achieve optimal drug deposition. In selected cases an α-adrenergic agonist may help to decongest the nose prior to taking the topical corticosteroid. Patients often worry about possible side-effects; nasal steroids can cause epistaxis but the amount used is insufficient to cause systemic effects.

If other therapy has failed, seasonal rhinitis and perennial rhinitis respond readily to a short course (maximum 2 weeks) of treatment with oral prednisolone 5–10 mg daily. Nasal polyps may respond to oral corticosteroids and their recurrence may be prevented by continuous use of topical corticosteroids.

Leukotriene antagonists

If there is no response to antihistamines or topical steroids, a leukotriene antagonist (e.g. montelukast 10 mg daily in the evening) may be helpful, especially in patients with a history of NSAID sensitivity or concomitant asthma.

Immunotherapy

This is used for patients with seasonal allergic rhinitis who have not responded to standard drugs. Both oral and injectable vaccines are available (see p. 63). Other forms of desensitizing vaccines are under development.

Sinusitis

See page 908.

Pharyngitis

The most common viruses causing pharyngitis are adenoviruses, of which there are about 32 serotypes. Endemic adenovirus infection causes the common sore throat, in which the oropharynx and soft palate are reddened and the tonsils are inflamed and swollen. Within 1–2 days the tonsillar lymph nodes enlarge. The disease is self-limiting and requires only symptomatic treatment without antibiotics.

Over several decades the proportion of sore throats due to bacterial infections, such as haemolytic streptococcus, has fallen. Many different pathogens have been implicated in pharyngitis but most do not require specific treatment. Persistent and severe tonsillitis should be treated with phenoxymethylpenicillin 500 mg four times daily or cefaclor 250 mg three times daily. Amoxicillin and ampicillin should be avoided if there is a possibility of infectious mononucleosis (see p. 524), as they are likely to cause drug rashes in this context.

Acute laryngotracheobronchitis

Acute laryngitis is an occasional but striking complication of upper respiratory tract infections, particularly those caused by parainfluenza viruses and measles. The condition is most severe in children under the age of 3 years. Inflammatory oedema extends to the vocal cords and the epiglottis, causing narrowing of the airway; there may be associated **tracheitis** or **tracheobronchitis**. The voice becomes hoarse, and there is a barking cough (croup) and audible stridor. Progressive airways obstruction may occur, with recession of the soft tissue of the neck and abdomen during inspiration and, in severe cases, central cyanosis. Steam inhalations are not helpful. Nebulized adrenaline (epinephrine) gives short-term relief. Oral or intramuscular corticosteroids (e.g. dexamethasone) should be given with oxygen and adequate fluids. If steroids are used, endotracheal intubation is rarely necessary. A tracheostomy is infrequently required.

Acute epiglottitis

Haemophilus influenzae type b (Hib) can cause life-threatening infection of the epiglottis, usually in children under 5 years of age. The child becomes extremely ill with a high fever, and severe airflow obstruction may rapidly occur. This is a life-threatening emergency and requires urgent endotracheal intubation and intravenous antibiotics (e.g. ceftazidime 25–150 mg/kg). Chloramphenicol (50–100 mg/kg) is also used in some countries. The epiglottis, which is red and swollen, should not be inspected until facilities to maintain the airways are available.

Other manifestations of Hib infection are meningitis, septic arthritis and osteomyelitis. A highly effective vaccine is now available, which is given to infants at 2, 3 and 4 months with their primary immunizations against diphtheria, tetanus and pertussis (DTP). In many countries, this programme has reduced death rates from Hib infections virtually to zero.

Influenza

The influenza virus belongs to the orthomyxovirus group and exists in two main forms, A and B. Influenza B is associated with localized outbreaks of mild disease, whereas influenza A causes worldwide pandemics (see p. 520).

Clinical features

The incubation period of influenza is usually 1–3 days. The illness starts abruptly with a fever, shivering and generalized aching in the limbs. This is associated with severe headache, soreness of the throat and a dry cough that can persist for several weeks. Diarrhoea occurs in 70% of cases of H5N1 ('bird flu'). Influenza infection can be followed by a prolonged period of debility and depression that may take weeks or months to clear.

Complications

Secondary bacterial infection is common following influenza virus infection, particularly with *Streptococcus pneumoniae* and *H.*

influenzae. Secondary pneumonia caused by *Staphylococcus aureus* is rarer but more serious, and carries a mortality of up to 20%. Post-infectious encephalomyelitis is rare after influenza infection.

Diagnosis and management

Laboratory diagnosis is not usually necessary in the community, but a definitive diagnosis can be established by demonstrating a four-fold increase in complement-fixing antibody or haemagglutinin antibody measured at onset and after 1–2 weeks, or by taking nasopharyngeal swabs. Viral swabs should be taken for hospital inpatients to facilitate infection control measures.

Management is by bed rest and paracetamol, with antibiotics to prevent secondary infection in those with chronic bronchitis or cardiac or renal disease. Neuraminidase inhibitors help to shorten the duration of symptoms in patients with influenza, if given within 48 hours of the first symptom. Inpatients should be cared for in a side room, with respiratory isolation measures in place to avoid cross-infection.

Prophylaxis

Protection by influenza vaccines is effective in only about 70% of people and lasts for about a year only. New vaccines have to be prepared to cover each change in viral antigenicity and are therefore in limited supply at the start of an epidemic. Nevertheless, routine vaccination is recommended for all individuals over 65 years of age and also for younger people with chronic heart disease, chronic lung disease (including asthma), chronic kidney disease or diabetes mellitus and for those who are immunosuppressed. Hospital and health service personnel should also be vaccinated. Influenza vaccine should be given to individuals who are allergic to egg protein with caution, as some types are manufactured in chick embryos; egg-free vaccines are now available.

Inhalation of foreign bodies

Children inhale foreign bodies, such as peanuts, more commonly than adults do. In adults, inhalation may occur after excess alcohol or under general anaesthesia (loose teeth or dentures).

When the foreign body is large, it may impact in the trachea. The person chokes and then becomes silent; death ensues unless the material is quickly removed. Guidelines for the management of choking should rapidly be followed (**Box 28.16**).

More often, impaction occurs in the right main bronchus and produces choking and persistent monophonic wheeze; it may lead to a suppurative pneumonia and/or lung abscess.

Acute and chronic cough

Cough is one of the most common respiratory symptoms reported by patients. **Acute cough** is often defined as one that lasts less than 3 weeks and **chronic cough** one that persists more than 8 weeks. The 'grey' area in between is often termed **subacute cough**.

Management of acute cough

Acute cough is often associated with upper respiratory tract infection, particularly in the winter months, and tends to settle after a few weeks (**Box 28.17**). However, any patient who has worrying symptoms or signs, such as haemoptysis, breathlessness, fever, weight loss, night sweats, chest pain or foreign body inhalation, should undergo urgent chest X-ray to look for lung cancer, pneumonia or tuberculosis, in particular. However, most acute cough is self-limiting and antibiotics are not indicated.

➕ Box 28.16 Sequence of steps for managing the adult victim who is choking

Suspect choking
- Be alert to choking, particularly if the victim is eating.

Encourage to cough
- Instruct the victim to cough.

Give back blows
- If cough becomes ineffective, give up to five back blows:
  - Stand to the side and slightly behind the victim.
  - Support the chest with one hand and lean the victim well forwards so that, when the obstructing object is dislodged, it comes out of the mouth rather than going further down the airway.
  - Give five sharp blows between the shoulder blades with the heel of your other hand.

Give abdominal thrusts
- If back blows are ineffective, give up to five abdominal thrusts:
  - Stand behind the victim and put both arms round the upper part of the abdomen.
  - Lean the victim forwards.
  - Clench your fist and place it between the umbilicus (navel) and the ribcage.
  - Grasp this hand with your other hand and pull sharply inwards and upwards.
  - Repeat up to five times.
  - If the obstruction is still not relieved, continue alternating five back blows with five abdominal thrusts.

Start cardiopulmonary resuscitation (CPR)
- Start CPR if the victim becomes unresponsive:
  - Support the victim as you lower them carefully to the ground.
  - Immediately activate the ambulance service.
  - Begin CPR with chest compressions.

(From resus.org.uk.)

❓ Box 28.17 Causes of cough

Cause	Example
Respiratory disease	Viral or bacterial infection, bronchospasm, chronic obstructive pulmonary disease, non-asthmatic eosinophilic asthma, bronchiolitis, malignancy, parenchymal disease (e.g. interstitial lung disease, bronchiectasis, cystic fibrosis, sarcoidosis), pleural disease, aspiration
Upper airways disease	Postnasal drip, sinusitis, inhaled foreign body, tonsillar enlargement
Cardiovascular disease	Heart failure, mitral stenosis
Gastro-oesophageal disease	Gastro-oesophageal reflux disease, also associated with laryngopharyngeal reflux
Neurological disease	Aspiration
Drugs and irritants	Angiotensin converting enzyme (ACE) inhibitors, cigarette smoke

Management of chronic cough

All patients with a chronic cough should have a chest X-ray and those with X-ray abnormalities should be investigated appropriately. If the chest X-ray is normal, then the five most likely diagnoses are undiagnosed asthma, postnasal drip, gastro-oesophageal reflux disease (see p. 1162), recent upper respiratory tract infection or smoking.

Spirometry should then be organized. If it reveals reversible airways obstruction, treatment is given as per asthma guidelines.

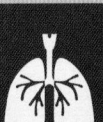

Otherwise, based on the history, patients should have a trial of treatment for the most likely cause:

- **nocturnal cough or wheeze:** a 2-week trial of oral or inhaled steroids
- **acid reflux:** an 8-week trial of a proton pump inhibitor
- **postnasal drip:** a trial of topical steroids
- **smoking:** smokers should be referred to the local smoking cessation service.

Ensure that the patient is not taking an angiotensin converting enzyme (ACE) inhibitor.

If a chronic cough does not settle after empirical treatment and the aetiology remains unclear, further investigations might include CT chest, bronchoscopy, bronchial provocation testing, oesophageal manometry and imaging of the sinuses. Referral to a specialist cough clinic may also be considered.

Further reading

Greiner AN, Hellings PW, Rotiroti G et al. Allergic rhinitis. *Lancet* 2011; 378:2112–2122.

National Institute for Health and Care Excellence. *NICE Guideline 120: Cough (Acute): Antimicrobial Prescribing*. NICE 2019; https://www.nice.org.uk/guidance/ng120.

Scadding GK, Kariyawasam HH, Scadding G et al. BSACI guidelines for the diagnosis and management of allergic and non-allergic rhinitis. *Clin Exp Allergy* 2017; 47:856–889.

https://www.worldallergy.org. *World Allergy Organization: education programmes and allergic disease resource centre.*

OBSTRUCTIVE RESPIRATORY DISEASE

Asthma

Asthma is a common chronic condition whose cause is incompletely understood. Symptoms include wheeze, chest tightness, cough and shortness of breath, often worse at night. Asthma commonly starts in childhood between the ages of 3 and 5 years and may either worsen or improve during adolescence. Classically, asthma has three characteristics:

- **airflow limitation**, which is usually reversible spontaneously or with treatment
- **airway hyper-responsiveness** to a wide range of stimuli (see later)
- **bronchial inflammation** with T lymphocytes, mast cells, eosinophils with associated plasma exudation, oedema, smooth muscle hypertrophy, matrix deposition, mucus plugging and epithelial damage.

In chronic asthma, inflammation may be accompanied by irreversible airflow limitation as a result of airway wall remodelling, which may involve large and small airways and mucus impaction.

Prevalence

In many countries the prevalence of asthma has increased since the mid-1980s. This increase is particularly marked in children and young adults, with up to 15% of the population being affected. Asthma is more common in developed countries, with some of the highest rates in the UK, New Zealand and Australia, and much lower rates in East Asia, Africa and Central and Eastern Europe. Long-term follow-up in developing countries suggests that asthma may become more frequent as individuals adopt a more 'Westernized' lifestyle but the environmental factors accounting for this remain unknown. Studies of occupational asthma suggest that a large proportion of the workforce (15–20%) may become asthmatic if exposed to potent sensitizers. Worldwide, asthma kills about 1000 people per day; approximately 300 million people have asthma and this figure is expected to rise to 400 million by 2025.

Classification

Asthma is a complex disorder. The current thinking is that symptoms can be caused by several different processes. Asthma can be classified according to its trigger factors, age of onset, inflammatory subtypes or response to therapy. There is considerable overlap between populations separated along these different dimensions and it is now increasingly common to describe clinical subtypes (or endotypes).

Many childhood-onset asthmatics have a wheezing illness with inhaled allergic triggers. Some 90% of children and 70% of adults with persistent asthma have positive skin-prick tests to common inhalant allergens such as dust mite, animal danders, pollens and fungi. Childhood-onset asthma is often accompanied by eczema (atopic dermatitis, see p. 660).

In some people with asthma, inhaled allergens are not relevant. This illness often starts in middle age and attacks are triggered by respiratory infections. Nevertheless, many patients with adult-onset asthma show positive allergen skin tests and, on close questioning, some of these will give a history of childhood respiratory symptoms suggesting that they have allergic asthma.

Non-atopic individuals may develop asthma in middle age from extrinsic causes, such as sensitization to occupational agents like toluene diisocyanate, intolerance to NSAIDs such as aspirin, or prescription of β-adrenoceptor-blocking agents that block the protective effect of endogenous catecholamines. Extrinsic causes must be considered in all cases of asthma and, where possible, avoided.

Other clinical phenotypes

Based on the clinical picture, other subtypes or endotypes of asthma are recognized, including 'brittle asthma' and steroid-resistant asthma. While eosinophilic airway inflammation is often present in asthma, there are also patients with eosinophilic bronchitis, who have sputum eosinophilia without wheeze. It remains unclear whether this is a pre-asthmatic state or whether anti-eosinophil treatment is helpful.

Aetiology

The major factors involved in the development of asthma and stimuli that can precipitate attacks are shown in **Fig. 28.18**.

Atopy and allergy

The term 'atopy' was coined in the early 1900s to describe a group of disorders, including asthma and hayfever, that appeared to run in families, have positive skin-prick tests to common inhalant allergens and have circulating allergen-specific antibodies. Allergen-specific IgE is present in 30–40% of the UK population, and elevated serum IgE levels are linked to airway hyper-responsiveness and the prevalence of asthma. Serum total IgE levels are affected by several genetic and environmental factors.

Genetic factors

There is no single gene for asthma but several, in combination with environmental factors, appear to influence its development. These include genes that affect the production of cytokines and IgE.

Environmental factors

Early childhood exposure to allergens and maternal smoking has a major influence on IgE production. Much interest focuses on the role of intestinal bacteria and childhood infections in shaping the immune system in early life. It has been suggested that growing up

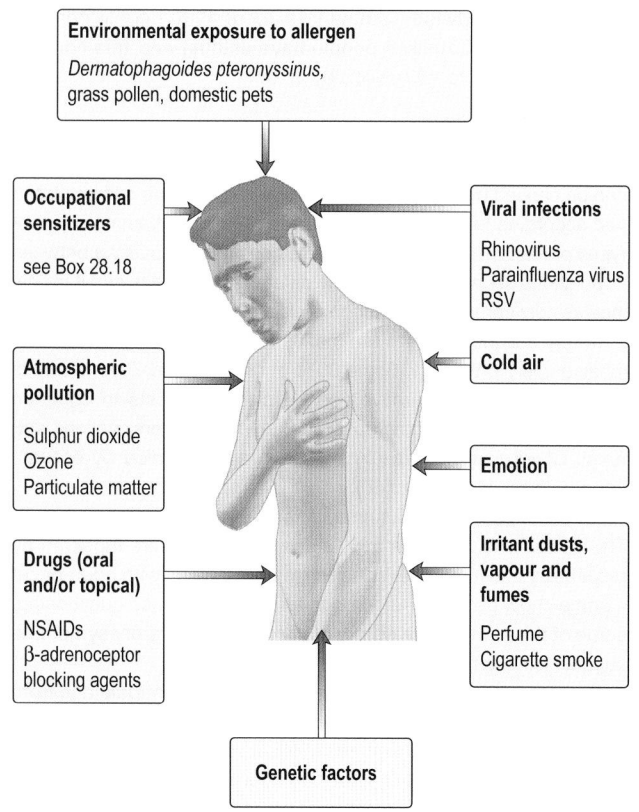

Environmental exposure to allergen

Dermatophagoides pteronyssinus,
grass pollen, domestic pets

Occupational sensitizers

see Box 28.18

Atmospheric pollution

Sulphur dioxide
Ozone
Particulate matter

Drugs (oral and/or topical)

NSAIDs
β-adrenoceptor blocking agents

Viral infections

Rhinovirus
Parainfluenza virus
RSV

Cold air

Emotion

Irritant dusts, vapour and fumes

Perfume
Cigarette smoke

Genetic factors

Fig. 28.18 Causes and triggers of asthma. NSAIDs, non-steroidal anti-inflammatory drugs; RSV, respiratory syncytial virus.

? Box 28.18 Occupational asthma	
Cause	**Source/occupation**
Low-molecular-weight (non-IgE-related)	
Isocyanates	Polyurethane varnishes Industrial coatings Spray painting
Colophony fumes	Soldering/welders Electronics industry
Wood dust	
Drugs	
Bleaches and dyes	
Complex metal salts, e.g. nickel, platinum, chromium	
High-molecular-weight (IgE-related)	
Allergens from animals and insects	Farmers, workers in poultry and seafood processing industry; laboratory workers
Antibiotics	Nurses, health industry
Latex	Health workers
Proteolytic enzymes	Manufacture (but not use) of 'biological' washing powders
Complex salts of platinum	Metal refining
Acid anhydrides and polyamine hardening agents	Industrial coatings

in a relatively 'clean' environment may predispose towards an IgE response to allergens (the 'hygiene hypothesis'). Conversely, growing up in a 'dirtier' environment may allow the immune system to avoid developing allergic responses, and early-life exposure to inhaled and ingested products of microorganisms, as occurs in livestock farming communities and developing countries, may reduce the subsequent risk of a child becoming allergic and/or developing asthma.

The allergens involved in allergic asthma are similar to those implicated in rhinitis, although pollens are relatively less implicated in asthma. Most allergic asthmatics are sensitized to house-dust mite allergens. Cockroach allergy has been implicated in asthma in inner-city children in the USA, while allergens from furry pets (especially cats) are increasingly common causes. The fungal spores from *Aspergillus fumigatus* cause a range of lung disorders, including asthma (see p. 993).

Precipitating factors

Occupational sensitizers

Over 250 materials encountered in the workplace can cause occupational asthma, which accounts for up to 15% of all asthma cases (**Box 28.18**). These are recognized occupational diseases in the UK and patients in insurable employment are eligible for statutory compensation, provided they apply within 10 years of leaving the occupation in which the asthma developed.

Asthma can be due to:

- low-molecular-weight compounds, e.g. reactive chemicals such as isocyanates and acid anhydrides that bond chemically to epithelial cells to activate them, as well as providing haptens recognized by T cells
- high-molecular-weight compounds, e.g. flour, organic dusts and other large protein molecules involving specific IgE antibodies.

Smoking increases the risk of developing some forms of occupational asthma. The proportion of employees developing occupational

asthma depends primarily on the level of exposure. Proper enclosure of industrial processes or appropriate ventilation greatly reduces the risk. Atopic individuals develop occupational asthma more rapidly when exposed to agents causing the development of specific IgE antibody. Non-atopic individuals can also develop asthma when exposed to such agents, but after a longer period of exposure.

Non-specific factors

Due to their AHR, patients with asthma will respond to a wide variety of non-specific direct and indirect stimuli, as well as reacting to specific allergens.

Cold air and exercise

Most asthmatics wheeze after prolonged exercise or inhalation of cold, dry air. Typically, the attack does not occur while exercising but afterwards. Exercise-induced wheeze is driven by release of histamine, prostaglandins (PGs) and leukotrienes (LTs) from mast cells, as well as stimulation of neural reflexes.

Atmospheric pollution and irritant dusts, vapours and fumes

Many patients with asthma experience worsening of symptoms on exposure to tobacco smoke, car exhaust fumes, solvents, strong perfumes or high concentrations of airborne dust. Major epidemics have been recorded when large amounts of allergens are released into the air, and asthma exacerbations increase during summer and winter air pollution episodes associated with climatic temperature inversions: in the presence of high concentrations of ozone, particulates and NO_2 in the summer and particulates, NO_2 and SO_2 in the winter.

Diet

Increased intake of fresh fruit and vegetables has been shown to be protective, possibly owing to the greater consumption of antioxidants or other protective molecules such as flavonoids. Genetic variation in antioxidant enzymes is associated with more severe asthma.

Emotion

Emotional factors influence asthma both acutely and chronically, but there is no evidence that patients with the disease are any more psychologically disturbed than their non-asthmatic peers. Patients at high risk of life-threatening attacks are understandably anxious.

Drugs

NSAIDs. NSAIDs, particularly aspirin and propionic acid derivatives, such as indometacin and ibuprofen, are implicated in triggering asthma in approximately 5% of patients. NSAID intolerance is especially prevalent in those with both nasal polyps and asthma, and is often associated with rhinitis and flushing on drug exposure.

Beta-blockers. The airways have a direct parasympathetic innervation that tends to produce bronchoconstriction. There is no direct sympathetic innervation of bronchial smooth muscle, so antagonism of parasympathetically induced bronchoconstriction is critically dependent on circulating adrenaline (epinephrine) acting through β_2-receptors on the surface of smooth muscle cells. Inhibition of this effect by non-selective β-adrenoceptor-blocking drugs, such as propranolol, leads to bronchoconstriction and airflow limitation, but only in asthmatic subjects. Selective β_1-adrenergic-blocking drugs, such as atenolol, may also induce attacks of asthma.

Clinical features

The principal symptoms of asthma are wheezing attacks and episodic shortness of breath. Symptoms are usually worst during the night, especially in uncontrolled disease. Cough is a frequent symptom that sometimes predominates, especially in children, in whom nocturnal cough can be a presenting feature. Attacks vary greatly in frequency and duration and may be precipitated by a wide range of triggers (see **Fig. 28.18**). Asthma is a major cause of impaired quality of life and has an impact on work and recreation, affecting both physical activities and emotions.

Investigations

There is no single satisfactory diagnostic test for all patients with asthma.

Lung function tests

PEFR measurements on waking, prior to taking a bronchodilator, before bed and after a bronchodilator are particularly useful in demonstrating the variable airflow limitation that characterizes the disease (see **Figs 28.13** and **28.14**). The diurnal variation in PEFR is a good measure of asthma activity and is of help in the longer-term assessment of the patient's disease and its response to treatment.

Spirometry is useful, especially in assessing reversibility. Asthma can be diagnosed by demonstrating a greater than 15% improvement in FEV_1 or PEFR following inhalation of a bronchodilator. The carbon monoxide (CO) transfer test is normal in asthma.

Histamine or methacholine bronchial provocation test

This was outlined on page 945.

Trial of corticosteroids

All patients who present with severe airflow limitation should undergo a formal trial of corticosteroids. Prednisolone 30 mg orally should be given daily for 2 weeks, with lung function measured before and immediately after the course. A substantial improvement in FEV_1 (>15%) confirms the presence of a reversible element and indicates that the administration of inhaled steroids will prove beneficial to the patient. If the trial is for 2 weeks or less, the oral corticosteroid can be withdrawn without tailing off the dose, and should be replaced by inhaled corticosteroids in those who have responded.

Exhaled nitric oxide

This test is a measure of airway inflammation and an index of corticosteroid response; it is used to assess the efficacy of corticosteroids.

Blood and sputum tests

Patients with asthma sometimes have increased numbers of eosinophils in peripheral blood ($>0.4 \times 10^9$/L) but sputum eosinophilia is a more specific diagnostic finding.

Chest X-ray

There are no diagnostic features of asthma on the chest X-ray, although overinflation is characteristic during an acute episode or in chronic severe disease. A chest X-ray may be helpful in excluding a pneumothorax, which can occur as a complication, or in detecting the pulmonary infiltrates associated with allergic bronchopulmonary aspergillosis.

Skin tests

Skin-prick tests should be performed in all cases of asthma to help identify allergic trigger factors. Allergen-specific IgE can be measured in serum if skin-prick test facilities are not available, the patient is taking antihistamines or no suitable allergen extracts are available.

Allergen provocation tests

Allergen inhalation challenge is a useful research tool; it is required when investigating patients with suspected occupational asthma but not in ordinary asthma.

Management

The **aims of treatment** are to:
- abolish symptoms
- restore normal or best possible lung function
- reduce the risk of severe attacks
- enable normal growth to occur in children
- minimize absence from school or employment.
  This involves:
- patient and family education about asthma
- patient and family participation in treatment
- avoidance of identified causes where possible
- use of the lowest effective doses of convenient medications to minimize short-term and long-term side-effects.

Many asthmatics join self-help groups in order to improve their understanding of the disease and to foster self-confidence and fitness.

Control of extrinsic factors

Where specific allergen triggers are identified, these should be avoided if possible. Sublingual allergen immunotherapy (SLIT) with house-dust mites has shown a reduction in the number of asthma attacks in children but is not recommended in adults. Active and passive smoking should be avoided, as should beta-blockers in either tablet or eye-drop form. Individuals intolerant to aspirin should avoid NSAIDs, although

Box 28.19 Inhaled therapy for asthma

Patients should be taught how to use inhalers and their technique should be checked regularly.

Use of a metered-dose inhaler
1. The canister is shaken.
2. The patient exhales to functional residual capacity (not residual volume), i.e. normal expiration.
3. The aerosol nozzle is placed to the open mouth.
4. The patient simultaneously inhales rapidly and activates the aerosol.
5. Inhalation is completed.
6. The breath is held for 10 sec if possible. Even with good technique, only 15% of the contents is inhaled and 85% is deposited on the wall of the pharynx and ultimately swallowed.

Spacers
These are plastic cones or spheres inserted between the patient's mouth and the inhaler. Some inhalers have a built-in spacer extension. These are designed to reduce particle velocity so that less drug is deposited in the mouth. Spacers also diminish the need for coordination between aerosol activation and inhalation. They are useful in children and the elderly, and reduce the risk of candidiasis.

they may tolerate cyclo-oxygenase-2 (COX-2) inhibitors. About one-third of individuals sensitized to occupational agents may be cured if they are kept permanently away from exposure.

Drug treatment

The mainstay of asthma therapy is use of inhaled therapeutic agents, delivered as aerosols or powders directly into the lungs (**Box 28.19**). The advantages of this method of administration are that drugs are delivered direct to the airways and first-pass metabolism in the liver is avoided; thus lower doses are necessary and systemic unwanted effects are minimized. To help those who cannot coordinate activation of the aerosol and inhalation, several breath-activated or dry powder devices have been developed. Patients vary in their ability to use such devices, and care should be taken to select an appropriate device and train the individual to use it properly.

Several national and international guidelines have been published on the treatment of asthma (**Fig. 28.19**), based on three principles:
- Asthma should be self-managed, with regular monitoring using a PEFR meter and an individual treatment plan that is discussed with each patient and written down.

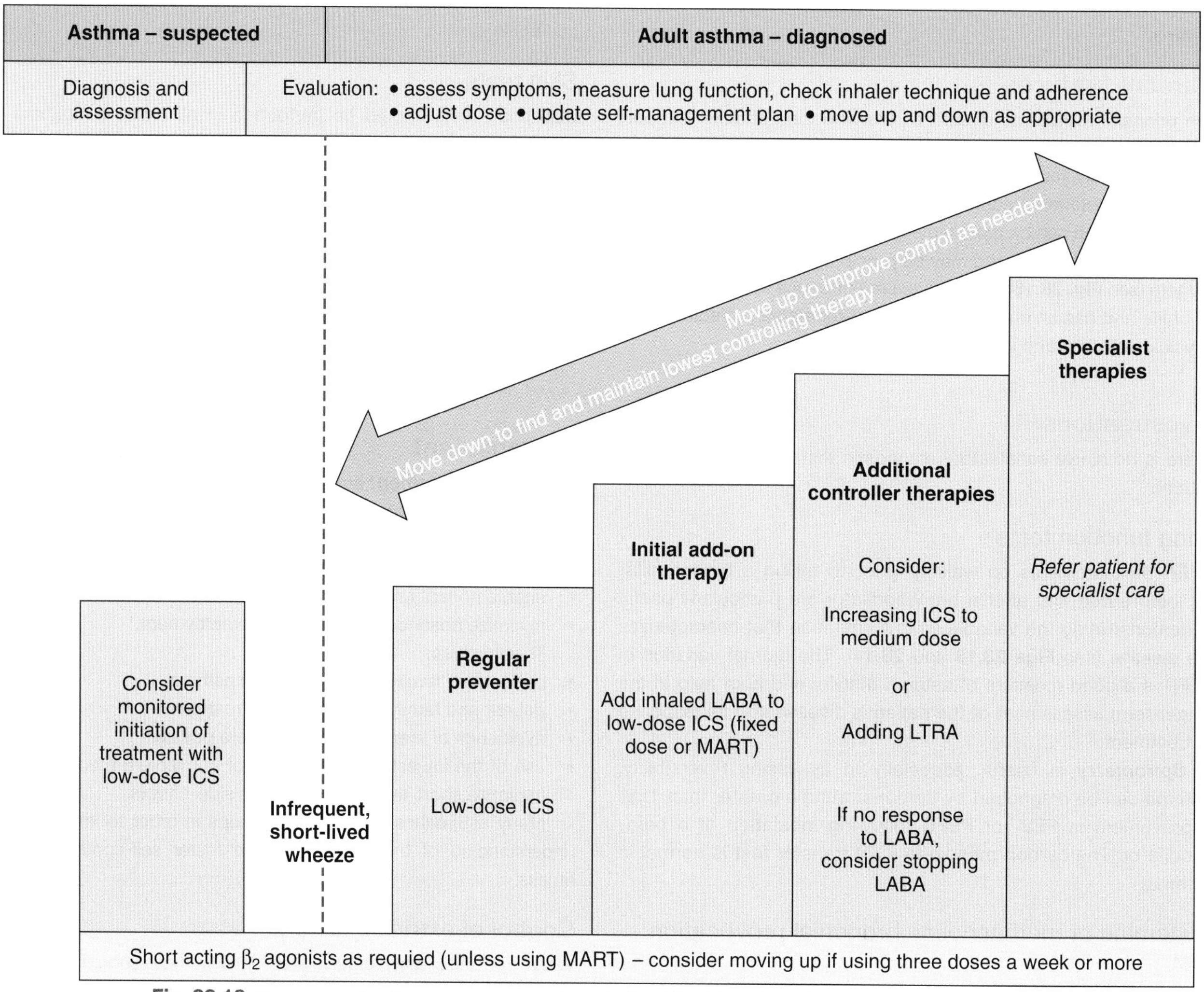

Asthma – suspected	Adult asthma – diagnosed
Diagnosis and assessment	Evaluation: • assess symptoms, measure lung function, check inhaler technique and adherence • adjust dose • update self-management plan • move up and down as appropriate

Move up to improve control as needed
Move down to find and maintain lowest controlling therapy

Consider monitored initiation of treatment with low-dose ICS

Infrequent, short-lived wheeze

Regular preventer

Low-dose ICS

Initial add-on therapy

Add inhaled LABA to low-dose ICS (fixed dose or MART)

Additional controller therapies

Consider:

Increasing ICS to medium dose

or

Adding LTRA

If no response to LABA, consider stopping LABA

Specialist therapies

Refer patient for specialist care

Short acting β₂ agonists as required (unless using MART) – consider moving up if using three doses a week or more

Fig. 28.19 Summary of asthma management in adults. ICS, inhaled corticosteroid; LABA, long-acting β agonist; LTRA, leukotriene receptor antagonist; MART, maintenance and reliever therapy. *(Scottish Intercollegiate Guidelines Network/British Thoracic Society. SIGN158: British Guideline on the Management of Asthma: A National Clinical Guideline. SIGN/BTS 2019; Fig. 2, p. 80.)*

- Asthma is an inflammatory disease, so anti-inflammatory (controller) therapy should be started, even in mild cases.
- Short-acting inhaled bronchodilators (e.g. salbutamol and terbutaline) should be used only to relieve breakthrough symptoms. Increased use of bronchodilator treatment to relieve increasing symptoms is an indication of deteriorating disease.

A list of drugs used in asthma is shown in **Box 28.20**. These are given in a stepwise fashion, as indicated in **Fig. 28.19**.

Beta₂-adrenoceptor agonists

Beta₂-adrenoceptor agonists are selective for the respiratory tract and do not stimulate the β_1 adrenoceptors of the myocardium. These drugs relax the bronchial smooth muscle and are very effective in relieving symptoms, but do not affect underlying airways inflammation.

- *Short-acting β agonists (SABAs)*, such as salbutamol 100 µg (called albuterol in the USA) or terbutaline 250 µg, can be taken as and when required, and should be prescribed as 'two puffs as required'.
- *Long-acting β_2-adrenoceptor agonists (LABAs)*, such as salmeterol or formoterol, are effective by inhalation for up to 12 hours and are given once or twice daily. They should be used in combination with an inhaled corticosteroid as fixed-dose combinations (e.g. salmeterol/fluticasone and formoterol/budesonide) in the same inhaler.

The mildest asthmatics with intermittent attacks are the only people who should rely on SABA treatment alone. Any patients using β_2-adrenoceptor agonists more than three times a week should be started on inhaled corticosteroids.

Inhaled corticosteroids

All patients who have regular persistent symptoms (even mild ones) need regular treatment with inhaled corticosteroids. Beclometasone dipropionate (BDP) is the most widely used inhaled steroid and is available in doses of 50, 100, 200 and 250 µg per puff. Other inhaled steroids include budesonide, fluticasone propionate, fluticasone furoate, mometasone furoate and triamcinolone.

Side-effects of inhaled steroids include oral thrush and hoarseness, and patients should be instructed to rinse their mouths out after using the inhaler. Subcapsular cataract formation is rare but can occur in the elderly. Osteoporosis is less likely than with oral

> ### *i* Box 28.20 Drugs used in asthma
>
> **Short-acting relievers**
> - Inhaled β_2 agonists (e.g. salbutamol (albuterol in USA), terbutaline)
>
> **Long-acting relievers/disease controllers**
> - Inhaled long-acting β_2 agonists (e.g. salmeterol, formoterol)
> - Inhaled corticosteroids (e.g. beclometasone, budesonide, fluticasone)
> - Compound inhaled long-acting β_2 agonists and corticosteroid (e.g. salmeterol and fluticasone)
> - Sodium cromoglicate
> - Leukotriene modifiers (e.g. montelukast, zafirlukast, zileuton)
>
> **Other agents with bronchodilator activity**
> - Inhaled antimuscarinic agents (e.g. ipratropium, oxitropium, aclidinium)
> - Theophylline preparations
> - Oral corticosteroids (e.g. prednisolone 40 mg daily)
>
> **Steroid-sparing agents**
> - Methotrexate
> - Ciclosporin
> - Intravenous immunoglobulin
> - Anti-IgE monoclonal antibody – omalizumab
> - Etanercept, infliximab, lebrikizumab

steroids but can occur with high-dose inhaled corticosteroids (beclometasone or budesonide >800 µg daily). In children, inhaled corticosteroids at doses above 400 µg daily have been shown to retard short-term growth but final heights are not affected. Inhaled corticosteroid use should be stepped down once asthma comes under control.

Oral corticosteroids and steroid-sparing agents

Oral corticosteroids are needed both for acute exacerbations and for longer-term use when other drug regimes have not controlled symptoms. The dose should be kept as low as possible to minimize side-effects. The effect of short-term treatment with prednisolone 30 mg daily is shown in **Fig. 28.14**. Some patients require continuing treatment with oral corticosteroids. Occasionally, low doses of methotrexate or ciclosporin are used as steroid-sparing agents in some steroid-dependent asthmatics but biologic monoclonal antibodies are now preferentially used in these patients.

Leukotriene receptor antagonists

This class of anti-asthma therapy targets the cysteinyl LT1 receptor. Montelukast, pranlukast (only available in South-east Asia) and zafirlukast are given orally and are effective in a subpopulation of asthma patients. However, it is not possible to predict which individuals will benefit; a 4-week trial of leukotriene receptor antagonist (LTRA) therapy is recommended before a decision is made to continue or stop. LTRAs should be tried in any patient who is not controlled on low to medium doses of inhaled steroids; their action is additive to that of LABAs. LTRAs are particularly useful in patients with aspirin-intolerant asthma. Because these drugs are orally active they are helpful in patients with asthma combined with rhinitis and in young children with asthma and/or virus-associated wheezing.

Antimuscarinic bronchodilators

Muscarinic receptors are found in the respiratory tract; large airways contain mainly M_3 receptors, whereas the peripheral lung tissue contains M_3 and M_1 receptors (see p. 931). A nebulized short-acting antimuscarinic agent, ipratropium, is used in acute severe exacerbations of asthma (**Box 28.21**). Short-acting inhaled antimuscarinic agents have not been shown to be of any benefit in patients who have asthma that is not controlled on standard therapy. Longer-acting antimuscarinics (tiotropium, aclidinium) can be tried in more severe cases.

Anti-inflammatory drugs

Sodium cromoglicate and nedocromil sodium prevent activation of many inflammatory cells, particularly mast cells, eosinophils and epithelial cells but not lymphocytes, by blocking a specific chloride channel, which in turn prevents calcium *influx*. These drugs are effective in patients with milder asthma but are not routinely used.

Monoclonal antibodies

Omalizumab, a recombinant humanized monoclonal antibody directed against IgE, chelates free IgE and downregulates the number and activity of mast cells and basophils. It is given subcutaneously every 2–4 weeks, depending on total serum IgE level and body weight. Although expensive, it is cost-effective in patients with frequent exacerbations requiring oral corticosteroids. Mepolizumab, reslizumab and benralizumab are newer monoclonal antibodies against interleukin-5 (IL-5) or its receptor. They have been shown to be effective in eosinophilic asthma and, similar to omalizumab, are cost-effective in patients who have recurrent exacerbations despite high-dose inhaled corticosteroids.

Currently in development is a wide range of other monoclonal antibody therapies against Th2 cytokine targets such as thymic stromal lymphopoietin (TSLP), thought to be important in asthma pathology.

Antibiotics

There is little evidence that antibiotics are helpful in managing patients with acute asthma. During acute exacerbations, yellow or green sputum containing eosinophils and bronchial epithelial cells may be coughed up. This is usually due to viral rather than bacterial infection and antibiotics are not required.

There is mixed evidence in severe asthma for long-term treatment with the macrolide antibiotic azithromycin, which has both anti-inflammatory and antibacterial actions.

Bronchial thermoplasty

Bronchial thermoplasty is a novel approach for moderate to severe persistent asthma. This bronchoscopic procedure uses radiofrequency radiation to heat the bronchial wall and reduce the mass of airway smooth muscle, decreasing bronchoconstriction. It is currently being evaluated.

Asthma attacks

Although these may occur spontaneously, asthma exacerbations are most commonly caused by lack of treatment adherence, respiratory virus infections associated with the common cold, and exposure to an allergen or triggering drug, e.g. an NSAID. Whenever possible, patients should have a written personalized plan that they can implement in anticipation or at the start of an exacerbation that includes the early use of a short course of oral corticosteroids. If the PEFR is >150 L/min, patients may improve dramatically on nebulized therapy and may not require hospital admission. Their regular treatment should be increased, to include treatment for 2 weeks with 30–60 mg of prednisolone, followed by substitution with an inhaled corticosteroid preparation. Short courses of oral prednisolone can be stopped abruptly without tailing down the dose.

Acute severe asthma

The term acute severe asthma is used to mean an exacerbation of asthma that has not been controlled by the use of standard medication.

Patients with acute severe asthma typically have:
- an inability to complete a sentence in one breath
- a respiratory rate of ≥25 breaths/min
- a tachycardia of ≥110 b.p.m. (pulsus paradoxus is not useful, as it is present in only 45% of cases)
- a PEFR of 33–50% of predicted normal or best.

Features of *life-threatening attacks* are:
- a silent chest, cyanosis or feeble respiratory effort
- exhaustion or altered level of consciousness
- bradycardia, hypotension or arrhythmia
- a PEFR of <33% of predicted normal or best (approximately 150 L/min in adults) or S_pO_2 of <92%.

Arterial blood gases should always be measured in asthmatic patients requiring admission to hospital, with particular attention paid to the P_aCO_2. *Pulse oximetry* is useful in monitoring oxygen saturation during the admission and can reduce the need for repeated arterial puncture.

Features suggesting *very severe life-threatening attacks* are:
- a high P_aCO_2 of >6 kPa
- severe hypoxaemia: P_aO_2 <8 kPa despite treatment with oxygen
- a low and/or falling arterial pH.

Management (see **Box 28.21**) consists of nebulized short-acting bronchodilators; nebulized antimuscarinics (e.g. ipratropium bromide) are also helpful. Intravenous hydrocortisone should be given together with prednisolone (40–60 mg daily) orally. If symptoms are not controlled, consider a single dose of intravenous magnesium sulphate (1.2 g–2 g infusion over 20 min).

Intravenous β_2-adrenoceptor agonists or aminophylline may be considered. Ventilation is required for patients who deteriorate despite this initial regimen. A chest X-ray is helpful to exclude pneumothorax and other causes of dyspnoea.

Further reading

Chung KF, Wenzel SE, Brozek JL et al. International ERS/ATS guidelines on definition, evaluation and treatment of severe asthma. *Eur Respir J* 2014; 43:343–373.
Scottish Intercollegiate Guidelines Network/British Thoracic Society. *SIGN 153: British Guideline on the Management of Asthma.* SIGN/BTS 2016; https://www.brit-thoracic.org.uk/.
Wong GWK. How should we treat patients with mild asthma? *N Engl J Med* 2019; 380:2064–2066.

Acute bronchitis

Acute bronchitis in previously healthy subjects is often viral. Bacterial infection with *Strep. pneumoniae* or *H. influenzae* is a common sequel to viral infections, and is more likely to occur in cigarette smokers or people with COPD.

The illness begins with an irritating, non-productive cough, together with discomfort behind the sternum. There may be associated chest tightness, wheezing and shortness of breath. Later the cough becomes productive, with yellow or green sputum. There is a mild fever and a neutrophil leucocytosis; wheeze with occasional crackles can be heard on auscultation. In otherwise healthy adults the disease improves spontaneously in 4–8 days without serious illness.

Antibiotics are often given (e.g. amoxicillin 250 mg three times daily), but it is not known whether they hasten recovery in otherwise healthy individuals and in most cases they should not be given.

Box 28.21 Treatment of acute severe asthma

At home
1. The patient is assessed. Tachycardia, a high respiratory rate and inability to speak in sentences indicate a severe attack.
2. If the peak expiratory flow rate (PEFR) is <150 L/min (in adults), an ambulance should be called.
3. Nebulized salbutamol 5 mg or terbutaline 10 mg is administered.
4. Hydrocortisone 200 mg i.v. is given.
5. Oxygen 40–60% is given if available.
6. Prednisolone 60 mg is given orally.

In hospital
1. The patient is reassessed.
2. Oxygen 40–60% is given.
3. The PEFR and O_2 saturation are measured.
4. Nebulized salbutamol 5 mg or terbutaline 10 mg is repeated and administered 4-hourly.
5. Nebulized ipratropium bromide 0.5 mg is added to nebulized salbutamol/terbutaline.
6. Hydrocortisone 200 mg i.v. is given.
7. Prednisolone is continued at 40–60 mg orally daily for at least 5 days.
8. Arterial blood gases are measured; if the P_aCO_2 is >8, ventilation may be required.
9. A chest X-ray is performed to exclude pneumothorax.
10. If there is no improvement, i.v. magnesium sulphate is given at 1.2–2 g over 20 min.
11. If there is still no improvement, urgent transfer to the intensive treatment unit is arranged.

Chronic bronchitis

Chronic bronchitis, one of the clinical syndromes of COPD (see next section), is classically defined as a daily productive cough for 3 months per year for 2 consecutive years.

Chronic obstructive pulmonary disease

Definition

Chronic obstructive pulmonary disease (COPD) has been described as 'a disease state characterized by airflow limitation that is not fully reversible. The airflow limitation is usually both progressive and associated with an abnormal inflammatory response of the lungs to noxious particles or gases.' COPD is an overarching diagnosis that brings together a variety of clinical syndromes (emphysema, small airways disease and chronic bronchitis) associated with airflow limitation and destruction of the lung parenchyma. There is resultant hyperinflation of the lungs, ventilation/perfusion mismatch, increased work of breathing and breathlessness.

The condition is associated with a number of co-morbidities, such as ischaemic heart disease, hypertension, diabetes, heart failure and cancer, suggesting that it may be part of a generalized systemic inflammatory process.

Epidemiology and aetiology

COPD is caused by long-term exposure to toxic particles and gases. In developed countries, cigarette smoking accounts for over 90% of cases. In developing countries, other factors are also implicated, such as inhalation of smoke from biomass heating fuels and cooking in poorly ventilated areas. Only 10–20% of smokers develop COPD, which suggests that there is an underlying individual susceptibility.

Urbanization, air pollution, socioeconomic class and occupation may also play a part in the aetiology but these effects are difficult to separate from that of smoking. Some animal studies suggest that diet could be a risk factor for COPD but this has not been proven in humans.

The economic burden of COPD is considerable. In the UK COPD causes approximately 18 million lost working days annually for men and 2.1 million lost working days for women, accounting for about 7% of all days of absence from work due to sickness. Nevertheless, the number of COPD admissions to UK hospitals has been falling steadily since the mid-1980s.

Pathophysiology

Pathologically, there is evidence of airways inflammation and structural changes within the airways and the lung parenchyma.

Structural changes

Structurally, there may be evidence of emphysema and small airways disease, with increased mucus-producing goblet cells in the bronchial mucosa, which may lead to chronic bronchitis (**Figs 28.20** and **28.21**). The physiological consequence of these changes is the development of airflow limitation.

Pathologically, there is evidence of both acute and chronic inflammation; endobronchial biopsies demonstrate a predominance of neutrophils, CD8-predominant lymphocytes and macrophages. This chronic inflammation results in scarring and fibrosis of the small airways. In addition, there is destruction of the alveolar walls, which results in emphysema. The phenotype of COPD will differ, depending on the predominance of small airways disease, emphysema or chronic bronchitis.

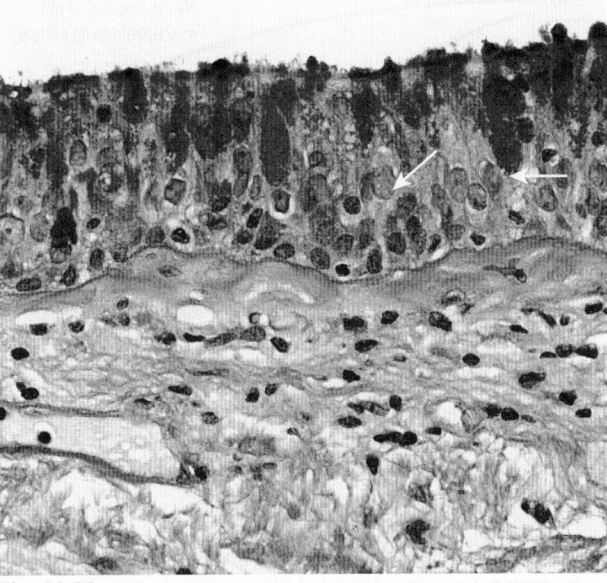

Fig. 28.20 Chronic obstructive pulmonary disease (COPD). Section of bronchial mucosa stained for mucus glands by periodic acid–Schiff (PAS) showing an increase in mucus-secreting goblet cells (arrowed). *(Courtesy of Dr J Wilson and Dr S Wilson, University of Southampton.)*

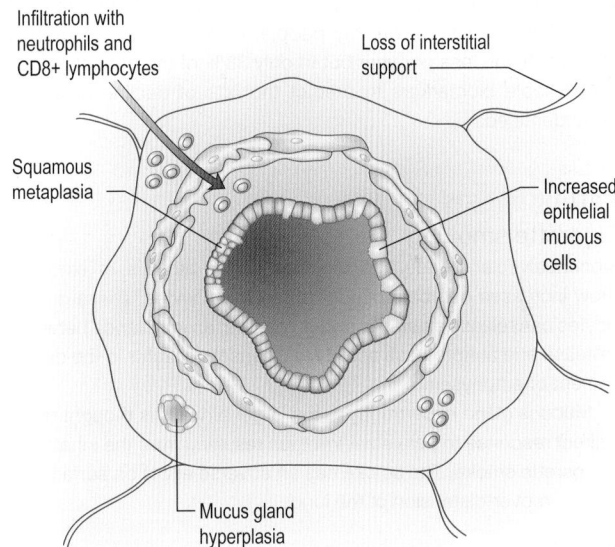

Fig. 28.21 Pathological changes in the airways in chronic obstructive pulmonary disease.

Emphysema

Emphysema is defined as abnormal and permanent enlargement of air spaces distal to the terminal bronchiole, accompanied by destruction of their walls. It is classified according to the distribution:

- *Centri-acinar emphysema.* Distension and damage of lung tissue are concentrated around the respiratory bronchioles, while the more distal alveolar ducts and alveoli tend to be well preserved. This form of emphysema is extremely common.
- *Pan-acinar emphysema.* This is less common but is the type associated with α_1-antitrypsin deficiency (see later). Distension and destruction affect the whole acinus, and in severe cases the lung is just a collection of bullae. Severe airflow limitation and mismatch occur.

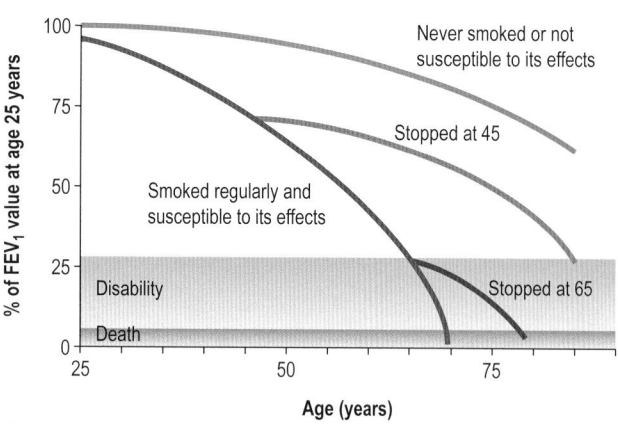

Fig. 28.22 Influence of smoking on airflow limitation. FEV_1, forced expiratory volume in 1 sec. *(From Fletcher CM, Peto R. The natural history of chronic airflow obstruction. Bri Med J 1977; 1:1645.)*

- *Irregular emphysema.* There is scarring and damage that affect the lung parenchyma patchily, independent of acinar structure.

  Emphysema leads to expiratory airflow limitation and air trapping. The loss of lung elastic recoil results in an increase in TLC. Premature closure of airways limits expiratory flow while the loss of alveoli decreases capacity for gas transfer.

  The *classic Fletcher and Peto studies* (**Fig. 28.22**) showed a loss of 50 mL per year in FEV_1 in patients with COPD compared with 20 mL per year in healthy people. A more recent study has shown a 40 mL loss per year but in only 38% of the patients studied. Reliable biomarkers to predict the rate of decline have not been identified.

Pathogenesis

Cigarette smoking

Bronchoalveolar lavage and biopsies of the airways of smokers show increased numbers of neutrophil granulocytes. These granulocytes can release elastases and proteases; an imbalance between protease and antiprotease activity is a causative factor in the development of emphysema.

Mucous gland hypertrophy in the larger airways is thought to be a direct response to persistent irritation resulting from the inhalation of cigarette smoke. The smoke has an adverse effect on surfactant, favouring over-distension of the lungs.

Infections

Respiratory infections are often the precipitating cause of acute exacerbations of the disease. It is less clear whether infection is responsible for the progressive airflow limitation that characterizes disabling COPD. Prompt use of antibiotics and routine vaccinations against influenza and pneumococci are appropriate.

Alpha₁-antitrypsin deficiency

Alpha₁-antitrypsin is a proteinase inhibitor produced in the liver; it is secreted into the blood and diffuses into the lung. Here it inhibits proteolytic enzymes such as neutrophil elastase, which are capable of destroying alveolar wall connective tissue. In α_1-antitrypsin deficiency, the protein accumulates in the liver, leading to low levels in the lung.

More than 75 alleles of the α_1-antitrypsin gene have been described. The three main phenotypes are MM (normal), MZ (heterozygous deficiency) and ZZ (homozygous deficiency). Hereditary

Box 28.22 COPD Assessment Test (CAT)

Minimal symptom statement	Score	Maximal symptoms	Score
I never cough	0 1 2 3 4 5 6	I cough all the time	
I have no phlegm at all	0 1 2 3 4 5 6	My chest is full of phlegm	
My chest doesn't feel tight at all	0 1 2 3 4 5 6	My chest feels very tight	
When I walk up a hill or one flight of stairs, I do not feel breathless at all	0 1 2 3 4 5 6	When I walk up a hill or one flight of stairs I am very breathless	
I am not limited doing any activities at home	0 1 2 3 4 5 6	I am very limited during activities at home	
I am confident leaving home despite my lung condition	0 1 2 3 4 5 6	I am not at all confident leaving home because of my lung condition	
I sleep soundly	0 1 2 3 4 5 6	I don't sleep soundly because of my lung condition	
I have lots of energy	0 1 2 3 4 5 6	I have no energy	
Total score			

(From Jones PW, Harding G, Berry P et al. Development and first validation of the COPD Assessment Test. Eur Respir J 2009; 34:648–654.)

deficiency of α_1-antitrypsin accounts for about 2% of UK emphysema cases. Deficiency can also cause liver disease (see p. 1302).

Clinical features

Symptoms

The characteristic symptoms of COPD are productive cough with white or clear sputum, wheeze and breathlessness. Individuals will be more prone to lower respiratory tract infections. Systemic effects include hypertension, osteoporosis, depression, weight loss and reduced muscle mass with general weakness and right heart failure.

Signs

In mild COPD there may be no signs or just quiet wheeze throughout the chest. In severe disease the patient is tachypnoeic, with prolonged expiration. The accessory muscles of respiration are used and there may be intercostal indrawing on inspiration and pursing of the lips on expiration (see p. 932). The cricosternal distance is reduced. Chest expansion is poor, the lungs are hyperinflated and there is loss of the normal cardiac and liver dullness.

Patients who remain responsive to CO_2 are usually breathless and rarely cyanosed. Heart failure and oedema are rare features, except as terminal events. In contrast, patients who become insensitive to CO_2 are often oedematous and cyanosed but not particularly breathless. Those with hypercapnia may have peripheral vasodilation, a bounding pulse, and a coarse flapping tremor of the outstretched hands. Severe hypercapnia causes confusion and progressive drowsiness. Papilloedema may be present but this is neither specific nor sensitive as a diagnostic feature.

Patients in the later stages may develop respiratory failure, pulmonary hypertension and cor pulmonale.

Diagnosis

This is usually clinical and based on a history of breathlessness and sputum production in a chronic smoker. In the absence of a history of cigarette smoking, asthma is a more likely explanation, unless there is a family history suggesting α_1-antitrypsin deficiency.

No individual clinical feature is diagnostic. The patient may have signs of hyperinflation and typical pursed lip respiration. There may be signs of over-inflation of the lungs (e.g. loss of liver dullness on percussion) but this also occurs in other diseases such as asthma. Conversely, centri-acinar emphysema may be present without signs of over-inflation. The chest may become 'barrel-shaped' but this can also result from osteoporosis of the spine in older men without emphysema.

The degree of breathlessness may be recorded using the Medical Research Council (MRC) dyspnoea score, while the COPD Assessment Test (CAT) is a patient scored symptom tool that measures the impact of the disease on the individual's health and wellbeing (**Box 28.22**).

Investigations

- **Lung function tests** show evidence of airflow limitation (see **Fig. 28.23**). The FEV_1:FVC ratio is reduced and the PEFR is low. In many patients the airflow limitation is partly reversible (usually a change in FEV_1 of <15%). Lung volumes may be normal or increased; carbon monoxide gas transfer factor is low when significant emphysema is present.
- **Chest X-ray** is often normal, even when disease is advanced. The classic features are over-inflation of the lungs with low, flattened diaphragms, and sometimes the presence of large bullae. Blood vessels may be 'pruned', with large proximal vessels and relatively little blood visible in the peripheral lung fields.
- **HRCT scans** are useful, particularly when the plain chest X-ray is normal.
- **Haemoglobin level and packed cell volume** can be elevated as a result of persistent hypoxaemia (secondary polycythaemia; see p. 356).
- **Blood gases** may be helpful to determine if there is any evidence of respiratory failure.
- **Sputum examination** may reveal *Strep. pneumoniae*, *H. influenzae* and *Moraxella catarrhalis*, which can cause infective exacerbations. Many acute episodes are viral in origin.
- **ECG** is often normal. If a patient has pulmonary hypertension secondary to COPD, the P wave is tall (P pulmonale), and there may be a right bundle branch block and evidence of right ventricular hypertrophy (see p. 1055).
- **Echocardiography** is useful to assess cardiac function where there is disproportionate dyspnoea.
- **α_1-Antitrypsin** levels and genotype are worth measuring in premature disease or life-long non-smokers.

Management

See **Fig. 28.23** for management strategies.

Smoking cessation

The single most useful measure is to persuade the patient to stop smoking. Even in advanced disease, this may slow down the rate of deterioration and prolong the time before disability and death occur (see **Fig. 28.22**). Smoke from burning biomass fuels in poorly ventilated homes should also be reduced.

Drug therapy

This is used both for the short-term management of exacerbations and for the long-term relief of symptoms. Many of the drugs used are similar to those employed in asthma (see p. 952).

> **Box 28.23 Classification of airflow limitation severity in COPD (based on post-bronchodilator FEV_1)**
>
> **In patients with FEV_1/FVC < 0.70:**
>
> | | | |
> |---|---|---|
> | GOLD 1: | Mild | $FEV_1 \geq 80\%$ predicted |
> | GOLD 2: | Moderate | $50\% \leq FEV_1 < 80\%$ predicted |
> | GOLD 3: | Severe | $30\% \leq FEV_1 < 50\%$ predicted |
> | GOLD 4: | Very severe | $FEV_1 < 30\%$ predicted |
>
> *(From Global Initiative for Chronic Obstructive Lung Disease (GOLD), 2016; www.goldcopd.com.)*

Bronchodilators

- **β-Adrenoceptor agonists.** Many patients with mild COPD feel less breathless after inhaling a β-adrenergic agonist such as salbutamol (200 µg every 4–6 h). In more severe airway limitation (moderate and severe COPD) a long-acting β_2 agonist should be used.
- **Antimuscarinic drugs.** Regular use of a LAMA (such as inhaled tiotropium) improves lung function, symptoms of dyspnoea and quality of life. Use of a LAMA does not prevent the decline in FEV_1.
- **Theophyllines.** Long-acting preparations of theophylline are of little benefit in COPD.

Phosphodiesterase type 4 inhibitors

Roflumilast is a phosphodiesterase inhibitor with anti-inflammatory properties. It is used as an adjunct to bronchodilators for maintenance treatment in those patients with an FEV_1 of less than 50% and chronic bronchitis.

Corticosteroids

Inhaled corticosteroids are recommended in patients with frequent exacerbations or a FEV_1 of less than 50% predicted. Demonstration of a blood eosinophilia may identify patients who are more likely to have a beneficial response to inhaled corticosteroid therapy. High-dose inhaled steroids are not advised, as their use is linked to increased rates of pneumonia.

Oral corticosteroids are prescribed in the context of an acute exacerbation.

Antibiotics

Prompt antibiotic treatment shortens exacerbations and should always be given in acute episodes, as it may prevent hospital admission and further lung damage. Patients can be given antibiotics to keep at home, starting them as soon as their sputum turns yellow or green.

In patients who experience frequent exacerbations, long-term treatment with macrolide antibiotics such as azithromycin has been shown to reduce exacerbations and improve quality of life.

Mucolytic agents

These reduce sputum viscosity and can reduce the number of acute exacerbations. A meta-analysis showed that mucolytics such as carbocysteine are useful in preventing COPD exacerbations in those who experience them frequently.

Oxygen therapy

Two controlled trials (chiefly in males) have shown improved survival with continuous administration of oxygen at 2 L/min via nasal prongs to achieve an oxygen saturation of more than 90% for large proportions of the day and night. Survival curves from these two studies are shown in **Fig. 28.24**. Only 30% of those not receiving long-term

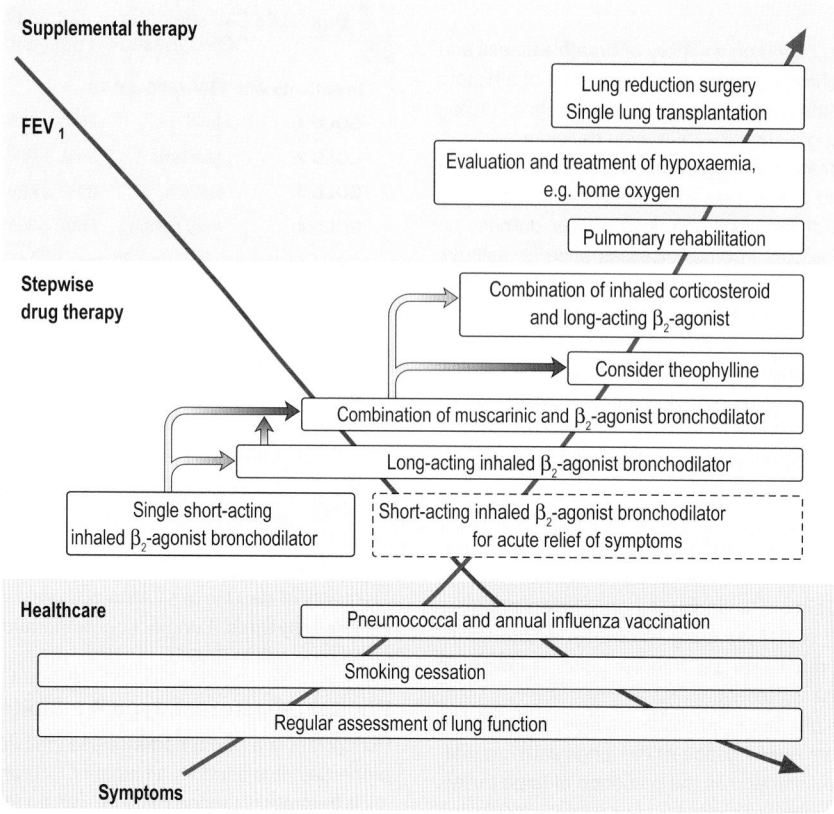

Fig. 28.23 Algorithm for the treatment of chronic obstructive pulmonary disease. The various components of management are shown as the forced expiratory volume in 1 sec (FEV$_1$) decreases and the symptoms become more severe. (*After Sutherland ER, Cherniack RM. Management of chronic obstructive pulmonary disease.* N Engl J Med *2004; 350:2689–2697. © 2004 Massachusetts Medical Society. All rights reserved.*)

oxygen therapy survived for more than 5 years. A fall in pulmonary artery pressure was achieved if oxygen was given for 15 hours daily, but substantial improvement in mortality was achieved only by the administration of oxygen for 19 hours daily. These results suggest that long-term continuous domiciliary oxygen therapy will benefit patients who have a:

- P_aO_2 of <7.3 kPa (55 mmHg) when breathing air; measurements should be taken on two occasions at least 3 weeks apart after appropriate bronchodilator therapy (**Box 28.24**)
- P_aO_2 of <8 kPa with secondary polycythaemia, nocturnal hypoxaemia, peripheral oedema or evidence of pulmonary hypertension
- carboxyhaemoglobin of <3% (i.e. patients who have stopped smoking).
  Domiciliary oxygen is best provided via an oxygen concentrator.

Pulmonary rehabilitation

Pulmonary rehabilitation courses are an essential part of management in COPD, and randomized control trials have shown them to improve symptoms of fatigue and dyspnoea, as well as exercise tolerance.

Additional measures

- **Vaccines.** Patients with COPD should receive a single dose of the polyvalent pneumococcal polysaccharide vaccine and yearly influenza vaccinations.

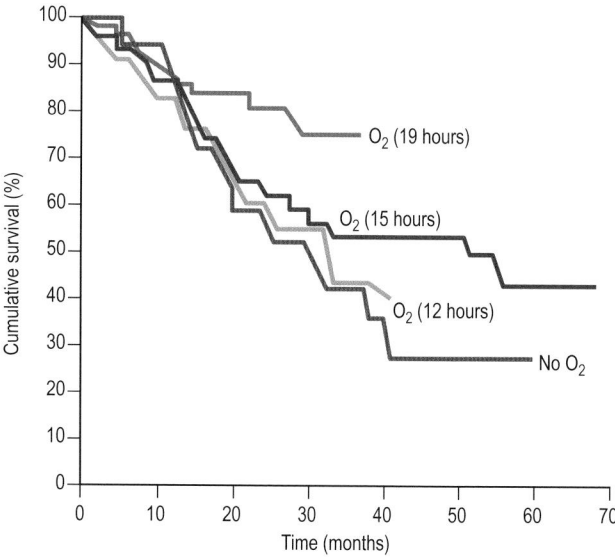

Fig. 28.24 Cumulative survival curves for patients receiving oxygen. Oxygen doses are in hours per day.

- **α_1-Antitrypsin replacement.** Weekly or monthly infusions of α_1-antitrypsin have been recommended for patients with serum levels <310 mg/L and abnormal lung function. Whether this modifies long-term progression remains to be determined.
- **Heart failure.** This should be treated (see p. 1073).

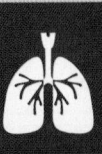

- *Secondary polycythaemia.* This requires venesection if the packed cell volume is >55%.
- *Sensation of breathlessness.* Short-acting sedation such as sublingual lorazepam or opiates may be a helpful palliative measure for intractable dyspnoea. Other useful adjuncts include breathing techniques and fan therapy.
- *Air travel.* Commercial aircraft are pressurized to the equivalent of 2000–2400 m altitude. In healthy people, this causes P_aO_2 to fall from 13.5 to 10 kPa, leading to a trivial 3% drop in oxygen saturation, but patients with moderate COPD may desaturate significantly. The desaturation associated with air travel can be simulated by breathing 15% oxygen at sea level. Patients whose saturation drops below 85% within 15 minutes should be advised to contact their airline to request supplemental oxygen during their flight.
- *Surgery.* Some patients have large emphysematous bullae that reduce lung capacity. Surgical bullectomy can enable adjacent areas of collapsed lung to re-expand, thereby restoring function. In addition, carefully selected patients with severe COPD (FEV_1 <1 L) have been treated with lung volume reduction surgery. Initial studies suggested that ventilation was improved and patients felt less breathless, although mortality was unchanged. However, a controlled trial in severe emphysema found increased mortality and no improvement in the patient's condition. *Single lung transplantation* (see p. 994) is used for end-stage emphysema.
- *Endobronchial valves.* These occlude airways of hyperinflated emphysematous lungs and effectively achieve lung volume reduction. In selected patients, studies have shown an improvement in quality of life and exercise tolerance.

COPD exacerbation

Acute exacerbations may be precipitated by a viral or bacterial infection. Patients may have symptoms of cough, acute bronchospasm and dyspnoea. Type I and type II respiratory failure may occur as a consequence of a COPD exacerbation.

Management consists of the following measures:
- *Airway, breathing and circulation.* These should be assessed (see Ch. 10).
- *Oxygen therapy.* COPD is by far the most common cause of respiratory failure. In managing respiratory failure, the main

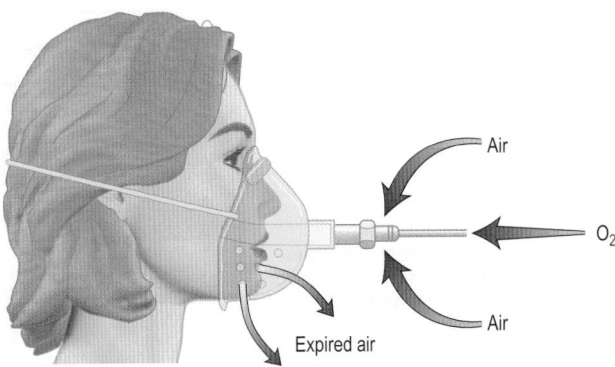

Fig. 28.25 'Fixed-performance' device for administration of oxygen to spontaneously breathing patients (Venturi mask). Oxygen is delivered through the injector of the Venturi mask at a given flow rate. A proportionate amount of air is entrained and the inspired oxygen can be predicted accurately. Masks are available that deliver 24%, 28% and 35% oxygen.

goal is to improve the P_aO_2 by continuous oxygen therapy. A fixed-percentage mask (Venturi mask, **Fig. 28.25**) is used to deliver controlled concentrations of oxygen. Initially, 24% oxygen is given, and the concentration of inspired oxygen can be gradually increased, provided the P_aCO_2 does not rise unacceptably. In type II respiratory failure, the P_aCO_2 is elevated and the patient is dependent on hypoxic drive. In this setting, giving additional oxygen will nearly always cause a further rise in P_aCO_2. Patients at risk of hypercapnia should be managed with oxygen therapy to maintain the saturations within a target range of 88–92%. It is important to monitor arterial blood gases closely if there is any risk of decompensated type II respiratory failure. If there is evidence of respiratory acidosis (pH <7.35 with an elevated P_aCO_2), despite medical management, the patient should be considered for non-invasive ventilation unless there are any contraindications (**Fig. 28.26**).
- *Corticosteroids, antibiotics and bronchodilators.* These should be administered in the acute phase of an exacerbation but decisions on long-term use should wait until the patient has recovered (see earlier).
- *Removal of retained secretions.* Patients should be encouraged to cough up secretions. Physiotherapy is helpful in achieving adequate chest clearance.

Type II respiratory failure in COPD

- *Respiratory support* (see p. 227). Non-invasive ventilation should be offered if a patient has a persistent respiratory acidosis with a pH of <7.35. Randomized controlled trials have demonstrated that non-invasive ventilation (NIV) reduces the need for intubation and lowers mortality. Indications and contraindications are shown in **Boxes 28.25** and **28.26**. Assisted ventilation with an endotracheal tube is occasionally necessary for patients with COPD who have severe respiratory failure but only when there is a clear precipitating factor and the overall prognosis is reasonable. Assessing the likelihood of reversibility in an acute setting can present a difficult ethical problem.

Prognosis of COPD

Predictors of a poor prognosis are increasing age and worsening airflow limitation: that is, decreasing FEV_1. A predictive index

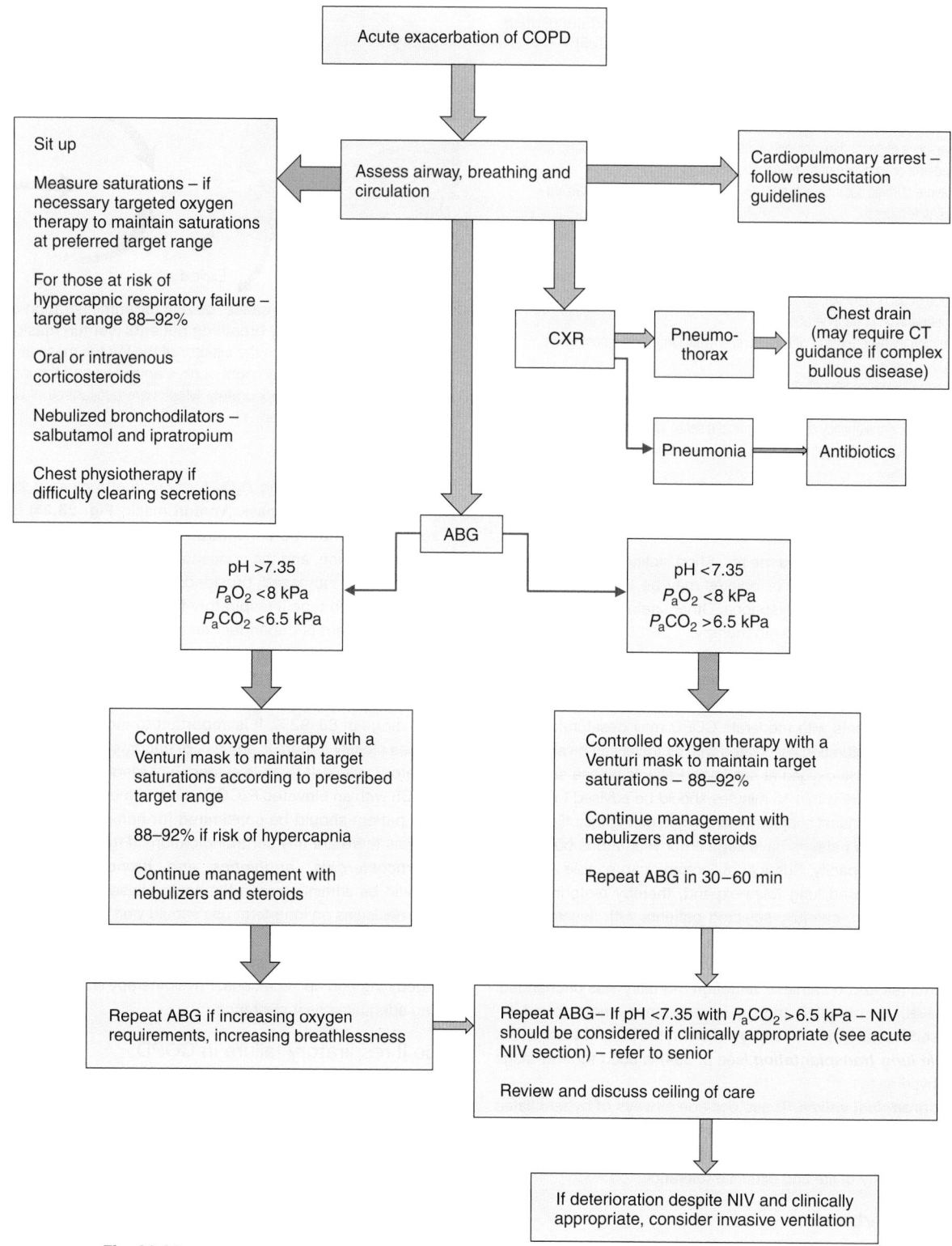

Fig. 28.26 Algorithm for the treatment of respiratory failure in COPD. BiPAP, bilevel positive airway pressure; CPAP, continuous positive airway pressure; CXR, chest X-ray. NIV, non-invasive ventilation.

(BODE, body mass index, degree of airflow obstruction, dyspnoea and exercise capacity) is shown in **Box 28.27**. A patient with a BODE index of 0–2 has a 4-year mortality rate of 10%, compared with 80% in someone with a BODE index of 7–10. This scoring tool may be useful in determining timing of referral for transplant consideration.

Obstructive sleep apnoea

Obstructive sleep apnoea (OSA) is a form of sleep-disordered breathing that is characterized by upper airway collapse resulting in obstructive apnoeas and hypopnoeas with desaturation. The prevalence of this condition is 3–5% of the population and it occurs most often in overweight, middle-aged men. The prevalence of OSA increases with

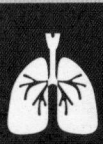

Box 28.25 Indications for non-invasive ventilation (NIV)

Conditions in which ward-based NIV is used	Clinical symptoms and biochemical markers
COPD, obesity	Respiratory rate >23 breaths/min pH <7.35 P_aCO_2 >6.5 kPa
Neuromuscular disease	Respiratory illness with respiratory rate >20 breaths/min if usual vital capacity <1 L, even if P_aCO_2 <6.5 kPa pH <7.35 P_aCO_2 >6.5 kPa

Box 28.26 Contraindications to ward-based non-invasive ventilation (NIV)

Absolute
- Severe facial deformity
- Facial burns
- Asthma
- Vomiting

Relative
- pH <7.15[a]
- pH <7.25 and additional adverse features[a]
- Glasgow Coma Scale score <8[a]
- Confusion or agitation[a]
- Cognitive impairment

[a]Consider NIV in a critical care setting.

Box 28.27 BODE index[a]

Variable	Points on BODE index			
	0	**1**	**2**	**3**
FEV$_1$ (% of predicted)	≥65	50–64	36–49	≤35
Distance walked in 6 min (m)	≥350	250–349	150–249	≤149
MMRC dyspnoea scale[b]	0–1	2	3	4
Body mass index	>21	≤21		

[a]*B*ody mass index, degree of airflow *o*bstruction, *d*yspnoea and *e*xercise capacity.
[b]Scores on the modified Medical Research Council (MMRC) dyspnoea scale range from 0 to 4, a score of 4 indicating that the patient is breathless when dressing.

age, menopause, obesity and endocrine conditions such as acromegaly and hypothyroidism. Obesity is increasing in developed countries and so the incidence of OSA is also predicted to rise. OSA can occur in children, particularly those with enlarged tonsils or trisomy 21. The major symptoms and their frequency are listed in **Box 28.28**.

Pathophysiology

During sleep, activity of the respiratory muscles is reduced, especially during rapid eye movement (REM) sleep when the diaphragm is virtually the only active muscle. Apnoeas occur when the airway at the back of the throat is sucked closed when breathing in during sleep. When the person is awake, this tendency is overcome by the action of opening muscles of the upper airway (the genioglossus and palatal muscles), but these become hypotonic during sleep (**Fig. 28.27**). Partial narrowing results in snoring, complete occlusion causes apnoea and critical narrowing causes hypopnoeas. Apnoea leads to hypoxia and increasingly strenuous respiratory efforts until

Box 28.28 Symptoms (%) of obstructive sleep apnoea

Loud snoring	95
Daytime sleepiness	90
Unrefreshed sleep	40
Restless sleep	40
Morning headache	30
Nocturnal choking	30
Reduced libido	20
Morning 'drunkenness'	5
Ankle swelling	5

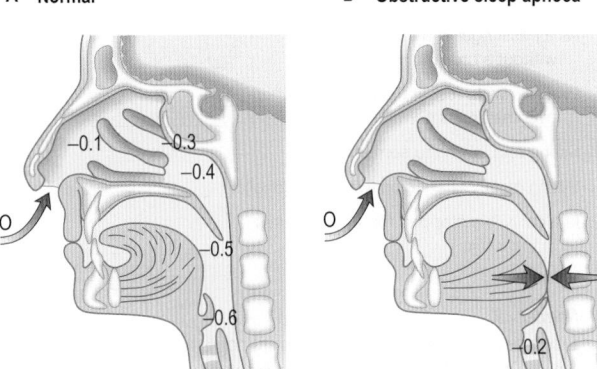

Fig. 28.27 Section through head, showing pressure changes in normal patients and those with obstructive sleep apnoea (OSA). **(A)** There is a pressure drop during inspiration as air is sucked through the turbinates. Changes are shown in kPa. **(B)** In OSA this is sufficient to collapse the pharynx (arrowed on right), obstructing inspiration.

the patient overcomes the resistance. The combination of central hypoxic stimulation and the effort to overcome obstruction wakes the patient from sleep. These awakenings are so brief that patients remain unaware of them but may be woken hundreds of times per night, leading to sleep deprivation with consequent daytime sleepiness and impaired intellectual performance.

Correctable factors occur in about one-third of cases and include:
- ***encroachment on pharynx*** – obesity, acromegaly, enlarged tonsils
- ***nasal obstruction*** – nasal deformities, rhinitis, polyps, adenoids
- ***respiratory depressant drugs*** – alcohol, sedatives, strong analgesics.

Diagnosis

Relatives often provide a good history of the snore–silence–snore cycle. Individuals may complain of poor concentration and of waking feeling unrefreshed. The Epworth Sleepiness Scale (**Box 28.29**) is a measure of excessive daytime sleepiness and may prompt investigation. The STOP BANG tool (**Box 28.30**) is also a useful screening tool and should flag appropriate patients to refer for further investigation. It may help discriminate OSA from simple snoring.

Investigations

If the diagnosis is suspected, further investigation is necessary to determine if there is sleep-disordered breathing. Many of these investigations can be performed at home, using overnight pulse oximetry, and monitoring the pulse and the oxygen level. Oximetry

---

ℹ️ **Box 28.29 Epworth sleepiness scale**

How likely are you to doze off or fall asleep in the following situations, in contrast to just feeling tired? This refers to your usual way of life in recent times. Even if you have not done some of these things recently, try to work out how they would have affected you. Use the following scale to choose the most appropriate number for each situation.

  0 = would never doze
  1 = slight chance of dozing
  2 = moderate chance of dozing
  3 = high chance of dozing

Situation	Chance of dozing
Sitting and reading	_____
Watching TV	_____
Sitting and inactive in a public place (theatre or meeting)	_____
As a passenger in a car for an hour without a break	_____
Lying down to rest in the afternoon when circumstances permit	_____
Sitting and talking to someone	_____
Sitting quietly after lunch (without alcohol)	_____
In a car, while stopped for a few minutes in the traffic	_____
TOTAL	_____

Normal <9

Excessive daytime somnolence >9 – causes include obstructive sleep apnoea. Other conditions causing excessive daytime somnolence include narcolepsy, restless leg syndrome and periodic limb movement disorder.

ℹ️ **Box 28.30 STOP BANG tool**

Question	Answer
Snoring – do you snore?	Yes/No
Tiredness – do you often feel tired, fatigued or sleepy?	Yes/No
Observed apnoeas	Yes/No
Pressure – do you have high blood pressure or are you on treatment for it?	Yes/No
Body mass index >35	Yes/No
Age >50 years	Yes/No
Neck size (≥male 43 cm, women ≥41 cm)	Yes/No
Gender – male	Yes/No

Obstructive sleep apnoea: low risk = yes to 0–2 questions, intermediate risk = yes to 3–4, high risk = yes to 5–8.

❓ **Box 28.31 Causes of chronic ventilatory failure**

Airflow obstruction
- Chronic obstructive pulmonary disease

Restrictive lung disease
- Obstructive sleep apnoea/obesity hypoventilation syndrome
- Kyphoscoliosis
- Thoracoplasty

Neuromuscular disease
- Post-polio syndrome
- Diaphragm palsy
- Motor neurone disease
- Myotonic dystrophy

Central causes
- Brain injury
- Multiple system atrophy

---

will demonstrate desaturations in a cyclical manner, which will give a typical sawtooth appearance. The oximetry desaturation index (ODI) measures the number of desaturations per hour, which can determine the severity of sleep apnoea and correlates with the apnoea–hypopnea index (see later).

Overnight oximetry will not differentiate between central and obstructive apnoeas. Multichannel sleep studies (nocturnal polygraphy), which measure body posture and movements, breathing rate and electroencephalography alongside pulse oximetry, are used where the diagnosis is uncertain.

Severity is defined by the number of episodes of apnoea or hypopnea per hour, which is known as the **apnoea–hypopnea index (AHI)**:
- AHI <5: normal
- AHI 5–15: mild OSA
- AHI 15–30: moderate OSA
- AHI >30: severe OSA.

Management

Management consists of correction of treatable factors, including encouraging weight loss and alcohol reduction. Patients who have OSA with associated daytime somnolence should be offered continuous positive airway pressure (CPAP) during sleep. CPAP splints the upper airway such that it cannot occlude. It improves symptoms, quality of life, daytime alertness and survival.

Chronic ventilatory failure

Ventilatory failure, also known as type II respiratory failure (see p. 224), is a failure of alveolar ventilation with associated hypercapnia. This can be the sequela of a number of conditions that result in an imbalance of the resistive load in the lungs (**Box 28.31**). Symptoms of hypercapnia include morning headaches, daytime somnolence, confusion, memory impairment and unsteadiness.

Domiciliary non-invasive ventilation

Home mechanical ventilation can be considered if a patient has persistent hypercapnia due to one of the conditions above. Patients typically use a portable ventilator overnight, which provides positive pressure support at different levels during inspiration and expiration. Home mechanical ventilation has been shown to improve survival in COPD patients who have persistent type II respiratory failure following an acute admission. There are no randomized trials of NIV in kyphoscoliosis; however, survival curves show improved survival where NIV is offered. In patients with neuromuscular disorders, home NIV has been shown to improve quality of life and prolong survival.

Further reading

Boucher RC. Muco-Obstructive Lung Diseases. *New Engl J Med* 2019; 380:1941–1953.

Jones PW, Harding G, Berry P et al. Development and first validation of the COPD Assessment Test. *Eur Respir J* 2009; 34:648–654.

Murphy PB, Rehal S, Arbane G et al. Effect of home non-invasive ventilation with oxygen therapy vs oxygen therapy alone on hospital readmission or death after an acute COPD exacerbation: a randomised controlled trial. *JAMA* 2017; 317:2177–2186.

Suissa S and Drazen JM. Making sense of Triple Inhaled Therapy for COPD. *New Engl J Med* 2018; 1723–1724

Zeng Z, Yang D, Huang X et al. Effect of carbocisteine on patients with COPD: a systematic review and meta-analysis. *Int J Chron Obstruct Pulmon Dis* 2017; 12:2277–2283.

https://goldcopd.org/. *Global Initiative for Chronic Obstructive Lung Disease (2019 Report)*.

https://www.brit-thoracic.org.uk. *British Thoracic Society guidelines for home oxygen use in adults (2015)*.

https://www.catestonline.org. *COPD Assessment Test (CAT)*.

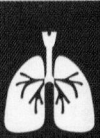

SMOKING

Prevalence

Cigarette smoking is declining in the Western world but remains a leading cause of preventable death. The World Health Organization (WHO) predicts that tobacco is responsible for the death of 7 million people each year. In 1974 in the UK, 51% of men and 41% of women smoked cigarettes – nearly half the adult population – whereas the annual population survey of 2015 showed that 17.2% of adults in the UK smoked.

Toxic effects

Cigarette smoke contains polycyclic aromatic hydrocarbons and nitrosamines, which are potent carcinogens. Smokers have an increase in neutrophils and macrophages in the airways. These inflammatory cells release proteases that are capable of destroying elastin and lead to lung damage. Pulmonary epithelial permeability increases, even in symptomless cigarette smokers, and correlates with the concentration of carboxyhaemoglobin in blood. This altered permeability may allow easier access into blood for carcinogens.

Dangers

Cigarette smoking is addictive and harmful to health (**Box 28.32**). Smoking 20 cigarettes daily for 20 years increases the lifetime risk of lung cancer by about ten times, compared to the risk in a life-long non-smoker. Smoking and asbestos exposure are synergistic risk factors for lung cancer, with a combined risk about 90 times that of unexposed non-smokers.

Environmental tobacco smoke ('passive smoking') has been shown to increase the frequency and severity of asthma attacks in children and may also raise the incidence of asthma. It is also associated with a small but definite increase in lung cancer. Worldwide, second-hand smoke was estimated to affect 40% of children, 33% of non-smoking males and 35% of non-smoking females in 2004. This caused 1% of all deaths worldwide and 0.7% of the total worldwide burden of disease in disability-adjusted life years (DALYs).

Smoking cessation

If the entire population could be persuaded to stop smoking, the effect on healthcare use would be enormous. National campaigns, bans on advertising and a substantial increase in the cost of cigarettes are the best ways of achieving this at the population level. Smoking bans in workplaces and public spaces have also helped. Meanwhile, active encouragement to stop smoking remains a useful approach for individuals. Smokers who want to quit should have access to smoking cessation clinics for behavioural support. Nicotine replacement therapy (NRT) and bupropion are effective aids to smoking cessation in those smoking more than 10 cigarettes per day. Both should be used only in smokers who commit to a target stop date, and the initial prescription should be for 2 weeks beyond the target stop date. NRT is the preferred choice; there is no evidence that combined therapy offers any advantage. Therapy should be changed after 3 months if abstinence is not achieved.

Varenicline is an oral partial agonist on the $\alpha_4\beta_2$ subtype of the nicotinic acetylcholine receptor. It stimulates the nicotine receptor and reduces withdrawal symptoms and also the craving for cigarettes. A 12-week course doubles the chances of smoking cessation. Electronic cigarettes (battery-operated vaporizers, e-cigarettes) are useful alternatives to tobacco smoking and there is evidence that they may be helpful in smoking cessation, although evidence regarding the long term safety of vaping is awaited.

Further reading

Christiani DC. Vaping induce acute lung injury. *N Engl J Med* 2020; 382:960–962.
Colditz GA. Smoke alarm – tobacco control remains paramount. *N Engl J Med* 2015; 372:665–666.
Gu D, Kelly TN, Wu X et al. Mortality attributable to smoking in China. *N Engl J Med* 2009; 360:150–159.
Oberg M, Jaakkola MS, Woodward A et al. Worldwide burden of disease from exposure to second-hand smoke: a retrospective analysis of data from 192 countries. *Lancet* 2008; 372:139–146.
Oncken C. Nicotine replacement for smoking cessation during pregnancy. *N Engl J Med* 2012; 366:846–847.

RESPIRATORY INFECTION

Pneumonia

Pneumonia is defined as inflammation of the substance of the lungs. It is usually caused by bacteria but can also be caused by viruses and fungi. Clinically, it usually presents as an acute illness with cough, purulent sputum, breathlessness and fever, together with physical signs or radiological changes compatible with consolidation of the lung (**Fig. 28.28**). However, it can present with more subtle symptoms, particularly in the elderly.

Pneumonia is usually *classified* by the setting in which the patient has contracted the infection, for example:
- *community-acquired pneumonia* in a person with no underlying immunosuppression or malignancy
- *hospital-acquired pneumonia* (sometimes called 'healthcare-associated pneumonia', reflecting the role of other institutions such as nursing homes)
- *aspiration pneumonia*, associated with the aspiration of food material or stomach contents into the lungs, and caused by impaired swallowing
- *pneumonia in immunocompromised patient*, acquired through either a genetic defect, immunosuppressive medication or acquired immunodeficiency, as in human immunodeficiency virus (HIV) infection
- *ventilator-acquired pneumonia*, acquired through mechanical ventilation on a critical care unit.

Community-acquired pneumonia

Community-acquired pneumonia (CAP) occurs across all ages but is more common at the extremes of age. *Streptococcus pneumoniae*

---

i | **Box 28.32 Dangers of cigarette smoking**

General
- Lung cancer
- Chronic obstructive pulmonary disease (COPD)
- Carcinoma of the oesophagus
- Ischaemic heart disease
- Peripheral vascular disease
- Bladder cancer
- An increase in abnormal spermatozoa
- Memory problems

Maternal smoking
- A decrease in birth weight of the infant
- An increase in fetal and neonatal mortality
- An increase in asthma

Passive smoking
- Risk of asthma, pneumonia and bronchitis in infants of smoking parents
- An increase in cough and breathlessness in smokers and non-smokers with COPD and asthma
- An increase in cancer risk

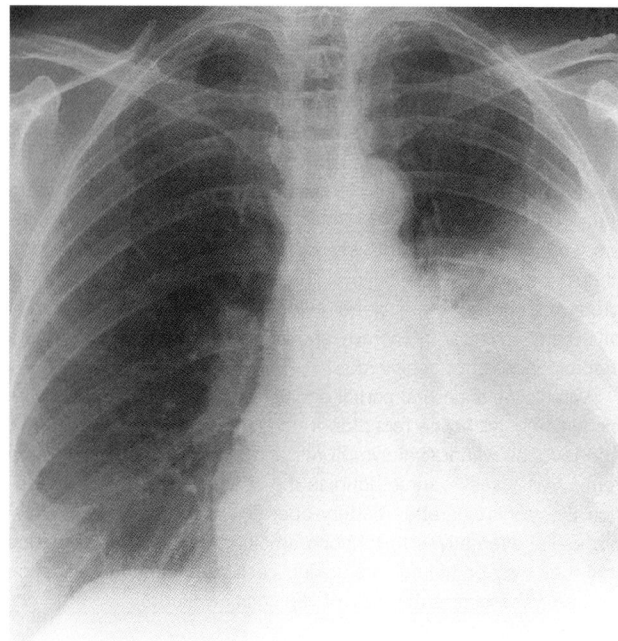

Fig. 28.28 Chest X-ray showing lobar pneumonia.

Box 28.33 Risk factors for community-acquired pneumonia

- *Age:* <16 or >65 years
- *Co-morbidities:* HIV infection, diabetes mellitus, chronic kidney disease, malnutrition, recent viral respiratory infection
- *Other respiratory conditions:* cystic fibrosis, bronchiectasis, chronic obstructive pulmonary disease, obstructing lesion (endoluminal cancer, inhaled foreign body)
- *Lifestyle:* cigarette smoking, excess alcohol, intravenous drug use
- *Iatrogenic:* immunosuppressant therapy (including prolonged corticosteroids)

---

is the most common cause overall; however, in 30–50% of cases no organism is identifiable, while in about 20% more than one organism is present. Infection can be localized, when the whole of one or more lobes is affected ('lobar pneumonia'), or diffuse, when the lobules of the lung are mainly affected, often due to infection centred on the bronchi and bronchioles ('bronchopneumonia'). Factors that increase the risk of developing CAP are shown in **Box 28.33**.

Clinical features

The clinical presentation varies according to the immune state of the patient and the infecting agent. Features include:
- *a dry or productive cough*, sometimes with haemoptysis
- *breathlessness*
- *fevers*, which, if swinging, may indicate empyema (see p. 965)
- *chest pain* may be experienced, commonly pleuritic in nature and due to inflammation of the pleura; a pleural rub may be heard early on in the illness
- *extrapulmonary features* (**Box 28.34**).

In the elderly, CAP can present with confusion or non-specific symptoms such as recurrent falls. CAP should always be considered in the differential diagnosis of sick elderly patients, given their frequently atypical presentation.

Initial assessment

The type and extent of investigations depend on the severity of the illness, which also guides where the patient should be managed

---

Box 28.34 Extrapulmonary features of community-acquired pneumonia

- *Myalgia, arthralgia and malaise* are common, particularly in infections caused by *Legionella* and *Mycoplasma*
- *Myocarditis and pericarditis* are cardiac manifestations of infection, most commonly in *Mycoplasma* pneumonia
- *Headache* is common in *Legionella* pneumonia. Meningoencephalitis and other neurological abnormalities also occur but are much less common
- *Abdominal pain, diarrhoea and vomiting* are common. Hepatitis can be a feature of *Legionella* pneumonia
- *Labial herpes simplex* reactivation is relatively common in pneumococcal pneumonia
- *Other skin rashes*, such as erythema multiforme and erythema nodosum, are found in *Mycoplasma* pneumonia. Stevens–Johnson syndrome (see p. 697) is a rare and potentially life-threatening complication of pneumonia

---

Box 28.35 CURB-65 score and other markers of severe community-acquired pneumonia

CURB-65
C: *Confusion* present (abbreviated mental test score <8/10)
U: (plasma) *Urea* level >7 mmol/L
R: *Respiratory rate* >30 breaths/min
B: systolic *Blood pressure* <90 mmHg; diastolic <60 mmHg
65: *age* >65
   1 point for each of the above:
- *Score 0–1:* Treat as outpatient
- *Score 2:* Admit to hospital
- *Score 3+:* Often require care in intensive treatment unit
   Mortality rates increase with increasing score.

Other markers
- *Chest X-ray:* more than one lobe involved
- *P_aO_2:* <8 kPa
- *Low albumin:* <35 g/L
- *White cell count:* <4 × 10^9/L or >20 × 10^9/L
- *Blood culture:* positive
- Other *co-morbidities*
- *Absence of fever* in the elderly

---

and predicts their outcome. Diagnostic microbiological tests are not needed in mild infection, which should be treated at home with standard oral antibiotics (amoxicillin, or clarithromycin for those with a history of penicillin allergy). Where patients have mild disease, chest X-ray is not routinely recommended unless they fail to improve after 48–72 hours.

Severity is commonly assessed by the **CURB-65** or the **CRB-65 score;** the CRB-65 score is used in the community where the serum urea level is not usually available (**Box 28.35**). These give a guide to the likely risk of fatal outcome but antibiotic choice must always be tempered by clinical assessment and judgement, taking into account other factors associated with increased rates of mortality (see **Box 28.27**).

Investigations

All patients admitted to hospital with suspected CAP should have a chest X-ray, blood tests and microbiological tests.

Chest X-ray

Radiological abnormalities can lag behind clinical signs. A normal chest X-ray on presentation should be repeated after 2–3 days if CAP is suspected clinically. The chest X-ray must be repeated 6 weeks later to rule out an underlying bronchial malignancy causing pneumonia due to bronchial obstruction.

Blood tests

Full blood count, serum creatinine and electrolytes, biochemistry and C-reactive protein (CRP) are helpful.

- *Strep. pneumoniae.* White cell count is usually $>15 \times 5^9$/L (90% leucocytosis neutrophils). Inflammatory markers are significantly elevated: erythrocyte sedimentation rate (ESR) >100 mm/h; CRP >100 mg/L.
- *Mycoplasma.* White cell count is usually normal. In the presence of anaemia, haemolysis should be ruled out (direct Coombs' test and measurement of cold agglutinins, see p. 965).
- *Legionella.* There is lymphopenia without marked leucocytosis, hyponatraemia, hypoalbuminaemia and high serum levels of liver aminotransferases.

Other tests

- *Sputum culture and blood cultures* are required for all patients who have moderate to severe CAP, ideally before antibiotics are administered. In *Strep. pneumoniae* infection, positive blood cultures indicate more severe disease with greater mortality.
- *Arterial blood gas analysis* is necessary if oxygen saturation is <94%.
- *An HIV test* should be offered to all patients with pneumonia since it is a common initial presenting illness in previously undiagnosed HIV infection.

General management

Initial management and assessment should follow the guidelines for management of sepsis (see p. 157), particularly when a patient appears to have a moderate to severe pneumonia. In general:

- *Oxygen.* Supplemental oxygen should be administered to maintain saturations between 94% and 98% (provided the patient is not at risk of carbon dioxide retention, due to loss of hypoxic drive in COPD). In patients with known COPD, oxygen saturations should be maintained between 88% and 92%.
- *Intravenous fluids.* These are required in hypotensive patients showing any evidence of volume depletion and hypotension.
- *Antibiotics.* The first dose of antibiotic should be administered *within 1 hour of identifying any high-risk criteria* and treatment should not be delayed while investigations are awaited. Parenteral antibiotics should be switched to oral once the temperature has settled for a period of 24h, provided there is no contraindication to oral therapy. If patients fail to respond to initial treatment, microbiological advice should be sought and alternative diagnoses considered. The antibiotic regimen should be adjusted specifically once culture and sensitivity results are available (**Fig. 28.29**).
- *Thromboprophylaxis.* If the patient is admitted for >12h, subcutaneous low-molecular-weight heparin should be prescribed and thromboembolus deterrent (TED) stockings should be fitted, unless contraindications exist.
- *Physiotherapy.* Chest physiotherapy is not needed unless sputum retention is an issue.
- *Nutritional supplementation.* Need is assessed by a dietician, particularly in severe disease.
- *Analgesia.* Simple analgesia, such as paracetamol or an NSAID, helps treat pleuritic pain, thereby reducing the risk of further complications due to restricted breathing because of pain (e.g. sputum retention, atelectasis or secondary infection).

Causes of a slow-resolving pneumonia are outlined in **Box 28.36**.

Prevention

Cigarette smoking is an independent risk factor for CAP; if the patient still smokes, cessation advice and support should be given.

Vaccination against influenza is recommended for at-risk groups. All patients over the age of 65 who have not previously been vaccinated and are admitted with CAP should have the pneumococcal vaccine before discharge from hospital.

Complications of pneumonia

See **Box 28.37**.

Parapneumonic effusion and empyema

Pleural effusions are common with pneumonia and complicate around one-third to one-half of cases of CAP. The majority of these are simple exudative effusions but empyema may also develop (purulent fluid in the pleural space). Early indications of empyema are ongoing fever and rising or persistently elevated inflammatory markers, despite appropriate antibiotic therapy.

Pleural aspiration should be performed under ultrasound guidance to make a diagnosis and fluid sent for Gram stain, culture, fluid protein, glucose and LDH (with comparison to serum levels). Light's criteria (see p. 973) can be applied to assess whether an effusion is transudative or exudative. An exudative effusion with pleural fluid pH of <7.2 is strongly suggestive of empyema. Pathogens are often detectable; sensitivity analysis will help guide antimicrobial therapy.

If an empyema develops, the fluid should be urgently drained to prevent further complications, such as development of a thick

---

? Box 28.36 Causes of slow-resolving pneumonia

Incorrect or incomplete antimicrobial treatment
- Underlying antibiotic resistance
- Inadequate dose/duration
- Non-adherence
- Malabsorption

Complication of community-acquired pneumonia
- Parapneumonic pleural effusion (exudative)
- Empyema
- Lung abscess

Underlying neoplastic lesion or other lung disease
- Obstructing lesion
- Bronchoalveolar cell carcinoma
- Bronchiectasis
- Tuberculosis

Alternative diagnosis
- Pulmonary thromboembolic disease
- Cryptogenic organizing pneumonia
- Eosinophilic pneumonia
- Pulmonary haemorrhage

---

i Box 28.37 Complications of pneumonia

General
- Respiratory failure
- Sepsis – multisystem failure

Local
- Pleural effusion
- Empyema
- Lung abscess
- Organizing pneumonia

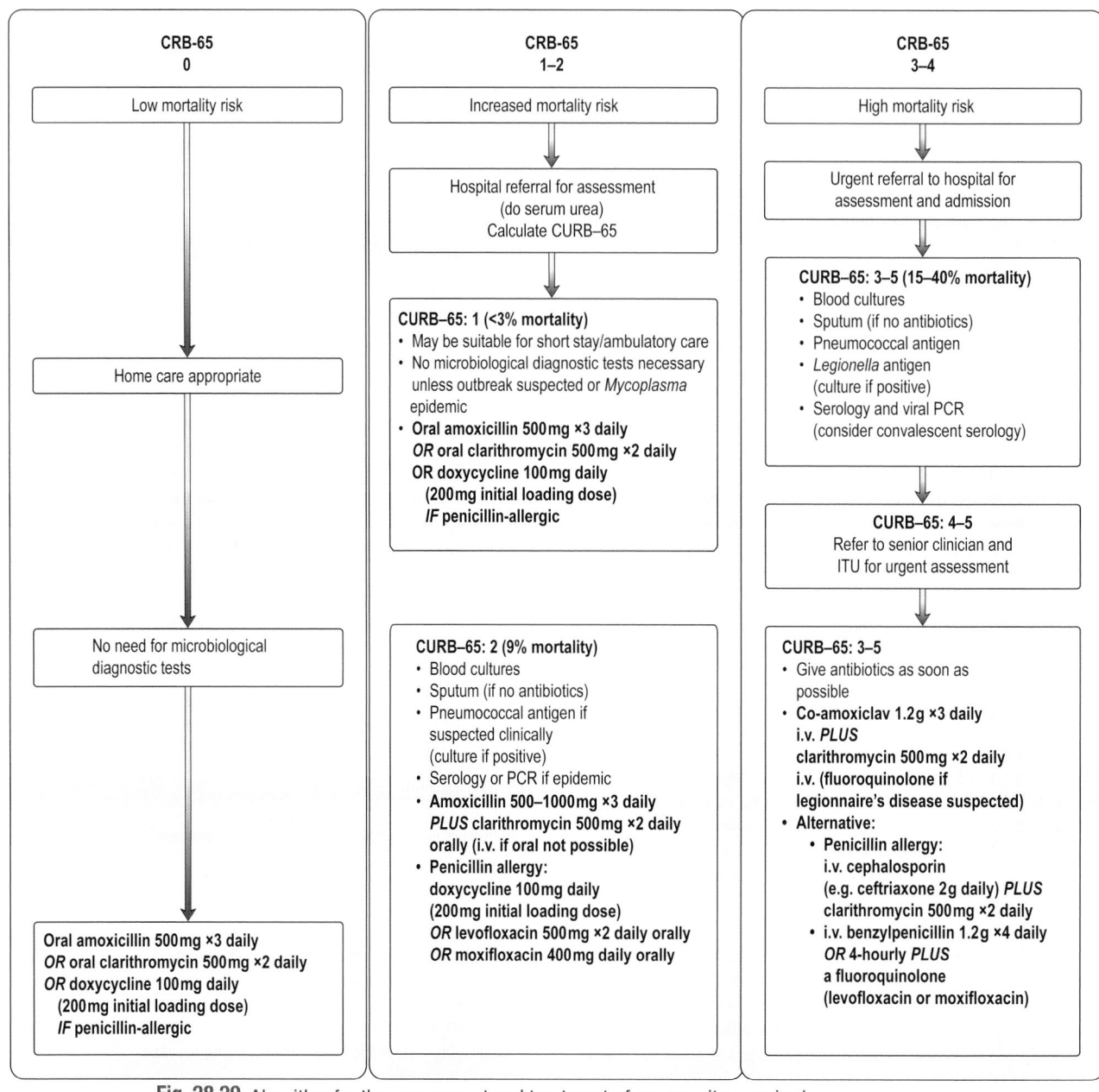

Fig. 28.29 Algorithm for the assessment and treatment of community-acquired pneumonia. CRB, confusion, respiratory rate, blood pressure (CURB includes urea); ITU, intensive treatment unit; PCR, polymerase chain reaction.

pleural rind or prolonged hospital admission. The presence of empyema further increases mortality risk. The duration of antibiotic administration will usually need to be extended. Whenever possible, the choice of antimicrobial should be guided by the results of cultures. Thoracic surgical intervention is necessary in severe cases.

Lung abscess

This term is used to describe severe localized suppuration within the lung associated with cavity formation visible on the chest X-ray or CT scan, often with a fluid level (which always indicates an air–liquid interface). There are several causes of lung abscess (**Box 28.38**). Clinical features usually include persisting or worsening pneumonia associated with the production of large quantities of sputum, which is often foul-smelling owing to the growth of anaerobic organisms. There is usually a swinging fever; malaise and weight loss frequently

occur. There may be few signs on physical examination, although clubbing occurs in chronic suppuration. Patients have a normocytic anaemia and raised inflammatory markers (ESR/CRP). CT scanning is essential and bronchoscopy can be undertaken to obtain samples or remove foreign bodies. Treatment should be guided by available culture results or clinical judgement, and is often prolonged (4–6 weeks). Surgical drainage is sometimes necessary.

Pneumonia in other settings

Hospital-acquired pneumonia

Hospital-acquired pneumonia (HAP) is defined as new onset of cough with purulent sputum, along with a compatible X-ray demonstrating consolidation, in patients who are beyond 2 days of their

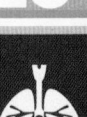

Causes
- Aspiration pneumonia
- Tuberculosis
- *Staphylococcus aureus* or *Klebsiella pneumoniae*
- Septic emboli usually containing staphylococci
- Inadequately treated community-acquired pneumonia
- Spread from an amoebic liver abscess
- Bronchial obstruction by an endoluminal cancer
- Foreign body inhalation

Common causative organisms
- *Klebsiella pneumoniae*
- *Staphylococcus aureus*
- Gram-negative enteric bacilli
- *Mycobacterium tuberculosis*
- *Streptococcus milleri*
- Anaerobic bacteria (post aspiration)
- *Haemophilus influenzae*

 Box 28.39 Organisms implicated in hospital-acquired pneumonia

- Gram-negative bacteria (*Pseudomonas* spp., *Escherichia* spp., *Klebsiella* spp.)
- Anaerobic bacteria (*Enterobacter* spp.)
- *Staphylococcus aureus* (including meticillin-resistant *Staph. aureus*)
- *Acinetobacter* spp.

initial admission to hospital or who have been in a healthcare setting within the last 3 months (including nursing or residential homes, as well as acute care facilities such as hospitals). HAP is the second most common form of hospital-acquired infection after urinary tract infections and carries a significant mortality risk, particularly in the elderly or those with co-morbidities such as stroke, respiratory disease or diabetes. In HAP, the causative organisms differ from those causing CAP (**Box 28.39**). Viral or fungal pathogens only affect immunocompromised hosts.

Ventilator-associated pneumonia

This occurs in the context of mechanical ventilation in a critical care setting. Often multidrug-resistant Gram-negative organisms (such as *Acinetobacter baumanii*) are responsible, requiring careful selection of an appropriate antibiotic in association with a clinical microbiologist.

Aspiration pneumonia

Acute aspiration of gastric contents into the lungs can produce an extremely severe and sometimes fatal illness owing to the intense destructiveness of gastric acid. This can complicate anaesthesia, particularly during pregnancy (Mendelson's syndrome). Because of the bronchial anatomy, the most usual sites for aspirated material to end up are the right middle lobe and the apical or posterior segments of the right lower lobe. Persistent pneumonia is often due to anaerobes and may progress to lung abscess or even bronchiectasis if protracted. It is vital to identify any underlying problem, as aspiration will recur without appropriate corrective measures.

Treatment should be directed specifically against positive cultures if available. If not, then co-amoxiclav is used for mild to moderate disease, which covers Gram-negative and anaerobic bacteria. Treatment needs to be escalated when there is a lack of response or cases are severe.

Pneumonia in immunocompromised patients

Patients who are immunosuppressed (either iatrogenically or due to a defect in host defences) are at risk not only from all the usual organisms that can cause pneumonia but also from opportunistic pathogens that would not be expected to cause disease. These opportunistic pathogens can be commonly occurring microorganisms (that are ubiquitous in the environment) or bacteria, viruses and fungi that are less common (see **Box 37.21**). The symptom pattern may resemble CAP or be more non-specific. A high degree of clinical suspicion is therefore necessary when assessing an ill patient who is immunocompromised.

Pneumocystis jirovecii pneumonia

Pneumocystis pneumonia is one of the most common opportunistic infections encountered in clinical practice. It affects patients on immunosuppressant therapy, such as long-term corticosteroids, monoclonal antibodies or methotrexate for autoimmune disease; those on anti-rejection medication after a solid organ or haemopoietic stem cell transplantation; and those infected with HIV. Individuals with CD4 counts of less than 200/mm^3 are at particular risk. *Pneumocystis jirovecii* is found in the air, and pneumonia arises from re-infection rather than reactivation of persisting organisms acquired in childhood.

Clinically, the pneumonia is associated with a high fever, breathlessness and dry cough. A characteristic feature on examination is rapid desaturation on exercise or exertion. The typical radiographic appearance is one of diffuse bilateral alveolar and interstitial shadowing beginning in the perihilar regions and spreading out in a butterfly pattern. Other chest X-ray appearances include localized infiltration, nodules, cavitation or a pneumothorax. Empirical treatment is justified in very sick high-risk patients; wherever possible, however, the diagnosis should be confirmed by indirect immunofluorescence on induced sputum or bronchoalveolar lavage fluid. First-line treatment of *Pneumocystis* pneumonia is with high-dose co-trimoxazole (see p. 1443), with adjunctive corticosteroids in patients with HIV infection.

Further reading

British Thoracic Society. 2015-Annotated BTS guideline for the management of CAP in adults (2009): Summary of recommendations; BTS 2015; https://brit.thoracic.org.uk/guidelines-and-quality-standards/community-acquired-pneumonia-in-adults-guidance/annotated-bts-guideline-for-the-management-of-cap-in-adults-2014/.
Jain S, Self WH, Wunderink S et al. Community-acquired pneumonia requiring hospitalization among US adults. *N Engl J Med* 2015; 373:415–427.
Lim WS, Baudouin SV, George RC et al. British Thoracic Society Guidelines for the management of community-acquired pneumonia in adults: update 2009. *Thorax* 2009; 64(Suppl III):iii1–iii55.
Loke YK, Kwok CS, Niruban A et al. Value of severity scales in predicting mortality from community-acquired pneumonia: systematic review and meta-analysis. *Thorax* 2010; 65:884–890.
Mansell A, Niederman LA. Aspiration pneumonia. *N Engl J Med* 2019; 380:651–663.
Musher DM, Thorner AR. Community acquired pneumonia. *N Engl J Med* 2014; 371:1619–1628.
National Institute for Health and Care Excellence. *Clinical Guideline 191: Pneumonia in Adults: Diagnosis and Management*. NICE 2014; https://www.nice.org.uk/guidance/cg191.
Wunderick RG, Waterer G. Advances in the causes and management of community acquired pneumonia in adults. *BMJ* 2017; 358:j2471.

Tuberculosis

Tuberculosis (TB) is one of the world's most common infectious diseases. It is caused by the bacterium *Mycobacterium tuberculosis*, which comes from the large *Mycobacteriaceae* family, members of which include *M. leprae*. It is estimated that one-third of the world's population is infected with tuberculosis (see also p. 503), with the majority of cases (around 65%) seen in Africa and Asia. There is

Box 28.40 Factors affecting prevalence and risk of developing tuberculosis in the developed world

Contact with high-risk groups
- Origination from a high-incidence country (defined as >40/100 000)
- Frequent travel to high-incidence areas

Immune deficiency
- HIV infection
- Corticosteroids or immunosuppressant therapy
- Chemotherapeutic drugs
- Nutritional deficiency (vitamin D)
- Diabetes mellitus
- Chronic kidney disease
- Malnutrition/body weight >10% below ideal body weight

Lifestyle factors
- Drug/alcohol misuse
- Homelessness/hostels/overcrowding
- Prison inmates

Genetic susceptibility
- Twin studies of gene polymorphisms

Box 28.41 Factors implicated in the reactivation of latent tuberculosis

- HIV co-infection
- Immunosuppressant therapy (chemotherapy/monoclonal antibody treatment), including corticosteroids
- Diabetes mellitus
- End-stage chronic kidney disease
- Malnutrition
- Ageing

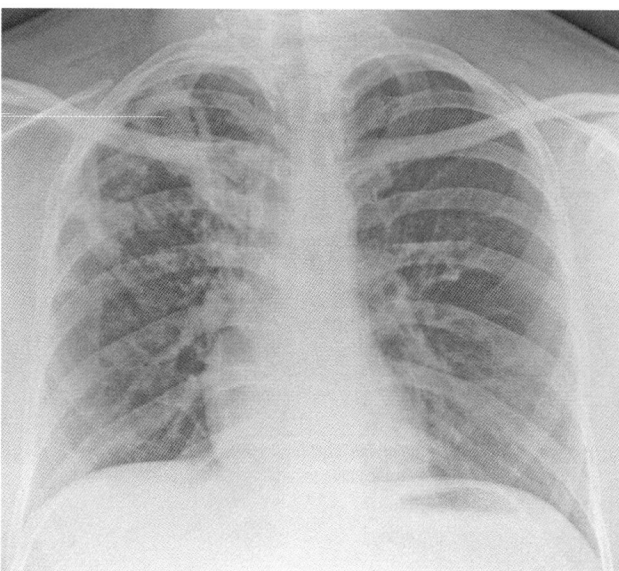

Fig. 28.30 Chest X-ray demonstrating patchy right mid and upper zone consolidation and a cavity at the right apex in a patient with tuberculosis.

a growing incidence of multidrug-resistant and extremely drug-resistant strains, which, together with HIV co-infection, places a huge health burden on resource-poor nations, with a high mortality from the two coexistent diseases. TB was responsible for 1.6 million deaths worldwide in 2017 and 20% of these were in HIV co-infected individuals. There are a number of factors affecting the prevalence and risk of developing TB (**Box 28.40**).

Pathogenesis

M. tuberculosis is an aerobic, intracellular pathogen. Due to their relative impermeability to acid-based dyes in the laboratory, these organisms are often termed 'acid-fast bacilli'. TB is an airborne infection spread by coughing via respiratory droplets. Only a small number of bacteria need to be inhaled for infection to develop, but not all those who are infected develop active disease.

Primary tuberculosis

'Primary TB' describes the first infection with TB. When the bacteria reach the alveolar macrophages, they are ingested and the subsequent inflammatory reaction results in tissue necrosis and formation of a granuloma. These granulomatous lesions consist of a central area of necrotic material called caseation, surrounded by epithelioid cells and Langhans giant cells.

Subsequently, the caseated areas heal completely and many become calcified. Some of these calcified nodules contain bacteria, which are contained by the immune system (and the hypoxic acidic environment created within the granuloma) and are capable of lying dormant for many years. This is known as the primary focus or the 'Ghon focus' of the disease. On a chest X-ray, the Ghon focus can be evident as a small, calcified nodule.

On initial contact with infection, less than 5% of patients develop active disease. This increases to 10% within the first year of exposure.

Reactivation tuberculosis

In the majority of people who are infected by *Mycobacterium* spp., the immune system contains the infection and the patient develops cell-mediated immune memory of the bacteria. This is termed 'latent TB'. The majority of active TB cases are due to reactivation of latent infection, where the initial contact usually occurred many years or decades earlier. Most patients are young and previously healthy but may have one or more risk factors implicated in the development

of active disease (**Box 28.41**). In patients with HIV infection, newly acquired TB is also common. The majority of active TB occurs in the lung, but extrapulmonary infection occurs with spread to the lymph nodes, particularly the cervical and intrathoracic chains, where it causes active disease in 20–25% (UK figures) and also via the bloodstream to more distant sites such as the brain, bones and skin.

Clinical features and diagnosis

The cardinal symptoms of TB are cough, haemoptysis and the systemic symptoms of fevers, night sweats and weight loss. However, in extrapulmonary sites, respiratory symptoms are often absent, and the systemic symptoms are often ignored by patients and medical practitioners alike.

In all cases of suspected TB, it is essential, depending on the site of disease, to obtain sputum, biopsy samples or fluid for microscopy, smear and culture, to obtain information on sensitivities. Tissue samples should also be sent for histopathological examination, either dry or in saline.

Pulmonary TB

Patients are frequently symptomatic with a productive cough and, occasionally, haemoptysis, along with systemic symptoms. Where there is laryngeal involvement, a hoarse voice and a severe cough are found. If disease involves the pleura, then pleuritic pain is a frequent presenting complaint.

The chest X-ray (**Fig. 28.30**) can show consolidation with or without cavitation, pleural effusion, or thickening or widening of the mediastinum caused by hilar or paratracheal adenopathy.

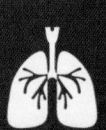

Serial sputum samples should be collected on at least three occasions (ideally, first thing in the morning); if the patient is unable to produce sputum, it may be necessary to organize an induced sputum or perform bronchoscopy to obtain samples.

Patients whose sputum is smear-positive for TB are considered to be infectious and should be isolated in hospital. Those who are smear-negative but subsequently culture-positive are less infectious and generally so not need to be isolated, although care should be taken when contacts include immunocompromised individuals.

Lymph node TB

The lymph nodes are the second most commonly affected organs. Extrathoracic nodes are more commonly involved than intrathoracic or mediastinal. Usually, presentation is with firm, non-tender enlargement of a cervical or supraclavicular node. The node becomes necrotic centrally and can liquefy and be fluctuant if peripheral. The overlying skin is frequently indurated or there can be sinus tract formation with purulent discharge, but characteristically there is no erythema ('cold abscess' formation). Nodes can typically be enlarged for several months prior to diagnosis. On CT imaging, the central area appears necrotic (**Box 28.42**). Samples should be obtained via either ultrasound-guided fine needle aspiration (FNA), core biopsy or, if necessary, removal of a whole node. All samples must be sent for AFB smear and culture, and cancer should be excluded on cytology. EBUS can be used to biopsy intrathoracic nodes.

Other forms of TB

Gastrointestinal TB

See page 1195.

TB of bone and spine

See pages 455 and 484.

Miliary TB

Miliary disease occurs through haematogenous spread of the bacilli to multiple sites, including the central nervous system (CNS) in 20% of cases. It often presents with systemic symptoms and the chest X-ray demonstrates multiple nodules, which appear like millet seeds: hence the term 'miliary'.

Other findings are liver and splenic microabscesses with deranged liver enzymes, cholestasis and gastrointestinal symptoms. All patients should have brain imaging (MRI), to look for evidence of cerebral disease, which can present as an asymptomatic brain tuberculoma.

Central nervous system TB

See page 870.

Pericardial TB

See page 1126.

Skin

See page 671.

Microbiological diagnosis

Once samples have been taken, the rapid identification of the presence of mycobacterium by stains is essential and should be performed within 24 hours; culture of the sample allows determination of the antibiotic sensitivity of the infecting strain.

Stains

Auramine–rhodamine staining is more sensitive (though less specific) than Ziehl–Neelsen; as a result, it is more widely used. It requires fluorescence microscopy and highlights bacilli as yellow–orange on a green background.

Culture

The majority of the developed world uses liquid/broth culture of mycobacteria in addition to solid media (Lowenstein–Jensen slopes or Middlebrook agar), as time to culture is shorter than for solid culture (1–3 weeks compared with 3–8 weeks). Using liquid culture in the presence of antimycobacterial drugs (usually first-line therapy) establishes the drug sensitivity for that strain and usually takes approximately 3 weeks.

Nucleic acid amplification and polymerase chain reaction

Nucleic acid amplification testing (NAAT) is increasingly used for rapid identification of MTb complex and is useful in differentiating between *M. tuberculosis complex* and non-tuberculous mycobacteria, as well as identifying TB in smear-negative sputum specimens. It works by using the polymerase chain reaction (PCR) to replicate and then identify mycobacterium DNA. Culture and staining are still necessary and should not be replaced by PCR. PCR is useful only at the initial stage of diagnosis, as it frequently remains positive despite treatment, due to the detection of dead organisms.

The identification of mycobacterial DNA is useful in facilitating rapid commencement of treatment and also rapid identification of drug resistance. Genetic mutations in bacterial DNA conferring rifampicin resistance are highly predictive of multidrug resistance. The development of a highly specific probe designed to detect this mutation thereby allows efficient identification of resistant disease and commencement of appropriate therapy sooner than waiting for cultures to complete (which may take up to 8 weeks).

Commercial kits, such as GeneXpert, are available that can reliably perform molecular testing in the field and take less than 2 hours to complete; they are now widely used in low- and middle-income countries to detect genetic mutations associated with rifampicin resistance.

More recently, in the UK, whole-genome sequencing (WGS) has begun to be used on a routine basis to identify different strains of mycobacterium and also detect drug resistance. This will start to replace routine culture and phenotypic testing in the near future.

Management

All patient should have routine blood tests and a viral hepatitis screen, and be offered an HIV test before treatment. Patients with active viral hepatitis are much more likely to develop a fatal drug-induced hepatitis and need careful monitoring and counselling. Those with fully sensitive TB require 6 months of treatment; the exception is TB infection of the CNS, for which the recommended duration is at least 12 months. Isoniazid, rifampicin, pyrazinamide and ethambutol are the first-line TB drugs, known as quadruple therapy. In CNS and pericardial disease, corticosteroids are used as an adjunct at treatment initiation to reduce long-term complications. **Box 28.43** summarizes the standard recommended regimens.

Enhanced case management, together with *directly observed therapy (DOT)*, is recommended where there are concerns about adherence to treatment or difficulties in taking medication (**Box 28.44**).

ℹ Box 28.42 Common sites of TB infection with radiological findings and diagnostic investigations

Radiology

Pulmonary, pleural and laryngeal TB

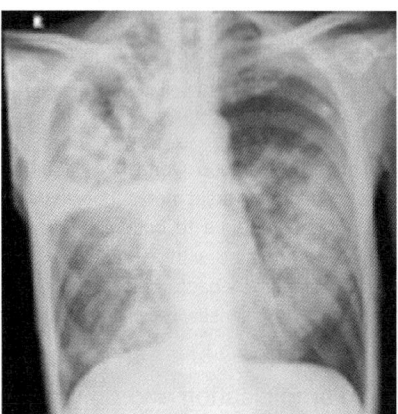

Chest X-ray of patient with suspected pulmonary TB

Miliary TB

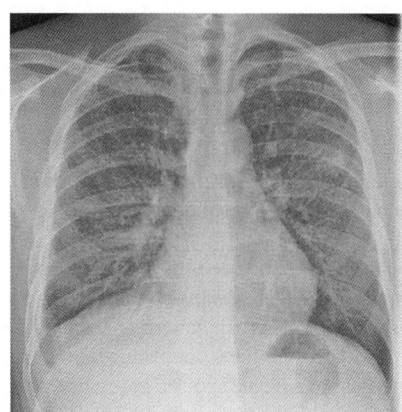

Chest X-ray of patient with miliary pulmonary changes

Central nervous system TB

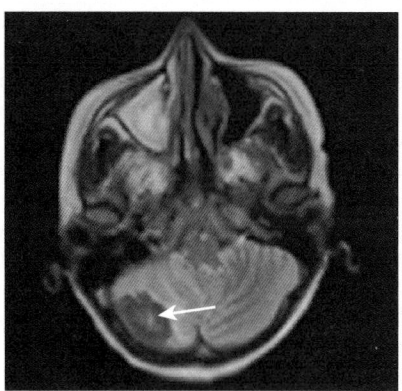

MRI head of patient with lesion in right cerebellum

Lymph node TB

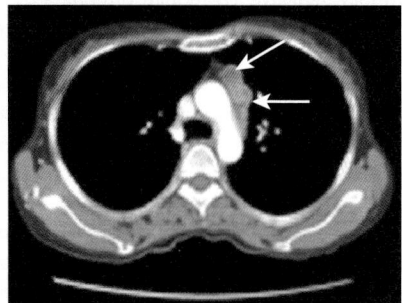

CT thorax with left anterior mediastinal nodes with necrotic centre

Investigations

Smear and culture of:
Sputum (≥2 samples increase diagnostic yield)
Induced sputum (inhaled hypertonic saline, which induces coughing): diagnostic yield comparable to bronchoscopic samples
Bronchoalveolar lavage fluid if cough unproductive and induced sputum not possible
Aspiration of pleural fluid and pleural biopsy
Gastric aspirates – can be useful in paediatric disease
Nasoendoscopic or bronchoscopic examination/biopsy of vocal cords with biopsy for smear/culture and histology in laryngeal disease

Blood cultures
Bronchoalveolar lavage fluid (usually smear-negative but culture-positive)
MRI head followed by lumbar puncture should be performed in all cases, unless contraindicated, to assess for central nervous system involvement (affects treatment duration), and sampling of other involved organs is often necessary

Ensure that patient and scans are discussed at neurology/neurosurgery MDT
Consider brain biopsy if concerns about diagnosis
Lumbar puncture if no contraindication – characteristics:
CSF protein may be very high (usually >2–3 g/L)
CSF glucose <½ blood glucose
CSF lymphocytosis

All samples should be sent for histocytopathological examination as well as culture and smear:
Fine needle aspiration or biopsy of an involved lymph node, usually under radiological guidance
Mediastinal nodal sampling (endobronchial ultrasound transbronchial needle aspiration, mediastinoscopy/mediastinotomy)

CSF, cerebrospinal fluid; MDT, multidisciplinary team meeting.

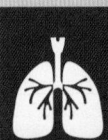

Box 28.43 Usual treatment and duration in fully sensitive tuberculosis

Site of disease	Duration of therapy	Drug choice
Pulmonary[a] Extrapulmonary (excluding CNS disease) Miliary (excluding CNS involvement)	6 months	Fully sensitive strain: 2HRZE + 4HR[b]
CNS TB	12 months	2HRZE + 10HR *Plus* Dexamethasone 0.3–0.4 mg/kg per day weaned over 8–12 weeks (or equivalent dose of prednisolone)
Latent TB	3 months *Or* 6 months	3RH *Or* 6H

[a]For pulmonary TB, 2HRZE + 4(HR)₃, i.e. 3 times weekly for 4HR, is acceptable.
[b]2HRZE + 4HR, 2 months of HRZE + 4 months of HR.
CNS, central nervous system; E, ethambutol; H, isoniazid; R, rifampicin; Z, pyrazinamide.

Box 28.44 Criteria for implementation of directly observed therapy (DOT) for tuberculosis

- Patients thought unlikely to comply:
  - History of serious mental illness
  - History of non-adherence to TB or other therapies
  - Previous TB treatment
- Multidrug-resistant TB
- Street-, shelter- or hostel-dwelling homelessness; 'sofa surfing'
- Prison history
- Substance misuse (recreational drugs and alcohol)

Unwanted effects of drug treatment

The most common side-effects of quadruple TB therapy are nausea, vomiting, rash and itching. An antiemetic or antihistamine can be prescribed to alleviate these symptoms, although in some cases treatment may need to be interrupted. This is a particular problem when liver function tests become deranged and there is concern about a drug-induced hepatitis, in which case it is often necessary to stop all four drugs and re-introduce one at a time. The drug should be stopped only if the serum bilirubin becomes elevated or if transferases are more than three times elevated.

Isoniazid can cause a polyneuropathy due to B₆ deficiency, as isoniazid interacts with pyridoxal phosphate; vitamin B₆, pyridoxine 10–25 mg daily, should be prescribed concomitantly to prevent this. Occasionally, isoniazid gives rise to allergic reactions, such as a skin rash and fever. Hepatitis occurs in less than 1% of cases but may lead to liver transplantation or death if the drug is continued.

Rifampicin induces liver enzymes, which may be transiently elevated in the serum of many patients. This also means that concomitant drug treatment may be made less effective and a careful review of a patient's therapy will need to be undertaken, particularly with antidepressants, anticoagulants and antiepileptics (see p. 259). Oral contraception will not be effective, so alternative birth-control methods should be used. Rifampicin stains body secretions red/pink and patients should be warned of the change in colour of their urine, tears (affecting contact lenses) and sweat. Thrombocytopenia has been reported.

Box 28.45 Factors associated with an increased risk of drug-resistant tuberculosis

- History of prior drug treatment of TB (particularly if unsupervised and self-administered)
- Co-infection with advanced HIV and previous TB treatment
- Infection acquired in a region with high rates of drug resistance
- Contact with a known case of resistant TB
- Failure to respond to empirical TB therapy despite documented adherence
- Exposure to multiple courses of fluoroquinolone antibiotics for presumed community-acquired pneumonia
- Healthcare workers exposed to cases of resistant TB

Pyrazinamide may cause hepatic toxicity but its most common side-effects are itching, rash and arthralgia; pyrazinamide reduces the renal excretion of urate and may precipitate hyperuricaemic gout.

Ethambutol can cause a dose-related optic retrobulbar neuritis that presents with colour blindness for green, reduction in visual acuity and a central scotoma. Patients should have their visual acuity and colour vision checked prior to treatment using Snellen and Ishihara charts. This condition usually reverses, provided the drug is stopped when symptoms develop; patients should therefore be warned of its effects. All patients prescribed the drug should be seen by an ophthalmologist prior to treatment and doses of 15 mg/kg should be used, with a maximum dose of 1.2 g.

Drug resistance

Mono- or multidrug resistance arises due to incomplete or incorrect drug treatment (acquired) and can be spread from person to person. Isoniazid monoresistance occurs in approximately 10% of TB cases in the UK. A risk assessment for drug resistance should be routinely performed (**Box 28.45**). The incidence of multidrug resistance in TB (resistance to both rifampicin and isoniazid, termed MDR-TB) is relatively low in developed countries (around 1%). Extremely drug-resistant disease (XDR-TB) is defined as high-level resistance to rifampicin, isoniazid, fluoroquinolones and at least one injectable agent such as amikacin, capreomycin or kanamycin.

TB in special situations
Mycobacterium bovis infection

Mycobacterium bovis infection occurs in humans who have consumed unpasteurized milk, farmers working with infected cows, and abattoir workers. TB due to *M. bovis* does not differ from ordinary TB in the chest but extrapulmonary sites of infection, such as lymph nodes, are more frequently involved. Immunosuppression is also a risk factor. The tuberculin test is positive. Treatment is with isoniazid, rifampicin and ethambutol; pyrazinamide resistance is common.

HIV co-infection

The increase in TB seen over recent decades has occurred to a considerable extent in association with the incidence of HIV infection, with high levels seen in Africa (particularly sub-Saharan), the Indian subcontinent and parts of Eastern Europe and Russia. The incidence of HIV infection in TB worldwide is around 10% and TB is responsible for about one-quarter of acquired immunodeficiency syndrome (AIDS)-related deaths.

Alongside the increased morbidity and mortality of co-infection, there are specific issues relating to the treatment of TB in HIV: namely, the incidence of drug interactions and intolerability, the increased risk of treatment toxicity and the higher incidence of drug resistance. TB/HIV infection should be managed by experts in TB (respiratory or infectious disease physicians) alongside HIV specialists.

Latent TB infection

Latent TB infection (LTBI) is diagnosed by demonstrating immune memory to mycobacterial proteins. Two types of test are available.

In the *tuberculin skin test ('Mantoux test')* a positive result is indicated by a delayed hypersensitivity reaction evident 48–72 hours after the intradermal injection of purified protein derivative (PPD), resulting in a raised, indurated lesion. False-negative (anergic) tuberculin skin tests (TSTs) are common in patients with immunosuppression due to HIV infection (CD4+ <200/mm^3), those taking immunosuppressant medications (chemotherapy, anti-TNF therapy, steroids), those at the extremes of age and those with active disease. False-positives occur due to cross-reactivity with non-tuberculous mycobacteria and bacille Calmette–Guérin (BCG) vaccination.

Interferon-gamma release assays (IGRAs) detect T-cell secretion of IFN-γ following exposure to *M. tuberculosis*-specific antigens (ESAT-6, CFP-10). Where a person has been previously infected or is currently infected with TB, activated T cells within their extracted whole blood secrete quantifiable levels of IFN-γ in response to re-exposure to TB-specific antigens. The test does not differentiate between active and latent infection. However, it is highly specific compared with the TST, has similar or better sensitivity, and requires only a single patient visit.

In certain groups with LTBI, *chemoprophylaxis* is offered to reduce the risk of active infection:

- household and close workplace contacts of patients with pulmonary and laryngeal TB
- health workers
- recent new migrant entrants from high-risk countries
- patients who are immunocompromised, such as those with HIV infection
- those about to commence treatment with biologic agents (such as infliximab)
- those due to have stem cell or solid organ transplants.

LTBI *treatment* is either with isoniazid and rifampicin for 3 months or with isoniazid monotherapy for 6 months.

BCG vaccination

BCG is a live attenuated vaccine derived from *M. bovis* that has lost its virulence. It has variable efficacy but is still recommended in certain situations in developed countries (but not the USA), though it is no longer offered routinely to all due to the lack of cost efficacy. In the UK it is still offered to all neonates in high-risk areas such as inner cities, although there are safety concerns in babies with HIV.

Non-tuberculous mycobacterial infection

Non-tuberculous mycobacteria (NTM) occur in soil and water, and are not usually pathogenic due to their lack of virulence. However, where there is a breach of the normal host defence mechanisms, certain strains have the potential to become pathogenic (**Box 28.46**). Factors associated with an increased risk of pulmonary NTM infection include structural lung disease such as COPD, bronchiectasis and cystic fibrosis, and immunosuppressive states such as HIV infection (see **Box 37.21**). Treatment is suggested if there is a compatible clinical picture, the organism is isolated from an invasive sample or an NTM is isolated from more than one sputum sample obtained at different times.

Further reading

Conradie F, Diacon AH, Ngubane N et al. Treatment of highly drug -resistant pulmonary tuberculosis. *N Engl J Med* 2020; 382:893–902.

---

i Box 28.46 Some non-tuberculous mycobacteria strains implicated in disease

Strain	Site of disease
M. avium intracellulare complex (MAC)	Pulmonary (nodular and interstitial infiltrates in middle lobe in women or fibrocavitary disease in middle-aged male smokers)
	Disseminated (usually in HIV)
	Hypersensitivity pulmonary disease ('hot-tub lung')
	Lymphadenitis in children
M. kansasii	Pulmonary (similar presentation to *Mycobacterium tuberculosis complex*, usually in middle-aged males)
	Disseminated disease (in HIV)
M. abscessus	Skin, soft tissue and bone disease
	Pulmonary (usually in bronchiectasis and older, non-smoking females)
M. chelonae	Skin, bone and soft tissue
	Pulmonary (similar to *M. abscessus*)
M. fortuitum	Pulmonary (similar to *M. abscessus*)
M. gordonae	Only rarely pathogenic (can be significant in immunocompromised host)
M. xenopi	Pulmonary (fibrocavitary disease in chronic obstructive pulmonary disease)
	Contaminated surgical instruments causing bone/soft tissue infection
M. malmoense	Pulmonary
	Lymph node
M. marinum	Soft tissue, skin and bone
M. szulgai	Pulmonary (similar to TB)

National Institute for Health and Care Excellence. *NICE Clinical Guideline NG33: Tuberculosis*. NICE 2016; https://www.nice.org.uk/guidance/ng33.
Tiberi S, du Plessis N, Walzl G et al. Tuberculosis: progress and advances in development of new drugs, treatment regimens, and host-directed therapies. *Lancet Infect Dis* 2018; 18:e199–210.
Walzl G, McNerney R, Du Plessis N et al. Tuberculosis: advances and challenges in development of new diagnostics and biomarkers. *Lancet Infect Dis* 2018; e183–198.
World Health Organization. *Global Tuberculosis Report 2019*; http://www.who.int/.

PLEURAL DISEASE

Pleural effusion

A pleural effusion is an excessive accumulation of fluid in the pleural space. It can be detected on X-ray when 300mL or more of fluid is present, and clinically when there is 500mL or more. The chest X-ray appearances (**Fig. 28.31**) range from obliteration of the costophrenic angle to dense homogeneous shadows occupying part or all of the hemithorax. Fluid below the lung (a subpulmonary effusion) can simulate a raised hemidiaphragm. Fluid in the fissures may resemble an intrapulmonary mass. The physical signs are are described in **Box 28.8**.

Diagnosis

This is by pleural aspiration (see p. 944), usually done under ultrasound guidance. The fluid that accumulates may be a transudate or an exudate (**Box 28.47**).

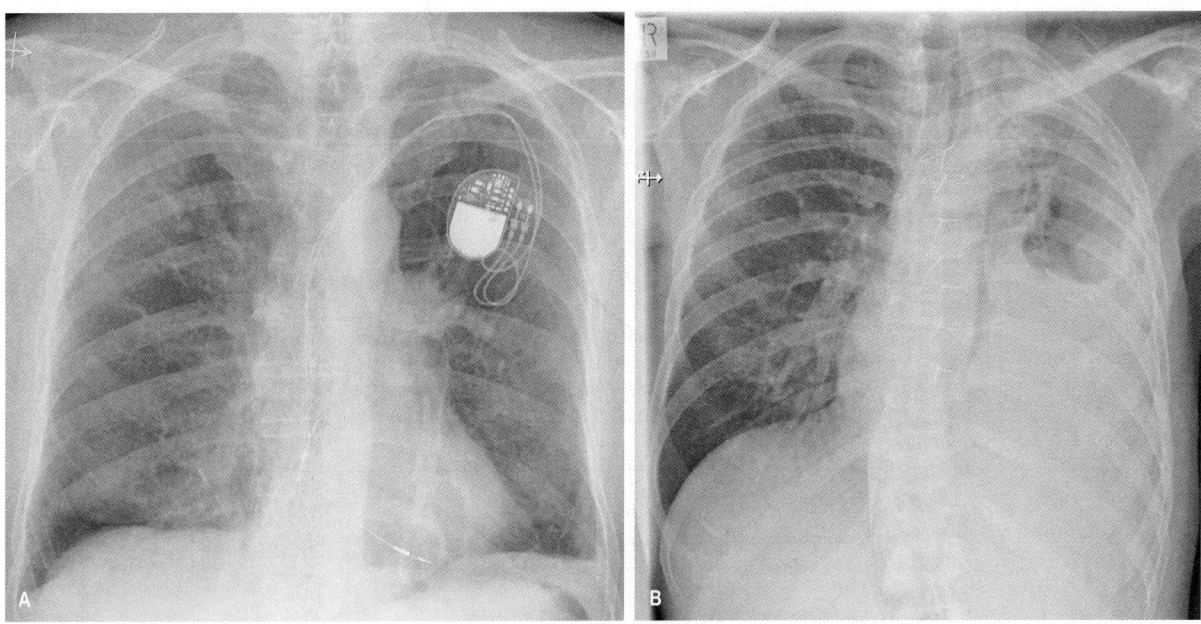

Fig. 28.31 Chest X-ray demonstrating pleural effusion. **(A)** Blunting of the left costophrenic angle due to a small left pleural effusion. There is a dual-lead pacemaker *in situ*. **(B)** A large left-sided pleural effusion.

> ⓘ **Box 28.47** Light's criteria to diagnose an exudative effusion
>
> - Pleural fluid protein : serum protein >0.5
> - Pleural fluid LDH : serum LDH >0.6
> - Pleural fluid LDH > ⅔ upper limit of normal for serum (105–333 IU/L)
>
> LDH, lactate dehydrogenase.
> *(Adapted from Light RW, Macgregor MI, Luchsinger PC et al. Pleural effusions: the diagnostic separation of transudates and exudates. Ann Intern Med 1972; 77:507–513.)*

Transudates

Effusions that are transudates can be bilateral but are often larger on the right side. The protein content is less than 30 g/L, the LDH is less than 200 IU/L and the fluid to serum LDH ratio is below 0.6. Causes include:

- heart failure
- hypoproteinaemia (e.g. nephrotic syndrome)
- constrictive pericarditis
- hypothyroidism
- ovarian tumours producing right-sided pleural effusion – Meigs' syndrome.

Exudates

The protein content of exudates is over 30 g/L and the LDH is more than 200 IU/L. Causes include:

- bacterial pneumonia (common)
- carcinoma of the bronchus – fluid may be blood-stained (common)
- pulmonary infarction
- TB
- autoimmune rheumatic diseases
- post-myocardial infarction syndrome (rare)
- acute pancreatitis (high amylase content) (rare)
- mesothelioma
- sarcoidosis (very rare)
- yellow-nail syndrome (effusion due to lymphoedema) (very rare)
- familial Mediterranean fever (very rare).

Pleural biopsy (see p. 944) may be necessary if the diagnosis has not been established by simple aspiration.

Management is of the underlying condition unless the fluid is purulent (empyema), in which case drainage is mandatory.

Management of malignant pleural effusions

Malignant pleural effusions that reaccumulate and are symptomatic can be aspirated to dryness followed by the instillation of a sclerosing agent such as tetracycline or talc. Effusions should be drained slowly since rapid shift of the mediastinum causes severe pain and occasionally shock. This treatment produces only temporary relief.

Chylothorax

This is caused by accumulation of lymph in the pleural space, usually resulting from leakage from the thoracic duct following trauma or infiltration by carcinoma.

Empyema

The presence of pus in the pleural space can be a complication of pneumonia. It requires urgent drainage (see p. 965).

Pneumothorax

'Pneumothorax' means air in the pleural space. Primary spontaneous pneumothoraces occur predominantly in young people. Traditionally, patients are tall, thin and male but shape, size and gender often do not follow this rule. Primary pneumothoraces are usually caused by rupture of a pleural bleb, usually apical, and are thought to be due to congenital defects in the connective tissue of the alveolar walls. Both lungs are affected with equal frequency.

Secondary pneumothoraces occur in conjunction with pre-existing lung disease such as COPD, infection and cystic fibrosis. Iatrogenic pneumothoraces are caused by instrumentation to the thorax, such as central venous line insertion, percutaneous or transbronchial lung biopsy, or trauma.

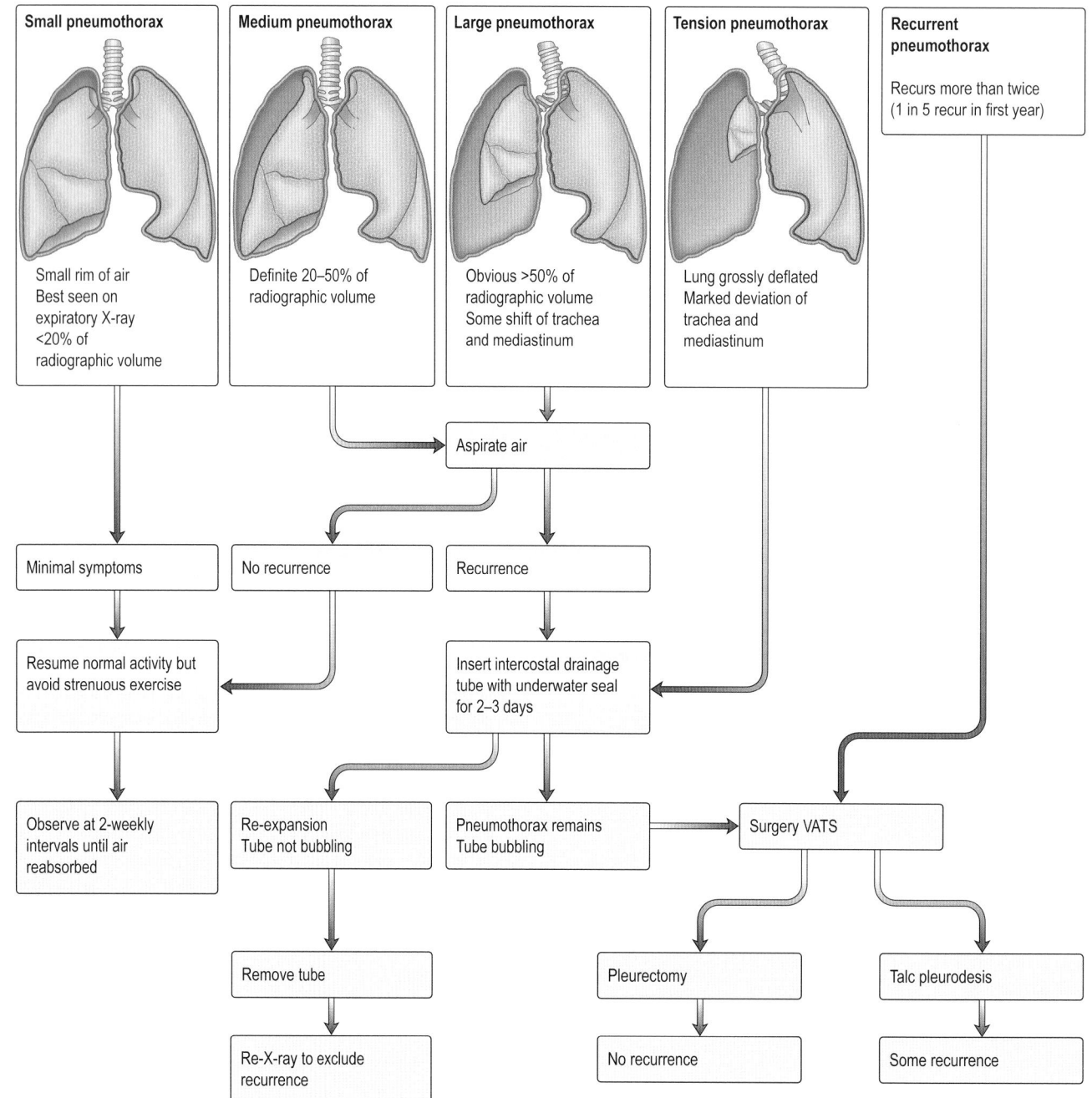

Fig. 28.32 Pneumothorax: an algorithm for management. Red: pneumothorax. VATS, video-assisted thoracoscopic surgery.

Clinical features

Patients commonly present with sudden onset of chest drain and breathlessness. On careful questioning, they may be discovered to have had a milder version of these symptoms in the past but not sought medical attention. In tension pneumothorax they may become shocked, and emergency decompression of the pneumothorax may be necessary using a 14–16 gauge needle in the second rib space in the mid-clavicular line.

Investigations

Plain chest X-ray is the baseline investigation and the size of pneumothorax should be recorded. There are several ways to measure: in North America the apex to cupola distance tends to be used, while UK guidelines recommend the pleura to edge of lung distance. If a patient's first pneumothorax resolves and there is no recurrence, cross-sectional imaging with a CT chest is unnecessary. However, if the chest is abnormal on resolution, a scan should be requested. With the common use of cannabis and other recreational drugs, bullae and associated emphysema are being more commonly seen in young people.

Management

Pneumothoraces can be managed in a number of ways (**Fig. 28.32**), depending on the cause and the severity of symptoms on presentation. Treatment includes simple observation, pleural aspiration, intercostal drain and surgical management, both in the more acute situation or electively.

- No flying for 1 week after complete resolution
- No diving
- Smoking cessation
- 30–50% chance of recurrence
- Future management: consider surgery

Box 28.49 Simple aspiration of pneumothorax

1. Explain the nature of the procedure and obtain consent.
2. Infiltrate 2% lidocaine down to the pleura in the second intercostal space in the mid-clavicular line.
3. Push a 3–4 cm 16-gauge cannula through the pleura.
4. Connect the cannula to a three-way tap and 50 mL syringe.
5. Aspirate up to 2.5 L of air. Stop if resistance to suction is felt or the patient coughs excessively.
6. Repeat the chest X-ray (in expiration) in the X-ray department.

- **Observation:** For patients with mild symptoms and a pneumothorax of <2 cm simple observation is enough. Patients can be discharged from the emergency department with instructions to return if their symptoms become worse. They should be advised not to fly until the pneumothorax has completely resolved and never to scuba dive unless they have had surgical pleurodesis (**Box 28.48**). They have a 30% chance of a recurrent pneumothorax. Patients often ask about sport and exercise, and while there are no real restrictions, apart from diving, they should generally rest for a few days before exercising in moderation and should avoid contact sports for a week or two. Outpatient follow-up should be arranged within 10 days.
- **Aspiration:** This can be considered in symptomatic patients with a pneumothorax of >2 cm, or 1 cm in a secondary pneumothorax. It is undertaken using a 16 French gauge needle attached to a three-way tap and a 50 mL syringe (**Box 28.49**). Generally, aspiration should not be attempted in most cases of traumatic pneumothorax. It should be followed by a repeat chest X-ray, discharge advice (as described) and outpatient follow-up.
- **Pleural intercostal drain:** If aspiration fails to inflate the lung satisfactorily, the patient is very breathless on admission, there is evidence of a tension pneumothorax or the cause is related to trauma, an intercostal drain should be inserted, normally in the mid-axillary line 4th intercostal space. The tube should be connected to an underwater drain and bottle, which are kept below the level of the patient's chest. It should be checked daily for evidence of infection at the insertion site and for kinks and leaks along its course.
- **Surgical pleurodesis and bleb resection:** An open surgical pleurodesis via thoracotomy or VATS procedure should be considered when the lung fails to re-inflate, or offered to patients electively.
- **Smoking:** Patients should be strongly advised to stop smoking both tobacco and recreational drugs. Cannabis, in particular, can cause marked emphysematous changes in younger people, which leads to subcutaneous blebs and bullae.
- **Psychological effects:** Medical staff underestimate the concern that patients often feel, knowing that they have a medical condition that can potentially recur at any time. Some become very anxious and often request surgical pleurodesis after their second or third recurrence.

Further reading

British Thoracic Society. Investigation of a unilateral pleural effusion in adults: British Thoracic Society pleural disease guideline 2010. *Thorax* 2010; 65(Suppl 2):ii4–ii17.

British Thoracic Society. Management of spontaneous pneumothorax: British Thoracic Society pleural disease guideline 2010. *Thorax* 2010; 65(Suppl 2):ii18–ii31.
Courtney Broaddus V. Clearing the air – a conservative option for spontaneous pneumothorax. *N Engl J Med* 2020; 382:469–470.

TUMOURS OF THE RESPIRATORY TRACT

Malignant tumours

Bronchial carcinoma

Bronchial carcinoma is the most common malignant tumour worldwide, causing around 1.76 million deaths annually. It is the fifth most frequent cause of death in the UK and is now the most common cause of cancer-related death in both men and women.

Cigarette smoking (including passive smoke exposure) accounts for 80% and 90% of lung cancer in men and women, respectively. There remains a higher incidence of bronchial carcinoma in urban compared with rural areas, even when allowance is made for cigarette smoking. Other aetiological factors include:

- **Environmental**: radon exposure, asbestos, polycyclic aromatic hydrocarbons and ionizing radiation; occupational exposure to arsenic, chromium, nickel, petroleum products and oils.
- **Host factors**: pre-existing lung disease such as pulmonary fibrosis; HIV infection; genetic factors.

Legislative control over smoking in public places in many parts of the world has been introduced to reduce ill health related to cigarette smoke.

Pathophysiology

Historically, lung cancers have been broadly divided into small-cell carcinoma and non-small-cell carcinoma, based on the histological appearances of the cells seen within the tumour. This distinction is necessary with respect to the behaviour of the tumour, providing prognostic information and determining best treatment. Non-small-cell carcinoma is further divided into a number of cell types (adenocarcinoma, squamous cell carcinoma, large-cell carcinoma (**Box 28.50**). A number of molecular characteristics have been described in the subtypes of cancer, which confer potential prognostic benefit and may result in the ability to deliver a more personalized therapy with targeted agents. The most common of these are activating mutations within epidermal growth factor receptor (*EGFR*), most commonly encountered in non-smokers, females and those of Asian origin, and the presence of anaplastic lymphoma kinase (*ALK*) fusion oncogene, again more commonly found in non-smokers or ex-smokers and younger patients (see p. 119).

Clinical features

The presentation and clinical course vary between the different cell types (see **Box 28.50**). Symptoms and signs may be different, depending on the extent and site of disease.

Common presenting features can be divided into those caused by direct/local tumour effects, metastatic spread and non-metastatic extrapulmonary features.

Local effects

- **Cough.** This is the most commonly encountered symptom in lung cancer. Because evidence suggests that this symptom is neglected by both patients and healthcare professionals, campaigns in the UK have highlighted the '3-week cough' as a symptom that merits a chest X-ray.

ℹ️ **Box 28.50** Lung cancer cell types and clinical features

Cell type	Incidence in UK (%)	Features
Non-small-cell carcinoma		
Squamous cell carcinoma	35	Remains the most common cell type in Europe
		Arises from epithelial cells, associated with production of keratin
		Occasionally cavitates with central necrosis
		Causes obstructing lesions of bronchus with post-obstructive infection
		Local spread common, metastasizes relatively late
Adenocarcinoma	27–30	Likely to become the most common cell type in the UK in the near future (most common cell type in the USA)
		Increasing incidence since 2005 possibly linked to low-tar cigarettes
		Originates from mucus-secreting glandular cells
		Most common cell type in non-smokers
		Often causes peripheral lesions on chest X-ray/CT
		Subtypes include bronchoalveolar cell carcinoma (associated with copious mucus secretion, multifocal disease)
		Metastases common: pleura, lymph nodes, brain, bones, adrenal glands
Large-cell carcinoma	10–15	Often poorly differentiated
		Metastasizes relatively early
Small-cell carcinoma	20	Arises from neuroendocrine cells (APUD cells)
		Often secretes polypeptide hormones
		Often arises centrally and metastasizes early

- **Breathlessness.** Central tumours occlude large airways, resulting in lung collapse and breathlessness on exertion. Many patients with lung cancer have coexistent COPD, which is also a cause of breathlessness. Patients may also develop a pleural effusion due to metastatic involvement of the pleura.
- **Haemoptysis.** Fresh or old blood is coughed up because of the tumour bleeding into an airway.
- **Chest pain.** Peripheral tumours invade the chest wall or pleura (both well innervated), resulting in sharp pleuritic pain. Large-volume mediastinal nodal disease often results in a characteristic dull central chest ache.
- **Wheeze.** This is monophonic when due to partial obstruction of an airway by tumour.
- **Hoarse voice.** Mediastinal nodal or direct tumour invasion of the mediastinum results in compression of the left recurrent laryngeal nerve.
- **Nerve compression.** Pancoast tumours in the apex of the lung invade the brachial plexus, causing C8/T1 palsy with small muscle wasting in the hand and weakness, as well as pain, radiating down the arm. An associated Horner's syndrome also occurs,

caused by compression of the sympathetic chain, with classic features of miosis, ptosis and anhidrosis.
- **Recurrent infections.** Tumour causing partial obstruction of an airway results in post-obstructive pneumonia.
- **Direct invasion of the phrenic nerve.** Bronchial carcinoma invading the phrenic nerve causes paralysis of the ipsilateral hemidiaphragm. It can involve the oesophagus, producing progressive dysphagia, and the pericardium, resulting in pericardial effusion and malignant dysrhythmias.
- **Superior vena caval obstruction.** See page 117.
- **Tracheal tumours.** These present with progressive dyspnoea and stridor. Flow–volume curves show dramatic reductions in inspiratory flow (see **Fig. 28.6C**).

Metastatic spread

Bronchial carcinoma commonly spreads to mediastinal, cervical and even axillary or intra-abdominal nodes. In addition, the liver, adrenal glands, bones, brain and skin are frequent sites for metastases:
- **Liver.** Common symptoms are anorexia, nausea and weight loss. Right upper quadrant pain radiating across the abdomen is associated with liver capsular pain.
- **Bone.** Bony pain and pathological fractures occur as a result of tumour spread. If the spine is involved, there is a risk of spinal cord compression (see p. 878), which requires urgent treatment.
- **Adrenal glands.** Metastases to the adrenals do not usually result in adrenal insufficiency and are generally asymptomatic.
- **Brain.** Metastases present as space-occupying lesions with subsequent mass effect and signs of raised intracranial pressure. Less common presentations include carcinomatous meningitis with cranial nerve defects, headache and confusion.
- **Malignant pleural effusion.** This presents with breathlessness and is commonly associated with pleuritic pain.

Non-metastatic extrapulmonary manifestations of bronchial carcinoma

discussed later Minor haematological extrapulmonary manifestations of lung cancer, such as normocytic anaemia and thrombocytosis, are reasonably common. Apart from finger clubbing and hypertrophic pulmonary osteoarthropathy (HPOA), most other non-metastatic complications are relatively rare. Approximately 10% of small-cell tumours produce ectopic hormones, giving rise to paraneoplastic syndromes (see **Box 6.9**).

Investigations

Investigations are necessary to:
- stage the extent of disease
- make a tissue diagnosis (to differentiate small-cell from non-small-cell lung cancer, as well as to detail the molecular characteristics – increasingly relevant with newer targeted biologic agents and immunotherapy)
- assess fitness to undergo treatment.

Staging and diagnosis
Chest X-ray

Plain chest X-rays may show obvious evidence of lung cancer or non-specific appearances (**Box 28.51**). In some cases the initial film is normal, either because the lesion is small or because disease is confined to central structures.

Computed tomography

CT indicates the extent of disease. Imaging should include the liver and adrenal glands, which are common sites for metastases. The

Box 28.51 Lung cancer presentations on chest X-ray

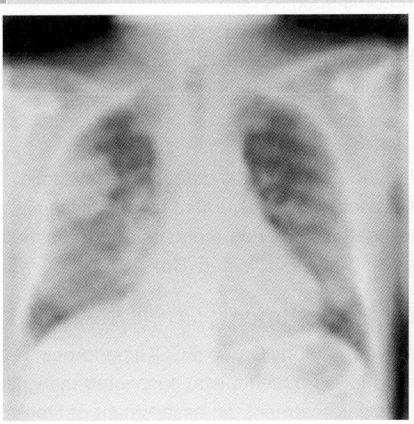

Mass lesion

Lesions visible if >1 cm in diameter. Spiculated, cavitating or smooth-edged. Often an incidental finding, usually asymptomatic if small. By the time symptoms are present, chest X-ray is almost always abnormal

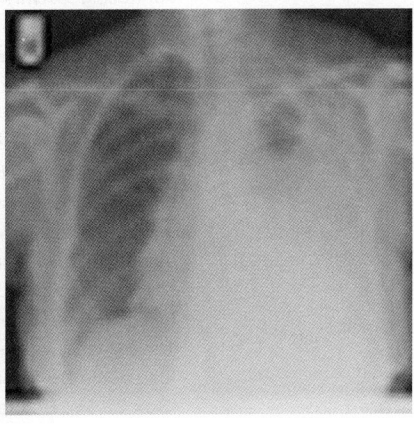

Pleural effusion

Usually unilateral; can obscure an underlying mass or pleural tumour. Mesothelioma and metastatic disease from other tumour sites are in the differential diagnosis

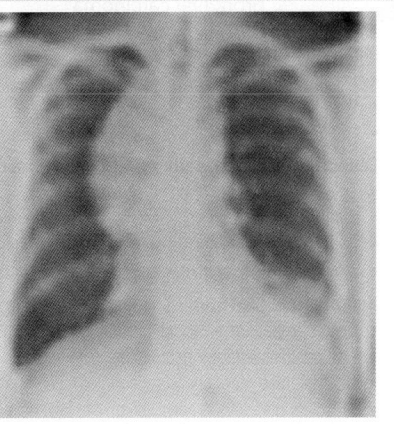

Mediastinal widening or hilar adenopathy

Lymphadenopathy evident on the plain film, manifested by splayed carina, hilar enlargement or paratracheal shadowing

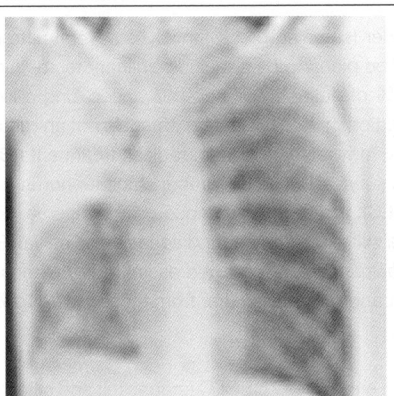

Slow-resolving consolidation

Tumour causes partial obstruction of a bronchus, resulting in retention of secretions, bacterial overgrowth and subsequent infection. (Persistent right upper lobe consolidation due to tumour in right upper lobe)

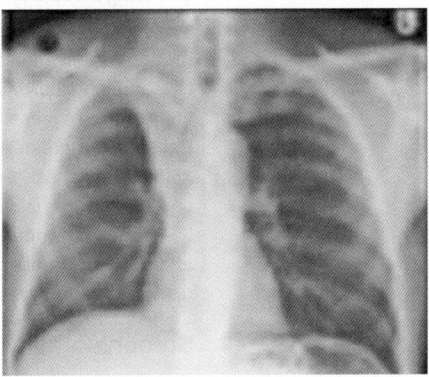

Collapse

Endoluminal tumour causes complete collapse of a lung and associated mediastinal shift, or collapse of a lobe or segment, resulting in volume loss on the affected side with raised hemidiaphragm/deviated trachea

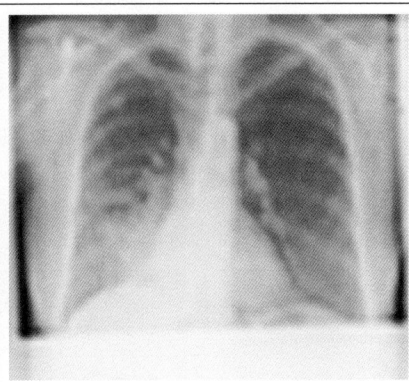

Reticular shadowing

Carcinoma spreads through the lymphatic channels of the lung to give rise to lymphangitis carcinomatosa; in bronchial carcinoma this is usually unilateral and associated with striking dyspnoea. Bilateral lymphangitis should prompt investigation for a primary site other than lung, such as breast, stomach or colon

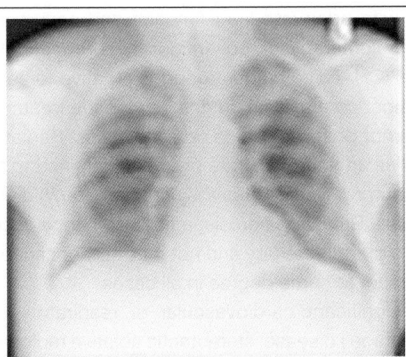

Normal

A normal film does not rule out an underlying tumour. A minority of tumours are confined to the central airways and mediastinum without obvious change on plain chest X-ray. Although investigation of isolated haemoptysis with a normal chest X-ray is often negative, a normal chest X-ray should not discourage further investigation, especially in smokers over the age of 40 years

Box 28.52 Non-metastatic extrapulmonary manifestations of bronchial carcinoma[a]

Metabolic (universal at some stage)
- Loss of weight
- Lassitude
- Anorexia

Endocrine (10%) (usually small-cell carcinoma)
- Ectopic adrenocorticotrophin syndrome
- Syndrome of inappropriate secretion of antidiuretic hormone (SIADH)
- Hypercalcaemia (usually squamous cell carcinoma)
- Rarer: hypoglycaemia, thyrotoxicosis, gynaecomastia

Neurological (2–16%)
- Encephalopathies – including subacute cerebellar degeneration
- Myelopathies – motor neurone disease
- Neuropathies – peripheral sensorimotor neuropathy
- Muscular disorders – polymyopathy, myasthenic syndrome (Eaton–Lambert syndrome)

Vascular and haematological (rare)
- Thrombophlebitis migrans
- Non-bacterial thrombotic endocarditis
- Microcytic and normocytic anaemia
- Disseminated intravascular coagulopathy
- Thrombotic thrombocytopenic purpura
- Haemolytic anaemia

Skeletal
- Clubbing (30%)
- Hypertrophic osteoarthropathy (± gynaecomastia) (3%)

Cutaneous (rare)
- Dermatomyositis
- Acanthosis nigricans
- Herpes zoster

[a]Percentage of all cases.

International Association for the Study of Lung Cancer (IASLC) has devised the most widely used staging definitions, based on CT imaging of tumour size (T), nodal involvement (N) and metastases (M), along with prognostic data (**Box 28.53**).

Using CT criteria, lymph nodes that are less than 1 cm in diameter are not classed as being enlarged, yet they can still contain malignant cells. With increasing size, the positive predictive value of CT in detecting malignant nodes grows; however, it cannot be assumed that enlarged nodes are definitely malignant and further staging tests should be performed if there are no distant metastases, and the primary tumour is thought to be eligible for curative treatment. These tests include direct sampling of affected nodes and PET-CT to assess distant spread of cancer.

If cerebral metastases are suspected, CT imaging of the brain should be performed.

PET-CT

See page 941.

Other imaging modalities

MRI is not useful for the diagnosis of primary lung tumours other than Pancoast tumours with nerve invasion or the assessment of chest wall involvement prior to surgery. MRI spine is required if there is any clinical suspicion of spinal cord compression. MRI brain may also be required to assess cerebral metastases.

Bone is a common site for metastatic deposits, and CT imaging of the primary tumour may demonstrate bony metastases. If the patient is describing bony pain that is not included in the CT imaging field, a **bone scan** may be helpful to demonstrate bony deposits. If these are identified, local radiotherapy may be helpful in controlling local symptoms such as pain.

Obtaining histology and cytology

Investigations for this purpose are listed in **Box 28.54**.

Other investigations

These include a full blood count for the detection of anaemia, and biochemistry to assess for liver involvement, hypercalcaemia and hyponatraemia. Investigations for non-metastatic extrapulmonary manifestations of cancer may be indicated (**Box 28.52**)

Assessing fitness for treatment

The Eastern Cooperative Oncology Group (ECOG) performance status should be recorded for all patients with suspected malignancy (**Box 28.55**). Before radical treatment, an assessment of fitness for treatment should be carried out. This work-up should include full lung function testing with transfer capacity, and if cardiovascular disease is present, cardiopulmonary exercise testing, stress echo or, occasionally, preoperative angiography may be required.

Management

Treatment of lung cancer (see also p. 119) involves several different modalities and should be planned by a multidisciplinary team. In the UK, approximately 75% of patients will have advanced lung cancer at the stage of presentation: hence radical treatment is not an option. Patient co-morbidities may also preclude radical treatment. **Box 28.56** shows the mean survival based on tumour stage for non-small-cell lung cancer (NSCLC), including squamous cell carcinoma: only 25–30% of patients are still alive 1 year after diagnosis and only 6–8% after 5 years. Small-cell carcinoma is staged as limited or extensive disease. The treatment and prognosis differ from those of NSCLC.

Surgery

Surgery is performed in early-stage NSCLC (stages I, II and selected IIIA) with curative intent. Many patients with stage III disease are treated with chemoradiation with a view to downstaging disease and rendering it amenable to surgical resection. Where surgical staging of resected lung cancer demonstrates nodal involvement, patients require adjuvant chemotherapy.

Radiation therapy with curative intent

In selected patients with adequate lung function and early-stage NSCLC, high-dose radiotherapy or continuous hyperfractionated accelerated regimens (CHART) provide a good alternative to surgical resection with almost comparable outcomes. It is the treatment of choice if surgery is not possible due to co-morbidities. Radiation pneumonitis (defined as an acute infiltrate precisely confined to the radiation area and occurring within 3 months of radiotherapy) develops in 10–15% of cases. Radiation fibrosis, a fibrotic change occurring within a year or so of radiotherapy and not precisely confined to the radiation area, occurs to some degree in all cases.

In patients with significant cardiovascular or respiratory co-morbidities and early stage I disease, stereotactic ablative radiotherapy (SABR) can be used. In the same patient group, radiofrequency ablation is used: this is an image-guided technique that uses heat to destroy small peripheral tumours. Data regarding long-term outcomes are unavailable as yet.

Palliative radiation treatment

Radiation therapy has a role in palliation of symptoms from lung cancer. Bone and chest wall pain from metastases or direct invasion, haemoptysis, occluded bronchi and superior vena caval obstruction

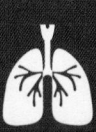

i Box 28.53 TNM staging system for lung cancer

Notation	Description
T – primary tumour	
TX	Primary tumour cannot be assessed, or tumour proven by the presence of malignant cells in sputum or bronchial washings, but not visualized by imaging or bronchoscopy
T0	No evidence of primary tumour
Tis	Carcinoma *in situ*[a]
T1	Tumour 3 cm or less in greatest dimension, surrounded by lung or visceral pleura, without bronchoscopic evidence of invasion more proximal than the lobar bronchus (i.e. not in the main bronchus); subtypes mi, a, b and c exist according to the tumour size.
T2	Tumour more than 3 cm but not more than 5 cm; or tumour with any of the following features:[b] • Involves main bronchus, regardless of distance to the carina but without involvement of the carina • Invades visceral pleura • Associated with atelectasis or obstructive pneumonitis that extends to the hilar region involving either part of or the entire lung
T2a	Tumour more than 3 cm but not more than 4 cm in greatest dimension
T2b	Tumour more than 4 cm but not more than 5 cm in greatest dimension
T3	Tumour more than 5 cm but not more than 7 cm in greatest dimension or one that directly invades any of the following: parietal pleura, chest wall (including superior sulcus tumours), phrenic nerve, parietal pericardium; or tumour nodule(s) in the same lobe as the primary
T4	Tumour more than 7 cm or of any size that invades any of the following: diaphragm, mediastinum, heart, great vessels, trachea, recurrent laryngeal nerve, oesophagus, vertebral body, carina; separate tumour nodule(s) in a different ipsilateral lobe to the primary
N – regional lymph nodes	
NX	Regional lymph nodes cannot be assessed
N0	No regional lymph node metastasis
N1	Metastasis in ipsilateral peribronchial and/or ipsilateral hilar lymph nodes and intrapulmonary nodes, including involvement by direct extension
N2	Metastasis in ipsilateral mediastinal and/or subcarinal lymph node(s)
N3	Metastasis in contralateral mediastinal, contralateral hilar, ipsilateral or contralateral scalene, or supraclavicular lymph node(s)
M – distant metastasis	
M0	No distant metastasis
M1	Distant metastasis
M1a	Separate tumour nodule(s) in a contralateral lobe; tumour with pleural nodules or malignant pleural or pericardial effusion[c]
M1b	Single extrathoracic metastasis in a single organ[d]
M1c	Multiple extrathoracic metastasis in a single or multiple organs

Resultant stage groupings

Occult carcinoma	TX	N0	M0
Stage 0	Tis	N0	M0
Stage IA[e]	T1	N0	M0
Stage IB	T2a	N0	M0
Stage IIA	T2b	N0	M0
Stage IIB	T1, T2a, b	N1	M0
	T3	N0	M0
Stage IIIA	T1, T2a, b	N2	M0
	T3	N1	M0
	T4	N0, N1	M0
Stage IIIB	T1, T2a, b	N3	M0
	T3, T4	N2	M0
Stage IIIC	T3, T4	N3	M0
Stage IV	Any T	Any N	M1
Stage IVA	Any T	Any N	M1a, M1b
Stage IVB	Any T	Any N	M1c

[a]Tis includes adenocarcinoma *in situ* and squamous carcinoma *in situ*.
[b]T2 tumours with these features are classified T2a if 4 cm or less or if size cannot be determined, and T2b if greater than 4 cm but not larger than 5 cm.
[c]Most pleural (pericardial) effusions with lung cancer are due to tumour. In a few patients, however, multiple microscopic examinations of pleural (pericardial) fluid are negative for tumour, and the fluid is non-bloody and is not an exudate. Where these elements and clinical judgement dictate that the effusion is not related to the tumour, the effusion should be excluded as a staging descriptor.
[d]This excludes involvement of a single non-regional node.
[e]Stage IA is split into three subclasses 1, 2 and 3 according to tumour size.
(Based on data from Goldstraw P, Crowley J, Chansky K et al.; International Association for the Study of Lung Cancer International Staging Committee; Participating Institutions. The IASLC Lung Cancer Staging Project: proposals for the revision of the TNM stage groupings in the forthcoming (8th) edition of the TNM classification of malignant tumours. J Thorac Oncol 2016; 2:706–714.)

respond favourably to irradiation in the short term. Radiotherapy is also given at the end of chemotherapy to consolidate treatment in small-cell lung cancer.

Chemotherapy, targeted therapy and immunotherapy

This is discussed on page 119–120. Adjuvant chemotherapy with radiotherapy improves response rate and extends median survival in NSCLC.

Targeted agents against EGFRs, tyrosine kinases and anaplastic lymphoma kinase (*ALK*) in NSCLC (in particular, adenocarcinoma) offer better outcomes in selected patients and can also be used where intravenous chemotherapy offers unacceptable toxicity or as second-line chemotherapy. Immunotherapy with checkpoint inhibitors and PDL-1 inhibitors modulates the immune response and offers another treatment option in appropriate patient groups. This is an emerging field and may have an impact on the prognosis of all types of lung cancer.

Laser therapy, cryotherapy and tracheobronchial stents

These techniques are used in the palliation of inoperable lung cancer in selected patients with tracheobronchial narrowing from intraluminal tumour, or extrinsic compression causing disabling breathlessness, intractable cough and complications including infection, haemoptysis and respiratory failure.

A *neodymium-Yag (Nd-Yag) laser* passed through a fibreoptic bronchoscope can be used to vaporize inoperable fungating intraluminal carcinoma involving short segments of trachea or main bronchus. Benign tumours, strictures and vascular lesions can also be treated effectively with immediate relief of symptoms.

Cryotherapy is an endobronchial technique by which a cryoprobe is passed through the bronchoscope. The cryoprobe

repeatedly freezes and thaws the tumour, which enables parts of it to be excised, restoring airway patency without causing bleeding. The excised tissue can be sent for histological analysis.

Tracheobronchial stents made of silicone or in the form of expandable metal springs are available for insertion into strictures caused by tumour, external compression, or weakening and collapse of the tracheobronchial wall.

Palliative care

Patients dying of cancer of the lung need attention to their overall wellbeing (see Ch. 7). Much can be done to render the individual's remaining life symptom-free and as active as possible. Patient and relatives both require psychological and emotional support, a task that should be shared between the respiratory team, oncology team, primary care team and nurses, social workers, hospital chaplains and doctors who together make up the palliative care team.

Mesothelioma

Mesothelioma describes a malignant tumour arising from the parietal or visceral mesothelial lining of the lung. These tumours are almost always related to asbestos exposure (see p. 996), and mesothelioma typically develops from pre-existing pleural plaque disease.

The number of cases of mesothelioma has increased progressively since the mid-1980s and has now reached 2500 deaths per year in the UK, which has the highest *per capita* death rate from this condition.

The most common presentation of mesothelioma is a pleural effusion, typically with persistent chest wall pain, which should raise the index of suspicion even if the initial pleural fluid or biopsy samples are non-diagnostic. CT/ultrasound-guided biopsy or VATS pleural biopsy is often needed to obtain sufficient tissue for diagnosis. Clinical trials of chemotherapy, sometimes combined with surgery, are under way but the outlook for most patients remains very limited.

Secondary tumours

Metastases in the lung are very common. They are usually detected on chest X-ray or CT in patients already diagnosed as having

---

> **_i_ Box 28.54 Investigations to obtain histology and cytology**
>
> - Fibreoptic bronchoscopy (**Fig. 28.33**)
> - Endobronchial ultrasound (**Fig. 28.34**)
> - CT/ultrasound-guided biopsy of lung lesions
> - Ultrasound-guided biopsy of lymph nodes, liver metastases or skin lesions
> - Ultrasound-guided pleural aspiration
> - Medical or video-assisted thoracoscopy
> - Mediastinoscopy

> **_i_ Box 28.55 Eastern Cooperative Oncology Group (ECOG) Performance Status**
>
> | Grade | Description |
> |---|---|
> | 0 | Fully active, able to carry out all pre-disease performance without restriction |
> | 1 | Restricted in physically strenuous activity but ambulatory and able to carry out work of a light or sedentary nature, e.g. light house work, office work |
> | 2 | Ambulatory and capable of all self-care but unable to carry out any work activities. Up and about more than 50% of waking hours |
> | 3 | Capable of only limited self-care. Confined to bed or chair for more than 50% of waking hours |
> | 4 | Completely disabled; cannot carry out any self-care; totally confined to bed or chair |
> | 5 | Dead |

> **_i_ Box 28.56 Survival in small-cell and non-small-cell cancer based on clinical stage[a]**
>
> | Stage[a] | 5-year survival (%) |
> |---|---|
> | IA1 | 92 |
> | IA2 | 83 |
> | IA3 | 77 |
> | IB | 68 |
> | IIA | 60 |
> | IIB | 53 |
> | IIIA | 36 |
> | IIIB | 26 |
> | IIIC | 13 |
> | IVA | 10 |
> | IVB | 0 |
>
> [a]See Box 28.53.
>
> *(Based on data from Goldstraw P, Crowley J, Chansky K et al.; International Association for the Study of Lung Cancer International Staging Committee; Participating Institutions. The IASLC Lung Cancer Staging Project: proposals for the revision of the TNM stage groupings in the forthcoming (8th) edition of the TNM classification of malignant tumours. J Thorac Oncol 2016; 2:706–714.)*

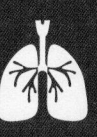

carcinoma but can be the first presentation. Typical sites for the primary tumour include the kidney, prostate, breast, bone, gastrointestinal tract, cervix or ovary.

Carcinoma, particularly of the stomach, pancreas and breast, can involve mediastinal glands and spread along the lymphatics of both lungs, leading to progressive and severe breathlessness (lymphangitis carcinomatosis). On the chest X-ray, bilateral lymphadenopathy is seen, together with streaky basal shadowing fanning out over both lung fields.

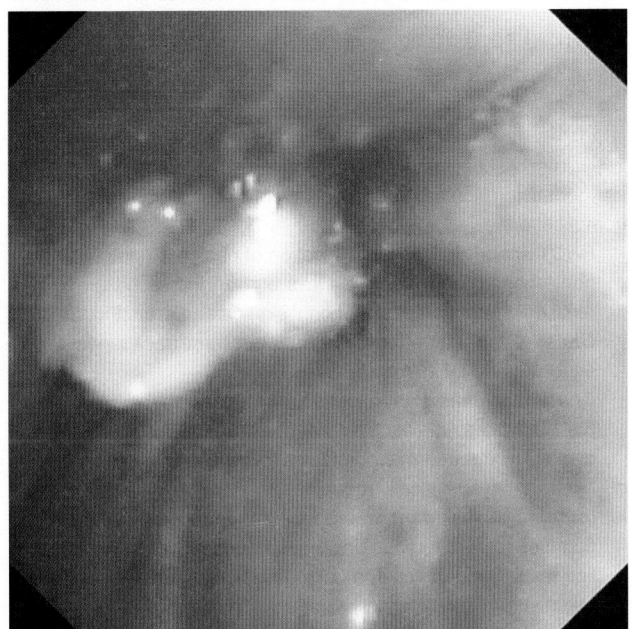

Fig. 28.33 Bronchoscopic view of a bronchial carcinoma obstructing a large bronchus.

Single pulmonary metastases can be removed surgically but, as CT scans usually show the presence of small metastases undetected on chest X-ray, detailed imaging, including PET scanning and assessment, is essential before undertaking surgery.

Solitary pulmonary nodules

A solitary pulmonary nodule is defined as a discrete lesion of less than 3 cm in diameter. The differential diagnoses for a solitary pulmonary nodule are:

- primary bronchial carcinoma
- pulmonary metastases
- inflammatory lesions, e.g. rounded pneumonia or abscess
- granuloma
- benign tumour of the lung, e.g. hamartoma
- rheumatoid nodules
- hydatid cyst.

With the increased use of CT scanning for other conditions, there has been greater incidental detection of asymptomatic, small, sub-centimetre nodules. The majority of these are benign; however, radiological follow-up should be arranged at intervals in line with recommended guidelines, determined by the size of the nodule in millimetres and the risk of developing malignancy. Scoring tools such as the Brock score are useful in assessing the risk of malignancy based on nodule characteristics and size.

Screening for lung cancer

A large trial carried out in the USA has demonstrated a 20% mortality benefit from low-dose helical CT screening for lung cancer in high-risk populations of smokers and ex-smokers between the ages of 55 and 74. A similar trial has been undertaken in the Netherlands and the UK. It is likely that low-dose CT screening will be employed in the future to detect cancer at an earlier stage so that curative treatment may be offered.

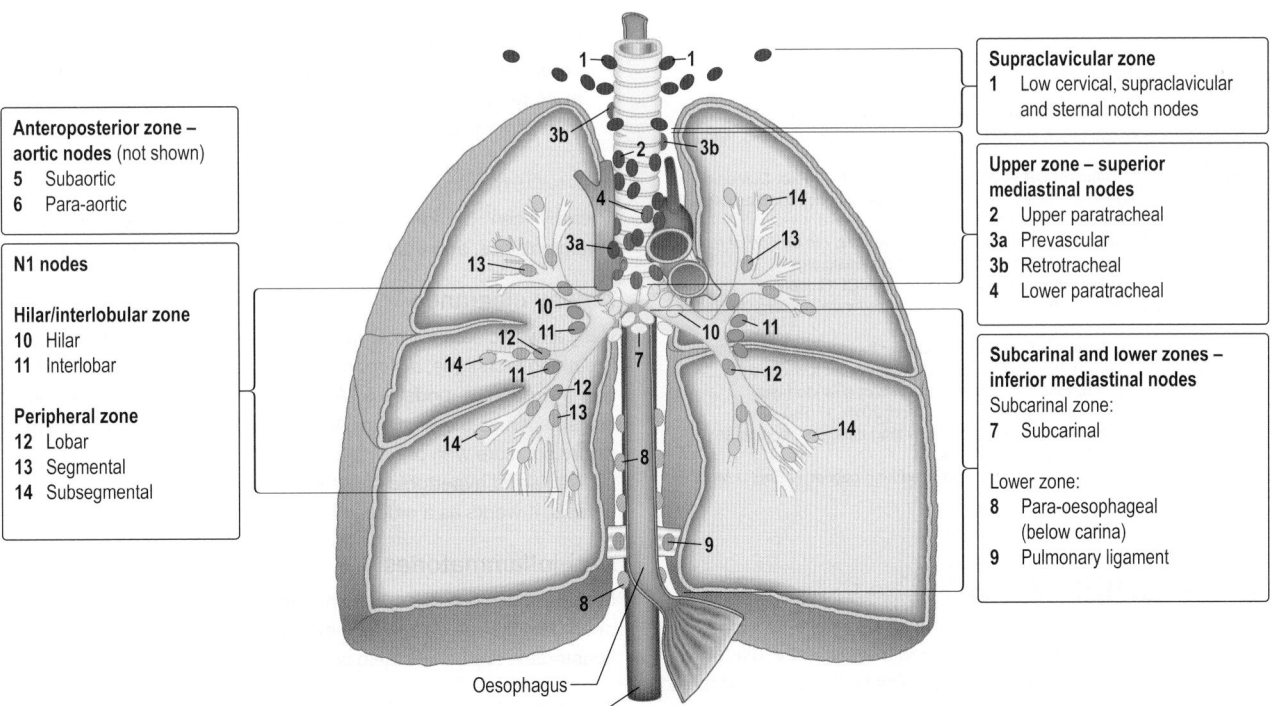

Anteroposterior zone – aortic nodes (not shown)
5 Subaortic
6 Para-aortic

N1 nodes

Hilar/interlobular zone
10 Hilar
11 Interlobar

Peripheral zone
12 Lobar
13 Segmental
14 Subsegmental

Supraclavicular zone
1 Low cervical, supraclavicular and sternal notch nodes

Upper zone – superior mediastinal nodes
2 Upper paratracheal
3a Prevascular
3b Retrotracheal
4 Lower paratracheal

Subcarinal and lower zones – inferior mediastinal nodes
Subcarinal zone:
7 Subcarinal

Lower zone:
8 Para-oesophageal (below carina)
9 Pulmonary ligament

Oesophagus
Aorta

Fig. 28.34 Lymph node stations commonly involved in lung cancer. These nodes are sampled during staging investigations.

Bronchial carcinoid tumours

These rare tumours are typically slow-growing, low-grade malignant neoplasms. They arise from neuroendocrine tumours and account for approximately 1% of all bronchial tumours. Many of these may be asymptomatic. Some patients will present with symptoms related to obstruction, recurrent infection or haemoptysis. The histological appearance may range from low-grade typical tumours to atypical tumours. Surgery is usually the treatment of choice, although patients will require long-term surveillance. As foregut derivatives, bronchial carcinoids produce adrenocorticotrophic hormone (ACTH) but do not usually produce the 5-hydroxytryptamine that is seen in midgut or hindgut carcinoid tumours. Staging of carcinoid tumours is the same as for NSCLC.

Benign tumours

Pulmonary hamartoma

This is the most common benign tumour of the lung and is usually seen on X-ray as a very well-defined round lesion 1–2 cm in diameter in the periphery of the lung. Growth is extremely slow but the tumour can reach several centimetres in diameter. Rarely, it arises from a major bronchus and causes obstruction.

Bronchial adenoma

This diverse group of benign tumours arises from mucus glands and ducts of the windpipe.

Cylindroma, chondroma and lipoma

These extremely rare tumours grow in the bronchus or trachea, causing obstruction.

Tracheal tumours

Benign tumours include squamous papilloma, leiomyoma and haemangiomas.

Further reading

Callister MEJ, Baldwin DR, Akram AR; British Thoracic Society. BTS guidelines for the investigation and management of pulmonary nodules. *Thorax* 2015; 70:suppl 2.
Field JK, Duffy SW, Baldwin DR et al. UK Lung Cancer RCT Pilot Screening Trial: baseline findings from the screening arm provide evidence for the potential implementation of lung cancer screening. *Thorax* 2016; 71:161–170.
International Association for the Study of Lung Cancer. *8th Edition of the TNM Classification for Lung Cancer*. IASLC 2017; www.iaslc.org.
National Institute for Health and Care Excellence. *NICE Guideline 122: Lung Cancer: Diagnosis and Management*. NICE 2019; http://www.nice.org.uk/guidance/ng122.
Patz Jr EF, Greco E, Gatsonis C et al. Lung cancer incidence and mortality in National Lung Screening Trial participants who underwent low-dose CT prevalence screening: a retrospective cohort analysis of a randomised, multicentre, diagnostic screening trial. *Lancet Oncol* 2016; 17:590–599.
Ru Zhao Y, Xie X, de Koning HJ et al. NELSON lung cancer screening study. *Cancer Imaging* 2011; 11 Spec No A:S79–84.
Schiller JH. A new standard of care for advanced lung cancer. *N Engl J Med*. 2018; 378:2135–2137.

BRONCHIECTASIS

Bronchiectasis describes abnormal and permanently dilated airways. The disease is characterized by a vicious circle of neutrophilic inflammation, recurrent infection and damage to the airway. This further impairs mucociliary clearance, and persistent inflammation leads to impairment of immunity.

Bronchiectasis is associated with a number of diseases but a cause will only be found in around 50% of cases. Little is known about the epidemiology and there is a wide variation in reported incidence. Bronchiectasis related to cystic fibrosis (see p. 983) is generally considered a separate entity.

Aetiology

The causes of bronchiectasis are listed in **Box 28.57**. Globally, TB is the leading cause. Bronchiectasis associated with other lung diseases – in particular, COPD – is becoming increasingly recognized.

Clinical features

These are shown in **Box 28.58**.

Investigations

The aims of investigation are to confirm the diagnosis, rule out an underlying cause, look for reversible factors and exclude complications.

- **HRCT scanning** is the investigation of choice. Characteristically, non-tapering 'tram track' airways and an increased bronchoarterial ratio termed the 'signet ring' sign can be seen (**Fig. 28.35**).
- **Chest X-ray** may often be normal but tram track airways, ring shadows and cysts may be seen.
- **Sputum examination** is useful for a focused antibiotic treatment plan, as well as the exclusion of non-tuberculous mycobacterial disease. Extended microbiological culture is often required and needs to be specifically requested.
- **Immune assessment** would include immunoglobulins and responses to Hib, tetanus and pneumococcal vaccines as baseline tests. Second-line immunological investigation by an immunologist may be necessary.
- **Sweat test and cystic fibrosis genetic assessment** (see p. 984) should be carried out for all patients under 40, but also for patients at any age where there is a high index of suspicion.
- **Nasal nitric oxide** is a useful test for screening for primary ciliary dyskinesia (PCD). It is very low in PCD. Further ciliary investigation in a specialist centre may be required.
- **Total IgE and** Aspergillus-**specific IgE or** Aspergillus **skin-prick testing** should be done to exclude allergic bronchopulmonary aspergillosis.

Management

Therapy can broadly be divided into airway clearance, anti-inflammatories, and treatment of infection and complications.

Airway clearance

Daily airway clearance therapies are advised. The activated cycle of breathing technique, **autogenic (self-)drainage** and postural drainage are popular modalities. A number of devices are available to assist, such as the Flutter or Acapella, which provide positive expiratory pressure with or without airway oscillation.

Nebulized hypertonic saline is also approved for use in bronchiectasis; it works as a mucoactive agent.

Anti-inflammatories

Long-term azithromycin has an immunomodulatory effect and has been demonstrated to reduce exacerbation frequency. Inhaled corticosteroids are beneficial to some patients.

Treatment of infection

Treatment of exacerbations usually lasts 2 weeks and is based on previously obtained microbiological information. When

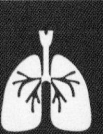

Congenital
- Deficiency of bronchial wall elements
- Pulmonary sequestration

Mechanical bronchial obstruction

Intrinsic
- Foreign body
- Inspissated mucus
- Post-tuberculous stenosis
- Tumour

Extrinsic
- Lymph node
- Tumour

Postinfective bronchial damage
- Bacterial and viral pneumonia, including pertussis, measles and aspiration pneumonia

Granuloma
- Tuberculosis, sarcoidosis

Diffuse diseases of the lung parenchyma
- e.g. Idiopathic pulmonary fibrosis

Immunological over-response
- Allergic bronchopulmonary aspergillosis
- Post-lung transplant
- Graft-versus-host disease

Immune deficiency

Primary
- Panhypogammaglobulinaemia
- Selective immunoglobulin deficiencies (IgA and IgG$_2$)

Secondary
- Human immunodeficiency virus and malignancy

Mucociliary clearance defects

Genetic
- Primary ciliary dyskinesia (Kartagener's syndrome with dextrocardia and situs inversus)
- Cystic fibrosis

Acquired
- Young's syndrome – azoospermia, sinusitis

---

i Box 28.58 Symptoms and signs in bronchiectasis

- *Cough*: usually persistent
- *Sputum production*: large amounts and purulent
- *Breathlessness*: as disease progresses
- *Haemoptysis*: usually a sign of infection; streaking is common but massive haemoptysis is a rare medical emergency
- *Infection*: usually characterized by increased sputum volume and increased purulence
- *Pleuritic chest pain*: can be a feature of infection, as well as fever and systemic upset
- *Coarse crackles*: heard on auscultation but examination can be normal
- *Clubbing*: especially in cystic fibrosis

Pseudomonas aeruginosa is being treated, dual therapy is often used where there are multi-resistant pathogens and where multiple antibiotic courses would be expected. High-dose ciprofloxacin (750 mg twice daily) is a useful oral drug for treatment of *Pseudomonas*. *H. influenzae* infection is common in bronchiectasis and usually responds to oral antibiotics such as amoxicillin, co-amoxiclav or doxycycline. Some multi-resistant species need intravenous cephalosporin treatment.

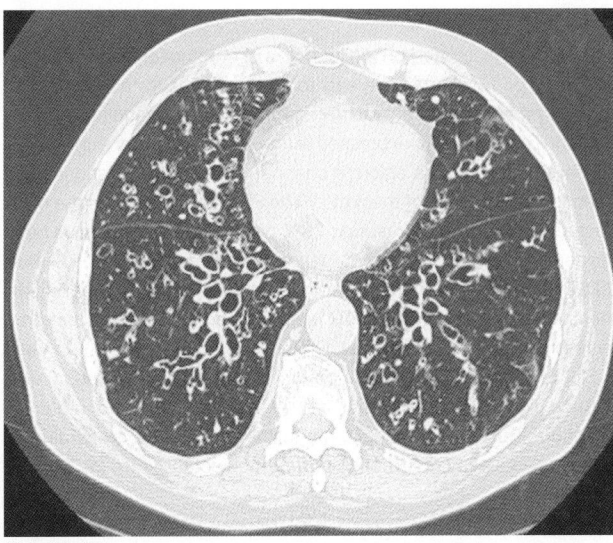

Fig. 28.35 CT scan showing bronchiectasis. Note the dilated bronchi with thickened wall, which are larger than adjacent arteries, giving a signet ring appearance.

Experience in cystic fibrosis has promoted the use of aggressive antibiotic strategies in bronchiectasis, with eradication therapy and chronic suppressive nebulized therapy with colistimethate or an aminoglycoside for *P. aeruginosa* (see p. 984).

Rotating oral antibiotic regimes are no longer recommended routinely. Long-term quinolones should be avoided.

Treatment of complications

- Pulmonary rehabilitation should be offered to patients with a reduced exercise capacity and breathlessness.
- Massive haemoptysis is a life-threatening medical emergency; treatment is resuscitation with airway protection until bronchial artery embolization can be performed to control the bleeding. If this is not successful, surgery may be required.
- Treatment of *Aspergillus* lung disease and non-tuberculous mycobacteria is covered on page 993.
- Respiratory failure should be treated with oxygen and non-invasive ventilation. Suitable patients should be referred to a transplant centre.
- Surgery is used for localized disease.

Prognosis

Prognosis is undefined and obviously quite variable, depending on disease severity. A low FEV$_1$ and infection with *P. aeruginosa* are associated with a poorer outcome.

Cystic fibrosis

Cystic fibrosis (CF) is an autosomal recessive condition. In the UK the birth prevalence is 1 in 2500 and the carrier rate is 1 in 25. Prevalence is a little lower in North America, rates being much lower in the non-Caucasian population. CF no longer causes most patients to die in childhood: survival has improved dramatically. The current expected median survival is now around 47 years. CF is a multisystem disease, although respiratory problems are usually the most prominent. A vicious circle of mucus stasis, inflammation and infection leads to respiratory failure and death in the majority of patients. Most individuals with CF also have pancreatic insufficiency.

Pathogenesis

The CF gene is located on the long arm of chromosome 7 at position 31.2 (see p. 18). Mutations lead to abnormalities in the production of the cystic fibrosis transmembrane conductance regulator (CFTR) protein. This protein is expressed in the apical membrane of epithelial cells and acts as a chloride channel. Over 1000 mutations have been identified, most of them rare. The F508del mutation is the most common, accounting for around 70% of cases. Mutations have been divided into different classes, depending on their effect on CFTR (**Box 28.59**). This classification is used therapeutically, with new CF treatments aimed at improving CFTR function. Ivacaftor was the first drug available for CF that improves CFTR function.

In the lungs, CFTR dysfunction leads to dehydrated airway surface liquid, mucus stasis, airway inflammation and recurrent infection. This process originates in the small airways, leading to progressive airway obstruction and bronchiectasis (**Fig. 28.36**).

Clinical features and complications

CF is a multisystem disease but in 90% of cases the eventual cause of death is related to respiratory disease. Pancreatic insufficiency occurs in the majority of patients and CF-related diabetes is becoming increasingly common as survival improves, occurring in up to 50% of older adults with CF. Liver disease occurs in around 20% of the CF population and can lead to cirrhosis in around 2%. Clinical manifestations and complications are summarized in **Box 28.60**.

Diagnosis

Most new CF diagnoses are currently made at newborn screening. The test involves measuring immunoreactive trypsinogen at the time of the neonatal heel-prick test. If the concentration is raised, formal testing is performed.

Aside from neonatal screening, diagnosis for children and adults is based on a combination of:
- Common clinical features (see **Box 28.60**).
- CFTR functional testing. The **sweat test (pilocarpine iontophoresis)** measures chloride concentration and is the test routinely performed. The normal range is <30 mmol/L, with borderline cases at 30–60 mmol/L. These cases often represent patients with a milder 'atypical' phenotype. In difficult cases, nasal potential difference can be measured.
- Confirmatory genetic testing.

Management

Patients with CF should be managed in a specialist centre by a multidisciplinary group of experienced healthcare professionals. They should be seen at least every 3 months and have an annual review. Lung function (FEV_1) and body mass index (BMI) should be recorded at every appointment, as they have prognostic importance.

Pulmonary disease

The aim of chronic pulmonary therapies is to reduce FEV_1 decline, daily symptoms and exacerbation frequency.
- **Airway clearance techniques** are a vital part of CF treatment regimens, taught to patients and their caregivers by specialist respiratory physiotherapists. Techniques include percussion, vibration, deep breathing and forced coughing; there is no consensus on the best type and patient choice is the main factor.
- **Nebulized therapy:**
  - Recombinant human DNase (rhDNase) works by lysing bacterial DNA and reducing sputum viscosity; it is advised for routine treatment from early childhood (regardless of disease status). There is clear evidence of improvement in lung disease and therapy may influence survival.
  - Hypertonic saline works as an osmotic agent to draw water to the cell surface and reduce sputum viscosity.
  - Inhaled mannitol also increases mucociliary clearance.
- **Anti-inflammatory treatment** with long-term azithromycin is widely used in CF and has an immunomodulatory effect.

Respiratory infection

Spread of respiratory infection is a great threat to CF patients. Clinics are microbiologically cohorted, patients are managed in single rooms and no patient social events are organized.

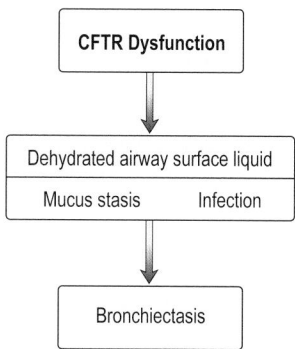

Fig. 28.36 Cystic fibrosis: pathogenesis of lung disease.

---

i Box 28.59 CFTR abnormalities in CF

Class	CFTR effect	Mutation example
I	Protein synthesis defect. No functional CFTR	G542X, R553X
II	Folding/trafficking defect. Does not reach apical membrane	F508del
III	Gating defect	G551D
IV	Conductance impairment due to narrow channel	R117H
V	Splicing defect	3849+10kbC>T
VI	Reduced stability	4326delTC

---

i Box 28.60 Clinical features and complications of cystic fibrosis

Respiratory
- Recurrent respiratory infection
- Chronic daily cough and sputum production
- Breathlessness
- Nasal polyps
- Haemoptysis (sometimes massive)
- Pneumothorax
- Respiratory failure and cor pulmonale
- Recurrent sinusitis

Gastrointestinal
- Failure to thrive in infancy and low body mass index in adults
- Meconium ileus in infancy
- Distal intestinal obstruction syndrome
- Steatorrhoea secondary to pancreatic insufficiency
- Cystic fibrosis-related liver disease and cirrhosis
- Increased risk of gastrointestinal malignancy

Other
- Cystic fibrosis-related diabetes
- Male infertility
- Osteoporosis
- Arthropathy

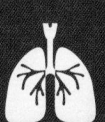

P. aeruginosa infection is common in patients with CF and is associated with accelerated lung function decline. Eradication is the treatment aim. A combination of nebulized colistimethate and oral ciprofloxacin, or inhaled tobramycin, can be given. Long-term nebulized suppression therapy with these medications is also used to improve respiratory health.

Other organisms, such as *Burkholderia cepacia*, meticillin-resistant *Staph. aureus* (MRSA) and *Stenotrophomonas maltophilia*, have been associated with worsening respiratory outcomes and so eradication regimes for these bacteria are being used. Non-tuberculous mycobacterial disease, in particular *M. abscessus*, can be associated with a rapid decline and active infection may preclude transplantation.

In exacerbations, intravenous antibiotic therapy is based on previous infection history. For *Pseudomonas*, a combination of a β-lactam antibiotic such as ceftazidime with an aminoglycoside such as tobramycin would be the first-line choice. *In vitro* sensitivities are less useful in CF. Many CF patients have a permanently implanted venous access device for delivery of intravenous therapy.

Advanced disease

Respiratory failure should be treated with oxygen and NIV. Patients should be referred for consideration of lung transplantation when FEV_1 falls to around 30% predicted. In end-stage disease, palliative care is an essential part of management. This can be challenging when patients are on an active waiting list for a lung transplant.

Non-respiratory complications

Pancreatic enzymes and vitamin supplements are used to treat patients with pancreatic insufficiency. Close attention is paid to diet and calorie supplementation. Overnight gastric feeding may be required to maintain BMI in some patients.

CF-related diabetes will often require treatment with insulin and is screened for at annual review. It is distinct from type 1 and type 2 diabetes. Osteoporosis is screened for and treated. Fertility treatment is available for men with CF who are infertile. Women with CF who become pregnant should be monitored very closely and deliver in a recognized CF centre.

The future

CFTR modulation has proved to be a major therapeutic advance, and studies of therapies for the F508del mutation are ongoing. Recently, lumacaftor (a CFTR corrector) in combination with ivacaftor has been shown to be beneficial in patients with p.Phe508del CFTR mutation. It is now widely available in the USA but not NICE-approved in UK, where it is given only as compassionate use. Trials are ongoing of triple therapy (using lumacaftor, ivacaftor and another agent that also improves CFTR function), which shows initial promise.

Further reading

Chambers JD, Chotirmall SH. Bronchiectasis: new therapies and new perspectives. *Lancet Respir Med* 2018; 6:715–726.
Elborn JS. Cystic fibrosis. *Lancet* 2016; 388:2519–2531.
Flume PA, Chalmers JD, Olivier KN. Advances in bronchiectasis: endotyping, genetics, microbiome, and disease heterogeneity. *Lancet* 2018; 392:880–890.
Grasemann H. Modulator therapy for cystic fibrosis. *N Engl J Med* 2017; 377:2085–2088.

INTERSTITIAL LUNG DISEASES

This heterogeneous group of conditions are also referred to as *diffuse parenchymal lung diseases* and account for about 15% of respiratory clinical practice. They are characterized by varying degrees of inflammation and fibrosis, initially affecting the interstitium of the lung and typically presenting with exertional dyspnoea, with or without cough. A classification is shown in **Fig. 28.37**.

Sarcoidosis

Sarcoidosis is a multisystem granulomatous disorder; it commonly affects young adults and typically presents with bilateral hilar lymphadenopathy, pulmonary infiltration and skin or eye lesions.

Epidemiology and aetiology

Sarcoidosis is a common disease of unknown aetiology that is often detected on routine chest X-ray. It is most common in Northern Europe (annual incidence 5–40/100 000) but uncommon in Japan (incidence 1–2/100 000). It occurs more frequently in Afro-Caribbean patients, who are also more likely to develop extrapulmonary or chronic disease. There is a female preponderance with a peak incidence in the third and fourth decades. There is no relation to any histocompatibility antigen but first-degree relatives (particularly Caucasians) have an increased risk of developing sarcoidosis.

Immunopathology

- Typical sarcoid granulomas consist of focal accumulations of epithelioid cells, macrophages and lymphocytes, mainly T cells.
- There is depressed cell-mediated reactivity to tuberculin; the Mantoux test is usually negative. There is overall lymphopenia; circulating T lymphocytes are low but B cells are slightly increased.
- Bronchoalveolar lavage shows a great increase in the overall number of cells; a lymphocytosis (particularly CD4+ T-helper cells) is common.
- Transbronchial biopsies show infiltration of the alveolar walls and interstitial spaces with leucocytes, mainly T cells, prior to granuloma formation.

Clinical features

Sarcoidosis can affect any organ (**Box 28.61**) but has a predilection for the lungs (involvement in up to 90%). Presentation may be with respiratory symptoms but it is not unusual for the diagnosis to be made incidentally on chest X-ray. Common extrathoracic manifestations include eye, skin or lymph node involvement, and constitutional upset with fatigue is a frequent and often refractory symptom.

A typical combination of bilateral hilar lymphadenopathy, erythema nodosum, arthralgia and fever is known as Löfgren's syndrome and usually resolves spontaneously without the need for treatment.

In less classic presentations, HRCT may initially suggest sarcoidosis but tissue biopsy of an affected organ is often sought for definitive diagnosis (the presence of non-caseating granulomas being diagnostic). Skin biopsy is comparatively non-invasive, and careful examination for infiltration of scars and tattoos amenable to sampling should be undertaken.

Pulmonary manifestations

Although pulmonary involvement may be an incidental finding, cough, exertional breathlessness and vague chest discomfort are common presentations. Even in symptomatic individuals the chest is often clear to auscultation, although wheeze may be evident if there is significant involvement of the airways with endobronchial disease. There are four radiological stages of lung involvement, which help inform prognosis:

- ***Stage 1:*** bilateral hilar lymphadenopathy alone (BHL) – 55–90% spontaneous remission.

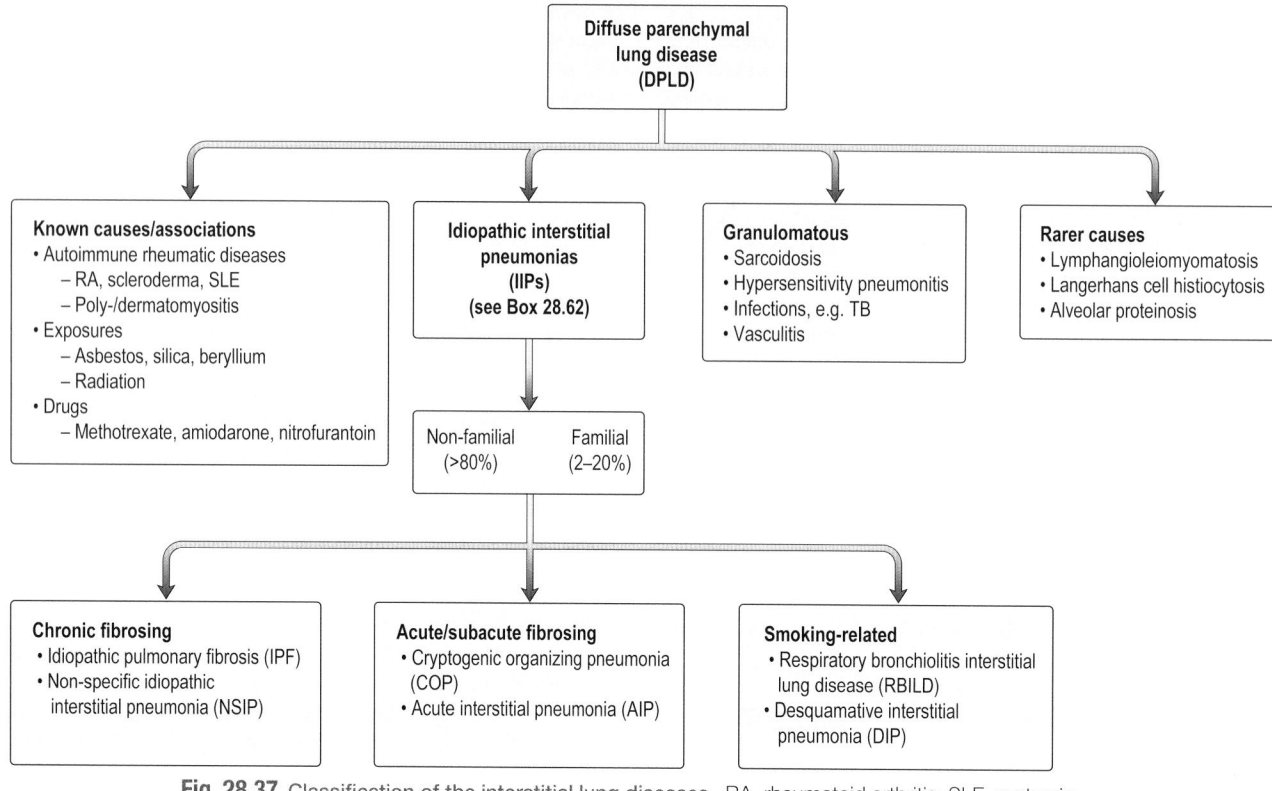

Fig. 28.37 Classification of the interstitial lung diseases. RA, rheumatoid arthritis; SLE, systemic lupus erythematosus; TB, tuberculosis.

- **Stage 2:** pulmonary infiltrates with BHL – 40–70% spontaneous remission.
- **Stage 3:** pulmonary infiltrates without BHL – 10–20% spontaneous remission.
- **Stage 4:** fibrosis.

Patients may present with any stage of disease and do not necessarily progress through the stages sequentially. Moreover, the extent of disease on chest X-ray does not correlate with the degree of impairment on pulmonary function testing.

Bilateral hilar lymphadenopathy

Symmetrical BHL is a characteristic feature of sarcoidosis and is usually asymptomatic. Occasionally, it is associated with a dull ache in the chest, malaise and a mild fever. The differential diagnosis of BHL includes:

- **Lymphoma:** this rarely affects the hilar lymph nodes in isolation.
- **Pulmonary TB:** hilar lymph nodes are usually enlarged asymmetrically.
- **Carcinoma of the bronchus** with malignant spread to the hilar lymph nodes: again, this is rarely symmetrical.

Pulmonary infiltration

Although the lung fields may appear normal on plain chest X-ray, the lung parenchyma is frequently involved, as shown by CT scanning (**Fig. 28.38**), transbronchial biopsy and bronchoalveolar lavage. Symptoms may be minimal (or even absent), despite quite marked radiographic abnormalities. Progressive disease may lead to irreversible fibrosis in up to 20% of cases. The principal differential diagnoses are TB, pneumoconiosis, idiopathic pulmonary fibrosis and hypersensitivity pneumonitis.

---

i **Box 28.61 Clinical presentations of sarcoidosis**

Constitutional
- Fever
- Weight loss
- Fatigue

Reticuloendothelial
- Splenomegaly
- Lymphadenopathy

Respiratory
- Stage 1–4 pulmonary involvement
- Cough
- Dyspnoea
- Wheeze

Hepatic
- Deranged liver function tests
- Hepatomegaly

Ocular
- Anterior uveitis
- Keratoconjunctivitis sicca

Hypercalcaemia/ hypercalciuria
- Hypercalciuria
- Nephrocalcinosis
- Calculi
- Tubulointerstitial nephritis

Cutaneous
- Erythema nodosum
- Lupus pernio

Neurological
- Cognitive dysfunction
- Headache
- Cranial nerve palsies
- Mononeuritis multiplex
- Peripheral neuropathy
- Seizures

Cardiac
- Arrhythmias
- Heart block
- Cardiomyopathy
- Sudden death

Extrapulmonary manifestations

Sarcoidosis can affect any organ. Cutaneous sarcoidosis and ocular sarcoidosis are the most common extrapulmonary presentations but cardiac and CNS involvement are the most important clinically.

Skin lesions

These occur in 10–30% of cases. Sarcoidosis is the most common cause of erythema nodosum (see p. 678). Lupus pernio (indurated

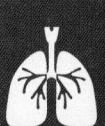

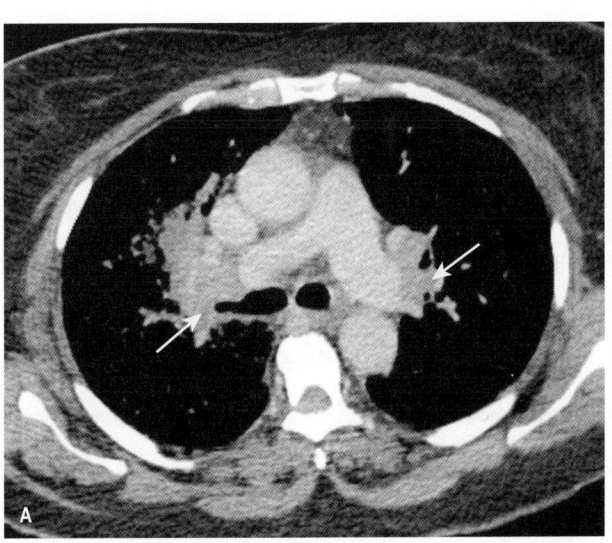

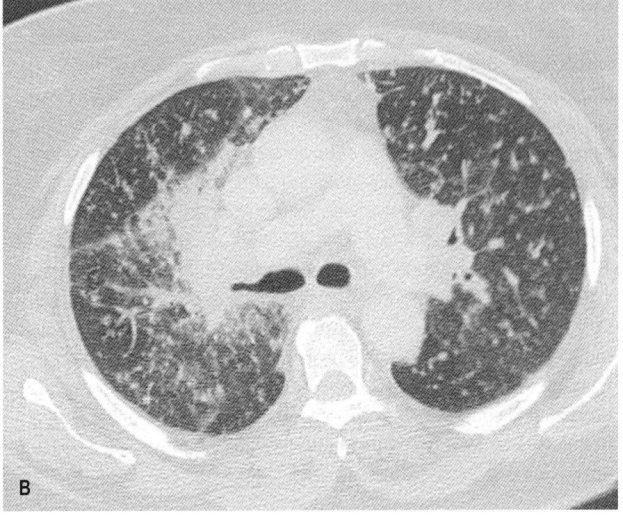

Fig. 28.38 CT chest showing sarcoidosis. **(A)** Soft tissue settings demonstrate bilateral hilar lymphadenopathy (arrowed). **(B)** Lung settings demonstrate multiple small nodules and reticulation in both lungs.

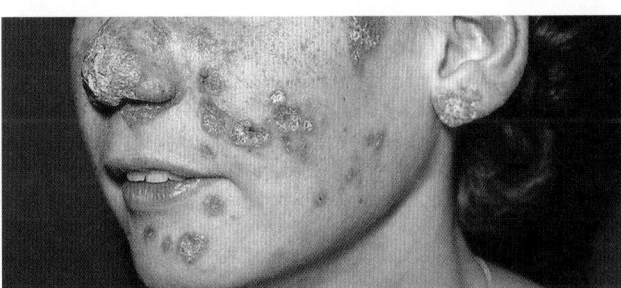

Fig. 28.39 The lupus pernio form of sarcoidosis. There are infiltrated violaceous plaques on the nose, cheeks, and ears. This girl had hoarseness owing to her laryngeal involvement with sarcoidosis and was left with severe scarring after treatment. *(From Paller AS, Mancini AJ. Hurwitz Clinical Pediatric Dermatology: A Textbook of Skin Disorders of Childhood and Adolescence, 5th edn. Elsevier Inc.; 2016; Fig. 25-20.)*

erythematous or violaceous papules or plaques, **Fig. 28.39**) may be seen over the face and ears.

Eye lesions

In 5% of patients, anterior or, less commonly, posterior uveitis presents with misting of vision, a painful, red eye or progressive loss of vision. Asymptomatic uveitis may be found in up to 25% of patients with sarcoidosis and ophthalmological assessment should be considered in all patients with a new diagnosis of sarcoidosis. Keratoconjunctivitis sicca and lacrimal gland enlargement also occur.

Metabolic manifestations

Hypercalcaemia and hypercalciuria can lead to the development of renal calculi, nephrocalcinosis and, ultimately, renal failure.

Central nervous system

CNS involvement is rare (2%) but can lead to severe neurological disease (see p. 868).

Bone and joint involvement

Arthralgia without erythema nodosum is seen in 5% of cases. Bone cysts with associated swelling, particularly affecting the digits, may be seen on X-ray.

Hepatosplenomegaly

Mild derangement of liver function tests is common and granulomas are seen in the majority of biopsy specimens, although these findings are rarely of clinical consequence. Progression to portal hypertension or liver failure is uncommon.

Renal involvement

Sarcoidosis classically causes a granulomatous tubulointerstitial nephritis, although kidney damage secondary to hypercalcaemia and stone formation may also be seen.

Cardiac involvement

Ventricular dysrhythmias, conduction defects and cardiomyopathy with congestive cardiac failure are rare (3%). Severity ranges from benign rhythm disturbance to sudden cardiac death. All patients with sarcoidosis should have an ECG at presentation.

Investigations

- **Imaging.** Chest X-ray is the initial modality for staging, followed by HRCT for assessment of parenchymal involvement. This may show nodules of up to 10 mm diameter that form a characteristic 'beading' appearance along airways, vessels and fissures; nodules may aggregate into larger nodules or masses of up to 3 cm; there may be increased reticulation due to septal thickening; in severe cases fibrotic honeycombing is seen.
- **Full blood count.** There may be a mild normochromic, normocytic anaemia with raised ESR.
- **Biochemistry.** Renal involvement is occasionally found and may require renal biopsy and first-line treatment. Hypercalcaemia occurs in 10–20% and hypercalciuria in 30–50%. Activated macrophages in lung and lymph nodes are able to hydroxylate vitamin D directly (independent of parathyroid hormone levels), leading to increased intestinal absorption of dietary calcium. Measurement of 24-hour urinary calcium excretion should be performed at presentation.
- **Serum ACE level.** This is elevated in over 75% of patients with untreated sarcoidosis. Raised (but lower) levels are also seen in patients with lymphoma, pulmonary TB, asbestosis and silicosis, limiting the diagnostic value of the test. The utility of serum ACE in monitoring disease activity and response to treatment is contentious.

- **Cardiac tests.** ECG and echocardiogram should be performed at presentation. If these raise concern about underlying cardiac sarcoidosis, then further investigation is with cardiac MRI.
- **Bronchoscopy.** Bronchoalveolar lavage typically shows a lymphocytosis with raised CD4:CD8 ratio. Transbronchial biopsy of the lung parenchyma is positive in up to 90% of cases of pulmonary sarcoidosis. Pulmonary non-caseating granulomas are found in approximately 50% of patients with extrapulmonary sarcoidosis who have a normal chest X-ray. If, in addition, endobronchial biopsy (EBUS) of thoracic lymph nodes is performed, this may significantly increase the yield, even if the macroscopic appearances are normal.
- **Lung function tests.** These show a restrictive lung defect with reduced gas transfer in patients with parenchymal infiltration or fibrosis. However, an obstructive defect may be seen in endobronchial disease and a mixed pattern is also possible. Lung function is usually normal in patients with isolated hilar adenopathy or extrapulmonary disease.

Prognosis and management

The natural history of sarcoidosis is unpredictable and varies from spontaneous remission to inexorable progression and death in a small number (1–5%). Even once remission has been achieved, relapses are common. Worse outcomes are seen in patients of Afro-Caribbean and Asian descent, and those presenting with extrathoracic disease. Systemic treatment is indicated for hypercalcaemia and extrathoracic major organ involvement, particularly neurological, cardiac or ocular disease resistant to topical therapy. Treatment of pulmonary sarcoidosis is less clear-cut, as spontaneous resolution is frequently seen, typically within the first 6 months. Moreover, although corticosteroids improve radiographic appearances, this is not consistently reflected in improved lung function tests. Treatment is therefore reserved for patients with troublesome symptoms, deteriorating lung function or radiological evidence of disease progression. First-line treatment is with prednisolone (or equivalent) 0.5 mg/kg for 4–6 weeks, gradually tapering to a maintenance dose for at least 12 months. Alternative immunosuppressants, including methotrexate, azathioprine and hydroxychloroquine, have been used in place of, or in addition to, prednisolone. Relapses are common on withdrawal of therapy. Lung transplantation should be considered for suitable patients with stage IV disease and respiratory failure.

Idiopathic interstitial pneumonias

The terminology used to describe the idiopathic interstitial pneumonias can be confusing but a distinction must be made between subgroups, as there are significant differences in terms of prognosis and treatment options. Clinical patterns usually link to particular histological subtypes; their classification is shown in **Box 28.62**.

Idiopathic pulmonary fibrosis

Idiopathic pulmonary fibrosis (IPF) is the most common of the idiopathic interstitial pneumonias. It is a progressive and ultimately fatal disease of unknown cause. There is significant worldwide variation in reported prevalence but the incidence appears to be increasing (6.8–8.8/100 000 in the USA). The onset is usually in the patient's sixties and is rare below the age of 50. Males are twice as likely to be affected.

Pathology

Usual interstitial pneumonia (UIP) is the histological finding in IPF. The key feature is a heterogenous appearance with areas of normal

---

> **i** | **Box 28.62 Classification of idiopathic interstitial pneumonias**

Clinical diagnosis	Pathological pattern
Idiopathic pulmonary fibrosis (IPF)	Usual interstitial pneumonia (UIP)
Desquamative interstitial pneumonia (DIP)	Desquamative interstitial pneumonia (DIP)
Respiratory bronchiolitis interstitial lung disease (RBILD)	Respiratory bronchiolitis interstitial lung disease (RBILD)
Acute interstitial pneumonia (AIP)	Diffuse alveolar damage (DAD)
Non-specific interstitial pneumonia (NSIP)	Non-specific interstitial pneumonia (NSIP)
Cryptogenic organizing pneumonia (COP)	Organizing pneumonia (OP)
Lymphoid interstitial pneumonia (LIP)	Lymphoid interstitial pneumonia (LIP)

(From ATS/ERS. American Thoracic Society/European Respiratory Society International multidisciplinary consensus classification of the idiopathic interstitial pneumonias. Am J Respir Crit Care Med 2002; 165:277.)

---

lung punctuated by areas of marked fibrosis, honeycombing mainly in subpleural areas and fibroblastic foci (dense proliferations of fibroblasts and myofibroblasts). The terms IPF and UIP are often used interchangeably but they are *not* synonymous, as UIP is also the primary histological finding in several other diffuse parenchymal lung diseases (e.g. pulmonary autoimmune rheumatic disease).

Pathogenesis

It is thought that repetitive injury to the alveolar epithelium, caused by currently unidentified environmental stimuli, leads to the activation of several pathways responsible for repair of the damaged tissue. However, in IPF, the wound healing mechanisms become uncontrolled, leading to over-production of fibroblasts and deposition of increased extracellular matrix in the interstitium with little inflammation. The structural integrity of the lung parenchyma is therefore disrupted: there is loss of elasticity and the ability to perform gas exchange is impaired, leading to progressive respiratory failure.

Clinical features

Patients typically present with insidious onset of progressive dyspnoea that may be accompanied by cough, with or without sputum production. Examination of the chest shows bi-basal end-inspiratory crackles and therefore it is not uncommon for patients to be mistakenly treated for heart failure or recurrent chest infections before the diagnosis of IPF is made. Finger clubbing is seen in 25–50% of cases.

Progressive respiratory failure may be complicated by pulmonary hypertension. Stepwise deterioration can occur due to pneumothorax, pulmonary embolism or intercurrent infection, but acute exacerbations with no identifiable cause are well recognized and are associated with increased mortality. An acute form (also known as Hamman–Rich syndrome) occasionally occurs and has a particularly poor prognosis.

Investigations

- **Respiratory function tests** usually show a restrictive pattern (FEV$_1$/FVC ratio >70%) with reduced lung volumes and gas transfer. However, spirometry may be normal in early disease and lung volumes can be preserved in the presence of coexisting emphysema.

- **Blood tests**, including antinuclear antibodies (ANA) and rheumatoid factor (RF), are performed to exclude autoimmune rheumatic disease but there is no specific serological test for IPF.
- **Chest X-ray** shows small-volume lungs with increased reticular shadowing at the bases but may be normal in early disease.
- **HRCT** is the imaging modality of choice. A confident diagnosis of IPF may be made in patients with:
  - **Basal distribution**: abnormalities are more pronounced at the bases.
  - **Subpleural reticulation**: reticulation is most evident in the lung peripheries.
  - **Traction bronchiectasis**: the fibrotic process distorts the normal lung architecture, pulling the airways open and causing bronchiectasis.
  - **Honeycombing**: there are basal layers of small, cystic airspaces with irregularly thickened walls composed of fibrous tissue (**Fig. 28.40**).
- **Bronchoalveolar lavage** is necessary only if an infective or malignant cause is suspected. A differential cell count may lend support to an alternative diagnosis: a lymphocytosis is suggestive of hypersensitivity pneumonitis, whereas a neutrophilic pattern (neutrophils >3%) is commonly seen in IPF.
- **Histological confirmation** is necessary in some patients. Surgical lung biopsy, usually via VATS, is the most reliable method for obtaining diagnostic histological samples; transbronchial biopsy can be undertaken bronchoscopically but only obtains small samples.

Differential diagnosis

The main differential diagnosis for IPF is an alternative interstitial lung disease. Other differentials for the chest X-ray appearances include interstitial pulmonary oedema, infection and lymphangitis carcinomatosa.

Prognosis and management

The median survival time for patients with IPF is 2–5 years. Serial lung function testing is used to monitor disease progression and a 10% decline in FVC or 15% decline in gas transfer (TLCO) in the first 6–12 months confers a worse prognosis. Periods of stability may be interspersed with spells of more accelerated decline but failure to recover back to baseline following these episodes is common. Mortality is increased following acute exacerbations.

Immunosuppression is generally avoided in IPF and steroids are no longer recommended in confirmed disease.

Pirfenidone, an antifibrotic agent, has been shown to slow the rate of FVC decline, with the most common side-effects being a reversible photosensitive rash and gastrointestinal disturbance. Other treatments include **nintedanib**, an intracellular inhibitor of tyrosine kinases.

Gastro-oesophageal reflux disease should be treated if symptomatic.

Even with treatment, IPF is a life-limiting disease and transplant assessment should be undertaken in accordance with local guidelines. All patients should have their need for supportive care evaluated with respect to oxygen therapy, pulmonary rehabilitation and palliative care input.

Other idiopathic interstitial pneumonias

These are described in **Box 28.63**.

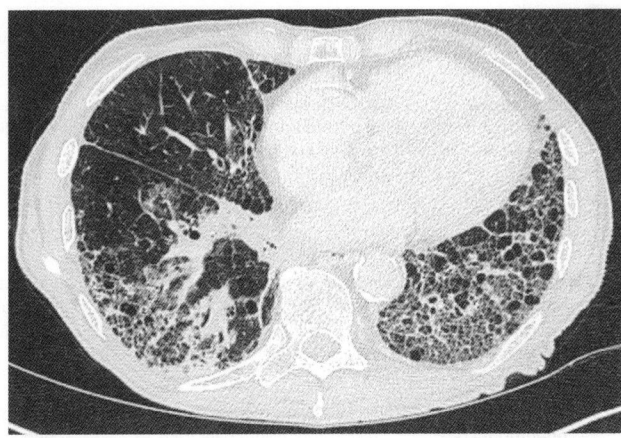

Fig. 28.40 CT chest demonstrating idiopathic pulmonary fibrosis. There is subpleural reticulation and honeycombing at both lung bases.

Hypersensitivity pneumonitis

Hypersensitivity pneumonitis (HP) is caused by an allergic reaction affecting the small airways and alveoli in response to an inhaled antigen or occasionally following ingestion of a causative drug. Common antigens are illustrated in **Box 28.64**.

One of the most common causes worldwide is farmer's lung, which can affect up to 9% of farmers in humid climates. Cigarette smokers have a lower risk of developing HP due to decreased antibody reaction to the antigen, but once established, smoking may lead to a more chronic or severe disease course.

Pathogenesis

Histological features include chronic inflammatory infiltrates and poorly defined interstitial granulomas, together with interstitial fibrosis and honeycomb change in chronic disease.

The allergic response to the inhaled antigen involves both cellular immunity and deposition of immune complexes, causing foci of inflammation through activation of complement via the classical pathway.

Clinical features

HP can be categorized according to the time course of symptoms, as determined by duration and intensity of exposure. Symptoms include weight loss, malaise, dyspnoea and cough. Auscultation reveals inspiratory squeaks due to bronchiolitis, and bilateral fine crackles. Wheeze is uncommon.

- **Acute:** symptom onset 4–6h following exposure. Fever is common and patients may be mistakenly diagnosed with a chest infection. Resolution occurs 24–48h following removal from the inciting antigen.
- **Subacute:** usually occurs with intermittent or lower-level exposure. Improvement is seen in weeks to months following removal from exposure.
- **Chronic:** usually no history of preceding acute symptoms. Insidious onset of respiratory and constitutional symptoms is typical. Finger clubbing may be present. Progression to irreversible fibrosis is associated with increased mortality.

? Box 28.63 Other idiopathic interstitial pneumonias (IIPs)

IIP	Presentation	HRCT	Pathology	Treatment
Desquamative interstitial pneumonia (DIP)	Middle-aged smokers Men > women Dyspnoea and cough over weeks to months	Widespread ground glass opacification	Alveolar spaces filled with pigmented macrophages (due to tobacco smoke)	Smoking cessation – may remit spontaneously Corticosteroids in severe or progressive disease ± additional immunosuppressants Response generally good
Respiratory bronchiolitis interstitial lung disease (RBILD)	Current or ex-smokers Similar to DIP	Centrilobular nodules Ground glass opacification	Pigmented macrophages in lumen of respiratory bronchioles	Smoking cessation No clear benefit with corticosteroids Outcome more favourable than in DIP
Acute interstitial pneumonia (AIP, Hamman–Rich syndrome)	Dyspnoea and progressive respiratory failure over days to weeks Often preceded by viral prodrome	Ground glass opacification Traction bronchiectasis Consolidation Septal thickening	Diffuse alveolar damage (DAD)	Pulsed i.v. methylprednisolone for 3 days followed by maintenance oral corticosteroids Additional immunosuppressants may be required Mortality 50–80%
Non-specific interstitial pneumonia (NSIP)	Similar to IPF but more indolent course May be associated with connective tissue disease	Similar to IPF but increased ground glass opacification, minimal honeycombing	Uniform inflammatory infiltrate with or without fibrosis (fibrotic vs cellular NSIP)	Corticosteroids ± additional immunosuppressants, e.g. azathioprine, cyclophosphamide Prognosis better with cellular form Outcome more favourable than in IPF
Cryptogenic organizing pneumonia (COP)	Influenza-like symptoms, dyspnoea, cough over weeks to months Secondary OP may be related to connective tissue, autoimmune disease or drugs	Bilateral flitting/migratory peripheral consolidation Variable ground glass opacification	Buds of connective tissue (Masson bodies) in alveoli and alveolar ducts	Usually rapidly responsive to corticosteroids but relapses common
Lymphoid interstitial pneumonia (LIP)	Commonly, middle-aged women Insidious dyspnoea, dry cough, systemic upset May be associated with connective tissue disease and HIV infection	Ground glass opacification Perivascular cysts	Interstitium infiltrated by lymphocytes, macrophages and plasma cells	Corticosteroids Anti-retrovirals in HIV Mortality up to 38%

HIV, human immunodeficiency virus; HRCT, high-resolution computed tomography; IPF, idiopathic pulmonary fibrosis.

? Box 28.64 Some causes of hypersensitivity pneumonitis

Disease	Situation	Antigens
Farmer's lung	Forking mouldy hay or any other mouldy vegetable material	Thermophilic actinomycetes, e.g. *Micropolyspora faeni* Fungi, e.g. *Aspergillus umbrosus*
Bird fancier's lung	Handling pigeons, cleaning lofts or budgerigar cages	Proteins present in the 'bloom' on the feathers and in excreta
Maltworker's lung	Turning germinating barley	*Aspergillus clavatus*
Humidifier fever	Contaminated humidifying systems in air conditioners or humidifiers in factories (especially in printing works)	Possibly a variety of bacterium or amoeba (e.g. *Naegleria gruberi*) Thermophilic actinomycetes
Mushroom worker's lung	Turning mushroom compost	Thermophilic actinomycetes
Cheese washer's lung	Mouldy cheese	*Penicillium casei* *Aspergillus clavatus*
Winemaker's lung	Mould on grapes	Botrytis

Investigations

A diagnosis can often be made by maintaining a high index of suspicion and taking a detailed exposure history. Identification of a culprit antigen in the context of typical clinical and radiological findings often makes lung biopsy unnecessary.

- **Chest X-ray** may be normal in acute and subacute disease. When present, abnormalities include diffuse small nodules and increased reticular shadowing.
- **HRCT** shows nodules with ground-glass opacity and evidence of air trapping. Increased reticulation and honeycomb change

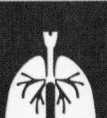

are seen in advanced disease. Abnormalities are most marked in the mid or upper zones.

- **Lung function tests** are not diagnostic. A restrictive ventilatory defect with decreased carbon monoxide gas transfer is seen in chronic disease.
- **Precipitating antibodies** are present in the serum. One-quarter of pigeon fanciers have precipitating IgG antibodies against pigeon protein and droppings in their serum, but only a small proportion have lung disease. Precipitating antibodies are therefore evidence of exposure, not disease.
- **Bronchoalveolar lavage** shows a lymphocytosis. A low CD4:CD8 ratio can help differentiate HP from sarcoidosis.
- **Lung biopsy** demonstrates a lymphocyte-rich infiltrate with varying degrees of fibrosis, depending on chronicity of disease.

Differential diagnosis

Although HP due to inhalation of the spores of *Micropolyspora faeni* is common among farmers (farmer's lung), it is probably more usual for these individuals to suffer from asthma related to inhalation of antigens from a variety of mites that infest stored grain and other vegetable material, such as *Lepidoglyphus domesticus, L. destructor* and *Acarus siro*.

Management

The key to successful treatment is avoidance of exposure to the inciting antigen (if known) and this may be achieved by changes in work practice. Pigeon fancier's lung is more difficult to control, as affected individuals remain strongly attached to their hobby. Prednisolone should be initiated in patients whose symptoms persist despite withdrawal from the causative antigen, and in severe disease. Established fibrosis will not resolve and, in some patients, the disease may progress inexorably to respiratory failure despite intensive therapy. Farmer's lung is a recognized occupational disease in the UK and sufferers are entitled to compensation, depending on their degree of disability.

Rare interstitial lung diseases

Langerhans cell histiocytosis

This rare disease is characterized histologically by proliferation of Langerhans cells. There is a wide variation in clinical presentation, from isolated lytic bone lesions to multisystem disease involving skin, lymph nodes and major organs (more commonly seen in young children). Pulmonary involvement occurs in 10% of cases and is strongly associated with cigarette smoking. Recurrent spontaneous pneumothorax is seen in up to 25% and is a common mode of presentation. HRCT shows characteristic interstitial thickening, nodules, cysts and honeycombing with mid and upper zone predominance, and this may be sufficient for diagnosis in a young smoker (typical age 20–40 years). Smoking cessation is essential. Various treatment strategies, including corticosteroids, chemotherapy agents and the purine analogue cladribine, have been used with variable success. Lung transplantation may be considered in advanced disease. Outcome varies from spontaneous remission to progressive end-stage fibrosis but overall 5-year survival is 75%.

Pulmonary lymphangioleiomyomatosis

Pulmonary lymphangioleiomyomatosis (LAM) is a rare disorder of premenopausal women, causing hamartomatous smooth muscle infiltration of the lungs. Extrapulmonary involvement, especially with

renal angiomyolipomas (hamartomas), is common. Some 15% of patients with pulmonary LAM have tuberous sclerosis. Presentation is with dyspnoea, chylous pleural effusions and pneumothorax. HRCT shows diffuse thin-walled cysts scattered throughout the lungs. Treatment with hormonal manipulation or oophorectomy has shown a variable response. Sirolimus (rapamycin) can be effective but lung transplantation may be necessary.

Pulmonary alveolar proteinosis

In this rare disease lipoproteinaceous material accumulates within the alveoli. It can be congenital but most cases are acquired and appear to have an autoimmune basis, with antibodies directed against the cytokine granulocyte-macrophage colony-stimulating factor (GM-CSF). The disease mostly affects men and presents with progressive exertional dyspnoea and cough. Inspiratory crackles are present in 50%. Diagnosis is made by bronchoalveolar lavage, which reveals a milky appearance and many large, foamy macrophages but few other inflammatory cells. Initial therapy is with whole-lung lavage.

Small-vessel vasculitides

The vasculitides are a group of autoimmune diseases that cause inflammation of the large, medium and small blood vessels. The small-vessel vasculitides associated with **anti-neutrophil cytoplasmic antibody** (**ANCA**) include granulomatosis with polyangiitis (GPA, formerly referred to as Wegener's granulomatosis), microscopic polyangiitis (MPA) and eosinophilic granulomatosis with polyangiitis (EGPA, formerly called Churg–Strauss syndrome). Staining for ANCA shows either a diffuse pattern (c-ANCA) with antibodies directed against proteinase 3 (PR3), or a perinuclear pattern (p-ANCA) with antibodies to myeloperoxidase (MPO) (see also p. 416). The respiratory tract and kidneys are frequently involved and the ESR is often markedly elevated (>100 mm/h).

Granulomatosis with polyangiitis

GPA typically affects older adults and is more common in Caucasians. The c-ANCA is usually positive with elevated PR3 antibodies. The ears and upper respiratory tract are frequently affected with bloody nasal discharge, crusting and destruction, sinusitis and otitis media. Evidence of glomerulonephritis should be sought on urinalysis (see p. 1352). Respiratory symptoms include cough, dyspnoea and pleuritic chest pain. Diffuse alveolar haemorrhage occurs in up to 45% and haemoptysis can be life-threatening. Thoracic imaging characteristically shows multiple nodules that often cavitate, areas of consolidation and ground-glass opacification (which may be due to pulmonary haemorrhage). Diagnosis should be confirmed with biopsy of the active site but it is sometimes necessary to initiate empirical treatment in acutely unwell patients. Initial immunosuppressant therapy is with a combination of glucocorticoids and cyclophosphamide, rituximab or methotrexate.

Microscopic polyangiitis

MPA is primarily associated with p-ANCA positivity. Presentation and treatment are similar to those of granulomatosis with polyangiitis. It is diagnosed on tissue biopsy, where the absence of granuloma formation differentiates it from GPA.

Eosinophilic granulomatosis with polyangiitis

EGPA classically presents in early adulthood with allergic rhinitis, asthma that is often difficult to control, and peripheral blood eosinophilia (>10%); it is ANCA-positive in up to 60% (usually p-ANCA). Systemic vasculitis subsequently develops, sometimes many years later. Involvement of skin (tender subcutaneous nodules, petechiae or purpuric lesions), peripheral nerves (mononeuritis multiplex), heart, kidneys and gastrointestinal tract may occur. The chest X-ray shows migratory patchy opacities that may be accompanied by nodules and pleural effusions. EGPA generally responds well to corticosteroids, although additional immunosuppressants are required for severe or refractory disease. Occasionally, EGPA is 'unmasked' when oral steroids are withdrawn in patients being treated for asthma.

Anti-glomerular basement membrane disease (Goodpasture's syndrome)

Anti-glomerular basement membrane (anti-GBM) disease is characterized by the triad of pulmonary haemorrhage, glomerulonephritis, and the presence of circulating antibodies directed against an antigen intrinsic to the basement membrane of both kidney and lung. Respiratory symptoms may precede the onset of glomerulonephritis by weeks or months. The chest X-ray shows transient patchy shadows due to intrapulmonary haemorrhage, although haemoptysis can vary from negligible to life-threatening. The carbon monoxide gas transfer is increased due to the presence of haemoglobin in the alveoli. The extent of renal recovery depends on early detection and treatment. Treatment is with plasmapheresis to remove circulating antibodies and immunosuppression (prednisolone and cyclophosphamide) to prevent further antibody production.

Diffuse alveolar haemorrhage

Bleeding into the alveolar spaces is associated with certain drugs, infections and autoimmune rheumatic diseases, including vasculitis, but can also occur without an identifiable precipitating cause. Haemoptysis may be minimal (or even absent), despite significant blood loss into the lungs. It is one of the relatively few causes of raised carbon monoxide gas transfer (K_{CO}, see p. 943). Gas exchange is impaired due to the presence of blood in the alveoli and patients may present with severe respiratory failure requiring intensive care support. Treatment is directed at the underlying cause, if known.

Pulmonary manifestations of autoimmune rheumatic diseases

Rheumatoid disease

The lungs can be affected by rheumatoid arthritis (RA) and also by some of the drugs used in its treatment (**Fig. 28.41**; see also **Box 18.32**).

- **Pleural effusions** are often unilateral and tend to be chronic. Low glucose content is typical but not specific.
- **Pulmonary fibrosis** occurring in RA has similar clinical features to the idiopathic form of the disease but often follows a more chronic course (see p. 443). In patients taking methotrexate, it is often impossible to determine whether fibrosis is due to the drug or the underlying disease; either way, methotrexate should be substituted for an alternative agent.
- **Rheumatoid nodules** appearing on the chest X-ray may be single or multiple, ranging in size from a few millimetres to a few centimetres. The nodules frequently cavitate. They usually produce no symptoms but can give rise to a pneumothorax or pleural effusion.
- **Obliterative bronchiolitis** causing concentric narrowing of the bronchioles is a rare disorder characterized by progressive breathlessness and irreversible airflow limitation. Response to

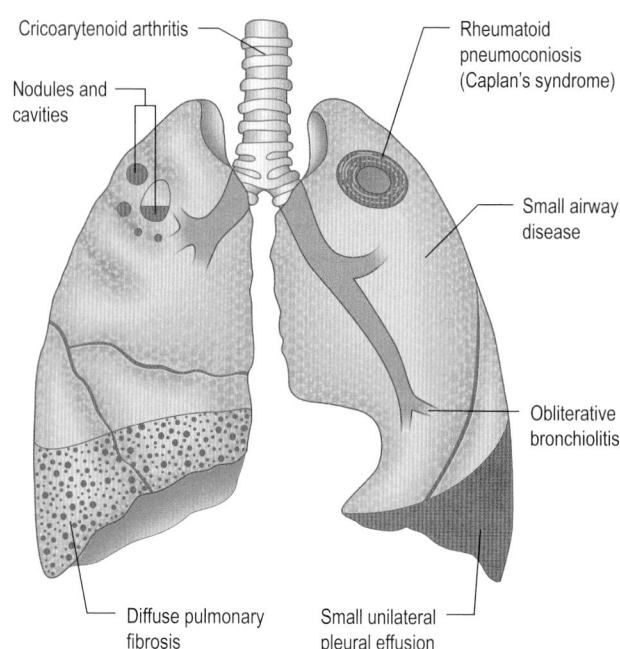

Cricoarytenoid arthritis

Nodules and cavities

Rheumatoid pneumoconiosis (Caplan's syndrome)

Small airway disease

Obliterative bronchiolitis

Diffuse pulmonary fibrosis

Small unilateral pleural effusion

Fig. 28.41 Respiratory manifestations of rheumatoid disease. Many drugs affect the lungs; see **Box 18.32**.

immunosuppressive therapy is generally poor but macrolide antibiotics may have a role.
- **Cricoarytenoid joint involvement** in RA gives rise to dyspnoea, stridor and hoarseness. Occasionally, severe obstruction necessitates tracheostomy.
- **Caplan's syndrome** is due to occupational dust inhalation in patients with RA; it occurs particularly in coal worker's pneumoconiosis but can by caused by exposure to other dusts, such as silica and asbestos. Typically, the chest X-ray shows rounded nodules 0.5–5.0 cm in diameter but progressive fibrosis can sometimes occur. These lesions may precede the development of arthritis. Rheumatoid factor is positive in the majority of patients.
- **Drugs** used in the treatment of RA can cause pulmonary problems, e.g. pneumonitis with methotrexate, gold and NSAIDs; fibrosis with methotrexate; bronchospasm with NSAIDs; infections with corticosteroids and methotrexate; and reactivation of TB with anti-TNF therapy.

Systemic lupus erythematosus

The most common respiratory manifestation is pleurisy, occurring in up to two-thirds of cases, with or without an effusion (see also p. 458), which is usually small and bilateral. Pneumonia also occurs, either because of infection or because of the disease process itself. In contrast to RA, diffuse pulmonary fibrosis is uncommon.

Systemic sclerosis

Some degree of lung involvement is present in the majority of cases of systemic sclerosis, and pulmonary complications are the leading cause of death (see p. 462). Interstitial fibrosis and pulmonary arterial hypertension are the most common pathologies. Serial lung function testing can aid early detection. Other complications include bronchiectasis and aspiration pneumonitis secondary to oesophageal dilation.

Pulmonary infiltration with eosinophilia

This is a group of allergic respiratory conditions, often directed against helminths or drugs; common types and characteristics are shown in **Box 28.65**. They range from simple pulmonary eosinophilia to the often fatal hypereosinophilic syndrome. **Simple pulmonary eosinophilia** is a relatively mild illness, with a slight fever and cough, and usually lasts for less than 2 weeks. If symptoms become more prolonged and there is an eosinophilia in the blood, it is then called **prolonged pulmonary eosinophilia**. In both conditions the chest X-ray shows either localized or diffuse opacities. The simple form is probably due to a transient allergic reaction in the alveoli. Many allergens have been implicated, including *Ascaris lumbricoides*, *Ancylostoma*, *Trichuris*, *Trichinella*, *Taenia* and *Strongyloides*. Drugs such as aspirin, penicillin, nitrofurantoin and sulphonamides have also been implicated. Often, however, no allergen is identified. The disease is self-limiting and no treatment is required, apart from withdrawing the identified cause. In the more chronic form, all unnecessary treatment should be withdrawn and corticosteroid therapy is indicated, with resolution of the disease over the ensuing weeks.

Asthmatic bronchopulmonary eosinophilia is characterized by the presence of asthma, transient fleeting shadows on the chest X-ray, and blood or sputum eosinophilia. By far the most common cause worldwide is allergy to *Aspergillus fumigatus* (see later), although *Candida albicans* and other mycoses may be the inciting allergen in a small number of patients. In many, no allergen can be identified. Whether these cases are intrinsic or driven by an unidentified extrinsic factor is uncertain. **Tropical pulmonary eosinophilia** is the term reserved for an allergic reaction to microfilaria from *Wuchereria bancrofti*.

Hypereosinophilic syndrome is characterized by eosinophilic infiltration in various organs, sometimes associated with an eosinophilic arteritis. The heart muscle is particularly involved, but pulmonary involvement in the form of a pleural effusion or interstitial lung disease occurs in about 40% of cases.

Diseases caused by *Aspergillus fumigatus*

The various types of lung disease caused by *A. fumigatus* are illustrated in **Fig. 28.42**.

The spores (diameter 5 mm) are readily inhaled and are present in the atmosphere throughout the year. *Aspergillus* can be grown from sputum in up to 15% of patients with chronic lung disease, in whom it does not produce active fungal disease. They are a cause of extrinsic asthma in atopic individuals.

Allergic bronchopulmonary aspergillosis (asthmatic pulmonary eosinophilia)

This rare disease is caused by a hypersensitivity reaction when the bronchi are colonized by *Aspergillus*. It can complicate asthma and cystic fibrosis. Proximal bronchiectasis occurs.

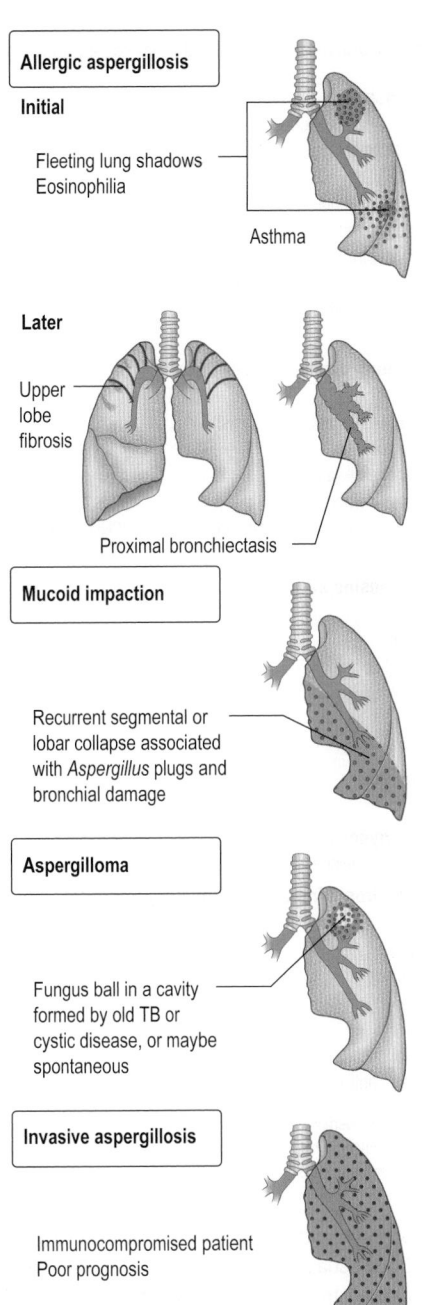

Fig. 28.42 Diseases caused by *Aspergillus fumigatus*.

Episodes of eosinophilic pneumonia present with a wheeze, cough, fever and malaise, associated with expectoration of firm sputum plugs containing the fungal mycelium. Occasionally, large mucus plugs obliterate the bronchial lumen, causing collapse of the lung. Left untreated, repeated episodes of eosinophilic pneumonia can result in progressive pulmonary fibrosis that usually affects the upper zones.

Box 28.65 Common types and characteristics of pulmonary infiltration with eosinophilia					
Disease	**Symptoms**	**Blood eosinophils (%)**	**Multisystem involvement**	**Duration**	**Outcome**
Simple pulmonary eosinophilia	Mild	10	None	<1 month	Good
Prolonged pulmonary eosinophilia	Mild/moderate	>20	None	>1 month	Good
Asthmatic bronchopulmonary eosinophilia	Moderate/severe	5–20	None	Years	Fair
Tropical pulmonary eosinophilia	Moderate/severe	>20	None	Years	Fair
Hypereosinophilic syndrome	Severe	>20	Always	Months/years	Poor

ⓘ Box 28.66 Some drug-induced respiratory reactions

Bronchospasm
- Penicillins, cephalosporins
- Sulphonamides
- Aspirin/NSAIDs
- Monoclonal antibodies, e.g. infliximab
- Iodine-containing contrast media
- β-Adrenoceptor-blocking drugs (e.g. propranolol)
- Non-depolarizing muscle relaxants
- Intravenous thiamine
- Adenosine

Interstitial lung disease and/or fibrosis
- Amiodarone
- Anakinra (IL-1 receptor antagonist)
- Nitrofurantoin
- Paraquat (weedkiller)
- Continuous oxygen
- Cytotoxic agents (many, particularly busulfan, CCNU, bleomycin, methotrexate)

Pulmonary eosinophilia
- Antibiotics:
  - Penicillin
  - Tetracycline
  - Sulphonamides, e.g. sulfasalazine
- NSAIDs
- Cytotoxic agents

Acute lung injury
- Paraquat

Pulmonary hypertension
- Fenfluramine, dexfenfluramine, phentermine

SLE-like syndrome including pulmonary infiltrates, effusions and fibrosis
- Hydralazine
- Procainamide
- Isoniazid
- Phenytoin
- ACE inhibitors
- Monoclonal antibodies

ACE, angiotensin-converting enzyme; CCNU, chloroethyl-cyclohexyl-nitrosourea (lomustine); IL-1, interleukin 1; NSAIDs, non-steroidal anti-inflammatory drugs; SLE, systemic lupus erythematosus.

The peripheral blood eosinophil count is usually raised and total levels of IgE are usually extremely high, at more than 1000 ng/mL (both that specific to *Aspergillus* and non-specific). Sputum may show eosinophils and mycelia. Treatment is with prednisolone 30 mg daily, which causes rapid clearing of the pulmonary infiltrates. Antifungal agents should be used in patients on high doses of steroids. The asthma component responds to inhaled corticosteroids, although these do not influence the occurrence of pulmonary infiltrates.

Aspergilloma and invasive aspergillosis

Aspergilloma is the growth of *A. fumigatus* within previously damaged lung tissue, where it forms a ball of mycelium within lung cavities. Typically, the chest X-ray shows a round lesion with an air 'halo' above it. The aspergilloma itself causes little trouble, though occasionally massive haemoptysis may occur, requiring resection of the area of damaged lung containing the aspergilloma. Treatment is with oral antifungal agents, although invasive aspergillosis is a well-recognized complication of immunosuppression and often requires intravenous antifungal therapy.

Drug- and radiation-induced respiratory reactions

Drugs affecting the respiratory system are shown in **Box 28.66**, together with the types of reaction they produce. Pulmonary infiltrates with fibrosis may result from a number of cytotoxic drugs used in the treatment of cancer. The most common cause of these reactions is bleomycin, in which case the pulmonary damage is dose-related. The most sensitive test is a decrease in carbon monoxide gas transfer, and therefore gas transfer should be measured repeatedly during treatment with the drug. The use of corticosteroids may help resolution.

Irradiation of the lung during radiotherapy can cause a radiation pneumonitis. Patients experience breathlessness and a dry cough. Radiation pneumonitis results in a restrictive lung defect. Corticosteroids should be given in the acute stage.

Further reading

Kousha M, Tadi R, Soubani AO. Pulmonary aspergillosis: a clinical review. *Eur Resp Rev* 2011; 20:156–174.
Muthiah MP, El Gamal A. Sarcoidosis. *BMJ Best Practice*; https://bestpractice.bmj.com/topics/en-gb/109.
Raghu G, Remy-Jardin M, Myers JL et al. Diagnosis of idiopathic pulmonary fibrosis. An official ATS/ERS/JRS/ALAT clinical practice guideline. *Am J Respir Crit Care Med* 2018; 198:e44–e68.
Travis WD, Costabel U, Hansell DM et al. An official American Thoracic Society/European Respiratory Society statement: update of the international multidisciplinary classification of the idiopathic interstitial pneumonias. *Am J Respir Crit Care Med* 2013; 188:733–748.

LUNG AND HEART–LUNG TRANSPLANTATION

Indications and donor selection

The main diseases treated by transplantation are:
- pulmonary fibrosis
- primary pulmonary hypertension
- cystic fibrosis
- bronchiectasis
- emphysema – particularly that caused by α_1-antitrypsin inhibitor deficiency
- Eisenmenger's syndrome.

Patients selected for transplantation are usually under 60 years and have a life expectancy of less than 18 months, with no underlying cancer and no serious systemic disease.

Organs are taken from donors under 40 years, with good cardiac and lung function, and chest measurements slightly smaller than those of the recipient. Matching for ABO blood group is essential but Rhesus blood group compatibility is not necessary. Since donor material is limited, single-lung transplantation is preferred to double-lung or heart–lung transplantation; this can be successfully undertaken in pulmonary fibrosis, pulmonary hypertension and emphysema. Bilateral lung transplantation is needed in infective conditions to prevent spillover of bacteria from the diseased lung to a single transplanted lung. Eisenmenger's syndrome requires heart–lung transplant.

Immunosuppression is with ciclosporin (the inhaled formulation has shown benefit) or tacrolimus, azathioprine or mycophenolate mofetil, and prednisolone.

Complications and their treatment

- **Early post-transplant pulmonary oedema** requires diuretics and ventilatory support.

- *Infections* are common, particularly within the first 3 months, and need prompt treatment:
  - bacterial pneumonia – antibiotics
  - cytomegalovirus infection – ganciclovir or valganciclovir (often given as prophylaxis in the early post-transplantation period)
  - herpes simplex virus – aciclovir
  - *Pneumocystis jirovecii* – co-trimoxazole (often given as prophylaxis).
- *Rejection*:
  - Early (first few weeks) – high-dose intravenous corticosteroids.
  - Late (after 3 months) – often produces the histological pattern of obliterative bronchiolitis. High-dose intravenous corticosteroids are sometimes effective in obliterative bronchiolitis.
- *Post-transplant lymphoproliferative disease* refers to a range of lymphomas seen in recipients of solid organ transplants; they may respond to rituximab, an anti-B-cell monoclonal antibody, or other forms of chemotherapy.

Prognosis

Several studies show a major improvement in overall quality of life after transplantation. One-year survival rates are around 80%, with a yearly mortality rate thereafter of about 10%. Death is due mainly to obliterative bronchiolitis. Overall survival varies with the original diagnosis but median survival is approximately 4 years.

OCCUPATIONAL LUNG DISEASE

Exposure to dusts, gases, vapours and fumes at work can cause several different types of lung disease:

- *acute bronchitis* and even *pulmonary oedema* from irritants such as sulphur dioxide, chlorine, ammonia or the oxides of nitrogen
- *pulmonary fibrosis* caused by mineral dust
- *occupational asthma* (see Box 28.18), now the most common industrial lung disease in the developed world
- *hypersensitivity pneumonitis* (see Box 28.64)
- *bronchial carcinoma* due to industrial agents (e.g. asbestos, polycyclic hydrocarbons, radon in mines).

The degree of fibrosis that follows inhalation of mineral dust varies. While iron (siderosis), barium (baritosis) and tin (stannosis) lead to dramatic, dense, nodular shadowing on the chest X-ray, their effect on lung function and symptoms is minimal. In contrast, exposure to silica or asbestos leads to extensive fibrosis and disability. Coal dust has an intermediate fibrogenic effect and used to account for 90% of all compensated industrial lung diseases in the UK.

Box 28.67 outlines how to take an occupational history in lung disease.

Coal-worker's pneumoconiosis

This disease is caused by coal dust particles approximately 2–5 μm in diameter that are retained in the small airways and alveoli of the lung. The incidence is related to total dust exposure, which is highest at the coal face, particularly if ventilation and dust suppression are poor. Improved ventilation and working conditions have reduced the risk of this disease.

Two very different syndromes result from the inhalation of coal.

Simple pneumoconiosis

This simply reflects the deposition of coal dust in the lung, which produces fine micronodular shadowing on the chest X-ray. It is

---

Box 28.67 Taking an occupational history

- Proceed chronologically. Most people cannot randomly remember, for example, what they might have been doing 20 years ago, or indeed, if asked in isolation, when they worked in a particular job. But if you start at the beginning of their life and work forward they find it much easier to remember (try it on yourself, starting with school examinations).
- Start by asking the patient how old they were when they left school, and what job or further education they went to; then ask them to continue through their life to the present day.
- Particularly for those who went on to further education, ask about holiday jobs (you might be surprised at their responses) and if they travelled overseas with their employment, especially if they were in the armed forces.
- Do not assume that all 80-year-olds are retired or that all young patients are in employment.

graded on the chest X-ray appearance according to standard categories set by the International Labour Office:

- *Category 1*: small round opacities definitely present but few in number
- *Category 2*: numerous small round opacities but normal lung markings still visible
- *Category 3*: very numerous small round opacities and normal lung markings partly or totally obscured.

There is considerable dispute about the effects of simple pneumoconiosis on respiratory function and symptoms. In many cases, symptoms may be due to COPD related to coexisting cigarette smoking but this is not always the case. Changes to UK workers' compensation legislation means that coal miners who develop COPD are compensated for their disability, regardless of their chest X-ray appearance.

Simple pneumoconiosis can progress to the development of progressive massive fibrosis (see next section). The latter virtually never occurs on a background of category 1 simple pneumoconiosis but does arise in about 7% of those with category 2 disease and in 30% of those with category 3 disease. Miners with category 1 pneumoconiosis are unlikely to receive compensation unless they also have evidence of COPD. Those with more extensive radiographic changes are compensated solely on the basis of their X-ray appearances.

Progressive massive fibrosis

In progressive massive fibrosis (PMF), patients develop round, fibrotic masses several centimetres in diameter, almost invariably situated in the upper lobes and sometimes having necrotic central cavities. Rheumatoid factor and antinuclear antibodies are both often present in the serum of patients with PMF, and also in those suffering from asbestosis or silicosis. Pathologically, there is apical destruction and disruption of the lung, resulting in emphysema and airway damage. Lung function tests show a mixed restrictive and obstructive ventilatory defect with loss of lung volume, irreversible airflow limitation and reduced gas transfer.

The patient with PMF suffers considerable effort dyspnoea, usually with a cough. The sputum may be black. The disease can progress (or even develop) after exposure to coal dust has ceased and may lead to respiratory failure.

Silicosis

Silicosis is caused by the inhalation of silica (silicon dioxide). While uncommon, it may still be encountered in stonemasons, sand-blasters, pottery and ceramic workers, and foundry workers involved in fettling (removing sand from metal castings made in sand-filled moulds). The dust is highly fibrogenic; a coal miner can remain healthy with 30 g of coal dust in the lungs but 3 g of silica is sufficient to kill. Silica seems particularly toxic to alveolar macrophages and readily initiates fibrogenesis. The chest X-ray appearances and clinical features of silicosis are similar to those of PMF but distinctive thin streaks of calcification may be seen around the hilar lymph nodes ('eggshell' calcification).

Diseases caused by asbestos

Asbestos is a mixture of silicates of iron, magnesium, nickel, cadmium and aluminium, and has the unique property of occurring naturally as a fibre. It is remarkably resistant to heat, acid and alkali, and has been widely used for roofing, insulation and fireproofing. Asbestos has been mined in southern Africa, Canada, Australia and Eastern Europe. Several different types of asbestos are recognized: about 90% of asbestos is chrysotile, 6% crocidolite and 4% amosite.

Chrysotile (white asbestos) is the softest asbestos fibre. Each fibre is often as long as 2 cm but only a few microns thick. It is less fibrogenic than crocidolite.

Crocidolite (blue asbestos) is particularly resistant to chemical destruction and exists in straight fibres up to 50 cm in length and 1–2 μm in width. Crocidolite is the type of asbestos most likely to produce asbestosis and mesothelioma.

Amosite (brown asbestos) was used in cement and pipe insulation and has sharp, needle-like fibres; exposure creates a higher risk of cancer in comparison with common chrysotile asbestos.

Exposure to asbestos occurred particularly in shipbuilding yards and in power stations, but it was used so widely that low levels of exposure were very common. There is a considerable time lag between exposure and development of disease, particularly mesothelioma (20–40 years). Regulations in the UK now prohibit the use of crocidolite and severely restrict the use of chrysotile. Careful dust control measures are enforced, which should eventually abolish the problem.

The risk of primary lung cancer (usually adenocarcinoma) is increased in people exposed to asbestos, even non-smokers. This risk is about 5–7-fold greater in those who have parenchymal asbestosis and about 1.5-fold in those with pleural plaques without parenchymal fibrosis. A synergistic relationship exists between asbestosis and cigarette smoking, the risk of bronchial carcinoma being about fivefold the risk attributable to smoking alone.

Diseases caused by asbestos are summarized in **Box 28.68**. Bilateral diffuse pleural thickening, asbestosis, mesothelioma (see p. 980) and asbestos-related carcinoma of the bronchus are all eligible for industrial injuries benefit in the UK.

Asbestosis

Asbestosis is defined as fibrosis of the lungs caused by asbestos dust, which may or may not be associated with fibrosis of the parietal or visceral layers of the pleura. It is a progressive disease characterized by breathlessness and accompanied by finger clubbing and bilateral basal end-inspiratory crackles. Minor degrees of fibrosis that are not seen on chest X-ray are often revealed on HRCT scan. No treatment is known to alter progress, though corticosteroids are often prescribed.

Byssinosis

This disease is caused by cotton dust; it occurs worldwide but is declining rapidly in areas where the number of people employed in cotton mills is falling. Typically, symptoms start on the first day back at work after a break (Monday sickness), with improvement as the week progresses. Tightness in the chest, cough and breathlessness occur within the first hour in dusty areas of the mill.

The exact nature of the disease and its aetiology remain disputed. Pure cotton does not cause the disease, and cotton dust has some effect on airflow limitation in all those exposed. Individuals with asthma are particularly badly affected by exposure to cotton dust. The most likely aetiology is constriction of the airways of the lung caused by endotoxins from bacteria present in raw cotton. There are no changes on the chest X-ray.

Box 28.68 Effects of asbestos on the lung

Effect	Exposure	Chest X-ray	Lung function	Symptoms	Outcome
Asbestos bodies	Light	Normal	Normal	None	Evidence of asbestos exposure only
Pleural plaques	Light	Pleural thickening (parietal pleura) and calcification (also in diaphragmatic pleura)	Mild restrictive ventilatory defect	Rare, occasional mild effort dyspnoea	No other sequelae
Effusion	First two decades following exposure	Effusion	Restrictive	Pleuritic pain, dyspnoea	Often recurrent
Bilateral diffuse pleural thickening	Light/moderate	Bilateral diffuse thickening (of both parietal and visceral pleura) >5 mm thick and extending over more than ¼ of chest wall	Restrictive ventilatory defect	Effort dyspnoea	May progress in absence of further exposure
Mesothelioma	Light (interval of 20–40 years from exposure to disease)	Pleural effusion, usually unilateral	Restrictive ventilatory defect	Pleuritic pain, increasing dyspnoea	Median survival 2 years
Asbestosis	Heavy (interval of 5–10 years from exposure to disease)	Diffuse bilateral streaky shadows, honeycomb lung	Severe restrictive ventilatory defect and reduced gas transfer	Progressive dyspnoea	Poor, progression in some cases after exposure
Asbestos-related carcinoma of the bronchus	The features of asbestosis, bilateral diffuse pleural thickening or bilateral pleural plaques plus those of bronchial carcinoma				Fatal

Berylliosis

Beryllium–copper alloy has a high tensile strength and is resistant to metal fatigue, high temperature and corrosion. It is used in the aerospace industry, atomic reactors and many electrical devices. When beryllium is inhaled, it can cause a systemic illness with a clinical picture similar to that of sarcoidosis. Clinically, there is progressive dyspnoea with pulmonary fibrosis. However, strict control of levels in the working atmosphere has made this disease a rarity.

Further reading

Cullinan P, Muñoz X, Suojalehto H et al. Occupational lung disease: from old and novel exposures to effective preventive strategies. *Lancet Respir Med* 2017; 5:445–455.
European Respiratory Society. *Occupational Lung Disease*; https://www.erswhitebook.org.

MISCELLANEOUS RESPIRATORY DISORDERS

Lung cysts

These can be congenital, bronchogenic or the result of a sequestrated pulmonary segment. Lung cysts therefore have a wide differential diagnosis, informed by the clinical presentation. Causes include:

- hydatid disease, which causes fluid-filled cysts
- lung abscesses (thin-walled cysts, found particularly in staphylococcal pneumonia)
- cavitating tuberculosis
- septic pulmonary infarction
- primary bronchogenic carcinoma or cavitating metastatic neoplasms
- paragonimiasis caused by the lung fluke *Paragonimus westermani*
- systemic conditions such as Birt–Hogg–Dubé syndrome.

Trauma

Trauma to the thoracic wall can cause penetrating wounds and lead to pneumothorax or haemothorax.

Rib fractures

Rib fractures are caused by trauma or coughing (particularly in the elderly), and can occur in patients with osteoporosis. Pathological rib fractures are due to metastatic spread (most often from carcinoma of the bronchus, breast, kidney, prostate or thyroid). Ribs can also become involved by a mesothelioma. Fractures may not be readily visible on a postero-anterior chest X-ray and so lateral X-rays and oblique views may be necessary.

Pain prevents adequate chest expansion and coughing, and this can lead to pneumonia.

Treatment is with adequate oral analgesia, or by local infiltration or an intercostal nerve block.

Two fractures in one rib can lead to a flail segment with paradoxical movement: that is, part of the chest wall moves inwards during inspiration. This can produce inefficient ventilation and may require intermittent positive-pressure ventilation, especially if several ribs are similarly affected.

Rupture of the trachea or a major bronchus

Rupture of the trachea or a major bronchus can occur during deceleration injuries, leading to pneumothorax, surgical emphysema, pneumomediastinum and haemoptysis. Surgical emphysema is caused by air leaking into the subcutaneous connective tissue; this can also arise after insertion of an intercostal drainage tube. A pneumomediastinum occurs when air leaks from the lung inside the parietal pleura and extends along the bronchial walls.

Rupture of the oesophagus

Rupture of the oesophagus (see p. 1170) leads to mediastinitis, usually with mixed bacterial infection. This is a serious complication of external injury, endoscopic procedures, bougienage or necrotic carcinoma, and requires broad-spectrum antibiotics.

Lung contusion

This causes widespread fluffy shadows on the chest X-ray owing to intrapulmonary haemorrhage. It may give rise to acute respiratory distress syndrome (see p. 232).

Kyphoscoliosis

Kyphoscoliosis may be congenital, due to disease of the vertebrae such as TB or osteomalacia, or due to neuromuscular disease such as Friedreich's ataxia or poliomyelitis. The respiratory effects of severe kyphoscoliosis are often more pronounced than might be expected and respiratory failure and death often occur in the fourth or fifth decade. The abnormality should be corrected at an early stage if possible. Positive airway pressure ventilation delivered through a tightly fitting nasal mask is the treatment of choice for respiratory failure (see p. 229).

Ankylosing spondylitis

Limitation of chest wall movement is often well compensated by diaphragmatic movement and so the respiratory effects of this disease are relatively mild (see also p. 448). It is occasionally associated with upper lobe fibrosis.

Pectus excavatum and pectus carinatum

Pectus excavatum causes few problems other than embarrassment about the deep vertical furrow in the chest, which can be corrected surgically. The heart is seen to lie well to the left on the chest X-ray. Pectus carinatum (pigeon chest) is often the result of rickets but is rarely seen in the West. No treatment is required.

Pleurisy

Pleurisy is pain arising from any disease of the pleura. The localized inflammation produces sharp localized pain, which is worse on deep inspiration, coughing and occasionally on twisting and bending movements. Common causes are pneumonia, pulmonary infarct and carcinoma. Rarer causes include rheumatoid arthritis and systemic lupus erythematosus.

Epidemic myalgia (Bornholm disease) is caused by infection with Coxsackie B virus. This illness is common in young adults in the late summer and autumn, and is characterized by an upper respiratory tract illness followed by pleuritic pain in the chest and upper abdomen with tender muscles. The chest X-ray remains normal and the illness clears within a week.

DISORDERS OF THE DIAPHRAGM

Diaphragmatic fatigue

The diaphragm can become fatigued if the force of contraction during inspiration exceeds 40% of the force it can develop in a maximal static effort. When this occurs acutely, in patients with exacerbations of COPD or cystic fibrosis, or in quadriplegics, positive-pressure ventilation is required. Further rehabilitation requires exercises to increase the strength and endurance of the diaphragm by breathing against resistance for 30 minutes a day.

Unilateral diaphragmatic paralysis

This is common and symptomless. The affected diaphragm is usually elevated and moves paradoxically on inspiration. It can be diagnosed by ultrasound when a sniff causes the paralysed diaphragm to rise and the unaffected diaphragm to descend. Causes include:

- surgery
- carcinoma of the bronchus with involvement of the phrenic nerve
- neurological disease, including poliomyelitis and herpes zoster
- trauma to the cervical spine, birth injury or subclavian vein puncture
- infection, such as TB, syphilis or pneumonia.

Bilateral diaphragmatic weakness or paralysis

This causes breathlessness in the supine position and may lead to sleep apnoea, with daytime headaches and somnolence. Tidal volume is decreased and respiratory rate increased. Vital capacity is substantially reduced when lying down and sniffing causes a paradoxical inward movement of the abdominal wall, best seen in the supine position. Causes include viral infections, multiple sclerosis, motor neurone disease, poliomyelitis, Guillain–Barré syndrome, quadriplegia after trauma, and rare muscle diseases. Treatment is either diaphragmatic pacing or night-time assisted ventilation.

Complete eventration of the diaphragm

This is a congenital condition (invariably left-sided) in which muscle is replaced by fibrous tissue. It presents as marked elevation of the left hemidiaphragm, sometimes associated with gastrointestinal symptoms. Partial eventration, usually on the right, causes a hump (often anteriorly) on the diaphragmatic shadow on X-ray.

Diaphragmatic hernias

These are most commonly through the oesophageal hiatus but occasionally occur anteriorly, through the foramen of Morgagni, posterolaterally through the foramen of Bochdalek, or at any site following traumatic tears.

Hiccups

Hiccups are due to involuntary diaphragmatic contractions with closure of the glottis and are extremely common. Occasionally, patients present with persistent hiccups. This can be as a result of diaphragmatic irritation (e.g. subphrenic abscess) or may have a metabolic cause (e.g. uraemia). Treatment for persistent hiccups is with gabapentin 300 mg or pregabalin 50 mg three times daily. The underlying cause should be treated, if known.

Further reading

McCool ED, Tzelepis GE. Dysfunction of the diaphragm. *N Engl J Med* 2012; 366:932–942.

MEDIASTINAL LESIONS

The mediastinum is defined as the region between the pleural sacs. It is additionally divided as shown in **Fig. 28.43**. Tumours

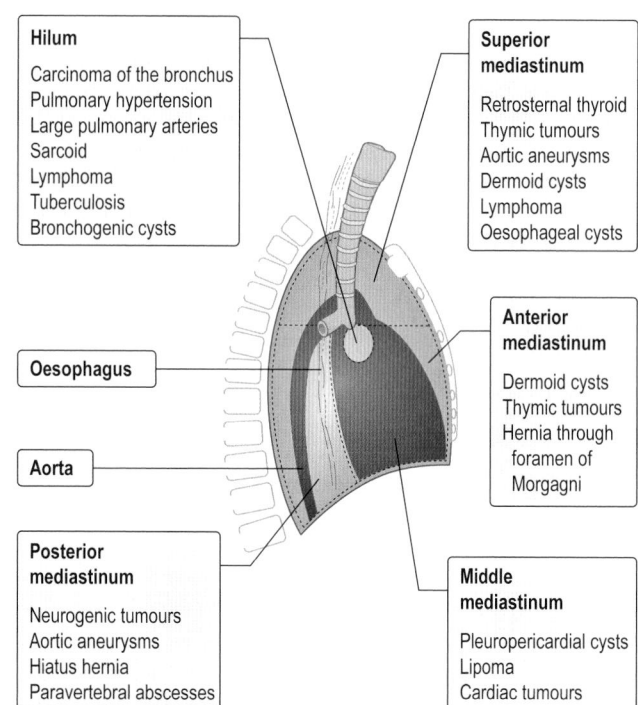

Hilum
Carcinoma of the bronchus
Pulmonary hypertension
Large pulmonary arteries
Sarcoid
Lymphoma
Tuberculosis
Bronchogenic cysts

Oesophagus

Aorta

Posterior mediastinum
Neurogenic tumours
Aortic aneurysms
Hiatus hernia
Paravertebral abscesses

Superior mediastinum
Retrosternal thyroid
Thymic tumours
Aortic aneurysms
Dermoid cysts
Lymphoma
Oesophageal cysts

Anterior mediastinum
Dermoid cysts
Thymic tumours
Hernia through foramen of Morgagni

Middle mediastinum
Pleuropericardial cysts
Lipoma
Cardiac tumours

Fig. 28.43 Subdivisions of the mediastinum and mass lesions.

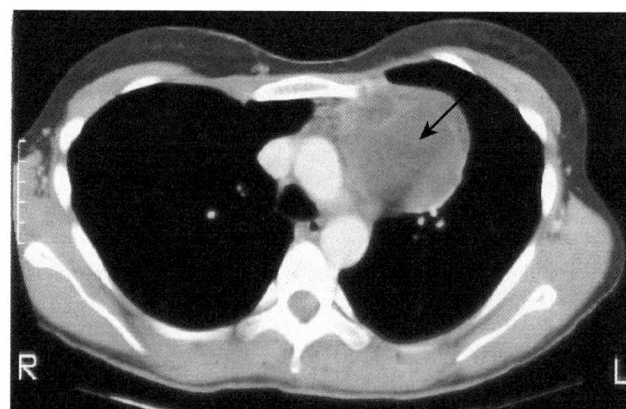

Fig. 28.44 CT scan of a dermoid cyst (arrowed) in the mediastinum.

affecting the mediastinum are rare. Masses are detected very accurately on CT, as well as on MRI scan (**Fig. 28.44**), and can be localized to the anterior, middle or posterior mediastinum. The position and characteristics of the lesion will help to determine the underlying aetiology.

Anterior mediastinum

Retrosternal or intrathoracic thyroid

The most common mediastinal mass is a retrosternal or intrathoracic thyroid, which is nearly always an extension of the thyroid present in the neck. Enlargement of the thyroid by a colloid goitre or malignant disease, or, rarely, in thyrotoxicosis, can cause displacement of the trachea and oesophagus to the opposite side. Symptoms of compression develop insidiously before producing the cardinal feature of dyspnoea. Flow–volume loops are useful to assess the physiological impact. Very occasionally, an intrathoracic

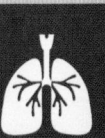

thyroid may cause dysphagia or hoarseness and vocal cord paralysis due to stretching of the recurrent laryngeal nerve. The treatment is surgical removal.

Thymic tumours (thymomas)

The thymus is large in childhood and occupies the superior and anterior mediastinum. It involutes with age but may be enlarged by cysts, which are rarely symptomatic, or by tumours, which may cause myasthenia gravis or compress the trachea or, rarely, the oesophagus. Surgery is the treatment of choice. Approximately half of the patients presenting with a thymic tumour have myasthenia gravis. Good's syndrome, a combined defect of humoral and cellular immunity, is seen in 10% of thymomas.

Middle mediastinum

- **Bronchogenic cyst** is a benign growth that is an embryological remnant.
- **Mediastinal lymphadenopathy** may be due to a number of conditions, including metastatic lesions, primary lung cancer, sarcoid, and infection such as tuberculosis. Lymphoma commonly presents with enlargement of the middle mediastinal nodes, and may represent both Hodgkin or non-Hodgkin disease (see pp. 399 and 401).
- **Pericardial cysts**, which may be up to 10 cm in diameter, are filled with clear fluid. Some 70% of them are situated anter-iorly in the cardiophrenic angle on the right side. Infection is rare and malignant change does not occur. The diagnosis may be made on MRI but needle aspiration may be required if there is any diagnostic uncertainty. No treatment is required but patients should be followed up, as an increase in cyst size suggests an alternative pathology and surgical excision is then advisable.
- **Vascular abnormalities** include aortic aneurysm and aortic dissection.
- **Tracheal tumours** were discussed earlier.

Posterior mediastinum

- **Embryological remnants** include neurogenic and neuroenteric cysts.
- **Oesophageal abnormalities**, e.g. oesophageal tumours and hiatus hernias, are seen here.

Significant websites

http://www.asthma.org.uk *Asthma UK.*
http://www.brit-thoracic.org.uk *British Thoracic Society.*
http://www.nhs.uk/live-well/quit-smoking *Good site for those wanting to stop smoking or to help patients to stop.*
http://www.thoracic.org *American Thoracic Society.*

Venous thromboembolic disease

Peter MacCallum and K. John Pasi

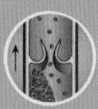

CORE SKILLS AND KNOWLEDGE

Venous thromboembolism (VTE) is common, affecting more than 5% of people during their lifetime. The risk increases with age. VTE presents as an acute episode of deep vein thrombosis (DVT) and/or pulmonary embolism (PE), and is frequently recurrent.

Patients with a suspected episode of VTE may present to their GP or directly to the hospital emergency department, or VTE may occur while care is being given to inpatients for other medical problems. Many clinical teams may therefore be involved in the initial diagnosis and management, but most commonly it is acute physicians who play a leading role. Haematologists often provide advice on acute management and frequently oversee long-term treatment, while some chest physicians have a particular interest in the management and long-term complications of PE.

Key learning objectives for VTE at undergraduate level include:

- being familiar with the main risk factors for VTE and recognizing its presenting clinical features
- knowing how to manage the acute stage following presentation with suspected VTE
- understanding the pharmacology of the different anticoagulants used to treat VTE, their use in clinical practice, and the management of anticoagulant-related bleeding.

Opportunities for learning about VTE include observing the work of a DVT diagnostic service (linked in many hospitals to the emergency department or acute medical unit), or attending an outpatient anticoagulant service, overseen in many hospitals by the haematology department.

INTRODUCTION

Pulmonary embolism (PE) is the third most common cause of cardiovascular death after acute myocardial infarction and stroke. As well as leading to PE, deep vein thrombosis (DVT) frequently results in the post-thrombotic syndrome, which is a major cause of long-term disability (see p. 1010). Venous thromboembolism (VTE, the term describing both conditions), is multicausal, often arising as a result of transient provoking factors, or in individuals with a heritable or acquired predisposition, but in up to 50% of people no cause can be established.

The clinician must be very familiar with VTE because:

- it is common, particularly in those admitted to hospital or those who have had surgery, suffered trauma or have other causes of reduced mobility
- it is life-threatening
- it is preventable: PE is the most common avoidable cause of death in patients admitted to hospital, and the single leading direct cause of death during pregnancy and the puerperium in the UK
- it can be difficult to diagnose: the clinical features and routine initial investigations, particularly for PE, are often non-specific, and this leads to diagnostic delays with potentially serious consequences
- its treatment can be hazardous: anticoagulant therapy, which may be long-term, is effective but carries the risk of major, even fatal, bleeding, and can be particularly challenging in patients with co-morbidities

- it is a significant cause of morbidity: long-term sequelae are frequent and significantly impair quality of life.

PATHOGENESIS OF THROMBOSIS

Thrombosis is the pathological process by which a localized solid mass of blood constituents (a blood clot or **thrombus**) forms within a blood vessel, mostly as a result of fibrin formation with a variable contribution from platelets and other cells. This differentiates it from physiological haemostasis, the process in which a fibrin-rich blood clot occurs outside the vessel-wall lining (or endothelium) as a result of injury. Thrombi form on, and are attached to, the vessel wall but fragments (**emboli**) may break off and occlude vessels downstream.

Arterial and venous thrombosis

Thrombosis can occur in both arteries and veins (for example, the usual cause of myocardial infarction is thrombosis within a coronary artery). The pathogenesis of thrombosis in these two sites is different, reflecting the different shear stresses in arteries and veins, and the contribution that rupture of atheromatous plaques makes to the initiation of arterial thrombosis. Arterial clots are described as white thrombi and venous clots as red thrombi, reflecting the contribution that platelets, as well as fibrin, make to the former, and fibrin and red cells to the latter. Thrombosis is thought to be the cause of about 25% of all deaths worldwide each year.

Factors influencing thrombosis

Thrombosis is considered to arise from the interplay between the three factors that make up Virchow's triad:

- changes in blood flow (stasis or turbulence)
- vessel wall dysfunction
- changes in blood components, leading to hypercoagulability.

The importance of the individual components of Virchow's triad varies between arterial and venous thrombosis:

- *Turbulence* and *vessel-wall dysfunction* caused by atheromatous plaques are factors in arterial thrombosis.
- *Stasis* and *hypercoagulability* are more relevant in the pathogenesis of venous thrombosis.

Further reading

Furie B, Furie BC. Mechanism of thrombus formation. *N Engl J Med* 2008; 359:938–949.

Wolberg AS, Rosendaal FR, Weitz JI et al. Venous thrombosis. *Nat Rev Dis Primers* 2015; 1:1–15.

DEFINITIONS

Most often, venous thrombosis originates in the deep veins of the leg: hence the term *deep vein thrombosis*. It is thought that the process starts within the pocket of one of the valves that line the veins, where flow may be turbulent and localized hypoxia may develop, resulting in endothelial dysfunction. The thrombus may remain localized to the leg veins or may embolize through the circulation to result in a *pulmonary embolus*. A minority (about 10%) of episodes of venous thrombosis arise in other sites, such as the upper limb, the cerebral venous sinuses and the splanchnic veins (hepatic, portal and mesenteric veins). Apart from upper limb venous thrombosis, these *unusual-site thromboses* are described further in relevant specialty-specific chapters.

If confined to the calf veins, the thrombus is called a *calf or distal DVT*. Untreated, the thrombus may extend proximally and, when it reaches the popliteal vein or above, is called a *proximal DVT*. Thrombi at this level are larger, and more likely to embolize and be transported with blood flow through the large veins of the pelvis and abdomen to the right atrium and ventricle. From there, they are pumped into the pulmonary arteries, which progressively divide into smaller arteries as they course through the lungs to supply the alveoli. The emboli stop in the pulmonary arteries, where they are no longer physically able to progress, and, in so doing, obstruct the flow of blood distally. It is thought to take at least several days for venous thrombi to become clinically evident.

EPIDEMIOLOGY AND RISK FACTORS

The annual incidence of VTE within the community is estimated at around 1 per 1000 per year overall and is age-dependent. VTE is uncommon in childhood, affects around 1 per 10000 young adults per year and 1 per 1000 middle-aged adults per year, and approaches an incidence of 1 in 100 elderly adults per year. Historical autopsy data suggest that about 10% of patients who died

> *i* **Box 29.1 Risk factors for venous thromboembolism**
>
> **Transient**
> - Surgery, especially major, lower limb/pelvis or cancer-related
> - Trauma, especially lower limb/pelvis
> - Active cancer
> - Acute medical admission
> - Immobilization (bed rest >3 days)
> - Plaster cast
> - Pregnancy/puerperium
> - Oestrogen administration (combined hormonal contraception, oral hormone therapy)
> - Recent long-haul travel (>4 h)
> - Central venous catheter
> - Heparin-induced thrombocytopenia
> - Superficial vein thrombosis
>
> **Persistent**
> - Increasing age
> - Body mass index >30 kg/m^2
> - Ethnicity
> - Previous episode of venous thromboembolism
> - Inflammatory conditions, e.g. inflammatory bowel disease, systemic lupus erythematosus, Behçet's syndrome
> - Nephrotic syndrome
> - Lower limb paresis, e.g. after stroke
> - Heritable thrombophilia (factor V Leiden, prothrombin gene mutation, deficiencies of antithrombin, protein C or protein S)
> - Antiphospholipid syndrome
> - Myeloproliferative neoplasms

in hospital did so from PE. Over 5% of people will develop one or more episodes of VTE during their lifetime. Clinically, about 60% of episodes of VTE present with DVT and the other 40% with PE, with or without accompanying features of DVT.

Risk factors for VTE are shown in **Box 29.1**. They can be divided into transient provoking factors (such as major surgery) and longer-term predisposing factors (such as obesity or heritable thrombophilias).

- *Stasis-related factors* include surgery, bed rest, plaster cast immobilization, pregnancy and long-haul travel.
- *Hypercoagulability* may be caused by cancer, surgery, pregnancy, and administration of oestrogens in combined hormonal contraception and hormone replacement, as well as the heritable thrombophilias.

Risk factors differ in the degree to which they increase the likelihood of VTE occurring:

- *Strong risk factors* increase the risk 10–50-fold and include major surgery, trauma and absolute bed rest.
- *Moderate risk factors* increase the risk 3–10-fold and include pregnancy, oestrogen therapy, and minor surgery under general anaesthesia. Most heritable thrombophilias also increase the risk 3–10-fold.
- *Weak risk factors* increase the risk up to 3-fold and include obesity and long-haul travel. For reasons that are not yet evident, the incidence of VTE is highest in people of African descent, intermediate in white people and lowest in Asians.

CLINICAL FEATURES

The typical features of *DVT* include pain and swelling in one leg. The leg may be red and warm to the touch. There may also be tenderness along the course of the deep veins and dilation of the superficial veins.

PE presents:

- In about 65% of cases, with pleuritic chest pain and breathlessness, sometimes accompanied by haemoptysis. Tachypnoea and tachycardia are typically present. Crackles and a pleural rub over a localized area of pulmonary infarction may be evident on auscultation.
- In another 25%, with isolated breathlessness, sometimes only evident on exertion.
- In the remaining 10%, with more severe features, including syncopal episodes, systolic hypotension or shock, and myocardial ischaemia with associated central chest pain. With this more severe presentation the patient is tachypnoeic, and has a tachycardia with peripheral shutdown, a raised jugular venous pulse (JVP) with a prominent α-wave, right ventricular heave, gallop rhythm and a widely split second heart sound. Cardiac arrest may occur, typically with pulseless electrical activity. The severity of presentation depends on both the thrombus burden and the individual's cardiopulmonary reserve.

At least one-third of patients presenting with DVT have clinically silent pulmonary emboli. About 70% of people presenting with symptomatic PE have an associated DVT that is symptomatic in about a quarter of cases.

DIAGNOSIS

Unfortunately, the differential diagnosis of suspected DVT or PE is very wide (**Box 29.2**), and most patients (>80%) who present with suspected VTE have the diagnosis excluded rather than confirmed. The clinical features are often non-specific and the majority of people who die from PE probably do so because earlier warning signs were missed rather than because of sudden collapse and death, or failure of treatment.

> ### ? Box 29.2 Differential diagnosis of venous thromboembolism
>
> **Deep vein thrombosis**
> - Ruptured Baker's cyst
> - Musculo-tendinous – trauma, haematoma, myositis, tendonitis
> - Superficial vein thrombosis
> - Post-thrombotic syndrome
> - Cellulitis
> - Osteoarthritis, osteomyelitis, synovitis, fracture, tumour
> - Acute arterial occlusion
> - Lymphoedema
> - Congestive cardiac failure and hypoalbuminaemia – usually cause bilateral leg swelling
>
> **Pulmonary embolism**
> - Chest infection/pneumonia
> - Exacerbation of chronic obstructive pulmonary disease
> - Asthma
> - Pneumothorax
> - Congestive cardiac failure
> - Acute coronary syndrome
> - Costochondritis
> - Musculoskeletal pain or rib fracture
> - Aortic dissection
> - Pericardial tamponade
> - Lung cancer
> - Primary pulmonary hypertension
> - Anxiety/hyperventilation

The challenge in the diagnostic investigation of suspected DVT and PE is therefore to identify, rapidly and accurately, when urgent treatment is required, and to distinguish these patients from those who do not have the condition, in whom unnecessary investigation and treatment would be potentially harmful.

Initial investigations

The initial investigations that might be undertaken because of chest pain or breathlessness are often non-diagnostic in patients with PE:

- *ECG* (**Fig. 29.1**): A right ventricular strain pattern may be seen, with T wave inversion in the inferior (II, III, AVF) and right precordial (V_1–V_4) leads. The classical ECG is of an 'S1Q3T3' pattern, with a prominent S wave in lead I and a prominent Q wave and inverted T wave in lead III, but this is present in only a minority of patients. It is more common to see a sinus tachycardia.
- *Chest X-ray*: This may be normal but more often shows non-specific abnormalities, including atelectasis, parenchymal abnormalities, cardiomegaly, elevation of the hemidiaphragm or a pleural effusion.
- *Arterial blood gas analysis*: Blood gases typically show hypoxia and hypocapnia, but again these are non-specific findings and are not always present.
- *Biomarkers of cardiac injury*: Plasma levels of brain natriuretic peptide (BNP) or its precursor, amino-terminal pro-BNP, may be elevated because of stretching of the right ventricle, and troponin may be increased because of right ventricular injury due to strain, but once again these findings are non-specific.

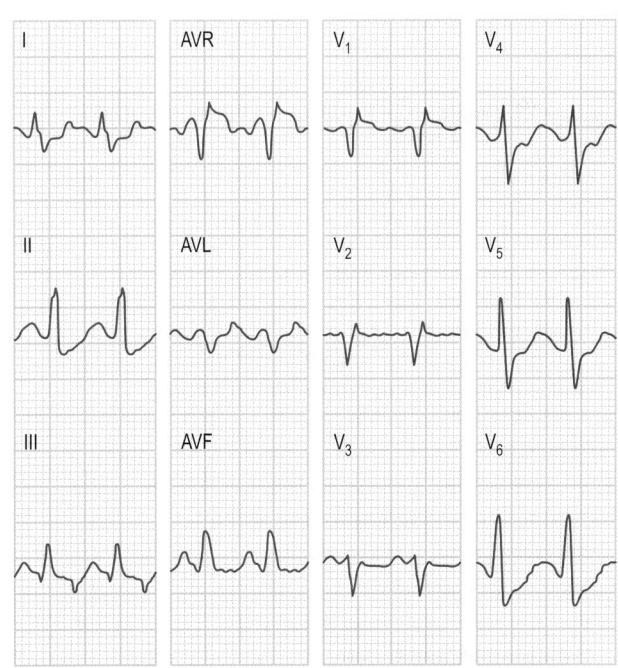

Fig. 29.1 Acute pulmonary embolism shown on a 12-lead ECG. There is an S wave in lead I, a Q wave in lead III and an inverted T wave in lead III (the S1, Q3, T3 pattern). There is sinus tachycardia (160 beats/min) and an incomplete right bundle branch block pattern (an R wave in AVR and V_1 and an S wave in V_6).

Diagnosis of DVT and PE

For patients in the UK, other than those with shock or hypotension due to suspected PE, the approach to the diagnosis of VTE recommended by the National Institute for Health and Care Excellence (NICE) is generally used.

Risk scoring

The diagnostic process starts with assessment of the clinical probability using a clinical prediction score that takes account of the individual patient's clinical features, the presence or absence of risk factors for VTE, and whether an alternative diagnosis is likely to explain the symptoms and signs. There are a number of clinical prediction scores available, and NICE recommends the modified two-level *Wells score* for DVT (**Box 29.3**) and the two-level **Wells score** for PE (**Box 29.4**); these categorize patients into groups that are likely or unlikely to have DVT or PE, respectively. Clinical prediction scores standardize clinical assessment and increase reproducibility among less experienced clinicians. However, in themselves, they do not confirm or exclude the diagnosis of VTE and further assessment is necessary.

Measurement of D-dimer

In those considered unlikely to have VTE based on the Wells score, the next step is D-dimer testing. D-dimer is a fibrin degradation product that can be measured quantitatively in plasma by highly sensitive laboratory tests, or qualitatively by point-of-care testing of whole blood. Raised levels indicate activation of the coagulation system but are not specific for VTE, as they are also seen, for example, with advanced age, infection, inflammation, postoperatively, in cancer and during pregnancy.

The value of D-dimer in VTE diagnosis is based on its high negative predictive value: that is, VTE is very unlikely in a patient who has a low pre-test probability of DVT or PE by the Wells score and in whom D-dimer, measured by a sensitive assay, falls below a predefined cut-off (typically quoted as 'normal'). Such patients do not need further diagnostic testing for VTE. With this approach it must be borne in mind that there is a small failure rate (<2% within 3 months) and that it does not absolutely exclude VTE.

In contrast, patients whose Wells score indicates that VTE is unlikely but whose D-dimer is raised (lies above the cut-off value) require formal radiological imaging to confirm or exclude VTE. Similarly, imaging is also required for all patients whose Wells score indicates that VTE is likely.

Imaging for DVT

The diagnosis of DVT is generally confirmed by ***ultrasonography*** of the deep venous system, which has long replaced the historical gold standard of venography, as it is quicker and non-invasive. At a minimum, ultrasonography involves examination of the proximal venous system. Typically, this includes compression of the popliteal and femoral veins by the ultrasound probe to determine whether the vein is compressible or not. This is usually supplemented by direct thrombus imaging with vein enlargement and assessment of blood flow by Doppler. Ultrasonography is very sensitive for proximal DVTs (>95%) but less so for distal DVTs (70%). In general terms, a positive scan will confirm the diagnosis. However, in those with a Wells score indicating that a DVT is likely, a negative scan, if limited to the proximal venous system, does not exclude the diagnosis, as it will not identify a proportion of patients who have a distal DVT. Further assessment of these patients is required (**Fig. 29.2**).

Alternatively, whole-leg ultrasonography can be performed. This avoids the need for repeat scanning but is more time-consuming and requires greater expertise.

The diagnosis of DVT in those with a prior event is often problematic because of the presence of residual vein occlusion, and expert radiological advice should be sought.

Imaging for PE

The approach to the diagnosis of PE is similar in principle (**Fig. 29.3**). When the Wells score indicates that a PE is unlikely, a negative D-dimer excludes the diagnosis without further investigation.

> *i* **Box 29.3 Wells score for deep vein thrombosis (DVT) (two-level)**

Clinical feature	Points
Active cancer (treatment on-going, within 6 months, or palliative)	1
Paralysis, paresis or recent plaster mobilization of the lower extremities	1
Recently bedridden for ≥3 days or major surgery within 12 weeks requiring general or regional anaesthesia	1
Localized tenderness along the distribution of the deep venous system	1
Entire leg swollen	1
Calf swelling at least 3 cm larger than asymptomatic side	1
Pitting oedema confined to the symptomatic leg	1
Collateral superficial veins (non-varicose)	1
Previously documented DVT	1
Alternative diagnosis at least as likely as DVT	−2
Clinical probability simplified score	
DVT *likely*	≥2
DVT *unlikely*	≤1

(From Wells PS, Anderson DR, Rodger M et al. Evaluation of D-dimer in the diagnosis of suspected deep-vein thrombosis. N Engl J Med 2003; 349:1227–1235.)

> *i* **Box 29.4 Wells score for pulmonary embolism (PE) (two-level)**

Clinical feature	Points
Clinical signs and symptoms of deep vein thrombosis (DVT) (minimum of leg swelling and pain with palpation of the deep veins)	3
Alternative diagnosis less likely than PE	3
Heart rate >100 beats/min	1.5
Immobilization (for >3 days) or surgery in the previous 4 weeks	1.5
Previous DVT/PE	1.5
Haemoptysis	1
Malignancy (on treatment, treated in the last 6 months, or palliative)	1
Clinical probability simplified score	
PE *likely*	>4
PE *unlikely*	≤4

(From Wells PS, Anderson DR, Rodger M et al. Derivation of a simple clinical model to categorize patients probability of pulmonary embolism: increasing the models utility with the SimpliRED D-dimer. Thromb Haemost 2000; 83:416–420.)

However, imaging is essential in those who either have a raised D-dimer level or are categorized as likely to have a PE based on their Wells score.

The most common imaging technique is *computed tomographic pulmonary angiography (CTPA)* (**Fig. 29.5**), which is widely available and sensitive, and can provide an alternative diagnosis when PE is excluded. The alternative is *ventilation–perfusion* ($\dot{V}/\dot{Q}$) *isotope lung scanning*, (**Fig. 29.6**). This test is performed in two stages:

- *a perfusion phase*, in which technetium-labelled albumin aggregates are injected intravenously and blood flow to the lungs is assessed
- *a ventilation phase*, in which patients inhale radiolabelled xenon or technetium to assess air delivery to the lungs.

A diagnosis of PE is made if there are mismatched defects in the perfusion scan, indicating impaired blood flow to the lungs, but normal ventilation because air entry to the lungs is normal. A normal $\dot{V}/\dot{Q}$ scan excludes the diagnosis of PE. This technique has the advantage of a lower radiation dose and is preferred in those with renal impairment and allergies to intravenous contrast agents. The disadvantages are that it is less readily available and the results are often non-diagnostic because other lung pathology can cause matched or smaller mismatched defects.

Timescale of investigation

Diagnostic testing for VTE should be performed urgently and completed within 24 hours of initial presentation. When imaging is required, a first dose of anticoagulant should be given if it is anticipated that it will take more than 1 hour to investigate a suspected PE and 4 hours for a suspected DVT.

The approaches described apply only to patients presenting to primary care or emergency departments. Inpatients and pregnant women should be regarded as high-risk and require appropriate imaging if DVT or PE is suspected (see p. 1457).

Emergency presentations

In the minority of patients with suspected PE who present with hypotension, mortality is high and prompt diagnosis is essential. If an urgent CTPA is not possible, a bedside transthoracic echocardiogram may be diagnostic, showing acute pulmonary hypertension and right ventricular dysfunction (see **Fig. 29.4**).

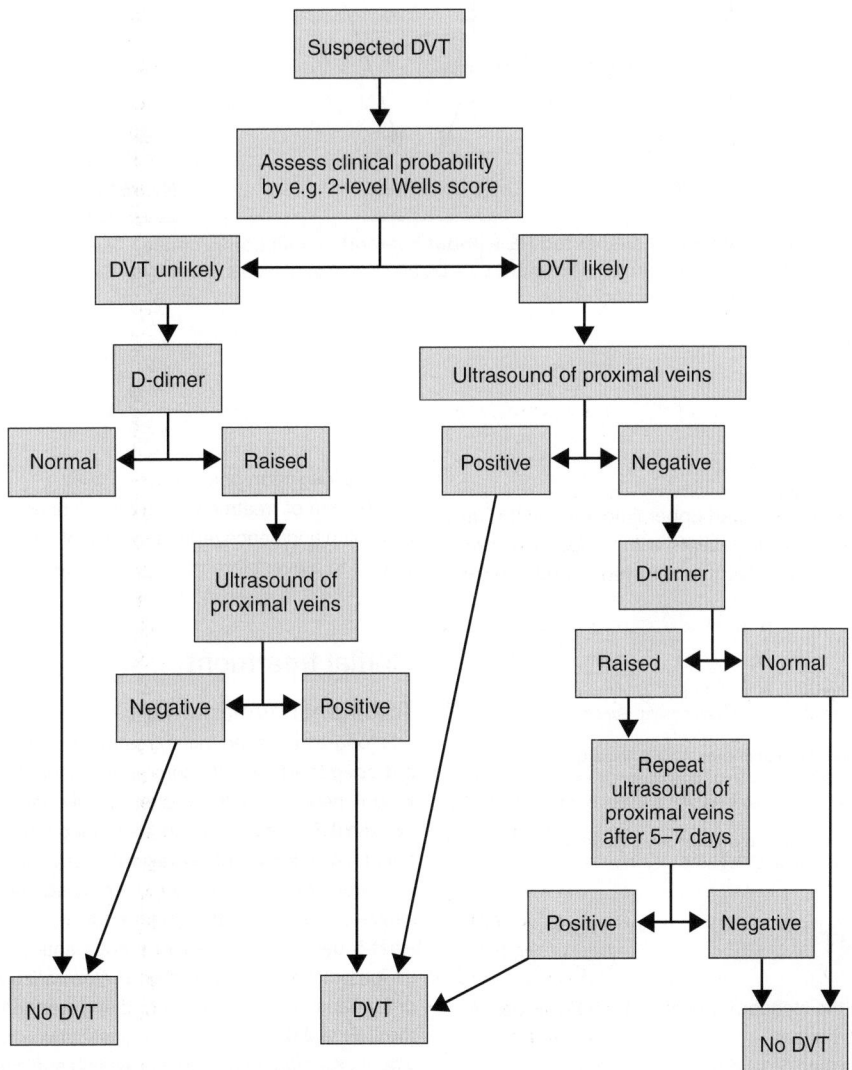

Fig. 29.2 Investigation of suspected DVT.

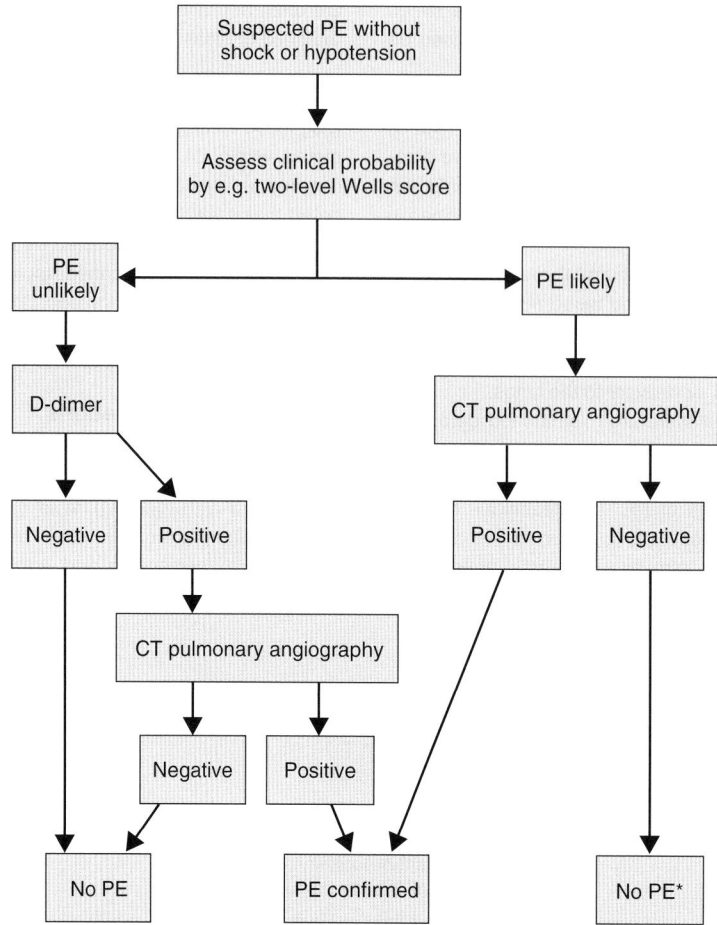

Fig. 29.3 Investigation of suspected PE without haemodynamic compromise. *In selected cases where clinical suspicion remains high it may be necessary to consider either bilateral lower limb ultrasonography or V/Q scan.

Upper limb DVT

The diagnostic algorithm for suspected upper limb venous thrombosis is less well established and patients with suggestive clinical features of arm pain and swelling typically require ultrasound imaging.

Further reading

Konstantinides S, Torbicki A, Agnelli G et al. 2014 ESC guidelines on the diagnosis and management of acute pulmonary embolism. *Eur Heart J* 2014; 33:3033–3080.
National Institute for Health and Care Excellence. *NICE Clinical Guideline 144: Venous Thromboembolic Diseases: Venous Thromboembolic Diseases: Diagnosis, Management and the Thrombophilia Testing*. NICE 2012; nice.org.uk/guidance/cg144.
Swan D, Hitchen S, Klok FA et al. The problem of under-diagnosis and over-diagnosis of pulmonary embolism. *Thromb Res* 2019; 177:122–129.

MANAGEMENT

Anticoagulant therapy is the standard treatment for VTE. It is traditionally divided into three phases:

- the acute phase, lasting 5–10 days
- a maintenance phase, lasting a minimum of 3 months
- a long-term phase beyond this.

The aim of treatment in the initial phase is to prevent thrombus extension and hence reduce the risk of embolization; the goal thereafter is to prevent thrombus recurrence.

Initial treatment

Traditional management

The long-established initial treatment of VTE involves a **parenteral anticoagulant**, most commonly subcutaneous low-molecular-weight heparin (LMWH); alternatively, intravenous unfractionated heparin (UFH) or subcutaneous fondaparinux may be used. In addition, an **oral vitamin K antagonist**, such as warfarin, is given.

Parenteral anticoagulants are used initially, as they provide almost immediate anticoagulant activity, whereas warfarin needs at least 5 days to provide therapeutic anticoagulation, as judged by its impact on the **International Normalized Ratio** (INR). Heparin or fondaparinux can be stopped and warfarin continued alone once the INR is 2.0 or more on 2 consecutive days, indicating that the vitamin K antagonist is now providing sufficient anticoagulation.

Anticoagulant agents are described on pages 1014–1016.

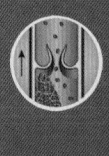

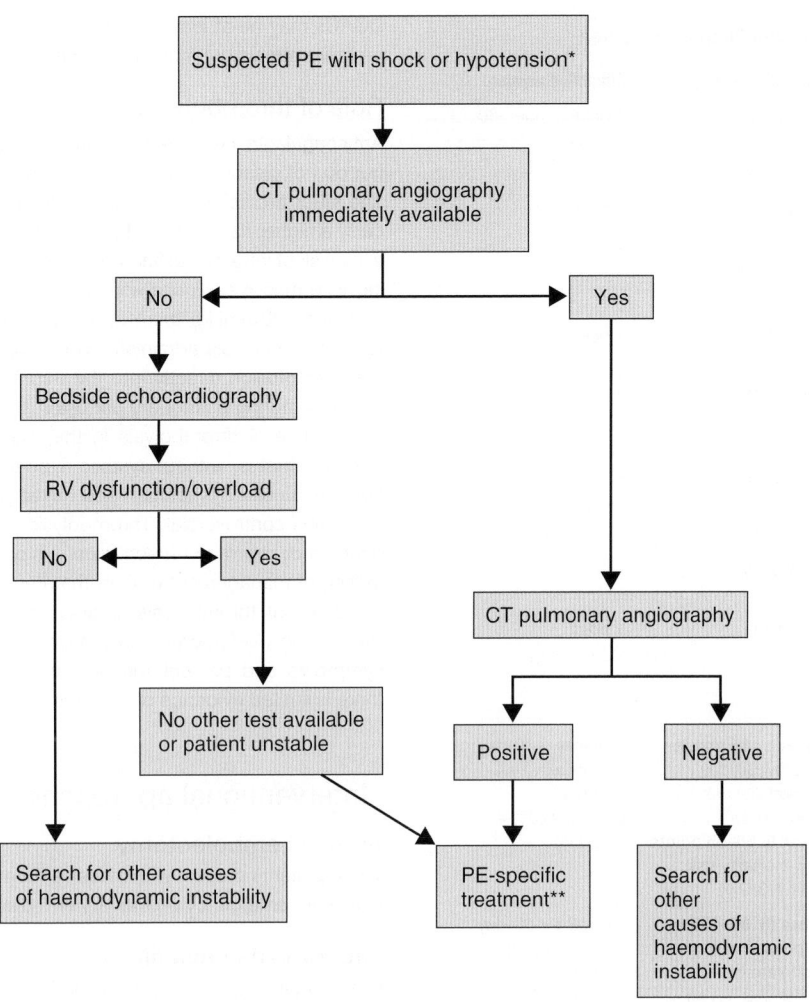

Fig. 29.4 **Investigation of patients with suspected PE and shock or hypotension (high-risk PE).** *Systolic blood pressure <90mmHg, or a systolic pressure drop >40mmHg for >15 minutes, if not caused by new-onset arrhythmia, hypovolaemia or sepsis. **Thrombolysis, surgical embolestomy or catheter-directed treatment. RV, right ventricle. *(From Konstantinides S, Torbicki A, Agnelli G et al. 2014 ESC Guidelines on the diagnosis and management of acute pulmonary embolism. Eur Heart J 2014; 33:3033-3080.)*

Direct oral anticoagulants

The introduction of the direct oral anticoagulants (DOACs) into clinical practice around 2010 has had a major impact on the management of VTE. Four DOACs are currently licensed for VTE treatment: three direct factor Xa inhibitors (apixaban, edoxaban and rivaroxaban) and one direct thrombin inhibitor (dabigatran). There are differences between them in the timing of their introduction, based on the large randomized clinical trials that led to approval for their use.

- *Edoxaban and dabigatran* are preceded by parenteral anticoagulation (such as LMWH) for 5 days prior to starting the DOAC alone: that is, there is a straight switch from LMWH to edoxaban or dabigatran on day 6 with no overlap.
- *Apixaban and rivaroxaban* do not require parenteral anticoagulation and the DOAC is used alone from the outset, albeit at a higher initial dose, for 7 and 21 days, respectively.

The different treatment models are shown in **Fig. 29.7** and the drugs are described further on pages 1014–1016.

Ambulatory care

Many patients with DVT can be managed on an outpatient basis, admission being reserved for those with a complex presentation or significant co-morbidities. Increasingly, too, low-risk PE can be managed on an outpatient basis or with early discharge after 24–48 hours. Low-risk patients can be identified using the **Pulmonary Embolism Severity Index (PESI)** or simplified PESI (**Box 29.5**); management as an outpatient or with early discharge might be considered for this group. Higher-risk patients need admission for close observation and administration of high-flow oxygen.

Special circumstances

A minority of patients warrant a different initial approach.

Pregnant women

Warfarin and the DOACs cross the placenta and should not be used in pregnancy, when LMWH is the treatment of choice. Warfarin causes embryopathy between the 6th and 12th weeks of pregnancy, with skeletal abnormalities including nasal hypoplasia and stippled epiphyses; later in pregnancy it causes bleeding in the fetus, with neurological abnormalities and a significant risk of intrauterine death. However, in women who become pregnant while taking warfarin, the drug is safe until the 6th week; it is therefore important to recognize pregnancy early and to switch by the 6th week to LMWH, which does not cross the placenta and is safe for

Box 29.5 Original and simplified PESI scores

Parameter	Original version	Simplified version
Age	Age in years	1 point (if age >80 years)
Male sex	+10 points	–
Cancer	+30 points	1 point
Chronic heart failure	+10 points	1 point
Chronic pulmonary disease	+10 points	
Pulse rate ≥110 beats/min	+20 points	1 point
Systolic blood pressure <100 mmHg	+30 points	1 point
Respiratory rate >30 breaths/min	+20 points	–
Temperature <36°C	+20 points	–
Altered mental status	+60 points	–
Arterial oxyhaemoglobin saturation <90%	+20 points	1 point

Risk strata[a]

	Class I: ≤65 points Very low 30-day mortality risk (0–1.6%)	**0 points** = 30-day mortality risk 1.0% (95% CI 0.0%–2.1%)
	Class II: 66–85 points Low mortality risk (1.7–3.5%)	
	Class III: 86–105 points Moderate mortality risk (3.2–7.1%)	**≥1 point** = 30-day mortality risk 10.9% (95% CI 8.5%–30.2%)
	Class IV: 106–125 points High mortality risk (4.0–11.4%)	
	Class V: >125 points Very high mortality risk (10.0–24.5%)	

[a]Based on the sum of points.
CI, confidence interval; PESI, Pulmonary Embolism Severity Index.
(From Konstantinides S, Torbicki A, Agnelli G et al. 2014 ESC Guidelines on the diagnosis and management of acute pulmonary embolism. Eur Heart J 2014; 33:3033–3080.)

the fetus. The consequence of exposure of the fetus to the DOACs is uncertain at this time. See page 1456 for further details of anticoagulation in pregnancy.

Breast-feeding mothers

Both warfarin and LMWH are safe for breast-feeding women but this has not been established for the DOACs, which should therefore be avoided (see also p. 1457).

Patients with cancer

Trials have shown that LMWH is more effective than warfarin in the treatment of VTE in patients with active cancer, who have a particularly high risk of recurrent thrombosis. Therefore, for many years LMWH has been the treatment of choice for cancer-associated thrombosis. Recent trial data suggest that, in the cancer setting,

DOACs may be at least as effective as LMWH in preventing recurrent thrombosis but may increase the risk of bleeding.

Role of thrombolysis

Anticoagulants help prevent thrombus extension and recurrence but do not dissolve blood clots, in contrast to thrombolytic agents. The latter are seldom used in the treatment of VTE because they carry a higher risk of major bleeding than anticoagulation, including a 2% risk of intracranial haemorrhage. However, in patients presenting with massive PE characterized by systolic hypotension (blood pressure ≤90 mmHg) there is a high risk of early death, and systemic thrombolysis administered intravenously, or occasionally by catheter infusion directly into the thrombus, may be life-saving by rapidly restoring pulmonary perfusion.

The role of thrombolysis in the management of intermediate-risk PE – that is, without systolic hypotension but with evidence of right ventricular dysfunction and raised pro-BNP or troponin levels – remains controversial. Thrombolysis – either systemic, catheter-directed or pharmaco-mechanical – is occasionally used in the rare setting of management of limb-threatening ilio-femoral vein thrombosis. Local thrombolysis is also sometimes used in non-limb-threatening ilio-femoral vein thrombosis in an attempt to reduce symptoms and prevent the post-thrombotic syndrome, although there is limited evidence of long-term benefit.

Interventional approaches

Surgical embolectomy

When patients present with massive PE and thrombolysis is contraindicated, emergency pulmonary embolectomy can be life-saving.

Inferior vena cava filters

Occasionally, patients with newly diagnosed VTE have a contraindication to anticoagulation – for example, active bleeding – or a major bleeding risk, such as the need for urgent surgery. In such settings an inferior vena cava (IVC) filter can be inserted by an interventional radiologist to prevent emboli from the deep veins in the leg reaching the lungs. Contraindications to anticoagulation are usually temporary, and anticoagulant treatment should be started as soon as it is safe to do so because filters do not entirely prevent pulmonary emboli and are independently associated with an increased risk of DVT. IVC filters do not reduce the risk of recurrent PE compared to anticoagulation alone. As IVC filters can give rise to complications that include migration and embolization, retrievable filters are preferred over permanent ones and they should be removed as soon as anticoagulation has been safely established.

Treatment duration

Anticoagulation needs to continue for a minimum of 3 months in all patients with proximal DVT or PE because earlier discontinuation is associated with a higher risk of recurrence. After 3 months, the decision as to whether to stop treatment or to continue anticoagulation long-term for secondary prevention should be made on an individual patient basis, taking account of the risks of recurrent thrombosis, bleeding and the person's own views.

Anticoagulants reduce the relative risk of recurrent thrombosis by 80–90% but carry a 1–3% absolute risk per year of major bleeding. Both recurrent thrombotic episodes and anticoagulant-associated

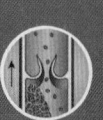

major bleeding carry a significant risk of morbidity and mortality. Therefore, the benefits of long-term anticoagulation potentially outweigh the risks of major bleeding in those at higher risk of recurrent thrombosis, whereas in others the risks of long-term treatment potentially outweigh the benefits.

Across all patients receiving anticoagulation for VTE, if anticoagulation is stopped after a minimum of 3 months, the risk of recurrent thrombosis is about 5% in the next year. It has been suggested that if the recurrence risk is greater than this, continuation of anticoagulation should be considered, whereas if the recurrence risk is less, anticoagulation should stop. As long as anticoagulation has been continued for at least 3 months, a longer duration of treatment does not appear to reduce the risk of recurrent thrombosis further on stopping anticoagulation.

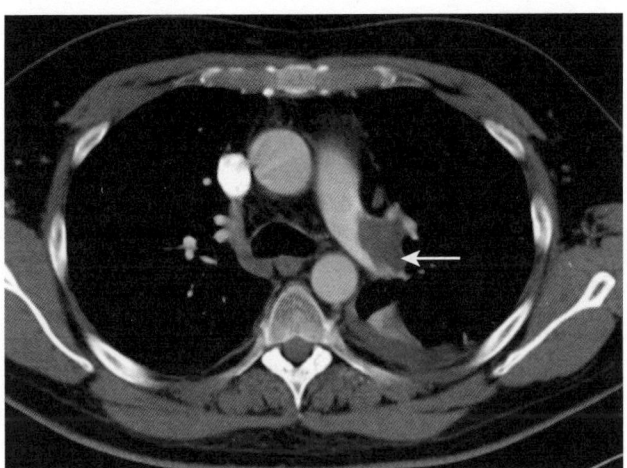

Fig. 29.5 **CT pulmonary angiography in pulmonary embolism.** The image is taken at the level of the main right and left pulmonary arteries, and shows a large thrombus (arrowed) in the left pulmonary artery.

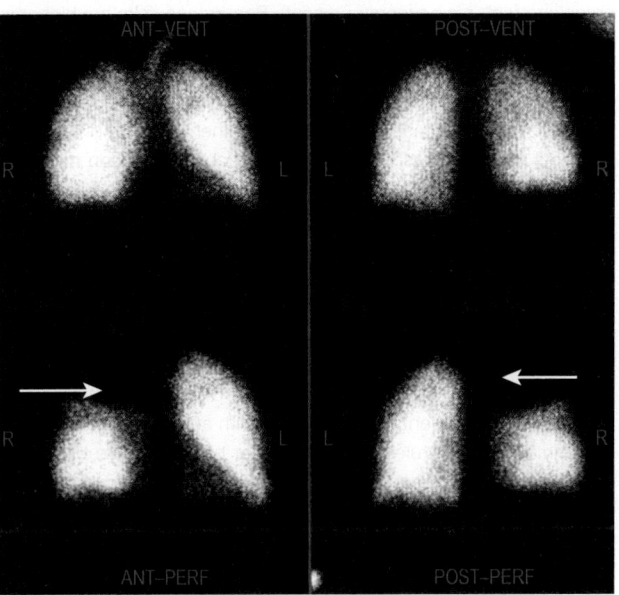

Fig. 29.6 **Radionuclide ventilation/perfusion scanning.** Ventilation (top) and perfusion (bottom) lung scans demonstrate an absence of perfusion in the right upper lobe: that is, probable pulmonary embolism (arrowed).

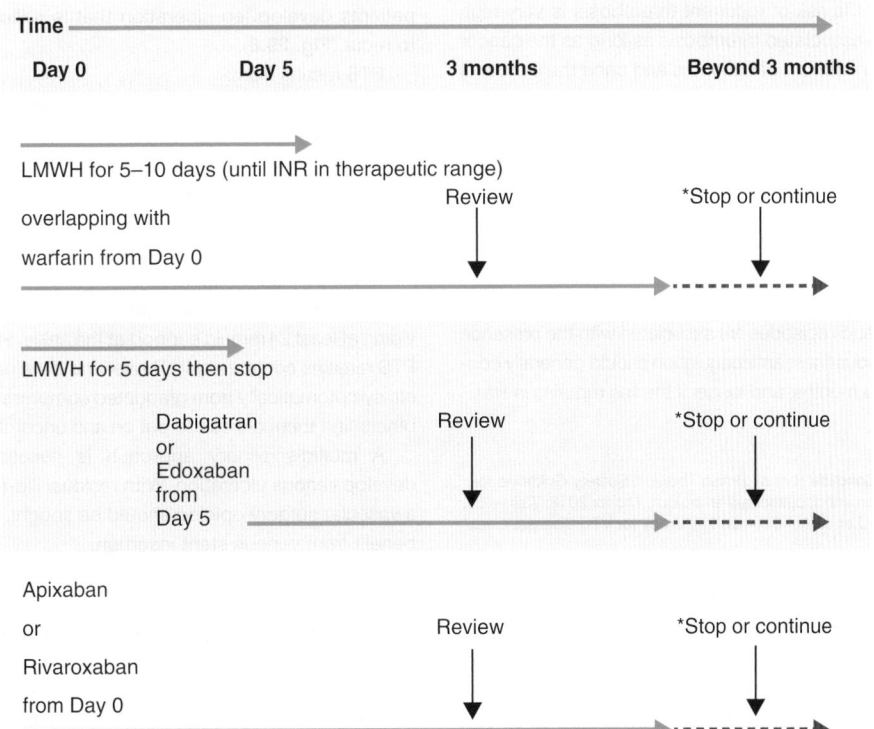

Fig. 29.7 **Models for anticoagulant management of newly diagnosed venous thromboembolism (VTE).** *The decision to stop or continue anticoagulation beyond 3 months is based on a balance of risks of VTE recurrence if anticoagulants are stopped, bleeding if anticoagulants continue and patient preference. INR, International Normalized Ratio; LMWH, low-molecular-weight heparin.

Risk of recurrence

Higher recurrence risks are seen in patients with unprovoked VTE episodes (about 10% at 1 year and 30% at 5 years) and in those with persisting risk factors. Lower recurrence risks are seen in those with transient provoking risk factors, and the stronger the transient provoking factor, the lower the recurrence risk (providing the transient provoking factor is no longer present). Recurrence risks are higher in males than in females, in those with second events, and in those with PE or proximal DVT as opposed to distal DVT. The risk of recurrent PE is higher in those whose initial presentation is with PE rather than with DVT. Since the case fatality of PE is higher than that of DVT, this suggests that the threshold for continuing anticoagulation might be lower in patients presenting with PE. Also relevant is the individual patient's cardiopulmonary reserve, since those with impaired reserve are less able to compensate for the acute circulatory effects of PE.

Accurate prediction of risk

A number of prediction rules have been devised to assist in the determination of risk of VTE recurrence in those with unprovoked VTE. These take into account a number of clinical features, and often the measurement of D-dimer 1 month after discontinuation of warfarin. Prediction rules for risk of major bleeding have been less well developed. Moreover, the VTE recurrence threshold for considering long-term anticoagulation may be different in patients on DOACs than those on warfarin.

Broadly, the approach in the UK for the treatment of unprovoked VTE is as outlined in NICE guidelines. These recommend consideration of long-term anticoagulation in those with unprovoked proximal DVT, and the offer of long-term anticoagulation to patients presenting with unprovoked PE.

Patients with persisting risk factors for recurrence should be considered for continuation of anticoagulation as long as the risk factor persists. For example, the risk of recurrent thrombosis is very high in patients with cancer-associated thrombosis as long as the cancer remains active. After a minimum of 6 months and once the cancer is in remission, anticoagulation can typically be discontinued.

In contrast, the risk of recurrence is lower following isolated calf vein thrombosis. In practice, most symptomatic distal DVTs are treated for 3 months and anticoagulation is then stopped. In those with a low risk of recurrence due, for example, to a transient provoking factor that has now resolved, it may be reasonable to reduce this duration to 6 weeks.

Treatment of upper limb DVT follows the same principles as for leg vein thrombosis. Many such episodes are associated with the presence of indwelling central venous lines; anticoagulation should generally continue for a minimum of 3 months, and longer if the line remains *in situ*.

Further reading

Howard LSGE, Barden S, Condliffe R et al. British Thoracic Society Guideline for the initial outpatient management of pulmonary embolism. *Thorax* 2018; 73:ii1–ii29.
Kearon C, Akl EA, Ornelas J et al. Antithrombotic therapy for VTE disease. *Chest* 2016; 149:315–352.
Konstantinides S, Torbicki A, Agnelli G et al. 2014 ESC Guidelines on the diagnosis and management of acute pulmonary embolism. *Eur Heart J* 2014; 33:3033–3080.
National Institute for Health and Care Excellence. *Clinical Guideline 144: Venous Thromboembolic Diseases: Diagnosis, Management and Thrombophilia Testing.* NICE 2012; nice.org.uk/guidance/cg144.

COMPLICATIONS

Mortality

Once VTE is diagnosed and treatment commenced, the short-term mortality rate is lower in patients presenting with DVT than with PE.

In those presenting with PE, the mortality rate by 1 month is around 5%, although at least half of these deaths are due to associated co-morbidities rather being directly caused by PE. Nevertheless, compared to those without VTE, mortality remains elevated in both the short and longer term, with observed mortality rates of 10–20% at 1 year; cancer is the leading cause of death.

Associated cancer

Cancer-associated thrombosis, the initial description of which is often attributed to Trousseau in the 19th century (Trousseau's syndrome), is common and 10–20% of all episodes of VTE are diagnosed in people with cancer. The pathogenesis is multifactorial and includes:
- hypercoagulability resulting directly from the cancer
- the added impact of surgery and/or chemotherapy
- reduced mobility
- use of indwelling central venous catheters that cause local catheter-associated thrombosis.

The combination of cancer and thrombosis carries a particularly poor prognosis. Up to 5% of patients who present with a seemingly unprovoked episode of VTE are diagnosed with cancer within 12 months.

Post-thrombotic syndrome

For many patients, quality of life after the diagnosis and initial treatment of VTE is adversely affected in the long term by development of the post-thrombotic syndrome (PTS). This occurs in about 40% of people following a proximal DVT. It causes symptoms of variable severity in the affected leg, including pain, swelling, heaviness, venous claudication on exercise, itching and discoloration. The symptoms may be persistent or intermittent, and reduce physical functioning and mobility. At its most severe, it leads to permanent skin damage with redness, hyperpigmentation, venous ectasia and skin fibrosis (lipodermatosclerosis), and 5–10% of patients develop leg ulceration that is difficult to treat and tends to recur (**Fig. 29.8**).

PTS results from:
- proximal venous occlusion with outflow obstruction
- damage to the venous valves that normally allow blood flow from superficial to deep and distal to proximal
- development of a collateral circulation
- venous hypertension
- capillary leakage
- localized inflammation.

The role of knee-length, graduated compression stockings, providing at least 24 mmHg support at the ankle, in the reduction of risk of PTS remains controversial. Those who develop PTS sometimes benefit symptomatically from graduated compression stockings, whereas others find them difficult to put on and uncomfortable to wear.

A multidisciplinary approach is necessary in patients who develop venous ulceration. With residual ilio-femoral vein occlusion, a vascular surgery opinion should be sought, as some patients may benefit from venous stent insertion.

Pulmonary hypertension

Following PE, up to 5% of patients remain persistently breathless due to chronic thromboembolic pulmonary hypertension (CTEPH). In this condition there is incomplete resolution of pulmonary emboli. The diagnosis should be suspected in those with persisting symptoms supported by follow-up perfusion lung scanning, CTPA showing evidence of residual occlusion, and echocardiography suggesting pulmonary hypertension. Assessment is undertaken by respiratory specialists and a proportion of patients can be successfully treated surgically with a pulmonary endarterectomy.

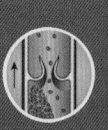

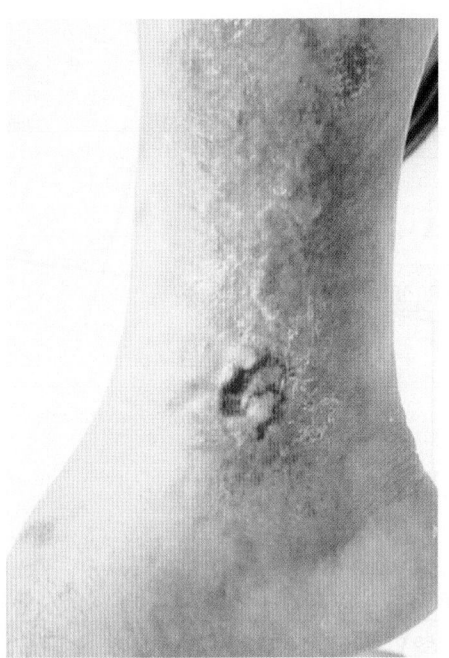

Fig. 29.8 Venous ulceration of the ankle. These ulcers, often with local venous-type staining of the local skin, are the result of poor venous drainage from the lower leg. Immobility, previous deep vein thrombosis and varicose veins may all contribute to their development. *(From Cross SS. Underwood's Pathology: A Clinical Approach, 7th edn, Elsevier Ltd, 2019, Fig. 13.17.)*

INVESTIGATION OF NEWLY DIAGNOSED VENOUS THROMBOSIS

General investigations

All patients with newly diagnosed unprovoked VTE should undergo a physical examination and have the following general tests:

- full blood count
- renal and liver function tests, including serum calcium
- clotting screen
- chest X-ray
- urinalysis.

Further assessment may be required, depending on the results of the initial assessment. In view of the frequency with which cancer is subsequently diagnosed in people with unprovoked VTE, the current recommendation from NICE is that, in patients aged over 40 years with unprovoked VTE, consideration should be given to further assessment, including a CT scan of the abdomen and pelvis and, in females, a mammogram. The benefit of this additional investigation is uncertain, however, as it has not been established that it improves survival.

Thrombophilia testing

Thrombophilia testing is often considered in patients with VTE but the indications remain controversial. In this context the term thrombophilia applies to a thrombotic tendency that can be identified in the laboratory. Thrombophilic tendencies can be either heritable or acquired.

Heritable thrombophilias

Heritable thrombophilias can be identified in about 20% of cases of VTE but do not play a significant role in arterial thrombosis. They can be divided into mutations that cause either gain of function of procoagulants or loss of function of anticoagulants.

Gain of function of procoagulants

Factor V Leiden results from a mutation in clotting factor V that causes activated clotting factor V (factor Va) to be resistant to inactivation by activated protein C, and thereby leads to an increase in thrombin generation. Heterozygous factor V Leiden is present in about 5% of individuals of European or Mediterranean origin but is not found in other ethnic groups such as those from eastern Asia. It increases the risk of VTE fivefold throughout life, and interacts synergistically with acquired risk factors such as combined hormonal contraceptives and pregnancy. Thus, the risk of thrombosis is increased about 30-fold in heterozygous V Leiden carriers on the combined oral contraceptive pill compared to non-carriers who are not on the combined oral contraceptive pill. However, because the absolute risk of VTE is low in young women, even a 30-fold increase in risk remains significantly below 0.5% per year for any single individual. Overall, factor V Leiden is present in about 20% of cases of VTE. Individuals who are homozygous for factor V Leiden are much less common but have a higher risk of thrombosis (about a 10-fold increase) than those who are heterozygous.

A *mutation in the 3' untranslated region of the prothrombin gene (G20210A)* causes levels of prothrombin to rise and increases the risk of VTE 2–3-fold throughout life. It is present in about 2% of Caucasians and in about 5% of people with VTE.

Loss of function of anticoagulants

The sites of action of the naturally occurring anticoagulants are shown in **Fig. 29.9**.

Antithrombin is a serine protease inhibitor (serpin) that functions as an anticoagulant by inhibiting predominantly thrombin and factor Xa reactions that are catalysed by heparin. Reduced antithrombin activity therefore leads to increased thrombin generation and activity, and thereby a predisposition to thrombosis. Heterozygous antithrombin deficiency is rare in the population but increases the risk of VTE about 10-fold. The disorder is identified by measurement of antithrombin activity rather than by genetic testing because multiple genetic mutations have been described. Some of these reduce synthesis of the antithrombin molecule, while others reduce the function of the synthesized protein due to conformational changes. Laboratory diagnosis is not straightforward because low antithrombin levels can also be acquired, for example, after acute illness, after surgery, with heparin therapy, in liver disease and in other disorders such as the nephrotic syndrome. Those with antithrombin deficiency often present at a young age and are more likely to have recurrent events. Because antithrombin is required for the action of heparin, those with antithrombin deficiency may be relatively resistant to heparin.

Protein C and protein S are vitamin K-dependent, naturally occurring anticoagulants. Together, they inhibit the activated forms of the clotting system co-factors, factor Va and factor; deficiency leads to an increase in thrombin generation and a predisposition to thrombosis. Heterozygous deficiencies of protein C and protein S are uncommon in the population and increase the risk of venous thrombosis at least fivefold. As with antithrombin deficiency, multiple genetic mutations have been described that affect either the synthesis or the function of the proteins. Diagnosis is therefore based on measurement of the activity or concentration of the proteins, and is often difficult because reduced levels can also be acquired due to, for example, acute illness, liver disease, warfarin or vitamin K deficiency, or, in the case of protein S, due to pregnancy

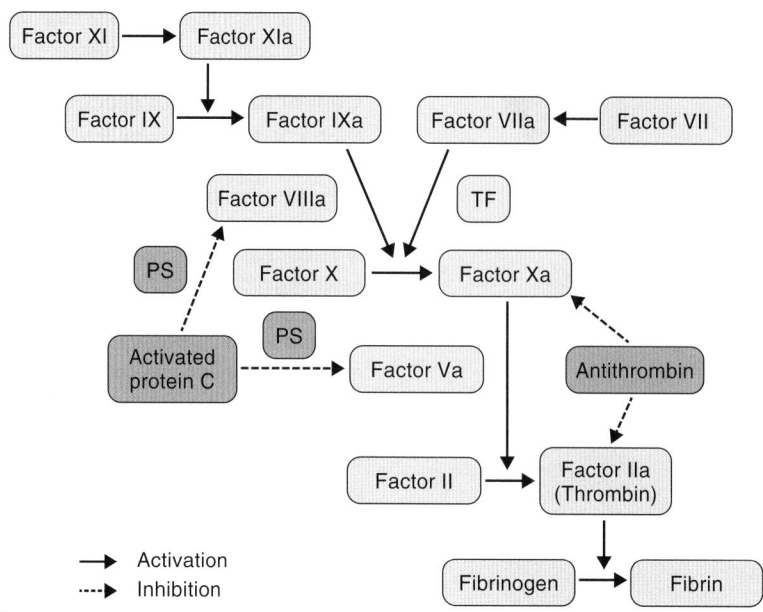

Fig. 29.9 Outline of the coagulation system, highlighting sites of action of the naturally occurring inhibitors of coagulation. Naturally-occurring anticoagulants are shown in blue. Activated protein C results from activation (not shown) of protein C by thrombin. PS, protein S; TF, tissue factor. *(From MacCallum P, Bowles L, Keeling D. Diagnosis and management of heritable thrombophilias. BMJ 2014; 349:g4387.)*

or oestrogen therapy. Very rarely, homozygous protein C or protein S deficiency may occur and present as neonatal purpura fulminans.

Management of heritable thrombophilias

In general, the more common heritable defects cause a milder clinical picture than those that are rare, such as antithrombin deficiency. The acute management of VTE is not affected by the presence or absence of heritable thrombophilia, and diagnosis of antithrombin, protein C and protein S deficiencies is problematic in the setting of acute VTE because levels of these proteins are often reduced either by the thrombosis itself or by the anticoagulants used in treatment. Moreover, for the most part, identification of a heritable thrombophilic defect does not influence the long-term management, since most defects do not influence the risk of recurrent VTE. Therefore, if a heritable thrombophilia is to be sought, it should preferably be once the acute stage is over and when the patient has completed a minimum of 3 months' anticoagulation, and their course of treatment either has finished or can be safely interrupted to allow measurement of naturally occurring anticoagulant levels. Testing for heritable thrombophilias might be considered in:

- those with unprovoked VTE who are planning to stop anticoagulation, particularly if they have a family history
- those who present with VTE under 50 years
- women of child-bearing age, for assistance with the management of future pregnancies
- those with unusual-site thromboses.

Acquired thrombophilia

Many risk factors for thrombosis cause an acquired hypercoagulable state, but in practice, from a laboratory angle, the main acquired thrombophilia is the antiphospholipid syndrome. Heparin-induced thrombocytopenia (HIT) is considered on page 1014.

Antiphospholipid syndrome

The antiphospholipid syndrome (APS) is an acquired prothrombotic disorder that has specific clinical and laboratory features. See page 459 for a full description, including diagnostic testing.

The diagnosis of APS should be considered in patients presenting with:

- **VTE at a young age** (<50 years), particularly if unprovoked or provoked by a minor risk factor.
- **Unusual-site venous thrombosis.**
- **Recurrent episodes of venous thrombosis**, particularly if anticoagulants are being given.
- **Arterial thrombosis** at a young age (<50 years) that is otherwise unexplained.
- **Pregnancy-related morbidity** – the loss of three or more embryos before the 10th week of gestation after exclusion of other causes such as chromosomal abnormalities, and/or one or more otherwise unexplained fetal deaths beyond the 10th week of gestation, and/or the premature birth of a morphologically normal neonate before the 34th week of gestation because of eclampsia, severe pre-eclampsia or placental insufficiency.
- **Incidentally detected abnormalities of clotting screens** performed for other reasons. The activated partial thromboplastin time (APTT) is typically prolonged; less often, the prothrombin time is. Although this would suggest a bleeding tendency, in practice it is a thrombotic tendency that is observed.

Recognition of APS in patients with VTE is associated with an increased risk of recurrent episodes. This may influence decisions on the duration of anticoagulation after an episode of VTE. There is emerging evidence that the DOACs may be less effective than warfarin in the prevention of recurrent thrombosis in APS.

Management of APS presenting with arterial thrombosis is controversial and there is ongoing debate as to whether the best approach is anticoagulation with warfarin, at either standard

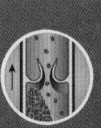

intensity (INR 2.0–3.0) or higher intensity (INR 3.0–4.0), and/or anti-platelet therapy.

Women with obstetric APS are generally managed throughout pregnancy with low-dose aspirin and a prophylactic dose of LMWH.

Further reading

Connors JM. Thrombophilia testing and venous thrombosis. *N Engl J Med* 2017; 377:1177–1187.

Schreiber K, Sciascia S, de Groot PG et al. Antiphospholipid syndrome. *Nat Rev Dis Primers* 2018; 4:17103.

PREVENTION

Between a third and a half of all episodes of VTE are provoked by surgery and/or admission to hospital, and mostly diagnosed in the three months after discharge. Studies in certain groups of patients, such as those undergoing major orthopaedic or cancer surgery, where routine postoperative screening for venous thrombosis has been undertaken, have reported incidences of asymptomatic DVT as high as 50%. As already stated, PE is the most common preventable cause of hospital-related death. Clinical trials have shown the benefit and cost-effectiveness of thromboprophylaxis in preventing symptomatic VTE in patients undergoing major surgery and in high-risk medical inpatients.

All adults admitted to hospital require formal assessment of their risks of VTE and of bleeding. The factors included in the UK Department of Health risk assessment tool are shown in **Box 29.6**.

Prophylactic measures can be considered as mechanical or pharmacological. Patients considered at risk of VTE who do not also have a bleeding risk are considered for pharmacological prophylaxis, with or without additional mechanical measures. Those who have a bleeding risk may be deemed unsuitable for pharmacological prophylaxis but may be considered for mechanical prophylaxis.

Mechanical prophylaxis

Measures include:

- early mobilization
- elevation of the legs
- use of anti-embolic stockings of knee or thigh length; these should not be used in peripheral arterial disease, stroke or situations where they could result in skin damage
- intermittent compression devices that can be applied to patients during surgery or on bed rest and aim to improve blood flow.

Pharmacological prophylaxis

This involves the prescription of anticoagulants in lower doses than those used in treatment. Most often, LMWH is used during hospital admission, and in some groups – for example, those undergoing major abdominal surgery for cancer – this is continued for a period following discharge. DOACs in low dose have been approved for VTE prevention following major hip and knee replacement surgery, and again these are continued for 2–5 weeks after surgery. Though traditionally not thought to be of benefit in VTE, aspirin has also been found to reduce the risk of venous thrombosis after major joint replacement surgery.

 Box 29.6 UK Department of Health risk assessment tool for venous thromboembolism (VTE) and bleeding

Patients at risk of VTE

- Medical patients expected to have ongoing reduced mobility relative to normal state
- Surgical patients

Thrombosis risk

Patient-related

- Active cancer or cancer treatment
- Age >60 years
- Dehydration
- Known thrombophilias
- Obesity (body mass index >30 kg/m²)
- One or more significant medical co-morbidities (e.g. heart disease; metabolic, endocrine or respiratory pathologies; acute infectious diseases; inflammatory conditions)
- Personal history or first-degree relative with a history of VTE
- Use of hormone replacement therapy
- Use of oestrogen-containing contraceptive therapy
- Varicose veins with phlebitis
- Pregnancy or <6 weeks postpartum

Admission-related

- Significantly reduced mobility for ≥3 days
- Hip or knee replacement
- Hip fracture
- Total anaesthetic + surgical time >90 min
- Surgery involving pelvis or lower limb with total anaesthetic + surgical time >60 min
- Acute surgical admission with inflammatory or intra-abdominal condition
- Critical care admission
- Surgery with significant reduction in mobility

Bleeding risk

Patient-related

- Active bleeding
- Acquired bleeding disorder (e.g. acute liver failure)
- Concurrent use of anticoagulants known to increase the risk of bleeding (e.g. warfarin with INR >2)
- Acute stroke
- Thrombocytopenia (platelets <75 × 10⁹/L)
- Uncontrolled systolic hypertension (≥230/120 mmHg)
- Untreated inherited bleeding disorders (e.g. haemophilia and von Willebrand's disease)

Admission-related

- Neurosurgery, spinal surgery or eye surgery
- Other procedure with high bleeding risk
- Lumbar puncture/epidural/spinal anaesthesia expected within the next 12 h
- Lumbar puncture/epidural/spinal anaesthesia within the previous 4 h

INR, International Normalized Ratio.

Further reading

National Institute for Health and Care Excellence. *NICE Guideline 89: Venous Thromboembolism in Over 16s: Reducing the Risk of Deep Vein Thrombosis or Pulmonary Embolism*. NICE 2018; https://www.nice.org.uk/guidance/ng89.

ANTICOAGULANT AGENTS

The physiological purpose of the coagulation system is to generate, rapidly and locally, the enzyme (or serine protease) ***thrombin***, which converts soluble circulating plasma fibrinogen into insoluble fibrin in response to vascular injury, and thereby helps secure ***haemostasis***.

This is achieved through a complex series of reactions on exposed cell surfaces and activated platelets, in which inactive circulating clotting factors become locally activated in a coordinated and sequential manner. Initiation follows the binding of circulating factor VII to tissue factor, a receptor expressed on subendothelial and adventitial cells, and leads to the generation of activated factor X (traditionally referred to as the **extrinsic system**, see p. 371). This, in turn, results in initial thrombin generation and subsequent amplification of the process through activation of the **intrinsic system**, leading to further activation of factor X and thrombin generation.

Venous thrombosis is characterized by the pathological formation of a localized fibrin-rich clot. Anticoagulants work by inhibiting the generation and/or activity of thrombin in different ways (**Figs 29.10** and **29.11**).

Parenteral anticoagulants

The main pharmacological properties of the parenteral anticoagulants used in the treatment and prevention of VTE are summarized in **Box 29.7**.

Heparin

Heparin is not a pure substance but a mixture of polysaccharides of different molecular weights of biological origin. In the UK, all heparins are derived from processed porcine gut mucosa. Heparins are destroyed in the stomach and must be administered parenterally. Heparin is an indirect anticoagulant because it does not work directly, but by binding through a specific pentasaccharide sequence to naturally occurring antithrombin in plasma, and inducing a conformational change that increases the inhibitory activity of antithrombin at least 1000-fold. The result is more rapid inhibition of several of the activated serine protease coagulation factors, particularly thrombin (factor IIa) and factor Xa. Heparins are classed as unfractionated heparin (UFH) or as low-molecular-weight heparin (LMWH).

Unfractionated (standard) heparin

For many years, UFH was the only form of heparin available for the treatment and prevention of VTE. In VTE treatment it is usually administered as an immediate-acting bolus injection, followed by an initially weight-based intravenous infusion. It is difficult to use in practice because it is necessary to monitor its effect on the APTT regularly and to adjust the rate of infusion to maintain the APTT ratio (APTT of patient sample compared to mid-point of the normal range) within a target range: typically, an APTT ratio of 1.5–2.5. UFH has a short half-life of 1 hour and, if necessary, can be rapidly reversed with a specific antidote, protamine sulphate. It is not excreted through the kidneys. It carries a small but significant risk of major bleeding, and of an uncommon but important immunologically mediated, prothrombotic adverse drug reaction, **heparin-induced thrombocytopenia** (HIT, see later). Its use nowadays in the treatment of VTE is largely restricted to particular high-risk settings where its short half-life, reversibility and lack of renal excretion are advantageous properties. UFH is rarely used for thromboprophylaxis because its short half-life means that it needs to be given two or three times daily by subcutaneous injection.

Low-molecular-weight heparin

LMWHs are the main type of heparin given nowadays because their favourable pharmacokinetic properties facilitate their use in clinical practice. LMWH is produced by the chemical or enzymatic degradation of unfractionated heparin, and results in polysaccharide chains of shorter length and molecular weight than UFH. Since long chains with at least 18 saccharides are required for inhibition of thrombin by antithrombin, whereas factor Xa is inhibited by shorter chains, the consequence is that, compared to UFH, the LMWHs inhibit factor Xa to a greater degree than thrombin. LMWH is administered by subcutaneous injection and peak activity is seen by 4 hours. The half-life of LMWH is longer than that of UFH at 4 hours. LMWH is excreted through the kidneys and caution is required in patients with renal impairment. Because of its better bioavailability than UFH, it has the major advantage of fixed, weight-based dosing, without the need for laboratory monitoring. As a result, the majority of patients with DVT and many with PE can be treated as outpatients without hospital admission. Further advantages of LMWH over UFH are that it is at least as safe and effective, and carries a lower risk of HIT. However, LMWH is only partially reversed by protamine sulphate.

In VTE treatment, standard practice for many years has been to give an initial subcutaneous injection of LMWH while awaiting confirmation of the radiological diagnosis of DVT or PE, and then continuing it with warfarin until the latter, with its slower onset of action, is providing sufficient anticoagulation for the LMWH to be stopped, a process that takes at least 5 days. During this time, LMWH is administered, often by the patients themselves, by subcutaneous injection once or twice daily. In certain groups, longer-term LMWH is preferred over oral anticoagulants:

- In pregnant women, LMWH is used throughout because it does not cross the placenta.
- In patients with cancer-associated thrombosis, LMWH is more effective than warfarin.

LMWH is also widely used as thromboprophylaxis in patients admitted to hospital or undergoing surgery, and has the advantages over UFH of once-daily administration and lower risk of HIT. LMWH (or an alternative anticoagulant) also may be used to reduce morbidity and mortality in acute coronary syndrome, where it is usually given twice daily.

Heparin-induced thrombocytopenia

An uncommon but important adverse effect of heparin administration in some patients is heparin-induced thrombocytopenia (HIT). Thrombocytopenia typically causes a bleeding tendency but that

---

Box 29.7 Pharmacological properties of parenteral anticoagulants

	Unfractionated (standard) heparin	Low-molecular-weight heparin	Fondaparinux
Source	Biological	Biological	Synthetic
Molecular weight (Da)	3000–30 000	2000–9000	1500
Target (via antithrombin)	Xa = IIa	Xa > IIa	Xa
Half-life	1 h	4 h	18 h
Monitoring test	APTT	Anti-factor Xa (not usually required)	Anti-factor Xa (not usually required)
Renal excretion	No	Yes	Yes
Antidote	Protamine sulphate	Protamine sulphate (partial reversal)	None

APTT, activated partial thromboplastin time; Da, Daltons

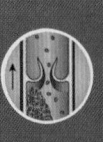

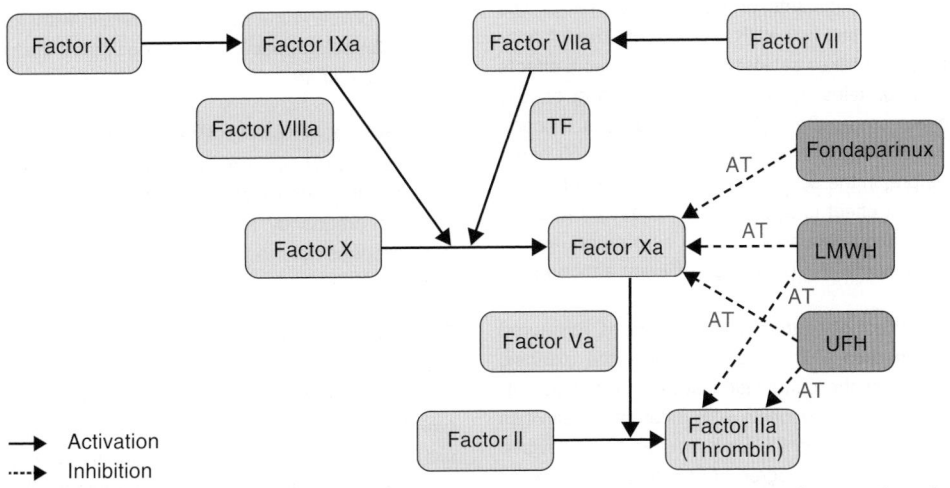

Fig. 29.10 **Sites of action of parenteral anticoagulants used in the treatment and prevention of venous thromboembolism.** AT, antithrombin; LMWH, low-molecular-weight heparin; TF, tissue factor; UFH, unfractionated heparin.

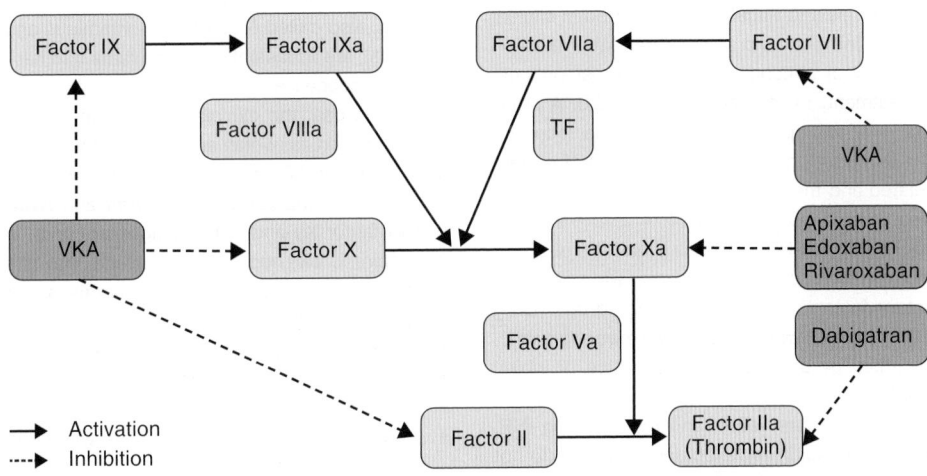

Fig. 29.11 **Sites of action of oral anticoagulants used in the treatment and secondary prevention of venous thromboembolism.** TF, tissue factor; VKA, vitamin K antagonist, e.g. warfarin.

seen in HIT is associated with a strong prothrombotic tendency due to activation of both platelets and the coagulation system. The disorder usually occurs 5–14 days after heparin exposure, with a greater than 30% fall in platelet count occurring over 1 or 2 days. The thrombocytopenia is usually mild to moderate and it is rare for the platelet count to fall below 20×10^9/L. HIT is immunologically mediated, with the development by the patient of immunoglobulin G (IgG) antibodies to a complex of heparin and platelet factor 4 (PF4) that is found in, and released from, platelet granules. Without prompt diagnosis and treatment, the risk of thrombosis, which can be either venous or arterial, is 50% over the next few days. The diagnosis is based on the clinical features, supplemented by laboratory confirmation of IgG antibodies to the heparin/PF4 complex.

If HIT is suspected and/or confirmed:
- Specialist advice should be sought.
- All heparin should be discontinued (including that used, for example, to flush indwelling lines).
- The allergic reaction should be noted on the drug chart.
- An alternative, non-heparin anticoagulant should be administered in view of the high rate of thrombosis.

The most common alternative anticoagulants used in this setting are ***danaparoid*** (a heparinoid), ***argatroban*** (an intravenously administered direct thrombin inhibitor) and ***fondaparinux***. Patients who develop HIT should not be re-exposed to heparin in future.

Fondaparinux

Unlike heparins, fondaparinux is a synthetic pentasaccharide. It binds to antithrombin, and because of its short chain length it inhibits only factor Xa and not thrombin. It is administered by subcutaneous injection and has a longer half-life than heparin at around 18 hours. It is renally excreted and cannot be used in those with significant renal impairment. Its effect is not reversed by protamine sulphate.

Oral anticoagulants

Vitamin K antagonists

These agents are indirect anticoagulants that inhibit the final stage of the synthesis of vitamin K-dependent proteins in the liver: namely, clotting factors II (prothrombin), VII, IX and X, and the naturally occurring anticoagulants, protein C and protein S. The main vitamin K antagonist used in the UK is *warfarin*. The full anti-coagulant effect of warfarin takes at least 5 days because it affects only synthesis of new proteins; those already circulating or fully formed in hepatocytes are unaffected and decline as a function of their half-lives, which vary from 6 hours (factor VII) to 60 hours (prothrombin). Therefore, in the setting of VTE treatment, where an immediate anticoagulant effect is desired, it is necessary to commence with a quick-acting anticoagulant such as heparin, and to continue the latter until warfarin is providing sufficient anticoagulation on its own.

The anticoagulant effect of vitamin K antagonists is measured using the *prothrombin time (PT)*, which measures the extrinsic and common pathways of the coagulation system. Because different laboratories use different reagents with different sensitivities and normal ranges to measure the PT, a system has been devised to standardize assessment of the degree of anticoagulation by the vitamin K antagonists. In this system the PT for each patient test (in comparison to the normal PT of the general population not on anti-coagulants) is converted to a standardized ratio, the *International Normalized Ratio (INR)*, and this enables comparison between results in different laboratories and target ranges defined in clinical trials to be adopted in routine clinical practice. The higher the INR is, the greater the intensity of anticoagulation. For most patients on warfarin for VTE treatment, the target INR is 2.0–3.0. A small proportion of patients – for example, those who have a recurrent VTE episode while the INR is in the target range – need to be more intensively anticoagulated and the new target range may be set at 3.0–4.0, reflecting greater prolongation of the PT.

Warfarin is metabolized in the liver and has a half-life of about 36 hours. It has a narrow therapeutic index and a wide range of interactions with dietary factors, alcohol and other drugs. Drug interactions can be either *pharmacokinetic* or *pharmacodynamic*. The former are represented by drugs that either induce or inhibit the metabolism of warfarin by the cytochrome P450 system, and thereby reduce or increase warfarin levels and the resulting INR. The latter are exemplified by aspirin and clopidogrel, which do not affect warfarin levels, but further increase the bleeding risk of warfarin through their antiplatelet effects. For reasons that are partly genetic, there is considerable variation between individuals in the dose of warfarin required for the same effect on the INR.

Monitoring warfarin therapy

The consequence of this is that, during the initial period of anticoagulation with warfarin and heparin, it is necessary to measure the INR frequently (almost daily) so that the dose of warfarin can be adjusted and heparin can be discontinued when the INR is in the target range for 2 consecutive days. Following this initial period, the frequency of INR monitoring can be reduced, but it remains necessary on a long-term basis at least every 8–12 weeks in patients whose INR control is stable, and more frequently in those with unstable INRs in order to allow appropriate dose adjustment: that is, a dose increase if the INR is below target and a dose reduction and/or omission if the INR is too high.

This process of INR monitoring is usually done either in hospital-based anticoagulant clinics or in general practice. A small number of motivated and trained patients self-test their INRs at home using point-of-care coagulometers. Patients starting warfarin must be fully counselled, and this should include information about the need to inform clinicians in advance of invasive procedures. This enables steps to be taken where necessary to interrupt warfarin several days beforehand (to allow for its long half-life), and consideration to be

given to covering the period off warfarin with, for example, LMWH, which can be stopped closer to the time of the procedure in view of its shorter half-life.

Pregnancy and breast-feeding

In general, warfarin should not be used in pregnancy because it crosses the placenta and is teratogenic between the 6th and 12th weeks of pregnancy, as well as causing fetal bleeding later in pregnancy. It does not cross into breast milk and therefore is safe during breast-feeding.

Risks of warfarin therapy

The main risk of warfarin is bleeding. Most bleeds are not major but can be a considerable nuisance for the patient. The risk of major bleeding is around 2% per year, and about 0.25% patients per year will have a fatal bleed, usually due to intracranial haemorrhage. Most bleeds occur when the INR is within the therapeutic range, but the higher the INR is, the greater the risk of a major bleed. Management of high INRs and of bleeding on warfarin is shown in **Box 29.8**.

Direct oral anticoagulants

DOACs, also called NOACs (non-vitamin K antagonist oral anticoagulants), are a class of anticoagulants that have been transforming clinical practice since their introduction around 2010. In view of their increasing use, the clinician should be aware of their pharmacological properties, which are very different to those of warfarin (**Box 29.9**). Four DOACs are currently licensed for treatment of VTE in the UK: three (*apixaban*, *edoxaban* and *rivaroxaban*) are inhibitors of factor Xa and one (*dabigatran*) is an inhibitor of factor IIa (thrombin). Unlike heparin and warfarin, they directly inhibit their target substrates. All are administered orally and peak levels are seen about 2 hours after ingestion.

- They have a wider therapeutic index than warfarin.
- There is no interaction with dietary factors or alcohol.
- There is limited interaction (compared to warfarin) with other drugs.
- They can be given in a fixed dose with no monitoring – a major clinical advantage.
- They are variably eliminated through the kidneys and have a half-life of around 12 hours.

 Box 29.8 Management of high INRs and bleeding on warfarin

INR >5.0, no bleeding
1. Withhold warfarin
2. Reduce maintenance warfarin dose
3. Investigate cause of elevated INR

INR >8.0, no bleeding or minor bleeding
1. Withhold warfarin
2. If no bleeding, give 1–5 mg oral vitamin K
3. If minor bleeding, give 1–3 mg intravenous vitamin K
4. Recheck INR within 24 h

Major bleeding
1. Withhold warfarin
2. Give four-factor prothrombin complex concentrate (PCC) 25–50 u/kg (fresh frozen plasma 15 mL/kg only if PCC not available)
3. Give 5 mg i.v. vitamin K
4. Recheck INR following administration of PCC
   In the event of bleeding, investigate local anatomical cause.

(From Keeling D, Baglin T, Tait C et al. and British Committee for Standards in Haematology. Guidelines on oral anticoagulation with warfarin – fourth edition. Br J Haematol 2011; 154:311–324.)

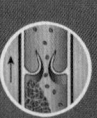

Box 29.9 Pharmacological properties of oral anticoagulants

	Warfarin	Apixaban	Edoxaban	Rivaroxaban	Dabigatran
Target	II, VII, IX, X	Xa	Xa	Xa	IIa
Peak effect	5 days (variable)	2 h	2 h	2 h	2 h
Approximate half-life	40 h	12 h	12 h	9 h	15 h
Renal elimination	No	25%	50%	33%	80%
Drug interactions	Multiple	P-gp 3A4	P-gp	P-gp 3A4	P-gp
Diet/alcohol interactions	Yes	No	No	No[a]	No
Monitoring	Yes	No	No	No	No
Measurement	INR	Anti-Xa	Anti-Xa	Anti-Xa	Dilute thrombin time
Reversal	Vitamin K Prothrombin complex concentrate	Andexanet (not currently licensed)	Andexanet (not currently licensed)	Andexanet (not currently licensed)	Idarucizumab

[a]Rivaroxaban should be taken with food to improve bioavailability.
INR, International Normalized Ratio; P-gp, inducers and inhibitors of P-glycoprotein; 3A4, inducers and inhibitors of cytochrome P450 3A4.

Clinical trials have shown they are as effective as heparin and warfarin in the treatment and secondary prevention of VTE. Overall, they carry a similar or lower risk of major bleeding, with a reduced risk of intracranial haemorrhage, partly offset by an increased risk of gastrointestinal haemorrhage.

Their use in the acute treatment of VTE has already been outlined. The combination of efficacy, safety, simplified dosing and avoidance of monitoring has led to a rapid increase in use of DOACs for VTE treatment and secondary prevention.

Special circumstances

DOACs cross the placenta and should not be used by pregnant women or those trying to conceive. Neither should they be used during breast-feeding. The Xa inhibitors are licensed for VTE treatment down to a creatinine clearance of 15 mL/min, although data are still limited in patients with a creatinine clearance of less than 30 mL/min, the lower limit for dabigatran. Significant interactions with certain drugs such as protease inhibitors and many antiepileptics preclude their use in some patients. They are also contraindicated in those with mechanical heart valve replacements, or moderate or severe mitral stenosis. Recent trials suggest that the DOACs are as effective as LMWH in the treatment of cancer-associated thrombosis. However, they increase the risk of gastrointestinal bleeding and LMWH remains the preferred option in patients with cancers where this is a risk.

Management of bleeding on DOACs

In the event of *major bleeding* on DOACs, management should, in general, follow established principles:

- The DOAC should be stopped.
- Supportive therapy, e.g. intravenous fluids and blood components like red cells, should be administered as appropriate.
- Consideration should be given to specialty-specific intervention, e.g. endoscopy.

In the event of *life-threatening bleeding*, specific antidotes are emerging as additional options. In the case of dabigatran, a monoclonal antibody, *idarucizumab*, which rapidly binds to and completely reverses dabigatran, is now widely available. An antidote to the inhibitors of factor Xa, *andexanet alfa*, is currently undergoing clinical evaluation.

Further reading

Elsebale MAT, van Es N, Langston A et al. Direct oral anticoagulants in patients with venous thromboembolism and thrombophilia: a systematic review and meta-analysis. *J Thromb Haemost* 2019; 17:645–656.
Greinacher A. Heparin-induced thrombocytopenia. *N Engl J Med* 2015; 373:252–261.
Nutescu EA, Burnett A, Fanikos J et al. Pharmacology of anticoagulants used in the treatment of venous thromboembolism. *J Thromb Thrombolysis* 2016; 41:15–31.

30

Cardiology

Nicholas H. Bunce, Robin Ray and Hitesh Patel

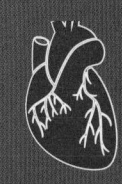

CORE SKILLS AND KNOWLEDGE

Heart disease remains the most common cause of death in the developed world and the third most common in low-income countries. Reducing this burden requires close collaboration between general practitioners, public health doctors, hospital specialists and allied health care professionals, with interventions including reducing smoking rates, encouraging healthy eating choices, promoting aerobic exercise, and targeting hypertension (Ch. 31) and dyslipidaemia (Ch. 24).

In the outpatient setting, patients with stable cardiac symptoms (e.g. exertional chest pain, palpitations or peripheral oedema) are evaluated, and those with established cardiological disease are followed up in order to optimize lifestyle factors and titrate medications.

Most cardiologists are trained in various interventional techniques (e.g. direct current cardioversion, coronary angiography or implantation of cardiac rhythm devices) and work closely with cardiac surgeons. Cardiologists also look after patients with emergency cardiac presentations (e.g. acute coronary syndromes or heart block), often on coronary care units.

Key skills in cardiology include:
- becoming familiar with the management of cardiac emergencies, including acute coronary syndrome and life-threatening rhythm disorders
- understanding cardiovascular risk reduction, and the management of chronic cardiological conditions such as heart failure and atrial fibrillation
- confidently interpreting electrocardiograms (ECGs) and echocardiogram reports, and understanding the role of different forms of invasive cardiac intervention.

Cardiology can be best learned by observing cardiology outpatient clinics, attending ward rounds on the coronary care unit, observing invasive procedures such as coronary angiography or DC cardioversion, and seeing patients in the community with general practitioners or specialist heart failure nurses.

CLINICAL SKILLS FOR CARDIOLOGY

History

A full cardiological history covers the relevant symptoms and risk factors for cardiac disease in detail and is focused on establishing the cause of symptoms. Is this patient's chest pain likely to originate in the heart? Is their breathlessness more likely to be due to heart failure, lung disease or something else? A fuller description of cardiac history-taking begins on page 1028 but **Box 30.1** provides a suggested structure to ensure that the relevant material is covered systematically.

 Box 30.1 History-taking in cardiac disease

Symptoms

Chest pain
Think anatomically, about the type of pain caused by disease in different structures within the chest:
- *Heart* – central, squeezing or crushing in nature, radiation to left arm or jaw, with associated sweating or nausea
- *Pericardium* – central, sharp in character, retrosternal, may radiate to back, worse sitting upright, associated viral symptoms or causative medication
- *Oesophagus* – central, burning or tight in nature, worse on lying flat, worse after eating, with associated burping, epigastric discomfort or altered taste
- *Pleural* – localized and often peripheral, sharp in nature, worse on deep inspiration or coughing, with associated cough, breathlessness or haemoptysis
- *Musculoskeletal* – often localized, intermittent and related to movement; possible trigger event (e.g. abnormal activity); reproducible on palpation or movement

Breathlessness
Identify severity (see **Box 30.23**) and likely cause:
- *Heart disease* – worse on lying flat, episodes of paroxysmal nocturnal dyspnoea, peripheral oedema
- *Lung disease* – associated respiratory symptoms, e.g. cough, wheeze, pleuritic pain or haemoptysis

Palpitations
These are usually episodic. Identify:
- *Nature of symptoms* – fast or slow, feelings of 'missing a beat', associated chest pain or tightness, breathlessness and dizziness
- *Pattern of symptoms* – duration of problem, frequency of attacks, associations with exercise, caffeine or alcohol intake
- *Severity of symptoms* – dizziness, pre-syncope or loss of consciousness

Dizziness or collapse
A full event history is required, ideally correlated by an eye-witness if there was a loss of consciousness, to try to diagnose the likely cause:
- *Possible vasovagal syncope* – intercurrent illness or dehydration, antihypertensive medication, emotion or physical exertion, preceding presyncopal symptoms, rapid recovery
- *Possible cardiac cause* (malignant dysrhythmia or valve disease) – preceding chest pain or palpitations, sudden loss of consciousness, lack of alternative explanation, family history of collapse or sudden death
- *Possible neurological cause* – neurological aura, abnormal movements, urinary incontinence, tongue-biting, post-ictal phase

Risk factors
- *Previous cardiovascular disease* – enquire about or look up previous investigations and interventions
- *Smoking* – quantified in pack years
- *Diabetes* – time since diagnosis, degree of glycaemic control
- *Hypertension* – time since diagnosis, degree of control, number of drugs required to control blood pressure
- *Hyperlipidaemia*
- *Chronic inflammatory disorders*
- *Family history of early-onset cardiovascular disease*
- *Cocaine use*

Functional baseline and disability
- *Accommodation* – where the patient lives and with whom
- *Physical activity* – fully active, limited by symptoms, house-, bed- or chair-bound
- *Symptom-related disability* – exertional chest pain or breathlessness (try to quantify – how far can they walk? Can they climb a flight of stairs?)
- *Level of care* – ranging from full functional independence to carer visits or full residential or nursing care

---

Examination

Many features of cardiovascular disease can be elicited on physical examination (see figure opposite). They include:
- Evidence of life-threatening cardiac disease requiring emergency resuscitation: shock, dysrhythmias, pulmonary oedema.
- Evidence of underlying conditions that contribute to cardiovascular disease (eg hyperlipidaemia or Marfan's syndrome)
- Evidence of heart failure
- Murmurs and specific signs associated with particular forms of valvular heart disease

ECG interpretation

The ECG is an essential bedside test in the investigation of all patients with cardiac disease. A full guide to understanding the science behind it and its interpretation begins on page 1033 but **Box 30.2** offers a systematic approach to ensure that abnormalities are not missed.

 Box 30.2 A systematic approach to interpreting the ECG

Step 1: Preliminaries
- Correct patient?
- Correct date and time?
- Standard speed (25 mm/sec)?
- Standard amplitude (10 mm/mV)?

Step 2: Heart structure
- Axis (left axis deviation if <−30 degrees, right axis deviation if >90 degrees)?
- Left ventricular hypertrophy (various criteria, see **Fig. 30.79**)?
- Evidence of atrial enlargement?

Step 3: Rate and rhythm
- Heart rate?
- Regular or irregular?
- Sinus rhythm (P–QRS–T)?
- Atrioventricular node delay (PR duration should be 120–200 ms)?
- Intraventricular conduction delay (QRS duration should be <120 ms)?
- Repolarization delay (QTc should be <450 ms)?

Step 4: Ischaemia
- Features include:
  - Q waves
  - ST elevation or depression
  - T-wave inversion
- Anatomical regions:
  - Anterior (V_1/V_2)
  - Septal (V_3/V_4)
  - Lateral (V_5/V_6)
  - Interior (II, III, AVF)
  - High lateral (I, AVL)

Step 5: Global features
- Pericarditis (global saddle-shaped ST elevation)?
- Electrolyte abnormalities, eg hyperkalaemia (peaked T waves)?
- Pre-excitation (upstroke before QRS complexes)?
- Rarer causes of global abnormalities include hypothermia, thyroid disease and drug effects.

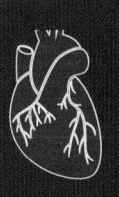

Examination

General
Breathless
Position - sitting up?
Colour - cyanosed
     (central)
     - pale
     - malar flush
     (mitral stenosis)
Pain
Obesity/cachexia
Signs of other conditions,
   e.g. Marfan's
Temperature
Sweating

Jugular venous pulsation
Height
Character

Carotid pulse
- Character
- Bruits

Blood pressure

Radial pulse
Rate
Rhythm
Volume

Hands
Splinter haemorrhages
Clubbing
Peripheral cyanosis
Tendon xanthomata
   (hyperlipidaemia)

Splinter haemorrhages

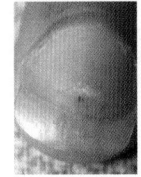

Xanthelasma

Mouth
Oral hygiene
Poor dentition

Precordium
Inspect - look for scars
Palpate - apex beat
       - thrills
       - ventricular heaves
Auscultate
- added sounds
- murmurs

Chest
Basal crackles

Abdomen
Hepatomegaly (pulsatile in
tricuspid incompetence)
Ascites
Aortic aneurysm

Legs
Oedema
Feel for peripheral pulses

Feet
Look for ischaemia
- Feel for pulses
- Temperature
Vasculitis rash

**Infective endocarditis,
septic embolization**

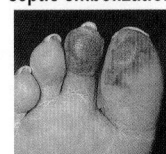

*(From Johnson RJ, Feehally J.
Comprehensive Clinical Nephrology,
2nd edn. St. Louis, Mosby; 2000,
with permission.)*

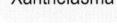

⑦ Box 30.3 Key conditions and learning objectives in cardiological disease

Condition	Patient contact	Additional learning objectives	Medications
Emergency			
Acute coronary syndrome (see p. 1084)	CCU MDT	ECG interpretation Observation of coronary angioplasty Cardiac rehabilitation class	Aspirin Thienopyridines Heparins Gp2b/3A inhibitors
Acute pulmonary oedema (see p. 1076)	CCU	Chest X-ray interpretation Observation of administration of CPAP	Furosemide Nitrates Morphine Dobutamine Milrinone
Symptomatic high-degree heart block (see p. 1053)	CCU	ECG interpretation Observation of temporary wire/pacemaker implantation	Atropine Isoprenaline Adrenaline (epinephrine)
Ventricular tachycardia/ ventricular fibrillation (see p. 1063)	CCU Attendance at cardiac arrest calls MDT	ECG interpretation Observation of emergency direct current defibrillation Observation of internal cardioverter–defibrillator implantation	Amiodarone Lidocaine Mexilitine
Tamponade/pericardial effusion (see p. 1126)	CCU	Echocardiographic features Observation of pericardial drain insertion	
Non-emergency			
Stable angina (see p. 1081)	Rapid access chest pain clinic General cardiology clinic MDT	Observation of stress echocardiography, cardiac CT coronary angiography, nuclear perfusion scans, coronary angiography	Beta-blockers Calcium-channel blockers Nitrates Potassium-channel activators Ivabradine Ranolazine
Atrial fibrillation/flutter (see p. 1059)	General cardiology clinic	ECG interpretation Attendance at cardioversion lists Observation of transoesophageal echocardiograms Observation of catheter ablation	Beta-blockers Calcium-channel blockers Digoxin Warfarin Direct-acting oral anticoagulants Flecainide Sotalol Amiodarone
Chronic heart failure (see p. 1071)	Heart failure clinics Nurse-led community heart failure clinics MDT	Observation of transthoracic echocardiograms	Beta-blockers Angiotensin-converting enzyme inhibitors Aldosterone receptor blockers Angiotensin receptor–neprilysin inhibitor Angiotensin II receptor blockers Diuretics Nitrates Hydralazine
Valve disease (see p. 1091)	General cardiology clinics Specialist valve clinics MDT Cardiology wards (for infective endocarditis)	Observation of transthoracic, stress and transoesophageal echocardiograms to assess valve lesions	Diuretics Vasodilators Antibiotics (for infective endocarditis)
Hypertension/dyslipidaemia (Ch. 24)	General cardiology clinics Hypertension clinic Lipid clinic	Attendance at lifestyle modification clinics led for dietary, exercise and smoking cessation instruction	Calcium-channel blockers Angiotensin-converting enzyme inhibitors Angiotensin II receptor blockers Aldosterone receptor blockers Thiazide diuretics Alpha-blockers Beta-blockers Statins Ezetimibe Fibrates PCSK9 inhibitors

CCU, coronary care unit; CPAP, continuous positive airways pressure; MDT, multidisciplinary team meeting; PCSK9, Proprotein convertase subtilisin/kexin type 9.

ANATOMY, PHYSIOLOGY AND EMBRYOLOGY OF THE HEART

Myocardial cells constitute 75% of the heart mass but only about 25% of the cell number. They are designed to perform two fundamental functions: initiation and conduction of electrical impulses and contraction. Although most myocardial cells are able to perform both these functions, the vast majority are predominantly contractile cells (myocytes) and a small number are specifically designed as electrical cells. The latter, collectively known as the conducting system of the heart, are not nervous tissue but modified myocytes lacking in myofibril components. They have the ability to generate electrical impulses, which are then conducted to the myocytes, leading to contraction by a process known as excitation–contraction coupling. The rate of electrical impulse generation and the force of myocardial contraction are modified by numerous factors, including autonomic input and stretch.

Three epicardial coronary arteries supply blood to the myocardium, and a more complex network of veins is responsible for drainage. In the face of continuous arterial pressure fluctuations, blood vessels, especially in the cerebral circulation, maintain constant tissue perfusion by a process known as *'autoregulation'*; blood vessel control is, however, complex, involving additional local and central mechanisms.

Conduction system of the heart

Sinus node (sinoatrial node)

The sinus node is a complex, spindle-shaped structure that lies in the lateral and epicardial aspects of the junction between the superior vena cava and the right atrium (**Fig. 30.1**). Physiologically, it generates impulses automatically by spontaneous depolarization of its membrane at a rate quicker than any other cardiac cell type. It is therefore the *natural pacemaker of the heart*.

A number of factors are responsible for the spontaneous decay of the sinus node cell membrane potential ('pacemaker potential'), the most significant of which is a small influx of sodium ions into the cells. This small sodium current has two components: the background inward (I_b) current and the 'funny' (I_f) current (or pacemaker current) (**Fig. 30.2**). The term 'funny' current denotes ionic flow through channels activated in *hyperpolarized* cells (–60 mV or greater), unlike other time- and voltage-dependent channels activated by *depolarization*. The rate of depolarization of the sinus node membrane potential is modulated by autonomic tone (i.e. sympathetic and parasympathetic input), stretch, temperature, hypoxia and blood pH, and responds to other hormonal influences (e.g. tri-iodothyronine and serotonin).

Atrial and ventricular myocyte action potentials

Action potentials in the sinus node trigger depolarization of the atrial myocytes and subsequently the ventricular ones. These cells have a different action potential from that of sinus node cells (see **Fig. 30.2**). Their resting membrane potential is a consequence of a small flow of potassium ions into the cells through open 'inward rectifier' channels (I_{K1}); at this stage, sodium and calcium channels are closed. The arrival of adjacent action potentials triggers the opening of voltage-gated, fast, self-inactivating sodium channels, resulting in a sharp depolarization spike. This is followed by a partial repolarization of the membrane due to activation of 'transient outward' potassium channels.

The plateau phase that follows is unique to myocytes and results from a small but sustained inward calcium current through L-type calcium channels (I_{CaL}) lasting 200–400 ms. This calcium influx is caused by a combined increase in permeability of the cell, especially the sarcolemmal membranes to calcium (**Fig. 30.3**). This plateau (or

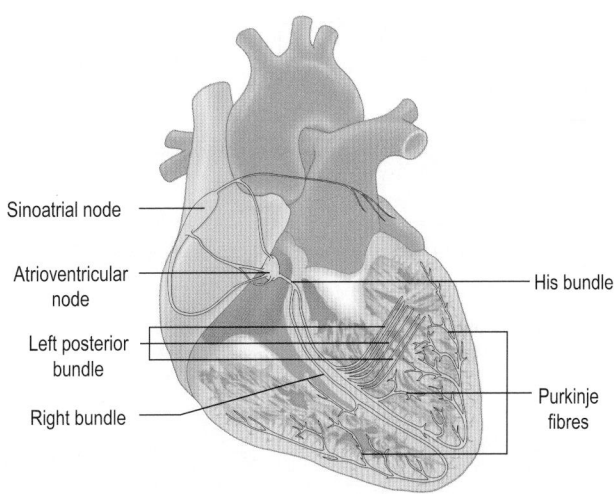

Fig. 30.1 The conducting system of the heart.

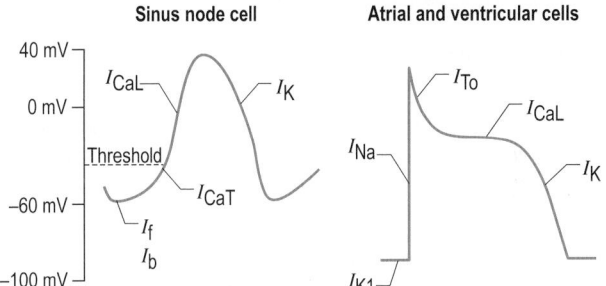

Fig. 30.2 Myocardial action potentials. I_b, background inward sodium current; I_{CaL}, long-lasting (or 'L'-type) calcium channel; I_{CaT}, transient (or 'T'-type) calcium channel; I_f, 'funny' current; I_K, delayed rectifier potassium current; I_{K1}, inward rectifier potassium current; I_{Na}, inward sodium current; I_{To}, transient outward potassium current.

refractory) phase in myocyte action potential prevents early reactivation of the myocytes and directly determines the strength of contraction. The gradual inactivation of the calcium channels activates delayed rectifier potassium channels (I_K), repolarizing the membrane. Atrial tissue is activated like a 'forest fire', but the activation peters out when the insulating layer between the atrium and the ventricle – the annulus fibrosus – is reached. Controversy exists about whether impulses from the sinoatrial (SA) node travel over specialized conducting 'pathways' in the atrium or over ordinary atrial myocardium.

Atrioventricular node, His bundle and Purkinje fibres

The depolarization continues to conduct slowly through the atrioventricular (AV) node. This is a small, bean-shaped structure that lies beneath the right atrial endocardium within the lower interatrial septum. The AV node continues as the His bundle, which penetrates the annulus fibrosus and conducts the cardiac impulse rapidly towards the ventricle. The His bundle reaches the crest of the interventricular septum and divides into the right bundle branch and the main left bundle branch.

The *right bundle branch* continues down the right side of the interventricular septum to the apex; from here, it radiates and divides to form the Purkinje network, which spreads throughout the subendocardial surface of the right ventricle. The *main left bundle branch* is a short structure, which fans out into many strands on the left side of the interventricular septum. These strands can be grouped into an anterior superior division (the anterior hemi-bundle) and a posterior inferior division (the posterior hemi-bundle). The anterior hemi-bundle supplies the subendocardial Purkinje network of the anterior and superior surfaces of the left ventricle, and the inferior hemi-bundle

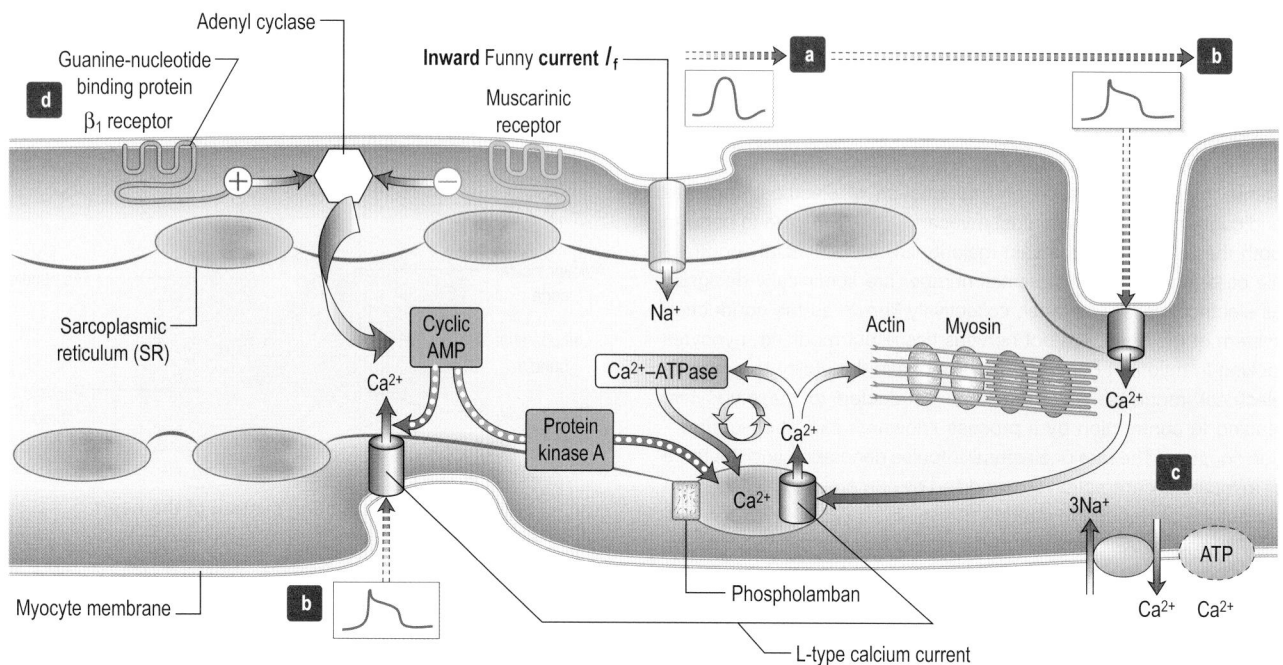

Fig. 30.3 The 'complete' cardiac cell. (a) *Spontaneous depolarization* in sinus node cells, due to sodium (Na) influx through the 'funny' current, generates the 'pacemaker' potential. **(b)** This activates other atrial and ventricular myocytes, triggering **action potentials** and activating L-type calcium (Ca) channels in the surface and transverse tubule membranes (at the top and bottom of the figure). **(c)** The resulting ***Ca influx*** acts on Ca-induced Ca release channels (RyR2) on the sarcoplasmic reticulum (SR); this causes the release of stored Ca, which acts on actin and myosin fibrils, leading to contraction. Ca reuptake pumps in the SR, regulated by phospholamban, replenish the stores; various exchange pumps also expel Ca from the cell. **(d)** *Autonomic input* has either a positive chronotropic/inotropic effect (β₁ receptors) or a negative chronotropic/inotropic effect (muscarinic receptors). AMP, adenosine monophosphate; ATPase, adenosine triphosphatase.

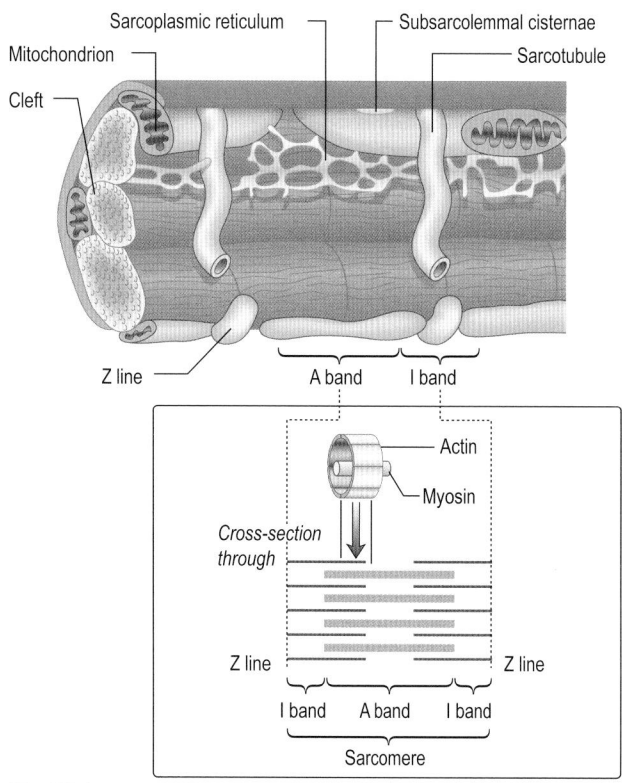

Fig. 30.4 The structure of a myofibril within a myocyte. The myofibrils are made up of a series of sarcomeres joined at the Z line.

supplies the inferior and posterior surfaces. Impulse conduction through the AV node is slow and depends on action potentials, largely produced by slow transmembrane calcium flux. In the atria, ventricles and His–Purkinje system, conduction is rapid and is due to action potentials generated by rapid transmembrane sodium diffusion.

Cellular basis of myocardial contraction–excitation–contraction coupling

Each myocyte, approximately 100 μm long, branches and interdigitates with adjacent cells. An intercalated disc permits electrical conduction to adjacent cells. Myocytes contain bundles of parallel myofibrils. Each myofibril is made up of a series of sarcomeres (**Fig. 30.4**). A sarcomere (the basic unit of contraction) is bound by two transverse Z lines, to each of which is attached a perpendicular filament of the protein actin. The actin filaments from each of the two Z bands overlap with thicker parallel protein filaments known as myosin. Actin and myosin filaments are attached to each other by cross-bridges that contain adenosine triphosphatase (ATPase), which breaks down adenosine triphosphate (ATP) to provide the energy for contraction.

Two chains of actin molecules form a helical structure with another molecule, tropomyosin, in the grooves of the actin helix; a further molecule, troponin, is attached to every seven actin molecules. During cardiac contraction, the length of the actin and myosin monofilaments does not change. Rather, the actin filaments slide between the myosin filaments when ATPase splits a high-energy bond of ATP. To supply the ATP, the myocyte (which cannot stop for a rest) has a very high mitochondrial density (35% of the cell volume). As calcium ions bind to troponin C, the activity of troponin I is inhibited, which induces a conformational change in tropomyosin.

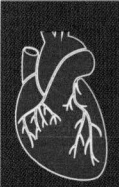

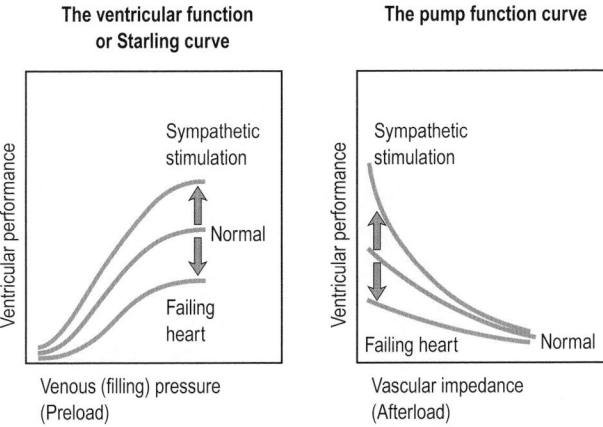

Fig. 30.5 The Frank–Starling mechanism. The effect on ventricular contraction of alteration in filling pressures and outflow impedance in the normal, failing and sympathetically stimulated ventricle is shown.

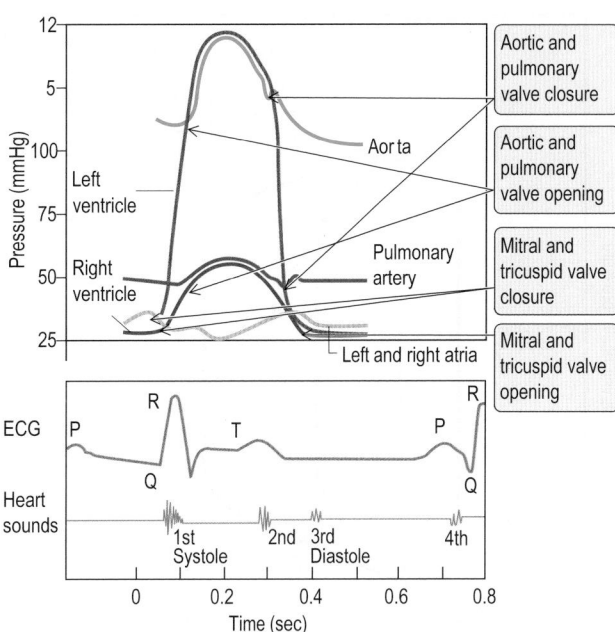

Fig. 30.6 The cardiac cycle.

This event unlocks the active site between actin and myosin, enabling contraction to proceed.

Calcium is made available during the plateau phase of the action potential when calcium ions enter the cell and are mobilized from the sarcoplasmic reticulum (SR) through the ryanodine receptor (RyR2) calcium-release channel (see p. 1121). RyR2 activity is regulated by the protein calstabin 2 and nitric oxide. The force of cardiac muscle contraction ('inotropic state') is thus regulated by the influx of calcium ions into the cell through calcium channels (see **Fig. 30.3**). T (transient) calcium channels open when the muscle is more depolarized, whereas L (long-lasting) calcium channels require less depolarization. The extent to which the sarcomere can shorten determines the stroke volume of the ventricle. It is maximally shortened in response to powerful inotropic drugs or severe exercise.

Starling's law of the heart

The contractile function of an isolated strip of cardiac tissue can be described by the relationship between the velocity of muscle contraction, the load that is moved by the contracting muscle, and the extent to which the muscle is stretched before contracting. As with all other types of muscle, the velocity of contraction of myocardial tissue is reduced by increasing the load against which the tissue must contract. However, in the non-failing heart, pre-stretching of cardiac muscle improves the relationship between the force and velocity of contraction (**Fig. 30.5**).

This phenomenon was described in the intact heart as an increase of stroke volume (ventricular performance) with an enlargement of the diastolic volume (preload), and is known as 'Starling's law of the heart' or the 'Frank–Starling relationship'. It has been transcribed into more clinically relevant indices. Thus, stroke work (aortic pressure × stroke volume) is increased as ventricular end-diastolic volume is raised. Alternatively, within certain limits, cardiac output rises as pulmonary capillary wedge pressure increases. This clinical relationship is described by the ventricular function curve (see **Fig. 30.5**), which also shows the effect of sympathetic stimulation.

Nerve supply of the myocardium

Adrenergic nerves supply atrial and ventricular muscle fibres, as well as the conduction system. Beta$_1$-receptors predominate in the heart, with both adrenaline (epinephrine) and noradrenaline (norepinephrine) having positive inotropic and chronotropic effects. Cholinergic nerves from the vagus supply mainly the SA and AV nodes via M$_2$ muscarinic receptors. The ventricular myocardium is sparsely innervated by the vagus. Under basal conditions, vagal inhibitory effects predominate over the sympathetic excitatory effects, resulting in a slow heart rate.

Adrenergic stimulation and cellular signalling

Beta$_1$-adrenergic stimulation enhances Ca^{2+} flux in the myocyte and thereby strengthens the force of contraction (see **Fig. 30.3**). Binding of catecholamines, such as noradrenaline, to the myocyte β$_1$-adrenergic receptor stimulates membrane-bound adenylate kinases. These enzymes enhance production of cyclic adenosine monophosphate (cAMP), which activates intracellular protein kinases; these, in turn, phosphorylate cellular proteins, including L-type calcium channels within the cell membrane. Beta$_1$-adrenergic stimulation of the myocyte also enhances myocyte relaxation.

The return of calcium from the cytosol to the SR is regulated by phospholamban (PL), a low-molecular-weight protein in the SR membrane. In its dephosphorylated state, PL inhibits Ca^{2+} uptake by the SR ATPase pump (see **Fig. 30.3**). However, β$_1$-adrenergic activation of protein kinase phosphorylates PL and blunts its inhibitory effect. The subsequently greater uptake of Ca^{2+} ions by the SR hastens Ca^{2+} removal from the cytosol and promotes myocyte relaxation.

The increased cAMP activity also results in phosphorylation of troponin I, an action that inhibits actin–myosin interaction and further enhances myocyte relaxation.

Cardiac cycle

The cardiac cycle (**Fig. 30.6**) consists of precisely timed rhythmic electrical and mechanical events that propel blood into the systemic and pulmonary circulations. The first event in the cardiac cycle is atrial depolarization (a P wave on the surface ECG), followed by right atrial and then left atrial contraction. Ventricular activation (the QRS complex on the ECG) follows after a short interval (the PR interval). Left ventricular contraction starts and, shortly thereafter, right ventricular contraction begins. The increased ventricular pressures exceed the atrial pressures and close first the mitral and then the tricuspid valves.

Until the aortic and pulmonary valves open, the ventricles contract with no change of volume (isovolumetric contraction). When ventricular pressures rise above the aortic and pulmonary artery

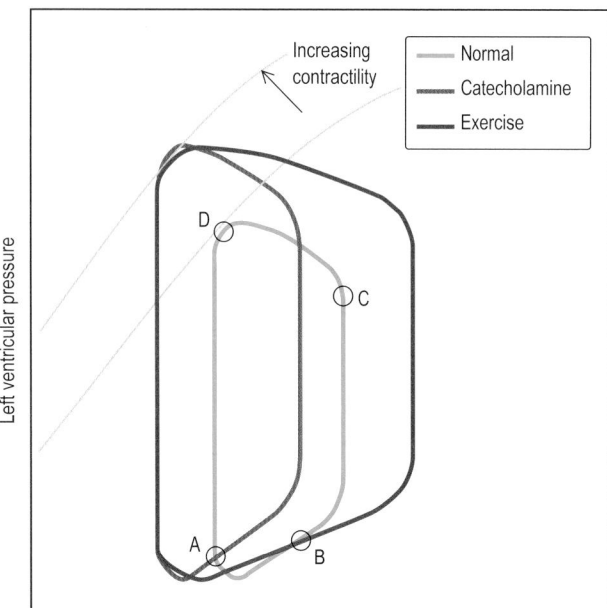

Fig. 30.7 Pressure–volume loop. AB, diastole: ventricular filling; **BC**, systole: isovolumetric ventricular contraction; **CD**, systole: ventricular emptying; **DA**, diastole: isovolumetric ventricular relaxation.

pressures the pulmonary valve and then the aortic valve open and ventricular ejection occurs. As the ventricles begin to relax, their pressures fall below the aortic and pulmonary arterial pressures, and aortic valve closure is followed by pulmonary valve closure. Isovolumetric relaxation then occurs. After the ventricular pressures have fallen below the right atrial and left atrial pressures, the tricuspid and mitral valves open. The cardiac cycle can be depicted graphically as the relationship between the pressure and volume of the ventricle (**Fig. 30.7**), illustrating the changing pressure–volume relationships in response to increased contractility and to exercise.

Coronary circulation

The coronary arterial system (**Fig. 30.8**) consists of the right and left coronary arteries. These arteries branch from the aorta, arising immediately above two cusps of the aortic valve. The right and left coronary arteries are unique in that they fill during diastole, when not occluded by valve cusps and when not squeezed by myocardial contraction. The right coronary artery arises from the right coronary sinus and courses through the right side of the AV groove, giving off vessels that supply the right atrium and the right ventricle. The vessel usually continues as the posterior descending coronary artery, which runs in the posterior interventricular groove and supplies the posterior part of the interventricular septum and the posterior left ventricular wall.

Within 2.5 cm of its origin from the left coronary sinus the left main coronary divides into the left anterior descending artery and the circumflex artery. The left anterior descending artery runs in the anterior interventricular groove and supplies the anterior septum and the anterior left ventricular wall. The left circumflex artery travels along the left AV groove and gives off branches to the left atrium and the left ventricle (marginal branches).

The sinus node and the AV node are supplied by the right coronary artery in about 60% and 90% of people, respectively. Therefore, disease in this artery may cause sinus bradycardia and AV nodal block. The majority of the left ventricle is supplied by the left coronary artery and disease in this vessel can cause significant myocardial dysfunction.

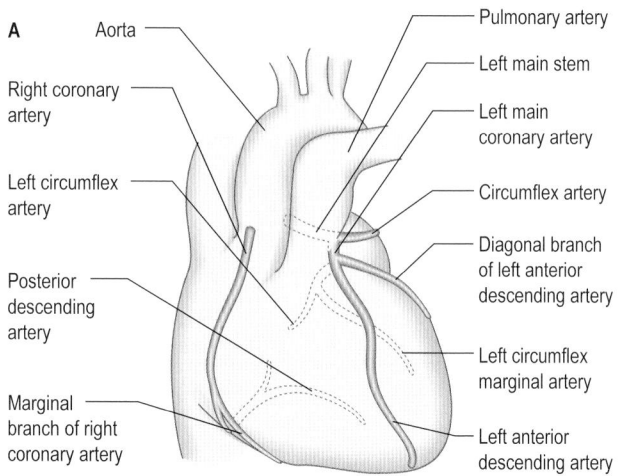

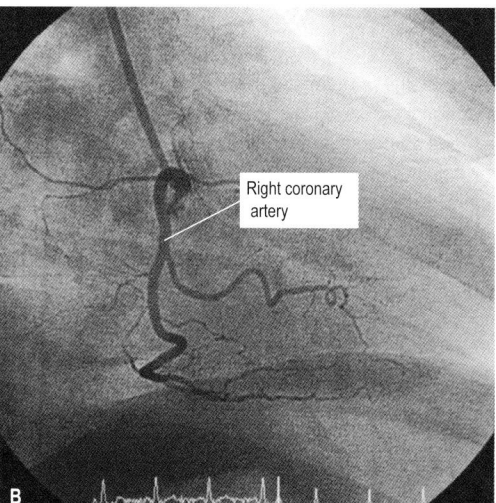

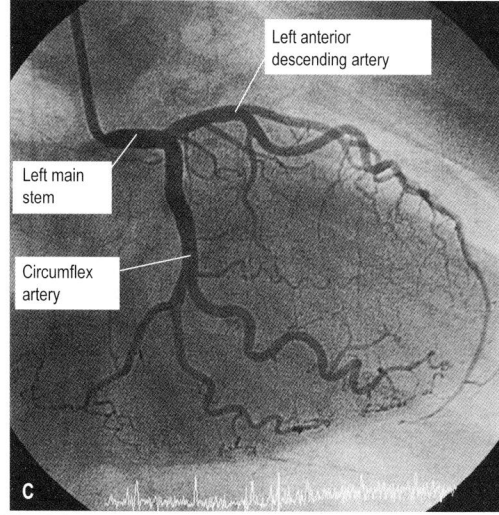

Fig. 30.8 The coronary circulation. (A) The normal coronary arterial anatomy. **(B)** Angiogram of the dominant right coronary system. **(C)** Angiogram of the left coronary system from the same patient (right anterior oblique projection).

Some blood from the capillary beds in the wall of the heart drains directly into the cavities of the heart via tiny veins but the majority returns by veins that accompany the arteries, to empty into the right atrium via the coronary sinus. An extensive lymphatic system drains into vessels that travel along the coronary vessels and then into the thoracic duct.

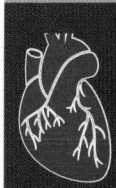

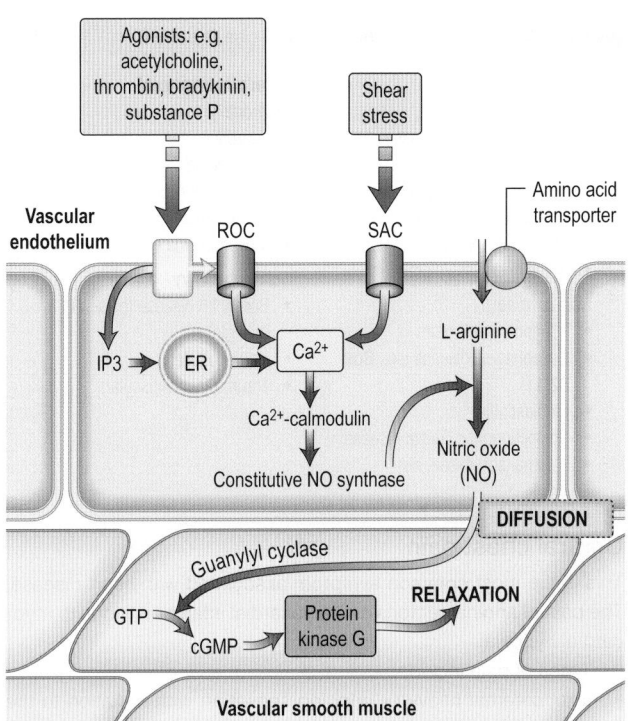

Fig. 30.9 The stimulus for production and function of nitric oxide (NO). Various stimuli lead to the production of NO via cytoplasmic calcium/calmodulin. NO triggers smooth muscle relaxation via the activation of guanylyl cyclase. cGMP, cyclic guanine monophosphate; ER, endoplasmic reticulum; GTP, guanine triphosphate; IP3, inositol triphosphate; ROC, receptor-operated Ca^{2+} channel; SAC, stretch-activated Ca^{2+} channel.

Blood vessel control and functions of the vascular endothelium

In functional terms the tunica intima with the vascular endothelium and the smooth-muscle-cell-containing tunica media are the main constituents of blood vessels. These two structures are closely inter-linked by a variety of mechanisms to regulate vascular tone. The central control of blood vessels is achieved via the neuroendocrine system. Sympathetic vasoconstrictor and parasympathetic vasodila-tor nerves regulate vascular tone in response to daily activity. Where neural control is impaired or in various pathological states, such as haemorrhage, endocrine control of blood vessels, mediated through adrenaline (epinephrine), angiotensin and vasopressin, takes over.

At a local level, tissue perfusion is maintained automatically and by the effect of various factors synthesized and/or released in the immediate vicinity. In the face of fluctuating arterial pressures, blood vessels vasoconstrict independently of nervous input when blood pressure drops, and vice versa. This process of **autoregulation** is a consequence of:

- the **Bayliss myogenic** response – the ability of blood vessels to constrict when distended
- the **vasodilator washout** effect – the vasoconstriction triggered by a decrease in the concentration of tissue metabolites.

The vascular endothelium is a cardiovascular endocrine organ, which occupies a strategic interface between blood and other tis-sues. It produces various compounds (e.g. nitric oxide (NO), prosta-cyclin (PGI₂), endothelin, endothelial-derived hyperpolarizing factor (EDHF), adhesion molecules, vascular endothelial growth factor (VEGF)), and has enzymes located on the surface, controlling the levels of circulating compounds such as angiotensin, bradykinin and serotonin. It has many regulatory roles.

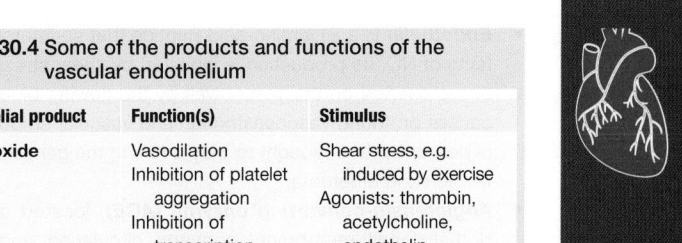

Box 30.4 Some of the products and functions of the vascular endothelium

Endothelial product	Function(s)	Stimulus
Nitric oxide	Vasodilation Inhibition of platelet aggregation Inhibition of transcription of adhesion molecules Inhibition of vascular smooth muscle proliferation	Shear stress, e.g. induced by exercise Agonists: thrombin, acetylcholine, endothelin, bradykinin, serotonin, substance P Inflammation/ endotoxin shock
Prostacyclin (PGI₂)	Vasodilation Inhibition of platelet aggregation	Agonist: thrombin Inflammation
Prostanoids	Vasoconstriction	Hypoxia
Endothelin	Vasoconstriction	Thrombin, angiotensin II, vasopressin Hypoxia *Note:* Inhibited by shear stress
Endothelial-derived hyperpolarizing factor	Vasodilation	Agonists: bradykinin, acetylcholine
Angiotensin-converting enzyme	Vasoconstriction	Expressed naturally
von Willebrand factor	Promotion of platelet aggregation Stabilization of factor VIII	Agonists: thrombin, adrenaline (epinephrine)
Adhesion molecules		
P, L, E selectins ICAM, VCAM, PECAM	Margination of white blood cells Binding and diapedesis of WBCs into vessel wall	Inflammatory mediators: histamine, thrombin, TNF, IL-6
Vascular endothelial growth factor (VEGF)	Angiogenesis Vasodilation Increase in vascular permeability	Pregnancy Hypoxia Inflammation, e.g. rheumatoid arthritis Trauma Tumours

ICAM, intracellular adhesion molecule; IL, interleukin; PECAM, platelet/endothelial cell adhesion molecule; TNF, tumour necrosis factor; VCAM, vascular cell adhesion molecule; WBC, white blood cell.

Vasomotor control

- **Nitric oxide** is a diffusible gas with a very short half-life; it is pro-duced in endothelial cells from the amino acid L-arginine via the action of the enzyme NO synthase (NOS), which is controlled by cytoplasmic calcium/calmodulin (**Fig. 30.9**). It is produced in re-sponse to various stimuli (**Box 30.4**), triggering vascular smooth muscle relaxation through activation of guanylate cyclase; this leads to an increase in the intracellular levels of cyclic 3,5-guanine monophosphate (cGMP). Its cardiovascular effects protect against atherosclerosis, high blood pressure, heart failure and thrombosis. NO is also the neurotransmitter in various 'nitrergic' nerves in the central and peripheral nervous systems and may play a role in the central regulation of vascular tone. The class of drugs used to treat erectile dysfunction, the phosphodiesterase (PDE₅) inhibitors, pre-vent the breakdown of cGMP and promote vasodilation.
- **PGI₂** is synergistic to NO and also plays a role in the local regula-tion of vasomotor tone.

- **Endothelin** is a 21-amino-acid peptide that counteracts the effects of NO. Its production is inhibited by shear stress – i.e. the stress exerted on the vessel wall by the flowing blood – and it causes profound vasoconstriction and vascular smooth muscle hypertrophy. It is thought to play a role in the genesis of hypertension and atheroma.
- **Angiotensin-converting enzyme (ACE)**, located on the endothelial cell membrane, converts circulating angiotensin I (synthesized by the action of renin on angiotensinogen) to angiotensin II, which has vasoconstrictor properties and leads to aldosterone release (see **Fig. 30.6**). Aldosterone promotes sodium absorption from the kidney and, together with the angiotensin-induced vasoconstriction, provides haemodynamic stability.
- **Other factors** that influence vasomotor tone include histamine (released by mast cells), bradykinin (synthesized from kininogen by the action of coagulation factor XIIa) and serotonin (released by platelets).

Anti- and prothrombotic mechanisms

PGI_2, produced from arachidonic acid in the endothelial cell membrane by the action of the enzyme cyclo-oxygenase, inhibits platelet aggregation. Low-dose aspirin prevents activation of the cyclo-oxygenase pathway in platelets but only to a degree that does not affect PGI_2 synthesis, unlike higher doses. Other antithrombotic agents, such as clopidogrel (an adenosine diphosphate (ADP) receptor antagonist) and glycoprotein IIb/IIIa inhibitors, achieve their effects by acting directly on platelet receptors. The antithrombotic effect of PGI_2 is aided by NO, affecting platelets via activation of guanylate cyclase. The endothelial cell membrane also produces other anticoagulant molecules, such as thrombomodulin, heparin sulphate and various fibrinolytic factors. Clinically used, fast-acting heparin preparations are identical to this naturally occurring molecule.

In addition to their ability to prevent clotting, endothelial cells also aid thrombosis. They are responsible for the production of von Willebrand factor through a unique organelle called the Weibel–Palade body, which not only acts as a carrier for factor VIII but also promotes platelet adhesion by binding to exposed collagen (see p. 367).

Further reading

Levick JR. *An Introduction to Cardiovascular Physiology*, 6th edn. London: Arnold; 2018.

CLINICAL APPROACH TO THE PATIENT WITH HEART DISEASE

Clinical features of heart disease

The following symptoms occur with heart disease:
- chest pain
- dyspnoea (breathlessness)
- palpitations
- syncope
- fatigue
- peripheral oedema.

The severity of cardiac symptoms or fatigue is classified according to the New York Heart Association (NYHA) grading of cardiac status (see **Box 30.23**). The differential diagnosis of chest pain is given in **Box 30.5**.

? Box 30.5 Differential diagnosis of chest pain

Central

Cardiac
- Ischaemic heart disease (infarction or angina)
- Coronary artery spasm
- Pericarditis/myocarditis
- Mitral valve prolapse
- Aortic aneurysm/dissection

Non-cardiac
- Pulmonary embolism
- Oesophageal disease (see **Box 32.11**)
- Mediastinitis
- Costochondritis (Tietze disease)
- Trauma (soft tissue, rib)

Lateral/peripheral

Pulmonary
- Infarction
- Pneumonia
- Pneumothorax
- Lung cancer
- Mesothelioma

Non-pulmonary
- Bornholm disease (epidemic myalgia)
- Herpes zoster
- Trauma (ribs/muscular)

Central chest pain

This is the most common symptom associated with heart disease. The pain of angina pectoris and myocardial infarction is due to myocardial hypoxia.

Types of pain include:
- a retrosternal heavy or gripping sensation with radiation to the left arm or neck that is provoked by exertion and eased with rest or nitrates – **angina** (see p. 1081)
- similar pain at rest – **acute coronary syndrome** (see p. 1084)
- severe, tearing chest pain radiating through to the back – **aortic dissection** (see p. 1130)
- sharp, central chest pain that is worse with movement or respiration but relieved with sitting forward – **pericarditis pain** (see p. 1125)
- sharp, stabbing, left submammary pain associated with anxiety – **da Costa's syndrome.**

Dyspnoea

Left ventricular failure causes dyspnoea due to oedema of the pulmonary interstitium and alveoli. This makes the lungs stiff (less compliant), thus increasing the respiratory effort required to ventilate them. **Tachypnoea** (increased respiratory rate) is often present owing to stimulation of pulmonary stretch receptors.

Orthopnoea refers to breathlessness on lying flat. Blood is redistributed from the legs to the torso, leading to an increase in central and pulmonary blood volume. The patient uses an increasing number of pillows to sleep.

Paroxysmal nocturnal dyspnoea (PND) is when a patient is woken from sleep fighting for breath. It is caused by the same mechanisms as orthopnoea. However, as sensory awareness is reduced during sleep, the pulmonary oedema can become quite severe before the patient is awoken.

Hyperventilation with alternating episodes of apnoea (**Cheyne–Stokes respiration**) occurs in severe heart failure.

If hypopnoea occurs rather than apnoea, the phenomenon is termed 'periodic breathing', but the two variations are known together as **central sleep apnoea syndrome (CSAS)**. This occurs due to malfunctioning of the respiratory centre in the brain, caused by poor cardiac output with concurrent cerebrovascular disease. The symptoms of CSAS, such as daytime somnolence and fatigue, are similar to those of obstructive sleep apnoea syndrome (OSAS, see p. 960) and there is considerable overlap with the symptoms of heart failure. CSAS is believed to lead to myocardial hypertrophy and fibrosis, deterioration in cardiac function and complex arrhythmias,

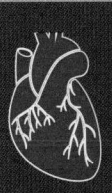

including non-sustained ventricular tachycardia, hypertension and stroke. Patients with CSAS have a worse prognosis than similar patients without CSAS.

Palpitations

These represent an increased awareness of the normal heart beat or the sensation of slow, rapid or irregular heart rhythms. The most common arrhythmias felt as palpitations are premature ectopic beats and paroxysmal tachycardias. A useful trick is to ask patients to tap out the rate and rhythm of their palpitations, as the different arrhythmias have different characteristics:

- **Premature beats (ectopics)** are felt by the patient as a pause followed by a forceful beat. This is because premature beats are usually followed by a pause before the next normal beat, as the heart resets itself. The next beat is more forceful, as the heart has had a longer diastolic period and therefore is filled with more blood before this beat.
- **Paroxysmal tachycardias** (see p. 1057) are felt as a sudden, racing heart beat.
- **Bradycardias** (see p. 1052) may be appreciated as slow, regular, heavy or forceful beats. Most often, however, they are simply not sensed. All palpitations can be graded by the NYHA cardiac status (see **Box 30.23**).

Syncope

Syncope is a transient loss of consciousness due to inadequate cerebral blood flow. The cardiovascular causes are listed in **Box 30.6**.

Vascular

- **A vasovagal attack** is a simple faint and is the most common cause of syncope. The mechanism begins with peripheral vasodilation and venous pooling of blood, leading to a reduction in the amount of blood returned to the heart. The near-empty heart responds by contracting vigorously, which, in turn, stimulates mechanoreceptors (stretch receptors) in the inferoposterior wall of the left ventricle. These, in turn, trigger reflexes via the central nervous system, which act to reduce ventricular stretch (i.e. further vasodilation and sometimes profound bradycardia), but this causes a drop in blood pressure and therefore syncope. These episodes are usually associated with a prodrome of dizziness, nausea, sweating, tinnitus, yawning and a sinking feeling. Recovery occurs within a few seconds, especially if the patient lies down.
- **Postural (orthostatic) hypotension** is a drop in systolic blood pressure of 20 mmHg or more on standing from a sitting or lying position. Usually, reflex vasoconstriction prevents a drop in pressure, but if this is absent or the patient is fluid-depleted or on vasodilating or diuretic drugs, hypotension occurs.

- **Postprandial hypotension** is a drop in systolic blood pressure of 20 mmHg or more, or the systolic blood pressure drops from over 100 mmHg to below 90 mmHg within 2 hours of eating. The mechanism is unknown but may involve pooling of blood in the splanchnic vessels. In normal people, this elicits a homeostatic response via activation of baroreceptors and the sympathetic system, peripheral vasoconstriction and an increase in cardiac output.
- **Micturition syncope** refers to loss of consciousness while passing urine.
- **Carotid sinus syncope** occurs when there is an exaggerated vagal response to carotid sinus stimulation, provoked by wearing a tight collar, looking upwards or turning the head.

Obstructive

The obstructive cardiac causes listed in **Box 30.6** all lead to syncope due to restriction of blood flow from the heart into the rest of the circulation, or between the different chambers of the heart.

Arrhythmias

Stokes–Adams attacks (see p. 1055) are a sudden loss of consciousness unrelated to posture and caused by intermittent high-grade AV block, profound bradycardia or ventricular standstill. The patient falls to the ground without warning, and is pale and deeply unconscious. The pulse is usually very slow or absent. After a few seconds the patient flushes brightly and recovers consciousness as the pulse quickens. Often there are no sequelae but patients may injure themselves during falls. Occasionally, a generalized convulsion may occur if the period of cerebral hypoxia is prolonged, leading to a misdiagnosis of epilepsy.

Fatigue

Fatigue may be a symptom of inadequate systemic perfusion in heart failure. Other contributing factors may include:
- poor sleep
- side-effects of medication, particularly beta-blockers
- electrolyte imbalance caused by diuretic therapy
- a systemic manifestation of infection, such as endocarditis.

Peripheral oedema

Heart failure results in salt and water retention due to renal underperfusion and consequent activation of the renin–angiotensin–aldosterone system (see p. 1346). This leads to dependent pitting oedema.

Further reading

Brignole M, Moya A, de Lange FJ et al. 2018 ESC Guidelines for the diagnosis and management of syncope. *Eur Heart J* 2018; 39:1883–1948.
National Institute for Health and Care Excellence. *NICE Clinical Guideline 109: Transient Loss of Consciousness ('Blackouts') in Over-16s.* NICE 2014; https://www.nice.org.uk/guidance/cg109.

? Box 30.6 Cardiovascular causes of syncope

Vascular
- Neurocardiogenic (vasovagal)
- Postural hypotension
- Postprandial hypotension
- Micturition syncope
- Carotid sinus syncope

Obstructive
- Aortic stenosis
- Hypertrophic cardiomyopathy
- Pulmonary stenosis
- Tetralogy of Fallot

- Pulmonary hypertension/embolism
- Atrial myxoma/thrombus
- Defective prosthetic valve

Arrhythmias
- Rapid tachycardias
- Profound bradycardias (Stokes–Adams)
- Significant pauses (in rhythm)
- Artificial pacemaker failure

Examination of the cardiovascular system

General examination

General features of the patient's wellbeing should be noted, as well as the presence of conjunctival pallor, obesity, jaundice and cachexia.

- **Clubbing** (see p. 937) is seen in congenital cyanotic heart disease, particularly Fallot's tetralogy, and also in 10% of patients with subacute infective endocarditis.

- **Splinter haemorrhages** are small, subungual linear haemorrhages that are frequently due to trauma but also seen in infective endocarditis.
- **Cyanosis** is a dusky blue discoloration of the skin (particularly at the extremities) or of the mucous membranes when the capillary oxygen saturation is below 85%. **Central cyanosis** (see p. 937) is seen with shunting of deoxygenated venous blood into the systemic circulation, as in the presence of a right-to-left heart shunt. **Peripheral cyanosis** is seen in the hands and feet, which are cold. It occurs in conditions associated with peripheral vasoconstriction and stasis of blood in the extremities, leading to increased peripheral oxygen extraction. Such conditions include congestive heart failure, circulatory shock, exposure to cold temperatures and abnormalities of the peripheral circulation, such as Raynaud's (see p. 1131).

Arterial pulse

The first pulse to be examined is the right radial pulse. A delayed femoral pulsation occurs because of a proximal stenosis, particularly of the aorta (coarctation).

Rate

The pulse rate should be between 60 and 80 beats per minute (b.p.m.) when an adult patient is lying quietly in bed.

Rhythm

The rhythm is regular, except for a slight quickening in early inspiration and a slowing in expiration (sinus arrhythmia).
- **Premature beats** occur as occasional or repeated irregularities superimposed on a regular pulse rhythm. Similarly, intermittent heart block is revealed by occasional beats dropped from an otherwise regular rhythm.
- **Atrial fibrillation** produces an 'irregularly irregular' pulse. This irregular pattern persists when the pulse quickens in response to exercise, in contrast to pulse irregularity due to ectopic beats, which usually disappears on exercise.

Character

- **Carotid pulsations** are not normally apparent on inspection of the neck but may be visible (Corrigan's sign) in conditions associated with a large-volume pulse, including high-output states (such as thyrotoxicosis, anaemia or fever), and in aortic regurgitation.
- A **'collapsing' or 'water hammer' pulse** (Fig. 30.10) is a large-volume pulse characterized by a short duration with a brisk rise and fall. This is best appreciated by palpating the radial artery with the palmar aspect of four fingers while elevating the patient's arm above the level of the heart. A collapsing pulse is characteristic of aortic valvular regurgitation or a persistent ductus arteriosus.
- A **small-volume pulse** is seen in cardiac failure, shock and obstructive valvular or vascular disease. It may also be present during tachyarrhythmias.
- A **plateau pulse** (see Fig. 30.10) is small in volume and slow in rising to a peak; it is due to aortic stenosis.
- An **alternating pulse** (**pulsus alternans**) (see Fig. 30.10) is characterized by regular alternate beats that are weak and strong. It is a feature of severe myocardial failure and is due to the prolonged recovery time of damaged myocardium; it indicates a very poor prognosis. It is easily noticed when taking the blood pressure because the systolic pressure may vary from beat to beat by as much as 50 mmHg.

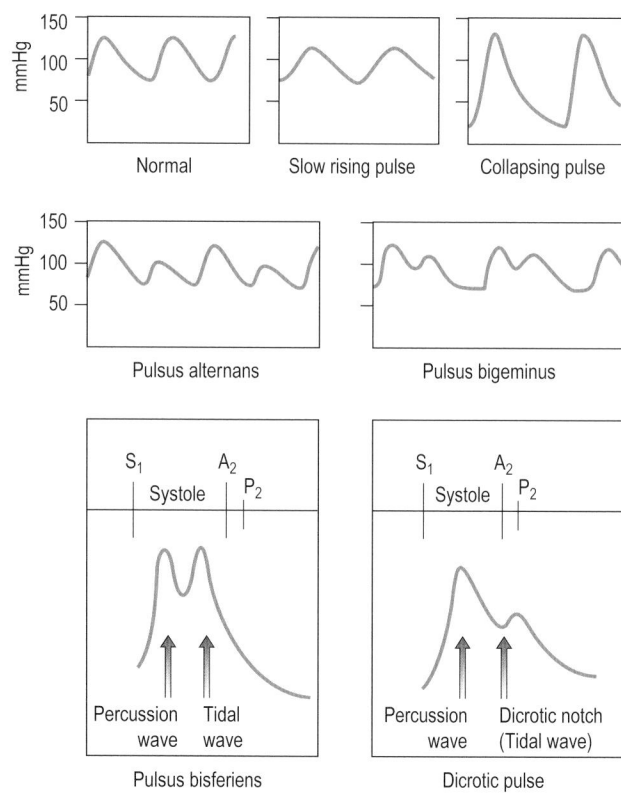

Fig. 30.10 Arterial waveforms. A_2, aortic component of the second heart sound; P_2, pulmonary component of the second heart sound; S_1, first heart sound.

- A **bigeminal pulse** (**pulsus bigeminus**) (see **Fig. 30.10**) is caused by a premature ectopic beat following every sinus beat. The rhythm is not regular because every weak pulse is premature.
- **Pulsus bisferiens** (see **Fig. 30.10**) is found in hypertrophic cardiomyopathy and in mixed aortic valve disease (regurgitation combined with stenosis). The first systolic wave is the 'percussion' wave, produced by transmission of the left ventricular pressure in early systole. The second peak is the 'tidal' wave, caused by recoil of the vascular bed. This normally happens in diastole (the dicrotic wave), but when the left ventricle empties slowly or is obstructed and cannot empty completely, the tidal wave occurs in late systole. The result is a palpable double pulse.
- A **dicrotic pulse** (see **Fig. 30.10**) results from an accentuated dicrotic wave. It occurs in sepsis and hypovolaemic shock, and after aortic valve replacement.
- **Paradoxical pulse** is a misnomer, as it is actually an exaggeration of the normal pattern. In normal subjects, the systolic pressure and the pulse pressure (the difference between the systolic and diastolic blood pressures) fall during inspiration. The normal fall of systolic pressure is less than 10 mmHg, and this can be measured using a sphygmomanometer. It is due to increased pulmonary intravascular volume during inspiration. In severe airflow limitation (especially severe asthma), there is an increased negative intrathoracic pressure on inspiration, which enhances the normal fall in blood pressure. In patients with cardiac tamponade, the fluid in the pericardium increases the intrapericardial pressure, thereby impeding diastolic filling of the heart. The normal inspiratory increase in venous return to the right ventricle is at the expense of the left ventricle, as both ventricles are confined by the accumulated pericardial fluid within the pericardial space. Paradox can occur via a similar mechanism in constrictive pericarditis but is less common.

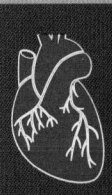

Box 30.7 Taking the blood pressure

Use a properly calibrated machine.
1. Take the blood pressure in the (right) arm with the patient relaxed and comfortable.
2. Wrap the sphygmomanometer cuff around the upper arm and place the inflation bag over the brachial artery.
3. Inflate the cuff until the pressure exceeds the arterial pressure – when the radial pulse is no longer palpable.
4. Position the diaphragm of the stethoscope over the brachial artery just below the cuff.
5. Slowly reduce the cuff pressure until sounds (Korotkoff sounds) can be heard (*phase 1*). This is the systolic pressure.
6. Allow the pressure to fall further until the Korotkoff sounds suddenly become muffled (*phase 4*).
7. Allow the pressure to fall still further until the sounds disappear (*phase 5*).
8. The diastolic pressure is usually taken as *phase 5* because this phase is more reproducible and nearer to the intravascular diastolic pressure. The Korotkoff sounds may disappear (*phase 2*) and reappear (*phase 3*) between the systolic and diastolic pressures. Do not mistake *phase 2* for the diastolic pressure or *phase 3* for the systolic pressure.

Blood pressure

The peak systemic arterial blood pressure is produced by transmission of left ventricular systolic pressure. Vascular tone and an intact aortic valve maintain the diastolic blood pressure. Instructions for taking the blood pressure are outlined in **Box 30.7**.

Jugular venous pressure

There are no valves between the internal jugular vein and the right atrium. Observation of the column of blood in the internal jugular system is therefore a good measure of right atrial pressure. The external jugular cannot be relied on because of its valves and because it may be obstructed by the fascial and muscular layers through which it passes; it can be used only if typical venous pulsation is seen, indicating no obstruction to flow.

Measurement of jugular venous pressure

See **Box 30.8**.

Elevation of the jugular venous pressure (JVP) occurs in *heart failure*. An elevated JVP also occurs in:
- constrictive pericarditis and cardiac tamponade (increases in inspiration – *Kussmaul's sign*)
- renal disease with salt and water retention
- over-transfusion or excessive infusion of fluids
- congestive cardiac failure
- superior vena cava obstruction.
 A reduced JVP occurs in hypovolaemia.

Jugular venous pressure wave

This consists of three peaks and two troughs (**Fig. 30.11**). The peaks are described as *a*, *c* and *v* waves and the troughs are known as *x* and *y* descents:
- *The a wave* is produced by atrial systole and is increased with right ventricular hypertrophy secondary to pulmonary hypertension or pulmonary stenosis. Giant cannon waves occur in complete heart block and ventricular tachycardia.
- *The x descent* occurs when atrial contraction finishes.
- *The c wave* occurs during the *x* descent and is due to transmission of right ventricular systolic pressure before the tricuspid valve closes.
- *The v wave* occurs with venous return filling the right atrium. Giant *v* waves occur in tricuspid regurgitation.

Box 30.8 Measurement of jugular venous pressure (JVP)

- The patient is positioned at about 45 degrees to the horizontal (between 30 and 60 degrees), wherever the top of the venous pulsation can be seen in a good light.
- The JVP is measured as the vertical distance between the manubriosternal angle and the top of the venous column.
- The normal JVP is usually <3 cmH$_2$O, which is equivalent to a right atrial pressure of 8 cmH$_2$O when measured with reference to a point midway between the anterior and posterior surfaces of the chest.
- The venous pulsations are not usually palpable (except for the forceful venous distension associated with tricuspid regurgitation).
- Compression of the right upper abdomen causes a temporary increase in venous pressure and makes the jugular venous pulse more visible (hepatojugular reflux).

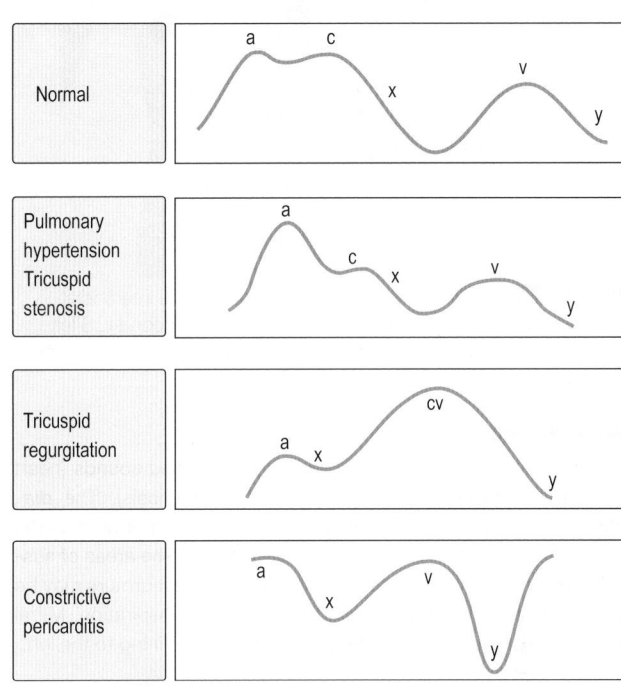

Fig. 30.11 Jugular venous waveforms.

- *The y descent* follows the *v* wave when the tricuspid valve opens. A steep *y* descent is seen in constrictive pericarditis and tricuspid incompetence.

Precordium

- With the patient at 45 degrees, the cardiac apex is located in the fifth intercostal space mid-clavicular line. Left ventricular dilation will displace the apex downwards and laterally. It may be impalpable in patients with emphysema, obesity, or pericardial or pleural effusions.
- *A tapping apex* is a palpable first sound and occurs in mitral stenosis.
- *A vigorous apex* may be present in diseases with volume overload, e.g. aortic regurgitation.
- *A heaving (sustained) apex* may occur with left ventricular hypertrophy – aortic stenosis, systemic hypertension and hypertrophic cardiomyopathy.
- *A double pulsation* may occur in hypertrophic cardiomyopathy.
- *A sustained left parasternal heave* occurs with right ventricular hypertrophy or left atrial enlargement.
- *A palpable thrill* may be felt overlying an abnormal cardiac valve, e.g. systolic thrill with aortic stenosis.

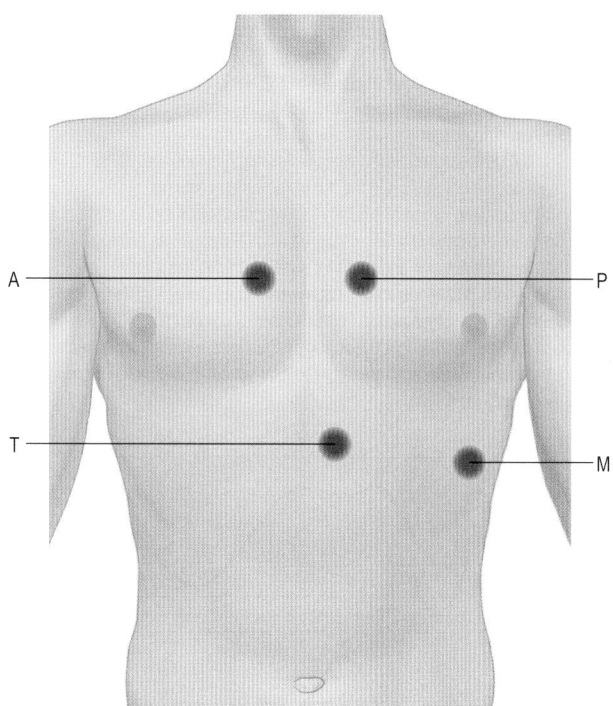

Fig. 30.12 Heart auscultation. Aortic area second intercostal space (ICS) right sternal edge (**A**). Pulmonary area second ICS left sternal edge (**P**). Mitral area fifth ICS mid-clavicular line (**M**). Tricuspid area fifth to fifth ICS left sternal edge (**T**).

Auscultation

The **bell** of the stethoscope is used for low-pitched sounds (heart sounds and mid-diastolic murmur in mitral stenosis). The **diaphragm** is used for high-pitched sounds (systolic murmurs, aortic regurgitation, ejection clicks and opening snaps). The areas of auscultation are shown in **Fig. 30.12**. Left-sided valve murmurs may be more prominent in expiration and right-sided in inspiration. Mitral murmurs may be more audible with the patient reclining to the left.

First heart sound (S1)

This is due to mitral and tricuspid valve closure. A loud S1 occurs in thin people, hyperdynamic circulation, tachycardias and mild to moderate mitral stenosis. A soft S1 occurs in obesity, emphysema, pericardial effusion, severe calcific mitral stenosis, mitral or tricuspid regurgitation, heart failure, shock, bradycardias and first-degree block.

Second heart sound (S2)

This is due to aortic and pulmonary valve closure. Physiological splitting of S2 occurs during inspiration in children and young adults.

Third and fourth heart sounds

These are pathological:
- *A third heart sound ('volume overload')* is due to rapid ventricular filling and is present in significant heart failure.
- *A fourth heart sound (pressure overload)* occurs in late diastole and is associated with atrial contraction. Causes include aortic stenosis, severe systemic hypertension and left ventricular outflow obstruction, as in hypertrophic cardiomyopathy, i.e. causes of significant left ventricular hypertrophy.

  Singly or together, they will produce a gallop rhythm.

Heart murmurs

These are due to turbulent blood flow and occur in hyperdynamic states or with abnormal valves. (Listen online on Student Consult.)

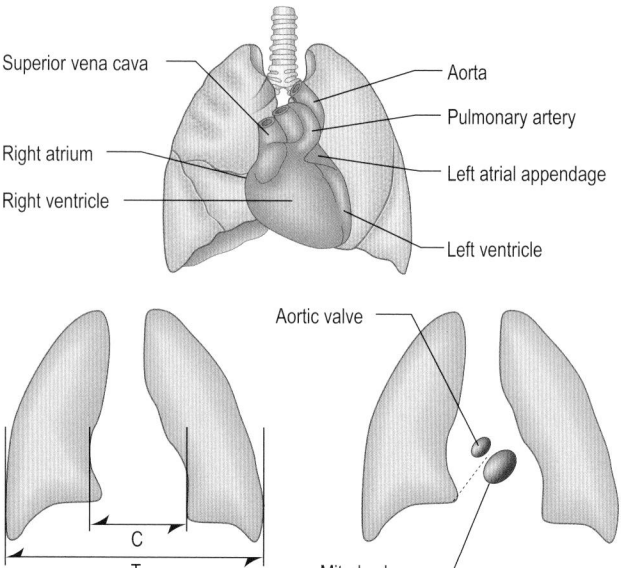

Fig. 30.13 The heart silhouette as it is seen on the chest X-ray. Measurements of the cardiothoracic ratio (CTR) and the location of the cardiac valves are also shown. The dotted line is an arbitrary line from the left hilum to the right cardiophrenic angle; a calcified aortic valve is seen above this line. $CTR = (C/T) \times 100\%$; normal CTR <50%.

Innocent or flow murmurs are soft, early systolic, short and non-radiating. They are heard frequently in children and young adults. Heart murmurs can be graded:
- 1/6: very faint; not always heard in all positions
- 2/6: quiet but not difficult to hear
- 3/6: moderately loud
- 4/6: loud with or without thrills
- 5/6: very loud with or without thrills; heard with the stethoscope partly off the chest
- 6/6: with or without thrills; heard with the stethoscope completely off the chest.

  The individual murmurs are discussed under valve disease (see p. 1091).

Cardiac investigations

Blood tests

These include:
- routine haematology
- serum creatinine and electrolytes
- liver biochemistry
- cardiac enzymes (troponin; creatine kinase, aspartate aminotransferase (AST) and lactate dehydrogenase (LDH) may also be elevated)
- thyroid function
- B-type natriuretic peptides (BNP).

Chest X-ray

Ideally, this is taken in the postero-anterior (PA) direction at maximum inspiration with the heart close to the X-ray film to minimize magnification with respect to the thorax. The cardiac structures and great vessels that can be seen are indicated in **Fig. 30.13**. An anteroposterior (AP) view is often taken in the emergency setting.

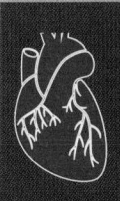

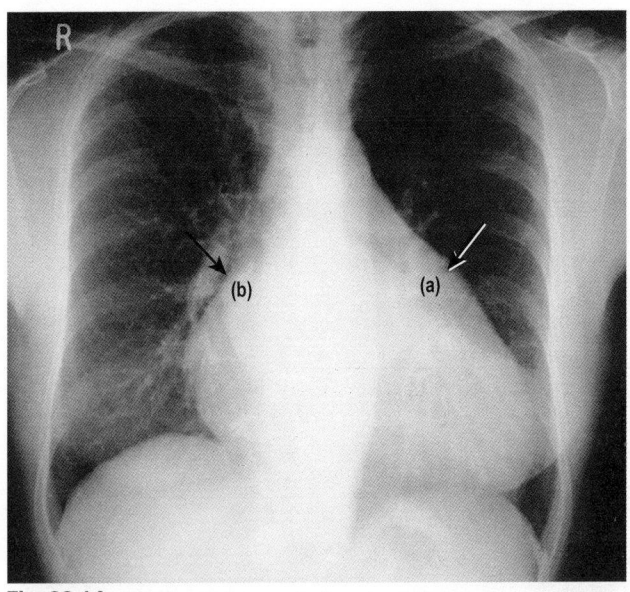

Fig. 30.14 A plain postero-anterior chest X-ray of a patient with mixed mitral valve disease. The left atrium (a) is markedly enlarged. Note the large bulge on the left heart border (left atrium). The 'double shadow' border of the right and left atria (b) is on the right side of the heart. There is cardiac (left ventricular) enlargement due to mitral regurgitation.

Heart size

Heart size can be reliably assessed only from the PA chest film. The maximum transverse diameter of the heart is compared with the maximum transverse diameter of the thorax measured from the inside of the ribs (the cardiothoracic ratio, CTR). The CTR is usually less than 50%, except in neonates, infants, athletes and patients with skeletal abnormalities such as scoliosis and funnel chest. A transverse cardiac diameter of more than 15.5 cm is abnormal. Pericardial effusion or cardiac dilation causes an increase in the ratio.

A **pericardial effusion** produces a globular heart (see **Fig. 30.120**). This enlargement may occur quite suddenly and, unlike in heart failure, there is no associated change in the pulmonary vasculature. The echocardiogram is more specific (see **Fig. 30.121**).

Certain patterns of specific chamber enlargement may be seen on the chest X-ray:

- **Left atrial dilation** leads to prominence of the left atrial appendage and a straightening or convex bulging of the upper left heart border, a double atrial shadow to the right of the sternum, and splaying of the carina because a large left atrium elevates the left main bronchus (**Fig. 30.14**). On a lateral chest X-ray, an enlarged left atrium bulges backwards, impinging on the oesophagus.
- **Left ventricular enlargement** causes an increase in the CTR and smooth elongation and increased convexity of the left heart border.
- **Right atrial enlargement** results in projection of the right border of the heart into the right lower lung field.
- **Right ventricular enlargement** causes an increase in the CTR and upward displacement of the apex of the heart because the enlarging right ventricle pushes the left ventricle leftwards, upwards and eventually backwards. Differentiation of left from right ventricular enlargement may be difficult using the shape of the left heart border alone, but the lateral view shows enlargement anteriorly for the right ventricle and posteriorly for the left ventricle.
- **Ascending aortic dilation or enlargement** is seen as a prominence of the aortic shadow to the right of the mediastinum between the right atrium and superior vena cava.

- **Dissection of the ascending aorta** is seen as a widening of the mediastinum on chest X-ray but an ultrasound/magnetic resonance imaging (MRI) should be performed.
- **Enlargement of the pulmonary artery** in pulmonary hypertension, pulmonary artery stenosis and left-to-right shunts produces a prominent bulge on the left-hand border of the mediastinum below the aortic knuckle.

Calcification

Calcification in the cardiovascular system occurs because of tissue degeneration. Calcification is visible on a lateral or a penetrated PA film but is best studied with computed tomography (CT) scanning.

Lung fields

- **Pulmonary plethora** results from left-to-right shunts (e.g. atrial or ventricular septal defects). It is seen as a general increase in the vascularity of the lung fields and as an increase in the size of hilar vessels (e.g. in the right lower lobe artery), which normally should not exceed 16 mm in diameter.
- **Pulmonary oligaemia** is a paucity of vascular markings and a reduction in the width of the arteries. It occurs in situations where there is reduced pulmonary blood flow, such as pulmonary embolism, severe pulmonary stenosis and Fallot's tetralogy.
- **Pulmonary hypertension** may result from pulmonary embolism, chronic lung disease or chronic left heart disease, e.g. left ventricular failure or mitral valve disease such as shunts due to a ventricular septal defect or mitral valve stenosis. In addition to the X-ray features of these conditions, the pulmonary arteries are prominent close to the hila but are reduced in size (pruned) in the peripheral lung fields. This pattern is usually symmetrical. Normal pulmonary capillary pressure is 5–14 mmHg at rest. Mild pulmonary capillary hypertension (15–20 mmHg) produces isolated dilation of the upper zone vessels.
- **Interstitial oedema** occurs when the pressure is between 21 and 30 mmHg. This manifests as fluid collections in the interlobar fissures, interlobular septa **(Kerley B lines)** and pleural spaces. This gives rise to indistinctness of the hilar regions and haziness of the lung fields.
- **Alveolar oedema** occurs when the pressure exceeds 30 mmHg, appearing as areas of consolidation and mottling of the lung fields (**Fig. 30.15**) and pleural effusions. Patients with longstanding elevation of the pulmonary capillary pressure have reactive thickening of the pulmonary arteriolar intima, which protects the alveoli from pulmonary oedema. Thus, in these patients, the pulmonary venous pressure may increase to well above 30 mmHg before frank pulmonary oedema develops.

Electrocardiography

The ECG is a recording of the electrical activity of the heart. It is the vector sum of the depolarization and repolarization potentials of all myocardial cells (see **Fig. 30.2**). At the body surface, these generate potential differences of about 1 mV, and fluctuations in these potentials create the familiar P–QRS–T pattern. At rest, the intracellular voltage of the myocardium is polarized at −90 mV compared with that of the extracellular space. This diastolic voltage difference occurs because of the high intracellular potassium concentration, which is maintained by the sodium–potassium pump despite the free membrane permeability to potassium. Depolarization of cardiac cells occurs when there is a sudden increase in the permeability of the membrane to sodium. Sodium rushes into the cell and the negative resting voltage is lost (phase 0 on **Fig. 30.38**). The depolarization of a myocardial cell causes the depolarization of adjacent cells and, in the healthy heart, the entire myocardium is depolarized

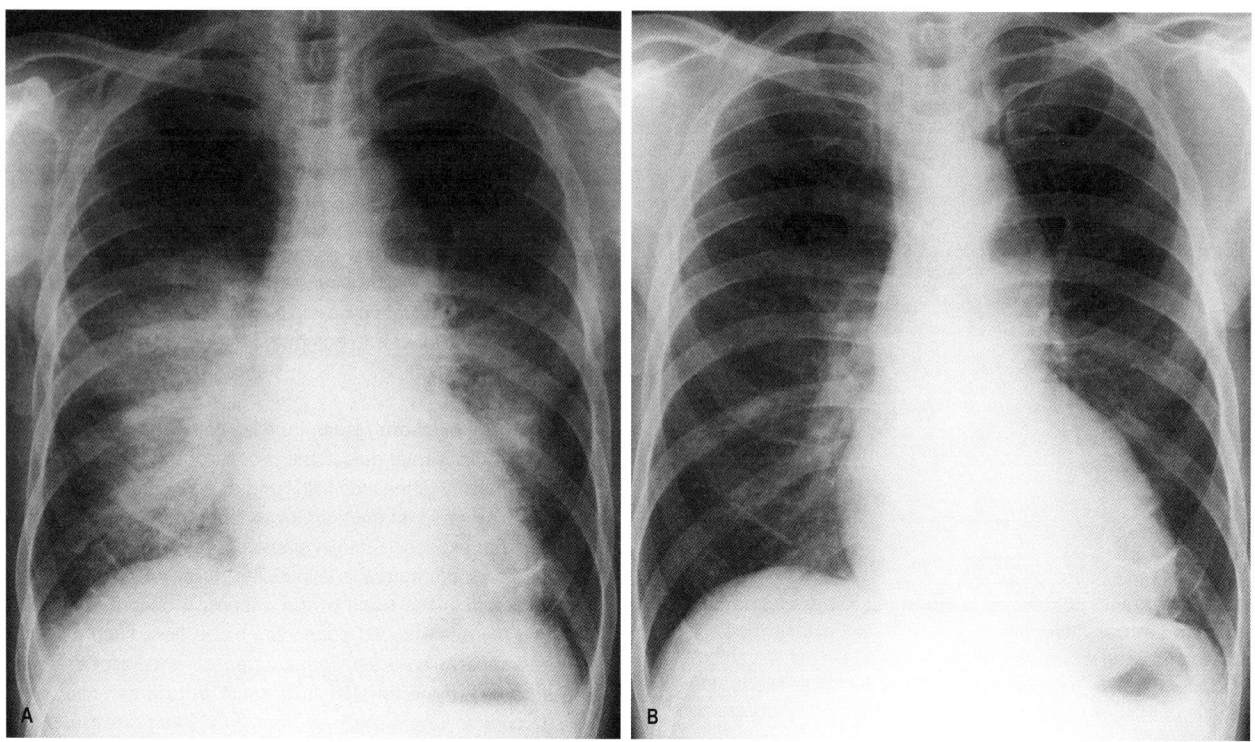

Fig. 30.15 **Acute pulmonary oedema: chest X-rays taken before and after treatment.**
(A) The X-ray taken when the oedema was present demonstrates hilar haziness, Kerley B lines, upper lobe venous engorgement, and fluid in the right horizontal interlobar fissure. **(B)** These abnormalities are resolved on the film taken after successful treatment.

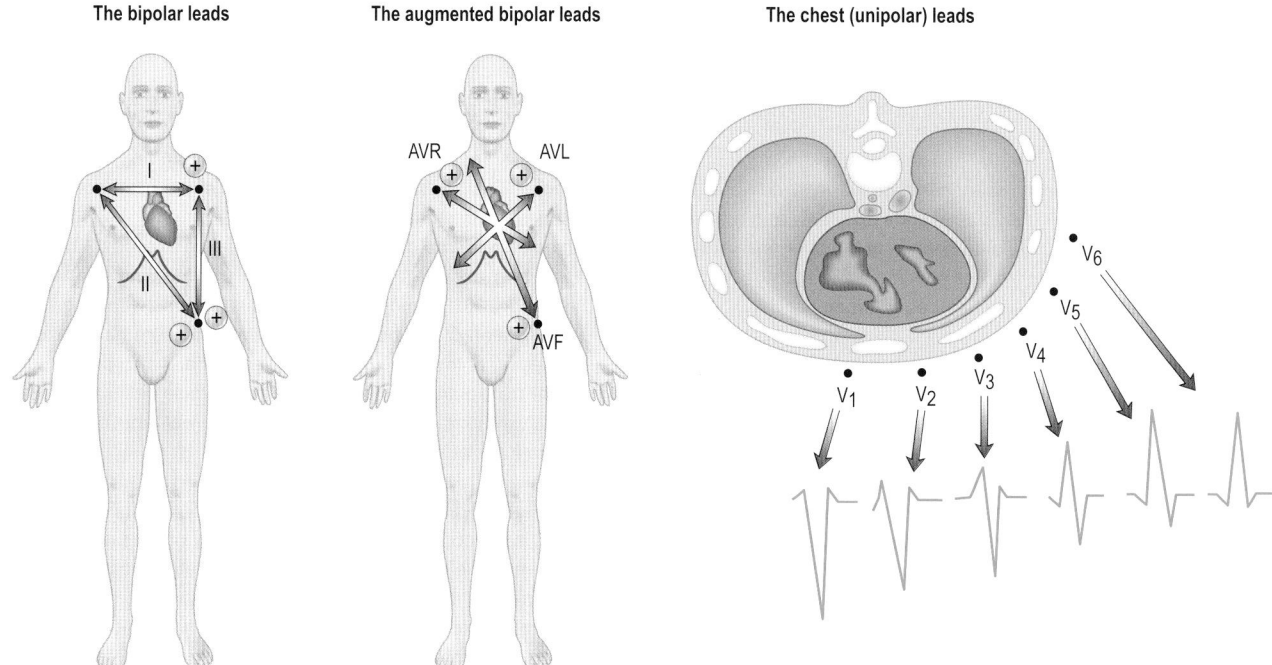

The bipolar leads   **The augmented bipolar leads**   **The chest (unipolar) leads**

Fig. 30.16 **The connections or directions that comprise the 12-lead electrocardiogram.**

in a coordinated fashion. During repolarization, cellular electrolyte balance is slowly restored (phases 1, 2 and 3). Slow diastolic depolarization (phase 4) follows until the threshold potential is reached. Another action potential then follows.

The ECG is recorded from two or more simultaneous points of skin contact (electrodes). When cardiac activation proceeds towards the positive contact, an upward deflection is produced on the ECG. Correct representation of a three-dimensional spatial vector requires recordings from three mutually perpendicular (orthogonal) axes. The shape of the human torso does not make this easy, so the practical ECG records 12 projections of the vector, called 'leads' (**Fig. 30.16**).

Six of the leads are obtained by recording voltages from the limbs (I, II, III, AVR, AVL and AVF). The other six leads record potentials between points on the chest surface and an average of the three limbs: RA, LA and LL. These are designated V_1–V_6 and aim to select activity from the right ventricle (V_1–V_2), interventricular septum (V_3–V_4) and left ventricle (V_5–V_6). Note that leads AVR and V_1 are oriented towards the cavity of the heart, leads II, III and AVF face the inferior surface, and leads I, AVL and V_6 face the lateral wall of the left ventricle. A V_4 on the right side of the chest (V_4R) is occasionally useful (e.g. for the diagnosis of right ventricular infarction).

Most ECG machines are simultaneous three-channel recorders, with output given either as a continuous strip or with automatic channel switching. Many ECG machines also analyse the recordings and print the analysis on the record. Usually, the machine interpretation is correct but many arrhythmias still defy automatic analysis.

ECG waveform

The shape of the normal ECG waveform (**Fig. 30.17**) has similarities, whatever the orientation. The first deflection is caused by atrial depolarization; it is a low-amplitude, slow deflection called a ***P wave***. The ***QRS complex*** reflects ventricular activation or depolarization, and is sharper and larger in amplitude than the P wave. An initial downward deflection is called the ***Q wave***. An initial upward deflection is called an ***R wave***. The ***S wave*** is the last part of ventricular activation. The ***T wave*** is another slow and low-amplitude deflection that results from ventricular repolarization.

The ***PR interval*** is the length of time from the start of the P wave to the start of the QRS complex. It is the time taken for activation to pass from the sinus node, through the atrium, AV node and His–Purkinje system, to the ventricle.

The ***QT interval*** extends from the start of the QRS complex to the end of the T wave. This interval represents the time taken to depolarize and repolarize the ventricular myocardium. The QT interval varies greatly with heart rate and is often represented as a corrected QT interval (or QTc) for a given heart rate. There are a number of formulae for derivation of QTc, but the most widely accepted are Bazett's formula and Fridericia's correction (**Box 30.9**).

An abnormally prolonged QTc can predispose to a risk of dangerous ventricular arrhythmias. Prolongation of the QT interval may be congenital or can occur in many acquired conditions (see **Box 30.18**).

The ***ST segment*** is the period between the end of the QRS complex and the start of the T wave. In the normal heart, all cells are depolarized by this phase of the ECG: that is, the ST segment represents ventricular repolarization.

A normal 12-lead ECG is shown in **Fig. 30.18**, and the normal values for the electrocardiographic intervals are indicated in **Box 30.9**. Leads that face the lateral wall of the left ventricle have predominantly positive deflections, and leads looking into the ventricular

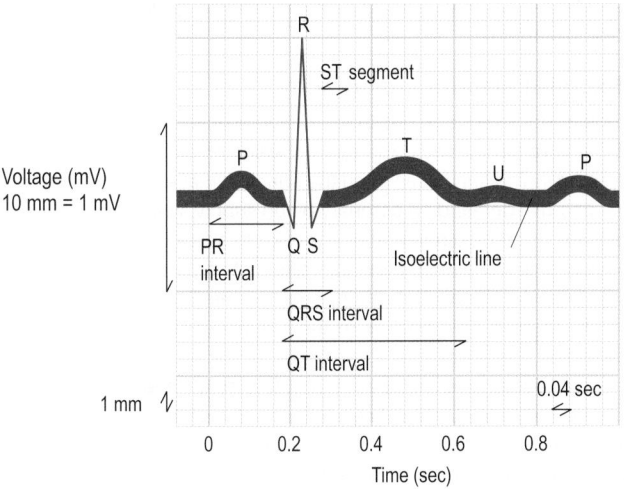

Fig. 30.17 The waves and elaboration of the normal electrocardiogram.

i Box 30.9 Normal ECG intervals	
Parameter	**Interval**
P wave duration	≤0.12 sec
PR interval	0.12–0.20 sec
QRS complex duration	≤0.10 sec
Corrected QT (QTc)	≤0.44 sec in males
	≤0.46 sec in females
$QT_{cB} = QT\sqrt[2]{(R-R)}$	Bazett's square root formula
$QT_{cF} = QT\sqrt[3]{(R-R)}$	Fridericia's cube root formula

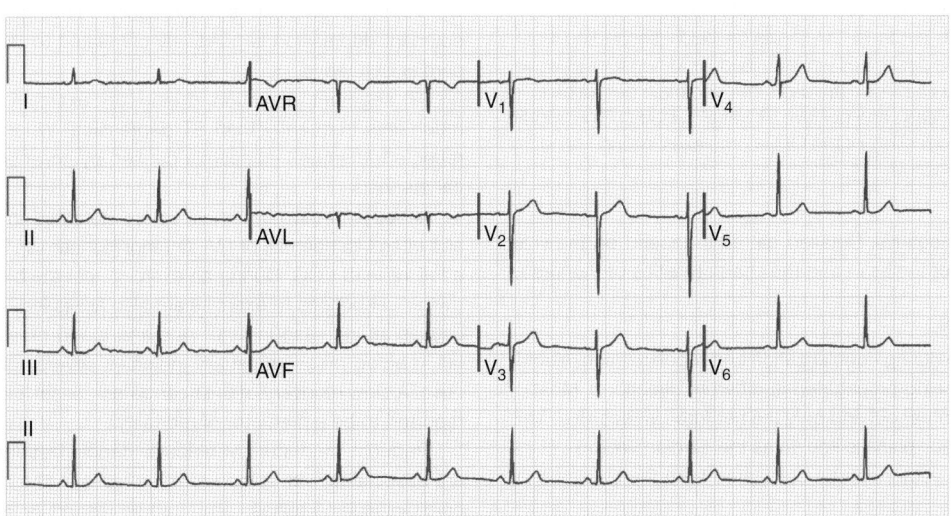

Fig. 30.18 A normal 12-lead electrocardiogram.

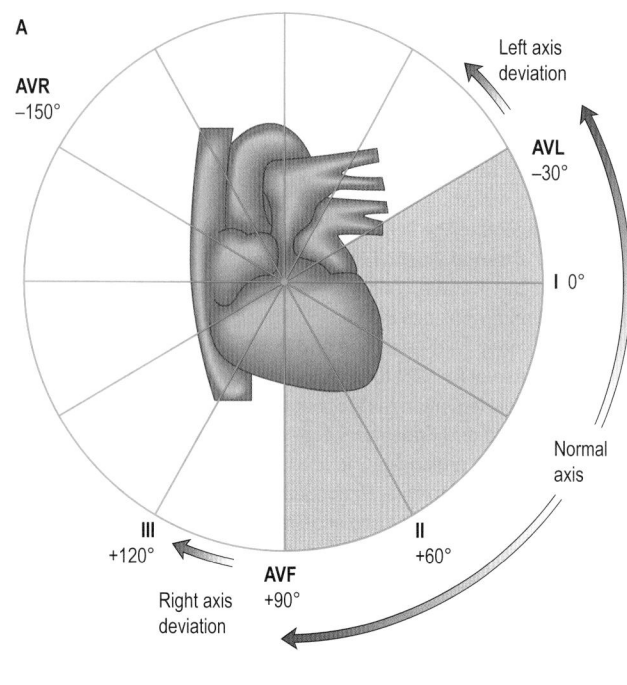

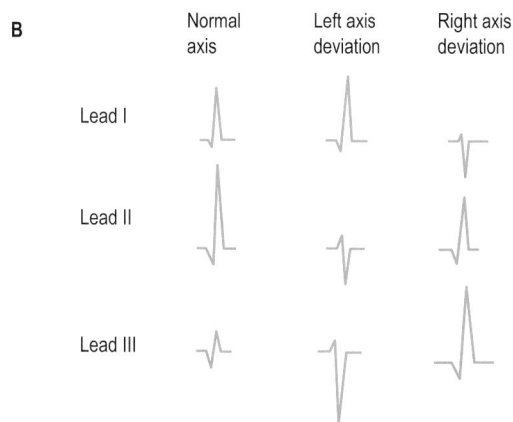

Fig. 30.19 Cardiac vectors. (A) The hexaxial reference system, illustrating the six leads in the frontal plane; for example, lead I is 0°, lead II is +60° and lead III is +120°. **(B)** Calculating the direction of the cardiac vector. In the first column, the QRS complex with zero net amplitude (i.e. when the positive and negative deflections are equal) is seen in lead III. The mean QRS vector is therefore perpendicular to lead III and is either −150° or +30°. Lead I is positive, so the axis must be +30°, which is normal. In left axis deviation (second column) the main deflection is positive (R wave) in lead I and negative (S wave) in lead III. In right axis deviation (third column) the main deflection is negative (S wave) in lead I and positive (R wave) in lead III. The frontal plane QRS axis is normal only if the QRS complexes in leads I and II are predominantly positive.

cavity are usually negative. Detailed patterns depend on the size, shape and rhythm of the heart and the characteristics of the torso.

Cardiac vectors

At any point in time during depolarization and repolarization, electrical potentials are being propagated in different directions. Most of these cancel each other out and only the net force is recorded. This net force in the frontal plane is known as the cardiac vector.

The mean QRS vector can be calculated from the six standard leads (**Fig. 30.19**):

- **Normal:** between −30° and +90°

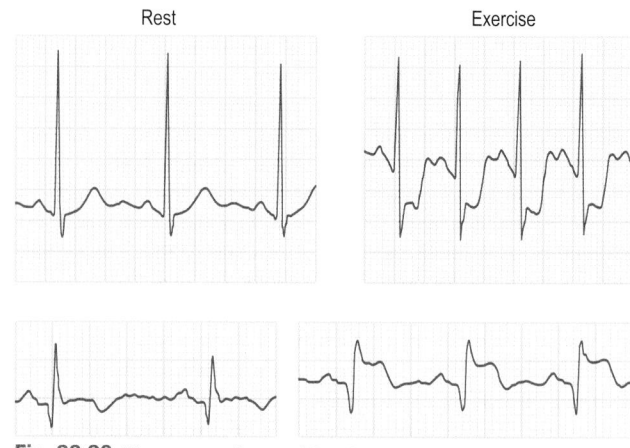

Fig. 30.20 Electrocardiographic changes during exercise testing. The upper traces show significant horizontal ST segment depression during exercise. The lower traces show ST elevation during exercise.

- **Left axis deviation:** between −30° and −90°
- **Right axis deviation:** between +90° and +150°.

Calculation of this vector is useful in the diagnosis of some cardiac disorders.

Exercise electrocardiography

This is less used than previously because of its low sensitivity. The ECG is recorded while the patient walks or runs on a motorized treadmill. The test is based on the principle that exercise increases myocardial demand on coronary blood supply, which may be inadequate during exercise, and at peak stress can result in relative myocardial ischaemia. Most exercise tests are performed according to a standardized method, such as the Bruce protocol. Normally, there is little change in the T wave or ST segment during exercise.

The patient's exercise capacity (the total time achieved) will depend on many factors; however, individuals who can exercise for less than 6 minutes generally have a poorer prognosis.

Myocardial ischaemia provoked by exertion results in ST segment depression (>1 mm) in leads facing the affected area. The form of ST segment depression provoked by ischaemia is characteristic: it either is planar or shows down-sloping depression (**Fig. 30.20**). Up-sloping depression is a non-specific finding. The degree of ST segment depression is positively correlated to the degree of myocardial ischaemia.

ST segment elevation during an exercise test is induced much less frequently than ST depression. When it does occur, it reflects transmural ischaemia caused by coronary spasm or critical stenosis.

Although most abnormalities are detected in lead V₅ (anterior and lateral ischaemia) or AVF (inferior ischaemia), it is best to record a full 12-lead ECG. During an exercise test the blood pressure and rhythm responses to exercise are also assessed. Exercise normally causes an increase in heart rate and blood pressure. A sustained fall in blood pressure usually indicates severe coronary artery disease. A slow recovery of the heart rate to basal levels has also been reported to be a predictor of mortality.

Frequent premature ventricular depolarizations during the test are associated with a long-term increase in the risk of death from cardiovascular causes, and further testing is required in these patients.

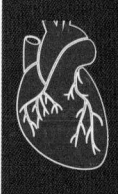

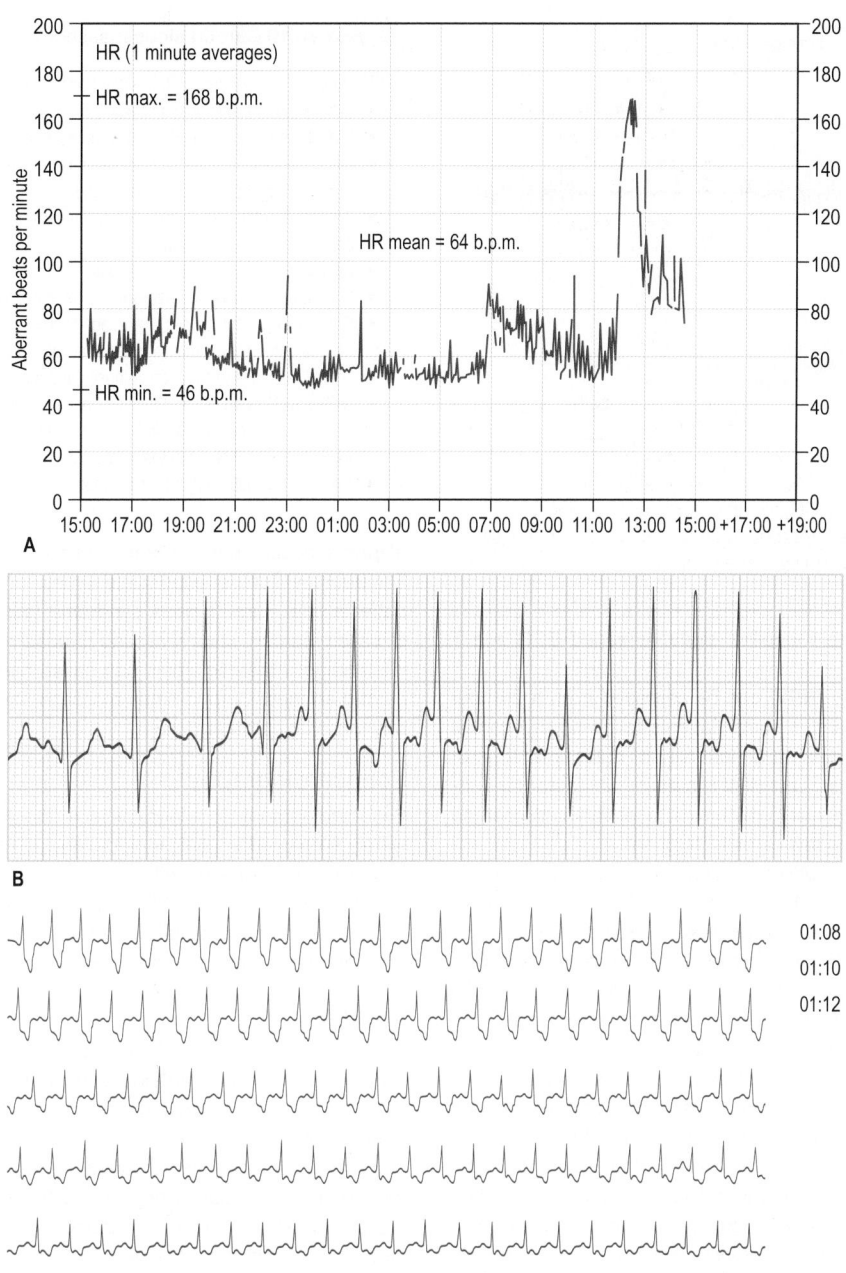

Fig. 30.21 Examples of Holter recordings. (A) A tachograph showing a sudden increase in heart rate (HR) between 11:00 and 13:00 h. **(B)** An ambulatory ECG record of the same patient, revealing supraventricular tachycardia. **(C)** An ambulatory ECG showing ST depression in a patient with silent myocardial ischaemia.

Twenty-four-hour ambulatory taped electrocardiography

This records transient changes, such as a brief paroxysm of tachycardia, an occasional pause in the rhythm or intermittent ST segment shifts (**Fig. 30.21**). A conventional 12-lead ECG is recorded in less than a minute and usually samples fewer than 20 complexes. In a 24-hour period, over 100 000 complexes are recorded. Such a large amount of data must be analysed by automatic or semi-automatic methods. This technique is called *Holter electrocardiography* after its inventor.

Event recording is another technique that is used to record less frequent arrhythmias. The patient is provided with a pocket-sized device that can record and store a short segment of the ECG. The device may be kept for several days or weeks until the arrhythmia is recorded. Most units of this kind will also allow transtelephonic ECG transmission so that the physician can determine the need for treatment or the continued need for monitoring.

A very small event recorder, known as an implantable loop recorder (ILR), can also be implanted subcutaneously, triggered by events or a magnet, and interrogated by the physician.

Other tests

Non-invasive methods that make use of digitalized Holter recordings to identify an increased risk of ventricular arrhythmias include

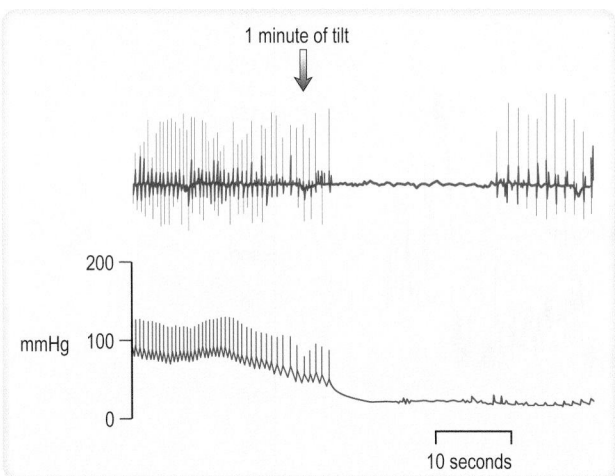

Fig. 30.22 Tilt test. The ECG (top trace) and arterial blood pressure (bottom trace) recorded during a tilt test. After 1 min of tilt, hypotension, bradycardia and syncope occur.

assessment of heart rate variability, signal-averaged ECG and T wave alternans.

- **Heart rate variability (HRV)** can be assessed from a 24-hour ECG. HRV is decreased in some patients following myocardial infarction and represents an abnormality of autonomic tone or cardiac responsiveness. Low HRV is a major risk factor for sudden death and ventricular arrhythmias in patients discharged from hospital following myocardial infarction.
- **Signal-averaged ECG (SAECG)** is a technique that requires amplification and averaging of abnormal low-amplitude signals that occur beyond the end of the QRS complex and extend well into the ST segment. These signals are therefore also known as late potentials and are too small to be detected on a surface ECG. They arise in areas of slow conduction in the myocardium, such as the border zone of an infarct, where re-entrant ventricular arrhythmias can originate.
- **T wave alternans (TWA)** is a valuable technique used as a non-invasive marker of susceptibility to ventricular arrhythmias and sudden cardiac death. TWA represents microvolt level changes in the morphology of the T waves in every other beat and can be detected during acute myocardial ischaemia using amplification techniques. Visible TWA on an ordinary surface ECG is quite a rare phenomenon, except in patients with long QT syndromes, particularly during emotion or exercise.

Tilt testing

Patients with suspected neurocardiogenic (vasovagal) syncope should be investigated by upright tilt testing. The patient is secured to a table that is tilted to +60 degrees to the vertical for 45 minutes or more. The ECG and blood pressure are monitored throughout. If neither symptoms nor signs develop, isoprenaline may be slowly infused or glyceryl trinitrate inhaled and the tilt repeated. A positive test results in hypotension, sometimes bradycardia (**Fig. 30.22**) and pre-syncope/syncope, and supports the diagnosis of neurocardiogenic syncope. If symptoms and signs appear, placing the patient flat can quickly reverse them. The effect of treatment can be evaluated by repeating the tilt test but it is not always reproducible. The overall sensitivity, specificity and reproducibility are low.

Carotid sinus massage

Carotid sinus massage (**Box 30.10**) may lead to asystole (>3 sec) and/or a fall in systolic blood pressure (>50 mmHg). This hypersensitive

Box 30.10 Carotid sinus massage

- Explain the procedure to the patient and obtain informed consent.
- Ensure that there is no significant carotid artery disease (carotid bruits).
- Provide continuous electrocardiographic monitoring.
- Place the patient in the supine position with the head slightly extended.
- Start with right carotid sinus massage.
- Apply firm rotary pressure to the carotid artery at the level of the third cervical vertebra for 5 sec.
- Alternatively, apply steady pressure.
- If there is no response, massage the left carotid sinus.
- Generally, right carotid sinus massage decreases the sinus node discharge, and left carotid sinus massage slows atrioventricular conduction.
- Do not massage both carotid sinuses at the same time.
- Single application of carotid sinus pressure may be effective in about 20–30% of patients with paroxysmal supraventricular tachycardias; multiple applications can terminate tachycardia in about 50% of patients.
- Asystole is a potential but rare complication.

response occurs in many of the normal (especially elderly) population but may also be responsible for loss of consciousness in some patients with carotid sinus syndrome (see p. 1052). In one-third of cases, carotid sinus massage is positive only when the patient is standing. Atherosclerosis can cause narrowing and stenosis of carotid arteries. Carotid sinus massage should thus be avoided in patients with carotid bruits.

Echocardiography

Echocardiography is a non-invasive diagnostic technique that is widely employed in clinical cardiology. It involves the use of ultrasound (either alone or with a contrast agent) to assess cardiac structure and function. A physician or technician performs the studies and a comprehensive examination takes 15–45 minutes. The ultrasound machines are either mobile on wheels or handheld.

Physics

Echocardiography uses transmitted ultrasound wavelengths of 1 mm or less, which correspond to frequencies of approximately 2 MHz or more (2 million cycles per second or more). At such high frequencies, the ultrasound waves can be focused into a 'beam' and aimed at a particular region of the heart. The waves are generated in very short bursts or pulses a few microseconds long by a crystal transducer, which also detects returning echoes and converts them into electrical signals.

When the handheld crystal transducer is placed on the body surface, the emitted ultrasound pulses encounter interfaces between various body tissues as they pass through the body. In crossing each interface, some of the wave energy is reflected, and if the beam path is approximately at right angles to the plane of the interface, the reflected waves return to the transducer as an echo. Since the velocity of sound in body tissues is almost constant (1550 m/s), the time delay for the echo to return measures the distance of the reflecting interface. Thus, if a single ultrasound pulse is transmitted, a series of echoes return, the first of which is from the closest interface.

Echocardiographic modalities
M-mode and two-dimensional echocardiography

M-mode echocardiography is a technique that details the changing motion of structures along the ultrasound beam with time. Thus, the motion of the interventricular septum during the cardiac cycle (either towards or away from the transducer placed on the chest wall) can be assessed and quantified. Stationary structures

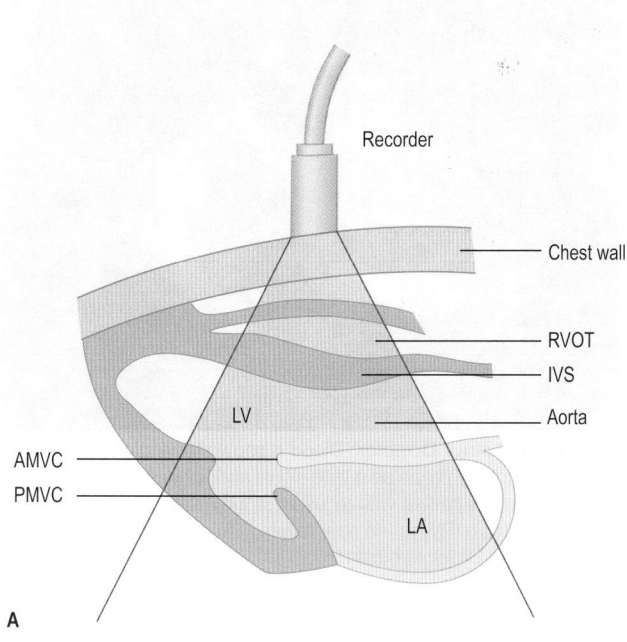

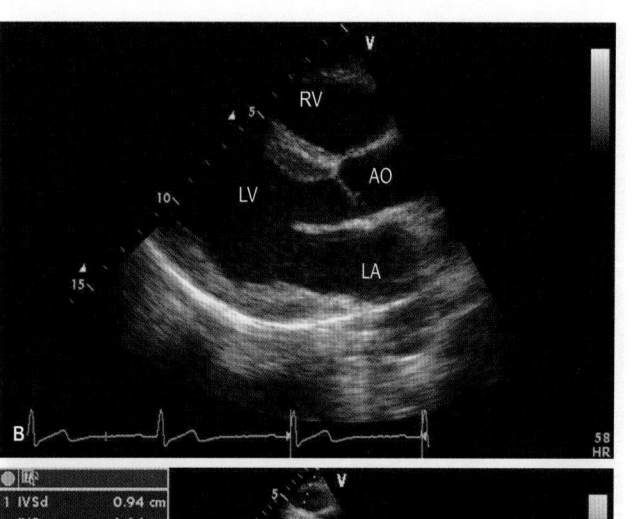

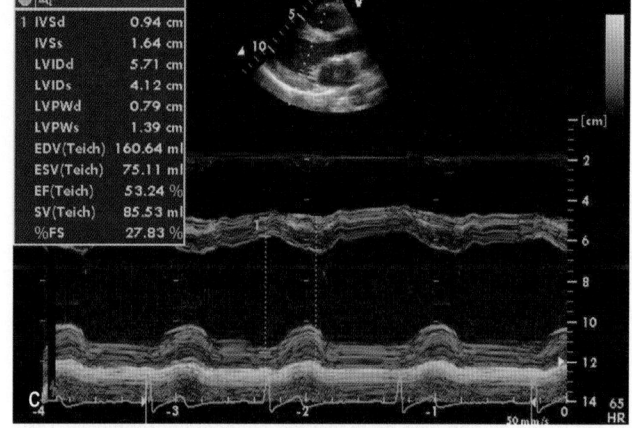

Fig. 30.23 Echocardiography. (A) Diagrammatic representations of the anatomy of the area scanned and of the echocardiogram. **(B)** Two-dimensional long-axis view from a normal subject. **(C)** M-mode recording from a normal subject with the ultrasound beam directed across the left ventricle, just below the mitral valve. AMVC, anterior mitral valve cusp; AO, aorta; IVS, interventricular septum; LA, left atrium; LV, left ventricle; PMVC, posterior mitral valve cusp; RV, right ventricle; RVOT, right ventricular outflow tract.

thus generate horizontal straight lines; the distances of these lines from the top of the screen indicate the depth of the structures, and movements, such as those of heart valves, are indicated by zigzag lines (**Fig. 30.23C**). Alternatively, a series of views from different positions can be obtained in the form of a two-dimensional image (cross-sectional 2-D echocardiography; **Fig. 30.23A,B**). This method is useful for delineating anatomical structures and for quantifying volumes of the cardiac chambers. M mode can be used to estimate left ventricular (LV) systolic function by comparing end-diastolic and end-systolic dimensions. For example, the percentage reduction in the left ventricular cavity size (fractional shortening, FS) is given by:

$$FS = \frac{LVDD - LVSD}{LVDD} \times 100\%$$

where LVDD is left ventricular diastolic diameter and LVSD is left ventricular systolic diameter, at the base of the heart. The normal range is 30–45%.

This method is easy to perform but is an inaccurate measure of *ejection fraction* (*EF*) because it does not take account of reduced regional function of the mid or apical myocardium – due to infarction, for example. For this reason, estimation of EF based on the difference in LV volumes from systole to diastole, derived from planimetered measurements of LV area in at least two planes, is more accurate. A normal EF is over 55%. This method is helpful in

assessing the response of the patient with heart failure to therapy. It also permits estimation of LV mass.

Three-dimensional echocardiography

Three-dimensional echocardiography is a novel development in cardiac imaging in which a volumetric dataset is acquired using a multiplane probe rotating around a fixed axis. Clinical uses include accurate volumetric assessment of ventricular function and mass, assessment of mitral and aortic valve disease, and assessment of adult congenital heart disease (**Fig. 30.24**).

Doppler echocardiography

Echocardiography imaging utilizes echoes from tissue interfaces. Using high amplification, it is also possible to detect weak echoes scattered by small targets, including those from red blood cells. Blood velocity in the heart chambers is typically much more rapid (>1 m/s) than the movement of myocardial tissue. If the blood is moving in the same direction as the direction of the ultrasound beam, the frequency of the returning echoes will be changed according to the Doppler phenomenon. The Doppler shift frequency is directly proportional to the blood velocity. Blood velocity data can be acquired and displayed in several ways.

Pulsed-wave (PW) Doppler extracts velocity data from the pulse echoes used to form a two-dimensional image and gives useful qualitative information. PW echoes can be specified from

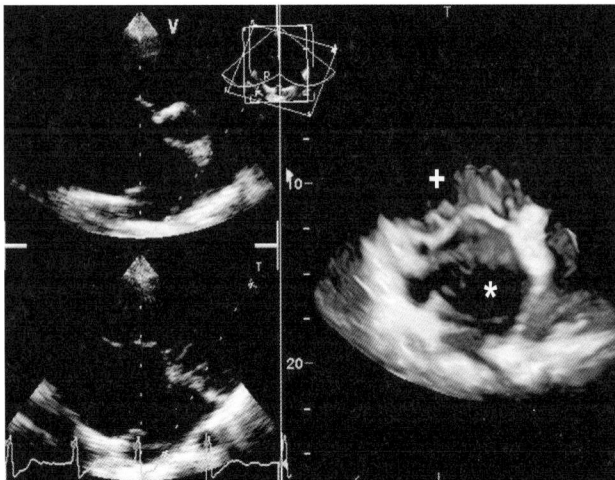

Fig. 30.24 Three-dimensional echocardiograph in a patient with an atrial septal defect (*). The mitral valve (+) and the left atrial anatomy are well delineated.

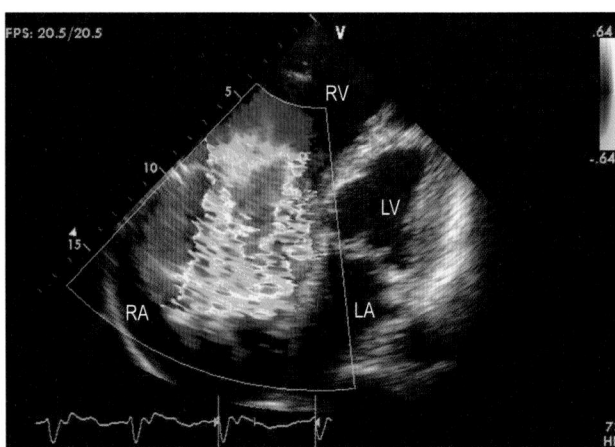

Fig. 30.25 Colour Doppler. Blood is shown flowing away from the echocardiography probe as a blue signal and towards the probe as a red signal. In this patient with tricuspid regurgitation, blood leaks from the right ventricle (RV) to the right atrium (RA) during cardiac systole. LA, left atrium; LV, left ventricle.

locations within an image identified by a sample volume cursor placed on the screen. Such information from the left ventricular outflow tract (LVOT) and right ventricular outflow tract provides the stroke distance, and is used to estimate cardiac output (CO) and also to quantify intracardiac shunts. Cardiac output can then be derived using the formula:

$$CO = \text{stroke volume} \times \text{heart rate}$$

Stroke volume is the stroke distance multiplied by the area of the LVOT, which can also be measured echocardiographically. PW Doppler of the flow across the mitral valve and into the left atrium through the pulmonary veins can be used as an element of the estimation of left ventricular filling pressure.

Colour flow Doppler imaging uses one colour for blood flowing towards the transducer and another colour for blood flowing away. This technique allows the direction, velocity and timing of the flow to be measured with a simultaneous view of cardiac structure and function. Colour flow Doppler is used to help assess valvular regurgitation (**Fig. 30.25**) and may be helpful in the assessment of coronary blood flow.

Continuous-wave (CW) Doppler collects all the velocity data from the path of the beam and analyses it to generate a spectral display. This is unlike PW Doppler, which provides information from a particular sample volume at one location along a line. Thus, CW Doppler does not provide any depth information.

The outline of the envelope of the spectral display is used to estimate the value of peak velocity throughout the cardiac cycle. CW Doppler is typically used to assess valvular obstruction, which then causes increased velocities. For example, normal flow velocities are of the order of 1 m/s across the normal aortic valve, but if there is a severe obstructive lesion, such as a severely stenotic aortic valve, velocities of 4 m/s or more can occur. These velocities are generated by the pressure gradient that exists across the lesion.

According to the Bernoulli equation, the pressure difference between two chambers is calculated as: 4 multiplied by the square of the CW Doppler velocity between chambers. Thus a velocity of 5 m/s across the aortic valve suggests a peak gradient of $4 \times 5 \times 5 = 100$ mmHg between the ascending aorta and the left ventricle. This equation has been validated in a wide variety of clinical situations, including valve stenoses, ventricular septal defects and intraventricular obstruction (as in hypertrophic cardiomyopathy). It

is often clinically unnecessary to resort to invasive methods such as cardiac catheterization to measure intracardiac pressure gradients.

Similarly, pulmonary artery (PA) systolic pressure and right ventricular diastolic pressure can be calculated using the Bernoulli equation. In this case, CW Doppler tracing of the tricuspid regurgitant jet is used to estimate the pressure gradient between the right ventricle and the right atrium. The PA systolic pressure is then calculated by adding the estimated right atrial pressure to the pressure gradient between the right ventricle and the right atrium.

Tissue Doppler is similar to PW Doppler. It measures myocardial tissue velocities within a particular sample volume placed on the image. Such velocities are of the order of 1 cm/s. Currently, tissue Doppler of the mitral annulus is used as part of the estimation of left ventricular filling pressure.

Other ultrasound modalities include harmonic power Doppler, pulse inversion Doppler and ultraharmonics, which are used to detect and amplify microsphere-specific signals as part of the echocardiographic assessment of myocardial perfusion.

Transoesophageal echocardiography

In transoesophageal echocardiography (TOE, see **Fig. 30.80**), a transducer mounted on a flexible tube is placed into the oesophagus. This involves the use of local anaesthesia and, sometimes, intravenous sedation. High-resolution images can be obtained because of the close proximity of the heart to the transducer in the oesophagus, and also because of the higher frequencies that are used relative to transthoracic imaging. TOE is most commonly used to assess valve structure and function (for reparability of mitral valve prolapse), the features and complications of infective endocarditis, and the aorta (for aortic dissection); it is also useful for seeking a cardiac source of embolus.

Wall motion stress echocardiography

Echocardiography can be used clinically to evaluate the patient for the presence of myocardial scars and reversible ischaemia. Since ultrasound cannot directly detect red blood cells in capillaries, myocardial wall motion is used as a surrogate for perfusion. Myocardial segments that demonstrate a change in function (defined as a change or reduction in thickening) from rest to stress can be assumed to be supplied by a flow-limiting stenosis in the epicardial artery or graft.

Stress for this indication needs to be inotropic to induce true ischaemia. Physiological stress includes treadmill exercise, which is complicated by the difficulty in obtaining reliable images rapidly as the patient comes off the treadmill, before heart rate reduces back to submaximal levels. Alternatively, pharmacological stress can be induced with dobutamine at graded doses. This is relatively safe but complications such as ventricular arrhythmia have been reported. This technique can also assess viability of the myocardium, and hibernating or stunned myocardium (see p. 1075).

Myocardial perfusion echocardiography

In order to assess myocardial perfusion by echocardiography (MPE), microspheres of similar size to red blood cells are used as an intravenous contrast agent. Microsphere-specific ultrasound modes, such as harmonic power Doppler, can be used for detection. MPE involves the use of intravenous contrast infusion to fill the myocardium. A pulse of ultrasound destroys microspheres within the capillaries (and not the left ventricular cavity), and the time taken to replenish the capillaries is a measure of myocardial blood flow. The time taken to fill should be significantly shorter at stress than at rest.

Contrast echo for left ventricular opacification

Intravenous contrast agents opacify the left ventricle and can define the endocardial border. Their clinical utility has reduced with the advent of harmonic imaging, which has improved image quality in patients who were previously 'difficult to image'.

Intravascular (coronary) ultrasound

Intravascular (coronary) ultrasound probes can be used to obtain images of proximal coronary arteries as part of a percutaneous transluminal coronary angioplasty (PTCA) procedure: for example, to assess adequacy of deployment of intracoronary stents.

Nuclear imaging

Nuclear imaging is used to detect myocardial infarction or to measure myocardial function, perfusion or viability, depending on the radiopharmaceutical and the imaging technique chosen. These data are particularly valuable when used in combination. All involve a significant radiation dose (see later).

Image type

Gamma cameras produce a planar image in which structures are superimposed, as in a standard X-ray. Single-photon emission computed tomography (SPECT) imaging uses similar raw data to construct tomographic images, just as a CT image is reconstructed from X-rays. This gives finer anatomical resolution but is technically demanding. These methods may be used with any of the radiopharmaceuticals.

Myocardial perfusion and viability

Thallium-201 is rapidly taken up by the myocardium, so an image taken immediately after injection reflects the distribution of blood flow to the myocardium. Areas of ischaemia or infarction receive less ^{201}Tl and appear dark. Between 2 and 24 hours after injection, ^{201}Tl is redistributed so that all cardiac myocytes contain a comparable concentration. Images obtained at this time show dark areas where the myocardium has infarcted but normal density in ischaemic areas. Comparison of early and late images is one method of predicting whether an ischaemic area of myocardium contains enough viable tissue to justify coronary

bypass or angioplasty. Technetium-99-labelled tetrofosmin (**Fig. 30.26**) is also taken up rapidly by cardiac myocytes but does not undergo redistribution. When this substance is injected during exercise, its distribution in the myocardium reflects the distribution of blood at the time of the exercise, even if the image is taken several hours later. This is a sensitive method of detecting myocardial viability. Images produced following injection of [99mTc]tetrofosmin during exercise can be compared to images produced following injection at rest to decide which areas of ischaemia are reversible (see p. 1075). In patients unable to exercise the heart can be stressed with drugs, such as dipyridamole or dobutamine.

Infarct imaging

Perfusion images produced using compounds labelled with ^{201}Tl or [99mTc]sestamibi show a myocardial infarction as a perfusion defect or 'cold spot'. These methods are sensitive for detecting and localizing the infarct but give no information about its age. [99mTc] Pyrophosphate is preferentially taken up by myocardium that has undergone infarction within the previous few days. Images are difficult to interpret because the isotope is also concentrated by bone and cartilage.

Cardiac computed tomography

Computed tomography (CT) is useful for assessment of the thoracic aorta and mediastinum. The development of 512-slice multidetector CT (MDCT) scanners has enabled accurate non-invasive imaging of the coronary arteries.

Coronary artery calcification

Calcium is absent in normal coronary arteries but is present in atherosclerosis and increases with age. Studies have demonstrated a positive correlation between calcification and the presence of coronary artery stenoses, although the relationship is non-linear. Electron beam CT (EBT) and MDCT scanners are used to obtain multiple thin axial slices through the heart and then the calcium score is calculated. The calcium score is based on the X-ray attenuation coefficient or CT number measured in Hounsfield units. Meta-analyses have demonstrated that a higher calcium score is associated with a higher event rate and higher relative risk ratios, although no study to date has shown a net effect on health outcomes of calcium scoring. The current National Institute for Health and Care Excellence (NICE) chest pain guidelines recommend the use of CT calcium scoring in patients with chest pain and a 10–29% likelihood of coronary artery disease (see p. 1082).

CT coronary angiography

CT coronary angiography (CTCA) is performed with a supine patient connected to a three-lead ECG for cardiac synchronization. The 64-slice MDCT scanners have a temporal resolution of 165–210 ms; image quality is optimal with a slow and steady heart rate (<65–70 b.p.m.), which can be obtained with the use of oral or intravenous beta-blockers. Sublingual nitroglycerin (0.4–0.8 mg dose) may improve visualization of the coronary artery lumen. A volume dataset containing the whole heart is acquired during a single breath-hold with the injection of 60–80 mL of iodinated contrast agent at 4–6 mL/sec. The radiation dose during the scan is 11–22 mSv but this can be reduced to 7–11 mSv with ECG-controlled dose modulation; this compares with 2.5–5.0 mSv for diagnostic coronary angiography and 15–20 mSv for SPECT. The volume dataset is then analysed with multiplanar reformatting for the presence of coronary artery stenoses (**Fig. 30.27**). Studies

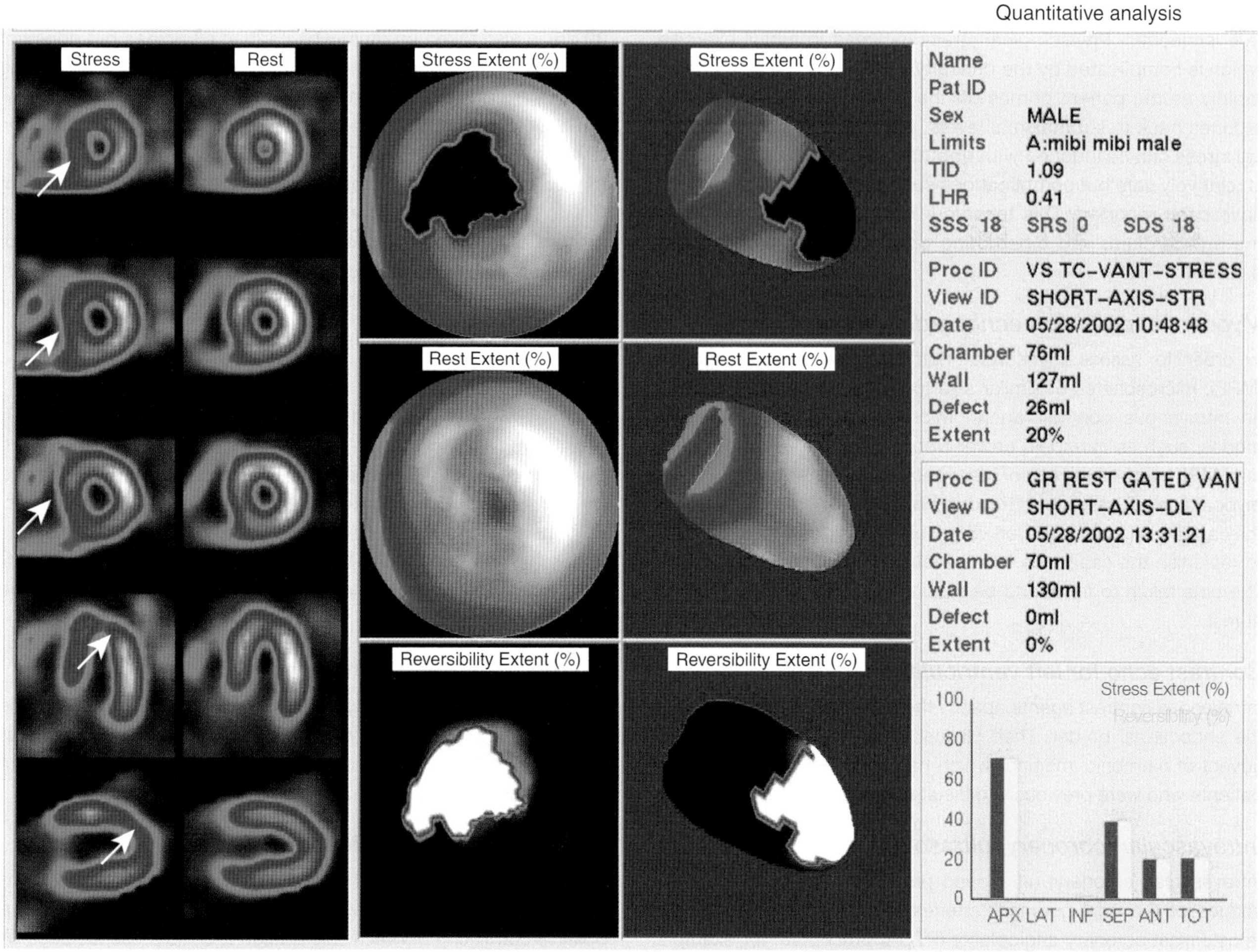

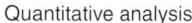

Fig. 30.26 Myocardial single-photon emission computed tomography (SPECT) study acquired with [⁹⁹ᵐTc]tetrofosmin tracer. *Left panel:* Three short-axis slices and a horizontal and a vertical axis plane of the left ventricle after stress and following a resting re-injection of tracer. The rest images demonstrate normal tracer uptake (orange signal) in the whole of the left ventricle. The stress images demonstrate reduced tracer uptake (arrows; purple-blue signal) in the anterior and septal walls, consistent with a significant stenosis in the left anterior descending artery. *Middle panel:* Polar maps of the whole myocardium can localize the ischaemic territory. *Right panel:* Quantitative analysis can help define the extent and reversibility of the ischaemia.

have reported high sensitivity (>85%) and specificity (>90%) for the detection of coronary artery disease, with a very high negative predictive value (>95%). CTCA may become part of an acute chest pain service in the emergency medicine department to exclude aortic dissection, pulmonary embolism and coronary artery disease. However, this technique does expose the patient to ionizing radiation.

Cardiovascular magnetic resonance

Cardiovascular magnetic resonance (CMR), a non-invasive imaging technique that does not involve harmful radiation, is increasingly used in the investigation of patients with cardiovascular disease.

CMR is usually performed with multiple breath-holds to minimize respiratory motion artefacts and cardiac gating to reduce blurring during the cardiac cycle. Several different sequences provide anatomical and functional information. Most sequences do not require a contrast agent but intravenous gadolinium may be needed for magnetic resonance angiography, myocardial perfusion, infarct and fibrosis imaging. The major contraindications are permanent pacemaker or defibrillator, intracerebral clips and significant

claustrophobia. Patients with coronary stents and prosthetic valves can be safely scanned.

Clinical use

The current indications for CMR are summarized in **Box 30.11**.

Congenital heart disease

CMR provides additional and complementary information to echocardiography in patients with congenital heart disease. Cine-imaging can accurately assess systemic and non-systemic ventricular function and mass. Extracardiac conduits, anomalous pulmonary venous return and aortic coarctations before and after repair can be studied by CMR, and the studies repeated for long-term follow-up without the risk of ionizing radiation.

Cardiomyopathies, pericardial disease and cardiac masses

In hypertrophic cardiomyopathy, CMR accurately defines the extent and distribution of myocardial hypertrophy and can be used in patients with suboptimal echocardiograms. Intravenous gadolinium can be

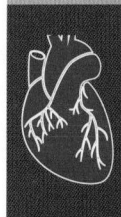

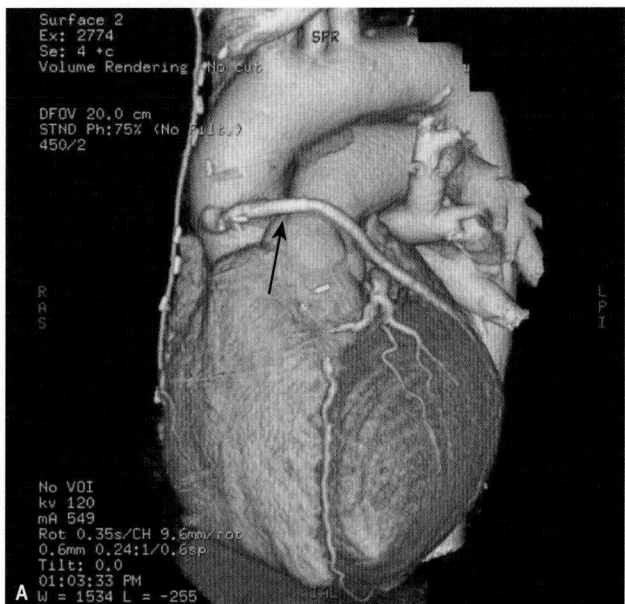

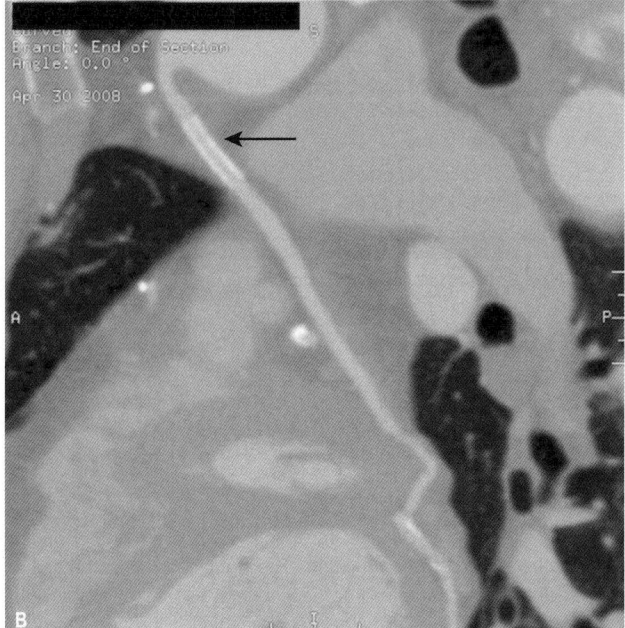

Fig. 30.27 Multislice computed tomography: coronary artery stent. (A) A volume-rendered image in a patient with coronary artery stent insertion (arrowed) in a saphenous vein graft to the native circumflex coronary artery. (B) The multiplanar reformatted image demonstrates stent patency (arrowed) and insertion of the graft to the circumflex coronary artery.

utilized to demonstrate regional myocardial fibrosis, which is associated with an adverse prognosis. In patients with suspected arrhythmogenic right ventricular cardiomyopathy, CMR is the imaging investigation of choice to detect global and regional wall motion abnormalities of the right ventricle and right ventricular outflow tract, and to detect fatty or fibro-fatty infiltration of the right and left ventricles. In constrictive pericarditis and restrictive cardiomyopathy, CMR can demonstrate the effects of the impaired ventricular filling common to both conditions (dilated right atrium and inferior vena cava) and can also determine the thickness of the pericardium (usually 4 mm in normal individuals) (**Fig. 30.28**). In patients with dilated cardiomyopathy, CMR can accurately quantify biventricular function and, with gadolinium, can demonstrate

- Congenital heart disease (CHD):
  - Anatomical assessment following echocardiography, particularly in patients with complex CHD or following surgical intervention
  - Follow-up/surveillance studies
  - Anomalous pulmonary or systemic venous return
  - Assessment of right or left ventricular function/dilation
- Cardiomyopathies/cardiac infiltration/pericardial disease
- Disease of the aorta, including aortic dissection, aneurysm, coarctation
- Valvular heart disease:
  - Quantification of stenosis and regurgitation
  - Accurate ventricular dimensions/function
  - Planimetry of valvular stenosis
- Coronary artery disease:
  - Left and right ventricular function
  - Wall motion assessment during dobutamine stress
  - Myocardial perfusion during adenosine stress
  - Coronary artery and coronary artery bypass graft imaging
  - Myocardial infarct imaging and viability assessment with dobutamine CMR or delayed enhancement
- Imaging of pulmonary vessels

myocardial fibrosis. In inflammatory and infiltrative conditions of the myocardium, such as myocarditis, sarcoidosis and amyloidosis (see p. 1357), CMR is increasingly used as a diagnostic investigation due to the different patterns of signal enhancement seen with gadolinium. In patients with thalassaemia, CMR can detect iron deposition within the myocardium and guide chelation therapy. CMR can be useful in patients with cardiac masses to differentiate benign from malignant tumours and to identify thrombus not visualized on echocardiography.

Diseases of the aorta

CMR is an excellent technique for assessing patients with aortic dissection and can detect the clinical features of an aortic dissection: the intimal flap, thrombosis in a false lumen, aortic regurgitation, pericardial effusion and aortic dilation. As it does not involve radiation or need contrast, CMR is an ideal method of surveillance of patients with dilated thoracic aortas or repaired coarctation.

Valvular heart disease

Valvular stenosis produces signal void on gradient-echo CMR. CMR can quantify the velocity across a stenosed valve using phase-contrast velocity mapping. Valvular regurgitation can be accurately quantified using phase-contrast velocity mapping across the valve, or by calculating the stroke volumes of the left and right ventricles, which are equal in the absence of significant regurgitation. However, in most patients, transthoracic and transoesophageal echocardiography should provide sufficient information.

Coronary artery disease

CMR can be used to evaluate coronary artery anatomy, left ventricular function, myocardial perfusion and viability in a 'one-stop' approach to the assessment of patients with coronary artery disease. Coronary artery anatomy and stenoses can be identified with ultra-fast breath-hold or respiratory-gated sequences with high accuracies. Global left ventricular function and wall motion abnormalities can be detected with cine-imaging performed at rest and during dobutamine stress. Myocardial perfusion can be assessed with gadolinium and first-pass imaging; ischaemia can be demonstrated with adenosine for coronary vasodilation. Myocardial viability can be determined using gadolinium and 'delayed enhancement' images. With these techniques, CMR is increasingly used to assess

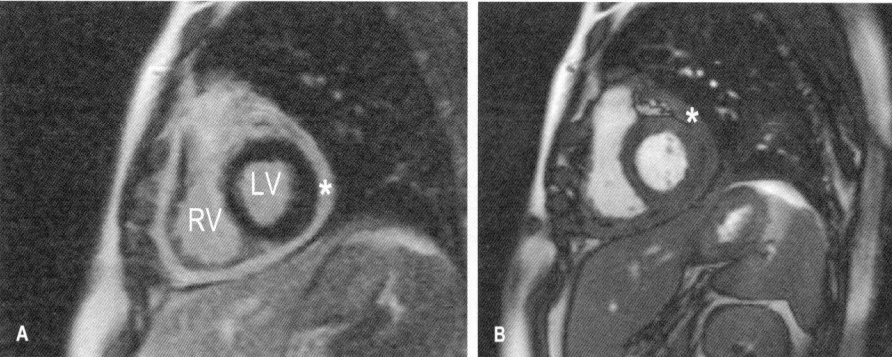

Fig. 30.28 Short-axis cardiac magnetic resonance (CMR) in a patient with constrictive pericarditis. Both images show thickening of the pericardium (*). LV, left ventricle; RV, right ventricle.

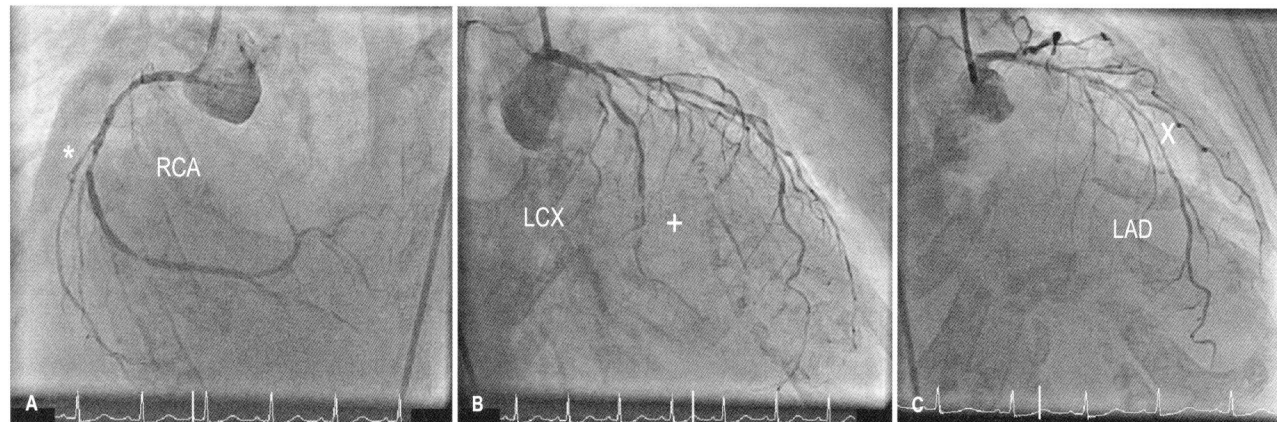

Fig. 30.29 Coronary angiogram (CMR) in a patient with type 2 diabetes mellitus and exertional breathlessness. (A) Diagnostic coronary angiography demonstrates a severe stenosis (*) in the right coronary artery (RCA). **(B)** There is a subtotally occluded (+) circumflex coronary artery (LCX). **(C)** A long diseased segment (X) is also seen in the left anterior descending coronary artery (LAD).

both ischaemia in patients with suspected coronary disease, and myocardial viability prior to revascularization in individuals with impaired cardiac function (**Figs 30.29** and **30.30**).

Pulmonary vessels

Magnetic resonance angiography (MRA) with gadolinium can provide high-quality images of the pulmonary veins, which can be fused with electrical data during pulmonary vein isolation for the treatment of atrial fibrillation.

Positron emission tomography

Positron emission tomography (PET) is based on detection of high-energy emissions caused by annihilation of positrons released from unstable isotopes. PET has several advantages over other techniques, such as improved spatial resolution, accurate quantification, and use of biological isotopes of carbon, nitrogen and oxygen. However, it is expensive and requires a cyclotron to produce the short-lived tracers. PET/CT has become a useful investigation in the detection of viable myocardium in patients who are suitable for revascularization.

Myocardial perfusion and ischaemia can be determined using PET with ^{13}N-ammonia or ^{15}oxygen with greater sensitivity than SPECT. Myocardial metabolism and viability can be detected with the use of ^{18}F-fluorodeoxyglucose (FDG), which the cardiac myocyte utilizes for energy production in the presence of reduced oxygen supply and blood flow. There may be reduced perfusion to infarcted or fibrotic myocardium, but also reduced FDG uptake. In hibernating myocardium, with viable but dysfunctional myocardium,

PET can demonstrate reduced myocardial perfusion but with preserved or increased FDG uptake.

Cardiac catheterization

Cardiac catheterization is the introduction of a thin radio-opaque tube (catheter) into the circulation. The right heart is catheterized by introducing the catheter into a peripheral vein (usually the right femoral or internal jugular vein) and advancing it through the right atrium and ventricle into the pulmonary artery. The pressures in the right heart chambers and in the pulmonary artery can be measured directly. An indirect measure of left atrial pressure can be obtained by 'wedging' a balloon-tipped catheter into the distal pulmonary artery (see **Fig. 10.15**). In this position the pressure from the right ventricle is obstructed by the catheter, and only the pulmonary venous and left atrial pressures are recorded. Left heart catheterization is usually performed via the right femoral or radial artery. A pigtail catheter is advanced up the aorta and manipulated through the aortic valve into the left ventricle. Pressure tracings are taken from the left ventricular cavity. The end-diastolic pressure is invariably elevated in patients with left ventricular dysfunction. A power injection of radio-opaque contrast material opacifies the left ventricular cavity (left ventriculography) and thereby assesses left ventricular systolic function. The catheter is then withdrawn across the aortic valve into the aorta and the 'pullback' gradient across the valve is measured. Aortography (a power injection into the aortic root) can be performed to assess the aortic root and the presence and severity of aortic regurgitation. Specially designed catheters are then used to engage the left and right

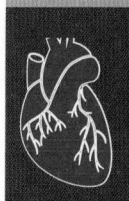

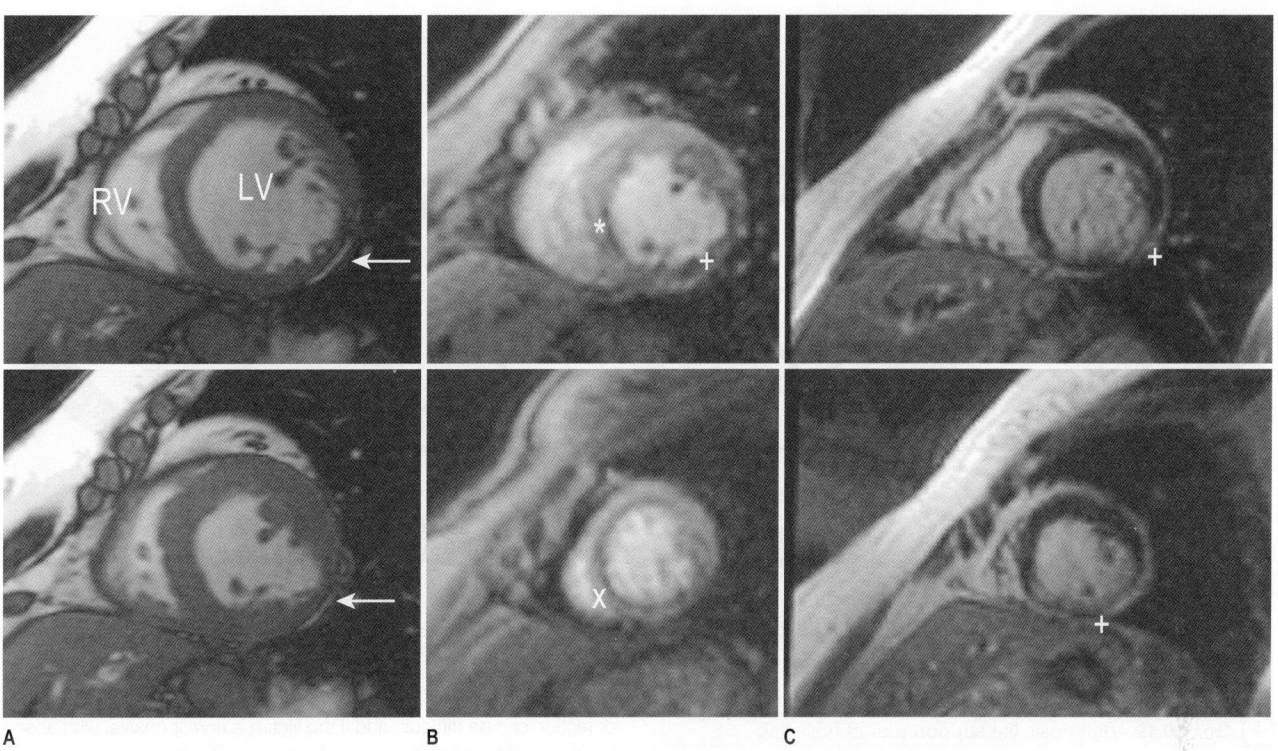

Fig. 30.30 Cardiac magnetic resonance (CMR). (A) Short-axis CMR FIESTA cine-imaging (diastole top, systole bottom) demonstrates thinning and hypokinesia of the inferolateral wall (arrowed) but preserved function of the rest of the myocardium. LV, left ventricle; RV, right ventricle. **(B)** First-pass perfusion CMR (mid top, apex bottom) demonstrates subendocardial perfusion defects in the inferolateral wall (+), infero-septum (*) and apical segments (X). **(C)** Delayed-enhancement CMR confirms a transmural myocardial infarction of the mid-apical infero-lateral wall (+) secondary to a previous infarction from the circumflex coronary artery, and demonstrates inducible ischaemia in the right and left coronary territories.

coronary arteries selectively, and contrast cine-angiograms are taken in order to define the coronary circulation and identify the presence and severity of any coronary artery disease. During the procedure, intracoronary nitrate or adenosine may be used to dilate the coronary arteries. During cardiac catheterization, blood samples may be withdrawn to measure the oxygen content. These estimations are used to quantify intracardiac shunts and measure cardiac output.

Further reading

Gongora CA, Bavishi C, Uretsky S et al. Acute chest pain evaluation using coronary computed tomography angiography compared with standard of care: a meta-analysis of randomised clinical trials. *Heart* 2018; 104:215.

Grayburn PA. Interpreting the coronary-artery calcium score. *N Engl J Med* 2012; 366:294–296.

Hundley WG, Bluemke DA, Finn JP et al.; American College of Cardiology Foundation Task Force on Expert Consensus Documents. ACCF/ACR/AHA/NASCI/SCMR 2010 expert consensus document on cardiovascular magnetic resonance: a report of the American College of Cardiology Foundation Task Force on Expert Consensus Documents. *Circulation* 2010; 121:2462–2508.

Quinones MA, Otto CM, Stoddard M et al. Recommendations for quantification of Doppler echocardiography: a report from the Doppler Quantification Task Force of the Nomenclature and Standards Committee of the American Society of Echocardiography. *J Am Soc Echocardiogr* 2002; 15:167–184.

http://bsecho.org/toe-minimum-dataset/. *Minimum dataset for a standard transoesophageal echocardiogram, British Society of Echocardiography Education Committee.*

THERAPEUTIC PROCEDURES

Cardiac resuscitation

Each year in the UK, there are approximately 100 000 unexpected deaths occurring within 24 hours of the development of cardiac symptoms. About half of these deaths are almost instantaneous. Most deaths are due to ventricular fibrillation or rapid ventricular tachycardia; a small proportion are caused by severe bradyarrhythmias. Coronary artery disease accounts for approximately 80% of sudden cardiac deaths in Western society. Transient ischaemia is suspected of being the major trigger factor; however, only a small proportion of survivors have clinical evidence of acute myocardial infarction.

When cardiac arrest occurs, basic life support must be started immediately. The longer the period of respiratory and circulatory arrest, the lower is the chance of restoring healthy life. The chain of survival (**Fig. 30.31**) includes:

- early recognition of cardiac arrest
- early activation of emergency services
- early cardiopulmonary resuscitation (CPR)
- early defibrillation and early advanced life support
- high-quality post-resuscitation care.

Basic life support

The first step in basic life support (BLS) is to ensure the safety of the victim and rescuer. The next is to ascertain that the victim is unresponsive by shaking them and shouting into one ear. If no response is obtained, help should be sought immediately prior to commencement of BLS. If the victim has absent or abnormal breathing, then cardiac arrest is confirmed and BLS should be started (**Box 30.12**).

Airway

Debris (e.g. blood and mucus) in the mouth and pharynx should be removed, as should loose or ill-fitting dentures. The airway should be opened gently by flexing the patient's neck and extending the

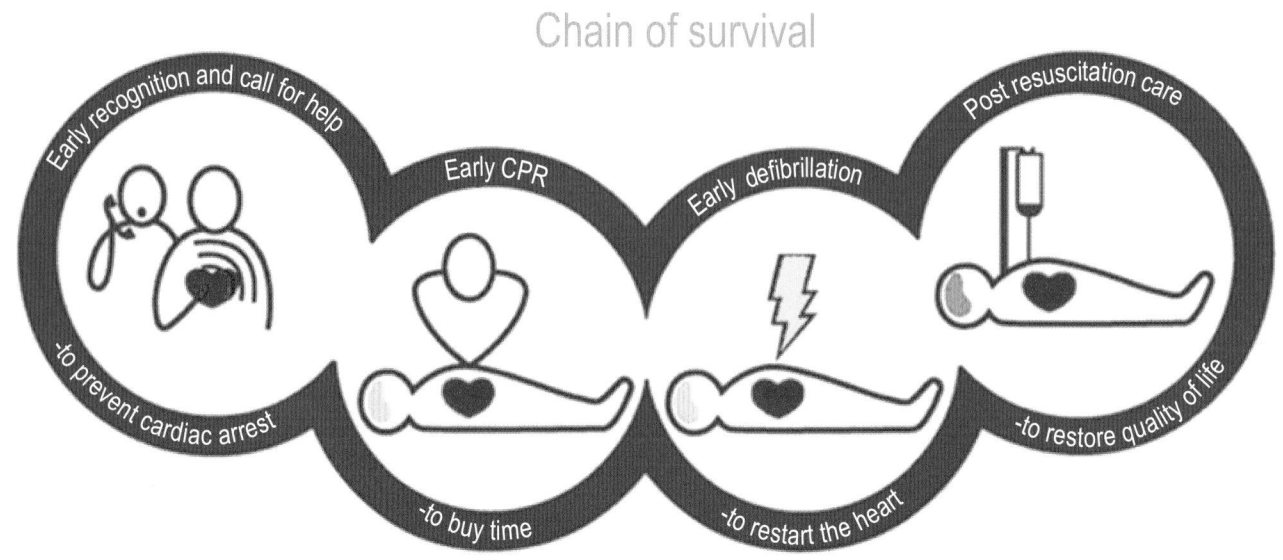

Fig. 30.31 Cardiopulmonary resuscitation chain of survival.

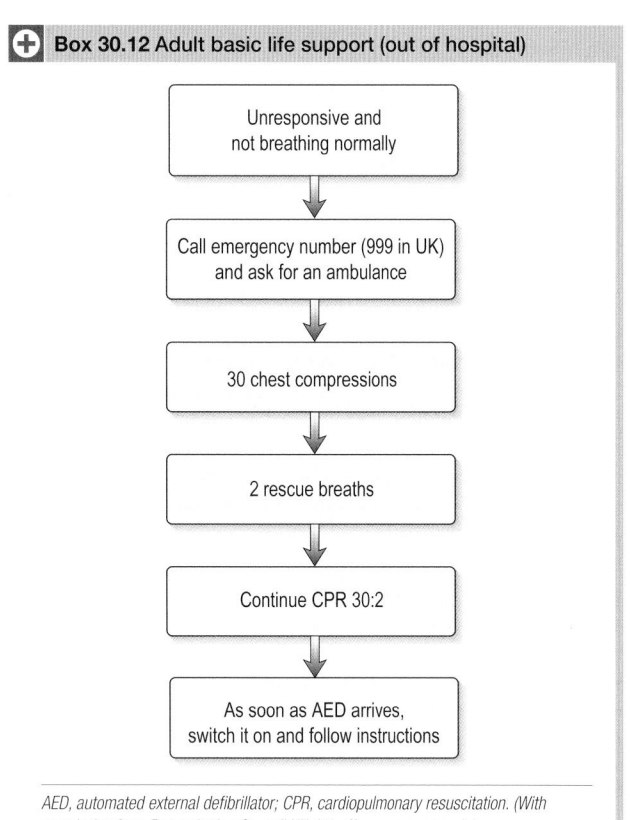

AED, automated external defibrillator; CPR, cardiopulmonary resuscitation. (With permission from Resuscitation Council UK; http://www.resus.org.uk.)

head ('sniffing the morning air' position). This manoeuvre is not recommended if a cervical spine injury is suspected. Any obstruction deep in the oral cavity or upper respiratory tract may need to be removed using abdominal and/or chest thrusts (Heimlich manoeuvre, see **Box 28.16**).

Circulation

Most adult cardiac arrest is due to a primary cardiac disorder, such as acute coronary syndrome, and results in circulatory collapse. Pulse detection can be difficult, and if the victim is unresponsive, with absent or abnormal breathing, external chest compression should be started immediately. The heel of one hand is placed over the centre of the patient's chest and the heel of the second hand is placed over the first with the fingers interlocked. The arms are kept straight and the sternum is rhythmically depressed by 5–6 cm at a rate of approximately 100–120 per minute, allowing for complete recoil between compressions. Chest compressions do not massage the heart. The thorax acts as a pump and the heart provides a system of one-way valves to ensure forward circulation. Respiratory and circulatory support is continued by providing two effective breaths for every 30 cardiac compressions (30:2 for one or two persons, 15:2 in paediatric patients). It is easier for the lay public to give compressions without interruption ('hands only CPR'). This maintains adequate cerebral and coronary perfusion pressures. The initiation of CPR by the lay public at the site of the arrest saves lives. There is evidence to suggest that if the person performing compressions tires, the quality of resuscitation deteriorates. Mechanical CPR devices are available but not yet widely used.

Breathing

After 30 compressions the rescuer opens the victim's airway by tilting the head backwards (**head tilt**) and pulling the chin forwards (**chin lift** or **jaw thrust**). The rescuer then pinches the victim's nostrils firmly, takes a deep breath and seals their lips around the mouth of the victim. Two effective breaths are given, each over 1 second. In paediatric patients, respiratory arrests are more common and patients should be given rescue breaths and a minute of CPR before a sole rescuer leaves the victim to seek help. CPR should not be interrupted to reassess the victim unless they start to show signs of life and begin to breathe normally.

Advanced cardiac life support

By the time effective life support has been established, more help should have arrived and advanced cardiac life support (ACLS) can begin. This consists of ECG monitoring, advanced airway management (endotracheal intubation or supraglottic airway tube) and establishment of an intravenous infusion in a large peripheral or central vein (an intraosseous needle may be used if intravenous

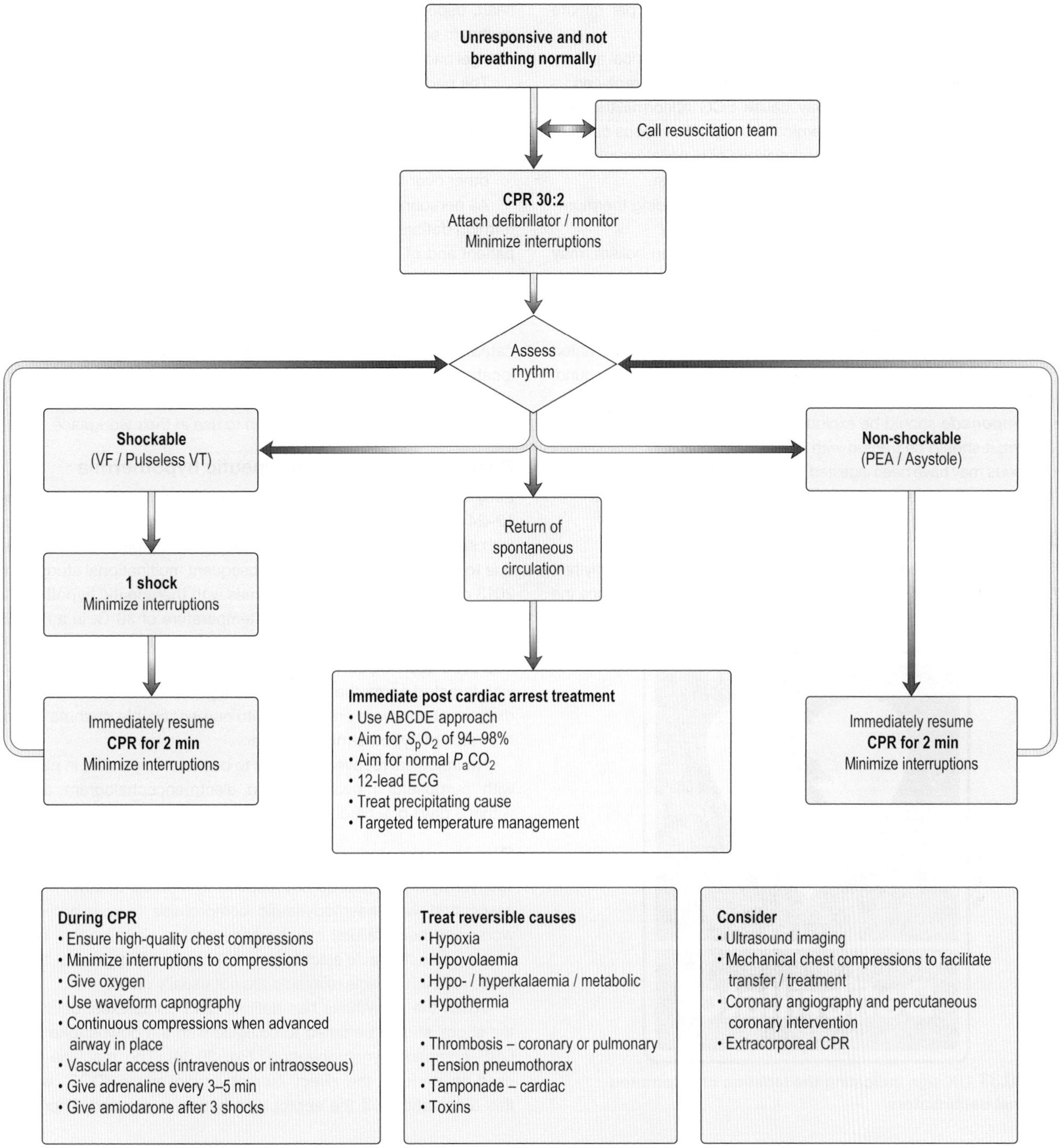

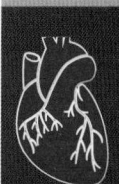

```
┌─────────────────────────┐
│   Unresponsive and not  │
│    breathing normally   │
└─────────────────────────┘
            │  ◄──────────►  ┌──────────────────────┐
            │                │ Call resuscitation team │
            ▼                └──────────────────────┘
┌─────────────────────────┐
│        CPR 30:2         │
│ Attach defibrillator / monitor │
│   Minimize interruptions │
└─────────────────────────┘
            │
            ▼
        ◇ Assess ◇
        ◇ rhythm ◇
```

| **Shockable** (VF / Pulseless VT) | Return of spontaneous circulation | **Non-shockable** (PEA / Asystole) |

| **1 shock** Minimize interruptions | | |

| Immediately resume **CPR for 2 min** Minimize interruptions | **Immediate post cardiac arrest treatment** • Use ABCDE approach • Aim for S_pO_2 of 94–98% • Aim for normal P_aCO_2 • 12-lead ECG • Treat precipitating cause • Targeted temperature management | Immediately resume **CPR for 2 min** Minimize interruptions |

During CPR	**Treat reversible causes**	**Consider**
• Ensure high-quality chest compressions • Minimize interruptions to compressions • Give oxygen • Use waveform capnography • Continuous compressions when advanced airway in place • Vascular access (intravenous or intraosseous) • Give adrenaline every 3–5 min • Give amiodarone after 3 shocks	• Hypoxia • Hypovolaemia • Hypo- / hyperkalaemia / metabolic • Hypothermia • Thrombosis – coronary or pulmonary • Tension pneumothorax • Tamponade – cardiac • Toxins	• Ultrasound imaging • Mechanical chest compressions to facilitate transfer / treatment • Coronary angiography and percutaneous coronary intervention • Extracorporeal CPR

Fig. 30.32 Adult advanced life support algorithm. ABCDE, Airway, Breathing, Circulation, Disability, Exposure; CPR, cardiopulmonary resuscitation; PEA, pulseless electrical activity; VF, ventricular fibrillation; VT, ventricular tachycardia. *(Reproduced with permission from the Resuscitation Council; http://www.resus.org.uk.)*

access is not possible). As soon as feasible, the cardiac rhythm should be established, as this determines which pathway of the European Resuscitation Council and the Resuscitation Council UK ACLS algorithm is followed (**Fig. 30.32**). This can be determined with an automated external defibrillator (AED), or the paddles or limb leads of a standard defibrillator.

If the ECG shows a shockable rhythm – ventricular fibrillation or pulseless ventricular tachycardia – then an unsynchronized shock of 150–200 J biphasic (360 J monophasic) is delivered without delay via paddles or self-adhesive pads, followed immediately by

2 minutes of CPR. For a non-shockable rhythm – asystole or pulseless electrical activity – minutes of CPR is delivered with 1 mg of intravenous adrenaline (epinephrine).

For both sides of the algorithm, it is vital to maintain CPR, ensure oxygenation and exclude or treat reversible causes – the *'four Hs and four Ts'*:

• *Hypoxia* should be minimized by ventilating the patient with oxygen and a bag-valve mask or advanced airway (endotracheal intubation or supraglottic airway tube), ensuring that there is bilateral air entry and chest expansion. With an advanced airway,

CPR should continue, with a ventilation rate of 10 per minute without interrupting cardiac massage.

- **Hypovolaemia** is a frequent cause of pulseless electrical activity due to haemorrhage. Intravenous volume should be replaced.
- **Hyper-** or **hypokalaemia** may cause ECG abnormalities and should be detected by biochemical testing. Intravenous calcium chloride may be helpful in hyperkalaemia or hypocalcaemia. Acidosis should be managed with effective ventilation.
- **Hypothermia** should be excluded with a low-reading thermometer and treated with external or internal warming.
- **Thromboembolism** and massive pulmonary embolism may cause pulseless electrical activity and patients should be considered for intravenous thrombolysis.
- **Tension pneumothorax** may occur during central venous cannulation or following chest trauma. Clinical diagnosis (deviated trachea, hyper-resonant chest, absent breath sounds, ultrasound) and needle thoracocentesis or thoracostomy may be required.
- **Tamponade** should be excluded with echocardiography; if present, it should be treated with pericardiocentesis.
- **Toxins** may have been ingested by accident or deliberate self-harm, and specific antidotes should be used in appropriate patients.

Defibrillation

This technique is used to convert ventricular fibrillation to sinus rhythm. When the defibrillator is discharged, a high-voltage field envelops the heart, depolarizing the myocardium and allowing an organized heart rhythm to emerge. Electrical energy is discharged through two paddles with gel pads or adhesive pads placed on the chest wall.

The paddles are placed in one of two positions:

- One paddle is placed to the right of the upper sternum and the other over the cardiac apex.
- One paddle is placed under the tip of the left scapula and the other over the anterior wall of the left chest.

All personnel should stand clear of the patient. The person performing defibrillation has responsibility for ensuring the safety of the patient and of the other people present. Conventional defibrillators employ a damped monophasic waveform. Biphasic defibrillators, which require less energy, are increasingly common. AEDs, which recognize ventricular fibrillation automatically, deliver a shock if indicated. These are available in some public places (in the UK, their location is signalled by a specific sign, **Fig. 30.33**). It is the responsibility of all healthcare practitioners to be familiar with the range of defibrillators they may be called on to use in their workplace.

Post resuscitation – therapeutic hypothermia

Early studies suggested that therapeutic hypothermia (32–34°C for 12–24 h) might improve outcomes in unconscious adult patients with spontaneous circulation after an out-of-hospital cardiac arrest due to ventricular fibrillation. A subsequent multinational study from 2013 demonstrated similar outcomes with therapeutic hypothermia at 33°C, compared to a targeted temperature of 36°C. In a French study from 2019, moderate hypothermia (33°C) was associated with improved neurological outcomes (but not mortality) when compared with targeted normothermia (37°C) in a group of out-of-hospital cardiac arrest survivors presenting with non-shockable rhythms. Thus, the value of hypothermia is unclear.

Neurological recovery appears to be more favourable in patients with purposeful movements and electroencephalogram activity within 3 days of a cardiac arrest.

Direct current cardioversion

Tachyarrhythmias that do not respond to medical treatment or are associated with haemodynamic compromise (e.g. hypotension, worsening heart failure) may be converted to sinus rhythm by the use of a transthoracic electric shock. A short-acting general anaesthetic is used. Muscle relaxants are not usually given.

When the arrhythmia has definite QRS complexes, delivery of the shock should be timed to coincide with the downstroke of the QRS complex (synchronization, **Fig. 30.34**). The machine being used to perform the direct current cardioversion (DCC) will do this automatically if the appropriate button is pressed. There is a

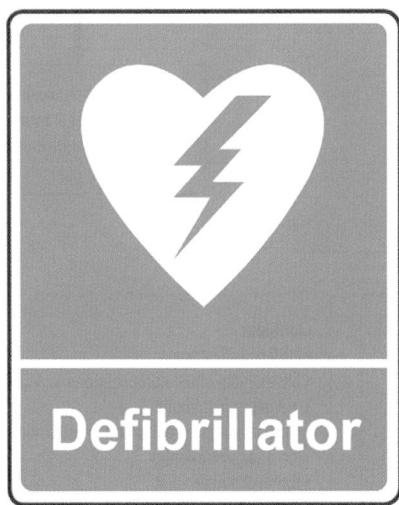

Fig. 30.33 UK sign indicating the location of automated external defibrillators.

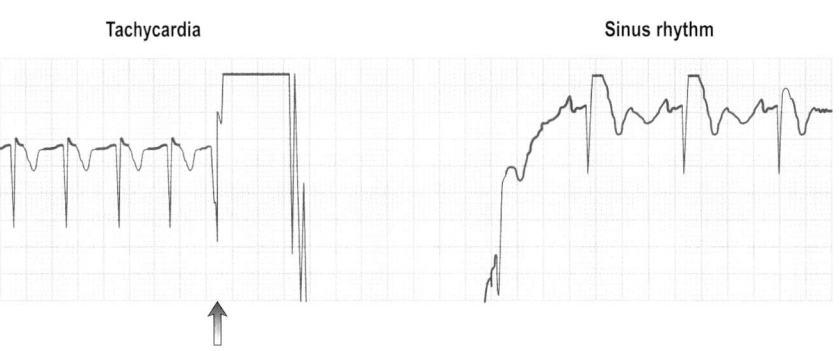

Tachycardia

Sinus rhythm

Synchronized DC shock

Fig. 30.34 Direct current (DC) cardioversion of a supraventricular tachycardia to sinus rhythm. The direct current shock is delivered synchronously with the QRS complex.

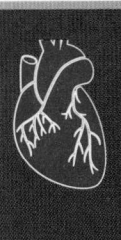

crucial difference between defibrillation and cardioversion: a non-synchronized shock is used to defibrillate. Accidental defibrillation of a patient who does not require it may itself precipitate ventricular fibrillation.

Typical indications for DCC include:

- atrial fibrillation
- atrial flutter
- sustained ventricular tachycardia
- junctional tachyarrhythmias.

If atrial fibrillation or flutter has been present for more than 48 hours, it is necessary to anticoagulate the patient adequately for 3 weeks before elective cardioversion to reduce the risk of embolization. The duration of anticoagulation after successful cardioversion for atrial fibrillation is a complex issue and depends on a number of factors: it should be given for at least 4 weeks after the procedure and may well be given for much longer.

Digoxin toxicity may lead to ventricular arrhythmias or asystole following cardioversion. Therapeutic digitalization does not increase the risks of cardioversion, but it is conventional to omit digoxin several days prior to elective cardioversion in order to be sure that toxicity is not present.

Cardiac enzyme levels may rise after a cardioversion.

Temporary pacing

Therapeutic cardiac pacing is employed in any patient with sustained symptomatic or haemodynamically compromising bradycardia. Bradycardias may be due to either a slow intrinsic heart rate (e.g. sinus node dysfunction) or AV block. Prophylactic cardiac pacing is employed in asymptomatic patients with either bradycardia or conduction abnormalities, as the risk of progression to symptomatic bradycardia justifies such a strategy.

Transvenous pacing is the preferred method in patients with symptomatic bradycardias. In summary, a thin (French gauge 5 or 6), bipolar pacing electrode wire is inserted via an internal jugular vein, a femoral vein or a subclavian vein and is positioned at the right ventricular apex using cardiac fluoroscopy. The energy needed for successful pacing (the pacing threshold) is assessed by reducing the energy until the pacemaker fails to stimulate the tissue (loss of capture). The output energy is then set at three times the threshold value to prevent inadvertent loss of capture. If the threshold increases above 5 V, the pacemaker wire should be resited. A temporary pacemaker unit (**Fig. 30.35A**) is almost always set to work 'on demand' – to fire only when a spontaneous beat has not occurred. The rate of temporary pacing is usually 60–80 per minute.

Transcutaneous pacing is the preferred method in selected patients with asymptomatic bradycardia or conduction abnormalities, and may be life-saving when a cardiac arrest is precipitated by bradycardia. In this method the myocardium is depolarized by current flow between two large adhesive electrodes positioned anteriorly and posteriorly on the chest wall. Transcutaneous pacing is uncomfortable for the conscious patient but can usually be tolerated until a temporary transvenous pacemaker is inserted.

Permanent pacing

Permanent pacemakers are fully implanted in the body and connected to the heart by one or two electrode leads (**Fig. 30.35B**). The pacemaker is powered by solid-state lithium batteries, which usually last 5–10 years. Pacemakers are 'programmable', in that their operating characteristics (e.g. the pacing rate) can be changed by a programmer that transmits specific electromagnetic signals through the skin. The pacemaker leads are passed transvenously to the right heart chambers. Leadless pacemakers have been developed

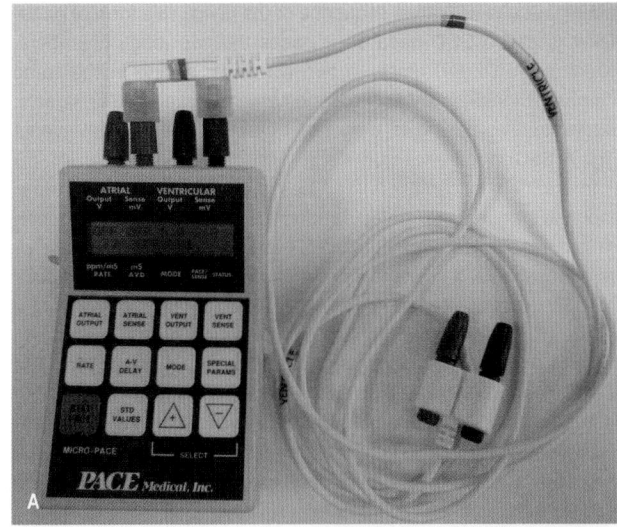

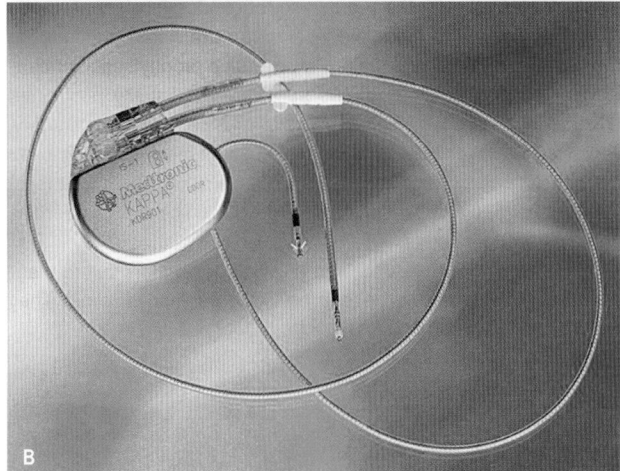

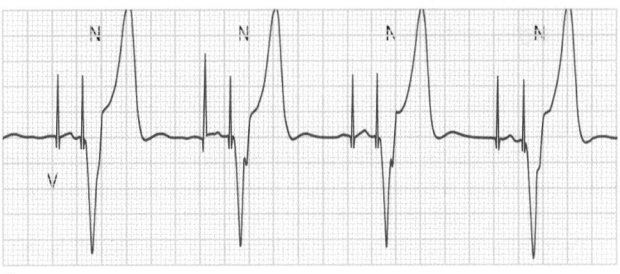

C

Fig. 30.35 Pacemakers. (A) A temporary pacemaker unit. **(B)** A permanent pacemaker with atrial and ventricular leads. **(C)** An electrocardiogram showing dual (atrial and ventricular) chamber pacing. A wide QRS complex results from abnormal activation of the ventricles from the right ventricular apex.

but are not recommended by NICE unless implanted as part of a research study.

Pacemakers are designed both to pace and to sense either the ventricles, the atria or, more commonly, both chambers. A single-chamber ventricular pacemaker is described as a 'VVI' unit because it paces the ventricle (V), senses the ventricle (V) and is inhibited (I) by a spontaneous ventricular signal. Occasionally (e.g. in symptomatic sinus bradycardia), an atrial pacemaker (AAI) may be implanted. Pacemakers that are connected to both the right atrium and ventricle ('dual-chamber' pacemakers) are used to simulate the natural pacemaker and activation sequence of the heart. This form of pacemaker is called DDD because it paces the two (dual) chambers, senses both (D) and reacts in two (D) ways: pacing in the same chamber is inhibited by spontaneous atrial and ventricular signals, and ventricular pacing is triggered by spontaneous atrial events (**Fig. 30.35C**).

In addition, pacemakers may be 'rate-responsive' (R). A rate-responsive pacemaker detects motion (level of vibration or acceleration), respiration or changes in QT interval; by employing one or more biosensors, it changes its rate of pacing so that it is appropriate to the level of exertion.

The choice of pacemaker mostly depends on the underlying rhythm abnormality and the general condition of the patient. For example, complete heart block in patients with sinus rhythm should be treated with a dual-chamber device in order to maintain AV synchrony, whereas inactive or infirm patients may not benefit from the most sophisticated units. Specialized biventricular pacemakers are used for the treatment of severe heart failure.

Permanent pacemakers are inserted under local anaesthetic using fluoroscopy to guide the insertion of the electrode leads via the cephalic or subclavian vein. Perioperative prophylactic antibiotics are routinely prescribed. The pacemaker is usually positioned subcutaneously in front of the pectoral muscle. Following surgery, which usually takes 60–90 minutes, the patient rests in bed for 6–12 hours before being discharged. Patients may not drive for at least 1 week after implantation, and must inform the licensing authorities and their motor insurers.

Complications are few but can prove to be very difficult to manage, and patients should be referred to the pacemaker clinic. They include the following:
- infection
- erosion
- pocket haematoma
- lead displacement
- electromagnetic interference.

Pericardiocentesis

A pericardial effusion is an accumulation of fluid between the parietal and visceral layers of pericardium. Fluid is removed for relief of symptoms that are due to haemodynamic embarrassment or for diagnostic purposes. This can be a technically difficult procedure, particularly in the acute setting, and should be performed in a cardiac laboratory. In an emergency, it can be performed at the bedside.

Pericardial aspiration or pericardiocentesis (**Fig. 30.36**) is performed by inserting a needle into the pericardial space, usually via a subxiphisternal route under ultrasound guidance. Certain effusions, particularly posterior ones, require surgical drainage under a general anaesthetic. If a large volume of fluid is to be removed, a wide-bore needle and cannula are inserted. The needle may be removed and the cannula left *in situ* to drain the fluid. Fluid that is removed is sent for chemical analysis, microscopy, including cytology, Gram stain and culture. If a reaccumulation of pericardial fluid is anticipated, the cannula may be left in place for several days, or an operation can be performed to cut a window in the parietal pericardium (fenestration) or to remove a large section of the pericardium.

Right-heart bedside catheterization

Bedside catheterization (see **Fig. 10.15**) of the pulmonary artery with a pulmonary artery balloon flotation catheter (Swan–Ganz catheter) is now rarely performed routinely, but may be required in patients with:
- cardiac failure

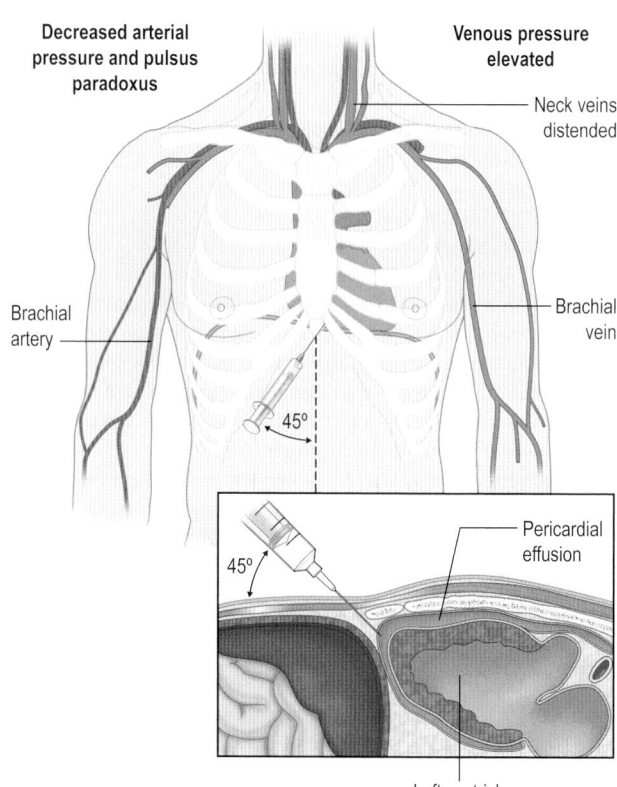

Fig. 30.36 Pericardiocentesis.

- cardiogenic shock
- doubtful fluid status.

Intra-aortic balloon pumping

This technique is used to assist the failing left ventricle temporarily. A catheter with a long, sausage-shaped balloon at its tip is introduced percutaneously into the femoral artery and manipulated under X-ray control so that the balloon lies in the descending aorta just below the aortic arch (**Fig. 30.37**). The balloon is rhythmically deflated and inflated with carbon dioxide gas. Using the ECG or intra-aortic pressure changes, the inflation is timed to occur during ventricular diastole to increase diastolic aortic pressure and, consequently, to improve coronary and cerebral blood flow. During systole the balloon is deflated, resulting in a reduction in the resistance to left ventricular emptying. Intra-aortic balloon pumping is used for circulatory support in the following acute situations:
- ***Acute heart failure.*** Balloon pumping is employed to improve cardiac output when there is a transient or reversible depression of left ventricular function, such as in a patient with severe mitral valve regurgitation who is awaiting surgical replacement of the mitral valve, or in a patient with a ventricular septal defect that is due to septal infarction. It may also be used to support patients awaiting heart transplantation.
- ***Unstable angina pectoris.*** Balloon pumping is utilized to treat unstable angina pectoris by improving coronary flow and decreasing myocardial oxygen consumption by reducing the 'afterload'. This technique may be successful, even when medical therapy has failed. It is followed by early angiography and appropriate definitive therapy, such as surgery or coronary angioplasty.

Balloon pumping should not be used when there is no remediable cause of cardiac dysfunction. It is also unsuitable in patients

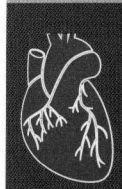

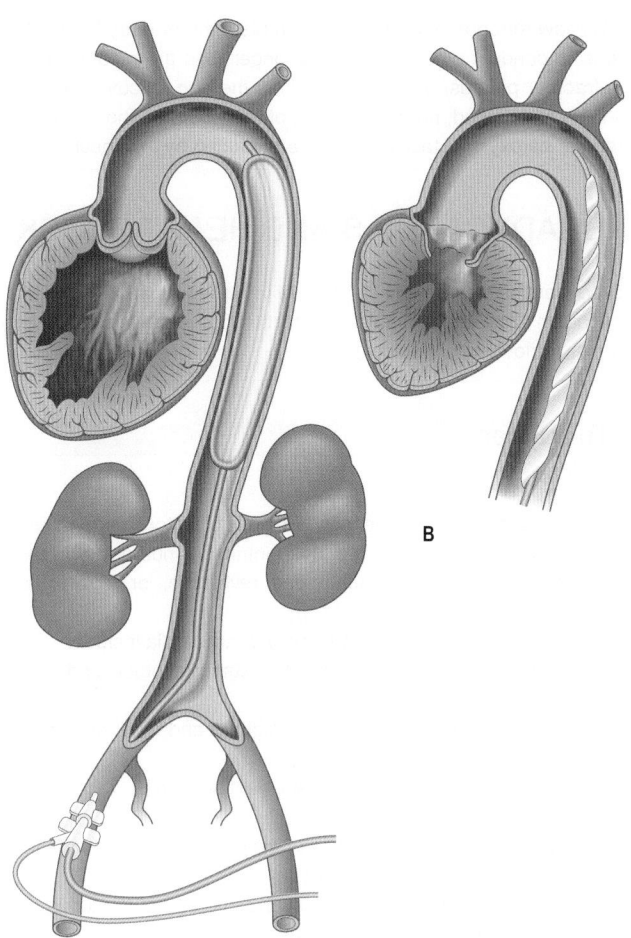

A

Fig. 30.37 Intra-aortic balloon pump. (A) The pump is inflated in the aorta during diastole. **(B)** The balloon is deflated during systole.

with severe aortic regurgitation, aortic dissection and severe peripheral vascular disease.

Complications of balloon pumping occur in about 20% of patients and include aortic dissection, leg ischaemia, emboli from the balloon, and balloon rupture. Embolic complications are reduced by anticoagulation with heparin.

Further reading

Nielsen N, Wettersley J, Cronberg T et al. Targeted temperature management at 33°C versus 36°C after cardiac arrest. *N Engl J Med* 2013; 369:2197–2206.
Soar J, Donnino MW, Maconochie I et al. 2018 International Consensus on Cardiopulmonary Resuscitation and Emergency Cardiovascular Care Science with Treatment Recommendations Summary. *Circulation* 2018; 133:194–206.
http://www.resus.org.uk. *Resuscitation Council (UK) Resuscitation Guidelines 2015*.

CARDIAC ARRHYTHMIAS

An abnormality of the cardiac rhythm is called a cardiac arrhythmia. Arrhythmias may cause sudden death, syncope, heart failure, chest pain, dizziness, palpitations or no symptoms at all. There are two main types of arrhythmia:

- **Bradycardia**: the heart rate is slow (<60 b.p.m. during the day or <50 b.p.m. at night).
- **Tachycardia**: the heart rate is fast (>100 b.p.m.).

Tachycardias are more symptomatic when the arrhythmia is fast and sustained. Tachycardias are subdivided into **supraventricular**

tachycardias, which arise from the atrium or the AV junction, and **ventricular tachycardias**, which arise from the ventricles.

Some arrhythmias occur in patients with apparently normal hearts; in others, arrhythmias originate from diseased tissue, such as scar, as a result of underlying structural heart disease. When myocardial function is poor, arrhythmias are more symptomatic and are potentially life-threatening.

Sinus node function

The normal cardiac pacemaker is the sinus node (see p. 1023) and, like most cardiac tissue, it depolarizes spontaneously.

The rate of sinus node discharge is modulated by the autonomic nervous system. Normally, the parasympathetic system predominates, resulting in slowing of the spontaneous discharge rate from approximately 100 to 70 b.p.m. A reduction of parasympathetic tone or an increase in sympathetic stimulation leads to tachycardia; conversely, increased parasympathetic tone or decreased sympathetic stimulation produces bradycardia. The sinus rate in women is slightly faster than in men. Normal sinus rhythm is characterized by P waves that are upright in leads I and II of the ECG (see **Fig. 30.18**) but inverted in lead AVR.

Sinus arrhythmia

Fluctuations of autonomic tone result in phasic changes of the sinus discharge rate. During inspiration, parasympathetic tone falls and the heart rate quickens; on expiration, the heart rate falls. This variation is normal, particularly in children and young adults. Typically, sinus arrhythmia results in predictable irregularities of the pulse.

Sinus bradycardia

A sinus rate of less than 60 b.p.m. during the day or <50 b.p.m. at night is known as sinus bradycardia. It is usually asymptomatic unless the rate is very slow. Sinus bradycardia is normal in athletes owing to increased vagal tone. Other causes may be divided into systemic or cardiac, and are discussed on page 1052.

Sinus tachycardia

Sinus rate acceleration to more than 100 b.p.m. is known as sinus tachycardia. Again, causes may be divided into systemic or cardiac, and are discussed on page 1057.

Mechanisms of arrhythmia production

Abnormalities of automaticity, which could arise from a single cell, and abnormalities of conduction, which require abnormal interaction between cells, account for both bradycardia and tachycardia. Sinus bradycardia is a result of abnormally slow automaticity while bradycardia due to AV block is caused by abnormal conduction within the AV node or the intraventricular conduction system. The mechanisms generating tachycardia are shown in **Fig. 30.38**.

Accelerated automaticity

The normal mechanism of spontaneous cardiac rhythmicity is slow depolarization of the transmembrane voltage during diastole until the threshold potential is reached and the action potential of the pacemaker cells takes off. This mechanism may be accelerated by increasing the rate of diastolic depolarization or changing the threshold potential (**Fig. 30.38A**). For example, sympathetic stimulation releases adrenaline (epinephrine), which enhances automaticity. Such changes are thought to produce sinus tachycardia, escape rhythms and accelerated AV nodal (junctional) rhythms.

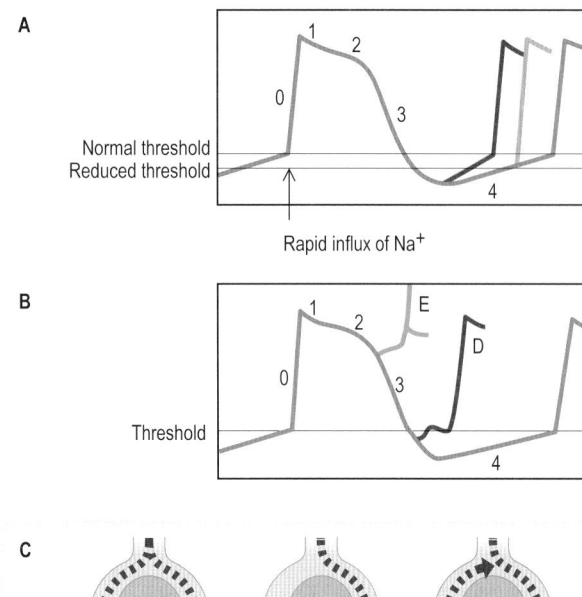

Fig. 30.38 Mechanisms of arrhythmogenesis. (A–B) Action potentials (i.e. the potential difference between intracellular and extracellular fluid) of ventricular myocardium after stimulation. **(A)** Increased (accelerated) automaticity due to reduced threshold potential or an increased slope of phase 4 depolarization (see p. 1033). **(B)** Triggered activity due to early (E) or delayed (D) 'after-depolarizations' reaching threshold potential. **(C)** Mechanism of circus movement or re-entry. In panel 1 the impulse passes down both limbs of the potential tachycardia circuit. In panel 2 the impulse is blocked in one pathway (α) but proceeds slowly down pathway β, returning along pathway α until it collides with refractory tissue. In panel 3 the impulse travels so slowly along pathway β that it can return along pathway α and complete the re-entry circuit, producing a circus movement tachycardia.

Triggered activity

Myocardial damage can result in oscillations of the transmembrane potential at the end of the action potential. These oscillations, called 'after-depolarizations', may reach threshold potential and produce an arrhythmia. If they occur before the transmembrane potential reaches its threshold (at the end of phase 3 of the action potential), they are called 'early after-depolarizations' (E in **Fig. 30.38B**). When they develop after the transmembrane potential is completed, they are called 'delayed after-depolarizations' (D in **Fig. 30.38B**).

The abnormal oscillations can be exaggerated by pacing, catecholamines, electrolyte disturbances, hypoxia, acidosis and some medications, which may then trigger an arrhythmia. The atrial tachycardias produced by digoxin toxicity are due to triggered activity. The initiation of ventricular arrhythmia in the long QT syndrome (see p. 1064) may be caused by this mechanism.

Re-entry (or circus movements)

The mechanism of re-entry (**Fig. 30.38C**) occurs when a 'ring' of cardiac tissue surrounds an inexcitable core (e.g. in a region of scarred myocardium). Tachycardia is initiated if an ectopic beat finds one limb refractory (α), resulting in unidirectional block, and the other limb excitable. Provided conduction through the excitable limb (β) is slow enough, the other limb (α) will have recovered and will allow retrograde activation to complete the re-entry loop. If the time to conduct around the ring is longer than the recovery times (refractory periods) of the tissue within the ring, circus movement will be maintained, producing a run of tachycardia. The majority of regular paroxysmal tachycardias are produced by this mechanism.

BRADYCARDIAS AND HEART BLOCK

Bradycardias may be due to failure of impulse formation (sinus bradycardia) or failure of impulse conduction from the atria to the ventricles (atrioventricular block).

Bradycardia

Sinus bradycardia

Sinus bradycardia is due either to extrinsic factors that influence a relatively normal sinus node, or to intrinsic sinus node disease. The mechanism can be acute and reversible, or chronic and degenerative.

Common **extrinsic causes** of sinus bradycardia include:
- hypothermia, hypothyroidism, cholestatic jaundice and raised intracranial pressure
- drug therapy with beta-blockers, digitalis and other antiarrhythmic drugs
- neurally mediated syndromes (see next section).

Common **intrinsic causes** include:
- acute ischaemia and infarction of the sinus node (as a complication of acute myocardial infarction)
- chronic degenerative changes, such as fibrosis of the atrium and sinus node (sick sinus syndrome).

Sick sinus syndrome or **sinoatrial disease** is usually caused by idiopathic fibrosis of the sinus node. Other causes of fibrosis, such as ischaemic heart disease, cardiomyopathy or myocarditis, can also cause the syndrome. Patients develop episodes of sinus bradycardia or sinus arrest (**Fig. 30.39B**), and commonly experience paroxysmal atrial tachyarrhythmias (tachy–brady syndrome) owing to diffuse atrial disease.

Neurally mediated syndromes

Neurally mediated syndromes are due to a reflex (Bezold–Jarisch) that may result in both bradycardia (sinus bradycardia, sinus arrest and AV block) and reflex peripheral vasodilation. These syndromes usually present as syncope or pre-syncope (dizzy spells).
- **Carotid sinus syndrome** occurs in the elderly and mainly leads to bradycardia. Syncope occurs (see p. 1029).
- **Neurocardiogenic (vasovagal) syncope** usually presents in young adults but may present for the first time in elderly patients (see p. 1029). It results from a variety of situations (physical and emotional) that affect the autonomic nervous system. The efferent output may be predominantly bradycardic, predominantly vasodilatory or mixed.
- **Postural orthostatic tachycardia syndrome (POTS)** is a sudden and significant increase in heart rate associated with normal or mildly reduced blood pressure and produced by standing. The underlying mechanism is a failure of the peripheral vasculature to constrict appropriately in response to orthostatic stress, which is compensated by an excessive increase in heart rate.

Many medications, such as antihypertensives, tricyclic antidepressants and neuroleptics, can be the cause of syncope, particularly in the elderly. Careful dose titration and avoidance of

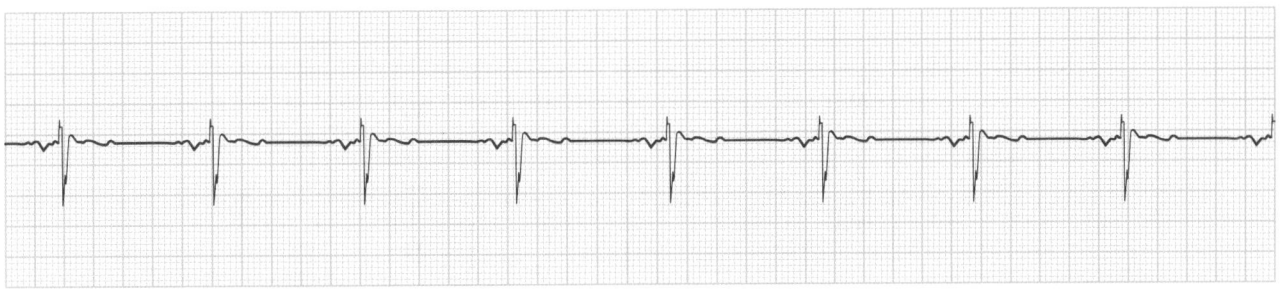

A

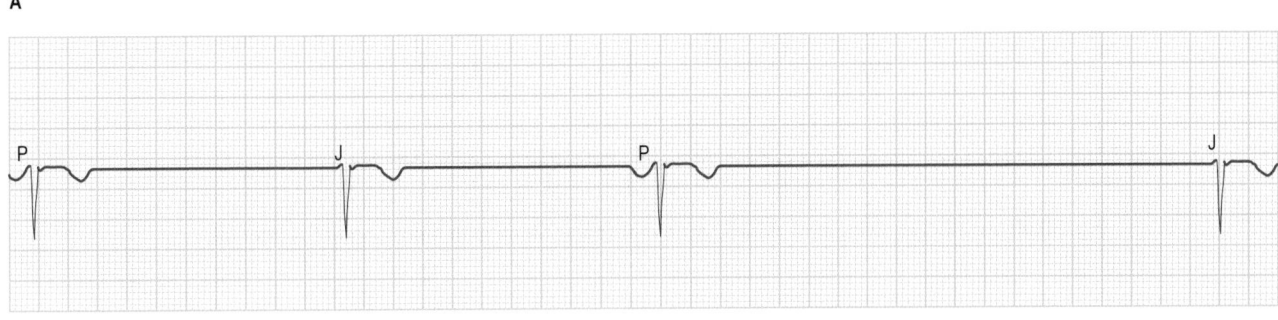

B

Fig. 30.39 Sinus node. (A) An ECG showing normal sinus rhythm (PR interval <0.2 sec). A P wave precedes each QRS complex. **(B)** A patient with sick sinus syndrome. The ECG shows sinus arrest (only occasional sinus P waves) and junctional escape beats (J). P waves are inverted in the cavity leads shown.

combination of two agents with the potential to cause syncope help to prevent iatrogenic syncope.

Management

The management of sinus bradycardia is first to identify and then, if possible, remove any extrinsic causes. Temporary pacing may be employed in patients with reversible causes until a normal sinus rate is restored, and in individuals with chronic degenerative conditions until a permanent pacemaker is implanted.

Chronic symptomatic sick sinus syndrome may require permanent pacing (DDD), with additional antiarrhythmic drugs (or ablation therapy) to manage any tachycardic element.

Patients with carotid sinus hypersensitivity (asystole >3 sec), especially if symptoms are reproduced by carotid sinus massage and life-threatening causes of syncope have been excluded, may benefit from pacemaker implantation.

Treatment options in vasovagal attacks include avoidance, if possible, of situations known to cause syncope in a particular patient, and sitting/lying down and applying counter-pressure manoeuvres (pushing the palms together or crossing the legs) if an attack threatens. Increased salt intake, compression of the lower legs with compression stockings, and drugs such as beta-blockers, alpha-agonists (e.g. midodrine) or myocardial negative inotropes (e.g. disopyramide) may be helpful.

In selected patients with 'malignant' neurocardiogenic syncope (syncope associated with injuries and demonstrated asystole), permanent pacemaker therapy is helpful. These patients benefit from dual-chamber pacemakers with a feature called 'rate drop response', which, once activated, paces the heart at a fast rate for a set period of time in order to prevent syncope.

Heart block

Heart block or conduction block may occur at any level in the conducting system. Block in either the AV node or the His bundle results in AV block, whereas block lower in the conduction system produces bundle branch block.

Atrioventricular block

There are three forms.

First-degree AV block

This is simple prolongation of the PR interval to more than 0.20 sec. Every atrial depolarization is followed by conduction to the ventricles but with delay (**Fig. 30.40**).

Second-degree AV block

This occurs when some P waves conduct and others do not. There are several forms (**Fig. 30.41**):

- **Mobitz I block** (Wenckebach block phenomenon) is progressive PR interval prolongation until a P wave fails to conduct. The PR interval before the blocked P wave is much longer than the PR interval after the blocked P wave.
- **Mobitz II block** occurs when a dropped QRS complex is not preceded by progressive PR interval prolongation. Usually, the QRS complex is wide (>0.12 sec).
- **2:1 or 3:1 (advanced) block** occurs when every second or third P wave conducts to the ventricles. This form of second-degree block is neither Mobitz I nor Mobitz II.

Wenckebach AV block in general is due to block in the AV node, whereas Mobitz II block signifies block at an infranodal level, such as the His bundle. The risk of progression to complete heart block is greater and reliability of the resultant escape rhythm is less with Mobitz II block. Therefore, pacing is usually indicated in Mobitz II block, whereas patients with Wenckebach AV block are usually monitored.

Acute myocardial infarction may produce **second-degree heart block**. In inferior myocardial infarction, close monitoring and transcutaneous temporary back-up pacing are all that is required. In anterior myocardial infarction, second-degree

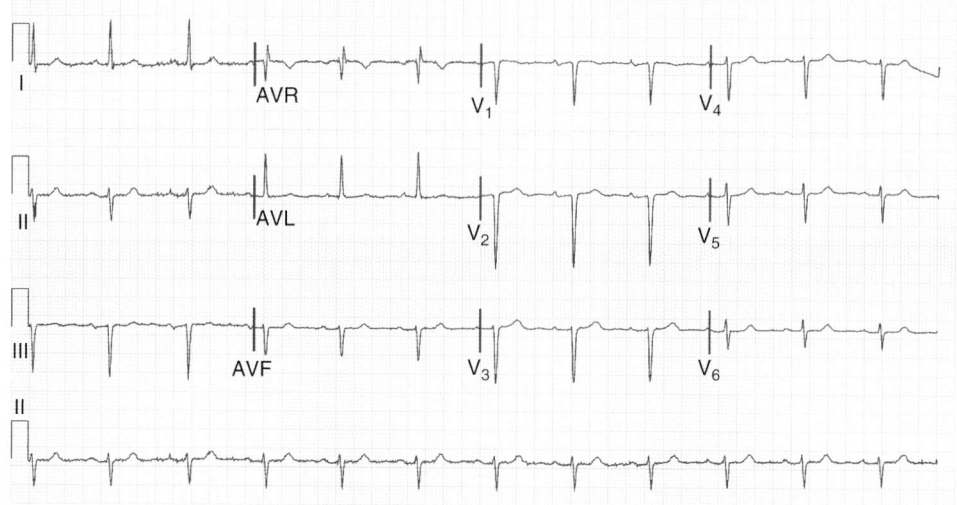

Fig. 30.40 An ECG showing first-degree atrioventricular block with a prolonged PR interval.

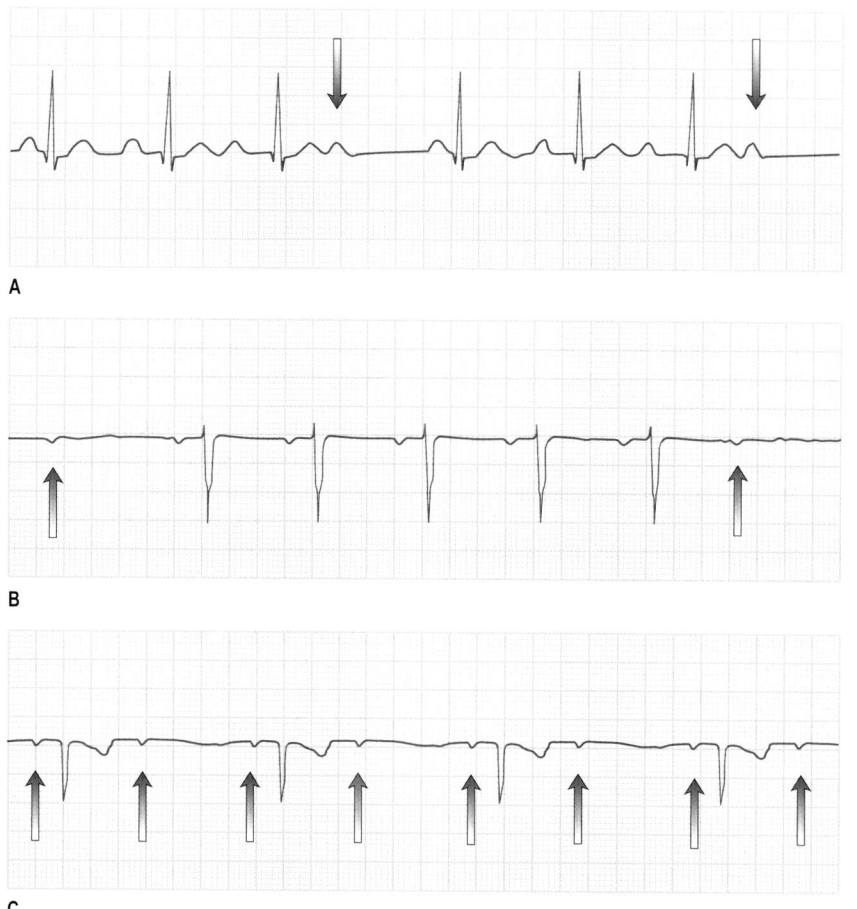

Fig. 30.41 **Three varieties of second-degree atrioventricular (AV) block.** **(A)** Wenckebach (Mobitz type I) AV block. The PR interval gradually prolongs until the P wave does not conduct to the ventricles (arrowed). **(B)** Mobitz type II AV block. The P waves that do not conduct to the ventricles (arrowed) are not preceded by gradual PR interval prolongation. **(C)** Two P waves to each QRS complex. The PR interval prior to the dropped P wave is always the same. It is not possible to define this type of AV block as type I or type II Mobitz block and it is, therefore, a third variety of second-degree AV block (arrows show P waves).

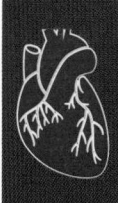

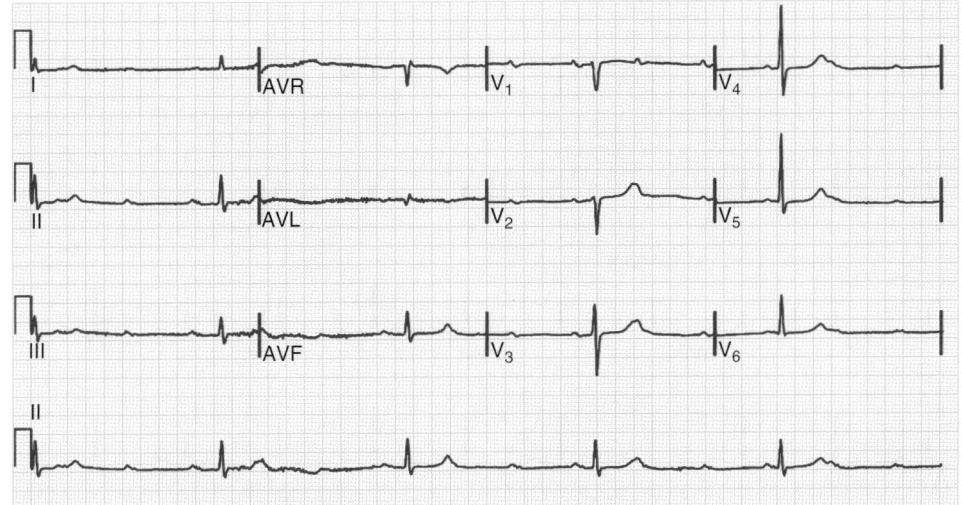

Fig. 30.42 Complete heart block. In this example, the QRS complexes are narrow (0.08 sec) and there is complete dissociation of atrial and ventricular complexes.

heart block is associated with a high risk of progression to complete heart block, and temporary pacing followed by permanent pacemaker implantation is usually indicated. Block either in the AV node or at an infranodal level may cause 2:1 heart block. Management depends on the clinical setting in which it occurs.

Third-degree (complete) AV block

Complete heart block occurs when all atrial activity fails to conduct to the ventricles (**Fig. 30.42**). In patients with complete heart block, the aetiology needs to be established (**Box 30.13**). In this situation, life is maintained by a spontaneous escape rhythm.

A narrow-complex escape rhythm (<0.12 sec QRS complex) originates from the His bundle and therefore implies that the region of block lies more proximally in the AV node. The escape rhythm occurs with an adequate rate (50–60 b.p.m.) and is relatively reliable. Treatment depends on the aetiology. Recent-onset, narrow-complex AV block that has transient causes may respond to intravenous atropine but temporary pacing facilities should be available for the management of these patients. Chronic narrow-complex AV block requires permanent pacing (dual-chamber; see p. 1049) if it is symptomatic or associated with heart disease. Pacing is also advocated for isolated, congenital AV block, even if asymptomatic.

Broad-complex escape rhythm (>0.12 sec) implies that the escape rhythm originates below the His bundle and therefore that the region of block lies more distally in the His–Purkinje system. The resulting rhythm is slow (15–40 b.p.m.) and relatively unreliable. Dizziness and blackouts (*Stokes–Adams attacks*) often occur. In the elderly it is usually caused by degenerative fibrosis and calcification of the distal conduction system (*Lev's disease*). In younger individuals a proximal progressive cardiac conduction disease due to an inflammatory process is known as *Lenegre's disease*. Sodium channel abnormalities have been identified in both syndromes. Broad-complex AV block may also be caused by ischaemic heart disease, myocarditis or cardiomyopathy. Permanent pacemaker implantation (see p. 1049) is indicated, as pacing considerably reduces the mortality. Because ventricular arrhythmias are not uncommon, an implantable cardioverter–defibrillator (ICD) may be

> **? Box 30.13 Causes of complete heart block**
>
> **Congenital**
> - Autoimmune (e.g. maternal SLE)
> - Structural heart disease (e.g. transposition of great vessels)
>
> **Idiopathic fibrosis**
> - Lev's disease (progressive fibrosis of distal His–Purkinje system in elderly patients)
> - Lenegre's disease (proximal His–Purkinje fibrosis in younger patients)
>
> **Ischaemic heart disease**
> - Acute myocardial infarct
> - Ischaemic cardiomyopathy
>
> **Non-ischaemic heart disease**
> - Calcific aortic stenosis
> - Idiopathic dilated cardiomyopathy
> - Infiltrations (e.g. amyloidosis, sarcoidosis, neoplasia)
>
> **Cardiac surgery**
> - e.g. Following aortic valve replacement, CABG, VSD repair
>
> **Iatrogenic**
> - Radiofrequency AV node ablation and pacemaker implantation
>
> **Drug-induced**
> - e.g. Digoxin, beta-blockers, non-dihydropyridine calcium-channel blockers, amiodarone
>
> **Infections**
> - Endocarditis
> - Lyme disease
> - Chagas' disease
>
> **Autoimmune rheumatic disease**
> - e.g. SLE, rheumatoid arthritis
>
> **Neuromuscular diseases**
> - e.g. Duchenne muscular dystrophy
>
> AV, atrioventricular; CABG, coronary artery bypass graft surgery; SLE, systemic lupus erythematosus; VSD, ventricular septal defect.

indicated in those with severe left ventricular dysfunction (>0.30 sec duration).

Bundle branch block

The His bundle gives rise to the right and left bundle branches. The left bundle subdivides into the anterior and posterior divisions of the left bundle. Various conduction disturbances can occur.

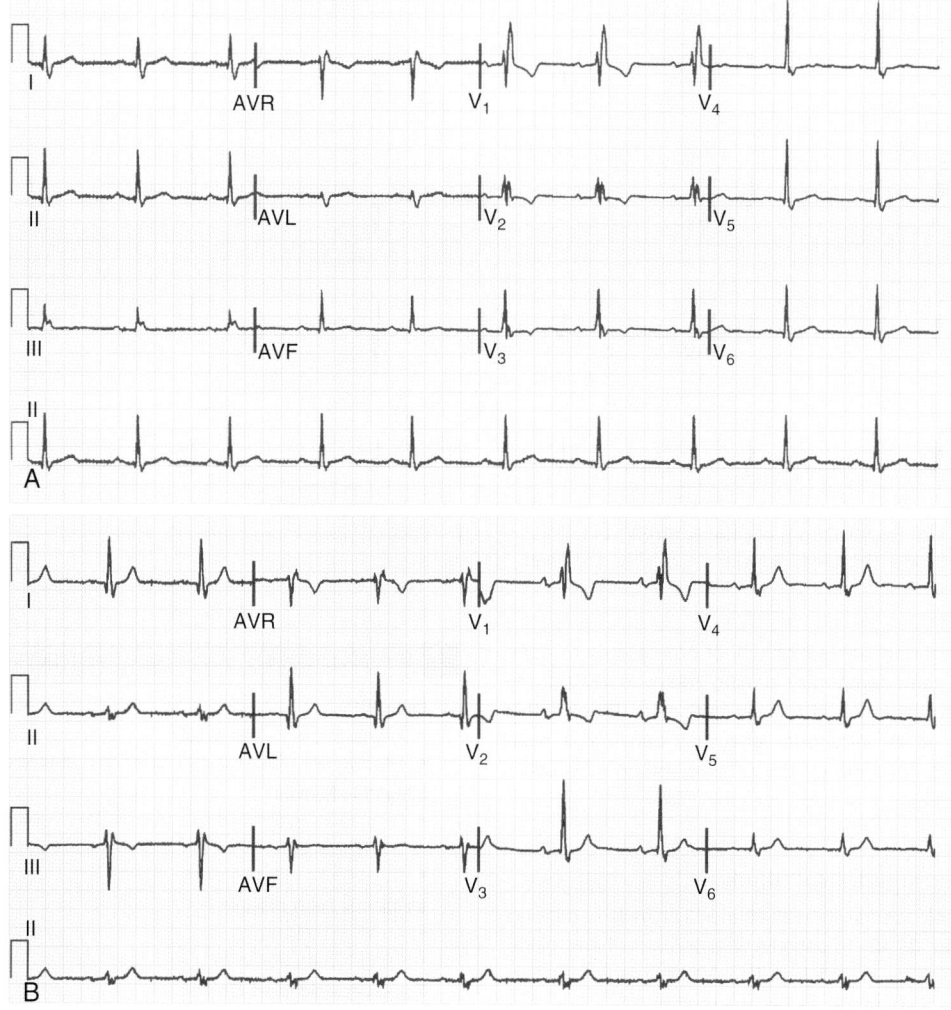

Fig. 30.43 Right bundle branch block versus bifascicular block. (A) A 12-lead ECG showing right bundle branch block. Note an rsR′ pattern with the tall R′ in lead V₁–V₂ and the broad S waves in leads I and V₅–V₆. **(B)** Compare with this ECG showing bifascicular block. In addition to right bundle branch block, note the left axis deviation and deep S waves in leads III and AVF, which are typical of left anterior hemiblock.

Bundle branch conduction delay

This produces slight widening of the QRS complex (up to 0.12 sec). It is known as incomplete bundle branch block.

Complete block of a bundle branch

This is associated with a wider QRS complex (≥0.12 sec). The shape of the QRS depends on whether the right or the left bundle is blocked.

    Right bundle branch block (**Fig. 30.43A**) produces late activation of the right ventricle. This is seen as deep S waves in leads I and V₆, and as a tall late R wave in lead V₁ (late activation moving towards right-sided leads and away from left-sided leads).

    Left bundle branch block (**Fig. 30.44**) produces the opposite: a deep S wave in lead V₁ and a tall late R wave in leads I and V₆. Because left bundle branch conduction is normally responsible for the initial ventricular activation, left bundle branch block also produces abnormal Q waves.

Hemiblock

Delay or block in the divisions of the left bundle branch produces a swing in the direction of depolarization (electrical axis) of the heart.

When the anterior division is blocked (left anterior hemiblock), the left ventricle is activated from inferior to superior. This produces a superior and leftward movement of the axis (left axis deviation). Delay or block in the postero-inferior division swings the QRS axis inferiorly to the right (right axis deviation).

Bifascicular block

Bifascicular block (see **Fig. 30.43B**) is a combination of a block of any two of the following: the right bundle branch, the left antero-superior division and the left postero-inferior division. Block of the remaining fascicle will result in complete AV block.

Clinical features of heart blocks

Bundle branch blocks are usually asymptomatic. Right bundle branch block causes wide but physiological splitting of the second heart sound. Left bundle branch block may cause reverse splitting of the second sound. Patients with intraventricular conduction disturbances may complain of syncope. This is due to intermittent complete heart block or to ventricular tachyarrhythmias. ECG monitoring and electrophysiological studies are needed to determine the cause of syncope in these patients.

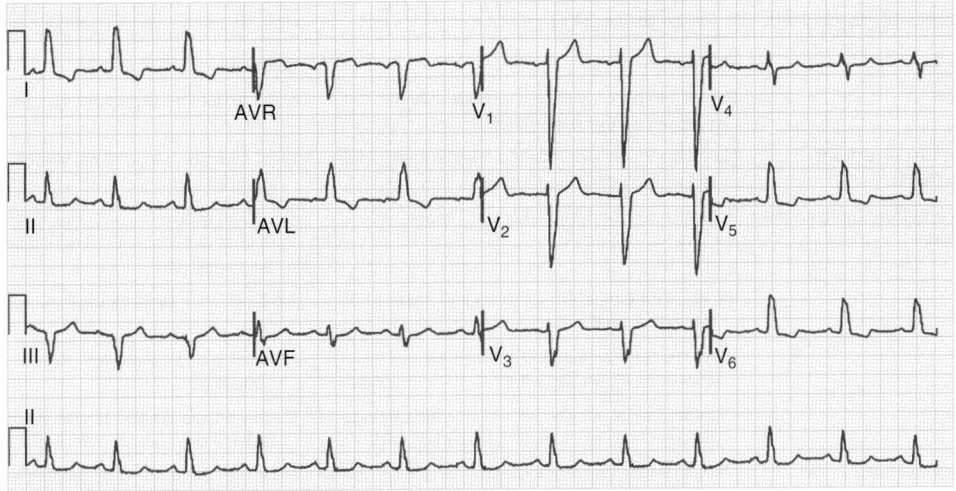

Fig. 30.44 A 12-lead ECG showing left bundle branch block. The QRS duration is more than 0.12 sec. Note the broad, notched R waves with ST depression in leads I, AVL and V6, and the broad QS waves in V1–V3.

Aetiology

Right bundle branch block occurs as an isolated congenital anomaly, present in 5% of healthy individuals, or is associated with cardiac or pulmonary conditions. Conditions commonly associated with right bundle branch block include congenital cardiac disorders, such atrial and ventricular septal defects, pulmonary stenosis and Fallot's tetralogy, pulmonary embolism, pulmonary hypertension, myocardial infarction, fibrosis of conduction tissue and Chagas' disease. Block in the right bundle alone does not tend to alter the electrical axis of the heart unless accompanied by right ventricular hypertrophy (RV overload) or coexistent fascicular block. The combination of right bundle branch block with left axis deviation is seen in patients with ostium primum atrial septal defects but more often signifies diffuse conduction tissue disease affecting the right bundle and the left anterior fascicle. Complete left bundle branch block is often associated with extensive left ventricular disease. The most common causes include aortic stenosis, hypertension, myocardial infarction and severe coronary disease, similar to the causes of complete heart block.

SUPRAVENTRICULAR TACHYCARDIAS

Supraventricular tachycardias (SVTs) arise from the atrium or the atrioventricular junction. Conduction is via the His–Purkinje system; therefore, the QRS shape during tachycardia is usually similar to that seen in the same patient during baseline rhythm. A classification of supraventricular tachycardia is given in **Box 30.14**. Some of these tachycardias are discussed in more detail in the sections that follow.

Inappropriate sinus tachycardia

Inappropriate sinus tachycardia is a persistent increase in resting heart rate unrelated to, or out of proportion with, the level of physical or emotional stress. It is found predominantly in young women. Sinus tachycardia due to intrinsic sinus node abnormalities, such as enhanced automaticity, or abnormal autonomic regulation of the heart with excess sympathetic and reduced parasympathetic input, is extremely rare.

In general, sinus tachycardia is a secondary phenomenon and the underlying causes need to be actively investigated. Depending on the clinical setting, acute causes include exercise, emotion, pain, fever, infection, acute heart failure, acute pulmonary embolism and hypovolaemia. Chronic causes include pregnancy, anaemia, hyperthyroidism and catecholamine excess. The underlying cause should be found and treated, rather than treating the compensatory physiological response. If necessary, beta-blockers may be used to slow the sinus rate – in hyperthyroidism, for example (see **Box 21.30**); ivabradine, an I_F (pacemaker current) blocker, may be useful when beta-blockade cannot be tolerated.

Atrioventricular junctional tachycardias

AV nodal re-entrant and AV re-entrant tachycardias are usually referred to as paroxysmal SVTs and are often seen in young patients with no or little structural heart disease, although congenital heart abnormalities can coexist in a small proportion of patients with these arrhythmias. The first presentation is commonly between ages 12 and 30, and the prevalence is approximately 2.5/1000.

In these tachycardias the AV node is an essential component of the re-entry circuit.

Atrioventricular nodal re-entrant tachycardia

Atrioventricular nodal re-entrant tachycardia (AVNRT) is twice as common in women. Clinically, the tachycardia often strikes suddenly without obvious provocation, but exertion, emotional stress, coffee, tea and alcohol may aggravate or induce it. An attack may stop spontaneously or may continue indefinitely until medical intervention.

In AVNRT, there are two functionally and anatomically different pathways predominantly within the AV node: one is characterized by a short effective refractory period and slow conduction, and the other has a longer effective refractory period and conducts faster. In sinus rhythm the atrial impulse that depolarizes the ventricles usually conducts through the fast pathway. If the atrial impulse (e.g. an atrial premature beat) occurs early when the fast pathway is still refractory, the slow pathway takes over in propagating the atrial impulse to the ventricles. It then travels back through the fast pathway, which has already recovered its excitability, thus initiating the most common 'slow–fast', or typical, AVNRT.

Box 30.14 Causes of supraventricular tachycardia (SVT)

Tachycardia	ECG features	Comment
Sinus tachycardia	P wave morphology similar to sinus rhythm; p waves always precede QRS	Need to determine underlying cause
Atrioventricular nodal re-entrant tachycardia (AVNRT)	No visible P wave, or inverted P wave immediately before or after QRS complex	Most common cause of palpitations in patients with normal hearts
Atrioventricular re-entrant tachycardia (AVRT) complexes	P wave visible between QRS and T wave	Due to an accessory pathway; if pathway conducts in both directions, ECG during sinus rhythm may be pre-excited
Atrial fibrillation	'Irregularly irregular' RR intervals and absence of organized atrial activity	Most common tachycardia in patients >65 years
Atrial flutter	Visible flutter waves at 300 b.p.m. (sawtooth appearance), usually with 2:1 AV conduction	Suspect in any patient with regular SVT at 150 b.p.m.
Atrial tachycardia	Organized atrial activity with P wave morphology different from sinus rhythm preceding QRS	Usually occurs in patients with structural heart disease or following extensive ablation within atria
Multifocal atrial tachycardia	Multiple P wave morphologies (≥3) and irregular RR intervals	Rare arrhythmia; most commonly associated with significant chronic lung disease
Accelerated junctional tachycardia	ECG similar to that in AVNRT	Rare in adults

The rhythm is recognized on ECG from normal regular QRS complexes, usually at a rate of 140–240/min (**Fig. 30.45A**). Sometimes, the QRS complexes will show typical bundle branch block. P waves either are not visible or are seen immediately before or after the QRS complex because of simultaneous atrial and ventricular activation. It is less common (5–10%) to observe a tachycardia when the atrial impulse conducts anterogradely through the fast pathway and returns through the slow pathway, producing a long RP′ interval ('fast–slow' or long RP′ tachycardia).

Atrioventricular re-entrant tachycardia

This large circuit comprises the AV node, the His bundle, the ventricle and an abnormal connection of myocardial fibres from the ventricle back to the atrium. It is called an accessory pathway or bypass tract and results from an incomplete separation of the atria and the ventricles during fetal development.

In contrast to AVNRT, atrioventricular re-entrant tachycardia (AVRT) is due to a macro re-entry circuit and each part of the circuit is activated sequentially. As a result, atrial activation occurs after ventricular activation and the P wave is usually seen clearly between the QRS and T waves (**Fig. 30.45B**).

Accessory pathways are most commonly situated on the left but may occur anywhere around the AV groove. The most common accessory pathways, known as **Kent bundles**, are in the free wall or septum. In about 10% of cases, multiple pathways occur. **Mahaim fibres** are atriofascicular or nodofascicular fibres that enter the ventricular myocardium in the region of the right bundle branch. Accessory pathways that conduct from the ventricles to the atria only are not visible on the surface ECG during sinus rhythm and are therefore 'concealed'. Accessory pathways that conduct bidirectionally usually are manifest on the surface ECG. If the accessory pathway conducts from the atrium to the ventricle during sinus rhythm, the electrical impulse can conduct quickly over this abnormal connection to depolarize part of the ventricles abnormally (pre-excitation). A pre-excited ECG is characterized by a short PR interval and a wide QRS complex that begins as a slurred part known as the δ **wave** (**Fig. 30.45C**). Patients with a history of palpitations and a pre-excited ECG have a condition known as Wolff–Parkinson–White (WPW) syndrome.

During AVRT, the AV node and ventricles are activated normally (**orthodromic AVRT**), usually resulting in a narrow QRS complex.

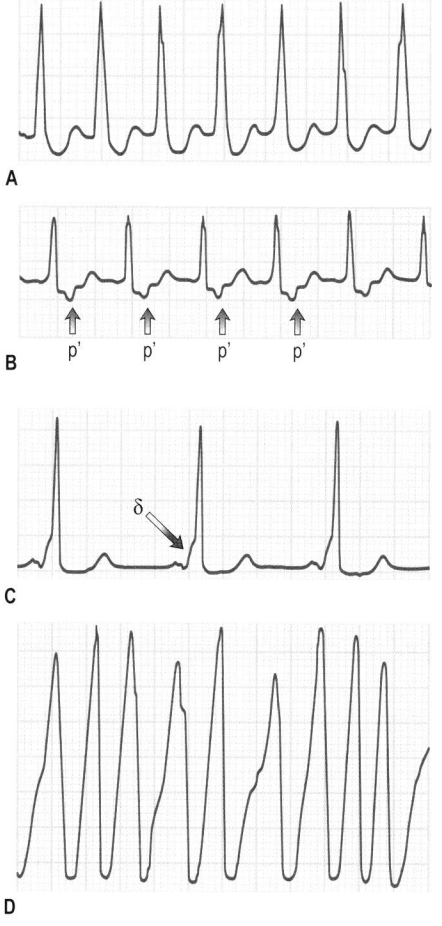

Fig. 30.45 Atrioventricular junctional tachycardia. (A) Atrioventricular nodal re-entrant tachycardia (AVNRT). The QRS complexes are narrow and the P waves cannot be seen. **(B)** Atrioventricular re-entrant tachycardia (AVRT) (Wolff–Parkinson–White syndrome, WPW). The tachycardia P waves (arrowed) are clearly seen after narrow QRS complexes. **(C)** An ECG taken in a patient with WPW syndrome during sinus rhythm. Note the short PR interval and the δ wave (arrowed). **(D)** Atrial fibrillation in the WPW syndrome. Note the tachycardia with broad QRS complexes and the fast and irregular ventricular rate.

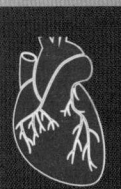

Less commonly, the tachycardia circuit can be reversed, with activation of the ventricles via the accessory pathway, and atrial activation via retrograde conduction through the AV node (*antidromic AVRT*). This results in a broad-complex tachycardia. These patients are also prone to atrial fibrillation.

During atrial fibrillation, the ventricles may be depolarized by impulses travelling over both the abnormal and the normal pathways. This results in pre-excited atrial fibrillation, a characteristic tachycardia that is typified by irregularly irregular broad QRS complexes (**Fig. 30.45D**). If an accessory pathway has a short antegrade effective refractory period (<250 ms), it may conduct to the ventricles at an extremely high rate and may cause ventricular fibrillation. The incidence of sudden death is 0.15–0.39% per patient-year and it may be a first manifestation of the disease in younger individuals. Verapamil and digoxin may allow a higher rate of conduction over the abnormal pathway and precipitate ventricular fibrillation. Therefore, neither verapamil nor digoxin should be used to treat atrial fibrillation associated with the WPW syndrome.

Clinical features of AVNRT and AVRT

The leading symptom of most SVTs, in particular AVNRT and AVRT, is rapid regular palpitations, usually with abrupt onset and sudden termination, which can occur spontaneously or be precipitated by simple movements. A common feature is termination by Valsalva manoeuvres. In younger individuals with no structural heart disease the rapid heart rate can be the main pathological finding.

Irregular palpitations may be due to atrial premature beats, atrial flutter with varying AV conduction block, atrial fibrillation or multifocal atrial tachycardia. In patients with depressed ventricular function, uncontrolled atrial fibrillation can reduce cardiac output and cause hypotension and congestive heart failure.

Other symptoms may include anxiety, dizziness, dyspnoea, neck pulsation, central chest pain and weakness. Polyuria may occur because of the release of atrial natriuretic peptide in response to increased atrial pressures during the tachycardia, especially during AVNRT and atrial fibrillation. Prominent jugular venous pulsations due to atrial contractions against closed AV valves may be observed during AVNRT.

Syncope has been reported in 10–15% of patients, usually just after initiation of the arrhythmia or in association with a prolonged pause following its termination. It is more common if the person is standing. However, in older patients with concomitant heart disease, such as aortic stenosis, hypertrophic cardiomyopathy and cerebrovascular disease, significant hypotension and syncope may result from moderately fast ventricular rates.

Management of AVNRT and AVRT

Acute management

In an emergency, distinguishing between AVNRT and AVRT may be difficult but is usually not critical, as both tachycardias respond to the same treatment. Patients presenting with SVTs and haemodynamic instability (e.g. hypotension, pulmonary oedema) require emergency cardioversion. If the patient is haemodynamically stable, vagal manoeuvres, including right carotid massage (see **Box 30.10**), the Valsalva manoeuvre and facial immersion in cold water, can be successfully employed.

If physical manoeuvres have not been successful, intravenous adenosine (initially 6 mg by i.v. push, followed by 12 mg if needed) should be tried. Adenosine is a very short-acting (half-life <10 sec), naturally occurring purine nucleoside that causes complete heart block for a fraction of a second following intravenous administration. It is highly effective at terminating AVNRT and AVRT or

unmasking underlying atrial activity, but rarely affects ventricular tachycardia. The side-effects of adenosine are very brief but may include chest pain, sense of impending doom, bronchospasm, flushing or heaviness of the limbs. Adenosine should be used with caution in patients with a history of asthma. An alternative treatment is verapamil 5–10 mg i.v. over 5–10 min or beta-blockers (esmolol, propranolol, metoprolol). Verapamil must not be given after beta-blockers *or* if the tachycardia presents with broad (>0.12 sec) QRS complexes.

Long-term management

Patients with suspected cardiac arrhythmias should always be referred to a cardiologist for electrophysiological evaluation and long-term management, as both pharmacological and non-pharmacological treatments, including ablation of an accessory pathway, are readily available. Verapamil, diltiazem and beta-blockers have proven efficacy in 60–80% of patients. Sodium-channel blockers (flecainide and propafenone), potassium repolarization current blockers (sotalol, dofetilide, azimilide) and the multichannel blocker amiodarone may also prevent the occurrence of tachycardia.

Refinement of catheter ablation techniques has rendered many AV junctional tachycardias entirely curable. Modification of the slow pathway is successful in 96% of patients with AVNRT, although a 1% risk of AV block is present. In AVRT, the target for catheter ablation is the accessory pathway(s). The success rate of ablation of a single accessory pathway is approximately 95%, with a recurrence rate of 5%, requiring a repeat procedure.

Atrial tachyarrhythmias

Atrial tachyarrhythmias, including atrial fibrillation, atrial flutter, atrial tachycardia and atrial ectopic beats, all arise from the atrial myocardium. They share similar aetiologies, of which the most commonly encountered in clinical practice are increasing age, myocardial infarction, hypertension, obesity, diabetes mellitus, hypertrophic cardiomyopathy, heart failure, valvular heart disease, myocarditis, pericarditis, cardiothoracic surgery, electrolyte imbalance, alcohol use, obstructive airway disease, chest infections and hyperthyroidism.

Atrial fibrillation

This is a common arrhythmia, occurring in 1–2% of the general population and 5–15% of patients over 75 years of age. It also occurs, particularly in a paroxysmal form, in younger patients. Any condition resulting in raised atrial pressure, increased atrial muscle mass, atrial fibrosis, or inflammation and infiltration of the atrium may cause atrial fibrillation.

Although rheumatic heart disease, alcohol intoxication and thyrotoxicosis are the 'classic' causes of atrial fibrillation, hypertension and heart failure are the most common causes in the developed world. Hyperthyroidism may provoke atrial fibrillation, sometimes as virtually the only feature of the disease, and thyroid function tests are mandatory in any patient with atrial fibrillation that is unaccounted for. Atrial fibrillation occurs in one-third of patients after cardiac surgery.

In some patients no cause can be found and this group is labelled as having 'lone' atrial fibrillation. The pathogenesis of 'lone', or 'idiopathic', atrial fibrillation is unknown but genetic predisposition or even specific genetically predetermined forms of the arrhythmia have been proposed. About 30–40% of patients with atrial fibrillation,

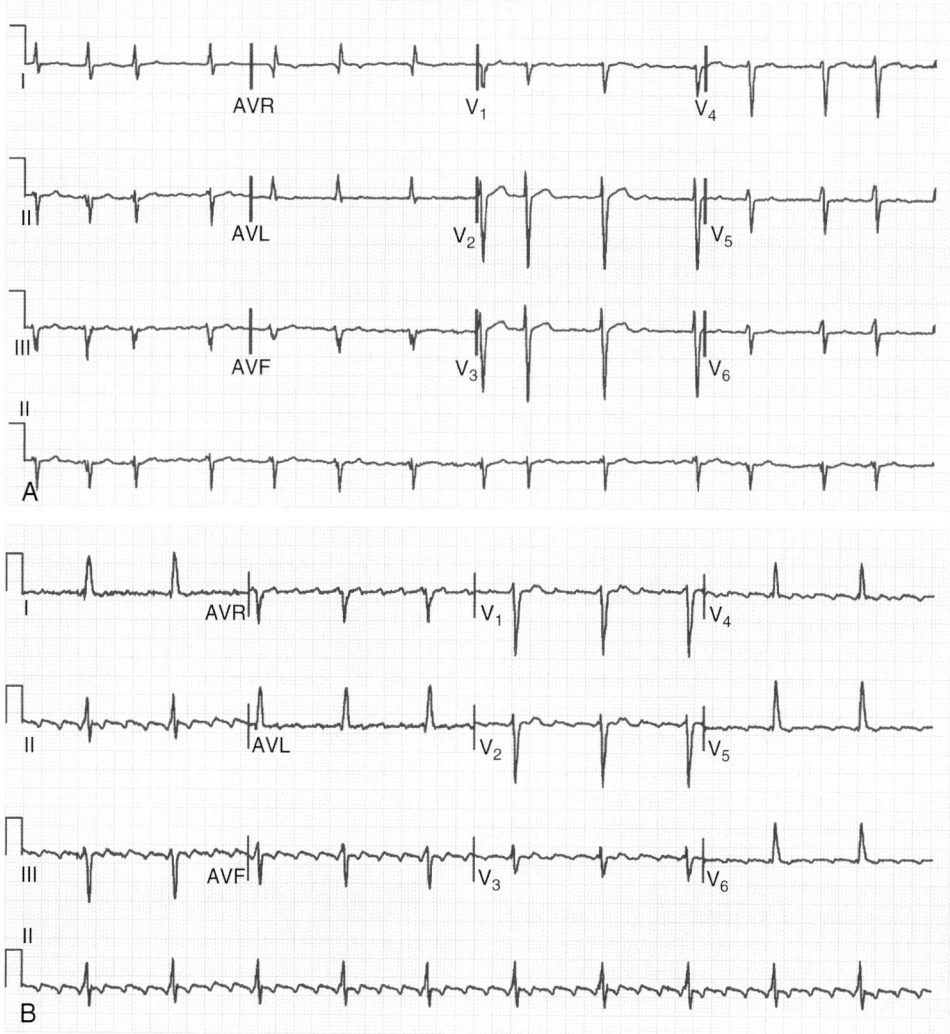

Fig. 30.46 Twelve-lead ECGs showing atrial fibrillation and atrial flutter. (A) Atrial fibrillation. Note the absolute rhythm irregularity. The ECG shows fine oscillations of the baseline (so-called fibrillation or *f* waves) and no clear P waves. **(B)** Atrial flutter, showing regular sawtooth-like atrial flutter waves (F waves) between QRS complexes. The flutter frequency is 300/min. Every fourth flutter wave is transmitted to the ventricles and the ventricular rate is therefore 75/min.

especially those who present at a young age, have at least one parent with the arrhythmia, and genes associated with the sodium channel, the potassium channel, gap junction proteins and right–left isomerism have been implicated. Gene defects linked to chromosomes 10, 6, 5 and 4 have been associated with familial atrial fibrillation.

Atrial fibrillation is maintained by continuous, rapid (300–600/min) activation of the atria by multiple meandering re-entry wavelets, often driven by rapidly depolarizing automatic foci, located predominantly within the pulmonary veins. The atria respond electrically at this rate but there is no coordinated mechanical action and only a proportion of the impulses are conducted to the ventricles. The ventricular response depends on the rate and regularity of atrial activity, particularly at the entry to the AV node, the refractory properties of the AV node itself, and the balance between sympathetic and parasympathetic tone.

Clinical features

Symptoms attributable to atrial fibrillation are highly variable. In some patients (about 30%) it is an incidental finding, while others attend hospital as an emergency with rapid palpitations, dyspnoea and/or chest pain following the onset of atrial fibrillation. Most patients with on-going atrial fibrillation experience some deterioration of exercise capacity or wellbeing, but this may be appreciated only once sinus rhythm is restored. When caused by rheumatic mitral stenosis, the onset of atrial fibrillation results in considerable worsening of cardiac failure.

The patient has an 'irregularly irregular' pulse, as opposed to a basically regular pulse with an occasional irregularity (e.g. extrasystoles) or recurring irregular patterns (e.g. Wenckebach block). The irregular nature of the pulse in atrial fibrillation is maintained during exercise.

The ECG shows fine oscillations of the baseline (so-called fibrillation or *f* waves) and no clear P waves (**Fig. 30.46A**). The QRS rhythm is rapid and irregular. Untreated, the ventricular rate is usually 120–180/min but it slows with treatment.

The clinical classification of atrial fibrillation includes:
- first detected – irrespective of duration or severity of symptoms
- paroxysmal – stops spontaneously within 7 days

- persistent – continuous >7 days
- longstanding persistent – continuous >1 year
- permanent – continuous, with a joint decision between the patient and the physician to cease further attempts to regain sinus rhythm.

The classification is helpful in choosing between rhythm restoration and rate control. Atrial fibrillation may be asymptomatic and the 'first detected episode' should not necessarily be regarded as the true onset.

Management

Acute management

When atrial fibrillation is due to an acute precipitating event, such as alcohol toxicity, chest infection or hyperthyroidism, the provoking cause should be treated. Strategies for the acute management of atrial fibrillation are:

- **Ventricular rate control**, achieved by drugs that block the AV node (see later).
- **Cardioversion**, achieved electrically by DC shock (see p. 1048), or medically by intravenous infusion of an antiarrhythmic drug such as flecainide, propafenone, vernakalant or amiodarone. Cardioversion can also be achieved by giving an oral agent (flecainide or propafenone) previously tested in hospital and found to be safe in a particular patient ('pill-in-pocket' approach).

The choice depends on:

- how well the arrhythmia is tolerated (is cardioversion urgent?)
- whether anticoagulation is required before considering elective cardioversion
- whether spontaneous cardioversion is likely (previous history? reversible cause?).

Conversion to sinus rhythm can be achieved by electrical DC cardioversion in about 80% of patients. Biphasic waveform defibrillation is more effective than conventional (monophasic) defibrillation, and biphasic defibrillators are now standard. To minimize the risk of thromboembolism associated with cardioversion, patients are fully anticoagulated with warfarin (International Normalized Ratio (INR) 2.0–3.0) or with a direct acting oral anticoagulant agent (DOAC) for 3 weeks before cardioversion (unless atrial fibrillation is of less than 48 hours' duration) and at least 4 weeks after the procedure. The patient is then assessed for the necessity for long-term anticoagulation based on their thromboembolic risk score (see later). If cardioversion is urgent and the patient is not on any anticoagulation, transoesophageal echocardiography is used to exclude the presence of atrial thrombus.

Long-term management

Two strategies are available:

- 'rate control' (AV nodal slowing agents **plus oral anticoagulation**)
- 'rhythm control' (antiarrhythmic drugs plus DC cardioversion **plus oral anticoagulation**).

Major randomized studies in patients predominantly over the age of 65 years (AFFIRM) or in patients with heart failure (AF-CHF) have shown that there is no net mortality or symptom benefit to be gained from one strategy compared with the other. Which strategy to adopt needs to be assessed for each individual patient. Factors to consider include the likelihood of maintaining sinus rhythm and the safety/tolerability of antiarrhythmic drugs in a particular patient.

Rhythm control

This is advocated for younger, symptomatic and physically active patients. **Recurrent paroxysms** may be prevented with oral medication. In general, patients with no significant heart disease can be treated with any class Ia, Ic or III antiarrhythmic drug, although it is recommended that amiodarone (because of its substantial extracardiac adverse effect profile) should be reserved until other drugs have failed. For patients with **heart failure** or **left ventricular hypertrophy** only amiodarone is recommended. Patients with **coronary artery disease** may be treated with sotalol or amiodarone. Patients with **paroxysmal atrial fibrillation** or with early **persistent atrial fibrillation** (little left atrial dilation) may be treated with left atrial ablation. The ectopic triggers for atrial fibrillation are generally found in the pulmonary veins, which can be isolated from the atria using radiofrequency or cryothermal energy. Occasionally, more extensive ablation within the left atrium is needed. These techniques are more successful than antiarrhythmic drugs and may represent a 'cure' in some patients. However, the procedure is invasive and carries some hazard of serious complications such as stroke, and bleeding in about 2% of cases. In the long term, recurrence is not uncommon and an apparently successful ablation does not remove the obligation for appropriate anticoagulation. Ablation has not been shown to improve long-term cardiovascular outcome but it does successfully treat symptoms due to atrial fibrillation.

Rate control

As a primary strategy, this is appropriate in patients who:

- have the permanent form of the arrhythmia associated with symptoms that can be further improved by slowing heart rate, or are older than 65 years with recurrent atrial tachyarrhythmias ('accepted' atrial fibrillation)
- have persistent tachyarrhythmias and have failed cardioversion(s) and serial prophylactic antiarrhythmic drug therapy, and in whom the risk/benefit ratio from using specific antiarrhythmic agents is shifted towards increased risk.

Rate control is usually achieved with a combination of **digoxin**, **beta-blockers** or **non-dihydropyridine calcium-channel blockers** (**verapamil** or **diltiazem**). Digoxin monotherapy may be sufficient for elderly, non-ambulant patients. In younger patients the effect of catecholamines easily overwhelms the vagotonic effect of digoxin and additional AV nodal slowing agents are needed. The ventricular rate response is generally considered to be controlled if the resting heart rate is below 110 b.p.m. but stricter control, between 60 and 80 b.p.m. at rest and below 110 b.p.m. during moderate exercise, may be needed if symptoms persist. To assess the adequacy of rate control, an ECG rhythm strip may be sufficient in an elderly patient but ambulatory 24-hour Holter monitoring and an exercise stress test (treadmill) are needed in younger individuals. Older patients with poor rate control despite optimal medical therapy should be considered for AV node ablation and pacemaker implantation (**'ablate and pace' strategy**). These patients usually experience a marked symptomatic improvement but require life-long anticoagulation because of the on-going risk of thromboembolism.

Anticoagulation

A scoring system known as CHA_2DS_2VASc is used (**Box 30.15**) as the first step in determining the need for anticoagulation.

Long-term prophylaxis against ischaemic stroke with oral anticoagulation must be balanced against the risk of haemorrhage. The HAS-BLED score is recommended by European, Canadian and UK (NICE) guidelines. A high HAS-BLED score identifies patients with a high risk of bleeding (**Box 30.16** and **Fig. 30.47**), and where risk factors exist, attempts may be made to modify them for instance by controlling hypertension and minimising alcohol intake.

Box 30.15 CHA$_2$DS$_2$-VASc scoring system for non-valvular atrial fibrillation

	Risk factors	Score/points
C	Congestive heart failure	1
H	Hypertension	1
A$_2$	Age ≥75	2
D	Diabetes mellitus	1
S$_2$	Stroke/TIA/thromboembolism	2
V	Vascular disease (aorta, coronary or peripheral arteries)	1
A	Age 65–74	1
Sc	Sex category: female	1

Annual risk of stroke

0 points = 0% risk: No prophylaxis
1 point = 1.3% risk: Consider anticoagulation in men
2+ points = 2.2% risk: Oral anticoagulant

TIA, transient ischaemic attack.

Box 30.16 HAS-BLED score for bleeding risk on oral anticoagulation in atrial fibrillation

Clinical characteristic	Score/points
Hypertension (systolic ≥160 mmHg)	1
Abnormal renal function	1
Abnormal liver function	1
Stroke in past	1
Bleeding	1
Labile INRs	1
Elderly: age ≥65 years	1
Drugs as well	1
Alcohol intake at same time	1

Yearly risk of developing major bleeding with anticoagulation rises with increasing score, from 1% with a score of 0 (low risk) to around >5% with a score of 3 or more (high risk).
INR, International Normalized Ratio.
(Adapted from European Society of Cardiology Clinical Practice Guidelines. Eur Heart J 2012; 33:2719–2747.)

When oral anticoagulation is required, either warfarin (dose adjusted to maintain an INR between 2.0 and 3.0) or one of the direct oral anticoagulants (the DOACs) can be used. These latter agents fall into two classes: direct thrombin inhibitors (e.g. dabigatran) and oral direct factor Xa inhibitors (e.g. rivaroxaban and apixaban). DOACs specifically block a single step in the coagulation cascade, in contrast to warfarin, which blocks several vitamin K-dependent factors (II, VII, IX and X). In comparison with warfarin, the DOACs have a rapid onset of action, shorter half-life and fewer food and drug interactions, and do not require INR testing. Trial data have shown them to be equally effective as, and maybe safer than, warfarin. Antiplatelet agents should not be used to reduce stroke risk. Percutaneous left atrial appendage occlusion (LAAO) may be offered where anticoagulation is contraindicated or not tolerated.

Atrial flutter

Atrial flutter is often associated with atrial fibrillation and frequently requires a similar initial therapeutic approach. Atrial flutter is usually an organized atrial rhythm with an atrial rate typically between 250

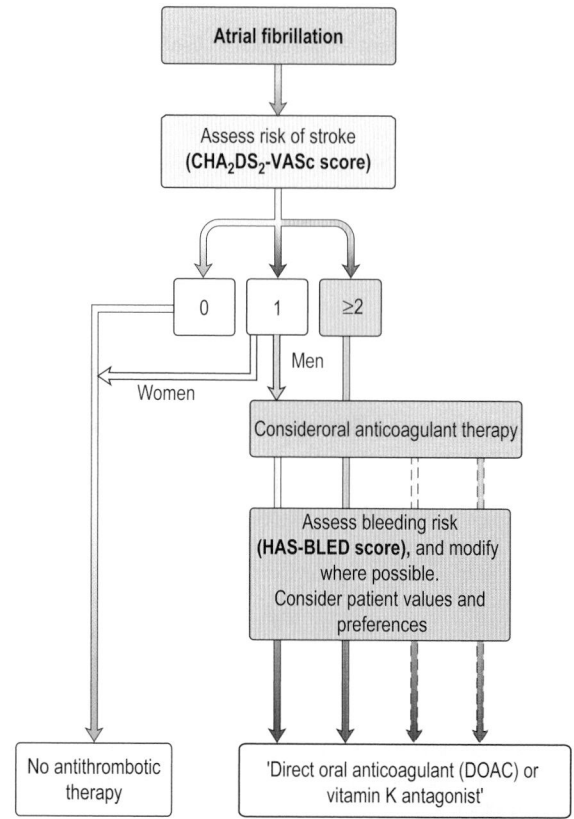

Fig. 30.47 Anticoagulation in atrial fibrillation. Based on *Atrial fibrillation: management* (2014) NICE Guidance CG180.

and 350 b.p.m. Typical, or isthmus-dependent, atrial flutter involves a macro re-entrant right atrial circuit around the tricuspid annulus. The wavefront circulates down the lateral wall of the right atrium, through the Eustachian ridge between the tricuspid annulus and the inferior vena cava, and up the interatrial septum, giving rise to the most frequent pattern, referred to as counter-clockwise flutter. Re-entry can also occur in the opposite direction (clockwise or reverse flutter).

The ECG shows regular sawtooth-like atrial flutter waves (F waves) between QRS complexes (see **Fig. 30.46B**). In typical counter-clockwise atrial flutter the F waves are negative in the inferior leads and positive in leads V$_1$ and V$_2$. In clockwise atrial flutter the deflection of the F waves is the opposite. If F waves are not clearly visible, it is worth trying to reveal them by slowing AV conduction by carotid sinus massage or by administering AV nodal blocking drugs such as adenosine or verapamil.

Symptoms are largely related to the degree of AV block. Most often, every second flutter beat conducts, giving a ventricular rate of 150 b.p.m. Occasionally, every beat conducts, producing a heart rate of 300 b.p.m. More often, especially when patients are receiving treatment, AV conduction block reduces the heart rate to approximately 75 b.p.m.

Management

Management of a symptomatic acute paroxysm is by electrical ***cardioversion***. Patients who have been in atrial flutter for more than 1–2 days should be treated in a similar manner to those with atrial fibrillation and ***anticoagulated*** for 3 weeks prior to cardioversion. Acute pharmacological cardioversion can be achieved using class

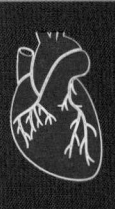

Ic (flecainide, propafenone) or certain class III antiarrhythmic agents (dofetilide, ibutilide; these have better efficacy than in atrial fibrillation but are not available in many countries).

Recurrent paroxysms may be prevented by *class III* antiarrhythmic agents (sotalol, amiodarone). *AV nodal blocking agents* may be used to control the ventricular rate if the arrhythmia persists. However, the treatment of choice for patients with recurrent atrial flutter is catheter *ablation* (see p. 1059), which permanently interrupts re-entry by creating a line of conduction block within the isthmus between the inferior vena cava and the tricuspid valve ring. This technique offers patients whose only arrhythmia is typical atrial flutter an almost certain chance of a cure, although the later occurrence of atrial fibrillation is not uncommon.

Atrial tachycardia

This is an uncommon arrhythmia. Its prevalence is believed to be less than 1% in patients with arrhythmias. It is usually associated with structural heart disease but in many cases it is referred to as idiopathic. Macro re-entrant tachycardia often occurs after surgery for congenital heart disease. Atrial tachycardia with block is often a result of digitalis poisoning.

The mechanisms of atrial tachycardia are attributed to enhanced automaticity, triggered activity or intra-atrial re-entry. Atrial re-entrant tachycardia is usually relatively slow (125–150 b.p.m.) and can be initiated and terminated by atrial premature beats. The P′P′ intervals are regular. The PR interval depends on the rate of tachycardia and is longer than in sinus rhythm at the same rate.

Automatic tachycardia usually presents with higher rates (125–250 b.p.m.) and is often characterized by a progressive increase in the atrial rate with onset of the tachycardia ('warm-up') and progressive decrease prior to termination ('cool-down'). Atrial tachycardia is typically caused by a focus that is frequently located along the crista terminalis in the right atrium, adjacent to a pulmonary vein in the left atrium, or around one of the atrial appendages. Automatic atrial tachycardia may also present as an incessant variety leading to tachycardia-induced cardiomyopathy. Short runs of atrial tachycardia may provoke more sustained episodes of atrial fibrillation.

Carotid sinus massage may increase AV block during tachycardia, thereby facilitating the diagnosis, but does not usually terminate the arrhythmia. Management options include *cardioversion*, *antiarrhythmic drug therapy* to maintain sinus rhythm, *AV nodal slowing agents* to control rate and, in selected cases, radiofrequency catheter *ablation*.

Atrial ectopic beats

These often cause no symptoms, although they may be sensed as an irregularity or heaviness of the heart beat. On the ECG, they appear as early and abnormal P waves and are usually, but not always, followed by normal QRS complexes. Treatment is not normally required unless the ectopic beats provoke more significant arrhythmias, when *beta-blockers* may be effective.

VENTRICULAR TACHYARRHYTHMIAS

Ventricular tachyarrhythmias can be discussed under the following headings:

- life-threatening ventricular tachyarrhythmias (sustained ventricular tachycardia, ventricular fibrillation, torsades de pointes)
- normal heart ventricular tachycardia
- non-sustained ventricular tachycardia

> **_i_   Box 30.17 ECG distinction between supraventricular tachycardia with bundle branch block and ventricular tachycardia**
>
> Ventricular tachycardia is more likely than supraventricular tachycardia with bundle branch block where there is:
> - a very broad QRS (>0.14 sec)
> - atrioventricular dissociation
> - a bifid, upright QRS with a taller first peak in V_1
> - a deep S wave in V_6
> - a concordant (same polarity) QRS direction in all chest leads (V_1–V_6)

- ventricular premature beats (ectopics).

Some of these conditions are cardiac channelopathies, congenital disorders caused by mutations that affect the function of cardiac ion channels and hence the electrical activity of the heart. They include Brugada's syndrome, congenital long QT syndrome, short QT syndrome, catecholaminergic polymorphic ventricular tachycardia (CPVT) and idiopathic ventricular fibrillation.

Sustained ventricular tachycardia

Sustained ventricular tachycardia (>30 sec) often results in *presyncope* (dizziness), *syncope*, *hypotension* and *cardiac arrest*, although it may be remarkably well tolerated in some patients. Examination reveals a pulse rate typically between 120 and 220 b.p.m. Usually, there are clinical signs of atrioventricular dissociation (i.e. intermittent cannon 'a' waves in the neck and variable intensity of the first heart sound).

The ECG shows a rapid ventricular rhythm with broad (often ≥0.14 sec), abnormal QRS complexes. AV dissociation may result in visible P waves, which appear to march through the tachycardia, capture beats (an intermittent narrow QRS complex owing to normal ventricular activation via the AV node and conducting system) and fusion beats (intermediate between ventricular tachycardia beat and capture beat).

SVT with bundle branch block may resemble ventricular tachycardia on the ECG. However, if a broad-complex tachycardia is due to SVT with either right or left bundle branch block, the QRS morphology should resemble a typical right bundle branch block or left bundle branch block pattern (see **Figs 30.43A** and **30.44**). Other ECG criteria to differentiate ventricular tachycardia from SVT with aberrancy are indicated in **Box 30.17**. Some 80% of all broad-complex tachycardias are due to ventricular tachycardia and the proportion is even higher in patients with structural heart disease. Therefore, in all cases of doubt, ventricular tachycardia should be diagnosed.

Management

Treatment may be urgent, depending on the haemodynamic situation. If the patient is haemodynamically compromised (e.g. hypotensive or pulmonary oedema), emergency DC cardioversion may be required. On the other hand, if the blood pressure and cardiac output are well maintained, intravenous therapy with beta-blockers (esmolol), class I drugs or amiodarone is usually used. DC cardioversion is necessary if medical therapy is unsuccessful.

Ventricular fibrillation

This involves very rapid and irregular ventricular activation with no mechanical effect. The patient is pulseless and becomes rapidly unconscious; respiration ceases (cardiac arrest). The ECG shows shapeless, rapid oscillations and there is no hint of organized complexes (**Fig. 30.48**). It is usually provoked by a ventricular ectopic beat. Ventricular fibrillation rarely reverses spontaneously. The only effective treatment is electrical defibrillation. Basic and advanced cardiac life support is needed (see p. 1045).

If the attack of ventricular fibrillation occurs during the first day or two of an acute myocardial infarction, it is probable that prophylactic therapy will be unnecessary. If the ventricular fibrillation was not related to an acute infarction, the long-term risk of recurrent cardiac arrest and sudden death is high.

Survivors of these ventricular tachyarrhythmias are, in the absence of an identifiable reversible cause (e.g. acute myocardial infarction, severe metabolic disturbance), at high risk of sudden death. Implantable cardioverter–defibrillators are first-line therapy in the management of these patients (see p. 1068).

Brugada's syndrome

This inheritable condition accounts for part of a group of patients with idiopathic ventricular fibrillation who have no evidence of causative structural cardiac disease. It is more common in young male adults and in South-east Asia. The diagnosis is made by identifying the classic ECG changes that may be present spontaneously or may be provoked by the administration of a class I antiarrhythmic (flecainide or ajmaline – principally used as a diagnostic agent in suspected Brugada patients): right bundle branch block with coved ST elevation in leads V_1–V_3 (**Fig. 30.49**). Atrial fibrillation may occur.

In 20% of cases, this is a monogenic inheritable condition associated with loss of sodium-channel function due to a mutation in the *SCN5A* gene. Recently, other mutations in the *SCN1B* gene, glycerol-3-phosphate dehydrogenase-1-like gene (*GPD1L*-type)

and genes related to calcium-channel subunits *CACNA1C* and *CACNB2* have also been implicated in the genesis of this syndrome. It can present with sudden death during sleep, resuscitated cardiac arrest and syncope, or the patient may be asymptomatic and diagnosed incidentally or during familial assessment. There is a high risk of sudden death, particularly in the symptomatic patient or those with spontaneous ECG changes. The only successful treatment is an ICD. Beta-blockade is not helpful and may be harmful.

Long QT syndrome

This describes an ECG where the ventricular repolarization (QT interval) is greatly prolonged. The causes of long QT syndrome are listed in **Box 30.18**.

Congenital long QT syndrome

Two major syndromes have been described, one that is (Jervell–Lange-Nielsen syndrome) and one that is not (Romano–Ward syndrome) associated with congenital deafness.

The molecular biology of the congenital long QT syndromes has been shown to be heterogeneous. It is usually a monogenic disorder and has been associated with mutations in cardiac potassium and

---

? Box 30.18 Causes of long QT syndrome

Congenital
- Jervell–Lange-Nielsen syndrome (autosomal recessive)
- Romano–Ward syndrome (autosomal dominant)

Acquired
Electrolyte abnormalities
- Hypokalaemia
- Hypomagnesaemia
- Hypocalcaemia

Drugs
- Quinidine, disopyramide
- Sotalol, amiodarone
- Tricyclic antidepressants, e.g. amitriptyline
- Phenothiazine drugs, e.g. chlorpromazine
- Antipsychotics, e.g. haloperidol, olanzapine
- Macrolides, e.g. erythromycin
- Quinolones, e.g. ciprofloxacin
- Methadone

Poisons
- Organophosphate insecticides

Miscellaneous
- Bradycardia
- Mitral valve prolapse
- Acute myocardial infarction
- Diabetes
- Prolonged fasting and liquid protein diets (long-term)
- Central nervous system diseases, e.g. dystrophia myotonica

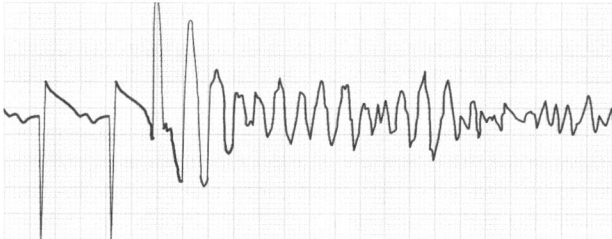

Fig. 30.48 Ventricular fibrillation. Two beats of sinus rhythm are followed by a ventricular ectopic beat that initiates ventricular fibrillation. The ST segment during sinus rhythm is elevated, owing to acute myocardial infarction in this case.

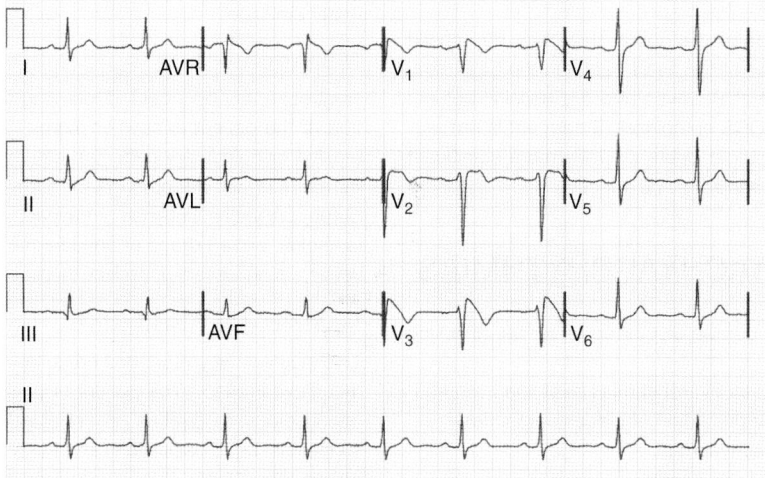

Fig. 30.49 The Brugada ECG. ST elevation (V1, V2, V3) with right bundle branch block.

sodium-channel genes. The different genes involved appear to correlate with different phenotypes (**Fig. 30.50A**) that can exhibit such variable penetrance that carriers may have completely normal ECGs. To date, thirteen long QT (LQT) subtypes have been identified but three major ones account for the majority of cases. These are:

- **LQT1** (*KCNQ1* gene mutation affecting the $I_{ks}\alpha$ subunit), in which the arrhythmia is usually provoked by exercise, particularly swimming
- **LQT2** (*KCNH2* gene mutation affecting the $I_{kr}\alpha$ subunit), in which arrhythmia provocation is associated with emotion and acoustic stimuli
- **LQT3** (*SCN5A* gene mutation affecting the $I_{Na}\alpha$ subunit), in which the arrhythmias occur during rest or when asleep.

It is likely that identification of the mutation involved will not only improve diagnostic accuracy, particularly with cascade screening in affected families, but also guide future therapy for the congenital long QT syndrome.

Acquired long QT syndrome

QT prolongation and torsades de pointes are usually provoked by bradycardia.

Clinical features

Patients with a long QT develop syncope and palpitations as a result of polymorphic ventricular tachycardia (torsades de pointes). They usually terminate spontaneously but may degenerate to ventricular fibrillation, resulting in sudden death.

Torsades de pointes is characterized on the ECG by rapid, irregular, sharp complexes that continuously change from an upright to an inverted position (**Fig. 30.50B**).

Between spells of tachycardia, or immediately preceding the onset of tachycardia, the ECG shows a prolonged QT interval; the corrected QT (see **Box 30.9**) is usually over 0.50 sec.

Management

Acute (acquired) long QT syndrome is treated as follows:
- Any electrolyte disturbance is corrected.
- Causative drugs are stopped.
- The heart rate is maintained with atrial or ventricular pacing.
- Magnesium sulphate 8 mmol (Mg^{2+}) is given over 10–15 min for acquired long QT.
- Intravenous isoprenaline may be effective when QT prolongation is acquired (isoprenaline is contraindicated for congenital long QT syndrome).

Long-term, congenital long QT syndrome is generally treated by beta-blockade, pacemaker therapy and, occasionally, left cardiac sympathetic denervation. LQT1 patients seem to respond well to beta-blockade while LQT3 patients are better treated with sodium-channel blockers. All long QT patients should avoid drugs known to prolong the QT interval. Patients who remain symptomatic despite conventional therapy, and those with marked QT prolongation or a strong family history of sudden death, usually need ICD therapy.

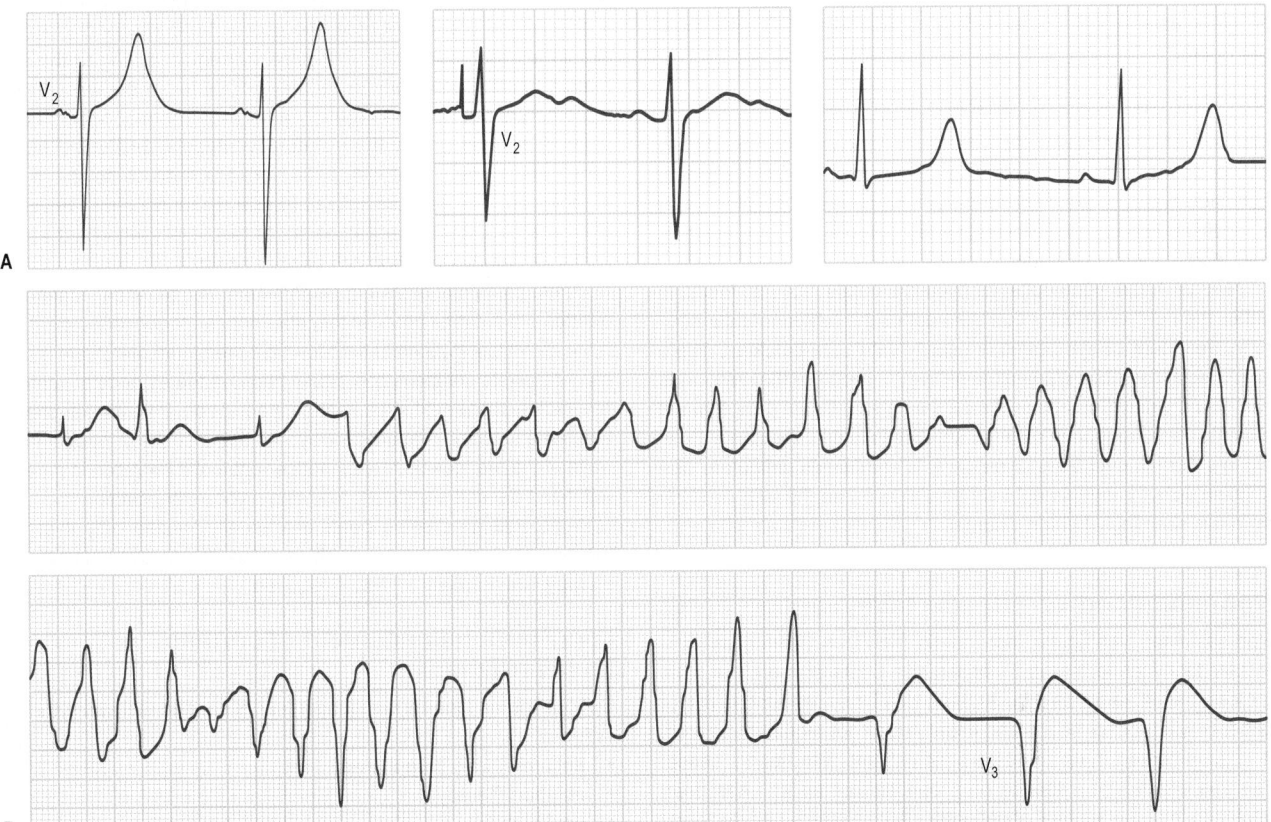

Fig. 30.50 Prolonged QT syndrome. (A) Three examples of a prolonged QT interval corresponding to three different types of long QT syndrome. **(B)** An ECG demonstrating a supraventricular rhythm with a long QT interval giving way to atypical ventricular tachycardia (torsades de pointes). The tachycardia is short-lived and is followed by a brief period of idioventricular rhythm.

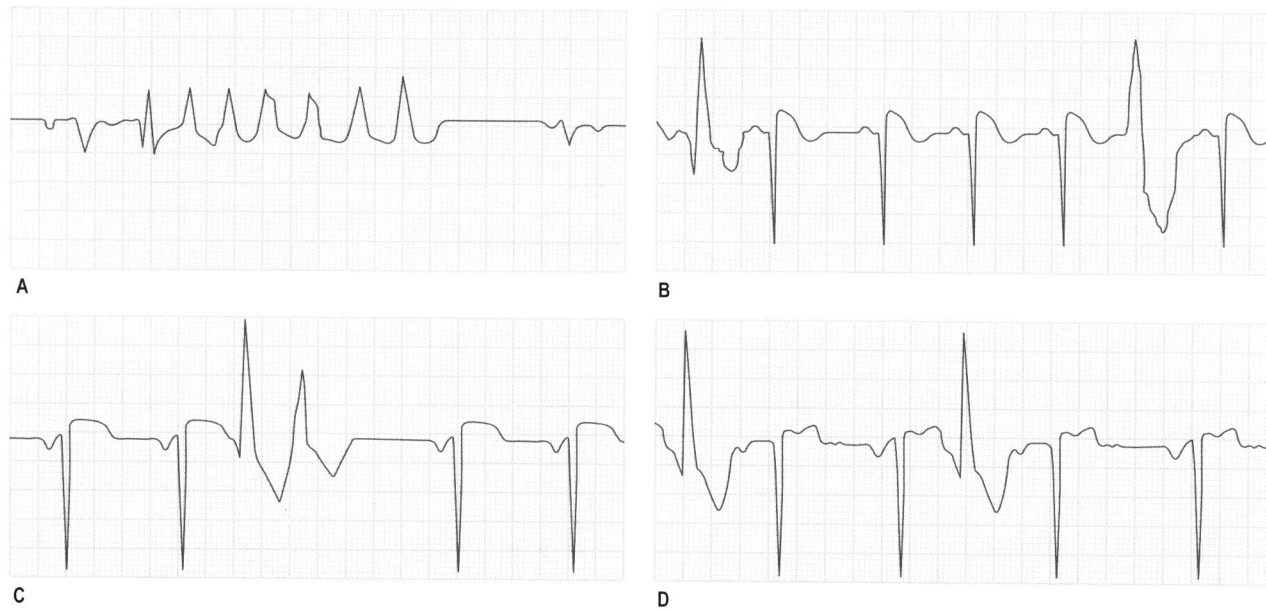

Fig. 30.51 Varieties of ventricular ectopic activity. **(A)** A brief run of ventricular tachycardia (*non-sustained ventricular tachycardia*) that follows previous ectopic activity. **(B)** Two ventricular ectopic beats of different morphology (multimorphological). **(C)** Two ventricular premature beats (VPBs) occurring one after the other (a pair or couplet of VPBs). **(D)** Frequently repetitive ventricular ectopic activity of a single morphology.

Short QT syndrome

Five types have been described; they are caused by genetic abnormalities that lead to faster repolarization. Ventricular arrhythmias and sudden death may occur and an ICD is the best treatment.

Normal heart ventricular tachycardia

Monomorphic ventricular tachycardia in patients with structurally normal hearts (idiopathic ventricular tachycardia) is usually a benign condition with an excellent long-term prognosis. Occasionally, it is incessant (so called Gallavardin's tachycardia) and, if untreated, may lead to cardiomyopathy.

Normal heart ventricular tachycardia arises from a focus in either the right ventricular outflow tract or the left ventricular septum. Treatment of symptoms is usually with beta-blockers. There is a special form of verapamil-sensitive tachycardia that responds well to non-dihydropyridine calcium antagonists. In symptomatic patients, radiofrequency catheter ablation is highly effective, resulting in a cure in over 90% of cases. It is sometimes difficult to distinguish arrhythmogenic right ventricular hypertrophy (see p. 1121) from this seemingly benign disorder.

Non-sustained ventricular tachycardia

Non-sustained ventricular tachycardia (NSVT) is defined as ventricular tachycardia that is 5 consecutive beats or more but lasts for less than 30 seconds (**Fig. 30.51A**). NSVT can be found in 6% of patients with normal hearts and usually does not require treatment. It is documented in up to 60–80% of patients with heart disease. There is insufficient evidence on prognosis but an ICD has been shown to improve survival of patients with particularly poor left ventricular function (ejection fraction ≤30%) by preventing arrhythmic death. Antiarrhythmic suppression of NSVT is not usually advocated but beta-blockers may improve quality of life in symptomatic individuals.

Ventricular premature beats (ectopics)

These may be uncomfortable, especially when frequent. The patient complains of extra beats, missed beats or heavy beats because it may be the premature beat, the post-ectopic pause or the next sinus beat that is noticed. The pulse is irregular owing to the premature beats. Some early beats may not be felt at the wrist. When a premature beat occurs regularly after every normal beat, 'pulsus bigeminus' may occur. If premature ventricular beats are highly symptomatic, treatment with beta-blockade may be helpful. If the ectopics are very frequent, left ventricular dysfunction may develop; if the ectopics stem from a single focus, especially when in the right ventricle, catheter ablation can be very effective.

These premature beats (**Fig. 30.51B–D**) have a broad (>0.12 sec) and bizarre QRS complex because they arise from an abnormal (ectopic) site in the ventricular myocardium. Following a premature beat, there is usually a complete compensatory pause because the AV node or ventricle is refractory to the next sinus impulse. Early 'R-on-T' ventricular premature beats (occurring simultaneously with the upstroke or peak of the T wave of the previous beat) may induce ventricular fibrillation in patients with heart disease, particularly following myocardial infarction.

Ventricular premature beats are usually treated only if symptomatic. Simple measures, such as reassurance and beta-blocker therapy, are normally all that is required.

Long-term management of cardiac tachyarrhythmias

Options for the long-term management of cardiac tachyarrhythmias include:

- antiarrhythmic drug therapy
- ablation therapy
- device therapy.

Antiarrhythmic drugs

Drugs that modify the rhythm and conduction of the heart are used to treat cardiac arrhythmias. Antiarrhythmic drugs may aggravate

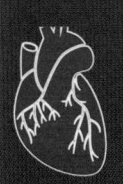

Box 30.19 Vaughan Williams classification of antiarrhythmic drugs

Class/action	Drugs
Class I	Membrane-depressant drugs (sodium-channel blockers)
Ia Lengthen action potential	Disopyramide
Ib Shorten action potential	Lidocaine, mexiletine
Ic No effect on action potential	Flecainide, propafenone
Class II Block β-adrenoceptors	Atenolol, acebutolol, bisoprolol, propranolol, esmolol
Class III Lengthen action potential	Amiodarone, dronedarone, sotalol, dofetilide, ibutilide, vernakalant
Class IV Reduce plateau phase of action potential	Calcium-channel blockers, e.g. verapamil, diltiazem
Other	Adenosine, digoxin

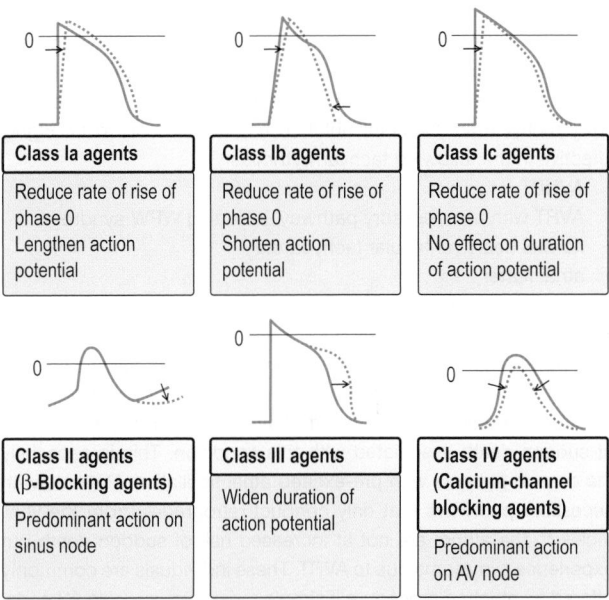

Fig. 30.52 **Vaughan Williams classification of antiarrhythmic drugs based on their effect on cardiac action potentials (see also Fig. 30.38).** (0 = 0 mV. The dotted curves indicate the effects of the drugs. AV, atrioventricular.)

or produce arrhythmias (proarrhythmia) and they may also depress ventricular contractility and must therefore be used with caution. They are classified according to their effect on the action potential (Vaughan Williams classification; **Box 30.19** and **Fig. 30.52**).

Class I drugs

These are membrane-depressant drugs that reduce the rate of entry of sodium into the cell (sodium-channel blockers). They may slow conduction, delay recovery or reduce the spontaneous discharge rate of myocardial cells. Class I agents have been found to increase mortality compared to placebo in post-myocardial infarction patients with ventricular ectopy (Cardiac Arrhythmia Suppression Trial (CAST) trials – class Ic agents) and in patients treated for atrial fibrillation (class Ia agent, quinidine). In view of this, class Ic agents, such as flecainide, and all other class I drugs should be reserved for patients who do not have significant coronary artery disease, left ventricular dysfunction or other forms of significant structural heart disease.

Class II drugs

These antisympathetic drugs prevent the effects of catecholamines on the action potential. Most are β-adrenoceptor antagonists. Cardioselective beta-blockers (β₁) include metoprolol, bisoprolol, atenolol and acebutolol. Beta-blockers suppress AV node conduction, which may be effective in preventing attacks of junctional tachycardia, and may help to control the ventricular rate during paroxysms of other forms of SVT (e.g. atrial fibrillation). In general, beta-blockers are anti-ischaemic and anti-adrenergic, and have proven beneficial effects in patients post myocardial infarction (by preventing ventricular fibrillation) and in those with congestive heart failure. It is therefore advisable to use beta-blocker therapy either alone or in combination with other antiarrhythmic drugs in patients with symptomatic tachyarrhythmias, particularly those with coronary artery disease.

Class III drugs

These prolong the action potential, usually by blocking the rapid component of the delayed rectifier potassium current (I_{Kr}), and do not affect sodium transport through the membrane. The drugs in this class are amiodarone and sotalol. Sotalol is also a beta-blocker.

Sotalol may result in acquired long QT syndrome and torsades de pointes. The risk of torsades is increased in the setting of hypokalaemia, and particular care should be taken in patients taking diuretic therapy. Amiodarone therapy, in contrast to most other antiarrhythmic drugs, carries a low risk of proarrhythmia in patients with significant structural heart disease, but its use may be limited due to toxic and potentially serious side-effects. Dronedarone is a multichannel-blocking drug that suppresses the recurrence of atrial fibrillation and reduces hospital admissions in patients with cardiovascular risk. However, it has proven harmful in patients with left ventricular dysfunction and is contraindicated in heart failure.

Vernakalant is a multichannel blocker that is approved for the rapid intravenous medical cardioversion of new-onset atrial fibrillation.

Class IV drugs

The non-dihydropyridine calcium-channel blockers are particularly effective at slowing conduction in nodal tissue. These drugs can prevent attacks of junctional tachycardia (AVNRT and AVRT) and may help to control ventricular rates during paroxysms of other forms of SVT (e.g. atrial fibrillation).

Clinical use of antiarrhythmic drugs

Antiarrhythmic drugs have not been shown to prolong life. Patient safety is the main factor in determining the choice of antiarrhythmic therapy, and proarrhythmic risks need to be carefully assessed prior to initiating therapy. As a generalization, class Ic agents are employed in patients with structurally normal hearts, and class III agents are used in those with structural heart disease, although exceptions exist.

Patients with structurally normal hearts and normal QT intervals, or those with implantable defibrillators, either are at very low risk of proarrhythmia or are protected from any life-threatening consequences; in these individuals, it is possible to persevere with drug therapy.

Catheter ablation

Catheter ablation (radiofrequency or cryoablation) is frequently employed in the management of symptomatic tachyarrhythmias.

Ablations are performed percutaneously by placing electrode catheters into the heart chambers, usually via femoral vessels. Successful ablation depends on accurate identification of either the site of origin of a focal tachycardia or a critical component of a macro re-entry tachycardia. Catheter ablation has been found to be highly effective in the following tachyarrhythmias:

- AVNRT
- AVRT with an accessory pathway, including WPW syndrome
- normal heart ventricular tachycardia
- atrial flutter
- atrial tachycardia
- paroxysmal atrial fibrillation (pulmonary vein isolation).

Symptomatic patients with a **pre-excited** ECG because of accessory pathway conduction (WPW syndrome) are advised to undergo catheter ablation as first-line therapy, owing to the risk of sudden death associated with this condition. This is especially the case in patients with pre-excited atrial fibrillation. Patients with accessory pathways that only conduct retrogradely from the ventricles to the atrium are not at increased risk of sudden death but experience symptoms due to AVRT. These individuals are commonly offered an ablation procedure if simple measures, such as AV nodal slowing agents, fail to suppress tachycardia. Asymptomatic patients with the WPW ECG pattern are now frequently offered an ablation procedure for prophylactic reasons. The main risk associated with accessory pathway ablation is thromboembolism in patients with left-sided accessory pathways. The success rate for catheter ablation of AVNRT and accessory pathways is more than 95%.

Patients with **normal hearts and documented ventricular tachycardia** should be referred for specialist evaluation. Unlike VT in patients with structural heart disease, normal heart VT is not associated with increased risk of sudden death and is easily cured by catheter ablation.

Catheter ablation is recommended in patients with **atrial flutter** that is not easily managed medically. Ablation of typical flutter is effective in 90–95% of cases. In the direct comparison of catheter ablation and antiarrhythmic therapy the rate of recurrence was significantly lower following ablation. **Atrial tachycardia**, especially in patients with structurally normal hearts, may also be cured by catheter ablation. In atrial fibrillation, adequate control of ventricular rates is sometimes not possible, despite optimal medical therapy. These patients experience a marked symptomatic improvement following AV node ablation (which leads to complete heart block) and pacemaker implantation.

In **younger patients** with structurally normal hearts, **atrial ectopic beats**, which commonly arise from a focus situated in the pulmonary veins, may trigger atrial fibrillation. Catheter ablation of this ectopic focus includes the application of radiofrequency energy around the pulmonary veins in order to abolish the connection between the sleeves of arrhythmogenic atrial myocardium surrounding or extending into the veins from the atrium (pulmonary vein isolation). The trigger is therefore eliminated and the arrhythmia does not recur. These techniques appear to be highly effective, especially in young patients with paroxysmal atrial fibrillation, normal atrial size and no underlying heart disease (70–80% long-term success), but are presently time-consuming procedures (4 h or more) and carry a risk of serious complications such as stroke, pericardial haemorrhage, pulmonary vein stenosis and atrio-oesophageal fistula in a small minority of patients (in experienced centres <2% altogether).

Implantable cardioverter–defibrillator

Life-threatening ventricular arrhythmias (ventricular fibrillation or rapid ventricular tachycardia with hypotension) result in death in up to 40% within 1 year of diagnosis. Large multicentre prospective trials, such as the Antiarrhythmics (amiodarone) Versus Implantable Defibrillator (AVID) trial, have proven that implantable defibrillators improve overall survival in patients who have experienced an episode of life-threatening ventricular tachyarrhythmia.

The implantable cardioverter–defibrillator (ICD) recognizes ventricular tachycardia or fibrillation and automatically delivers pacing or a shock to the heart to cause cardioversion to sinus rhythm. Modern ICDs are only a little larger than a pacemaker and the generator is implanted in a pectoral position (**Fig. 30.53**), although in younger patients a subcutaneous device may be appropriate. The device may have leads to sense and pace both the right atrium and ventricle, and the lithium batteries employed are able to provide energy for over 100 shocks, each of around 30 J. ICD discharges are painful if the patient is conscious. However, ventricular tachycardia may often be terminated by overdrive pacing the heart, which is painless. The ICD is superior to all other treatment options at preventing sudden cardiac death. The use of this device has cut the sudden death rate in patients with a history of serious ventricular arrhythmias to approximately 2% per year. However, the majority of these people have significant structural heart disease and overall cardiac mortality due to progressive heart failure remains high. As a result, the ICD is now first-line therapy in the secondary prevention of sudden death.

ICDs are also employed in the primary prevention of sudden cardiac death. The chances of surviving an out-of-hospital cardiac arrest are as low as 10%. Therefore, selected patients who have never experienced a spontaneous episode of life-threatening ventricular tachyarrhythmia but who are assessed to be at high risk of sudden death are advised to undergo ICD implantation. In two large primary prevention ICD trials, Multicenter Automated Defibrillator Implantation Trial (MADIT II) and Sudden Cardiac Death in Heart Failure Trial (SCD-HeFT), therapy with an ICD reduced mortality by 23–31% on top of conventional treatment, which included revascularization, beta-blockers and ACE inhibitors. ICD combined with cardiac resynchronization therapy may improve both symptoms and life expectancy of patients with any degree of heart failure (the COMPANION, CARE-HF and MADIT-CRT trials).

The following groups of patients may merit prophylactic ICD placement for primary prevention:

- Patients with heart failure with a left ventricular ejection fraction of 35% or less and NYHA functional class below IV (see **Box 30.23**). In such patients who also have left bundle branch block (QRS >120 ms), there is additional benefit in combining ICD with cardiac resynchronization therapy (CRT-D; see p. 1075).
- Those with a familial condition and high risk of sudden death, such as dilated and hypertrophic cardiomyopathy, long QT syndrome, Brugada's syndrome or other channelopathies, who have a strong family history of sudden cardiac death and arrhythmogenic right ventricular dysplasia.

Further reading

Brignole M, Arruchio A, Baron-Esquivias G et al. 2013 ESC Guidelines on cardiac pacing and cardiac resynchronization therapy: the task force on cardiac pacing and resynchronization therapy of the European Society of Cardiology (ESC). Developed in collaboration with the European Heart Rhythm Association (EHRA). *Eur Heart J* 2013; 34:2281–2329.

Kirchhof P, Benussi S, Kotecha D et al. 2016 ESC Guidelines for the management of atrial fibrillation developed in collaboration with EACTS. *Eur Heart J* 2016; 37:2893–2962.

National Institute for Health and Care Excellence. *NICE Clinical Guideline 180: Atrial Fibrillation: Management*. NICE 2014; https://www.nice.org.uk/CG180.

National Institute for Health and Care Excellence. *NICE Technology Appraisal 314: Implantable Cardioverter Defibrillators and Cardiac Resynchronisation Therapy for Arrhythmias and Heart Failure*. NICE 2014; https://www.nice.org.uk/guidance/ta314.

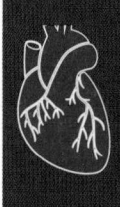

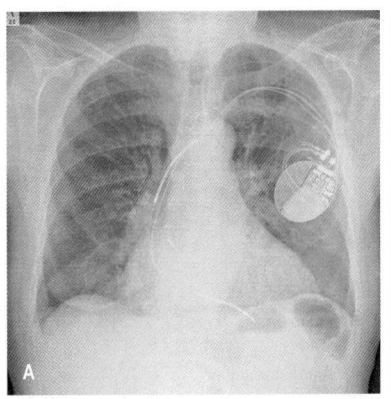

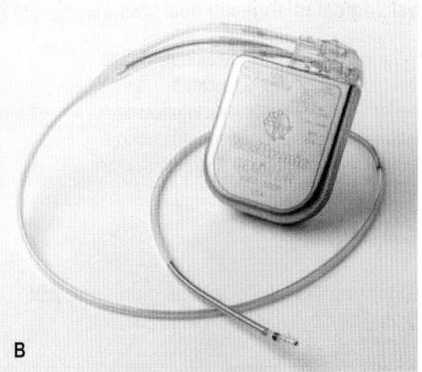

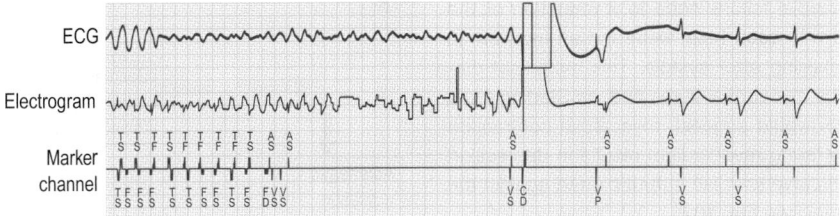

Fig. 30.53 Implantable cardioverter–defibrillator. **(A)** X-ray of a 'dual-chamber' defibrillator in a left pectoral position with atrial and ventricular leads. **(B)** Medtronic GEM® III DR defibrillator. **(C)** ECG showing the termination of ventricular fibrillation by a direct current shock at 20 J. The electrogram, recorded internally from the ventricular lead of an ICD, reveals chaotic ventricular activity consistent with ventricular fibrillation. This is confirmed by an electrocardiogram (lead V_2). The marker channel demonstrates that the device detects ventricular fibrillation correctly (FS, fibrillation sensing, lower line) and delivers an appropriate shock (CD) that terminates the arrhythmia and restores normal sinus rhythm (VS, ventricular sensing, lower line). Incidentally, atrial fibrillation is also detected before shock delivery (upper line on the marker channel).

National Institute for Health and Care Excellence. *NICE Interventional Procedures Guidance 603: Subcutaneous Implantable Cardioverter Defibrillator Insertion for Preventing Sudden Cardiac Death.* NICE 2017; https://www.nice.org.uk/guidance/ipg603.
Priori SG, Blomström-Lundqvist C, Mazzant A et al. 2015 ESC Guidelines for the management of patients with ventricular arrhythmias and the prevention of sudden cardiac death. *Eur Heart J* 2015; 36:2793–2867.
Priori SG, Wilde AA, Horie M et al. Executive summary: HRS/EHRA/APHRS expert consensus statement on the diagnosis and management of patients with inherited primary arrhythmia syndromes. *Europace* 2013; 15:1389–1406.

HEART FAILURE

Heart failure is a complex syndrome that can result from any structural or functional cardiac disorder that impairs the ability of the heart to function as a pump to support a physiological circulation. Worldwide, the incidence of heart failure is variable but increases with advancing age, with approximately 26 million people affected. In the UK, overall incidence is about 2 in 1000. The prognosis of heart failure has improved over the past 10 years with evidence-based therapy, but the mortality rate remains high and approximately 50% of patients are dead at 5 years. Heart failure is the leading cause of medical hospital admissions in over 65-year-olds and accounts for 5% of admissions to hospital medical wards. The cost of managing heart failure in the UK exceeds £1 billion per year. Coronary artery disease is the most common cause of heart failure in Western countries.

The causes of heart failure are shown in **Box 30.20**.

Pathophysiology

There are a number of changes affecting the heart and peripheral vascular system in response to the haemodynamic changes

> **?** **Box 30.20 Causes of heart failure**
>
> **Main causes**
> - Ischaemic heart disease (35–40%)
> - Cardiomyopathy (dilated) (30–34%)
> - Hypertension (15–20%)
>
> **Other causes**
> - Cardiomyopathy (undilated): hypertrophic, restrictive (amyloidosis, sarcoidosis)
> - Valvular heart disease (mitral, aortic, tricuspid)
> - Congenital heart disease (atrial septal defect, ventricular septal defect)
> - Alcohol and drugs (chemotherapy – trastuzumab, imatinib)
> - Hyperdynamic circulation (anaemia, thyrotoxicosis, haemochromatosis, Paget's disease)
> - Right heart failure (right ventricular infarct, pulmonary hypertension, pulmonary embolism, chronic obstructive pulmonary disease)
> - Arrhythmias (atrial fibrillation, bradycardia (complete heart block, sick sinus syndrome))
> - Pericardial disease (constrictive pericarditis, pericardial effusion)
> - Infections, e.g. myocarditis, Chagas' disease

associated with heart failure (**Box 30.21**). These physiological changes are compensatory and maintain cardiac output and peripheral perfusion. However, as heart failure progresses, these mechanisms are overwhelmed and become pathological. The development of pathological peripheral vasoconstriction and sodium retention in heart failure by activation of the renin–angiotensin–aldosterone system entails a loss of beneficial compensatory mechanisms and represents cardiac decompensation. Factors involved are venous return, outflow resistance, contractility of the myocardium, and salt and water retention.

Venous return (preload)

In the intact heart, myocardial failure leads to a reduction of the volume of blood ejected with each heart beat and an increase in the volume of blood remaining after systole. This increased diastolic volume stretches the myocardial fibres and, as Starling's law of the heart (see p. 1025) would suggest, myocardial contraction is restored. However, the failing myocardium results in depression of the ventricular function curve (cardiac output plotted against the ventricular diastolic volume) (see **Fig. 10.8**).

Mild myocardial depression is not associated with a reduction in cardiac output because it is maintained by an increase in venous pressure (and hence diastolic volume). However, the proportion of blood ejected with each heart beat (ejection fraction) is reduced early in heart failure. Sinus tachycardia also ensures that any reduction of stroke volume is compensated for by the increase in heart rate; cardiac output (stroke volume × heart rate) is therefore maintained.

When there is more severe myocardial dysfunction, cardiac output can be maintained only by a large increase in venous pressure and/or marked sinus tachycardia. The increased venous pressure contributes to the development of dyspnoea, owing to the accumulation of interstitial and alveolar fluid, and ascites with hepatic enlargement and dependent oedema from increased systemic venous pressure. However, the cardiac output at rest may not be much depressed, but myocardial and haemodynamic reserve is so compromised that a normal increase in cardiac output cannot be produced by exercise. In very severe heart failure the cardiac output at rest is depressed, despite high venous pressures. The inadequate cardiac output is redistributed to maintain perfusion of vital organs, such as the heart, brain and kidneys, at the expense of the skin and muscle.

Outflow resistance (afterload)

Outflow resistance (afterload) (see **Fig. 30.5**) is the load or resistance against which the ventricle contracts. It is formed by:
- pulmonary and systemic resistance
- physical characteristics of the vessel walls
- the volume of blood that is ejected.

An increase in afterload decreases the cardiac output, resulting in a further increase of end-diastolic volume and dilation of the ventricle, which further exacerbates the problem of afterload. This is expressed by Laplace's law: the tension of the myocardium (T) is proportional to the intraventricular pressure (P) multiplied by the radius of the ventricular chamber (R) – that is, $T \propto PR$.

Myocardial contractility (inotropic state)

The state of the myocardium also influences performance. The sympathetic nervous system is activated in heart failure via baroreceptors as an early compensatory mechanism, which provides inotropic support and maintains cardiac output. Chronic sympathetic

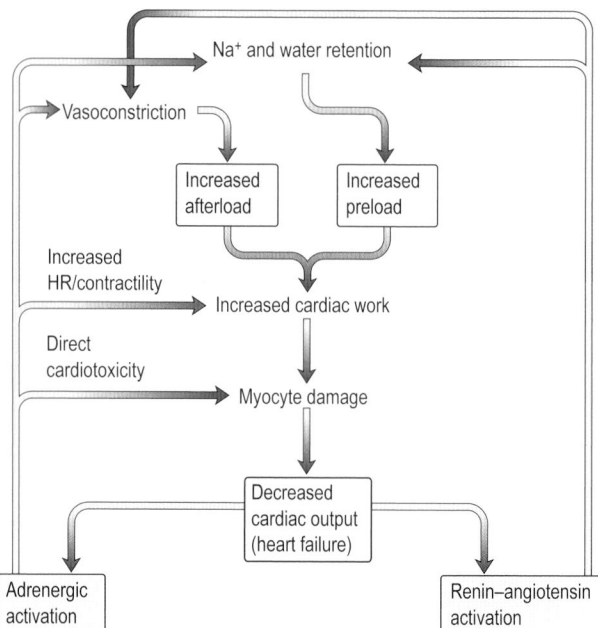

Fig. 30.54 The compensatory physiological response to heart failure. Chronic activation of the renin–angiotensin and adrenergic systems results in a 'vicious circle' of cardiac deterioration that further exacerbates the physiological response. HR, heart rate.

activation, however, has deleterious effects by further increasing neurohormonal activation and myocyte apoptosis. This is compensated by a downregulation of β-receptors. Increased contractility (positive inotropism) can result from increased sympathetic drive and this is a normal part of the Frank–Starling relationship (see **Fig. 30.5**). Conversely, myocardial depressants (e.g. hypoxia) decrease myocardial contractility (negative inotropism).

Neurohormonal and sympathetic system activation: salt and water retention

The increase in venous pressure that occurs when the ventricles fail leads to retention of salt and water, and their accumulation in the interstitium, producing many of the physical signs of heart failure. Reduced cardiac output also leads to diminished renal perfusion, activating the renin–angiotensin system and enhancing salt and water retention (see **Fig. 36.6**), which further increases venous pressure (**Fig. 30.54**). The retention of sodium is, in part, compensated by the action of circulating atrial natriuretic peptides and antidiuretic hormone (see p. 176).

Myocardial remodelling in heart failure

Left ventricular remodelling is a process of progressive alteration of ventricular size, shape and function owing to the influence of mechanical, neurohormonal and possibly genetic factors in several clinical conditions, including myocardial infarction, cardiomyopathy, hypertension and valvular heart disease. Its hallmarks include hypertrophy, loss of myocytes and increased interstitial fibrosis. Remodelling continues for months after the initial insult, and the eventual change in the shape of the ventricle becomes responsible for the impairment of overall function of the heart (**Fig. 30.55A**). In cardiomyopathy, the process of progressive ventricular dilation or hypertrophy takes place without ischaemic myocardial injury or infarction (**Fig. 30.55B**).

Abnormal calcium homeostasis

Calcium ion flux within myocytes plays a pivotal role in the regulation of contractile function. Excitation of the myocyte cell membrane

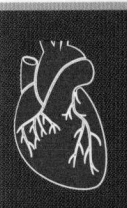

A Ventricular remodelling after acute infarction

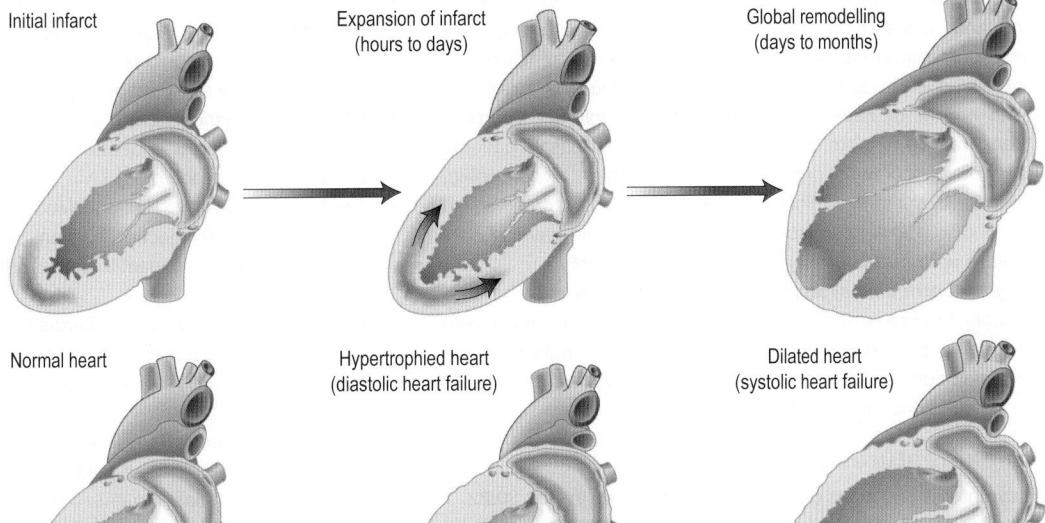

Initial infarct　　Expansion of infarct (hours to days)　　Global remodelling (days to months)

B Ventricular remodelling in diastolic and systolic heart failure

Normal heart　　Hypertrophied heart (diastolic heart failure)　　Dilated heart (systolic heart failure)

Fig. 30.55 Ventricular remodelling. (A) In ischaemic (myocardial infarction) heart failure. **(B)** In non-ischaemic heart failure (e.g. in cardiomyopathy).

causes the rapid entry of calcium into myocytes from the extra-cellular space via calcium channels. This triggers the release of intracellular calcium from the sarcoplasmic reticulum and initiates contraction (see **Fig. 30.3**). Relaxation results from the uptake and storage of calcium by the sarcoplasmic reticulum (see **Fig. 30.9**), controlled by changes in nitric oxide. In heart failure, there is a pro-longation of the calcium current in association with prolongation of contraction and relaxation.

Natriuretic peptides (ANP, BNP and CNP)

- ***Atrial natriuretic peptide (ANP)*** is released from atrial myo-cytes in response to stretch. ANP induces diuresis, natriuresis, vasodilation and suppression of the renin–angiotensin system. Levels of circulating ANP are increased in congestive cardiac failure and correlate with functional class, prognosis and haemo-dynamic state.
- ***B-type natriuretic peptide (BNP)*** is predominantly secreted by the ventricles in response to increased myocardial wall stress. N-terminal (NT)-proBNP is an inactive protein that is cleaved from proBNP to release BNP. Both BNP and NT-proBNP are in-creased in patients with heart failure, and levels correlate with ventricular wall stress and the severity of heart failure. BNP and NT-proBNP are good predictors of cardiovascular events and mortality, although monitoring levels are not routinely used to guide heart failure management.
- ***C-type natriuretic peptide (CNP)***, which is limited to vascular endothelium and the central nervous system, has similar effects to those of ANP and BNP.

Endothelial function in heart failure

The endothelium has a central role in the regulation of vasomotor tone. In patients with heart failure, endothelium-dependent vaso-dilation in peripheral blood vessels is impaired and may be one mechanism of exercise limitation. The cause of abnormal endo-thelial responsiveness relates to abnormal release of both nitric oxide and vasoconstrictor substances, such as endothelin (ET).

The activity of nitric oxide, a potent vasodilator, is blunted in heart failure. ET secretion from a variety of tissues is stimulated by many factors, including hypoxia, catecholamines and angiotensin II. The plasma concentration of ET is elevated in patients with heart failure, and levels correlate with the severity of haemodynamic disturbance.

ET has many actions that potentially contribute to the patho-physiology of heart failure: vasoconstriction, sympathetic stimu-lation, renin–angiotensin system activation and left ventricular hypertrophy. Acute intravenous administration of ET antagonists improves haemodynamic abnormalities in patients with congestive cardiac failure, and oral ET antagonists are being developed.

Antidiuretic hormone (vasopressin)

Antidiuretic hormone (ADH) is raised in severe chronic heart failure, particularly in patients on diuretic treatment. A high ADH concentra-tion precipitates hyponatraemia, which is an ominous prognostic indicator.

Clinical syndromes of heart failure

There are many causes of heart failure (see **Box 30.20**) that can present suddenly, with acute heart failure (AHF), or more insidiously, with chronic heart failure (CHF). One common classification of heart failure uses the left ventricular ejection fraction (LVEF):

- ***Heart failure with reduced ejection fraction (HFREF)*** (ejection fraction <40%) is commonly caused by ischaemic heart disease but can also occur with valvular heart disease and hypertension. It is only in this group of patients that heart failure therapies have been demonstrated to have benefit with reduced morbidity and mortality.
- ***Heart failure with preserved left ventricular ejection fraction (HFPEF)*** is a syndrome consisting of symptoms and signs of heart failure with an ejection fraction of >50%. There is increased stiffness in the ventricular wall and decreased left ventricular

compliance, leading to impairment of diastolic ventricular filling and hence decreased cardiac output. Echocardiography may demonstrate an increase in left ventricular wall thickness, increased left atrial size and abnormal left ventricular relaxation with normal or near-normal left ventricular volume. **Diastolic heart failure** is more common in elderly hypertensive patients but may occur with primary cardiomyopathies (hypertrophic, restrictive, infiltrative). Those patients in the grey zone with an LVEF of 40–50% have recently been classified as having **heart failure with mid-range ejection fraction (HFmrEF)**.

- **Right ventricular systolic dysfunction (RVSD)** may be secondary to chronic left-sided heart disease but can occur with primary and secondary pulmonary hypertension, right ventricular infarction, arrhythmogenic right ventricular cardiomyopathy and adult congenital heart disease.

Clinical features of heart failure

The symptoms and signs of heart failure are shown in **Box 30.22**.

The NYHA classification of heart failure (**Box 30.23**) can be used to describe the symptoms of heart failure and limitation of exercise capacity, and is useful for assessing response to therapy.

Diagnosis of heart failure

The diagnosis of heart failure should be based on a detailed history, clinical findings, natriuretic peptide levels and objective evidence of cardiac dysfunction using measures of left ventricular structure and function (usually echocardiography). The underlying cause of heart failure should be established in all patients (**Box 30.24** and **Fig. 30.56**).

Investigations in heart failure

- **Blood tests.** Full blood count, serum creatinine and electrolytes, liver biochemistry, cardiac enzymes (eg troponin) in acute heart failure, BNP or NT-proBNP, and thyroid function should be measured.
- **Chest X-ray.** Look for cardiomegaly, pulmonary congestion with upper lobe diversion, fluid in fissures, Kerley B lines and pulmonary oedema.

- **ECG.** Identify ischaemia, ventricular hypertrophy or arrhythmia.
- **Echocardiography.** Assess cardiac chamber dimension, systolic and diastolic function, regional wall motion abnormalities, valvular disease and cardiomyopathies.
- **Stress echocardiography.** Assess viability in dysfunctional myocardium – dobutamine identifies contractile reserve in stunned or hibernating myocardium.
- **Nuclear cardiology.** Radionucleotide angiography (RNA) can quantify ventricular ejection fraction; SPECT or PET can demonstrate myocardial ischaemia and viability in dysfunctional myocardium.
- **Cardiac MRI (CMR).** Assess cardiac structure and function and viability in dysfunctional myocardium with the use of dobutamine for contractile reserve or with gadolinium for delayed enhancement ('infarct imaging').
- **Cardiac catheterization.** This technique is employed for the diagnosis of ischaemic heart failure (and suitability for revascularization) and for measurement of pulmonary artery pressure, left atrial (wedge) pressure, left ventricular end-diastolic pressure.

> *i* **Box 30.24 Diagnosis of heart failure (European Society of Cardiology guidelines)**

Diagnosis of HF-REF requires three conditions to be satisfied
1. Symptoms typical of heart failure
2. Signs typical of heart failure
3. Reduced LV ejection fraction

Diagnosis of HF-PEF requires four conditions to be satisfied
1. Symptoms typical of heart failure
2. Signs typical of heart failure
3. Normal or only mildly reduced LV ejection fraction and LV not dilated
4. Relevant structural heart disease (LV hypertrophy/left atrial enlargement) and/or diastolic dysfunction

HF-REF = heart failure and a reduced ejection fraction; HF-PEF = heart failure with 'preserved' ejection fraction; LV = left ventricular.

> *i* **Box 30.22 Clinical features of heart failure**

Symptoms
- Exertional dyspnoea
- Orthopnoea
- Paroxysmal nocturnal dyspnoea
- Fatigue

Signs
- Tachycardia
- Elevated jugular venous pressure

- Cardiomegaly
- Third and fourth heart sounds
- Bi-basal crackles
- Pleural effusion
- Peripheral ankle oedema
- Ascites
- Tender hepatomegaly

> *i* **Box 30.23 New York Heart Association (NYHA) classification of heart failure**

Class	Features
Class I	No limitation. Normal physical exercise does not cause fatigue, dyspnoea or palpitations
Class II	Mild limitation. Comfortable at rest but normal physical activity produces fatigue, dyspnoea or palpitations
Class III	Marked limitation. Comfortable at rest but gentle physical activity produces marked symptoms of heart failure
Class IV	Symptoms of heart failure occur at rest and are exacerbated by any physical activity

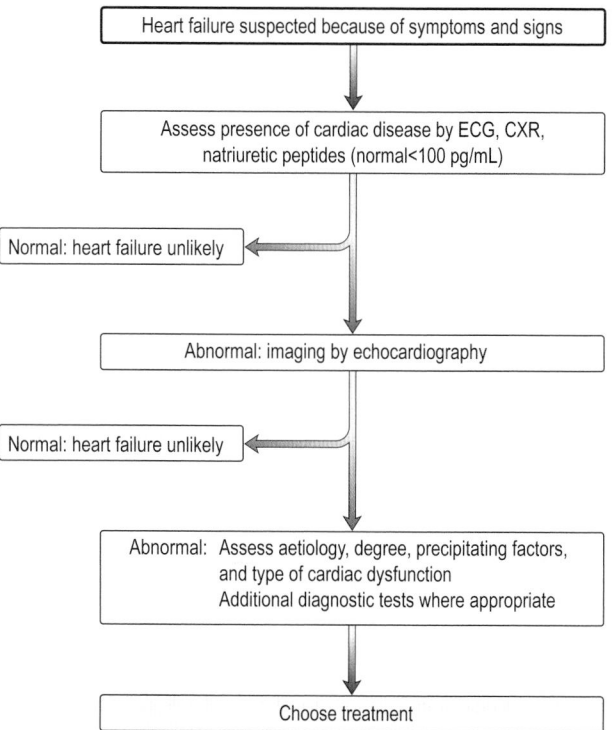

Fig. 30.56 Algorithm for the diagnosis of heart failure. *(Based on the European Society of Cardiology and NICE guidelines.)*

- **Cardiac biopsy.** This is used for diagnosis of cardiomyopathies, such as amyloid (see p. 1357), and for follow-up of transplanted patients to assess rejection.
- **Cardiopulmonary exercise testing.** Peak oxygen consumption (VO_2) is predictive of hospital admission and death in heart failure. A 6-minute exercise walk is an alternative.
- **Ambulatory 24-hour ECG monitoring (Holter).** This is used in patients with suspected arrhythmia, and may be employed in those with severe heart failure or inherited cardiomyopathy to determine whether a defibrillator is appropriate (non-sustained ventricular tachycardia).

Management of heart failure

Management is aimed at relief of symptoms, prevention and control of disease leading to cardiac dysfunction and heart failure, retarding of disease progression, and improvement in quality and length of life.

Measures to prevent heart failure include cessation of smoking, alcohol and illicit drugs, effective treatment of hypertension, diabetes and hypercholesterolaemia, and pharmacological therapy following myocardial infarction.

The management of heart failure requires any factor aggravating the failure to be identified and treated. Similarly, the cause of heart failure must be elucidated and, where possible, corrected. Community nursing programmes to help with drug compliance and detect early deterioration may prevent acute hospitalization.

General lifestyle advice

- **Education.** Effective counselling of patients and family, emphasizing weight monitoring and dose adjustment of diuretics, may prevent hospitalization. This is usually guided by primary care physicians and specialist community heart failure nurses.
- **Dietary modification.** Salt restriction is required, and foods rich in salt or salt added in cooking and at the table should be avoided. In severe heart failure, fluid restriction is necessary and patients may need to weigh themselves daily. Alcohol has a negative inotropic effect and heart failure patients should moderate consumption.
- **Smoking.** Smoking should be stopped with help from anti-smoking clinics if necessary (see p. 963).
- **Physical activity, exercise training and rehabilitation.** Low-level endurance exercise (e.g. 20–30 min walking 3–5 times per week or 20 min cycling at 70–80% of peak heart rate 5 times per week) is actively encouraged in patients with compensated heart failure in order to reverse 'deconditioning' of peripheral muscle metabolism. Strenuous isometric activity should be avoided. For hospitalized patients with exacerbations of congestive cardiac failure, limiting activity reduces the demands on the heart. Prolonged bed rest may, lead to the development of deep vein thrombosis (DVT); this can be avoided by daily leg exercises, low-dose subcutaneous heparin and elastic support stockings.
- **Vaccination.** It is recommended that patients with heart failure be vaccinated against pneumococcal disease and influenza (see p. 948).
- **Sexual activity.** Patients taking nitrate medication should not take concomitant phosphodiesterase type 5 inhibitors (e.g. sildenafil), as they may induce profound hypotension.
- **Driving.** Driving of cars and motorcycles may continue, provided that there are no symptoms that distract the driver's attention. Symptomatic heart failure or an LVEF of less than 40% disqualifies patients from driving large lorries and buses in the UK.

Monitoring

The clinical condition of a person with heart failure fluctuates; lengthy and repeated hospital admissions are common, with an average inpatient stay of between 5 and 10 days. Monitoring of clinical status is necessary and this responsibility should be shared between primary and secondary healthcare professionals.

Essential monitoring includes assessment of:

- functional capacity (e.g. NYHA functional class, exercise tolerance test, echocardiography)
- fluid status (body weight, clinical assessment, and serum creatinine and electrolytes)
- cardiac rhythm (ECG, Holter monitoring).

Multidisciplinary team approach

Heart failure care should be delivered by a multidisciplinary team with an integrated approach across the healthcare community. The team should involve specialist healthcare professionals: cardiologist or physician with a specialist interest in heart failure, heart failure nurse, dietician, pharmacist, occupational therapist, physiotherapist and palliative care adviser. Understanding the information needs of patients and carers is vital. Good communication is essential for best clinical management, and should include advice on anxiety, depression and 'end-of-life' issues.

Drug management

Box 30.25 lists the drugs used in heart failure. **Fig. 30.57** shows the stages of heart failure and the treatment options.

Diuretics

These act by promoting the renal excretion of salt and water by blocking tubular reabsorption of sodium and chloride (see p. 178). Loop diuretics (e.g. furosemide and bumetanide) and thiazide diuretics (e.g. bendroflumethiazide, hydrochlorothiazide) should be given in patients with fluid overload. Although diuretics provide symptomatic relief of dyspnoea and improve exercise tolerance, there is limited evidence that they affect survival. In severe heart failure patients, the combination of a loop and thiazide diuretic may be required, including the use of metolazone. Serum electrolytes and renal function must be monitored regularly (risk of hypokalaemia and hypomagnesaemia).

Angiotensin-converting enzyme inhibitors

The use of ACE inhibitors in patients with heart failure has been demonstrated in multiple large randomized controlled trials (CONSENSUS, SOLVD) to improve symptoms and reduce mortality significantly. ACE inhibitors also benefit patients with asymptomatic heart failure following myocardial infarction. Thus, ACE inhibitors improve survival in patients in all functional classes (NYHA I–IV) and are recommended in all patients at risk of developing heart failure. The main adverse effects of ACE inhibitors are cough, hypotension, hyperkalaemia and renal dysfunction. Contraindications to their use include renal artery stenosis, pregnancy and previous angio-oedema. In patients with heart failure, ACE inhibitors should be introduced at a low initial dose and gradually titrated, with regular monitoring of blood pressure and renal function.

Angiotensin II receptor antagonists

The angiotensin II receptor antagonists (ARAs; candesartan, losartan, valsartan) are indicated as second-line therapy in patients intolerant of ACE inhibitors. Unlike ACE inhibitors, they do not affect bradykinin metabolism and do not produce a cough. The CHARM Alternative Trial showed that candesartan reduced the risk of heart failure hospitalization compared to placebo in patients intolerant of ACE inhibitors. Other trials (Val-HeFT and ELITE II) have assessed other ARAs. Valsartan and a neprilysin inhibitor, sacubitril, in combination have demonstrated their promise in the treatment of heart failure.

i **Box 30.25 Drugs used in heart failure**

Drug	Dose (initial/maximum)	Precautions
ACE inhibitors/ARAs		
Ramipril	1.25–2.5 mg daily/10 mg daily	Monitor renal function and use with caution if baseline serum creatinine >250 μmol/L or baseline blood pressure <90 mmHg
Enalapril	2.5 mg daily/10 mg ×2 daily	
Captopril	6.25 mg ×3 daily/50 mg ×3 daily	
Candesartan	4 mg daily/32 mg daily	
Lisinopril	2.5–5 mg daily/20–40 mg daily	
Perindopril	2 mg daily/8–16 mg daily	
Valsartan	80 mg daily/320 mg daily	
Losartan	50 mg daily/100 mg daily	
Beta-adrenoceptor-blocking drugs		
Bisoprolol	1.25 mg daily/10 mg daily	Use with caution in obstructive airways disease, bradyarrhythmias
Carvedilol	3.125 mg ×2 daily/50 mg ×2 daily	Avoid in acute heart failure until patient is cardiovascularly stable
Metoprolol succinate (CR/XL)	12.5–25 mg daily/200 mg daily	
Nebivolol	1.25 mg daily/10 mg daily	
ARNIs		
Angiotensin receptor neprilysin inhibitor Sacubitril/valsartan	24/26–49/51 mg ×2 daily/ 97/103 mg × daily	Monitor renal function, check for hyperkalaemia. Discontinue ACE inhibitor 3 days prior to starting, discontinue ARA the day of starting.
Diuretics		
Furosemide	20–40 mg daily/250–500 mg daily	Monitor renal function and check for hypokalaemia and hypomagnesaemia
Bumetanide	0.5–1.0 mg daily/5–10 mg daily	
Bendroflumethiazide	2.5 mg daily/10 mg daily	Rarely need more than 2.5 mg daily. Reduced efficacy when eGFR<30 mL/min/1.73 m^2)
Metolazone	2.5 mg daily/10 mg daily	Use in severe heart failure
Aldosterone antagonists		
Spironolactone	12.5–25 mg daily/50 mg daily	Monitor renal function, check for hyperkalaemia, gynaecomastia with spironolactone
Eplerenone	25 mg daily/50 mg daily	
Cardiac glycosides		
Digoxin	0.125–0.25 mg daily (reduce dose in elderly or in renal impairment)	Use with caution in renal impairment or conduction disease, and with amiodarone
Vasodilators		
Isosorbide dinitrate	20–40 mg ×3 daily	
Hydralazine	37.5–75 mg ×3 daily	
I_F Channel blocker		
Ivabradine	5 mg daily/7.5 mg ×2 daily	Use with caution in sick sinus syndrome; AV block

ACE, angiotensin-converting enzyme; ARA, angiotensin II receptor antagonist; AV, atrioventricular.

Beta-blockers

Beta-blockers have been shown to improve functional status and reduce cardiovascular morbidity and mortality in patients with heart failure. Several trials (CIBIS, CIBIS II, MERIT-HF, COMET) have assessed the effects of beta-blockers in varying degrees of heart failure. Bisoprolol and carvedilol reduce mortality in any grade of heart failure. Nebivolol is used in the treatment of stable mild to moderate heart failure in patients over 70 years old. In patients with significant heart failure beta-blockers are started at a low dose and gradually increased, with monitoring of heart rate and blood pressure.

Aldosterone antagonists

The aldosterone antagonists spironolactone and eplerenone have been shown to improve survival in patients with heart failure. In the RALES study, spironolactone reduced total mortality by 30% in severe heart failure. However, gynaecomastia or breast pain occurred in 1 in 10 men taking spironolactone. In EPHESUS, eplerenone given to patients with an acute myocardial infarction and heart failure reduced total mortality by 15% and sudden cardiac death by 21%, with no gynaecomastia.

Angiotensin receptor neprilysin inhibitor

Angiotensin receptor neprilysin inhibitors (ARNIs) are a new class of drug that produce dual inhibition of the angiotensin (AT$_1$) receptor and the natriuretic system. The PARADIGM-HF trial studied sacubitril/valsartan in patients with established symptomatic heart failure and reduced ejection fraction, and demonstrated superiority over ACE inhibitor therapy in lowering morbidity and mortality.

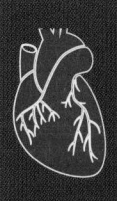

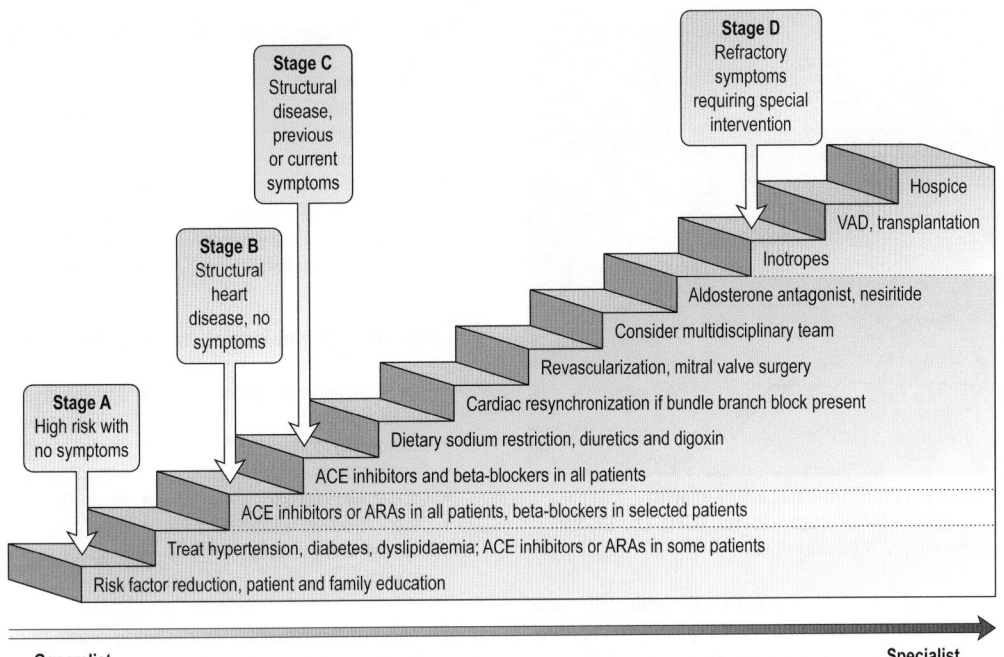

Fig. 30.57 Stages of heart failure and treatment options for systolic heart failure. ACE, angiotensin-converting enzyme; ARA, angiotensin II receptor antagonist; VAD, ventricular assisted device.

Cardiac glycosides

Digoxin is a cardiac glycoside that is indicated in patients in atrial fibrillation with heart failure. It is infrequently used as add-on therapy in symptomatic heart failure patients already receiving ACE inhibitors and beta-blockers. Although the DIG study demonstrated that digoxin reduced hospital admissions in patients with heart failure, a subanalysis in the ROCKET AF trial suggested that mortality may, in fact, be increased.

Vasodilators and nitrates

The combination of hydralazine and nitrates reduces preload and afterload, and is used in patients intolerant of ACE inhibitors or ARAs. The Veterans Administration Cooperative Study demonstrated that it improved survival in patients with chronic heart failure. The A-HeFT trial showed that the same combination reduced mortality and hospitalization for heart failure in black patients with heart failure.

Inotropic and vasopressor agents

Intravenous inotropes and vasopressor agents (see **Box 30.29**) are used in patients with acute heart failure and severe haemodynamic compromise. Although they produce haemodynamic improvements, they have not been shown to improve long-term mortality when compared with placebo.

Other medications

In hospital, all patients require prophylactic anticoagulation. Heart failure is associated with a fourfold increase in the risk of stroke. Oral anticoagulants are recommended in patients with atrial fibrillation and in those with sinus rhythm and a history of thromboembolism, left ventricular aneurysm or thrombus. In people with known ischaemic heart disease, antiplatelet therapy (aspirin, clopidogrel) and statin therapy should be continued. Arrhythmias are common in heart failure and are implicated in sudden death. Although treatment of complex ventricular arrhythmias might be expected to improve survival, there is no evidence to support this and it may increase mortality. In SCD-HeFT, amiodarone showed no benefit compared

to placebo in patients with impaired left ventricular function and mild to moderate heart failure (whereas an ICD reduced mortality by 23% compared to placebo). Patients with heart failure and symptomatic ventricular arrhythmias should be assessed for suitability for an ICD.

Ivabradine selectively decreases heart rate without affecting blood pressure by inhibiting the I_F channels in the sinoatrial node (see p. 1023). An elevated heart rate in patients with heart failure is associated with worse cardiovascular outcomes. The SHIFT study reported a reduction in cardiovascular death and heart failure hospitalization in patients in sinus rhythm with chronic heart failure and left ventricular dysfunction (LVEF ≤35%). Ivabradine can be used in patients in sinus rhythm with an elevated heart rate despite beta-blocker treatment or in those who are unable to tolerate beta-blockers.

Non-pharmacological treatment
Revascularization

While coronary artery disease is the most common cause of heart failure, the role of revascularization in patients with heart failure is unclear. Patients with angina and left ventricular dysfunction have a higher mortality from surgery (10–20%), but have the most to gain in terms of improved symptoms and prognosis. Factors that must be considered before recommending surgery include symptoms, age, co-morbidities and evidence of reversible myocardial ischaemia.

Hibernating myocardium and myocardial stunning

'Hibernating' myocardium can be defined as reversible left ventricular dysfunction due to chronic coronary artery disease that responds positively to inotropic stress and indicates the presence of viable heart muscle that may recover after revascularization. It is caused by reduced myocardial perfusion, which is just sufficient to maintain viability of the heart muscle. Myocardial hibernation results from repetitive episodes of cardiac stunning that occur, for example, with repeated exercise in a patient with coronary artery disease.

Myocardial stunning is reversible ventricular dysfunction that persists following an episode of ischaemia when the blood flow has returned to normal: that is, there is a mismatch between flow and function.

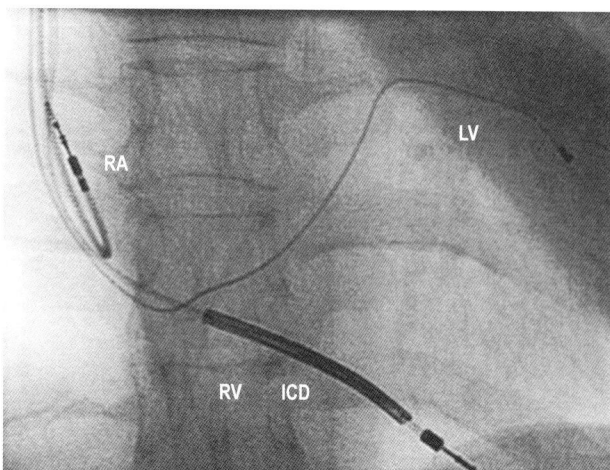

Fig. 30.58 Implanted biventricular pacemaker with implantable cardioverter–defibrillator device (CRT-D). LV, left ventricle; RA, right atrium; RV, right ventricle.

The prevalence of hibernating myocardium in patients with coronary artery disease can be estimated from the frequency of improvement in regional abnormalities in wall motion after revascularization; it is thought to be 33% of such patients. Techniques to try to identify hibernating myocardium include stress echocardiography, nuclear imaging, CMR and PET.

The clinical relevance of the hibernating and stunned myocardium is that ventricular dysfunction due to these mechanisms may be wrongly ascribed to myocardial necrosis and scarring, which seems untreatable, whereas reversible hibernating and stunned myocardium responds to coronary revascularization.

Cardiac resynchronization therapy or implantable cardioverter–defibrillator

Cardiac resynchronization therapy (CRT) entails simultaneous pacing of both ventricles (biventricular pacing) using a lead placed in the right ventricle and another in the coronary sinus to pace the left ventricle (**Fig. 30.58**). It is an effective therapy in addition to optimal medical treatment in patients with significant left ventricular impairment and a prolonged QRS interval (left bundle branch block). Resynchronization may reverse the process of ventricular remodelling, reduce functional mitral regurgitation and improve left ventricular function. The CARE-HF and COMPANION trials reported symptomatic benefit and a reduction in heart failure events and mortality following CRT implantation in patients with heart failure in NYHA classes III and IV. Similar findings have been noted in more recent trials in patients with mild heart failure or no symptoms.

Most patients with heart failure who receive CRT also meet the criteria for use of an ICD and should receive a combined device (CRT-D). Patients with end-stage heart failure (NYHA IV) or other co-morbidities that may significantly reduce lifespan are generally not candidates for an ICD.

Cardiac transplantation

Cardiac transplantation has become the treatment of choice for younger patients with severe intractable heart failure, whose life expectancy is less than 6 months. With careful recipient selection the expected 1-year survival for patients following transplantation is over 90%, and 75% at 5 years. Irrespective of survival, quality of life is dramatically improved for the majority. The availability of heart transplantation is limited.

Heart allografts do not function normally, as cardiac denervation results in a high resting heart rate, loss of diurnal blood pressure variation and impaired renin–angiotensin–aldosterone regulation. Some patients develop a 'stiff heart' syndrome, caused by rejection,

- Allograft rejection:
  - 'Humoral'
  - 'Vascular'
  - 'Cell-mediated'
- Infections:
  - Early: hospital-acquired organisms – staphylococci; Gram-negative bacteria
  - Late (2–6 months): opportunistic (toxoplasmosis, cytomegalovirus, fungi, *Pneumocystis*)
- Allograft vascular disease
- Hypertension
- Hypercholesterolaemia
- Malignancy

- Age >60 years (some variations between centres)
- Alcohol/drug misuse
- Uncontrolled psychiatric illness
- Uncontrolled infection
- Severe renal/liver failure
- High pulmonary vascular resistance
- Systemic disease with multiorgan involvement
- Treated cancer in remission but with <5 years' follow-up
- Recent thromboembolism
- Other disease with a poor prognosis

denervation and ischaemic injury during organ harvest and implantation. Transplantation of an inappropriately small donor heart can also result in elevated right and left heart pressure.

The complications of heart transplantation are summarized in **Box 30.26**. Many (infection, malignancy, hypertension and hyperlipidaemia) are related to immunosuppression. Allograft coronary atherosclerosis is the major cause of long-term graft failure and is present in 30–50% of patients at 5 years. It is due to a 'vascular' rejection process in conjunction with hypertension and hyperlipidaemia.

There are specific contraindications to cardiac transplantation (**Box 30.27**); notably, high pulmonary vascular resistance and active malignancy are absolute contraindications.

Acute heart failure

Acute heart failure (AHF) occurs with the rapid onset of symptoms and signs of heart failure secondary to abnormal cardiac function, causing elevated cardiac filling pressures. This leads to severe dyspnoea, and fluid accumulates in the interstitium and alveolar spaces of the lung (pulmonary oedema). AHF is the leading cause of hospital admission in people above the age of 65 years; it has a poor prognosis, with a 60-day mortality rate of nearly 10% and a rate of death or rehospitalization of 35% within 60 days. In patients with *acute pulmonary oedema*, the in-hospital mortality rate is 12% and by 12 months this rises to 30%. Poor prognostic indicators include a high (>16 mmHg) pulmonary capillary wedge pressure, low serum sodium concentration, increased left ventricular end-diastolic dimension on echo and low oxygen consumption.

The aetiology of AHF is similar to that of chronic heart failure:
- *Ischaemic heart disease* patients present with an acute coronary syndrome or develop a complication of myocardial infarction, such as papillary muscle rupture or ventricular septal defect requiring surgical intervention.
- *Valvular heart disease* patients also present with AHF due to valvular regurgitation in endocarditis or prosthetic valve thrombosis. A thoracic aortic dissection may produce severe aortic regurgitation.
- *Hypertension* patients present with episodes of 'flash' pulmonary oedema despite preserved left ventricular systolic function.
- *Acute and chronic kidney disease* both involve fluid overload and reduced renal excretion, which will produce pulmonary oedema.
- *Atrial fibrillation* is frequently associated with AHF and may require emergency cardioversion.

Several clinical syndromes of AHF can be defined (**Box 30.28**). In a clinical environment, both the Killip score (based on a

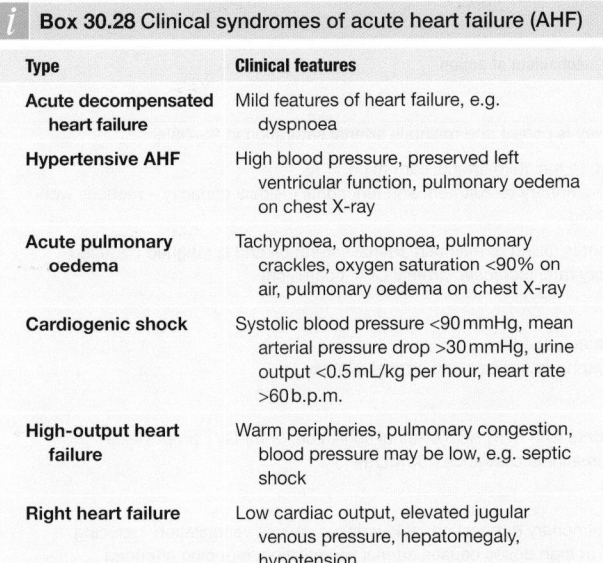

Box 30.28 Clinical syndromes of acute heart failure (AHF)

Type	Clinical features
Acute decompensated heart failure	Mild features of heart failure, e.g. dyspnoea
Hypertensive AHF	High blood pressure, preserved left ventricular function, pulmonary oedema on chest X-ray
Acute pulmonary oedema	Tachypnoea, orthopnoea, pulmonary crackles, oxygen saturation <90% on air, pulmonary oedema on chest X-ray
Cardiogenic shock	Systolic blood pressure <90 mmHg, mean arterial pressure drop >30 mmHg, urine output <0.5 mL/kg per hour, heart rate >60 b.p.m.
High-output heart failure	Warm peripheries, pulmonary congestion, blood pressure may be low, e.g. septic shock
Right heart failure	Low cardiac output, elevated jugular venous pressure, hepatomegaly, hypotension

(Modified from the European Society of Cardiology.)

cardiorespiratory clinical assessment, see p. 1090) and Forrester classification (based on right catheterization findings) provide therapeutic and prognostic information.

Pathophysiology

The pathophysiology of AHF is similar to that of chronic heart failure with activation of the renin–angiotensin–aldosterone axis and sympathetic nervous system. In addition, prolonged ischaemia (e.g. in acute coronary syndromes) results in myocardial stunning (see p. 1075), which exacerbates myocardial dysfunction but may respond to inotropic support. If myocardial ischaemia persists, the myocardium may exhibit hibernation (persistently impaired function due to reduced coronary blood flow), which may recover with successful revascularization.

Diagnosis

In a person presenting with symptoms and signs of heart failure, a structured assessment should result in the clinical diagnosis of AHF and direct initial treatment to stabilize the patient. Initial investigations performed in the accident and emergency department should include the following:

- **A 12-lead ECG** will identify acute coronary syndromes, left ventricular hypertrophy, atrial fibrillation, valvular heart disease and left bundle branch block.
- **A chest X-ray** may demonstrate cardiomegaly, pulmonary oedema, pleural effusions or non-cardiac disease.
- **Blood investigations** should include serum creatinine and electrolytes, full blood count, blood glucose, cardiac enzymes and troponin, C-reactive protein (CRP) and D-dimer.
- **Plasma BNP** or **NT-proBNP** (BNP >100 pg/mL or NT-proBNP >300 pg/mL) is suggestive of heart failure.
- **TTE** should be performed without delay to confirm the diagnosis of heart failure (see p. 1038) and possibly identify the cause.

If the baseline investigations confirm AHF, then treatment should be commenced.

Management

The goals of treatment in a patient with AHF include:

- immediate relief of symptoms and stabilization of haemodynamics (short-term benefits)
- reduction in length of hospital stay and hospital re-admissions
- reduction in mortality from heart failure.

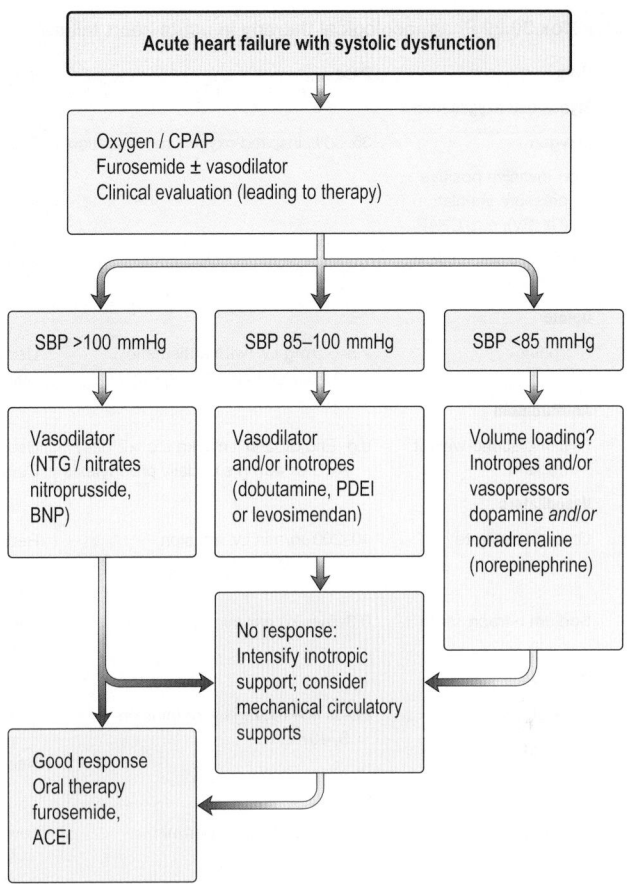

Key:
ACEI = Angiotensin-converting enzyme inhibitor
BNP = B-type natriuretic peptide, e.g. nesiritide
CPAP = Continuous positive airway pressure
NTG = Nitroglycerine (glyceryl trinitrate)
PDEI = Phosphodiesterase inhibitor
SBP = Systolic blood pressure

Fig. 30.59 Algorithm for the management of acute heart failure with systolic dysfunction. (*From Nieminen MS, Böhm M, Cowie MR et al. Executive summary of the guidelines on the diagnosis and treatment of acute heart failure: the Task Force on Acute Heart Failure of the European Society of Cardiology. Eur Heart J 2005; 26:384–416, Fig. 6, with permission from Oxford University Press and the European Society of Cardiology.*)

Patients with AHF should be managed in a high-dependency area with regular measurement of temperature, heart rate, blood pressure and cardiac monitoring. All require prophylactic anticoagulation with low-molecular-weight heparin.

Individuals with haemodynamic compromise may need arterial lines for invasive blood pressure monitoring and arterial gas sampling, central venous cannulation (intravenous medication, inotropic support, monitoring of central venous pressure) and pulmonary artery catheterisation (calculation of cardiac output/index, peripheral vasoconstriction and pulmonary wedge pressure).

Initial therapy (**Fig. 30.59** and **Box 30.29**) includes oxygen and diuretics (e.g. i.v. furosemide 50 mg). If intravenous nitrates (e.g. glyceryl trinitrate infusion 10–200 µg/min) are required (e.g. concomitant myocardial ischaemia, severe hypertension), careful monitoring

i   **Box 30.29 Pharmacological therapy in acute heart failure**

Drug	Dose	Indications/mechanism of action
Myocardial oxygenation		
Oxygen	35–50% inspired oxygen concentration	Ensure airway is patent and maintain arterial saturation at 95–98%
Non-invasive positive pressure ventilation (NIPPV), e.g. CPAP		Use if failing to maintain arterial saturation Increases pulmonary recruitment and functional residual capacity – reduces work of breathing
Intubation/mechanical ventilation		Use if patient is failing to maintain arterial saturation and is fatigued (reduced respiratory rate, increased arterial CO_2, confusion)
Opiate		
Morphine	2.5–5.0 mg i.v. (with antiemetic metoclopramide 10 mg i.v.)	Use in agitated patient Relieves dyspnoea, venous and arterial dilation
Antithrombin		
Low-molecular-weight heparin	e.g. Enoxaparin 1 mg/kg s.c. ×2 daily ACS or 40 mg s.c. daily prophylaxis	Use in patients with AHF, ACS or atrial fibrillation, or for DVT prophylaxis Caution if creatinine clearance <30 mL/min
Vasodilators		
Glyceryl trinitrate	10–200 µg/min i.v. infusion	Reduces pulmonary congestion; at low doses causes venodilation, reducing preload; at high doses causes arterial vasodilation, reducing afterload Ensure BP >85–90 mmHg
Sodium nitroprusside	0.3–5 µg/kg per min i.v. infusion	Use in severe AHF where there is predominantly high afterload, e.g. hypertensive AHF Needs arterial BP monitoring for profound hypotension
Diuretic		
Furosemide	Bolus 40–100 mg i.v. or infusion 5–40 mg/h	Low doses produce vasodilation, reduce right atrial pressure and PCWP, and promote diuresis Need to monitor sodium, potassium and creatinine
Inotropes		
Dopamine	Low dose <2 µg/kg per min	Low dose acts on peripheral dopamine receptors to produce vasodilation (renal, splanchnic, coronary, cerebrovascular) and may improve diuresis although evidence of significant improvements in outcomes is lacking
	Medium dose >2 µg/kg per min	Medium dose acts on β-receptors to increase myocardial contractility and cardiac output
	High dose >5 µg/kg per min	High dose acts on α-receptors, causing vasoconstriction and increasing total peripheral resistance (increases afterload, PAP)
Dobutamine	2–20 µg/kg per min (patients on beta-blockers may need high dose)	Stimulates β1 and β2-receptors, producing vasodilation. Increases heart rate and cardiac output, and also diuresis as haemodynamics are improved
Milrinone	Bolus 25–75 µg/kg over 10–20 min then 0.375–0.75 µg/kg per min	Inhibits phosphodiesterase and maintains cAMP Increases cardiac output and stroke volume, reduces PAP/PCWP/total peripheral resistance/BP
Levosimendan	Bolus 12–24 µg/kg over 10 min then 0.05–2 µg/kg per min	Positive inotropic drug with vasodilator effects by increasing sensitivity of contractile proteins to calcium and opening potassium channels Increases cardiac output and reduces PCWP
Vasopressors		
Noradrenaline (norepinephrine)	0.2–1.0 µg/kg per min	Stimulates α-receptors Increases total peripheral resistance and BP
Adrenaline (epinephrine)	Bolus 1 mg at resuscitation then 0.05–0.5 µg/kg per min	Stimulates α, β1- and β2-receptors Increases cardiac output, heart rate, total peripheral resistance and BP
Cardiac glycoside		
Digoxin	0.5 mg i.v. repeated after 2–6 h	Inhibits myocardial sodium/potassium ATPase, leading to increased calcium and sodium exchange Increases cardiac output and slows AV conduction Use in AF; avoid in ACS

ACS, acute coronary syndrome; AF, atrial fibrillation; AHF, acute heart failure; ATPase, adenosine triphosphatase; AV, atrioventricular; BP, blood pressure; cAMP, cyclic adenosine monophosphate; CPAP, continuous positive airway pressure; DVT, deep venous thrombosis; i.v., intravenous; PAP, positive airway pressure; PCWP, pulmonary capillary wedge pressure; s.c., subcutaneous.

of the blood pressure is mandatory. Inotropic support (see p. 222) with dobutamine, phosphodiesterase inhibitors or levosimendan can be added in patients who do not respond to initial therapy.

Nesiritide (recombinant human B-type natriuretic peptide) can also be used in AHF as a bolus injection followed by an infusion.

Patients with profound hypotension may require inotropes and vasopressors to improve haemodynamic status and alleviate symptoms but these have not been shown to improve mortality.

Non-invasive continuous positive airway pressure/positive pressure ventilation (CPAP/NIPPV; see p. 229) has been shown to provide earlier improvement in dyspnoea and respiratory distress than standard oxygen via mask; mortality is, however, unaffected.

Mechanical assist devices

Mechanical assist devices can be used in patients who fail to respond to standard medical therapy but in whom there is either

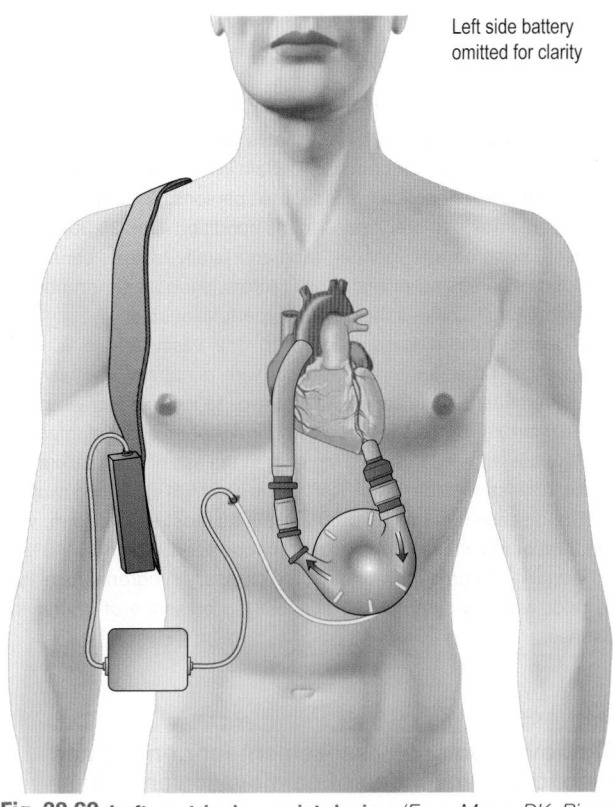

Left side battery omitted for clarity

Fig. 30.60 Left ventricular assist device. (*From Moser DK, Riegel B. Cardiac Nursing. Philadelphia: Saunders; 2007, p. 981, with permission of Elsevier.*)

transient myocardial dysfunction with likelihood of recovery (e.g. post anterior myocardial infarction treated with coronary angioplasty) or as a bridge to cardiac surgery, including transplantation.

Ventricular assist devices

Ventricular assist devices (VADs; **Fig. 30.60**) are mechanical systems that replace or help the failing ventricles in delivering blood around the body. A left ventricular assist device (LVAD) receives blood from the left ventricle and delivers it to the aorta; a right ventricular assist device (RVAD) receives blood from the right ventricle and delivers it to the pulmonary artery. The devices can be extracorporeal (suitable for short-term support) or intracorporeal (suitable for long-term support as a bridge to transplantation or as destination therapy in patients with end-stage heart failure who are not candidates for transplantation). The main problems with VADs include thromboembolism, bleeding, infection and device malfunction.

Further reading

Ellison DH, Felker GM. Diuretic treatment in heart failure. *N Engl J Med* 2017; 377:1964–1975

Ponikowski P, Voors AA, Anker SD et al. 2016 ESC Guidelines for the diagnosis and treatment of acute and chronic heart failure: The Task Force for the diagnosis and treatment of acute and chronic heart failure of the European Society of Cardiology (ESC). *Eur J Heart Failure* 2016; 37:2129–2200.

CORONARY ARTERY DISEASE

Myocardial ischaemia occurs when there is an imbalance between the supply of oxygen (and other essential myocardial nutrients) and the myocardial demand for these substances.

Coronary blood flow to a region of the myocardium may be reduced by a mechanical obstruction that is due to:

- atheroma
- thrombosis
- spasm
- embolus
- coronary ostial stenosis
- coronary arteritis (e.g. in systemic lupus erythematosus).

There can be a decrease in the flow of oxygenated blood to the myocardium that is due to:

- anaemia
- carboxyhaemoglobulinaemia
- hypotension, causing decreased coronary perfusion pressure.

A higher demand for oxygen may occur owing to an increase in cardiac output (e.g. thyrotoxicosis) or myocardial hypertrophy (e.g. from aortic stenosis or hypertension).

Myocardial ischaemia most commonly arises as a result of obstructive coronary artery disease (CAD) in the form of coronary atherosclerosis. In addition to this fixed obstruction, variations in the tone of smooth muscle in the wall of a coronary artery may add another element of dynamic or variable obstruction.

CAD is the largest single cause of death in the UK and many parts of the world. In 2010, cardiovascular diseases were the UK's biggest killer, accounting for nearly 180000 deaths. CAD was responsible for 1 in 5 male deaths and 1 in 10 female deaths (approximately 80000 deaths). Sudden cardiac death is a prominent feature of CAD, 1 in every 6 coronary attacks presenting with sudden death as the first, last and only symptom.

Pathophysiology of coronary atherosclerosis

Coronary atherosclerosis is a complex inflammatory process characterized by the accumulation of lipid, macrophages and smooth muscle cells in intimal plaques in the large and medium-sized epicardial coronary arteries. The vascular endothelium plays a critical role in maintaining vascular integrity and homeostasis. Mechanical shear stresses (e.g. from morbid hypertension), biochemical abnormalities (e.g. elevated low-density lipoprotein (LDL), diabetes mellitus), immunological factors (e.g. free radicals from smoking), inflammation and genetic alteration may contribute to the initial endothelial 'injury' or dysfunction, which is believed to trigger atherogenesis.

The **development of atherosclerosis** follows endothelial dysfunction, with increased permeability to and accumulation of oxidized lipoproteins, which are taken up by macrophages at focal sites within the endothelium to produce lipid-laden foam cells. Macroscopically, these lesions are seen as flat yellow dots or lines on the endothelium of the artery and are known as **'fatty streaks'**. The 'fatty streak' progresses with the appearance of extracellular lipid within the endothelium (**'transitional plaque'**). Release of cytokines, such as platelet-derived growth factor and transforming growth factor beta (TGF-β), by monocytes, macrophages or the damaged endothelium promotes further accumulation of macrophages, as well as smooth muscle cell migration and proliferation. The proliferation of smooth muscle with the formation of a layer of cells covering the extracellular lipid separates it from the adaptive smooth muscle thickening in the endothelium. Collagen is produced in larger and larger quantities by the smooth muscle and the whole sequence of events cumulates as an **'advanced or raised fibrolipid plaque'**. The 'advanced plaque' may grow slowly and encroach on the lumen, or become unstable, undergo thrombosis and produce an obstruction (**'complicated plaque'**).

Two different mechanisms are responsible for thrombosis on the plaques (**Fig. 30.61**):

- ***The first process*** is superficial endothelial injury, which involves denudation of the endothelial covering over the plaque. Subendocardial connective tissue matrix is then exposed and platelet adhesion occurs because of reaction with collagen. The thrombus is adherent to the surface of the plaque.
- ***The second process*** is deep endothelial fissuring, which involves an advanced plaque with a lipid core. The plaque cap tears (ulcerates, fissures or ruptures), allowing blood from the lumen to enter the inside of the plaque itself. The core with lamellar lipid surfaces, tissue factor (which triggers platelet adhesion and activation) produced by macrophages and exposed collagen is highly thrombogenic. Thrombus forms within the plaque, expanding its volume and distorting its shape. Thrombosis may then extend into the lumen.

A 50% reduction in luminal diameter (producing a reduction in luminal cross-sectional area of approximately 70%) causes a haemodynamically significant stenosis. At this point, the smaller distal intramyocardial arteries and arterioles are maximally dilated (coronary flow reserve is near zero), and any increase in myocardial oxygen demand provokes ischaemia.

CAD gives rise to a wide variety of clinical presentations, ranging from relatively stable angina through to the acute coronary syndromes of unstable angina and myocardial infarction (**Fig. 30.62**). **Fig. 30.63** shows a plaque rupture.

Risk factors for coronary artery disease

CAD is an atherosclerotic disease that is multifactorial in origin, giving rise to the risk factor concept. Certain living habits promote atherogenic traits in genetically susceptible persons. A number of 'risk' factors are known to predispose to the condition (**Box 30.30**). Some of these, such as age, gender, race and family history, cannot be modified, whereas other major risk factors, such as serum cholesterol, smoking habits, diabetes and hypertension, can.

Atherosclerotic disease manifest in one vascular bed is often advanced in other territories. Patients with peripheral vascular disease (intermittent claudication) have a two- to fourfold increased risk of CAD, stroke or heart failure. Following initial myocardial infarction (MI), there is a three- to sixfold increase in the risk of heart failure and stroke. After stroke, the risk of heart failure and MI is increased twofold.

The disease can be asymptomatic in its most severe form, with 1 in 3 myocardial infarctions going unrecognized. Some 30–40% of individuals who present with an acute coronary syndrome have had no prior warning symptom to suggest the presence of underlying disease.

Diagnosis

Cardiovascular risk assessment for primary and secondary prevention of cardiovascular disease

Primary prevention can be defined as prevention of the atherosclerotic disease process and ***secondary prevention*** as treatment of the atherosclerotic disease process (i.e. treatment of the disease or its complications). The objective of prevention is to reduce the incidence of first or recurrent clinical events due to CAD, ischaemic stroke and peripheral artery disease.

In the UK, NICE guidelines recommend that primary care should use the QRISK®3 risk assessment tool (see Further reading) to identify people who are likely to be at high risk (10-year risk of cardiovascular disease ≥10%).

Lipids

A full lipid profile should be obtained, including total cholesterol, high-density lipoprotein (HDL) cholesterol, non-HDL cholesterol and triglyceride concentrations. Patients with a total cholesterol concentration of more than 7.5 mmol/L and a family history of premature coronary heart disease may have ***familial hypercholesterolaemia***.

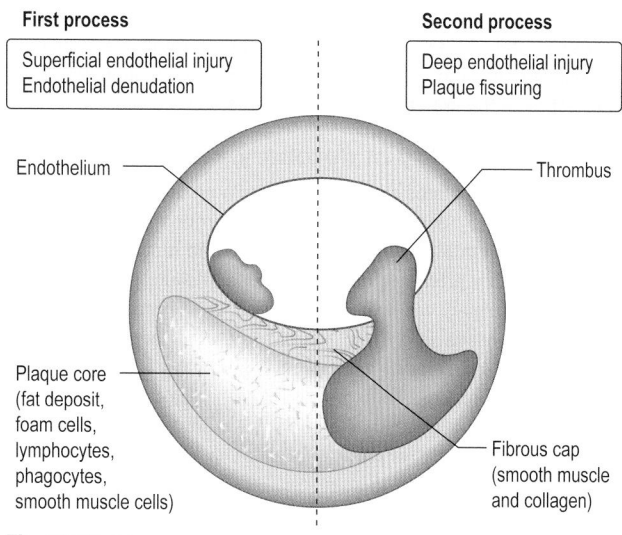

Fig. 30.61 **Mechanisms underlying the development of thrombosis on plaques.**

First process
Superficial endothelial injury
Endothelial denudation

Second process
Deep endothelial injury
Plaque fissuring

Endothelium
Thrombus
Plaque core (fat deposit, foam cells, lymphocytes, phagocytes, smooth muscle cells)
Fibrous cap (smooth muscle and collagen)

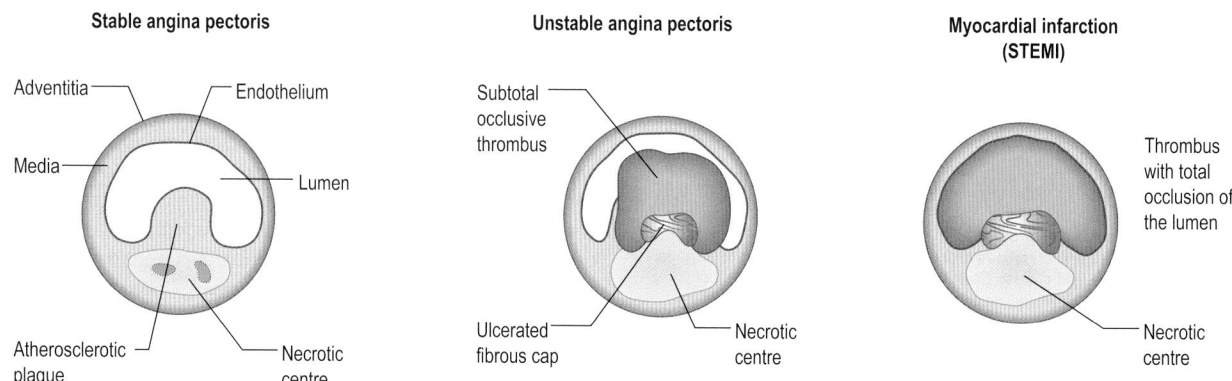

Stable angina pectoris
Adventitia
Endothelium
Media
Lumen
Atherosclerotic plaque
Necrotic centre

Unstable angina pectoris
Subtotal occlusive thrombus
Ulcerated fibrous cap
Necrotic centre

Myocardial infarction (STEMI)
Thrombus with total occlusion of the lumen
Necrotic centre

Fig. 30.62 **Mechanisms underlying the development of thrombosis on plaques in various clinical syndromes.** Relationship between the state of the coronary artery vessel wall and the various syndromes. STEMI, ST-elevation myocardial infarction.

Lifestyle modifications

Patients should eat a diet with a reduced fat intake (≤30% of total energy intake, saturated fats ≤7% total energy intake) and a dietary cholesterol intake of less than 300 mg/day. Saturated fats should be replaced by monounsaturated and polyunsaturated fats (rapeseed and olive oils). People should aim to reduce their intake of sugar and food products that contain refined sugars (e.g. fructose), and to eat at least five portions of fruit and vegetables per day, two portions of fish per week, and four to five portions of unsalted nuts, seeds and legumes per week. The weekly exercise recommendations are 150 minutes or more of moderate-intensity aerobic activity or 75 minutes of vigorous-intensity aerobic activity. Weight/body mass index (BMI) should be <25 kg/m² (see p. 1247). In the UK the recommendation is not to drink more than 14 units per week (men and women), ideally spread evenly over 3 or more days, and smoking should be discontinued. Blood pressure and diabetes should be managed according to NICE guidelines in the UK.

Statin treatment

Atorvastatin 20 mg is recommended for the primary prevention of cardiovascular disease in people with a 10-year risk of cardiovascular disease of 10% or higher. In patients with established cardiovascular disease, NICE recommends atorvastatin 80 mg, unless there are potential drug interactions, a high risk of adverse effects or a different patient preference.

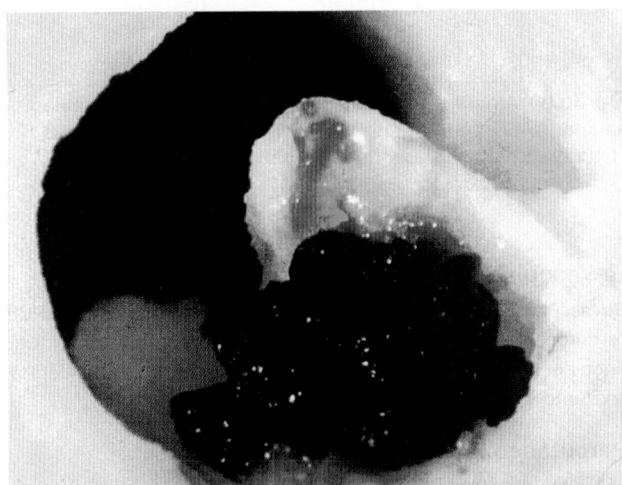

Fig. 30.63 Acute coronary thrombus. Cross-section (×30) of the epicardial coronary artery, demonstrating a rupture of the shoulder region of the plaque with a luminal thrombus.

> **Box 30.30 Risk factors for coronary disease**
>
> **Fixed**
> - Age
> - Male sex
> - Positive family history
> - Deletion polymorphism in the angiotensin-converting enzyme (*ACE*) gene (DD)
>
> **Potentially changeable**
> - Hyperlipidaemia
> - Cigarette smoking
> - Hypertension
> - Diabetes mellitus
>
> - Lack of exercise
> - Blood coagulation factors – high fibrinogen, factor VII
> - Elevated C-reactive protein
> - Homocysteinaemia
> - Obesity
> - Gout
> - Soft water
> - Drugs, e.g. contraceptive pill, nucleoside analogues, cyclo-oxygenase 2 (COX-2) inhibitors, rosiglitazone
> - Heavy alcohol consumption

ANGINA

Myocardial ischaemia in patients with stable CAD occurs when there is a mismatch between blood supply and metabolic demand. This results in regional wall motion abnormalities, ST–T changes on the 12-lead ECG and cardiac ischaemic pain – angina. Ischaemic metabolites, including adenosine, stimulate nerve endings and produce pain.

Epidemiology

The prevalence of angina increases with age in both sexes: in women it is 5–7% at 45–64 years as opposed to 10–12% at 65–84 years, while in men it is 4–7% at 45–64 years as opposed to 12–14% at 65–84 years. The annual mortality rate ranges from 1.2% to 2.4% and there is an annual incidence of cardiac death of 0.6–1.4%. Risk factors include hypertension, hyperlipidaemia, diabetes mellitus, sedentary lifestyle, obesity, smoking and family history.

Diagnosis

The diagnosis of angina is largely based on the clinical history.

- **Classical angina** or **typical angina** is characterized by chest pain:
  - 'Heavy', 'tight' or 'gripping' central or retrosternal pain may radiate to the jaw and/or arms.
  - Pain occurs with exercise or emotional stress.
  - Pain eases rapidly with rest or with GTN.
- **Atypical angina** is described by NICE as chest pain with 2 out of 3 of the features above.
- **Non-angina chest pain** is described by NICE as chest pain with 1 out of 3 of the features above.
- **Stable angina** can be classified according to the Canadian Cardiovascular Society guidelines (**Box 30.31**).
- **Unstable angina** refers to angina of recent onset (<24 h) or deterioration in previous stable angina, with symptoms frequently occurring at rest: that is, **acute coronary syndrome.**
- **Refractory angina** refers to patients with severe coronary disease in whom revascularization is not possible and angina is not controlled by medical therapy.
- **Vasospastic** or **variant (Prinzmetal's) angina** refers to angina that occurs without provocation, usually at rest, as a result of coronary artery spasm. It occurs more frequently in women. Characteristically, there is ST segment elevation on the ECG during the pain.
- **Microvascular angina** patients have exercise-induced angina but normal or unobstructed coronary arteries (on coronary angiography, CTCA). Intracoronary acetylcholine may cause coronary spasm. Whilst they have a good prognosis, they are often highly symptomatic and can be difficult to treat. In women with

---

> **Box 30.31 Canadian Cardiovascular Society functional classification of angina**
>
> | Class | Description |
> | --- | --- |
> | Class I | No angina with ordinary activity; angina with strenuous activity |
> | Class II | Angina during ordinary activity, e.g. walking up hills, walking rapidly upstairs, with mild limitation of activities |
> | Class III | Angina with low levels of activity, e.g. walking 50–100 m on the flat, walking up one flight of stairs, with marked restriction of activities |
> | Class IV | Angina at rest or with any level of exercise |

i **Box 30.32** Initial investigations in stable angina

Laboratory tests
- Full blood count
- Thyroid function tests
- Fasting glucose
- HbA_{1c} (see p. 710)
- Fasting lipid profile
- Glomerular filtration rate
- Troponin if unstable

12-lead ECG
- Exclude coronary syndrome, pathological Q waves, left ventricular hypertrophy, left bundle branch block

Echocardiography
- Regional wall motion abnormalities
- Left ventricular ejection fraction
- Diastolic function
- Alternative causes of chest pain

Ambulatory ECG
- Paroxysmal arrhythmia
- Vasospastic angina

Chest X-ray
- Atypical presentation
- Pulmonary disease
- Heart failure

this syndrome, the myocardium shows an abnormal metabolic response to stress, consistent with the suggestion that the myocardial ischaemia results from abnormal dilator responses of the coronary microvasculature to stress.

Examination

There are usually no abnormal findings in angina. Signs to suggest anaemia, thyrotoxicosis or hyperlipidaemia (e.g. lipid arcus, xanthelasma, tendon xanthoma) should be sought. It is essential to exclude aortic stenosis (i.e. slow-rising carotid impulse and ejection systolic murmur radiating to the neck) as a possible cause of the angina. The blood pressure should be taken to identify coexistent hypertension. BMI or waist circumference should be measured.

Investigations

Patients with suspected angina should have initial investigations (**Box 30.32**). The diagnosis of stable angina can be made on clinical assessment alone *or* by clinical assessment combined with anatomical (cardiac catheterization or CTCA) or functional imaging (SPECT, stress echocardiography, stress MRI).

Patients *without known CAD* presenting with chest pain can be categorized as having typical angina, atypical angina or non-anginal chest pain.

- Patients with **typical or atypical angina** or patients with **non-anginal chest pain but with ST changes or Q waves** should be referred for 64-slice (or above) CTCA.
- If the results from CTCA are inconclusive, the patient should be referred for non-invasive functional tests (SPECT, stress echocardiography, stress MRI).
- If stable angina cannot be diagnosed in patients with known coronary artery disease, non-invasive functional tests would be appropriate.
- Patient with **non-anginal chest pain** (more likely if the pain is continuous, unrelated to exertion, exacerbated by respiration, or associated with dizziness, palpitations or difficulty in swallowing) and a normal ECG should be considered for alternative diagnoses and investigated appropriately.

Management of stable angina

Patients should be informed of the nature of their condition and reassured that the prognosis is good (annual mortality <2%). Lifestyle management should be instigated, as for prevention of CAD. The stable angina algorithm in **Fig. 30.64** should be used to guide initial patient management, while **Box 30.33** outlines pharmacological therapy.

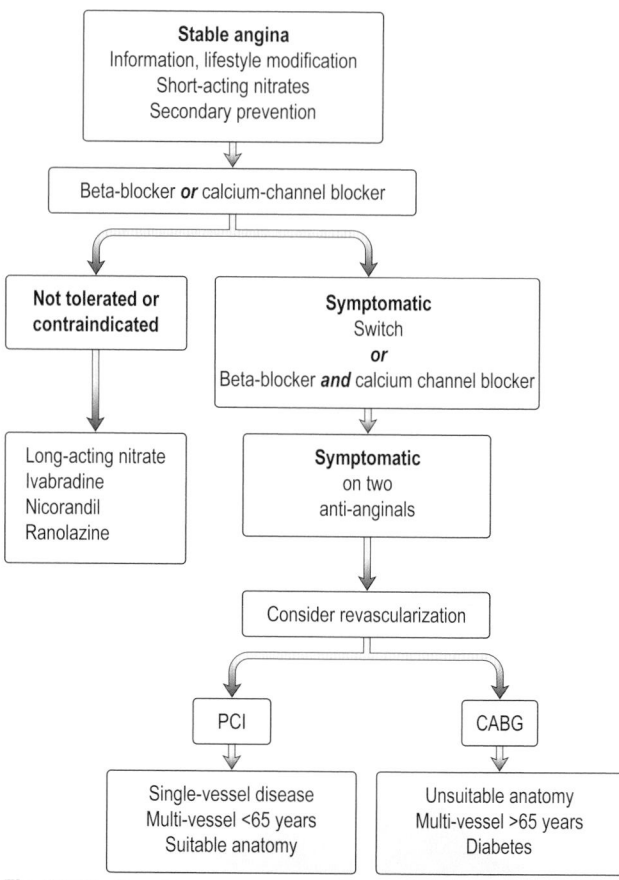

Fig. 30.64 Algorithm for management of patients with stable angina. CABG, coronary artery bypass grafting; PCI, percutaneous coronary intervention. (*From National Institute for Health and Care Excellence. Clinical Guideline CG126L: Management of Stable Angina. NICE July 2011, with permission.*)

Revascularization

Revascularization with percutaneous coronary intervention (PCI) or coronary artery bypass surgery is indicated for patients with ongoing angina symptoms despite appropriate medical therapy and/or to improve prognosis.

Percutaneous coronary intervention

PCI is the process of dilating a coronary artery stenosis by introducing an inflatable balloon and metallic stent (**Fig. 30.65**) into the arterial circulation via the femoral, radial or brachial artery (**Fig. 30.66**); the radial artery is the best (see later). Fractional flow reserve (FFR) measurement can be used to assess the severity of a stenosis prior to PCI. An FFR of more than 0.80 treated medically (i.e. no stent) is associated with improved patient outcomes. Complications of PCI include bleeding, haematoma, dissection and pseudo-aneurysm from the arterial puncture site, although use of the radial artery reduces these risks and is the standard technique in the UK. Serious complications include acute myocardial infarction (2%), stroke (0.4%) and death (1%). **Bare metal stents** (BMSs) are associated with a 20–30% risk of coronary artery restenosis within 6–9 months of implantation. First-generation **drug-eluting stents** (DESs) with **sirolimus** and **paclitaxel** reduced restenosis but suffered from late and very late stent thrombosis. Second-generation DESs (with thinner struts and biodegradable or biocompatible polymers) demonstrated better safety and efficacy, and are recommended for most patients (BMSs may be preferred in patients requiring anticoagulation and

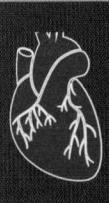

Box 30.33 Pharmacological therapy in stable angina

Drug	Dose	Indications/mechanism of action/cautions
Vasodilators		
Glyceryl trinitrate	0.3–1.0 mg sublingual 2.0–3.0 mg buccal	Prophylaxis and treatment of angina – rapid onset Repeat after 5 min if symptomatic Vasodilation (causes headache and flushing)
Isosorbide mononitrate	10–60 mg ×2 daily (slow-release preparations available)	Prophylaxis of angina Side-effects – headache and flushing Contraindicated with phosphodiesterase type 5 inhibitors
Beta-blocker		
Bisoprolol	2.5–10 mg daily	Inhibits β-adrenoceptors, reduces heart rate and BP, reduces myocardial oxygen consumption Caution – COPD, acute heart failure, AV conduction Side-effects – fatigue, peripheral vasoconstriction (cold peripheries), sexual dysfunction, bronchospasm
Calcium-channel blockers		
Verapamil (phenylalkylamines)	80–120 mg ×3 daily (or 240–480 mg daily slow-release)	Inhibit calcium channels in myocardium, cardiac conductive tissue and vascular smooth muscle Diltiazem and verapamil – contraindicated in severe bradycardia, left ventricular failure with pulmonary congestion, second- or third-degree AV block Side-effects – constipation (verapamil), ankle oedema (amlodipine, diltiazem), reflex tachycardia (amlodipine)
Diltiazem (benzothiapines)	60–120 mg ×3 daily (longer-acting preparations available)	
Amlodipine (dihydropyridines)	5–10 mg daily	
Other anti-anginal drugs		
Ivabradine	2.5–7.5 mg ×2 daily	Inhibits pacemaker I_f current in SA node Use in sinus rhythm ± beta-blocker Side-effects – bradycardia, phosphenes Contraindications – sick sinus syndrome, AV block
Nicorandil	5–30 mg ×2 daily	Activates ATP-sensitive potassium channels and has nitrate properties – peripheral and coronary vasodilation Use as adjunctive therapy Side-effects – headache, flushing, oral ulceration
Ranolazine	375–750 mg ×2 daily	Inhibits late sodium channels into cardiac cells Use as adjunctive therapy Metabolized by cytochrome P450 3A4 Side-effects – constipation, dizziness, lengthened QT
Event-reducing drugs		
Antiplatelet	Aspirin 75-100 mg daily	Reversible inhibition of platelet COX-1 and thromboxane production
	Clopidogrel 75 mg daily	Thienopyridine that antagonizes platelet ADP receptor P2Y12. Use in aspirin intolerance
ACE inhibitor or ARB	Enalapril 10 mg daily	Indicated if treating other condition, e.g. hypertension, heart failure, chronic kidney disease
Statins	Atorvastatin 80 mg daily	Use to reduce LDL cholesterol to <1.8 mmol/L

ACE, angiotensin-converting enzyme; ADP, adenosine diphosphate; ARB, angiotensin receptor blocker; ATP, adenosine triphosphate; AV, atrioventricular; BP, blood pressure; COPD, chronic obstructive pulmonary disease; COX-1, cyclo-oxygenase-1; LDL, low-density lipoprotein; SA, sinoatrial.

early surgery). Dual antiplatelet therapy (aspirin and a P2Y12 inhibitor, e.g. clopidogrel) should continue for 6–12 months.

Coronary artery bypass grafting

With CABG, autologous veins or arteries are anastomosed to the ascending aorta and to the native coronary arteries distal to the area of stenosis (**Fig. 30.67**). Improved graft survival can be obtained with *in situ* internal mammary and gastroepiploic arteries grafted on to the stenosed coronary artery, compared to vein grafts. Operative mortality is well below 1% in patients with normal left ventricular function.

PCI versus CABG

The heart team (made up of interventional and non-interventional cardiologists, cardiac surgeons, cardiac anaesthetists and intensivists) should review whether patients should continue with medical therapy or be referred for PCI or CABG. The STS score and/or EuroSCORE II

(see Further reading) can be utilized to determine in-hospital mortality and morbidity in patients referred for surgery. The SYNTAX score should be used for complex CAD to determine long-term mortality and morbidity in patients referred for PCI. In the current European Society of Cardiology (ESC) guidelines for revascularization (see Further reading), PCI is preferred to CABG in patients with single- or double-vessel disease not involving the proximal left anterior descending (LAD) or left main stem (LMS) vessel. CABG and PCI are both appropriate in patients with proximal LAD stenosis, LMS or three-vessel disease (without diabetes mellitus) and a low SYNTAX score (0–22). CABG is preferred to PCI in patients with three-vessel disease and diabetes or elevated SYNTAX score (>22) and in patients with LMS and SYNTAX score of more than 22. Patient clinical characteristics (severe co-morbidities, reduced life expectancy, porcelain aorta (heavily calcified), need for additional surgery to the aorta or valves) may alter the modality of revascularization.

Patients with intractable angina

Some patients remain symptomatic despite medication and are not suitable for (further) revascularization. These individuals need a pain management programme.

Further reading

Mehran R, Baber U, Sharma SK et al. Ticagrelor with or without Aspirin in High-Risk Patients after PCI. *N Engl J Med* 2019; 381:2032–2042.

National Institute for Health and Care Excellence. *NICE Clinical Guideline 95: Chest Pain of Recent Onset: Assessment and Diagnosis*. NICE 2010; https://www.nice.org.uk/guidance/cg95.

National Institute for Health and Care Excellence. *NICE Clinical Guideline 126: Stable Angina: Management*. NICE 2011; https://www.nice.org.uk/guidance/cg126.

Neumann FJ, Sousa-Uva M, Ahlsson A et al. 2018 ESC/EACTS Guidelines on myocardial revascularization. *Eur Heart J* 2019; 40:87–165.

Scottish Intercollegiate Guidelines Network. *SIGN National Clinical Guideline 151: Management of Stable Angina*. SIGN 2018; https://www.sign.ac.uk/assets/sign151.pdf.

Xaplanteris P, Fournier S, Pijls, NHJ et al. Five-Year Outcomes with PCI Guided by Fractional Flow Reserve. *N Engl J Med* 2018; 379:250–259.

http://riskcalc.sts.org/stswebriskcalc/calculate. *Society of Thoracic Surgeons (STS) score.*

http://www.euroscore.org/calc.html. *EuroSCORE II.*

http://www.syntaxscore.com/calculator/start.htm. *SYNTAX score.*

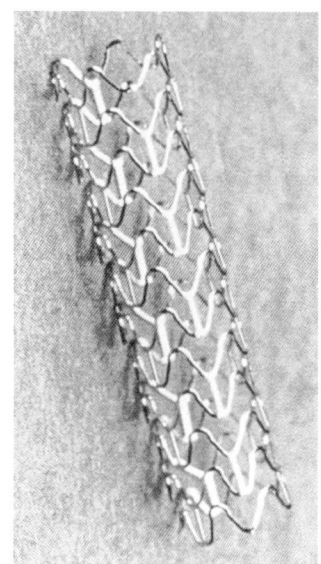

Fig. 30.65 An intracoronary stent.

ACUTE CORONARY SYNDROMES

Acute coronary syndromes (ACSs) include:

- *ST-elevation myocardial infarction (STEMI)*
- *non-ST-elevation myocardial infarction (NSTEMI)*
- *unstable angina (UA).*

The difference between UA and NSTEMI is that, in the latter, there is occluding thrombus, which leads to myocardial necrosis and a rise in serum troponins or creatine kinase-MB (CK-MB). Myocardial infarction (MI) occurs when cardiac myocytes die due to myocardial ischaemia. It can be diagnosed on the basis of appropriate clinical history, 12-lead ECG and elevated biochemical markers: troponin I and T, and CK-MB.

There are five types of MI:

- *type 1 – spontaneous MI with ischaemia* due to a primary coronary event, e.g. plaque erosion/rupture, fissuring or dissection
- *type 2 – MI secondary to ischaemia* due to increased oxygen demand or decreased supply, such as in coronary spasm,

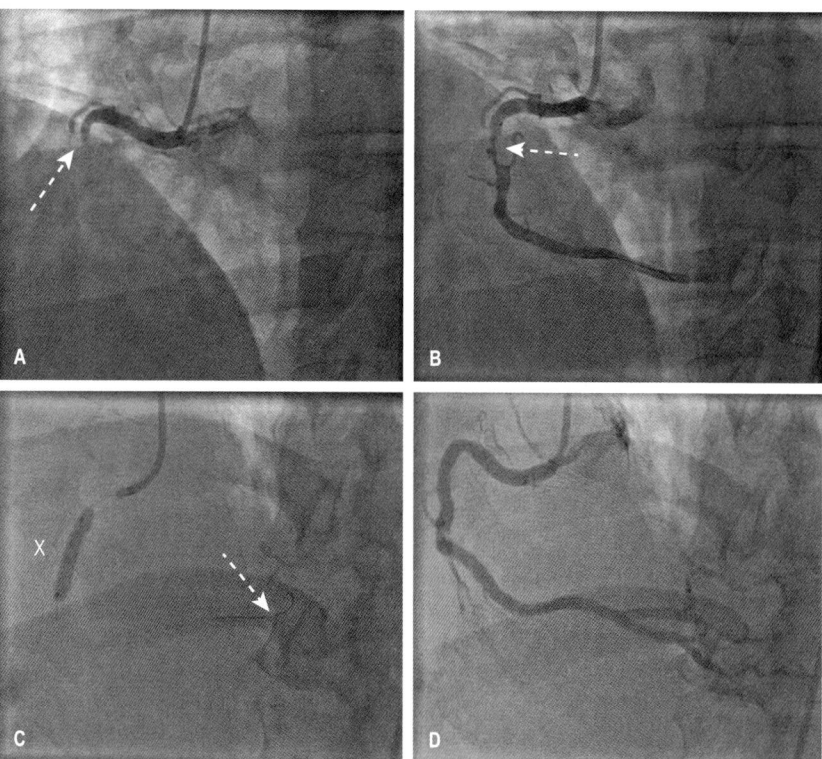

Fig. 30.66 Percutaneous transluminal coronary angioplasty (PTCA). (A) Coronary angiography demonstrates an occluded right coronary artery (arrowed). (B) A soft wire passed through the guide catheter reopens the artery but a severe stenosis remains (arrowed). (C) A balloon (X) is inflated to dilate the stenosis. The soft guidewire can be seen in the distal posterior descending artery (arrowed). (D) The right coronary artery has now been successfully reopened with good antegrade flow.

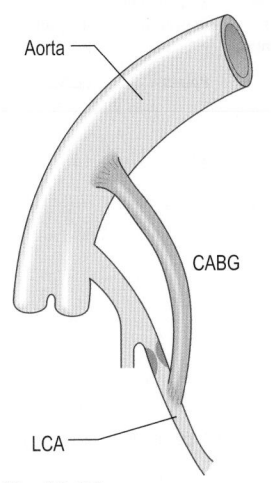

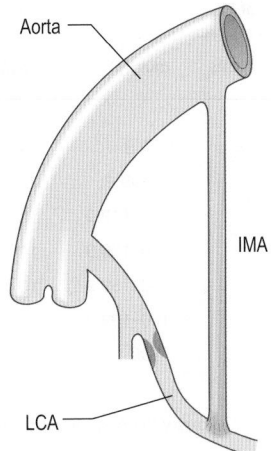

Fig. 30.67 Relief of coronary obstruction by surgical techniques: coronary artery bypass grafting (CABG) and internal mammary arterial implantation (IMA). In both of these examples the graft bypasses a coronary obstruction in the left coronary artery (LCA).

coronary embolism, anaemia, arrhythmias, hypertension or hypotension

- *type 3 – diagnosis of MI in sudden cardiac death*
- *type 4a – MI related to PCI*
- *type 4b – MI related to stent thrombosis*
- *type 5 – MI related to CABG.*

Pathophysiology

The mechanism that is common to all ACSs is rupture or erosion of the fibrous cap of a coronary artery plaque. This leads to platelet aggregation and adhesion, localized thrombosis, vasoconstriction and distal thrombus embolization. The presence of a rich lipid pool within the plaque and a thin, fibrous cap is associated with an increased risk of rupture. Thrombus formation and the vasoconstriction produced by platelet release of serotonin and thromboxane A_2 result in myocardial ischaemia due to reduction of coronary blood flow.

Clinical features

Patients with an ACS may complain of a new onset of **chest pain**, chest pain at rest or a deterioration of pre-existing angina. However, some present with atypical features, including indigestion, pleuritic chest pain or dyspnoea. Physical examination can detect alternative diagnoses, such as aortic dissection, pulmonary embolism or peptic ulceration. In addition, it can also identify adverse clinical signs, such as hypotension, basal crackles, fourth heart sounds and cardiac murmurs.

Investigations

Electrocardiogram

Although the 12-lead ECG may be normal, ST depression and T-wave inversion are highly suggestive of an ACS, particularly if associated with anginal chest pain. The ECG should be repeated when the patient is in pain and continuous ST-segment monitoring is recommended. With a STEMI, complete occlusion of a coronary vessel will result in a persistent ST elevation or left bundle branch block pattern, although transient ST elevation is seen with coronary vasospasm or Prinzmetal's angina.

i **Box 30.34 Relationship between troponin I and risk of death in acute coronary syndrome**

Serum troponin levels (ng/mL)	Mortality at 42 days (% of patients)
0 to <0.4	1.0
0.4 to <1.0	1.7
1.0 to <2.0	3.4
2.0 to <5.0	3.7
5.0 to <9.0	6.0
>9.0	7.5

(Adapted from Antman EM, Tanasijevic MJ, Thompson B et al. Cardiac-specific troponin I levels to predict the risk of mortality in patients with acute coronary syndromes. N Engl J Med 1996; 335:1342–1349.)

i **Box 30.35 TIMI risk score in acute coronary syndrome (NSTEMI/UA)**

Risk factor	Score
Age >65 years	1
>3 CAD risk factors – hypertension, hyperlipidaemia, family history, diabetes, smoking	1
Known CAD (coronary angiography stenosis >50%)	1
Aspirin use in the last 7 days	1
Severe angina (>2 episodes of rest pain in 24 h)	1
ST deviation on ECG (horizontal ST depression or transient ST elevation >1 mm)	1
Elevated cardiac markers (CK-MB or troponin)	1
Total score	

0–1: rate of death/MI in 14 days 3%; rate of death/MI/urgent revascularization 4.75%
2: 3%; 8.3%
3: 5%; 13.2%
4: 7%; 19.9%
5: 12%; 26.2%
6–7: 19%; 40.9%

CAD, coronary artery disease; CK-MB, creatine kinase MB; MI, myocardial infarction; NSTEMI, non-ST-elevation myocardial infarction; TIMI, Thrombolysis in Myocardial Infarction; UA, unstable angina.

Biochemical markers

The cardiac troponin complex is made up of three distinct proteins (I, T and C), which are situated with tropomyosin on the thin actin filament that forms the skeleton of the cardiac myofilament. Troponin T attaches the complex to tropomyosin, troponin C binds calcium during excitation–contraction coupling, and troponin I inhibits the myosin binding site on the actin. 'Highly sensitive' troponin assays can now detect troponins in normal people. There are many different assays and results should be interpreted in the context of the clinical picture and the ECG. A negative predictive value of 99.4% has been shown for a serum troponin below 5 ng/L; this has been shown to be consistent across a wide group of patients. If the initial troponin assay is negative, it should be repeated 3 hours later. The troponin assay provides prognostic information: that is, a high serum troponin level carries an increased mortality risk in ACS (**Box 30.34**). It also defines which patients may benefit from aggressive medical therapy and early coronary revascularization.

NSTEMI and unstable angina

Risk stratification

Both the Thrombolysis in Myocardial Infarction (TIMI) score (**Box 30.35**) and the Global Registry of Acute Coronary Events (GRACE)

Age		Findings at initial hospital presentation		Findings during hospitalization		History of CCF	History of MI	Systolic BP		Elevated cardiac enzymes	ST segment depression	No in-hospital PCI
Age (years)	Points	Resting heart rate (b.p.m.)	Points	Initial serum creatinine (mg/dL)	Points	Points	Points	(mmHg)	Points	Points	Points	Points
≤29	0	≤49.9	0	0–0.39	1	24	12	≤79.9	24	15	11	14
30–39	0	50–69.9	3	0.4–0.79	3			80–99.9	22			
40–49	18	70–89.9	9	0.8–1.19	5			100–119.9	18			
50–59	36	90–109.9	14	1.2–1.59	7			120–139.9	14			
60–69	55	110–149.9	23	1.6–1.99	9			140–159.9	10			
70–79	73	150–199.9	35	2–3.99	15			160–199.9	4			
80–89	91	≥200	43	>4	20			≥200	0			
≥90	100											

BP, blood pressure; CCF, congestive cardiac failure; GRACE, Global Registry of Acute Coronary Events; MI, myocardial infarction; PCI, percutaneous coronary intervention.

Syndrome type/ timeframe	Risk category (tertiles)	GRACE risk score	Deaths (%)
NSTEMI-ACS			
In hospital	Low	≤108	<1
	Intermediate	109–140	1–3
	High	>140	>3
Post discharge to 6 months	Low	≤88	<3
	Intermediate	89–118	3–8
	High	>118	>8
STEMI-ACS			
In hospital	Low	49–125	<2
	Intermediate	126–154	2–5
	High	155–319	>5
Post discharge to 6 months	Low	27–99	<3
	Intermediate	100–127	3–8
	High	128–263	>8

ACS, acute coronary syndrome; GRACE, Global Registry of Acute Coronary Events; NSTEMI, non-ST-elevation myocardial infarction; STEMI, ST-elevation myocardial infarction. *(From http://www.outcomes-umassmed.org/grace/grace_risk_table.aspx.)*

prediction score can be used in patients with ACS to define risk. The GRACE score is based on age, heart rate, systolic blood pressure, serum creatinine and the Killip score (**Boxes 30.36** and **30.37**).

Investigations and management

All patients require immediate management of their chest pain, as outlined on page 1088 and in **Box 30.38**.

Antiplatelet drugs

The platelet is a key part of the thrombosis cascade involved in ACS. Rupture of the atheromatous plaque exposes the circulating platelets to adenosine diphosphate (ADP), thromboxane A_2 (TxA_2), adrenaline (epinephrine), thrombin and collagen tissue factor. This causes platelet activation, with thrombin as an especially potent stimulant of such activity. Platelet activation stimulates the expression of glycoprotein (GP) IIb/IIIa receptors on the platelet surface.

These receptors bridge fibrinogen between adjacent platelets, causing platelet aggregates (see **Fig. 16.32**). ACS patients should be treated with dual antiplatelet agents:

- **aspirin 300 mg** loading dose then 75-100 mg daily *and*
- an ADP-receptor antagonist
  - **clopidogrel 300–600 mg** loading then 75 mg daily *or*
  - **prasugrel 60 mg** loading then 10 mg daily *or*
  - **ticagrelor 180 mg** loading then 90 mg twice daily.

Antithrombin drugs

An antithrombin should be added to dual antiplatelets in patients with ACS. **Unfractionated heparin (UFH)** requires frequent monitoring; the low-molecular-weight heparin **enoxaparin** appears to be superior and can be given subcutaneously twice daily. **Bivalirudin** is a direct thrombin inhibitor that reversibly binds to thrombin and inhibits clot-bound thrombin. In the ACUITY trial, bivalirudin appeared as effective as heparin plus GPIIb/IIIa inhibitors in reducing ischaemic events in patients pre-treated with a thienopyridine and undergoing diagnostic angiography or percutaneous intervention, but with less bleeding. **Fondaparinux** is a synthetic pentasaccharide that selectively binds to antithrombin; this inactivates factor Xa, resulting in strong inhibition of thrombin generation and clot formation. It does not inactivate thrombin and has no effect on platelets.

Activated glycoprotein (GP) IIb/IIIa receptors on platelets bind to fibrinogen, initiating platelet aggregation. Receptor antagonists (abciximab, eptifibatide, tirofiban) have been developed that are powerful inhibitors of platelet aggregation. However, their use in ACS patients should be restricted to patients with heavy thrombus burden identified during coronary angiography and for complications during PCI (e.g. distal embolization).

Anti-ischaemia agents

In patients with no contraindications (asthma, AV block, acute pulmonary oedema) beta-blockers are administered orally, to reduce myocardial ischaemia by blocking circulating catecholamines. This will lower the heart rate and blood pressure, reducing myocardial oxygen consumption. The dose can be titrated to produce a resting heart rate of 50–60 b.p.m. In patients with on-going angina, nitrates should be given either sublingually or intravenously. They effectively reduce preload and produce coronary vasodilation. However, tolerance can become a problem and patients should be weaned off intravenous administration if symptoms resolve.

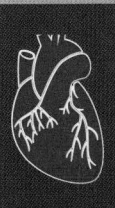

Box 30.38 Pharmacological therapy in acute coronary syndrome

Drug	Dose	Notes
Antiplatelet drugs		
Aspirin	150–300 mg chewable or soluble aspirin, then 75-100 mg orally daily	Caution if active peptic ulceration
Clopidogrel	300 mg orally loading dose, then 75 mg orally daily	Caution: increased risk of bleeding; avoid if CABG planned
Prasugrel	60 mg oral loading dose, then 10 mg orally daily (5 mg daily if <60 kg or >75 years old)	
Ticagrelor	Initially 180 mg, then 90 mg ×2 daily	
Antithrombin drugs		
Heparin	5000 units i.v. bolus, then 0.25 units/kg per hour	Measure anticoagulant effect with APTT at 6 h
Low-molecular-weight heparins, e.g. enoxaparin	1 mg/kg s.c. ×2 daily	Risk of bleeding
Bivalirudin	0.75 mg/kg i.v. bolus, then 1.75 mg/kg per hour for 4 h post PCI	
Fondaparinux	2.5 mg s.c. daily, for up to 8 days	
Rivaroxaban	Oral 2.5–10 mg daily	
Glycoprotein IIB/IIIA inhibitors[a]		
Abciximab	0.25 mg/kg i.v. bolus, then 0.125 µg/kg per min up to 10 µg/min i.v. ×12 h	Indicated if coronary intervention likely within 24 h
Eptifibatide	180 µg/kg i.v. bolus, then 2 µg/kg per min ×18 h	Indicated in high-risk patients managed without coronary intervention or during PCI
Tirofiban	25 µg/kg over 5 min, then 0.15 µg/kg per min for up to 18 h	Indicated in high-risk patients managed without coronary intervention or during PCI
Analgesia		
Diamorphine or morphine	2.5–5.0 mg i.v.	Prescribe with antiemetic, e.g. metoclopramide 10 mg i.v.
Myocardial energy consumption		
Atenolol	5 mg i.v. repeated after 15 min, then 25–50 mg orally daily	Avoid in asthma, heart failure, hypotension, bradyarrhythmias
Metoprolol	5 mg i.v. repeated to a maximum of 15 mg, then 25–50 mg orally ×2 daily	
Coronary vasodilation		
Glyceryl trinitrate	2–10 mg/h i.v./buccal/sublingual	Maintain systolic BP >90 mmHg
Plaque stabilization/ventricular remodelling		
HMG-CoA reductase inhibitors (statins)		
Rosuvastatin	20–40 mg orally	Combine with dietary advice and modification
Pravastatin	20–40 mg orally	
Atorvastatin	80 mg orally	
ACE inhibitors		
Ramipril	2.5–10 mg orally	Monitor renal function
Lisinopril	5–10 mg orally	

[a]Not now used in patients pre-treated with clopidogrel and aspirin prior to coronary intervention. ABG, arterial blood gases; ACE, angiotensin-converting enzyme; APTT, activated partial thromboplastin time; BP, blood pressure; CABG, coronary artery bypass graft; COPD, chronic obstructive pulmonary disease; i.v., intravenous; PCI, percutaneous coronary intervention; s.c., subcutaneous.

Plaque stabilization/remodelling

HMG-CoA reductase inhibitor drugs (statins) and ACE inhibitors are routinely administered to patients with ACS. These agents may produce plaque stabilization, improve vascular and myocardial remodelling, and reduce future cardiovascular events. Starting the drugs while the patient is still in hospital increases the likelihood of these individuals receiving secondary drug therapy.

Coronary angiography and intervention

Very high-risk patients require urgent coronary angiography (<2 h). This includes those individuals with persistent or recurrent chest pain not responding to medical therapy, clinical signs of heart failure or haemodynamic instability or cardiogenic shock, or life-threatening arrhythmias (ventricular fibrillation, ventricular tachycardia).

High-risk patients with rising or falling cardiac troponin levels, dynamic ST- or T-wave changes, or elevated GRACE scores (>140) require coronary angiography within 24 h.

Intermediate-risk patients with diabetes mellitus, renal impairment (estimated glomerular filtration rate <60), LVEF below 40% or congestive cardiac failure, early post infarction angina, previous PCI or CABG, or a GRACE score of over 109 but less than 140 require coronary angiography within 72 h.

Box 30.39 TIMI risk score in ST elevation myocardial infarction (STEMI)

Risk factor	Score
Age >65 years	2
Age >75 years	3
History of angina	1
History of hypertension	1
History of diabetes	1
Systolic BP <100 mmHg	3
Heart rate >100 b.p.m.	2
Killip score II–IV	2
Weight >67 kg	1
Anterior MI or LBBB	1
Delay to treatment >4 h	1

Total score

0: risk of death at 30 days 0.8%
1: 1.6%
2: 2.2%
3: 4.4%
4: 7.3%
5: 12.4%
6: 16.1%
7: 23.4%
8: 26.8%
9–16: 35.9%

BP, blood pressure; LBBB, left bundle branch block; MI, myocardial infarction; TIMI, Thrombolysis in Myocardial Infarction.

Low-risk patients can be managed initially with medical therapy but an invasive strategy with cardiac catheterization is preferred in most patients.

ST elevation myocardial infarction (STEMI)

Myocardial infarction occurs when cardiac myocytes die due to prolonged myocardial ischaemia. In Europe, approximately 1.8 million people die annually from ischaemic heart disease.

Pathophysiology

Rupture or erosion of a vulnerable coronary artery plaque can produce prolonged occlusion of a coronary artery, leading to myocardial necrosis within 15–30 minutes. The subendocardial myocardium is initially affected but, with continued ischaemia, the infarct zone extends through to the subepicardial myocardium, producing a transmural Q wave MI. Early reperfusion may salvage regions of the myocardium, reducing future mortality and morbidity.

The in-hospital mortality rate is between 6% and 14%. Several risk factors can be identified that predict death rate at 30 days (TIMI STEMI score, **Box 30.39**).

Clinical features

Any patient presenting with severe chest pain lasting more than 20 minutes may be suffering from MI. The pain does not usually respond to sublingual glyceryl trinitrate, and opiate analgesia is required. The pain may radiate to the left arm, neck or jaw. However, in some patients, particularly elderly or diabetic ones, the symptoms may be atypical and include dyspnoea, fatigue, pre-syncope or syncope. Autonomic symptoms are common and on examination the patient may be pale and clammy, with marked sweating. In addition, the pulse may be thready with significant hypotension, bradycardia or tachycardia.

Box 30.40 Typical ECG changes in myocardial infarction (STEMI)

Infarct site	Leads showing ST elevation
Anterior	
Small	V_3–V_4
Extensive	V_2–V_5
Anteroseptal	V_1–V_3
Anterolateral	V_4–V_6, I, AVL
Lateral	I, AVL
Inferior	II, III, AVF
Posterior	V_1, V_2 reciprocal changes, i.e. ST depression
Subendocardial	Any lead
Right ventricle	VR_4

Investigations

Electrocardiography

An ECG in patients with chest pain should be performed within 10 minutes of first contact with the emergency medical team (ambulance or emergency department). The baseline ECG is rarely normal, but if it is, it should be repeated every 15 minutes, while the patient remains in pain. Continuous cardiac monitoring is required because of the high likelihood of significant cardiac arrhythmias. ECG changes (**Box 30.40**) are usually confined to the ECG leads that 'face' the infarction. The presence of new ST elevation (due to opening of the K+ channels) of 0.2 mV or more at the J-point in leads V_1–V_3 and 0.1 mV or more in other leads suggests anterior MI (**Fig. 30.68**). An inferior wall MI is diagnosed when ST elevation is seen in leads II, III and AVF (**Fig. 30.69**). Lateral MI produces changes in leads I, AVL and V_5/V_6. In patients with a posterior MI, there may be ST depression in leads V_1–V_3 with a dominant R wave, and ST elevation in lead V_5/V_6. New, or presumed new, left bundle branch block is compatible with coronary artery occlusion requiring urgent reperfusion therapy. It may not be possible to exclude MI in patients with a paced rhythm or right bundle branch block, and patients with symptoms compatible with MI should be triaged in the MI pathway. The evolution of the ECG during the course of STEMI is illustrated in **Fig. 30.70**.

Blood tests and other imaging

Blood samples should be taken for cardiac troponin I or T levels, although treatment should not be deferred until the results are available. Full blood count, serum electrolytes, glucose and lipid profile should be obtained. Transthoracic echocardiography (TTE) may be helpful to confirm an MI, as wall-motion abnormalities are detectable early in STEMI. TTE may detect alternative diagnoses, such as aortic dissection, pericarditis or pulmonary embolism.

Management

Early medical management

Initial assessment involves rapid triage for chest pain (*note that time is muscle*) and referral for reperfusion therapy (primary PCI or thrombolysis). Initial medical therapy includes oxygen (if saturations are <90%), intravenous opioids (morphine if in pain) and aspirin (300 mg) (see **Box 30.38**).

Primary percutaneous coronary intervention (PCI)

The preferred reperfusion therapy for STEMI in interventional cardiology centres is primary PCI with a target of 60 minutes for wire

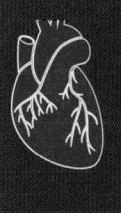

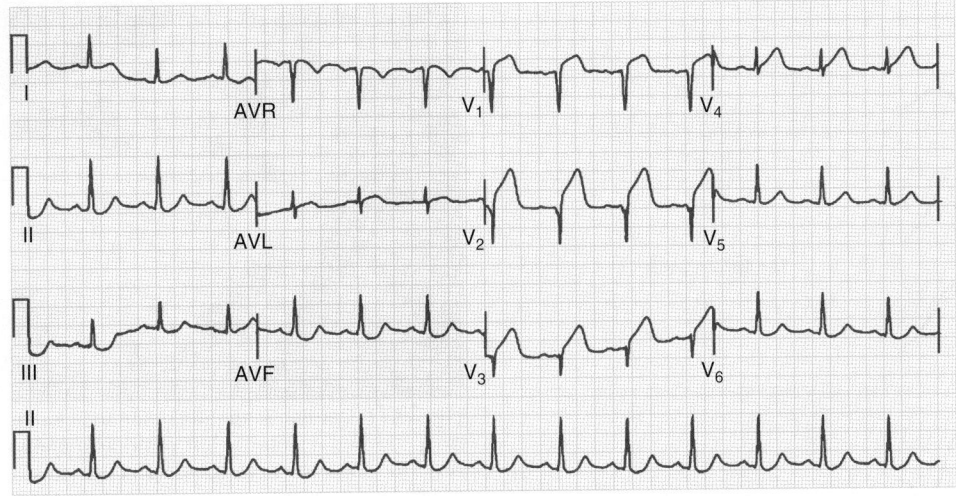

Fig. 30.68 An acute anteroseptal myocardial infarction, shown by a 12-lead ECG. Note the ST segment elevation and pathological Q waves in leads V₁-V₃. Ischaemic changes with ST segment depression are also seen in the inferior leads (II, III and AVF).

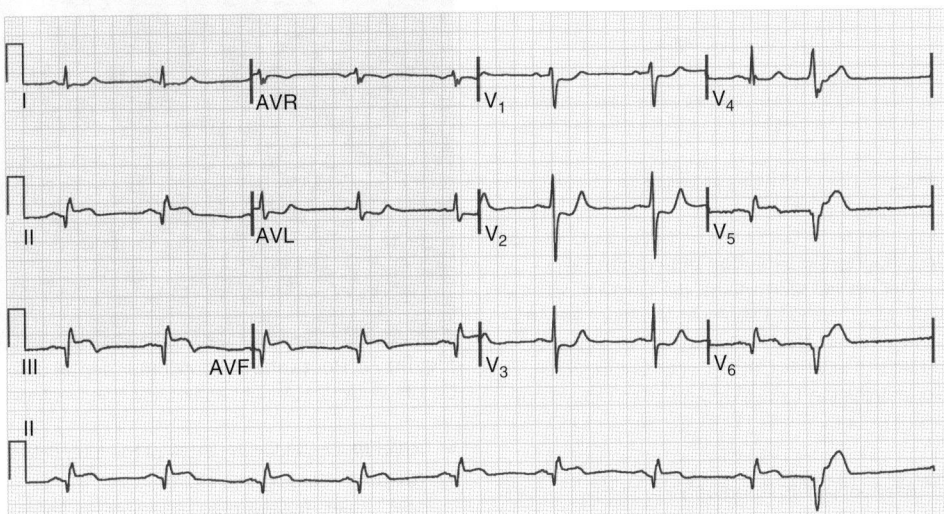

Fig. 30.69 An acute inferior wall myocardial infarction, shown by a 12-lead ECG. Note the raised ST segment and Q waves in the inferior leads (II, III and AVF).

crossing of the culprit vessel. Recent updated ESC guidelines recommend performing complete revascularization during the index hospital admission. Data from the RIVAL and RIFLE STEACS studies demonstrate that radial access is the preferred route, as this reduces complications and may improve survival. Primary PCI performed with drug eluting stents is preferred to bare metal stents. Routine thrombus aspiration is not recommended. Dual antiplatelet therapy is with aspirin and an ADP-receptor blocker (prasugrel or ticagrelor). Anticoagulant options include unfractionated heparin, enoxaparin or bivalirudin. The routine use of GP IIb/IIIa inhibitors is no longer recommended.

Thrombolysis

Thrombolytic agents (see p. 370) enhance the breakdown of occlusive thromboses by the activation of plasminogen to form plasmin. Thrombolysis is appropriate if primary PCI is not deliverable within 120 minutes of STEMI diagnosis. A meta-analysis showed that thrombolysis within 6 hours of STEMI or left bundle branch block

MI prevented 30 deaths in every 1000 patients treated. Between 7 and 12 hours, 20 in every 1000 deaths were prevented. After 12 hours the benefits are limited, and there is evidence to suggest less benefit for older patients, possibly because of the increased risk of strokes. The target for reperfusion therapy is less than 10 minutes delivery of bolus therapy. For patients who fail to reperfuse by 60–90 minutes, as demonstrated by 50% resolution of the ST-segment elevation, re-thrombolysis or referral for rescue coronary angioplasty is recommended. The contraindications to thrombolysis are provided in **Box 30.41**. Aspirin and clopidogrel are recommended in patients undergoing thrombolysis. Anticoagulant options include unfractionated heparin, enoxaparin or fondaparinux.

Coronary artery bypass surgery

Cardiac surgery is usually reserved for the complications of MI, such as ventricular septal defect or mitral regurgitation. Operative mortality is highest in the first 72 hours after STEMI.

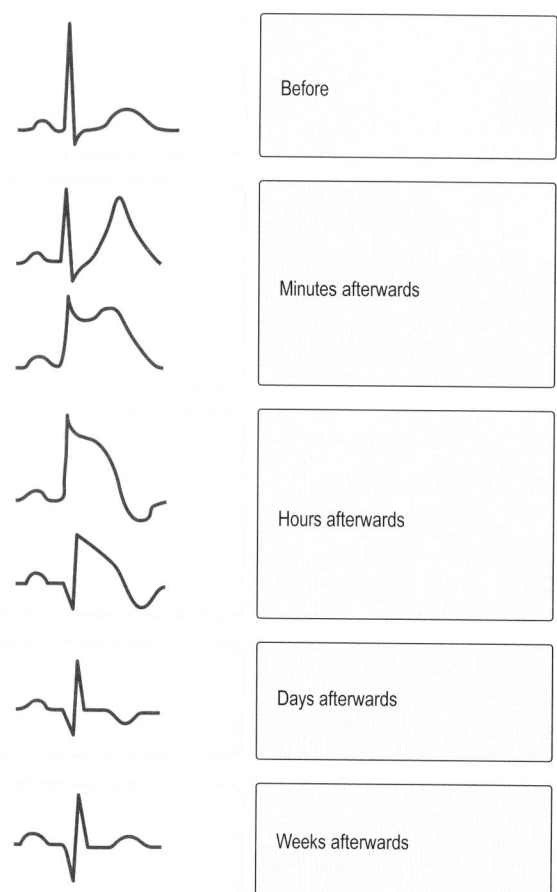

	Before
	Minutes afterwards
	Hours afterwards
	Days afterwards
	Weeks afterwards

Fig. 30.70 Electrocardiographic evolution of myocardial infarction (STEMI). After the first few minutes, the T waves become tall, pointed and upright, and there is ST segment elevation. After the first few hours, the T waves invert, the R-wave voltage is decreased and Q waves develop. After a few days, the ST segment returns to normal. After weeks or months the T wave may return to upright but the Q wave remains.

Box 30.41 Contraindications to thrombolysis

Absolute contraindications
- Haemorrhagic stroke or stroke of unknown origin at any time
- Ischaemic stroke in the preceding 3 months
- Central nervous system damage/neoplasm/vascular malformation
- Recent major trauma/surgery/head injury (within the preceding 3 weeks)
- Gastrointestinal bleeding within the last month
- Known bleeding disorder
- Aortic dissection

Relative contraindications
- Ischaemic stroke in the preceding 3 months
- Oral anticoagulant therapy
- Pregnancy or within 1 week postpartum
- Non-compressible vascular punctures
- Traumatic resuscitation
- Refractory hypertension (systolic blood pressure >180 mmHg)
- Advanced liver disease
- Internal bleeding, e.g. active peptic ulcer
- Dementia

Complications of myocardial infarction

Heart failure

Cardiac failure post STEMI is a poor prognostic feature that necessitates medical and invasive therapy to reduce the death rate. The Killip classification is used to assess patients with heart failure post MI:
- *Killip I* – no crackles and no third heart sound
- *Killip II* – crackles in <50% of the lung fields or a third heart sound

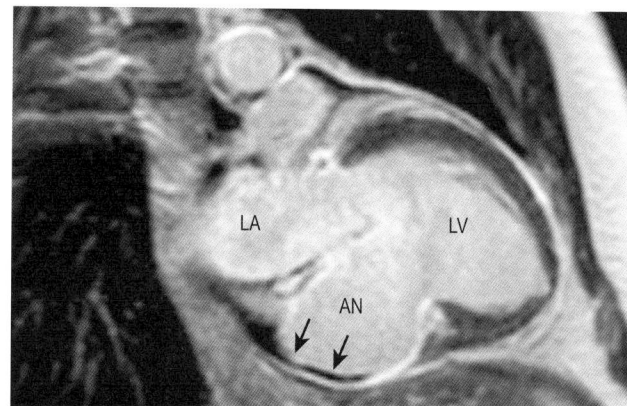

Fig. 30.71 Cardiac magnetic resonance image (vertical long axis) showing an inferior left ventricular aneurysm (arrowed, AN). The aneurysm was successfully resected surgically. LA, left atrium; LV, left ventricle.

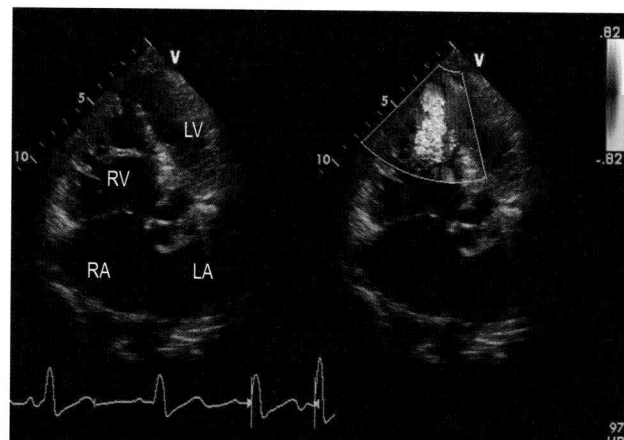

Fig. 30.72 Post-infarct ventricular septal defect. LA, left atrium; LV, left ventricle; RA, right atrium; RV, right ventricle.

- *Killip III* – crackles in >50% of the lung fields
- *Killip IV* – cardiogenic shock.

Mild heart failure may respond to intravenous furosemide 40–80 mg i.v., with glyceryl trinitrate administration if the blood pressure is satisfactory. Oxygen is required, with regular oxygen monitoring. ACE inhibitors can be given within 24–48 hours if the blood pressure is satisfactory. Patients with severe heart failure may require Swan–Ganz catheterization to determine the pulmonary wedge pressure. Intravenous inotropes, such as dopamine or dobutamine, are used in severe heart failure. If the patient is in cardiogenic shock, revascularization with or without mechanical circulatory support may be required.

Myocardial rupture and aneurysmal dilation

Rupture of the free wall of the left ventricle is usually an early, catastrophic and fatal event. The patient will have a haemodynamic collapse, then an electromechanical cardiac arrest. A subacute rupture may allow for pericardiocentesis, followed by surgical repair of the rupture. Aneurysmal dilation of the infarcted myocardium (**Fig. 30.71**) is a late complication that may require surgical repair.

Ventricular septal defect

A ventricular septal defect VSD (**Fig. 30.72**) may occur in 1–2.0% of patients with STEMI and may be associated with delayed or failed fibrinolysis. However, mortality is very high and there is a 12-month non-operated mortality of 92%. An intra-aortic balloon pump and coronary angiography may allow patient optimization prior to surgery.

Mitral regurgitation

Severe mitral regurgitation can occur early in the course of STEMI. Three mechanisms may be responsible and a TOE may be necessary to confirm the aetiology:

- severe left ventricular dysfunction and dilation, causing annular dilation of the valve and subsequent regurgitation
- myocardial infarction of the inferior wall, producing dysfunction of the papillary muscle that may respond to coronary intervention
- myocardial infarction of the papillary muscles, producing sudden severe pulmonary oedema and cardiogenic shock (intra-aortic balloon pump, coronary angiography and early surgery may improve patient survival).

Cardiac arrhythmias

Ventricular tachycardia and ventricular fibrillation are common in STEMI, particularly with reperfusion. Cardiac arrest requires defibrillation. Ventricular tachycardia should be treated with intravenous beta-blockers (metoprolol 5 mg, esmolol 50–200 μg/kg per min), lidocaine 50–100 mg, or amiodarone 900–1200 mg/24 h. If the patient is hypotensive, synchronized cardioversion may be performed. Ensure that the serum potassium is over 4.5 mmol/L. Refractory ventricular tachycardia or fibrillation may respond to magnesium 8 mmol/L over 15 min i.v.

Atrial fibrillation occurs frequently, and treatment with beta-blockers and digoxin may be required. Cardioversion is possible but relapse is common.

Bradyarrhythmias can be treated initially with atropine 0.5 mg i.v. repeated up to six times in 4 h. Temporary transcutaneous or transvenous pacemaker insertion may be necessary in patients with symptomatic heart block.

Conduction disturbances

These are common following MI. AV block may occur during acute MI, especially of the inferior wall (the right coronary artery usually supplies the SA and AV nodes). When associated with haemodynamic compromise, heart block may need treatment with atropine or a temporary pacemaker. Such blocks may last for only a few minutes but frequently continue for several days. Permanent pacing may need to be considered if heart block persists for over 2 weeks.

Post-MI pericarditis and Dressler's syndrome

See page 1126.

Post-ACS lifestyle modification

After recovery from an ACS, patients should be encouraged to participate in a cardiac rehabilitation programme that provides education and information appropriate to their requirements. An exercise programme forms part of the rehabilitation.

- Dietary recommendations include calorie control of obesity, increased fruit and vegetables, reduced *trans* and saturated fats, and reduced salt intake in patients with hypertension.
- Alcohol consumption should be maintained within safe limits (≤14 units per week for both men and women), avoiding binge drinking.
- Patients should be physically active (30 min of moderate aerobic exercise 5 times per week).
- Patients should stop smoking (nicotine patches and buprenorphine are safe).
- A healthy weight (BMI <25 kg/m^2) should be maintained.

- Blood pressure should be reduced to a systolic measurement <140 mmHg.
- Patients with diabetes should be treated to maintain HbA_{1c} <7% (53 mmol/mol).

Post-ACS drug therapy and assessment

Extensive clinical trial evidence has been gathered in post-MI patients, demonstrating that a range of pharmaceuticals is advantageous in reducing mortality over the following years. Therefore, after MI, most patients should be taking most of the following medications:

- aspirin 75 mg daily
- ADP-receptor blocker
- oral beta-blocker to maintain heart rate <60 b.p.m.
- proton pump inhibitor for patients at high risk of bleeding while on dual antiplatelet therapy
- ACE inhibitor or angiotensin receptor blocker, particularly if LVEF is <40%
- high-intensity statin with target LDL cholesterol <1.8 mmol/L
- aldosterone antagonist, if there is clinical evidence of heart failure and LVEF is <40%; the serum creatinine is <221 μmol/L (men) or <177 μmol/L (women); and the serum potassium is <5.0 mEq/L.

Patients with permanent atrial fibrillation receiving medical therapy or CABG should be treated with dual therapy: aspirin or clopidogrel with anticoagulation warfarin or a DOAC.

Patients with permanent atrial fibrillation receiving stenting should be assessed for their bleeding risk using the HAS-BLED score (see **Box 30.16**):

- If this is 0–2, they can receive triple therapy for 6 months (aspirin and clopidogrel and warfarin) and then dual therapy (aspirin or clopidogrel with anticoagulation warfarin or a DOAC).
- If it is over 2, they can receive triple therapy for 4 weeks (aspirin and clopidogrel and warfarin) and then dual therapy (aspirin or clopidogrel with anticoagulation warfarin or a DOAC) for a further 11 months.

Further reading

Berry JD, Dyer A, Cal X et al. Lifetime risks of cardiovascular disease. *N Engl J Med* 2012; 366:321–329.
Ibanez B, James S, Agewall S et al. 2017 ESC Guidelines for the management of acute myocardial infarction in patients presenting with ST-segment elevation. The Task Force for the management of acute myocardial infarction in patients presenting with ST-segment elevation of the European Society of Cardiology (ESC). *Eur Heart J* 2018; 39:119–177.
Montalescot G, Sechtem U, Achenbach S et al. 2013 ESC guidelines on the management of stable coronary artery disease. *Eur Heart J* 2013; 34:2949–3003.
Roffi M, Patrono C, Collet JP et al. 2015 ESC Guidelines for the management of acute coronary syndromes in patients presenting without persistent ST-segment elevation: Task Force for the Management of Acute Coronary Syndromes in Patients Presenting without Persistent ST-Segment Elevation of the European Society of Cardiology (ESC). *Eur Heart J* 2016; 37:267–315.
Shah AS, Anand A, Sandoval Y et al. High-sensitivity cardiac troponin I at presentation in patients with suspected acute coronary syndrome: a cohort study. *Lancet* 2015; 386:2481–2488.
Thygesen K, Alpert JS, Jaffe AS et al. Fourth universal definition of myocardial infarction (2018). *Eur Heart J* 2019; 40:237–269.
https://qrisk.org/three/. QRISK®3-2018 Cardiovascular disease risk assessment tool.

VALVULAR HEART DISEASE

MITRAL VALVE

The mitral valve consists of the fibrous annulus, anterior and posterior leaflets, chordae tendineae and the papillary muscles (**Fig. 30.73**).

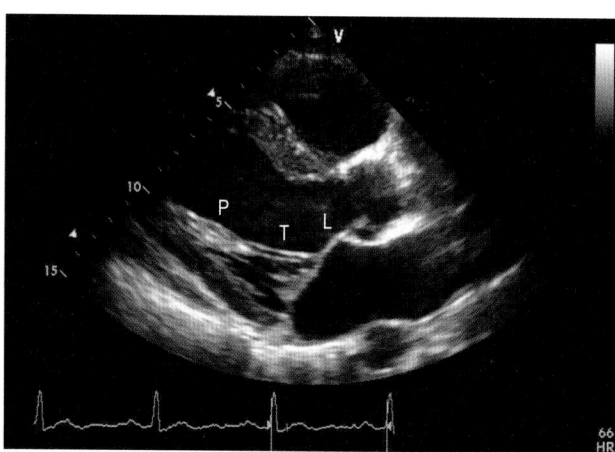

Fig. 30.73 Mitral valve apparatus – parasternal long axis.
L, leaflets; P, papillary muscle; T, chordae tendineae.

Mitral stenosis

Mitral stenosis is commonly due to rheumatic heart disease following previous rheumatic fever due to infection with a group A β-haemolytic streptococcus; in low- to medium-income countries this affects nearly 20 million people. The condition is more common in women than men. Inflammation leads to commissural fusion and a reduction in mitral valve orifice area, causing the characteristic doming pattern seen on echocardiography. Over many years the condition progresses to valve thickening, cusp fusion, calcium deposition, a severely narrowed (stenotic) valve orifice and progressive immobility of the valve cusps.

Other causes of mitral stenosis include:

- congenital mitral stenosis
- Lutembacher's syndrome (the combination of acquired mitral stenosis and an atrial septal defect)
- mitral annular calcification, rarely; this may lead to mitral stenosis if extensive, particularly in elderly patients and those with end-stage renal disease
- carcinoid tumours metastasizing to the lung, or primary bronchial carcinoid.

Pathophysiology

When the normal valve orifice area of 4–6 cm^2 is reduced to less than 1 cm^2, severe mitral stenosis is present. In order for sufficient cardiac output to be maintained, the left atrial pressure increases and left atrial hypertrophy and dilation occur. Consequently, pulmonary venous, pulmonary arterial and right heart pressures also increase. The increase in pulmonary capillary pressure is followed by the development of pulmonary oedema, particularly when the rhythm deteriorates to atrial fibrillation with tachycardia and loss of coordinated atrial contraction. This is partially prevented by alveolar and capillary thickening and pulmonary arterial vasoconstriction (reactive pulmonary hypertension). Pulmonary hypertension leads to right ventricular hypertrophy, dilation and failure, with subsequent tricuspid regurgitation.

Clinical features

Symptoms

Usually, there are no symptoms until the valve orifice is moderately stenosed (area <2 cm^2). In Europe, this does not usually occur until several decades after the first attack of rheumatic fever, but in low- to medium-income countries severe stenosis may occur at 10–20 years of age.

Progressively **severe dyspnoea** develops from the elevation in left atrial pressure, vascular congestion and interstitial pulmonary oedema. A cough productive of blood-tinged, frothy sputum or frank haemoptysis may occur. The development of pulmonary hypertension eventually leads to **right heart failure** and its symptoms of weakness, fatigue and abdominal or lower limb swelling.

The large left atrium predisposes to **atrial fibrillation**, giving rise to symptoms such as palpitations. Atrial fibrillation may result in **systemic emboli**, most commonly to the cerebral vessels, producing neurological sequelae, but mesenteric, renal and peripheral emboli are also seen.

Signs

See the 'Clinical memo' in **Fig. 30.74**.

Face

Severe mitral stenosis with pulmonary hypertension is associated with the so-called mitral facies or malar flush. This is a bilateral, cyanotic or dusky pink discoloration over the upper cheeks, which is due to arteriovenous anastomoses and vascular stasis.

Pulse

A small-volume pulse is typical in mitral stenosis. This may be regular early on in the disease process (patient in sinus rhythm), but as the disease progresses, an 'irregularly irregular' pulse (atrial fibrillation) may occur and may cause symptomatic clinical deterioration.

Jugular veins

Right heart failure may develop, leading to jugular venous distension. When pulmonary hypertension or tricuspid stenosis is present, the 'a'-wave will be prominent, provided that atrial fibrillation has not supervened.

Palpation

There is a tapping impulse felt parasternally on the left side. This is the result of a palpable first heart sound combined with left ventricular backward displacement produced by an enlarging right ventricle. A sustained parasternal impulse due to right ventricular hypertrophy may also be felt.

Auscultation

Auscultation (see **Fig. 30.74**) reveals a loud first heart sound if the mitral valve is pliable but this will not occur in calcific mitral stenosis. As the valve suddenly opens with the force of the increased left atrial pressure, an 'opening snap' will be heard. This is followed by a low-pitched, 'rumbling', mid-diastolic murmur, best heard with the bell of the stethoscope held lightly at the apex and the patient lying on the left side in expiration. If the patient is in sinus rhythm, the murmur becomes louder at the end of diastole as a result of atrial contraction (pre-systolic accentuation). Pulmonary hypertension may result in pulmonary valvular regurgitation, which causes an early diastolic murmur in the pulmonary area, known as a Graham Steell murmur.

Investigations

Chest X-ray

The chest X-ray may show left atrial enlargement with straightening of the left heart border and a 'double shadow' on the border of the right and left atria (see **Fig. 30.14**). Late in the course of the disease a calcified mitral valve may be seen on a penetrated or lateral view. Pulmonary vascular congestion and enlargement of the main pulmonary arteries may also be apparent in severe disease.

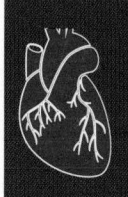

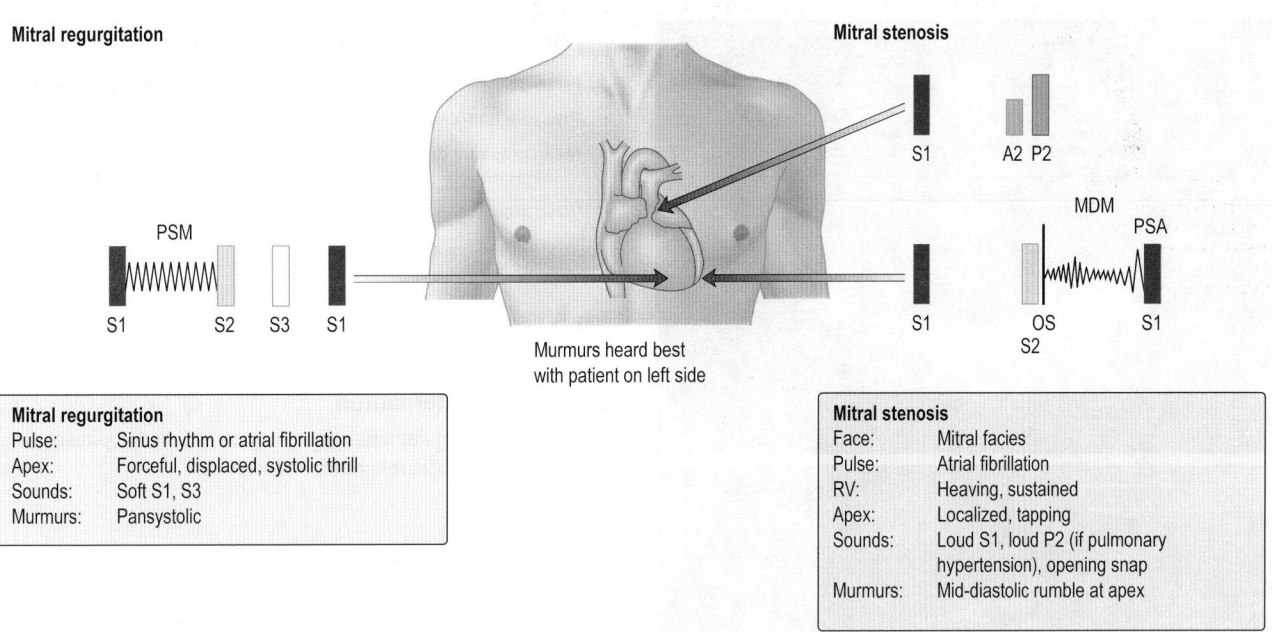

Mitral regurgitation

Mitral stenosis

Murmurs heard best
with patient on left side

Mitral regurgitation	
Pulse:	Sinus rhythm or atrial fibrillation
Apex:	Forceful, displaced, systolic thrill
Sounds:	Soft S1, S3
Murmurs:	Pansystolic

Mitral stenosis	
Face:	Mitral facies
Pulse:	Atrial fibrillation
RV:	Heaving, sustained
Apex:	Localized, tapping
Sounds:	Loud S1, loud P2 (if pulmonary hypertension), opening snap
Murmurs:	Mid-diastolic rumble at apex

Fig. 30.74 Features associated with mitral regurgitation and mitral stenosis. A2, aortic component of the second heart sound; MDM, mid-diastolic murmur; OS, opening snap; P2, pulmonary component of the second heart sound (loud with pulmonary hypertension); PSA, pre-systolic accentuation; PSM, pansystolic murmur; RV, right ventricle; S1, first heart sound; S2, second heart sound; S3, third heart sound.

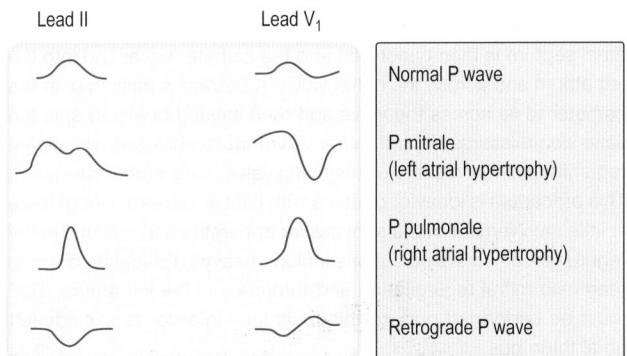

Fig. 30.75 A bifid P wave, as seen on the ECG in mitral stenosis (P mitrale). Other P wave abnormalities are also shown for comparison.

ECG

In sinus rhythm the ECG may show a bifid P wave owing to delayed left atrial activation (**Fig. 30.75**). However, atrial fibrillation is frequently present. As the disease progresses the ECG features of right ventricular hypertrophy (right axis deviation and, perhaps, tall R waves in lead V_1) may develop (**Fig. 30.76**).

Echocardiogram

TTE is able to determine left atrial size and the degree of thickening, calcification and mobility of the mitral leaflets, as well as the degree of commissural fusion (**Fig. 30.77**). The severity of the mitral stenosis (**Box 30.42**) can be defined by mitral valve area on two-dimensional echocardiography, with continuous wave (CW) Doppler to measure the pressure half-time (the time taken for the pressure to halve from the peak value) and mean pressure drop across the valve. CW Doppler may also be used to estimate pulmonary artery pressure through measurement of the degree of tricuspid regurgitation.

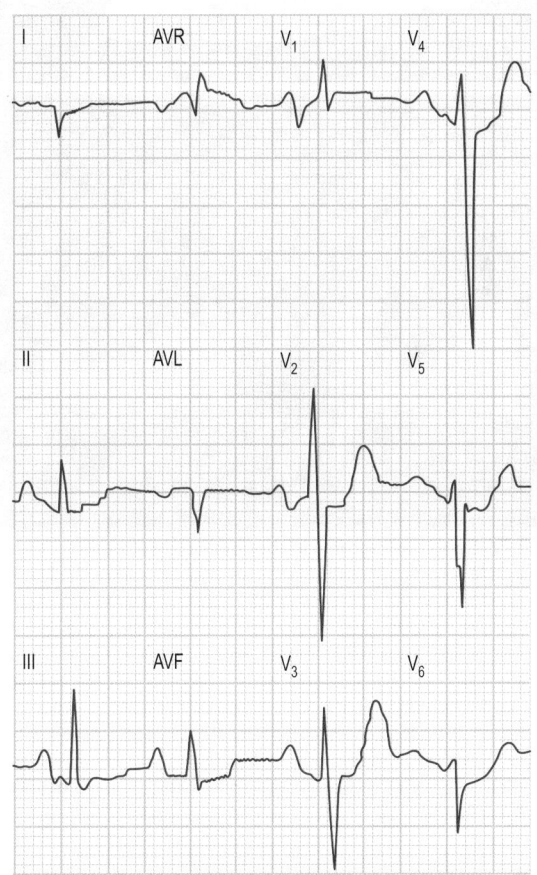

Fig. 30.76 Severe mitral stenosis, shown by a 12-lead ECG. Note the right axis deviation (frontal plane axis = +120°), the left atrial conduction abnormality (large terminal negative component of the P wave in V_1) and the right ventricular hypertrophy (R wave in V_1 and right axis deviation).

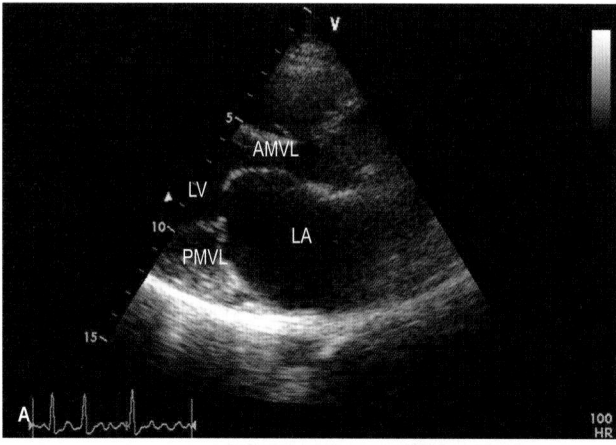

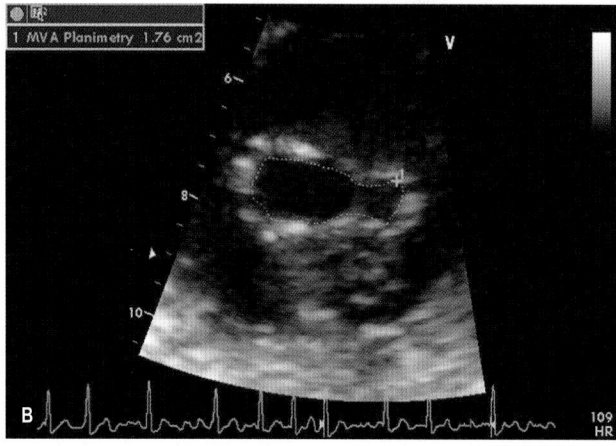

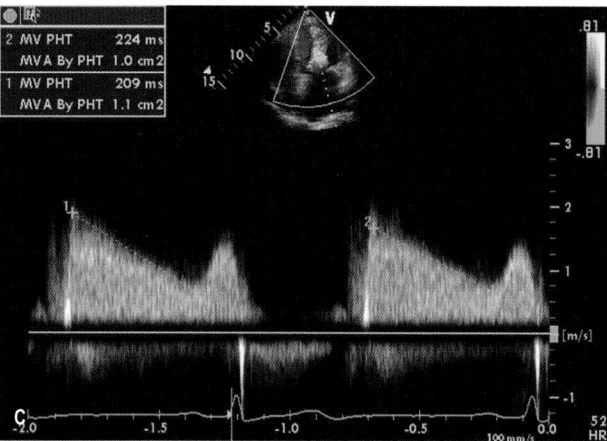

Fig. 30.77 Echocardiograms in rheumatic mitral valve disease. (A) A two-dimensional long-axis view, showing an enlarged left atrium and the 'hooked' appearance of the mitral valve leaflets, resulting from commissural fusion. **(B)** A magnified short-axis view, showing the mitral valve orifice as seen from the left atrium. The orifice area can be planimetered to assess the severity; in this case, it is 1.5 cm², indicating moderately severe disease. **(C)** A continuous-wave (CW) Doppler recording, showing the slow rate of decay of flow velocity from the left atrium to the left ventricle during diastole. It is also possible to derive the valve orifice area from the velocity decay rate. AMVL, anterior mitral valve leaflet; LA, left atrium; LV, left ventricle; PMVL, posterior mitral valve leaflet.

TOE is performed to detect the presence of left atrial thrombus (see p. 1040) or to carry out a detailed assessment prior to consideration of surgical or percutaneous intervention. The Wilkins score is an echocardiographic assessment of the mitral valve (leaflet mobility, valve thickening, valve calcification and subvalvular apparatus)

Parameter	Normal	Mild	Moderate	Severe
Pressure half-time (ms)	40–70	71–139	140–219	>219
Mean pressure drop (mmHg)		<5.0	5–10	>10
Valve area (cm²)	4.0–6.0	1.5–2.0	1.0–1.5	<1.0

(Source: British Society of Echocardiography.)

and is also used to determine suitability for percutaneous mitral valvuloplasty.

Cardiac catheterization

Left and right heart catheterization may be required in patients with severe mitral stenosis referred for intervention.

Management

Early symptoms of mitral stenosis, such as mild dyspnoea, can usually be treated with low doses of diuretics. The onset of atrial fibrillation requires treatment with beta-blockers or DC cardioversion and anticoagulation to prevent atrial thrombus and systemic embolization. Patients with severe mitral stenosis who develop persistent symptoms or pulmonary hypertension are appropriate for intervention. There are four operative measures.

Trans-septal balloon valvotomy

A catheter is introduced into the right atrium via the femoral vein under local anaesthesia in the cardiac catheter laboratory. The interatrial septum is then punctured and the catheter advanced into the left atrium and across the mitral valve. A balloon is passed over the catheter to lie across the valve and then inflated briefly to split the valve commissures. As with other valvotomy techniques, significant regurgitation may result, necessitating valve replacement (see later). This procedure is ideal for patients with pliable valves in whom there is little involvement of the subvalvular apparatus and minimal mitral regurgitation. Contraindications include heavy calcification or more than mild mitral regurgitation and thrombus in the left atrium. TOE must be performed prior to this technique in order to exclude left atrial thrombus.

Closed valvotomy

This operation is advised for patients with mobile, non-calcified and non-regurgitant mitral valves. The fused cusps are forced apart by a dilator introduced through the apex of the left ventricle and guided into position by the surgeon's finger inserted via the left atrial appendage. Cardiopulmonary bypass is not needed for this operation. Closed valvotomy may produce a good result for 10 years or more. The valve cusps often re-fuse and another operation may eventually be necessary.

Open valvotomy

This operation is often preferred to closed valvotomy. The cusps are carefully dissected apart under direct vision. Cardiopulmonary bypass is required. Open dissection reduces the likelihood of causing traumatic mitral regurgitation.

Mitral valve replacement

Replacement of the mitral valve is necessary if:
- mitral regurgitation is also present
- there is a badly diseased or calcified stenotic valve that cannot be re-opened without producing significant regurgitation

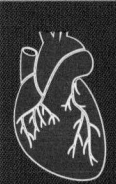

- there is severe mitral stenosis and thrombus in the left atrium despite anticoagulation.

  Artificial valves (see p. 1102) may work successfully for more than 20 years. Anticoagulants are generally necessary to prevent the formation of thrombus, which might obstruct the valve or embolize.

Mitral regurgitation

Mitral regurgitation can occur due to abnormalities of the valve leaflets, the annulus, the chordae tendineae or papillary muscles, or the left ventricle. The most frequent causes of mitral regurgitation are degenerative (myxomatous) disease, ischaemic heart disease, rheumatic heart disease and infectious endocarditis. Mitral regurgitation is also seen in diseases of the myocardium (dilated and hypertrophic cardiomyopathy), rheumatic autoimmune diseases (e.g. systemic lupus erythematosus), collagen diseases (e.g. Marfan's and Ehlers–Danlos syndromes) and disorders caused by drugs, including centrally acting appetite suppressants (fenfluramine) and dopamine agonists (cabergoline).

Pathophysiology

Regurgitation into the left atrium produces left atrial dilation but little increase in left atrial pressure if the regurgitation is long-standing, as the regurgitant flow is accommodated by the large left atrium. With acute mitral regurgitation the normal compliance of the left atrium does not allow much dilation and the left atrial pressure rises. Thus, in acute mitral regurgitation the left atrial *v*-wave is greatly increased and pulmonary venous pressure rises, leading to pulmonary oedema. Since a proportion of the stroke volume is regurgitated, the stroke volume increases to maintain the forward cardiac output and the left ventricle therefore enlarges.

The Carpentier classification (**Fig. 30.78**) uses mitral leaflet motion to divide patients into different classes according to the mechanism of regurgitation, which can be useful when considering surgical intervention.

Clinical features

Symptoms

Mitral regurgitation can be present for many years and the cardiac dimensions greatly increased before any symptoms occur.

- *Dyspnoea* and *orthopnoea* develop because of pulmonary venous hypertension that arises as a direct result of the mitral regurgitation and secondarily as a consequence of left ventricular failure.
- *Fatigue* and *lethargy* develop because of the reduced cardiac output.

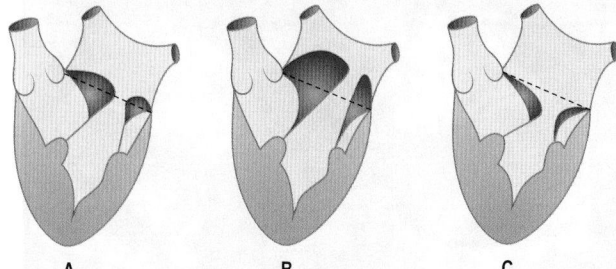

Fig. 30.78 Carpentier classification of mitral regurgitation and its causes. (A) Normal leaflet motion. **(B)** Increased leaflet motion/prolapse. **(C)** Restricted leaflet motion. (*Reproduced from Tuladhar SM, Punjabi PP. Surgical reconstruction of the mitral valve.* Heart *2006; 92:1373–1377, with permission.*)

- In the late stages of the disease the symptoms of *right heart failure* also occur and eventually lead to congestive cardiac failure.
- *Cardiac cachexia* may develop.
- Thromboembolism is less common than in mitral stenosis but *subacute infective endocarditis* is much more common.

Signs

See **Fig. 30.74**.

The physical signs of uncomplicated mitral regurgitation are:

- *Laterally displaced (forceful) diffuse apex beat* and a *systolic thrill* (if severe).
- *Soft first heart sound*, owing to the incomplete apposition of the valve cusps and their partial closure by the time ventricular systole begins.
- *Pansystolic murmur*, due to the occurrence of regurgitation throughout the whole of systole, being loudest at the apex but radiating widely over the precordium and into the axilla.
- *Mid-systolic click*, which may be present with a floppy mitral valve (see later); it is produced by the sudden prolapse of the valve and the tensing of the chordae tendineae that occurs during systole. This may be followed by a late systolic murmur owing to some regurgitation.
- *Prominent third heart sound* (S3), owing to the sudden rush of blood back into the dilated left ventricle in early diastole (sometimes a short mid-diastolic flow murmur may follow the third heart sound).

The signs related to atrial fibrillation, pulmonary hypertension and left and right heart failure develop later in the disease. The onset of atrial fibrillation has a much less dramatic effect on symptoms than in mitral stenosis.

Investigations

Chest X-ray

The chest X-ray may show left atrial and left ventricular enlargement. There is an increase in the cardiothoracic ratio and valve calcification may be present.

ECG

The ECG shows the features of left atrial delay (bifid P waves) and left ventricular hypertrophy (**Fig. 30.79**), as manifested by tall R waves in the left lateral leads (e.g. leads I and V_6) and deep S waves in the right-sided precordial leads (e.g. leads V_1 and V_2). (Note that S in V_1 plus R in V_5 or R in V_6 >35mm indicates left ventricular hypertrophy.) Left ventricular hypertrophy occurs in about 50% of patients with mitral regurgitation. Atrial fibrillation may be present.

Echocardiogram

The echocardiogram (**Fig. 30.80**) shows a dilated left atrium and left ventricle. There may be specific features of chordal or papillary muscle rupture. The severity of regurgitation can be assessed with the use of colour Doppler, looking at the narrowest jet width (vena contracta) and area, and calculating the regurgitant fraction, volume or orifice area. Useful information regarding the severity of the condition can be obtained indirectly by observing the dynamics of ventricular function. *TOE* can be helpful to identify structural valve abnormalities before surgery (see **Fig. 30.80**) and intraoperative TOE can aid assessment of the efficacy of valve repair.

Cardiac catheterization

Left and right heart catheterization is appropriate for patients referred for surgical repair or replacement.

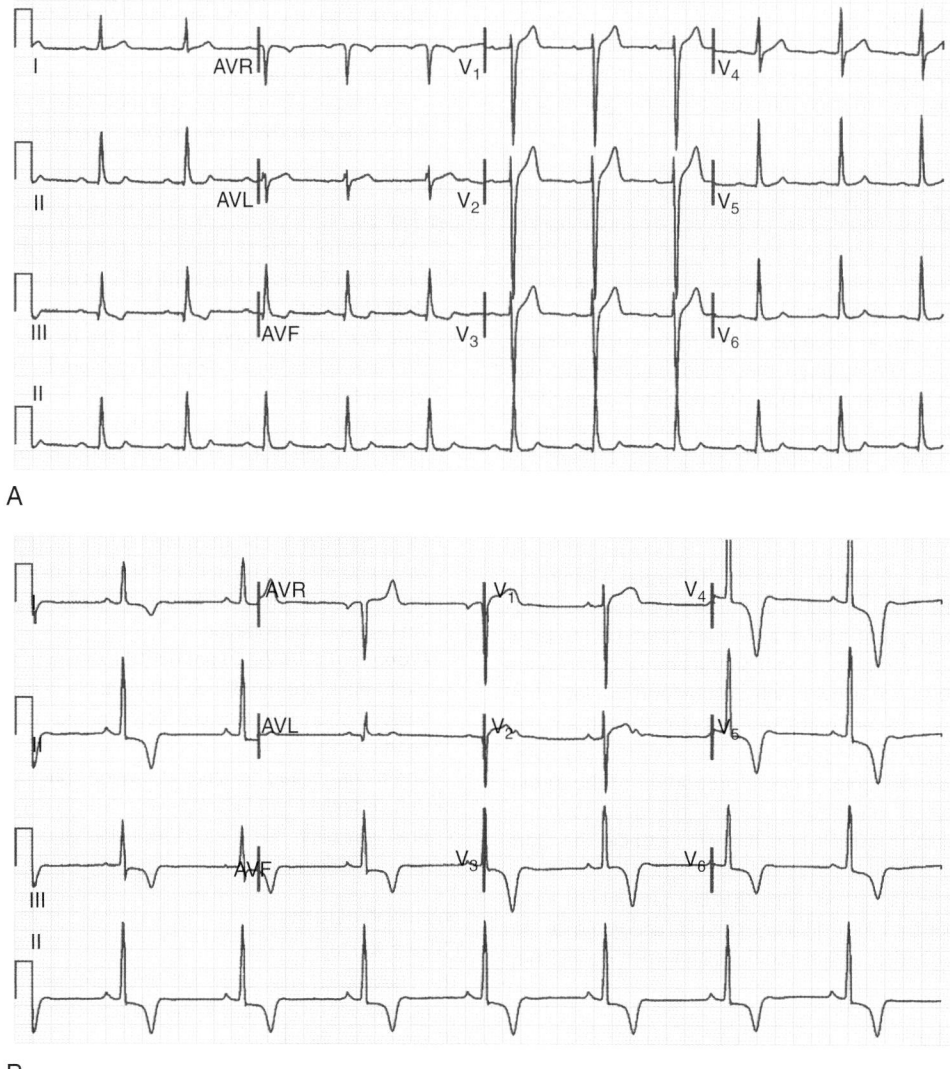

A

B

Fig. 30.79 Left ventricular hypertrophy, shown in 12-lead ECGs. (A) Note the size of the S wave seen in V_1 (26 mm); S in V_1 + R in V_6 = >35 mm. **(B)** Left ventricular hypertrophy in a patient with hypertrophic cardiomyopathy, with additional repolarization changes of deep T-wave inversion in leads V_3–V_6 and leads I, II, III and AVF.

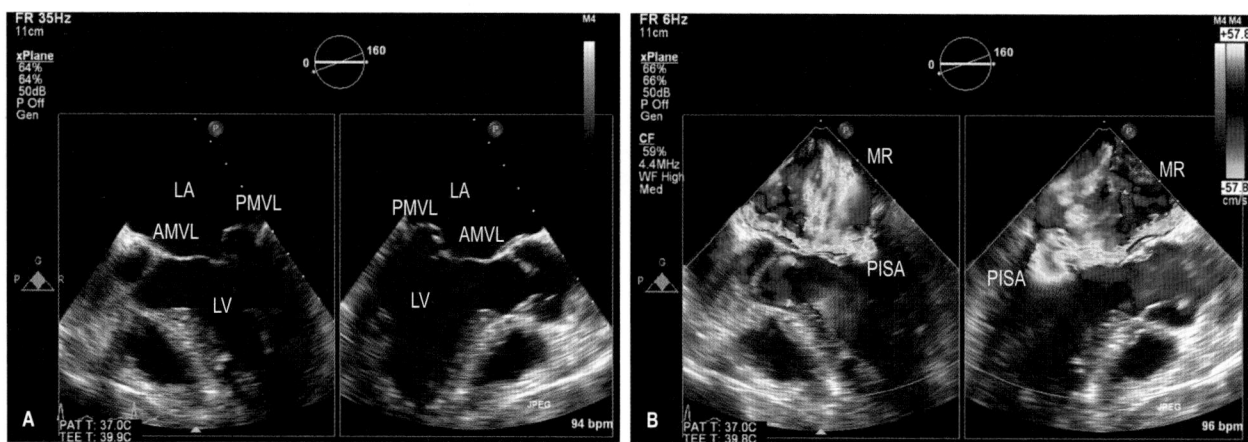

Fig. 30.80 Mitral regurgitation. (A) Transoesophageal echocardiography with marked prolapse of part of the posterior mitral valve leaflet (PMVL). **(B)** Image A with colour Doppler demonstrating severe mitral regurgitation (MR) into the left atrium (LA). AMVL, aortic mitral valve leaflet; LV, left ventricle; PISA, proximal isovelocity surface area.

Management

Mild to moderate mitral regurgitation can be managed conservatively by following the patient with serial echocardiograms. Prophylaxis against endocarditis is discussed on page 1106.

Current ESC guidelines recommend surgical intervention in patients with symptomatic severe mitral regurgitation, LVEF of more than 30% and end-diastolic dimension of less than 55 mm, and in asymptomatic patients with left ventricular dysfunction (end-systolic dimension >45 mm and/or ejection fraction of <60%). Surgery should also be considered in patients with asymptomatic severe mitral regurgitation with preserved left ventricular function and atrial fibrillation and/or pulmonary hypertension. The advantages of surgical intervention are diminished in more advanced disease. (*Sudden torrential mitral regurgitation, as seen with chordal or papillary muscle rupture or infective endocarditis, necessitates emergency mitral valve replacement.*) When patients are not suited to surgical intervention or when surgery will be performed at a later date, management involves treatment with diuretics, ACE inhibitors and possibly anticoagulants. A percutaneous mitral valve repair (MitraClip) may be appropriate in selected patients unsuitable for cardiac surgery.

Prolapsing (billowing) mitral valve

This is also known as Barlow's syndrome or floppy mitral valve. It is due to excessively large mitral valve leaflets, an enlarged mitral annulus, abnormally long chordae or disordered papillary muscle contraction. Histology may demonstrate myxomatous degeneration of the mitral valve leaflets. Prolapsing mitral valve is more commonly seen in young women than in men or older women, and has a familial incidence. Its cause is unknown but it is associated with connective tissue disorders (Marfan's syndrome, Ehlers–Danlos syndrome and pseudoxanthoma elasticum).

AORTIC VALVE

Aortic stenosis

Aortic stenosis is a chronic progressive disease that limits left ventricular outflow, leading to symptoms of chest pain, breathlessness, syncope and pre-syncope, and fatigue.

Aortic valve stenosis includes calcific stenosis of a trileaflet aortic valve, stenosis of a congenitally bicuspid valve and rheumatic aortic stenosis.

Calcific aortic valvular disease (CAVD) is the most common cause of aortic stenosis and occurs mainly in the elderly. This is an inflammatory process involving macrophages and T lymphocytes, initially with thickening of the subendothelium and adjacent fibrosis. The lesions contain lipoproteins, which calcify, increasing leaflet stiffness and reducing systolic opening. This can occur in a tri- or bileaflet aortic valve. Risk factors for CAVD include old age, male sex, elevated lipoprotein(a) and LDL cholesterol, hypertension, diabetes and smoking.

Bicuspid aortic valve (BAV) (**Fig. 30.81**) is the most common form of congenital heart disease, occurring in 1–2% of live births; in about 9% of cases it is familial. Patients with familial bicuspid valve tend to present at an earlier age. BAV is associated with aortic coarctation, root dilation and, potentially, aortic dissection, and patients should have regular follow-up echocardiography.

Rheumatic fever can produce progressive fusion, thickening and calcification of the aortic valve. In rheumatic heart disease, the

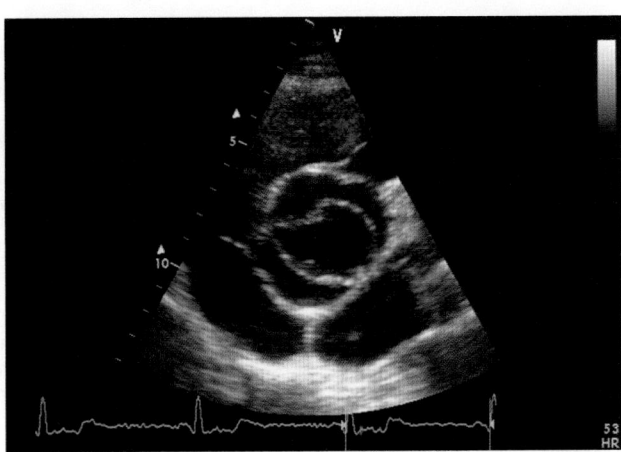

Fig. 30.81 **Bicuspid aortic valve.**

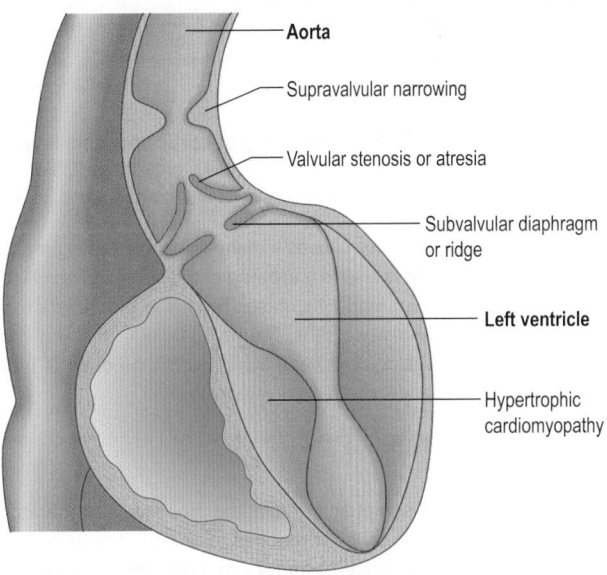

Aorta

Supravalvular narrowing

Valvular stenosis or atresia

Subvalvular diaphragm or ridge

Left ventricle

Hypertrophic cardiomyopathy

Fig. 30.82 **Several forms of left ventricular outflow tract obstruction.**

aortic valve is affected in about 30–40% of cases and there is usually associated mitral valve disease.

Other causes of valvular stenosis include chronic kidney disease, Paget's disease of bone, previous radiation exposure and systemic lupus erythematosus. *Valvular aortic stenosis* should be distinguished from other causes of obstruction to left ventricular emptying (**Fig. 30.82**), which include:

- supravalvular obstruction – a congenital fibrous diaphragm above the aortic valve, often associated with learning difficulties and hypercalcaemia (Williams' syndrome)
- subvalvular aortic stenosis – a congenital condition in which a fibrous ridge or diaphragm is situated immediately below the aortic valve
- hypertrophic cardiomyopathy – septal muscle hypertrophy obstructing left ventricular outflow.

Pathophysiology

Obstructed left ventricular emptying leads to increased left ventricular pressure and compensatory left ventricular hypertrophy. In turn, this results in relative ischaemia of the left ventricular myocardium and consequent angina, arrhythmias and left ventricular failure. The obstruction to left ventricular emptying is relatively more severe on

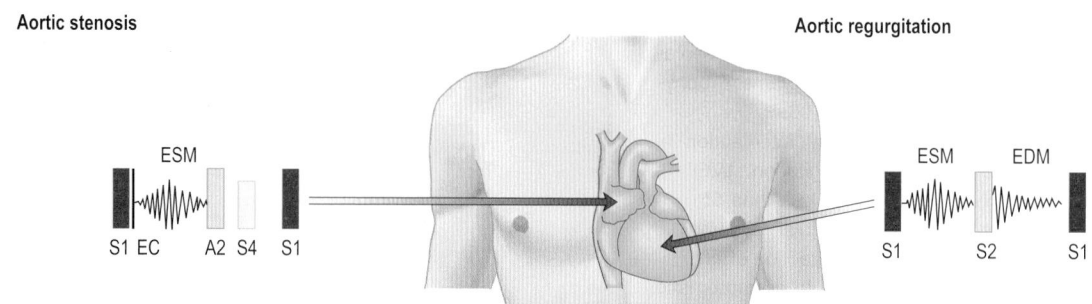

Fig. 30.83 Features of aortic stenosis and aortic regurgitation. EC, ejection click; EDM, early diastolic murmur; LSE, left sternal edge; ESM, ejection systolic murmur; A2, aortic component of the second heart sound; S1, first heart sound; S4, fourth heart sound.

exercise. Normally, exercise causes a many-fold increase in cardiac output, but when there is severe narrowing of the aortic valve orifice, the cardiac output can hardly increase. Thus, the blood pressure falls, coronary ischaemia worsens, the myocardium fails and cardiac arrhythmias develop. Left ventricular systolic function is typically preserved in patients with aortic stenosis.

Clinical features

Symptoms

There are usually no symptoms until aortic stenosis is moderately severe (when the aortic orifice is reduced to one-third of its normal size). At this stage, *exercise-induced syncope, angina* and *dyspnoea* develop. When symptoms occur, the prognosis is poor: on average, death occurs within 2–3 years if there has been no surgical intervention.

Signs

See **Fig. 30.83**.

Pulse

The carotid pulse is small-volume and slow-rising or plateau in nature (see p. 1030).

Precordial palpation

The apex beat is not usually displaced because hypertrophy (as opposed to dilation) does not produce noticeable cardiomegaly. However, the pulsation is sustained and obvious. A double impulse is sometimes felt because the fourth heart sound or atrial contraction ('kick') may be palpable. A systolic thrill may be felt in the aortic area.

Auscultation

The most obvious auscultatory finding in aortic stenosis is an ejection systolic murmur that is usually 'diamond-shaped' (crescendo–decrescendo). The murmur is usually longer when the disease is more severe, as a longer ejection time is needed. The murmur is usually rough in quality and best heard in the aortic area. It radiates into the carotid arteries and also the precordium. The intensity of the murmur is not a good guide to the severity of the condition because

it is lessened by a reduced cardiac output. In severe cases the murmur may be inaudible.

Other findings include:

- *systolic ejection click*, unless the valve has become immobile and calcified
- *soft or inaudible aortic second heart sound* when the aortic valve becomes immobile
- *reversed splitting of the second heart sound* (splitting on expiration) (see p. 1032)
- *prominent fourth heart sound*, caused by atrial contraction and heard unless coexisting mitral stenosis prevents this.

Investigations

Chest X-ray

The chest X-ray usually reveals a relatively small heart with a prominent, dilated, ascending aorta. This occurs because turbulent blood flow above the stenosed aortic valve produces so-called 'post-stenotic dilation'. The aortic valve may be calcified. The cardiothoracic ratio increases when heart failure occurs.

ECG

The ECG shows left ventricular hypertrophy and left atrial delay. A left ventricular 'strain' pattern due to 'pressure overload' (depressed ST segments and T-wave inversion in leads orientated towards the left ventricle, i.e. leads I, AVL, V_5 and V_6) is common when disease is severe. Usually, sinus rhythm is present but ventricular arrhythmias may be recorded.

Echocardiogram

Echocardiography readily demonstrates the thickened, calcified and immobile aortic valve cusps, and the presence of left ventricular hypertrophy; it can be used to determine the severity of aortic stenosis (**Box 30.43** and **Fig. 30.84**). TOE is rarely indicated.

Cardiac catheterization

Cardiac catheterization is rarely necessary since all of this information can be gained non-invasively with echocardiography and CMR. Coronary angiography is required before surgery is recommended.

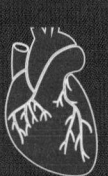

CMR and cardiac CT

These techniques are indicated for assessing the thoracic aorta for the presence of aneurysm, dissection or coarctation but are rarely needed.

Management

In patients with aortic stenosis, symptoms are a good index of severity and all symptomatic, appropriate patients should have *aortic valve replacement*. Patients with a BAV and ascending aorta of over 50 mm or expanding at more than 5 mm per year should be considered for surgical intervention. Asymptomatic patients should be under regular review for assessment of symptoms and echocardiography. Surgical intervention for asymptomatic people with severe aortic stenosis is recommended in those with:

- symptoms or hypotension during an exercise test
- an LVEF of less than 50%
- moderate to severe stenosis undergoing CABG, surgery of the ascending aorta or other cardiac valve.
  - peak velocity through the aortic valve >5.5 m/s
  - Systolic pulmonary artery pressure >60 mmHg
  - Rapid increase in velocity through the valve at >0.3 m/s/year

Antibiotic prophylaxis against infective endocarditis is discussed on page 1106. Provided that the valve is not severely deformed or heavily calcified, critical aortic stenosis in childhood or adolescence can be treated by valvotomy (performed under direct vision by the surgeon or by balloon dilation using X-ray visualization). This produces temporary relief from the obstruction. Aortic valve replacement will usually be needed a few years later. Balloon dilation (valvuloplasty) has been tried in adults, especially in the elderly, as an alternative to surgery. Generally, results are poor and such treatment is reserved for patients unfit for surgery or as a 'bridge' to surgery (as systolic function will often improve).

Percutaneous valve replacement

A novel treatment for patients unsuitable for surgical aortic valve replacement is transcatheter aortic valve implantation (TAVI), with a balloon expandable stent valve. Valve implantation has been shown to be successful (86%) with a procedural mortality of 2% and 30-day mortality of 12%. Good results have been reported in follow-up studies, and this technique may replace the need for surgery.

Aortic regurgitation

Aortic regurgitation can occur in diseases affecting the aortic valve, such as endocarditis, and diseases affecting the aortic root, such as Marfan's syndrome (**Box 30.44**).

Pathophysiology

Aortic regurgitation is reflux of blood from the aorta through the aortic valve into the left ventricle during diastole. If net cardiac output is to be maintained, the total volume of blood pumped into the aorta must increase and, consequently, left ventricular size must enlarge. Because of the aortic runoff during diastole, diastolic blood pressure falls and coronary perfusion is decreased. In addition, the larger left ventricular size is mechanically less efficient, so that the demand for oxygen is greater and cardiac ischaemia develops.

Clinical features
Symptoms

In aortic regurgitation, significant symptoms occur late and do not develop until *left ventricular failure* develops. *Angina pectoris* may arise. Varying grades of *dyspnoea* occur, depending on the extent of left ventricular dilation and dysfunction. *Arrhythmias* are relatively uncommon.

Signs

See **Fig. 30.83**. The signs of aortic regurgitation are many and are due to the hyperdynamic circulation, reflux of blood into the left ventricle and increased left ventricular size.

The pulse is bounding or collapsing (see p. 1030). The following signs, which are rare, also indicate a hyperdynamic circulation:

- *Quincke's sign* – capillary pulsation in the nail beds

> **ⓘ Box 30.43 Echocardiographic severity of aortic stenosis**

Parameter	Normal	Mild	Moderate	Severe
Peak velocity (m/s)	<1.7	1.7–2.9	3.0–4.0	>4.0
Peak pressure drop (mmHg)		<36	36–64	>64
Mean pressure drop (mmHg)		<25	25–40	>40
Valve area (cm²)	>2.0	1.5–2.0	1.0–1.4	<1.0

(Source: British Society of Echocardiography.)

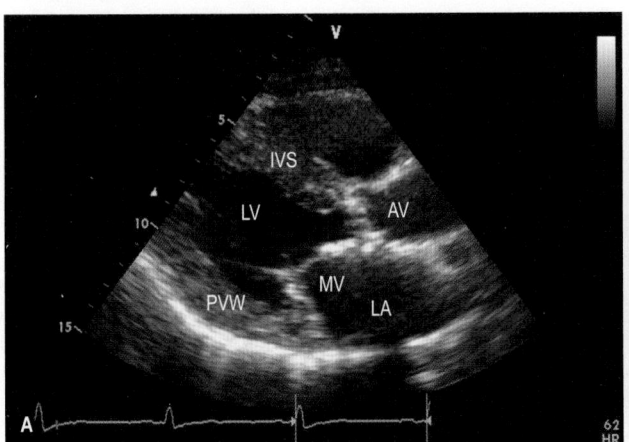
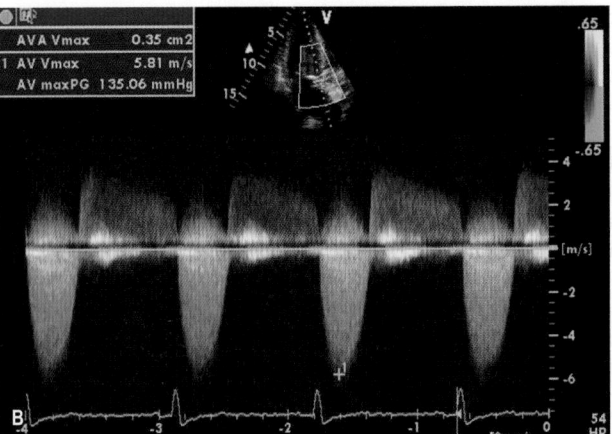

Fig. 30.84 Cardiac echograms. (A) Two-dimensional echocardiogram (long-axis view) in a patient with calcific aortic stenosis. The calcium in the valve generates abnormally intense echoes. There is some evidence of associated left ventricular hypertrophy. **(B)** Continuous-wave (CW) Doppler signals obtained from the right upper parasternal edge, where the high-velocity jet from the stenotic valve is coming towards the transducer. AV, aortic valve; IVS, interventricular septum; LA, left atrium; LV, left ventricle; MV, mitral valve; PVW, posterior ventricular wall.

Box 30.44 Causes and associations of aortic regurgitation

? Box 30.44 Causes and associations of aortic regurgitation

Acute aortic regurgitation
- Acute rheumatic fever
- Infective endocarditis
- Dissection of the aorta
- Ruptured sinus of Valsalva aneurysm
- Failure of prosthetic valve

Chronic aortic regurgitation
- Rheumatic heart disease
- Syphilis

- Arthritides:
  - Reactive arthritis
  - Ankylosing spondylitis
  - Rheumatoid arthritis
- Hypertension (severe)
- Bicuspid aortic valve
- Aortic endocarditis
- Marfan's syndrome
- Osteogenesis imperfecta

- ***de Musset's sign*** – head nodding with each heart beat
- ***Duroziez's sign*** – a to-and-fro murmur heard when the femoral artery is auscultated with pressure applied distally (if found, it is a sign of severe aortic regurgitation)
- ***pistol shot femorals*** – a sharp bang heard on auscultation over the femoral arteries in time with each heart beat.

The apex beat is displaced laterally and downwards and is forceful in quality. On auscultation, there is a high-pitched early diastolic murmur best heard at the left sternal edge in the fourth intercostal space with the patient leaning forwards and the breath held in expiration. Because of the volume overload there is commonly an ejection systolic flow murmur. The regurgitant jet can impinge on the anterior mitral valve cusp, causing a mid-diastolic murmur (Austin Flint rumble).

Investigations

Chest X-ray

The chest X-ray features are those of left ventricular enlargement and, possibly, dilation of the ascending aorta. The ascending aortic wall may be calcified in syphilis, and the aortic valve calcified if valvular disease is responsible for the regurgitation.

ECG

The ECG appearances are those of left ventricular hypertrophy due to 'volume overload': tall R waves and deeply inverted T waves in the left-sided chest leads, and deep S waves in the right-sided leads. Normally, sinus rhythm is present.

Echocardiogram

The echocardiogram (**Fig. 30.85**) demonstrates vigorous cardiac contraction and a dilated left ventricle. The aortic root may also be enlarged. Diastolic fluttering of the mitral leaflets or septum occurs in severe aortic regurgitation (producing the Austin Flint rumble). The severity of aortic regurgitation is assessed with a combination of colour Doppler (extent of the regurgitant jet, width of the vena contracta; **Fig. 30.85**) and CW Doppler (diastolic flow reversal in the descending thoracic aorta, pressure half-time). TOE may provide additional information about the valves and aortic root.

Cardiac catheterization

Cardiac catheterization is appropriate for patients requiring valvular intervention, although CTCA or CT angiography may be an alternative in younger patients.

CMR and cardiac CT

These techniques may be indicated for assessing the thoracic aorta in cases of aortic dilation or dissection. CMR can be used to quantify regurgitant volume.

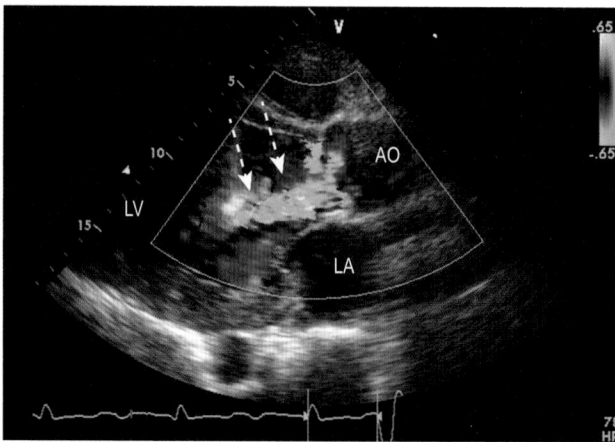

Fig. 30.85 Aortic regurgitation: colour Doppler. A regurgitant jet (green) can be seen passing retrogradely into the left ventricle from the aorta. AO, aorta; LA, left atrium; LV, left ventricle.

Management

The underlying cause of aortic regurgitation (e.g. syphilitic aortitis or infective endocarditis) may require specific treatment. Patients with acute aortic regurgitation may need treatment with vasodilators and inotropes. ACE inhibitors are useful in patients with left ventricular dysfunction and beta-blockers may slow aortic dilation in Marfan's patients. Because symptoms do not develop until the myocardium fails and because the myocardium does not recover fully after surgery, operative valve replacement may be performed before significant symptoms occur.

Aortic surgery is indicated in:
- acute severe aortic regurgitation, e.g. endocarditis
- symptomatic patients (dyspnoea, NYHA class II–IV, angina) with chronic severe aortic regurgitation
- asymptomatic patients with an LVEF of ≤50%
- asymptomatic patients with an LVEF of >50% but with a dilated left ventricle (end-diastolic dimension >70 mm or systolic dimension >50 mm)
- those undergoing CABG or surgery of the ascending aorta or other cardiac valve.

Both mechanical prostheses and tissue valves are used. Tissue valves are preferred in the elderly and in cases where anticoagulants must be avoided, but are contraindicated in children and young adults because of the rapid calcification and degeneration of the valves.

Antibiotic prophylaxis against infective endocarditis (see p. 1106) is not recommended.

TRICUSPID VALVE

Tricuspid stenosis

This uncommon valve lesion, which is seen much more often in women than in men, is usually due to rheumatic heart disease and is frequently associated with mitral and/or aortic valve disease. Tricuspid stenosis is also seen in the carcinoid syndrome.

Pathophysiology

Tricuspid valve stenosis results in a reduced cardiac output, which is restored towards normal when the right atrial pressure increases. The resulting systemic venous congestion produces hepatomegaly, ascites and dependent oedema.

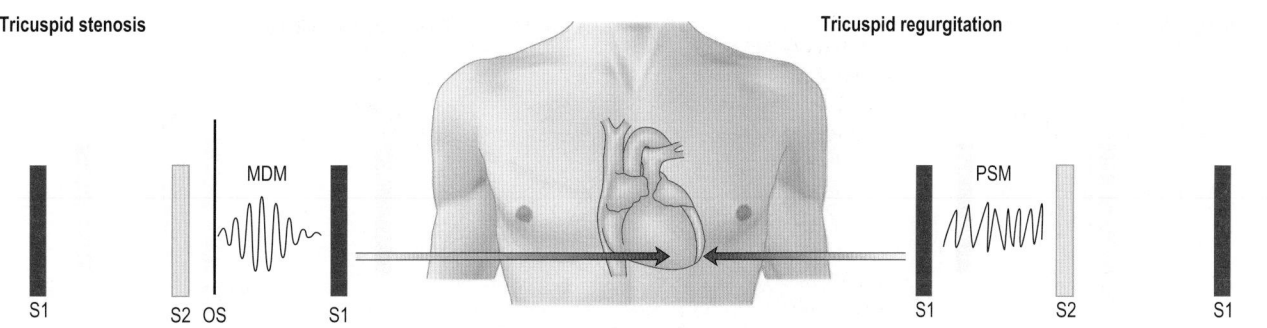

Fig. 30.86 Features of tricuspid stenosis and tricuspid regurgitation. MDM, mid-diastolic murmur; OS, opening snap; PSM, pansystolic murmur; S1, first heart sound; S2, second heart sound.

Clinical features

Symptoms

Patients with tricuspid stenosis are likely to have left side rheumatic valve disease that may be the main driver of symtoms. Symptoms of prominent tricuspid stenosis include abdominal pain (hepatomegaly), abdominal distension (ascites) and peripheral oedema.

Signs

See **Fig. 30.86**. The patient remains in sinus rhythm, which is unusual, and there is a prominent jugular venous *a*-wave. This pre-systolic pulsation may also be felt over the liver. There is usually a rumbling mid-diastolic murmur, which is heard best at the lower left sternal edge and is louder on inspiration. It may be missed because of the murmur of coexisting mitral stenosis. A tricuspid opening snap may occasionally be heard. Hepatomegaly, abdominal ascites and dependent oedema may be present.

Investigations

On the chest X-ray there may be a prominent right atrial bulge. On the ECG, the enlarged right atrium is shown by peaked, tall P waves (>3 mm) in lead II. The echocardiogram may show a thickened and immobile tricuspid valve but this is not so clearly seen as an abnormal mitral valve.

Management

Medical management consists of diuretic therapy and salt restriction. Tricuspid valvotomy is occasionally possible but tricuspid valve replacement is often necessary. Usually, other valves also need replacement because tricuspid valve stenosis is rarely an isolated lesion.

Tricuspid regurgitation

Functional tricuspid regurgitation (see **Fig. 30.25**) may occur whenever the right ventricle dilates: for example, in cor pulmonale, MI or pulmonary hypertension.

Organic tricuspid regurgitation may occur with rheumatic heart disease, infective endocarditis, carcinoid syndrome, Ebstein's anomaly (a congenitally malpositioned tricuspid valve) and other congenital abnormalities of the AV valves.

Clinical features

The valvular regurgitation gives rise to high right atrial and systemic venous pressures. Patients may experience the symptoms of **right heart failure** (see p. 1092).

Signs (see **Fig. 30.86**) include a large jugular venous '*cv*'-wave and a palpable liver that pulsates in systole. Usually, a right ventricular impulse may be felt at the left sternal edge, and there is a blowing pansystolic murmur, best heard on inspiration at the lower left sternal edge. Atrial fibrillation is common.

Investigations

An **echocardiogram** shows dilation of the right ventricle with thickening of the valve.

Management

Functional tricuspid regurgitation usually disappears with medical management. Severe organic tricuspid regurgitation may require operative repair of the tricuspid valve (annuloplasty or annuloplication). Very occasionally, tricuspid valve replacement may be necessary. In intravenous drug users with infective endocarditis of the tricuspid valve, surgical removal of the valve is recommended to eradicate the infection. This is usually well tolerated in the short term. The insertion of a prosthetic valve for this condition is sometimes necessary.

PULMONARY VALVE

Pulmonary stenosis

This is usually a congenital lesion but may rarely result from rheumatic fever or from the carcinoid syndrome. Congenital pulmonary stenosis may be associated with Fallot's tetralogy, Noonan's syndrome or congenital rubella syndrome. Pulmonary stenosis may be valvular, subvalvular or supravalvular.

Clinical features

The obstruction to right ventricular emptying results in right ventricular hypertrophy, which, in turn, leads to right atrial hypertrophy. Severe **pulmonary obstruction** may be incompatible with life but lesser degrees of obstruction give rise to **fatigue**, **syncope** and the

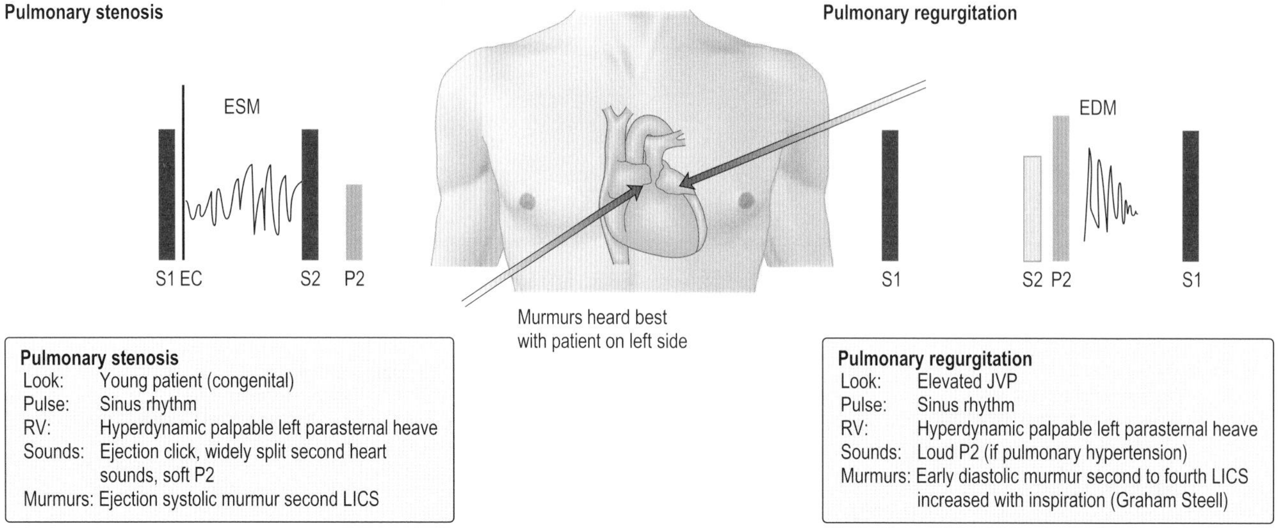

Pulmonary stenosis

ESM

S1 EC   S2 P2

Murmurs heard best
with patient on left side

Pulmonary regurgitation

EDM

S1   S2 P2   S1

Pulmonary stenosis
Look: Young patient (congenital)
Pulse: Sinus rhythm
RV: Hyperdynamic palpable left parasternal heave
Sounds: Ejection click, widely split second heart
          sounds, soft P2
Murmurs: Ejection systolic murmur second LICS

Pulmonary regurgitation
Look: Elevated JVP
Pulse: Sinus rhythm
RV: Hyperdynamic palpable left parasternal heave
Sounds: Loud P2 (if pulmonary hypertension)
Murmurs: Early diastolic murmur second to fourth LICS
          increased with inspiration (Graham Steell)

Fig. 30.87 **Features of pulmonary stenosis and pulmonary regurgitation.** EC, ejection click; EDM, early diastolic murmur; ESM, end-systolic murmur; ICS, intercostal space; LICS, left intercostal space; JVP, jugular venous pulse; P2, pulmonary component of the second heart sound; S1, first heart sound; S2, second heart sound.

symptoms of **right heart failure**. Mild pulmonary stenosis may be asymptomatic.

Physical signs (**Fig. 30.87**) are characterized by a harsh midsystolic ejection murmur, best heard on inspiration, to the left of the sternum in the second intercostal space. This murmur is often associated with a thrill. The pulmonary closure sound is usually delayed and soft. There may be a pulmonary ejection sound if the obstruction is valvular. A right ventricular fourth sound and a prominent jugular venous *a*-wave are present when the stenosis is moderately severe. A right ventricular heave (sustained impulse) may be felt.

Investigations

The chest X-ray usually shows a prominent pulmonary artery owing to post-stenotic dilation. The ECG demonstrates both right atrial and right ventricular hypertrophy, although it may sometimes be normal, even in severe pulmonary stenosis. A Doppler echocardiogram is the investigation of choice.

Management

Management of severe pulmonary stenosis requires pulmonary valvotomy (balloon valvotomy or direct surgery).

Pulmonary regurgitation

This is the most common acquired lesion of the pulmonary valve. It results from dilation of the pulmonary valve ring, which occurs with pulmonary hypertension (Graham Steell murmur). It may also occur following tetralogy of Fallot repair. It is characterized by a decrescendo diastolic murmur, beginning with the pulmonary component of the second heart sound that is difficult to distinguish from the murmur of aortic regurgitation ('Clinical memo', **Fig. 30.87**). Pulmonary regurgitation usually causes no symptoms and treatment is rarely necessary.

PROSTHETIC VALVES

There is no ideal replacement for our own normally functioning, native heart valves. There are two options for valve prostheses: mechanical (**Fig. 30.88**) or tissue (bioprosthetic).

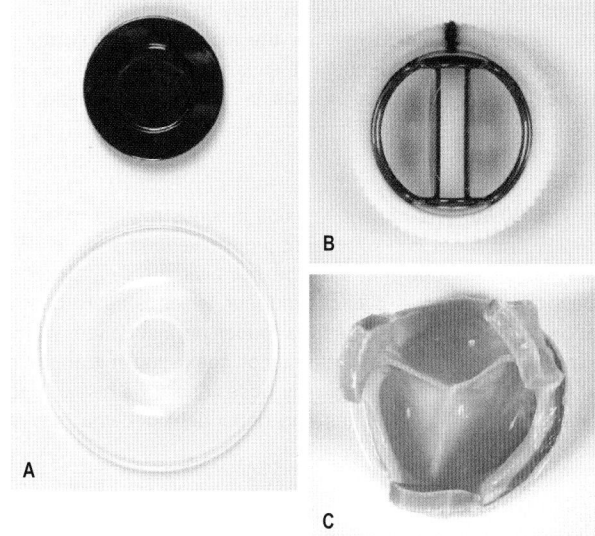

Fig. 30.88 **Prosthetic valves.** **(A)** Björk–Shiley mechanical prosthetic valve. **(B)** St Jude double tilting disc. **(C)** Aortic valve tissue prosthesis (aortic view).

The valves consist of two basic components: an opening to allow blood to flow through and an occluding mechanism to regulate the flow. Mechanical prostheses rely on artificial occluders: a ball and cage (Starr–Edwards), tilting disc (Björk–Shiley) or double tilting disc (St Jude). Tissue prostheses are derived from human (homograft) or porcine or bovine (xenograft) sources. A valve replacement from within the same patient (i.e. pulmonary to aortic valve position) is termed an autograft.

Mechanical versus tissue valves

Mechanical valves, being artificial structures, are more durable than their tissue counterparts, which tend to degenerate after 10 years. However, artificial structures are more thrombogenic. Mechanical valves require formal anticoagulation for the lifetime of the prosthesis. The target INR is determined by what type of valve is inserted,

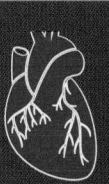

where it is positioned, and whether the patient has additional risk factors for thromboembolism (mitral, tricuspid, pulmonary valve disease; previous thromboembolism; atrial fibrillation; left atrial diameter >50 mm; mitral stenosis; LVEF <35%; hypercoagulable state, see p. 1002):

- **low-thrombogenicity valve** (Carbomedics (aortic position), Medtronic Hall, St Jude Medical (without silzone)): INR 2.5 without and 3.0 with additional risk factors
- **medium-thrombogenicity valve** (Björk–Shiley, other bileaflet valves): INR 3.0 without and 3.5 with additional risk factors
- **high-thrombogenicity valve** (Lillehei–Kaster, Omniscience, Starr–Edwards): INR 3.5 without and 4.0 with additional risk factors.

Tissue valves require anticoagulation for a limited postoperative period only, while the suture lines endothelialize (the ESC recommends 3 months with a target INR of 2.5, although some centres use low-dose aspirin 75–100 mg daily); it can then be discontinued unless another risk factor for thromboembolism (e.g. atrial fibrillation) persists. There is currently no role for direct oral anticoagulants (DOACs).

On auscultation, tissue valve heart sounds are comparable to those of a native valve. Mechanical valve heart sounds are generally louder and both opening and closing sounds can be heard.

Complications

All prostheses carry a risk of infection. Prosthetic valve endocarditis is associated with significant morbidity and mortality; prevention is the cornerstone of management. Patient education about antibiotic prophylaxis is vital and should be reinforced at clinic visits. Details of antibiotic prophylaxis indicated in patients undergoing different types of interventional procedures are given on p. 161 and in **Box 8.7**. Additional prophylaxis indicated in patients at higher risk of endocarditis are discussed on p. 1106. This must be borne in mind when managing a patient with a prosthetic heart valve and steps should be taken to minimize the risk involved. The prosthetic valve occluding mechanism can be interrupted by vegetations but also by thrombosis and calcification, resulting in either stenosis or regurgitation. The prosthesis can become detached from the valve ring, resulting in a **para-prosthetic leak**. Evidence of structural failure can be detected by simple auscultation, with echocardiography as the initial investigation of choice. TTE is non-invasive but scattering of echoes by mechanical valves makes assessment difficult. TOE provides alternative views and higher image resolution, making it the investigation of choice when prosthetic valve endocarditis is suspected.

Interruption of anticoagulant therapy

For minor surgical procedures, including dental extraction and diagnostic endoscopy, anticoagulation should not be interrupted, although the target INR should be reduced to 2.0. Percutaneous arterial puncture is safe with an INR below 2.0, although radial catheterization may be possible at higher INR levels. For major surgical procedures, anticoagulation should be discontinued 5 days before the procedure and intravenous unfractionated heparin or subcutaneous low-molecular-weight heparin commenced when the INR is below 2.0.

Pregnancy and prosthetic heart valves

The types of valve prosthesis for use in women of childbearing age are as follows:

- **Bioprosthetic valves** are preferable during pregnancy, as they are less thrombogenic and do not require anticoagulation. How-

ever, valve degradation in women of childbearing age has been shown to be as high as 50% at 10 years and 90% at 15 years; women with a bioprosthetic valve may require redo valve surgery.
- **Mechanical heart valves** have excellent durability but are thrombogenic and require life-long anticoagulation with warfarin. Pregnancy is a hypercoagulable state due to increased levels of fibrinogen and factors VII, VIII and X, decreased levels of protein S activity, venous hypertension and stasis.

Pregnancy in women with a mechanical heart valve is associated with increased maternal mortality (1–4%) due to valve thrombosis because safe anticoagulation in these patients is complex. Warfarin crosses the placenta and is associated with a 5–12% risk of embryopathy during the first trimester. Warfarin also has an anticoagulant effect in the fetus, which may lead to spontaneous fetal intracranial haemorrhage. Many women will choose unfractionated heparin or low-molecular-weight heparin, as these drugs do not cross the placenta or cause fetal embryopathy. However, unfractionated heparin may not provide consistent therapeutic anticoagulation during pregnancy and there is a high incidence (25%) of valve thrombosis. Low-molecular-weight heparin provides a more consistent anticoagulant effect when given twice daily, with dose adjustment to maintain anti-Xa levels of 0.8–1.2 U/mL 4 hours after administration.

Further reading

Baumgartner H, Falk V, Bax JJ et al. 2017 ESC/EACTS Guidelines for the management of valvular heart disease. *Eur Heart J* 2017; 38:2739–2791.
Lancellotti P, Vannan MA. Timing of intervention in aortic stenosis. *N Engl J Med* 2020; 382:191–193
Nishimura RA, Holmes DR. Treatment after TAVR — discordance and clinical implications. *N Engl J Med* 2020; 382:193–194

INFECTIVE ENDOCARDITIS

Infective endocarditis is an endovascular infection of cardiovascular structures, including cardiac valves, atrial and ventricular endocardium, large intrathoracic vessels and intracardiac foreign bodies, such as prosthetic valves, pacemaker leads and surgical conduits. The annual incidence in the UK is 6–7/100 000 but higher in developing countries. Without treatment, mortality approaches 100%; even with treatment, there is significant morbidity and mortality.

Aetiology

Endocarditis is usually the consequence of two factors: the presence of organisms in the bloodstream, and abnormal cardiac endothelium that facilitates their adherence and growth.

Bacteraemia may arise for patient-specific reasons (poor dental hygiene, intravenous drug use, soft tissue infections) or may be associated with diagnostic or therapeutic procedures (dental treatment, intravascular cannulae, cardiac surgery or permanent pacemakers).

Damaged endocardium promotes platelet and fibrin deposition, which allows organisms to adhere and grow, leading to an infected vegetation. Valvular lesions may create non-laminar flow, and jet lesions from septal defects or a patent ductus arteriosus result in abnormal vascular endothelium. Aortic and mitral valves are most commonly involved in infective endocarditis; intravenous drug users are the exception, as right-sided lesions are more common in these patients.

Organisms

Common organisms and the sources of infection are shown in **Fig. 30.89**.

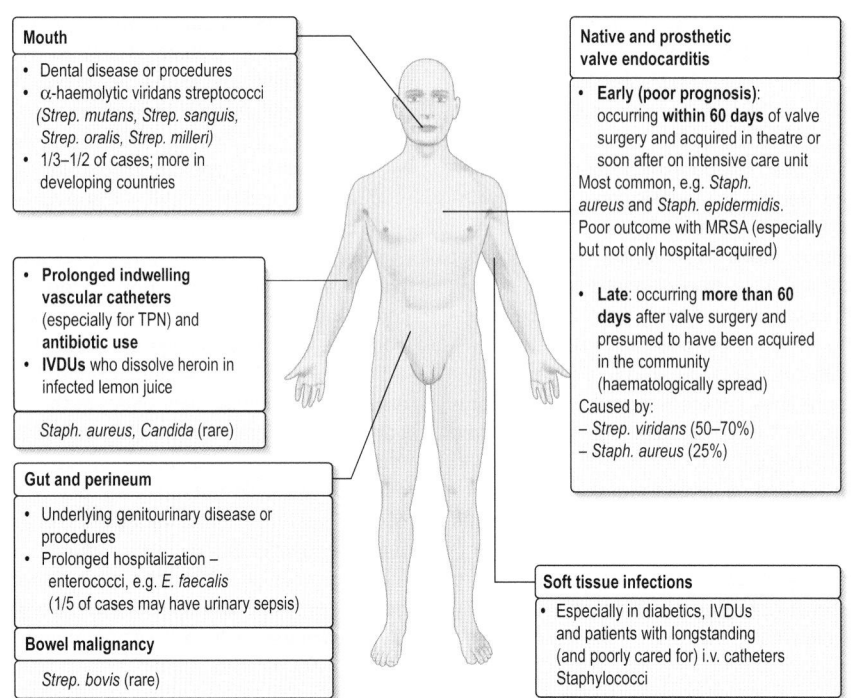

Mouth
- Dental disease or procedures
- α-haemolytic viridans streptococci (*Strep. mutans, Strep. sanguis, Strep. oralis, Strep. milleri*)
- 1/3–1/2 of cases; more in developing countries

- **Prolonged indwelling vascular catheters** (especially for TPN) and **antibiotic use**
- **IVDUs** who dissolve heroin in infected lemon juice

Staph. aureus, Candida (rare)

Gut and perineum
- Underlying genitourinary disease or procedures
- Prolonged hospitalization – enterococci, e.g. *E. faecalis* (1/5 of cases may have urinary sepsis)

Bowel malignancy

Strep. bovis (rare)

Native and prosthetic valve endocarditis
- **Early (poor prognosis):** occurring **within 60 days** of valve surgery and acquired in theatre or soon after on intensive care unit
  Most common, e.g. *Staph. aureus* and *Staph. epidermidis*. Poor outcome with MRSA (especially but not only hospital-acquired)
- **Late**: occurring **more than 60 days** after valve surgery and presumed to have been acquired in the community (haematologically spread)
  Caused by:
  – *Strep. viridans* (50–70%)
  – *Staph. aureus* (25%)

Soft tissue infections
- Especially in diabetics, IVDUs and patients with longstanding (and poorly cared for) i.v. catheters Staphylococci

Fig. 30.89 Infective endocarditis: aetiology and sources of infection. IVDU, intravenous drug user; MRSA, meticillin-resistant *Staphylococcus aureus*; TPN, total parenteral nutrition.

> **ℹ Box 30.45 Modified Duke criteria for endocarditis**[a]
>
> **Major criteria**
> - A positive blood culture for infective endocarditis, as defined by the recovery of a typical microorganism from two separate blood cultures in the absence of a primary focus (*viridans* streptococci, *Abiotrophia* species and *Granulicatella* species; *Streptococcus bovis*, HACEK group[b], or community-acquired *Staphylococcus aureus* or enterococcus species) *or*
> - A persistently positive blood culture, defined as the recovery of a microorganism consistent with endocarditis either from blood samples obtained more than 12h apart or from all three or a majority of four or more separate blood samples, with the first and last obtained at least 1 h apart *or*
> - A positive serological test for Q fever, with an immunofluorescence assay showing phase 1 immunoglobulin G antibodies at a titre >1:800 *or*
> - Echocardiographic evidence of endocardial involvement:
>   – an oscillating intracardiac mass on the valve or supporting structures, in the path of regurgitant jets, or on implanted material in the absence of an alternative anatomical explanation *or*
>   – an abscess *or*
>
> - New partial dehiscence of a prosthetic valve *or*
> - New valvular regurgitation
>
> **Minor criteria**
> - Predisposition: predisposing heart condition or intravenous drug use
> - Fever: temperature ≥38°C (100.4°F)
> - Vascular phenomena: major arterial emboli, septic pulmonary infarcts, mycotic aneurysm, intracranial haemorrhage, conjunctival haemorrhages, Janeway lesion
> - Immunological phenomena: glomerulonephritis, Osler nodes, Roth spots, rheumatoid factor
> - Microbiological evidence: a positive blood culture but not meeting a major criterion as noted earlier, or serological evidence of an active infection with an organism that can cause infective endocarditis[c]
> - Echocardiogram: findings consistent with infective endocarditis but not meeting a major criterion as noted earlier
>
> [a]The diagnosis of infective endocarditis is definite when: (1) a microorganism is demonstrated by culture of a specimen from a vegetation, an embolism or an intracardiac abscess; (2) active endocarditis is confirmed by histological examination of the vegetation or intracardiac abscess; (3) two major clinical criteria, one major and three minor criteria, or five minor criteria are met. [b]HACEK denotes *Haemophilus* species, *Actinobacillus actinomycetemcomitans, Cardiobacterium hominis, Eikenella corrodens* and *Kingella kingae*. [c]Excluded from this criterion is a single positive blood culture for coagulase-negative staphylococci or other organisms that do not cause endocarditis. Serological tests for organisms that cause endocarditis include tests for *Brucella, Coxiella burnetii, Chlamydia, Legionella* and *Bartonella* species.
> (After Raoult D, Abbara S, Jassal DS et al. Case records of the Massachusetts General Hospital. Case 5–2007. A 53-year-old man with a prosthetic aortic valve and recent onset of fatigue, dyspnea, weight loss, and sweats. N Engl J Med 2007; 356:715. ©2007 Massachusetts Medical Society. All rights reserved.)

Rare causes

These include the HACEK group of organisms, which tend to run a more insidious course (**Box 30.45**).

Culture-negative endocarditis

This accounts for 5–10% of endocarditis cases. The usual cause is prior antibiotic therapy (good history-taking is vital) but some cases are due to a variety of fastidious organisms that fail to grow in normal blood cultures. These include *Coxiella burnetii*

(the cause of Q fever), *Chlamydia* species, *Bartonella* species (organisms that cause trench fever and cat scratch disease) and *Legionella*.

Clinical features

The clinical presentation of infective endocarditis (**Box 30.46**) is dependent on the organism and the presence of predisposing cardiac conditions. Infective endocarditis may occur as an acute, fulminating infection but also as a chronic or subacute illness with low-grade fever and non-specific symptoms. A high index of clinical

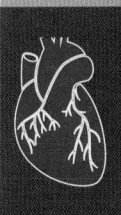

Box 30.46 Clinical features of infective endocarditis

Clinical feature	Approximate %
General	
Malaise	95
Clubbing	10
Cardiac	
Murmurs	90
Cardiac failure	50
Arthralgia	25
Pyrexia	90
Skin lesions	
Osler nodes	15
Splinter haemorrhages	10
Janeway lesions	5
Petechiae	50
Eyes	
Roth spots	5
Conjunctival splinter haemorrhages	Rare
Splenomegaly	40
Neurological	
Cerebral emboli	20
Mycotic aneurysm	10
Renal	
Haematuria	70

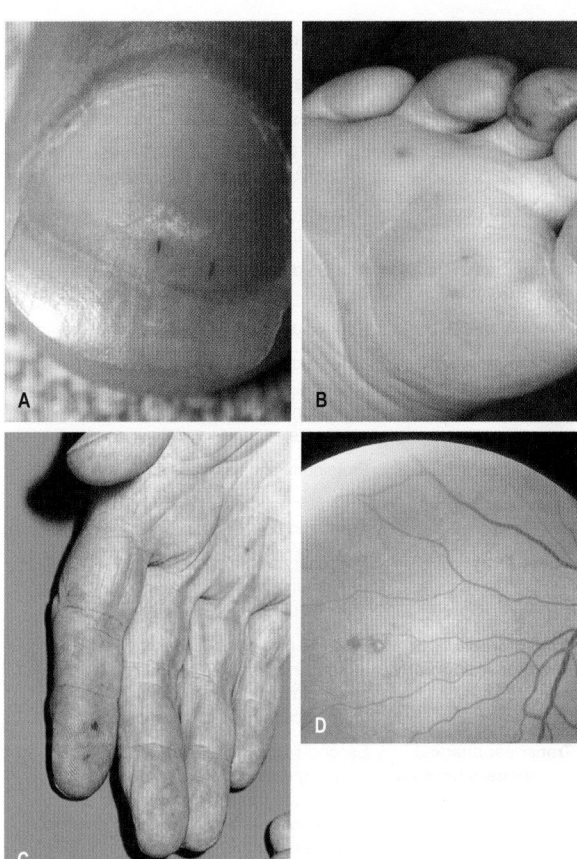

Fig. 30.90 Infective endocarditis. (A) Splinter haemorrhages. **(B)** Janeway lesions. **(C)** Osler nodes. **(D)** Roth spots. (*A, B From Moser DK, Riegel B.* Cardiac Nursing. *Philadelphia: Saunders; 2007, p. 1127, with permission from Elsevier. C From Forbes CD, Jackson WF.* Color Atlas and Text of Clinical Medicine, *3rd edn. St Louis: Mosby; 2003, p. 232; © Elsevier. D. Courtesy of Professor Ian Constable.*)

suspicion is required to identify patients with infective endocarditis and certain criteria should alert the physician.

High clinical suspicion

- New valve lesion/(regurgitant) murmur.
- Embolic event(s) of unknown origin.
- Sepsis of unknown origin.
- Haematuria, glomerulonephritis and suspected renal infarction.
- 'Fever' plus:
  - Prosthetic material inside the heart
  - Other high predisposition for infective endocarditis, e.g. intravenous drug use
  - Newly developed ventricular arrhythmias or conduction disturbances
  - First manifestation of congestive cardiac failure
  - Positive blood cultures (with typical organism)
  - Cutaneous (Osler, Janeway) or ophthalmic (Roth) lesions (**Fig. 30.90**)
  - Peripheral abscesses (renal, splenic, spine) of unknown origin
  - Predisposition and recent diagnostic/therapeutic interventions known to result in significant bacteraemia.

Low clinical suspicion

- Fever plus none of the above.

Diagnosis

The criteria for the clinical diagnosis of endocarditis have been established – the modified Duke criteria (see **Box 30.45**).

Investigations

The mainstays of diagnosis of infective endocarditis are blood cultures and echocardiography, performed in order to identify the organism, ensure appropriate therapy and monitor the patient's response to therapy (**Box 30.47**). Echocardiography is an extremely useful tool if used appropriately but is not an appropriate screening test for patients with just a fever or an isolated positive blood culture where there is a low pre-test probability of endocarditis. A negative echocardiogram does not exclude a diagnosis of endocarditis and TOE and CT-PET may be required, particularly in cases of suspected prosthetic valve infection.

Management

The location of the infection means that prolonged courses of antibiotics are usually required. The combination of antibiotics may be synergistic in eradicating microbial infection and minimizing resistance. Blood cultures should be taken prior to empirical antibiotic therapy (but this should not delay therapy in unstable patients). Antibiotic treatment should continue for 4–6 weeks. Typical therapeutic regimens are shown in **Box 30.48** but advice on specific therapy should be sought from the local microbiology department, according to the organism identified and current sensitivities. Serum levels of gentamicin and vancomycin need to be monitored to ensure adequate therapy and prevent toxicity. In patients with penicillin allergy, one of the glycopeptide antibiotics, vancomycin or teicoplanin, can be used. Penicillins, however, are fundamental to the therapy of bacterial endocarditis; allergies therefore

ⓘ **Box 30.47 Investigations and findings in endocarditis**

Investigation	Findings and notes
Blood cultures	Three sets from different venepuncture sites
Serological tests	Consider in culture-negative cases for *Coxiella*, *Bartonella*, *Legionella*, *Chlamydia*
Full blood count	Reduced haemoglobin, increased white cells, increased or reduced platelets
Serum creatinine and electrolytes	Increased urea and creatinine
Liver biochemistry	Increased serum alkaline phosphatase
Inflammatory markers	Increased erythrocyte sedimentation rate and C-reactive protein (CRP reduces in response to therapy and increases with relapse)
Urine	Proteinuria and haematuria
Electrocardiogram	PR prolongation/heart block is associated with aortic root abscess
Chest X-ray	Pulmonary oedema in left-sided disease, pulmonary emboli/abscess in right-sided disease
Transthoracic echocardiography	First-line non-invasive imaging test with sensitivity of 60–75%; demonstrates vegetations, valvular dysfunction, ventricular function, abscesses
Transoesophageal echocardiography	Second-line invasive imaging test with greater sensitivity (>90%) and specificity; useful in suspected aortic root abscess and essential in prosthetic valve endocarditis

ⓘ **Box 30.48 Antibiotics in endocarditis[a]**

Clinical situation	Suggested antibiotic regimen to start [b,c,d]
Clinical endocarditis, culture results awaited, no suspicion of staphylococci	Penicillin 1.2 g 4-hourly, gentamicin 80 mg 12-hourly
Suspected staphylococcal endocarditis (intravenous drug user, recent intravascular devices or cardiac surgery, acute infection)	Vancomycin 1 g 12-hourly, gentamicin 80–120 mg 8-hourly
Streptococcal endocarditis (penicillin-sensitive)	Penicillin 1.2 g 4-hourly, gentamicin 80 mg 12-hourly
Enterococcal endocarditis (no high-level gentamicin resistance)	Ampicillin/amoxicillin 2 g 4-hourly, gentamicin 80 mg 12-hourly
Staphylococcal endocarditis[e]	Vancomycin 1 g 12-hourly *or*
	Flucloxacillin 2 g 4-hourly *or*
	Benzylpenicillin 1.2 g 4-hourly *plus*
	Gentamicin 80–120 mg 8-hourly

[a]Adapted from British Society for Antimicrobial Chemotherapy (BSAC) guidelines. [b]Optimum choice of therapy needs close liaison with microbiology/infectious diseases departments. All antibiotics given i.v. [c]Monitor vancomycin and gentamicin levels, and adjust if necessary. [d]Choice of antibiotic for staphylococci depends on sensitivities. [e]MRSA can affect valves.

seriously compromise the choice of antibiotics. It is essential to confirm the nature of a patient's allergy to ensure that the appropriate treatment is not withheld needlessly. Anaphylaxis would be much more influential on antibiotic choice than a simple gastrointestinal disturbance.

Persistent fever

Most patients with infective endocarditis should respond within 48 hours of initiation of appropriate antibiotic therapy, as evidenced by a resolution of fever, reduction in serum markers of infection, and relief of systemic symptoms of infection. Failure of these factors to occur needs to be taken very seriously. The following should be considered:

- perivalvular extension of infection and possible abscess formation
- drug reaction (the fever should resolve promptly after drug withdrawal)
- hospital-acquired infection (i.e. venous access site, urinary tract infection)
- pulmonary embolism (secondary right-sided endocarditis or prolonged hospitalization).

In such cases, samples for culture should be taken from all possible sites and evidence sought of the above causes. A change of antibiotic dosage or regimen should be avoided unless there are positive cultures or a drug reaction is suspected. Emergence of bacterial resistance is uncommon. Close liaison with the microbiology department is recommended and a cardiothoracic surgical opinion should be sought.

Surgery

Decisions about surgical intervention in patients with infective endocarditis should be made after joint consultation between the cardiologist and cardiothoracic surgeon, taking into account patient-specific features (age, non-cardiac morbidities, presence of prosthetic material or cardiac failure) and infective endocarditis features (infective organism, vegetation size, presence of perivalvular infection, systemic embolization).

Prevention

In 2015 the ESC produced guidelines for the management of infective endocarditis. They identified three groups of patients who could be considered at highest risk of developing infective endocarditis and who suffered significant morbidity and mortality complications from it:

- those who have prosthetic valves (including transcatheter devices) or material used for valve repair
- those with a previous episode of IE
- those with uncorrected cyanotic congenital heart disease or who have received palliative shunts. Patients who have successful corrective surgery are at high risk for the first 6 months postoperatively.

The ESC recommends that these groups should receive antibiotic prophylaxis during high-risk procedures. This includes dental procedures that involve manipulation of the gingival or periapical part of the teeth or perforation of the oral mucosa. (The American Heart Association also considers that cardiac transplant patients with valvular heart disease should be included as highest-risk patients.)

The ESC also provided additional recommendations applicable to all patients with valvular heart disease (including the highest-risk patients). These include:

- regular dental check-ups (6 months for the highest-risk groups and 12 months for all others)
- disinfection of wounds and eradication of chronic bacterial carriage (skin, urine)
- curative antibiotics for any focus of bacterial infection
- no self-medication with antibiotics
- strict infection control during at-risk procedures

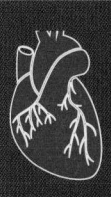

Fetal circulation

- Pulmonary vein
- Ductus arteriosus
- Aorta
- Pulmonary vein
- Superior vena cava
- Lungs (unexpanded)
- Crista dividens
- Foramen ovale
- RA
- RV
- LA
- LV
- PA
- Inferior vena cava
- Ductus venosus
- Liver
- Sphincter in ductus venosus
- Portal vein
- Inferior vena cava
- Descending aorta
- Umbilical vein
- Umbilical arteries

Normal heart after birth

- To lungs
- Pulmonary veins from lungs
- AO
- PA
- LA
- Mitral valve
- Aortic valve
- Superior vena cava
- Atrial septum
- RA
- LV
- Tricuspid valve
- Inferior vena cava
- RV
- Pulmonary valve
- Ventricular septum

Oxygen saturation of blood

| High | Medium | Low |

Fig. 30.91 **Anatomy showing the circulation.** AO, aorta; LA, left atrium; LV, left ventricle; PA, pulmonary artery; RA, right atrium; RV, right ventricle.

- avoidance of piercing or tattoos
- limitation of the usage of infusion catheters, preferring peripheral versus central catheters; peripheral catheters should be changed every 3–4 days.

Further reading

Duval Z, Hoen B. Prophylaxis for infective endocarditis: let's end the debate. *Lancet* 2015; 385:1164–1165.
Habib G, Lancellotti P, Antunes MJ et al. 2015 ESC Guidelines for the management of infective endocarditis: The Task Force for the Management of Infective Endocarditis of the European Society of Cardiology (ESC). *Eur Heart J* 2015; 36:3075–3128.
Hoen B, Duval X. Infective endocarditis. *N Engl J Med* 2013; 368:1425–1433.
Thornhill MH. Impact of the NICE guidelines recommending cessation of antibiotic prophylaxis for prevention of infective endocarditis: before and after study. *Br Med J* 2011; 342:2392.

CONGENITAL HEART DISEASE

Fetal circulation

Oxygenated blood and nutrients are supplied to the developing fetus via the placenta and the umbilical vein (**Fig. 30.91**). Half of that blood is directed to the fetal ductus venosus and carried to the inferior vena cava; the other half enters the liver. Blood moves from the inferior vena cava to the right atrium of the heart. In the fetus there is an opening between the right and left atrium (the foramen ovale) and most of the blood flows from the right into the left atrium, bypassing the pulmonary circulation. This blood goes into the left ventricle and is pumped through the aorta into the fetal body. Some of the blood flows from the aorta through the internal iliac arteries to the umbilical arteries and re-enters the placenta, where carbon dioxide and other waste products from the fetus are taken up and enter the woman's circulation.

Some of the blood from the right atrium does not enter the left atrium, but rather enters the right ventricle and is pumped into the pulmonary artery. In the fetus there is a connection between the pulmonary artery and the aorta, the ductus arteriosus, which directs most of this blood away from the lungs. With the first breath after delivery, the lungs expand, vascular resistance in the pulmonary arteries falls, more blood moves from the right atrium to the right ventricle and pulmonary arteries, and oxygenated blood travels back to the left atrium through the pulmonary veins. The decrease in right atrial pressure and relative increase in left atrial pressure result in closure of the foramen ovale.

The ductus arteriosus usually closes off within 1 or 2 days of birth, completely separating the left and right systems. The umbilical vein and the ductus venosus close off within 2–5 days of birth, leaving behind the ligamentum teres and the ligamentum venosus of the liver, respectively.

Adult congenital heart disease

Heart defects are the most common birth defect and affect approximately 1% of babies born in the UK. As a result of improved medical and surgical management, the majority of those born with congenital cardiac disease are surviving into late adulthood, having families and leading active lifestyles. Patients with congenital heart disease require ongoing multidisciplinary specialist care and surveillance, as many need further intervention, surgery and electrophysiological input in adulthood. In the UK the majority of these patients will be reviewed in designated specialist centres at intervals, depending on clinical need; however, non-specialists often look after them in local hospitals and all physicians should therefore have a practical understanding of congenital heart disease.

Ventricular septal defect

Ventricular septal defect (VSD) is the most common congenital cardiac malformation. The haemodynamic consequences of the VSD are dependent on the defect and resultant shunt size. In

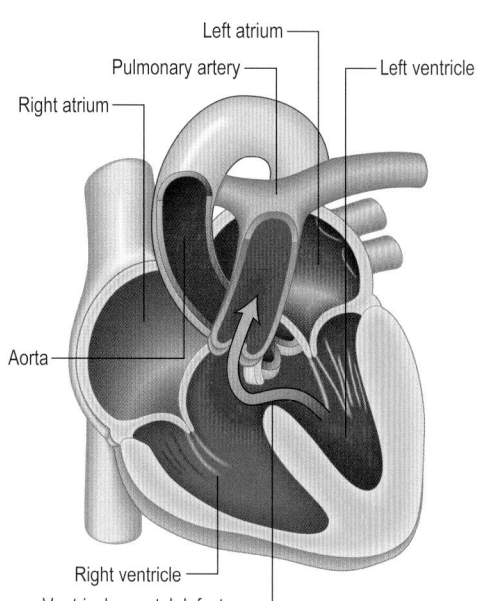

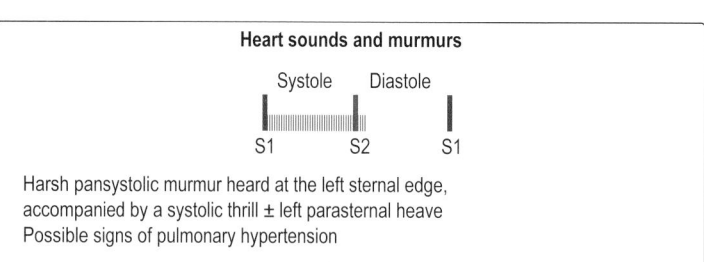

Left atrium

Pulmonary artery — Left ventricle

Right atrium

Aorta

Right ventricle

Ventricular septal defect

Heart sounds and murmurs

Systole   Diastole

S1   S2   S1

Harsh pansystolic murmur heard at the left sternal edge, accompanied by a systolic thrill ± left parasternal heave
Possible signs of pulmonary hypertension

Pathophysiology

- Left-to-right shunt
- When the left ventricle contracts, it ejects some blood into the aorta and some across the ventricular septal defect into the right ventricle and pulmonary artery
- **Small** VSDs ('maladie de Roger'): loud and sometimes long systolic murmur
- **Moderate** VSDs: loud, 'tearing' pansystolic murmur
- **Large** VSDs: cause pulmonary hypertension and soft murmur Eisenmenger's complex may result

Fig. 30.92 Ventricular septal defect (VSD). Pathophysiology and auscultatory findings.

an otherwise structurally normal heart, left ventricular pressure is higher than right and blood will shunt from left to right through a VSD (**Fig. 30.92**).

- In small defects the shunt velocity is high and the actual volume of blood shunting across the defect is small with no haemodynamic consequence.
- In larger defects the shunt, which is directed into the right ventricular outflow tract and the pulmonary vasculature and then back to the left heart, may lead to dilation of the *left atrium and left ventricle*, and this is an indication for intervention or repair.
- In large, non-restrictive defects, a large volume of blood shunts into the pulmonary vasculature, leading to remodelling of the pulmonary vessels and pulmonary hypertension. Eventually, when the right ventricular pressure becomes suprasystemic (higher than left), blood starts to shunt from right to left, causing cyanosis. This is referred to as *Eisenmenger's syndrome.*

Clinical features

- *Restrictive VSDs* ('maladie de Roger') are often found incidentally, as patients are asymptomatic. These defects are associated with a loud pansystolic murmur. The majority close spontaneously by the age of 10 years.
- *Large (non-restrictive) VSDs* usually present with heart failure symptoms in childhood and eventually lead to pulmonary hypertension and Eisenmenger's syndrome. As pressures equalize, the murmur becomes softer. With established Eisenmenger's syndrome, patients will be cyanosed and have evidence of clubbing.

Investigations and treatment

A small VSD produces no abnormal X-ray or ECG findings. This is often a clinical diagnosis and echocardiography is used to confirm the VSD and assess for left heart dilation. If there is none, these lesions are managed conservatively and the only risk is an increased risk of endarteritis or endocarditis.

In larger defects, echocardiography is used to assess the size and location of the VSD and its haemodynamic consequences. VSDs can occur just below the pulmonary and aortic valves, or in the perimembranous or muscular septum. Interventional options are either surgical repair or device closure. Closure (surgical or interventional)

is offered for a significant shunt causing left atrial and ventricular enlargement with no evidence of irreversible pulmonary hypertension.

Atrial septal defect

The diagnosis of an atrial septal defect (ASD) is often made in adulthood, as patients remain asymptomatic through childhood and clinical signs can be subtle.

There are three main types of ASD (**Fig. 30.93**):

- S*ecundum defects* (most common type): located in the midseptum (fossa ovalis).
- *Sinus venosus defects*: located in the superior part of the septum near the superior vena cava (superior sinus venosus defect), or the inferior part of the septum near the inferior vena cava (inferior sinus venosus defect) entry point.
- *Ostium primum (atrioventricular septal) defects* (15%): located in the lower part of atrial septum at the level of, and often involving, the atrioventricular valves.

An ASD with a significant left-to-right shunt causes right heart volume overload and right atrial and ventricular dilation. This may lead to arrhythmia, which is often the presenting symptom, along with breathlessness and exercise intolerance. There is raised pulmonary pressure due to increased blood flow through the pulmonary vessels, but significant pulmonary vascular disease develops in less than 5% of patients.

Clinical features

The clinical findings in a patient with an ASD and significant shunt might be a flow murmur from increased blood flow across the pulmonary valve and a fixed, split second heart sound (see **Fig. 30.93**).

Investigations and treatment

- *Chest X-ray* may demonstrate prominent pulmonary arteries and cardiomegaly due to right heart dilation.
- *ECG* may show right bundle branch block and right axis deviation. Some patients with late diagnosis may have atrial arrhythmia.
- *Echocardiography* is used to confirm the diagnosis; it demonstrates the defect in the septum. The shunt direction is evaluated with colour Doppler. The right atrium and ventricle are assessed for dilation and the pulmonary pressure is measured. It is also

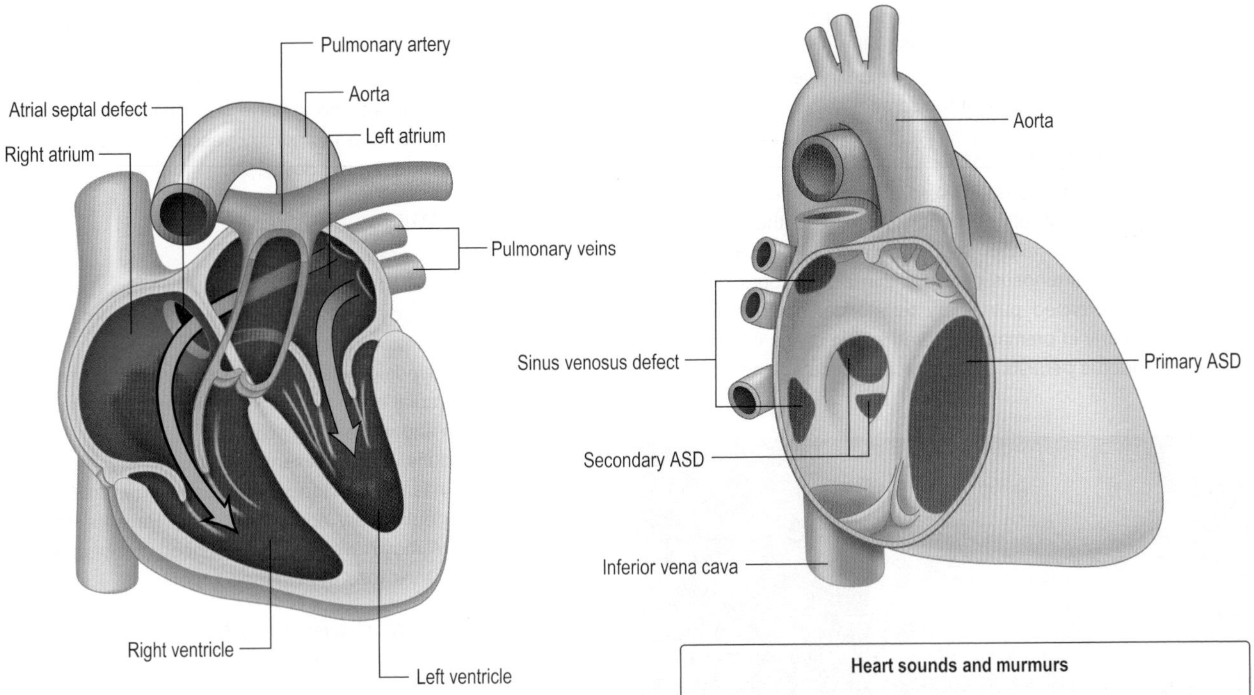

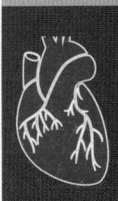

Pulmonary artery

Aorta

Atrial septal defect

Left atrium

Right atrium

Pulmonary veins

Aorta

Sinus venosus defect

Primary ASD

Secondary ASD

Inferior vena cava

Right ventricle

Left ventricle

Pathophysiology

- Left-to-right shunt through the defect in the interatrial septum
- Dilation of the pulmonary artery resulting from the shunt
- The murmur is produced by increased flow across the pulmonary valve and an increased stroke volume

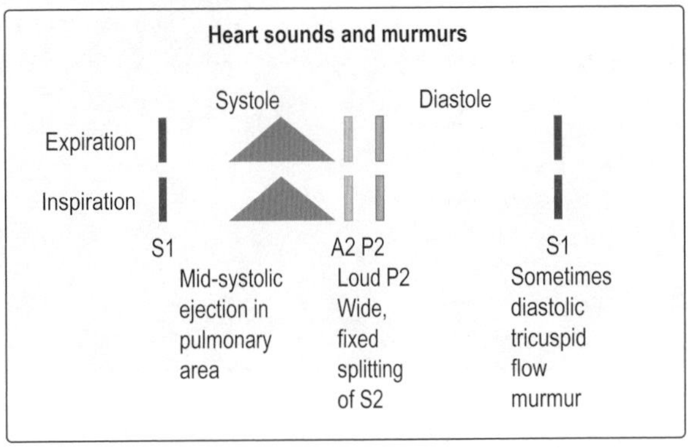

Heart sounds and murmurs

	Systole	Diastole
Expiration		
Inspiration		

S1

A2 P2

S1

Mid-systolic ejection in pulmonary area

Loud P2 Wide, fixed splitting of S2

Sometimes diastolic tricuspid flow murmur

Fig. 30.93 Atrial septal defect (ASD). Pathophysiology and auscultatory findings.

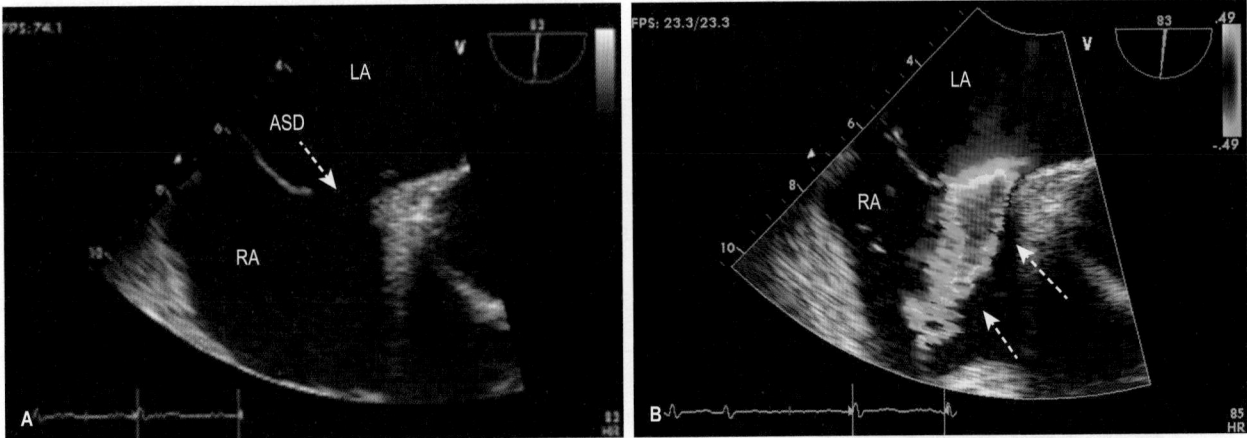

Fig. 30.94 Ostium secundum atrial septal defect (ASD, arrowed) in a young girl. (A) The defect is shown in a two-dimensional echocardiogram subcostal four-chamber view. **(B)** Colour Doppler can demonstrate the left-to-right shunt. LA, left atrium; RA, right atrium.

important to assess the left heart, as if there is significant left ventricular or mitral pathology, this needs to be considered when considering whether and how to close the defect (**Fig. 30.94**). TOE may be helpful if the images are not clear, and guides device closure of the ASD.

- **CMR and CT** are helpful for assessing anomalous pulmonary venous drainage and confirming sinus venous defects.

Closure of an ASD is indicated if there is a significant left-to-right shunt, resulting in right atrial and ventricular enlargement with normal pulmonary vascular resistance and oxygen saturations.

Secundum defects can often be closed with a device by an interventionalist if the defect is not too large and there are adequate rims of atrial septal tissue (**Fig. 30.95**). All other ASDs are closed surgically, and if there is anomalous pulmonary venous drainage, it is redirected to the left atrium at the same time.

Patent ductus arteriosus

A patent ductus arteriosus (PDA) is a persistent communication between the proximal left pulmonary artery and the descending aorta, resulting in a continuous left-to-right shunt (**Fig. 30.96**). Normally, the ductus arteriosus closes within a few hours of birth in response to decreased pulmonary resistance; however, in some cases (particularly in premature babies and in cases with maternal rubella) the ductus persists. Indometacin (a prostaglandin inhibitor)

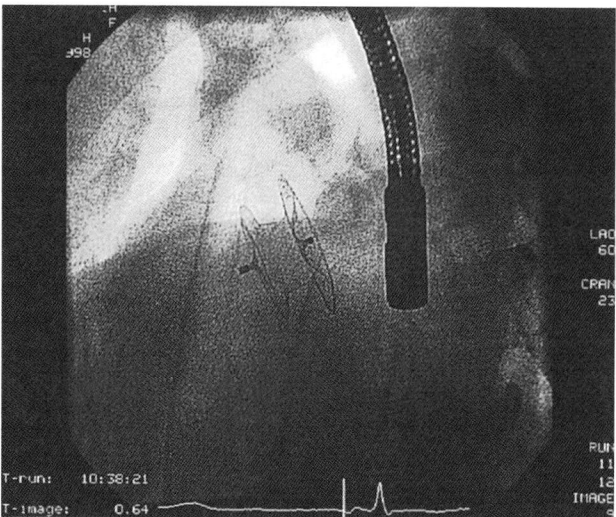

Fig. 30.95 Angiographic appearance of a fully deployed atrial septal defect (ASD) closure device. The device bridges the ASD and wedges against the surfaces of the right and left atrial septa, occluding flow. The metal object in frame is the distal end of a transoesophageal echocardiography probe. (*Courtesy of Dr D Ward, St George's, University of London.*)

is given to stimulate duct closure. The shunt size is dependent on the size of the duct and the pressure difference between the pulmonary arteries and aorta. If the left-to-right shunt is significant, it will result in left heart volume overload. Those with large unrestrictive defects may present with congestive heart failure in infancy and, if untreated, may develop pulmonary vascular disease; with time, Eisenmenger's syndrome will develop.

Clinical features

In adults, PDAs are graded as:
- **Silent:** tiny PDA, no murmur – incidental finding on echo.
- **Small:** no haemodynamic effect or significant shunt but audible systolic or continuous murmur.
- **Moderate:** bounding pulses (wide pulse pressure) and continuous murmur radiating to the back; displaced apex beat from left heart dilation and volume overload.
- **Large:** in adults these present with pulmonary hypertension; the murmur has often disappeared due to equalized pressures between the pulmonary artery and aorta. Patients with Eisenmenger's PDA may have more pronounced clubbing and lower saturations in their toes than in their fingers.

Investigations and treatment

- **Chest X-ray** in an adult with a significant left-to-right shunt will show enlarged pulmonary arteries and an increased cardiothoracic ratio (left heart dilation).
- **ECG** may demonstrate left atrial abnormality (broad p waves) and high-voltage QRS complexes related to left heart overload. If there is right axis deviation and a tall R in V_1, this may represent established Eisenmenger's syndrome.
- **Echocardiography** colour and continuous wave Doppler imaging of the proximal pulmonary arteries may demonstrate the shunt. Echocardiography may show a dilated left atrium and left ventricle if there is a significant left-to-right shunt. Pulmonary pressure can be assessed. If there is pulmonary hypertension, the right ventricle will be hypertrophied.
- **A right heart catheter study** may be necessary in the adult who is diagnosed with a PDA and significantly raised pulmonary pressure to estimate the shunt and pulmonary vascular resistance.

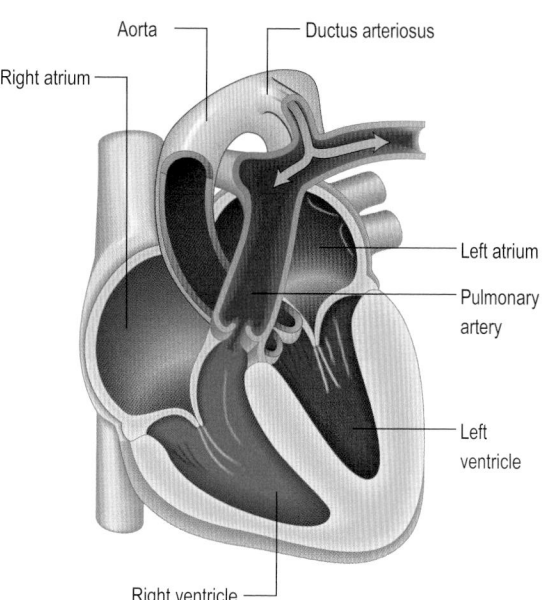

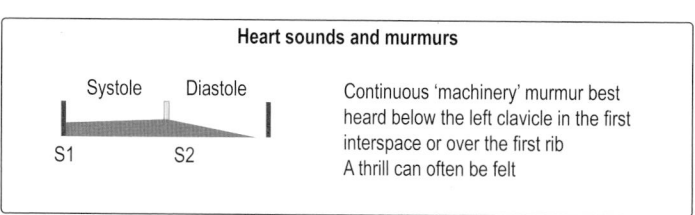

Heart sounds and murmurs

Systole   Diastole

S1   S2

Continuous 'machinery' murmur best heard below the left clavicle in the first interspace or over the first rib
A thrill can often be felt

Pathophysiology
- Left-to-right shunt
- Some of the blood from the aorta crosses the ductus arteriosus and flows into the pulmonary artery
- The murmur is produced by the turbulent aortic-to-pulmonary artery shunting in both systole and diastole
- Dilation of the pulmonary artery, left atrium and left ventricle
- As pulmonary hypertension (Eisenmenger's reaction) develops, the murmur becomes quieter, may be confined to systole or may even disappear, causing central cyanosis

Fig. 30.96 Patent ductus arteriosus. Pathophysiology and auscultatory findings.

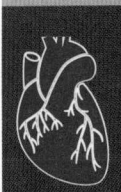

Life expectancy is normal in silent PDAs and patients who have had appropriate and timely closure of a PDA. Indications for intervention (usually with percutaneous devices) include left ventricular dilation with significant shunt and no significant pulmonary vascular disease (assessed by pulmonary vascular resistance at right heart catheter). Small defects may predispose to endarteritis and should be considered for device closure unless clinically silent.

Coarctation of the aorta

A coarctation of the aorta is a narrowing of the aorta at, or just distal to, the insertion of the ductus arteriosus (distal to the origin of the left subclavian artery; **Fig. 30.97**). Rarely, it can occur proximal to the left subclavian. In 80% of cases the aortic valve is bicuspid. There is an association with circle of Willis aneurysms (affecting approximately 10%). Severe narrowing of the aorta encourages the formation of a collateral arterial circulation involving the intercostal arteries.

Coarctation of the aorta can be asymptomatic for many years. Adults with undetected coarctation may present with hypertension, headaches, nosebleeds and, in severe coarctation, *claudication* and cold legs may be present.

Clinical features

Physical examination of patients with significant coarctation reveals hypertension in the upper limbs and weak, delayed (radio-femoral delay) pulses in the legs. If coarctation is present in the aorta, proximal to the left subclavian artery, there will be asynchronous radial pulses in right and left arms and often the arch itself is hypoplastic and the blood pressure in the right arm is higher than in the left. For heart sounds and murmurs in coarctation of aorta, see **Fig. 30.97**. Those who have had surgery to correct coarctation may have a thoracotomy scar.

Investigations and treatment

- **Chest X-ray** may reveal a dilated aorta indented at the site of the coarctation. This kink in the aortic contour in the upper left mediastinum is shaped like a number 3 and known as the '3 sign'. In adults, tortuous and dilated collateral intercostal arteries may cause rib notching.

- **ECG** may demonstrate left ventricular hypertrophy.
- **Echocardiography** of suprasternal aortic arch windows can be difficult in adults but may demonstrate turbulence in the descending aorta. Continuous Doppler of the descending aorta in significant coarctation will show high-velocity flow and slow diastolic runoff (diastolic tail) due to the obstruction.
- **CT and MRI** (**Fig. 30.98**) demonstrate the coarctation and the proximity to the aortic branch vessels, which needs to be considered in intervention. MRI is preferable for surveillance, as it does not use radiation. If the aortic valve is bicuspid, it is also important to obtain images of the ascending aorta for associated aortopathy.

Intervention/repair

Intervention is indicated if there is a peak–peak gradient across the coarctation of more than 20 mmHg in the cardiac catheter laboratory or greater than 50% luminal narrowing with associated hypertension or left ventricular hypertrophy. If there is significant collateralization, there may be minimal gradient, even in the setting of significant coarctation. In neonates, coarctation is treated with surgical repair. In older children and adults, balloon dilation and stenting is the preferred option. Balloon dilation is preferred for re-coarctation.

Tetralogy of Fallot

Tetralogy of Fallot (**Fig. 30.99**) consists of:
- a large, malaligned VSD
- an overriding aorta
- right ventricular outflow tract obstruction
- right ventricular hypertrophy.

The term tetralogy of Fallot represents a spectrum of disease: some patients will have only mild pulmonary stenosis, whereas the more severe extreme is pulmonary atresia in which the pulmonary vasculature can also develop abnormally. Symptoms depend on the degree of pulmonary stenosis but the majority of patients with tetralogy present in childhood. In infancy, cyanosis usually develops due to increased right-sided pressures, resulting in a right-to-left shunt. Fallot's spells are episodes of severe cyanosis noted in children due to spasm of the subpulmonary muscle; these can be relieved by increasing systemic

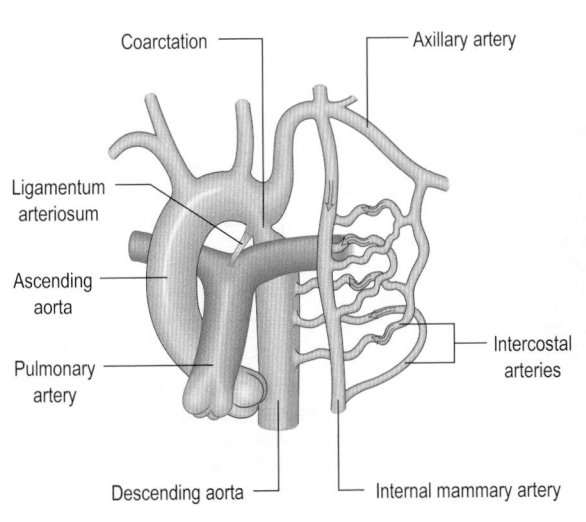

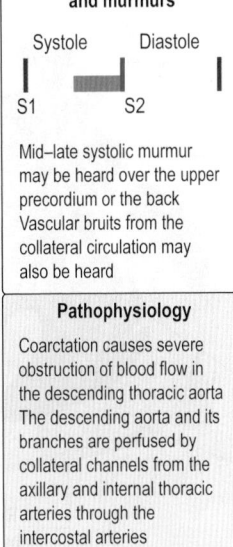

Heart sounds and murmurs

Systole   Diastole

S1   S2

Mid–late systolic murmur may be heard over the upper precordium or the back Vascular bruits from the collateral circulation may also be heard

Pathophysiology

Coarctation causes severe obstruction of blood flow in the descending thoracic aorta The descending aorta and its branches are perfused by collateral channels from the axillary and internal thoracic arteries through the intercostal arteries

Labels: Coarctation, Axillary artery, Ligamentum arteriosum, Ascending aorta, Pulmonary artery, Intercostal arteries, Descending aorta, Internal mammary artery

Fig. 30.97 Coarctation of the aorta. Pathophysiology and auscultatory findings.

resistance using postural manoeuvres, such as squatting. In babies with severe pulmonary stenosis, systemic-to-pulmonary artery shunts (i.e. a Blalock–Taussig subclavian-to-pulmonary artery shunt) may have been used initially to increase pulmonary blood flow until the pulmonary arteries are large enough for repair. The majority of adults with tetralogy of Fallot will have undergone complete repair but repair in childhood will often leave them with significant pulmonary regurgitation, which is generally well tolerated into early adulthood; the majority, however, will need pulmonary valve replacement with time.

The overall survival of those who have had operative repair is excellent. Many patients with repaired tetralogy of Fallot lead unlimited active lives. They do require ongoing specialist follow-up as, in those with transannular patch repair (surgical or interventional), pulmonary valve replacements are needed during follow-up and late

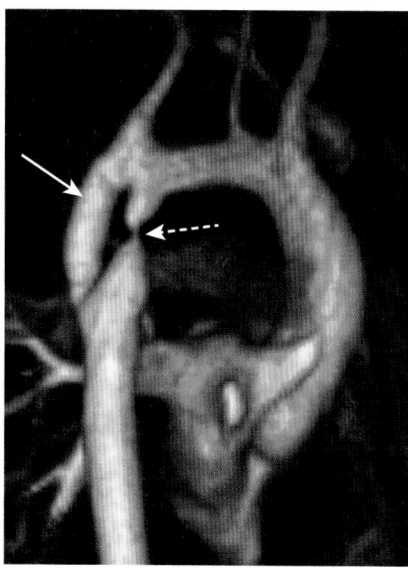

Fig. 30.98 Severe aortic coarctation in an adult. The coarctation is shown on cardiac magnetic resonance angiography. The solid arrow indicates the jump bypass graft; the dotted arrow indicates severe aortic coarctation.

complications include ventricular and atrial arrhythmias, heart failure and sudden death.

Transposition of the great arteries

In transposition of the great arteries (TGA) the right atrium connects to the morphological right ventricle, which gives rise to the aorta, and the left atrium connects to the morphological left ventricle, which gives rise to the pulmonary artery (**Fig. 30.100**). This is incompatible with life, as blood circulates in two parallel circuits: that is, deoxygenated blood from the systemic venous return passes into the right heart and then, via the aorta, back to the systemic circulation. Babies with transposition are born cyanosed and rely on an ASD, VSD or PDA allowing oxygenated and deoxygenated blood to be mixed. In those without an adequate shunt an atrial septostomy is performed: a Rashkind's balloon is deployed to dilate the foramen ovale and is used to maintain saturations at 50–80% until a definitive procedure can be performed.

The majority of adult patients with TGA who were born between the 1960s and mid-1980s will have had an 'atrial switch' operation. In this procedure, systemic venous blood was baffled across into the left atrium and then pumped via the left ventricle into the pulmonary artery; the pulmonary venous (oxygenated blood) returning to the left atrium was redirected via a baffle into the right atrium and right ventricle, and into the aorta. This palliation allowed patients a good quality of life into their fourth decade, but the right ventricle remains the systemic ventricle and with time starts to fail. Atrial arrhythmia is also common in this group.

The first arterial switch procedure was performed in 1975 and it is now routinely performed in babies with TGA in the first 2 weeks of life. The aorta is reconnected to the left ventricle and the pulmonary artery is connected to the right ventricle. The coronary arteries are re-implanted. Late complications include coronary complications, narrowing of the pulmonary arteries, which are stretched around the aorta, and neovalvular regurgitation.

Congenitally corrected transposition of the great arteries

In congenitally corrected transposition of the great arteries (ccTGA), systemic venous return to the right atrium enters a

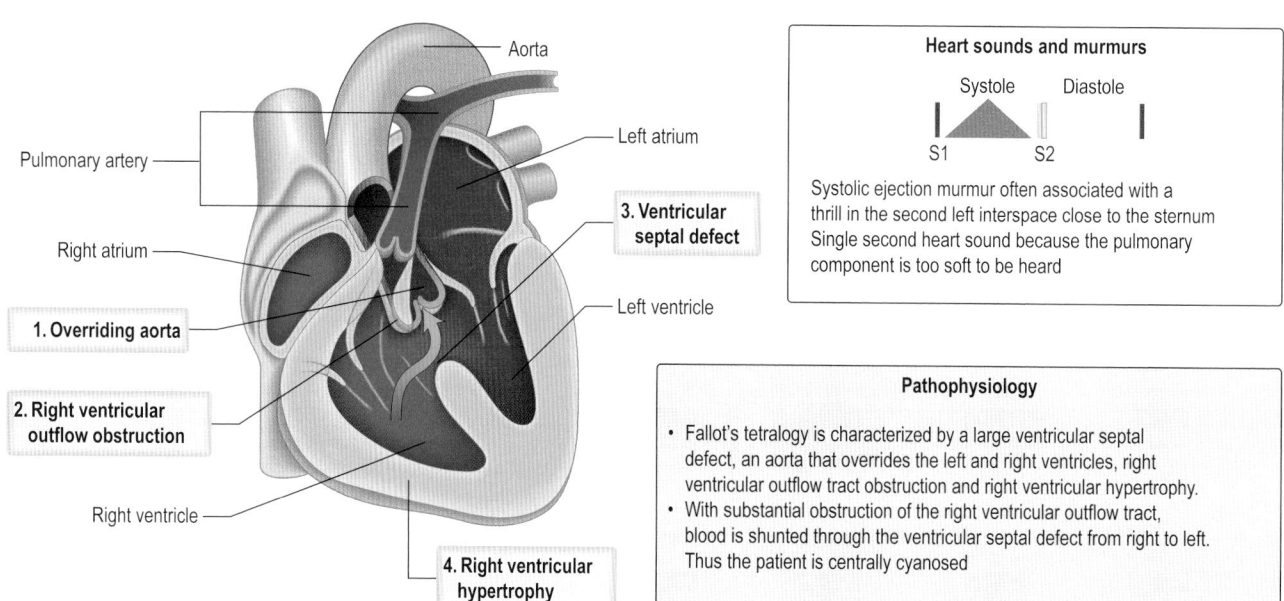

Aorta

Pulmonary artery

Left atrium

Right atrium

3. Ventricular septal defect

1. Overriding aorta

Left ventricle

2. Right ventricular outflow obstruction

Right ventricle

4. Right ventricular hypertrophy

Heart sounds and murmurs

Systole   Diastole

S1   S2

Systolic ejection murmur often associated with a thrill in the second left interspace close to the sternum
Single second heart sound because the pulmonary component is too soft to be heard

Pathophysiology

• Fallot's tetralogy is characterized by a large ventricular septal defect, an aorta that overrides the left and right ventricles, right ventricular outflow tract obstruction and right ventricular hypertrophy.
• With substantial obstruction of the right ventricular outflow tract, blood is shunted through the ventricular septal defect from right to left. Thus the patient is centrally cyanosed

Fig. 30.99 Fallot's tetralogy. Pathophysiology and auscultatory findings.

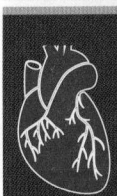

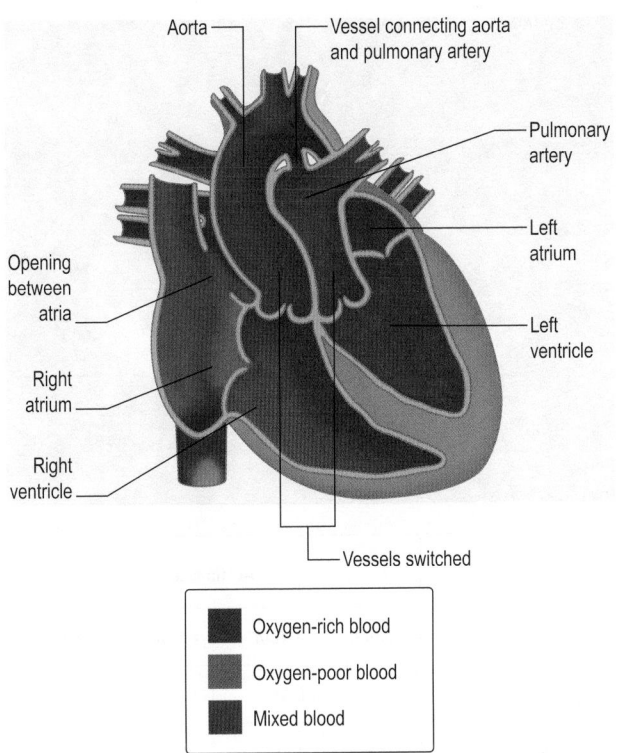

Fig. 30.100 **Transposition of the great arteries.**

Legend:
- Oxygen-rich blood
- Oxygen-poor blood
- Mixed blood

Labels on diagram: Aorta; Vessel connecting aorta and pulmonary artery; Pulmonary artery; Left atrium; Left ventricle; Opening between atria; Right atrium; Right ventricle; Vessels switched

morphological left ventricle, which pumps deoxygenated blood into the pulmonary arteries. Pulmonary venous blood returns to the left atrium and then, via the morphological right ventricle, to the aorta. The circulation is physiologically corrected and these babies are not typically cyanosed, but the systemic circulation is supported by a morphological right ventricle. ccTGA is often associated with cardiac lesions:

- systemic (tricuspid) AV valve abnormalities with valve insufficiency
- VSD
- subpulmonary stenosis
- complete heart block
- WPW syndrome
- dextrocardia.

Some patients with ccTGA may live a normal life, while others develop progressive tricuspid regurgitation and systemic ventricular failure or require pacemaker insertion (the AV node is abnormal, leading to heart block).

Further reading

Baumgartner H, Bonhoeffer P, De Groot NM et al. ESC Guidelines for the management of grown-up congenital heart disease. *Eur Heart J* 2010; 31:2915–2957.
Gatzoulis M, Webb G, Daubney P, eds. *Diagnosis and Management of Adult Congenital Heart Disease*, 3rd edn. Elsevier; 2016.

MARFAN'S SYNDROME

Marfan's syndrome (MFS) is a connective tissue disorder with autosomal dominant inheritance pattern and a prevalence estimated at 1:5000. One-quarter of cases are not inherited and are due to *de novo* mutations. In 1991 it was established that MFS is caused by a mutation in the *FBN1* gene on chromosome 15q21. The *FBN1* gene encodes for

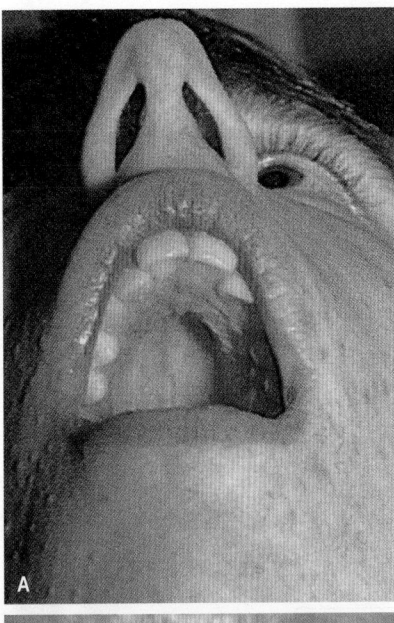

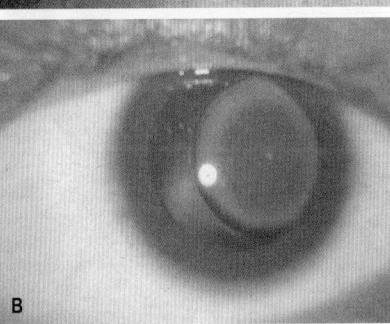

Fig. 30.101 **Marfan's syndrome. (A)** High arched palate. **(B)** Eye lens dislocation. (*From Forbes CD, Jackson WF. Color Atlas and Text of Clinical Medicine, 3rd edn. St Louis: Mosby; 2003, p. 134, © Elsevier.*)

a protein known as fibrillin-1. Fibrillin-1 is a component of structures called microfibrils, which are part of the extracellular matrix.

Diagnosis

Despite the finding of a causative gene, there is no specific definitive test for MFS. Diagnosis requires a complete medical and family history, examination, relevant investigations and, in equivocal cases, genetic analysis. This syndrome can affect the eyes, lungs, skeletal system and cardiovascular system (**Figs 30.101** and **30.102**). The diagnosis is currently made using the Modified Ghent Criteria (**Box 30.49**). The findings of aortic root aneurysm (ectopia lentis) lens dislocation or a family history of MFS are major criteria in the diagnosis of MFS in these guidelines.

Management

The management of patients with MFS requires multidisciplinary input from geneticists, cardiologists, cardiothoracic, vascular and orthopaedic surgeons, ophthalmologists and physiotherapists, among others.

Cardiovascular surveillance and management

The primary cause of death in MFS is cardiovascular. In the 1970s the mean age of death was reported to be 32 years, but survival has significantly improved with better means of assessing for this condition and with prophylactic aortic root replacement for those with

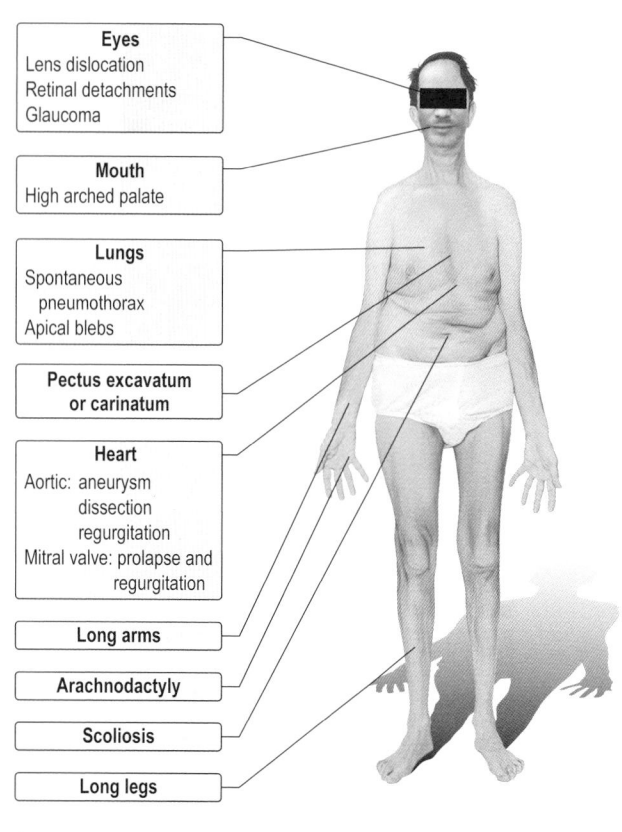

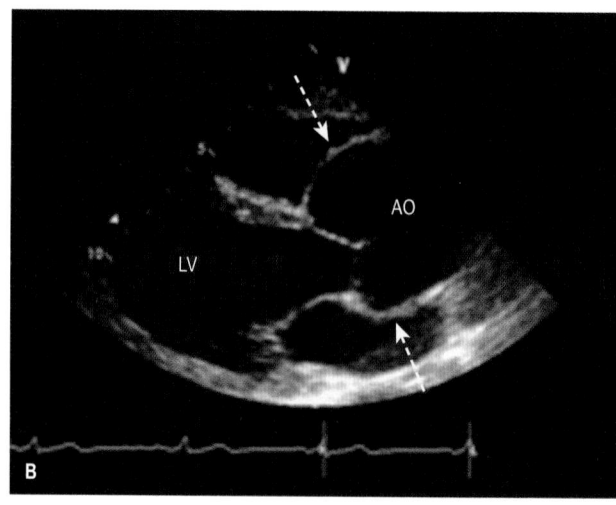

Yearly risk	Aortic size			
	> 3.5cm	> 4cm	> 5cm	> 6cm
Rupture	0.0%	0.3%	1.7%	3.6%
Dissection	2.2%	1.5%	2.5%	3.7%
Death	5.9%	4.6%	4.8%	10.8%
Any of the above	7.2%	5.3%	6.5%	14.1%

C

Fig. 30.102 Marfan's syndrome. (A) Photograph of a 63-year-old man. **(B)** Two-dimensional longitudinal echocardiogram revealing dilatation of the aortic root (arrows). **(C)** Yearly risk of complications based on aortic size. LV, left ventricle; AO, aorta

dilated ascending aortas. Patients with MFS are followed up with serial cardiovascular imaging, tailored to the specific cardiovascular findings of the individual. Yearly follow-up of aortic dimensions is recommended; however, patients with a cross-sectional diameter of more than 4.5 cm on the initial scan or a growth rate of 0.5 cm or more per year require more frequent (6-monthly) measurements. Echocardiography is readily available and useful for assessing the aortic sinuses, sinotubular junction and part of the ascending aorta, as well as valvular and left ventricular function, which may be impaired in MFS. Cross-sectional imaging (CT or MRI) is necessary to assess the arch and descending aorta, which can also be involved. These modalities give more readily reproducible images to monitor interval change and may be preferred for this purpose in patients approaching the need for surgical intervention.

The current indication (European and American guidelines) for prophylactic root replacement in patients with MFS is an aortic root measuring 5 cm (or 4.5 cm in those with a family history of dissection). An aneurysm of 6 cm or more in the descending aorta qualifies the patient for an open surgical repair, with surgery preferred over endovascular stenting due to fragility of the vasculature.

Medical therapy

- **Beta-blockers.** These are considered standard therapy for patients with aortic dilation and MFS; however, the evidence base for their use is conflicted, and composed of small series and only one randomized control led trial of 70 patients.

- **Angiotensin receptor blockers (ARBs).** Deficiency of fibrillin-1 leads to excessive activation of the TGF cytokine. Mouse model studies have shown that dysregulation of TGF-β leads to aortic aneurysms and mitral valve prolapse, and that TGF-β antagonism rescued this phenotype. ARBs specifically inhibit TGF-β. In one randomized controlled trial, there was no difference between ARB therapy and beta-blockers over a three year period in terms of aortic dilation progression or cardiovascular events. Further research with randomized controlled trials is still required, to help establish the relative effectiveness of the various medications used in MFS.

Lifestyle

Contact sports and strenuous and isometric exertion should be avoided but moderate cardiovascular exercise is encouraged. Patients with Marfan's are excluded from joining the military.

Pregnancy

All women with MFS should have preconceptual assessment and counselling. There is a 50% chance of their child being affected and they need to be made aware of the options for pre-implantation genetic diagnosis (*in vitro* fertilization pregnancy where embryos can be assessed for the *FBN* mutation prior to implantation) and prenatal diagnosis (amniocentesis and chorionic villus sampling). Women having MFS with or without aortic dilation are at increased risk of aortic dissection. This is estimated at 1% if the aortic root measures

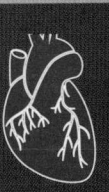

 Box 30.49 Modified Ghent Criteria for Marfan's syndrome (MFS)

No family history of MFS
- Aortic root dilation Z-score ≥2 AND ectopia lentis = MFS
- Aortic root dilation Z-score ≥2 AND *FBN1* = MFS
- Aortic root dilation Z-score ≥2 AND systemic score ≥7 points* = MFS
- Ectopia lentis AND *FBN1* with known aortic root dilation = MFS

Family history of MFS
- Ectopia lentis = MFS
- Systemic score ≥7 points* = MFS
- Aortic root dilation Z-score ≥2 above 20 years old, ≥3 below 20 years old = MFS

* Systemic features	Score
Wrist AND thumb sign	3
Wrist OR thumb sign	1
Pectus carinatum (protrusion of chest wall)	2
Pectus excavatum (indentation of chest wall) or chest asymmetry	1
Hindfoot deformity	2
Pes planus (flat foot)	1
Spontaneous pneumothorax	2
Dural ectasia	2
Protrusio acetabuli	2
Scoliosis or thoracolumbar kyphosis	1
Reduced elbow extension	1
3/5 facial features (dolichocephaly, enophthalmos, down-slanting palpebral fissure, malar hypoplasia, retrognathia)	1
Skin striae	1
Severe myopia	1
Mitral valve prolapse	1
Reduced upper segment/lower segment (<0.85 whites, <0.78 blacks AND increased arm span/height >1.05).	1
	Maximum total 20 points; score ≥7 indicates systemic involvement

less than 4 cm and 10% if it is over 4 cm. Pregnancy should be discouraged in women with aortic dimensions of more than 4.5 cm and they should be offered prophylactic root replacement prior to pregnancy. Current recommendations are that echocardiography should be performed every 6–8 weeks throughout pregnancy and the postpartum period. Blood pressure should be regularly monitored and hypertension treated aggressively. ARBs are teratogenic and women planning pregnancy should be converted to beta-blockers.

Further reading

Lacro RV, Dietz HC, Sleeper LA et al. Atenolol versus losartan in choldren and young adults with Marfan's syndrome. *N Engl J Med* 2014; 371:2061–2071
Loeys BL, Dietz HC, Braverman AC et al. The revised Ghent nosology for the Marfan syndrome. *J Med Genet* 2010; 47:476–485.

PULMONARY HEART DISEASE

The normal mean pulmonary artery pressure (mPAP) at rest is 14 ± 3 mmHg with an upper limit of normal of 20 mmHg. The normal values for mPAP, mean capillary wedge pressure (mPCWP) and cardiac output (CO) are 12 ± 2 mmHg, 6 ± 2 mmHg and 5 L/min, respectively. The fall in pressure across the lung circulation is known as the transpulmonary gradient and reflects the difference between mPAP and mPCWP. The normal transpulmonary gradient is 6 ± 2 mmHg.

The ***pulmonary vascular resistance*** (PVR) is calculated by the formula:

$$\frac{mPAP - mPCWP}{CO}$$

It is normally about 1.5 mmHg/L per min (1.5 Wood units). Approximately 60% of the body's endothelial surface is in the lungs and the lungs normally offer a low resistance to blood flow. This is because the media of the pre-capillary pulmonary arterioles is thin, as compared with their more muscular systemic counterparts that have to respond constantly to postural changes under the influence of gravity. The fact that the lung circulation normally offers a low resistance to flow explains the preferential passage of blood through the lungs in specific forms of congenital heart disease, which may eventually lead to remodelling of the lung circulation and pulmonary hypertension.

Pulmonary hypertension

Pulmonary hypertension (PH) is defined as an mPAP of more than 25 mmHg at rest, as measured on right heart catheterization. The clinical classification of PH is provided in **Box 30.50**.

Pathophysiology

The different groups are characterized by variable amounts of hypertrophy, proliferation and fibrotic changes in distal pulmonary arteries (pulmonary arterial hypertension, PAH; pulmonary veno-occlusive disease, PVOD; pulmonary hypertension, PH, due to left heart disease; PH due to lung disease and/or hypoxia). Pulmonary venous changes are seen in PVOD and PH groups due to left heart disease, and the vascular bed may be destroyed in emphysematous or fibrotic areas seen in lung disease. In chronic thromboembolic pulmonary hypertension (CTEPH), organized thrombi are seen in the elastic pulmonary arteries. Patients with PH with unclear and/or multifactorial mechanisms have variable pathological findings.

Patients with progressive PH develop right ventricular hypertrophy, dilation, heart failure and death.

Pulmonary artery hypertension
Epidemiology

A French registry of 674 patients with PAH identified 39.2% with idiopathic pulmonary artery hypertension (IPAH), 3.9% with familial (or heritable) disease, 9.5% with drug and toxin (anorexigens) causes, 15.3% with autoimmune rheumatic disease, 11.3% with congenital heart disease, 10.4% with portal hypertension and 6.2% with HIV-associated disease. In familial or heritable PAH, mutations in the bone morphogenetic protein receptor type 2 (*BMPR2*) gene are detected in over 70% of cases; other mutations are seen in patients with hereditary haemorrhagic telangiectasia (Osler–Weber–Rendu syndrome).

Drugs and toxins known to cause PAH include fenfluramine, dexfenfluramine, toxic rapeseed oil and the anorectic agents aminorex and benfluorex.

Clinical features

Patients with PAH may present with symptoms of dyspnoea, fatigue, weakness, angina, syncope or abdominal distension. Clinical signs of PAH and right heart hypertrophy include a left parasternal heave,

> ℹ **Box 30.50** Clinical classification of pulmonary hypertension[a]
>
> | Group | Aetiological classification | Subtypes |
> |---|---|---|
> | 1 | Pulmonary arterial hypertension (PAH) | 1.1 Idiopathic
1.2 Heritable
1.2.1 *BMPR2*
1.2.2 *ALK1, ENG, SMAD9, CAV1, KCNK3*
1.2.3 Unknown
1.3 Drugs and toxins
1.4 Associated with:
1.4.1 Connective tissue disease[b]
1.4.2 HIV infection
1.4.3 Portal hypertension
1.4.4 Congenital heart disease
1.4.5 Schistosomiasis |
> | 1′ | Pulmonary veno-occlusive disease (PVOD) and/or pulmonary capillary haemangiomatosis | |
> | 1″ | Persistent pulmonary hypertension of the newborn (PPHN) | |
> | 2 | Pulmonary hypertension due to left heart disease | 2.1 Systolic dysfunction
2.2 Diastolic dysfunction
2.3 Valvular disease
2.4 Congenital/acquired left heart inflow/outflow tract obstruction and congenital cardiomyopathies |
> | 3 | Pulmonary hypertension due to lung diseases and/or hypoxia | 3.1 Chronic obstructive pulmonary disease
3.2 Interstitial lung disease
3.3 Other pulmonary disease with mixed restrictive and obstructive pattern
3.4 Sleep-disordered breathing
3.5 Alveolar hypoventilation disorders
3.6 Chronic exposure to high altitude
3.7 Developmental abnormalities |
> | 4 | Chronic thromboembolic pulmonary hypertension (CTEPH) | |
> | 5 | Pulmonary hypertension with unclear and/or multifactorial mechanisms | 5.1 Haematological disorders: chronic haemolytic anaemia, myeloproliferative disorders, splenectomy
5.2 Systemic disorders: sarcoidosis, pulmonary histiocytosis, lymphangioleiomyomatosis
5.3 Metabolic disorders: glycogen storage disease, Gaucher's disease, thyroid disorders
5.4 Others: tumoral obstruction, fibrosing mediastinitis, chronic renal failure on dialysis, segmental pulmonary hypertension |
>
> [a]5th World Symposium on Pulmonary Hypertension, Nice, 2013. [b]Now called 'autoimmune rheumatic disease'. *ALK1*, activin-like receptor kinase-1; *BMPR*, bone morphogenetic protein receptor type II; *CAV1*, caveolin-1; *ENG*, endoglin; HIV, human immunodeficiency virus; *KCNK3*, potassium channel super-family K member-3; *SMAD9*, mothers against decapentaplegic 9.
> *(From Simonneau G, Gatzoulis MA, Adatia I et al. Updated clinical classification of pulmonary hypertension. J Am Coll Cardiol 2013; 62:D34–41.)*

a loud P2 heart sound, a soft pansystolic murmur with tricuspid regurgitation or early diastolic murmur with pulmonary regurgitation. Right heart failure leads to jugular venous distension, ascites, peripheral oedema and hepatomegaly. Clinical signs of associated diseases, such as systemic sclerosis or chronic liver disease, should be sought.

Investigations

- **Routine blood tests** include full blood count, renal and liver biochemistry, thyroid function tests, and serological assays for underlying autoimmune rheumatic diseases, HIV and hepatitis.
- **Chest X-ray** shows enlargement of the pulmonary arteries and the major branches, with marked tapering (pruning) of peripheral arteries. The lung fields are usually lucent and there may be right atrial and right ventricular enlargement. The chest X-ray may facilitate the diagnosis of PH due to left heart or chronic lung disease.
- **ECG** shows right ventricular hypertrophy and right atrial enlargement (P pulmonale).
- **Echocardiography** (**Fig. 30.103**) with tricuspid regurgitation can be used for determination of PAP using the simplified Bernoulli

equation (PAP = $4 \times$ (tricuspid regurgitation velocity)^2 + estimated right atrial pressure). Right atrial pressure can be assumed at 5–10 mmHg unless there is significant dilation of the inferior vena cava with reduced respiratory variation. mPAP = $0.61 \times$ PA systolic pressure + 2 mmHg (although the Bernoulli equation may not be accurate in cases of severe tricuspid regurgitation).
- **CMR** may be useful in adult congenital heart disease and in assessing right ventricular function on serial assessment.
- **Abdominal liver ultrasound** is useful to exclude liver cirrhosis and portal hypertension.
- **Right heart catheterization** may be indicated as part of the clinical assessment to confirm the diagnosis (elevated PAP), determine the pulmonary wedge pressure (PWP), calculate the cardiac output, and assess for pulmonary vascular resistance and reactivity. In PAH, a vasodilator challenge (inhaled nitric oxide, intravenous adenosine or epoprostenol) should be performed to identify patients who might benefit from vasodilator therapies. A responder is defined as a reduction in mean PAP of 10 mmHg or more to reach an absolute mPAP of 40 mmHg or less with increased or unchanged cardiac output. These vasodilator challenges are not recommended in patients with other types of PH (types 2–5).

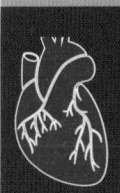

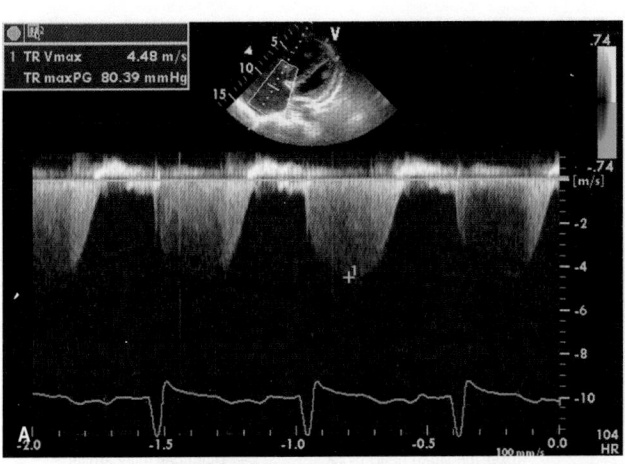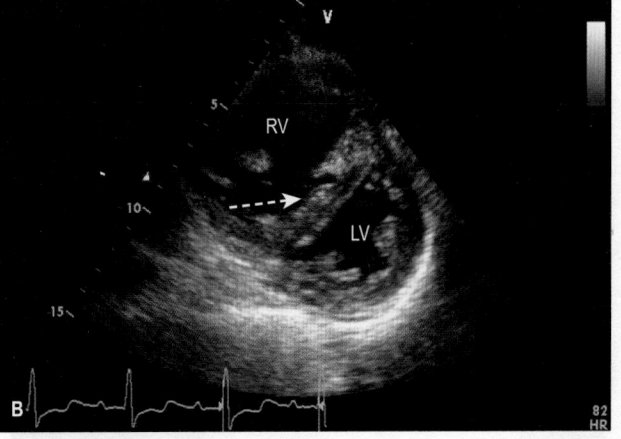

Fig. 30.103 Pulmonary hypertension. (A) Continuous wave Doppler echocardiography demonstrating markedly elevated tricuspid regurgitation velocity consistent with pulmonary hypertension. **(B)** Parasternal short-axis echocardiogram with a dilated right ventricle **(RV)** and septal flattening (arrowed) in a patient with pulmonary hypertension. LV, left ventricle.

Management

- **Physical activity.** Patients should be encouraged to remain physically active but avoid exertion that precipitates severe dyspnoea, chest pain or pre-syncope.
- **Pregnancy.** Patients with PAH have a very high mortality rate during pregnancy (30–50%) and should be counselled against conception. Contraception may include barrier methods, progesterone-only pill or Mirena coil.
- **Travel.** During plane travel, supplementary oxygen at 2 L/min may be appropriate for patients with reduced functional class and with resting hypoxia of less than 8 kPa.
- **Vaccination.** Vaccination should be given for influenza and pneumococcal pneumonia.
- **Elective surgery.** Epidural anaesthesia may be preferable to a general anaesthetic.
- **Oral anticoagulation.** There is evidence to support the use of oral anticoagulation in patients with IPAH, heritable PAH and PAH due to anorexigens. The European target INR is 2.0–3.0.
- **Diuretics.** These are used in patients with right heart failure and fluid overload.
- **Digoxin.** This may be helpful in patients with tachyarrhythmias.
- **Calcium-channel blockers.** These can be effective in high doses in selected patients with IPAH who demonstrate a response to a vasodilator challenge. Right heart catheterization should be repeated in 3–4 months to assess response to therapy.
- **Prostanoids.** Prostacyclin is a potent vasodilator that also inhibits platelet aggregation and cell proliferation. Synthetic prostacyclins are generally short-acting compounds requiring continuous intravenous or subcutaneous infusion or regular aerosol inhalation. They provide symptomatic relief and can improve exercise capacity; **epoprostenol** can improve survival in patients with both IPAH and associated pulmonary arterial hypertension. Oral **selexipag** has been approved by the US Food and Drug Administration for PAH treatment.
- **Endothelin receptor antagonists.** Endothelin-1 is a potent vasoconstrictor and mitogen that binds to endothelin A and B receptors in the pulmonary vasculature. Both dual antagonists (**bosentan**) and selective A receptor antagonists (**sitaxentan**, **ambrisentan**) can improve symptoms, exercise capacity and haemodynamics in patients with IPAH.
- **Phosphodiesterase type 5 inhibitors.** These produce vasodilation in the pulmonary vasculature and reduce cellular proliferation. **Sildenafil** and **tadalafil** have been demonstrated to provide symptomatic relief and improve exercise capacity in patients with IPAH.
- **Balloon atrial septostomy.** This technique may be considered as palliative therapy in severe cases of PH.
- **Lung transplantation.** This is used in patients with an adverse prognosis, although the 5-year survival following transplantation may be only 40–50%.

Other pulmonary hypertension groups

Left-sided heart disease (systolic and diastolic heart failure) and valvular heart disease are frequently associated with PH, as is advanced chronic obstructive pulmonary disease (see p. 956), pulmonary fibrosis and emphysema. Following acute pulmonary embolism, 0.5–2.0% of patients will develop chronic thromboembolic pulmonary hypertension (CTEPH).

MYOCARDIAL AND ENDOCARDIAL DISEASE

CARDIAC TUMOURS

Primary cardiac tumours are rare and three-quarters of these are benign.

Atrial myxomas are the most common. Most are sporadic but some are familial or part of a multi-system syndrome (Carney complex – hyperpigmented skin lesions with extracardiac tumours). Histologically, they are benign, polypoid, gelatinous structures. Most are solitary and occur in the left atrium (75%), attached by a pedicle to the atrial septum. The tumour may obstruct the mitral valve or may be a site of thrombi, which can embolize. The mean age of presentation is 50 years and there is a female predominance. Patients may be asymptomatic or present with dyspnoea, syncope or a mild fever. Physical signs include a loud first heart sound, a tumour 'plop' (a loud third heart sound produced as the pedunculated tumour comes to an abrupt halt), a mid-diastolic murmur and/or signs of embolization. Echocardiography, CT and CMR are appropriate to

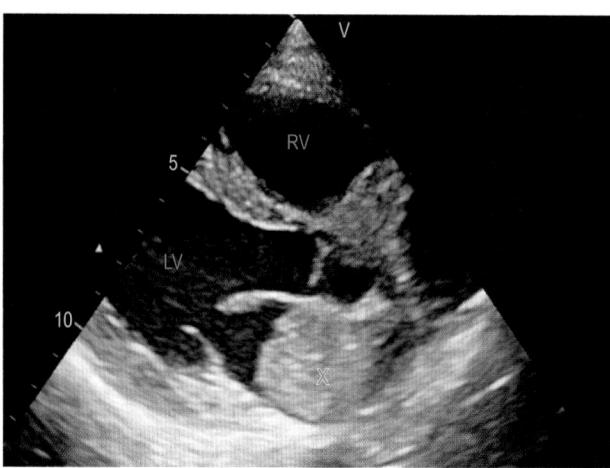

Fig. 30.104 Atrial myxoma shown by a two-dimensional echocardiogram (long-axis view). The myxoma (X) is an echo-dense mass obstructing the mitral valve orifice. It was removed surgically. LV, left ventricle; LA, left atrium.

confirm the diagnosis (**Fig. 30.104**) prior to cardiac surgery. Because of local recurrence, long-term surveillance is recommended.

Other benign cardiac tumours include lipoma, papillary fibro-elastoma, fibroma, haemangioma and rhabdomyoma.

Malignant primary cardiac tumours include angiosarcoma, undifferentiated sarcoma, rhabdomyosarcoma (children), osteosarcoma and leiomyosarcoma. Primary cardiac lymphoma typically occurs in the right heart.

Metastatic spread (**secondary cardiac tumours**) is 20–40 times more common. Direct invasion can occur with bronchogenic, breast and oesophageal carcinoma. There may be haematogenous or lymphatic spread with lymphoma, leukaemia, transvenous renal cell carcinoma, hepatoma and adrenal tumours. Pericardial effusions are common and pericardiocentesis may be required for diagnosis or for cases with cardiac tamponade.

MYOCARDIAL DISEASE

Myocardial disease that is not due to ischaemic, valvular or hypertensive heart disease, or a known infiltrative, metabolic/toxic or neuromuscular disorder, may be caused by:
- an acute or chronic inflammatory pathology (myocarditis)
- idiopathic myocardial disease (cardiomyopathy).

Myocarditis

Acute inflammation of the myocardium has many causes (**Box 30.51**). In North America and Europe the most common causes of inflammation are viruses (enteroviruses, adenoviruses, human herpes virus-6, Epstein–Barr virus, cytomegalovirus, hepatitis C and parvovirus B19). Chagas' disease, due to *Trypanosoma cruzi*, which is endemic in South America, is one of the most common causes of myocarditis worldwide. Additionally, toxins (including prescribed drugs), physical agents, hypersensitivity reactions and autoimmune conditions may also cause myocardial inflammation.

Pathology

In the acute phase, myocarditic hearts are flabby with focal haemorrhages; in chronic cases, they are enlarged and hypertrophied.

? Box 30.51 Causes of myocarditis

- Idiopathic
- Infective:
  - Viral: coxsackievirus, adenovirus, cytomegalovirus, echovirus, influenza, polio, hepatitis, HIV
  - Parasitic: *Trypanosoma cruzi, Toxoplasma gondii* (a cause of myocarditis in the newborn or immunocompromised)
  - Bacterial: streptococcus (most commonly, rheumatic carditis), diphtheria (toxin-mediated heart block common)
  - Spirochaetal: Lyme disease (heart block common), leptospirosis
  - Fungal
  - Rickettsial
- Toxic:
  - Drugs: those causing hypersensitivity reactions, e.g. methyldopa, penicillin, sulphonamides, antituberculous, modafinil
  - Radiation: may cause myocarditis but pericarditis is more common
- Autoimmune:
  - An autoimmune form with autoactivated T cells and organ-specific antibodies may occur
  - Giant cell myocarditis
- Alcohol
- Hydrocarbons

? Box 30.52 Causes of sudden cardiac death

Coronary artery disease
- Acute myocardial infarction – STEMI
- Chronic ischaemic heart disease
- Following coronary artery bypass surgery
- Following successful resuscitation for cardiac arrest
- Congenital anomaly of coronary arteries
- Coronary artery embolism
- Coronary arteritis

Non-coronary artery disease
- Hypertrophic cardiomyopathy
- Dilated cardiomyopathy (ischaemic or idiopathic)
- Arrhythmogenic right ventricular cardiomyopathy
- Congenital long QT syndrome
- Brugada's syndrome
- Valvular heart disease (aortic stenosis, mitral valve prolapse) ± infective endocarditis
- Cyanotic heart disease (tetralogy of Fallot, transposition)
- Acyanotic heart disease (ventricular septal defect, patent ductus arteriosus)

STEMI, ST elevation myocardial infarction.

Histologically (**Fig. 30.105**), an inflammatory infiltrate is present – lymphocytes predominating with viral causes, polymorphonuclear cells with bacterial causes, and eosinophils with allergic and hypersensitivity causes.

Clinical features

Myocarditis typically presents in young adult patients. Presentation may vary from mild fatigue, palpitations, chest pain and dyspnoea through to fulminant congestive cardiac failure. Physical examination reveals soft heart sounds, a prominent third sound and often a tachycardia. A pericardial friction rub may be heard.

Investigations

- **ECG** may demonstrate diffuse ST- and T-wave abnormalities (concave ST elevation) and arrhythmias. AV block may be seen with Lyme disease, sarcoid, giant-cell myocarditis and Chagas' disease (see later).

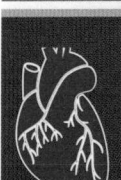

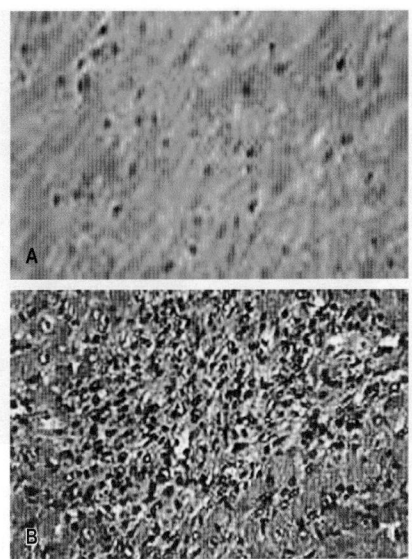

Fig. 30.105 Myocardial biopsies. (A) Normal myocardium. **(B)** Myocarditis, with increased interstitial inflammatory cells.

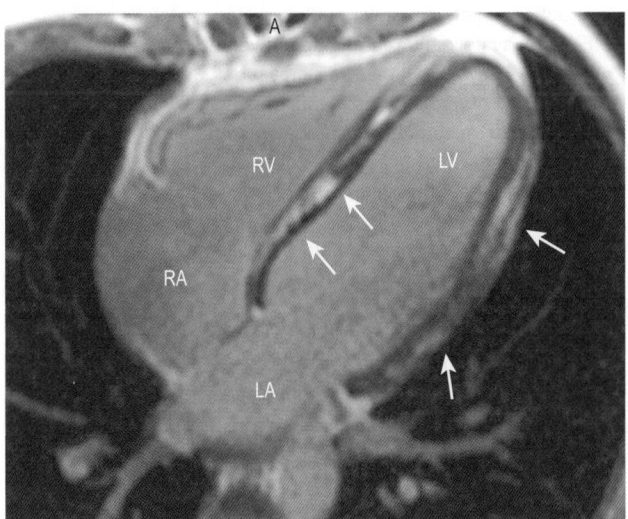

Fig. 30.106 Acute myocarditis. There is patchy mid-wall and epicardial myocardial enhancement (arrowed) with gadolinium. A, anterior chest wall; LA, left atrium; LV, left ventricle; RA, right atrium; RV, right ventricle.

- **Echocardiography** is required and may reveal normal or reduced bi-ventricular function with resting regional wall motion abnormalities.
- **Blood tests** include ESR and CRP, which are frequently elevated in the acute presentation. Cardiac troponin and creatine kinase levels will also be elevated. Viral serology is not usually helpful.
- **CMR** is recommended to confirm the diagnosis. Patients with acute myocarditis may demonstrate myocardial oedema on T2-weighted images and patchy myocardial enhancement with gadolinium (**Fig. 30.106**).
- **Endomyocardial biopsy** is considered the gold standard for the diagnosis of myocarditis although its use is reserved for selected patients (fulminant presentation or clinical deterioration) as this is an invasive test performed in specialised units.
- **Coronary angiography** is frequently performed to exclude acute ischaemia as the cause of the patient's presentation.

Management

Myocarditis resolves within a few weeks in the majority of patients, although a small percentage of patients deteriorate and may require urgent transfer to a cardiac centre with access to extracorporeal membrane oxygenation and/or cardiac transplantation. Bed rest is recommended in the acute phase of the illness and athletic activities should be avoided for 6 months. Heart failure should be treated in the usual way (see p. 1073).

Giant cell myocarditis

This severe form of myocarditis is characterized by the presence of multinucleated giant cells within the myocardium. The cause is unknown but it may be associated with sarcoidosis, thymomas and autoimmune disease. The disease has a rapidly progressive course and a poor prognosis. Immunosuppression is recommended.

Chagas' disease

Chagas' disease (see p. 568) is caused by the protozoon *Trypanosoma cruzi* and is endemic in South America, where upwards of 20 million people are infected. Acutely, features of myocarditis are present with fever and congestive heart failure. Chronically, there is progression to a dilated cardiomyopathy with a propensity towards heart block and ventricular arrhythmias. Treatment is discussed on page 569. Amiodarone is helpful for the control of ventricular arrhythmias; heart failure is treated in the usual way.

Cardiomyopathy

Cardiomyopathies are a group of diseases of the myocardium that affect the mechanical or electrical function of the heart. The ESC provides a classification system according to morphological and functional differences:
- hypertrophic cardiomyopathy (HCM)
- arrhythmogenic cardiomyopathy (ACM)
- dilated cardiomyopathy (DCM)
- restrictive cardiomyopathies (RCM)
- unclassified.

Patients can be further divided into familial (genetic) and non-familial subtypes.

Hypertrophic cardiomyopathy

HCMs include a group of inherited conditions that produce hypertrophy of the myocardium in the absence of an alternative cause (e.g. aortic stenosis or hypertension). It is the most common cause of sudden cardiac death in young people and affects 1 in 500 of the population. The majority of cases are familial autosomal dominant and are due to mutations in the genes encoding sarcomeric proteins (**Fig. 30.107**). The most common causes of HCM are mutations of the β-myosin heavy chain *MYH7* and myosin-binding protein C *MYBPC3*.

There are non-sarcomeric protein mutations in genes that control cardiac metabolism that result in glycogen storage diseases (Danon's, Pompe's and Fabry's diseases) and cause cardiac hypertrophy that may be indistinguishable from inherited HCM on echocardiography.

Clinical features

HCM is characterized by myocardial hypertrophy that frequently involves the interventricular septum, and by disorganization ('disarray') of cardiac myocytes and myofibrils. Some 25% of patients have dynamic left ventricular outflow tract obstruction due to the

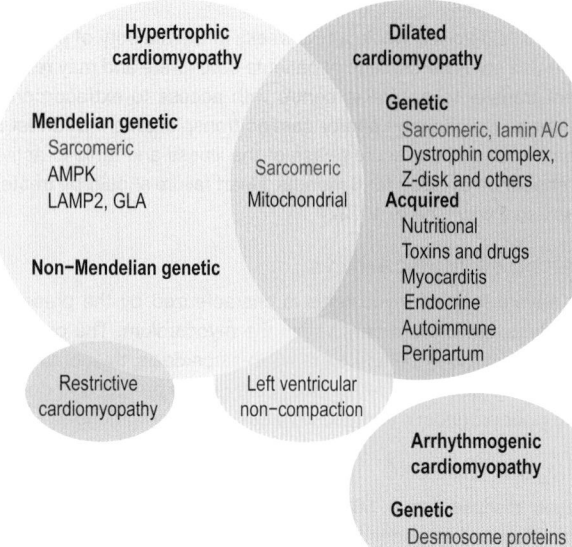

Fig. 30.107 Cardiomyopathy: clinical categories and genetic basis. Hypertrophic and dilated cardiomyopathies share the same genes, as do the less common restrictive cardiomyopathy and left ventricular non-compaction. Arrhythmogenic cardiomyopathy (ACM) is genetically different. AMPK, adenosine monophosphate-activated kinase; GLA, galactosidase A; LAMP2, lysosomal assisted membrane protein 2; TMEM43, transmembrane protein 43. *(From Watkins H, Ashrafian H, Redwood C. Inherited cardiomyopathies. N Engl J Med 2011; 364:1643–1656, with permission.)*

combined effects of hypertrophy, systolic anterior motion of the anterior mitral valve leaflet and rapid ventricular ejection. The salient clinical and morphological features of the disease vary according to the underlying genetic mutation. For example, marked hypertrophy is common with β-myosin heavy chain mutations, whereas mutations in troponin T may be associated with mild hypertrophy but a high risk of sudden death. The hypertrophy may not manifest before completion of the adolescent growth spurt, making the diagnosis difficult in children. HCM due to myosin-binding protein may not manifest until the sixth decade of life or later.

Symptoms

- Many cases are asymptomatic and are detected by family screening of an affected individual or by a routine ECG examination.
- Chest pain, dyspnoea, syncope or pre-syncope (typically with exertion), cardiac arrhythmias and sudden death are seen.
- Sudden death occurs at any age but the highest rates (up to 6% per annum) occur in adolescents or young adults. Risk factors for sudden death are discussed later.
- Dyspnoea occurs due to impaired relaxation of the heart muscle or the left ventricular outflow tract obstruction that occurs in some patients. The systolic cavity remains small until the late stages of disease, when progressive dilation may occur. If a patient develops atrial fibrillation, there is often a rapid deterioration in clinical status due to the loss of atrial contraction and the tachycardia, resulting in elevated left atrial pressure and acute pulmonary oedema.

Signs

- Double apical pulsation (forceful atrial contraction producing a fourth heart sound).

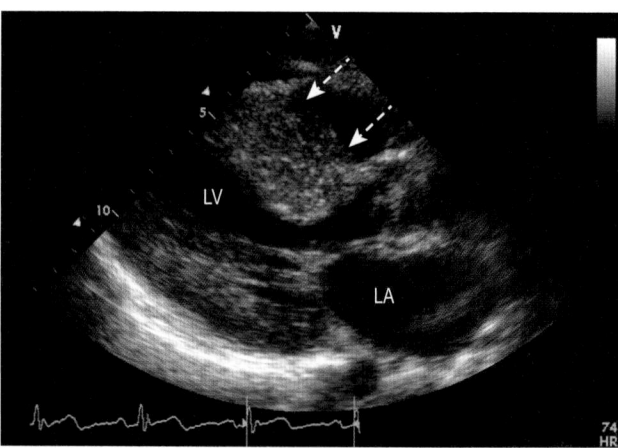

Fig. 30.108 Hypertrophic cardiomyopathy. A two-dimensional echocardiogram (short-axis view). The grossly thickened interventricular septum is shown, resulting in a small left ventricular cavity. This condition is associated with an abnormal anterior motion of the mitral valve during systole (arrowed). LA, left atrium; LV, left ventricle.

- Jerky carotid pulse because of rapid ejection and sudden obstruction to left ventricular outflow during systole.
- Ejection systolic murmur due to left ventricular outflow obstruction late in systole; it can be increased by manoeuvres that decrease afterload, such as standing or Valsalva, and decreased by manoeuvres that increase afterload and venous return, such as squatting.
- Pansystolic murmur due to mitral regurgitation (secondary to systolic anterior motion).
- Fourth heart sound (if not in atrial fibrillation).

Investigations

- **ECG** abnormalities in HCM include left ventricular hypertrophy (see **Fig. 30.79**), ST- and T-wave changes, and abnormal Q waves, especially in the inferolateral leads.
- **Echocardiography** is usually diagnostic. In classical HCM, there is asymmetric left ventricular hypertrophy (involving the septum more than the posterior wall), systolic anterior motion of the mitral valve, and a vigorously contracting ventricle (**Fig. 30.108**). However, any pattern of hypertrophy may be seen, including concentric and apical hypertrophy.
- **CMR** can detect both the hypertrophy and abnormal myocardial fibrosis (**Fig. 30.109**) and can differentiate between HCM and infiltrative cardiomyopathies.
- **Genetic analysis**, where available, may confirm the diagnosis and provide prognostic information for the patient and relatives.

Management

The management of HCM includes treatment of symptoms and prevention of sudden cardiac death in the patient and relatives.

Risk factors for sudden death are:

- massive left ventricular hypertrophy (>30 mm on echocardiography)
- family history of sudden cardiac death (<50 years old)
- non-sustained ventricular tachycardia on 24-hour Holter monitoring
- prior unexplained syncope
- abnormal blood pressure response on exercise (flat or hypotensive response).

The presence of these cardiac risk factors is associated with an increased risk of sudden death (**Box 20.52**), and patients with two

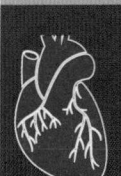

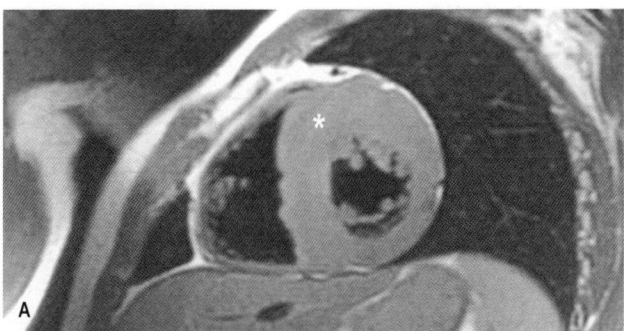

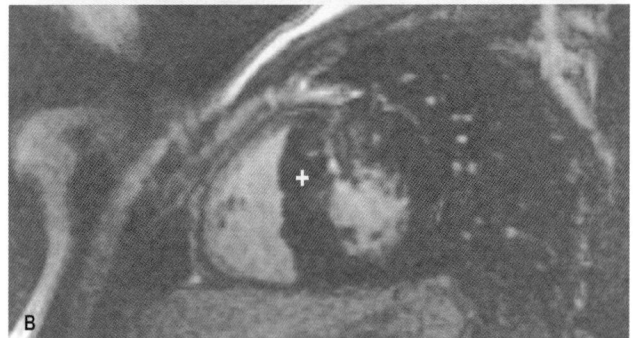

Fig. 30.109 Cardiac magnetic resonance imaging in a patient with hypertrophic cardiomyopathy. (A) Turbo spin-echo demonstrates marked thickening of the basal to mid-anterior wall and septum (*). **(B)** Inversion recovery image post gadolinium demonstrates regional fibrosis with enhancement (+).

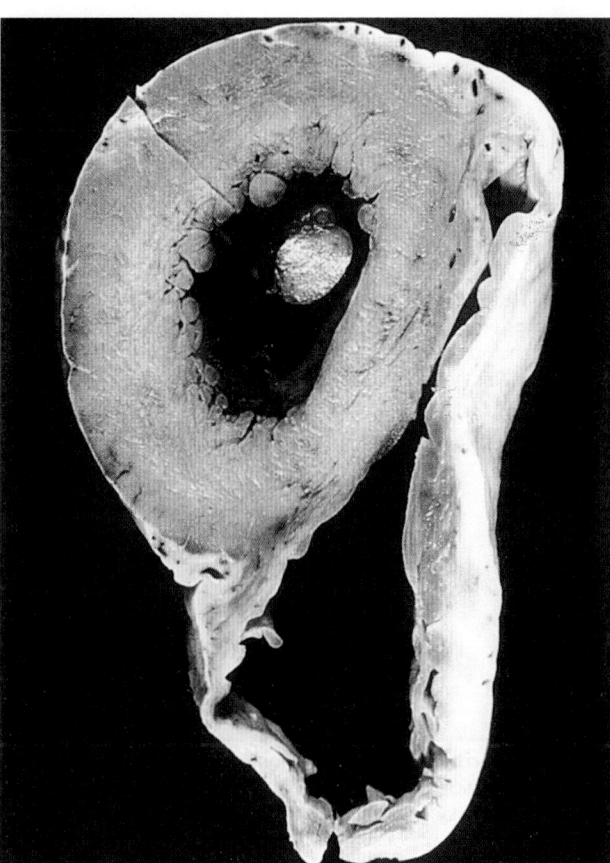

Fig. 30.110 Gross pathological specimen demonstrating thinning and fibro-fatty replacement of the right ventricular free wall from a patient with arrhythmogenic cardiomyopathy. *(From Basso C, Thiene G, Corrado D et al. Arrhythmogenic right ventricular cardiomyopathy. Dysplasia, dystrophy, or myocarditis? Circulation 1996; 94:983–991, with permission.)*

or more should be assessed for ICD insertion. When the risk is less, amiodarone is an appropriate alternative.

Chest pain and dyspnoea are treated with beta-blockers and verapamil, either alone or in combination. An alternative agent is disopyramide if patients have left ventricular outflow tract obstruction. In some individuals with significant left outflow obstruction and symptoms, dual-chamber pacing is necessary. Alcohol (non-surgical) ablation of the septum has been investigated and appears to give good results in reduction of outflow tract obstruction and subsequent improvement in exercise capacity. This procedure carries risks, including the development of complete heart block and MI. Occasionally, surgical resection of septal myocardium may be indicated. Vasodilators should be avoided because they may aggravate left ventricular outflow obstruction or cause refractory hypotension.

Arrhythmogenic cardiomyopathy/ arrhythmogenic right ventricular cardiomyopathy

Arrhythmogenic cardiomyopathy (ACM) is an uncommon (1 in 1000–5000 population) inherited condition that predominantly affects the right ventricle with fatty or fibro-fatty replacement of myocytes, leading to segmental or global dilation (**Fig. 30.110**). Left ventricular involvement has been reported in up to 75% of cases. The fibro-fatty replacement leads to ventricular arrhythmia and risk of sudden death in its early stages, and right ventricular or biventricular failure in its later stages.

Autosomal dominant ACM has been mapped to mutations in genes coding for desmosomal proteins. These are the cardiac ryanodine receptor RyR2 (see p. 1024; also responsible for familial catecholaminergic polymorphic ventricular tachycardia, CPVT), desmoplakin, plakophilin-2 and mutations altering the regulatory sequences of the TGF-β gene.

There are two recessive forms: **Naxos disease** (associated with palmoplantar keratoderma and woolly hair), which is due to a mutation in junctional plakoglobin, and **Carvajal's syndrome**, due to a mutation in desmoplakin.

Clinical features

Most patients are asymptomatic. Symptomatic ventricular arrhythmia, syncope or sudden death occurs. Occasionally, presentation is with symptoms and signs of right heart failure, although this is more common in the later stages of the disease. Some patients may be detected through family screening, although frequently the morphological appearance of the right ventricle is normal, despite significant cardiac arrhythmias.

Investigations and diagnosis

- **ECG** is usually normal but may demonstrate T-wave inversion in the precordial leads related to the right ventricle (V_1–V_3). Small-amplitude potentials occurring at the end of the QRS complex (epsilon waves) may be present (**Fig. 30.111**) and incomplete or complete right bundle branch block is sometimes seen. Signal-averaged ECG may indicate the presence of late potentials and the delayed depolarization of individual muscle cells; 24-hour Holter monitoring may demonstrate frequent extrasystoles of right ventricular origin or runs of non-sustained ventricular tachycardia.

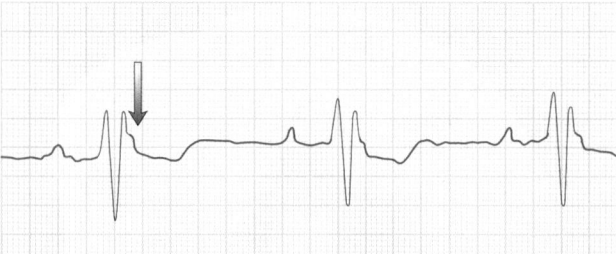

Fig. 30.111 Electrocardiogram from an adult with arrhythmogenic cardiomyopathy. The ECG demonstrates right bundle branch block and precordial T-wave insertion, with epsilon waves visible at the terminal of the QRS complex (arrowed).

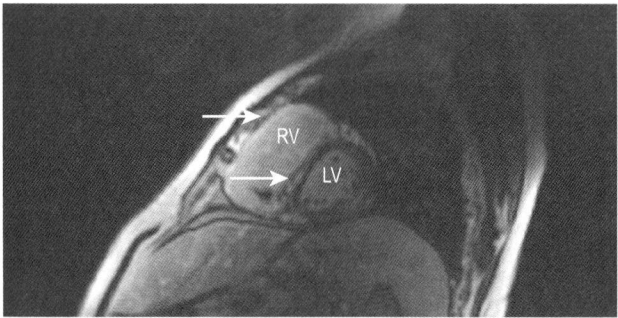

Fig. 30.112 Arrhythmogenic cardiomyopathy (ACM). Inversion recovery magnetic resonance image post gadolinium demonstrates marked hyper-enhancement (arrowed) in the right ventricular free wall and inferoseptum consistent with fibro-fatty replacement in right ventricle (RV) and left ventricle (LV).

- **Echocardiography** is frequently normal but with more advanced cases may demonstrate right ventricular dilation and aneurysm formation; there may be left ventricular dilation.
- **CMR** can assess the right ventricle more accurately and in some cases can demonstrate fibro-fatty infiltration (**Fig. 30.112**).
- **Genetic testing** may soon be the diagnostic 'gold standard'.

Clinical diagnosis is made using Task Force Criteria, which include:

- structural abnormalities of the right ventricle and right ventricular outflow tract (dilation and abnormal wall motion on echocardiography or MRI)
- fibro-fatty replacement of myocytes on tissue biopsy
- repolarization and conduction abnormalities on ECG or signal-averaged ECG
- ventricular tachycardia or frequent ventricular extrasystoles on Holter monitoring
- family history of ACM in a first- or second-degree relative
- premature sudden death (<35 years) due to ACM.

Management

Beta-blockers are first-line treatment for patients with non-life-threatening arrhythmias. Amiodarone or sotalol is used for symptomatic arrhythmias but for refractory or life-threatening arrhythmias an ICD is required. Occasionally, cardiac transplantation is indicated for either intractable arrhythmia or cardiac failure.

Dilated cardiomyopathy

Dilated cardiomyopathy (DCM) has a prevalence of 7–12 in 100 000 and is characterized by dilation of the ventricular chambers and systolic dysfunction with preserved wall thickness.

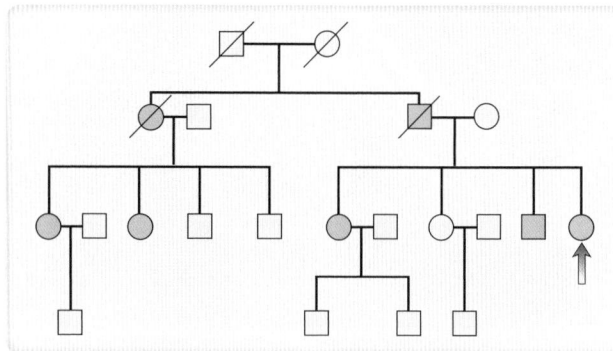

Fig. 30.113 Pedigree of a family with dilated cardiomyopathy. Blue symbols are affected family members. The arrow indicates the index case.

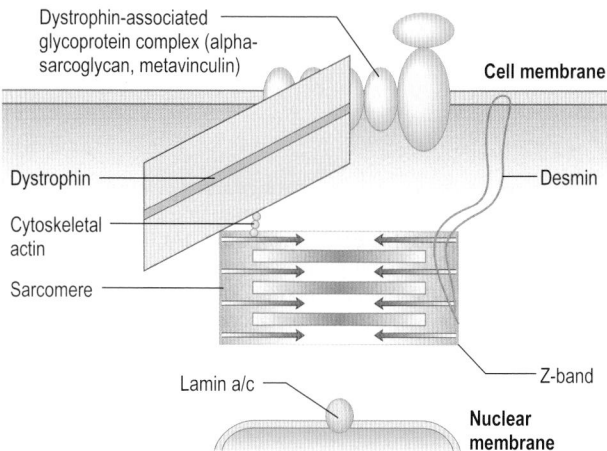

Fig. 30.114 Myocyte proteins implicated in dilated cardiomyopathy.

Familial DCM is predominantly autosomal dominant and can be associated with over 20 abnormal loci and genes (**Fig. 30.113**). Many of these are genes encoding cytoskeletal or associated myocyte proteins (dystrophin in X-linked cardiomyopathy; actin, desmin, troponin T, β-myosin heavy chain, sarcoglycans, vinculin and lamin a/c in autosomal dominant DCM; **Fig. 30.114**). Many of these have prominent associated features, such as skeletal myopathy or conduction system disease, and therefore differ from the majority of cases of DCM.

Sporadic DCM can be caused by multiple conditions:
- myocarditis: Coxsackievirus, adenoviruses, erythroviruses, HIV, bacteria, fungi, mycobacteria, parasitic (Chagas' disease)
- toxins: alcohol, chemotherapy, metals (cobalt, lead, mercury, arsenic)
- autoimmune disorders
- endocrine disorders
- neuromuscular disorders.

Clinical features

DCM can present with heart failure, cardiac arrhythmias, conduction defects, thromboembolism or sudden death. Increasingly, evaluation of relatives of DCM patients is allowing identification of early asymptomatic disease, prior to the onset of these complications. Clinical evaluation should include a family history and construction of a pedigree where appropriate.

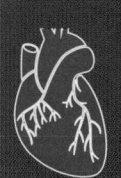

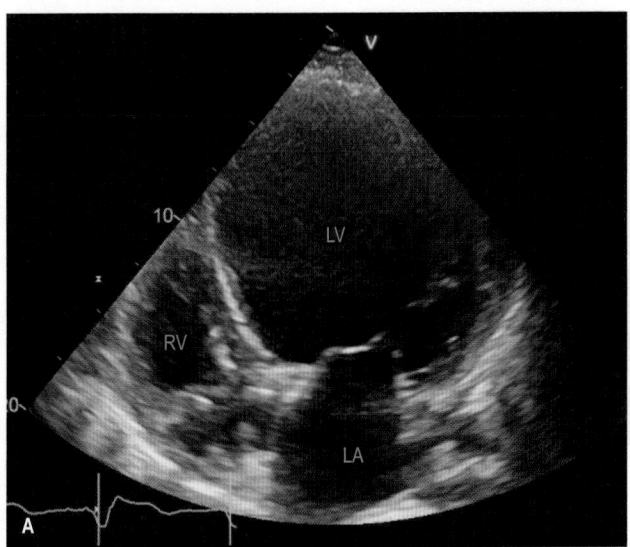

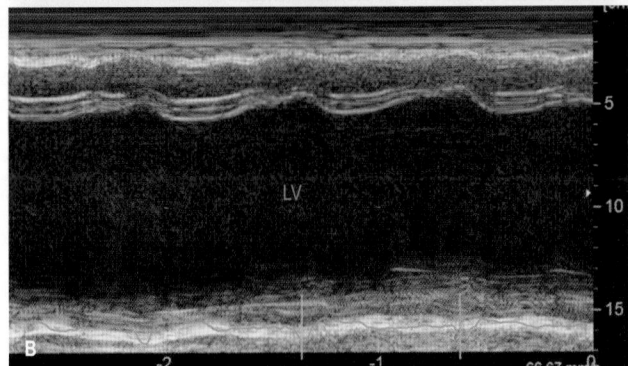

Fig. 30.115 Dilated cardiomyopathy. (A) Two-dimensional (apical four-chamber view) echocardiogram. The heart has a 'globular' appearance with all four chambers dilated. **(B)** M mode echocardiogram. The extremely impaired left ventricular function can be appreciated by comparing the systolic shortening fraction with that of **Figure 30.23**. LA, left atrium; LV, left ventricle; RA, right atrium.

Investigations

- **ECG** may demonstrate diffuse non-specific ST-segment and T-wave changes. Sinus tachycardia, conduction abnormalities and arrhythmias (i.e. atrial fibrillation, ventricular premature contractions or ventricular tachycardia) are also seen.
- **Echocardiogram** reveals dilation of the left and/or right ventricle with poor global contraction function (**Fig. 30.115**).
- **CMR** may demonstrate other aetiologies of left ventricular dysfunction (e.g. previous MI) or show abnormal myocardial fibrosis (**Fig. 30.116**).
- **Coronary angiography** or CTCA should be performed to exclude coronary artery disease in all individuals at risk (generally, patients >40 years, or younger if symptoms or risk factors are present).
- **Biopsy** is not normally indicated outside specialist care.

Management

Treatment consists of the conventional management of heart failure with the option of cardiac resynchronization therapy and ICDs in patients with NYHA III/IV grading. Cardiac transplantation is appropriate for certain patients.

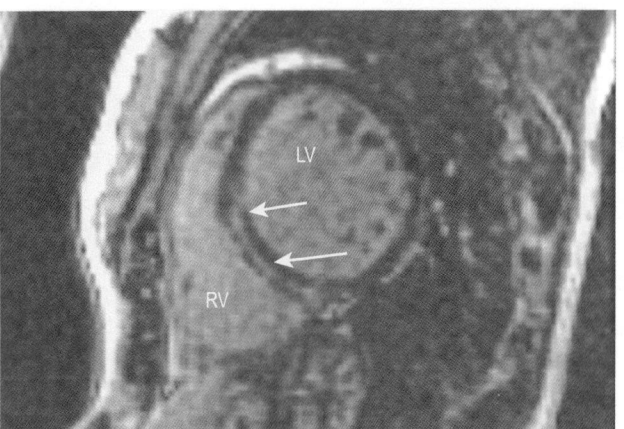

Fig. 30.116 Dilated cardiomyopathy. Inversion recovery magnetic resonance scan post gadolinium demonstrates septal mid-wall hyper-enhancement (arrowed) consistent with fibrosis in a patient with dilated cardiomyopathy. LV, left ventricle; RV, right ventricle.

Left ventricular non-compaction

Left ventricular non-compaction (LVNC) is associated with a sponge-like appearance of the left ventricle. The condition predominantly affects the apical portion of the left ventricle and may be associated with congenital heart abnormalities. LVNC is diagnosed by echocardiography, CMR or left ventricular angiography. The natural history is unresolved but includes congestive cardiac failure, thromboembolism, cardiac arrhythmias and sudden death. Familial and spontaneous cases have been described.

Primary restrictive non-hypertrophic cardiomyopathy

In this rare condition there is normal or decreased volume of both ventricles with bi-atrial enlargement, normal wall thickness, normal cardiac valves and impaired ventricular filling with restrictive physiology but near-normal systolic function. The restrictive physiology produces symptoms and signs of heart failure. Conditions associated with this form of cardiomyopathy include amyloidosis (most common, see p. 1358), sarcoidosis, Loeffler's endocarditis and endomyocardial fibrosis; in the latter two conditions there is myocardial and endocardial fibrosis, associated with eosinophilia. The idiopathic form of restrictive cardiomyopathy may be familial.

Clinical features

Patients with restrictive cardiomyopathy may present with dyspnoea, fatigue and embolic symptoms. On clinical examination there will be elevated JVP with diastolic collapse (Friedreich's sign) and elevation of venous pressure with inspiration (Kussmaul's sign), hepatic enlargement, ascites and dependent oedema. Third and fourth heart sounds may be present.

Investigations

- **ECG** may demonstrate low-voltage QRS and ST-segment and T-wave abnormalities.
- **Echocardiography** shows symmetrical myocardial thickening and often a normal systolic ejection fraction, but impaired ventricular filling. In amyloid patients the myocardium typically appears speckled with absent radial thickening, as demonstrated by 'tramlines' on M-mode echocardiography (**Fig. 30.117**).
- **CMR** may show abnormal myocardial fibrosis in amyloidosis or sarcoidosis.

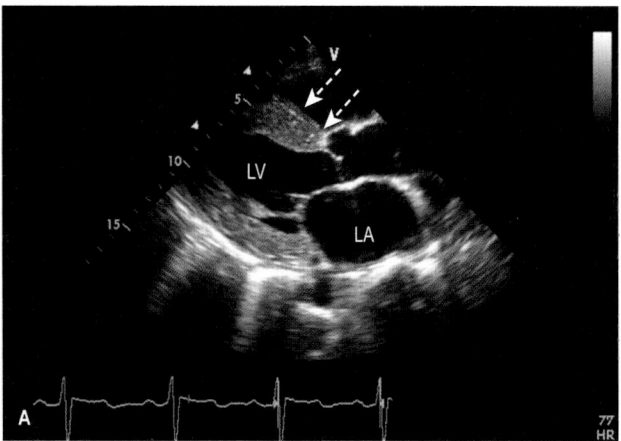
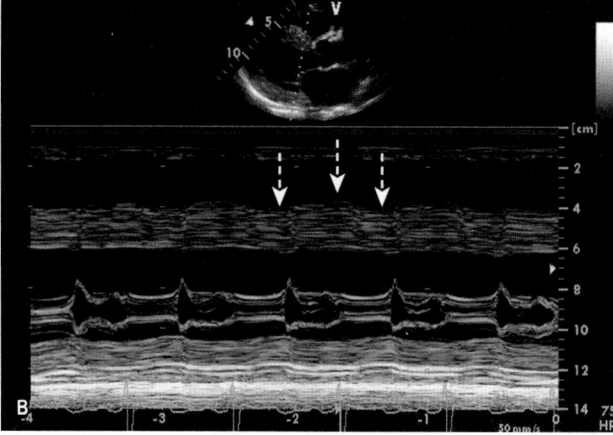

Fig. 30.117 Cardiac amyloidosis. (A) Parasternal long-axis echocardiogram demonstrating left ventricular hypertrophy with reduced systolic function. The septum has a speckled appearance (arrowed). LA, left atrium; LV, left ventricle. **(B)** M-mode echocardiogram demonstrates reduced septal thickening with a 'tramline' appearance (arrowed). These features are suggestive of cardiac amyloid – confirmed on cardiac biopsy.

- ***Cardiac catheterization*** and haemodynamic studies may help distinguish between restrictive cardiomyopathy and constrictive pericarditis, although volume loading may be required.
- ***Endomyocardial biopsy*** is often useful in this condition, in contrast to other cardiomyopathies, and may permit a specific diagnosis, such as amyloidosis, to be made.

Management

There is no specific treatment. Cardiac failure and embolic manifestations should be treated. Cardiac transplantation is necessary in some severe cases, especially the idiopathic variety. Management of primary amyloidosis is discussed elsewhere (p. 1358). However, patients with cardiac amyloidosis have a worse prognosis than those with other forms of the disease, and the disease often recurs after transplantation. Liver transplantation may be effective in familial amyloidosis (due to production of mutant pre-albumin) and may lead to reversal of the cardiac abnormalities.

Acquired cardiomyopathies
Stress (Tako-tsubo/octopus pot/apical ballooning syndrome) cardiomyopathy

Patients with this condition present acutely with chest pain and breathlessness associated with ECG changes and elevated cardiac biomarkers consistent with acute MI. Diagnostic coronary angiography typically demonstrates unobstructed coronary arteries, with characteristic akinesia of the mid-apical segments of the left ventricle on ventriculography or echocardiography, and preserved basal function (**Fig. 30.118**). The pathophysiology is uncertain but disease may be due to transient catecholamine excess, coronary vasospasm, abnormalities of the coronary microcirculation and hypertrophy of the basal septum. The syndrome is more common in middle-aged to elderly women. Severe cases may have cardiogenic shock and pulmonary oedema. Patients with a significant left ventricular gradient may respond to cautious beta-blockade. Complete recovery of function is usual within 4–6 weeks but there are recurrences.

Peripartum cardiomyopathy

This rare condition affects women in the last trimester of pregnancy or within 5 months of delivery. It presents as a dilated cardiomyopathy, is more common in obese, multiparous women over 30 years old, and is associated with pre-eclampsia. Nearly half of patients

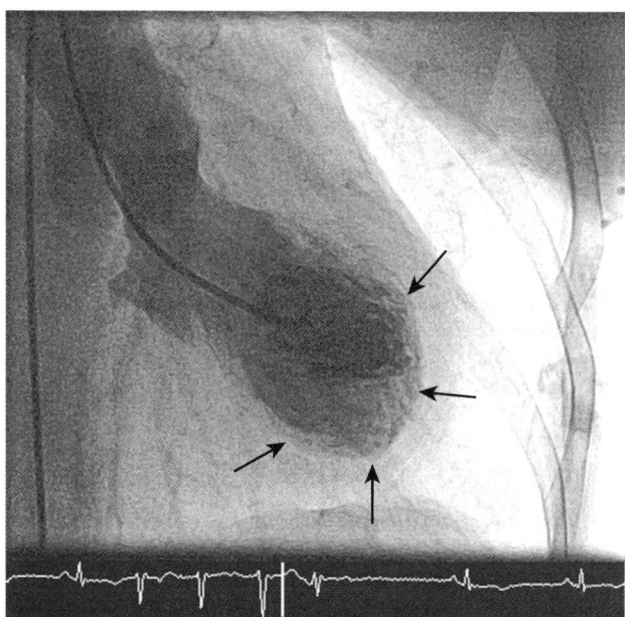

Fig. 30.118 Tako-tsubo cardiomyopathy. Left ventricular angiography in a patient admitted with chest pain following emotional stress demonstrates apical ballooning (arrowed) consistent with Tako-tsubo cardiomyopathy. Diagnostic coronary angiography showed normal coronary arteries.

will recover to normal function within 6 months but in some it can cause progressive heart failure and sudden death.

Tachycardia cardiomyopathy

Prolonged periods of supraventricular or ventricular tachycardia will lead to dilated cardiomyopathy. Cardioversion and ablation may be necessary to restore sinus rhythm and allow for recovery of cardiac function.

Further reading

Caforio AL, Pankuweit S, Arbustini E et al. Current state of knowledge on aetiology, diagnosis, management, and therapy of myocarditis: a position statement of the European Society of Cardiology Working Group on Myocardial and Pericardial Diseases. *Eur Heart J* 2013; 34:2636–2648.

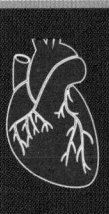

PERICARDIAL DISEASE

The pericardium acts as a protective covering for the heart. It consists of an outer fibrous pericardial sac and an inner serous pericardium; the latter is made up of the inner visceral epicardium that lines the heart and great vessels, and its reflection, the outer parietal pericardium that lines the fibrous sac. The normal amount of pericardial fluid is 20–49 mL and this fluid lubricates the surface of the heart. Presentations of pericardial disease include:

- acute, incessant and chronic pericarditis
- pericardial effusion and cardiac tamponade
- constrictive pericarditis
- pericardial masses.

? **Box 30.53 Aetiology of pericarditis**

I. Infectious pericarditis
  – Viral (Coxsackievirus, echovirus, mumps, herpes, HIV)
  – Bacterial (staphylococcal, streptococcal, pneumococcal and meningococcal infections, *Haemophilus influenzae*, mycoplasmosis, borreliosis, chlamydia)
  – Tuberculous
  – Fungal (histoplasmosis, coccidioidomycosis, candidiasis)
II. Post-myocardial infarction pericarditis
  – Acute myocardial infarction (early)
  – Dressler's syndrome (late)
III. Malignant pericarditis
  – Primary tumours of the heart (mesothelioma)
  – Metastatic pericarditis (breast and lung carcinoma, lymphoma, leukaemia, melanoma)
IV. Uraemic pericarditis
V. Myxoedematous pericarditis
VI. Chylopericardium
VII. Autoimmune pericarditis
  – Collagen-vascular (rheumatoid arthritis, rheumatic fever, systemic lupus erythematosus, scleroderma)
  – Drug-induced (procainamide, hydralazine, isoniazid, doxorubicin, cyclophosphamides)
VIII. Post-radiation pericarditis
IX. Post-surgical pericarditis
  – Post-pericardiotomy syndrome
X. Post-traumatic pericarditis
XI. Familial and idiopathic pericarditis

Acute pericarditis

This term refers to inflammation of the pericardium, which may account for 5% of accident and emergency presentations with chest pain. The condition is more common in men, particularly young adults. Acute pericarditis has numerous aetiologies (**Box 30.53**), although, in most cases, a cause is not identified (idiopathic).

Clinical features and investigations

There are four common clinical features of acute pericarditis:

- **chest pain** that may be pleuritic, exacerbated by movement and relieved by sitting forwards
- **pericardial friction rub**
- **ECG abnormalities** with widespread concave-upwards (saddle-shaped) ST elevation (**Fig. 30.119**), reciprocal ST depression in leads AVR and V_1, and PR segment depression
- **pericardial effusion** (**Fig. 30.120**).

A clinical diagnosis of acute pericarditis can be made with two out of four of these features.

Inflammatory blood tests will be elevated (**CRP, ESR, white cell count**) and can be used to monitor disease resolution. Cardiac troponin and creatine kinase may be elevated in cases with myopericarditis. Chest X-ray may demonstrate cardiomegaly in patients with a large pericardial effusion.

Management and treatment

In 70–90% of cases acute pericarditis is self-limiting. Most patients can be treated with aspirin 750–1000 mg 3 times daily or ibuprofen 600–800 mg 3 times daily for 1–2 weeks, together with colchicine (0.5 mg twice daily for 3 months). Corticosteroids should be reserved for patients with a known immune cause, as their use is associated with an increased rate of recurrence. High-risk patients (fever >38°C, subacute onset, large effusion, tamponade, lack of response to therapy) should be admitted for treatment. Activity should be restricted until the inflammatory markers are normalized. Competitive athletes are advised to avoid exercise for at least 3 months.

Incessant or chronic pericarditis

About 20% of cases of acute pericarditis go on to develop idiopathic relapsing pericarditis, which may be incessant (recurring within 6 weeks) or chronic (lasting >3 months). The first-line treatment is non-steroidal anti-inflammatory drugs (NSAIDS) or aspirin

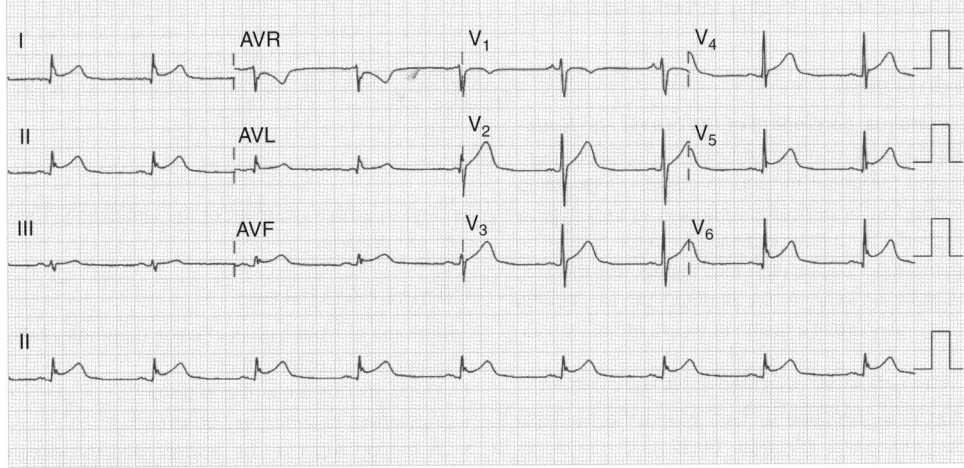

Fig. 30.119 Electrocardiogram associated with acute pericarditis. Note the diffuse, concave, raised ST segments seen in most leads.

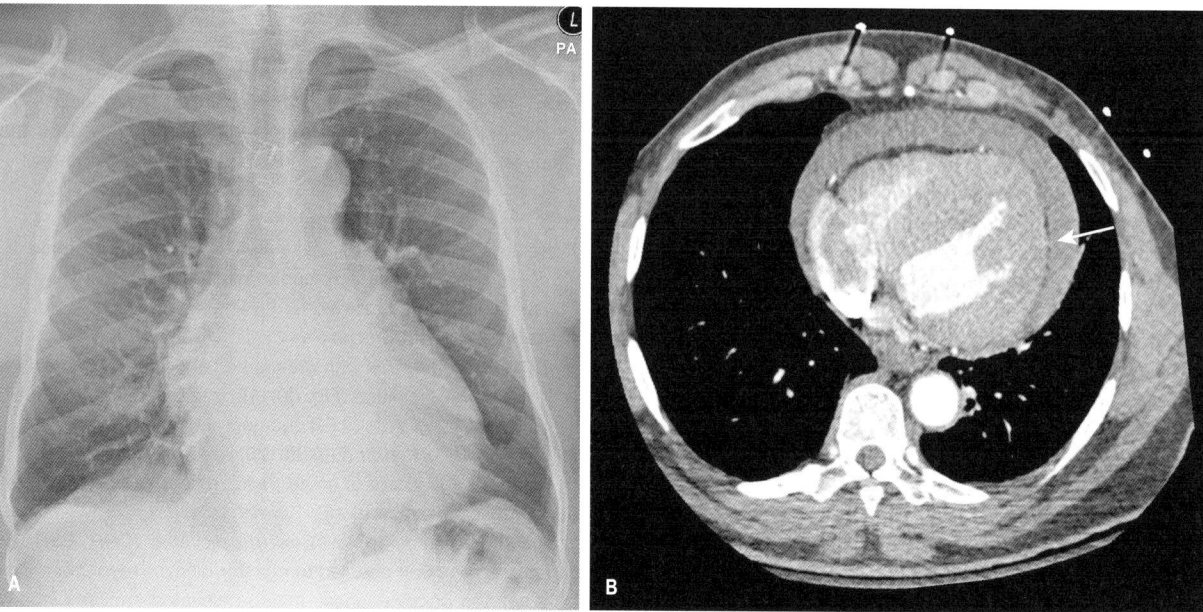

Fig. 30.120 Pericardial effusion. **(A)** Note the globular appearance to the cardiac silhouette on chest X-ray. **(B)** CT scan confirms the circumferential pericardial effusion (arrowed). Note the absence of pericardial calcification that is a feature of chronic pericardial disease.

with colchicine for up to 6 months. In resistant cases oral corticosteroids may be effective, and in some patients pericardiectomy may be appropriate. CT or CMR may be helpful in demonstrating thickened (>4 mm) or inflamed pericardium.

Tuberculous pericarditis

This is uncommon (<5%) in the developed world but may account for over 50% of cases in developing countries and over 90% in patients with HIV. Tuberculous pericarditis usually presents with chronic low-grade fever, particularly in the evening, associated with features of acute pericarditis, dyspnoea, malaise, night sweats and weight loss. Pericardial aspiration is often required to make the diagnosis. Constrictive pericarditis is a frequent outcome. Treatment is as for pulmonary tuberculosis (see p. 969) with added prednisolone 60 mg daily for 2–6 weeks.

Post-cardiac injury syndromes

This includes pericarditis following MI (Dressler's syndrome), cardiac surgery or trauma. An autoimmune reaction is triggered by myocardial or pericardial damage, leading to pericarditis. Recurrences are common.

Malignant pericarditis

Carcinoma of the bronchus, *carcinoma of the breast* and *Hodgkin's lymphoma* are the most common causes of malignant pericarditis. Leukaemia and malignant melanoma are also associated with pericarditis. A substantial pericardial effusion is very typical and is due to obstruction of lymphatic drainage from the heart. The effusion is often haemorrhagic. Radiation and therapy for thoracic tumours may cause radiation injury to the pericardium, resulting in serous or haemorrhagic pericardial effusion and pericardial fibrosis.

Pericardial effusion and cardiac tamponade

A pericardial effusion is a collection of fluid within the potential space of the serous pericardial sac (**Fig. 30.121**); it commonly accompanies an episode of acute pericarditis. When a large volume collects in this space, ventricular filling is compromised,

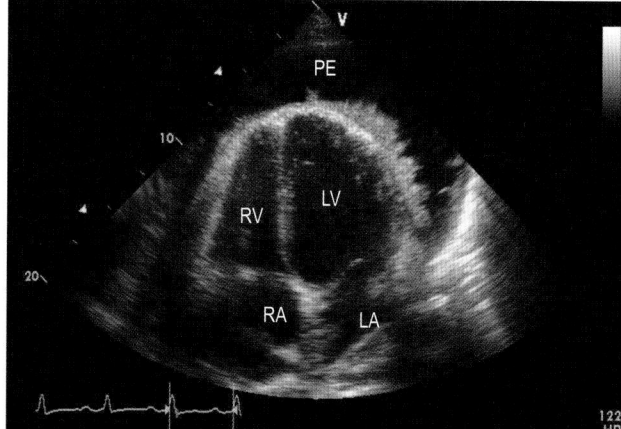

Fig. 30.121 Two-dimensional echocardiogram (short-axis view) from a patient with a large pericardial effusion associated with pulmonary tuberculosis. The exudate is seen between the visceral and parietal layers of the pericardium and would give a false impression of cardiomegaly on a chest X-ray. Note the multiple fibrous strands within the effusion, showing that it is consolidating and will probably lead to constriction of cardiac function. LA, left atrium; LV, left ventricle; PE, pericardial effusion; RA, right atrium; RV, right ventricle.

leading to embarrassment of the circulation. This is known as cardiac tamponade.

Clinical features

Symptoms of a pericardial effusion commonly reflect the underlying pericarditis. On examination:
- Heart sounds are soft and distant.
- Apex beat is commonly obscured.
- A friction rub may be evident due to pericarditis in the early stages, but this becomes quieter as fluid accumulates and pushes the layers of the pericardium apart.

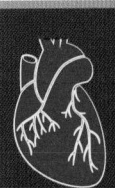

- Rarely, the effusion may compress the base of the left lung, producing an area of dullness to percussion below the angle of the left scapula (Ewart's sign).
- As the effusion worsens, signs of cardiac tamponade may become evident:
  - raised JVP with sharp x descent
  - Kussmaul's sign (rise in JVP/increased neck vein distension during inspiration)
  - pulsus paradoxus (an exaggeration in the normal variation in pulse pressure seen with inspiration, such that there is a drop in systolic blood pressure of ≥10 mmHg)
  - reduced cardiac output.

Investigations

- ***ECG*** reveals low-voltage QRS complexes (<0.5 mV in limb leads) with sinus tachycardia and there may be electric alternans (alteration of QRS amplitude or axis between beats).
- ***Chest X-ray*** (see **Fig. 30.120A**) shows a large, globular or pear-shaped heart with sharp outlines. Typically, the pulmonary veins are not distended.
- ***Echocardiography*** (see **Fig. 30.121**) is the most useful technique for demonstrating the effusion and looking for evidence of tamponade: late diastolic collapse of the right atrium, early diastolic collapse of the right ventricle, ventricular septum displacement into the left ventricle during inspiration, diastolic flow reversal in the hepatic veins during expiration, and dilated inferior vena cava with <50% reduction during inspiration.
- ***Cardiac CT or MRI*** is helpful if loculated pericardial effusions are suspected (post cardiac surgery).
- ***Pericardiocentesis*** is the removal of pericardial fluid with an aseptic technique under echocardiographic guidance (see **Fig. 30.36**). It is indicated when a tuberculous, malignant or purulent effusion is suspected.
- ***Pericardial biopsy*** may be needed if tuberculosis is suspected and pericardiocentesis is not diagnostic.

Other tests may be needed to identify underlying causes: for example, blood cultures or autoantibody screen.

Management

An underlying cause should be sought and treated if possible. Most pericardial effusions resolve spontaneously. However, when the effusion collects rapidly, tamponade may result. Pericardiocentesis is then indicated to relieve the pressure; a drain may be left in place temporarily to allow sufficient release of fluid. Pericardial effusions may re-accumulate, most commonly due to malignancy (in the UK). This may require pericardial fenestration: that is, creation of a window in the pericardium to allow the slow release of fluid into the surrounding tissues. This procedure may be performed either transcutaneously under local anaesthetic or using a conventional surgical approach.

Constrictive pericarditis

Certain causes of pericarditis, such as tuberculosis, haemopericardium, bacterial infection and rheumatic heart disease, result in the pericardium becoming thick, fibrous and calcified. This may also develop late after open heart surgery, and fibrosis also occurs with the use of dopamine agonists, such as cabergoline and pergolide. In many cases these pericardial changes do not cause any symptoms. If, however, the pericardium becomes so inelastic as to interfere with diastolic filling of the heart, constrictive pericarditis is said to have developed. As these changes are chronic, allowing the body time to compensate, this condition is not as immediately life-threatening as cardiac tamponade, in which the circulation is more acutely embarrassed.

Constrictive pericarditis should be distinguished from restrictive cardiomyopathy (see p. 1123). The two conditions are very similar in their presentation but the former is fully treatable, whereas most cases of the latter are not. In the later stages of constrictive pericarditis, the subepicardial layers of myocardium may undergo fibrosis, atrophy and calcification.

Clinical features

The symptoms and signs of constrictive pericarditis occur due to:
- reduced ventricular filling (similar to cardiac: Kussmaul's sign, sharp, pulsus paradoxus; different to tamponade: raised JVP with deep y descent or Friedreich's sign)
- systemic venous congestion (ascites, dependent oedema, hepatomegaly and raised JVP)
- pulmonary venous congestion (dyspnoea, cough, orthopnoea, paroxysmal nocturnal dyspnoea)
  Less commonly, the cause may be:
- reduced cardiac output (fatigue, hypotension, reflex tachycardia)
- rapid ventricular filling (a 'pericardial knock' is heard in early diastole at the lower left sternal border)
- atrial dilation (30% of cases have atrial fibrillation).

Investigations

- ***Chest X-ray*** shows a relatively small heart in view of the symptoms of heart failure. Pericardial calcification may be present in up to 50%. A lateral chest film may be useful for detecting calcification that is missed on a postero-anterior film. However, a calcified pericardium is not necessarily a constricted one.
- ***ECG*** reveals low-voltage QRS complexes with generalized T-wave flattening or inversion.
- ***Echocardiography*** shows thickened, calcified pericardium and small ventricular cavities with normal wall thickness. Doppler studies may be useful.
- ***CT and CMR*** are used to assess pericardial anatomy and thickness (≥4 mm) (see **Fig. 30.28**).
- ***Endomyocardial biopsy*** may be helpful in distinguishing constrictive pericarditis from restrictive cardiomyopathy in difficult cases.
- ***Cardiac catheterization*** will usually reveal equal end-diastolic pressures in the left and right ventricles, owing to pericardial constriction.

Restrictive cardiomyopathy is a close mimic of constrictive pericarditis and all the above tests may help to distinguish the two conditions.

Management

The treatment for chronic constrictive pericarditis is complete resection of the pericardium. This is a risky procedure with a high complication rate due to the presence of myocardial atrophy in many cases at the time of surgery. Thus, early pericardiectomy is suggested in non-tuberculous cases, before severe constriction and myocardial atrophy have developed.

In cases of tuberculous constriction, the presence of pericardial calcification implies chronic disease. Early pericardiectomy with antituberculous drug cover is used in these cases. If there is no calcification, a course of antituberculous therapy should be attempted first. If the patient's haemodynamic state remains static or deteriorates after 4–6 weeks of therapy, pericardiectomy is recommended.

Further reading

Adler Y, Charron P, Imazio M et al. 2015 ESC Guidelines for the diagnosis and management of pericardial diseases: The Task Force for the Diagnosis and Management of Pericardial Diseases of the European Society of Cardiology (ESC). *Eur Heart J* 2015; 36:2921–2964.
Bogaert J, Francone M. Cardiovascular magnetic resonance in pericardial diseases. *J Cardiovasc Magn Reson* 2009; 11:14.
Welch TD. Constrictive pericarditis: diagnosis, management and clinical outcomes. *Heart* 2018; 104:725–731.

PERIPHERAL VASCULAR DISEASE

PERIPHERAL ARTERIAL DISEASE

Peripheral vascular disease (PVD) is commonly caused by atherosclerosis and usually affects the aorto-iliac or infra-inguinal arteries. It is present in 7% of middle-aged men and 4.5% of middle-aged women, but the mortality associated with coexisting cardiovascular and cerebrovascular disease means that only a proportion of patients with PVD progress to losing their leg.

Limb ischaemia

Limb ischaemia may be classified as chronic or acute.

Chronic lower limb ischaemia

Common risk factors are:
- smoking
- diabetes
- hypercholesterolaemia
- hypertension.

Premature atherosclerosis in patients aged below 45 years may be associated with thrombophilia and hyperhomocysteinaemia.

Clinical features

Symptoms

Peripheral arterial disease can be described using the Fontaine classification:
- Stage I: asymptomatic
- Stage II: intermittent claudication
- Stage III: rest pain/nocturnal pain
- Stage IV: necrosis/gangrene.

Patients with *intermittent claudication* complain of exertional discomfort, most commonly in the calf, which is relieved by rest. Patients with aorto-iliac disease may experience pain in the buttock, hip or thigh and may notice erectile dysfunction. The 'claudication distance' may be reproducible.

Patients with *rest pain* experience severe, unremitting pain in the foot, which stops a patient from sleeping. It is partially relieved by dangling the foot over the edge of the bed or standing on a cold floor.

Patients with severe PVD or critical lower limb ischaemia may have ulceration or *necrosis* of the tissue (*gangrene*).

Signs

The lower limbs are cold with dry skin and lack of hair. Pulses may be diminished or absent. Ulceration may occur in association with dark discoloration of the toes or gangrene. The abdomen should be examined for a possible aortic aneurysm.

Differential diagnosis

Symptoms may be confused with those of:
- spinal canal claudication (when all pulses are present)
- osteoarthritis of the hip/knee (knee pain often at rest)
- peripheral neuropathy (associated with numbness and tingling)
- popliteal artery entrapment (young patients who may have normal pulses)
- venous claudication (bursting pain on walking with a previous history of a DVT)
- fibromuscular dysplasia
- Buerger's disease (young males, heavy smokers).

Investigations

An estimation of the anatomical level of disease may be possible with the examination of pulses. The severity of disease is indicated by the *ankle/brachial pressure index* (ABPI). This is a measurement of the cuff pressure at which blood flow is detectable by Doppler in the posterior tibial or anterior tibial artery compared to the pressure in the brachial artery (ankle/brachial pressure). Intermittent claudication is associated with an ABPI of 0.5–0.9, while values less than 0.5 are associated with critical limb ischaemia. The sensitivity of the test may be improved by a fall in ABPI after exercise. If the arteries are heavily calcified and incompressible, commonly where there is coexisting renal or diabetic disease, the ABPI will be falsely elevated. In these patients toe pressure values are more sensitive. Diagnostic imaging includes the following options:
- *Duplex ultrasound using B-mode ultrasound and colour Doppler* is usually the first-line investigation and can provide an accurate anatomical map of the lower limbs with sensitivity of 87% and specificity of 94% compared to formal angiography.
- *Contrast-enhanced MR angiography* provides excellent imaging of both legs with a single contrast injection without exposure to ionizing radiation, and is commonly used to assess the extent of disease prior to planned intervention.
- *CT angiography* is an effective alternative to MR angiography where MR is contraindicated, although extensive calcification may obscure stenoses. CT angiography requires ionizing radiation and iodinated contrast media.
- *Digital subtraction angiography (DSA)* provides an arterial map (**Fig. 30.122**) but requires peripheral arterial cannulation and exposes the individual to iodinated contrast; it should be reserved for use in patients immediately prior to intervention.

Management

Medical

All patients need aggressive risk factor management, as PVD also puts them at significant risk of ischaemic heart disease and cerebrovascular disease. Those with diabetes require careful glycaemic control and regular review by a chiropodist.

A supervised exercise programme should be offered to all patients with intermittent claudication, where they are encouraged to undergo aerobic exercise for at least 2 hours per week, up to the point of maximal pain.

Naftidrofuryl oxalate is a vasodilator agent that inhibits vascular and platelet 5-hydroxytryptamine$_2$ (5-HT$_2$) receptors and can reduce lactic acid levels. At a dose of 1–200 mg three times a day, it may increase walking distance and improve quality of life. It should be considered for a trial period of 3–6 months when patients are reluctant to undergo interventional treatment and supervised exercise has proved insufficient to control symptoms.

Surgical and radiological

Vascular intervention for stable claudication is not generally recommended, except when symptoms are severe or disabling. *Percutaneous transluminal angioplasty* is the first option and is carried out via a catheter inserted into the femoral artery. The long-term

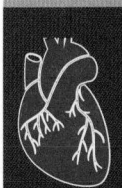
has previously reported symptoms of claudication. Thrombus may also form in normal vessels in individuals who are hypercoagulable because of malignancy or thrombophilia defects. Prosthetic or venous grafts may also thrombose either *de novo* or secondary to a developing stenosis in the graft or the native vessels. Popliteal aneurysms may thrombose or embolize distally.

Acute upper limb ischaemia may be caused by similar processes or occur secondary to external compression with a cervical rib/band.

Investigations

Investigations are similar to those described for chronic lower limb disease.

Management

Medical

Management is dependent on the degree of ischaemia. Patients showing improvement may be treatable with heparin and appropriate treatment of the underlying cause. Those with emboli following MI or atrial fibrillation need long-term warfarin.

Surgical and radiological

Patients with mild to moderate ischaemic symptoms who have an occluded graft may need graft thrombolysis. Intra-arterial thrombolysis may reveal an underlying stenosis within a graft or native vessel that could be treated with angioplasty. Patients with an embolus may benefit from its surgical removal (embolectomy). A bypass graft may be required after occlusion of a popliteal aneurysm or acute-on-chronic lower limb arterial disease. When an ischaemic limb is revascularized, the sudden improvement in blood flow can cause reperfusion injury, with release of toxic metabolites into the circulation. In muscle compartments the consequent oedema may lead to a 'compartment syndrome', which requires fasciotomies (release of the fascia to prevent muscle damage). An amputation may be warranted in unreconstructable or severe ischaemia. In patients dying from other causes, acute limb ischaemia may occur as a 'terminal event' and intervention may then be inappropriate.

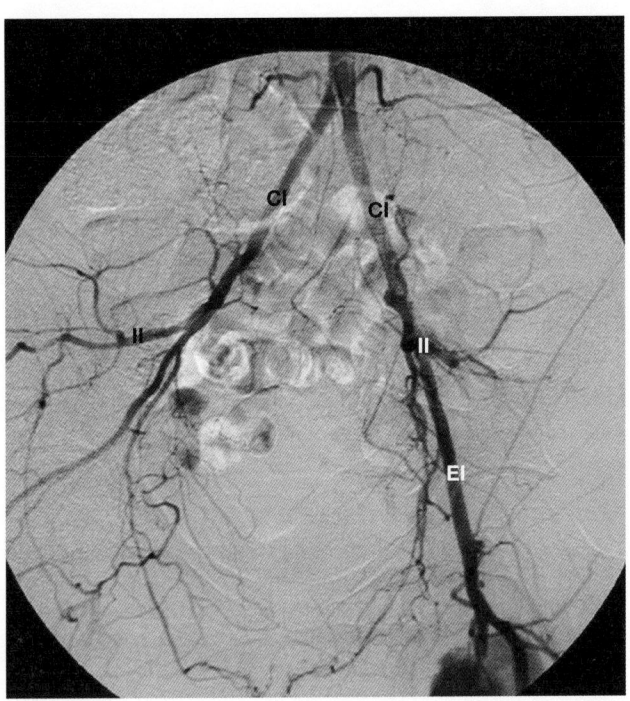

Fig. 30.122 Angiogram showing occlusion of the right external iliac artery. CI, common iliac; EI, external iliac; II, internal iliac.

patency rates decrease as the angioplasty becomes more distal. Overall results of angioplasty appear to be similar to those achieved with a continued exercise programme. Arterial stents may be deployed in recurrent iliac disease, and drug-eluting stents allowing long-term patency are also used. **Bypass procedures** may be performed using Dacron, polytetrafluoroethylene (PTFE) or autologous veins. Bypasses to distal vessels have poorer long-term patencies. Prosthetic grafts have equal patencies in above-knee bypasses but are inferior to veins in bypasses below the knee. In severe ischaemia with unreconstructable arterial disease, an **amputation** may be necessary. An amputation commonly leads to loss of independence, with only 70% of below-knee and 30% of above-knee amputees achieving full mobility.

Acute lower limb ischaemia

Clinical features

Symptoms

Patients complain of the 'five Ps': *pain*, the fact that the leg looks white (*pallor*), *paraesthesia*, *paralysis* and the sensation that it is *perishingly* cold. The pain is unbearable and normally requires opioids for relief.

Signs

The limb is cold, with mottling or marbling of the skin. Pulses are diminished or absent. Sensation in and movement of the leg are reduced in severe ischaemia. Patients may develop a compartment syndrome with pain in the calf on compression.

Aetiology

Acute limb ischaemia (ALI) may occur because of embolic or thrombotic disease. **Embolic disease** is commonly due to cardiac thrombus and cardiac arrhythmias such as atrial fibrillation. Emboli may also occur secondary to aneurysm thrombus or thrombus on atherosclerotic plaques. Emboli from atrial myxomas are rare.

ALI is more often due to **thrombotic disease**. Acute thrombus usually forms on a chronic atherosclerotic stenosis in a patient who

Aneurysmal disease

Aneurysms are defined as a permanent dilation of the artery to twice the normal diameter and may be classified as true or false. In true aneurysms the arterial wall forms the wall of the aneurysm. The arteries most frequently involved are the abdominal aorta, the iliac, popliteal and femoral arteries, and the thoracic aorta (in decreasing frequency). In false aneurysms (pseudoaneurysms) the surrounding tissues form the wall of the aneurysm. False aneurysms can occur following femoral artery puncture. A haematoma is formed because of inadequate compression of the entry site and continued bleeding into the surrounding compressed soft tissue forms the wall of this aneurysm.

Abdominal aortic aneurysm

Abdominal aortic aneurysms (AAAs) occur most commonly below the renal arteries (infra-renal). The incidence increases with age, AAAs being present in 5% of the population over 60 years of age. They arise five times more frequently in men, and in 1 in 4 male children of an affected individual. Aneurysms may occur secondary to atherosclerosis, infection (syphilis, *Escherichia coli*, *Salmonella*) and trauma, or may be genetic (Marfan's or Ehlers–Danlos syndrome).

Screening

In England and Wales the prevalence of AAA is 3–4% of men aged 65 years or more, and approximately 6000 deaths occur each year from a ruptured aortic aneurysm. The mortality rate for elective surgery is 3.5% or lower, compared to 50% for an emergency repair. There are fixed risk factors – age, male gender, strong family history – and modifiable risk factors – smoking, hypertension, hypercholesterolaemia.

The UK recommendation is that screening should be offered to men aged 65–74 years, who receive an abdominal ultrasound.

- **Normal** or **<3cm** aortas do not require treatment or further scans.
- **Small (3–4.4cm)** aortas require annual ultrasound surveillance and GP review to optimize lifestyle.
- **Medium (4.5–5.4cm)** aortas require quarterly ultrasound surveillance and cardiovascular secondary prevention therapy.
- **Large (≥5.5cm)** aortas are referred for assessment and possible elective repair.

Screening of female patients is *not* recommended, as the prevalence is much lower.

Clinical features

Symptoms

Most aneurysms are asymptomatic and are found on routine abdominal examination or plain X-ray, or during urological investigations. Rapid expansion or rupture of an AAA may cause **severe pain** (epigastric pain radiating to the back). A ruptured AAA causes **hypotension**, **tachycardia**, **profound anaemia** and **sudden death**. The symptoms of rupture may mimic renal colic, diverticulitis and severe lower abdominal or testicular pain. Gradual erosion of the vertebral bodies may cause non-specific back pain. The aneurysm may embolize distally causing acute limb ischaemia. Inflammatory aneurysms can obstruct adjacent structures, such as the ureter, duodenum and vena cava. Rarely, aneurysms can present with severe haematemesis secondary to an aortoduodenal fistula.

Signs

The aorta is retroperitoneal and in overweight patients there may be no overt signs. An aneurysm is suspected if a pulsatile, expansile abdominal mass is felt. The presence of an AAA should alert a clinician to the possibility of popliteal aneurysms. Patients may present with 'trash feet', dusky discoloration of the digits secondary to emboli from the aortic thrombus.

Management

As with any operation, treatment of an asymptomatic aneurysm depends on the balance of operative risk and conservative management. The UK Small Aneurysm Trial showed that patients with infra-renal AAAs did best with an operation if the aneurysm was:

- ≥5.5cm in diameter
- expanding at a rate of >1cm/year
- symptomatic.

Medical

Aneurysmal disease needs careful control of hypertension, smoking cessation and lipid-lowering medication. Patients with AAAs of less than 5.5cm are followed up by regular ultrasound surveillance.

Surgical and endovascular intervention

Intervention to treat AAA can be performed by open aneurysm repair, hand-assisted or total laparoscopic repair, or endovascular stent insertion (via the femoral or iliac arteries). The Endovascular Aneurysm Repair (EVAR) studies (stent versus open surgical repair) and EVAR 2 (stent versus medical therapy in patients unsuitable for open repair) investigated the role of endovascular stents in patients with an AAA of 5.5cm or more on CT. In EVAR, the 30-day mortality rate was 1.7% with stenting versus 4.7% with surgery ($p=0.009$) but the long-term mortality rate was similar in both groups at 4 years. In EVAR 2, the 30-day mortality rate with stenting was 9%. Long-term mortality rate was similar in both stent and medical therapy groups. Current UK guidance recommends surgical repair rather than EVAR for unruptured aneurysms, although this is presently being reviewed. EVAR has a more prominent role in treating ruptured aneurysms, especially in older and frailer patients.

Prognosis

After repair, patients with an AAA should return to normal activity within a few months.

Thoraco-abdominal aneurysm

The ascending, arch or descending thoracic aorta may become aneurysmal. Ascending thoraco-abdominal aneurysms (TAAs) occur most commonly in patients with Marfan's syndrome or hypertension. Descending or arch TAAs occur secondary to atherosclerosis and are now rarely due to syphilis.

Clinical features

Most aneurysms are asymptomatic and are found on routine chest X-ray or cardiological investigation. Rapid expansion may cause severe pain (chest pain radiating to the upper back) and rupture is associated with hypotension, tachycardia and death. Chest symptoms from expansion may include stridor (compressed bronchial tree), haemoptysis (aortobronchial fistula) and hoarseness (compression of the recurrent laryngeal nerve). Aorto-oesophageal fistula is an uncommon cause of haematemesis.

Investigations

- **CT or MRI scan** is used for assessment of a TAA.
- **Aortography** may be helpful for assessing the position of the key branches in relation to the aneurysm.
- **TOE** can be useful for identifying an aortic dissection.

Management

If the aneurysm is bigger than 6cm, then operative repair or stenting may be appropriate, but these procedures can be technically difficult and carry a high risk of mortality and paraplegia. EVAR is, at present, the procedure of choice for isolated descending thoracic aneurysms.

Acute aortic syndromes

Acute aortic syndromes include aortic dissection, intramural haematoma (IMH) and penetrating aortic ulcers. Aortic dissection usually begins with a tear in the intima. Blood penetrates the diseased medial layer and then cleaves the intimal laminal plain, leading to dissection. IMH is considered a precursor of dissection, in which there is rupture of the vasa vasorum in the aortic media with aortic wall infarction. IMH is typically in the descending thoracic aorta. Deep penetrating aortic plaques may lead to IMH, dissection or ulceration/perforation. There is a predisposition to aortic dissection in patients with autoimmune rheumatic disorders and Marfan's and Ehlers–Danlos syndromes.

Aortic dissection can be classified according to the timing of diagnosis from the origin of symptoms: acute, less than 2 weeks; subacute, 2–8 weeks; and chronic, more than 8 weeks, with

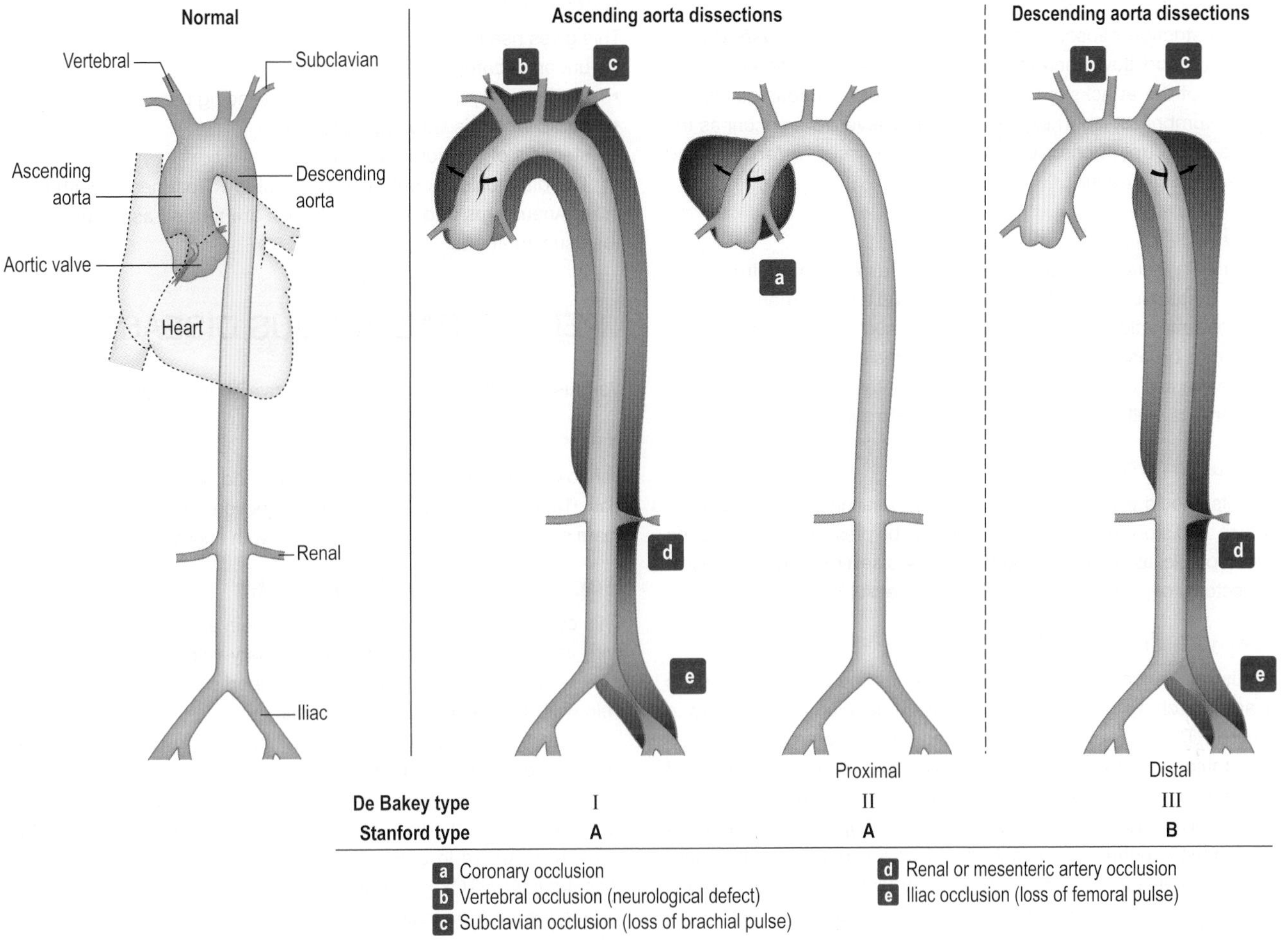

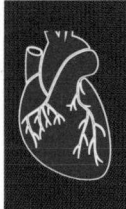

Normal

Vertebral — — Subclavian

Ascending aorta — — Descending aorta

Aortic valve —

Heart

— Renal

— Iliac

Ascending aorta dissections

Descending aorta dissections

De Bakey type	I	II	III
Stanford type	A	A	B
		Proximal	Distal

a Coronary occlusion
b Vertebral occlusion (neurological defect)
c Subclavian occlusion (loss of brachial pulse)
d Renal or mesenteric artery occlusion
e Iliac occlusion (loss of femoral pulse)

Fig. 30.123 Classification of aortic aneurysms.

mortality and extension decreasing with time. It can also be classified anatomically:

- **Type A** involves the aortic arch and aortic valve proximal to the left subclavian artery origin. This category includes De Bakey type I (extends to the abdominal aorta) and De Bakey type II (localized to the ascending aorta).
- **Type B** involves the descending thoracic aorta distal to the left subclavian artery origin. This category includes De Bakey type III (**Fig. 30.123**).

Clinical features

Symptoms

Most patients present with a sudden onset of severe and central **chest pain** that often radiates to the back and down the arms, mimicking MI. The pain is often described as tearing in nature and may be migratory.

Signs

Patients may be shocked and may have neurological symptoms secondary to loss of blood supply to the spinal cord. They may develop aortic regurgitation, coronary ischaemia and cardiac tamponade. Distal extension may produce acute kidney failure, acute lower limb ischaemia or visceral ischaemia. Peripheral pulses may be absent.

Investigations

The mediastinum may be widened on chest X-ray; urgent CT scan, TOE or MRI will confirm the diagnosis (see **Fig. 30.102**).

Management

At least 50% of patients are hypertensive and may require urgent antihypertensive medication to reduce blood pressure to below 120 mmHg; intravenous beta-blockers (labetalol, metoprolol) and vasodilators (GTN) are used. Type A dissections should undergo surgery (arch replacement) if the patient is fit enough, as medical management carries a high mortality (50% within 2 weeks). Type B dissections carry a better prognosis and have a survival rate of 89% at 1 month; initially, these patients should be managed medically unless they develop complications. Endovascular intervention with stents may be indicated in individuals with rapidly expanding dissections (>1 cm/year), critical diameter (>5.5 cm), refractory pain or malperfusion syndrome, blunt chest trauma, penetrating aortic ulcers or IMH. Patients will require long-term follow-up with CT or MRI.

Other types of peripheral arterial disease

Raynaud's phenomenon or Raynaud's disease

Raynaud's phenomenon consists of spasm of the digital arteries, usually precipitated by cold and relieved by heat. If there is no underlying cause, it is known as Raynaud's disease. This affects 5% of the population, mostly women. The disorder is usually bilateral and fingers are affected more commonly than toes.

Clinical features

Vasoconstriction causes skin **pallor** followed by **cyanosis** due to sluggish blood flow, then redness secondary to hyperaemia. The duration of the attacks is variable but they can sometimes last for hours. Numbness, a burning sensation and severe pain occur as the fingers warm up. In chronic, severe disease tissue, **infarction** and **digital loss** can occur.

Diagnosis

Primary Raynaud's disease needs to be differentiated from secondary treatable causes leading to Raynaud's phenomenon. These are the rheumatic autoimmune disorders, such as systemic sclerosis. It can be associated with atherosclerosis or occupations that involve the use of vibrating tools. Ergot-containing drugs and beta-blockers, as well as smoking, can aggravate symptoms.

Management

Patients should avoid cold provocation by wearing gloves and warm clothes, and stop smoking. Vasodilators can be prescribed but are often unacceptable, as cerebral vasodilation causes severe headaches. Sympathectomy or prostacyclin infusion can be helpful in severe disease.

Takayasu's disease

This is rare, except in Japan. It is known as the pulseless disease or aortic arch syndrome. It is of unknown aetiology and occurs in females. There is a vasculitis involving the aortic arch, as well as other major arteries. A systemic illness is also present, with pain and tenderness over the affected arteries. Absent peripheral pulses and hypertension are common. Corticosteroids help the constitutional symptoms. Eventually, heart failure and strokes may occur but most patients survive for at least 5 years. Treatment may involve a surgical bypass to improve perfusion of the affected areas.

Thromboangiitis obliterans (Buerger's disease)

This disease, involving the small vessels of the lower limbs, occurs in young men who smoke. Although sometimes clinically indistinguishable from atheromatous disease, pathologically there is inflammation of the arteries and sometimes veins, which may indicate a separate disease entity. Clinically, it presents with severe claudication and rest pain, leading to gangrene. A thrombophlebitis is sometimes present. Treatment is as for all peripheral vascular disease but patients must stop smoking.

Cardiovascular syphilis

This gives rise to:
- uncomplicated aortitis
- aortic aneurysms, usually in the ascending part
- aortic valvulitis with regurgitation
- stenosis of the coronary ostia.

The diagnosis is confirmed by serology. Treatment is with penicillin. Aneurysms and valvular disease are treated as necessary by the usual methods.

PERIPHERAL VENOUS DISEASE

Venous thromboembolic disease is covered in Chapter 29.

Varicose veins

Varicose veins are a common problem and sometimes give rise to pain. They may be treated by surgery, injection with ultrasound-guided foam sclerotherapy, or thermal ablation with endovenous lasers.

Superficial thrombophlebitis

This commonly affects the saphenous vein and is often associated with varicosities. Occasionally, the axillary vein is involved, usually as a result of trauma. There is local superficial inflammation in the vein wall, with secondary thrombosis.

The clinical picture is of a painful, tender, cord-like structure with associated redness and swelling.

The condition usually responds to symptomatic treatment with rest, elevation of the limb and analgesics (e.g. NSAIDs). The Comparison of Arixtra in Lower Limb Superficial Vein Thrombosis with Placebo (CALISTO) trial demonstrated that a 45-day course of subcutaneous fondaparinux (2.5 mg daily), compared with placebo, significantly decreased the rate of thromboembolic events (pulmonary embolism and DVT) from 1.3% to 0.2%, and limited the extension of superficial vein thrombosis to the saphenofemoral junction from 3.4% to 0.3% with no increased risk of bleeding.

Significant websites

http://www.achd-library.com *Nevil Thomas Adult Congenital Heart Library*.
http://www.americanheart.org *American Heart Association*.
http://www.dh.gov.uk *UK National Service Framework: Coronary Heart Disease (2000)*.
http://www.ecglibrary.com/ecghome.html *ECG tracings library*.
http://www.erc.edu *European Resuscitation Council*.
http://www.resus.org.uk *Resuscitation Council (UK)*.

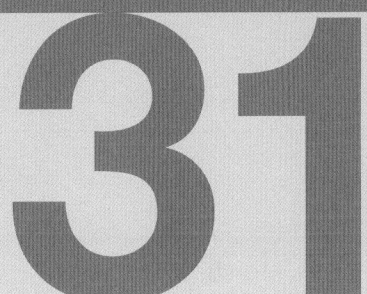

31

Hypertension

Vikas Kapil

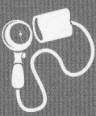

CORE SKILLS AND KNOWLEDGE

Hypertension is a major cardiovascular risk factor affecting one-third of the adult population. It should be managed as part of a comprehensive cardiovascular risk reduction strategy, while also assessing for hypertensive end-organ damage and ruling out secondary causes. Treatment involves modifying lifestyle to improve diet and body weight, and making use of a range of antihypertensive medications.

Most hypertension is managed in primary care. However, young patients with hypertension, or patients who have uncontrolled hypertension despite taking three or more antihypertensives, should be referred for expert evaluation. Doctors may subspecialize in the management of hypertension after completing training in clinical pharmacology, cardiology, renal medicine or another medical specialty.

Key skills in hypertension include:

- diagnosing appropriately, and placing this in the context of an individual's overall cardiovascular risk
- screening for secondary causes of hypertension and seeking evidence of end-organ damage
- understanding the evidence-based guidelines for treating hypertension, and becoming familiar with the main classes of drug used.

Gaining experience in the practical management of hypertension is best done during primary care attachments: for instance, by observing patients undergoing annual blood pressure medication reviews with their general practitioner. Attending a specialist hypertension clinic in a secondary or tertiary care setting gives an interesting insight into secondary causes and more severe phenotypes of hypertension.

INTRODUCTION

Raised blood pressure (BP) is the leading risk factor for death worldwide, outstripping tobacco smoking, poor sanitation and infectious diseases. It is a leading risk factor for atrial fibrillation, stroke, myocardial infarction and end-stage kidney disease. It is such a powerful predictor of these cardiovascular events that modern drug therapies are licensed for cardiovascular protection simply on evidence of sustained BP reduction.

Hypertension refers to the **persistent elevation of BP in the systemic arterial circulation**. It is the most common chronic health condition for which patients receive medication from their primary care doctor and is associated with 1 in 10 of all primary care appointments. It affects one-third of adults and this number continues to rise in all populations. Annual drug costs related to hypertension are well in excess of £1 billion in the UK.

Hypertension is diagnosed against threshold levels of BP from the evidence gathered from large multicentre, multinational studies.

However, given the continuous relationship between BP and cardiovascular disease (**Fig. 31.1**) and renal morbidity, there is a trend towards basing treatment on even lower thresholds, and towards using total **cardiovascular risk** (see p. 751) to guide decisions on whether lowering BP is of benefit in individual patients. The majority of patients with hypertension are managed in primary care, with specialist hospital services usually reserved for evaluation of secondary causes, or for those patients with problematic BP phenotypes (see p. 1136) or medication intolerances.

Despite the wide availability of diagnostics (i.e. BP monitors) and proven treatments (i.e. medications), reduction of BP in hypertensive patients to target levels is less than 50% in most populations and remains the focus of renewed efforts on an international, national and local scale.

Hypertension is a disease of **ageing**. It is rare in children and adolescents, and a diagnosis in those under 30 years of age requires careful evaluation of possible underlying secondary causes (see p. 1136). Due to age-related stiffening in large arterial structure

1133

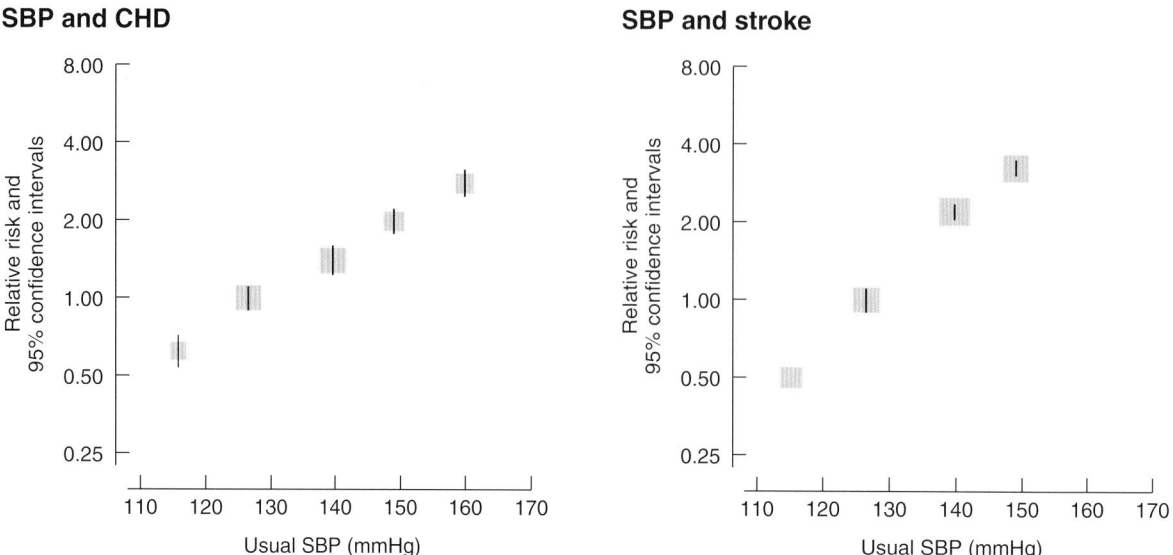

Fig. 31.1 The relationship between blood pressure and cardiovascular morbidity. CHD, coronary heart disease; SBP, systolic blood pressure. (Jackson et al. Lancet 2005; 365: 434-441.)

(arteriosclerosis), BP tends to increase throughout middle and later life. Female sex hormones appear to protect against raised BP, as women have lower BP levels at all ages until menopause, when both prevalence of hypertension and achieved BP levels approximate to those of men. Hypertension is more common in certain ethnic groups (black African, African–Caribbean) and is also associated with urbanized and migrant populations, although an unequivocal explanation for these phenomena is not agreed.

CLINICAL APPROACH TO THE PATIENT WITH HYPERTENSION

Hypertension is largely asymptomatic, though it is associated with increased prevalence of headaches, epistaxis and, less commonly, other neurological symptoms such as visual disturbance and dizziness. Furthermore, in the absence of a hypertensive emergency syndrome (see p. 1144), symptoms related to raised BP are not an indication for treatment. Indeed, antihypertensive therapy is more likely to be the cause of adverse symptoms, such as postural intolerance. History and examination should seek out identifiable causes of raised BP and asymptomatic organ damage.

There are four key considerations in the clinical assessment of patients with hypertension (**Fig. 31.2**) that can be determined through history, examination and investigations:

- What is the true BP level?
- Is there an identifiable reason for high BP?
- Does the BP level require lowering?
- Are there compelling reasons to use certain therapeutic approaches above others?

History

This should cover:

- symptoms of hypertension or secondary causes
- lifestyle issues: weight, alcohol excess, stimulant recreational drug use, tobacco smoking, exercise, stressors (work and personal)

- family history
- pregnancy
- adherence to antihypertensives.

Examination and investigations

These should include:

- 'out-of-office' BP level
- asymptomatic organ damage: eyes, kidneys, heart (**Fig. 31.2**)
- exclusion of secondary causes where relevant
- estimation of total cardiovascular risk.

MEASUREMENT OF BLOOD PRESSURE

Due to the non-continuous, pulsatile blood flow maintained by the cardiac cycle, BP is represented by two numbers: systolic (peak arterial pressure during cardiac contraction) and diastolic (lowest arterial pressure during cardiac relaxation). It is presented as *systolic pressure/diastolic pressure in mmHg* (millimetres of mercury). BP is dynamic and has patterns of variability over seconds (related to breathing, sympathetic activation), minutes (exertion), hours (wake–sleep, circadian hormonal patterns) and the longer term (seasonal). Therefore, the measurement of BP and its use to determine the treatment of hypertension are inherently imprecise and a single measure may not reliably represent the usual (real) BP and its contribution to overall cardiovascular risk. As with any biological variable, the true usual BP is better approximated with multiple measurements at each assessment, and sometimes over several different assessment episodes, before decisions are made regarding changes in treatment.

BP can be measured in several different locations on the body, though readings are traditionally taken in the non-dominant arm. Initially, the BP may be checked in both arms; if there is a significant difference (usually considered to be >10 mmHg), then the arm with the higher BP is used for subsequent measurements.

It is important to measure BP in the correct manner. Methodological variation can falsely and hugely over- or underestimate BP.

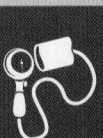

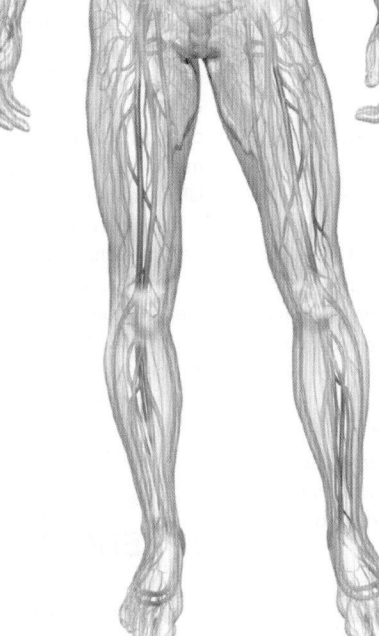

History
- duration of hypertension
- symptoms (headaches, vision, epistaxis – usually asymptomatic)
- co-morbidities (diabetes, CKD, CAD, stroke, gout)
- family history, particularly young hypertension and cardio-renal events
- hypertensive disorders of pregnancy, active attempt to become pregnant
- Secondary causes - see Box 31.2

Examination
- Target organ disease:
  - fundoscopy
  - cardiac palpation and auscultation
- Secondary causes - see Box 31.2

Investigations
- Target organ disease
  - urine reagent strip testing and ACR
  - eGFR
  - ECG
- CV risk - lipids
          - Hba$_{1c}$
- Secondary causes - see Box 31.2

Measurement
- Office   - correct technique
           - >1 reading
- Out-of-office   - ambulatory
                  - home

Thresholds (mmHg)
Under 80 years: >140 or >90 (office) or >135 or >85 (ambulatory or home)
Over 80 years: >160 or >90 (office) or >150 or >85 (ambulatory or home)

Target (mmHg)
- In UK, <140/90 if <80 years and <150/90 if >80 years)
- Growing international trend to aim for <130/80 in all patients if tolerated

Aims of the examination:
- Seeking signs of end organ damage and dysfunction including retinal disease, heart failure, stroke and chronic kidney disease
- Assessing associated cardiovascular risk factors - blood glucose, stigmata of hyperlipidaemia
- In the younger adult - looking for rarer secondary causes e.g. Cushingoid features, acromegaly, renal masses.

Fig. 31.2 Clinical assessment in hypertension. ACR, albumin:creatinine ratio; CAD, coronary artery disease; CKD, chronic kidney disease; CV, cardiovascular; eGFR, estimated glomerular filtration rate.

For static measurements (office/surgery, home), BP should be measured in the seated position after 5 minutes' uninterrupted rest, with the back supported and the legs uncrossed. The BP bladder should encircle at least 80% of the upper arm circumference and should be placed at the level of the heart; the arm should be supported (**Fig. 31.3**).

Although the unit of BP is still 'millimetres of mercury' (mmHg), mercuric sphygmomanometers are obsolete. Modern monitors are usually electronic, oscillometric devices that are automated and have been validated against mercuric devices or intra-arterial BP catheters.

One situation where auscultatory (i.e. using a cuff and stethoscope to listen over the brachial artery) methods are still preferred is in **atrial fibrillation** (see p. 1059), where variations in pulse volume and rapid variation in BP due to variable left

ventricular filling time lead to inaccuracies when oscillometric BP machines are used, especially when ventricular rates are uncontrolled. In particular, diastolic BP tends to be poorly estimated in this situation.

Office/surgery measurement

This refers to measurement of the BP by a healthcare professional in a healthcare setting, such as a primary care surgery or hospital outpatient department. This is the most established method of measurement and all clinical trials of antihypertensive drugs have used it to assess for inclusion and for titration towards target.

It is established practice to take more than two sequential BP readings and to use either the mean or the lowest of these to represent office BP.

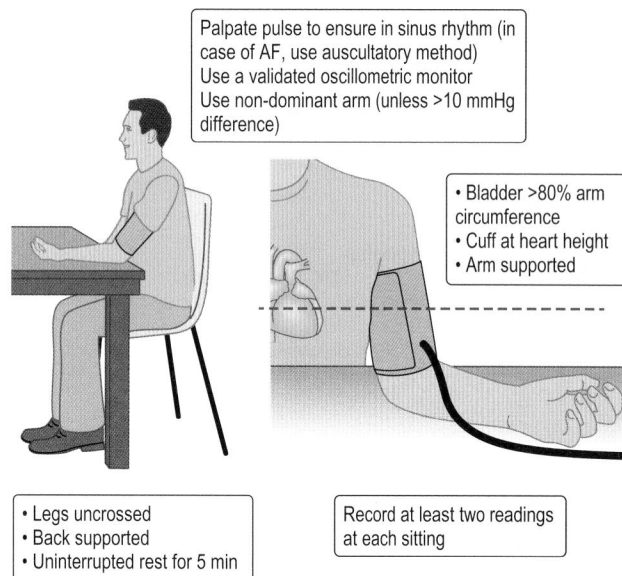

Palpate pulse to ensure in sinus rhythm (in case of AF, use auscultatory method)
Use a validated oscillometric monitor
Use non-dominant arm (unless >10 mmHg difference)

• Bladder >80% arm circumference
• Cuff at heart height
• Arm supported

• Legs uncrossed
• Back supported
• Uninterrupted rest for 5 min

Record at least two readings at each sitting

Fig. 31.3 The correct way to measure blood pressure. AF, atrial fibrillation.

Issues with this approach include:
• a requirement for healthcare professionals and setting (expense, time)
• a requirement for multiple visits to obtain sufficient data for decision-making (expense, time)
• a 'white coat effect': for most people, BP measured by healthcare professionals is approximately 5/5 mmHg higher than at home, though there is inter-individual variation in the magnitude
• the fact that home and ambulatory BP measurements are more predictive of cardiovascular events, as patients do not live in healthcare settings.

Although office BP is no longer recommended as the sole measure for diagnosis in many guidelines, it is still advocated for on-going monitoring and medication titration, as no cardiovascular outcome trials have used out-of-office readings to adjust treatment.

Home measurement

This is measurement of BP at home by the patients themselves, using the same type of machine as in the clinic. It is a type of 'out-of-office' BP measurement and is closely approximated to daytime ambulatory BP. It is particularly useful for:
• identification of different BP phenotypes
• engagement of patients in healthcare and shared decision-making
• long-term monitoring of BP between healthcare visits.

Current recommendations suggest that BP is measured on two or more occasions in sequence, in the morning prior to medicines and again in the evening for 4–7 days. The initial day's readings are discarded and the rest of the values are averaged to calculate home BP. This BP is highly predictive of cardiovascular events and tends to be approximately 5/5 mmHg lower than that measured in the clinic.

Issues with this approach include:
• a requirement for patients to obtain their own machine (expense)
• a requirement for training
• the lack of objective readings (i.e. the measurements are often patient-reported averages, rather than independent evaluations).

Box 31.1 Phenotypes of hypertension and corresponding BP measurements

Phenotype/ method	Office BP	Out-of-office BP	Cardiovascular risk
Normotension	Normal	Normal	Lowest
White coat hypertension	High	Normal	Intermediate
Masked hypertension	Normal	High	Intermediate
Hypertension	High	High	Highest

Ambulatory measurement

Ambulatory BP monitors are portable, oscillometric devices that measure BP discontinuously throughout a 24-hour period, most commonly every 20–30 minutes during waking hours and every 30–60 minutes during sleep.

The large number of readings that this provides gives an accurate estimate of true BP. The 24-hour mean of the sequence of daytime and nocturnal BP measurements is more predictive of cardiovascular events than both home and office BP measurements. Ambulatory BP monitoring is now recommended in the UK instead of office BP for diagnosis, and is recommended as a complementary strategy to office BP in most other high-income health economies.

Similar to home BP, ambulatory BP allows in a single measurement:
• improved diagnostic accuracy over office BP
• identification of different BP phenotypes.

Daytime ambulatory BP is 5–10/5 mmHg lower than office BP in the same patient. Issues with this approach include dislike of repeated BP measurement, especially at night.

PHENOTYPES OF HYPERTENSION

The measurement techniques described can describe different phenotypes of hypertension (**Box 31.1**). Although both *white coat hypertension* and *masked hypertension* represent intermediate cardiovascular risk phenotypes, masked hypertension is treated using out-of-office values to guide treatment, while antihypertensives are not recommended for use in white coat hypertension, despite elevated cardiovascular risk, due to a current lack of evidence.

There are other common phenotypes of hypertension:

Isolated systolic hypertension

Due to age-related arterial stiffening, systolic BP continues to rise in patients above 50 years of age, with a corresponding reduction in diastolic BP. This widening *pulse pressure* (the difference between systolic and diastolic BP, usually <50 mmHg) is associated with increased vascular damage. Drug treatment in isolated systolic hypertension is the same as for combined hypertension (where both systolic and diastolic BP are elevated), though care is needed not to reduce diastolic BP below 60 mmHg, which could cause problems with coronary blood flow (largely due to diastolic flow/pressure). Aortic valve incompetence can also cause an isolated systolic phenotype, though this is normally apparent on cardiac auscultation and/or echocardiography.

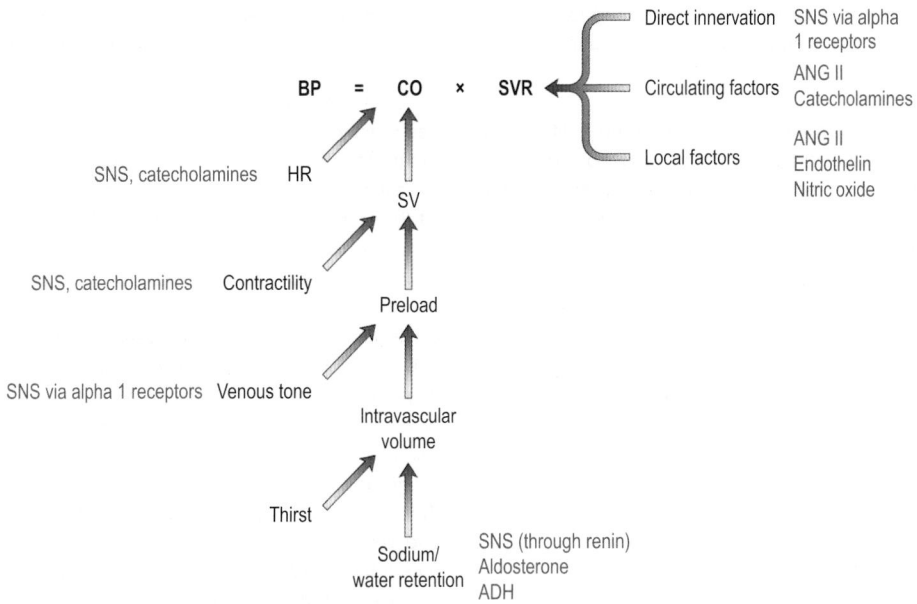

Fig. 31.4 The main mechanisms affecting BP. ANGII, angiotensin II; CO, cardiac output; HR, heart rate; SNS, sympathetic nervous system; SVR, systemic vascular resistance.

Orthostatic hypotension

This refers to a sustained fall in BP within 3 minutes of assuming an upright position of either more than 20 mmHg systolic or more than 10 mmHg diastolic BP. It is more common in older age, and in conditions associated with **autonomic neuropathies,** such as diabetes mellitus and Parkinson's disease. It is typically asymptomatic, although it can cause postural intolerance or instability, **dizziness** and falls. It should be actively screened for in those with typical symptoms or risk factors. Most guidelines recommend using the standing BP as the true BP value for guiding treatment.

Variable blood pressure

Although BP is a highly dynamic variable, the degree of variability is exaggerated in some patients. This is often due to disorders of the autonomic nervous or endocrine system. Reliable assessment is achieved only through a combination of repeated short-term (ambulatory) and long-term (home) methodologies. Management of BP levels in such patients is often complex and best performed in specialist clinics.

CAUSES OF RAISED BLOOD PRESSURE

Up to 90% of patients have no singular identifiable cause of their elevated BP; this is called **primary hypertension** (preferred to the historical term, 'essential hypertension', see later). Advances in genomic research have increased our understanding of polygenic effects on BP (see p. 30). We now know that several hundred genes are individually associated with prevalent BP levels but that each one contributes only small amounts (perhaps 0.5–1 mmHg). Combined, however, they may account for 60% of the BP level in any one person. As such, a family history of hypertension is common, though a family history of hypertension or strokes at unusually young ages should instigate careful evaluation for secondary causes. While there are a large number of distinct genetic influences on BP regulation, for the purposes of clinical assessment and management the main mechanisms affecting BP are **vascular volume and tone**, and **cardiac output** (**Fig. 31.4**). The remaining effects on BP (up to 40%) are mediated by environmental (e.g. temperature, noise) and lifestyle stressors (e.g. diet).

Sudden development of severe hypertension or worsening of previously good control should alert healthcare professionals to the need for careful evaluation of adherence, and for consideration of lifestyle and secondary causes of hypertension if adherence is confirmed. Adherence issues and causes of secondary hypertension should also be borne in mind in patients with **resistant hypertension** (usually defined as uncontrolled BP despite three separate, guideline-recommended antihypertensives).

Lifestyle-related issues

Diet

Relevant **dietary** information provided by patients is often inaccurate. Nevertheless, some clear dietary patterns are associated with raised BP:
- high salt intake
- low vegetable and fruit intake
- high saturated fat intake
- high simple carbohydrate intake
- excessive liquorice (inhibits an enzyme that normally prevents cortisol from activating the mineralocorticoid receptor).

Lack of exercise

Both cardiovascular and strength training forms of **exercise** are associated with lower BP values, along with other health benefits.

Population interventions

In view of the potential effects of these lifestyle issues, together with those associated with obesity (see later), population approaches are increasingly being taken to reduce BP, including:
- public health education drives to:
  - reduce salt and body weight
  - increase exercise

- regulatory approaches to reducing salt in processed foods
- consideration of sugar taxes and minimum alcohol unit pricing.

Drugs

Many patients with hypertension will have other co-morbidities that require additional pharmacological treatment, and consideration should therefore be given to the possible interference of these other drugs with BP control. Both over-the-counter medicines, such as non-steroidal anti-inflammatory drugs (NSAIDs), and recreational drugs, such as alcohol and sympathomimetic stimulants, should be taken into account, as patients may not mention them when a history is being taken unless specific enquiry is made.

Commonly implicated drugs that raise BP include:

- alcohol
- stimulant, recreational drugs
- oral contraceptive pill
- NSAIDs
- corticosteroids
- calcineurin inhibitors
- vascular endothelial growth factor inhibitors
- some antidepressants (e.g. venlafaxine).

Secondary hypertension

Hypertension can have an identifiable singular cause, removal or reversal of which leads to normalization of BP. These are *secondary causes* of hypertension, and are broadly categorised into renal, vascular, endocrine and neural problems (**Box 31.2**). Together, these are present in only 10% of all hypertensive patients (though this proportion is higher in those under 30 years of age). The most common causes of secondary hypertension are largely thought to be *primary hyperaldosteronism* (increased salt/water retention), *obstructive sleep apnoea* and *obesity* (the last two causing sympathetic overdrive), though the precise proportions ascribed to these and other causes vary in different studies due to advances in evaluation and diagnostics.

Although it is not usually considered a secondary cause, *pregnancy* can be associated with raised BP. The normal physiological response to pregnancy is an increase in circulating volume that is offset by significant vasodilation, leading to lower BP, particularly in the second trimester. However, in some pregnant women, defects in placental formation or vascularity lead to pregnancy-induced hypertension and/or *pre-eclampsia* (see p. 1454). Hypertension associated with pregnancy often improves within a few months of the infant's delivery but women with hypertensive disorders of pregnancy are more likely to develop hypertension earlier in life than age-matched controls. The history should establish whether women of child-bearing age are actively trying to become pregnant, as many of the first-line drugs are not recommended in this situation (see **Box 31.6**).

THRESHOLDS AND TARGETS IN HYPERTENSION

Primary hypertension used to be termed 'essential' as, in the 19th century, raised BP was largely thought to be an appropriate physiological adaptation. However, with the advent of randomized clinical trials and modern therapeutics, evidence has grown that lowering BP is beneficial, reducing both cardiorenal events and overall mortality.

The first Veterans Administration Cooperation study randomized patients with a diastolic BP of 115–129 mmHg to active or placebo treatments. By modern standards, this would be considered to be severe hypertension, yet we know of the benefit of lowering BP only from these and subsequent trials.

Since around 1990, the threshold for diagnosis of hypertension has mostly been an office BP of more than 140 mmHg systolic or more than 90 mmHg diastolic (whichever is *worse*). Treatment has largely been reserved for those with **grade 2 hypertension** (**Box 31.3**), as there is a large evidence base for lowering BP with medications in these patients. For **grade 1 hypertension**, it has been usual practice to persevere with lifestyle changes to lower BP and to recommend immediate treatment for those with an overall elevated cardiovascular risk (>1% per year, using validated cardiovascular risk equations), or evidence of organ injury due to hypertension (hypertensive target organ damage). Drug therapy is advocated, however, if BP fails to normalize after a 3–12-month period of best-tolerated lifestyle changes.

For the most part, then, the target has been an office BP of less than 140/90 mmHg, with stricter targets for patients with diabetes and proteinuric chronic renal disease (<130/80 mmHg). However, recent trials such as SPRINT and meta-analysis of other trials have suggested that there is incremental benefit in targeting all patients to a BP below 130/80 mmHg; this is reflected in most international guidelines, though not currently in those produced by the National Institute for Health and Care Excellence (NICE) in the UK.

In older people (over 80 years), there is less evidence for treating mild hypertension, and most guidelines recommend treating only moderate (i.e. grade 2) hypertension. Some guidelines (e.g. NICE) suggest a lax target office BP of below 150/90 mmHg in patients diagnosed over 80 years of age. However, age is often used incorrectly as a surrogate for frailty, and although there is good reason to lower BP cautiously and judiciously in the frail elderly or in those at increased risk of falls or postural hypotension, there is a similar trend in some up-to-date international guidelines, such as those of the European Society of Cardiology (ESC) and the European Society of Hypertension (ESH), to reduce office BP to below 130/80 mm Hg in biologically fit elderly patients, if tolerated.

There are additional considerations relating to these values. As mentioned, there has been a consistent shift to using out-of-office methods, preferably ambulatory, for diagnosis. Because these methods avoid any white coat effect, the thresholds for diagnosis are based on different numerical values, usually considered to be 5–10/5 mmHg lower than in the office.

Further reading

The SPRINT Research Group. A randomized trial of intensive versus standard blood-pressure control. *N Engl J Med* 2015; 373:2103–2116.
Williams B, Mancia G, Spiering W et al. 2018 ESC/ESH Guidelines for the management of arterial hypertension. *Eur Heart J* 2018; 39:3021–3104.

HYPERTENSIVE TARGET ORGAN DAMAGE

Hypertension can cause structural or functional changes in the heart, kidney and central nervous system that may be regarded as intermediate end-points with respect to reducing absolute clinical end-points of myocardial infarction, heart failure, end-stage renal disease and strokes.

Eyes

Direct ophthalmoscopy (fundoscopy) of the dilated eye is recommended in most guidelines for evaluation of hypertensive vascular changes. The most commonly used grading classification is the

? Box 31.2 Drivers/secondary causes of hypertension

System	Causes	History	Examination	Investigations	Management
Lifestyle	Diet	Dietary history		24 h urinary sodium excretion (as a guide and to track improvement in salt intake)	Dietary advice
	Lack of exercise	<30 min/day moderate-intensity exercise			Exercise advice
Drugs	Alcohol	Alcohol history, features of alcohol dependence	May have signs of chronic liver disease	Only if indicated for underlying liver disease	Alcohol reduction <14 units/week
	BP-increasing medications	Medication history, including supplements, recreational and over-the-counter		Use of reference sources to identify BP-increasing medications	Cessation, switching where possible
	Poor adherence to antihypertensives	Validated adherence questionnaires Open, non-judgemental attitude		Urine or plasma qualitative drug monitoring	Shared decision-making, single-pill combinations
Metabolic	Obesity	Recent weight gain	Body mass index >30		Weight loss advice, bariatric surgery
Vascular	Coarctation of aorta		Unequal arm–arm or arm–leg pulses or BP Cardiac murmur or abdominal bruit	MR or CT angiography of whole aorta	Surgery, angioplasty of conservative
Renal	Renal artery stenosis	Sudden deterioration in renal function with ACE inhibitor/ARB Flash pulmonary oedema with normal cardiac function	Abdominal bruit	MR or CT renal angiogram	Balloon angioplasty ± stenting
	Chronic kidney disease	Childhood UTIs Features of vasculitis/GN (see p. 1360)	Ballotable renal masses (PKD) Vasculitic rash	Urine dipstick and ACR eGFR Renal ultrasound Immunological tests (if GN likely) Renal biopsy (if GN likely)	Treatment of BP Treatment of underlying inflammatory renal disease
Endocrine	Primary hyperaldosteronism	Weakness, fatigue		Low K, raised aldosterone:renin MRI/CT adrenal ± adrenal vein sampling	Laparoscopic adrenalectomy if unilateral secretion
	Hypercortisolaemia	Weight gain, fatigue	Centripetal weight distribution, hirsutism, pigmented striae	Low-dose dexamethasone suppression (cortisol should normally be low)	Laparoscopic adrenalectomy or pituitary surgery, depending on source
	Phaeochromocytoma	Palpitations, sweating, BP surges, dizziness, pallor, anxiety	Associated with neurofibromatosis-1	Plasma metanephrines MIBG scan/MRI chest/abdomen/pelvis to localize	Surgery after sufficient alpha blockade
	Acromegaly	Sweating, skin tags, growth of soft tissues, visual disturbance	Large hands, feet, interdental separation, bitemporal hemianopia	Serum IGF-1	Pituitary surgery
	Thyroid (both hypo- and hyperthyroidism)	Weight gain, tiredness (hypothyroidism) Irritability, weight loss (hyperthyroidism)	Pretibial myxoedema, slow relaxing reflex (hypothyroidism) exophthalmos, acropachy (hyperthyroidism)	Serum TSH	Thyroxine replacement (hypothyroidism) or thyroid blockade/surgery (hyperthyroidism)
Respiratory	Obstructive sleep apnoea (p. 960)	Daytime somnolence (Epworth score), snoring, nocturnal sweating, morning headaches	Large neck, Mallampati score 3 or 4	Overnight oximetry (screening) Sleep study	Weight loss Mandibular advancement device CPAP
Neurological	Autonomic failure	Postural intolerance, thermoregulatory issues, parkinsonism	Variable BP Supine hypertension with normal or low BP sitting, standing	24 h BP: nocturnal hypertension Autonomic function testing	Symptom-based, nocturnal medication if supine hypertension
Obstetric	Pregnancy	Secondary amenorrhoea Visual disturbance, oedema, headaches, seizures (for PET/eclampsia only)	Fundal palpation	Urine or serum β-hCG	Pregnancy-safe medicines Delivery of fetus

ACE, angiotensin-converting enzyme; ACR, albumin:creatinine ratio; ARB, angiotensin II receptor blocker; CPAP, continuous positive airways pressure; CT, computed tomography; eGFR, estimated glomerular filtration rate; GN, glomerulonephritis; hCG, human chorionic gonadotrophin; IGF-1, insulin-like growth factor 1; MIBG, meta-iodobenzylguanidine; MRI, magnetic resonance imaging; PET, positron emission tomography; PKD, polycystic kidney disease; TSH, thyroid stimulating hormone; UTI, urinary tract infection.

Description	Office BP (mmHg)		Daytime ambulatory or home BP (mmHg)	
	Systolic BP	Diastolic BP	Systolic BP	Diastolic BP
Normal BP	<130	<80	n/a	n/a
High-normal BP	130–139	80–89	n/a	n/a
Grade 1 hypertension	140–159	90–99	135–149	85–94
Grade 2 hypertension	160–179	100–109	150–169	95–104
Severe hypertension	>180	>110	>170	>105
Isolated systolic hypertension	>140	<90	>135	<85

Keith–Wagener–Barker system, comprising four distinct ophthalmic hypertensive phenotypes (*retinopathy*). More recent evaluation, however, has suggested combining the two milder phenotypes, leaving three grades to consider (**Fig. 31.5**):

- *Mild:* Generalized arteriolar narrowing, focal arteriolar narrowing, arteriovenous nicking (modest association with cardiovascular and cerebral events).
- *Moderate:* Haemorrhage (blot, dot or flame-shaped), micro-aneurysm, cotton-wool spot, hard exudate, or a combination of these signs (strong association with cardiovascular and cerebral events).
- *Severe:* Signs of moderate retinopathy plus papilloedema (swelling of optic head) (strong association with cardiovascular events, stroke and death).

Heart

The heart is a muscle and hypertrophy may occur in response to increased workload. Left ventricular remodelling is initially a compensatory phenomenon to reduce wall stress but eventually leads to a pathogenic increase in left ventricular mass.

Hypertensive left ventricular hypertrophy is usually asymptomatic but can be detected as a thrusting apex beat on precordial palpation. It is also sometimes detected on standard 12-lead electrocardiography (ECG), demonstrating various patterns of increased voltages in the chest leads and T-wave abnormalities (see **Fig. 30.79**). There are many different scoring systems for ECG criteria for diagnosing left ventricular hypertrophy; all are quite insensitive (20–50%) but specificity is better (>90%), which means that if criteria are positive, true left ventricular hypertrophy is likely to be present.

ECGs are recommended in all hypertensive patients, as they are widely available and cheap, and do not require much in the way of additional training to interpret, especially as modern ECG machines have in-built reporting algorithms. However, cardiac imaging, using transthoracic echocardiography and cardiac MRI, is more sensitive and specific than ECG (when compared to autopsy data), though access, cost and need for additional trained staff to conduct and report these tests limit their wide utility and acceptance in all hypertensive patients. These cardiac imaging modalities can estimate the actual mass of the left ventricle; this is indexed to height and weight, and has sex-specific normal values.

Kidney

Kidney disease is both a cause and a consequence of hypertension. Early hypertensive kidney damage is most easily detectable through an increase in microalbuminuria on urine test strips or as an increased laboratory albumin : creatinine ratio. Estimates of glomerular filtration rate (GFR), based on serum creatinine and demographic criteria, are also obtained, especially as several antihypertensive medications are potentially nephrotoxic. However, there is usually an initial reduction in GFR associated with chronic BP-lowering from any cause, and this usually reflects intra-renal haemodynamic changes rather than intrinsic renal damage; it is therefore common practice to allow GFR to reduce by up to 10% on initiation of antihypertensive therapy. More regular follow-up is mandated to ensure that this does not indicate progressive renal decline.

TREATMENT

Meta-analyses of large-scale RCTs have shown that a 10/5 mmHg reduction in BP is associated with a 15% reduction in all-cause mortality, 35% reduction in stroke, 40% reduction in heart failure and 20% reduction in myocardial infarction. Hypertension is treated to reduce these major cardiovascular and renal events. For this reason, treatment of hypertension without managing other modifiable cardiovascular risk factors (raised cholesterol, diabetes mellitus, tobacco smoking, obesity) is suboptimal. Cardiovascular risk scores, such as QRISK2®, are useful for integrating all of these risk factors, to judge when there is benefit in treating hypertensive patients. Ten-year risk estimates are less useful than lifetime risk estimates in young patients, given the powerful role of age in all cardiovascular risk scores.

Lifestyle changes

These are recommended for all hypertensive patients, irrespective of grade or duration of disease. The BP reductions accompanying such lifestyle changes are complementary and similar in magnitude (compared to half-standard monotherapy) to those achieved by antihypertensive medications (**Box 31.4**).

Bariatric surgery is indicated for those with hypertension and a body mass index (BMI) of more than 35 kg/m², but it is not commonly performed without the additional co-morbidity of type 2 diabetes. Recent data confirm the profound BP-lowering effect of such surgery, which may be due to additional gut hormonal changes postoperatively, in addition to expected weight loss.

Drug treatment

A single antihypertensive medication at standard dose reduces BP by about 9/5 mmHg in mild hypertension. Although patients with mild hypertension may achieve control with monotherapy, those with moderate or worse hypertension invariably require several drugs in combination. Greater effects are obtained by combining medications from different classes, targeting different mechanisms. Three antihypertensives at half-standard dose reduce BP by 20/11 mmHg. Most *adverse effects* with antihypertensives, in keeping with most pharmaceuticals, are type A adverse reactions (see p. 258) and are thus dose-dependent. Keeping doses to a minimum but combining different classes minimizes the chances of adverse effects and maximizes the likelihood of effectively lowering BP to target levels.

As mentioned, *adherence* is increasingly recognized as a key barrier to achieving BP control. Although there are different validated measures to assess this, such as the Morisky-8 Medication

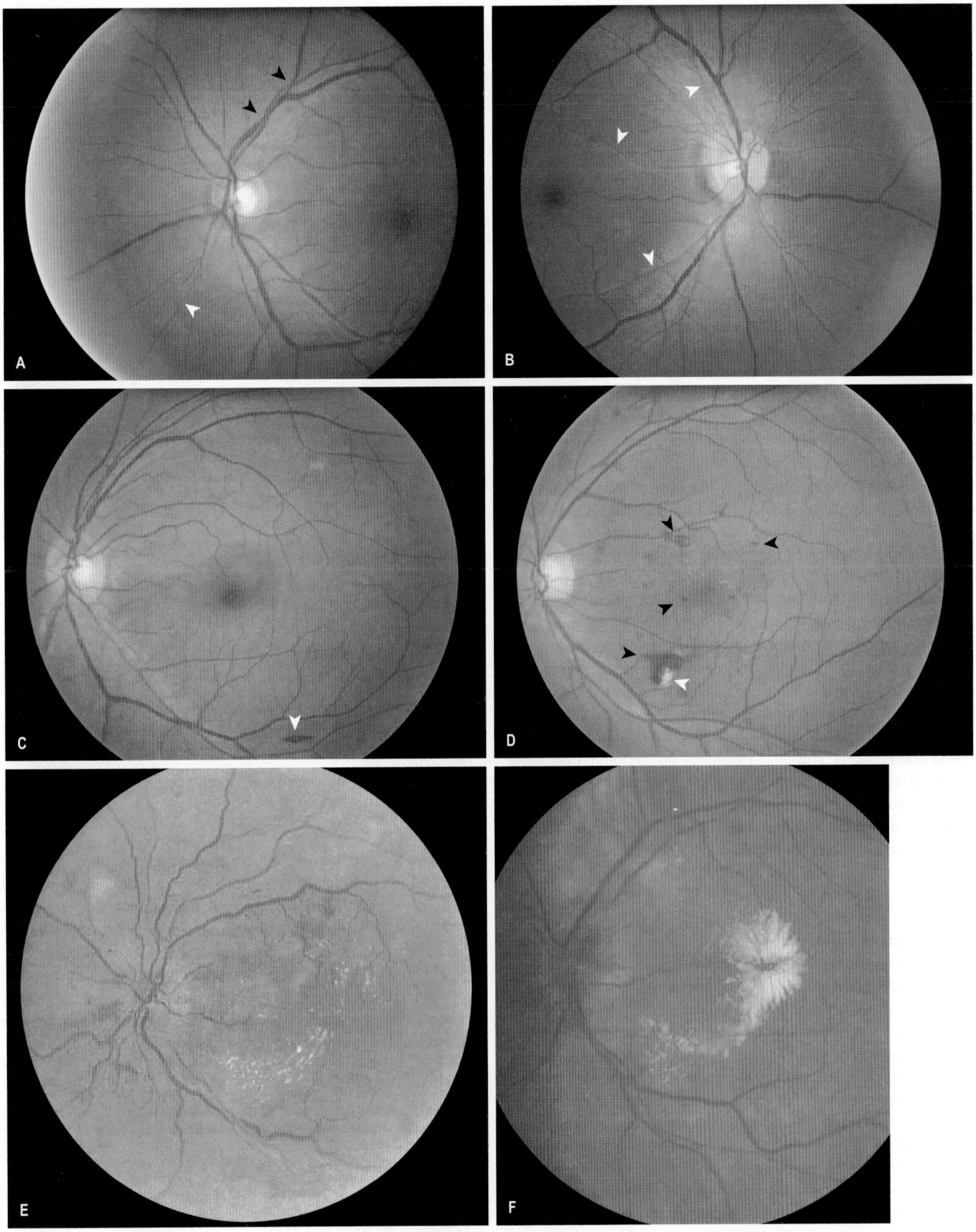

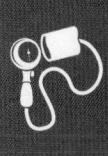

Fig. 31.5 Hypertensive retinopathy. **(A–B)** Examples of *mild hypertensive retinopathy*. **(A)** Arteriovenous nicking (black arrows) and focal narrowing (white arrow). **(B)** Opacification (silver or copper wiring) of arteriolar wall (white arrows). **(C–D)** Examples of *moderate hypertensive retinopathy*. **(C)** A flame-shaped retinal haemorrhage (white arrow). **(D)** A cotton-wool spot (white arrow), retinal haemorrhages and microaneurysms (black arrows). **(E–F)** *Severe hypertensive retinopathy*. **(E)** Exudates and flame haemorrhages in grade 3 retinopathy. **(F)** Signs of malignant hypertension in grade 4 disease, with a swollen optic disc and macular exudate. *(A–D From Schachat AP, Sadda SVR, Hinton DR et al. Ryan's Retina, 6th edn. Elsevier Inc., 2018, Figs 52.1 and 52.2; E–F from Innes JA, Dover AR, Fairhurst K. Macleod's Clinical Examination, 14th edn. Elsevier Ltd, 2018, Fig. 8.18CD.)*

Lifestyle change	Expected mean BP reduction
Regular cardiovascular exercise (30 min daily)	5 mmHg
Weight reduction if overweight (body mass index >25 kg/m²)	1 mmHg/kg
Increased intake of fruits and vegetables, reduced intake of saturated fat	10 mmHg
Dietary salt reduction <6 g day	5 mmHg
Alcohol <2 units daily	3 mmHg

Please answer each question, based on your personal experience with your medications. Note that there is no right or wrong answer.

1. Do you sometimes forget to take your medications?		No	Yes
2. People sometimes miss taking their medications for reasons other than forgetting. Thinking over the past 2 weeks, were there any days when you did not take your medications?		No	Yes
3. Have you ever cut back or stopped taking your medications without telling your doctor because you felt worse when you took it?		No	Yes
4. When you travel or leave home, do you sometimes forget to bring along your medications?		No	Yes
5. Did you take your medications yesterday?		No	Yes
6. When you feel that your health condition is under control, do you sometimes stop taking your medications?		No	Yes
7. Taking medications every day is a real inconvenience for some people. Do you ever feel hassled about sticking to your treatment plan?		No	Yes
8. How often do you have difficulty remembering to take all your medications?	Never/rarely	1
	Once in a while	0
	Sometimes	0
	Usually	0
	All the time	0

'No' answers to questions 1–4, 6 and 7, a 'Yes' answer to question 5 and 'Never/rarely' to question 8 score 1. A score of 8 suggests good adherence. Score of 7 or less suggests poor adherence and is associated with poorer BP control. *(Adapted from Morisky DE, Ang A, Krousel-Wood M et al. Predictive validity of a medication adherence measure in an outpatient setting.* J Clin Hypertens *2008; 10:348–354.)*

Adherence Scale (**Box 31.5**), along with prescription refill rate (whether patients receive a resupply at the right time to have therapy every day), modern drug analytical techniques on plasma or urine have demonstrated that question-/refill-based assessment correlates poorly to objective evidence of measurable drug in biological matrices. From these newer techniques, it appears that up to two-thirds of patients in specialist care do not take some or any of their antihypertensive medications. There are no easy solutions to such covert non-adherence but keeping an open, non-judgemental approach can facilitate the volunteering of this information and then shared-decision making can determine how best to proceed and what patients want for their own health.

In view of this, and with evidence that suggests there is an elevated cardiovascular risk when control is achieved over protracted (>6 months) timeframes, guidelines have recently tended to abandon monotherapy and suggest starting with a combination of medicines to achieve BP control effectively and rapidly. Current ESH/ESC guidelines have taken this further and have used evidence that single-pill combinations of two or more antihypertensive medications improve adherence to suggest that most patients should be started on single-pill combination therapy.

There are numerous classes of antihypertensive medication available and their key features are described in **Box 31.6**.

Most guidelines recommend choosing one (or two) of the following three classes of drugs, as initial therapy:

- angiotensin-converting enzyme (ACE) inhibitors/angiotensin II receptor blockers (ARBS),
- calcium channel blockers
- thiazide-like diuretics.

Current UK NICE guidelines use age and ethnicity as surrogates for plasma renin activity. Older and black African ancestries are associated with low renin status and so have reduced responsiveness to drugs ACEIs and ARBs as monotherapy: hence calcium-channel blockers are recommended in these groups. Younger white patients are recommended to start on an ACEI or ARB. These are largely thought to be interchangeable, except that ARBs are better tolerated, with less cough and angio-oedema.

There is clear evidence from the PATHWAY-2 study that spironolactone is the best fourth-line drug, in preference to beta- or alpha-blockers, though it is unlicensed for this indication in most countries and patients should be appropriately counselled. Once a patient is on three or four drugs and remains uncontrolled (**resistant hypertension**), they should be referred for specialist assessment.

In keeping with the view that reduction in total cardiovascular risk is paramount, cholesterol-lowering therapy, most commonly with small doses of potent statins, is recommended in all patients with a total cardiovascular risk of more than 1% per year. This threshold may not be reached in younger patients due to the power of age in the risk calculators, and so a more long-term view of risk reduction should be taken in these patients. Although low-dose aspirin has been used in **primary cardiovascular prevention** for many decades, contemporary large-scale trials have not demonstrated a net benefit on mortality, even in patients with diabetes, with any gains from reduction in cardiovascular events offset by increases in bleeding events. Given these data, aspirin is no longer recommended in any patient group for primary prevention.

Further reading

Ettehad D, Emdin CA, Kiran A et al. Blood pressure lowering for prevention of cardiovascular disease and death: a systematic review and meta-analysis. *Lancet* 2016; 387:957–967.

Morisky DE, Ang A, Krousel-Wood M et al. Predictive validity of a medication adherence measure in an outpatient setting. *J Clin Hypertens* 2008; 10:348–354.

Williams B, MacDonald TM, Morant M et al. Spironolactone versus placebo, bisoprolol, and doxazosin to determine the optimal treatment for drug-resistant hypertension (PATHWAY-2): a randomised, double-blind, crossover trial. *Lancet* 2015; 386:2059–2068.

https://www.qrisk.org/three/. *Cardiovascular risk score calculator.*

Future approaches

Poor hypertension control rates are apparent with available prescribed medicines, largely due to adherence issues rather than

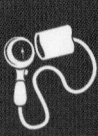

? Box 31.6 Main classes of antihypertensive agent and their key features

Class	Mechanism	Adverse effects	Compelling indication	Compelling contra-indication	Monitoring	Example
Angiotensin-converting enzyme (ACE) inhibitor	Reduce angiotensin II vasoconstriction	Cough Angio-oedema Hyperkalaemia		Bilateral RAS Angio-oedema	eGFR, K	Ramipril 2.5–10 mg daily
Angiotensin II receptor blockers (ARB)	Reduce angiotensin II vasoconstriction	Hyperkalaemia		Bilateral RAS	eGFR, K	Losartan 25–100 mg daily
Dihydropyridine calcium-channel blocker (DHP CCB)	Peripheral vasodilation	Constipation, headache, oedema	Nifedipine/amlo-dipine recommended for use in pregnancy			Amlodipine 5–10 mg daily
Non-DHP CCB	Peripheral vasodilation	Constipation, bradycardia		High grade atrioventricular block Bradycardia	Heart rate	Verapamil 120–480 mg daily
Thiazide-like diuretic	Vasodilation, salt/water loss	Hyponatraemia, hypokalaemia, hyperuricaemia, hyperglycaemia	Heart failure	Gout	Serum electrolytes, HbA$_{1c}$, urate	Indapamide 1.5–2.5 mg daily
Potassium-sparing diuretic	Salt/water loss	Hyponatraemia, hyperkalaemia, gynaecomastia	Primary hyperaldosteronism Resistant hypertension	eGFR <30 mL/min K >5.0 mmol/L	Serum electrolytes	Spironolactone 25–50 mg daily
Beta-blocker	Vasodilation through renin inhibition, sympatholysis	Bradycardia, sleep disturbance, bronchospasm	Heart failure with reduced ejection fraction Ischaemic heart disease Labetalol licensed in pregnancy	Asthma High-grade atrioventricular block Bradycardia	Heart rate	Bisoprolol 2.5–10 mg daily
Alpha-blocker	Venodilation	Postural hypotension, urine incontinence, oedema	Suspected phaeochromocytoma Benign prostatic hypertrophy	Urinary incontinence Postural hypotension Heart failure		Doxazosin 1–8 mg twice daily
Central	Sympatholysis	Depression, drowsiness, dry mouth	Methyldopa licensed in pregnancy	Mood disorders Heart failure with reduced ejection fraction	Rebound hypertension on cessation	Methyldopa 250–500 mg 3 times daily

eGFR, estimated glomerular filtration rate; K, potassium; RAS, renin–angiotensin system.

ineffectiveness of the drugs. Nevertheless, patients are keen to explore medicine-free mechanisms to lower BP.

Neural sympathetic signalling has a key role in vascular homeostasis, with effects mediated via afferent renal and aortic/carotid baroreceptor functions. Novel interventional approaches to alter this signalling are currently under evaluation to improve BP in both medicine-naive and treated hypertensive patients. The most advanced, in terms of regulatory pathways and evidence base, is renal sympathetic denervation. This group of procedures uses modern endovascular catheter-based approaches to the renal sympathetic nerves, which lie on the outside of the renal artery. Catheters can then deliver energy (radio-frequency, ultrasound) or neurotoxins (such as alcohol) across the renal artery wall to reach the sympathetic nerves and abrogate afferent signalling to the vasomotor centres, thus reducing total sympathetic drive and BP. Although the technological advancements are impressive and there is evidence of robust BP-lowering using modern out-of-office measurements, the magnitude of these effects is similar to that of antihypertensive monotherapy and thus most patients will still require drug therapy to control BP in the long term. Furthermore, these are new technologies: the long-term safety of the procedures is not clear, as regards

the renal artery or otherwise, and there are no outcome studies investigating cardiac, renal, stroke or death end-points using any technology apart from drugs.

Further reading

Schlaich MP. Renal sympathetic denervation: a viable option for treating resistant hypertension. *Am J Hypertens* 2017; 30:847–856.

Townsend RR, Mahfoud F, Kandzari DE et al. Catheter-based renal denervation in patients with uncontrolled hypertension in the absence of antihypertensive medications (SPYRAL HTN-OFF MED): a randomised, sham-controlled, proof-of-concept trial. *Lancet* 2017; 390:2160–2170.

MANAGING BLOOD PRESSURE IN HOSPITAL

Perioperative period

Preoperative

Uncontrolled hypertension is a common reason for cancellation of elective surgical procedures. Patients with severely elevated BP (>180/110 mmHg) are associated with greater perioperative harm, such as myocardial injury, though there is no clear evidence that reducing BP acutely in the preoperative period to controlled levels is beneficial. Patients with uncontrolled BP (evidence of chronic poor control of >160/100 mmHg in treated patients, or opportunistic measurements in pre-assessment in previously normotensive patients of >180/110 mmHg) are commonly referred back to their primary care doctor for adequate management of hypertension prior to elective procedures, though this is not a reason to delay necessary emergency surgical intervention. Although ACEIs and ARBs are often withheld arbitrarily for 24 hours preoperatively, it is usual to continue antihypertensive medications throughout the perioperative period unless there is documented hypotension or other related issues, such as withholding nephrotoxic antihypertensives if there is acute kidney injury.

Intraoperative

Sympathetic activation during induction of anaesthesia can cause elevation of BP by 30 mmHg, with far larger responses in patients with untreated hypertension. Subsequently, with maintenance of anaesthesia, BP tends to fall due to the direct sympatholytic and vasodilating actions of anaesthetic drugs and loss of baroreflex regulation of BP. Patients with pre-existing uncontrolled hypertension are more likely to experience intraoperative BP lability (i.e. hypotension or hypertension), which is a risk factor for myocardial ischaemia and injury. Intraoperative hypertension is most commonly associated with inadequate analgesia or depth of anaesthesia, though it is prudent and recommended to exclude serious problems with airway, oxygen delivery and breathing first.

Postoperative

Pain and (inadvertent) omission of antihypertensive medications are the most common reasons for postoperative hypertension. Once these factors have been corrected, there are no data to support the further active lowering of BP in the postoperative period without evidence of acute end-organ damage, though it is usual practice to try to keep BP below 180/110 mmHg, in part to reduce the risk of problems with postoperative haemostasis.

Blood pressure on the wards

Patients with hypertension are often admitted to hospital for other medical reasons. Various factors can contribute to acute elevations of BP, such as antihypertensive medication omission, drug-induced hypertension (see earlier), anxiety, pain, bladder distension, recreational drug withdrawal and neurological injury. In the absence of a hypertensive emergency or other co-morbidity that requires acute BP management (e.g. to facilitate thrombolysis in acute stroke), uncontrolled BP does not require immediate management.

However, as with most phenotypes, there is a threshold value that makes most healthcare professionals anxious about increased cerebral and cardiovascular risk, even in inpatients, and it is therefore common for BPs consistently above 180/110 mmHg to be treated, where there is no other clear precipitant. There is no role for short-acting drugs, such as sublingual glyceryl trinitrate (GTN) or nifedipine, and titration of standard chronic therapies with on-going monitoring is preferred.

Hypertensive emergencies

Only a small subset of patients with significantly elevated BP (usually >180/120 mmHg) have signs or symptoms of acute target-organ damage, termed hypertensive emergencies. The rate and magnitude of any increase in BP may be more important than the absolute level of BP in determining the severity of organ injury; this is key in obstetric medicine, where the usual BP in younger women may be verging on hypotensive (90–110/60–70 mmHg), and pre-eclampsia may develop with a BP over 140/90 mmHg.

In all hypertensive emergencies, intravenous antihypertensive medication therapy is indicated to cause rapid reduction of BP, as this is thought to minimize on-going organ damage and prevent or reduce the risk of morbidity and mortality. The timing, magnitude and other considerations related to the management of these conditions are considered in **Box 31.7**.

Referral to specialist care

The majority of hypertensive patients are managed in primary care. Apart from the clear indications related to hypertensive emergencies described earlier, there are other reasons to mandate referral to specialist secondary care:

- Patients taking ≥3 drugs with uncontrolled hypertension (resistant hypertension).
- Suspected secondary causes:
  - Young age (<30–40 years)
  - Historical features (i.e. obstructive sleep apnoea, phaeochromocytoma)
  - Examination findings (i.e. abdominal bruit suggesting renal artery stenosis)
  - Sudden change in BP.
- Target organ damage detected with normal BP values.
- Intolerance of medicines preventing guideline-based treatment.
- Symptomatic hypertension or hypotension.
- Labile or highly variable BP.
- Mild hypertension when it is not clear whether a patient would benefit from BP-lowering.

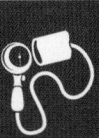

Box 31.7 Management of hypertensive emergencies

Presentation/ syndrome	History	Examination	Investigation of choice	Target/timeframe	First line therapies	Notes
Malignant hypertension	Visual disturbance, headache	Moderate–severe retinopathy		25% MAP reduction within a few hours	i.v. Labetalol, nicardipine (with retinopathy only, some consider oral atenolol sufficient)	Often associated with acute kidney injury, due to fibrinoid small-artery necrosis
Hypertensive encephalopathy	Visual disturbance, headache, seizures, confusion, coma	Often features moderate–severe retinopathy	MRI brain: posterior fossa oedema (PRES)	Immediate MAP reduction by 25%	i.v. Labetalol, nicardipine	
Acute aortic dissection	Tearing chest pain	Unequal arm pulses or BP Aortic valve incompetence	CT angiogram aorta, trans-oesophageal echo: dissection flap visible	Immediate SBP reduction to 100–120 mmHg *and* heart rate to 50–60 beats/min	i.v. Labetalol Once rate control is adequate, vasodilators can be added (GTN, nicardipine)	Patients with Marfan's or proximal aorta syndromes more commonly proceed to early surgery
Acute pulmonary oedema	Shortness of breath	Bibasal crackles, elevated jugular venous pressure	Chest X-ray: interstitial oedema	Immediate SBP reduction to <140 mmHg	i.v. GTN, diamorphine	Loop diuretics are also vasodilating and lower BP
Acute coronary syndrome	Chest pain	Diaphoretic	ECG: ST/T-wave changes Serum troponin elevated	Immediate SBP reduction to <140 mmHg	i.v. GTN, labetalol	
Pre-eclampsia	Oedema, visual disturbance, abdominal pain	Oedematous New proteinuria on string reagent testing		Immediate SBP reduction to <160 and DBP to <105 mmHg	i.v. Labetalol, nicardipine	i.v. Magnesium used to prevent/treat eclamptic seizures

CT, computed tomography; DBP, diastolic blood pressure; ECG, electrocardiography; GTN, glyceryl trinitrate; MAP, mean arterial pressure; MRI, magnetic resonance imaging; PRES, posterior reversible encephalopathy syndrome; SBP, systolic blood pressure.

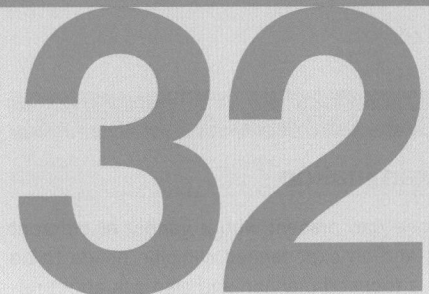

Gastroenterology

Noor Jawad and Charlotte Skinner

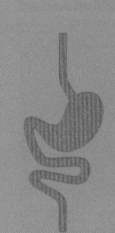

CORE SKILLS AND KNOWLEDGE

Gastrointestinal disease is common throughout the world. The WHO estimates that diarrhoeal illnesses alone caused 1.4 million deaths in 2016. Gastrointestinal disease accounts for approximately 10% of primary care appointments, and colorectal cancer is the third commonest cancer globally.

Gastroenterologists care for patients in inpatient settings (e.g. for those with acute flares of inflammatory bowel disease or gastrointestinal bleeding), outpatient clinics (for long-term management of chronic gastrointestinal conditions, or diagnosis of newly presenting patients), and they provide diagnostic, therapeutic and screening endoscopy services. Gastroenterology research is a fertile area with many exciting new therapies and technologies appearing in recent years, and gastroenterologists may also be active in medical education or hospital management.

Key skills in gastroenterology include:

- managing and investigating acute and chronic gastrointestinal bleeding
- understanding different treatment strategies for inflammatory bowel disease, including the role for biological agents and surgical treatment
- developing an understanding of functional gastrointestinal disease and how to help patients suffering with problems such as irritable bowel syndrome.

There are many opportunities to gain the knowledge and skills to successfully manage patients with gastrointestinal diseases, including reviewing patients on general gastroenterology wards, attending general and specialist outpatient clinics, observing endoscopic procedures and attending multidisciplinary team (MDT) meetings. MDTs commonly exist for upper and lower gastrointestinal cancers and inflammatory bowel disease, and allow the discussion of patients by gastroenterologists, radiologists, histopathologists, surgeons, oncologists and nurse specialists.

CLINICAL SKILLS FOR GASTROENTEROLOGY

 Box 32.1 History-taking in gastroenterology

Symptoms of upper gastrointestinal disease
- **Dysphagia** – distinguish between a likely *neurological cause* (often high in mouth or pharynx, worse with swallowing liquids, often speech involvement), and a likely *anatomical cause* (lower down in chest or upper abdomen, worse with larger and more solid food boluses).
- **Dyspepsia** – often a non-specific symptom, but establish the relationship with food ingestion posture – symptoms of reflux disease are worsened by both.
- **Early satiety** – may be a symptom of stomach cancer
- **Nausea and vomiting** – these may be mediated by central causes, but a close relationship with food (e.g. projectile vomiting after eating) suggests a pyloric stricture.
- **Haematemesis** – vomiting of fresh red blood should be treated as a medical emergency. Vomiting of altered blood (sometimes described as 'coffee grounds') is more difficult to evaluate, but should still be taken seriously. Haematemesis after a prolonged bout of vomiting may suggest a Mallory–Weiss tear.
- **Melaena** – this describes the passage of thick, black, 'tarry' altered blood from the rectum and indicates upper gastrointestinal bleeding – a medical emergency.

Symptoms of lower gastrointestinal disease
- **Change in bowel habit** – while constipation is often a symptom of inadequate diet or physical exercise, unexplained loosening of stool, particularly if persistent, may be an symptom of colonic diseases, including cancer and colitis.
- **Rectal bleeding** – fresh blood dripping after passing stool, or present on wiping, suggests anorectal disease including haemorrhoids. Blood mixed with stool may indicate colitis or colonic malignancy.
- **Tenesmus** – a feeling of incomplete rectal emptying after defecation suggests anorectal pathology such as a tumour.

'Red flag' symptoms suggestive of malignancy
- Progressive weight loss.
- Anorexia.
- Symptoms of anaemia from chronic blood loss.

Past medical history
- Gastrointestinal disease.
- Autoimmune disease.
- Abdominal surgery.

Drug history
- All prescription drugs.
- Non-steroidal anti-inflammatories, over-the-counter drugs and herbal remedies.
- Recent courses of antibiotics.

Social history
- Smoking.
- Alcohol consumption.

History and examination

Gastrointestinal disease can present with a variety of different symptoms and signs and an experienced clinician needs to be able to elicit these in a focused manner, and also ask about relevant risk factors (**Box 32.1**). The figure opposite illustrates signs of common gastrointestinal diseases to be found on examination.

Visualizing the bowel

The different types of endoscopy are discussed fully on page 1158. **Box 32.3** illustrates the ability of different techniques of endoscopy (including contrast techniques in ERCP) to visualize different parts of the gastrointestinal and biliary tract. Most are readily available in the majority of units, although capsule endoscopy and balloon enteroscopy remain more specialist procedures. All except capsule endoscopy allow biopsies to be taken and a range of therapeutic procedures to be performed.

 Box 32.2 Core knowledge in gastroenterology

The 'top ten' presentations
- Acute upper GI bleed
- Dysphagia
- Dyspepsia
- Abdominal pain
- Malabsorption
- Diarrhoea
- Iron-deficiency anaemia
- Rectal bleeding
- Constipation
- Tenesmus

The 'top ten' conditions
- Functional bowel disorders
- Peptic ulcer disease
- Gastro-oesophageal reflux disease
- Oesophageal cancer
- Gastric cancer
- Coeliac disease
- Inflammatory bowel disease

- Infectious diarrhoea
- Colorectal cancer
- Diverticulosis

The 'top ten' medications
- Proton pump inhibitors and H$_2$ receptor antagonists
- *Helicobacter pylori* eradication regimens
- Anti-emetics
- 5-aminosalicylic acids
- Oral and intravenous steroids
- Azathioprine and methotrexate
- Anti-tumour necrosis factor antibodies
- Oral iron preparations
- Antispasmodics
- Antibiotics for infectious diarrhoea, and when to use them

i **Box 32.3 Endoscopy techniques**

Oesophagogastro-duodenoscopy (OGD)	Endoscopic retrograde cholangiopancreatography (ERCP)	Capsule endoscopy	Balloon enteroscopy	Proctoscopy	Flexible sigmoidoscopy	Colonoscopy

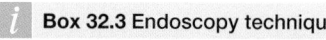

Face
Conjunctival pallor

Mouth
Angular stomatitis (malnutrition)
Oral ulcers (Crohn's)
Glossitis (inflammation of the tongue) can be due to iron-deficiency anaemia, B12 deficiency or malabsorption

Neck
Cervical and clavicular lymphadenopathy
Virchow's node (enlarged left supraclavicular lymph node) which is a sentinel lymph node for gastric cancer

Hands
Koilonychia (spoon-shaped nails, associated with iron-deficiency anaemia)
Clubbing

Hernial orifices
Signs of incarcerated hernia if intestinal obstruction is suspected

Digital examination of the rectum
Haemorrhoids
Anorectal cancer
Empty rectum (intestinal obstruction)
Full rectum (constipation)
Blood on finger (malignancy or colitis)

Legs
Pyoderma gangrenosum or erythema nodosum (both seen in inflammatory bowel disease)

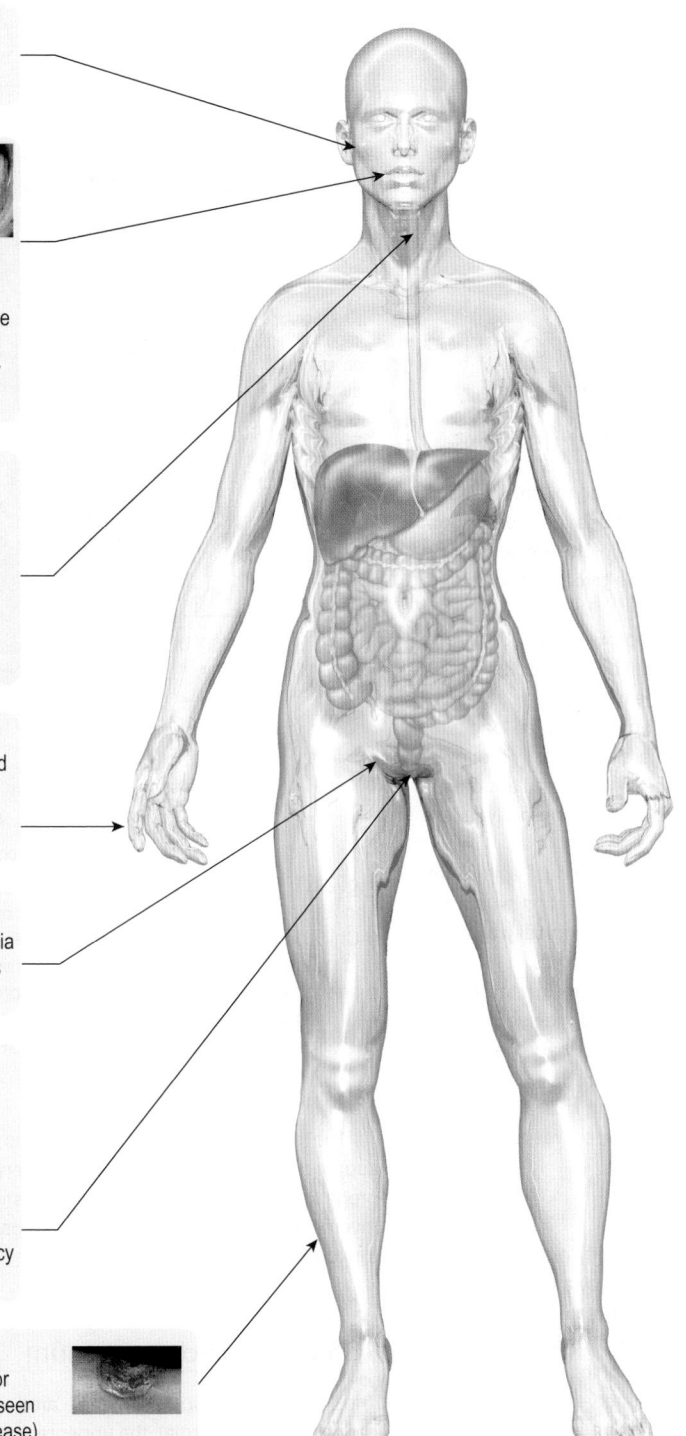

General features
Cachexia
Jaundice
Pallor

Observation chart
Tachycardia or shock (in acute bleeding)

Abdomen
Inspection
- scars
- abdominal distension

Abdomen
Soft touch palpation
- abdominal tenderness
- masses

Abdomen
Deeper palpation
- masses
- hepatomegaly
- splenomegaly

Abdomen
Percussion
- shifting dullness (ascites)
- suprapubic dullness (distended bladder)
- hepatomegaly
- splenomegaly

Abdomen
Auscultation
- generally not of great value
- absent bowel sounds in peritonism
- high pitched or 'tinkling' in intestinal obstruction

INTRODUCTION

The gastrointestinal tract has many functions, such as digestion, absorption and excretion, as well as the synthesis of hormones, growth factors and cytokines. In addition, a complex enteric nervous system controls its function and communicates with the central and peripheral nervous systems. Finally, as the gastrointestinal tract is the part of the body containing the largest source of foreign antigens, it has very well-developed arms of both the innate and the acquired immune systems. The intestinal microbiota exerts a range of beneficial functions aiding nutrition, absorption and the development of a mature immune system. Disruption of the composition and diversity of the microbiota is associated with the development of gastrointestinal and systemic disease.

ANATOMY AND PHYSIOLOGY OF THE GASTROINTESTINAL TRACT

Mouth, oropharynx and oesophagus

The oral cavity extends from the lips to the pharynx and contains the tongue, teeth and gums. Its primary functions are mastication, swallowing and speech. The **pharynx** consists of the nasal, oral and laryngeal sections. The latter is the part of the throat that connects to the oesophagus.

The **oesophagus** is a muscular tube approximately 20 cm long that connects the pharynx to the stomach just below the diaphragm. Its only function is to transport food from the mouth to the stomach. In the upper portion of the oesophagus, both the outer longitudinal layer and inner circular muscle layers are striated. In the lower two-thirds of the oesophagus, including the thoracic and abdominal parts containing the lower oesophageal sphincter, both layers are composed of smooth muscle.

The oesophagus is lined by stratified squamous epithelium, which extends distally to the squamocolumnar junction where the oesophagus joins the stomach, recognized endoscopically by a zigzag ('Z') line, just above the most proximal gastric folds.

The oesophagus is separated from the pharynx by the **upper oesophageal sphincter** (UOS), which is normally closed due to tonic activity of the nerves supplying the cricopharyngeus. The **lower oesophageal sphincter** (LOS) consists of a 2–4-cm zone in the distal end of the oesophagus that has a high resting tone and, assisted by the diaphragmatic sphincter, is largely responsible for the prevention of gastric reflux.

Swallowing

During swallowing, the bolus of food is voluntarily moved from the mouth to the pharynx. This process is mediated by a complex reflex involving a swallowing centre in the dorsal motor nucleus of the vagus in the brainstem. Once activated, the swallowing centre neurones send pre-programmed discharges of inhibition followed by excitation to the motor nuclei of the cranial nerves. This results in initial relaxation, followed by distally progressive activation of neurones to the oesophageal smooth muscle and LOS. Pharyngeal and oesophageal peristalsis mediated by this swallowing reflex causes **primary peristalsis**. **Secondary peristalsis** arises as a result of stimulation by a food bolus in the lumen, mediated by a local intra-oesophageal reflex. **Tertiary contractions** indicate pathological non-propulsive contractions resulting from aberrant activation of local reflexes within the myenteric plexus.

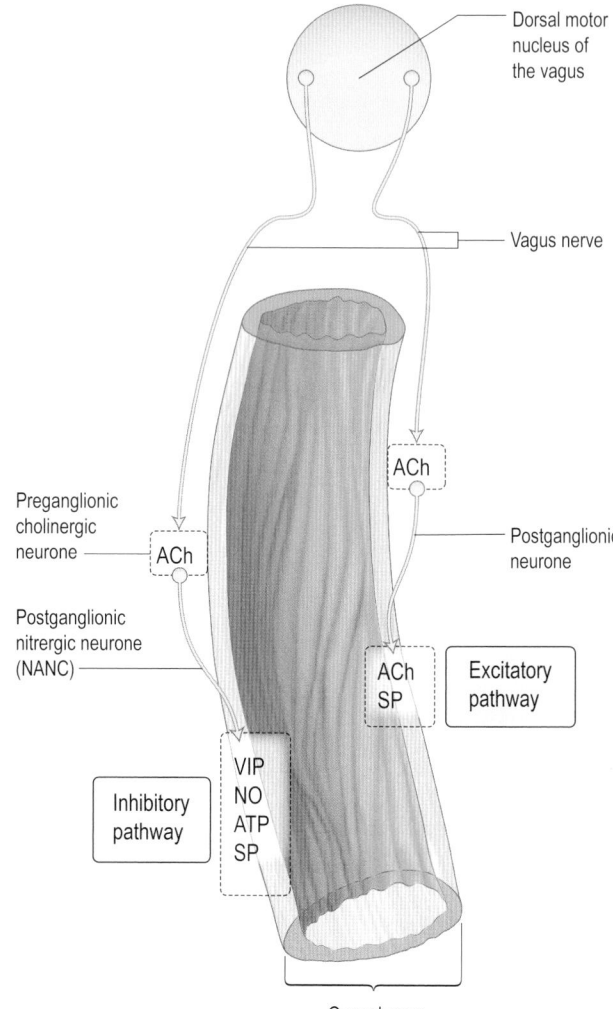

Fig. 32.1 Innervation of the oesophagus. The excitatory pathway consists of vagal preganglionic neurones releasing acetylcholine (ACh), connecting to postganglionic neurones that release ACh and substance P (SP). The inhibitory pathway consists of vagal preganglionic neurones releasing ACh, connecting to postganglionic neurones that release nitric oxide (NO), vasoactive intestinal peptide (VIP), adenosine triphosphate (ATP) and SP.

The smooth muscle of the thoracic oesophagus and LOS is supplied by vagal autonomic motor nerves consisting of extrinsic preganglionic fibres and intramural postganglionic neurones in the myenteric plexus (**Fig. 32.1**). There are parallel excitatory and inhibitory pathways.

Stomach and duodenum

The stomach occupies a small area immediately distal to the oesophagus (the cardia), the upper region (the fundus, under the left diaphragm), the mid-region or body and the antrum, which extends to the pylorus (see **Fig. 32.10**). It serves as a reservoir where food can be retained and broken up before being actively expelled into the proximal small intestine.

The smooth muscle of the wall of the stomach has three layers: outer longitudinal, inner circular and innermost oblique layers. There are two sphincters: the gastro-oesophageal sphincter and the pyloric sphincter. The latter is largely made up of a thickening of the circular muscle layer and controls the exit of gastric contents into the duodenum.

The duodenum has outer longitudinal and inner circular smooth muscle layers. It is C-shaped and the pancreas sits in the concavity. It terminates at the duodenojejunal flexure, where it joins the jejunum.

- The ***mucosal lining*** of the stomach can stretch in size with feeding. The greater curvature of the undistended stomach has thick folds or rugae. The mucosa of the upper two-thirds of the stomach contains ***parietal cells***, which secrete hydrochloric acid, and ***chief cells***, which secrete pepsinogen (which initiates proteolysis). There is often a colour change at the junction between the body and the antrum of the stomach, which can be seen macroscopically and confirmed by measuring surface pH.
- The ***antral mucosa*** secretes bicarbonate and contains mucus-secreting cells and ***G cells***, which secrete gastrin, stimulating acid production. There are two major forms of gastrin, G17 and G34, depending on the number of amino-acid residues. G17 is the major form found in the antrum. Somatostatin, a suppressant of acid secretion, is also produced by specialized antral cells (***D cells***).
- ***Mucus-secreting cells*** are present throughout the stomach and secrete mucus and bicarbonate. The mucus is made of glycoproteins called mucins.
- The ***'mucosal barrier'***, made up of the plasma membranes of mucosal cells and the mucus layer, protects the gastric epithelium from damage by acid and, for example, alcohol, aspirin, nonsteroidal anti-inflammatory drugs (NSAIDs) and bile salts. Prostaglandins stimulate secretion of mucus, and their synthesis is inhibited by aspirin and NSAIDs, which inhibit cyclo-oxygenase (see p. 1176).
- The ***duodenal mucosa*** has villi like the rest of the small bowel, and also contains Brunner's glands, which secrete alkaline mucus. This, along with the pancreatic and biliary secretions, helps to neutralize the acid secretion from the stomach when it reaches the duodenum.

Physiology

Acid secretion is central to the functionality of the stomach; factors controlling acid secretion are shown in **Fig. 32.2**. Acid is not essential for digestion but does prevent some food-borne infections. It is under neural and hormonal control, and both stimulate acid secretion through the direct action of histamine on the parietal cell. Acetylcholine and gastrin also release histamine via the enterochromaffin cells. Somatostatin inhibits both histamine and gastrin release, and therefore acid secretion.

Other major gastric functions are:
- reservoir for food
- emulsification of fat and mixing of gastric contents
- secretion of intrinsic factor
- absorption (of only minimal importance).

Gastric emptying depends on many factors. There are osmoreceptors in the duodenal mucosa, which control gastric emptying by local reflexes and the release of gut hormones. In particular, intraduodenal fat delays gastric emptying by negative feedback through duodenal receptors.

Small intestine anatomy

The small intestine extends from the duodenum to the ileocaecal valve. It is 3–6 m in length, and 300 m² in surface area. The upper

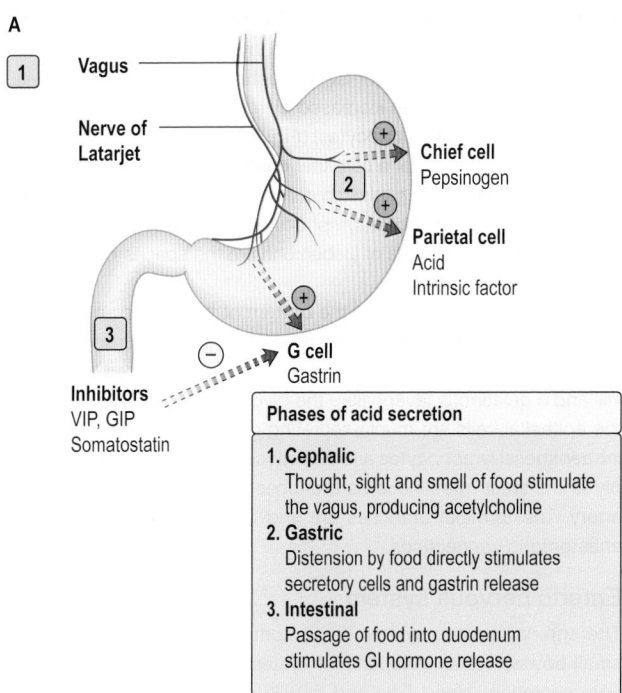

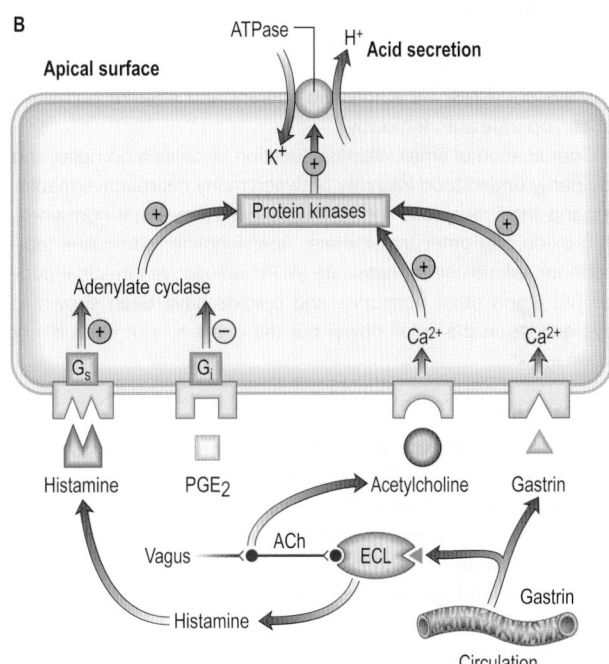

Fig. 32.2 Pathophysiology of acid secretion. (A) Control of acid secretion. **(B)** Mechanisms involved in acid secretion. Histamine stimulates the G_s protein via the H_2 receptors and acts via cyclic adenosine monophosphate (cAMP). Prostaglandin E_2 (PGE_2) activates the G_i protein and *inhibits* acid secretion. Acetylcholine (ACh) acts via the vagus M_3 receptors. ACh also acts via the enterochromaffin cell (ECL). Gastrin acts via the cholecystokinin B (CCKBB)–gastrin receptor, increasing the intracellular free calcium, and also via the ECL cell, stimulating histamine. Gs and Gi, stimulating and inhibiting G-proteins; GIP, gastric inhibitory polypeptide; VIP, vasoactive intestinal polypeptide.

40% is the duodenum and jejunum; the remainder is the ileum. Its surface area is enormously increased by circumferential mucosal folds that bear multiple finger-like projections called villi. On the villi, the surface area is further increased by microvilli on the luminal side of the epithelial cells (enterocytes) (**Fig. 32.3**).

Each villus consists of a core that contains blood vessels, lacteals (lymphatics) and cells (e.g. plasma cells and lymphocytes). The lamina propria contains plasma cells, lymphocytes, macrophages, eosinophils and mast cells. The crypts of Lieberkühn are the spaces between the bases of the villi.

Enterocytes are formed at the bottom of the crypts and migrate toward the tops of the villi, where they are shed. This process takes 3–4 days. On its luminal side, the enterocyte is covered by microvilli and a gelatinous layer called the glycocalyx. Scattered between the epithelial cells are mucin-secreting goblet cells and occasional intraepithelial lymphocytes and Paneth cells. Most of the blood supply to the small intestine is via branches of the superior mesenteric artery. The terminal branches are end arteries; there are no local anastomotic connections.

Enteric nervous system

The enteric nervous system (ENS) controls the functioning of the small bowel; it is an independent system that coordinates absorption, secretion, blood flow and motility. It is estimated to contain 10^8 neurones (as many as the spinal cord), organized in two major ganglionated plexuses: the *myenteric plexus* between the muscular layers of the intestinal wall, and the *submucosal plexuses* associated with the mucosa. The ENS communicates with the central nervous system (CNS) via autonomic afferent and efferent pathways but can operate autonomously.

Coordination of small intestinal function involves a complex and only partly understood interplay between many neuroactive mediators and their receptors, ion channels, gastrointestinal hormones, nitric oxide and other transmitters. Acetylcholine, adrenaline (epinephrine), adenosine triphosphate (ATP), vasoactive intestinal peptide (VIP), and other hormones and opioids have been shown to have actions in the small bowel but the exact role of each is not yet clear.

Gut motility

The contractile patterns of the small intestinal muscular layers are primarily determined by the ENS. The CNS and gut hormones also have a modulatory role in motility. The interstitial cells of Cajal, which lie within the smooth muscle, appear to govern rhythmic contractions.

During fasting, a distally migrating sequence of motor events, termed the migrating motor complex (MMC), occurs in a cyclical fashion. The MMC consists of:
- a period of motor quiescence (*phase I*)
- a period of irregular contractile activity (*phase II*)
- a short (5–10-min) burst of regular phasic contractions (*phase III*).

Each MMC cycle lasts for approximately 90 minutes. In the duodenum, phase III is associated with increased gastric, pancreatic and biliary secretions. The role of the MMC is unclear, but the strong phase III contractions propel secretions, residual food and desquamated cells towards the colon. It is named the 'intestinal housekeeper'.

After a meal, the MMC pattern is disrupted and replaced by irregular contractions. This seemingly chaotic pattern lasts typically for 2–5 hours after feeding, depending on the size and nutrient content of the meal. The irregular contractions of the fed pattern have a mixing function, moving intraluminal contents to and fro and aiding the digestive process.

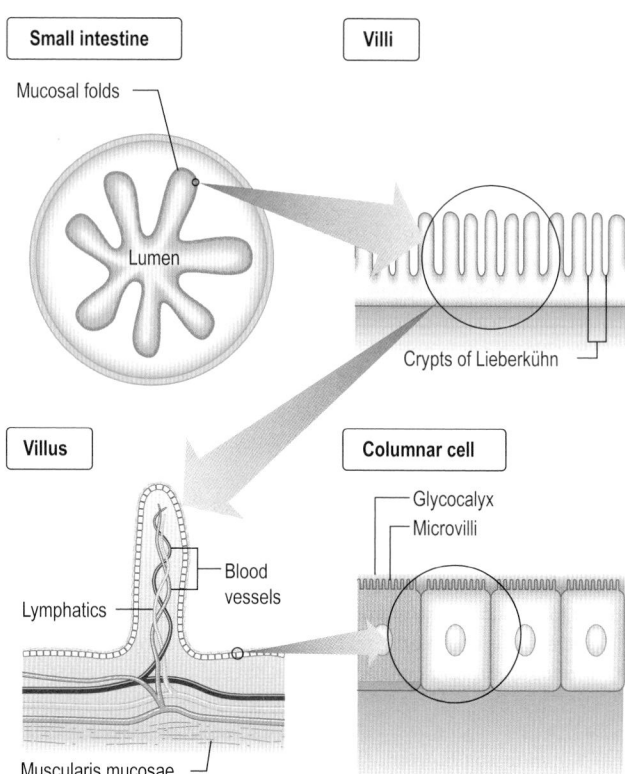

Fig. 32.3 Structure of the small intestine.

Neuroendocrine peptide production

The hormone-producing cells of the gut are scattered diffusely throughout its length and also occur in the pancreas.

Gut hormones play a part in the regulation and integration of the functions of the small bowel and other metabolic activities, including appetite. Their actions are complex and interactive, both with each other and with the ENS (**Box 32.4**).

Small intestine physiology

In the small bowel, digestion and absorption of nutrients and ions takes place, as does the regulation of fluid absorption and secretion. The epithelial cells of the small bowel form a physical barrier that is selectively permeable to ions, small molecules and macromolecules. Digestive enzymes, such as proteases and disaccharidases, are produced by intestinal cells and expressed on the surface of microvilli; others, such as lipases produced by the pancreas, are associated with the glycocalyx. Some nutrients are absorbed most actively in specific parts of the small intestine: iron and folate in the duodenum and jejunum, and vitamin B_{12} and bile salts in the terminal ileum, where they have specific receptors.

General principles of absorption
Simple diffusion

This process is non-specific, requires no carrier molecule or energy, and takes place if there is a concentration gradient from the intestinal lumen (high concentration) to the bloodstream (low concentration). Vitamin B_{12} can be absorbed from the jejunum by this means.

Facilitated diffusion

Absorption takes place down a concentration gradient but a membrane carrier protein is involved, conferring specificity on the process. Fructose transport is an example.

> **i** **Box 32.4** Gut regulatory peptides

Peptide	Localization	Main actions
Gastrin/cholecystokinin family		
Cholecystokinin (CCK): multiple forms from CCK8 (8 amino acids) to CCK83; 8, 33 and 58 are predominant Terminal 5 amino acids same as gastrin	Duodenum and jejunum (I cells) Enteric nerves CNS	Causes gall bladder contraction and sphincter of Oddi relaxation. Trophic effects on duodenum and pancreas. Pancreatic secretion (minor role) Role in satiety – acting on CNS
Gastrin	G cells in gastric antrum and duodenum	Stimulates acid secretion. Trophic to mucosa
Secretin-glucagon family		
Secretin	Duodenum and jejunum (S cells)	Stimulates pancreatic bicarbonate secretion
Glucagon	Alpha cells of pancreas	Opposes insulin in blood glucose control
Vasoactive intestinal polypeptide (VIP)	Enteric nerves	Intestinal secretion of water and electrolytes. Neurotransmitter. Splanchnic vasodilation, stimulates insulin release
Glucose-dependent insulinotropic peptide (GIP)	Duodenum (K cells) Gastric antrum Ileum	Release by intraduodenal glucose causes greater insulin release by islets than i.v. glucose (incretin effect)
Glucagon-like peptide-1 (GLP-1)	Ileum and colon (L cells)	Incretin. Stimulates insulin synthesis. Trophic to islet cells. Inhibits glucagon secretion and gastric emptying Stimulates growth of enterocytes
Glicentin	L cells, A cells	Stimulates insulin secretion and gut growth, inhibits gastric secretion
Growth hormone-releasing factor (GHRF)	Small intestine	Unclear
Pancreatic polypeptide family		
Pancreatic polypeptide (PP)	Pancreas (PP cells)	Inhibits pancreatic and biliary secretion
Peptide YY (PYY)	Ileum and colon (L cells)	Inhibits pancreatic exocrine secretion. Slows gastric and small bowel transit ('ileal brake'). Reduces food intake and appetite
Neuropeptide Y (NPY)	Enteric nerves	Stimulates feeding. Regulates intestinal blood flow
Other		
Motilin	Whole gut	Increases gastric emptying and small bowel contraction
Ghrelin	Stomach	Stimulates appetite, increases gastric emptying
Obestatin	Stomach and small intestine	Opposes ghrelin
Oxyntomodulin	Colon	Inhibits appetite
Gastrin releasing-polypeptide (bombesin)	Whole gut and pancreas	Stimulates pancreatic exocrine secretion and gastric acid secretion
Somatostatin	Stomach and pancreas (D cells) Small and large intestine	Inhibits secretion and action of most hormones
Substance P	Enteric nerves	Enhances gastric acid secretion, smooth muscle contraction
Neurotensin	Ileum	Affects gut motility. Increases jejunal and ileal fluid secretion
Insulin	Pancreatic β cells	Increases glucose utilization
Chromogranins	Neuroendocrine cells	Precursor for other regulatory peptides that inhibit neuroendocrine secretion

Active transport

Absorption occurs via a specific carrier protein, powered by cellular energy, allowing a substance to be transported against a concentration gradient. Many carrier proteins are powered by ion gradients across the enterocyte wall. For example, glucose crosses the enterocyte microvillous membrane from the lumen into the cell against a concentration gradient by using a **co-transporter** carrier molecule. This is the sodium/glucose co-transporter, SGLT1 (**Fig. 32.4**). The process is powered by the energy derived from the flow of Na^+ ions from a high concentration outside the cell to a low concentration inside. The sodium gradient across the cell wall is maintained by a separate ATP-consuming Na^+/K^+ exchanger in the basolateral membrane. Glucose leaves the cell on the serosal side

by facilitated diffusion via a sodium-independent carrier (GLUT-2) in the basolateral membrane.

Another active transport mechanism operates for Na^+ absorption in the ileum using an Na^+/H^+ **exchange** mechanism, powered by the outwardly directed gradient of H^+ across the cell membrane.

Absorption of nutrients in the small intestine
Carbohydrate

Dietary carbohydrate consists mainly of starch, with some sucrose and a small amount of lactose. Starch is a polysaccharide made up of numerous glucose units. In order to have a nutrient value, starch must be digested into smaller oligo-, di- and finally monosaccharides, which may then be absorbed.

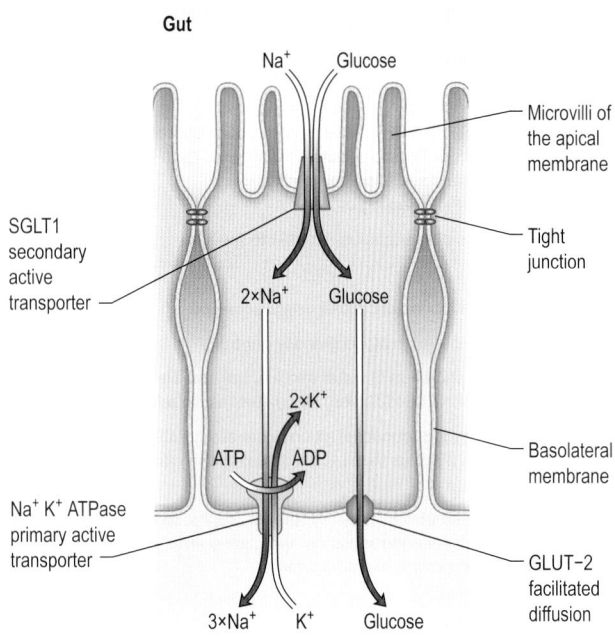

Gut

Na⁺   Glucose

Microvilli of the apical membrane

SGLT1 secondary active transporter

Tight junction

2×Na⁺   Glucose

2×K⁺

ATP   ADP

Basolateral membrane

Na⁺ K⁺ ATPase primary active transporter

GLUT–2 facilitated diffusion

3×Na⁺   K⁺   Glucose

Intercellular space

Fig. 32.4 Transcellular uptake of glucose across the intestinal epithelia. Glucose is co-transported across the apical membrane with sodium ions by the sodium-dependent glucose transporter (SGLT). This is secondary active transport, as the sodium is travelling down its electrochemical gradient. The sodium gradient is maintained by the primary active transport of sodium across the basolateral membrane by the Na⁺/K⁺ ATPase (thus intracellular Na⁺ is kept low). Transcellular transport of glucose is achieved by facilitated diffusion across the basolateral membrane as glucose is moved down its concentration gradient by GLUT-2.

Polysaccharide hydrolysis begins in the mouth and is catalyzed by salivary amylase, though the majority takes place under the action of pancreatic amylase in the upper intestine. The breakdown products of starch digestion are maltose and maltotriose, together with sucrose and lactose. These are further hydrolysed on the microvillous membrane by specific oligo- and disaccharidases to form glucose, galactose and fructose. These monosaccharides are then able to be transported across the enterocytes into the blood (see **Fig. 32.4**).

Protein

Dietary protein is digested by pancreatic proteolytic enzymes to amino acids and peptides prior to absorption. These enzymes are secreted by the pancreas as pro-enzymes and transformed to active forms in the lumen. Protein in the duodenal lumen stimulates the enzymatic conversion of trypsinogen to trypsin, and this, in turn, activates the other pro-enzymes, chymotrypsin and elastase.

These enzymes break down protein into oligopeptides. Some di- and tripeptides are absorbed intact by carrier-mediated processes, while the remainder are broken down into free amino acids by peptidases on the microvillous membranes of the enterocytes, prior to absorption into the cell by a variety of amino acid and peptide carrier systems.

Fat

Dietary fat consists mainly of triglycerides with some cholesterol and fat-soluble vitamins. Fat is emulsified by mechanical action

in the stomach. Bile containing the amphipathic detergents, bile acids and phospholipids enters the duodenum following gall bladder contraction. These substances act to solubilize fat and promote hydrolysis of triglycerides in the duodenum by pancreatic lipase to yield fatty acids and monoglycerides. Bile acids, phospholipids and the products of fat digestion cluster together with their hydrophilic ends on the outside to form aggregations called mixed micelles. Trapped in the centre of the micelles are the hydrophobic monoglycerides, fatty acids and cholesterol. At the cell membrane, the lipid contents of the micelles are absorbed, while the bile salts remain in the lumen. Inside the cell, the monoglycerides and fatty acids are re-esterified to triglycerides. The triglycerides and other fat-soluble molecules (e.g. cholesterol, phospholipids) are then incorporated into chylomicrons to be transported into the lymph.

Any unabsorbed lipids that reach the ileum delay gastric emptying via peptide YY, which is secreted by the ileum (called the '**ileal brake**'). This delay allows more time for absorption of lipids in the small intestine.

Medium-chain triglycerides (MCTs, fatty acids of chain length 6–12) are transported via the portal vein with a small amount of long-chain fatty acid. Patients with pancreatic exocrine or bile salt insufficiency can therefore supplement their fat absorption with MCTs.

Bile salts are not absorbed in the jejunum, so the intraluminal concentration in the upper gut is high. They pass down the intestine to be absorbed in the terminal ileum and are transported back to the liver. This enterohepatic circulation prevents excess loss of bile salts (see p. 1266).

The pathophysiology of fat absorption is shown in **Fig. 32.5**. Interference with absorption can occur at all stages, as indicated, giving rise to steatorrhoea (>17 mmol or 6 g of faecal fat per day).

Water and electrolytes

Large amounts of water and electrolytes, partly dietary but mainly from intestinal secretions, are absorbed, coupled with absorption of monosaccharides, amino acids and bicarbonate in the upper jejunum. Water and electrolytes are also absorbed paracellularly (between the enterocytes) down electrochemical and osmotic gradients. Additional water and electrolytes are absorbed in the ileum and colon, where active sodium transport is not coupled to solute absorption. Secretion of fluid and electrolytes occurs together to maintain the normal functioning of the gut. Secretory diarrhoea (see p. 1185) can occur because of defects in intestinal secretory mechanisms.

Water-soluble vitamins, essential metals and trace elements

These are all absorbed in the small intestine. Vitamin B₁₂ (see p. 335) and bile salts are absorbed by specific transport mechanisms in the terminal ileum; malabsorption of both these substances often occurs following ileal resection.

Calcium

Calcium absorption is discussed on page 474.

Iron

Iron absorption is discussed on page 329.

Response of the small bowel to antigens and pathogens

The small bowel has a number of mechanisms to prevent colonization and invasion by pathogens while simultaneously preventing

A

| Absorption | | Malabsorption (steatorrhoea) |

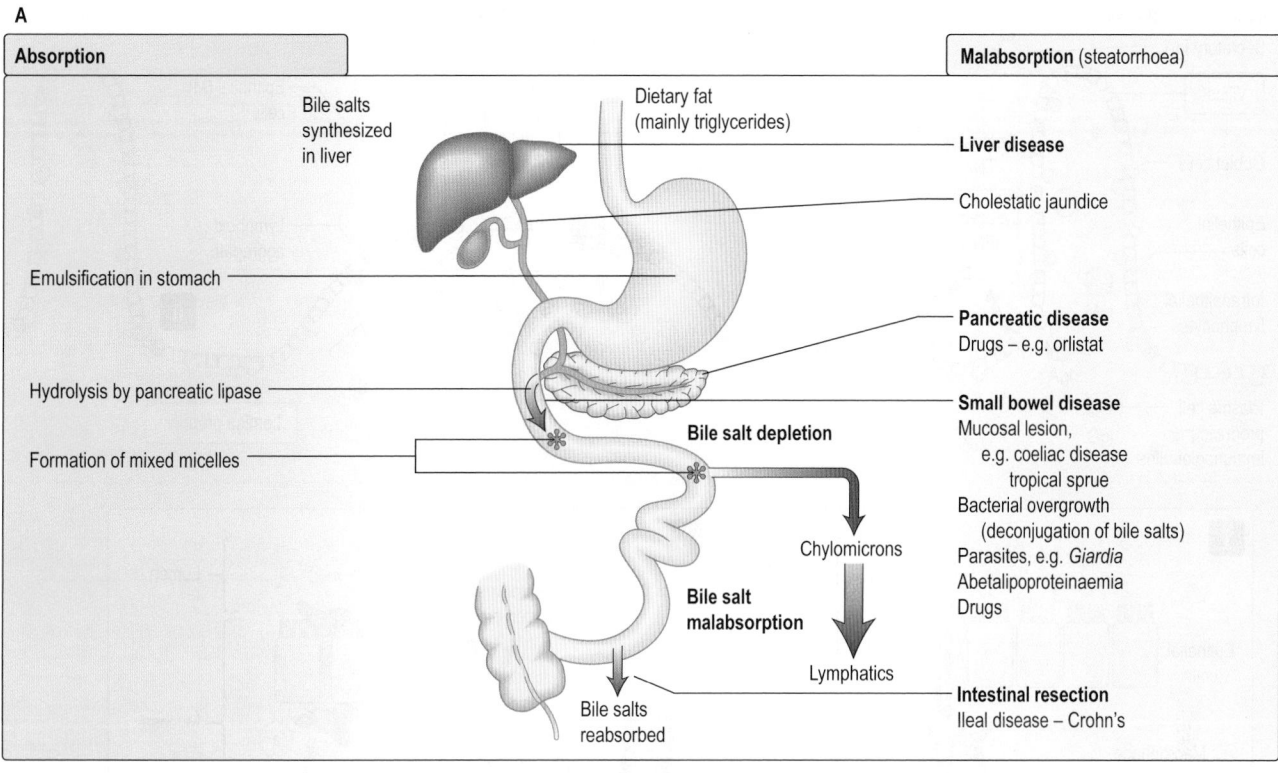

Bile salts synthesized in liver

Dietary fat (mainly triglycerides)

Liver disease

Cholestatic jaundice

Emulsification in stomach

Pancreatic disease
Drugs – e.g. orlistat

Hydrolysis by pancreatic lipase

Small bowel disease
Mucosal lesion,
 e.g. coeliac disease
  tropical sprue
Bacterial overgrowth
 (deconjugation of bile salts)
Parasites, e.g. *Giardia*
Abetalipoproteinaemia
Drugs

Formation of mixed micelles

Bile salt depletion

Chylomicrons

Bile salt malabsorption

Lymphatics

Bile salts reabsorbed

Intestinal resection
Ileal disease – Crohn's

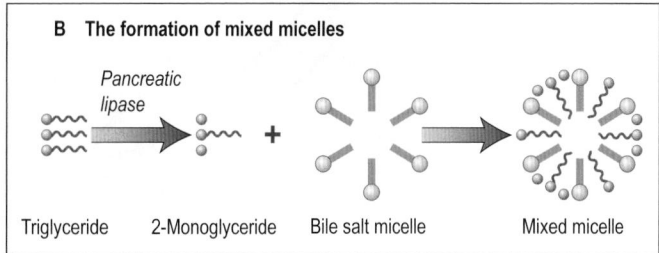

B   The formation of mixed micelles

Pancreatic lipase

Triglyceride   2-Monoglyceride   +   Bile salt micelle   Mixed micelle

Fig. 32.5 **Fat absorption in the small intestine. (A)** The pathophysiology of fat absorption. Diseases impairing fat absorption, that may therefore cause steatorrhoea, are shown on the right of the diagram. **(B)** The formation of mixed micelles.

inappropriate responses to foreign antigens or the indigenous bacterial population. At the same time, commensal bacteria maintain the integrity of the small bowel and play a major role in host physiology.

Mechanisms

Physical defence

- The mucus layer.
- Continuous shedding of surface epithelial cells.
- The physical movement of the luminal contents.
- Colonization resistance – the ability of the indigenous microbiota to outcompete pathogens for a survival niche in the gut.

Innate chemical defence

- **Enzymes** such as lysozyme and phospholipase A_2, secreted by Paneth cells at the base of the crypts, help ensure an infection-free environment in the gut, even in the presence of commensal bacteria.
- **Antimicrobial peptides** are secreted from enterocytes and Paneth cells in response to pathogenic bacteria. These include **defensins**, which are 15–20 amino-acid peptides with potent activity against a broad range of pathogens, includ-

ing Gram-positive and Gram-negative bacteria, fungi and viruses.

- **Trefoil peptides** are a family of small proteins secreted by goblet cells. They consist of a three-loop structure with intra-chain disulphide bonds, which makes the molecules highly resistant to digestion. Their actions include stabilization of mucus, promotion of cell migration to injured areas, and promotion of repair. Three trefoil factors (TFFs) are found in humans (TFF1, TFF2 and TFF3), all of which have been implicated in the response to gastrointestinal injury in experimental models. Their molecular mode of action is not yet known.

Innate immunological defence

- **Humoral defence**. IgA is the principal mucosal antibody. It mediates mucosal immunity by agglutinating and neutralizing pathogens in the lumen and preventing colonization of the epithelial surface (**Fig. 32.6**). IgA is secreted from immunocytes in the lamina propria as dimers joined by a protein called the 'joining chain' (J-chain); in this form, it is known as polymeric IgA (pIgA). This pIgA is internalized by endocytosis at the basolateral membrane of enterocytes. It crosses the cell as a complex of pIgA/pIgAR and is secreted on to the mucosal surface.

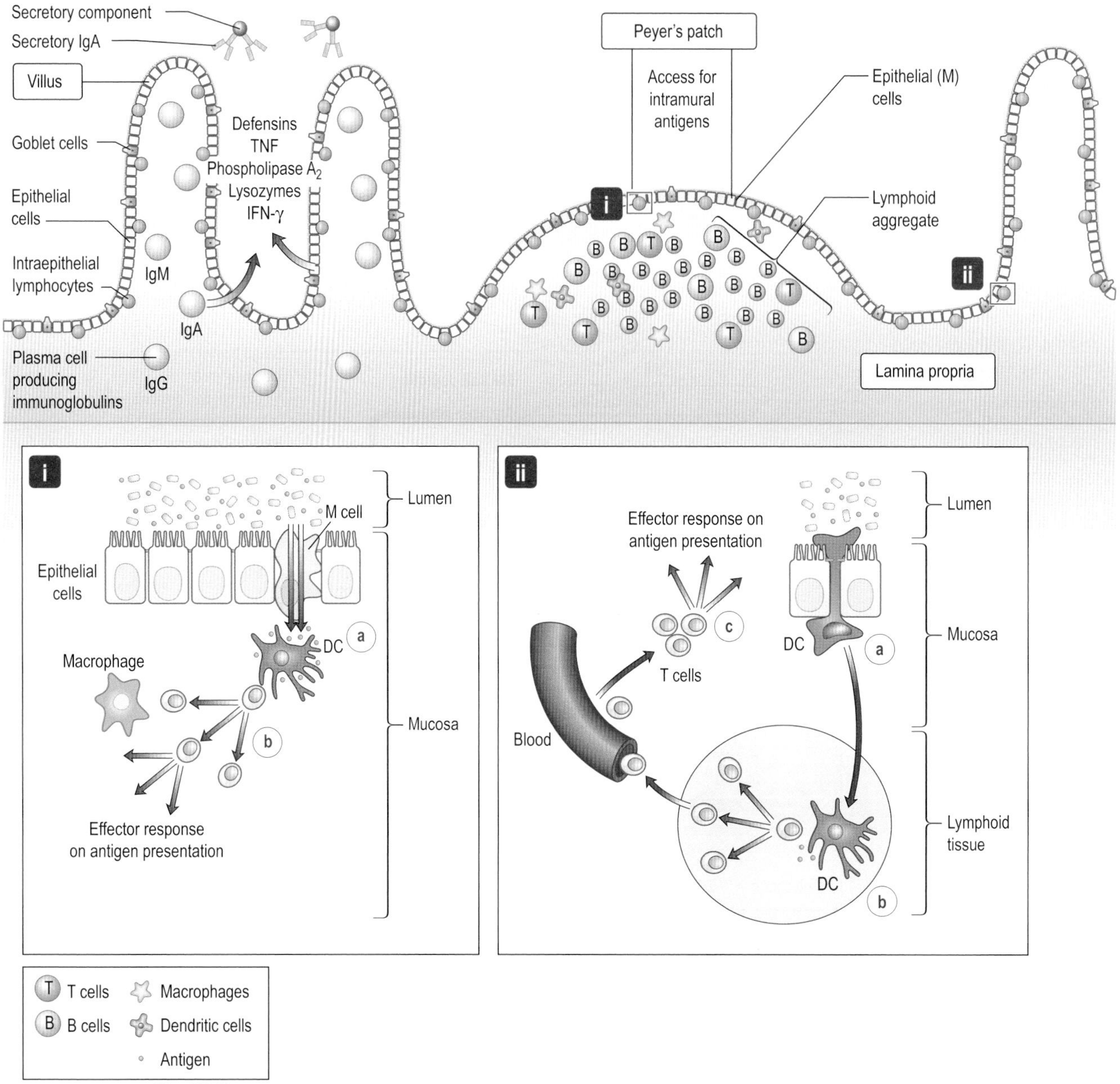

Secretory component

Secretory IgA

Villus

Goblet cells

Epithelial cells

Intraepithelial lymphocytes

Plasma cell producing immunoglobulins

Defensins
TNF
Phospholipase A$_2$
Lysozymes
IFN-γ

IgM

IgA

IgG

Peyer's patch

Access for intramural antigens

Epithelial (M) cells

Lymphoid aggregate

Lamina propria

i

ii

i   Lumen

M cell

Epithelial cells

Macrophage

DC   a

b

Effector response on antigen presentation

Mucosa

ii   Lumen

Effector response on antigen presentation

T cells

Blood

DC   a

c

Mucosa

Lymphoid tissue

DC   b

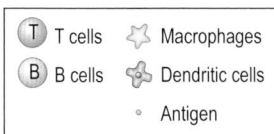

(T) T cells   ☆ Macrophages

(B) B cells   ⚛ Dendritic cells

    ° Antigen

Fig. 32.6 Small intestinal mucosa with a Peyer's patch, showing the gut-associated lymphoid tissue (GALT). Inset i: (a) Specialized 'M' cells within a lymphoid follicle pass antigen to underlying antigen-presenting cells (APCs), such as dendritic cells (DCs). (b) DCs present antigen to T cells, resulting in activation and effector responses. Inset ii: (a) DCs pass dendrites through epithelial tight junctions to sample luminal antigen. (b) DCs traffic to the mesenteric lymph node and present antigen to naive T cells, which differentiate into effector or regulatory subtypes and are imprinted with a gut homing integrin. (c) On subsequent antigen presentation, activated T cells home to lamina propria and exert a regulatory or inflammatory effect, depending on their phenotype. IFN-γ, interferon-gamma; Ig, immunoglobulin; TNF, tumour necrosis factor.

- **B-cell sensitization.** Antigens from the lumen of the bowel are transported by M cells and dendritic cells in the follicle-associated epithelium (FAE). This covers Peyer's patches in the 'dome' region that contain abundant virgin B cells, helper T cells and antigen-presenting cells. Activated B cells then produce IgA locally and are programmed to home back to the lamina propria. They travel through mesenteric lymph nodes and then via the thoracic duct to the blood and back to the small bowel and other mucosal surfaces (such as the airways), where they undergo terminal differentiation into plasma cells. Homing back to the gut is facilitated by the

$\alpha4\beta7$-integrin on gut-derived lymphocytes binding to MAdCAM-1, uniquely expressed on blood vessels in the gut.
- **Cellular defence.** T lymphocytes also provide host defence and initiate, activate and regulate adaptive immune responses. **Intestinal T lymphocytes** occur principally in three major compartments:
  - *Organized gut-associated lymphoid tissue (GALT)*, such as Peyer's patches, where mucosal T cell responses are generated, and after which cells leave the organized lymphoid tissue and home back to the mucosa.

- *The lamina propria*, containing mostly CD4 cells.
- The *surface epithelium*, where these lymphocytes are known as intraepithelial lymphocytes (IELs) and are mostly CD8 cells. T cells are sensitized to antigen in the Peyer's patch lymphoid tissue in a similar fashion to B cells, and pass through mesenteric lymph nodes into the thoracic duct and into the circulation, homing back to the small bowel to end up in the lamina propria or the epithelium. It is probable that IELs are cytotoxic cells, capable of killing virally or bacterially infected epithelial cells. CD4 cells in the lamina propria of healthy individuals are highly activated cells, probably protecting against low-grade infections, since loss of these cells, as in HIV infection, leads to colonization of the gut by protozoa such as cryptosporidia.

The gut microbiome

The relationship between the hundred thousand billion microbes in the human gut and the host is only beginning to be appreciated. New molecular sequencing techniques have allowed the identification and classification of the gut microbiota. The use of metabonomics has aided the assessment of its functional output. There is increasing evidence that a reduction in the diversity of the gut microbiota is associated with a range of conditions, including inflammatory bowel disease and metabolic syndrome. Germ-free mice have essentially no mucosal immune system, showing that the abundant and activated immune system seen in healthy individuals is driven by the flora, without adverse effects. Bacteria also release chemical signals, such as lipopolysaccharide (LPS) and lipoteichoic acid, which are recognized by Toll-like receptors (TLRs) (see p. 47) present on a variety of intestinal cells, priming repair processes and enhancing the ability of the epithelium to respond to injury.

Oral tolerance

The immune system must guard against pathogens and toxins while avoiding an excessive response to the multiplicity of food antigens and commensal bacteria. The mechanisms by which tolerance occurs are multiple, including maintenance of barrier function to prevent excess antigen uptake, active inhibition via regulatory T cells, and promotion of tolerogenic rather than immunogenic T-cell responses by dendritic cells. All of these are likely to play a role in diseases such as coeliac disease, caused by an excessive T-cell response to gluten, or Crohn's disease, where tolerance to the indigenous bacterial population is defective.

Colon and rectal anatomy

The large intestine starts at the caecum, on the posterior medial wall of which is the appendix.

The **colon** is made up of ascending, transverse, descending and sigmoid parts, which join the rectum at the rectosigmoid junction (**Fig. 32.7**). The muscle wall consists of an inner circular layer and an outer longitudinal layer. The outer layer is incomplete, coming together to form the taeniae coli, which produce the haustral pattern seen in the normal colon.

The mucosa of the colon is lined with epithelial cells and goblet cells. There are crypts but no villi, so that the surface is flat. A variety of cells, mainly lymphocytes and macrophages, are found in the lamina propria.

The blood supply to the colon is from the superior and inferior mesenteric vessels. The colon is innervated mainly by the enteric

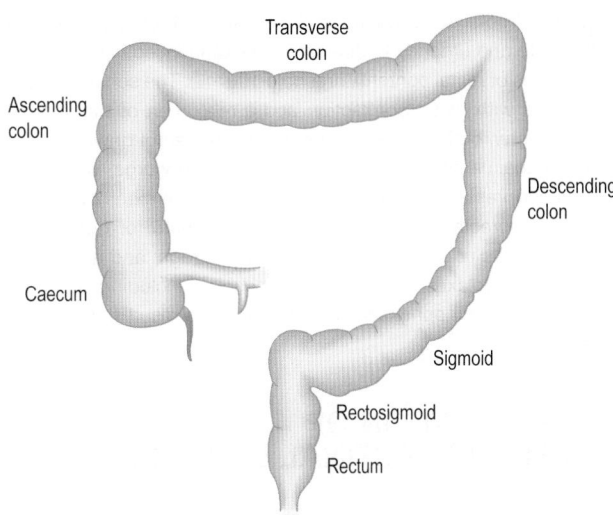

Fig. 32.7 Structure of the large intestine.

i	Box 32.5 Input and output of water and electrolytes in the gastrointestinal tract over 24 hours			
		Water (mL)	**Sodium (mmol)**	**Potassium (mmol)**
Input				
Diet		1500	150	80
Gastrointestinal secretions		7500	1000	40
Totals		9000	1150	120
Output				
Faeces		150	5	12
Ileostomy (adapted)		500–1000	60–120	4

nervous system with input from the parasympathetic and sympathetic pathways. Spinal afferent neurones from the dorsal root ganglia innervate the entire colon.

The **rectum** is about 12 cm long. Its interior is divided by three crescentic circular muscles that produce shelf-like folds. These are the rectal valves, which can be seen at sigmoidoscopy. The anal canal has an internal and an external sphincter.

Physiology of the colon

The main roles of the colon are the absorption of water and electrolytes (**Box 32.5**) and the propulsion of contents from the caecum to the anorectal region. Approximately 1.5–2 L of fluid pass the ileocaecal valve each day. Absorption is stimulated by short-chain fatty acids, which are produced predominantly in the right colon by the anaerobic metabolism of dietary fibre by bacterial polysaccharidase enzyme systems. Colonic contents are mixed, aiding absorption by non-propagative segmenting muscular contractions. High-amplitude propagative colonic contractions cause propulsion. Peristalsis is induced by the release of serotonin (5-HT) from neuroendocrine cells in response to luminal distension. Serotonin activates the HT_4 receptors, which, in turn, results in the activation of sensory (calcitonin gene-related peptide, CGRP) neurones. Normal colonic transit time is 24–48 hours with normal stool weights of up to 250 g/day.

Physiology of defecation

The role of the rectum and anus in defecation is complex. The rectum is normally empty. Stool is propelled into the rectum by propagated colonic contractions. A sensation of fullness, a desire to defecate and urgency to defecate are experienced with increasing volumes of rectal content (threshold 100 mL). The sensations are associated with rectal contraction and a relaxation of the internal anal sphincter, both of which serve to push the stool down into the proximal anal canal. This increases the defecatory urge, which can only be suppressed by vigorous contraction of the external sphincter and puborectalis. If conditions are appropriate for defecation, the subject sits or squats, contracts the diaphragm and abdominal muscles, and relaxes the pelvic floor muscles, including puborectalis, and the anal sphincter muscles, with the result that stool is expelled.

INVESTIGATION OF GASTROINTESTINAL DISEASE

Routine haematology and biochemistry, followed by endoscopy and radiology, are the principal investigations.

Blood tests

All patients undergoing investigation for gastrointestinal disease should have routine blood tests. These include a full blood count, serum creatinine and electrolytes, liver function tests and clotting. This basic screen checks for anaemia, elevated/depleted white cell or platelet counts, electrolyte disturbances and clotting abnormalities which can be present in several gastrointestinal diseases.

Stool tests

Stool tests are vital investigation for GI disease. Stool should always be sent for microscopy, culture and sensitivities (MCS) in order to exclude infection in patients presenting with diarrhoea. For patients who have travelled abroad recently it can be useful to also look for stool ova, cysts and parasites to check for infections such a giardiasis, amoebiasis or tapeworm. **Faecal calprotectin** is a protein found in stool during intestinal inflammation (e.g. IBD or infection). It is commonly used in outpatients both diagnostically (it is 93% sensitive and 96% specific for inflammatory bowel disease in adults) and for monitoring disease activity. Below 100 μg/g is within normal limits and a level higher than 200 μg/g is suggestive of inflammatory bowel disease or an infective colitis. It should not be used in older patients where malignancy is suspected.

Endoscopy

Video endoscopes relay colour images to a high-definition television monitor. The tip of the endoscope can be angulated in all directions, and channels in the instrument are used for air insufflation, water injection, suction, and the passage of accessories such as biopsy forceps or brushes for obtaining tissue, snares for polypectomy and needles for injection therapies.

- **Oesophagogastroduodenoscopy** (**OGD**, 'gastroscopy') is the investigation of choice for upper gastrointestinal disorders with the possibility of therapy and mucosal biopsy. Findings include reflux oesophagitis, gastritis, ulcers and cancer. Therapeutic OGD is used to treat upper gastrointestinal haemorrhage and both benign and malignant obstruction. The mortality for diagnostic endoscopy is 0.001% with significant complications in 1:10000, usually when performed as an emergency (e.g. gastrointestinal haemorrhage).

Box 32.6 Gastroscopy and colonoscopy

- Explain the procedure to the patient, including benefits and risks.
- Discuss the need for sedation.
- Obtain written informed consent.

Gastroscopy

- The patient should be fasted for at least 4 h.
- Give oxygen and monitor oxygen saturation with an oximeter.
- Give lidocaine throat spray or sedation (midazolam ± opiate if required).
- Pass the gastroscope to the duodenum under direct vision.
- Examine during insertion and withdrawal.
- Gastroscopy takes 5–15 min, depending on the indication and findings.
- Withhold fluid and food until local anaesthetic/sedation wears off.
- Complications are rare but beware of over-sedation, perforation and aspiration.
- The patient must be accompanied home if sedation has been given.

Colonoscopy

- Stop oral iron a week before the procedure.
- Restrict the diet to low-residue foods for 48 h; clear fluids only for 24 h.
- Use a local bowel-cleansing regime, usually starting 24 h beforehand (e.g. two sachets of sodium picosulfate with magnesium citrate and 2–4 bisacodyl tablets, or macrogols 2–4 L, or local alternative; more if constipated).
- Give oxygen and monitor O_2 levels.
- Give sedation (midazolam ± opiate) if required by the patient.
- Pass the colonoscope to the caecum or ileum under direct vision.
- Examine in detail during withdrawal.
- Colonoscopy takes 15–30 min, depending on the colon anatomy, indication and findings.
- Withhold fluid and food until sedation wears off.
- Observe the patient for at least an hour after sedation has been given.
- Complications are rare but beware of over-sedation, perforation and aspiration.
- The patient must be accompanied home if sedation has been given.

For patients on antiplatelet therapy and anticoagulants (including antithrombotic agents), see Veitch AM, Vanbiervliet G, Gershlick AH et al. *Endoscopy in patients on antiplatelet or anticoagulant therapy including direct oral anticoagulants. British Society of Gastroenterology (BSG) and European Society of Gastrointestinal Endoscopy (ESGE) guidelines.* Gut *2016; 65:374–389.*

Box 32.7 Proctoscopy

- The proctoscope is passed into the anus and the obturator is removed.
- The patient strains down as the proctoscope is removed.
- Haemorrhoids are seen as purplish veins in the left lateral, right posterior or right anterior position.
- Fissures may also be seen, but pain often prevents the procedure from being performed.

- **Colonoscopy** allows good visualization of the whole colon and terminal ileum. Biopsies can be obtained and polyps removed. Benign strictures can be dilated and malignant strictures stented. Cancer, polyps and diverticular disease are the most common significant findings. Perforation occurs in 1:1000 examinations but this is higher (up to 2%) after polypectomy and endoscopic mucosal resection (**Box 32.6**).
- **Proctoscopy** (**Box 32.7**) is performed in all patients with a history of bright red rectal bleeding to look for anorectal pathology such as haemorrhoids; a rigid sigmoidoscope is too narrow and long to enable adequate examination of the anal canal.
- **Sigmoidoscopy**, either flexible or rigid, is part of the routine hospital examination in cases of diarrhoea and in patients with lower

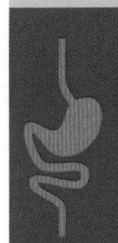

abdominal symptoms such as a change in bowel habit or rectal bleeding. *Rigid sigmoidoscopy* can visualize the distal 20–25 cm of large bowel, whereas *flexible sigmoidoscopy* (*FS*) can reach up to the splenic flexure (60 cm), and is typically performed in the endoscopy unit after evacuation of the distal colon using an enema or suppository.

- *Balloon enteroscopy*, either double- or single-balloon, can examine the small bowel from the duodenum to the ileum, adopting both cranial and caudal approaches, and using specialized enteroscopes in expert centres.
- *Capsule endoscopy* is used for the evaluation of obscure gastrointestinal bleeding (after negative gastroscopy and colonoscopy) and for the detection of small bowel tumours and occult inflammatory bowel disease. It should be avoided if strictures are suspected.
- *pH studies, impedance monitoring and manometry* are all discussed in more detail in the upper gastrointestinal disease section.

Imaging

Plain X-rays

Plain X-rays of the chest and abdomen are chiefly used in the investigation of an acute abdomen. Interpretation depends on analysis of gas shadows inside and outside the bowel. Plain films are particularly useful where obstruction or perforation is suspected, to exclude toxic megacolon in colitis, and to assess faecal loading in constipation. Calcification may be seen with gall-bladder stones and in chronic pancreatitis, though computed tomography is more sensitive for both.

Ultrasound

Ultrasonography involves no radiation and is the first-line investigation for abdominal distension: for example, in ascites, a mass or suspected inflammatory conditions. It can show dilated, fluid-filled loops of bowel in obstruction, and thickening of the bowel wall. It can be used to guide biopsies or percutaneous drainage. In an acute abdomen, ultrasound can diagnose cholecystitis, appendicitis, enlarged mesenteric glands and other inflammatory conditions.

Computed tomography

Computed tomography (CT) involves a significant dose of radiation (approximately 10 millisieverts). Modern multislice fast scanners and techniques, involving intraluminal and intravenous contrast, enhance diagnostic capability. Intraluminal contrast may be positive (Gastrografin or Omnipaque) or negative (usually water). The bowel wall and mesentery are well seen after intravenous contrast, especially with negative intraluminal contrast. Clinically unsuspected diseases of other abdominal organs are quite often also revealed (**Fig. 32.8A**).

CT is widely used as a first-line investigation for the acute abdomen. It is sensitive for small volumes of gas from a perforated viscus, as well as leakage of contrast from the gut lumen. Inflammatory conditions, such as abscesses, appendicitis, diverticulitis, Crohn's disease and its complications, are well demonstrated. In high-grade bowel obstruction, CT is usually diagnostic of both the presence and the cause of the obstruction.

CT is widely used in cancer staging and as guidance for biopsy of tumour or lymph nodes.

CT pneumocolon/CT colonography (virtual colonoscopy) after CO_2 insufflation into a previously cleansed colon provides an alternative to colonoscopy for diagnosis of colonic mass lesions (see **Fig. 32.8B**). It is being evaluated as a screening test for colon pathology with sensitivities of over 90% for polyps larger than 10 mm.

Magnetic resonance imaging

Magnetic resonance imaging (MRI) uses no radiation and is particularly useful in the evaluation of rectal cancers and of abscesses and fistulae in the perianal region. It is also useful in small bowel disease (MR enteroclysis) and in hepatobiliary and pancreatic disease.

Positron emission tomography

Positron emission tomography (PET) relies on detection of the metabolism of fluorodeoxyglucose. It is used for staging oesophageal, gastric and colorectal cancer and in detecting metastatic and recurrent disease. PET/CT adds additional anatomical information.

Contrast studies

These include barium swallow examination, double-contrast barium meal and small-bowel follow through or meal. *Absorbable water-soluble (Gastrografin or Omnipaque) contrast agents* should be used in preference to barium when perforation is suspected anywhere in the gut. These are useful examinations for the upper GI tract and small bowel but do rely on good technique. They are gradually being superseded by other modalities of imaging, particularly MRI.

Radioisotopes

Radionuclides are used to a varying degree, depending on availability and expertise. Some of the more common indications are measuring the rate of gastric emptying, demonstration of a Meckel's diverticulum, evaluation of neuroendocrine tumours, assessment of bile salt malabsorption (SeHCAT scan) or detection of bacterial overgrowth. These will be explored in more detail in the relevant sections.

FUNCTIONAL GASTROINTESTINAL DISORDERS

There is a large group of gastrointestinal disorders that are termed 'functional' because symptoms occur in the absence of any demonstrable abnormalities in the digestion and absorption of nutrients, fluid and electrolytes, and no structural abnormality can be identified in the gastrointestinal tract, although there may be discernible abnormalities in neuromuscular function, such as dysmotility and visceral hypersensitivity, which are not routinely investigated.

Pathophysiology and brain–gut interactions

People with functional gastrointestinal disorders (FGIDs) are characterized by having a greater gastrointestinal motility response to life events than normal subjects. There is, however, a poor association between measured gastrointestinal motility changes and symptoms in many of the FGIDs. Patients with FGID have been shown to have abnormalities in visceral sensation and to have a lower pain threshold when tested with balloon distension (visceral hyperalgesia). Visceral hypersensitivity possibly relates to:

- altered receptor sensitivity at the viscus itself

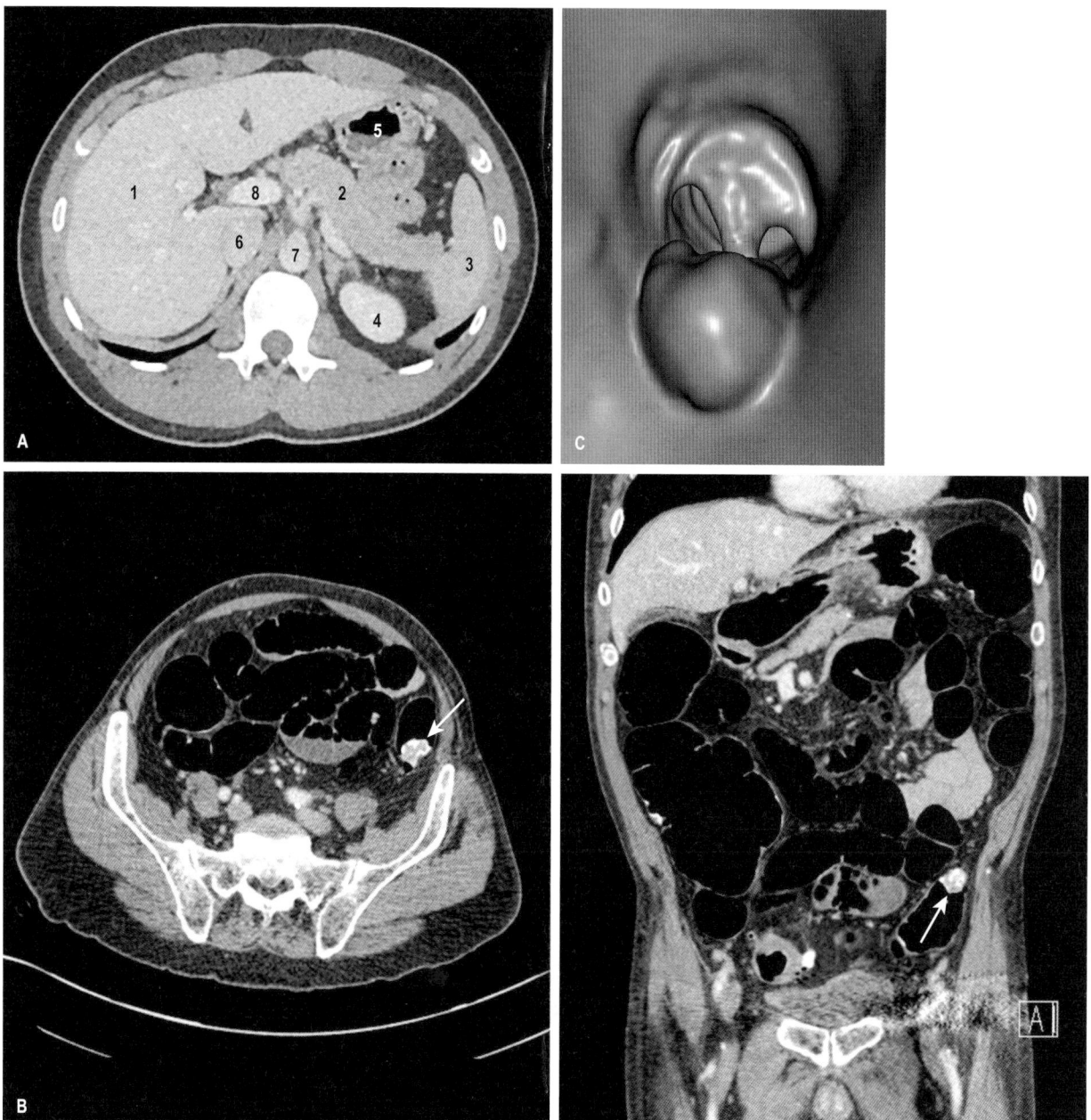

Fig. 32.8 Computed tomography in gastrointestinal disease. **(A)** Annotated axial CT image of the abdomen. (1) Liver; (2) pancreas; (3) spleen; (4) left kidney; (5) stomach; (6) inferior vena cava; (7) aorta; (8) portal vein. **(B)** Axial and coronal CT colonography images demonstrate a stalked polyp in the distal descending colon (arrows). (C) 3D view of the polyp demonstrated in (B).

• increased excitability of the spinal cord dorsal horn neurones
• altered central modulation of sensations.

A systematic review of published studies suggests that 10% of patients who experience an acute infective gastroenteritis develop a degree of FGID. It is not clear whether this is caused by post-infectious bile salt malabsorption, alterations in the mucosal immune system or the use of antibiotics to treat the index infection.

The brain–gut axis describes a combination of intestinal motor, sensory and activities (**Fig. 32.9**). Thus, extrinsic (e.g. vision, smell) and intrinsic (e.g. emotion, thought) information can affect gastrointestinal sensation because of the neural connections from higher centres. Conversely, viscerotropic events can affect central pain perception, mood and behaviour.

Psychological stress can exacerbate gastrointestinal symptoms, and psychological disturbances are more common in patients with FGIDs. These disturbances alter attitude to illness, promote healthcare seeking, and often lead to a poor clinical outcome. They have psychosocial consequences with poor quality of life at home and work. Early in life, genetic and environmental influences (e.g. family attitudes towards bowel training, verbal or sexual abuse, exposure to an infection) may affect psychosocial development (susceptibility to life stress, psychological state, coping skills, development of social support) or the development of gut dysfunction (abnormal motility or visceral hypersensitivity). Therefore, FGID should be regarded as a dysregulation of brain–gut function.

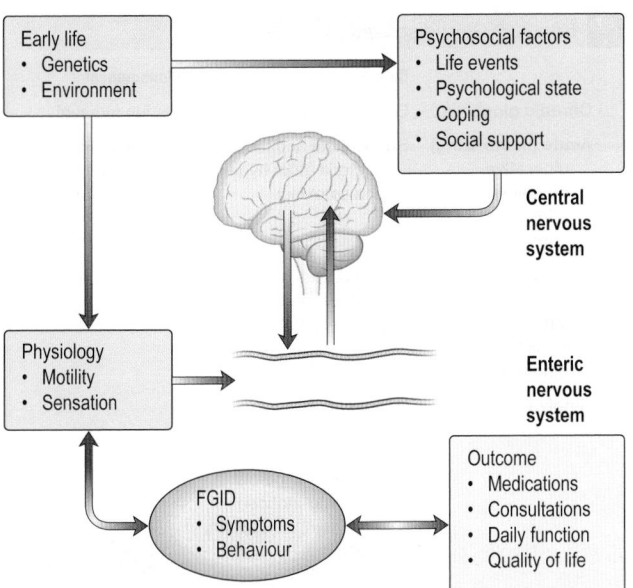

Fig. 32.9 A biopsychosocial conceptualization of the pathogenesis and clinical expression of functional gastrointestinal disorders (FGIDs). *Genetic, environmental and psychological factors may interact to cause dysregulation of brain–gut function. (Modified from Drossman DA. The functional gastrointestinal disorders and the Rome III process. Gastroenterology 2006; 130:1377–1390, with permission from Elsevier.)*

MOUTH

Recurrent aphthous ulceration

Idiopathic aphthous ulceration is common and affects up to 25% of the population. Recurrent painful round or ovoid mouth ulcers are seen with inflammatory halos. They are more common in females and non-smokers, usually appear first in childhood, and tend to reduce in number and frequency before the age of 40. Other family members may be affected. There is no sign of systemic disease.

- **Minor aphthous ulcers** are the most common; they are less than 10 mm diameter, have a grey/white centre with a thin erythematous halo, and heal within 14 days without scarring. They rarely affect the dorsum of the tongue or hard palate.
- **Major aphthous ulcers** (>10 mm diameter) often persist for weeks or months and heal with scarring.

The cause is not known. Deficiencies of iron, folic acid or vitamin B_{12} (with or without gastrointestinal disorders) are sometimes found but are not causally linked. Secondary causes, such as Crohn's disease, should be excluded (**Box 32.8**).

There are no specific effective therapies. Sufferers should avoid oral trauma, and acidic foods or drinks that cause pain. Topical (1% triamcinolone) or systemic corticosteroids may lessen the duration and severity of the attacks. Chlorhexidine gluconate or tetracycline mouthwash, dapsone, colchicine, thalidomide and azathioprine have all been used with variable effect.

Neoplasia (squamous cell carcinoma)

Malignant tumours of the mouth account for 1% of all malignant tumours in the UK. The majority develop on the floor of the mouth or lateral borders of the tongue. Early lesions may be painless, but

- Idiopathic aphthous ulceration (most common)
- Gastrointestinal disease:
  - Inflammatory bowel disease
  - Coeliac disease
- Infection:
  - Viral – herpes simplex virus (HSV), human immunodeficiency virus (HIV), Coxsackie
  - Fungal – candidiasis
  - Bacterial – syphilis, tuberculosis
- Systemic disease:
  - Reactive arthritis (see p. 450)
  - Behçet's syndrome
  - Systemic lupus erythematosus
- Trauma:
  - E.g. dentures
- Neoplasia:
  - E.g. squamous cell carcinoma
- Drugs:
  - In erythema multiforme major, toxic epidermal necrolysis
  - Chemotherapy, antimalarials
- Skin disease:
  - Pemphigoid
  - Pemphigus
  - Lichen planus

advanced tumours are easily recognizable as hard, indurated ulcers with raised and rolled edges. Aetiological agents include tobacco, heavy alcohol consumption and the areca nut. Human papillomavirus 16 causes some oral cancers. Pre-malignant lesions include leucoplakia (single adherent white patch), lichen planus, submucous fibrosis and erythroplakia (a red patch).

Management

Treatment is by surgical excision, which may require extensive neck dissection to remove involved lymph nodes and/or radiotherapy. Ablative treatment with photodynamic therapy is being pioneered for early lesions.

Pigmented neoplastic lesions

These include melanotic naevi on the hard palate and buccal mucosa. These are rarer in the mouth than on the skin. Malignant melanomas are rare, but more common in males, and occur mainly on the upper jaw. The 5-year survival is only 5%.

Non-neoplastic lesions

Oral white patches

Transient white patches either are due to *Candida* infection or are very occasionally found in systemic lupus erythematosus. Local causes include mechanical, irritative or chemical trauma from drugs (e.g. ill-fitting dentures or aspirin). Oral candidiasis in adults is seen following therapy with broad-spectrum antibiotics or inhaled steroids, and in people with diabetes, patients who are seriously ill or those who are immunocompromised.

Persistent white patches can be due to **leucoplakia**, which is associated with alcohol and (particularly) smoking; it is premalignant. A biopsy should always be taken; histology shows alteration in the keratinization and dysplasia of the epithelium. Treatment is unsatisfactory. Isotretinoin possibly reduces disease progression. **Oral lichen planus** presents as white striae, which can rarely extend into the oesophagus.

Oral pigmented lesions

Racial pigmentation is scattered and symmetrically distributed. Amalgam tattoo is the most common form of localized oral pigmentation and consists of blue–black macules involving the gingivae; it results from dental amalgam sequestering into the tissues. Diseases causing pigmentation include Peutz–Jeghers syndrome and Addison's disease. Heavy metals (e.g. lead, bismuth and mercury) and drugs (e.g. phenothiazines and antimalarials) all cause pigmentation of the gums.

Tongue

The tongue may be affected by inflammatory or malignant processes, with similar lesions to those described above.

Glossitis

Glossitis is a red, smooth, sore tongue associated with vitamin B_{12}, folate, iron, riboflavin and nicotinic acid deficiency. It is also seen in infections due to *Candida*.

Geographic tongue

A geographic tongue is an idiopathic condition occurring in 1–2% of the population and may be familial. There are erythematous areas surrounded by well-defined, slightly raised irregular margins. The lesions are usually painless and the patient should be reassured.

Gums

The gums (gingivae) are the mucous membranes covering the alveolar processes of the mandible and the maxilla. Diseases of the gum are shown in **Box 32.9**.

Teeth

Dental caries occur as a result of bacterial damage to tooth structures leading to tooth decay and 'cavities'. The main cause in humans is *Streptococcus mutans*, which is cariogenic only in the presence of dietary sugar. Dental caries can progress to pulpitis and pulp necrosis, and spreading infection can cause dentoalveolar abscesses. If there is soft tissue swelling, antibiotics (e.g. amoxicillin or metronidazole) should be prescribed prior to dental intervention.

Erosion of the teeth can result from exposure to acid (e.g. in bulimia nervosa) or, very occasionally, from severe gastro-oesophageal reflux disease.

SALIVARY GLANDS

Diseases of the salivary glands are shown in **Box 32.10**.

PHARYNX AND OESOPHAGUS

Gastro-oesophageal reflux disease

Epidemiology and pathophysiology

Gastro-oesophageal reflux disease (GORD) is common with a prevalence of 10–20% in the developed world. It is more common in the Western world than in Asia. There are a number of lifestyle

---

? Box 32.9 Gum diseases

	Cause	Management
Chronic gingivitis	Bacterial plaque	Plaque removal
Acute (necrotizing) ulcerative gingivitis (Vincent's angina)	Spirochaete and fusiform bacteria (poor hygiene and smoking)	Oral metronidazole 200 mg 3 times daily for 3 days Chlorhexidine mouthwash
Desquamative gingivitis (smooth red atrophic gingivae)	Lichen planus or mucous membrane pemphigoid	Confirmation with biopsy
Gingival swelling	Inflammation (e.g. pregnancy, scurvy) infiltrations (leukaemia) or fibrous hyperplasia (e.g. drug-induced – phenytoin, ciclosporin, nifedipine)	

? Box 32.10 Diseases of the salivary glands

- Dry mouth (xerostomia):
  - Sjögren's syndrome
  - Drugs (e.g. antimuscarinic, anti-parkinsonian, lithium, tricyclics, monoamine oxidase inhibitors (MAOIs))
  - Radiotherapy
  - Psychogenic
  - Dehydration
- Acute sialadenitis:
  - Viral (e.g. mumps)
  - Bacterial (e.g. *Staphylococcus*, *Streptococcus*)
- Salivary duct obstruction:
  - Calculus
- Sarcoidosis (see p. 985)
- Neoplasms (3% of all tumours worldwide):
  - Pleomorphic adenoma (15% become malignant and can cause VII lower motor neurone signs)

---

risk factors as well as possible genetic factors, and the cardinal clinical feature is heartburn. Psychosocial factors are often determinants of symptom severity, with heartburn increased during times of stress. Factors associated with GORD are shown in **Box 32.11**.

The underlying cause of GORD is reflux of gastric acid, pepsin, bile and duodenal contents back into the oesophagus. This can be influenced by many factors that overcome the innate defence mechanisms, primarily the lower oesophageal sphincter (LOS). Between swallows, the muscles of the oesophagus are relaxed, except for those of the two sphincters. The LOS in the distal oesophagus remains closed because of the unique property of the muscle, and relaxes when swallowing is initiated (see p. 1150). ***Transient lower (o)esophageal sphincter relaxations*** (TLESRs) are part of normal physiology, but occur more frequently in patients with GORD, allowing gastric acid to flow back into the oesophagus (**Fig. 32.10**). Increased abdominal pressure (pregnancy) and low LOS pressure also predispose to GORD.

Other anti-reflux mechanisms involve the intra-abdominal segment of the oesophagus, which acts as a flap valve. In addition, the mucosal rosette, formed by folds of the gastric mucosa, and the crural diaphragm at the LOS, which contracts and acts like a pinchcock, prevent acid reflux. A hiatus hernia can impair this mechanism

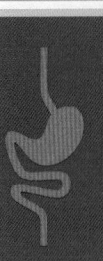

> **Box 32.11 Factors associated with gastro-oesophageal reflux**
>
> - Pregnancy or obesity
> - Fat, chocolate, coffee or alcohol ingestion
> - Large meals
> - Cigarette smoking
> - Drugs – antimuscarinic, calcium-channel blockers, nitrates
> - Systemic sclerosis
> - Treatment for achalasia
> - Hiatus hernia

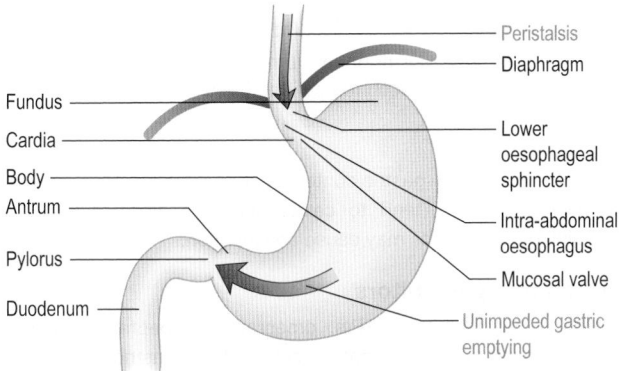

Fig. 32.10 The main anti-reflux mechanisms. These are shown on the right.

> **Box 32.12 Hiatus hernia**
>
> **Sliding hiatus hernia**
> The oesophageal–gastric junction and part of the stomach 'slide' through the hiatus so that it lies above the diaphragm.
> - Present in 30% of people over 50 years
> - Produces no symptoms – any symptoms are due to reflux
>
> **Rolling or para-oesophageal hernia**
> Part of the fundus of the stomach prolapses through the hiatus alongside the oesophagus.
> - The lower oesophageal sphincter remains below the diaphragm and remains competent
> - Occasionally, severe pain occurs due to volvulus or strangulation

(**Box 32.12**). Normally, the oesophagus is also 'cleared' rapidly of refluxate by secondary peristalsis, gravity and salivary bicarbonate.

The clinical features of reflux occur when the anti-reflux mechanisms fail, allowing acidic gastric contents to make prolonged contact with the lower oesophageal mucosa. The sphincter relaxes transiently, independently of a swallow, after meals, and this is the cause of almost all reflux in normal subjects and in and about two-thirds of GORD patients.

The role of the **acid pocket** in GORD has gained more credence in the last 5 years. Food and fluid generally increase the gastric pH, but the acid pocket is an area of unbuffered gastric acid that accumulates postprandially in the proximal stomach. It serves as a reservoir for acid reflux, particularly in individuals with a hiatus hernia where the distal oesophagus is supradiaphragmatic, especially on lying flat. This can be specifically targeted with an antacid–alginate combination.

Clinical features

Heartburn is the major feature. This is a burning chest pain that is aggravated by bending, stooping and lying down, all of which

> **Box 32.13 Classic features of the pain of gastro-oesophageal reflux and cardiac ischaemia**
>
> **Reflux pain: burning, worse on bending, stooping or lying down**
> - Seldom radiates to the arms
> - Worse with spicy food, hot drinks or alcohol
> - Relieved by antacids
>
> **Cardiac ischaemic pain**
> - Gripping or crushing
> - Radiates to neck or left arm
> - Worse with exercise
> - Accompanied by dyspnoea

promote acid exposure. The patient typically complains of pain on eating spicy food or drinking hot liquids or alcohol.

The correlation between heartburn and oesophagitis is poor. Some patients have mild oesophagitis but severe heartburn, while others have severe oesophagitis in the absence of symptoms, and can present with haematemesis or iron deficiency anaemia from chronic blood loss.

Differentiation of cardiac and oesophageal pain can be difficult; 20% of cases seen in emergency departments have GORD (**Box 32.13**). A trial of antacid therapy is often useful, resolving reflux-induced pain, before progressing to 24-hour pH studies only if symptoms persist.

Regurgitation of food and acid into the mouth occurs, particularly on bending or lying flat. This can lead to excess salivation in the mouth, commonly known as water-brash. Aspiration pneumonia is unusual without an accompanying obstruction, but cough and asthma can occur and respond slowly (1–4 months) to a proton pump inhibitor (PPI).

Laryngopharyngeal reflux disease (LPRD) is the transport of gastric contents into the larynx and pharynx, usually, although not exclusively, in the context of GORD. Heartburn may be one of the associated symptoms but cough, hoarse voice, postnasal drip and asthma are more frequently seen, but are not common.

Diagnosis and investigations

The **clinical** diagnosis can usually be made without investigation. Unless there are alarm signs, especially dysphagia (see p. 901), patients under the age of 45 years can safely be treated initially without investigations. If investigation is required, there are two aims:

- **Assess oesophagitis and hiatal hernia by endoscopy.** If there is oesophagitis (**Fig. 32.11**) or Barrett's oesophagus (see p. 1165), reflux is confirmed.
- **Intraluminal monitoring** (**Fig. 32.12**). Intraluminal pH monitoring or impedance combined with manometry is helpful if there is no response to PPIs and should always be performed to confirm reflux before surgery. Ambulatory 24-hour pH monitoring consists of passing a nasgogastric tube with a pH probe at its tip which is placed at the level of the LOS. This allows measurements of acid exposure and is worn for 24 hours. Some centres now offer a wireless probe (known as a Bravo capsule) which is clipped to the lower oesophagus without the need for an NG tube. This then gradually detaches and is passed in the stool. A composite score of the various parameters measured is then calculated, with a score higher than 14.72 indicating reflux. This is known as a DeMeester score. There should also be a good correlation between reflux (pH <4.0) and symptoms. Impedance testing is when a catheter is used to measure the resistance to flow of 'alternating current' in the contents of the oesophagus. It can also be helpful to assess oesophageal dysmotility as a potential cause of the symptoms, leading to impaired oesophageal clearance.

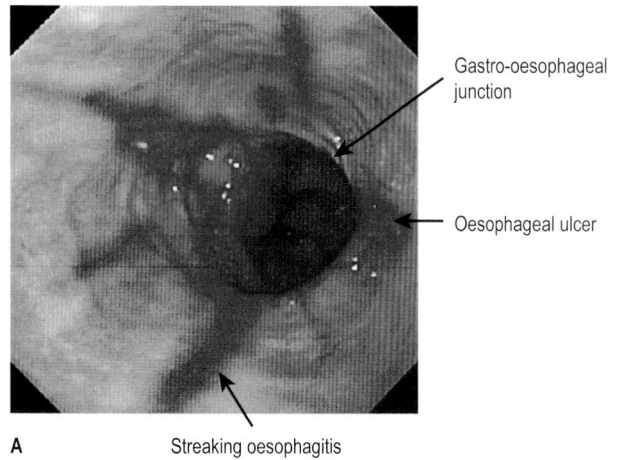

Gastro-oesophageal junction

Oesophageal ulcer

A   Streaking oesophagitis

Grade A

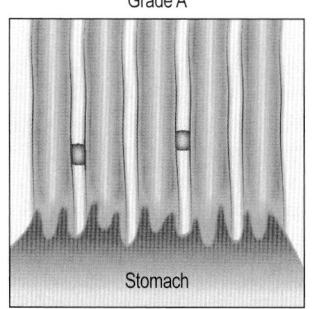

Stomach

Grade B

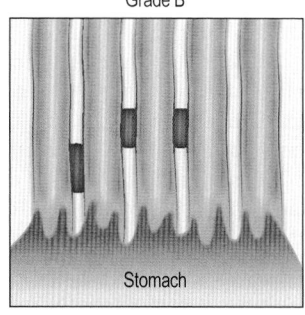

Stomach

Grade C

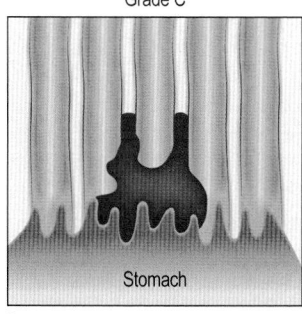

Stomach

Grade D

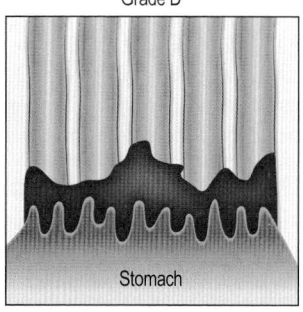

Stomach

B

Fig. 32.11 Oesophagitis. **(A)** Oesophagitis seen on endoscopy. **(B)** Los Angeles classification of oesophagitis. **Grade A** = mucosal breaks confined to the mucosal folds, each no longer than 5 mm. **Grade B** = at least one mucosal break longer than 5 mm confined to the mucosal fold but not continuous between two folds. **Grade C** = mucosal breaks that are continuous between the tops of mucosal folds but not circumferential. **Grade D** = extensive mucosal breaks engaging at least 75% of the oesophageal circumference.

Management

Approximately half of patients with reflux symptoms in primary care can be treated successfully with simple antacids, loss of weight and raising the head of the bed at night. Precipitating factors should be avoided, with dietary measures, reduction in alcohol and caffeine consumption, and cessation of smoking. These measures are simple to say but difficult to carry out, though they are useful in mild disease in compliant patients.

Drugs

Alginate-containing antacids

Alginate-containing antacids (10 mL three times daily) are the most frequently used 'over-the-counter' agents for GORD. They form a

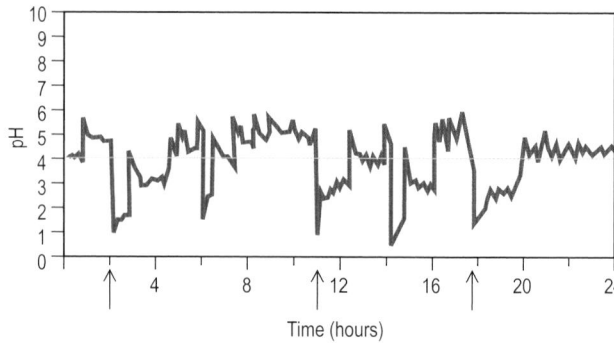

Fig. 32.12 Twenty-four-hour intraluminal pH monitoring. Five reflux episodes (pH <4) occurred but only three produced symptoms (arrowed).

gel or 'foam raft' with gastric contents to reduce reflux. Magnesium-containing antacids tend to cause diarrhoea while aluminium-containing compounds may cause constipation.

Proton pump inhibitors

Proton pump inhibitors (PPIs; omeprazole, rabeprazole, lansoprazole, pantoprazole, esomeprazole) inhibit gastric hydrogen/potassium-adenosine triphosphatase. PPIs reduce gastric acid secretion by up to 90% and are the drugs of choice for all but mild cases. Most patients with GORD will respond well, with approximately 60% symptom-free after 4 weeks of a once-daily PPI. Patients with severe symptoms may need twice-daily PPIs and prolonged treatment, often for years. Once oesophageal sensitivity has normalized, a lower dose, e.g. omeprazole 20 mg, may be sufficient for maintenance. Long-term PPI prescription is not uncommon, and although some recent data have suggested side-effects such as osteoporosis, and an increase in gastrointestinal infections such as *Clostridium difficile*, these are uncommon and tend to occur in at-risk patients.

Patients who do not respond to a PPI and have continuing symptoms with a normal endoscopy are described as having ***non-erosive reflux disease (NERD)*** (**Fig. 32.13**). These patients are usually female and often the symptoms are functional, although a small group have a 'hypersensitive' oesophagus, giving discomfort with only slight changes in pH. Isomers of some of the original PPIs (e.g. dexlansoprazole) have the benefit of more effective gastric acid inhibition over a longer time period, as their metabolism of the active metabolite is slower.

H₂-receptor antagonists

H_2-receptor antagonists (e.g. cimetidine, ranitidine, famotidine and nizatidine) are frequently used for acid suppression if antacids fail, as they can easily be obtained. They can be used in conjunction with PPIs for patients with more severe GORD.

Dopamine antagonist prokinetic agents

The dopamine antagonist prokinetic agents metoclopramide and domperidone are occasionally helpful, as they enhance peristalsis and speed gastric emptying, but there are few data to substantiate this. The role of domperidone has been limited still further following reports of serious cardiac side-effects.

Endoluminal gastroplication

In this endoscopic procedure, multiple plications or pleats are made below the gastro-oesophageal junction. Randomized controlled trials have shown benefit with reduction in heartburn, acid reflux

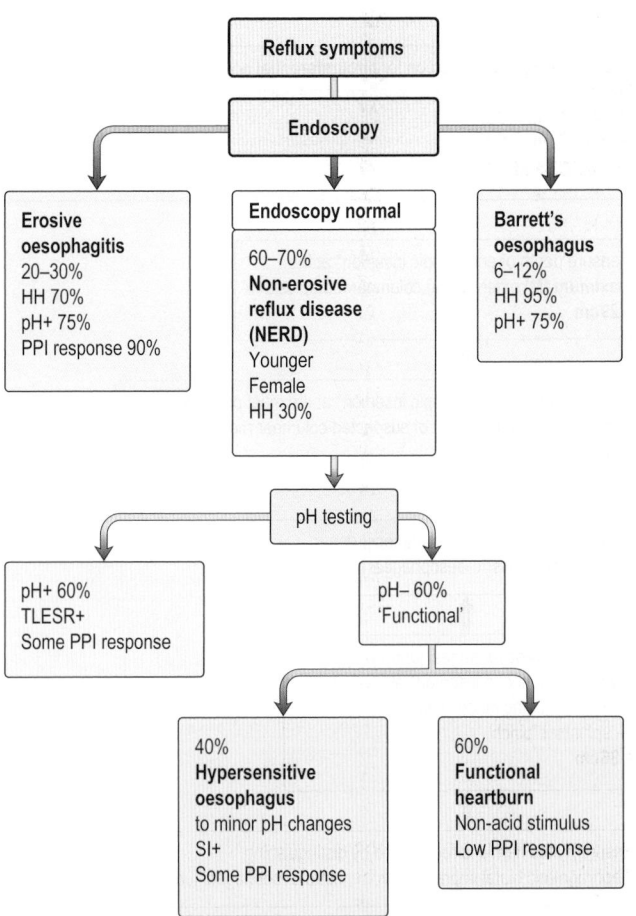

Fig. 32.13 Outcome of patients with reflux symptoms. HH, hiatus hernia; pH+, meets standard criteria for excessive acid reflux on intraluminal testing; pH−, does not meet standard criteria for excessive acid reflux; PPI, proton pump inhibitor; SI+, symptom index; TLESR, transient lower (o)esophageal sphincter relaxation.

episodes and PPI usage, but not sustained improvements in the oesophageal pH measurements.

Surgery

Surgery should never be performed for a hiatus hernia alone. The best predictors of a good surgical result are typical reflux symptoms with documented acid reflux, which correlates with symptoms and response to a PPI. With such highly selected cases in experienced hands, the laparoscopic Nissen fundoplication has a satisfaction rate of over 90% at 5 years, and available 10-year data show satisfaction rates remain high at 88%. Current surgical techniques return the oesophagogastric junction to the abdominal cavity, mobilize the gastric fundus, close the diaphragmatic crura snugly and involve a short, tension-free fundoplication.

The **_Linx reflux management system_** consists of a row of magnets that increase LOS closure pressure, allowing food passage during swallowing; it is inserted laparoscopically. Improvement in quality of life with no PPI therapy has been shown but further studies are necessary. Patients cannot have an MRI study with the device _in situ_.

Indications for operation are not clear-cut but include intolerance to medication, the desire for freedom from medication, the expense of therapy and concern about long-term side-effects.

The most common cause of mechanical fundoplication failure is recurrent hiatus hernia.

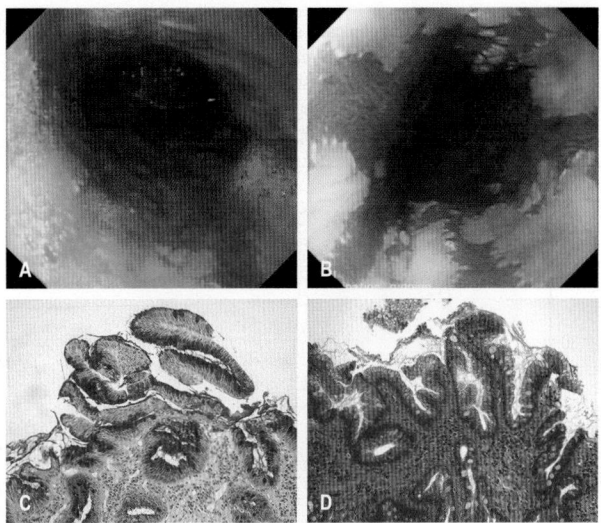

Fig. 32.14 Barrett's oesophagus. (A) Endoscopic picture of Barrett's oesophagus. (B) Endoscopic narrow band imaging of Barrett's mucosa. (C) Alcian blue staining of Barrett's mucosa highlighting the blue-staining goblet cells. (D) Haematoxylin and eosin staining of Barrett's columnar mucosa.

Patients with oesophageal dysmotility unrelated to acid reflux, those with no response to PPIs and those with underlying functional bowel disease should rarely have surgery.

Complications of gastro-oesophageal reflux disease

Peptic stricture

Since the advent of PPIs, peptic strictures have become far less common. They usually occur in patients over the age of 60 and present with intermittent dysphagia for solids, which worsens gradually over a long period. Mild cases may respond to PPIs alone. More severe cases need endoscopic dilation and long-term PPI therapy. Surgery is required if medical treatment fails.

Barrett's oesophagus

Barrett's oesophagus (**Fig. 32.14**) is a condition in which part of the normal oesophageal squamous epithelium is replaced by metaplastic columnar mucosa to form a segment of 'columnar-lined oesophagus' (CLO). It is a complication of GORD and there is almost always a hiatus hernia present.

Diagnosis and classification

The diagnosis is made if endoscopy shows proximal displacement of the squamocolumnar mucosal junction and biopsy demonstrates columnar lining above the proximal gastric folds (>1 cm); intestinal metaplasia is no longer a requirement of the British Society of Gastroenterology definition but is central to the American College of Gastroenterology guidelines. Barrett's oesophagus may be seen as a continual circumferential sheet, as finger-like projections extending upwards from the squamocolumnar junction or as islands of columnar mucosa interspersed with areas of squamous mucosa. The Prague classification (**Fig. 32.15**) is used for recording the endoscopic distribution, stating both the length of circumferential CLO (C measurement) and the maximum length (M measurement), the distance from the top of the gastric folds to the most proximal tongue of the columnar mucosa.

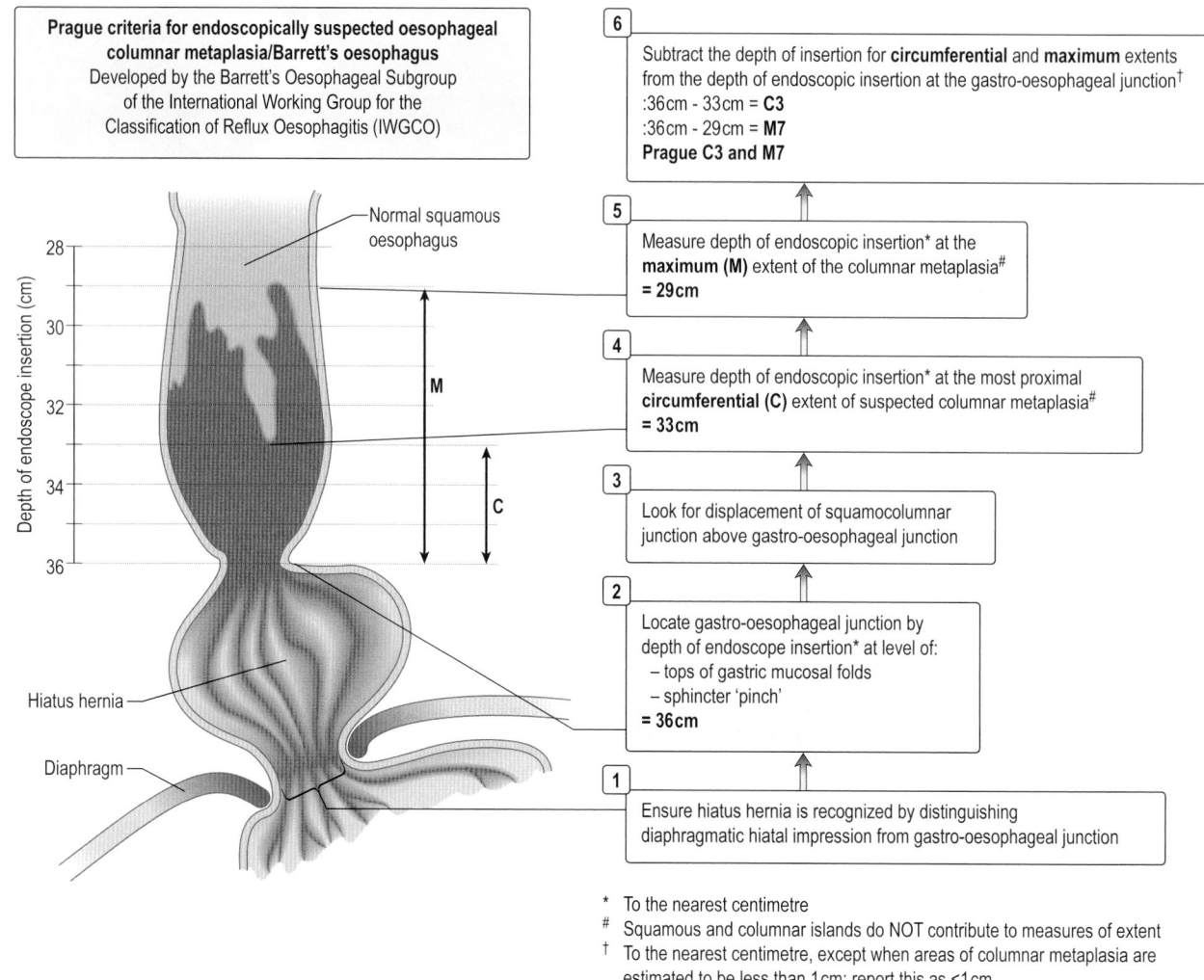

Prague criteria for endoscopically suspected oesophageal columnar metaplasia/Barrett's oesophagus
Developed by the Barrett's Oesophageal Subgroup of the International Working Group for the Classification of Reflux Oesophagitis (IWGCO)

6 Subtract the depth of insertion for **circumferential** and **maximum** extents from the depth of endoscopic insertion at the gastro-oesophageal junction†
:36cm - 33cm = **C3**
:36cm - 29cm = **M7**
Prague C3 and M7

5 Measure depth of endoscopic insertion* at the **maximum (M)** extent of the columnar metaplasia# = 29cm

4 Measure depth of endoscopic insertion* at the most proximal **circumferential (C)** extent of suspected columnar metaplasia# = 33cm

3 Look for displacement of squamocolumnar junction above gastro-oesophageal junction

2 Locate gastro-oesophageal junction by depth of endoscope insertion* at level of:
– tops of gastric mucosal folds
– sphincter 'pinch'
= **36cm**

1 Ensure hiatus hernia is recognized by distinguishing diaphragmatic hiatal impression from gastro-oesophageal junction

Normal squamous oesophagus
Hiatus hernia
Diaphragm

*   To the nearest centimetre
\#   Squamous and columnar islands do NOT contribute to measures of extent
†   To the nearest centimetre, except when areas of columnar metaplasia are estimated to be less than 1cm: report this as <1cm

Fig. 32.15 The Prague criteria for endoscopically suspected oesophageal columnar metaplasia/Barrett's oesophagus.

Central obesity increases the risk of Barrett's by 4.3 times. Long-segment (>3cm) and short-segment (<3cm) Barrett's is found, respectively, in 5% and 15% of patients undergoing endoscopy for reflux symptoms. Barrett's is also often found incidentally in endoscoped patients without reflux symptoms. It is most common in middle-aged obese men. The major concern is that approximately 0.12–0.5% of Barrett's patients develop oesophageal adenocarcinoma per year; the majority, probably, through a gradual transformation from intestinal metaplasia to low-grade then high-grade dysplasia, before invasive adenocarcinoma. Barrett's increases the chance of developing oesophageal adenocarcinoma 30- to 50-fold in early studies but recent studies have shown the risk to be much lower and closer to a 1% lifetime risk in the typical patient.

Because of the poor correlation between Barrett's oesophagus and symptoms, screening is not recommended; however, in the absence of high-quality trial evidence, endoscopic surveillance is recommended by some. This involves inspection of the oesophageal mucosa with a high-definition gastroscope, and the taking of targeted biopsies of any focally abnormal tissue in addition to random biopsies from all four quadrants (every 1–2cm) of the CLO. The interval between endoscopies is determined by the length of the CLO and the degree of cellular disturbance within it (**Fig. 32.16**). High-grade dysplasia (HGD) is usually associated with endoscopically visible nodules or ulceration, optimally visualized with a high-definition endoscope. Chromo-endoscopy (the topical application of stains or pigments via the endoscope), narrow band and autofluorescence imaging may aid the diagnosis of dysplasia and carcinoma. Endoscopic technology has improved the detection of pre-malignant lesions, enabling their removal by either endoscopic mucosal resection (EMR) or endoscopic submucosal dissection, therefore preventing surgical oesophagectomy.

If **low-grade dysplasia** is found on endoscopic surveillance, a repeat endoscopy with quadrantic biopsies every 1cm is usually performed within 6months, while on high-dose proton pump inhibition. Recent guidelines now suggest that if low-grade dysplasia persists then these patients should be offered endoscopic ablation therapy or 6-monthly surveillance.

If **high-grade dysplasia** is found, it is usually in the context of an endoscopically visible lesion, which, if nodular, is removed by endoscopic mucosal resection for more accurate histological staging. If high-grade dysplasia is detected in the absence of any endoscopically visible lesion, high-dose proton pump inhibition is started and repeat biopsies taken within 3months. Endoscopic ultrasound is frequently used to stage this patient group more accurately, in order to exclude cancer and associated significant lymphadenopathy.

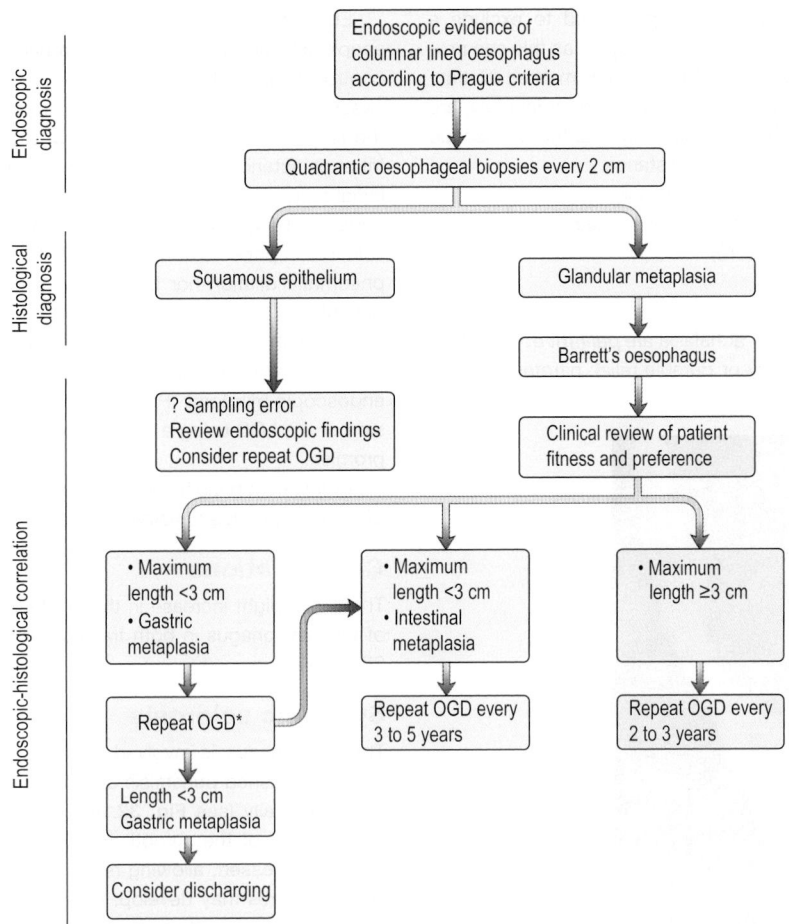

Fig. 32.16 endoscopic flowchart:

Endoscopic diagnosis

Endoscopic evidence of columnar lined oesophagus according to Prague criteria

Quadrantic oesophageal biopsies every 2 cm

Histological diagnosis

Squamous epithelium

Glandular metaplasia

Barrett's oesophagus

Endoscopic-histological correlation

? Sampling error
Review endoscopic findings
Consider repeat OGD

Clinical review of patient fitness and preference

- Maximum length <3 cm
- Gastric metaplasia

- Maximum length <3 cm
- Intestinal metaplasia

- Maximum length ≥3 cm

Repeat OGD*

Repeat OGD every 3 to 5 years

Repeat OGD every 2 to 3 years

Length <3 cm
Gastric metaplasia

Consider discharging

* Interval depends on the degree of clinical confidence about diagnosis (accuracy of endoscopic report and number of biopsies)

Fig. 32.16 British Society of Gastroenterology (BSG) Guidelines for surveillance.

Radiofrequency ablation (RFA) has superseded photodynamic therapy as the technique of choice for endoscopic treatment of dysplasia within Barrett's segments following removal of any nodular lesions, returning the oesophagus to squamous lining. The benefit of RFA in low-grade dysplasia is currently under evaluation.

Motility disorders

Achalasia

Achalasia is characterized by oesophageal aperistalsis and impaired relaxation of the lower oesophageal sphincter. The lower oesophageal pressure is elevated in more than half of patients.

Clinical features

The incidence of achalasia is 1:100000 and is equal in males and females. It occurs at all ages but is rare in childhood. Patients usually have a long history of intermittent dysphagia, characteristically for both liquids and solids from the onset. Regurgitation of food from the dilated oesophagus occurs, particularly at night, and aspiration pneumonia is a complication. Spontaneous chest pain occurs and is said to be due to oesophageal 'spasm'; it may be misdiagnosed as cardiac pain. Dysphagia may be mild and accepted by the patient as normal; weight loss is usually minimal.

Pathogenesis

The aetiology of achalasia is unknown, with autoimmune, viral and neurodegenerative aetiologies all being postulated. A similar clinical picture is seen in chronic Chagas' disease (American trypanosomiasis; see p. 568), where there is damage to the neural plexus of the gut.

Histopathology shows inflammation of the myenteric plexus of the oesophagus with reduction of ganglion cell numbers. Cholinergic innervation appears to be preserved. Reduction in nitric oxide synthase-containing neurones has been shown by immunohistochemical staining. Pharmacological studies in patients with achalasia support the selective loss of *inhibitory*, nitrergic neurones.

Differential diagnosis

The differential diagnosis of achalasia worldwide includes genetic syndromes, infectious diseases, neoplasms and chronic inflammatory conditions.

Investigations

- *Chest X-ray* shows a dilated oesophagus, sometimes with a fluid level seen behind the heart. The fundal gas shadow is absent.
- *Barium swallow* shows lack of peristalsis and often synchronous contractions in the body of the oesophagus, sometimes with dilation. The lower end shows a 'bird's beak' due to failure of the sphincter to relax (**Fig. 32.17**).

- *Oesophagogastroduodenoscopy* is performed to exclude a carcinoma at the lower end of the oesophagus, as this can produce a similar X-ray appearance. When there is marked dilation, a 24-h liquid-only diet and a washout, prior to endoscopy, are useful to remove food debris. In true achalasia, the endoscope passes through the LOS with little resistance.
- *CT scan* excludes distal oesophageal cancer.
- *Manometry* shows aperistalsis of the oesophagus and failure of relaxation of the LOS (**Fig. 32.18**).

Management

All current forms of treatment for achalasia are *palliative*. Drug therapy rarely produces satisfactory or durable relief; nitrates or sildenafil can be tried initially.

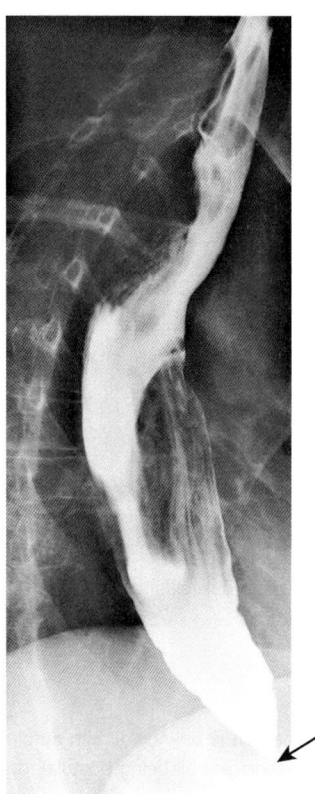

Fig. 32.17 Barium swallow demonstrating achalasia. The oesophagus is dilated and tapers inferiorly with a 'bird-beak' (arrow) appearance at the gastro-oesophageal junction.

Endoscopic and surgical therapies are equally effective. Endoscopic dilation of the LOS, using a pneumatic balloon under X-ray control, weakens the sphincter and is initially successful in 80% of cases. About 50% of patients require a second or third dilation in the first 5 years. There is a low but significant risk of perforation. Intrasphincteric injection of botulinum toxin A produces satisfactory initial results but the effects wear off within months. Further injections can be given. It is safer and simpler than dilation, so may be valuable in patients at risk of death if a perforation occurs. Neither pneumatic dilation nor botulinum toxin works as well in younger patients.

Surgical division of the LOS, Heller's operation, usually performed laparoscopically, is the surgical treatment of choice. Per oral endoscopic myotomy (POEM) is a novel technique, which is a division of the LOS using a gastroscope. The early results show great promise.

Reflux oesophagitis complicates all procedures and aperistalsis of the oesophagus remains.

Complications

There is a slight increase in the incidence of squamous carcinoma of the oesophagus in both treated and untreated cases (7% after 25 years).

Systemic sclerosis

The oesophagus is involved in almost all patients with this disease. Diminished peristalsis and oesophageal clearance, detected manometrically (see **Fig. 32.18**) or by barium swallow, is due to replacement of the smooth muscle by fibrous tissue. LOS pressure is decreased, allowing reflux with consequent mucosal damage. Strictures may develop. Initially, there are no symptoms, but dysphagia and heartburn occur as the oesophagus becomes more severely involved. Similar motility abnormalities may be found in other autoimmune rheumatic disorders, particularly if Raynaud's phenomenon is present. Treatment is as for reflux disease (see p. 1162) and benign stricture.

Diffuse oesophageal spasm

This is a severe form of oesophageal dysmotility that can sometimes produce retrosternal chest pain and dysphagia. It can accompany GORD. Swallowing is accompanied by bizarre and marked contractions of the oesophagus without normal peristalsis (see **Fig. 32.18**). On barium swallow, the appearance may be that of a 'corkscrew' oesophagus. However, asymptomatic oesophageal 'dysmotility' is not infrequent, particularly in patients over the age of 60 years.

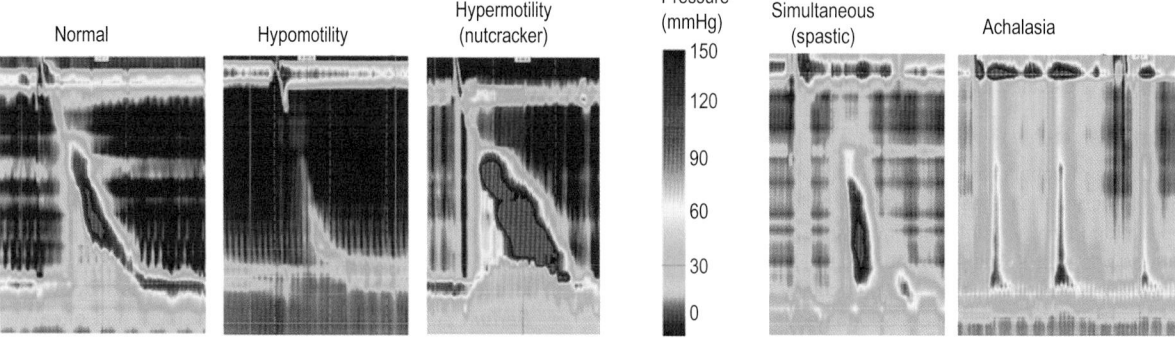

Fig. 32.18 High-resolution manometry of the oesophagus. Results are shown in the normal subject and in patients with hypomotility, hypermotility, simultaneous (spastic) contractions and achalasia. Changes in colour reflect changes in pressure.

A variant of diffuse oesophageal spasm is the 'nutcracker' oesophagus, which is characterized by very high-amplitude peristalsis (pressures >200 mmHg) within the oesophagus. Chest pain is more common than dysphagia.

Management

True oesophageal spasm producing severe symptoms is uncommon and treatment is often difficult. PPIs may be successful if reflux is a factor. Antispasmodics, nitrates, calcium-channel blockers and γ-aminobutyric acid (GABA) receptor agonists (e.g. baclofen) are used. Occasionally, balloon dilation or even longitudinal oesophageal myotomy is necessary.

Miscellaneous motility disorders

Abnormalities of motility that occasionally produce dysphagia are found in the elderly, and in diabetes mellitus, myotonic dystrophy, oculopharyngeal muscular dystrophy and myasthenia gravis, as well as neurological disorders involving the brainstem.

Other oesophageal disorders

Oesophageal diverticulum

Diverticula occur:

* immediately **above** the upper oesophageal sphincter (pharyngeal pouch – Zenker's diverticulum; see p. 912)
* near the **middle** of the oesophagus (traction diverticulum due to inflammation, or associated with diffuse oesophageal spasm or mediastinal fibrosis)
* just above the **lower** oesophageal sphincter (epiphrenic diverticulum – associated with achalasia).

Usually detected incidentally on a barium swallow performed for other reasons, these are often asymptomatic. Dysphagia and regurgitation can occur with a pharyngeal pouch, becoming more problematic as the diverticula increase in size (see p. 901). These can be treated surgically and endoscopically.

Rings and webs

An oesophageal web is a thin, membranous tissue flap covered with squamous epithelium. Most acquired webs are located anteriorly in the postcricoid region of the cervical oesophagus and are well seen on barium swallow. They may produce dysphagia. In the **Plummer–Vinson syndrome** (or **Paterson–Brown–Kelly syndrome**), a web is associated with chronic iron deficiency anaemia, glossitis and angular stomatitis. This rare syndrome affects mainly women and its aetiology is not understood. The web may be difficult to see at endoscopy and is often ruptured unintentionally by the passage of the endoscope. Dilation of the web is rarely necessary. Iron is given for the iron deficiency.

Lower oesophageal rings

Lower oesophageal rings are of two types:

* **Mucosal (Schatzki's ring, also called B ring)** is located at the squamocolumnar mucosal junction and is common (**Fig. 32.19**). It is associated with a characteristic history of intermittent bolus obstruction.
* **Muscular (A ring)** is located proximal to the mucosal ring and is uncommon. It is covered by squamous epithelium and may cause dysphagia.

Management for these rings is usually with reassurance and dietary advice, but dilation is occasionally necessary. After a single dilation, 68% of patients with Schatzki's rings are symptom-free at

1 year and 35% remain symptom-free after 2 years, but only 11% are symptom-free at 3 years. Many also respond to oral PPI, either alone or with dilation.

Benign oesophageal stricture

Peptic stricture (**Fig. 32.20**) secondary to reflux is the most common cause of benign strictures (for treatment, see p. 1165). They also occur after the ingestion of corrosives, radiotherapy, sclerotherapy of varices and prolonged nasogastric intubation. Dysphagia is usually treated by endoscopic dilation. Surgery is sometimes required.

Oesophageal infections

Infection is a cause of painful swallowing and is seen particularly in immunosuppressed (e.g. on chemotherapy) and debilitated patients, and in those with acquired immunodeficiency syndrome (AIDS). Infection can occur with:

* *Candida*
* herpes simplex
* cytomegalovirus
* *Mycobacterium tuberculosis*.

It is occasionally difficult to distinguish between these disorders on oesophagoscopy, as only widespread ulceration is seen. In candidiasis, the characteristic white plaques are frequently found; oral candidiasis is not always present. The diagnosis of *Candida* infection can be confirmed by examining a direct smear taken at endoscopy, but often infections are mixed and cultures and biopsies must be performed. Tuberculosis causes deep ulceration with associated mediastinal lymphadenopathy.

Management

Most patients on large doses of immunosuppressive agents are treated prophylactically for candidiasis with nystatin, fluconazole or

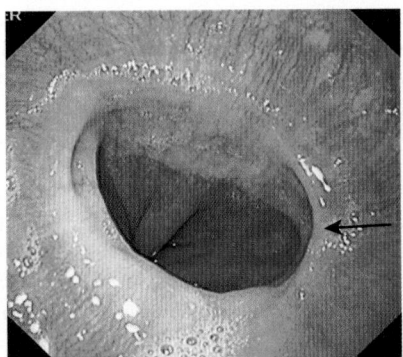

Fig. 32.19 Schatzki's ring. Endoscopic view.

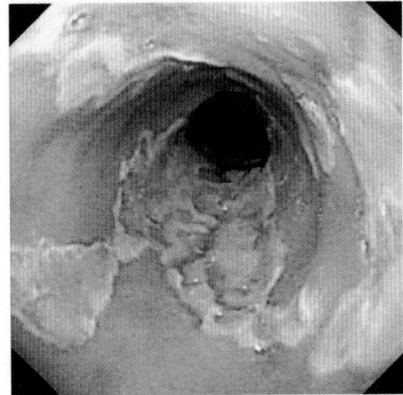

Fig. 32.20 Benign oesophageal reflux stricture. Endoscopic view.

amphotericin. Antifungal or antiviral treatment is prescribed appropriately for other infections.

Mallory–Weiss syndrome

This is described on page 1184.

Eosinophilic oesophagitis

Eosinophils can be seen in the oesophageal mucosa (which is usually devoid of eosinophils microscopically) due to a variety of causes, such as eosinophilic (or allergic) oesophagitis and GORD.

Eosinophilic oesophagitis (**Fig. 32.21**) is increasingly recognized but its pathogenesis is unknown. There may be a personal or family history of allergic disorders, such as food allergy, eczema or asthma.

Patients present with a long history of dysphagia, food impaction, 'heartburn' and oesophageal pain caused by the eosinophil-induced oesophageal inflammation. Usually, the patient is male and white, and has an average age at diagnosis of 35, but eosinophilic oesophagitis is becoming more common in children.

Typical endoscopic abnormalities include mucosal furrowing, loss of vascular pattern due to a thickened mucosa, plaques of eosinophilic surface exudate and prominent circular folds, but the oesophagus may appear macroscopically normal. Reflux oesophagitis and Schatzki's rings may coexist. Endoscopic forceps biopsies should be taken throughout the oesophagus for histology and eosinophil numbers calculated.

The eosinophilic infiltration of the oesophagus due to **reflux disease** tends to have a different microscopic appearance and fewer eosinophils.

Management

First-line treatment is with topical steroids, such as swallowing fluticasone spray or budesonide syrup. If this is not effective, systemic steroids or empirical elimination diets may also be used (dietary treatment is more beneficial in children). A cohort of patients respond to PPIs in the absence of GORD. Dilation is sometimes necessary, with a risk of perforation of 2%.

Oesophageal perforation

Oesophageal perforation most commonly occurs at the time of endoscopic dilation and, rarely, following insertion of a nasogastric tube, gastroscope or transoesophageal echoprobe. Patients with malignant, corrosive or post-radiotherapy strictures are more likely to perforate than those with a benign peptic stricture.

Management

This normally involves placement of an expanding covered oesophageal stent, which usually seals the hole. A water-soluble contrast X-ray is performed after 2–3 days to check the perforation has sealed.

Oesophageal rupture

'**Spontaneous**' oesophageal rupture occurs with violent vomiting (Boerhaave's syndrome), producing severe chest pain and collapse in typical cases. Diagnosis can be difficult because classic symptoms are absent in about one-third of cases, and delays in presentation for medical care are common. Rupture may follow alcohol ingestion. A chest X-ray shows a hydropneumothorax. The diagnosis is made with a water-soluble contrast swallow or on CT. The mortality rate is approximately 35%, making it the most lethal perforation of the gastrointestinal tract. The best outcomes are associated with early diagnosis and definitive surgical management within 12 hours of rupture. If intervention is delayed longer than 24 hours, the mortality rate (even after surgery) rises to above 50%, and to nearly 90% after 48 hours.

Oesophageal tumours

Cancer of the oesophagus

This is the sixth most common cancer worldwide. Squamous cancers occurring in the middle third account for 40% of tumours, and for 15% in the upper third. Adenocarcinomas occur in the lower third of the oesophagus and at the cardia, and represent approximately 45% of tumours. Primary small cell cancer of the oesophagus is extremely rare.

Epidemiology and aetiology

Squamous cell carcinoma

The geographic variation in incidence is greater than for any other carcinoma – often in regions very close to one another. Squamous cell carcinoma (SCC) is common in Ethiopia, China, South and East Africa, and the Caspian regions of Iran. By contrast, North, Central and West Africa have low rates.

In the UK, the incidence is 5–10 per 100 000 and SCC represents 2.2% of all malignant disease. The incidence is decreasing, in contrast to that of adenocarcinoma. SCC of the oesophagus is more common in men (2 : 1). Risk factors are shown in **Box 32.14**.

High levels of alcohol consumption increase the risk of squamous cell cancer of the oesophagus, while tobacco use is associated with an increased incidence of both squamous cell and adenocarcinomas of the oesophagus. Smoking, obesity and low

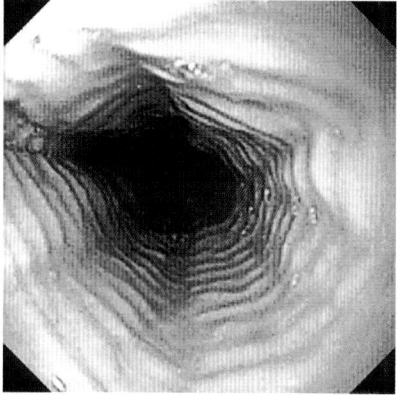

Fig. 32.21 Eosinophilic oesophagitis.

> *i* **Box 32.14 Risk factors for cancer of the oesophagus**
>
> **Squamous cell carcinoma**
> - Tobacco smoking
> - High alcohol intake
> - Plummer–Vinson syndrome
> - Achalasia
> - Corrosive strictures
> - Coeliac disease
> - Breast cancer treated with radiotherapy
> - Tylosis[a]
>
> **Adenocarcinoma**
> - Longstanding heartburn
> - Barrett's oesophagus
> - Tobacco smoking
> - Obesity
> - Breast cancer treated with radiotherapy
> - Older age
>
> [a]Tylosis is a rare autosomal dominant condition with hyperkeratosis of the palms and soles.

fruit and vegetable consumption are implicated in approximately 9 in 10 squamous cell cancers of the oesophagus.

Diets rich in fibre, carotenoids, folate, vitamin C and non-starchy vegetables probably decrease the risk of oesophageal cancer, whereas diets high in saturated fat, cholesterol and refined cereals have been associated with an increased risk. Red and processed meat intake has been associated with an increased risk of both oesophageal SCC and adenocarcinoma. Conversely, fish and white meat consumption have been inversely associated with risk of oesophageal SCC in case–control studies from Italy, Switzerland and Uruguay.

Adenocarcinoma

These tumours primarily arise in columnar-lined epithelium in the lower oesophagus (see p. 1165). The incidence of this tumour is increasing in Western industrialized countries. It currently accounts for more than 70% of all new oesophageal cancer diagnoses. Extension of an adenocarcinoma of the gastric cardia into the oesophagus can present with the same symptoms. Previous reflux symptoms increase the risk up to eightfold and the risk is proportional to their severity.

Clinical features

Carcinoma of the oesophagus occurs mainly in those aged 60–70 years. Dysphagia is progressive and unrelenting. Initially, there is difficulty in swallowing solids but, typically, dysphagia for liquids follows within weeks. Impaction of food causes pain but more persistent pain implies infiltration of adjacent structures.

The lesion may be ulcerative, proliferative or scirrhous, extending variably around the wall of the oesophagus to produce a stricture. Direct invasion of the surrounding structures and metastases to lymph nodes are more common than disseminated metastases. Weight loss, due to the dysphagia as well as to anorexia, is frequent. Oesophageal obstruction eventually causes difficulty in swallowing saliva, coughing and aspiration into the lungs.

Weight loss, anorexia and lymphadenopathy are the most common physical signs.

Investigations
Diagnosis

- **Endoscopy** provides histological proof of the carcinoma (**Fig. 32.22A**).
- **Barium swallow** can be useful where the differential diagnosis of dysphagia includes a motility disorder such as achalasia (see **Fig. 32.22B**).

Staging

The TNM staging system is used (see p. 1179); it is similar to the one used for gastric cancer. Tumour invasion of the wall of the oesophagus (T), presence of tumour in lymph nodes (N) and metastases (M)

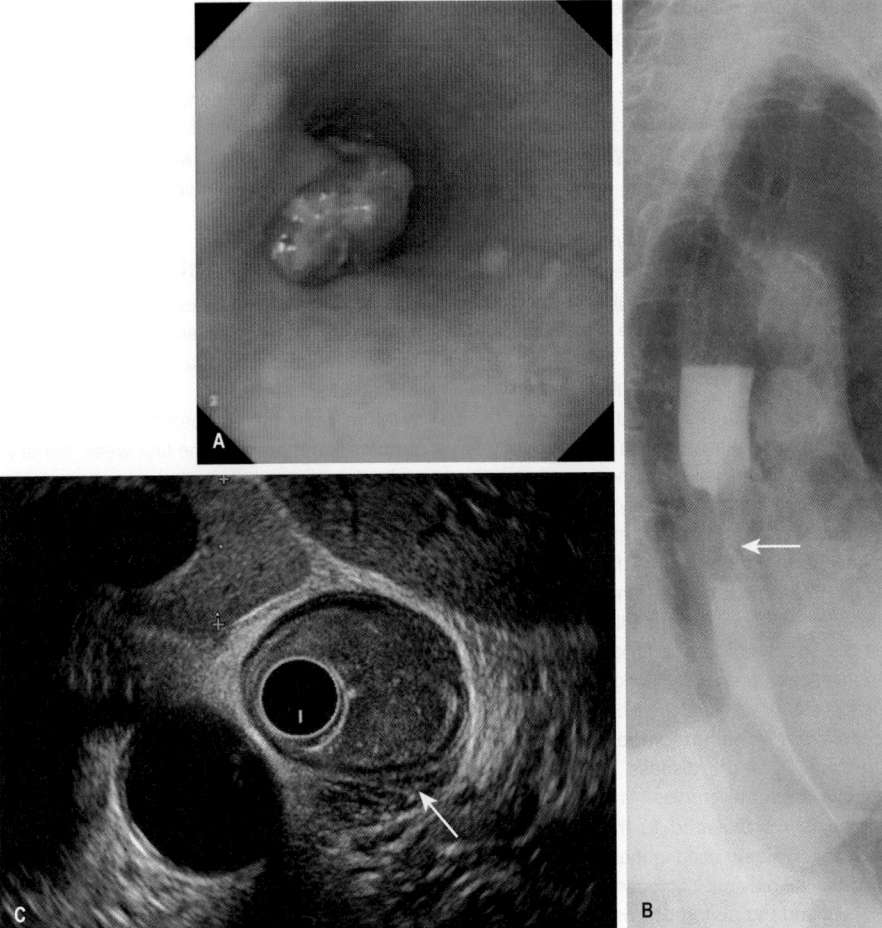

Fig. 32.22 Carcinoma of the oesophagus. (A) Endoscopic image. **(B)** Barium swallow demonstrating a tight stricture in the mid-oesophagus (arrow) due to oesophageal cancer. **(C)** Endoscopic ultrasound. The central concentric circles are the probe. The arrow points to a break in the muscle layer and the soft tissue mass of the carcinoma.

are combined into stage categories. Tumours arising in the cervical, thoracic or abdominal oesophagus, including those that arise from within 5 cm from the gastro-oesophageal junction, share the same TNM staging criteria, but recent reclassification has differentiated between **squamous** and **adenocarcinoma** cancers.

- **CT scan** of the thorax and upper abdomen shows the volume of the tumour, local invasion, peritumoral and coeliac lymph node involvement, and metastases in the lung and elsewhere.
- **MRI** is equivalent to CT in local staging but not as good for pulmonary metastases.
- **Endoscopic ultrasound** has an accuracy rate of nearly 90% for assessing depth of tumour and infiltration, and of 80% for staging lymph node involvement. It is useful if CT has not already demonstrated that a cancer is too advanced for surgery. A fine-needle aspiration (FNA) of lymph nodes improves staging accuracy. Accurate T staging is necessary, as cancers confined to the superficial mucosa can be removed endoscopically (see **Fig. 32.22C**).
- **Laparoscopy** is useful if the tumour is at the cardia, to look for peritoneal and node metastases.
- **PET** after fluorodeoxyglucose is used principally to confirm distant metastases suspected on CT.

Management

Although oesophageal SCC and adenocarcinoma are undoubtedly two different disease processes with independent tumour biology, the majority of trial data do not discriminate between the two. The influence of histology on treatment is therefore unclear and varies around the globe.

Treatment is dependent on the age and performance status of the patient and the stage of the disease, with approximately 40% of all patients still alive 1 year after diagnosis. Five-year survival with stage 1 disease is 80% (T_1/T_2, N_0, M_0), stage 2 is 30%, stage 3 is 18% and stage 4 is 4%. Some 70% of patients present with stage 3 or greater disease, so that overall survival is 40% at 1 year and around 15% at 5 years. Management should be undertaken by multidisciplinary teams, including gastroenterologists, upper gastrointestinal surgeons, oncologists, palliative care physicians and dieticians.

- **Surgery** provides the best chance of a cure but should only be used when imaging (see above) has shown that the tumour has not infiltrated outside the oesophageal wall. Less than 40% of patients will have potentially resectable disease at the time of presentation. Patients must be evaluated preoperatively, particularly with regard to performance status (see p. 1179), and surgery should be undertaken in designated units. Poor outcome data from surgery alone have challenged its role as monotherapy and it is more often used in conjunction with neo-adjuvant (preoperative) and adjuvant (postoperative) treatment. The role of surgery in early oesophageal SCC is less clear. As mentioned previously, endoscopic mucosal resection may be appropriate for early mucosal disease.
- **Preoperative ('neo-adjuvant') chemoradiation therapy** may benefit patients with stage 2b and 3 disease. Prolongation of survival has been shown in some studies. In the USA, neo-adjuvant chemoradiotherapy is preferred to the neo-adjuvant chemotherapy alone that is typically used in the UK.
- **Palliative therapy** is often the only realistic possibility. Dilation is only of short-term benefit and the perforation risk is higher than for benign strictures. Combination of endoscopic dilation with laser or brachytherapy (see p. 115) prolongs luminal patency and gives as good, if not better, functional results than stenting.

Insertion of an expanding metal stent allows liquids and soft foods to be eaten.
- **Chemoradiation alone** is sometimes given but evidence of benefit is poor, except in early-stage SCC.
- **Nutritional support**, as well as support for the patient and their family, is vital in this distressing condition.

Other oesophageal tumours

Most other tumours are rare. **Gastrointestinal stromal tumours** (see p. 124) and **leiomyomas** (both submucosal tumours) are found usually by chance; 10% cause dysphagia or bleeding. Surgical removal is performed for symptomatic lesions or those over 3 cm, which are more likely to harbour malignancy. Small, benign tumours are relatively common and often do not require treatment.

Kaposi's sarcoma is found in the oesophagus as well as the mouth (see p. 1448) and hypopharynx in patients with AIDS.

Functional oesophageal disorders

The criteria for diagnosis rest mainly on compatible symptoms. However, pathological gastro-oesophageal reflux and eosinophilic oesophagitis may need to be excluded (see p. 1170).

Globus

This presents as:
- persistent or intermittent sensation of a lump or foreign body in the throat
- occurrence of the sensation between meals
- absence of dysphagia and pain on swallowing (odynophagia).

Management is with explanation and reassurance, and a trial of anti-reflux therapy. Antidepressants may be tried.

Functional chest pain of presumed oesophageal origin

This is characterized by episodes of mainly midline chest pain, not burning in nature, that are potentially of oesophageal origin and occur in the absence of a cardiological cause, gastro-oesophageal reflux and achalasia.

More than half of patients will respond to high-dose acid-suppression therapy in the first week; some will respond to nitrates and calcium-channel blockers.

Antidepressant therapy, e.g. amitriptyline or the selective serotonin reuptake inhibitor (SSRI) citalopram, have been shown to be effective.

Further reading

Furuta GT, Katzka DA. Eosinophilic esophagitis. *N Engl J Med* 2015; 373: 1640–1648.
Hvid-Jensen F, Pedersen L, Drewes AM et al. Incidence of adenocarcinoma among patients with Barrett's esophagus. *N Engl J Med* 2011; 365:1375–1383.
Kahrilas PJ, McColl K, Fox M et al. The acid pocket: a target for treatment in reflux disease? *Am J Gastroenterol* 2013; 108:1058–1064.
NICE. Gastro-oesophageal refleux disease and dyspepsia in adults: investigation and management. *Clinical guideline 184, 2014 (updated 2019)*. https://www.nice.org.uk/guidance/CG184.
Pophali P, Halland M. Barrett's oesophagus: diagnosis and management. *BMJ* 2016; 353:i2373.
Richter JE, Boeckxstaens GE. Management of achalasia: surgery or pneumatic dilation. *Gut* 2011; 60:869–876.
Rustgi AK, El-Serag HB. Esophageal carcinoma. *N Engl J Med* 2014: 371: 2499–2509.
Werner VB, Hakanson B, Martinek et al. Endoscopic or surgical myotomy in patients with idiopathic achalasia. *N Engl J Med* 2019 381;2219–2229.

STOMACH AND DUODENUM

Gastritis and gastropathy

'*Gastritis*' indicates inflammation associated with mucosal injury (although the term is often used loosely by endoscopists to describe 'redness'), and '*gastropathy*' indicates epithelial cell damage and regeneration without inflammation.

Gastritis

Several classifications of gastritis (e.g. Sydney classification) have been proposed but are controversial due to lack of correlation between endoscopic and histological findings. *H. pylori* infection is the most common cause of gastritis, with autoimmune gastritis being seen in 5% of cases; the remaining causes include viruses (e.g. cytomegalovirus and herpes simplex), duodenogastric reflux and specific causes, e.g. Crohn's, more common in children than adults. Chronic inflammation, particularly if induced by *H. pylori*, can lead to gastric intestinal metaplasia, a precursor to gastric cancer. The role of surveillance in these patients is unclear.

Autoimmune gastritis

This affects the fundus and body of the stomach (pangastritis), leading to atrophic gastritis and loss of parietal cells, with achlorhydria and intrinsic factor deficiency causing the clinical syndrome of 'pernicious anaemia' (see p. 334). Metaplasia, usually of the intestinal type, is almost always in the context of atrophic gastritis. Serum autoantibodies to gastric parietal cells are common and non-specific; antibodies to intrinsic factor are rarer and more significant (see p. 334).

Gastropathy

Gastropathy is usually caused by irritants (drugs, NSAIDs and alcohol), bile reflux and chronic congestion. Acute erosive/haemorrhagic gastropathy can also be seen after severe stress (stress ulcers); secondary to burns (Curling ulcers), trauma, shock or renal failure; and in portal hypertension (called portal gastropathy). The underlying mechanism for these ulcers is unknown but may be related to an alteration in mucosal blood flow.

Helicobacter pylori infection

Helicobacter pylori is a slow-growing, spiral, Gram-negative, flagellate, urease-producing bacterium (**Fig. 32.23**), which plays a major role in gastritis and peptic ulcer disease. It colonizes the mucous layer in the gastric antrum, but is also found in the duodenum in areas of gastric metaplasia. *H. pylori* is found in greatest numbers under the mucous layer in gastric pits, where it adheres specifically to gastric epithelial cells. It is protected from gastric acid by the juxtamucosal mucous layer, which traps bicarbonate secreted by antral cells, and ammonia produced by bacterial urease.

Epidemiology

The prevalence of *H. pylori* is high in developing countries (80–90% of the population) and much lower (20–50%) in developed countries. Infection rates are highest in lower-income groups. Infection is usually acquired in childhood; although the exact route is uncertain, it may be faecal–oral or oral–oral. The incidence increases with age, probably due to acquisition in childhood when hygiene was poorer (cohort effect) rather than infection in adult life, which is most likely far less than 1% per year in developed countries.

Pathogenesis

The pathogenetic mechanisms are not fully understood, with the majority of the colonized population remaining asymptomatic throughout their life. *H. pylori* is highly adapted to the stomach environment, exclusively colonizing gastric epithelium and inhabiting the mucous layer, or just beneath. It adheres by a number of adhesion molecules including BabA, which binds to the Lewis antigen expressed on the surface of gastric mucosal cells and causes gastritis in all infected subjects. Damage to the gastric epithelial cell is caused by the release of enzymes and the induction of apoptosis through binding to class II major histocompatibility complex (MHC) molecules. The production of urease enables the conversion of urea to ammonium and chloride, which are directly cytotoxic. Ulcers are most common when the infecting strain expresses *CagA* (cytotoxic-associated protein) and *VacA* (vacuolating toxin) genes secondary to a more pronounced inflammatory and immune response. Expression of *CagA* and *VacA* is associated with greater induction of interleukin 8 (IL-8), a potent mediator of gastric inflammation. Genetic variations in the host are also thought to be involved; for example, polymorphisms leading to increased levels of IL-1β are associated with atrophic gastritis and cancer.

Results of *H. pylori* infection

- Inflammation (antral gastritis and gastric intestinal metaplasia).
- Peptic ulcers (duodenal and gastric).
- Gastric cancer (see p. 1178).

Antral gastritis

Antral gastritis is the usual effect of *H. pylori* infection. It is normally asymptomatic, although patients without ulcers do sometimes experience relief of dyspeptic symptoms after *Helicobacter* eradication. Chronic antral gastritis causes hypergastrinaemia due to gastrin release from antral G cells. The subsequent increase in acid output is usually asymptomatic but can lead to duodenal ulceration.

Duodenal ulcer

The prevalence of *H. pylori* infection in patients with duodenal ulcers (DUs; **Fig. 32.24A**) is falling and in the developed world is now between 50% and 75%, whereas duodenal ulceration was once rare in the absence of *H. pylori* infection. This has been attributed to a decrease in prevalence of the bacterium and an increase in NSAID use. Eradication of the infection improves ulcer healing and decreases the incidence of recurrence.

The precise mechanism of duodenal ulceration is unclear, as only 15% of patients infected with *H. pylori* (50–60% of the adult population worldwide) develop duodenal ulcers. Factors that have been implicated include increased gastrin secretion, smoking, bacterial virulence and genetic susceptibility.

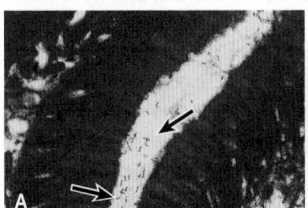
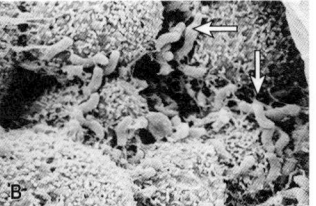

Fig. 32.23 *Helicobacter pylori*. **(A)** Organisms (arrowed) are shown on the gastric mucosa (cresyl fast violet (modified Giemsa stain). **(B)** Scanning electron microscopy, showing the spiral-shaped bacterium (arrowed). *(A, Courtesy of Dr Alan Phillips, Department of Paediatric Gastroenterology, Royal Free Hospital.)*

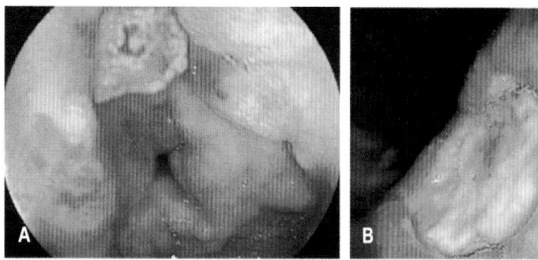

Fig. 32.24 Endoscopic views in *Helicobacter pylori* infection. **(A)** Duodenal ulcer with inflamed duodenal folds. **(B)** Benign gastric ulcer.

Gastric ulcer

Gastric ulcers (GUs; see **Fig. 32.24B**) are associated with a gastritis affecting the body as well as the antrum of the stomach (pangastritis), causing parietal cell loss and reduced acid production. The ulcers are thought to occur because of a reduction of gastric mucosal resistance due to cytokine production caused by the infection, or perhaps because of alterations in gastric mucus.

Peptic ulcer disease

A **peptic ulcer** consists of a break in the superficial epithelial cells penetrating down to the muscularis mucosa of either the stomach or the duodenum; there is a fibrous base and an increase in inflammatory cells. **Erosions**, by contrast, are superficial breaks in the mucosa alone. DUs are most commonly found in the duodenal cap; the surrounding mucosa appears inflamed, haemorrhagic or friable (duodenitis). GUs are most commonly seen on the lesser curve near the incisura, but can be found in any part of the stomach.

Epidemiology of peptic ulcer disease

DUs affect approximately 10% of the adult population and are 2–3 times more common than GUs.

Ulcer rates are declining rapidly for younger men and increasing for older individuals, particularly women. Both DUs and GUs are common in the elderly. There is considerable geographical variation, with peptic ulcer disease being more prevalent in developing countries related to the high *H. pylori* infection. In the developed world, the percentage of NSAID-induced peptic ulcers is increasing as the prevalence of *H. pylori* declines.

Clinical features of peptic ulcer disease

The characteristic feature of peptic ulcer is recurrent, burning epigastric pain. It has been shown that if a patient points with a single finger to the epigastrium as the site of the pain, this is strongly suggestive of peptic ulcer disease. The relationship of the pain to food is variable and, on the whole, not helpful in diagnosis. The pain of a DU classically occurs at night (as well as during the day) and is worse when the patient is hungry, but this is not reliable. The pain of both GUs and DUs may be relieved by antacids.

Nausea may accompany the pain; vomiting is infrequent but can relieve the pain. Anorexia and weight loss may occur, particularly with GUs. Persistent and severe pain suggests complications, such as penetration into other organs. Back pain suggests a penetrating posterior ulcer. Severe ulceration can occasionally be symptomless, as many who present with acute ulcer bleeding or perforation have no preceding ulcer symptoms.

Untreated, the symptoms of a DU relapse and remit spontaneously. The natural history is for the disease to remit over many years due to the onset of atrophic gastritis and a decrease in acid secretion.

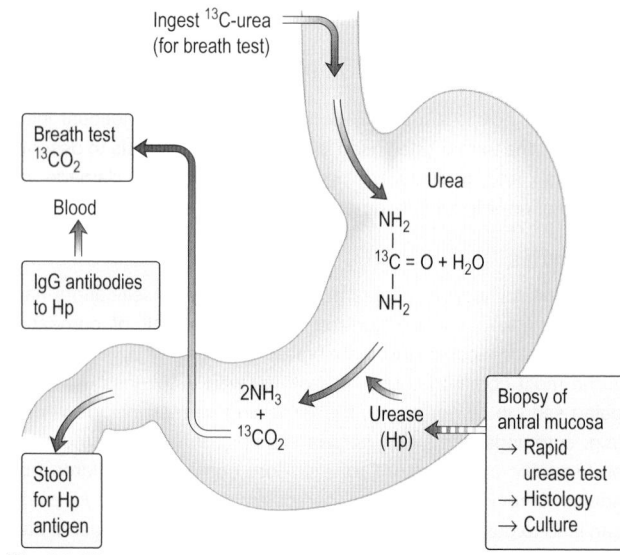

Fig. 32.25 Metabolism of urea by *Helicobacter pylori* (Hp). The different tests available for the detection of *H. pylori* are shown.

Epigastric tenderness is common in both ulcer and non-ulcer dyspepsia.

Diagnosis of *Helicobacter pylori* infection

Diagnosis of *H. pylori* is necessary if the clinician plans to treat a positive result. This is usually in the context of active peptic ulcer disease, previous peptic ulcer disease or mucosa-associated lymphoid tissue (MALT) lymphoma, or to 'test and treat' patients with dyspepsia under the age of 55 with no alarm symptoms (i.e. weight loss, anaemia, dysphagia, vomiting or family history of gastrointestinal cancer). **Examination** is usually unhelpful.

Non-invasive methods

- **Serological tests** detect immunoglobulin G (IgG) antibodies and are reasonably sensitive (90%) and specific (83%). They have been used in diagnosis and in epidemiological studies. IgG titres may take up to 1 year to fall by 50% after eradication therapy and therefore are not useful for confirming eradication or the presence of a current infection. Antibodies can also be found in the saliva but tests are not as sensitive or specific as serology.
- **^{13}C-Urea breath test** (**Fig. 32.25**) is a reliable test for *H. pylori* and can be used as a screening test. The measurement of $^{13}CO_2$ in the breath after ingestion of ^{13}C-urea requires a mass spectrometer. The test is sensitive (90%) and specific (96%), but the sensitivity can be improved by ensuring the patient has not taken antibiotics in the 4 weeks before the test and PPIs in the previous 2 weeks.
- **Stool antigen test** has superceded breath testing as the method used to determine *H. pylori* status. A specific immunoassay, using monoclonal antibodies for the qualitative detection of *H. pylori* antigen, is now widely available. The overall sensitivity is 97.6% and specificity is 96%. The test is useful in the diagnosis of *H. pylori* infection and for monitoring efficacy of eradication therapy. Patients should be off PPIs for 2 weeks but can continue with H_2-blockers. Newer stool antigen tests are being developed that can be performed in the clinic setting, although at present the sensitivity and specificity are not as good as for those performed in the laboratory.

Invasive methods (endoscopy)

- ***Biopsy urease test (Campylobacter-like organism – CLO test).*** Gastric biopsies, usually antral unless additional material is needed to exclude proximal migration, are added to a substrate containing urea and phenol red. If *H. pylori* is present, the urease enzyme that the bacteria produce splits the urea to release ammonia, which raises the pH of the solution and causes a rapid colour change (yellow to red). This enables patients' *H. pylori* status to be determined before they leave the endoscopy suite. The test may be falsely negative if patients are taking PPIs or antibiotics at the time.
- ***Histology.*** *H. pylori* can be detected histologically on routine (Giemsa) stained sections of gastric mucosa obtained at endoscopy. The sensitivity is reduced if a patient is on PPIs, but less so than with the urease test. Sensitivity can be improved with immunohistochemical staining using an anti-*H. pylori* antibody.
- ***Culture.*** Biopsies obtained can be cultured on a special medium, and *in vitro* sensitivities to antibiotics can be tested. This technique is typically used for patients with refractory *H. pylori* infection to identify the appropriate antibiotic regimen; routine culture is rare.

Investigation of suspected peptic ulcer disease

- ***Patients under 55 years of age***, with typical symptoms of peptic ulcer disease who test positive for *H. pylori*, can start eradication therapy without further investigation.
- ***Older patients*** require endoscopic diagnosis (see **Fig. 13.24**) and exclusion of cancer. All gastric ulcers must be biopsied to exclude an underlying malignancy and should be followed up endoscopically until healing has taken place.
- All patients with 'alarm symptoms' should undergo endoscopy:
  - iron deficiency anaemia
  - weight loss
  - anorexia
  - haematemesis/melaena
  - persistent vomiting
  - epigastric mass.

Management
Eradication therapy

Current recommendations are that all patients with duodenal and gastric ulcers should have *H. pylori* eradication therapy if the bacteria are present. Many patients have incidental *H. pylori* infection with no GU or DU. On balance, whether all such patients should have eradication therapy is controversial.

The increase in the prevalence of GORD and adenocarcinoma of the lower oesophagus in the last few years is currently unexplained, but has been postulated to be linked to eradication of *H. pylori*; this seems unlikely but is not disproven.

Depending on local antibacterial resistance patterns, standard eradication therapies in the developed world are successful in approximately 90% of patients. Re-infection is very uncommon (1%) in developed countries. In developing countries, re-infection is more common, compliance with treatment may be poor and metronidazole resistance is high (>50%, as it is frequently used for parasitic infections), so failure of eradication is common.

There are many regimens for eradication, but all must take into account that:
- Good compliance is essential.
- There is a high incidence of resistance to metronidazole and clarithromycin, particularly in some populations. Clarithromycin resistance has doubled in Europe in the last decade.

- Oral metronidazole has frequent side-effects.
- Bismuth chelate is unpleasant to take, even as tablets.

Metronidazole, clarithromycin, amoxicillin, tetracycline and bismuth are the most widely used agents. Resistance to amoxicillin (1–2%) and tetracycline (<1%) is low, except in countries where they are available without prescription, where resistance may exceed 50%. Quinolones (such as ciprofloxacin), furazolidone and rifabutin are also used when standard regimens have failed ('rescue therapy'). None of these drugs is effective alone; eradication regimens therefore usually comprise two antibiotics, given with powerful acid suppression in the form of a PPI. Bismuth-containing quadruple therapy is advocated as first-line treatment because of increasing clarithromycin resistance; the standard clarithromycin-based triple therapy has been replaced as the treatment of choice in areas where resistance is high.

Example regimens

- Omeprazole 20 mg + clarithromycin 500 mg and amoxicillin 1 g – all twice daily.
- Omeprazole 20 mg + metronidazole 400 mg and clarithromycin 500 mg – all twice daily.

These should be given for 7 or 14 days. Two-week treatments increase the eradication rates but increased side-effects may reduce compliance.

In ***eradication failures*** and in areas of clarithromycin resistance, bismuth chelate (120 mg 4 times daily), metronidazole (400 mg 3 times daily), tetracycline (500 mg 4 times daily) and a PPI (20–40 mg twice daily) for 14 days is used. Sequential courses of therapy are also used in such cases (5 days of PPI and amoxicillin, followed by a 5-day period of PPI with clarithromycin and tinidazole). With the increase in clarithromycin resistance, many are using this quadruple therapy for initial treatment.

Prolonged therapy with a PPI after a course of PPI-based 7-day triple therapy is not necessary for ulcer healing in most *H. pylori*-infected patients. The effectiveness of treatment for uncomplicated duodenal ulcer should be assessed symptomatically. If symptoms persist, breath or stool testing should be performed to check eradication (off PPI therapy).

Patients with a risk of bleeding or those with complications, such as haemorrhage or perforation, should always have a ^{13}C-urea breath test or stool test for *H. pylori* 6 weeks after the end of treatment to be sure that eradication has been successful. Long-term PPIs may be necessary if a rebleed would be likely to be fatal.

General measures

Stopping smoking should be strongly encouraged, as smoking slows mucosal healing.

Patients with gastric ulcers should be routinely re-endoscoped at 6 weeks to confirm mucosal healing and exclude an underlying gastric cancer. Repeat biopsies may be necessary.

Complications of peptic ulcer disease
Haemorrhage
See page 1181.

Perforation

The frequency of perforation of peptic ulceration is decreasing, partly because of medical therapy. DUs perforate more commonly than GUs, usually into the peritoneal cavity; perforation into the lesser sac also occurs. Detailed management of perforation is described on page 1222. Laparoscopic surgery is usually performed to close the perforation and drain the abdomen. Conservative management using nasogastric suction, intravenous fluids and antibiotics is occasionally used in elderly and very sick patients.

Gastric outlet obstruction

The obstruction may be pre-pyloric, pyloric or duodenal. The obstruction occurs either because there is an active ulcer with surrounding oedema or because the healing of an ulcer has been followed by scarring. However, obstruction due to peptic ulcer disease and gastric malignancy are now uncommon; Crohn's disease or external compression from a pancreatic carcinoma is a more common cause. Adult hypertrophic pyloric stenosis is a very rare cause.

After gastric outlet obstruction, the stomach becomes full of gastric juice and ingested fluid and food, giving rise to the main symptom of vomiting, usually without pain, as the characteristic ulcer pain has abated owing to healing.

Vomiting is infrequent, projectile and large in volume; the vomitus contains particles of previous meals. On examination of the abdomen, there may be a succussion splash. The diagnosis is made by endoscopy but can be suspected from the nature of the vomiting; by contrast, psychogenic vomiting is frequent, small-volume and usually noisy.

Severe or persistent vomiting causes loss of acid from the stomach and a hypokalaemic metabolic alkalosis (see p. 201). Vomiting will often settle with intravenous fluid and electrolyte replacement, gastric drainage via a nasogastric tube, and potent acid suppression therapy. Endoscopic dilation of the pyloric region is useful, as is luminal stenting, and overall, 70% of patients can be managed without surgery.

Surgical treatment and its long-term consequences

Once the mainstay of treatment, surgery is now used in peptic ulcer disease only for complications including:
- recurrent uncontrolled haemorrhage
- perforation, which is oversewn.

No other procedure, such as gastrectomy or vagotomy, is required.

In the past, two types of operation were performed: a partial gastrectomy or a vagotomy. In the latter, either a truncal vagotomy with a pyloroplasty or gastro-jejunostomy was performed, or highly selective vagotomy or proximal gastric vagotomy, which did not require a bypass procedure.

Long-term complications of surgery, which are still seen occasionally, include:
- **Recurrent ulcer.** If this occurs, check for *H. pylori*; rule out Zollinger–Ellison syndrome (see p. 1336). Malignancy needs to be excluded in all cases.
- **Dumping.** This term describes a number of upper abdominal symptoms (e.g. nausea and distension associated with sweating, faintness and palpitations) that occur in patients following gastrectomy or gastroenterostomy. It is due to 'dumping' of food into the jejunum, causing rapid fluid shifts from plasma to dilute the high osmotic load with reduction of blood volume. The symptoms are usually mild and patients adapt to them. It is rare for it to be a long-term problem, and if so, the symptoms usually have a functional element. Hypoglycaemia can also occur.
- **Diarrhoea.** This was chiefly seen after vagotomy. Recurrent severe episodes occurred in about 1% of patients. Antidiarrhoeals are the usual treatment.
- **Nutritional complications.** In the long term, almost any gastric surgery, but particularly gastrectomy, may be followed by:
  - iron deficiency, due to poor absorption
  - folate deficiency, usually due to poor intake
  - vitamin B_{12} deficiency, due to intrinsic factor deficiency
  - weight loss, usually due to reduced intake.

Other H. pylori-associated diseases

- **Gastric adenocarcinoma.** The incidence of distal (but not proximal) gastric cancer parallels that of *H. pylori* infection in countries with a high incidence of gastric cancer. Serological studies show that people infected with *H. pylori* have a higher incidence of distal gastric carcinoma (see p. 1178).
- **Gastric B-cell lymphoma.** Over 70% of patients with gastric B-cell lymphomas (MALT) have *H. pylori*. *H. pylori* gastritis has been shown to contain the clonal B cell that eventually gives rise to the MALT lymphoma (see p. 1180).

NSAIDs, Helicobacter and ulcers

Aspirin and other NSAIDs deplete mucosal prostaglandins by inhibiting the cyclo-oxygenase (COX) pathway, which leads to mucosal damage. Cyclo-oxygenase occurs in two main forms: COX-1, the constitutive enzyme; and COX-2, inducible by cytokine stimulation in areas of inflammation. COX-2-specific inhibitors have less effect on the COX-1 enzyme in the gastric mucosa; they still produce gastric mucosal damage but less than with other conventional NSAIDs. Their use is limited by concern regarding cardiovascular side-effects.

Some 50% of patients taking regular NSAIDs will develop gastric mucosal damage and approximately 30% will have ulcers on endoscopy. Only a small proportion of patients have symptoms (about 5%) and only 1–2% have a major problem: that is, gastrointestinal bleed or perforation. Because of the large number of patients on NSAIDs, including low-dose aspirin for vascular prophylaxis, this is a significant problem, particularly in the elderly.

H. pylori and NSAIDs are independent and synergistic risk factors for the development of ulcers. In a meta-analysis, the odds ratio (OR) for the incidence of peptic ulcer was 61.1 in patients infected with *H. pylori* and also taking NSAIDs, compared with uninfected controls not taking NSAIDs.

Management

- Stop the ingestion of NSAIDs.
- Give a PPI.
- Start *H. pylori* eradication therapy if the patient is *H. pylori*-positive.

In many people with severe arthritis, stopping NSAIDs may not be possible. Therefore use:
- **An NSAID** with low GI side-effects at the lowest dose possible. If there is no cardiovascular risk, a COX-2 NSAID can be used (see p. 431).
- **Prophylactic cytoprotective therapy**, e.g. PPI or misoprostol (a synthetic analogue of prostaglandin E_1 800 µg/day) for all high-risk patients, i.e. over 65 years, those with a peptic ulcer history, particularly with complications, and those on corticosteroid or anticoagulant therapy. PPIs reduce the risk of endoscopic duodenal and gastric ulcers and are better tolerated than misoprostol, which causes diarrhoea.

Gastroparesis

Gastroparesis results when there is delayed gastric emptying. There are a number of known causes such as:
- diabetes
- amyloidosis
- scleroderma
- parkinsonism
- multiple sclerosis
- stress

- medications (tricyclic antidepressants, dopamine agonists, calcium-channel blockers, octreotide, cyclosporine, glucagon-like peptide agonists, phenothiazines)
- post-surgical
- idiopathic.

Symptoms include nausea, vomiting, early satiety, fullness, bloating and upper abdominal pain.

Investigation should exclude mechanical obstruction thus all patients with suspected delayed gastric emptying should undergo an OGD. Further imaging may then be needed with either CT/MRI or a barium meal. Once obstruction has been ruled out, the diagnosis of delayed gastric emptying is confirmed by scintigraphy. This is a nuclear medicine scan that determines the rate of gastric emptying. The patient must fast overnight before eating an isotope-labelled meal. The residual content of the stomach is then measured at 4 hours with more than 10% considered abnormal. Gastroduodenal manometry can help to differentiate between myopathic (amyloid, scleroderma) and neuropathic (diabetes) causes.

Management is directed at relief of symptoms and correction of nutritional deficiencies. Improvement of gastric emptying can sometimes be achieved by medical or surgical treatments, such as pro-motility agents (metoclopramide, domperidone or erythromycin) or gastric pacemaker insertion. A diet of frequent, small, low-fibre meals can help symptoms in a number of patients. In diabetics, glycaemic control is helpful.

Dyspepsia

'Indigestion' is common: 80% of the population will suffer from this symptom at some time. Dyspepsia is an inexact term used to describe a number of upper abdominal symptoms such as heartburn, acidity, pain or discomfort, nausea, wind, fullness or belching. Patients who use the term 'indigestion' may also be describing lower gastrointestinal symptoms such as constipation or the presence of undigested vegetable material in the stool, so obtaining a precise history is necessary.

Features of dyspepsia that are suggestive of serious diseases such as cancer are known as *'alarm' symptoms*. They include:

- dysphagia
- weight loss
- vomiting
- anorexia
- haematemesis or melaena.

Patients aged 55 years or over who demonstrate these features have a higher possibility of significant gastrointestinal pathology and should be investigated on an urgent basis. However, most patients with dyspepsia can be managed in primary care without need for referral to a gastroenterologist. See the current NICE guideline algorithm for managing a patient with dyspepsia (https://www.nice.org.uk/guidance/cg184).

Cyclical vomiting syndrome

This syndrome is characterized by typical bouts of intense vomiting lasting for hours to days, separated by periods with no symptoms. It can occur in children or adults. There is a link to migraine headaches but the cause is not known. In some cases, provocative triggers can be identified; for example, there is a specific syndrome associated with frequent cannabis use – cannabinoid hyperemesis syndrome.

Diagnosis of cyclical vomiting syndrome is by recognition of the pattern of symptoms and ruling out of other causes.

Management

Treatment is with antiemetics and intravenous rehydration and electrolyte replacement during bouts, with avoidance of triggers where these are known. Prophylactic treatment of migraine, when it coexists, may help.

Nausea and vomiting

Nausea is the sensation of being about to vomit, which can occur with or without vomiting. It can be more unpleasant and disabling for patients than vomiting alone. There are two central areas that are responsible for triggering nausea and vomiting. The nucleus tractus solitarius in the medulla, which acts as a central pattern generator for vomiting, and the area postrema in the floor of the fourth ventricle. This contains the 'chemoreceptor trigger zone', which has five different receptors:

- 5-HT receptors
- histamine H1 receptors
- muscarinic receptors
- dopamine D2 receptors
- substance P (neurokinin-1-neuropeptide).

Substances such as opioids, hormones, ketoacids and urea can all stimulate the CTZ directly as they are carried in the bloodstream.

Nausea and vomiting can be caused by a huge number of varied conditions, infections, medications and toxins. The choice of antiemetic depends on the cause of the vomiting and the side-effect profile of the antiemetic (**Box 32.15**).

---

i **Box 32.15 Commonly used antiemetic drugs**

Antiemetic class	Drugs	When to use	Side-effects
Antihistamines	Cyclizine Promethazine	Motion sickness Vestibular nausea	IV cyclizine can be addictive.
Dopamine-R antagonists	Prochlorperazine Chlorpromazine (phenothiazines)	Post-chemotherapy	Extra-pyramidal reactions – avoid in Parkinson's
	Haloperidol	Palliative	QT prolongation
	Metoclopramide	Gastroenteritis Migraine Postoperative	Increased gastric emptying Tardive dyskinesia with prolonged use
Serotonin receptor antagonists (5-HT$_3$)	Ondansetron	Chemotherapy-induced (1st-line)	Constipation Headache Dizziness
Glucocorticoids	Dexamethasone	Chemotherapy-induced (in combo with 5-HT$_3$ RA)	Steroid side-effect profile

Gastric tumours

Adenocarcinoma

Gastric cancer is currently the fourth most common cancer found worldwide and the second leading cause of cancer-related mortality. The incidence increases with age (peak incidence 50–70 years), and it is rare under the age of 30 years. The highest incidence of the disease is found in Eastern Asia, Eastern Europe and South America. The incidence in men is twice that in women and varies throughout the world, being high in Japan (M: 53/100 000, F: 21.3/100 000) and Chile, and relatively low in the USA (M: 7/100 000, F: 2.9/100 000). In the UK, carcinoma of the stomach (**Fig. 32.26**) is the eighth most common cancer (M: 16/100 000, F 9/100 000). The overall worldwide incidence of gastric carcinoma is falling, even in Japan, probably due to reductions in the incidence of *Helicobacter* and, before this, improvements in food storage. However, the incidence of proximal gastric cancers is increasing in the West and they have very similar demographic and pathological features to Barrett's-associated oesophageal adenocarcinoma.

Epidemiology and pathogenesis

- **H. pylori infection** and distal gastric cancer are strongly linked. *H. pylori* is recognized by the International Agency for Research in Cancer (IARC) as a group 1 (definite) gastric carcinogen. *H. pylori* infection causes chronic gastritis, which eventually leads to atrophic gastritis and pre-malignant intestinal metaplasia (**Fig. 32.27**). Much of the earlier epidemiological data (i.e. the increase of cancer in lower socioeconomic groups) can be explained by the intrafamilial spread of *H. pylori*. Epstein–Barr virus is detected in 2–16% of gastric cancers worldwide, but its role in aetiology is not well understood.
- **Dietary factors** may also be involved (as both initiators and promoters) and have separate roles in carcinogenesis. Diets high in salt probably increase the risk. Dietary nitrates can be converted into nitrosamines by bacteria at neutral pH; nitrosamines are known to be carcinogenic in animals but the evidence in human carcinogenesis is limited. Nitrosamines are also present in the stomach of patients with achlorhydria, who have an increased cancer risk.
- **Tobacco smoking** is associated with an increased incidence of stomach cancer.
- **Genetic abnormality** is also a factor. The most common abnormality is a loss of heterozygosity (LOH) of tumour suppressor genes such as *p53* (in 50% of cancers, as well as in

pre-cancerous states) and the gene encoding adenomatous polyposis coli (*APC*) (in over one-third of gastric cancers). These abnormalities are similar to those found in colorectal cancers. Some rare families with diffuse gastric cancer have been shown to have mutations in the E-cadherin gene (*CDH-1*). There is a higher incidence of gastric cancer in blood group A patients.

- **First-degree relatives** of patients with gastric cancer have 2–3-fold increased relative risk of developing the disease, but this may be environmental rather than inherited.
- **Pernicious anaemia** carries a small increased risk of gastric carcinoma due to the accompanying atrophic gastritis.
- **Partial gastrectomy** (postoperative stomach) carries an increased risk of gastric cancer, whether performed for a GU or DU; this is probably due to untreated *H. pylori* infection.

Screening

Earlier diagnosis has been advocated in an attempt to improve the poor prognosis of gastric cancer. (Screening is discussed on p. 102.) Although the incidence of gastric cancer is falling in Japan, where aggressive screening by barium studies is followed by endoscopy if there is doubt, there is no evidence that screening has had an effect on overall mortality. Similarly, early investigation of dyspepsia has had little effect on mortality, possibly because of the relatively low prevalence of cancer.

Early gastric cancer

Early gastric cancer is defined as a carcinoma that is confined to the mucosa or submucosa, regardless of the presence of lymph node

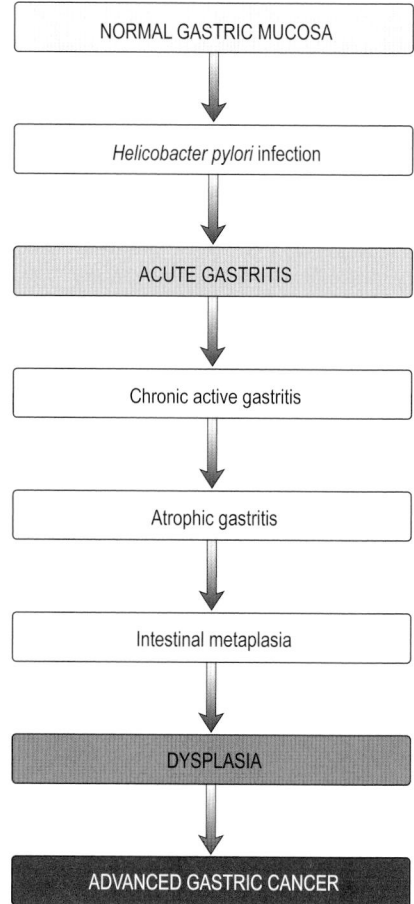

Fig. 32.27 Flow diagram showing the development of gastric cancer associated with *H. pylori* infection.

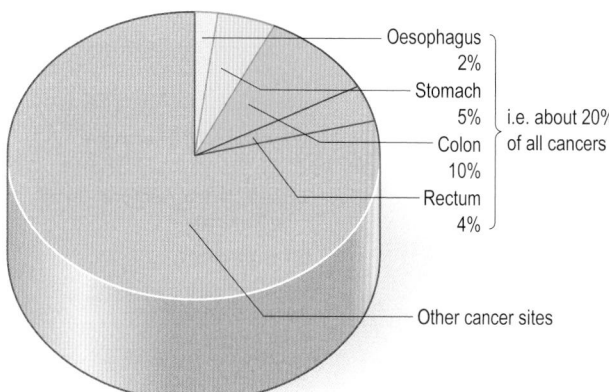

Fig. 32.26 Relative contribution of gastrointestinal sites to all cancers.

metastases. It is associated with 5-year survival rates of approximately 90%, but many of these patients would have survived 5 years without treatment. In Japan, mass screening with mobile units has increased the proportion of early gastric cancers (EGC) diagnosed. In a large series of patients from the UK with gastric cancer, only 0.7% were identified as having EGC. They are usually detected by chance, as although EGC exists in Western populations, endoscopists do not readily recognize it at present.

Pathology

There are two major types of gastric cancer:
- **Intestinal** (**type 1**) with well-formed glandular structures (differentiated). The tumours are polypoid or ulcerating lesions with heaped-up, rolled edges. Intestinal metaplasia is seen in the surrounding mucosa, often with *H. pylori*. This type is more likely to involve the distal stomach and occur in patients with atrophic gastritis. It has a strong environmental association.
- **Diffuse** (**type 2**) with poorly cohesive cells (undifferentiated) that tend to infiltrate the gastric wall. It may involve any part of the stomach, especially the cardia, and has a worse prognosis than the intestinal type. Loss of expression of the cell adhesion molecule E-cadherin is the key event in the carcinogenesis of diffuse gastric cancers. Unlike type 1 gastric cancers, type 2 cancers have similar frequencies in all geographic areas and occur in a younger population.

Some 50% of gastric cancers in Western countries occur in the proximal stomach.

Clinical features

Symptoms

Around 50% of patients with EGC discovered at screening have no symptoms. Most patients with carcinoma of the stomach have advanced disease at the time of presentation. The most common symptom of advanced disease is epigastric pain, indistinguishable from the pain of peptic ulcer disease; it may be relieved by food and antacids. The pain can vary in intensity but may be constant and severe, and there may also be nausea, anorexia and weight loss. Vomiting is frequent and can be severe if the tumour encroaches on the pylorus. Dysphagia can occur with tumours involving the fundus. Gross haematemesis is unusual but anaemia from occult blood loss is frequent. No pattern of symptoms is suggestive of EGC.

Widely spreading submucosal gastric cancer causes diffuse thickening and rigidity of the stomach wall and is called '*linitis plastica*'.

Patients can present at a late stage with malignant ascites or jaundice due to liver involvement. Metastases also occur in bone, brain and lung, producing appropriate symptoms.

Signs

Weight loss is often the dominant feature. Nearly 50% of patients have a palpable epigastric mass with abdominal tenderness. A palpable lymph node is sometimes found in the supraclavicular fossa (Virchow's node, usually on the left side), and metastases are present in up to one-third of patients at presentation. This cancer is the most frequently associated with dermatomyositis (see p. 462) and acanthosis nigricans.

Diagnosis

Gastroscopy (**Fig. 32.28**) allows biopsies to be taken for histological assessment. Positive biopsies can be obtained in almost all cases of obvious carcinoma, but a negative biopsy does not necessarily rule out the diagnosis. For this reason, 8–10 biopsies should be taken from suspicious lesions. Diffuse type gastric cancer infiltrates the submucosa and muscularis propria and can be undetected on endoscopy; multiple deep biopsies help.

Staging

- ***CT scan of the chest and abdomen*** with a gastric water load can demonstrate gastric wall thickening, lymphadenopathy and lung and liver secondaries, but has limited ability to determine the depth of local tumour invasion.
- ***Endoscopic ultrasound*** is useful for local staging to demonstrate the depth of penetration of the cancer through the gastric wall and extension into local lymph nodes. It complements CT and ultrasound but is most relevant to confirm that a cancer is confined to the superficial mucosa, before endoscopic resection.
- ***Laparoscopy*** is useful in patients being considered for surgery to exclude serosal disease.
- ***PET and CT/PET*** can be helpful in further delineation of the cancer.

The TNM classification is used. The tumour grade (T) indicates depth of tumour invasion, N denotes the presence or absence of lymph nodes, and M indicates presence or absence of metastases. TNM classification is then combined into stage categories 0–4. At presentation, two-thirds of patients are at stage 3 or 4: that is, advanced disease (**Box 32.16**). The histological grade of the tumour also determines survival.

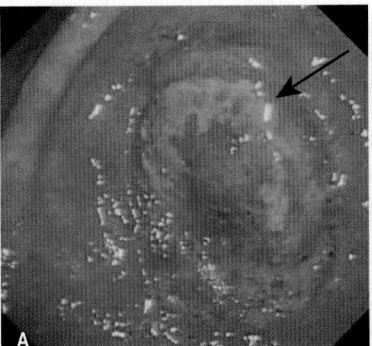
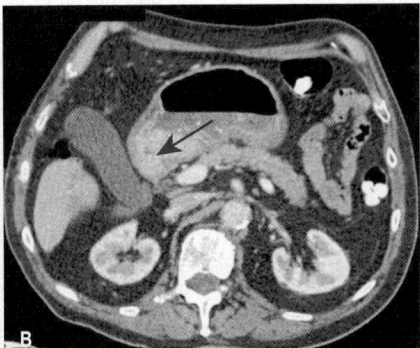
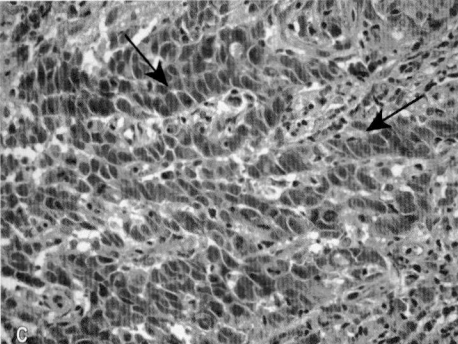

Fig. 32.28 Carcinoma of the stomach. **(A)** Endoscopic picture showing a large, irregular ulcer with rolled edges (arrowed). **(B)** Axial CT scan (ulcer arrowed). **(C)** Histopathology showing an adenocarcinoma (arrowed).

Stage	TNM[a] stage	5-year survival (%)
1	T1N0M0, T1N1M0 or T2N0M0	88
2	T1N2M0, T2N1M0 or T3N0M0	65
3a	T2N2M0, T3N1M0 or T4N0M0	35
3b	T3N2M0	35
4	T4N1–3M0, TxN3M0 or TxNxM1[b]	5

[a]T, tumour; N, nodes; M, metastases.
[b]Tx indicates any T stage; Nx, any N stage.

Management

As with all cancers, treatment is discussed with a multidisciplinary team. Early non-ulcerated mucosal lesions can be removed endoscopically by either endoscopic mucosal resection or endoscopic submucosal dissection.

Surgery remains the most effective form of treatment if the patient is an operative candidate. Careful selection has reduced the numbers undergoing surgery and has improved the overall surgical 5-year survival rates to around 30%. Five-year survival rates in 'curative' operations are as high as 50%. Surgery, combined chemoradiotherapy and treatment of advanced disease are described on page 124. The multinational MAGIC trial demonstrated the benefits of perioperative chemotherapy with epirubicin, cisplatin and infusional 5-fluorouracil (ECF) (see p. 124), where 5-year survival in operable gastric and lower oesophageal adenocarcinomas increased from 23% to 36%. An alternative regimen is oral epirubicin, oxaliplatin and capecitabine. Despite the improved results, the overall survival rate for a patient with gastric carcinoma has not dramatically improved, with a maximum 5-year survival rate of 10% overall. Palliative care, with relief of pain and counselling, is usually required.

Gastrointestinal stromal tumours

Gastrointestinal stromal tumours (GISTs) are a subset of gastrointestinal mesenchymal tumours of varying differentiation. They are usually asymptomatic and found by chance but occasionally they can ulcerate and bleed. There are 200–900 new cases each year in the UK. GISTs mostly affect people between 55 and 65 years of age.

These tumours were previously classified as gastrointestinal leiomyomas, leiomyosarcomas, leiomyoblastomas or schwannomas. Truly benign leiomyomas do occur, mainly in the oesophagus, but GISTs are now recognized as a distinct group of mesenchymal tumours and comprise about 80% of gastrointestinal mesenchymal tumours. They are of stromal origin and are thought to share a common ancestry with the interstitial cells of Cajal. They have varying differentiation, with mutations occurring in the cellular proto-oncogene *KIT* (which leads to activation and cell-surface expression of the tyrosine kinase KIT (CD 117)) in 80%, and also in platelet-derived growth factor receptor-α (PDGFRA) in up to 10% of patients.

Management

Treatment is surgical as far as possible. These tumours generally grow slowly but may be malignant. Imatinib, a tyrosine kinase inhibitor (see p. 113), is chosen for unresectable or metastatic disease, and is now used as adjunctive therapy after surgical removal of the primary in the absence of metastatic disease. Some patients are resistant to this; sunitinib can be used as an alternative agent over a short time period.

Primary gastric lymphoma

Mucosa-associated lymphatic tissue (MALT) lymphomas are indolent B-cell marginal zone lymphomas that primarily involve sites other than lymph nodes (gastrointestinal tract, thyroid, breast or skin). They constitute about 10% of all types of non-Hodgkin's lymphoma (NHL).

Aetiology

About 90% of cases are due to *H. pylori* infection. Chromosome abnormalities t(1;14)(p22; q32) and t(11;18)(q21; q21) have also been noted in this form of NHL.

Clinical features

Most patients are diagnosed in their 60s with stage I or stage II disease outside the lymph nodes. Patients have stomach pain, ulcers or other localized symptoms, but rarely have systemic complaints such as fatigue or fever.

Management

Eradication of *H. pylori* infection may resolve cases of local gastric involvement. After standard eradication regimens, 50% of patients show resolution at 3 months. Other patients may resolve after 12–18 months of observation. Stage III or IV disease is treated with surgery or chemotherapy with or without radiation. The prognosis is good, with an estimated 90% 5-year survival.

Gastric polyps

Gastric polyps are found in about 1% of endoscopies, usually by chance. They rarely produce symptoms, but larger lesions can result in anaemia or haematemesis.

Endoscopic biopsy is the usual approach to diagnosis and treatment is possible polypectomy based on histological finding. Occasional large or multiple polyps may require surgery.

- **Hyperplastic polyps** are by far the most common type. Most are smaller than 2 cm. The polyps are rarely pre-malignant, but may be accompanied by pre-malignant atrophic gastritis.
- **Adenomatous polyps** are usually solitary lesions in the antrum. Approximately 3% progress to gastric cancer, especially if greater than 2 cm in diameter, but they are not a common cause of gastric cancer (compare this with colorectal cancer).
- **Cystic gland polyps** contain microcysts that are lined by fundic-type parietal and chief cells. They are located in the fundus and body of the stomach. They are found in otherwise normal subjects, but are especially common in familial polyposis syndromes and patients on PPIs. Their malignant potential is negligible, although low-grade dysplasia is seen in the absence of familial adenomatous polyposis coli (FAP), and high-grade dysplasia exclusively in its presence.
- **Inflammatory fibroid polyps** are benign spindle cell tumours infiltrated by eosinophils. Excision of these polyps is indicated because of their propensity to enlarge and cause obstruction.

Further reading

Heinrich MC, Rankin C, Blanke CD. Correlation of long-term results of imatinib in advanced gastrointestinal stromal tumor with next-generation sequencing results. *JAMA Oncol* 2017; 3:944–952.
Malfertheiner P, Bazzoli F, Delchier JC et al. *Helicobacter pylori* eradication with a capsule containing bismuth subcitrate potassium, metronidazole, and tetracycline given with omeprazole versus clarithromycin-based triple therapy: a randomised, open-label, non-inferiority, phase 3 trial. *Lancet* 2011; 377: 905–913.
Crowe SE. *Helicobacter pylori* infection. *N Engl J Med* 2019; 380:1158–1165.

ACUTE AND CHRONIC GASTROINTESTINAL BLEEDING

Acute upper gastrointestinal bleeding

GI bleeds are one of the most common medical emergencies (>4 unit transfused). Incidence is 1.33/1000 population, or 85 000 cases/ year. In the 2015 NCEPOD report on the management of GI haemorrhage, 40% of patients in the study population, who received treatment for acute upper GI bleeding, were inpatients being treated for another condition when they had an acute upper GI bleed.

The cardinal features are haematemesis (the vomiting of blood) and melaena (the passage of black tarry stools, the black colour being due to blood altered by passage through the gut). Melaena can occur with bleeding from any lesion proximal to the right colon. Rarely, melaena can also result from bleeding from the right colon.

Following a bleed from the upper gastrointestinal tract, unaltered blood can appear *per rectum*, but the bleeding must be massive and is almost always accompanied by shock. The passage of dark blood and clots without shock is most often due to lower gastrointestinal bleeding. Of note, stool may be frankly bloody or maroon with massive or brisk upper GI bleeding.

Aetiology

Peptic ulceration is the most common cause of serious and life-threatening gastrointestinal bleeding (**Fig. 32.29** and **Box 32.17**). The relative incidence of causes depends on the patient population; overall, incidence has fallen. In the developing world, haemorrhagic

viral infections (see **Box 20.37**) can cause significant gastrointestinal bleeding.

Drugs

Aspirin (even 75 mg/day) and other NSAIDs can produce ulcers and erosions. These agents are also responsible for gastrointestinal haemorrhage from both duodenal and gastric ulcers, particularly in the elderly. They are available over the counter in the UK and patients may not be aware that they are taking aspirin or an NSAID. Corticosteroids in the usual therapeutic doses have no influence on gastrointestinal haemorrhage. The estimated relative risks of glucocorticoids alone for gastrointestinal adverse effects, including GI bleeding, vary from 1.1 (not significant) to 1.5 (marginally significant). However, the combination of glucocorticoids and NSAIDs results in a synergistic increase in the incidence of gastrointestinal haemorrhage. Anticoagulants and antiplatelet agents do not cause acute gastrointestinal haemorrhage *per se*, but bleeding from any cause is greater if the patient is anticoagulated.

Clinical approach to the patient with acute upper GI bleeding

All cases with a recent (i.e. within 48 hours) significant gastrointestinal bleed should be seen in hospital. In many, no immediate

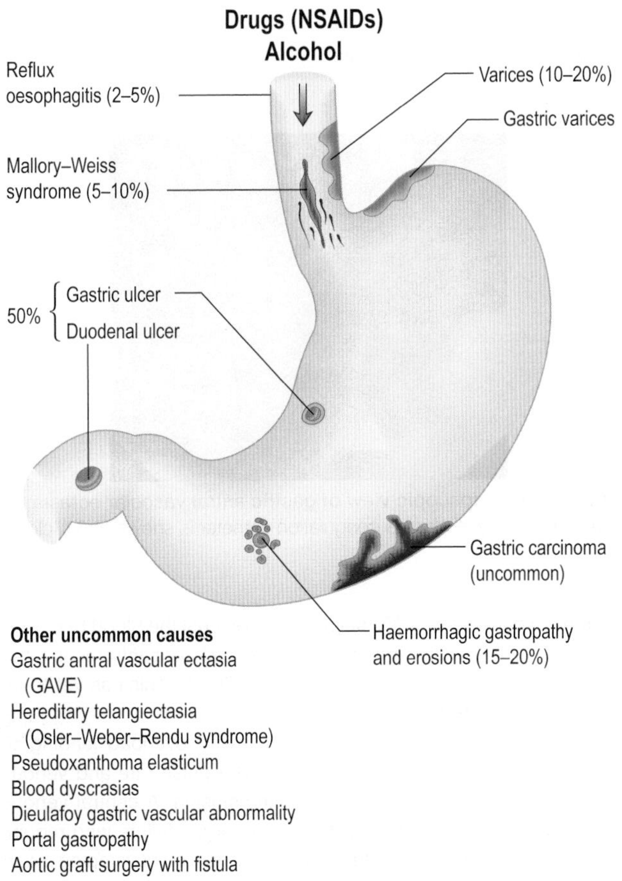

Drugs (NSAIDs) Alcohol

Reflux oesophagitis (2–5%)

Varices (10–20%)

Gastric varices

Mallory–Weiss syndrome (5–10%)

50% { Gastric ulcer / Duodenal ulcer

Gastric carcinoma (uncommon)

Haemorrhagic gastropathy and erosions (15–20%)

Other uncommon causes
Gastric antral vascular ectasia (GAVE)
Hereditary telangiectasia (Osler–Weber–Rendu syndrome)
Pseudoxanthoma elasticum
Blood dyscrasias
Dieulafoy gastric vascular abnormality
Portal gastropathy
Aortic graft surgery with fistula

Fig. 32.29 Causes of upper gastrointestinal haemorrhage. The approximate frequency is also given. NSAID, non-steroidal anti-inflammatory drug.

> ⊕ **Box 32.17** Overview of emergency assessment of severe upper gastrointestinal bleeding in adults
>
> **Major causes**
> - Peptic ulcer, oesophagogastric varices, arteriovenous malformation, tumour, oesophageal (Mallory–Weiss) tear
>
> **Clinical features**
> *History*
> - Use of: non-steroidal anti-inflammatory drugs (NSAIDs), aspirin, anticoagulants, antiplatelet agents
> - Alcohol misuse; previous gastrointestinal (GI) bleed; liver disease; coagulopathy
>
> *Symptoms and signs*
> Abdominal pain; haematemesis or 'coffee ground' emesis; passing melaena/tarry stool (stool may be frankly bloody or maroon with massive or brisk upper GI bleeding)
>
> **Examination**
> - Tachycardia, orthostatic blood pressure changes suggest moderate to severe blood loss; hypotension suggests life-threatening blood loss (hypotension may be late finding in healthy younger adult)
> - Rectal examination is performed to assess stool colour (melaena versus haematochezia versus brown)
> - Significant abdominal tenderness accompanied by signs of peritoneal irritation (e.g. involuntary guarding) suggests perforation
>
> **Management**
> - Obtain type and crossmatch for haemodynamic instability, severe bleeding, or high-risk patient
> - Obtain Hb (may be inaccurate with acute severe haemorrhage), PLT count, PT with INR, AST, ALT, albumin and creatinine
> - Closely monitor airway, clinical status, observations, cardiac rhythm, urine output
> - Do NOT give patient anything by mouth
> - Establish two large bore i.v. lines (16-gauge or larger)
> - Provide supplemental oxygen
> - Treat hypotension initially with rapid, bolus infusions of isotonic crystalloid
> - Monitored bed or ITU depending on the severity of bleeding
>
> ALT, alanine aminotransferase; AST, aspartate aminotransferase; INR, international normalized ratio; PLT, platelet count; PT, prothrombin time.

Box 32.18 Rockall risk assessment score in non-variceal upper gastrointestinal haemorrhage

Variable	Score			
	0	**1**	**2**	**3**
Age (years)	<60	60–79	>79	–
Circulation	BP >100 mmHg	BP >100 mmHg	BP <100 mmHg	–
	Pulse <100 beats/min	Pulse >100 beats/min	Pulse >100 beats/min	
Co-morbidity	None	–	Cardiac disease, any other major co-morbidity	Chronic kidney disease, liver failure, disseminated malignancy
Endoscopic diagnosis	Mallory–Weiss tear, no lesion	All other diagnoses	Malignancy of the upper gastrointestinal tract	–
Major SRH	None, or dark spots	–	Blood in the upper gastrointestinal tract, adherent clot or spurting vessel	–

BP, blood pressure (systolic); SRH, stigmata of recent haemorrhage.

treatment is required, as there has been only a small amount of blood loss. Approximately 85% of patients stop bleeding spontaneously within 48 hours.

Scoring systems have been developed to assess the risk of rebleeding or death.

Boxes 13.18 and **13.19** show the Rockall score, which is based on clinical and endoscopy findings. The Blatchford score uses the level of plasma urea, haemoglobin and clinical markers, but not endoscopic findings, to determine the need for intervention such as blood transfusion or endoscopy in gastrointestinal bleeding. Incorporation of a validated risk score for upper gastrointestinal bleeding into routine clinical practice facilitates optimal triage decisions.

The following factors affect the risk of rebleeding and death:
- age
- evidence of co-morbidity, e.g. cardiac failure, ischaemic heart disease, chronic kidney disease and malignant disease
- presence of the classical clinical features of shock (pallor, cold peripheries, tachycardia and low blood pressure)
- endoscopic diagnosis, e.g. Mallory–Weiss tear, peptic ulceration, gastric antral vascular ectasia (GAVE; **Fig. 32.30**)
- endoscopic stigmata of recent bleeding, e.g. adherent blood clot, spurting vessel
- clinical signs of chronic liver disease.

Bleeding associated with liver disease is often severe and recurrent if it is from varices. Liver failure can develop.

Management

Immediate management

This is shown in **Box 32.20**. In addition, stop NSAIDs, aspirin, clopidogrel and warfarin if patients are taking them (**Boxes 32.21** and **32.22**). Stopping antiplatelets can be dangerous and may produce thrombosis; discuss this urgently with a cardiologist.

Many hospitals have multidisciplinary specialist teams with agreed protocols and the latter should be followed. Patients should be managed in monitored beds or ITU depending on the severity of bleeding. Oxygen should be given and the patient should be kept nil by mouth until an endoscopy has been performed.

Patients with large bleeds and clinical signs of shock require urgent resuscitation. Details of the management of shock are given in **Fig. 10.24**.

Blood volume

See **Box 32.23**. The major principle is to restore the blood volume rapidly to normal via two or more large-bore intravenous cannulae;

Box 32.19 Rockall scores post-endoscopy

Rockall score	Predicted probabilities	
	Rebleeding risk (%)	**Mortality (%)**
0	5	0
1	3	0
2	5	0
3	11	3
4	14	5
5	24	11
6	33	17
7	44	27
8+	42	41

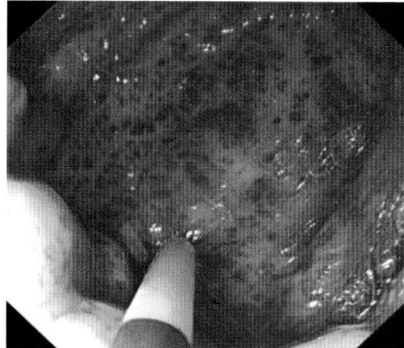

Fig. 32.30 Endoscopic view of gastric antral vascular ectasia (GAVE). An argon plasma coagulation catheter is shown at 6 o'clock.

plasma expanders or 0.9% saline are given until the blood becomes available (see p. 221). Transfusion of red cell concentrates is used with a proposed transfusion threshold of 70 g/L. This has yet to be universally adopted.

Transfusion must be monitored to avoid overload leading to heart failure, particularly in the elderly. The pulse rate and venous pressure are guides to adequacy of transfusion. A central venous pressure line is inserted for patients with organ failure who require blood transfusion, and in those most at risk of developing heart failure.

Haemoglobin levels are generally a poor indicator of the need to transfuse because anaemia does not develop immediately as

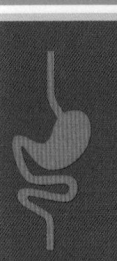

an indication of the risk of rebleeding and death (see **Box 32.19**). **Box 32.24** shows medical treatment prior to endoscopy.
  At first endoscopy:

- Varices should be treated, usually with banding.
- Stenting is also used for bleeding varices but is not yet widely available (see p. 1294). It is an alternative to a Sengstaken tube.
- Bleeding ulcers and those with stigmata of recent bleeding should be treated using two or three haemostatic methods: injection with adrenaline (epinephrine) and thermal coagulation (with heater probe, bipolar probe, or laser or argon plasma coagulation) or endoscopic clipping; dual and triple therapy is more effective than monotherapy in reducing rebleeding. Haemostatic powders have recently been developed that can be sprayed through a catheter during gastroscopy. These are useful in the more difficult bleeds, such as cancer-related bleeding and challenging ulcers.
- Antral biopsies should be taken to look for *H. pylori*. A positive biopsy urease test is valid but a negative test is not reliable. If the urease test is negative, gastric histology should always be performed.
  Balloon tamponade may be performed as a temporizing measure for patients with uncontrollable haemorrhage likely due to varices using any of several devices (e.g. Sengstaken–Blakemore tube). Tracheal intubation is necessary if such a device is to be placed; ensure proper device placement prior to inflation to avoid oesophageal rupture.

Drug therapy

After diagnosis at endoscopy, an intravenous PPI (e.g. omeprazole 80 mg followed by infusion 8 mg/h for 72 h) should be given to all patients with actively bleeding ulcers or ulcers with a visible vessel, as it reduces rebleeding rates and the need for surgery.

  Tranexamic acid is an antifibrinolytic agent that has been studied in patients with upper GI bleeding. A meta-analysis that included eight randomized trials of tranexamic acid in patients with upper GI bleeding found a benefit with regard to mortality but not with regard to bleeding, surgery, or transfusion requirements.

Uncontrolled or repeat bleeding

Endoscopy should be repeated to assess the bleeding site and to treat, if possible. Embolization by an interventional radiologist may

haemodilution has not taken place. In most patients, the bleeding stops, albeit temporarily, so that further assessment can be made.

Endoscopy

Endoscopy will usually diagnose, stratify risk and enable therapy to be performed if needed. Endoscopy should be carried out as soon as possible after the patient has been resuscitated. Patients with Rockall scores of 0 or 1 pre-endoscopy may be candidates for immediate discharge (see below) and outpatient endoscopy the following day, depending on local policy.

  Endoscopy can detect the cause of the haemorrhage in 80% or more of cases. In patients with a peptic ulcer, if the stigmata of a recent bleed are seen (i.e. a spurting vessel, active oozing, fresh or organized blood clot or black spots), the patient is more likely to rebleed. Calculation of the post-endoscopy Rockall score gives

be necessary if the bleeding persists. If this is not available locally or is unsuccessful, surgery is used to control the haemorrhage primarily.

Discharge policy

The patient's age, diagnosis on endoscopy, co-morbidity, the presence or absence of shock and the availability of support in the community should be taken into consideration. In general, all patients who are haemodynamically stable and have no stigmata of recent haemorrhage on endoscopy (Rockall score pre-endoscopy 0, post-endoscopy <1) can be discharged from hospital within 24 hours. All shocked patients and patients with co-morbidity need longer inpatient observation.

Specific conditions

Oesophageal varices

These are discussed on page 1294.

Mallory–Weiss tear

This is a linear mucosal tear occurring at the oesophagogastric junction and produced by a sudden increase in intra-abdominal pressure. It often follows a bout of coughing or retching, and is classically seen after alcoholic 'dry heaves'. There may, however, be no antecedent history of retching. Most bleeds are minor and discharge is usual within 24 hours. The haemorrhage may be large but most patients stop spontaneously. Early endoscopy confirms diagnosis and allows therapy such as clipping if necessary. Surgery with oversewing of the tear is rarely needed.

Chronic peptic ulcer

Eradication of *H. pylori* is started as soon as possible (see p. 1175). A PPI is continued for 4 weeks to ensure ulcer healing. Eradication of *H. pylori* should always be checked in a patient who has bled, and long-term acid suppression is given if *H. pylori* eradication cannot be achieved. If bleeding is not controlled, the patient should either undergo angiography and embolization or be referred directly for surgery.

Gastric carcinoma

Most of these patients do not have large bleeds but surgery is occasionally necessary for uncontrolled or repeat bleeding. Usually, surgery can be delayed until the patient has been fully evaluated (see p. 1178). Oozing from gastric cancer is very difficult to control endoscopically. Radiotherapy can occasionally be successful but its effects are not immediate.

Bleeding after percutaneous coronary intervention

In the era of ever more aggressive percutaneous coronary intervention (PCI), the list of antithrombotic medication grows longer: glycoprotein IIb/IIIa inhibitors, unfractionated heparin, low-molecular-weight heparin, fondaparinux and platelet inhibitors (e.g. clopidogrel, prasugrel and ticagrelor). Taken in addition to the oral anticoagulants that this group of patients are often taking, these give rise to a gastrointestinal bleeding rate of approximately 2% of patients undergoing PCI (who are on antiplatelet therapy, e.g. clopidogrel), and there is a high mortality of 5–10%. It has become increasingly evident in this patient group that gastroscopy should be performed on an urgent basis and not deferred for days or weeks. A bolus of intravenous PPI is administered, followed by an infusion; platelet infusion is given to counter the effect of clopidogrel. Management is difficult, as cessation of antiplatelet therapy has a high risk of acute stent thrombosis and also an associated high

> **Box 32.25 Take-home messages for upper gastrointestinal bleeding**
>
> - Endoscopy for unstable patients with severe upper gastrointestinal (GI) bleeding immediately after resuscitation
> - Offer endoscopy within 24 hours of admission to all other patients with upper GI bleeding
> - Interventional radiology (IR) to all patients who rebleed after endoscopy
> - Surgery if IR not available
> - Consider early transjugular intrahepatic portosystemic shunt (TIPS) in varices

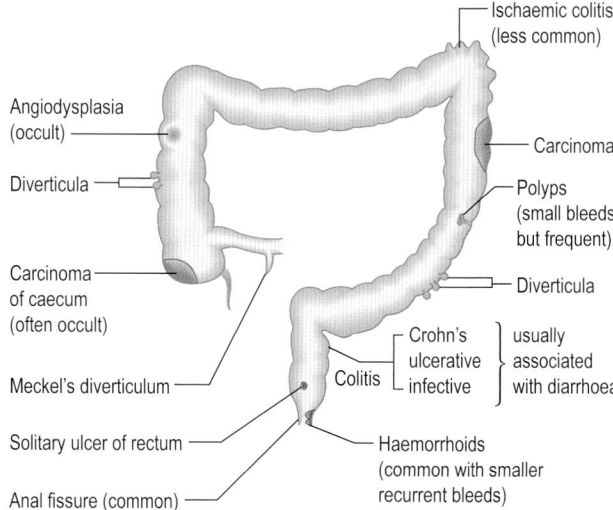

Fig. 32.31 Causes of lower gastrointestinal bleeding. The sites shown are illustrative – many of the lesions can be seen in other parts of the colon.

mortality. Using a risk assessment score (e.g. Blatchford), a reasonable approach is to stop all antiplatelet therapy in high-risk patients but continue it in low-risk ones. Co-prescribed proton pump inhibition does not decrease the antiplatelet effect of clopidogrel, as was first thought. These patients should be under the combined care of a cardiologist and a gastroenterologist.

See **Box 32.25** for take-home messages for the management of upper GI bleeding.

Prognosis

The mortality from gastrointestinal haemorrhage has not changed from 5–12% over the years, despite many changes in management, mainly because of a demographic shift to more elderly patients with co-morbidity. The lowest mortality rates are achieved in dedicated medical/surgical gastrointestinal units.

Acute lower gastrointestinal bleeding

Massive bleeding from the lower gastrointestinal tract is rare and is usually due to diverticular disease or ischaemic colitis. Common causes of small bleeds are haemorrhoids and anal fissures (**Fig. 32.31**).

Management

Most acute lower gastrointestinal bleeds start and stop spontaneously. The few patients who continue bleeding and are haemodynamically unstable need resuscitation using the same principles as for upper gastrointestinal bleeding (see p. 1181). Surgery is rarely required.

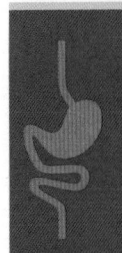

A diagnosis is made using the history and examination, including rectal examination and the following investigations as appropriate:

- **Proctoscopy** (e.g. anorectal disease, particularly haemorrhoids)
- **Flexible sigmoidoscopy or colonoscopy** (e.g. inflammatory bowel disease, cancer, ischaemic colitis, diverticular disease, angiodysplasia)
- **Video capsule endoscopy** (Fig. 32.32)
- **Angiography** to seek vascular abnormality (e.g. angiodysplasia). The yield of angiography is low, so it is a test of last resort.

Isolated episodes of rectal bleeding in the young (<45 years) usually only require rectal examination and flexible sigmoidoscopy because the probability of a significant proximal lesion is very low, unless there is a strong family history of colorectal cancer at a young age. Individual lesions are treated as appropriate.

Chronic gastrointestinal bleeding

Patients with chronic bleeding usually present with iron deficiency anaemia (see p. 330).

Chronic blood loss producing iron deficiency anaemia in men, and in women after the menopause, is always due to bleeding from the gastrointestinal tract. The primary concern is to exclude cancer, particularly of the stomach or right colon, and coeliac disease. Occult stool tests are unhelpful.

Diagnosis

Chronic blood loss can occur with any lesion of the gastrointestinal tract that produces acute bleeding (see **Figs 32.29** and **32.31**). However, oesophageal varices usually bleed overtly and rarely present as chronic blood loss. Although uncommon in developed countries, hookworm is the most common worldwide cause of chronic gastrointestinal blood loss.

History and examination may indicate the most likely site of the bleeding, but if no clue is available, it is usual to investigate both the upper and lower gastrointestinal tract endoscopically at the same session ('top and tail'), especially in males and postmenopausal females:

- **Upper gastrointestinal endoscopy** is usually performed first. Duodenal biopsies should always be taken to diagnose coeliac disease, even if coeliac serology has been performed.
- **Colonoscopy** follows and any lesion should be biopsied or removed, though it is unsafe to assume that colonic polyps are the cause of chronic blood loss.
- **Unprepared CT** scanning is a reasonable test to look for colon cancer in frail patients.
- **CT colonography** can be used as an alternative to colonoscopy.

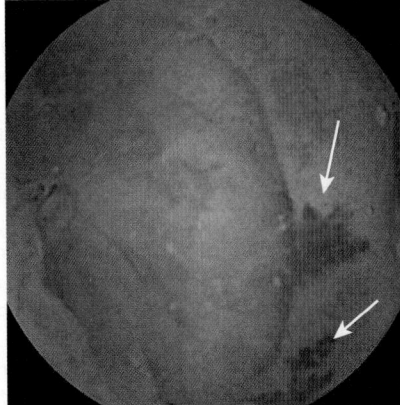

Fig. 32.32 Angiodysplastic lesions (arrows) seen on video capsule endoscopy.

If gastroscopy, colonoscopy and duodenal biopsy have not revealed the cause, investigation of the small bowel is necessary. **Capsule endoscopy** is the diagnostic investigation of choice but currently has no therapeutic ability. Positive diagnostic yield varies from 60% to 85%, depending on series. Bleeding lesions can be identified and later treated with balloon-assisted enteroscopy.

Occasionally, intravenous technetium-labelled colloid may be used to demonstrate a potential bleeding site in a Meckel's diverticulum.

Management

The cause of the bleeding should be dealt with, if found. Oral iron is given to treat anaemia (see p. 332), although intravenous infusions are occasionally required. Some patients will require maintenance with regular transfusion as a last resort.

Further reading

Bennett C, Klingenberg SL, Langholz E et al. Tranexamic acid for upper gastrointestinal bleeding. *Cochrane Database Syst* 2014; Issue 11. Art. No.: CD006640.
Blatchford O, Murray WR, Blatchford M. A risk score to predict need for treatment for upper-gastrointestinal haemorrhage. *Lancet* 2000; 356: 1318–1321.
Herbert FC, Carson JL. Transfusion threshold of 7 g per deciliter – the new normal. *N Engl J Med* 2014; 371:1459–1461.
Laine L. Timing of endoscopy in patients hospitalized with upper gastrointestinal bleeding. *N Engl J Med* 2020; 382:1361–1363.
Pennazio M, Spada C, Eliakim R et al. Small-bowel capsule endoscopy and device-assisted enteroscopy for diagnosis and treatment of small-bowel disorders: European Society of Gastrointestinal Endoscopy (ESGE) Clinical Guideline. *Endoscopy* 2015; 47:352–376.
https://www.bsg.org.uk/resource/bsge-acute-upper-gi-bleed-care-bundle.html. *British Society of Gastroenterology acute upper GI bleed care bundle*.

SMALL INTESTINE

Diarrhoea

The word 'diarrhoea' comes from the Greek meaning 'to flow through'. It is a very common manifestation of GI disease with many causes. There are many definitions but commonly it is accepted as being more than three loose stools in 24 hours.

Pathophysiology

Osmotic diarrhoea

The gut mucosa acts as a semipermeable membrane and fluid enters the bowel if there are large quantities of non-absorbed hypertonic substances in the lumen. This occurs because the patient:

- has ingested a non-absorbable substance (e.g. a purgative, such as magnesium sulphate or magnesium-containing antacid)
- has generalized malabsorption, so that high concentrations of solute (e.g. glucose) remain in the lumen
- has a specific absorptive defect (e.g. disaccharidase deficiency or glucose-galactose malabsorption).

The volume of diarrhoea produced by these mechanisms is reduced by the absorption of fluid by the ileum and colon. The diarrhoea stops when the patient stops eating or the malabsorptive substance is discontinued.

Secretory diarrhoea

In this disorder, there is both active intestinal secretion of fluid and electrolytes, and decreased absorption. The mechanism of intestinal secretion is shown in **Fig. 32.33A**.

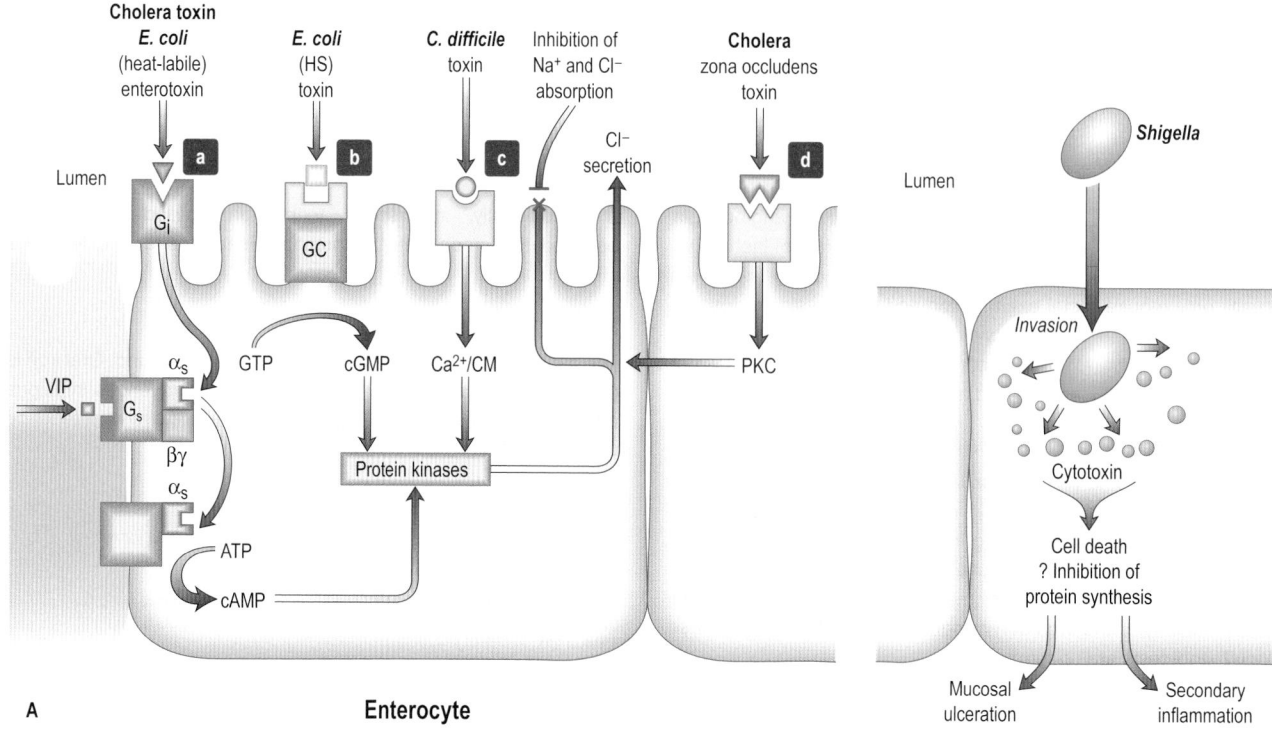

Fig. 32.33 Mechanisms of diarrhoea. **(A)** Small intestinal secretion of water and electrolytes. (a) *Cholera toxin* binds to its receptor (monosialoganglioside G_i) via fimbria (toxin co-regulated pili) on its β-subunit. This activates the $α_s$ subunit (of the G_s protein), which in turn dissociates and activates cyclic AMP (cAMP). The increase in cAMP activates intermediates (e.g. protein kinase and Ca^{2+}), which then act on the apical membrane, causing Cl^- secretion (with water) and inhibition of Na^+ and Cl^- absorption. *Heat-labile E. coli enterotoxin* shares a receptor with cholera toxin. (b) *Heat-stable (HS) E. coli toxin* binds to its own receptor and activates guanylate cyclase (cGMP), producing the same effect on secretion. (c) *Clostridium difficile* activates the protein kinases via Ca^{2+}/calmodulin (Ca^{2+}/CM). (d) *Zona occludens toxin* is the product of the *ZOT* gene, which loosens tight junctions and is required for function of the cholera toxin. It has enterotoxic activity, producing secretion. Cholera and *E. coli* cause these effects without invasion of the cell. **(B)** Colonic mucosal cell. This demonstrates one of the mechanisms by which an invasive pathogen (e.g. *Shigella*) acts. Following penetration, the pathogens generate cytotoxins, which leads to mucosal ulceration and cell death. ATP, adenosine triphosphate; G, G protein consisting of subunits α, β, γ; GC, guanyl cyclase; GMP, guanosine monophosphate; GTP, guanosine triphosphate; i, inhibitory; PKC, protein kinase C; s, stimulatory; VIP, vasoactive intestinal polypeptide.

Common causes of secretory diarrhoea are:

- enterotoxins (e.g. cholera, *E. coli* thermolabile or thermostable toxin, *C. difficile* toxin)
- hormones (e.g. vasoactive intestinal peptide in Verner–Morrison syndrome; see p. 1336)
- bile salts (in the colon) following ileal resection
- fatty acids (in the colon) following ileal resection
- some laxatives (e.g. docusate sodium).

Inflammatory diarrhoea (mucosal destruction)

Diarrhoea occurs because of damage to the intestinal mucosal cell so that there is a loss of fluid and blood (**Fig. 32.33B**). In addition, there is defective absorption of fluid and electrolytes. Causes are usually infective (e.g. dysentery due to *Shigella*) or inflammatory (IBD).

Abnormal motility

Diabetic, post-vagotomy and hyperthyroid diarrhoea are all due to abnormal motility of the upper gut. Symptoms may be exacerbated by small bowel bacterial overgrowth.

Acute diarrhoea

Acute diarrhoea is defined as lasting less than 14 days. The cause is usually infectious, most commonly viral in children but sometimes bacterial (usually more severe cases). Common infectious causes include:

- Viral infection, e.g. norovirus or rotavirus
- *E. coli* food poisoning (causes a secretory diarrhoea)
- Food poisoning from *Salmonella*, *Campylobacter* or *Staphylococcus* bacteria
- *Clostridium difficile* infection (usually due to recent course of antibiotics)
- Contaminated food or water ('traveller's diarrhoea'), often *Giardia* or *Entamoeba histolytica*.

Clinical features associated with acute diarrhoea include fever, abdominal pain and vomiting. Stools are usually loose and watery but can also be bloody. If the diarrhoea is severe then dehydration can occur, especially in very young or elderly patients.

The key investigation is to send a stool sample to try to isolate an organism. **Stool microscopy culture sensitivities (MCS)** should be sent in all patients. Samples for **C. difficile toxin** should be sent in at risk patients (elderly, nursing home residents, recent antibiotic

Box 32.26 Common antibiotic regimens for acute diarrhoea

Infection	Antibiotic
Empirical therapy	Ciprofloxacin p.o. 500 mg twice daily for 5 days
Salmonella/Shigella	Ciprofloxacin p.o. 500 mg twice daily for 5 days
Campylobacter	Clarithromycin p.o. 500 mg twice daily for 5 days
Clostridium difficile	Metronidazole p.o. 400 mg three times daily for 10–14 days OR Vancomycin p.o. 125–250 mg four times daily for 10–14 days

use). Stool for ova, cysts and parasites should be sent in the following cases:

- persistent diarrhoea (>14 days <30 days)
- men who have sex with men
- immunocompromised patients
- recent travel abroad
- if suspecting giardiasis/amoebiasis/cryptosporidium.

Management of acute diarrhoea usually focuses on volume repletion, usually with oral rehydration solutions that contain water, salt and sugar. In severe cases of dehydration, patients may need to be admitted to hospital for intravenous fluid resuscitation. Antibiotics are not usually empirically given unless it is a particularly severe case or complications develop (**Box 32.26** lists common antibiotic regimens). Antimotility agents (e.g. codeine phosphate or loperamide) should be avoided if possible.

Indications for antibiotic treatment include:

- severe/prolonged symptoms (>5 days)
- systemic signs of infection
- extremes of age
- immunocompromise
- presence of complications
- bloody or mucoid stools.

Chronic diarrhoea

This is defined as diarrhoea present for longer than 30 days. Causes are listed in **Box 32.27**.

A thorough history is important including the onset, timeframe and severity of symptoms. Important points to address are any associated features such as bloody stools, abdominal pain, weight loss, steatorrhoea, recent changes in medication, food/other triggers and a full past medical history. A full examination is needed.

Initial investigations should include:

- full blood count, serum creatinine and electrolytes, thyroid function
- coeliac screen (tissue transglutaminase (TTG) or endomysial antibodies (EMA) antibodies)
- faecal calprotectin (see p. 1158 for more information)
- stool MCS, *C. difficile* toxin.

If the above do not reveal a cause then patients should undergo a flexible sigmoidoscopy. In the following circumstances, however, patients should undergo a full colonoscopy:

- iron deficiency anaemia
- abnormal faecal calprotectin with a suspicion of IBD
- older patients where screening for polyps and colorectal cancer would be advantageous.

Further investigations include bowel imaging (CT abdomen, MRI small bowel, pancreatic CT), video capsule endoscopy, SeHCAT scan and lactose hydrogen breath tests; the choice will depend

Box 32.27 Causes of chronic diarrhoea

Common causes
- Irritable bowel syndrome
- Microscopic colitis
- Inflammatory bowel disease
- Colonic cancer
- Medications
- Diet
- Bile acid diarrhoea
- Pancreatic insufficiency
- Coeliac disease
- Overflow diarrhoea

Infrequent causes
- Radiation enteritis
- Lymphoma
- Diabetes

- Faecal incontinence
- Small bowel overgrowth
- Hyperthyroidism
- Small bowel resection
- Mesenteric ischaemia
- Chronic pancreatitis

Rare causes
- VIPoma
- Carcinoid
- Gastrinoma
- Whipple's disease
- Amyloidosis
- Tropical sprue
- Addison's disease

Box 32.28 Take-home messages for patients presenting with diarrhoea

	Acute diarrhoea	Chronic diarrhoea
Length	<14 days	>30 days
Common causes	Unknown Viral illness Bacterial if severe	Irritable bowel syndrome, inflammatory bowel disease, medications, overflow diarrhoea, diet, coeliac
Key investigations	Stool MCS OCP if risk factors	Coeliac screen Faecal calprotectin Flexible sigmoidoscopy Imaging
Management	Volume repletion Antibiotics only if severe/ complications	Treat cause

MCS, microscopy culture and sensitivities; OCP, ova, cysts and parasites.

on the individual patient's symptoms. Management of chronic diarrhoea involves treating the underlying cause and this will be discussed in more detail later. See **Box 32.28** for a summary of take-home messages for the patient.

Irritable bowel syndrome

Irritable bowel syndrome (IBS) is the most common functional gastrointestinal disorder. In Western populations, up to 1 in 5 people report symptoms consistent with IBS. Approximately 50% will consult their doctors and, of these, up to 30% will be referred by their doctor to a hospital specialist. Up to 40% of all patients seen in specialist gastroenterology clinics will have IBS. Estimates in the UK put the annual cost of IBS to healthcare resources as £45.6 million; in the USA, the cost is higher at $8 billion. In the UK, approximately one-quarter of IBS patients take time off work for periods ranging from 7 to 13 days each year.

The factors that determine whether an IBS sufferer in the community seeks medical advice include higher illness attitude scores and higher anxiety and depression scores than non-consulters. Consulters perceive that their symptoms are more severe than those of non-consulters, and consulting behaviour may be determined by the number of presenting symptoms. Female consulters outnumber male consulters by a factor of 2–3 to 1.

IBS – a multisystem disorder

IBS patients suffer from a number of non-intestinal symptoms (**Box 32.29**), which may be more intrusive than the classical features. IBS coexists with chronic fatigue syndrome (see p. 770), fibromyalgia (see p. 430) and temporomandibular joint dysfunction.

The biopsychosocial conceptualization of the pathogenesis and clinical expression of FGIDs is particularly relevant to IBS (see **Fig. 32.9**), and **Box 32.30** lists some common factors that have been shown to trigger IBS symptoms. Infectious diarrhoea precedes the onset of IBS symptoms in 7–30% of patients. Whether this is a factor for all patients or just a small subgroup remains controversial. Risk factors in these patients have been shown to include female sex, severity and duration of diarrhoea, pre-existing adverse life events and high hypochondriacal anxiety and neurotic scores at the time of the initial illness. Symptoms of anxiety and depression are more common in IBS patients, and stress or adverse life events often precede the onset of chronic bowel symptoms.

Diagnosis

Diagnostic criteria (Rome IV 2016) state that, in the preceding 3 months, there should be at least 1 day per week in the last 3 months of recurrent abdominal pain associated with two or more of the following:
1. Related to defecation.
2. Onset associated with a change in frequency of stool.
3. Onset associated with a change in form (appearance) of stool.

These are useful for comparative studies. Subgroups of IBS patients can be identified according to the criteria listed in **Box 32.31**.

The decision as to whether to investigate and the choice of investigations should be based on clinical judgement. Pointers to the need for thorough investigation are the presence of the above symptoms in association with rectal bleeding, nocturnal pain, fever and weight loss, and a clinical suspicion of organic diarrhoea. A raised stool calprotectin or lactoferrin would suggest inflammation needing further investigation.

Management

Current strategies for the treatment of IBS include therapies target central and end-organ pathways (**Box 32.32**); these are not mutually exclusive.

Patients with IBS are often worried that their symptoms are due to a serious disease such as cancer. Alarm symptoms much be investigated when present. However, a positive diagnosis of IBS with an explanation of the symptoms and reassurance is often helpful and may require no further investigation or treatment. It is helpful to establish and maintain a good clinician–patient relationship from the beginning. **Box 32.32** shows the overall management strategies used in IBS for those with severe and longstanding

Box 32.31 Subtyping irritable bowel syndrome by predominant stool pattern

Type	Description
IBS with constipation (IBS-C)	Hard lumpy stools >25% and loose (mushy) or watery stools <25% of bowel movements
IBS with diarrhoea (IBS-D)	Loose (mushy) or watery stools >25% and hard or lumpy stools <25% of bowel movements
Mixed IBS (IBS-M)	Hard or lumpy stools >25% and loose (mushy) or watery stools >25% of bowel movements
Unsubtyped IBS	Insufficient abnormality of stool consistency to meet criteria for IBS-C, D or M

Box 32.32 Approaches to the management of the irritable bowel syndrome

Treatment modality	Action
End-organ treatment	
Exploration of dietary triggers	Refer to dietician
High-fibre diet ± fibre supplements for constipation, low FODMAP diet for bloating	Refer to dietician
Alteration of microbiota	Rifaximin has shown short-term benefit in IBS patients without constipation (target I and II trials) Pro- and prebiotics
Anti-diarrhoeal drugs for bowel frequency	Loperamide Codeine phosphate Co-phenotrope ^aEluxadoline
Constipation	5-HT$_4$ receptor agonist, e.g. prucalopride
Smooth muscle relaxants for pain	Mebeverine hydrochloride Dicycloverine hydrochloride Peppermint oil
Central treatment	
Explanation of physiology and symptoms	At consultation (leaflets with diagrams help)
Psychotherapy	Refer to clinical psychologist (see p. 771)
Hypnotherapy	
Cognitive behavioural therapy	Refer to psychiatrist
Antidepressants	Functional diarrhoea – clomipramine Diarrhoea-predominant IBS – tricyclic group, e.g. amitriptyline Constipation-predominant IBS – SSRI, e.g. paroxetine

^aEluxadoline – a μ- and κ-opioid receptor agonist and δ-opioid receptor antagonist.
FODMAP, fermentable oligo-, di- and monosaccharides and polyols; SSRI, selective serotonin reuptake inhibitor.

Box 32.29 Non-gastrointestinal features of irritable bowel syndrome

Gynaecological symptoms
- Painful periods (dysmenorrhoea)
- Pain following sexual intercourse (dyspareunia)

Urinary symptoms
- Frequency
- Urgency
- Passing urine at night (nocturia)
- Incomplete emptying of bladder

Other symptoms
- Joint hypermobility
- Back pain
- Headaches
- Bad breath, unpleasant taste in the mouth
- Poor sleeping
- Fatigue

Box 32.30 Some factors that can trigger onset of irritable bowel symptoms

- Affective disorders, e.g. depression, anxiety
- Psychological stress and trauma
- Gastrointestinal infection
- Antibiotic therapy
- Sexual, physical or verbal abuse
- Pelvic surgery
- Eating disorders

problems. Lifestyle and dietary modifications should be the mainstay of management for patients with mild–moderate symptoms with pharmacologic therapy used adjunctively for those who fail to respond or who have more severe symptoms.

Pain/gas/bloat syndrome/midgut dysmotility

Disordered motility and visceral sensation that predominantly affects the small intestine or midgut results in symptoms of pain and bloating without altered defecation. Other symptoms include postprandial fullness, nausea and, on occasions, anorexia and weight loss.

Management of patients with pain/gas/bloat syndrome is not easy, and in some, pain can be chronic and severe. The main approaches are summarized below:

- Narcotics should always be avoided.
- Central and end-organ-targeted treatment approaches should be combined: for example, the SSRI paroxetine combined with a prokinetic agent, such as domperidone, or a smooth muscle relaxant, such as *mebeverine.*
- Small bowel bacterial overgrowth can be a contributory feature that can be treated with non-absorbed antibiotics such as *rifaximin,* however this is expensive and cheaper antibiotics such as doxycycline can also offer symptomatic benefit.
- Research has highlighted the benefit of altering the fermentable components of the diet. A diet with reduced fermentable oligo-, di- and monosaccharides and polyols (low *FODMAP*) will exclude a range of food types, including garlic, onions, specific beans, fructose-containing fruit, wheat-containing products, and certain natural and synthetic sweeteners. Small sham-diet-controlled clinical trials have shown significant benefit in patients with functional symptoms but long-term randomized controlled studies are necessary.
- The role of **probiotics** for management of IBS patients is not yet clear. A recent meta-analysis found some evidence for the efficacy of various probiotics in helping with symptoms such as pain, bloating and flatulence but with varying methodological limitations in most of the studies. Two studies found that *Bifidobacterium infantis* versus placebo led to symptomatic improvement in patients with IBS. It is likely that future work will focus on subgroups of patients, particularly those with diarrhoea-predominant IBS, and aim to correct the microbiome on an individual level according to the particular alterations of the compositional flora rather than give a generic probiotic.

Some patients with pain/gas/bloat syndrome have particularly severe and chronic symptoms, which may be nocturnal. A small subgroup of these has been shown to have manometric features consistent with a diagnosis of **chronic idiopathic intestinal pseudo-obstruction (CIIP)**, and specifically of an enteric neuropathy. Full-thickness small intestinal biopsies confirm this diagnosis by showing a deficiency of α actin staining in the inner circular layer of smooth muscle. More appropriately, these patients should be considered as having a gastrointestinal neuromuscular disorder of the gut. About 10% of these individuals are subsequently found to have an underlying autoimmune overlap disorder (see p. 463).

Management of patients with neuromuscular disorders of the gut requires a multidisciplinary approach, with an emphasis on the management of pain, psychological state and nutrition. Patients with underlying autoimmune rheumatic disorders may benefit from primary treatment of these. Patients with intestinal failure as a result of CIIP need long-term parenteral nutrition.

Functional diarrhoea

In this form of functional bowel disease, symptoms occur in the absence of abdominal pain. They commonly include:

- the passage of several stools in rapid succession, usually first thing in the morning; no further bowel action may occur that day, or defecation takes place only after meals
- a first stool of the day that is usually formed, the later ones being mushy, looser or watery
- urgency of defecation
- anxiety, and uncertainty about bowel function with restriction of movement (e.g. travelling)
- exhaustion after defecation.

Chronic diarrhoea without pain is caused by many diseases that are indistinguishable by history from functional diarrhoea. Features that are atypical of a functional disorder (e.g. large-volume stools, rectal bleeding, nutritional deficiency and weight loss) call for more extensive investigations.

Treatment of functional diarrhoea is with **loperamide**, often combined with a tricyclic antidepressant prescribed at night (e.g. clomipramine 10–30 mg).

Purgative abuse

This is most commonly seen in females who surreptitiously take high-dose purgatives and are often extensively investigated for chronic diarrhoea. The diarrhoea is usually of high volume (>1 L daily) and patients may have a low serum potassium. Biochemical analysis of the stool may help diagnose laxative abuse. Management is difficult, as most patients deny purgative ingestion. Purgative abuse often occurs in association with eating disorders and patients may need psychiatric help.

Malabsorption

In many small bowel diseases, malabsorption of specific substances occurs, but these deficiencies do not usually dominate the clinical picture. An example is Crohn's disease, in which malabsorption of vitamin B_{12} can be demonstrated, but this is not usually the major problem; diarrhoea and general ill-health are the major features.

The major disorders of the small intestine that cause malabsorption are shown in **Box 32.33**.

Coeliac disease (gluten-sensitive enteropathy)

Coeliac disease is an autoimmune condition in which there is inflammation of the mucosa of the upper small bowel that improves when gluten is withdrawn from the diet and relapses when gluten is reintroduced. Gluten is the entire protein content of the cereals wheat, barley and rye. Up to 1% of many populations are affected, though most have clinically silent disease.

? **Box 32.33** Disorders of the small intestine causing malabsorption

- Coeliac disease
- Dermatitis herpetiformis
- Tropical sprue
- Bacterial overgrowth
- Intestinal resection
- Whipple's disease
- Radiation enteropathy
- Parasite infestation (e.g. *Giardia intestinalis*)

Aetiology

The aetiology of coeliac disease is multifactorial with both genetic and environmental factors needed for the disease to manifest. Prolamins (gliadin from wheat, hordeins from barley, secalins from rye) are the damaging factors in these patients. These proteins are resistant to digestion by pepsin and chymotrypsin because of their high glutamine and proline content, and remain in the intestinal lumen, triggering the immune responses that result in coeliac disease. Gliadin peptides pass through the epithelium (para- and/or intracellularly) and are deaminated by tissue transglutaminase, which increases their immunogenicity. Gliadin peptides then bind to antigen-presenting cells, which interact with CD4+ T cells in the lamina propria via HLA class II molecules DQ2 or DQ8. These T cells produce pro-inflammatory cytokines, particularly interferon-γ. CD4+ T cells also interact with B cells to produce endomysial and tissue transglutaminase antibodies. Gliadin peptides also cause release of IL-15 from enterocytes, activating intraepithelial lymphocytes with a natural killer cell marker. This inflammatory cascade releases metalloproteinases and other mediators, which contribute to the villous atrophy and crypt hyperplasia that are typical of the disease.

The mucosa of the proximal small bowel is predominantly affected, the mucosal damage decreasing in severity towards the ileum as gluten is digested into smaller 'non-toxic' fragments.

Genetic factors

There is an increased incidence of coeliac disease within families but the exact mode of inheritance is unknown; 10–15% of first-degree relatives will have the condition, although it may be asymptomatic. The concordance rate in identical twins is about 70%.

HLA-DQ2 (DQAI*0501, DQBI*0201) and HLA-DQ8 (DQAI*0301, DQBI*0302) are associated with coeliac disease. Over 90% of patients will have HLA-DQ2, compared with 20–30% of the general population. Studies in twins and siblings indicate that HLA genes are responsible for less than 50% of the genetic cause of the disease. Many unaffected people also carry these genes, so other factors must also be involved. Non-HLA genes may also contribute to coeliac disease: for example, chromosome regions 19p13.1, 11q, 5q31–33 and 6q21–22. The *CD28/CTLA4/ILO5* gene cluster has also shown linkage with coeliac disease.

Environmental factors

Breast-feeding and the age of introduction of gluten into the diet are significant. Rotavirus infection in infancy also increases the risk; adenovirus-12, which has sequence homology with α-gliadin, was suspected as a causative agent but this is now thought to be unlikely.

Clinical features

Coeliac disease can present at any age. In infancy, it sometimes appears after weaning on to gluten-containing foods. The peak period for diagnosis in adults is in the fifth decade, with a female preponderance. Many patients are asymptomatic (silent) and come to attention because of routine blood tests: for example, a raised MCV, or iron deficiency in pregnancy. The symptoms are very variable and often non-specific; they include tiredness and malaise, often associated with anaemia.

Gastrointestinal symptoms may be absent or mild. Coeliac disease should be tested for in all patients with symptoms suggestive of irritable bowel syndrome. Diarrhoea or steatorrhoea, abdominal pain and weight loss suggest more severe disease. Mouth ulcers and angular stomatitis are frequent and can be intermittent. Infertility and neuropsychiatric symptoms of anxiety and depression can occur.

Rare complications include tetany, osteomalacia or gross malnutrition with peripheral oedema. Long-term problems include osteoporosis, which occurs even in patients on long-term gluten-free diets. Neurological symptoms, such as paraesthesia, ataxia (due to cerebellar calcification), muscle weakness or a polyneuropathy occur; the prognosis for these symptoms is variable. There is an increased incidence of atopy and autoimmune disease, including thyroid disease, type 1 diabetes and Sjögren's syndrome. Other associated diseases include:

- inflammatory bowel disease
- primary biliary cholangitis
- chronic liver disease
- interstitial lung disease
- epilepsy
- IgA deficiency is more common than in the general population.
  Physical signs are usually few and non-specific, and are related to anaemia and malnutrition.

Diagnosis

Small bowel biopsy is still considered to be the 'gold standard' for positive diagnosis and is therefore desirable in all but the most clear-cut cases, because treatment involves a life-long diet that is both expensive and socially limiting. However, with the increasing accuracy of serological tests, it is no longer necessary to take duodenal biopsies for suspected coeliac disease in patients without antibodies. For example, in patients undergoing endoscopy for iron deficiency anaemia with negative coeliac serology, the pretest value of small bowel histology is less than 0.03%.

If biopsies are to be taken, 4–6 forceps biopsies should be taken from the second part of the duodenum and the bulb because the disease is sometimes patchy and it can be difficult to orientate endoscopic biopsies for histological section. Endoscopic signs, including absence of mucosal folds, mosaic pattern of the surface and scalloping of mucosal folds, are often present; however, their absence is not conclusive because they are markers of relatively severe disease. Patients must be consuming gluten at the time of the endoscopy for the test to be diagnostic.

Histology

Histological changes are of variable severity and are graded using the Marsh–Oberhuber classification (**Box 32.34**) with types 2 and 3 being diagnostically supportive of coeliac disease. Villous atrophy can be caused by other conditions (e.g. tropical sprue, common variable immunodeficiency, non-coeliac enteropathy), but coeliac disease is the most common cause of subtotal villous atrophy.

Serology

Indications for testing include fatigue, persistent diarrhoea, folate or iron deficiency, unexplained abnormal liver biochemistry, a family history of coeliac disease and associated autoimmune disease.

> ### Box 32.34 Marsh–Oberhuber classification for histological changes in coeliac disease
>
> | Marsh grade | Histological appearance |
> | --- | --- |
> | 0 | Normal mucosa |
> | 1 | Increased intraepithelial lymphocytes |
> | 2 | Crypt hyperplasia |
> | 3a | Partial villous atrophy |
> | 3b | Subtotal villous atrophy |
> | 3c | Total villous atrophy |
> | 4 | Hypoplasia of small bowel architecture |

The most sensitive tests are for endomysial (EMA) and tissue transglutaminase (tTG) antibodies (95% sensitivity). Titres of either of these correlate with the severity of mucosal damage and so they can be used for dietary monitoring. Standard tests use IgA class antibodies. Selective IgA deficiency occurs in 2.5% of coeliac disease patients but only 0.25% of normals. In a few cases, this may render these tests falsely negative. In situations in which CD is strongly suspected in a patient negative for EMA antibodies, IgA levels should be measured; if low, IgG-based tests should then be used (e.g. deaminated gliadin peptide (DGP) antibody).

HLA typing

HLA-DQ2 is present in 90–95% of coeliac disease patients and HLA-DQ8 in about 8% – most of the rest. The *absence* of both alleles has a high negative predictive value for coeliac disease. HLA typing can be useful for risk assessment: for example, in patients already on a gluten-free diet, in whom serology would be negative.

Other investigations

- *Haematology.* Mild or moderate anaemia is present in 50% of cases. Folate deficiency is common, often causing macrocytosis. Vitamin B_{12} deficiency is rare. Iron deficiency, due to malabsorption of iron and increased loss of desquamated cells, is common. A blood film may therefore show microcytes and macrocytes (i.e. a dimorphic picture), as well as hypersegmented polymorphonuclear leucocytes and Howell–Jolly bodies (see p. 356) due to splenic atrophy.
- *Biochemistry.* In *severe cases*, biochemical evidence of osteomalacia may be seen (low calcium and high phosphate) and there is hypoalbuminaemia.
- *Imaging.* A small bowel barium follow-through or MRI enteroclysis may show dilation of the small bowel with slow transit. Folds become thicker, and in severe disease, total effacement is seen. Imaging is mainly used when a complication, such as lymphoma, is suspected.
- *Bone densitometry.* Dual energy X-ray absorptiometry (DXA) should be performed on all patients because of the risk of osteoporosis.
- *Capsule endoscopy* (see p. 1158). This is used to look for gut abnormalities when a complication is suspected.

Management

Replacement minerals and vitamins, such as iron, folic acid, calcium and vitamin D, may be needed initially to replace body stores.

Management is with a gluten-free diet for life. Dietary elimination of wheat, barley and rye usually produces a clinical improvement within days or weeks. Morphological improvement often takes months, especially in adults. Oats are tolerated by most people with CD but must not be contaminated with flour during their production. Meat, dairy products, fruits and vegetables are naturally gluten-free and are all safe.

Gluten-free products can be expensive, unless subsidized by national health services; however, this is slowly improving as gluten-free diets are becoming more popular amongst the general population in the industrialized world. Patient support organizations, such as the Coeliac Society (UK), are valuable as information sources and for advice about diet, recipes and gluten-free processed foods. Referral to a dietician for help with what to eat can be very beneficial for some patients. Despite advice, many patients do not keep to a strict diet but maintain good health. The long-term effects of this low gluten intake are uncertain but osteoporosis can occur, even in treated cases.

The usual cause of *failure to respond* to the diet is poor compliance. Dietary adherence can be monitored by serial tests for EMA and tTG. If clinical progress is suboptimal, then a repeat intestinal biopsy should be taken. If the diagnosis is equivocal on the diagnostic mucosal biopsy, or if the patient has already started on a gluten-free diet, then a gluten challenge, i.e. re-introduction of oral gluten, with evidence of jejunal morphological change, can confirm the diagnosis.

Patients should have *pneumococcal vaccinations* (because of splenic atrophy) once every 5 years (see p. 357).

Complications

A few patients do not improve on a strict diet and are said to have *non-responsive coeliac disease*. Many of these patients are still ingesting gluten. A few of the others may have concomitant problems, such as microscopic colitis, inflammatory bowel disease, small bowel bacterial overgrowth or lactase deficiency.

A very small percentage will have the rare complication of *refractory coeliac disease* (RCD):

- Type 1 RCD – the lymphocytes are normal and the T-cell receptors are polyclonal; 5-year survival is 93%.
- Type 2 – there are abnormal clonal lymphocytes with loss of CD8 and CD3 surface markers. The 5-year survival rate is 40–60%.

Very rarely, enteropathy-associated *T-cell lymphoma (EATCL)* (8–20% 5-year survival) or ulcerative jejunitis can occur as part of a spectrum of neoplastic T-cell disorders.

Ulcerative jejunitis presents with fever, abdominal pain, perforation and bleeding.

Diagnosis of these conditions is with MRI or barium studies, but laparoscopy with full-thickness small bowel biopsies is often required. Steroids and immunosuppressive agents, such as azathioprine, are used in ulcerative jejunitis.

The incidence of *carcinoma of the oesophagus and small bowel adenocarcinoma*, as well as that of extragastrointestinal cancers, is also increased. Malignancy seems to be unrelated to the duration of the disease but the incidence is reduced by a gluten-free diet.

Dermatitis herpetiformis

This is an uncommon, blistering, subepidermal eruption of the skin associated with a gluten-sensitive enteropathy (see also p. 687). Rarely, gross malabsorption occurs, but usually the jejunal morphological abnormalities are not as severe as in coeliac disease. The inheritance and immunological abnormalities are the same as for coeliac disease. The skin condition responds to *dapsone* but a gluten-free diet improves both the enteropathy and the skin lesion, and is recommended for long-term benefit.

Non-coeliac gluten intolerance

There is a recognized group of patients who are sensitive to dietary wheat and gluten-containing foods but do not have coeliac disease, in so far as their coeliac serology is negative and duodenal biopsies are normal. These patients have a range of symptoms, including diarrhoea, bloating and abdominal pain, which improve on avoidance of gluten. The mechanism is not yet clear.

Tropical sprue

This condition presents with chronic diarrhoea and malabsorption, and occurs in residents of or visitors to tropical areas where the disease is endemic: most of Asia, some Caribbean islands, Puerto Rico and parts of South America. Epidemics occur, lasting up to 2 years; in some areas, repeated epidemics are seen at varying intervals of up to 10 years.

The term tropical sprue is reserved for severe malabsorption (of two or more substances) accompanied by diarrhoea and malnutrition. A mild degree of malabsorption, sometimes following an enteric infection, is quite common in the tropics; it is usually asymptomatic and is sometimes called tropical malabsorption.

Aetiology

The aetiology is unknown but is likely to be infective because the disease occurs in epidemics and patients improve on antibiotics. A number of agents have been suggested but none has been unequivocally shown to be responsible. Different agents could be involved in different parts of the world.

Clinical features

These vary in intensity and consist of diarrhoea, anorexia, abdominal distension and weight loss. The onset is sometimes acute and occurs either a few days or many years after being in the tropics. Epidemics can break out in villages, affecting thousands of people at the same time. The onset can also be insidious, with chronic diarrhoea and evidence of nutritional deficiency. The clinical features of tropical sprue vary in different parts of the world, particularly as different criteria are used for diagnosis.

Diagnosis

Acute infective causes of diarrhoea must be excluded (**Box 32.35**), particularly *Giardia*, which can produce a syndrome very similar to tropical sprue. Malabsorption should be demonstrated, particularly of fat and vitamin B_{12}. The jejunal mucosa is abnormal, showing some villous atrophy (partial villous atrophy). In most cases, the lesion is less severe than that found in coeliac disease, although it affects the whole of the small bowel. Mild mucosal changes can be seen in asymptomatic individuals in the tropics.

Management

Many patients improve when they leave the sprue area and take folic acid (5 mg daily). Most patients also require an antibiotic to ensure a complete recovery (usually tetracycline 1 g daily for up to 6 months).

Severely ill patients require resuscitation with fluids and electrolytes for dehydration, and nutritional deficiencies should be corrected. Vitamin B_{12} (1000 μg) is also given to all acute cases.

Prognosis

The prognosis is excellent. Mortality is usually associated with water and electrolyte depletion, particularly in epidemics.

Bacterial overgrowth

The gut contains many resident bacteria in the terminal ileum and colon. Anaerobic bacteria, e.g. *Bacteroides*, bifidobacteria, are 100–1000 times more abundant than aerobic bacterial (facultative anaerobes), such as *Escherichia, Enterobacter* and *Enterococcus*. This gut microflora has major functions, including metabolic ones, such as fermentation of non-digestible dietary residues into short-chain fatty acids as an energy source in the colon.

The microflora that influences epithelial cell proliferation is involved in the development and maintenance of the immune system and protects the gut mucosa from colonization by pathogenic bacteria. Bacteria also initiate vitamin K production.

The upper part of the small intestine is almost sterile, containing only a few organisms derived from the mouth. Gastric acid kills some ingested organisms and intestinal motility keeps bacterial counts in the jejunum low. The normal terminal ileum contains faecal-type organisms, mainly *Escherichia coli* and anaerobes, and the colon has abundant bacteria.

Bacterial overgrowth is normally found in association with a structural abnormality of the small intestine, such as a stricture or diverticulum, although it can occur occasionally in the elderly without such an abnormality. *E. coli* and/or *Bacteroides*, both in concentrations of greater than 10^6/mL, are found as part of a mixed flora. These bacteria are capable of deconjugating and dehydroxylating bile salts, so that unconjugated and dehydroxylated bile salts can be detected in small bowel aspirates.

Clinical features

The clinical features of overgrowth are chiefly diarrhoea and steatorrhoea. There may also be symptoms caused by the underlying small bowel pathology. Steatorrhoea (see p. 1154) occurs because of conjugated bile salt deficiency. Some bacteria can metabolize vitamin B_{12} and interfere with its binding to intrinsic factor, leading to mild B_{12} deficiency (see p. 334); it is rarely severe enough to produce a neurological deficit. Some bacteria produce folic acid, giving a high serum folate. Bacterial overgrowth has only minimal effects on the absorption of other substances. Confirmation of bacterial overgrowth is with the hydrogen breath test:

- ***Hydrogen breath test.*** Bacteria are present in the oral cavity so the mouth should be rinsed out with an antiseptic mouthwash beforehand. The appearance of a breath hydrogen peak after ***oral glucose*** is used to estimate mouth-to-caecum transit time. An earlier rise in the breath hydrogen after glucose indicates bacterial breakdown in the small intestine.

? Box 32.35 Causes of diarrhoea

Non-infective causes
- Inflammatory bowel disease
- Radiation proctitis or colitis
- Behçet's disease
- Diverticular disease
- Ischaemic colitis
- Gastrointestinal lymphoma
- Carcinoma of the colon (change in bowel habit)
- Malabsorption
- Gut resection
- Bile acid malabsorption
- Drugs – many, including:
  - Laxatives
  - Metformin
  - Anti-cancer drugs
  - Statins
  - Proton pump inhibitors
- Faecal impaction with overflow
- Irritable bowel syndrome and functional diarrhoea
- Endocrine causes:
  - Zollinger–Ellison syndrome
  - VIPoma
  - Somatostatinoma
  - Glucagonoma
  - Carcinoid syndrome
  - Thyrotoxicosis
  - Medullary carcinoma of thyroid
  - Diabetic autonomic neuropathy

- Factitious diarrhoea:
  - Purgative abuse
  - Dilutional diarrhoea

Infective causes
- Bacterial, e.g.
  - *Campylobacter jejuni*
  - *Salmonella* spp.
  - *Shigella*
  - *Escherichia coli* (see p. 541)
  - Staphylococcal enterocolitis
  - *Bacillus cereus*
  - *Clostridium perfringens, C. botulinum, C. difficile*
  - Gastrointestinal tuberculosis
- Viral, e.g.
  - Rotavirus
- Fungal, e.g.
  - Histoplasmosis
- Parasitic, e.g.
  - Amoebic dysentery (*Entamoeba histolytica*)
  - Schistosomiasis
  - *Giardia intestinalis*

This test is simple to perform and does not involve radioisotopes. However, interpretation is often difficult, and sensitivity and specificity are low.

Management

If possible, the underlying lesion should be corrected (e.g. a stricture should be resected). Where this is not possible, rotating courses of antibiotics are necessary, such as metronidazole, a tetracycline or ciprofloxacin. The response to antibiotics is unpredictable.

Bile acid malabsorption

Bile is released from the gall bladder after eating and is essential for fat digestion. In a healthy gut, most of the bile is reabsorbed in the small intestine and recycled (enterohepatic bile acid circulation). However, this reabsorption is interrupted in some patients leading to more bile passing through into the colon. The increased concentration of bile acids in the colon leads to diarrhoea by reducing absorption of water and electrolytes as well as increasing secretion and colonic motility. Causes include:

- Crohn's disease with ileal disease
- ileal resection
- HIV infection
- idiopathic/primary bile acid diarrhoea
- post-infective gastroenteritis
- post-cholecystectomy.

Diagnosis is made by either a trial of medication or with a SeHCAT scan. This is carried out by giving oral **SeHCAT** (a synthetic taurine conjugate) and measuring the retention of the bile acid by whole-body counting at 7 days. Patients are managed by giving bile acid sequestrants such as cholestyramine or colesevelam. These bind and inactivate the action of bile acids in the colon.

Lactose intolerance

This is a clinical syndrome where ingestion of lactose causes symptoms such as diarrhoea, abdominal pain, bloating and flatulence. This is occasionally due to lactase deficiency but can also be due to secondary lactose malabsorption (usually due to underlying intestinal disease). There is a high incidence of lactase deficiency in many parts of the world (e.g. the Mediterranean countries and parts of Africa and Asia). There can be variability in symptoms amongst patients and a crossover with IBS symptoms. Formal diagnostic testing involves giving an oral dose of 50 g of lactose and serial measurement of blood glucose over 2 hours.

Small intestinal resection

Small intestinal resection is usually well tolerated, but massive resection leaving less than 1 m of small bowel in continuity is followed by the **short bowel syndrome**. The effects of resection depend on the amount and location of the resection and the presence or absence of the colon. Resection of the jejunum is better tolerated than ileal resection, where there is less adaptation, probably due to low levels of glucagon-like peptide 2 (GLP-2), which is a specific growth hormone for the enterocyte. Patients with an anatomically short small bowel after surgical resection should have close follow-up to ensure they do not become depleted of electrolytes or develop malnutrition. Management will depend on investigations, but might include the use of loperamide and codeine to reduce small intestinal transit time, high-dose PPI therapy to reduce gastric secretion, oral rehydration solution and, where necessary, parenteral electrolyte and calorie replacement.

Ileal resection

The ileum is the site of specific mechanisms for the absorption of bile salts and vitamin B_{12}. Relatively small resections lead to malabsorption of these substances. Loss of the ileal brake (see p. 1154) leads to diarrhoea. Removal of the ileocaecal valve increases the incidence of diarrhoea (**Fig. 32.34**).

The following occur after ileal resection:

- **Bile-salt-induced diarrhoea.** Bile salts and fatty acids enter the colon and cause malabsorption of water and electrolytes (see p. 1185).
- **Steatorrhoea and gallstone formation.** Increased bile salt synthesis can compensate for loss of approximately one-third of the bile salts in the faeces. Greater loss than this results in decreased micelle formation and steatorrhoea, and lithogenic bile and gallstone formation.
- **Oxaluria and oxalate stones.** Bile salts in the colon cause increased oxalate absorption with oxaluria, leading to urinary stone formation.
- **B_{12} deficiency.** Low serum B_{12}, macrocytosis and other effects of B_{12} deficiency are seen.

Investigations

These include imaging of the small bowel measurement of B_{12}, and a bile salt retention (SeHCAT) test (see above). A hydrogen breath test may show rapid transit (p. 1192). Many patients require B_{12} replacement and some need a low-fat diet if there is steatorrhoea. Diarrhoea is often improved by colestyramine, which binds bile salts and reduces the level of diarrhoeogenic bile salts in the colon.

Jejunal resection

The ileum can compensate for loss of jejunal absorptive function. Jejunal resection may lead to gastric hypersecretion with high gastrin levels; the exact mechanism is unclear. Structural and functional

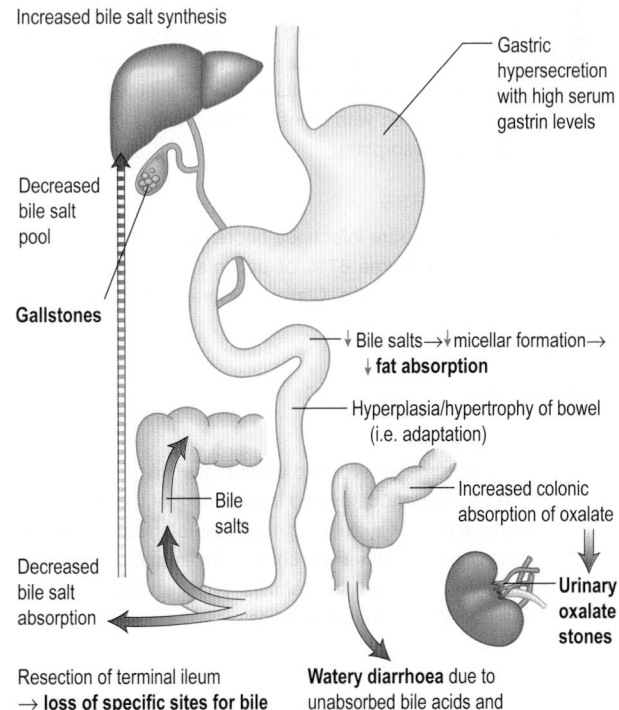

Increased bile salt synthesis

Gastric hypersecretion with high serum gastrin levels

Decreased bile salt pool

Gallstones

↓ Bile salts → ↓ micellar formation → ↓ **fat absorption**

Hyperplasia/hypertrophy of bowel (i.e. adaptation)

Bile salts

Increased colonic absorption of oxalate

Decreased bile salt absorption

Urinary oxalate stones

Resection of terminal ileum → **loss of specific sites for bile salt and B_{12} absorption**

Watery diarrhoea due to unabsorbed bile acids and hydroxy fatty acids

Fig. 32.34 The effects of resecting the distal small bowel.

intestinal adaptation takes place over the course of a year, with an increase in the absorption per unit length of bowel in both jejunum and ileum.

Massive intestinal resection (short bowel syndrome)

Intestinal failure results from obstruction, dysmotility, surgical resection, congenital defect, or disease-associated loss of absorption. It is characterized by the inability to maintain protein-energy, fluid, electrolyte or micronutrient balance. This most often occurs following resection for Crohn's disease, mesenteric vessel occlusion (see p. 1196), radiation enteritis (see later) or trauma. There are two common situations.

Shortened small intestine ending at a terminal small bowel stoma

The major problem is sodium and fluid depletion; the majority of patients with 100 cm or less of jejunum remaining will require parenteral supplements of fluid and electrolytes, often with nutrients. Sodium losses can be minimized by increasing salt intake, restricting hypotonic fluids between meals, and administering oral glucose–electrolyte mixture with a sodium concentration of 90 mmol/L. Jejunal transit time can be increased and stomal effluent loss reduced by treatment with the somatostatin analogue octreotide, often used in combination with a PPI, loperamide and codeine phosphate. There is no benefit from a low-fat diet, but fat assimilation can be increased on treatment with colestyramine and synthetic bile acids.

Teduglutide, a GLP-2 analogue, reduces stomal output and the number of days of parenteral nutrition.

Shortened small intestine in continuity with colon

Because of the absorptive capacity of the colon for fluid and electrolytes, only a small proportion of these patients require parenteral supplementation. Unabsorbed fat results in impairment of colonic fluid and electrolyte absorption, and so patients should be on a low-fat diet. A high carbohydrate intake is advised, as unabsorbed carbohydrate is metabolized anaerobically to short-chain fatty acids (SCFAs), which are absorbed; they also stimulate fluid and electrolyte absorption in the colon and act as an energy source (1.6 kcal/g). Patients are often treated with colestyramine to reduce diarrhoea and colonic oxalate absorption.

Whipple's disease

Whipple's disease is a rare infectious bacterial disease caused by *Tropheryma whipplei*. Some 87% of patients are males, and are usually white and middle-aged. Clinical features can progress over many years and can include:
- arthritis and arthralgia
- weight loss
- diarrhoea or steatorrhoea
- abdominal pain
- systemic symptoms of fever and weight loss
- peripheral lymphadenopathy and involvement of the heart, lung, joints and brain occur, simulating many neurological conditions.

Blood tests show features of chronic inflammation and malabsorption. Endoscopy typically shows pale, shaggy duodenal mucosa with eroded, red, friable patches.

Diagnosis

Diagnosis is made by small bowel biopsy. Periodic acid–Schiff (PAS)-positive macrophages are present but are non-specific. On electron microscopy, the characteristic trilaminar cell wall of *T.*

whipplei can be seen within macrophages. *T. whipplei* antibodies can be identified by immunohistochemistry. A confirmatory polymerase chain reaction (PCR)-based assay is available.

Management

Treatment is with antibiotics that cross the blood–brain barrier, such as 160 mg trimethoprim and 800 mg sulfamethoxazole (cotrimoxazole) daily for 1 year. This is preceded by a 2-week course of streptomycin and penicillin or ceftriaxone. Treatment periods of less than 1 year are associated with relapse in about 40%. If left untreated, it can be fatal.

Radiation enteritis

Radiation of more than 40 Gy will damage the intestine. The chronic effects of radiation are muscle fibre atrophy, ulcerative changes due to ischaemia, and obstruction due to radiation-induced fibrotic strictures.

Pelvic irradiation is frequently used for gynaecological and urinary tract malignancies, and so the ileum and rectum are the areas most often involved.

At the time of the irradiation, there may be nausea, vomiting, diarrhoea and abdominal pain, usually improving within 6 weeks of completion of therapy.

Chronic radiation enteritis is diagnosed if symptoms persist for 3 months or more. The prevalence is higher than 15% of patients receiving radiotherapy that includes the abdomen. Abdominal pain due to obstruction is the main symptom. Malabsorption can be due to bacterial overgrowth in dilated segments and mucosal damage. Many patients suffer from increased bowel frequency. **Management** is symptomatic, although often unsuccessful in chronic radiation enteritis. Surgery should be avoided if possible, being reserved for obstruction or perforation. Hyperbaric oxygen has been shown to be beneficial but this is not available in many centres.

Acute radiation damage to the rectum produces a **radiation proctitis** with diarrhoea and tenesmus, with or without blood. Local steroids sometimes help initially. When the acute phase heals, mucosal telangiectases form and may cause persistent bleeding. If there is resistant anaemia, these can be treated with argon plasma coagulation or, under a light anaesthetic, by packing the rectum with a formalin-soaked swab for 2 minutes, both of which destroy the telangiectases.

Parasite infestation

- **Giardia intestinalis** (see p. 572) not only produces diarrhoea but also can produce malabsorption with steatorrhoea. Minor changes are seen in the jejunal mucosa and the organism can be found in the jejunal fluid or mucosa.
- **Cryptosporidiosis** (see p. 573) can also produce malabsorption.
- **HIV infection** causes patients to be particularly prone to parasitic infestation (**Box 32.36**).

Other causes of malabsorption

- **Drugs that bind bile salts** (e.g. colestyramine) and some antibiotics (e.g. neomycin) produce steatorrhoea.
- **Orlistat** is used in obesity to reduce fat absorption by inhibiting gastric and pancreatic lipase, so causing diarrhoea and steatorrhoea. A low-fat diet is also necessary, which leads to weight loss.
- **Thyrotoxicosis** causes diarrhoea, rarely with steatorrhoea, owing to increased gastric emptying and increased motility.
- **Zollinger–Ellison syndrome** is described on page 1336.
- **Intestinal lymphangiectasia** produces diarrhoea and, rarely, steatorrhoea.

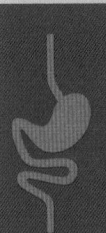

Box 32.36 Gastrointestinal problems in patients with AIDS

Symptoms	Causes
Mouth/oesophagus	
Dysphagia	Herpes simplex virus (HSV)
Retrosternal discomfort	Cytomegalovirus (CMV)
Oral ulceration	Candidiasis
Small bowel/colon	
Chronic diarrhoea Steatorrhoea Weight loss	**Parasites:**
	Entamoeba histolytica
	Giardia intestinalis
	Blastocystis hominis
	Isospora belli
	Microsporidia
	Cyclospora cayetanensis
	Viruses:
	Cytomegalovirus, herpes simplex virus, adenovirus
	Bacteria:
	Salmonella
	Campylobacter
	Shigella
	Mycobacterium avium-intracellulare
	Non-infective enteropathy – cause unknown
Rectum/colon	
Bloody diarrhoea	Bacterial infection (e.g. *Shigella*)
Any site	
Weight loss Diarrhoea	**Neoplasia:**
	Kaposi's sarcoma
	Lymphoma
	Squamous carcinoma
	Infection – disseminated, e.g.
	Mycobacterium avium-intracellulare
	Anti-retroviral therapy (ART)

- *Lymphoma* that has infiltrated the small bowel mucosa causes malabsorption.
- *Diabetes mellitus* (see p. 732) causes diarrhoea, malabsorption and steatorrhoea, sometimes due to bacterial overgrowth from autonomic neuropathy that leads to small bowel stasis.
- *Hypogammaglobulinaemia*, which is seen in a number of conditions including lymphoid nodular hyperplasia, causes steatorrhoea due either to an abnormal jejunal mucosa or to secondary infestation with *Giardia intestinalis*.

Miscellaneous intestinal diseases

Protein-losing enteropathy

Protein-losing enteropathy refers to intestinal conditions that lead to protein loss, and usually manifest with hypoalbuminaemia. The causes include:

- Crohn's disease
- tumours
- Ménétrier's disease, a condition with giant rugal folds (**Fig. 32.35**)

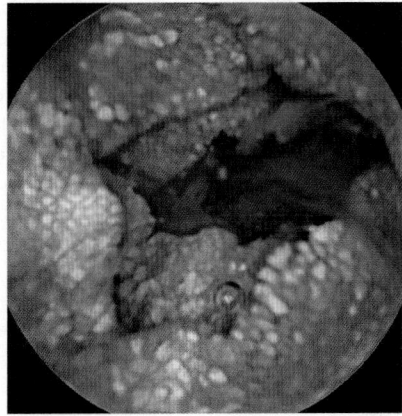

Fig. 32.35 Protein-losing enteropathy showing giant rugal folds.

- coeliac disease
- lymphatic disorders (e.g. lymphangiectasia).

Usually, protein-losing enteropathy forms a minor part of the generalized disorder but, occasionally, hepatic synthesis of albumin cannot compensate for the protein loss, and peripheral oedema dominates the clinical picture. Confirmation of the diagnosis is by measurement of α_1-antitrypsin clearance. It does not require an isotope. Alpha$_1$-antitrypsin is a large molecule (>50 000 daltons), which is resistant to proteolysis. Simultaneous measurements of serum and stool concentration (24-h collection) are made. The treatment is that of the underlying disorder.

Meckel's diverticulum

This is the most common congenital abnormality of the gastrointestinal tract, affecting 2–3% of the population. The diverticulum projects from the wall of the ileum approximately 60 cm from the ileocaecal valve. It is usually symptomless. However, 50% contain gastric mucosa that secretes hydrochloric acid, and peptic ulcers can occur and may bleed (see p. 1181) or perforate.

Acute inflammation of the diverticulum also occurs and is indistinguishable clinically from acute appendicitis. Rarely, there is obstruction from an associated band.

Management is surgical removal, often laparoscopically.

Tuberculosis

Tuberculosis (TB; see also p. 967) can affect the intestine, as well as the peritoneum (see p. 1223). In developed countries, most patients are from ethnic minority groups, or are immunocompromised because of HIV or drugs. Intestinal TB is due to reactivation of primary disease caused by *Mycobacterium tuberculosis*. Bovine TB occurs in areas where milk is unpasteurized and is rare in Western countries.

Clinical features

These are abdominal pain, weight loss, anaemia, fever with night sweats, obstruction, right iliac fossa pain or a palpable mass. The ileocaecal area is most commonly affected, but the colon – and, rarely, other parts of the gastrointestinal tract – can be involved. One-third of patients present acutely with intestinal obstruction or generalized peritonitis; 50% have X-ray evidence of pulmonary TB.

Diagnosis

Differential diagnosis includes Crohn's disease and caecal carcinoma.

- *Small bowel follow-through* may show transverse ulceration, and diffuse narrowing of the bowel with shortening of the caecal pole.

- *Ultrasound, MRI or CT* shows additional mesenteric thickening and lymph node enlargement.
- *Histology and culture of tissue* is desirable but not always possible. Specimens can be obtained by colonoscopy or laparoscopy but laparotomy is required in some cases. The histological findings include chronic inflammation with caseating granuloma. Acid-fast bacilli may be seen on dedicated stains. However, the histology is not always distinguishable from that of Crohn's disease.

Management

Drug treatment is similar to that for pulmonary TB (see p. 969). Treatment should be started if there is a high degree of suspicion.

Amyloidosis

Systemic amyloidosis may affect any part of the gastrointestinal tract (see p. 1357). Rectal biopsy may be diagnostic. Occasionally, amyloid deposits occur as polypoid lesions. The symptoms depend on the site of involvement; amyloidosis in the small intestine gives rise to diarrhoea.

Autoimmune rheumatic diseases

Systemic sclerosis (see p. 460) most commonly affects the oesophagus (see p. 992), although the small bowel and colon are often found to be involved if investigated. There may be no symptoms of this involvement, but diarrhoea and steatorrhoea can occur due to bacterial overgrowth caused by reduced motility, dilation and the presence of diverticula.

Intestinal ischaemia

Intestinal ischaemia results from occlusion of arterial inflow, occlusion of venous outflow or failure of perfusion; these factors may act alone or in combination and usually occur in the elderly.

- *Arterial inflow occlusion* can be caused by atheroma, thrombosis and embolism (cardiac arrhythmia), including cholesterol emboli (see p. 1372), aortic disease (occluding ostia of mesenteric vessels) or vasculitis (see p. 464), thromboangiitis and Takayasu's syndrome.
- *Venous outflow occlusion* occurs in 5–15% of cases, usually in sick patients with circulatory failure.
- *Infarction without occlusion* can occur due to reduced cardiac output, hypotension and shock, causing reduced intestinal blood flow.

Acute small intestinal ischaemia

An embolus from the heart in a patient with atrial fibrillation is the most common cause and usually occludes the superior mesenteric artery. Patients present with sudden abdominal pain and vomiting, with a distended and tender abdomen and absent bowel sounds. The patient is hypotensive and ill. Surgery is necessary to resect the gangrenous bowel. Mortality is high (up to 90%) and is related to coexisting disease, the development of multiorgan failure (MOF; see p. 219) and massive fluid and electrolyte losses in the postoperative period. Survivors may go on to develop nutritionally inadequate short bowel syndrome (see p. 1194).

Ischaemic colitis

See page 1211.

Chronic small intestinal ischaemia

This is due to atheromatous occlusion or cholesterol emboli of the mesenteric vessels, and is found particularly in the elderly. Good collateral circulation can minimize clinical effects. The characteristic symptom is postprandial abdominal pain and weight loss. Loud bruits may be heard but, as these are heard in normal subjects, they are of doubtful significance. The diagnosis is made using angiography.

Eosinophilic gastroenteritis

In this condition of unknown aetiology there is eosinophilic infiltration and oedema of any part of the gastrointestinal mucosa. The gastric antrum and proximal small intestine are usually involved, hosting either a localized lesion (eosinophilic granuloma) or diffuse sheets of eosinophils in the serosal and submucosal layers. There is an association with asthma, eczema and urticaria.

The condition occurs mainly in the third decade. The clinical presentation depends on the site of gut involvement. Abdominal pain, nausea and vomiting, and upper gastrointestinal bleeding occur. Peripheral eosinophilia is present in only 20% of patients. Endoscopic biopsy is useful for making the diagnosis histologically. Radiology may demonstrate mass lesions.

Treatment is with corticosteroids for the widespread infiltration, particularly if peripheral eosinophilia is present.

In some adults, the condition appears to be allergic (allergic gastroenteritis) and is associated with peripheral eosinophilia and high levels of plasma and tissue IgE. The relationship of eosinophilic oesophagitis (see p. 1170) to eosinophilic gastroenteritis is unclear.

Intestinal lymphangiectasia

Dilation of the lymphatics may be primary or secondary to lymphatic obstruction, such as occurs in malignancy or constrictive pericarditis. Hypoproteinaemia with ankle oedema is the main feature. The rare primary form may be detected incidentally as dilated lacteals on a jejunal biopsy or it can produce steatorrhoea of varying degrees. White-tipped villi are seen on capsule endoscopy. Serum immunoglobulin levels are reduced, with low circulating lymphocytes. Management is with a low-fat diet, mid-chain triglycerides and fat-soluble vitamin supplements as required. Octreotide has a dramatic effect in a few primary cases, although the mechanism of action is unknown.

Abetalipoproteinaemia

This rare congenital disorder is due to a failure of apo B-100 synthesis in the liver and apo B-48 in the intestinal cell, so that chylomicrons are not formed. This leads to fat accumulation in the intestinal cells, lending a characteristic histological appearance to the jejunal mucosa. Clinical features include acanthocytosis (spiky red cells owing to membrane abnormalities), a form of retinitis pigmentosa, and mental and neurological abnormalities. The latter can be prevented by vitamin E injections.

Tumours of the small intestine

The small intestine is relatively resistant to the development of neoplasia and only 3–6% of all gastrointestinal tumours and less than 1% of all malignant lesions occur here. The reason for the rarity of tumours is unknown. Explanations include the fluidity and relative sterility of small bowel contents and the rapid transit time, reducing the time of exposure to potential carcinogens. It is also possible that the high population of lymphoid tissue and secretion of IgA in the small intestine protect against malignancy.

Adenocarcinoma and lymphoma

Adenocarcinoma of the small intestine is rare and found most frequently in the duodenum (in the periampullary region) and in the jejunum. It is the most common tumour of the small intestine, accounting for up to 50% of primary tumours.

Lymphomas are most frequently found in the ileum. These are of the non-Hodgkin's type and must be distinguished from peripheral or nodal lymphomas involving the gut secondarily.

In developed countries, the most common type of lymphoma is the B cell type arising from MALT. These lymphomas tend to be annular or polypoid masses in the distal or terminal ileum, whereas most T cell lymphomas are ulcerated plaques or strictures in the proximal small bowel.

A tumour similar to Burkitt's lymphoma also occurs and commonly affects the terminal ileum of children in North Africa and the Middle East.

Predisposing factors for adenocarcinoma and lymphoma

Coeliac disease

There is an increased incidence of lymphoma of the T cell type and adenocarcinoma of the small bowel, as well as an unexplained increase in all malignancies, both in the gastrointestinal tract and elsewhere. The reason for the local development of malignancy is unknown. It is now accepted that coeliac disease is a pre-malignant condition but there is no association with the length of the symptoms. Management with a gluten-free diet can reduce the risk of both lymphoma and carcinoma.

Crohn's disease

There is a small increase in the incidence of adenocarcinoma of the small bowel in Crohn's disease.

Immunoproliferative small intestinal disease

Immunoproliferative small intestinal disease (IPSID) is a rare B cell disorder in which there is proliferation of plasma cells in the lamina propria of the upper small bowel, producing truncated monoclonal heavy chains, without associated light chains. The α heavy chains are found in the gut mucosa on immunofluorescence and can also be detected in the serum. IPSID usually occurs in countries surrounding the Mediterranean, but it has also been found in developing countries in South America and the Far East. It predominantly affects people in lower socioeconomic groups in areas with poor hygiene and a high incidence of bacterial and parasitic infection of the gut. IPSID presents as a malabsorptive syndrome associated with diffuse lymphoid infiltration of the small bowel and neighbouring lymph nodes, progressing in some cases to a lymphoma. The condition has also been documented in the developed world.

Clinically, patients present with abdominal pain, diarrhoea, anorexia, weight loss and symptoms of anaemia. There may be a palpable mass, and an ultrasound followed by an MRI scan may detect a mass lesion. Endoscopic biopsy is useful where lesions are within reach. Ultrasound and CT may show bowel wall thickening and the involvement of lymph nodes, which is common with lymphoma. Wireless capsule endoscopy can be used where obstruction by the capsule is not likely, but cannot deliver histology.

Management of small intestinal tumours

Adenocarcinoma

Most patients are treated surgically with a segmental resection. The overall 5-year survival rate is 20–35%; this varies with the histological grade and the presence or absence of lymph node involvement. Radiotherapy and chemotherapy are used in addition.

IPSID

If there is no evidence of lymphoma, antibiotics, such as tetracycline, should be tried initially. In the presence of lymphoma, combination chemotherapy is used; in one series, the 3–5-year survival rate was 58%.

Lymphoma

Most patients require surgery and radiotherapy with chemotherapy for more extensive disease. The prognosis varies with the type. The 5-year survival rate for T cell lymphomas is 25% but is better for B cell lymphomas, varying from 50% to 75%, depending on the grade of lymphoma.

Carcinoid tumours

These originate from the enterochromaffin cells (APUD cells) of the intestine. They make up 10% of all small bowel neoplasms, the most common sites being the appendix and terminal ileum. It is often difficult to be certain histologically whether a particular tumour is benign or malignant. A total of 10% of carcinoid tumours in the appendix present as acute appendicitis, secondary to obstruction. Surgical resection of the tumour is usually performed.

Most carcinoids do not secrete hormones or vasoactive compounds, and may present with liver enlargement due to metastases.

Carcinoid syndrome occurs in only 5% of patients with carcinoid tumours and only when there are liver metastases. Patients complain of spontaneous or induced bluish-red flushing, predominantly on the face and neck, sometimes leading to permanent changes with telangiectases.

Gastrointestinal symptoms consist of abdominal pain and recurrent watery diarrhoea. Cardiac abnormalities are found in 50% of patients and take the form of pulmonary stenosis or tricuspid incompetence. Examination of the abdomen reveals hepatomegaly. The tumours secrete a variety of biologically active amines and peptides, including serotonin (5-hydroxytryptamine, 5-HT), bradykinin, histamine, tachykinins and prostaglandins. The diarrhoea and cardiac complications are probably caused by 5-HT itself, but the cutaneous flushing is thought to be produced by one of the kinins, such as bradykinin. This is known to cause vasodilation, bronchospasm and increased intestinal motility.

Diagnosis of carcinoid syndrome

- *Ultrasound examination* confirms the presence of liver secondary deposits.
- *Urine* shows a high concentration of 5-hydroxyindoleacetic acid (5-HIAA), which is the major metabolite of 5-HT.
- *Serum chromogranin A* is raised in nearly all hindgut tumours and 80–90% of symptomatic foregut and midgut tumours.

Management of carcinoid syndrome

Treatment is with octreotide and lanreotide; both are octapeptide somatostatin analogues that inhibit the release of many gut hormones. They alleviate flushing and diarrhoea, and can control a carcinoid crisis. Interferon and other chemotherapeutic regimens also occasionally reduce tumour growth, but have not been shown to increase survival.

Most patients survive for 5–10 years after diagnosis.

Peutz–Jeghers syndrome

This consists of mucocutaneous pigmentation (circumoral in 95% of patients, and on the hands in 70% and feet in 60%) and gastrointestinal polyps. It has an autosomal dominant inheritance. The gene *STK11* (also known as *LKB1*) that is responsible for Peutz–Jeghers syndrome codes for a serine protein kinase and can be used for genetic analysis. The brown buccal pigment is characteristic of the condition. The polyps, which are hamartomas, can occur anywhere in the gastrointestinal tract but are most frequent in the small bowel. They may bleed or cause small bowel obstruction or intussusception (50% of patients).

Management

Management is by endoscopic polypectomy. Balloon enteroscopy may be necessary to reach all the small bowel polyps. Bowel resection should be avoided if possible, but may be necessary in patients presenting with gangrenous bowel due to intussusception. Follow-up is with yearly pan-endoscopy. There is an increased incidence of gastrointestinal cancers. Non-gastrointestinal cancers also occur with increased frequency, so yearly screening for uterine, ovarian and cervical cancer should start in the teens, and breast and testicular screening by the age of 20.

Other tumours

Adenomas, lipomas and stromal tumours (see p. 1180) are rarely found and are usually asymptomatic and picked up incidentally. They occasionally present with iron deficiency anaemia. In familial adenomatous polyposis (FAP), duodenal adenomas form in one-third of patients and may progress to adenocarcinoma. This is the most common cause of death in FAP patients who have been treated by prophylactic colectomy.

Further reading

Abrahams C, Medzhitov R. Interactions between the host innate immune system and microbes in inflammatory bowel disease. *Gastroenterology* 2011; 140:1720–1728.

Aikou S, Ohmoto Y, Gunji T. Tests for serum levels of trefoil factor family proteins can improve gastric cancer screening. *Gastroenterology* 2011; 141:837–845.

Fenollar F, Puéchal X, Raoult D. Whipple's disease (review). *N Engl J Med* 2007; 356:55–66.

Lundin KE, Sollid LM. Advances in coeliac disease. *Curr Opin Gastroenterol* 2014; 30:154–162.

Malamut G, Cellier C. Refractory celiac disease. *Expert Rev Gastroenterol Hepatol* 2014; 8:323–328.

Mooney PD, Hadjivassiliou M, Sanders DS. Coeliac disease. *BMJ* 2014; 348:g1561.

INFLAMMATORY BOWEL DISEASE

Two major forms of inflammatory bowel disease (IBD) are recognized:
- Crohn's disease (CD), which can affect any part of the gastrointestinal tract
- Ulcerative colitis (UC), which affects only the colon.

There is a degree of overlap between these two conditions in their aetiopathogenesis, clinical features, histological and radiological abnormalities; in 10% of cases of IBD causing colitis, a definitive diagnosis of either UC or CD is not possible and the diagnosis is termed colitis of undetermined type (indeterminate colitis). It is clinically useful to distinguish between UC and CD because of differences in their management, although, in reality, they may represent two aspects of the same disease.

Another form of colitis related to microscopic inflammation is termed microscopic colitis; this is subdivided into lymphocytic and collagenous types (see p. 1208). The distinction between this and IBD is the absence of macroscopic evidence of inflammation.

Epidemiology

- The incidence of CD varies from country to country but is approximately 4–10 per 100 000 annually, with a prevalence of 25–100/100 000.

- The incidence of UC is stable at 6–15/100 000 annually, with a prevalence of 80–150/100 000.

Although both conditions have a worldwide distribution, the highest incidence rates and prevalence have been reported from Northern Europe, the UK and North America. Both race and ethnic origin affect the incidence and prevalence of CD and UC. Thus, in North America, prevalence rates of CD are lower in Hispanic and Asian people (4.1/100 000 and 5.6/100 000, respectively) compared with white individuals (43.6/100 000). Jewish people are more prone to IBD than any other ethnic group. Prevalence rates also change after migration; thus there is an increasing incidence of CD in the UK-born children of migrants from South-east Asia. Recent studies suggest that the incidence of both CD and UC is increasing in traditional low-prevalence areas such as South-east Asia.

Approximately 25% of patients are diagnosed before their 18th birthday and there is evidence that disease commencing in youth is more extensive and more aggressive than that occurring in older patients.

Aetiology and pathogenesis

Although the aetiology of IBD is unknown, it is increasingly clear that IBD represents the interaction between several co-factors: genetic susceptibility, the environment, the intestinal microbiota and host immune response (**Fig. 32.36**).

Genetic factors

CD and UC are complex polygenic diseases and having a positive family history is the largest independent risk factor for development of IBD. Up to 1 in 5 patients with CD and 1 in 6 patients with UC will have a first-degree relative with the disease. The monozygotic and dizygotic twin concordance rates for CD are 20–50% and 10%, respectively.

Genome-wide association studies have identified multiple susceptibility loci, and many of the underlying risk variants have been identified. The major genetic factors for CD include the *NOD2* (*CARD 15*) gene (nucleotide oligomerization domain 2), the autophagy genes and the Th17 pathway (IL-23–type 17 helper T cells). The NOD2 protein on chromosome 16 is an intracellular sensor of bacterial peptidoglycan, present in bacterial cell walls (see below). NOD2 is expressed in epithelial cells, macrophages and endothelial cells. Individuals who are homozygote or compound heterozygote for one of several mutations in the *NOD2* gene have a significantly increased risk of developing ileal CD. Likewise, mutations in the autophagy genes *ATG16L1* and *IRGM* (immunity-related GTP-ase M-protein) and IL-23 receptor gene increase CD risk, and mutations in genes associated with the mucosal barrier increase UC risk. However, the presence of IBD-associated genes in many unaffected individuals and the failure of the approximately 71 genetic susceptibility loci identified thus far to explain more than around one-fifth of the genetic risk of CD highlight the complexity of the genetic basis of IBD. Specific genetic defects in the IL-10 receptor pathway are associated with a severe form of extremely early-onset colitis and perianal disease in children.

Apart from susceptibility, HLA genes on chromosome 6 also appear to have a role in modifying the disease. The *DRB*0103* allele is linked to a particularly aggressive course of UC and the need for surgery, as well as with colonic CD. *DRB*0103* and *MICA*010* are associated with perianal disease, and *DRB*0701* with ileal CD. For the extraintestinal disease complications and HLA links, see page 1202.

Environmental and other factors

- ***Smoking.*** Patients with CD are more likely to be smokers, and smoking has been shown to exacerbate CD and increase the risk

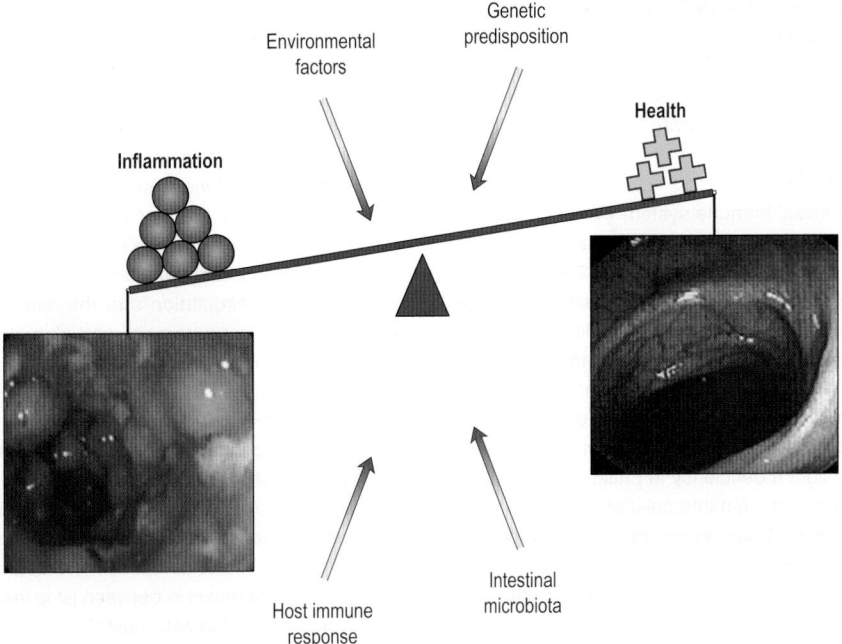

Fig. 32.36 The aetiopathogenesis of inflammatory bowel disease.

of disease recurrence after surgery. By contrast, there is an increased risk of UC in non- or ex-smokers and nicotine has been shown to be an effective treatment in one small clinical trial.

- **NSAIDs.** NSAID ingestion is associated with both the onset of IBD and flares of disease in patients with an established diagnosis.
- **Hygiene.** Poor and large families living in crowded conditions have a lower risk of developing CD. A 'clean' environment may not expose the intestinal immune system to pathogenic or non-pathogenic microorganisms such as helminths, which seems to alter the balance between effector and regulatory immune responses.
- **Nutritional factors.** Many foods and food components have been suggested as playing a role in the aetiopathogenesis of IBD (e.g. high sugar and fat intake) but, unfortunately, the results of numerous studies designed to define risk have been equivocal. However, breast-feeding may provide protection against the development of IBD in offspring.
- **Psychological factors.** Factors such as chronic stress and depression seem to increase relapses in patients with quiescent disease.
- **Appendicectomy.** This appears to be 'protective' against the development of UC, particularly if performed for appendicitis or for mesenteric lymphadenitis before the age of 20. It also influences the clinical course of UC, with a lower incidence of colectomy and reduced need for immunosuppressive therapy. By contrast, appendicectomy may increase the risk of development of CD.

Intestinal microbiota

The gut is colonized by 10 times more bacterial organisms than there are host cells, there being 300–400 distinct bacterial species within each host intestine. The intestinal microbiota plays a crucial role in perpetuating intestinal inflammation, in both animal models of disease and patients with IBD. The number of mucosal adherent bacteria is increased in patients with CD compared to healthy subjects, and diversion of the bacterial component of the faecal stream induces clinical remission. However, there is also evidence of an immunoregulatory role for the commensal microbiota, which protects against intestinal inflammation and upregulates epithelial defence mechanisms in animal models of colitis.

Mechanisms by which the intestinal microbiota may relate to the aetiology of IBD include:

- **Intestinal dysbiosis.** There is an alteration in the bacterial flora in patients with CD. Although results vary due to differences in both the patient groups studied and the microbiological method utilized, the most consistent finding in patients with IBD is a reduced diversity of microbial species. In addition, higher concentrations of *Bacteroides* and *E. coli*, and lower concentrations of bifidobacteria and *Faecalibacterium prausnitzii* have been reported in faecal and mucosal samples from patients with CD compared to healthy controls. Lower concentrations of *F. prausnitzii* have been found in patients with active compared with quiescent disease, and low levels of this organism in CD resection specimens predict subsequent endoscopic disease recurrence.
- **Specific pathogenic organisms.** It has been shown that there is increased *E. coli* adherence to the ileal epithelial cells in CD, with evidence of invasion into the mucosa. *E. coli*'s type 1 pili adhere to a protein called carcinoembryonic antigen-related cell adhesion molecule 6 (CEACAM6). Many authors have also suggested a link between CD and *Mycobacterium paratuberculosis* (MAP), although recent PCR-based studies have failed to confirm this and therapeutic trials of anti-*Mycobacterium tuberculosis* (MTB) therapy were not effective.
- **Bacterial antigens.** Bacteria exert their influence by the interaction of ligands such as peptidoglycan-polysaccharides (PG-PS) and lipopolysaccharides (LPS) with host pattern recognition receptors such as the Toll-like receptor family (cell surface) and the NOD family (intracellular).
- **Defective chemical barrier or intestinal defensins** (see p. 1155). Evidence suggests a decrease in human α defensin-1 (HD-1) in the mucosa of both CD and UC, and a lack of induction of HD-2, HD-3 and HD-5 in CD.

- **Impaired mucosal barrier function.** This may explain the presence of unusual and potentially pathogenic bacteria, such as MAP, *Listeria* and mucosal adherent *E. coli*. However, their presence does not necessarily imply causation of the disease, and they may reflect previous disease activity.

Intestinal immune system

IBD occurs when the mucosal immune system exerts an inappropriate response to luminal antigens, such as bacteria, which may enter the mucosa via a leaky epithelium (**Fig. 32.37**). Bacterial ligands interact with the innate and acquired mucosal immune system via Toll-like receptors expressed on both epithelial and antigen-presenting cells. Deficiencies occur in the clearance of invading bacteria by aspects of the innate immune system, such as neutrophils, which may allow inappropriate activation of the acquired immune system. In keeping with the genetic susceptibility loci identified, these findings highlight a deficiency in patients with IBD in a component of the inflammasome (an intracellular danger sensor of the innate immune system that can trigger caspase-1-dependent processing of inflammatory mediators, such as IL-1β and IL-18). In addition, individual bacterial species have distinct immunological effects mediated by dendritic cells (DCs), which sample bacteria from the intestinal lumen and direct the subsequent functional differentiation of naive T cells into effector or regulatory populations.

IBD is associated with an imbalance in the relative numbers of intestinal homing effector (Th1 and Th17) and regulatory T cell populations, which disturbs the normal tolerance to the luminal antigenic load.

The pro-inflammatory cytokines released by these activated effector T cells stimulate macrophages to secrete pro-inflammatory cytokines, such as tumour necrosis factor-alpha (TNF-α), IL-1 and IL-6 in large quantities. These mechanisms result in increased adhesion molecule expression on the intestinal vascular endothelium, which facilitates the recruitment of leucocytes from the circulation and the release of chemokines, all of which lead to tissue damage and also attract more inflammatory cells in a vicious circle.

Pathology

CD is a chronic inflammatory condition that may affect any part of the gastrointestinal tract from the mouth to the anus but has a particular tendency to affect the terminal ileum and ascending colon (ileocolonic disease) (**Fig. 32.38**). The disease can involve one small area of the gut, such as the terminal ileum, or multiple areas with relatively normal bowel in between (skip lesions). It may also involve the whole of the colon (total colitis), sometimes without macroscopic small bowel involvement. It is also associated with the development of perianal fistulae and fissures (**Box 32.37**).

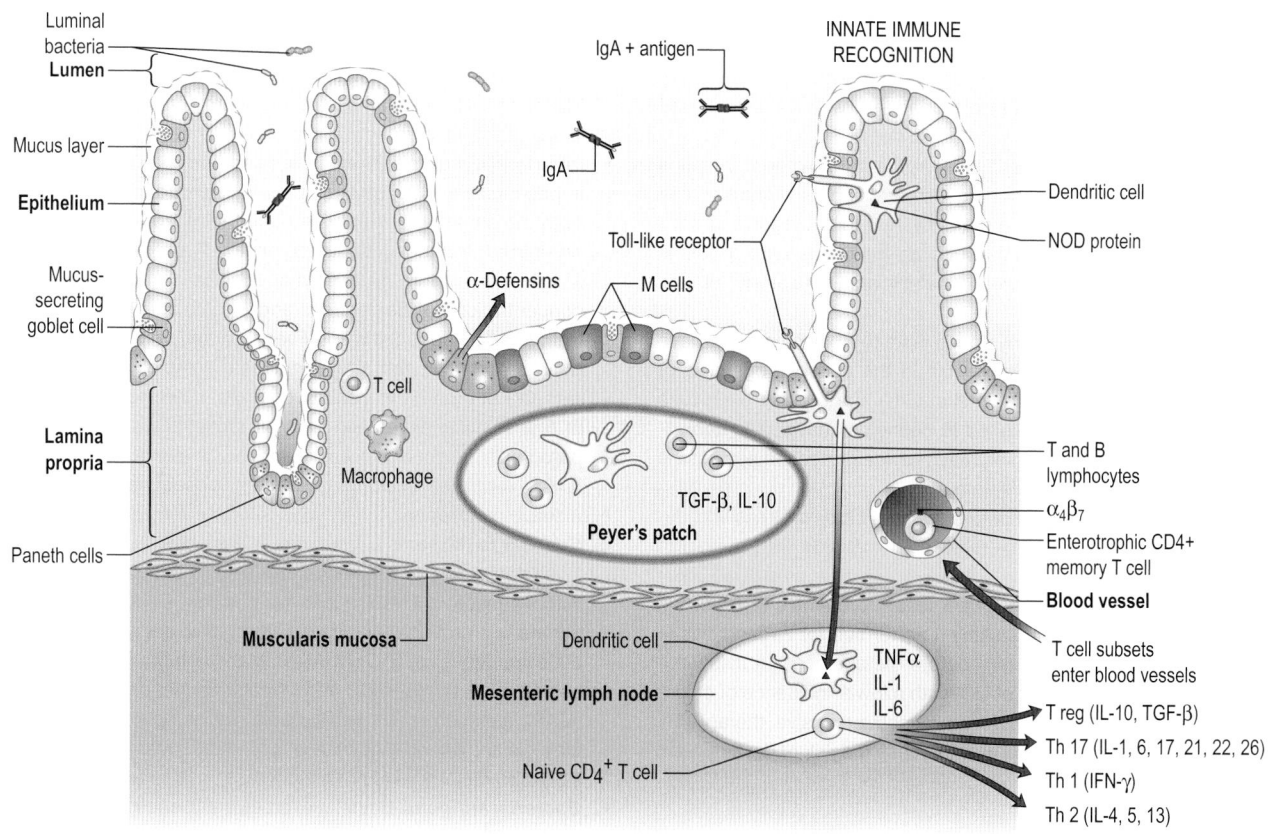

Fig. 32.37 Cellular intestinal processes involved in inflammatory bowel disease. Bacterial ligands attach to the epithelium and antigen-presenting cells (e.g. dendritic cells and macrophages) via Toll-like receptors and the NOD protein. The dendritic cells migrate to the Peyer's patches and mesenteric lymph nodes. They present antigens to naive T cells, releasing a number of cytokines that cause damage. The T-cell subsets enter the blood vessels, where the enterotropic molecules α4-β7 are induced and allow homing back to the gut, causing further damage. IFN-γ, interferon-gamma; IL, interleukin; TGF-β, transforming growth factor-beta; TNF-α, tumour necrosis factor-alpha. *(Modified from Abraham C, Cho JH. Inflammatory bowel disease. N Engl J Med 2009; 361:2066–2078.)*

UC can affect the rectum alone (proctitis), can extend proximally to involve the sigmoid and descending colon (left-sided colitis), or may involve the whole colon (extensive colitis) (**Fig. 32.39**). In a few of these patients, there is also inflammation of the distal terminal ileum (backwash ileitis).

Macroscopic changes

In *CD*, the involved bowel is usually thickened and is often narrowed. Deep ulcers and fissures in the mucosa produce a cobblestone appearance. Intra-abdominal fistulae and abscesses may be seen, which reflect penetrating disease. An early feature is aphthoid ulceration in the colon, usually seen at colonoscopy (**Fig. 32.40**); later, larger and deeper ulcers appear in a patchy distribution, again producing a cobblestone appearance.

In *UC*, the mucosa looks reddened and inflamed, and bleeds easily (friability). In severe disease, there may be extensive ulceration, with the adjacent mucosa appearing as post-inflammatory (pseudo-) polyps.

In *fulminant colonic disease* of either type, most of the mucosa is lost, leaving a few islands of oedematous mucosa (mucosal islands), and toxic dilation occurs. On healing, the mucosa can return to normal, although there is usually some residual scarring.

Microscopic changes

In *CD*, the inflammation extends through all layers (transmural) of the bowel, whereas in UC superficial inflammation limited to the mucosa is seen. In CD, there is an increase in chronic inflammatory cells and lymphoid hyperplasia, and in 50–60% of patients, granulomas are present. These granulomas are non-caseating epithelioid cell aggregates with Langhans' giant cells.

In *UC*, the mucosa shows a chronic inflammatory cell infiltrate in the lamina propria. Crypt abscesses and goblet cell depletion are also seen.

These two diseases can usually be differentiated not only on the basis of clinical and radiological data but also on the histological differences seen in the rectal and colonic mucosa obtained by biopsy (**Box 32.38**).

It is occasionally not possible to distinguish between the two disorders, particularly if biopsies are obtained in the acute phase, and such patients are considered to have indeterminate colitis. Serological testing for anti-neutrophil cytoplasmic antibodies

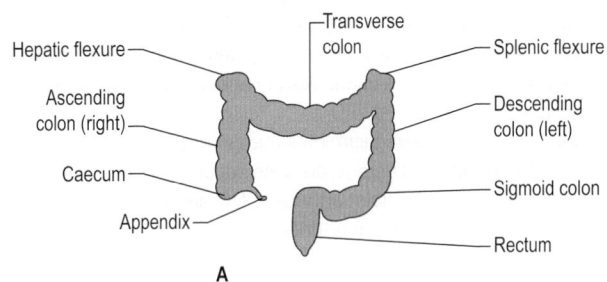

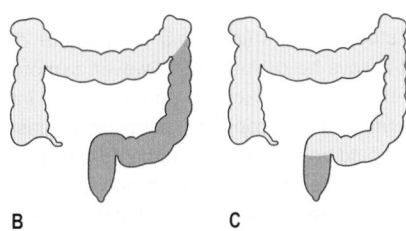

Fig. 32.39 Sites of ulcerative colitis (Montreal classification). **(A)** *Extensive colitis (E3)*: pancolitis, total colitis: entire colon and rectum inflamed. **(B)** *Distal colitis (E2)*: left-sided colitis: rectum, sigmoid and descending colon inflamed. **(C)** *Proctitis (E1)*: rectum only inflamed.

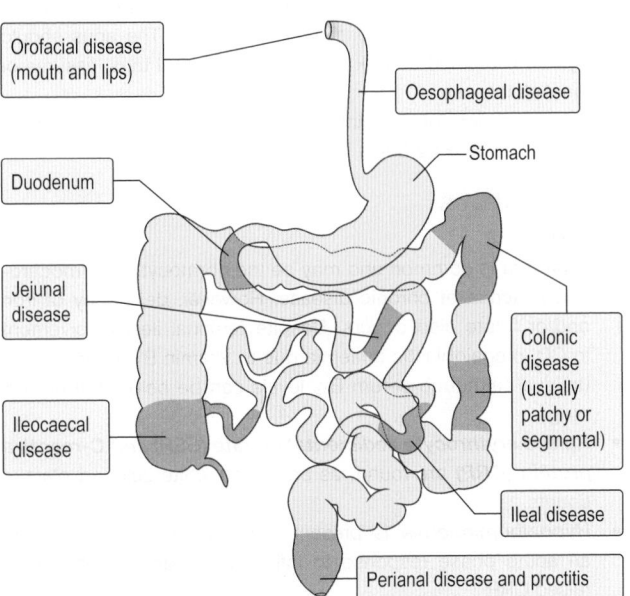

Fig. 32.38 Sites of Crohn's disease.

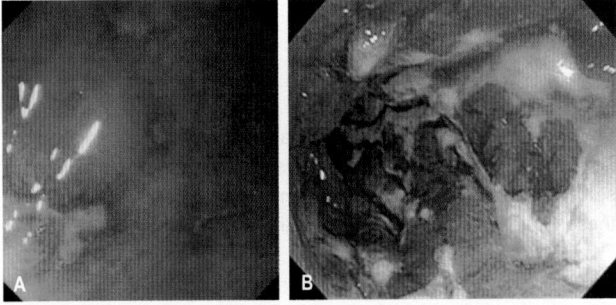

Fig. 32.40 Crohn's disease: colonoscopic appearances. **(A)** Aphthoid ulcers typical of Crohn's disease. **(B)** Deep, serpiginous ulceration in colonic Crohn's disease.

i   **Box 32.38 Histological differences between Crohn's disease and ulcerative colitis**

Histological feature	Crohn's disease	Ulcerative colitis
Inflammation	Deep (transmural) patchy	Mucosal continuous
Granulomas	++	Rare
Goblet cells	Present	Depleted
Crypt abscesses	+	++

(ANCA) in UC and anti-*Saccharomyces cerevisiae* antibodies (ASCA) in CD may be of value in differentiating the two conditions (see below), although an exact diagnosis can sometimes be made only after examining a surgical colectomy specimen. Occasionally, examination of the colectomy specimen still does not lead to a diagnosis of CD or UC and the patient is labelled as having indeterminate colitis.

Extraintestinal manifestations

These occur with both diseases (**Box 32.39**). Joint complications are most common; the peripheral arthropathies are classified as:

- *Type 1 (pauciarticular)* attacks are acute and self-limiting (<10 weeks), and occur with IBD relapses; they are associated with other extraintestinal manifestations of IBD activity.
- *Type 2 (polyarticular)* arthropathy lasts longer (months to years), is independent of IBD activity and usually associated with uveitis.

Joint and other extragastrointestinal manifestations of IBD are shown in **Box 32.39**. There is an association of HLA *DRB1*0103* with pauciarticular large-joint arthritis in UC and CD, and HLA-B44 with small-joint symmetrical arthritis. HLA-B27 is associated with sacroiliitis.

Differential diagnosis

Alternative causes of diarrhoea should be excluded (see **Box 32.35**) and stool cultures (including *Clostridium difficile* toxin assay) must always be performed. However, symptoms persisting beyond 5 days are unlikely to be caused by infective gastroenteritis. Stool microscopy for parasitic diseases such as amoebiasis should be carried out in patients with a relevant travel history. CD should be considered in all individuals with evidence of vitamin malabsorption (e.g. megaloblastic anaemia) or malnourishment, as well as in children with reduced growth velocity. Ileocolonic tuberculosis (see p. 1195) is common in developing countries, such as India, which makes a diagnosis of CD difficult. Microscopy and culture for TB of any available tissue is essential in these countries. A therapeutic trial of anti-TB therapy may be required. Lymphomas can occasionally involve the ileum and caecum, although they are rare in the patient population at risk from IBD.

Crohn's disease

Clinical features

The major symptoms are diarrhoea, abdominal pain and weight loss. Constitutional symptoms of malaise, lethargy, anorexia, nausea, vomiting and low-grade fever may be present and in 15% of these patients there are no gastrointestinal symptoms. Reduced growth velocity and delayed puberty may be the main presenting features in children. Despite the recurrent nature of this condition, some patients have an almost normal lifestyle. However, patients with extensive disease have frequent recurrences and progress from inflammatory to stricturing and penetrating disease. Approximately 50% of patients will require an intestinal resection within 5 years of diagnosis.

Clinical features are very variable and depend partly on the region of the bowel that is affected. The disease may present insidiously or acutely. Abdominal pain can be colicky, suggesting obstruction, but it usually has no special characteristics and sometimes in colonic disease only minimal discomfort is present. Diarrhoea occurs in 80% of all cases and in colonic disease it usually contains blood, making it difficult to differentiate from UC. Steatorrhoea can be present in small bowel disease. Diarrhoea can also be due to bile acid malabsorption, occurring as a consequence of ileal resection or ileal disease.

CD can also present as an emergency with acute right iliac fossa pain mimicking appendicitis. If laparotomy is undertaken, an oedematous, reddened terminal ileum is found. Other causes of an acute ileitis include infections such as *Yersinia* and TB.

CD is complicated by anal and perianal disease, and this is the presenting feature in 25% of cases, often preceding colonic and small intestinal symptoms (see **Box 32.37**). Enteric fistulae – for example, to bladder, vagina or abdominal wall – occur in 20–40% of cases.

Examination

Physical signs are few, apart from loss of weight and signs of malnutrition. Aphthous ulceration of the mouth is often seen. Abdominal examination may be normal, although tenderness and/or a right iliac fossa mass are occasionally found. The mass is due either to inflamed loops of bowel that are matted together or to an abscess, which may also cause psoas muscle irritation. The anus should always be examined to look for oedematous anal tags, fissures or perianal abscesses.

The presence of extraintestinal features of IBD should be assessed (see **Box 32.39**).

Investigations

Blood tests

- *Anaemia* is common and may be the normocytic, normochromic anaemia of chronic disease. However, deficiency of iron and/or folate also occurs. Despite terminal ileal involvement in CD, megaloblastic anaemia due to vitamin B_{12} deficiency is unusual, although serum B_{12} levels can be below the normal range.
- *Raised erythrocyte sedimentation rate (ESR) and C-reactive protein (CRP)* are found, as are raised white cell and platelet counts.
- *Hypoalbuminaemia* is present in severe disease as part of an acute phase response to inflammation associated with a raised CRP.
- *Liver biochemistry* may be abnormal.
- *Blood cultures* are required if septicaemia is suspected.
- *Serological tests* may reveal negative perinuclear ANCA (pANCA) and positive ASCA (see p. 1201).

Stool tests

Stool cultures, including *C. difficile* toxin assay, should always be performed if diarrhoea is present. Microscopy for parasites is essential in patients with a relevant travel history. Faecal calprotectin and

---

> **ℹ** **Box 32.39 Extragastrointestinal manifestations of inflammatory bowel disease**
>
> - Eyes:
>   - Uveitis
>   - Episcleritis, conjunctivitis
> - Joints:
>   - Type I (pauciarticular) arthropathy
>   - Type II (polyarticular) arthropathy
>   - Arthralgia
>   - Ankylosing spondylitis
>   - Inflammatory back pain
>
> - Skin:
>   - Erythema nodosum
>   - Pyoderma gangrenosum
> - Liver and biliary tree:
>   - Sclerosing cholangitis
>   - Fatty liver
>   - Chronic hepatitis
>   - Cirrhosis
>   - Gallstones
> - Nephrolithiasis
> - Venous thrombosis

lactoferrin are raised in active intestinal disease. Faecal calprotectin is useful for disease monitoring in IBD.

Endoscopy and radiological imaging

- **Colonoscopy** is performed if colonic involvement is suspected, except in patients presenting with severe disease (in whom a limited unprepared sigmoidoscopy should be carried out). The findings vary from mild, patchy, superficial (aphthoid) ulceration to more widespread, larger and deeper ulcers that produce a cobblestone appearance (see **Fig. 32.40**). Endoscopic assessment of the terminal ileum is essential in all patients with suspected CD. Two biopsies should be performed in five areas, including the rectum and terminal ileum.
- **Upper gastrointestinal endoscopy** is required to exclude oesophageal and gastroduodenal disease in patients with relevant symptoms and is increasingly being performed in all patients at diagnosis to define the extent of disease accurately as a guide to prognosis.
- **Small bowel imaging** is mandatory in patients with suspected CD. The technique used will depend on availability and local expertise. Techniques include barium follow-through, CT scan with oral contrast, small bowel ultrasound or MRI enteroclysis. An asymmetrical alteration in the mucosal pattern with deep ulceration, and areas of narrowing or structuring may be found. Although disease is commonly confined to the terminal ileum (**Fig. 32.41**), other areas of the small bowel can be involved, and skip lesions with normal bowel are seen between affected sites. Axial imaging allows the diagnosis of extraintestinal sepsis in patients presenting acutely and is therefore preferred in this situation.
- **Ultrasound scanning** provides a convenient radiation-free method for assessing disease activity in the ileum and colon and can be performed by appropriately trained gastroenterologists at the bedside.
- **Perianal MRI or endoanal ultrasound** is used to evaluate perianal disease.
- **Capsule endoscopy** is used in CD patients when radiological examination is normal. A patency capsule assessment is often performed first to exclude strictures of the small bowel that would constitute a contraindication to subsequent capsule endoscopy.
- **Radionuclide scans** with indium- or technetium-labelled leucocytes are used in some centres to identify small intestinal and colonic disease inflammation and to localize extraintestinal abscesses.

Disease activity

This can be assessed using simple parameters such as haemoglobin, white cell count, inflammatory markers (raised ESR, CRP and platelet count) and serum albumin. Formal clinical activity indices (e.g. CD Activity Index or Harvey Bradshaw Index) are used in research studies. Faecal calprotectin or lactoferrin has the potential to be a simple, cheap, non-invasive marker of disease activity in IBD and these tests are of value in predicting response to and failure of treatment.

Medical management of Crohn's disease

See **Box 32.40**.

General considerations

The aims of management are to induce and then maintain clinical remission and to achieve mucosal healing in order to prevent disease progression and complications. Alternative causes for symptoms, such as gastroenteritis, extraintestinal sepsis, stricture formation, functional gastrointestinal disease or bile salt malabsorption, must be excluded before commencing immunosuppressive therapy. Patients with mild symptoms and no evidence of extensive disease may require symptomatic treatment only. Cigarette smoking should be stopped. Anaemia, if due to vitamin B_{12}, folic acid or iron deficiency, should be treated with the appropriate replacement. Patients who are intolerant of oral iron should receive an intravenous iron infusion. Most patients can be treated as outpatients, although severe attacks may require admission, and prophylaxis for thromboembolism (see p. 1013) should be given to all inpatients.

Induction of remission

Glucocorticosteroids

These are commonly used to induce remission in moderate and severe attacks of CD (oral prednisolone 30–60 mg/day). Mild to moderate ileocaecal disease should be treated with controlled-release corticosteroids, such as budesonide, which has reduced systemic availability and is associated with a lower frequency and intensity of steroidal side-effects.

Overall remission/response rates vary from 60% to 90%, depending on type, site and extent of disease. Steroids should be avoided in patients with penetrating intestinal disease or perianal sepsis.

Aminosalicylates

These have been used but there is little evidence to support their efficacy in CD.

Antibiotics

Antibiotics (ciprofloxacin and metronidazole) are used for treating secondary complications of CD (e.g. abscess and perianal disease).

Exclusive enteral nutrition

This is the traditional treatment for moderate to severe attacks of CD in paediatric practice, but is under-utilized in adults due to issues with compliance to the diet. If administered as the sole source of nutrition for 28 days, rates of induction of remission are similar to those obtained with steroids. Relapse rates are high, however, particularly in those with colonic involvement.

Refractory or fulminant disease

Patients with symptoms that do not respond to conventional therapy should be re-assessed to exclude an alternative diagnosis such as a stricture or penetrating abscess. In patients with disease limited to the terminal ileum, surgical resection may be appropriate. In those with more extensive disease, remission should be induced with an anti-TNF agent, either as monotherapy or preferably in combination with an immunosuppressant such as azathioprine (see below).

Maintenance of remission

All patients require regular monitoring to exclude persistent intestinal inflammation. Patients with disease that has a good prognosis (older age at diagnosis, no perianal disease, limited ulceration at index investigations, non-smoker) may not require maintenance therapy. Patients with disease that has a poor prognosis (young age at diagnosis, extensive small bowel disease, deep colonic ulceration, perianal/rectal disease, smoker) or that flares up after induction therapy is withdrawn require long-term maintenance immunosuppression. The goal of maintenance therapy is to prevent

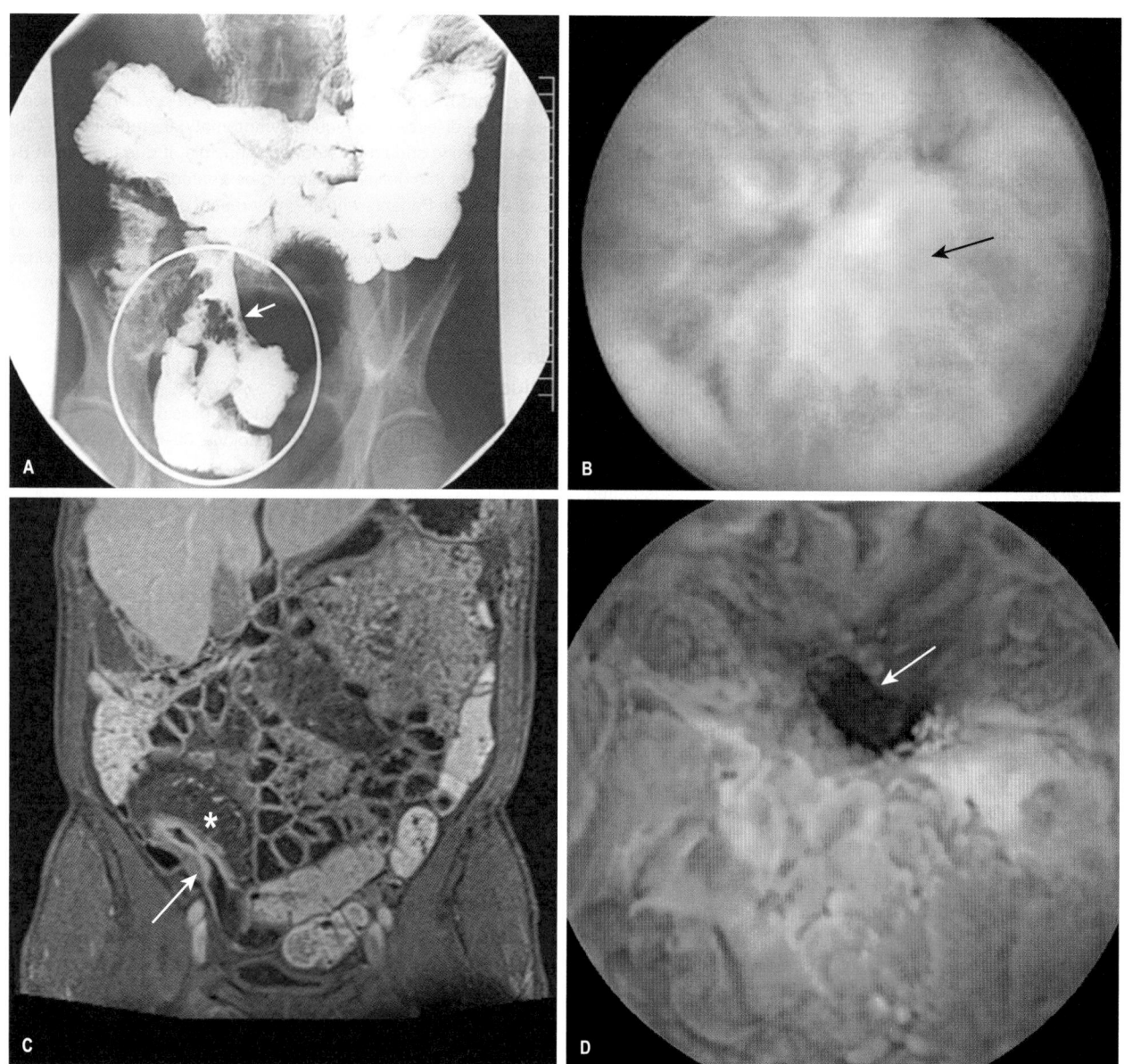

Fig. 32.41 Imaging of the small bowel in Crohn's disease. **(A)** Barium follow-through showing an ulcerated stricture (arrowed), pre-stenotic dilation and separation of the small bowel loops due to fibro-fatty proliferation. Small bowel follow-through has generally been superseded by small bowel MRI. **(B)** Capsule endoscopy picture of an ileal ulcer in a patient with Crohn's disease (arrowed). **(C)** Post-contrast T1 fat-suppressed coronal image from an MRI enterography examination demonstrates bowel wall thickening of the terminal ileum and mucosal hyperenhancement consistent with active inflammation (arrow). There is also fibrofatty proliferation (*) adjacent to the inflamed bowel consistent with chronic disease and, therefore, the overall appearances represent chronic active Crohn's disease. **(D)** Capsule endoscopy showing an ileal Crohn's disease stricture (arrowed).

> *i* **Box 32.40 Options for the medical treatment of Crohn's disease**
>
> **Induction of remission**
> - Oral or i.v. glucocorticosteroids
> - Enteral nutrition
> - Anti-tumour necrosis factor (TNF) antibodies
>
> **Maintenance of remission**
> - Azathioprine, mercaptopurine, methotrexate
> - Anti-TNF antibodies
>
> **Perianal disease**
> - Surgical drainage of sepsis
> - Ciprofloxacin and metronidazole
> - Azathioprine
> - Anti-TNF antibodies

disease progression, as well as to reduce the need for corticosteroids, which are associated with a high burden of side-effects. Therapies that induce mucosal healing result in better outcomes. All maintenance therapies require careful monitoring to ensure optimal disease control and prevent side-effects. If there is ongoing evidence of disease activity, adherence should be confirmed and dose optimization or therapy escalation undertaken.

Conventional maintenance therapies

These include *azathioprine* (AZA; 2.5 mg/kg per day), *mercaptopurine* (MP; 1.5 mg/kg per day) and *methotrexate* (25 mg **once a**

week until remission, then reduced to 15 mg per week) (see **Box 32.40**). Long-term treatment with these drugs is necessary, as the rate of relapse on discontinuation is high. Patient education regarding side-effects and appropriate monitoring for complications is essential and may increase adherence. The key enzyme involved in AZA and MP metabolism is thiopurine methyl transferase (TPMT). This enzyme has a significant genetic variation and deficiencies can result in high circulating levels of thioguanine nucleotides with an increased risk of bone marrow depression. Assays of TPMT activity are available and should be performed before treatment. TPMT deficiency is not the only cause of bone marrow depression so 3-monthly blood counts should be performed on all patients. Metabolite measurement can be undertaken to assess adherence and ensure optimal dosing.

Anti-TNF agents

These have clear evidence of benefit in the induction and maintenance of remission in patients with CD. They are indicated in patients with disease refractory to conventional immunosuppressive therapy. Early use of anti-TNF therapy is indicated in selected patients with disease that has a poor prognosis (see above). They are also used to treat complex perianal/rectal disease once sepsis has been drained. Available anti-TNF agents include **infliximab** (a chimeric anti-TNF-α IgG1 monoclonal antibody), **adalimumab** (a fully humanized anti-TNF IgG1 monoclonal antibody) and **certolizumab pegol** (a PEGylated Fab′ fragment of a humanized anti-TNF antibody). They neutralize soluble TNF-α, bind to membrane-bound TNF-α and induce immune cell apoptosis, although the exact mechanism of action is not defined. In clinical trials, they have been shown to exert a steroid-sparing effect and bring about complete mucosal healing in up to one-third of patients in the long term. This results in a reduced need for hospital admission and surgery. These agents should always be used on a regular basis as maintenance therapy, as they are less effective and induce anti-drug antibodies if used episodically. In patients who are naive to azathioprine, combination therapy increases efficacy and reduces immunogenicity. Their use should be limited to clinicians experienced in the management of CD, as they are associated with significant complications, including opportunistic infections (such as TB), demyelination and malignancy.

Novel biological therapies

Novel therapies for the treatment of CD include the anti-α4β7 integrin therapy, vedolizumab, which acts to reduce leucocyte recruitment to the inflamed intestine. This is used in patients with moderately to severely active Crohn's disease who are intolerant to an anti-TNF or in whom it is contraindicated, or in those patients who have had an inadequate response or lost response to an anti-TNF-α agent. Therapies that target the IL-12/IL-23 pathway, such as ustekinumab, are currently used to treat moderate to severely active Crohn's disease, in those patients who cannot have, or have had an inadequate response to, an anti-TNF-α agent. Risankizumab is a human monoclonal antibody that targets the p19 subunit of interleukin-23, currently in phase 3 trials for patients with moderately to severely active Crohn's disease. Recent preliminary studies using the oral anti-sense oligonucleotide, mongersen, have shown promise for the treatment of active Crohn's disease. This agent binds to, and causes degradation of, *SMAD7* messenger RNA, thereby restoring TGF-β1 signalling and decreasing the production of pro-inflammatory markers. Phase 3 studies are underway. Ozanimod is an oral agonist of the sphingosine-1-phosphate receptor subtypes 1 and 5 that decreases circulating activated lymphocytes, currently in phase 3 trials for the treatment of moderately to severe Crohn's disease.

Advances in mucosal immunology have highlighted a variety of targets to resolve the inflammation and symptoms of the disease. Numerous investigational therapies concentrate on inhibiting, suppressing or altering T-cell differentiation.

Surgical management of Crohn's disease

Studies prior to the introduction of biological agents suggest that up to 80% of patients will require an operation at some time during the course of their disease. Nevertheless, surgery should be avoided if possible and only minimal resections undertaken, as recurrence (15% per year) is almost inevitable without prophylactic maintenance therapy. The *indications for surgery* are:

- failure of medical therapy, with acute or chronic symptoms producing ill-health
- complications (e.g. toxic dilation, obstruction, perforation, abscesses, enterocutaneous fistula)
- failure to grow in children despite medical treatment
- presence of perianal sepsis; an examination is performed under anaesthetic, the sepsis is drained, and a seton is inserted to ensure ongoing drainage.

In patients with small bowel disease some strictures can be widened (stricturoplasty), whereas others require resection and anastomosis. It is essential to consider postoperative maintenance therapy in patients undergoing ileocolonic resection and anastomosis. All patients should refrain from smoking. There is some evidence that a 3-month course of metronidazole reduces relapse rates. Patients with a high risk of relapse (previous surgery, smoker, penetrating disease at the time of index surgery) should be evaluated for maintenance immunosuppressive therapy. Patients should undergo an ileocolonoscopy to assess the anastomosis for disease recurrence 6 months after surgery, when further therapy can be agreed with the patient.

When colonic CD involves the entire colon and the rectum is spared or minimally involved, a subtotal colectomy and ileorectal anastomosis may be performed. An eventual recurrence rate of 60–70% in the ileum, rectum or both is to be expected; however, two-thirds of these patients retain a functional rectum for 10 years. If the whole colon and rectum are involved, a panproctocolectomy with an end ileostomy is the standard operation. CD patients are not suitable for a pouch operation (see p. 1207), as recurrence in the pouch is high.

Problems associated with ileostomies include:

- mechanical problems
- dehydration, particularly if there is a short length of small bowel remaining
- psychosexual problems
- erectile dysfunction in men and reduced fecundity in women (due to prior pelvic surgery)
- recurrence of CD.

Prognosis

The majority of patients have inflammatory disease at diagnosis, although up to 20% will present with complicated disease, including strictures and penetrating disease. If disease is left untreated, its natural history is progression from inflammatory to stricturing and penetrating disease that may require surgery. Up to 50% of patients will require a surgical resection within the first 5 years of disease. The goal of therapy is to target early aggressive therapy at those patients with a poor prognosis. However, predicting disease prognosis at diagnosis is not easy. Features that imply a poor prognosis include young age at diagnosis (<20 years of age), extensive small bowel disease, complex perianal disease and deep ulceration at index colonoscopy.

Ulcerative colitis

Clinical features

The major symptom in UC is diarrhoea with blood and mucus, sometimes accompanied by lower abdominal discomfort. General features include malaise, lethargy and anorexia with weight loss, although these features are not as severe as with CD. Aphthous ulceration in the mouth may be seen. The disease can be mild, moderate or severe (**Box 32.41**), and in most patients runs a course of remissions and exacerbations. Disease extent is defined as limited to the rectum (proctitis), left-sided or extensive (see **Fig. 32.39**).

Proctitis is characterized by the frequent passage of blood and mucus, urgency and tenesmus. There are normally few constitutional symptoms and the stool, when passed, may be solid. Patients are nevertheless greatly inconvenienced by the frequency of defecation.

In an acute attack of left-sided or extensive UC, patients have bloody diarrhoea, passing up to 10–20 liquid stools per day. Diarrhoea also occurs at night, with urgency and incontinence that is severely disabling for the patient. Patients with an acute severe flare of colitis (see **Box 32.40**) require urgent admission for intensive therapy.

Toxic megacolon is a serious complication associated with acute severe colitis. The plain abdominal X-ray shows a dilated, thin-walled colon with a diameter of more than 6 cm; it is gas-filled and contains mucosal islands (**Fig. 32.42**). It is a particularly dangerous stage of advanced disease, with impending perforation and a high mortality (15–25%). Urgent surgery is required in all patients in whom toxic dilation has not resolved within 48 hours, with intensive therapy as above. The differential diagnosis includes an infectious colitis, e.g. with *C. difficile* and cytomegalovirus.

Examination

In general, there are no specific signs in UC. The abdomen may be slightly distended or tender to palpation. Tachycardia and pyrexia are signs of severe colitis and mandate admission. The anus is usually normal. Rectal examination will reveal the presence of blood. Sigmoidoscopy is usually abnormal, showing an inflamed, bleeding, friable mucosa. Very occasionally, rectal sparing occurs, with normal proctoscopy.

Investigations

Blood tests

- **White cell and platelet counts** are commonly raised in moderate to severe attacks, and iron deficiency anaemia is present.
- **ESR and CRP** are often raised; liver biochemistry may be abnormal, with hypoalbuminaemia occurring in severe disease.
- **pANCA** may be positive. This is contrary to CD, where pANCA is usually negative (see p. 1202).

Stool tests and *C. difficile* toxin

These should always be performed to exclude infective causes of colitis. Stool microscopy to exclude amoebiasis is mandated in patients with a relevant travel history. Faecal calprotectin/lactoferrin will be elevated.

Colonoscopy

Endoscopy with mucosal biopsy is the 'gold standard' investigation for the diagnosis of UC. Colonoscopy also allows assessment of disease activity and extent. In patients with long-term colitis, chromoendoscopy is used to diagnose dysplasia. Full colonoscopy should not be performed in severe attacks of disease for fear of perforation; instead, a limited unprepared flexible sigmoidoscopy should be used to confirm diagnosis.

Imaging

A plain abdominal X-ray is essential in patients suffering acute severe attacks to exclude colonic dilation. However, the extent of disease is not reliably assessed using this investigation. Other imaging modalities are rarely used in the assessment of patients with UC, as endoscopy is preferred. However, inflammation of the colonic wall is detected on ultrasound, as is the presence of free fluid within the abdominal cavity.

Medical management of ulcerative colitis

Wherever possible, patients with IBD should be managed in patient-focused IBD clinics with access to a full multidisciplinary team. The mainstay of treatment for mild and moderate disease of any extent is an aminosalicylate, which acts topically in the colonic lumen. The

---

> **i** **Box 32.41 Definition and management of a severe attack of ulcerative colitis**
>
> **Definition**
> - Stool frequency: >6 stools/day with blood +++
> - Fever: >37.5°C
> - Tachycardia: >90 beats/min
> - Erythrocyte sedimentation rate: >30 mm/h
> - Anaemia: <100 g/L haemoglobin
> - Albumin: <30 g/L
>
> **Management**
> - Admit to hospital
> - Exclude enteric infection
> - Confirm diagnosis with unprepared limited flexible sigmoidoscopy
> - Assess fluid status
> - Give prophylactic anticoagulation
> - I.v. hydrocortisone 100 mg, 4 times daily
> - Monitor daily:
>   – Stool frequency
>   – Abdominal X-ray
>   – Bloods (FBC/CRP/albumin)

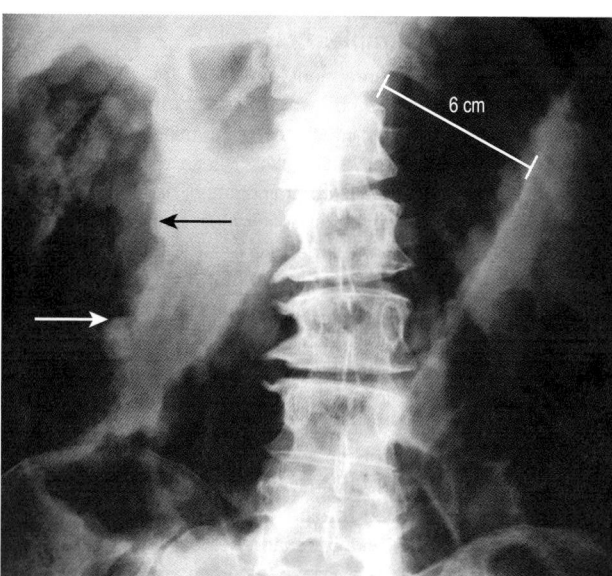

Fig. 32.42 Plain abdominal X-ray showing toxic dilation. The arrows indicate mucosal islands.

active moiety of these drugs is 5-aminosalicylic acid (5-ASA), which is absorbed in the small intestine. Therefore, the various amino-salicylate preparations are designed to deliver the active 5-ASA to the colon. This is achieved by binding of 5-ASA with an azo bond to sulfapyridine (sulfasalazine), 4-aminobenzoyl-β-alanine (balsalazide) or to 5-ASA itself (olsalazine), coating with a pH-sensitive polymer, packaging of 5-ASA in microspheres, or a combination of these. The azo bonds are broken down by colonic bacteria to release 5-ASA within the colon.

The mode of action of 5-ASA in IBD is unknown, although it may involve the intracellular peroxisome proliferator-activated receptor (PPAR)-γ signalling pathway. The aminosalicylates have been shown to be effective in inducing remission in mild to moderately active disease, and maintaining remission in all forms of disease. There is also evidence that they are chemopreventive for UC-associated colorectal cancer. 5-ASA can rarely cause renal disease.

Proctitis

Rectal 5-ASA suppositories are the first-line treatment. Topical steroids are less effective than 5-ASA preparations. Oral 5-ASA can be added to increase remission rates. Some cases of proctitis do not respond to 5-ASA treatment and require oral prednisolone.

Left-sided colitis

Topical 5-ASA enemas are the first-line treatment. The addition of an oral 5-ASA will increase remission rates. Patients who do not respond to this or have worsening symptoms require oral prednisolone.

Extensive colitis

Patients with mild to moderate symptoms can be treated with an oral 5-ASA at an adequate dose. The additional of a 5-ASA enema increases remission rates. Patients who do not respond to this or have worsening symptoms require oral prednisolone.

Refractory/severe colitis of any extent

Patients with colitis that is refractory to standard conventional therapies should be investigated to ensure adherence to therapy, confirm active colitis and exclude infection, including biopsies to exclude reactivation of CMV colitis. *They should then receive biological therapy with either an anti-TNF agent (infliximab, adalimumab or golimumab) or an anti-integrin therapy (vedolizumab), or tofacitinib, an oral inhibitor of Janus kinase 1-3, which became available in 2018 for the treatment of adults with moderately to severely active UC.*

Patients with severe colitis (see **Box 32.41**) and those who do not respond to oral prednisolone should be admitted to hospital and treated initially with hydrocortisone 100 mg i.v. 6-hourly, with s.c. low-molecular-weight heparin to prevent thromboembolism. Investigations to confirm the diagnosis and exclude enteric infection (see above) should be performed and full supportive therapy administered (intravenous fluids, and nutritional support via the enteral route if required). The incidence of concomitant *C. difficile* infection in patients admitted for severe colitis is increasing. This is associated with a significant increase in morbidity and must be excluded. The clinical status of patients should be monitored daily (fever, tachycardia, stool frequency), and daily FBC, CRP, and urea and electrolytes should be performed. Repeat abdominal X-rays are required if patients are not improving. Success or failure of medical treatment of a severe attack of UC must be judged by an experienced gastroenterologist and colorectal surgeon. If patients have not responded to intravenous steroids within 3 days, either salvage medical therapy or surgery is required. If patients respond to intravenous steroids, they should be switched to oral prednisolone after approximately 5 days, which they can be weaned off over 8–10 weeks. All patients who have been admitted for severe colitis should commence long-term maintenance therapy with a thiopurine (azathioprine/mercaptopurine).

Salvage therapy

Salvage therapy to avoid colectomy is required for patients with a CRP higher than 45 mg/L or more than eight bowel motions after 3 days of intravenous hydrocortisone. Continuing steroid therapy alone in this situation will delay the inevitable colectomy and increase mortality. Salvage medical therapies with clear evidence of benefit in controlled clinical trials are intravenous ciclosporin 2 mg/kg per day as a continuous infusion or infliximab induction and maintenance therapy. Patients with extensive ulceration may require higher doses of induction infliximab. Patients with a low albumin level have been shown to have a lower response rate to salvage therapy. These agents should only be used by experienced gastroenterologists who are part of a multidisciplinary team with colorectal surgeons. Patients should be weaned off steroids rapidly, once salvage therapy has commenced, to reduce morbidity. Those who respond should be treated with oral ciclosporin or further infliximab infusions, as appropriate, while maintenance thiopurine therapy is commenced.

Novel therapies

Alicaforsen is an inhibitor of intracellular adhesion molecule-1. Alicaforsen enemas have demonstrated efficacy in the treatment of distal ulcerative colitis as well as pouchitis in clinical trials. An autologous stem cell transplantation trial in refractory Crohn's disease – low intensity therapy evaluation (ASTIClite) is currently underway. It is looking to assess whether stem cell transplantation, with a low intensity treatment regimen, can reduce the symptoms and activity of Crohn's disease and enhance quality of life, compared to current standard care. The trial will also assess the safety of the procedure, explore the mechanisms involved in immune reconstitution and whether patients who do experience recurrent disease after the stem cell transplant will respond to treatments that had not worked previously. Finally, the trial aims to assess the long-term safety and efficacy in patients undergoing stem cell transplantation over a minimum of a further 4 years.

Surgical management of ulcerative colitis

While the treatment of UC remains primarily medical, surgery continues to have a central role because it may be life-saving, is curative and eliminates the long-term risk of cancer. The main indications for surgery are severe colitis that fails to respond to medical therapy, and chronic active therapy-refractory disease. Other indications are listed in **Box 32.42**. In expert centres, laparoscopic surgery is often used to improve postoperative pain, recovery time and cosmesis.

---

i | **Box 32.42 Indications for surgery in ulcerative colitis**

Fulminant acute attack	Chronic disease
• Failure of medical treatment	• Incomplete response to medical treatment/steroid-dependent
• Toxic dilation	
• Haemorrhage	• Dysplasia on surveillance colonoscopy
• Imminent perforation	

In acute disease, subtotal colectomy with end ileostomy and preservation of the rectum is the operation of choice. At a later date, a number of surgical options are available and are best carried out in a specialist colorectal centre. These include proctectomy with a permanent ileostomy; to avoid a permanent ileostomy, an ileo-anal pouch procedure can be performed (**Fig. 32.43**). The ileo-anal pouch is anastomosed to the anus at the dentate line following excision of the remaining rectum. One-third of patients, however, will experience '***pouchitis***', inflammation of the pouch mucosa with clinical symptoms of diarrhoea, bleeding, fever and, at times, exacerbation of extracolonic manifestations (**Fig. 32.44**). The incidence of pouchitis is twice as high in patients with primary sclerosing cholangitis and is also raised in patients with a positive ANCA and backwash ileitis prior to colectomy. Two-thirds of pouchitis cases will recur as either acute relapsing or chronic unremitting forms. The mainstay of treatment is antibiotics (metronidazole with or without ciprofloxacin). Treatment is not always satisfactory and steroids may be required. The probiotic VSL#3 has been shown to be effective in preventing the onset of pouchitis and in maintaining remission in patients with antibiotic-treated pouchitis to induce mucosal healing.

Course and prognosis

One-third of patients with distal inflammatory proctitis due to UC will develop more proximal disease, with 5–10% developing total colitis. One-third of patients with UC will have a single attack and the others will follow a relapsing course. One-third of patients with UC will undergo colectomy within 20 years of diagnosis.

Cancer in inflammatory bowel disease

Patients with UC and extensive Crohn's colitis have an increased incidence of developing dysplasia and subsequent colon cancer. The risk of dysplasia is related to the extent and duration of disease, as well as the presence of untreated mucosal inflammation. A family history of colorectal cancer and the presence of primary sclerosing cholangitis also increase the risk. Appropriate colonoscopic screening strategies according to guidelines are used by many, although evidence for overall benefit is still uncertain. A 40-year analysis of colonoscopy surveillance for neoplasia in UC, conducted at St Mark's Hospital in the UK, suggested that surveillance may have a significant role in reducing the risk of advanced and interval colorectal cancer.

Mortality in inflammatory bowel disease

Population-based studies demonstrate that mortality in UC is similar to that in the general population. The two exceptions are patients with severe colitis, who have a slightly higher mortality in the first year after diagnosis, and patients aged over 60 at the time of diagnosis. Although it is currently unclear whether there is a slightly higher overall mortality in patients with CD, those with extensive jejunal and ileal disease and those with gastric and duodenal disease have been shown to have a relatively higher mortality.

Microscopic colitis

Patients with this group of disorders present with chronic or fluctuating watery diarrhoea. Although the macroscopic features on colonoscopy are normal, the histopathological findings on biopsy are abnormal. There are three distinct forms of microscopic inflammatory colitis:

- ***Microscopic UC.*** There is a chronic inflammatory cell infiltrate in the lamina propria, with deformed crypt architecture and goblet cell depletion, with or without crypt abscesses. Treatment is as for UC; many patients respond to treatment with aminosalicylates alone.
- ***Microscopic lymphocytic colitis.*** There is surface epithelial injury, prominent lymphocytic infiltration in the surface epithelium and increased lamina propria mononuclear cells.
- ***Microscopic collagenous colitis.*** There is a thickened subepithelial collagen layer (>10 μm) adjacent to the basal membrane, and increased infiltration of the lamina propria with lymphocytes and plasma cells, and surface epithelial cell damage. It is

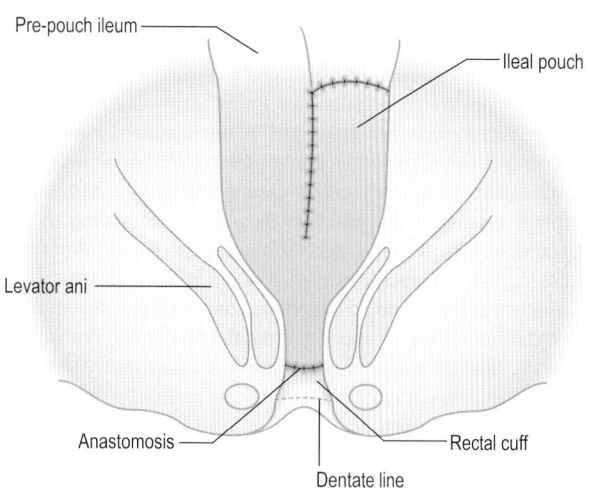

Fig. 32.43 An ileo-anal pouch for ulcerative colitis.

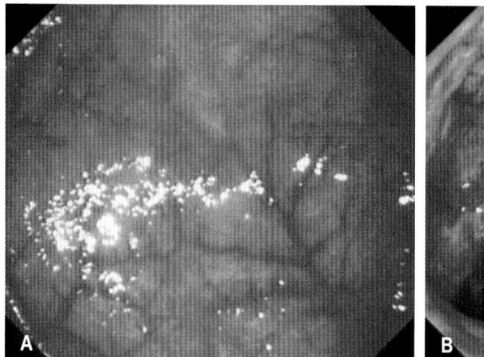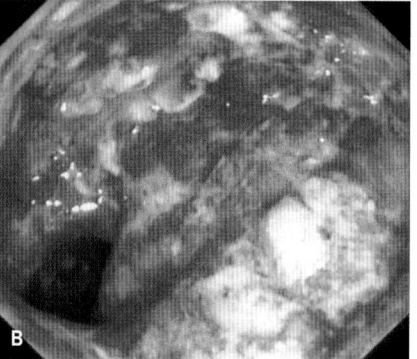

Fig. 32.44 Pouchitis: fibreoptic sigmoidoscopic appearances. **(A)** Mild changes. **(B)** Severe haemorrhagic ulceration.

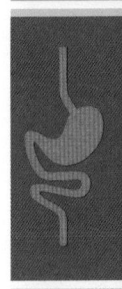
predominantly a disorder of middle-aged or elderly females, and is associated with a variety of autoimmune disorders (arthritis, thyroid disease, limited cutaneous scleroderma and primary biliary cirrhosis).

The incidence of both microscopic lymphocytic and collagenous colitis is increased in patients with coeliac disease and this must be excluded. Treatment of microscopic and collagenous colitis is usually with budesonide. There is also evidence of benefit for aminosalicylates, bismuth-containing preparations and, if refractory, prednisolone and azathioprine. A small number of patients with microscopic lymphocytic and collagenous colitis have coexisting bile acid malabsorption and can thus respond to cholestyramine. Prognosis is good.

Further reading

Ananthakrishnan AN. Epidemiology and risk factors for IBD. *Nat Rev Gastroenterol Hepatol* 2015; 12:205–217.

Choi CH, Rutter MD, Askara A et al. Forty-year analysis of colonoscopic surveillance programme for neoplasia in ulcerative colitis: an updated overview. *Am J Gastroenterol* 2015; 110:1022–1034.

Ek WE, D'Amato M, Halfvarson J. The history of genetics in inflammatory bowel disease. *Ann Gastroenterol* 2014; 27:294–303.

Feagan BG, Sandborn WJ, Gasink C et al. Ustekinumab as Induction and Maintenance Therapy for Crohn's Disease. *N Eng J Med* 2016; 375:1945–1960.

Lamb CA, Kennedy NA, Raine T et al. British Society of Gastroenterology consensus guidelines on the management of inflammatory bowel disease in adults. *Gut* 2019; 0:1–106.

Monteleone G, Neurath MF, Ardizzone S. Mongersen, an oral *SMAD7* antisense oligonucleotide, and Crohn's disease. *N Engl J Med* 2015; 372: 1104–1113.

Ungaro R, Mehandru S, Allen PB et al. Ulcerative colitis. *Lancet* 2016; 389;1756–1770.

COLON AND RECTUM

Constipation

'Constipation' is a very common symptom, particularly in women and the elderly. A consensus definition used in research (the Rome IV criteria) defines constipation as having two or more of the following for at least 3 months:

- infrequent passage of stools (<3/week),
- straining >25% of time,
- passage of hard stools (Bristol stool chart form 1–2) in >25% defecations
- incomplete evacuation and sensation of anorectal blockage in >25% defecations
- manual manoeuvres to facilitate >25% defecations (digital evacuation, support of the pelvic floor).

Other symptoms include abdominal bloating and/or discomfort (undistinguishable from the irritable bowel syndrome), as well as local and perianal pain. The causes of constipation are shown in **Box 32.43**.

Diagnosis

This relies on the history. When there has been a recent change in bowel habit in association with other significant symptoms (e.g. rectal bleeding), a colonoscopy or CT of the pneumocolon is indicated. By these means, gastrointestinal causes, such as colorectal cancer and narrowed segments due to diverticular disease, can be excluded.

Constipation can be classified into three broad categories but there is much overlap:

- normal transit through the colon (59%)
- defecatory disorders (25%)

- slow transit (13%).
Defecatory disorders with slow transit can occur together (3%).

Normal-transit constipation

In normal-transit constipation, stool traverses the colon at a normal rate, the stool frequency is normal and yet patients believe they are constipated. This is likely to be due to perceived difficulties of evacuation or the passage of hard stools. Patients may complain of abdominal pain or bloating. Normal-transit constipation can be distinguished from slow-transit constipation by undertaking marker studies of colonic transit. Capsules containing 20 radio-opaque shapes are swallowed on days 1, 2 and 3 and an abdominal X-ray obtained 120 hours after ingestion of the first capsule. Each capsule contains shapes of different configuration and the presence of more than 4 shapes from the first capsule, 6 from the second and 12 from the third denotes moderate to severe slow transit (**Fig. 32.45**).

Defecatory disorders

A 'paradoxical' contraction, rather than the normal relaxation of puborectalis and the external anal sphincter and associated muscles during straining, may prevent evacuation (pelvic floor dyssynergia, anismus). These are mainly due to dysfunction of the anal sphincter and pelvic floor. An anterior rectocele is a common problem where there is a weakness of the rectovaginal septum, resulting in protuberance of the anterior wall of the rectum with trapping of stool if the diameter is more than 3 cm. In some patients, the mucosa of the anterior rectal wall prolapses downwards during straining (see p. 1214), impeding the passage of stool, while in others there may be a higher mucosal intussusception.

In some patients, the rectum can become unduly sensitive to the presence of small volumes of stool, resulting in the urge to pass frequent amounts of small-volume stool and the sensation of incomplete evacuation.

The defecatory disorders can often be characterized by performing evacuation proctography and tests of anorectal physiology.

? Box 32.43 Causes of constipation

General
- Inadequate fibre intake
- Immobility

Metabolic/endocrine
- Diabetes mellitus
- Hypercalcaemia
- Hypothyroidism
- Porphyria

Functional
- Irritable bowel syndrome
- Idiopathic slow transit

Drugs
- Opiates
- Antimuscarinics
- Calcium-channel blockers, e.g. verapamil
- Antidepressants, e.g. tricyclics
- Iron

Neurological
- Spinal cord lesions
- Parkinson's disease

Psychological
- Depression
- Anorexia nervosa
- Repressed urge to defecate

Gastrointestinal disease
- Intestinal obstruction and pseudo-obstruction
- Colonic disease, e.g. carcinoma, diverticular disease
- Aganglionosis, e.g. Hirschsprung's disease, Chagas' disease
- Painful anal conditions, e.g. anal fissure

Defecatory disorders
- Rectal prolapse, mucosal prolapse intussusception and solitary rectal ulcer syndrome
- Large rectocele
- Pelvic floor dyssynergia/anismus
- Megarectum

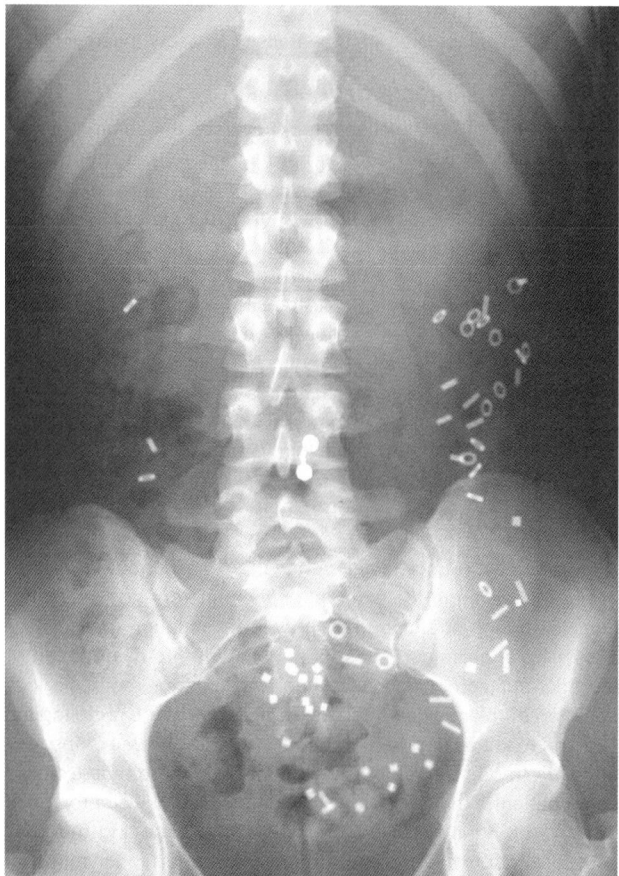

Fig. 32.45 Slow-transit constipation. Frontal abdominal X-ray taken on day 6 after ingestion of capsules, each containing 20 radio-opaque shapes, which were administered daily on days 1, 2 and 3. All the markers are retained, confirming the diagnosis of severe slow-transit constipation.

Slow-transit constipation

Slow-transit constipation occurs predominantly in young women who have infrequent bowel movements (usually less than once a week). The condition often starts at puberty and the symptoms include an infrequent urge to defecate, bloating, abdominal pain and discomfort. Some patients with severe slow-transit constipation have delayed emptying of the proximal colon and others a failure of 'meal-stimulated' colonic motility. Histopathological abnormalities have been demonstrated in the colons of some patients with severe slow-transit constipation, and some patients have coexisting disorders of small intestinal motility, consistent with a diagnosis of chronic idiopathic intestinal pseudo-obstruction (see p. 1223).

Management

Any underlying cause should be treated. In patients with normal and slow-transit constipation, the main focus should be directed towards increasing the fibre content of the diet in conjunction with increasing fluid intake.

The use of laxatives should be restricted to cases where symptoms impact on the patient's quality of life. The types of laxatives available are listed in **Box 32.44**. *Osmotic laxatives* act by increasing the colonic inflow of fluid and electrolytes; this acts not only to soften the stool but also to stimulate colonic contractility. The *polyethylene glycols (macrogols)* have the advantage over the

> **Box 32.44 Laxatives and enemas**
>
> **Bulk-forming laxatives**
> - Dietary fibre
> - Wheat bran
> - Methylcellulose
> - Mucilaginous gums – sterculia
> - Mucilaginous seeds and seed coats, e.g. ispaghula husk
>
> **Stimulant laxatives**
> (Stimulate motility and intestinal secretion)
> - Phenolphthalein
> - Bisacodyl
> - Anthraquinones – senna and dantron (only for the terminally ill)
> - Docusate sodium
> - Methylnaltrexone (for opioid-induced constipation)
> - Lubiprostone
> - Prucalopride
> - Linaclotide
> - Sodium picosulfate
>
> **Osmotic laxatives**
> - Magnesium sulphate
> - Lactulose
> - Macrogols
>
> **Suppositories**
> - Bisacodyl
> - Glycerol
>
> **Enemas**
> - Arachis oil
> - Docusate sodium
> - Hypertonic phosphate
> - Sodium citrate

synthetic disaccharide lactulose in that they are not fermented anaerobically in the colon to gas that can distend the colon and cause pain. The osmotic laxatives are preferred to the stimulatory laxatives, which act by stimulating colonic contractility and by causing intestinal secretion. *Prucalopride* is a high-affinity 5-HT$_4$ agonist that increases colonic transit and is an effective therapy for refractory constipation.

Linaclotide, a minimally absorbed peptide agonist of guanylate cyclase-C receptor, works by activating the cystic fibrosis transmembrane conductance regulator to stimulate chloride secretion and increase gastrointestinal fluid secretion. Significant benefit over placebo has been shown in clinical trials. *Lubiprostone* is an orally active agonist for type 2 chloride channels and therefore also increases gastrointestinal fluid secretion.

Patients with defecatory disorders should be referred to a specialist centre, as surgery may be indicated: for example, for anterior rectocele or internal anal mucosal intussusception. Anterior mucosal prolapse can be treated by injection, and those with pelvic floor dyssynergia (anismus) can benefit from biofeedback therapy.

Miscellaneous colonic conditions

Clostridium difficile-associated diarrhoea and pseudomembranous colitis

Clostridium difficile infection (CDI) is a common hospital-acquired infection and can be a significant cause of morbidity, especially amongst the elderly. It frequently occurs following antibiotic therapy due to disruption of the normal gut flora. The following antibiotics are particularly associated with CDI:

- fluoroquinolones
- clindamycin
- cephalosporins
- penicillins
- (macrolides and co-trimoxazole are less frequently associated).

Clinical features include profuse diarrhoea, which can lead to hypovolaemia and shock if severe. The white blood cell count is often significantly elevated and endoscopically there may be pseudomembranous colitis (severe inflammation of the bowel wall lining). Complications include ileus, toxic megacolon and bowel perforation. If megacolon or perforation is suspected then patients should have urgent imaging (X-ray or CT).

Diagnosis is made with a positive test for *C. difficile* toxin A and B. A positive test for glutamate dehydrogenase (GDH) antigen is not necessarily indicative of active infection, simply that the patient is a carrier of the pathogen.

Treatment

Initial treatment regimens are covered on page 1186. For recurrent or refractory CDI, antibiotics such as rifaximin or fidaxomicin can be useful. However, recently faecal microbiota transplantation (FMT) has become increasingly common. For this procedure, a solution of donor stool is given to the patient either through a nasogastric tube or via flexible sigmoidoscopy. The donor stool has been carefully selected from a centralized stool bank where all donors have had their blood and stool extensively screened for infection.

Megacolon

The term 'megacolon' is used to describe a number of congenital and acquired conditions in which the colon is dilated. In many instances, it is secondary to chronic constipation; in some parts of the world, Chagas' disease is a common cause.

In all young patients with megacolon, Hirschsprung's disease should be excluded. In this condition, which presents in the first years of life, an aganglionic segment of the rectum (megarectum) gives rise to constipation and subacute obstruction. Occasionally, Hirschsprung's disease affecting only a short segment of the rectum can be missed in childhood. A preliminary rectal biopsy is performed and stained for ganglion cells in the submucosal plexus. In doubtful cases, a full-thickness biopsy should be obtained. A frozen section is stained for acetylcholinesterase, which is elevated in Hirschsprung's disease. Manometric studies show failure of relaxation of the internal sphincter, which is diagnostic of Hirschsprung's disease. This condition can be successfully treated surgically.

Treatment of other causes of a megacolon is similar to that of slow-transit constipation, but saline washouts and manual removal of faeces are sometimes required.

Faecal incontinence

Of the healthy population over the age of 65, 7% experience a degree of incontinence. Incontinence is classified as minor (inability to control flatus or liquid stool, causing soiling) or major (frequent and inadvertent evacuation of stool of normal consistency); see **Box 32.45** for common causes. Obstetric injury is a common cause and sphincter defects have been found in up to 30% of primiparous women. Endoanal ultrasonography or pelvic MRI is the investigation of choice in the assessment of anal sphincter damage (**Fig. 32.46**). Neurophysiological investigation of pudendal nerve function, anal sensation and anal sphincter function may be required to elicit the cause of the problem.

Initial ***management*** of minor incontinence is bowel habit regulation. Loperamide is the most potent antidiarrhoeal agent, which also increases internal sphincter tone.

Biofeedback is effective in some people with faecal incontinence associated with impaired function of the puborectalis muscle and the external anal sphincter. Sacral spinal nerve stimulation has been shown to be effective in the treatment of patients with a functionally deficient but morphologically intact external anal sphincter. Surgery may be required for anal sphincter trauma and should only be carried out in specialist centres.

> **?** **Box 32.45 Aetiology of faecal incontinence**
>
> - Congenital:
>   - e.g. surgery for imperforate anus
> - Anal sphincter dysfunction:
>   - Structural damage: surgery – anorectal, vaginal hysterectomy; obstetric injury during childbirth; trauma; radiation; perianal Crohn's disease
>   - Pudendal nerve damage: childbirth
>   - Perineal descent: prolonged straining at stool
> - Rectal prolapse
> - Faecal impaction with overflow diarrhoea
> - Severe diarrhoea:
>   - e.g. ulcerative colitis, functional diarrhoea, irritable bowel syndrome
> - Neurological and psychological disorders:
>   - Spinal trauma (S2–S4)
>   - Spina bifida
>   - Stroke
>   - Multiple sclerosis
>   - Diabetes mellitus (with autonomic involvement)
>   - Dementia
>   - Psychological illness

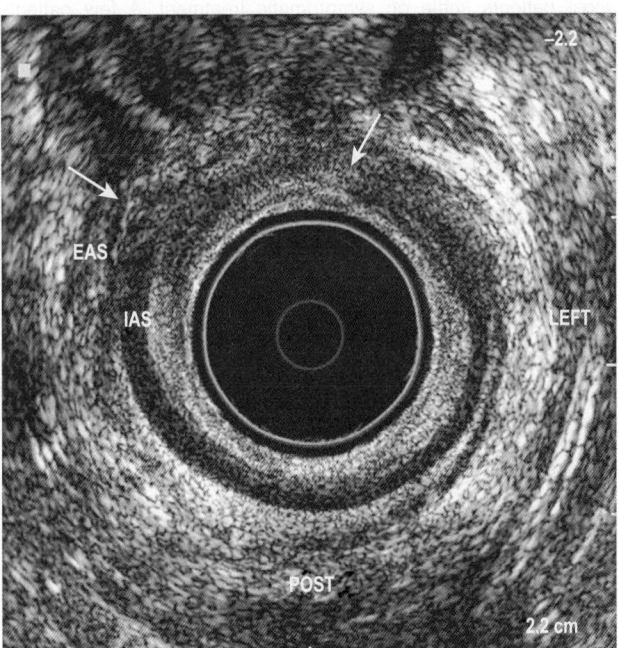

Fig. 32.46 Endoanal ultrasound scan. Axial mid-canal image, showing a large tear between 10 and 1 o'clock (arrowed) following vaginal delivery, involving the external anal sphincter (EAS) and internal anal sphincter (IAS), resulting in faecal incontinence. *(Courtesy of Professor Clive Bartram, Princess Grace Hospital, London.)*

Ischaemic disease of the colon (ischaemic colitis)

Occlusion of branches of the superior mesenteric artery (SMA) or inferior mesenteric artery (IMA), often in the older age group, commonly presents with sudden onset of abdominal pain and the passage of bright red blood *per rectum*, with or without diarrhoea. There may be signs of shock and evidence of underlying cardiovascular disease. The anatomy of the vascular supply to the colon results in a watershed area at the splenic flexure, which is therefore the most common site affected. This condition has also been described in women taking the contraceptive pill, patients on nicorandil, and those with thrombophilia and small- or medium-vessel vasculitis.

Examination

On examination, the abdomen may be distended and tender. A straight abdominal X-ray often shows thumb-printing (a characteristic sign of ischaemic disease) at the splenic flexure. Patients are likely to display signs of cardiovascular shock and may have a lactic acidosis.

Differential diagnosis and investigations

The differential diagnosis includes other causes of acute colitis. Patients often require an urgent CT scan to exclude perforation. An unprepared flexible sigmoidoscopy is the diagnostic investigation of choice; biopsies showing epithelial cell apoptosis and lamina propria fibrosis are characteristic. A colonoscopy should be performed when the patient has fully recovered to exclude the formation of a stricture at the site of disease and confirm mucosal healing. Patients without evidence of underlying cardiovascular disease should be screened for thrombophilia and vasculitis.

Management

Most patients settle on symptomatic treatment. A few patients show progressive signs of peritonism and imminent perforation, and require urgent surgery.

Diverticular disease

Diverticula are frequently found in the colon and occur in 50% of patients over the age of 50 years. They are most frequent in the sigmoid, but can be present throughout the whole colon.

Terminology:

- *diverticulosis* indicates the presence of diverticula
- *diverticulitis* implies that these diverticula are inflamed
- *diverticular colitis* refers to crescentic inflammation on the folds in areas of diverticulosis.

It is perhaps better to use the more general term *diverticular disease*, as it is often difficult to be sure whether the diverticula are inflamed. The precise mechanism of diverticula formation is not known. There is thickening of the muscle layer and, because of high intraluminal pressures, pouches of mucosa extrude through the muscular wall through weakened areas near blood vessels to form diverticula. An alternative explanation is cholinergic denervation with increasing age, which leads to hypersensitivity and increased uncoordinated muscular contraction. Diverticular disease seems to be related to the low-fibre diet eaten in developed countries and is rare in rural Africa.

Diverticulitis occurs when faeces obstruct the neck of the diverticulum, causing stagnation and allowing bacteria to multiply and produce inflammation. This can then lead to bowel perforation (peridiverticulitis), abscess formation, fistulae into adjacent organs, haemorrhage and even generalized peritonitis.

Clinical features and investigations

Diverticular disease is asymptomatic in 95% of cases and is usually discovered incidentally on colonoscopy or barium enema examination. No treatment other than advice to increase dietary fibre is required in those patients. In symptomatic patients, intermittent left iliac fossa pain or discomfort and an erratic bowel habit commonly occur, which are difficult to differentiate from the irritable bowel syndrome. In severe disease, luminal narrowing results in severe pain and constipation. In the absence of clinical signs of acute diverticulitis, a colonoscopy or 'virtual colonoscopy' (see p. 1159) is the investigation of choice (**Fig. 32.47**). Barium enema combined with flexible sigmoidoscopy is also used.

Management

Management of uncomplicated symptomatic disease is with a well-balanced (soluble and insoluble) fibre diet (20 g/day), with smooth muscle relaxants if required. Antibiotics and admission to hospital are not required for uncomplicated disease.

Acute diverticulitis

The pathophysiology of diverticulitis is associated with altered gut motility, increased luminal pressure and a disordered colonic microenvironment. Acute diverticulitis most commonly affects diverticula in the sigmoid colon. It presents with severe pain in the left iliac fossa, often accompanied by fever and constipation. These symptoms and signs are similar to those of appendicitis but are located on the left side. On examination, the patient is often febrile with a tachycardia. *Abdominal examination* shows tenderness, guarding and rigidity on the left side of the abdomen. A palpable tender mass is sometimes felt in the left iliac fossa.

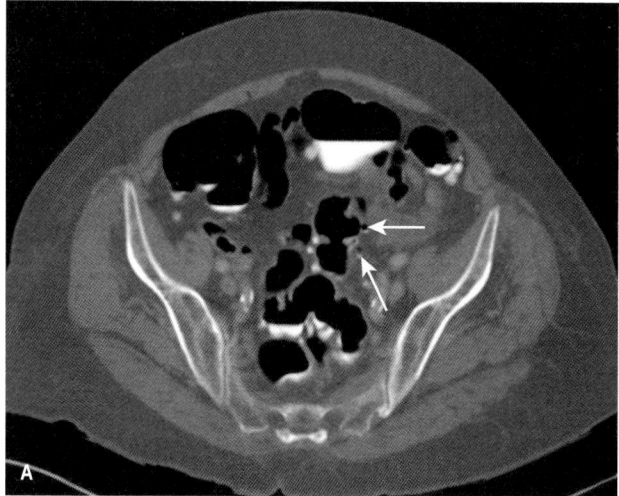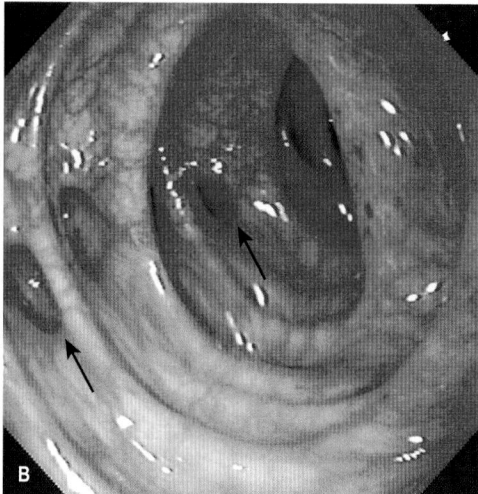

Fig. 32.47 Diverticular disease. **(A)** Axial CT colonography image demonstrating diverticular disease (diverticulosis) of the sigmoid colon (arrows). **(B)** Diverticula (arrowed) seen on colonoscopy.

Investigations

- **Blood tests** often reveal a polymorphonuclear leucocytosis. The ESR and CRP are raised.
- **CT colonography** (**Fig. 32.48**) will show colonic wall thickening, diverticula and often pericolic collections and abscesses. There is usually a streaky increased density extending into the immediate pericolic fat with thickening of the pelvic fascial planes. These findings are diagnostic of acute diverticulitis (95% sensitivity and specificity) and differ from those of malignant disease. Sigmoidoscopy and colonoscopy are not performed during an acute attack.
- **Ultrasound examination** is often more readily available and is cheaper. It can demonstrate thickened bowel and large pericolic collections, but is less sensitive than CT.

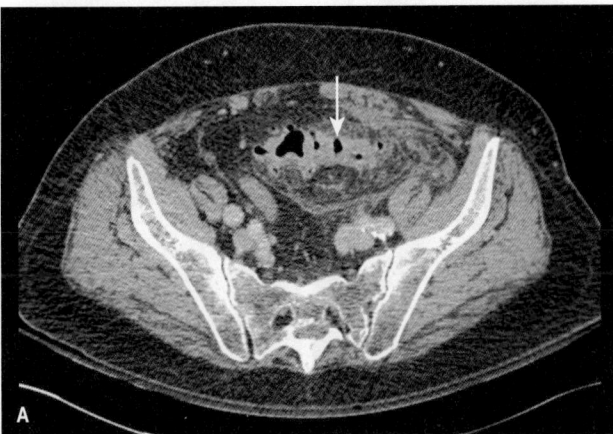

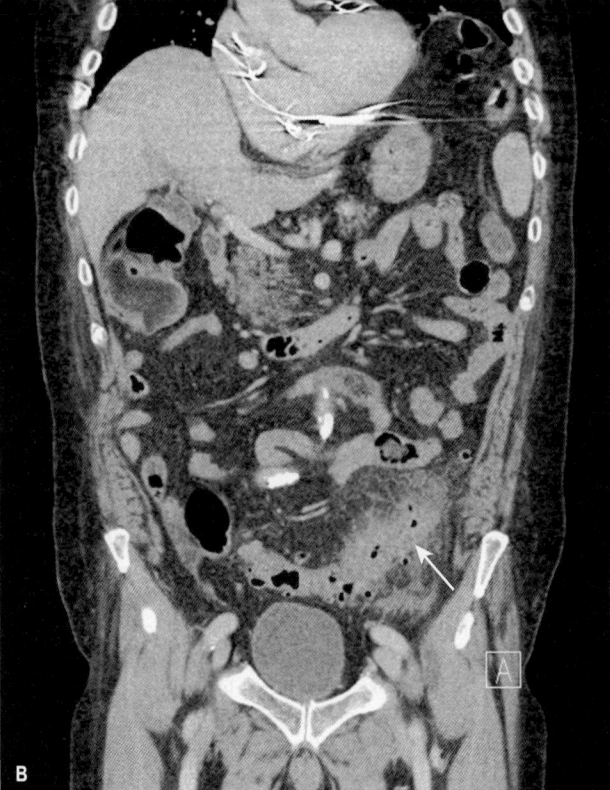

Fig. 32.48 CT colonography. Axial (**A**) and coronal (**B**) CT images demonstrate bowel wall thickening involving the sigmoid colon at the site of diverticular disease and inflammation of the adjacent mesenteric fat consistent with acute diverticulitis (arrow).

Management

Mild attacks can be treated on an outpatient basis using oral antibiotics such as ciprofloxacin and metronidazole. Patients with signs of systemic upset (fevers, tachycardia), significant abdominal pain or co-morbidity require bowel rest, intravenous fluids and intravenous antibiotic therapy. Recent large trials of 5-ASA therapy have shown minor benefit in preventing recurrent diverticulitis. Repeat attacks often require surgery.

Complications of diverticular disease

- **Perforation** usually occurs in association with acute diverticulitis, and can lead to formation of a paracolic or pelvic abscess or generalized peritonitis. Surgery may be required.
- **Fistula formation** into the bladder, causing dysuria or pneumaturia, or into the vagina, causing discharge.
- **Intestinal obstruction** (see p. 1222), usually after repeated episodes of acute diverticulitis.
- **Bleeding** is sometimes massive. In most cases, the bleeding stops and the cause of the bleeding can be established by colonoscopy and sometimes angiography. In rare cases, emergency segmental colectomy is required.
- **Mucosal inflammation** occurs in areas of diverticula, giving the appearance of a segmental colitis at endoscopy that may resemble Crohn's disease.

Anorectal disorders

Pruritus ani

Pruritus ani, or an itchy bottom, is common. Perianal excoriation results from scratching. Usually, the condition results from haemorrhoids or overactivity of sweat glands. **Management** consists of enhancing toilet hygiene, keeping the area dry and avoiding the use of perfumed moisturizing creams. Secondary causes include threadworm (*Enterobius vermicularis*) infestation, fungal infections (e.g. candidiasis) and perianal eczema, which should be treated appropriately.

Haemorrhoids

Haemorrhoids (primary – internal; second degree – prolapsing; third degree – prolapsed) usually cause rectal bleeding, discomfort and pruritus ani. Patients may notice red blood on their toilet paper and blood on the outside of their stools. They are the most common cause of rectal bleeding (see **Fig. 32.31**). Diagnosis is made by inspection, rectal examination and proctoscopy.

Management

If symptoms are minor, no treatment is required apart from advice about avoiding constipation. Suppositories containing a local anaesthetic and corticosteroids are helpful. If symptoms are more severe, rubber band ligation or injection of a sclerosant can be used. Haemorrhoidal artery ligation operation (HALO) uses Doppler ultrasound to identify and ligate feeding arteries to the haemorrhoids and is being used more frequently in place of surgery.

Anal fissures

An anal fissure is a tear in the sensitive skin-lined lower anal canal distal to the dentate line, which produces pain on defecation. It can be an isolated primary problem in young to middle-aged adults or may occur in association with Crohn's disease or ulcerative colitis, in which case perianal abscesses and anal fistulae can complicate the fissure.

Diagnosis can usually be made on the history alone and confirmed on perianal inspection. Rectal examination is often not possible because of pain and sphincter spasm. The spasm not only causes pain but also impairs wound healing. In severe cases, proctoscopy and sigmoidoscopy should be performed under anaesthesia to exclude other anorectal disease. Initial treatment is with local anaesthetic gel and stool softeners. Use of 0.4% glyceryl trinitrate and 2% diltiazem ointments is of benefit. Botulinum toxin is used in chronic fissures but lateral subcutaneous internal sphincterotomy is also employed for severe cases.

Fistula in ano and anorectal abscesses

The anatomy of perianal fistulae may be simple or complex (**Fig. 32.49**). The fistulae usually present as abscesses and heal after the abscess is incised. In other cases, a small, discharging pilonidal sinus may be noted by the patient.

Endoanal ultrasonography, MRI and/or examination under anaesthetic are usually required to define the primary and any secondary tracks, exclude sepsis and detect any associated disease, such as Crohn's disease and tuberculosis. Management is with surgical incision and drainage with antibiotics.

Rectal prolapse, intussusception and solitary rectal ulcer syndrome

All these conditions are thought to be related, rectal prolapse being the unifying pathology. Some patients with solitary rectal ulcer syndrome (SRUS) do not have prolapse but strain excessively and ulcerate the anterior rectal wall, which is forced into the anus during attempts at defecation. Constipation and chronic straining may be precipitating causes. Patients commonly present with slight bleeding and mucus on defecation, tenesmus and a sensation of anal obstruction.

SRUS is commonly located on the anterior wall of the rectum within 13 cm of the anal verge, and is sometimes difficult to distinguish from cancer and Crohn's disease during endoscopic examination. SRUS has typical histological features of non-specific inflammatory changes with bands of smooth muscle extending into the lamina propria.

Asymptomatic SRUS should not be treated. Symptomatic patients should be advised to stop straining and measures should be taken to soften the stool. If rectal prolapse can be demonstrated during defecation, this should be repaired; in severe cases, surgical treatment by rectopexy may be indicated. Surgical treatment for complete rectal prolapse is also required.

Colonic tumours

Colon polyps and polyposis syndromes

A colonic polyp is an abnormal growth of tissue projecting from the colonic mucosa. Polyps range from a few millimetres to several centimetres in diameter and are single or multiple, pedunculated, sessile or 'flat' (**Fig. 32.50**).

Many histological types of polyp are found in the colon (**Box 32.46**). However, adenomas are the precursor lesions in most cases of colon cancer.

Classification of colorectal polyps

Classification is summarized in **Box 32.46**.

Sporadic adenomas

An adenoma is a benign, dysplastic tumour of columnar cells or glandular tissue. Adenomas have tubular, tubulovillous or villous

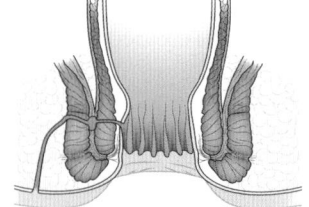 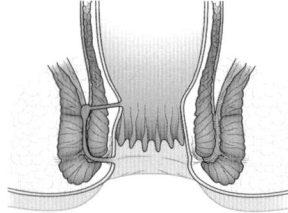

Transsphincteric fistula   Intersphincteric fistula

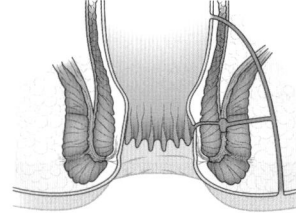 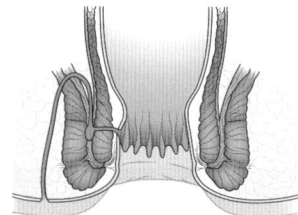

Extrasphincteric fistula   Suprasphincteric fistula

A

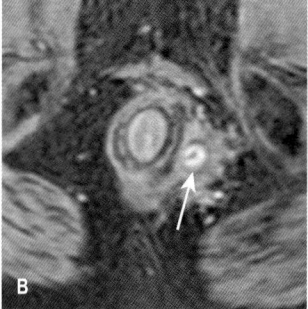 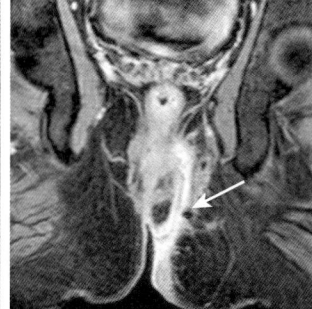

B

Fig. 32.49 Perianal fistulae. (A) Common sites. **(B)** Fistulae and sepsis in Crohn's disease (arrowed). An MRI of the pelvis showing a complex extrasphincteric horseshoe tract with extension to the ischio-anal fossae (right; arrowed).

morphology. The vast majority of adenomas are not inherited and are termed 'sporadic'. Although many sporadic adenomas do not become malignant in the patient's lifetime, they have a tendency to progress to cancer via increasing grades of dysplasia due to progressive accumulation of genetic changes (adenoma–carcinoma sequence). Factors favouring malignant transformation in colorectal polyps, and the relation between adenoma size and likelihood of cancer, are shown in **Box 32.47**.

The progression from benign polyp to cancer is shown in **Fig. 32.51**.

The likelihood of an adenoma being present increases with age; it is rare before the age of 30 years. By the age of 60–70, 5% of asymptomatic subjects will have a polyp equal to or longer than 1 cm, or cancer with no symptoms, and up to 50% will have at least one small (less than 1 cm) adenoma. Removal of polyps at colonoscopy and subsequent surveillance reduce the risk of development of colon cancer by approximately 80%. Techniques such as chromoscopy, using dye spray or narrow band imaging, are being used to assist in their detection (flat adenomas account for approximately 12% of all adenomas).

Polyps in the rectum and sigmoid often present with rectal bleeding. More proximal lesions rarely produce symptoms and most are diagnosed on barium enema, CT colonography or on colonoscopy performed for screening or for other reasons. Large

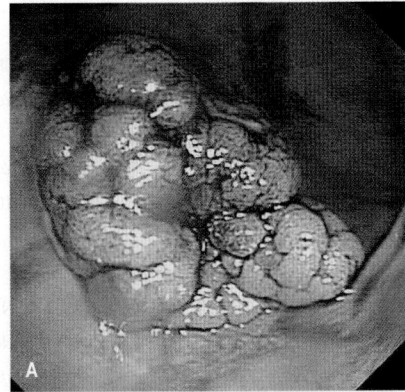

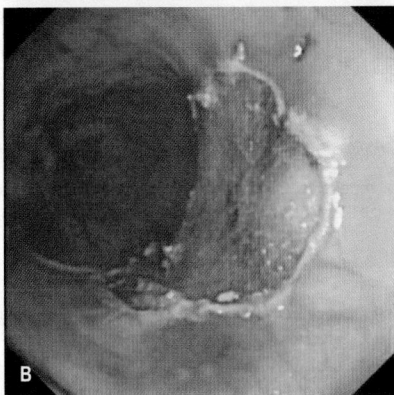

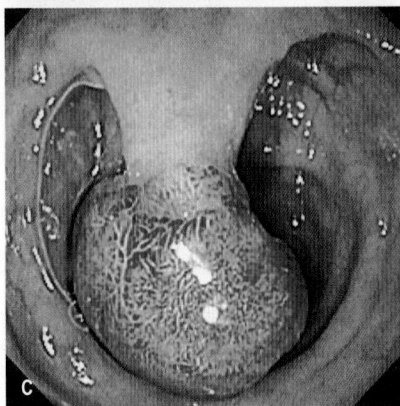

Fig. 32.50 Colonoscopic appearance of sessile and pedunculated polyps. **(A)** A sessile flat polyp with Indigo carmine. **(B)** Colon after resection of a sessile polyp. **(C)** A large pedunculated polyp.

villous adenomas can present with profuse diarrhoea with mucus and hypokalaemia.

Once a polyp has been found, it is almost always possible to remove it endoscopically. Surveillance guidelines dictate the frequency of repeat investigations:

- at 5 years, if 1 or 2 adenomas <1 cm are found
- at 3 years, if there are 3–4 small adenomas or at least 1 that is >1 cm
- at 1 year, if there are ≥5 small adenomas or there are ≥3, at least 1 of which is >1 cm.

If any doubt exists about the completeness of excision of any polyp, then an earlier repeat examination is suggested.

Sessile serrated adenomas

Serrated polyps form a heterogeneous group of colorectal lesions that includes the benign hyperplastic polyps (HPs), and the pre-malignant sessile serrated adenoma (SSA) and traditional serrated adenoma (TSA). They are characterized by the saw-tooth appearance of the crypt epithelium. It is now recognized that approximately 30% of colorectal cancers (particularly those in the right colon) originate from these lesions. Progression of serrated polyps is thought to occur via a distinct pathway from the adenoma–carcinoma sequence, with involvement of *BRAF* gene mutations and gene promoter hypermethylation (CpG island methylator phenotype, or CIMP; see p. 1217). Microsatellite instability can be detected in both the adenoma–carcinoma and the serrated pathways. Endoscopic resection of SSAs and TSAs with appropriate surveillance is recommended.

Inherited polyposis syndromes

About 5% of colorectal cancers have a well-defined single-gene basis.

Familial adenomatous polyposis

Familial adenomatous polyposis (FAP) is an autosomal dominant condition arising from germline mutations of the *APC* gene, located on chromosome 5q21–q22. More than 825 different mutations have been identified. Penetrance is virtually 100%. It is characterized by the presence of hundreds to thousands of colorectal and duodenal adenomas. The mean age of adenoma development is 16 years; the average age at which colorectal cancer develops is 39 years. Tracing and screening of relatives are essential, and affected individuals should be offered a prophylactic colectomy. Surgical options include colectomy and ileorectal anastomosis, which requires lifelong surveillance of the rectal stump, or a restorative proctocolectomy or pouch procedure with complete removal of rectal mucosa.

Cystic gland polyps, predominantly in the proximal stomach, and duodenal adenomas are frequently found in FAP, as well as other extraintestinal lesions such as osteomas, epidermoid cysts and desmoid tumours. The duodenal adenomas may progress to cancer and are the most common cause of death in colectomized patients with FAP. Congenital hypertrophy of the retinal pigment epithelium (CHRPE) occurs in many families with FAP. Other cancers in FAP include thyroid, pancreatic and hepatoblastomas.

APC gene mutations can be found in about 80% of families with FAP. Once the mutation has been identified in an index case, other family members can be tested for the mutation, and screening can then be directed at mutation carriers. If a mutation cannot be found in a known FAP case, all family members should undergo clinical screening with regular colonoscopy.

Attenuated FAP may be missed as it presents later (average age 44 years) and has fewer polyps (<100), which tend to occur on the right side of the colon rather than on the left. It may be indistinguishable from sporadic cases but the gene mutation is in the *APC* germline.

MYH-associated polyposis

MUT Y homologue-associated polyposis (MYH-AP) is an autosomal recessive inherited syndrome of multiple colorectal adenomas and cancer. *MYH* is a base-excision-repair gene that corrects oxidative DNA damage. MYH-AP may account for 7–8% of families with the FAP phenotype in whom *APC* mutations cannot be found. Subjects with multiple adenomas or an FAP phenotype without *APC* mutations and with a family history compatible with a recessive pattern of inheritance should be tested for MYH-AP.

Lynch syndrome

In Lynch syndrome (previously called hereditary non-polyposis colon cancer, HNPCC), polyps are formed in the colon and may

> *i* **Box 32.46 Classification of colorectal polyps and polyposis syndromes**

Histology	Polyposis syndrome	Defective gene	Inheritance	CRC risk
Hyperplastic	Hyperplastic polyposis	*BRAF*		Yes
Hamartoma	Juvenile polyposis	*MADH4* or *BMPR1A*	AD	10–70%
	Peutz–Jeghers syndrome	*STK11*	AD	Yes
	Cowden's syndrome	*PTEN*	AD	10%?
	Lhermitte–Duclos disorder	*PTEN*	AD	
	Bannayan–Riley–Ruvalcaba syndrome	*PTEN*	AD	
Inflammatory	None	None		No
Lymphoid	Benign lymphoid polyposis	Unknown		No
Adenoma	FAP	*APC*	AD	100%
	AFAP			Yes
	Gardner's syndrome			Yes
	Turcot's syndrome			Yes
	MYH-AP	*MYH-AP*	AR	
Adenoma	Lynch syndrome (HNPCC)	Mismatch repair genes (*MSH-2, MLH-1*)	AD	70–80%

AD, autosomal dominant; AFAP, attenuated FAP; APC, adenomatous polyposis coli; AR, autosomal recessive; CRC, colorectal cancer; FAP, familial adenomatous polyposis; HNPCC, hereditary non-polyposis colorectal cancer; MLH-1, MutL homologue 1; MSH-2, MutS homologue 2; MYH-AP, MUT Y homologue-associated polyposis; PTEN, phosphatase and tensin homologue.

> *i* **Box 32.47 Factors affecting risk of malignant change in an adenoma**

Factor	Higher risk	Lower risk
Size	>1.5 cm	<1 cm
Type	Sessile or flat	Pedunculated
Histology	Severe dysplasia	Mild dysplasia
	Villous architecture	Tubular architecture
	Squamous metaplasia	
Number	Multiple polyps	Single polyp

progress rapidly to colon cancer. It affects 1 : 5000 people, causing 3–10% of colorectal cancer cases.

The disease is caused by a mutation in one of the DNA mismatch repair genes, usually *hMSH2* or *hMLH1*, although others (*hMSH6, PMS1* and *PMS*) have been reported. Mismatch repair genes are responsible for maintaining the stability of DNA during replication. Inheritance is autosomal dominant. The defect in function of the mismatch repair mechanism causes naturally occurring, highly repeated, short DNA sequences known as microsatellites to be shorter or longer than normal, a phenomenon called microsatellite instability (MSI).

Onset of cancer is earlier than in sporadic cases, at age 40–50 or younger. Tumours have a predilection for the right colon, in contrast to sporadic cases. In contrast to FAP, the lifetime risk of colon cancer (penetrance of the gene) in mutation carriers is 70–80%. Other cancers are also more common in Lynch syndrome: stomach, small intestine, bladder, skin, brain and hepatobiliary system. Female patients are at risk for endometrial and ovarian cancer.

The diagnosis is made from the family history of colon cancer at a young age and the presence of associated cancers in the family. These are formalized in the various editions of the Amsterdam and the Bethesda criteria (**Box 32.48**).

Turcot's syndrome

This consists of FAP or Lynch syndrome (HNPCC) with brain tumours.

> *i* **Box 32.48 Diagnostic criteria for Lynch syndrome**
>
> **Modified Amsterdam criteria**
> - One individual diagnosed with CRC (or extracolonic Lynch tumours) before age 50 years
> - Two affected generations
> - Three affected relatives, one a first-degree relative of the other two
> - FAP excluded
> - Tumours verified by pathological examination
>
> **Bethesda guidelines**
> - CRC diagnosed in patient who is younger than 50 years
> - Presence of synchronous, metachronous CRC, or other Lynch tumours, irrespective of age
> - CRC with the MSI-H histology diagnosed in a patient who is younger than 60 years
> - CRC diagnosed in one or more first-degree relative with a Lynch-related tumour, with one of the cancers being diagnosed under the age 50 years
> - CRC diagnosed in two or more first- or second-degree relatives with Lynch-related tumours, irrespective of age
>
> CRC, colorectal cancer; MSI-H, microsatellite instability – high.

Gardner's syndrome

This involves, in addition to FAP, desmoid tumours, osteomas of the skull and other lesions.

Hamartomatous polyps

These are commonly large and stalked. The inherited syndromes show autosomal dominant inheritance and include:

- ***Juvenile polyps***, which occur mainly in children and teenagers, and are found mainly in the colon; histologically, they show mucus retention cysts. Most are sporadic, but a syndrome of juvenile polyposis is defined as: >3–5 juvenile colonic polyps, juvenile polyps throughout the gastrointestinal tract, or any number of polyps with a family history. This is an autosomal dominant condition and the relevant gene has been identified (see **Box 32.46**). The polyps are a cause of bleeding and intussusception in the first decade of life. There is also an increased risk of colonic cancer (relative risk (RR) of 34), and surveillance and removal of polyps must be undertaken.

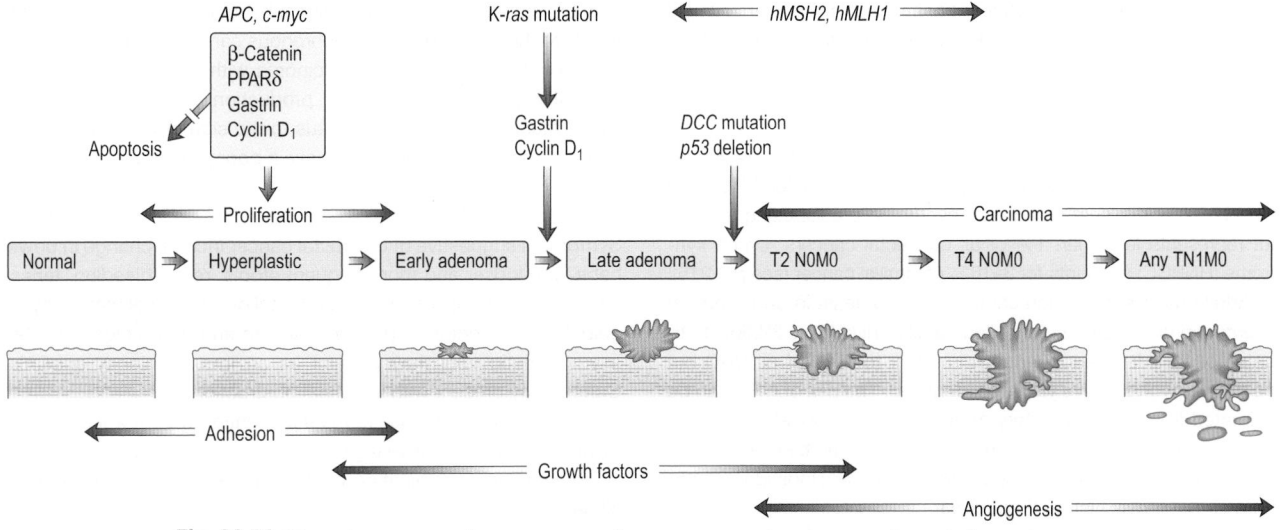

Fig. 32.51 The adenoma–carcinoma progression sequence, showing genetic mutations at different stages. APC, adenomatous polyposis coli; PPARδ, peroxisome proliferator-activated receptor delta.

- **Peutz–Jeghers syndrome** (see p. 1197).
- **PTEN hamartoma–tumour syndrome** (PHTS), which includes Cowden's syndrome, Bannayan–Riley–Ruvalcaba syndrome and all syndromes caused by germline phosphatase and tensin homologue (*PTEN*) mutations. Cowden's (multiple hamartoma) syndrome is associated with characteristic skin stigmata, and by intestinal polyps regarded as hamartomas but with a mixture of cell types. These patients have an increased risk of various extraintestinal malignancies (thyroid, breast, uterine and ovarian). These syndromes are uncommon and together account for less than 1% of colon cancer cases.

Colorectal carcinoma

Colorectal cancer (CRC) is the third most common cancer worldwide and the second most common cause of cancer death in the UK.

Each year approximately, 40 000 new cases are diagnosed in England and Wales (68% colon, 32% rectal cancer), and CRC is registered as the cause of death in about half this number. The prevalence rate per 100 000 (at all ages) is 53.5 for men and 36.7 for women. The incidence increases with age; the average age at diagnosis is 60–65 years. Approximately 20% of patients in the UK have distant metastases at diagnosis. The disease is much more common in Westernized countries than in Asia or Africa.

Factors related to risk of colorectal cancer are shown in **Box 32.49**.

Genetics

Most colorectal cancers develop as a result of progression from normal mucosa to adenoma to invasive cancer. This progression is controlled by the accumulation of abnormalities in a number of critical growth-regulating genes and can be divided into three main pathways:

- **Chromosomal instability (CIN).** CIN is the most common cause of conventional adenomas throughout the colon. This pathway involves the sequential accumulation of genetic mutations in tumour suppressor genes, usually initiated by a mutation in the gene encoding adenomatous polyposis coli (*APC*).

_i_ Box 32.49 Risk factors in colorectal cancer

Increased risk
- Increasing age
- Animal fat (saturated) and red meat consumption
- Sugar consumption
- Colorectal polyps
- Family history of colon cancer or colonic polyps
- Chronic inflammatory bowel disease
- Obesity (body and abdominal)
- Smoking
- Alcohol misuse
- Acromegaly
- Abdominal radiotherapy
- Ureterosigmoidostomy

Decreased risk
- Vegetable, garlic, milk, calcium consumption
- Exercise (colon only)
- Aspirin (including low-dose) and other NSAIDs

NSAIDs, non-steroidal anti-inflammatory drugs.

- **CpG island methylator phenotype.** CpG island methylator phenotype (CIMP) tumours arise via the serrated neoplasia pathway and have a marked predilection for the proximal colon. Following an initiating genetic mutation in the genes encoding *BRAF* or *KRAS*, these lesions progress via *epigenetic* silencing of tumour suppressor and mismatch repair (MMR) genes by promoter methylation (p. 1215). This pathway is epitomized by the serrated polyposis syndrome. The stepwise accumulation of genetic mutations in onco- and tumour suppressor genes that underpins the SCRC carcinogenesis pathway is well established and has significantly altered worldwide clinical practice. For example, mutations in KRAS appear to have importance as predictive factors for lack of response to certain oncological therapies. Activating KRAS mutations, which are identified in approximately 40–45% of CRCs, are associated with resistance to treatments that target the epidermal growth factor receptor (EGFR), such as cetuximab and panitumumab.
- **Microsatellite instability.** Microsatellite instability (MSI) tumours are also more commonly located in the proximal colon. They arise from defective DNA repair through inactivation of mismatch repair genes, epitomized by the germline mutation of MMR genes seen in Lynch syndrome (HNPCC).

This molecular classification can help to distinguish clinical characteristics, such as patient demographics, tumour distribution, response to therapy and prognosis.

Cancer families

A family history of CRC confers an increased risk to relatives. Family history is, next to age, the most common risk factor for CRC. FAP (**Fig. 32.52**) is the best-recognized syndrome predisposing to CRC but represents less than 1% of all colorectal cancers. Lynch syndrome (HNPCC) accounts for 3–10% of familial cancer (see p. 1215).

Additionally, some colon cancers arise, at least in part, from an inherited predisposition, so-called familial risk (**Box 32.50**). Estimates of their frequency range from 10% to 30% of all CRC but the genes involved have yet to be identified. The risk of CRC can be estimated from a family history matched with empirical risk tables, so that appropriate advice regarding screening can be offered.

Most CRCs are, however, sporadic and occur in individuals without a strong family history (**Fig. 32.53**).

Pathology

CRC, which usually takes the form of a polypoid mass with ulceration, spreads by direct infiltration through the bowel wall. It involves

lymphatics and blood vessels with subsequent spread, most commonly to the liver and lung. Synchronous cancers are present in 2% of cases. Histology is adenocarcinoma with variably differentiated glandular epithelium and mucin production. 'Signet ring' cells, in which mucin displaces the nucleus to the side of the cell, are relatively uncommon and generally have a poor prognosis.

Clinical features

Symptoms suggestive of colorectal cancer include change in bowel habit with looser and more frequent stools, rectal bleeding, tenesmus and symptoms of anaemia. A rectal or abdominal mass may be palpable. Cancers arising in the caecum and right colon are often asymptomatic until they present as an iron deficiency anaemia. Cancer may present with intestinal obstruction.

Patients aged over 35–40 years presenting with new large bowel symptoms should be investigated. Digital examination of the rectum is essential and examination of the colon should be performed in all cases.

Investigations

- **Colonoscopy** is the 'gold standard' for investigation and allows biopsy for histology. Biopsy of the tumour is mandatory, usually at endoscopy (**Fig. 32.54**).
- **Double-contrast barium enema** can visualize the large bowel but has now been superseded by CT colonography.
- **Endoanal ultrasound and pelvic MRI** are used for staging rectal cancer.
- **Chest, abdominal and pelvic CT** scanning evaluate tumour size, local spread, and liver and lung metastases, contributing to tumour staging.
- **PET scanning** is useful for detecting occult metastases and for evaluation of suspicious lesions found on CT or MRI.
- **MRI** is also useful for evaluating suspicious lesions found on CT or ultrasound, especially in the liver.
- **Serum carcinoembryonic antigen** (**CEA**) is of little use for primary diagnosis and should not be performed as a screening test. It is useful for follow-up; rising levels suggest recurrence.
- **Faecal occult blood (FOB) tests** are used for mass population screening.

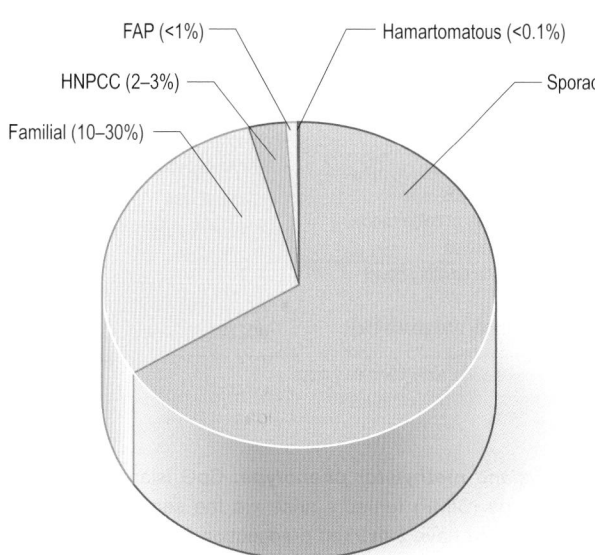

Fig. 32.52 Percentages of colon cancer according to family risk. FAP, familial adenomatous polyposis; HNPCC, hereditary non-polyposis colorectal cancer (Lynch syndrome).

FAP (<1%)
Hamartomatous (<0.1%)
HNPCC (2–3%)
Sporadic
Familial (10–30%)

Box 32.50 Lifetime risk of colorectal cancer (CRC) in first-degree relatives of a CRC patient

Individuals affected	Risk
Population risk	1 in 50
One first-degree relative affected (any age)	1 in 17
One first-degree and one second-degree relative affected	1 in 12
One first-degree relative affected (age <45)	1 in 10
Two first-degree relatives affected	1 in 6
Autosomal dominant pedigree	1 in 2

(From Houlston RS, Murday V, Harocopos C et al. Screening and genetic counselling for relatives of patients with colorectal cancer in a family cancer clinic. Br Med J 1990; 301:366–368.)

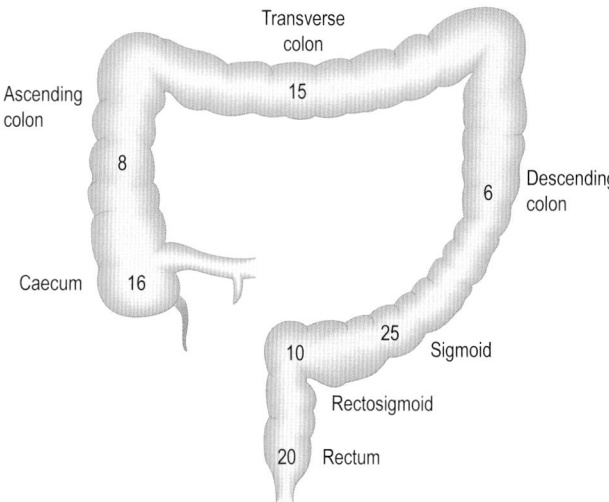

Transverse colon
Ascending colon
15
8
Descending colon
6
Caecum
16
25
10
Sigmoid
Rectosigmoid
20 Rectum

Fig. 32.53 Distribution of sporadic colorectal cancer. Only 60% are in the range of flexible sigmoidoscopy.

Management

Management should be undertaken by multidisciplinary teams working in specialist units. About 80% of patients with CRC undergo surgery (often laparoscopically). The operative procedure depends on the cancer site. Long-term survival relates to the stage of the primary tumour and the presence of metastatic disease. There has been a gradual move from using Dukes' classification to the TNM classification system (see **Box 28.53**). Long-term survival is only likely when the cancer is completely removed by surgery with adequate clearance margins and regional lymph node clearance.

- *Total mesorectal excision (TME)* is required for rectal cancers and removes the entire package of mesorectal tissue surrounding the cancer. A low rectal anastomosis is then performed. Abdomino-perineal excision, which requires a permanent colostomy, is reserved for very low tumours within 5 cm of the anal margin. TME combined with preoperative radiotherapy reduces local recurrence rates in rectal cancer to around 8% and improves survival. Pre- or postoperative chemotherapy reduces local recurrence rates but had no effect on survival in a recent study.
- *Segmental resection* and restorative anastomosis, with removal of the draining lymph nodes as far as the root of the mesentery, is used for cancer elsewhere in the colon. Surgery in patients with obstruction carries greater morbidity and mortality. Where technically possible, preoperative decompression by endoscopic stenting with a mesh-metal stent relieves obstruction, so surgery can be elective rather than emergency, and is probably associated with a decrease in morbidity and mortality.
- *Local transanal surgery* is very occasionally used for early superficial rectal cancers.
- *Surgical or ablative treatment of liver and lung metastases* prolongs life where treatment is technically feasible and the patient is fit enough to undergo the treatment.

- *Radiotherapy is not helpful* for colonic cancers proximal to the rectum because of difficulties in delivering a sufficient dose to the tumour without excess toxicity to adjacent structures, particularly the small bowel.
- *Adjuvant postoperative chemotherapy* improves disease-free survival and overall survival in stage III colon cancer (see p. 125). Those with stage II tumours and advanced features such as vascular invasion may also benefit. Genetic testing for KRAS mutations can help target appropriate chemotherapy regimens.

Management of *advanced colorectal cancer* is discussed on page 124.

Follow-up

All patients who have surgery should have a total colonoscopy performed before surgery to look for additional lesions. If total colonoscopy cannot be achieved before surgery, a second 'clearance' colonoscopy within 6 months of surgery is essential. Patients with stage II or III disease should be followed up with regular colonoscopy and CEA measurements; rising levels of CEA suggest recurrence. Annual CT scanning of the chest and abdomen to detect operable liver metastases should be performed for up to 3 years post surgery.

Screening for CRC

- *FOB tests* have been studied as a screening test for colorectal cancer. Several large randomized studies have demonstrated a reduction in cancer-related mortality of 15–33%. Immunologically based FOB tests are superior to the conventional guaiac-based systems. The disadvantage of screening with FOB is its relatively low sensitivity, which means many negative colonoscopies. In FOB test screen-positive patients in the UK National Bowel Cancer Screening Programme (NHS BCSP), about 10% have cancer, 40% have adenomas and the colon is normal in 50%. Faecal immunochemical tests (FIT) for blood – FIT for haemoglobin are more specific than guaiac tests because FIT detects only human globin and therefore does not detect upper gastrointestinal bleeding (since the globin is digested in transit). Additionally, foods with peroxidase activity do not produce a positive reaction. FIT has replaced FOBt in the bowel cancer screening programme in the UK since April 2018.
- *Flexible sigmoidoscopy* screening has been shown to reduce the mortality from CRC, but not overall mortality.
- *Colonoscopy* is the 'gold standard' technique for examination of the colon and rectum and is the investigation of choice for high-risk patients. Universal screening strategies have been implemented in the UK for subjects between 60 and 69 who have a positive FOB. Cancer has been detected in 8–12% of patients, 75% of which was located in the left colon; 72% of detected cancers are at an 'early' stage (10% polyp cancer, 32% stage I and 30% stage II).
- *CT colonography* ('virtual colonoscopy', see **Fig. 32.8**) is increasingly being used.

Further reading

Atkin WS, Edwards R, Kralj-Hans I et al and UK Flexible Sigmoidoscopy Trial Investigators. Once-only flexible sigmoidoscopy screening in prevention of colorectal cancer: a multicentre randomised controlled trial. *Lancet* 2010; 375:1624–1633.
Camilleri M, Bharucha AE. Behavioural and new pharmacological treatments for constipation: getting the balance right. *Gut* 2010; 59:1288–1296.
Cunningham D, Atkin W, Lenz HJ et al. Colorectal cancer. *Lancet* 2010; 375:1030.
Markowitz SD, Bertagnolli MM. Molecular origins of cancer: molecular basis of colorectal cancer. *N Engl J Med* 2009; 361:2449–2460.

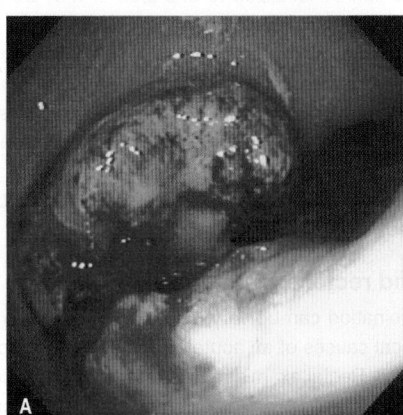
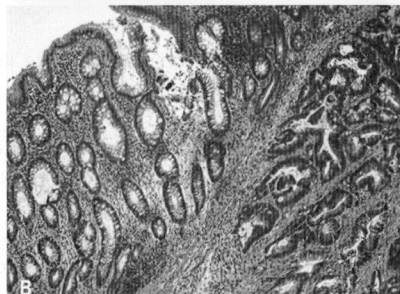

Fig. 32.54 Carcinoma in the ascending colon. Colonoscopic appearance of a large irregular ulcer. (B) Histopathology showing an adenocarcinoma.

Morris AM, Regenbogen SE, Hardiman KM et al. Sigmoid diverticulitis: a systematic review. *JAMA* 2014; 311:287–297.
National Institute for Health and Care Excellence. *NICE Clinical Guideline 49: Faecal Incontinence: The Management of Faecal Incontinence.* NICE 2007; http://www.nice.org.uk/guidance/CG49.
Norton C. Treating faecal incontinence with bulking-agent injections. *Lancet* 2011; 377:971–972.
Tursi A. Diverticular disease: what is the best long-term treatment? Nature Reviews. *Gastroenterol Hepatol* 2010; 7:77–78.
http://www.bsg.org.uk. *British Society of Gastroenterology.*

THE ACUTE ABDOMEN

This section deals with the acute abdominal conditions that cause the patient to be hospitalized within a few hours of the onset of pain (**Box 32.51**). If they are recognized quickly as an emergency, a reduction in morbidity and mortality can be achieved. Although a specific diagnosis should be attempted, the immediate problem in management is to decide whether an 'acute abdomen' exists and whether surgery is required.

Diagnosis

History

This should include previous operations, any gynaecological problems and presence of any concurrent medical condition.

Pain

The onset, site, type and subsequent course of the pain should be determined as accurately as possible. In general, the pain of an acute abdomen can be either constant (usually owing to inflammation) or colicky (because of a blocked 'tube'). The inflammatory nature of a constant pain will be supported by a raised temperature, tachycardia and/or a raised white cell count. If these are normal, then other causes (e.g. musculoskeletal, aortic aneurysm), even rare ones (e.g. porphyria), should be considered. Colicky pain can be due to an obstruction of the gut, biliary system, urogenital system or uterus. These cases will probably require conservative management initially, along with analgesics. If a colicky pain becomes a constant pain, then inflammation of the organ may have supervened (e.g. strangulated hernia, ascending cholangitis or salpingitis).

A **sudden onset** of pain suggests:

- perforation (e.g. of a duodenal ulcer)
- rupture (e.g. of an ectopic pregnancy)
- torsion (e.g. of an ovarian cyst)
- acute pancreatitis
- infarction (e.g. mesenteric).

? Box 32.51 Common causes of acute abdominal pain

Diagnosis	%[a]
Non-specific abdominal pain	35
Acute appendicitis	30
Gall bladder disease	10
Gynaecological disorders	5
Intestinal obstruction	5
Perforated ulcer/dyspepsia	5
Renal colic	2
Urinary tract infection	2
Diverticular disease	2
Other diagnoses	4

[a]Percentages are approximate and vary in different communities.

Back pain suggests:

- pancreatitis
- rupture of an aortic aneurysm
- renal tract disease.

Inflammatory conditions (e.g. appendicitis) produce a more gradual onset of pain. With peritonitis, the pain is continuous and may be made worse by movement. Many inflammatory conditions can progress to those listed as having a sudden onset due to complications.

Vomiting

Vomiting may accompany any acute abdominal pain but, if persistent, suggests an obstructive lesion of the gut. The character of the vomit should be asked about. Does it contain blood, bile or small bowel contents?

Other symptoms

Any change in bowel habit or of urinary frequency should be documented and, in females, a gynaecological history, including last menstrual period, should be taken.

Physical examination

The general condition of the person should be noted. Do they look ill or shocked? Large volumes of fluid may be lost from the vascular compartment into the peritoneal cavity or into the lumen of the bowel, giving rise to hypovolaemia: that is, a pale, cold skin, a weak, rapid pulse and hypotension.

The abdomen

- **Inspection.** Look for the presence of scars, distension or masses.
- **Palpation.** The abdomen should be examined gently for sites of tenderness and the presence or absence of guarding. Guarding is involuntary spasm of the abdominal wall and indicates peritonitis. This can be localized to one area or may be generalized, involving the whole abdomen.
- **Bowel sounds.** Increased high-pitched, tinkling bowel sounds indicate fluid obstruction; this occurs because of fluid movement within the dilated bowel lumen. Absent bowel sounds suggest peritonitis. In an obstructed patient, absent bowel sounds may be due to strangulation, ischaemia or ileus. It is essential for the hernial orifices to be examined if intestinal obstruction is suspected.

Vaginal and rectal examination

Vaginal examination can be very helpful, particularly in diagnosing gynaecological causes of an acute abdomen (e.g. a ruptured ectopic pregnancy). Rectal examination is less helpful, as localized tenderness may be due to any cause; it may show blood on the glove.

Other observations

- **Temperature.** Fever is more common in acute inflammatory processes.
- **Urine.** Examine for:
  - blood – suggests urinary tract infection or renal colic
  - glucose and ketones – ketoacidosis can present with acute pain
  - protein and white cells – to exclude acute pyelonephritis.
- **Medical causes.** These should be borne in mind (**Box 32.52**).

Investigations

- **Blood count.** A raised white cell count occurs in inflammatory conditions.

Box 32.52 Medical causes of acute abdomen

- Referred pain:
  - Pneumonia
  - Myocardial infarction
- Functional gastrointestinal disorders
- Renal causes:
  - Pelviureteric colic
  - Acute pyelonephritis
- Metabolic causes:
  - Diabetes mellitus
  - Acute intermittent porphyria
- Lead poisoning
- Familial Mediterranean fever
- Haematological causes:
  - Haemophilia and other bleeding disorders
  - Henoch–Schönlein purpura
  - Sickle cell crisis
  - Polycythaemia vera
  - Paroxysmal nocturnal haemoglobinaemia
- Vasculitis

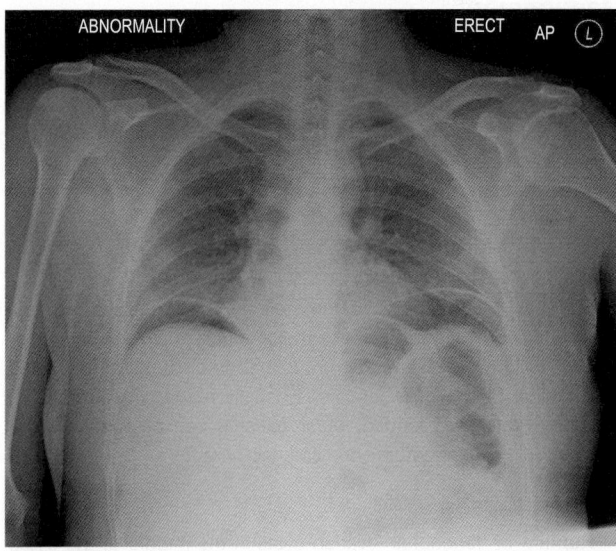

Fig. 32.55 Erect chest radiograph demonstrating free gas under the diaphragm (pneumoperitoneum).

- **Serum amylase.** High levels (more than five times normal) indicate acute pancreatitis. Raised levels below this can occur in any acute abdomen and should not be considered diagnostic of pancreatitis.
- **Serum electrolytes.** These are not particularly helpful for diagnosis but are useful for general evaluation of the patient.
- **Pregnancy test.** A urine dipstick is used for women of childbearing age.
- **X-rays.** An erect chest X-ray is useful to detect air under the diaphragm caused by a perforation (**Fig. 32.55**). Dilated loops of bowel or fluid levels are suggestive of obstruction on abdominal X-ray (**Fig. 32.56**).
- **Ultrasound.** This is useful in the diagnosis of acute cholangitis, cholecystitis and aortic aneurysm, and in expert hands is reliable in the diagnosis of acute appendicitis. Gynaecological and other pelvic causes of pain can be detected.
- **CT scan.** Spiral CT of the abdomen and pelvis is the most accurate investigation in most acute emergencies. It should be used more often to avoid unnecessary laparotomies.
- **Laparoscopy.** This is used increasingly as a diagnostic tool prior to proceeding with surgery, particularly in men and women over the age of 50 years. In addition, therapeutic procedures, such as appendicectomy, can be performed.

Acute appendicitis

This is a common surgical emergency and affects all age groups. Appendicitis should always be considered in the differential diagnosis if the appendix has not been removed.

Acute appendicitis mostly occurs when the lumen of the appendix becomes obstructed with a faecolith; however, in some cases, there is only generalized acute inflammation. If the appendix is not removed at this stage, gangrene occurs with perforation, leading to a localized abscess or to generalized peritonitis.

Clinical features

Most patients present with abdominal pain; in many, it starts vaguely in the centre of the abdomen, becoming localized to the right iliac fossa in the first few hours. Nausea, vomiting, anorexia and occasional diarrhoea can occur.

Examination of the abdomen usually reveals tenderness in the right iliac fossa, with guarding due to the localized peritonitis. There may be a tender mass in the right iliac fossa. Although raised white cell counts, ESR and CRP are helpful, other laboratory tests can be less valuable. An ultrasound scan can detect an inflamed appendix and can also indicate an appendix mass or other localized lesion. CT is highly sensitive (98.5%) and specific (98% negative predictive value; 99.5% positive predictive value), and reduces the incidence of removal of a 'normal' appendix. With the use of these

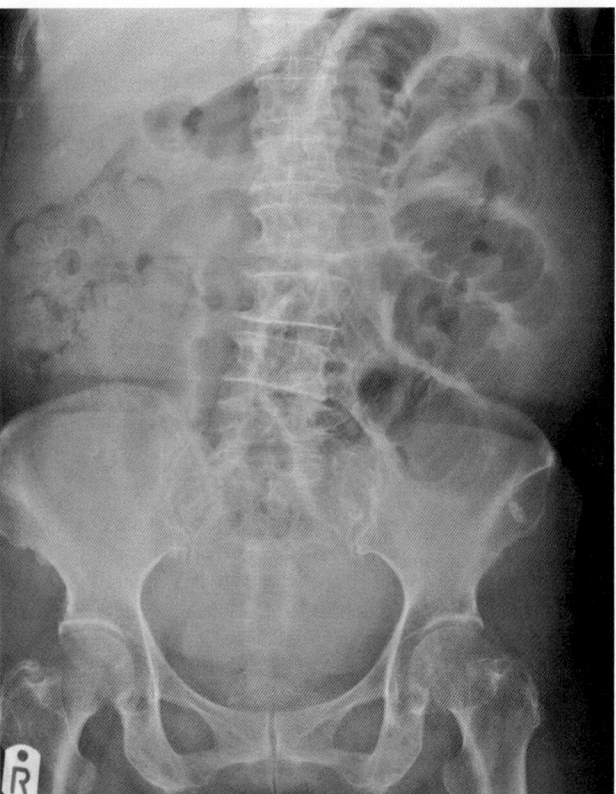

Fig. 32.56 Abdominal radiograph demonstrating multiple dilated loops of small bowel consistent with small bowel obstruction.

investigations, the incidence of 'normal' appendix histology has fallen to 15–20%.

Differential diagnosis

- Non-specific mesenteric lymphadenitis – may mimic appendicitis.
- Acute terminal ileitis due to Crohn's disease or *Yersinia* infection.
- Gynaecological causes:
  - inflamed Meckel's diverticulum
  - functional bowel disease.

Management

The appendix is removed by laparoscopic surgery. If an appendix mass is present, the patient is usually treated conservatively with intravenous fluids and antibiotics. The pain subsides over a few days and the mass usually disappears over a few weeks. Interval appendicectomy is recommended at a later date to prevent further acute episodes.

Gynaecological causes of an acute abdomen

Ruptured ectopic pregnancy

The fallopian tube is the most common extrauterine site of implantation. Delayed diagnosis is the major cause of morbidity. Most patients will present with recurrent low abdominal pain associated with vaginal bleeding. Diagnosis is usually made with abdominal and transvaginal ultrasound. Most patients can be managed by laparoscopic salpingostomy or salpingectomy.

Ovarian causes

- Rupture of 'functional' ovarian cysts in the middle of the cycle (Mittelschmerz).
- Torsion or rupture of ovarian cysts.

Acute salpingitis

Most cases are associated with sexually transmitted infection. Patients commonly present with bilateral low abdominal pain, a fever and vaginal discharge. In the *Fitz-Hugh–Curtis syndrome*, *Chlamydia* infection tracks up the right paracolic gutter to cause a perihepatitis. Patients can present with acute right hypochondrial pain, fever and mildly abnormal liver biochemistry.

Acute peritonitis

Localized peritonitis

There is virtually always some degree of localized peritonitis with all acute inflammatory conditions of the gastrointestinal tract (e.g. acute appendicitis, acute cholecystitis). Pain and tenderness are largely features of this localized peritonitis. The treatment is for the underlying disease.

Generalized peritonitis

This is a serious condition, resulting from irritation of the peritoneum owing to infection (e.g. perforated appendix) or from chemical irritation due to leakage of intestinal contents (e.g. perforated ulcer). In the latter case, superadded infection gradually occurs; *E. coli* and *Bacteroides* are the most common organisms.

The peritoneal cavity becomes acutely inflamed, with production of an inflammatory exudate that spreads throughout the peritoneum, leading to intestinal dilation and paralytic ileus.

Clinical features

In perforation, the onset is sudden with acute, severe abdominal pain, followed by general collapse and shock. The patient may improve temporarily, only to become worse later as generalized toxaemia occurs.

When peritonitis is secondary to inflammatory disease, the onset is less rapid, the initial features being those of the underlying disease.

Investigations

Investigations should always include an erect chest X-ray. X-ray is used to detect free air under the diaphragm, and serum amylase is measured to diagnose acute pancreatitis, which is treated conservatively. Imaging with ultrasound and/or CT should always be performed for diagnosis.

Management

Peritonitis is treated surgically after adequate resuscitation and the re-establishment of a good urinary output. This includes insertion of a nasogastric tube, intravenous fluids and antibiotics. Surgery has a two-fold objective:

- peritoneal lavage of the abdominal cavity
- specific treatment of the underlying condition.

Complications

Any delay in the treatment of peritonitis produces more profound toxaemia and septicaemia, which may lead to the development of multiorgan failure (see p. 219). Local abscess formation can occur and should be suspected if a patient continues to remain unwell postoperatively, with a swinging fever, high white cell count and continuing pain. Abscesses are commonly pelvic or subphrenic, and can be localized and drained using ultrasound and CT scanning techniques.

Intestinal obstruction

Most intestinal obstruction is due to a mechanical block. Sometimes the bowel does not function, leading to a paralytic ileus. This occurs temporarily after most abdominal operations and with peritonitis. The most common cause in adults is adhesions (**Box 32.53**).

Obstruction of the bowel leads to bowel distension above the block, with increased secretion of fluid into the distended bowel. Bacterial contamination takes place in the distended stagnant bowel. In strangulation, the blood supply is impeded, leading to gangrene, perforation and peritonitis unless urgent treatment of the condition is undertaken.

Clinical features

The patient complains of abdominal colic, vomiting and constipation without passage of wind. In upper gut obstruction the vomiting is profuse, but in lower gut obstruction it may be absent.

Examination of the abdomen reveals distension with increased bowel sounds. Marked tenderness suggests strangulation, and urgent surgery is necessary. Examination of the hernial orifices and rectum must be performed. X-ray of the abdomen reveals distended loops of bowel proximal to the obstruction. Fluid levels are seen in small bowel obstruction on an erect film. In large bowel obstruction, the caecum and ascending colon are distended. An instant, water-soluble Gastrografin enema without air insufflation may help to demonstrate the site of the obstruction. CT can localize the lesion accurately and is the investigation of choice.

Management

Initial management is by resuscitation with intravenous fluids (mainly 0.9% saline with potassium) and decompression. Many cases will settle on conservative management, but an increasing temperature, raised pulse rate, increasing pain and a rising white cell count require urgent scanning and possible exploratory laparotomy.

? Box 32.53 Causes of intestinal obstruction

Small intestinal obstruction	Colonic obstruction
- Adhesions (80% in adults)	- Carcinoma of the colon
- Hernias	- Sigmoid volvulus
- Crohn's disease	- Diverticular disease
- Intussusception	
- Obstruction due to extrinsic involvement by cancer	

Laparotomy with removal of the obstruction will be necessary in some cases of small bowel obstruction. If the bowel is gangrenous owing to strangulation, gut resection will be required. A few patients (e.g. those with Crohn's disease) may have recurrent episodes of incomplete intestinal obstruction that can be managed conservatively. In large bowel obstruction due to malignancy, a self-expanding metal stent can be used, followed by elective surgery. In critically ill patients, a defunctioning colostomy may be needed. Volvulus of the sigmoid colon can be managed by the passage of a flexible sigmoidoscope or a rectal tube to un-kink and deflate the bowel, but recurrent volvulus may require sigmoid resection.

Acute colonic pseudo-obstruction

A clinical picture mimicking mechanical obstruction may develop in patients who do not have a mechanical cause. In more than 80% of cases, it complicates other clinical conditions, such as:

- intra-abdominal trauma, pelvic, spinal and femoral fractures
- postoperative states (abdominal, pelvic, cardiothoracic, orthopaedic, neurosurgical)
- intra-abdominal sepsis
- pneumonia
- metabolic disorders (e.g. electrolyte disturbances, malnutrition, diabetes mellitus, Parkinson's disease)
- drugs – opiates (particularly after orthopaedic surgery), antidepressants, antiparkinsonian drugs.

Patients present with rapid and progressive abdominal distension and pain. X-ray shows a gas-filled large bowel. Management is of the underlying problem (e.g. withdrawal of opiate analgesia), together with a trial of intravenous neostigmine therapy. Patients should be monitored and consideration should be given to surgery if the diameter of the caecum exceeds 14 cm.

PERITONEUM

Anatomy and physiology

The peritoneal cavity is a closed sac lined by mesothelial cells; these produce surfactant, which acts as a lubricant within the peritoneal cavity. The cavity contains <100 mL of serous fluid containing <30 g/L of protein.

The mesothelial cells lining the diaphragm have gaps that allow communication between the peritoneum and the diaphragmatic lymphatics. Approximately one-third of fluid drains through these lymphatics, the remainder through the parietal peritoneum. These mechanisms allow particulate matter to be removed rapidly from the peritoneal cavity.

Complement activation is an early defence mechanism and is followed rapidly by upregulation of the peritoneal mesothelial cells and migration of polymorphonuclear neutrophils and macrophages into the peritoneum.

Mast cells release potent mediators of inflammation, including histamine and eicosanoids, and interact with T cells to generate an immune response.

The peritoneum-associated lymphoid tissue includes the omental milky spots, the lymphocytes within the peritoneal cavity and the draining lymph nodes. B cells with a unique CD5+ are common. This defence system plays a major role in localizing peritoneal infection.

Disorders affecting the peritoneum

Conditions that can affect the peritoneum are shown in **Box 32.54**.

> **?** **Box 32.54** Diseases of the peritoneum

Infective (bacterial) peritonitis
- Secondary to gut disease, e.g. appendicitis
- Perforation of any organ
- Chronic peritoneal dialysis
- Spontaneous, usually in ascites with liver disease
- Tuberculosis

Neoplasia
- Secondary deposits (e.g. from ovary, stomach)
- Primary mesothelioma

Vasculitis
- Rheumatic autoimmune disease
- Polyserositis (e.g. familial Mediterranean fever)

Peritonitis can be acute or chronic, as seen in TB. Most cases of infective peritonitis are secondary to gastrointestinal disease, but it occurs occasionally without intra-abdominal sepsis in ascites due to liver disease. Very rarely, fungal and parasitic infections (e.g. amoebiasis, candidiasis) can also cause primary peritonitis. Peritonitis is discussed further on page 1222.

The peritoneum can be involved by secondary malignant deposits, and the most common cause of ascites in a young to middle-aged woman is an ovarian carcinoma.

A *subphrenic abscess* is usually secondary to infection in the abdomen and is characterized by fever, malaise, pain in the right or left hypochondrium and shoulder-tip pain. An erect chest X-ray may show gas under the diaphragm, impaired movement of the diaphragm on screening and/or a pleural effusion. Ultrasound is usually diagnostic. Percutaneous catheter drainage inserted under CT or ultrasound guidance and antibiotics constitute highly successful therapy.

Ascites is associated with all diseases of the peritoneum. The fluid that collects is an exudate with a high protein content. It is also seen in liver disease. The mechanism, causes and investigation of ascites are discussed on page 1295.

Peritoneal adhesions

Adhesions form as a result of abdominal or pelvic surgery, or inflammation in the abdominoperitoneal cavity. They cause a variety of conditions, including adhesive small bowel obstruction (ASBO), chronic abdominal pain, complications during future surgery, and female infertility when they involve the fallopian tubes or ovaries. There is no satisfactory medical or surgical treatment and so surgical techniques have been developed to minimize peritoneal injury,

Retroperitoneal fibrosis (peri-aortitis)

This is a rare condition, in which there is a marked fibrosis over the posterior abdominal wall and retroperitoneum. It is associated with raised serum IgG4 levels (see p. 65) and is described on page 1379.

Tuberculous peritonitis

This is the second most common form of abdominal TB. Three subgroups can be identified: wet, dry and fibrous.

- In patients with the *wet* type, ascitic fluid should be examined for protein concentration (>20 g/L) and tubercle bacilli (rarely found).
- In the *dry* form, patients present with subacute intestinal obstruction, which is due to tuberculous small bowel adhesions.
- In the *fibrous* form, patients present with abdominal pain, distension and ill-defined, irregular, tender abdominal masses.

The diagnosis of peritoneal TB can be supported by findings on ultrasound or CT screening (mesenteric thickening and lymph node enlargement). A histological diagnosis is not always required before instituting treatment. In some patients, careful laparoscopy (to avoid perforation) may have to be performed, and rarely laparotomy.

Management

Drug treatment is similar to that for pulmonary TB (see p. 969) and should be supervised by chest physicians who have experience in dealing with contacts.

Bibliography

Feldman M, Friedman LS, Brandt LL. *Sleisenger and Fordtran's Gastrointestinal and Liver Disease*, 10th edn. Philadelphia: WB Saunders; 2015.

Significant websites

http://www.bsg.org.uk *British Society of Gastroenterology.*
http://www.coeliac.co.uk *Coeliac UK.*
http://www.corecharity.org.uk *Gastric ulcer and GORD.*
https://www.crohnsandcolitis.org.uk *Crohn's and Colitis UK.*

Nutrition

Marinos Elia, Susan A. Lanham-New and Klaartje Kok

CORE SKILLS AND KNOWLEDGE

Nutrition is a crucial but easily overlooked contributor to health. While more than half of the adult population in developed countries are overweight or obese, malnutrition or specific nutritional deficiencies may affect those with inadequate diet or with malabsorption syndromes. It is estimated that over one-third of adults over the age of 65 are at risk of malnutrition when they are admitted to hospital. Despite significant progress in eradicating extreme poverty globally, there are still parts of the developing world where malnutrition is a major population problem, often complicated by micronutrient deficiencies.

In well-resourced settings, dieticians monitor for malnutrition in inpatients, and recommend dietary supplements or clinically assisted nutrition to address this. This is especially relevant where patients cannot swallow, such as for patients who have suffered a stroke, of in those who are hypercatabolic (for instance during critical illness). Gastroenterologists with an interest in nutrition often advise in cases of malabsorption or where parenteral feeding is required.

Key skills in nutrition include:
- developing an awareness of patients at risk of malnutrition, and understanding the role of dietary supplements and clinically assisted nutrition in addressing this
- being aware of syndromes associated with specific micronutrient deficiencies
- understanding the consequences of obesity for health, and different ways of helping patients to lose weight.

Opportunities for learning about nutrition include shadowing dieticians reviewing patients in the community or as inpatients, attending specialist nutrition ward rounds led by gastroenterologists, or through attending obesity and bariatric surgery outpatient clinics.

INTRODUCTION

Nutrition is essential in health. Diseases in many organs have adverse effects on food intake and metabolism, leading to nutrition-related conditions associated with increased morbidity and mortality. Conversely, food intake determines health and plays a major role in diseases like cardiovascular disease, diabetes and cancer. There is no universally accepted definition of malnutrition, but a reasonable definition is as follows: 'Malnutrition is a state of nutrition in which a deficiency, excess or imbalance of energy, protein and other nutrients causes measurable adverse effects on tissue/body form (body shape, size and composition) and function, and on clinical outcome.'

In developing countries, the lack of food and poor usage of the available food, often in association with ongoing inflammatory processes, result in what has traditionally been called protein–energy malnutrition (PEM). However, micro nutrient deficiencies often accompany PEM and they may contribute to its development. Worldwide, in 2011, 165 million children under 5 years of age were affected by stunting, and at least 52 million by wasting. Obesity has also been a growing problem in developing countries and the combination of stunting with obesity has been increasing. In developed countries, excess food is available, and overweight and obesity are the most common nutritional problems. However, under-nutrition (often referred to as 'malnutrition') continues to remain a major clinical and public health problem worldwide.

Diet and disease are inter-related in many ways:

- **Excess energy intake contributes to a number of diseases**, including ischaemic heart disease and diabetes, particularly when high in animal (saturated) fat content.
- **There is a relationship between food intake and cancer**, as found in many epidemiological studies. An excess of energy-rich foods (i.e. those containing fat and sugar), often combined with physical inactivity, plays a role in the development of certain cancers, while diets high in vegetables and fruits reduce the risk of most epithelial cancers. Numerous carcinogens, intentional additions (e.g. nitrates for preserving foods) or accidental contaminants (e.g. moulds producing aflatoxin and fungi) may also be involved in the development of cancer.
- **The proportion of processed foods eaten may affect the development of disease.** Some processed convenience foods have a high sugar and fat content and therefore predispose to dental caries and obesity, respectively. They also have a low fibre content, and dietary fibre can help in the prevention of a number of diseases (see p. 1230).
- **Long-term under-nutrition is implicated in disease** by some epidemiological studies; for example, low growth rates *in utero* are associated with high death rates from cardiovascular disease in adult life.

In the UK, dietary reference values for food, energy and nutrients are stated as **reference nutrient intakes** (RNIs), on the basis of data from the Food and Agriculture Organization (FAO-WHO), United Nations University (UNU) expert committee and elsewhere. The RNI is sufficient, or more than sufficient, to meet the nutritional needs of 97.5% of healthy people in a population. Most people's daily requirements are less than this, and so an **estimated average requirement (EAR)** is also given, which will certainly be adequate for most. A lower reference nutrient intake (LRNI), which fails to meet the requirements of 97.5% of the population, is also given. The RNI figures quoted in this chapter are for the age group 19–50 years. These represent values for healthy subjects and are not always appropriate for patients with disease.

WATER AND ELECTROLYTE BALANCE

Water and electrolyte balance is dealt with fully in Chapter 9. About 1 L of water is required in the daily diet to balance insensible losses but much more is usually drunk, the kidneys being able to excrete large quantities. The daily RNI for sodium is 70 mmol (1.6 g) but daily sodium intake varies in the range 90–440 mmol (2–10 g). These are needlessly high intakes of sodium, which are thought to play a role in causing hypertension (see Ch. 31). The World Health Organization (WHO) also recommends at least 90 mmol (3.5 g) potassium, which would reduce blood pressure and cardiovascular risk of stroke and coronary artery disease.

DIETARY REQUIREMENTS

Energy

Food is necessary to provide the body with energy **(Fig. 33.1)**. The SI unit of energy is the joule (J), and 1 kJ = 0.239 kcal. The conversion factor of 4.2 kJ, equivalent to 1.00 kcal, is used in clinical nutrition.

Energy balance

Energy balance is the difference between energy intake and energy expenditure. Weight gain or loss is a simple but accurate way of indicating differences in energy balance.

Energy requirements

There are two approaches to assessing energy requirements for subjects who are weight-stable and close to energy balance:

- assessment of energy intake
- assessment of total energy expenditure.

Energy intake

Energy intake can be estimated from dietary surveys and, in the past, this has been used to decide daily energy requirements. However, measurement of energy expenditure gives a more accurate assessment of requirements.

Energy expenditure

Daily energy expenditure **(Fig. 33.2)** is the sum of:

- the basal metabolic rate (BMR)
- the thermic effect of food eaten
- occupational activities
- non-occupational activities.

Total energy expenditure can be measured using a double-labelled water technique. Water containing the stable isotopes ^2H and ^{18}O is given orally. As energy is expended, carbon dioxide and water are produced. The difference between the rates of loss of the two isotopes is used to calculate the carbon dioxide production, which is then used to calculate energy expenditure. This can be done on urine samples over a 2–3-week period with the subject ambulatory. The technique is accurate, but it is expensive and requires the availability of a mass spectrometer. An alternative tracer technique for measuring total energy expenditure is to estimate CO_2 production by isotopic dilution. A subcutaneous infusion of labelled bicarbonate is administered continuously by a minipump, and urine is collected to measure isotopic dilution by urea, which is formed from CO_2. Other methods for estimating energy expenditure, such as heart rate monitors or activity monitors, are also available but are less accurate.

Basal metabolic rate can be calculated by measuring oxygen consumption and CO_2 production, but it is more usually taken from

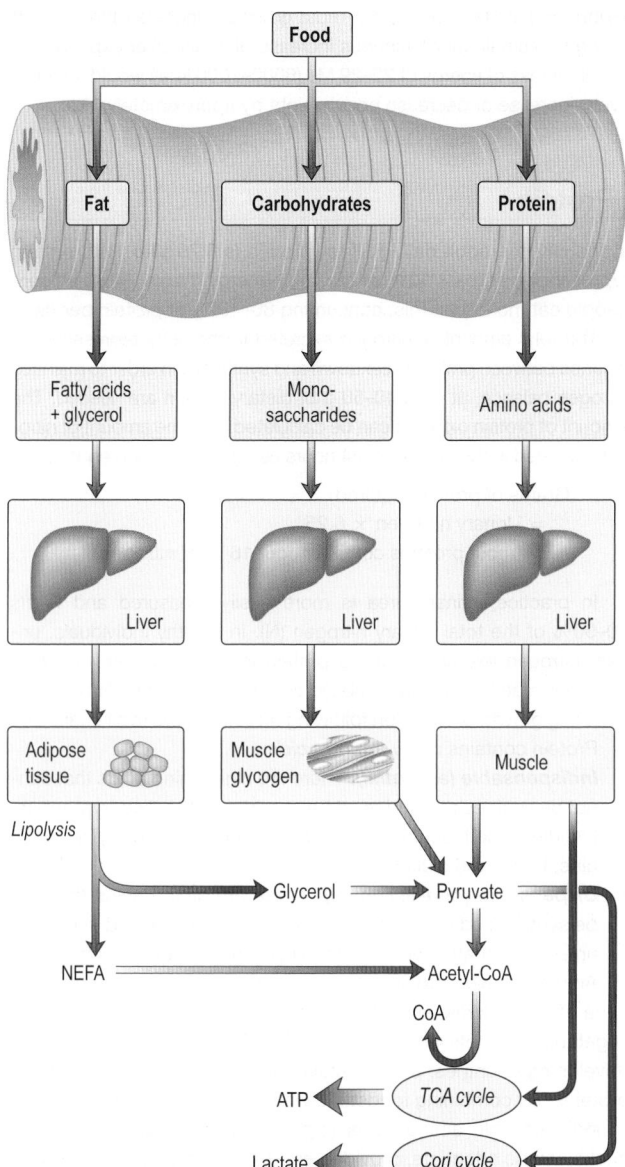

Fig. 33.1 The production of energy from the main constituents of food. Alcohol produces up to 5% of total calories but the variation between individuals is wide. One mol of glucose produces 36 mol of adenosine triphosphate (ATP). CoA, coenzyme A; NEFA, non-esterified fatty acids; TCA, tricarboxylic acid.

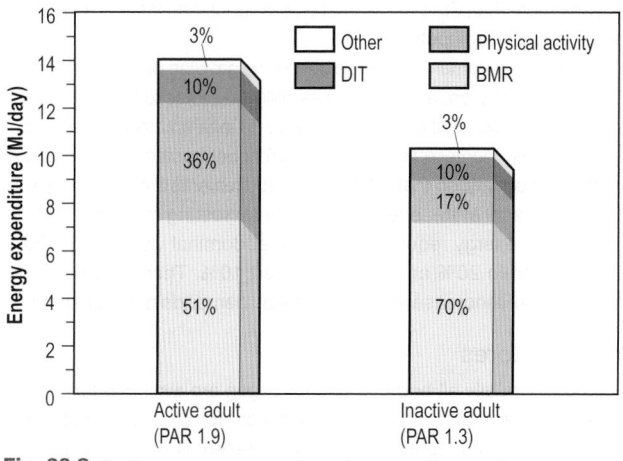

Fig. 33.2 Daily energy expenditure in an active and a sedentary 70-kg adult. BMR, basal metabolic rate; DIT, dietary-induced thermogenesis; PAR, physical activity ratio.

i **Box 33.1** Equations for the prediction of basal metabolic rate (BMR) (in MJ/day)

Age range (years)	Equation for predicting BMR[a]	95% confidence limits
Men		
10–17	$0.0740 \times (wt) + 2.754$	±0.88
18–29	$0.0630 \times (wt) + 2.896$	±1.28
30–59	$0.0480 \times (wt) + 3.653$	±1.40
60–74	$0.0499 \times (wt) + 2.930$	N/A
75+	$0.0350 \times (wt) + 3.434$	N/A
Women		
10–17	$0.0560 \times (wt) + 2.898$	±0.94
18–29	$0.0620 \times (wt) + 2.036$	±1.00
30–59	$0.0340 \times (wt) + 3.538$	±0.94
60–74	$0.0386 \times (wt) + 2.875$	N/A
75+	$0.0410 \times (wt) + 2.610$	N/A

[a]Body weight (wt) in kg.
(Data from Department of Health, 1991.)

standardized tables **(Box 33.1)** that only require knowledge of the subject's age, weight and sex.

The *physical activity ratio* (PAR) is expressed as multiples of the BMR for both occupational and non-occupational activities of varying intensities **(Box 33.2)**.

Total daily expenditure

= BMR × [Time in bed + (Time at work × PAR)
+ Non−occupational time × PAR)]

Thus, for example, to determine the daily energy expenditure of a 73-year-old, 50-kg female doctor, with a BMR of 4805 kJ/day, who spends one-third of a day sleeping, working and engaged in non-occupational activities, the latter at a PAR of 2.1, the following calculation ensues:

$$= (4805 \, kJ/day) \times [0.3 \times 1.7) + 0.3 \times 2.10)]$$
$$= 6919 \, kJ \, (1655 \, kcal/day)$$

i **Box 33.2** Physical activity ratio (PAR) for various activities (expressed as multiples of basal metabolic rate)

Activity	PAR
Professional/housewife	1.7
Domestic helper/salesperson	2.7
Labourer	3.0
Reading/eating	1.2
Household/cooking	2.1
Gardening/golf	3.7
Jogging/swimming/football	6.9

In the UK, the estimated 'average' daily energy requirement is:
- for a 55-year-old female – 8100 kJ (1940 kcal)
- for a 55-year-old male – 10 600 kJ (2550 kcal).

This is at present made up of about 50% carbohydrate, 35% fat, 15% protein ± 5% alcohol. In developing countries, however, carbohydrate may be more than 75% of the total energy input, and fat less than 15% of the total energy input.

Energy requirements increase during the growing period, with pregnancy and lactation, and sometimes following infection or trauma. In general, the increased BMR associated with inflammatory or traumatic conditions is counteracted or more than counteracted by a decrease in physical activity, so that total energy requirements are not increased.

In the basal state, energy demands for resting muscle are 20% of the total energy required, those for abdominal viscera 35–40%, those for brain 20% and those for heart 10%. There can be more than a 50-fold increase in muscle energy demands during exercise.

Energy stores

Although virtually all body fat and glycogen are available for oxidation, less than half the protein is available for oxidation. **Fig. 33.3** shows that fat accounts for the largest reserves of energy in both lean and obese subjects. The size of the stores determines survival during starvation.

Body weight

Body weight depends on energy balance. Intake depends not only on food availability but also on a number of complex interrelationships that include the stimulus of good food, the role of hunger, metabolic changes (e.g. hypoglycaemia), and the pleasure and habit of eating. Some people are able to keep their body weight constant within a few

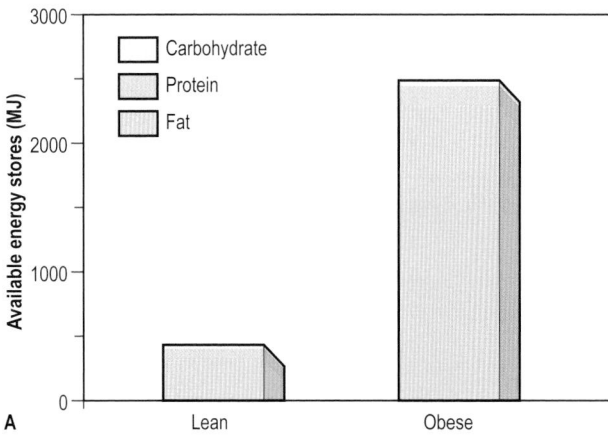

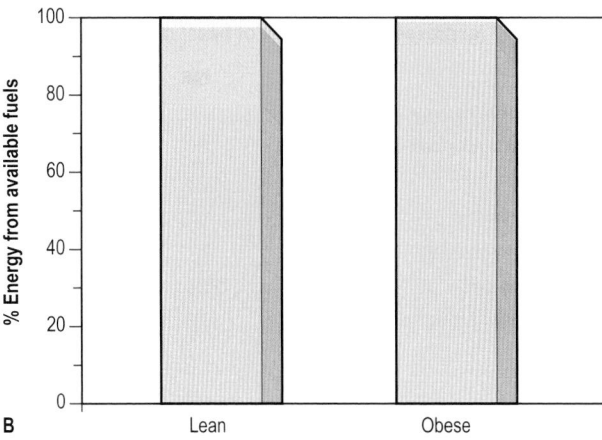

Fig. 33.3 Available energy reserves from different fuels.
Values are shown for a lean hypothetical 70-kg adult and an obese 140-kg adult. **(A)** Expressed in MJ. **(B)** Expressed as a percentage of the total.

kilograms for many years, but most gradually increase their weight owing to a small but continuous increase of intake over expenditure. A gain or loss of energy of 25–29 MJ (6000–7000 kcal) would, respectively, increase or decrease body weight by approximately 1 kg.

Protein

In the UK, the adult daily RNI for protein is 0.75 g/kg, with protein representing at least 10% of the total energy intake. Most affluent people eat more than this, consuming 80–100 g of protein per day.

The total amount of nitrogen excreted in the urine represents the balance between protein breakdown and synthesis. In order to maintain nitrogen balance, at least 40–50 g of dietary protein are needed. The amount of protein oxidized can be calculated from the amount of nitrogen excreted in the urine over 24 hours using the following equation:

$$\text{Grams of protein required} = \text{Urinary nitrogen} \times 6.25$$
$$(\text{most proteins contain about } 16\% \text{ of nitrogen})$$

In practice, urinary urea is more easily measured and forms 80–90% of the total urinary nitrogen (N). In healthy individuals, urinary nitrogen excretion reflects protein intake. However, excretion does not match intake in catabolic conditions (negative N balance), or during growth or repletion following an illness (positive N balance).

Protein contains many *amino acids*:

- *Indispensable (essential).* There are nine amino acids that cannot be synthesized and must be provided in the diet: tryptophan, histidine, methionine, threonine, isoleucine, valine, phenylalanine, lysine and leucine.
- *Dispensable (non-essential).* These are amino acids that can be synthesized in the body (some may still be needed in the diet unless adequate amounts of their precursors are available).

Animal proteins (e.g. in milk, meat and eggs) contain a good balance of all the indispensable amino acids, but many proteins from vegetables are deficient in at least one indispensable amino acid. In developing countries, protein intake derives mainly from vegetable proteins. By combining foodstuffs with different low concentrations of indispensable amino acids (e.g. maize with legumes), protein intake can be adequate, provided enough vegetables are available.

Loss of protein from the body (negative N balance) occurs not only because of inadequate protein intake, but also because of inadequate energy intake. When there is loss of energy from the body, more protein is directed towards oxidative pathways and, eventually, gluconeogenesis for energy.

Role of amino acids

- *Glutamine* is quantitatively the most significant amino acid in the circulation and in inter-organ exchange.
- *Alanine* is released from muscle; it is deaminated and converted into pyruvic acid before entering the citric acid cycle.
- *Homocysteine* is a sulphur-containing amino acid that is derived from methionine in the diet. A raised plasma concentration is an independent risk factor for vascular disease.

Amino acids are utilized to synthesize products other than protein or urea. For example:

- *Glycine* is required for haem production.
- *Tyrosine* is required for melanin and thyroid hormones.
- *Glutamine, aspartate and glycine* are required for nucleic acid bases.
- *Glutamate, cysteine and glycine* are required for glutathione, which is part of the defence system against free radicals.

Box 33.3 The main fatty acids in foods

Fatty acid	No. of carbon atoms : no. of double bonds	Position of double bonds[a]
Saturated		
Lauric	C12:0	
Myristic	C14:0	
Palmitic	C16:0	
Stearic	C18:0	
Monounsaturated		
Oleic	C18:1	*n*-9
Elaidic	C18:1	*n*-9 *trans*
Polyunsaturated		
Linoleic	C18:2	*n*-6
α-Linolenic	C18:3	*n*-3
Arachidonic	C20:4	*n*-6
Eicosapentaenoic	C20:5	*n*-3
Docosahexaenoic	C22:6	*n*-3

[a]Positions of the double bonds (designated either *n* as here or ω) are shown counted from the methyl end of the molecule. All double bonds are in the *cis* position except that marked *trans*.

Box 33.4 Dietary sources of fatty acids

Type of acid	Sources
Saturated fatty acids	Mainly animal fat
n-6 fatty acids	Vegetable oils and other plant foods
n-3 fatty acids	Vegetable foods, rapeseed oil, fish oils
trans fatty acids	Hydrogenated fat or oils, e.g. in margarine, cakes, biscuits

Fat

Dietary fat is chiefly in the form of triglycerides, which are esters of glycerol and free fatty acids. Fatty acids vary in chain length and in saturation **(Box 33.3)**. The hydrogen molecules related to the double bonds can be in the *cis* or the *trans* position; most natural fatty acids in food are in the *cis* position **(Box 33.4)**.

The ***essential fatty acids*** (EFAs) are linoleic and α-linolenic acid, both of which are precursors of prostaglandins. Eicosapentaenoic and docosahexaenoic acid are also necessary, but can be made to a limited extent in the tissues from linoleic and linolenic acid, and thus a dietary supply is not essential.

Synthesis of triglycerides, sterols and phospholipids is very efficient. Even with low-fat diets, subcutaneous fat stores can be normal.

Dietary fat provides 37 kJ (9 kcal) of energy per gram. A high-fat intake has been implicated in the causation of:

- cardiovascular disease
- cancer (e.g. breast, colon and prostate)
- obesity
- type 2 diabetes.

The data on causation are largely epidemiological and disputed by many. Nevertheless, it is often suggested that the consumption of saturated fatty acids should be reduced, accompanied by an increase in monounsaturated fatty acids, such as those in olive oil (the 'Mediterranean diet'), or polyunsaturated fatty acids. Any increase in polyunsaturated fats should not, however, exceed 10% of the total food energy, particularly as this requires a big dietary change.

Trans fats (partly hydrogenated fatty acids)

Increased consumption of hydrogenated vegetable and fish oils in margarines has led to increased *trans* fatty acid consumption. *Trans* fatty acids (also called *trans* fats) behave as if they were saturated fatty acids, increasing circulating low-density lipoprotein (LDL) and decreasing high-density lipoprotein (HDL) cholesterol concentrations, which, in turn, raise the risk of cardiovascular disease. In most countries, nutrition labels for all conventional foods and supplements must indicate the *trans* fatty acid content. The usage of *trans* fatty acids from partially hydrogenated oils has now been banned in many countries.

Polyunsaturated fatty acids

The ***n-6 polyunsaturated fatty acids (PUFAs)*** are components of membrane phospholipids, influencing membrane fluidity and ion transport. They also have antiarrhythmic, antithrombotic and anti-inflammatory properties, all of which are potentially helpful in preventing cardiovascular disease.

The ***n-3 PUFAs*** increase circulating HDL cholesterol and lower triglycerides, both of which might reduce cardiovascular risk. Some of the actions of *n*-3 PUFAs are mediated by a range of leukotrienes and eicosanoids, which differ in pattern and functions from those produced from *n*-6 PUFAs.

Epidemiological studies and clinical intervention studies suggest that *n*-3 PUFAs may have effects in the secondary prevention of cardiovascular disease and all-cause mortality (e.g. a 20–30% reduction in mortality from cardiovascular disease, according to some studies). The benefits, which have been noted as early as 4 months after intervention, have been attributed largely to the antiarrhythmic effects of *n*-3 PUFAs, but some work suggests that *n*-3 PUFAs, administered as capsules, can be rapidly incorporated into atheromatous plaques, stabilizing them and preventing rupture. Whether these effects are due directly to *n*-3 PUFAs or other changes in the diet is still debated.

Recommendations for fat intake

The British Nutrition Foundation and the American Heart Association presently recommend a two-fold increase of the current intake of total *n*-3 PUFAs (a several-fold increase in the intake of fish oils, and a 50% increase in the intake of α-linolenic acid). Implementing this recommendation will mean either a major change in the dietary habits of populations that eat little fish, or ingestion of capsules containing fish oils. Some government agencies have warned of the hazards of eating certain types of fish, which increase the risk of mercury poisoning and possibly other toxicities.

The current recommendations for fat intake for the UK are shown in **Box 33.5**.

Cholesterol

Cholesterol is found in all animal products. Eggs are particularly rich in cholesterol, which is virtually absent from plants. The average daily intake in the UK is 300–500 mg. Cholesterol is also synthesized (see **Fig. 34.5**), and only very high or low dietary intakes will significantly affect blood levels.

Essential fatty acid deficiency

Essential fatty acid deficiency may accompany PEM, and it has been clearly defined as a clinical entity in patients on long-term parenteral nutrition given glucose, protein and no fat. Alopecia, thrombocytopenia, anaemia and dermatitis occur within weeks, with an increased ratio of triene (*n*-9) to tetraene (*n*-6) in plasma fatty acids.

i **Box 33.5 Recommended healthy dietary intake**

Dietary component	Approximate amounts (% of total energy unless otherwise stated)	General hints
Total carbohydrate	55 (55–75)	Increase fruit, vegetables, beans, pasta, bread
Free sugar	10 (<10)*	Decrease sugary drinks
Protein	15 (10–15)	Decrease red meat (see 'Fat' below)
Total fat	30 (15–30)	Increase vegetable, olive and fish oil and decrease animal fat
Saturated fatty acids	10 (<10)	
Cis-monounsaturated fatty acids	20	Mainly oleic acid (*n*-6)
Cis-polyunsaturated fatty acids	6	Both *n*-6 and *n*-3 PUFAs
Approximate amounts		
Cholesterol	<300 (<300) mg/day	Decrease meat and eggs
Salt	<6 (<5) g/day	Decrease prepared meats and do not add extra salt to food
Total dietary fibre	30 (>25) g/day	Increase fruit, vegetables and wholegrain foods

Values in parentheses are goals for the intake of populations, as given by the World Health Organization (including populations who are already on low-fat diets). Some of the extreme ranges are not realistic short-term goals for developed countries, e.g. 75% of total energy from carbohydrate and 15% fat. When total energy intake is 2500 kcal (10 500 kJ) per day, 55% of intake comes from carbohydrate (344 g, i.e. 1376 kcal (5579 kJ)) and 30% from fat (83 g, i.e. 747 kcal (3137 kJ)). PUFAs, polyunsaturated fatty acids.
*Recent recommendations suggest <5% of total energy consumption.

Carbohydrate

Carbohydrates are readily available in the diet, providing 17 kJ (4 kcal) per gram of energy (15.7 kJ (3.75 kcal) per gram monosaccharide equivalent). Carbohydrate intake comprises:

- polysaccharide starch
- disaccharides (mainly sucrose)
- monosaccharides (glucose and fructose).

Carbohydrate is cheap, compared with other foodstuffs; a great deal is therefore eaten, usually more than required. WHO suggests that sugar intake should be less than 5% of a person's total energy consumption.

Dietary fibre

Dietary fibre, which is largely **non-starch polysaccharide** (NSP; entirely NSP according to some authorities), is often removed in the processing of food. This leaves highly refined carbohydrates, such as sucrose, which contribute to the development of dental caries and obesity. Lignin is included in dietary fibre in some classification systems but it is not a polysaccharide. It is only a minor component of the human diet.

The principal classes of NSP are:

- cellulose
- hemicelluloses
- pectins
- gums.

None of these is digested by gut enzymes. However, NSP is partly broken down in the gastrointestinal tract, mainly by colonic bacteria, producing gas and volatile fatty acids, e.g. butyrate.

All plant food, when unprocessed, contains NSP, so that all unprocessed food eaten will increase the NSP content of the diet. Bran, the fibre from wheat, provides an easy way of adding additional fibre to the diet; it increases faecal bulk and is helpful in the treatment of constipation.

The average daily intake of NSP in the diet is approximately 16 g. NSP deficiency is accepted as an entity by many authorities and it is suggested that the total NSP be increased to up to 30 g daily. This could be achieved by increased consumption of bread, potatoes, fruit and vegetables, with a reduction in sugar intake in order not to increase total calories. Each extra gram of fibre daily adds approximately 3–5 g to the daily stool weight. Pectins and gums have also been added to food to slow down monosaccharide absorption, and this is particularly useful in type 2 diabetes.

Eating a diet rich in plant foods (fruits, vegetables, cereals and whole grain – the main sources of dietary fibre) is broadly recommended for general health promotion, including protection against ischaemic heart disease, stroke and certain types of cancers. This has been attributed to a lipid-lowering effect and to the presence of protective substances, such as vitamin and non-vitamin antioxidants and other vitamins such as folic acid, which is linked to homocysteine metabolism, a risk factor for cardiovascular disease. Fermentation of fibre in the colon may protect against the development of colonic cancer. However, associated lifestyle factors, such as low physical activity, may also help explain some of those associations.

Health promotion

Many chronic diseases – particularly obesity, diabetes mellitus and cardiovascular disease – cause premature mortality and morbidity, and are potentially preventable by dietary change. This is a global problem; for example, obesity affects 1 in 9 adults in the world, and the body mass index (BMI) is now similar in high- and middle-income groups. Reduction in salt and fat intake, combined with exercise and stopping smoking, would have a major effect on the health of the population.

Box 33.5 suggests the composition of the 'ideal healthy diet'. The values given are based on the principle of:

- reducing total fat in the diet, particularly saturated fat
- increasing consumption of fish, which contains *n*-3 (or ω-3) PUFAs
- increasing intake of wholegrain cereals and green and orange vegetables and fruits, leading to an increase in fibre and antioxidants.

Reductions in dietary sodium and cholesterol have also been suggested. There would be no disadvantage in this, and most studies have suggested some benefit.

Fortification of foods

Fortification of foods with specific nutrients is common. In the UK, **margarine** and **milk** are fortified with vitamins A and D, **flour** with calcium, iron, thiamine and niacin, and **breakfast cereals** with several vitamins and iron.

Nutrient goals and dietary guidelines

The interests of the individual are often different from those associated with government policy. A distinction needs to be made between nutrient goals and dietary guidelines:

- **Nutrient goals** refer to the national intakes of nutrients that are considered appropriate for optimal health in the population.

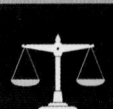

- **Dietary guidelines** refer to the dietary methods used to achieve these goals.

Since dietary habits vary in different countries, dietary guidelines may also differ, even when the nutrient goals are the same. Nutrient goals are based on scientific information that links nutrient intake to disease. Although the information is incomplete, it includes evidence from a wide range of sources, including experimental animal studies, clinical studies, and both short-term and long-term epidemiological studies.

Further reading

Black RE, Victora CG, Walker SP et al. Maternal and child undernutrition and overweight in low-income and middle-income countries. *Lancet* 2013; 382:427–451.
Bosch J, Gerstein HC, Dagenais GR et al. n-3 fatty acids and cardiovascular outcomes in patients with dysglycemia. *N Engl J Med* 2012; 367:309–318.
Panel on Dietary Reference Values of the Committee on Medical Aspects of Food Policy. *Dietary Reference for Food Energy and Nutrients for the United Kingdom (Report 41DOH).* London: HMSO; 1991.
Roncaglioni MC, Tombesi M, Avanzini F et al. n-3 fatty acids in patients with multiple cardiovascular risk factors. *N Engl J Med* 2013; 368:1800–1808.
Scientific Advisory Committee on Nutrition 2011. *Dietary Reference Values for Energy.* London: Stationery Office; 2012.

PROTEIN–ENERGY MALNUTRITION

Developed countries

Starvation uncomplicated by disease is relatively uncommon in developed countries, although some degree of under-nourishment is seen in very poor areas. Most nutritional problems occurring in the population at large are due to eating wrong combinations of foodstuffs, such as an excess of refined carbohydrate or a diet low in fresh vegetables. Under-nourishment associated with disease is common in hospitals and nursing homes, and **Box 33.6** gives a list of conditions in which malnutrition is often seen. Surgical complications, with sepsis, are a common cause. Many patients are admitted to hospital under-nourished, and a variety of chronic conditions predispose to this state **(Box 33.7)**.

Most of the weight loss, leading to malnutrition, is due to **poor intake secondary to the anorexia associated with the underlying condition**. Disease may also contribute by causing malabsorption and increased catabolism, which is mediated by complex changes in cytokines, hormones, side-effects of drugs, and immobility. The elderly are particularly at risk of malnutrition because they often suffer from diseases and psychosocial problems, such as social isolation or bereavement (see **Box 33.7**).

Pathophysiology of starvation

In the first 24 h following low dietary intake, the body relies for energy on the breakdown of hepatic glycogen to glucose **(Fig. 33.4)**. Hepatic glycogen stores are small and therefore gluconeogenesis is soon necessary to maintain glucose levels. Gluconeogenesis takes place mainly from pyruvate, lactate, glycerol and amino acids, especially alanine and glutamine. The majority of protein breakdown takes place in muscle, with eventual loss of muscle bulk.

Lipolysis, the breakdown of the body's fat stores, also occurs. It is inhibited by insulin, but the level of this hormone falls off as starvation continues. The stored triglyceride is hydrolysed by lipase to glycerol, which is used for gluconeogenesis, and also to nonesterified fatty acids, which can be used directly as a fuel or oxidized in the liver to ketone bodies.

Adaptive processes take place as starvation continues, to prevent the body's available protein being completely utilized. There is a decrease in metabolic rate and total body energy expenditure. Central nervous metabolism changes from glucose as a substrate to ketone bodies. Gluconeogenesis in the liver decreases, as does protein breakdown in muscle, both of these processes being inhibited directly by ketone bodies. Most of the energy at this stage

---

> **i** **Box 33.6 Common conditions associated with protein–energy malnutrition**

- Sepsis
- Trauma
- Surgery, particularly of the gastrointestinal tract with complications
- Gastrointestinal disease, particularly involving the small bowel

- Dementia
- Malignancy
- Any very ill patient
- Severe chronic inflammatory diseases
- Psychosocial: poverty, social isolation, anorexia nervosa, depression

---

> **i** **Box 33.7 Nutritional consequences of disease and the underlying risk factors (physical/psychosocial problems)**

Risk factors	Consequence
Underlying disease	
Almost any moderate/severe chronic disease	Anorexia, increased requirements for some nutrients, and other effects initiated below (depending on condition)
Recovery from severe acute/subacute disease	
Physical problems	
Muscle weakness (respiratory and peripheral muscles) and/or incoordination Severe arthritis in hands and arms	} Problems with shopping, cooking and eating
Swallowing problem (neurological causes), painful or obstructive conditions of mouth and GIT	Inadequate food intake, and/or risk of aspiration pneumonia
GIT symptoms (e.g. nausea, vomiting, diarrhoea, jaundice)	Food aversion, malabsorption (small bowel disease), anorexia
Sensory deficit (e.g. impaired sight, hearing and other deficits)	Difficulties in shopping, cooking and/or decreased intake of food
Psychosocial problems	
Loneliness, depression, bereavement, confusion, living alone, poverty, alcoholism, drug addiction	Self-neglect, inadequate intake of food or quality of food
Multiple drug use (polypharmacy)	Indication of severe disease or multiple physical and psychosocial problems; drugs may lead to confusion, sedation, depression and GIT side-effects (including malabsorption of nutrients)

GIT, gastrointestinal tract.

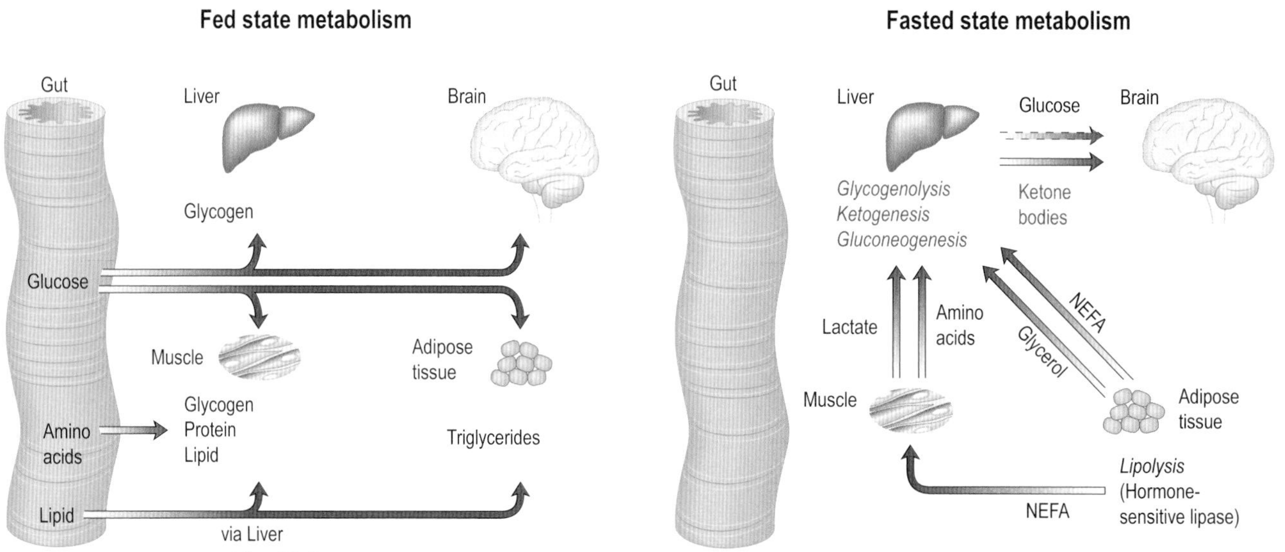

Fed state metabolism

Fasted state metabolism

Fig. 33.4 Metabolism in the fed and the fasted state. NEFA, non-esterified fatty acids.

comes from adipose tissue, with some gluconeogenesis from amino acids, particularly from alanine in the liver and glutamine in the kidney.

The **metabolic response to prolonged starvation** differs between lean and obese individuals. One of the major differences concerns the proportion of energy derived from protein oxidation, which determines the proportion of weight loss from lean tissues. This proportion may be up to three times smaller in obese subjects than lean subjects. It can be regarded as an adaptation that depends on the composition of the initial reserves (see **Fig. 33.3**). This means that deterioration in body function is more rapid in lean subjects, and survival time shorter in lean subjects (approximately 2 months) compared with the obese (in whom it can be at least several months).

Following trauma or shock, some of the adaptive changes do not take place. Glucocorticoids and cytokines (see below) stimulate the ubiquitin–proteasome pathway in muscle, which is responsible for accelerated proteolysis in muscle in many catabolic illnesses. In starvation, there is a decrease in BMR, while in inflammatory and traumatic disease, there is often an increase in BMR. These changes all result in continuing gluconeogenesis with massive muscle breakdown, and further reduction in survival time.

Regulation of metabolism

Tissue metabolism is regulated by multiple coordinated processes. Some are rapid, involving nerves, whilst others are slower, involving circulating substrates and hormones. Factors include:

- **Circulating substrate concentrations.** The uptake and metabolism of ketone bodies, which serve as the major fuel for the brain during prolonged starvation, are primarily determined by the circulatory concentration, which can increase up to 5 mmol/L or more. The liver is responsible for the production of ketone bodies, which is, in turn, controlled by the availability of fatty acids derived from adipose tissue. Substrates may also compete with each other for metabolism; e.g. glucose competes with non-esterified fatty acids for uptake and metabolism in muscle and heart (the glucose–fatty acid cycle), and this is independent of hormones.
- **Blood flow.** The delivery of substrates to tissues depends not only on their circulating concentration but also on the blood flow

to tissues. In many tissues, there is coupling between metabolic activity and blood flow, with arterioles regulating blood flow to the tissue according to demand; e.g. blood flow to muscle increases during exercise.

- **Signals.** Hormones and other signals, such as cytokines (see below), regulate intracellular metabolism.

Insulin/glucagon ratios in the fed and fasted state

In the fed state, insulin/glucagon ratios are high. Insulin promotes synthesis of glycogen, protein and fat, and inhibits lipolysis and gluconeogenesis.

In the fasted state, insulin/glucagon ratios are low. Glucagon acts mainly on the liver and has no action on muscle. It increases glycogenolysis and gluconeogenesis, as well as increasing ketone body production from fatty acids. It also stimulates lipolysis in adipose tissue. Catecholamines have a similar action to glucagon but also affect muscle metabolism. These agents both act via cyclic adenosine monophosphate (cAMP) to stimulate lipolysis, producing free fatty acids that can then act as a major source of energy.

Proportion of lean to fat tissue

During weight loss uncomplicated by disease, the proportion of lean to fat tissue loss (or proportion of energy derived from protein metabolism) is greater in lean than overweight/obese individuals.

During acute disease, loss of lean tissue, which is associated with protein oxidation, can be particularly rapid. Hormones such as corticosteroids, pro-inflammatory cytokines and insulin resistance are all involved.

Role of cytokines

The metabolic response to trauma, injury and inflammation depends on the balance between *pro*-inflammatory (e.g. tumour necrosis factor, TNF; interleukin-2, IL-2) and *anti*-inflammatory cytokines (e.g. IL-10), and the production of many of these cytokines is influenced by genetic polymorphisms. Since many chronic diseases, including atherosclerosis, have an inflammatory component, these changes have wide-reaching metabolic implications.

Cytokines such as IL-1, IL-6 and TNF play a significant role in regulating metabolism. In acute diseases, they contribute to the

---

Box 33.8 Keys to detecting chronic protein–energy malnutrition (PEM) in developed countries

1. Body mass index (BMI)
   – Probable chronic PEM: <18.5 kg/m²
   – Possible chronic PEM: 18.5–20 kg/m²
   – Little or no risk of chronic PEM: >20 kg/m²
   In patients with oedema or dehydration the BMI may be somewhat misleading.
2. Weight loss in previous 3–6 months
   – >10%: high risk of developing PEM
   – 5–10%: possible risk of developing PEM
   – <5%: low/no risk of developing PEM
3. Acute disease effect
   – Diseases that have resulted or are likely to result in no dietary intake for >5 days (e.g. prolonged unconsciousness, persistent swallowing problems after a stroke, or prolonged ileus after abdominal surgery): high risk of malnutrition

---

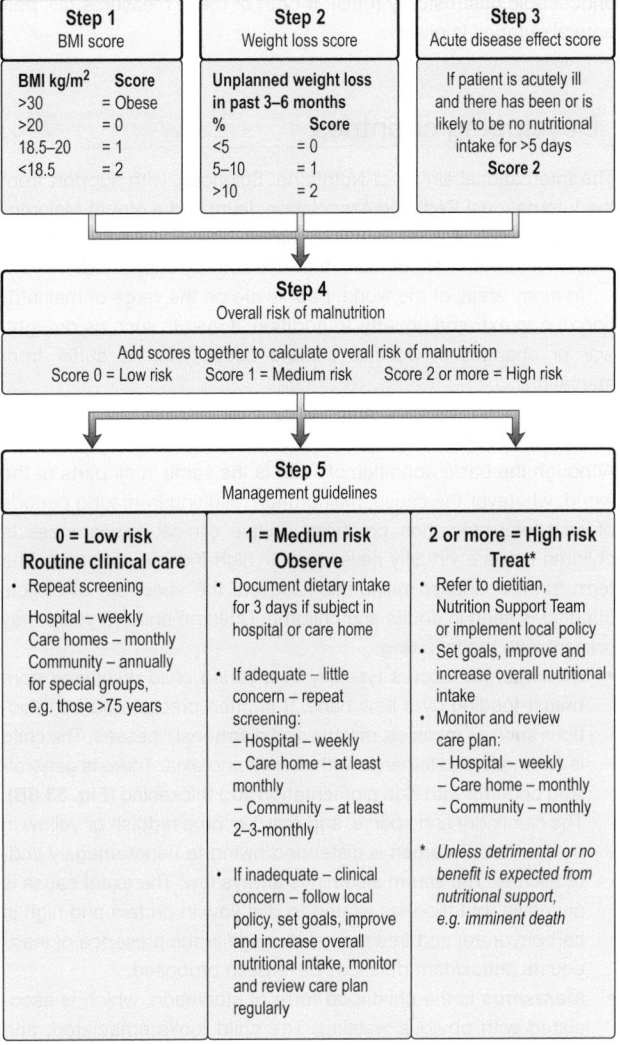

Fig. 33.5 **Malnutrition Universal Screening Tool (MUST).** BMI, body mass index. *(With permission from the British Association for Parenteral and Enteral Nutrition (BAPEN), at: http://www.bapen.org.uk.)*

---

catabolic process, glycogenolysis and acute phase protein synthesis. TNF, which inhibits lipoprotein lipase, is one of a number of 'cachexia factors' in patients with cancer.

It is unclear how these cytokines interact with central feeding pathways to cause anorexia. However, in animal models of both cancer and inflammatory bowel disease, many peripheral and central mediators of appetite are involved. For example, neuropeptide Y levels in the hypothalamus are often inappropriately low, so there is a reduced drive to feed.

Clinical features

Patients are sometimes seen with loss of weight or malnutrition (failure to thrive in children) as the primary symptom. Mostly, however, malnourishment is only seen as an accompaniment of some other disease process, such as malignancy. Severe malnutrition is seen mainly with advanced organic disease or after surgical procedures followed by complications. Three key features that help in the detection of chronic protein–energy malnutrition (PEM) in adults are listed in **Box 33.8**.

Other factors that may suggest PEM include:

- history of decreased food intake/loss of appetite
- clothes becoming loose-fitting (weight loss) and a general appearance indicating obvious wasting
- physical and psychosocial disturbances likely to have contributed to the weight loss.

The factors listed in **Box 33.8** act as a link between detection and management (see also **Fig. 33.5**, the Malnutrition Universal Screening Tool). If the underlying physical or psychosocial problems are not addressed adequately, treatment may not be successful.

PEM leads to a depression of the immunological defence mechanism, resulting in a decreased resistance to infection. It also detrimentally affects muscle strength and fatigue, reproductive function (e.g. in anorexia nervosa, which is common in adolescent girls; see p. 797), wound healing and psychological function (depression, anxiety, hypochondriasis, loss of libido).

In children, growth failure is a key element in the diagnosis of PEM. WHO standards for optimal growth in children of 0–4 years have been adopted by developing and developed countries. They aim to reflect optimal rather than prevailing growth in both developed and developing countries, since they involved a healthy pregnancy and children born to non-smoking, relatively affluent mothers who breast-fed their children exclusively or predominantly

for the first 6 months of life. The general principles of management of severe PEM in children are similar in developed and developing countries but resources are required to manage the problems once they have been identified (see p. 1236).

Management

When malnutrition is obvious and the underlying disease cannot be corrected at once, some form of nutritional support is necessary (see also p. 1253). Nutrition should be given enterally if the gastrointestinal tract is functioning adequately. This can be done most easily by encouraging the patient to eat more often and by giving a high-calorie supplement. If this is not possible, a liquefied diet may be given intragastrically via a fine-bore tube or by a percutaneous endoscopic gastrostomy (PEG). If both of these measures fail, parenteral nutrition is given.

Developing countries

The International Union of Nutritional Sciences, with support from the International Pediatric Association, launched a global Malnutrition Task Force in 2005 to ensure that an integrated system of prevention and treatment of malnutrition is actively supported.

In many areas of the world, people are on the verge of malnutrition due to extreme poverty. In addition, if events such as drought, war or changes in political climate occur, millions suffer from starvation.

Clinical features

Although the basic condition of PEM is the same in all parts of the world, whatever the cause, malnutrition resulting from long periods of near-total starvation produces unique clinical appearances in children that are virtually never seen in high-income countries. The term 'protein–energy malnutrition' covers the spectrum of clinical conditions seen in adults and children. Children under 5 years may present with the following:

- **Kwashiorkor** occurs typically in a young child displaced from breast-feeding by a new baby. It is often precipitated by infections such as measles, malaria and diarrhoeal illnesses. The child is apathetic and lethargic with severe anorexia. There is generalized oedema with skin pigmentation and thickening **(Fig. 33.6B)**. The hair is dry and sparse, and may become reddish or yellow in colour. The abdomen is distended owing to hepatomegaly and/or ascites. The serum albumin is always low. The exact cause is unknown, but theories related to diet (low in protein and high in carbohydrate) and free radical damage in the presence of inadequate antioxidant defences have been proposed.
- **Marasmus** is the childhood form of starvation, which is associated with obvious wasting. The child looks emaciated, and there is obvious muscle wasting and loss of body fat. There

is no oedema. The hair is thin and dry **(Fig. 33.6A)**. The child is not as apathetic or anorexic as with kwashiorkor. Diarrhoea is frequently present and signs of infection must be looked for carefully.

The **WHO classification of severe malnutrition (Box 33.9)** makes no distinction between kwashiorkor and marasmus because the approach to treatment is similar in both. The WHO classification of chronic under-nutrition in children is based on standard deviation (SD) scores. Thus, children with an SD score between −2 and −3 (between 3 and 2 SD scores below the median, corresponding to a value between 0.13 and 2.3 centiles) can be regarded as being at moderate risk of under-nutrition; below an SD score of −3, there is a risk of severe malnutrition. A low weight-for-height is a measure of thinness (wasting when pathological) and a low height-for-age is a measure of shortness (stunting when pathological). Those with oedema and clinical signs of severe malnutrition are classified as having oedematous malnutrition.

Starvation in adults may lead to extreme loss of weight, depending on the severity and duration. They may crave food, are apathetic, and complain of cold and weakness with a loss of subcutaneous fat and muscle wasting. The WHO classification is based on BMI, with a value less than $18.5\,kg/m^2$ indicating malnutrition (severe malnutrition if $<16.0\,kg/m^2$).

Severely malnourished adults and children are very susceptible to respiratory and gastrointestinal infections, leading to an increased mortality in these groups.

Investigations

These are not always practicable in certain settings in the developing world.

- **Blood tests** may demonstrate the following results:
  - Anaemia due to folate, iron and copper deficiency is often present, but the haematocrit may be high owing to dehydration.
  - Eosinophilia suggests parasitic infestation.
  - Electrolyte disturbances are common.
  - Malarial parasites should be sought.
  - Human immunodeficiency (HIV) tests should be performed.

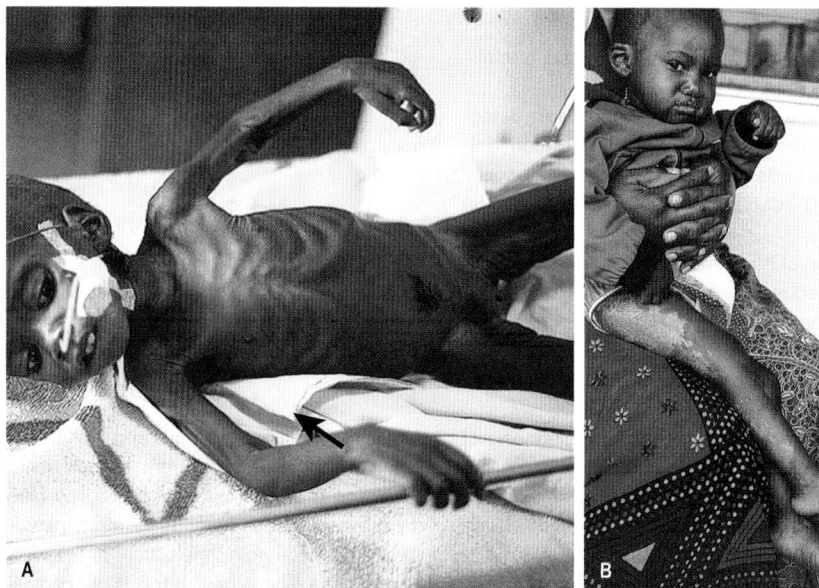

Fig. 33.6 Malnourished children. (A) Marasmus. **(B)** Kwashiorkor. *(Courtesy of Dr Paul Kelly.)*

- **Stools** should be examined for parasitic infestations.
- **Chest X-ray** may reveal tuberculosis, which is common and easily missed if a chest X-ray is not performed.

Management

Management must involve the provision of protein and energy supplements and the control of infection. The approach to the treatment of children is described below. Adults do not usually suffer such severe malnutrition but the same general principles of treatment should be followed.

Resuscitation and stabilization

The severely ill child will require:

- correction of fluid and electrolyte abnormalities, avoiding intravenous therapy, if possible, because of the danger of fluid overload
- treatment of shock

Box 33.9 Classification of childhood malnutrition

	Moderate malnutrition	Severe malnutrition[a]
Symmetrical oedema	No	Yes: oedematous malnutrition[b]
Weight-for-height SD score	−3 to −2 (70–79%)[c]	<−3 (<70%)[c] (severe wasting)[d]
Height-for-age SD score	−3 to −2 (85–89%)[c]	<−3 (<85%)[c] (severe stunting)

[a]The diagnoses are not mutually exclusive. [b]Older classifications use the terms kwashiorkor and marasmic kwashiorkor instead. [c]Percentage of the median National Centre for Health Statistics/WHO reference. [d]Called marasmus (without oedema) in the Wellcome classification and grade II in the Gomez classification.

Box 33.10 Infections seen in PEM in developing countries

- Diarrhoea
  - Bacteria
  - Protozoa
  - Helminths
- Malaria
- Tuberculosis
- HIV infection
- Measles
- Respiratory infections

- treatment of hypoglycaemia (blood glucose <3 mmol/L), hypothermia (reduce heat loss, and provide additional heat if necessary) and infection (antibiotics) – these often coexist.

The standard WHO **oral hydration solution** has a high sodium and low potassium content and is not suitable for severely malnourished children. Instead, the rehydration solution for malnutrition (ReSoMal) is recommended. It is commercially available but can also be produced by modification of the standard WHO oral hydration solution.

Infection is common (**Box 33.10**). Diarrhoea is often due to bacterial or protozoal overgrowth; metronidazole is very effective and is often given routinely. Parasites are also common and, as facilities for stool examination are usually not available, mebendazole 100 mg twice daily should be given for 3 days. In high-risk areas, antimalarial therapy is given. A recent study in Malawi suggests that the addition of antibiotics to therapeutic regimens for uncomplicated severe acute malnutrition in children less than 5 years of age is associated with a significant improvement in recovery and mortality.

Large doses of **vitamin A** are also given because deficiency of this vitamin is common. After the initial resuscitation, further stabilization over the next few days is undertaken, as indicated in **Box 33.11**.

Re-feeding

This needs to be planned carefully. During the initial management of the acute situation, a balanced diet with sufficient protein and energy is given to maintain a steady state. Large increases in energy can lead to heart failure, circulatory collapse and death (**re-feeding syndrome**). Initial feeding involves the administration of feeds that are low in osmolarity and low in lactose. WHO recommendations are 100 kcal/kg per day; 1.0–1.5 g protein/kg per day; and 130 mL liquid/kg per day (100 mL/kg per day if the child has marked oedema). Attempts should be made to give the feeds slowly and frequently (e.g. 2-hourly during days 1–2; 3-hourly during days 3–5; and 4-hourly thereafter), although anorexia is often a problem and can be exacerbated by excessive feeding. If necessary, fluids and food should be given by nasogastric tube. The child is then gradually weaned to liquids and then solids by mouth. All severely malnourished children have vitamin and mineral

Box 33.11 Timeframe for the management of the child with severe malnutrition (10-step approach recommended by WHO)

Management	Stabilization		Rehabilitation	Follow-up
	Days 1–2	Days 3–7	Weeks 2–6	Weeks 7–26
1. Treat or prevent hypoglycaemia	→→→→→			
2. Treat or prevent hypothermia	→→→→→			
3. Treat or prevent dehydration	→→→→→			
4. Correct electrolyte imbalance	→→→→→→→→→→→→→→→→			
5. Treat infection	→→→→→→→→→→			
6. Correct micronutrient deficiencies	Without iron		With iron →→→→→→	
7. Begin feeding	→→→→→→→→→→			
8. Increase feeding to recover lost weight			→→→→→→→→→→→→→→→→→	
9. Stimulate emotional and sensorial development			→→→→→→→→→→→→→→→→→→	
10. Prepare for discharge			→→→→→→→	

deficiencies. Although anaemia is common, the WHO recommends giving iron only after the child develops a good appetite and starts gaining weight, because of concern about detrimental effects during the acute phase of illness (iron is a pro-oxidant). The child should be given daily micronutrient supplements for at least 2 weeks. These should include a multivitamin supplement with folic acid, zinc and copper.

Rehabilitation

Gradually, as the child improves, more energy can be given, and during rehabilitation, weight gain is achieved by providing extra energy and protein ('catch-up weight gain'). Children who have been severely ill need constant attention right through the convalescent period, as home conditions are often poor and feeds are refused. Sensory stimulation and emotional support are major components of management during both the stabilization and the rehabilitation phases. The treatment of underlying chronic infective conditions, such as HIV, malaria and tuberculosis, is also necessary.

Care setting

In some parts of the world where malnutrition is widespread, there are not enough hospitals or therapeutic feeding centres to cope with the problem; this emphasizes the need for outpatient and community-based programmes, although these require investment and time to build to full capacity. The programmes may involve the use of ready-to-use therapeutic foods, such as energy-dense pastes with minerals and vitamins, without the need to add water, which could potentially contaminate the food.

Prognosis

Children with extreme malnutrition have a mortality of over 50%. By careful management, this can be reduced significantly to less than 10%, depending on the availability of facilities and trained staff. Treatment of underlying disease is essential. Brain development takes place in the first years of life, a time when severe PEM is frequently seen. There is evidence that intellectual impairment and behavioural abnormalities occur in severely affected children. Physical growth is also impaired. Probably both of these effects can be alleviated if it is possible to maintain a high standard of living with a good diet and freedom from infection over a long period.

Prevention

Prevention of PEM depends not only on the availability of adequate nutrients but also on the education of both governments and individuals in the importance of good nutrition and immunization **(Box 33.12)**. Short-term programmes are useful for acute shortages of food, but long-term programmes involving improved agriculture are equally necessary. Bad feeding practices and infections are more prevalent than actual shortage of food in many areas of the world. However, good surveillance is necessary to avoid periods of famine.

> **i** **Box 33.12 Prevention of protein–energy malnutrition – GOBIF (a WHO priority programme)**
>
> - **G**rowth monitoring: the WHO has a simple growth chart that the mother keeps
> - **O**ral rehydration, particularly for diarrhoea
> - **B**reast-feeding supplemented by food after 6 months
> - **I**mmunization: against measles, tetanus, pertussis, diphtheria, polio and tuberculosis (see also **Box 20.20**)
> - **F**amily planning

Food supplements (and additional vitamins) should be given to 'at-risk' groups by adding high-energy food (e.g. milk powder, meat concentrates) to the diet. Pregnancy and lactation are times of high energy requirement and supplements have been shown to be beneficial.

Further reading

Black RE, Victora CG, Walker SP et al. Maternal and child undernutrition and overweight in low-income and middle-income countries. *Lancet* 2013; 382: 427–451.
Cawood AL, Elia M, Stratton RJ. Systematic review and meta-analysis of the effects of high protein oral nutritional supplements. *Ageing Res Rev* 2012; 11:278–296.
Collins PF, Elia M, Stratton RJ. Nutritional support and functional capacity in chronic obstructive pulmonary disease: a systematic review and meta-analysis. *Respirology* 2013; 18:616–629.
Elia M. Multidisciplinary input is essential in the care of malnourished people. *Guidelines in Practice* 2013; 16:42–50.
Mehler PS, Brown C. Anorexia nervosa - medical complications. *Journal of eating disorders* 2015; 3:11.
Trehan I, Goldbach HS, Lacey N et al. Antibiotics as part of the management of severe acute malnutrition. *N Engl J Med* 2013; 368:425–435.
World Health Organization. *Guideline: Updates on the Management of Severe Acute Malnutrition in Infants and Children.* WHO: Geneva; 2013.
Wright CM, Williams AF, Ellman D et al. Using the new UK-WHO growth charts. *Br Med J* 2010; 340:647–650 (charts and supporting materials: http://www.growthcharts.rcpch.ac.uk).

VITAMINS

Deficiencies due to inadequate intake associated with PEM **(Box 33.13)** are commonly seen in developing countries. This is not, however, invariable. For example, vitamin A deficiency is not seen in Jamaica, but is common in PEM in Hyderabad, India. In the West, deficiency of vitamins is less common but prominent in the specific groups shown in **Box 33.14**. The widespread use of vitamins as 'tonics' is unnecessary. Toxicity from excess fat-soluble vitamins is occasionally seen.

FAT-SOLUBLE VITAMINS

Vitamin A

Vitamin A (retinol) is part of the family of retinoids, which is present in food and the body as esters combined with long-chain fatty acids. The richest food source is liver, but it is also found in milk, butter, cheese, egg yolks and fish oils. Retinol or carotene is added to margarine in the UK and other countries.

Beta-carotene is the main carotenoid found in green vegetables, carrots and other yellow and red fruits. Other carotenoids, lycopene and lutein, are probably of little quantitative importance as dietary precursors of vitamin A.

Beta-carotene is cleaved in the intestinal mucosa by carotene dioxygenase, yielding retinaldehyde, which can be reduced to retinol. Between one-quarter and one-third of dietary vitamin A in the UK is derived from retinoids. Nutritionally, $6\,\mu g$ of β-carotene is equivalent to $1\,\mu g$ of preformed retinol; vitamin A activity in the diet is given as retinol equivalents.

Function

Retinol is stored in the liver and is transported in plasma bound to an α-globulin, retinol-binding protein (RBP). Vitamin A has several metabolic roles:

- Retinaldehyde in its *cis* form is found in the opsin proteins in the rods (rhodopsin) and cones (iodopsin) of the retina (see p. 913).

i **Box 33.13 Fat-soluble and water-soluble vitamins: UK reference nutrient intake (RNI) and lower reference nutrient intake (LRNI) fo[r] men aged 19–50 years[a]**

Vitamin	RNI/day (sufficient)	LRNI/day (insufficient)	Major clinical features of deficiency	Dietary sources
Fat-soluble				
A (retinol)	700 µg	300 µg	Xerophthalmia, night blindness, keratomalacia, follicular hyperkeratosis	Oily fish, liver, dairy products (provitamin A carotenoids – carrots, dark green, leafy vegetables, corn, tomatoes)
D (cholecalciferol)	No dietary intake required	10 µg (living indoors)	Rickets, osteomalacia	Oily fish, fortified breakfast cereals and margarine, eggs, milk
K	(1 µg/kg body weight; safe and adequate)[b]		Coagulation defects	Green, leafy vegetables, liver, cheese, certain fruits (kiwi fruit, rhubarb)
E (α-tocopherol)	(15 mg)[c]		Neurological disorders, e.g. ataxia	Plant oils (soya, palm oil), animal fats, nuts, seeds, vegetables, wheatgerm
Water-soluble				
B_1 (thiamine)	0.4 mg/1000 kcal[d]	0.23 mg/1000 kcal[d]	Beriberi, Wernicke–Korsakoff syndrome	Wide range of animal and vegetable products. Fortified cereals, flour and bread, unrefined cereals, grain, nuts, legumes, organ meats
B_2 (riboflavin)	1.3 mg	0.8 mg	Angular stomatitis	Dairy products (major source), cereals grains, meat, fish, broccoli, spinach
Niacin	6.6 mg/1000 kcal	4.4 mg/1000 kcal	Pellagra	Meat, cereals
B_6 (pyridoxine)	15 µg/g of dietary protein	11 µg/g of dietary protein	Polyneuropathy	Meat, cereals
B_{12} (cobalamin)	1.5 µg	1.0 µg	Megaloblastic anaemia, neurological disorders	Meat, fortified breakfast cereals, eggs
Folate	200 µg	100 µg	Megaloblastic anaemia	Widely distributed in animal (especially liver) and plant foods (e.g. vegetables)
C (ascorbic acid)	40 mg	10 mg	Scurvy	Fresh vegetables, citrus fruits, strawberries, spinach, tomatoes

[a]Values vary with age and sex. For women, values are generally the same or lower than for men, except during pregnancy and lactation, when they are generally higher than for men. [b]No RNI. [c]No official RNI in the UK because the amount varies, depending on the polyunsaturated fatty acid content of the diet; 15 mg is the value from the National Academy of Sciences, USA. [d]Thiamine requirements are related to energy metabolism.

? Box 33.14 Some causes of vitamin deficiency in developed countries

Decreased intake
- Alcohol dependency: chiefly B vitamins (e.g. thiamine)
- Small bowel disease: chiefly folate, occasionally fat-soluble vitamins
- Vegans: vitamin D (if no exposure to sunlight), vitamin B_{12}
- Elderly with poor diet: chiefly vitamin D (if no exposure to sunlight), folate
- Anorexia from any cause: chiefly folate

Decreased absorption
- Ileal disease/resection: only vitamin B_{12}
- Liver and biliary tract disease: fat-soluble vitamins
- Intestinal bacterial overgrowth: vitamin B_{12}
- Oral antibiotics: vitamin K

Miscellaneous
- Long-term enteral or parenteral nutrition: usually vitamin supplements are given
- Renal disease: vitamin D
- Drug antagonists (e.g. methotrexate interfering with folate metabolism)

Light causes retinaldehyde to change to its *trans* isomer, and this leads to changes in membrane potentials that are transmitted to the brain.

- Retinol and retinoic acid are involved in the control of cell proliferation and differentiation.
- Retinyl phosphate is a co-factor in the synthesis of most glycoproteins containing mannose.

---

i **Box 33.15 Classification of xerophthalmia by ocular signs**

Ocular signs	Classification
Night blindness	XN
Conjunctival xerosis	XIA
Bitot's spot	X2
Corneal xerosis	X2
Corneal ulceration/keratomalacia <⅓ corneal surface	X3A
Corneal ulceration/keratomalacia >⅓ corneal surface	X3B
Corneal scar	XS
Xerophthalmic fundus	XF

(From WHO/UNICEF/IVACG 1988.)

Vitamin A deficiency

Worldwide, vitamin A deficiency and xerophthalmia (see below) are major causes of blindness in young children, despite intensive preventive programmes.

Xerophthalmia has been classified by the WHO **(Box 33.15)**. Impaired adaptation, followed by night blindness, is the first effect. There is dryness and thickening of the conjunctiva and the cornea (xerophthalmia occurs as a result of keratinization). Bitot's spots – white plaques of keratinized epithelial cells – are found on the conjunctiva of

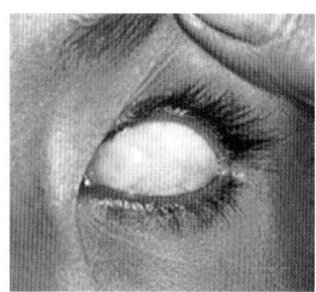

Fig. 33.7 Vitamin A deficiency. Blindness due to vitamin A deficiency and corneal scarring. *(Courtesy of Ehrnstrom P. In: Bolognia J, Jorrizzo J, Rapini R (eds). Dermatology, 2nd edn. St Louis: Mosby; 2008: Fig. 51.6.)*

young children with vitamin A deficiency. These spots can, however, be seen without vitamin A deficiency, possibly caused by exposure. Corneal softening, ulceration and dissolution (keratomalacia) eventually occur, superimposed infection is a frequent accompaniment and both lead to blindness **(Fig. 33.7)**. In PEM, retinol-binding protein is reduced, along with other proteins. This suggests vitamin A deficiency, although body stores are not necessarily reduced.

Vitamin A in malnourished children

Vitamin A supplementation (single oral dose of 60 mg retinol palmitate) appears to improve morbidity and mortality from measles. It has also been suggested that similar supplementation reduces morbidity and/or mortality from diarrhoeal diseases and respiratory infections, and improves growth.

Diagnosis

In parts of the world where deficiency is common, diagnosis is made on the basis of the clinical features, and deficiency should always be suspected if any degree of malnutrition is present. Blood levels of vitamin A will usually be low, but the best guide to diagnosis is a response to replacement therapy.

Management

Urgent treatment with retinol palmitate 30 mg orally should be given on two successive days. In the presence of vomiting and diarrhoea, 30 mg of vitamin A is given intramuscularly. Associated malnutrition must be treated, and superadded bacterial infection should be treated with antibiotics. Referral for specialist ophthalmic treatment is necessary in severe cases.

Prevention

Most Western diets contain enough dairy products and green vegetables, but vitamin A is added to foodstuffs (e.g. margarine) in some countries. Vitamin A is not destroyed by cooking.

In some developing countries, vitamin A supplements are given at the time a child attends for measles vaccination. Food fortification programmes are another approach. Education of the population is necessary and people should be encouraged to grow their own vegetables. In particular, pregnant women and children should be encouraged to eat green vegetables and yellow fruits.

Other effects of vitamin A

In a chronically malnourished population, maternal repletion with vitamin A before, during and after pregnancy may improve lung function in the offspring at 9–13 years. It may also reduce maternal mortality. Administration of vitamin A to young children at risk of deficiency reduces mortality, although to a lesser extent than previously thought. The effect of β-carotene in cardiovascular and other diseases is discussed below in the section entitled 'Dietary antioxidants' (see p. 1242). Retinoic acid and some synthetic retinoids are used in dermatology (see **Box 20.9**).

Possible adverse effects

- **High intakes of vitamin A.** Chronic ingestion of retinol can cause liver and bone damage, hair loss, double vision, vomiting, headaches and other abnormalities. Single doses of 300 mg in adults or 100 mg in children can be harmful.
- **Retinol is teratogenic.** The incidence of birth defects in infants is high with vitamin A intakes of more than 3 mg a day during pregnancy. In pregnancy, extra vitamin A or consumption of liver is not recommended in the UK. However, β-carotene is not toxic.

Vitamin D

Vitamin D is discussed in more detail on pages 483–444, where the most common manifestations of deficiency are outlined (rickets and osteomalacia). Vitamin D status is assessed by measurement of 25-hydroxyvitamin D in the serum. Vitamin D receptors are distributed widely in human tissues but their function in many non-musculoskeletal tissues still remains poorly understood. Vitamin D status has been linked to a wide range of diseases, including:

- cardiovascular disorders (ischaemic heart disease, heart failure, hypertension)
- respiratory disorders (chest infections)
- renal disorders (progression of renal disease)
- endocrine disorders (type 1 and type 2 diabetes)
- neuropsychiatric disorders (depression, cognitive deficits)
- cancer (e.g. prostate, breast, colon) and mortality from various causes.
- multiple sclerosis (see p. 864).

It has therefore been suggested that vitamin D may have a role in global health, and not just the health of the musculoskeletal system. Studies of the relationship between vitamin D serum levels (25-hydroxyvitamin D) and the risk of the conditions listed above have led to different definitions of the optimal level of 25-hydroxyvitamin D for adequate status. This also implies that there are different requirements for vitamin D in different diseases. However, randomized controlled trials (RCTs) of vitamin D supplementation have not been as promising in averting some of these conditions as might have been anticipated from the observational relationships. Reduced circulating concentrations of vitamin D can result not only from lack of exposure to sunlight and a poor diet, but also from inflammation, smoking and obesity.

Vitamin K

Vitamin K is found as phylloquinone (vitamin K_1) in green, leafy vegetables, dairy products, and rapeseed and soya bean oils. Intestinal bacteria can synthesize the other major form of vitamin K, menaquinone (vitamin K_2), in the terminal ileum and colon. Vitamin K is absorbed in a similar manner to other fat-soluble substances in the upper small gut. Some menaquinones must also be absorbed, as this is the major form found in the human liver.

Function

Vitamin K is a co-factor that is necessary for the production not only of blood clotting factors (II, VII, IX and X, and other proteins involved in coagulation), but also of proteins that are necessary for the formation of bone.

Vitamin K is a co-factor for the post-translational carboxylation of specific protein-bound glutamate residues in γ-carboxyglutamate (Gla). Gla residues bind calcium ions to phospholipid templates, and this action on factors II, VII, IX and X, and on proteins C and S, is required for coagulation to take place.

Bone osteoblasts contain three vitamin K-dependent proteins: osteocalcin, matrix Gla protein and protein S, which have a role in bone matrix formation. Osteocalcin contains three Gla residues, which bind tightly to the hydroxyapatite matrix, depending on the degree of carboxylation; this leads to bone mineralization. There is, however, no convincing evidence that vitamin K deficiency or antagonism affects bone other than rapidly growing bone.

Vitamin K deficiency

Vitamin K deficiency results in inadequate synthesis of clotting factors, which leads to an increase in the prothrombin time and haemorrhage. It has also been linked to bone health, but there is inadequate evidence to support the routine use of vitamin K to prevent osteoporosis and reduce fracture risk. Deficiency occurs in the newborn, in cholestatic jaundice, and with concomitant use of vitamin K antagonists.

The newborn

Deficiency occurs in the newborn owing to:
- poor placental transfer of vitamin K
- the fact that there is little vitamin K in breast milk
- the lack of hepatic stores of menaquinone (no intestinal bacteria in the neonate).

Deficiency leads to a haemorrhagic disease of the newborn, which can be prevented with prophylactic vitamin K. Vitamin K (phytomenadione 1 mg, i.m.) is given to all neonates after the risks have been discussed with parents and consent has been obtained.

Cholestatic jaundice

When bile flow into the intestine is interrupted, malabsorption of vitamin K occurs, as no bile salts are available to facilitate absorption and the prothrombin time increases. This can be corrected by giving 10 mg of phytomenadione intramuscularly. (Note that an increased prothrombin time caused by liver disease does not respond to vitamin K injection, there being no shortage of vitamin K – just poor liver function.) In patients with chronic cholestasis (e.g. primary biliary cholangitis), oral therapy with a water-soluble preparation, menadiol sodium phosphate 10 mg daily, is used.

Concomitant vitamin K antagonists

Oral anticoagulants, such as warfarin, antagonize vitamin K. Antibacterial drugs also interfere with the bacterial synthesis of vitamin K.

Vitamin E

Vitamin E includes eight naturally occurring compounds that may be divided into tocopherols and tocotrienols. The most active compound and the most widely available in food is the natural isomer d-d-α-tocopherol (or RRR-α-tocopherol), which accounts for 90% of vitamin E in the human body. Vegetables and seed oils, including soya bean, saffron, sunflower, cereals and nuts, are the main sources. Animal products are poor sources of the vitamin. Vitamin E is absorbed with fat, transported in the blood largely in LDLs.

An individual's vitamin E requirement depends on the intake of polyunsaturated fatty acids (PUFAs). Since this varies widely, no daily requirement is given in the UK. The requirement stated in the USA is approximately 7–10 mg/day, but average diets contain much more than this. If PUFAs are taken in large amounts, more vitamin E is required.

Function

The biological activity of vitamin E results principally from its anti-oxidant properties. In biological membranes, it contributes to membrane stability. It protects cellular structures against damage from a number of highly reactive oxygen species, including hydrogen peroxide, superoxide and other oxygen radicals. Vitamin E may also affect cell proliferation and growth.

Vitamin E deficiency

The first deficiency to be demonstrated was a haemolytic anaemia described in premature infants. Infant formulations now contain vitamin E.

Deficiency is seen only in children with abetalipoproteinaemia (see p. 1196) and in patients on long-term parenteral nutrition. The severe neurological deficit (gross ataxia) can be prevented with vitamin E injections.

Plasma or serum levels of α-tocopherol can be measured and should be corrected for the level of plasma lipids by expressing the value as milligrams per milligram of plasma lipid.

Epidemiological data and clinical trials

Animals fed an atherogenic diet supplemented with α-tocopherol develop far fewer new atheromatous lesions than those fed an atherogenic diet alone; there may be regression of existing lesions.

There is also evidence for vitamin E intake and blood α-tocopherol levels as an independent risk factor for the development of ischaemic heart disease in healthy, well-nourished individuals eating a Western diet. This has been shown in comparisons of different communities in the WHO 'MONICA' observational study.

Randomized trials involving vitamin E supplementation have produced conflicting results, possibly due to factors such as short duration of treatment, use of suboptimal doses or lack of concurrent administration of vitamin C. There are very few trials to assess the role of vitamin E in prevention of peripheral vascular disease and cancer.

WATER-SOLUBLE VITAMINS

Water-soluble vitamins are non-toxic and relatively cheap; they can therefore be given in large amounts if a deficiency is possible. The daily requirements for water-soluble vitamins are given in **Box 33.13**.

Thiamine (vitamin B_1)

Function

Thiamine diphosphate, often called thiamine pyrophosphate (TPP), is an essential co-factor, particularly in carbohydrate metabolism.

TPP is involved in the oxidative decarboxylation of acetyl coenzyme A (CoA) in mitochondria. In formation of acetyl CoA (from pyruvate) and in the Krebs cycle, TPP is the key enzyme for the decarboxylation of α-ketoglutarate to succinyl CoA. TPP is also the co-factor for transketolase, a key enzyme in the hexose monophosphate shunt.

Thiamine is found in many foodstuffs, including cereals, grains, beans and nuts, as well as pork and duck. It is often added to food (e.g. in cereals) in developed countries. The dietary requirement (see **Box 33.13)** depends on energy intake, more being required if the diet is high in carbohydrates.

Following absorption, thiamine is found in all body tissues, the majority being in the liver. Body stores are small and signs of deficiency quickly develop with inadequate intake.

There is no evidence that a high oral intake is dangerous but ataxia has been reported after high parenteral therapy.

Thiamine deficiency

Thiamine deficiency is seen:
- As **beriberi**, where the only staple food consumed is polished rice.
- In **chronic alcohol-dependent patients** who are consuming virtually no food at all.
- In **starved patients** (e.g. with carcinoma of the stomach), and in severe prolonged hyperemesis gravidarum, anorexia nervosa and prolonged total starvation in healthy subjects (e.g. fasts for political reasons). It can also occur in patients given parenteral nutrition with little or no thiamine, as large doses of glucose increase requirements for thiamine and can precipitate deficiency (e.g. during re-feeding).

Beriberi

This is now confined to the poorest areas of South-east Asia. It can be prevented by eating under-milled or parboiled rice, or by fortification of rice with thiamine. The prevention of beriberi needs a general increase in overall food consumption so that the staple diet is varied and includes legumes and pulses, which contain a large amount of thiamine. There are two main clinical types of beriberi, which, surprisingly, only rarely occur together.
- **Dry beriberi** usually presents insidiously with a symmetrical polyneuropathy. The initial symptoms are heaviness and stiffness of the legs, followed by weakness, numbness, and pins and needles. The ankle jerk reflexes are lost and eventually all the signs of polyneuropathy that may involve the trunk and arms are found (see p. 891). Cerebral involvement occurs, producing the picture of the Wernicke–Korsakoff syndrome (p. 891). In endemic areas, mild symptoms and signs may be present for years without unduly affecting the patient.
- **Wet beriberi** causes oedema. Initially, this is of the legs, but it can extend to involve the whole body, with ascites and pleural effusions. The peripheral oedema may mask the accompanying features of dry beriberi.

Thiamine deficiency impairs pyruvate dehydrogenase with accumulation of lactate and pyruvate, producing peripheral vasodilatation and eventually oedema. The heart muscle is also affected and heart failure occurs, causing a further increase in the oedema. Initially, there are warm extremities, a full, fast, bounding pulse and a raised venous pressure ('high-output state'), but eventually heart failure advances and a poor cardiac output ensues. The electrocardiogram may show conduction defects.

Infantile beriberi occurs, usually acutely, in breast-fed babies at approximately 3 months of age. The mothers show no signs of thiamine deficiency but presumably their body stores must be virtually nil. The infant becomes anorexic, develops oedema and has some degree of aphonia. Tachycardia and tachypnoea develop and, unless treatment is instituted, death occurs quickly.

Diagnosis

In endemic areas, the diagnosis of beriberi should always be suspected; if it is in doubt, treatment with thiamine should be instituted. A rapid disappearance of oedema after thiamine (50 mg i.m.) is diagnostic. Other causes of oedema must be considered (e.g. renal or liver disease), and the polyneuropathy is indistinguishable from that due to other causes. The diagnosis is confirmed by measurement of the circulating thiamine concentration or transketolase activity in red cells using fresh heparinized blood.

Management

Thiamine 50 mg i.m. is given for 3 days, followed by 50 mg of thiamine daily by mouth. The response in wet beriberi is seen in hours, providing a dramatic improvement, but in dry beriberi improvement is often slow to occur. In most cases, all the B vitamins are given because of multiple deficiency. Infantile beriberi is treated by giving thiamine to the mother, which is then passed on to the infant via the breast milk.

Thiamine deficiency in people with alcohol dependence or acute illness

In the developed world, alcohol-dependent people and those with severe acute illness receiving high-carbohydrate infusions without vitamins are the only major groups to suffer from thiamine deficiency. Rarely, they develop wet beriberi, which must be distinguished from alcoholic cardiomyopathy. More usually, however, thiamine deficiency presents with polyneuropathy or with the **Wernicke–Korsakoff syndrome**.

This syndrome, which consists of dementia, ataxia, varying ophthalmoplegia and nystagmus (see p. 891), presents acutely and should be suspected in all heavy drinkers. If treated promptly, it is reversible; if left, it becomes irreversible. It is a major cause of dementia in the USA.

Urgent treatment with thiamine 250 mg i.m. or i.v. infusion once daily is given for 3 days, often combined with other B-complex vitamins. Anaphylaxis can occur. Thiamine must always be given before any intravenous glucose infusion.

Riboflavin

Riboflavin is widely distributed throughout all plant and animal cells. Good sources are dairy products, offal and leafy vegetables. Riboflavin is not destroyed appreciably by cooking but is destroyed by sunlight. It is a flavo-protein that is a co-factor for many oxidative reactions in the cell.

There is no definite deficiency, although many communities have low dietary intakes. Studies in volunteers taking a low-riboflavin diet have produced:
- angular stomatitis or cheilosis (fissuring at the corners of the mouth)
- a red, inflamed tongue
- seborrhoeic dermatitis, particularly involving the face (around the nose) and the scrotum or vulva.

Conjunctivitis with vascularization of the cornea and opacity of the lens has also been described. It is probable, however, that many of the above features are due to multiple deficiencies rather than lack of riboflavin itself.

Riboflavin 5 mg daily can be tried for the above conditions, usually given as the vitamin B complex.

Niacin

This is the generic name for the two chemical forms, nicotinic acid and nicotinamide, the latter being found in the two pyridine nucleotides, nicotinamide adenine dinucleotide (NAD) and nicotinamide adenine dinucleotide phosphate (NADP). Both act as hydrogen acceptors in many oxidative reactions, and in their reduced forms (NADH and NADPH) act as hydrogen donors in reductive reactions. Many oxidative steps in the production of energy require NAD and NADP.

Niacin is found in many foodstuffs, including plants, meat (particularly offal) and fish. Niacin is lost when bran is removed from cereals, but is added to processed cereals and white bread in many countries.

Niacin can be synthesized in humans from tryptophan, 60 mg of tryptophan being converted to 1 mg of niacin. The amount of niacin in food is given as the 'niacin equivalent', which is equal to the amount of niacin plus one-60th of the tryptophan content. Eggs and cheese contain tryptophan.

Kynureninase and kynurenine hydroxylase, key enzymes in the conversion of tryptophan to nicotinic acid, are both B_6 and riboflavin-dependent, and deficiency of these B vitamins can also produce pellagra.

Pellagra

This is rare but is found in people who eat virtually only maize: for example, in parts of Africa. Maize contains niacin in the form of niacytin, which is biologically unavailable and has a low content of tryptophan. In Central America, pellagra has always been rare because maize (for the cooking of tortillas) is soaked overnight in calcium hydroxide, which releases niacin. Many of the features of pellagra **(Fig. 33.8)** can be explained purely by niacin deficiency, but some are probably due to multiple deficiencies, including deficiencies of proteins and of other vitamins.

Clinical features

The classical features are dermatitis, diarrhoea and dementia. Although this is an easily remembered triad, not all features are always present and the mental changes are not a true dementia.

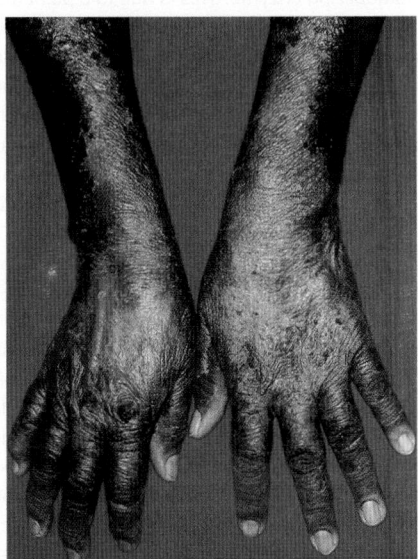

Fig. 33.8 Pellagra. Hyperpigmentation with desquamation of the dorsal aspects of the hands and forearms. *(From Bolognia JL, Jorrizzo JL, Schaffer JV (eds). Dermatology, 3rd edn. St Louis: Mosby; 2012, with permission.)*

- *Dermatitis.* In the areas of skin exposed to sunlight, there is redness initially, followed by cracks with occasional ulceration. Chronic thickening, dryness and pigmentation develop. The lesions are always symmetrical and often affect the dorsal surfaces of the hands. The perianal skin and vulva are frequently involved. Casal's necklace or collar is the term given to the skin lesion around the neck, which is confined to this area by the clothes worn.
- *Diarrhoea.* This is often a feature but constipation is occasionally seen. Other gastrointestinal manifestations include a painful, red, raw tongue, glossitis and angular stomatitis. Recurring mouth infections occur.
- *Dementia.* This occurs in chronic disease. In milder cases, there are symptoms of depression, apathy and sometimes thought disorders. Tremor and an encephalopathy frequently occur. Hallucinations and acute psychosis are also seen with more severe cases.

Pellagra may also occur in the following circumstances:

- *Isoniazid therapy.* This can lead to a deficiency of vitamin B_6, which is needed for the synthesis of nicotinamide from tryptophan. Vitamin B_6 is now given concomitantly with isoniazid.
- *Hartnup's disease*, a rare inborn error in which basic amino acids, including tryptophan, are not absorbed by the gut. There is also loss of this amino acid in the urine.
- *Generalized malabsorption* (rare).
- *Alcohol-dependent patients* who eat little.
- *Very-low-protein diets*
- *Carcinoid syndrome and phaeochromocytomas.* In these disorders, tryptophan metabolism is diverted away from the formation of nicotinamide to form amines.

Diagnosis and management

In endemic areas, diagnosis and management are based on the clinical features, remembering that other vitamin deficiencies can produce similar changes (e.g. angular stomatitis). Nicotinamide (approximately 300 mg daily by mouth) is given, with a maintenance dose of 50 mg daily, and produces a dramatic improvement in the skin and diarrhoea. Mostly, however, vitamin B complex is given, as other deficiencies are often present.

An increase in the protein content of the diet, and treatment of malnutrition and other vitamin deficiencies, are essential.

Vitamin B_6

Vitamin B_6 exists as pyridoxine, pyridoxal and pyridoxamine, and is found widely in plant and animal foodstuffs. Pyridoxal phosphate is a co-factor in the metabolism of many amino acids. Dietary deficiency is extremely rare. Some drugs (e.g. isoniazid, hydralazine and penicillamine) interact with pyridoxal phosphate, producing B_6 deficiency. The polyneuropathy occurring after isoniazid usually responds to vitamin B_6.

Sideroblastic anaemia may respond to vitamin B_6 (see p. 332).

A polyneuropathy has occurred after high doses (>200 mg) given over many months.

Biotin and pantothenic acid

Biotin is involved in a number of carboxylase reactions. It occurs in many foodstuffs and the dietary requirement is small. Deficiency is extremely rare and is confined to a few people who consume raw eggs, which contain an antagonist (avidin) to biotin. It has also been reported in patients receiving long-term parenteral nutrition without adequate amounts of biotin. It causes a dermatitis that responds to biotin replacements.

Pantothenic acid is widely distributed in all foods and deficiency in humans has not been described.

Vitamin C

Ascorbic acid is a powerful reducing agent that controls the redox potential within cells. It is involved in the hydroxylation of proline to hydroxyproline, which is necessary for the formation of collagen. The failure of this biochemical pathway in vitamin C deficiency accounts for virtually all of the clinical effects seen.

Humans, along with a few other animals (e.g. primates and the guinea-pig), are unusual in not being able to synthesize ascorbic acid from glucose.

Vitamin C is present in all fresh fruit and vegetables. Unfortunately, ascorbic acid is easily leached out of vegetables when they are placed in water and it is also oxidized to dehydro-ascorbic acid during cooking or exposure to copper or alkalis. Potatoes are a good source, as many people eat a lot of them, but vitamin C is lost during storage.

It has been suggested that ascorbic acid in high dosage (1–2 g daily) will prevent the common cold. While there is some scientific support for this, clinical trials have shown no significant effect. Vitamin C supplements have also been advocated to prevent atherosclerosis and cancer, but again a clear benefit has not been demonstrated.

Vitamin C deficiency is seen mainly in infants fed boiled milk and in people who do not eat vegetables, such as those consuming rice-only diets.

Scurvy

In adults, the early symptoms of vitamin C deficiency may be non-specific, with weakness and muscle pain. Other features are shown in **Box 33.16**. Parafollicular haemorrhages and corkscrew hairs **(Fig. 33.9)** occur. In infantile scurvy, there is irritability, painful legs,

---

> **Box 33.16 Clinical features of vitamin C deficiency (scurvy)**
>
> - Keratosis of hair follicles with 'corkscrew' hair
> - Perifollicular haemorrhages
> - Swollen, spongy gums with bleeding and superadded infection, loosening of teeth
> - Spontaneous bruising
> - Spontaneous haemorrhage
> - Anaemia
> - Failure of wound healing

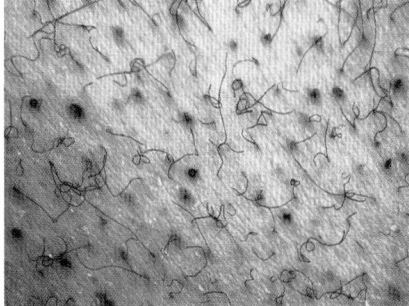

Fig. 33.9 Scurvy. Corkscrew hairs and perifollicular haemorrhage on the lower extremity. *(From Bolognia JL, Jorrizzo JL, Schaffer JV (eds). Dermatology, 3rd edn. St Louis: Mosby; 2012, with permission.)*

---

anaemia and characteristic subperiosteal haemorrhages, particularly into the ends of long bones.

Diagnosis

The anaemia is usually hypochromic but, occasionally, a normochromic or megaloblastic anaemia is seen. The type of anaemia depends on whether iron deficiency (owing to decreased absorption or loss due to haemorrhage) or folate deficiency (folate being largely found in green vegetables) is present.

Plasma ascorbic acid is very low in obvious deficiency and a vitamin C level of below 11 µmol/L (0.2 mg/100 mL) indicates vitamin C deficiency. The leucocyte-platelet layer (buffy coat) of centrifuged blood corresponds to vitamin C concentrations in other tissues. The normal level of leucocyte ascorbate is $1.1–2.8\,pmol/10^6$ cells.

Management

Initially, the patient is given 250 mg of ascorbic acid daily and encouraged to eat fresh fruit and vegetables. Subsequently, 40 mg daily will maintain a normal exchangeable body pool of about 900 mg (5.1 mmol).

Prevention

Orange juice should be given to bottle-fed infants. The intake of breast-fed infants depends on the mother's diet. In the elderly, eating adequate fruit and vegetables is the best way to avoid scurvy. Careful surveillance of the elderly, particularly those who live alone, is necessary. Ascorbic acid supplements should be necessary only occasionally.

Vitamin B$_{12}$ and folate

These are dealt with on page 334 and daily requirements are shown in **Box 33.13**.

Folate

In many developed countries, up to 15% of the population have a partial deficiency of 5,10-methylene tetrahydrofolate reductase, a key folate-metabolizing enzyme. This is due to a point mutation and is associated with an increase in neural tube defects and hyperhomocysteinaemia, which has been linked to cardiovascular disease. Autoantibodies against folate receptors have been found in serum from women who have had a pregnancy complicated by neural tube defects. However, the role of this in the pathogenesis is unclear.

In the USA and some other countries, enriched cereals are fortified with folic acid 1.4 mg/kg of grain to increase daily intake.

DIETARY ANTIOXIDANTS

Free radicals are generated during inflammatory processes, radiotherapy, smoking and in the course of a wide range of diseases. They may cause uncontrolled damage of multiple cellular components, the most sensitive of which are unsaturated lipids, proteins and DNA, and they also disrupt the normal replication process. They have been implicated as a cause of a wide range of diseases, including malignant, acute inflammatory and traumatic diseases, cardiovascular disease, neurodegenerative conditions such as Alzheimer's disease, senile macular degeneration, and cataract. Defence against uncontrolled damage by free radicals is provided by antioxidant enzymes (e.g. catalase, superoxide dismutase) and antioxidants, which may be endogenous (e.g. glutathione) or exogenous (e.g. vitamins C and E, carotenoids). A possible causal link between lack of antioxidants and cardiovascular disease has emerged from epidemiological studies, although several RCTs have not confirmed this.

Epidemiology

Dietary intake

- A high intake of fruits and vegetables has been linked to a reduced risk of heart disease, cerebrovascular disease and total cardiovascular morbidity and mortality.
- A high intake of nuts (rich in vitamin E) and dietary components, such as red wine, onions and apples (rich in flavonoids), which are strong scavengers of free radicals, has also been linked to a reduced risk of cardiovascular disease.
- The seasonal variation in cardiovascular disease, which is higher in winter, has been related to a decreased intake of fresh fruit and vegetables at that time of year.
- The decline in cardiovascular disease in the USA since the 1950s has been associated with a simultaneous increase in the intake of fresh fruit and vegetables.

Status of antioxidant nutrients

The level of antioxidant nutrients in the circulation has been reported to be inversely related to cardiovascular morbidity and mortality, the extent of atherosclerosis as assessed by intra-arterial ultrasound, and clinical signs of ischaemic heart disease. The tissue content of lycopene, a marker of vegetable intake, has been reported to be low in patients with myocardial infarction.

Antioxidants, especially vitamin E, have been shown to prevent the initiation and progression of atherosclerotic disease in animals. They also reduce the oxidation of LDL in the arterial wall *in vitro*. Oxidation of LDL is an initial event in the atherosclerotic process (see p. 1079). However, these epidemiological studies show an association rather than a causal link, and RCTs comparing the antioxidant against a control group are necessary.

The results of *RCTs* (see also p. 72) have been formally evaluated through a series of systematic reviews and meta-analyses.

- For ***primary or secondary prevention*** of cardiovascular disease, intervention with β-carotene, α-tocopherol (vitamin E) and ascorbic acid (vitamin C) has demonstrated no significant benefit.
- Vitamin E or β-carotene given in, for example, stroke and fatal and non-fatal myocardial infarction has also not yielded benefits.
- There is a report of increased risk of intracerebral and subarachnoid haemorrhage in healthy individuals receiving carotene and α-tocopherol.
- A meta-analysis has shown a small but significant overall increased risk of cardiovascular death and all-cause mortality in individuals treated with β-carotene (compared with the control group).
- There is an increased risk of developing lung cancer when large doses of β-carotene are administered to subjects with a history of heavy smoking.
- Although administration of antioxidant nutrients has been proposed in a wide range of acute (e.g. critical illness, pancreatitis) and chronic diseases, the evidence base from RCTs is generally not strong.
- In some cases, improvement in indices of free radical damage has been demonstrated (e.g. in acute inflammatory conditions), but with little evidence of clinical benefit.

Epidemiological studies are also confounded by other associated variables, such as eating a low-fat diet or undertaking more

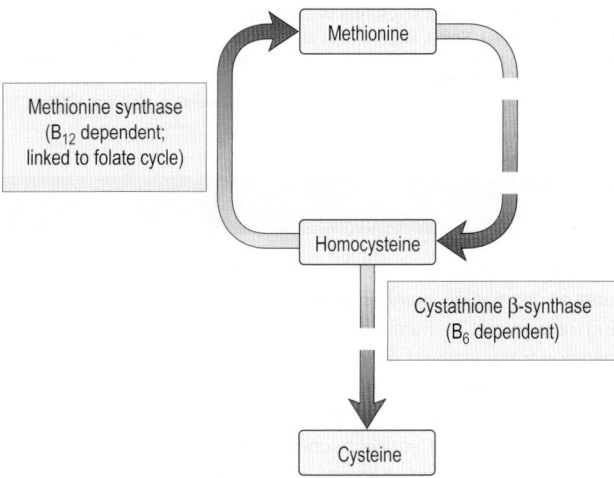

Fig. 33.10 Homocysteine metabolism.

exercise. The latter may be more valuable in the causal pathway than the intake of antioxidants. Diets rich in fresh fruit and vegetables also contain a range of antioxidants that were not tested in the clinical trials. Therefore, the results of large-scale RCTs using various combinations and doses of antioxidant nutrients are awaited. In the meantime, the policy of encouraging 'healthy' behaviour, which includes increased physical activity and a varied diet rich in fresh fruit and vegetables, and nuts, is still generally recommended both for the population as a whole and for those at risk of cardiovascular disease.

HOMOCYSTEINE, CARDIOVASCULAR DISEASE AND B VITAMINS

The circulating concentration of the amino acid homocysteine is an independent risk factor for cardiovascular disease. A high concentration is related to ischaemic heart disease, stroke, thrombosis, pulmonary embolism, coronary artery stenosis and heart failure. The strength of the association is similar to that in smoking or hyperlipidaemia.

Proposed mechanisms, based on experimental evidence, by which homocysteine detrimentally affects vascular function, include:

- the direct damaging effects of homocysteine on endothelial cells of blood vessels
- an increase in blood vessel stiffness
- an increase in blood coagulation.

Homocysteine is not found in food, but results from metabolism within the body, which depends on folic acid, vitamin B_{12} and pyridoxine (vitamin B_6) **(Fig. 33.10)**. Deficiency of one or more of these vitamins is common in the elderly, which would increase the concentration of homocysteine. If an elevated homocysteine concentration were causally linked to cardiovascular disease, then it should be possible to lower the risk by administering one or more of these vitamins to decrease the homocysteine concentration. However, several studies suggest that lowering homocysteine concentrations in this way does not reduce the risk of cardiovascular disease.

Further reading

Awasthi S, Peto R, Read S et al. Vitamin A supplementation every 6 months with retinol in 1 million pre-school children in north India: DEVTA, a cluster-randomised trial. *Lancet* 2013; 381:1469–1477.
Institute of Medicine. *Dietary Reference Intakes for Thiamin, Riboflavin, Niacin, Vitamin B6, Folate, Vitamin B12, Pantothenic Acid, Biotin, and Choline.*

Washington DC: National Academies Press; 2000.

Marti-Carvajal AJ, Sola I, Lathyris D et al. Homocysteine-lowering interventions for preventing cardiovascular events. *Cochrane Database of Systematic Reviews (Online)* 2013; 1:CD006612.

Welsh P, Sattar N. Vitamin D and chronic disease prevention. *Br Med J* 2014; 348:g228.

MINERALS

A number of minerals have been shown to be essential in animals, and an increasing number of deficiency syndromes are becoming recognized in humans. Long-term total parenteral nutrition allowed trace element deficiency to be studied in controlled conditions; now trace elements are always added to long-term parenteral nutrition regimens. It is highly probable that trace-element deficiency is also a frequent accompaniment of all PEM states, but this is difficult to study because of multiple deficiencies. Sodium, potassium, magnesium and chloride are discussed in Chapter 9. Reference nutrient intake (RNI) values are shown in **Box 33.17**. However, in disease, the requirements of specific nutrients may increase (e.g. sodium potassium, magnesium and zinc in patients with persistent diarrhoea or other gastrointestinal fluid losses) or decrease (e.g. phosphate, potassium and sodium in chronic kidney disease).

Iron

Iron deficiency (see also p. 330) is common worldwide, affecting both developing and developed countries. It is particularly prevalent in women of reproductive age. Dietary iron overload is seen in South African men who cook and brew in iron pots.

Copper

Copper deficiency

Menkes' kinky hair syndrome is a rare condition caused by malabsorption of copper. The Menkes' disease gene (*ATP7A*) encodes a copper-transporting ATPase and has a homology to the gene in Wilson's disease. Infants with this sex-linked recessive abnormality develop growth failure, mental retardation, bone lesions and brittle hair. Anaemia and neutropenia also occur. This condition, which serves as a model for copper deficiency, supports the idea that some of the clinical features seen in PEM are due to copper deficiency. Breast and cow's milk are low in copper, and supplementation is occasionally necessary when first treating PEM.

Copper toxicity

This occurs in Wilson's disease; see page 862.

Zinc

Zinc is involved in many metabolic pathways, often acting as a coenzyme; it is essential for the synthesis of RNA and DNA. In young children in developing countries, death attributable to zinc deficiency is lower than previously thought. One study found significant improvements when extra zinc was provided with several other micronutrients.

Box 33.17 Daily reference nutrient intake (RNI) values for some elements

Element	Daily RNI	Dietary sources
Sodium	1.6 g (70 mmol)	Mostly in processed food (e.g. meat products, bread and cereal) but contribution from added salt
Chloride	2.5 g (70 mmol)	As for sodium
Potassium	3.5 g (90 mmol)	Vegetables, fruit, juices, meat and milk
Calcium	700 mg (17.5 mmol)[a]	In many foodstuffs; two-thirds of intake comes from milk and milk products, and only 5% from vegetables[b]
Phosphate	550 mg (17.5 mmol)	All natural foods, e.g. milk, meat, bread, cereals
Magnesium	300 mg (12.3 mmol) for men / 270 mg (10.9 mmol) for women	Milk, bread, cereal products, potatoes and other vegetables
Iron	160 µmol (8.7 mg) for men / 260 µmol (14.8 mg) for women	Meat, bread, flour, cereal products, potatoes and vegetables
Copper	1.2 mg (19 µmol)	Shellfish, legumes, cereals and nuts
Zinc	9.5 mg (145 µmol) for men / 7 mg (110 µmol) for women	Widely available in food
Iodine	140 µg (1.1 µmol)	Milk, meat and seafoods
Fluoride	None	Little fluoride in food except sea fish and tea (tea provides 70% of daily intake)
Selenium	75 µg (0.9 µmol) for men / 60 µg (0.8 µmol) for women	Cereals, fish, meat, cheese, eggs, milk

[a]UK value; a substantially higher value is recommended in the USA.
[b]In the UK, most flour is fortified.

Zinc deficiency

Acrodermatitis enteropathica is an inherited disorder caused by malabsorption of zinc. Infants develop growth retardation, severe diarrhoea, hair loss and a skin rash, which can occur anywhere on the body but is most often found around the mouth, genitalia and hands (a similar rash occurs in adults suffering from zinc deficiency due to other causes; see below). There are also associated *Candida* and bacterial infections **(Fig. 33.11)**. This condition provides a model for zinc deficiency. Zinc supplementation results in a complete cure. Zinc deficiency probably also plays a role in PEM and in many diseases in children in the developing world. Zinc supplementation has been demonstrated as being of some benefit in, for example, the prevention of diarrhoeal diseases and acute respiratory infections; it also improves growth.

Levels of zinc have also been shown to be low in some patients with malabsorption or skin disease, and in patients with the acquired immunodeficiency (AIDS), but its exact role in these

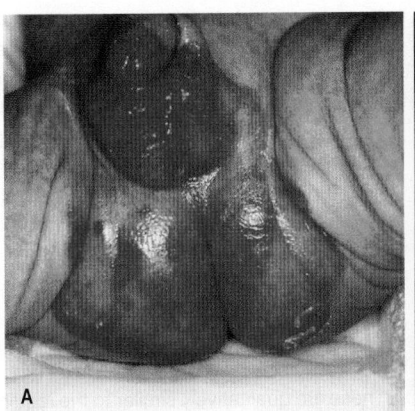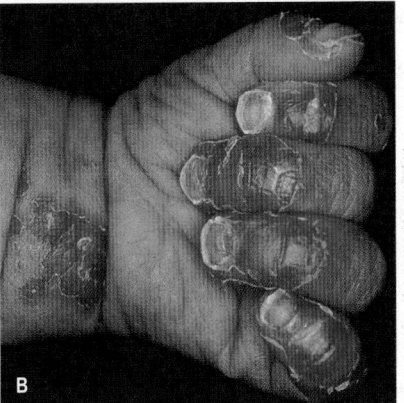

Fig. 33.11 **Zinc deficiency (genetic).** **(A)** Erythema and erosions. **(B)** Crusting and desquamation. *(From Bolognia JL, Jorrizzo JL, Schaffer JV (eds). Dermatology, 3rd edn. St Louis: Mosby; 2012, with permission.)*

situations is disputed. Zinc has low toxicity, but high zinc levels from water stored in galvanized containers interfere with iron and copper absorption. Conversely, administration of copper or iron to treat deficiencies such as iron deficiency anaemia can precipitate zinc deficiency. Wound healing is impaired with moderate zinc deficiency and is improved by zinc supplements. Impaired taste and smell, hair loss and night blindness are also features of severe zinc deficiency.

Iodine

Iodine exists in foodstuffs as inorganic iodides, which are efficiently absorbed. Iodine is a constituent of the thyroid hormones (see **Box 21.25**).

Iodine deficiency

Many areas throughout the world lack iodine in the soil, and so iodine deficiency, which impairs brain development, is a WHO priority. Two billion people worldwide (one-third of whom are children) have insufficient iodine intake. Endemic goitre **(Fig. 33.12)** occurs in remote areas where the daily intake is below 70 μg, and in those parts 1–5% of babies are born with congenital hypothyroidism (with severe stunting, learning difficulty and a goitre). In these areas, iodized oil should be given intramuscularly to all reproductive women every 3–5 years. Salt iodization is now practised in many countries and is a simple, cost-effective way to prevent deficiency.

Fluoride

In areas where the level of fluoride in drinking water is less than 1 part per million (0.7–1.2 mg/L), dental caries is relatively more prevalent. Fluoridation of the water provides 1–2 mg daily, resulting in a reduction of about 50% of tooth decay in children. There is little fluoride in food. Fluoride-containing toothpaste may add up to 2 mg/day.

Excessive fluoride intake in areas where the water fluoride level is above 3 mg/L can result in fluorosis, in which there is infiltration into the enamel of the teeth, producing pitting and discoloration.

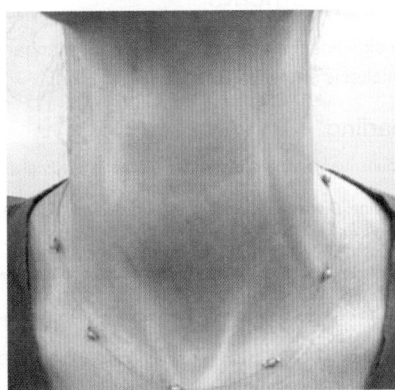

Fig. 33.12 **Goitre due to iodine deficiency.** *(From Dhillon RS, East CA. Ear, Nose and Throat and Head and Neck Surgery, 4th edn. Elsevier; 2013, with permission.)*

Selenium

Clinical deficiency of selenium is rare, except in areas of China where Keshan disease, a selenium-responsive cardiomyopathy, occurs. Selenium deficiency may also cause a myopathy. Interactions between selenium and viruses have also been implicated. Toxicity has been described with very high intakes.

Calcium

Calcium absorption (see also p. 474) from the gastrointestinal tract is vitamin D-dependent. Some 99% of body calcium is in the skeleton.

Increased calcium is required in pregnancy and lactation, when dietary intake must be increased. Calcium deficiency is usually due to vitamin D deficiency.

Phosphate

Phosphates (see also p. 192) are present in all natural foods, and dietary deficiency has not been described. Patients taking large amounts of aluminium hydroxide can, however, develop phosphate

i Box 33.18 Other trace elements

Element	Deficiency
Chromium	Glucose intolerance
Cobalt	Anaemia (vitamin B$_{12}$)
Manganese	Skin rash, ?osteoporosis, ?mood
Molybdenum	?(case study involving parenteral nutrition)
Nickel	?Animals only

deficiency owing to binding in the gut lumen. It can also be seen in total parenteral nutrition. Symptoms include anorexia, weakness and osteoporosis.

Other trace elements

The possible significance of chromium, cobalt, manganese, molybdenum and nickel is shown in **Box 33.18**.

Further reading

Bauer DC. Calcium supplements and fracture prevention. *N Engl J Med* 2013; 369:1537–1543.
Institute of Medicine. *Dietary Reference Intakes for Vitamin A, Vitamin K, Arsenic, Chromium, Copper, Iodine, Iron, Manganese, Molybdenum, Silicon, Vanadium, and Zinc*. Washington DC: Institute of Medicine; 2001.
Kotchen TA, Cowley AW, Jr, Frohlich ED. Salt in health and disease – a delicate balance. *N Engl J Med* 2013; 368:1229–1237.
Loscalzo J. Keshan disease, selenium deficiency, and selenoproteome. *N Engl J Med* 2014; 370; 18:1756–1760.
Pearce SHS, Cheetam TD. Diagnosis and management of vitamin D deficiency. *Br Med J* 2010; 340:141–147.
Pitta AG, Chung M, Trikalinos T et al. Systematic review: vitamin D and cardiometabolic outcomes. *Ann Intern Med* 2010; 152:307–314.
Soofi S, Cousens S, Iqbal SP et al. Effect of provision of daily zinc and iron with several micronutrients on growth and morbidity among young children in Pakistan: a cluster-randomised trial. *Lancet* 2013; 382:29–40.

NUTRITION AND AGEING

Early origins of health and disease in older adults

A low birth weight (and/or length) is associated with reduced height, as well as reduced mass and fat-free mass in adult life. These relationships are independent of genetic factors; the smaller of identical twins becomes a shorter and lighter adult.

Relationships have also been reported between growth of the fetus and a variety of diseases and risk factors for disease in adults and older people. These include cardiovascular disease (especially ischaemic heart disease), hypertension, diabetes, and even obesity and fat distribution. However, the strength of association for some of these conditions is weak. Animal studies involving dietary modifications (e.g. protein and zinc, even within the normal range) during pregnancy or in early postnatal life have clearly demonstrated effects, such as on rates of hypertension. The effects can not only persist through the lifetime of the offspring, but also be passed through to their offspring.

The extent to which these findings apply to humans is uncertain and the mechanisms are poorly understood. Since relationships have been reported between cardiovascular disease in old age and growth in the first few years of life, as well as starvation during puberty, it is likely that cumulative environmental stresses, including nutritional stress, from the time of implantation of the fertilized egg, to fetal and postnatal growth and development, and into adult life, summate to produce an overall disease risk **(Fig. 33.13)**. Although high birth weight and length are associated with a reduced risk of cardiovascular disease in later life, they may also be associated with an increased risk of cancer.

Nutritional requirements in the elderly

These are qualitatively similar to the requirements of younger adults; the diet should contain approximately the same proportions of nutrients, and essential nutrients are still needed. However, the RNIs stated earlier (see **Boxes 33.13** and **33.17**) are intended for healthy people without disease; specific requirements in disease, which is common in older people, are less well defined. Furthermore, the extent to which muscle loss is due to ageing, malnutrition and disease continues to be debated, as do the boundaries between sarcopenia, cachexia, malnutrition and frailty. *Sarcopenia* is defined as loss of skeletal muscle bulk, accompanied by decreased strength; unlike cachexia, it occurs without an underlying illness. Sarcopenia leads to disability with an increase in falls (see Ch 15).

Maintenance of physical activity continues to be necessary for overall health, regardless of age. However, energy expenditure by the elderly is less, so they have a lower energy requirement. For people aged 60 and above, irrespective of age, the daily energy requirement has been set at approximately 1.5 × BMR. Because they have reduced fat-free mass – from an average of 60 kg to 50 kg in men, and from 40 kg to 35 kg in women – their BMR is reduced.

Nutritional deficits in the elderly are common and may be due to many factors, such as dental problems, depression and lack of motivation. Significant malnourishment in developed countries is usually secondary to social problems or disease. In elderly people who are in institutions, multiple nutrient deficiencies are common. Vitamin D supplements (colecalciferol 20 µg (800 units) daily) may be required because of poor diet, and elderly people may not receive adequate exposure to sunlight. Owing to the high prevalence of osteoporosis in elderly people, an increased daily calcium intake (1–1.5 g/day) is often recommended.

Further reading

Ali S, Garcia JM. Sarcopenia, cachexia and aging: diagnosis, mechanisms and therapeutic options – a mini-review. *Gerontology* 2014; 60:294–305.
Boyd-Kirkup JD, Green CD, Wu G et al. Epigenomics and the regulation of aging. *Epigenomics* 2013; 5:205–227.
Chatterji S, Byles J, Cutler D et al. Health, functioning, and disability in older adults – present status and future implications. *Lancet* 2015; 385: 563–570.
Clegg A, Young J, Iliffe S et al. Frailty in elderly people. *Lancet* 2013; 381: 752–762.
Cruz-Jentoft AJ, Landi F. Sarcopenia. *Clin Med* 2014; 14:183–186.
Mathers CD, Stevens GA, Boerma T et al. Causes of international increases in older age life expectancy. *Lancet* 2015; 385:540–548.
Prince MJ, Wu F, Guo Y et al. The burden of disease in older people and implications for health policy and practice. *Lancet* 2015; 385:549–562.
Xi H, Li C, Ren F et al. Telomere, aging and age-related diseases. *Aging Clin Exp Res* 2013; 25:139–146.

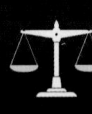

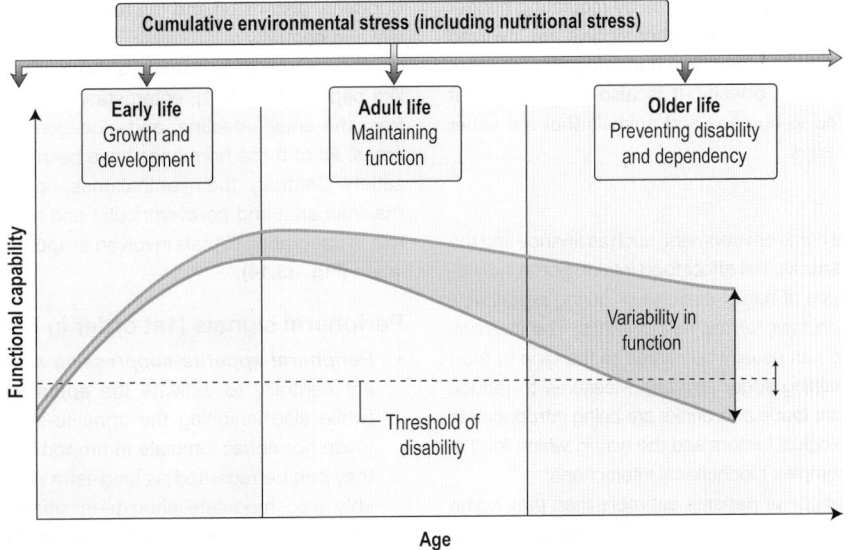

Fig. 33.13 Nutrition and ageing. Nutrition is a contributory cause of the variability in function during the lifespan. Appropriate nutrition may improve function, or delay deterioration below the threshold of disability and dependence.

OBESITY

Obesity is almost invariable in developed countries and almost all people accumulate some fat as they get older. The WHO acknowledges that obesity (BMI >30 kg/m^2) is a worldwide problem that also affects many developing countries. Obesity implies an excess storage of fat and this can most easily be detected by looking at the undressed patient. Not all obese people eat more than the average person but all obviously eat more than they need.

The present obesity epidemic is mainly due to changes in lifestyle behaviour (although genetic factors may be involved in some individuals). There has been a trebling in the prevalence of obesity over the last three decades in the UK, as well as a vast increase in developing countries. The growing obesity problem in humans has affected children, adults and older people. Clinical and public health interventions require a multi-level approach: for example, by altering the cumulative environmental experience during the lifespan. Strategies to prevent and treat obesity in children can influence obesity in adults, and this in turn influences obesity in old age. Ultimately, all depend on changing energy balance through effects on food intake and/or energy expenditure.

Most patients suffer from simple obesity, but in certain conditions, obesity is an associated feature **(Box 33.19)**. Even in the latter situation, the intake of calories must have exceeded energy expenditure over a prolonged period of time. Hormonal imbalance is often incriminated in women (e.g. after the menopause or when taking contraceptive pills), but most weight gain in such cases is usually small and due to water retention.

Pathophysiology
Genetic and environmental factors
These have always been difficult to separate in the study of obesity but there is little doubt that the recent obesity 'epidemic', which has developed over a few decades, is predominantly due to changes in lifestyle (various environmental factors) and unlikely to be caused by rapid changes in the gene pool over this period of time. This is

---

Box 33.19 Conditions in which obesity is an associated feature

- Genetic syndromes associated with hypogonadism (e.g. Prader–Willi, Laurence–Moon–Biedl)
- Hypothyroidism
- Cushing's syndrome
- Stein–Leventhal syndrome
- Drug-induced disorders (e.g. with corticosteroids)
- Hypothalamic damage (e.g. due to trauma, tumour)

---

consistent with the view that evolution during times of limited food resources has tended to defend more against under-nutrition than over-nutrition. However, observational studies in both monozygotic and dizygotic twins, reared together or apart, suggest that strong genetic influences account for the difference in BMI later in life, and that the influence of the childhood environment is weaker. These observations also showed that weight gain did not occur in all pairs of twins, suggesting that environmental factors operate.

A search for genetic factors led to the identification of a putative gene, first in the obese (*ob ob*) mouse and now in humans. The ***ob gene*** was shown to be expressed solely in both white and brown adipose tissue. The *ob* gene is found on chromosome 7 and produces a 16 kDa protein called leptin. In the *ob ob* mouse, a mutation in the *ob* gene leads to production of a non-functioning protein. Administration of normal leptin to these obese mice reduces food intake and corrects the obesity. A similar situation has been described in a very rare genetic condition that causes obesity in humans, in which leptin is not expressed.

In massively obese subjects, leptin mRNA in subcutaneous adipose tissue is 80% higher than in controls. Plasma levels of leptin are also very high, correlating with the BMI. Weight loss due to food restriction decreases plasma levels of leptin. However, in contrast to the *ob ob* mouse, the leptin structure is normal, and abnormalities in leptin are not the prime cause of human obesity.

Leptin secreted from fat cells was thought to act as a feedback mechanism between the adipose tissue and the brain, acting as a 'lipostat' (adipostat), and controlling fat stores by regulating hunger and satiety (see below). However, many other signals are involved and the human genome map has identified hundreds of genes that correlate with the presence of obesity. It is also interesting that obesity is largely restricted to humans and animals that are either domesticated or living in zoos.

Food intake

Many factors related to the home environment, such as finance and the availability of sweets and snacks, will affect food intake. Some individuals eat more during periods of heavy exercise or during pregnancy, and are unable to return to their former eating habits. The increase in obesity in social class 5 can usually be related to the type of food consumed (i.e. food containing sugar and fat). Measures to reduce the sugar content in popular foods and drinks are being introduced in various countries. Psychological factors and the way in which food is presented may override complex biochemical interactions.

It has been shown that obese patients eat more than they admit to eating, and over the years, a very small daily excess of intake over expenditure can lead to a large accumulation of fat. For example, a 44 kJ (10.5 kcal) daily excess would lead to a 10 kg weight gain over 20 years.

Control of appetite

Appetite is the desire to eat and this usually initiates food intake. Following a meal, satiation occurs. This depends on gastric and duodenal distension and the release of many substances peripherally and centrally.

Following a meal, cholecystokinin (CCK), bombesin, glucagon-like peptide 1 (GLP-1), enterostatin and somatostatin are released from the small intestine, and glucagon and insulin from the pancreas. All of these hormones have been implicated in the control of satiety. Centrally, the hypothalamus – particularly the lateral hypothalamic area and paraventricular and arcuate nuclei – plays a key role in integrating signals involved in appetite and body weight regulation **(Fig. 33.14)**.

Peripheral signals (1st order in Fig. 33.14)

- *Peripheral appetite-suppressing signals. Leptin* and *insulin* act centrally to activate the *appetite-suppressing pathway* (while also inhibiting the appetite-stimulating pathway). Since these hormones circulate in proportion to adipose tissue mass, they can be regarded as long-term signals, although they probably also modulate short-term signals (insulin also responds acutely to meal ingestion). *Peptide YY (PYY)* is produced by the L cells of the large bowel and distal small bowel in proportion to the energy ingested. The release of this rapidly responsive (short-acting) signal begins shortly after food intake, suggesting that the initial response involves neural pathways, before ingested nutrients reach the site of PYY production. PYY is thought to reduce appetite, at least partly through inhibition of the *appetite-stimulating pathway (NPY/AgRP-expressing*

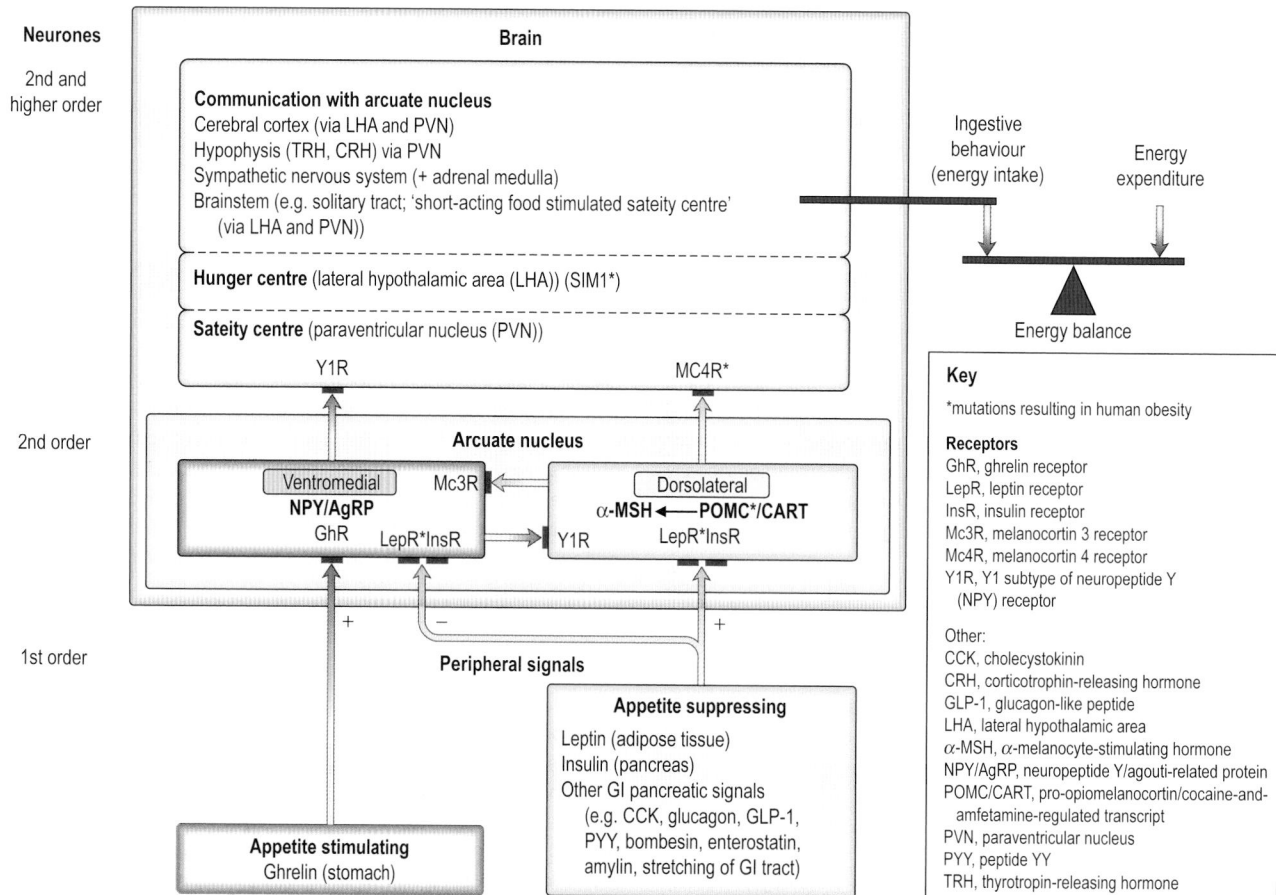

Fig. 33.14 Peripheral signals and central pathways involved in the control of food intake. The stimulatory (orange) and suppressive (green) signals and pathways are shown. In the arcuate nucleus, POMC is converted to melanocortins, including α-MSH, through the action of prohormone convertase. The solid red areas represent receptors for a variety of signals (see list in the key).

neurones). There are a large number of other peripheral appetite-suppressing signals, including GLP-1 and oxyntomodulin, which, like PYY, are produced by the gut in a nutrient-dependent manner.

- **Peripheral appetite-stimulating signals.** Ghrelin is a 28-amino-acetylated peptide produced by the oxyntic cells of the fundus of the stomach. It is the first known gastrointestinal tract peptide that stimulates appetite by activating the central appetite-stimulating pathway. The circulatory concentration is high before a meal and is reduced rapidly by ingestion of a meal or glucose (compare PYY, which increases after a meal). It may also act as a long-term signal, as its circulating concentration in weight-stable individuals is inversely related to BMI over a wide range (compare insulin and leptin, which are positively related to BMI; see below). Ghrelin is also increased in several situations in which there is a negative energy balance, such as long-term exercise, very-low-calorie diets, anorexia nervosa, and both cancer and cardiac cachexia (an exception is vertical banded gastric bypass surgery, where its concentration is low rather than high). The peptide, obestatin, produced by the same gene that encodes ghrelin, counteracts the increase in food intake induced by ghrelin.

Central pathways (2nd order in Fig. 33.14)

There are two main pathways in the arcuate nucleus:

- The **central appetite-stimulating (orexigenic) pathway** in the ventromedial part of the arcuate nucleus, which expresses **neuropeptide Y (NPY)** and **agouti pathway-related protein (AgRP)**. Animal studies suggest that this pathway also decreases energy expenditure.
- The **central appetite-suppressing pathway (anorexigenic pathway or leptin–melanocortin pathway)** in the dorsolateral part of the arcuate nucleus, which expresses pro-opiomelanocortin/cocaine-and-amfetamine-regulated transcript (**POMC/CART**). In this pathway, α-melanocyte-stimulating hormone (α-MSH), formed by cleavage of POMC by prohormone convertase (PC1), exerts its appetite-suppressing effect via the melanocortin-4 receptors (Mc4R) in areas of the brain that regulate food intake and autonomic activity. Animal studies suggest that this pathway also increases energy expenditure.

These pathways interact with each other and feed into the lateral hypothalamus, which communicates with other parts of the brain, and influence the autonomic nervous system and ingestive behaviour.

These central pathways are in turn influenced by a variety of peripheral signals, which can also be classified as appetite-stimulating or appetite-suppressing.

Other factors

The single gene mutations affecting the appetite-suppressing pathway in humans, e.g. leptin, leptin receptor, *POMC*, *Mc4R*, *PC1* and *SIM1*, are rare and recessive, with the exception of *Mc4R*, which is common and dominant with incomplete penetrance. It appears that the **Mc4R mutation** accounts for 2–6% of human obesity. Affected individuals are obese without disturbances in pituitary function or resting energy expenditure, although children tend to be tall. However, these mutations are of little significance, as obesity is predominantly polygenic in origin (the human obesity gene map has already identified several hundreds of candidate genes).

The **endocannabinoid system** is also involved in both central and peripheral regulation of food intake and control of energy balance. There are two receptors: endocannabinoid (CB₁) in the brain

and CB₂ in the periphery. CB₁ receptors are located in the cerebral cortex, cerebellum and hippocampus.

The control of appetite is extremely complex. To take just one signal, leptin, as an example, there can be leptin resistance, in which obese individuals have high circulating leptin but appetite is not reduced. In contrast, in acute starvation, leptin concentrations decrease to lower levels than could be expected from the prevailing adipose tissue mass. It is known that cytokines, such as TNF and IL-2, which are elevated in a wide range of inflammatory and traumatic conditions, also suppress appetite, although the exact pathways involved are not entirely clear. Finally, a range of transmitters in the central nervous system appear to affect appetite:

- appetite inhibitors: dopamine, serotonin, γ-aminobutyric acid
- appetite stimulators, e.g. opioids.

Energy expenditure

Basal metabolic rate

Basal metabolic rate (BMR) in obese subjects is higher than in lean subjects, which is not surprising since obesity is associated with an increase in lean body mass.

Physical activity

Obese patients tend to expend more energy during physical activity, as they have a larger mass to move. On the other hand, many obese patients decrease their amount of physical activity. The energy expended on walking at 3 miles/hour is only 15.5 kJ/min (3.7 kcal/min); therefore, a mild to moderate increase in physical activity plays only a small part in losing weight. Nevertheless, because increased body fat develops insidiously over many years, any change in energy balance is helpful.

Thermogenesis

About 10% of ingested energy is dissipated as heat and is unconnected with physical activity. This dietary-induced thermogenesis has been reported to be lower in obese and post-obese subjects than in lean subjects. This would tend to favour energy deposition in obesity and those predisposed to obesity. However, other reports have identified no difference in dietary-induced thermogenesis between lean and obese subjects.

When stimulated by cold or food, brown adipose tissue in animals dissipates the energy derived from ingested food into heat. This can be a major component of overall energy balance in small mammals but the effect is likely to be very small and of doubtful clinical significance in adult humans, even though brown adipose tissue is found in humans. The principal receptors mediating catecholamine-stimulated lipolysis in brown adipose tissue, and to a lesser extent at other sites, are the β₃-adrenergic receptors. Drugs with β₃-adrenergic activities have been developed but side-effects have limited their use.

Clinical features

Most patients recognize the problem posed by their weight, but feel trapped and unable to take steps to address it. Many symptoms are related to psychological problems or social pressures.

The degree of obesity can be assessed by comparing the patient with tables of ideal weight for height, calculating the BMI **(Box 33.20)** and measuring skinfold thickness. The latter should be measured over the middle of the triceps muscle; normal values are 20 mm in a man and 30 mm in a woman. A central distribution of body fat (a waist/hip circumference ratio of >1.0 in men and >0.9 in women) is associated with a higher risk of morbidity and

Box 33.20 BMI ranges used to classify degrees of overweight and associated risk of co-morbidities

WHO classification	BMI (kg/m²)	Risk of co-morbidities
Overweight	25–30	Mildly increased
Obese	**>30**	
Class I	30–35	Moderate
Class II	35–40	Severe
Class III	>40	Very severe

BMI, body mass index; WHO, World Health Organization.

 Box 33.21 Conditions and complications associated with obesity

- Depression and anxiety
- Osteoarthritis of knees and hips
- Varicose veins
- Hiatus hernia
- Gallstones
- Postoperative complications
- Low back pain
- Obstructive sleep apnoea
- Hypertension
- Breathlessness
- Ischaemic heart disease
- Stroke
- Diabetes mellitus (type 2)
- Hyperlipidaemia
- Menstrual abnormalities
- Increased cancer risk
- Heart failure
- Non-alcoholic fatty liver disease
- Increased morbidity and mortality

mortality than a more peripheral distribution of body fat (waist/hip ratio <0.85 in men and <0.75 in women). This is because fat located centrally, especially inside the abdomen, is more sensitive to lipolytic stimuli, with the result that the abnormalities in circulating lipids are more severe.

Box 33.21 shows the conditions and complications that are associated with obesity. The relationship between cardiovascular disease (hypertension or ischaemic heart disease), hyperlipidaemia, smoking, physical exercise and obesity is complex. Difficulties arise in interpreting mortality figures because of the number of factors involved. Many studies do not differentiate between the types of physical exercise taken nor do they take into account the cuff-size artefact in the measurement of blood pressure (an artefact will occur if a large cuff is not used in patients with a large arm). Nevertheless, obesity almost certainly plays a part in all of these diseases and should be treated. An exception is that stopping smoking, even if accompanied by weight gain, is more beneficial than any of the other factors. Physical fitness is also helpful, and there is some evidence to suggest that a fit obese person may have a similar cardiovascular risk to a leaner, unfit person, or even a lower risk.

Morbidity and mortality

Obese patients are at risk of early death, mainly from diabetes, coronary heart disease and cerebrovascular disease. The greater the obesity, the higher are the morbidity and mortality rates. For example, men who are 10% overweight have a 13% increased risk of death, while the increase in mortality for those 20% overweight is 25%. The rise is less in women, and in men over 65, obesity is not an independent risk factor. Weight reduction reduces this mortality and therefore should be strongly encouraged. The benefits are probably greater in more obese subjects **(Box 33.22)**.

 Box 33.22 Potential benefits from loss of 10 kg in 100-kg patients with co-morbidities

Mortality
- 20–25% fall in total mortality
- 30–40% fall in diabetes-related deaths
- 40–50% fall in obesity-related cancer deaths

Blood pressure
- Fall of about 10 mmHg (systolic and diastolic)

Diabetes
- Reduction in risk of developing diabetes by >50%
- 30–50% fall in fasting blood glucose
- 15% fall in HbA$_{1c}$

Serum lipids
- 10% fall in total cholesterol
- 15% fall in LDL cholesterol
- 30% fall in triglycerides
- 8% increase in HDL cholesterol

HbA$_{1c}$, haemoglobin A$_{1c}$; HDL, high-density lipoprotein; LDL, low-density lipoprotein.

Metabolic syndrome

There are two classification systems, which are shown in **Box 33.23**. The differences are as follows:

- A large waist is an absolute requirement for the International Diabetes Federation (IDF) but not for the Adult Treatment Panel 3 National Cholesterol Education Programme (ATP III NCEP).
- The IDF criteria use lower cut-off values for waist circumference (close to values for people with a BMI of 25 kg/m²) and lower fasting blood glucose concentrations.

This means that the prevalence of metabolic syndrome will be higher using the IDF criteria, and that the IDF criteria will identify at-risk patients at an earlier stage. This could lead to further investigations following on from the initial screening, and earlier institution of preventative as well as therapeutic measures.

Overweight/central obesity and insulin resistance, which causes glucose and lipid disturbances including non-alcoholic fatty liver disease, seem to form the basis of many features of the metabolic syndrome. Early treatment of obesity and the metabolic syndrome can prevent the development of clinical diabetes and its complications.

The metabolic syndrome is a combination of risk factors (see **Box 33.23**). Its overall role in the prediction of the risk of cardiovascular disease has been questioned, as the sum of the combined risk factors involved in the syndrome does not offer more than the individual factors added together.

Management

Dietary control

This largely depends on a reduction in calorie intake. The most common diets allow a daily intake of approximately 4200 kJ (1000 kcal), although this may need to be nearer 6300 kJ (1500 kcal) for someone engaged in physical work. Very-low-calorie diets are also advocated by some, usually over shorter periods of time, but unless they are accompanied by changes in lifestyle, weight regain is likely. Patients must realize that prolonged dieting is necessary for large amounts of fat to be lost. Furthermore, a permanent change in eating habits is required to maintain the new low weight. It is relatively easy for most people to lose the first few kilograms but long-term success in moderate obesity is poor (no more than 10%). Most obese people oscillate in weight; they often regain the lost weight but many manage to lose weight again. This 'cycling' in body weight may play a role in the development of coronary artery disease.

Many dietary regimens aim to produce a weight loss of approximately 1 kg/week. Weight loss will be greater initially owing to accompanying protein and glycogen breakdown and consequent water loss. After 3–4 weeks, further weight loss may be very small because only adipose tissue is broken down and there is less accompanying water loss.

Patients must understand the principles of energy intake and expenditure, and the best results are obtained in educated, well-motivated patients. Constant supervision by healthcare professionals or close relatives, or through membership of a slimming club, helps to encourage compliance. It is essential to establish realistic aims. A 10% reduction in weight (see **Box 33.22**), is a realistic initial aim.

An increase in exercise will increase energy expenditure and should be encouraged – provided there is no contraindication – since weight control is usually not achieved without exercise. The effects of exercise are complex and not entirely understood. However, exercise alone will usually produce little long-term benefit. On the other hand, there is evidence to suggest that, in combination with dietary therapy, it can prevent weight being regained. In addition, regular exercise (30 min daily) will improve general health.

The diet should contain adequate amounts of protein, vitamins and trace elements **(Box 33.24)**.

A balanced diet, attractively presented, is of much greater value and is safer than any of the slimming regimens often advertised in magazines.

A wide range of diets are available, including low-fat or low-carbohydrate diets, and some suit certain individuals better than others. The following general statements can be made about them:

- All low-calorie diets produce loss of body weight and fat, irrespective of dietary composition. Short-term weight loss is faster on low-carbohydrate diets, as a result of greater loss of body water, which is regained after the end of dietary therapy.
- Very-low-fat diets are often low in vitamins E and B_{12}, and in zinc. Very-low-carbohydrate diets may be nutritionally inadequate and may lead to deficiencies.
- Low-fat diets decrease LDL triglycerides and increase HDL, whereas low-carbohydrate diets produce a greater decrease in HDL and triglyceride, with no change in LDL.
- There are some potential long-term concerns with low-carbohydrate diets (high in fat and protein), including increased risk of osteoporosis, renal stones and atheroma (due to high intake of saturated fat, high *trans* fat and cholesterol, and the

lack of fruits, vegetables and whole grains), but long-term studies are lacking.
- Low-energy-density diets, often bulky and rich in fibre and complex carbohydrates, may be more satiating but they are often less palatable than high-energy-dense diets, which may affect long-term compliance.
- Liquids, such as soft drinks, appear to be less satiating than solid foods.
- A study has shown that Mediterranean and low-carbohydrate diets are as effective as a low-fat diet for weight loss.

Behavioural modification

The aim of behavioural modification is to encourage the patient to take personal responsibility for changing lifestyle, which will determine dietary habits and physical activity. Family therapy may also be useful, especially when it involves obese children, but can be time-consuming and expensive. Cognitive behavioural therapy is even more time-consuming and expensive.

Drug therapy

Drugs can be used in the short term (e.g. up to 3 months and then reviewed), as an adjunct to the dietary regimen, but they do not substitute for strict dieting. The pancreatic lipase inhibitor, orlistat, is the only drug licensed specifically for weight loss in the UK.

Centrally acting drugs include:

- Drugs acting on both *serotoninergic and noradrenergic pathways*, e.g. sibutramine (now withdrawn in Europe due to side-effects). Other drugs are being evaluated.
- *Cannabinoid-1 receptor blockers*, e.g. rimonabant (now withdrawn due to depression/suicide risk), acting on the endocannabinoid system.
- *Drugs acting on the noradrenergic pathways.* These do suppress appetite but all have been withdrawn, at least in the UK, because of cardiovascular side-effects.

Peripherally acting drugs are as follows:

- *Orlistat* is an inhibitor of pancreatic and gastric lipases. It reduces dietary fat absorption and aids weight loss. Weight regain occurs after the drug is stopped. It has been used continuously in a large-scale trial for up to 2 years. Patients complain of diarrhoea during treatment and, to avoid this, take a low-fat diet, resulting in weight loss.
- *GLP-1* receptor agonists suppress appetite; injections have been used to treat obesity (see Fig. 33.14) and type 2 diabetes mellitus (see p. 719).
- *Sodium-glucose cotransporter-2 (SGLT-2) inhibitors* such as canagliflozin are used to treat diabetes, and have also been demonstrated to reduce body weight and improve cardiovascular outcomes (see p. 719).

A systematic review of long-term pharmacotherapy concluded that there was a paucity of long-term studies with anti-obesity agents, and that in weight loss trials of 1 year's duration, these agents appear to be only modestly effective in promoting weight loss (about 3 or 4 kg greater weight loss, respectively, than the control group). Other randomized trials show that a combination of lifestyle modification and pharmacotherapy produces greater weight loss than either treatment alone, but the withdrawal of several anti-obesity drugs from the market suggests that a pharmacotherapeutic 'magic bullet' to treat obesity without substantial short-term and long-term effects is not yet available.

Surgical management (bariatric surgery, metabolic surgery)

Surgery is now performed laparoscopically in patients with morbid obesity (BMI >40 kg/m²), or in patients with a BMI higher than 35 kg/m² and obesity-related complications, after conventional lifestyle approaches have failed. Fitness for surgery should be checked, especially in older people. Some centres may insert a balloon into the stomach to initiate weight loss prior to bariatric surgery for morbid obesity. A variety of gastrointestinal surgical procedures have been used, which fall into three main groups (Fig. 33.15):

- **Restrictive procedures**, which restrict the ability to eat (e.g. adjustable gastric banding, vertical banded gastroplasty and sleeve gastroplasty).
- **Malabsorptive procedures**, which reduce the ability to absorb nutrients (e.g. biliopancreatic diversion and Roux-en-Y gastric bypass). The malabsorptive procedures cause nutrient deficiencies, malnutrition and, in some cases, anastomotic leaks and the dumping syndrome (e.g. with the duodenal switch).
- **Restrictive plus malabsorptive procedures** (e.g. duodenal switch, Roux-en-Y gastric bypass, intragastric balloon).

The procedures all have advantages and disadvantages, and there is controversy about the procedure of choice for specific groups of patients. The restrictive procedures are more straightforward than the complex bypass procedures. The adjustable gastric banding procedure is attractive in concept, especially since it can be undertaken laparoscopically with a lower perioperative mortality (<0.3%) than the other procedures (approximately 1%); it can, however, be associated with erosion and slippage of the band, as well as problems with the port, making repeat operations a frequent requirement (>10% of cases). The sleeve gastrectomy is associated with heartburn and greater risk of weight regain, but a biliary pancreatic diversion (duodenal switch) can be added later.

Postoperatively, there is a need to monitor nutrient status carefully and to provide supplements of vitamins and minerals (including iron and calcium), as nutrient deficiencies are common. Weight loss following the combined restrictive and malabsorptive procedures tends to be greater than with either procedure alone.

A systematic analysis of several bariatric surgical procedures concluded that, in comparison to non-surgical treatments, they produced significantly more weight loss (23–37 kg), which was maintained up to 8 years and associated with improvement in quality of life and co-morbidities. There is now evidence showing that the risk of myocardial infarction, stroke, cardiovascular events and mortality is reduced by about half compared to non-surgical controls over a follow-up period of 2–15 years. Although fertility is improved after bariatric surgery, women are advised to delay pregnancy for a year or more after rapid and substantial weight loss, while the safety of pregnancy is being elucidated. A recent study has shown a reduction in risk of gestational diabetes and earlier than expected birth but the benefits and risks of bariatric surgery still need further study. The commissioning of specialist obesity services should be multidisciplinary and should not focus on the surgical treatment only.

Liposuction, the removal of large amounts of fat by suction, does not deal with the underlying problem and weight regain frequently occurs. There appears to be no reduction in cardiovascular risk factors with the procedure.

Prevention

Preventing obesity must always be the goal because most obese people find it difficult to maintain any weight loss they manage to achieve. All health professionals must be aware of the dangers of obesity and encourage children, and young as well as older adults, from gaining too much weight. A small gain each year over a long period produces an obese individual for whom treatment is difficult. Public health policies should consider the creation of public places to encourage physical activity and fitness, education about the benefits of losing weight or not gaining it, and changes in food composition (alternatives to high-fat, high-energy-dense foods and sugar reduction).

Since the present obesity epidemic has resulted from lifestyle changes, it is appropriate to promote lifestyle changes, not only as

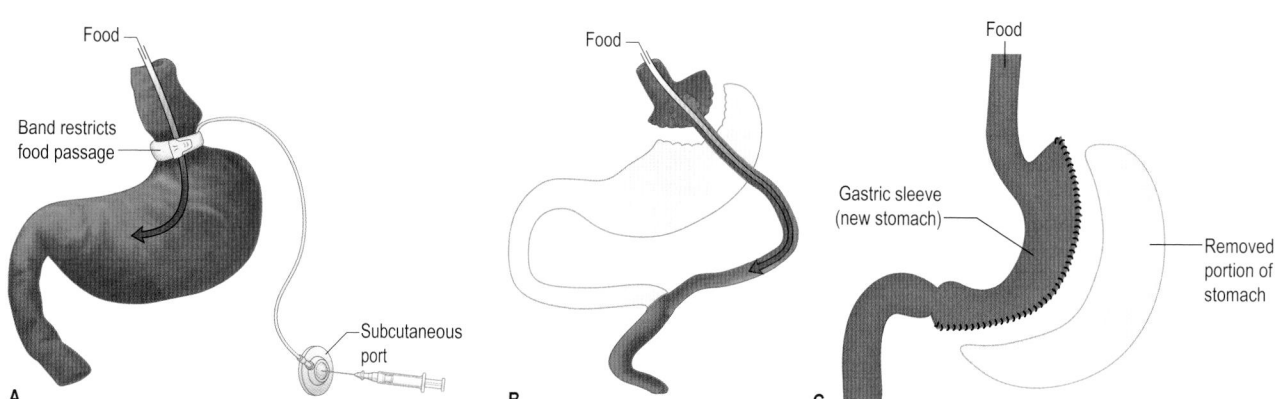

Fig. 33.15 Examples of surgical procedures to treat morbid obesity. (A) Restrictive procedure: gastric banding with a subcutaneous port attached to the anterior abdominal wall so that fluid can be injected into the adjustable band around the upper stomach. **(B)** Restrictive plus malabsorptive procedure: Roux-en-Y gastric bypass, in which food passes through a small stomach pouch and bypasses the proximal small bowel. **(C)** Gastric sleeve.

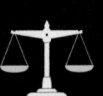

the first-line therapy for most overweight and obese individuals, but also in the prevention of overweight and obesity. Lifestyle modification may include reducing the proportion of time spent in physical inactivity (for instance, watching television); building physical activity into daily routines (for instance, through cycling to work), and encouraging patterns of healthy eating.

Further reading

Caprio S. Calories from soft drinks – do they matter? *N Engl J Med* 2012; 367:1462–1463.

Casazza K, Pate R, Allison DB. Myths, presumptions, and facts about obesity. *N Engl J Med* 2013; 368:2236–2237.

Caughey AB. Bariatric surgery before pregnancy. *N Engl J Med* 2015: 372; 877–878.

Choban P, Dickerson R, Malone A et al. A.S.P.E.N. Clinical guidelines: nutrition support of hospitalized adult patients with obesity. *J Parenter Enteral Nutr* 2013; 37:714–744.

Hawkes C, Smith TG, Jewell J et al. Smart food policies for obesity prevention. *Lancet* 2015; 385:2410–2421.

Huang TT-K, Cawley JH, Ashe M et al. Mobilisation of public support for policy actions to prevent obesity. *Lancet* 2015; 385:2422–2431.

Kwok CS, Pradhan A, Khan MA et al. Bariatric surgery and its impact on cardiovascular disease and mortality: a systematic review and meta-analysis. *Int J Cardiol* 2014; 173:20–28.

Ozanne SE. Epigenetic signatures of obesity. *N Engl J Med* 2015; 372: 973–974.

Roberto CA, Swinburn B, Hawkes C et al. Patchy progress of obesity prevention: emerging examples, entrenched barriers, new thinking. *Lancet* 2015; 385:2400–2409.

Stein J, Stier C, Raab H et al. Review article: The nutritional and pharmacological consequences of obesity surgery. *Aliment Pharmacol Ther* 2014; 40:582–609.

NUTRITIONAL SUPPORT

Support in the hospital patient

Nutritional support is recognized as being necessary in many hospitalized patients. The pathophysiology and hallmarks of malnutrition have been described earlier (see p. 1231) but malnutrition is often not immediately clinically apparent. Screening tools can be used to identify adults who are malnourished or at risk of malnutrition. The Malnutrition Universal Screening Tool (MUST score) is widely used (see Fig. 33.5) to identify patients that require nutritional support. In the UK, up to 40% of patients are malnourished on acute admission to hospital and up to 70% of patients are malnourished on discharge. Here, the forms of nutritional support that are available are discussed, along with special nutritional requirements in some diseases.

Principles

Some form of nutritional supplementation is required in those patients who cannot eat, should not eat, will not eat or cannot eat enough. All patients should be screened for malnutrition on admission and the findings linked to a care plan, preferably under the supervision of a trained multidisciplinary team, including a dietician. Plans are discussed with patients and consent is taken for any invasive procedure (e.g. nasogastric tube, parenteral nutrition). If the patient is unable to give consent, the healthcare team should act in the patient's best interest, considering any previously expressed wishes of the patient and views of the family. It is usually necessary to provide nutritional support for:

- all severely malnourished patients on admission to hospital

- moderately malnourished patients who, because of their physical illness, are not expected to eat for more than 5 days
- normally nourished patients expected not to eat for more than 5 days or expected to eat less than half their intake for more than 8–10 days.

Enteral rather than parenteral nutrition should be used if the gastrointestinal tract is functioning normally.

In the *re-feeding syndrome*, the shifts of water and electrolytes that occur during parenteral and enteral nutrition can be life-threatening. Carbohydrate intake stimulates insulin release, which leads to cellular uptake of phosphate, potassium and magnesium. **Complications** include hypophosphataemia, hypokalaemia, hypomagnesaemia and fluid overload because of sodium retention (decreased renal excretion of sodium and water). Biochemical abnormalities can result in cardiac arrhythmias and respiratory insufficiency, and are associated with a raised mortality. Any electrolyte deficiency should be replaced and monitored, and patients who have eaten little or nothing for more than 5 days should initially receive no more than 50% of their energy requirements (National Institute for Health and Care Excellence (NICE) guidelines). Patients at risk of the re-feeding syndrome should be given high potency vitamins daily for 10 days and oral or enteral thiamine 50 mg 4 times daily for 10 days, along with multivitamins.

Nutritional requirements for adults

The exact nutrient requirements in many disease states are not clearly defined and vary with the stage and severity of disease, as well as nutritional status. The optimal protein and energy intakes needed to produce the best clinical outcomes in acute critical illness continue to be debated. The following general guidance is provided for specific nutrients or groups of nutrients:

- *Fluid.* Typical requirements are approximately 2–3 L/day (>60 years = 30 mL/kg, 18–60 years = 35 mL/kg). Requirements are increased in patients with large-output stomas, nasogastric aspirates, diarrhoea and fever. Requirements are reduced in patients with oedema, hepatic failure and renal failure.
- *Energy.* Typical requirements are approximately 7.5–10.0 MJ/day (1800–2400 kcal/day). Disease increases resting energy expenditure but decreases physical activity. Extra energy is given for repletion and reduced energy for obesity.
- *Protein.* Typical requirements are 9–15 g N/day (56–94 g protein/day) or 0.15–0.25 g N/kg per day (0.94–1.56 g protein/kg per day). Extra protein may be needed in severely catabolic conditions, such as extensive burns, sepsis and major trauma.
- *Major minerals.* Typical requirements for sodium and potassium are 60–100 mmol/day (1.0–1.5 mmol/kg). Requirements are increased in patients with gastrointestinal effluents. The excretion of these minerals in various effluents can provide an indication of the additional requirements (see **Box 9.12**). Requirements may be lower in patients with fluid overload (or those with hypernatraemia and hyperkalaemia). The requirements for calcium and magnesium are higher in enteral than in parenteral nutrition because only a proportion of these minerals is absorbed by the gut.
- *Trace elements.* For trace elements such as iodine, fluoride and selenium, which are well absorbed, the requirements are similar in enteral and parenteral nutrition. For other trace elements, such as iron, zinc, manganese and chromium, the requirements in parenteral nutrition are substantially lower than in enteral nutrition **(Fig. 33.16)**.

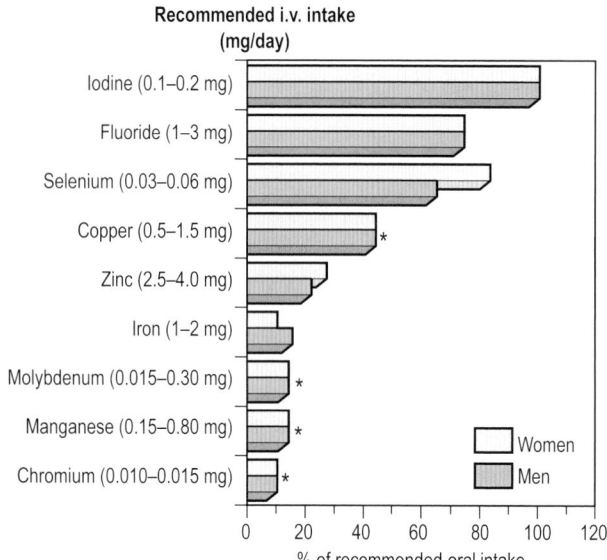

Recommended i.v. intake
(mg/day)

Fig. 33.16 Trace elements. Recommended intravenous intake in absolute values and as a percentage of recommended oral intake. *Trace elements for which there is too little information to establish a recommended value for dietary oral intake; the midpoint of estimated safe and adequate oral intake is shown.

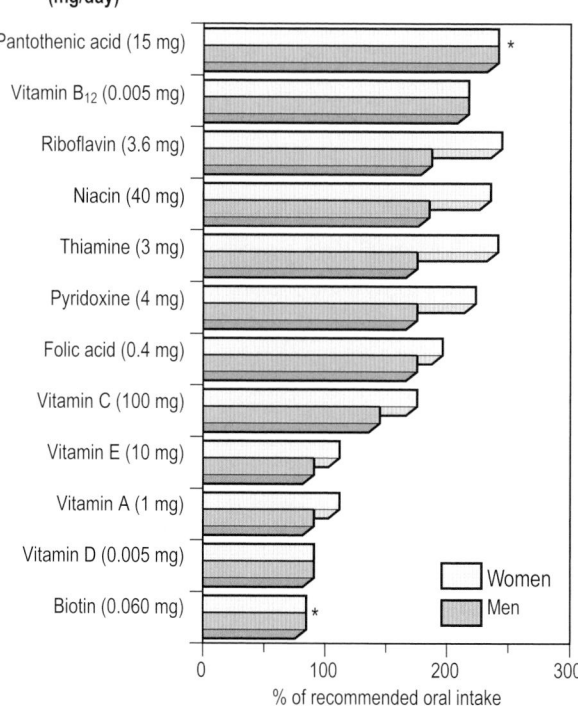

Recommended i.v. intake
(mg/day)

Fig. 33.17 Vitamins. Recommended intravenous intake in absolute values and as a percentage of recommended oral intake. *Vitamins for which there is too little information to establish recommended dietary oral intake; the midpoint of estimated safe and adequate oral intake is shown.

- *Vitamins.* Many vitamins are given in greater quantities in patients receiving parenteral nutrition than in those receiving enteral nutrition **(Fig. 33.17)**. This is because patients on parenteral nutrition may have increased requirements, partly because of severe disease, partly because they may already have depleted pools of vitamins, and partly because some vitamins degrade during storage. Vitamin K is usually absent from parenteral nutrition regimens and therefore it may need to be administered separately.

Enteral nutrition

In enteral nutrition, feeds can be given by various routes:
- By mouth (food can be supplemented with solid or liquid supplements with multiple benefits).
- By fine-bore nasogastric tube **(Box 33.25)**.
- By percutaneous endoscopic gastrostomy (PEG). This is useful for patients who need enteral nutrition for a prolonged period (e.g. >30 days), such as those with swallowing problems following a head injury, or elderly people after a stroke. A catheter is placed percutaneously into the stomach under endoscopic control **(Fig. 33.18)**.
- By needle catheter jejunostomy. In this technique, a fine catheter is inserted into the jejunum at laparotomy and brought out through the abdominal wall.

Diet formulation

A polymeric diet with whole protein and fat can be used **(Box 33.26)**, except in patients with severely impaired gastrointestinal function, who may require a pre-digested (i.e. semi-elemental/ elemental) diet. In these patients, the nitrogen source is purified low-molecular-weight peptides or amino acid mixtures, the fat sometimes being given partly as medium-chain triglycerides (MCTs).

 Box 33.25 Insertion of a nasogastric tube

Explain the procedure to the patient and obtain consent.
Procedure
- Insert a fine-bore tube intranasally with a wire stylet.
- Confirm the position of the tube in the stomach by aspiration of gastric contents (check pH).
- Check by X-ray if aspiration is unsuccessful or pH >5.5. Care should be taken in patients on strong acid suppressants such as proton pump inhibitors.

Problems
- No satisfactory way of keeping nasogastric tubes in place (up to 60% come out).

Main complications
- Regurgitation and aspiration into bronchus.
- Blockage of the nasogastric tube.
- Gastrointestinal side-effects, the most common being diarrhoea.
- Metabolic complications of feeding, including hyperglycaemia and hypokalaemia, as well as low levels of magnesium, calcium and phosphate.

Management of enteral nutrition

Daily amounts of fluid vary between 1.5 and 2.5 L, but small amounts are started in patients with suspected poor gastric emptying and severe malnutrition (to avoid the re-feeding syndrome).

Hypercatabolic patients require a high supply of nitrogen (0.25–0.35 g/kg daily) and often will not achieve positive nitrogen balance until the primary injury is resolved.

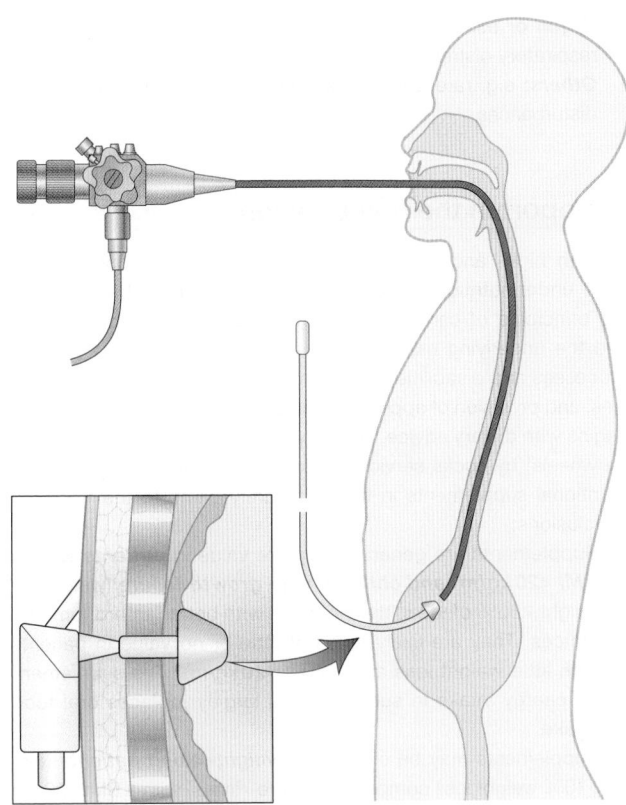

Fig. 33.18 Percutaneous endoscopic gastrostomy (PEG).

> *i*   **Box 33.26** Standard enteric diet, providing 8.4 MJ/day
> (= 2000 kcal/day)
>
> **Energy**
> - Carbohydrate as glucose polymers (49–53% of total energy). Fat as triglycerides (30–35% of total energy)
>
> **Nitrogen**
> - Whole protein (10–14 g of nitrogen/day). Additional electrolytes, vitamins and trace elements
>
> **Features**
> - Ratio of energy to nitrogen kJ : g = 620 : 1 (kcal : g = 150 : 1) Osmolality = 285–300 mOsm/kg

The success of enteral feeding depends on careful supervision of the patient, with monitoring of weight, biochemistry and diet charts.

Parenteral nutrition

This should only be used if the enteral route cannot be used. The need for major improvements in the practice of parenteral nutrition in UK hospitals has been emphasized by the National Confidential Enquiry into Patient Outcome and Death (NCEPOD). This included a requirement for improvements at every level: assessment, monitoring and follow-up, including appropriate care of lines to avoid catheter-related sepsis and documentation.

Peripheral parenteral nutrition

Specially formulated mixtures for peripheral use are available; these have a low osmolality (<800 mosmol/L) and contain lipid emulsions. Heparin and corticosteroids can be added to the infusion and local

> **Box 33.27** Subclavian vein catheter placement for parenteral nutrition
>
> This should be performed only by experienced clinicians under aseptic conditions in an operating theatre.
>   Explain the procedure to the patient and obtain consent.
> - Place the patient supine with 5° of head-down tilt to avoid air embolism.
> - Infiltrate the skin below the midpoint of the right clavicle with 1–2% lidocaine and make a 1 cm skin incision.
> - Insert a 20-gauge needle on a syringe beneath the clavicle and first rib, angling it towards the tip of a finger held in the suprasternal notch.
> - When blood is aspirated freely, use the needle as a guide to insert the cannula through the skin incision and into the subclavian vein.
> - Advance the catheter so that its tip lies in the distal part of the superior vena cava.
> - Create a skin tunnel under local anaesthetic using an introducer inserted through a point about 10 cm below and medial to the incision and passed upwards to the incision.
> - Pass the proximal end of the catheter (with hub removed) backwards through the introducer so that it emerges 10 cm below the clavicle; suture it to the chest wall.
> - Now suture the original infraclavicular entry incision.

application of glyceryl trinitrate patches reduces the occurrence of thrombophlebitis and prolongs catheter life.
- A peripheral cannula can be inserted into a mid-arm vein (20 cm) and can be left for up to 5 days.
- A longer (60 cm), peripherally inserted central catheter (PICC) placed into an antecubital fossa vein has its distal end lying in a central vein; here, there is less risk of thrombophlebitis and hyperosmolar solutions can be given. With careful management, PICCs can be used for up to a month or so.

Peripheral parenteral nutrition is often preferred initially, allowing time to consider the necessity for insertion of a central venous catheter.

Parenteral nutrition via a central venous catheter

A silicone catheter is placed into a central vein, usually adopting an infraclavicular approach to the subclavian vein **(Box 33.27)**. The skin-entry site should be dressed carefully and not disturbed unless there is a suggestion of catheter-related sepsis.

Complications of catheter placement include central vein thrombosis, pneumothorax and embolism, but one of the most common problems is catheter-related sepsis. Organisms, mainly staphylococci, enter along the side of the catheter, leading to septicaemia. Sepsis can be prevented by ensuring careful and sterile placement of the catheter, not removing the dressing over the catheter entry site, and not giving other substances (e.g. blood products, antibiotics) via the central vein catheter.

Sepsis should be suspected if the patient develops fever and leucocytosis. In two-thirds of cases, organisms can be grown from the catheter tip after removal. Treatment involves removal of the catheter and appropriate systemic antibiotics.

Nutrients

With parenteral nutrition, it is possible to provide sufficient nitrogen for protein synthesis and calories to meet energy requirements. Electrolytes, vitamins and trace elements are also necessary. All these substances are infused simultaneously.

Nitrogen source

Most patients receive at least 11–15 g N/day, in the form of synthetic L-amino acids.

Energy source

Energy is supplied by glucose, with additional calories provided by a fat emulsion. Fat infusions give a greater number of calories in a smaller volume than can be provided by carbohydrate. Fat infusions are not hypertonic and they also prevent essential fatty acid deficiency, which has been reported in long-term parenteral nutritional regimens without fat emulsions. Deficiency causes a scaly skin, hair loss and a delay in healing.

Electrolytes, vitamins and trace elements

Initially, the electrolyte status should be monitored daily and electrolyte solutions given as appropriate. Fat- and water-soluble vitamins and minerals, including trace elements, should be given routinely (see **Figs 33.16** and **33.17**).

Management of parenteral nutrition

Peripheral parenteral nutrition is administered via 3-L bags over 24 hours, the constituents being premixed under sterile conditions. **Box 33.28** shows the composition that provides 9 g of nitrogen and 7206 kJ (1700 kcal) in 24 hours.

For a *central venous parenteral nutrition regimen*, most hospitals now use premixed 3-L bags. A standard parenteral nutrition regimen that provides 14 g of nitrogen 9305 kJ (2250 kcal) over 24 hours is also given in **Box 33.28**.

Monitoring includes:
- *Blood tests.* Plasma electrolytes and glucose are checked daily (at least initially); full blood count, liver biochemistry and function, calcium and phosphate twice weekly; and magnesium, zinc and triglycerides weekly.
- *Nutritional status.* Weight and skinfold thickness are monitored on a weekly basis if appropriate calipers are available. Daily weight changes reflect changes in fluid balance.
- *Nitrogen balance assessment* (see p. 1228). This requires complete collections of urine.

Complications

- *Mechanical*: insertional trauma and catheter-related (see above).
- *Metabolic*: e.g. hyperglycaemia (insulin therapy is often necessary), fluid and electrolyte disturbances, hypercalcaemia, nutrient deficiencies (if inadequately provided).

> ℹ **Box 33.28 Examples of parenteral nutrition regimens**[a]
>
> **Peripheral**
>
> *Nitrogen*
> - L-amino acids 9 g/L: 1 L
>
> *Energy*
> - Glucose 20%: 1 L
> - Lipid 20%: 0.5 L
> - + Trace elements, electrolytes, water-soluble and fat-soluble vitamins, heparin 1000 U/L and hydrocortisone 100 mg; insulin is added if required. Nitrogen 9 g, non-protein calories 7206 kJ (1700 kcal)
>
> **Central**
>
> *Nitrogen*
> - L-amino acids 14 g/L: 1 L
>
> *Energy*
> - Glucose 50%: 0.5 L
> - Glucose 20%: 0.5 L
> - + Lipid 10% as either Intralipid or Lipofundin: 0.5 L; fractionated soya oil 100 g/L, soya oil 50 g, medium-chain triglycerides 50 g/L
> - + Electrolytes, water-soluble and fat-soluble vitamins, trace elements; heparin and insulin may be added if required. Nitrogen 14 g, non-protein calories 9305 kJ (2250 kcal)

- *Organ or tissue dysfunction*: e.g. abnormal liver dysfunction, respiratory distress and metabolic bone disease.
- *Others*: e.g. rare allergic reactions to lipid, and psychological disturbances.

Support in the home patient

In both high- and low-income countries, there is considerably more under-nutrition in the community than in hospital. However, the principles of care are very similar: detection of malnutrition and the underlying risk factors; treatment of underlying disease processes and disabilities; correction of specific nutrient deficiencies; and provision of appropriate nutritional support. This typically begins with dietary advice, and may involve the provision of 'meals on wheels' by social services. A systematic review of the use of nutritional supplements in the community came to the following conclusions:

- Supplements are generally of more value in *patients with a BMI <20 kg/m^2 and children with growth failure* (weight for height <85% of ideal) than in those with better anthropometric indices. They are likely to be of little or no value in patients with little weight loss and a BMI >20 kg/m^2. The supplemental energy intake in such subjects largely replaces oral food intake.
- Supplements may be of value in *weight-losing patients* (e.g. >10% weight loss compared with pre-illness) with a BMI >20 kg/m^2, and in *children with deteriorating growth performance* without chronic protein–energy under-nutrition.
- The functional benefits vary according to the patient group. In patients with *chronic obstructive airways disease*, the observed functional benefits were increases in respiratory muscle strength, handgrip strength, and walking distance/duration of exercise. In the *elderly*, the benefits were reduction in number of falls, or increase in activities of daily living, and reduction in pressure ulcer surface area. In patients with *HIV/AIDS*, there were changes in immunological function and improved cognition. Patients with *liver disease* experienced a lower incidence of severe infections and had a lower frequency of hospitalization.
- *Acceptability and compliance* are likely to be better when a choice of supplements (of type, flavour, consistency) and the schedule are decided in conjunction with the patient and/or carer. Adjustments to these may be necessary when there is a change in patterns of daily activities, disease status, and 'taste fatigue' with prolonged use of the same supplement.
- Nutritional *counselling and monitoring* are recommended before and after the start of supplements (see below).

Some patients receive enteral tube feeding or parenteral nutrition at home. Indeed in developed countries, enteral tube feeding occurs more frequently at home than in hospital.

Home enteral nutrition

In adults, the most common reason for starting home tube feeding is for swallowing difficulties. This involves patients with neurological disorders, such as motor neurone disease, multiple sclerosis and Parkinson's disease, but the most common single diagnosis is cerebrovascular disease. Approximately 2% of patients who have had a stroke in the UK receive home enteral tube feeding (HETF). However, in a British Nutrition survey of patients with these disorders (apart from Parkinson's), only 15% in total were able to return to oral feeding after 1 year.

The swallowing capabilities of patients should be assessed regularly in order to avoid unnecessary tube feeding. The patients and/or carers should have adequate training, contacts with appropriate health professions, and a reliable delivery service for feeds and ancillary equipment. They should also be clear about how to manage simple problems associated with the feeding tube, which is usually a gastrostomy rather than a nasogastric tube.

Home parenteral nutrition

Home parenteral nutrition is practised much less frequently, and usually comes under the supervision of specialist centres. The potential value of intestinal transplantation in patients with long-term intestinal failure is still being assessed.

Further reading

Boateng AA, Sriram K, Meguid MM et al. Refeeding syndrome: treatment considerations based on collective analysis of literature case reports. *Nutrition* 2010; 26:156–167.
Casaer MP, Van den Berghe G. Nutrition in the acute phase of critical illness. *N Engl J Med* 2014; 370:2450–2451.
Elia M. Multidisciplinary input is essential in the care of malnourished people. *Guidelines in Practice* 2013; 16:42–50.
Malone A. Clinical guidelines from the American Society for Parenteral and Enteral Nutrition: best practice recommendations for patient care. *J Infus Nurs* 2014; 37:179–184.
Mirtallo JM. Consensus of parenteral nutrition safety issues and recommendations. *J Parenter Enteral Nutr* 2012; 36:62S.

FOOD ALLERGY AND FOOD INTOLERANCE

Many people ascribe their various symptoms to food, and many such sufferers are seen and started on exclusion diets. The scientific evidence that food does harm is weak, in most instances, although adverse reactions to food certainly exist. These can be divided into those that involve immune mechanisms (**food allergy**) and those that do not (**food intolerance**).

Food allergy

Food allergy, which is estimated to affect up to 5–7% of young children and 1–2% of adults (with a rising prevalence), may be mediated by immunoglobulin E (IgE) or not mediated by IgE (T cell-mediated). The IgE-mediated reactions tend to occur early after a food challenge (within minutes to an hour). Adults tend to be allergic to fish, shellfish and peanuts, while children tend to be allergic to cow's milk, egg white, wheat and soy. Peanuts are very allergenic and peanut allergy persists throughout life. The following conditions can result from food allergy:

- *Acute hypersensitivity.* An example is urticaria, vomiting or diarrhoea after eating nuts, strawberries or shellfish. These IgE-mediated reactions do not usually produce clinical problems, as the patients have already learned to avoid the suspected food. Inadvertent ingestion of the incriminating food can sometimes occur, leading to angio oedema or anaphylaxis (see p. 668).
- *Eczema and asthma.* These tend to affect young children; they are often due to egg and are IgE-mediated.
- *Rhinitis and asthma.* These have been produced by foods such as milk and chocolate, mainly in atopic subjects.
- *Chronic urticaria.* This has been treated successfully by an exclusion diet.
- *Food-sensitive enteropathy.* This may manifest itself as coeliac disease (gluten (wheat) sensitive enteropathy) and cow's milk enteropathy (in infants); it is T cell-mediated.

Food intolerance

- *Migraine.* This sometimes follows the intake of foods such as chocolate, cheese and alcohol, which are rich in certain amines, such as tyramine. Patients on monoamine oxidase inhibitors, which are involved in the metabolism of these amines, are particularly vulnerable.
- *Irritable bowel syndrome.* In some patients, this seems to be related to ingestion of certain food items, such as wheat, but the mechanisms are not clearly defined.
- *Chinese restaurant syndrome.* Monosodium glutamate, a flavour enhancer used in cooking Chinese food, may produce dizziness, faintness, nausea, sweating and chest pains.
- *Lactose intolerance.* Patients develop abdominal bloating and diarrhoea following ingestion of lactose, which is present in milk (see p. 1193). This is probably the most common form of food intolerance worldwide, and may be genetic in origin.
- *Phenylketonuria.* This can also be classified as a form of food intolerance; it is due to lack of phenylalanine hydroxylase, which is necessary for the metabolism of phenylalanine present in dietary protein.

A number of other inborn errors of metabolism can also be regarded as forms of food intolerance.

Food intolerance may be caused by a constituent of food (e.g. the histamine in mackerel or canned food, or the tyramine in cheeses); by chemical mediators released by food (e.g. histamine may be released by tomatoes or strawberries); or by toxic chemicals found in food (e.g. the food additive tartrazine). Many other additives and compounds with certain E numbers have been implicated as causing reactions but the evidence is poor.

There is little or no evidence to suggest that diseases such as arthritis, behavioural and affective disorders, and Crohn's disease are due to ingestion of a particular food. Multiple vague symptoms, such as tiredness or malaise, are also not caused by food allergy, and psychiatric evaluation may be indicated (see p. 772).

Management

- The history may help to delineate the causative agent, particularly when the effects are immediate.
- Skin-prick testing with allergen and measurement in the serum of antigen or antibodies do not generally correlate with symptoms and are usually misleading.
- Diagnostic exclusion diets are sometimes used but are time-consuming. They can occasionally be of value in identifying a particular food that is causing problems.
- Dietary challenge consists of the food and the test being given sublingually or by inhalation in an attempt to reproduce the symptoms. Again, this may be helpful in a few cases.
- Most people who have acute reactions to food realize it and stop eating the food; they do not require medical attention. In the remainder of patients, a small minority seem to be helped by modifying their diet but there is no good scientific evidence to support these exclusion diets. A recent study showed that the introduction of peanuts decreased the frequency of peanut allergy in children at high risk of developing this allergy, and modulated immune responses to peanuts.
- Increasing evidence suggests that many children with milk and egg allergies are able to tolerate the food when heat-modified, and this may speed up resolution of the allergy.
- There is no good evidence to recommend that pregnant or breast-feeding women should change their diet to prevent allergies in infants at high risk or normal risk.

Further reading

de Silva D, Geromi M, Halken S et al. Primary prevention of food allergy in children and adults: systematic review. *Allergy* 2014; 69:581–589.

de Silva D, Geromi M, Panesar SS et al. Acute and long-term management of food allergy: systematic review. *Allergy* 2014; 69:159–167.

Gruchalla RS, Sampson HA. Preventing peanut allergy through early consumption. *N Engl J Med* 2015; 372:875–877.

Longo G, Berti I, Burks AW et al. IgE-mediated food allergy in children. *Lancet* 2013; 382:1656–1664.

Nwaru BI, Hickstein L, Panesar SS et al. The epidemiology of food allergy in Europe: a systematic review and meta-analysis. *Allergy* 2014; 69:62–75.

Perry TT, Pesek RD. Clinical manifestations of food allergy. *Pediatr Ann* 2013; 42:96–101.

ALCOHOL

Although alcohol is not a nutrient, it is consumed in large quantities all over the world. In many countries, alcohol consumption is a major medical and social problem (see p. 790). It increases morbidity and mortality in a variety of ways, including effects on heart disease, stroke, cancers, liver and neurological/psychiatric problems, and is associated with nutritional deficiencies and abnormal metabolism of drugs.

Ethanol (ethyl alcohol) is oxidized, in the steps shown in **Box 33.29**, to acetaldehyde. Acetaldehyde is then converted to acetate, 90% in the liver mitochondria. Acetate is released into the blood and oxidized by peripheral tissues to carbon dioxide and water.

Alcohol dehydrogenases are found in many tissues and it has been suggested that enzymes present in the gastric mucosa may contribute substantially to ethanol metabolism.

Ethanol itself produces 29.3 kJ/g (7 kcal/g), but many alcoholic drinks also contain sugar, which increases their calorific value. For example, 1 pint of beer provides about 1045 kJ (250 kcal), so heavy drinkers will be unable to lose weight if they continue to drink.

Effects of excess alcohol consumption

Excess consumption of alcohol leads to two major problems, both of which can be present in the same patient:

- alcohol dependence syndrome (see p. 790)
- physical damage to various tissues.

Each unit of alcohol (defined as 10 mL (7.9 g) of pure ethanol) corresponds to about half a pint of normal beer, one single measure of spirit or half a glass of wine **(Fig. 33.19)**. An intake of less than 14 units per week is generally considered to be safe. All the long-term effects of excess alcohol consumption are due to excess ethanol, irrespective of the type of alcoholic beverage; that is, beer and spirits are no different in their long-term effects. Short-term effects, such as hangovers, depend on additional substances, particularly other alcohols such as isoamyl alcohol, which are known as congeners. Brandy and bourbon contain the highest percentage of congeners.

The amount of alcohol that produces damage varies and not everyone who drinks heavily will suffer physical damage. For example, only 20% of people who drink heavily develop cirrhosis of the liver. The effect of alcohol on different organs of the body is not the same; in some patients, the liver is affected; in others, the brain or muscle. The differences may be genetically determined.

Thiamin deficiency contributes to neurological (confusion, Wernicke–Korsakoff syndrome; see p. 891) and some of the non-neurological manifestations (cardiomyopathy). The susceptibility of different organs to damage is variable and the figures given in **Box 33.30** are provided only as a guide to sensible drinking. Heavy drinkers who persist for many years are at greater risk than heavy sporadic drinkers.

Liver disease

In general, the effects of a given intake of alcohol seem to be worse in women. The following figures are for men and should be reduced by about 30% for women:

- **High risk:** 160 g ethanol per day (20 single drinks)
- **Medium risk:** 80 g ethanol per day (10 single drinks)
- **Little risk:** 40 g ethanol per day (5 single drinks).

Alcohol consumption in pregnancy

Women are advised not to drink alcohol at all during pregnancy because consumption of even small amounts of alcohol can lead to fetal growth restriction and may also increase the risk of miscarriage. The fetal alcohol syndrome is characterized by mental retardation, dysmorphic features and growth impairment; it occurs in fetuses of alcohol-dependent women.

A summary of the physical effects of alcohol is given in **Box 33.31**. Details of these diseases are discussed in the relevant

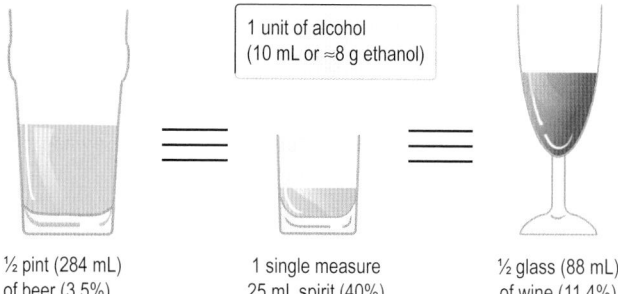

Fig. 33.19 Measures containing 1 unit of alcohol. The percentage refers to the proportion of alcohol by volume (vol/vol). The alcohol content of beers, spirits and wines can vary substantially.

---

i **Box 33.30 Guide to sensible alcohol drinking**

Weekly maximum
- 14 units for both men and women

To help achieve this
- Use a standard measure
- Do not drink during the daytime
- Have alcohol-free days each week

Remember
- Health can be damaged without being 'drunk'. Regular heavy intake is more harmful than occasional binges
- Do not drink to 'drown sorrows'
- In the UK, the drink-before-driving limit of alcohol in the blood is 800 mg/L
- 1 unit of alcohol is eliminated per hour; therefore spread drinking time
- Food decreases absorption and therefore results in a lower blood alcohol level
- 4–5 units are sufficient to put the blood alcohol level over the legal driving limit in a 70 kg man (less in a lighter person)

---

i **Box 33.29 The main pathways of ethanol oxidization**

Alcohol dehydrogenase

$$CH_3CH_2OH + NAD^+ \xrightarrow{ADH} CH_3CHO + NADH + H^+ \qquad [1]$$
$$\text{(ethanol)} \qquad\qquad\qquad \text{(acetaldehyde)}$$

Liver microsomal ethanol oxidizing system (MEOS)
- Includes the specific P450 enzyme, CYP2EI, which is induced by ethanol

$$CH_3CH_2OH + NADPH + H^+ + O_2 \xrightarrow{MEOS} CH_3CHO + NADP + 2H_2O \qquad [2]$$

Box 33.31 Physical effects of excess alcohol consumption

Central nervous system
- Epilepsy (see p. 852)
- Wernicke–Korsakoff syndrome (see p. 891)
- Polyneuropathy (see p. 891)

Muscles
- Acute or chronic myopathy

Cardiovascular system
- Cardiomyopathy (see p. 1119)
- Beriberi heart disease (see p. 1240)
- Cardiac arrhythmias
- Hypertension

Metabolism
- Hyperuricaemia (gout)
- Hyperlipidaemia
- Hypoglycaemia
- Obesity

Endocrine system
- Pseudo–Cushing's syndrome

Respiratory system
- Chest infections

Gastrointestinal system
- Acute gastritis (including bleeding; see p. 1181)
- Carcinoma of the oesophagus or large bowel
- Pancreatic disease
- Liver disease (fatty liver, hepatitis, cirrhosis; see p. 1303)

Haemopoiesis
- Macrocytosis (due to direct toxic effect on bone marrow or folate deficiency)
- Thrombocytopenia
- Leucopenia

Bone
- Osteoporosis
- Osteomalacia

---

chapters. The effects of alcohol withdrawal are discussed on page 791.

Specific public health and clinical guidance on prevention and management of alcohol-related disorders has been produced by NICE. The clinical guidelines specifically address alcohol withdrawal, Wernicke's encephalopathy, and both alcohol-related liver and pancreatic disease.

Further reading

National Institute for Health and Care Excellence. *NICE Clinical Guideline 115: Alcohol-use Disorders: Diagnosis, Assessment and Management of Harmful Drinking and Alcohol Dependence.* NICE 2011; http://www.nice.org.uk/guidance/cg115.
Stewart S, Swain S. Assessment and management of alcohol dependence and withdrawal in the acute hospital: concise guidance. *Clin Med* 2012; 12:266–271.

Bibliography

Elia M, Ljungqvist O, Stratton RJ et al. *Clinical Nutrition*, 2nd edn. Oxford: Wiley–Blackwell, 2013 (part of Nutrition Society textbook bundle; available at http://eu.wiley.com).

Significant websites

http://www.ajcn.org/ American Journal of Clinical Nutrition.
http://www.ama-assn.org/ *American Medical Association; assessment and management of adult obesity.*
http://www.fao.org/ *Food and Agriculture Organization; autonomous body within the United Nations aiming to improve health through nutrition and agricultural productivity, especially in rural populations.*
http://www.www.food.gov.uk *Food Standards Agency. UK information on food safety and hygiene, news and alerts, and business guidance.*
https://foodinsight.org/ *International Food Information Council; non-profit organization communicating science-based information on health, nutrition and food safety for the public good.*
http://www.nature.com/ejcn/ European Journal of Clinical Nutrition.
http://www.nature.com/ijo International Journal of Obesity.
https://www.nice.org.uk/search?q=obesity *NICE; various publications related to obesity.*
https://www.nice.org.uk/search?q=alcohol *NICE; various publications related to prevention and treatment of alcohol-related problems.*
http://jn.nutrition.org/ Journal of Nutrition.
http://www.nutritioncare.org/ Journal of Parenteral and Enteral Nutrition.
http://www.nutritionsociety.org/publications/ British Journal of Nutrition.
http://www.nhlbi.nih.gov/health/educational/ *National Heart, Lung and Blood Institute: Aim for a Healthy Weight.*
http://www.who.int/nut *WHO recommendations and intervention programmes for nutrient-related diseases.*
http://www.who.int/nutgrowthdb/ *World Health Organization; provides information on worldwide nutritional issues, resources and research.*

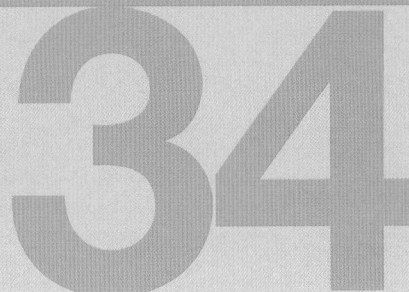

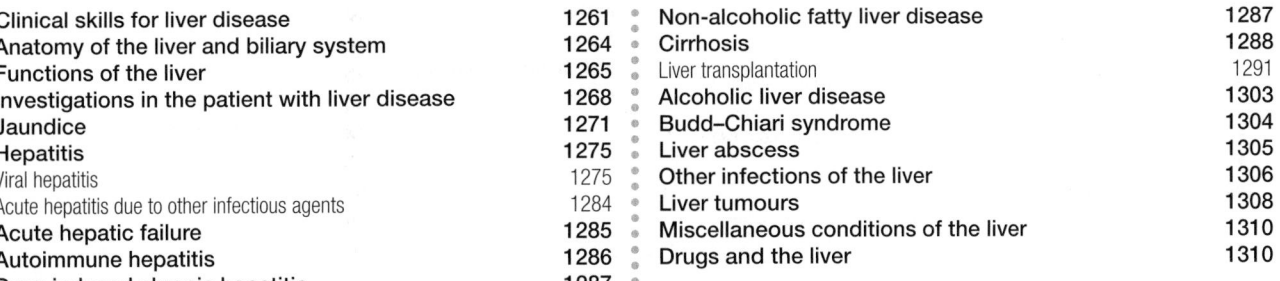

34

Liver disease

Graham Foster and Alastair O'Brien

CORE SKILLS AND KNOWLEDGE

Liver disease is common and its incidence is rising, predominantly because of viral hepatitis in developing countries, and alcohol and obesity in developed ones. It remains a major cause of mortality and morbidity, with death occurring secondary to cirrhosis and hepatocellular carcinoma.

Hepatologists divide their time between inpatient work (decompensated chronic liver disease and acute liver failure may both require intensive inpatient management) and clinic work (managing patients with stable liver disease and diagnosing patients newly referred from primary care). Many also perform procedures such as endoscopic retrograde cholangiopancreatography (ERCP); and some subspecialize in the management of alcohol cessation, viral hepatitis or liver transplantation.

Key skills in hepatology include:

- managing patients with decompensated chronic liver disease, including variceal bleeding, ascites and encephalopathy, and those presenting with acute liver failure
- appreciating the role of history, examination, imaging, blood tests and liver biopsy in the diagnosis of patients newly presenting with evidence of liver disease
- understanding the natural history of hepatitis B and C infection and how to use the recently licensed and older medications available for their management.

Opportunities to learn hepatology include attending ward rounds on inpatient liver units, participating in outpatient hepatology clinics, observing the work of specialist nurses who manage patients with chronic liver disease in the community, learning how to perform paracentesis safely on medical day units, and watching ERCP procedures being performed.

CLINICAL SKILLS FOR LIVER DISEASE

History

Both acute and chronic liver disease are often asymptomatic, especially in the early stages. Taking a history in hepatology involves not only asking about symptoms but also establishing the presence of common risk factors for liver disease to help establish a diagnosis (**Box 34.1**).

Asking about alcohol

This requires gentleness and tact (**Box 34.2**). Patients often underestimate their alcohol intake or degree of dependence. This history should be non-judgemental, and help should be offered through referral to alcohol support services if patients express a desire to become abstinent.

Examination

In acute liver disease there may be few signs, apart from jaundice and an enlarged liver. In the cholestatic phase of the illness, pale stools and dark urine are present.

The figure on p. 1263 illustrates the many signs associated with chronic liver disease, although physical examination is occasionally normal in patients with advanced disease.

Investigations

A detailed overview of the diagnostic investigations used in liver disease begins on page 1268. **Fig. 34.1** illustrates how these investigations may be employed in an outpatient setting for a patient referred from primary care with raised liver transaminases.

Box 34.1 Taking a history in liver disease

Symptoms of acute liver disease
- May be asymptomatic and anicteric
- Symptomatic disease, often viral, producing malaise, anorexia and fever
- Jaundice (see later), often appearing as the illness progresses

Symptoms of chronic liver disease
- Non-specific symptoms, particularly weakness, anorexia and fatigue
- Right hypochondrial pain due to liver distension
- Abdominal distension due to ascites
- Ankle swelling due to fluid retention
- Haematemesis and melaena from variceal haemorrhage
- Pruritus due to cholestasis – often an early symptom of primary biliary cholangitis (PBC)
- Endocrine dysfunction: gynaecomastia, loss of libido and amenorrhoea
- Confusion and drowsiness due to hepatic encephalopathy

Past medical history
- Any previous disease affecting the liver, biliary tract, pancreas or gut
- Heart failure
- History of autoimmune disease
- Features of metabolic syndrome: obesity, diabetes, gout, hypercholesterolaemia

Medications
- Recent antibiotic use (several cause cholestasis)
- Paracetamol overdose
- Full medication history, establishing whether any cause liver damage

Family history
- History of jaundice, liver disease or specific diseases such as haemochromatosis

Alcohol use
- Take a detailed history (see later)

Risk factors for viral hepatitis
- Childhood spent in countries where hepatitis B or C is endemic
- Contaminated needles – unsafe tattoos, injecting drug use
- High-risk unprotected sexual activity

Box 34.2 Taking an alcohol history in patients with liver disease

Extent of use
- Preferred type of alcohol (beer, wine, spirits); strength where relevant ('super-strength' beers can be up to 10% ethanol)
- Daily consumption (in cans, bottles or glasses, subsequently converted to units)
- Number of abstinent days per week
- Frequency of consuming >8 units on one occasion
- Duration of alcohol use, and changing use over this time

Degree of dependence
- Number of times alcohol has interfered with regular activities (e.g. going to work)
- Number of times the person has been unable to stop drinking once they have started

- Need for a morning drink to 'get going'
- Feelings of guilt about alcohol consumption
- Concern on the part of family and friends about alcohol use
- Injuries to self or others caused by alcohol

Views on abstinence
- Awareness of risks of current level of alcohol use (if this exceeds target levels)
- Willingness to cut down versus abstaining completely
- Previous attempts to give up
- Previous experiences of support groups, including Alcoholics Anonymous, and cognitive behavioural therapy
- Sources of support: family members, close friends, social or religious groups

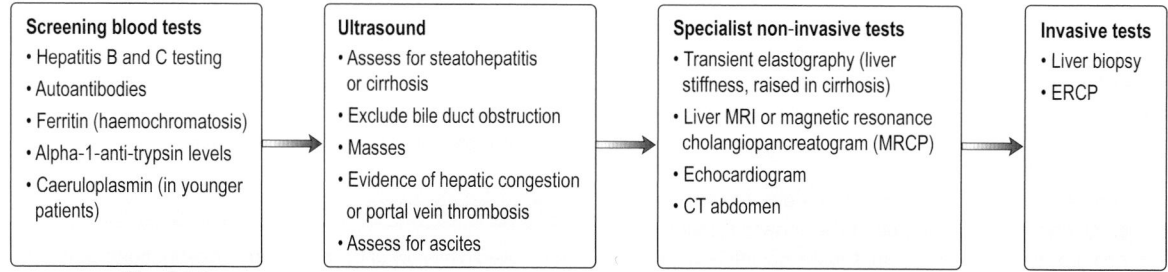

Screening blood tests
- Hepatitis B and C testing
- Autoantibodies
- Ferritin (haemochromatosis)
- Alpha-1-anti-trypsin levels
- Caeruloplasmin (in younger patients)

Ultrasound
- Assess for steatohepatitis or cirrhosis
- Exclude bile duct obstruction
- Masses
- Evidence of hepatic congestion or portal vein thrombosis
- Assess for ascites

Specialist non-invasive tests
- Transient elastography (liver stiffness, raised in cirrhosis)
- Liver MRI or magnetic resonance cholangiopancreatogram (MRCP)
- Echocardiogram
- CT abdomen

Invasive tests
- Liver biopsy
- ERCP

Fig. 34.1   Use of diagnostic investigations in an outpatient setting. This scheme would be appropriate for a patient referred from primary care with raised liver transferases.

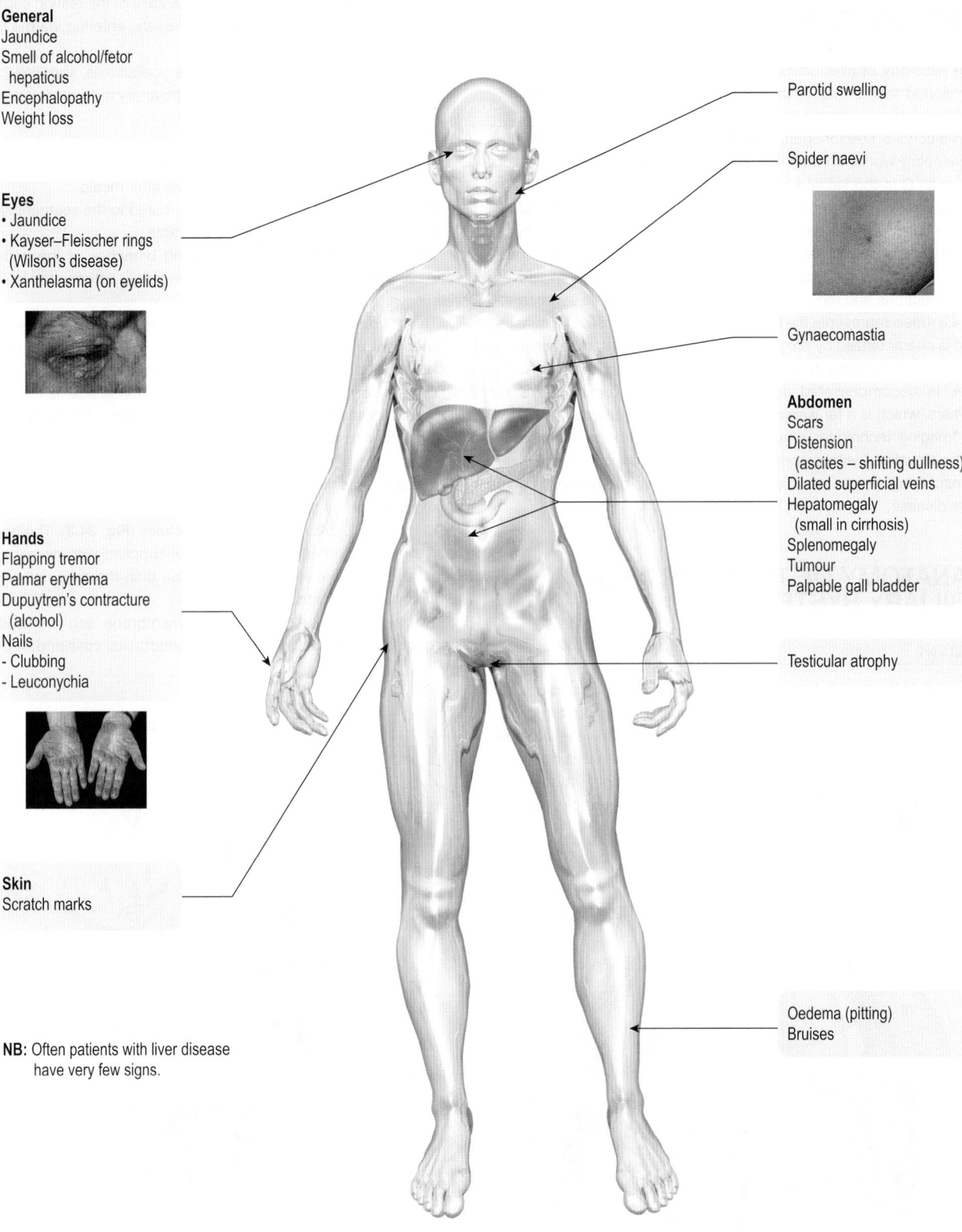

General
Jaundice
Smell of alcohol/fetor
  hepaticus
Encephalopathy
Weight loss

Eyes
• Jaundice
• Kayser–Fleischer rings
  (Wilson's disease)
• Xanthelasma (on eyelids)

Hands
Flapping tremor
Palmar erythema
Dupuytren's contracture
  (alcohol)
Nails
- Clubbing
- Leuconychia

Skin
Scratch marks

NB: Often patients with liver disease
  have very few signs.

Parotid swelling

Spider naevi

Gynaecomastia

Abdomen
Scars
Distension
  (ascites – shifting dullness)
Dilated superficial veins
Hepatomegaly
  (small in cirrhosis)
Splenomegaly
Tumour
Palpable gall bladder

Testicular atrophy

Oedema (pitting)
Bruises

INTRODUCTION

The aetiology of liver disease differs from region to region. In the developed world, liver inflammation is most often due to obesity, the metabolic syndrome (non-alcoholic fatty liver disease, NAFLD), non-alcoholic steatohepatitis (NASH) and alcohol excess. In the developing world, chronic viral infection with either hepatitis B or hepatitis C is the leading cause of liver mortality. In England, liver disease is the fifth most common cause of premature mortality. Globally, about half a billion people suffer from chronic viral hepatitis. Health education and the improvement in public health, along with vaccination programmes, should help to stop the spread of viral infections and reduce risk factors for the metabolic syndrome.

Cirrhosis represents the final common pathway for liver diseases and is characterized by progressive fibrosis of the liver parenchyma, which leads to portal hypertension and deterioration of liver function. In decompensated cirrhosis the median overall survival is 2 years, which is a far worse prognosis than for many cancers.

Imaging techniques enable the liver, biliary tree and pancreas to be visualized with precision, resulting in earlier diagnosis. Liver transplantation is an established therapy for both acute and chronic liver disease.

ANATOMY OF THE LIVER AND BILIARY SYSTEM

Liver

The liver is the body's largest internal organ (1.2–1.5 kg) and is situated in the right hypochondrium. A functional division into the larger right lobe (containing caudate and quadrate lobes) and the left lobe is made by the middle hepatic vein. The liver is further subdivided into eight segments (**Fig. 34.2**) by divisions of the right, middle and left hepatic veins. Each segment has its own portal pedicle, permitting individual segment resection at surgery.

The hepatic blood supply constitutes 25% of the resting cardiac output and is delivered via two main vessels, entering via the liver hilum (porta hepatis):
- **The hepatic artery**, a branch of the coeliac axis, supplies 25% of the hepatic blood flow. The hepatic artery autoregulates flow, ensuring a constant total blood flow.
- **The portal vein** drains most of the gastrointestinal tract and the spleen. It supplies 75% of hepatic blood flow. The normal portal pressure is 5–8 mmHg; flow increases after meals.

The blood from these vessels is distributed to the segments and flows into the sinusoids via the portal tracts.

Blood leaves the sinusoids, entering branches of the hepatic vein, which join into three main branches before entering the inferior vena cava.

The **caudate lobe** is an autonomous segment, as it receives an independent blood supply from the portal vein and hepatic artery, and its hepatic vein drains directly into the inferior vena cava.

Lymph, formed mainly in the perisinusoidal space, is collected in lymphatics that are present in the portal tracts. These small lymphatics enter larger vessels, which eventually drain into the portal system.

The **acinus** is the functional hepatic unit. This consists of parenchyma supplied by the smallest portal tracts containing portal vein radicles, hepatic arterioles and bile ductules (**Fig. 34.3**). The hepatocytes near this triad (zone 1) are well supplied with oxygenated blood and are more resistant to damage than the cells nearer the terminal hepatic (central) veins (zone 3).

The **sinusoids** lack a basement membrane and are loosely surrounded by specialist fenestrated endothelial cells and Kupffer

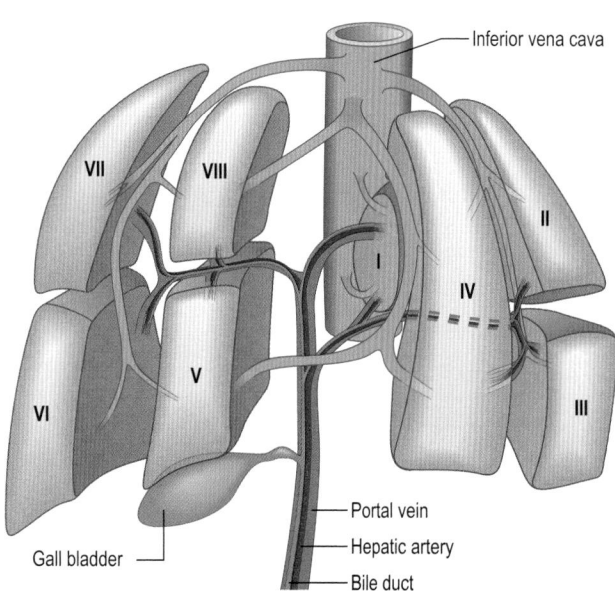

Fig. 34.2 Segmental anatomy of the liver. The eight hepatic segments are shown: I, caudate lobe; II–IV, left hemiliver; V–VIII, right hemiliver.

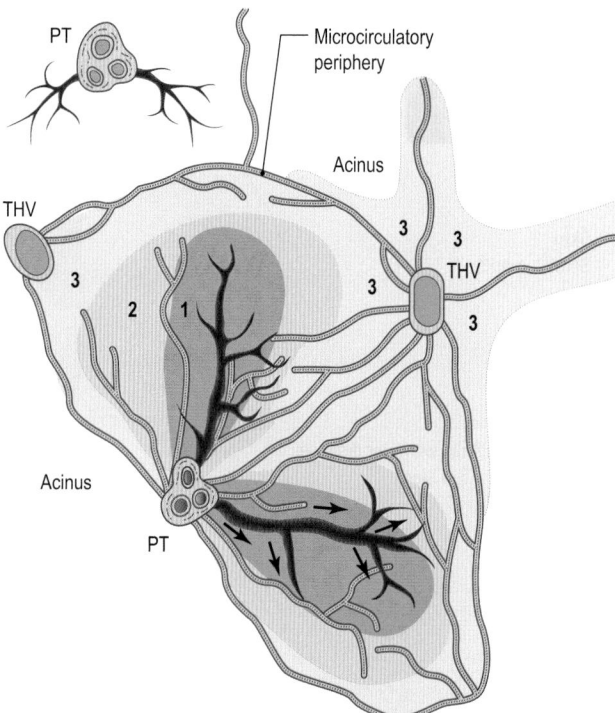

Fig. 34.3 The acinus. Zones 1, 2 and 3 represent areas supplied by blood, zone 1 being best oxygenated. Zone 3 is supplied by blood remote from afferent vessels and is in the microcirculatory periphery of the acinus. The perivascular area (the star-shaped green area around the terminal hepatic venule, THV) is formed by the most peripheral parts of zone 3 and is made up of several adjacent acini; it is the least well oxygenated area. PT, portal triad.

cells (phagocytic cells). Sinusoids are separated by plates of liver cells (hepatocytes). The subendothelial space between the sinusoids and hepatocytes is the space of Disse, which contains a matrix of basement membrane constituents and stellate cells (see **Fig. 34.21**).

Stellate cells store retinoids in their resting state and contain the intermediate filament, desmin. When activated (to myofibroblasts), they are contractile and regulate sinusoidal blood flow. Endothelin and nitric oxide play a major role in modulating stellate cell contractility. Stellate cells are activated by a wide variety of inflammatory cytokines (such as tumour necrosis factor-alpha, TNF-α); once activated, they generate extracellular matrix proteins, including collagen, leading to fibrosis and eventually cirrhosis. Under appropriate conditions, stellate cells can also produce proteases that degrade the extracellular matrix, leading to reversal of fibrosis. The balance between collagen production and degradation is critical to the progression of liver scarring and cirrhosis development/resolution (see p. 1289).

Biliary system

Bile canaliculi form a network between the hepatocytes. These join to form thin bile ductules near the portal tract, which, in turn, enter the bile ducts in the portal tracts. These then combine to form the right and left hepatic ducts, which leave each liver lobe. The hepatic ducts join at the porta hepatis to form the common hepatic duct. The cystic duct connects the gall bladder to the lower end of the common hepatic duct. The gall bladder lies under the right lobe of the liver and stores and concentrates hepatic bile; its capacity is approximately 50 mL. The common bile duct is formed at the junction of the cystic and common hepatic ducts and is 8 mm in diameter or less, passing through the head of the pancreas, and narrowing at its lower end to pass into the duodenum. The common bile duct and pancreatic duct open into the second part of the duodenum, most often through a common channel at the ampulla of Vater, which contains the muscular sphincter of Oddi. This contracts rhythmically and prevents all of the bile from entering the duodenum, by maintaining a higher pressure than the gall bladder in the fasting state.

FUNCTIONS OF THE LIVER

Protein metabolism

See also page 1228.

Synthesis and storage

The liver is the principal site of synthesis of all circulating proteins, apart from γ-globulins (produced in the reticuloendothelial system). The liver receives amino acids from the intestine and muscles and, by controlling the rate of gluconeogenesis and transamination, regulates plasma levels. Plasma contains 60–80 g/L of protein, mainly albumin, globulin and fibrinogen.

Albumin has a half-life of 16–24 days, and 10–12 g is synthesized daily. Its main functions are to maintain intravascular oncotic (colloid osmotic) pressure, and to transport water-insoluble substances such as bilirubin, hormones, fatty acids and drugs. Reduced synthesis of albumin over prolonged periods produces hypoalbuminaemia and is seen in chronic liver disease and malnutrition. Hypoalbuminaemia is also found in hypercatabolic states (e.g. trauma, burns

and sepsis) and in diseases associated with an excessive loss (e.g. nephrotic syndrome or protein-losing enteropathy).

Transport or carrier proteins, such as transferrin and caeruloplasmin, acute phase and other proteins (e.g. α_1-antitrypsin and α-fetoprotein) are also produced in the liver.

The liver also synthesizes all coagulation factors (except for one-third of factor VIII) – that is, fibrinogen, prothrombin, factors V, VII, IX, X and XIII, proteins C and S, and antithrombin (see pp. 368–369), as well as components of the complement system. The liver stores large amounts of certain vitamins, particularly A, D and B$_{12}$, lesser amounts of others (vitamin K and folate), and minerals – iron in ferritin and haemosiderin, and copper.

Degradation (nitrogen excretion)

Amino acids are degraded by transamination and oxidative deamination to produce ammonia, which is then converted to urea and excreted by the kidneys. This is the major pathway for the elimination of nitrogenous waste. Failure of this process occurs in severe liver disease.

Carbohydrate metabolism

Glucose homeostasis and maintenance of blood sugar are major functions of the liver. It stores approximately 80 g of glycogen. In the immediate fasting state, blood glucose is maintained either by glucose release from glycogen breakdown (glycogenolysis) or by synthesis of new glucose (gluconeogenesis). Sources for gluconeogenesis are lactate, pyruvate, amino acids from muscles (mainly alanine and glutamine), and glycerol from lipolysis of fat stores. In prolonged starvation, ketone bodies and fatty acids are used as alternative sources of fuel as body tissues adapt to a lower glucose requirement (see p. 1231).

Lipid metabolism

Fats are insoluble in water and are transported in plasma as protein–lipid complexes (lipoproteins). These are discussed in detail on page 744.

The liver has a major role in the metabolism of lipoproteins. It synthesizes very-low-density lipoproteins (VLDLs) and high-density lipoproteins (HDLs). HDLs are the substrate for lecithin-cholesterol acyltransferase (LCAT), which catalyses the conversion of free cholesterol to cholesterol ester (see later). Hepatic lipase removes triglyceride from intermediate-density lipoproteins (IDLs) to produce low-density lipoproteins (LDLs), which are degraded by the liver after uptake by specific cell-surface receptors (see **Fig. 24.3**).

Triglycerides are mainly of dietary origin but are also formed in the liver from circulating free fatty acids (FFAs) and glycerol, and incorporated into VLDLs. Oxidation or *de novo* synthesis of FFAs occurs in the liver, depending on availability of dietary fat.

Cholesterol may be of dietary origin but most is synthesized from acetyl-coenzyme A (acetyl-CoA) in the liver, intestine, adrenal cortex and skin. It either occurs as free cholesterol or is esterified with fatty acids; this reaction is catalysed by LCAT. This enzyme is reduced in severe liver disease, increasing the ratio of free cholesterol to ester, which alters membrane structures. One result of this is the red cell abnormalities (e.g. target cells) seen in chronic liver disease. Phospholipids (e.g. lecithin) are synthesized in the liver. The complex interrelationships between protein, carbohydrate and fat metabolism are shown in **Fig. 34.4**.

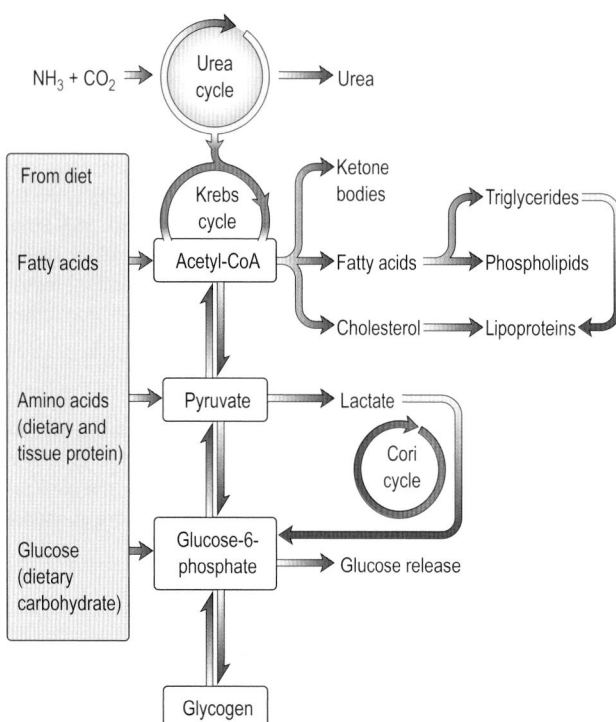

Fig. 34.4 Interrelationships of protein, carbohydrate and lipid metabolism in the liver.

Formation of bile

Bile secretion and bile acid metabolism

Bile consists of water, electrolytes, bile acids, cholesterol, phospholipids and conjugated bilirubin. Two processes are involved in bile secretion across the canalicular membrane of the hepatocyte – **bile salt-dependent** and **bile salt-independent** processes – each contributing about 230 mL/day. Another 150 mL/day is produced by bile ductule epithelial cells.

Bile formation requires uptake of bile acids and other organic and inorganic ions across the basolateral (sinusoidal) membranes by multiple transport proteins (sodium taurocholate co-transporting polypeptide (NTCP) and sodium-independent organic anion-transporting polypeptide 2 (OATP2); **Fig. 34.5**). This process is driven by sodium/potassium adenosine triphosphatase (Na$^+$/K$^+$-ATPase) in the basolateral membranes. Intracellular transport across hepatocytes is partly through microtubules and partly by cytosol transport proteins.

Bile acids are also synthesized in hepatocytes from cholesterol, the rate-limiting step being those catalysed mainly by cholesterol-7α-hydroxylase and the P450 enzymes (CYP7A1 and CYP8B1).

The farnesoid X bile acid receptor blocks bile acid formation from cholesterol and also regulates the transport proteins (NTCP, OATP2) that increase bile acid uptake by the liver. It is a target for a new class of therapeutic drugs, farnesoid X receptor (FXR) agonists.

The canalicular membrane contains multispecific organic anion transporters, mainly ATPase-dependent (ATP binding cassette), the multidrug-resistant protein 2 (MRP2), multidrug-resistant protein 3 (MDR3) and the bile salt excretory pump (BSEP), which carry a broad range of compounds including bilirubin diglucuronide, glucuronidated and sulphated bile acids, and other organic anions against a concentration gradient into the biliary canaliculus. Na$^+$ and water follow the passage of bile salts by diffusion across the tight junction between hepatocytes (a bile salt-dependent process). In the bile salt-independent process, water flow is due to other osmotically active solutes such as glutathione and bicarbonate.

Secretion of a bicarbonate-rich solution is stimulated mainly by secretin and inhibited by somatostatin. This involves several membrane proteins, including the Cl$^-$/HCO$_3^-$ exchanger and the cystic fibrosis transmembrane conductance regulator that controls Cl$^-$ secretion, and water channels (aquaporins) in cholangiocyte membranes.

The bile acids are excreted into bile and pass via the common bile duct into the duodenum. The two primary bile acids – cholic acid and chenodeoxycholic acid (see **Fig. 34.5**) – are conjugated with glycine or taurine, which increases their solubility. Intestinal bacteria convert these acids into secondary bile acids, deoxycholic and lithocholic acid. **Fig. 34.6** shows the enterohepatic circulation of bile acids.

The average total bile flow is 600 mL/day. During fasting, half flows into the duodenum and half is diverted into the gall bladder. The gall bladder mucosa absorbs 80–90% of the water and electrolytes but is impermeable to bile acids and cholesterol. Following a meal, the I cells of the duodenal mucosa secrete cholecystokinin, which stimulates contraction of the gall bladder and relaxation of the sphincter of Oddi, allowing bile to enter the duodenum. An adequate bile flow is dependent on bile salts being returned to the liver by the enterohepatic circulation.

Bile acids act as detergents; their main function is lipid solubilization. Bile acid molecules have both a hydrophilic and a hydrophobic end. In aqueous solutions they form micelles, with their hydrophobic (lipid-soluble) ends in the centre. Micelles are expanded by cholesterol and phospholipids (mainly lecithin), forming mixed micelles.

Bile acid receptors in liver disease

Bile acids have been identified as crucial cell signalling molecules that regulate multiple biological processes. Bile acids are endogenous ligands for FXR and TGR5, a G-protein coupled receptor. Gain- and loss-of-function studies have demonstrated that both are involved in the regulation of lipid and carbohydrate metabolism and inflammatory responses. These receptors may therefore be potential targets for treatment of NAFLD, and phase III trials of the FXR agonist obeticholic acid are nearing completion in NASH (see p. 1288). Furthermore, obeticholic acid has been approved for the second-line treatment of PBC following trial results demonstrating an improvement in liver blood tests. Finally, obeticholic acid showed potential beneficial effect for primary sclerosing cholangitis and a long-term multicentre study is ongoing. In cirrhotic animal models, this drug reduced both portal hypertension and gut bacterial translocation. However, hepatic decompensation, liver failure and death have been reported when Child B or C cirrhosis patients are dosed more frequently than recommended and so it remains uncertain whether it will emerge as a treatment for portal hypertension.

Bilirubin metabolism

Bilirubin is produced mainly from the breakdown of mature red cells by Kupffer cells in the liver and reticuloendothelial system; 15% of bilirubin is formed from catabolism of other haem-containing proteins, such as myoglobin, cytochromes and catalases.

Normally, 250–300 mg (425–510 mmol) of bilirubin are produced daily. The iron and globin are removed from haem and reused. Biliverdin is formed from haem and reduced to form bilirubin. The bilirubin produced is unconjugated and water-insoluble, due to internal hydrogen bonding, and is transported to the liver

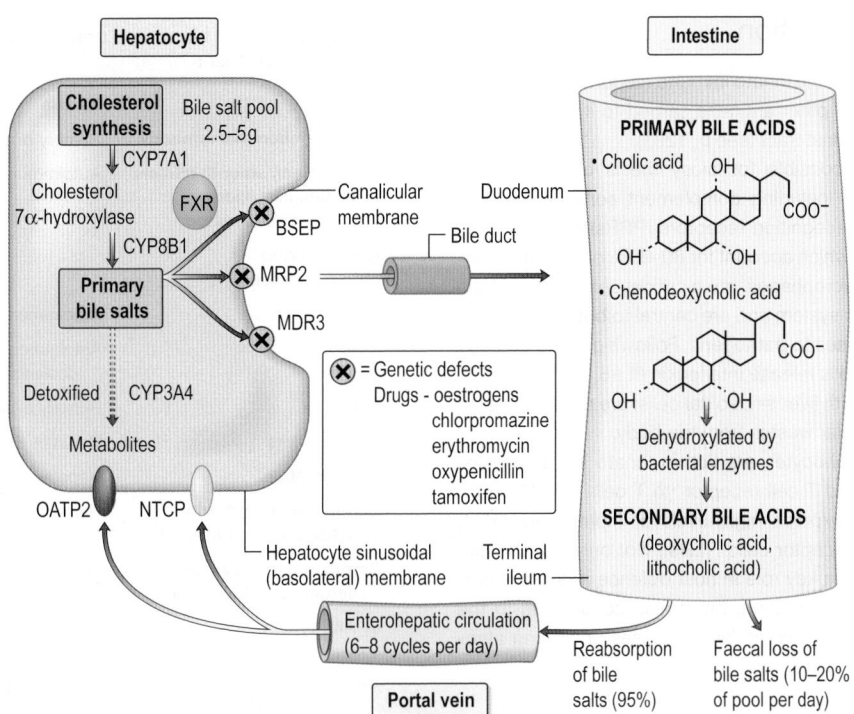

Fig. 34.5 Cholesterol synthesis and its conversion to primary and secondary bile acids. All bile acids are normally conjugated with glycine or taurine. BSEP, bile salt export pump; FXR, nuclear farnesoid X receptor; MDR3, multidrug-resistant protein 3; MRP2, multidrug-resistant protein 2; NTCP, sodium taurocholate co-transporting polypeptide; OATP2, sodium-independent organic anion-transporting polypeptide 2.

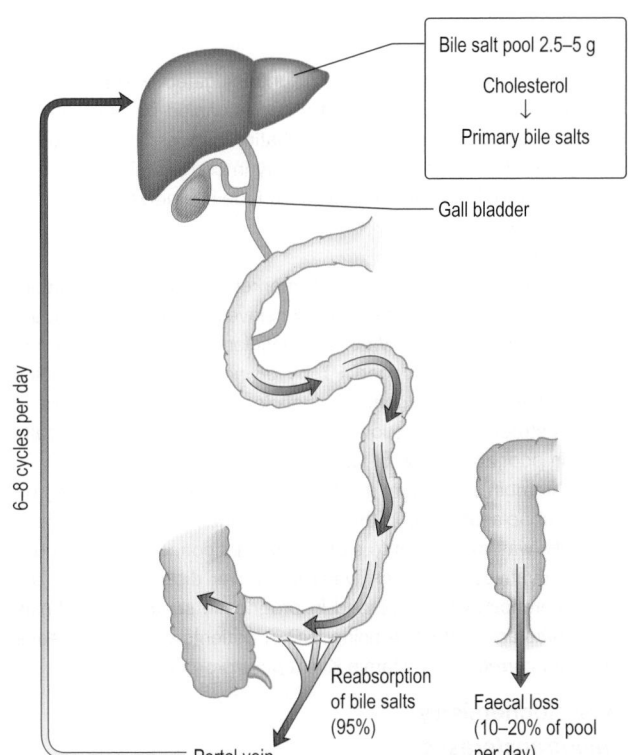

Fig. 34.6 Recirculation of bile acids. The bile salt pool is relatively small and the entire pool recycles 6–8 times via the enterohepatic circulation. Synthesis of new bile acids compensates for faecal loss.

attached to albumin. Bilirubin dissociates from albumin and is taken up by hepatic cell membranes and transported to the endoplasmic reticulum by cytoplasmic proteins, where it is conjugated with glucuronic acid and excreted into bile. The microsomal enzyme uridine diphosphoglucuronosyl transferase catalyses the formation of bilirubin monoglucuronide and then diglucuronide. This conjugated bilirubin is water-soluble; it is actively secreted into biliary canaliculi and excreted into the intestine within bile (see **Fig. 16.5**). It is not absorbed from the small intestine because of its large molecular size. In the terminal ileum, bacterial enzymes hydrolyse the molecule, releasing free bilirubin, which is then reduced to urobilinogen; some of this is excreted in the stools as stercobilinogen. The remainder is absorbed by the terminal ileum, passes to the liver via the enterohepatic circulation, and is re-excreted into bile. Urobilinogen bound to albumin enters the circulation and is excreted in urine via the kidneys. When hepatic excretion of conjugated bilirubin is impaired, a small amount is strongly bound to serum albumin and is not excreted by the kidneys; it accounts for persisting hyperbilirubinaemia after cholestasis has resolved.

Hormone and drug inactivation

The liver catabolizes hormones such as insulin, glucagon, oestrogens, growth hormone, glucocorticoids and parathyroid hormone. It is also the prime target organ for many hormones (e.g. insulin). It is the major site for the metabolism of drugs (see p. 1310) and alcohol (see p. 1258). Fat-soluble drugs are converted to water-soluble substances that facilitate their excretion in the bile or urine. Cholecalciferol is converted to 25-hydroxycholecalciferol.

Immunological function

The liver plays a key role in the innate immune response and acts as a 'sieve' for bacterial and other antigens carried to it by the portal vein from the gastrointestinal tract (see p. 1291).

Hepatocytes are responsible for biosynthesis of 80–90% of innate immune proteins, including complement components and many secreted pattern-recognition receptors (PRRs) expressed by host cells. Kupffer cells, which account for 80–90% of the total population of fixed tissue macrophages, are a critical component of the mononuclear phagocytic system and are central to both the hepatic and the systemic responses to pathogens. Following stimulation by endotoxin, the Kupffer cells release interleukin (IL)-6, IL-8 and TNF-α, and, in combination with liver sinusoidal cells, are responsible for the elimination of molecular wastes from the body.

In addition, liver lymphocytes are rich in innate immune cells, including natural killer and T cell receptor $\gamma\delta$ T cells. Finally, non-parenchymal liver cells express high levels of membrane-bound PRRs, such as Toll-like receptor cells (TLRs). Not only does innate immunity in the liver play a key role in host defence against microbial infection and tumour formation, but it also contributes to the pathogenesis of acute and chronic liver diseases, including alcoholic liver disease (see p. 1303).

Further reading

Dooley JS, Lok ASF, Garcia-Tsao G et al (eds). *Sherlock's Diseases of the Liver and Biliary System*, 13th edn. Hoboken: Wiley–Blackwell; 2018.
Li Y, Jadhav K, Zhang Y. Bile acid receptors in non-alcoholic fatty liver disease. *Biochem Pharmacol* 2013; 86:1517–1524.

INVESTIGATIONS IN THE PATIENT WITH LIVER DISEASE

Investigative tests can be divided into:

- **Blood tests:**
  - Liver 'function' tests: serum albumin and bilirubin; prothrombin time (PT).
  - Liver biochemistry: serum aspartate (AST) and alanine aminotransferases (ALT) – an increase reflects hepatocellular damage; serum alkaline phosphatase (ALP) and gamma-glutamyl transpeptidase (γ-GT) – an increase reflects cholestasis; total protein.
  - Viral markers.
  - Additional blood investigations: haematological, biochemical, immunological, markers of liver fibrosis and genetic analysis.
- *Imaging techniques* – to define gross anatomy.
- *Liver biopsy* – for histology.

Blood tests ordered for 'liver function' are usually processed by an automated multichannel analyser to produce serum levels of bilirubin, aminotransferases, ALP, γ-GT and total proteins. These routine tests are markers of liver damage but not actual tests of 'function' *per se*. Subsequent investigations are often based on these tests.

Blood tests

Useful blood tests for certain liver diseases are shown in **Box 34.3**.

Liver function tests

Serum albumin

This is a marker of synthetic function and is useful for gauging the severity of chronic liver disease: a falling serum albumin is a bad prognostic sign. In acute liver disease, initial albumin levels may be normal. Interpretation of a low albumin can be difficult when other

> **Box 34.3 Useful blood and urine tests for certain liver diseases**
>
> | Test | Disease |
> | --- | --- |
> | Anti-mitochondrial antibody | Primary biliary cholangitis |
> | Anti-nuclear, smooth muscle (actin), liver/kidney microsomal antibody | Autoimmune hepatitis |
> | Raised serum immunoglobulins: | |
> | IgG | Autoimmune hepatitis |
> | IgG4 | Autoimmune hepatitis/ cholangiopathy and pancreatitis |
> | IgM | Primary biliary cholangitis |
> | Viral markers | Hepatitis A, B, C, D, E and others |
> | α-Fetoprotein | Hepatocellular carcinoma |
> | Serum iron, transferrin saturation, serum ferritin | Hereditary haemochromatosis |
> | Serum and urinary copper, serum caeruloplasmin | Wilson's disease |
> | α_1-Antitrypsin | α_1-Antitrypsin deficiency (cirrhosis ± emphysema) |
> | Anti-nuclear cytoplasmic antibodies (ANCA) | Primary sclerosing cholangitis |
> | Markers of liver fibrosis (see p. 1269) | Non-alcoholic fatty liver disease |
> | | Hepatitis C |
> | Genetic analyses | e.g. *HFE* gene (hereditary haemochromatosis), α_1-antitrypsin |

causes of hypoalbuminaemia (e.g. malnutrition, urinary protein loss or sepsis) are present.

Bilirubin

Serum bilirubin is normally almost all unconjugated. In liver disease, increased serum bilirubin is usually accompanied by other abnormalities in liver biochemistry. Differentiation between conjugated or unconjugated bilirubin is necessary only in congenital disorders of bilirubin metabolism (see later) or to exclude haemolysis.

Prothrombin time

Prothrombin time (PT) is also a marker of synthetic function. Because of its short half-life, it is a sensitive indicator of both acute and chronic liver disease. Vitamin K deficiency should be excluded as the cause of a prolonged PT by giving an intravenous bolus (10 mg) of vitamin K. Vitamin K deficiency commonly occurs in biliary obstruction, as the low intestinal concentration of bile salts results in poor absorption of vitamin K.

Prothrombin times vary in different laboratories, depending on the thromboplastin used in the assay. The international normalized ratio (INR) was developed to standardize anticoagulation with coumarin derivatives but is very variable in liver disease and causes large differences when included in prognostic scores for cirrhosis across different centres. A rising INR in patients with liver disease that is not corrected by vitamin K is a poor prognostic sign.

Liver biochemistry

Aminotransferases

These enzymes (often referred to as transaminases) are contained in hepatocytes and leak into the blood with liver cell damage. Two enzymes are measured:

- **Aspartate aminotransferase** (AST) is primarily a mitochondrial enzyme (80%; 20% in cytoplasm) and is also present in heart, muscle, kidney and brain. High levels are seen in hepatic necrosis, myocardial infarction, muscle injury and congestive cardiac failure.
- **Alanine aminotransferase** (ALT) is a cytosol enzyme, more specific to the liver, so that a rise occurs only with liver disease. The ALT:AST ratio is a useful clinical indicator:
- In viral hepatitis, ALT is greater than AST unless cirrhosis is present, in which case AST is greater than ALT.
- In alcoholic liver disease and steatohepatitis, the AST is often greater than the ALT.
- In patients with viral hepatitis, an AST:ALT ratio of more than 1 indicates cirrhosis.
- In patients with liver disease without cirrhosis, in whom AST is greater than ALT, alcohol or obesity is the most likely aetiological agent.

Alkaline phosphatase

Alkaline phosphatase (ALP) is present in hepatic canalicular and sinusoidal membranes, and also in bone, intestine and placenta. If necessary, its origin can be determined by electrophoretic separation of isoenzymes or bone-specific monoclonal antibodies. In clinical practice, if the γ-GT is also abnormal, the ALP is presumed to come from the liver.

Serum ALP is raised in both intrahepatic and extrahepatic cholestatic disease of any cause, due to increased synthesis. In cholestatic jaundice, levels may be 4–6 times the normal limit. Raised levels also occur with hepatic infiltrations (e.g. metastases) and in cirrhosis, frequently in the absence of jaundice.

Gamma-glutamyl transpeptidase

This is a microsomal enzyme present in liver and also in many tissues. Its activity can be induced by numerous drugs such as phenytoin, warfarin and rifampicin, and by alcohol. If the ALP is normal, a raised serum γ-GT can be a useful guide to alcohol intake (see p. 790). However, mild elevations of γ-GT are common, even with minimal alcohol consumption, and it is also raised in fatty liver disease. In the absence of other liver function test abnormalities, a slightly raised γ-GT can safely be ignored. In cholestasis, the γ-GT rises in parallel with the ALP, as it has a similar pathway of excretion.

Total proteins and globulin fraction

The globulin fraction is often raised in autoimmune hepatitis; if it falls, it indicates successful therapy.

Viral markers

Viruses are a major cause of liver disease. Virological studies have a key role in diagnosis; markers are available for most common viruses that cause hepatitis.

Haematological tests

A full blood count may show thrombocytopenia. Thrombocytopenia is a common finding in cirrhosis and is often aggravated by alcohol-induced bone marrow suppression. A low platelet count (below the lower limit of normal – 150×10^9/L) should be regarded as indicative of cirrhosis, unless another cause can be found. In alcohol excess, red blood cells are often macrocytic.

Biochemical tests

- **α₁-Antitrypsin** enzyme deficiency can produce cirrhosis.
- **α-Fetoprotein** is normally produced by the fetal liver. Its reappearance in increasing and high concentrations in adults

indicates hepatocellular carcinoma. Increased concentrations in pregnancy in blood and amniotic fluid suggest fetal neural tube defects. Blood levels are also slightly raised with regenerative liver tissue in patients with hepatitis, chronic liver disease and also teratomas.
- **Urinary copper** is raised, and serum copper and caeruloplasmin are low in Wilson's disease (see p. 1301).

Immunological tests

Serum immunoglobulins

Increased γ-globulins are thought to result from reduced phagocytosis by sinusoidal and Kupffer cells of the gut-absorbed antigens. These antigens then stimulate antibody production in the spleen, lymph nodes and portal tract lymphoid and plasma cell infiltrates. In PBC the predominant raised serum immunoglobulin is IgM, while in autoimmune hepatitis it is IgG. IgG4 is raised in autoimmune pancreatitis/cholangitis (see p. 1330 and **Box 3.10**).

Serum autoantibodies

- **Anti-mitochondrial antibody (AMA)** in serum is found in over 95% of patients with PBC (see p. 1298). Several different AMA subtypes are described, depending on their antigen specificity, and are also found in autoimmune hepatitis and other autoimmune diseases. AMA is demonstrated by an immunofluorescent technique and is neither organ- nor species-specific. The M2 subtype is specific for PBC.
- **Nucleic, smooth muscle (actin), liver/kidney microsomal antibodies** can be found in serum, often in high titre, in patients with autoimmune hepatitis. These serum antibodies are also present in other autoimmune conditions and other liver diseases.
- **Anti-nuclear cytoplasmic antibodies (ANCA)** can be found in the serum of patients with primary sclerosing cholangitis (see p. 1299).

Markers of liver fibrosis

Fibrosis plays a key role in the outcome of many chronic liver diseases, and accurate assessment of fibrosis is critical for the appropriate management of many liver disorders. A variety of systems have been developed to assess the extent of liver fibrosis and these range from algorithms of varying degrees of complexity that use standard haematological and biochemical tests, to novel biomarkers. Simple algorithms include the **APRI** (**a**spartate aminotransferase to **p**latelet **r**atio **i**ndex) score, while more complex commercial tests include the **fibrotest algorithm**. Novel biomarker-based algorithms include those based on measurements of hyaluronic acid, procollagen III amino terminal peptide and tissue inhibitor of metalloproteinase I (TIMP-1), all combined in the **enhanced liver fibrosis (ELF) test**. In general, these markers have been developed for chronic hepatitis C but they are often successfully applied to other liver disorders. The current assays have a high sensitivity/specificity for the detection or absence of cirrhosis but are less effective at detecting intermediate levels of fibrosis. Combining mechanical non-invasive fibrosis tests, such as transient elastography (see p. 1270), with fibrosis markers allows many patients to avoid a liver biopsy to assess fibrosis.

Genetic analysis

These tests are performed routinely for haemochromatosis (*HFE* gene) and for α₁-antitrypsin deficiency. Markers are also available for the most frequent abnormal genes in Wilson's disease (see p. 1301).

Imaging techniques

Ultrasound examination

This non-invasive, safe and relatively cheap technique involves analysis of the reflected ultrasound beam detected by a probe moved across the abdomen. The normal liver appears as a relatively homogeneous structure. The gall bladder, common bile duct, pancreas, portal vein and other structures in the abdomen can be visualized. ***Abdominal ultrasound*** is useful in:

- Detection of extrahepatic obstruction (the bile duct is usually dilated, particularly in advanced disease). Note that opiates may cause biliary dilation without obstruction, and so scans in injecting drug users often show extrahepatic biliary dilation.
- Assessment of a jaundiced patient (to exclude obstruction) (see p. 1273).
- Assessment of hepatomegaly/splenomegaly.
- Detection of gallstones (see **Fig. 35.2**).
- Assessment of focal liver disease – lesions >1 cm.
- Assessment of portal and hepatic vein patency.
- Assessment of the hepatic parenchyma – diffuse fatty infiltration often leads to a 'bright' appearance on ultrasound but experience is required to distinguish this from normal variation.
- Identification of cirrhosis – in advanced cirrhosis, the liver edge is irregular and the spleen is often enlarged. Note that a normal ultrasound does not exclude cirrhosis.
- Assessment of lymph node enlargement.

Other abdominal masses can be delineated and biopsies obtained under ultrasonic guidance.

Colour Doppler ultrasound

This will demonstrate vascularity within a lesion, and the direction of portal and hepatic vein blood flow.

Hepatic stiffness (transient elastography)

Using an ultrasound transducer, a vibration of low frequency and amplitude is passed through the liver, the velocity of which correlates with hepatic stiffness. Stiffness (measured in kPa) increases with worsening liver fibrosis (sensitivity and specificity 80–95%, compared to liver biopsy). Elastography can reliably exclude cirrhosis and, in cirrhosis, increasing liver stiffness is associated with a higher risk of complications. Elastography is less effective for determining lesser degrees of fibrosis but, particularly when combined with non-invasive fibrosis tests (see earlier), it can be used to exclude cirrhosis reliably. It cannot be employed in the presence of ascites and morbid obesity, and is affected by inflammatory tissue and congestion.

Acoustic radiation force impulse is incorporated into standard B mode ultrasonography and has similar physical principles to transient elastography.

Computed tomography examination

Computed tomography (CT), during or immediately after intravenous contrast, shows both arterial and portal venous phases of enhancement, enabling more precise characterization of a lesion and its vascular supply (**Fig. 34.7**). Retrospective analysis of data allows multiple overlapping slices to be obtained with no increase in the radiation dose, providing excellent visualization of the size, shape and density of the liver, pancreas, spleen, lymph nodes and lesions in the porta hepatis. Multiplanar and three-dimensional reconstruction in the arterial phase can create a CT angiogram, often making formal invasive angiography unnecessary. CT also provides guidance for biopsy. It has advantages over ultrasound in detecting calcification and is useful in obese subjects, although

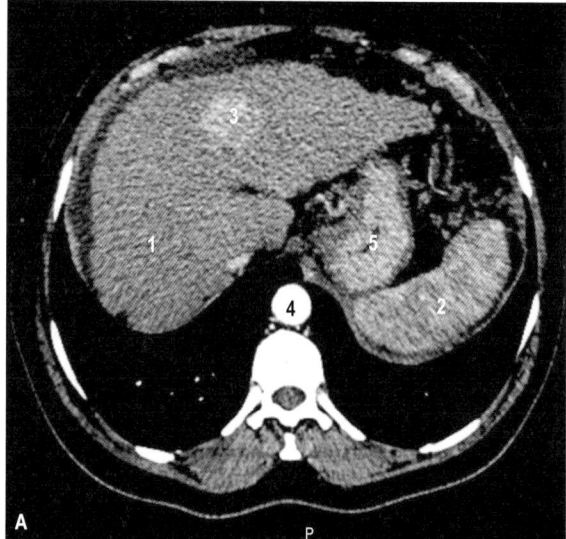

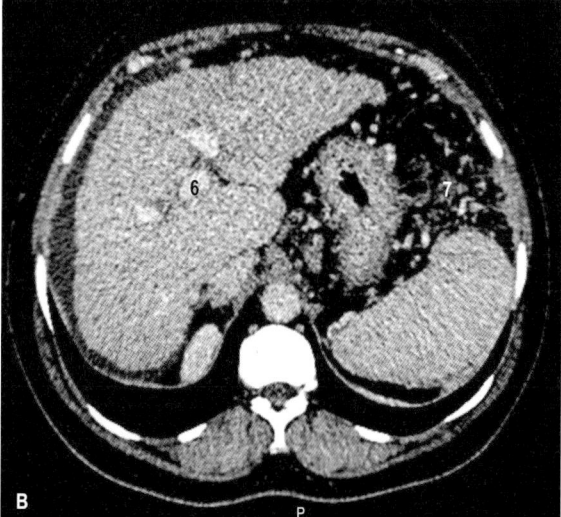

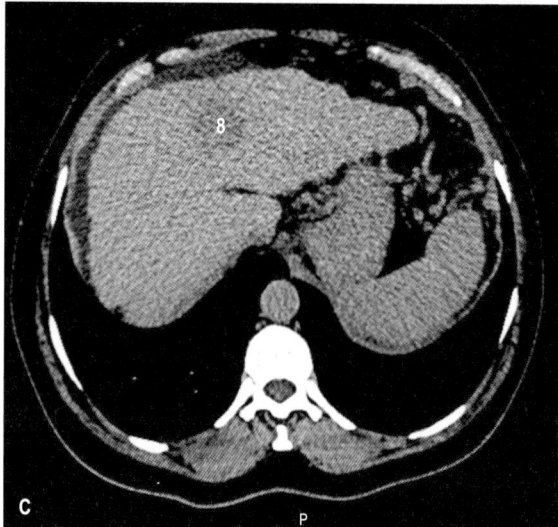

Fig. 34.7 Triple phase liver CT showing a hepatocellular carcinoma. The liver has an irregular contour consistent with cirrhosis and there are splenic and gastric varices. The arterial phase **(A)** demonstrates an enhancing lesion, which is poorly seen on the portal venous phase **(B)** but demonstrates washout on the delayed phase imaging **(C)** consistent with hepatocellular carcinoma. (1) Liver; (2) spleen; (3) lesion; (4) aorta; (5) stomach; (6) portal vein; (7) varices; (8) washout of lesion.

ultrasound is usually the first imaging modality to be used to investigate liver disease.

Magnetic resonance imaging

Magnetic resonance imaging (MRI) produces cross-sectional images in any plane within the body and does not involve radiation. It is the most sensitive investigation for focal liver disease but can also assess fibrosis. Diffuse liver disease alters the T1 and T2 characteristics. Other fat-suppression modes, such as **short T1 inversion recovery (STIR)**, allow good differentiation between haemangiomas and other lesions. Contrast agents such as intravenous gadolinium, which allow further characterization of lesions, are suitable for those with iodine allergy, and provide angiography and venography of the splanchnic circulation. Use of these agents has superseded direct arteriography.

Magnetic resonance cholangiopancreatography

Magnetic resonance cholangiopancreatography (MRCP) involves the manipulation of data acquired by MRI. A heavily T2-weighted sequence enhances visualization of the 'water-filled' bile ducts and pancreatic ducts to produce high-quality images of ductal anatomy. This non-invasive technique is replacing diagnostic (but not therapeutic) endoscopic retrograde cholangiopancreatography (see p. 1325) and is usually the next test to be applied if a biliary abnormality is present on ultrasound examination.

Radionuclide imaging – scintiscanning

In a ^{99m}Tc-IODIDA scan, technetium-labelled iododiethyl IDA is taken up by the hepatocytes and excreted rapidly into the biliary system. Its main uses are in the diagnosis of:

- acute cholecystitis
- jaundice due to either biliary atresia or hepatitis in the neonatal period.

Endoscopy

Upper gastrointestinal endoscopy is used for diagnosis and treatment of varices, detection of portal hypertensive gastropathy, and detection of associated lesions such as peptic ulcers. Colonoscopy may show portal hypertensive colopathy. Capsule endoscopy can identify small intestinal varices.

Endoscopic retrograde cholangiopancreatography

Endoscopic retrograde cholangiopancreatography (ERCP) outlines the biliary and pancreatic ducts (see p. 1325).

Angiography

This is performed by selective catheterization of the coeliac axis and hepatic artery. It outlines the hepatic vasculature and the abnormal vasculature of hepatic tumours, but spiral CT and MRI have replaced diagnostic angiography. The portal vein can be demonstrated with increased definition using subtraction techniques that have replaced splenoportography (by direct splenic puncture).

In **digital vascular imaging** (DVI), contrast given intravenously or intra-arterially can be detected in the portal system using computerized subtraction analysis.

Hepatic venous cannulation allows abnormal hepatic veins to be diagnosed in patients with Budd–Chiari syndrome and is also used to measure portal pressure indirectly. There is a 1:1 relationship of occluded (by balloon) hepatic venous pressure with portal pressure in patients with alcoholic or viral-related cirrhosis. The height of portal pressure has prognostic value for survival in cirrhosis: a difference of the occluded minus the free hepatic venous pressure (hepatic venous

---

> *i* **Box 34.4** Indications for and contraindications to liver biopsy
>
> **Diagnosis**
> - Multiple parenchymal liver diseases
> - Abnormal liver tests of unknown aetiology
> - Fever of unknown origin
> - Focal or diffuse abnormalities on imaging studies (rarely for hepatocellular carcinoma)
> - Unexplained hepatomegaly
> - Drug-related liver disease
> - Post liver transplant
>
> **Prognosis**
> - Staging of known parenchymal liver disease, e.g. hepatitis B/C, non-alcoholic fatty liver disease, primary biliary cholangitis, autoimmune hepatitis, primary sclerosing cholangitis
> - Haemochromatosis and alcohol-induced liver disease
>
> **Management**
> - Development of treatment plans based on histological analysis
>
> **Usual contraindications to percutaneous needle biopsy**
> - Uncooperative patient
> - Prolonged INR (>1.5)
> - Platelets $<60 \times 10^9$/L
> - Ascites
> - Extrahepatic cholestasis
>
> INR, International normalized ratio.

pressure gradient, HVPG) of 20% or more from baseline values, or below 12 mmHg, has been associated with protection from rebleeding and prevention of other complications of cirrhosis.

Liver biopsy

Histological examination of the liver is valuable in the differential diagnosis of diffuse or localized parenchymal disease and its severity. Liver biopsy can be performed on a day-case basis. The indications and contraindications are shown in **Box 34.4**. The mortality rate is less than 0.02% when the technique is performed by experienced operators.

Liver biopsy guided by ultrasound or CT is performed under a local anaesthetic via a percutaneous approach in the right intercostal space. A transjugular approach is used when liver histology is essential for management but coagulation abnormalities or ascites prevent the percutaneous approach.

Most **complications** of liver biopsy occur within 24 hours (usually in the first 2 hours). They are often minor and include abdominal or shoulder pain that settles with analgesics. Minor intraperitoneal bleeding can occur but this settles spontaneously. Rare complications include major intraperitoneal bleeding, haemothorax and pleurisy, biliary peritonitis, haemobilia and transient septicaemia. Haemobilia produces biliary colic, jaundice and melaena within 3 days of the biopsy.

Further reading

Tripodi A, Mannucci PM. The coagulopathy of chronic liver disease. *N Engl J Med* 2011; 365:147–156.

JAUNDICE

Jaundice (icterus) is detectable clinically when the serum bilirubin is over 50 μmol/L (3 mg/dL). It may be divided into:

- **haemolytic jaundice** – increased bilirubin load for the liver cells
- **congenital hyperbilirubinaemias** – defects in conjugation
- **cholestatic jaundice** – including hepatocellular (parenchymal) liver disease and large duct obstruction.

Haemolytic jaundice

The increased breakdown of red cells (see **Fig. 16.5**) leads to an increase in production of bilirubin. The resulting jaundice is usually mild (serum bilirubin of 68–102 µmol/L, or 4–6 mg/dL), as normal liver function can easily manage the increased bilirubin. Unconjugated bilirubin is not water-soluble and therefore does not pass into urine: hence 'acholuric jaundice'. Urinary urobilinogen is increased.

The causes are those of haemolytic anaemia (p. 338), and clinical features of anaemia, jaundice, splenomegaly, gallstones and leg ulcers may be seen.

Investigations show haemolysis and elevated unconjugated bilirubin, but normal serum ALP, transferases and albumin. Serum haptoglobulins are low.

Congenital hyperbilirubinaemias (non-haemolytic)
Unconjugated types
Gilbert's syndrome

This is the most common familial unconjugated hyperbilirubinaemia and affects 2–7% of the population. It is asymptomatic and usually detected incidentally with a raised bilirubin (17–102 µmol/L, or 1–6 mg/dL). All other liver biochemistry is normal and there are no signs of liver disease. There is a family history of jaundice in 5–15% of patients. Most patients have reduced levels of UDP-glucuronosyl transferase (UGT-1) activity; this is the enzyme that conjugates bilirubin with glucuronic acid.

Mutations occur in the gene (UGT1A1 promoter region) encoding this enzyme, with an expanded nucleotide repeat consisting of two extra bases in the upstream 5′ promoter element. This abnormality appears to be required for the syndrome to occur but is not in itself sufficient for clinical manifestation (phenotypic expression).

Establishing the diagnosis is necessary to provide reassurance and prevent unnecessary investigations. The raised unconjugated bilirubin is diagnostic and rises on fasting and during mild illness. The reticulocyte count is normal, excluding haemolysis, and no treatment is necessary.

Crigler–Najjar syndrome

This is very rare. Only patients with type II (autosomal dominant) disease, with a decrease in, rather than absence (type I – autosomal recessive) of, UGT survive into adult life. Liver histology is normal. Transplantation is the only effective treatment.

Conjugated types
Dubin–Johnson and Rotor's syndromes

Dubin–Johnson and Rotor's syndromes (autosomal recessive) are due to defects in hepatic bilirubin handling. The prognosis is good in both. In the Dubin–Johnson syndrome the liver is black owing to melanin deposition.

Benign recurrent intrahepatic cholestasis

This is rare and presents in early adulthood. Recurrent attacks of acute cholestasis occur without progression to chronic liver disease. Jaundice, severe pruritus, steatorrhoea and weight loss develop. Serum γ-GT is normal. Benign recurrent intrahepatic cholestasis may be associated with intrahepatic cholestasis of pregnancy (see p. 1455). Genetic testing is available and there are two forms: BRIC1 is caused by mutations in the *ATP8B1* gene and BRIC2 by mutations in the *ABCB11* gene. Both are autosomal recessive. Treatment includes medications to manage symptoms and occasionally specialized therapies, such as nasobiliary drainage, to shorten episodes.

Progressive familial intrahepatic cholestasis syndromes

Progressive familial intrahepatic cholestasis (PFIC) syndromes are a heterogeneous group of autosomal recessive conditions defined by defective secretion of bile acids (see **Figs 34.5** and **35.1**).
- In **type 1** (PFIC1), with cholestasis in the first weeks of life, the γ-GT is normal.
- In **type 2** (PFIC2), there is frequently a non-specific giant cell hepatitis that progresses to cholestasis; again, γ-GT is normal.
- In **type 3** (PFIC3), deficient canalicular phosphatidylcholine transport and accumulation of toxic bile acids cause liver damage, which can lead to cirrhosis.
  Liver transplantation is the only cure for these syndromes.

Cholestatic jaundice (acquired)

This condition can be divided into extrahepatic and intrahepatic cholestasis. The causes are shown in **Fig. 34.8**.

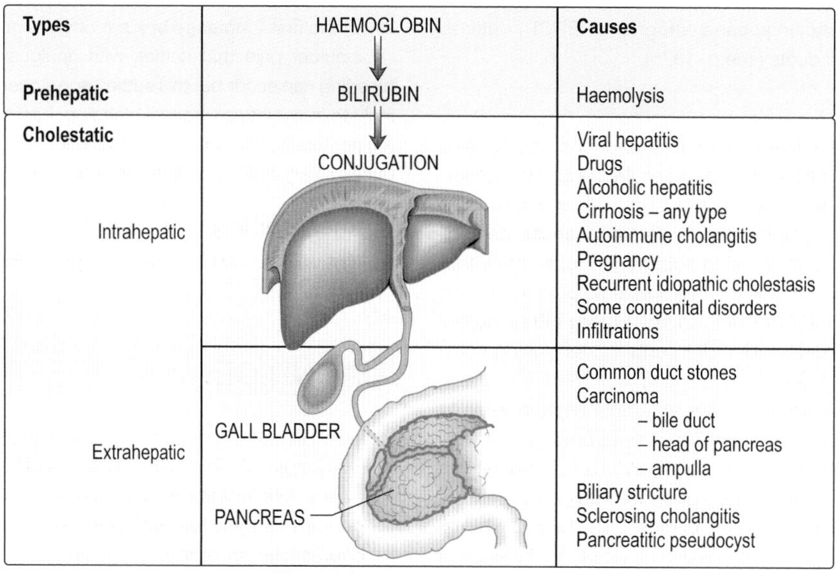

Types	HAEMOGLOBIN	Causes
Prehepatic	BILIRUBIN	Haemolysis
Cholestatic	CONJUGATION	Viral hepatitis Drugs Alcoholic hepatitis Cirrhosis – any type Autoimmune cholangitis Pregnancy Recurrent idiopathic cholestasis Some congenital disorders Infiltrations
Intrahepatic		

Extrahepatic	GALL BLADDER
	PANCREAS
		Common duct stones
		Carcinoma
		   – bile duct
		   – head of pancreas
		   – ampulla
		Biliary stricture
		Sclerosing cholangitis
		Pancreatitic pseudocyst

Fig. 34.8 Causes of jaundice.

- **Extrahepatic cholestasis** is due to large duct obstruction of bile flow at any point in the biliary tract distal to the bile canaliculi.
- **Intrahepatic cholestasis** occurs because of failure of bile secretion, which may be caused by intrinsic defects in bile secretion or inflammation in the intrahepatic ducts.

Clinically, in both types, there is jaundice with pale stools and dark urine, and the serum bilirubin is conjugated. However, intrahepatic and extrahepatic cholestatic jaundice must be differentiated, as their clinical management is entirely different.

Differential diagnosis of jaundice

Jaundice (see p. 1263) may occur in previously healthy people who have an acute hepatic illness or may develop in patients with cirrhosis who have 'decompensated'. The management of decompensated cirrhosis is described on page 1290 but all patients with jaundice should be questioned closely about risk factors for chronic liver disease to determine whether this is a true acute presentation rather than an 'acute on chronic' illness. The history often gives a clue to the diagnosis. Certain causes of jaundice are more likely in particular categories of people. For example, a young person is more likely to have infectious hepatitis, so questions should be asked about drug and alcohol misuse, and sexual behaviour. An elderly person with gross weight loss is more likely to have a carcinoma. All patients may complain of malaise. Abdominal pain occurs in patients with biliary obstruction by gallstones, and sometimes with an enlarged liver there is pain resulting from distension of the capsule.

Questions should be appropriate to the particular situation, and the following aspects of the history should be covered:

- **Country of origin.** The incidence of hepatitis B virus (HBV) and hepatitis C virus (HCV) infection is increased in many parts of the world (see pp. 1277 and 1282).
- **Duration of illness.** A history of jaundice with prolonged weight loss in an older patient suggests malignancy. A short history, particularly with a prodromal illness of malaise, suggests an infectious hepatitis.
- **Recent outbreak of jaundice.** An outbreak in the community suggests hepatitis A virus (HAV).
- **Intravenous drug use, or recent injections or tattoos.** These all increase the chance of HBV and HCV infection.
- **Men having sex with men.** There is an increased chance of HBV and HCV infection.
- **Female sex workers.** There is an increased chance of HBV infection.
- **Medical treatment in the developing world.** There is an increased risk of HBV and HCV due to poorly sterilized equipment or administration of unscreened blood or blood products.
- **Alcohol consumption.** A history of drinking habits should be taken, although many patients often understate their consumption.
- **Drugs (particularly those taken in the previous 2–3 months).** Many drugs, including over-the-counter and herbal preparations, cause jaundice (see p. 1310).
- **Travel.** Certain areas have a high risk of HAV infection, as well as hepatitis E virus (HEV), but HAV is common in the UK and HEV is common in travellers to the Indian subcontinent.
- **Family history.** Patients with, for example, Gilbert's disease may have family members who experience recurrent jaundice.
- **Recent surgery.** Surgery on the biliary tract or for carcinoma is relevant.
- **Environment.** People engaged in recreational activities in rural areas, as well as farm and sewage workers, are at risk for leptospirosis, hepatitis E and exposure to chemicals.
- **Fevers or rigors.** These are suggestive of cholangitis or possibly a liver abscess.

> **?** **Box 34.5** Causes of hepatomegaly

Apparent
- Low-lying diaphragm
- Riedel's lobe
- Cirrhosis (early)

Inflammation
- Hepatitis
- Schistosomiasis
- Abscesses (pyogenic or amoebic)

Cysts
- Hydatid
- Polycystic

Metabolic
- Fatty liver
- Amyloid deposition
- Glycogen storage disease

Haematological
- Leukaemias
- Lymphoma
- Myeloproliferative disorders
- Thalassaemia

Tumours
- Primary and secondary carcinoma

Venous congestion
- Heart failure
- Constrictive pericarditis
- Hepatic vein occlusion

Biliary obstruction
- (Particularly extrahepatic)

Clinical features

The signs of acute and chronic liver disease should be looked for (see p. 1263). Certain additional signs may be helpful:

- **Hepatomegaly.** A smooth, tender liver is seen in hepatitis and in extrahepatic obstruction, but a knobbly, irregular liver suggests metastases or cirrhosis. Causes of hepatomegaly are shown in **Box 34.5.**
- **Splenomegaly.** This indicates portal hypertension when signs of chronic liver disease are present. The spleen can also be 'tipped' occasionally in viral hepatitis. In alcoholic cirrhosis, in particular, the spleen may not be grossly enlarged and may not be palpable.
- **Ascites.** This is found in cirrhosis but can also be due to other causes (see **Box 34.21**).
- **Palpable gall bladder.** This occurs with a carcinoma of the pancreas obstructing the bile duct.
- **Generalized lymphadenopathy.** This suggests a lymphoma.
- **Cold sores** are often seen with a herpes simplex virus hepatitis.

Investigations

Jaundice is not itself a diagnosis and the cause should always be sought. The two most useful tests are the **viral markers** (for HAV, HBV and HCV), and an ultrasound examination. Liver biochemistry confirms the jaundice and may help in the diagnosis.

An **ultrasound examination** should always be performed to exclude an extrahepatic obstruction and to diagnose any features compatible with chronic liver disease. Ultrasound will demonstrate:

- the size of the bile ducts, which are dilated in biliary obstruction (**Fig. 34.9**)
- the level of the obstruction
- the cause of the obstruction in virtually all patients with tumours and in 75% of patients with gallstones.

The pathological diagnosis of any mass lesion can be made by fine-needle aspiration cytology (sensitivity approximately 60%) or by needle biopsy (sensitivity approximately 90%).

A flow diagram for the general investigation of the jaundiced patient is shown in **Fig. 34.10**.

Liver biochemistry

In hepatitis, serum AST and ALT tend to be high early in the disease, with only a small rise in serum ALP. Conversely, in extrahepatic obstruction, the ALP is high, with a smaller rise in aminotransferases. However, these findings alone cannot be relied on to make a diagnosis in an individual case. The PT is often prolonged in long-standing liver disease and the serum albumin is low.

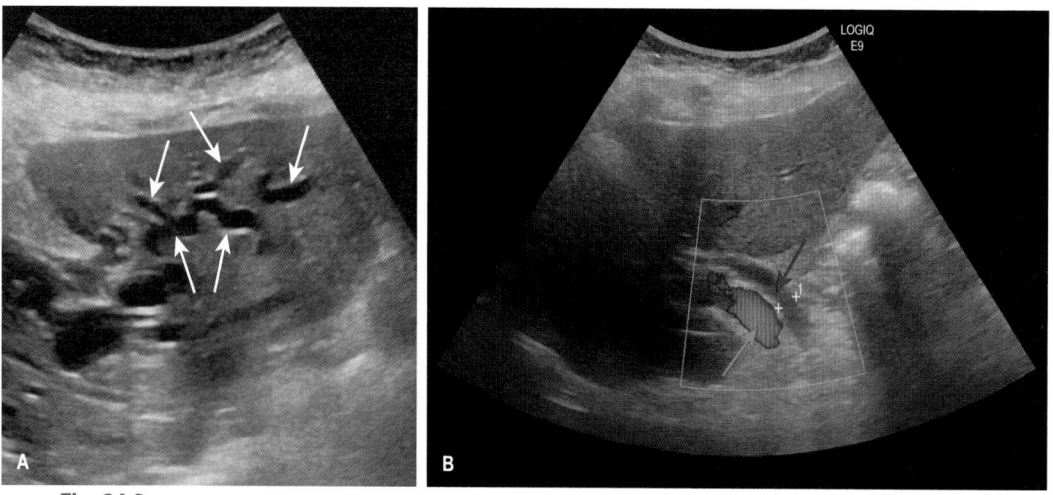

Fig. 34.9 Liver ultrasound. (A) Markedly dilated intrahepatic ducts (arrowed). **(B)** A dilated common bile duct (red arrow). A duct with a diameter of 6 mm or less is normal; however, it can be of larger calibre and still not represent pathology in some circumstances, such as in elderly patients and after cholecystectomy. Several factors must therefore be considered when deciding what is normal for a patient. Normal colour flow is demonstrated in the portal vein (green arrow).

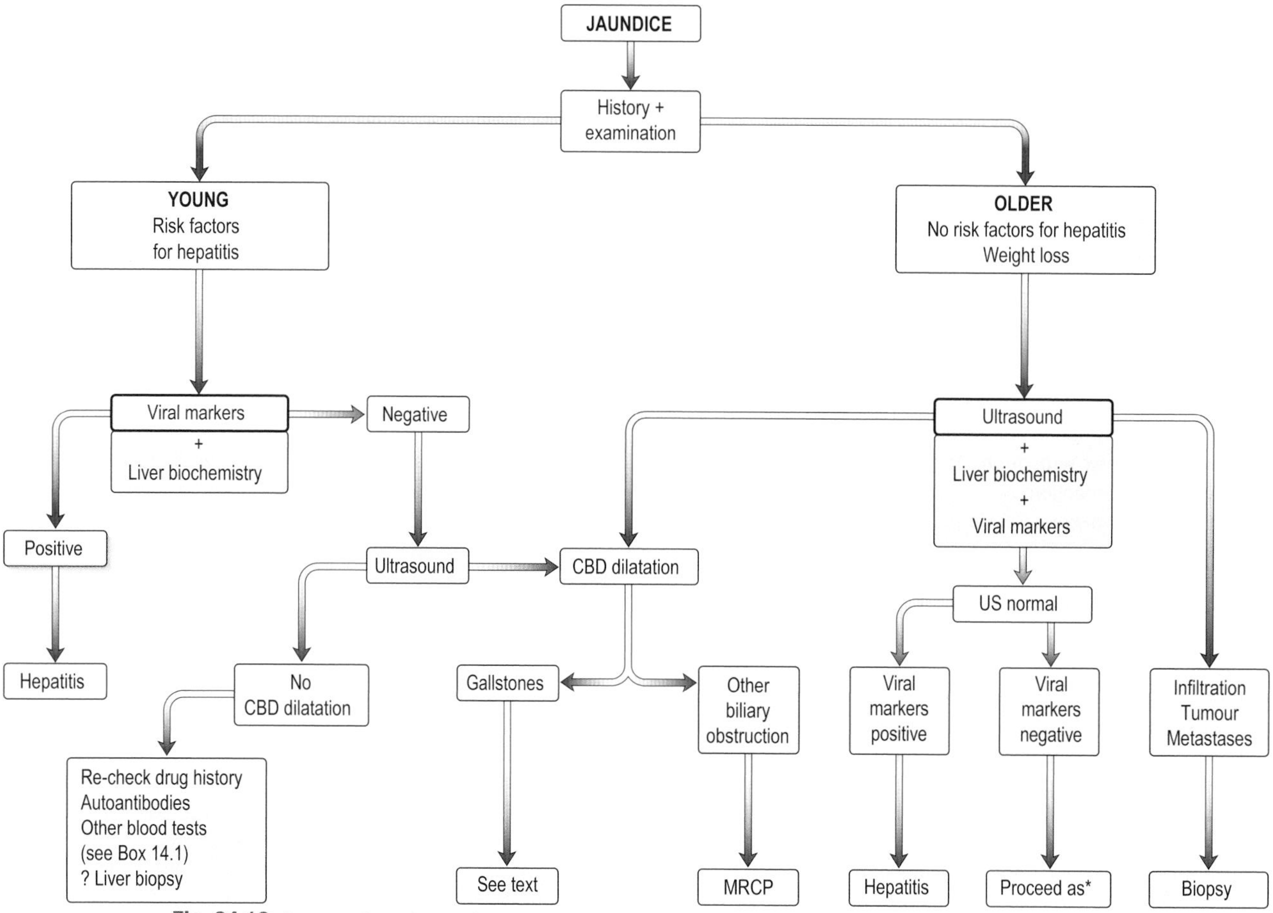

Fig. 34.10 Approach to the patient with jaundice. CBD, common bile duct; MRCP, magnetic resonance cholangiopancreatography; US, ultrasound. * Proceed as in bottom left box (Re-check drug history...)

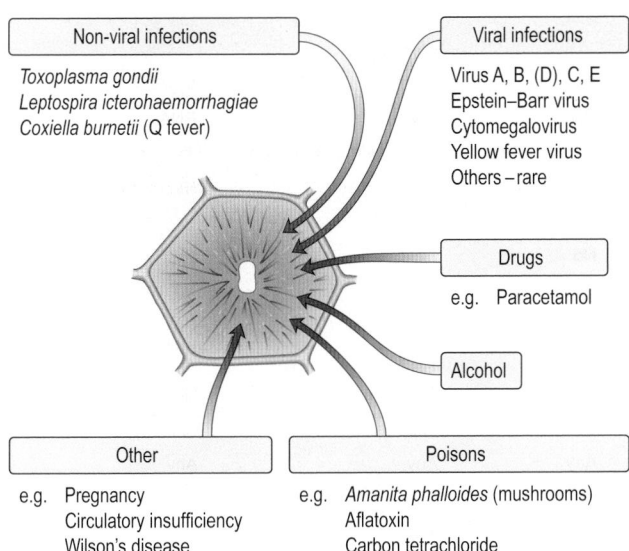

Non-viral infections

Toxoplasma gondii
Leptospira icterohaemorrhagiae
Coxiella burnetii (Q fever)

Viral infections

Virus A, B, (D), C, E
Epstein–Barr virus
Cytomegalovirus
Yellow fever virus
Others – rare

Drugs

e.g. Paracetamol

Alcohol

Other

e.g. Pregnancy
Circulatory insufficiency
Wilson's disease

Poisons

e.g. *Amanita phalloides* (mushrooms)
Aflatoxin
Carbon tetrachloride

Fig. 34.11 Some causes of acute parenchymal damage.

Haematological tests

In haemolytic jaundice the bilirubin is raised and the other liver biochemistry is normal. A raised white cell count may indicate infection (e.g. cholangitis). A leucopenia often occurs in viral hepatitis, while abnormal mononuclear cells suggest infectious mononucleosis (Epstein–Barr virus) and a Monospot test should be performed.

Other blood tests

These include tests to confirm the presence of specific causes of acute or chronic liver disease, e.g. AMA for PBC. HIV status should be established.

HEPATITIS

- *Acute parenchymal liver damage* can be caused by many agents (**Fig. 34.11**).
- *Chronic hepatitis* is defined as any hepatitis lasting for 6 months or longer and is classified according to the aetiology (**Box 34.6**). Chronic viral hepatitis is the principal cause of chronic liver disease, cirrhosis and hepatocellular carcinoma worldwide.

Acute hepatitis
Pathology

Although some histological features are suggestive of the aetiological factor, most changes are non-specific. Hepatocytes show degenerative changes (swelling, cytoplasmic granularity, vacuolation) and undergo necrosis (becoming shrunken, containing eosinophilic Councilman bodies). The distribution of these changes may vary with aetiology but necrosis is usually maximal in zone 3. The extent of the damage is very variable between individuals, even when they are affected by the same agent; at one end of the spectrum, single and small groups of hepatocytes die (spotty or focal necrosis), while at the other end, there is multiacinar necrosis involving a substantial part of the liver (massive hepatic necrosis) and resulting in acute hepatic failure. Between these extremes, there is limited confluent necrosis with collapse of the reticulin framework, leading to linking (bridging) between the central veins, between the central veins and portal tracts, and between the portal

Box 34.6 Causes of chronic hepatitis

- Metabolic:
  - Non-alcoholic fatty liver disease
- Alcohol-induced
- Viral:
  - Hepatitis B ± hepatitis D
  - Hepatitis C
  - Hepatitis E (immunosuppressed)
- Drugs:
  - (e.g. Methyldopa, isoniazid, ketoconazole, nitrofurantoin)
- Autoimmune
- Hereditary:
  - Wilson's disease, haemochromatosis.
  Unusual causes include infections (syphilis, tuberculosis, various tropical infections), infiltrative diseases, including amyloidosis and lymphoma, and ingestion of toxins.

tracts. The extent of the inflammatory infiltrate is also variable but portal tracts and lobules are infiltrated mainly by lymphocytes. Other variable features include cholestasis in zone 3 and fatty change, the latter being prominent in hepatitis due to alcohol or certain drugs.

Chronic hepatitis
Pathology

The pathological features are often diagnostic. Chronic inflammatory cell infiltrates, comprising lymphocytes, plasma cells and sometimes lymphoid follicles, are usually present in the portal tracts. The amount of inflammation varies from mild to severe. In addition, there may be:

- loss of definition of the portal/periportal limiting plate – interface hepatitis (damage is due to apoptosis rather than necrosis)
- lobular change, focal lytic necrosis, apoptosis and focal inflammation
- confluent necrosis
- fibrosis, which may be mild, bridging (across portal tracts) or severe cirrhosis.

The overall severity of the hepatitis is judged by the degree of hepatitis and inflammation (grading), and the severity of fibrosis or cirrhosis (staging). In chronic viral hepatitis there are various scoring systems. For example, the **Knodell scoring system** (histological activity index) uses the sum of four factors (periportal or bridging necrosis, intralobular degeneration and focal necrosis, portal inflammation and fibrosis). The **Ishak score** stages fibrosis from 0 (none) to 6 (cirrhosis). The **METAVIR system** has four stages. Scoring systems are used for drug trials and for assessing progression of disease, but are not quantitative measures of fibrosis and different systems may be used for different diseases (for example, the **Brunt scoring system** is usually applied to NAFLD, and the METAVIR system is reserved for hepatitis C).

Viral hepatitis

The differing features of the common forms of viral hepatitis are summarized in **Box 34.7**. Two different patterns are recognized: acute hepatitis with rapid onset of infection and, usually, rapid resolution; and chronic viral hepatitis, which is asymptomatic and often detected on routine blood tests or during screening for infection. Hepatitis A always and hepatitis E usually cause acute infections, while hepatitis B, C and D may cause acute or chronic disease.

	A	**B**	**C**	**D**	**E**
Virus	RNA	DNA	RNA	RNA	RNA
	27 nm	42 nm	Approx. 50 nm	36 nm (with HBsAg coat)	27–35 nm
	Picornaviridae	*Hepadnaviridae*	*Flaviviridae*	*Deltaviridae*	*Hepeviridae*
Spread					
Faeco-oral	Yes	No	No	No	Yes
Blood/blood products	Rare	Yes	Yes	Yes	No
Vertical	No	Yes	Rare	Occasional	No
Saliva	Yes	Yes	Yes	? No	?
Sexual	Rare	Yes	Yes (rare)	Rare	No
Incubation	Short (2–3 weeks)	Long (1–5 months)	Long	Intermediate	Short
Age	Young	Any	Any	Any	Any
Carrier state	No	Yes	Yes	?	No
Chronic liver disease	No	Yes	Yes	Yes	No[a]
Liver cancer	No	Yes	Yes	Yes	No
Mortality (acute)	<0.5%	<1%	<1%	<1%	1–2% (pregnant women 10–20%)
Immunization					
Passive	Normal immunoglobulin serum i.m. (0.04–0.06 mL/kg)	Hepatitis B immunoglobulin (HBIg)	No	No	No
Active	Vaccine	Vaccine	No	HBV vaccine to prevent co-infection	Vaccine

[a]Chronic hepatitis in immunosuppressed patients. HBsAg, hepatitis B surface antigen.

Hepatitis A

Epidemiology

Hepatitis A is common worldwide, often occurring in epidemics. The disease is usually seen in the autumn and affects children and young adults. Spread of infection is mainly by the faeco-oral route and arises from ingestion of contaminated food or water (e.g. shellfish). Overcrowding and poor sanitation facilitate spread, and outbreaks of infection have occurred in men who have sex in men. There is no carrier state. In the UK it is a notifiable disease.

Hepatitis A virus

Hepatitis A virus (HAV) is a picornavirus (**Fig. 34.12**). It has a single serotype, as only one epitope is immunodominant. It replicates in the liver, is excreted in bile, and then excreted in the faeces for about 2 weeks before the onset of clinical illness and for up to 7 days after. The disease is maximally infectious just before the onset of jaundice. HAV particles can be demonstrated in the faeces by electron microscopy.

Clinical features

The viraemia causes the patient to feel unwell, with non-specific symptoms that include nausea and anorexia. Many recover at this stage and remain anicteric. An anicteric infection is common in children and confers lifetime immunity. In the developing world, improvements in hygiene have reduced early infection and, paradoxically, led to an increase in symptomatic infection in exposed adults.

After 1 or 2 weeks, some patients become jaundiced and symptoms often improve. Persistence of nausea, vomiting or any mental confusion warrants assessment in hospital. As the jaundice deepens, the urine becomes dark and the stools are pale. The liver is moderately enlarged and the spleen may be palpable. Occasionally, tender lymphadenopathy is seen, with a transient rash in some cases. Thereafter, the jaundice lessens and, in the

A HAV virion

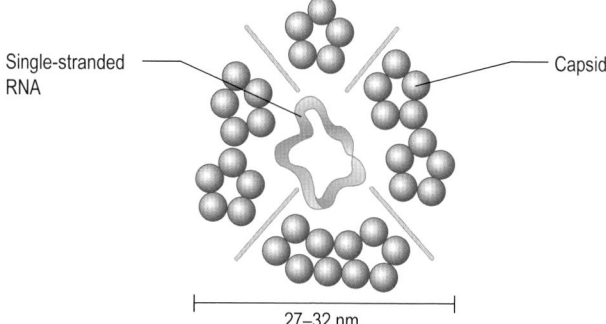

Single-stranded RNA — Capsid

27–32 nm

B HAV genome

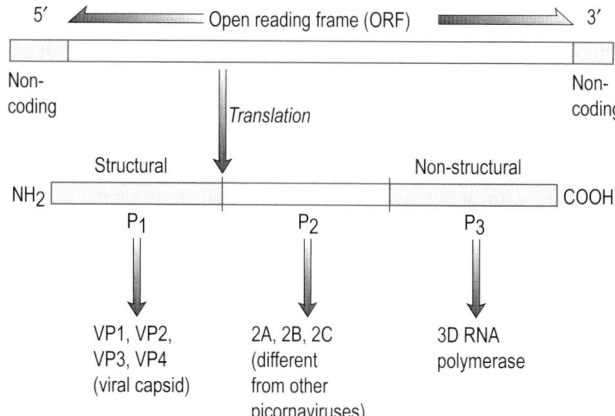

Fig. 34.12 Hepatitis A. (A) The hepatitis A (HAV) virion consists of four polypeptides (VP1–VP4), which form a tight protein shell, or capsid, containing the RNA. The major antigenic component is associated with VP1. **(B)** Arrangement of the HAV genome.

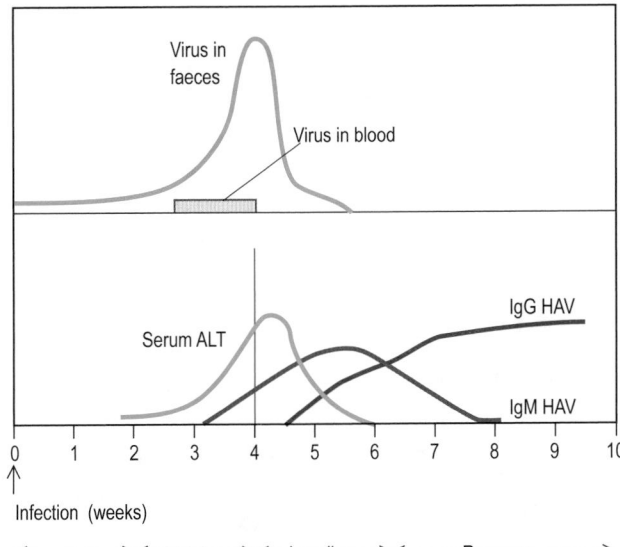

Fig. 34.13 Hepatitis A virus (HAV): sequence of events after exposure. ALT, alanine aminotransferase; Ig, immunoglobulin.

majority of cases, the illness is over within 3–6 weeks. Extrahepatic complications are rare but include arthritis, vasculitis, myocarditis and acute kidney injury. A biphasic illness occasionally occurs, with the return of jaundice and, classically, a more severe 'second phase', which is cholestatic (cholestatic viral hepatitis) with an increase in the ALP rather than the aminotransferases; thus, it runs a prolonged course of 7–20 weeks. Rarely, the disease may be very severe with acute hepatitis, liver coma and death; this is more common in the elderly. The typical sequence of events after HAV exposure is shown in **Fig. 34.13**.

Investigations

Liver biochemistry

- **Prodromal stage**: The serum bilirubin is usually normal. A raised serum AST or ALT, which can sometimes be over many thousands, precedes the jaundice.
- **Icteric stage**: The serum bilirubin reflects the level of jaundice. Serum AST reaches a maximum 1–2 days after the appearance of jaundice, and may rise above 500 IU/L. Serum ALP is usually less than 300 IU/L.

After the jaundice has subsided, the aminotransferases may remain elevated for some weeks and occasionally for up to 6 months.

Haematological tests

There is leucopenia with a relative lymphocytosis. Very rarely, there is a Coombs'-positive haemolytic anaemia or an associated aplastic anaemia. The PT is prolonged in severe cases. The erythrocyte sedimentation rate (ESR) is raised.

Viral markers: antibodies to HAV

IgG antibodies are common in the general population over the age of 50 years but an anti-HAV IgM means an acute infection. In areas of high prevalence, most children have antibodies by the age of 3 years following asymptomatic infection.

Other tests

Further tests are not necessary in the presence of an IgM antibody but liver biochemistry must be followed to establish a return to normal levels.

Differential diagnosis

Differentiation must be made from all other causes of jaundice, but in particular from other types of viral and drug-induced hepatitis.

Prognosis

The prognosis is excellent, with most patients making a complete recovery. The mortality in young adults is 0.1% but increases with age. Death is due to acute hepatic necrosis.

There is no reason to stop alcohol consumption, other than for the few weeks when the patient is ill. Patients may complain of debility for several months following resolution of the symptoms and biochemical parameters. This is known as the post-hepatitis syndrome and treatment is by reassurance. HAV hepatitis never progresses to chronic liver disease.

Management

There is no specific treatment, and rest and dietary measures are unhelpful. Corticosteroids have no benefit. Admission to hospital is not usually necessary.

Prevention

Control of hepatitis depends on good hygiene. The virus is resistant to chlorination but is killed by boiling water for 10 minutes.

Active immunization

A formaldehyde-inactivated HAV vaccine is given to people travelling frequently to endemic areas, patients with chronic liver disease, those with haemophilia, and workers in frequent contact with hepatitis cases (e.g. in residential institutions for patients with learning difficulties). Community outbreaks can be interrupted by vaccination. A single dose produces antibodies that persist for at least 1 year, with immunity lasting beyond 10 years. This obviates the need for a booster injection in healthy individuals.

Passive immunization

Normal human immunoglobulin (0.02 mL/kg i.m.) is used if exposure to HAV is for less than 2 weeks. HAV vaccine should also be given.

Hepatitis B

Epidemiology

The hepatitis B virus (HBV) is present worldwide and there are an estimated 220 million carriers. The UK and the USA have a low carrier rate (0.5–2%) but this rises to 10–20% in parts of Africa and the Middle and Far East.

Vertical transmission from mother to child, usually during parturition or soon after birth, and rarely *in utero*, is the usual means of transmission worldwide, although in Africa transmission from other infected children is common during the early childhood years. HBV is not transmitted by breast-feeding.

Horizontal transmission occurs, particularly in children, through minor abrasions or close contact with other children, and HBV can survive on household articles, such as toys or toothbrushes, for prolonged periods. Childhood chronic HBV is associated with very high levels of viral replication (up to 10^{10} IU/mL), ensuring that high levels of virus are present in minute amounts of blood and thus facilitating viral spread.

HBV spread also occurs by the intravenous route (e.g. by transfusion of infected blood or blood products, or by contaminated needles employed by drug users, tattooists or acupuncturists) or by close personal contact, such as during sexual intercourse, particularly in men who have sex with men. The virus can be found in semen and saliva.

Hepatitis B virus

The complete infective virion or Dane particle is a 42 nm particle comprised of an inner core or nucleocapsid (27 nm), surrounded by an outer envelope of surface protein (hepatitis B surface antigen, HBsAg). This surface coat is produced in excess by the infected hepatocytes and can exist separately from the whole virion in serum and body fluid as 22 nm particles or tubules.

The HBV genome is variable, and genetic sequencing can be used to define the different HBV genotypes, A–H. There is a strong correlation between genotypes and geographical areas. **Genotype A** is found in north-west Europe, North America and Central Africa; **B** in South-east Asia (including China, Taiwan and Japan); **C** in South-east Asia; **D** in southern Europe, India and the Middle East; **E** in West Africa; **F** in South and Central America, in American Indians and in Polynesia; **G** in France and the USA; and **H** in Central and South America. These genotypes may influence the chance of responding to interferon treatment (A more than B; C more than D) but all genotypes respond equally well to nucleoside analogues.

The core or nucleocapsid is formed of core protein (HBcAg), containing incompletely double-stranded circular DNA and DNA polymerase/reverse transcriptase. One strand is almost a complete circle and contains overlapping genes that encode both structural proteins (pre-S, surface (S), core (C)) and replicative proteins (polymerase (P) and X). The other strand is variable in length. DR1 and DR2 are direct repeats necessary for HBV synthesis during viral replication (**Fig. 34.14**).

HBeAg is a protein formed via specific self-cleavage of the precore/core gene product, which is secreted separately by the cell.

Hepatitis B mutants

Mutations occur in the various reading frames of the HBV genome (**Fig. 34.14**). These mutants can emerge in patients with chronic HBV infection (escape mutants) or can be acquired by infection.

HBsAg mutants are produced by alterations in the 'a' antigenic determinants of the HbsAg proteins, usually with a substitution of glycine for arginine at position 145. This results in changes in the antibody-binding domain and may render the vaccine ineffective. In patients with some HBV genotypes (particularly genotype D), a mutation in the **pre-core region**, when a guanosine (G) to adenosine (A) change creates a stop codon (TAG), prevents the production of HBeAg (the secreted form of HBcAG) but the synthesis of HBcAg is unaffected. This mutation may be associated with HBeAg-negative disease but other mutations in the core promoter region of the virus also give rise to HBeAg-negative disease. To detect infectivity in HBeAg-negative disease, HBV DNA must always be measured, as no HBeAg will be present.

DNA polymerase mutants occur, particularly following treatment with the first generation of directly acting antiviral drugs, such as lamivudine.

Pathogenesis

Pre-S$_1$ and pre-S$_2$ regions are involved in attachment to the hepatocyte receptor – the sodium taurocholate co-transporting polypeptide (NTCP). After penetration into the cell the virus loses its coat and the virus core is transported to the nucleus without processing. The transcription of HBV into messenger RNA takes place when the HBV DNA is converted into a closed circular form (cccDNA), which acts as a template for RNA transcription. The transcribed RNA is then reverse-transcribed by the viral polymerase protein to HBV DNA, which is circularized and packaged. Hence HBV, like HIV, replicates via reverse transcription that introduces errors into the replication cycle (reverse transcriptase enzymes are error-prone) but allows production of viral DNA that can integrate into the host

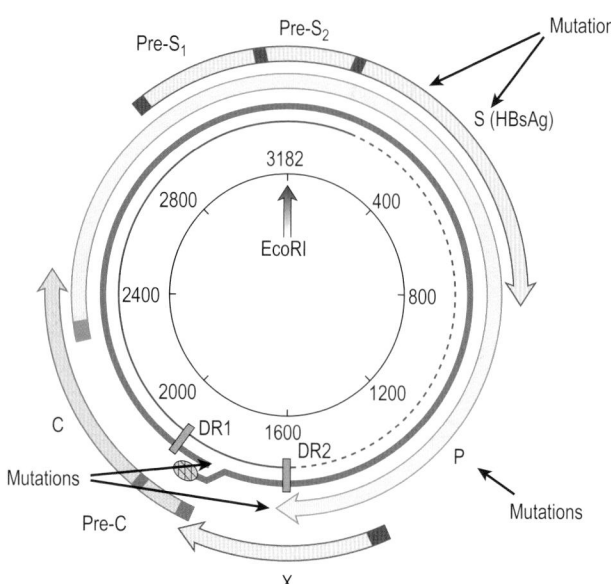

Fig. 34.14 Hepatitis B virus (HBV) genome. The viral DNA is partially double-stranded (red incomplete circle and blue circle). The long strand (blue) encodes seven proteins from four overlapping reading frames (S, surface (Pre-S$_1$, Pre-S$_2$, S); c, core (Pre-C, C); P, polymerase (P); and X gene (X)). EcoRI restriction enzyme-binding site is included as a reference point. DR, direct repeat; HBsAg, hepatitis B surface antigen.

ℹ️ Box 34.8 Hepatitis B virus (HBV) proteins

HBV protein	Significance
Core	Protein of core particle; forms nucleocapsids
Pre-core (HBeAg)	Pre-core/core cleaves to HBeAg; good marker of active replication and role in inducing immunotolerance
Surface (HBsAg)	Envelope protein of HBV; basis of current vaccine
Pre-S$_2$ Pre-S$_1$	HBV binding and entry into hepatocytes
Polymerase	Viral replication
X protein	Transcriptional and transactivator activity

genome. Unsurprisingly, some drugs (e.g. lamivudine and tenofovir) that are active against the HIV polymerase also have effects on the HBV polymerase.

Translation into HBV proteins (**Box 34.8**), as well as replication of the genome, takes place in the endoplasmic reticulum; the proteins are then packaged together and exported from the cell. There is excess production of non-infective HBsAg particles, which are extruded into the circulation.

The HBV is not usually directly cytopathic (although high replication levels in immunosuppressed individuals can lead to direct toxicity) and liver damage is produced by the host immune response.

HBV-specific cytotoxic CD8 T cells recognize the viral antigen via human leucocyte antigen (HLA) class I molecules on the infected hepatocytes. However, suppressor or regulatory T cells inhibit these cytotoxic cells, leading to viral persistence and chronic HBV infection. Th1 responses (IL-2, interferon-gamma) are thought to be associated with viral clearance, and Th2 (IL-4, 5, 6, 10, 13) responses with the development of chronic infection and disease severity. Viral persistence in patients with a very poor cell-mediated

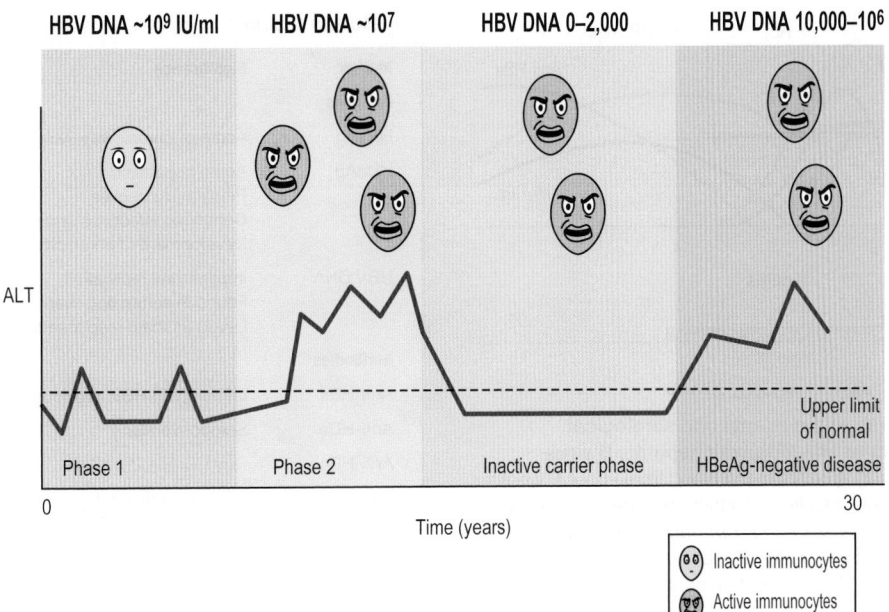

Fig. 34.15 Natural history of childhood-acquired hepatitis B virus (HBV). Phase 1 HBeAg-positive chronic HBV infection: early disease is characterized by high-level viraemia with HBeAg (the secreted form of HBcAg) and a minimal immune response, not leading to any significant liver damage. **Phase 2** HBeAg-positive chronic HBV infection: fluctuating liver function tests (tests of alanine aminotransferase, ALTs) and ongoing liver damage that may lead to cirrhosis. Treatment in this phase may lead to seroconversion. In many, the immunoactive phase is followed by a period of immune control **(the 'inactive carrier' phase)**, when host immune responses suppress viral replication, leading to low-level HBV DNA (<2000 IU/mL), absence of HBeAg and normal ALTs. In some patients the virus is eventually cleared, with the loss of HBsAg; in many, however, viral reactivation occurs with viral mutations, leading to **HBeAg-negative disease** with high levels of viral replication (HBV DNA $10^5/10^6$) and ALT in the absence of HBeAg. Note that, in this phase, fluctuating ALTs may lead to misdiagnosis, and so the ALTs and HBV DNA should be tested four times a year to establish the diagnosis in patients who are HBeAg-negative.

response leads to an asymptomatic, inactive, chronic HBV infective state. However, a better response results in continuing hepatocellular damage, with the development of chronic hepatitis.

Chronic HBV infection progresses through a series of four distinct phases (**Fig. 34.15**).

- **Phase 1 HBeAg-positive chronic HBV infection.** The natural history of childhood-acquired HBV is shown in the figure. In this first early phase there is high-level viral replication, with HBeAg, which is not associated with an immune-mediated liver injury response and does not cause liver damage. This was previously called the 'immunotolerant phase' of HBV but it is now clear that an immune response does develop, although why this does not lead to an obvious hepatitis has not yet been established. Management is not indicated but close follow-up is required. This phase matures into the next adolescent phase.

- **Phase 2 HBeAg-positive chronic HBV infection.** During adolescence, liver damage often develops, with fluctuating raised transferases (ALT) in the presence of high levels of HBeAg-positive infection. This was previously termed the 'immunoactive phase' but it is now recognized that the change from 'inactive' to 'active' disease is complex and not simply related to changes in immune tolerance. In some patients, this disease phase will progress to cirrhosis and therapy is therefore indicated to reduce the development of fibrosis. Management in this phase may lead to seroconversion from HBeAg-positive to HBeAg-negative.

- **Phase 3 HBeAg-negative chronic HBV infection.** In many patients the disease evolves to a quiescent phase (previously termed the 'inactive carrier' phase), when host immune

responses suppress viral replication, leading to low-level HBV DNA (<2000 IU/mL), absence of HBeAg and normal ALTs. In some patients the virus is eventually cleared with the loss of HBsAg.

- **Phase 4 HBeAg-negative chronic HBV infection.** In a proportion of patients with inactive HBV, disease will reactivate as they age, and this final phase is characterized by high-level viral replication (HBV DNA $10^5/10^6$) but negative HBeAg and raised ALT. In this phase, fluctuating ALT levels may lead to misdiagnosis and so liver function and HBV DNA should be tested four times a year to establish the diagnosis in patients who are HBeAg-negative. This disease phase is often associated with viral mutations (see earlier). Therapy for HBeAg-negative disease is indicated to prevent disease progression.

Hepatocellular carcinoma (HCC) can develop at all stages of disease but is more common in those with high levels of HBV DNA.

Immunosuppression, such as occurs during chemotherapy, aggravates all phases of HBV and a particular problem is seen in patients with HBeAg-negative, inactive disease, where the presence of normal liver biochemistry provides a false sense of security. HBV reactivation is common in such patients and has a high mortality. It is essential for all those due to receive chemotherapy to be screened for HBsAg, and those who have chronic HBV should receive prophylactic antiviral therapy, such as tenofovir or entecavir. Profound immunosuppression, such as occurs during bone marrow transplantation or rituximab therapy, can lead to disease reactivation in patients who have lost all traces of HBV, and in those with evidence of HBV exposure (i.e. those with antibodies against hepatitis B – anti-hepatitis B core or anti-hepatitis B surface antibodies) consideration of prophylactic therapy or close monitoring is required.

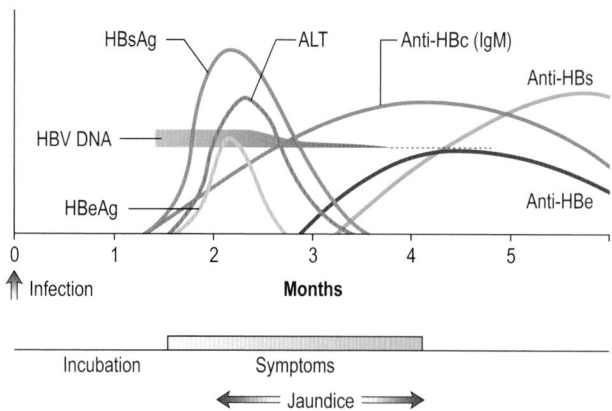

Fig. 34.16 Time course of the events and serological changes following acute infection with hepatitis B virus (HBV). *Antigens:* HBsAg appears in the blood from about 6 weeks to 3 months after an acute infection and then disappears. HBeAg rises early and usually declines rapidly. *Antibodies:* Anti-HBs appears late and indicates immunity. Anti-HBc is the first antibody to appear and high titres of IgM anti-HBc suggest an acute and continuing viral replication. It persists for many months. IgM anti-HBc may be the only serological indicator of recent HBV infection in a period when HBsAg has disappeared and anti-HBs is not detectable in the serum. Anti-HBe appears after the anti-HBc and its appearance relates to a decreased infectivity: that is, a low risk. ALT, alanine aminotransferase.

Clinical features of acute hepatitis B infection

The sequence of events following acute HBV infection is shown in **Fig. 34.16**. However, in many, the infection is subclinical. When HBV infection is acquired perinatally, an acute hepatitis does not usually occur and chronic infection develops. In adults, an acute infection is common and the virus is cleared in approximately 99% of patients. The clinical picture is the same as that found in HAV infection, although the illness may be more severe. In addition, a serum sickness-like immunological syndrome may be seen. This consists of rashes (e.g. urticaria or a maculopapular rash) and polyarthritis affecting small joints in up to 25% of cases in the prodromal period. Fever is usual. Extrahepatic immune complex-mediated conditions, such as an arteritis or glomerulonephritis, are occasionally seen.

Investigations

These are generally the same as for hepatitis A.

Specific tests

The markers for HBV are shown in **Box 34.9**. HBsAg is looked for initially; if it is found, a full viral profile is performed. In acute infection, as HBsAg may be cleared rapidly and anti-HBc IgM is diagnostic, patients must be tested for both HBsAg and anti-core antibodies if HBV is suspected. HBV DNA is the most sensitive index of viral replication.

Prognosis

The majority of patients recover completely, acute hepatic failure occurring in up to 1%. Some patients go on to develop chronic hepatitis and the outcome depends on several factors, chiefly the age of the patient.

Management of acute hepatitis

This is mainly symptomatic. However, patients should have their HBV markers monitored. Several experts suggest that entecavir

Box 34.9 Significance of viral markers in hepatitis B

Marker	Significance
Antigens	
HBsAg	Acute or chronic infection
HBeAg	Acute hepatitis B Persistence implies: Continued infectious state Development of chronicity
HBV DNA	Implies viral replication Found in serum and liver Levels indicate response to antiviral treatment
Antibodies	
Anti-HBs	Immunity to HBV; previous exposure; vaccination
Anti-HBe	Seroconversion
Anti-HBc	
IgM	Acute hepatitis B (high titre) Chronic hepatitis B (low titre)
IgG	Past exposure to hepatitis B (HBsAg-negative)

or tenofovir should be given for the persistent presence of HbeAg beyond 12 weeks, and in some patients who are very ill.

Prevention

Prevention depends on vaccination. In countries that do not vaccinate all citizens, prevention depends on avoiding risk factors (see earlier). These include not sharing needles and having safe sex. Vertical transmission is discussed later. Infectivity is highest in those with the e antigen and/or HBV DNA in their blood.

Immunization

Vaccination is obligatory in most developed countries (the UK recently added HBV to the childhood vaccination schedule), as well as countries with high endemicity, and has been shown to reduce mortality and morbidity. In countries that do not have a universal vaccination policy, groups at high risk are vaccinated. These include all healthcare personnel; members of emergency and rescue teams; morticians and embalmers; children in high-risk areas; people with haemophilia; patients in some psychiatric units; patients with chronic kidney disease/on dialysis units; long-term travellers; men who have sex with men, bisexual men and sex workers; and intravenous drug users.

Active and passive (combined) prophylaxis with vaccination and immunoglobulin should be given to healthcare staff with accidental needlestick injury; all newborn babies of HBsAg-positive mothers; and regular sexual partners of HBsAg-positive patients who have been found to be HBV-negative.

For adults, a dose of 500 IU of specific hepatitis B immunoglobulin (HBIg) (200 IU for newborns) is given; the vaccine (i.m.) is given at another site.

Prevention of mother-to-child transmission of HBV offers the potential to arrest transmission of this infection but the logistics of delivering the vaccine in a timely manner to babies born to high-risk mothers in developing countries (such as rural Africa and China) have, so far, prevented an effective campaign.

Active immunization

This is with a recombinant yeast vaccine, produced by insertion of a plasmid containing the gene of HBsAg into a yeast.

Dosage regimen

Three injections (at 0, 1 and 6 months) are given into the deltoid muscle; this gives short-term protection in over 90% of patients. People who are over 50 years of age or clinically ill and/or immuno-compromised (including those with human immunodeficiency virus (HIV) infection or acquired immunodeficiency syndrome (AIDS)) have a poor antibody response; more frequent and larger doses are required. Antibody levels should be measured at 7–9 months after the initial dose in all at-risk groups. Antibody levels fall steadily after vaccination, and booster doses may be required after approximately 3–5 years. It is not cost-effective to check antibody levels prior to active immunization. There are few side-effects from the vaccine.

Chronic hepatitis B virus infection

Following an acute HBV infection, which may be subclinical, approximately 1–10% of patients will not clear the virus and will develop a chronic HBV infection. The features are described on page 1280.

Investigations

These may show a moderate rise in aminotransferases but infection with normal aminotransferases is common. The serum bilirubin is often normal. HBsAg and HBV DNA are found in the serum, sometimes with HBeAg.

Histologically, there is a full spectrum of changes, from near normal with only a few lymphocytes and interface hepatitis to full-blown cirrhosis. HBsAg may lend a 'ground-glass' appearance to the cytoplasm on haematoxylin and eosin staining, and this can be confirmed on orcein staining or, more specifically, immunohisto-chemical staining. HBcAg can also be demonstrated in hepatocytes by appropriate immunohistochemical staining.

Management of chronic hepatitis B

Indications for therapy are similar to those for HBeAg-positive and negative patients with chronic hepatitis. **Three criteria** are used: serum HBV DNA levels, serum ALT levels and histological grade and stage. Increasingly, non-invasive assessment of liver fibrosis by, for example, transient elastography is replacing liver biopsy:

- **Patients with moderate to severe active necroinflammation** and/or fibrosis in the liver, with HBV DNA above 2000 IU/mL (approximately 10 000 copies/mL) and/or ALT above the upper limit of normal, are usually offered therapy. Age and co-morbidities also affect the decision to treat and the choice of agents.
- **If cirrhosis is present**, treatment should be given, independent of ALT or HBV DNA levels. Patients with decompensated cirrhosis can also be treated with oral antiviral agents but liver transplantation may be required.

All patients, regardless of disease phase, need long-term follow-up, as transition to an active phase is common; the lifetime risk of malignancy is increased in all patients who are HBsAg-positive, and men over 40 and women over 50 should be offered 6-monthly ultrasound screening.

Aim of therapy

The goals are to prevent disease progression and, ideally, eliminate HBsAg.

- **Interferon** is an immunostimulator that induces an immune response, leading to prolonged remission after discontinuation of therapy.
- **Oral nucleotides** suppress viral replication and are used for prolonged periods of time.

 Box 34.10 Factors predictive of a sustained response to treatment in chronic hepatitis B

Duration of disease
- Short

Liver biochemistry
- High serum aminotransferases

Histology
- Active liver disease (mild to moderate)

Viral levels
- Low HBV DNA levels

Other
- Absence of immunosuppression
- Female gender
- Acquisition in adulthood
- Delta virus negative
- Rapidity of response to oral therapy

In patients receiving long-term oral antiviral agents, liver fibrosis regresses. Even those with cirrhosis may recover, and the liver may remodel and lose all traces of fibrosis.

Antiviral agents

Interferon, entecavir and tenofovir are the most commonly used drugs.

Pegylated interferon-alfa-2a (180 µg once a week s.c.) is most often used in patients who are HBeAg-positive with active disease. Some patients (25–45%, depending on genotype – A and B respond best) lose HBeAg and move to the 'inactive' HBeAg-negative phase of disease. A proportion then goes on to lose HBsAg some years after treatment discontinuation. Patients with higher serum aminotransferase values (three times the upper limit of normal), who are younger and have viral loads below 10^7 IU/mL, respond best to treatment. Patients with concomitant HIV respond poorly and those with cirrhosis should not receive interferon. Response can be assessed during therapy by measuring the serum levels of HBsAg: if these fall after 3 months, a favourable outcome is likely, and most doctors stop therapy after 3 months if the HBsAg level remains unchanged. In patients with HBeAg-negative HBV, pegylated interferon-alfa-2a is occasionally used, as it offers a finite duration of therapy. A proportion of patients with active disease (high ALT, increased HBV DNA) convert to inactive disease, and response can be assessed by an early decline in HBsAg.

Side-effects of treatment include an acute influenza-like illness occurring 6–8 hours after the first injection. This usually disappears after subsequent injections but malaise, headaches and myalgia are common; depression, reversible hair loss and bone marrow depression and infection may also occur.

Oral antiviral therapy for HBV (entecavir and tenofovir) is very effective and almost all compliant patients respond with a decrease in HBV DNA to undetectable levels and a reduction in liver inflammation (**Box 34.10**). Both HBeAg-positive and HBeAg-negative patients respond equally well. Long-term viral suppression has been shown to reverse fibrosis, and even patients with cirrhosis respond with reversion of fibrosis. Resistance is rarely seen with third-generation drugs, and older, more resistance-prone drugs, like **lamivudine**, are no longer recommended. A small proportion of patients develop an immune response leading to loss of HBeAg and, very rarely, loss of HBsAg. However, the majority of patients who commence oral antiviral agents will require very prolonged treatment, perhaps life-long. Studies are in progress to determine whether antiviral therapy can ever be safely discontinued. **Entecavir** and **tenofovir** are the drugs of choice for HBV, and both agents are associated with very few side-effects and an excellent response. Combination therapy has little benefit and a single drug should be used. New treatments that target alternative steps in the viral life cycle (e.g. polymerization of the core protein) or augment the immune response (e.g. 'checkpoint inhibitors', see p. 113) are under evaluation, as they carry the possibility of finite therapy with loss of HBsAg).

Prognosis

The clinical course of hepatitis B is very variable; treatments have improved survival, stopped progression of fibrosis and enabled regression of fibrosis. Established cirrhosis is associated with a poor prognosis. **Hepatocellular carcinoma (HCC)** is a frequent association and is one of the most common carcinomas in HBV-endemic areas such as the Far East. Surveillance for HCC must continue, even when HBV DNA is negative in patients who have HBsAg and are not treated, and also in those rendered negative by therapy. The incidence of HCC is being reduced by routine HBV vaccination of all children.

Hepatitis D

This is caused by the hepatitis D virus (HDV or delta virus), an incomplete RNA particle enclosed in a shell of HBsAg; it belongs to the *Deltaviridae* family. The virus is unable to replicate on its own but is activated by the presence of HBV. It is common in some parts of the world, including Eastern Europe (Romania, Bulgaria), North Africa and the Brazilian rainforest. Hepatitis D viral infection can occur either as a co-infection or as a superinfection.

- **Co-infection** of HDV and HBV is clinically indistinguishable from an acute icteric HBV infection but a biphasic rise of serum aminotransferases may be seen. **Diagnosis** is confirmed by finding serum IgM anti-HDV in the presence of IgM anti-HBc. IgM anti-delta appears at 1 week and disappears by 5–6 weeks (occasionally 12 weeks), when serum IgG anti-delta is seen. The HDV RNA is an early marker of infection. The infection may be transient but the clinical course is variable.
- **Superinfection** results in an acute flare-up of previously quiescent chronic HBV infection. A rise in serum AST or ALT may be the only indication of infection. **Diagnosis** is made by finding HDV RNA or serum IgM anti-HDV at the same time as IgG anti-HBc. Active HBV DNA synthesis is reduced by delta superinfection and patients are usually negative for HBeAg with low HBV DNA.

Acute hepatic failure can follow both types of infection but is more common after co-infection. HDV RNA in the serum and liver can be measured and is found in acute and chronic HDV infection.

Chronic hepatitis D

This is a relatively infrequent chronic hepatitis but spontaneous resolution is rare. Between 60% and 70% of patients will develop cirrhosis, and more rapidly than with HBV infection alone. In 15% the disease is rapidly progressive, with development of cirrhosis in only a few years. The diagnosis is made by finding anti-delta antibody in a patient with chronic liver disease who is HBsAg-positive. It can be confirmed by finding HDV in the liver or HDV RNA in the serum by reverse transcription polymerase chain reaction (PCR).

Management

Treatment of patients with active liver disease (raised ALT levels and/or inflammation on biopsy) is with pegylated interferon-alfa-2a for 12 months, although response rates are very low.

Hepatitis C
Epidemiology

An estimated 70 million people are infected with this virus worldwide. The prevalence rate of infection ranges from 0.4% in Europe and 1–3%

in Southern Europe (possibly linked to intramuscular injections of vaccines or other medicines) to 6% in Africa; in Egypt, the rates are as high as 19%, owing to parenteral antimony treatment for schistosomiasis. The virus is transmitted by blood and blood products, and was common in people with haemophilia treated before screening of blood products was introduced. The incidence in intravenous drug users is high (40–60%). The low rate of HCV infection in high-risk groups – such as men who have sex with men, sex workers and attendees at sexually transmitted infection clinics – suggests a limited role for sexual transmission. Vertical transmission from a healthy mother to child can occur but is rare (approximately 5%). Other routes of community-acquired infection (e.g. close contact) are extremely rare. In 20% of cases the exact mode of transmission is unknown.

Hepatitis C virus (HCV)

Hepatitis C virus (HCV) is a single-stranded RNA virus of the *Flaviviridae* family. The RNA genome is approximately 10 kb in length, encoding a polyprotein product consisting of structural (capsid and envelope) and non-structural viral proteins (**Fig. 34.17**). Comparisons of subgenomic regions, such as E1, NS4 or NS5, have allowed variants to be classified into six genotypes, which have differing geographical distributions. Variability is distributed throughout the genome, with the non-structural gene of different genotypes showing 30–50% nucleotide sequence disparity. Genotypes 1a and 1b account for 70% of cases in the USA and 50% in Europe, while genotype 3 is common in the Indian subcontinent and genotype 4 is prevalent in Egypt. There is a rapid change in envelope proteins, making it difficult to develop a vaccine. Antigens from the nucleocapsid regions have been used to develop enzyme-linked immunosorbent assays (ELISAs). The current assay, ELISA-3, incorporates antigens NS3, NS4 and NS5 regions.

Clinical features

Most acute infections are asymptomatic, about 10% of patients having a mild influenza-like illness with jaundice and a rise in serum aminotransferases. Most patients will not be diagnosed until they present, years later, with evidence of abnormal transferase values at health checks or with chronic liver disease.

Investigations

Investigation is by evaluation of HCV, RNA and HCV antibodies; HCV RNA can be detected from 1 to 8 weeks after infection. Anti-HCV tests are usually positive 8 weeks from infection. Patients with acute HCV infection should be tested on several occasions, as many have fluctuating viraemia during the first few months of infection, with periods of undetectable HCV RNA followed by virological relapse. Viral clearance is confirmed by multiple tests for HCV RNA over a period of many months.

Management

In acute infection, most experts recommend a period of monitoring for a few weeks with serial assessments of HCV RNA. If the viral load is falling, treatment may not be required, but the patient should be observed for several months to confirm true viral clearance. If the HCV RNA level does not decline, therapy is indicated. Needle-stick injuries must be followed and treated early, although the vast majority (>97%) do not go on to develop viraemia. For the treatment of patients with co-infection with HIV, see page 1445.

Prognosis

Some 85–90% of asymptomatic patients develop chronic liver disease. A higher percentage of symptomatic patients 'clear' the virus, with only 48–75% going on to chronic liver disease.

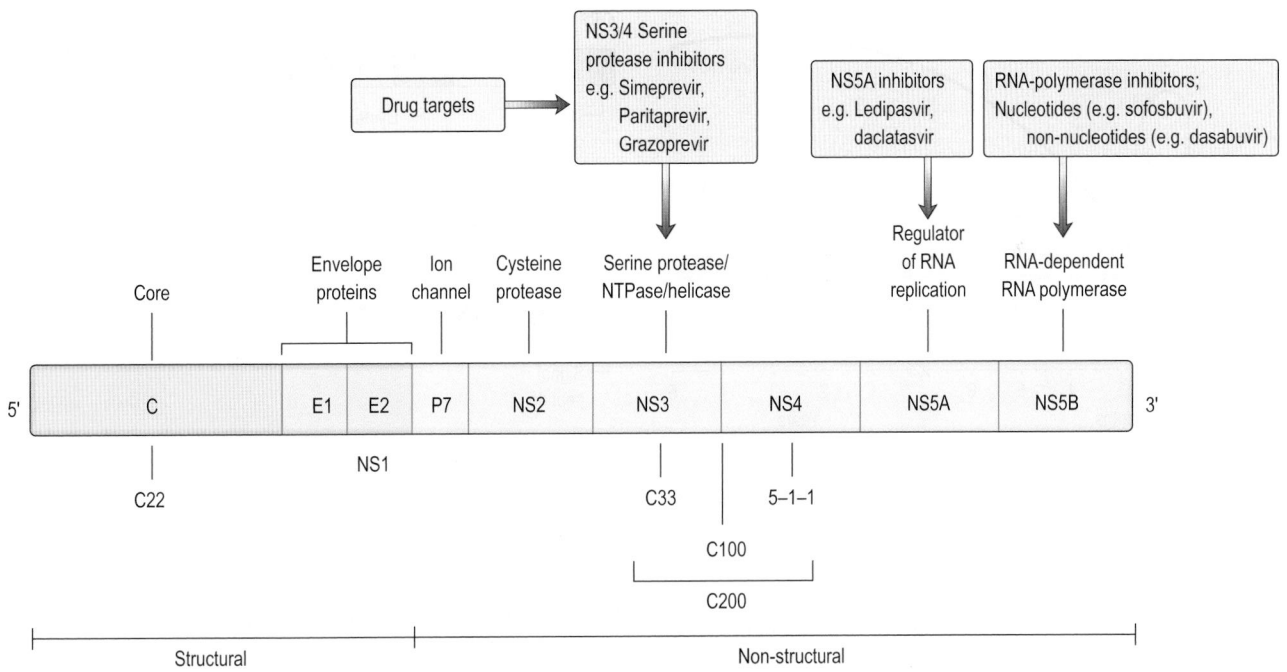

Fig. 34.17 Hepatitis C virus. This is a single-stranded RNA virus with viral proteins. Targets for recent drugs are shown. C, core; E, envelope; NS, non-structural.

Chronic hepatitis C infection

Pathogenesis

As with hepatitis B infection, cytokines in the Th2 phenotypes are profibrotic and cause the development of chronic infection. A dominant CD4 Th2 response, with a weak CD8 interferon-gamma response, may lead to rapid fibrosis. Th1 cytokines are antifibrotic and thus a dominant CD4 Th1 and CD8 cytolytic response may cause less fibrosis.

Clinical features

Patients with chronic HCV infection are usually asymptomatic, the disease only being discovered following a routine biochemical test when mild elevations in the aminotransferases (usually ALT) are noticed (50%). The elevation in ALT may be minimal and fluctuating (**Fig. 34.18**), and some patients have a persistently normal ALT (25%), the disease being detected by checking HCV antibodies (e.g. in blood donors). Non-specific malaise and fatigue are common in chronic infection and often reverse following viral clearance. Extrahepatic manifestations are seen, including arthritis, cryoglobulinaemia with or without glomerulonephritis, and porphyria cutanea tarda. There is a higher incidence of diabetes, and associations with lichen planus, sicca syndrome and non-Hodgkin lymphoma.

Chronic HCV infection causes slowly progressive fibrosis that leads, over decades, to cirrhosis. After 20 years of infection, 16% of patients have developed cirrhosis; the proportion that will ultimately develop cirrhosis after a lifetime of infection remains unknown but is likely to be higher than the proportions reported after short-term follow-up. Factors associated with rapid progression of HCV fibrosis include excess alcohol consumption, co-infection with HIV, obesity, diabetes and infection with genotype 3. Once cirrhosis has developed, some 3–4% per year will develop decompensated cirrhosis and approximately 1% will develop liver cancer. Unlike HBV infection, HCV rarely causes liver cancer in the absence of cirrhosis. In most parts of the world, HCV was spread (either by injection drug use or by poorly sterilized medical devices) in the 1970s. Given the slow development of cirrhosis, current mathematical models of disease burden predict a massive increase in HCV-related end-stage liver disease over the next decade.

Investigations

Diagnosis is made by finding HCV antibody in the serum using third-generation ELISA-3 tests. A proportion of patients with spontaneous clearance will have undetectable HCV RNA in the serum (measured by PCR) but most individuals who are antibody-positive will be viraemic. The level of viraemia varies from a few thousand to many millions of viral copies per millilitre, although current practice is to present viral load measurements in international units (IU). Disease progression and treatment outcome are not influenced by the viral load.

The HCV genotype should be characterized in patients who are to be given treatment (see next section), and assessment of fibrosis (by either liver biopsy or non-invasive methods) is required in those who would prefer to defer therapy. Cirrhosis should be excluded in all patients who have been infected for more than 20 years and a liver biopsy or non-invasive marker should be used.

Management

The aim of treatment is to eliminate the HCV RNA from the serum in order to:
- stop the progression of active liver disease
- prevent the development of HCC.

A clinical cure is determined by a sustained virological response (SVR), defined by a negative HCV RNA by PCR 6 months after the end of therapy. Additional public health benefits may accrue from a reduction in the pool of infected people, and campaigns to eliminate HCV in populations at high risk of infection (such as people who inject drugs) are under way.

Antiviral agents

Treatment for HCV infection is now based on direct-acting antiviral agents that are administered orally. These drugs target enzymes in

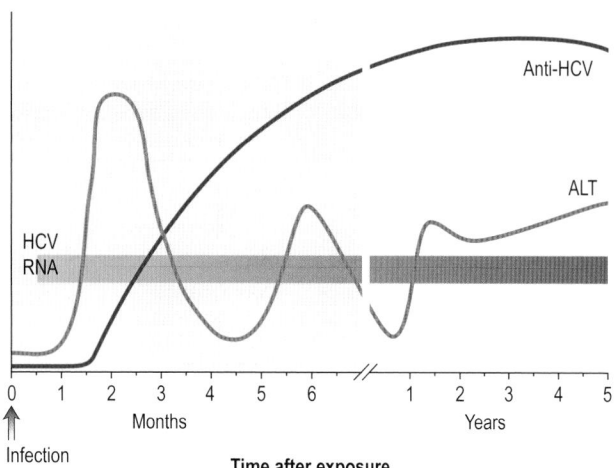

Fig. 34.18 Time course of the events and serological changes seen following infection with hepatitis C virus. ALT, alanine aminotransferase.

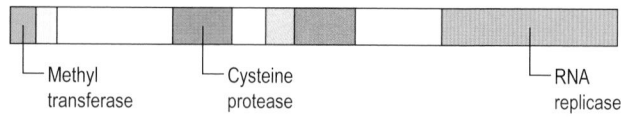

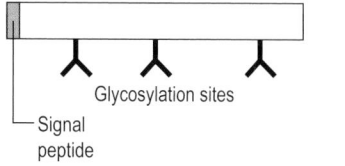

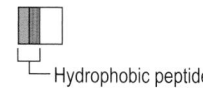

Fig. 34.19 Hepatitis E genome. A single-stranded RNA genome with three open reading frames (ORFs).

the virus – usually the polymerase, NS5a protein or NS3/4 protease. Therapy may involve a nucleotide inhibitor of the polymerase (sofosbuvir) combined with an NS5a inhibitor. This combination may be pan-genotypic (sofosbuvir/velpatasvir) or specific for genotypes 1 and 4 (sofosbuvir/ledipasvir), and involves a single tablet given once a day for 8–12 weeks. An alternative strategy is to use a protease inhibitor-based regimen (either glecaprevir or grazoprevir) combined with an NS5a inhibitor. Glecaprevir is combined with pibrentasvir and involves three tablets a day for 8 weeks in patients without cirrhosis or for 12 weeks in those with cirrhosis. The regimen is effective in all viral genotypes. Grazoprevir is combined with elbasvir and is used as a single tablet that is taken for 12 weeks and is effective in patients with genotypes 1 and 4. All of the treatment regimens eliminate virus in more than 95% of patients; in the very few who do not respond to therapy a 'rescue' treatment involving sofosbuvir/velpatasvir and the pan-genotypic protease inhibitor voxilaprevir is licensed and eliminates virus in over 90% of patients. Following viral clearance, liver fibrosis progression is halted and may even reverse, but in patients with cirrhosis the risk of liver cancer persists (albeit at a reduced level). Patients who do not have cirrhosis can be discharged from follow-up after successful therapy, defined as undetectable virus 12 weeks after discontinuation of treatment.

The extraordinary effectiveness of the oral antiviral regimens against HCV, combined with their excellent safety programme, has led to campaigns to identify and treat all patients with HCV, and the World Health Organization has a goal of eliminating HCV by 2030. If this can be achieved, it will represent the first time that a viral infection has been controlled without an effective vaccine.

Hepatitis E

Hepatitis E virus (HEV) is an RNA virus (Hepeviridae family; **Fig. 34.19**); it causes disease that is clinically very similar to hepatitis A. It is enterally transmitted, usually by contaminated water, with 30% of dogs, pigs and rodents carrying the virus. Epidemics have been seen in many developing countries, and sporadically in developed countries, in patients who have had contact with farm animals or have travelled abroad. In some developing countries, zoonotic infection from contaminated pork has led to acute HEV infection becoming relatively common. It has a mortality from fulminant hepatic failure of 1–2%, which rises to 20% in pregnant women. There is no carrier state and

infection does not progress to chronic liver disease, except in some immunosuppressed patients. An ELISA for IgG and IgM anti-HEV is available for diagnosis. HEV RNA can be detected in the serum or stools by PCR. Prevention and control depend on good sanitation and hygiene; a vaccine has been developed and used successfully in China. Over the last few years it has become clear that HEV infection is common in many domestic animals, particularly pigs. Contamination of meat is not uncommon and acute infection with HEV is now the most common cause of acute viral hepatitis in the UK and many EU countries. The infection with animal-derived HEV is usually less aggressive than the water-borne infections in the Indian subcontinent and the symptoms and outcomes are similar to those of hepatitis A infection. A large proportion of the adult population in England have evidence of infection with hepatitis E, suggesting that subclinical infection is common. In patients who are immunocompromised, HEV infection may lead to chronic infection, which is treated by reduction of the immunosuppression and/or introduction of the broad-spectrum antiviral agent ribavirin.

Hepatitis non-A–E

Approximately 10–15% of acute viral hepatitides cannot be typed and are described as hepatitis non-A–E. GB agent (hepatitis G virus, HGV) and transfusion-transmitted virus (TTV) agents have not been documented as causing disease in humans.

Acute hepatitis due to other infectious agents

Abnormal liver biochemistry is frequently found in a number of acute infections. The abnormalities are usually mild and have no clinical significance.

Infectious mononucleosis

Infectious mononucleosis (see also p. 524) is due to the Epstein–Barr (EB) virus. Mild jaundice, associated with minor abnormalities of liver biochemistry, is extremely common but 'clinical' hepatitis is rare. Hepatic histological changes occur within 5 days of onset; the sinusoids and portal tracts are infiltrated with large mononuclear cells but the liver architecture is preserved. A Paul–Bunnell or Monospot test is usually positive, and atypical lymphocytes are present in the peripheral blood. Treatment is symptomatic.

Cytomegalovirus

Cytomegalovirus (CMV; see also p. 524) can cause acute hepatitis, usually a 'glandular fever-type syndrome', in healthy individuals but is more severe in those with an impaired immune response. Only the latter need treatment with valganciclovir or ganciclovir.

CMV DNA is positive in blood; CMV IgM is also positive but there are false-positive reactions. Liver biopsy shows intranuclear inclusions and giant cells.

Herpes simplex

Very occasionally, the herpes simplex virus (see also p. 513) causes a generalized acute infection, particularly in the immunosuppressed patient and occasionally in pregnancy. Aminotransferases are usually massively elevated. Liver biopsy shows extensive necrosis. Aciclovir is used for treatment.

Toxoplasmosis

The clinical picture in toxoplasmosis (see also p. 570) is similar to that of infectious mononucleosis, with abnormal liver biochemistry, but the Paul–Bunnell test is negative.

Yellow fever

Yellow fever (see also p. 531) is a viral infection carried by the mosquito *Aedes aegypti*; it can cause acute hepatic necrosis. There is no specific treatment.

Further reading

European Association for the Study of the Liver. EASL Clinical Practice Guidelines: management of chronic hepatitis B infection. *J Hepatol* 2017; 67:370–398.

European Association for the Study of the Liver. EASL recommendations of treatment of hepatitis C 2018. *J Hepatol* 2018; 69:461–511.

Lawitz E, Reau N, Hinestrosa F et al. Efficacy of sofosbuvir velpatasvir, and GS-9857 in patients with genotype-1 hepatitis C virus infection in an open-label, phase 2 trial. Gastroenterology 2016; 151:795–798

National Institute for Health and Care Excellence. *NICE Clinical Guideline 165: Hepatitis B (Chronic): Diagnosis and Management of Chronic Hepatitis B in Children, Young People and Adults.* NICE 2013, updated 2017; https://www.nice.org.uk/guidance/cg165.

Razavi H, Waked I, Sarrazin C et al. The present and future disease burden of hepatitis C virus (HCV) infection with today's treatment paradigm. *J Viral Hepatitis* 2014; 21(Supplement S1):34–59.

Visvanathan K, Dusheiko G, Giles M et al. Managing HBV in pregnancy. *Gut* 2016; 65:340–350.

Wedemeyer H, Yurdaydin C, Dalekos GN et al, for the HIDIT Study Group. Peginterferon plus adefovir versus either drug alone for hepatitis delta. *N Engl J Med* 2011; 364:322–331.

World Health Organization. Combating hepatitis B and C to reach elimination by 2030. Advocacy brief 2016, available from https://www.who.int/hepatitis/publications/hep-elimination-by-2030-brief/en/

ACUTE HEPATIC FAILURE

Acute liver failure (ALF) is defined as acute liver injury with encephalopathy and deranged coagulation (INR >1.5) in a patient with a previously normal liver. The time intervals are variable. The time of development of jaundice to encephalopathy varies from 7 days

Box 34.11 Causes of acute hepatic failure

Viruses
- HAV, HBV, (HDV), HEV; rarely, HCV
- Cytomegalovirus
- Haemorrhagic fever viruses
- Herpes simplex virus
- Paramyxovirus
- Epstein–Barr virus

Drugs (examples)
- Paracetamol (acetaminophen)
- Antibiotics (ampicillin–clavulanate, ciprofloxacin, doxycycline, erythromycin, isoniazid, nitrofurantoin, tetracycline)
- Antidepressants (amitriptyline, nortriptyline)
- Antiepileptics (phenytoin, valproate)
- Anaesthetic agents (halothane)
- Lipid-lowering medications (atorvastatin, lovastatin, simvastatin)
- Immunosuppressive agents (cyclophosphamide, methotrexate)
- NSAIDs
- Salicylates (as a result of Reye's syndrome, see p. 1310)
- Disulfiram, flutamide, gold, propylthiouracil
- Illicit drugs (e.g. 'ecstasy' or cocaine)
- Herbal/alternative medicines (ginseng, pennyroyal oil, *Teucrium polium* chaparral or germander tea, kawa kawa)

Toxins
- *Amanita phalloides* mushroom toxin
- *Bacillus cereus* toxin
- Cyanobacteria toxin
- Organic solvents (e.g. carbon tetrachloride)
- Yellow phosphorus

Hepatic failure in pregnancy
- Acute fatty liver of pregnancy (AFLP)
- HELLP (*h*aemolysis, *e*levated *l*iver enzymes, *l*ow *p*latelets)

Vascular causes
- Ischaemic hepatitis
- Budd–Chiari syndrome
- Hepatic sinusoidal obstruction syndrome
- Portal vein thrombosis
- Hepatic arterial thrombosis (consider post transplant)

Metabolic causes
- α_1-antitrypsin deficiency
- Fructose intolerance
- Galactosaemia
- Lecithin–cholesterol acyltransferase deficiency
- Reye's syndrome
- Tyrosinaemia
- Wilson's disease

Malignancies
- Primary (usually HCC, rarely cholangiocarcinoma)
- Secondary (extensive hepatic metastases or infiltration)

Miscellaneous
- Adult-onset Still's disease
- Heatstroke
- Primary graft non-function in liver transplant

HAV/HBV/HCV/HDV/HEV, hepatitis A/B/C/D/E virus; HCC, hepatocellular carcinoma; NSAIDs, non-steroidal anti-inflammatory drugs.

(hyper-acute) to 8–28 days (acute) and 21–26 weeks (subacute). Occasionally, patients may have previous liver damage: for example, D virus superinfection in a previous carrier of HBsAg, Budd–Chiari syndrome or Wilson's disease.

ALF is a rare but often life-threatening syndrome that is due to acute hepatitis from many causes (**Box 34.11**). These causes vary throughout the world; most involve viral hepatitis but paracetamol overdose is common in the UK (50% of cases). HCV does not usually cause acute hepatic failure, although exceptional cases have been reported from Japan and India.

Histologically, there is multiacinar necrosis involving a substantial part of the liver. Severe fatty change is seen in pregnancy (see p. 1455) and Reye's syndrome (p. 1310), or following intravenous tetracycline administration.

Clinical features

Examination shows a jaundiced patient with a small liver and signs of hepatic encephalopathy. The mental state varies from slight drowsiness, confusion and disorientation (grades I and II) to unresponsive coma (grade IV) with convulsions. Fetor hepaticus is common but ascites and splenomegaly are rare. Fever, vomiting, hypotension and hypoglycaemia occur. Neurological examination shows spasticity and hyper-reflexia; plantar responses remain flexor until late. Cerebral oedema develops in 80% of patients with ALF but is far less common with subacute failure; its consequences, intracranial hypertension and brain herniation, account for about 25% of the causes of death. Other complications include bacterial and fungal infections, gastrointestinal bleeding, respiratory arrest, kidney injury (hepatorenal syndrome and acute tubular necrosis) and pancreatitis.

Investigations

- Routine tests (see p. 1268).
- There is hyperbilirubinaemia, high serum aminotransferases and low levels of coagulation factors, including prothrombin and factor V. Aminotransferases are not useful indicators of the course of the disease, as they tend to fall along with the albumin with progressive liver damage.
- An electroencephalogram (EEG) is sometimes helpful in grading the encephalopathy.
- Ultrasound will define liver size and may indicate underlying liver pathology.

Management

There is no specific treatment but patients should be managed in a specialized unit. Transfer criteria to such units are shown in **Box 34.12**. Supportive therapy, as for hepatic encephalopathy, is necessary (see p. 1297). When signs of raised intracranial pressure (which may be measured directly) are present, 20% mannitol (1 g/kg body weight) should be infused intravenously; this dose may need to be repeated. Dexamethasone is not of value. Hypoglycaemia, hypokalaemia, hypomagnesaemia, hypophosphataemia and hypocalcaemia should be anticipated and corrected with a 10% glucose infusion (checked by 2-hourly dipstick testing), potassium, calcium, phosphate and magnesium supplements. Hyponatraemia should be corrected with hypertonic saline. Coagulopathy is managed with intravenous vitamin K, platelets, blood or fresh frozen plasma. Haemorrhage may be a problem and patients are given a proton pump inhibitor (PPI) to prevent gastrointestinal bleeding. Prophylaxis against bacterial and fungal infection is routine, as infection is a frequent cause of death and may preclude liver transplantation. Suspected infection should be treated immediately with suitable antibiotics. Renal and respiratory failure should be treated as necessary. Liver transplantation has been a major advance for patients with ALF. It is difficult to judge the timing or the necessity for transplantation, but there are guidelines based on validated prognostic indices of survival (see later).

Prognosis

In mild cases (grades I and II encephalopathy with drowsiness and confusion), two-thirds of patients will survive. The outcome

of severe cases (grades III and IV encephalopathy with stupor or deep coma) is related to aetiology. In specialist units, 70% of patients with paracetamol overdosage and grade IV coma will survive, as will 30–40% patients with HAV or HBV hepatitis. Poor prognostic variables indicating a need to transplant the liver are shown in **Box 34.13**.

Further reading

Bernal W, Wendon J. Acute liver failure. *N Engl J Med* 2013; 369:2525–2534.

AUTOIMMUNE HEPATITIS

Autoimmune hepatitis (AIH) is a progressive inflammatory liver condition with a 75% female preponderance. Approximately 40% of AIH patients have a family history of autoimmune disease (e.g. pernicious anaemia, thyroiditis or coeliac disease), and at least 20% have concomitant autoimmune diseases or will develop them during follow-up.

Pathogenesis

The pathogenesis of AIH is incompletely understood, although evidence increasingly demonstrates that genetic susceptibility, molecular mimicry and impaired immunoregulatory networks contribute to the initiation and perpetuation of the autoimmune attack. Liver damage is thought to be mediated primarily by T cell-mediated events (CD4+ T cells) against liver antigens, producing a progressive necro-inflammatory process that leads to fibrosis and cirrhosis. However, no clear trigger mechanism has been found.

Clinical features

There are two peaks in presentation. In the peri- and postmenopausal group, patients may be asymptomatic, or present with fatigue and abnormalities in liver biochemistry or the presence of chronic liver disease on examination. In the teens and early twenties, the disease (often type II) presents as an acute hepatitis with jaundice and very high aminotransferases, which do not improve with time. This age group often has clinical features of cirrhosis and patients who are ill may also have features of an autoimmune disease, such as fever, migratory polyarthritis, glomerulonephritis, pleurisy, pulmonary infiltration or lung fibrosis.

There are rare overlap syndromes with primary biliary cholangitis and primary sclerosing cholangitis, existing concomitantly or developing consecutively.

Box 34.12 Transfer criteria to specialized units for patients with acute liver injury

- INR >3.0
- Presence of hepatic encephalopathy
- Hypotension after resuscitation with fluid
- Metabolic acidosis
- Prothrombin time (seconds) > interval (hours) from overdose (paracetamol cases)

INR, International normalized ratio.

Box 34.13 Poor prognostic variables in acute hepatic failure indicating liver transplantation

Non-paracetamol (acetaminophen) causes

Three of the following five:

- Drug or A–E hepatitis
- Age <10 and >40 years
- Interval from onset of jaundice to encephalopathy >7 days
- Serum bilirubin >300 μmol/L
- Prothrombin time >50 sec (or >100 sec in isolation)

Paracetamol overdose

- Arterial pH <7.3 (after resuscitation, 7.25 on acetylcysteine)

  or

- Serum creatinine >300 μmol/L *and*
- Prothrombin time >100 sec *and*
- Grade III–IV encephalopathy

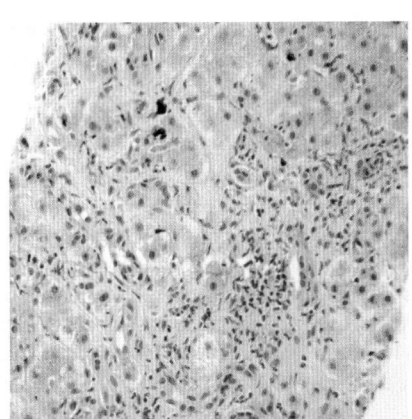

Fig. 34.20 Chronic active hepatitis. Note the inflammation with interface hepatitis (haematoxylin and eosin, ×10).

Investigations

Liver biochemistry

The serum aminotransferases are high, with lesser elevations in the ALP and bilirubin. The serum γ-globulins are high: frequently twice normal, particularly the IgG. The biochemical pattern is similar in both types.

Haematology

A mild normochromic normocytic anaemia with thrombocytopenia and leucopenia is present, even before portal hypertension and splenomegaly. The PT is often high.

Autoantibodies

Two types of autoimmune hepatitis have been recognized:
- **Type I with antibodies** (titres >1:80):
  - anti-nuclear (ANA)
  - anti-smooth muscle (anti-actin).
- **Type II with antibodies**: anti-liver/kidney microsomal (anti-LKM1). The main target is cytochrome P4502D6 (CYP2D6) on liver cell plasma membranes.
- A third type of AIH (AIH-3) was proposed, positive for anti-soluble liver antigen (SLA) and negative for conventional autoantibodies. However, subsequent studies showed that anti-SLA is also present in typical cases of AIH-1 and AIH-2. Patients positive for anti-SLA only, and therefore having *bona fide* AIH-3, are rare. Approximately 13% of patients lack the autoantibodies listed.

Liver biopsy

Since transferases and IgG levels do not reflect disease activity, liver biopsy is mandatory to confirm the diagnosis and evaluate disease severity. The biopsy (**Fig. 34.20**) commonly shows chronic active hepatitis with inflammation and interface hepatitis. This reflects the changes of chronic hepatitis described on page 1275. The amount of interface hepatitis is variable but tends to be high in untreated patients. Lymphoid follicles are less often seen than in hepatitis C, and plasma cell infiltration is frequent. Fibrosis is present in all but the mildest forms of the disease and approximately one-third of patients have cirrhosis at presentation.

Management

Prednisolone 30 mg is given daily for at least 2 weeks, followed by slow reduction to a maintenance dose of 5–15 mg daily. Azathioprine should be added, 1–2 mg/kg daily, as a steroid-sparing agent and, in some, as sole long-term maintenance therapy. Levels of thiopurine methyltransferase (TPMT) should be obtained before treatment is started (see p. 1204). Other agents that have been used in resistant cases include budesonide (in non-cirrhotic patients), mycophenolate, ciclosporin and tacrolimus.

Prognosis

Steroid and azathioprine therapy induce remission in over 80%; indeed, this response forms part of the diagnostic criteria. Treatment is life-long in most, although withdrawal may be considered after 2–3 years of biochemical remission. Those with initial cirrhosis are more likely to relapse following withdrawal and require indefinite therapy. Liver transplantation is performed if treatment fails, although the disease may recur. HCC occurs less frequently than with viral-induced cirrhosis. The risk of malignancy associated with chronic low-dose azathioprine therapy has been reported to be 1.4 times normal.

Further reading

Mieli-Vergani G, Vergani D, Czaja AJ et al. Autoimmune hepatitis. *Nat Rev Dis Primers* 2018; 4:18017.
Terziroli Beretta-Piccoli B, Mieli-Vergani G, Vergani D. Autoimmune hepatitis: standard treatment and systematic review of alternative treatments. *World J Gastroenterol* 2017; 23:6030–6048.

DRUG-INDUCED CHRONIC HEPATITIS

Several drugs can cause a chronic hepatitis similar to autoimmune hepatitis (see **Box 34.25**). Patients are often female, present with jaundice and hepatomegaly, and have raised serum aminotransferases and globulin levels. Improvement follows drug withdrawal but exacerbations can occur with re-introduction. Isoniazid, amiodarone and methotrexate can cause chronic histological changes. With rare exceptions, patients with pre-existing chronic liver disease are not more susceptible to drug injury.

CHRONIC HEPATITIS OF UNKNOWN CAUSE

As increasing numbers undergo routine blood tests, mild elevations in serum aminotransferases and γ-GT are commonly found. Many will have no symptoms or signs of liver disease. All known aetiological agents should be excluded, risk factors for NAFLD evaluated, and tests carried out to exclude liver diseases. Liver biopsy should be performed if the elevation in aminotransferases (>100 IU/L) persists for over a year but often only non-specific changes are found.

NON-ALCOHOLIC FATTY LIVER DISEASE

Non-alcoholic fatty liver disease (NAFLD) is now the most common cause of chronic liver disease in many developed countries. It is often detected on routine abdominal ultrasound examination, and steatosis is found in up to one-third of these patients. NAFLD is a spectrum of liver diseases comprised of non-alcoholic fatty liver (NAFL) and non-alcoholic steatohepatitis (NASH). Whereas NAFL has negligible risk of progression, 10–30% of NASH patients may develop cirrhosis or HCC. NAFL and NASH have traditionally been considered as two separate clinical entities, rather than two points on a disease continuum. However, studies that have evaluated sequential liver biopsies are challenging this notion and have found that both patients with NAFL and those with NASH have the potential to develop progressive liver disease, suggesting that

NAFL, NASH and fibrosis progression are a continuum rather than separate diagnoses. Indeed, one large study showed no difference in liver-related adverse events between definite NASH and severe steatosis. However, patients with advanced fibrosis at presentation were much more likely to progress than those without, and these patients therefore require follow-up. In this cohort, complications of cirrhosis were the third most common cause of death, following cardiovascular events and non-hepatic malignancies.

Risk factors for NAFLD are obesity, hypertension, type 2 diabetes and hyperlipidaemia, such that NAFLD is considered to be the liver component of the metabolic syndrome (see p. 1250). Most patients are asymptomatic, although hepatomegaly may be present. Mild increases in serum aminotransferases and/or γ-GT (with ALT greater than AST) are frequently the sole liver biochemical abnormality. Despite the high prevalence of NAFLD, well-defined screening recommendations are currently lacking.

Pathogenesis

Histological changes follow a spectrum similar to that of alcohol-induced hepatic injury, and range from simple fatty change to fat and inflammation (NASH), fibrosis and cirrhosis.

Oxidative stress injury and other factors lead to lipid peroxidation in the presence of fatty infiltration and inflammation. Fibrosis may then occur, enhanced by insulin resistance, which induces connective tissue growth factor.

Investigations

- *Ultrasound* demonstration of steatosis in the absence of other injurious causes, such as alcohol, usually provides the diagnosis.
- *Liver biopsy* allows staging of the disease. Although no definitive guidelines exist, many clinicians perform a biopsy if a diagnosis of NASH or advanced fibrosis is considered likely.
- *Elastography* (see p. 1270) is used to evaluate the degree of fibrosis but may not be technically possible in the morbidly obese.

Management

- All NAFLD patients require *lifestyle advice* aimed at weight loss, increased physical activity and attention to cardiovascular risk factors. Calorie restriction is recommended, aimed at losing 0.5–1 kg per week until target weight is achieved. A reduction of more than 7–9% in body weight has been associated with reduced steatosis, hepatocellular injury and hepatic inflammation. However, less than 15% of patients will achieve significant long-term weight loss.
- *Orlistat*, an enteric lipase inhibitor causing malabsorption of dietary fat, is used with a low-fat diet as an adjunct in subjects with a body mass index (BMI) of more than 30 kg/m^2. The effects are modest and only those achieving a greater than 5% loss of body weight in 3 months should continue orlistat, and then for only 1 year, as fat-soluble vitamin deficiency may occur.
- *Pioglitazone* or vitamin E may be used for those with biopsy-proven NASH, when lifestyle intervention has failed. Meta-analysis data demonstrated that pioglitazone significantly improved liver steatosis, inflammation and, to a lesser degree, fibrosis. However, it is associated with weight gain and reports of congestive cardiac failure, bladder cancer and reduced bone density. Conversely, pioglitazone reduces death, myocardial infarction and stroke in diabetes patients. The risks and benefits to each patient should be evaluated accordingly and pioglitazone is infrequently used in clinical practice.

- *Vitamin E* (800 IU/day) is an antioxidant that improves steatohepatitis. A meta-analysis showed an increase in all-cause mortality at doses over 400 IU/day, and an increased risk of haemorrhagic stroke and prostate cancer has also been reported. Again, this is not frequently used.
- Weight loss following *bariatric surgery* leads to reduced steatosis, steatohepatitis and fibrosis. The optimum technique is unknown and long-term data are lacking, although initial concerns about worsening fibrosis have not been borne out. Bariatric surgery should be avoided in those with advanced cirrhosis and portal hypertension, but gastric bypass and sleeve gastrectomy (p. 1250) have been shown to achieve weight loss and improve obesity-related co-morbidities in Child–Pugh A cirrhotic patients.

Hepatocellular carcinoma

The yearly cumulative incidence of HCC is 2.6% in patients with NASH cirrhosis and ultrasound surveillance should therefore be performed 6-monthly. Hyperinsulinaemia and obesity are risk factors for many malignancies and HCC can occur in NAFL/NASH patients in the absence of cirrhosis.

Liver transplantation

NASH cirrhosis is the most rapidly growing indication for transplantation in the US, the leading cause in women and the second leading cause overall. Survival is comparable to that in other indications, and although recurrence occurs post transplant (4–25%), it does not appear to have an impact on graft survival. Patients frequently have multiple cardiovascular risk factors that must be managed aggressively. UK guidelines suggest that bariatric surgery could be considered at transplantation for the morbidly obese.

New treatments for NASH

There has been substantial industry investment in pharmacotherapies for NASH, with the pipeline currently crowded at mid-stage. However, there are several phase III studies that are due to complete in the early 2020s and all of these agents showed potential clinical benefit in phase II trials. They include elafibranor, a dual peroxisome proliferator-activated receptor (PPAR)α/δ agonist; obeticholic acid, the FXR agonist; cenicriviroc, a dual antagonist of C-C chemokine receptor types 2 and 5; selonsertib, an apoptosis signal-regulating kinase 1 inhibitor; and liraglutide, a glucagon-like peptide. It is highly likely that the landscape of treatments for NASH will change substantially by 2025.

However, it is imperative to tackle obesity at source: for example, through public health campaigns, taxation of high-sugar food, reduction in processed food within the diet, education, increased activity and vegetable consumption. Prevention of obesity, especially in children and adolescents, will most likely be far superior to the effects of these drugs.

Further reading

Hardy T, Anstee QM, Day CP. Nonalcoholic fatty liver disease: new treatments. *Curr Opin Gastroenterol* 2015; 31:175–183.
Noureddin M, Anstee QM, Loomba R. Review article: emerging anti-fibrotic therapies in the treatment of non-alcoholic steatohepatitis. *Aliment Pharmacol Ther* 2016; 43:1109–1123.

CIRRHOSIS

In cirrhosis, the liver architecture is diffusely abnormal and interferes with liver blood flow and function; this leads to the clinical manifestations of portal hypertension and liver failure.

If the cause of fibrosis is eliminated (e.g. through treatment of viral hepatitis), resolution (complete reversal to near-normal liver architecture) of early fibrosis can occur. In cirrhosis, regression (improvement, not reversal) occurs, which improves clinical outcomes. Antifibrotic therapies are emerging (including stem cell transplant strategies) but currently liver transplantation is the only available treatment for liver failure.

Pathology

The characteristic features of cirrhosis are regenerating nodules separated by fibrous septa, and loss of lobular architecture within the nodules (**Fig. 34.22A–C**). Two types are described:

- *Micronodular cirrhosis.* Regenerating nodules are usually <3 mm in size with uniform involvement of the liver; often caused by alcohol or biliary tract disease.
- *Macronodular cirrhosis.* The nodules are of variable size and normal acini may be seen within larger nodules; often caused by chronic viral hepatitis.

A mixed picture with small and large nodules occurs occasionally. Symptoms and signs are described on page 1263.

Investigations

Investigations aim to assess the severity and type of liver disease.

Severity

- *Liver function.* Serum albumin and PT are the best indicators of liver function; the outlook is poor if the albumin level is <28/L. The degree to which the PT is prolonged is commensurate with disease severity.
- *Liver biochemistry.* This may be normal, depending on the severity of disease. In most cases, there is a slight elevation in the serum ALP and serum aminotransferases. In decompensated cirrhosis, all biochemistry is deranged.
- *Serum electrolytes.* A low sodium indicates severe liver disease due to a defect in free water clearance or excess diuretic therapy.
- *Serum creatinine.* An elevated concentration of >130 μmol/L is a marker of poor prognosis.
- *Biomarkers.* In the Enhanced Liver Fibrosis (ELF) test, which assesses fibrosis, a value of <7.7 indicates none to mild, 7.7–9.8 moderate and ≥9.8 severe disease.

In addition, a serum α-fetoprotein of >200 ng/mL is strongly suggestive of HCC.

Type

This can be determined by:

- viral markers
- serum autoantibodies
- serum immunoglobulins
- iron indices and ferritin
- copper and caeruloplasmin (see p. 1301)
- α₁-antitrypsin (see p. 1302).
- genetic markers.

Serum copper and serum α₁-antitrypsin should always be measured in young cirrhotics. Total iron-binding capacity (TIBC) and ferritin should be measured to exclude hereditary haemochromatosis; genetic markers are also available (see p. 1300).

Imaging

- *Ultrasound examination* can demonstrate changes in the size and shape of the liver. Fatty change and fibrosis produce a diffusely increased echogenicity. In established cirrhosis, there may be marginal nodularity of the liver surface and distortion

---

Box 34.14 Causes of cirrhosis

Common
- Alcohol
- Hepatitis B ± D
- Hepatitis C
- Non-alcoholic fatty liver disease (NAFLD)

Others
- Primary biliary cholangitis
- Secondary biliary cirrhosis
- Autoimmune hepatitis
- Hereditary haemochromatosis

- Hepatic venous congestion
- Budd–Chiari syndrome
- Wilson's disease
- Drugs (e.g. methotrexate)
- α₁-antitrypsin deficiency
- Cystic fibrosis
- Galactosaemia
- Glycogen storage disease
- Veno-occlusive disease
- Idiopathic (cryptogenic)
- ? Other viruses

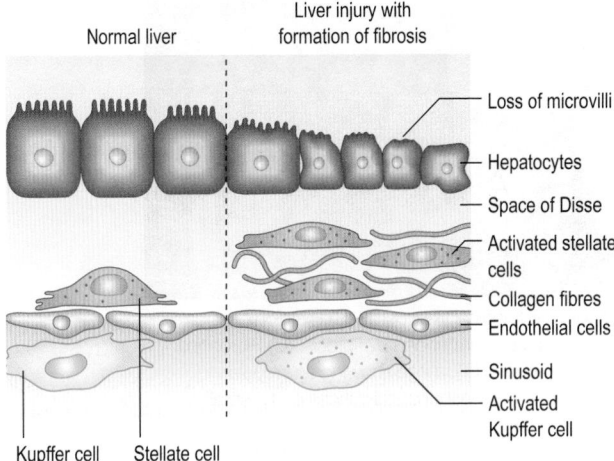

Normal liver

Liver injury with formation of fibrosis

- Loss of microvilli
- Hepatocytes
- Space of Disse
- Activated stellate cells
- Collagen fibres
- Endothelial cells
- Sinusoid
- Activated Kupffer cell

Kupffer cell   Stellate cell

Fig. 34.21 Pathogenesis of fibrosis. The normal liver is shown on the left. Activation of the stellate cell is followed by proliferation of fibroblasts and deposition of collagen.

Aetiology

Causes of cirrhosis are shown in **Box 34.14**. Alcohol is currently the most common cause in the West but is likely to be superseded by NAFLD; viral infection is the most common aetiological factor worldwide. All patients with cirrhosis must be investigated to exclude treatable causes (e.g. viral hepatitis, Wilson's disease and so on).

Pathogenesis

Although the liver has a remarkable capacity to adapt to injury through tissue repair, chronic injury results in inflammation, matrix deposition, necrosis and angiogenesis, all of which lead to fibrosis (**Fig. 34.21**). Liver injury causes necrosis and apoptosis, releasing cell contents and reactive oxygen species (ROS). This activates hepatic stellate cells and tissue macrophages through the CC-chemokine ligand 2–CC-chemokine receptor 2 (CCL2–CCR2) axis (see p. 1264). These cells phagocytose necrotic and apoptotic cells and secrete pro-inflammatory mediators, including transforming growth factor-beta (TGF-β); this leads to transdifferentiation of stellate cells to myofibroblasts and platelet-derived growth factor (PDGF), which stimulates myofibroblast proliferation. Macrophages degrade scar matrix by secretion of matrix metalloproteinases (MMPs), but this is inhibited by concurrent myofibroblast and macrophage production of tissue inhibitors of metalloproteinases (TIMPs). This results in progressive matrix deposition and scar accumulation. Increased gut permeability and hepatic lipopolysaccharide–Toll-like receptor 4 (LPS–TLR4) signalling also promotes fibrogenesis. Repetitive or chronic injury and inflammation perpetuate this process.

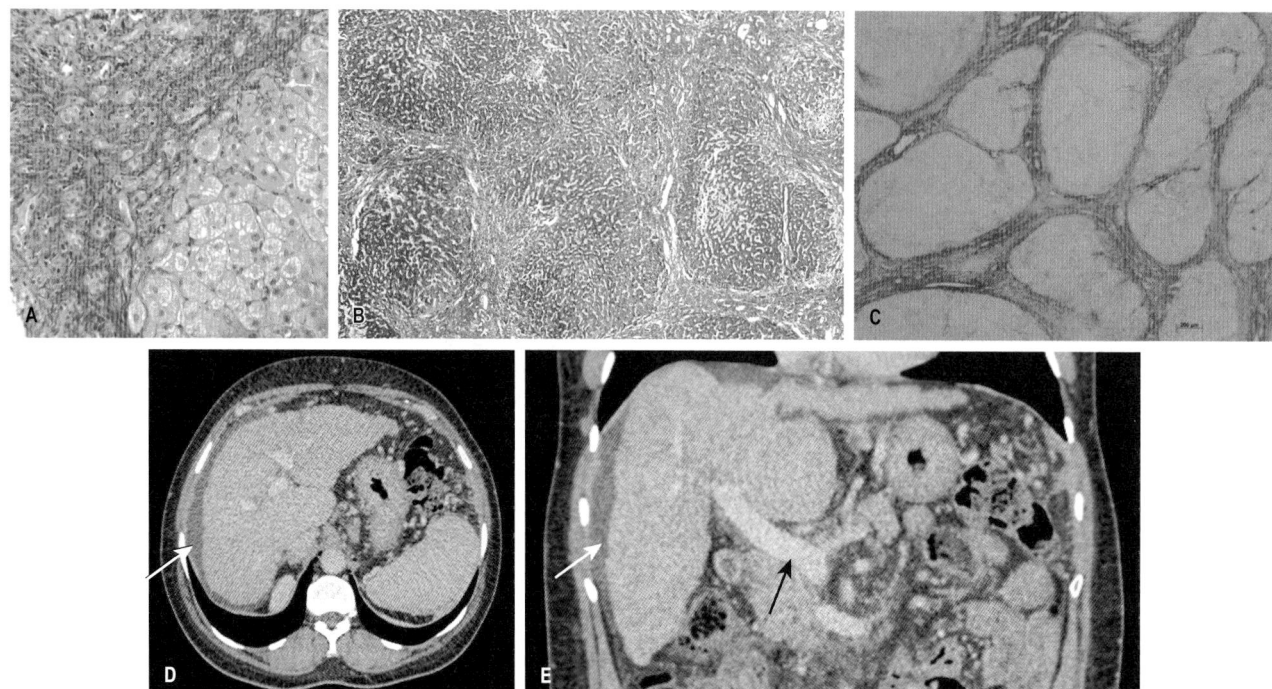

Fig. 34.22 Pathology of cirrhosis. (A) Haematoxylin and eosin histological view (×10). **(B)** Histological appearance (Giemsa stain) showing nodules of liver tissue of varying size, surrounded by fibrosis. **(C)** Picrosirius red stain of collagen used for morphometric evaluation of fibrosis. **(D)** Axial CT image showing an irregular contour of the liver consistent with cirrhosis. There are splenic, gastric and oesophageal varices and a small volume of ascites (arrowed). **(E)** Coronal CT image of the liver demonstrates an irregular contour to the liver consistent with cirrhosis. The portal vein is patent (black arrow). There is small-volume ascites (white arrow).

of the arterial vascular architecture. The patency of the portal and hepatic veins can be evaluated. Ultrasound is useful for detecting HCC.
- **Transient elastography** is increasingly used to avoid liver biopsy (see p. 1270). Technical limitations preclude its use in patients with ascites or morbid obesity but it is suitable for most. If the reading is high (>25), portal hypertension is likely, and some experts recommend that endoscopy to identify varices should be restricted to patients with high fibroscan scores.
- **CT scanning** (see p. 1270) is also helpful. **Fig. 34.22D–E** shows hepatosplenomegaly and the dilated collaterals seen in chronic liver disease. Arterial phase contrast-enhanced scans are useful for detecting HCC.
- **Endoscopy** is performed for the detection and treatment of varices and portal hypertensive gastropathy. If identified, varices can be treated by banding or injection sclerotherapy. Colonoscopy is occasionally carried out for colopathy.
- **MRI scanning** is useful in the diagnosis of both malignant and benign tumours such as haemangiomas. MR angiography can demonstrate the vascular anatomy, and MR cholangiography the biliary tree.

Liver biopsy

This remains the 'gold standard' for confirming the type and severity of liver disease. Adequate samples, in terms of length and number of complete portal tracts, are necessary for diagnosis and staging/grading of chronic viral hepatitis; in macronodular cirrhosis, the core of liver may fragment, causing sampling errors. Immunocytochemical stains can identify viruses, bile ducts, angiogenic structures and oncogenic markers. Chemical measurement of iron and copper is necessary to confirm a diagnosis of iron overload or Wilson's

disease. Digital image analysis of picrosirius red staining can be used to quantitate collagen in biopsy specimens (see **Fig. 34.22C**).

Management

Management is that of the complications of decompensated cirrhosis. Patients should undergo 6-monthly ultrasound to screen for the early development of HCC (see p. 1308), as all therapeutic strategies work best with small, single tumours.

Treatment of the underlying cause may arrest or reverse cirrhosis. Patients with compensated cirrhosis should lead a normal life. Those at risk should receive hepatitis A and B vaccination. The only dietary restriction is reduction of salt intake (≤2 g sodium per day). Alcohol should be avoided, as should aspirin and non-steroidal anti-inflammatory drugs (NSAIDs), which may precipitate gastrointestinal bleeding or renal impairment.

Prognosis

Prognosis is extremely variable. In general, the 5-year survival rate is approximately 50%, depending on the stage at which diagnosis is made. Poor prognostic indicators are shown in **Box 34.15**. Development of any complication usually worsens the prognosis.

There are a number of prognostic classifications based on modifications of Child's grading (A, B and C; **Box 34.16**) and the Model for End-stage Liver Disease (MELD; **Box 34.17**); these focus on serum bilirubin, creatinine and the INR, which is widely used as a predictor of mortality in patients awaiting liver transplantation. Modifications of the MELD score (e.g. UKELD) are used in some countries.

Acute-on-chronic liver failure

Acute-on-chronic liver failure (ACLF) refers to the condition of patients hospitalized for an acute complication of cirrhosis accompanied by organ failure(s); it has a high short-term mortality. ACLF is believed to be distinct from traditional decompensated cirrhosis, based not only on the presence of organ failure(s) and high mortality rate, but also on younger age, alcohol aetiology, higher prevalence of certain precipitating events (e.g. bacterial infections or active alcohol excess), and a higher level of systemic inflammation. It is estimated to occur in 31% of patients hospitalized with an acute complication of cirrhosis.

Liver assist devices

As the liver has great potential to regenerate, extracorporeal liver support devices may allow patients with liver failure to be bridged to recovery or even liver transplantation. Current approaches include the use of biological devices that contain hepatocytes and those that function as detoxification devices, and artificial liver support systems. However, no device is currently available routinely.

Gut–liver axis

The liver is exposed to gut-derived bacterial components that have little consequence in health, as an effective gut barrier limits the amount of bacterial components transported to the liver. In advanced liver disease the intestinal barrier function is compromised due to changes in gut motility, an increase in intestinal permeability, and suppression of gut immunological functions. This leads to bacteria and bacterial components (eg lipopolysaccharide) entering the portal circulation and being transported to the liver, activating Toll-like receptors and producing an inflammatory response. This cross-talk between the intestinal microbiota and the liver is referred to as the gut–liver axis; it is seen as a key pathophysiological mechanism in the progression of liver disease and development of the complications of cirrhosis. Antibiotics and non-selective beta-blockers intercept the gut–liver axis by **blocking bacterial translocation**, which is likely to account for their beneficial effects in reducing portal pressure, variceal haemorrhage and spontaneous bacterial peritonitis. However, absorbable antibiotics will lead to the selection of resistant bacteria. Rifaximin, a poorly absorbed antibiotic used for encephalopathy, specifically affects the gut flora and has a low risk for inducing resistance; it may therefore have a role in this indication.

Further reading

Leckie P, Davenport A, Jalan R. Extracorporeal liver support. *Blood Purif* 2012; 34:158–163.
Madsen BS, Havelund T, Krag A. Targeting the gut–liver axis in cirrhosis: antibiotics and non-selective β-blockers. *Adv Ther* 2013; 30:659–670.
Moreau R, Jalan R, Gines P et al and the CANONIC Study Investigators of the EASL–CLIF Consortium. Acute-on-chronic liver failure is a distinct syndrome that develops in patients with acute decompensation of cirrhosis. *Gastroenterology* 2013; 144:1426–1437.
Pellicoro A, Ramachandran P, Iredale JP et al. Liver fibrosis and repair: immune regulation of wound healing in a solid organ. *Nat Rev Immunol* 2014; 14:181–194.

Liver transplantation

This is the only established treatment for advanced liver disease. Shortage of donors is a major problem in all developed countries and in some, such as Japan or South Korea, living related donors form the majority.

Indications

These include:
- *acute liver disease*: acute hepatic failure of any cause (see p. 1286)
- *chronic liver disease*: usually for complications of cirrhosis that are no longer responsive to therapy.

The timing of transplantation depends on donor availability. All patients with end-stage cirrhosis (Child's grade C; MELD score ≥20; UKELD score ≥49) and those with debilitating symptoms should be referred to a transplant centre. In addition, specific extrahepatic complications of cirrhosis, even with preserved liver function, such as hepatopulmonary syndrome and porto-pulmonary hypertension, can be reversed by transplantation.
- *Primary biliary cholangitis.* Patients should be transplanted when their serum bilirubin is persistently >100 µmol/L or when they have symptoms such as intractable pruritus.
- *Chronic hepatitis B if HBV DNA-negative* or levels are falling with effective therapy. Following transplantation, recurrence of hepatitis is prevented by hepatitis B immunoglobulin and nucleoside analogues in combination.
- *Chronic hepatitis C.* Following the introduction of the directly acting antiviral drugs, rates of transplantation for HCV have fallen substantially; for example, a reduction from 10.5% in 2013 to 4.7% in 2016 was seen in the UK

- *Autoimmune hepatitis.* In patients who have failed to respond to medical treatment, the disease can recur.
- *Alcoholic liver disease.* Well-motivated patients who have stopped drinking without improvement of liver disease are offered a transplant, with frequent counselling. It has been shown that transplantation may represent life-saving treatment in patients with severe alcoholic hepatitis who are not responding to medical therapy. However, further studies are awaited. Early liver transplantation is an emerging therapy for acute severe alcoholic hepatitis, and multiple small studies have demonstrated that 'highly selected' patients have comparable 1- and 3-year survival to those with chronic liver disease following transplantation. However, not all caregivers agree that the usual expectation of demonstrated alcohol abstinence prior to transplantation should be waived and further data are needed.
- *Primary metabolic disorders.* Examples are Wilson's disease, hereditary haemochromatosis and α_1-antitrypsin deficiency.
- *NASH cirrhosis.* In view of the increasing rates of obesity, this is highly likely to become the most frequent indication for transplantation.
- *Other conditions*, such as primary sclerosing cholangitis, polycystic liver disease and metabolic diseases such as primary oxaluria.

Contraindications

Absolute contraindications include active sepsis outside the hepatobiliary tree, malignancy outside the liver, liver metastases (except neuroendocrine) and a lack of psychological commitment on the part of the patient.

Relative contraindications are mainly anatomical considerations that make surgery more difficult, such as extensive splanchnic venous thrombosis. With exceptions, patients aged 70 years or over are not usually given a transplant. In HCC the recurrence rate is high, unless there are fewer than three small (<3 cm) lesions or a solitary nodule of less than 5 cm (Milan criteria).

Preparation for surgery

Pre-transplant work-up includes confirmation of the diagnosis, ultrasound and cross-sectional imaging, and radiological demonstration of the hepatic arterial and biliary trees, as well as assessment of cardiorespiratory and renal status. In view of the ethical and financial implications of transplantation, regular psychosocial and possibly psychiatric support is vital.

The donor should be ABO-compatible (HLA matching is not necessary) and have no evidence of active sepsis, malignancy, or HIV, HBV or HCV infection. Younger donors (<50 years) experience better graft function. The donor liver is cooled and stored on ice; its preservation time may be up to 20 hours. The recipient operation takes approximately 8 hours and rarely requires a large blood transfusion. Cadaveric donor livers (from heart-beating or non-heart-beating donors) may consist of whole graft, split grafts (for two recipients) or reduced grafts. Live donors may be healthy individuals or patients with, for example, familial amyloid polyneuropathy, whose livers can be transplanted into others (domino transplant). The mortality of right lobe donors is between 1 in 200 and 1 in 400. Recent advances in devices for storing donated liver prior to transplantation may allow livers to be used that were previously considered unsuitable.

The operative mortality is very low and most postoperative deaths occur in the first 3 months. Sepsis and haemorrhage can be serious complications. Opportunistic infections occur owing to immunosuppression. Various immunosuppressive agents have been used: tacrolimus – alone or in combination with azathioprine or mycophenolate mofetil – steroids, sirolimus and micro-emulsified ciclosporin are the most common.

Rejection

- *Acute or cellular rejection* usually occurs 5–10 days post transplant; it can be asymptomatic or there may be a fever. On biopsy, a pleomorphic portal infiltrate is seen with prominent eosinophils, bile duct damage and endothelialitis of the blood vessels. This responds well to immunosuppressive therapy.
- *Chronic ductopenic rejection* is seen between 6 weeks and 9 months post transplant, with disappearing bile ducts (vanishing bile duct syndrome, VBDS), and an arteriopathy with narrowing and occlusion of the arteries. Early ductopenic rejection is rarely reversed by immunosuppression and often requires retransplantation.
- *Graft-versus-host disease* is extremely rare.

Prognosis

Elective liver transplantation in low-risk patients has a 90% 1-year survival and a 70–85% 5-year survival. Patients require life-long immunosuppression, although doses can be reduced over time without significant problems. Future strategies to reduce immunosuppression requirements after transplant may include infusion of autologous regulatory T cells. HCV cirrhosis, primary sclerosing cholangitis and HCC are conditions in which long-term survival after transplantation is compromised by disease recurrence.

Further reading

Artzner T, Michard B, Besch C et al. Liver transplantation for critically ill cirrhotic patients: overview and pragmatic proposals. *World J Gastroenterol* 2018; 24:5203–5214.
Lucey MR. Liver transplantation for alcoholic liver diseases. *Nat Rev Gastroenterol Hepatol* 2014; 11:300–307.

Complications and effects of cirrhosis

These are shown in **Box 34.18**.

Portal hypertension

The portal vein is formed by the union of the superior mesenteric and splenic veins. Normal pressure is 5–8 mmHg with only a small gradient across the liver to the hepatic vein, in which blood is returned to the heart via the inferior vena cava. Portal hypertension is classified according to the site of obstruction:

- *pre-hepatic* – blockage of the portal vein before the liver
- *intrahepatic* – distortion of the liver architecture, either pre-sinusoidal (e.g. schistosomiasis) or post-sinusoidal (e.g. cirrhosis)
- *post-hepatic* – venous blockage outside the liver (rare).

As portal pressure rises above 10–12 mmHg, the compliant venous system dilates and collaterals form within the systemic venous system. The main sites of collaterals are the gastro-oesophageal junction, rectum, left renal vein, diaphragm, retroperitoneum and the anterior abdominal wall via the umbilical vein.

The collaterals at the gastro-oesophageal junction (varices) are superficial and tend to rupture. Portosystemic anastomoses at other sites rarely cause symptoms. Rectal varices are frequently found (30%) if looked for and can be differentiated from haemorrhoids, which are lower in the anal canal. The microvasculature of the gut becomes congested, giving rise to portal hypertensive gastropathy and colopathy, in which there is punctate erythema and erosions, which can bleed.

> **Box 34.18 Complications and effects of cirrhosis**
>
> - Portal hypertension and gastrointestinal haemorrhage
> - Ascites
> - Portosystemic encephalopathy
> - Hepatocellular carcinoma
> - Bacteraemias, infections
> - Renal failure
> - Hepatopulmonary syndrome

> **Box 34.19 Causes of portal hypertension**
>
> **Prehepatic**
> - Portal vein thrombosis
>
> **Intrahepatic**
>
> *Pre-sinusoidal*
> - Schistosomiasis; sarcoidosis
> - Primary biliary cholangitis
>
> *Sinusoidal*
> - Cirrhosis (e.g. alcoholic)
> - Partial nodular transformation
> - Congenital hepatic fibrosis
>
> *Post-sinusoidal*
> - Veno-occlusive disease
> - Budd–Chiari syndrome
>
> **Post-hepatic**
> - Right heart failure (rare)
> - Constrictive pericarditis
> - Inferior vena cava obstruction

Pathophysiology

Following liver injury and fibrogenesis, the contraction of activated myofibroblasts (mediated by endothelin, nitric oxide and prostaglandins) contributes to increased resistance to blood flow. This increased resistance leads to portal hypertension and opening of portosystemic anastomoses in both pre-cirrhotic and cirrhotic livers. Neo-angiogenesis also occurs. The hyperdynamic circulation of cirrhosis (caused by nitric oxide, cannabinoids and glucagon) leads to peripheral and splanchnic vasodilation. This, combined with plasma volume expansion due to sodium retention (see p. 1295), has a significant effect on maintaining portal hypertension.

Aetiology

The most common cause is cirrhosis (**Box 34.19**). Others are described here.

Pre-hepatic causes

Extrahepatic blockage due to portal vein thrombosis can be caused by congenital portal venous abnormalities, neonatal sepsis of the umbilical vein or inherited prothrombotic conditions, such as factor V Leiden or primary myeloproliferative disorders with or without *JAK2* mutations (see p. 394).

Patients present with gastrointestinal bleeding, often at a young age. They have normal liver function and prognosis following bleeding is therefore excellent.

The portal vein blockage can be identified by ultrasound with Doppler imaging; CT and MR angiography are also used.

Treatment for variceal bleeding is usually repeated endoscopic therapy or non-selective beta-blockade. Splenectomy is performed only if there is isolated splenic vein thrombosis. Anticoagulation prevents further thrombosis and intestinal infarction, and does not increase the risk of bleeding.

Intrahepatic causes

Cirrhosis is by far the most common cause but others include:

- **Non-cirrhotic portal hypertension** is characterized by mild portal tract fibrosis on liver histology. The aetiology is unknown but arsenic, vinyl chloride, anti-retroviral therapy and other toxins have been implicated. A similar disease is frequently found in India. The liver lesion does not progress and prognosis is good.

- **Schistosomiasis** with extensive pipe-stem fibrosis occurs in endemic areas such as Egypt and Brazil. Often there is concomitant liver disease, such as HCV infection, which was transmitted by non-sterile equipment.
- **Other causes** include congenital hepatic fibrosis, and nodular regenerative hyperplasia and partial nodular transformation.

Post-hepatic causes

Prolonged severe heart failure with tricuspid incompetence or constrictive pericarditis can cause portal hypertension. The Budd–Chiari syndrome is described on page 1304.

Clinical features

Patients are often asymptomatic, the only clinical evidence being splenomegaly, although features of chronic liver disease may exist (see p. 1263).

Variceal haemorrhage

Approximately 90% of patients with cirrhosis will develop gastro-oesophageal varices over 10 years but only one-third of these will bleed. Bleeding is likely to occur with large varices, or in those with red signs at endoscopy, and in severe liver disease.

Management

Management can be divided into:
- the active bleeding episode
- prevention of rebleeding
- prophylactic measures to prevent the first haemorrhage.

Despite the therapeutic techniques available, prognosis ultimately depends on the severity of the underlying liver disease; overall 6-week mortality from variceal haemorrhage is 15–25%, reaching 50% in Child's grade C.

Initial management of acute variceal bleeding

See **Fig. 34.23**, and also the general management of gastrointestinal haemorrhage on page 1181.

Resuscitation

- **Assess** the patient: pulse, blood pressure and conscious state.
- Insert a **large-bore intravenous line** and obtain **blood** for group and crossmatching, haemoglobin, PT/INR, serum creatinine and electrolytes, liver biochemistry and blood cultures.
- **Restore blood volume** with plasma expanders or, if possible, blood transfusion. See the treatment of shock for more detail (p. 221). Prompt correction, but not over-correction, of hypovolaemia is necessary in cirrhosis patients, as their baroreceptor reflexes are diminished. A target haemoglobin of 80 g/L is sufficient and this lessens the likelihood of early rebleeding.
- Perform an **ascitic tap**.
- Monitor for alcohol withdrawal and treat with lorazepam or oxazepam (the half-life of chlordiazepoxide will increase in advanced liver disease, amplifying the risk of adverse events). Give intravenous thiamine.
- Start prophylactic antibiotics. These treat and prevent infection, and reduce early rebleeding and mortality.

Urgent endoscopy

Endoscopy (**Fig. 34.24**) should be performed to confirm the diagnosis and to exclude bleeding from other sites (e.g. gastric ulceration) and portal hypertensive gastropathy/gastric antral vascular ectasia (GAVE). The latter describes chronic gastric congestion, punctate erythema and gastric erosions, which may contribute to

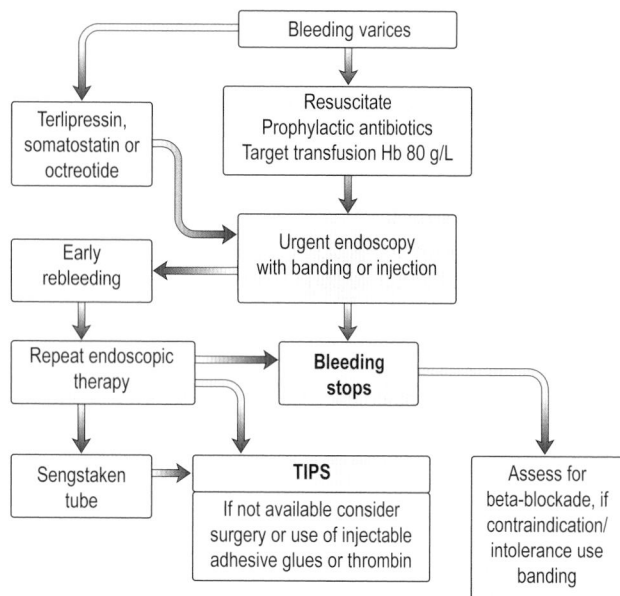

Fig. 34.23 **Management of gastrointestinal haemorrhage due to oesophageal varices.** Hb, haemoglobin; TIPS, transjugular intrahepatic portosystemic shunt.

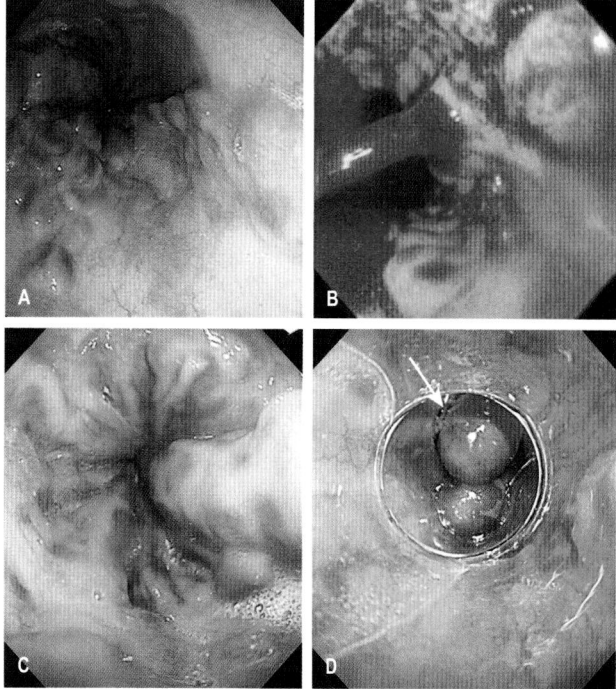

Fig. 34.24 **Endoscopic views of oesophageal varices.** **(A)** Gross varices. **(B)** Blood spurting from a varix. **(C)** Following a recent bleed. **(D)** Varices with a band in place (arrowed). *(A, C and D, Courtesy of Dr Peter Fairclough.)*

chronic anaemia. Portal hypertensive gastropathy and GAVE are distinct entities; management of portal hypertensive gastropathy is centred on reduction in portal pressures with beta-blockers, whereas treatment of GAVE is endoscopic and uses various ablative techniques.

Variceal banding or injection sclerotherapy

Banding of oesophageal varices is performed by mounting a band on the tip of the endoscope, sucking the varix into the end of the

scope, and dislodging the band over the varix using a trip-wire mechanism.

Between 15% and 20% of bleeding comes from gastric varices, which are associated with a greater mortality (up to 40%); endoscopic injection of cyanoacrylate is the best treatment.

Overall, haemostasis is achieved in 80–90% of patients. Best practice is to perform the endoscopy with the patient under general anaesthetic to provide appropriate airway support, and with critical care support.

Injection sclerotherapy is now rarely performed for oesophageal varices.

Other measures
Vasoconstrictor therapy

This is used to restrict portal inflow by splanchnic arterial constriction and has shown benefit when used in combination with endoscopic techniques.

- **Terlipressin.** This is the only vasoconstrictor proven to reduce mortality. The dose is 2 mg 6-hourly, reducing to 1 mg 4-hourly after 48 hours if a prolonged regimen is required (up to 5 days). Terlipressin should not be given to patients with ischaemic heart disease. The patient may complain of abdominal colic, and may defecate and have facial pallor owing to generalized vasoconstriction. If haemostasis has been achieved at endoscopy, there is probably little added benefit with this therapy, and treatment should be tapered accordingly.
- **Somatostatin.** This has few side-effects. Infusion of 250–500 µg/h reduces bleeding and is reserved for patients with contraindications to terlipressin.

A recent prospective, multicentre study showed that haemostatic effects and safety at day 5 of treatment did not differ significantly between terlipressin, somatostatin and octreotide when utilized as adjuvants to endoscopic treatment.

Balloon tamponade

Balloon tamponade is used if endoscopic therapy has failed or if there is exsanguinating haemorrhage. The usual balloon tube is a four-lumen Sengstaken–Blakemore, which should be left in place for no more than 12 hours and removed in the endoscopy room prior to follow-up endoscopy. The tube is passed into the stomach and the gastric balloon inflated with air and pulled back. It should be positioned in close apposition to the gastro-oesophageal junction to prevent the cephalad variceal blood flow to the bleeding point. The oesophageal balloon should be inflated only if bleeding is not controlled by the gastric balloon alone.

Haemostasis is achieved in up to 90%. However, the balloon may cause serious complications, such as aspiration pneumonia, oesophageal rupture and mucosal ulceration. The procedure is also very unpleasant for the patient.

A self-expanding covered metal stent (Danis), which has a wire loop to enable removal and is introduced orally or endoscopically, can be placed over the varices. This is effective and has the advantages that it does not impair swallowing, cannot be removed by uncooperative patients and allows post-endoscopic investigation. The stent is removed 7 days after insertion. A randomized trial in 28 patients showed that oesophageal stents may have greater efficacy with less adverse events than balloon tamponade in the control of variceal bleed following endoscopic failure.

Additional management of the acute episode

- **Measures to prevent encephalopathy.** Portosystemic encephalopathy (PSE) can be precipitated by a large bleed (blood contains protein). Management is as outlined on page 1297.

- **Nursing.** Patients require high-dependency/intensive care nursing. They should remain nil by mouth until bleeding has stopped.
- **Reduction in acid secretion.** Ranitidine may be preferable to PPIs, as it lessens the risk of *Clostridium difficile* infection; PPIs are widely used, however. Sucralfate 1 g four times daily can reduce oesophageal ulceration following endoscopic therapy.

Management of an acute rebleed

Rebleeding occurs in approximately 15–20% within 5 days. The source should be established by endoscopy and sometimes takes the form of ulceration or slippage of a ligation band. Endoscopy should be performed once only to control *re*bleeding. If haemostasis cannot be achieved, then transjugular intrahepatic portocaval shunting will be necessary.

Transjugular intrahepatic portocaval shunt

Transjugular intrahepatic portocaval shunt (TIPS) is used when bleeding cannot be controlled either acutely or following a rebleed. Under X-ray guidance, a guidewire is passed from the jugular vein into the liver and the portal vein. After balloon expansion of the tract between the hepatic and portal veins, an expandable, covered metal shunt is placed over the wire to form a channel between the systemic and portal venous systems. It reduces the hepatic sinusoidal and portal vein pressure by creating a total shunt. There is an increased risk of portal systemic encephalopathy. Stent stenosis or thrombosis is far less frequent now that 'covered' stents are used, as opposed to the 'bare metal' stents employed previously. Collaterals arising from the splenic or portal veins can be selectively embolized.

A recent observational study in 671 patients validated the survival benefit of 'pre-emptive' TIPS (within 72 hours of admission) in those with cirrhosis and acute variceal haemorrhage, and at high risk for treatment failure. Most of the benefit was seen in patients with Child–Pugh class C disease. However, widespread implementation of this approach represents a significant challenge for many healthcare systems, and despite strong supporting evidence, most centres have not adopted it at present.

Emergency surgery

This is performed very rarely when other measures fail. Oesophageal transection and ligation of the feeding vessels to the bleeding varices or acute portosystemic shunt surgery is performed.

Prevention of recurrent variceal bleeding (secondary prophylaxis)

The risk of bleeding recurring without prophylaxis is 60–80% over a 2-year period, with an approximate mortality of 20% per episode.

Prophylactic long-term measures
Non-selective beta-blockade

Oral propranolol or carvedilol to reduce the resting pulse rate by 25% decreases portal pressure. Portal inflow is reduced by a decrease in cardiac output (β_1) and by blockade of β_2 vasodilator receptors on the splanchnic arteries, leaving an unopposed vasoconstrictor effect. Significant reduction of hepatic venous pressure gradient (HVPG, measured by hepatic vein catheterization) is associated with very low rates of rebleeding, particularly if below 12 mmHg. Data have emerged demonstrating that additional α_1-adrenergic blockade, causing vasodilation with carvedilol, may increase the number of patients with a reduction in HVPG compared to propranolol.

Endoscopic treatment

Repeated courses of banding at 2-weekly intervals lead to obliteration of varices. This markedly reduces rebleeding, most instances occurring before the varices have been fully obliterated. Between 30% and 40% of varices return per year, so follow-up endoscopy should be performed at 1–3 months after obliteration and then every 6–12 months. Complications of banding include oesophageal ulceration, mediastinitis and, rarely, strictures.

Combination therapy reduces overall bleeding compared to endoscopic therapy alone but with no overall improvement in mortality. A pragmatic approach is therefore to give combination therapy to those who can tolerate beta-blockade, and band ligation alone to those who cannot.

Surgery

- **Surgical portosystemic shunting** is associated with an extremely low risk of rebleeding and is used if TIPS is not available. Hepatic encephalopathy is a significant complication. The 'shunts' are usually an end-to-side portocaval anastomosis or a selective distal splenorenal shunt (Warren shunt).
- **Devascularization procedures**, including oesophageal transection, do not produce encephalopathy and can be used when there is splanchnic venous thrombosis.
- **Liver transplantation** (see p. 1291) is the best option when there is poor liver function.

Prophylactic measures (primary prophylaxis)

Patients with cirrhosis and significant varices that have not bled should be prescribed non-selective beta-blockers. This reduces the chances of upper gastrointestinal bleeding by approximately 50%, may increase survival and is cost-effective. If there are contraindications, variceal banding is an option. Two large-scale trials were due to start in the UK in 2020 and aimed to clarify the best approach for primary prophylaxis. It was anticipated that these studies would complete by 2026.

Ascites

Ascites, fluid within the peritoneal cavity, is a common complication of cirrhosis. Several factors underlie its pathogenesis:

- **Sodium and water retention** results from peripheral arterial vasodilation (secondary to nitric oxide, atrial natriuretic peptide and prostaglandins), which causes a reduction in the effective blood volume. This reduction activates the sympathetic nervous system and the renin–angiotensin system, promoting salt and water retention (see **Fig. 9.6**).
- **Portal hypertension** exerts a local hydrostatic pressure, leading to increased hepatic and splanchnic production of lymph, and transudation of fluid into the peritoneal cavity.
- **Low serum albumin** (due to poor liver function) may further contribute by reducing plasma oncotic pressure.

In patients with ascites, urine sodium excretion rarely exceeds 5 mmol in 24 hours. Loss of sodium from extrarenal sites accounts for approximately 30 mmol in 24 hours. Under these circumstances, a normal daily sodium intake of 120–200 mmol results in a positive sodium balance of approximately 90–170 mmol in 24 hours (equivalent to 600–1300 mL of fluid retained).

Clinical features

Abdominal swelling may develop over days or several weeks. Precipitating factors include continued excessive alcohol consumption, infection/sepsis, development of an HCC or splanchnic vein thrombosis. Mild abdominal pain and discomfort are common but, if more severe, should raise the suspicion of SBP (see later). Respiratory distress and difficulty eating accompany tense ascites.

The presence of fluid is confirmed clinically by demonstrating shifting dullness. Many patients also have peripheral oedema. A pleural effusion (usually right-sided) may infrequently be found and arises from the passage of ascites through congenital diaphragmatic defects.

Investigations

A diagnostic aspiration of 10–20 mL of fluid should be obtained for:

- **Cell count.** A neutrophil count >250 cells/mm^3 is indicative of an underlying (usually spontaneous) bacterial peritonitis.
- **Gram stain and culture.**
- **Protein measurement.** A high serum–ascites albumin gradient of >11 g/L suggests portal hypertension, while a low gradient of <11 g/L is associated with non-liver disease-related abnormalities of the peritoneum, such as neoplasia (**Box 34.20**).
- **Cytology.** A search should be made for malignant cells.
- **Amylase.** Pancreatic ascites should be excluded.
  The differential diagnosis of ascites is listed in **Box 34.21**.

Management

The aim is both to reduce sodium intake and to increase renal sodium excretion, producing a net reabsorption of fluid from the ascites into the circulating volume. The maximum rate at which ascites can be mobilized is 500–700 mL in 24 hours (see later).

- **Serum electrolytes, creatinine and estimated glomerular filtration rate (eGFR).** Check on alternate days; weigh the patient and measure urinary output daily.
- **Bed rest.** This will cause a diuresis by improving renal perfusion but is rarely helpful.
- **Dietary sodium restriction.** It is possible to reduce sodium intake to 40 mmol in 24 hours and still maintain an adequate protein and calorie intake with a palatable diet.
- **Drugs.** Many contain significant amounts of sodium (up to 50 mmol daily). Examples include antacids and antibiotics (particularly penicillins and cephalosporins). Sodium-retaining drugs (NSAIDs, corticosteroids) should be avoided.
- **Fluid restriction.** This is unnecessary unless the serum sodium is <128 mmol/L (see later).
- **Diuretics.** The diuretic of choice is the aldosterone antagonist spironolactone, starting at 100 mg daily. Chronic administration produces gynaecomastia. Eplerenone 25 mg once daily does not cause gynaecomastia.

The aim of diuretic therapy should be to produce a net loss of fluid approaching 700 mL in 24 hours (0.7 kg weight loss, or 1.0 kg if peripheral oedema is present). Although 60% of patients respond on this regimen, the spironolactone can be increased gradually to 400 mg

daily if necessary, providing there is no hyperkalaemia. Urinary sodium may be used to titrate the dose. A loop diuretic, such as furosemide 20–40 mg or bumetanide 0.5 mg or 1 mg daily, is added if response is poor. These loop diuretics have several potential disadvantages, including hyponatraemia, hypokalaemia and volume depletion.

Diuretics should be temporarily discontinued if a rise in serum creatinine occurs, representing over-diuresis and hypovolaemia, or if there is hyperkalaemia or worsening encephalopathy. Hyponatraemia almost always represents haemodilution secondary to a failure to clear free water (usually a marker of reduced renal perfusion), and diuretics should be stopped if the sodium falls below 128 mmol/L. Vaptans (see p. 180), vasopressin V_2-receptor antagonists that increase free water clearance, have a small beneficial effect on hyponatraemia and ascites but do not affect mortality, complications of cirrhosis or renal failure; routine use in cirrhosis cannot be recommended.

Paracentesis

This is used when symptomatic tense ascites needs to be relieved or diuretic therapy is insufficient to control accumulation of fluid. The main complications are hypovolaemia and renal dysfunction (post-paracentesis circulatory dysfunction), predominantly due to an accentuation of the arteriolar vasodilation already present in these patients; this is more likely when more than 5 L are removed and with worse liver function. In patients with normal renal function and without hyponatraemia, this is overcome by infusing albumin (8 g/L of ascitic fluid removed). In practice, up to 20 L can be removed over 4–6 hours, with albumin infusion.

Shunts

A TIPS may be inserted to treat resistant ascites, providing there is no spontaneous portosystemic encephalopathy and there is minimal disturbance of renal function. Frequency of paracentesis and diuretic use is reduced and nutrition is enhanced. Survival may also improve.

A peritoneo-bladder conduit, by means of an implantable, rechargeable, battery-powered pump, has been developed for use in patients with advanced cirrhosis and resistant ascites (Alfapump). This removes ascites from the peritoneal cavity into the urinary bladder, to be eliminated through urination. Early studies have shown a reduction in the need for large-volume paracentesis but several complications, including pain and infection, occur.

Box 34.21 Causes of ascites according to type of ascitic fluid

Straw-coloured
- Malignancy (most common cause)
- Cirrhosis
- Infective:
  - Tuberculosis
  - Following intra-abdominal perforation – any bacterium may be found (e.g. *Escherichia coli*)
  - Spontaneous in cirrhosis
- Hepatic vein obstruction (Budd–Chiari syndrome) – protein level high in fluid
- Chronic pancreatitis
- Congestive cardiac failure
- Constrictive pericarditis

- Meigs' syndrome (ovarian tumour)
- Hypoproteinaemia (e.g. nephrotic syndrome)

Chylous
- Obstruction of main lymphatic duct (e.g. by carcinoma) – chylomicrons are present
- Cirrhosis

Haemorrhagic
- Malignancy
- Ruptured ectopic pregnancy
- Abdominal trauma
- Acute pancreatitis

Box 34.20 Serum–ascites albumin gradient

High serum–ascites albumin gradient (>11 g/L)	Low serum–ascites albumin gradient (<11 g/L)
• Portal hypertension, e.g. hepatic cirrhosis	• Peritoneal carcinomatosis
• Hepatic outflow obstruction	• Peritoneal tuberculosis
• Budd–Chiari syndrome	• Pancreatitis
• Hepatic veno-occlusive disease	• Nephrotic syndrome
• Tricuspid regurgitation	
• Constrictive pericarditis	
• Right-sided heart failure	

(Modified from Chung RT, Iafrate AJ, Amrein PC et al. Case records of the Massachusetts General Hospital. N Engl J Med 2006; 354:2166–2175.)

In patients requiring end-of-life care, insertion of a long-term abdominal drain (LTADs) may allow ascites management outside of a hospital setting. Although not formally evaluated in cirrhosis, they have been used successfully in patients whose ascites is due to malignancy.

Spontaneous bacterial peritonitis

Spontaneous bacterial peritonitis (SBP) represents a serious complication that is an indication for referral for transplant assessment; it occurs in up to 18% of patients with ascites who have undergone decompensation. The infecting organisms gain access to the peritoneum by haematogenous spread; most are *Escherichia coli*, *Klebsiella* or enterococci. The condition should be suspected in any patient with ascites who deteriorates, as pain and pyrexia are frequently absent. Diagnostic aspiration should always be performed. A raised neutrophil count in ascites is sufficient evidence alone to start immediate treatment. A broad-spectrum antibiotic is used, with subsequent alteration according to culture results *in combination with infusions of human albumin solution*. Evidence has emerged that non-selective beta-blockers should be stopped following diagnosis of SBP, as prescription increases the risk of renal impairment. Mortality is 10–15%. Recurrence is common (70% within a year) and secondary prevention – for example, with norfloxacin 400 mg daily – prolongs survival. Primary prophylaxis of SBP in patients with ascites protein below 10 g/L or severe liver disease may prevent hepatorenal syndrome and improve survival.

Portosystemic encephalopathy

Portosystemic encephalopathy (PSE) is a chronic neuropsychiatric syndrome that is secondary to cirrhosis. Acute encephalopathy can occur in acute hepatic failure (see p. 1285). PSE can arise in portal hypertensive patients due to spontaneous 'shunting', or in those with surgical or TIPS shunts.

Pathogenesis

In cirrhosis, the portal blood bypasses the liver via collaterals, and 'toxic' metabolites pass directly to the brain to produce encephalopathy. Ammonia-induced alteration of brain neurotransmitter balance, especially at the astrocyte–neurone interface, is considered to be the leading pathophysiological mechanism. Ammonia is produced by the breakdown of protein by intestinal bacteria. Other implicated substances are free fatty acids and mercaptans; accumulation of false neurotransmitters (octopamine) or activation of the γ-aminobutyric acid (GABA) inhibitory neurotransmitter system may also be responsible. Increased blood levels of aromatic amino acids (tyrosine and phenylalanine) and reduced branched-chain amino acids (valine, leucine and isoleucine) also occur. The factors precipitating PSE are shown in **Box 34.22**.

Clinical features

An acute onset often has a precipitating factor (**Box 34.22**). The patient becomes increasingly drowsy and comatose.

Chronically, there is a disorder of personality, mood and intellect, with a reversal of normal sleep rhythm. These changes may fluctuate and a collateral history should be obtained. The patient is irritable, confused and disorientated, and has slow, slurred speech. General features include nausea, vomiting and weakness. There is hyper-reflexia and increased tone. Coma occurs as the encephalopathy becomes more marked. Convulsions are very rare, and if they do occur, other causes must be considered.

Signs include:
- fetor hepaticus (a sweet smell to the breath)

> **ⓘ Box 34.22** Factors precipitating portosystemic encephalopathy
>
> - High dietary protein
> - Gastrointestinal haemorrhage
> - Constipation
> - Infection, including spontaneous bacterial peritonitis
> - Fluid and electrolyte disturbance due to diuretic therapy or paracentesis
> - Drugs (e.g. any central nervous system depressant)
> - Portosystemic shunt operations, TIPS
> - Any surgical procedure
> - Progressive liver damage
> - Development of hepatocellular carcinoma
>
> TIPS, transjugular intrahepatic portocaval shunt.

- a coarse flapping tremor seen when the hands are outstretched and wrists hyperextended (asterixis)
- constructional apraxia, with the patient being unable to write or draw a five-pointed star, for example
- decreased mental function, which can be assessed by using the serial sevens test or a trail-making (or connection) test.

Investigations

Diagnosis is clinical.

Additional investigations
- **EEG** shows a decrease in the frequency of the normal α-waves (8–13 Hz) to 1.5–3 Hz. These changes occur before coma supervenes.
- **Visual evoked responses** (see p. 830) also detect subclinical encephalopathy.
- **Arterial blood ammonia** can be useful for the differential diagnosis of coma and for following a patient with PSE, but is not always available.

Management
- **Identify and remove the possible precipitating cause**, such as cerebral depressant drugs, constipation or electrolyte imbalance due to over-diuresis.
- **Give purgation and enemas** to empty the bowels of nitrogenous substances. Lactulose (10–30 mL three times daily) is an osmotic purgative that reduces the colonic pH and limits ammonia absorption. Lactilol (β-galactoside sorbitol 30 g daily) is metabolized by colonic bacteria and is comparable in efficacy.
- **Maintain nutrition**, if necessary via a fine-bore nasogastric tube, and do not restrict protein for more than 48 hours.
- **Give antibiotics.** Rifaximin is a poorly absorbed semisynthetic antibiotic based on rifamycin that has a beneficial effect on secondary prevention of PSE. Metronidazole (200 mg four times daily) may be effective acutely. Neomycin should be avoided.
- **Stop or reduce diuretic therapy.**
- **Give intravenous fluids** as necessary (beware of too much sodium).
- **Treat infection.**
- **Increase protein** in the diet to the limit of tolerance as encephalopathy improves.
- **Embolize collaterals.** In selected patients, embolization of collaterals that bypass the liver may improve liver blood flow and reduce encephalopathy but careful case selection is mandatory.

Prognosis

Acute encephalopathy in acute hepatic failure has a very poor prognosis associated with that of the disease itself. In cirrhosis, chronic PSE adversely affects prognosis but the course is very variable. Very rarely with chronic portosystemic shunting, an organic syndrome with cerebellar signs or choreoathetosis develops, as well as myelopathy leading to a spastic paraparesis due to demyelination. These patients require referral to a liver transplant centre.

Renal failure (hepatorenal syndrome)

The hepatorenal syndrome typically occurs in patients with advanced cirrhosis, portal hypertension, jaundice and ascites. The urine output is low with a low urinary sodium concentration, a maintained capacity to concentrate urine (i.e. intact tubular function) and almost normal renal histology. The renal failure is therefore described as 'functional'. It is often precipitated by over-vigorous diuretic therapy, NSAIDs, diarrhoea, paracentesis and infection, particularly SBP.

The mechanism is similar to that of ascites, with extreme peripheral vasodilation leading to decreased effective blood volume and consequent hypotension (see p. 1295). This causes increased plasma renin, aldosterone, noradrenaline (norepinephrine) and vasopressin, leading to renal vasoconstriction. There is an increased pre-glomerular vascular resistance that causes blood to be directed away from the renal cortex. This leads to a reduced GFR and plasma renin remains high. Salt and water retention occurs, with reabsorption of sodium from the renal tubules.

Eicosanoids have been incriminated in the pathogenesis, supported by precipitation of the syndrome by inhibitors of prostaglandin synthase, such as NSAIDs.

Diuretic therapy should be stopped and intravascular hypovolaemia corrected, preferably with albumin. Terlipressin or noradrenaline with intravenous albumin improves renal function in approximately 50%. Liver transplantation is the best option. In patients who are candidates for transplantation, haemodialysis can be used as a bridging option but is frequently difficult to perform, and survival is generally limited by the severity of the hepatic failure.

Hepatopulmonary syndrome

This is hypoxaemia in patients with advanced liver disease due to intrapulmonary vascular dilation with no evidence of primary pulmonary disease. The patients have features of cirrhosis with spider naevi and clubbing, as well as cyanosis. Most are asymptomatic, but with more severe disease become breathless on standing. Transthoracic echocardiography shows intrapulmonary shunting and arterial blood gases confirm hypoxaemia. These changes are improved with liver transplantation.

Porto-pulmonary hypertension

This occurs in 1–2% of patients with cirrhosis and portal hypertension. It may respond to medical therapy (e.g. intravenous epoprostenol, or oral bosentan and sildenafil). Severe pulmonary hypertension is a contraindication to liver transplantation.

Primary hepatocellular carcinoma

This is discussed on page 1308.

Further reading

Hadjihambi A, Khetan V, Jalan R. Pharmacotherapy for hyperammonemia. *Expert Opin Pharmacother* 2014; 15:1685–1695.
Kimer N, Krag A, Moller S et al. Systematic review with meta-analysis: the effects of rifaximin in hepatic encephalopathy. *Aliment Pharmacol Ther* 2014; 40:123–132.
Rodriguez-Roisin R, Krowka MJ. Hepatopulmonary syndrome. *N Engl J Med* 2008; 358:2378–2387.

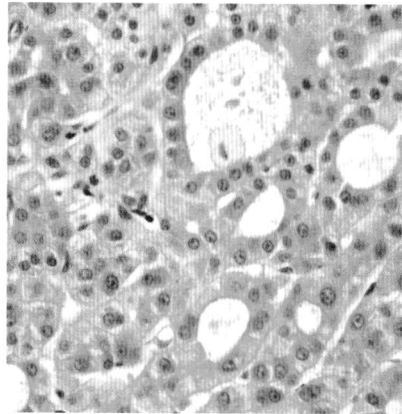

Fig. 34.25 Primary biliary cholangitis. Portal tract inflammation with lymphocytes and plasma cells (haematoxylin and eosin, ×10).

Turon F, Casu S, Hernández-Gea V et al. Variceal and other portal hypertension related bleeding. *Best Pract Res Clin Gastroenterol* 2013; 27:649–664.
Wijdicks EFM, Hepatic encephalopathy New Engl J Med 216;375:1660-1670

Types of cirrhosis

Alcoholic cirrhosis

This is discussed on page 1303.

Primary biliary cholangitis

Primary biliary cholangitis (PBC; **Fig. 34.25**) is a chronic disorder with progressive destruction of small interlobular bile ducts, leading to cirrhosis. Women aged 40–50 years constitute 90% of patients. PBC is diagnosed increasingly frequently in its milder forms. The prevalence is approximately 7.5 per 100 000, with a 1–6% increase in first-degree relatives. PBC has been called 'chronic non-suppurative destructive cholangitis', a term more descriptive of the early lesion, which emphasizes the fact that true cirrhosis occurs only in the later stages.

Aetiology

The aetiology is unknown but an immunological basis is well described. Serum anti-mitochondrial antibodies (AMA) are found in almost all patients. The mitochondrial antigen M2 is specific to PBC and five M2-specific antigens have been identified. The presence of AMA in high titre is unrelated to the clinical or histological picture and its role in pathogenesis is unclear. Antibodies against nuclear antigens, such as anti-gp210, are present in 50% of patients and correlate with progression towards liver failure.

It seems likely that an environmental factor acts on a genetically predisposed host via molecular mimicry, initiating autoimmunity. *E. coli* and *Novosphingobium aromaticivorans* antibodies are present in high titre.

Synthesis of IgM is increased, thought to be due to failure of the switch from IgM to IgG antibody synthesis. No specific associated class II major histocompatibility complex (MHC) loci have been found.

Clinical features

Asymptomatic patients are discovered on routine examination or screening, and may have hepatomegaly, a raised serum ALP or autoantibodies.

Pruritus is often the earliest symptom. Fatigue, which is frequently disabling, may accompany the pruritus, particularly in progressive cases. When jaundice appears, hepatomegaly is usually

present. Pigmented xanthelasma on eyelids or deposits of cholesterol in the creases of the hands may be seen.

Associated disorders

Autoimmune disorders (e.g. Sjögren's syndrome, scleroderma, thyroid disease) occur with increased frequency. Keratoconjunctivitis
sicca (dry eyes and mouth) is seen in 70% of cases. Renal tubular acidosis, membranous glomerulonephritis, coeliac disease and
interstitial pneumonitis are also associations.

Investigations

- *Mitochondrial antibodies* – measured routinely by ELISA (in
  titres >1 : 160) – are present in over 95% of patients; M2 antibody
  is 98% specific. Other non-specific antibodies (e.g. anti-nuclear
  factor and smooth muscle) may also be present.
- *High serum alkaline phosphatase* is often the only liver
  biochemistry abnormality.
- *Serum cholesterol* is raised.
- *Serum IgM* may be very high.
- *Ultrasound* can show a diffuse alteration in liver architecture.
- *Liver biopsy* shows characteristic histological features of a
  portal tract infiltrate, mainly of lymphocytes and plasma cells;
  approximately 40% have granulomas. Most of the early changes
  are in zone 1. Later, there is damage to and loss of small bile
  ducts with ductular proliferation. Portal tract fibrosis and,
  eventually, cirrhosis are seen.
  Hepatic granulomas are also seen in sarcoidosis, tuberculosis,
  schistosomiasis, drug reactions, brucellosis and parasitic infestation (e.g. strongyloidiasis).

Differential diagnosis

The classical picture presents little difficulty with diagnosis (and can
be confirmed by biopsy, although this is necessary only in doubtful
cases). A group of patients with the histological changes of PBC but
the serology of autoimmune hepatitis are termed as having autoimmune cholangitis and respond to steroids and azathioprine.

In the jaundiced patient, extrahepatic biliary obstruction should
be excluded by ultrasound or MRCP.

Management

- *Ursodeoxycholic acid* (10–15 mg/kg) improves bilirubin
  and aminotransferase levels. It should be given early in the
  asymptomatic phase, as these patients benefit, whereas no
  benefit is achieved in advanced disease. In patients who do
  not respond to ursodeoxycholic acid, obeticholic acid may
  be considered, but this drug is associated with increases in
  cholesterol and may exacerbate itching.
- *Steroids* improve biochemical and histological disease but
  cause osteoporosis and other side-effects, and so should not
  be used.
- Malabsorption of *fat-soluble vitamins (A, D and K)* occurs and
  supplementation is required.
- *Bisphosphonates* are needed for osteoporosis. Despite
  raised serum lipid concentrations, PBC is not associated
  with an increased cardiovascular disease risk, and strategies
  for prevention of vascular events should be tailored to the
  individual.
- Pruritus is difficult to control; *colestyramine* is helpful, although
  unpalatable. *Rifampicin*, and *naloxone* and *naltrexone* (opioid
  antagonists) have been shown to be of benefit. Intractable
  pruritus can be relieved by plasmapheresis or a molecular
  absorbent recirculating system (MARS).

- The lack of effective medical therapy has made PBC a major
  indication for *liver transplantation* (see p. 1291).
- Fatigue is common and can be severely debilitating; there is no
  proven therapy and transplantation does not improve symptoms.
  Modafinil, used for narcolepsy, has shown promise but has yet
  to be evaluated in randomized studies; it may cause significant
  side-effects and has addictive potential.

Complications

Complications are those of cirrhosis. In addition, osteoporosis and,
rarely, osteomalacia and a polyneuropathy occur.

Prognosis

Prognosis is very variable. Asymptomatic patients and those presenting with pruritus only will survive for more than 20 years. Symptomatic patients with jaundice have a more rapidly progressive
course and may die of liver failure or bleeding varices within 5 years.
Liver transplantation should therefore be offered when the serum
bilirubin is persistently above 100 µmol/L.

Primary sclerosing cholangitis

Primary sclerosing cholangitis (PSC) is a chronic cholestatic liver
disease characterized by fibrosing inflammatory destruction of both
the intra- and extrahepatic bile ducts. In 75% of patients, PSC is
associated with inflammatory bowel disease (usually ulcerative colitis); it is not unusual for PSC to predate the onset of inflammatory
bowel disease. The causes are unknown but genetic susceptibility
to PSC is associated with the HLA-A1-B8-DR3 haplotype. The autoantibody pANCA (anti-neutrophil cytoplasmic antibody) is found in
the serum of 60% of cases. Seventy per cent of patients are men
and the average age of onset is approximately 40 years. Secondary
PSC is seen in patients with HIV and cryptosporidium (see p. 1444),
and may follow ketamine misuse.

Clinical features

With increasing screening of patients who have inflammatory bowel
disease, PSC is detected at an asymptomatic phase with abnormal
liver biochemistry, usually a raised serum ALP. Symptomatic presentation is usually with fluctuating pruritus, jaundice and cholangitis.

Diagnosis

The typical biliary changes associated with PSC may be identified
by MRCP. The cholangiogram characteristically shows irregularity of
calibre of both intra- and extrahepatic ducts, although either may be
involved alone (**Fig. 34.26**).

Pathology

Histology can be contributory; it shows inflammation of the intrahepatic biliary radicles with associated scar tissue, classically
described as having the appearance of 'onion skin'. These changes
range from minor inflammatory infiltrates to the level of established
cirrhosis.

Management

PSC is a slowly progressive lesion (symptoms and biochemical
tests may fluctuate), which ultimately leads to liver cirrhosis and
associated decompensation. Recurrent cholangitis may be a feature before the onset of cirrhosis. Cholangiocarcinoma occurs in up
to 15% of patients (see pp. 1308 and 1322).

The only proven treatment is liver transplantation. Ursodeoxycholic acid, a bile acid, has been evaluated extensively but there
is no evidence of benefit. High-dose therapy (30 mg/kg) may be

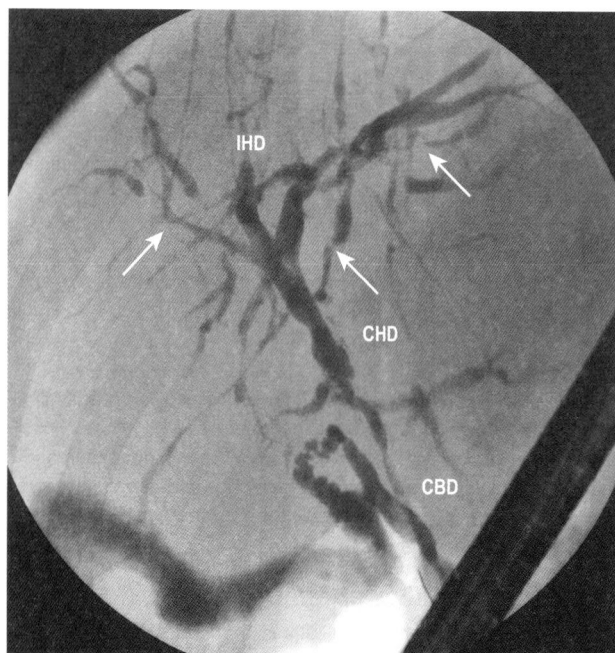

Fig. 34.26 Primary sclerosing cholangitis. An endoscopic cholangiogram showing the typical features of primary sclerosing cholangitis. There are calibre irregularities of the intrahepatic ducts (IHD). There is also minor stricturing of the extrahepatic ducts at the confluence between the common bile duct (CBD) and the common hepatic duct (CHD).

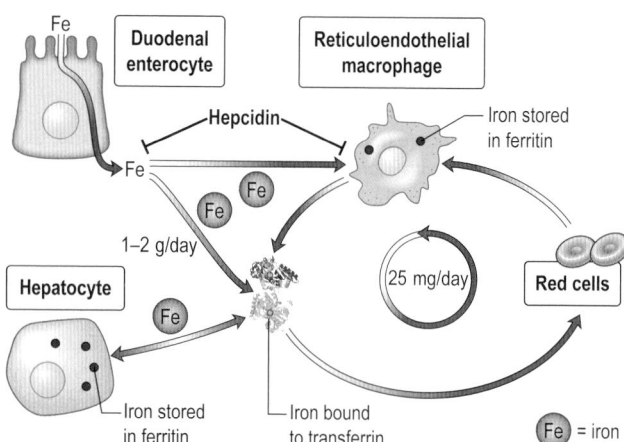

Fig. 34.27 The circulation of iron from the duodenal enterocyte to and from the liver, red cells and reticuloendothelial macrophages. Some 1–2 g of iron is absorbed from the intestine (see **Fig. 16.8**) and circulates bound to transferrin. The reticuloendothelial cells clear old erythrocytes and release iron to circulate and be stored as ferritin in the liver. The liver is the major site of production of the peptide hormone hepcidin. Hepcidin blocks release of iron from the erythrocytes and macrophages by degrading the iron exporter transferrin. Fe, iron. *(Modified from Fleming RE, Ponka P. Iron overload in human disease. N Engl J Med 2012; 366:348–359, with permission.)*

deleterious. In a small minority the dominant lesion is sited in the extrahepatic ducts (see **Fig. 34.26**). Such lesions may be amenable to endoscopic biliary intervention with balloon dilation and temporary stent placement (see p. 1321).

Secondary biliary cirrhosis

Cirrhosis can result from prolonged (for months) large-duct biliary obstruction. Causes include bile duct strictures, gallstones and sclerosing cholangitis. An ultrasound examination and MRCP, sometimes followed by ERCP or percutaneous transhepatic cholangiography (where the ducts are cannulated under ultrasound guidance through the skin) if cannulation is difficult, are performed to outline the ducts, and any remedial cause is treated.

Hereditary haemochromatosis

Hereditary haemochromatosis (HH; see also p. 1269) is an inherited disease characterized by excess iron deposition in various organs, leading to eventual fibrosis and functional organ failure. There are four main types of inherited disorder:

- **type 1** HFE: the **HFE** gene (mutation C282Y) is the most common and is on chromosome 6
- **type 2A**: the juvenile **HJV** gene (mutation G320V); **type 2B**: the juvenile **HAMP** gene (mutation 93delG)
- **type 3** TfR2: the **TfR2** gene (mutation Y250X)
- **type 4** ferroportin: the **SLC40A1** gene (mutation V162del).

All are transmitted by an autosomal recessive gene, apart from the ferroportin iron overload, which is dominantly transmitted.

HH has a prevalence in Caucasians (homozygotes) of 1 in 400, but very variable phenotypic expression and a heterozygote (carrier) frequency of 1 in 10. It is the most common single-gene disorder in Caucasians.

Aetiology

Between 85% and 90% of patients with overt HH are homozygous for the Cys 282 Tyr (C282Y mutation): that is, type 1 *HFE*. A second mutation (His 63 Asp, H63D) occurs in about 25% of the population and is in complete linkage disequilibrium with Cys 282 Tyr.

Another form of haemochromatosis (type 3) occurs in southern Europe and is associated with TfR2, a transferrin receptor isoform. The other types, ferroportin-related (type 4) and juvenile forms (2A and 2B), are much rarer.

Dietary intakes of iron and chelating agents (ascorbic acid) may be relevant. Iron overload may be present in alcoholics; alcohol excess *per se* does not cause HH, although there is a history of excess alcohol intake in 25% of patients.

Mechanism of damage

The *HFE* gene protein interacts with the transferrin receptor 1, which is a mediator in intestinal iron absorption (see **Fig. 16.8**). Iron is taken up by the mucosal cells inappropriately, exceeding the binding capacity of transferrin.

Hepcidin, a protein synthesized in the liver (**Fig. 34.27**), is central to the control of iron absorption; it is increased in iron deficiency states and decreased with iron overload. The mutations described disrupt hepcidin expression, thereby internalizing ferroportin and leading to uninhibited iron overload.

Hepatic expression of the hepcidin gene is decreased in HFE haemochromatosis, facilitating liver iron overload. Excess iron is then gradually taken up by the liver and other tissues over a long period. It seems likely that it is the iron itself that precipitates fibrosis.

Pathology

In symptomatic patients the total body iron content is 20–40 g, compared with 3–4 g in a normal person. The iron content is particularly increased in the liver (**Fig. 34.28**) and pancreas (50–100 times normal) but is also higher in other organs (e.g. endocrine glands, heart and skin).

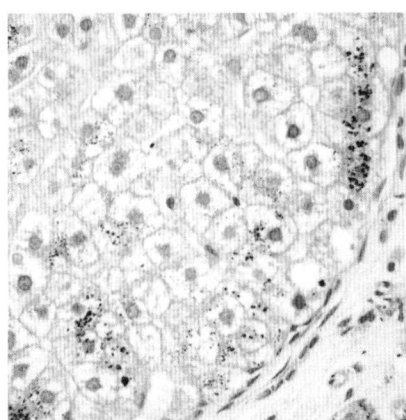

Fig. 34.28 Cirrhotic nodule in haemochromatosis. Note the iron overload (blue) (Perls, ×25).

In established cases the liver shows extensive iron deposition and fibrosis. Early in the disease, iron is deposited in the periportal hepatocytes (in pericanalicular lysosomes). Later, it is distributed widely throughout all acinar zones, biliary duct epithelium, Kupffer cells and connective tissue. Cirrhosis is a late feature.

Clinical features

The course of the disease depends on a number of factors, including gender, dietary iron intake, presence of associated hepatotoxins (especially alcohol) and genotypes. Overt clinical manifestations occur more frequently in men; the reduced incidence in women is probably explained by physiological blood loss and a smaller dietary intake of iron. Most affected individuals present in the fifth decade. The classic triad of bronze skin pigmentation (due to melanin deposition), hepatomegaly and diabetes mellitus is present only in cases of gross iron overload.

Hypogonadism secondary to pituitary dysfunction is the most common endocrine feature. Deficiency of other pituitary hormones is also found but symptomatic endocrine deficiencies, such as loss of libido, are very rare. Cardiac manifestations, particularly heart failure and arrhythmias, are common, especially in younger patients. Calcium pyrophosphate is deposited asymmetrically in both large and small joints (chondrocalcinosis), leading to an arthropathy. The exact relationship of chondrocalcinosis to iron deposition is uncertain.

Complications

Some 30% of people with cirrhosis will develop primary hepatocellular carcinoma (HCC). HCC has been described only very rarely in non-cirrhotic patients in whom the excess iron stores have been removed. Early diagnosis is vital.

Investigations

Homozygotes

- **Serum iron** is elevated (>30 μmol/L) in 90% with a reduction in the TIBC and a transferrin saturation of >45%.
- **Serum ferritin** is elevated (usually >500 μg/L or 240 nmol/L).
- **Liver biochemistry** is often normal, even with established cirrhosis.

Heterozygotes

Heterozygotes may have normal biochemical tests or modest increases in serum iron transferrin saturation (>45%) or serum ferritin (usually >400 μg/L).

Genetic testing

If iron studies are abnormal, genetic testing is performed.

Liver biopsy

This is not required for diagnosis but is useful to establish the extent of tissue damage, assess tissue iron and measure the hepatic iron concentration (>180 μmol/g dry weight of liver indicates haemochromatosis).

Mild degrees of parenchymal iron deposition in patients with other forms of cirrhosis, particularly if due to alcohol, can often cause confusion with true homozygous HH.

Magnetic resonance imaging

MRI shows a dramatic reduction in the signal intensity of the liver and pancreas owing to the paramagnetic effect of ferritin and haemosiderin. A highly T2-weighted, gradient recalled echo (GRE) technique detects all clinically relevant liver iron overload (>60 μmol/g of liver). In secondary iron overload (haemosiderosis), which involves the reticuloendothelial cells, the pancreas is spared, enabling distinction between these two conditions.

Management
Venesection

This prolongs life and may reverse tissue damage; the risk of malignancy still remains if cirrhosis is present. All patients should have excess iron removed as rapidly as possible. This is achieved using venesection of 500 mL performed twice weekly for up to 2 years: that is, 160 units with 250 mg of iron per unit, which equals 40 g removed. During venesection, serum iron and ferritin and the mean corpuscular volume (MCV) should be monitored. These fall only when available iron is depleted. Three or four venesections per year are required to prevent re-accumulation of iron. Serum ferritin should remain within the normal range.

Manifestations of the disease usually improve or disappear, except for diabetes, testicular atrophy and chondrocalcinosis. The requirements for insulin often diminish in diabetic patients. Testosterone replacement is frequently helpful.

In the rare patient who cannot tolerate venesection (because of severe cardiac disease or anaemia), chelation therapy with desferrioxamine, either intermittently or continuously by infusion, has been successful in removing iron.

Screening

In all cases of HH, all first-degree family members must be screened to detect early and asymptomatic disease. *HFE* mutation analysis is performed with measurement of transferrin saturation and serum ferritin.

In the general population, serum iron and transferrin saturation are the best and cheapest tests available.

Wilson's disease (progressive hepatolenticular degeneration)

Dietary copper is normally absorbed from the stomach and upper small intestine. Copper is transported to the liver loosely bound to albumin; in the liver, it is incorporated into apocaeruloplasmin, forming caeruloplasmin, a glycoprotein synthesized in the liver, and secreted into the blood. The remaining copper is normally excreted in the bile and excreted in faeces.

Wilson's disease is a very rare inborn error of copper metabolism that results in copper deposition in various organs, including the liver, the basal ganglia of the brain and the cornea. It is potentially treatable and all young patients with liver disease must be screened for this condition.

Aetiology

Wilson's disease is an autosomal recessive disorder with a molecular defect within a copper-transporting ATPase encoded by a gene (designated *ATP7B*) located on chromosome 13. It affects between 1 in 30 000 and 1 in 100 000 individuals. Over 300 mutations have been identified, the most frequent being His 1069 Gly (H1069Q), found in approximately 50% of Caucasian patients; compound heterozygotes are common. This mutation is rare in India and Asia. Wilson's disease occurs worldwide, particularly in countries where consanguinity is common. There is a failure of both incorporation of copper into pro-caeruloplasmin, which leads to low serum caeruloplasmin, and biliary excretion of copper. There is a low serum caeruloplasmin in over 80% of patients but this is not the cause of the copper deposition. The precise mechanism for the failure of copper excretion is not known.

Pathology

The liver histology is not diagnostic and varies from that of chronic hepatitis to macronodular cirrhosis. Stains for copper show a periportal distribution but this can be unreliable (see later). The basal ganglia are damaged and show cavitation, the kidneys demonstrate tubular degeneration, and erosions are seen in bones.

Clinical features

Children usually present with hepatic problems, whereas young adults have more neurological problems, such as tremor, dysarthria, involuntary movements and eventually dementia. The liver disease varies from episodes of acute hepatitis, especially in children (which can go on to acute hepatic failure), to chronic hepatitis or cirrhosis.

Typical signs are those of chronic liver disease with neurological signs of basal ganglia involvement (see p. 862). A specific sign is the Kayser–Fleischer ring, caused by copper deposition in Descemet's membrane in the cornea. It appears as a greenish-brown pigment at the corneoscleral junction and frequently requires slit-lamp examination for identification. It may be absent in young children.

Investigations

- **Serum copper and caeruloplasmin** are usually reduced but can be normal.
- **Urinary copper** is usually increased to 100–1000 μg in 24 h (1.6–16 μmol); normal levels are <40 μg (0.6 μmol).
- **Liver biopsy** aids diagnosis, which depends on measurement of the amount of copper in the liver (>250 μg/g dry weight), although high levels of copper are also found in the liver in chronic cholestasis.
- **Haemolysis and anaemia** may be present.
- **Genetic analysis** is limited but selected exons are screened according to population groups.

Management

- Lifetime treatment with **penicillamine**, 1–1.5 g daily, is effective in chelating copper. If treatment is started early, clinical and biochemical improvement can occur. Urinary copper levels should be monitored and the drug dose adjusted downwards after 2–3 years. Serious side-effects of the drug occur in 10% and include skin rashes, leucopenia, skin changes and renal damage.
- **Trientine** (1.2–1.8 g/day) and **zinc acetate** (150 mg/day) are used as maintenance therapy and for asymptomatic cases. All siblings and children of patients should be screened (*ATP7B*

mutation analysis is useful) and treatment with zinc is given, even in the asymptomatic, if there is evidence of copper accumulation. A diet low in copper (i.e. excluding chocolate and peanuts) is advised.

Prognosis

Early diagnosis and effective treatment have improved the outlook. Neurological damage is, however, permanent. Acute hepatic failure or decompensated cirrhosis should be treated by liver transplantation.

Alpha₁-antitrypsin deficiency

A deficiency of α_1-antitrypsin (α_1-AT, see also p. 956) is sometimes associated with liver disease and pulmonary emphysema (particularly in smokers). Part of a family of serine protease inhibitors, or serpin superfamily, α_1-AT is a glycoprotein. Deficiency of α_1-AT is a genetic disorder and 1 in 10 northern Europeans carries an abnormal gene.

The protein is a 394-amino acid 52 kDa acute phase protein that is synthesized in the liver and constitutes 90% of the serum α_1-globulin seen on electrophoresis. Its main role is to inhibit the proteolytic enzyme, neutrophil elastase.

The gene is located on chromosome 14. The genetic variants of α_1-AT are characterized by their electrophoretic mobilities as medium (M), slow (S) or very slow (Z). The normal genotype is protease inhibitor MM (PiMM), the homozygote for Z is PiZZ, and the heterozygotes are PiMZ and PiSZ. S and Z variants are due to a single amino acid replacement of glutamic acid at positions 264 and 342 of the polypeptide, respectively. This results in decreased synthesis and secretion of the protein by the liver as protein–protein interactions occur between the reactive centre loop of one molecule and the β-pleated sheet of a second (loop sheet polymerization).

How this causes liver disease is uncertain. It is postulated that failure of secretion of the abnormal protein leads to an accumulation in the liver, leading to liver damage.

Clinical features

The majority of patients with clinical disease are homozygotes with a PiZZ phenotype. Some may present in childhood and a few require transplantation. Approximately 10–15% of adult patients will develop cirrhosis, usually over the age of 50 years, and 75% will have respiratory problems. Approximately 5% of patients die of their liver disease. Heterozygotes (e.g. PiSZ or PiMZ) may develop liver disease but the risk is small.

Investigations

- **Serum α_1-antritrypsin** is low, at 10% of the normal level in the PiZZ phenotypes, and 60% of normal in the S variant.
  Histologically, periodic acid–Schiff (PAS)-positive, diastase-resistant globules that contain α_1-AT are seen in periportal hepatocytes. Fibrosis and cirrhosis can be present.

Management

There is no treatment, apart from managing the complications of liver disease. Patients with hepatic decompensation should be assessed for liver transplantation and should stop smoking.

Further reading

Andrews NC. Closing the iron gate. *N Engl J Med* 2012; 366:376–377.
Bacon BR, Adams PC, Kowdley KV et al. Diagnosis and management of hemochromatosis: 2011 practice guideline by the American Association for the Study of Liver Diseases. *Hepatology* 2011; 54:328–343.

European Association for the Study of the Liver. EASL Clinical Practice Guidelines: Wilson disease. *J Hepatol* 2012; 56:671–685.
Hirschfield GM, Karlsen TH, Lindor KD et al. Primary sclerosing cholangitis. *Lancet* 2013; 382:1587–1599.
Pietrangelo A. Hereditary haemochromatosis: pathogenesis, diagnosis, and treatment. *Gastroenterology* 2010; 139:393–408.
Selmi C, Bowlus CL, Gershwin ME et al. Primary biliary cirrhosis. *Lancet* 2011; 377:1600–1609.

ALCOHOLIC LIVER DISEASE

This section describes the pathology and clinical features of alcoholic liver disease. The amounts needed to produce liver damage, alcohol metabolism and other clinical effects of alcohol are described on pages 1258–1259.

Ethanol is metabolized in the liver by two pathways, resulting in an increase in the NADH/NAD ratio. The altered redox potential causes increased hepatic fatty acid synthesis with decreased fatty acid oxidation; both events lead to hepatic accumulation of fatty acid, which is then esterified to glycerides.

The changes in oxidation–reduction also impair carbohydrate and protein metabolism and are the cause of the centrilobular necrosis of the hepatic acinus that is typical of alcohol damage. TNF-α release from Kupffer cells causes the release of reactive oxygen species, leading in turn to tissue injury and fibrosis.

Acetaldehyde is formed by the oxidation of ethanol, and its effect on hepatic proteins may well be a factor in producing liver cell damage. The exact mechanism of alcoholic hepatitis and cirrhosis is unknown, but since only 10–20% of people who drink heavily will develop cirrhosis, a genetic predisposition is recognized. Immunological mechanisms have also been proposed, with the release of cytokines, particularly IL-8, which is a neutrophil chemoattractant; infiltration with neutrophils is a feature of alcoholic hepatitis.

Alcohol can enhance the effects of the toxic metabolites of drugs (e.g. paracetamol) on the liver, as it induces microsomal metabolism via the microsomal ethanol oxidizing system (MEOS; see p. 1258).

Pathology

Alcohol can produce a wide spectrum of liver disease, from fatty change to hepatitis and cirrhosis.

Fatty liver

The metabolism of alcohol invariably produces fat in the liver (**Fig. 34.29**), mainly in zone 3. This is minimal with small amounts of alcohol, but with larger amounts the cells become swollen with fat (steatosis). There is no liver cell damage. The fat disappears on stopping alcohol. Steatosis is also seen in NAFLD (see p. 1287).

In some cases, collagen is laid down around the central hepatic veins (perivenular fibrosis) and this can sometimes progress to cirrhosis without a preceding hepatitis. Alcohol directly affects stellate cells, transforming them into collagen-producing myofibroblast cells (see p. 1264).

Alcoholic hepatitis

In addition to fatty change, there is infiltration by polymorphonuclear leucocytes and hepatocyte necrosis, mainly in zone 3. Dense cytoplasmic inclusions called Mallory bodies are sometimes seen in hepatocytes, and giant mitochondria are also a feature. Mallory bodies are suggestive of, but not specific for, alcoholic damage, as they can be found in other liver disease, such as Wilson's disease and primary biliary cholangitis. If alcohol consumption continues, alcoholic hepatitis may progress to cirrhosis.

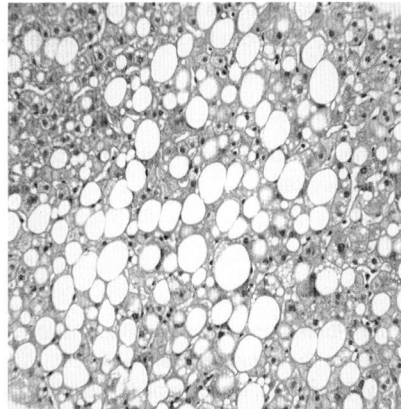

Fig. 34.29 Liver steatosis. (Haematoxylin and eosin, x10.)

Alcoholic cirrhosis

This is classically of the micronodular type but a mixed pattern is also seen accompanying fatty change; evidence of pre-existing alcoholic hepatitis may be present.

Clinical features

Fatty liver

There are often no symptoms or signs. Vague abdominal symptoms of nausea, vomiting and diarrhoea are due to the more general effects of alcohol on the gastrointestinal tract. Hepatomegaly, sometimes huge, can occur, together with other features of chronic liver disease.

Alcoholic hepatitis

The clinical features vary in degree:
- The patient may be well, with few symptoms, the hepatitis being apparent only on the liver biopsy in addition to fatty change.
- Mild to moderate symptoms of ill-health, occasionally with mild jaundice, may occur. Signs include all the features of chronic liver disease. Liver biochemistry is deranged and the diagnosis is made on liver histology.
- In the severe case, often superimposed on alcoholic cirrhosis, the patient is ill, with jaundice and ascites. Abdominal pain is frequently present and a high fever is associated with the liver necrosis. On examination there is deep jaundice, hepatomegaly, sometimes splenomegaly, and ascites with ankle oedema. The signs of chronic liver disease are also present.

Alcoholic cirrhosis

This represents the final stage of liver disease from alcohol use. Nevertheless, patients can be very well with few symptoms. On examination, there are usually signs of chronic liver disease (p. 1263). The diagnosis is confirmed by liver biopsy.

The patient usually presents with one of the complications of cirrhosis. In many cases there are features of alcohol dependency (see p. 790), as well as evidence of involvement of other systems, such as polyneuropathy.

Investigations

Fatty liver

An elevated MCV often indicates heavy drinking. Liver biochemistry shows mild abnormalities with elevation of both serum aminotransferase enzymes. The γ-GT level is a useful test for determining whether the patient is taking alcohol. With severe fatty infiltration, marked changes in all liver biochemical parameters can occur.

Ultrasound or CT will demonstrate fatty infiltration, as will liver histology. Elastography (p. 1270) can be used to estimate the degree of fibrosis.

Alcoholic hepatitis

Investigations show a leucocytosis with markedly deranged liver biochemistry and elevated:

- serum bilirubin
- serum AST and ALT
- serum ALP
- PT.

A **low serum albumin** may also be found. Rarely, hyperlipidaemia with haemolysis (**Zieve syndrome**) may occur.

Liver biopsy, if required, is performed by the transjugular route because of the prolonged PT.

Alcoholic cirrhosis

Investigations are as for cirrhosis in general.

Management and prognosis

General management

All patients should stop drinking alcohol. Delirium tremens (a withdrawal symptom) is treated with diazepam. Intravenous thiamine should be given empirically to prevent Wernicke–Korsakoff encephalopathy. Bed rest is necessary, along with a diet high in protein and vitamin supplements. Parenteral nutrition is sometimes required. Patients must be advised to participate in alcohol cessation programmes. The likelihood of abstention is dependent on many factors, particularly social and family ones.

Fatty liver

The patient is advised to stop drinking alcohol; the fat will disappear and the liver biochemistry usually returns to normal. Small amounts of alcohol can be drunk subsequently, as long as patients are aware of the problems and can control their consumption.

Alcoholic hepatitis

In severe cases the alcoholic hepatitis leads to acute decompensation and the patient requires admission to hospital. Nutrition must be maintained with enteral feeding, if necessary, and vitamin supplementation given. Steroid therapy has been widely used in patients with a discriminant function score of more than 32 but a multicentre UK study from 2005, which included over 1000 patients, suggested that there was no survival benefit.

Discriminant function (DF)

$$DF = [4.6 \times \text{prothrombin time above control in seconds}] + \text{bilirubin (mg/dL)}$$

Bilirubin mmol/L ÷ 17 to convert to mg/dL.
Severe = >32.

The response to steroid therapy can also be evaluated by the Lille score (>0.45 indicates poor response to steroids, which can therefore be stopped) and the Glasgow score (**Boxes 34.23 and 34.24**). A Glasgow score of more than 9 indicates that steroids are necessary because at above 9 the 28-day mortality is 75%, while at below 9 it is 50%. The MELD score (see **Box 34.17**) is also used but does not indicate which patients need steroid therapy.

Infection must be excluded or concomitantly treated. Treatment for encephalopathy and ascites is commenced. Antifungal prophylaxis should also be used.

> **Box 34.23 Lille score for alcoholic hepatitis**
>
> (*Calculator at* http://www.lillemodel.com)
> $R = 3.19 - (0.101 \times \text{age in years}) + (0.147 \times \text{albumin on admission in g/L}) + (0.0165 \times \text{change in bilirubin level from day 0 to day 7 in } \mu\text{mol/L}) - (0.206 \times \text{renal insufficiency [0 if absent, 1 if present]}^a) - (0.0065 \times \text{bilirubin day 0 in } \mu\text{mol/L}) - (0.0096 \times \text{INR})$
> **Score** $= \text{EXP}(-R)/[1+\text{EXP}(-R)]$
> A score of <0.16 indicates a 96% chance of survival at 28 days; ≥0.56 indicates a 55% chance of survival at 28 days.
>
> ---
> aCreatinine >115 μmol/L. INR, international normalized ratio.

> **Box 34.24 Glasgow alcoholic hepatitis score**
>
> | Score | 1 | 2 | 3 |
> |---|---|---|---|
> | **Age** | <50 | >50 | |
> | **White cell count** (× 10⁹/L) | <15 | >15 | |
> | **Urea** (nmol/L) | <5 | >5 | |
> | **Bilirubin** (μmol/L) | <125 | 125–250 | >250 |
> | **INR** | <1.5 | 1.5–2.0 | >2.0 |
>
> Poor prognosis = total score >9.

INR, international normalized ratio.

Patients are advised to stop drinking for life, as this is undoubtedly a pre-cirrhotic condition. The prognosis is variable: despite abstinence, liver disease is progressive in many patients but abstinence significantly improves survival. Granulocyte-colony stimulating factor (G-CSF) for 5 days improves 90-day survival in preliminary studies.

In severe cases the mortality is at least 50%; with a PT twice normal, progressive encephalopathy and acute kidney injury, the mortality approaches 90%. Early transplantation for patients with severe alcoholic hepatitis has a survival rate of 78%, compared with 32% of those not transplanted. Unfortunately, many return to drinking.

Alcoholic cirrhosis

The management of cirrhosis is described on page 1290. Again, all patients are advised to stop drinking for life. Abstinence from alcohol results in an improvement in prognosis, with a 5-year survival of 90%, but with continued drinking this falls to 60%. In advanced disease (i.e. jaundice, ascites and haematemesis) the 5-year survival rate falls to 35%, most of the deaths occurring in the first year. Liver transplantation results in good survival; recurrence of cirrhosis due to recidivism is rare. Patients often sign a contract with their clinicians regarding their abstinence, both before and after transplantation.

A trial of abstention to establish whether liver disease can improve is mandatory but transplantation should not be denied if the patient continues to deteriorate. Specific follow-up regarding alcohol use is recommended.

HCC is a complication, particularly in men.

Further reading

Thursz MR, Richardson P, Allison M et al. Prednisolone or pentoxifylline for alcoholic hepatitis. *N Engl J Med* 2015; 372:1619–1628.

BUDD–CHIARI SYNDROME

In this condition there is obstruction to the venous outflow of the liver owing to occlusion of the hepatic vein. In one-third of patients the cause is unknown but specific causes include hypercoagulability states (e.g. paroxysmal nocturnal haemoglobinuria, polycythaemia vera) or thrombophilia (see p. 1011), the contraceptive pill and leukaemia. Other causes include occlusion of the hepatic vein owing to posterior abdominal wall sarcomas, renal or adrenal tumours, HCC, hepatic infections (e.g. hydatid cyst), congenital venous webs, radiotherapy or trauma to the liver.

Clinical features

The acute form presents with abdominal pain, nausea, vomiting, tender hepatomegaly and ascites (a fulminant form occurs particularly in pregnant women). In the chronic form there is enlargement of the liver (particularly the caudate lobe), mild jaundice, ascites, a negative hepatojugular reflux, and splenomegaly with portal hypertension.

Investigations

Investigations show a high protein content in the ascitic fluid and characteristic liver histology with centrizonal congestion, haemorrhage, fibrosis and cirrhosis. Ultrasound, CT or MRI will demonstrate hepatic vein occlusion with diffuse abnormal parenchyma on contrast enhancement. The caudate lobe is spared because of its independent blood supply and venous drainage. There may be compression of the inferior vena cava. Pulsed Doppler sonography or colour Doppler is useful, as it shows abnormalities of flow in the hepatic vein. Thrombophilia screening is mandatory. Multiple defects of coagulation occur. Thrombosis of the portal vein is present in 2% of patients.

Differential diagnosis

A similar clinical picture can be produced by inferior vena caval obstruction, right-sided cardiac failure or constrictive pericarditis, and appropriate investigations should be performed.

Management

In the *acute situation*, thrombolytic therapy can be given. Ascites should be treated, as should any underlying cause (e.g. polycythaemia). Congenital webs should be treated radiologically or resected surgically. A TIPS is the treatment of choice, as caval compression does not prejudice its efficacy. Surgical portocaval shunts are reserved for those who fail this treatment, providing there is no caval obstruction or severe caval compression when a caval stent can be inserted. Liver transplantation is the first-choice treatment for *chronic* Budd–Chiari syndrome and for the fulminant form. Life-long anticoagulation is mandatory following TIPS and transplantation.

Prognosis

The prognosis depends on the aetiology but the reported life expectancy is 3 years after the first symptoms. However, a step-wise approach to therapy, as described earlier, can lead to a 5-year survival rate of nearly 85%.

Further reading

Mancuso A. An update on management of Budd–Chiari syndrome. *Ann Hepatol* 2014; 13:323–326.
Valla DC. Budd–Chiari syndrome/hepatic venous outflow tract obstruction. *Hepatol Int* 2018; 12(Suppl 1):168–180.

HEPATIC SINUSOIDAL OBSTRUCTION SYNDROME

Hepatic sinusoidal obstruction syndrome (SOS, previously known as veno-occlusive disease) is due to injury of the hepatic veins and presents clinically like the Budd–Chiari syndrome. It was originally described in Jamaica, where ingestion of toxic pyrrolizidine alkaloids in bush tea (made from plants of the genera *Senecio*, *Heliotropium* and *Crotalaria*) caused damage to the hepatic veins, but it can be seen in other parts of the world. It also occurs as a complication of chemotherapy and total body irradiation, used before allogeneic bone marrow transplantation. The development of SOS after bone marrow transplantation carries a high mortality. Treatment is supportive, with control of ascites and hepatocellular failure. TIPS has been used in a few cases. Defibrotide is recommended for prophylactic use before bone marrow transplantation in children and adults with a high risk of SOS (e.g. pre-existing hepatic disease or prior treatment with gemtuzumab ozogamicin).

FIBROPOLYCYSTIC DISEASES

These diseases are usually inherited and lead to the presence of cysts or fibrosis in the liver, kidney and occasionally the pancreas, and other organs.

Polycystic disease of the liver

Multiple cysts can occur in the liver as part of autosomal dominant polycystic disease of the kidney (see p. 1405). These cysts are usually asymptomatic but occasionally cause abdominal pain and distension. Liver function is normal and complications such as oesophageal varices are very rare. The prognosis is excellent and depends on the kidney disease.

Solitary cysts

These are usually found by chance during imaging and are mainly asymptomatic.

Congenital hepatic fibrosis

In this rare condition the liver architecture is normal but there are broad collagenous fibrous bands extending from the portal tracts. Congenital hepatic fibrosis is often inherited as an autosomal recessive condition but can also occur sporadically. It usually presents in childhood with hepatosplenomegaly, and portal hypertension is common. It may present later in life and can be misdiagnosed as cirrhosis.

A wedge biopsy of the liver may be required to confirm the diagnosis. The outlook is good and the condition should be distinguished from cirrhosis. Patients who bleed do well after endoscopic therapy of varices (or a portocaval anastomosis) because of their good liver function.

Congenital intrahepatic biliary dilation (Caroli's disease)

In this rare, non-familial disease there are saccular dilations of the intrahepatic or extrahepatic ducts. It can present at any age (although it usually does so in childhood) with fever, abdominal pain and recurrent attacks of cholangitis with Gram-negative septicaemia. Jaundice and portal hypertension are absent. Diagnosis is by ultrasound, percutaneous transhepatic cholangiography and MRCP. There is an increased risk of biliary malignancy.

LIVER ABSCESS

Pyogenic abscess

Pyogenic abscesses are uncommon; they may be single or multiple. The most common used to be a portal pyaemia from intra-abdominal sepsis (e.g. appendicitis or perforations) but nowadays the aetiology is not known in many cases. In the elderly, biliary sepsis is a common cause. Other causes include trauma, bacteraemia and direct extension from, for example, a perinephric abscess.

The most common organism is *E. coli. Streptococcus milleri* and anaerobic organisms such as *Bacteroides* are often seen. Others include *Enterococcus faecalis*, *Proteus vulgaris* and *Staphylococcus aureus*. Often the infection is mixed.

Clinical features

Some patients present with malaise lasting several days or even months. Others can present with fever, rigors, anorexia, vomiting, weight loss and abdominal pain. In these patients, a Gram-negative septicaemia with shock can occur. On examination there may be little of note; alternatively, the patient may be toxic, febrile and jaundiced. In such patients the liver is tender and enlarged, and there may a pleural effusion or a pleural rub in the right lower chest.

Investigations

Patients are often investigated for 'pyrexia of unknown origin' and most investigations will be normal.
- **Serum bilirubin** is raised in 25% of cases.
- **Normochromic normocytic anaemia** may occur, usually accompanied by a polymorphonuclear leucocytosis.
- **Serum ALP, ESR and CRP** are often raised.
- **Serum vitamin B$_{12}$** is very high, as it is stored in and subsequently released from the liver.
- **Blood cultures** are positive in only 30% of cases.

Imaging

Ultrasound is useful for detecting abscesses. A CT scan may be of value in complex and multiple lesions (**Fig. 34.30**). A chest X-ray will show elevation of the right hemidiaphragm, with a pleural effusion in the severe case. Depending on age, imaging of the colon may be necessary to find the source of infection.

Management

Aspiration of the abscess should be attempted under ultrasound control. Antibiotics should initially cover Gram-positive, Gram-negative and anaerobic organisms until the causative organism is identified.

Further drainage via a large-bore needle under ultrasound control or surgically may be necessary if resolution is difficult or slow. Any underlying cause must be treated.

Prognosis

The overall mortality depends on the nature of the underlying pathology but has been reduced to approximately 16% with needle aspiration and antibiotics. A unilocular abscess in the right lobe has the best prognosis. Scattered multiple abscesses have a very high mortality, with only 1 in 5 patients surviving.

Amoebic abscess

This occurs worldwide and must be considered in patients travelling from endemic areas. *Entamoeba histolytica* (see p. 571) can be carried from the bowel to the liver in the portal venous system, leading to portal inflammation with the development of multiple microabscesses and, eventually, single or multiple large abscesses.

Clinically, the onset is usually gradual but may be sudden. There is fever, anorexia, weight loss and malaise. There is often no history of dysentery. On examination the patient looks ill and has tender hepatomegaly and signs of an effusion or consolidation in the base of the right side of the chest. Jaundice is unusual.

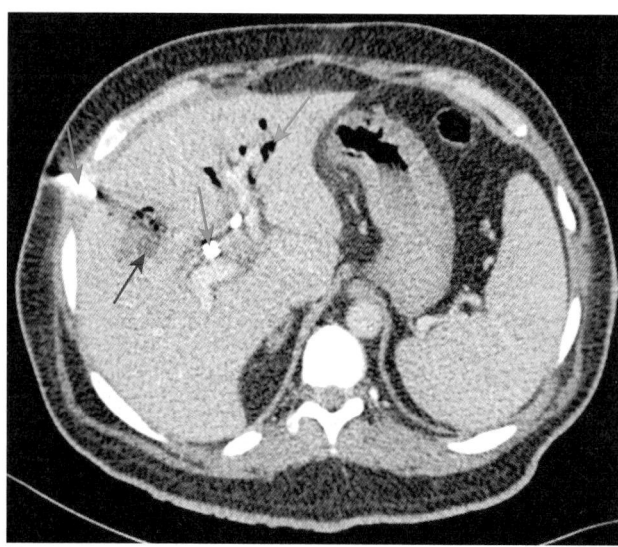

Fig. 34.30 Axial CT image demonstrating a fluid- and gas-containing lesion consistent with a liver abscess (red arrow). The patient has an external biliary drain in situ (green arrows) and there is gas in the biliary tree (aerobilia) (blue arrow).

Investigations

These are as for pyogenic abscess, plus:
- **Serological tests for amoeba** (e.g. haemagglutination, amoebic complement fixation test, ELISA). These are always positive, particularly if there are bowel symptoms; they remain positive after a clinical cure and therefore do not indicate current disease. A repeat negative test, however, is good evidence against an amoebic abscess.
- **Diagnostic aspiration of fluid** looking like anchovy sauce.

Management

Metronidazole 800 mg three times daily is given for 10 days. Aspiration is used in patients failing to respond, in those with multiple and sometimes large abscesses, and in those with abscesses in the left lobe of the liver or impending rupture.

Complications

Complications include rupture, secondary infection and septicaemia.

OTHER INFECTIONS OF THE LIVER

Schistosomiasis

Schistosoma mansoni and *S. japonicum* affect the liver but *S. haematobium* rarely does so (see also p. 578). During their life cycle the ova reach the liver via the venous system and obstruct the portal branches, producing granulomas, fibrosis and inflammation, but not cirrhosis.

Clinical features and investigations

Clinically, there is hepatosplenomegaly and portal hypertension, which is particularly severe with *S. mansoni*. In Egypt there is frequently concomitant chronic hepatitis C infection.

Investigations show a raised serum ALP, and ova can be found in the stools (centrifuged deposits) and in rectal and liver biopsies. Skin tests and other immunological tests often give false results and may also be positive because of past infection.

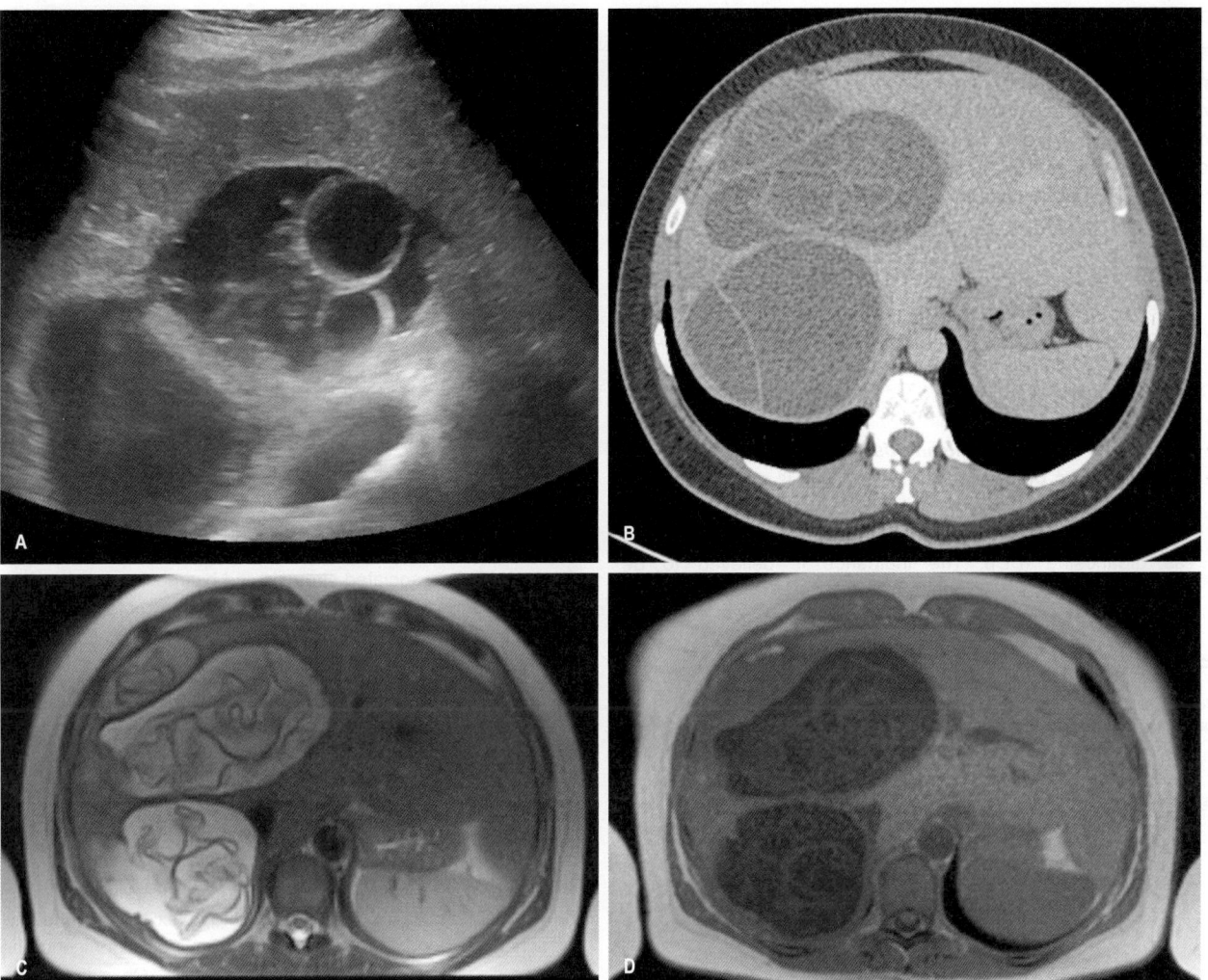

Fig. 34.31 Multimodality imaging from the same patient demonstrating hydatid cysts containing multiple daughter cysts. **(A)** Ultrasound. **(B)** CT. **(C)** T2-weighted MRI. **(D)** T1-weighted MRI.

Management

Treatment is with praziquantel, but fibrosis still remains with a potential risk of portal hypertension, characteristically pre-sinusoidal due to intense portal fibrosis.

Hydatid disease

Cysts caused by *Echinococcus granulosus* are single or multiple. They usually occur in the lower part of the right lobe. The cyst has three layers: an outside layer derived from the host, an intermediate laminated layer, and an inner germinal layer that buds off brood capsules to form daughter cysts (see also p. 581).

Clinical features and investigations

Clinically, there may be no symptoms or there may be a dull ache and swelling in the right hypochondrium.

Investigations show a peripheral eosinophilia in 30% of cases and usually a positive hydatid complement fixation test or haemagglutination (85%). Plain abdominal X-ray may show calcification of the outer coat of the cyst. Ultrasound and CT scan demonstrate cysts and may show diagnostic daughter cysts within the parent cyst (**Fig. 34.31**).

Management

Medical treatment (e.g. with albendazole 10 mg/kg, which penetrates into large cysts) results in cysts becoming smaller. Puncture, aspiration, injection, re-aspiration (PAIR) has been used since the 1980s. Fine-needle aspiration is undertaken under ultrasound control with chemotherapeutic cover. Surgery can be performed with removal of the cyst intact, if possible, after first sterilizing the cyst with alcohol, saline or cetrimide. Chronic calcified cysts can be left; there have been no well-designed clinical trials for any therapy.

Complications and prognosis

These include rupture into the biliary tree or other organs, or intraperitoneally, with spread of infection. The prognosis without any complications is good, although there is always a risk of rupture. *Preventative measures* include deworming pet dogs and preventing pets from eating infected carcasses, as well as veterinary control programmes.

Echinococcus multilocularis causes alveolar echinococcosis and is almost exclusively a hepatic disease, with a high mortality if not treated. Early diagnosis enables radical surgery and then continued chemosuppression.

Acquired immunodeficiency syndrome

The liver is often involved in AIDS and is a significant cause of morbidity or mortality. HIV itself is not the cause of the liver abnormalities. Clinical hepatomegaly is common (60% of patients). The following are seen, although less frequently in areas where antiretroviral therapy (ART) is available:

- **Pre-existing/coincidental viral hepatitis.** The hepatitis (HBV, HCV, HDV) progresses more rapidly and is a leading cause of death.
- **Neoplasia.** Kaposi's sarcoma and non-Hodgkin lymphoma may be seen, and there is an increased risk of HCC.
- **Opportunistic infection** (e.g. *Mycobacterium tuberculosis*, *M. avium-intracellulare*, *Cryptococcus*, *Candida albicans*, toxoplasmosis).
- **Drug hepatotoxicity.**
- **Secondary sclerosing cholangitis** (see p. 1444).
- **Non-cirrhotic portal hypertension.** This is associated with ART and is more common in people who have had profound immunosuppression and received early nucleotides, such as didanosine (DDI). The incidence is believed to be declining with the introduction of early ART and less toxic drugs.

Further reading

Joshi D, O'Grady J, Dieterich D et al. Increasing burden of liver disease in patients with HIV infection. *Lancet* 2011; 377:1198–1209.

LIVER DISEASE IN PREGNANCY

See page 1455.

LIVER TUMOURS

Secondary liver tumours

The most common liver tumour is a secondary (metastatic) tumour, particularly from the gastrointestinal tract (from the distribution of the portal blood supply), breast or bronchus. Secondary liver tumours are usually multiple.

Clinical features

These are variable but usually include weight loss, malaise, upper abdominal pain and hepatomegaly, with or without jaundice.

Investigations

Ultrasound is the primary investigation, with CT or MRI to define metastases and look for a primary. The serum ALP is almost invariably raised.

Management

This will depend on the site of the primary and the burden of liver metastases. The best results are obtained in colorectal cancer with few hepatic metastases. If the primary tumour is removed and hepatic resection is performed, reasonable survival rates are possible. Chemotherapy is used, particularly with breast cancer. Radiofrequency ablation of the metastases is an alternative to surgery. Thermal therapy and cryotherapy are also used.

Primary malignant tumours

Primary liver tumours may be benign or malignant, but the most common are malignant.

Hepatocellular carcinoma

Hepatocellular carcinoma (HCC) is the fifth most common cancer worldwide.

Aetiology

Carriers of HBV and HCV have an extremely high risk of developing HCC. In areas where HBV is prevalent, 90% of patients with this cancer are positive for HBV. Cirrhosis is present in approximately 80% of these people. The development of HCC is related to the integration of viral HBV DNA into the genome of the host hepatocyte (see p. 1278), and to the degree of viral replication (>10 000 copies/mL). The risk of HCC in HCV is higher than in HBV (and even higher with both HBV and HCV), despite no viral integration. Unlike in HBV infection, cirrhosis is always present in HCV. Primary liver cancer is also associated with other forms of cirrhosis, such as alcoholic cirrhosis, NAFLD-associated cirrhosis and haemochromatosis. Males are affected more than females. Other aetiological factors are aflatoxin (a metabolite of a fungus found in groundnuts) and androgenic steroids, and there is a weak association with the contraceptive pill.

Pathology

The tumour either is single or occurs as multiple nodules throughout the liver. Histologically, it consists of cells resembling hepatocytes. It can metastasize via the hepatic or portal veins to the lymph nodes, bones and lungs.

Clinical features

The clinical features include weight loss, anorexia, fever, an ache in the right hypochondrium and ascites. The rapid development of these features in a cirrhotic patient is suggestive of HCC. On examination, an enlarged, irregular, tender liver may be felt. Increasingly, due to surveillance, HCC is found without symptoms in patients with cirrhosis.

Investigations

- Routine liver biochemistry, full blood count, serum creatinine and electrolytes.
- **Serum α-fetoprotein** may be raised but is normal in at least a third of patients.
- **Ultrasound** scans show filling defects in 90% of cases.
- **Enhanced CT scans** (**Fig. 34.32**) identify HCC but it is difficult to confirm the diagnosis in lesions smaller than 1 cm. An **MRI** scan can help to delineate lesions further.
- **Tumour biopsy** (**Fig. 34.33**), particularly under ultrasonic guidance, is now used less frequently for diagnosis, as imaging techniques show characteristic appearances (hypervascularity of the nodule and lack of portal vein washout) and because seeding along the biopsy tract can occur.

Management and prognosis

See page 126.

Prevention

Persistent HBV infection, usually acquired after perinatal infection, is a strong risk factor for HCC in many parts of the world, such as South-east Asia. Widespread vaccination against HBV is being used and this has reduced the annual incidence of HCC in Taiwan.

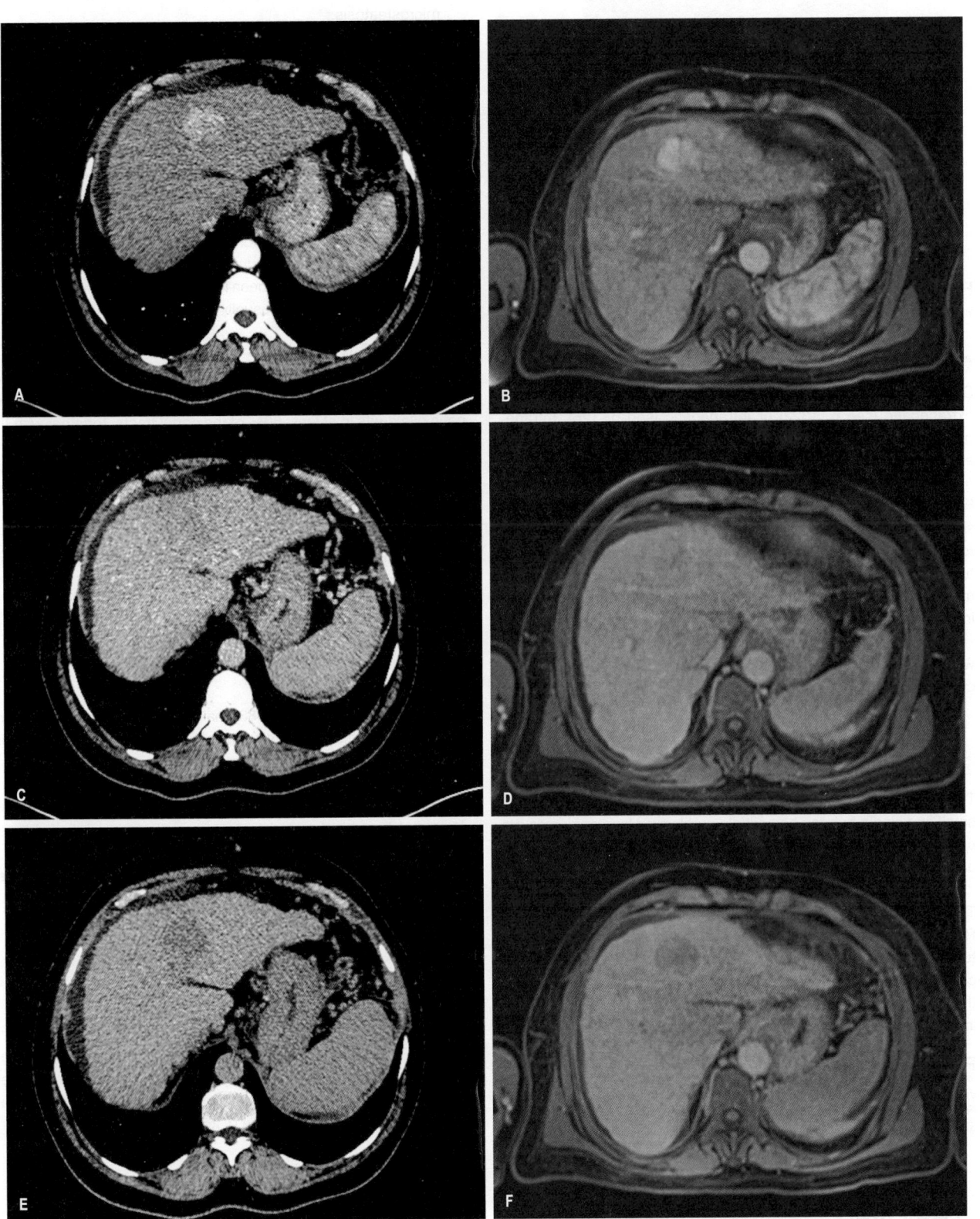

Fig. 34.32 Hepatocellular carcinoma (HCC). Two cases of HCC on **(A–C)** multiphasic contrast-enhanced CT and **(D–F)** MRI. HCC classically demonstrates enhancement on the arterial phase imaging (A, D) and washout on more delayed phases of imaging. In both cases there is subtle washout on the portal venous phase imaged (B, E) with more definite washout on the delayed phase imaging (C, F).

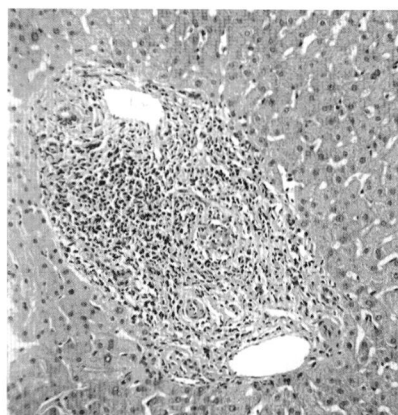

Fig. 34.33 Hepatocellular carcinoma. (Haematoxylin and eosin, ×25.)

Cholangiocarcinoma

Cholangiocarcinomas are increasing in incidence and can be extrahepatic (see p. 1322) or intrahepatic (see p. 126). Intrahepatic adenocarcinomas arising from the bile ducts account for approximately 10% of primary tumours of the liver and biliary tract. They are not associated with cirrhosis or hepatitis B. In the Far East, they may be associated with infestation with *Clonorchis sinensis* or *Opisthorchis viverrini*. The clinical features are similar to those of primary HCC, except that jaundice is frequent with hilar tumours, and cholangitis is more common. There is an increased association with inflammatory bowel disease and primary sclerosing cholangitis (see p. 1299).

Surgical resection is rarely possible and patients usually die within 6 months. Transplantation is contraindicated, outside of specialized protocols.

Benign tumours

The most common benign tumour is a **haemangioma**. It is usually small and single but can be multiple and large. Haemangiomas are usually found incidentally on ultrasound, CT or MRI, and have characteristic appearances. They require no treatment.

Hepatic adenomas are associated with oral contraceptives. They can present with abdominal pain or intraperitoneal bleeding. Resection is required only for symptomatic patients, those with tumours of more than 5 cm in diameter, and those in whom discontinuation of oral contraception does not result in shrinkage of the tumour. Immunohistochemical characteristics are helpful for indicating malignant potential, which is far more common in men.

Further reading

Villanueva A. Hepatocellular carcinoma. *N Engl J Med* 2019;380:1450–1462.
Forner A, Llovet JM, Bruix J et al. Hepatocellular carcinoma. *Lancet* 2012; 379:1245–1255.

MISCELLANEOUS CONDITIONS OF THE LIVER

Hepatic mitochondrial injury syndromes

These syndromes, in which there is mitochondrial damage with inhibition of β-oxidation of fatty acids, can be categorized as having the following causes:

- **Genetic**, with abnormalities that include medium-chain acyl-coenzyme A dehydrogenase deficiency, leading to microsteatosis.
- **Toxins** leading to liver failure, which include aflatoxin and cerulide (produced by *Bacillus cereus*); the latter causes food poisoning (see p. 542).
- **Drugs** (e.g. i.v. tetracycline, valproic acid and nucleoside reverse-transcriptase inhibitors), which can produce a fatal microsteatosis.
- **Idiopathic**, the best known being fatty liver of pregnancy (see p. 1455) and Reye's syndrome. The latter, caused by inhibition of β-oxidation and uncoupling of oxidative phosphorylation in mitochondria, leads in children to an acute encephalopathy and diffuse microvesicular fatty infiltration of the liver. Aspirin ingestion and viral infections have been implicated as precipitating agents. Mortality is about 50%, usually due to cerebral oedema.

Idiopathic adult ductopenia

This unexplained condition is characterized by pruritus and cholestatic jaundice. Histology of the liver shows a decrease in intrahepatic bile ducts in at least 50% of the portal tracts, together with the features of cholestasis and marked fibrosis or cirrhosis. In most, the disease is progressive and the only treatment is liver transplantation.

Indian childhood cirrhosis

This condition of children is seen in the Indian subcontinent. The cause is unknown. Eventually, there is development of a micronodular cirrhosis with excess copper in the liver.

Hepatic porphyrias

These are dealt with on page 755.

Cystic fibrosis

Cystic fibrosis (see also p. 983) mainly affects the lung and pancreas, but patients can develop fatty liver, cholestasis and cirrhosis. The aetiology of the liver involvement is unclear.

Coeliac disease

Abnormal liver biochemical tests are common in coeliac disease (see also p. 1190) and return to normal with a gluten-free diet. A tissue transglutaminase test should be performed if hepatic causes are not found when investigating abnormal liver biochemistry.

DRUGS AND THE LIVER

Drug metabolism

The liver is the major site of drug metabolism. Drugs are converted from fat-soluble to water-soluble substances that can be excreted in the urine or bile. This metabolism of drugs is mediated by a group of mixed-function enzymes (see p. 253).

Drug hepatotoxicity

Many drugs impair liver function. When abnormal liver biochemical tests are found, drugs should always be considered as a cause, particularly when other causes have been excluded. Damage to the liver by drugs (drug-induced liver injury, DILI) is usually classified as being either predictable (or dose-related) or non-predictable (not dose-related) (see p. Box 12.9). However, there is considerable overlap and at least *six mechanisms* may be involved in the production of damage:

1. disruption of intracellular calcium homeostasis
2. disruption of bile canalicular transport mechanisms
3. formation of non-functioning adducts (enzyme–drug), which may then lead to
4. presentation on the surface of the hepatocyte as new immunogens (attacked by T cells)
5. induction of apoptosis
6. inhibition of mitochondrial function, which prevents fatty acid metabolism and accumulation of both lactate and reactive oxygen species.

The predominant mechanism or combination of mechanisms determines the type of liver injury: that is, hepatitic, cholestatic or immunological (skin rashes, fever and arthralgia, i.e. serum sickness syndrome). Eosinophilia and circulating immune complexes and antibodies are occasionally detected.

When a small amount of hepatotoxic drug whose effect is dose-dependent (e.g. paracetamol) is ingested, a large proportion of it undergoes conjugation with glucuronide and sulphate, while the remainder is metabolized by microsomal enzymes to produce toxic derivatives that are immediately detoxified by conjugation with glutathione. If larger doses are ingested, the former pathway becomes saturated and the toxic derivative is produced at a faster rate. Once the hepatic glutathione is depleted, large amounts of the toxic metabolite accumulate and produce damage (see p. 265).

The 'predictability' of drugs to produce damage can, however, be affected by metabolic events preceding their ingestion. For example, chronic alcohol users may become more susceptible to liver damage because of the enzyme-inducing effects of alcohol, or ill or starving patients may become susceptible because of the depletion of hepatic glutathione produced by starvation. Many other factors, such as environmental or genetic effects, may be involved in determining the 'susceptibility' of certain patients to certain drugs.

The incidence of drug hepatotoxicity is 14 per 100 000 population with a 6% mortality. It is the most common cause of acute liver failure in the USA. Liver transplantation is used.

Hepatitic damage

The type of damage produced by various drugs is shown in **Box 34.25**. Most reactions occur within 3 months of starting the drug. Monitoring liver biochemistry in patients on long-term treatment, such as anti-tuberculosis therapy, is mandatory. If a drug is suspected of causing hepatic damage, it should be stopped immediately. Liver biopsy is of limited help in confirming the diagnosis, but occasionally, hepatic eosinophilia or granulomas may be seen. Diagnostic challenge with subtherapeutic doses of the drug is sometimes required after the liver biochemistry has returned to normal, to confirm the diagnosis.

Individual drugs

Paracetamol

In high doses, paracetamol produces liver cell necrosis (see earlier). The toxic metabolite binds irreversibly to liver cell membranes. Overdosage is discussed on page 265.

Steroid compounds

Cholestasis is caused by natural and synthetic oestrogens, as well as methyltestosterone. These agents interfere with canalicular

Box 34.25 Liver damage produced by some drugs

Types of liver damage	Drugs	
Zone 3 necrosis	Carbon tetrachloride	Salicylates
	Amanita mushrooms	Piroxicam
	Paracetamol	Cocaine
Zone 1 necrosis	Ferrous sulphate	
Microvesicular fat	Sodium valproate	Tetracyclines
Steatohepatitis	Amiodarone	Nifedipine
	Synthetic oestrogens	
Fibrosis	Methotrexate	Vitamin A
	Other cytotoxic agents	Retinoids
	Arsenic	
Vascular		
Sinusoidal dilation	Contraceptive drugs	Anabolic steroids
Peliosis hepatis	Azathioprine	Anabolic steroids, e.g. danazol
	Oral contraceptives	
Veno-occlusive	Pyrrolizidine alkaloids (*Senecio* in bush tea)	Cytotoxics – cyclophosphamide
Acute hepatitis	Isoniazid	Cytotoxic drugs
	Rifampicin	Clonazepam
	Methyldopa	Disulfiram
	Atenolol	Niacin
	Enalapril	Volatile liquid anaesthetics, e.g. halothane
	Verapamil	
	Ketoconazole	
		Infliximab
Chronic hepatitis	Methyldopa	Fenofibrate
	Nitrofurantoin	Isoniazid
General hypersensitivity	Sulphonamides, e.g. Sulfasalazine Co-trimoxazole Fansidar	Allopurinol Anti-thyroid, e.g. Propylthiouracil Carbimazole
	Penicillins, e.g. Flucloxacillin Ampicillin Amoxicillin Co-amoxiclav	Quinine, e.g. quinidine Diltiazem Anticonvulsants, e.g. phenytoin
	NSAIDs, e.g. Salicylates Diclofenac	
Canalicular cholestasis	Sex hormones	Fucidin
	Ciclosporin	Cimetidine/ranitidine
	Chlorpromazine	Nitrofurantoin
	Haloperidol	Imipramine
	Erythromycin	Azathioprine
	Flucloxacillin	Oral hypoglycaemics
Biliary sludge	Ceftriaxone	
Sclerosing cholangitis	Hepatic arterial infusion of 5-fluorouracil	
Hepatic tumours	Pills with high hormone content (adenomas)	
Hepatocellular carcinoma	Contraceptive pill	Danazol
Nodular regenerative hyperplasia	Azathioprine	Some anti-retroviral therapies

NSAID, non-steroidal anti-inflammatory drug. *Note:* Anti-HIV drugs, e.g. maraviroc, cause hepatic dysfunction.

biliary flow by blocking MRP2 and MDR3 (see **Fig. 34.5**) and cause a pure cholestasis.

Cholestasis is rare with the contraceptive pill because of the low dosage used. However, the contraceptive pill is associated with an increased incidence of gallstones, hepatic adenomas (rarely, HCCs), the Budd–Chiari syndrome and peliosis hepatis. The latter condition, which also occurs with anabolic steroids, consists of dilation of the hepatic sinusoids to form blood-filled lakes.

Phenothiazines

Phenothiazines (e.g. chlorpromazine) can produce a cholestatic picture owing to a hypersensitivity reaction. This occurs in 1% of patients, usually within 4 weeks of starting the drug. Typically, it is associated with a fever and eosinophilia. Recovery occurs on stopping the drug.

Anti-tuberculous chemotherapy

Isoniazid produces elevated aminotransferases in 10–20% of patients. Hepatic necrosis with jaundice occurs in a smaller percentage. The hepatotoxicity of isoniazid is related to its metabolites and is dependent on acetylator status. Rifampicin produces hepatitis, usually within 3 weeks of starting the drug, particularly in patients on high doses. Pyrazinamide produces abnormal liver biochemical tests and, rarely, liver cell necrosis.

Amiodarone

This leads to a steatohepatitis histologically, and liver failure if the drug is not stopped in time.

Sodium valproate

This causes mitochondrial injury with microvesicular steatosis. Intravenous carnitine should be used as an antidote.

Drug prescribing for patients with liver disease

The metabolism of drugs is impaired in severe liver disease (with jaundice and ascites), as the removal of many drugs depends on liver blood flow and the integrity of the hepatocyte. In general, therefore, the effect of drugs is prolonged by liver disease and also by cholestasis. This is further accentuated by portosystemic shunting, which diminishes the first-pass extraction of drugs. With hypoproteinaemia, there is decreased protein binding of some drugs, and bilirubin competes with many drugs for the binding sites on serum albumin. In patients with portosystemic encephalopathy, care must be taken in prescribing drugs with a central depressant action, such as narcotics like codeine and anxiolytics. Other common drugs to be avoided in cirrhosis include angiotensin-converting enzyme (ACE) inhibitors (which cause hepatorenal failure) and NSAIDs (which cause bleeding).

Further reading

Björnsson E. Review article: drug-induced liver injury in clinical practice. *Aliment Pharmacol Ther* 2010; 32:3–13.
Hoofnagel JH, Bjornesson E. Drug induced liver injury. N Engl J Med 2019;381;264-273

Bibliography

Ryder SD, Chapman RW (eds). Liver disorders: Parts 1 and 2. *Medicine* 2011; 39:507–634.
Williams R, Aspinall R, Bellis M et al. Addressing liver disease in the UK. *Lancet* 2014; 384:1953–1997.

35

Biliary tract and pancreatic disease

Christopher Wadsworth

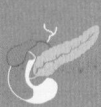

CORE SKILLS AND KNOWLEDGE

In developed countries, up to 15% of the adult population have gallstones, which are the leading cause of hepatobiliary disease; although in many they do not cause symptoms, acute pancreatitis and ascending cholangitis are serious conditions with a significant mortality. Cancers of the pancreas and gallbladder are not uncommon, and often present late.

Patients with diseases of the biliary tract and pancreas may be cared for as inpatients and outpatients by either gastroenterologists or hepatologists, depending on local services, with complex disease being looked after in specialist centres where there is hepatobiliary surgical, radiological and endoscopic support. Endoscopic retrograde cholangiopancreatography (ERCP) and endoscopic ultrasound (EUS) are core procedures, allowing a range of interventions including stone extraction, stent placement and direct biopsy of lesions.

Key skills in this field include:
- managing emergency conditions, such as ascending cholangitis and acute pancreatitis
- being aware of the need for vigilance in the early diagnosis of pancreatic cancer and cholangiocarcinoma.

Opportunities for learning about biliary tract and pancreatic disease include searching out, interviewing and examining inpatients with these conditions (who may be cared for on general surgical or gastrointestinal wards), observing ERCP and EUS procedures, and seeking to understand any treatment strategies employed. Attending an upper gastrointestinal surgical clinic and acute surgical on call, a surgical list to observe a laparoscopic cholecystectomy, and an upper gastrointestinal multidisciplinary team meeting may all prove useful.

INTRODUCTION

Biliary and pancreatic disease places a major burden on healthcare systems worldwide. In the West, acute pancreatitis and gallstone disease are the two most common gastrointestinal causes of urgent hospital admission. Pancreatic and biliary tree neoplasms carry a poor prognosis, pose significant diagnostic challenges and are increasing in incidence.

Patients with upper abdominal pain (acute or chronic), cholestasis (painless or painful) or insidious onset of weight loss commonly present in primary and secondary care. Such presentations can represent major underlying pathology and should warrant prompt and appropriate investigation.

Key skills for managing pancreatobiliary disease include the ability to:
- recognize patterns of liver enzyme derangement, including cholestasis
- manage severe sepsis complicating biliary disease
- select a rational imaging modality for upper abdominal pain
- recognize and manage nutritional deficiency in patients with acute and chronic pancreatitis
- recognize and institute management of diabetes that is due to pancreatitis (see Box 23.4).

Management of pancreatobiliary disease may require the appropriate use of
- antibiotics in the management of biliary sepsis
- pancreatic enzyme supplements
- fat-soluble vitamin supplements (vitamins A, D and K)
- proton pump inhibitors to improve pancreatic enzyme function
- chemotherapy drugs in the management of pancreatic adenocarcinoma.

Ultrasound, computed tomography (CT) and magnetic resonance imaging (MRI) technology enables the biliary tree and pancreas to be visualized with increasing resolution. Widespread use of such imaging has led to improved diagnosis but also to a burgeoning need to characterize and manage incidental, small, often asymptomatic lesions, particularly in the pancreas.

Endoscopic diagnosis of pancreatobiliary disease has been enhanced by improvements in EUS technology, and the re-emergence of direct cholangioscopy for visualization of the bile duct. Therapeutic endoscopy and laparoscopic surgery are now widely available and permit a minimally invasive approach to the management of almost all gallstone disease, and to the resection or palliation of pancreatobiliary cancer.

GALL BLADDER AND BILIARY SYSTEM

The structure and function of the biliary system and the formation of bile are discussed on pages 1265 and 1266.

BILIARY SYSTEM

Bile canaliculi form a network between the hepatocytes. These join to form thin bile ductules, which, in turn, enter the bile ducts in the portal tracts. These then combine to form the right and left hepatic ducts, which leave each liver lobe. The hepatic ducts join at the porta hepatis to form the common hepatic duct. The cystic duct connects the gall bladder to the lower end of the common hepatic duct. The gall bladder lies under the right lobe of the liver, and stores and concentrates hepatic bile; its capacity is approximately 50 mL. The common bile duct (CBD) is formed at the junction of the cystic and common hepatic ducts, and is 8 mm or less in diameter, passing through the head of the pancreas and narrowing at its lower end to pass into the duodenum. The CBD and pancreatic duct open into the second part of the duodenum, most often through a common channel at the ampulla of Vater, which contains the muscular sphincter of Oddi. This contracts rhythmically and prevents all of the bile from entering the duodenum, by maintaining a higher pressure than the gall bladder in the fasting state.

Gallstones

Gallstone disease represents a major cause of patient morbidity, particularly in the Western world, and has a major impact on healthcare economics. Gallstones may be present at any age but are unusual before the third decade. Their prevalence is strongly influenced by both age and gender. There is a progressive increase in the presence of gallstones with age and the prevalence is 2–3 times higher in women than in men, although this difference is less marked in the sixth and seventh decades. At this age the prevalence ranges between 20% and 30%. The increase in life expectancy is reflected in a greater burden of symptomatic gallstone disease. There are considerable racial differences, gallstones being more common in Scandinavians, South Americans and Native North Americans but less so in Asian and African groups. These racial differences may reflect both genetic and dietary factors. Some of these differences are being eroded by the adoption of Western diets containing high cholesterol in countries with emerging economies.

Pathogenesis

Types of gallstone

The large majority of gallstones are of two types: cholesterol stones (containing >50% of the sterol) and, less frequently, pigment stones, predominantly composed of calcium bilirubinate or polymer-like complexes with calcium, copper and some cholesterol.

Cholesterol gallstones

This type of stone accounts for 85% of gallstones in the Western world. The formation of cholesterol stones is the consequence of cholesterol crystallization from gall bladder bile. This is dependent on three factors:

- cholesterol supersaturation of bile
- crystallization-promoting factors within bile
- motility of the gall bladder.

The majority of cholesterol is derived from hepatic uptake from dietary sources. However, hepatic biosynthesis may account for up to 20%. The rate-limiting step in cholesterol synthesis is β-hydroxy-β methyl glutaryl CoA (HMG-CoA) reductase, which catalyses the first step: that is, the conversion of acetate to mevalonate.

- The cholesterol formed is co-secreted with phospholipids into the biliary canaliculus as unilamellar vesicles.
- Cholesterol will crystallize into stones only when the bile is supersaturated with cholesterol relative to the bile salt and phospholipid content. This can occur as a consequence of excess cholesterol secretion into bile, which, in some instances, has been shown to be due to an increase in HMG-CoA reductase activity.
- Increased secretion of cholesterol into bile has also been associated with insulin resistance and the metabolic syndrome (see p. 1250).
- A high-cholesterol diet increases biliary cholesterol secretion and decreases bile salt synthesis and the bile salt pool in cholesterol gallstone subjects but not in controls.

These findings suggest that increased intestinal uptake of the sterol could play a role in gallstone pathogenesis. In support of this observation, pharmacological inhibition of cholesterol absorption prevents gallstone formation in a mouse model. Ezetimibe is a highly selective intestinal cholesterol absorption inhibitor, suppressing the uptake of dietary and biliary cholesterol across the brush border membrane of the enterocyte. This may offer a potential therapy for the management/prevention of gallstone formation in patients.

While cholesterol supersaturation of bile is essential for cholesterol stone formation, many individuals in whom such supersaturation occurs will never develop stones. It is the balance between cholesterol crystallizing and solubilizing factors that determines whether cholesterol will crystallize out of solution. A number of lipoproteins have been reported as putative crystallizing factors.

Statins are effective in the treatment of hypercholesterolaemia by competitively inhibiting HMG-CoA reductase. There is emerging evidence that statins reduce cholesterol secretion into bile and, by doing so, promote gallstone dissolution. The prevalence of gallstone disease in patient groups taking statins for the management of hypercholesterolaemia appears to be reduced.

Leptin (see p. 1247) has been shown to increase cholesterol secretion into bile. Elevated levels of leptin during rapid weight loss may account for the increased incidence of cholesterol gallstones.

An alternative mechanism of supersaturation is a decreased bile salt content, which may occur as a consequence of bile salt loss (e.g. terminal ileal resection or ileal involvement with Crohn's disease).

The *composition of the bile salt pool* may also influence the ability to maintain cholesterol in solution. There is evidence that an increased proportion of deoxycholic acid (a hydrophobic bile acid) in the bile acid pool may predispose to cholesterol stone formation. This has been linked with slow colonic transit, during which cholic acid, the primary bile acid, may undergo microbial enzyme metabolism, yielding deoxycholic acid, which is then absorbed back into the bile salt pool (see **Fig. 34.5**).

Evidence from *epidemiological*, family and twin studies points to the role of genetic factors in gallstone formation. A number of lithogenic genes have been identified, which may interact with environmental factors. The process of bile formation is maintained by a network of adenosine triphosphate-binding cassette (ABC) transporters in the hepatocyte canalicular membrane, which enables biliary secretion of cholesterol, bile salts and phospholipids. This process is regulated by the nuclear receptors farnesoid X receptor (FXR) and liver X receptor (LXR). Loss-of-function mutations in specific ABC transporter genes have been associated with cholesterol gallstones secondary to bile salt and phospholipid deficiencies within the nascent bile (**Fig. 35.1**). However, monogenic susceptibility appears uncommon. There are rare cases in which a single

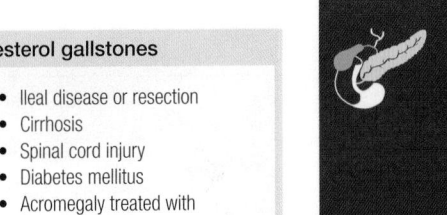

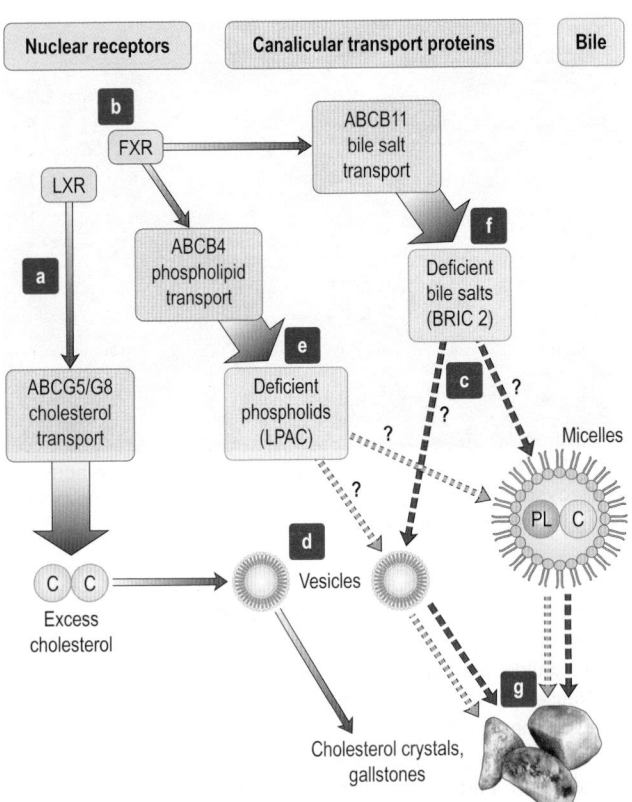

Fig. 35.1 Nascent bile formation at the hepatocytic canalicular membrane, biliary cholesterol solubilization and gallstone formation. (a) ABCG5/G8 transports cholesterol into bile (regulated by nuclear receptor LXR). **(b)** ABCB11 and ABCB4 transport bile salts and phosphatidylcholine into bile (regulated by nuclear receptor FXR). **(c)** Bile cholesterol is solubilized in mixed micelles or contained in cholesterol–phospholipid vesicles. **(d)** Most gallstones are caused by excess biliary cholesterol secretion and subsequent crystallization from supersaturated vesicles (continuous lines). **(e)** Low phospholipid (PL)-associated cholelithiasis (LPAC) occurs if there is deficient phospholipid in bile due to function mutations in gene *ABCB4*. **(f)** Benign recurrent intrahepatic cholestasis (BRIC) type 2 is characterized by deficient bile salts in bile due to function mutations in gene *ABCB11*. **(g)** In both LPAC and BRIC type 2 there is an increased risk of gallstone formation.

missense mutation of the multidrug-resistant (*MDR3*) gene has been associated with extensive intra- and extrahepatic cholelithiasis at an early age (<40 years).

Gall bladder motility represents a further factor that may influence the cholesterol crystallization from supersaturated bile. There is evidence from animal models that gall bladder stasis leads to cholesterol crystallization mediated by hypersecretion of mucin. Abnormalities of gall bladder motility have been suggested as factors in such circumstances as pregnancy, multiparity and diabetes, as well as octreotide-related gall bladder stones (see p. 638). Recognized risk factors for cholesterol gallstones are shown in **Box 35.1**.

Bile pigment stones

The pathogenesis of pigment stones is entirely independent of cholesterol gallstones. There are two main types of pigment gallstone: black and brown.

Black pigment gallstones are composed of calcium bilirubinate and a network of mucin glycoproteins that interlace with salts, such as calcium carbonate and/or calcium phosphate. These

stones range in colour from deep black to very dark brown and have a glass-like cross-sectional surface on fracturing. Because hyperbilirubinaemia is the critical risk factor, black stones are associated with all major **haemolytic anaemias**, such as spherocytosis, sickle cell disease and thalassaemia, and also with subclinical haemolysis from prosthetic valve replacements, malaria, hypersplenism from hepatic cirrhosis, and foot trauma in long-distance runners. An increased prevalence of black pigment gallstones is also seen in Gilbert's syndrome (see p. 1272), which is associated with enhanced biliary secretion of monoglucuronosyl bilirubin.

There is evidence that bile salt loss into the colon (consequent on ileal resection or ileal disease) promotes solubilization and colonic reabsorption of bilirubin. This enhances the enterohepatic circulation and biliary secretion of bilirubin with the formation of gallstones. Pigment stones have also been linked with bacterial colonization of the biliary tree. Some pigment stones have been shown to contain bacteria, many of which produce glucuronidase and phospholipase, factors that are known to facilitate stone formation. It is speculated that this subclinical bacterial colonization of the bile duct is responsible for pigment stone formation.

Brown pigment stones are usually of a muddy hue and, on cross-section, seem to have alternating brown and tan layers. These stones are composed of calcium salts of fatty acids, as well as calcium bilirubinate. They are almost always found in the presence of bile stasis and/or biliary infection. Brown stones can form in any part of the biliary tree secondary to chronic stasis and the presence of anaerobic bacterial infection.

The **Oriental hepatolithiasis syndrome (recurrent pyogenic cholangitis)** is the most serious manifestation of pigment stone disease. Biliary strictures are formed, possibly due to nematode or fluke infestation within the extrahepatic and intrahepatic bile ducts. *Ascaris lumbricoides*, *Clonorchis sinensis* and *Opisthorchis viverrini* are the parasites most commonly recognized with this condition. Brown stones may also be the cause of recurrent bile duct stones following cholecystectomy, and are also found in the intrahepatic bile ducts in stenosing biliary disease such as Caroli's syndrome and primary sclerosing cholangitis.

Clinical features

The majority of gallstones are asymptomatic and remain so during a person's lifetime. Gallstones are increasingly detected as an incidental finding at the time of either abdominal radiography or ultrasound scanning (**Fig. 35.2**). Over a 10–15-year period, approximately 20% of these stones will be the cause of symptoms and 10% will involve severe complications. Once gallstones have become symptomatic, there is a strong trend towards recurrent complications, often of increasing severity. Gallstones do not cause dyspepsia, fat intolerance, flatulence or other vague upper abdominal symptoms.

The clinical syndromes associated with gallstones are shown in **Fig. 35.3**.

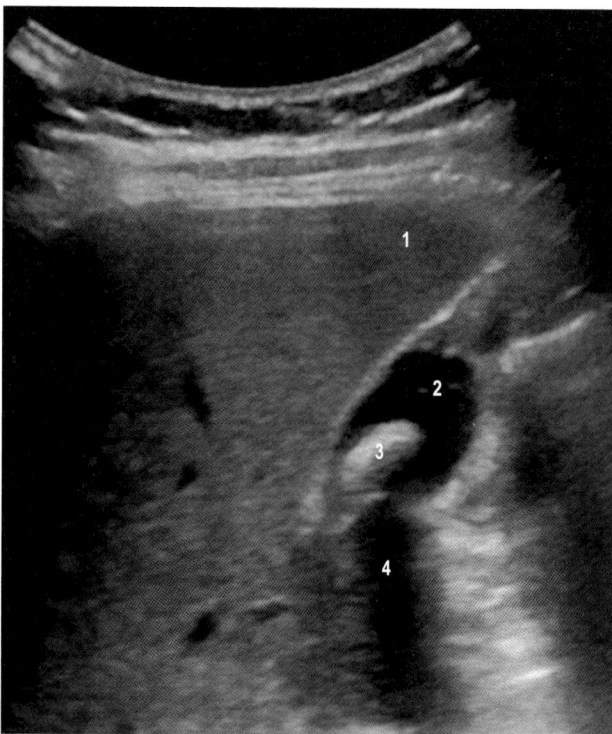

Fig. 35.2 Abdominal ultrasound image demonstrating a gallstone in the gallbladder. This is casting an acoustic shadow, as the ultrasound waves are unable to travel through the gallstone; the structures beneath are therefore not seen. **(1)** Liver; **(2)** gallbladder; **(3)** gallstone; **(4)** acoustic shadow.

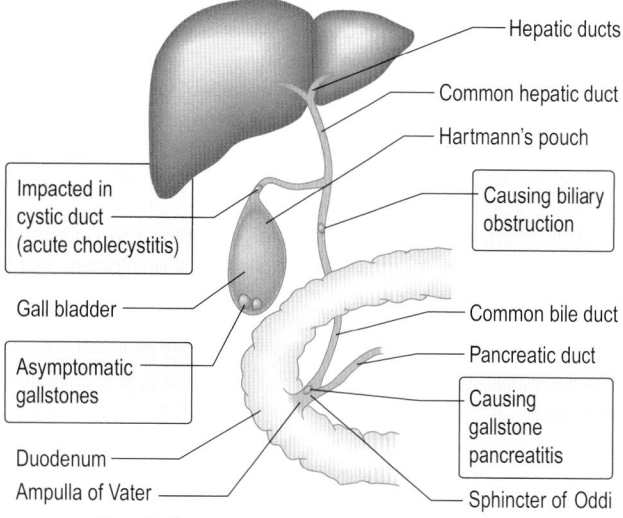

Fig. 35.3 Clinical presentation of gallstones.

Biliary colic

Biliary colic is the term used for the pain associated with the temporary obstruction of the cystic or common bile duct by a stone usually migrating from the gall bladder. Despite the term 'colic', the pain of stone-induced ductular obstruction is of sudden onset, severe but constant (not like a 'colic'), and has a crescendo characteristic. Some patients relate the symptoms to over-indulgence with food, particularly when this has a high fat content. The most common time of day for such an episode is in the mid-evening, lasting until the early hours of the morning.

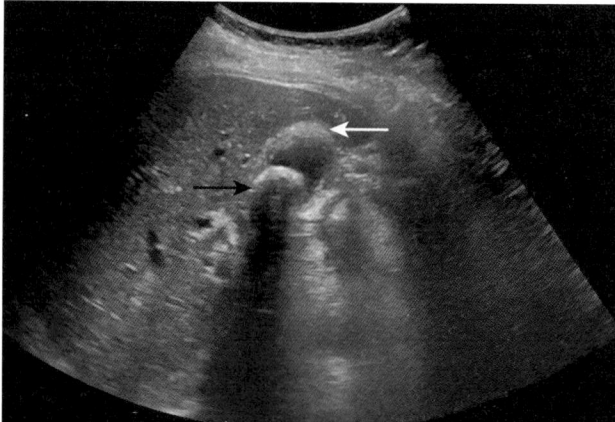

Fig. 35.4 Abdominal ultrasound image demonstrating acute cholecystitis. There is gallbladder wall thickening (white arrow) and a large gallstone (black arrow).

The initial site of pain is usually the epigastrium but there may be a right upper quadrant component. Radiation may occur over the right shoulder and right subscapular region.

Nausea and vomiting frequently accompany the more severe attacks. The attack may be terminated spontaneously after a number of hours or by the administration of opiate analgesia. More protracted pain, particularly when associated with fevers and rigors, suggests secondary complications such as cholecystitis, cholangitis or gallstone-related pancreatitis (see later).

Acute cholecystitis

The initial event in acute cholecystitis is the obstruction of gall bladder emptying. In 95% of cases a gall bladder stone can be identified as the cause (**Fig. 35.4**). Such obstruction results in an increase of gall bladder glandular secretion, leading to progressive distension that, in turn, may compromise the vascular supply to the gall bladder.

There is also an inflammatory response secondary to retained bile within the gall bladder. Infection is a secondary phenomenon following this sequence of obstructive, inflammatory and vascular events.

The initial clinical features of an episode of cholecystitis are similar to those of biliary colic described earlier. Over a number of hours, however, there is progression with severe localized right upper quadrant abdominal pain corresponding to parietal peritoneal involvement in the inflammatory process. The pain is associated with tenderness and muscle guarding or rigidity. This is frequently manifest by Murphy's sign, consisting of pain on taking a deep breath when the examiner's fingers are on the approximate location of the gall bladder. Occasionally, the gall bladder can become distended by pus (an empyema) and, rarely, an acute gangrenous cholecystitis develops, which can perforate, with generalized peritonitis.

Investigations

Biliary colic as a consequence of a stone in the neck of the gall bladder or cystic duct is unlikely to be associated with significant abnormality of laboratory tests. ***Abdominal ultrasound scan*** is the single most useful investigation for the diagnosis of gallstone-related disease (see **Fig. 35.2**).

Acute cholecystitis is usually associated with a moderate leucocytosis and raised inflammatory markers (e.g. C-reactive protein, CRP). Serum bilirubin, alkaline phosphatase and aminotransferase

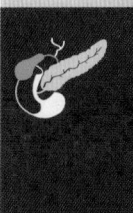

levels may be marginally elevated in the presence of cholecystitis alone, even in the absence of bile duct obstruction. More significant elevation of the bilirubin and alkaline phosphatase is in keeping with bile duct obstruction. Abdominal ultrasound has a positive predictive value of 92% and a negative predictive value of 95% in patients with a clinical history of acute cholecystitis and Murphy's sign. Look for:

- *gallstones* within the gall bladder, particularly when these are obstructing the gall bladder neck or cystic duct
- *focal tenderness* over the underlying gall bladder
- *thickening of the gall bladder wall*, which may also be seen with hypoalbuminaemia, portal hypertension and acute viral hepatitis.

Gallstones are a common finding in an ageing population, and in the absence of specific symptoms great care should be taken when determining whether the gallstones are responsible for any symptoms.

Differential diagnosis

Typical cases of biliary colic are usually suspected on the clinical history. The differential diagnosis includes irritable bowel syndrome (spasm of the hepatic flexure), carcinoma of the right side of the colon, atypical peptic ulcer disease, renal colic and pancreatitis.

The differential diagnosis of acute cholecystitis includes a number of other conditions marked by severe right upper quadrant pain and fever: for example, acute episodes of pancreatitis, perforated peptic ulceration or an intrahepatic abscess. Conditions above the right diaphragm, such as basal pneumonia, as well as myocardial infarction, may mimic the clinical picture on occasion.

Management

Cholecystectomy

Cholecystectomy is the treatment of choice for virtually all patients with symptomatic gall bladder stones. In patients admitted with specific gallstone-related complications (see later), cholecystectomy should be carried out during the period of that admission to prevent the risk of recurrence. For those presenting with pain alone, an elective procedure can be planned but the waiting time should be minimized to avoid the high risk of recurrent symptoms (approximately 30% over 4 months) and the need for another hospital admission.

Cholecystectomy should not be performed in the absence of typical symptoms just because stones are found on investigation. There is an ongoing debate as to whether prophylactic cholecystectomy is justified in young patients found to have small stones. Such patients have a long period over which they may develop symptomatic disease and small stones are an independent risk factor for the potentially serious complication of gallstone pancreatitis. The most recent guidance available does not recommend prophylactic surgery.

The laparotomy approach to cholecystectomy has now been replaced by the laparoscopic technique. Postoperative pain is minimized with only a short period of ileus and the early ability to mobilize the patient. Laparoscopic cholecystectomy can be safely carried out on a day-care basis in an elective setting in otherwise fit patients. This has considerable cost benefits over open cholecystectomy, which is now reserved for a small proportion of patients with contraindications, such as extensive previous upper abdominal surgery, ongoing bile duct obstruction or portal hypertension.

In approximately 5% of cases, a laparoscopic cholecystectomy is converted to an open operation because of technical difficulties: in particular, adhesions in the right upper quadrant or difficulty in identifying the biliary anatomy.

Acute cholecystitis

The initial management is conservative, consisting of keeping the patient nil by mouth, and administering intravenous fluids, opiate analgesia and intravenous antibiotics. Bacteria that are commonly associated with cholecystitis include *Escherichia coli*, *Bacteroides fragilis*, *Klebsiella*, *Enterococcus* and *Pseudomonas* species. Antibiotic selection is dictated by local policy and is guided by the severity of any associated sepsis and the result of any blood culture. Options include extended-spectrum cephalosporins (e.g. ceftriaxone) in combination with metronidazole, piperacillin/tazobactam or imipenem/meropenem.

Cholecystectomy is usually delayed for a few days to allow the symptoms to settle but can then be carried out quite safely in the majority of cases.

When the clinical situation fails to respond to this conservative management, particularly if there is increasing pain and fever, an empyema or gangrene of the gall bladder may have occurred. In this circumstance, urgent imaging (transabdominal ultrasound or CT scan) is required to define the pathology. Surgical intervention is usually needed, although a radiologically placed gall bladder drain can be used as a temporizing measure for the management of an empyema. The placement of a drain is the best option in patients who are considered unfit for early surgery (because of ongoing sepsis or significant co-morbidity).

Specific complications of cholecystectomy

These include a biliary leak, either from the cystic duct or the gall bladder bed. Injury to the bile duct itself occurs in up to 0.5% of laparoscopic operations and may have serious long-term sequelae in the form of a bile duct stricture and secondary biliary liver injury. Injuries to the extrahepatic biliary tree are more likely with variant duct anatomy, such as a low cystic duct insertion or draining of the cystic duct into the right posterior ducts rather than the CBD. There is an overall mortality of 0.2% associated with cholecystectomy.

Stone dissolution and shock wave lithotripsy

These non-surgical techniques for the management of gall bladder stones are used infrequently but still have a role in a few highly selected patients who may not be fit for cholecystectomy or have declined the surgical option.

Stone dissolution

Pure or near-pure cholesterol stones can be solubilized by increasing the bile salt content of bile. Most experience is with oral ursodeoxycholic acid. The approach requires long-term therapy and the recurrence rate of gallstones is high when therapy is stopped. Additional pharmacological tools for treating cholesterol gallstones include cholesterol-lowering agents that inhibit hepatic cholesterol synthesis (statins) or intestinal cholesterol absorption (ezetimibe), or drugs acting on specific nuclear receptors involved in cholesterol and bile acid homeostasis (see p. 1266).

Extracorporeal shock wave lithotripsy

A shock wave can be directed either radiologically or by ultrasound on to gall bladder stones. This technique was highly successful but only in a restricted patient population. The cystic duct requires patency for stone fragments to pass. Recurrence rates are high but may be reduced by the pharmacological approaches discussed earlier.

Post-cholecystectomy syndrome

This refers to right upper quadrant pain, often biliary in type, which occurs a few months after the cholecystectomy but may be delayed for a number of years. The patients often comment that the pain is identical to that for which the original operation was carried out. In many cases, this syndrome is related to a functional large bowel disorder with colonic spasm at the hepatic flexure (hepatic flexure syndrome). It may be speculated that a functional gut disorder may have been responsible for the original pain that led to the cholecystectomy. In a small proportion of patients the pain is the result of a retained CBD stone; in a further subsection sphincter of Oddi dysfunction is a potential cause.

Sphincter of Oddi dysfunction

Sphincter of Oddi dysfunction (SOD) is a clinical syndrome of biliary or pancreatic pain and is caused by either:

- sphincter of Oddi stenosis, e.g. following prior instrumentation or passage of stones; *or*
- sphincter of Oddi hypertension.

A full history of the type of pain is performed, as well as an assessment of serum liver biochemistry and amylase during, and between, episodes of pain.

Biliary SOD

In *type I* disease, patients have biliary-type pain with *both* raised serum bilirubin, alkaline phosphatase or aminotransferases during episodes *and* a distended CBD on imaging.

In *type II* disease, patients have biliary-type pain and *either* abnormal liver biochemistry during episodes *or* a distended CBD.

In *type III* disease, there is recurrent biliary-type pain but no abnormality in the liver biochemistry and a normal-calibre CBD.

Management is as follows:

- Type I SOD usually responds to endoscopic sphincterotomy.
- Type II SOD sometimes responds to endoscopic sphincterotomy.
- Type III SOD does not respond to endoscopic sphincterotomy and therefore this should not be performed.

Pancreatic SOD

In *type I* disease, patients have recurrent pancreatic pain, a raised serum amylase and a dilated pancreatic duct.

In *type II* disease, patients have recurrent pancreatic pain with *either* transient hyperamylasaemia *or* a dilated pancreatic duct.

In *type III* disease, patients have pain but neither an elevated amylase nor a dilated pancreatic duct.

Management is as follows:

- Types I and II SOD may respond to endoscopic sphincterotomy.
- Type III SOD with pain only does not respond to endoscopic sphincterotomy.

Common bile duct stones

The classical features of CBD stones are biliary colic, fever and jaundice (acute cholangitis). This triad is present only in a minority of patients. Abdominal pain is the most common symptom and has the typical features of biliary colic (see earlier). Jaundice is a variable accompaniment and is almost always preceded by abdominal pain. A patient with bile duct stones may experience sequential episodes of pain, only some of which are accompanied by jaundice. In contrast to malignant bile duct obstruction, the level of jaundice associated with CBD stones characteristically tends to fluctuate. In the elderly or immunocompromised patient, cholangitis may present with very non-specific symptoms, and only associated abnormal liver biochemistry may point to the diagnosis.

Fever is present only in a minority of cases but indicates biliary sepsis and sometimes associated septicaemia. The presence of such biliary sepsis is a significant adverse prognostic factor.

A minority of patients with bile duct stones are discovered incidentally during imaging for gall bladder disease or other intra-abdominal pathology. Some 15% of patients undergoing cholecystectomy will have stones within the bile duct that are detected only at the time of operative cholangiography. The frequency of asymptomatic bile duct stones resulting in complications is not well documented. It is likely that many such stones will pass into the duodenum without causing symptoms. However, the potential for serious complication is well recognized; in most circumstances, incidentally identified bile duct stones are removed (see later).

Examination

If the patient is examined between episodes, there may be no abnormal physical finding. During a symptomatic episode the patient may be jaundiced with a fever and associated tachycardia. There is tenderness in the right upper quadrant, varying from mild to extremely severe.

More widespread abdominal tenderness extending from the epigastrium to the left upper quadrant, associated with distension, may indicate associated stone-related pancreatitis (see later).

Investigations

Laboratory tests

- **Full blood count** is usually normal in the presence of uncomplicated bile duct stones.
- **An elevated neutrophil count** and raised inflammatory markers (erythrocyte sedimentation rate (ESR) and CRP) are frequent accompaniments of cholangitis.
- **The raised serum bilirubin** tends to be mild and often transient. Very high concentrations of bilirubin (>200 μmol/L) almost always reflect complete bile duct obstruction.
- **Serum alkaline phosphatase and γ-glutamyl transpeptidase** are similarly elevated in proportion to the degree of hyperbilirubinaemia.
- **Aminotransferase levels** are usually mildly elevated, but with complete bile duct obstruction there may be very marked rises to 10–15 times the normal value. The alanine aminotransferase is characteristically higher than the aspartate aminotransferase. These high levels may lead to an initial misdiagnosis of a hepatitic process.
- **Serum amylase levels** are often mildly elevated in the presence of bile duct obstruction but are markedly so if stone-related pancreatitis has occurred.
- **Prothrombin time** may be prolonged if bile duct obstruction has occurred and is sustained over several days; this reflects decreased absorption of vitamin K.

Imaging

- **Transabdominal ultrasound** is the initial imaging technique of choice. **Bile duct obstruction** is characterized by dilation of intrahepatic biliary radicles, which are usually readily detected by the ultrasound scan. It may, however, not be possible to identify the cause of obstruction. Stones situated in the distal CBD are poorly visualized by transabdominal ultrasound and up to 50% are missed. The detection of stones within the gall bladder is poorly predictive of the cause of bile duct obstruction. Asymptomatic gallstones are common (up to 15%) in patients who are 65 years and older. Conversely, in 5–10% of patients with bile duct stones, no calculi can be seen within the gall bladder.

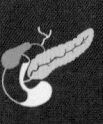

- *Magnetic resonance cholangiography (MRC)* delineates the fluid column within the biliary tree and is a sensitive technique for the detection of CBD stones in the presence of a dilated duct. The technique may be less accurate in the absence of duct dilation (see the role of EUS, later) (**Fig. 35.5**).
- *CT scanning* is an alternative way to detect bile duct dilation. Opaque stones are more readily identifiable within the bile duct than radiolucent cholesterol stones. CT scanning also provides a means of excluding other causes of bile duct obstruction, such as carcinoma of the head of the pancreas.
- *EUS* (**Fig. 35.6**) has enabled high-resolution imaging of the CBD, gall bladder and pancreas, although, unlike the preceding imaging techniques, it is an invasive procedure. The EUS probe in the duodenum is in close proximity to the distal CBD and hence can identify the majority of stones at this level. This technique is particularly useful for identifying small calculi (microcalculi) in a non-dilated CBD.
- *Endoscopic retrograde cholangiography (ERC).* In experienced hands, visualization of the CBD will be successful in 98% of cases, providing good documentation of bile duct stones (**Fig. 35.7**; see also **Fig. 35.5**). However, small stones can still be missed. ERC is an invasive procedure with recognized risks. In almost all circumstances, this is a therapeutic tool used to remove the stones that have been identified by the less invasive investigations described earlier.

Differential diagnosis

Cholangitis may occur independently of gallstones in any condition associated with impaired biliary drainage. It is commonly linked with primary abnormalities of the biliary tree, such as sclerosing cholangitis and Caroli's syndrome (a congenital disorder leading to ectasia/dilation of the intrahepatic bile ducts). Cholangitis may also complicate post-traumatic or surgery-associated bile duct strictures. It is unusual in malignant bile duct obstruction unless

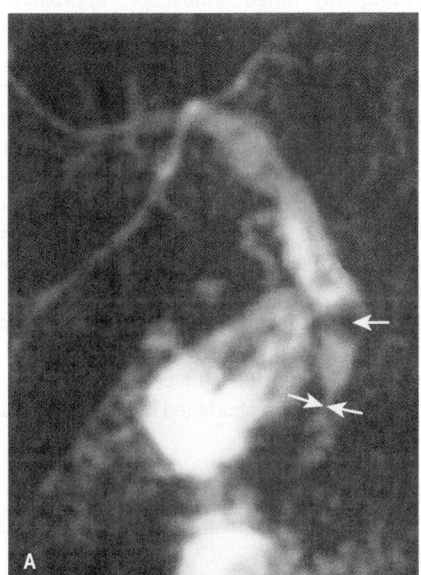
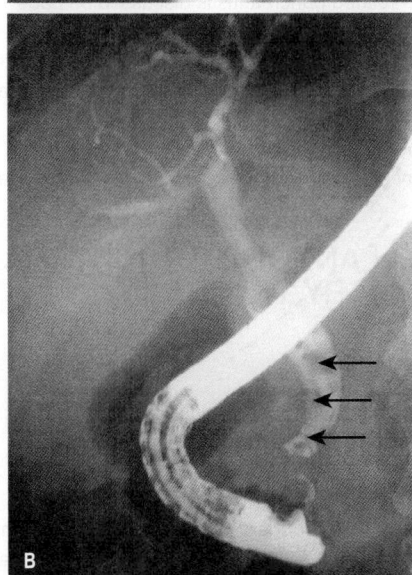

Fig. 35.5 A patient presenting with abdominal pain and jaundice. (A) A magnetic resonance cholangiogram (MRC) shows evidence of a distal common bile duct stricture (bottom arrows) with a stone in the bile duct proximal to this (top arrow). **(B)** An endoscopic retrograde cholangiopancreatogram (ERCP) in the same patient confirms the details identified in the MRC scan. The stones (arrowed) were removed at the time of the ERCP after initial dilation of the stricture.

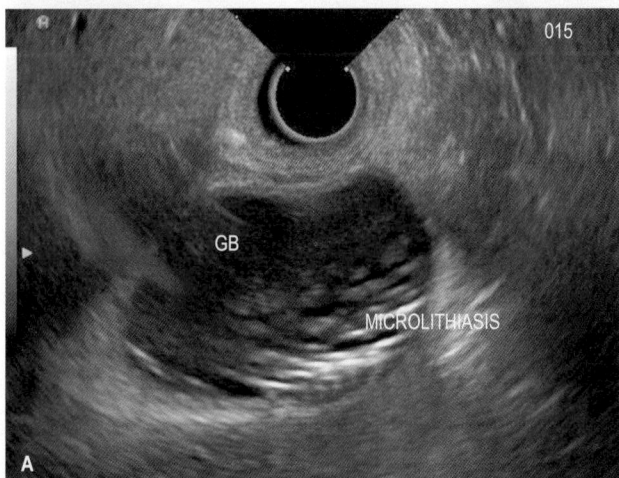
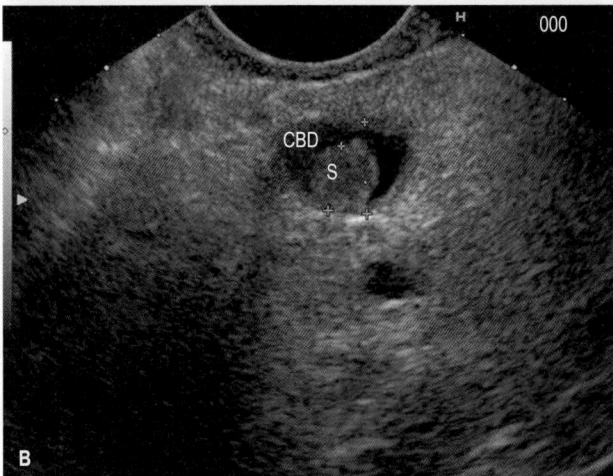

Fig. 35.6 An endoscopic ultrasound scan with the probe in the first part of the duodenum. (A) The gall bladder (GB) and multiple small, echo-poor stones within (microlithiasis). The patient had presented with recurrent episodes of unexplained abdominal pain. **(B)** The common bile duct (CBD) and a stone (S) clearly identified within the lumen.

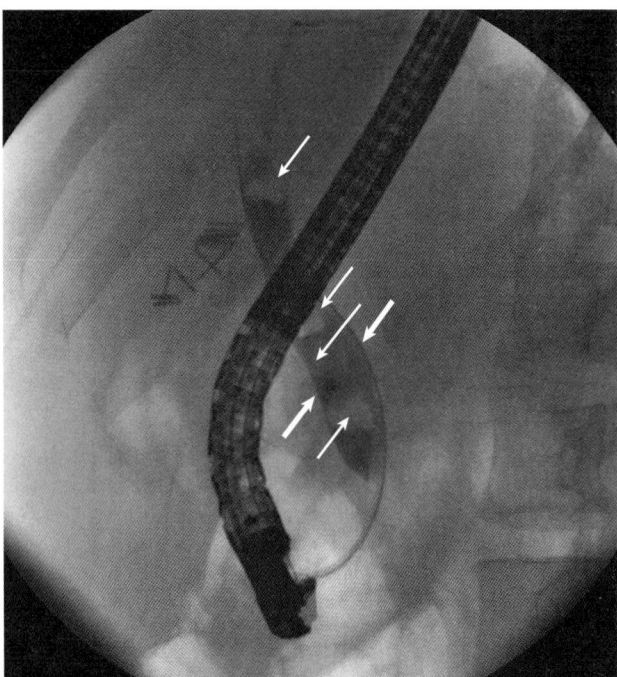

Fig. 35.7 An endoscopic retrograde cholangiopancreatogram (ERCP) carried out in a patient with abdominal pain, fluctuating jaundice and fever. The cholangiogram shows a dilated common bile duct (between thick arrows) and multiple stones within (arrowed). These stones were removed at the time of ERCP by means of balloon and basket retrieval. Note the multiple clips to the left of the upper bile duct, which were placed at a prior laparoscopic cholecystectomy.

there has been prior endoscopic or surgical intervention. Jaundice may also be a feature of acute cholecystitis in the absence of bile duct stones. A stone impacted in the neck of the gall bladder (Hartmann's pouch) or the cystic duct itself may compress and obstruct the bile duct (Mirizzi's syndrome). CBD stones may produce pain, but in the absence of jaundice, the differential diagnosis is that of biliary colic (see earlier).

Management

Acute cholangitis has a high morbidity and mortality, particularly in the elderly or those with serious co-morbidity. Successful management depends on intravenous antibiotics (as for acute cholecystitis) and urgent bile duct drainage. In most circumstances the latter is achieved by the endoscopic retrograde approach (ERCP, see earlier). Access to the bile duct is achieved by sphincterotomy and thereafter the stones can be removed by either balloon or basket catheters. In the severely ill patient a plastic stent (a small tube prosthesis) can be inserted into the bile duct to maintain bile drainage without the need to remove the stones, hence minimizing the time required to complete the procedure. The residual stones can then be cleared and the stent removed endoscopically when the patient has recovered from the acute episode. If endoscopic drainage is not available or is prevented by an inability to access the second part of the duodenum, a radiologically placed percutaneous biliary drain represents an alternative management option. Surgical drainage during an acute cholangitic episode has been associated with a high mortality and has been replaced by the endoscopic or percutaneous approach.

Urgent endoscopic bile duct clearance is also indicated in some patients with acute gallstone pancreatitis but only when this

coexists with persisting bile duct obstruction (see later). Patients who have retained CBD stones after a previous cholecystectomy are also optimally managed by endoscopic clearance.

Patients shown to have CBD stones as well as gall bladder stones may be treated using different approaches:

- ***At the time of laparoscopic cholecystectomy***, which can also include exploration of the CBD via the cystic duct or via direct choledochotomy. By using these techniques the surgeon can extract stones from the CBD. The skills and time required for bile duct exploration are considerably greater than those for laparoscopic cholecystectomy alone. This single-procedure approach minimizes the length of hospital admission. Concerns around an increased risk of bile duct injury with bile duct exploration have not been confirmed in controlled studies.
- ***An independently timed endoscopic approach***, either immediately before or after the cholecystectomy. Removal of CBD stones by this method is preferred in the UK. Large bile duct stones (>10 mm) may present a significant challenge to endoscopic removal. Mechanical lithotripsy facilitates stone fragmentation and removal into the duodenum. Extracorporeal shock wave stone fragmentation has been used but is not widely available. The recently increased availability of endoscopic cholangioscopy (direct visualization of the bile duct) has facilitated intraductal shock wave lithotripsy, utilizing electrohydraulic or laser probes.
- ***A combined laparoscopic and endoscopic approach***, in which an ERC and duct clearance are carried out under the same anaesthetic used for the laparoscopic cholecystectomy. This approach leads to a shortened hospital stay and the use of only one anaesthetic.

Complications of gallstones

- Acute cholecystitis and acute cholangitis are discussed on page 1316.
- Gallstone-related pancreatitis is discussed on page 1329.
- Gallstones can occasionally erode through the wall of the gall bladder into the intestine, giving rise to a biliary enteric fistula. Passage of a gallstone through to the small bowel can give rise to an ileus or true obstruction.
- There is little evidence that gallstones are associated with an increased risk of adenocarcinoma of the gall bladder (see p. 1322).

MISCELLANEOUS CONDITIONS OF THE BILIARY TRACT

Gall bladder

There are a number of non-calculous conditions of the gall bladder, some of which have been associated with symptoms.

Acalculous cholecystitis

Almost 10% of gall bladders removed for biliary symptoms are shown to have chronic inflammation within the wall but an absence of gallstones. Such cases are described as acalculous cholecystitis. In many instances the gall bladder inflammation is minor and of doubtful significance. In some cases, chemical inflammation of the gall bladder may occur from reflux of pancreatic enzymes back into the biliary tree, usually through the common channel at the ampulla of Vater. Bacterial and viral infections of the gall bladder have been recognized as a cause of acalculous cholecystitis. The decision to carry out cholecystectomy in the absence of defined gall bladder

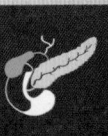
stones should be guided by the specific features of the history and by evidence of a diseased gall bladder wall on ultrasound scanning.

A distinct subtype of acalculous cholecystitis is characterized by severe necroinflammation of the gall bladder and generally occurs in an elderly and already critically ill group of patients, usually after major trauma or surgery. Around 20% of these patients develop inflammatory masses with subsequent cholestasis and jaundice; gall bladder perforation is a frequent complication. Morbidity and mortality are very high, and aggressive management of sepsis with antibiotics and cholecystostomy (percutaneous gall bladder drainage) or urgent cholecystectomy is required.

Cholesterolosis of the gall bladder

In cholesterolosis, cholesterol and other lipids are deposited in macrophages within the lamina propria of the gall bladder wall. These may be diffusely situated, giving a granular appearance to the gall bladder wall, or on occasion may be more discrete, giving a polypoid appearance (see later). Cholesterolosis of the gall bladder may coexist with gallstones but also occurs independently. Some degree of gall bladder cholesterolosis is found in up to 26% of laparoscopic cholecystectomy specimens, and as an incidental finding in up to 12% of autopsies in an elderly population. Interestingly, in contrast to cholelithiasis, rates are equal in men and women. It is doubtful whether isolated gall bladder cholesterolosis is a cause of symptoms.

Adenomyomatosis of the gall bladder

Adenomyomatosis is a gall bladder abnormality characterized by hyperplasia of the mucosa, thickening of the muscle wall and multiple intramural diverticula (the so-called 'Rokitansky–Aschoff sinuses').

The condition is usually detected as an incidental finding during investigation for possible gall bladder disease. It has been suggested that this condition is secondary to increased intraluminal gall bladder pressure but this is not proven. Gallstones frequently coexist, particularly when the adenomyomatosis is in a segmental distribution, but there is no evidence to support a direct relationship. It is unlikely that adenomyomatosis alone is a cause of biliary symptoms and it is not considered a pre-malignant state.

Chronic cholecystitis

There are no symptoms or signs that can conclusively be shown to be due to chronic cholecystitis. Symptoms attributed to this condition are vague, such as indigestion, upper abdominal discomfort or distension. There is no doubt that gall bladders studied histologically can show signs of chronic inflammation and, occasionally, a small, shrunken gall bladder is found either radiologically or on ultrasound examination. However, these findings can be seen in asymptomatic people and therefore this clinical diagnosis should not be made. Most patients with chronic right hypochondrial pain suffer from functional bowel disease (see p. 1159).

Extrahepatic biliary tract

Primary sclerosing cholangitis

In up to 40% of patients with primary sclerosing cholangitis (PSC; see also p. 1187) the clinical course is influenced by a dominant hilar or distal biliary stricture. This is relevant in those patients who do not have established advanced liver involvement, in whom maintenance of bile flow may protect the liver from secondary biliary injury. Drainage with a surgical hepaticojejunostomy has been beneficial

in some cases, but outcomes of such restricted surgery in PSC are generally inferior to those of orthotopic liver transplantation. Repeated endoscopic balloon dilation of the dominant stricture, with or without temporary short-term stenting, has been associated with sustained improvement in jaundice and even prolonged transplant-free survival. A significant minority of dominant strictures in PSC, particularly those at the hilum, represent development of an associated cholangiocarcinoma (see later). Development of cholangiocarcinoma in this context carries a very poor prognosis and surgical resection is rarely feasible. A benign dominant stricture in a non-cirrhotic patient, with recurrent cholangitis, refractory jaundice and pruritus, may be an indication for orthotopic liver transplantation. Conversely, superadded cholangiocarcinoma is currently an absolute contraindication to liver transplantation in most healthcare systems.

Autoimmune cholangitis

Immunoglobulin (Ig) G4-associated cholangitis is the biliary manifestation of a multisystem fibro-inflammatory disorder in which affected organs have a characteristic lymphoplasmacytic infiltrate rich in IgG4-positive cells (see p. 65). The original description of this condition was in the context of autoimmune pancreatitis and around 70% of these patients have evidence of IgG4 cholangiopathy (see p. 1330). However, IgG4 cholangiopathy can exist in the absence of pancreatic involvement.

The large majority of cases are recognized in middle-aged or elderly men. Presentation is varied, depending on the systems involved, but may include abdominal pain and jaundice. Both intra- and extrahepatic biliary strictures may be seen and the findings may be misinterpreted as representing cholangiocarcinoma or PSC. The diagnosis relies on clinical suspicion, confirmation of an elevated serum IgG4 level, a typical lymphocytoplasmic infiltrate on histological examination of involved tissue, and clinical response to glucocorticosteroid treatment. The condition is almost always responsive to steroids but can lead to hepatic failure.

Biliary cysts (choledochal malformation)

Cystic malformations may occur anywhere in the biliary tree, although they are most commonly extrahepatic. The resulting dilation of the bile duct may be of saccular, diverticular or fusiform configuration. In many cases there is an associated abnormal pancreatobiliary junction – a congenital malunion where the pancreatic duct drains directly into the CBD. The majority of symptomatic cases present in childhood with features of cholangitis, jaundice or a palpable mass. The formation of stones and sludge within the cystic segment may predispose to acute relapsing pancreatitis. In adult life, choledochal cysts may be a differential diagnosis in patients presenting with symptoms suggestive of bile duct stones. Extrahepatic bile duct cysts must be fully resected to avoid recurrent biliary sepsis, as well as reducing the risk (approximately 15%) of subsequent cholangiocarcinoma.

Benign bile duct strictures

Benign strictures are a recognized complication of biliary surgery. They may result from inadvertent direct stapling of the duct, or may be a secondary consequence of ischaemic injury (often in association with a bile duct leak). Strictures may also occur at the level of any bile duct anastomosis, either enteric or duct-to-duct. Biliary stricturing is also a rare complication of major trauma to the right upper quadrant. The inflammation and fibrosis of chronic pancreatitis commonly impinge on the intrapancreatic CBD (see later). This can result in cholestasis, jaundice and cholangitis.

In most cases, initial therapy includes endoscopic balloon dilation of the stricture and temporary bile duct stenting (see later). This may provide definitive management, but in some cases, surgical intervention with hepaticojejunostomy is required.

Haemobilia

Haemobilia describes blood in the biliary tree. This may be a consequence of liver trauma or a complication of liver surgery. Biopsy of the liver and erosion of a gallstone or hepatobiliary tumour into adjacent structures are also well-recognized causes. The end result is a fistula between a hepatic blood vessel and a bile duct.

Haemobilia may be a cause of significant gastrointestinal blood loss and should be suspected when melaena is accompanied by right-sided upper abdominal pain and jaundice, particularly in the context of recent hepatobiliary intervention. However, the bleeding may occur without any overt biliary symptoms. If the diagnosis is suspected, bleeding may be managed by occlusion of the feeding blood vessel by radiological embolization. Some patients will require surgery to control the bleeding point.

Tumours of the biliary tract

Gall bladder polyps

Polyps of the gall bladder are a common finding, being seen in approximately 4% of all patients referred for hepatobiliary ultrasonography. The vast majority of these are small (<5 mm) and non-neoplastic; they are inflammatory in origin or composed of cholesterol deposits (see earlier). Adenomas are the most common benign neoplasm of the gall bladder. Only a proportion of these have cancerous potential. The only reliable predictor of malignant risk is polyp size (>10 mm). Cholecystectomy is recommended for any polyp of 10 mm or larger in diameter.

Carcinoma of the gall bladder

Adenocarcinoma of the gall bladder represents 1% of all cancers. The mean age of occurrence is the early sixties, with a female-to-male ratio of 3:1. Gall bladder stones are often found in association with gall bladder cancer; gallstones have been suggested as an aetiological factor but this relationship remains unproven. Diffuse calcification of the gall bladder (porcelain gall bladder), considered to be the end-stage of chronic cholecystitis, has been associated with cancer of the gall bladder and is an indication for early cholecystectomy. Adenomatous polyps of the gall bladder in excess of 10 mm in diameter are also recognized as pre-malignant lesions (see earlier).

Carcinoma of the gall bladder may be detected incidentally at the time of planned cholecystectomy for gallstones; in such circumstances, resection of an early lesion may be curative. Radical surgery with negative resection margins offers the only potential cure. However, early lymphatic spread to the liver and adjacent biliary tract precludes curative resection in more advanced lesions. Palliative chemotherapy treatment may be given, usually with either 5-fluorouracil (5-FU)-based regimes, or gemcitabine (a nucleoside analogue) and cisplatin (a platinum-containing anticancer drug), with some evidence of a modest improvement in survival. A small proportion of cases are sensitive to radiotherapy. However, the generally advanced stage of disease at presentation means that the overall 5-year survival is less than 5%.

Cholangiocarcinoma

Cancers of the biliary tree (see also p. 1310) are classified as intrahepatic (above the hilum of the liver) or extrahepatic (involving the

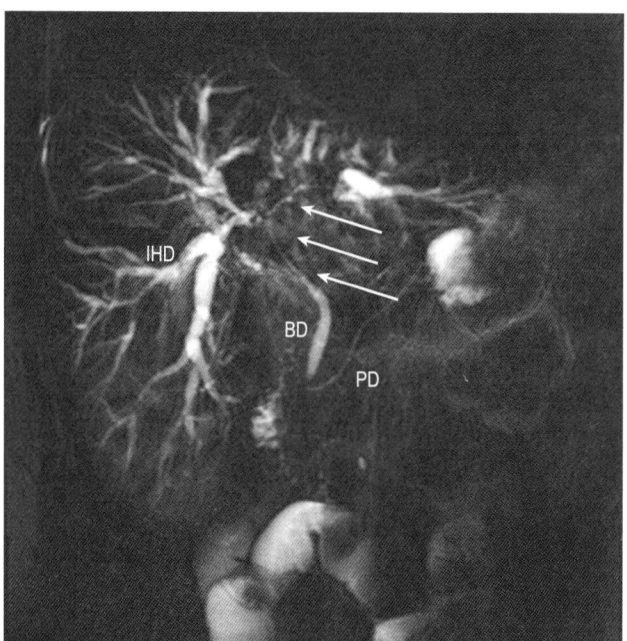

Fig. 35.8 Magnetic resonance cholangiopancreatography (MRCP) image of hilar cholangiocarcinoma extending into the left main duct. There is a normal-calibre distal bile duct (BD) and pancreatic duct (PD). The common hepatic duct and left main duct are strictured (arrowed). There is marked intrahepatic duct (IHD) dilation.

hilum or bile duct distal to the hilum). The latter are classified either on the TMN classification or on the site of the lesion (Bismuth–Corlette classification of biliary strictures). These malignancies represent approximately 1% of all cancers. A number of associations have been identified, such as that with choledochal malformation (see earlier) and that with primary sclerosing cholangitis (see p. 1321). Chronic infection of the biliary tree with parasitic liver flukes, particularly *Opisthorchis viverrini* or *Clonorchis sinensis*, has also been strongly implicated in areas where they are endemic. Extrahepatic bile duct malignancy usually presents with jaundice and may be confirmed on imaging tests, initially ultrasound and thereafter CT and, in particular, magnetic resonance cholangiopancreatography (MRCP; **Fig. 35.8**). Typical findings are of a bile duct stricture with proximal biliary dilation, with or without a visible mass. Histopathological diagnosis often proves difficult because the malignant cells are few in number and contained within a dense stroma. Endoscopically obtained cytology specimens have only 30% sensitivity. This yield can be enhanced by using additional endoscopic sampling techniques, such as transpapillary biopsy, and analytical enhancements, such as fluorescent *in situ* hybridization and digital image analysis. The recent application of direct endoscopic cholangioscopy has enabled direct visualization of biliary lesions and targeted biopsy.

Cholangiocarcinoma is often detected at a late stage and is characterized by early perineural, vascular and lymphatic spread. In a minority of cases, complete surgical resection is feasible, offering the only chance of cure. Cholangiocarcinoma of the CBD may be amenable to a limited bile duct resection. Very distal lesions require a pancreatoduodenectomy (Whipple procedure), and perihilar lesions frequently require partial hepatic resection in addition to biliary resection. In some international centres, extensive neoadjuvant chemoradiation therapy, followed by liver transplantation, has been used to cure localized hilar cholangiocarcinoma. Results from this emerging technique show promise, but cholangiocarcinoma remains an absolute contraindication to liver transplantation in most healthcare systems worldwide due to early disease recurrence.

The majority of patients with cholangiocarcinoma are treated palliatively with biliary decompression (see later) and gemcitabine- and cisplatin-based chemotherapy regimens.

Secondary malignant involvement of the biliary tree

Carcinoma of the head of the pancreas frequently presents with CBD obstruction and jaundice. Metastases to the bile duct from distant cancers are uncommon. Melanoma is the most frequent neoplasm to do so. Infiltration of the bile duct is not uncommon in disseminated lymphoma. Other carcinomas that may give rise to bile duct metastases, in order of frequency, are those arising in the lung, breast and colon, as well as those from the pancreas (metastatic as compared to direct infiltration).

Management
Palliation of malignant bile duct obstruction

All patients must be fully staged for operability using the imaging techniques described earlier. However, in the greater proportion of patients the treatment is palliative. Relief of bile duct obstruction has been shown to improve quality of life considerably and, with pain control, is the mainstay of effective palliation. Effective biliary decompression is also critical in jaundiced patients who wish to proceed with palliative chemotherapy. In recent years, endoscopic techniques have allowed the insertion of stents into the biliary tree to re-establish bile flow. The initial use of plastic stents has largely been replaced by self-expanding metal stents that have considerably longer periods of patency (**Fig. 35.9**). In the small proportion of

patients in whom bile duct drainage is not possible endoscopically, the percutaneous route offers an alternative method of stent placement under radiological control.

Further reading
Razumilava N, Gores GJ. Cholangiocarcinoma. *Lancet* 2014; 383:2168–2179.
Valle JW, Borbath I, Khan SA Huguet et al, on behalf of the ESMO Guidelines Committee. Biliary cancer: ESMO Clinical Practice Guidelines for diagnosis, treatment and follow-up. *Ann Oncol* 2016; 27(suppl. 5):v28–v37.

PANCREAS

Anatomy and function
Structure

The pancreas extends retroperitoneally across the posterior abdominal wall from the second part of the duodenum to the spleen. Anatomically, it is divided into a head, which rests within the concavity of the duodenum; a body, lying behind the base of the stomach; and a tail, which ends abutting the spleen. The neck of the pancreas lies between the body and head, and is in front of the superior mesenteric artery and vein. The head of the pancreas surrounds these two vessels. An uncinate process emerges from the lower part of the head, lying behind the superior mesenteric artery. The pancreas consists of exocrine and endocrine cells. The exocrine pancreas comprises 98% of the parenchyma.

The functional unit of the exocrine pancreas is composed of an acinus and its draining ductule. A ductule from the acinus drains into interlobular (intercalated) ducts, which, in turn, drain into the main pancreatic ductal system. The main pancreatic duct itself joins the CBD to enter the duodenum as a short single duct at the ampulla of Vater.

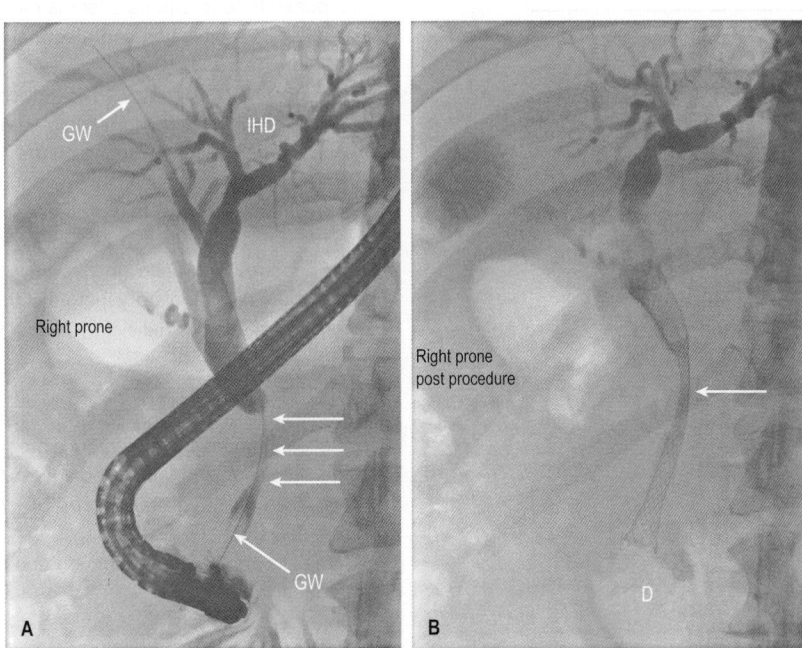

Fig. 35.9 **An endoscopic retrograde cholangiopancreatogram in a patient presenting with painless jaundice.** **(A)** There is a tight stricture in the mid-common bile duct extending proximally over 4 cm (extent defined by arrows). The intrahepatic ducts (IHD) proximally are dilated. A guidewire (GW) has been placed endoscopically across the stricture. **(B)** A self-expanding metal stent has been placed across the stricture and released. The stent is compressed at the level of the stricture (arrowed) but will open fully over 24 h. The contrast in the intrahepatic ducts has largely drained through the stent. The distal margin of the stent is in the duodenum (D).

The endocrine component is scattered throughout the gland in the form of pancreatic islets (of Langerhans).

Exocrine function

The pancreatic acinar cells are responsible for the production of digestive enzymes. These include amylase, lipase, colipase, phospholipase and the proteases (trypsin and chymotrypsin). These enzymes are stored within the acinar cells in secretory granules and are released by exocytosis (**Fig. 35.10**). The enzymes released by the acinar cells are transported into the duodenum by a high-volume pancreatic secretion, the majority of which is produced by the ductal cells. This fluid has a high concentration of bicarbonate, which neutralizes the gastric acid that has emptied into the duodenum. The neutralization of gastric acid is essential to facilitate pancreatic enzyme activity, which is pH-dependent (requiring a neutral pH).

After ingestion of a meal, pancreatic exocrine secretion is regulated by cephalic, gastric and intestinal stimuli. The cephalic phase is stimulated by behavioural cues related to the sight, smell and taste of food. The input from these sensory stimuli is integrated in the central nervous system at the dorsal vagal complex, and the output is transmitted to the exocrine pancreas via the vagus nerve. The gastric phase of pancreatic secretion results from the effects of

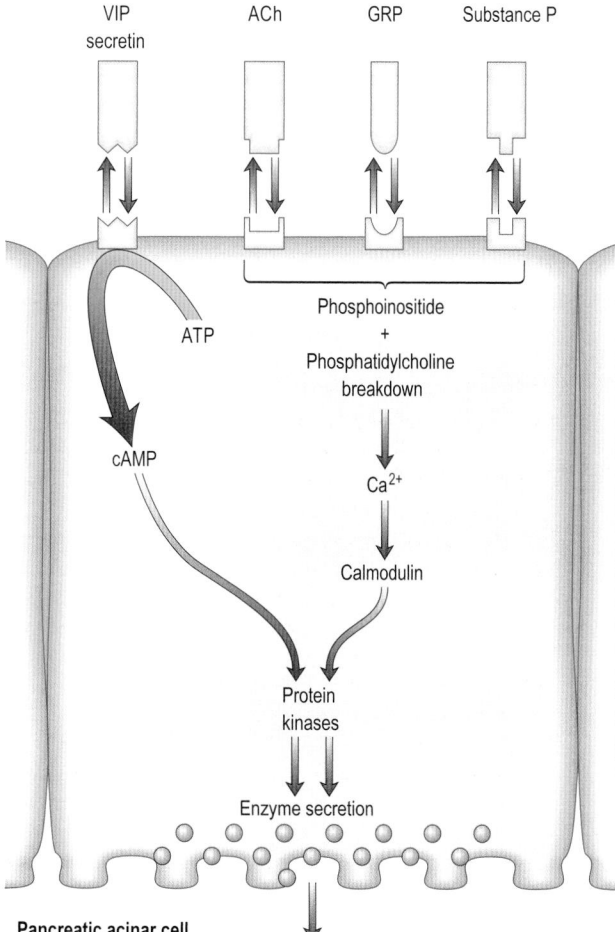

Fig. 35.10 Stimulation of digestive enzyme secretion from the acinar cell. G-protein-coupled receptors have been identified for vasoactive intestinal peptide (VIP), secretin, acetylcholine (ACh), gastrin-releasing polypeptide (GRP) and substance P. There are no cholecystokinin (CCK) receptors in humans. ATP, adenosine triphosphate; cAMP, cyclic adenosine monophosphate.

the meal in the stomach. The major stimulus of pancreatic secretion in the gastric phase is gastric distension, which causes secretion of an enzyme-rich fluid with little secretion of water and bicarbonate. This phase is also under vagal control. The intestinal phase of pancreatic secretion starts when protein, fat and gastric acid from the stomach enter the duodenum and continues for the duration of the digestive period. It is mediated by both hormones and enteropancreatic vagovagal reflexes. Feedback regulatory events eventually terminate pancreatic secretion.

- **Cholecystokinin (CCK)** plays a major role in meal-stimulated digestive enzyme secretion during the intestinal phase of pancreatic secretion. The hormone is produced in specialized gut endocrine cells (I cells) of the mucosa of the small intestine and is secreted in response to intraluminal food. There are no CCK receptors in human pancreatic cells, and CCK acts via receptors on vagal afferent fibres to stimulate pancreatic secretion.
- **Secretin** is also released from specialized enteroendocrine cells of the small intestine during a meal and, in particular, during duodenal acidification. Secretin has a direct effect on the pancreatic acinar cells, as well as the ductal cells. There is also a vagal-mediated secretory response. Secretin action is mediated via G-coupled receptors and calcium-mediated enzyme release. Secretin results in a bicarbonate-rich pancreatic secretion.

The efficiency of the digestive phase of pancreatic secretion requires a negative feedback mechanism to bring the process to a close. Completion of the postprandial secretory phase involves both neural and hormonal control.

- **Pancreatic polypeptide** is released from the islet cells of the pancreas in response to a meal and has an inhibitory effect on acinar enzyme secretion, via both a local effect and central receptors.
- **Somatostatin**, present within the pancreas, stomach and central nervous system, also has an inhibitory effect. It is released in response to food and its effect is mediated by both direct pancreatic acinar inhibition and a central nervous system inhibitory component.
- **Peptide YY (PYY)**, contained in endocrine cells of the distal small intestine is released by nutrients within the ileum and inhibits pancreatic secretion by acting on the acinar cells themselves, as well as centrally via the inhibitory regulation of vagal nerve.

There is also evidence that proteases within the duodenal lumen also have a negative feedback effect on acinar secretion. The gut-related peptides leptin and ghrelin, as well as influencing appetite behaviour, are also regulatory factors in the exocrine function of the pancreas. This effect is believed to occur via hypothalamic centres.

Endocrine pancreas

This consists of hormone-producing cells arranged in nests or islets (islets of Langerhans). The hormones produced are secreted directly into the circulation and there is no access to the pancreatic ductular system. There are **five main types of islet cell** corresponding to different secretory components:

- Beta cells are the most common and are responsible for insulin production.
- Alpha cells produce glucagon.
- D cells produce somatostatin.
- PP cells produce pancreatic polypeptide.
- Enterochromaffin cells produce serotonin.

A number of other hormones have been identified within the endocrine pancreas, including gastrin-releasing peptide, neuropeptide Y and galanin. These are believed to be neurotransmitters active in the neuro-gastrointestinal axis.

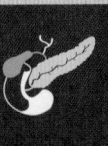

Investigations

Assessment of exocrine function

Pancreatic exocrine function is assessed in the investigation of patients with possible chronic pancreatic disease. Clinically evident fat malabsorption does not occur until there has been an 85–90% reduction in pancreatic lipase and is therefore a very late manifestation of pancreatic disease.

Direct tests of pancreatic function

These tests rely on the analysis of a duodenal aspirate following pancreatic stimulation, using either naso-duodenal tube or endoscopic aspiration. The original test involved pancreatic stimulation with the oral administration of a specified meal (Lundh meal) then replaced with intravenous secretin and cholecystokinin. The aspirate was assessed for pancreatic enzymes and bicarbonate production. These procedures are invasive and require meticulous technique, and are now rarely used.

Non-invasive indirect tests of pancreatic function

Faecal tests

- **Faecal elastase** is an enzyme produced in the pancreas; as it is not degraded in the intestine, it has high concentrations within the faeces. Diminished levels are seen in moderate and severe pancreatic insufficiency. This assay has replaced the faecal chymotrypsin test. It is unaffected by the administration of oral pancreatic enzyme supplements. However, as it relies on the concentration of elastase within the stool sample, it can render false low results in the context of diarrhoea, or water contamination during sample collection.
- **Faecal fat estimation.** This is rarely performed.

Oral pancreatic function tests

- **N-benzoyl-L-tyrosyl-p-aminobenzoic acid** (basis of the PABA test) and **fluorescein dilaurate** are oral compounds utilized in pancreatic function tests. They are digested by pancreatic enzymes, releasing substrates that are excreted and measured in the urine. Both tests are commercially available and have good sensitivity in moderate to severe pancreatic exocrine failure.

Clinical application of pancreatic function tests

While the invasive duodenal aspiration tests represent the most sensitive and specific means of assessing pancreatic function, they are very rarely used outside specialized centres. The non-invasive tests are widely available but are highly sensitive only in the detection of severe pancreatic insufficiency. The faecal elastase test (in a commercially available form) provides similar sensitivity and specificity, and is the test of choice as a screening tool for pancreatic insufficiency.

Pancreatic imaging

Imaging (see p. 1270) has a pivotal role in the investigation and management of pancreatic disease, which covers the spectrum of acute, chronic and malignant conditions.

- **A plain abdominal X-ray** may show the calcification associated with chronic pancreatitis, particularly when alcohol is the aetiology.
- **Transabdominal ultrasound** of the pancreas usually offers reasonable views of the pancreas; it is a useful screening investigation for inflammation or neoplasia, and is reasonably sensitive for detection of gallstone disease in a patient with pancreatitis. Views may be limited by overlying bowel gas, and ultrasound

should not be relied on in the exclusion of pancreatic neoplasia if clinical suspicion exists.

- **CT scan** with contrast enhancement and following a specific pancreatic protocol remains the 'gold standard' imaging technique for the investigation of pancreatic disease.
- **MRI scanning** represents an alternative to CT. MRCP gives clear definition of the pancreatic duct, as well as the biliary tree. Gallstones (including microcalculi) may also be identified in the biliary tree using MRI/MRCP.
- **Endoscopic ultrasound (EUS)** is very useful for identifying distal CBD stones, which may be the cause of an episode of acute pancreatitis. EUS can identify the early changes of chronic pancreatitis before these are evident with other imaging methods. There is also an increasing role for this technique to stage the operability of pancreatic adenocarcinoma, particularly with respect to vascular invasion. EUS is now considered the imaging technique of choice for investigating cystic lesions of the pancreas (see later). The technique allows fine-needle biopsy, as well as the therapeutic option of cyst drainage. EUS is a sensitive means of detecting small pancreatic tumours, particularly those of neuroendocrine origin.
- **Endoscopic retrograde cholangiopancreatography (ERCP)** is an invasive procedure and, while having a good safety profile, is associated with a small risk of serious adverse events: in particular, the precipitation of acute pancreatitis. The availability of MRCP and EUS has provided alternative means of defining pancreatic pathology. ERCP has an increasing therapeutic role in pancreatic disease (see later).
- [18F]**Fluorodeoxyglucose positron emission tomography (FDG-PET)/CT and** [68]**gallium-DOTATATE PET/CT** are scintigraphic techniques with a high diagnostic accuracy in patients with suspected neuroendocrine tumours, including those of the pancreas. They are also useful in defining the location of a neuroendocrine tumour, identifying multifocal small lesions, evaluating treatment options and detecting metastatic disease.

In summary, an initial transabdominal ultrasound, supplemented by CT, provides sufficient diagnostic information for most inflammatory and neoplastic conditions of the pancreas. MRI and MRCP are now widely available and provide additional information, particularly with respect to pancreatic ductular and biliary anatomy. EUS is a useful, albeit more invasive, tool for the investigation of both benign and malignant disease of the pancreas, and facilitates fine-needle aspiration and biopsy of targetable lesions.

PANCREATITIS

Classification

Pancreatitis is divided into **acute** and **chronic**. By definition, acute pancreatitis is a process that occurs on the background of a previously normal pancreas and can return to normal after resolution of the episode. Nevertheless, acute alcoholic pancreatitis occurs only in chronic misuse of alcohol. In chronic pancreatitis there is continuing inflammation with irreversible structural changes.

In practice, the differentiation between acute and chronic pancreatitis may be difficult. Any of the causes of acute pancreatitis, if untreated, may result in recurrent episodes, classified as **acute relapsing pancreatitis** and eventually bringing about permanent structural changes. In other cases, recurrent episodes of acute pancreatitis may represent exacerbations of an underlying chronic process.

Acute pancreatitis

Acute pancreatitis is a syndrome of inflammation of the pancreatic gland initiated by any acute injury. The causes of acute pancreatitis are listed in **Box 35.2**. In the Western world, gallstones and alcohol account for the vast majority of episodes. Alcohol also causes chronic pancreatitis (see later). The severity of the pancreatitis may range from mild and self-limiting to extremely severe, with extensive pancreatic and peripancreatic necrosis, as well as haemorrhage. In the most severe form (approximately 10% of cases) the mortality is between 40% and 80%.

Pathogenesis

This is still not completely understood. A precipitating event, such as gallstones or alcohol, is thought to induce the acute episode. Whatever the nature of the initiating insult, the pancreatic inflammatory response is secondary to the premature and exaggerated activation of digestive enzymes, principally trypsin, within the pancreas itself. In severe cases the subsequent cascade of autodigestion, microvascular injury, systemic inflammatory response and bacterial translocation can result in a devastating outcome.

Gallstone pancreatitis

The inducing effect is obstruction to pancreatic drainage at the ampulla by a stone or associated oedema. In this pathological situation, trypsinogen is cleaved (by cathepsin B) to trypsin, and trypsin degradation by chymotrypsin C is impaired and quickly overwhelmed. Intracellular calcium also increases and may also cause early activation of trypsinogen with upregulation of nuclear factor kappa B, leading to extensive acinar cell damage.

Alcohol-induced pancreatitis

There is evidence that alcohol interferes with calcium homeostasis in pancreatic acinar cells. In addition, activation of pancreatic stellate cells by acetaldehyde occurs, with production of collagen and then matrix proteins.

Clinical features

Acute pancreatitis is a differential diagnosis in any patient with upper abdominal pain. The pain usually begins in the epigastrium, accompanied by nausea and vomiting. As inflammation spreads throughout the peritoneal cavity, the pain becomes more intense. Involvement of the retroperitoneum frequently leads to back pain.

The patient may give a history of previous similar episodes or be known to have gallstones. An attack may follow an alcoholic binge. However, in many cases, there are no obvious aetiological factors.

Physical examination at the time of presentation may show little more than a patient in pain with some upper abdominal tenderness but no systemic abnormalities. In severe disease the patient has a tachycardia and hypotension, and is oliguric. Abdominal examination may show widespread tenderness with guarding, as well as reduced or absent bowel sounds. Specific clinical signs that support a diagnosis of severe necrotizing pancreatitis include periumbilical (**Cullen's sign**) and flank bruising (**Grey Turner's sign**). In patients with gallstone aetiology the clinical picture may also include jaundice or cholangitis.

Diagnosis

Blood tests

- **Serum amylase** is an extremely sensitive test if it is three times the upper limit of normal when measured within 24 h of the onset of pain. A number of other conditions may occasionally cause a very elevated amylase (**Box 35.3**). Amylase levels gradually fall back towards normal over the next 3–5 days. With a late presentation the serum amylase level may give a false-negative result.
- **Urinary amylase** levels may be diagnostic, as they remain elevated over a longer period of time.
- **Serum lipase** levels are also raised in acute pancreatitis and remain elevated for a longer period of time than amylase levels. However, overall, the accuracy of serum lipase is not significantly greater than that of amylase and it is technically more difficult to measure.
- **CRP level** is useful in assessing disease severity and prognosis.
- **Other baseline investigations** include a full blood count, serum creatinine and electrolytes, blood glucose, liver biochemistry, plasma calcium and arterial blood gases. These are documented at presentation and then repeated at 24 and 48 h, providing a basis for assessing the severity of an attack (see later).

Radiology

- An erect **chest X-ray** is mandatory to exclude gastroduodenal perforation, which also raises the serum amylase (see **Box 35.3**). A supine abdominal film may show gallstones or pancreatic calcification.
- An **abdominal ultrasound scan** is used as a screening test to identify a possible biliary (gallstone) cause of pancreatitis. Gallstones are difficult to detect in the distal CBD but dilated intrahepatic ducts may occur in the presence of bile duct obstruction. Stones within the gall bladder are not sufficient to justify a diagnosis of gallstone-related pancreatitis. The ultrasound may also demonstrate pancreatic swelling and necrosis, as well as peripancreatic fluid collections if present. In severe pancreatitis the pancreas may be difficult to visualize because of gas-filled loops of bowel.

? Box 35.2 Causes of acute pancreatitis

Common
- Gallstones
- Alcohol
- Iatrogenic (post-ERCP, surgery)
- Idiopathic (<10%)

Less common
- Trauma
- Infections, e.g. mumps, Coxsackie B, HIV, adenovirus
- Pancreatic tumours
- Hereditary
- Congenital pancreatic abnormalities, e.g. pancreas divisum
- Metabolic, e.g. hypercalcaemia, hypertriglyceridaemia
- Venom, e.g. scorpion stings, spider

- Sphincter of Oddi dysfunction (see p. 1318)
- Miscellaneous
- Drugs (see next section)

Drugs
- Azathioprine/mercaptopurine
- Didanosine
- Oestrogens
- Antibiotics, e.g. tetracycline
- Valproic acid
- Furosemide
- Sulphonamides
- Aminosalicylates
- Corticosteroids
- Metronidazole
- ACE inhibitors

ACE, angiotensin-converting enzyme; ERCP, endoscopic retrograde cholangiopancreatography; HIV, human immunodeficiency virus.

? Box 35.3 Elevation of serum amylase unrelated to pancreatitis

Leakage of upper gastrointestinal contents into the peritoneum
- Upper gastrointestinal perforation
- Biliary peritonitis
- Intestinal infarction

Inherited abnormalities of amylase
- Macroamylasaemia

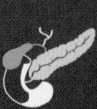

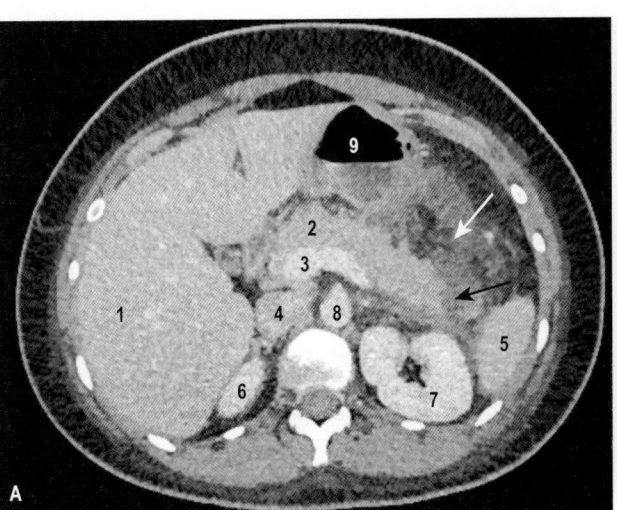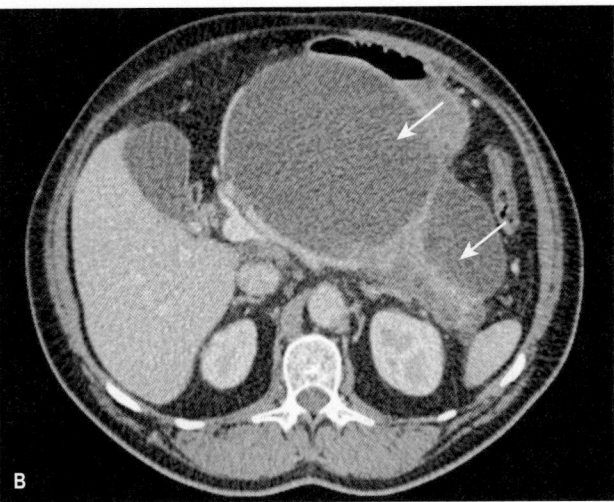

Fig. 35.11 Acute pancreatitis. (A) Abdominal CT demonstrating features of acute pancreatitis. There is marked inflammatory change/free fluid surrounding the pancreas and a focal area of necrosis in the pancreatic tail. (1) Liver; (2) pancreas; (3) portal vein; (4) inferior vena cava; (5) spleen; (6) right kidney; (7) left kidney; (8) aorta; (9) stomach. **(B)** Abdominal CT in a patient who presented with acute pancreatitis a few weeks prior to the scan demonstrating large pseudocysts (arrowed).

- **Contrast-enhanced CT scanning** is essential in all but the mildest attacks of pancreatitis. It should be performed after 72 h to assess the extent of pancreatic necrosis. CT provides very valuable prognostic information. Later, repeated CT scans can detect other complications, including fluid collections, abscess formation and pseudocyst development (**Fig. 35.11**).
- **MRI (MRCP)** assesses the degree of pancreatic damage and identifies gallstones within the biliary tree. MRI is particularly useful to differentiate between fluid and solid inflammatory masses.
- **ERCP** is used as a treatment measure to remove bile duct stones in selected cases of gallstone-related pancreatitis (see later).

Assessment of disease severity

The majority of cases of acute pancreatitis are mild and run a short, self-limiting course. However, approximately 25% follow a more complicated course and in 10% this is life-threatening. The revised Atlanta criteria define mild, moderately severe or severe pancreatitis and are summarized in **Box 35.4**; they require assessment of organ failure using the Modified Marshall scoring system (**Box 35.5**). In practice, patients with moderately severe acute pancreatitis should be managed as having severe disease until sustained improvement is seen.

In severe cases, mortality may be as high as 80%. The initial clinical course is marked by a systemic inflammatory response syndrome (SIRS), haemodynamic instability and multiple organ failure. The consequences of SIRS, including respiratory and acute kidney injury, account for most of the mortality within the first 7 days of an episode of severe acute pancreatitis. After 7 days the majority of deaths are linked to delayed complications, such as sepsis due to infected collections or haemorrhage due to inflammatory effects on major vessels.

Accurate identification of patients likely to progress to severe pancreatitis permits appropriate monitoring and intensive care to be put in place. Early clinical assessment has been shown to have poor sensitivity for predicting a severe attack. Similarly, individual laboratory tests have very limited value. Therefore, multiple factors have been used to develop clinical scoring systems. The **Glasgow and Ranson scoring systems** (**Boxes 35.6** and **35.7**) are based on such parameters and have been shown to have 80% sensitivity

---

i   Box 35.4 Severity of acute pancreatitis: revised Atlanta criteria 2013

Mild
- Absence of organ failure
- Absence of local complications

Moderate/severe
- Local complication and/or transient organ failure (<48 h)

Severe
- Persistent organ failure (>48 h), defined by the modified Marshall score for the evolution of organ failure (see **Box 35.5**)

---

for predicting a severe attack, although only after 48 h from presentation. The **Acute Physiology and Chronic Health Evaluation (APACHE) II score** has been extensively adopted as a means of assessing the severity of a wide spectrum of illness. It is based on common physiological and laboratory values, patient age and the presence or absence of a number of other chronic health problems, including obesity (**Box 35.8**). This scoring system appears to have a high sensitivity and can be applied as early as 24 h after onset of symptoms. There is evidence that obesity affects the outcome of an episode of pancreatitis, perhaps because adipose tissue is a substrate for activated enzyme activity, worsening the inflammatory reaction. All scoring systems for predicting the severity of acute pancreatitis have proven to have modest utility in clinical practice. However, systematic classification tools can guide consistent clinical assessment and are certainly necessary in clinical studies and audit of outcomes.

Management

The initial management of acute pancreatitis is similar for all causes. A multiple factor scoring system (ideally, APACHE II with a modification for obesity) should be used at the end of the first 24 h after presentation to allow identification of patients with a predicted severe attack. This should be repeated at 48 h to identify a further subgroup who appear to be moving into the severe category. These patients should be managed on a high-dependency or intensive care unit and the case should be discussed with a specialist pancreatic unit at an early stage. Even patients outside the severe category may require considerable supportive care.

Box 35.5 Modified Marshall scoring system[a]

Score system	0	1	2	3	4
Respiratory PO_2/F_iO_2	>400	301–400	201–300	101–200	≤101
Renal Serum creatinine (μmol/L)	134	134–169	170–310	311–439	>439
Cardiovascular Systolic blood pressure (mmHg)	>90	<90 Fluid-responsive	<90 Not fluid-responsive	<90 pH <7.3	<90 pH <7.2

[a]A score of ≥2 in any system defines the presence of organ failure.

Box 35.6 Glasgow prognostic criteria in acute pancreatitis[a]

Criteria	Measurement
Age	>55 years
White blood cell count	>15 × 10⁹/L
Blood glucose	>10 mmol/L
Serum urea	>16 mmol/L
Serum albumin	<30 g/L
Serum aminotransferase	>200 U/L
Serum calcium	<2 mmol/L
Serum lactate dehydrogenase	>600 U/L
P_aO_2	<8.0 kPa (60 mmHg)

[a]More than three positive factors during the first 48 h suggests severe pancreatitis and a poorer prognosis.

Box 35.8 Acute Physiology and Chronic Health Evaluation (APACHE) II scoring system[a]

Physiological
- Temperature
- Heart rate
- Respiratory rate
- Mean arterial pressure
- Glasgow Coma Scale score
- Presence of acute kidney injury
- Age
- Organ insufficiency
- Immunocompromise

Laboratory
- Oxygenation (P_aO_2)
- Arterial pH
- Serum:
  - Sodium
  - Potassium
  - Creatinine
  - Haematocrit
  - White blood cell count

[a]APACHE is applied within 24 h of admission. Score can range from 0 to 71 (normal to abnormal). Higher scores correspond to more severe disease and a higher risk of death. Body mass index (BMI) is an additional parameter that can be added specifically in assessing severity of acute pancreatitis.

Box 35.7 Ranson criteria in pancreatitis

Criteria	Measurement
At admission	
Age	>55 years
White blood cell count	>16 × 10⁹/L
Blood glucose	>11 mmol/L
Serum lactate dehydrogenase	>600 U/L
Serum aminotransferase	>250 U/L
Within 48 h	
Haematocrit fall	>10%
Serum aminotransferase	>200 U/L
Serum calcium	<2 mmol/L
Serum urea increase	>1.8 mmol/L
Base deficit	>4 Meq/L
P_aO_2	<8.0 kPa (60 mmHg)

Early fluid losses in acute pancreatitis may be large, requiring well-maintained intravenous access and a urinary catheter to monitor circulating volume and renal function. Arterial and central venous catheterization may be necessary to facilitate close monitoring of haemodynamic status and permit repeat sampling of arterial blood gases.

- **Nasogastric suction.** This prevents abdominal distension and vomitus, and hence the risk of aspiration pneumonia.
- **Baseline arterial blood gases.** These are a key predictive factor for severity of an episode and determine the need for continuous oxygen administration.
- **Prophylactic antibiotics.** Controlled data for the use of antibiotics are available but the results are not uniform in showing

benefit, particularly in demonstrating improved mortality. There is some evidence that the β-lactam imipenem reduces the incidence of infected pancreatic necrosis. Antibiotics should usually be reserved for cases where cholangitis or infected necrotic tissue is strongly suspected and, if possible, the choice should be guided by blood culture results.

- **Analgesia requirements.** Tramadol or another opiate is the drug of choice for immediate post-presentation pain control. Unless there is prompt resolution of pain, a patient-controlled system of administration is indicated to provide continuous and adequate pain relief. Fentanyl has been used widely for this application. There is a theoretical risk that morphine and diamorphine might exacerbate pancreatic ductular hypertension by causing sphincter of Oddi contraction. Although there are no clinical data to support this risk, some clinicians avoid these drugs in acute pancreatitis.
- **Feeding.** In a severe episode there is little likelihood of oral nutrition for a number of weeks. Total parenteral nutrition has been associated with a high risk of infection and has been replaced by enteral nutrition. In the absence of gastroparesis, most patients will tolerate nasogastric administration of feed without exacerbation of pain. In those with gastroparesis or poorly tolerated nasogastric feeding (exacerbation of pain or precipitation of nausea and vomiting), post-pyloric feeding should be instituted by the endoscopic placement of a nasojejunal tube.
- **Anticoagulation.** Low-molecular-weight heparin should be given for prophylaxis of deep vein thrombosis.

In a small proportion of patients, multiorgan failure will develop in the first few days after presentation, reflecting the extent of SIRS. Such patients may require positive-pressure ventilation and renal support (see p. 220).

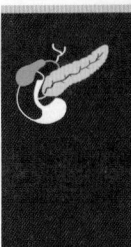

Gallstone-related pancreatitis

In patients with gallstone-related pancreatitis and associated bile duct obstruction (particularly when complicated by cholangitis), endoscopic intervention with sphincterotomy and stone extraction is the treatment of choice. In the absence of bile duct obstruction, sphincterotomy and stone extraction are of proven benefit only when the episode of pancreatitis is predicted to be severe. In less severe cases of gallstone-related pancreatitis the presence of residual bile duct stones can be assessed electively by MRCP or EUS in the recovery phase of the acute episode; if stones are present, they can be removed by ERCP. To prevent a recurrent episode of gallstone pancreatitis, cholecystectomy should be carried out as soon as feasible after the acute episode has resolved.

Complications

These are listed **Box 35.9**. After the first 7 days, the prognosis of acute pancreatitis is most closely related to the extent of pancreatic necrosis. This can be most accurately assessed by contrast-enhanced CT, which should be carried out in all patients with severe disease after the first week. Extensive necrosis (>50% of the pancreas) is associated with a high risk of further complicated disease, frequently requiring surgical intervention.

In this minority of patients with extensive necrosis of the pancreatic and peripancreatic tissues, superimposed infection is associated with a greatly increased risk of mortality. A 'step-up', minimally invasive approach is now preferred, with open surgical debridement avoided if at all possible. Long courses of antibiotics are given, and percutaneous drainage and EUS-guided endoscopic necrosectomy are used to clear infected collections. The aims of such interventions are to control infection, evacuate devitalized tissues (the culture medium for invasive infection) and promote conditions for healing.

The best outcomes from intervention are achieved when debridement is delayed until at least 4 weeks after the onset of pancreatitis. When the damaged area has been walled off and liquefaction has begun, a pseudocyst develops. If necessary, acute sepsis may be controlled by percutaneous drainage of collections in the first instance.

Prognosis

The vast majority of patients with a mild to moderate episode of acute pancreatitis will make a full recovery with no long-term sequelae. Recurrent episodes of pancreatitis may occur, particularly if there has been any long-term pancreatic ductular damage. Patients with more severe acute pancreatitis may develop pancreatic insufficiency with respect to both exocrine (malabsorption) and endocrine function (diabetes); both of these carry their own significant, life-long morbidity.

Chronic pancreatitis

Aetiology

In developed countries, alcohol is reported to be the only aetiological factor in 60–80% of cases. There is a sizeable list of other reported aetiological factors, which can be categorized into toxic–metabolic, genetic, autoimmune, recurrent acute or severe acute pancreatitis, obstruction and idiopathic causes (**Box 35.10**).

Pathogenesis

There is increasing evidence that an increase in activated trypsin within the pancreas is a common pathway for the development of chronic pancreatitis. This may occur as a result of premature activation of trypsinogen to trypsin, or of impaired inactivation/clearance

> **i** **Box 35.9 Complications of acute pancreatitis**
>
> **Systemic**
> - Systemic inflammatory response syndrome (SIRS)
> - Multiorgan dysfunction
>
> **Pancreas**
> - Pancreatic fluid collections
> - Necrosis ± infection
> - Pancreatic abscess
> - Pancreatic pseudocyst (after 4–6 weeks)
>
> **Lungs**
> - Pleural effusion
> - Acute respiratory distress syndrome (ARDS) – hypoxia
> - Pneumonia
>
> **Kidney**
> - Acute kidney injury
>
> **Gastrointestinal tract**
> - Gastrointestinal bleeding from gastric or duodenal erosions
> - Paralytic ileus
>
> **Hepatobiliary**
> - Jaundice
> - Common bile duct obstruction
> - Portal vein thrombosis
>
> **Metabolic**
> - Hypoglycaemia
> - Hyperglycaemia
> - Hypocalcaemia
>
> **Haematological**
> - Disseminated intravascular coagulation (DIC)

> **?** **Box 35.10 Causes of chronic pancreatitis**
>
> - Alcohol
> - Chronic kidney disease
> - Hereditary:
>   - Cystic fibrosis
>   - Trypsinogen and inhibitory protein defects
> - Tropical chronic pancreatitis
> - Obstructive
> - Trauma
> - Idiopathic
> - Hypercalcaemia
> - Recurrent acute pancreatitis
> - Autoimmune (immunoglobulin G4)

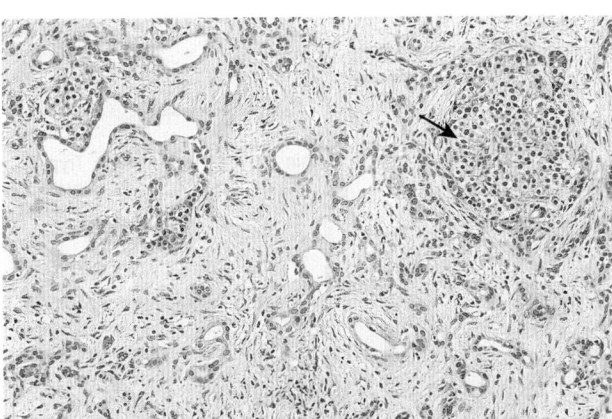

Fig. 35.12 Histology of chronic pancreatitis. There is considerable loss of acini and replacement by fibrosis. Inflammatory cells are relatively inconspicuous at this late stage. Islets of Langerhans (one is arrowed) sometimes escape destruction but their loss can result in diabetes mellitus. *(From Underwood JC (ed.). General and Systematic Pathology, 4th edn. Edinburgh: Churchill Livingstone; 2004, with permission.)*

of the activated enzyme from the pancreas. It is believed that the increased or prolonged intrapancreatic enzyme activity leads to the precipitation of proteins within the duct lumen in the shape of plugs. These then form a nidus for calcification and cause ductal obstruction, leading to ductal hypertension and further pancreatic damage (**Fig. 35.12**).

In the case of alcohol-related chronic pancreatitis, ethanol increases intracellular calcium, promoting trypsinogen activation to trypsin, as well as diminishing the protective inactivation pathway. The observation that the vast majority of people drinking excess alcohol do not develop pancreatitis suggests that the disease process is a complex interaction of different mechanisms. It is proposed that the alcohol is only one factor that interacts with other environmental and/or genetic influences (see later).

Genetic aspects of chronic pancreatitis

A number of genetic factors have been identified that influence the process of trypsin activation and inactivation. Cationic trypsinogen is the major form of trypsinogen produced in the pancreas and is encoded by the *PRSS1* gene (**Fig. 35.13**). Gain-of-function mutations of this gene are recognized as the major factor in hereditary pancreatitis, an autosomal dominant condition with high penetrance.

Calcium levels within the pancreas have a role in the process of activation and inactivation of trypsinogen/trypsin and are, in part, modulated by the calcium-sensing receptor (CASR). Mutations coding for this receptor have been associated with pancreatitis and are believed to facilitate the damaging effects of alcohol on the pancreas.

The serine protease inhibitor Kazal type 1 (*SPINK-1*) is a specific trypsin inhibitor and is co-secreted with trypsinogen by the acinar cells. Loss-of-function mutations of the *SPINK-1* gene have been associated with the development of chronic pancreatitis and identified, in particular, as a factor in the development of tropical pancreatitis (almost certainly interacting with environmental triggers).

Chymotrypsin C is produced in trace amounts by the acinar cells and has also been shown to have a role in trypsin degradation. Loss-of-function mutations of the encoding gene have been identified in patients with chronic pancreatitis.

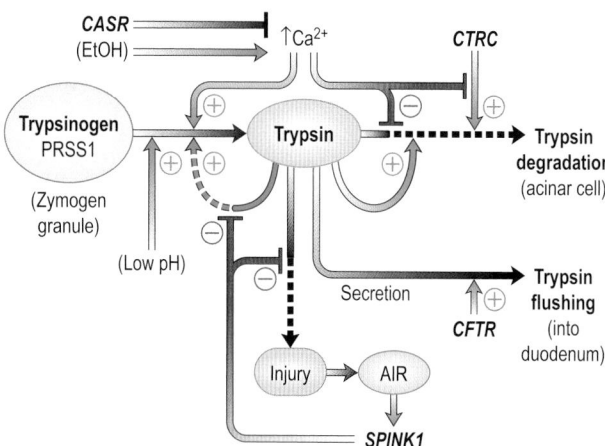

Fig. 35.13 Genetic factors in trypsinogen activation and trypsin inactivation. Early activation of trypsinogen to trypsin within the pancreas is crucial in the development of pancreatitis. Trypsinogen activation is promoted by cationic trypsinogen mutations (PRSS1+), active trypsin, high calcium (Ca²⁺) and low pH. Calcium levels are regulated in part by calcium-sensing receptor (CASR) and dysregulated by ethanol (EtOH). Active trypsin degradation is facilitated by *CTRC* and by other active trypsin molecules, but blocked by high calcium. Active trypsin within the pancreas leads to pancreatic injury, which causes an acute inflammatory response (AIR). AIR upregulates expression of serine protease inhibitor Kazal 1 (*SPINK1*), which blocks active trypsin and therefore prevents further activation of trypsinogens and limits further tissue injury. Cystic fibrosis transmembrane conductance regulator (*CFTR*) represents an extra-acinar cell mechanism to eliminate trypsin by flushing it out of the pancreatic duct and into the duodenum. *(Adapted from Whitcomb DC. Genetic aspects of pancreatitis.* Ann Rev Med *2010; 61:413–424.)*

The cystic fibrosis transmembrane conductance regulator (*CFTR*) is expressed on the apical surface of the acinar cells and is responsible for maintaining a high-volume, bicarbonate-rich pancreatic secretion. This high-volume secretion is responsible for flushing the activated trypsin into the duodenum. The homozygote or complex heterozygote *CFTR* mutations associated with the cystic fibrosis disease state are almost always manifest by perinatal/early pancreatic exocrine failure (see p. 1332). An increased frequency of a single *CFTR* mutation in patients with idiopathic chronic pancreatitis has been identified.

The identification of a genetic component to the development of chronic pancreatitis has led to speculation that, in many cases, the evolution of the disease is dependent on the complex interaction of gene–gene and gene–environmental factors.

Autoimmune chronic pancreatitis

Two types of autoimmune chronic pancreatitis (ACP) have been identified. The ***most common variant (type 1)*** is seen predominantly in middle-aged men and is associated with raised serum and tissue levels of IgG4. Other autoantibodies, including those directed towards nuclear and smooth muscle antigens, are also observed. Extrapancreatic tissue involvement is common, including the biliary tree (autoimmune cholangitis; see earlier), as well as thyroid, salivary gland and renal tissue (see p. 1378). In all these disorders there is a raised serum IgG4 level and, pathologically, there is a dense lymphoplasmacytic infiltrate with many IgG4-positive plasma cells, a mild to moderate eosinophil infiltrate and an obliterative phlebitis in some organs. ACP is one of the few settings in which the pathogenesis of the disease may be independent of the activated trypsin pathways.

The ***second variant (type 2)*** tends to occur in early midlife with an equal sex distribution and does not have the autoimmune markers or IgG4-positive cells. Some 30% of cases are associated with inflammatory bowel disease. Disease is much more likely to be restricted to the pancreas and lacks the associations with other organ/tissue involvement seen with the type 1 variant. The hallmark of both types of autoimmune pancreatitis is evidence of responsiveness to steroids (see later).

The presentation of autoimmune pancreatitis is varied, particularly in type 1, in which extrapancreatic disease may predominate. Abdominal pain and weight loss are common features; jaundice may be an early symptom, both secondary to bile duct obstruction by the inflamed head of pancreas, and a manifestation of the cholangitis seen in type 1 cases.

Clinical features

Epigastric pain is the most common presentation of chronic pancreatitis, often radiating into the back. The pattern of pain may be episodic, with short periods of severe pain, or is chronic and unremitting. For those with an alcohol-related aetiology, exacerbations of the pain may follow further alcohol excess, although this is not a uniform relationship. Alcohol excess or meals with a high fat content may also lead to exacerbations of pain, independent of the aetiology.

During periods of abdominal pain, anorexia is common and weight loss may be severe. This is particularly so in those patients with chronic, unremitting symptoms. Exocrine insufficiency may develop at any time and occasionally malabsorption is the presenting feature in the absence of abdominal pain. Diabetes occurs in approximately 30% of cases and is usually a late event in the disease process, almost always following the development of exocrine insufficiency. Jaundice secondary to obstruction of the CBD during

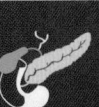

its course through the fibrosed head of the pancreas may also occur and may be a presenting feature in a small proportion of patients.

Investigations

The extent to which investigations are required is dependent on the clinical setting.

- **Serum amylase and lipase** levels may be elevated, but in advanced disease there may not be sufficient residual acinar tissue to produce this elevation.
- **Serum IgG4 levels** should be measured in those cases with suspected autoimmune pancreatitis.
- **Faecal elastase** level will be abnormal in the majority of patients with moderate to severe pancreatic disease.
- **Gene mutation analysis** should be carried out in selected cases when the aetiology is uncertain. This is most relevant in patients presenting below the age of 40. Common mutations of the *PRSS1*, *SPINK-1* and *CFTR* encoding genes are available via reference centres.
- **Transabdominal ultrasound scan** is frequently used for initial assessment.
- **Contrast-enhanced CT scanning** provides a more detailed assessment. In the presence of pancreatic calcification and a dilated pancreatic duct, the diagnosis of chronic pancreatitis can be readily established (**Fig. 35.14**). This may be much more difficult when these features are not present.
- **MRI with MRCP** is utilized to define more subtle abnormalities of the pancreatic duct, which may be seen in non-dilated chronic pancreatitis. Administration of intravenous secretin during an MRCP can afford dynamic images of pancreatic duct distension that offer an indirect measure of pancreatic exocrine function.
- **MRCP** has replaced diagnostic ERCP.
- **EUS** is used increasingly when doubt about the diagnosis remains after the imaging described, or specifically when complications of chronic pancreatitis, including pseudocyst formation and the possible development of malignancy, need assessment.

Differential diagnosis

The differential diagnosis is that of pancreatic malignancy. Carcinoma of the pancreas can reproduce many of the symptoms and imaging abnormalities that are commonly seen with chronic pancreatitis. The diagnosis of malignancy should be considered in patients with a short history when there is a localized pancreatic mass. Considerable difficulties may arise when a malignancy develops on the background of established chronic pancreatitis (the latter being a recognized pre-malignant lesion).

High-quality imaging is able to define malignant features with a localized mass lesion, local invasion and lymph node enlargement. EUS with fine-needle biopsy provides the most accurate assessment of a potential mass lesion.

Management

In patients with alcohol-related chronic pancreatitis, long-term abstinence is likely to be of benefit, although this has been difficult to prove. Tobacco smoking is also an independent risk factor for chronic pancreatitis and pancreatic cancer, and smoking cessation is strongly recommended. Autoimmune pancreatitis is steroid-responsive and failure to respond would put the diagnosis in question. Relapse is common when the steroids are withdrawn, and long-term immunomodulators (e.g. azathioprine) may be required.

Abdominal pain

For short-term flare-ups of pain, a combination of a non-steroidal anti-inflammatory drug (NSAID) and an opiate (tramadol) is usually sufficient for symptomatic relief. In patients with chronic unremitting pain, this may be inadequate and also risks opiate dependence.

Tricyclic antidepressants (e.g. amitriptyline) and membrane-stabilizing agents (e.g. pregabalin) are used for chronic pain and reduce the need for opiates. Coeliac axis nerve block may produce good pain relief but is unreliable in its efficacity and duration of action. In the majority of patients, some spontaneous improvement in pain control occurs with time. After a 6–10-year period, some 60% of patients will become pain-free. For recurrent severe or debilitating chronic pain, both endoscopic and surgical intervention has been used. Such intervention is indicated in patients with a dilated pancreatic duct upstream of a pancreatic duct stricture or stone. The endoscopic approach has centred on improving duct drainage by removing intraductal stones and duct stenting to maintain patency. Extracorporeal shock wave lithotripsy has been used to fragment stones within the head of the pancreas.

Surgical intervention usually involves a duct drainage procedure, which can be combined with partial resection of the diseased pancreas. Trials have reported improved pain control following surgical intervention, as compared with the endoscopic approach. However, many patients have a high level of debility (and often continued alcohol excess) and are unsuitable for major surgery due to co-morbidity or technical factors such as the presence of varices within the operative field. In such circumstances, endoscopic therapy is justified as a first measure and there is no evidence that this adversely influences subsequent surgery.

Malabsorption

The steatorrhoea associated with pancreatic insufficiency may be high, with up to 30 mmol of fat lost per 24 h. This will usually improve with pancreatic enzyme supplements. Current preparations are presented in the form of microspheres, which reduce the problems of acid degradation in the stomach. An acid suppressor (H_2-receptor antagonist or proton pump inhibitor) is also given. Despite this, a proportion of patients continue to malabsorb, usually reflecting the inadequate mixing of the pancreatic supplements with the food, as well as the low pH in the duodenum secondary to inadequate pancreatic bicarbonate production. There is no justification to reduce fat intake below the recommended levels of a normal diet, as this will contribute to the malnutrition seen in patients with chronic

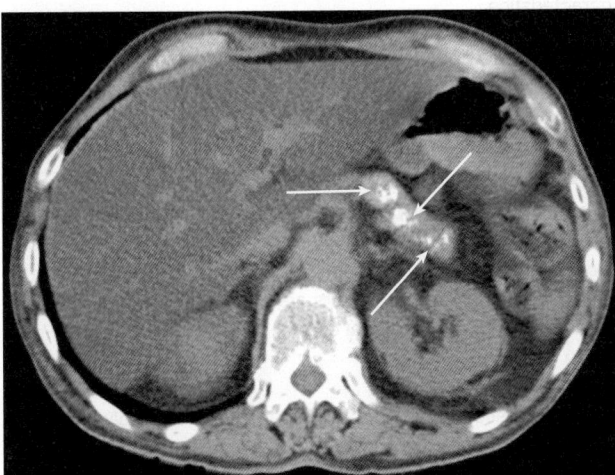

Fig. 35.14 Contrast-enhanced CT scan in a patient with chronic pancreatitis. Multiple calcific densities (arrowed) are demonstrated along the line of the main pancreatic duct.

pancreatitis. Dietetic input is valuable for the management of malabsorption and also for monitoring and alleviating the malnutrition that is often seen secondary to abdominal pain and food aversion.

Diabetes

Diabetes associated with pancreatic endocrine failure may be difficult to control, with a rapid progression from oral hypoglycaemic agents to an insulin requirement. Labile blood sugar levels are a common problem secondary to inadequate glucagon production by the damaged pancreas.

Autoimmune pancreatitis

Most patients respond to glucocorticoid therapy, e.g. prednisolone 40 mg daily for 4–6 weeks. Relapses are treated with azathioprine.

Specific complications

The most common structural complication of chronic pancreatitis is a **pancreatic pseudocyst**, a fluid collection surrounded by granulation tissue (see p. 505). These usually occur in relationship to a period of enhanced inflammatory activity within the pancreas giving abdominal pain but may develop silently during what would appear to be a stable phase. Intra- or retroperitoneal rupture, bleeding or cyst infection may occur. The larger cysts may occlude nearby structures, including the duodenum and the bile duct. In pseudocysts less than 6 cm in diameter, spontaneous resolution can be anticipated. In larger cysts that have been present for a period in excess of 6 weeks, resolution is less common and a long-term complication rate of approximately 30% can be anticipated. Many pseudocysts are closely opposed to the posterior wall of the stomach or duodenum, and can be successfully drained endoscopically using EUS to identify the optimum drainage site. A direct fistula is created between the pseudocyst lumen and the gastric or duodenal lumen, which is then kept patent by the insertion of removable stents. This approach will be successful in approximately 75% of cases. Surgical drainage is required for failures of endoscopic therapy or in circumstances where the pseudocyst anatomy does not allow endoscopic access.

Ascites and, occasionally, **pleural effusions** can be a direct consequence of chronic pancreatitis when there has been disruption of the main pancreatic duct. A high amylase level in the ascites or pleural fluid confirms the aetiology. Such disruptions of the main pancreatic duct require surgical intervention or ERCP and pancreatic duct stent placement.

There is an increased risk of **pancreatic cancer** in patients with chronic pancreatitis. The risk of malignancy is closely related to the duration of the inflammatory process. The highest incidence has been reported in hereditary pancreatitis, with a 50-fold increase and a lifetime risk as high as 40%. This reflects the early onset (in childhood) of the disease. Increases of 20–30-fold have been described in patients carrying other gene mutations and early onset of disease. The lifetime risk of malignancy in other causes of chronic pancreatitis, such as alcohol, which develop much later, is 10–15%. Cancer surveillance programmes have been proposed for the very high-risk groups (hereditary pancreatitis and other causes of early-onset disease), usually starting around the age of 40 years and relying on yearly imaging and tumour marker measurement.

Cystic fibrosis

Some 85% of people with cystic fibrosis (see p. 983) will have pancreatic exocrine failure, and in the majority of these this will develop *in utero* or the perinatal period. Malabsorption and failure to thrive are common presentations in the perinatal period and first year of life, and diabetes will develop subsequently in 30% of these patients during their lifetime.

In the remaining 15% of cases there is sufficient pancreatic exocrine secretion, which may persist throughout the patient's lifetime. This reflects residual *CFTR* function and is associated with class IV and V mutations. The patients tend to present later in life and have less severe pulmonary involvement, although this is not uniform. Some of these cases will progress to pancreatic exocrine insufficiency at variable times in the course of their disease. A small proportion develop symptomatic pancreatitis as part of this process.

The **management** of pancreatic exocrine insufficiency in cystic fibrosis is necessary to optimize growth and overall nutrition. **Pancreatic enzyme supplements** are closely titrated against the level of steatorrhoea. **Fat intake** should be maintained to avoid nutritional deficit. A daily **lipase intake** of up to 10 000 units/kg body weight is required. The efficacy of the supplements may be improved by the use of a **proton pump inhibitor**. These drugs reduce the risk of acid denaturation of the enzymes and also prevent acidification of the duodenum, which also impairs the enzymes' activity. Despite optimization of the use of enzyme supplements, a degree of fat malabsorption may persist. This reflects other luminal abnormalities of fat absorption in cystic fibrosis that are related to viscous mucus, small bowel bacterial colonization, and poor mixing of the food bolus with bile.

Further reading

Braganza JM, Lee SH, McCloy RF et al. Chronic pancreatitis. *Lancet* 2011; 377:1184–1197.
Kamisawa T, Zen Y, Pillai J et al. IgG4-related disease. *Lancet* 2015; 385: 1460–1471.
Lankisch PG, Apte M, Banks PA. Acute pancreatitis. *Lancet* 2015; 386:85–96.
National Institute for Health and Care Excellence. NICE Guideline NG104: Pancreatitis. NICE 2018; https://www.nice.org.uk/guidance/ng104/evidence/full-guideline-pdf-6535536157.

PANCREATIC CANCER

The many types of pancreatic cancer can be divided into two main groupings. The vast majority of cases (about 99%) occur in the exocrine component of the pancreas. There are several subtypes of exocrine pancreatic cancer but their diagnosis and treatment have much in common. A small minority of pancreatic cancers arise in the endocrine tissue of the pancreas and have different clinical characteristics.

Pancreatic adenocarcinoma

The incidence of pancreatic cancer in the West has been estimated at approximately 10 cases per 100 000, with no increase over the last 20 years. The diagnosis is rarely made in persons younger than 40 years of age, and the median age at diagnosis is 71 years. Approximately 60% of patients with this condition are male. It is the eighth leading cause of death from cancer in men and the ninth leading cause of death from cancer in women throughout the world. Some 96% of pancreatic cancers are adenocarcinoma in type and the large majority are of ductal origin.

Aetiology

Smoking is associated with a twofold increase. Excessive intake of alcohol or coffee and excessive use of aspirin have also been implicated. There is an increased incidence of pancreatic cancer among patients with a history of diabetes and chronic pancreatitis. The risk of developing pancreatic cancer is most marked in those patients with a genetic mutation predisposing to chronic pancreatitis (there is a 50 times increased risk in the presence of a *PRSS-1* mutation; see **Fig. 35.13**). Although it is estimated that 5–10% of pancreatic cancers have an inherited component, the genetic basis for familial aggregation has not been identified in most cases. A subgroup of such high-risk kindreds carry germline mutations of DNA repair genes, such as *BRCA2* and the partner and localizer of *BRCA2*. Among people with a known family history of pancreatic cancer in a first-degree relative, the relative risk of pancreatic cancer developing is increased by a factor of 2, 6 and 30 in people with one, two and three affected family members, respectively (**Box 35.11**).

Pathogenesis

Data suggest that pancreatic cancer results from the successive accumulation of gene mutations (**Fig. 35.15**). The cancer originates in the ductal epithelium and evolves from pre-malignant lesions to fully invasive cancer. The lesion called *pancreatic intraepithelial neoplasia (PanIN)* is the best-characterized histological precursor of pancreatic cancer. The progression from minimally dysplastic epithelium (PanIN grades 1A and 1B) to more severe dysplasia (grades 2 and 3) and finally to invasive carcinoma is paralleled by the successive accumulation of mutations. More than 90% of cases of PanIN of all grades have *KRAS* mutations. The mutational inactivation of the *CDKN2A*, *p53* and *SMAD* family member (*SMAD4*) tumour suppressors is detected with increasing frequency in type 2 and type 3 lesions of PanIN, suggesting that they are rate-limiting events for tumour progression. Exome-sequencing studies have identified additional loss-of-function mutations encoding components of the SWI/SNF nucleosome remodelling complex, which

are cumulatively detected in approximately 10–15% of pancreatic adenocarcinomas, as well as other, less frequent alterations.

A small percentage of pancreatic adenocarcinomas arise from cystic lesions, including **intraductal papillary mucinous neoplasm (IPMN)** and **mucinous cystic neoplasia** (see later). There is evidence that these cystic neoplasms demonstrate a similar multistep genetic and histological progression to invasive adenocarcinoma, although there are recognized differences in the mutational events that occur.

Clinical features

Approximately two-thirds of pancreatic cancers are located in the head of the pancreas, and the remainder in the body and tail (**Fig. 35.16**). Patients with pancreatic cancer most commonly present with abdominal pain, anorexia and weight loss. Many have experienced low-grade symptoms for a number of months before they present for investigation. New onset of depressive symptoms has also been identified as an early manifestation. In many cases the onset of these non-diagnostic symptoms is at a stage when there is already advanced local or metastatic disease. The pain associated with pancreatic cancer frequently radiates through into the back and, in some cases, is partially relieved by leaning forwards. Jaundice is a common, and maybe an early, manifestation of tumours of the ampulla and pancreatic head. This reflects the occlusion or compression of the distal CBD as it traverses the head of pancreas before entering the duodenum at the level of the ampulla. The patient may have noticed pale stools, dark urine and itching associated with bile duct obstruction in the absence (or prior to the onset) of detectable jaundice. Diabetes is present in at least 50% of patients with pancreatic cancer and may predate any other manifestation of disease. The obstruction of the pancreatic duct by the cancer may also lead to symptoms of malabsorption and overt steatorrhoea. An episode of symptomatic pancreatitis may, on occasion, be the presenting clinical picture. Other unusual presenting features can include thromboembolic phenomena, polyarthritis and skin nodules. These manifestations, distant to the tumour itself, have not been fully explained but may precede the development of a detectable pancreatic mass lesion by many months.

Signs

At the time of first presentation, there may be an absence of physical signs. Evidence of weight loss is common. Jaundice may be present, with associated scratch marks prompted by pruritus. In a proportion of cases the gall bladder will be palpable (***Courvoisier's sign***)

Box 35.11 Relative risks of pancreatic cancer in patients with a family history or associated gene mutations	
Risk factor	**Relative risk**
Familial pancreatic cancer	
Two first-degree relatives affected	18
Three first-degree relatives affected	57
Hereditary pancreatic cancer syndromes	
BRCA2 mutation	5.9
Familial atypical multiple mole melanoma (FAMMM)	16
Peutz–Jeghers syndrome	36
Hereditary pancreatitis	50

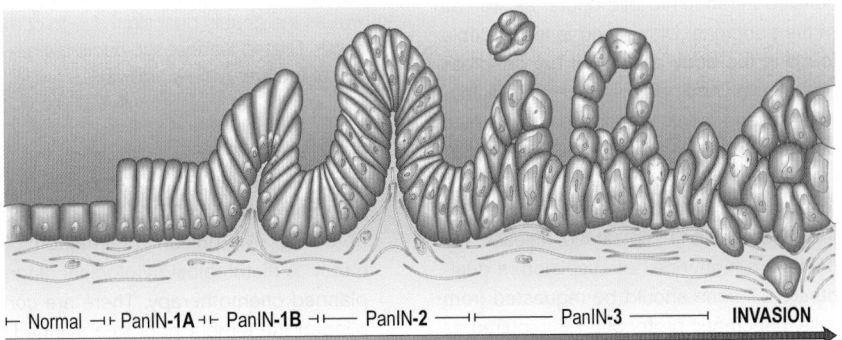

Fig. 35.15 Genetic model for the development of pancreatic ductal adenocarcinoma. The stages indicate histological progression with specific gene alterations. PanIN, pancreatic intraepithelial neoplasia. *(Modified from Maitra A, Adsay NV, Argani P et al. Multicomponent analysis of the pancreatic adenocarcinoma progression model using a pancreatic intraepithelial neoplasia tissue microarray. Mod Pathol 2003; 16:902–912, with permission from the Nature Publishing Group.)*

← Normal → PanIN-1A → PanIN-1B → PanIN-2 → PanIN-3 → **INVASION**

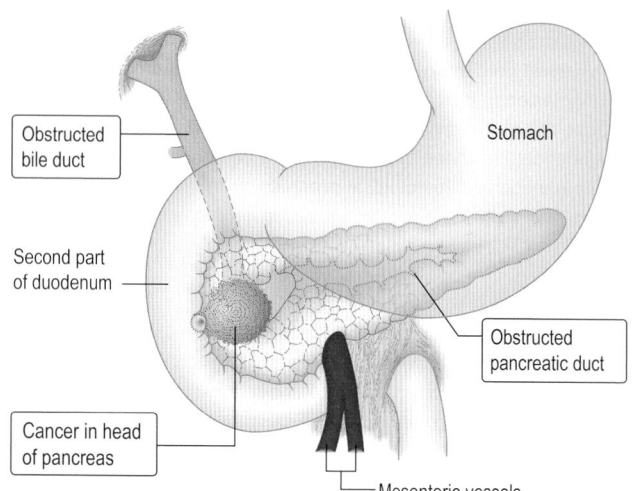

Fig. 35.16 **Carcinoma of the head of the pancreas.** The close relationship of a carcinoma of the head of pancreas to the surrounding structures.

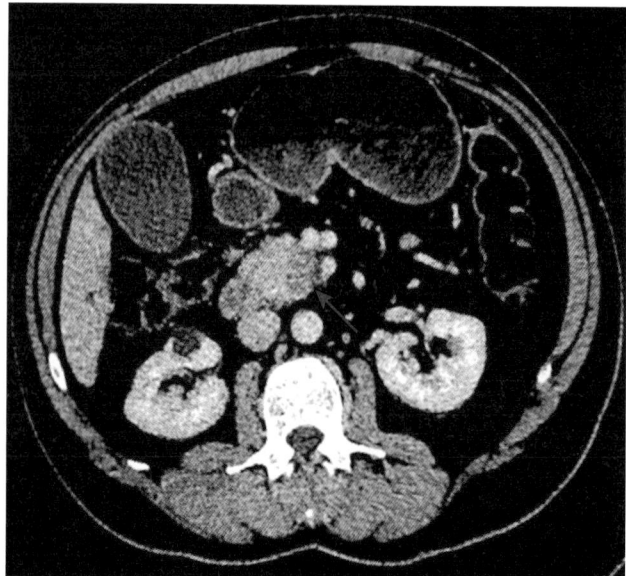

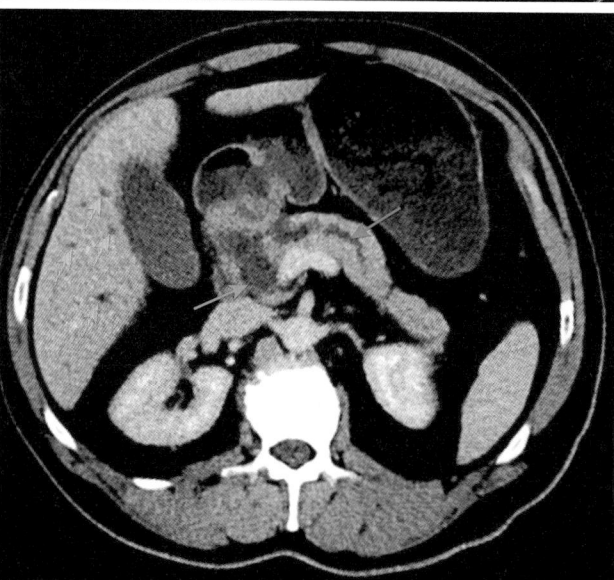

Fig. 35.17 **Axial CT images demonstrating pancreatic cancer. (A)** An image through the pancreatic head demonstrates a low-attenuation lesion in the head of the pancreas that is contacting the superior mesenteric artery and superior mesenteric vein (arrowed). **(B)** A more superior image demonstrates dilation of both the pancreatic duct (green arrow) and common bile duct (blue arrow) (known as the double duct sign) due to compression of the ducts by the mass. Dilated intrahepatic ducts are also visible in the imaged portion of the liver (yellow arrows).

secondary to an obstructed bile duct (or cystic duct). A palpable epigastric or central abdominal mass may be present as a reflection of advanced local disease. Liver metastases may be reflected in hepatomegaly.

Diagnosis and investigations

Patients with pancreatic adenocarcinoma frequently present for investigation at a late stage of tumour development, precluding curative surgery. In many cases, symptoms have been present for a number of months but have not led to investigation that is specifically aimed at confirming/excluding a pancreatic cancer. To improve outcome from this cancer there is increasing emphasis on earlier diagnosis. This is focused on targeted investigation in patients recognized as high-risk (see earlier). More emphasis is also placed on earlier referral for investigation in patients over the age of 40 who have low-grade symptoms that persist after initial assessment and empirical therapy. The upper gut symptoms frequently prompt referral for an upper gastrointestinal endoscopy. In most cases, this will not add diagnostic information and it is essential that a negative endoscopy does not delay further investigation – in particular, imaging.

- **Transabdominal ultrasound** is the initial imaging investigation in the majority of patients. In the presence of bile duct obstruction this will confirm dilated intrahepatic bile ducts, as well as a mass in the head of the pancreas. Ultrasound is less reliable when the cancer is found in the body and tail of the pancreas because of overlying bowel gas, and has a sensitivity of detection of 60%. A negative transabdominal ultrasound scan should not be considered as excluding the diagnosis.
- **Contrast-enhanced CT scan** should confirm the presence of a mass lesion in most cases of pancreatic adenocarcinoma (**Fig. 35.17**). Lymph node involvement and metastatic disease will also be identified. If there is a high index of suspicion, a dual-phase pancreatic protocol CT scan should be requested from the outset. A high-quality pancreatic protocol CT is required as a staging procedure prior to planned curative surgery. Extending the CT to the chest will exclude pulmonary metastases.
- **EUS** is the most sensitive (>85%) non-surgical procedure for the detection of pancreatic cancer (**Fig. 35.18**). In most cases, it does not add to the diagnostic and staging information pro-

vided by the CT scan. However, the procedure is valuable for the definition of small (<2 cm) lesions of the pancreas, which may be missed on CT. EUS is now the approach of choice for obtaining cytological confirmation of the underlying malignancy. A histological/cytological diagnosis is essential prior to planned chemotherapy. There are concerns that needle sampling of the tumour prior to a planned curative resection might lead to cancer cell seeding. This has been reported as a rare event (1–2%).

- **MRI and PET scanning** are useful techniques in a small proportion of patients when the local tumour or possibility of metastases has not been adequately defined.

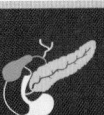

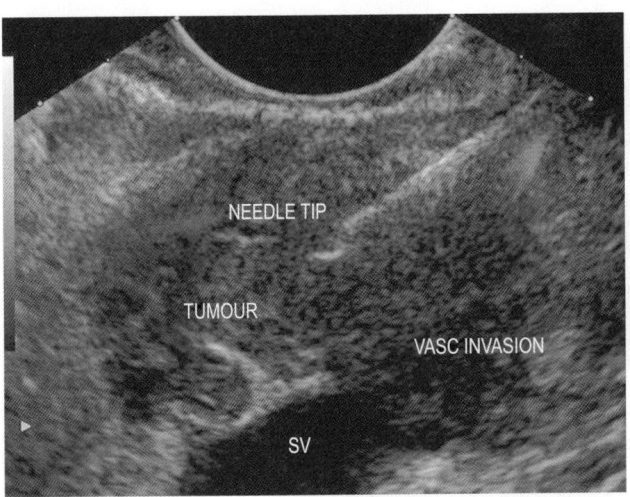

Fig. 35.18 An endoscopic ultrasound scan with the probe in the distal stomach in a patient with pancreatic cancer. The patient presented with intractable periumbilical pain. A mass lesion of the pancreatic body is defined (tumour). There is invasion by the lesion into the splenic vein (SV, vasc invasion). The line of a transendoscopic needle is seen (needle tip), which has been placed under the guidance of the ultrasound probe to obtain a needle aspirate for cytological diagnosis.

- **Several tumour markers** have been evaluated for the diagnosis and monitoring of pancreatic cancer. The CA19–9 has reasonable sensitivity (80%) but a high false-positive rate. In individual patients, single values of these tumour markers may be of little help but a progressive elevation over time is often diagnostic; in such circumstances, tumour marker levels can be used to monitor response to treatment.

Differential diagnosis

The diagnosis should not be difficult in the presence of painless jaundice or epigastric pain radiating into the back with progressive weight loss. Unfortunately, many patients present with very minor symptoms, including pain, change in bowel habit and weight loss. Imaging, particularly abdominal CT, should be performed if pancreatic cancer is suspected. IgG4-related autoimmune pancreatitis is now recognized as a differential diagnosis in patients presenting with abdominal pain, jaundice and an abnormal pancreas on imaging (localized or diffuse enlargement; see earlier). Pancreatic cancer may rarely present with recurrent episodes of typical acute pancreatitis.

Management

The 5-year survival rate for carcinoma of the pancreas is approximately 3%. Some 90% of patients with a diagnosis of pancreatic adenocarcinoma will have a cause of death directly related to the disease. Surgical intervention represents the only chance of long-term survival. Approximately 20% of all cases have a localized tumour suitable for resection, but in an elderly population, many have co-morbid factors that preclude such major surgery. Assessment of the primary tumour and involvement of local vessels, including the coeliac artery, superior mesenteric artery and vein, portal vein and hepatic artery, is critical in determining resectability. Strategies for management are optimally defined as part of a multidisciplinary team approach.

When treatment is considered to be of curative intent, a pancreatoduodenectomy (**Whipple procedure**) is required to remove tumours of the head and neck of the pancreas. Tumours of the body and tail are resected as part of a distal pancreatectomy, which is increasingly carried out by the laparoscopic approach. Adjuvant and neo-adjuvant chemotherapy (fluorouracil or gemcitabine) has been used in those undergoing attempted curative resection, with some evidence of improved survival. There is early evidence that more intensive multidrug regimes (the addition of irinotecan and oxaliplatin) may further improve outcome but at the expense of increased drug toxicity. Radiotherapy has been evaluated as adjuvant treatment but does not have an established role.

In the large majority of cases, therapy is considered non-curative. Chemotherapy (see earlier) is widely used in this setting, with increasing emphasis on multidrug regimens (see p. 126). The mainstay of palliative therapy is attention to detail in managing the generalized and specific complications of pancreatic cancer.

- **Pain** is a debilitating feature in many cases. Management is best directed by dedicated pain teams. Opiates are a mainstay. There is some evidence that early intervention with coeliac axis block may have benefits.
- **Nutritional deficit** is a frequent feature at presentation and may be exacerbated by chemotherapy. Early dietetic support may alleviate this. Malabsorption is common with pancreatic cancer and can be managed by the introduction of pancreatic enzyme supplementation. The adverse metabolic effects of diabetes can be avoided by early detection and management.
- **Obstructive jaundice** will occur at some stage in 70% of cases and is frequently associated with anorexia and nausea, as well as pruritus. Endoscopic placement of endoprostheses (stents) offers excellent palliation (see p. 1323).
- **Duodenal obstruction** is seen in up to 20% of cases, particularly when the tumour is situated in the head or uncinate process of the pancreas. Endoscopic stenting is the treatment of choice with excellent palliation. Surgical bypass is an option in selected cases.

Pancreatic cystic neoplasms

Cystic lesions of the pancreas are common. Around 75% will be pseudocysts (see p. 1332) but, of the remainder, the majority are true cystic neoplasms. Careful characterization of lesions with CT and MRI, and discussion in a specialist pancreatic multidisciplinary team, are crucial. There is a high potential for the development of malignancy in true cystic neoplasms and therefore resection is generally recommended. The decision to operate may be difficult in patients with small (<3 cm) lesions of the head of the pancreas (in the absence of confirmed malignancy at presentation) and in those with significant co-morbidity. An initially conservative approach with follow-up imaging may be justified. Differentiation between pseudocysts and true cystic neoplasms may be difficult, even with multiple imaging techniques. EUS and fine-needle aspiration are frequently helpful in characterizing cystic lesions of the pancreas. EUS appearance (**Fig. 35.19**), cytology, and the measurement of cyst fluid carcinoembryonic antigen and amylase may help to categorize cystic lesions and identify malignant change.

Serous cystadenomas are composed of multiple small, cystic cavities lined by cuboidal, glycogen-rich, mucin-poor cells. These lesions tend to occur in an elderly age group and are often an asymptomatic finding. Malignant transformation in a serous cystadenoma is extremely rare and so surgical resection is rarely required. Larger serous cystadenomas may cause local compressive complications, including pain, which may warrant surgical resection.

Solid pseudopapillary neoplasms are rare lesions, usually found in women in their fourth decade; they may occur anywhere

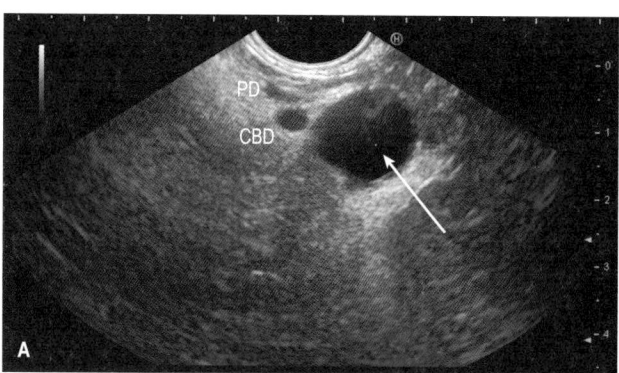
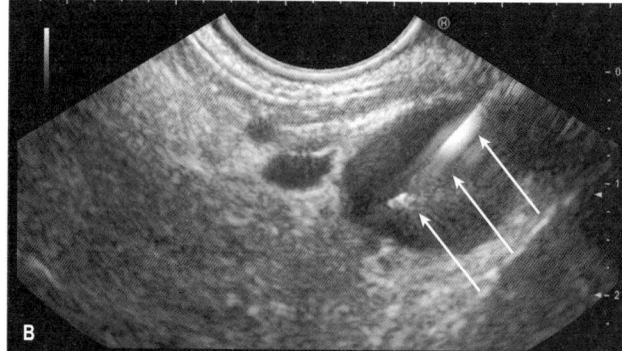

Fig. 35.19 Linear endoscopic ultrasound images. (A) A cystic lesion (arrowed) in the head of the pancreas; the common bile duct (CBD) and pancreatic duct (PD) are also visible. The lesion is an intraductal papillary mucinous neoplasm. **(B)** The same lesion being sampled by fine needle aspiration for cytology, fluid amylase and fluid carcinoembryonic antigen estimation. The needle is arrowed.

in the pancreas. Resection is required, as around 20% show malignant features on histological examination.

Mucinous cystadenomas are almost exclusively found in women, usually in the fifth or sixth decade, and are sited in the pancreatic body and tail. Multilocular cysts are lined by tall, mucin-synthesizing cells. Around 20% of these lesions are malignant at the time of presentation and the majority appear to have malignant potential. Surgical resection is generally mandated.

Intraductal papillary mucinous neoplasm (IPMN) is a pancreatic cystic neoplasm that can arise in either the main pancreatic duct (main duct IPMN) or its side branches (branch duct IPMN). The majority are found in men between the ages of 60 and 70. Presentation is usually with pancreatic pain but branch duct IPMN is often an incidental finding. IPMNs are slowly progressive but carry a significant malignant potential. Generally, all main duct IPMNs and large branch duct IPMNs should be resected. Small branch duct IPMNs have a much lower malignant potential and are generally kept under radiological surveillance.

Cystic degeneration of a pancreatic adenocarcinoma or pancreatic neuroendocrine tumour can occur.

Pancreatic neuroendocrine tumours

Pancreatic neuroendocrine tumours (NETs) are thought to arise from the cells of the islets of Langerhans and can secrete a variety of active hormones, most frequently insulin. Pancreatic NETs have increased in incidence over the last two decades, reaching an incidence of 4–5/1 000 000 population. They represent a heterogeneous group of tumours with varying symptomology, tumour biology and prognosis. Between 25% and 50% of the patients present with symptoms related to hormones released from the tumour. The remainder have 'non-functioning' tumours that may be an incidental finding or present with symptoms related to tumour bulk, such as obstruction, jaundice, bleeding or abdominal mass. The increasing incidence of pancreatic NETs has been attributed to the widespread use of high-resolution cross-sectional imaging, leading to incidental detection of asymptomatic lesions.

In addition to insulin and glucagon, pancreatic NETs may synthesize ectopic hormones that are not usually found in the pancreas, such as gastrin, adrenocorticotrophin, vasoactive intestinal peptide and growth hormone. While many pancreatic endocrine tumours are multihormonal, one peptide tends to predominate and is responsible for any clinical syndrome (see later). Non-functioning pancreatic NETs often contain peptide hormone on immunostaining but this remains functionally inactive. The majority of endocrine neoplasia

pancreatic tumours are malignant in their behaviour. Between 10% and 15% of pancreatic NETs are linked to an inherited syndrome, such as the multiple endocrine neoplasia type 1 (MEN-1) or von Hippel–Lindau (VHL) syndrome (see p. 1407).

Clinical syndromes

Insulinoma is described on page 647.

A *gastrinoma* accounts for approximately 1 in 1000 cases of duodenal ulcer disease. The ulceration results from hypersecretion of gastric acid secondary in response to high serum gastrin concentrations, secreted by the pancreatic tumour (Zollinger–Ellison syndrome). Recurrent severe duodenal ulceration occurs, with only a partial response to acid suppression. The diagnosis is confirmed by an elevated gastrin level. High-dose proton pump inhibitors are used to suppress symptoms.

A *VIPoma* is an endocrine pancreatic tumour producing vasoactive intestinal polypeptide (VIP). This causes secretory diarrhoea secondary to the stimulation of adenyl cyclase within the enterocyte (Verner–Morrison or watery diarrhoea syndrome). The clinical syndrome is one of profuse watery diarrhoea, hypokalaemia and a metabolic acidosis. To produce the syndrome, the tumours are usually in excess of 3 cm in diameter.

Glucagonomas are rare α-cell tumours that are responsible for a syndrome of migratory necrolytic dermatitis, weight loss, diabetes mellitus, deep vein thrombosis, anaemia and hypoalbuminaemia. The diagnosis is made by measuring pancreatic glucagon in the serum.

Somatostatinomas are rare malignant D-cell tumours of the pancreas. These tumours cause diabetes mellitus, gallstones and diarrhoea/steatorrhoea. They can be diagnosed by high serum somatostatin levels.

Investigations

Diagnosis is based on a combination of biochemical and histopathological markers. The biochemical diagnosis includes measurement of circulatory chromogranin A or specific hormones such as gastrin, insulin, glucagon and VIP. The histopathology includes features such as positive staining for chromogranin A and specific hormones such as gastrin, pro-insulin and glucagon.

Tumour localization depends on cross-sectional imaging, including CT and MRI scanning. The majority of NETs express somatostatin receptors, and a radiolabelled somatostatin analogue (such as octreotide) provides a means of tumour localization using scintigraphy. PET scanning with ^{18}F-FDG-PET/CT or ^{68}Ga-DOTATATE PET/CT is now widely used in the localization of primary disease and any metastases.

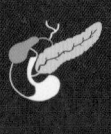

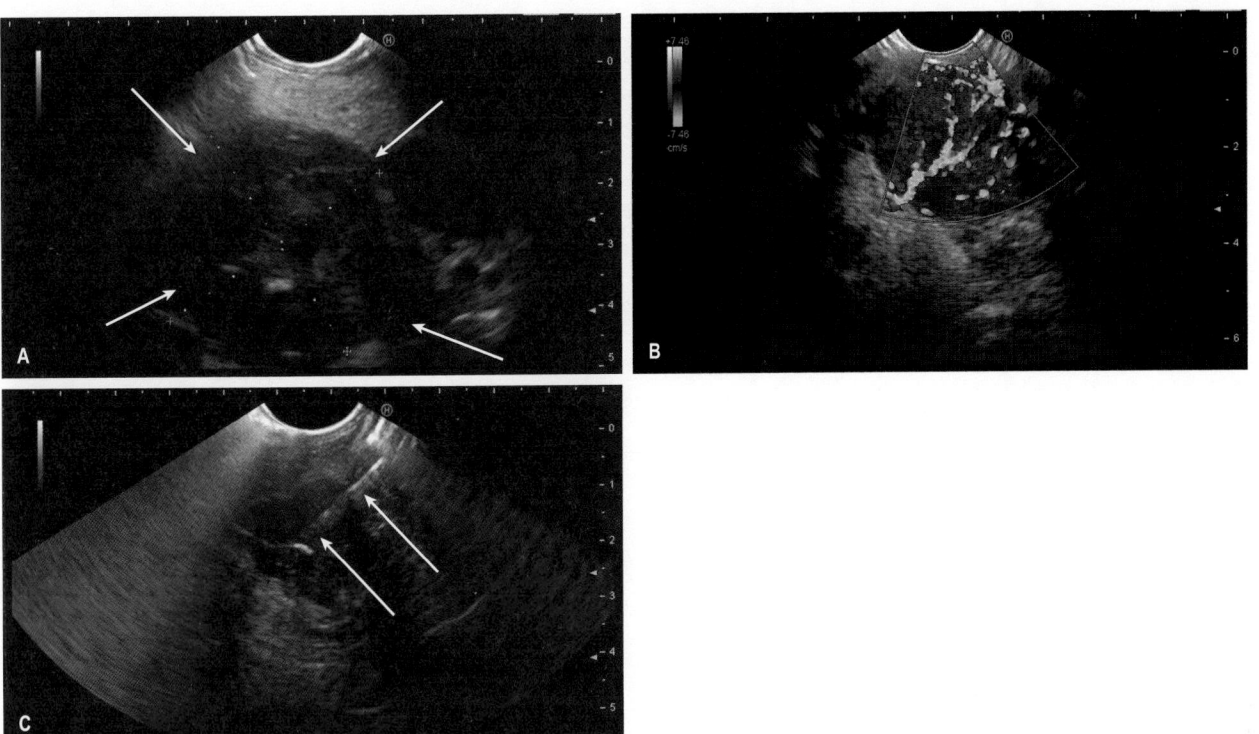

Fig. 35.20 Linear endoscopic ultrasound images. **(A)** A heterogeneous solid mass (arrowed) in the head of the pancreas with some central calcification. **(B)** Doppler study demonstrating the vascularity of the lesion. **(C)** Endoscopic ultrasound-guided fine needle aspiration (arrowed) of the same lesion, which confirmed the presence of a neuroendocrine tumour.

Identification of the primary and possibly metastatic lesions may be difficult despite multiple imaging techniques. EUS is the most sensitive means of detecting small primary NETs in the pancreas. It also offers the opportunity to undertake fine needle aspiration sampling of lesions, affording a cytopathological diagnosis **(Fig. 35.20)**.

Management

Treatment of pancreatic NETs requires a multidisciplinary approach and depends on the presence or absence of metastatic (usually hepatic) disease. Where possible, surgical resection of the primary lesion is the optimal management of pancreatic endocrine tumours, as it offers the only possible cure. The propensity of many endocrine tumours to metastasize early precludes a cure in many cases. Debulking of the tumour, including liver metastases, is frequently carried out to facilitate systemic treatment.

Somatostatin analogues, such as octreotide and lanreotide, are used to control hormonal-related symptoms and also have a tumour-modulating effect. There is some evidence that somatostatin analogues combined with interferon-alfa also control tumour proliferation. Radionuclide therapy using somatostatin analogues has proven benefit in patients with tumours that express a high content of somatostatin receptors.

The ***chemotherapeutic agents*** streptozotocin, 5-fluorouracil and doxorubicin produce partial remission in approximately 40% of cases. Recent advances include the introduction of tyrosine kinase and the mammalian target of rapamycin (mTOR) inhibitors. Pancreatic NETs show a very high degree of vascularization, as well as abundant production and secretion of growth factors. There is preliminary evidence of benefit from anti-angiogenesis therapy utilizing vascular endothelial growth factor (VEGF) antagonists.

In patients with extensive liver metastasis, occlusion of the arterial blood flow by hepatic arterial embolization may control hormone-related symptoms. In most cases the tumours are slowly progressive and may allow a reasonable quality of life for many years.

Further reading

Ryan DP, Hong TS, Bardeesy N. Pancreatic adenocarcinoma. *N Engl J Med* 2014; 371:1039–1049.

Significant websites

https://www.bsg.org.uk *British Society of Gastroenterology guidelines.*
https://www.emedicine.medscape.com *Cholecystitis and cholelithiasis.*
https://www.gastrohep.com *Resources for gastroenterology, hepatology and endoscopy.*
https://www.gi.org *American College of Gastroenterology guidelines.*
https://www.nice.org.uk *Guidelines and service standards.*
https://www.ueg.eu/education *Online learning in gastroenterology.*

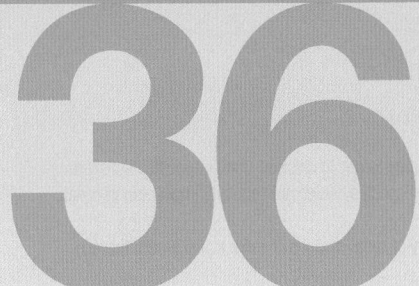

36

Kidney and urinary tract disease

M. Magdi Yaqoob and Neil Ashman

CORE SKILLS AND KNOWLEDGE

Renal disease is common: acute kidney injury (AKI) affects around 20% of hospitalized patients, and 10–15% of the general population meet the criteria for chronic kidney disease (CKD). The kidney is often involved in systemic conditions such as diabetes, hypertension, autoimmune disorders, haematological malignancies and infections, including human immunodeficiency virus (HIV) and viral hepatitis.

Renal physicians work in lifetime partnership with patients, their families and colleagues, including nurses, therapists, counsellors, nutritionists, technicians and pharmacists, in a multidisciplinary fashion. General nephrology is provided in secondary care, as patients with renal conditions such as CKD or nephrotic syndrome are managed in renal outpatients, and patients with AKI are investigated in general or renal-specific inpatient wards. Specialist services are offered in tertiary care. Renal physicians manage immunosuppression during and after kidney transplantation, and supervise peritoneal and haemodialysis to offer personalized, life-sustaining treatment that mixes physics with physiology. Nephrologists need to be general physicians, comfortable with complexity but able to understand and treat a wide variety of non-renal conditions in patients with CKD.

Key skills in renal medicine include:

- becoming comfortable with diagnosing the cause of AKI and managing its complications
- understanding CKD: its causes, complications and progression
- being familiar with the principles of dialysis and transplantation.

Opportunities for learning renal medicine include attending renal outpatient clinics, seeking out and assessing patients with AKI presenting to the hospital emergency department or acute admissions unit, and spending time with doctors or allied health professionals in specialist centres helping patients receiving renal replacement therapy (RRT).

CLINICAL SKILLS FOR NEPHROLOGY

History

In its early stages, renal disease is often asymptomatic and may be diagnosed incidentally. History-taking in renal medicine (**Box 36.1**) should be tailored to the individual patient, with the focus on either diagnostic or management questions as appropriate to the clinical context.

A diagnostic approach to unexplained renal disease

The approach to thinking about the causes of unexplained renal dysfunction presented in **Box 36.2** is especially relevant in AKI but is also relevant in CKD, especially when there is superimposed AKI or a rapid deterioration in kidney function.

1339

Box 36.1 History-taking in kidney and urinary tract disease

Assessing the likely duration of renal dysfunction
- Duration of any symptoms present (see next section)
- Previous occasions on which urinalysis or measurement of urea and creatinine might have been performed, e.g. pre-employment or insurance medical examinations or new patient checks in general practice
- Urine volume:
  - Oliguria is a powerful symptom of sudden kidney injury
  - Slowly progressive kidney disease can see urine volume actually increase, as failing tubular function leads to a salt- and water-wasting state. As concentrating ability in the tubules fails, urine volume increases through the day and night, and so polyuria and nocturia are useful symptoms to suggest the length of time for which CKD has been present

Symptoms of uraemia
Symptoms are common when the serum urea concentration exceeds 40 mmol/L but many patients develop uraemic symptoms at lower levels. Symptoms are generally non-specific but may include:
- malaise, loss of energy
- loss of appetite, loss of weight
- insomnia
- nocturia and polyuria
- itching
- nausea and vomiting
- 'restless legs' syndrome
- bone pain
- peripheral oedema
- symptoms due to anaemia
- amenorrhoea in women
- erectile dysfunction in men.

In more advanced uraemia, these symptoms become more severe and central nervous system symptoms are common, including mental slowing and clouding of consciousness, or in severe cases seizures and myoclonic twitching

Risk factors for renal disease
- Take a thorough *past medical history*, focusing particularly on diseases that commonly affect the kidney: diabetes, hypertension, systemic inflammatory diseases, blood-borne viruses, myeloma
- Ask about all *medications* the patient is using or has used in the past, remembering in particular known nephrotoxic agents (such as non-steroidal anti-inflammatory drugs, NSAIDs), which the patient may have obtained over the counter and therefore may forget to disclose unless specifically asked), and traditional and herbal remedies, which are regularly implicated in renal disease
- Ask about a *family history* of renal disease or renal replacement therapy (RRT)
- Ask about *recent ill health* – conditions such as sepsis or dehydration can cause renal hypoperfusion and pre-renal AKI
- Ask about symptoms of *urinary tract obstruction* (see p. 1477)
- Ask about symptoms of *systemic inflammatory or malignant conditions*: fever, malaise, rashes, eye inflammation, hair thinning, nasal discharge, haemoptysis and others

Experience of RRT (where relevant):
Patients with advanced CKD
- What do they understand about their diagnosis?
- Would they wish to be considered for RRT or prefer a supportive/palliative approach to their disease?
- What is their lifestyle, and what form of RRT would offer them the best quality of life?

Patients receiving dialysis
- How are they coping with the treatment?
- Are there any symptoms relating to anaemia or CKD mineral and bone disease?
- Is transplantation feasible? (It is usually best to have considered the medical prospects of achieving transplantation before discussing the options with patients)

Kidney transplant recipients
- How is their general health?
- Any symptoms of opportunistic infections?
- How are they coping with their immunosuppressant medication? Any missed doses?
- Can their lifestyle be optimized to increase the likely survival of their graft?

Quantification of proteinuria

Quantifying the level of urinary protein is necessary in a number of renal conditions (see p. 1349). This is often done initially using a urine dipstick and then quantified using one of the three measures shown in **Box 36.3**. There is a rough equivalence between methods if proteinuria is non-selective (i.e. if protein is excreted in the urine in the same proportions as it is found in blood).

In healthy people there should be virtually no urinary albumin (uACR <2.5 mg/mmol for men, <3.5 mg/mmol for women); even very low levels above this threshold (not detectable by dipstick testing) indicate increased cardiovascular risk.

High levels of proteinuria (uPCR >200 mg/mmol) generally indicate glomerular disease, and uPCR >350 mg/mmol indicates nephrotic syndrome if other symptoms are present (hypoalbuminuria and fluid overload).

Box 36.2 Causes of unexplained renal dysfunction

Pre-renal causes
- Intercurrent illness, including systemic infection or sepsis in particular
- Vomiting, diarrhoea and dehydration
- Concurrent use of antihypertensives or diuretics, especially angiotensin-converting enzyme (ACE) inhibitors and angiotensin receptor blockers

Intrarenal causes
- History of disease with associated renal manifestations, e.g. cast nephropathy in myeloma
- Nephrotoxic medications
- Symptoms suggestive of a systemic inflammatory disease
- Presence of proteinuria (see above)

Post-renal causes
- Symptoms of urinary tract obstruction
- Complete anuria
- History of a condition liable to progress to causing urinary tract obstruction: benign or malignant prostate disease, bladder or pelvic cancer
- Bladder distension or hydronephrosis on ultrasound

Box 36.3 Quantifying the level of urinary protein

24-hour urine protein collection (g/24 h)	Urine protein:creatinine ratio (uPCR, mg/mmol)	Urinary albumin: creatinine ratio (uACR, mg/mmol)
1	100	70
2	200	150
3	300	200
4+	400+	300+

Examination

There are few physical signs specific to uraemia, although some of the features shown on the figure in **grey boxes** are often observed. The **yellow boxes** indicate signs related to RRT in patients with established end-stage renal disease, and may tell a story of treatment modalities previously received. Frequently, there are physical signs of peritoneal dialysis, haemodialysis and transplantation to be found (see also p. 170).

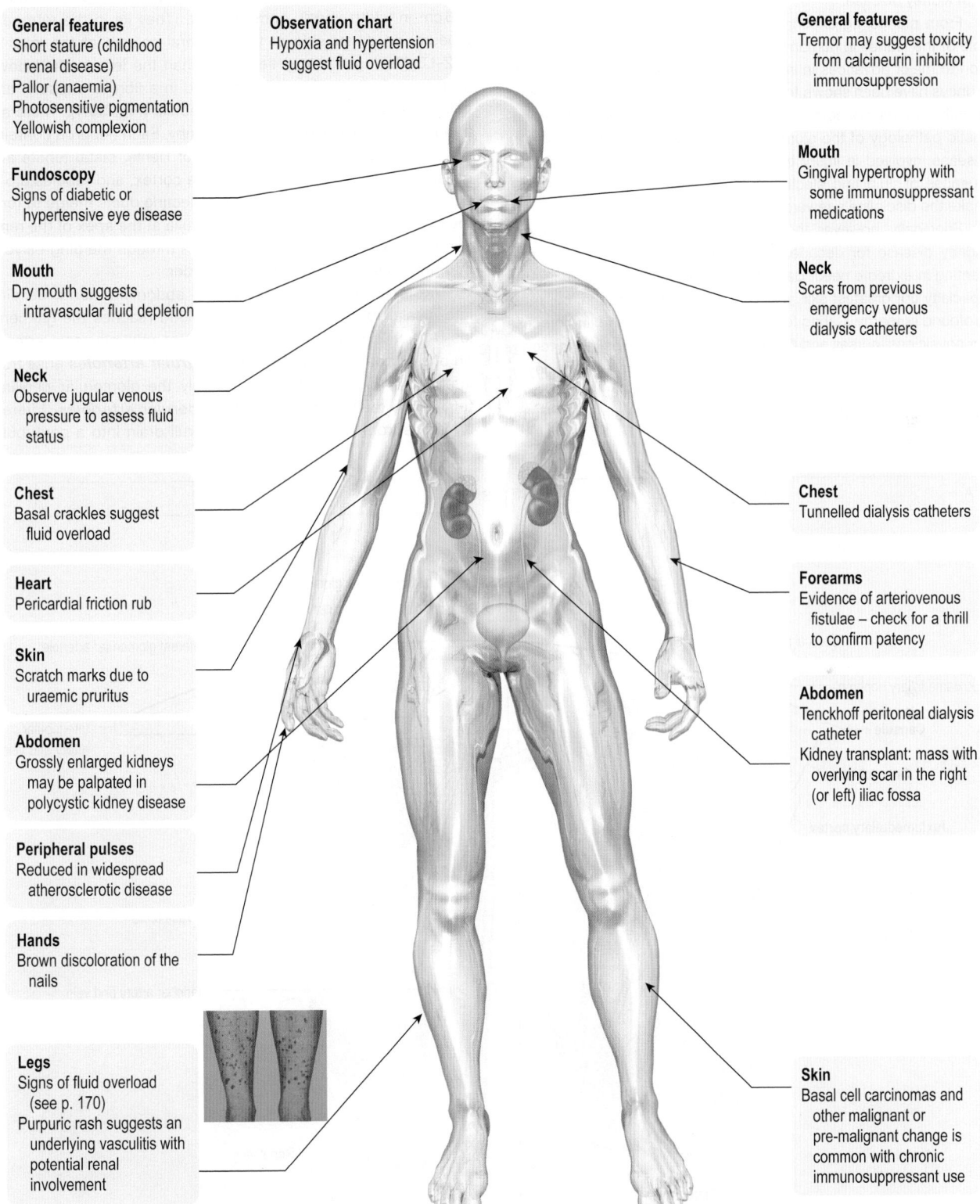

General features
Short stature (childhood renal disease)
Pallor (anaemia)
Photosensitive pigmentation
Yellowish complexion

Fundoscopy
Signs of diabetic or hypertensive eye disease

Mouth
Dry mouth suggests intravascular fluid depletion

Neck
Observe jugular venous pressure to assess fluid status

Chest
Basal crackles suggest fluid overload

Heart
Pericardial friction rub

Skin
Scratch marks due to uraemic pruritus

Abdomen
Grossly enlarged kidneys may be palpated in polycystic kidney disease

Peripheral pulses
Reduced in widespread atherosclerotic disease

Hands
Brown discoloration of the nails

Legs
Signs of fluid overload (see p. 170)
Purpuric rash suggests an underlying vasculitis with potential renal involvement

Observation chart
Hypoxia and hypertension suggest fluid overload

General features
Tremor may suggest toxicity from calcineurin inhibitor immunosuppression

Mouth
Gingival hypertrophy with some immunosuppressant medications

Neck
Scars from previous emergency venous dialysis catheters

Chest
Tunnelled dialysis catheters

Forearms
Evidence of arteriovenous fistulae – check for a thrill to confirm patency

Abdomen
Tenckhoff peritoneal dialysis catheter
Kidney transplant: mass with overlying scar in the right (or left) iliac fossa

Skin
Basal cell carcinomas and other malignant or pre-malignant change is common with chronic immunosuppressant use

INTRODUCTION

Nephrology has evolved over the last five decades from a peripheral to a major medical specialty, tasked with developing care strategies for over 10% of the world population who are believed to be living with kidney disease.

From pioneering experiments demonstrating the extraordinary role of the kidney in human physiology and blood pressure regulation to major advances in immunology and genomic medicine, the kidneys have been shown to maintain our internal environment, and to influence all systems when failing. The striking and oddly aesthetic pathology of the glomerulus, an array of local and systemic disease involved in injury to the kidney, and the complex consequences of fluid and electrolyte shifts and disorders (see Ch. 9) make the discipline a rewardingly broad and challenging one.

Principally, however, the men, women and children living with kidney disease for decades, clustered in families and often presenting in extreme need, demand of all clinicians who come to the specialty our greatest skill, and where this is not enough, our most profound empathy. Caring for kidney disease is a humbling process for physicians, nurses and therapists, where we are asked to recognize the extraordinary courage of our patients literally every day or second day on dialysis. Our relationships with patients stretch for entire careers, always asking us to think beyond a single consultation or admission.

ANATOMY AND PHYSIOLOGY OF THE KIDNEY AND URINARY TRACT

Functional anatomy

The *kidneys* are paired organs, 11–14 cm in length in adults, 5–6 cm in width and 3–4 cm in depth. They lie in the retroperitoneum, on either side of the vertebral column at the level of T12–L3 (the right kidney lies lower than the left, pushed down by the liver). Each kidney is enclosed in a fibrous capsule, and has an outer cortex and an inner medulla (**Fig. 36.1**). There are about 1 million *nephrons* in each kidney. Each nephron contains a glomerulus, proximal tubule, loop of Henle, distal tubule and collecting duct. All glomeruli lie in the cortex, and tubules dip in and out of the medulla, where the collecting ducts merge to form the ducts of Bellini, emptying at a papilla at the apex of the renal pyramid into a calyx. Urine then flows through merging calyces into the renal pelvis, ureters and bladder.

The renal arteries branch off the abdominal aorta, dividing into smaller branches until arterial blood reaches the glomerulus. About 25% of people have dual or multiple renal arteries on one or both sides. *Afferent glomerular arterioles* arise from interlobular branch arteries to supply the glomerular capillary tuft, which drains into *efferent glomerular arterioles*. Efferent arterioles from (outer) cortical glomeruli drain into a peritubular

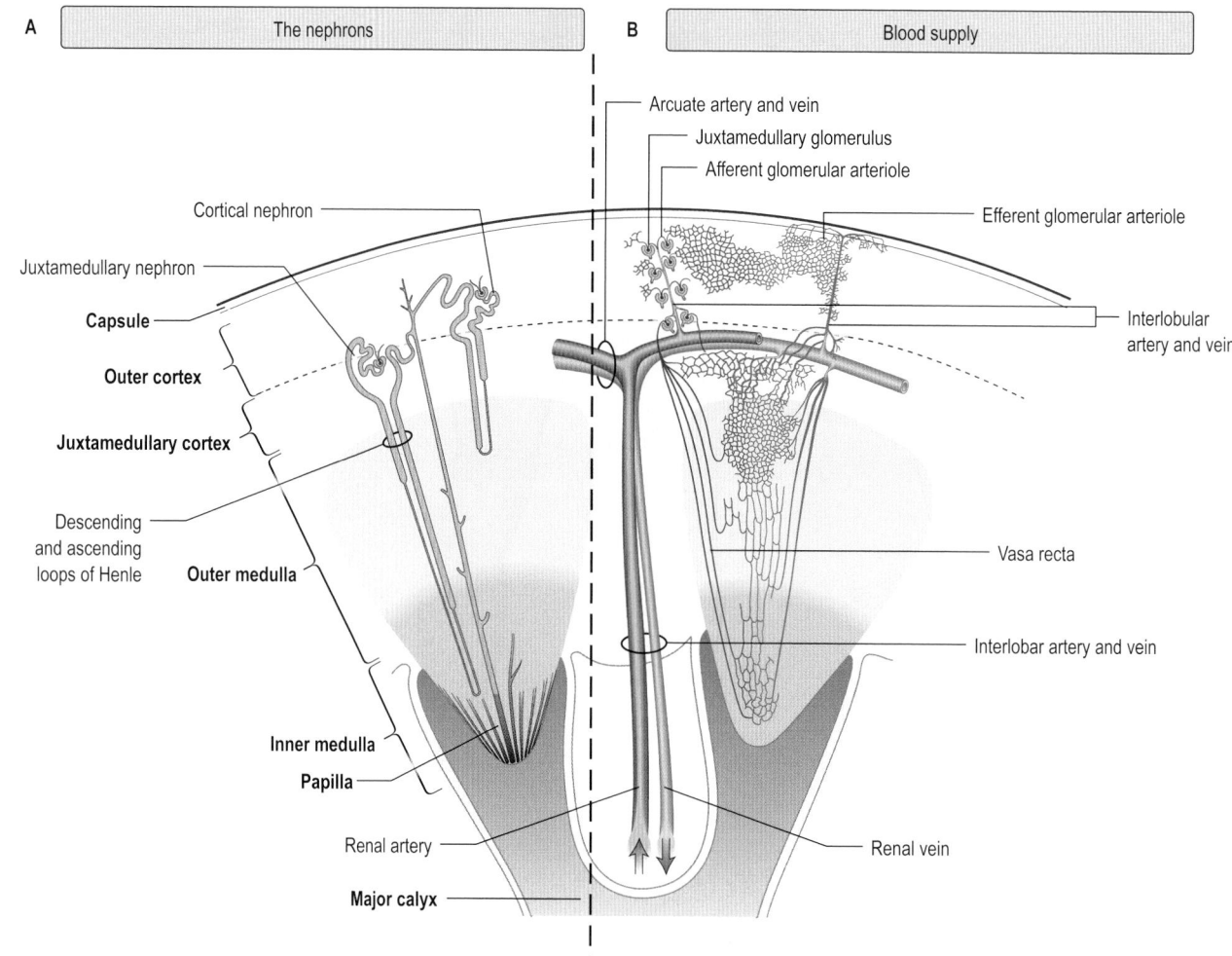

Fig. 36.1 Functional anatomy of the kidney. **(A)** The nephrons. **(B)** Arterial and venous supply. *(After Standring S (ed.). Gray's Anatomy, 41st edn. London: Elsevier; 2016.)*

capillary network within the renal cortex and then into increasingly large and more proximal branches of the renal vein. By contrast, blood from the (inner) juxtamedullary glomeruli passes via vasa recta in the medulla and returns via the cortex to renal veins that drain into the inferior vena cava.

The renal capsule and ureters are innervated via T10–12 and L1 nerve roots, and renal pain is felt over the corresponding dermatomes.

Nephron

A ball of capillaries makes up the glomerular tuft, enclosed by Bowman's capsule, a chamber lined with specialized **parietal epithelial cells** that marks the origin of the tubule (**Fig. 36.2**). The tuft, held together and regulated by **mesangial cells**, then serves as the filtration barrier, allowing filtrate from plasma to move into the urinary (Bowman's) space. The rate of glomerular filtration is influenced by changes in the contractile tone in either the afferent or the efferent arterioles; for example, efferent vasoconstriction will increase the transglomerular capillary pressure, and increase filtration.

Glomerular capillaries are lined with **endothelial cells**, fenestrated with 60–80 nm pores and covered with charged glycocalyx. The glomerular basement membrane (GBM), about 300 nm thick and made of type IV collagen, laminin and heparin sulphate, separates endothelium from podocytes (or visceral epithelial cells). Podocytes anchor on to the GBM by means of an extensive trabecular network of foot processes, and hang into Bowman's space. The interdigitating foot processes of podocytes then form the 40 nm filtration slit, a narrow potential space traversed by a protein 'zipper' that may prevent the passage of larger molecules (such as albumin) into the urinary space, and regulates the architecture and function of podocytes.

Mesangial cells (thought to be related to macrophages) sit within the tuft, able to contract and relax to control blood flow and the filtration surface area along the glomerular capillaries in response to a host of mediators. They also secrete the **mesangial matrix**, which provides the scaffolding for glomerular capillaries.

The **renal tubules** are lined by epithelial cells, which alter the composition of filtrate to form urine eventually. Proximal tubular cells have a luminal brush border to increase (by 30-fold) the surface area exposed to filtrate, rich in transporters and channels. The loop of Henle is lined with squamous cells, which are more permeable to water than solute, and cuboidal epithelium, when the reverse is true. The distal tubule regulates electrolytes and pH through cuboidal epithelium, and the cortical portion of the collecting ducts contains two cell types with different functions: principal cells (sodium, potassium and water) and intercalated cells (acid–base; see p. 175). Finally, resident interstitial fibroblast-like cells in the renal cortex produce erythropoietin in response to hypoxia (see p. 1347).

Juxtaglomerular apparatus

The juxtaglomerular apparatus regulates flow and filtration in each individual nephron. Columnar epithelium in the macula densa (**Fig. 36.3**) senses the concentration of tubular fluid sodium (higher filtrate flow means more delivered sodium), triggering adenosine-mediated vasoconstriction of the afferent arteriole to drop glomerular filtration (so-called tubulo–glomerular feedback). Juxtaglomerular cells secrete renin, able to induce aldosterone release, allowing the apparatus to monitor flow, and respond when necessary to drop glomerular filtration rate (GFR) and retain salt to maintain fluid balance.

Further reading

Ingelfinger JR. Tackling Tsc to promote nephrogenesis. *N Engl J Med* 2018; 379:2476–2478.

Physiology

A **hydrostatic pressure gradient** of approximately 10 mmHg (a capillary pressure of 45 mmHg minus 10 mmHg of pressure within Bowman's space and 25 mmHg of plasma oncotic pressure) provides the driving force for ultrafiltration of virtually protein-free and fat-free fluid across the glomerular filter into Bowman's space and so into the renal tubule (**Fig. 36.4**).

The **ultrafiltration rate** (GFR) varies with age and sex but is approximately 120–130 mL/min per 1.73 m² surface area in adults. This means that, each day, ultrafiltration of 170–180 L of water and unbound small-molecular-weight constituents of blood occurs. If these large volumes of ultrafiltrate were excreted unchanged as urine, it would be necessary to drink huge amounts of water and salts to stay in balance.

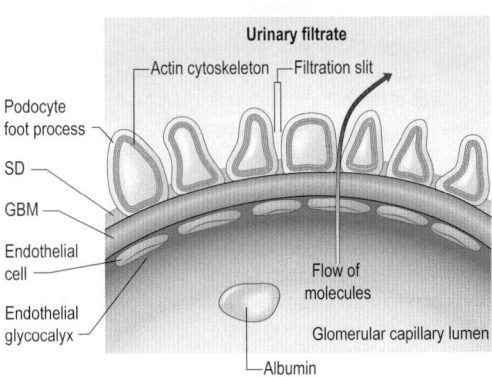
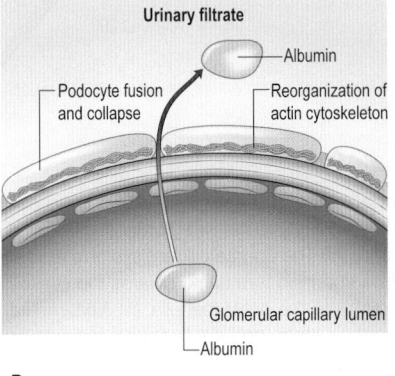
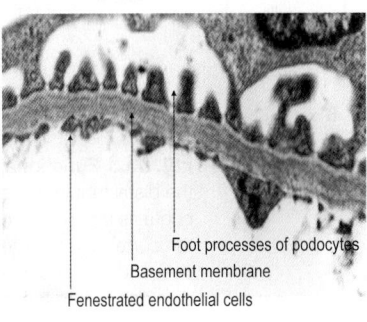

Fig. 36.2 The glomerular filtration barrier. (A) Blood enters the glomerular capillaries and is filtered across the endothelium and the glomerular basement membrane (GBM), and through the filtration slits between podocyte foot processes to produce the primary urine filtrate. In healthy glomeruli, this barrier restricts the passage of macromolecules. The proteins that form the slit diaphragm (SD) are essential for the normal functioning of the filtration barrier. **(B)** Loss of these proteins, either genetically or by acquired means, leads to foot process effacement, breakdown of the barrier and leakage of albumin (this is central to the pathophysiology of glomerular diseases such as those presenting with nephrotic syndrome). **(C)** Electron micrograph of the normal filtration barrier. *(A, B, Adapted from Quaggin S. Sizing up sialic acid in glomerular disease.* J Clin Invest *2007; 117:1480–1483.)*

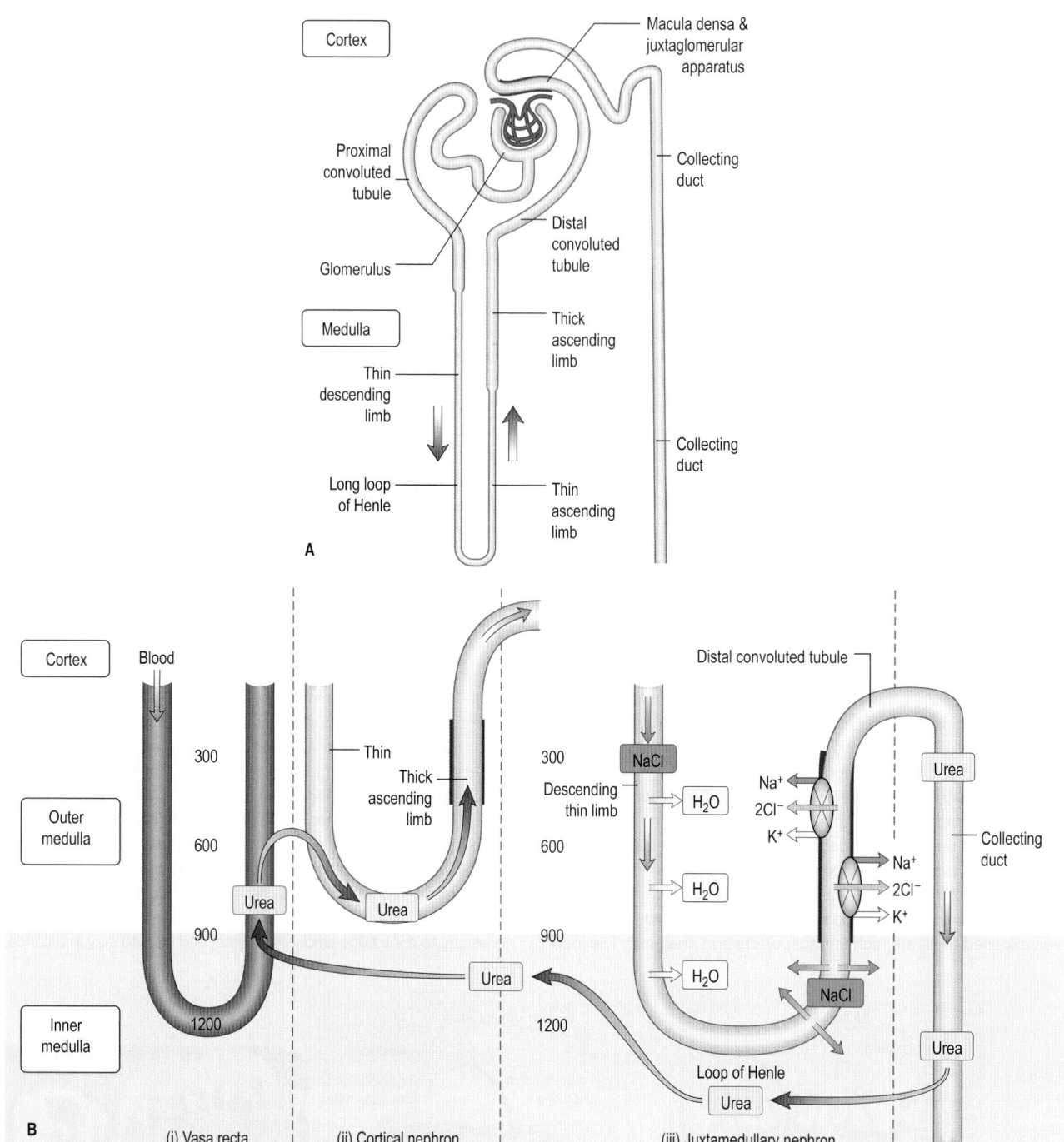

Fig. 36.3 Functional anatomy of the nephron. (A) Principal parts of the nephron. The point where the distal tubule is in close proximity to its own glomerulus is called the juxtaglomerular apparatus. This contains the macula densa. **(B)** The countercurrent system. (i) Vasa recta: these vessels descend from the cortex into the medulla and then turn back towards the cortex. (ii) Cortical nephron: these have short descending limbs extending into the outer medulla. (iii) Juxtamedullary nephron: the descending limb dips deeply into the hypertonic inner medulla. Numbers indicate approximate osmolalities.

Absorption of solutes

Essential electrolytes and other blood constituents, such as glucose and amino acids, are absorbed from filtrate in transit along the long course of the nephron (see **Fig. 36.3**).

Sodium filters freely, and 60–80% of filtered sodium (and water) is reabsorbed in the late proximal tubule, where the apical membrane Na^+/H^+ exchanger (NHE3) trades hydrogen ions into the lumen for absorbed sodium, with anionic chloride (Cl^-) accompanying sodium to maintain electric neutrality. Secreted H^+ allows bicarbonate (HCO_3^-), formed from water and CO_2 by cellular and luminal carbonic anhydrase, to exit the basolateral membrane with absorbed Na^+. Recently, sodium–glucose co-transporters 1 and 2 (SGLT 1 and 2) have generated a lot of interest because of the use of their inhibitors in the treatment of diabetes. SGLT 2 is a predominant proximal

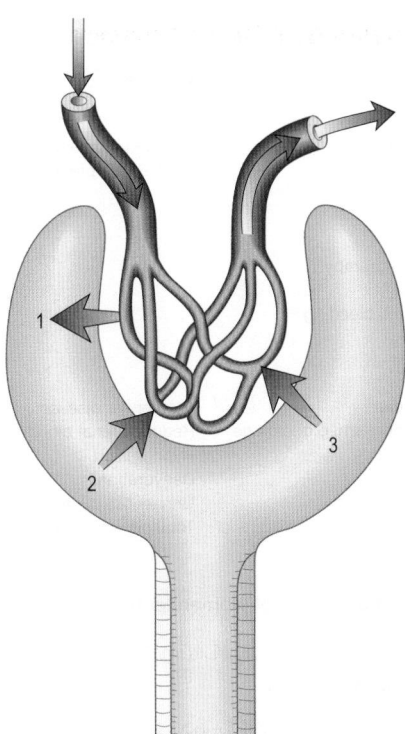

Fig. 36.4 **Pressures controlling glomerular filtration.** (1) Capillary hydrostatic pressure (45 mmHg). (2) Hydrostatic pressure in Bowman's space (10 mmHg). (3) Plasma protein oncotic pressure (25 mmHg). Arrows (1, 2, 3) indicate the direction of a pressure gradient.

tubular transporter that adsorbs glucose and sodium. SGLT 2 inhibitors promote glycosuria and natriuresis, with excellent safety and efficacy in diabetes patients. Around 25% of Na^+ is then absorbed in the thick ascending limb of the loop of Henle, as NaCl by the $Na^+/K^+/2Cl^-$ co-transporter (NKCC). The remaining 5% is absorbed by the thiazide-sensitive NaCl co-transporter and the epithelial sodium channel (ENaC), in the principal cell of the collecting duct. Of the recommended allowance of <6 g/day of *salt* (equivalent to around 2 g Na^+), around 5–10% will be excreted in urine, stool and sweat.

Potassium is freely filtered at the glomerulus, largely reabsorbed in the proximal tubule, and secreted in the distal tubule and collecting ducts. A clinical consequence of this is that the ability to eliminate unwanted potassium is less dependent on GFR than is the elimination of urea or creatinine. Virtually all bicarbonate, glucose and amino acids (see **Fig. 36.3B**) are absorbed in the proximal tubule, making use of the large surface area of this segment of the nephron.

The proximal tubule has a maximal absorptive capacity for many compounds. For instance, if blood glucose levels are elevated above the normal range, the amount filtered (filtered load = GFR × plasma concentration) may exceed the maximal absorptive capacity of the proximal tubule and glucose will 'spill over' into the urine as glycosuria. Inherited or acquired defects in tubular function may also lead to incomplete absorption of a *normal* filtered load, and substances such as glucose (renal glycosuria), amino acids, phosphate, sodium, potassium and calcium will appear in the urine, either singly or in combination. Examples include cystinuria (a defect of a specific amino acid transporter, p. 336) or Fanconi's syndrome (see p. 1369).

Other compounds filtered and reabsorbed or secreted to a variable extent include urate, many organic acids, and many drugs or their metabolic breakdown products. The more tubular secretion of a compound that occurs, the less dependent elimination is on the GFR.

Absorption of water

Urine is concentrated by the countercurrent multiplier mechanism in the loop of Henle, the medullary interstitium, medullary blood vessels (vasa recta) and, finally, the collecting ducts (see p. 175). Sodium and urea in water flow as filtrate into the descending loop, permeable to water and impermeable to sodium. In the thick ascending limb (impermeable to water), active absorption of sodium by the $Na^+/K^+/2Cl^-$ co-transporter into the interstitium increases the tissue osmolarity. Because of the hairpin nature of the loop, water from the permeable descending limb enters the interstitium by osmosis, where the vasa recta return fluid to the circulation. Constant active absorption of sodium in the ascending loop multiplies this process over time, and the solute concentration at the tip of the loop is fourfold that of extracellular fluid. By this mechanism, salt and water are returned to the circulation. Filtrate entering the collecting duct is increasingly concentrated by the action of antidiuretic hormone (ADH, or vasopressin), leading to the release of intracellular aquaporin water channels, which insert themselves across the apical membrane. Water then enters the cell along an osmotic gradient. When the effect of ADH wears off, water channels return to the cell cytoplasm (see **Fig. 9.8**). The final urine volume is 1–2 L daily.

Glomerular filtration rate

In health the GFR remains constant owing to intrarenal regulatory mechanisms. In disease (e.g. a reduction in intrarenal blood flow, damage to or loss of glomeruli, or obstruction to the free flow of ultrafiltrate along the tubule) the GFR will fall. The ability to eliminate wastes and to regulate the volume and composition of body fluid will decline. This is measured as a rise in the plasma urea or creatinine, or as a reduction in measured GFR.

The concentration of urea or creatinine in plasma represents the dynamic equilibrium between production and elimination. In healthy subjects there is an enormous reserve of renal excretory function, and serum urea and creatinine do not rise above the normal range until there is a reduction of 50–60% in the GFR (**Fig. 36.5**). Thereafter, the level of urea depends on both the GFR and its production rate (**Box 36.4**). The latter is heavily influenced by protein intake and tissue catabolism. The level of creatinine is much less dependent on diet but is more related to age, sex and muscle mass. Once it is elevated, serum creatinine is a better guide to GFR than urea and is widely used to monitor further deterioration in the GFR.

Measuring or estimating the GFR

If a substance is filtered, and then unmodified by the tubules as it passes along the nephron, the concentration of that substance per mL will be the same in blood and urine. Accurate calculations of the GFR, particularly in cases where the urea and creatinine may be in the normal range or near normal, can be assessed by cystatin C and creatinine clearance. Cystatin C, a freely filtered low-molecular-weight protein, is a more accurate marker of kidney function than creatinine, though measurement has not widely entered clinical practice as yet.

Daily production of creatinine (principally from muscle cells) is fairly constant and little affected by protein intake. Serum creatinine and excreted (urinary) creatinine vary little throughout the day, allowing measurement of the *creatinine clearance*. Urine is collected over 24 hours for measurement of total urinary creatinine, paired with a single plasma creatinine measured during the 24-hour period. Creatinine clearance is calculated as $U \times V/P$, where U = urine concentration of creatinine, V = rate of urine flow in mL/

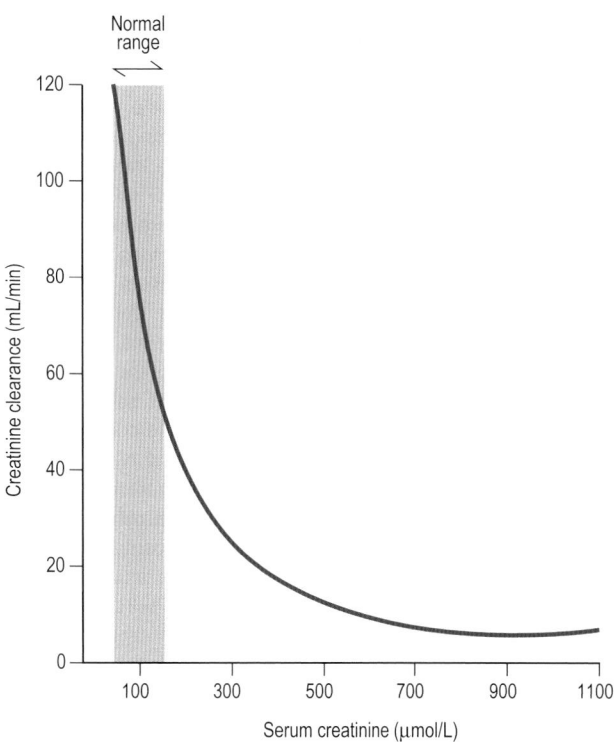

Fig. 36.5 Creatinine clearance versus serum creatinine. Note that the serum creatinine does not rise above the normal range until there is a reduction of 50–60% in the glomerular filtration rate (creatinine clearance).

min, and P = plasma concentration of creatinine. Normal ranges are 90–140 mL/min in men and 80–125 mL/min in women.

Alternatives for quantifying the true GFR include measuring iohexol or inulin clearance, or radio-isotope (^{51}Cr-EDTA) GFR. Neither is practical for daily clinical practice.

Estimated or calculated GFR – the eGFR

Measurement of GFR is cumbersome and time-consuming, and may be inaccurate if 24-hour urine collections are incomplete. Several formulae predict creatinine clearance or GFR from serum creatinine and patient characteristics, often derived from large trials. Variables include age, weight, gender and ethnicity. Commonly used equations are displayed in **Box 36.5**. All have their shortcomings, and are less accurate the closer a GFR is to normal (so patients with seemingly abnormal calculated GFRs may have normal kidney function). Of the equations, the CKD-EPI is more accurate than the modification of diet in renal disease (MDRD) study equation overall and is most reliable for predicting eGFR above 60 mL/min/1.73 m².

All these equations have not, however, been fully validated across all ranges of renal impairment, weights or body mass index (BMI), or in all ethnic groups. However, for monitoring patients with acute or chronic kidney disease, the convenience and ease of the eGFR has led to its widespread adoption.

Drugs, toxins, proteins and the kidney

A substantial fraction of prescription drugs is handled and eliminated by the kidney. Many of these medications (e.g. penicillins, cephalosporins, diuretics, NSAIDs and antivirals) circulate in the plasma as small organic anions, and are actively eliminated in the proximal tubule by a specific organic anion transporter (OAT) system.

---

i Box 36.4 Factors influencing serum urea levels

Production	Elimination
Increased by	
High-protein diet	Elevated glomerular filtration
Increased catabolism	rate, e.g. pregnancy
Surgery	
Infection	
Trauma	
Corticosteroid therapy	
Tetracyclines	
Gastrointestinal bleeding	
Cancer	
Decreased by	
Low-protein diet	Glomerular disease
Reduced catabolism, e.g. old age	Reduced renal blood flow
Liver failure	Hypotension
	Dehydration
	Urinary obstruction
	Tubulointerstitial nephritis

---

i Box 36.5 Estimation of glomerular filtration rate (GFR)

To convert creatinine values in µmol/L to mg/dL, multiply by 0.0113.

Cockcroft–Gault equation

$$\text{Creatinine clearance} = \frac{(140 - \text{age}) \times \text{weight (kg)} \times \text{constant}}{\text{Serum creatinine [µmol/L]}}$$

Constant = 1.23 for males and 1.04 for women.

Modification of diet in renal disease (MDRD) equation
Calculation of estimated GFR by four variables:

$$\text{Estimated GFR} \left(\text{mL/min/1.73m}^2 \right) = 32788 \times (S_{Cr})^{-1.154} \times (\text{age})^{-0203}$$
$$\times \text{constant} \, (0.742 \text{ if female}) \times (1.210 \text{ if black African})$$

CKD Epidemiology (CKD-EPI) Collaboration equation
GFR (mL/min/1.73 m²) = 141 × min (serum creatinine/κ, 1)α × max (serum creatinine/κ, 1)$^{-1.209}$ × 0.993^{Age} × 1.018 [if female] × 1.159 [if black]
where κ is 0.7 for females and 0.9 for males, α is −0.329 for females and −0.411 for males, min indicates the minimum or serum creatinine/κ or 1, and max indicates the maximum of serum creatinine/κ or 1.

(Adapted from MacGregor MS, Boag DE, Innes A. Chronic kidney disease. QJM 2006; 99:365–375.)

The kidney is also a major site for the catabolism (and so elimination) of many small-molecular-weight proteins and polypeptides, including many hormones such as insulin, parathyroid hormone (PTH) and calcitonin, by endocytosis carried out by the megalin–cubilin complex in the brush border of proximal tubular cells. In CKD the metabolic clearance of these substances is reduced and their half-life is prolonged. This accounts, for example, for the reduced insulin requirements of patients with diabetes as their renal function declines.

Endocrine function

Renin–angiotensin system

(See **Fig. 36.6**.) The *juxtaglomerular apparatus (JGA)* regulates flow and filtration in each individual nephron. Columnar epithelium in the macula densa (see **Fig. 36.3**) senses the concentration of tubular fluid sodium (higher filtrate flow means more delivered sodium), triggering purinergic or adenosine-mediated vasoconstriction of the afferent arteriole to drop glomerular filtration (tubuloglomerular feedback).

Pro-renin, synthesized by specialized arteriolar smooth muscle cells in the JGA, is cleaved into the active proteolytic enzyme, renin.

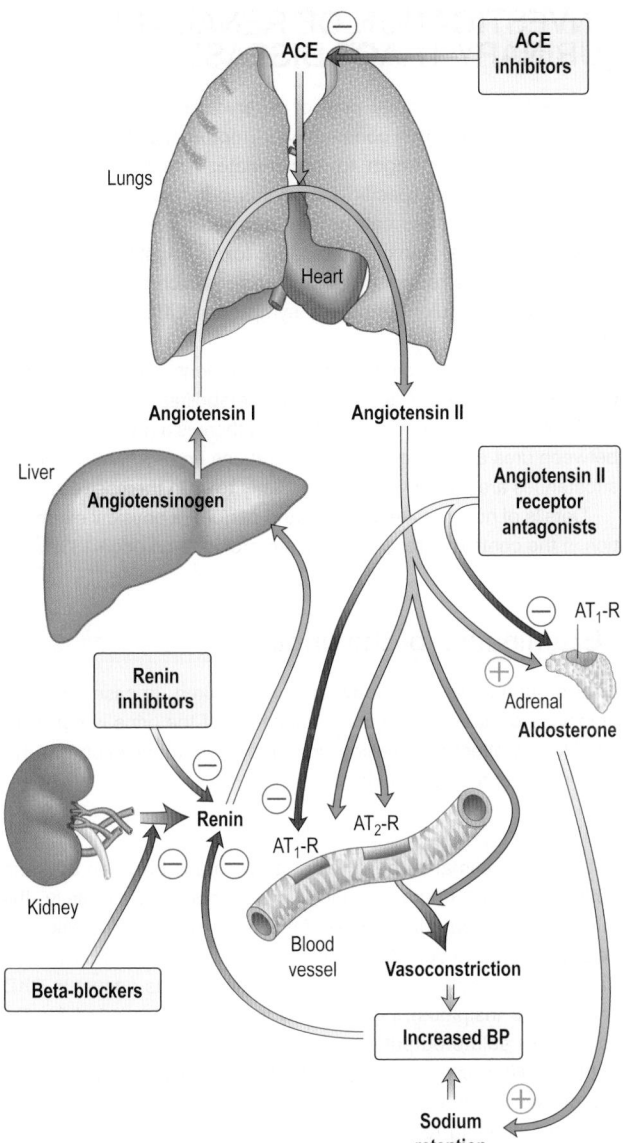

Fig. 36.6 The renin–angiotensin–aldosterone system. Angiotensin-converting enzyme (ACE) inhibitors and angiotensin II antagonists can inhibit this system. BP, blood pressure.

Active renin is stored in the JGA, and released in response to a falling intravascular volume, pressure or increased fluid losses via the kidney. These are 'sensed' as:

- pressure changes in the afferent arteriole or changes in sympathetic tone
- chloride and osmotic concentration in the distal tubule via the macula densa (see **Fig. 36.3A**) – **tubuloglomerular feedback**
- local prostaglandin and nitric oxide release.

In the blood, renin converts angiotensinogen to inactive angiotensin I, which is further cleaved by angiotensin-converting enzyme (ACE, present in lung and vascular endothelium) into active **angiotensin II (AII)**, which has two major actions (mediated by two types of receptor, AT_1 and AT_2). When AII binds the AT_1 subtype (found in the heart, blood vessels, kidney, adrenal cortex, lung and brain), AII:

- causes rapid, powerful vasoconstriction
- stimulates the adrenal zona glomerulosa to increase aldosterone production (over hours or days), leading to sodium (and water) absorption in the collecting duct

- causes vasoconstriction of efferent (but also, to a lesser extent, afferent) renal arterioles, resulting in increase of glomerular capillary pressure to maintain GFR.

In diabetes mellitus, with absorption of excessively filtered glucose and sodium via SGLT-1 and SGLT-2 in the proximal tubules, sodium delivery is reduced at the JGA, which leads to activation of the renin–angiotensin axis and causes increased GFR; this is known as hyperfiltration of diabetes. The renin–angiotensin system can be blocked at several points with renin inhibitors, ACE inhibitors and angiotensin II receptor antagonists (AII-RAs). These are useful agents in the treatment of hypertension and heart failure (see pp. 1140 and 1073) but have differences in action: ACE inhibitors also block kinin production while AII-RAs are specific for AT_1 receptors.

Erythropoietin

Erythropoietin (EPO) (see also p. 325) is the major stimulus for erythropoiesis, the synthesis of red cells. It is a glycoprotein produced principally by fibroblast-like cells in the renal interstitium.

- Under **hypoxic** conditions, both the α and the β subunits of hypoxia inducible factor 2 (HIF-2) are expressed, forming a heterodimer and causing erythropoietin gene transcription. Once formed, erythropoietin binds to its receptors on erythroid precursor cells, to maintain normal red cell synthesis.
- Under **normal oxygen** conditions, only the HIF-2-β subunit is constitutively expressed. The α subunit undergoes proline hydroxylation in the presence of iron and oxygen. The hydroxylated HIF-2-α subunit binds to von Hippel–Lindau protein, with the activating ubiquitination and subsequent degradation of HIF-2-α via proteasomes, so that no erythropoietin is transcribed.

This and other hydroxylation steps have an absolute requirement for molecular oxygen; this forms the basis of oxygen sensing.

Loss of renal substance, with decreased erythropoietin production, results in a normochromic, normocytic anaemia. Conversely, erythropoietin secretion may be increased, with resultant polycythaemia, in people with polycystic renal disease, benign renal cysts or renal cell carcinoma.

Recombinant human erythropoietin is used routinely in clinical practice to treat the anaemia associated with chronic kidney disease. HIF stabilizers are compounds that are being used orally to promote endogenous erythropoietin production in the treatment of anaemia of CKD.

Vitamin D metabolism

Naturally occurring vitamin D (cholecalciferol, see also p. 474) requires hydroxylation in the liver at position 25 and again by a renal 1α-hydroxylase enzyme to produce the metabolically active 1,25-dihydroxycholecalciferol $(1,25\text{-}(OH)_2D_3)$.

Activity of 1α-hydroxylase is decreased by fibroblast growth factor 23 (FGF23), produced by osteocytes in response to high phosphate to promote phosphaturia by downregulation of the sodium–phosphate co-transporter in the proximal tubule, and also to decrease intestinal phosphate absorption by inhibiting activation of vitamin D. FGF23 is increasingly recognized as a possible mediator of bone mineral disease in CKD.

Activity of 1α-hydroxylase is increased by:

- high plasma levels of PTH
- low serum phosphate
- low $1,25\text{-}(OH)_2D_3$.

Both 1,25-dihydroxycholecalciferol and 25-hydroxycholecalciferol are degraded in part by being hydroxylated at position 24 by 24-hydroxylase. The activity of this enzyme is reduced by PTH and increased by $1,25\text{-}(OH)_2D_3$ (which therefore promotes its own inactivation).

Reduced 1α-hydroxylase activity in diseased kidneys leads to relative deficiency of $1,25\text{-}(OH)_2D_3$. As a result, gastrointestinal calcium and, to a lesser extent, phosphate absorption are reduced and bone mineralization is impaired. Reduced gut calcium absorption leads to hypocalcaemia, which is sensed by a specific calcium-sensing receptor (CaSR) on parathyroid glands, and in turn induces release of PTH. Receptors for $1,25\text{-}(OH)_2D_3$ are also found on parathyroid glands, and reduced receptor binding alters the set-point for release of PTH when plasma calcium falls. This combination contributes to the (common) secondary hyperparathyroidism seen in patients with CKD, even of modest degree.

Autocrine function

Prostaglandins

Prostaglandins are unsaturated, oxygenated fatty acids, derived from the enzymatic metabolism of arachidonic acid, mainly by constitutively expressed cyclo-oxygenase-1 (COX-1) or inducible COX-2. COX-1 is highly expressed in the collecting duct, while COX-2 expression is restricted to the macula densa. Both COX isoforms finally convert arachidonic acid into PGE_2 in the collecting duct (leading to a natriuresis/diuresis), prostacyclin (PGI_2) and thromboxane A_2, a vasoconstrictor, mainly synthesized in the glomerulus.

These all maintain renal blood flow and GFR in the face of vasoconstrictors such as angiotensin II, catecholamines and α-adrenergic stimulation. Inhibition of prostaglandin synthesis by NSAIDs results in a fall in GFR, sometimes sufficiently severe to cause AKI, particularly in the elderly, with volume depletion, or where ACE inhibitors or AII-RAs are also being used.

Nitric oxide and the kidney

Nitric oxide (see **Fig. 10.21**), a molecular gas, is formed by the action of three isoforms of nitric oxide synthase (NOS), all of which are expressed in the kidney: eNOS is found in vessels, nNOS mainly in the macula densa and inner medullary collecting duct, and iNOS in several tubule segments. Nitric oxide binds soluble guanylate cyclase, enhancing the synthesis of cyclic guanosine monophosphate (cGMP) from guanosine triphosphate (GTP), and mediates the following physiological actions in the kidney:

- regulation of renal perfusion and glomerular pressure
- natriuresis, by inhibiting Na^+/K^+-ATPase and NHE3
- antagonism of ADH
- modulation of tubuloglomerular feedback (see p. 1343).

Further reading

de Boer IH, Kahn SE. SGLT2 inhibitors – sweet success for diabetic kidney disease? *J Am Soc Nephrol* 2017; 28: 7–10.

Gupta N, Wish JB. Hypoxia-inducible factor prolyl hydroxylase inhibitors: a potential new treatment for anemia in patients with CKD. *Am J Kidney Dis* 2017; 69: 815–826.

Shih HM, Wu CJ, Lin SL. Physiology and pathophysiology of renal erythropoietin-producing cells. *J Formos Med Assoc* 2018; 117:955–963.

White CA, Allen CM, Akbari A et al. Comparison of the new and traditional CKD-EPI GFR estimation equations with urinary inulin clearance: a study of equation performance. *Clin Chim Acta* 2019; 488:189–195.

INVESTIGATION OF RENAL AND URINARY TRACT DISEASE

The kidneys have a great deal of reserve; as a result, the early stages of CKD are often completely asymptomatic, even as renally cleared metabolites begin to accumulate. It is not clear which metabolites lead to specific symptoms but they are thought to be products of protein catabolism (nitrogenous waste products). These metabolites, also called uraemic toxins, must be of relatively small molecular size, since haemodialysis, which clears only relatively small molecules, improves symptoms. Little else is known with certainty.

Serum urea and creatinine concentrations are measured in CKD as surrogates of accumulating metabolites (uraemic toxins) because their measurement is easy, and there is a rough correlation between urea and creatinine concentrations and symptoms. These substances are not, however, particularly toxic in themselves.

Details of how to take a history and perform a physical examination in the context of renal disease are provided on page 1339.

Examination of the urine

Unless urine is visibly bloody (or cola-coloured, in cases of myoglobinuria or haemoglobinuria), inspection of the urine is not helpful. Cloudy, offensive-smelling urine may denote infection but this should be confirmed on culture.

Volume

In temperate climates, healthy adults will pass between 800 and 2500 mL per 24 hours (roughly 1 mL/kg per hour). Usually, the minimum urine output capable of maintaining solute excretion for health (without accumulation in the body) is around 650 mL per day. If the kidney loses concentrating capacity (as occurs in CKD or diabetes insipidus), higher urine volumes are needed for the same daily solute output, and urine outputs may rise well above 2500 mL. **Nocturia** is a symptom of kidney disease, as patients without the ability to concentrate solute into a small urine volume will wake needing to pass urine during the night. High daily volumes are also seen with glycosuria or increased protein catabolism following surgery, as the solute load requiring excretion is higher.

Dipsticks (chemical testing) and urine microscopy

Dipsticks are cheap and hugely helpful in investigating suspected kidney disease, using reagents fixed on pads that change colour on reacting with specific elements in urine.

Specific gravity and osmolality

Urine specific gravity (SG, where <1.008 is dilute and >1.020 is concentrated) is a measure of the weight of dissolved particles in urine, so urine osmolality reflects the number of such particles. Measurement of urine SG or osmolality can be helpful in confirming loss of concentrating ability (as might be seen when tubular function fails in acute tubular necrosis or CKD). It can also be helpful in oliguric patients, when a high SG might suggest pre-renal AKI, as opposed to established acute tubular necrosis (see p. 1389).

Urinary pH

Measurement of urinary pH (usually 5.5–6.5) is helpful only in the investigation and treatment of renal tubular acidosis (see p. 199).

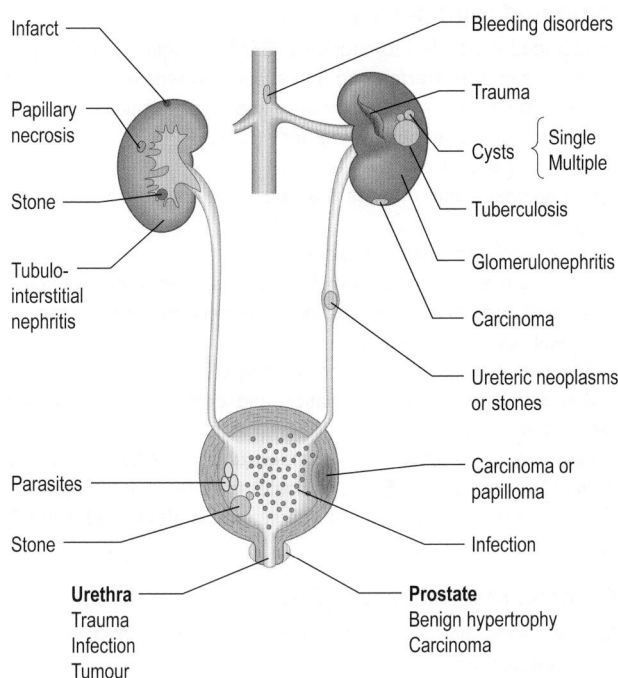

Fig. 36.7 Sites and causes of bleeding from the urinary tract.

Blood

Haematuria may originate from anywhere in the urinary tract. Once it is found on dipstick, a mid-stream sample may be spun at 2000 rpm and examined for red cells or casts on microscopy. Red cells (usually 1–2 per high-power field) are described as dysmorphic (altered in shape) if they originate from the early nephron (glomerular bleeding), and may be accompanied by red-cell casts. Casts are cylindrical bodies, moulded in the shape of the distal tubular lumen. Red-cell casts – even if only single – always indicate glomerular disease. A dipstick that is strongly positive for haematuria with no red cells seen on microscopy might suggest haemoglobinuria or myoglobinuria.

Bleeding may come from any site within the urinary tract (**Fig. 36.7**):

- *Overt bleeding from the urethra* is suggested when blood is seen at the start of voiding and then the urine becomes clear.
- *Blood diffusely present* throughout the urine comes from the bladder or above.
- *Blood only at the end of micturition* suggests bleeding from the prostate or bladder base.

Women will commonly have dipstick-positive haematuria during a period; it is usually worth repeating testing after menstruation.

Protein

Proteinuria is one of the most common signs of renal disease: normal individuals excrete less than 30 mg per day. Dipsticks will detect proteinuria from around 50–150 mg/L, and may be designed to test for either albuminuria or proteinuria. If two separate urine samples find proteinuria on dipstick testing, a random urine protein:creatinine ratio (uPCR) should be measured. This convenient test has largely replaced formal (timed) 24-hour urine collections for proteinuria; an alternative is the albumin:creatinine ratio (ACR). As albumin is usually the dominant protein lost in the urine, patients who have albuminuria always have proteinuria (and the urine PCR will be

higher than the urine ACR). Confusingly, the terms are often used interchangeably. For people with diabetes the urine ACR has particular prognostic significance and is usually the preferred screening test (see p. 730) for the *microalbuminuria* found in early diabetic kidney disease.

Both tests are expressed as mg protein/mmol creatinine. Generally, an ACR of 2.5–20 mg/mmol corresponds to albuminuria of 30–300 mg daily (crudely, multiply the result by a factor of 15 – so an ACR of 50 mg/mmol = 750 mg/day albuminuria). Similarly, a uPCR of 3–30 mg/mmol corresponds to 30–300 mg daily (multiplying by a factor of 10 for this test – so a PCR of 50 mg/mmol = 500 mg proteinuria per day). The uPCR assay is relatively cheap and identifies patients whose proteinuria is of tubular and glomerular origin. ACR or PCR levels independently predict all-cause and cardiovascular mortality in the general population in addition to better risk stratifications of patients with CKD for future renal outcomes. Pyrexia, exercise and adoption of the upright posture (*postural proteinuria*) all increase urinary protein output but are benign. Proteinuria may associate with coarse granular casts seen on urine microscopy. *Urine electrophoresis and immunofixation* may detect light chains, which can be present in myeloma without a detectable serum paraprotein.

Electrolytes

Urinary electrolytes are unhelpful in CKD. The use of urinary sodium concentration in the distinction between pre-renal and intrinsic renal disease is discussed on page 1388.

Glucose

Renal glycosuria is uncommon, so that a positive test for glucose might prompt consideration of diabetes mellitus. Dipsticks for glucose are very sensitive, however.

Bacteria and pus cells

Dipstick tests for bacteriuria are based on the detection of *nitrite* produced from the reduction of urinary nitrate by bacteria, and also on the detection of leucocyte esterase, an enzyme specific for neutrophils. Both tests have limitations, particularly in the elderly. When positive, a mid-stream sample should be sent for microscopy, culture and sensitivities (MC&S).

Urine microscopy

(See p. 1348.) White blood cells (WBCs) may be seen on microscopy, as may bacteria. A measurement of 10 WBCs/mL or more in fresh mid-stream urine samples is abnormal and suggests urinary tract infection (UTI). Not all pyuria is UTI, though; pus cells are seen with renal stones, tubulointerstitial nephritis, papillary necrosis, tuberculosis and interstitial cystitis. White cell casts may be seen with (and are more characteristic of) acute pyelonephritis.

Granular casts are formed from abnormal cells within the tubular lumen and indicate active renal disease. Red-cell casts are highly suggestive of glomerulonephritis.

Blood and quantitative tests

The use of serum urea, creatinine and GFR as measures of renal function is discussed on page 1345. Other quantitative tests of disturbed renal function are described under the relevant disorders, as are specific diagnostic tests. Most assessments of kidney disease might include the tests described here.

Serum biochemistry

- Urea, electrolytes, bicarbonate and creatinine, with a calculation of eGFR.
- Electrophoresis and immunofixation with serum free light chains for myeloma.
- Calcium, phosphate, alkaline phosphatase, with or without intact PTH, liver function, creatine kinase and lactate dehydrogenase.
- Blood glucose and HbA_{1C}, which estimate chronic diabetic control.

Haematology

- Full blood count, blood film and ESR.
- Tests for sickle cell disease, when relevant.

Immunology

- *Complement components* may be low in active renal disease due to systemic lupus erythematosus (SLE), mesangiocapillary glomerulonephritis, post-streptococcal glomerulonephritis and cryoglobulinaemia.
- *Autoantibody screening* is useful in detection of SLE (see p. 457), scleroderma (p. 460), granulomatosis with polyangiitis and microscopic polyangiitis (p. 991), and Goodpasture's syndrome (p. 992). Anti-phospholipase A2 receptor antibodies are positive in membranous nephropathy.
- *Cryoglobulins* are measured in unexplained glomerular disease, particularly mesangiocapillary glomerulonephritis.
- *Antibodies to streptococcal antigens* (antistreptolysin O titre (ASOT), anti-DNAse B) are sought if post-streptococcal glomerulonephritis is possible.
- *Antibodies to hepatitis B and C* may point to polyarteritis or membranous nephropathy (hepatitis B) or to cryoglobulinaemic renal disease (hepatitis C).
- *Antibodies to HIV* raise the possibility of HIV-associated renal disease.

Imaging techniques

Ultrasonography

Ultrasound of the kidneys and bladder is safe and non-invasive, avoiding ionizing radiation and intravascular contrast medium. In renal diagnosis, it is the imaging method of choice for:

- assessing renal size and symmetry (normal-sized kidneys with abnormal function suggest an acute cause, as kidneys scar as they fail, and may shrink in length and volume)
- ruling out obstruction, either of the bladder and ureters (with unilateral or bilateral hydronephrosis), or of the kidney itself (where pelvicalyceal dilation may suggest high ureteric or pelvic disease)
- characterizing renal masses as cystic (either simple cysts or polycystic kidneys), or complex and solid (benign and malignant renal tumours, or infected collections)
- guiding interventions aimed at relieving obstruction (percutaneous nephrostomy)
- confirming renal vein patency, and suggesting (but not proving) renal artery disease, in the case of *Doppler ultrasonography (duplex)*
- looking for bladder tumours or stones; a scan obtained after voiding (post-micturition) allows bladder emptying to be assessed.

Computed tomography

Unenhanced computed tomography (CT) is the first-line investigation for cases of **ureteric colic** and suspected renal calculi. It has superseded excretion urography (also known as intravenous urography (IVU) or intravenous pyelography (IVP)).

CT is also used to:

- characterize renal masses that are indeterminate at ultrasonography
- stage renal and bladder tumours
- evaluate the retroperitoneum for tumours, retroperitoneal fibrosis (peri-aortitis) and other causes of ureteric obstruction
- assess severe renal trauma
- visualize the renal arteries and veins by CT angiography.

Disadvantages include radiation and contrast nephrotoxicity (see p. 1350).

Positron emission tomography (PET), using ^{18}F-fluorodeoxyglucose (FDG), is useful for detection of infection (e.g. in a cyst), inflammation or tumours, and is often used with CT (PET/CT).

Magnetic resonance imaging

Magnetic resonance imaging (MRI) is used as an alternative to CT with no irradiation:

- to stage prostate (and also renal and bladder) cancer
- to reconstruct the anatomy of the renal arteries using magnetic resonance **angiography** (MRA) with gadolinium as contrast medium; in experienced hands, its sensitivity and specificity approach those of renal angiography.

The Food and Drug Administration (FDA) advises not using gadolinium in patients with renal insufficiency because of the development of nephrogenic systemic fibrosis (see p. 681).

Plain X-ray

A plain radiograph of the abdomen may be useful to identify renal calcification or radiodense calculi in the kidney, renal pelvis and the line of the ureters or bladder (**Fig. 36.8**).

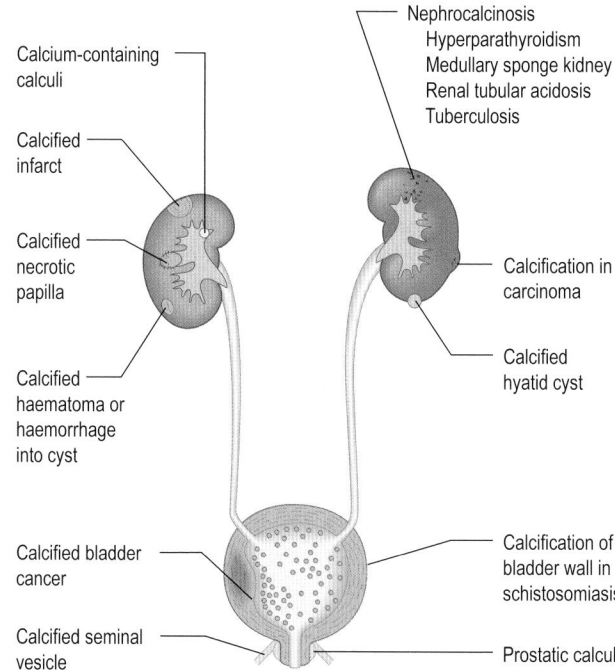

Fig. 36.8 Calcification in the renal tract. Calculi can occur at any site.

Labels in figure:
- Calcium-containing calculi
- Calcified infarct
- Calcified necrotic papilla
- Calcified haematoma or haemorrhage into cyst
- Calcified bladder cancer
- Calcified seminal vesicle
- Nephrocalcinosis / Hyperparathyroidism / Medullary sponge kidney / Renal tubular acidosis / Tuberculosis
- Calcification in carcinoma
- Calcified hyatid cyst
- Calcification of bladder wall in schistosomiasis
- Prostatic calculi

Antegrade pyelography

Antegrade pyelography (**Fig. 36.9**) involves percutaneous puncture of a pelvicalyceal system with a needle and the injection of contrast medium to outline the pelvicalyceal system and ureter to the level of obstruction. Drains can be sited and stents placed during the procedure.

Micturating cystourethrography

After bladder catheterization, contrast is instilled into the bladder. The catheter is then removed and the patient screened during voiding to check for vesico-ureteric reflux and to study the urethra and bladder emptying. Micturating cystourethrography (MCUG) is used in children with recurrent infection. It is rarely appropriate in adults, as with bladder wall hypertrophy in adulthood, vesico-ureteric reflux tends to disappear.

Aortography or renal arteriography

Conventional or digital subtraction angiography (DSA) is used diagnostically, and also in cases of suspected renal artery stenosis, to allow therapeutic renal artery balloon angioplasty and stenting. Complications include cholesterol embolization (see p. 1372) and contrast-induced kidney damage (contrast nephropathy).

Renal scintigraphy

Isotope studies are helpful for dynamic or static investigation of perfusion or excretion. Following venous injection of a bolus of tracer, emissions from the kidney can be recorded by gamma camera. Technetium-labelled diethylenetriaminepenta-acetic acid (^{99m}Tc-DTPA) is excreted by glomerular filtration and can be used to confirm renal perfusion (e.g. in renal artery stenosis, see p. 1371). Dimercaptosuccinic acid labelled with technetium (^{99m}Tc-DMSA) is filtered by the glomerulus and then binds to proximal tubular cells.

Static studies are useful to assess the relative contribution in function of asymmetric kidneys, and to highlight 'photon-deficient' areas (where isotope is not seen), suggestive of scars or infarction, when compared to healthy tissue uptake. Mercapto-acetyltriglycine (MAG3) labelled with technetium (^{99m}Tc) is excreted by renal tubular secretion, so resistance to flow in the pelvis or ureter (with obstruction) prolongs the parenchymal transit of tracer with a delay in emptying the pelvis. On whole-kidney renograms, the time–activity curve fails to fall after an initial peak, or continues to rise (**Fig. 36.10**), confirming hold-up to flow. Furosemide may be given to exaggerate urine output and emphasize the delay, in order to aid diagnosis.

Transcutaneous renal biopsy

Renal biopsy (**Box 36.6**) is carried out under ultrasound control in specialized centres and requires interpretation by an experienced pathologist. It is helpful in the investigation of the nephritic and nephrotic syndromes, acute and chronic kidney disease, haematuria after urological investigations and renal graft dysfunction. Native renal biopsy material must be examined by conventional histochemical staining, by electron microscopy, and by immunoperoxidase or immunofluorescence. Techniques like *in situ* hybridization and polymerase chain reaction (PCR) analysis are also widely used in renal biopsy specimens.

The complications of transcutaneous renal biopsy are shown in **Box 36.7**.

Glomerular disease is usually described by kidney biopsy findings. Commonly used terms are shown in **Box 36.8**.

THE GLOMERULUS AND GLOMERULAR DISEASE

A glomerulus consists of a collection of capillaries seated within Bowman's capsule in the urinary space. Blood flows in via the afferent arteriole and exits via the efferent arteriole. Filtrate leaves Bowman's space and moves into the proximal tubule. The capillary tuft is supported by mesangial cells and mesangial matrix. Filtrate moves from

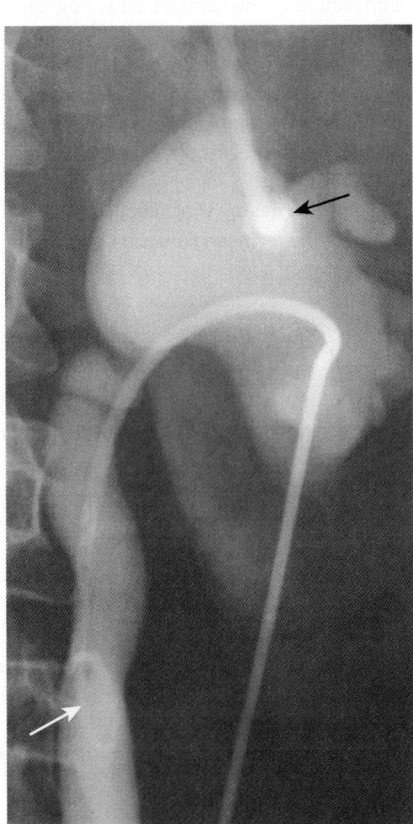

Fig. 36.9 Antegrade pyelography via percutaneous catheter (black arrow) of obstructed system. A percutaneous drainage catheter (white arrow) has been inserted.

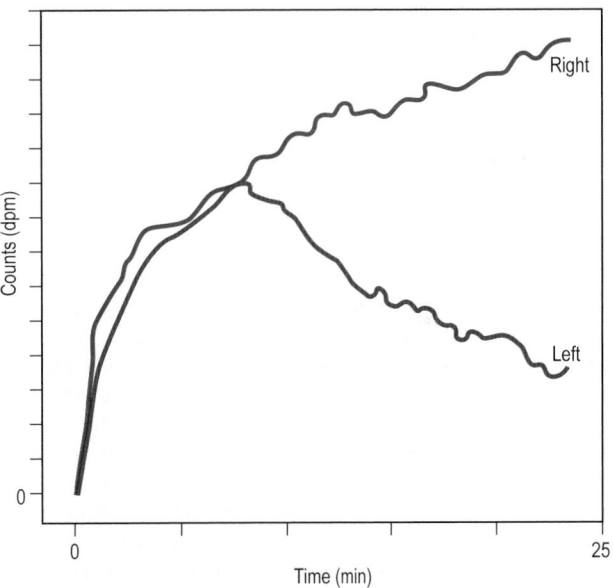

Fig. 36.10 Dynamic scintigram. Note the progressive rise of the right kidney curve to a plateau (in contrast to the normal left kidney curve), owing to urinary tract obstruction on the right side.

Box 36.6 Transcutaneous renal biopsy

Before biopsy

- Perform a coagulation screen; it must be normal.
- Group and save the serum for cross-matching.
- Give the patient a full explanation of what is involved and obtain consent.

During biopsy

- Ask the patient to lie prone with a hard pillow under the abdomen.
- Localize the kidney by ultrasound.
- Inject local anaesthetic along the biopsy track.
- Instruct the patient to hold a breath when the biopsy is performed.

After biopsy

- Apply pressure dressing to the biopsy site and ask the patient to rest in bed for 8–24 h.
- Maximize fluid intake to prevent clot colic.
- Check the pulse and blood pressure regularly.
- Advise the patient to avoid heavy lifting or gardening for 2 weeks.

---

i **Box 36.7 Complications of transcutaneous renal biopsy**

- Macroscopic haematuria – up to 10%
- Pain in the flank, sometimes referred to the shoulder tip
- Perirenal haematoma
- Arteriovenous aneurysm formation – about 20%, almost always of no clinical significance
- Profuse haematuria demanding blood transfusion – 1–3%
- Profuse haematuria demanding occlusion of the bleeding vessel at angiography or nephrectomy – approximately 1 in 400
- Introduction of infection
- Mortality rate of about 0.1%

---

i **Box 36.8 Glomerular disease: commonly used terms**

- ***Focal:*** some, but not all, glomeruli show the lesion
- ***Diffuse*** (global)***:*** most of the glomeruli (>75%) contain the lesion
- ***Segmental:*** only a part of the glomerulus is affected (most focal lesions are also segmental, e.g. focal segmental glomerulosclerosis)
- ***Global:*** all of the glomerulus is symmetrically involved
- ***Proliferative:*** an increase in cell numbers due to hyperplasia of one or more of the resident glomerular cells with or without inflammation
- ***Membrane alterations:*** capillary wall thickening due to deposition of immune deposits or alterations in basement membrane
- ***Crescent formation:*** epithelial cell proliferation with mononuclear cell infiltration in Bowman's space

the capillary lumen into the urinary space across the glomerular filter (see p. 1343). Three elements are involved in allowing or preventing filtration: endothelium, the GBM and podocytes (**Fig. 36.11**).

Filtration barrier (slit diaphragm)

The glomerular filtration barrier (see **Fig. 36.2**) consists of the fenestrated endothelium, the GBM and the terminally differentiated visceral epithelial cells known as podocytes. Podocytes attach to the GBM by foot processes via adhesion molecules, such as $\alpha_3\beta_1$ and dystroglycans. Adjacent podocytes are joined laterally via their foot process by slit diaphragms, which bridge across the filtration slits. The various proteins comprising the slit diaphragm include nephrin, CD2-associated protein (CD2AP), canonical transient receptor potential channel 6 (TRPC6), podocin, P-cadherin, α- and β-catenin, and zonula occludens-1 (ZO-1). They co-localize within the subcellular domain to function as a molecular sieve. These proteins, in addition to providing structural support to the cytoskeletal proteins like filamentous actin, also have signalling functions in order to maintain the normal function of podocytes. Abnormalities in any of these proteins result in the

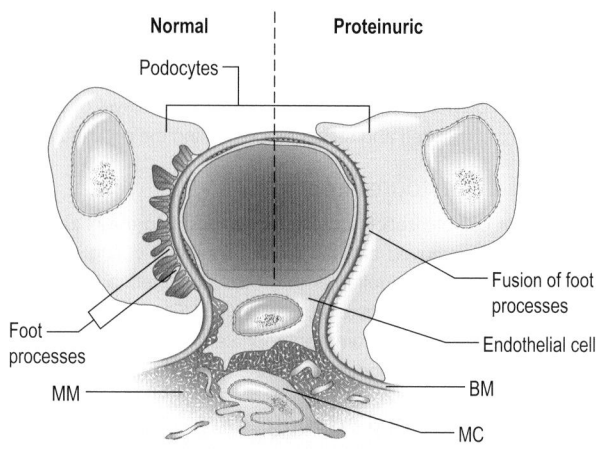

Fig. 36.11 A normal (left) and a proteinuric (right) glomerulus. A capillary loop shows normal glomerular morphology on the left with a podocyte with pseudopodia (foot processes). In the proteinuric diagram (right), there is fusion of the foot processes, which is characteristic of many diseases. BM, basement membrane; MC, mesangial cell; MM, mesangial matrix.

breakdown of the filtration barrier with consequent torrential leak of macromolecules.

Podocyte changes

The podocyte structure (see earlier) is maintained by actin, which supports the cytoskeleton (see **Fig. 36.2**). A rearrangement of the fluid actin cytoskeleton leads to foot process effacement (flattening). As the architecture of the filtration slit is now disrupted, albumin leaks into the urine; recovery of the cytoskeleton reverses proteinuria. The cytoskeleton can be altered by:

- abnormalities of cytoskeletal proteins like α-actinin-4, which causes hereditary focal segmental glomerular sclerosis
- injury to or abnormalities of slit diaphragm proteins
- changes in the GBM itself
- direct injury to podocytes by viral infection, drugs, toxins or the local activation of the renin–angiotensin system.

Glomerular disease

Glomerular disease is the third most common cause (after diabetes and hypertension) of end-stage kidney disease (ESKD) in Europe and the USA, accounting for some 10–15% of such patients. These are diseases in which:

- there may be an immunologically mediated inflammatory injury to glomeruli, or structural or functional glomerular damage without inflammation
- renal interstitial damage is a regular accompaniment
- the kidneys are involved symmetrically
- secondary mechanisms of glomerular injury may come into play following an initial immune insult, such as fibrin deposition, platelet aggregation, neutrophil infiltration and free radical-induced damage
- haemodynamic consequences of a primary injury may further disturb glomerular function
- renal lesions may be part of a generalized disease (e.g. SLE).

Describing glomerular disease

The nomenclature relating to glomerular disease can be confusing, as descriptive terms (as seen on histology) overlap with clinical syndromes and more recent molecular insights into the pathogenesis of disease. If there is predominant inflammation on histology, glomerular disease may be described as a *glomerulonephritis*. If inflammation is absent, *glomerulopathy* is more correct. There remains much overlap between the two, and the terms are often (wrongly) used interchangeably. It may be better to think about glomerular disease in terms of the predominant compartment involved, where the GBM separates podocytes from mesangial and endothelial cells.

- **Podocytes** (in the urinary compartment) are principally involved in glomerular diseases (usually glomerulopathies) that present as the *nephrotic syndrome*, where proteinuria is often heavy.
- **Endothelial and mesangial cells** (in the endocapillary compartment) are principally involved in glomerular disease presenting as *nephritis* (glomerulonephritis), where haematuria, proteinuria and often hypertension are equally evident.
- Podocytes, endothelial and mesangial cells may be equally involved where a glomerulonephritis presents with heavy proteinuria and the nephrotic syndrome as well.

Clinical classification of glomerular disease is also often used, although there is no complete correlation between histopathological types and clinical features. Four major glomerular syndromes are often described:

- *Nephrotic syndrome:* massive proteinuria (>3.5 g/day), hypoalbuminaemia, oedema, lipiduria and hyperlipidaemia. Podocyte malfunction or injury is often causative.
- *Glomerulonephritis (nephritic syndrome):*
  - *Acute glomerulonephritis:* abrupt onset of glomerular haematuria (red blood cell casts or dysmorphic red blood cells), non-nephrotic-range proteinuria, oedema, hypertension and transient renal impairment, *or*
  - *Rapidly progressive glomerulonephritis:* features of acute nephritis, focal necrosis with or without crescents, and rapidly progressive renal failure over weeks.
- *Mixed nephritic/nephrotic presentations:* where glomerulonephritis is part of a systemic disease (e.g. lupus nephritis, cryoglobulinaemia and Henoch–Schönlein purpura), a nephritic syndrome is often associated with the nephrotic syndrome.
- *Asymptomatic haematuria, proteinuria* or both.

Investigation of glomerular diseases is shown in **Box 36.9**.

Nephrotic syndrome

Nephrotic syndrome is characterized by:
- hypoalbuminaemia
- >3.5 g proteinuria/day
- dyslipidaemia
- salt and water retention, leading to oedema.

Pathophysiology

Hypoalbuminaemia

Loss of urinary protein (largely albumin) of the order of 3.5 g or more daily in an adult may lead to hypoalbuminaemia. Normal dietary protein intake in the UK is around 70 g daily and the normal liver can synthesize albumin at a rate of 10–12 g daily. How, then, does a daily urinary protein loss of 3.5 g result in hypoalbuminaemia? This can be partly explained by increased catabolism of reabsorbed protein, largely albumin, in the proximal tubules, even though the rate of albumin synthesis is increased.

Box 36.9 Investigation of glomerular diseases

Investigations	Positive findings
Urine microscopy	Red cells, red-cell casts
Urinary protein	Nephrotic or sub-nephrotic-range proteinuria
Serum urea	May be elevated
Serum creatinine	May be elevated
Culture (throat swab, discharge from ear, swab from inflamed skin)	Nephritogenic organism (not always)
Antistreptolysin-O titre	Elevated in post-streptococcal nephritis
C3 and C4 levels	May be reduced
Antinuclear antibody (ANA)	Present in significant titre in systemic lupus erythematosus
Antinuclear cytoplasmic antibody (ANCA)	Positive in some vasculitides
Anti-glomerular basement membrane (anti-GBM)	Positive in Goodpasture's syndrome
Cryoglobulins	Increased in cryoglobulinaemia
Chest X-ray	Cardiomegaly, pulmonary oedema (not always)
Renal imaging	Usually normal
Renal biopsy	Any glomerulopathy

Proteinuria

Proteinuria occurs partly because structural damage to the glomerular barrier (podocytes, basement membrane, fenestrated endothelium and endothelial charge) allows the passage of more and larger molecules. The filtration slit between podocytes and normal podocyte architecture, and interdigitating podocyte foot processes are critical to maintaining a barrier to protein loss into the urinary space, as is a functional GBM and healthy capillary endothelium (and its charge).

Hyperlipidaemia

This is a consequence of increased synthesis of lipoproteins (such as apolipoprotein B, C-III lipoprotein (a)), as a direct consequence of a low plasma albumin. Low-density lipoprotein (LDL) increases, partly due to upregulation of a liver serine protease, *pro-protein convertase subtilisin kexin-9 (PCSK9)*, which causes internalization of LDL receptors. Very-low-density lipoprotein (VLDL) and/or intermediate-density lipoprotein (IDL) fractions increase, with no change (or a decrease) in high-density lipoprotein (HDL) (the LDL:HDL cholesterol ratio increases). There is also reduced clearance of the principal triglycerides bearing lipoprotein (chylomicrons and VLDL), as high plasma levels of free fatty acid (FFA) trigger release of appropriately sialylated angiopoietin-like 4 (ANGPTL4) protein from adipose tissue, heart and skeletal muscles, inhibiting lipoprotein lipase and resulting in hypertriglyceridaemia.

Oedema in hypoalbuminaemia

See page 177.

Management

General measures

- *Initial management* should be with dietary sodium restriction and a loop diuretic (e.g. furosemide or bumetanide). Unresponsive patients require furosemide 40–120 mg daily (or more) with the addition of amiloride (5 mg daily; monitor serum potassium concentration regularly). Nephrotic patients may malabsorb diuretics (as well as other drugs) owing to gut mucosal oedema, and intravenous administration may be needed initially. Patients are sometimes hypovolaemic, and moderate oedema may have to be accepted in order to avoid postural hypotension.

- **Normal protein intake** is advisable. A high-protein diet (80–90 g protein daily) increases proteinuria and can be harmful in the long term.
- **Hypercoagulable states** predispose to venous thrombosis. The hypercoagulable state is due to loss of clotting factors (e.g. antithrombin) in the urine and an increase in hepatic production of fibrinogen. Prolonged bed rest should be avoided, as thromboembolism is very common (particularly in membranous nephropathy). Long-term prophylactic anticoagulation may be indicated, and if renal vein thrombosis occurs, permanent anticoagulation is required.
- **Sepsis** is a major cause of death in nephrotic patients. The increased susceptibility to infection is partly due to loss of immunoglobulin in the urine. Pneumococcal infections are particularly common and pneumococcal vaccine should be given. Early detection and aggressive treatment of infections, rather than long-term antibiotic prophylaxis, constitute the best approach.
- **Lipid abnormalities** are responsible for an increase in the risk of cardiovascular disease in patients with proteinuria. Treatment of hypercholesterolaemia starts with an HMG-CoA reductase inhibitor (a statin).
- Lastly, **ACE inhibitors and/or angiotensin II receptor antagonists** (AII-RAs) are indicated for their antiproteinuric properties in all types of glomerulonephropathy, but most especially the nephrotic syndrome. These drugs reduce proteinuria by lowering glomerular capillary filtration pressure (a fall in efferent tone decreases the transglomerular capillary pressure, and so protein loss into the urinary space); blood pressure and renal function should be monitored regularly.

Specific measures

Treat the underlying cause of any urinary protein leak. **Box 36.10** shows the glomerular lesions commonly associated with the nephrotic syndrome.

Causes of nephrotic syndrome

Minimal-change nephropathy (minimal-change disease)

In minimal-change nephropathy (MCN; also called minimal-change disease, MCD), glomeruli appear normal on light microscopy (**Fig. 36.12**).

Box 36.10 Glomerulopathies associated with the nephrotic syndrome

Primary glomerular disease	Secondary glomerular disease
Nephrotic syndrome	
Minimal-change nephropathy	Amyloidosis
Congenital nephrotic syndrome	Diabetic nephropathy
Focal segmental glomerular sclerosis	
Membranous nephropathy	
Mixed nephrotic/nephritic	
Mesangiocapillary glomerulonephritis	Systemic lupus erythematosus
Mesangial proliferative glomerulonephritis	Cryoglobulinaemic disease
	Henoch–Schönlein syndrome
	Idiopathic fibrillary glomerulopathy
	Immunotactoid glomerulopathy
	Fibronectin glomerulonephropathy

On electron microscopy, fusion of the foot processes of podocytes is seen, consistent with a disrupted podocyte actin cytoskeleton (see **Fig. 36.2B**). Neither immune complexes nor anti-GBM antibody can be demonstrated by immunofluorescence on glomerular staining for antibody.

Immature differentiating CD34 stem cells (rather than mature T lymphocytes) appear to be responsible for the pathogenesis of MCN. Podocyte function is also affected by interleukin 13 (IL-13), the production of vascular endothelial growth factor (VEGF), or the upregulation of vascular hyposialylated-angiopoietin-like 4 (ANG-PTL4), secreted by the podocytes.

Many drugs have been implicated in MCN, including NSAIDs, lithium, antibiotics (cephalosporins, rifampicin, ampicillin), bisphosphonates and sulfasalazine. Atopy is present in 30% of cases of MCN, and allergic reactions can trigger the nephrotic syndrome. Infections, such as hepatitis C virus, HIV and tuberculosis, are rarer causes.

Clinical features

MCN is most common in children, particularly boys, and is responsible for the large majority of cases of nephrotic syndrome in childhood. Proteinuria is usually 'highly selective', where albumin, but not higher-molecular-weight proteins such as immunoglobulins, is lost in the urine. Oedema is usual and in children this may present predominantly around the face. The condition accounts for 20–25% of cases of adult nephrotic syndrome. It is often regarded as a condition that does not lead to CKD (but see focal segmental glomerulosclerosis below).

Management

- Manage symptoms with general measures (see earlier).
- High-dose corticosteroid therapy with prednisolone 60 mg/m² daily (up to a maximum of 80 mg/day) for a maximum of 4–6 weeks, followed by 40 mg/m² every other day for a further 4–6 weeks, reverses proteinuria in more than 95% of children. Response rates in adults are significantly lower and response may occur only after many months (12 weeks with daily steroid therapy and 12 weeks of maintenance with alternate-day therapy). Spontaneous remission also occurs and steroid therapy should, in general, be withheld if urinary protein loss is insufficient to cause hypoalbuminaemia or oedema. In both children and adults, if remission lasts for 4 years after steroid therapy, further relapse is very rare.
- Two-thirds of children relapse after steroid therapy and further courses of corticosteroids are required. One-third of these patients regularly relapse on steroid withdrawal, so that

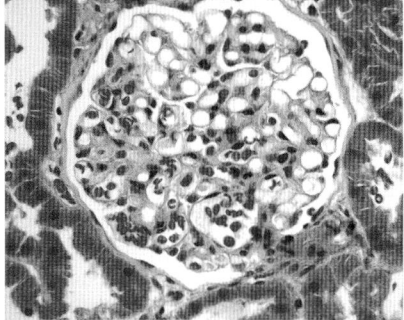

Fig. 36.12 Normal glomerulus on light microscopy in minimal-change nephropathy.

a second-line agent should be added after repeat induction with steroids.

- Ciclosporin or tacrolimus may be effective (with or without steroids) but must be continued long-term to prevent relapse on stopping treatment. The antiproteinuric effect of these calcineurin inhibitors is normally attributed to its immunosuppressive action but may result from the stabilization of the actin cytoskeleton in kidney podocytes. Ciclosporin inhibits the calcineurin-mediated dephosphorylation of synaptopodin (a regulator of actin cytoskeleton) and protects it from cathepsin L-mediated degradation. These results have shed new light on the role of calcineurin signalling in proteinuric kidney diseases. Excretory function and ciclosporin and tacrolimus trough blood levels must be monitored regularly, as both drugs are potentially nephrotoxic.

- Rituximab, a depleting monoclonal antibody directed against CD20 and present on B lymphocytes, is showing promise in reducing the number of recurrences in frequently relapsing disease, and also in minimizing the immunosuppressant burden in corticosteroid-dependent disease.

- Cyclophosphamide 1.5–2.0 mg/kg daily is given for 8–12 weeks with prednisolone 7.5–15 mg/day. This increases the likelihood of long-term remission. Steroid-unresponsive patients may also respond to cyclophosphamide. No more than two courses of cyclophosphamide should be prescribed in children because of the risk of side-effects, which include future infertility (azoospermia and premature ovarian failure).

- In corticosteroid-dependent children, the anthelminthic agent levamisole 2.5 mg/kg to a maximum of 150 mg on alternate days is also useful in maintenance of remission. Levamisole's mode of action is attributable to its direct effects on podocytes by inducing expression of glucocorticoid receptor (GR) and activated GR signalling in podocytes.

Congenital nephrotic syndrome

Congenital nephrotic syndrome (Finnish type) is an autosomal recessively inherited disorder due to mutations in the gene coding for a transmembrane protein, nephrin; it occurs at a frequency of 1 per 8200 live births in Finland. Nephrin is a critical element of the filtration slit, and its loss of function results in massive proteinuria shortly after birth. The disorder can be diagnosed *in utero*, as increased α-fetoprotein in amniotic fluid is a common feature. This condition is characterized by relentless progression to ESKD.

Other inherited nephrotic syndromes involve mutations in other genes that encode other podocyte proteins, such as podocin, α-actinin 4 and Wilms' tumour suppressor gene. Congenital nephrotic syndrome patients are steroid-resistant. Mutation analysis in steroid-resistant nephrotic syndrome (SRNS) has identified more than 30 recessive or dominant genes, revealing that the encoded proteins are essential for glomerular function. Mutation analysis could be offered to all individuals who manifest with SRNS before the age of 25 years, for diagnosis and for exploration of possible therapies, as it may permit personalized treatment options based on genetic causation by way of 'precision medicine'.

Focal segmental glomerulosclerosis

Focal segmental glomerulosclerosis (FSGS) describes a sclerotic glomerular lesion that affects some (but not all) glomeruli, and some (but not all) segments of each tuft.

- **Primary FSGS** is an unusual primary cause of the nephrotic syndrome.

- **Secondary FSGS** looks similar on light microscopy. Although proteinuria may be heavy, hypoalbuminaemia is *unusual*.

Primary focal segmental glomerulosclerosis

This disease of unknown aetiology usually presents as massive proteinuria (usually non-selective), haematuria, hypertension and renal impairment. The associated nephrotic syndrome is often resistant to steroid therapy. All age groups are affected. It usually recurs in transplanted kidneys, sometimes within days of transplantation, and particularly in patients with aggressive primary renal disease.

Aetiology of primary FSGS

A circulating permeability factor causes the increased protein leak; plasma from patients increases membrane permeability in isolated glomeruli. Kidneys transplanted into murine models of FSGS develop the lesion, but kidneys from FSGS-prone mice transplanted to a normal strain are protected. Removal of this factor by plasmapheresis results in transient amelioration of proteinuria. The identity of the permeability factor remains unknown but recent findings suggest that cardiotrophin-like cytokine 1 is a likely candidate in FSGS. Soluble urokinase-like plasminogen activator receptor (SuPAR) was initially thought to be involved but now appears less likely to be causative, based on recent experimental and clinical evidence.

Pathology

Segmental glomerulosclerosis is seen on light microscopy, which later progresses to global sclerosis. The deep glomeruli at the corticomedullary junction are affected first. These may be missed on transcutaneous biopsy, leading to a mistaken diagnosis of MCN (see p. 1354). A pathogenetic link may exist between MCN and FSGS, as a proportion of cases classified as having the former condition develop progressive CKD, which is unusual. Electron microscopy demonstrates primarily foot process effacement, occasionally in a patchy distribution. The degree of podocyte foot process effacement on electron microscopy can help distinguish between 'primary' and 'secondary' FSGS. If severe foot process effacement is present in normal and sclerosed glomeruli on electron microscopy, primary FSGS is more likely (this is not the case if foot process effacement is largely localized to sclerosed glomeruli alone).

Five histological variants of FSGS exist:

- In **classic FSGS** (**Fig. 36.13A**) the involved glomeruli show sclerotic segments in any location of the glomerulus.

- The **glomerular tip lesion** is characterized by segmental sclerosis, at the tubular pole of all the affected glomeruli at a very early stage (tip FSGS, **Fig. 36.13B**). These patients have a more favourable response to steroids and disease runs a more benign course.

- In **collapsing FSGS** (**Fig. 36.13C**), podocytes are usually enlarged and coarsely vacuolated with wrinkled and collapsed capillary walls. Collapsing FSGS is commonly seen in young black people with HIV infection, and is known as HIV-associated nephropathy (HIVAN; see later).

- The **perihilar variant** (**Fig. 36.13D**) consists of perihilar sclerosis and hyalinosis in more than 50% of segmentally sclerotic glomeruli. It is frequently observed with secondary FSGS.

- The **cellular variant** (**Fig. 36.13E**) is characterized by at least one glomerulus with segmental hypercellularity (proliferation) that occludes the capillary lumen.

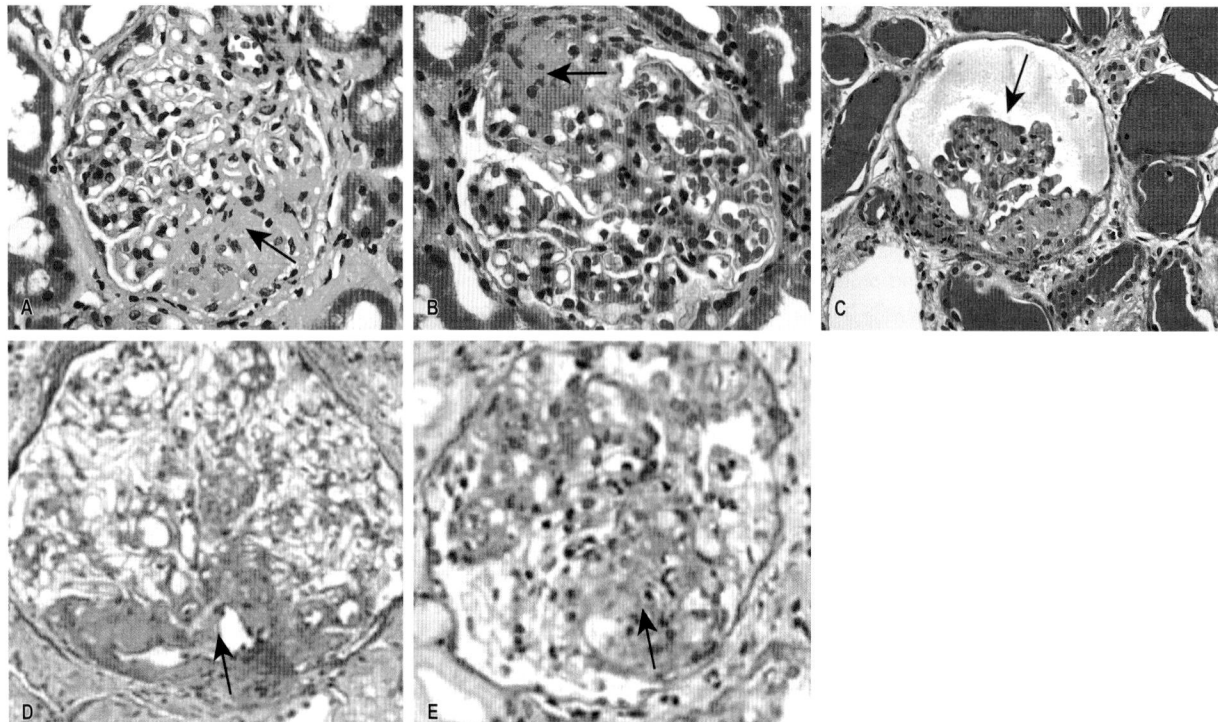

Fig. 36.13 Focal segmental glomerulosclerosis (FSGS). **(A)** Classic FSGS showing sclerotic segments in the glomerulus. **(B)** Glomerular tip lesions showing segmental sclerosis at the pole of the glomerulus. **(C)** Collapsing FSGS. **(D)** FSGS perihilar variant. **(E)** FSGS cellular variant. Arrows show the sclerotic segment in each light micrograph.

Management

- **Prednisolone** 0.5–2 mg/kg per day is used in most patients and continued for 6 months before the patient is considered resistant to therapy, which is common.
- **Ciclosporin or tacrolimus** may be effective in reducing or stopping urinary protein excretion. Relapse after reducing or stopping drug is very common, so that long-term use is required.
- **Cyclophosphamide**, **chlorambucil** or **azathioprine** is used as second-line therapy in adults. In patients with FSGS with mesangial hypercellularity and tip lesion, cyclophosphamide 1–1.5 mg/kg per day with 60 mg of prednisolone for 3–6 months, followed by prednisolone and azathioprine, can be used as maintenance therapy.

About 50% of patients progress to ESKD within 10 years of diagnosis, particularly those who are resistant to therapy. The recurrence of this renal lesion following renal transplantation is very high with a poor renal prognosis. Plasmapheresis or immunoabsorption has been the mainstay of treatment in patients with post-transplant recurrence but has had modest results. Anti-CD80 antibodies (abatacept), used in rheumatology, have been tried with some success in patients with podocyte upregulation of CD80. Adrenocorticotrophic hormone (ACTH) gel applied topically has been used successfully in refractory cases of post-transplant FSGS.

Secondary FSGS

Secondary FSGS with similar glomerular changes is seen as a **secondary phenomenon** when the number of functioning nephrons is reduced for any reason. Here, FSGS represents the common final glomerular lesion seen in response to subsequent haemodynamic glomerular strain. As nephrons fail, increased flow through the remaining nephrons leads to glomerular hypertrophy and hyperfiltration, and hydraulic injury, with the secondary changes of FSGS. It is also described as remnant nephropathy (see p. 1393). Associations include:

- **reduced nephron number** (e.g. nephrectomy, hypertension, gross obesity, ischaemia, sickle nephropathy, reflux nephropathy, chronic allograft nephropathy, IgA nephropathy, and scarring following renal vasculitis)
- **mutations** in specific podocyte genes
- **viruses**, e.g. HIV type 1, erythrovirus B19, cytomegalovirus, Epstein–Barr virus and simian virus 40
- **drugs** such as heroin, all interferons, anabolic steroids, lithium, sirolimus, pamidronate and calcineurin inhibitors, e.g. ciclosporin, which can also cause FSGS
- **APOL1 gene mutations** on chromosome 22 as G1/G2 renal disease variant (acquired to give protection against African trypanosomiasis) in patients of African ancestry, which makes them susceptible to FSGS in response to insults such as hypertension, SLE and HIV.

HIV-associated nephropathy

In HIV-associated nephropathy (HIVAN), glomeruli are characteristically 'collapsed' on light microscopy (see **Fig. 36.13C**); podocytes are enlarged, hyperplastic and coarsely vacuolated, containing protein absorption droplets and overlying capillaries with varying degrees of wrinkling and collapse of the walls. Direct podocyte HIV-1 infection is associated with loss of podocyte-specific markers such as Wilms' tumour factor and synaptopodin in HIVAN. HIVAN presents with nephrotic-range proteinuria, oedema and CKD, which can be rapid in progression. Anti-retroviral therapy

(ART) may reverse the renal lesions, and restores renal function if treatment is commenced early.

Membranous glomerulopathy

Autoimmune membranous glomerulopathy occurs mainly in adults and predominantly in men. It presents with asymptomatic proteinuria or frank nephrotic syndrome. Microscopic haematuria, hypertension and/or renal impairment may accompany the nephrotic syndrome. As in other glomerular disease, hypertension and a greater degree of renal impairment are poor prognostic signs. In membranous glomerulopathy, one-third of patients undergo spontaneous or therapy-related remission. About 40% develop CKD, usually in association with persistent nephrotic-range proteinuria. Younger people, females and those with asymptomatic proteinuria of modest degree at the time of presentation do best.

Pathogenesis

A majority of patients (75%) with idiopathic or autoimmune membranous nephropathy have been found to have immunoglobulin G4 (IgG4)-type autoantibodies against M type phospholipase A_2 receptor (PLA$_2$R), a glycoprotein constituent of normal glomeruli. PLA$_2$R is present in normal human podocytes and in immune deposits in patients with idiopathic membranous nephropathy, indicating that it could be a major autoantigen in this disease; it is linked to human leucocyte antigen (HLA)-DQA1. Antibodies against a novel podocyte antigen, thrombospondin type 1 domain-containing 7A (THSD7A), have been identified in 3% of PLA$_2$R-positive and 10% of PLA$_2$R-negative patients with membranous nephropathy, associated in membranous glomerulopathy with underlying malignancy.

In secondary membranous nephropathy, where no detectable anti-PLA$_2$R or anti-THSD7A antibodies (or glomerular antigen staining) can be found, glomerular histology is identical to that seen in autoimmune disease. Causes include:

- drugs (e.g. penicillamine, gold, NSAIDs, probenecid, mercury, captopril)
- other autoimmune disease (e.g. SLE, thyroiditis)
- infections (e.g. hepatitis B, hepatitis C, schistosomiasis, *Plasmodium malariae*)
- cancers (e.g. carcinoma of the lung, colon, stomach, breast and lymphoma)
- other causes (e.g. sarcoidosis, sickle cell disease).

On light microscopy, capillary loops appear thick. Using a periodic acid–Schiff or silver stain (which highlights basement membrane), 'spikes' of basement membrane are visible. On electron microscopy, small, electron-dense deposits in the subepithelial aspects of the capillary walls are seen, encircled by perpendicular basement membrane spikes. Uniform granular capillary wall deposits of PLA$_2$R antigen and IgG subclasses (IgG4 is predominant in idiopathic membranous nephropathy), as well as complement C3, are seen on immunofluorescence. Late in the disease, deposits are completely surrounded by basement membrane and are undergoing resorption, which appears as uniform thickening of the capillary basement membrane on light microscopy (**Fig. 36.14**).

Management

As many as one-third or more of patients will undergo spontaneous remission if watched for at least 6–12 months, particularly if kidney function is normal, anti-PLA$_2$R antibodies are low in titre and proteinuria is modest. In general, patients with heavier proteinuria,

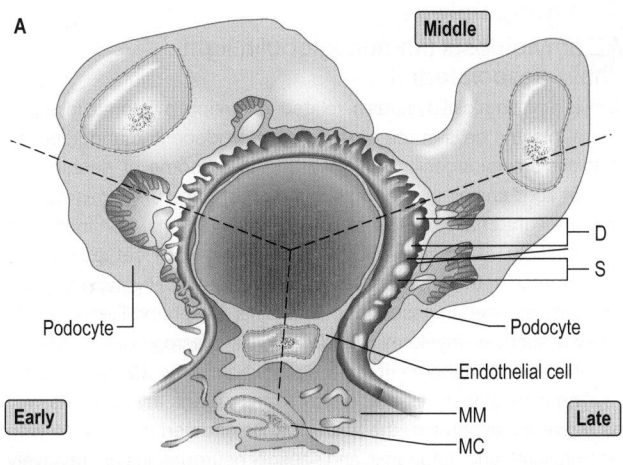

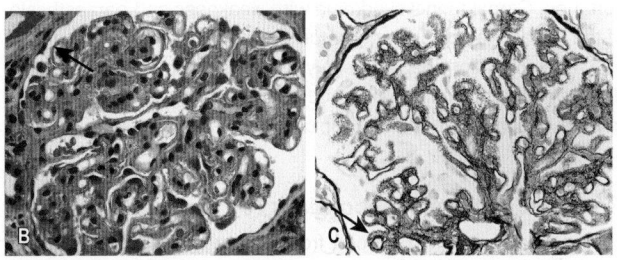

Fig. 36.14 Membranous glomerulopathy. (A) Membranous nephropathy showing the early, middle and late stages. D, subepithelial deposits; MC, mesangial cell; MM, mesangial matrix; S, spikes. **(B)** Light microscopy of membranous nephropathy showing thickened basement membrane (arrowed). **(C)** Silver stain showing spikes (arrowed) in membranous nephropathy. *(A, After Marsh FP.* Postgraduate Nephrology. *Oxford: Butterworth Heinemann; 1985.)*

progressive renal dysfunction and a high titre of anti-PLA$_2$R antibodies are considered for early treatment.

- All patients should receive ACE inhibition at the maximum tolerated dose, anticoagulation, diuretics and a statin if indicated.
- Rituximab, an anti-CD20 antibody (which ablates B lymphocytes), is effective in inducing remission, maintaining or improving renal function, and reducing proteinuria; few significant adverse affects have been shown in the short term.
- The alkylating agents cyclophosphamide (1.5–2.5 mg/kg per day for 6–12 months with 1 mg/kg per day of oral prednisolone on alternate days for the first 2 months) and chlorambucil (0.2 mg/kg per day in months 2, 4 and 6, alternating with oral prednisolone 0.4 mg/kg per day in months 1, 3 and 5) are both effective.
- Ciclosporin or tacrolimus is of use, though relapse is common and treatment courses are longer.
- Oral corticosteroids are of no benefit alone but may be additive.

Amyloidosis

Amyloidosis is a systemic disorder of protein folding, in which normally soluble proteins or fragments are deposited extracellularly as abnormal insoluble fibrils (usually β-pleated sheets that are resistant to proteolysis), causing progressive organ dysfunction and death.

The disease may be acquired or inherited. Classification is based on the nature of the precursor plasma proteins (at least 20) that form the fibrillar deposits. The most common forms are AL amyloidosis (where abnormal protein may be derived from light chains or immunoglobulin) and AA amyloidosis (where deposits form from serum amyloid A protein). The renal consequences are similar, even if systemic features differ.

Pathophysiology

AL amyloidosis (immunoglobulin light chain-associated)

This is a plasma cell dyscrasia, related to multiple myeloma, in which clonal plasma cells in the bone marrow produce immunoglobulins that are amyloidogenic. This may be the outcome of destabilization of light chains owing to substitution of particular amino acids into the light chain variable region. There is a clonal dominance of amyloid light (AL) chains – either the dominant κ or γ isotype – which are excreted in the urine (as Bence Jones protein). This type of amyloid may be seen in association with other lymphoproliferative disorders, such as myeloma, Waldenström's macroglobulinaemia or non-Hodgkin lymphoma. It rarely occurs before the age of 40 years.

The clinical features are related to the organs involved. As well as nephrotic syndrome, the heart may be affected (presenting with heart failure), and autonomic and sensory neuropathies are relatively common. Carpal tunnel syndrome with weakness and paraesthesia of the hands may be an early feature.

On examination, hepatomegaly and, rarely, splenomegaly, cardiomyopathy, polyneuropathy and bruising may be seen. Macroglossia occurs in about 10% of cases and periorbital purpura in 15%.

Reactive systemic (secondary AA) amyloidosis

This is due to amyloid formed from serum amyloid A (SAA), an acute-phase protein that rises in response to inflammatory stimuli in a similar way to C-reactive protein (CRP). It is, therefore, related to chronic inflammatory disorders and chronic infection.

Clinical features depend on the nature of the underlying disorder. Chronic inflammatory disorders include rheumatoid arthritis, inflammatory bowel disease and untreated familial Mediterranean fever. In developing countries, it is still associated with infectious diseases such as tuberculosis, bronchiectasis and osteomyelitis. In higher-income countries, it is often seen in injecting drug users, who may have chronic skin abscesses and sinus formation related to injection sites. AA amyloidosis often presents with nephrotic syndrome, CKD, hepatomegaly and splenomegaly. Macroglossia is not a feature and cardiac involvement is rare.

Familial amyloidoses

These are autosomally dominant transmitted diseases where the mutant protein forms amyloid fibrils, starting usually in middle age. The most common form is due to a mutant transthyretin, leading to transthyretin-associated amyloidosis (ATTR). Transthyretin is a tetrameric protein with four identical subunits, which functions as a transport protein for thyroxine and retinol-binding protein, and is mainly synthesized in the liver. Over 80 amino acid substitutions have been described; for example, a common substitution is that of methionine for valine at position 30 (Met 30) in all racial groups, and alanine for threonine (Ala 60) in the English and Irish. These substitutions destabilize the protein, which precipitates following stimulation, and can cause nephrotic syndrome, although more commonly other problems, including polyneuropathy or cardiomyopathy, predominate.

Clinically, peripheral sensorimotor and autonomic neuropathy is common, with symptoms of autonomic dysfunction, diarrhoea and weight loss. Renal disease is less prevalent than with AL amyloidosis. Macroglossia does not occur. Cardiac problems are usually those of conduction. There may be a family history of unidentified neurological disease.

Other hereditary systemic amyloidoses include various familial amyloid polyneuropathies (e.g. Portuguese, Icelandic, Dutch). The

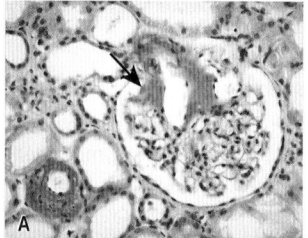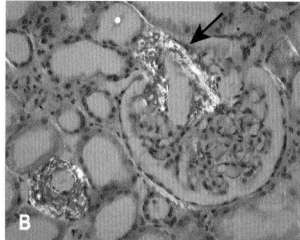

Fig. 36.15 Amyloid. **(A)** Light microscopy of eosinophilic amyloid deposits (arrowed). **(B)** Congo red stain under polarized light showing apple green refringence.

brain is a common site of amyloid deposition (see p. 881), although it is not directly affected in any form of acquired systemic amyloidosis. Intracerebral and cerebrovascular amyloid deposits are seen in Alzheimer's disease.

Diagnosis

The diagnosis can often be made clinically when features of amyloidosis are present elsewhere. On imaging, the kidneys are often large. Scintigraphy with radiolabelled serum amyloid P (SAP), a technique for quantitatively imaging amyloid deposits *in vivo*, is used to detect the rate of regression or progression of amyloidosis over a period of time.

Renal biopsy is necessary in all suspected cases of renal involvement. Widespread eosinophilic deposits are seen in the mesangium, capillary loops and arteriolar walls. Deposits stain pink, with green bi-refringence under polarized light with Congo red (**Fig. 36.15**). On electron microscopy the characteristic fibrils of amyloid can be seen. Amyloid consisting of immunoglobulin light chains (AL amyloid) can be identified by immunohistochemistry in only 40% of cases, as compared to almost 100% of patients with protein found in secondary amyloid (AA amyloid). If the primary presentation of amyloidosis is with non-renal disease, or if renal histology cannot be obtained, amyloid deposits can be seen in tissues obtained from the rectum, gums, abdominal fat or myocardium.

A paraproteinaemia and light chains in the urine may be seen in AL amyloidosis, along with a possible increase in plasma cells on bone marrow biopsy. In secondary or reactive amyloidosis, there will be an underlying inflammatory disorder. Genetic testing for inherited amyloidosis should be undertaken where there is a relevant family history.

Management

Treatments that reduce production of the amyloidogenic protein can improve organ function and survival:

- Myeloma-directed therapy (such as bortezemib or rituximab) is used to treat AL amyloidosis, with or without stem cell transplantation.
- In AA amyloidosis, production of serum amyloid A can sometimes be decreased by treatment of the underlying inflammatory condition but cannot be completely suppressed. Colchicine may help in familial Mediterranean fever.
- In ATTR amyloidosis, where transthyretin is predominantly synthesized in the liver, liver transplantation (causing a complete disappearance of the mutant protein from the blood) is considered as the definitive therapy.

Renoprotective measures should be started (see **Box 36.12**), as should relevant treatment started for nephrotic syndrome and heart failure. As renal failure progresses, the success of dialysis and

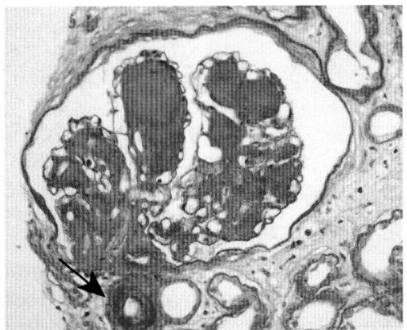

Fig. 36.16 Diabetes mellitus. Advanced diabetic glomerulopathy and arteriolar sclerosis (arrowed).

kidney transplantation depends on the extent of amyloid deposition in extrarenal sites, especially the heart.

Diabetic nephropathy

Diabetic renal disease is the leading cause of ESKD in the Western world, arising largely as a complication of type 2 diabetes mellitus. Diabetic kidney disease occurs in about 20–30% of both type 1 and type 2 diabetics (see p. 729); the natural history is similar from the onset of proteinuria, and the histological lesion is the same. Risk factors for nephropathy include poor glycaemic control, hypertension, male gender, ethnicity and social deprivation.

Pathology

Pathophysiology is fully discussed on page 730. Glomerular hyperfiltration (the GFR increases to >150 mL/min per m^2) and initial enlargement of kidney volume occur as local vasoactive factors increase flow. The GBM thickens and the mesangium expands. Progressive depletion of podocytes (see p. 1352) from the filtration barrier (through apoptosis or detachment) results in podocyturia early in the disease. Proteinuria evolves as filtration pressures rise and the filter is compromised. Later, glomerulosclerosis develops with nodules (Kimmelstiel–Wilson lesion) and hyaline deposits in the glomerular arterioles (**Fig. 36.16**). Mesangial expansion and hyalinosis are partly due to amylin (β-islet-specific amyloid protein) deposits, with increasing proteinuria.

The Renal Pathology Society has developed a consensus classification combining type 1 and type 2 diabetic nephropathies (**Box 36.11**). This discriminates lesions by various degrees of severity for use in international clinical practice.

Management

Lifestyle changes (cessation of smoking, attention to salt intake, weight loss and increased exercise) are necessary to prevent progression of any diabetic complication.

- *Aim for good (intensive) glycaemic control.* If achieved for even a limited period, this reduces the incidence of ESKD and other microvascular complications in the long term (the so-called 'legacy' effect' in both type 1 and type 2 diabetes mellitus). SGLT2 inhibitors (dapagliflozin, canagliflozin and empagliflozin) and glucagon-like peptide-1 (GLP-1) agonists such as liraglutide, semaglutide and dulaglutide (safe in renal impairment) have been shown to have specific cardiac (particularly heart failure) and renoprotective effects, in addition to controlling blood glucose.
- *Control dyslipidaemia.*
- *Control blood pressure* to <130/80 mmHg with ACE inhibitors or AII-RAs; these should be used once microalbuminuria develops, even if blood pressure control is good.

i **Box 36.11** Renal Pathology Society classification of types 1 and 2 diabetic nephropathy

Class	Name
I	Isolated glomerular basement membrane thickening (>395 nm in females, >430 nm in males). No evidence of mesangial expansion, mesangial matrix increase, or global glomerulosclerosis involving >50% of glomeruli
IIa	Mild mesangial expansion
IIb	Severe mesangial expansion (in a severe lesion, >25% of the total mesangium contains areas of expansion larger than the mean area of a capillary lumen)
III	Nodular intercapillary glomerulosclerosis (≥1 Kimmelstiel–Wilson lesion(s)) and <50% global glomerulosclerosis
IV	Advanced diabetic glomerulosclerosis and >50% global glomerulosclerosis

i **Box 36.12** Renoprotection

Goals of treatment
- Blood pressure <130/80 mmHg
- Proteinuria <0.3 g/24 h

Treatment measures
Patients with chronic kidney disease and proteinuria >1 g/24 h:
- Angiotensin-converting enzyme inhibitor increasing to maximum dose
  - Angiotensin receptor antagonist if goals are not achieved[a]
- Addition of diuretic to prevent hyperkalaemia and help to control blood pressure
  - Addition of calcium-channel blocker (verapamil or diltiazem) if goals are not achieved

Additional management
- Statins to lower cholesterol to <4.5 mmol/L
- Smoking cessation (threefold higher rate of deterioration in chronic kidney disease)
- Treatment of diabetes (HbA$_{1c}$ <7%, 53 mmol/mol)
- Normal protein diet (0.8–1 g/kg body weight)

[a]In type 2 diabetes start with angiotensin receptor antagonist.

As in other kidney diseases, however, nearly the entire course of renal injury in diabetes is clinically silent. The aim of medical intervention during this silent phase is to slow GFR decline over time (**Box 36.12**). Despite intensified metabolic and blood pressure control, many still go on to develop ESKD.

Other interventions with a less robust evidence base include:

- *Pentoxyphylline* (previously used for peripheral vascular disease) slows the rate of GFR decline and proteinuria (by putatively reducing the production of tumour necrosis factor-alpha, TNF-α). This interesting observation requires external validation.
- *Atrasentan* (a selective endothelin A receptor (ET$_A$R) antagonist combined with renin–angiotensin system inhibitors) is similarly generally safe and effective in reducing residual albuminuria. This could ultimately translate into improved renal outcomes in patients with type 2 diabetic nephropathy but this needs confirmation in long-term follow-up studies.

Isolated proteinuria without haematuria

In asymptomatic patients this is often an incidental finding. It is usually found below 1 g/day with normal renal function. Over 50% of these patients have (benign) postural proteinuria, although it may be an early sign of a serious glomerular lesion such as membranous glomerulopathy, IgA nephropathy, FSGS, diabetic nephropathy or amyloidosis (see earlier). Mild and transient proteinuria may also accompany a febrile illness, congestive heart failure or infectious diseases with no clinical renal significance.

Glomerulonephritis (asymptomatic, acute and rapidly progressive)

Glomerulonephritis (GN) is immunologically mediated, with involvement of cellular immunity (T lymphocytes, macrophages/dendritic cells), humoral immunity (antibodies, immune complexes, complement) and other inflammatory mediators (including cytokines, chemokines and the coagulation cascade). The immune response can be directed against known target antigens, particularly when GN complicates infections, cancers or drugs. The underlying antigenic target is more often unknown. Primary GN may occur in genetically susceptible individuals (usually determined by major histocompatibility complex (MHC) genes like *HLA-A1*, *B8*, *DR2* and *DR3*), following environmental insults. Circulating autoantibodies and/or abnormalities in serum complement, and glomerular deposition of antibodies, immune complexes, complement and fibrin characterize the condition. GN may present as:

- asymptomatic urinary abnormalities
- acute nephritis (nephritic syndrome)
- rapidly progressive glomerulonephritis.

The same underlying histology may often present in any of these ways, and these should be seen as clinical syndromes on a spectrum rather than as distinct diseases.

Asymptomatic urinary abnormalities

Haematuria with or without sub-nephrotic-range proteinuria in an asymptomatic patient may lead to the early discovery of potentially serious glomerular disease such as SLE, Henoch–Schönlein purpura, post-infectious GN or idiopathic hypercalciuria in children. Asymptomatic haematuria is also the primary presenting manifestation of a number of specific glomerular diseases discussed below.

Acute nephritis (nephritic syndrome)

This classically presents as:

- haematuria (macroscopic or microscopic) – with red-cell casts on urine microscopy
- proteinuria
- hypertension
- oedema (periorbital, leg or sacral)
- temporary oliguria and uraemia.

Nephritis can present indolently or incidentally, and is usually distinguished from rapidly progressive glomerulonephritis by the lack of cellular necrosis (and crescent formation) in the glomeruli seen on biopsy, and the rate at which renal decline evolves. These syndromes should be seen as a continuum.

Rapidly progressive glomerulonephritis

Rapidly progressive glomerulonephritis (RPGN) is a syndrome with glomerular haematuria (red blood cell casts or dysmorphic red blood cells), rapidly developing acute kidney failure over weeks to months and focal glomerular necrosis (**Fig. 36.17**) with or without glomerular crescent development on renal biopsy. The 'crescent' is an aggregate of macrophages and epithelial cells in Bowman's space. RPGN can develop with immune deposits (anti-GBM or immune complex

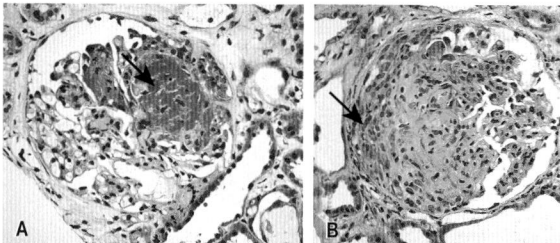

Fig. 36.17 Rapidly progressive glomerulonephritis (RPGN). Arrows show 'crescents' with aggregates of macrophages and epithelial cells in Bowman's space. **(A)** Focal necrotizing glomerulonephritis. **(B)** Crescentic glomerulonephritis.

> ***i*** **Box 36.13 Types of rapidly progressive glomerulonephritis (RPGN)**
>
> **Linear immunofluorescent pattern (see Fig. 36.20A)**
> - Idiopathic anti-GBM antibody-mediated RPGN
> - Goodpasture's syndrome
>
> **Granular immunofluorescent pattern (immune complex-mediated RPGN; see Fig. 36.20B)**
> - Idiopathic immune complex-mediated RPGN
> - Associated with other primary GN:
>   – Mesangiocapillary GN (type II > type I)
>   – IgA nephropathy
>   – Membranous glomerulopathy
> - Associated with secondary GN:
>   – Post-infectious GN
>   – Systemic lupus erythematosus
>   – Henoch–Schönlein syndrome
>   – Cryoglobulinaemia
>
> **Negative immunofluorescent pattern (pauci-immune RPGN)**
> - ANCA-associated systemic vasculitides
>
> ANCA, anti-neutrophil cytoplasmic antibody; GBM, glomerular basement membrane; IgA, immunoglobulin A.

---

type, e.g. SLE) or without immune deposits (pauci-immune, e.g. anti-proteinase 3 (PR3) and or anti-myeloperoxidase–antineutrophil cytoplasmic antibodies (MPO-ANCA)-positive vasculitides). It can also develop as an idiopathic primary glomerular disease, or can be superimposed on secondary glomerular diseases such as IgA nephropathy, membranous GN and post-infective GN. It can be classified based on the pattern of immune complex deposition in glomeruli (seen on immunofluorescence): that is, linear, granular and negative immunofluorescent patterns (**Box 36.13**).

Post-streptococcal glomerulonephritis

Post-streptococcal glomerulonephritis (PSGN) occurs in childhood. An acute nephritis follows 1–3 weeks after a streptococcal infection. Streptococcal throat infection, otitis media or cellulitis can all be responsible. The infecting organism is a Lancefield group A β-haemolytic streptococcus of a nephritogenic type. The latent interval between infection and the development of symptoms and signs of renal involvement reflects the time taken for immune complex formation and deposition and glomerular injury to occur. PSGN is now rare in developed countries. Renal biopsy shows diffuse, florid, acute inflammation in the glomerulus (without necrosis but occasionally with cellular crescents), with neutrophils and deposition of IgG and complement (**Fig. 36.18**). Similar biopsy findings may be seen in ***non-streptococcal post-infectious glomerulonephritis*** (**Box 36.14**).

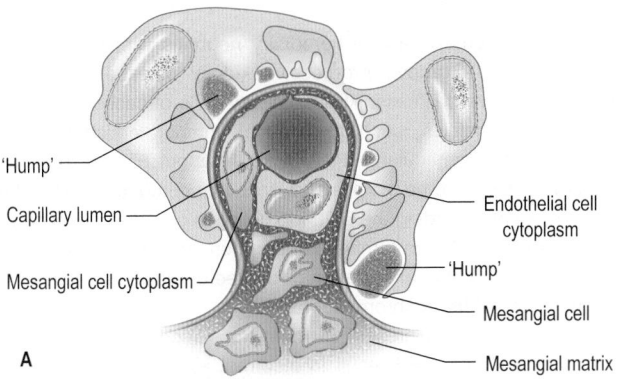

'Hump'

Capillary lumen

Mesangial cell cytoplasm

Endothelial cell cytoplasm

'Hump'

Mesangial cell

Mesangial matrix

A

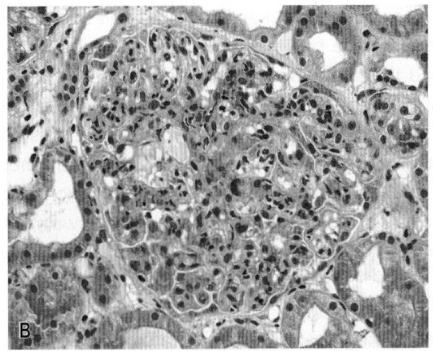

B

Fig. 36.18 Post-streptococcal glomerulonephritis. **(A)** Large aggregates of immune material ('humps') in the extracapillary area. There is an increase in mesangial matrix and mesangial cells, with occlusion of the capillary lumen by endothelial cell cytoplasm, leucocytes and mesangial cell cytoplasm. **(B)** Light microscopy showing acute inflammation of the glomerulus with neutrophils. *(After Marsh FP. Postgraduate Nephrology. Oxford: Butterworth Heinemann; 1985.)*

Management

Aim for good blood pressure control, diuretics and salt restriction for oedema, and dialysis as necessary. If recovery is slow, corticosteroids may be helpful. The prognosis is usually good in children. A small number of adults develop hypertension and/or CKD later in life. Therefore, in older patients, an annual blood pressure check and measurement of serum creatinine are required. Evidence in support of long-term penicillin prophylaxis after the development of GN is lacking. In non-streptococcal post-infectious GN, prognosis is equally good if the underlying infection is eradicated.

Glomerulonephritis with infective endocarditis

GN occurs rarely in patients with infective endocarditis or infected ventriculoperitoneal shunts (**shunt nephritis**). Histological appearances resemble those of post-infectious GN but lesions are usually focal and segmental. Crescentic GN with AKI has been described, particularly with *Staphylococcus aureus* infection. Appropriate antibiotic therapy or surgical eradication of infection in fulminant cases usually results in a return of normal renal function.

GN also occurs in association with **visceral abscesses** (mainly pulmonary) and is indistinguishable from post-infectious GN. Complement levels are normal and immune deposits are absent on biopsy. Antibiotic therapy and surgical drainage of the abscess result in complete recovery of renal function in approximately 50% of patients.

Box 36.14 Diseases commonly associated with the acute nephritic syndrome

- Post-streptococcal glomerulo-nephritis
- Non-streptococcal post-infectious glomerulonephritis, e.g. *Staphylococcus*, pneumo-coccus, *Legionella*, syphilis, mumps, varicella, hepatitis B and C, echovirus, Epstein–Barr virus, toxoplasmosis, malaria, schistosomiasis, trichinosis
- Infective endocarditis
- Shunt nephritis
- Visceral abscess
- Systemic lupus erythematosus (see p. 457)
- Henoch–Schönlein syndrome (see p. 1367)
- Cryoglobulinaemia (see p. 1368)

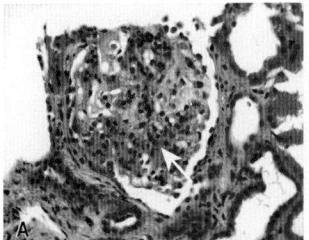

A

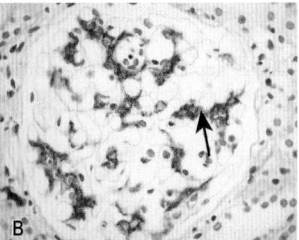

B

Fig. 36.19 IgA nephropathy. **(A)** Light microscopy showing mesangial cell proliferation (arrowed) and increased matrix. **(B)** IgA deposits (arrowed) on immunoperoxidase staining.

IgA nephropathy

IgA nephropathy (**Fig. 36.19**) has replaced PSGN as the most common form of GN worldwide. Demographic and family studies support the existence of a genetic contribution to the pathogenesis of IgA nephropathy but results from genetic association studies of candidate genes are inconsistent. A genome-wide analysis study conducted in European patients showed a strong association on chromosome 6p in the region of the MHC/DQ and HLA-B loci.

Histology

There is a focal and segmental proliferative GN with mesangial deposits of polymeric IgA1. In some cases, IgG, IgM and C3 are also seen in the glomerular mesangium. Superimposed crescent formation is frequent, particularly following macroscopic haematuria associated with upper respiratory tract infection.

An Oxford histological classification for IgA nephropathy is shown in **Box 36.15**. The features have prognostic significance and should be taken into account for predicting outcome independent of the clinical features, both at the time of presentation and during follow-up.

Pathogenesis

The disease may be a result of a number of events, including:

- exaggerated bone marrow and tonsillar IgA1 immune response to viral or other antigens
- an abnormality in O-linked galactosylation in the hinge region of the IgA1 molecule
- functional abnormalities of two IgA receptors: CD89 expressed on blood myeloid cells and the transferring receptor (CD71) on mesangial cells
- circulating immune complexes composed of a glycan-specific IgG and a galactose-deficient IgA1 antibody.

IgA-rich immune complexes deposited in the glomerular mesangium induce mesangial cell activation and proliferation, and matrix synthesis and deposition. Removal of these complexes by bacterial proteases attenuates injury, and it is thought that glycan-specific

Histological variable	Description	Class
Mesangial hypercellularity	Average mesangial hypercellularity[a] >0.5	M1
	Average mesangial hypercellularity <0.5	M0
Segmental glomerulosclerosis	Part of glomerular tuft involved in sclerosis	S1
	No segmental glomerulosclerosis	S0
Endocapillary hypercellularity	Hypercellularity present and results in luminal narrowing	E1
	No hypercellularity	E0
Tubular atrophy/ interstitial fibrosis	Percentage of cortical area involved:	
	>50	T2
	26–50	T1
	0–25	T0

[a]Mesangial hypercellularity is scored 0 for glomeruli with <4 mesangial cells per mesangial area; 1 for those with 4–5 cells; 2 for 6–7 cells; and 3 for ≥8 cells. Scores obtained for all glomeruli are then averaged.

autoantibodies, rather than IgA1 itself, play a key role in the pathogenesis. Up to 50% of patients exhibit elevated serum IgA (polyclonal). Several diseases are associated with IgA deposits, including Henoch–Schönlein purpura, chronic liver disease, malignancies (especially carcinoma of bronchus), seronegative spondyloarthritis, coeliac disease, mycosis fungoides and psoriasis.

Clinical features

IgA nephropathy tends to occur in children and young males, presenting with asymptomatic microscopic haematuria or recurrent macroscopic haematuria following an upper respiratory or gastrointestinal viral infection. Proteinuria occurs and 5% of cases can be nephrotic. The prognosis is usually good, especially in those with normal blood pressure, normal renal function and absence of proteinuria at presentation. Surprisingly, recurrent macroscopic haematuria is a good prognostic sign, although this may be due to 'lead-time bias' (see p. 102), as patients with overt haematuria come to medical attention at an earlier stage of their illness. The risk of eventual development of ESKD is about 25% in those with proteinuria of more than 1 g per day, elevated serum creatinine, hypertension, *ACE* gene polymorphism (DD isoform) and tubulointerstitial fibrosis on renal biopsy.

Management

All patients, with or without hypertension and proteinuria, should receive an ACE inhibitor or an AII-RA, to reduce proteinuria and preserve renal function.
- Patients with proteinuria of >1–3 g/day, mild glomerular changes and normal renal function may be treated with steroids, aiming to reduce proteinuria and stabilize function.
- In patients with higher-risk progressive disease with proteinuria of >750 mg/day and eGFR falling to <60 mL/min, prednisolone alone or with cyclophosphamide for 3 months, followed by maintenance with prednisolone, has failed to demonstrate any benefit.
- Tonsillectomy can reduce proteinuria and haematuria in those with recurrent tonsillitis.

Alport's syndrome

Alport's syndrome is a rare hereditary nephritis with haematuria, proteinuria (<1–2 g/day), progressive kidney disease and high-frequency nerve deafness. Approximately 15% of cases may have ocular abnormalities, such as bilateral anterior lenticonus, and macular and perimacular retinal flecks. In about 85% of patients with Alport's syndrome there is an X-linked inherited mutation in the *COL4α5* gene encoding the COL4α5 collagen chain, a critical component of the GBM. In female carriers, penetrance is variable and depends on the type of mutation or degree of mosaicism following hybridization of the X chromosome.

These mutations present as post-translational defects in α3, α4 and α5 chains, and result in incorrect assembly or folding of monomers; defective monomers are rapidly degraded. Over time the basement membrane undergoes selective proteolysis, and glomerular membranes thicken unevenly, split and ultimately deteriorate. Although the basement membrane is abnormal, podocyte function and the slit diaphragm are unaffected, and so proteinuria in Alport's syndrome is often mild and is the result of glomerular sclerosis, rather than primary loss of slit pores. In some patients with Alport's syndrome and carriers, a thin basement membrane, as seen in benign familial haematuria, is the only abnormality detected on histology. For this reason the boundary between Alport's and benign familial haematuria has become increasingly vague.

Management

The disease is progressive and accounts for some 5% of cases of ESKD in childhood or adolescence. Patients with mild CKD can be treated with ACE inhibitors to attenuate proteinuria. Exciting experimental evidence suggests that mesenchymal stem cells can transdifferentiate into podocytes, repair basement abnormalities and slow the rate of progression.

Thin GBM disease

This condition is inherited in autosomal dominant fashion and typically presents with persistent microscopic glomerular haematuria (red blood cell casts or dysmorphic red blood cells). The diagnosis is made on renal biopsy, which shows thinning of the glomerular capillary basement membrane on electron microscopy. The condition was under-diagnosed and is much more common than previously believed. The prognosis for renal function is usually very good but some patients develop renal insufficiency over decades. No treatment is of known benefit.

Anti-GBM glomerulonephritis

Anti-GBM glomerulonephritis (**Fig. 36.20A**), characterized by linear capillary loop staining with IgG and C3 and extensive crescent formation, accounts for 15–20% of all cases of RPGN, although overall represents less than 5% of all forms of GN. This condition is rare, with an incidence of 1 per 2 million in the general population. About two-thirds of these patients have *Goodpasture's syndrome* with associated lung haemorrhage (see p. 992). The remainder have a renal restricted anti-GBM RPGN, which is seen in patients over 50 years and affects both genders equally.

Anti-GBM antibodies (detected by enzyme-linked immunosorbent assay, or ELISA) are present in serum and are directed against the *non-collagenous (NCI) component* of α3 (IV) collagen of the basement membrane. Anti-GBM GN never occurs in patients with Alport's syndrome; although it can develop after patients with Alport's receive a kidney transplant, anti-GBM alloantibodies evolve in response to the 'foreign' α3, α4, α5 (IV) collagen network absent in a patient's own kidneys.

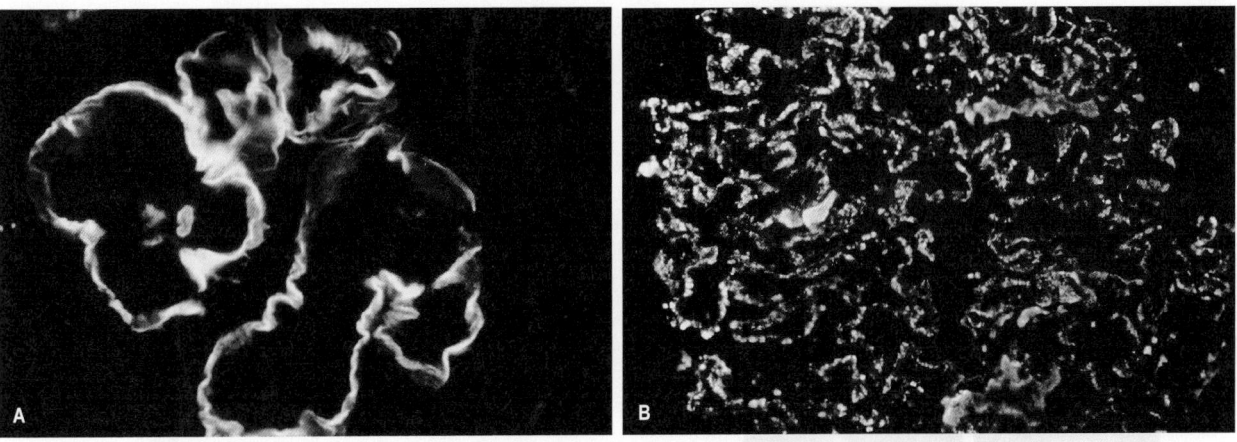

Fig. 36.20 Immunofluorescence. **(A)** Anti-glomerular basement membrane antibody (anti-GBM) deposition in a linear pattern typical of Goodpasture's syndrome. **(B)** Immune complex deposition in a diffuse granular pattern.

The thymus expresses α3 (IV) NCI peptides that eliminate autoreactive CD4+ helper T cells, but a few such cells escape deletion and are kept in check by circulating regulatory (Treg) cells. Breakdown of this peripheral tolerance (the mechanism of which is unknown) results in autoreactive CD4+ cells producing anti-GBM antibodies. These antibodies are very specific: antibodies against α1, α2 and α3 NCI domains do not cause RPGN. Since the α3 (IV) NCI epitope is hidden within the α3, α4 and α5 (IV) promoter, it is presumed that an environmental factor, such as exposure to hydrocarbons or tobacco smoke, is required in order to reveal cryptic epitopes to the immune system.

The mechanism of renal injury is complex. When anti-GBM antibody binds basement membrane, it activates complement and proteases, and results in disruption of the filtration barrier and Bowman's capsule, causing proteinuria and the formation of crescents. Crescent formation is facilitated by IL-12 and interferon-gamma, which are produced by resident and infiltrating inflammatory cells.

Management involves:
- *plasma exchange* to remove circulating anti-GBM antibodies
- *steroids* to suppress inflammation from antibody already deposited in the tissue
- *cyclophosphamide* to suppress further antibody synthesis.

The *prognosis* is directly related to the extent of glomerular damage (measured by percentage of glomeruli containing crescents, serum creatinine and need for dialysis) at the initiation of treatment. When oliguria occurs or serum creatinine rises above 600–700 ′mol/L, renal failure is usually irreversible. Once the active disease is treated, this condition, unlike other autoimmune diseases, does not follow a remitting/relapsing course. If left untreated, autoantibodies diminish spontaneously within 3 years and autoreactive T cells cannot be detected in convalescent patients. This is suggestive of re-establishment of peripheral tolerance, which coincides with re-emergence of regulatory CD25+ cells in the peripheral blood; these play a key role in inhibiting the autoimmune response. The emergence and persistence of these regulatory cells may underlie the 'single hit' nature of this condition.

ANCA-positive small-vessel vasculitis

(See also p. 464.) Inflammation and necrosis of the blood vessel wall occurs in many primary vasculitic disorders. The small-vessel vasculitides affecting the kidney include:
- granulomatosis with polyangiitis (GPA)
- microscopic polyangiitis (MPA)

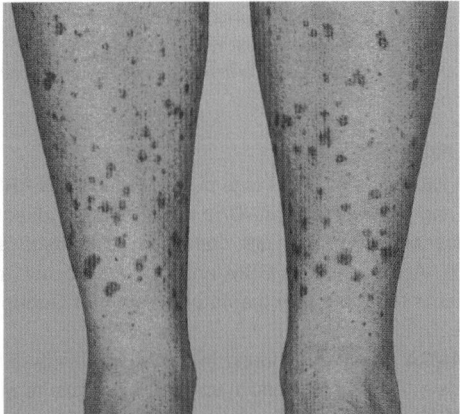

Fig. 36.21 Vasculitic rash.

- renal-limited vasculitis (without systemic features)
- eosinophilic granulomatosis with polyangiitis (which is frequently ANCA-negative).

The ANCA-associated small-vessel vasculitides are GPA, MPA and renal-limited vasculitis. GPA and MPA share a common pathology with focal necrotizing lesions, which affect many different vessels and organs:
- in the lungs, a capillaritis may cause lung haemorrhage
- within the glomerulus of the kidney, crescentic GN and/or focal necrotizing lesions may cause AKI (see **Fig. 36.17**)
- in the dermis, there may be a purpuric rash or vasculitic (**Fig. 36.21**) ulceration.

Renal histology is regarded as a 'gold standard' for diagnosis and prognostication of ANCA-associated GN. A consensus group proposed a new classification around four general categories of lesions:
- *focal* (≥50% normal glomeruli not affected by the disease process)
- *crescentic* (≥50% of glomeruli with cellular crescents)
- *mixed* (a heterogeneous glomerular phenotype in which no glomerular feature predominates)
- *sclerotic* (≥50% of glomeruli with global sclerosis).

This system has been shown to have a prognostic value for 1- and 5-year renal outcomes and may guide therapy.

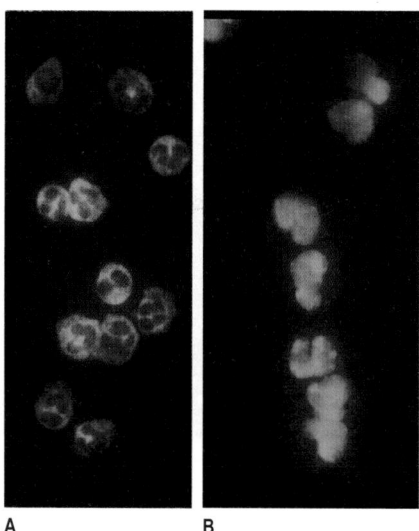

Fig. 36.22 Antineutrophil cytoplasmic antibody (ANCA)-positive glomerulonephritis: immunofluorescence. (A) Cytoplasmic ANCA (cANCA). (B) Perinuclear ANCA (pANCA). *(From Schrier RW. The Schrier Atlas of Diseases of the Kidney, Vol. IV: Systemic Diseases and the Kidney. 1999; Wiley–Blackwell, with permission.)*

Pathogenesis

There are two forms of ANCA (see p. 416; **Fig. 36.22**): PR3-ANCA (cANCA) and MPO-ANCA (pANCA). If ELISA and indirect immunofluorescence techniques are combined, diagnostic specificity is 99%. ANCA and anti-GBM antibodies do occur together; such patients tend to follow the natural history of Goodpasture's syndrome.

- **PR3-ANCA positivity** is found in the large majority (>90%) of patients with active GPA and in up to 50% of patients with MPA.
- **Anti-MPO positivity** is present in the majority of patients with renal-limited vasculitis and in a variable number of cases of MPA. There is some evidence to suggest that ANCAs are pathogenic and not just markers of disease; for example, development of drug-induced ANCA is associated with vasculitic lesions in humans. Eosinophilic GPA may have either anti-MPO or anti-PR3 ANCA.
- **Positivity for both types of ANCA** antibodies occurs in up to 10% of patients, who have a variable clinical course but a worse renal outcome.
- **Drugs** (e.g. propylthiouracil, hydralazine, minocycline, penicillamine) may induce vasculitis associated (most commonly) with MPO-ANCA, often in very high titres. Cases of drug-induced ANCA-associated vasculitis present with constitutional symptoms, arthralgia and cutaneous vasculitis. Crescentic GN and lung haemorrhage also occur.

Both ANCA autoantigens are present in immature neutrophil granules. In contrast to the normally silenced state of these two genes in mature neutrophils of healthy subjects, *PR3* and *MPO* are aberrantly expressed in mature neutrophils of patients with ANCA vasculitis due to unsilencing of both antigens because of epigenetic modifications.

- It is unclear how and why **autoimmunity** causes the formation of ANCA antibodies. Patients with anti-PR3 have autoantibodies to a peptide translated from the antisense DNA strand of PR3 (complementary PR3; cPR3). This suggests that autoimmunity is initiated via a response against a peptide that is antisense or complementary to the autoantigen, which then induces anti-

idiotypic antibodies (autoantibodies) that cross-react with the autoantigen.
- Infection by fimbriated bacteria (Gram-negative pathogens such as *Escherichia coli*, *Klebsiella pneumoniae* and *Proteus mirabilis*) can, through molecular mimicry, trigger cross-reactive autoimmunity to lysosomal membrane protein 2 (LAMP-2), a membrane protein co-localized with PR3 and MPO in the intracellular vesicles of neutrophils.

Management

The sooner treatment is instituted, the greater chance there is of recovery of renal function.

- **High-dose oral corticosteroids** and **intravenous pulsed cyclophosphamide** are of benefit in inducing remission. The best indicators of adverse prognosis are pulmonary haemorrhage and severity of renal failure at presentation.
- **Rituximab** is equally effective in inducing remission in ANCA-associated vasculitides in the short term (6–12 months), with similar adverse event rates. Rituximab may be a therapeutic option in patients who cannot tolerate cyclophosphamide, and in those whose disease is poorly controlled and who relapse while on cyclophosphamide.

Fulminant disease requires intensification of immunosuppression with adjuvant plasma exchange or intravenous pulsed methylprednisolone (1 g/day for 3 consecutive days). In the PEXIVAS study of more than 700 patients with severe ANCA-positive RPGN, with or without lung haemorrhage, the addition of plasma exchange neither saved lives nor avoided ESKD. This study also demonstrated that lower-dose oral glucocorticoids than conventionally used significantly reduced serious infection rates without less effective disease control.

- Once remission has been achieved, azathioprine can be substituted for cyclophosphamide, which was more effective than mycophenolate in a head-to-head comparison trial. Use of rituximab every 3 months in fixed dose has been shown to be superior to azathioprine in the maintenance of remission.
- Colonization of the upper respiratory tract with *Staph. aureus* increases the risk of relapse, and treatment with sulfamethoxazole/trimethoprim reduces the relapse rate.
- Relapse after complete withdrawal of immunosuppression occurs relatively frequently, and long-term, relatively low-dose immunosuppression may be necessary.
- Up to 25% of patients with PR3-ANCA harbour antibodies against human plasminogen and/or tissue plasminogen activator. Their presence has been correlated with venous thromboembolic events and fibrinoid necrotic glomerular lesions, suggesting functional interference with fibrinolysis. However, a formal role for anticoagulation in patients with ANCA-associated GN remains uncertain.

Mixed nephritic and nephrotic syndrome

Injury involves mesangial cells, endothelium, the basement membrane and podocytes in this heterogeneous group of conditions.

Mesangiocapillary (membranoproliferative) glomerulonephritis

Mesangiocapillary (membranoproliferative) glomerulonephritis (MCGN) is an uncommon descriptive lesion that has three subtypes with similar clinical presentations: nephrotic syndrome, haematuria, hypertension and renal impairment. They also produce similar

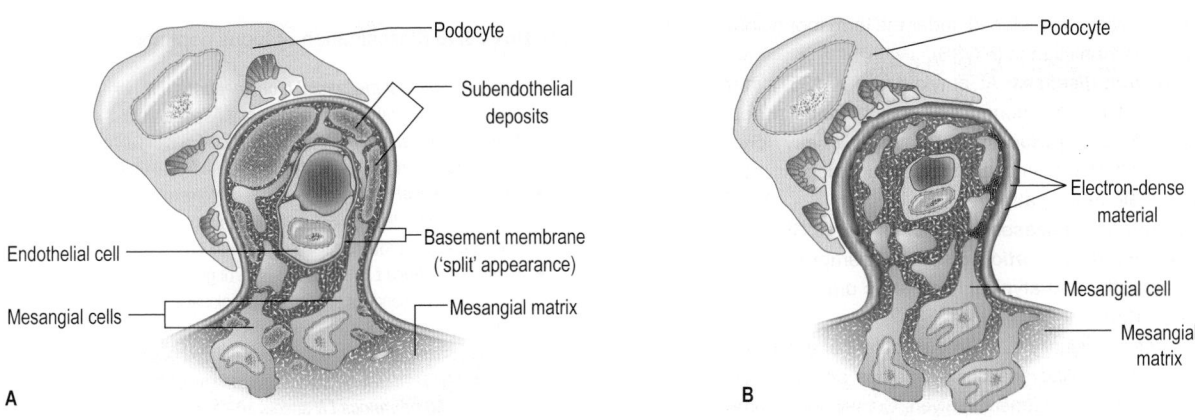

Fig. 36.23 Mesangiocapillary glomerulonephritis (MCGN). **(A)** Type 1 MCGN showing expanded mesangial matrix and mesangial cells, thickened capillary wall, large subendothelial deposits and formation of a new layer of basement membrane (tramline effect). **(B)** Type 2 MCGN showing a variable glomerular appearance; very electron-dense material has replaced Bowman's capsule, tubular basement membrane and part of the capillary. There is some proliferation of mesangial cells. *(After Marsh FP. Postgraduate Nephrology. Oxford: Butterworth–Heinemann; 1985.)*

microscopic findings, although the pathogenesis may be different. Electron microscopy defines:

- **Type 1 MCGN:** involves mesangial cell proliferation, with mainly subendothelial immune deposition and apparent splitting of the capillary basement membrane, giving a 'tramline' effect. It can be associated with persistently reduced plasma levels of C3 and normal levels of C4, and activation of the classical complement cascade. It is often idiopathic but occurs with chronic infection (abscesses, infective endocarditis, infected ventriculoperitoneal shunt) or cryoglobulinaemia secondary to hepatitis C infections (**Fig. 36.23A**).

- **Type 2 MCGN, or C3 nephropathy:** demonstrates mesangial cell proliferation with electron-dense, linear (ribbon-like) intramembranous deposits that usually stain for C3 only (**Fig. 36.23B**). This **dense deposit disease** may be idiopathic, or associated with factor H deficiency and partial lipodystrophy (loss of subcutaneous fat on the face and upper trunk). Alternatively, **C3 nephropathy** presents with low C3 levels (as in type 1 MCGN), due in this case to activation of the alternative pathway of the complement cascade, where loss-of-function mutations in complement factor H or other such factors allow uncontrolled alternative pathway activation. Autoantibodies to the C3 convertase enzyme (C3 nephritic factor) are present. In patients of Cypriot origin, an autosomal dominant inherited heterozygous duplication in the *CFHR5* gene (CFHR5 nephropathy) leads to a similar presentation.

- **Type 3 MCGN** has features of both type 1 and type 2 disease. Complement activation appears to be via the final common pathway of the cascade.

Most patients eventually go on to develop ESKD over several years. C3 nephropathy, particularly with an underlying genetic cause, recurs in a high proportion of renal transplant patients, usually within the first year but is less common in type 1 disease (25%).

Management

In idiopathic MCGN (**all age groups**) with normal renal function and non-nephrotic-range proteinuria, no specific therapy is required. Good blood pressure control, ideally with an ACE inhibitor, is of benefit.

In **children** with the nephritic syndrome and/or impaired renal function, a trial of steroids may be warranted (alternate-day prednisolone 40 mg/m^2 for a period of 6–12 months). If no benefit is seen,

this treatment is discontinued. Regular follow-up, with control of blood pressure, use of agents to reduce proteinuria and correction of lipid abnormalities, is necessary.

In **adults** with the nephritic syndrome and/or renal impairment, aspirin (325 mg) or dipyridamole (75–100 mg) daily, or a combination of the two, may be given for 6–12 months. Again, if no benefits are seen, the treatment should be stopped. Treatment to slow the rate of progression of CKD is instituted (see p. 1398). In C3 nephropathy due to loss-of-function mutation in complement factor H, anti-C5 antibody (eculizumab) has been used successfully in several patients and in recurrence following transplantation.

IgM nephropathy

This disorder is characterized by increased mesangial cellularity in most of the glomeruli, associated with granular immune deposits of IgM and complement. People present with episodic or persistent haematuria and the nephrotic syndrome. Unlike in minimal-change disease, the prognosis is not uniformly good, as steroid response is only 50%. Between 10% and 30% develop progressive renal insufficiency with evidence of secondary FSGS (see p. 1355) on repeat biopsy.

C1q nephropathy

C1q nephropathy is very similar to IgM nephropathy in terms of presenting features and microscopic appearance, with the exception of C1q deposits in the mesangium. Sometimes it is misdiagnosed as lupus nephritis, particularly in people with negative serology (so-called 'seronegative lupus'). The distinguishing features are intense C1q staining and absence of tubuloreticular inclusions (attributable to high circulating interferon-alfa) on electron microscopy.

Monoclonal gammopathy of renal significance

A monoclonal gammopathy of undetermined significance (MGUS, see p. 408) occurs in asymptomatic people with a paraprotein or M-band (often incidentally) detected in blood. Renal (usually glomerular) disease is increasingly recognized in association, related to deposition or precipitation of monotypic whole immunoglobulin or light chains in the kidney. Renal injury is driven by a clonal B-cell or plasma cell population.

The following are included under the term monoclonal gammopathy of renal significance (MGRS):

- **deposition diseases:** AL amyloid (see p. 1357), immunotactoid and fibrillary GN, monoclonal immunoglobulin deposition diseases (MIDDs, including light chain and heavy chain DD), proliferative GN with monoclonal immunoglobulin deposition and light chain tubulopathy
- **precipitation diseases:** cryoglobulinaemic GN
- **complement activation diseases:** paraprotein-associated C3 nephropathy and atypical haemolytic uraemic syndrome (HUS, see p. 1368).

Diagnosis is usually made in the context of a detectable paraprotein and characteristic renal biopsy findings, and progression to ESKD is common unless treatment is given. Conventional immunosuppression is of no benefit, but clone-directed therapy with bortezomib, rituximab or potentially daratumumab offers better outcomes.

Idiopathic fibrillary glomerulopathy

In this rare condition, microfibrillary structures are seen in the mesangium and glomerular capillary wall, visible on electron microscopy, and staining is positive for a specific marker, DNAJB9. Fibrils are larger than in amyloidosis (20–30 nm as opposed to 10 nm in diameter) and do not stain with Congo red. Patients present with proteinuria, mostly in the nephrotic range (60%), and microscopic haematuria (70%), hypertension and CKD (50%) that may progress rapidly; 40–50% develop ESKD within 2–6 years. No treatment is known to be of benefit.

Immunotactoid glomerulopathy

In this disorder, microtubules that are much larger (30–40 nm in diameter) than the fibrils in fibrillary glomerulopathy are seen on electron microscopy. The majority of patients have circulating paraproteins, or monoclonal immunoglobulin deposition is seen in the glomeruli on immunofluorescence microscopy. A lymphoproliferative disease is the underlying cause in over 50% of cases. The clinical presentation and course are similar to those of fibrillary glomerulopathy. Complete or partial remission of the nephrotic syndrome can be achieved with chemotherapy in 80% of patients.

Fibronectin glomerulopathy

This is also a form of glomerulonephritis due to fibrillar deposits, which, unlike amyloidosis but like fibrillary glomerulonephritis and immunotactoid glomerulopathy, is negative for Congo red staining. It is inherited as an autosomal dominant disorder and is associated with the massive deposition of fibronectin, a large dimeric glycoprotein consisting of two similar subunits (approximately 250 kDa in weight). The possible genetic abnormality in this disorder is a loss-of-function mutation in uteroglobin.

It presents with varying degrees of proteinuria seen first between the ages of 20 and 40, followed by hypertension, microscopic haematuria, and slow progression to ESKD in most patients.

Systemic lupus erythematosus (lupus nephritis)

Overt renal disease occurs in at least one-third of systemic lupus erythematosus (SLE) patients and, of these, 25% reach ESKD within 10 years (see also p. 458). Histologically, almost all patients will have changes. **Box 36.16** shows the progression of the histological findings and the clinical picture from classes I to VI.

Serial renal biopsies show that in approximately 25% of patients, histological appearances change from one class to another during the inter-biopsy interval. Immune deposits in the

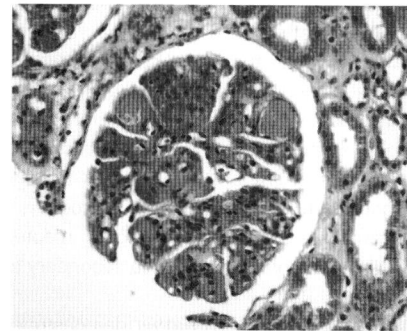

Fig. 36.24 Lupus nephritis type IV – a diffuse proliferative nephritis. There is proliferation of endothelial and mesangial cells.

glomeruli and mesangium are characteristic of SLE (tubuloreticular structure in glomerular endothelial cells) and stain positive for IgG, IgM, IgA and the complement components C3, C1q and C4 on immunofluorescence.

Pathophysiology

SLE is known to be a multifactorial autoantigen-driven, T-cell-dependent and B-cell-mediated autoimmune disorder.

- Lupus nephritis typically associates with multiple circulating autoantibodies to cellular antigens (particularly anti-dsDNA, anti-Ro) and with complement activation, which leads to reduced serum levels of C3, C4 and (particularly) C1q.
- C1q is the first component of the classical pathway of the complement cascade (see p. 44) and is involved in the activation of complement and clearance of self-antigens generated during apoptosis.
- Although self DNA was thought to be the inciting autoantigen, nucleosomes (structures comprising DNA and histone, generated during apoptosis) are more likely to be antigenic.
- Nucleosome-specific T cells, antinucleosome antibodies and nephritogenic immune complexes are generated.
- T-helper 2 (Th2) cells, with basophils and B-cell survival factors (such as BLyS), enhance B-cell differentiation and survival, and stimulated nucleic acid-binding receptors promote the production of autoreactive antibodies.

- Positively charged histone components of the nucleosome bind to the negatively charged heparan sulphate of the GBM, targeting an inflammatory reaction to the kidney.
- Inflammation stimulates complement activation, mesangial cell proliferation, mesangial matrix expansion and recruitment of inflammatory leucocytes.

The extraglomerular renal features of lupus nephritis include tubulointerstitial nephritis (75% of patients), renal vein thrombosis and renal artery stenosis. Thrombotic manifestations are associated with autoantibodies to phospholipids (anticardiolipin or lupus anticoagulant, see p. 459), and may present as infarction of glomerular segments, thrombotic microangiopathy or vasculitis.

Management

Initial management depends on the clinical presentation but hypertension and oedema should always be treated. Disease activity, kidney biopsy and histology, as well as the presence or absence of extrarenal manifestations of lupus, guide therapy. **Type I lupus nephritis** requires no specific treatment. **Type II** usually runs a benign course but some patients are treated with hydroxychloroquine and/or steroids alone.

- There have been a number of clinical trials with immunosuppressive agents in **types III, IV and V** lupus nephritis. Outcomes are affected by ethnicity, clinical characteristics, irreversible damage (on renal biopsy), initial response to treatment and the future frequency of renal flares.
- Steroids and high-dose intravenous cyclophosphamide or mycophenolate mofetil (MMF) may be used as induction therapy. In white populations, low-dose cyclophosphamide is a good alternative to high-dose cyclophosphamide, as it is similarly effective and associated with less toxicity.
- MMF is as effective as high-dose intravenous cyclophosphamide in the induction phase with a similar safety profile, but cyclophosphamide may be inferior to MMF in black and Hispanic people, possibly because of poor tolerance.
- Most patients respond to induction therapy. Remission is maintained with MMF (superior to azathioprine) or azathioprine, which is similar in effectiveness to ciclosporin in reducing the risk of relapse.
- B-cell depletion with rituximab (anti-CD20) has been used in some patients, with favourable results over the short term. However, controlled trials have not shown consistent results. It might be useful in severe, refractory lupus nephritis.

Prognosis

Treatment leading to the normalization of proteinuria, hypertension and renal dysfunction indicates a good prognosis. The prognosis is better in patients with types I, II and V disease. Glomerulosclerosis (type VI) usually predicts ESKD.

Cryoglobulinaemic renal disease

Cryoglobulins (CGs) are individual or mixed immunoglobulins and complement components, which precipitate reversibly in the cold. Three types are recognized:

- **Type I** is characterized by a cryoprecipitable immunoglobulin of a single monoclonal type, as is found in multiple myeloma and lymphoproliferative disorders.
- **Types II and III** cryoglobulinaemias are mixed types. In each, an antiglobulin is bound to the Fc portion of polyclonal IgG. In type II the antiglobulin is usually monoclonal IgM with rheumatoid factor activity, often associated with hepatitis C virus infection but also with other causes listed later. In type III the antiglobulin

is polyclonal IgM. Type II cryoglobulinaemias account for 40–60% cases, while 40–50% of all CG cases are of type III.

Glomerular disease is more common in type II than in type III cryoglobulinaemia. In approximately 30% of these 'mixed' cryoglobulinaemias, no underlying or associated disease is found (essential cryoglobulinaemia). Recognized associations include viral infections (hepatitis B and C, HIV, cytomegalovirus, Epstein–Barr infection), fungal and spirochaetal infections, malaria and infective endocarditis, and autoimmune rheumatic diseases (SLE, rheumatoid arthritis and Sjögren's syndrome). Glomerular pathological changes resemble those of MCGN (see **Fig. 36.23**).

Presentation is usually in the fourth or fifth decade of life, and women are more frequently affected than men. Systemic features include purpura, arthralgia, leg ulcers, Raynaud's phenomenon, evidence of systemic vasculitis, a polyneuropathy and hepatic involvement. The glomerular disease typically presents as asymptomatic proteinuria, microscopic haematuria or both, but presentation with an acute nephritic and nephrotic syndrome (most commonly) or features of CKD also occurs.

Complement is consumed, cryoglobulins can be detected, and protein electrophoresis, rheumatoid factor, autoantibodies and antiviral antibodies or mRNA of hepatitis C, depending on the associated disorder, should be sought.

The underlying cause should be treated; as hepatitis C virus infection is the most common cause, antivirals, such as directly acting antiviral agents, are highly efficacious. Intensive plasma exchange or cryofiltration has been used in selected cases where vasculitis is limb-, organ- or life-threatening to achieve rapid removal of cryoglobulins. Uncontrolled studies of the anti-CD20 chimeric monoclonal antibody rituximab, which depletes B cells, appear promising.

Immunoglobulin A vasculitis (Henoch-Schonlein syndrome)

This clinical syndrome comprises a characteristic skin rash, abdominal colic, joint pain and GN. Approximately 30–70% have clinical evidence of renal disease with haematuria and/or proteinuria. The renal disease is usually mild but the nephrotic syndrome and AKI can occur. The renal lesion is a focal segmental proliferative glomerulonephritis, sometimes with mesangial hypercellularity. In more severe cases, epithelial crescents may be present. Immunoglobulin deposition is mainly IgA in the glomerular mesangium distribution, similar to IgA nephropathy. There is no treatment of proven benefit; steroid therapy is ineffective and management is usually supportive. In crescentic GN, aggressive immunosuppression has been tried but with variable outcome.

Other glomerular disorders

Fabry's disease

This X-linked lysosomal storage disease results from a deficiency of the enzyme α-galactosidase. Glycosphingolipids (globotriaosylceramide) accumulate in many cells; in the kidney, podocytes are affected. Systemic features include angiokeratomas in the skin, cardiovascular disease, neuropathies and proteinuric progressive CKD. Enzyme replacement with agalsidase (α-galactosidase) slows progression and injury to the heart, kidney and skin. In certain cases migalastat, an oral molecular chaperone, is effective.

Sickle nephropathy

Sickle disease or trait is complicated relatively commonly by papillary sclerosis or necrosis, nephrogenic diabetes insipidus and incomplete renal tubular acidosis. Glomerular lesions are rare and can sometimes be traced to hepatitis B or C infection acquired through repeated blood transfusions. Occasionally, proteinuria or nephrotic syndrome with progressive renal insufficiency is seen without prior infection, particularly in *APOL1* G1/G2 gene variant. Rarely, membranous GN or mesangiocapillary GN with IgG deposits occurs in association. No form of effective therapy is known.

Glomerulopathy associated with pre-eclampsia

Patients with pre-eclampsia present with hypertension and proteinuria, often of rapid onset, which usually disappears after delivery. The glomerular lesion is characterized by marked endothelial swelling and obliteration of capillary lumina. The renal lesion may not be reversible and 30% of patients have changes for 6 months or more. In severe cases, associated with cortical necrosis, there may be a microangiopathic haemolytic anaemia. Normal placental development, regulated by angiogenic factors like vascular endothelial growth factor (VEGF) and by placental growth factors, does not occur in pre-eclampsia. Implantation is abnormal, in part due to a soluble fms-like tyrosine kinase (sFlt1) receptor, an antagonist of placental growth factor and specifically of VEGF, which is upregulated in the placenta of patients with pre-eclampsia. High circulating levels of these receptors antagonize angiopoietic factors and cause endothelial dysfunction. Excessive free radical generation in the placenta of pre-eclamptic patients is due to upregulation of NADPH oxidase activity, caused by generation of an angiotensin II receptor agonist antibody in some patients.

Paraneoplastic glomerulonephritis

A rare complication of malignancy, paraneoplastic GN is usually misdiagnosed as idiopathic GN. A number of cancers involve the kidney:

- ***Thymoma or Hodgkin lymphoma:*** polarization of the immune response towards a Th2 profile and possibly excessive production of IL-13 leads to the development of minimal change disease, mesangiocapillary GN or membranous nephropathy.
- ***B-cell lymphoma and leukaemia:*** these may induce injury through the presence of monoclonal immunoglobulin, cryoglobulin, and possibly hepatitis C virus infection.
- ***Polycythaemia vera, essential thrombocythaemia or primary myelofibrosis:*** severe thrombocytosis may induce FSGS, possibly due to elevated levels of platelet-derived growth factor.
- ***Myelodysplastic syndromes:*** autoimmunity causes a variety of glomerulonephritides.
- ***Epithelial carcinoma:*** glomerular inflammatory cells and subepithelial immune IgG1- and IgG2-containing complexes are usually present and may aid in the diagnosis of paraneoplastic membranous nephropathy.

Further reading

Noris M, Remuzzi G. Glomerular diseases dependent on complement activation, including atypical hemolytic uremic syndrome, membranoproliferative glomerulonephritis, and C3 glomerulopathy: core curriculum 2015. *Am J Kidney Dis* 2015; 66:359–375.

Ren S, Wu C, Zhang Y et al. An update on clinical significance of use of THSD7A in diagnosing idiopathic membranous nephropathy: a systematic review and meta-analysis of THSD7A in IMN. *Ren Fail* 2018; 40:306–313.

Suwanchote S, Rachayon M, Rodsaward P et al. Anti-neutrophil cytoplasmic antibodies and their clinical significance. *Clin Rheumatol* 2018; 37:875–884.

Trotter K, Clark MR, Liarski VM. Overview of pathophysiology and treatment of human lupus nephritis. *Curr Opin Rheumatol* 2016; 28:460–467.

KIDNEY INVOLVEMENT IN OTHER DISEASES

Polyarteritis nodosa

Classical polyarteritis nodosa (PAN) is a multisystem disorder (see also p. 465). Aneurysmal dilation of medium-sized arteries presents as hypertension, polyneuropathy and ischaemic infarction of a number of organs (including skin, gut, heart and brain). Aneurysms may be seen on renal arteriography. The condition is more common in men and in the elderly; typically, patients are ANCA-negative. PAN may be associated with drug use and hepatitis B infection. This form of polyangiitis is linked with slowly progressive CKD, often accompanied by severe hypertension. Rapidly progressive kidney failure is rare. Treatment with immunosuppression is less effective than it is for microscopic polyangiitis.

Systemic sclerosis (scleroderma)

Systemic sclerosis (scleroderma, SSc; see p. 460) is a chronic multisystem disease characterized by fibrosis and vasculopathy of the skin and visceral organs. Plasmacytoid dendritic cells appear to produce high plasma levels of CXCL4, which associated with both skin and lung fibrosis, as well as with pulmonary arterial hypertension in patients with SSc.

Some 10% of SSc patients develop scleroderma renal crisis, characterized by accelerated hypertension, rapidly progressive kidney failure and proteinuria. On kidney biopsy, 'onion skinning' in arcuate and interlobular arteries is seen and results from vessel intimal proliferation, fibrin thrombi and fibrinoid necrosis. The treatment of choice is ACE inhibitors, which have led to a remarkable improvement in outcomes in scleroderma renal crisis. Death is now rarely due to renal failure, though fewer than 30% of patients progress to ESKD.

Haemolytic uraemic syndrome

Haemolytic uraemic syndrome (HUS) is characterized by intravascular haemolysis with red cell fragmentation (microangiopathic haemolysis), thrombocytopenia and AKI due to thrombosis in small arteries and arterioles (**Fig. 36.25**). These features are also seen in disseminated intravascular coagulation but coagulation tests are typically normal in HUS.

Diarrhoea-associated HUS

Diarrhoea-associated HUS (D+ HUS) often follows a febrile illness, particularly gastroenteritis associated with *E. coli*, notably strain O157. The latter produces verocytotoxin (or shiga toxin), with a pathogenic A unit that inhibits protein synthesis and initiates

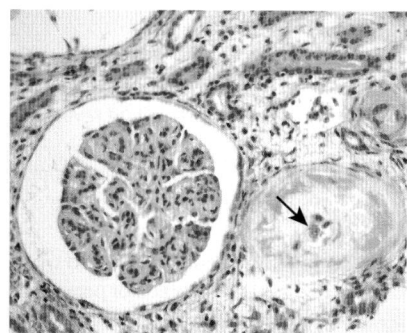

Fig. 36.25 Typical haemolytic uraemic syndrome (HUS) renal lesion – light microscopy. The arrow shows microthrombi.

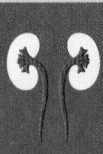

endothelial damage. B units facilitate entry of the A unit into the endothelial cells by binding to a receptor (Gb3) on the endothelial cell. Toxins are transported to and into endothelial cells from the gut on neutrophils. Most patients with D+ HUS recover renal function but commonly require supportive care, including fluid and electrolyte balance, antihypertensives, nutritional support and dialysis. Plasmapheresis is not beneficial. About 5% die during the acute episode, 5% develop ESKD and 30% exhibit evidence of long-term damage with persistent proteinuria. Antibiotic and antimotility agents for diarrhoea increase the risk of HUS and its complications.

Atypical HUS

Atypical HUS (aHUS) is a complement-driven illness, often related to a deficiency of complement factor H (CFH) or complement factor I (CFI). Factor H is a soluble protein produced by the liver, which regulates the activity of the alternative complement activation pathway; in particular, it protects host cell surfaces from complement-mediated damage. In some families with aHUS a mutation has been traced to another complement regulatory protein, CD46 (previously known as membrane co-factor protein, MCP). This protein is highly expressed in the kidney and normally prevents glomerular C3 activation. A loss-of-function mutation in CD46 results in unopposed complement activation and development of HUS. Functional deficiency of these factors can be acquired due to autoantibody formation, either as an isolated phenomenon or as part of an autoimmune disease such as SLE. A loss-of-function mutation in thrombomodulin (a membrane-bound anticoagulant glycoprotein) has been identified as an alternative complement pathway. Rarely, gain-of-function mutations can affect genes encoding the alternative pathway C3 convertase components, CFB and C3.

Management of aHUS

Treatment is often difficult, and severe hypertension and recurrence are frequent. The course of the disease is often indolent and progressive.

- Plasmapheresis or plasma infusion is used at initiation of therapy in the majority of patients, often until diagnosis is clear.
- C5 activation is one of the critical steps in the activation of complement cascade. **Eculizumab**, a monoclonal humanized anti-C5 antibody, has transformed outcomes, both at acute presentation and in prevention of recurrence (in native kidneys and in transplants).
- Liver transplantation is a potentially curative treatment in patients harbouring CFH and CFI mutations.

Sporadic cases of aHUS

These can be associated with pregnancy, SLE, scleroderma, malignant hypertension, metastatic cancer, HIV infection and various drugs, including oral contraceptives, ciclosporin, tacrolimus, chemotherapeutic agents (e.g. cisplatin, mitomycin C, bleomycin) and heparin. Management is supportive, with removal of the offending agent or specific treatment of the underlying cause. There is no evidence in favour of plasma infusion or plasmapheresis in these sporadic cases but it is tried, usually as a last resort.

Streptococcus pneumoniae produces an enzyme (possibly neuroaminidase) that can expose an antigen (Thomsen antigen) present on red blood cells, platelets and glomeruli. Antibodies to the antigen result in an antigen–antibody reaction and can lead to HUS and anaemia. The improved outcome is due to increasing awareness of this complication, judicious use of (washed) blood products and avoidance of plasma infusion or plasmapheresis.

Metabolism-associated HUS

Cobalamin C disease is a hereditary disorder of vitamin B_{12} metabolism that may cause HUS and multiple organ damage in infants and, rarely, adults. It is caused by mutations in a gene encoding the methylmalonic aciduria and homocystinuria type C protein (*MMACHC*). The resulting deficiency in methylcobalamin causes hyperhomocysteinaemia, decreased plasma methionine levels and methylmalonic aciduria.

Abnormal cobalamin C metabolism is associated with platelet activation, generation of reactive oxygen species, endothelial dysfunction, increased tissue factor expression, coagulation activation and HUS.

Parenteral hydroxocobalamin is the principal treatment for infants.

Thrombotic thrombocytopenic purpura

Thrombotic thrombocytopenic purpura (TTP; see p. 374) is characterized by microangiopathic haemolysis, renal failure and evidence of neurological disturbance. Young adults are most commonly affected. Wherever TTP or HUS is suspected, the serum activity of *ADAMTS13* should be measured. *ADAMTS13* activity is reduced in TTP, but normal in HUS and other conditions that cause thrombotic microangiopathy.

Antiphospholipid syndrome

In the antiphospholipid syndrome (APS; see p. 459) the binding of antiphospholipid antibodies (aPL) to beta 2 glycoprotein I (β2GPI) induces endothelial cell–leucocyte adhesion and thrombus formation through the inhibition of endothelial nitric oxide synthase (eNOS).

The central feature of APS is recurrent thrombosis (both venous and arterial) and early pregnancy loss in the presence of antiphospholipid antibodies. Antibodies may be primary, or secondary to infection (HIV, hepatitis C) or autoimmune disease (SLE). Some 50% have renal involvement with proteinuria. Thrombotic microangiopathy is a rare but well-recognized presentation. In some cases a lupus nephritis-like lesion (usually mesangiocapillary GN) is seen. The only proven treatment for APS is systemic anticoagulation. Use of steroids or plasmapheresis is reserved for patients with APS and life-threatening renal involvement with thrombotic microangiopathy. Treatment is variably successful (30–70%).

Multiple myeloma

AKI is relatively common in myeloma, occurring in 20–30% of affected individuals at the time of diagnosis, and is mainly due to the nephrotoxic effects of the abnormal immunoglobulins. It is often irreversible and may present as:

- **light chain cast nephropathy** – intratubular deposition of light chains, particularly kappa chains, which characteristically appear on renal histology as fractured casts with a giant cell reaction (Fig. 36.26)
- **AL amyloidosis** – deposition of amyloid fibrils of light chains (Congo red-positive)
- **light chain deposition disease** – nodular glomerulosclerosis with granular deposits of usually lambda light chains (Congo red-negative)
- **plasma cell infiltration** – often an incidental finding at postmortem
- **Fanconi's syndrome** – tubular toxicity due to light chains
- **hypercalcaemic nephropathy** – bone resorption causing hypercalcaemia

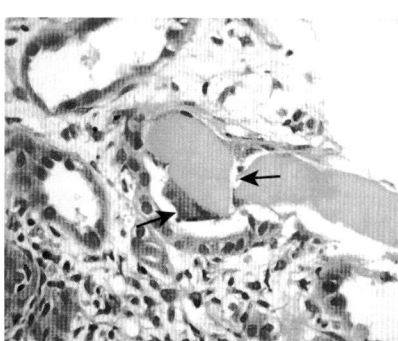

Fig. 36.26 Cast nephropathy in a patient with multiple myeloma. Light microscopy showing a characteristic fractured cast and giant cell reaction (arrowed).

- *hyperuricaemic nephropathy* – tumour lysis causing tubular crystallization of uric acid
- *radiocontrast nephropathy* – interaction between light chains and radiocontrast.

Treatment of the underlying myeloma is key to recovery (see p. 409). If a patient with cast nephropathy and severe AKI remains dialysis-dependent, the prognosis is poor. Commencement of effective bortezomib-based chemotherapy, which decreases light chain production, and a high-cut-off haemodialysis have shown some promise in relapsed myeloma.

Further reading

Bu F, Zhang Y, Wang K et al. Genetic analysis of 400 patients refines understanding and implicates a new gene in atypical hemolytic uremic syndrome. *J Am Soc Nephrol* 2018; 29:2809–2819.
Saha M, McDaniel JK, Zheng XL. Thrombotic thrombocytopenic purpura: pathogenesis, diagnosis and potential novel therapeutics. *J Thromb Haemost* 2017; 15:1889–1900.

HYPERTENSION AND THE KIDNEY

Hypertension can be the cause or the result of renal disease. It is often difficult to differentiate between the two on clinical grounds. Routine tests (see p. 1134) should be performed on all hypertensive patients, though renal imaging is usually unnecessary.

The *mechanisms* responsible for normal regulation of arterial blood pressure and the development of essential primary hypertension are unclear (see p. 1137). One basic concept is that long-term regulation of arterial pressure is closely linked to the ability of the kidneys to excrete sufficient salt to maintain normal sodium balance, extracellular fluid volume and normal blood volume at normotensive arterial pressures. Cross-transplantation experiments suggest that hypertension travels with the kidney, as hypertension develops in the normotensive recipient of a kidney genetically programmed for hypertension. Similarly, patients with ESKD due to hypertension become normotensive after receiving a kidney transplant from normotensive donors, provided the new kidney functions well.

One renal factor contributing to future hypertension is the total number of nephrons per kidney ('nephron dose'). People with hypertension and normal renal function have a significantly reduced number of nephrons in each kidney, and individual nephrons are enlarged as a result of glomerular hyperfiltration (see p. 1359). Where hypertension is more common (as it is in black or Hispanic men and women), increased glomerular volume is found (a surrogate marker for reduced nephron number).

Whether reduced nephron number is genetic or environmental in origin is unclear. Changes in the intrauterine environment may lead to poor renal growth (and reduced renal volume, suggesting lower nephron number) before birth, low birth weight and hypertension in adult life.

Excess renal sympathetic activity may also contribute. Strategies to achieve bilateral renal sympathetic denervation were hugely effective in patients with refractory hypertension in uncontrolled studies; to date, this benefit has not been borne out by a well-controlled trial.

Essential hypertension

In essential hypertension, arteriosclerosis of major renal arteries and changes in the intrarenal vasculature (nephrosclerosis) occur. Arterial pressure is a product of cardiac output and systemic vascular resistance (SVR). The compliance of systemic arteries is, then, a critical component; 'stiff' (sclerotic) arteries cannot modulate pressure surges in systole, and systolic pressures rise. Over time, vessels (and the kidney) remodel:

- In small vessels and arterioles, intimal thickening with reduplication of the internal elastic lamina occurs and the vessel wall becomes hyalinized.
- In large vessels, concentric reduplication of the internal elastic lamina and endothelial proliferation produce an 'onion skin' appearance.
- Reduction in size of both kidneys occurs; this may be asymmetrical if one major renal artery is more affected than the other.
- The proportion of sclerotic (scarred) glomeruli is increased, compared with that in age-matched controls.

Renal function does deteriorate with these changes but severe CKD is unusual in white people (1 in 10000). In people of black African descent, by contrast, hypertension much more often results in the development of CKD, with a fourfold higher incidence of ESKD compared to that in white people. This difference in incidence of hypertensive renal disease may be due to overestimation of the diagnosis on clinical grounds, a higher incidence of hypertension (usually salt-sensitive), reduced nephron number and a higher frequency of susceptibility alleles for ESKD in the (West) African than the European gene pool.

A genome-wide study found statistically stronger associations between two independent sequence variants in the apolipoprotein L1 gene *(APOL1)* and non-diabetic nephropathy in African–Americans, in hypertension-attributed ESKD. These kidney disease risk variants most likely arose due to the positive selection for evolutionary advantage that these variants in *APOL1* conferred against trypanosomal infection and protection from African sleeping sickness. These observations provide some evidence, similar to findings in sickle cell anaemia, that natural selection might protect from one disease but allow another one to develop.

In accelerated or malignant-phase hypertension:

- Arteriolar fibrinoid necrosis occurs, probably as a result of plasma entering the media of the vessel through splits in the intima. It is prominent in afferent glomerular arterioles.
- Fibrin deposition within small vessels is often associated with thrombocytopenia and red cell fragmentation seen on the peripheral blood film (microangiopathic haemolytic anaemia).

Microscopic haematuria, proteinuria (usually of modest degree – 1–3 g daily) and progressive CKD occur. If disease is untreated, fewer than 10% of patients survive 2 years.

Management

The management of hypertension is described on page 1140. If treatment is begun before CKD has developed, the prognosis for renal function is good, despite an initial fall in eGFR due to haemodynamic effects. Stabilization or improvement in renal function, with healing of intrarenal arteriolar lesions and resolution of microangiopathic haemolysis, occurs with effective treatment of malignant-phase hypertension.

Renal hypertension

Hypertension commonly complicates bilateral renal disease such as chronic GN, bilateral reflux nephropathy, polycystic disease and analgesic nephropathy. Two main mechanisms are responsible:

- activation of the renin–angiotensin–aldosterone system
- retention of salt and water as excretory function declines, leading to an increase in blood volume and blood pressure.

As CKD progresses, salt and water overload becomes ever more involved in driving high blood pressure.

Hypertension occurs earlier, is more common and tends to be more severe in patients with glomerular disease (GN) than in those with tubulointerstitial diseases such as reflux or analgesic nephropathy.

Management is described on page 1140. Meticulous control of blood pressure may prevent ongoing or new vascular or parenchymal changes, and further deterioration of renal function. There is good evidence that ACE inhibitors offer additional renoprotective benefits for the same degree of blood pressure control than other agents. In a study of African-Americans with hypertension, intensive blood pressure control (130/78 mmHg) was not superior to standard control (141/86 mmHg) in the prevention of ESKD. However, in the same study, patients with proteinuria benefited more from intensive blood pressure control. The presence of the *APOL1* risk allele was associated with rapid decline of GFR, irrespective of achieved blood pressure or baseline proteinuria.

Renovascular disease

Renal ischaemia, or a fall in perfusion pressures in the afferent glomerular arterioles, leads to increased production and release of renin from the juxtaglomerular apparatus (see p. 1343). This, in turn, causes a consequent increase in angiotensin II, a potent vasoconstrictor, which also triggers aldosterone secretion, stimulates thirst and leads to vascular smooth muscle hypertrophy and fibrosis in the kidney.

In renal artery stenosis, narrowing of the renal artery or arteries causes a fall in renal perfusion pressure on the distal side of the stenosis; in each affected kidney, angiotensin release occurs and local salt and water reabsorption is increased. Urine from the ischaemic kidney is more concentrated, with a lower sodium concentration than urine from an unaffected kidney. GFR is decreased on the ischaemic side as well.

Narrowing of the renal arteries (renal artery stenosis) is caused by one of two pathologies: **atherosclerotic renovascular disease** or **fibromuscular dysplasia**.

Atherosclerotic renovascular disease

Atherosclerotic renovascular disease (ARVD) is a common cause of hypertension and CKD due to ischaemic nephropathy. Its incidence increases with age:

- 5% in those under 60 years of age
- 16% in those over 60 years of age.

In most patients the atherosclerotic lesion is ostial (within 1 cm of the origin of the renal artery) and usually associated with symptomatic atherosclerotic vascular disease elsewhere. Patients with peripheral vascular disease (39%), coronary artery disease (10–29%), congestive cardiac failure (34%) and aortic aneurysm (38%) are at high risk of developing significant renal artery stenosis.

Many patients are asymptomatic and are discovered incidentally during investigation for other conditions. Aortography experience from the USA shows that 11% of asymptomatic patients have significant unilateral stenosis and 4% have bilateral disease. ARVD results in hypertension (present in 50%), sodium retention (ankle and flash pulmonary oedema), proteinuria (usually in the subnephrotic range) and decreased GFR. Beyond the stenosis, affected kidneys demonstrate changes histologically, with vascular sclerosis, tubular atrophy, interstitial fibrosis with inflammatory cellular infiltrate, atubular glomeruli, cholesterol emboli and secondary FSGS changes. These changes are often described as 'ischaemic nephropathy'. The affected kidney loses volume (as fibrosis replaces normal tissue) and becomes smaller on ultrasound measurement. These morphological changes are responsible for the associated fall in GFR; the arterial stenosis itself drives hypertension.

Renovascular disease should be considered in:

- patients with hypertension and/or CKD with abdominal or other audible bruits
- patients with renal asymmetry, particularly where ultrasound suggests >1.5 cm difference in length
- recurrent flash pulmonary oedema without cardiopulmonary disease
- progressive CKD in patients with evidence of generalized atherosclerosis.

Management

The **aims of treatment** are to prevent decline in renal function and to reverse salt and water overload. Most patients with ARVD will die a cardiovascular death and modifiable risk factors should be addressed. All patients with ARVD should be managed with a combination of aspirin, statins and optimal control of blood pressure as prophylaxis against progression of atherosclerosis. Hypertension should be controlled, ideally with an ACE inhibitor. This is the paradox of ARVD: angiotensin drives the renal and cardiac events, so ACE inhibition is ideal medical therapy. However, because ACE inhibitors will cause a fall (often significant) in renal perfusion beyond the stenosis, ACE inhibitors can cause AKI in patients with bilateral, haemodynamically significant ARVD.

Renal artery stenosis can also progress to occlusion, particularly in patients with stenosis of more than 75%, as shown by serial angiography. Revascularization offers definitive treatment of stenotic lesions in ARVD:

- **Options in renal artery stenosis** include transluminal angioplasty to dilate the stenotic region, insertion of stents across the stenosis (sometimes the only endoscopic option when the stenosis occurs close to the origin of the renal artery from the aorta, making angioplasty technically difficult or impossible), reconstructive vascular surgery and nephrectomy.
- **Indications for revascularization** are vessels with stenosis of >75% and recurrent flash pulmonary oedema, drug-resistant severe hypertension, ARVD affecting a solitary functioning kidney, patients with cardiac failure needing ACE inhibitors, unexplained progressive CKD and dialysis-dependent renal failure.

In a number of trials, renal artery stenting did not confer a significant benefit with respect to the prevention of clinical events (cardiovascular events, progressive renal insufficiency or the need for

RRT) when added to comprehensive, multifactorial medical therapy in people with atherosclerotic renal artery stenosis and hypertension or CKD. Up to 30% of renal artery interventions will be complicated by atheroembolism, which may lead to further functional deterioration.

Prognosis

Mortality is high because of other associated co-morbidities, and ARVD patients have generalized endothelial dysfunction. ARVD patients with ESKD have higher death rates than those with other causes of ESKD. Five-year survival is only 18% in patients with ESKD due to ARVD.

Fibromuscular dysplasia of the renal arteries

Fibromuscular dysplasia (FMD) is often asymptomatic, occurring in younger women with hypertension. It is far less common than ARVD. FMD affects many arterial beds, including the carotid and coronary arteries. Renal function is often normal.

MRA (gadolinium-enhanced) reveals a characteristic string of beads appearance in the mid-renal artery (rather than affecting the ostium, as seen in ARVD).

Angioplasty (occasionally with stent insertion) or, rarely, surgery was offered to affected individuals. Cure rates were only 36% and 54%, respectively, in a study of over 2000 patients (defining cure as blood pressure <140/90 mmHg without treatment), and the blood pressure outcome was strongly age-related. Procedural complications were common: 12% after angioplasty and 17% after surgery. Current medical antihypertensive therapy is very effective in this group and angioplasty is now not usually performed.

Screening for renovascular disease

- **Radionuclide studies** (see p. 1351) can demonstrate decreased renal perfusion on the affected side. In unilateral renal artery stenosis a disproportionate fall in isotope uptake occurs on the affected side after administration of captopril. A completely normal result makes renovascular disease unlikely.
- **Doppler ultrasound** is sensitive but highly operator-dependent and time-consuming. Higher renal artery velocity on Doppler may mean a higher pressure differential across a stenosis. Doppler also describes the intrarenal vascular resistance, which can be valuable in predicting the success of revascularization procedures. A resistive index of >80 is a predictor of poor response following intervention.
- **MRA** can be used to visualize the renal arteries and there is a good – though not perfect – correlation between MRA findings and those of renal arteriography.
- **CT scannng** permits non-invasive imaging of the renal arteries. It is much less expensive than MRA but does expose the patient to ionizing radiation and to contrast injection, and is less reliable than MRA.
- **Renal arteriography** (see p. 1351) is used to confirm the diagnosis of renal arterial disease. It also allows therapeutic intervention if needed at diagnosis.

Further reading

Chang AR, Lóser M, Malhotra R et al. Blood pressure goals in patients with chronic kidney disease: a review of evidence and guidelines. *Clin J Am Soc Nephrol* 2019; 14:161–169.
Cooper CJ, Murphy TP, Cutlip DE et al and CORAL Investigators. Stenting and medical therapy for atherosclerotic renal-artery stenosis. *N Engl J Med* 2014; 370:13–22.

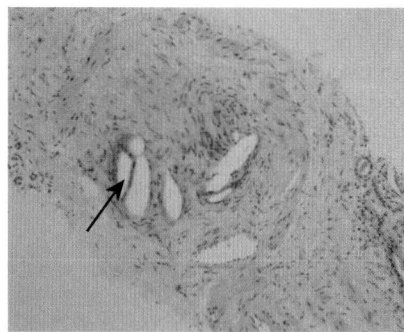

Fig. 36.27 Renal cholesterol emboli showing the characteristic cholesterol biconvex clefts (arrowed).

Malhotra R, Craven T, Ambrosius WT et al; SPRINT Research Group. Effects of intensive blood pressure lowering on kidney tubule injury in CKD: a longitudinal subgroup analysis in SPRINT. *Am J Kidney Dis* 2019; 73:21–30.
Parsa A, Kao WH, Xie D et al. and AASK Study Investigators; CRIC Study Investigators. APOL1 risk variants, race, and progression of chronic kidney disease. *N Engl J Med* 2013; 369:2183–2196.

OTHER VASCULAR DISORDERS OF THE KIDNEY

Renal artery occlusion

This occurs from thrombosis *in situ*, usually in a severely damaged atherosclerotic vessel, or more commonly from embolization, such as in atrial fibrillation. Both lead to renal infarction, either of a wedge of kidney or of the whole kidney. Occlusion of a small branch artery may produce no effect but occlusion of larger vessels results in dull flank pain, macroscopic haematuria and varying degrees of CKD. Intra-arterial thrombolytic therapy has been tried with mixed results.

Cholesterol embolization (atheroembolic renal disease)

Showers of cholesterol-rich atheromatous material from ulcerated plaques reach the kidney from the aorta and/or renal arteries, particularly after catheterization of the abdominal aorta or attempts at renal artery angioplasty. Anticoagulants and thrombolytic agents also precipitate non-traumatic cholesterol embolization. Renal failure from cholesterol emboli may be acute or slowly progressive. Clinical features include fever, eosinophilia, back and abdominal pain, and evidence of embolization elsewhere, such as to the retina or digits. The diagnosis can be confirmed by renal biopsy (**Fig. 36.27**). It is more common in males, the elderly (>70 years) and patients with cardiovascular disease. Over 80% have abnormal renal function at baseline. Atheroembolic renal disease occurs spontaneously in 25% of cases. The 2-year mortality is 30% and a similar percentage of patients develop CKD. Baseline co-morbidities – that is, reduced renal function, presence of diabetes, history of heart failure, acute/subacute presentation and gastrointestinal tract involvement – are significant predictors of event occurrence. The risk of dialysis and death is 50% lower among those receiving statins.

Renal vein thrombosis

This is usually of insidious onset, occurring in patients with the nephrotic syndrome, with a renal cell carcinoma, and in thrombophilia (see p. 1011) with an increased risk of venous thrombosis. Anticoagulation is indicated.

Type of renal stone	Percentage of stones
Calcium oxalate usually with calcium phosphate	65
Calcium phosphate alone	15
Magnesium ammonium phosphate (struvite)	10–15
Uric acid	3–5
Cystine	1–2

? **Box 36.18** Causes of urinary tract stones

- Dehydration
- Hypercalcaemia
- Hypercalciuria
- Hyperoxaluria
- Hyperuricaemia and hyperuricosuria
- Infection
- Cystinuria
- Primary renal disease (polycystic kidneys, medullary sponge kidneys, renal tubular acidosis)
- Drugs (see text)

RENAL CALCULI AND NEPHROCALCINOSIS

Renal and vesical calculi

Nephrolithiasis, or renal stones, usually occurs in the upper urinary tract. It is very common worldwide, with a lifetime risk of about 10%.

Most stones are composed of calcium oxalate and phosphate; these are more common in men (**Box 36.17**). Mixed infective stones, which account for about 15% of all calculi, are twice as common in women as in men. The overall male to female ratio of stone disease is 2:1.

Stone disease is frequently recurrent and more than 50% of patients will experience a second stone within 10 years of their first. The risk of recurrence increases if a metabolic or structural abnormality predisposing to stone formation is present and is not modified by treatment. Nephrolithiasis is not a benign condition; observational studies show an association with an increased risk of ESKD, bone diseases, hypertension and myocardial infarction.

Aetiology

Stones form because solute concentrations exceed saturation, often in the context of a trigger or nidus to crystallize around. Inhibitors of crystal formation prevent stone formation in normal urine, despite the concentrations of stone-forming substances exceeding maximum solubility in water. Factors predisposing to stone formation in these so-called 'idiopathic stone-formers' are:

- *Chemical composition of urine* that favours stone crystallization.
- *A concentrated urine* resulting from dehydration (particularly in those who are living or working in a hot climate or environment).
- *Impairment of inhibitors that prevent crystallization* in normal urine. These inhibitors include inorganic magnesium, pyrophosphate and citrate. Organic inhibitors include glycosaminoglycans and nephrocalcin (an acidic protein of tubular origin). Tamm–Horsfall protein may have a dual role in both inhibiting and promoting stone formation; it usually inhibits crystallization of urinary oxalate but in an undersialylated form promotes stone formation.

Recognized risk factors for stone formation are listed in **Box 36.18**.

Stones may be single or multiple, and vary enormously in size from minute, sand-like particles to staghorn calculi or large stone concretions in the bladder. They may be located within the renal parenchyma or within the collecting system. Stones regularly cause obstruction, leading to hydronephrosis; a combination of obstruction and infection often causes lasting damage to the kidney.

Hypercalcaemia

If the GFR is normal, hypercalcaemia almost invariably leads to hypercalciuria. Common causes of systemic hypercalcaemia leading to stone formation are:

- primary hyperparathyroidism (see p. 644)
- vitamin D ingestion
- sarcoidosis.

Hypercalciuria

This is by far the most common metabolic abnormality detected in calcium stone-formers. Approximately 8% of men excrete more than 7.5 mmol of calcium per day. Calcium stone formation is more common in this group, although the cut-off is entirely arbitrary. In women, a 24-hour calcium excretion of more than 6.25 mmol tends to make stone formation more likely.

About 90% of ionized calcium filtered by the kidney is reabsorbed in the tubule, controlled largely by PTH. Causes of hypercalciuria include:

- hypercalcaemia
- high dietary intake of calcium
- excessive resorption of calcium from the skeleton, such as occurs with prolonged immobilization or weightlessness
- idiopathic hypercalciuria.

Idiopathic hypercalciuria is a common risk factor for the formation of stones, and can be thought of as accelerated calcium transport, with enhanced gut uptake, and increased urine excretion of calcium.

Hyperoxaluria

There are two inborn errors of glyoxylate metabolism that cause increased endogenous oxalate biosynthesis and are inherited in an autosomal recessive manner:

- *type 1:* alanine–glyoxylate aminotransferase deficiency
- *type 2:* glyoxylate reductase hydroxypyruvate reductase deficiency.

In both types, calcium oxalate stone formation occurs. The prognosis is poor, as widespread calcium oxalate crystal deposition in the kidneys leads to CKD in the late teens or early twenties. Successful liver transplantation has been shown to cure the metabolic defect.

Much more common causes of mild hyperoxaluria are:

- excess ingestion of foodstuffs high in oxalate, such as spinach, rhubarb and tea
- dietary calcium restriction, with compensatory increased absorption of oxalate
- gastrointestinal disease (e.g. Crohn's), usually with an intestinal resection, associated with increased absorption of oxalate from the colon.

Dehydration secondary to fluid loss from the gut also plays a part in stone formation.

Hyperuricaemia and hyperuricosuria

Uric acid stones account for 3–5% of all stones in the UK but in Israel the proportion is as high as 40%. Uric acid is the endpoint of purine

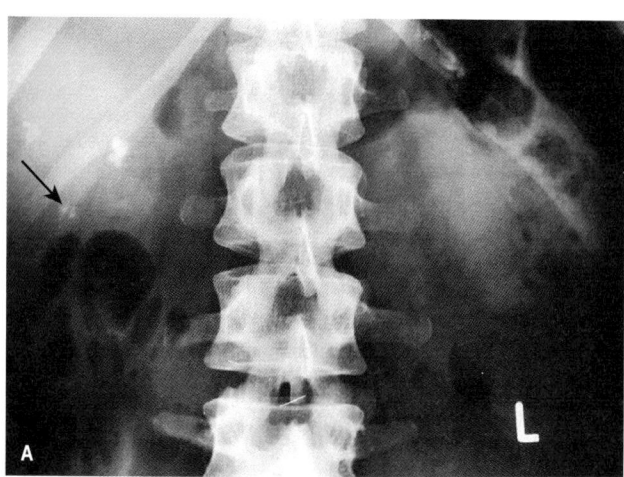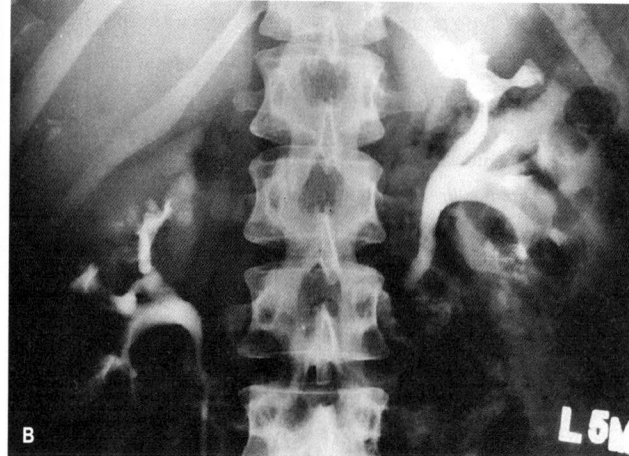

Fig. 36.28 Medullary sponge kidney. (A) Plain film showing 'spotty' calcification in the renal areas (arrowed). **(B)** After injection of contrast the calcification is shown to be small calculi in the papillary zones.

metabolism. Hyperuricaemia (see p. 452) can occur as a primary defect in idiopathic gout and as a secondary consequence of increased cell turnover: for example, in myeloproliferative disorders. Increased uric acid excretion occurs in these conditions and stones will develop in some patients. Some uric acid stone-formers have hyperuricosuria (>4 mmol/24 h on a low-purine diet), without hyperuricaemia.

Dehydration alone may also cause uric acid stones to form. Patients with ileostomies are at particular risk, both from dehydration and from the fact that loss of bicarbonate from gastrointestinal secretions results in the production of an acid urine (uric acid is more soluble in an alkaline medium than in an acid one).

Some patients with calcium stones also have hyperuricaemia and/or hyperuricosuria; it is believed that the calcium salts precipitate on an initial nidus of uric acid in such patients.

Urinary tract infection

Mixed infective stones are composed of magnesium ammonium phosphate together with variable amounts of calcium. Such struvite stones are often large, forming a cast of the collecting system (staghorn calculus). These stones are usually due to urinary tract infection with organisms such as *Proteus mirabilis* that hydrolyse urea, with formation of the strong base ammonium hydroxide. The availability of ammonium ions and the alkalinity of the urine favour stone formation. An increased production of mucoprotein from infection also creates an organic matrix on which stone formation can occur.

Cystinuria

Cystinuria results in the formation of cystine stones (about 1–2% of all stones).

Primary renal disease

- **Polycystic renal disease** (see p. 1405) shows a high prevalence of stone disease.
- **Medullary sponge kidney** involves dilation of the collecting ducts that leads to urinary stasis and calcification (**Fig. 36.28**). Approximately 20% of these patients have hypercalciuria and a similar proportion have a renal tubular acidification defect.
- **Renal tubular acidosis**, either inherited and acquired, is associated with nephrocalcinosis and stone formation. Persistently alkaline urine and reduced urinary citrate excretion lead to stone formation, as calcium and citrate form a *soluble* complex in urine.

> **Box 36.19 Clinical features of urinary tract stones**
>
> - Asymptomatic
> - Pain: renal colic
> - Haematuria
> - Urinary tract infection
> - Urinary tract obstruction

Drugs

Some drugs promote calcium stone formation (e.g. loop diuretics, antacids, glucocorticoids, theophylline, vitamins D and C, acetazolamide); some promote uric acid stones (e.g. thiazides, salicylates); and some precipitate into stones (e.g. indinavir, triamterene, sulfadiazine).

Clinical features

Most people with urinary tract calculi are asymptomatic.

- Pain is the most common symptom and may be sharp or dull, constant, intermittent or colicky (**Box 36.19**).
- If the urinary tract is obstructed, fluids or diuretics (including alcohol) make the pain worse as peristaltic flow increases.
- Exertion may cause mobile calculi to move, precipitating pain and, occasionally, haematuria.
- Ureteric colic occurs when a stone enters the ureter and either obstructs it or causes spasm during its passage down the ureter. Classically, pain radiates from the flank to the iliac fossa, testis or labia (in the distribution of the first lumbar nerve root). Pallor, sweating and vomiting often occur and the patient is restless, trying to obtain relief from the pain. Haematuria often occurs. Untreated, the pain of ureteric colic typically subsides after a few hours.

When urinary tract obstruction and infection are present, the features of acute pyelonephritis or of a Gram-negative septicaemia may dominate the clinical picture.

Calcified papillae may mimic ordinary calculi, so that causes of papillary necrosis such as analgesic abuse should be considered (see p. 1386).

Bladder stones

Bladder stones (**Box 36.20**) are usually associated with bacteriuria and present with frequency, dysuria and haematuria; severe introital or perineal pain may occur if trigonitis is present.

A calculus at the bladder neck or an obstruction in the urethra may cause bladder outflow obstruction, resulting in anuria and painful bladder distension.

Investigations

- **Dipsticks** are used to test for red cells, protein and glucose.
- **Chemical analysis** should be employed for passed stones.
- **A mid-stream specimen of urine** should be taken for microscopy (crystals) and culture.
- **Serum urea, electrolyte, creatinine (eGFR) and calcium levels** should be measured.
- **Ultrasonography** shows kidney stones and renal pelvis dilation well but ureteric stones can be missed.
- **Computed tomography of kidneys, ureters and bladder (CT-KUB)** is the best diagnostic test available and has a sensitivity of >95%. It involves radiation and in young patients many physicians perform ultrasonographs as the first investigation.

A normal CT excludes the diagnosis of pain due to calculous disease. The CT-KUB appearances in a patient with acute left ureteric obstruction are shown in **Fig. 36.29**.

Pure uric acid stones are radiolucent and show as a filling defect after injection of contrast medium if excretion urography is performed. Uric acid stones are readily seen on CT scanning (**Fig. 36.30**). Mixed infective stones in which organic matrix predominates are barely radio-opaque.

Management

Renal colic is painful. Analgesia with an NSAID, such as diclofenac 75 mg i.m., compares favourably with opiates such as diamorphine or pethidine. Stones of less than 0.5 cm diameter usually pass spontaneously, particularly if hydration is maintained (patients that can drink should aim for over 2.5 L intake). Alpha-blockers (e.g. tamsulosin) were thought to help expulsion of distal ureteral stones of less than 6 mm in size (alpha receptors are predominantly present in the distal ureter and detrusor) but a randomized controlled trial has shown no benefit.

Stones of more than 1 cm diameter usually need urological or radiological intervention. Extracorporeal shock-wave lithotripsy (ESWL) will fragment most stones, which then pass spontaneously. Ureteroscopy with a YAG laser can be used for larger stones. Percutaneous nephrolithotomy is also used. Open surgery is rarely needed.

Investigation of the cause of stone formation

In an elderly patient who has had a single episode with one stone, only limited investigation is required. Younger patients and those with recurrent stone formation need detailed investigation.

- **Renal imaging** excludes structural abnormalities of the urinary tract.
- **Urine culture** excludes significant bacteriuria.
- **Chemical analysis** is performed on any stone passed (required in the diagnosis of cystinuria or uric acid stone formation).
- **Serum calcium** is investigated if hypercalcaemia is present (see p. 1375).
- **Serum urate concentration** is often, but not invariably, elevated in uric acid stone-formers.
- **A screening test for cystinuria** should be carried out by adding sodium nitroprusside to a random unacidified urine sample; a purple colour indicates that cystinuria may be present. Urine chromatography is required to define the diagnosis precisely.
- **Urinary calcium, oxalate and uric acid output** should be measured in two consecutive, carefully collected 24 hour urine samples. After aliquots are withdrawn for estimation of uric acid, the urine is acidified to prevent crystallization of calcium salts on the walls of the container, which would give falsely low results for urinary calcium and oxalate.
- **Plasma bicarbonate** is low in renal tubular acidosis. The finding of a urine pH that does not fall below 5.5 in the face of metabolic acidosis is diagnostic of this condition (see p. 199).

Prevention of recurrent stones

- All idiopathic stone-formers, where no metabolic abnormality is present, should maintain a high intake of fluid throughout the day and night to ensure a daily urine volume of 2–2.5 L. This reduces saturation of solute.

? Box 36.20 Bladder stones

Occur where stasis, infection and a nidus for stone formation come together:
- Bladder outflow obstruction (e.g. urethral stricture, neuropathic bladder, prostatic obstruction)
- Presence of a foreign body (e.g. catheters, non-absorbable sutures)

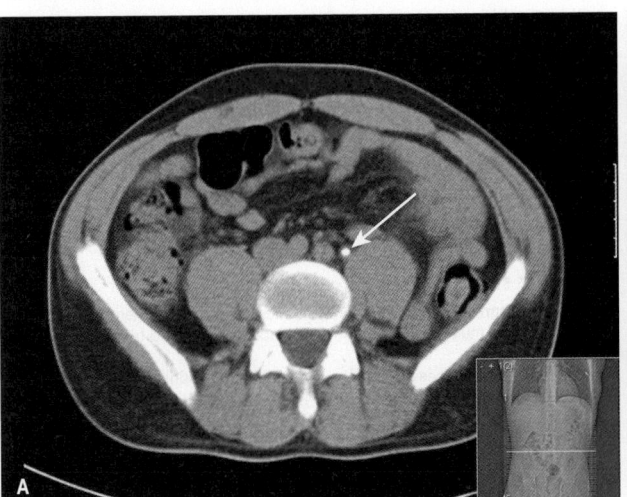
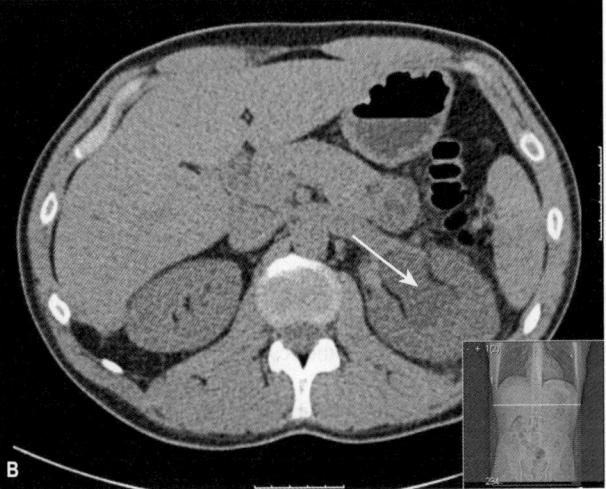

Fig. 36.29 Computed tomography of kidneys, ureters and bladder (CT-KUB) in ureteric stone obstruction. **(A)** Left ureteric calculus (arrowed). **(B)** A dilated renal pelvis (arrowed) proximal to the ureteric stone in A.

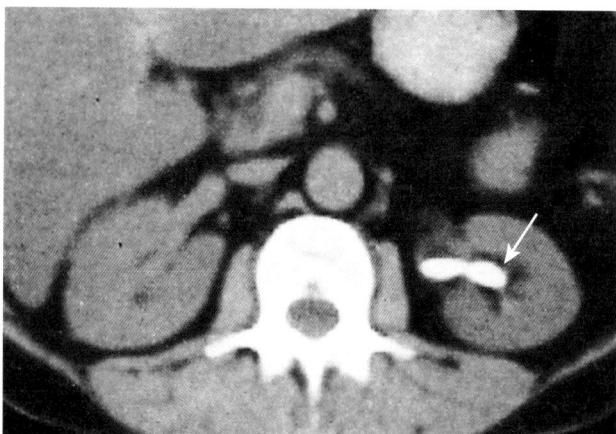

Fig. 36.30 CT scan showing a uric acid stone. The stone appears as a bright lesion in the left kidney (arrowed).

- With idiopathic hypercalciuria, dietary calcium restriction is inappropriate, as restriction results in hyperabsorption of oxalate. Foods rich in oxalate should be avoided (nuts, spinach, chocolate, rhubarb). Patients who live in a hard-water area may benefit from drinking softened water.
- Salt intake should be limited to 50 mmol/day (calcium excretion increases by 0.6 mmol/day for every 100 mmol Na⁺ in the urine).
- If hypercalciuria stone formation persists, a thiazide diuretic (e.g. bendroflumethiazide 2.5 or 5 mg each morning) reduces urinary calcium excretion. This indirect effect is due to mild volume contraction resulting in increased calcium absorption in the proximal renal tubule.
- Reduction of animal proteins to 50 g/day is also advisable.
- Where mixed infective stones recur, long-term, low-dose prophylactic antibiotics may prevent bacteriuria.
- Uric acid stones can be prevented by the long-term use of allopurinol or febuxostat to maintain the serum urate and urinary uric acid excretion in the normal range. Uric acid is more soluble at alkaline pH, and long-term sodium bicarbonate supplementation to maintain an alkaline urine is an alternative approach in those few patients unable to take allopurinol (see p. 1387). However, alkalinization of the urine facilitates precipitation of calcium oxalate and phosphate.

Cystine stones can be prevented and indeed will dissolve slowly with a high fluid intake. To achieve this, up to 5 L of water is drunk in each 24 hours. Patients need to wake twice during the night to drink 500 mL or more of water. Understandably, many patients cannot tolerate this regimen. Alkalinization to a pH of 7 requires high doses of potassium citrate or bicarbonate. An alternative option is long-term use of the chelating agent penicillamine; this causes cystine to be converted to the more soluble penicillamine–cysteine complex. Side-effects include drug rashes, blood dyscrasias and immune complex-mediated glomerulonephritis. However, it is especially effective in promoting dissolution of cystine stones already present. Other cystine-binding drugs include captopril and tiopronin.

Monogenic hyperoxaluria can be managed with oral high-dose pyridoxine if type 1 (though no response will occur with type 2). Unfortunately, there is currently no proven pharmacotherapy for effective treatment of the more common form of 'idiopathic' hyperoxaluria present in up to 40% of stone-formers. Probiotic *Oxalobacter formigenes* has shown some promise.

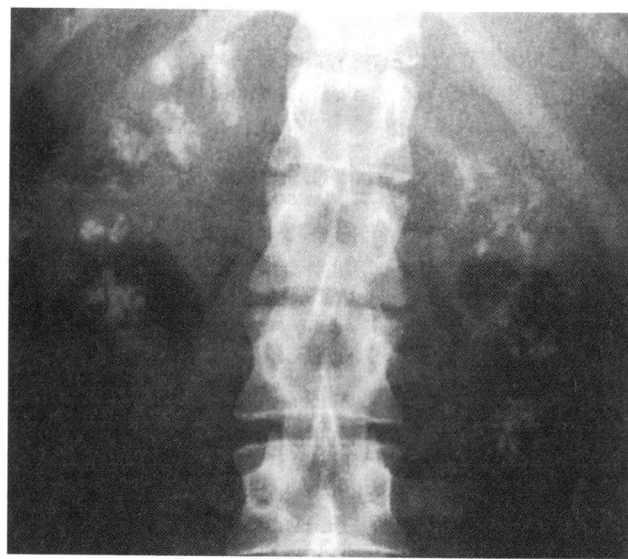

Fig. 36.31 X-ray showing nephrocalcinosis.

> **? Box 36.21 Causes of nephrocalcinosis**
>
> **Mainly cortical (rare)**
> - Renal cortical necrosis (tramline calcification)
>
> **Mainly medullary**
> - Hypercalcaemia (primary hyperparathyroidism, hypervitaminosis D, sarcoidosis)
> - Renal tubular acidosis (inherited and acquired)
> - Primary hyperoxaluria
> - Medullary sponge kidney
> - Tuberculosis

Nephrocalcinosis

The term 'nephrocalcinosis' means diffuse renal parenchymal calcification that is detectable radiologically (**Fig. 36.31**). The condition is typically painless. Hypertension and CKD commonly occur. The main causes of nephrocalcinosis are listed in **Box 36.21**.

Dystrophic calcification occurs following renal cortical necrosis. In **hypercalcaemia and hyperoxaluria**, deposition of calcium oxalate results from the high concentration of calcium and oxalate within the kidney.

In **renal tubular acidosis** (see p. 199), failure of urinary acidification and a reduction in urinary citrate excretion both favour calcium phosphate and oxalate precipitation, since precipitation occurs more readily in an alkaline medium and the calcium-chelating action of urinary citrate is reduced.

Management and prevention of nephrocalcinosis consist of treating the cause.

Further reading

Pickard R, Starr K, MacLennan G et al. Medical expulsive therapy in adults with ureteric colic: a multicentre, randomised, placebo-controlled trial. *Lancet* 2015; 386:341–349.
Zisman AL. Effectiveness of treatment modalities on kidney stone recurrence. *Clin J Am Soc Nephrol* 2017; 12:1699–1708.

URINARY TRACT OBSTRUCTION

Urinary tract obstruction can occur at any point between the kidney and the urethral meatus. Obstruction can be partial or complete, and

Within the lumen
- Calculus
- Blood clot
- Sloughed papilla (diabetes; analgesia misuse; sickle cell disease or trait)
- Tumour of renal pelvis, ureter or bladder

Within the wall
- Pelviureteric neuromuscular dysfunction (congenital, 10% bilateral)
- Ureteric stricture (tuberculosis, especially after treatment; calculus; after surgery)
- Ureterovesical stricture (congenital; ureterocele; calculus; schistosomiasis)
- Congenital megaureter
- Congenital bladder neck obstruction
- Neuropathic bladder
- Urethral stricture (calculus; gonococcal; after instrumentation)
- Congenital urethral valve
- Pin-hole meatus

Pressure from outside
- Pelviureteric compression (bands; aberrant vessels)
- Tumours (e.g. retroperitoneal tumour or glands; carcinoma of colon; tumours in pelvis, e.g. carcinoma of cervix)
- Diverticulitis
- Aortic aneurysm
- Retroperitoneal fibrosis (peri-aortitis, eg IgG4 disease)
- Accidental ligation of ureter
- Retrocaval ureter (right-sided obstruction)
- Prostatic obstruction
- Phimosis

leads to delayed transit of urine, rising urinary tract (and intrarenal) pressure, and – if obstructing both kidneys – eventual renal impairment.

Aetiology

Obstructing lesions may lie within the lumen, in the wall of the urinary tract or outside the wall, causing obstruction by external pressure. Obstruction causing dilation of the renal pelvis and/or ureter is known as hydronephrosis. The major causes of obstruction are shown in **Box 36.22**. In children, obstruction usually results from congenital abnormalities or urethral valves. In young women, pelvic tumours, pregnancy or stones cause obstruction. In younger men, stones are the dominant cause, but bladder outflow obstruction (prostatic disease) dominates later in life.

Pathophysiology

Urine continues to be formed despite obstruction to flow. This leads to:
- progressive rise in intraluminal pressure
- dilation proximal to the site of obstruction
- compression and thinning of the renal parenchyma, eventually reducing it to a thin rim and resulting in a decrease in the size of the kidney.

Acute obstruction is followed by transient renal arterial vasodilation succeeded by vasoconstriction, probably mediated mainly by angiotensin II and thromboxane A_2. Ischaemic interstitial damage mediated by free oxygen radicals and inflammatory cytokines compounds the damage induced by compression of the renal substance.

Clinical features

Symptoms

Loin pain occurs, which can be dull or sharp, and constant or intermittent. Pain is made worse if urine flow and volume increase, as the collecting system distends. A high fluid intake or diuretics, including alcohol and coffee, may provoke pain.

Complete anuria is strongly suggestive of complete bilateral obstruction or complete obstruction of a single kidney.

Polyuria may occur in partial obstruction, as rising pressures impair renal tubular concentrating capacity; intermittent anuria and polyuria indicate intermittent complete obstruction.

Infection is a major complication and may give rise to malaise, fever and septicaemia.

Bladder outflow obstruction may occur with few symptoms. Hesitancy, narrowing and diminished force of the urinary stream, terminal dribbling (lower urinary tract symptoms, or LUTS) and a sense of incomplete bladder emptying are typical features (see p. 1480). Infection is common (and may precipitate acute retention) with frequency, urgency, urge incontinence, dysuria and the passage of cloudy, smelly urine. Acute bladder retention causes significant discomfort and distress, though in the elderly may present as confusion and agitation alone.

Signs

On abdominal palpation, loin tenderness may be present, and occasionally an enlarged hydronephrotic kidney is palpable. In acute or chronic retention the enlarged bladder can be felt or percussed. Examination of the genitalia, rectum and vagina is performed, since prostatic obstruction and pelvic malignancy are common causes of urinary tract obstruction. However, the apparent size of the prostate on digital examination is a poor guide to the presence of prostatic obstruction.

Investigations

- **Urinalysis** is performed for haematuria.
- **A mid-stream sample of urine for MC&S** is assessed to exclude infection.
- **Routine biochemical investigations** may show a raised serum urea or creatinine (or a reduced eGFR), hyperkalaemia, or anaemia of chronic disease. Prostate-specific antigen may be abnormal (see p. 1480).
- **Ultrasonography** (see p. 1350) is the investigation of choice to confirm or rule out upper urinary tract dilation. Ultrasound cannot distinguish a baggy, low-pressure, unobstructed system from a tense, high-pressure, obstructed one, so that false-positive scans are seen. Stones in the ureter can be missed.
- **Plain abdominal X-ray** may detect radiolucent stones/calcification but can miss stones lying over the bone.
- **CT scanning** has a high sensitivity and can visualize uric acid (radiolucent) stones as small as 1 mm, as well as details of the obstruction. CT also allows detection of local mass lesions or lymphadenopathy.
- **Excretion urography** is now seldom used. A characteristic delayed nephrogram is seen on the obstructed side (owing to a reduction in the GFR). With time, the nephrogram on the affected side becomes denser than normal, owing to the prolonged nephron transit time, and the site of obstruction with proximal dilation is seen (**Fig. 36.32**).
- **Radionuclide studies** (see p. 1351) have a role in longstanding obstruction to differentiate true obstructive nephropathy from retention of tracer in a baggy, low-pressure, unobstructed pelvicalyceal system.
- **Antegrade pyelography and ureterography** (see p. 1351) define the site and cause of obstruction. This technique can be combined with drainage of the collecting system by percutaneous needle nephrostomy.

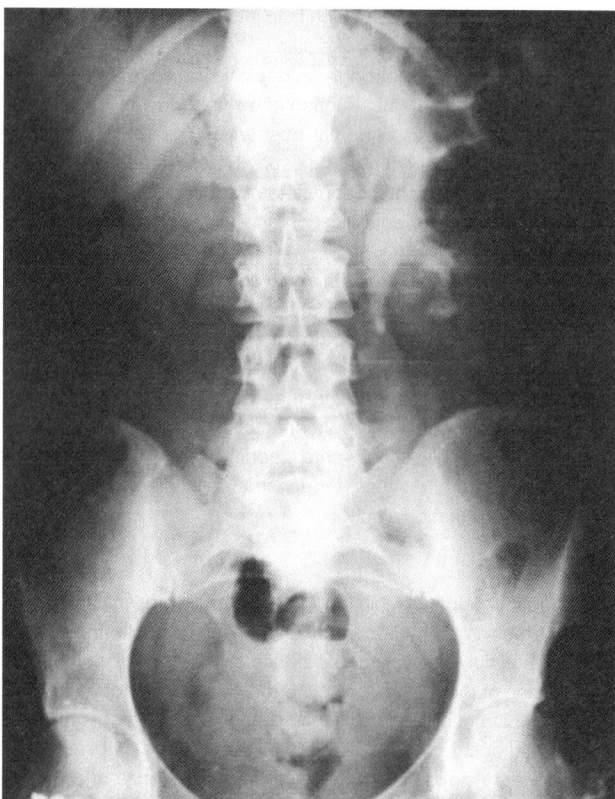

Fig. 36.32 Intravenous urographic X-ray taken 24 hours after injection of contrast. A delayed nephrogram and pyelogram are shown on the left side, with dilation of the system to the level of the block. By this time, contrast medium has disappeared from the normal right side.

- *Retrograde ureterography* (see p. 1350) offers the option of relieving ureteric obstruction from below at the time of examination. In obstruction due to neuromuscular dysfunction at the pelviureteric junction or retroperitoneal fibrosis, the collecting system may fill normally from below.
- *Cystoscopy, urethroscopy and urethrography* can visualize obstructing lesions within the bladder and urethra directly. Urethrography involves introducing contrast medium into the bladder by catheterization or suprapubic bladder puncture, and taking X-ray films during voiding to show obstructing lesions in the urethra. It is of particular value in the diagnosis of urethral valves and strictures.

Management

Treatment aims to:
- relieve the obstruction
- treat the underlying cause
- prevent and treat infection
- preserve renal function.

An obstructed and infected urinary tract is a medical emergency; delay can lead to septicaemia.
- Bladder catheterization offers rapid relief of outflow tract obstruction. If a urinary catheter cannot be passed urethrally, a suprapubic catheter should be placed.
- Obstructed and hydronephrotic kidneys can be relieved by placing a percutaneous nephrostomy under ultrasound guidance.
- It is also possible to relieve obstructed ureters by cystoscopic (retrograde) stenting.

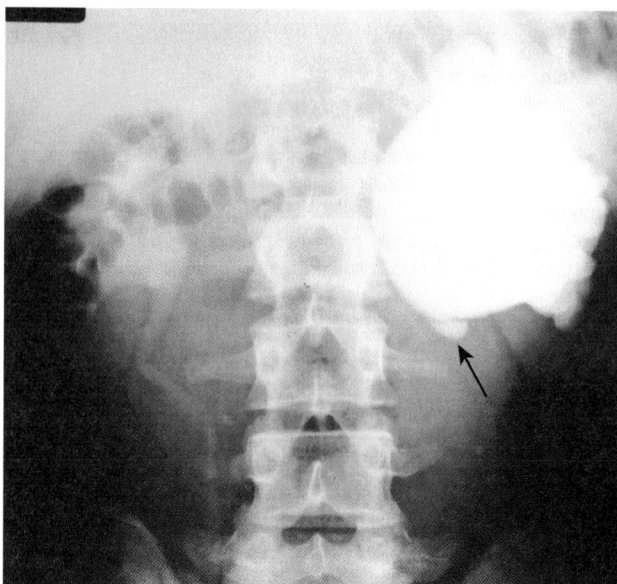

Fig. 36.33 X-ray showing left pelviureteric junction obstruction (arrowed).

In contrast, with partial urinary tract obstruction, particularly if spontaneous relief is expected – such as by passage of a calculus – there is no immediate urgency. *Surgical management* depends on the cause of the obstruction (see later) and local expertise. Dialysis may be required in the ill patient prior to surgery.

Post-obstructive diuresis

This occurs after relief of the obstruction at any site in the urinary tract. Massive diuresis may occur following relief of bilateral obstruction, as prior sodium and water retention, the osmotic effect of retained solutes and defective renal tubular reabsorptive capacity correct. This diuresis is associated with increased blood volume and high levels of atrial natriuretic peptide (ANP). The diuresis is usually self-limiting, but a minority of patients develop severe sodium, water and potassium depletion needing intravenous replacement. In milder cases, oral salt and potassium supplements, together with a high water intake, are sufficient.

Specific causes of obstruction

Calculi

These are discussed on page 1373.

Pelviureteric junction obstruction

A functional disturbance in peristalsis of the collecting system, without any mechanical obstruction, causes pelvic hydronephrosis (**Fig. 36.33**). In patients with recurrent loin pain or progressive kidney damage, surgical correction by open or percutaneous pyeloplasty is indicated.

Obstructive megaureter

This childhood condition may become evident only in adult life. It results from the presence of a region of defective peristalsis at the lower end of the ureter adjacent to the ureterovesical junction. The condition is more common in males. It presents with urinary tract infection, flank pain or haematuria. The diagnosis is made on imaging with ultrasound, CT or, if necessary, ascending ureterography.

Excision of the abnormal portion of ureter with re-implantation into the bladder is always indicated in children and in adults when the condition is associated with evidence of progressive deterioration in renal function, bacteriuria that cannot be controlled by medical means, or recurrent stone formation.

Retroperitoneal fibrosis (chronic peri-aortitis)

Retroperitoneal fibrosis (RPF) is a descriptive term used when inflammatory fibrotic tissue encases the aorta and ureters; it has a number of underlying causes. RPF is three times more common in men than in women and is an IgG4-related disease (see p. 65).

Extraluminal ureteric obstruction leads to unilateral or bilateral obstruction. The condition may extend from the level of the second lumbar vertebra to the pelvic brim. In up to 15% of patients the fibrotic process can extend outside the retroperitoneum, consistent with it being a systemic condition. Mediastinal fibrosis, Riedel fibrosing thyroiditis, sclerosing cholangitis, fibrotic orbital pseudotumour, fibrotic arthropathy, and pleural, pericardial and lung fibrosis have been reported with increasing frequency in IgG4-related disease.

RPF is thought to be either an autoallergic response to leakage of material, probably ceroid, from atheromatous plaques, producing an inflammatory reaction, or a systemic autoimmune disease. There is an association with HLA-DRB1*03, an allele linked to various autoimmune diseases. RPF is possibly initiated as a vasa vasorum vasculitis in the aortic wall, which is often seen in chronic peri-aortitis. This inflammatory process can cause medial wall thinning and promote atherosclerosis, and also extends into the surrounding retroperitoneum with a fibro-inflammatory reaction typical of chronic peri-aortitis. The autoimmune reaction to plaque antigens could be an epiphenomenon of this immune-mediated process. Activating antibodies against fibroblasts (detectable in one-third of patients) have also been implicated in the pathogenesis, as has the presence of **IgG4-bearing plasma cells**; the latter is a common finding in autoimmune chronic pancreatitis, a disorder sometimes associated with idiopathic retroperitoneal fibrosis. In addition, several infiltrating B cells show clonal or oligoclonal immunoglobulin heavy chain rearrangement. These findings raise the possibility of RPF being a primary B-cell disorder.

Aetiology of RPF

Causes are many:
- **Idiopathic** (in 60–70%).
- **Secondary** causes include:
  - drugs (methysergide, lysergic acid, ergot-derived dopamine receptor agonists (cabergoline, bromocriptine, pergolide), ergotamine, methyldopa, hydralazine, beta-blockers)
  - malignancy (carcinomas of the colon, prostate, breast, stomach, carcinoid, Hodgkin and non-Hodgkin lymphomas, sarcomas)
  - infection (tuberculosis, syphilis, histoplasmosis, actinomycosis, fungal infections)
  - surgery/radiotherapy (lymph node resection, colectomy, hysterectomy, aortic aneurysm repair).

Recognized associations include untreated abdominal aortic aneurysm, smoking and asbestosis.

Clinical features and investigation of RPF

RPF may present with malaise, low back pain, weight loss, testicular pain, claudication and haematuria.

Laboratory tests show normochromic anaemia, CKD, raised ESR and CRP, and increased serum IgG4 levels. **Imaging** with ultrasound will show a poorly circumscribed peri-aortic mass. The test of choice is contrast-enhanced CT, which will show the mass,

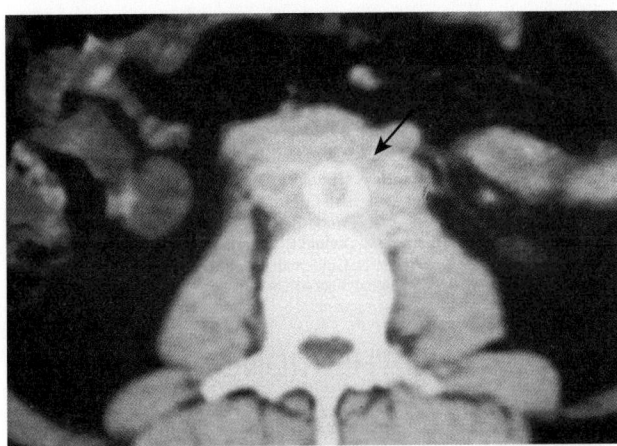

Fig. 36.34 Retroperitoneal fibrosis (peri-aortitis). Note the large mass (arrowed) surrounding the abdominal aorta on this CT scan.

lymph nodes and tumour (**Fig. 36.34**). MRI will demonstrate similar findings but does not require contrast. FDG-PET, a functional imaging modality, assesses the metabolic activity of the retroperitoneal mass; it also allows whole-body imaging and can detect occult malignant or infectious foci, particularly in secondary RPF.

Management of RPF

A biopsy is performed to exclude an underlying infection, lymphoma or carcinoma. Initial management may involve decompressing obstructed ureters by stenting (anterograde or retrograde). Corticosteroids may reverse the obstructing inflammatory tissue, if only as a holding measure before definitive treatment of the underlying cause. Rituximab is effective in cases of proven IgG4-related disease. Response to treatment and disease activity are assessed by serial measurements of ESR and eGFR, and repeat FDG-PET scans can also monitor disease.

Obstruction is relieved surgically by ureterolysis. A long-term ureteric stent or stents can be used with chronic corticosteroid therapy, but regular (usually 6-monthly) changes of the stent(s) are required if the peri-aortic mass does not regress.

Relapse after withdrawal of steroid therapy may occur and treatment may need to be continued for years. Mycophenolate or tamoxifen is also effective. Long-term follow-up is mandatory.

Benign prostatic hypertrophy

Benign prostatic hypertrophy (see p. 1480) is a common cause of urinary tract obstruction.

Prognosis of urinary tract obstruction

The prognosis depends on the cause and the stage at which obstruction is relieved. Four factors influence the rate at which kidney damage occurs, its extent, and the degree and rapidity of recovery of renal function after relief of obstruction:
- whether obstruction is partial or complete
- the duration of obstruction
- the presence or absence of infection
- the site of obstruction.

Complete obstruction for several weeks will lead to irreversible or only partially reversible kidney damage. If complete obstruction lasts several months, irreversible destruction of the affected kidney occurs. Partial obstruction carries a better prognosis, depending on its severity. Bacterial infection with obstruction rapidly increases kidney damage. Obstruction at or below the bladder neck leads to hypertrophy and trabeculation of the bladder without a rise in pressure within the upper urinary tract, in which case the kidneys are protected from the effects of back-pressure.

Further reading

Stone JH, Zen Y, Deshpande V. IgG4-related disease. *N Engl J Med* 2012; 366:539–551.
Yaqoob MM, Bennett-Richards K, Junaid I. Retroperitoneal fibrosis. In: Turner N, Lameire N, Goldsmith GJ et al (eds). *Oxford Textbook of Clinical Nephrology*, 4th edn. Oxford: Oxford University Press; 2016; pp. 2861–2864.
Yaqoob MM, Bennett-Richards K, Junaid I. The patient with urinary tract obstruction. In: Turner N, Lameire N, Goldsmith GJ et al (eds). *Oxford Textbook of Clinical Nephrology*, 4th edn. Oxford: Oxford University Press; 2016; pp. 2854–2860.

DRUGS AND THE KIDNEY

The kidney eliminates many drugs, as well as the (often active) products of drug metabolism in the liver. Dosing requires some thought with CKD, particularly in the elderly. Many drugs can further impair renal function, either over time, or acutely if hypovolaemia occurs (with vomiting or diarrhoea, for example), where a prescribed drug (such as an ACE inhibitor) prevents an appropriate response.

Drug-induced impairment of renal function

Renal perfusion falls with drugs that cause:
- hypovolaemia, e.g.:
  - loop diuretics such as furosemide, especially in elderly patients
  - renal salt and water loss, such as from hypercalcaemia induced by vitamin D therapy (since hypercalcaemia adversely affects renal tubular salt and water conservation)
- decrease in cardiac output, which impairs renal perfusion (e.g. beta-blockers)
- decrease in renal blood flow (e.g. ACE inhibitors, particularly in the presence of renovascular disease).

Drugs may directly damage the kidney:
- ***Acute tubular necrosis produced by direct nephrotoxicity*** from prolonged or high-dose treatment with aminoglycosides (e.g. gentamicin, amikacin), amphotericin B, tenofovir, cisplatin or calcineurin inhibitors. The combination of aminoglycosides with loop diuretics is particularly nephrotoxic.
- ***Crystal nephropathies*** caused by antivirals such as aciclovir and indinavir.
- ***Acute tubulointerstitial nephritis*** (see p. 1385), a cell-mediated hypersensitivity nephritis occurring with many drugs, including penicillins, cephalosporins, proton pump inhibitors, diuretics, sulphonamides and NSAIDs (which have many other effects on the kidney; **Box 36.23**).
- ***Chronic tubulointerstitial nephritis*** due to drugs (see p. 1386).
- ***Membranous glomerulonephritis***, e.g. penicillamine, gold, anti-TNF (see p. 1357).
- Retroperitoneal fibrosis with urinary tract obstruction – can result from the use of drugs (see p. 1379).

Using drugs in patients with impaired renal function

See **Box 36.24**.

Absorption

Absorption can be unpredictable in uraemia, as gastric emptying may be delayed, and nausea and vomiting are frequent.

 Box 36.23 Non-steroidal anti-inflammatory drugs and the kidney

Problem	Cause
Sodium and water retention	Reduction of prostaglandin production
Acute tubulointerstitial nephritis	Hypersensitivity reaction
Nephrotic syndrome	Membranous glomerulopathy
Analgesic nephropathy	Papillary necrosis after chronic use
Acute kidney injury	Acute tubular necrosis
Hyperkalaemia	Decreased renal excretion of K^+

 Box 36.24 Safe prescribing in kidney disease

Safe prescribing in CKD demands knowledge of the clinical pharmacology of the drug and its metabolites in normal individuals and in uraemia. The clinician should ask the following questions when prescribing, and discuss them with the patient:
1. *Is treatment mandatory?* Unless it is, it should be withheld.
2. *Can the drug reach its site of action?* For example, there is little point in prescribing the urinary antiseptic nitrofurantoin in severe CKD since bacteriostatic concentrations will not be attained in the urine.
3. *Is the drug's metabolism altered in uraemia?*
4. *Will accumulation of the drug or metabolites occur?* Even if accumulation is a potential problem, owing to the drug or its metabolites being excreted by the kidneys, it is not necessarily an indication to change the drug given. The size of the loading dose will depend on the size of the patient and is unrelated to renal function. Avoidance of toxic levels of drug in blood and tissues subsequently requires the administration of normal doses of the drug at longer time intervals than usual, or in smaller doses at the usual time intervals.
5. *Is the drug toxic to the kidney?*
6. *Are the effective concentrations* of the drug in biological tissues similar to the toxic concentrations? Should blood levels of the drug be measured?
7. *Will the drug worsen the uraemic state* by means other than nephrotoxicity, e.g. steroids, tetracycline?
8. *Is the drug a sodium or potassium salt?* These are potentially hazardous in uraemia.

Not surprisingly, adverse drug reactions are more than twice as common in patients with CKD as in normal individuals. Elderly patients, in whom unsuspected CKD is common, are particularly at risk. Attention to the above and titration of the dose of drugs employed should reduce the problem.

The dose may be titrated by:
- observation of its clinical effect, e.g. hypotensive agents
- early detection of toxic effects
- measurement of drug levels in the blood, e.g. gentamicin levels.

Metabolism

The rate of drug metabolism by the kidney is reduced as a result of:
- ***Reduced drug catabolism.*** Insulin, for example, is in part catabolized by the normal kidney. In renal disease, insulin catabolism is reduced. For this reason, the insulin requirements of diabetics decline as renal function deteriorates.
- ***Reduced conversion of a precursor to a more active metabolite.*** An example is the conversion of 25-hydroxycholecalciferol to the more active $1,25\text{-}(OH)_2D_3$. The 1α-hydroxylase enzyme responsible for this conversion is located in the kidney. In renal disease, production of the enzyme declines and deficiency of $1,25\text{-}(OH)_2D_3$ results.

Protein binding

Reduced protein binding of a drug potentiates its activity and increases the potential for toxic side-effects. Hypoalbuminaemia (in the nephrotic syndrome) leads to increased free drug, as do uraemic toxins binding to albumin (occupying drug-binding sites). Measurement of total plasma concentration (albumin-bound and free drug) of such drugs can give misleading results. For example, more free phenytoin than albumin-bound phenytoin is present in CKD, for the same total plasma concentration seen in healthy individuals – and lower levels will control seizures in patients with CKD.

Volume of distribution

Salt and water overload or depletion may occur in patients with renal disease. This affects the concentration of drug obtained from a given dose.

End-organ sensitivity

The renal response to drug treatment may be reduced in renal disease. For example, mild thiazide diuretics have little diuretic effect in patients with severe CKD.

Renal elimination

In CKD, drugs eliminated by the kidneys are no longer excreted normally. Water-soluble drugs, such as gentamicin, which are poorly absorbed from the gut, typically given by injection and not metabolized by the liver, give rise to far more problems than lipid-soluble drugs such as propranolol, which are well absorbed and principally metabolized by the liver.

Drugs affecting protein anabolism and catabolism

Tetracyclines, with the exception of doxycycline, have a catabolic effect. Increased nitrogenous waste products are not well cleared and uraemia may be more marked. Corticosteroids also have a catabolic effect and may lead to a disproportionate increase in urea compared to creatinine when used in high doses in CKD.

Problem patients

Particular problems are presented by patients with rapidly changing renal function, such as those with evolving AKI or recovering acute tubular necrosis. In addition, drugs may be removed by dialysis and haemofiltration, which will affect the dosage required.

URINARY TRACT INFECTION

Urinary tract infection (UTI) is common, particularly in women, most often occurring in a normal urinary tract and usually as cystitis; half of all women will experience a UTI in their lifetime. Most UTIs occur in isolation (**Fig. 36.35**). It is uncommon in men and children; when diagnosed, it often occurs in an abnormal urinary tract. Between 1% and 2% of patients presenting in primary care will have a UTI. UTI is not always uncomplicated; recurrent infection causes considerable morbidity, and infection can lead to life-threatening Gram-negative septicaemia and kidney failure.

Aetiology and pathogenesis

Infection is most often caused by bacteria from a patient's own bowel flora (**Box 36.25**) and usually ascends up the urethra. In women the short urethra makes ascending infection more likely. Rarely, infection may arise from the bloodstream or lymphatics, or by direct extension (e.g. from a vesicocolic fistula).

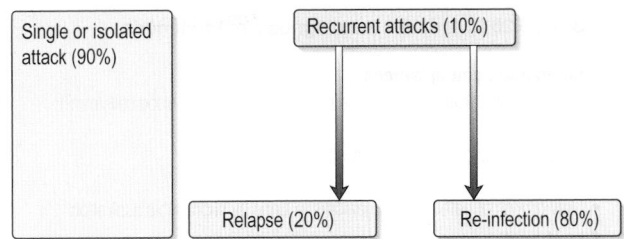

Fig. 36.35 The natural history of urinary tract infection.

| Single or isolated attack (90%) | Recurrent attacks (10%) |
| Relapse (20%) | Re-infection (80%) |

Box 36.25 Organisms causing urinary tract infection in domiciliary practice

Organism	Approximate frequency (%)
Escherichia coli and other 'coliforms'	70
Proteus spp.	12
Staphylococcus saprophyticus or *epidermidis*[a]	10
Enterococcus faecalis[b]	6
Pseudomonas spp.	5
Klebsiella spp.	4

[a]More common in young women (20–30%).
[b]More common in hospital practice.

Bacterial virulence

How well an organism adheres to urothelium determines its virulence. The presence of flagella (for motility), aerobactin (used to acquire iron), haemolysin (to form pores) and, above all, the presence of fimbriae (adhesins that attach organisms to the perineum and urothelium) on the bacterial cell surface make *E. coli* such a common pathogen.

Innate host defence

Innate host defence prevents UTI in the following ways:
- **Neutrophils.** Bacterial adhesins activate receptors, e.g. Toll receptor 4, on the mucosal surface, resulting in IL-8 production and expression of its receptor, CXCR1, on neutrophil surfaces. Activation of neutrophils is essential for bacterial killing.
- **Urine osmolality and pH.** Urinary osmolality >800 mOsm/kg and low or high pH reduce bacterial survival.
- **Complement.** Complement activation with mucosal IgA production by uroepithelium (acquired immunity) plays a major role in defence against UTI.
- **Commensal organisms.** Eradication of commensal organisms such as lactobacilli, corynebacteria, streptococci and bacteroides by spermicidal jelly or antibiotics results in overgrowth of *E. coli*.
- **Urine flow.** Good urine flow and normal micturition wash out bacteria. Urine stasis promotes UTI.
- **Uroepithelium.** Mannosylated Tamm–Horsfall proteins, present in the mucus and glycocalyx covering uroepithelium, have antibacterial properties and interfere with bacterial binding to uroepithelium. Cranberry juice and blueberry juice contain a large-molecular-weight factor (pro-anthrocyanidins) that prevents binding of *E. coli* to the uroepithelium.
- **Blood group antigens.** Women who are non-secretors of ABH blood group antigens are 3–4 times more likely to have recurrent UTIs.

> *i* **Box 36.26 Criteria for the diagnosis of bacteriuria**
>
> **Symptomatic young women**
> - $\geq 10^2$ coliform organisms/mL urine plus pyuria (>10 white blood cells/mm³)
>   *or*
> - $\geq 10^5$ any pathogenic organism/mL urine
>   *or*
> - Any growth of pathogenic organisms in urine by suprapubic aspiration
>
> **Symptomatic men**
> - $\geq 10^3$ pathogenic organisms/mL urine
>
> **Asymptomatic patients**
> - $\geq 10^5$ pathogenic organisms/mL urine on two occasions

Risk factors

- Female gender, especially postmenopausal women.
- New sexual activity, particularly in young women.
- Indwelling urinary catheter or instrumentation of the urinary tract.
- Urinary tract stones.
- Urinary tract stasis (incomplete bladder emptying).
- Diabetes mellitus or immunosuppression.
- Dementia.

Clinical features

The most typical symptoms of (lower) UTI are:
- frequency of micturition by day and night
- dysuria (painful voiding)
- suprapubic pain and tenderness
- haematuria
- smelly urine.

These are the symptoms of bladder and urethral inflammation, or 'cystitis'. Loin pain and tenderness, with fever, chills, night sweats and rigors, suggest extension of infection to the pelvis and kidney, known as pyelitis or pyelonephritis. Localization of the site of infection on the basis of symptoms alone is unreliable.

UTI can also present with few or no symptoms (particularly in the immunocompromised), or even with abdominal pain, fever or haematuria in the absence of frequency or dysuria. In the elderly, new confusion may be the only symptom of UTI. In small children, who cannot complain of dysuria, symptoms are often 'atypical'. The possibility of UTI must always be considered in the fretful, febrile, sick child who fails to thrive.

Diagnosis

Uncomplicated UTIs in younger women (age ≤65) can be diagnosed in those without known urinary tract abnormalities, recent urinary tract instrumentation, or systemic illness if they exhibit at least two of three cardinal symptoms – dysuria, urgency or frequency – along with an absence of vaginal discharge. Neither urine dipstick testing for leucocyte esterase nor urine culture enhances diagnostic sensitivity. Telephone-based protocols have outcomes similar to those of surgery-based diagnosis and treatment, and such methods are often preferred by patients. Patients with histories of uncomplicated UTIs can be taught to self-diagnose and initiate therapy.

Otherwise, diagnosis is based on culture of a clean-catch midstream specimen of urine and the presence or absence of pyuria. The criteria for the diagnosis of UTI, particularly in symptomatic women, are shown in **Box 36.26**. Most Gram-negative organisms reduce nitrates to nitrites and produce a red colour in the reagent square. False-negative results are common. Dipsticks that detect significant pyuria depend on the release of esterases from leucocytes. Dipstick tests that are positive for both nitrite and leucocyte

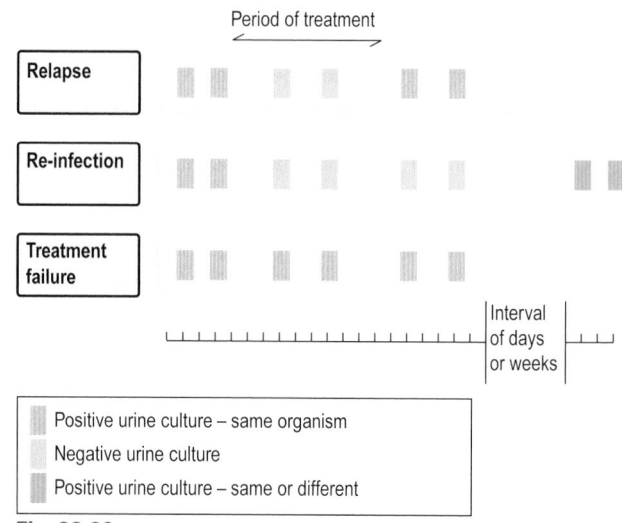

Fig. 36.36 A comparison of re-infection, relapse and treatment failure in urinary tract infection.

esterase are highly predictive of acute infection (sensitivity of 75% and specificity of 82%).

Re-infection may be distinguished from relapsing infection in the following ways:
- ***Relapse*** is diagnosed by recurrence of bacteriuria with the same organism within 7 days of completion of antibacterial treatment. Treatment failure may suggest (**Fig. 36.36**) associated stones, scarred kidneys, polycystic disease or bacterial prostatitis.
- ***Re-infection*** is when bacteriuria is absent after treatment for at least 14 days, usually longer, followed by recurrence of infection with the same or different organisms. This is not due to failure to eradicate infection but is the result of re-invasion of a susceptible tract with new organisms. Approximately 80% of recurrent infections are due to re-infection.

Where culture is negative and symptoms persist, consider:
- ***Abacteriuric frequency or dysuria ('urethral syndrome').*** This is caused by bladder trauma after intercourse; vaginitis, atrophic vaginitis or urethritis in the elderly; and *Chlamydia* infection and tuberculosis in symptomatic young women with 'sterile pyuria'.
- ***Interstitial cystitis.*** This is uncommon but distressing, affecting women over the age of 40. Patients present with frequency, dysuria and often severe suprapubic pain but cultures are sterile. Cystoscopy shows typical inflammatory changes with ulceration of the bladder base. It is now thought to be an autoimmune disorder. Treatments include oral prednisolone, bladder instillation of sodium cromoglicate or dimethyl sulphoxide, and bladder stretching under anaesthesia. Unfortunately, relief of symptoms can be difficult to achieve.
- ***Predominant frequency*** and passage of small volumes of urine ('irritable bladder'). These may occur after previous UTI.

Natural history

Serious morbidity is unusual. However, renal scarring can result from recurrent UTI, and dissemination of infection as septicaemia can be fatal. In patients with a ***normal urinary tract (with normal renal imaging)***, outcomes are very good, and persistent or recurrent infection seldom results in serious kidney damage (uncomplicated UTI). In those with ***abnormal urinary tracts*** (stones or stasis), recurrence is more common and outcomes are less good. The combination of infection and obstruction results in severe, sometimes rapid, kidney damage (obstructive pyonephrosis) and is

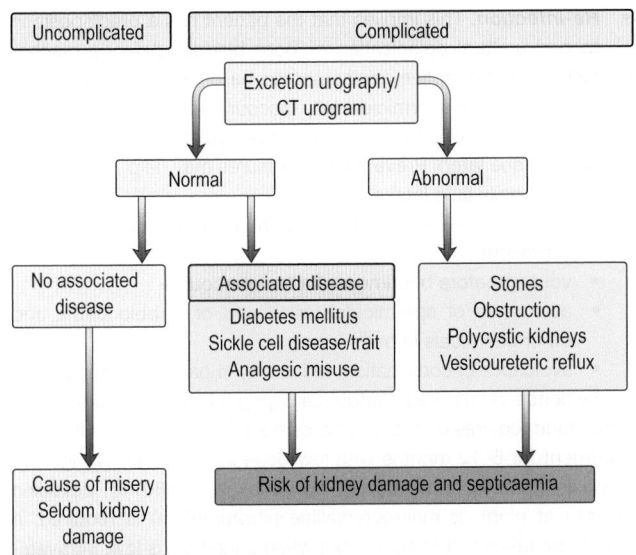

Fig. 36.37 Complicated versus uncomplicated urinary tract infection.

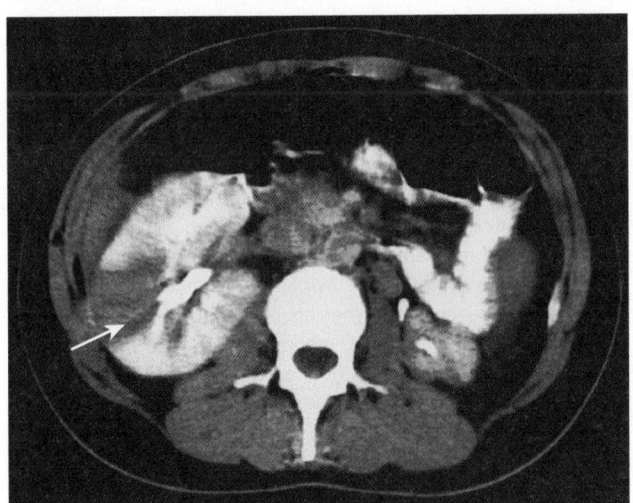

Fig. 36.38 Computed tomogram showing a wedge-shaped area of renal cortical loss (arrowed) following acute pyelonephritis.

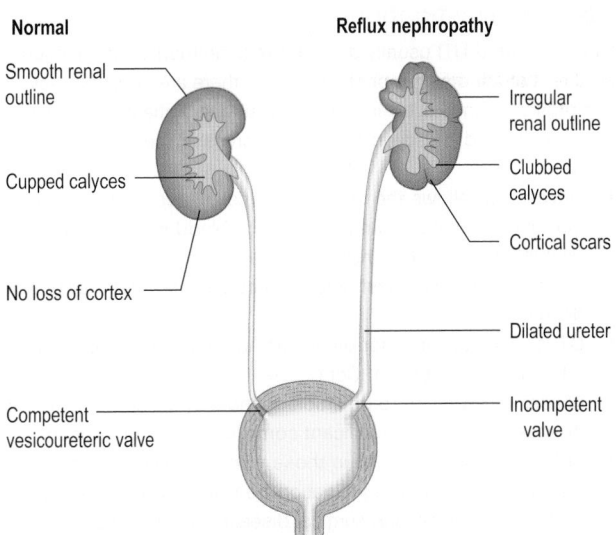

Fig. 36.39 Findings in patients with reflux nephropathy compared with normal individuals.

a major cause of Gram-negative septicaemia from *Pseudomonas* and *Enterobacter* spp. Complicated and uncomplicated infection is compared in **Fig. 36.37**.

Acute pyelonephritis

Fever, loin pain with tenderness and significant bacteriuria usually imply infection of the kidney (acute pyelonephritis). Small renal cortical abscesses and streaks of pus in the renal medulla are often present. Histologically, there is focal infiltration by polymorphonuclear leucocytes and many polymorphs in tubular lumina.

Although, with antibiotics, significant permanent kidney damage in adults with normal urinary tracts is rare, CT scanning can show wedge-shaped areas of inflammation in the renal cortex (**Fig. 36.38**), where renal function will be impaired.

Reflux nephropathy

This was called chronic pyelonephritis or atrophic pyelonephritis, resulting from a combination of:

• vesicoureteric reflux

• infection acquired in infancy or early childhood.

Normally, the vesicoureteric junction acts as a one-way valve (**Fig. 36.39**), urine entering the bladder from above; the ureter is shut off during bladder contraction, thus preventing reflux of urine. In some infants and children – possibly even *in utero* – this valve mechanism is incompetent, bladder voiding being associated with variable reflux of a jet of urine up the ureter. A secondary consequence is incomplete bladder emptying, as refluxed urine returns to the bladder after voiding. This latter event predisposes to infection, and the reflux of infected urine leads to kidney damage.

Typically, there is papillary damage, tubulointerstitial nephritis and cortical scarring in areas adjacent to 'clubbed calyces'.

Diagnosis is based on CT scan of the kidneys, which shows irregular renal outlines, clubbed calyces and a variable reduction in renal size. The condition may be unilateral or bilateral, and may affect all or part of the kidney.

Reflux usually ceases around puberty with growth of the bladder base (a thickened bladder wall is able to prevent reflux with bladder contraction). Damage already done persists and progressive renal fibrosis and further loss of function occur in severe cases, even though there is no further infection.

Reflux nephropathy cannot occur in the absence of reflux – it does not begin in adult life. Consequently, women with bacteriuria and a normal urogram can be reassured that kidney damage will not develop.

Chronic reflux nephropathy acquired in infancy predisposes to hypertension in later life and, if severe, is a relatively common cause of ESKD in childhood or adult life. Meticulous early detection and control of infection, with or without ureteral re-implantation to create a competent valve, can prevent further scarring and allow normal growth of the kidneys. No proof exists, however, that re-implantation surgery confers long-term benefit.

Continuous antibiotic prophylaxis (CAP), compared with no treatment, significantly reduces the risk of symptomatic UTI in children with chronic reflux nephropathy but at the expense of increased risk for developing antimicrobial-resistant bacterial strains. CAP does not have a significant impact on the occurrence of new renal scarring.

Special investigations

Uncomplicated UTI usually does not require imaging. If infection is recurrent or affects men or children, or if there are unusually severe symptoms, it should be investigated further. Patients with diabetes mellitus and those on immunosuppression benefit from early imaging.

- **Ultrasound** allows the detection of calculi, obstruction, abnormal urinary anatomy and incomplete bladder emptying (post-micturition scan). It is helpful in the assessment of suspected pyelonephritis or an obstructed, infected kidney that may require drainage.
- **CT** is more sensitive for diagnosis and follow-up of complicated renal tract infection. Contrast-enhanced CT allows different phases of excretion to be studied, and can define the extent of disease and identify significant complications or obstruction.
- **MRI** is particularly useful in those with iodinated contrast allergies, offering an ionizing radiation-free alternative in the diagnosis of both medical and surgical diseases of the kidney.
- **Nuclear medicine** has a limited role in the evaluation of UTI in adults. Its main role is in the assessment of renal function and detection of scars by DMSA scan, often prior to surgery.

Management

Management of a single isolated attack

- **The most appropriate antibiotic choices** are trimethoprim–sulfamethoxazole (160/800 mg twice daily for 3–7 days) or nitrofurantoin (100 mg twice daily for 5–7 days). Fluoroquinolones offer no advantage in terms of cure rates; β-lactam antibiotics, such as amoxicillin–clavulanate, are less effective than the first-line recommendations. Most patients who delay antibiotic treatment to encourage spontaneous resolution eventually receive antibiotics and have longer times to resolution. Men with uncomplicated UTIs should be treated as above but for 7–14 days.
- **Shorter 3–5-day courses** with amoxicillin (250 mg three times daily), trimethoprim (200 mg twice daily) or an oral cephalosporin are also used, and modified in light of the result of urine culture and sensitivity testing, and/or the clinical response.
- **Single-shot treatment** with 3 g of amoxicillin or 1.92 g of co-trimoxazole is used for patients with bladder symptoms of more than 36 hours' duration who have no previous history of UTI.
- **A high (2 L daily) fluid intake** should be encouraged during treatment and for some subsequent weeks. Urine culture should be repeated 5 days after treatment.
- **If the patient is acutely ill with high fever, loin pain and tenderness** (acute pyelonephritis), antibiotics are given intravenously, e.g. aztreonam, cefuroxime, ciprofloxacin or gentamicin, switching to a further 7 days' treatment with oral therapy as symptoms improve. Intravenous fluids may be required to achieve a good urine output.
- **In patients presenting for the first time with high fever, loin pain and tenderness**, urgent renal ultrasound examination is required to exclude an obstructed pyonephrosis. If this is present, it should be drained by percutaneous nephrostomy (see p. 1350).

Management of recurrent infection

Pre-treatment and post-treatment urine cultures are necessary to confirm the diagnosis and to establish whether recurrent infection is due to relapse or re-infection.

- **Relapse.** A search should be made for a cause (e.g. stones or scarred kidneys), and treatment modified if possible. Intense or prolonged treatment may be required. If this fails, long-term antibiotics are necessary.

- **Re-infection.** This implies that the patient has a predisposition to peri-urethral colonization or poor bladder defence mechanisms. Contraceptive advice should be offered and the use of a diaphragm or spermicidal jelly discouraged. Atrophic vaginitis should be identified in postmenopausal women, who should be treated (see later). Preventative measures may help:
  - a 2 L daily fluid intake
  - voiding at 2–3-hour intervals, with double micturition if reflux is present
  - voiding before bedtime and after intercourse
  - avoidance of spermicidal jellies and of bubble baths and other chemicals in bath water
  - avoidance of constipation, which may impair bladder emptying.

Evidence of impaired bladder emptying on excretion urography/ultrasound requires urological assessment. If UTI continues to recur, treatment for 6–12 months with low-dose alternating monthly prophylaxis (trimethoprim 100 mg, co-trimoxazole 480 mg, cefalexin 125 mg at night or macrocrystalline nitrofurantoin) is required; it should be taken last thing at night when urine flow is low. Intravaginal oestrogen therapy has been shown to produce a reduction in the number of episodes of UTI in postmenopausal women. Cranberry juice is said to reduce the risk of symptoms and re-infection by 12–20% but studies are limited.

Urinary infections in the presence of an indwelling catheter

Colonization of the bladder by a pathogen is common after a urinary catheter has been *in situ* for more than a few days, partly due to organisms forming biofilms. So long as the bladder catheter is in place, antibiotics are likely to be ineffective and will encourage the development of resistant organisms. The patient should be treated only if there are symptoms or evidence of infection. The catheter should always be replaced. When changing catheters, a single dose of antibiotic (e.g. gentamicin) is recommended.

Infection by *Candida* is a frequent complication of prolonged bladder catheterization. Treatment should be reserved for patients with evidence of invasive infection and those who are immunosuppressed. The catheter should be removed or replaced. In severe infections, continuous bladder irrigation with amphotericin 50 ´g/mL is useful.

Bacteriuria in pregnancy

Pregnant women should have their urine cultured, as 2–6% have asymptomatic bacteriuria (see p. 1460). Usually harmless in non-pregnant women, bacteriuria in pregnancy can lead to acute pyelonephritis and in late pregnancy may trigger pre-term labour. Ureteric dilation in response to hormonal changes may allow ascending infection. *Bacteriuria must always be treated and shown to be eradicated.* Re-infection may require prophylactic therapy. Tetracycline, trimethoprim, sulphonamides and quinolones are contraindicated in pregnancy. Amoxicillin and ampicillin, nitrofurantoin and oral cephalosporins may be used safely in pregnancy.

Bacterial prostatitis

Bacterial prostatitis is a relapsing infection that presents as perineal pain, recurrent epididymo-orchitis and prostatic tenderness, with pus in expressed prostatic secretions. Treatment is for 4–6 weeks with drugs that penetrate into the prostate, such as trimethoprim or ciprofloxacin. Long-term, low-dose treatment may be required. Prostadynia (prostatic pain in the absence of active infection) may persist long after the infection. Amitriptyline and carbamazepine may alleviate the symptoms.

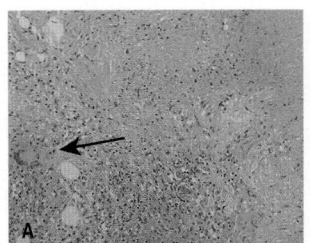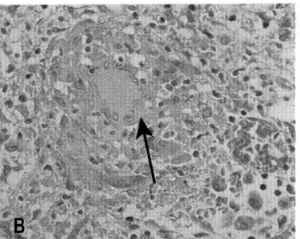

Fig. 36.40 Renal tuberculosis. **(A)** Caseating granulomatous interstitial nephritis showing multinuclear giant cell (arrowed). **(B)** Ziehl–Neelsen staining showing mycobacteria (arrowed).

Renal carbuncle

Renal carbuncle is an abscess in the renal cortex caused by a blood-borne staphylococcus, usually from a boil or carbuncle of the skin. It presents with a high, swinging fever, loin pain and tenderness, and fullness in the loin. The urine shows no abnormality, as the abscess does not communicate with the renal pelvis, more often extending into the perirenal tissue. Staphylococcal septicaemia is common. Diagnosis is by ultrasound or CT scanning. Treatment involves antibacterial therapy with flucloxacillin and surgical drainage.

Tuberculosis of the urinary tract

Tuberculous infection is on the increase worldwide, partly due to the reservoir of infection in susceptible HIV-infected individuals and the emergence of drug-resistant strains. Tuberculosis of the urinary tract presents with frequency, dysuria or haematuria. Cortical lesions result from haematogenous spread in the primary phase of infection. Most heal, but in some, infection persists and spreads to the papillae, with the formation of cavitating lesions and the discharge of mycobacteria into the urine. Infection of the ureters and bladder commonly follows, with the potential for development of ureteral strictures and a contracted bladder. Rarely, cold abscesses may form in the loin. In males, the disease may present with testicular or epididymal discomfort and thickening.

Diagnosis depends on constant awareness, especially in patients with sterile pyuria. Imaging may show cavitating lesions in the renal papillary areas, commonly with calcification. There may also be evidence of ureteral obstruction with hydronephrosis. Culture of mycobacteria from early morning urine samples is not straightforward. Imaging may be normal in diffuse interstitial renal tuberculosis, when diagnosis is made instead by renal biopsy, which demonstrates caseating granulomata with multinucleate giant cells and acid-fast bacilli on Ziehl–Neelsen staining (**Fig. 36.40**). Some patients present late with small, unobstructed kidneys, when the diagnosis is easy to miss.

Treatment is as for pulmonary tuberculosis (see p. 969). Renal ultrasonography and/or CT scanning should be carried out 2–3 months after initiation of treatment, as ureteric strictures may first develop in the healing phase.

Xanthogranulomatous pyelonephritis

This is an uncommon chronic interstitial infection of the kidney, most often due to *Proteus*, in which there is fever, weight loss, loin pain and a palpable enlarged kidney. It is usually unilateral and associated with staghorn calculi and UTI. CT scanning shows up intrarenal abscesses as lucent areas within the kidney. Nephrectomy is the treatment of choice; antibacterial treatment rarely, if ever, eradicates the infection.

Box 36.27 Common causes of acute tubulointerstitial nephritis

- Drugs (70%):
  - Antibiotics: cephalosporins, ciprofloxacin, erythromycin, penicillin, rifampicin, sulphonamides
  - Analgesics: non-steroidal anti-inflammatory drugs
  - Diuretics: furosemide, thiazides
  - Miscellaneous: allopurinol, carbamazepine, cimetidine, phenytoin, proton pump inhibitors, valproate
- Infection (15%):
  - Viruses, e.g. hantavirus
  - Bacteria, e.g. streptococci
- Idiopathic (8%)
- Tubulointerstitial nephritis with uveitis (TINU) (5%)
- Systemic inflammatory disorders, e.g.:
  - Systemic lupus erythematosus (2%)
  - IgG4-related disorder

Further reading

Chapagain A, Dobbie H, Sheaff M et al. Presentation, diagnosis, and treatment outcome of tuberculous-mediated tubulointerstitial nephritis. *Kidney Int* 2011; 79:671–677.
Hooton TM. Uncomplicated urinary tract infection. *N Engl J Med* 2012; 366:1028–1037.
Johnson JR, Rosso TA. Acute pyelonephritis in adults. *N Engl J Med* 2020;378:48–59.
Wise GJ, Schlegel PN. Sterile pyuria. *N Engl J Med* 2015; 372:1048–1054.

TUBULOINTERSTITIAL NEPHRITIS

Diseases of the kidney primarily affect the glomeruli, vasculature, or the substance of the renal parenchyma, made up of tubules and the interstitium. Tubular and interstitial injury and recovery tend to go hand in hand.

Acute tubulointerstitial nephritis

In approximately 70% of cases, acute tubulointerstitial nephritis (TIN) is a hypersensitivity reaction to drugs (**Box 36.27**), most commonly penicillins, NSAIDs or proton pump inhibitors.

Drug-induced acute TIN

Patients may be wholly asymptomatic (with impaired renal function found incidentally), or present with fever, arthralgia, skin rashes and acute oliguric or non-oliguric kidney injury. Many have eosinophilia and eosinophiluria. Renal histology shows an intense interstitial cellular infiltrate, often including eosinophils, with variable tubular necrosis (**Fig. 36.41**). Rarely, NSAIDs can cause a glomerular minimal-change lesion in addition to TIN and disease presents as the nephrotic syndrome. Treatment involves stopping the offending drug. High-dose prednisolone (60 mg daily) may reduce risk of dialysis-requiring AKI or shorten time to recovery. Most patients make a good recovery in terms of kidney function, but some may be left with significant interstitial fibrosis and CKD.

Infection causing acute TIN

Acute pyelonephritis leads to inflammation of the tubules, producing a neutrophilic cellular infiltrate. TIN can complicate systemic infections with viruses (Hantavirus, Epstein–Barr virus, HIV, measles, adenovirus), bacteria (*Legionella*, *Leptospira*, streptococci, *Mycoplasma*, *Brucella*, *Chlamydia*) and others (*Leishmania*, *Toxoplasma*). Hantavirus causes haemorrhagic fever with TIN and can be fatal. In immunocompromised patients, such as those who have had renal transplantation, cytomegalovirus, polyoma (BK) and herpes simplex

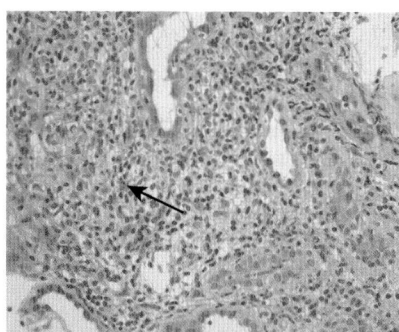

Fig. 36.41 Tubulointerstitial nephritis showing diffuse interstitial infiltrate with red staining eosinophils (arrowed).

virus can cause acute TIN in the renal graft. Treatment involves eradication of infection with appropriate antibiotics or antiviral agents; in renal transplantation, the immunosuppressive regimen is modified.

Acute TIN as part of multisystem inflammatory diseases

Several non-infectious inflammatory disorders, such as Sjögren's syndrome or SLE, can cause acute or chronic TIN rather than glomerulonephritis. Sjögren's syndrome may additionally present as renal tubular acidosis. Sarcoidosis presents as granulomatous TIN in up to 20% of patients. Associated hypercalcaemia causes AKI. These heterogeneous conditions with TIN generally respond to steroids.

TIN with uveitis syndrome

Patients with tubulointerstitial nephritis with uveitis (TINU) syndrome present with uveitis, an acute TIN, weight loss, anaemia and a raised ESR of unknown cause. It is common in childhood but has been reported in adulthood, and is more frequently found in women. It may be associated with autoantibodies directed against modified CRP. A prolonged course of steroids leads to improvement in both renal function and uveitis.

Chronic tubulointerstitial nephritis

The major causes of chronic TIN are given in **Box 36.28**. Patients present with any of polyuria, nocturia, proteinuria (usually slight, <1 g daily) or uraemia. Chronic TIN may be linked with papillary necrosis (ischaemic damage to the papillae, which then slough into the calyces and urine) when associated with longstanding analgesic use, diabetes mellitus, sickle cell disease or trait. Microscopic or overt haematuria or sterile pyuria also occurs, and occasionally a sloughed papilla may cause ureteric colic or produce acute ureteric obstruction. Histologically, a generalized chronic inflammatory cellular infiltration of the interstitium with tubular atrophy and generalized interstitial oedema or fibrosis is present, and in many cases no cause is found.

IgG4-related TIN is distinguished by very low concentrations of complement and increased serum IgG4. This may lead to immune complex formation.

The radiological appearances must be distinguished from those of reflux nephropathy (**Fig. 36.42**) or obstructive uropathy.

Tubular damage to the medullary area of the kidney leads to defects in urine concentration and sodium conservation with polyuria and salt wasting. Fibrosis progressing into the cortex leads to loss of excretory function and urea.

Analgesic nephropathy

The chronic consumption of large amounts of analgesics (classically, phenacetin but now NSAIDs) leads to chronic TIN and papillary

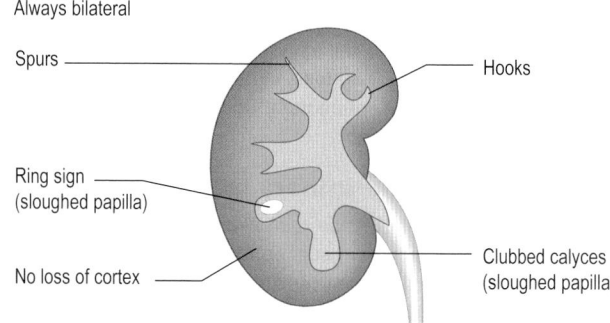

Box 36.28 Causes of chronic tubulointerstitial nephritis

Drugs and toxins, e.g.
- All causes of acute tubulointerstitial nephritis, e.g. analgesics
- Ciclosporin
- 5-aminosalicylates
- Cadmium, lead, titanium
- Irradiation

Systemic disease, e.g.
- Diabetes mellitus
- Sickle cell disease or trait
- Systemic lupus erythematosus/ vasculitis
- Sarcoidosis
- IgG4-related disease

Metabolic, e.g.
- Hyperuricaemia
- Nephrocalcinosis
- Hyperoxaluria

Infection, e.g.
- Human immunodeficiency virus
- Epstein–Barr virus

Miscellaneous
- Hypertension
- Balkan nephropathy
- Herbal nephropathy
- Alport's syndrome

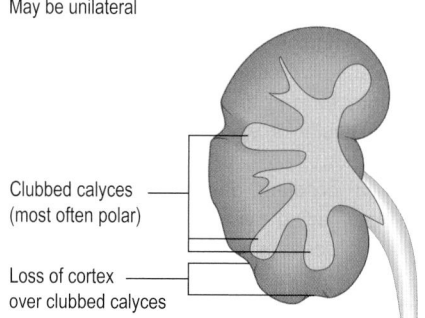

Papillary necrosis
Always bilateral

Spurs

Hooks

Ring sign (sloughed papilla)

No loss of cortex

Clubbed calyces (sloughed papilla)

Reflux nephropathy
May be unilateral

Clubbed calyces (most often polar)

Loss of cortex over clubbed calyces

Fig. 36.42 A comparison of the radiological appearances of papillary necrosis and reflux nephropathy.

necrosis. Analgesic nephropathy is more common in women and typically presents in middle age. Presentation may be with anaemia, CKD, UTIs, haematuria or urinary tract obstruction (owing to sloughing of a renal papilla). Salt- and water-wasting renal disease may occur. Chronic analgesic use also predisposes to the development of uroepithelial tumours. Diagnosis is usually made on clinical grounds combined with the non-pathognomonic appearance on imaging (such as ultrasonography or CT scan), which demonstrates smallish, irregularly outlined kidneys.

Patients should be encouraged to avoid NSAIDs, and, if necessary, dihydrocodeine or paracetamol may be offered as a reasonable alternative (this may stop further damage and even achieve an improvement). The development of flank pain or an unexpectedly rapid deterioration in renal function should prompt ultrasonography to screen for urinary tract obstruction due to a sloughed papilla.

Balkan nephropathy

Balkan nephropathy is a chronic TIN endemic in areas along the tributaries of the River Danube. Inhabitants of the low-lying plains, which are subjected to frequent flooding and where the water supply comes from shallow wells, are affected, whereas the disease does not occur in hillside villages where surface water provides the supply. Chronic dietary poisoning by aristolochic acid is thought to be responsible for Balkan nephropathy and the urothelial cancers that accompany the diagnosis. The disease is insidious in onset, with mild proteinuria progressing to ESKD in 3 months to 10 years. There is no treatment.

Chinese herb nephropathy

Chinese herbal medicines may contain aristolochic acid, produced as a result of fungal contamination of the product. Histology is similar to that of Balkan nephropathy but the clinical course is aggressive, with relentless progression to ESKD and a high incidence of uroepithelial tumours.

Other forms of chronic TIN

These are rare (see **Box 36.28**). Diagnosis of all forms depends on a history of drug ingestion or industrial exposure to nephrotoxins. In patients with unexplained renal impairment with normal-sized kidneys, renal biopsy must always be undertaken to exclude a treatable TIN, such as granulomatous TIN due to *renal sarcoidosis* (**Fig. 36.43**), which may be the first presentation of sarcoidosis (see p. 985). Renal sarcoidosis generally responds rapidly to steroids.

Hyperuricaemic nephropathy

Acute hyperuricaemic nephropathy (see p. 118), as part of tumour lysis syndrome, causes AKI in patients with very high serum urate concentrations. It may occur prior to treatment of haematological malignancies but more often supervenes after treatment. As the abundant tumour cells lyse in response to chemotherapy, large amounts of nucleoprotein are released with increased uric acid production. Renal failure is due to intrarenal and extrarenal obstruction caused by deposition of uric acid crystals in the collecting ducts, pelvis and ureters.

There may be flank pain or colic, and oliguria or anuria with increasing uraemia. Plasma urate levels are over 0.75 mmol/L and may be as high as 4.5 mmol/L. *Diagnosis* is based on the hyperuricaemia and the clinical setting. Ultrasound may demonstrate extrarenal obstruction due to stones but may be unremarkable.

Allopurinol 100–200 mg three times daily for 5 days is given prior to and throughout treatment with radiotherapy or cytotoxic drugs. A high rate of urine flow must be maintained by oral or parenteral fluid, and the urine kept alkaline by the administration of sodium bicarbonate and acetazolamide, since uric acid is more soluble in an alkaline than an acid medium. Febuxostat, a non-purine analogue inhibitor of xanthine oxidase, can be used if allopurinol cannot be tolerated and eGFR is more than 30 mL/min. *Rasburicase*, a recombinant urate oxidase (see p. 1392), and *pegloticase*, a pegylated uricase, are successfully used to lower serum urate concentrations rapidly for both treatment and prevention. In severely oliguric or anuric patients, dialysis is required to lower the plasma urate.

There is no convincing direct evidence for *chronic hyperuricaemia nephropathy*. However, a few observational studies have suggested that elevated levels of uric acid independently increase the risk for new-onset CKD, and that plasma urate reduction with allopurinol has a beneficial effect in slowing the rate of progression of CKD.

Further reading

Kamisawa T, Zen Y, Pillais S et al. IgG4-related disease. *Lancet* 2015; 385:1460–1471.

ACUTE KIDNEY INJURY

Acute kidney injury (AKI) is defined as follows:

- There is an abrupt deterioration in renal function, usually over hours or days.
- It is usually (but not always) reversible over days or weeks.

AKI may cause sudden, life-threatening biochemical disturbances as a medical emergency. Oliguria is often a feature. The distinction between AKI and CKD, or even acute-on-chronic kidney disease, is not always obvious. AKI is usually recognized by a falling urine output and rising serum urea and creatinine, or both. In some situations, urea and creatinine are less accurate predictors of deteriorating renal function (**Box 36.29**).

AKI may result from:

- *pre-renal* causes (reduced kidney perfusion leads to a falling GFR)
- *renal* parenchymal disorders (injury to glomerulus, tubule or vessels)
- *post-renal* causes (urinary tract obstruction – functioning kidneys cannot excrete urine with back-pressure affecting function).

The Acute Dialysis Quality Initiative group proposed the *RIFLE classification* (*r*isk, *i*njury, *f*ailure, *l*oss, *e*nd-stage renal disease) to define AKI better, using either an increase in serum creatinine or a decrease in urine output. RIFLE describes three levels of renal dysfunction (R, I, F) and two outcome measures (L, E). These criteria

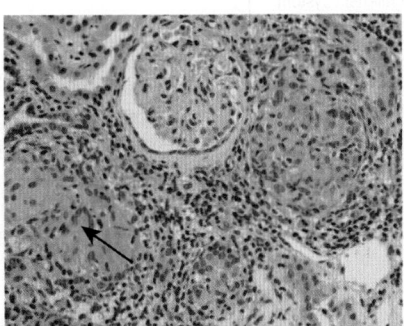

Fig. 36.43 Granulomatous tubulointerstitial nephritis. The granuloma consists of both giant cells (arrowed) and epithelioid cells. These findings are characteristic of renal sarcoid but can be seen with any cause (drug or infection) of interstitial nephritis.

?	Box 36.29 Causes of altered serum urea and creatinine concentration other than altered renal function	
Decreased concentration		**Increased concentration**
Urea		
Low protein intake		Corticosteroid treatment
Liver failure		Tetracycline treatment
Sodium valproate treatment		Gastrointestinal bleeding
Creatinine		
Low muscle mass		High muscle mass
		Red meat ingestion
		Muscle damage (rhabdomyolysis)
		Decreased tubular secretion (e.g. therapy with cimetidine or trimethoprim)

indicate an increasing degree of renal damage and have a predictive value for mortality.

The Acute Kidney Injury Network (AKIN) proposed a modification of the original RIFLE criteria to include less severe AKI and a time constraint of 48 hours, and gives a correction for volume status before classification.

- 'R' in RIFLE is **stage 1** (a serum creatinine rise of ≥26.4 μmol/L: i.e. a 1.5-fold increase within 48 hours).
- 'I' is **stage 2**: i.e. a 2–3-fold increase in serum creatinine.
- 'F' is **stage 3**: i.e. an increase in serum creatinine of >300% (equal to ≥354 μmol/L).

Urine output data are the same.

Using the same criteria of serum creatinine and urine output, a more recent classification (the Kidney Diseases: Improving Global Outcomes (KDIGO) classification) is shown in **Box 36.30**.

Epidemiology

Using the KDIGO definition, 1 in 5 adults and 1 in 3 children worldwide experience AKI during a hospital episode of care.

- Community-acquired AKI on admission to hospital affects approximately 5% in the UK (superimposed on CKD in half of these patients).
- Severe AKI (creatinine >500 μmol/L, often requiring dialysis) affects about 130–140 per million population per year.
- About 25% of patients with sepsis and 50% of patients with septic shock will have AKI.

ℹ️ Box 36.30 KDIGO[a] classification of acute kidney injury

Stage	Serum creatinine concentration (SCr)	Urine output criteria
1	SCr 1.5–1.9 times baseline OR ≥26.5 μmol/L (0.3 mg/dL) increase	<0.5 mL/kg/h for 6–12 h
2	SCr 2–2.9 times baseline	<0.5 mL/kg/h for 6–12 h
3	SCr 3 times baseline OR Initiation of renal replacement therapy OR In patients <18 years, decrease in eGFR to <35 mL/min per 1.73 m²	Anuria for ≥12 h

[a]Kidney Diseases: Improving Global Outcomes.

Outcomes vary: uncomplicated AKI carries a good prognosis, with mortality rates of less than 5–10%. In contrast, AKI complicating non-renal organ system failure (in the intensive treatment unit (ITU) setting) is associated with mortality rates of 50–70%, which have not changed for several decades. Sepsis-related AKI has a significantly worse prognosis than AKI in the absence of sepsis.

Approaching AKI

Pre-renal AKI

Falling renal blood flow leads to a falling GFR. This might be due either to changes in the circulation, or to intrarenal vasomotor changes that drop glomerular perfusion pressures. Common causes of a falling effective circulating volume include (**Box 36.31**):

- hypovolaemia of any cause, including dehydration or haemorrhage
- hypotension without hypovolaemia, including cirrhosis or septic shock
- low cardiac output, including cardiac failure or cardiogenic shock
- combinations of the above.

Common intra-renal causes include: NSAIDs, ACE inhibitors (**Fig. 36.44**), amphotericin B and calcineurin inhibitors, often in the context of added changes in renal blood flow.

Usually, the kidney maintains glomerular filtration close to normal, despite wide variations in renal perfusion pressure and volume status – so-called 'autoregulation' (prostaglandins, nitric oxide and angiotensin acting on afferent and efferent arterioles). Once autoregulation fails, GFR drops and AKI develops. Over time, reduced

---

❓ Box 36.31 Causes of hypovolaemia

- Dehydration
- Reduced intake (nil by mouth, confusion)
- Gut losses (vomiting, nasogastric tube losses, diarrhoea)
- Renal losses (diuretics, hyperglycaemia)
- Burns, sweating
- Haemorrhage
- Third space losses (pancreatitis, peritonitis, bowel obstruction)
- Systemic vasodilation (septic shock, cirrhosis)
- Cardiac failure or shock (myocardial infarction, arrhythmias, cardiomyopathy, tamponade)

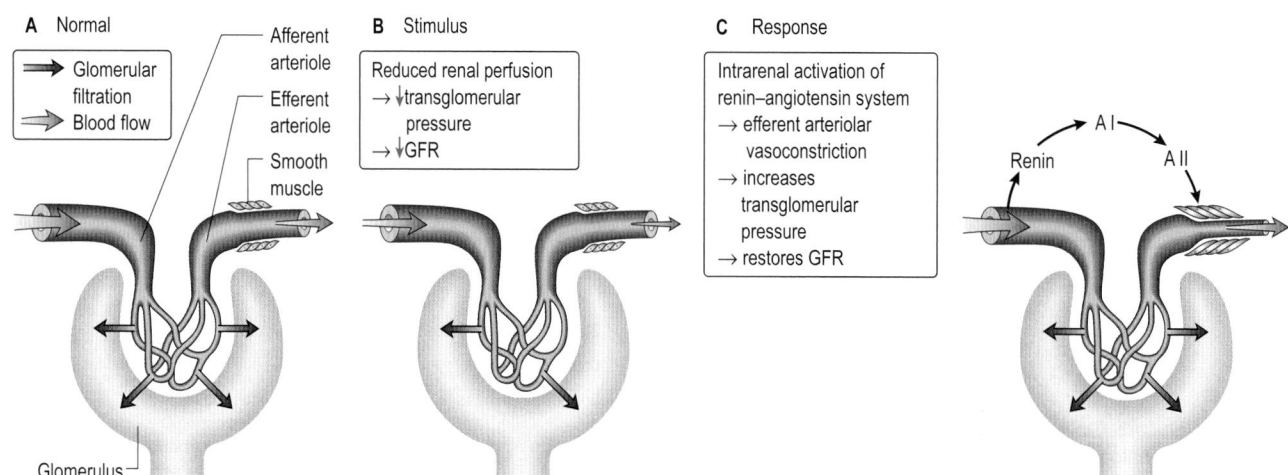

Fig. 36.44 Glomerular dynamics. Effect of the renin–angiotensin system. AI, angiotensin I; AII, angiotensin II; GFR, glomerular filtration rate.

Box 36.32 Criteria for distinction between pre-renal and intrinsic causes of renal dysfunction

Criteria	Pre-renal	Intrinsic
Urine specific gravity	>1.020	<1.010
Urine osmolality (mOsm/kg)	>500	<350
Urine sodium (mmol/L)	<10	>20
$Fe_{Na} = \frac{U_{Na}}{P_{Na}} + \frac{U_{Cr}}{P_{Cr}} \div 100$	<1%	>1%

Cr, creatinine; Fe, fractional excretion; Na, sodium; P, plasma; U, urine.

Box 36.33 Distinguishing causes of shock on clinical examination

	Hypovolaemia	Low cardiac output	Vasodilation
Hypotension	Postural hypotension	Hypotension	Hypotension
Peripheries	Cool	Cool	Warm
Jugular venous pressure	Low	Raised	Low

blood flow may lead to established parenchymal injury, but if renal perfusion is corrected early, AKI will resolve fully.

A few simple biochemical measures have long been used to prove pre-renal AKI (**Box 36.32**). Urine specific gravity or osmolality will rise, as solutes are concentrated into smaller urine volumes (the kidney is retaining fluid to improve renal blood flow). Urine sodium will be low, as salt is retained for the same reason. The fractional excretion of sodium (FE_{Na}) is a more reliable measure of sodium retention. None of these measures is reliable on its own and laboratory tests are no substitute for clinical assessment (**Box 36.33**).

Management of pre-renal AKI

This largely depends on the underlying cause. Most cases of AKI have an element of hypovolaemia, so prompt fluid resuscitation is most often indicated. When there is uncertainty as to the volume status of a patient, a fluid challenge of 250 mL crystalloid will often prove whether hypotension is fluid-responsive. Crystalloids and particularly balanced solutions such as plasmalyte and Ringer's lactate are the recommended resuscitative fluid, as normal saline can lead to hyperchloraemic acidosis. Colloids such as hydroxyethyl starch are contraindicated, as they can lead to worsening AKI. Heart rate, blood pressure and urine output will all guide response to resuscitation. For cardiogenic shock and septic shock, see page 218.

Post-renal AKI

Obstruction of the urinary tract may occur at any point from the calyces to the external urethral orifice but commonly takes the form of bladder outflow obstruction (prostate disease in men) or bilateral ureteric obstruction (stones or tumours). The causes and presentation of urinary tract obstruction are dealt with on page 1377. Almost every case of unexplained AKI should result in an ultrasound to exclude obstruction, as, once this is relieved (and if acute), renal function will return to baseline.

Renal parenchymal AKI

This is most commonly (80–90%) due to *acute tubular necrosis* (ATN; see later and **Box 36.34**). Almost any cause of pre-renal AKI, if prolonged to the point at which renal autoregulation fails (see

Box 36.34 Some causes of acute tubular necrosis

- Haemorrhage
- Burns
- Diarrhoea and vomiting, fluid loss from fistulae
- Pancreatitis
- Diuretics
- Myocardial infarction
- Congestive cardiac failure
- Endotoxic shock
- Snake bite
- Myoglobinaemia
- Haemoglobinaemia (due to haemolysis, e.g. in falciparum malaria, 'blackwater fever')
- Hepatorenal syndrome
- Radiological contrast agents (see p. 1391)
- Drugs, e.g. aminoglycosides, non-steroidal anti-inflammatory drugs, angiotensin-converting enzyme inhibitors, platinum derivatives
- Abruptio placentae
- Pre-eclampsia and eclampsia

earlier), will lead to ischaemic ATN. If not ischaemic, then ATN usually results from direct tubular toxins. As a result, ATN is common in hospital practice. Other causes of parenchymal AKI include:
- Disease affecting the intrarenal arteries and arterioles, as well as glomerular capillaries, such as a vasculitis (see p. 1363), accelerated hypertension, cholesterol embolism, HUS, TTP, pre-eclampsia and crescentic glomerulonephritis.
- Acute TIN (see p. 1385). This also occurs when renal tubules are acutely obstructed by crystals, e.g. after rapid lysis of certain malignant tumours following chemotherapy (acute hyperuricaemic nephropathy).
- Acute bilateral suppurative pyelonephritis or pyelonephritis of a single kidney, which can cause acute uraemia.

Acute tubular necrosis

Acute tubular necrosis (ATN) (see **Box 36.34**) occurs due to:
- sustained under-perfusion and reduced renal blood flow of renal tubules, leading to tubular cell death (hence the name), *or*
- nephrotoxins causing direct injury and cell death in renal tubules.

Factors involved in the development of ATN include:
- ***Intrarenal microvascular vasoconstriction with falling delivery of O_2 and increasing tubular hypoxia:***
  - vasoconstriction in response to endothelin, adenosine, thromboxane A_2, leukotrienes and sympathetic nerve activity
  - impaired vasodilation due to reduced sensitivity to nitric oxide, prostaglandins (PGE_2), acetylcholine and bradykinin.
- ***Increased endothelial and vascular smooth muscle cell structural damage:***
  - increased leucocyte–endothelial adhesion, vascular congestion and obstruction, leucocyte activation and inflammation.
- ***Tubular cell injury.*** Ischaemic injury results in rapid depletion of intracellular ATP stores, resulting in cell death either by necrosis or apoptosis, with:
  - increased cytosolic cell calcium concentration
  - induction of nitric oxide synthases with increased production of nitric oxide, causing cell death
  - increased production of intracellular proteases such as calpain, which cause proteolysis of cytoskeletal proteins and cell wall collapse
  - tubular obstruction by desquamated viable or necrotic cells and casts
  - loss of cell polarity, i.e. integrins located on the basolateral side of the cell are translocated to the apical surface, which, when combined with other desquamated cells, forms casts, with tubular obstruction and back-leak of tubular fluid.

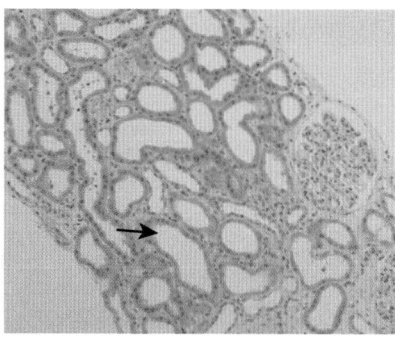

Fig. 36.45 Acute tubular necrosis. Effacement and loss of the proximal tubule brush border, patchy loss of tubular cells and focal areas of proximal tubule dilation (arrowed).

- **Tubular cellular recovery.** Tubular cells have the capacity to regenerate rapidly and to reform the disrupted tubular basement membrane, which explains the reversibility of ATN. Multiple growth factors, including insulin-like growth factor 1, epidermal growth factor and hepatocyte growth factor, and their receptors are upregulated during the regenerative process after injury.

Once established, renal blood flow is much reduced in ATN, particularly blood flow to the renal cortex. Ischaemic tubular damage contributes to a reduction in glomerular filtration as glomeruli contract through afferent arteriolar spasm, filtrate leaks back towards the glomerulus, and tubular obstruction evolves (**Fig. 36.45**).

Oliguria is common in the early stages; non-oliguric AKI is usually the result of a less severe renal insult. Recovery of renal function typically occurs after 7–21 days, although recovery is delayed by continuing sepsis. The use of intravenous mannitol, furosemide or 'renal-dose' dopamine is not supported by controlled trial evidence.

Emergency investigation of AKI

The aim is to define the AKI syndrome – pre-renal, renal or post-renal – and decide if the deterioration in function is all acute or acute-on-chronic kidney disease.

Pre-renal, renal or post-renal AKI?

Pre-renal AKI is diagnosed largely on clinical examination, and assessing the volume status is vital; it can be difficult to distinguish pre-renal and renal AKI (particularly since prolonged renal hypoperfusion will lead to ATN). Bladder outflow obstruction is ruled out by clinical examination (a large palpable bladder suggests longstanding outflow obstruction), after inserting a urethral catheter (or flushing of an existing catheter) and draining large urine volumes, or on ultrasound of the kidneys and bladder. Absence of upper tract dilation on renal ultrasonography will, with very rare exceptions, rule out urinary tract obstruction.

Other investigations are as follows:
- Urinalysis, urine microscopy, particularly for red cells and red-cell casts (indicative of glomerulonephritis), and urine culture. Urine should be tested for free haemoglobin and myoglobin, where appropriate. uPCR is helpful if parenchymal disease is possible.
- In AKI, it takes 48–72 h before creatinine rises in the plasma; by that time, cell injury is well established and irreversible. Urinary and plasma biomarkers (e.g. kidney injury molecule 1, neutrophil gelatinase-associated lipocalin, insulin-like growth factor-binding protein 7 and tissue inhibitor of metalloproteinases-2) rise within a few hours of AKI and may allow earlier treatment.

- Blood tests include measurement of serum urea, electrolytes, creatinine, calcium, phosphate, albumin, alkaline phosphatase and urate concentrations, as well as a full blood count and examination of the peripheral blood film where necessary. Coagulation studies, blood cultures and measurements of nephrotoxic drug blood levels should be carried out.

Acute or chronic uraemia?

The distinction between AKI and longstanding CKD depends on the history and duration of symptoms (a long history of nocturia suggests progressive tubular failure). Previous urinalysis or measurement of renal function is often vital in understanding the length of renal injury. Rapid changes in creatinine or GFR over days or weeks suggest an acute process.

Ultrasound is key; renal size (measured as the pole-to-pole length) and reflectivity (or echogenicity) are helpful, as small, scarred (increased echogenicity) kidneys suggest a longstanding process. The reverse is not true; the kidney may remain normal in size in diabetes and amyloidosis, for instance.

An anaemia of chronic disease, hyperparathyroidism or renal osteodystrophy also suggests CKD.

Management of AKI

Early specialist review is advisable. Often unwell, patients with AKI should be monitored in a high-dependency setting.

General measures

Good nursing, infection control and physiotherapy are vital. Fluid balance, as intake and output (particularly urine output), will be key to recovery. Daily measurements of weight and lying and standing blood pressure, medication review to withhold nephrotoxins, collateral history and past results will all form part of the management plan.

Hyperkalaemia

This may be life-threatening, leading to cardiac dysrhythmias, particularly ventricular fibrillation. Treatment is outlined in **Box 9.20**.

Intravenous sodium bicarbonate reduces potassium, as it corrects acidosis; it should not be used in volume-overloaded patients, however, because the sodium content may trigger or exacerbate pulmonary oedema. Rapid correction of acidosis in a hypocalcaemic patient may also trigger tetany (the ionized calcium fraction falls as albumin binding increases with a normalizing pH). Ion exchange resins such as patiromer and ZS-9 can be used to prevent chronic hyperkalaemia, but in many patients hyperkalaemia will be controlled only by dialysis or haemofiltration.

Pulmonary oedema

Unless a diuresis can be induced with intravenous furosemide, dialysis or haemofiltration will be required.

Sepsis

Infection needs to be treated promptly, avoiding nephrotoxic antibiotics. Use of prophylactic antibiotics or barrier nursing is not usually recommended.

Use of drugs

Nephrotoxins must be avoided and all drug dosing requires thought; GFR may be changing on a day-by-day basis and dose modification needs to follow. There is a particular risk with anticoagulants (oral and heparins; see pp. 1013–1017).

Fluid and electrolyte balance

Twice-daily clinical assessment is needed. In general, once the patient is euvolaemic, daily fluid intake should equal urine output plus losses from the gut (including nasogastric loss) plus an allowance of 500 mL daily for insensible loss. Febrile patients will require an additional allowance.

Replacement fluid may be a balanced replacement solution, 0.9% saline (e.g. burns, pancreatitis) or 4% albumin. There are no significant differences between them with respect to death rates, organ failure, need for RRT or duration of hospitalization.

Large-volume fluid infusion or changes in daily weight (reflecting changes in fluid balance) make more regular review necessary. When overload is present, loop diuretics may be useful. Non-oliguric patients with AKI fare better than oliguric patients. However, conversion of oliguria to non-oliguria has not been shown to decrease mortality, and diuretics have not been demonstrated to prevent AKI or improve outcomes.

Nutrition

Salt and potassium should be restricted. Protein intake is sometimes limited to approximately 40 g daily (0.5 g/kg per day) to avoid the need for RRT, but this poses the risk of a negative nitrogen balance. Patients on RRT are managed on a 70 g protein (and not >1.5 g/kg per day) diet, with hypercatabolic individuals requiring a greater nitrogen intake. Ideally, nutrition should be by mouth or nasogastric tube, or, as a last resort, by parenteral feeding (with sustained bowel dysfunction of more than 14 days).

Renal replacement therapy – haemodialysis and haemofiltration

The main indications for blood purification and/or fluid removal are:

- symptomatic uraemia (including pericarditis or tamponade)
- hyperkalaemia not controlled by conservative measures
- pulmonary oedema unresponsive to diuresis
- severe acidosis
- for removal of drugs causing the AKI, e.g. gentamicin, lithium, severe aspirin overdose.

Contemporary RRT options include intermittent haemodialysis or haemodiafiltration (HDF), continuous venovenous haemofiltration (CVVHF) or peritoneal dialysis. It is not clear when to start RRT; however, several trials have questioned the wisdom of early initiation because it fails to improve outcome and in up to 30% of cases dialysis appeared unnecessary because of renal recovery without RRT. There are no data to favour haemodialysis or CVVHF as a superior mode of therapy in AKI. However, there is a consensus that in haemodynamically unstable patients, particularly those on the ITU, continuous treatments like CVVHF are more widely used for systemically unwell patients with AKI. Fluids (including nutrition, blood products or antibiotics) can be administered as volume is ultrafiltered off, preventing swings in volume and delivering more cardiovascular stability. More RRT is not necessarily better; two large trials have failed to show a survival benefit with augmented doses of RRT in critically ill patients.

Haemodialysis is explained on page 1398. CVVHF achieves blood flow using a blood pump to draw and return blood (hence, venovenous) from the lumen of a dual-lumen catheter placed in the jugular, subclavian or femoral vein. Ultrafiltrate (plasma in this case) is continually removed from the patient, usually at rates of up to 1000 mL/h, combined with simultaneous infusion of replacement solution. For instance, in a fluid-overloaded patient, filtrate might be removed at 1000 mL/h and replaced at a rate of 900 mL/h, achieving a net fluid removal of 100 mL/h.

Peritoneal dialysis is also used in the management of AKI, mainly in resource-poor countries. It has low efficiency (removing solutes slowly and less completely), and is not appropriate for patients with intra-abdominal causes or complications of their AKI. Increasing intra-abdominal pressure as peritoneal dialysis fluid is instilled can compromise lung function as well.

Management of the recovery phase

Usually, after 1–3 weeks, renal function improves, with an increase in urine output and better kidney function. If it has been required, dialysis or haemofiltration can be discontinued. A characteristic recovery phase, with a large-volume diuresis, develops as GFR recovers ahead of renal tubular reabsorptive capacity for sodium, potassium and water. Intravenous fluids are often needed to support patients, with replacement sodium chloride and potassium. Typically, the diuretic phase lasts for only a few days.

Other causes of AKI

Rhabdomyolysis

Rhabdomyolysis, or 'crush syndrome', occurs when skeletal muscle injury provokes the release of intracellular myoglobin, a direct tubular toxin leading to ATN. Causes include trauma, compartment syndrome, excessive exertion (marathon runners), status epilepticus and muscle toxins (statins, malaria and antimalarials, and snake and insect venom). Rapid rises in potassium, phosphate and lactate accompany elevated muscle enzymes (aspartate aminotransferase, AST); characteristically, creatine phosphokinase (CK) is massively elevated. Early and vigorous fluid resuscitation is vital (injured muscle sequesters large amounts of fluid, causing hypovolaemic shock). Inflamed, injured muscle may become ischaemic in compartments, and a careful examination for typical 'woody-hard' muscle compartments may suggest a need for fasciotomies to release at-risk muscle. Sodium bicarbonate used to alkalinize the urine may limit myoglobin-induced injury.

A similar syndrome can arise with massive haemolysis, where the tubular toxin is haemoglobin rather than myoglobin. As cell breakdown is on a far smaller scale, the biochemical derangements seen with muscle injury may be absent.

Acute cortical necrosis

Renal hypoperfusion results in diversion of blood flow from the cortex to the medulla, with a drop in GFR. Medullary ischaemic damage is largely reversible because tubular cells have the capacity for regeneration. In contrast, glomerular ischaemic injury does not heal with regeneration but with scarring – glomerulosclerosis. Prolonged cortical ischaemia may lead to irreversible loss of renal function termed 'cortical necrosis'. This may be patchy or complete. Any cause of ATN, if sufficiently severe or prolonged, may lead to cortical necrosis. Cortical necrosis occurs more commonly where the vasculature and endothelium have been damaged (with or without coagulopathy), such as with HUS and with complications of pregnancy.

Contrast nephropathy

In patients with impaired renal function, iodinated radiological contrast media may be nephrotoxic, possibly by causing renal vasoconstriction and by exerting a direct toxic effect on renal tubules. The effect is dose-dependent and more commonly seen in procedures that require large amounts of contrast, such as angiography with or without angioplasty. In many patients the effect is mild, transient and fully reversible. However, it is not benign; even a transient elevation of creatinine following contrast administration is associated with long-term consequences (an increased risk of cardiac events, ESKD and mortality). Risk factors include:

- associated hypovolaemia
- more advanced CKD
- cardiac failure
- diabetic nephropathy
- nephrotoxins (ACE inhibitors, NSAIDs in particular, and the presence of a paraprotein band).

Diabetes *per se* is not a risk factor. However, metformin can precipitate a lactic acidosis; it should be stopped if creatinine is over 130 μmol/L and not restarted until renal function returns to the baseline level.

Prevention is key: minimize the dose of contrast administered, use an iso-osmolar or low-osmolality contrast medium, and ensure patients are pre-hydrated with 1 L of 0.9% saline or 1 L of sodium bicarbonate 1.4% peri-procedure and up to 8–12 h post-procedure, avoiding volume overload in susceptible patients. One trial confirmed that fluid administration guided by left end-diastolic pressure was safe and more effective in the prevention of contrast-induced AKI among high-risk patients undergoing cardiac catheterization.

N-acetylcysteine (a potent antioxidant) given 48 h prior to radiological intervention may be of borderline benefit at best. Dopamine, theophylline (an adenosine antagonist) and prophylactic haemodialysis (removing contrast agent from the circulation) are of no benefit.

Acute phosphate nephropathy

Administration of oral sodium phosphate solution as bowel preparation for gastrointestinal investigations is a cause of AKI. Oral phosphate solution is contraindicated in patients with CKD, congestive heart failure, gastrointestinal obstruction, and pre-existing electrolyte disorders like hypercalcaemia. Renal biopsy shows abundant calcium phosphate deposits. Treatment is usually supportive and dialysis is carried out if necessary, with good renal recovery.

Tumour lysis syndrome

Tumour lysis syndrome (see p. 118) complicates the first treatment of lymphoproliferative tumours; it can occur spontaneously and be found with other cancers. Chemotherapy (or even steroids), causing rapid death of malignant cells, sees the release of intracellular and membrane products, including uric acid, potassium and phosphate. A high filtered uric acid load leads to an obstructive crystal uropathy; serum urate may be 4- or 5-fold the upper limit of normal. The danger is hyperkalaemia; at-risk patients should be pre-hydrated to maintain a good urine output (allowing large urinary potassium losses), and xanthine oxidase inhibitors such as allopurinol may prevent uric acid formation. Rasburicase, a recombinant urase oxidase that does not occur in primates, oxidizes uric acid to soluble allantoin; urate levels can be undetectable after administration.

Hepatorenal syndrome

The renal failure observed in hepatorenal syndrome results from profound renal vasoconstriction with histologically normal kidneys (see p. 1298). It only occurs once portal hypertension and ascites have complicated liver disease. Patients are not hypovolaemic, and renal recovery is usually observed after successful liver transplantation.

Further reading

Cavanaugh C, Perazella MA. Urine sediment examination in the diagnosis and management of kidney disease: core curriculum 2019. *Am J Kidney Dis* 2019; 73:258–272.
Moore PK, Hsu RK, Liu KD. Management of acute kidney injury: core curriculum 2018. *Am J Kidney Dis* 2018; 72:136–148.

CHRONIC KIDNEY DISEASE

The term 'chronic kidney disease' (CKD) has replaced terms like chronic renal failure or insufficiency. CKD is a descriptive term and is used for deteriorating kidney function of any underlying cause. CKD implies longstanding (>3 months), potentially progressive impairment in renal function. However, in most cases of stage 1–3 CKD, kidney function does not continue to decline over time, and patients do not die as a direct result of kidney disease.

In many cases, there is no effective means to reverse the underlying disease process. There are exceptions where reversal is likely:

- relief of urinary tract obstruction
- immunosuppressive therapy for glomerulonephritis or systemic vasculitis
- treatment of accelerated hypertension
- correction of critical narrowing of renal arteries.

In many other cases of CKD, even if the underlying diagnosis cannot be fully treated, the rate of deterioration in renal function can be slowed (see p. 1398). A list of causes of CKD is given in **Box 36.35**.

Staging and prevalence

CKD is staged according to the National Kidney Foundation's Kidney Disease Outcomes Quality Initiative (K/DOQI) and endorsed by International Kidney Disease: Improving Global Outcomes (KDIGO). Staging is intended to reflect patient prognosis and outcomes (**Fig. 36.46**). If this MDRD-GFR-based system is used (see p. 1346), high prevalences of CKD are now found in population-based surveys, particularly in elderly patients. CKD has an elevated global

---

? Box 36.35 Causes of chronic kidney disease

Congenital and inherited disease
- Polycystic kidney disease (adult and infantile forms)
- Medullary cystic disease
- Tuberous sclerosis
- Oxalosis
- Cystinosis
- Congenital obstructive uropathy

Glomerular disease

Primary glomerulonephritides
- Including focal glomerulosclerosis

Secondary glomerular disease
- Systemic lupus, polyangiitis, granulomatosis with polyangiitis, amyloidosis, diabetic glomerulosclerosis, accelerated hypertension, haemolytic uraemic syndrome, thrombotic thrombocytopenic purpura, systemic sclerosis, sickle cell disease

Vascular disease
- Hypertensive nephrosclerosis (common in people of black African descent)

- Renovascular disease
- Small- and medium-sized-vessel vasculitis

Tubulointerstitial disease
- Tubulointerstitial nephritis – idiopathic, due to drugs (especially nephrotoxic analgesics), immunologically mediated
- Reflux nephropathy
- Tuberculosis
- Schistosomiasis
- Nephrocalcinosis
- Multiple myeloma (myeloma kidney)
- Balkan nephropathy
- Renal papillary necrosis (diabetes, sickle cell disease and trait, analgesic nephropathy)
- Chinese herb nephropathy

Urinary tract obstruction
- Calculus disease
- Prostatic disease
- Pelvic tumours
- Retroperitoneal fibrosis
- Schistosomiasis

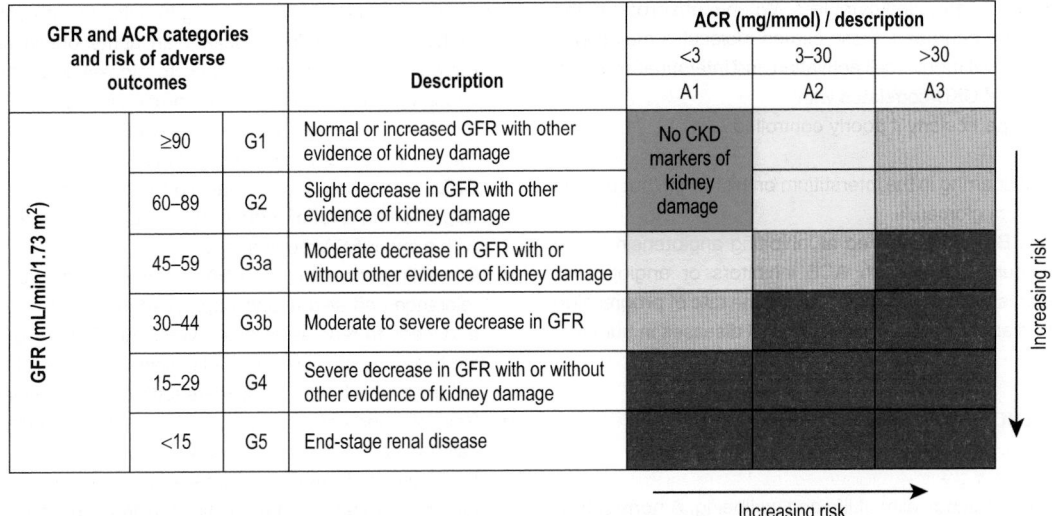

GFR and ACR categories and risk of adverse outcomes			Description	ACR (mg/mmol) / description		
				<3	3–30	>30
				A1	A2	A3
GFR (mL/min/1.73 m²)	≥90	G1	Normal or increased GFR with other evidence of kidney damage	No CKD markers of kidney damage		
	60–89	G2	Slight decrease in GFR with other evidence of kidney damage			
	45–59	G3a	Moderate decrease in GFR with or without other evidence of kidney damage			
	30–44	G3b	Moderate to severe decrease in GFR			
	15–29	G4	Severe decrease in GFR with or without other evidence of kidney damage			
	<15	G5	End-stage renal disease			

Increasing risk →

↓ Increasing risk

Fig. 36.46 Classification of chronic kidney disease (CKD) using glomerular filtration rate (GFR) and albumin:creatinine (ACR) categories. *(Adapted with permission from Kidney Disease: Improving Global Outcomes (KDIGO) CKD Work Group. KDIGO 2012 clinical practice guideline for the evaluation and management of chronic kidney disease. Kidney Int 2013; Suppl. 3:1–150.)*

prevalence, consistently estimated at between 11% and 15%, with the majority at stage 3 (**Box 36.36**).

Staging is increasingly complex:

- Patients are staged both on eGFR (with a prefix G) and albuminuria (with a prefix A), reflecting the fact that both of these parameters correlate with progressive renal impairment and cardiovascular risk. For instance a patient may be staged as having G3bA3 disease.
- Stage 3 CKD has been divided into two stages (3a and 3b) in recognition of the increased cardiovascular complications seen with more advanced disease.
- It has been advocated that cystatin C (see p. 1346), a more accurate marker of GFR, be used in patients with stage 3 CKD to better stratify risk in this group.
- Confusingly, patients with stage G2 CKD are not thought to have disease unless there is other evidence of kidney damage; this might include haematuria, proteinuria, structurally abnormal kidneys, inherited kidney disease or biopsy changes consistent with kidney disease.

Diagnosis of CKD is becoming more likely as people live longer. There is wide geographical variation in the incidence, prevalence and causes of CKD across the globe. For instance, the most common cause of GN in sub-Saharan Africa is malaria. Schistosomiasis is a common cause of CKD due to urinary tract obstruction in parts of the Middle East, including southern Iraq.

The incidence of ESKD varies between ethnic groups, being 3–4 times as common in people of black African descent in the UK and USA as it is in the white population, and hypertensive nephropathy is a much more frequent cause of ESKD in this group. The prevalence of diabetes mellitus, and hence of diabetic nephropathy, is higher in some Asian groups than in white people. Age is also of relevance: CKD caused by atherosclerotic renal vascular disease is much more common in the elderly than in the young. Over 70% of all cases of CKD are due to diabetes mellitus, hypertension and atherosclerosis.

Progression

CKD tends to progress to ESKD, although the rate of progression may be slow. The speed of decline tends to depend on the

i **Box 36.36 Prevalence of CKD**

CKD stage	Age in years (% of population affected)			
	<65	65–74	75–84	≥85
3	1.4	15.4	29.4	30.9
4	0.04	0.4	1.3	2.4
5	0.03	0.2	0.1	0.1
Total	**1.5**	**15.9**	**30.9**	**33.4**

underlying nephropathy and on control of blood pressure. Patients with chronic glomerular diseases tend to deteriorate more quickly than those with chronic tubulointerstitial nephropathies. Regardless of cause, there may be common pathways to progression in CKD:

- Each kidney has roughly a million nephrons. In CKD, when many nephrons have failed and scarred, the burden of filtration falls to fewer functioning nephrons.
- Functioning ('remnant') nephrons experience increased flow per nephron (hyperfiltration), as renal blood flow has not changed, and adapt with glomerular hypertrophy and reduced arteriolar resistance.
- Increased flow, increased pressure and increased shear stress set in motion a vicious circle of raised intraglomerular capillary pressure and strain, which accelerates remnant nephron failure.
- Increased flow and strain may be detected as new or increasing proteinuria.

Angiotensin II produced locally modulates intraglomerular capillary pressure and GFR, causing vasoconstriction of postglomerular arterioles, and increasing the glomerular hydraulic pressure and filtration fraction (see **Fig. 36.44**). In addition, it indirectly upregulates transforming growth factor-beta (TGF-β), a potent fibrogenic cytokine, increasing collagen synthesis and epithelial cell transdifferentiation to myofibroblasts that contribute to excessive matrix formation. Angiotensin II also upregulates plasminogen activator inhibitor-1 (PAI-1), which inhibits matrix proteolysis by plasmin, with accumulation of excessive matrix and scarring in both the glomeruli and interstitium.

Proteinuria itself may be harmful in the tubulointerstitium. Albumin, in disease, may appear in the urinary space carrying bound fatty acids, growth factors and cytokines. When reabsorbed in the proximal tubule and degraded, these carried molecules may themselves cause proximal tubular cell activation and interstitial scarring.

The prognosis of CKD correlates with:

- hypertension, particularly if poorly controlled
- proteinuria
- the degree of scarring in the interstitium on histology (but not the changes seen in glomeruli).

Therapy (see **Box 36.12**) aimed at inhibiting angiotensin II and reducing proteinuria mainly with ACE inhibitors or angiotensin-receptor antagonists offers benefit in slowing the rate of progression of CKD in both diabetic and non-diabetic renal diseases in humans.

Complications of CKD

Anaemia

Anaemia in CKD impairs quality of life and wellbeing. A normochromic, normocytic anaemia develops by a number of mechanisms:

- **Erythropoietin deficiency** – this is the most significant mechanism.
- **Increased blood loss** – there may be occult gastrointestinal bleeding, repeated blood sampling, blood loss during haemodialysis, or platelet dysfunction.
- **Bone marrow toxins** – these are retained in CKD, or there is fibrosis secondary to hyperparathyroidism.
- **Haematinic deficiency** – there may be decreased iron, vitamin B_{12} or folate.
- **Increased red-cell destruction** – red cells have a shortened lifespan in uraemia, and haemodialysis itself may cause a degree of haemolysis.
- **ACE inhibitors** – these may cause anaemia in CKD, probably by interfering with the control of endogenous erythropoietin release.

Management

Synthetic (recombinant) human erythropoiesis-stimulating agents (ESAs; epoetin-α or β, or the longer-acting darbepoetin-α) have transformed the management of renal anaemia. ESAs can be given subcutaneously or by intravenous injection, at a starting dose of 50 U/kg of epoetin-α three times weekly, or darbepoetin 30 μg weekly. Supplemental intravenous iron may promote a response to erythropoietin and can be given prior to starting ESAs. Haemoglobin is then measured every 2 weeks, and the dose adjusted to maintain a target haemoglobin of 100–120 g/L (see later). As hypertension can be a significant side-effect in 30% of patients new to ESAs, blood pressure should be monitored in the first 6 months, and treated if rising. Peripheral resistance increases in all patients, owing to loss of hypoxic vasodilation and to an increase in blood viscosity. The rare complication of encephalopathy with fits, transient cortical blindness and hypertension can complicate treatment.

Targets and treatment are as follows:

- **Target haemoglobin** is between 100 and 120 g/L. Studies in pre-dialysis CKD patients have not shown any outcome benefits in those treated to achieve higher haemoglobin targets (>120 g/L).
- Patients who **fail to respond** to 300 U/kg weekly of epoetin-α should be screened to exclude associated iron deficiency, bleeding, malignancy, infection, inflammation, or formation of anti-erythropoietin neutralizing antibodies.
- The increased demand for iron by the bone marrow is enormous when an ESA is started. Functional iron deficiency (poor mobilization of iron, despite adequate iron stores with ferritin

>500 μg/L) is a common finding in patients with chronic inflammation. Synthesis of hepcidin, an acute phase reactant produced by the liver in response to cytokines (particularly IL-6), inhibits gastrointestinal iron absorption (see p. 329) and sequesters iron in the liver, preventing its release. Intravenous (rather than oral) iron supplements optimize the response to ESAs in CKD. A trial has shown that high-dose intravenous iron and a target ferritin level of around 400 μg/L were safe and associated with a lower ESA requirement.

- Correcting anaemia with ESAs improves quality of life, exercise tolerance and sexual and cognitive function in dialysis patients, and leads to regression of left ventricular hypertrophy. By avoiding blood transfusion, the risk is minimized of sensitization to HLA antigens, which may complicate future renal transplantation.
- Several reports of anti-erythropoietin antibody-mediated pure red-cell aplasia in patients receiving subcutaneous ESA therapy (particularly epoetin-α) have been described. Changes in the manufacturing process of the pre-filled syringes used to deliver ESAs have reduced the number of these cases; the rubber stoppers interacted with the drug vehicle to act as an immunological adjuvant, stimulating anti-erythropoietin antibody production in hosts.

Several novel ESAs are in clinical trials. An engineered peptide that stimulates the erythropoietin receptor has been withdrawn because of anaphylaxis in a few patients. Oral agents that inhibit prolyl hydroxylase and prolong the life of hypoxia inducible factor (HIF) 1α, a transcription factor for endogenous production of erythropoietin, have shown promise and will be available to use in near future.

CKD mineral and bone disorder

Once called 'renal osteodystrophy' but now more appropriately described as a mineral and bone disorder, CKD-MBD encompasses:

- changes in calcium, phosphorus, PTH, FGF23 and vitamin D metabolism
- the various forms of bone disease that may develop alone or in combination in CKD
- the vascular consequences, such as arterial stiffness and calcification, that accompany it.

Altered bone morphology might be described in CKD (**Fig. 36.47**) as:

- hyperparathyroid bone disease
- osteomalacia
- osteoporosis
- osteosclerosis
- adynamic bone disease.

Most patients with CKD are found on bone biopsy to have mixed bone disease. CKD-MBD is almost universal by late stage 3 CKD. Vascular calcification is common in CKD patients; it is speculated that vascular smooth muscle cells, modulated by uraemia and/or phosphate, differentiate to an osteoblast-like phenotype, able to synthesize and deposit matrix, which is then mineralized. Calcified vessel walls become increasingly stiff and non-compliant (leading to left ventricular hypertrophy over time), cardiac valves calcify, and soft-tissue calcium is deposited widely. There is an association between vascular calcification and mortality in CKD but a causal link has not yet been proved.

Pathogenesis of CKD-MBD

Phosphate excretion falls in the very early stages of CKD. Retained phosphate then results in the release of FGF23 and other phosphaturic agents by osteocytes as a compensatory mechanism (see p. 192). FGF23 causes phosphaturia to bring the plasma phosphate

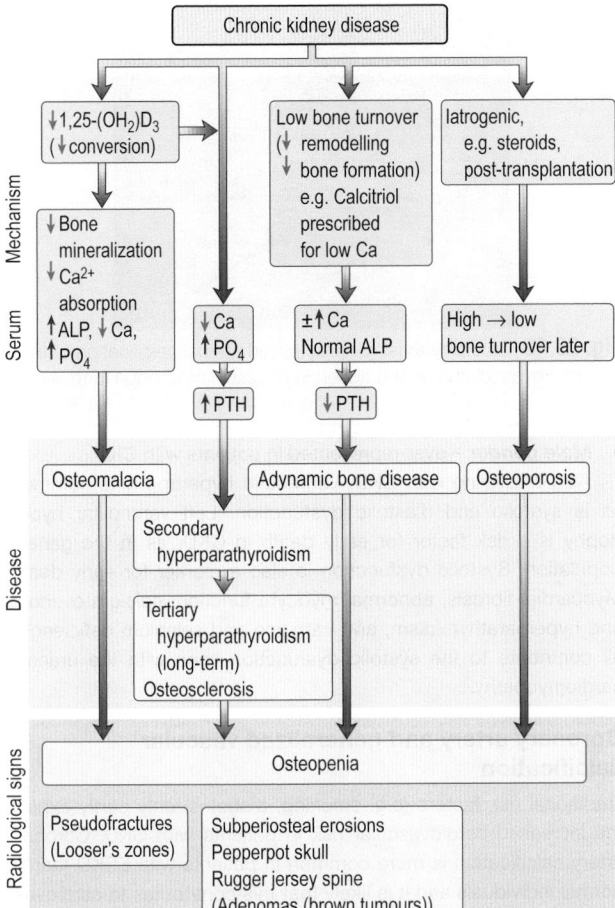

Fig. 36.47 Chronic kidney disease mineral and bone disorder (CKD-MB). Pathogenesis and radiological features of renal bone disease. ALP, alkaline phosphatase; PTH, parathyroid hormone.

This 'secondary' hyperparathyroidism leads to increased osteoclastic activity, cyst formation and bone marrow fibrosis (osteitis fibrosa cystica). The typical biochemical findings are hypocalcaemia, hyperphosphataemia, an elevated PTH and a raised serum alkaline phosphatase (as a marker of increased bone turnover). Radiologically, digital subperiosteal erosions and a 'pepperpot skull' are seen. Longstanding secondary hyperparathyroidism ultimately leads to hyperplasia of the glands with autonomous or **tertiary hyperparathyroidism**. PTH release now occurs independently of calcium or 1,25-$(OH)_2D_3$ control, and high turnover in bone leads to hypercalcaemia.

Longstanding hyperparathyroidism causes increased bone density (**osteosclerosis**), seen particularly in the spine, where alternating bands of sclerotic and porotic bone give rise to a characteristic 'rugger jersey' appearance on X-ray.

Deficiency of 1,25-$(OH)_2D_3$ and hypocalcaemia can also result in impaired mineralization of osteoid (**osteomalacia**).

'Adynamic bone disease' describes a state in which both bone formation and resorption are depressed and the skeleton becomes inert. Bone turnover is reduced, usually where there is overtreatment with active vitamin D, low PTH (after surgical parathyroidectomy), accumulation of aluminium used as a phosphate binder, or diabetes. There may be hypercalcaemia, particularly if calcium intake is high (excess calcium cannot be laid down in bone); the serum alkaline phosphatase is normal and the PTH is low. X-rays and dual X-ray absorptiometry (DXA) scans show osteopenia. No treatment is of proven benefit.

Osteoporosis is commonly found in CKD, often after transplantation and the use of corticosteroids. Monitoring is with yearly DXA scanning.

Management of CKD-MBD

The aim is to keep serum calcium and phosphate in the normal range as CKD progresses, and once dialysis is needed, to control PTH within 2- to 3-fold the upper limit of normal. This is to ensure that bone turnover continues and adynamic bone does not develop. The less well understood goal is to limit vascular calcification as well, by maintaining good bone health and avoiding calcium exposure.

Calcium, phosphate and PTH should be measured 3-monthly, and some would use imaging to define the extent of vascular calcification (e.g. by X-ray of the lumbar spine or of the abdomen). Treatment and targets, then, aim to reduce phosphate (and preferably limit calcium load), and to control PTH and achieve a normal calcium.

Reduction of phosphate and limiting of calcium load

- **Dietary restriction.** This is seldom effective alone because so many foods are phosphate-rich. Phosphate-restricted diets lead to protein malnutrition.
- **Gut phosphate binders.** Sevelamer carbonate, lanthanum carbonate, calcium carbonate and calcium acetate all reduce phosphate absorption and serum phosphate levels when taken with meals. Sevelamer (unlike calcium-containing binders) attenuates vascular calcification and lowers cholesterol levels by 10%; it has not been shown to reduce mortality. Generally, however, adherence to phosphate binders is poor.
- **Aluminium-containing gut phosphate binders.** These are very effective but absorption of aluminium poses the risk of aluminium bone disease and development of cognitive impairment. They are rarely used in developed countries but are still employed in developing countries because they are extremely cheap.

level to within the normal range. FGF23 also downregulates renal 1α-hydroxylase, reducing the action of activated vitamin D in increasing intestinal absorption of phosphate. Despite consistently elevated levels of FGF23, phosphate levels in blood will once again rise as CKD progresses. Elevated FGF23 levels are the strongest independent predictor of mortality in patients with CKD. This underscores the necessity of controlling phosphate levels during the very early stages of CKD.

As CKD progresses, **secondary hyperparathyroidism** develops:

- Decreased renal production of 1α-hydroxylase results in reduced conversion of 25-$(OH)_2D_3$ to the more metabolically active 1,25-$(OH)_2D_3$ (1,25-dihydroxycholecalciferol).
- 1,25-$(OH)_2D_3$ deficiency results in reduced gut calcium absorption and a fall in calcium.
- Reduced activation of vitamin D receptors in the parathyroid glands by 1,25-$(OH)_2D_3$ increases the release of PTH.
- Calcium-sensing receptors, expressed in the parathyroid glands, react rapidly to acute changes in extracellular calcium concentrations, and a low calcium triggers increased PTH release.
- Retained phosphate also indirectly lowers ionized calcium (and probably directly via a putative but unrecognized phosphate receptor), resulting in increased PTH synthesis and release.
- PTH promotes reabsorption of calcium from bone and increased proximal renal tubular reabsorption of calcium. This mechanism attempts to reverse the hypocalcaemia caused by 1,25-$(OH)_2D_3$ deficiency and phosphate retention.

- **Tenapanor**, a minimally absorbed, small-molecule inhibitor of the sodium/hydrogen exchanger isoform 3 (NHE3), inhibits both sodium and water transport locally in the gastrointestinal tract, as well as phosphate transport by indirectly inhibiting paracellular absorption of phosphate. It also downregulates intestinal phosphate transporters Na/Pi2b and reduces absorption directly. Clinically, the role of inhibitors of phosphate absorption has not yet been determined.

Control of PTH and achievement of normal calcium

- **Calcitriol (1,25-dihydroxycholecalciferol), vitamin D analogues** such as alfacalcidol, or novel vitamin D metabolites (22-oxacalcitriol, paricalcitol, doxercalciferol). These are given orally to suppress PTH once the level is three times or more above the upper limit of normal. Newer vitamin D analogues, such as paricalcitol (19-nor-1,25 dihydroxyvitamin D_2), may be less likely to lead to hypercalcaemia, but their usefulness over the conventional but less expensive calcitriol or alfacalcidol remains to be established.
- **Calcimimetic agents** (e.g. cinacalcet and etelcalcetide, calcium-sensing receptor agonists, see p. 645). These have also been tried in established secondary hyperparathyroidism with successful suppression of PTH levels and lowering of calcium × phosphate product. Calcimimetics act by activating the calcium-sensing receptor, leading the parathyroid to respond as though serum calcium levels were high, reducing PTH synthesis and release. The long-term safety and efficacy of these agents have been confirmed; however, a controlled trial to assess potential survival benefits on treatment was non-conclusive.

Calciphylaxis

Also known as calcific uraemic arteriolopathy, this is a rare but serious life-threatening complication in CKD patients. It presents as painful skin patches, plaques and ulcers, with non-healing eschars, panniculitis and dermal necrosis. The characteristic feature on histology is vascular calcification and superimposed small-vessel thrombosis (**Fig. 36.48**). Risk factors include hyperparathyroidism, elevated serum phosphate, morbid obesity and warfarin use (by inhibiting vitamin K-dependent carboxylation and activation of calcification inhibitor matrix gla protein). Control of hyperparathyroidism is with either surgical intervention or a calcimimetic agent, aiming to drop both calcium and phosphate to low–normal ranges. Sodium thiosulfate (an antioxidant) and bisphosphonates have been tried with variable success. Despite treatment, subsequent infection escalates the risk, as patients are often already frail, and many die within a year of diagnosis.

Cardiovascular disease

CKD is a major risk factor for cardiovascular disease, and the greatly increased (16-fold) incidence of cardiovascular disease in CKD compared with the normal population has a significant impact on life expectancy. Sudden cardiac death, myocardial infarction, cardiac failure, stroke and peripheral vascular disease all occur in excess as GFR declines (and the presence of proteinuria adds further to this risk). Renal transplantation reverses the risk seen with stage 5 CKD.

Risk factors

- **Hypertension** – very common in CKD.
- **Diabetes mellitus** – the most common cause of CKD.
- **Dyslipidaemia** – universal in uraemic patients.
- **Smoking** – as common as in the general population.

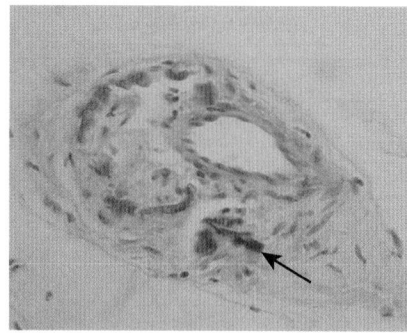

Fig. 36.48 Calciphylaxis. Characteristic arterial calcification of the skin microvasculature in the absence of vasculitic change (arrowed).

- **Male gender** – over-represented in patients with CKD.

Also clustering with CKD, ventricular hypertrophy is common, as is systolic and diastolic dysfunction. Left ventricular hypertrophy is a risk factor for early death in CKD, as in the general population. Systolic dysfunction is also a marker for early death. Myocardial fibrosis, abnormal myocyte function, calcium overload and hyperparathyroidism, and carnitine and selenium deficiencies all contribute to the systolic dysfunction seen with the uraemic cardiomyopathy.

Coronary artery and generalized vascular calcification

Traditional risk factors (e.g. smoking, diabetes) only partly explain the increased cardiovascular risk in patients with CKD. Coronary artery calcification is more common in patients with ESKD than in normal individuals and it is likely that this contributes to cardiovascular mortality. Peripheral vessel calcification **increases vascular stiffness (reduced compliance)**, which manifests as increased pulse pressure, increased pulse wave velocity, and an increased afterload with advancing left ventricular hypertrophy. Risk factors related to calcification include:

- **A raised (calcium × phosphate) product**, which promotes calcification.
- **Hyperparathyroidism**, which increases intracellular calcium.
- **Uraemia**, which leads to loss of constitutive inhibitors of calcification, with vascular smooth muscle cells acquiring osteoblast-like characteristics.
- **Inflammation**, which further inhibits fetuin (a glycoprotein synthesized by liver, and a potent inhibitor of vascular calcification).

Plain abdominal X-ray (demonstrating 'pipe-stem' calcification of large arteries), electron beam or multislice CT of the coronaries, and vascular Doppler can all identify and quantify vascular calcification.

Risk factor modification is similar to that undertaken in patients without CKD, although clear evidence of benefit is less obvious.

Other cardiovascular risk factors

Hyperhomocysteinaemia, *Chlamydophila pneumoniae* infection, malnutrition, inflammation, insulin resistance, oxidative stress and elevated endogenous inhibitor of nitric oxide synthase and asymmetric dimethyl arginine (ADMA) all contribute to increased cardiovascular events. High ADMA levels in uraemia are caused, in part, by oxidative stress and can possibly explain the 52% increase in the risk of death and 34% increase in the risk of cardiovascular events in uraemic patients. The use of antioxidants, vitamin E or acetylcysteine has been associated with a significant reduction in all-cause and cardiovascular mortality. However, trials to reduce levels of homocysteine with folic acid, B_6 and B_{12} supplementation have been unsuccessful.

The conclusion from a study of heart and renal protection (SHARP) in over 9500 CKD patients was that around one-quarter of all heart attacks, strokes and revascularizations could be avoided in CKD by using a combination of ezetimibe and simvastatin to lower blood cholesterol. This combination did not, however, confer any survival advantage or prevent the development of ESKD.

Pericarditis

This is common and occurs in two clinical settings:

- Uraemic pericarditis is a feature of severe, pre-terminal uraemia or of under-dialysis. Haemorrhagic pericardial effusion and atrial arrhythmias are often associated. There is a danger of pericardial tamponade, and anticoagulants should be used with caution. Pericarditis may resolve with intensive dialysis.
- Dialysis pericarditis occurs as a result of an intercurrent illness or surgery in a patient receiving apparently adequate dialysis.

Skin disease

Pruritus (itching) is common and is caused by:

- accumulating nitrogenous waste products of protein catabolism (itching improves following dialysis)
- hypercalcaemia and hyperphosphataemia, or an elevated calcium × phosphate product
- hyperparathyroidism (even if calcium and phosphate levels are normal)
- iron deficiency.

In dialysis patients, inadequate dialysis is a treatable cause of pruritus. However, for many, the cause of itching is unknown and no effective treatment exists.

Many patients with CKD suffer from dry skin, for which simple aqueous creams are helpful. CKD may also cause porphyria cutanea tarda, a blistering, photosensitive skin rash. This results from a decrease in hepatic uroporphyrinogen decarboxylase combined with decreased clearance of porphyrins in the urine or by dialysis. Pseudoporphyria, a condition similar to porphyria cutanea tarda but without enzyme deficiency, is also seen in CKD with increased frequency.

Nephrogenic systemic fibrosis

Nephrogenic systemic fibrosis (NSF) is a systemic fibrosing skin disorder seen only in patients with moderate to severe CKD (eGFR <30 mL/min), particularly those on dialysis. Gadolinium-containing contrast agents, which are excreted exclusively by the kidney, have been implicated in the causation of over 95% of cases of NSF (see p. 1350).

The *diagnosis* is based on biopsy of an involved site, showing proliferation of dermal fibrocytes with excessive collagen deposition. Special testing may show gadolinium.

NSF is chronic and unremitting, with 30% having no improvement, 20% having modest improvement and 30% dying. No single or combination therapy offers benefit, except for improving renal function following transplantation. *Prevention* is key and so gadolinium-based contrast agents should be avoided in patents with an eGFR below 30 mL/min or those on dialysis.

Gastrointestinal complications

Decreased gastric emptying and an increased risk of reflux oesophagitis, gastritis and peptic ulceration are all common (hypergastrinaemia increases as GFR declines); gastrointestinal tract bleeding is more frequently seen as a result. Constipation is particularly common in patients on continuous ambulatory peritoneal dialysis (CAPD).

Acute pancreatitis occurs more frequently, though elevations of serum amylase of up to three times normal may be found in CKD without any evidence of pancreatic disease, owing to retention of high-molecular-weight forms of amylase normally excreted in the urine.

Metabolic abnormalities
Gout

Urate is retained as GFR declines, and many drugs used to manage CKD increase the risk of gout. Nephrotoxic NSAIDs are less useful in treatment, though colchicine is helpful for the acute attack. Reduced-dose allopurinol or febuxostat is effective in the prevention of further attacks.

Insulin

Insulin is catabolized by, and to some extent excreted via, the kidneys. Moreover, renal glucose production is diminished with progressive CKD. For these reasons, insulin requirements in diabetic patients decrease as CKD progresses. By contrast, end-organ resistance to insulin is a feature of advanced CKD, resulting in modestly impaired glucose tolerance. Insulin resistance may contribute to hypertension and lipid abnormalities.

Lipid metabolism

Abnormalities in lipid metabolism are common in CKD and include:

- impaired clearance of triglyceride-rich particles
- hypercholesterolaemia (particularly in advanced CKD).

The situation is further complicated in ESKD, when regular heparinization (in haemodialysis), excessive glucose absorption (in CAPD) and immunosuppressive drugs (in transplantation) may all contribute to lipid abnormalities.

Endocrine abnormalities

These include:

- Hyperprolactinaemia, which may present with galactorrhoea in men as well as women.
- Decreased serum testosterone levels (only seldom below the normal level). Loss of libido, erectile dysfunction and decreased spermatogenesis are common.
- Menstrual irregularities, oligomenorrhoea or amenorrhoea (very few women on dialysis will have periods), which are common, as is loss of libido (see p. 584).
- Complex abnormalities of growth hormone secretion and action, resulting in impaired growth in uraemic children (pharmacological treatment with recombinant growth hormone and insulin-like growth factor is used).
- Altered protein binding (and increased thyroid-binding globulin loss with proteinuria). These make thyroid function tests difficult to interpret. Thyroid-stimulating hormone (TSH) is the best test of thyroid function. True hypothyroidism occurs with increased frequency in CKD.

Posterior pituitary gland function is normal in CKD.

Muscle dysfunction

Uraemia appears to interfere with muscle energy metabolism but the mechanism is uncertain. Decreased physical fitness (cardiovascular deconditioning) also contributes.

Nervous system abnormalities

Uraemia affects the *central nervous system* as depressed cerebral function, a decreased seizure threshold, asterixis, tremor and myoclonus. Anxiety, depression and impaired cognition also occur. In people with profound uraemia, and high blood urea prior to their first dialysis, the sudden correction of urea can cause **dialysis disequilibrium** (urea does not equilibrate rapidly across the blood–brain barrier and, as blood urea falls on dialysis in advance of central nervous system urea, rapid movement of water into the higher-urea environment within the central nervous system leads to osmotic cerebral swelling and even fits). This can be avoided by correcting uraemia gradually by short, repeated haemodialysis treatments or by the use of peritoneal dialysis.

Increased circulating catecholamines lead to downregulation of α-receptors, impaired baroreceptor sensitivity and impaired efferent vagal function in the **autonomic nervous system**. Overactivity of the sympathetic nervous system may contribute to the hypertension seen in CKD. These abnormalities correct to some extent with regular dialysis and resolve after successful renal transplantation.

Peripherally, median nerve compression in the carpal tunnel is common, usually due to β_2-microglobulin-related amyloidosis (see p. 1400). Advanced uraemia leads to a symmetrical polyneuropathy (which may recur in inadequately dialysed patients).

Management of CKD

General measures

- As always, make a diagnosis, and treat any modifiable underlying cause.
- Address cardiovascular risk factors: in particular, smoking cessation, exercise and weight loss.
- Avoid nephrotoxic drugs (see later).
- Arrange systematic follow-up, depending on the stage of CKD, to identify those most likely to progress **early.**

As stage 3 CKD progresses to stage 4 CKD, attention should be paid to correcting the complications described earlier: anaemia, CKD-MDB and metabolic abnormalities. Primary prevention of cardiovascular disease is a major part of CKD management at this stage.

Renoprotection

The multidrug approach to chronic nephropathies has been formalized in an international protocol (see **Box 36.12**).

Correction of specific complications

Hyperkalaemia often responds to dietary restriction of potassium intake. Drugs that cause potassium retention (see p. 187) should be stopped. Occasionally, it may be necessary to prescribe ion-exchange resins to remove potassium in the gastrointestinal tract. Two new orally active drugs, patiromer and sodium zirconium cyclosilicate, have been successful in controlling hyperkalaemia in phase 3 trials and are now available for use in clinical practice. Emergency treatment of severe hyperkalaemia is described on page 188.

Correction of acidosis helps to address hyperkalaemia in CKD and may also decrease muscle catabolism. Sodium bicarbonate supplements are effective (4.8 g (57 mmol) of Na^+ and HCO_3^- daily), without significant risk of oedema or hypertension. Correction of metabolic acidosis with sodium bicarbonate at a mean dose of 1.8 g/day also reduces the rate of decline of GFR (slowing progression) in advanced (stage 4 and 5) CKD. Calcium carbonate, also used as a calcium supplement and phosphate binder, has a beneficial effect on acidosis.

Drug therapy should be reviewed and nephrotoxins avoided in patients with CKD. These include:

- tetracyclines (with the possible exception of doxycycline)

- drugs excreted by the kidneys, such as gentamicin; these should be prescribed only in the absence of any alternative, and drug levels monitored if feasible
- NSAIDs
- potassium-sparing agents, such as spironolactone and amiloride; these pose particular dangers, as do artificial salt substitutes, all of which contain potassium.

Antibiotics, anticoagulants (particularly anti-thrombin oral anticoagulants, which currently lack a practical monitoring measurement of effect), beta-blockers, oral hypoglycaemics, insulin, antidepressants and analgesics (especially opioids, which can accumulate, leading to an opiate narcosis) often need dose adjustment when prescribed for patients with CKD.

Early referral

Patients need time to adjust to the demands of CKD and its treatment, and to absorb information. Those who share in the decisions about their care, who are able to understand and choose treatments, make the best transition to dialysis or transplantation. As GFR declines below 20 mL/min per 1.73 m², a dedicated team should counsel patients as to their diet, review medication, encourage risk factor modification, and support them to RRT (or the choice not to undertake dialysis).

If the patient opts for regular haemodialysis, an arteriovenous fistula should be fashioned well in advance of the need for dialysis (when serum creatinine is in the order of 400–500´mol/L in non-diabetics, and at an even earlier stage in diabetics with poorer vasculature). Such fistulae require several weeks to mature and become usable for vascular access. Veins required for future arteriovenous fistulae should not be rendered useless by cannulation (**Fig. 36.49**). Patients choosing peritoneal dialysis might have a buried catheter placed and left subcutaneously for some time, able to be externalized on the day dialysis starts.

Where suitable, patients should be offered and prepared for **preemptive living donor transplantation** as the best option for RRT.

Renal replacement therapy

About 3 million people worldwide either are treated by haemodialysis or peritoneal dialysis, or live with a functioning renal transplant. In the UK, around 53 000 people receive treatment for ESKD; around

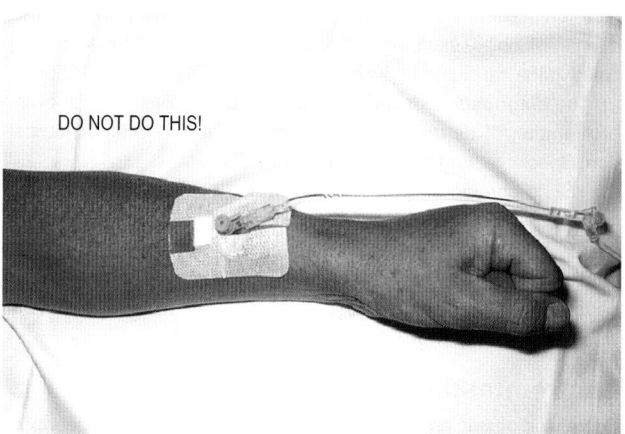

Fig. 36.49 Intravenous cannula in exactly the WRONG place. The cannula is shown in a right-handed patient with CKD, who will, in future, need a left (non-dominant arm) radiocephalic fistula.

50% have been transplanted, 42% are on haemodialysis and 8% are on peritoneal dialysis.

Dialysis aims to mimic the excretory function of normal kidneys by:

- eliminating (nitrogenous and small molecular) wastes
- maintaining normal electrolyte concentrations
- preventing systemic acidosis
- maintaining a normal extracellular volume.

Initiation of dialysis

It is not widely agreed *when* to start dialysis in patients with stage 5 CKD, and trials have suggested that early initiation is not associated with improved survival or clinical outcomes. There is a general tendency to start dialysis at an eGFR close to 10 mL/min but this decision is best shared with an individual patient, taking into account symptoms and life plans.

An informed choice

Many people, particularly if they are frail or living with other co-morbidities, will choose not to undergo RRT if able to make a shared, informed decision with their physician and families. For some, the *quantity* of extended life offered by dialysis is not matched by the perceived impact on the *quality* of their lives. For others, events and complications of dialysis can make the daily experience of treatment difficult to endure, and they may choose to withdraw from dialysis. Support through their last illness, good symptom control and respect for the individual's informed choices can allow patients a comfortable end of life after a period of long illness.

A difficult choice

Across the globe, RRT (like other treatments) can be an expensive option. For many societies, health resources may be allocated to other pressing priorities, or may be available for a defined time period only, or one form of RRT may be preferred over others. The drive for more cost-effective and low-technology solutions to treat renal failure is a pressing need for the specialty worldwide.

Haemodialysis

Basic principles

Anticoagulated blood from a patient is pumped around an extra-corporeal circuit and through a biocompatible, semipermeable membrane (the dialyser, or 'artificial kidney') before being returned to the circulation. In the dialyser, ultrapure dialysate flowing in the opposite direction is in close contact with blood. Small solutes (but not cells and larger-molecular-weight proteins) can cross the membrane, and move by diffusion down a concentration gradient (**Fig. 36.50**). A transmembrane pressure allows controlled fluid removal by ultrafiltration (and with fluid, more solute removal by convection).

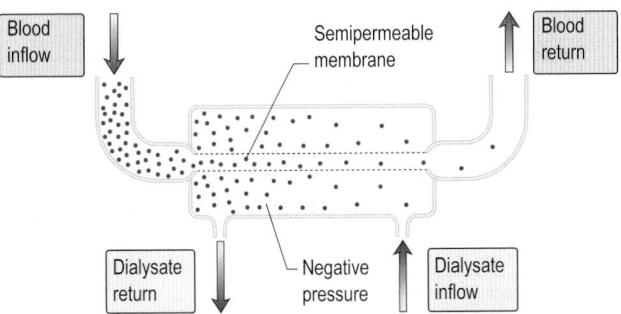

Fig. 36.50 Changes across a semipermeable dialysis membrane.

Over a standard 4-hour session, up to 80 L of blood (at around 300 mL/min) is circulated through the dialyser; even so, this provides an equivalent GFR of only 10–12 mL/min per m². **Box 36.37** describes a typical dialysate; dialysis is individually prescribed for any particular patient to obtain optimal results.

Access

Effective dialysis needs blood flows of between 250 and 450 mL/min. In order to achieve this, a surgically fashioned arteriovenous fistula (AVF, **Fig. 36.51**) is formed, using the radial or brachial artery and the cephalic vein. Large-bore needles are inserted into the arterialized vein of the AVF to take blood to and from the dialysis machine. In patients with poor-quality veins or arterial disease (e.g. diabetes mellitus), synthetic arteriovenous grafts offer an alternative.

For many, an AVF is not an immediate or appropriate solution, and a *semi-permanent dual-lumen venous catheter* can be inserted under a skin tunnel into the jugular or femoral vein. Although

i Box 36.37 Range of concentrations in routinely available final dialysates used for haemodialysis	
Dialysate	**Range of concentration (mmol/L)**
Sodium	130–145
Potassium	0.0–4.0
Calcium	1.0–1.6
Magnesium	0.25–0.85
Chloride	99–108
Bicarbonate	35–40
Glucose	0–10

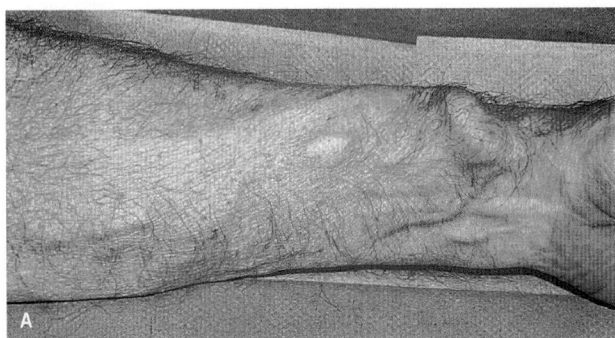

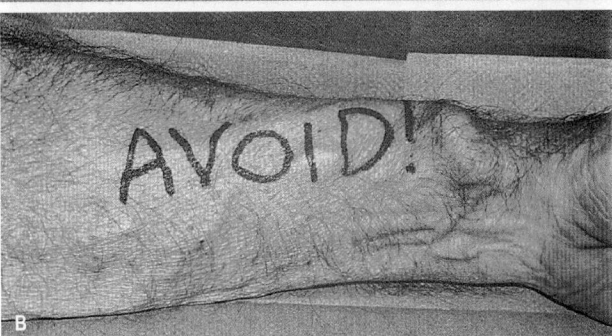

Fig. 36.51 Arteriovenous (radiocephalic) fistula. **(A)** Fistula in the left forearm. **(B)** One way of reminding the anaesthetic, nursing and surgical teams about the presence of an existing arteriovenous fistula in a haemodialysis patient about to undergo surgery. In particular, the fistula should not be compressed during surgery, to avoid thrombosis within it.

easy to place and offering immediate use, there is a significant risk of bloodstream infection (with a foreign body directly accessing the circulation), catheter malfunction (thrombosis), or venous stenosis or occlusion.

For urgent dialysis a temporary (and untunnelled) large-bore, double-lumen dialysis catheter may be inserted into a central vein – usually the subclavian, jugular or femoral vein.

Aims

- *Maintain euvolaemia* – the ideal (or 'dry') weight. Fluid gains (in kilograms) between each dialysis session are the sum of fluid intake less fluid losses over a 48-hour interdialytic interval. A patient who is anuric (with no urine output) who drinks 2 L/day will gain 4 kg if no insensible or stool losses occur. If a patient is weighed before and after each session (with the post-dialysis weight described as the 'dry' weight), dialysis can deliver long-term volume and blood pressure control.
- *Maintain electrolytes* in balance. A low dialysate potassium (of 1–3 mmol/L) allows rapid control of hyperkalaemia and a negative potassium balance (of 1–2 mmol/kg per session) over a treatment. Dialysate sodium is carefully controlled to prevent large fluid shifts (at 137–141 mmol/L, although this can be individualized), and calcium fixed to mimic the ionized fraction (and prevent net calcium gain during dialysis).
- *Prevent acidosis.* Dialysate is buffered with bicarbonate at (for example) 36 mmol/L. This will diffuse into blood to correct acidosis during treatment.
- *Balance frequency and duration with quality of life.* Between 4 and 5 h of treatment three times a week is considered 'adequate' to maintain volume and solute balance over time. Shorter or less frequent dialysis is usually sufficient only if a patient has considerable *residual renal function* (usually assessed by measuring 24- or 48-h urine volumes and clearances, then adding this to the dialysis clearance). Recent evidence is pointing towards more frequent dialysis (up to 5–6 dialysis sessions per week) or longer treatment duration (6–8 h three times weekly) as offering more benefit in terms of quality of life, solute clearance and cardiovascular health. However, it is less popular among patients and associated with early loss of residual renal function and vascular access loss.
- *Deliver enough dialysis* (adequacy). The size, number and nature of 'uraemic toxins' are not clear, and the only true measure of adequacy is patient mortality and morbidity. Symptoms of under-dialysis are non-specific and include insomnia, itching and fatigue (despite adequate correction of anaemia), restless legs and a peripheral sensory neuropathy. Formal measures using urea as a surrogate calculate the urea reduction ratio (URR, targeting >65% per session) or the eKt/V (where K is the dialyser clearance, t is the duration of dialysis in minutes, and V is the urea distribution volume estimated as total body water) as minimum thresholds required for well-nourished dialysis patients dialysed three times per week. It is unclear whether a higher eKt/V (more dialysis than is thought of as adequate) associates with better outcomes; initial trial data suggest not.

Specific complications

- Access (either AVF or catheter) malfunction, thrombosis or bleeding.
- Bloodstream infections, which may disseminate to soft tissue (septic arthritis), cardiac valves (endocarditis) or spinal column (vertebritis).
- Dialysis disequilibrium, when dialysis is initiated with too rapid early urea removal. Subsequent movement of fluid towards the higher urea seen across the blood–brain barrier can cause cerebral oedema and fitting.
- Intradialytic hypotension (where too rapid fluid removal exceeds refill of the circulation from the extravascular space).
- Dialysis-related amyloidosis, where failure of clearance of β_2-microglobulin, a molecule of 11.8 kDa, leads to amyloid deposits, median nerve compression in the carpal tunnel, a dialysis arthropathy, bone cysts and fractures, pseudotumours and gastrointestinal bleeding.

Haemofiltration

Haemofiltration differs from haemodialysis in that there is no dialysate; rather, plasma water (along with suspended solutes) is removed by convection across a high-flux semipermeable membrane. Substitution fluid (with the desired biochemical composition) is then infused to replace (large) fluid losses (**Fig. 36.52**). Haemofiltration may be preferred in the acute setting, where haemodynamic instability is common (particularly on ITUs). Modern dialysis machines have built-in facilities to generate online ultra-pure water, which has minimized the cost of the procedure. It has also given the clinician the option to use this technique either as haemofiltration or in combination with dialysis as *haemodiafiltration* (HDF) to increase middle molecule clearance (e.g. β_2-microglobulin) and prevent long-term dialysis complications such as dialysis-related amyloidosis, particularly in young, highly sensitized, non-transplantable patients. Post-hoc analysis of several trials has suggested that HDF with a convection component of more than 20 L per session is associated with survival advantage.

Peritoneal dialysis

Peritoneal dialysis uses the peritoneal membrane as a semipermeable membrane, avoiding the need for extracorporeal circulation of blood. It is a very simple, low-technology (yet effective) treatment compared to haemodialysis (**Fig. 36.53**).

- A soft catheter is placed through a skin tunnel into the peritoneal cavity through the midline of the anterior abdominal wall (**Fig. 36.54**).
- Dialysate is run into the peritoneal cavity, usually under gravity.
- Urea, creatinine, phosphate and other uraemic toxins pass into the dialysate down their concentration gradients.
- Water (with solutes) is attracted into the peritoneal cavity by osmosis, depending on the osmolarity of the dialysate. This is determined by the glucose or polymer (icodextrin) content of the dialysate (**Box 36.38**). More hypertonic solutions (rising from around 1.5% to 4% glucose) will improve fluid removal.
- The fluid is exchanged regularly to repeat the process.

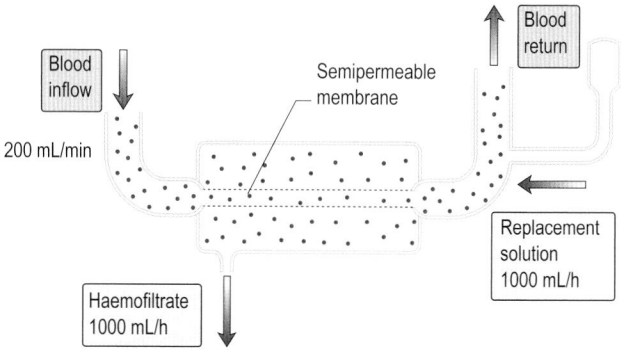

Fig. 36.52 Principles of haemofiltration.

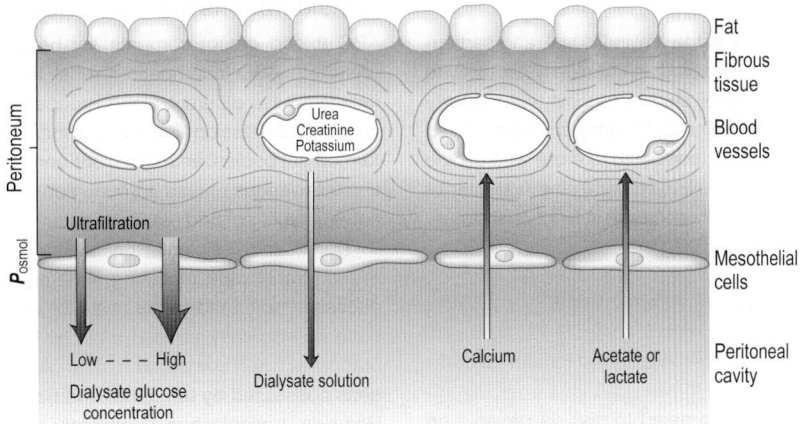

Fig. 36.53 Principles of peritoneal dialysis. Water is attracted into the peritoneal cavity, depending on the osmolarity of the dialysate.

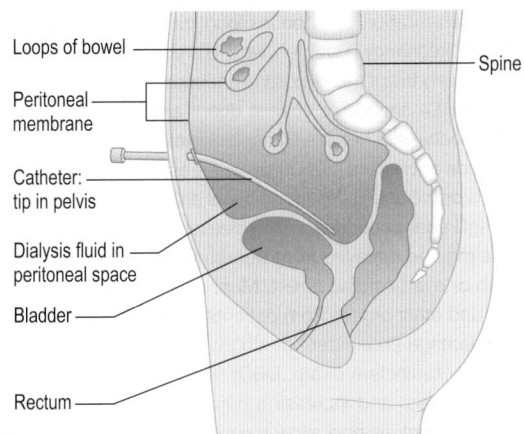

Fig. 36.54 The siting of a Tenckhoff peritoneal dialysis catheter.

> **Box 36.38 Range of concentrations in routinely available CAPD dialysates**

Dialysate	Range of concentration (mmol/L)
Sodium	130–134
Potassium	0
Calcium	1.0–1.75
Magnesium	0.25–0.75
Chloride	95–104
Lactate	35–40
Glucose[a]	77–236
Total osmolality	356–511 mOsm/kg

[a]Glucose content is often expressed as g/dL of anhydrous glucose (e.g. 1.36% = 77 mmol/L). An even more hypertonic dialysate (6.36%) is available for acute (intermittent) peritoneal dialysis. CAPD, continuous ambulatory peritoneal dialysis.

***Continuous ambulatory peritoneal dialysis* (*CAPD*)** has dialysate present within the peritoneal cavity continuously, except during an exchange (done 3–5 times a day using a sterile no-touch technique to connect 1.5–3 L bags of dialysate to the peritoneal catheter; each exchange takes 20–40 minutes.

***Automated peritoneal dialysis* (or *nightly intermittent peritoneal dialysis*)** has a simple exchange machine performing continuous low-volume exchanges each night while the patient is asleep.

> **? Box 36.39 Some causes of CAPD peritonitis[a]**

Cause	Approximate % of cases
Staphylococcus epidermidis	40–50
Escherichia coli, Pseudomonas and other Gram-negative organisms	25
Staphylococcus aureus	15
Mycobacterium tuberculosis	2
Candida and other fungal species	2

[a]In approximately 20%, no bacteria are found. CAPD, continuous ambulatory peritoneal dialysis.

Sometimes dialysate is left in the peritoneal cavity during the day in addition, to increase the time during which biochemical exchange is taking place.

Specific complications

- Bacterial peritonitis, presenting as fever, abdominal pain and a cloudy peritoneal dialysate effluent (>100 cells/mm³ on microscopy is suggestive) progressing to frank peritonitis, occurs at the rate of about one episode for every 2 patient-years. Once peritoneal effluent is sent for culture, empirical antibiotic treatment is started. Common causative organisms are listed in **Box 36.39.**
- Catheter exit site infections may progress to skin tunnel infections and peritonitis.
- Constipation may impair flow of dialysate in and out of the pelvis.
- Hernias are caused by raised intra-abdominal pressure, and dialysate 'leaks' into the pleural cavity or scrotum (down a patent processus vaginalis).
- Sclerosing peritonitis is a potentially fatal complication of CAPD, where long-term patients develop progressive thickening of the peritoneal membrane. This occurs in association with adhesions and strictures, turning the small bowel into a mass of matted loops and causing repeated episodes of small bowel obstruction.

Adequacy

Most clinicians aim for a weekly *Kt/V* of 2.0 (see earlier), coupled with a creatinine clearance of 60 L per week. Once patients stop passing urine (and have no residual renal function), peritoneal dialysis inadequacy becomes common, and a switch in technique to haemodialysis may be required.

Dialysis in the frail

Dialysis can prolong life but the benefit to any individual, and particularly to frail patients, varies widely. Outcomes in frail elderly people who are undergoing dialysis are poor. Small studies suggest that mortality or quality-of-life outcomes do not differ significantly among selected patients who elect to undergo dialysis, compared to those who decide against dialysis. In one study, over 50% died within the first year of initiating dialysis and around 30% had a decrease in functional status.

Renal transplantation

Successful renal transplantation offers the potential for almost complete rehabilitation in ESKD.

- Survival is significantly better compared to dialysis patients on transplant waiting lists.
- Transplantation allows freedom from dietary and fluid restrictions.
- Anaemia and infertility are corrected.
- Any need for parathyroidectomy is reduced.

It is the treatment of choice for any *appropriate* patients with ESKD. However, the supply of donor organs (in the UK, 44 per million population per year) is exceeded by demand. Donor organs are a scarce and valuable resource that must be used optimally.

Kidney transplantation involves the anastomosis of an explanted human kidney, usually either from a deceased donor or from a living related or unrelated donor, on to the iliac vessels of the recipient (**Fig. 36.55**). The donor ureter is placed into the recipient's bladder. Unless the donor is genetically identical (i.e. an identical twin), immunosuppressive treatment is needed, for as long as the transplant remains in place, to prevent rejection. Patient and graft survival has steadily improved with:

- more appropriate patient selection and assessment
- better donor–recipient compatibility
- improvements in surgical techniques
- more efficient immunosuppressive regimens.

Some 80% of grafts now survive for 5–10 years in the best centres, and 50% for 10–30 years. However, the half-life of renal allografts is still 13–16 years. The three most common causes of late graft loss are death of patients with a functioning graft, recurrence of the original (or new) renal disease, and chronic allograft nephropathy.

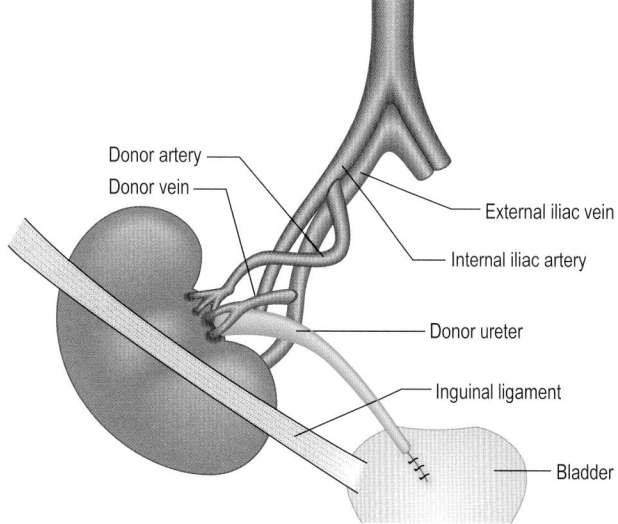

Donor artery
Donor vein
External iliac vein
Internal iliac artery
Donor ureter
Inguinal ligament
Bladder

Fig. 36.55 Anatomy of a renal transplant operation.

Considerations in successful kidney transplantation

ABO (blood group) compatibility between donor and recipient is preferred. ABO-incompatible renal transplants (where donor and recipient have different blood groups) are successful with directed immunosuppression (including immunoadsorption to remove preformed antibodies, anti-CD20 antibodies to remove B lymphocytes, and intravenous pooled immunoglobulins for immunomodulation or anti-idiotypic antibodies).

Donor and recipient HLA mismatches should ideally be minimized. Nationwide matching schemes for kidneys retrieved from deceased donors form the basis for kidney transplant offers. Complete compatibility at A, B and DR loci offers the best long-term outcomes when compared to multiply mismatched organs (i.e. antigens possessed by the donor and not possessed by the recipient). However, transplanting completely mismatched kidneys, particularly with living donation, is routine and results are as good as, if not better than, properly matched deceased donor kidneys.

Pre-formed (historical) anti-HLA antibodies in recipients, resulting from either sensitization from prior blood transfusions, kidney transplants or past pregnancy in women, tend to predict less good outcomes. This is particularly true if these existing antibodies are donor-specific (or recipient anti-HLA antibodies against donor antigens). Transplantation can still be successful but pre-transplant strategies are necessary to minimize these antibodies (with plasmapheresis, intravenous immunoglobulin and/or the anti-B cell monoclonal antibody rituximab or newly described IgG endopeptidase, which cleaves off IgG).

Organs may be retrieved from donors who have sustained brainstem death or even cardiac arrest. Most countries allow the removal of kidneys and other organs from patients who have suffered irretrievable brain damage ('brainstem death') while the heart is still beating (donation after brainstem death, DBD; see p. 236). Due to the shortage of solid organs and increasing numbers of patients waiting for them, several countries now allow the retrieval of organs after cardiac death (donation after cardiac death, DCD), with comparable results to 'heart-beating' donations. Increasing use is also made of expanded criteria donors (ECDs) aged over 60 years, or those between 55 and 59 years but with co-morbidity such as hypertension, diabetes, pre-retrieval AKI and intracranial haemorrhage as a cause of death.

Living related or unrelated donation offers the best kidney outcomes. Potential living donors undergo comprehensive preoperative evaluation to ensure that they will come to no harm through donating a kidney to another person. Recent evidence suggests that live donors carry a statistically increased risk of CKD/ESKD post donation but the inherent risk is too low for it to be of clinical significance. Young women donors are at increased risk of gestational hypertension or preeclampsia in subsequent pregnancies, though without any ill-effects on their children. As a result, all living donors should be consented carefully and monitored regularly.

Timing transplantation so that it takes place prior to dialysis initiation (pre-emptive transplantation) offers benefits to both recipient and graft.

Immunosuppression for transplantation

Long-term inhibition of the recipient immune system is needed to prevent immune-mediated injury to grafts recognized as non-self. This is almost universally the case, except where living related donation from an identical twin occurs. Some degree of immunological tolerance does develop and the risk of rejection is highest in the first 3 months after transplantation. In the early months, rejection episodes occur in less than 20% of cadaver kidney recipients on current immunosuppression protocols, and most cases are reversible. A combination of immunosuppressive drugs is usually used (**Box 36.40**). Individualizing

Box 36.40 Immunosuppressive drugs used in renal transplantation

Class	Mechanism of action	Examples	Clinical role	Side-effects
Calcineurin inhibitors	Disrupt T-cell signalling	Ciclosporin Tacrolimus	Mainstay of most regimens	Nephrotoxicity (monitor levels), hypertension, diabetes, hirsutism, virilization
Inhibitors of purine synthesis	Inhibit purine synthesis and hence active proliferation of cells (especially lymphocytes)	Azathioprine Mycophenolate mofetil (MMF)	Used in most regimens	Neutropenia, pancytopenia, deranged LFTs (azathioprine), diarrhoea (MMF) Interaction with allopurinol (azathioprine)
Steroids	Inhibit cytokine-regulated T-cell signalling	Prednisolone (oral) Methylprednisolone (i.v.)	Used in most regimens. Dose tapers over first few weeks I.v. methylprednisolone used on induction and to treat acute rejection	Multiple, including osteoporosis, hypertension, diabetes, weight gain, poor wound healing, lipid abnormalities
Rapamycin (Sirolimus)	Inhibits cytokine-dependent cell proliferation		Role still being explored Alternative to calcineurin inhibitors	Delayed graft function, myelosuppression, impaired wound healing, thrombocytopenia Levels should be monitored
Anti-CD25 antibodies	Monoclonal antibody, blocking the IL-2 receptor	Daclizumab Basiliximab	Given on induction Usually used in patients with medium to high risk of rejection	Well tolerated
Antibodies causing T-cell depletion	Target and destroy T cells	Anti-thymocyte globulin (ATG) = polyclonal OKT3 = monoclonal anti-CD3 antibody	For steroid-resistant rejection (7–10-day course) May be used as induction agent for patients at high risk of rejection	Severe T-cell depletion (risk of sepsis) Late development of malignancy, esp. lymphoma
Anti-CD52 antibody	Depletes both T and B cells	Alemtuzumab	Used as induction agent	Over-immunosuppression, risk of sepsis and malignancy in longer term Long-term outcome data awaited
Anti-B7 antibody	Prevents engagement of B7 and CD28 Blocks co-stimulatory signal	Belatacept	Has been tried with success in maintenance regimens instead of calcineurin inhibitors	Relatively high but mild rejection High incidence of post-transplant lymphoma in EBV-negative patients
Anti-C5a antibody	Inhibits complement activation by blocking activated C5	Eculizumab	Success in acute antibody-mediated rejections Atypical HUS post transplant	Infections, particularly meningococcal meningitis. Patients should be vaccinated against meningitis prior to its use

EBV, Epstein–Barr virus; HUS, haemolytic uraemic syndrome; IL-2, interleukin 2; LFTs, liver function tests.

immunosuppression to a specific recipient remains an inexact science, and preventing the complications of over-immunosuppression is as necessary as preventing rejection. Therapeutic drug monitoring is useful in delivering the most intense immunosuppression in the early post-transplant phase and allows lower target ranges further out.

Early complications

Early (technical) failure
Occlusion or stenosis of the arterial anastomosis, occlusion of the venous anastomosis and urinary leaks owing to damage to the lower ureter or to defects in the anastomosis between ureter and recipient bladder can occur, despite best surgical technique.

Acute tubular necrosis
Delayed graft function (DGF) resulting from ATN is the most common cause of deceased donor graft dysfunction (up to 40–50%), particularly in kidneys from DCD or ECD donors (see earlier). Hypotension or loss of cardiac output will have an understandable impact on the retrieved organ. A prolonged 'cold ischaemia time' (the period during which the retrieved organ is cooled on ice in transit and awaits implantation) also leads to delayed graft function due to ATN. Finally, calcineurin inhibitors used to prevent rejection are themselves nephrotoxic where high peak and trough concentrations cause tubular injury. Kidneys transported on a perfusion machine, and controlled hypothermia in deceased donors prior to organ retrieval, have been associated with improvements in DGF rates.

Acute rejection
Acute rejection is seen in between 10% and 30% of transplant recipients and usually presents with declining renal function within the first 3 months. Renal biopsy (**Fig. 36.56A**) can confirm the diagnosis and also assesses the severity and type of rejection, but sampling errors do occur. Urinary measurement of RNA is also being used to detect acute cellular rejection (T-cell or antibody-mediated, with or without endothelial injury – so-called 'vascular rejection').

Cellular rejection may respond to high-dose intravenous corticosteroids, increased or switched calcineurin inhibition, or the use

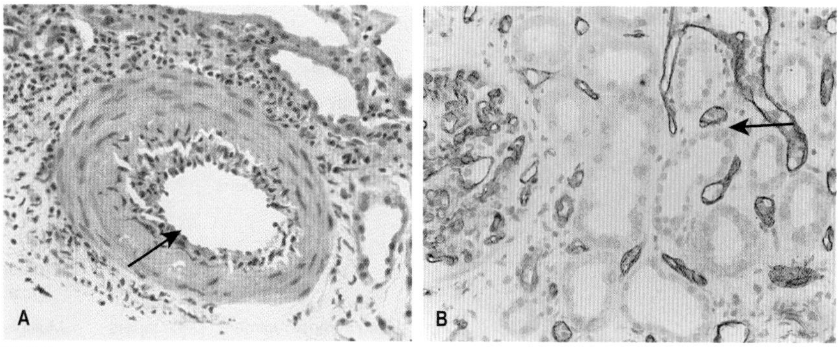

Fig. 36.56 Histology of kidney in rejection. **(A)** Acute vascular rejection: the mononuclear inflammatory cell infiltrate is limited to the expanded intima and does not involve the entire vascular wall as in systemic vasculitis. The arrow indicates endothelialitis. **(B)** Antibody-mediated rejection: an acute tubular necrosis with capillary glomerulitis and peritubular and glomerular capillary C4d positivity (arrowed).

of T-cell-depleting agents such as anti-thymocyte globulin (ATG) or anti-CD52 antibody (Campath). Antibody-mediated rejection (diagnosed by the presence of circulating donor-specific anti-HLA antibodies and evidence of complement activation on renal biopsy by C4d staining, **Fig. 36.56B**) is usually treated empirically by a combination of intravenous immunoglobulin (to neutralize and promote the clearance of anti-HLA antibodies), plasmapheresis (to remove antibodies) and anti-CD20 antibody administration (to deplete B lymphocytes), with variable success.

More than one rejection within the first 3 months, vascular and/or antibody-mediated rejection, delayed rejection (requirement of dialysis within the first week after transplantation), and failure of serum creatinine to return to baseline (<130 μmol/L) after a rejection episode are associated with worse long-term outcome.

Infection

- Bacterial infections occur early (<1 month postoperatively) and involve the urinary tract, wounds and chest.
- Cytomegalovirus infection develops weeks or months after transplantation in 70% of cytomegalovirus-seronegative recipients receiving grafts from a seropositive donor, and in patients receiving biological agents (antibodies) as induction or therapy for rejection, unless prophylaxis with valganciclovir is given. Opportunist infections, such as those with *Pneumocystis jiroveci*, occur and prophylactic co-trimoxazole is given in the early months. These infections also arise in the months after transplantation and are associated with heavier immunosuppressant burdens.
- Polyomavirus infection (**BK nephropathy**) causes an often aggressive TIN that may lead to graft loss. The only existing therapy is minimization of immunosuppression in the hope of spontaneous viral clearance.

Late complications

- **Post-transplantation lymphoproliferative disorders**, often associated with Epstein–Barr virus, are more frequent malignancies in patients who received profound immunosuppression. Immunization is minimized and standard chemotherapy offered, with mixed outcomes.
- **Immunosuppressive therapy** increases the risk of skin tumours, including basal and squamous cell carcinoma. Other cancers that occur at increased frequency include renal, cervical and vaginal malignancies.
- **Cardiovascular disease** causes 50% of patient deaths after transplantation. Increased hypertension, obesity, diabetes, insu-

lin resistance and lipid disorders all play a role, as does an often long history of CKD.
- **Post-transplant osteoporosis** may occur as a result of steroid use.
- **Recurrent renal disease** is surprisingly common. Primary FSGS often recurs and causes early graft loss. Mesangiocapillary GN, diabetic nephropathy and IgA nephropathy also commonly recur, with variable effects on long-term graft survival.

Most grafts fail eventually through lasting immunological injury, the toxicities of immunosuppressant drugs, or even both. A common histological finding is interstitial fibrosis and tubular atrophy, a lesion once called chronic allograft nephropathy. There is a growing understanding of the role of subclinical chronic antibody-mediated rejection due to existing or *de novo* donor-specific antibodies, but non-immunological factors play an important part as well. Progressive irreversible decline in graft function is associated with mild to modest proteinuria (<3 g/day), and interventions to change this trajectory currently lack evidence of benefit.

Renal transplantation in HIV patients

Modern anti-retroviral therapy (ART) offers patients with HIV infection a near-normal life expectancy. However, an increasing number develop ESKD, and HIV was considered to be a contraindication to renal transplantation. However, a study of outcomes for 150 HIV-infected patients undergoing renal transplantation has shown that kidney transplantation is safe and effective in these individuals, at least in the short term. The patients in the study had CD4+ T-cell counts of 200 cells/mm³ or more, and undetectable plasma levels of HIV type 1 RNA while on stable ART during the 16 weeks before renal transplantation. Median follow-up was 1.7 years. Survival rates at 1 year (95%) and 3 years (88%) were worse in HIV-infected patients than in the general population of kidney transplant recipients, but better than those in patients aged 65 years and over. Many rejection episodes were glucocorticoid-resistant, suggesting an aggressive response to donor antigens.

Further reading

Levin A, Tonelli M, Bonventre J et al; ISN Global Kidney Health Summit participants. Global kidney health 2017 and beyond: a roadmap for closing gaps in care, research, and policy. *Lancet* 2017; 390:1888–1917.

Loupy A, Lefaucheur C. Antibody-mediated rejection of solid-organ allografts. *N Engl J Med* 2018; 379:1150–1160.

Siu JHY, Surendrakumar V, Richards JA et al. T cell allorecognition pathways in solid organ transplantation. *Front Immunol* 2018; 9:2548.

Steiner RW. The risks of living kidney donation. *N Engl J Med* 2016; 374:479–481.

Webster AC, Nagler EV, Morton RL et al. Chronic kidney disease. *Lancet* 2017; 389:1238–1252.

CYSTIC RENAL DISEASE

Solitary or multiple renal cysts are common, especially with advancing age; 50% of those over 50 years of age have one or more such cysts. They have no special significance, except in the differential diagnosis of renal tumours (see p. 1406). These cysts are often asymptomatic and are found on ultrasound examination performed for some other reason. Occasionally, they may cause pain and/or haematuria if large, or bleeding may occur into the cyst. Cystic degeneration (the formation of multiple cysts that enlarge with time) occurs regularly in the non-functioning kidneys of patients with ESKD treated by dialysis and/or transplantation. These acquired cysts have malignant potential.

Autosomal dominant polycystic kidney disease

Autosomal dominant polycystic kidney disease (ADPKD) is an inherited disorder that usually presents in adulthood. It is characterized by the development of multiple renal cysts, variably associated with extrarenal (mainly hepatic and cardiovascular) abnormalities. ADPKD is by far the most common inherited nephropathy, with a prevalence rate ranging from 1:400 to 1:1000 in white populations. It accounts for 3–10% of all patients commencing regular dialysis in the West.

Mutations in *PKD1* (on chromosome 16) are responsible for 85% of cases, with mutations in *PKD2* (on chromosome 4) accounting for the remainder. These genetic abnormalities are distinct from the autosomal recessive form of polycystic disease (due to mutations in the *PKHD1* gene on chromosome 6p21.1-p12), which is often lethal in early life.

PKD1 encodes polycystin 1, involved in cell–cell and/or cell–matrix interactions. *PKD2* encodes polycystin 2, which functions as a calcium ion channel. The polycystin complex occurs in cilia, responsible for sensing flow in the tubule. Disruption of the polycystin pathway results in reduced cytoplasmic calcium, which, in principal cells (see p. 196) of the collecting duct, causes defective ciliary signalling and disoriented cell division, leading to cyst formation. Extra-renal manifestations include an increased level of intracranial aneurysms and polycystic liver disease, which can be severe and associated with significant morbidity. Mis-sense mutations in *GANAB*, encoding glucosidase II subunit α (GIIα), have been discovered to be associated with combined ADPKD and polycystic liver disease. The *GANAB* gene product GIIα is an absolute requirement for maturation and surface and ciliary localization of the ADPKD proteins (PKD1 and PKD2).

Progressive loss of renal function is usually attributed to mechanical compression, apoptosis of the healthy tissue and reactive fibrosis. Renal function declines at a variable rate, depending on the growth and size of cysts; patients with rapidly growing cysts on MRI lose renal function more rapidly. Strategies to slow the growth rate of cysts have been very effective in preserving renal function in animal models. These therapies include the vasopressin V_2 receptor inhibitors (vaptans, to reduce cyclic adenosine monophosphate (cAMP) in the principal cells), roscovitine (a cyclin-dependent kinase inhibitor) and antiproliferative therapy with sirolimus (mammalian target of rapamycin (mTOR) inhibitor).

Clinical features

Presenting symptoms occur from any point in the second decade onwards:

- loin pain and/or haematuria from haemorrhage into a cyst, cyst infection or urinary tract stone formation
- loin or abdominal discomfort as the size of the kidneys increases

- subarachnoid haemorrhage associated with berry aneurysm rupture
- complications of hypertension
- complications of associated liver cysts (occur in around 50%)
- symptoms of uraemia and/or anaemia associated with CKD.

Complications and associations

- Pain from large cysts can be difficult to manage; surgical decompression is of some benefit in about two-thirds of affected patients.
- Cyst infection is most effectively treated with lipophilic antibiotics that penetrate into infected cysts and are active against Gram-negative bacteria, such as co-trimoxazole and fluoroquinolones.
- Renal calculi occur in 10–20% and are often composed of uric acid and are radiolucent (see **Fig. 36.30**).
- Hypertension is an early and very common feature of ADPKD. Intrarenal activation of the renin–angiotensin system is thought to be contributory, so ACE inhibitors are logical first-line agents in treatment. Early control of blood pressure is essential as left ventricular hypertrophy is common, and cardiovascular complications are a major cause of death in ADPKD.
- Progressive CKD is the most serious complication of ADPKD. At glomerular filtration rates below 50 mL/min, the rate of decline in GFR averages 5 mL/min each year, which is more rapid than in other primary renal disorders. The probability of being alive without requiring dialysis or transplantation by the age of 70 years is in the order of 30%. Survival rates on regular haemodialysis and after renal transplantation in ADPKD are better than those in patients with other primary renal diseases.
- Approximately 30% of patients have hepatic cysts, occasionally massive enlargement of the polycystic liver with pain, infection and, more rarely, compression of the bile duct, portal vein or hepatic venous outflow.
- Some 10% of ADPKD patients have an asymptomatic intracranial aneurysm (see p. 845). The prevalence is twice as high if a family history of aneurysms or intracranial haemorrhage is present. Screening for intracranial aneurysm in ADPKD is recommended for patients aged 18–40 years who have a positive family history.
- Mitral valve prolapse is found in 20% of individuals with ADPKD.

Diagnosis and screening

Physical examination commonly reveals large, irregular kidneys and possibly hepatomegaly. Definitive diagnosis is established by ultrasound examination (**Fig. 36.57** and **Box 36.41**). However, such renal imaging techniques may be equivocal, especially in subjects under the age of 15 years. A number of conditions can mimic the clinical and radiological appearance of ADPKD (**Box 36.42**).

The children and siblings of patients with established ADPKD should, in general, be offered screening. Affected individuals should have regular blood pressure checks and should be offered genetic counselling. Gene linkage analysis can be utilized in many families.

Management

No definitive therapy is yet available. Potential strategies include:

- ***Vasopressin receptor antagonists***, which act by inhibiting cAMP in principal cells, reduce cyst growth and slow the rate of progression of renal failure; they have been approved for use in patients with annual rate of decline of eGFR of >3 mL/min. Reversible liver toxicity requires close monitoring.

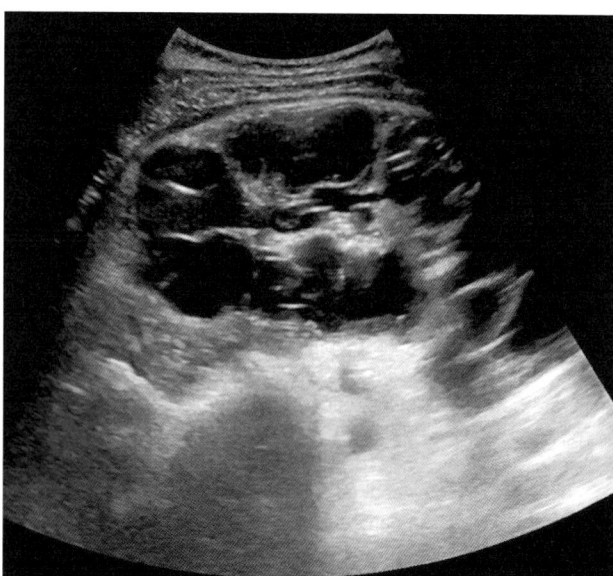

Fig. 36.57 Ultrasound image of a polycystic kidney. There is almost complete replacement of normal renal tissue.

> ℹ **Box 36.41 Ultrasonographic diagnostic criteria for testing individuals at risk of autosomal dominant polycystic kidney disease (ADPKD)**
>
> In at-risk individuals, a diagnosis of ADPKD is established if patients meet the following criteria:
> - 15–39 years: ≥3 cysts (unilateral or bilateral)
> - 40–59 years: ≥2 cysts in each kidney
> - ≥60 years: ≥4 cysts in each kidney
>   ADPKD is excluded in patients meeting the following criteria:
> - ≥40 years: <2 cysts
> - 30–39 years: 0 cysts (this excludes ADPKD in 98% of cases).
>   At <30 years, a negative renal ultrasound scan does not exclude a diagnosis of ADPKD; other imaging techniques, such as CT and MRI, may be useful and molecular genetic testing might be needed.

- **Octreotide**, a long-acting somatostatin analogue (which also inhibits cAMP), has been beneficial in halting the growth of both liver and renal cysts. However, in a recent study the somatostatin analogue lanreotide did not slow decline in kidney function in more than 300 patients with later-stage ADPKD (eGFR 30–60 mL/min) over 2.5 years of follow-up, despite a significant effect on the rate of htTKV growth.
- In the HALT-PKD study A, patients with early PKD and eGFR >60 mL/min, when randomized to a low blood pressure group (95/60–110/75 mmHg), had slower annualized increase in total kidney volume and lower albuminuria and left ventricular mass index, compared to the standard blood pressure group (120/70–130/80 mmHg). In late-stage PKD (eGFR 25–60 mL/min), adding an angiotensin receptor blocker to an ACE inhibitor (dual blockade) did not confer additional benefit at 5–8-year follow-up.
- Two studies of mTOR inhibitors, e.g. rapamycin, in PKD were essentially negative for the primary end-point of cyst growth and preservation of renal function.

Medullary cystic disease ('juvenile nephronophthisis')

Juvenile nephronophthisis develops early in childhood and is inherited in an autosomal recessive manner. Mutations in the genes *NPHP1–4*, encoding nephrocystin and inversin (both co-localized in

> ℹ **Box 36.42 Conditions that clinically and radiologically mimic polycystic kidney disease**
>
> - *Tuberous sclerosis*: includes lymphangiomyomatosis and lymphangioleiomyomatosis, and can be associated with the *TSC2–PKD1* contiguous gene syndrome
> - *Von Hippel–Lindau syndrome*
> - *Multicystic dysplastic kidney*: a non-heritable unilateral syndrome or a systemic syndrome (e.g. prune belly syndrome)
> - *Juvenile nephronophthisis* and medullary cystic kidney disease: can be autosomal recessive (presenting in the second decade of life) or autosomal dominant (presenting in the third to fourth decades)
> - *Glomerulocystic kidney disease*: involves the expansion of Bowman's space and is autosomal dominant
> - *Acquired cystic disease*: involves end-stage kidney disease and hypokalaemia
> - *Renal-cell carcinoma*: involves cystic changes

the cilia of the renal tubules) lead to multiple cyst formation. Polyuria, polydipsia and growth retardation result from impaired tubular function. A similar condition developing later in childhood (medullary cystic disease) is inherited as an autosomal dominant trait but sporadic cases occur in both conditions. The dominant histological findings are interstitial inflammation and tubular atrophy, with later development of medullary cysts.

Diagnosis is based on family history and renal biopsy, the cysts rarely being visible on imaging.

Medullary sponge kidney

Medullary sponge kidney is an uncommon cystic condition presenting as intermittent renal colic, the passage of small stones and haematuria. Although it is most often sporadic, a few affected families have been reported. Dilation of the collecting ducts in the papillae occurs, sometimes with cystic change. In severe cases the medullary area has a sponge-like appearance. The condition may affect one or both kidneys, or only part of one kidney. Cyst formation is commonly associated with the development of small calculi within the cyst. In about 20% of patients there is associated hypercalciuria or renal tubular acidosis (see p. 199). Hemi-hypertrophy of the skeleton has been described in this condition.

CT or IVU (see **Fig. 36.28**) is diagnostic. Renal function is usually well maintained and CKD is unusual, except where obstructive nephropathy develops owing to the presence of stones in the pelvis or ureters.

Further reading

Ghata J, Cowley BD, Jr. Polycystic kidney disease. *Compr Physiol* 2017; 7:945–975.

Ingelfinger JR. Tolvaptan and autosomal dominant polycystic kidney disease. *N Engl J Med* 2017; 377:1988–1989.

Meijer E, Visser FW, van Aerts RMM et al. Effect of lanreotide on kidney function in patients with autosomal dominant polycystic kidney disease: the DIPAK 1 Randomized Clinical Trial. *JAMA* 2018; 320:2010–2019.

TUMOURS OF THE KIDNEY AND GENITOURINARY TRACT

Renal cell carcinoma

Renal cell carcinomas (RCCs) arise from proximal tubular epithelium. They are the most common renal tumour in adults (accounting for 1–2% of all malignancies) and affect men more often than women (2 : 1). They usually present after 50 years of age (and rarely before the age of 40).

RCCs are highly vascular tumours; microscopically, most are composed of large cells containing clear cytoplasm.

Clinical features

- RCCs are often asymptomatic and discovered incidentally.
- Haematuria, loin pain and a mass in the flank occur.
- Malaise, anorexia and weight loss may be present (30%).
- Some 5% of patients have polycythaemia (see p. 355).
- Around 30% of patients have hypertension (due to secretion of renin by the tumour) and anaemia, due to depression of erythropoietin in approximately the same number.
- Pyrexia occurs in about 20% of patients.
- Approximately one-third present with metastases.
- Rarely, a left-sided varicocele may be associated with left-sided tumours that have invaded the renal vein and caused obstruction to drainage of the left testicular vein.

Diagnosis

Ultrasound may demonstrate a solid lesion. CT scanning is used to identify the renal lesion and involvement of the renal vein or inferior vena cava. MRI is better than CT for tumour staging. Urine cytology for malignant cells is of no value. The ESR is usually raised. Liver biochemistry may be abnormal, returning to normal after surgery.

Management

Medical management of RCC is discussed on page 127. A nephrectomy is performed unless bilateral tumours are present or the contralateral kidney functions poorly, in which case conservative surgery, such as partial nephrectomy, may be indicated. If metastases are present, nephrectomy may still be warranted, since regression of metastases has been reported after removal of the main tumour mass.

Von Hippel–Lindau (VHL) disease is an autosomal dominant disorder presenting with bilateral RCCs, retinal and cerebellar haemangioblastomas, phaeochromocytomas, pancreatic neuroendocrine tumours and renal cysts. VHL protein acts as a tumour suppressor by tagging hypoxia-inducible gene products (VEGF, TGF) for degradation. Inactivating mutations of the *VHL* gene lead to uncontrolled angiogenesis and neoplasia. Mutations of the same tumour suppressor gene are responsible for RCC and VHL.

Nephroblastoma (Wilms' tumour)

Seen within the first 3 years of life, Wilms' tumour presents as an (occasionally bilateral) abdominal mass, rarely with haematuria. Diagnosis is established by ultrasound, CT and MRI. A combination of nephrectomy, radiotherapy and chemotherapy has much improved survival rates, even in children with metastatic disease. Overall, the 5-year survival rate is 90%.

Urothelial tumours

The calyces, renal pelvis, ureter, bladder and urethra are lined by transitional cell epithelium. Transitional cell cancers account for about 3% of deaths from all forms of malignancy. These tumours are uncommon below the age of 40 years, but more common in men (the male : female ratio is 4 : 1). Bladder tumours are about 50 times as common as those of the ureter or renal pelvis. Predisposing factors include:

- cigarette smoking
- exposure to industrial carcinogens such as β-naphthylamine and benzidine (workers in the petroleum, chemical, cable and rubber industries are at particular risk) or ingestion of aristolochic acid, found in some herbal weight-loss preparations

- exposure to drugs (e.g. phenacetin, cyclophosphamide)
- chronic inflammation (e.g. schistosomiasis, usually associated with squamous carcinoma).

Clinical features

Painless haematuria is the most common presenting symptom (80%) of bladder malignancy, although pain may occur owing to clot retention. Symptoms suggestive of UTI develop in the absence of significant bacteriuria. In patients with bladder cancer, pain also results from local nerve involvement. Presenting symptoms may result from local metastases. Flank pain may occur with urinary tract obstruction in ureteric lesions.

Investigations

- Urine cytology for malignant cells.
- Urinary tumour markers.
- Cystoscopy to assess the tumour burden and for biopsy.
- CT or MRI of the pelvis.

Management

Medical management of urothelial and testicular tumours is discussed on pages 127 and 129, respectively.

DISEASES OF THE PROSTATE GLAND

Benign enlargement of the prostate gland

Benign prostatic enlargement is discussed in detail on page 1480.

Prostatic carcinoma

The pathogenesis, diagnosis and prognosis of prostate cancer are described on page 1480. Management of early disease is outlined on page 1481 and that of later-stage disease on page 128.

THE URINARY TRACT IN THE ELDERLY

Progressive sclerosis of glomeruli occurs with ageing and this, together with the development of atheromatous renal vascular disease, accounts for the progressive reduction in GFR seen as people age. A GFR of 50–60 mL/min (about half the normal value for a young adult) may be regarded as 'normal' in patients over 80 years of age. The reduction in muscle mass often seen with ageing may mask this deterioration in renal function, as creatinine falls despite a falling GFR. Accurate estimation of GFR in the elderly is necessary, particularly when prescribing drugs wholly or partly excreted by the kidney.

Urinary tract infections

UTIs are common in the elderly, where impaired bladder emptying (due to prostatic disease in men) or a neuropathic bladder (especially common in women) is frequently found. Symptoms may be atypical, with confusion, incontinence, nocturia, smelly urine or a vague change in wellbeing with little in the way of dysuria more common (see p. 1374).

Urinary incontinence

See page 312.

Further reading

Tonelli M, Riella M. Chronic kidney disease and the ageing population. *Lancet* 2014; 383:1278–1279.

Bibliography

Cameron JS, Davison AM, Grunfeld JP et al (eds). *Oxford Textbook of Clinical Nephrology*. Oxford: Oxford University Press; 2004.
Current Opinion in Nephrology and Hypertension. A monthly journal with review articles, each issue devoted to one or two topics.

Journal of the American Society of Nephrology. The highest-impact journal in nephrology with bi-monthly self-assessment programme (SAP) supplements.
Kidney International. The major journal associated with the International Society of Nephrology – monthly with original and review articles.
Nephrology, Dialysis, Transplantation. The major European journal devoted to the subject, with review articles, editorial comments and original papers.

Significant websites

http://www.kidney.org.uk *UK charity run by and for patients.*
http://www.tinkershop.net/nephro.htm *Nephrology calculator.*

37 Sexually transmitted infections and human immunodeficiency virus

Janet D. Wilson and Jane Anderson

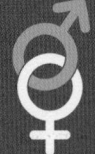

CORE SKILLS AND KNOWLEDGE

Sexually transmitted infections (STIs) are among the most common causes of illness in the world and remain endemic in all societies. They rank among the top five disease categories for which adults seek healthcare worldwide.

Major advances in the treatment of human immunodeficiency virus (HIV) infection have led the global prevalence to increase, even as rates of new infection fall. In those parts of the world with consistent access to effective anti-retroviral therapy, HIV infection has been transformed from a progressively debilitating life-limiting illness characterized by opportunistic infections, into a chronic condition requiring life-long multidisciplinary care.

In many countries the medical specialty of Genitourinary Medicine encompasses sexual health, contraception, HIV care and some public health functions. The specialty is multidisciplinary and holistic; doctors work closely with nurses, health advisers, psychologists, microbiologists, virologists, pharmacists and public health clinicians.

Key skills in this specialty include:

- taking a sexual history and obtaining information for partner notification
- performing a sexual health examination and STI investigations, and correctly interpreting the results
- understanding the principles of anti-retroviral therapy and the holistic approach to outpatient management of HIV infection
- assessing patients with HIV and severe immunosuppression, recognizing important opportunistic infections and acquired immunodeficiency syndrome (AIDS)-defining conditions
- discussing prevention interventions to ensure that people can avoid acquiring or transmitting STIs and HIV.

The best place to experience the outpatient care of people with STIs is in the sexual health clinic, and of those living with HIV in the HIV outpatient clinic. Inpatients with HIV – for example, people presenting with late-stage HIV infection and opportunistic infections – offer opportunities to learn about this spectrum of disease.

CLINICAL SKILLS FOR STI AND HIV CARE

History

Patients presenting with possible STIs or HIV are frequently anxious, embarrassed and concerned about confidentiality. Staff must be alert to these issues and respond sensitively. The clinical setting must ensure privacy and reinforce confidentiality. The clinical history is, of course, tailored to the particular presentation encountered, but many of the points in **Box 37.1** are likely to be relevant.

Examination in the sexual health clinic

Explain the purpose of the examination and obtain consent. Ensure that the clinic door is locked, a chaperone is present, and a good light source is available (**Figs 37.1** and **37.2**).

 Box 37.1 Taking a clinical history in patients with an STI or HIV

Symptom history relevant to STIs
- STIs may be asymptomatic or present with primarily genital symptoms, the most common being:
  - Urethral discharge in males
  - Vaginal discharge in females
  - Lower abdominal pain in females
  - Genital lumps
  - Genital ulceration
  - Genital itching
  - Rectal symptoms
- Systemic symptoms of fever, skin rash, joint pains and eye symptoms may also be present

Symptom history relevant to HIV
- Acute HIV infection:
  - Fever
  - Malaise
  - Myalgia
  - Lethargy
  - Sore throat
  - Maculopapular rash
- Advanced HIV with immunosuppression:
  - Systemic symptoms: fever, weight loss, anorexia
  - Symptoms related to HIV end-organ damage: cognitive impairment, skin disease, weight loss and gastrointestinal disturbance, symptoms of heart or kidney failure
  - Symptoms of immunosuppression and associated infection/malignancy: fever, cough, breathlessness, diarrhoea, skin changes
- A thorough 'review of systems' (see p. 3) is often helpful

Sexual history
- Number and types of recent sexual contacts, with dates
- Gender of partners
- Regular or casual sexual contact with the partner; if regular, how long the couple has been having sex
- Use of condoms
- Any known symptoms or STI diagnosis in the partner
- Sexual practices, e.g. insertive or receptive vaginal, insertive or receptive anal, insertive or receptive pharyngeal, and insertive or receptive oroanal sex
- Whether the patient has ever paid, or has been paid, for sex
- Country of origin of any sexual partners

Previous history of STIs and ongoing risk exposure
- Previous STIs, including dates and treatment received
- HIV testing and results
- Hepatitis A and B, and human papillomavirus (HPV) vaccination status
- Risk factors for ongoing acquisition of HIV and STIs:
  - Frequent partner change
  - Unprotected sex
  - Use of drugs and/or alcohol to a level that reduces safer sex
  - Men having sex with men (MSM)
  - Sexual partners from countries with high HIV prevalence
- Offer risk reduction advice and make patients aware of post-exposure HIV prophylaxis following sexual exposure (PEPSE) and pre-exposure prophylaxis (PrEP, see p. 1449)

Wider history
- Full general medical history
- Full drug history, including recent antibacterial or antiviral treatment
- In women, a menstrual, obstetric and cervical cytology screening history, as well as details of current contraception
- Any past or current history of drug or alcohol misuse

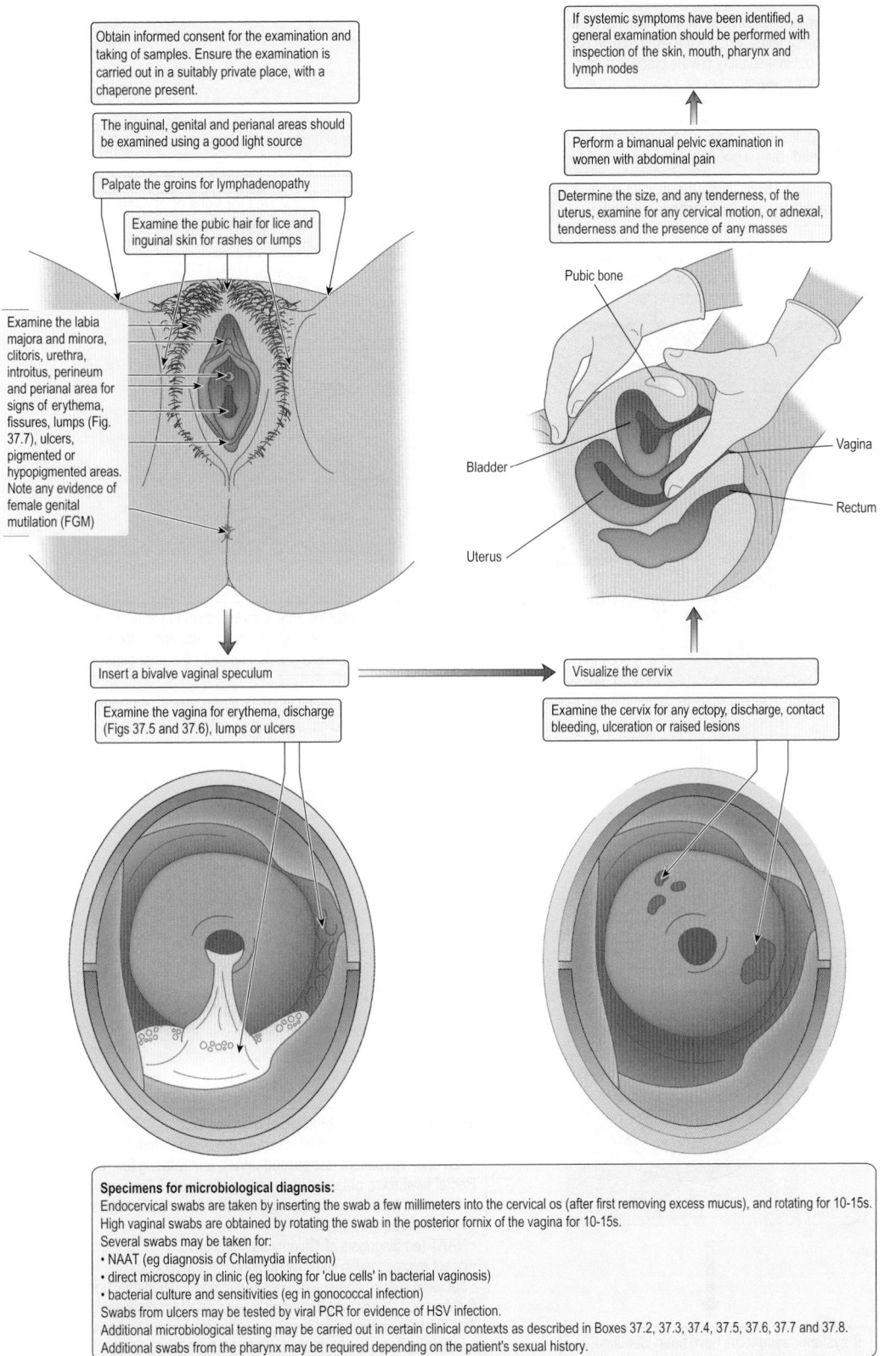

Obtain informed consent for the examination and taking of samples. Ensure the examination is carried out in a suitably private place, with a chaperone present.

The inguinal, genital and perianal areas should be examined using a good light source

Palpate the groins for lymphadenopathy

Examine the pubic hair for lice and inguinal skin for rashes or lumps

Examine the labia majora and minora, clitoris, urethra, introitus, perineum and perianal area for signs of erythema, fissures, lumps (Fig. 37.7), ulcers, pigmented or hypopigmented areas. Note any evidence of female genital mutilation (FGM)

If systemic symptoms have been identified, a general examination should be performed with inspection of the skin, mouth, pharynx and lymph nodes

Perform a bimanual pelvic examination in women with abdominal pain

Determine the size, and any tenderness, of the uterus, examine for any cervical motion, or adnexal, tenderness and the presence of any masses

Pubic bone

Bladder

Uterus

Vagina

Rectum

Insert a bivalve vaginal speculum

Examine the vagina for erythema, discharge (Figs 37.5 and 37.6), lumps or ulcers

Visualize the cervix

Examine the cervix for any ectopy, discharge, contact bleeding, ulceration or raised lesions

Specimens for microbiological diagnosis:
Endocervical swabs are taken by inserting the swab a few millimeters into the cervical os (after first removing excess mucus), and rotating for 10-15s. High vaginal swabs are obtained by rotating the swab in the posterior fornix of the vagina for 10-15s.
Several swabs may be taken for:
• NAAT (eg diagnosis of Chlamydia infection)
• direct microscopy in clinic (eg looking for 'clue cells' in bacterial vaginosis)
• bacterial culture and sensitivities (eg in gonococcal infection)
Swabs from ulcers may be tested by viral PCR for evidence of HSV infection.
Additional microbiological testing may be carried out in certain clinical contexts as described in Boxes 37.2, 37.3, 37.4, 37.5, 37.6, 37.7 and 37.8.
Additional swabs from the pharynx may be required depending on the patient's sexual history.

Fig. 37.1 Female genital examination. HSV, herpes simplex virus, NAAT, nucleic acid amplification testing; PCR, polymerase chain reaction.

Obtain informed consent for the examination and taking of samples. Ensure the examination is carried out in a suitably private place, with a chaperone present.

The inguinal and genital areas should be examined using a good light source

Palpate the groins for lymphadenopathy

Examine the pubic hair for lice and inguinal skin for rashes or lumps

The skin of the penile shaft (retracting the prepuce if present) should be examined for rashes, lumps or ulcers (Fig. 37.8)

The scrotal contents should be palpated, noting any tenderness or lumps, as well as the consistency of the testes

Examine the urethral meatus

Inspect for erythema and discharge (Fig. 37. 4)

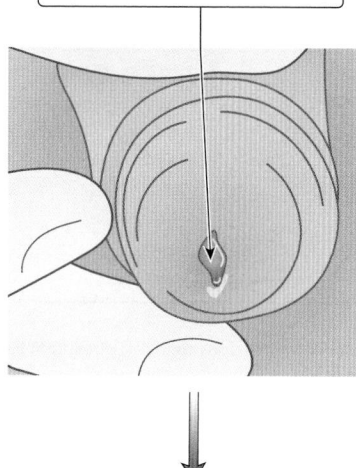

If systemic symptoms have been identified, a general examination should be performed with inspection of the skin, mouth, pharynx and lymph nodes

The perianal area should be examined using a good light source

Examine the perianal area for signs of erythema, fissures, lumps, ulcers, pigmentation or hypopigmentation

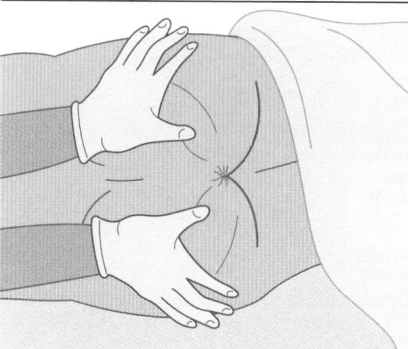

Insert a proctoscope in patients with symptoms of rectal pain, bleeding and discharge, and in those with perianal warts extending into the anal canal

Examine the rectal mucosa for erythema, discharge, contact bleeding, ulceration or raised lesions

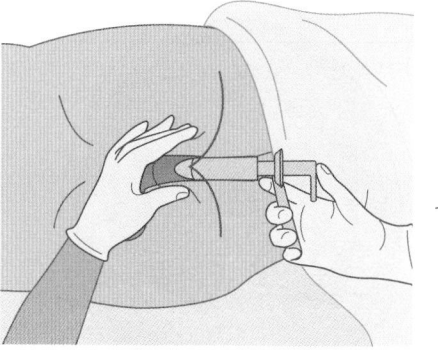

Specimens for microbiological diagnosis:
Urethral swabs are taken by inserting the swab 2-4cm into the urethra (at least 2h after the patient last passed urine), and rotating for 10-15s.
Rectal swabs are obtained by inserting the swab 2-3cm into the rectum, rotating for a few seconds and leaving in place for up to 30s to absorb organisms.
Several swabs may be taken for:
• NAAT (eg diagnosis of Chlamydia infection)
• direct microscopy in clinic (eg looking for gonococcus)
• bacterial culture and sensitivities (eg in gonococcal infection)
Swabs from ulcers may be tested by viral PCR for evidence of HSV infection.
Additional microbiological testing may be carried out in certain clinical contexts as described in Boxes 37.2, 37.4, 37.5, 37.6 37.7 and 37.8.
Additional swabs from the pharynx may be required depending on the patient's sexual history.

Fig. 37.2 Male genital examination and perianal examination in both sexes. HSV, herpes simplex virus, NAAT, nucleic acid amplification testing; PCR, polymerase chain reaction.

SEXUALLY TRANSMITTED INFECTIONS

INTRODUCTION

The World Health Organization (WHO) estimates that more than 1 million people acquire an STI every day. Each year, there are an estimated 376 million new infections with one of the four major curable STIs (chlamydia, gonorrhoea, syphilis and trichomoniasis) in adults aged 15–49 throughout the world. These included 6.3 million cases of syphilis, 87 million of gonorrhoea, 127 million of chlamydia and 156 million of trichomoniasis. The estimates suggest that the vast majority of these infections are in low-income countries. The pattern of STIs is usually different in high-income countries: for example, in England in 2018, the most common STIs were chlamydia (218 095; 49% of all new STI diagnoses), genital warts (57 318; 13%), gonorrhoea (56 259; 13%) and genital herpes (33 867; 8%). The highest prevalence of STIs is in young people, men who have sex with men (MSM) and bisexual men, and black and ethnic minority populations. STIs are associated with high-risk sexual behaviour, frequent partner change and inconsistent use of condoms. Increased travel (both within and between countries), recreational drug use and alcohol are also implicated.

Despite their high global incidence and substantial morbidity, STIs remain neglected in clinical practice, public health and research. There have been rapid increases in antimicrobial resistance in *Neisseria gonorrhoeae* and *Mycoplasma genitalium*, with the possibility of untreatable cases in the near future. STIs often coexist and the inflammation caused by one STI can increase the risk of acquisition of others; most infections also increase the acquisition and transmission of HIV.

ASYMPTOMATIC STI SCREENING

All STIs can be asymptomatic and multiple infections frequently coexist; hence many people without symptoms attend sexual health clinics to seek sexual health checks and advice. Sexual health checks offer public health, as well as individual, benefits because treatment of asymptomatic infections reduces the period of infectivity, prevents long-term complications and reduces onward transmission.

Increasingly, sexual health clinics are making asymptomatic sexual health checks available online, as routine examination of those with no symptoms yields few additional diagnoses. An electronic medical history is self-completed, to confirm the absence of symptoms, as well as a sexual history and risk assessment for STIs, HIV and other blood-borne viruses, to determine which investigations are needed. The self-sampling kit is posted out to the person with instructions of how to take the samples and package them safely. These are then posted back to the service for testing and the results are returned electronically.

The minimum investigations, even if the person is asymptomatic, are tests for chlamydia, gonorrhoea (including samples from extra-genital sites if indicated by the sexual history), syphilis and HIV. HIV antibody testing should be performed on an 'opt-out' basis. If it is declined, the reasons why should be documented. Screening for hepatitis viruses should be performed in those at increased risk, as indicated later.

INVESTIGATION OF STIs

Although the history and examination will guide investigations, remember that multiple infections may coexist and may be asymptomatic. Tests for all STIs are indicated in any patient with a known STI or in those who have been in contact with an STI. The recommended investigations for the different clinical presentations are shown in **Boxes 37.2–37.8** and the recommended tests for specific infections are indicated in the following sections.

Screening for hepatitis A and vaccination

A test for antibodies to hepatitis A (with vaccination if negative) should be performed in:

- MSM
- people who inject drugs
- people with chronic hepatitis B or C
- people living with HIV.

Screening for hepatitis B and vaccination

The recommended screening test in those who have not been immunized is immunoglobulin G (IgG) anti-hepatitis B core (anti-HBc), which is a marker of past infection, and/or hepatitis B surface antigen (HBsAg), which identifies currently infected individuals. Screening is recommended for:

- sexual partners of those who are HBsAg-positive
- MSM and their sexual partners
- people who have been sexually assaulted
- sex workers
- people who inject drugs and their sexual partners
- individuals or those with a sexual partner from countries with intermediate or high prevalence of chronic hepatitis B (defined as 2% or more and including all countries outside Western Europe, North America and Australasia)

? Box 37.2 Causes of urethral discharge

- Urethritis in men usually presents with a urethral discharge and dysuria
- Urethritis is usually divided into gonococcal (due to *N. gonorrhoeae*) or non-gonococcal (NGU)

Infective causes
- *Chlamydia trachomatis*[a]
- *Mycoplasma genitalium*[b]
- *Ureaplasma urealyticum*
- *Neisseria gonorrhoeae*
- *Trichomonas vaginalis* (TV)[c]
- Herpes simplex virus (HSV)[c]
- Urinary tract infection (UTI)[d]
- Adenoviruses (often associated with conjunctivitis)[c]

Non-infective causes
- Non-specific urethritis (where no cause can be identified)
- Physical or chemical trauma
- Urethral stricture

Questions that help discriminate between causes
- Colour of discharge?
- Any dysuria, urinary frequency, nocturia or haematuria?
- Any testicular pain or swelling?
- Any other symptoms, e.g. genital sores or rash, sore eyes?

Investigations
- Microscopy of urethral discharge, nucleic acid amplification test (NAAT) and culture for *N. gonorrhoeae*, NAAT for *C. trachomatis*, NAAT for M. genitalium, serology for syphilis and HIV
- Tests for TV and HSV are not usually performed routinely
- There is no commercial tests available for *U. urealyticum*
- A mid-stream specimen of urine (MSU) should be taken if symptoms are suggestive of UTI

[a]Most common cause of NGU. [b]Second most common cause of NGU. [c]Rarer causes of NGU. [d]Most frequent non-sexually transmitted cause of NGU.

❓ Box 37.3 Causes of vaginal discharge

Infective causes

Vaginal infections
- Bacterial vaginosis (BV)[a]
- *Candida albicans*[a]
- *Trichomonas vaginalis* (TV)[b]

Cervical infections
- *Chlamydia trachomatis*
- *Neisseria gonorrhoeae*
- Herpes simplex virus

Non-infective causes
- Physiological discharge/cervical ectopy[c]
- Cervical polyps
- Neoplasms
- Retained products (e.g. of conception, tampons)
- Chemical irritation

Questions that help discriminate between causes
- Does the discharge have an offensive odour?
- Any vulval itching or soreness?
- Any other symptoms, e.g. dysuria, intermenstrual or postcoital bleeding, abdominal pain?

Investigations
- Microscopy of vaginal discharge for BV, candida and TV, culture for candida, nucleic acid amplification test (NAAT; if available) or culture for TV, NAAT for *N. gonorrhoeae* and *C. trachomatis*, serology for syphilis and HIV

[a]The most common causes of altered vaginal discharge but *C. trachomatis* and *N. gonorrhoeae* infections must also be considered. [b]The most common cause worldwide but rarer in high-income countries. [c]Also a common cause (diagnosis usually made on the basis of exclusion of infective causes).

❓ Box 37.4 Causes of lower abdominal pain

Infective causes
- Pelvic inflammatory disease (PID)[a,b]
  - *Chlamydia trachomatis*[c]
  - *Neisseria gonorrhoeae*
  - *Mycoplasma genitalium*
  - Bacterial vaginosis (BV)
- Urinary tract infection (UTI)

Non-infective causes
- Ectopic pregnancy
- Acute appendicitis
- Endometriosis
- Irritable bowel syndrome
- Neoplasms
- Torsion or haemorrhage of ovarian cyst

Questions that help discriminate between causes
- Site, character and duration of pain?
- Any vaginal discharge, postcoital or intermenstrual bleeding, or deep dyspareunia?
- Date of last menstrual period (LMP) and contraception used? Is pregnancy possible?
- Any dysuria, urinary frequency, nocturia or haematuria?
- Any nausea, vomiting, diarrhoea or constipation?

Investigations
- Microscopy of vaginal discharge for BV and TV, nucleic acid amplification test (NAAT; if available) or culture for TV, NAAT and culture for *N. gonorrhoeae*, NAAT for *C. trachomatis*, NAAT for M. genitalium, serology for syphilis and HIV
- A pregnancy test should be performed, as ectopic pregnancy is a differential diagnosis
- A mid-stream specimen of urine (MSU) should be taken if symptoms are suggestive of UTI

[a]Most common in young (under 25 years) sexually active women. [b]Symptoms of abnormal vaginal discharge and/or abnormal bleeding are usually present with PID, and BV is also often present. [c]The most common cause of PID.

❓ Box 37.5 Causes of genital lumps

Infective causes
- Human papillomavirus (HPV; anogenital warts)[a,b]
- Molluscum contagiosum
- *Sarcoptes scabiei* (scabies – excoriated lesions)[c]
- *Treponema pallidum*
  - Secondary condylomata lata[d]

Non-infective causes
- Normal anatomical variants (e.g. papillae, sebaceous glands and skin tags)
- Sebaceous cysts
- Neoplasms

Questions that help discriminate between causes
- Where are the lumps?
- Are they single or multiple?
- Are they itchy or painful?
- How long have they been present?
- Are there any lumps or rashes elsewhere on the skin?

Investigations
- Nucleic acid amplification test (NAAT) for *Neisseria gonorrhoeae* and NAAT for *Chlamydia trachomatis*, serology for syphilis and HIV
- Diagnoses of anogenital warts and molluscum contagiosum are made on clinical appearances; HPV testing is not appropriate for diagnosing anogenital warts

[a]Most common infective causes, followed by molluscum contagiosum. [b]Lumps present on the mucous membranes are more likely to be anogenital warts, as molluscum contagiosum does not occur there. [c]Can present with excoriated papules on the genital area due to excessive scratching. [d]Moist papules present in secondary syphilis – rare but easily misdiagnosed as anogenital warts.

❓ Box 37.6 Causes of genital ulceration

Infective causes
- Herpes simplex virus (HSV) types 1 and 2[a]:
  - Primary
  - Recurrent
- *Treponema pallidum*[b]:
  - Primary chancre
  - Secondary mucous patches
  - Tertiary gumma
- Herpes zoster[c]
- Lymphogranuloma venereum (LGV)[d]
- Chancroid[d]
- Donovanosis (granuloma inguinale)[d]

Non-infective causes
- Trauma
- Aphthous ulceration (e.g. as in Behçet's syndrome)[e]
- Lichen sclerosus
- Erosive lichen planus
- Fixed drug eruptions
- Stevens–Johnson syndrome
- Crohn's disease
- Neoplasms

Questions that help distinguish between causes
- Are the ulcers painful?
- Are they single or multiple?
- How long have they been present?
- Is there any external dysuria?
- Are there any ulcers or rash elsewhere on the skin?
- Are there any systematic symptoms?

Investigations
- Ulcer swab for HSV polymerase chain reaction (PCR). Some laboratories also test these swabs for *T. pallidum* using PCR. Nucleic acid amplification test (NAAT) for *Neisseria gonorrhoeae*, NAAT for *Chlamydia trachomatis*, serology for syphilis and HIV. Syphilis serology should be repeated after the 3-month window period if appropriate
- In men who have sex with men (MSM), consider an ulcer swab for *C. trachomatis* and NAAT with genotyping for LGV if positive

[a]Most common cause of multiple painful ulcers. [b]Syphilis ulcers are usually single and non-painful. [c]Much rarer than HSV and characterized by unilateral presentation. [d]LGV rare except in MSM; chancroid and donovanosis extremely rare. [e]Most common non-infective cause; usually, there is a history of similar lesions in the mouth.

Box 37.7 Causes of genital itching

Infective causes
- *Candida albicans*[a]
- *Trichomonas vaginalis* (TV)
- *Phthirus pubis* (pubic lice)[b]
- *Sarcoptes scabiei* (scabies)[c]

Non-infective causes[d]
- Irritant dermatitis
- Genital eczema
- Lichen sclerosus
- Lichen planus

Questions that help distinguish between causes
- Site and duration of itching?
- Any vaginal discharge, offensive odour or vulval swelling?
- Any itching or rash elsewhere on the skin, or any known skin problems?

Investigations
- Microscopy of vaginal discharge for candida and TV, culture for candida, nucleic acid amplification test (NAAT; if available) or culture for TV, NAAT for *Neisseria gonorrhoeae* and *Chlamydia trachomatis*, serology for syphilis and HIV

[a]The most frequent symptom in females is vulval itching rather than vaginal discharge. [b]Relatively rare but easily visible in the hair area. [c]Can cause genital itching and may present with excoriated papules due to excessive scratching. [d]Genital dermatoses are common causes of genital itching and are frequently misdiagnosed as candida.

Box 37.8 Causes of rectal symptoms

- Symptoms of proctitis are rectal pain, mucopurulent anal discharge, rectal bleeding, constipation and tenesmus
- Proctoscopy may reveal mucosal erythema, oedema, contact bleeding and a mucopurulent discharge, with ulceration in severe cases

Infective causes

Rectal infections
- *Neisseria gonorrhoeae*[a]
- *Chlamydia trachomatis*[a]
- Lymphogranuloma venereum (LGV)[b]
- Herpes simplex virus (HSV)[c]
- *Treponema pallidum*[c]

Intestinal infections
- *Shigella* spp.[b]
- *Campylobacter* spp.
- *Entamoeba histolytica*
- *Salmonella* spp.
- *Escherichia coli*
- *Cryptosporidium* spp.

Non-infective causes
- Ulcerative colitis
- Crohn's disease
- Neoplasms

Questions that help distinguish between causes
- Any irritation or pain around the anus or in the rectum?
- Any discharge or bleeding from the anus?
- Any abdominal pain, diarrhoea or blood in the stool?
- Any feeling of incomplete bowel evacuation or constipation?
- Any systemic symptoms?

Investigations
- Microscopy of a rectal smear, rectal culture and nucleic acid amplification test (NAAT) for *N. gonorrhoeae*, NAAT for *C. trachomatis*, serology for syphilis and HIV. If positive for *C. trachomatis*, genotyping for LGV should be requested
- If there is severe proctitis, a swab for HSV and *T. pallidum* polymerase chain reaction (PCR) should be performed
- LGV should be considered in MSM with suspected inflammatory bowel disease, as the clinical presentation can be very similar
- Cultures for enteric pathogens should be performed if symptoms of enteritis are present

[a]Most common causes of proctitis in women and MSM. [b]Outbreaks occurring in Europe in MSM. [c]Rarer causes than *N. gonorrhoeae* and *C. trachomatis*; mainly seen in MSM.

- needle-stick injury recipients
- people with chronic hepatitis C or people living with HIV
- those born to a mother infected with hepatitis B.

Patients who are negative and have ongoing increased risk should be offered vaccination.

Screening for hepatitis C

Screening for antibodies to hepatitis C is recommended in:
- sexual partners of hepatitis C virus (HCV)-positive people
- people who inject drugs
- MSM who are taking, or are eligible for, pre-exposure prophylaxis (PrEP) for HIV (see p. 1449)
- those who have additional risk factors, e.g. sex associated with trauma or injury, history of recreational drug use or rectal lymphogranuloma venereum (LGV)
- sex workers
- individuals from countries with intermediate or high prevalence of chronic hepatitis C (as defined earlier for hepatitis B)
- needle-stick injury recipients
- people with chronic hepatitis B or people living with HIV
- those born to a mother infected with HCV.

Investigations for symptomatic patients

These will depend on clinical presentation but should always include tests for chlamydia, gonorrhoea, syphilis and HIV. The recommended investigations for these presentations are shown in **Boxes 37.2–37.8**.

MANAGEMENT, PREVENTION AND CONTROL

The treatment of specific conditions is covered in the appropriate sections. Most sexual health clinics give directly observed therapy where possible or dispense medication directly to the patient to improve adherence in order to prevent onward transmission.

Tracing the sexual partners of patients (partner notification) is crucial in controlling the spread of STIs. The aims are to identify and treat those with infections (particularly those with asymptomatic infections) in order to break the chain of transmission. Also, appropriate antibiotic therapy is usually offered to recent sexual partners of those known to have an active infection (epidemiological treatment). Interviewing people about their sexual partners requires considerable tact and sensitivity, and specialist health advisers are available in sexual health clinics.

Many STI diagnoses are in young people (16–24 years). Prevention starts with education and information. People begin sexual activity at ever younger ages and education programmes need to include school pupils, as well as young adults. Education of health professionals is also crucial. Primary public health programmes aimed at informing groups most at risk of STIs, such as MSM, sex workers, young people and some black and minority ethnic groups, in order to modify sexual behaviour, should be implemented at local and national levels. Vaccination against hepatitis A and B, and human papillomavirus (HPV), should also be given to those at increased risk. Secondary interventions include the prompt diagnosis and appropriate management of STIs in order to reduce complications and onward transmission. The National Chlamydia Screening Programme (NCSP) in England aims to provide earlier detection and treatment for chlamydia by providing easy access for under-25-year-olds to chlamydia testing in community settings.

Reducing the numbers of sexual partners, avoiding overlapping relationships, using condoms correctly and consistently, and avoiding sex if symptoms are present can reduce the risks of acquiring and transmitting an STI. For those who change their sexual partners frequently, regular sexual health checks (approximately 3-monthly) are advisable. Once people develop symptoms, they should be encouraged to seek medical advice as soon as possible to reduce complications and spread to others.

Further reading

Gottlieb SL, Johnston C. Future prospects for new vaccines against sexually transmitted infections. *Curr Opin Infect Dis* 2017; 30:77–86.
Mercer CH, Tanton C, Prah P et al. Changes in sexual attitudes and lifestyles in Britain through the life course and over time: findings from the National Surveys of Sexual Attitudes and Lifestyles (Natsal). *Lancet* 2013; 382:1781–1794.
Rowley J, Vander Hoorn S, Korenromp E et al. Chlamydia, gonorrhoea, trichomoniasis and syphilis: global prevalence and incidence estimates, 2016. *Bull World Health Org* 2019; 97:548–562.
Sonnenberg P, Clifton S, Beddows S et al. Prevalence, risk factors, and uptake of interventions for sexually transmitted infections in Britain: findings from the National Surveys of Sexual Attitudes and Lifestyles (Natsal). *Lancet* 2013; 382:1795–1806.
Unemo M, Bradshaw CS, Hocking JS et al. Sexually transmitted infections: challenges ahead. *Lancet Infect Dis* 2017; 17:e235-279.

SPECIFIC INFECTIONS

HIV/AIDS

This is discussed on page 1425.

Hepatitis B

This is discussed on page 1277. Sexual contacts should be screened and immunized if they are not immune.

Chlamydia trachomatis

Chlamydia trachomatis (CT) is the most common STI in the UK; up to 10% of sexually active people below the age of 25 years are infected. It infects the urethra, endocervix, rectum, pharynx and conjunctiva. As up to 80% of women and 50% of men may be asymptomatic, it is frequently unrecognized and therefore untreated. Pelvic inflammatory disease, the main complication of CT, can result in tubal infertility, ectopic pregnancy and chronic pelvic pain, causing significant morbidity and cost to health services.

Clinical features

The exact incubation period is unclear but is thought to be between 7 and 21 days.

In men, CT can cause an anterior urethritis with a mucopurulent urethral discharge (worse on waking, when there may be crusting at the meatus) and dysuria. The infection can ascend along the vas deferens, leading to epididymo-orchitis.

In women, the most common site of infection is the endocervix but the urethra can also be infected. Symptoms may include increased vaginal discharge, dysuria, postcoital or intermenstrual bleeding, and lower abdominal pain. Examination of the cervix may reveal mucopurulent cervicitis and/or contact bleeding. Ascending infection into the uterus and fallopian tubes causes endometritis and acute salpingitis (pelvic inflammatory disease). In pregnancy, CT is associated with preterm birth, postpartum infection, and neonatal mucopurulent conjunctivitis and pneumonia due to vertical transmission during vaginal delivery.

Rectal infection, through receptive anal sex, may be asymptomatic but can cause proctitis. Reactive arthritis (see p. 450) can occur with CT infection, particularly in human leucocyte antigen (HLA)-B27-positive individuals.

Diagnosis

Nucleic acid amplification tests (NAATs) are the diagnostic tests of choice for CT, as they have sensitivities of 90–99%. In men, first-voided urine (FVU) samples or urethral swabs, and in women vulvo-vaginal swabs (VVSs) or endocervical swabs, are used. Self-taken VVSs are as sensitive at detecting CT as clinician-taken VVSs but

FVU samples in women are less sensitive than VVSs and endocervical swabs. The advantage of male FVU samples and self-taken VVSs is that they are non-invasive (meaning they can be obtained by the patient without the need for an examination), so are ideal for asymptomatic chlamydia screening.

MSM who practise receptive anal sex and receptive oral sex should have rectal and pharyngeal swabs for CT NAAT performed.

Management

Doxycycline 100 mg twice daily for 7 days is the recommended regimen for uncomplicated infection; azithromycin 1 g stat, followed by 500 mg daily for 2 days, is used if doxycycline is contraindicated. Azithromycin is recommended in pregnant or lactating women in WHO, USA, UK and Australian guidelines but the manufacturers advise use only if adequate alternatives are not available. Doxycycline is contraindicated in pregnancy. Longer courses of antibiotics are required for complicated infections (see pelvic inflammatory disease and epididymo-orchitis later). Epidemiological treatment pending test results is usually offered to those who have had recent sex with someone who has confirmed CT infection, as the infection rate can be up to 50%. Abstinence from sex for at least 7 days, or until treatment is completed, should be advised. Sexual contacts must be traced, notified and treated, as many infections are asymptomatic.

A follow-up consultation (possibly by telephone) should assess adherence to therapy and partner notification. A routine test of cure is not necessary after treatment, except in pregnant women or where symptoms persist or re-infection is suspected. NAATs may remain positive for some time after treatment, as they detect non-viable organisms, so a test of cure should be deferred until 6 weeks after the start of treatment.

Gonorrhoea

Neisseria gonorrhoeae is a Gram-negative intracellular diplococcus (**Fig. 37.3**), which infects the urethra, endocervix, rectum, pharynx and conjunctiva. Up to 50% of infected women and 10% of infected men are asymptomatic. Co-infection with CT is common, occurring in 20% of men and 40% of women with gonococcal infection (GC).

Clinical features

The incubation period is 2–14 days, most symptoms in males occurring between 2 and 5 days.

In men, GC can cause anterior urethritis with mucopurulent or purulent urethral discharge and dysuria (**Fig. 37.4**). The discharge can be profuse, causing staining of underwear. Complications include ascending infection, leading to epididymo-orchitis.

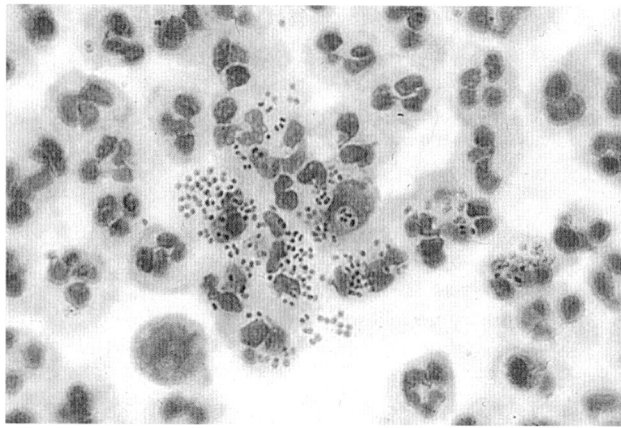

Fig. 37.3 *Neisseria gonorrhoeae*. Gram-negative intracellular diplococci. *(Courtesy of Dr B. Goh.)*

In women, symptoms may include increased vaginal discharge, dysuria, postcoital or intermenstrual bleeding, and lower abdominal pain. Examination of the cervix may reveal mucopurulent or purulent cervicitis and/or contact bleeding. Complications include Bartholin's abscesses, and ascending infection into the uterus and fallopian tubes causes endometritis and acute salpingitis (pelvic inflammatory disease). In pregnancy, GC is associated with preterm birth, postpartum infection, and neonatal purulent conjunctivitis due to vertical transmission during vaginal delivery.

Rectal infection, through receptive anal sex, may be asymptomatic but can cause proctitis. GC septicaemia (disseminated gonococcal infection, DGI) is a rare complication presenting as fever, tenosynovitis, arthritis and characteristic erythematous skin lesions with necrotic centres.

Diagnosis

NAATs are the diagnostic test of choice for *N. gonorrhoeae*, as they have better sensitivity than culture. However, as *N. gonorrhoeae* antimicrobial resistance is increasing, and ceftriaxone-resistant isolates have been identified in the UK and globally, culture on selective media should be performed prior to any treatment for GC being given. In men, FVU samples or urethral swabs, and in women VVSs or endocervical swabs, are the specimens of choice for GC NAATs. Self-taken VVSs are as sensitive at detecting GC as clinician-taken VVSs. FVU samples in women should not be used, as they are less sensitive than VVSs and endocervical swabs. As male FVU samples and self-taken VVSs are non-invasive, they are ideal for asymptomatic screening. MSM who practise receptive anal sex and receptive oral sex should have rectal and pharyngeal swabs for GC NAATs taken. A urethral swab in men, an endocervical swab in women, and rectal and pharyngeal swabs in both are the specimens to use for culture.

Microscopy of Gram-stained urethral and endocervical secretions may demonstrate intracellular, Gram-negative diplococci, allowing rapid diagnosis. The sensitivity ranges from 90–95% in urethral specimens from symptomatic men to 37–50% in endocervical specimens. Microscopy should not be used for pharyngeal specimens. The sensitivity of blood and synovial fluid cultures is poor, so NAATs from the genital tract, rectum and pharynx remain the tests of choice for investigations of DGI.

Management

Treatment should be given to those who have positive microscopy, a positive NAAT or a positive culture for GC. Antibiotic-resistant strains of *N. gonorrhoeae* are increasing and so culture should have been taken prior to treatment. When antimicrobial susceptibility is not known prior to treatment, single-dose ceftriaxone 1 g i.m. is recommended in the UK. If confirmed susceptibility is known in advance of treatment, ciprofloxacin 500 mg single dose should be used. If there is a history of penicillin anaphylaxis or established cephalosporin allergy, spectinomycin 2 g i.m. with azithromycin 2 g, or gentamicin 240 mg i.m. with azithromycin 2 g, should be used. Both of these regimens can be used in pregnancy. Longer courses of antibiotics are required for complicated infections (see pelvic inflammatory disease and epididymo-orchitis later). Epidemiological treatment (treatment based on known exposure) pending test results can be offered to those who have had sex within the past 14 days with someone who has confirmed GC infection. Abstinence from sex for at least 7 days, or until treatment has been completed, should be advised. All sexual contacts should be notified, tested, and treated if positive.

A follow-up assessment and test of cure using GC NAAT should take place 14 days after treatment.

Non-gonococcal urethritis and *Mycoplasma genitalium*

Non-gonococcal urethritis (NGU) in men is characterized by a urethral discharge and dysuria. There are a number of causes, many of which are sexually transmitted; the most common of these is *C. trachomatis*, which was discussed earlier. Up to 25% of NGU is caused by *Mycoplasma genitalium* (Mgen). Other causes are *Ureaplasma urealyticum*, *Trichomonas vaginalis* (TV), adenoviruses, and herpes simplex viruses (HSV) 1 and 2, in that order of frequency. Studies investigating the aetiology of NGU have consistently identified no known cause in over 60% of cases. Non-sexually transmitted causes of NGU may be urinary tract infections (UTIs) and strictures.

Clinical features

The incubation period is usually 2–3 weeks. The main symptom is a mucopurulent urethral discharge (worse on waking, when there may be crusting at the meatus). Dysuria is common but not universal. Discomfort or itching within the urethra may be present.

Diagnosis

Microscopy of Gram-stained urethral secretion showing five or more polymorphonuclear leucocytes per high-power (×1000 oil-immersion lens) field is diagnostic. Men who are symptomatic but have no objective evidence of urethritis should be re-examined and tested after holding their urine overnight. NAAT for *N. gonorrhoeae*, *C. trachomatis* and *M. genitalium* should be performed in all men with symptoms of urethritis, on an FVU sample. Mgen-positive specimens should be tested for macrolide resistance mutations. Testing for TV and HSV is not routinely performed and there is no commercial test available for *U. urealyticum*. A mid-stream specimen of urine (MSU) should be taken if symptoms are suggestive of a UTI (urinary frequency, nocturia, urgency, haematuria).

Management

First-line therapy for NGU is doxycycline 100 mg twice daily for 7 days. Abstinence from sex for at least 7 days should be advised. All sexual contacts should be notified, tested and treated. Follow-up is indicated only if CT or Mgen is confirmed or if symptoms persist.

Recurrent/persistent NGU

This is defined as persistent or recurrent symptomatic urethritis occurring 30–90 days following treatment of acute NGU, and occurs in 10–20% of cases. The aetiology is probably multifactorial but Mgen and TV are likely causes. It is necessary to ensure that there is still objective evidence of urethritis, that there was good adherence

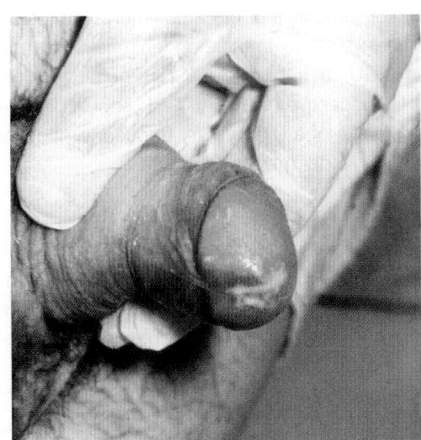

Fig. 37.4 *Neisseria gonorrhoeae.* Mucopurulent urethral discharge.

to NGU treatment with sexual abstinence, and that sexual partners were also treated. If there is no objective evidence of urethritis, patients should be reassured and further antibiotic therapy avoided. Subsequent treatment needs to cover *M. genitalium* and TV. The recommended treatment is azithromycin 1 g orally as a single dose, followed by 500 mg daily for 2 days with metronidazole 400 mg twice daily for 5–7 days. This should be started within 2 weeks of finishing the doxycycline if the patient is Mgen-positive and macrolide-sensitive. If the patient is Mgen-positive and macrolide-resistant, or if treatment with azithromycin has failed, moxifloxacin 400 mg daily for 10 days should be given. Current sexual partners of those infected with Mgen should also be tested (using a VVS in women) and treated with the same antibiotic regimen as their sexual partner. Abstinence from sex until both have finished their treatment should be advised. All who were Mgen-positive should have a test of cure 5 weeks after the start of treatment.

Pelvic inflammatory disease

Pelvic inflammatory disease (PID) results when infections ascend from the cervix or vagina into the upper genital tract. It is most frequent in young (under 25 years) sexually active women. It includes endometritis, salpingitis, tubo-ovarian abscess and pelvic peritonitis. *C. trachomatis* and *N. gonorrhoeae* account for about 25% of UK cases and *M. genitalium* for 10–13% of cases. Anaerobes have also been implicated in the aetiology. Even in women with laparoscopically proven PID, often no bacterial cause is found. PID has serious long-term sequelae due to tubal damage and pelvic adhesions, resulting in tubal infertility, increased risk of ectopic pregnancy and chronic pelvic pain. The risk of sequelae increases with more severe and multiple episodes of PID. Tubal infertility occurs in 10–12% of women after one episode of PID and increases to 50–60% after three or more episodes. The risk of ectopic pregnancy is increased 6–10-fold, and abdominal or pelvic pain for longer than 6 months occurs in 18% of women.

Clinical features

The onset of symptoms often occurs in the first part of the menstrual cycle. Lower abdominal pain, usually bilateral, is the most common symptom, with increased vaginal discharge, irregular bleeding, deep dyspareunia and dysuria being present in some women. There may be a mucopurulent cervical discharge with contact bleeding. Lower abdominal tenderness and adnexal and cervical motion tenderness on bimanual examination are the most common signs.

Diagnosis

The diagnosis is usually made on the clinical findings of lower abdominal pain, with supportive symptoms of increased vaginal discharge and abnormal bleeding, and cervical motion and/or adnexal tenderness on bimanual examination. However, such a clinical diagnosis has a specificity of only 65–70%. The differential diagnosis includes ectopic pregnancy, acute appendicitis, endometriosis, UTI and irritable bowel disease.

Investigations should include microscopy of Gram-stained vaginal discharge (for bacterial vaginosis, BV) and of an endocervical specimen (for evidence of inflammatory cells and intracellular, Gram-negative diplococci suggestive of gonorrhoea), NAAT and culture for *N. gonorrhoeae*, and NAAT for *C. trachomatis* and *M. genitalium.* A pregnancy test should be performed on all women suspected of having PID, as ectopic pregnancy is a differential diagnosis. An MSU should be taken if symptoms are suggestive of a UTI (urinary frequency, nocturia, urgency, haematuria).

Management

Early diagnosis and treatment reduce the risk of long-term sequelae and so empirical treatment should be started before microbiology results are known. A broad-spectrum antibiotic regimen is needed to cover the main bacterial causes. The recommended first-line treatment is single-dose ceftriaxone 1 g by intramuscular injection, with doxycycline 100 mg twice daily and metronidazole 400 mg twice daily for 14 days. Alternatives are ofloxacin 400 mg twice daily and metronidazole 400 mg twice daily for 14 days; or moxifloxacin 400 mg daily for 14 days (this should be first-line if the patient is Mgen-positive). Abstinence from sex for at least 14 days should be advised. All sexual contacts should be notified, tested and treated.

Those with moderate or severe clinical findings should be reviewed within 2–3 days to ensure that they are improving on treatment. Lack of response requires further investigation and possible admission for intravenous therapy and/or surgical intervention. All women should be reviewed after 2–4 weeks in order to assess symptom resolution, adherence to therapy and partner notification.

Epididymo-orchitis

Acute epididymo-orchitis is a clinical syndrome consisting of pain, swelling and inflammation of the epididymis that can extend into the testis. It is caused mainly by extension of infection from the urethra or the bladder. In men under 35 years, *C. trachomatis* and *N. gonorrhoeae* are the main causes and *M. genitalium* also appears to be implicated. In men over 35 years, it is more commonly a complication of a UTI. Mumps is another cause of epididymo-orchitis in non-immune men. The most common differential diagnosis is torsion of the spermatic cord, which is a urological emergency.

Clinical features

The typical presentation is subacute onset of unilateral scrotal pain and swelling. There may also be symptoms of a urethral discharge and dysuria but these are often absent. On examination, there is tenderness and usually palpable swelling of the epididymis. There may also be some tenderness and swelling of the testicle, with oedema and erythema of the overlying scrotal skin. A urethral discharge may be present.

Diagnosis

The diagnosis is usually made on the clinical findings described. The main differential diagnosis is testicular torsion.

Investigations

These include a NAAT and culture for *N. gonorrhoeae* and a NAAT for *C. trachomatis* and *M. genitalium*. If microscopy of Gram-stained urethral secretions shows 5 or more polymorphonuclear leucocytes per high-power (×1000 oil-immersion lens) field, this indicates the diagnosis of NGU. If intracellular Gram-negative diplococci are present, this is suggestive of GC. An MSU should be taken if symptoms are suggestive of a UTI (urinary frequency, nocturia, urgency, haematuria) and in older men.

Management

As empirical treatment should be started before microbiology results are known, a broad-spectrum antibiotic regimen is needed to cover the main bacterial causes. In younger men, where an STI is the likely diagnosis, the recommended regimen is single-dose ceftriaxone 1 g i.m. with doxycycline 100 mg twice daily for 14 days. If the patient is Mgen-positive, moxifloxacin 400 mg daily for 14 days should be given. Where a UTI is the more likely diagnosis, ofloxacin 200 mg twice daily for 14 days should be prescribed. Abstinence from sex for at least 14 days should be advised. All sexual contacts should be notified, tested and treated.

Patients are reassessed after 3 days if there is no improvement in their symptoms, as this requires further investigations. All should be seen after 2 weeks in order to assess symptom resolution, adherence to therapy and partner notification.

Bacterial vaginosis

Bacterial vaginosis (BV) is the most frequent cause of vaginal discharge among women of childbearing age. A BV prevalence of 9% was reported in women attending general practice for cervical cytology screening and in 15% of pregnant women in the UK. BV develops when the normal lactobacilli-dominant vaginal flora are replaced by an overgrowth of other bacteria, including *Gardnerella vaginalis*, anaerobes, mycoplasmas and *Mobiluncus* spp. It is not regarded as a sexually transmitted disease. BV in pregnancy is associated with an increased risk of miscarriage and preterm birth. It also increases the risk of acquisition and transmission of HIV. Up to 50% of women with BV have no symptoms. It is not necessary to look for or treat asymptomatic BV.

Clinical features

The symptoms are an increased vaginal discharge and offensive fishy odour. On examination, there is a creamy-white homogeneous discharge, which may be slightly frothy (due to the volatile amine production by the bacteria, which is responsible for the characteristic odour) (**Fig. 37.5**). Visible inflammatory changes are not seen with BV.

Diagnosis

The most accurate method of diagnosis is microscopy of Gram-stained vaginal discharge, as the characteristic pattern of the BV bacteria is easily distinguished from the normal lactobacilli-dominant vaginal flora. It is possible to diagnose BV just on clinical criteria but this is less specific. All three of the following should be present for the diagnosis to be made:

- characteristic creamy-white homogeneous vaginal discharge
- raised vaginal pH of >4.5 (measured using narrow-range pH paper)
- characteristic fishy odour (which can be released by mixing the vaginal discharge with 10% potassium hydroxide).

Many of the clinical symptoms and signs of BV are similar to those of TV and so women with recurrent BV should have a TV NAAT to ensure they do not have undiagnosed TV.

Management

The recommended treatment is oral metronidazole 400 mg twice daily for 7 days. A single dose of metronidazole 2 g can also be used but this is less effective. Alternative topical treatments are intravaginal metronidazole 0.75% gel for 5 nights, or intravaginal clindamycin 2% cream for 7 nights. High-dose metronidazole should be avoided in pregnancy but the 7-day oral course can be safely prescribed, as can either of the intravaginal regimens.

BV recurrences are frequent, with about 50% of women experiencing a recurrence within 12 months of completing metronidazole therapy. Simultaneous treatment of the male partner does not reduce the rate of recurrence, and treatment of male partners is not indicated.

Candidiasis

Candida is a ubiquitous organism and is not classified as an STI. Vulvovaginal *Candida* infection is extremely common; about 75% of women have at least one episode of symptomatic candidiasis in their lifetime. Predisposing factors for symptomatic infection include pregnancy, diabetes, the use of broad-spectrum antibiotics and corticosteroids, and immunosuppression. *Candida albicans* causes 90% of vaginal yeast infections, with *Candida glabrata* and other *Candida* species causing the remainder. Male sexual partners of women with candidiasis can contract transient penile colonization (and may develop penile rashes) following sex due to direct inoculation from the vagina.

Clinical features

In women, the main symptom is vulval itching, which is present in nearly all symptomatic women. An increased thick, white vaginal discharge, vulval burning, external dysuria and superficial dyspareunia may also be present. On examination, vulval erythema, fissuring and oedema may be present. There may be the typical white, curdy, adherent plaques on the vaginal walls (**Fig. 37.6**) but the discharge may be minimal.

In men, there may be a transient penile irritation and rash immediately following sex, but some men experience more persistent balanoposthitis. On examination, there may be erythema of the foreskin and glans penis, or a spotty, red, itchy rash on the glans, with an accumulation of white discharge under the foreskin. In severe cases, there may be fissuring and phimosis of the foreskin.

Diagnosis

Microscopy of a Gram-stained vaginal smear, or a subpreputial smear, identifies the fungal pseudohyphae and spores in 50% of cases of candidiasis. Culture of vaginal, or subpreputial, swabs has almost 100% sensitivity. Diabetes should be excluded in men with severe balanoposthitis.

Management

There are a number of short-course oral and intravaginal antifungal agents available, all with efficacies of 80–85%. Recommended treatments are the oral triazole drugs, such as fluconazole 150 mg as a single dose or itraconazole 200 mg twice daily for 1 day, and

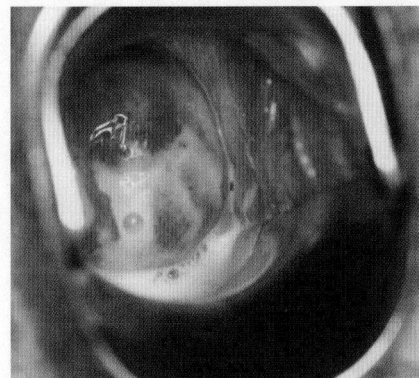

Fig. 37.5 Bacterial vaginosis. Homogenous creamy-white vaginal discharge, which may be slightly frothy and adherent to the vaginal walls.

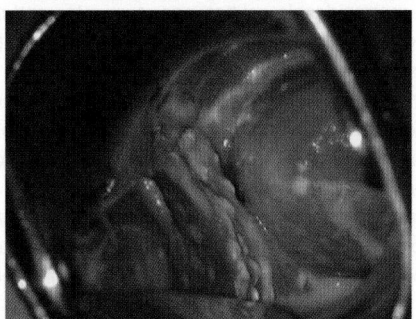

Fig. 37.6 Candidiasis. Adherent plaques of discharge on the vaginal walls.

intravaginal imidazole pessaries or creams, such as clotrimazole pessary 500 mg as a single dose, miconazole vaginal ovule 1.2 g as a single dose or econazole pessary 150 mg nightly for 1–3 nights. These treatments can be supplemented with antifungal cream applied to the vulva. Males can be treated with either oral therapy or topical antifungal cream. Nystatin pessaries 200 000 units nightly for 14 nights are the treatment of choice for *C. glabrata* and other non-*albicans* yeasts. Intravaginal treatments are safe in pregnancy but oral therapies should not be used.

Recurrent candidiasis (four or more symptomatic episodes in 1 year) occurs in up to 5% of healthy women of reproductive age. It frequently requires weekly oral fluconazole 150 mg, or clotrimazole pessary 500 mg, for up to 6 months in order to prevent recurring symptoms. There is no evidence that treatment of male partners reduces recurrences in women, so male partners do not need treatment unless they also have symptoms.

Trichomoniasis

Trichomonas vaginalis (TV) infection is the most common STI worldwide but it is much rarer in Western Europe and Australasia. The organism is a flagellated protozoon that is sexually transmitted. In women, it infects the vagina and urethra; in men, it infects the urethra and subpreputial sac. Nearly all infected men are asymptomatic, as are 10–50% of women. TV in pregnancy is associated with an increased risk of preterm birth and low birth weight, and it increases the risk of acquisition of HIV.

Clinical features

In women, the most common symptoms are an increased purulent vaginal discharge and malodour. There may also be vulval pruritus, external dysuria and dyspareunia. On examination, there may be vulval erythema with inflamed vaginal mucosa. The discharge is yellow or grey and frothy, and can be profuse. The cervix may have multiple small haemorrhagic areas, which have given rise to the description 'strawberry cervix'.

In men, the majority have no symptoms, although they may complain of urethral discharge, irritation and dysuria.

Diagnosis

Phase-contrast microscopy of vaginal discharge identifies the motile protozoa in up to 50% of infected females. The sensitivity of microscopy of urethral discharge in males is much lower. Culture will detect 70–80% of infections but NAATs are the diagnostic tests of choice with VVSs in women, and FVU in males, detecting over 90% of infections.

Management

The treatment of choice is metronidazole 400 mg twice daily for 7 days. Single-dose metronidazole 2 g can be used but it is less effective. As TV infects areas beyond the vagina (e.g. the urethra), intravaginal metronidazole gel has poor cure rates and should not be used. High-dose metronidazole should be avoided in pregnancy but the 7-day oral course can be safely prescribed.

Abstinence from sex for at least 7 days should be advised. All sexual contacts should be notified, tested and treated. Tests of cure are recommended only if the patient remains symptomatic following treatment or if symptoms recur.

Occasionally, TV can become resistant to metronidazole and other nitroimidazoles. This is usually relative rather than absolute and may be overcome by high-dose metronidazole or tinidazole therapy.

Human papillomavirus – anogenital warts

Anogenital warts are painless, benign, epithelial tumours and constitute a common STI. The causative agent is human papillomavirus (HPV) types 6 and 11. Genital HPV infection is acquired by direct skin-to-skin contact during sex with a person who has either clinical or subclinical infection. Subclinical infection is very common in young, sexually active people, with rates of up to 20%. Anogenital warts are the 'tip of the iceberg', occurring in only about 1% of those with subclinical infection.

Warts due to HPV 6 and 11 do not undergo malignant transformation. The main oncogenic HPV types are 16 and 18. These lead to subclinical infection, not genital warts, and cause the majority of cases of cervical and other anogenital cancers (see p. 530). Neonates may acquire HPV from an infected birth canal, which may result either in anogenital warts or in laryngeal papillomatosis.

Clinical features

Anogenital warts have a long incubation period; the average is 3 months but it can extend to years. The warts first appear at sites of trauma during sex. In males, this is around the prepuce and glans; from there, they can spread to the urethra and down the penile shaft. In women, they usually start at the fourchette and then spread to the vulva and perineum (**Fig. 37.7**). Perianal lesions are common in both sexes but more common in MSM. Warts on mucous membranes tend to be soft and non-keratinized, whereas those on the hair-bearing skin tend to be firm and keratinized. Warts tend to increase in size and number during pregnancy or in immunosuppressed patients.

Diagnosis

The diagnosis is made on the clinical appearances. HPV testing is not appropriate for diagnosing anogenital warts. The main differential diagnoses are molluscum contagiosum and the condylomata lata of secondary syphilis. Atypical lesions should be biopsied, particularly in older patients, as pre-malignant and malignant lesions can look similar to warts. Investigations should include NAAT for *N. gonorrhoeae* and *C. trachomatis*, and serology for syphilis and HIV, as co-infection with other STIs is common.

Management

There are a number of treatments available for anogenital warts but all of them have significant failure and relapse rates. The choice of treatment depends on the number, type and distribution of lesions. Topical podophyllotoxin (0.5% solution or 0.15% cream used twice daily for 3 consecutive days per week) acts as a cytotoxic agent and is useful for non-keratinized warts; keratinized warts respond better to ablative therapy, such as cryotherapy or

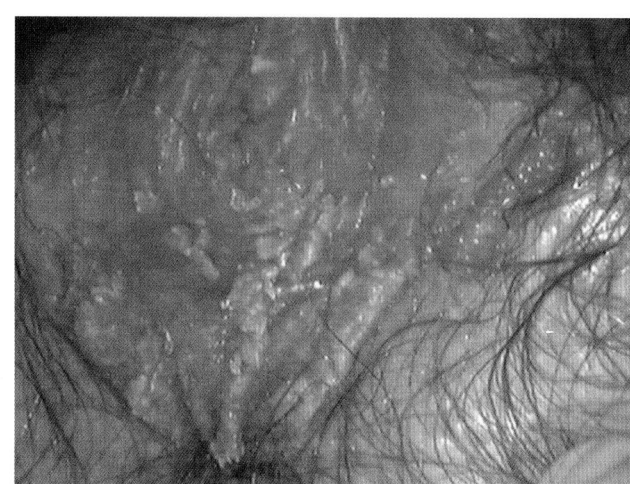

Fig. 37.7 Genital warts on the fourchette and perineum.

electrocautery. Imiquimod enhances the local immune response when applied to skin infected with HPV (5% cream used daily, three times a week) and is effective in both types of wart. Podophyllotoxin and imiquimod have the advantage of being self-applied home therapies.

Podophyllotoxin and imiquimod should not be used in pregnancy. Pregnant women, those co-infected with HIV and those with other causes of immunosuppression may have a poorer response to treatment.

The use of condoms should be advised in new relationships, as they protect against the transmission of HPV infection and genital warts. Current sexual partners may have undetected genital warts so may benefit from a sexual health assessment.

Follow-up is recommended in order to monitor the response to treatment and to assess the need for any change of therapy.

Prevention and vaccination

There are very effective vaccines against HPV:
- A bivalent vaccine protects against HPV types 16 and 18, which are the most common high-risk types.
- A quadrivalent vaccine protects against types 6, 11, 16 and 18, which covers the most common high-risk types and those that cause genital warts.
- A vaccine protecting against nine virus types, which contains the same HPV antigens as the quadrivalent vaccine plus five additional high-risk types (31, 33, 45, 52 and 58) is also available.

They are given over 6 months in three divided doses and have excellent safety profiles, with almost 100% serological response that is maintained over a number of years. Vaccination is most beneficial in those who have not yet been exposed to HPV infection; hence most national vaccination programmes target those aged 12–13 years. All programmes vaccinate girls and some also include boys.

The best evidence of the effect of HPV vaccination is from Australia, where there has been a school-based quadrivalent HPV vaccination programme in girls since 2007 and boys since 2013. There has been a rapid reduction of 90% in genital warts and 50% in high-grade cervical lesions.

Molluscum contagiosum

Molluscum contagiosum (see p. 672) is a large DNA virus. It causes small (typically 2–5 mm in diameter), benign, smooth papules with central umbilication. It is spread via direct skin-to-skin contact. When it is transmitted sexually, the lesions are usually multiple and present on the labia majora, penile shaft, pubic region, lower abdomen and upper inner thighs.

Diagnosis

The diagnosis is made on the characteristic clinical appearance. As this is a sexually acquired condition, investigations for other STIs should include NAAT for *N. gonorrhoeae* and *C. trachomatis*, and serology for syphilis and HIV.

Management

Molluscum infection is often self-limiting, resolving naturally. Treatment options, if required, are cryotherapy, podophyllotoxin cream or imiquimod cream. The creams have the advantage of being self-applied home therapies. Podophyllotoxin and imiquimod should be avoided in pregnancy. Patients should be advised about the risks of auto-inoculation of the virus and discouraged from shaving or waxing the pubic hair in order to prevent further spread. No routine follow-up or partner notification is required, unless any other STIs are identified.

Herpes simplex

Genital herpes (see also p. 514) is the most common cause of genital ulceration in all countries worldwide. The peak incidence for primary infection is in 16–24-year-olds. Women acquire the infection more frequently than men, probably because of the larger surface area of susceptible mucous membrane on the vulva. Transmission occurs from the mucous membrane of a person who is shedding herpes simplex virus (HSV), many of whom will be asymptomatic. Only about 20% of people with serological evidence of genital herpes give a clinical history of herpes, suggesting that many individuals have subclinical infection.

Genital herpes can be due to HSV type 1 or type 2. It is possible to be co-infected with both. HSV-1 infection may be spread from an infected genital tract or from orolabial lesions via orogenital sex. HSV-2 is almost always transmitted via genital-to-genital contact. In the UK, more than 50% of primary HSV is due to HSV-1.

During the primary infection, the virus ascends the peripheral sensory nerves supplying the area of inoculation and establishes latency in the dorsal root ganglia, thus allowing future reactivation and recurrences.

Clinical features

The ***initial episode*** is the first occurrence of either HSV-1 or HSV-2. This is subdivided as described here, depending on whether or not the person has had prior exposure to the other HSV type.

Primary genital infection is the first ever exposure to either HSV type 1 or 2. It typically presents with multiple painful, shallow ulcers (**Fig. 37.8**). There is usually tender inguinal lymphadenopathy and systemic symptoms of viraemia, including fever, myalgia and headache. In women, external dysuria and vulval pain are the main symptoms. Ulcers may be present on the cervix and can have the appearance of a malignancy. Rectal infection may lead to severe proctitis with pain and bleeding (this is mainly seen in MSM). The lesions start to heal over a period of 10–21 days, even without treatment. Neurological complications can include aseptic meningitis and autonomic neuropathy leading to urinary retention. However, primary infection can be asymptomatic.

Non-primary genital infection occurs in people with previous HSV-1 or HSV-2 who then acquire the other type of genital HSV. There is some cross-protection from the prior HSV infection, resulting in a milder illness than in primary infection. Non-primary genital infections are more likely to be asymptomatic than primary infections.

Recurrent genital herpes is due to reactivation of previous HSV-1 or HSV-2 infection. HSV-2 recurs more frequently than HSV-1. The median recurrence rate in the subsequent year

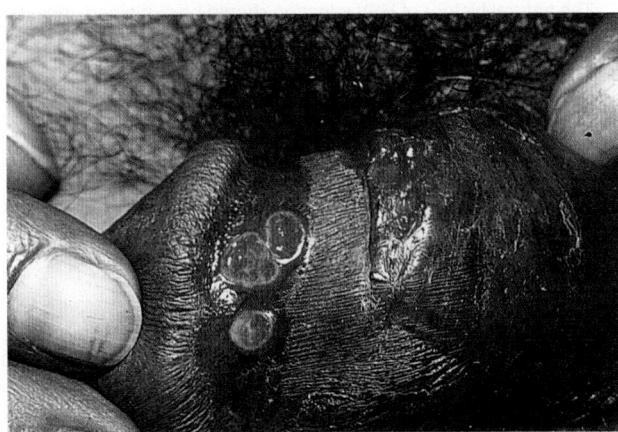

Fig. 37.8 Herpes simplex rash on the penis. *(Courtesy of Dr B. Goh.)*

following a primary or non-primary infection is about one recurrence for HSV-1 and about four recurrences for HSV-2. The recurrences may be preceded by a prodrome of tingling, itching or pain in the area. On examination, there are usually a few ulcers confined to a small area and systemic symptoms are rare. Recurrences are not always noticed and asymptomatic, subclinical viral shedding can occur. However, all of these reactivated episodes are potentially infectious. Long-term studies show that symptomatic recurrences and subclinical viral shedding gradually decrease with time.

The clinical presentation of primary infection in immunosuppressed patients (including those with HIV and pregnant women) is usually more severe, with increased frequency of symptomatic and subclinical recurrences. Rarely, the infection can disseminate, causing a systemic life-threatening condition.

Genital herpes increases the acquisition and transmission of HIV and is a significant attributable risk in the spread of HIV. Many people with recurrent HSV develop psychological and psychosexual problems, and fear rejection on disclosure of their infection to sexual partners.

Diagnosis

HSV DNA detection using polymerase chain reaction (PCR) on a swab taken from the ulcer is the diagnostic method of choice. This can distinguish between HSV-1 and HSV-2. Tests for other STIs should be performed, including NAAT for *N. gonorrhoeae* and *C. trachomatis*, and serology for syphilis and HIV.

Blood tests for HSV type-specific antibodies can be used to diagnose prior HSV-1 and HSV-2 infections when the clinical history is suggestive of genital herpes but confirmation by HSV DNA detection has not been possible. The presence of HSV-2 antibodies is indicative of genital herpes but the presence of HSV-1 antibodies cannot differentiate between genital and orolabial infections.

Management

Initial episode

Saltwater bathing or sitting in a warm bath is soothing and may allow women to pass urine more comfortably. Topical anaesthetic agents can also be used to ease micturition. Recommended antiviral therapies are aciclovir 400 mg three times daily, valaciclovir 500 mg twice daily or famciclovir 250 mg three times daily, all for 5 days. Aciclovir is the drug of choice in pregnancy and breastfeeding. If lesions are already healing, antiviral therapy will have little added effect. Secondary bacterial infection occasionally occurs and should be treated.

The natural history of HSV infection should be explained, including recurrences, subclinical viral shedding, and the potential for sexual transmission with both of these infections. Patients should be advised to avoid sex during the prodrome and recurrences. Subclinical viral shedding is most common during the first 12 months following initial HSV-2 infection and in those with frequent symptomatic recurrences. Condoms and suppressive treatment reduce the risk of transmission from subclinical viral shedding but neither completely prevents it. Consequently, disclosure should be advised in all relationships.

Recurrence

The appropriate management will depend on the number and severity of recurrences. As recurrences tend to be less severe and self-limiting, they can sometimes be managed with saltwater bathing and topical anaesthetic agents.

Episodic treatment

When recurrences are infrequent but severe, episodic antiviral therapy, started early by the patient, will reduce the duration and severity but will not reduce the number of recurrences. Recommended episodic regimens are aciclovir 400 mg three times daily, valaciclovir 500 mg twice daily or famciclovir 250 mg three times daily, all for 5 days. Shorter-course therapies are also effective: aciclovir 800 mg three times daily for 2 days, famciclovir 1 g twice daily for 1 day or valaciclovir 500 mg twice daily for 3 days can be used.

Suppressive treatment

In those with six or more recurrences per year, long-term suppressive therapy is effective at stopping or reducing the recurrences. The decision whether to start suppressive treatment depends on the number of recurrences and the inconvenience of taking daily treatment. Recommended regimens are aciclovir 400 mg twice daily, valaciclovir 500 mg daily or famciclovir 250 mg twice daily for a maximum of 12 months. Therapy should then be discontinued in order to assess the frequency of recurrences. If they are still frequent, suppressive treatment can be restarted.

Frequent recurrences are associated with psychological and psychosexual morbidity; support and counselling are often needed.

HSV in pregnancy

The main risk of HSV in pregnancy is vertical transmission. Despite antiviral treatment, neonatal HSV has high mortality and high morbidity in those who survive. The primary episode of genital HSV in late pregnancy poses the highest risk of transmission, and caesarean section should be the recommended mode of delivery for all, but particularly for women within 6 weeks of the expected delivery date. Women who present with an initial episode of HSV in the third trimester should continue with daily suppressive aciclovir 400 mg three times daily (increased due to the altered pharmacokinetics of the drug in pregnancy) until delivery. Those presenting with an initial episode of HSV in the first or second trimester can be given suppressive aciclovir from 36 weeks' gestation. This reduces recurrences and subclinical viral shedding, and therefore the need for a caesarean section.

The risk of neonatal herpes with recurrent HSV is small, even if lesions are present at the time of delivery. The Royal College of Obstetricians and Gynaecologists in the UK suggests that caesarean section is not indicated in such women, but daily suppressive aciclovir from 36 weeks' gestation should be considered.

Syphilis

Syphilis is a chronic systemic disease caused by *Treponema pallidum* (TP), a motile spirochaete. It is mainly transmitted by direct contact with an infectious lesion and enters the new host through breaches in squamous or columnar epithelium, usually during sex. Primary infection of non-genital sites may occur but is rare. It can also be transmitted by infected blood products or from mother to child during pregnancy; hence syphilis is classified as acquired or congenital. **Acquired syphilis** is further subdivided into primary, secondary and early latent (all also referred to as early or infectious syphilis, and indicating that infection has been acquired during the last 2 years), late latent (infection for more than 2 years) and tertiary syphilis (the most destructive stage, which includes cardiovascular and neurological syphilis and gummatous lesions of any organ). **Congenital syphilis** is also further subdivided into early (diagnosed within the first 2 years of life) and late (diagnosed over the age of 2).

The incidence varies significantly with geographical location. It is more common in low- and middle-income countries; in high-income countries, it is mainly confined to MSM and is increasing. For instance, diagnoses of infectious syphilis in England between 2008 and 2017 increased by 148% and most cases were in MSM. However, syphilis still affects large numbers of pregnant women worldwide. It was estimated that, in 2016, 988 000 pregnant women were infected worldwide with syphilis, resulting in over 350 000 adverse birth outcomes, including 200 000 stillbirths and newborn deaths.

Clinical features

Primary syphilis

Between 9 and 90 days (mean 21 days) after exposure, a papule develops at the site of inoculation. This ulcerates to become a painless, firm ulcer (chancre). There is usually also a painless regional lymphadenopathy. The primary lesion may go unnoticed, especially if it is on the cervix or within the rectum. Healing occurs spontaneously within 2–6 weeks.

Secondary syphilis

This occurs in 25% with untreated primary syphilis. Between 6 and 10 weeks after the appearance of the primary lesion, constitutional symptoms, including fever, sore throat, malaise and arthralgia, may appear due to septicaemia. Hence, any organ may be affected, and hepatitis, nephritis, arthritis, meningitis, uveitis, interstitial keratitis and retinal involvement have all been described.

Common signs include:

- widespread skin rash (present in 75%), which can involve the whole body, including the palms and soles – typically, a non-itchy, maculopapular rash that may have a coppery colour (**Fig. 37.9**)
- generalized lymphadenopathy (present in 50%)
- condylomata lata, which are moist, wart-like plaques found in the perianal area and other moist body sites
- mucosal lesions in the mouth and on the genitalia presenting as distinct mucous patches or becoming confluent to form 'snail-track ulcers'.

Without treatment, the symptoms and signs of secondary syphilis resolve but may recur, especially in the first year of infection.

Latent syphilis

Latent syphilis is diagnosed on the basis of reactive syphilis serology in someone who has no symptoms and has not been treated. It is divided into early latent (defined as within 2 years of infection acquisition, or within 1 year in the USA) and late latent syphilis (present for 2 or more years), as sexual transmission can occur in early latency but not in late latent disease. Latent syphilis may persist for years or may even be life-long.

Tertiary syphilis

About one-third of people with untreated latent syphilis will develop tertiary syphilis within 2–30 or more years of contracting the infection. Gummatous syphilis (with inflammatory, granulomatous, destructive lesions) is the most benign and commonly involves the skin and bones, but lesions can occur in any organ. Cardiovascular syphilis causes aortitis, aortic regurgitation, aneurysm of the ascending aorta and stenosis of the coronary artery ostia. Neurosyphilis causes chronic meningovascular damage and endarteritis of the small vessels of the brain and spinal cord, presenting as 'general paralysis of the insane' and tabes dorsalis.

Syphilis in pregnancy and congenital syphilis

Syphilis can be transmitted transplacentally at any stage of pregnancy. The risk of transmission is dependent on the stage of maternal infection and can be up to 100% in early syphilis, and even up to 10% with late infection. The WHO estimates that untreated early syphilis in pregnancy results in rates of second-trimester miscarriage or stillbirth of 25%, preterm birth before 32 weeks' gestation of 13%, neonatal death of 11% and congenital syphilis among the infants born of 20%. Detection and treatment of syphilis early in pregnancy prevent congenital syphilis and neonatal death at term, and reduce adverse pregnancy outcomes.

Signs of early congenital syphilis occur in the neonatal period and include a rash, condylomata lata, mucous patches, nasal discharge, hepatosplenomegaly and periostitis. Late syphilis (occurring after 2 years of age) can present with neurological or gummatous lesions but also includes the 'stigmata of congenital syphilis', resulting from early damage to developing structures, particularly teeth and bones. These are Hutchinson's teeth, sabre tibia, bossing of the frontal and parietal bones, and saddle nose.

Diagnosis

T. pallidum cannot be cultured but it can be identified by dark-ground microscopy of secretions from a primary chancre or condylomata lata; however, sensitivity is dependent on highly skilled microscopists. Some laboratories are able to test swabs for TP using PCR but serological testing remains the main laboratory diagnosis.

Most laboratories use a treponemal enzyme immunoassay (EIA) to detect IgG and IgM as a screening test. If this is positive, a further treponemal test and a non-treponemal test are performed.

Treponemal tests

T. pallidum haemagglutination (TPHA) and *T. pallidum* particle agglutination (TPPA) assays are highly specific for treponemal disease but usually remain positive for life, even after treatment, so are unable to differentiate between prior treated infection and re-infection.

Non-treponemal tests

The Venereal Disease Research Laboratory (VDRL) and rapid plasma reagin (RPR) tests become positive within 3–4 weeks of the primary infection. They are quantifiable tests that can be used to monitor treatment response and evidence of re-infection. They are not specific to syphilis and false-positive results may occur in other conditions, particularly in other infections and autoimmune diseases.

Examination of the cerebrospinal fluid (CSF) for evidence of neurosyphilis is indicated in those patients with positive syphilis serology who demonstrate neurological signs and symptoms.

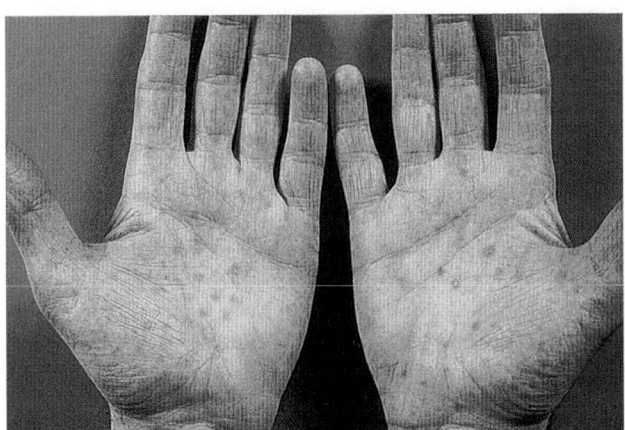

Fig. 37.9 Rash of secondary syphilis on the palms. *(Courtesy of Dr B. Goh.)*

Management

Treponemocidal levels of an antibiotic are required for at least 7 days in early syphilis to cover the slow division time of the organism (30 h). In late syphilis, treponemes may divide even more slowly and so longer therapy is required. Ideally, a long-acting penicillin should be given intramuscularly.

Early syphilis (primary, secondary and early latent)

- Benzathine penicillin G 2.4 MU i.m. single dose.
  In penicillin allergy:
- Doxycycline 100 mg twice daily for 14 days.

The **Jarisch–Herxheimer reaction** is caused by release of inflammatory cytokines and occurs in 50% of patients with primary syphilis and up to 90% with secondary syphilis. It occurs about 8 hours after the injection and usually consists of mild fever, malaise and headache lasting several hours.

Late latent, cardiovascular and gummatous syphilis

- Benzathine penicillin G 2.4 MU i.m. three doses at weekly intervals.
  In penicillin allergy:
- Doxycycline 100 mg twice daily for 28 days.

Neurosyphilis

- Procaine penicillin 2.4 MU i.m. daily plus probenecid 500 mg orally four times daily for 14 days.
  In penicillin allergy:
- Doxycycline 200 mg twice daily for 28 days.

Pregnancy

- Penicillin can be safely used in pregnancy but doxycycline should not be used.

Syphilis and HIV

The diagnosis and management of syphilis in HIV-co-infected patients remain unaltered; however, if disease is untreated, it may advance more rapidly than in HIV-negative patients and there is a higher incidence of neurosyphilis.

Prognosis and follow-up

Those being treated for early syphilis should abstain from sex for at least 14 days and sexual contacts must be traced and investigated. There should be regular follow-up within the first year using repeat VDRL/RPR titres to establish the 'fourfold fall', which demonstrates adequately treated syphilis.

The prognosis of syphilis depends on the stage at which the infection is treated. Early syphilis has an excellent outlook, but once permanent damage has occurred in tertiary syphilis, the damage will not be reversed, although further progression will be halted.

Lymphogranuloma venereum

Lymphogranuloma venereum (LGV) is an STI caused by the invasive serovars, L1, L2 and L3, of *Chlamydia trachomatis*. It is endemic in several tropical areas, including southern Africa, India, South-east Asia and the Caribbean, where it accounts for 2–10% of genital ulcer disease. It used to be rare in Western Europe but since 2003 has become endemic among MSM, particularly those with HIV. It is frequently associated with other STIs and acute hepatitis C infection. The main presentation in MSM is with rectal symptoms; genital infections are rarely seen. LGV should be considered in MSM with suspected inflammatory bowel disease, as the clinical presentation can be very similar and the histological findings of LGV proctitis are similar to those of other causes of granulomatous proctitis, such as Crohn's disease.

Clinical features

There are three clinical stages. The primary lesion may be transient and is frequently unnoticed. In the genital area, it takes the form of a painless papule or shallow ulcer appearing at the area of inoculation, 7–30 days after exposure. The main presentation in MSM is proctitis with symptoms of rectal pain, mucopurulent discharge, rectal bleeding, constipation and tenesmus. Some also report systemic symptoms, such as fever and malaise.

The secondary lesions are enlarged, tender regional lymph nodes. With genital LGV, they are usually unilateral and affect the inguinal and femoral nodes. When both are involved, the 'groove sign' develops due to the inguinal ligament separating the two enlarged lymph node systems. The nodes may become matted with bubo formation, which may rupture.

The tertiary stage is a chronic inflammatory response with tissue destruction. In the rectum, it can cause fistulae, strictures and granulomatous fibrosis, mimicking Crohn's disease. There may also be scarring of the genital area, and destruction of local lymph nodes can lead to genital lymphoedema.

Diagnosis

A swab should be taken from the genital ulcer base, or from the rectal mucosa, for *C. trachomatis* NAAT. If this is positive, genotyping for LGV should be performed. Testing for the other causes of genital ulcers (see **Box 37.5**) or rectal symptoms (see **Box 37.8**) should include a swab for HSV and TP PCR, and serology for syphilis, which should be repeated after the 3-month window period. A NAAT for *N. gonorrhoeae* and *C. trachomatis* on FVU, or a VVS, and serology for HIV should be performed, and serology for hepatitis C should be considered in MSM in view of the frequent co-infection of acute hepatitis C with LGV.

Management

First-choice treatment is doxycycline 100 mg twice daily for 21 days or erythromycin 500 mg four times daily for 21 days. Patients should be advised to abstain from sex until completion of treatment. Sexual contacts should be notified, examined, tested and treated. Follow-up should continue until all symptoms and signs have resolved, which is usually by 3–6 weeks.

Chancroid

Chancroid is caused by *Haemophilus ducreyi*. It used to be one of the most common causes of genital ulcers worldwide but its incidence has now decreased markedly. It is extremely rare in high-income countries.

Clinical features

Chancroid has a short incubation period of 4–7 days. Tender papules develop at the site of inoculation, which rupture into painful, ragged-edged ulcers with necrotic bases that bleed easily. The usual sites of infection are the prepuce and glans penis in men and the labia minora and fourchette in women. There is often painful inguinal lymphadenopathy, which can develop into large buboes that suppurate.

Diagnosis and management

Detection of *H. ducreyi* DNA using PCR is the most sensitive diagnostic test but there are no commercial assays available for this. A 'probable diagnosis' may be made if the patient has the appropriate clinical picture, without evidence of syphilis or HSV.

Testing for the other causes of genital ulcers should be undertaken (see **Box 37.5**) and should include an ulcer swab for HSV and TP PCR, an ulcer swab for *C. trachomatis* NAAT with genotyping for LGV if positive, and serology for syphilis, which should be repeated after the 3-month window period. A NAAT for *N. gonorrhoeae* and *C. trachomatis* on FVU, or a VVS, and serology for HIV should also be performed.

Single-dose regimens include ceftriaxone 250 mg i.m. or azithromycin 1 g orally. Multiple-dose regimens are ciprofloxacin 500 mg twice daily for 3 days or erythromycin 500 mg four times daily for 7 days. Multiple-dose regimens should be used in HIV patients, as treatment failures have been reported with single-dose therapy. Patients should be advised to abstain from sex for at least 7 days and be followed up at 3–7 days, when the ulcers should be healing. HIV-infected patients should be monitored closely, as healing may be slower. Sexual partners should be notified, examined, tested and treated epidemiologically, as asymptomatic carriage has been reported.

Donovanosis

Donovanosis (also known as granuloma inguinale) is exceedingly rare and is confined to a few countries in South-east Asia, southern Africa, parts of India and Brazil. It is caused by *Klebsiella granulomatis*.

Clinical features

Nodules at the site of inoculation develop into friable, non-painful ulcers or hypertrophic lesions that increase in size. There is enlargement of the inguinal lymph nodes, which may ulcerate.

Diagnosis and management

The diagnosis is made on the presence of Donovan bodies using Giemsa or Silver stains in scrapings or biopsies of the lesions. Donovan bodies are the encapsulated intracellular Gram-negative rods of *K. granulomatis* visible within mononuclear cells. Screening for all other STIs should be undertaken.

Antibiotic treatment should be given for a minimum of 3 weeks and until the lesions have healed. Regimens include azithromycin 1 g weekly or 500 mg daily, or doxycycline 100 mg twice daily. Patients should be advised to abstain from sex for at least 3 weeks and be followed up until the lesions have fully resolved. Sexual partners should be notified, examined and treated if necessary.

Pediculosis pubis

The pubic louse (*Phthirus pubis*) is able to attach tightly to the pubic and coarse body hair. It can also attach to eyelashes and eyebrows. It is host-specific and is transferred by close bodily contact. Although infestation may be asymptomatic, the most common complaint is of itch due to hypersensitivity to the louse bites.

Diagnosis and management

Lice may be seen on the pubic and body hairs. They resemble small scabs or freckles but can be seen moving. The eggs (nits) are laid at the hair base and are strongly adherent to the hairs. Screening for other STIs should include NAAT for *N. gonorrhoeae* and *C. trachomatis*, and serology for syphilis and HIV.

Treatment should be applied to all areas of the body, including facial hair if present. Permethrin 1% should be left on for 10 minutes and malathion 0.5% should be left on for 12 hours. A second application is usually advised after 7 days. Permethrin is safe

in pregnancy. Sexual partners should be examined and treated if infected.

Scabies

This is discussed on page 674.

Further reading

British Association for Sexual Health and HIV (BASHH). *BASHH Clinical Effectiveness Guidelines*. BASHH; http://www.bashh.org/.
Brunham RC, Gottlieb SL, Paavonen J. Pelvic inflammatory disease. *N Engl J Med* 2015; 372:2039–2208.
Chow EP, Danielewski JA, Fehler G et al. Human papillomavirus in young women with *Chlamydia trachomatis* infection 7 years after the Australian human papillomavirus vaccination programme: a cross-sectional study. *Lancet Infect Dis* 2015; 15:1314–1323.
Hofstetter AM, Rosenthal SL, Stanberry LR. Current thinking on genital herpes. *Curr Opin Infect Dis* 2014; 27:75–83.
Jensen JS. *Mycoplasma genitalium*: yet another challenging STI. *Lancet Infect Dis* 2017; 17:795–796.
Korenromp EL, Rowley J, Alonso M et al. Global burden of maternal and congenital syphilis and associated adverse birth outcomes – estimates for 2016 and progress since 2012. *PLOS One* 2019; 14:e0211720; https://doi.org/10.1371/journal.pone.0211720.
Merin A, Pachankis JE. The psychological impact of genital herpes stigma. *J Health Psychol* 2011; 16:80–90.
Unemo M, Jensen JS. Antimicrobial-resistant sexually transmitted infections: gonorrhoea and *Mycoplasma genitalium*. *Nat Rev Urol* 2017; 14:139–152.

HUMAN IMMUNODEFICIENCY VIRUS AND ACQUIRED IMMUNODEFICIENCY SYNDROME

EPIDEMIOLOGY AND PATHOGENESIS

Epidemiology

Since the first description of AIDS in 1981 and identification of the causative organism, HIV, in 1983, more than 78 million people are estimated to have been infected and 39 million people have died. At the latest estimate, 36.9 million people worldwide were living with HIV infection (representing 0.8% of adults aged 15-49 years), of whom 21.7 million are accessing anti-retroviral therapy (ART). Highly active ART has dramatically reduced mortality for those who are able to access care, transforming HIV from a universally fatal infection into a long-term, manageable condition, with a consequent rise in global prevalence. Effective ART also reduces onward transmission, and since 2001 new infections globally have fallen by 38%; there is, however, considerable geographical diversity, with infection rates continue to rise in Eastern Europe and parts of Central Asia. HIV is a major contributor to the global burden of disease, being the leading cause of disability-adjusted life-years for people aged 30–45 years and the leading cause of death for women aged 15–49 years.

In 2014 the United Nations Programme on HIV/AIDS (UNAIDS) established new global targets for a scale-up in HIV treatment to help end the AIDS epidemic by 2030. These '90-90-90' ambitions are that:

- 90% of all people living with HIV know their HIV status
- 90% of people with diagnosed HIV infection receive sustained ART
- 90% of all people receiving ART achieve viral suppression.

HIV in sub-Saharan Africa

Sub-Saharan Africa remains the region most seriously affected by the HIV epidemic. While southern and eastern Africa is home to 6.2% of the global population, this figure includes over half of the world's population living with HIV, and 43% of new HIV infections each year occur in this region. Swaziland has the world's highest prevalence of HIV, with 27.2% of adults aged 15–49 infected. In sub-Saharan Africa, HIV infection is almost twice as common in young women (average prevalence 3.2%) than in men (1.6%). The reasons behind this are complex. The predominant route of HIV transmission in the region is through heterosexual sexual intercourse.

Despite the scale of the challenge faced in this region, progress is being made towards the '90-90-90' goals, with an estimated 2.9 million people initiating anti-retroviral agents (ARVs) in the region in 2017.

HIV in high-income countries

Although the rate of new diagnoses is falling in many higher-income countries, the prevalence of HIV is rising: for example, there has been a decline in new diagnoses in the UK since 2015, with 4363 people newly diagnosed in 2017, but falling death rates and continuing new infections mean that the total number of people living with HIV continues to rise. In 2017, 101 600 people in the UK were estimated to be living with HIV; of these, 92% had received the diagnosis and 98% of those diagnosed were on treatment, of whom 97% were virally suppressed.

The fall in new infection rates is due to a combination of factors, including increased and repeat testing, rapid initiation of effective therapy for those testing HIV-positive, and greater use of pre-exposure prophylaxis (PrEP) for those who are HIV-negative but at significant risk of acquiring the virus (see p. 1449). Of those diagnosed with HIV in the UK, MSM and heterosexual populations from sub-Saharan Africa are the two largest groups of people living with the disease; 30% are women. As mortality rates fall, the population living with HIV is becoming older, with more than 1 in 3 now aged 50 years and over.

Late diagnosis is the most common cause of HIV-related morbidity and mortality in the UK. Although the number of people diagnosed late (with a CD4 count of <350 cells/mL within 3 months of diagnosis) has declined from 52% in 2004 to 43% in 2017, this figure remains stubbornly high. Reducing late diagnosis and undiagnosed HIV through wider testing access, particularly in those patients presenting with clinical conditions that are associated with HIV and those living in areas with a high HIV serum prevalence, is critical to both individual and public health.

The changing face of the epidemic

With effective ART, increasing numbers of people with HIV are living with long-term, sustained viral suppression. In countries where ART is consistently accessible, AIDS-defining illnesses have given way to non-communicable conditions as the major health problems for people with HIV. Although chronic health conditions accumulate in general through life, higher levels of multimorbidity occur in people with HIV at a younger age than in those who are HIV-negative, and frailty and its associated disabilities also appear to occur at a younger age. Leading causes of hospital admission of people with HIV in Europe in 2017 included respiratory illness, psychiatric conditions, and cardiovascular, renal and neurological disorders. Data from the UK show that 75% of those living with HIV have at least one other long-term condition, including mental health problems, hypertension, lipid disorders and diabetes. The prevention, identification and treatment of co-morbidities through an integrated, outcomes-focused, person-centred approach are now central to HIV care.

Pathology

Whom to test for HIV infection, and where to do it, are summarized in **Box 37.9**.

Routes of acquisition

Despite the fact that HIV can be isolated from a wide range of body fluids and tissues, the majority of infections are transmitted sexually via semen, cervical secretions and blood. The most significant marker for transmission risk is the HIV viral load, which is highest in acute infection and reduced by effective ART. HIV-associated stigma and discrimination, gender-based violence and, in some countries of the world, the legal position for those at especially high risk can all impede access to appropriate services and increase the risks of transmission and acquisition of HIV.

Sexual intercourse (vaginal and anal)

Globally, heterosexual intercourse accounts for the vast majority of infections, and coexistent STIs, especially those causing genital ulceration, enhance transmission. Passage of HIV appears to be more efficient from men to women, and to the receptive partner in anal intercourse, than vice versa. Once the viral load is consistently reduced below the limit of detection by effective ART, HIV cannot be transmitted to sexual partners. Male circumcision has been shown to reduce both acquisition and transmission. In the UK, sex between men accounts for over half of the new diagnoses reported but there is a consistent rate of heterosexual transmission. In Central and sub-Saharan Africa, the epidemic has always been heterosexual, and more than half of HIV-positive adults in these regions are women. South-east Asia and the Indian subcontinent are experiencing an explosive epidemic, driven by heterosexual intercourse and a high incidence of other STIs.

Vertical transmission (transplacental, perinatal, breast-feeding)

Vertical transmission is the most common route of HIV infection in children. European studies suggest that, with no intervention, 15% of babies born to HIV-positive mothers are likely to acquire HIV, although rates of up to 40% have been reported from Africa and the USA. Increased vertical transmission is associated with an advanced stage of infection in the mother, maternal viral load, prolonged and premature rupture of membranes, and chorioamnionitis. Transmission can occur *in utero*, although the majority of infections take place perinatally. Breast-feeding has been shown to double the risk of vertical transmission in the pre-treatment era, but with considerable reduction in risk when women are using effective ART. In high-income countries, interventions to reduce vertical transmission, including screening for infection in pregnancy, use of ARVs and avoidance of breast-feeding, have led to a dramatic fall in the numbers of infected children. In the UK the risk of vertically transmitted infection is 1:1000. The lack of access to these interventions in the resource-poor countries where 90% of infections occur is a major global issue.

Contaminated blood, blood products and organ donations

Screening of blood and blood products was introduced in 1985 in Europe and North America. Prior to this, HIV infection was associated with the use of clotting factors (for haemophilia) and with blood transfusions. In some parts of the world where blood products may not be screened and in areas where the rate of new HIV infections is very high, transfusion-associated transmission continues to occur.

Contaminated needles (intravenous drug misuse, injections and needle-stick injuries)

The practice of sharing needles and syringes for intravenous drug use continues to be a major route of HIV transmission in parts of South-east Asia, Latin America and Eastern Europe. Successful education and needle exchange schemes can reduce the rate of transmission by this route. Iatrogenic transmission from re-use of needles and syringes in low- and middle-income countries is reported. Healthcare workers have a risk of approximately 0.3% following a single needle-stick injury with known HIV-positive blood, although data were obtained before widespread use of effective ART and the associated reduction in viral load.

There is no evidence that HIV is spread by social or household contact or by blood-sucking insects such as mosquitoes and bed bugs.

The virus

HIV belongs to the lentivirus group of the retrovirus family. There are two types, HIV-1 and HIV-2. HIV-1 is the most frequently occurring strain globally. HIV-2 is almost entirely confined to West Africa, although there is some spread to Europe, particularly France and Portugal. HIV-2 has only 40% structural homology with HIV-1 and, although associated with immunosuppression and AIDS, appears to take a more indolent course than HIV-1. Many of the drugs that are used in HIV-1 are ineffective in HIV-2. The structure of HIV is shown in **Fig. 37.10**.

Retroviruses are characterized by possession of the enzyme reverse transcriptase, which allows viral RNA to be transcribed into DNA and then incorporated into the host cell genome. Reverse transcription is an error-prone process with a significant rate of mis-incorporation of bases. This, combined with a high rate of viral

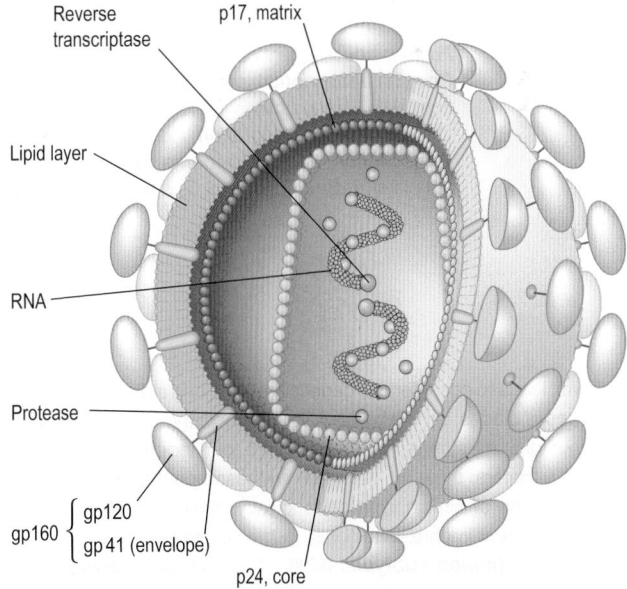

Fig. 37.10 Structure of HIV. Two molecules of single-stranded RNA are shown within the nucleus. The reverse transcriptase polymerase converts viral RNA into DNA (a characteristic of retroviruses). The protease includes integrase (p32 and p10). The p24 (core protein) levels can be used to monitor HIV disease. p17 is the matrix protein; gp120 is the outer envelope glycoprotein, which binds to cell surface CD4 molecules; and gp41, a transmembrane protein, influences infectivity and cell fusion capacity.

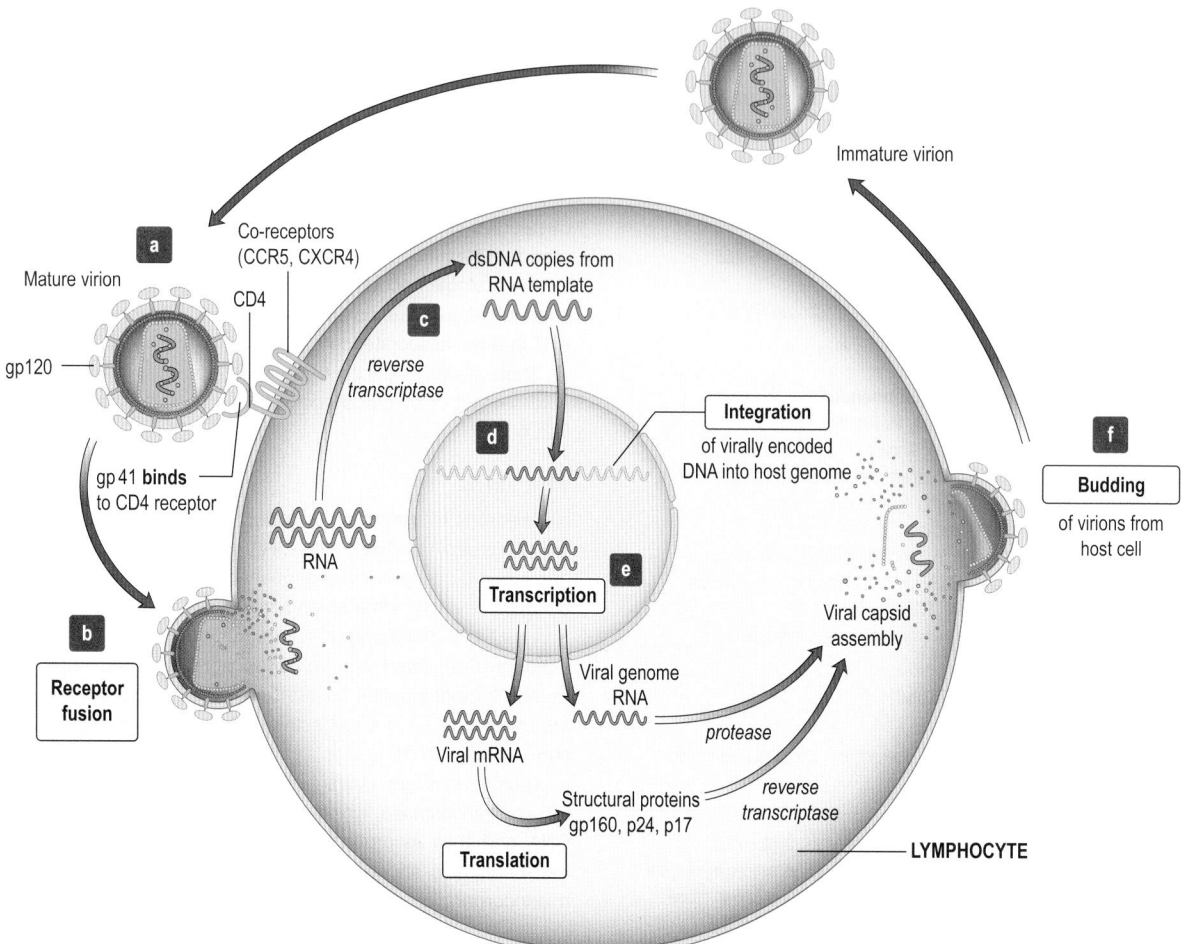

Fig. 37.11 HIV entry and replication in CD4 T lymphocytes. (a) *Binding*: the virus binds to host CD4 receptor molecules via the envelope glycoprotein gp120 and co-receptors CCR5 and CXCR4. (b) *Fusion*: a subsequent conformational change results in fusion between *gp41* and the cell membrane. (c) *Reverse transcription*: entry of the viral capsid is followed by uncoating of the RNA. DNA copies are made from both RNA templates. DNA polymerase from the host cell leads to the formation of double-stranded DNA (dsDNA). (d) *Integration*: in the nucleus, virally encoded DNA is inserted into the host genome. (e) *Transcription*: regulatory proteins control transcription (an RNA molecule is now synthesized from the DNA template). (f) *Budding*: the virus is re-assembled in the cytoplasm and budded out from the host cell.

turnover, leads to considerable genetic variation and a diversity of viral subtypes or clades. On the basis of DNA sequencing, HIV-1 is divided into four distinct strains, which represent four independent cross-species transfers: three (M, N and O) are based on the chimpanzee-related strains of simian immunodeficiency virus (SIV) and one (P) may represent chimpanzee to gorilla to human transmission.

- *Group M (major) subtypes* (98% of infections worldwide) exhibit a high degree of diversity, with subtypes (or clades), denoted A–K. There is a predominance of subtype B in Europe, North America and Australia, but areas of Central and sub-Saharan Africa have multiple M subtypes, clade C being the most common. Recombination of viral material generates an array of circulating recombinant forms (CRFs), which increase the genetic diversity and are becoming more common.
- *Group N (new)* is mostly confined to parts of west Central Africa (e.g. Gabon).

- *Group O (outlier) subtypes* are highly divergent from group M and are largely confined to small numbers that are centred on Cameroon.
- *Group P*, related to gorilla strains of SIV, has been identified from a patient from Cameroon.

Pathogenesis

The interrelationship between HIV and the host immune system is the basis of the pathogenesis of HIV disease. At the time of initial exposure, the virus is transported by dendritic cells from mucosal surfaces to regional lymph nodes, where permanent infection is established, usually by one 'founder virus'. The host cellular receptor that is recognized by HIV surface glycoprotein gp120 is the CD4 molecule, which defines the cell populations that are susceptible to infection (**Fig. 37.11**). The interaction between CD4 and HIV gp120 surface glycoprotein, together with host chemokine CCR5 or CXCR4 co-receptors, is responsible for HIV entry into cells. Although CCR5 CD4 memory T lymphocytes within all body systems are susceptible to infection and depletion, those found in the gastrointestinal tract are heavily infected early in the process. These lymphocytes become rapidly depleted, leading to compromised mucosal immune function, and thus allowing microbial lipopolysaccharides to enter the circulation. HIV infection that is independent of CD4 receptors can occur in astrocytes and renal epithelial cells, leading to end-organ damage.

Studies of viral turnover have demonstrated a virus half-life in the circulation of about 6 hours. To maintain observed levels of plasma viraemia, 10^8–10^9 virus particles need to be released and cleared daily. Virus production by infected cells lasts for about 2 days and is probably limited by the death of the cell, owing to direct HIV effects. This links HIV replication to the process of CD4 destruction and depletion. Progressive loss of activated CD4 T lymphocytes due to killing by CD8 cells is a key factor in the immunopathogenesis of HIV. Natural killer cells are involved in the host immune response, although escape mutations within the virus population compromise their antiviral effects. The production of neutralizing antibodies, which, in some people, can be against several viral subtypes, occurs at about 12 weeks after infection.

Resulting cell-mediated immunodeficiency leaves the host open to infections with intracellular pathogens, while coexisting antibody abnormalities predispose to infections with capsulated bacteria. HIV is associated with immune activation, a long-term inflammatory state, which is a key driver of disease progression. T-cell activation is observed from the earliest stages of infection, which, in turn, leads to an increase in the numbers of susceptible CD4-bearing target cells that can become infected and destroyed. This inflammatory state is associated with HIV itself, with co-pathogens such as cytomegalovirus, and with the translocation of microbial products, in particular lipopolysaccharides, from the gut into the systemic circulation following HIV destruction of normal mucosal immunity. Raised levels of inflammatory cytokines and coagulation system activation occur. These inflammatory responses may remain, despite effective ART, and play a role in HIV-associated end-organ damage, as well as raising the risks of myocardial infarction and some malignancies.

Further reading

Jones A, Cremin I, Abdullah F et al. Transformation of HIV from pandemic to low-endemic levels: a public health approach to combination prevention. *Lancet* 2014; 384:272–279.

National AIDS Trust. *HIV and Black African Communities in the UK*. London: National AIDS Trust; 2014.

Public Health England. Progress Towards Ending the HIV Epidemic in the United Kingdom: 2018 Report; https://assets.publishing.service.gov.uk/government/uploads/system/uploads/attachment_data/file/759408/HIV_annual_report_2018.pdf.

Punyacharoensin N, Edmunds WJ, De Angelis D et al. Modelling the HIV epidemic among MSM in the United Kingdom: quantifying the contributions to HIV transmission to better inform prevention initiatives. *AIDS* 2015; 29:339–349.

CLINICAL FEATURES OF UNTREATED HIV INFECTION

The features of HIV infection can be divided into the early/acute and long-term phases. The spectrum of disorders associated with HIV infection is broad and is the result of direct HIV effects, HIV-associated immune dysfunction and the drugs used to treat the condition, as well as coexisting morbidity and co-infections. With early intervention using effective ART, the majority of people with HIV in high-income settings begin treatment while asymptomatic,

---

Box 37.10 AIDS-defining conditions

- Candidiasis of bronchi, trachea or lungs
- Candidiasis, oesophageal
- Cervical carcinoma, invasive
- Coccidioidomycosis, disseminated or extrapulmonary
- Cryptococcosis, extrapulmonary
- Cryptosporidiosis, chronic intestinal (1-month duration)
- Cytomegalovirus (CMV) disease (other than liver, spleen or nodes)
- CMV retinitis (with loss of vision)
- Encephalopathy, HIV-related
- Herpes simplex, chronic ulcers (1-month duration), or bronchitis, pneumonitis or oesophagitis
- Histoplasmosis, disseminated or extrapulmonary
- Isosporiasis, chronic intestinal (1-month duration)
- Kaposi's sarcoma
- Lymphoma, Burkitt
- Lymphoma, immunoblastic (or equivalent term)
- Lymphoma (primary) of brain
- *Mycobacterium avium-intracellulare* complex or *M. kansasii*, disseminated or extrapulmonary
- *Mycobacterium tuberculosis*, any site
- *Mycobacterium*, other species or unidentified species, disseminated or extrapulmonary
- *Pneumocystis jirovecii* pneumonia
- Pneumonia, recurrent
- Progressive multifocal leucoencephalopathy
- *Salmonella* septicaemia, recurrent
- Toxoplasmosis of brain
- Wasting syndrome, due to HIV

Box 37.11 Summary of the Centers for Disease Control (CDC) classification of HIV infection

Absolute CD4 count (/mm³)	A — Asymptomatic or persistent generalized lymphadenopathy or acute seroconversion illness	B — HIV-related conditions,[a] not A or C	C — Clinical conditions listed in AIDS surveillance case definition (see Box 37.10)
>500	A1	B1	C1
200–499	A2	B2	C2
<200	A3	B3	C3

[a]Examples of category B conditions include bacillary angiomatosis, candidiasis (oropharyngeal), constitutional symptoms, oral hairy leukoplakia, herpes zoster involving more than one dermatome, idiopathic thrombocytopenic purpura, listeriosis, pelvic inflammatory disease, especially if complicated by tubo-ovarian abscess, peripheral neuropathy.

---

before the onset of significant immunosuppression, and therefore progression to an AIDS-defining event is now uncommon. Without treatment, immunosuppression progresses and the patient becomes susceptible to an increasing range of opportunistic infections and tumours, certain of which meet the criteria for the diagnosis of AIDS (**Box 37.10**).

Several HIV classification systems exist, the two most frequently used being the WHO and Centers for Disease Control (CDC) classification (**Box 37.11**). Their major application is in public health monitoring and surveillance rather than in routine clinical care. The CDC classification (Stages 0–3) includes a combination of HIV-positive laboratory results, the CD4 count and the presence of clinical AIDS-defining conditions. Immunological and clinical markers in combination with a positive HIV antibody test are incorporated in the WHO classification system.

Early HIV infection: incubation, seroconversion and acute illness

Early infection refers to the 6-month period following HIV acquisition, and is marked by rapid viral replication resulting in high levels of HIV circulating in the plasma and genital tract, and consequently by high infectiousness. This time is increasingly recognized as a key period for intervention, both to reduce long-term sequelae and to cut onward transmission.

The 2–4 weeks immediately following infection may be silent, both clinically and serologically. In a number of people, a self-limiting acute viral illness, which may be confused with glandular fever, occurs 3–6 weeks after exposure. Symptoms include fever, arthralgia, myalgia, lethargy, lymphadenopathy, sore throat, mucosal ulcers and, occasionally, a transient, faint pink, maculopapular rash. Neurological symptoms are common and include headache, photophobia, myelopathy, neuropathy and, in rare cases, encephalopathy. The illness lasts up to 3 weeks and recovery is usually complete.

This is a crucial point at which to make a diagnosis of HIV; however, HIV is frequently not considered in the differential diagnosis in patients presenting with such non-specific, viral symptoms.

Laboratory abnormalities in the early phase of infection include lymphopenia with atypical reactive lymphocytes noted on the blood film, thrombocytopenia and raised liver transferases. CD4 lymphocytes may be markedly depleted and the CD4:CD8 ratio reversed. With increasingly sensitive assays, a majority of people with HIV develop detectable antibodies within the first 2–4 weeks of early infection. However, antibodies to HIV may be absent during the earliest stages of infection, although the level of circulating viral RNA is high and p24 core protein may be detectable. NAAT assays of HIV RNA may be diagnostic 7 days before a p24 antigen test and 12 days before a sensitive HIV antibody test. If early or acute HIV infection is suspected but standard diagnostic tests are negative, repeat testing in 7 days and referral for expert advice is recommended.

Clinical latency

The rate of clinical progression of untreated HIV is variable. The majority of people with HIV infection are asymptomatic for a substantial but variable length of time. However, the virus continues to replicate and the person remains infectious. Most people with HIV have a gradual decline in CD4 count over a period of approximately 10 years before progression to symptomatic disease or AIDS (**Fig. 37.12**). Others progress much more rapidly, with continued high levels of viral RNA and a rapid decline in CD4 count over 2–5 years. Other 'long-term non-progressors' may continue with a normal CD4 count over many years. Within this group, a small subpopulation of 'elite controllers' maintain a viral load of less than 2000 copies/mL, or even have undetectable levels or virus, without therapy.

Older age is associated with more rapid progression. Gender and pregnancy *per se* do not appear to influence the rate of progression, although women may fare less well for a variety of reasons. A subgroup of patients with asymptomatic infection have ***persistent generalized lymphadenopathy*** (PGL), defined as lymphadenopathy (>1 cm) at two or more extra-inguinal sites for more than 3 months in the absence of causes other than HIV infection. The nodes are usually symmetrical, firm, mobile and non-tender. There

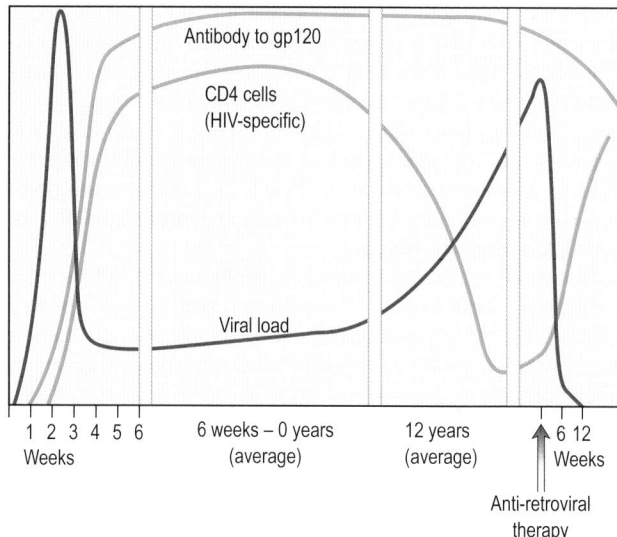

Fig. 37.12 The immune response to HIV (seroconversion).

may be associated splenomegaly. The architecture of the nodes shows hyperplasia of the follicles and proliferation of the capillary endothelium. Biopsy is rarely indicated. The presence of PGL does not seem to affect disease progression, although as the disease progresses, nodes may disappear.

Symptomatic HIV infection

As HIV infection progresses, the viral load rises, the CD4 count falls and the patient develops an array of symptoms and signs. The clinical picture is due to:

- the direct result of HIV causing end-organ damage
- the result of HIV-associated immunosuppression.

End-organ effects of HIV

Neurological disease

Infection of the nervous tissue occurs at an early stage and clinical neurological involvement increases as HIV advances. Manifestations include ***AIDS dementia complex*** (***ADC***), ***sensory polyneuropathy*** and ***aseptic meningitis*** (see p. 871). These conditions have become much less common since the introduction of ART. The pathogenesis is thought to be due both to the release of neurotoxic products by HIV itself and to cytokine abnormalities secondary to immune dysregulation.

ADC has varying degrees of severity, ranging from mild memory impairment and poor concentration through to severe cognitive deficit, personality change and psychomotor slowing. Changes in affect are common and depressive or psychotic features may be present. The spinal cord may show vacuolar myelopathy histologically. In severe cases, computed tomography (CT) scanning of the brain shows atrophic change of varying degrees. Magnetic resonance imaging (MRI) changes consist of white-matter lesions of increased density on T2-weighted sections. Electroencephalography (EEG) shows non-specific changes consistent with encephalopathy. The CSF is usually normal, although the protein concentration may be raised. Patients with mild neurological dysfunction may be unduly sensitive to the effects of other insults, such as fever, metabolic

aSee also page 676.

> ### i Box 37.12 Some mucocutaneous manifestations of HIV infectiona
>
> **Skin**
> - Dry skin and scalp
> - Onychomycosis
> - Seborrhoeic dermatitis
> - Tinea: cruris, pedis
> - Pityriasis: versicolor, rosea
> - Folliculitis
> - Acne
> - Molluscum contagiosum
> - Warts
> - Herpes zoster: multidermatomal disseminated
> - Papular pruritic eruption
> - Scabies
> - Ichthyosis
> - Kaposi's sarcoma
>
> **Mucous membranes**
> - Candidiasis: oral, vulvovaginal
> - Oral hairy leukoplakia
> - Aphthous ulcers
> - Herpes simplex: genital, oral, labial
> - Periodontal disease
> - Warts: oral, genital

disturbance or psychotropic medication, any of which may lead to a marked deterioration in cognitive functioning.

Sensory polyneuropathy is seen in advanced HIV infection, mainly in the legs and feet, although the hands may also be affected. Severe forms cause intense pain, usually in the feet, which disrupts sleep, impairs mobility and generally reduces quality of life.

Autonomic neuropathy may also occur, with postural hypotension and diarrhoea. Autonomic nerve damage is found in the small bowel.

ARVs that penetrate the central nervous system (CNS) can lead to significant improvements in cognitive function in many patients with ADC. They may also have a neuroprotective role.

Eye disease

Eye pathology may occur in the later stages of infection. The most serious condition is cytomegalovirus retinitis (see p. 525), which is sight-threatening. Retinal cotton wool spots due to HIV *per se* are rarely troublesome but can be confused with cytomegalovirus retinitis. Anterior uveitis can present as acute red eye associated with rifabutin therapy for mycobacterial infections in HIV. Steroids used topically are usually effective but modification of the dose of rifabutin is required to prevent relapse. *Pneumocystis* infection, toxoplasmosis, syphilis and lymphoma can all affect the retina and the eye may be the site of first presentation.

Mucocutaneous manifestations

The skin is a common site for HIV-related pathology (**Box 37.12**), as the function of dendritic and Langerhans cells, both target cells for HIV, is disrupted. Delayed-type hypersensitivity, a good indicator of cell-mediated immunity, is frequently reduced or absent, even before clinical signs of immunosuppression appear. Pruritus is a common complaint at all stages of HIV. Generalized dry, itchy, flaky skin is typical and the hair may become thin and dry. An intensely pruritic papular eruption favouring the extremities may be found, particularly in patients from African backgrounds. Eosinophilic folliculitis presents with urticarial lesions, particularly on the face, arms and legs.

Drug reactions with cutaneous manifestations are frequent, rashes developing notably to sulphur-containing drugs, among others (see **Fig. 22.31**). Recurrent aphthous ulceration, which is severe and slow to heal, may impair the patient's ability to eat. Biopsy may be indicated to exclude other causes of ulceration. Topical steroids are useful and resistant cases may respond to thalidomide. In addition to these conditions, the skin is a common site of opportunistic infections (see p. 676).

Haematological complications

These are common in advanced HIV infection.
- *Lymphopenia* progresses as the CD4 count falls.
- *Anaemia of chronic HIV infection* is usually mild, normochromic and normocytic.
- *Neutropenia* is common and usually mild.
- *Isolated thrombocytopenia* may occur early in infection and be the only manifestation of HIV for some time. Platelet counts are often moderately reduced but can fall dramatically to 10–20×10^9/L, producing easy bleeding and bruising. Circulating antiplatelet antibodies lead to peripheral destruction. Megakaryocytes are increased in the bone marrow but their function is impaired. Effective ART usually produces a rise in platelet count. Thrombocytopenic patients undergoing dental, medical or surgical procedures may need therapy with human immunoglobulin, which gives a transient rise in platelet count, or with platelet transfusion. Steroids are best avoided.
- *Pancytopenia* occurs because of underlying opportunistic infection or malignancies, in particular *M. avium-intracellulare* (MAI), disseminated cytomegalovirus and lymphoma.
- *Other complications* involve myelotoxic drugs, which include lamivudine (anaemia, neutropenia), ganciclovir (neutropenia), systemic chemotherapy (pancytopenia) and co-trimoxazole (agranulocytosis).

Gastrointestinal effects

Weight loss and diarrhoea are common in people with advanced untreated HIV infection (see **Box 32.36**). Wasting is a common feature of advanced HIV infection, which, although originally attributed to direct HIV effects on metabolism, is frequently a consequence of anorexia. There is a small increase in resting energy expenditure in all stages of HIV, but weight and lean body mass usually remain normal during periods of clinical latency when the patient is eating normally.

HIV enteropathy with varying degrees of villous atrophy has been described with chronic diarrhoea when no other pathogen has been found. Hypochlorhydria is reported in patients with advanced HIV disease and may have consequences for drug absorption and bacterial overgrowth in the gut. Rectal lymphoid tissue cells are the targets for HIV infection during penetrative anal sex and may be a reservoir for infection to spread through the body.

Renal complications

HIV-associated nephropathy (HIVAN; see p. 1356*)*, although rare, can cause significant renal impairment, particularly in more advanced disease. It is most frequently seen in black male patients and can be exacerbated by heroin use. It causes a collapsing variant of focal segmental glomerulosclerosis, along with a tubulopathy due to direct viral infection of tubular cells. The course is usually relentlessly progressive and renal replacement therapy is often required.

Other renal pathology seen in HIV includes *HIV-immune complex kidney disease (HIVICK)*, which can present with a range of glomerular abnormalities, **IgA nephropathy** and **thrombotic microangiopathy (TMA)**.

Many *nephrotoxic drugs* are used in the management of HIV-associated pathology: for example, foscarnet, amphotericin B, pentamidine and sulfadiazine. Tenofovir is associated with Fanconi's syndrome (see p. 337).

Respiratory complications

The upper airway and lungs serve as a physical barrier to airborne pathogens and any damage will decrease the efficiency of protection, leading to an increase in upper and lower respiratory tract infections. The sinus mucosa may also function abnormally in HIV infection and is frequently the site of chronic inflammation. Response to antibacterial therapy and topical steroids is usual but some patients require surgical intervention. A similar process is seen in the middle ear, which can lead to chronic otitis media.

Lymphoid interstitial pneumonitis (LIP) is well described in paediatric HIV infection but is uncommon in adults. There is an infiltration of lymphocytes, plasma cells and lymphoblasts in alveolar tissue. Epstein–Barr virus may be present. The patient presents with dyspnoea and a dry cough, which may be confused with *Pneumocystis* infection (see p. 1443). Reticular nodular shadowing is seen on chest X-ray. Therapy with steroids may produce clinical and histological benefit in some patients.

Endocrine complications

Various endocrine abnormalities have been reported, including reduced levels of testosterone and abnormal adrenal function. The latter assumes clinical significance in advanced disease when intercurrent infection superimposed on borderline adrenal function precipitates clear adrenal insufficiency, requiring replacement doses of gluco- and mineralocorticoid. Cytomegalovirus is also implicated in adrenal-deficient states.

Cardiac complications

A recent systematic review and meta-analysis showed that people living with HIV are twice as likely to develop cardiovascular disease as the general population Although lipid dysregulation has been associated with ARV medication, the observation has been made that high-density lipoprotein (HDL) levels are lower in those with untreated HIV infection than in HIV-negative controls. In a large international study (SMART), ischaemic heart disease was more common in those who took intermittent ARV therapy than in those who maintained viral suppression. Cardiomyopathy has been associated with HIV and may lead to congestive cardiac failure, although, in the ART era, cardiomyopathy related to ischaemic disease is becoming more common. Lymphocytic and necrotic myocarditis has been described. In cases of diagnostic uncertainty, ventricular biopsy can be undertaken to ensure that other treatable causes of myocarditis are excluded.

Conditions associated with HIV immunodeficiency

Immunodeficiency (see p. 59) allows the development of opportunistic infections (**Box 37.13**; see also **Box 37.21**). These are diseases caused by organisms that are not usually considered pathogenic, by known pathogens with unusual presentations, and by tumours that may have an oncogenic viral aetiology. Susceptibility increases as the patient becomes more immunosuppressed, and CD4 T-lymphocyte numbers are used as markers to predict the risk of infection. Patients with CD4 counts of more than 200 cells/mm^3 are at low risk for the majority of **AIDS-defining conditions** (see **Box 37.10**), while a hierarchy of thresholds for specific infectious risks can be constructed as the CD4 count falls.

Mechanisms of this increasing susceptibility to infection include:
- defective T-cell function against protozoa, fungi and viruses

---

i Box 37.13 Major HIV-associated pathogens

Protozoa
- *Toxoplasma gondii*
- *Cryptosporidium parvum*
- *Microsporidia* spp.
- *Leishmania donovani*
- *Isospora belli*

Viruses
- Cytomegalovirus
- Herpes simplex
- Varicella zoster
- Human papillomavirus
- Human herpes virus-8
- JC polyomavirus

Fungi and yeasts
- *Pneumocystis jirovecii*
- *Cryptococcus neoformans*

- *Candida* spp.
- Dermatophytes *(Trichophyton)*
- *Aspergillus fumigatus*
- *Histoplasma capsulatum*
- *Coccidioides immitis*

Bacteria
- *Salmonella* spp.
- *Mycobacterium tuberculosis*
- *M. avium-intracellulare*
- *Streptococcus pneumoniae*
- *Staphylococcus aureus*
- *Haemophilus influenzae*
- *Moraxella catarrhalis*
- *Rhodococcus equii*
- *Bartonella quintana*
- *Nocardia*

- impaired macrophage function against intracellular bacteria such as *Mycobacteria* and *Salmonella*
- defective B-cell immunity against capsulated bacteria such as *Streptococcus pneumoniae* and *Haemophilus*.

Many of the organisms causing clinical disease are ubiquitous in the environment or are already carried by the patient.

Diagnosis in an immunosuppressed patient may be complicated by a lack of typical signs, as the inflammatory response is impaired. Examples are lack of neck stiffness in cryptococcal meningitis or minimal clinical findings in early *Pneumocystis jirovecii* pneumonia. Multiple pathogens may coexist. Indirect serological tests are frequently unreliable. Specimens should be obtained from the appropriate site for examination and culture in order to make a diagnosis.

In an individual patient, the clinical consequences of HIV-related immune dysfunction will depend on at least three factors:
- **Microbial exposure of the patient throughout life.** Many clinical episodes represent reactivation of previously acquired infection, which has been latent. Geographical factors determine the microbial repertoire of an individual patient. Those organisms requiring intact cell-mediated immunity for their control are most likely to cause clinical problems.
- **Pathogenicity of organisms encountered.** High-grade pathogens, such as *Mycobacterium tuberculosis*, *Candida* and the herpesviruses, are clinically relevant, even when immunosuppression is mild, and will thus occur earlier in the course of HIV infection. Less virulent organisms occur at later stages of immunodeficiency.
- **Degree of immunosuppression of the host.** When patients are severely immunocompromised (CD4 count <100 cells/mm^3), disseminated infections with organisms of very low virulence, such as MAI and *Cryptosporidium*, are able to establish themselves. These infections are very resistant to treatment, mainly because there is no functioning immune response to clear organisms. This hierarchy of infection allows for appropriate intervention with prophylactic drugs.

CLINICAL APPROACH TO THE PATIENT WITH HIV

HIV testing

HIV testing may be carried out in a number of settings (see p. 1449), and infection is diagnosed either by detection of virus-specific antibodies (anti-HIV) or by direct identification of viral material. Modern 'fourth-generation' tests, which are now the standard of care in many countries, test for anti-HIV antibodies and the p24 antigen simultaneously.

Detection of anti-HIV antibodies

This is the most commonly used marker of infection. The routine tests used for screening are based on enzyme-linked immunosorbent assay (ELISA) techniques, which may be confirmed with Western blot assays. Up to 3 months (mean 6 weeks) may elapse from initial infection to antibody detection (serological latency, or the 'window period'). These antibodies to HIV have no protective function and persist for life. As with all IgG antibodies, anti-HIV will cross the placenta. All babies born to HIV-positive women will thus have the antibody at birth. In this situation, anti-HIV antibody is not a reliable marker of active infection, and will be gradually lost over the first 18 months of life in uninfected babies.

A serological testing algorithm for recent HIV seroconversions (STARHS) can be used to identify recently acquired infection. A highly sensitive ELISA that is able to detect HIV antibodies 6–8 weeks after infection is used on blood from patients with a positive oral fluid test, in parallel with a less sensitive (detuned) test that identifies later HIV antibodies within 130 days. A positive result on the sensitive test and a negative 'detuned' test are indicative of recent infection, while positive results on both tests point to an infection that is more than 130 days old. The major application of this is in epidemiological surveillance and monitoring.

Detection of viral p24 antigen

The p24 antigen (p24ag) is a protein from the HIV viral capsid that can be detected in blood shortly after infection, but which has usually disappeared by 8–10 weeks after exposure (see **Fig. 37.12**). It can be a useful marker in individuals who have been infected recently but have not had time to mount an antibody response. Anti-p24 antibodies (anti-p24) can be detected from the earliest weeks of infection and through the asymptomatic phase. It is frequently lost as the disease progresses.

Genome detection assays

Nucleic acid-based assays that amplify and test for components of the HIV genome are available. These assays are used to aid the diagnosis of HIV in the babies of HIV-positive mothers or in situations where serological tests may be inadequate, such as in early infection when antibody may not be present, or in subtyping HIV variants for medico-legal reasons. (See the discussion of viral load monitoring on p. 1434.)

Isolation of virus in culture

This is a specialized technique available in some laboratories as a diagnostic aid and a research tool.

Initial assessment

People are newly diagnosed with HIV in many different settings and need to be transferred rapidly to effective specialist care. All those with a new diagnosis of HIV should be reviewed by an HIV clinician within 2 weeks of diagnosis, or earlier if the patient is symptomatic or has other acute needs. A full medical history, physical examination and laboratory evaluation should be undertaken in all newly diagnosed patients to determine the stage of infection and the presence of co-morbidities and co-infections, and to assess

---

> **i** **Box 37.14** Baseline assessment investigations for a newly diagnosed asymptomatic patient with HIV infection
>
> **History of all other coexisting conditions, including sexual, psychiatric and reproductive health**
> - Knowledge and beliefs about HIV, including treatment and transmission
> - Full drug history, including recreational substances
> - Vaccination history
> - Social circumstances, including relationships, disclosure and support
> - General physical examination, including weight, height, body mass index, blood pressure and waist circumference
>
> **Haematology**
> - Full blood count, differential count and film
>
> **Biochemistry**
> - Serum, liver and renal function, including estimated glomerular filtration rate (eGFR)
> - Fasting serum lipid profile, total cholesterol, high-density lipoprotein (HDL) cholesterol
> - Fasting blood glucose
> - Serum bone profile
> - Urinalysis
> - Dipstick for blood, protein and glucose
> - Urine protein : creatinine ratio
>
> **Immunology**
> - Lymphocyte subsets (repeat to confirm baseline within 1–3 months)
> - Human leucocyte antigen (HLA)-B*5701 status
>
> **Virology**
> - HIV antibody (confirmatory)
> - HIV viral load
> - HIV genotype and subtype determination
> - Hepatitis A immunoglobulin G
> - Hepatitis B surface antigen and full profile
> - Hepatitis C antibody (followed by hepatitis C RNA testing if antibody-positive, and confirmation of antibody-positive status if RNA-negative)
>
> **Microbiology**
> - Toxoplasmosis serology
> - Syphilis serology
> - Tuberculosis status
> - Screen for other sexually transmitted infections
>
> **Other**
> - Cervical cytology
> - Chest X-ray if indicated
> - 10-year cardiovascular risk assessment
> - Fracture risk assessment

overall physical, mental and sexual health. The initial assessment should also include details of the patient's socioeconomic situation, relationships, family and social support networks, and substance misuse, together with contact tracing and partner notification. Specialist advice should be sought if there are children who require testing. Baseline investigations will depend on the clinical setting, but those appropriate for an asymptomatic person in the UK are shown in **Box 37.14**.

Genotype determination

Viral genotype analysis is recommended for all newly diagnosed patients with HIV. Clear genotype variations exist within HIV; not only are there variations between viral subtypes but also well-identified point mutations are associated with resistance to ARVs. New infections with drug-resistant variants of HIV may be seen. The most appropriate sample is the one closest to the time of diagnosis and the results are used to guide the selection of ART agents.

Monitoring

Patients are regularly monitored, depending on clinical, virological and treatment stage.

For people with HIV who have chosen not to initiate therapy, monitoring should take place 2–4 times per year, with longer intervals for those with higher CD4 counts, to assess progression of the infection and to discuss treatment options.

For people starting therapy and those on established effective therapy, monitoring is described on page 1438.

Immunological monitoring

Absolute numbers (and relative proportions) of **CD4 lymphocytes** are monitored. The absolute CD4 count and its percentage of total lymphocytes fall as HIV progresses. These figures bear a relationship to the risk of occurrence of HIV-related pathology, and patients with counts of less than 200 cells/mm^3 are at greatest risk. Rapidly falling CD4 counts and those at or below 350 cells/mm are an indication for immediate initiation of ART. Factors other than HIV (e.g. smoking, exercise, intercurrent infections and diurnal variation) also affect CD4 numbers. Once the patient is virologically stable on ART with a CD4 above 350 cells/mm, CD4 counts are performed at approximately yearly intervals. For those not taking ART, 4–6-monthly intervals are appropriate, unless values are approaching critical levels for intervention, in which case they are performed more frequently.

Virological monitoring

The HIV **viral load (HIV RNA)** is monitored, which has both prognostic and therapeutic value. HIV replicates at a high rate throughout the course of infection, many billions of new virus particles being produced daily. The rate of viral clearance is relatively constant in any individual and thus the level of viraemia is a reflection of the rate of virus replication.

Three **HIV RNA assays for viral load** are in current use:
- branched-chain DNA (bDNA)
- reverse transcription polymerase chain reaction (RT-PCR)
- nucleic acid sequence-based amplification (NASBA).

Results are given in copies of viral RNA/mL of plasma, or converted to a logarithmic scale, and there is good correlation between tests. The most sensitive test is able to detect as few as 20 copies of viral RNA/mL. Transient increases in viral load are seen following immunizations (e.g. for influenza and pneumococcus) or during episodes of acute intercurrent infection (e.g. tuberculosis), and viral load measurements should not be carried out within a month of these events.

By about 6 months after seroconversion to HIV, the viral set-point for an individual is established and there is a correlation between HIV RNA levels and long-term prognosis, independent of the CD4 count. Those patients with a viral load consistently above 100 000 copies/mL have a 10 times higher risk of progression to AIDS over the ensuing 5 years than those with counts consistently below 10 000 copies/mL.

HIV RNA is the standard marker of anti-retroviral treatment efficacy (see later). Both duration and magnitude of virus suppression are pointers to clinical outcome. The aim of therapy is to secure long-term virological suppression, and a rising viral load in a patient whose adherence is assured indicates drug failure.

Baseline measurements are followed by repeat estimations at intervals of 4–6 months. Following initiation of ART or changes in therapy, a reduction in viral load should be seen by 4 weeks, reaching a maximum at 10–12 weeks, when repeat viral load testing should be carried out (see **Fig. 37.12**).

Monitoring other aspects of health

Regular assessment is needed to monitor for intercurrent medical problems, medications, vaccinations, recreational drug use, sexual history, reproductive decision-making, cervical cytology and social situation, including support networks, employment, benefits and accommodation. Depression and anxiety are common among people living with HIV and can have a deleterious impact on health-related quality of life, as well as adherence to medication regimens, meaning that mood and cognitive function should be routinely and regularly assessed. Psychological support may be needed, not only for the patient but also for family, friends and carers.

Regular reviews of sexual and reproductive health, together with advice on reducing the risk of HIV transmission, must be provided and future sexual practices discussed. Information is required to allow people to make informed choices about childbearing. The implications for sexual partners and existing family members should be considered and diagnostic testing offered as necessary.

Regular monitoring of weight, body mass index, metabolic and bone markers, blood pressure and cardiovascular risk is required. Dietary assessment and advice should be freely accessible. General health promotion advice on smoking, alcohol, diet, drug misuse and exercise should be given, particularly in light of the increased risk of cardiovascular and metabolic co-morbidities associated with HIV and its treatment.

Further reading

Angus B, Brook G, Awosusi F et al. *BHIVA Guidelines for the Routine Investigation and Monitoring of Adult HIV-1-positive Individuals 2016 (2019 Interim Update).* London: British HIV Association; 2019.

Deeks SG, Lewin SR, Havlir DV. The end of AIDS: HIV infection as a chronic disease. *Lancet* 2013; 382:1525–1533.

Justice A, Falutz J. Aging and HIV: an evolving understanding. *Curr Opin HIV AIDS* 2014; 9:291.

May MT, Gompels M, Delpech V et al. Impact on life expectancy of HIV-1 positive individuals of CD4+ cell count and viral load response to antiretroviral therapy: UK cohort study. *AIDS* 2014; 28:1193–1202.

MANAGEMENT OF HIV-POSITIVE PATIENTS

Effective ART has transformed clinical outcomes for people with HIV, extending life expectancy towards that of the general population, bringing down morbidity and cutting onward transmission. Current management strategies aim to maximize wellbeing with sustained viral-suppressive therapy within a long-term condition model, with appropriate attention to the prevention and treatment of HIV-associated co-morbidities (**Box 37.15**).

With access and adherence to potent, tolerable ARVs within a managed clinical setting, life expectancy for people with HIV approaches that of the general population. Nevertheless, there is still no cure for HIV and patients live with a chronic, potentially infectious and sometimes unpredictable condition. Limitations on ART efficacy include the inability of existing drugs to clear HIV from certain intracellular pools, the occurrence of drug side-effects, adherence requirements, complex drug–drug interactions and the emergence of resistant viral strains. Even with complete viral suppression, ART does not fully restore health, and treated infection is associated with a variety of complications and co-morbidities, including cardiovascular disease, some cancers and impaired mental health. Measures

---

Box 37.15 An approach to sick HIV-positive patients

Potential problems
- Adverse drug reactions
- Drug–drug interactions
- Presentation or complications of malignancy
- Immune reconstitution phenomenon
- Infection in an immunocompromised host
- Acute opportunistic infections
- Organic or functional brain disorders
- Non-HIV-related pathology

Full medical history
- Anti-retroviral drugs, recreational drugs, prophylaxis, travel, previous HIV-related pathology, potential sources of infectious agents (food hygiene, pets, contacts with acute infections, contact with tuberculosis, sexually transmitted infections)
- Secure confidentiality; ask the patient who is aware of the HIV diagnosis

Full physical examination
- Signs of adverse drug reactions, e.g. skin rashes, oral ulceration
- Signs of disseminated sepsis
- Clinical evidence of immunosuppression, e.g. oral candida, oral hairy leukoplakia
- Focal neurological signs and/or meningism
- Evidence of altered mental state – organic or functional
- Examine:
    - Genitalia, e.g. herpes simplex, syphilis, gonorrhoea
    - Fundi, e.g. cytomegalovirus retinitis
    - Mouth
- Lymphadenopathy

Immediate investigations[a]
- Full blood count and differential count
- Liver and renal function tests
- Plasma glucose
- Blood gases, including acid–base balance
- Blood cultures, including specimens for mycobacterial culture
- Microscopy and culture of available/appropriate specimens: stool, sputum, urine, cerebrospinal fluid
- Malaria screen in recent travellers from endemic areas
- Serological tests for cryptococcal antigen, toxoplasmosis; save serum for viral studies
- Chest X-ray
- CT/MRI scan of brain if there are focal neurological signs and *always* before lumbar puncture

[a]Lymphocyte subsets and HIV viral load assays may yield misleading results during intercurrent illness.

---

of health-related quality of life are consistently lower among people living with HIV than in the general population.

Anti-retroviral drugs

The treatment of HIV using ART (**Box 37.16**) continues to evolve and improve. Increased potency, reduced toxicity, greater convenience of formulation, and availability of compounds with different mechanisms of action, coupled with a better understanding of drug resistance, have combined to improve HIV clinical and virological outcomes consistently. An increase in the numbers of compounds available and the high risk of drug–drug interactions combine to make HIV treatment complex, and better clinical outcomes have been closely linked to physician expertise and the numbers of patients under direct care. With increasing numbers of compounds now available as generics, some drug costs are falling, and commissioners are increasingly focusing on the cost-effectiveness of the newer agents to justify their use. Regularly updated treatment

guidelines are produced in the UK by the British HIV Association (BHIVA) and in the USA by the Department of Health and Human Services (DHHS). The most up-to-date versions can be found on their websites (see Further reading) and the current version must be used in all circumstances.

The key practical principles of prescribing ARVs are given in **Box 37.17**.

When to start ART

ART should be offered to everyone who is HIV-positive, irrespective of CD4 count, and started as soon as the patient is ready, which may be at the time of diagnosis. The move away from CD4-guided treatment initiation is based on clinical trial data demonstrating benefits of ART on morbidity and mortality, even when CD4 counts are above 500, together with the impact of effective therapy on reducing onward transmission.

- In patients with an AIDS-defining condition or an opportunistic infection, ART should be initiated within 2 weeks of starting treatment for intercurrent conditions.
- For people with primary HIV infection, treatment should be started immediately.

The evidence that treatment reduces infectiousness should be discussed with all patients with HIV. Their full involvement in therapeutic decision-making is essential for success. Various national guidelines and treatment frameworks exist (e.g. guidelines from BHIVA and the DHHS, recommendations from the International Antiviral Society, IAS). Laboratory marker data, including viral load, genotype, CD4 counts, co-morbidities and current medications, together with individual circumstances, underpin therapeutic decision-making. In situations where therapy is recommended but the patient elects not to start, more intensive clinical and laboratory monitoring is advisable.

Although the benefits of ART in HIV infection are indisputable, treatment is likely to be life-long and requires a long-term commitment to high levels of adherence. With newer agents and improved formulations, many of the difficulties associated with earlier ART regimens have markedly diminished. The major risks of therapy include short- and longer-term side-effects, drug–drug interactions and the potential for development of resistant strains of virus. Special situations (co-infection with hepatitis B and C, seroconversion, pregnancy, post-exposure prophylaxis) in which ARV agents may be used are described on page 1440.

Which drugs to start

The drug regimen used for starting therapy must be individualized to suit each patient's needs, clinical situation and lifestyle. Treatment is always initiated with three drugs: two nucleoside/nucleotide reverse transcriptase inhibitors (NRTIs) in combination, and a third agent – either an integrase inhibitor, a boosted protease inhibitor or a non-nucleoside reverse transcriptase inhibitor (NNRTI, **Box 37.18**; see also **Box 37.16**). The availability of fixed-dose co-formulations reduces pill burden, increases convenience and facilitates adherence.

Nucleoside/nucleotide reverse transcriptase inhibitors

Nucleoside reverse transcriptase inhibitors (NRTIs) are nucleoside analogues that inhibit the synthesis of DNA by reverse transcription and also act as DNA chain terminators. They were the first group of agents to be used against HIV and need to be phosphorylated intracellularly for activity to occur. Nucleotide reverse transcriptase inhibitors (NtRTIs), such as tenofovir, have a similar mechanism of

Box 37.16 Anti-retroviral drugs (ARVs) commonly used in clinical practice

Drug class	Drugs	Comments
Nucleoside and nucleotide reverse transcriptase inhibitors (NRTIs)	Tenofovir, abacavir, lamivudine, emtricitabine	Tenofovir associated with renal dysfunction Abacavir associated with hypersensitivity reactions in at-risk individuals (HLA-B*5701) Abacavir plus lamivudine should only be used when baseline VL is <100 000 copies/mL The combination of tenofovir plus emtricitabine is a preferred first-line regimen in most regions
Non-nucleoside reverse transcriptase inhibitors (NNRTIs)	Efavirenz, nevirapine[a], etravirine, rilpivirine	Efavirenz can cause central nervous system toxicity (usually time-limited) Nevirapine can cause severe hepatotoxicity in patients with higher CD4 cell counts (>250 cells/mm^3 for women and >400 cells/mm^3 for men) Rilpivirine should be used only when baseline VL is <100 000 copies/mL Etravine is given twice daily and has generally been used as a second-line regimen
Integrase inhibitors or integrase strand transfer inhibitors (INSTIs)	Raltegravir, dolutegravir, elvitegravir	Integrase inhibitors are generally well tolerated and have fewer adverse effects than other ARV classes Raltegravir is taken twice daily Elvitegravir requires boosting by cobicistat
Protease inhibitors	Fosamprenavir, atazanavir, darunavir, lopinavir, saquinavir (ritonavir)	Most protease inhibitors are extensively metabolized by the cytochrome P450 3A system; ritonavir is generally given at low doses (100–200 mg per day) to inhibit P450 and boost the co-administered protease inhibitors Most protease inhibitors are associated with hyperlipidaemia and other metabolic abnormalities such as insulin resistance Long-term protease inhibitor exposure has been associated with increased risk of cardiovascular disease
CCR5 inhibitors	Maraviroc	Maraviroc is active only in patients who do not have virions that use CXCR4 for cell entry. A specialized assay is therefore needed to screen for co-receptor tropism. By contrast with other ARVs, maraviroc binds to a host rather than a viral target
Fusion inhibitors	Enfuvirtide	Enfuvirtide must be given subcutaneously twice daily and is very expensive; generally used only in patients who have no other therapeutic options

[a]Some drugs, such as zidovudine, stavudine and nevirapine, are generally used in low-income countries because of cost considerations. These are not recommended as preferred agents in resource-rich regions in view of their potential toxic effects. HLA, human leucocyte antigen; VL, viral load.
(Modified from Volberding PA, Deeks SG. Antiretroviral therapy and management of HIV infection. Lancet 2010; 376:49–62.)

Box 37.17 Prescribing anti-retroviral drugs (ARVs): practice points

Characteristics of ARVs	Practice points
Adherence for the long term is key to success	Make treatment decisions in partnership with the patient. Check for any factors that may compromise accurate adherence Ensure that the proposed drug regimen fits with lifestyles Clarify that the patient is fully conversant with the requirements and understands the reasons for strict adherence Check access to appropriate storage conditions for some agents
Should not be stopped suddenly	Make sure that mechanisms are in place to ensure adequate drug supplies, e.g. regular clinic appointments, repeat prescriptions, home delivery of medications Beware unexpected time away from home, e.g. holidays, intercurrent hospital admissions, immigration detention, police detention If there is an urgent medical indication to stop, obtain advice from specialist physician or pharmacist
Can be compromised by the introduction of other medications, including other ARVs and vice versa	Take care with direct-acting antiviral (DAA) therapies in hepatitis C (expert advice required) Be careful with enzyme inducers, e.g. rifampicin, rifabutin, warfarin and nevirapine, which reduce the effective levels of some ARVs Remember that methadone levels may be reduced by efavirenz Note that some ARVs block the metabolism of other agents, which may reach toxic levels, e.g. steroids, statins Always check potential interactions before adding new agents; see www.hiv-druginteractions.org Remember that therapeutic drug monitoring may be necessary
Can interact adversely with some herbal, complementary and recreational agents	Note that herbal remedies that induce cytochrome P450, e.g. St John's wort and Chinese herbal remedies, reduce levels of some ARVs Check potential interactions before adding new agents; see www.hiv-druginteractions.org Remember that therapeutic drug monitoring is necessary
May produce additive toxicities when given with other medications	For example, note that corticosteroid (inhaled and systemic) levels may be elevated, statins may cause increased muscle toxicity, there may be increased hepatotoxicity with anti-tuberculosis medication, and increased myelosuppression with chemotherapy or high-dose co-trimoxazole
Are associated with a range of adverse drug reactions, which may be confused with other pathology	For example, note that rash, fever, nausea and diarrhoea may all be caused by intercurrent pathology and/or ARVs
May exacerbate co-morbidities	Examples include hepatic dysfunction due to hepatitis B and C, cardiovascular risk, osteoporosis

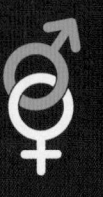

action but require only two intracellular phosphorylation steps for activity, as opposed to the three steps for nucleoside analogues.

Usually, two drugs of this class are combined to provide the 'backbone' of an ART regimen. Several fixed-dose NRTI combinations are available, which helps reduce the pill burden. The choice of which two NRTIs should form the backbone of therapy is influenced by efficacy, toxicity and ease of administration. The availability of the once-daily, one-tablet, fixed-dose combinations, including Truvada (tenofovir/emtricitabine) and Kivexa (abacavir/lamivudine), has led to the prescription of one of these as the two-NRTI backbone for the majority of patients who are naive to medication. Kivexa should be used only in those who are HLA-B*5701-negative. Data comparing Truvada and Kivexa in naive patients have demonstrated the non-inferiority of Kivexa at viral levels of less than 100 000 copies/mL. In patients with high viral levels, Kivexa should be reserved for use when Truvada is contraindicated. NRTIs have been associated with mitochondrial toxicity (see p. 1440), as a consequence of their effect on the human mitochondrial DNA polymerase, and this can lead to kidney and bone disease with long-term use.

Tenofovir alafenamide (TAF) is a prodrug of tenofovir. Its use results in lower plasma concentrations of tenofovir (the active drug) than the traditional tenofovir formulation (tenofovir disoproxil fumarate, TDF) while achieving virological non-inferiority; this reduces the potential for renal and bone toxicity. Many different fixed-dose formulations incorporating TAF and other anti-retroviral drugs are now available.

Non-nucleoside analogues

Non-nucleoside reverse transcriptase inhibitors (NNRTIs) interfere with reverse transcriptase by direct binding to the enzyme. They are generally small molecules that are widely disseminated throughout the body and have a long half-life. They affect cytochrome P450 and consequently have a wide-range of drug–drug interactions. They are ineffective against HIV-2, and the level of cross-resistance across the class is very high. All have been associated with rashes and elevation of liver enzymes. Second-generation NNRTIs, such as etravirine and rilpivirine, which have fewer adverse effects, have some activity against viruses resistant to other compounds of the NNRTI class.

Having demonstrated very good durability over time, and potency at low CD4 counts and in high viral loads, **efavirenz** is now recommended as an alternative rather than a preferred option in the UK due to its CNS side-effects, such as dysphoria, insomnia and an association with increased risk of suicide. **Rilpivirine** has been directly compared with efavirenz and shown to be virologically superior and better tolerated when used in patients with a viral load below 100 000 copies/mL. On this basis the British guidelines have moved rilpivirine from an alternative to a preferred third agent. Rilpivirine must be taken with food and has interactions with acid-reducing agents; proton pump inhibitors are contraindicated.

Etravirine is a second-generation NNRTI with some activity against drug-resistant strains, and is useful in the treatment of ART-experienced patients. Rash is the most common adverse effect.

Nevirapine, although safe and effective for those already established on therapy, is no longer a preferred option for those starting ART in the UK. The small risk of serious hepatic or cutaneous toxicity is now unjustified in light of the wide choice of other effective agents. If it is being considered, it must not be used in women with a CD4 count above 250 cells/mm^3 or men with a CD4 count of more than 400 cells/mm^3, as there is an increased risk of hepatotoxicity and rash.

Protease inhibitors

Protease inhibitors (PIs) act competitively on the HIV aspartyl protease enzyme, which is involved in the production of functional viral proteins and enzymes. As a consequence, viral maturation is impaired and immature dysfunctional viral particles are produced. Most of the PIs are active at very low concentrations and, *in vitro*, are found to have synergy with reverse transcriptase inhibitors. However, there are differences in toxicity, pharmacokinetics, resistance patterns and also cost, which influence prescribing. Cross-resistance can occur across the PI group.

Clinically significant interactions with the cytochrome P450 system are used to therapeutic advantage, by 'boosting' blood levels of PI through blocking drug breakdown using small doses of ritonavir or cobicistat. This increases the half-life of the active drug, allowing greater drug exposure, fewer pills, enhanced potency and a minimized risk of resistance. The disadvantages include a greater pill burden, other drug–drug interactions and increased risk of lipid abnormalities, particularly raised fasting triglycerides. PIs have been linked with abnormalities of fat metabolism and control of blood sugar, and some have been associated with deterioration in clotting function in people with haemophilia.

In general, PIs have a higher genetic barrier to resistance than other drug classes, and newer PIs such as darunavir have activity against viruses resistant to the older drugs in the class.

Boosted **atazanavir** and **darunavir** are most commonly used as first-line therapy. Each can cause gastrointestinal disturbance and lipid abnormalities. Atazanavir increases unconjugated bilirubin levels and may produce icterus. **Symtuza** is a once-daily, fixed-dose single tablet containing darunavir, cobicistat, emtricitabine and tenofovir alafenamide, and is the first PI-based single-tablet regimen to reach the market.

Integrase strand transfer inhibitors

Integrase strand transfer inhibitors (INSTIs) act as selective inhibitors of HIV integrase, which blocks viral replication by preventing insertion of HIV DNA into the human DNA genome. Several are in clinical use and are effective in treatment of both drug-experienced and drug-naive patients, with tolerability and safety profiles that are superior to those of NNRTIs and PIs. For these reasons, INSTIs such as raltegravir and dolutegravir are increasingly chosen as the third agent in ARV regimens.

Raltegravir, the first licensed compound in this drug class, has high anti-HIV activity for both treatment-naive and treatment-experienced patients, with a favourable side-effect profile and few drug interactions. **Dolutegravir**, a second-generation INSTI with a good side-effect profile, has a higher genetic barrier to resistance than raltegravir and can be dosed once daily. Dolutegravir is associated with a small increase in creatinine as it blocks tubular secretion. A fixed-dose tablet of dolutegravir co-formulated with abacavir and lamivudine (Triumeq) is available.

Elvitegravir is metabolized via the cytochrome P450 pathway, requiring co-administration of a cytochrome-P450 blocker to secure adequate plasma concentrations, thus increasing the drug–drug interaction potential. Single-tablet co-formulations exist with tenofovir, emtricitabine and cobicistat (Stribild). **Bictegravir** is the newest in the INSTI class with potency against strains with integrase resistance.

Co-receptor blockers

Maraviroc is a chemokine receptor antagonist that blocks the cellular CCR5 receptor entry by CCR5 tropic strains of HIV. These strains are found in earlier HIV infection and, with time, adaptations (against which maraviroc is ineffective) allow the CXCR4 receptor to become the more dominant form. The drug is metabolized by cytochrome P450 (3A), giving the potential for drug–drug interactions. Tropism assays to establish that the patient is carrying a CCR5 tropic virus are required before treatment is used.

Fusion inhibitors

Enfuvirtide is the only licensed compound in this class of agents. It is an injectable peptide derived from HIV gp41 that inhibits gp41-mediated fusion of HIV with the target cell. It is synergistic with NRTIs and PIs. Although resistance to enfuvirtide has been described, there is no evidence of cross-resistance with other drug classes. Because it has an extracellular mode of action there are few drug–drug interactions. Side-effects relate to the subcutaneous route of administration in the form of injection site reactions.

Post attachment inhibitors

Ibalizumab, a humanized monoclonal antibody administered intravenously, blocks HIV cell entry, which has been shown to be effective in people with multidrug-resistant HIV, for which it is licensed. It requires intravenous administration every 14 days.

Monitoring therapy

Success rates for initial therapy using modern ARVs are very high: by 4 weeks of therapy the viral load should have dropped by at least 1 log10 copies/mL, and by 12–24 weeks should be fully suppressed (<50 copies/mL). Patients are reviewed 2–4 weeks after starting therapy to check for adverse drug effects and ensure good adherence. The viral load is measured at 1, 3 and 6 months after starting ART and a suboptimal response at any time point demands a full assessment and possible change in therapy.

Once clinically stable and virologically suppressed on therapy, the viral load should be routinely measured every 6 months. CD4 count should be repeated at 3 months after starting ART and then every 3–4 months. Once the viral load is below 50 copies/mL and the CD4 count has been above 350 cells/mm³ for at least 12 months, monitoring frequency may fall to 6-monthly or even longer (**Box 37.19**).

Box 37.19 Monitoring patients on anti-retroviral therapy (ART)

Clinical history
- Assessment of adherence to medication
- Evidence of ART toxicity or intolerance
- Documentation of any new clinical conditions occurring since last assessment
- Drug history, including all co-medications (prescribed, recreational, over-the-counter, complementary and herbal)

Physical examination
- Blood pressure
- Weight
- HIV viral load
- Lymphocyte subsets
- Full blood count

- Urinalysis if tenofovir is being used
- Liver and renal function
- Fasting lipid profile
- Fasting blood glucose or HbA₁

Additional investigations (depending on the clinical picture)
- HIV genotype if there is evidence of virological failure
- Therapeutic drug level monitoring in certain situations
- Dual-energy X-ray absorptiometry (DEXA) scan and calculation of FRAX score (see **Box 19.8**)
- Cardiovascular risk assessment

Impaired immunological recovery is seen when treatment is initiated in advanced infection (a low CD4 count and late diagnosis) and in older adults.

Regular clinical assessment (6–12-monthly) should include review of adherence to, and tolerability of, the regimen, weight, blood pressure and urinalysis. Patients should be monitored for drug toxicity and co-morbidities, including full blood count and liver, renal and bone profile, with a metabolic assessment that includes fasting lipids and HbA₁C.

Drug resistance

Resistance to ARVs (**Box 37.20**) results from mutations in the protease, reverse transcriptase and integrase genes of the virus. HIV has a rapid turnover, with 10^8 replications occurring per day. The error rate is high, resulting in genetic diversity within the population of virus in an individual, which will include drug-resistant mutants. When drugs only partially inhibit virus replication, there will be a selection pressure for the emergence of drug-resistant strains. The rate at which resistance develops depends on the frequency of pre-existing variants and the number of mutations required. Resistance to most NRTIs and PIs occurs with an accumulation of mutations, while a single-point mutation will confer high-level resistance to NNRTIs. There is evidence for the transmission of HIV strains that are resistant to all or some classes of drug. Studies of primary HIV infection have shown prevalence rates of between 2% and 20%. Prevalence of primary mutations associated with drug resistance in chronically infected patients not on treatment ranges from 3% to 10% in various studies.

HIV anti-retroviral drug resistance testing is routine clinical management in patients at diagnosis and before starting therapy, and for whom therapy is failing. The tests are based on PCR amplification of the virus and give an indirect measure of drug susceptibility in the predominant variants. Such assays are limited by both the starting concentration of virus and their ability to detect minority strains.

For results to be useful in situations where therapy is failing, samples must be analysed when the patient is on therapy, as once the selection pressure of therapy is withdrawn, wild-type virus becomes the predominant strain and resistance mutations present earlier may no longer be detectable.

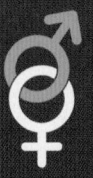

Databases containing nearly all published HIV (among others) and protease sequences, with their associated resistance patterns, are maintained in real time by Stanford University (see Further reading).

Phenotypic assays provide a more direct measure of susceptibility but the complexity of the assays limits availability.

Drug interactions

Drug therapy in HIV is complex and the potential for clinically relevant drug interactions is substantial. Both PIs and NNRTIs are able to inhibit and induce cytochrome P450 variably, influencing both their own metabolic rates and those of other drugs. Both inducers and inhibitors of cytochrome P450 are sometimes prescribed simultaneously. Induction of metabolism may result in subtherapeutic ARV levels, with the risk of treatment failure and development of viral resistance, while inhibition can raise drug levels to toxic values and precipitate adverse reactions.

Conventional (e.g. rifamycins) and complementary therapies (e.g. St John's wort) affect cytochrome P450 activity and may precipitate substantial drug interactions. Therapeutic drug monitoring (TDM), indicating peak and trough plasma levels, may be useful in certain settings.

Potential interactions can be checked using the online tool maintained by Liverpool University (see Further reading).

Other commonly prescribed medications may affect other classes of ART by different mechanisms – for instance, INSTI levels may be reduced by antacids, which seem to affect drug absorption; however, there is a lower risk of drug–drug interactions with INSTIs, as they largely are metabolized via glucuronidation.

Adherence

Patients' beliefs about their personal need for medicines and their concerns about treatment affect how and whether they take them. Adherence to treatment is pivotal to success. Levels of adherence of below 95% have been associated with poor virological and immunological responses with older compounds having poor absorption and low bioavailability; however, the newer ARVs are more forgiving. For some compounds, trough levels are barely adequate to suppress viral replication, and missing even a single dose will result in plasma drug levels falling dangerously low. Patchy adherence facilitates the emergence of drug-resistant variants, which, in time, will lead to virological treatment failure.

Factors implicated in poor adherence may be associated with the medication, the patient or the provider:

- **_Medication-related factors_** include side-effects, the degree of complexity and pill burden, and the inconvenience of the regimen.
- **_Patient factors_** include the level of motivation and commitment to the therapy, psychological wellbeing, level of available family and social support, and health beliefs. Supporting adherence is a key part of clinical care.
- **_Provider factors_** include the level of education patients are given about their condition and treatment, which is a fundamental requirement for good adherence, as is education of clinicians in adherence support techniques.

The acceptability and tolerability of the regimen, together with an assessment of adherence, should be documented at each visit. Provision of acute and ongoing multidisciplinary support for adherence within clinical settings should be universal. Medication-alert devices may be useful for some patients.

Treatment failure

Failure of ART – that is, persistent viral replication causing immunological deterioration and eventual clinical evidence of disease progression – is caused by a variety of factors, such as poor adherence, limited drug potency, and food or other medication that may compromise drug absorption. There may be drug interactions or limited penetration of drug into sanctuary sites such as the CNS, permitting viral replication. Side-effects and other patient-related elements contribute to poor adherence.

Changing therapy

A rise in viral load, new clinical events that imply progression of HIV infection or the development of new co-morbidities are all reasons to review therapy. Virological failure – that is, two consecutive viral loads of over 400 copies/mL in a previously fully suppressed patient – requires investigation. Viral genotyping should be used to help select future therapy, choosing at least two new agents to which the virus is fully sensitive. If a new suitable treatment option is available, it should be started as soon as possible.

Treatment failure in highly treatment-experienced patients poses considerable challenges but new classes of ARV, with activity against drug-resistant strains of HIV, make long-term virological suppression a realistic objective, even in heavily pre-treated patients.

If the patient has a viral load below the limit of detection and a change needs to be made because of intolerance of a particular drug, then a switch should be made to another sensitive drug within the same class. Simplification of complex regimens may be considered if adherence is problematic.

Stopping therapy

ARVs may have to be stopped if there is, for example, cumulative toxicity or potential drug interactions with medications needed to deal with another more pressing problem. If adherence is poor, stopping completely may be preferable to continuing with inadequate dosing, in order to reduce the development of viral resistance. Poor quality of life and the views of the patient should be discussed.

The NRTIs efavirenz and nevirapine have long half-lives and, depending on the other components of the regimen, may need to be stopped *before* the other drugs in the mixture to reduce the risk of drug resistance. If this is not possible, a boosted PI may be used for several weeks, either as a substitute for the NNRTI or as monotherapy, to cover the period of subtherapeutic levels.

Complications and long-term safety of ART

As efficacy and tolerability of ARVs have improved and longevity for people with HIV has increased, long-term safety has become increasingly important. Side-effects can be a problem in ART (see **Box 37.16**). Some are acute and associated with initiation of medication, while others emerge after longer-term exposure to drugs.

Allergic reactions

Allergic reactions occur with greater frequency in people with HIV infection and have been documented with all the ARVs. Abacavir is associated with a potentially fatal hypersensitivity reaction, strongly linked to the presence of HLA-B*5701, usually within the first 6 weeks of treatment. There may be a discrete rash and often a fever, coupled with general malaise and gastrointestinal and respiratory symptoms. The diagnosis is clinical and symptoms resolve when abacavir is withdrawn. Rechallenge with abacavir can be fatal and is contraindicated. In the UK, routine screening for the HLA-B*5701 allele has reduced the incidence of abacavir hypersensitivity. Allergies to NNRTIs (often in the second or third week of treatment) usually present with a widespread maculopapular pruritic rash, often with a fever and disordered liver biochemical tests. Reactions can resolve, even with continuing therapy, but drugs should be stopped immediately in any patient with mucous membrane involvement or severe hepatic dysfunction.

Lipodystrophy and metabolic syndrome

A syndrome of lipodystrophy occurs in patients with HIV on ART, comprising characteristic morphological changes and metabolic abnormalities. The main characteristics include:

- a loss of subcutaneous fat in the arms, legs and face (lipoatrophy)
- deposition of visceral, breast and local fat
- raised total cholesterol, HDL cholesterol and triglycerides
- insulin resistance with hyperglycaemia.

The syndrome is potentially associated with increased cardiovascular morbidity. The highest incidence occurs in those taking combinations of NRTIs and PIs. The older drugs, stavudine and zidovudine, are associated with the lipoatrophy component of the process. Dietary advice and increase in exercise may improve some of the metabolic problems and help body shape. Statins and fibrates are recommended to reduce circulating lipids. Simvastatin is contraindicated, as it has high levels of drug interactions with PIs.

Mitochondrial toxicity and lactic acidosis

Mitochondrial toxicity, mostly involving the older drugs stavudine and didanosine, in the nucleoside analogue class, leads to raised lactate and lactic acidosis, which has, in some cases, been fatal. NRTIs inhibit gamma-DNA polymerase and other enzymes that are necessary for normal mitochondrial function. Symptoms are often vague and insidious, and include anorexia, nausea, abdominal pain

and general malaise. Venous lactate is raised and the anion gap is typically widened. This is a serious condition, requiring immediate cessation of ART and provision of appropriate supportive measures until normal biochemistry is restored. All patients should be alerted to the possible symptoms and encouraged to attend hospital promptly.

Bone metabolism

A variety of bone disorders have been reported in HIV: in particular, low bone mineral density (BMD) and fragility fractures. The prevalence of these conditions has varied widely in different studies. Although untreated HIV is believed to have a direct impact on bone metabolism, a fall in BMD has been associated with starting ART and is most noticeable in tenofovir-containing regimens. This may be due to direct effects of the drug on bone or an indirect renal-mediated effect. Tenofovir alafenamide appears to have far less effect on bone health. Fracture risk using the FRAX score (see **Box 19.8**) should be assessed at baseline in all patients over 50 years of age and postmenopausal women, or in the presence of other risk factors.

Immune reconstitution inflammatory syndrome

Paradoxical inflammatory reactions (immune reconstitution inflammatory syndrome, IRIS) may occur on initiating ART. This usually occurs in people who have been profoundly immunosuppressed and begin therapy. As their immune system recovers, they are able to mount an inflammatory response to a range of pathogens, which can include exacerbation of symptoms with new or worsening clinical signs. Examples include unusual mass lesions or lymphadenopathy associated with mycobacteria, including deteriorating radiological appearances associated with tuberculosis infection. Inflammatory retinal lesions in association with cytomegalovirus, deterioration in liver function in chronic hepatitis B carriers, and vigorous vesicular eruptions with herpes zoster have also been described. To avoid this situation, certain pathogens, in particular *M. tuberculosis* and *Cryptococcus*, should be treated for several weeks to reduce the microbiological burden before ARVs are initiated.

Specific therapeutic situations

Acute HIV infection

ART should be started immediately in patients presenting with acute HIV. This stage of disease may represent a unique opportunity for therapy, as there is less viral diversity and the host immune capacity is still intact. There is evidence to show that the viral load can be reduced substantially by effective therapy at this point. People with severe symptoms during primary HIV infection may gain a clinical improvement on ARVs.

Pregnancy

In the UK the mother-to-child HIV transmission rate is 1% for all women diagnosed prior to delivery and 0.1% for women on ART with a viral load of less than 50 copies/mL. Management of HIV-positive pregnant women requires close collaboration between obstetric, medical and paediatric teams. The management aim is to deliver a healthy, uninfected baby to a healthy mother without prejudicing the future treatment options of the mother. Although considerations regarding the pregnancy must be factored into clinical decision-making, pregnancy *per se* is not a contraindication to providing optimum HIV-related care for the woman. HIV-positive women are still advised against breast-feeding, although with effective suppressive ART the risk of transmission is extremely small. Delivery by caesarean section reduced the risk of vertical transmission in the pre-ART era, but if the woman is on effective ART and the labour is uncomplicated, vaginal delivery carries no additional risk. Women conceiving on an effective ART regimen should continue on their medication. For women naive to therapy who require treatment of their own HIV, whether pregnant or not, triple therapy is the regimen of choice. Risk of vertical transmission increases with viral load. Although the fetus will be exposed to drugs, the chances of reducing the viral load, and hence preventing infection, are greatest with a potent triple therapy regimen in the mother. In this situation, **treatment** should start as soon as possible and continue during delivery. The baby should receive zidovudine for 4 weeks postpartum and the mother should remain on ARVs with appropriate monitoring and support.

For the small numbers of women who do not wish to take ART treatment for their own health, ART, initiated at the beginning of the second trimester if the baseline viral load is above 30 000 HIV RNA copies/mL, should be offered to reduce transmission to the fetus, and consideration should be given to starting earlier if the viral load is above 100 000 HIV RNA copies/mL.

Post-exposure prophylaxis

The time taken for HIV infection to become established after exposure offers an opportunity for prevention. Animal models provide support for the use of triple ARVs for post-exposure prophylaxis (PEP) but there are no prospective trials to inform the best approach and each situation should be evaluated on a case-by-case basis to estimate the potential risk of infection and potential treatment benefit.

Healthcare workers may be treated following occupational exposure to HIV, as may those exposed sexually. The risk of acquisition of HIV following exposure is dependent on the risk that the source is HIV-positive (this is often unknown in a sexual exposure) and the risk of transmission of the particular exposure. PEP may be useful up to 72 hours after possible exposure. In the UK the standard regimen is Truvada plus raltegravir, although this may be varied depending on what is known about the source. When the source patient is known to have an undetectable HIV viral load (<200 copies HIV RNA/mL), PEP is not recommended.

Treatment is given for 4 weeks and the recipient should be monitored for toxicity. The at-risk patient should be tested for established HIV infection before PEP is dispensed. Rapid point-of-care tests are particularly useful in this setting. PEP following sexual exposure should not be seen as a substitute for other methods of prevention, although people with HIV and a fully suppressed viral load are not infectious. PreP is discussed on page 1449.

Towards cure

Current therapy, although effective, is life-long, expensive and complex. There is increasing interest in the possibilities of a cure for HIV: either a 'functional' cure, which would mean long-term control of the virus without the use of drugs, or a 'sterilizing' cure, which would require all HIV-containing cells to be eliminated. Several reports of successful interventions exist. These include two patients with HIV infection who underwent stem-cell transplants for treatment of coexisting malignancies, as well as aggressive interventions very early in the course of the infection, which may allow immune function to be preserved. Ways are being explored in which latently infected T cells could be purged. The possibilities are being studied of making cells resistant to new HIV infection, using gene manipulation to alter the CCR5 receptor that mediates viral entry into the cell.

Despite some early encouraging results, it is clear that there is still a very long way to go and, at least for the moment, there is no realistic alternative to life-long ART.

Further reading

Ananworanich J, Fauci AS. HIV cure research: a formidable challenge. *J Virus Erad* 2015; 1:1–3.
British HIV Association. *British HIV Association Standards of Care for People Living with HIV 2013.* London: BHIVA; 2012.
British HIV Association. *British HIV Association Guidelines for the Management of HIV Infection in Pregnant Women 2012.* London: BHIVA; 2012.
Deeks SG, Hunt PW. Antiretroviral therapy: stubborn limitations persist. *Lancet* 2014; 384:214–216.
Fidler S, Anderson J, Azad Y et al. Position statement on the use of antiretroviral therapy to reduce HIV transmission, January 2013: the British HIV Association (BHIVA) and the Expert Advisory Group on AIDS (EAGA). *HIV Med* 2013; 14:259–262.
Lewin SR, Deeks SG, Barré-Sinoussi F. Towards a cure for HIV – are we making progress? *Lancet* 2014; 384:209–211.
Waters L, Ahmed N, Angus B et al. *British HIV Association Guidelines for the Treatment of HIV-1-positive Adults with Antiretroviral Therapy 2015 (2016 Interim update).* London: BHIVA; 2016; https://www.bhiva.org/file/RVYKzFwyxpgil/treatment-guidelines-2016-interim-update.pdf.
http://hivdb.stanford.edu. *Stanford University HIV drug resistance database.*
http://www.aidsinfo.nih.gov/guidelines. *US Department of Health and Human Services guidelines on the use of ARVs in HIV-1-infected adults and adolescents.*
http://www.hiv-druginteractions.org. *Potential HIV drug interactions can be checked using the online tool maintained by Liverpool University.*

SPECIFIC CONDITIONS ASSOCIATED WITH HIV INFECTION

The treatment of opportunistic infections in immunosuppressed patients is most commonly seen either in regions of the world where ART is not available, in previously undiagnosed patients who are diagnosed late and have presented with advanced infection (<200 CD4+ cells/mL), or in patients not adhering to prescribed treatment.

In parallel, the types of infection seen in the context of HIV have altered, with fewer episodes of the 'classic' opportunistic infections, such as *Pneumocystis* pneumonia and cytomegalovirus, but an increase in community-acquired infections such as *Strep. pneumoniae* and *Haemophilus influenzae* (**Box 37.21**).

Immune reconstitution with ART may produce unusual responses to opportunistic pathogens and confuse the clinical picture. Thus, prevention and treatment of opportunistic infections remain integral parts of the management of HIV infection.

Prevention of opportunistic infection in patients with HIV

Avoidance of infection

Exposure to certain organisms can be avoided in those known to be HIV-positive and immunosuppressed. Attention to food hygiene will reduce exposure to *Salmonella*, toxoplasmosis and *Cryptosporidium*, and protected sexual intercourse will reduce exposure to HSV, hepatitis B and C viruses, and papillomaviruses. Cytomegalovirus-negative patients should be given cytomegalovirus-negative blood products. Travel-related infection can be minimized with appropriate advice.

Immunization strategies

Guidance on the appropriate use of vaccines in HIV (**Box 37.22**) is available from BHIVA (see Further reading). Immunization may not be as effective in immunosuppressed HIV-positive individuals.

Hepatitis A and B vaccines should be given to those without natural immunity who are at risk, particularly if there is coexisting liver pathology, such as hepatitis C.

? Box 37.21 Some causes of opportunistic pneumonia in immunocompromised patients[a]

Pathogen	Affected patient population	Clinical and radiographic features
Pneumocystis jirovecii	Impaired cell-mediated immunity: HIV infection CD4 <200 cells/mm^3, long-term corticosteroid use, immunosuppressant drugs	*Pneumocystis* pneumonia Perihilar ground-glass shadowing, cysts
Non-tuberculous mycobacterial species	Impaired cell-mediated immunity: HIV infection CD4 usually <200 cells/mm^3 Structural lung disease: bronchiectasis, cystic fibrosis, severe COPD	Varied clinical presentation (see p. 972): Non-specific fevers, cough, malaise Lymphadenopathy or hepatosplenomegaly CT findings: nodules, cavitation, thickened airways, 'tree-in-bud' small airways
Nocardia spp.	Impaired cell-mediated immunity: HIV infection CD4 usually <150 cells/mm^3, chronic corticosteroid use, post-solid-organ transplantation, post-stem-cell transplantation Structural lung disease: bronchiectasis, cystic fibrosis, severe COPD	Acute, subacute or chronic pneumonia Multiple radiographic presentations including lobar infiltrates, abscesses, cavities, pleural effusion, pulmonary nodules
Aspergillus spp. *Zygomycetes* spp. *Penicillium* spp.	Prolonged neutropenia: post-chemotherapy for haematological malignancy, post-stem-cell transplant (myeloablative transplants are at particular risk) Impaired cell-mediated immunity: graft-versus-host disease, immunosuppressant therapy Chronic granulomatous disease	Invasive fungal pneumonia characterized by cough ± haemoptysis, pleuritic pain and fevers CT findings are any of: cavitating consolidation, 'tree-in-bud', nodules with ground-glass halo and, in later stages, air-crescent sign (caused by lung necrosis)
Cryptococcus spp.	Impaired cell-mediated immunity: HIV infection CD4 usually <200 cells/mm^3, chronic corticosteroid use, post-solid-organ transplantation, post-stem-cell transplantation	Non-specific respiratory symptoms of fever, cough, breathlessness Usually associated with neurological involvement but isolated pulmonary disease does occur Progresses to disseminated disease in immunocompromised patients CT findings are any of: cavities, nodules, infiltrates
Histoplasma capsulatum	Impaired cell-mediated immunity: HIV infection CD4 usually <50 cells/mm^3	Fever, fatigue, weight loss Cough and dyspnoea are the most common respiratory symptoms Chest X-ray can be normal in disseminated disease CT findings: diffuse reticular/reticulonodular infiltrates, miliary infiltrates, occasionally mediastinal lymphadenopathy
Coccidioides *Paracoccidioides* *Blastomyces*	Impaired cell-mediated immunity: HIV infection CD4 usually <50 cells/mm^3	Often presents as disseminated disease (chest X-ray frequently normal) Focal or diffuse pneumonia CT findings: diffuse reticulonodular infiltrates, consolidation, nodules (multiple or single), cavities, mediastinal lymphadenopathy
Cytomegalovirus (uncommon – usually presents with retinitis or colitis)	Impaired cell-mediated immunity: HIV infection CD4 usually <50 cells/mm^3, post-transplantation on immunosuppressant therapy	Cough, dyspnoea and fever CT findings: reticular or ground-glass opacities, alveolar infiltrates, nodules/nodular opacities, pleural effusions
Respiratory syncytial virus, human metapneumovirus, influenza, parainfluenza	Impaired cell-mediated immunity: HIV infection CD4 usually <200 cells/mm^3, chronic corticosteroid use, post-solid-organ transplantation, post-stem-cell transplantation	Cough, dyspnoea and fever CT findings: ground-glass opacification, air-space shadowing, 'tree-in-bud', airway dilation and wall thickening
Toxoplasma gondii	Impaired cell-mediated immunity: HIV infection CD4 usually <100 cells/mm^3	Isolated pulmonary or disseminated disease Dry cough, fever, dyspnoea CT findings: appearance similar to those of *Pneumocystis jirovecii* or fungal pneumonia; pleural effusion

[a]COPD, chronic obstructive pulmonary disease; CT, computed tomography.

Chemoprophylaxis

In the absence of a normal immune response, many opportunistic infections are hard to eradicate using antimicrobials and the recurrence rate is high. Primary and secondary chemoprophylaxis can be used to reduce the incidence of some opportunistic infections. Advantages must be balanced against the potential for toxicity, drug interactions and cost, with each medication added to what are often complex drug regimens.

- Primary prophylaxis is effective in reducing the risk of *Pneumocystis jirovecii*, toxoplasmosis and MAI.
- Primary prophylaxis is *not* normally recommended against cytomegalovirus, herpesviruses or fungi.

With the introduction of ART and immune reconstitution, ongoing chemoprophylaxis can be discontinued in those patients with CD4 counts that remain consistently above 200 cells/mm^3. In areas where effective ART may not be available, long-term secondary

> *i* **Box 37.22 Use of vaccines in HIV-infected adults**

Vaccine	Type	Indications[a]
Hepatitis A	Inactivated	Non-immune, at-risk patients
Hepatitis B	Subunit	All non-immune patients
Human papilloma virus	Virus-like particle	Age and sex criteria
Influenza	Inactivated	All patients on a yearly basis
Meningococcus	Conjugated or recombinant protein	At-risk groups, age criteria
Pneumococcus	Conjugated and polysaccharide	Conjugated vaccine for all groups, polysaccharide additionally for at-risk groups
Pertussis	Acellular multicomponent	Pregnant women
Measles, mumps and rubella (MMR)	Live attenuated	All non-immune patients
Varicella (chickenpox)	Live attenuated	All non-immune patients
Herpes zoster (shingles)	Live attenuated	At-risk groups (age criteria)

[a]Vaccination regimens are different in HIV-positive patients from those in the general population because of suboptimal immune responses requiring higher or more frequent dosage. Live attenuated viruses should not be given to patients with CD4 counts of <200 cells/mL, and should be used with caution in those with CD4 counts of <350 cells/mL.
(Modified from British HIV Association guidelines on the use of vaccines in HIV-positive adults: summary of recommendations; https://www.bhiva.org/file/PYnNXxGAUfVeD/2015-Summary-of-recommendations.pdf.)

prophylaxis still has a role. Other less severe but recurrent infections may also warrant prophylaxis (e.g. herpes simplex, candidiasis).

Fungal infections

Pneumocystis jirovecii infection

Pneumocystis jirovecii most commonly causes pneumonia (see p. 967) but can cause disseminated infection. It is not usually seen until patients are severely immunocompromised with a CD4 count below 200 cells/mm³. The introduction of effective ART and primary prophylaxis in patients with CD4 counts of less than 200 cells/mm³ has significantly reduced the incidence in the UK. The organism damages the alveolar epithelium, which impedes gas exchange and reduces lung compliance.

The onset is often insidious over a period of weeks, with a prolonged period of increasing shortness of breath (usually on exertion), non-productive cough, fever and malaise. ***Clinical features*** on examination include tachypnoea, tachycardia, cyanosis and signs of hypoxia. Fine crackles are heard on auscultation, although in mild cases there may be no auscultatory abnormality. In early infection, the chest X-ray is normal but the typical appearances are of bilateral perihilar interstitial infiltrates, which can progress to confluent alveolar shadows throughout the lungs. High-resolution CT scans of the chest demonstrate a characteristic ground-glass appearance, even when there is little to see on the chest X-ray. The patient is usually hypoxic and desaturates on exercise. Definitive diagnosis rests on demonstrating the organisms in the lungs via

bronchoalveolar lavage or by PCR amplification of the fungal DNA from a peripheral blood sample. As the organism cannot be cultured *in vitro*, it must be directly observed either with silver staining or with immunofluorescent techniques.

Treatment should be instituted as early as possible. First-line therapy for severe infection (P_aO_2 <8 kPa or type 2 respiratory failure) is with intravenous co-trimoxazole (120 mg/kg daily in divided doses) for 21 days. Up to 40% of patients receiving this regimen will develop some adverse drug reaction, including a typical allergic rash. If the patient is sensitive to co-trimoxazole, intravenous pentamidine (4 mg/kg per day) or dapsone and trimethoprim is given for the same duration. Atovaquone or a combination of clindamycin and primaquine is also used. In severe disease, systemic corticosteroids reduce mortality and should be added. Continuous positive airways pressure (CPAP) or mechanical ventilation (see p. 229) is required if the patient remains severely hypoxic or develops diaphragmatic fatigue. Pneumothorax may complicate the clinical course in an already severely hypoxic patient. If ART is not already being given, it should be initiated early in the course of infection. In patients with milder disease, therapy may be given orally and steroids are not indicated.

Secondary prophylaxis is required when the CD4 count remains below 200 cells/mm³, to prevent relapse, the usual regimen being co-trimoxazole 960 mg three times a week. Patients sensitive to sulphonamide are given dapsone, pyrimethamine or nebulized pentamidine. The last protects only the lungs and does not penetrate the upper lobes particularly efficiently; hence, if relapses occur on this regimen, they may be either atypical or extrapulmonary.

Cryptococcosis

The most common presentation of cryptococcal infection (see p. 560) in the context of HIV is meningitis, although pulmonary and disseminated infections can also occur. The organism, *Cryptococcus neoformans*, is widely distributed, often in bird droppings, and is usually acquired by inhalation. The onset may be insidious with non-specific fever, nausea and headache. As the infection progresses, the conscious level is impaired and changes in affect may be noted. Fits or focal neurological presentations are uncommon. Neck stiffness and photophobia may be absent, as these signs depend on the inflammatory response of the host, which, in this setting, is abnormal.

Diagnosis is made on examination of the CSF (perform a CT scan before lumbar puncture to exclude space-occupying pathology). Indian ink staining shows the organisms directly and CSF cryptococcal antigen is positive at variable titre. It is unusual for the cryptococcal antigen to become negative after treatment, although the levels should fall substantially. Cryptococci can also be cultured from CSF and/or blood.

Factors associated with a poor prognosis include a high organism count in the CSF, a low white cell count in the CSF, and an impaired consciousness level at presentation.

Initial ***treatment*** is usually with intravenous liposomal amphotericin B (4.0 mg/kg per day) with or without flucytosine as induction, although intravenous fluconazole (400 mg daily) is useful if renal function is impaired or if amphotericin side-effects are troublesome. Steroids should be avoided. Following 2 weeks of intravenous amphotericin/flucytosine, therapy should be continued with fluconazole for up to 8 weeks.

Patients diagnosed with cryptococcal disease should receive ART, starting at approximately 2 weeks after commencement of cryptococcal treatment, to minimize the risk of IRIS. Long-term maintenance therapy with fluconazole should be continued for up to 1 year and until the viral load is suppressed and the CD4 count is consistently above 100 cells/mm³.

Candidiasis

Mucosal infection with *Candida*, particularly in the mouth (see p. 559), is common in immunosuppressed HIV-positive patients. *Candida albicans* is the usual organism, although *C. krusei* and *C. glabrata* also occur. Pseudomembranous candidiasis, consisting of creamy plaques in the mouth and pharynx, is easily recognized, but erythematous *Candida* appears as reddened areas on the hard palate or as atypical areas on the tongue. Angular cheilitis can occur in association with either form. Vulvovaginal *Candida* may be difficult to treat. Oesophageal *Candida* infection produces odynophagia (see p. 1172).

Fluconazole or itraconazole is the agent of choice for **treatment**. Disseminated *Candida* is uncommon in the context of HIV infection, but if present, fluconazole is the preferred drug; amphotericin, voriconazole or caspofungin can also be used. *C. krusei* may colonize patients who have been treated with fluconazole, as it is fluconazole-resistant. Amphotericin is useful in the treatment of this infection, and an attempt to type *Candida* from clinically azole-resistant patients should be made. The most successful strategy for managing HIV-positive patients with candidiasis is effective ART.

Aspergillosis

Infection with *Aspergillus fumigatus* (see p. 993) is rare in HIV, unless there are coexisting factors, such as lung pathology, neutropenia, transplantation or glucocorticoid use. Spores are air-borne and ubiquitous. Following inhalation, lung infection proceeds to haematogenous spread to other organs. Sinus infection occurs.

Voriconazole is the preferred **treatment**, with liposomal amphotericin B (3 mg/kg i.v. daily) as an alternative. Caspofungin is also effective.

Histoplasmosis, blastomycosis, coccidioidomycosis and *Penicillium marneffei* infection

These fungal infections are geographically restricted but should be considered in HIV-positive patients who have travelled to areas of high risk. The most common manifestation is with pneumonia, which may be confused with *Pneumocystis jirovecii* in its presentation (see earlier), although systemic infection is reported, particularly with *Penicillium*, which can also produce papular skin lesions. **Treatment** is with amphotericin B.

Protozoal infections

Toxoplasmosis

Toxoplasma gondii (see p. 571) most commonly causes encephalitis and cerebral abscess in the context of HIV, usually as a result of reactivation of previously acquired infection. The incidence depends on the rate of seropositivity to toxoplasmosis in the particular population. High antibody levels are found in France (90% of the adult population). About 25% of the adult UK population is seropositive to *Toxoplasma*.

Clinical features include a focal neurological lesion and convulsions, fever, headache and possible confusion. Examination reveals focal neurological signs in more than 50% of cases. Eye involvement with chorioretinitis may also be present. In most, but not all, cases of *Toxoplasma*, serology is positive. Typically, contrast-enhanced CT

scan of the brain shows multiple ring-enhancing lesions. A single lesion on CT may be found to be one of several on MRI. A solitary lesion on MRI, however, makes a diagnosis of toxoplasmosis unlikely.

Diagnosis is by characteristic radiological findings on CT and MRI. Single photon emission computed tomography (SPECT) may also be helpful for differentiating toxoplasmosis from primary CNS lymphoma. In most cases, an empirical trial of anti-toxoplasmosis therapy is instituted; if this leads to radiological improvement within 3 weeks, it is considered diagnostic. The differential diagnosis includes cerebral lymphoma, tuberculoma or focal cryptococcal infection.

Treatment is with pyrimethamine for at least 6 weeks (loading dose 200 mg, then 50 mg daily), combined with sulfadiazine and folinic acid. Clindamycin and pyrimethamine or atovaquone may be used in patients allergic to sulphonamide.

ART should be initiated as soon as the patient is clinically stable, approximately 2 weeks after acute treatment has begun, to minimize the risk of IRIS.

Cryptosporidiosis

Cryptosporidium parvum (see p. 573) can cause a self-limiting acute diarrhoea in an immunocompetent individual. In HIV infection it can cause severe and progressive watery diarrhoea, which may be associated with anorexia, abdominal pain, and nausea and vomiting. In the era of ART, the infection is rare. Cysts attach to the epithelium of the small bowel wall, causing secretion of fluid into the gut lumen and failure of fluid absorption. It is also associated with sclerosing cholangitis (see p. 1299). The cysts are seen on stool specimen microscopy using Kinyoun acid-fast stain and are readily identified in small bowel biopsy specimens. Nitazoxanide and paromomycin may have some effect; however, immune restoration with effective ART is the treatment of choice and usually leads to remission.

Microsporidiosis

Enterocytozoon bieneusi and *Septata intestinalis* are causes of diarrhoea. Spores can be detected in stools using a trichrome or fluorescent stain that attaches to the chitin of the spore surface. ART and immune restoration constitute the **treatment** of choice and can have a dramatic effect.

Leishmaniasis

Leishmaniasis (see p. 570) occurs in immunosuppressed HIV-positive individuals who have been in endemic areas, which include South America, tropical Africa and much of the Mediterranean. Symptoms are frequently non-specific, with fever, malaise, diarrhoea and weight loss. Splenomegaly, anaemia and thrombocytopenia are significant findings. Amastigotes may be seen on bone marrow biopsy or splenic aspirates. Serological tests exist for *Leishmania* but they are not reliable in this setting.

Treatment is with liposomal amphotericin, the drug of choice, and ART once the patient is stable. Relapse is common without ART, in which case long-term secondary prophylaxis may be given.

Viral infections

Hepatitis B and C virus co-infection with HIV

Because of the comparable routes of transmission of hepatitis viruses (see pp. 1277 and 1282) and HIV, co-infection is common, particularly in MSM, drug users and those infected by blood products. A higher prevalence of hepatitis viruses is found in those with HIV infection than in the general population. Globally, estimates suggest that 5–15% of people with HIV have chronic hepatitis B virus (HBV) infection and about one-third have hepatitis C virus (HCV) infection. In the UK, 6.9% of adults with HIV are also estimated to be HbSAg positive. A global epidemic of acute hepatitis C has been observed over the past decade among HIV-positive MSM.

As treatment advances have improved HIV prognosis, hepatitis virus co-infection has become an increasingly significant cause of morbidity and mortality, making the management of HIV and hepatitis co-infection a key aspect of clinical care.

All those with newly diagnosed HIV should be screened for hepatitis A, B and C; for those without evidence of immunity, hepatitis A and B vaccines should be provided.

Patients with HIV and hepatitis co-infection are more likely to have rapid liver disease progression than people with mono-infection. In all patients with chronic HCV/HIV and HBV/HIV infections, liver disease should be staged (see p. 1275). For those who are likely to have cirrhosis, appropriate monitoring for complications of portal hypertension and HCV screening should be performed. Patients with HIV and liver disease should be jointly managed by clinicians from HIV and hepatitis backgrounds. For people with end-stage liver disease, care should be based in specialist centres, ideally with links to a transplant unit.

In co-infected patients, the hepatotoxicity associated with certain ARVs may be potentiated. Advice on alcohol use and safer sexual practices should be given to all co-infected patients.

Hepatitis B infection

Hepatitis B infection (see p. 1277) does not appear to influence the natural history of HIV or responses to anti-HIV treatment; however, in HIV co-infected patients, there is a significantly reduced rate of hepatitis B e antigen (HBeAg) clearance, the HBV viral load is higher, and the risk of developing chronic infection is increased. In those with resolved or controlled hepatitis B infection, disease may reactivate. Liver disease occurs most commonly in those with high HBV DNA levels indicative of continuing replication. In HBV infection, detection and quantification of HBV DNA act as a marker of viral activity and are predictive of response to treatment. Baseline HBV resistance testing may guide interventions in those previously exposed to antiviral drugs.

Decisions about whether HBV and/or HIV require **treatment** must be based on assessment of both viruses. All treatments for HBV that include agents with concomitant anti-HIV activity, including tenofovir and emtricitabine, must be used within an effective anti-HIV regimen. UK guidelines recommend that ART inclusive of anti-HBV-active agents should be initiated in all co-infected patients with a CD4 count of less than 500 cells/mm^3, with evidence of fibrotic liver damage or with active HBV replication. Patients with a CD4 of 500 cells/mm^3 or more, an HBV DNA of less than 2000 IU/mL, and minimal or no evidence of fibrosis can be given the option to commence treatment or to be monitored not less than 6-monthly with HBV DNA and measurement of alanine aminotransferase (ALT), and at least yearly for evidence of fibrosis. Initiation of ART may result in a flare of HBV, resulting from the improved immune function.

Hepatitis C infection

Hepatitis C is associated with more rapid progression of HIV infection and the CD4 responses to ART in co-infected patients may be blunted. Hepatitis C progression is both more likely and more rapid in the presence of HIV infection, and the hepatitis C viral load tends to be elevated. The drug-related hepatotoxicity may be worse in those with HCV co-infection. Assessment of co-infected patients requires full clinical and laboratory evaluation and staging of both

infections. For HCV, both viral load and genotype will influence therapeutic decision-making.

Treatment is a rapidly changing and complex field with the arrival of potent direct-acting antivirals (DAAs) for the treatment and cure of hepatitis C.

All HIV/HCV co-infected patients should commence ART. If HCV therapy is planned, ART should be started first in most instances, ideally 4–6 weeks before starting treatment for HCV.

The drug options for treatment of HCV in individuals with co-infection are similar to the choices for those infected with HCV alone (see p. 1283), and are dependent on stage of disease, HCV genotype and co-administered ART. The introduction of DAAs for HCV has changed the treatment landscape. The latest HCV agents are given for 12 weeks, with response rates of more than 90%.

When DAAs are chosen, there is some restriction on ARV choice due to drug–drug interactions. Careful selection of the most effective combination of antivirals is required and expert opinion should be sought. Online information resources (see Further reading) provide data on possible interactions.

All those with HIV/HCV co-infection who defer treatment should undergo hepatic elastography (see p. 1270) or an alternative non-invasive form of monitoring at least annually.

Acute hepatitis C has increased in people with HIV, particularly MSM, and recognized epidemics have been reported in a number of countries, including the UK. UK guidelines recommend that patients without a decrease of 2^{log10} in HCV RNA at week 4 post diagnosis of acute infection, or with a positive HCV RNA at week 12 post diagnosis of acute infection, be offered therapy. Immune responses to HCV do not protect against re-infection, and high rates of re-infection have been reported following both therapeutic and spontaneous clearance. Patients who initially clear HCV but have evidence of re-emergent virus should be assessed for relapse or re-infection; relapse is treated as for chronic HCV and re-infection is managed as for acute hepatitis C.

Cytomegalovirus infection

Cytomegalovirus (CMV, see p. 524) has been the cause of considerable morbidity in HIV-positive individuals, especially in the later stages of disease when the CD4 count is consistently below 100 cells/mm^3. The availability of ART has dramatically altered the epidemiology, as a majority of patients start ARVs before they are at risk for CMV disease. The major problems encountered are retinitis, colitis, oesophageal ulceration, encephalitis and pneumonitis. CMV infection is associated with an arteritis, which may be the major pathogenic mechanism. CMV also causes polyradiculopathy and adrenalitis.

CMV retinitis

This occurs once the CD4 count is below 50 cells/mm^3. Although usually unilateral to begin with, the infection may progress to involve both eyes. Presenting features depend on the area of retina involved (loss of vision being most common with macular involvement) and include floaters, loss of visual acuity, field loss and scotomata, orbital pain and headache.

Examination of the fundus (**Fig. 37.13**) reveals haemorrhages and exudates, which follow the vasculature of the retina (so-called 'pizza pie' appearances). The features are highly characteristic and the diagnosis is made clinically. Retinal detachment and papillitis may occasionally occur. If untreated, retinitis spreads within the eye, destroying the retina within its path. Routine fundoscopy should be carried out on all HIV-positive patients to look for evidence of early infection. Any patient with symptoms of visual disturbance should

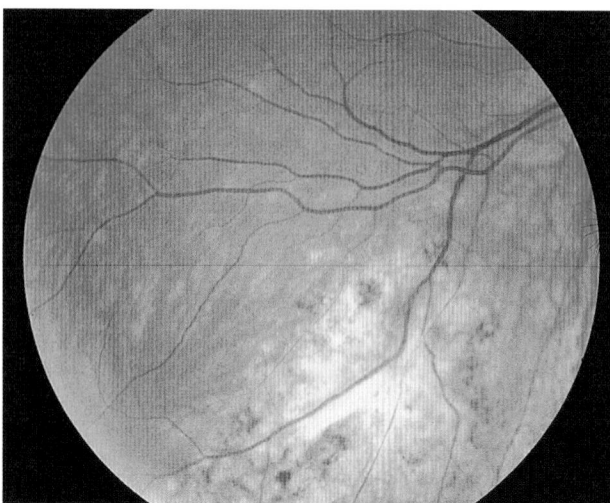

Fig. 37.13 Untreated cytomegalovirus retinitis.

have a thorough examination with pupils dilated; if no evident pathology is seen, a specialist ophthalmological opinion should be sought.

Treatment for CMV should be started as soon as possible, with either oral valganciclovir (900 mg twice daily), intravenous ganciclovir (5 mg/kg twice daily) or intravenous foscarnet (90 mg/kg twice daily), given for at least 3 weeks or until retinitis is quiescent. If immunosuppression is not reversed, reactivation is common, leading to blindness. The major side-effect of ganciclovir is myelosuppression, and foscarnet is nephrotoxic. Maintenance therapy may be required until ART is instituted and has improved immune competence. Valganciclovir, an oral prodrug of ganciclovir, has some long-term benefit when used as maintenance therapy, but a lower efficacy than intravenous ganciclovir. Ganciclovir can be given directly into the vitreous cavity but regular injections are required. A sustained-release implant of ganciclovir can be surgically inserted into the affected eye. Cidofovir is available for use when the drugs described are contraindicated. It has renal toxicity.

CMV gastrointestinal conditions

CMV colitis usually presents with abdominal pain, often generalized or in the left iliac fossa, diarrhoea that may be bloody, generalized abdominal tenderness and a low-grade fever. Dilated large bowel may be seen on abdominal X-ray. Sigmoidoscopy shows a friable or ulcerated mucosa; histology shows the characteristic 'owl's eye' cytoplasmic inclusion bodies (see **Fig. 20.14**).

Treatment is with intravenous ganciclovir (5 mg/kg twice daily) for 14–28 days; when the patient is stable, optimization of ART improves symptoms and the histological changes are reversed. Restoration of immune competence with ART removes the need for maintenance therapy.

Other sites along the gastrointestinal tract are also prone to CMV infection: for example, ulceration of the oesophagus, usually in the lower third, causes odynophagia. CMV can also cause hepatitis.

CMV neurological conditions

CMV encephalopathy has clinical similarities to that caused by HIV itself, although it tends to be more aggressive in its course. **CMV polyradiculopathy** can affect the lumbosacral roots, leading to muscle weakness and sphincter disturbance. The CSF demonstrates an increase in white cells, which, surprisingly, are almost all neutrophils. Although progression may be arrested by anti-CMV

medication, functional recovery may not occur. Diagnosis may be based on MRI and CSF PCR. *Treatment* is with ganciclovir. ART should be started after anti-CMV treatment.

Herpesvirus infection

Herpes simplex primary infection (see p. 1421) occurs with greater frequency and severity, presenting in an ulcerative rather than vesicle form in profoundly immunosuppressed individuals. Genital, oral and occasionally disseminated infection is seen. Viral shedding may be prolonged in comparison with immunocompetent patients.

Varicella zoster virus infection

Varicella zoster can occur at any stage of HIV but tends to be more aggressive and longer-lasting in the more immunosuppressed patient. Multidermatomal zoster may occur.

Treatment with aciclovir is usually effective. Frequent recurrences need suppressive therapy. Aciclovir-resistant strains (usually due to thymidine kinase-deficient mutants) in HIV-positive patients have become more common. Such strains may respond to foscarnet.

Herpesvirus 8 (**HHV-8**) is the causative agent of Kaposi's sarcoma (see p. 1448).

Epstein–Barr virus infection

Patients with HIV have been shown to have high levels of Epstein–Barr virus (EBV) colonization (see p. 524). There are increased EBV titres in oropharyngeal secretions and high levels of EBV-infected B cells. The normal T-cell response to EBV is depressed in HIV. EBV is strongly associated with primary cerebral lymphoma and non-Hodgkin lymphoma (see later). Oral hairy leukoplakia caused by EBV is a sign of immunosuppression first noted in HIV but now also recognized in other conditions. It appears intermittently on the lateral borders of the tongue or the buccal mucosa as a pale, ridged lesion. Although it is usually asymptomatic, patients may find it unsightly and occasionally painful. The virus can be identified histologically and on electron microscopy. There is a variable response to *treatment* with aciclovir.

Human papillomavirus infection

Human papillomavirus (HPV; see p. 672) produces genital, plantar and occasionally oral warts, which may be slow to respond to therapy and recur repeatedly. HPV is associated with the more rapid development of cervical and anal intraepithelial neoplasia, which in time may progress to squamous cell carcinoma of the cervix or rectum in HIV-positive individuals. HPV vaccination should be given (see p. 530).

Polyomavirus infection

JC virus, a member of the papovavirus family, which infects oligodendrocytes, causes progressive multifocal leucoencephalopathy (PML, see p. 529). This leads to demyelination, particularly within the white matter of the brain. The features are of progressive neurological and/or intellectual impairment, often including hemiparesis or aphasia. The condition is usually inexorably progressive but a stuttering course may be seen. Radiologically, the lesions are usually multiple and confined to the white matter. They do not enhance with contrast and do not produce a mass effect. MRI (**Fig. 37.14**) is more sensitive than CT and reveals enhanced signal on T2-weighted images of the lesions. MRI appearances and JC virus detection by PCR in a CSF sample are usually sufficient for diagnosis and avoid the need for a tissue diagnosis requiring brain biopsy. There is no specific *treatment*. Effective ART is the only intervention that has been shown to deliver both clinical and radiological remission.

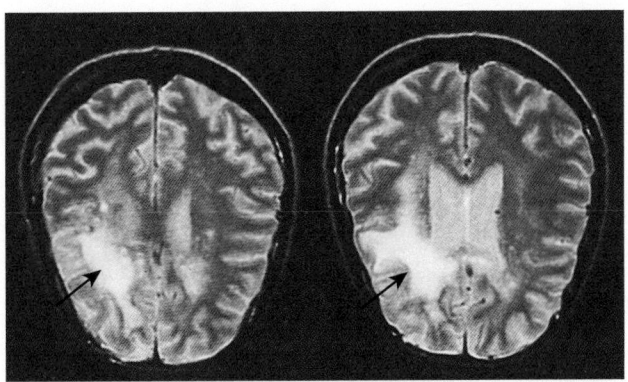

Fig. 37.14 MRI scans showing progressive multifocal leucoencephalopathy.

Bacterial infections

Bacterial infection in HIV is common. Cell-mediated immune responses normally control infection against intracellular bacteria, such as mycobacteria. The abnormalities of B-cell function associated with HIV lead to infections with encapsulated bacteria, as reduced production of IgG2 cannot protect against the polysaccharide coat of such organisms. These functional abnormalities may be present well before there is a significant decline in CD4 numbers and so bacterial sepsis may be seen at early stages of HIV infection. *Strep. pneumoniae, H. influenzae* and *Moraxella catarrhalis* infections are examples. Bacterial infection is often disseminated and, although usually amenable to standard antibiotic therapy, may reoccur. Long-term prophylaxis is required if recurrent infection is frequent.

Mycobacterium tuberculosis infection

Many parts of the world that have a high prevalence of tuberculosis (TB, see p. 967), such as Africa, also have high rates of HIV infection, both of which are increasing. The respiratory transmission of TB means that both HIV-positive and HIV-negative people are being infected. TB can cause disease when there is only minimal immunosuppression and thus often appears early in the course of HIV infection. HIV-related TB frequently represents reactivation of latent TB, but there is also clear evidence of newly acquired infection and hospital-acquired spread in HIV-positive populations.

The pattern of disease differs with immunosuppression:

- Patients with relatively well-preserved CD4 counts have a clinical picture similar to that seen in HIV-negative patients with pulmonary infection.
- In more advanced HIV disease, atypical pulmonary presentations occur, which are often extrapulmonary, affecting lymph nodes, bone marrow or liver. TB bacteraemia may be present.

Diagnosis depends on demonstrating the organisms in appropriate tissue specimens. The response to tuberculin testing is blunted in HIV-positive individuals and is unreliable. Sputum microscopy may be negative, even in pulmonary infection, and culture techniques are the best diagnostic tool.

M. tuberculosis infection usually responds well to standard **treatment** regimens, although the duration of therapy may be extended, especially in extrapulmonary infection. Multidrug-resistant and extensive drug-resistant TB (see p. 971) is a problem, particularly in the USA, where it is developing into a health danger. Cases from HIV units in the UK have been reported. Compliance with anti-tuberculous therapy needs to be emphasized. Treatment

of TB (see later) is not curative and long-term isoniazid prophylaxis may be given. In patients from TB-endemic areas, primary prophylaxis may prevent the emergence of infection.

Drug–drug interactions between anti-retroviral and anti-tuberculous medications are complex and are a consequence of enzyme induction or inhibition. Rifampicin is a potent inducer of cytochrome P450, which is also the route for metabolism of anti-HIV PIs. Using both drugs together results in a reduction in circulating PI with reduced efficacy and increased potential for drug resistance. Some PIs themselves block cytochrome P450, which leads to potentially toxic levels of rifampicin and problems such as uveitis and hepatotoxicity. The NNRTI class also interacts variably with rifamycins, requiring dose alterations. Additionally, there are overlapping toxicities between ART regimens and anti-tuberculous drugs: in particular, hepatotoxicity, peripheral neuropathy and gastrointestinal side-effects. Rifabutin has a weaker effect on cytochrome P450 and may be substituted for rifampicin. Dose adjustments must be made for drugs used in this situation to take account of these interactions.

Paradoxical inflammatory reactions (IRIS, see p. 1440), which can include exacerbation of symptoms, new or worsening clinical signs, and deteriorating radiological appearances, have been associated with the improvement of immune function seen in HIV-positive patients starting ART in the face of *M. tuberculosis* infection. They are most commonly seen in the first few weeks after initiation of ART in patients recovering from TB and can last several weeks or months. The syndrome does not reflect inadequate TB therapy and is not confined to any particular combination of ARVs. It is vital to exclude new pathology in this situation. However, delaying ART increases the risks of further opportunistic events. Allowing at least 2 weeks of anti-tuberculous therapy before commencing ART allows some reduction in the burden of mycobacteria. If the CD4 count is below 100 cells/mm^3, then ARVs should be started at about 2 weeks of anti-tuberculous medication. If the CD4 count is over 200 cells/mm^3, initiation of ART may be delayed for at least 6 weeks after the start of anti-tuberculous therapy.

Mycobacterium avium-intracellulare infection

Atypical mycobacteria, particularly *M. avium-intracellulare* (MAI), generally appear only in the very late stages of HIV infection when patients are profoundly immunosuppressed. MAI is a saprophytic organism of low pathogenicity that is ubiquitous in soil and water. Entry may be via the gastrointestinal tract or lungs with dissemination via infected macrophages.

The major ***clinical features*** are fevers, malaise, weight loss, anorexia and sweats. Dissemination to the bone marrow causes anaemia. Gastrointestinal symptoms may be prominent with diarrhoea and malabsorption. At this stage of disease, patients frequently have other concurrent infections, so differentiating MAI is difficult on clinical grounds. Direct examination and culture of blood, lymph node, bone marrow or liver indicate the diagnosis most reliably.

MAI is typically resistant to standard anti-tuberculous ***treatments***, although ethambutol may be useful. Drugs such as rifabutin in combination with clarithromycin or azithromycin reduce the burden of organisms and, in some, ameliorate symptoms. A common combination is ethambutol, rifabutin and clarithromycin. Addition of amikacin to a drug regimen may produce a good symptomatic response. Primary prophylaxis with rifabutin or azithromycin may delay the appearance of MAI, but no corresponding increase in survival has been shown.

Infections due to other organisms

Influenza virus A (IVA) is no more frequent in HIV-positive people, but has been associated with an increased severity and complication rate, in particular when CD4 counts are low. Oral oseltamivir 75 mg twice daily for 5 days should be used as treatment. People with HIV should be vaccinated annually against IVA. Prophylaxis with oseltamivir is used in unvaccinated individuals with a CD4 count below 200 cells/mm³.

Salmonellae (non-typhoidal, see p. 540) are much less frequent pathogens in HIV infection if effective ART is being used. They are able to survive within macrophages, this being a major factor in their pathogenicity. Organisms are usually acquired orally and frequently cause disseminated infection. Gastrointestinal disturbance may be disproportionate to the degree of dissemination, and once the pathogen is in the bloodstream, any organ may be infected. *Salmonella* osteomyelitis and cystitis have been reported. Diagnosis is from blood and stool cultures. Despite increasing reports of resistance, a majority of isolates are sensitive to oral ciprofloxacin 500 mg twice daily for 5 days. Education on food hygiene should be provided.

Skin conditions, such as folliculitis, abscesses and cellulitis, are common and are usually caused by *Staph. aureus*. Periodontal disease, which may be necrotizing, causes pain and damage to the gums. It is more common in smokers but no specific causative agent has been identified. Therapy is with local debridement and systemic antibiotics.

Strongyloides (see p. 577), a nematode found in tropical areas, may cause a hyper-infection syndrome in HIV-positive patients. Larvae are produced, which invade through the bowel wall and migrate to the lung and occasionally to the brain. Albendazole or ivermectin may be used to control infection. Gram-negative septicaemia can develop.

Scabies (see p. 674) may be much more severe in HIV infection. It may be widely disseminated over the body and appear as atypical, crusted papular lesions known as 'Norwegian scabies', from which mites are readily demonstrated. Superadded staphylococcal infection may occur. Treatment with conventional agents, such as lindane, may fail and ivermectin has been used to good effect in some patients.

Neoplasms

HIV infection is associated with an increased risk of cancer, the most tightly linked being Kaposi's sarcoma, non-Hodgkin lymphoma and cervical cancer, which are AIDS-defining illnesses. Other cancers that have an association with infectious agents, such as liver and anal cancer and Hodgkin lymphoma, although not AIDS-defining, are significantly more common in HIV-positive patients. Patterns are changing and there has been a marked reduction in AIDS-defining malignancy in association with effective ART. The increased longevity of people with HIV increases the risks for development of cancers that are associated with older age. Some data suggest that ART may provide some prevention benefits for non-AIDS-defining malignancies.

Kaposi's sarcoma

Kaposi's sarcoma (KS, see p. 692) in association with HIV (epidemic KS) behaves more aggressively than that associated with HIV-negative populations (endemic KS). The incidence has fallen significantly since the introduction of ART. Human herpesvirus 8 (HHV-8)

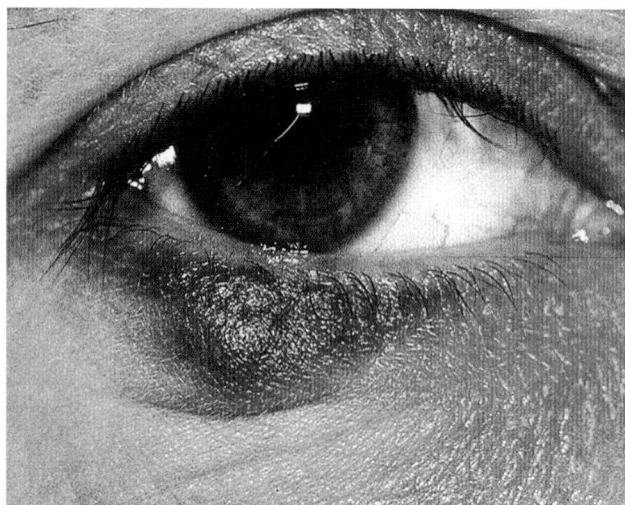

Fig. 37.15 Kaposi's sarcoma of the eyelid.

is involved in the pathogenesis. KS skin lesions are characteristically pigmented and well circumscribed, occurring in multiple sites. KS is a multicentric tumour consisting of spindle cells and vascular endothelial cells, which together form slit-like spaces in which red blood cells become trapped. This process is responsible for the characteristic purple hue of the tumour. In addition to the skin lesions, KS affects lymphatics and lymph nodes, the lung and gastrointestinal tract, giving rise to a wide range of symptoms and signs. Most patients with visceral involvement also have skin or mucous membrane lesions. Visceral KS carries a worse prognosis than disease confined to the skin. KS is seen around the eye (**Fig. 37.15**), particularly in the conjunctivae, which can cause periorbital oedema.

ART leads to regression of lesions. Local radiotherapy gives good results in skin lesions and is helpful in lymph node disease. In aggressive disease, systemic chemotherapy is indicated.

Lymphoma

A significant proportion of patients with HIV develop lymphoma, mostly of the non-Hodgkin, large B-cell type (see p. 401). These are frequently extranodal and often affect the brain, lung and gastrointestinal tract. Many of these tumours are strongly associated with EBV, with evidence of expression of latent gene nuclear antigens such as EBNA 1–6, some of which are involved in the immortalization of B cells and drive a neoplastic pathway.

HIV-associated lymphomas are frequently very aggressive. Patients often present with systemic 'B' syndromes and progress rapidly, despite chemotherapy. Primary cerebral lymphoma is variably responsive to radiotherapy but overall carries a poor prognosis. Lymphomas occurring early in the course of HIV infection tend to respond better to therapy and carry a better prognosis, occasionally going into complete remission.

Cervical carcinoma

Women with HIV are at increased risk of cervical cancer caused by oncogenic subtypes of HPV. Annual cervical cytology is indicated to monitor for pre-malignant changes.

Further reading

Bichoupan K, Dieterich D, Martel-Laferrière V. HIV-hepatitis C virus co-infection in the era of direct-acting antivirals. *Curr HIV/AIDS Rep* 2014; 11: 241–249.

Boulware DR, Meya DB, Muzoora C et al. Timing of antiretroviral therapy after diagnosis of cryptococcal meningitis. *N Engl J Med* 2014; 370:2487–2498.

Bradshaw D, Matthews G, Danta M. Sexually transmitted hepatitis C infection: the new epidemic in MSM? *Curr Opin Infect Dis* 2013; 26:66–72.
Munteanu DI, Rockstroh JK. New agents for the treatment of hepatitis C in patients co-infected with HIV. *Therapeut Adv Infect Dis* 2013; 1:71–80.
Wilkins E, Nelson M, Agarwal K et al. British HIV Association guidelines for the management of hepatitis viruses in adults infected with HIV 2013. *HIV Med* 2013; 14(S4):1–71.
http://www.euro.who.int/. *Guidelines on the management of hepatitis C and HIV co-infection.*
http://www.hep-druginteractions.org. *Potential hepatitis drug interactions can be checked using the online tool maintained by Liverpool University.*

PREVENTION AND CONTROL OF HIV INFECTION

HIV is now a manageable chronic condition with a life expectancy that can match that of the general population, in those who start effective ART early enough. Initiating treatment when infection is more advanced compromises clinical outcomes, and is the most important predictor of morbidity and mortality. In 2017 in the UK:

- an estimated 8% of people with HIV were undiagnosed
- 43% of people newly diagnosed with HIV were diagnosed late (CD4 count below the threshold to start therapy, <350 cells/mm³)
- 23% had a CD4 count <200 cells/mm³ at the time of diagnosis, putting them at high risk of HIV-associated pathology (see **Fig. 37.12**).

Expanding HIV testing

Expansion of testing is a key intervention to achieve good clinical outcomes and a reduction in the rate of new infections. UK Guidelines on HIV testing from BHIVA and the National Institute for Health and Care Excellence (NICE) include clinical settings in which HIV testing should be universally offered, together with a list of clinical situations and diagnoses (indicator conditions) that are highly predictive of HIV infection and in which HIV testing should be recommended (see **Box 37.9**). Testing should be recommended for all new registrants in primary care and for patients admitted to acute medical care in areas where HIV seroprevalence is over 2/1000 population.

An increasing array of point-of-care HIV antibody tests are available that are sensitive and specific and easy to use, can test either blood or oral fluids, and give results within minutes. Home sampling approaches, with specimens sent to a central laboratory and results given over the telephone, have been shown to increase testing rates in some populations, and changes in legislation have allowed the sale of home testing kits for HIV in the UK.

However, because of a significant false-positive rate, it is crucial for all reactive point-of-care tests to be followed up with confirmatory serological assays, and for appropriate arrangements to be made to ensure that patients who are found to be HIV-positive have rapid routes into specialist care. HIV testing also offers the opportunity for appropriate prevention interventions for people who test HIV-negative.

Strategies for reducing HIV transmission

HIV is a completely preventable infection, yet new HIV infection continues to arise. Combinations of behavioural, biomedical and structural approaches are required, with interventions appropriate for the particular population at risk. Models of the epidemic in the UK suggest that a majority of new infections are transmitted from people who are unaware of their HIV status or have recently acquired HIV. Reduction of the high rates of undiagnosed infection through scaling-up of testing and early initiation of effective treatment is therefore central to an effective prevention response.

For those at high risk of acquisition, an additional emphasis on the need for repeat testing is required, as those with early infection and a high viral load are particularly infectious. Vaccine development has been hampered by the genetic variability of the virus and the complex immune response that is required from the host, with disappointing results from trials of candidate agents.

Consistent condom use and education for behaviour change have been key strategies. Provision of clean injecting equipment for people who inject drugs has been successful in those countries where it has been implemented.

Medically performed circumcision has been shown in African studies of HIV-negative heterosexual men to reduce the female-to-male transmission of HIV by at least 50%. A more modest reduction in HIV incidence in HIV-negative women following circumcision of HIV-positive male partners has been demonstrated but only at 2 years after the procedure.

Use of effective ART by people with HIV has been demonstrated to reduce onward transmission substantially: for instance, the Partner and Partner 2 studies reported zero transmissions during condomless sex from a positive partner on fully suppressive ART to their HIV-negative partner. These data have been used to support the message 'U=U' (undetectable equals untransmittable) campaign, reinforcing the benefits of testing and early treatment.

Partner notification schemes are helpful but can be sensitive and controversial. Availability and accessibility of confidential HIV testing provide an opportunity for individual health education and risk reduction to be discussed.

Pre-exposure prophylaxis

The use of ARVs by people who are HIV-negative prior to potential exposure (pre-exposure prophylaxis, PrEP) typically consists of oral tenofovir–emtricitabine (TDF-FTC), taken either daily or on demand prior to potential exposure to HIV. When used consistently, it has been shown to be highly successful and safe, in both MSM and heterosexual men and women, with up to a 90% reduction in the risk of HIV acquisition. On the basis of these results, PrEP, with appropriate safety monitoring, is recommended as an effective HIV prevention strategy; however, work is still ongoing to scale up access for all those who could benefit from PrEP within the National Health Service in England.

Global strategies

Understanding and changing behaviour is crucial but notoriously difficult, especially in areas like sex, HIV and AIDS, which carry many taboos. Stigma, poverty, punitive legislation, social unrest and war all contribute to the spread of HIV. Ongoing investment in and prioritization of HIV requires political will – not always readily available – if the progress that has been made is to be sustained.

Further reading

Brady M, Rodger A, Asboe D et al. *BHIVA/BASHH Guidelines on the Use of HIV Pre-exposure Prophylaxis (PrEP) 2018.* London: British HIV Association and British Association for Sexual Health and HIV; 2018.
McCormack SM, Gafos M, Desai M et al. Biomedical prevention: state of the science. *Clin Infect Dis* 2014; 59(Suppl 1):S41–46.
Mayer KH. Antiretroviral chemoprophylaxis: new successes and questions. *Lancet* 2015; 385:2236–2237.
Rodger AJ, Cambiano V, Bruun T et al. Risk of HIV transmission through condomless sex in serodifferent gay couples with the HIV-positive partner taking suppressive antiretroviral therapy (PARTNER): final results of a multicentre, prospective, observational study. *Lancet* 2019; 393:2428–2438.
http://www.BHIVA.org.uk. *British HIV Association guidance on the appropriate use of vaccines in HIV.*

Bibliography

Aral S, Fenton KA, Lipshutz JA. *The New Public Health and STD/HIV Prevention: Personal, Public and Health Systems Approaches*. New York: Springer; 2013.

Ferreira A, Young T, Mathews C et al. Strategies for Partner Notification for Sexually Transmitted Infections, Including HIV *(Cochrane Review)*. Chichester: Cochrane Library; 2013; issue 10.

Fowler N. *AIDS: Don't Die of Prejudice*. London: Bite Back; 2014.

Maartens G, Celum C, Lewin SR. HIV infection: epidemiology, pathogenesis, treatment, and prevention. *Lancet* 2014; 384:258–271.

Smith CJ, Ryom L, Weber R et al. Trends in underlying causes of death in people with HIV from 1999 to 2011 (D:A:D): a multicohort collaboration. *Lancet* 2014; 384:241–248.

World Health Organization. *Consolidated Guidelines on HIV Prevention, Diagnosis, Treatment and Care for Key Populations*. Geneva: WHO; 2014.

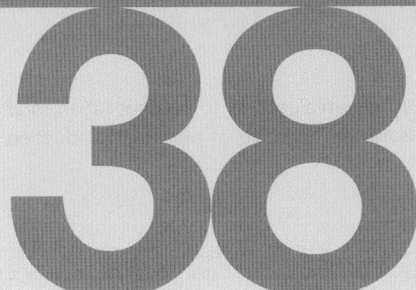

38

Obstetric medicine

Catherine Nelson-Piercy

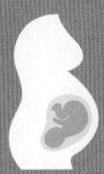

CORE SKILLS AND KNOWLEDGE

Obstetric medicine refers to the care of pregnant women with medical problems. These include the 10% of women who enter pregnancy with pre-existing diseases (such as asthma, epilepsy, hypertension and diabetes), as well as those with diseases that arise acutely in pregnancy (such as pneumonia and venous thrombosis).

Obstetric medicine is a new and growing medical specialty, comprised of physicians who specialize in providing care to pregnant women with medical problems, and who increasingly work alongside specialist obstetricians (who have also received specialist training in obstetric medicine), specialist obstetric anaesthetists and midwives. Historically (and currently in many centres without an obstetric physician), this care was provided by general obstetricians alongside general adult physicians. Training programmes in most medical specialties require trainees to learn about the care of patients within the specialty in the context of

pregnancy. General practitioners also have a crucial role, as they provide continuity of care before and after the pregnancy.

Special skills necessary for physicians to practise obstetric medicine include:

- an in-depth knowledge of which medications and radiological investigations are compatible with pregnancy and breast-feeding
- the ability to take a detailed obstetric history and a grasp of its relevance to chronic medical disease
- an understanding of how to interpret blood results and other investigations in pregnancy.

Opportunities to learn obstetric medicine may arise by completing training attachments in obstetrics and gynaecology, by attending obstetric medicine multidisciplinary team meetings or clinics, if they exist, and by seeking out pregnant women who are under close surveillance because of coexisting medical problems. There is now a post CCT credential in obstetric medicine available through RCP London.

CLINICAL SKILLS FOR OBSTETRIC MEDICINE

History

Many symptoms are normal in pregnancy. These include fatigue, nausea, vomiting, palpitations, breathlessness, gastro-oesophageal reflux, constipation and oedema. A careful history is required to discriminate breathlessness due to pathology such as a pulmonary

embolism from that which is physiological. Typically, pathological symptoms may arise suddenly, differ from those experienced in previous pregnancies or be particularly severe. Even with significant experience, differentiating pathological from physiological symptoms in pregnancy can be challenging.

Examination

Physiological changes occurring in pregnancy are illustrated in the figure opposite. They contribute to the production of signs accompanying all normal pregnancies, including a relative resting tachycardia of up to 100 beats/min, relative hypotension (a systolic blood pressure of 90 mmHg is not unusual) and oedema.

Investigations

Blood tests need interpreting based on pregnancy normal ranges, which differ from those outside pregnancy because of underlying changes in physiology. Serum creatinine falls below 70 μmol/L,

there is a physiological anaemia related to haemodilution, and alkaline phosphatase is raised because of placental production (**Box 38.1**).

Screening

Healthcare systems vary as to which screening tests are carried out during pregnancy, according to the local prevalence of different diseases and the availability of resources. **Box 38.2** describes tests routinely performed in the UK. Clinic appointments are usually made at booking (generally 8–12 weeks' gestation), and then at 16, 20, 25, 28, 31, 34, 36, 38, 40, 41 and 42 weeks of gestation in healthy women, with fetal ultrasound at 12 and 20 weeks.

i **Box 38.1 Normal haematological values in pregnancy**

Test	Normal range in pregnancy	Normal range in general population
Haemoglobin (Hb)	110–140 g/L	115–155 g/L
Mean corpuscular volume (MCV)	80–100 fL	80–96 fL
White cell count (WCC)	$6–16 \times 10^9$/L	$4–11 \times 10^9$/L
Platelets	$150–400 \times 10^9$/L	$150–400 \times 10^9$/L
Sodium	130–140 mmol/L	135–146 mmol/L
Potassium	3.3–4.1 mmol/L	3.5–5.0 mmol/L
Urea	<4.5 mmol/L	2.5–6.7 mmol/L (8–25 mg/dL)
Creatinine	<70 μmol/L	79–118 μmol/L (0.6–1.5 mg/dL)
Bilirubin	<16 μmol/L	<17 μmol/L (0.3–1.5 mg/dL)
Aspartate aminotransferase (AST)	10–30 U/L	12–40 U/L
Alanine aminotransferase (ALT)	6–32 U/L	<40 U/L
Alkaline phosphatase (ALP)	30–418 U/L	39–117 U/L
Albumin	28–37 g/L	35–50 g/L

i **Box 38.2 Screening tests in pregnancy**

Confirmation of pregnancy
- Urine beta-human chorionic gonadotrophin (β-hCG) testing kits are highly sensitive for confirming pregnancy in the context of a missed period (and need not be repeated if a woman has performed a test that has proved positive at home)
- A serum β-hCG level is not used in routine practice for diagnosing pregnancy but is used in managing certain conditions, including ectopic pregnancy and molar pregnancy

Infectious diseases
- Human immunodeficiency virus (HIV), hepatitis B and syphilis are screened for as early as possible in pregnancy so that treatment can be instituted to reduce the risk of transmission to the fetus

Obesity
- Body mass index (BMI) is calculated from height and weight measured at the booking visit
- Lifestyle advice to encourage healthy behaviour is given at this point and repeated throughout pregnancy

Hypertension and pre-eclampsia
- Blood pressure measurement and urine dipstick examination are performed at each antenatal appointment
- Women with hypertension or proteinuria are monitored much more closely; renal and liver function is measured

Anaemia
- A full blood count is measured at booking and at the 28-week visit
- Haemoglobin targets are lower during pregnancy
- General iron, folate and vitamin B_{12} concentrations are also measured if anaemia is diagnosed

Gestational diabetes mellitus (GDM)
- An oral glucose tolerance test (OGTT) is offered to high-risk women, including those with previous GDM, previous high-birth-weight babies, or a family history of type 2 diabetes

Blood group and Rhesus status
- Blood group is recorded, in case there is a transfusion requirement during labour
- Women who are Rhesus-negative are offered anti-D in the third trimester to prevent formation of Rhesus antibodies (from transfer of Rhesus-positive blood from a Rhesus-positive baby), which may cause haemolytic disease of the newborn in a subsequent pregnancy (see p. 353)

Screening for inherited diseases
- Thalassaemia and sickle-cell screening is offered in all pregnancies to those at high risk; the main purpose is to identify (via partner screening if the woman is a carrier) the risk of disease in the fetus, which can be confirmed by chorionic villous sampling

Screening for fetal chromosomal abnormalities
- See page 15

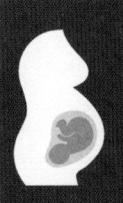

Physiological changes in pregnancy

Haematology
↑ Plasma volume (by 50%)
↓ Haemoglobin
↓ Platelets
↑ Fibrinogen (by 50%)
↑ Clotting factors VIII, IX, X
Venous stasis (L>R)

Respiratory
↑ Oxygen consumption
   (by 20%)
↑ Minute ventilation
   (by 40–50%)
↑ PO_2
↓ PCO_2
↓ Forced vital capacity (third
trimester)

Cardiac
↑ Cardiac output (by 40%)
↑ Stroke volume
↑ Heart rate (by 10–20 b.p.m.)
↓ Blood pressure (↓ in first
   and second trimesters)
↓ Systemic vascular
   resistance (by 25–30%)
↓ Serum colloid osmotic
   pressure (by 10–15%)

Renal
↑ Renal blood flow
   (by 60–80%)
↑ Glomerular filtration rate
   (by 55%)
↑ Protein excretion (up to
   300 mg / 24 h)
↓ Serum creatinine
   (max = 70 μmol/L)
Glycosuria
Physiological
   hydronephrosis (R>L)

Gastroenterology
↓ Gut motility
↑ Alkaline phosphatase
↓ Albumin (by 20–40%)

Endocrine
Impaired glucose tolerance
Insulin resistance
↑ Prolactin (10-fold)
↑ Cortisol
↑ Renin, angiotensin,
   aldosterone

General
Fatigue
Weight gain
Nausea/vomiting
Constipation
Breathlessness
Palpitations
Ankle oedema

Skin
Palmar erythema
Dry skin
Telangiectasia
Pruritus (in 20%)

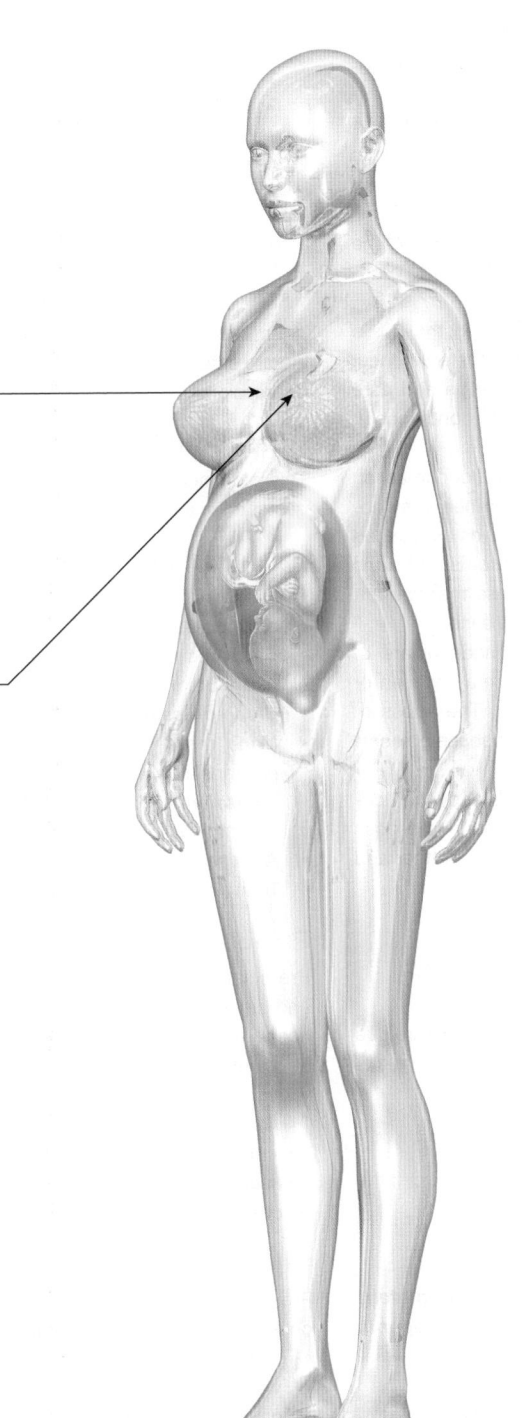

INTRODUCTION

The prevalence of medical conditions that complicate pregnancy is increasing, partly because:

- women in Western countries are delaying childbearing until they are older
- 50% of pregnant women are now overweight or obese, resulting in more patients with diabetes, hypertension and associated co-morbidities
- women with chronic medical diseases, such as congenital heart disease, diabetes, chronic kidney disease (CKD) and cystic fibrosis now survive into their childbearing years because of better medical care
- widening access to assisted conception services, including the use of donor eggs, means that age is no longer a barrier to pregnancy.

Maternal death (during or soon after pregnancy) in the UK is now more often due to medical complications than obstetric ones. Confidential enquiries show that inadequate knowledge and care are implicated in one-quarter of deaths from medical conditions in pregnancy.

The anatomical and physiological changes that occur as an adaptation to normal pregnancy can result in a number of symptoms and signs. These overlap with the clinical features associated with diseases outside pregnancy. Most of the symptoms and signs are benign, but clinicians need to be aware of those that warrant further investigation and may be associated with disease.

Women with pre-existing disease should be made aware of the normal adaptation to pregnancy, as symptoms may worsen or improve, depending on the body system involved. The stress of pregnancy may also result in previously subclinical disease presenting for the first time.

Infectious diseases are a major problem in pregnancy, particularly in low- and middle-income countries (see individual diseases in Chapter 20). There is increased mortality in both the mother and the fetus.

HYPERTENSIVE DISORDERS

During normal pregnancy, there is a reduction in blood pressure due to a fall in systemic vascular resistance; this is maximal by weeks 22–24.

Chronic/pre-existing hypertension

This is present at the initial booking visit or before 20 weeks, or if the patient is already taking medication for hypertension.

Management

- **Angiotensin-converting enzyme (ACE) inhibitors, angiotensin II receptor blockers (ARBs) and chlorothiazide agents** that are associated with congenital abnormalities should be discontinued.
- **Dietary salt** intake should be kept low (2 g or 100 mmol daily).
- **Aspirin** 75 mg should be given from 12 weeks until birth to women at moderate or high risk of pre-eclampsia (see later).
- **Oral labetalol** is first-line therapy during pregnancy. Second-line agents are methyldopa and nifedipine. Treatment may be required for several weeks postpartum.
- **Target blood pressure** is <135 mmHg systolic and <85 mmHg diastolic. Delivery should be considered after 34 weeks gestation and before 38 weeks gestation. Difficulty controlling the blood pressure is an indication for delivery.

> **i** | **Box 38.3 Risk factors for pre-eclampsia**
>
> - Age >40 years
> - Obesity: body mass index (BMI) >30
> - Family history
> - Primiparity
> - Multiple pregnancy
> - Previous pre-eclampsia
> - Long birth interval
> - Hydrops with a large placenta
> - Hydatidiform mole
> - Triploidy (particular association with pre-eclampsia of very
>
>   early onset – before 24 weeks' gestation)
> - Medical disorders:
>   - Pre-existing hypertension
>   - Renal disease (even without renal impairment)
>   - Diabetes mellitus (pre-existing or gestational)
>   - Antiphospholipid syndrome
>   - Autoimmune rheumatic diseases
>   - Sickle cell disease

In **breast-feeding**, ACE inhibitors, beta-blockers and nifedipine are safe. Methyldopa should be avoided because of the risk of depression.

Gestational hypertension

This is defined as blood pressure of >140/90 mmHg after 20 weeks' gestation in a previously normotensive woman.

Investigations and management

- **Blood tests**, including full blood count, serum creatinine and electrolytes, calcium, liver biochemistry and liver function tests. Estimated glomerular filtration rate (eGFR) is not validated for use in pregnancy.
- **Blood pressure measurements** once a week.
- **Urine tests** for protein, as there is an increased risk of pre-eclampsia developing.
- **Treatment of moderate hypertension** (159–150/109–100 mmHg) with oral labetalol.
- **Admission to hospital** if blood pressure is ≥160/110 mmHg. Treatment may be required for several weeks postpartum.

Pre-eclampsia

Pre-eclampsia is a common direct (obstetric) cause of maternal and perinatal death, and a significant cause of maternal and neonatal morbidity. The risk factors are shown in **Box 38.3**. It is a heterogeneous multisystem endothelial disorder that has widespread effects.

There is good evidence that low-dose aspirin is beneficial in patients with a moderate to high risk of developing pre-eclampsia; it is safe in pregnancy and is usually stopped 10 days to 4 weeks before delivery.

Clinical features

Pre-eclampsia varies in severity, timing, progression and order of onset of different clinical features. Symptoms include:

- severe headache
- visual blurring or flashing
- nausea and vomiting
- severe epigastric or right upper quadrant pain
- rapidly progressive oedema of the hands, feet and face.

Signs include new hypertension at more than 20 weeks, oedema and proteinuria (>0.3 g/24 h or urinary protein : creatinine ratio >30 mg/mmol on a 'spot' sample); these are the most common manifestations of pre-eclampsia. Hyper-reflexia may be seen.

Pre-eclampsia (including eclampsia) may present ante-, intra- or postpartum. Postpartum disease is more likely to be associated with symptoms. Complications and crises are shown in **Box 38.4**.

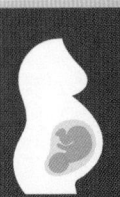

Box 38.4 Complications and crises seen in pre-eclampsia

- Eclampsia
- HELLP syndrome (*h*aemolysis, *e*levated *l*iver enzymes, *l*ow *p*latelets)
- Pulmonary oedema
- Placental abruption
- Cerebral haemorrhage
- Cortical blindness
- Disseminated intravascular coagulation
- Acute kidney injury
- Hepatic rupture
- Transient left ventricular systolic or diastolic dysfunction

Investigations

- *Full blood count* – thrombocytopenia.
- *Serum electrolytes and creatinine* – to monitor for acute kidney injury (AKI).
- *Liver biochemistry* – raised transaminases.
- *Urine protein:creatinine ratio.*
- *Ultrasound fetus* – for fetal growth.
- *Soluble fms-like tyrosine kinase-1/placental growth factor (sFlt-1/PlGF) ratio* – a novel immunoassay recommended by the National Institute for Health and Care Excellence (NICE) to rule out pre-eclampsia, following clinical assessment.

Management

Patients should be admitted and monitored for hypertension with regular blood pressure measurements (4 times daily) and blood tests (2–3 weekly).

Close fetal monitoring is required because of the risks of placental insufficiency and intrauterine growth restriction.

Delivery is the only cure for pre-eclampsia and this may be indicated for either fetal or maternal reasons. The recurrence risk of pre-eclampsia is increased with early-onset disease.

Women whose pregnancy has been complicated by pre-eclampsia are significantly more likely to develop hypertension, ischaemic heart disease, cerebrovascular disease and CKD in later life.

If a patient develops eclampsia (convulsions or coma) and/or HELLP syndrome (see next section), she should be admitted to a critical care or high-dependency unit and may require intravenous hydralazine, labetalol and, if suffering convulsions, magnesium sulphate (4 g over 5 min then maintenance 1 g/h) and prompt delivery. Patients should be given steroids (betamethasone 12 mg i.m. for fetal lung maturation, repeated at 24 h if delivery is likely within 7 days).

HELLP

HELLP is a syndrome describing *h*aemolysis, *e*levated *l*iver enzymes and *l*ow *p*latelets (<100 × 10⁹/L) in a pregnant woman. It is a form of severe pre-eclampsia, more common in multiparous women, and can occur in the second and third trimesters or postpartum. The haemolysis is due to a microangiopathic haemolytic anaemia (see p. 355). Hypertension and proteinuria may be absent or mild. Clinically, patients complain of epigastric/right upper quadrant pain, nausea, vomiting and jaundice (5%). If symptoms are severe, prompt delivery is necessary and is advised in all patients who are beyond 34 weeks' gestation.

Further reading

Bartsch E, Medcalf KE, Park AL et al. Clinical risk factors for pre-eclampsia determined in early pregnancy: systemic review and meta analysis of large cohort studies. *BMJ* 2016; 353:i1753.

National Institute for Health and Care Excellence. *NICE Clinical Guideline 133: Hypertension in Pregnancy: diagnosis and management*. NICE 2019; http://www.nice.org.uk/guidance/ng133.

LIVER DISEASE

Liver function is not impaired in pregnancy. Any liver disease (see Ch. 34), from whatever cause, can occur incidentally and coincide with pregnancy. For example, viral hepatitis accounts for 40% of all cases of jaundice during pregnancy. Pregnancy does not necessarily exacerbate established liver disease but it is uncommon for women with advanced liver disease to conceive.

The following effects are seen:

- Plasma and blood volumes increase during pregnancy but the hepatic blood flow remains constant.
- The proportion of cardiac output delivered to the liver therefore falls from 35% to 29% in late pregnancy; drug metabolism can thus be affected.
- The size of the liver remains constant.
- Liver biochemistry remains unchanged, apart from a rise in serum alkaline phosphatase from the placenta (up to 3–4 times increased), and a decrease in total protein and albumin concentration owing to increased plasma volume.
- Triglycerides and cholesterol levels rise, and caeruloplasmin, transferrin, α_1-antitrypsin and fibrinogen levels are elevated owing to increased hepatic synthesis.
- During pregnancy and particularly postpartum, there is a tendency to hypercoagulability, and acute Budd–Chiari syndrome (see p. 1304) can occur.

There are a number of liver diseases that complicate pregnancy: hyperemesis gravidarum, intrahepatic cholestasis and acute fatty liver.

Hyperemesis gravidarum

Pathological vomiting during pregnancy can be associated with liver dysfunction and jaundice. Liver dysfunction resolves when vomiting subsides.

Intrahepatic cholestasis of pregnancy

This condition of unknown aetiology usually presents with pruritus alone in the third trimester. It has a familial tendency and there is a higher prevalence in Scandinavia, Chile and Bolivia.

Investigations

Liver biochemistry shows raised aminotransferases, which occasionally can be very high. The hallmark is raised serum bile acids but serum bilirubin and gamma-glutamyl transferase (γ-GT) may also be slightly raised. Jaundice is rare. Liver biopsy is not indicated but would show centrilobular cholestasis.

Management and prognosis

Treatment is symptomatic with ursodeoxycholic acid 1–2 g daily in divided doses. Prognosis is usually excellent for the mother but there is increased fetal loss, which has been shown to correlate with higher (>100 μmol/L) bile acid levels. The condition resolves after delivery. Recurrent cholestasis may occur during subsequent pregnancies or with the ingestion of oestrogen-containing oral contraceptive pills.

Acute fatty liver of pregnancy

Acute fatty liver of pregnancy (AFLP) is a rare but serious condition occurring in the third trimester and affecting 1 in 6000–20 000 pregnancies. It is more common in women with multiple gestations. Patients present with abdominal pain, vomiting and jaundice. Polyuria and thirst due to diabetes insipidus may occur because of reduced breakdown of placentally derived vasopressinase. AKI

---

i **Box 38.5 Pregnancy-associated risks of different cardiac diseases**

Low risk
- Uncomplicated small or mild pulmonary stenosis, patent ductus arteriosus, mitral valve prolapse
- Successfully repaired ASD, VSD, patent ductus arteriosus
- Atrial and ventricular ectopic beats

Small increased risk of mortality/moderate increased risk of morbidity
- Unrepaired ASD, VSD
- Repaired tetralogy of Fallot
- Most arrhythmias

Moderate increased risk of mortality or severe morbidity
- Mild LV dysfunction (LVEF >45%), hypertrophic cardiomyopathy
- Repaired coarctation
- Most native or tissue valve disease (except those with extremely high risk)

Significant increased risk of mortality or severe morbidity
- Mechanical valves
- Systemic RV with good or mildly impaired ventricular function

- Fontan circulation
- Unrepaired cyanotic congenital heart disease

Extremely high risk of mortality or severe morbidity
- Pulmonary arterial hypertension
- Severe systemic ventricular dysfunction – left ventricular ejection fraction <30% (New York Heart Association (NYHA) class III/IV; see Box 30.23)
- Previous peripartum cardiomyopathy with any residual LV impairment
- Severe mitral stenosis/symptomatic aortic stenosis
- Severe aortic (re)coarctation
- Systemic RV with moderate or severely decreased ventricular function
- Aortic root >4.5 cm in Marfan's syndrome
- Turner syndrome with ASI >25 mm/m^2
- Tetralogy of Fallot >50 mm
- Ascending aorta >5 cm with bicuspid aortic valve
- Vascular Ehlers–Danlos syndrome
- Fontan circulation with any complication

ASD, atrial septal defect; LV, left ventricular; RV, right ventricle; VSD, ventricular septal defect. ASI, aortic size index

---

and lactic acidosis are commonly seen. In fulminant AFLP patients, encephalopathy, coagulopathy and hypoglycaemia can occur. AFLP may be associated with features of pre-eclampsia.

Investigations
- Full blood count.
- Serum electrolytes and creatinine.
- Serum glucose ↓.
- Serum uric acid ↑
- Liver biochemistry – shows hepatocellular damage (raised serum aminotransferases and raised bilirubin).
- Coagulopathy.
- *Liver biopsy* – rarely performed and not necessary for diagnosis but would show fine droplets of fat (microvesicular) in the hepatocytes with a little necrosis.

Management
Treatment is as for acute liver failure (see p. 1286). N-acetyl cysteine is safe in pregnancy. Immediate delivery may save both the baby and the mother. Early diagnosis and treatment have reduced the mortality to less than 20%.

CARDIAC DISEASE

Cardiac disease, both congenital and acquired, is commonly encountered in pregnancy and is mostly benign. Many women experience palpitations and breathlessness due to awareness of physiological sinus tachycardia, ventricular premature/ectopic beats and increased minute ventilation.

Cardiac disease, predominantly acquired, is the most common cause of maternal death in the UK. The main conditions causing severe morbidity and mortality are as follows:
- *Myocardial infarction* in pregnant women is more often due to coronary artery dissection or thrombus than in non-pregnant women. Intervention with primary angioplasty and coronary artery stenting is appropriate.
- *Peripartum cardiomyopathy* is defined as the development of heart failure with left ventricular ejection fraction (LVEF) <45% at the end of pregnancy or in the months following de-

livery, where no other cause of heart failure is found. It is a dilated cardiomyopathy (see p. 1122) and is more common in obese and multiparous women. It should be treated with conventional heart failure therapy (including thromboprophylaxis), except that ACE inhibitors and ARBs are withheld until after delivery. Nearly half of these patients will recover to normal within 6 months.
- *Pulmonary hypertension* (see p. 115) and fixed pulmonary vascular resistance are dangerous and often (10–20%) fatal in pregnancy.

A number of serious cardiac conditions constituting absolute or relative contraindications to pregnancy are shown in **Box 38.5** and include a dilated aortic root of more than 4.5 cm, severe left heart obstruction from critical mitral or aortic stenosis, and severe impairment of left ventricular function.

Women with significant heart disease need multidisciplinary care in a specialist centre by obstetricians, cardiologists and anaesthetists who have expertise in the care of heart disease in pregnancy. Agreed management plans should be documented.

If *pregnancy is contraindicated*, then appropriate contraceptive advice is essential. The levels of risk associated with pregnancy for individual conditions are summarized in **Box 38.5**, based on the European Society of Cardiology guidelines.

Pregnancy and prosthetic heart valves
See page 1103.

Any strategy for anticoagulation for a pregnant woman with a mechanical heart valve is associated with risks to the mother and/or fetus. *Pre-pregnancy counselling* is essential, explaining that warfarin is the safest option for the mother but associated with a 5% risk of warfarin embryopathy and increased risks of miscarriage, stillbirth and fetal intracranial haemorrhage. The alternative is full anticoagulant doses of low-molecular-weight heparin (LMWH), given twice daily and titrated upwards in pregnancy, based on *regular monitoring of anti-factor Xa* levels.

Further reading
Task Force for the Management of Cardiovascular Diseases during Pregnancy of the European Society of Cardiology (ESC). ESC Guidelines on the management of cardiovascular diseases during pregnancy. *Eur Heart J* 2018; 39:3165–3241.

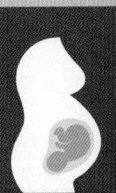

> ### *i* Box 38.6 Risk factors for venous thromboembolism in pregnancy
>
> - Previous venous thromboembolism
> - Thrombophilia
> - Active medical disease, e.g. inflammatory bowel disease, systemic lupus erythematosus, pyelonephritis, nephrotic syndrome
> - Age >35 years
> - Obesity (body mass index >30 kg/m²) either before pregnancy or in early pregnancy
> - Parity ≥3 (a woman becomes 'para 3' after her third delivery)
> - Smoking
> - Gross varicose veins (symptomatic or above the knee or with associated phlebitis, oedema/skin changes)
>
> - Dehydration, hyperemesis gravidarum, ovarian hyperstimulation syndrome
> - Paraplegia, immobility
> - Multiple pregnancy
> - Current pre-eclampsia
> - Caesarean section .
> - Prolonged labour (>24 h)
> - Mid-cavity rotational operative delivery
> - Stillbirth
> - Preterm birth
> - Postpartum haemorrhage (>1 L/requiring transfusion)
> - Surgery in pregnancy or the puerperium

THROMBOEMBOLIC DISEASE

Pulmonary embolism is the most common direct cause of death in pregnancy and the puerperium. Pregnancy and especially the puerperium are associated with a sixfold increased risk of thrombosis. Although the risks are highest after emergency caesarean section, women with risk factors (**Box 38.6**) are at risk antenatally, especially if admitted to hospital, and after vaginal delivery.

Diagnosis

Objective diagnosis of deep vein thrombosis (DVT) and pulmonary embolism (PE) must be made in those with a suggestive history and risk factors. ***D-dimers*** are not useful in pregnancy, as the levels are often raised. DVT is much more common in the left leg (ratio 9 : 1) than the right in pregnancy because the gravid uterus compresses the left common iliac vein, which lies under the right common iliac artery. ***Ventilation/perfusion (V̇/Q̇) scans*** and computed tomography ***pulmonary angiograms (CTPAs)*** are associated with negligible radiation to the fetus and are safe, but V̇/Q̇ scans are preferred, as they do not irradiate the maternal breast and increase the risk of breast cancer.

Management

Treatment of venous thromboembolism (VTE) in pregnancy involves:
- larger doses of LMWHs, e.g. enoxaparin
- avoidance of warfarin and new oral anticoagulants
- continuance of LMWH for the rest of the pregnancy and the puerperium.

  Decisions regarding thromboprophylaxis in pregnancy relate to past history of VTE, the presence of thrombophilia and other risk factors (see **Box 38.6**).

  Women with previous VTE should receive antenatal and postnatal thromboprophylaxis with LMWH. This should begin as early in pregnancy as possible. LMWH and warfarin are safe in lactating mothers.

Further reading
Royal College of Obstetricians and Gynaecologists. *Green-top Guideline no. 37a: Thrombosis and Embolism during Pregnancy and the Puerperium, Reducing the Risk*. RCOG 2015; http://www.rcog.org.uk/.
Royal College of Obstetricians and Gynaecologists. *Green-top Guideline no. 37b: Thrombosis and Embolism during Pregnancy and the Puerperium: Acute Management*. RCOG 2015; http://www.rcog.org.uk/.

RESPIRATORY DISEASE

Asthma

The treatment of asthma (see p. 949) in pregnant women does not differ from that in the non-pregnant patient. Pregnancy itself does not usually influence the severity of asthma. For the majority of women, asthma has no adverse effect on pregnancy outcome.
- Poorly controlled severe asthma presents more of a risk to the fetus than the medication used to prevent or treat it. This small risk is minimized with good control.
- Education and reassurance, ideally prior to pregnancy, concerning the safety of asthma medications during pregnancy are integral parts of management.
- Decreasing or stopping inhaled anti-inflammatory therapy during pregnancy causes a deterioration in disease control.
- Inhaled, oral and intravenous steroids, inhaled, nebulized and intravenous short- and long-acting β_2-agonists, and the leukotriene receptor antagonist montelukast are safe to use in pregnancy and while breast-feeding. Early data for omalizumab would suggest no adverse effects in pregnancy but there are no pregnancy data available for the newer biologic agents.
- Effective control of the disease process and its accompanying symptoms is a priority. An increase in the dose or frequency of inhaled steroids should be the first step if symptoms are not optimally controlled on the current dose of inhaled steroids and the inhaler technique is good.

Pneumonia

The bacteria that cause pneumonia (see p. 963) are no different in pregnancy. Chest X-rays are safe in pregnancy. Most antibiotics are safe to use in pregnancy and during lactation. Aminoglycosides should not be used unless essential and tetracycline/doxycycline should not be given. Varicella and influenza A pneumonia may be fatal in pregnancy and active steps must be taken to prevent chickenpox infection. Non-immune pregnant women exposed to varicella in pregnancy should be given varicella zoster immunoglobulin (VZIG). If a pregnant woman does contract chickenpox, she should be treated with aciclovir as soon as possible.

All pregnant women should receive immunization against seasonal influenza and influenza A H1N1.

Tuberculosis

Tuberculosis (TB) is particularly common in Asia and Africa. A chest X-ray should be performed if TB is suspected and the advice of a respiratory physician should be sought. Extrapulmonary TB is as common as pulmonary TB in pregnancy. The diagnosis must be confirmed bacteriologically, which may necessitate bronchoscopy or biopsy, which unfortunately is often delayed because of inappropriate reluctance to perform invasive investigations in pregnancy. The neonate should be given bacille Calmette–Guérin (BCG) vaccination.

Sarcoidosis

The course of sarcoidosis is unaltered by pregnancy. Flare-up of the disease is more likely postpartum. Erythema nodosum may occur in a normal pregnancy. Serum ACE is not reliable for the diagnosis of sarcoidosis in pregnancy. Systemic steroids should be used if indicated (see p. 988).

Cystic fibrosis

Women with cystic fibrosis often reach childbearing age with adequate lung function, or will have received a lung transplant and be able to consider pregnancy. Pre-pregnancy counselling, with consideration of lung function and concomitant diabetes, is required. Joint care with a cystic fibrosis centre should be maintained throughout pregnancy. Pregnancy outcome is related to pre-pregnancy lung function. Perinatal outcome is usually good but preterm delivery rates are high. Maternal outcome is variable, and worse in the presence of pulmonary hypertension. Specialist dietary advice with additional energy supplements should be given. Chest physiotherapy can and should be continued in pregnancy and infective exacerbations should be treated aggressively. There is an increased risk of gestational diabetes.

Severe restrictive lung disease

Women with severe lung disease are better able to tolerate pregnancy than women with severe cardiac insufficiency. If the forced vital capacity (FVC) is over 1 L, a successful pregnancy is usually possible but individual assessment is necessary. Immunosuppression for diffuse parenchymal lung disease should be continued in pregnancy. Respiratory diseases complicated by pulmonary hypertension have a poor prognosis in pregnancy.

NEUROLOGICAL DISEASE

Epilepsy
Birth defects

The overall risk of birth defects in babies of mothers who take one antiepileptic drug (AED) is around 7%, compared with 3% in women without epilepsy. The risk with lamotrigine and levetiracetam appears to be low. In most women, the frequency of seizures is not altered in pregnancy, provided there is compliance with AEDs. Free drug levels tend to fall in pregnancy and increased doses of AEDs, particularly lamotrigine, may be required. The risk to the fetus of uncontrolled seizures is greater than the risks of continuing AED treatment; poorly controlled epilepsy and recurrent seizures are associated with adverse outcomes for the fetus, such as an increased risk of *s*udden *u*nexplained *d*eath in *ep*ilepsy (SUDEP). If drugs cannot be safely stopped, monotherapy is preferable at the minimum effective dose. Sodium valproate is associated with a higher rate of serious malformations (e.g. neural tube defects) and long-term neurodevelopmental defects (e.g. a reduced IQ, increased risk of autism spectrum disorder and attention deficit disorder, ADHD), and should be stopped or substituted if necessary prior to conception.

Management

Counselling before conception is essential. Folic acid (5 mg/day) supplements should be taken before conception and throughout the first trimester. Antenatal screening for congenital abnormalities is necessary.

Breast-feeding

Mothers taking AEDs need not, in general, be discouraged from breast-feeding, though manufacturers are often hesitant in assuring that there is no risk to the baby.

Contraception

AEDs which induce hepatic enzymes (e.g. carbamazepine, phenytoin and phenobarbital) reduce the efficacy of oral contraceptives. A combined contraceptive pill containing a higher dose of oestrogen or the progesterone-only pill provides greater contraceptive security. An intrauterine device or barrier method of contraception is often used in preference to oral contraceptives.

Migraine

Migraine can occur as a pregnancy-related phenomenon in women without a prior history of migraine. Those with pre-existing migraine often improve in pregnancy. Hemiplegic migraine, particularly aura without headache, can mimic transient ischaemic attacks (TIAs). Ergotamine should be avoided in pregnancy. Sumatriptan may be used to treat migraine. Low-dose aspirin, beta-blockers, tricyclic antidepressants and pizotifen are used for prophylaxis. Greater occipital nerve (GON) injections are safe in pregnancy.

Multiple sclerosis

Pregnancy has no effect on the long-term prognosis of multiple sclerosis. Relapses are less likely during pregnancy but more likely in the postpartum period. Prophylactic treatments, such as interferon beta, glatiramer and natalizumab, are usually avoided in pregnancy and breast-feeding, but benefit may outweigh risk for some women. Discontinuation of natalizumab may result in flare-ups in pregnancy and is not advised, but the injections can be spaced and interrupted in late pregnancy to avoid excessive transfer to the fetus. All women should receive vitamin D supplements of at least 2000 units daily. Those with disability may require extra help during pregnancy and while caring for the infant following delivery. There is no contraindication to epidural anaesthesia, except that documentation of pre-existing neurological deficit in the legs is necessary to avoid any postpartum exacerbation of multiple sclerosis being inappropriately attributed to the regional block.

Myasthenia gravis

The course of myasthenia gravis in pregnancy is unpredictable, but in women with stable disease pregnancy outcome is usually normal. Postpartum exacerbations occur in 30% of women. Usual immunosuppressant therapy with steroids, azathioprine, IVIG and calcineurin inhibitors should be continued. Plasmapheresis is not contraindicated in pregnancy. Increased doses of long-acting anticholinesterases may be required. Many drugs should be avoided in myasthenia gravis and an experienced obstetric anaesthetist should be consulted. Transient neonatal myasthenia gravis may develop in up to 10% of neonates born to myasthenic mothers due to transplacental passage of immunoglobulin G acetylcholine receptor antibodies.

Stroke

The risks of arterial ischaemic stroke, cerebral venous thrombosis and intracranial haemorrhage are increased, particularly in the puerperium. In pregnant women, the prevalence of haemorrhagic stroke equals that of ischaemic stroke, in contrast to non-pregnant women, in whom ischaemic stroke is more common (>75% of strokes). Causes of stroke in pregnancy are listed in **Box 38.7**.

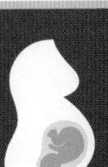

Ischaemic
- Cardiac causes, e.g. arterial emboli or arrhythmias
- Peripartum cardiomyopathy (see p. 1124)
- Paradoxical embolus (in situations causing increased right atrial pressure compared with left) through an atrial septal defect or patent foramen ovale
- Aortic/carotid artery dissection
- Antiphospholipid syndrome
- Sickle-cell disease

Haemorrhagic
- Pre-eclampsia/eclampsia

Depression

Depression in pregnancy and the puerperium is discussed on page 777.

ENDOCRINE DISEASE

Diabetes mellitus

Pre-existing diabetes during pregnancy and gestational diabetes are discussed on page 739.

Thyroid and parathyroid disease
Thyrotoxicosis

Untreated thyrotoxicosis (see p. 614) is dangerous for both the mother and her fetus, increasing the risk of miscarriage, fetal growth restriction and preterm delivery. Graves' disease affects about 0.2% of pregnancies and often improves during pregnancy, but there is a risk of flare-up postpartum. Both carbimazole and propylthiouracil (PTU) cross the placenta, and in high doses may cause fetal hypothyroidism and goitre. The lowest possible maintenance dose of antithyroid drug should be used. Guidelines advise avoidance of carbimazole in the first trimester, due to the risk of teratogenesis. PTU is usually not given because of the risk of liver failure in the general population, but may be used specifically in women planning pregnancy or in the first trimester. Women do not need to be swapped from one antithyroid drug to another before or during pregnancy; they should remain on whichever drug is controlling their disease. For those with good control of thyrotoxicosis on doses of carbimazole of less than 15 mg/day or PTU less than 150 mg/day, the maternal and fetal outcome is usually good and unaffected by the thyrotoxicosis. Women may safely breast-feed on these doses of antithyroid drugs. Beta-blockers are safe to use in the short term, if required for control of thyrotoxic symptoms. Neonatal or fetal thyrotoxicosis due to transplacental passage of thyroid-stimulating antibodies is rare, but occurs most commonly in women with active disease in pregnancy and those with high levels of thyroid-stimulating antibodies.

Hypothyroidism

Hypothyroidism (see p. 611) affects about 1% of pregnancies. Untreated hypothyroidism is associated with infertility, an increased rate of miscarriage, and fetal loss. For those on adequate replacement therapy, maternal and fetal outcome is usually good and is unaffected by the hypothyroidism. Very little thyroxine crosses the placenta and the fetus is not at risk of thyrotoxicosis from maternal thyroxine replacement therapy. Provided they are euthyroid at the beginning of pregnancy, most women do not usually require any adjustment to thyroxine dose during pregnancy or in the puerperium. Any dose increase should be based on thyroid function tests, interpreted using reference ranges for pregnancy (4.0 mU/L is taken as the upper limit for thyroid-stimulating hormone (TSH) after 7 weeks' gestation). There is no evidence to support older recommendations for a target TSH of less than 2.5 mU/L.

Subclinical hypothyroidism affects 5% of the general population and is more common in women, particularly those who have anti-thyroid antibodies. Studies fail to demonstrate a consistent association between any adverse pregnancy outcome and subclinical hypothyroidism in pregnancy, and there is insufficient evidence that thyroxine replacement in subclinical hypothyroidism benefits pregnancy outcome.

Postpartum thyroiditis is more common in women with a family history of hypothyroidism, thyroid peroxidase antibodies and type 1 diabetes. Presentation is usually between 3 and 4 months postpartum. Disease may present with symptoms of hyper- or hypothyroidism but a high index of suspicion is needed. The condition is caused by a destructive autoimmune lymphocytic thyroiditis. Most patients recover spontaneously and treatment is not always required. Postpartum thyroiditis often recurs and is a significant predictor of future hypothyroidism.

Hyperparathyroidism

Hypercalcaemia may be improved by pregnancy and the fetal demand for calcium. The risks to the mother are from acute pancreatitis and hypercalcaemic crisis, especially postpartum, when maternal transfer of calcium to the fetus stops abruptly. There is an increased risk of miscarriage, intrauterine death and preterm labour. Fetal mortality rates are up to 40% when the maternal hypercalcaemia is severe (>3.5 mmol/L). Up to 25% of women with hyperparathyroidism develop hypertension or pre-eclampsia. The risk to the neonate is from tetany and hypocalcaemic convulsions, caused by suppression of fetal parathyroid hormone (PTH) by high maternal calcium levels. Acute neonatal hypocalcaemia usually presents 5–14 days after birth but may be delayed by up to 1 month if the infant is breast-fed. The ideal treatment is surgery and this may be safely performed in pregnancy, though it is usually delayed until the second trimester.

Further reading
Alexander EK, Pearce EN, Brent GA et al. Guidelines of the American Thyroid Association for the diagnosis and management of thyroid disease during pregnancy and the postpartum. *Thyroid* 2017; 27:315–389.

Pituitary disease
See page 592.

Prolactinomas

Prolactinomas are the most common pituitary tumours encountered in pregnancy but rarely cause problems. The prolactin level should not be measured during pregnancy, as it is invariably raised. Those with microprolactinomas usually have no problems in pregnancy. The risk of tumour enlargement during pregnancy is increased with macroprolactinomas. Dopamine receptor agonists are safe for use in pregnancy and are usually continued in women with macroprolactinomas. Visual fields should be measured in each trimester in those with macroprolactinomas. If tumour enlargement is suspected, magnetic resonance imaging (MRI) of the pituitary is indicated. If women with macroprolactinomas wish to breast-feed, their dopamine receptor agonists may be discontinued in the last few weeks of pregnancy and during breast-feeding, but serial visual field examinations and pituitary MRI are required, and cabergoline or bromocriptine should be re-introduced if there is concern regarding tumour expansion.

Diabetes insipidus

Established or subclinical diabetes insipidus (DI, see p. 641) may worsen in pregnancy due to increased vasopressinase production by the placenta, or decreased vasopressinase breakdown by the liver. Extended fluid deprivation tests should be avoided in pregnancy and close observation with paired urine and plasma osmolality measurements may be sufficient to exclude DI. Desmopressin is safe for use in pregnancy for diagnosis or treatment of DI. Transient DI may occur in pregnancy and is often associated with acute fatty liver of pregnancy and, more rarely, with pre-eclampsia and HELLP syndrome (see p. 1455).

Hypopituitarism

Hypopituitarism (see p. 595) is rare in pregnancy but may be caused by:
- pituitary surgery
- radiotherapy
- pituitary or hypothalamic tumours
- pituitary haemorrhage
- postpartum pituitary infarction (Sheehan's syndrome)
- lymphocytic hypophysitis.

Sheehan's syndrome usually presents after delivery following postpartum haemorrhage and may lead to partial or complete pituitary failure. There may be a delay in diagnosis, as the symptoms may be attributed to the postpartum state. **Lymphocytic hypophysitis** is an uncommon autoimmune disorder due to extensive infiltration of the anterior pituitary by chronic inflammatory cells, predominantly lymphocytes, causing pituitary expansion. Anti-pituitary antibodies have been described and this condition is associated with autoimmune thyroiditis or adrenalitis in 20% of cases. It is most common in late pregnancy and the postpartum period. It presents with features suggestive of an expanding pituitary tumour and 85% of cases have endocrine hypofunction.

Adrenal disease

See also page 598.

Conn's syndrome and hyperaldosteronism

This is rare in pregnancy but hypertension, particularly in the absence of a positive family history, and hypokalaemia are indications for screening. High levels of progesterone in pregnancy may antagonize aldosterone and ameliorate the hypokalaemia. Renin and aldosterone levels are increased in pregnancy, and diagnosis requires the use of pregnancy-specific normal ranges. Hypertension is controlled in the usual way with labetalol, methyldopa or nifedipine, and hypokalaemia is treated with potassium supplementation or potassium-sparing diuretics. Amiloride is safe to use in pregnancy and high doses (e.g. 20 mg) may be needed. Spironolactone, which is used as a potassium-sparing diuretic in Conn's syndrome outside pregnancy, should be avoided: it may cause feminization of a male fetus because it is an antiandrogen. Surgery for adrenal adenomas can usually be safely deferred until after delivery.

Phaeochromocytoma and paraganglioma

Phaeochromocytoma and paraganglioma (see p. 608) are rare but dangerous causes of hypertension in pregnancy. Women with hypertension associated with unusual features of palpitations, anxiety, sweating or headache should be screened. Management involves adequate α-blockade with phenoxybenzamine to control hypertension, followed by β-blockade, if required, to control tachycardia. Alpha-blockade is imperative prior to delivery. Surgical removal is the only cure, and optimal timing of tumour resection depends on the point of gestation at which the diagnosis is made. There is an increasing vogue to delay tumour resection until the puerperium.

RENAL DISEASE

Urinary tract infection

See page 1381.

Bacteriuria in pregnancy

The urine of all pregnant women must be cultured, as 2–6% have asymptomatic bacteriuria. While asymptomatic bacteriuria in the non-pregnant female seldom leads to acute pyelonephritis and often does not require treatment, acute pyelonephritis frequently occurs in pregnancy under these circumstances. Failure to treat may thus result in severe symptomatic pyelonephritis later in pregnancy, with the possibility of preterm labour. *Therefore, bacteriuria must always be treated and be shown to be eradicated.* Re-infection may require prophylactic therapy. Tetracycline, sulphonamides and 4-quinolones must be avoided in pregnancy. Trimethoprim should be avoided in the first trimester. Amoxicillin, nitrofurantoin and cephalosporins may safely be used in pregnancy.

Chronic kidney disease

Women with CKD are at increased risk of pre-eclampsia, fetal growth restriction (FGR), preterm delivery and caesarean section; their perinatal mortality rate is increased. These obstetric complications and the risk of permanent deterioration in renal function are increased by the presence and severity of any renal impairment or hypertension.

In women with **moderate or severe renal impairment** (CKD stage 3–5, GFR 15–45 mL/min/1.73 m^2), 60–90% of infants are born preterm and there is a risk of accelerated decline in renal function of 20–50% in the mother.

An increase in the degree of proteinuria is very common in pregnancy and does not necessarily imply pre-eclampsia or worsening renal disease.

Management

Management should include regular monitoring of blood pressure, renal function and fetal wellbeing. In view of the increased risk of pre-eclampsia, treatment is with low-dose aspirin (75 mg daily from week 12 to delivery), especially in those with hypertension and renal impairment or a previous poor obstetric history.

Renal transplantation

If graft function is normal, pregnancy outcome is excellent and there is no adverse long-term effect on renal allograft function or survival. The chance of successful pregnancy outcome is reduced and the risk of long-term deterioration in graft function increased with poor baseline graft function. Pregnancy outcome is optimal in those without hypertension, proteinuria or recent episodes of graft rejection.

The doses of immunosuppressive drugs are maintained at pre-pregnancy levels. Prednisolone, azathioprine, ciclosporin and tacrolimus are safe for use in pregnancy without any reported increase in the risk of congenital malformations. Mycophenolate mofetil and sirolimus are contraindicated. Prophylactic antibiotics should be given for recurrent urinary tract infection and to cover any surgical procedure. The risks of pre-eclampsia, graft rejection, FGR, preterm delivery and infection are increased. Caesarean section is required only for obstetric indications but the rate is increased.

Acute kidney injury

Because serum creatinine falls in pregnancy, AKI is defined as an abrupt deterioration in renal function with a serum creatinine of more than 90 μmol/L. Mild degrees of AKI are not uncommon, particularly in the immediate postpartum period. The most common underlying causes are:

- **infection**: septic abortion, puerperal sepsis, acute pyelonephritis
- **blood loss**: postpartum haemorrhage, placental abruption
- **volume contraction**: pre-eclampsia, eclampsia, hyperemesis gravidarum, diarrhoea
- **post-renal failure**: ureteric damage or obstruction
- **drugs**: NSAIDs, antibiotics (e.g. aminoglycosides).

Women with pre-eclampsia are particularly prone to pulmonary oedema and therefore management protocols include fluid restriction, even in the presence of oliguria. If these patients develop AKI, this is usually rapidly reversible on recovery and less dangerous than pulmonary oedema, which may result if the AKI is treated with repeated fluid challenges. In this respect, therefore, the management of AKI differs from that outside pregnancy.

SKIN DISORDERS

Common skin changes that occur in pregnancy include striae (see p. 679), spider naevi, melasma (pigmentation on the face) and linea nigra (midline pigmentation on the abdomen). A shift in maternal immune profile from predominantly Th1 to Th2 may underlie the tendency for atopic dermatitis to develop or worsen during pregnancy. Psoriasis usually improves. Up to 20% of pregnant women will develop pruritus, which is most common on the lower legs. Intrahepatic cholestasis (see pp. 1272 and 1455) of pregnancy should be excluded by performing liver function tests and measuring bile acid levels.

The specific dermatoses of pregnancy are classified as shown in **Box 38.8**.

Further reading

Vaughan Jones S, Ambros-Rudolph C, Nelson-Piercy C. Skin diseases in pregnancy. *Br Med J* 2014; 348:g3489.

RHEUMATIC DISEASE

Some 50% of women with rheumatoid arthritis go into remission in pregnancy and 50% will flare during the postpartum period. Many disease-modifying anti-rheumatic drugs (DMARDs) are not contra-indicated in pregnancy. Women should take advice from their rheumatologist and obstetrician *prior* to conception. **Box 38.9** shows the use of drugs for rheumatoid arthritis in pregnancy.

Further reading

Flint J, Panchal S, Hurrell A et al. BSR and BHPR guideline on prescribing drugs in pregnancy and breastfeeding – Part I: standard and biologic disease modifying anti-rheumatic drugs and corticosteroids. *Rheumatology* 2016; 55:1693–1697.
Götestam Skorpen C, Hoeltzenbein M, Tincani A et al. The EULAR points to consider for use of antirheumatic drugs before pregnancy, and during pregnancy and lactation. *Ann Rheum Dis* 2016; 75:795–810.

PRESCRIBING IN PREGNANCY

Many clinicians are understandably reluctant to prescribe drugs for pregnant women. This relates mainly to concern regarding teratogenic risk. The following general principles should be remembered:

- **Older generic drugs.** Use older generic drugs within each class, since there are likely to be more data on use in pregnancy.
- **Dosages.** Resist the temptation to prescribe lower doses. Pregnant women usually need *higher* doses because of increased renal and liver clearance.

_i_ **Box 38.8 Classification of specific dermatoses of pregnancy**

Dermatosis	Description	Management
Atopic eruption of pregnancy Atopic eczema Prurigo of pregnancy	See p. 660 Usually starts on abdomen in third trimester but may persist for some months after delivery Clustered excoriated papules (prurigo-like lesions) occur on abdomen and extensor surfaces of limbs Cause unknown Can recur in subsequent pregnancies	Topical steroids and oral antihistamines
Pruritic folliculitis of pregnancy	Itchy folliculitis, looks similar to steroid-induced 'acne' Not associated with any increased maternal or fetal risk	Topical benzoyl peroxide; hydrocortisone cream helps relieve symptoms
Polymorphic eruption of pregnancy (pruritic urticated papules of pregnancy)	A relatively common, intensely itchy rash that starts on abdomen, often within striae, in third trimester Associated with multiple births Uncomfortable but harmless	Symptomatic topical therapy and antihistamines helpful until after delivery, when rash resolves
Pemphigoid gestationis	A rare disease analogous to bullous pemphigoid (see p. 686) Associated with prematurity and stillbirth; transplacental passage of pathogenic immunoglobulin G (IgG) antibodies can lead to transient blistering in the neonate Often starts around umbilicus with itchy, inflamed papules; then blistering appears and eruption may become generalized Onset in the first or second trimester; typically flares postpartum Diagnosis confirmed with direct immunofluorescence (see p. 686) Recurrences may occur with subsequent pregnancies and oral contraceptive pill, which should be avoided	Systemic steroid therapy required

---

_i_ Box 38.9 Drug use during pregnancy in treatment of rheumatoid arthritis

- *Paracetamol*: the oral analgesic of choice
- *Oral NSAIDs and selective COX-2 inhibitors*: can be used after implantation up until 30 weeks' gestation if symptoms justify their use
- *Corticosteroids*: may be used to control disease flares (main maternal risks are hypertension, glucose intolerance and osteoporosis)
- *DMARDs*:
  - *May be used*: sulfasalazine, hydroxychloroquine, azathioprine or ciclosporin if required to control inflammation
  - *Must be avoided*: mycophenolate mofetil, methotrexate, leflunomide and

cyclophosphamide; women should not conceive while taking mycophenolate mofetil, methotrexate or leflunomide
- *Biological agents*: good safety data during pregnancy for infliximab, adalimumab, etanercept and certolizimab pegol
- Safety for newer agents not yet established
- *Contraindicated in breast-feeding*: methotrexate, leflunomide, cyclophosphamide mycophenolate mofetil

COX-2, cyclo-oxygenase 2; DMARDs, disease-modifying anti-rheumatic drugs; NSAIDs, non-steroidal anti-inflammatory drugs.

- *Disease control.* Control of underlying diseases, such as arthritis, inflammatory bowel disease, epilepsy, asthma and thyrotoxicosis, with appropriate drug therapy is likely to reduce adverse fetal and neonatal outcomes, including preterm birth and growth restriction.
- *Treatment for unfamiliar diseases.* Always ask the specialist physician, 'What would you do if this woman was not pregnant?' Then assess the risks of this strategy in pregnancy.
- *Risks to the fetus.* These must be balanced against potential benefits to the mother (and therefore indirectly the fetus).

The *teratogenic potential* of some drugs classified as *'absolutely contraindicated'* (see Box 12.6) is sufficiently high to justify discussion of termination of a pregnancy following inadvertent exposure: these include mycophenolate mofetil, sodium valproate and thalidomide. For others, there are theoretical reasons to avoid their use in pregnancy, but they carry a low risk of teratogenesis

and therefore there is no justification for termination (e.g. rubella vaccine, simvastatin, ACE inhibitors).

For drugs that are *'relatively contraindicated'*, there are situations in which use is appropriate and where no safer alternative exists: for example, warfarin in women with prosthetic heart valves or AEDs in women with epilepsy.

- *Beta-blockers* should not be used as first-line treatment for hypertension, but may be indicated to control tachyarrhythmias, for migraine prophylaxis, thyrotoxicosis and mitral stenosis, and in those at risk of aortic dissection.
- *Diuretics* should be avoided in the treatment of hypertension but are appropriate in the treatment of pulmonary oedema.

Further reading

National Institute for Health and Care Excellence. *NICE Clinical Guideline 192: Antenatal and Postnatal Mental Health: Clinical Management and Service Guideline.* NICE 2018; https://www.nice.org.uk/guidance/cg192/chapter/1-Recommendations.

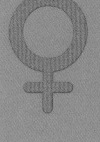

Women's health

Edward W. S. Mullins and Lesley Regan

CORE SKILLS AND KNOWLEDGE

Women experience specific illnesses related to their physiology and reproductive health, as well as having increased rates of common mental illnesses relative to men. About 1 in 20 women aged between 30 and 49 years consult their doctor each year because of menstrual problems, and 1 in 6 couples experience subfertility. Women in the UK will have a median of 1.8 children in their lifetime and 1 in 3 will have an abortion, although globally there are huge disparities in both of these rates.

The majority of gynaecological disorders are dealt with in primary care; referral is required if initial treatments have been ineffective or are contraindicated, or if gynaecological cancer is suspected. Outpatient services are often provided in one-stop Rapid Access Clinics, which allow a consultation, ultrasound and procedures such as hysteroscopy or colposcopy to be performed on the same day. Specialist clinics often employ specialist nurses to improve continuity of care and perform procedures.

Key skills in women's health include:

- taking a gynaecological history and performing speculum and bimanual examinations
- understanding contraception: the benefits and risks of different forms, and the physiological effects and drug interactions of hormonal preparations
- being familiar with the presentations of and treatment strategies for the common gynaecological cancers.

Experience of the conditions covered in this chapter can be gained in general gynaecological and antenatal clinics, early pregnancy and emergency gynaecology units, and a multitude of specialist clinics, including those for suspected gynaecological cancers, menopause and fertility disorders.

CLINICAL SKILLS FOR WOMEN'S HEALTH

History

Ensure that you have a confidential area in which to take a history and conduct an examination. You will need to ask direct but sensitive questions about intimate issues, and women may not feel comfortable talking about these in front of family members or friends (**Box 39.1**).

Examination

The vaginal (bimanual) examination and the speculum examination (**Fig. 39.1**) are crucial for diagnosing the cause of a number of gynaecological symptoms, including vaginal discharge, intra- or postmenopausal bleeding, and dyspareunia. First of all, consider the preliminaries listed in **Box 39.2**. Because these examinations may represent invasive, intimate and potentially uncomfortable experiences for a woman, it is essential to gain competence on pelvic training simulators.

Box 39.1 Taking a gynaecological history

Periods
- Age when periods began and stopped (if postmenopausal)
- Any significant changes in periods during that time
- Last menstrual period (LMP)
- Heavy or painful periods: most importantly, as perceived by the woman herself, but also gauged by semi-objective measures, e.g. whether she needs to take days off work, and the frequency with which sanitary towels require changing
- Regularity of periods: usual length of cycle and duration of bleeding

Pregnancies
- Outcomes of all pregnancies, beginning with the first and working chronologically; ask sensitively, as there may have been adverse outcomes and difficult decisions. Avoid confusing gravida/parity jargon; a chronological list is more useful

Medical history
- Past medical and surgical history
- Personal and family history of gynaecological and breast disorders
- Current and past medications: in women of childbearing age, focus on those that can affect pregnancy, e.g. sodium valproate

Cervical cancer risk factors
- Uptake of cervical screening; if so, date and outcomes of last screening. N.B. Women in same-sex relationships are also at risk of cervical cancer

- History of human papillomavirus (HPV) vaccination in younger women: introduced in the UK in 2008 for girls aged 12–13; extended to boys of the same age in 2018, chiefly to achieve herd immunity and reduce transmission to women

Sexual history
- All sexual partners and types of intercourse in the preceding 6 months
- Any history of sexually transmitted infections (STIs) and pelvic infections
- Current and past use of contraception

As appropriate
- Any history of sexual abuse or non-consensual sexual activity:
  - If the abuse or incident occurred recently, a forensic medical examination may be required to collect samples to support future criminal prosecution. An example of good practice exists in London, where the Havens provide a 24-hour service to organize this (see 'Further reading')
  - If the abuse or incident occurred some time ago, establish whether the woman has reported it to the police; if not, offer her support to do so now if she wishes. Also consider the need for psychological support
- Any history of female genital mutilation (FGM):
  - Ask all women who have grown up in countries where the practice is widespread, chiefly in Africa and the Middle East. The different types of FGM are listed in **Box 39.7**; they are linked to various health problems later in life

---

Box 39.2 Preliminaries to a vaginal or speculum examination

- Ensure that the environment is comfortable and private.
- Wash your hands.
- Introduce yourself (name and role) to the patient, confirming their details.
- Make sure that a chaperone is present (ideally, a female chaperone should support a male clinician) and record their name in the notes.
- Explain the proposed procedure clearly and answer any questions that the patient may have.
- Obtain explicit consent; explain that the patient may change her mind at any time.

- Ask whether there is any possibility that the patient might be pregnant.
- Put on gloves.
- Ask the patient to remove her underwear and lie on the examination couch with her heels drawn to her buttocks and her knees out to the sides (the modified lithotomy position).
- Provide a sheet or modesty blanket and ensure that the door is closed and locked.

Bimanual examination	Speculum examination
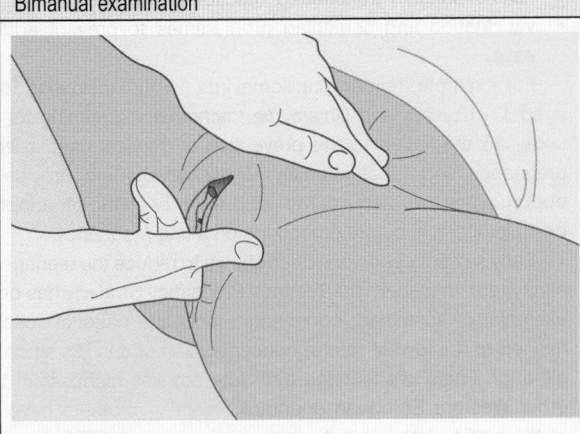	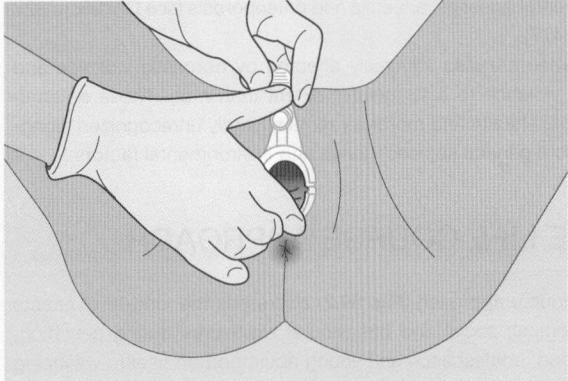

Bimanual examination

- Inspect vulva:
  - Ulcers
  - Vaginal discharge
  - Masses (malignant or abscesses)
- Enter vagina using two lubricated fingers
- Assess vagina (including the fornices) for masses or irregularities
- Assess cervix:
  - Masses
  - Os (open/closed)
  - Pain on palpation – 'cervical excitation'
- Assess uterus:
  - Place second hand on lower abdomen
  - Use internal fingers in posterior fornix to push uterus upwards and palpate between hands
  - Assess size, shape and position
- Assess adnexa:
  - Place internal fingers into left lateral fornix
  - Place other hand to palpate deeply in left iliac fossa
  - Move internal fingers towards other hand to assess for tenderness and masses
  - Repeat on right
- Close the encounter:
  - Stop examination, remove gloves
  - Offer paper towels and encourage patient to dress
  - Summarize findings and next steps
  - Document procedure and chaperone identity

Speculum examination

- Inspect vulva (see left)
- Insert speculum:
  - Warn patient you will now insert speculum
  - Lubricate speculum (if possible, also warm metal speculums)
  - Part labia using thumb and first finger of non-dominant hand
  - Insert the speculum sideways, rotate 90 degrees once inside (so handle faces upwards)
  - Open speculum blades and visualize cervix
  - Tighten locking nut to hold blades open
- Assess cervix:
  - Os (open/closed)
  - Ulcers
  - Masses
  - Discharge
- Perform any necessary diagnostic procedures:
  - Swabs for conventional culture or nucleic acid amplification tests (NAATs)
  - Smear test for cytology
- Remove speculum:
  - Loosen locking nut
  - Partially close blades, taking care not to trap vaginal wall between blades
  - Rotate 90 degrees and withdraw speculum
- Close the encounter (see left)
- Ensure all samples are sent for appropriate tests

Fig. 39.1 Bimanual and speculum examination.

INTRODUCTION

Women are affected by both general and gender-specific medical problems. They have predictable long-term reproductive healthcare needs and more frequent interactions with health services than men. Some 82% of women born in 1971 will have one or more children during their lives; this has decreased from almost 89% of women born in 1944. In addition to complications relating to pregnancy and childbirth (see Ch. 38), and to genital tract and breast cancers (see p. 1474 and p. 121), women also have a higher lifetime risk of common mental illnesses, anaemia and osteoporosis (see Ch. 25, p. 327 and p. 477).

Women are also adversely affected by domestic violence and sexual violence to a far greater extent than men. These determinants of ill-health and morbidity remain largely unrecognized alongside more general socioeconomic and environmental factors.

THE LIFE COURSE APPROACH

A life course approach (**Fig. 39.2**) addresses the long-term effects of biological, social and behavioural exposures during gestation, childhood, adolescence and young adulthood on health, wellbeing and disease in later life and across generations. This perspective recognizes that early life events can have an impact on long-term outcomes, that the circumstances of pregnancy can have an impact on the health of the offspring, and that early interventions may reduce the risk and severity of disease.

Women's reproductive and sexual health needs are largely predictable across their lifespan. The vast majority want to enjoy healthy sexual relationships and to control their own fertility.

Sexual health education

Relationships and sex education became statutory in primary and secondary schools in the UK from September 2019. It provides information on:
- what a healthy relationship should feel like
- consent, empowering girls to say no to unwanted attention and how to seek help if they are concerned
- optimal methods of contraception to avoid unplanned pregnancy
- risks of sexually transmitted infections (STIs, see Ch. 37)
- vaccination and screening programmes to prevent adult disease.

For example, human papillomavirus (HPV) vaccination for girls aged 11–13 years and *Chlamydia trachomatis* screening for those under 25 are linked to the prevention of cervical cancer, ectopic pregnancy and tubal infertility. These encounters provide early opportunities to discuss the long-term benefits of adopting a healthier lifestyle before embarking on a first pregnancy.

Early sex education has been shown to reduce the teenage pregnancy rate. In the UK, the Teenage Pregnancy Strategy has been an exemplar of sustained, coordinated local and national action and has led to the lowest rate of conceptions in under-18s since 1969, although England's teenage birth rate remains higher than that in other Western European countries. Teenage mothers have some of the worst obstetric outcomes, besides which 90% drop out of school and 20% become pregnant again in their teenage years.

Pre-pregnancy counselling

Forty per cent of pregnancies in the UK are unplanned and opportunities to provide general preconceptual advice on diet, weight,

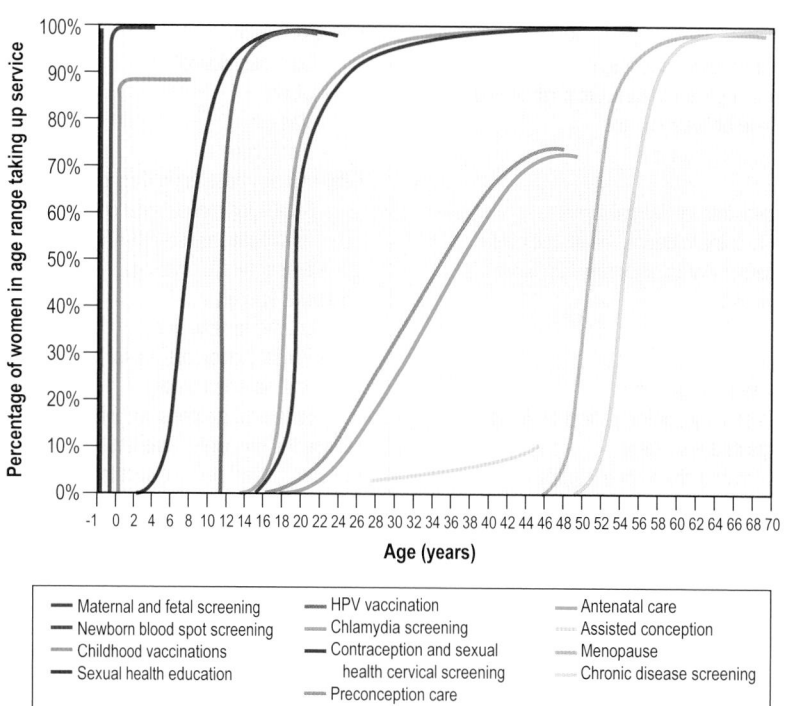

Fig. 39.2 The life course approach: major health issues specifically affecting women as they age. HPV, human papillomavirus. *(After Royal College of Obstetricians and Gynaecologists. SEC Opinion Paper 27; August 2011.)*

exercise, smoking, alcohol use and folic acid intake are often missed until women become pregnant. Pre-pregnancy counselling allows a review of general health and recent medication, and ensures that a management plan for the pregnancy is in place.

The 2018 MBRRACE-UK report into maternal mortality in 2014–16 (see 'Further reading, p. 1474) highlighted the fact that 68% of women who died were known to have identified pre-existing medical or mental health problems before they became pregnant, and 66% of the increased risk of maternal deaths in the UK could be attributed to these co-morbidities.

Around 20% of women in the UK now remain childless, either by choice or otherwise. A smaller, but growing, number of women are pursuing assisted conception, such as *in vitro* fertilization (IVF), to overcome their age-related decline in fertility, of which the British Fertility Society has highlighted that few women are aware. These women are at increased risk of serious complications during pregnancy due to medical co-morbidities. Access to IVF is recommended by the National Institute for Health and Care Excellence (NICE) but is currently restricted by many primary healthcare providers; local referral criteria and available funding are a source of inequality.

The physiological response to pregnancy

Complications in pregnancy that arise due to a woman's physiological response to pregnancy can reveal information about her future risk of disease. For example:

- *Pre-eclampsia* and *hypertension* in pregnancy resolve after delivery but are associated with higher cardiovascular mortality in later life (pre-eclampsia is associated with an odds ratio of 2.0 for cardiovascular disease).
- Roughly 50% of women with *gestational diabetes* will develop type 2 diabetes within 10 years, and children born of diabetic pregnancies are more likely to develop diabetes. These women should be screened annually for diabetes and placed on a diabetes risk register in primary care.
- *Teenage pregnancies* and *premature deliveries* repeat across generations.
- Perinatal *mental illness* affects 1 in 5 women and is the leading direct cause of maternal death up to 1 year postnatally; it is associated with low birth weight and impaired intellectual development, as measured by lower IQ at age 3 years.

Pregnancy should be viewed as the Healthcare Opportunity of Two Lifetimes (HOOTL, **Fig. 39.3**), which offers major potential for population health gain and is the first step on the way to tackling and interrupting the cross-generational transmission of ill-health.

The postnatal visit

The postnatal visit is an ideal time to plan future healthcare needs for mother and baby, and can have a positive impact on lifestyle issues such as obesity, exercise, dental health, contraception, smoking and drug misuse. Review of the recent pregnancy will provide valuable information on the risk of future morbidity and provides an opportunity for prevention of diabetes, cardiovascular disease and recurrent pregnancy complications.

The normal menstrual cycle

Definitions and some disorders

- *Puberty* (see p. 632). The mean age of menarche is 12.8 years but it may take several years for the menstrual cycle to establish a regular pattern. The initial cycles are usually anovulatory and frequently unpredictable.
- *Precocious puberty* (see p. 636). This is defined as menses or breast development before the age of 8 years.
- *Delayed puberty* (see p. 636). This is defined as the absence of secondary sex characteristics after 14 years. It may be due to a central defect (including anorexia, excessive exercise, chronic illness or pituitary tumour) or to a failure of gonadal function (Turner's syndrome, XX gonadal dysgenesis).
- *Amenorrhoea* (see p. 628). This is defined as primary in a girl who fails to menstruate by 16 years of age, and secondary when the menses stop for more than 6 months in a normal female who is not pregnant, lactating or menopausal.
- *Menorrhagia.* This is defined as menses with abnormally heavy or prolonged bleeding.
- *Premenstrual syndrome (PMS)* (see p. 772). This is extremely common. In 5–15%, the severity of the progesterone-induced bloating, weight gain, mastalgia, headaches, depression and irritability in the luteal phase are so debilitating that lifestyle and personal relationships are adversely affected. Treatment success, using lifestyle modifications, hormonal preparations, cognitive behavioural therapy, selective serotonin reuptake inhibitors (SSRIs) and surgery, is highly variable.

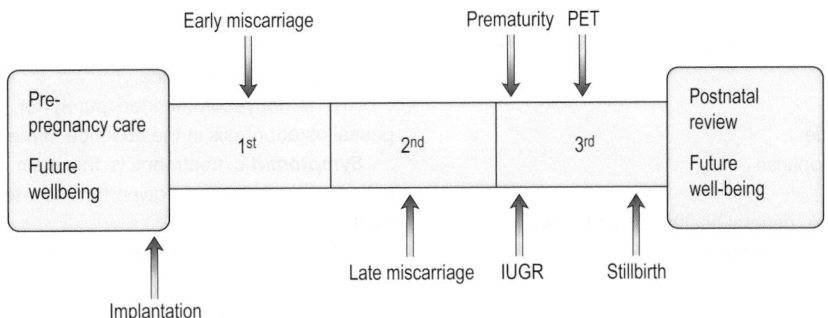

Fig. 39.3 The Healthcare Opportunity of Two Lifetimes (HOOTL). IUGR, intrauterine growth retardation; PET, pre-eclampsia.

- *Premature ovarian insufficiency (POI)* (see p. 628). This is defined as cessation of periods before 40 years of age and occurs in 1% of women.
- *Menopause.* The average age of menopause among Western women is 51 (see below).
- *Postmenopausal bleeding (PMB).* The majority of cases of PMB are due to benign atrophic vaginitis and respond to topical oestrogens. Approximately 10% of cases of PMB will have some sort of pathology, such as atypical hyperplasia or cancer, requiring staging and usually surgical clearance of the uterus and ovaries, with or without adjuvant therapy. Investigation is by ultrasound to assess endometrial thickness, proceeding to tissue sampling when it exceeds 3–5 mm. Women on tamoxifen for breast disease may have irregular, thickened and cystic endometrium, and require hysteroscopy and directed tissue biopsy.

Menopause

The menopause, or cessation of periods, naturally occurs at about the age of 45–55 years. Female life expectancy has increased significantly over the last century, with many women now living into their eighties or nineties. During the fifth decade, follicle stimulating hormone (FSH) concentrations and then luteinizing hormone (LH) concentrations begin to rise, probably as follicle supply diminishes. Oestrogen levels fall and the menstrual cycle becomes disrupted. Most women notice a gradual change to irregular, scanty periods, although sudden amenorrhoea or menorrhagia occurs in some. Eventually, the menopausal pattern of low oestradiol levels with grossly elevated LH and FSH levels (usually >50 and >25 U/L, respectively) is established. Premature menopause may also occur as a result of surgery, or of radiotherapy to the ovaries, or due to ovarian disease.

Clinical features

In women over 45 years, the following can be diagnosed without laboratory tests:
- perimenopause based on vasomotor symptoms and irregular periods
- menopause in women who have not had a period for at least 12 months and are not using hormonal contraception
- menopause based on symptoms in women without a uterus

   Features of oestrogen deficiency are hot flushes (which occur in most women and can be disabling), vaginal dryness and atrophy of the breasts. There may also be loss of libido, loss of self-esteem, non-specific aches and pains, sleep disturbance, irritability, depression, loss of concentration, and weight gain.

   Women show a rapid loss of bone density in the 10 years following the menopause (osteoporosis; see p. 477), and the premenopausal protection against ischaemic heart disease disappears.

Management

Explanation should include:
- the stages of the menopause
- common symptoms
- lifestyle changes to help general health and wellbeing
- the benefits and risks of treatments
- the long-term implications of menopause
   Treatment options include:
- hormonal, e.g. hormone replacement therapy
- non-hormonal, e.g. clonidine
- non-pharmaceutical, e.g. cognitive behavioural therapy.

> **ℹ Box 39.3 Risks and benefits of hormone replacement therapy (HRT)[a]**
>
> **Potential benefits**
> - *Symptomatic improvement in most menopausal symptoms* for the majority of women. Oestrogen-deficient symptoms respond well to oestrogen replacement; the vaguer general symptoms may or may not improve. Vaginal symptoms also respond to local oestrogen preparations.
> - *Protection against fractures of wrist, spine and hip, secondary to osteoporosis* (~24–33%) (see p. 477), owing to protection of predominantly trabecular bone (see p. 473).
> - *Significant reduction in the risk of large bowel cancer* (~33%).
> - *Possible increase in general wellbeing*, although hopes for a reduction in the incidence of Alzheimer's disease have not been confirmed.
>
> **Potential risks**
> - *Significant increase in the risk of breast cancer* (+26%) but no change in breast cancer mortality. This is primarily a risk of combined oestrogen–progesterone HRT. Some studies suggest that breast cancers diagnosed on HRT are easier to treat effectively.
> - *Significant increase in the risk of endometrial cancer* when unopposed oestrogens are given to women with a uterus.
> - *Significant increase in the risk of ischaemic heart disease* (+29%) and *stroke* (+41%).
> - *Inconvenience of withdrawal bleeds*, unless a hysterectomy has been performed or regimens used that include continuous oestrogen and progesterone.
>
> [a]Percentages are from the Women's Health Initiative (WHI) study of 16 600 women.

Hormone replacement therapy

Symptomatic patients should usually be treated but the previous widespread use of hormone replacement therapy (HRT) has been thrown into doubt by a number of large prospective studies that have reported in recent years. The overall benefits and risks are dependent on whether oestrogen alone or oestrogen and progesterone are combined, and are summarized in the most recent NICE guidance (**Box 39.3**). Absolute risks and benefits for individual women clearly depend on their background risk of a specific disease, and there is as yet no evidence on the relative risks of different hormone preparations or routes of administration (oral, transdermal or implant), excepting a lower risk of venous thromboembolism with transdermal preparations. Overall, the Women's Health Initiative (WHI) study estimated that, over 5 years of treatment, one extra woman in every 100 would develop an illness that would not have occurred, had she not been taking HRT. However, the decision about whether or not a woman takes HRT is now very much an individual one and is based on:
- the severity of the woman's menopausal symptoms
- her personal risk of conditions that may be prevented or made more likely by HRT
- individual patient choice.

   HRT is not recommended purely for prevention of postmenopausal osteoporosis in the absence of menopausal symptoms.

   Symptomatic treatment is the main indication, with the lowest effective dose being given for short-term rather than long-term treatment.

   Selective oestrogen receptor modulators (SERMs, e.g. raloxifene) offer a potentially attractive combination of positive oestrogen effects on bone and cardiovascular system with no effects on oestrogen receptors of uterus and breast, and a possible reduction in breast cancer incidence; long-term outcome studies are still awaited, however.

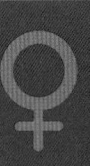

The Women's Health Initiative and Million Women Study suggested an association between longer-term usage of HRT and an increased risk of breast cancer, stroke and venous thromboembolism, but this has recently been challenged. The incidence of ischaemic heart disease increases after the menopause but this is 10 years later than in men.

Further reading

Chlebowski RT, Schwartz AG, Wakelee H et al. Oestrogen plus progestin and lung cancer in postmenopausal women (Women's Health Initiative trial): a post-hoc analysis of a randomised controlled trial. *Lancet* 2009; 374:1243–1251.

Manson JE, Chlebowski RT, Stefanick ML et al. Menopausal hormone therapy and health outcomes during the intervention and extended poststopping phases of the Women's Health Initiative randomized trials. *JAMA* 2013; 310:1353–1368.

National Institute for Health and Care Excellence. *NICE Clinical Guideline NG23: Menopause: Diagnosis and Treatment.* NICE 2015; https://www.nice.org.uk/guidance/ng23.

Palmert MR, Dunkel L. Delayed puberty. *N Engl J Med* 2012; 336:443–453.

Royal College of Obstetricians and Gynaecologists. *Why Should We Consider a Life Course Approach to Women's Health Care?* Scientific Impact Paper No. 27. London: RCOG; 2011.

https://www.ons.gov.uk/peoplepopulationandcommunity/birthsdeathsandmarriages/conceptionandfertilityrates/bulletins/conceptionstatistics/2017. *UK Office for National Statistics.*

https://www.thehavens.org.uk/referrals/how-do-i-refer/. *A 24-hour service in the UK that organizes forensic medical examination to collect samples to support future criminal prosecution of an attacker.*

Contraception

Control of fertility has positive effects on a woman's health and wellbeing. Those who lack access to contraceptive methods are at increased risk of mortality and morbidity, due to obstetric complications and the consequences of illegal abortion. More than 30% of maternal deaths and 10% of child mortality can be prevented by ensuring a 2-year interval between each pregnancy.

Women require expert advice about the safest and most suitable methods of contraception available to them at different ages. In general, contraception is extremely safe, although some methods do have rare but serious side-effects. The combined oestrogen–progestogen pill also protects against both ovarian and endometrial cancer, and many hormonal methods help control heavy or painful periods. Barrier methods prevent STIs and protect against cervical cancer.

The efficacy of any contraceptive method depends on how it works and how easy it is to use. A wide choice of contraception options is now available. They include barrier methods (condoms, diaphragms), the combined oestrogen–progestogen or progestogen-only pill, long-acting progestogen injection or implant, and intrauterine systems. Each has its advantages and disadvantages.

Hormonal contraception

Hormonal contraception (delivered by several routes, including pills, transdermal patches, subdermal implants and intrauterine coils) provides either a combination of oestrogen and progesterone, or progesterone alone, with different risk and benefit profiles:

- **Combined oestrogen and progesterone contraceptives** act to prevent ovulation, make the endometrium hostile to implantation, and alter the cervical mucus. They are highly effective but only if used correctly and consistently. Minor side-effects may lead to discontinuation and include headaches, mood swings, bloating, weight gain and breast tenderness. The more significant risks relate to cardiovascular disease, including venous thromboembolism (three- to fivefold increase), myocardial infarction and stroke (rare). These preparations are contraindicated in many women, including those at high risk of cardiovascular disease and venous thromboembolism.
- **Progestogen-only preparations** avoid the side-effects of oestrogen and are suitable for women who are breast-feeding, are older,

are smokers and have cardiovascular risks (hypertension, diabetes). They act on cervical mucus and the endometrium, but higher-dose preparations also inhibit ovulation. Common side-effects include irregular bleeding, simple ovarian cysts, breast tenderness and acne.

Preparations of hormonal contraception include:

The combined oral contraceptive pill

The combined oestrogen–progestogen pill is widely used for contraception and has a low failure rate (<1 per 100 woman-years). 'Pills' contain 20–40 µg of oestrogen, usually ethinylestradiol, together with a variable amount of one of several progestogens. The mechanism of action is twofold:

- suppression by oestrogen of gonadotrophins, thus preventing follicular development, ovulation and luteinization
- progestogen effects on cervical mucus, making it hostile to sperm, and on tubal motility and the endometrium.

Side-effects of these preparations are shown in **Box 39.4**. Most of the serious ones are rare and are less common with typical modern 20–30 µg oestrogen pills, although evidence suggests that thromboembolism may be slightly more common with 'third-generation pills' containing desogestrel and gestodene (approximately 30/100 000 woman-years compared with 15/100 000 on older pills and 5/100 000 on no treatment). While some problems require immediate cessation of the pill, other milder side-effects must be judged against the hazards of pregnancy occurring with inadequate contraception, especially if other effective methods are not practicable or acceptable.

Hazards of the combined pill are increased in smokers, the obese and those with other risk factors for cardiovascular disease (e.g. hypertension, hyperlipidaemia, diabetes), especially in women aged over 35 years (avoid if over 50 years).

The 'mini-pill'

The 'mini-pill' (progestogen-only, usually norethisterone) is less effective than the combined pill but is suitable for women who are breast-feeding, are older, are smokers, have other cardiovascular risk factors or cannot tolerate the combined pill because of side-effects such as loss of libido (see **Box 39.4**).

Long-acting reversible contraceptiion

Long-acting reversible contraceptive (LARC) methods, such as implants, injectables and intrauterine devices, all have lower failure rates than user-dependent contraception and tend to have better continuation rates as they cannot be easily abandoned. They have also been shown to be more cost-effective than oral contraceptives. LARC methods generally deliver progesterone-only contraception, and include:

- Subdermal implants (e.g. Nexplanon), which are inserted in the upper arm using local anaesthetic and last for 3 years. They are a highly effective method of long-term contraception and offer a rapid return of fertility after removal. Irregular bleeding is common.
- Injectables (e.g. Depo-Provera), which are given intramuscularly and are effective for 12 weeks. Side-effects include weight gain, irregular periods or amenorrhoea, and delays in return of fertility of up to 6 months.
- Intrauterine systems (e.g. the Mirena coil, which is effective for 5 years – see later).

Barrier methods

Condoms, diaphragms, spermicides and sponges, which require users to remember to employ them correctly every time they have sexual intercourse, have the highest failure rates but offer protection against STIs.

> ### i Box 39.4 Adverse effects and drug interactions of oral contraceptives (mixed oestrogen–progesterone combinations)
>
> **General**
> - Weight gain
> - Loss of libido
> - Pigmentation (chloasma)
> - Breast tenderness
> - Increased growth rate of some malignancies
>
> **Cardiovascular**
> - Increased blood pressure[a]
> - Deep vein thrombosis[a]
> - Myocardial infarction
> - Stroke (migraine is a risk factor)
>
> **Gastrointestinal**
> - Nausea and vomiting
> - Abnormal liver biochemistry
> - Gallstones increased
> - Hepatic tumours
>
> **Nervous system**
> - Headache
> - Migraine[a]
> - Depression[a]
>
> **Malignancy**
> - Increase in cancer of the breast (but reduced risk of ovarian and endometrial cancer)
>
> **Gynaecological**
> - Amenorrhoea
> - 'Spotting'
> - Cervical erosion
>
> **Haematological**
> - Increased clotting tendency
>
> **Endocrine/metabolic**
> - Mild impairment of glucose tolerance
> - Worsened lipid profile, though variable
>
> **Drug interactions[b]**
> - Antibiotics
> - Barbiturates
> - Carbamazepine
> - Phenytoin
> - Rifampicin
> - St John's wort
>
> [a]Common reasons for stopping oral contraceptives.
> [b]Reduced contraceptive effect owing to enzyme induction.

> ### i Box 39.5 Practical classification of miscarriage
>
> | Type of miscarriage | Ultrasound findings | Clinical presentation |
> |---|---|---|
> | Biochemical pregnancy | Uterine cavity empty | PV bleeding 'late period' after positive pregnancy test |
> | Threatened miscarriage | Intrauterine pregnancy | PV bleeding and pain Speculum: cervical os closed |
> | Inevitable miscarriage | Intrauterine pregnancy | PV bleeding and pain Speculum: cervical os open |
> | Incomplete miscarriage | Retained products of conception in cavity | PV bleeding and pain Speculum: cervical os open ± products in cervical os |
> | Complete miscarriage | Uterine cavity empty, no retained products | Pain and PV bleeding resolved Speculum: cervical os closed |
> | Missed miscarriage | Fetal pole present >7 mm, no heartbeat present; or gestation sac >25 mm if no fetal pole | ± PV bleeding and pain |
>
> PV, *per vaginam*.

Intrauterine contraceptive devices

Intrauterine contraceptive devices (IUDs) are a highly effective and increasingly popular method of contraception that is independent of intercourse and user compliance. The device is inserted into the uterine cavity by trained healthcare personnel and a thread is left protruding from the cervix into the vagina, which allows the IUD to be removed by traction.

Copper IUDs are cheap, licensed for 5–10 years of use and cause less menstrual disruption than the older plastic models. They have a toxic effect on both egg and sperm before fertilization occurs.

Levonorgestrol-releasing intrauterine systems (e.g. Mirena) are licensed for contraception, the treatment of heavy menstrual bleeding, and use as part of HRT regimens. The duration of use is 3–5 years, depending on the device, during which time many women become amenorrhoeic. Irregular vaginal spotting is common initially but may resolve. Some women complain of greasier skin, breast tenderness and mood swings but these symptoms often settle with time.

Emergency contraception

Emergency contraception can be used following unprotected intercourse. Levonorgestrol is available over the counter in the UK and needs to be taken within 72 hours. Ulipristal acetate can be used up to 120 hours after intercourse but is available on prescription only. Insertion of a copper IUD within 5 days is highly effective.

Permanent contraception

This may be achieved by male or female sterilization but both carry a late failure rate, quoted as 1:2000 and 1:200, respectively. Male vasectomy can be carried out under local anaesthetic.

MISCARRIAGE

Miscarriage is a pregnancy that ends spontaneously before the fetus reaches a viable gestational age. The term includes all pregnancy losses between the time of conception and 24 weeks of gestation. Sporadic miscarriage is the most common complication of pregnancy and the majority of cases are due to random genetic abnormalities in the embryo or fetus. The incidence of clinically recognized miscarriage is generally quoted as 15–20%, but the total number of very early conceptions that are lost is in the region of 50%. The miscarriage rate decreases with advancing gestation, reaching 10% by 8 weeks and 3% after a heartbeat is seen on ultrasound scan. By 13 weeks (the start of the second trimester), no more than 1% of viable pregnancies are lost.

Maternal age at conception and previous reproductive history are strong and independent risk factors for miscarriage. The risk of fetal loss rises steeply after the age of 35 years, reaching 75% by 45 years, as the increase in poor-quality oocytes leads to chromosomally abnormal conceptions. Delayed childbearing has resulted in increased rates of miscarriage, ectopic pregnancy, stillbirth and other later complications of pregnancy. Less common factors contributing to early pregnancy loss are uterine abnormalities, infections, medical/endocrine disorders and exposure to drugs and chemicals.

The different types of miscarriage can be classified by the clinical presentation and the results of investigations (**Box 39.5**). Vaginal bleeding in early pregnancy is common and the differential diagnosis includes:

- a threatened, inevitable or incomplete miscarriage
- bleeding from a viable pregnancy
- ectopic pregnancy
- lower genital tract pathology
- trophoblastic disease.

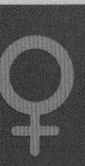

Sensitive home pregnancy testing kits have identified many biochemical pregnancies that fail to implant successfully and resolve spontaneously as a delayed and/or heavy menstrual period.

A detailed clinical history must be taken and examination performed in women presenting with vaginal bleeding in pregnancy:

- *Speculum examination* (see p. 1464) assesses the state of the cervix and excludes lower genital tract pathology such as cervical polyps or ectropion.
- *Transvaginal ultrasound* determines the location, gestation, nature and viability of the pregnancy. It also offers the woman valuable reassurance if fetal heart activity can be shown.

Bleeding and pain associated with products of conception that are distending the cervical canal can be very severe, and should be promptly removed with sponge forceps. Serial measurements of serum beta-human chorionic gonadotrophin (β-HCG) levels may be necessary when the site of pregnancy is unknown.

Severe pain localized to either iliac fossa and peritonism are suggestive of ectopic pregnancy and may warrant urgent laparoscopic assessment and treatment. However, many ectopic gestations resolve spontaneously by being resorbed or miscarried from the tube into the peritoneal cavity.

Management

This depends on clinical presentation and patient choice. Most miscarriages can be managed expectantly, although urgent surgical evacuation may be required if the bleeding becomes heavy.

- *Follow-up urinary pregnancy test or pelvic scan* confirms whether the miscarriage is complete.
- *Prostaglandins* (oral or vaginal misoprostol) to induce uterine contractions and expulsion are cheap and effective.
- *Subsequent surgical evacuation of the uterus* is required for a small number of women.

The recommended first-line management for miscarriage in the UK is expectant for 7–14 days, although the initial choice of strategy depends on the woman's preference, her risk of haemorrhage, previous adverse events and evidence of infection. Medical management of miscarriage in the UK is with 800 μg misoprostol; mifepristone is no longer routinely used. Surgical management of miscarriage (or evacuation of the retained products of conception, ERPC) can be performed by suction under general anaesthesia or by manual vacuum aspiration (MVA) under local anaesthesia. It is associated with a small but definite morbidity, including uterine perforation, cervical trauma, intrauterine adhesion formation and postoperative pelvic infection.

Recurrent miscarriage

Recurrent miscarriage (RM), the loss of three or more consecutive pregnancies, affects 1–2% of women trying to conceive and is associated with significant psychological morbidity. Investigation includes a search for parental translocations and for anatomical, infective, endocrine, immune and thrombophilic causes. Most cases remain unexplained, which conveys a good prognosis for future pregnancy outcome.

Currently, the most treatable cause of RM is the antiphospholipid syndrome (see p. 459), which is present in 15–20% of all women with RM. When it is managed with low-dose aspirin and heparin, a live birth rate of more than 75% can be achieved.

Women with a history of recurrent miscarriage are at greater risk of pre-eclampsia, fetal growth restriction and prematurity when they achieve a successful pregnancy because all of these problems are determined by the quality and depth of early implantation. These patients are also more likely to suffer strokes at an earlier age than women with no miscarriage history.

Miscarriages can cause acute anxiety, depression, denial, anger, blame, severed relationships and a sense of loss and inadequacy. Compassionate counselling services and access to support groups for women who have experienced pregnancy loss are needed.

Stillbirths

Various definitions exist for stillbirth as distinct from miscarriage, and generally are based on gestational age (varying from 20 to 28 weeks). The World Health Organization (WHO) defines stillbirth as a pregnancy loss with a fetal weight of 1000 g or more, an assumed equivalent of 28 weeks' gestation. Worldwide, there were 2.6 million third-trimester stillbirths in 2015. Although there was a reduction in maternal and child mortality, both targeted in the Millennium Development Goals (MDGs, see p. 278), the number of stillbirths annually remains high, sadly with little reduction in the past decade. Intrapartum losses are extremely high, at 1.3 million, many of which are preventable.

Further reading

Lancet Series 1, 2, 3. Ending preventable stillbirths. *Lancet* 2016; 387:374, 387, 604.
https://www.npeu.ox.ac.uk/downloads/files/mbrrace-uk/reports/MBRRACE-UK%20Perinatal%20Surveillance%20Full%20Report%20for%202016%20-%20June%202018.pdf. *MBRRACE-UK Perinatal Mortality Surveillance Report: UK Perinatal Deaths for Births from January to December 2016.*

HEAVY MENSTRUAL BLEEDING

Heavy menstrual bleeding (HMB) accounts for 1 in 5 gynaecology clinic consultations and is the most common cause of iron deficiency anaemia. Objective methods to quantify menstrual blood loss are inaccurate and therefore clinical assessment, based on the woman's perception of blood loss and how it impacts on her quality of life, is needed. Periods characterized by the passage of large blood clots, severe pain or flooding that prevents the woman leaving home require investigation and management. The 2018 NICE guidance provides clear and practical advice on assessment and management (see 'Further reading').

Briefly, it is necessary to take a detailed menstrual and general medical history. On examination, signs of anaemia should be sought. Abdominal and pelvic examination is carried out to exclude pelvic masses, visualize the cervix, perform a smear if needed, and take swabs if infection is suspected. Investigations to consider are:

- *full blood count and iron studies* – to assess the need for iron replacement and, in extreme cases, blood transfusion
- *a haematological opinion* – if the history is consistent with a coagulation disorder
- *ultrasound scan* – if a pelvic mass is palpated or the bleeding pattern suggests endometrial pathology
- *endometrial biopsy* (at the outpatient clinic or at hysteroscopy in women aged >45 years) – for irregular or intermenstrual bleeding and where drug therapy fails
- *ultrasound and haematological investigation* – young women presenting with menorrhagia from their first period.

Selecting the most appropriate treatment for HMB involves patient preference, risk/benefit analysis of the available options, the woman's fertility and contraceptive requirements, and any contraindications to medical or surgical therapies.

Management

First-line medical therapies

Choice depends on women's preference and the presence of fibroids and any co-morbidities. Strategies include:

- **Levonorgestrel intrauterine system** (LNG-IUS or Mirena coil). This has revolutionized the treatment of HMB. It results in a 95% reduction in blood loss (30% of women are amenorrhoeic within 1 year of insertion), is an effective contraceptive, improves dysmenorrhoea and has few side-effects. It should be considered in the majority of women with HMB as an alternative to surgical treatment. Some women are troubled by irregular bleeding and persistent spotting for the first 3–9 months after insertion.
- **Tranexamic acid.** This antifibrinolytic agent is associated with a 50% reduction in HMB.
- **Mefenamic acid.** This non-steroidal anti-inflammatory drug (NSAID) is associated with a 25% reduction in bleeding and is taken during the menses.
- **Combined oral contraceptive pill.** This has the added advantage of providing effective contraception but may be contraindicated in women with risk factors for thromboembolism or breast cancer, smokers over the age of 35 and the obese.
- **Oral progestogens.** Taken on days 6–26 of the menstrual cycle, these may regulate the bleeding pattern, but are not contraceptive and can cause breakthrough bleeding.
- **Ulipristal acetate.** This can be added to the choice of strategies in women with fibroids >3 cm, acknowledging the risk of rare but serious liver injury.

Gonadotrophin-releasing hormone (GnRH) agonist drugs act on the pituitary and result in amenorrhoea. They are suitable only for short-term use because they produce a hypo-oestrogenic state that predisposes to osteoporosis.

Surgical treatments

Surgical treatments for HMB should generally be offered only when medical treatments have failed and when women have completed their family.

- **Endometrial ablation techniques.** These destroy the endometrial lining to a depth that prevents cyclical regeneration. The second-generation microwave and thermal ablation techniques are highly successful in treating HMB and are undertaken as day-case procedures.
- **Hysterectomy.** Removal of the uterus may be via abdominal, vaginal or laparoscopic routes, depending on the size of the uterine body, the degree of laxity of the pelvic muscular floor and the skill set of the surgeon. Histology of the uterus is normal in about 40% of cases. The vaginal and laparoscopic surgical procedures usually mean shorter hospital stays and a faster return to normal activities.

Uterine fibroids (leiomyomata)

These are the most common solid pelvic tumours in women of reproductive age. The prevalence increases with age and is higher in Afro-Caribbean women. Heavy and/or prolonged periods, pressure symptoms due to the pelvic mass, and reproductive dysfunction are common presenting symptoms. The mechanism(s) by which fibroids cause HMB are poorly understood but submucosal lesions within the uterine cavity are particularly troublesome.

Management

Treatment is surgical excision, with magnetic resonance-guided focused ultrasound or uterine artery embolization (UAE), for which the uterine arteries are selectively catheterized via a femoral approach and microbeads are injected until flow is demonstrably reduced. There is a small risk of menopause where the ovarian circulation arises dominantly from the uterine arteries; this should be screened for with angiography prior to embolization. Pregnancy after UAE carries an increased risk of abnormal placental implantation and generally this approach should be considered only if future pregnancy is not intended.

GnRH agonists can be used to alleviate HMB as a short-term measure or to shrink the overall size and vascularity of the fibroids prior to surgery.

Recent data on the incidence of sarcoma within fibroids (0.05–0.29%) has led to changes in counselling for non-hysterectomy management of fibroids: after laparoscopic myomectomy, fibroids are morcellated to allow removal, and the risks of sarcoma must be presented in a balanced way when considering management.

ABORTION/TERMINATION OF PREGNANCY

Unintended pregnancy is common and abortion is one of the most frequently performed gynaecological procedures. One in three women will have an abortion in their lifetime. However, abortion remains a controversial subject, mostly related to cultural, moral and religious beliefs.

Every year, an estimated 210 million pregnancies occur worldwide: 80 million are unplanned and 50 million are terminated by abortion, 20 million of them illegally. Where abortion for unintended pregnancy is illegal, it is invariably unsafe and frequently has tragic sequelae. Approximately 70 000 maternal deaths occur each year due to unsafe abortion, 99% of them in developing countries.

In developed countries that have legalized abortion, the procedure is extremely safe. The risk of death from an early surgical termination of pregnancy is less than 1 per 100 000, which is far lower than the maternal mortality associated with a full-term pregnancy. Abortion was legalized in the UK in 1967 and 95% of the 190 000 procedures performed yearly are for Clause C of the Abortion Act, which states that the pregnancy has not exceeded its 24th week and that continuance of the pregnancy would involve risk, greater than if the pregnancy were terminated, of injury to the physical or mental health of the pregnant woman. Only 1% of abortions are done because of a risk that the child would be born handicapped.

Induced abortion can be undertaken surgically under local or general anaesthesia or using drug regimens that induce miscarriage. The type of procedure is generally dictated by the gestation of the pregnancy, availability of methods and the wishes of the woman concerned. The earlier an abortion is performed, the safer it is. Currently, 91% of abortions in the UK are carried out before 13 weeks' gestation.

Early medical abortion (before 9 weeks' gestation), using misoprostol to expel the products, achieves a complete abortion in over 80% of cases. Asthma and cardiac disease are contraindications to medical abortion. Most women remain in the clinical facility for 4–6 hours after the misoprostol insertion to abort the pregnancy, but some units support women so that they can remain at home during an early medical abortion. UK legislation passed in 2018 allows misoprostol to be taken at home for abortion, and clinical service change will probably follow.

Surgical abortions before 14 weeks are usually performed as suction terminations under general anaesthesia. Preoperative priming of the cervix with oral or vaginal misoprostol reduces the risk of

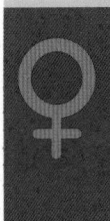

cervical trauma and haemorrhage. Early abortions before 7 weeks can be performed with an MVA syringe under local anaesthesia.

With modern early abortion techniques and routine screening for pelvic infection in high-risk women, the risk of future subfertility is extremely low. Later medical and surgical abortions are associated with more complications: in particular, incomplete procedures, pelvic infection and trauma to the genital tract. Contraception should be discussed before the abortion and started immediately after the procedure to avoid a further unplanned pregnancy.

Many women are emotionally vulnerable following an abortion. Feelings of guilt and regret are frequently mixed with relief that the ordeal is over. There is no evidence of an increase in serious psychiatric disease after abortion. Psychological problems can be minimized with careful counselling before the procedure and access to post-abortion support services.

URINARY INCONTINENCE

Urinary incontinence (UI) is common and has a negative impact on a woman's quality of life. One in three women over the age of 60 years suffers from some urinary leakage and the majority are too embarrassed to seek help, despite the fact that the symptoms can often be alleviated by simple, non-pharmacological interventions. As the average age of populations in developing countries continues to rise, UI will become an even more prevalent problem, placing an increasingly large demand on healthcare resources.

NICE guidelines offer a simple classification of female UI (**Box 39.6**). Other factors that may predominate, especially in elderly women, such as functional incontinence secondary to immobility, are discussed on page 312.

Lifestyle interventions, including weight loss, smoking cessation, caffeine reduction and timed fluid restriction, can alleviate the symptoms of UI significantly. Physiotherapy and bladder retraining may be helpful in cases of stress and urgency, respectively, and also for mixed UI. In postmenopausal women, oestrogen deficiency exaggerates many urinary symptoms, and topical vaginal or systemic HRT is a treatment option.

Referral for specialist management may include detailed assessment of the pelvic floor and any prolapse, urinary tract imaging and urodynamic evaluation where appropriate. Discussion of further management is based on the type of incontinence, the woman's preferences and future fertility wishes.

DOMESTIC ABUSE AND VIOLENCE

Domestic violence is the cause of considerable hidden morbidity and mortality. One in four women in England and Wales experience some form of domestic abuse or violence – whether it be psychological, physical, sexual, financial or emotional – during their lifetime. One in ten women experience rape. Domestic violence accounts for one-third of violent crimes, and the cost of domestic violence in human and economic terms is enormous: an estimated £23 billion per annum in the UK alone.

There are several groups of people who are more vulnerable to becoming victims. Around 30% of domestic abuse begins or escalates during pregnancy. After road accidents, domestic abuse is the second leading cause of trauma during pregnancy, and pregnant women are more likely to have multiple sites of injury. The prevalence among women requesting a termination of pregnancy is six times higher than among women attending antenatal clinics. The disabled are also at greater risk of abuse: the odds of being a victim of violence are twofold higher in people with a physical disability and threefold higher in those with a mental illness. Sex workers, trafficked women and certain ethnic groups also have a higher prevalence of domestic violence.

Victims of domestic abuse are significantly more likely to commit suicide. Domestic violence and abuse are serious health concerns, and healthcare professionals are particularly well placed to identify abuse and intervene, as the victims frequently present to departments of Emergency Medicine, Psychiatry, and Obstetrics and Gynaecology. Healthcare professionals have a role to play in tackling the problem and are often the first and only point of contact to whom the isolated and vulnerable victim reaches out. All healthcare workers need to be trained to recognize the signs of violence and abuse, use targeted questioning, and know how to act and refer to ensure the women's safety.

The key actions to reduce violence against women and girls are shown in **Fig. 39.4**.

Female genital mutilation

A cultural form of violence against women commonly seen in obstetric and gynaecological practice is female genital mutilation (FGM). A classification of FGM is shown in **Box 39.7**. In recent years the problems associated with FGM have become apparent in the UK. FGM was made illegal in the Female Genital Mutilation Act 2003; however, the only prosecution in the UK to date involved a doctor, who was found not guilty. It is estimated that 21 000 young women are at risk of FGM.

FGM has wide-ranging physical sequelae. Acutely, these include severe pain, abscess formation, sepsis, tetanus, haemorrhage,

---

i **Box 39.6 Classification of urinary incontinence (UI) in women**

- *Stress UI* is involuntary urine leakage on effort or exertion, or on sneezing or coughing.
- *Urgency UI* is involuntary urine leakage accompanied or immediately preceded by urgency (a sudden compelling desire to urinate that is difficult to delay).
- *Mixed UI* is involuntary urine leakage associated with both urgency and exertion, effort, sneezing or coughing.
- *Overactive bladder (OAB)* is defined as urgency that occurs with or without urgency UI, and usually with frequency and nocturia.

Protection – delivering an effective criminal justice system:
Investigation; prosecution; victim support and protection; perpetrator programmes

Provision – helping women and girls to continue with their lives:
Effective advice and support; emergency and acute services; refuges and safe accommodation

Prevention – changing attitudes and preventing violence:
Awareness-raising campaigns; safeguarding and educating children and young people; early identification/intervention and training

Fig. 39.4 Key actions to reduce violence against women and girls. *(After National Institute for Health and Care Excellence. NICE Public Health Guidance 50: Domestic Violence and Abuse: Multi-Agency Working. NICE 2014.)*

ⓘ Box 39.7 Classification of female genital mutilation

Type	Definition
I	Partial or total removal of the clitoris and/or the prepuce (clitoridectomy)
II	Partial or total removal of the clitoris and the labia minora, with or without excision of the labia majora (excision)
III	Narrowing of the vaginal orifice with creation of a covering seal by cutting and appositioning the labia minora and/or the labia majora, with or without excision of the clitoris (infibulation)
IV	All other harmful procedures to the female genitalia for non-medical purposes, e.g. pricking, piercing[a], incising, scraping and cauterizing

[a]Piercing is part of this WHO classification but its legal status is unclear in the UK.
(From Royal College of Obstetricians and Gynaecologists. Female Genital Mutilation and its Management. *Green-top Guideline no. 53, 2015; https://www.rcog.org.uk/globalassets/documents/guidelines/gtg-53-fgm.pdf.)*

urinary retention and blood-borne virus transmission. Chronically, dyspareunia, chronic pain, dysmenorrhoea, urinary tract infection and urinary outflow obstruction, post-traumatic stress disorder and difficulty conceiving all complicate FGM. In a subsequent pregnancy, the chances of caesarean section, postpartum haemorrhage, stillbirth and neonatal death are all higher.

Further reading

Faculty of Sexual and Reproductive Healthcare, Royal College of Obstetricians and Gynaecologists. *The UK Medical Eligibility Criteria for Contraceptive Use 2016.* London: RCOG; 2016; http://ukmec.pagelizard.com/2016.
Knight M, Bunch K, Tuffnell D et al (eds). *Saving Lives, Improving Mothers' Care: Lessons Learned to Inform Maternity Care from the UK and Ireland Confidential Enquiries into Maternal Deaths and Morbidity 2014–16;* https://www.npeu.ox.ac.uk/downloads/files/mbrrace-uk/reports/MBRRACE-UK%20Maternal%20Report%202018%20-%20Web%20Version.pdf.
National Institute for Health and Care Excellence. *NICE Clinical Guideline 171: Urinary Incontinence in Women: Management.* NICE 2013; https://www.nice.org.uk/guidance/cg171.

National Institute for Health and Care Excellence. *NICE Guideline 88: Heavy Menstrual Bleeding: Assessment and Management.* NICE 2018; https://www.nice.org.uk/guidance/ng88.
National Institute for Health and Care Excellence. *NICE Public Health Guidance 50: Domestic Violence and Abuse: Multi-Agency Working.* NICE 2014; https://www.nice.org.uk/guidance/ph50.
National Institute for Health and Care Excellence and British Medical Association Board of Science. *Domestic Abuse – Updated BMA Policy Report.* London: BMA; 2014.
Royal College of Obstetricians and Gynaecologists. *Female Genital Mutilation and its Management.* Green-top Guideline no. 53. London: RCOG; 2015; https://www.rcog.org.uk/globalassets/documents/guidelines/gtg-53-fgm.pdf.
Royal College of Obstetricians and Gynaecologists. *The Care of Women Requesting Induced Abortion.* Evidence-based Clinical Guideline no. 7. London: RCOG; 2011.
Royal College of Obstetricians and Gynaecologists. *The Investigation and Treatment of Couples with Recurrent First-trimester and Second-trimester Miscarriage.* Green-top Guideline no. 17. London: RCOG; 2011.

GYNAECOLOGICAL CANCERS

The most common genital tract tumours found in women are ovarian, endometrial and ovarian cancers (see p. 130). Each presents different challenges:

- ovarian cancer tends to present late and non-specifically, and most cases require specialist surgery and chemotherapy
- endometrial cancer is linked to increased peripheral androgen conversion to oestriol in adipose tissue and incidence will continue to increase with obesity
- cervical cancer can be screened for and there is now a vaccine for the causative agent – HPV.

An outline of these cancers is presented in **Box 39.8**. Suspected cancers should be referred urgently to secondary care, usually to a rapid access gynaecology or colposcopy clinic where diagnostic imaging and histology can be obtained, often on the same day.

Further reading

https://bgcs.org.uk/professionals/guidelines.html. *British Gynaecological Cancer Society guidelines.*
https://www.cancerresearchuk.org/about-cancer/type and https://www.cancerresearchuk.org/health-professional/cancer-statistics/statistics-by-cancer-type. *Cancer Research UK.*

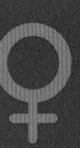

Box 39.8 Key clinical characteristics of cervical, endometrial and ovarian cancer

	Cervical	Endometrial	Ovarian
Incidence UK (annual)	3100	9000	7300
5-year survival (all stages)	65%	79%	46%
Peak rate of cases (age group)	25–29 years	75–79 years	75–79 years
Risk factors	HPV	Obesity, diabetes, endometrial hyperplasia	*BRCA1/2* mutations, obesity, hormone replacement therapy
General population screening in UK	Women aged 25–49 years invited every 3 years, then every 5 years until age 64, for cervical cytology and HPV testing	No	No UKCTOCS negative primary outcome for mortality reduction from screen but possible delayed benefit; longer follow-up data required
Presenting symptoms	Postcoital bleeding Intermenstrual bleeding Painful sex Vaginal discharge Pelvic pain	Postmenopausal bleeding Intermenstrual bleeding Vaginal discharge	Early satiety Loss of appetite Abdominal pain Abdominal bloating or increased size Urinary frequency Fatigue Unexplained weight loss Change in bowel habit
Modal stage at presentation	1	1	1 (31%), 3 (31%)
Diagnosis prior to definitive treatment	Cervical biopsy	Endometrial biopsy – pipelle, curettage	Ultrasound pelvis, CA125, CT
Surgery	Up to stage 2A or for palliative reasons 1A1: possible LLTEZ, radical trachelectomy for fertility preservation in small stage 1 tumours, otherwise radical hysterectomy	Majority: hysterectomy, BSO (most laparoscopic), radical hysterectomy, ± omentectomy if ≥ stage 2	Majority: 1aUSO = staging biopsies, otherwise TAH, BSO, omentectomy + required excision to achieve complete debulking; may require interval debulking
Chemotherapy	Chemoradiotherapy may be considered as an alternative to surgery up to stage 2A in some cases; adjuvant in stage 1B2 to 4A Agents: cisplatin, carboplatin, paclitaxel, topotecan	If high-grade or type 2 (see below) Agents: paclitaxel, carboplatin, cisplatin, doxorubicin, cyclophosphamide	May require neoadjuvant chemotherapy; majority will require adjuvant chemotherapy Agents: paclitaxel, carboplatin, gemcitabine, etoposide, doxorubicin, trabectedin, cyclophosphamide, topotecan
DXT	As above	Usually after surgery. Stage 1/2 if high-grade	Rarely used
Subtypes	Squamous cell carcinoma Adenocarcinoma Adenosquamous carcinoma Small cell carcinoma	Endometroid adenocarcinoma (type 1) Serous carcinoma (type 2) Clear cell carcinoma (type 2) Uterine sarcoma (type 2) Uterine carcinosarcoma (type 2)	Epithelial ovarian: serous, endometroid, clear cell, mucinous, undifferentiated Teratoma (germ cell) Granulosa tumours Borderline ovarian tumours Primary peritoneal Fallopian tube

BSO, bilateral salpingo-oophorectomy; CT, computed tomography; DXT, deep X-ray therapy; HPV, human papillomavirus; LLETZ, large loop excision of transformation zone; TAH, total abdominal hysterectomy; UKCTOCS, United Kingdom Collaborative Trial of Ovarian Cancer Screening; USO, unilateral salpingo-oophorectomy.
(From Cancer Research UK 2015 data.)

40

Men's health

Frank Chinegwundah and Damiete Harry

CORE SKILLS AND KNOWLEDGE

Men, like women, suffer with all manner of health problems, but there are particular disparities between the sexes in the rates of many common disorders. This chapter begins by surveying these differences and the particular health needs of men. It goes on to cover a range of disorders specific to the male urogenital tract, including diseases of the prostate, penis and testes. These disorders are common, especially benign and malignant prostate disease in middle-aged and older men.

Some patients are looked after in primary care but urologists manage others in secondary care, commonly in an outpatient setting but also as inpatients in emergency situations. Much of urological surgery is performed as a day-case procedure, and urologists are supported by nurse specialists in delivering services.

Key skills to develop include:
- history-taking for lower urinary tract symptoms
- examination of the prostate gland
- urinary catheterization, which is a core skill for all doctors.

Key medications in urology include alpha-blockers (e.g. tamsulosin), and hormonal drugs to treat symptomatic prostate disease (5-α-reductase inhibitors such as finasteride).

Key urological emergencies that all doctors need to recognize include testicular torsion, acute urinary retention, paraphimosis and priapism.

CLINICAL SKILLS FOR MEN'S HEALTH

History

Lower urinary tract symptoms (LUTS) are commonly said to fall into two distinct groups – storage and voiding – and carefully eliciting the nature of a patient's problems may suggest the underlying disorder (**Box 40.1**).

- *Storage LUTS* are caused by disorders that affect the storage of urine, and suggest irritation or inflammation of the lining of the bladder. Causes include lower urinary tract infection (UTI), other forms of cystitis, sexually transmitted infections, bladder stones and prostatitis.
- *Voiding LUTS* are caused by disorders that affect the voiding of urine, with benign and malignant prostate diseases the most common causes. Chronic urinary retention caused by neurological problems (e.g. multiple sclerosis) is often asymptomatic, as there is abnormal sensation of bladder fullness; it may be detected only on abdominal palpation or imaging. The passing of frequent, small volumes of urine should always raise the possibility of urinary retention with 'overflow' voiding, particularly if it is accompanied by lower abdominal pain and tenderness, and a palpable bladder.

---

i **Box 40.1 Lower urinary tract symptoms (LUTS)**

Storage LUTS
- *Dysuria*: pain or burning on urination
- *Frequency*: the passing of small volumes of urine at frequent intervals
- *Urgency*: a sudden urge to pass urine
- *Urge incontinence*: urgency leading to involuntary loss of urine
- *Nocturia*: waking at night to pass urine

Voiding LUTS
- *Hesitancy*: a longer than usual wait for urine flow to begin
- *Weak stream*
- *Intermittency*: urine flow that stops and starts
- *Terminal dribbling*: weak urine flow continues after an attempt is made to stop
- *Straining*: the need to increase abdominal pressure in order to urinate

Examination

A urologist is able to estimate the size of the prostate gland by comparing the prostate volume on ultrasound or magnetic resonance imaging (MRI) with what is felt on digital rectal examination (DRE, **Fig. 40.1**). A fleshy-feeling prostate is likely to be benign, whereas a hard, craggy gland is more likely to be malignant.

Investigations: bladder scanning

Portable bladder scanners use basic ultrasound technology to allow the volume of urine in a patient's bladder to be assessed at the bedside by ward staff not trained in formal diagnostic ultrasound scanning. Although individual models vary, generally use is very simple (**Fig. 40.2** and **Box 40.2**). Such scanners are often available on wards and can be used for:
- diagnosing urinary retention
- assessing successful voiding after a trial without catheter
- assessing whether a patient's bladder empties completely after voiding.

A bladder volume of more than 150 mL after attempted voiding is considered significant. In acute urinary retention, volumes of more than 1 L may be seen, and urgent urethral catheterization is required (**Box 40.3** and **Fig. 40.3**).

Box 40.2 Bladder scanning

- Switch on the bladder scanner.
- Apply aqueous gel to the head of the transducer.
- Palpate the symphysis pubis and place the scanner 3 cm above this, pointing down into the pelvis.
- Hold the transducer steady while pressing the scanning button; this will reveal the bladder volume on screen.
- Repeat the procedure three times, with slight alterations in the position of the transducer.
- Record the highest volume in the patient's medical record.

Box 40.3 Male catheterization

- Obtain consent
- Employ an aseptic no-touch technique.
- Clean the glans penis with an antiseptic solution.
- Instil lidocaine anaesthetic gel into the urethra.
- After 5 min, insert an appropriately sized catheter (generally 14F/16F/18F) through the external urethral meatus. When the catheter is inserted to the hilt, urine drains out.
- Inflate the catheter balloon with 10 mL saline and withdraw the catheter until the balloon is snug against the bladder neck.
- Note the volume of urine drained.
- Replace the foreskin, if present, over the glans penis.

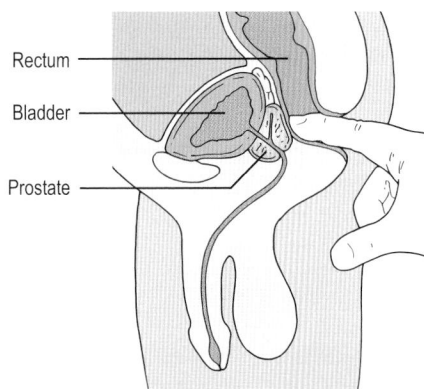

Fig. 40.1 Digital rectal examination (DRE). A gloved, lubricated index finger is inserted into the rectum to feel the prostate, which lies anteriorly. *(From Scully C. Scully's Handbook of Medical Problems in Dentistry, 2016, Elsevier, with permission.)*

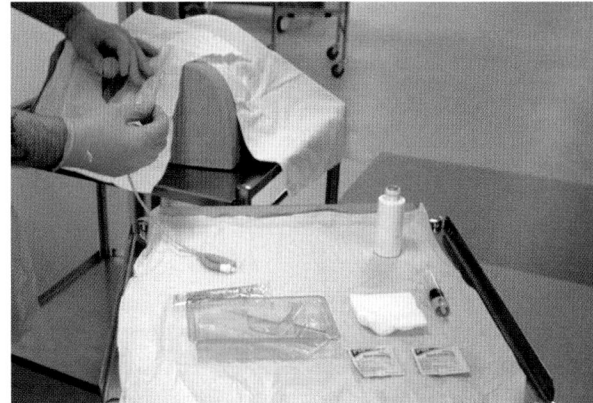

Fig. 40.3 Male catheterization of a mannequin. *(From O'Neill P et al. (eds). Macleod's Clinical OSCEs, 2016, Elsevier, with permission.)*

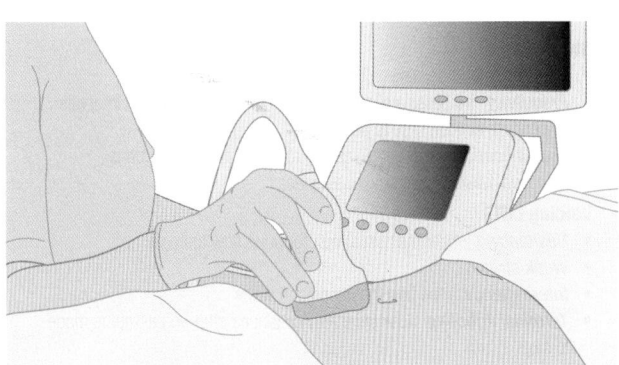

Fig. 40.2 Portable bladder scanner.

INTRODUCTION

Disparities between men's and women's health

In high-income countries there remain stark disparities between men's and women's health. These differences are highlighted in data from England and Wales (**Box 40.4**).

Men are their own worst enemies

Many of the health disparities between the sexes can be attributed to the fact that men have lower levels of health literacy than women, and are therefore less likely to acknowledge problems, seek help, or utilize resources such as a general practitioner or pharmacist. It is suggested that fear of having illness confirmed, with the potential perceived loss of masculinity, results in men maintaining an appearance of being in control and bearing up, instead of being honest, reporting symptoms, seeking help and accepting interventions.

These UK trends are seen in most parts of the world, where health outcomes among boys and men continue to be substantially worse than those among girls and women. Globally, women live an average of 6 years longer, ranging from 5.3 years longer in sub-Saharan Africa to >10 years longer in Russia. Despite these differences, few countries have addressed the burden that men's ill-health creates by adopting national, male-centred strategies. Advocates of such concerted global action point to the huge transformative impacts that these changes might bring socially and economically. Closing the gap would benefit all of the world's population, regardless of gender, as male ill-health has significant effects on the psychological wellbeing of women too, as well as the health, finances and social cohesiveness of the family.

Further reading

Baker P, Dworkin SL, Tong S et al. The men's health gap: men must be included in the global health equity agenda. *Bull World Health Org* 2014; 92: 618–620.
White A, McKee M, Richardson N et al. Europe's men need their own health strategy. *Br Med J* 2011; 343:d739.

SPECIFIC DISEASES OF MEN

The top five causes of male deaths, according to the UK Office for National Statistics (2017), are dementia and Alzheimer's disease, ischaemic heart disease, cerebrovascular disease, chronic respiratory disease and lung cancer. Prostate cancer is, however, the most common cancer in UK males, followed by lung and colorectal cancers.

DISEASES OF THE PROSTATE GLAND

Prostatitis

Prostatitis describes inflammation of the prostate gland. It can be divided into acute prostatitis, which is uncommon, and the much more common chronic prostatitis.

Acute prostatitis

This presents with the symptoms of a severe UTI, including dysuria, frequency, malaise, fever and genital region pain. The prostate is found to be swollen and tender on digital rectal examination. Infectious agents include various gram negative organisms responsible for urinary tract infection, and organisms that cause sexually transmitted infection such as *Chlamydia trachomatis* and *Neisseria gonorrhoeae*. Hospital admission is required for antibiotic treatment. If the condition is left untreated, sepsis may result.

Chronic prostatitis

Chronic disease may affect up to 10–15% of men. Most of these patients have chronic non-bacterial prostatitis, termed chronic prostatitis or chronic pelvic pain syndrome. A diagnosis can be made if symptoms have been present for more than 3 months. The condition generally occurs in men aged 30–50 years. Typically, the clinical features wax and wane over several years but may include a combination of pain, urinary symptoms and sexual dysfunction, with pain being the main feature. It may be experienced in the penis, scrotum, perineum or anus. Voiding difficulties are common. There may be erectile dysfunction and/or pain on ejaculation.

The cause is unknown. Investigations are undertaken to exclude other diagnoses.

Management is difficult. Options include antibiotics (even where there is no microbiologically proven infection), alpha-blockers such as tamsulosin, 5-alpha-reductase inhibitors such as finasteride, non-steroidal anti-inflammatory drugs (NSAIDs) and prostate massage under general anaesthesia. Dietary manipulation may be of value, as may stress reduction. A chronic pain specialist may be involved. Many men seek complementary therapies.

Box 40.4 Health disparities between the sexes (England and Wales, 2015)

Mortality
- Mortality rates are higher for men than for women in every age group under the age of 85 years. In 2015, age-standardized mortality rates (ASMRs) were 1156.4 and 863.8 deaths per 100 000 population for men and women, respectively.
- Men are more likely than women to die prematurely: 19% of all male deaths but only 12% of women's deaths were in those under 65 years.
- This difference is accentuated in the 15–34 age group, where 67% of all deaths were male, representing 1.65% of all male deaths but only 0.75% of female deaths.

Cancer
- The biggest single cause of death in men and women remains cancer. It accounts for nearly one-third of all male deaths but only one-quarter of female deaths.

Mental health and suicide
- 1 : 8 men in the UK suffer from one of the common mental health conditions, compared to 1 : 5 women.
- However, men are 50% more likely than women to be detained under the Mental Health Act and treated compulsorily. Men are far less likely to access psychological therapies than women.
- Men account for 76% of all suicides; suicide is the single biggest cause of death in men under 35 years.
- Research suggests that men have less access to the social support of friends, relatives and the wider community.

Alcohol, illicit drugs and crime
- Men are three times more likely to become problem drinkers; alcohol dependence affects 8.7% of men compared to 3.3% of women.
- Men are more likely to use, and to also die from, illicit drugs: 4.2% of men but only 1.4% of women report frequent drug use.
- Men make up 95% of the prison population, committing 86% of violent crime.

Benign enlargement of the prostate gland

Benign prostatic enlargement occurs most often in men over the age of 60 years. The aetiology is not established but the condition is unknown when there is hypogonadism, confirming the androgen dependency of the condition. Microscopically, hyperplasia affects the glandular and connective tissue elements of the prostate. Enlargement of the gland stretches and distorts the urethra, obstructing bladder outflow.

Clinical features

Frequency of urination, usually first noted as nocturia, is a common early symptom. Difficulty or delay in initiating urination, with variability and reduced forcefulness of the urinary stream and post-void dribbling, are often present (voiding LUTS). Acute retention of urine (see later) or retention with overflow incontinence may occur. Occasionally, severe haematuria results from rupture of prostatic veins or is a consequence of bacteriuria or stone disease.

Examination and investigations

Abdominal examination for bladder enlargement is performed, together with a digital rectal examination (DRE); a benign prostate characteristically feels smooth. Investigations should include:
- urine culture
- measurement of serum prostate-specific antigen (PSA)
- renal function tests
- ultrasound
- measurement of the urinary flow rate.

Pressure-flow studies (urodynamics or cystometry) are not routinely indicated.

Management

The severity of symptoms is assessed by the self-administered International Prostate Symptom Score, which is based on seven questions about urinary symptoms and one concerning quality of life. Management is outlined in **Box 40.5**.

If surgery is needed, minimally invasive day-case procedures include the insertion of implants to maintain urethral patency (e.g. the Urolift system), and transurethral needle ablation of the prostate in which low-frequency radio waves are used to induce necrosis in the enlarged prostate gland.

Deterioration in renal function or the development of upper tract dilation usually requires surgery.

_i_ Box 40.5 Management of benign prostatic enlargement

Patients with mild symptoms
- Lifestyle change alone, e.g. attention to the amount and types of fluid ingested

Patients with moderate symptoms
- Alpha-blockers, e.g. tamsulosin, which relaxes prostate and bladder smooth muscle tone
- 5-α-reductase inhibitors, e.g. finasteride, which blocks the conversion of testosterone to dihydrotestosterone, the androgen primarily responsible for prostatic growth and enlargement
- Combination therapy, e.g. an alpha-blocker and an anti-cholinergic drug for a concomitant overactive bladder

Surgical treatment
- Transurethral resection of the prostate (TURP)
- Laser therapy (enucleation or vaporization)
- Open prostatectomy for a very large prostate gland: now uncommon in moderate- and high-income countries due to the availability of holmium laser enucleation

---

In acute retention or retention with overflow, the priorities are to relieve pain and catheterize (and drain) the bladder. If urethral catheterization is impossible, a suprapubic catheter can be placed.

Prostate cancer

Prostatic carcinoma accounts for 7% of all cancers in men and is the sixth most common cancer in the world. Malignant change within the prostate becomes increasingly common with advancing age. By 80 years, 80% of men have malignant foci within the gland but most of these appear to lie dormant. Histologically, the tumour is almost invariably an adenocarcinoma.

Prostate cancer is the most common male-specific cancer in the UK. Some 47 000 men develop it every year, representing 1 in every 8 men, with deaths running at 12 000 per year. It is particularly common in men aged over 50 years, in men with a family history of prostate or breast cancer, and in black men (where the risk is 1 in 4).

Pathogenesis

Genetic studies have shown that the homeobox gene *HOXB13* predisposes to prostate cancer. Genome-wide association studies have identified over 100 single-nucleotide polymorphisms (SNPs) associated with it. The *BRCA2* gene, associated with breast cancer in women, confers a 5–7 times higher risk.

Clinical features and diagnosis

Most men with early prostate cancer do not have any symptoms. The diagnosis is suggested by the finding of a raised serum prostate-specific antigen (PSA) and/or an abnormal-feeling prostate gland on DRE. Where there are symptoms, they are similar to those of a benignly enlarged prostate gland: namely, features of urinary voiding (slow flow and hesitancy) and urinary storage (frequency and urgency).

A serum PSA level of more than 3 ng/mL is abnormal but a measurement of between 3 and 10 ng/mL can be due to benign hypertrophy, prostatitis or cancer. Levels of more than 10 ng/mL suggest malignant disease.

Investigations include a multiparametric MRI (mpMRI) scan of prostate, followed in most instances by a prostate biopsy. Currently, this most commonly takes the form of a transrectal ultrasound-guided biopsy (**Fig. 40.4**), but this is being superseded in several centres by transperineal ultrasound-guided biopsy, which has better diagnostic accuracy and carries a reduced risk of sepsis.

Prostate cancer commonly metastasizes to bone. These metastases appear as osteosclerotic lesions on X-ray and are also detected by isotopic bone scans.

Prognosis

The histological appearances are graded according to the combined Gleason score (**Fig. 40.5**). Together with the serum PSA level, and accurate staging of the local extent of disease with pelvic MRI (dynamic contrast) and transrectal ultrasound, this score can identify prognostic groups (**Box 40.6**). Treatment decisions must balance the age and performance status of the patient with the predicted behaviour of the cancer (future developments in gene profiling will allow better prognostication). This allows the selection of patients with a good prognosis for non-aggressive treatment; they may reasonably choose to be kept under an active surveillance programme.

About 95% of men in England diagnosed with prostate cancer between 50 and 69 years of age survive their disease for 5 years or more, and overall prostate cancer survival is improving.

Management

See **Figure 40.6**.

Localized disease

Patients with disease localized to the prostate that requires treatment can be managed by curative surgery (typically, robotically assisted radical prostatectomy), external beam radiotherapy, or brachytherapy (with radioactive iodine implants), which all achieve equivalent survival

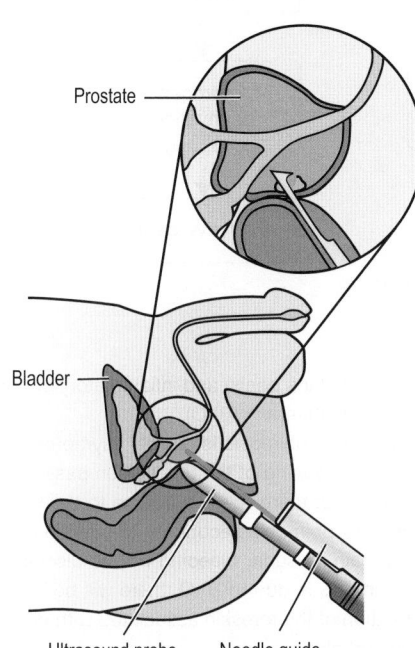

Fig. 40.4 Transrectal ultrasound-guided biopsy of the prostate
Prior to the biopsy the patient is given prophylactic antibiotics. An ultrasound probe is introduced into the rectum to visualize the prostate. Using ultrasound as a guide, local anaesthetic is then infused into the tissue surrounding the prostate. This allows for core biopsies to be taken from the prostate comfortably. *(From Pagana K et al. Mosby's Canadian Manual of Diagnostic and Laboratory Tests, 2nd Canadian edn, 2019, Elsevier, with permission.)*

rates but differ in the spectrum of unwanted side-effects, including incontinence and sexual dysfunction. Radiotherapy tends to be used more frequently in older patients who wish to avoid surgery.

In the UK, treatment options are determined jointly by multi-disciplinary clinical teams and informed patients. A key priority is the avoidance of unnecessary overtreatment (the rate of which has fallen to 8% in the UK, according to the National Prostate Cancer Audit 2017).

Discussion between patients and clinicians are vital to enable a treatment choice that is most appropriate to the patient's circumstances. In many with lower-risk disease (combined Gleason scores of 6 or less, **Box 40.7**), localized prostate cancer may be managed expectantly using the strategy of active surveillance, in which regular PSA tests are supplemented with repeat mpMRI and repeat prostatic biopsies, to establish whether the cancer is becoming more aggressive and thus warrants active therapy.

Traditionally, therapies with curative intent have targeted the whole gland. However, there is developing interest in focal therapies for prostate cancer, along the lines of a 'lumpectomy' for breast cancer. High-intensity focused ultrasound and cryotherapy are just two of the technologies used to ablate the part of the prostate harbouring the cancer.

> *i* **Box 40.6 Prostate cancer: prognostic factors**
>
> **At initial diagnosis**
> - Clinical stage
> - Biopsy Gleason grade
> - Serum PSA level
>
> **Post surgery**
> - Surgical/pathological stage
> - Surgical margins
> - Extracapsular spread, extension to seminal vesicles or lymph nodes
>
> **Metastatic, hormone-resistant disease**
> - Performance status
> - Serum PSA
> - Haemoglobin, albumin, alkaline phosphatase and lactate dehydrogenase level
>
> PSA, prostate-specific antigen.

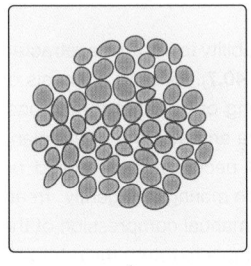 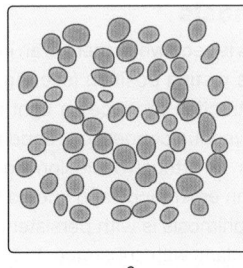 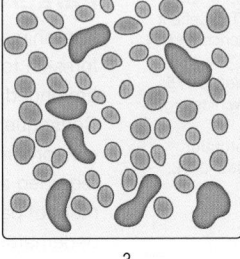 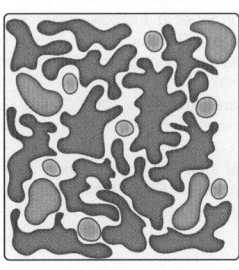 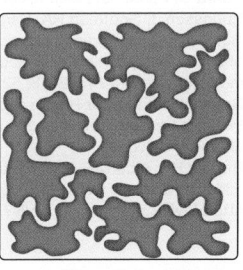

| 1 | 2 | 3 | 4 | 5 |

Well differentiated → Moderately differentiated → Poorly differentiated Anaplastic →

Fig. 40.5 Gleason's Pattern Scale. The Gleason is a grading scale that runs from 1 to 5, the number indicating the extent of differentiation of the adenocarcinoma cells of the prostate. Due to the multifocal and heterogenous nature of prostate cancer, the Gleason score is calculated by adding together the two most prevalent grades. For example, Gleason 3 + 4 = 7 would mean that the most dominant cell type is Gleason 3, followed by Gleason 4, and the two combined give an overall value of Gleason 7. An overall Gleason score of 2–6 is considered as well differentiated, Gleason 7 is moderately differentiated and 8–10 is poorly differentiated. **(1)** Small, uniform glands. **(2)** More space (stroma) between glands. **(3)** Distinct infiltration of cells from glands at margins. **(4)** Irregular masses of neoplastic cells with few glands. **(5)** Lack of/occasional glands, sheets of cells. *(Redrawn after Kirby RS, Brawer MK, Denis LJ (eds), Prostate Cancer: Fast Facts, 3rd edn. Abingdon: Health Press; 2001.)*

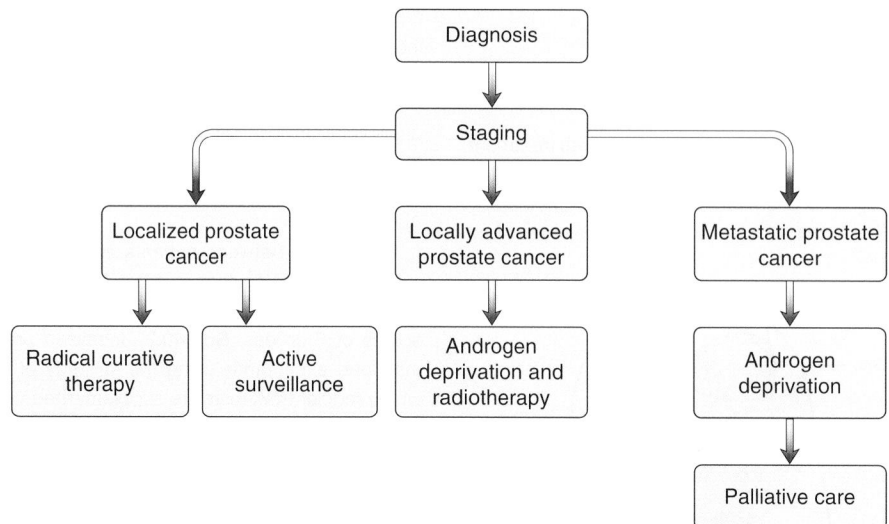

Fig. 40.6 Management of prostate cancer.

> ℹ **Box 40.7** High- and low-risk prostate cancer

Risk	PSA	TNM stage[a]	Gleason score
Low	<10	T1 or T2	6
High	>20	T3 or T4	≥4 + 3 = 7

[a]See **Box 6.12**. PSA, prostate-specific antigen.

Locally advanced and metastatic disease

Management of prostate cancer in cases where surgery is not possible is discussed on page 128. It is based around endocrine therapy to achieve androgen blockade, alongside systemic chemotherapy.

Screening

See Chapter 14 for a review of the evidence for prostate cancer screening.

Further reading

Attard G, Parker C, Eeles RA et al. Prostate cancer. *Lancet* 2016; 387:70–82.

Hugosson J, Godtman RA, Carlsson SV et al. Eighteen-year follow-up of the Göteborg Randomized Population-based Prostate Cancer Screening Trial: effect of sociodemographic variables on participation, prostate cancer incidence and mortality. *Scand J Urol* 2018; 52:27–37.

National Institute for Health and Care Excellence. *NICE Clinical Guideline 175: Prostate Cancer: Diagnosis and Management.* NICE 2014; https://www.nice.org.uk/guidance/cg175.

Richter HE, Albo ME, Zyczynski HM et al. Retropubic versus transobturator midurethral slings for stress incontinence. *N Engl J Med* 2010; 362:2066–2076.

https://www.npca.org.uk/. *UK National Prostate Cancer Audit 2017.*

DISEASES OF THE PENIS

Benign diseases of the penis

Phimosis

Phimosis is a condition in which the contracted foreskin (prepuce) has a tight, narrow orifice and cannot be retracted over the glans of the penis (**Fig. 40.7**). A physiological phimosis is present at birth, but through penile growth, erection and accumulation of epithelial debris (smegma) under the foreskin, separation occurs, enabling the foreskin to be retracted. By the age of 17, only 1% of boys will have a phimosis. Pathological phimosis is caused by recurrent balanitis (inflammation of the glans penis) and inflammatory conditions such as balanitis xerotica obliterans (BXO).

While physiological phimosis is usually asymptomatic, patients may present with ballooning of the foreskin on passing urine. If the man is sexually active, there may be trauma to the foreskin during coitus. Pathological phimosis secondary to infection or inflammation may cause pain, dysuria, bleeding or pus discharge from the orifice. If the phimosis is due to BXO, there will be hypopigmentation or discoloration of the foreskin associated with pruritic plaques on the foreskin and glans.

In adults, phimosis is usually pathological and any associated infection should be treated. The main treatment in adults is circumcision but children should be managed as conservatively as possible. Corticosteroid cream, in addition to antibiotics, is effective for treating underlying balanitis and softening the phimosis. The indications for circumcision in children are BXO, recurrent balanitis and recurrent UTIs in those with urinary tract abnormalities (e.g. vesico-ureteric reflux, posterior urethral valves or neuropathic bladder dysfunction).

Paraphimosis

Paraphimosis is seen when there is an inability to return the retracted foreskin to its resting position (see **Fig. 40.7**). Existing phimosis or prolonged retraction produces a tight ring of tissue at the corona. Consequent venous congestion, oedema and swelling of the glans can progress to arterial occlusion and necrosis. This should be regarded as an emergency and should be managed urgently. Treatment of paraphimosis is with persistent manual compression of the oedematous glans with subsequent attempts to return the retracted foreskin to its normal position. Should this manoeuvre fail, a dorsal slit or circumcision is the definitive management.

Malignant disease of the penis

Penile cancer

Over 95% of penile malignancies are squamous cell carcinomas arising from the epithelium of the inner prepuce or the glans. In industrialized countries, penile cancer is uncommon, with an overall incidence of around 1/100 000 males in Europe and the USA. In contrast, in some other parts of the world such as South America,

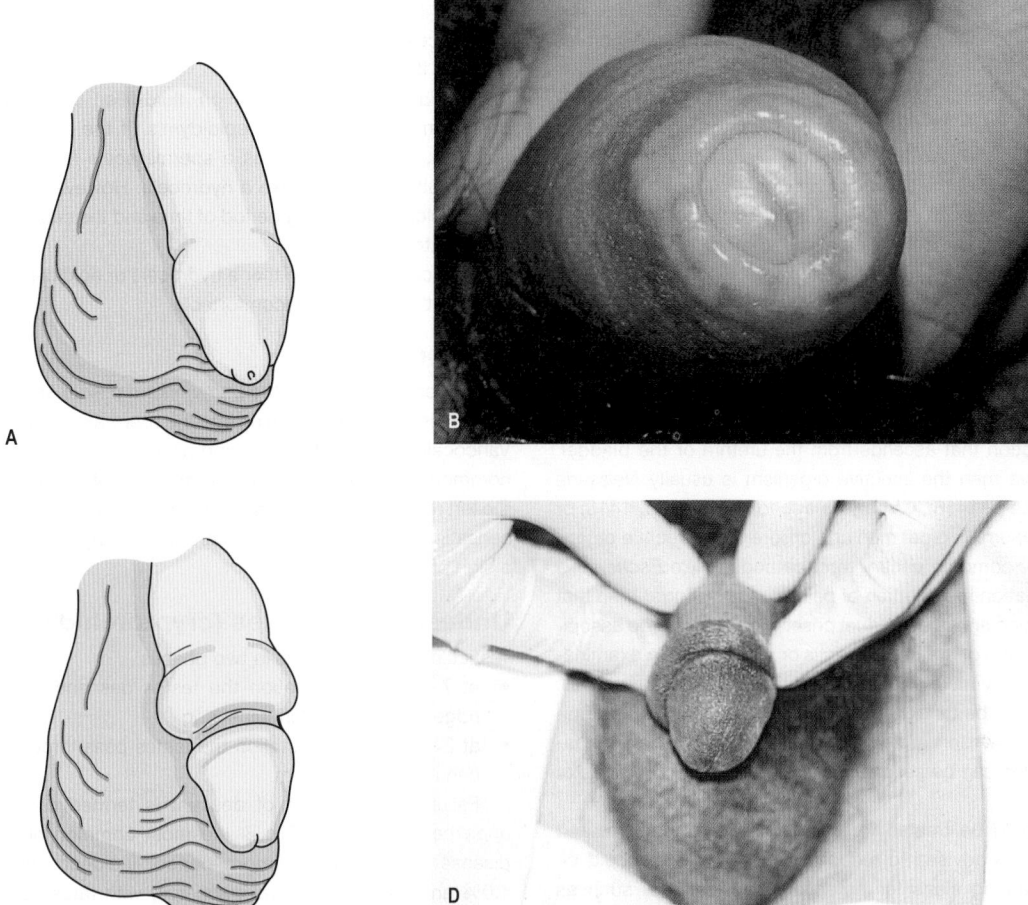

Fig. 40.7 Phimosis and paraphimosis. (A) Phimosis: the foreskin has a narrow opening that is not large enough to permit retraction over the glans. **(B)** Phimosis: lesions on the prepuce secondary to infection cause swelling, and retraction of the foreskin may be impossible. Circumcision is usually required. **(C)** Paraphimosis: the foreskin is retracted over the glans but cannot be reduced to its normal position. Here it has formed a constricting band around the penis. **(D)** This oedematous foreskin is the result of paraphimosis. *(From Roberts JR, Hedges JR. Clinical Procedures in Emergency Medicine, 5th edn. Philadelphia: Saunders; 2009.)*

South-east Asia and parts of Africa, the incidence is much higher and can account for 1–2% of malignant disease in men. Penile cancer is common in regions with a high prevalence of human papillomavirus (HPV); some cases are attributed to HPV-related carcinogenesis, most commonly HPV subtypes 6, 16 and 18. It is not linked to human immunodeficiency virus (HIV) infection or acquired immunodeficiency syndrome (AIDS). Other known risk factors are phimosis, chronic penile inflammation (BXO or balanitis), smoking and multiple sexual partners. Neonatal circumcision dramatically reduces the frequency of penile cancer.

The aims of treatment of the primary tumour are complete tumour removal with as much organ preservation as possible, without compromising oncological control. Local recurrence has little influence on long-term survival, so organ preservation strategies are justified (European Association of Urology (EAU) guidelines 2018, see 'Further reading'). Radiotherapy and laser ablation are organ-preserving management options in patients with superficial disease. Radiotherapy and chemotherapy are most often used in the palliative setting. Chemotherapy is frequently cisplatin-based and is usually based on fluorouracil or a taxane.

TESTICULAR AND SPERMATIC CORD DISEASE

Benign diseases of the testicle

Testicular torsion

Testicular torsion is the lateral to medial (inward) twisting of the spermatic cord. This results in strangulation of the blood supply to the testis and the epididymis, and is a time-sensitive true urological emergency. Testicular torsion occurs most often in the neonatal period and around puberty (peak incidence at 13–15 years of age). These patients usually present with a short history (less than 12 h) of severe, sudden-onset hemi-scrotal pain, which sometimes wakes them from sleep and can radiate to the groin, loin or epigastrium. The pain is associated with nausea and vomiting, and an altered, broad-based 'cowboy' gait. On examination, there may be an absent cremasteric reflex (unreliable in older children and adults), and the testicle may be high-riding and in a horizontal position. The testicle itself can be swollen and tense, and is exquisitely tender. Elevation of the testicle does not ameliorate the symptoms (negative Prehn's sign).

Diagnosis is usually based on the clinical presentation alone. Doppler ultrasound cannot rule out the presence of testicular torsion and delays definitive treatment, so should not be relied on for diagnosis in acute presentations.

Management is immediate surgical exploration in patients presenting with less than 24 hours of pain. Delay can result in permanent ischaemic damage to the testicle. Detorsion and bilateral orchidopexy (fixation of the testicle to prevent recurrent torsion) are performed in the presence of a viable testicle. If the testicle is non-viable, orchidectomy and contralateral orchidopexy are carried out.

Epididymitis and orchitis

Epididymitis is an acute or chronic inflammatory condition of the epididymis. It often involves the testicle and as such is referred to as *epididymo-orchitis*. Patients who present acutely can have symptoms that mimic testicular torsion. Epididymitis is usually caused by a bacterial infection that ascends from the urethra or the bladder. In sexually active men the infective organism is usually *Neisseria gonorrhoeae* (see p. 1416), *Chlamydia trachomatis* (see p. 1416) or a coliform bacterium. In older men and children the infective organisms are usually common urinary tract pathogens like *Escherichia coli*. On presentation the duration of pain is usually longer than that of testicular torsion and is of gradual onset. The pain can be associated with symptoms of urethritis, cystitis or prostatitis. On examination the patient may have a fever and appear systemically unwell. The epididymis will be tender and swollen on palpation. The hemiscrotum is often swollen and warm to the touch, and erythematous skin changes can be seen. Urinalysis may also show signs of infection.

Patients should be treated for the most likely organism, and scrotal elevation is advised to reduce swelling. Advice should be provided on warning signs for potential complications, such as abscess formation, infarction of testis, chronic pain, chronic infection and infertility. In patients with parotid swelling, a viral mumps orchitis should be considered (see p. 525) and a thorough vaccination history taken.

Hydrocele and epididymal cyst

A *hydrocele* is an abnormal collection of fluid within the tunica vaginalis of the scrotum or along the spermatic cord (**Fig. 40.8**). It is usually painless but the testicle is difficult to palpate due to the tense fluid collection. The superior margin of the hydrocele is palpable. The fact that the clinician can 'get above' the lump differentiates a hydrocele from an inguinal hernia. It is also possible to transilluminate it.

Epididymal cysts are benign, fluid-filled cystic swellings that arise from the head of the epididymis. If the cyst contains spermatozoa, it is referred to as a spermatocele (see **Fig. 40.8**). It is often multiloculated, unlike a hydrocele. However, a spermatocele too develops over a long period of time and the superior margin can be palpated.

Surgical excision of either a hydrocele or epididymal cyst is indicated if it is large and uncomfortable.

Varicocele

A varicocele is dilation of the pampiniform plexus of veins surrounding the testis and extending up into the spermatic cord (see **Fig. 40.8**). Varicoceles are usually small and asymptomatic. They occur more commonly on the left side due to drainage of the gonadal vein into the left renal vein. When symptomatic, patients describe a dragging sensation or a dull ache in the scrotum. Rarely, a varicocele can be a sign of renal malignancy.

Undescended testes (cryptorchidism)

Testicular descent occurs in two phases:
- at 7–8 weeks' gestation the testes descend from the genital ridge to the internal inguinal ring
- at 24–28 weeks' gestation the testes pass through the inguinal canal into the scrotum.

Failure at any stage of descent is termed cryptorchidism or undescended testes. This is the most common endocrinological disease in the male newborn period. Incidence varies between 1.0% and 4.6% in full-term neonates, with rates as high as 45% in preterm neonates (EAU guidelines, see 'Further reading'). These patients have an eight-fold higher risk of testicular cancer and a 4% life-long risk of cancer in the intra-abdominal testis. They have reduced fertility, although this improves if orchidopexy is performed before 2 years of age. They are also at increased risk of testicular torsion and inguinal hernia formation.

Malignant disease of the testicle

Testicular germ cell tumours

Testicular cancer represents 1% of male neoplasms and 5% of urological tumours, with 3–10 new cases occurring per 100 000 males per year in Western societies. It is the most common solid cancer in young men in Western populations (see p. 129).

Clinical features

Most men usually present with a painless unilateral testicular or scrotal mass. Up to 27% can have pain or a dragging sensation as their first symptom. A detailed history will uncover the 11% of cases that present with back and flank pain due to metastases and the 7% that present with gynaecomastia, if the tumour secretes human chorionic gonadotropin (hCG).

Of note, 10% of cases of testicular cancer can mimic epididymo-orchitis. On encountering these acutely presenting patients, it is imperative to carry out a general abdominal examination, looking for supraclavicular lymphadenopathy and a palpable abdominal mass.

Investigations and management

These are described on page 129.

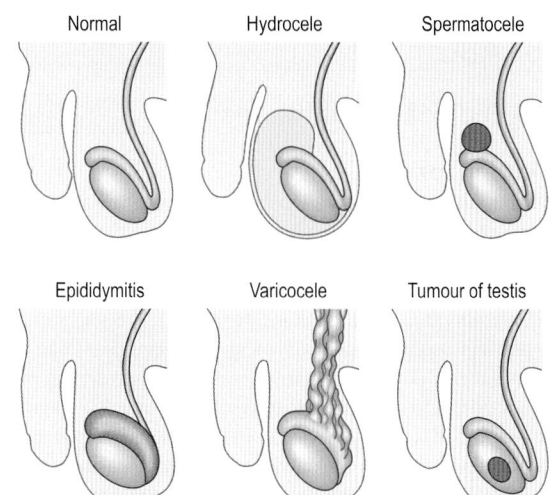

Fig. 40.8 Diseases of the testicle. *(From Innes JA, Dover AR, Fairhurst K (eds),* Macleod's Clinical Examination, *14th edn, 2018, Elsevier, with permission.)*

Normal   Hydrocele   Spermatocele

Epididymitis   Varicocele   Tumour of testis

? Box 40.8 Common causes of erectile dysfunction

- Vascular, e.g. complicating peripheral vascular disease, especially in smokers and the obese; often associated with systemic cardiovascular disease
- Neurogenic, e.g. in diabetic neuropathy or spinal cord lesions
- Anatomical
- Hormonal, e.g. in hypogonadism or hyperprolactinaemia
- Drug-induced, e.g. beta-blockers
- Psychogenic

Self-examination

While there are no data to demonstrate that screening for testicular cancer by regular self-examination saves lives, it seems sensible, and is widely recommended, that men examine their testes once a month. Most testicular cancers come to light when a swelling is noticed.

Further reading

Rosen A, Jayram G, Drazer M et al. Global trends in testicular cancer incidence and mortality. *Eur Urol* 2011; 60:374–379.
https://uroweb.org/guideline/penile-cancer/. *EAU guidelines for penile cancer.*
https://uroweb.org/guideline/paediatric-urology/#1. *EAU guidelines for paediatric urology.*

LACK OF LIBIDO AND ERECTILE DYSFUNCTION

Lack of libido is a loss of sexual desire. In some instances this is due to low serum testosterone levels, but more commonly the testosterone is normal and reduced libido is attributed to psychological factors or lifestyle stresses. *Erectile dysfunction* is a complex phenomenon that is defined as the persistent inability to attain and maintain an erection sufficient to permit satisfactory sexual performance (EAU guidelines 2018, see 'Further reading'). Low libido and erectile dysfunction may occur together or separately, and each can precipitate the other. Both are common symptoms in hypogonadism, but most people with either symptom have normal hormone levels and in many patients there is no definable organic cause.

Erectile dysfunction may affect a person's physical and psychosocial health, and can have a significant impact on the quality of life of patients and their partners. Common causes are listed in **Box 40.8.**

The presence of nocturnal emissions and frequent satisfactory morning erections make hormonal disease unlikely. Psychogenic erectile dysfunction is commonly a diagnosis of exclusion. In addition to the various aetiologies considered individually, in most cases there is more than one pathological element and often a psychological component.

Management

A detailed medical and sexual history should be obtained from the patient and, if available, their partner. This should be followed by physical examination of the genitourinary system and the suspected aetiological system - for instance, checking peripheral pulses in the legs. Laboratory tests should be performed according to the patient's history and risk factors.

Modifiable or reversible risk factors, such as lifestyle choices (e.g. smoking, obesity or lack of exercise), can be tackled first, and offending drugs should be stopped if possible. Treatment or management of underlying systemic disease, such as diabetes mellitus, hypertension and the causes of hypogonadism, can also have a positive effect on the management of erectile dysfunction.

First-line therapies

The treatment algorithm for erectile dysfunction is a delicate balance between the invasiveness and efficacy of any given intervention. The mainstay of first-line therapy is an oral phosphodiesterase type 5 inhibitor (PDE5I), such as sildenafil, tadalafil, vardenafil and avanafil. These drugs cause smooth muscle relaxation and thus increase penile arterial blood flow, which enables a man to achieve an erection. The time from ingestion of medication to effectiveness can vary, depending on which medication is prescribed, but is generally between 15 and 60 minutes. PDE5Is are contraindicated in any patient using any form of organic nitrate (e.g. nitroglycerine, isosorbide mononitrate or isosorbide dinitrate). They are also contraindicated in anyone who has had a myocardial infarction, stroke or life-threatening arrhythmia in the preceding 6 months. Their use is also contraindicated in resting hypotension (blood pressure <90/50 mmHg), hypertension (blood pressure >170/100 mmHg), unstable angina, angina with sexual intercourse and severe congestive heart failure.

Vacuum erection devices provide passive engorgement of the corpora cavernosa. A constrictor ring is then placed at the base of the penis to retain blood within the corpora. This non-invasive option is contraindicated in patients with bleeding disorders or those on anticoagulation. It can be offered to well-informed patients who have infrequent sexual intercourse and co-morbidities requiring non-invasive, drug-free management of erectile dysfunction.

Topical and intra-urethral alprostadil application is the last of the first-line therapies. Topical alprostadil is applied to the glans and absorbed via the urethral meatus. An alprostadil pellet can also be administered intra-urethrally as an alternative.

Second-line therapies

Patients who do not respond to oral drugs or other first-line therapies may be offered intracavernous alprostadil injections. Intracavernous administration of vasoactive drugs was the first medical treatment developed for erectile dysfunction. Dedicated outpatient training for a patient or his partner by a specialist member of the urology team is needed to ensure correct technique.

Third-line therapies

The surgical implantation of a penile prosthesis may be considered in patients who do not respond to pharmacotherapy or who prefer a permanent solution.

If no organic disease is found or if there is clear evidence of psychological problems, the couple should receive psychosexual counselling.

PRIAPISM

A priapism is a long-lasting painful erection. Without prompt resolution, permanent damage to the penile tissue occurs, resulting in permanent erectile dysfunction. It thus constitutes a urological emergency. Priapism most commonly affects people with sickle cell disease. Other causes include some treatments for erectile dysfunction, blood disorders and recreational drugs. Treatment in the first instance is by insertion of a needle into a corpus cavernosum to withdraw blood.

Further reading

Shamloul R, Ghanem H. Erectile dysfunction. *Lancet* 2013; 381:153–165.
https://uroweb.org/guideline/male-sexual-dysfunction/. *EAU guidelines for erectile dysfunction and lack of libido.*

THE AGEING MALE

In the male, there is no sudden 'change of life' and no direct equivalent of the female menopause. However, there is a progressive loss of sexual function with reduction in morning erections and frequency of intercourse.

The age of onset varies widely. Typically, overall testicular volume diminishes and sex hormone binding globulin (SHBG) and gonadotrophin levels gradually rise, but other men present with low or borderline testosterone without elevation of luteinizing hormone/ follicle stimulating hormone (LH/FSH). Low testosterone certainly increases the risk of osteoporosis and, in some studies, is associated with increased cardiovascular risk. It remains unclear to what extent general symptoms of lack of energy, drive, muscle strength and general wellbeing may relate to these hormonal changes; a recent trial of testosterone replacement showed no benefit for general symptoms, although there was an improvement in sexual function. Loss of libido and erectile dysfunction are, however, common symptoms, even when hormone levels are normal, and long-term outcome studies of testosterone replacement are still awaited. Therefore, the decision to offer testosterone replacement to an ageing male is currently based on full clinical and biochemical assessment and thorough discussion of the potential risks (including prostate disease), as well as benefits. If testosterone is unequivocally low (<7 pmol/L) and there are symptoms specific to androgen deficiency (low libido, erectile dysfunction and loss of early morning erections), most authorities would recommend replacement. However, few would treat if testosterone is over 12 pmol/L with normal LH/FSH. Clinically, a large proportion of cases are in the borderline range (7–12 pmol/L), which can lead to difficulties in reaching a firm diagnosis. There is an increasing move towards measuring fasting testosterone levels, as food intake may decrease testosterone, leading to an incorrect diagnosis of androgen deficiency.

General measures to keep healthy include:
- eating a good diet containing fruit and vegetables
- taking regular exercise
- keeping below the maximum 'safe' drinking level of 14 units per week
- maintaining a healthy weight
- engaging in physical check-ups, such as blood pressure assessment.

The authors advocate regular PSA blood tests from the age of 45 years but acknowledge that this is controversial. Making use of other screening opportunities, such as those for bowel cancer and aortic aneurysm, is also recommended.

Environmental medicine

Michael L. Clark and Parveen J. Kumar

CORE SKILLS AND KNOWLEDGE

There are numerous ways in which environmental factors affect health. Much of the focus of this chapter is on specific conditions associated with exposure to extreme environmental conditions including heat, cold, altitude, ionizing radiation and smoke inhalation. Doctors specializing in treating such conditions include emergency medicine physicians and those with special interests in expedition medicine, military medicine or disaster relief.

Environmental exposures alter rapidly as a result of climate change, natural disasters, political crises and war. As well as addressing the needs of individual patients experiencing illness, a fuller response to the threats of environmental disease requires political action and combined interventions with a range of other agencies in society and internationally. Further discussion of such topics can be found in Chapter 13, Global health and Chapter 14, Public health.

Key things to understand from this chapter include:

- the emergency management of illness arising from extreme environmental exposure
- the role of medical professionals in relief efforts to populations affected by natural disasters.

AIR POLLUTION

Epidemiology

Air pollution is one of the biggest problems facing the world. It has become a public health emergency as it leads to chronic diseases and exacerbates respiratory, cardiac and other medical problems. According to the World Health Organization, air pollution causes over 7 million premature deaths per year, mainly from heart disease, stroke, chronic obstructive pulmonary disease, lung cancer, and acute respiratory infections in children. Annually, pollution is the cause of 1.6 million deaths in China, 1.24 million in India in 2017 and 135 000 in Pakistan, and figures are rising. There are 29 000 deaths each year in the UK due to air pollution. It is also the single largest environmental risk in Europe, causing 800 000 premature deaths. It has been estimated that air pollution kills more people in a year than malaria and HIV combined, and about ten times more deaths than road accidents in some countries. Atmospheric air pollution, due to the burning of coal for energy and heat, has been a feature of urban living in high-income countries for at least two centuries.

Air pollution consists of black smoke and sulphur dioxide (SO_2) and, from combustion of hydrocarbon fuels in motor vehicles, nitrogen oxides (NO and NO_2), diesel particulates, polyaromatic hydrocarbons and ozone, a secondary pollutant generated by photochemical reactions in the atmosphere. Levels of NO_2 can be high in poorly ventilated kitchens and living rooms where gas is used for cooking and in open fires.

Particulate matter consists of coarse particles (10–2.5 μm in aerodynamic diameter), produced by construction work and farming, and fine particles (<2.5 μm) generated from burning fossil fuels. Fine particulates ($PM_{2.5}$) remain airborne for long periods and are carried into rural areas. Several respiratory and cardiac problems are exacerbated by these very small particles.

The World Health Organization (WHO) global air-quality guidelines suggest 24-hour values of <25 μg/m³ for $PM_{2.5}$ for the short term and 10 μg/m³ in the long term. In Europe, 70% of the particulates present in urban air result from the combustion of diesel fuel, providing a background concentration of 3–5 μg/m³.

Deaths from respiratory and cardiovascular disease occur mainly in older populations; air pollution mainly causes bronchitis in children. Pollution from motor vehicles has been linked to increased hospital admissions, reduced lung function in children and younger adults, and an increase in lung cancer (polyaromatic hydrocarbons). Although it has been proposed that air pollution may cause asthma and other allergic diseases, there is no current evidence for this (**Box 41.1**). However, air pollution does adversely affect lung development in teenagers, while both NO_2 and ozone enhance the nasal and lung airway responses to inhaled allergens in people with established allergic disease.

Management

When air quality is poor, patients with asthma are advised to avoid exercising outdoors and to increase their anti-inflammatory medication (i.e. inhaled corticosteroids). Short- and long-term measures

Box 41.1 Air pollutants and their health effects

Pollutant	Average concentration	Poor air quality	Susceptible individuals	Mechanisms of health effects
Sulphur dioxide (SO_2)	5–15 ppb	>125 ppb	Patients with asthma	Bronchoconstriction through neurogenic mechanism
Ozone (O_3)	10–30 ppb	>90 ppb	All affected, particularly during exercise	Restrictive lung defect Airway inflammation Enhanced response to allergen
Nitrogen dioxide (NO_2)	25–40 ppb	>100 ppb	Allergic individuals	Airway inflammation Enhanced response to allergen
Particulate matter				
PM_{10}	25–30 μg/m³	>65 μg/m³	Elderly Allergic individuals	Airway and alveolar inflammation Enhanced selective production of the allergy antibody (IgE)
$PM_{2.5}$	3–5 μg/m³	>10 μg/m³	Those with cardiac and respiratory disease	Airway inflammation

ppb, parts per billion.

are required to reduce air pollution, particularly diesel particulates (which are predicted to increase as more diesel engines are used). Such measures include increased motor engine efficiency, catalytic converters, diesel particulate traps and decreased reliance on cars and trucks.

Further reading

Beelen R, Raaschou-Nielsen O, Stafoggia M et al. Effects of long-term exposure to air pollution on natural-cause mortality: an analysis of 22 European cohorts within the multicenter ESCAPE project. *Lancet* 2014; 383:785–795.
Editorial. Short-lived climate pollutants: a focus for hot air. *Lancet* 2015; 386: 1707.
Holgate ST. 'Every breath we take: the lifelong impact of air pollution' – a call for action. *Clin Med (Lond)* 2017; 17:8–12.

HEAT INJURY

Body core temperature (T_{Core}) is maintained at 37°C by the thermoregulatory centre in the hypothalamus, which integrates information from skin temperature sensors with core temperatures from receptors in the brain and in the walls of large blood vessels.

Heat is produced by cellular metabolism and is dissipated through the skin by both vasodilation and sweating, and in expired air via the alveoli. When the environmental temperature (T_{Env}) is higher than 32.5°C, profuse sweating occurs. The elderly, whose ability to adjust physiologically to heat is reduced due to diminished thermoregulatory capacity, and the chronically ill are more easily affected. The rising global temperature has given rise to heat waves and increased mortality particularly in these groups.

Sweat evaporation is the principal mechanism for controlling T_{Core} following exercise or in response to an increase in T_{Env}.

Heat acclimatization takes place over several weeks. The sweat volume increases and the sweat salt content falls. Increased evaporation of sweat reduces T_{Core}.

Heat cramps

Painful muscle cramps, usually in the legs, often occur in fit people when they exercise excessively, especially in hot weather. Cramps are probably due to low extracellular sodium caused by excess intake of water over salt. They can be prevented by increasing dietary salt. They respond to combined salt and water replacement, and in the acute stage to stretching and muscle massage. T_{Core} remains normal.

Heat exhaustion

At any environmental temperature (especially with T_{Env} of >25°C), and with a high humidity, strenuous exercise in clothing that inhibits sweating, such as a wetsuit or military uniform, can cause an elevation in T_{Core} in less than 15 minutes. Weakness/exhaustion, cramps, dizziness and syncope, with T_{Core} higher than 37°C, define heat exhaustion. Elevation of T_{Core} is more critical than water and sodium loss. Heat exhaustion may progress to heat stroke, a serious emergency (see below).

Management

Reduce (T_{Env}) if possible and cool the patient with sponging and fans. Give O_2 by mask.

Other causes of high T_{Core}, such as malaria, should be ruled out and appropriately treated.

Oral rehydration with *both* salt and water (25 g of salt per 5 L of water/day) is given in the first instance, with adequate replacement thereafter. In severe heat exhaustion, intravenous fluids are needed. Monitor serum sodium and correct secondary potassium loss.

Heat stroke

Heat stroke is an acute life-threatening situation in which T_{Core} rises above 41°C. The diagnosis is based on a triad of hyperthermia, neurological symptoms and heat exposure or strenuous exercise. There is headache, nausea, vomiting and weakness, progressing to confusion, seizures, coma and death. The skin *feels* intensely hot to the touch. Sweating is often absent but not invariably so.

Heat stroke can develop in acclimatized people in hot, humid, windless conditions, even without exercise. Sweating may be limited by prickly heat (plugging or rupture of the sweat ducts, leading to a pruritic, papular, erythematous rash).

Excessive exercise in inappropriate clothing, such as exercising on land in a wetsuit, can lead to heat injury in temperate climates. Diabetes, alcohol and drugs, such as antimuscarinics, diuretics and phenothiazines, can contribute. Heat stroke can lead to a fall in cardiac output, lactic acidosis and intravascular coagulation.

Prevention

Acclimatization, fluids, avoidance of inappropriate clothing and common sense are required.

Management

The major aim of treatment is to reduce the temperature below 40.5° as soon as possible. Delay only for essential cardiopulmonary

resuscitation. No pharmacological agents are effective in lowering core temperature.

- Reduce T_{Env} if possible.
- Arrange cold water immersion if facilities are available. Otherwise, cool the patient with sponging, icepacks or fanning.
- Give O_2 by mask.
- Move the patient to a medical facility. Manage in intensive care: monitor cardiac output and respiration; measure biochemistry, clotting and muscle enzymes.
- Give fluids intravenously so the intravascular volume remains normal.

Prompt treatment is essential and can be curative, even with a T_{Core} higher than 40.5°C. Morbidity and mortality are directly related to the duration of the high T_{Core}.

Complications are hypovolaemia, intravascular coagulation, cerebral oedema, rhabdomyolysis, and renal and hepatic failure.

Further reading

Epstein Y, Yanovich R. Heatstroke. *N Engl J Med* 2019; 380:2449–2459.
Hajat S, O'Connor M, Kosatsky T. Health effects of hot weather: from awareness of risk factors to effective health protection. *Lancet* 2010; 375:856–863.

COLD INJURY

Cold injury may be divided into hypothermia, which is whole-body cooling, and peripheral cold injury (**Box 41.2**).

Hypothermia

Hypothermia occurs in many settings.

At home. Hypothermia can occur when T_{Env} is less than 8°C, if there is poor heating, inadequate clothing and poor nutrition. Depressant drugs, such as hypnotics, as well as alcohol, hypothyroidism or intercurrent illness also contribute. Hypothermia is commonly seen in the poor, frail and elderly. The elderly have a diminished ability to sense cold and may have little insulating fat.

Neonates and infants become hypothermic rapidly because of a relatively large surface area in proportion to subcutaneous fat.

Outdoors on land. Hypothermia is a prominent cause of death in climbers, skiers and polar travellers, and in wartime. Wet, cold conditions with wind chill, physical exhaustion, injuries and inadequate clothing are contributory. Babies and children are at risk because they cannot take action to warm themselves.

Cold water immersion. Dangerous hypothermia can develop following immersion for more than 30 minutes to 1 hour in water temperatures of 15–20°C. In T_{Water} below 12°C, limbs rapidly become numb and weak. Recovery takes place gradually, over several hours following rescue.

> *i* **Box 41.2 Cold injury**
>
> - ***Hypothermia*** – classification by temperature (T_{Core}):
>   – Mild: 32–35°C
>   – Moderate: 28–32°C. Risk of arrhythmias and cardiac arrest
>   – Severe: <28°C. Frequently lethal
> - ***Peripheral cold injury*** includes:
>   – ***Frostbite***: the local cold injury that follows freezing of tissue
>   – ***Non-freezing cold injury***: the damage – usually to feet – following prolonged exposure to a T_{Env} between 0° and 5°C, usually in damp conditions

Clinical features

Mild hypothermia (T_{Core} <32°C) causes shivering and initially intense discomfort. However, the hypothermic subject, though alert, may not act appropriately to rewarming: for example, by huddling, wearing extra clothing or exercising. As the T_{Core} falls below 32°C, severe hypothermia causes impaired judgement – including lack of awareness of cold – and drowsiness and coma. Death follows, usually from ventricular fibrillation.

Diagnosis

Diagnosis is straightforward, if a low-reading thermometer is available. If not, rapid clinical assessment is reliable. Someone who *feels* icy to the touch – abdomen, groin, axillae – is *probably* substantially hypothermic. If the person is clammy, uncooperative or sleepy, T_{Core} is almost certainly below 32°C.

Sequelae

Pulse rate and systemic blood pressure fall. Cardiac output and cerebral blood flow are low in hypothermia and can fall further if the upright position is maintained or the thorax restrained by a harness, or by hauling during evacuation. This is why helicopter and lifeboat winch rescues are often carried out with a stretcher rather than a chest harness.

Respiration becomes shallow and slow. Muscle stiffness develops; tendon reflexes become sluggish, then absent. As coma ensues, pupillary and other brainstem reflexes are lost; pupils are fixed and may be dilated in severe hypothermia. Metabolic changes are variable, with either metabolic acidosis or alkalosis. Arterial PO_2 may appear normal: that is, falsely high.

There is shift of the oxygen dissociation curve (see p. 206) to the left because of the reduction in temperature of haemoglobin. Thus, if an arterial blood sample from a hypothermic patient is analysed at 37°C, the PO_2 will be falsely high. Within the range 37–33°C, this factor is around 7% per degree centigrade. Many blood gas machines also calculate the arterial saturation; this too will be falsely high. When a patient is monitored using a pulse oximeter, the level of arterial oxygen saturation (S_aO_2) will, however, be correct, but if S_aO_2 is then converted by calculation to P_aO_2, a downward correction must be applied – simply due to hypothermia.

Bradycardia with 'J' waves (above the isoelectric line at the junction of the QRS complex and ST segment; **Fig. 41.1**) are pathognomonic of hypothermia. Prolongation of PR and QT intervals and the QRS complex also occurs. Ventricular dysrhythmia (tachycardia/fibrillation) or asystole is the usual cause of death.

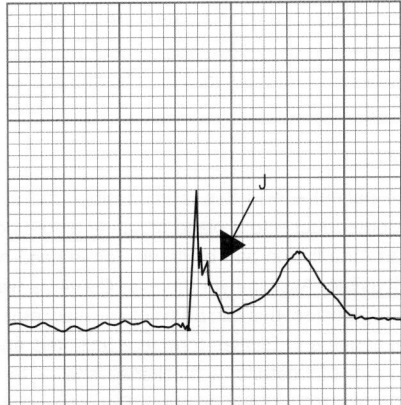

Fig. 41.1 Electrocardiogram showing J waves in hypothermia.

Management

- Maintain the patient horizontal or slightly head-down.
- Rewarm gradually.
- Correct metabolic abnormalities.
- Anticipate and treat dysrhythmias.
- Check for hypothyroidism (see p. 611).

If the patient is awake, with a core temperature of more than 32°C, place in a warm room, use a foil wrap and give warm fluids orally. Outdoors, add extra dry clothing, huddle together and use a warmed sleeping bag. Rewarming may take several hours. Avoid alcohol: this adds to confusion, boosts confidence factitiously, causes peripheral vasodilation and further heat loss, and can precipitate hypoglycaemia.

Severe hypothermia

In severe hypothermia (<28°C), people look dead. Always exclude hypothermia before diagnosing brainstem death (see p. 236). Warm gradually, aiming at a 1°C/hour increase in T_{Core}. Direct mild surface heat from an electric blanket can be helpful. Treat any underlying condition promptly, such as sepsis. Monitor all vital functions. Correct dysrhythmias. Check for sedative drugs.

Give warm intravenous fluids slowly. Correct metabolic abnormalities. Hypothyroidism, if present, should be treated with liothyronine. Various methods of artificial rewarming exist: inhaled warm humidified air, gastric or peritoneal lavage, and haemodialysis. These are rarely used. Extracorporeal membrane oxygenation (ECMO) is used in specialized centres with improved survival. Hypothermia is frequently lethal when T_{Core} falls below 30°C. Survival with full recovery has, however, been recorded with a T_{Core} of <16°C.

Prevention

Hypothermia in the field can often be prevented by forethought and action. For the elderly, improved home heating and insulation, central heating in bedrooms and electric blankets are helpful in cold spells. This can be expensive and unaffordable for some people, so supplemental finance is required.

Peripheral cold injury

Frostbite

Ice crystals form within skin and superficial tissues when the temperature of the tissue (T_{Tissue}) falls to −3°C: T_{Env} generally must be below −6°C. Wind chill is frequently a factor. Typically, fingers, toes, nose and ears become frostbitten.

Frostbitten tissue is pale, greyish and initially doughy to the touch. Later, tissue freezes hard, looking like meat from a freezer. Frostbite can easily occur when working or exercising in low temperatures and typically develops without the patient's knowledge. Hands or feet that have lost their feeling are at risk of cold injury.

Management

Transport the patient – or if this is impossible, make them walk, even on frostbitten feet – to a place of safety before commencing warming. Warm the frozen part by immersion in hand-hot water at 39–42°C, if feasible. Assess hypothermia. Continue warming until obvious thawing occurs; this can be painful. Vasodilator drugs have no part in management. Blisters form in a few days and, depending on the depth of frostbite, a blackened shell – the **carapace** – develops as blisters regress or burst. Dry, non-adherent dressings and aseptic precautions are essential, though hard to achieve.

Frostbitten tissues are anaesthetic and at risk from further trauma and infection. Recovery takes place over many weeks and may be incomplete. Surgery may be needed, but should be avoided in the early stages.

Chilblains

These are small, purplish itchy inflammatory lesions, occurring on toes and fingers. They occur in cold, wet conditions. They are more common in women and heal in 7–14 days. Prevention is by keeping warm and wearing gloves and warm footwear.

Non-freezing cold injury

Non-freezing cold injury (NFCI; trench foot) describes tissue damage following prolonged exposure, usually for several hours or more, at T_{Env} around or slightly above freezing, but without frostbite. Wet socks and boots are the usual cause. There is severe vasoconstriction, and blotchiness of the lower limbs, with pain and oedema on rewarming. Recovery usually follows over several weeks. There may be a prolonged late susceptibility to cold. NFCI is a prominent cause of morbidity in troops operating in low temperatures and is a subsequent cause of litigation.

Prevention of frostbite and NFCI is largely by education and common sense: avoid damp feet and wet boots. Always carry spare dry socks, gloves and headgear.

Further reading

Morrison G. Management of acute hypothermia. *Medicine* 2017; 45 (3):135–138.
Resuscitation Council (UK). Resuscitation in special circumstances. In: *Advanced Life Support*, 7th edn. London: Resuscitation Council UK 2016; 145–148.
Sheridan RL, Goldstein MA, Stoddard FJ Jr et al. Case records of the Massachusetts General Hospital. Case 41-2009. A 16-year-old boy with hypothermia and frostbite. *N Engl J Med* 2009; 361:2654–2662.
Wira CR, Becker JU, Martin G et al. Anti-arrhythmic and vasopressor medications for the treatment of ventricular fibrillation in severe hypothermia: a systematic review of the literature. *Resuscitation* 2008; 78:21–29.

HIGH ALTITUDE

The partial pressure of atmospheric oxygen – and hence alveolar and arterial oxygen – falls in a near-linear relationship as barometric pressure drops with increasing altitude (**Fig. 41.2**).

Commercial aircraft are pressurized to around 2400 m (lowering the oxygen saturation by 3–4%). This trivial reduction is not noticed by healthy individuals.

On land, below 3000 m there are few clinical effects. The resulting hypoxaemia causes breathlessness only in those with severe cardiorespiratory disease. Above 3000–3500 m, hypoxia causes a spectrum of related syndromes that affect high-altitude visitors, principally climbers, trekkers, skiers and troops (**Box 41.3**), especially when they exercise. These conditions occur largely during acclimatization, a process that takes several weeks; once completed, this can enable humans to live – permanently, if necessary – up to about 5600 m. At greater heights, although people can survive for days or weeks, deterioration due to chronic hypoxia is inevitable.

The world's highest railway runs to Lhasa in Tibet, reaching altitudes of over 5000 m. Emergency oxygen is provided in the carriages. Roads at similar altitudes in Central Asia are used extensively but since road passengers do not exercise, serious altitude-related illnesses are unusual. Climbing the world's highest summits is just possible without supplementary oxygen, though it is often used on peaks above 7500 m. At the summit of Mount Everest (8848 m), the barometric pressure is 34 kPa (253 mmHg). An acclimatized mountaineer has an alveolar PO_2 of 4.0–4.7 kPa (30–35 mmHg) – near

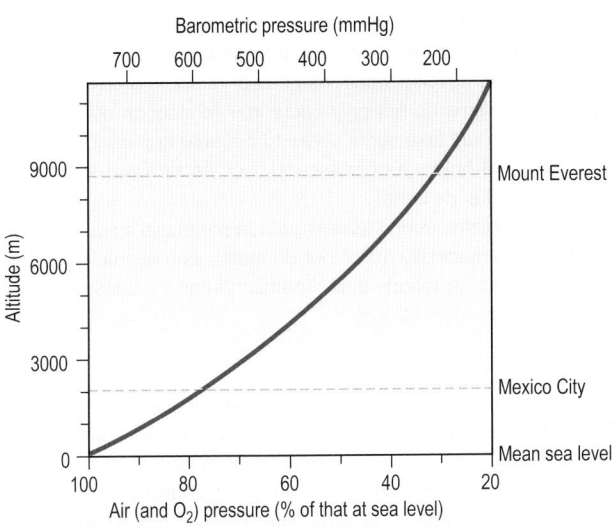

Fig. 41.2 The decrease in oxygen and barometric pressure with increasing altitude.

<table>
<tr><td></td></tr>
</table>

i **Box 41.3 Conditions caused by sustained hypoxia**

Condition	Incidence (%)	Usual altitude (m)
Acute mountain sickness	70	3500–4000
Acute pulmonary oedema	2	4000
Acute cerebral oedema	1	4500
Retinal haemorrhage	50	5000
Deterioration	100	≥6000
Chronic mountain sickness	Rare	3500–4000

humans' absolute physiological limit. In 2007, arterial blood samples from acclimatized doctors on Everest at altitude 8400 m, breathing air, showed an average PO_2 of 24.6 mmHg (3.3 kPa).

Acute mountain sickness

Acute mountain sickness (AMS) describes malaise, nausea, headache and lassitude that affect the majority of people for a few days, above 3500 m. Following arrival at this altitude, there is usually a latent interval of 6–36 hours before symptoms begin. Treatment is rest, with analgesics if necessary. Recovery is usually spontaneous over several days.

Prophylactic treatment with acetazolamide, a carbonic anhydrase inhibitor and respiratory stimulant, is of some value in preventing AMS. Acclimatizing – that is, ascending gradually – provides better and more natural prophylaxis.

In the minority, more serious sequelae – high-altitude pulmonary oedema and high-altitude cerebral oedema – develop.

High-altitude pulmonary oedema

Predisposing factors include youth, rapidity of ascent, heavy exertion and severe AMS. Breathlessness, occasionally with frothy blood-stained sputum, indicates established oedema. Unless treated rapidly, this leads to cardiorespiratory failure and death. Milder forms are common. Breathlessness at rest should raise the suspicion of pulmonary oedema.

High-altitude cerebral oedema

Cerebral oedema is the result of an abrupt increase in cerebral blood flow that occurs even at modest altitudes of 3500–4000 m.

It is unusual below 4500 m, and occurs typically in the first 2 weeks, during acclimatization. Cerebral oedema can also develop suddenly in well-acclimatized climbers above 7000 m. Headache is followed by drowsiness, ataxia and papilloedema, with coma and death if brain oedema progresses.

Management

Any but the milder forms of AMS require urgent treatment. Oxygen should be given by mask if available, and descent should take place as quickly as possible. Nifedipine reduces pulmonary hypertension and is used in pulmonary oedema. Dexamethasone is effective in reducing brain oedema. Portable pressure bags inflated by a foot pump are widely used; the patient is enclosed in the bag.

Retinal haemorrhage

Small flame haemorrhages within the retinal nerve fibre layer are common above 5000 m and usually symptomless. Rarely, a haemorrhage will cover the macula, causing painless loss of central vision. Recovery is usual.

Deterioration

Prolonged residence between 6000 and 7000 m leads to weight loss, anorexia and listlessness after several weeks. Above 7500 m, the effects of deterioration become apparent over several days, although it is possible to survive for a week or more at altitudes near 8000 m without supplementary oxygen.

Chronic mountain sickness

Chronic mountain sickness occurs in long-term residents at high altitudes, usually after several decades, and is seen in the Andes and in Central Asia.

Headache, polycythaemia, lassitude, cyanosis, finger clubbing, congested cheeks and ear lobes, and right ventricular enlargement develop. Chronic mountain sickness is gradually progressive.

Coronary artery disease and hypertension are rare in high-altitude native populations.

Further reading

Grocott MP, Martin DS, Levett DZ et al. Arterial blood gases and oxygen content in climbers on Mount Everest. *N Engl J Med* 2009; 360:140–149.
Imray CH, Grocott MP, Wilson MH et al. Extreme, expedition and wilderness medicine. *Lancet* 2015; 386:2520–2525.
Wilson MH, Habig K, Wright C et al. Pre-hospital emergency medicine. *Lancet* 2015; 386:2526–2534.
http://www.thebmc.co.uk. *Union Internationale des Associations d'Alpinisme (UIAA) Mountain Medicine Data Centre leaflets, available from British Mountaineering Council, 177–179 Burton Road, Manchester M20 2BB, UK.*
http://www.wms.org. *Wilderness Medical Society Information, PO Box 2463, Indianapolis, Indiana 462206, USA.*

DIVING

Free diving by breath-holding is possible to around 5 m, or with practice to greater depths. Air can be supplied to divers by various methods.

A **snorkel** provides air to a depth of about 0.5 m; inspiratory effort is the limiting factor. At depths of more than 0.5 m – that is, with a longer snorkel tube, forced negative-pressure ventilation can cause pulmonary capillary damage with haemorrhagic alveolar oedema.

Scuba divers – recreational sports divers descending to 30 m – carry bottled compressed air or a nitrogen–oxygen mixture.

Commercial divers who work at great depths breathe helium–oxygen or nitrogen–oxygen mixtures, delivered by hose from the surface.

Ambient pressures at various depths are shown in **Box 41.4**.

Water depth (m)	Pressure	
	Atmospheres	mmHg
0	1	760
10	2	1520
50	6	4560
90	10	7600

Problems during descent

Middle ear barotrauma (squeeze) is common and is due to an inability to equalize pressure in the middle ear; Eustachian tube blockage is the usual cause. Pain and hearing loss occur, sometimes with tympanic membrane rupture and acute vertigo.

Sinus squeeze is intense local pain due to blockage of the nasal and paranasal sinus ostia.

Management is by holding the nostrils closed and swallowing, or similar manoeuvres, as well as use of decongestants. Diving with a respiratory or sinus infection should be avoided.

Oxygen narcosis

Pure oxygen is not used for diving because of oxygen toxicity. Lung atelectasis, endothelial cell damage and pulmonary oedema occur when alveolar oxygen pressure exceeds 1.5 atmospheres, at depths of around 5 m. At around 10 m, the central nervous system (CNS) becomes affected: apprehension, nausea and sweating are followed by muscle twitching and generalized convulsions.

Nitrogen narcosis

When compressed air is breathed below 30 m, the narcotic effects of nitrogen begin to impair brain function. Poor judgement is hazardous; this also occurs with nitrogen–oxygen mixtures in recreational diving. Nitrogen narcosis is avoided by replacing air with helium–oxygen mixtures, enabling descent to 700 m. At these extreme depths, the direct effect of pressure on neurones can cause tremor, hemiparesis and cognitive impairment.

Problems during and following ascent

Free divers who breath-hold often hyperventilate deliberately prior to plunging in. This drives off CO_2, reducing the stimulus to inspire. During the subsequent breath-hold, P_aCO_2 rises and P_aO_2 falls. On surfacing, decompression lowers P_aO_2 further. This can lead to syncope, known as a *shallow water blackout*. Since loss of consciousness can take place in the water, this can lead to fatalities.

Decompression sickness

Decompression sickness (the bends) is caused by the release of bubbles of nitrogen or helium and follows too rapid a return to the surface. Decompression tables indicate the duration for safe return from a given depth to the surface. In general, no decompression is necessary for diving above 30 m; at 30–60 m, decompression is necessary.

Bends can be mild (*type 1, non-neurological bends*), with skin irritation and mottling and/or joint pain. *Type 2, neurological bends*, are more serious and involve the development of cortical blindness, hemiparesis, sensory disturbances or cord lesions.

If bubbles form in pulmonary vessels, divers experience retrosternal discomfort, breathlessness and cough, known as **the chokes**. These develop within minutes or hours of a dive. Decompression problems do not only occur immediately on reaching the surface; they may take some hours to become apparent. Over the subsequent 24 hours, further ascent, such as air travel, can occasionally provoke the bends.

Other problems during ascent include paranasal sinus pain and nosebleeds – medically minor but dramatic, with excruciating pain and a mask full of bloody fluid. Toothache can be caused by gas bubbles within rotten fillings.

Management

All but the mildest forms of decompression sickness, such as skin mottling alone, require recompression in a pressure chamber, following strict guidelines. Recovery is usual. A long-term problem is aseptic necrosis of the hip due to nitrogen bubbles causing infarction. Focal neurological damage may persist, but complaints of fatigue and poor concentration are issues compounded by litigation that commonly follows diving accidents. Objective, evidence-based assessments are essential.

Lung rupture, pneumothorax and surgical emphysema

These emergencies occur when divers breath-hold during emergency ascents after gas supplies become exhausted. There is dyspnoea, cough and haemoptysis. Pneumothorax and surgical emphysema resolve with 100% oxygen. Air embolism can also occur and is treated with recompression.

Further reading

Brubakk A, Neuman TS. *Bennett and Elliott's Physiology and Medicine of Diving,* 5th edn. London: WB Saunders; 2002.

Edmonds C, Thomas B, McKewzie B et al. *Diving Medicine for Scuba Divers,* 4th edn; 2012; Manly, Australia: Carl Edmonds.

Lynch JH, Bove AA. Diving medicine: a review of current evidence. *J Am Board Fam Med* 2009; 22:399–407.

http://www.diversalertnetwork.org/. *Divers Alert Network (DAN).*

DROWNING

Drowning is defined as a process resulting in primary respiratory impairment from submersion or immersion in a liquid medium. Terms such as 'near-drowning and 'wet drowning' should not be used.

Drowning is a common cause of accidental death worldwide. In the UK, some 40% of drownings occur in children under 5 years of age. Drowning can also follow a seizure or a myocardial infarct. Exhaustion, alcohol, drugs and hypothermia all contribute to deaths following submersion.

Fresh or seawater aspiration destroys pulmonary surfactant, leading to alveolar collapse, ventilation/perfusion mismatch and hypoxaemia. Aspiration of hypertonic seawater (5% NaCl) pulls additional fluid into the alveoli with further ventilation/perfusion mismatch. In practice, there is little difference between saltwater and freshwater aspiration. In both, severe hypoxaemia develops rapidly. Severe metabolic acidosis develops in the majority of survivors.

Management and prognosis

Clearance of the airway and ventilation are the major requirements for submerged people, and bystanders should start resuscitation immediately once the person is stable on land. Rescue breaths and chest compression come before the initiation of standard

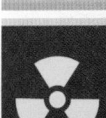

cardiopulmonary resuscitation as used in cardiac arrest (see p. 1045). Patients have survived for up to 30 minutes under water without suffering brain damage – and sometimes for longer periods if T_{Water} is near 10°C. Survival is probably related to the protective role of the **diving reflex**; submersion causes bradycardia and vasoconstriction. Oxygen consumption is also decreased by hypothermia.

Resuscitation should always be attempted, even with absent pulse and fixed dilated pupils. Patients frequently make a dramatic recovery. All survivors should be admitted to hospital for intensive monitoring, as acute respiratory distress syndrome (ARDS) can develop during the subsequent 48 hours.

Recovery is frequently complete if consciousness is regained within several minutes of commencing resuscitation but poor if a patient remains stuporose or in coma at 30 minutes.

Prevention

This includes making sure that all people can swim, particularly young children. Any water can be dangerous, and swimming should only be undertaken in supervised areas.

Further reading

Szpilman D, Bierens JJ, Handley AJ et al. Drowning. *N Engl J Med* 2012; 366:2102–2110.
Vanden Hoek TL, Morrison LJ, Shuster M et al. Part 12: Cardiac arrest in special situations: 2010 American Heart Association Guidelines for Cardiopulmonary Resuscitation and Emergency Cardiovascular Care. *Circulation* 2010; 122:S829.

IONIZING RADIATION

Ionizing radiation is either penetrating (X-rays, γ-rays or neutrons) or non-penetrating (α- or β-particles). Penetrating radiation affects the skin and deeper tissues, while non-penetrating radiation affects the skin alone. All radiation effects depend on the type of radiation, the distribution of dose and the dose rate.

Dosage is measured in **joules per kilogram** (J/kg): 1 J/kg = 1 gray (1 Gy) = 100 rads.

Radioactivity is measured in **becquerels** (Bq); 1 Bq is defined as the activity of a quantity of radioactive material in which one nucleus decays per second; 3.7×10^{10} Bq = 1 **curie** (Ci), the older, non-SI unit.

Radiation differs in the density of ionization it causes. Therefore, a dose-equivalent called a **sievert** (Sv) is used. This is the absorbed dose weighted for the damaging effect of the radiation. The annual background radiation is approximately 2.5 mSv. A chest X-ray delivers 0.02 mSv and CT of the abdomen/pelvis about 10 mSv (see **Box 6.5**).

A cumulative risk of cancer following repeated imaging procedures has been established and X-ray exposures should be reduced if possible.

Excessive exposure to ionizing radiation follows accidents in industry, nuclear power plants and hospitals, and deliberate nuclear explosions designed to eliminate populations – and exceptionally, by poisoning, with polonium, for example.

Mild acute radiation sickness

Nausea, vomiting and malaise follow doses of approximately 1 Gy. Lymphopenia occurs within several days, followed 2–3 weeks later by a fall in all white cells and platelets.

Acute radiation sickness

Many systems are affected; the extent depends on the dose of radiation (**Box 41.5**).

_i_ Box 41.5 Systemic radiation effects

Acute effects
- Haemopoietic syndrome
- Gastrointestinal syndrome
- CNS syndrome
- Radiation dermatitis

Delayed effects
- Infertility
- Teratogenesis
- Cataract
- Neoplasia:
  - Acute myeloid leukaemia
  - Thyroid
  - Salivary glands
  - Skin
  - Others

Haemopoietic syndrome

Absorption of 2–10 Gy is followed by transient vomiting in some individuals, followed by a period of improvement. Lymphocytes are particularly sensitive to radiation damage; severe lymphopenia develops over several days. A decrease in granulocytes and platelets follows 2–3 weeks later, since no new cells are formed in the marrow. Thrombocytopenia develops with bleeding and frequent overwhelming infections; there is a high mortality.

Gastrointestinal syndrome

Doses higher than 6 Gy cause vomiting several hours after exposure. This then stops, only to recur some 4 days later, accompanied by diarrhoea. The villous lining of the intestine becomes denuded. Intractable bloody diarrhoea follows, with dehydration, secondary infection and sometimes death.

CNS syndrome

Exposures of more than 30 Gy are followed rapidly by nausea, vomiting, disorientation and coma. Death due to cerebral oedema can follow, usually within 36 hours.

Radiation dermatitis

Skin erythema, purpura, blistering and secondary infection occur. Total loss of body hair is a bad prognostic sign and usually follows an exposure of more than 5 Gy.

Late effects of radiation exposure

Survivors of the nuclear bombing of Hiroshima and Nagasaki in 1945 provided data on long-term radiation effects. Risks of acute myeloid leukaemia and cancer, particularly of skin, thyroid and salivary glands, increase. Infertility, teratogenesis and cataract are also late sequelae, developing years after exposure.

Major nuclear power plant accidents

Two high-level nuclear accidents have occurred: the first in 1986 in Chernobyl in the Ukraine (part of the Soviet Union at the time), and the second in 2011 in Fukushima in Japan.

In Chernobyl, 30 people died in the first 3 months due to radiation and other factors. The majority of the people in the area received variable doses of radiation and the long-term consequences are still occurring, including the high incidence of cancer, particularly of the thyroid. However, the long-term effects on mortality are said to be enormously higher than originally thought and will keep increasing.

In the Fukushima disaster, which occurred following an earthquake that generated tsunamis along the east coast of Japan, radiation release was 10–30% of that released in Chernobyl. There were no immediate deaths due to radiation and the long-term effect of radiation is thought likely to be small.

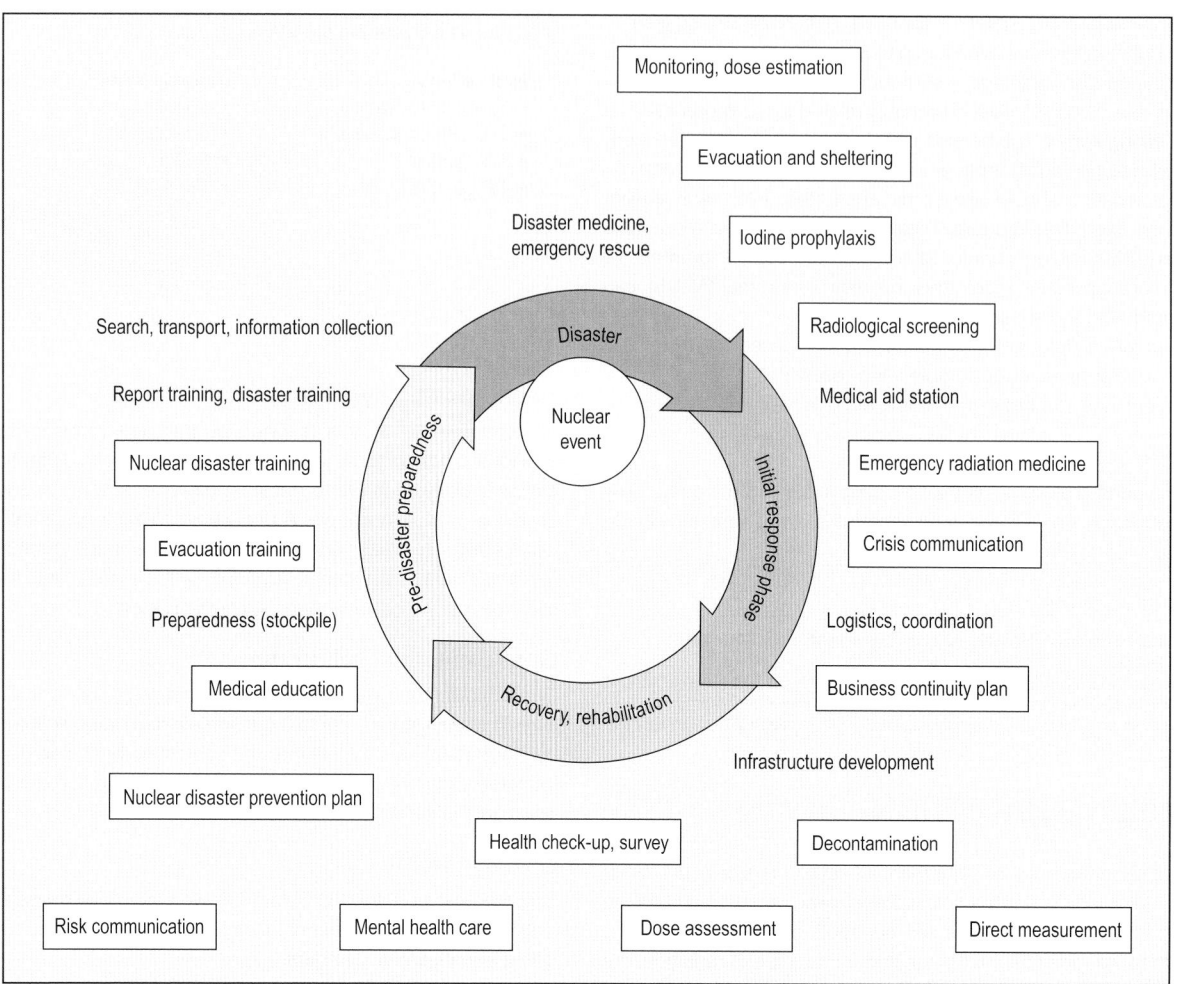

Fig. 41.3 General disaster and nuclear disaster cycle. The measures shown in boxes refer to a programme specifically for a nuclear disaster. Those not in boxes are measures required for any large-scale disaster. *(From Ohtsuru A, Tanigawa K, Kumagai A et al. Nuclear disasters and health: lessons learned, challenges, and proposals. Lancet 2015; 386:489–499, with permission.)*

The major problems caused by both disasters relate to psychological and social effects, as a result of the populations' evacuation and removal from their homes for years following the accidents, as well as a general concern about the effects of radiation on themselves and their children.

Fig. 41.3 shows the measures needed in a nuclear disaster.

Therapeutic radiation

The sequelae of therapeutic radiation – early, early-delayed and late-delayed radiation effects – are discussed on page 116. Focusing techniques are used to target radiation towards the field being treated, so that radiosensitive structures, such as the ovaries, are protected by shielding.

Management

Acute radiation sickness is an emergency. Absorption of the initial radiation dose can be reduced by removing contaminated clothing.

Management is largely supportive: prevention and treatment of infection, haemorrhage and fluid loss. Harvesting of blood products is sometimes carried out.

Accidental ingestion of, or exposure to, bone-seeking radio-isotopes (e.g. ^{90}strontium and ^{137}caesium) is treated with chelating agents, such as EDTA and massive doses of oral calcium.

Radio-iodine contamination should be treated immediately with potassium iodide to block radio-iodine absorption by the thyroid.

Further reading

Christodouleas JP, Forrest RD, Ainsley CG et al. Short-term and long-term health risks of nuclear-power-plant accidents. *N Engl J Med* 2011; 364:2334–2341.
Clancey G, Chhem R. Hiroshima, Nagasaki and Fukushima. *Lancet* 2015; 386:405–406.
Ohtsuru A, Tanigawa K et al. A nuclear shadow from Hiroshima and Nagasaki to Fukushima. *Lancet* 2015; 386:403.

ELECTRIC SHOCK

Electric shock can produce:

- ***Pain and psychological sequelae.*** The common domestic electric shock is typically painful, but rarely fatal or followed by serious sequelae. Nevertheless, it is an unpleasant and intensely frightening experience. A brief, immediate jerking episode can occur, which is not an epileptic seizure. There is usually no lasting neurological, cardiac or skin damage.
- ***More serious effects.*** These are distinctly rare following accidents in the home or in industry, but claims by survivors following industrial accidents are frequently made.

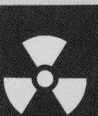

- ***Cardiac, neurological and muscle damage.*** Ventricular fibrillation, muscular contraction and spinal cord damage *can* follow a major shock.
- ***Electrical burns.*** These are commonly restricted to the skin. Muscle necrosis and spinal cord damage can also occur.
- ***Electrocution.*** This means death following ventricular fibrillation, either accidentally, or deliberately as a method of execution. In the USA, at executions, an initial voltage of more than 2000 volts was applied for some 15 seconds in the electric chair, causing loss of consciousness and ventricular fibrillation, before the voltage was lowered. The T_{Core} during the execution process would sometimes reach higher than 50°C, leading to severe damage to internal organs.

LIGHTNING STRIKE

This describes cloud-to-ground lightning originating in thunderstorms. Human tissues are directly damaged by the high-voltage DC current of more than 10 million volts that lasts only for a few milliseconds. The result is cardiac arrest due to asystole.

Fern-shaped burns are seen on the skin. The victim's clothes explode off the body and the person is pulseless, not breathing and in coma. The only chance of survival at this stage is bystander cardiopulmonary resuscitation. The mortality is high and those who survive are left with variable CNS damage.

Further reading

Davis C, Engeln A, Johnson E et al. Wilderness Medical Society practice guidelines for the prevention and treatment of lightning injuries. *Wilderness Environ Med* 2012; 23:260.

INHALED SMOKE

Smoke is air containing toxic and/or irritant gases and carbon particles, coated with organic acids, aldehydes and synthetic materials. Carbon monoxide, sulphur dioxide, sulphuric and hydrochloric acids, and other toxins may also be present. The highly toxic polyvinyl chloride is no longer used in household goods. Air pollution is discussed on page 1487.

On smoke inhalation, patients become breathless and tachypnoeic immediately. Choking and stridor may require intubation. Pulmonary oedema and hypoxia can be fatal.

Breathing through a wet towel or clothing is the best emergency treatment. Remove the victim from the scene as rapidly as possible. Give oxygen and arrange intensive therapy unit (ITU) support.

Prevention. Smoke alarms, regularly checked, should be installed in every household.

Further reading

Sheridan RL. Fire related inhalation injury. *N Engl J Med* 2016; 375:464–469.

Index